Brief Contents

Resources available on thePoint®

Fundamentals of Nursing

The Art and Science of Person-Centered Care

Tenth Edition

Carol Taylor, PhD, MSN, RN, FAAN
Professor of Nursing
Georgetown University School of Nursing and Health Studies
Washington, DC

Pamela Lynn, EdD, MSN, RN
Associate Professor
Frances M. Maguire School of Nursing and Health Professions
Gwynedd Mercy University
Gwynedd Valley, Pennsylvania

Jennifer L. Bartlett, PhD, RN-BC, CNE, CHSE
Associate Professor
Georgia Baptist College of Nursing of Mercer University
Atlanta, Georgia

Wolters Kluwer

Philadelphia • Baltimore • New York • London
Buenos Aires • Hong Kong • Sydney • Tokyo

Vice President, Nursing Segment: Julie K. Stegman
Director, Nursing Education and Practice Content: Jamie Blum
Senior Acquisitions Editor: Jonathan Joyce
Senior Development Editor: Julie M. Vitale
Developmental Editor: Kelly Horvath
Senior Content Editing Associate: Devika Kishore
Editorial Coordinator: Erin E. Hernandez
Senior Production Project Manager: David Saltzberg
Marketing Manager: Greta Swanson
Manager, Graphic Arts & Design: Stephen Druding
Art Director, Illustration: Jennifer Clements
Manufacturing Coordinator: Margie Orzech-Zeranko
Prepress Vendor: Aptara, Inc.

10th Edition

11 10 9 8 7 6 5 4 3
Printed in Mexico

Library of Congress Cataloging-in-Publication Data
Names: Taylor, Carol (Carol R.), author. | Lynn, Pamela (Pamela Barbara), 1961- author. | Bartlett, Jennifer L., author.
Title: Fundamentals of nursing : the art and science of person-centered care / Carol Taylor, Pamela Lynn, Jennifer L. Bartlett.
Description: Tenth edition. | Philadelphia, PA : Wolters Kluwer, 2023. | Includes bibliographical references and index.
Identifiers: LCCN 2022021674 (print) | LCCN 2022021675 (ebook) | ISBN 9781975168155 (hardcover) | ISBN 9781975168162 (ebook)
Subjects: MESH: Nursing Care | Nursing Process | Patient-Centered Care | BISAC: MEDICAL / Nursing / Fundamentals & Skills | MEDICAL / Education & Training
Classification: LCC RT41 (print) | LCC RT41 (ebook) | NLM WY 100.1 | DDC 610.73–dc23/eng/20220625
LC record available at https://lccn.loc.gov/2022021674
LC ebook record available at https://lccn.loc.gov/2022021675

shop.lww.com

QUADM0825

We jointly dedicate this special 10th edition written during the COVID-19 pandemic and the 2020–2021 Years of the Nurse and the Midwife, honoring the 200th anniversary of the birth of Florence Nightingale. We dedicate this text to all nurses everywhere who continue to care for society's most vulnerable and to the educators preparing the next generation of nurses to continue this service. May we always earn recognition as the most trusted profession.

—Carol, Pam, and Jennifer

A SPECIAL NOTE FROM THE AUTHOR TEAM

This text and every element in the teaching–learning package have been revised during a time that none of us could have envisioned. We have written and rewritten numerous chapters too often to count as new developments within our global community, country, and profession commanded our attention and begged to be brought to yours! Never have we been prouder to be nurses, and never have the demands on our expertise, energy, commitment, and resilience been greater. We recently read that nurses today need dedication, strength, grit, resilience, innovation, and kindness. We would add love, love for humanity, including love for self. So what are some of these new developments?

- As the American Nurses Association celebrated its 125th anniversary, it released the fourth edition of its *Scope and Standards of Practice* in May 2021. A major revision, this edition includes a new definition of nursing which references the art and science of caring, human functioning, compassionate presence, and recognition of the connection of all humanity.
- Earlier in 2021, the American Association of Colleges of Nursing released the re-envisioned *Essentials* that define competency requirements for baccalaureate and graduate nursing program graduates. These will revolutionize how nurses are prepared for entry-level and advanced roles.
- The National Council of State Boards of Nursing (NCSBN) announced the new Next Generation NCLEX (NGN) promising to incorporate the assessment of clinical judgment utilizing new evaluation model and question design.
- Simultaneously, the National Academies of Sciences, Engineering, and Medicine released *The Future of Nursing 2020–2030: Charting a Path to Achieve Health Equity.* This report outlines and affirms the role nurses can play in creating healthy communities for all. Understanding the dramatic changes the health care industry is undergoing, this report summarizes the challenges health care and the nursing profession are likely to face in the future and discusses steps for overcoming them, including how nurses can:
  - Work over the next decade to reduce health disparities and promote equity
  - Address rising costs through more equitable care delivery
  - Use technology to maximize reaching vulnerable populations
  - Prioritize patient- and family-centered care
- The COVID-19 pandemic continues to stretch every sector of health care, including our nurse leaders and front-line caregivers, to dig deep and give all they have to meet daunting demands for care.
- Disparities in health care, for far too long, have gone unacknowledged. Diversity, inclusion, and equity require active engagement.
- Similarly, climate change is no longer a theory, as massive fires, flooding, drought, and other climate extremes ravage the globe. What every nurse can do to promote environmental health and essential contributions.

AUTHORS AND CONTRIBUTORS

AUTHORS

Carol Taylor, PhD, MSN, RN, FAAN
Chapters 1, 2, 3, 4, 5, 6, 7, 10, 11, 12, 13, 15, 16, 17, 18, 19, 20, 21, 42, 44, 45, 47

Pamela Lynn, EdD, MSN, RN
Chapters 8, 9, 26, 27, 29, 32, 34, 35, 37, 38, 39, 40, 41

Jennifer L. Bartlett, PhD, RN-BC, CNE, CHSE
Chapters 14, 22, 23, 24, 25, 28, 30, 31, 33, 36, 43, 46

CONTRIBUTORS

Teri Capriotti, DO, MSN, CRNP, RN
Clinical Professor
Villanova University
M. Louise Fitzpatrick College of Nursing
Villanova, Pennsylvania
Contributor to Chapter 20

Meredith Mackenzie Greenle, DO
Clinical Professor
Villanova University
M. Louise Fitzpatrick College of Nursing
Villanova, Pennsylvania
Contributor to Chapter 20

Andrea R. Mann, MSN, RN, CNE
Professor of Practice
Gwynedd Mercy University
Frances M. Maguire School of Nursing and Health Professions
Gwynedd Valley, Pennsylvania
Practicing for NCLEX

Humberto Reinoso, PhD, FNP-BC, ENP-BC
Assistant Professor & Nurse Practitioner Coordinator
Georgia Baptist College of Nursing of Mercer University
Atlanta, Georgia
PICOT in Practice: Asking Clinical Questions

REVIEWERS

Karen Arca-Contreras, DNP, RN-BC
Assistant Professor of Nursing
College of Staten Island
Staten Island, New York

Rita Bergevin, MA, RN-BC, CWCN
Clinical Instructor
University of North Carolina at Chapel Hill, School of Nursing
Chapel Hill, North Carolina

Barbara Blozen, EdD, MA, RN-BC, CNL
Professor of Nursing
New Jersey City University
Jersey City, New Jersey

Deborah Byrne, PhD, RN, CNE
Assistant Professor of Nursing
La Salle University
Philadelphia, Pennsylvania

Adeline Chu, PhD, ME, BSN
Clinical Assistant Professor
University of Washington, School of Nursing
Seattle, Washington

Ashleigh Clark, MS
Assistant Professor of Nursing
McNeese State University
Sulphur, Louisiana

Gina Galosi, DNP, RNC-OB, CNE
Assistant Professor
Thomas Jefferson University
Philadelphia, Pennsylvania

Kimberly F. Gibson, RN
Practical Nursing Instructor
Tennessee College of Applied Technology at Athens
Athens, Tennessee

Tish Gill, DNP, MSN, RN, CNE
Assistant Professor of Nursing
Temple University
Philadelphia, Pennsylvania

Kristen Mathieu Gonzalez, DNP, MSN/Ed, RN
Assistant Clinical Professor
Northeastern University
Burlington, Massachusetts

Susan Growe, DNP, RN, COI
Assistant Professor of Nursing
Nevada State College
Las Vegas, Nevada

Katherine Howard, MS, RN-BC, CNE
Instructor of Nursing
Middlesex County College
Edison, New Jersey

Colby Philip Hunsberger, DNP, MSN, RN
Instructor of Nursing
Clarion University
Clarion, Pennsylvania

Heather LaPoint, PhD, RN, CNE, CCRN-K
Assistant Professor of Nursing
State University of New York at Plattsburgh
Plattsburgh, New York

Bridget Maley, PhD, RN
Assistant Professor
New York City College of Technology
Brooklyn, New York

Hyacinth Martin
Professor of Nursing
Borough of Manhattan Community College
New York, New York

Maria Fatima Martinez, DNP, RN, CNE, CMS-BC
Assistant Professor of Nursing
Oak Point University
Oak Brook, Illinois

Tina M. Mathers, MSN, MBA, RN
Assistant Professor of Nursing
The University of Texas Medical Branch School of Nursing
Galveston, Texas

Darci McCall, PhD, MSN, RNC-OB, C-EFM
Clinical Associate Professor, School of Nursing
Boise State University
Boise, Idaho

Sara McPherson, PhD, RN, CNE
Director, UIC Nursing-Springfield Campus
Clinical Assistant Professor
Department of Biobehavioral Nursing Science
University of Illinois at Chicago
Springfield, Illinois

Egan Monroe
South College
Knoxville, Tennessee

Bethany Nasser, PhD, MS, BSN
Assistant Professor of Nursing
Endicott College
Beverly, Massachusetts

Kimberlie Noyes, MSN, APRN, FNP-C
Assistant Professor of Nursing
Finger Lakes Community College
Canandaigua, New York

Mary Owens
Assistant Professor
Mercy College of Health Sciences
Des Moines, Iowa

Rebecca Toothaker, PhD, RN
Associate Professor of Nursing
Bloomsburg University
Bloomsburg, Pennsylvania

Geraldine Tyrell, DNP, MSN, BSN
Director of the Department of Nursing
Bethel College
Newton, Kansas

Sharon Wexler, PhD
Professor
Pace University
White Plains, New York

Nadine Wodaski, DNP, MSN-Ed, CNS, BSN
Assistant Professor of Nursing
University of Detroit Mercy
Detroit, Michigan

Heather Zonts, PhD, RN, CNE
BSN Program Chair
Assistant Professor of Nursing
Mount Aloysius College
Cresson, Pennsylvania

PREFACE

Today's competitive, market-driven health care environment is challenging the very nature of professional nursing practice. *Fundamentals of Nursing: The Art and Science of Person-Centered Care, Tenth Edition*, promotes nursing as an evolving art and science, directed to human health and well-being. It challenges students to cultivate the Quality and Safety Education for Nurses (QSEN) and blended competencies they will need to serve patients and the public well. Our aim is to prepare nurses who combine the highest level of scientific knowledge and technical skill with responsible, caring practice. We want to challenge students to identify and master the cognitive and technical skills required of a nurse. But we also intentionally integrate other core content including interprofessional/intraprofessional/interpersonal communication, ethical comportment, legal regulations and standards, population health principles, and a systems-based perspective to facilitate the development of the student nurse as a member of the profession. We refuse to allow love of humanity, accountability, caring relationships, compassionate presence, and advocacy to become relics of a bygone era.

Those new to nursing can quickly become overwhelmed by the demands placed on the nurse's knowledge, technical competence, interpersonal skills, and commitment. Therefore, much care has gone into the selection of both the content in this edition and the manner of its presentation. We strive to capture the unique essence of both the art and science of nursing, distilling what the person beginning the study and practice of nursing needs to know. We invite students to identify with the profession, to share in its pride, and to respond to today's challenges competently, enthusiastically, and accountably. The Gallop Poll for 2021 noted that nurses earned the most trusted professional distinction for the 20th year. We hope to provide an opportunity for students to appreciate how their individual, unique talents contribute to and strengthen the profession of nursing.

LEARNING EXPERIENCE

This text and the entire Taylor Suite have been created with the student's experience in mind. Care has been taken to appeal to all learning styles. The student-friendly writing style ensures that students will comprehend and retain information. The updated art program and strong features enhance understanding of important concepts. The textbook features, interrelated Fundamentals products, and associated CoursePoint resources have been intentionally developed and integrated to provide a consistent, cohesive learning experience.

ORGANIZATION

Fundamentals of Nursing: The Art and Science of Person-Centered Care, Tenth Edition, is organized into seven units. Ideally, the text is followed sequentially, but every effort has been made to respect the differing needs of diverse curricula and students. Thus, each chapter stands on its own merit and may be read independently of others. Nursing Concepts lists in each chapter opener highlight connections to fundamental nursing concepts and support ease of identification, especially for concept-based nursing programs.

Unit I, Foundations of Thoughtful, Person-Centered Nursing Practice

Unit I opens with a description of contemporary nursing. Successive chapters introduce content foundational to nursing practice: theory, research, and evidence-based practice; health, illness, and disparities; health of the individual, family, community and environment; cultural diversity; values, ethics, and advocacy; legal dimensions of nursing practice; communication; teaching and counseling; and leadership, managing, and delegating.

Unit II, Health Care Delivery

Unit II is completely revised in light of the continuing changes in health care delivery. The new content highlights nurses' expanding roles in care coordination as partnerships are forged with patients, families, local and global communities, and the populations we serve. Chapters address the variety of community-based health care settings; continuity of care as the patient enters a health care facility, is transferred within the facility, and is discharged into another setting within the community; and care provided within the home. This unit highlights ANA's Principles for Health System Transformation, IHI's quadruple aim, new information on Reliability Care Accountability Matrix, and updated health care reform information that emphasizes nurses' contributions.

Unit III, Processes of Thoughtful, Person-Centered Practice

Unit III offers a thoroughly revised and detailed, step-by-step guide to each component of the nursing process with practical guidelines and examples included in each chapter. Each chapter concludes with a section on "Reflective

Practice Leading to Personal Learning" that invites readers to look at their experience with each step of the nursing process, understand it, and learn from it. The goal is always to invite reflection on how we can improve our thoughtful, person-centered practice.

Chapter 13 offers a careful introduction to thoughtful, person-centered practice with expanded content on theories of caring, clinical reasoning, clinical judgment, decision making, and reflective practice. Separate chapters address the nursing process as a whole: Quality and Safety Education for Nurses (QSEN) and blended competencies, clinical reasoning, clinical judgment, assessing, diagnosing/problem identification, outcome identification and planning, implementing, and evaluating. Chapter 14 is a new chapter dedicated exclusively to clinical judgment that describes new features in the text. Chapter 16, previously focused on nursing diagnoses, now has a new focus on analyzing and hypothesizing to identify patient problems and needs. Chapter 20 includes expanded content on privacy guidelines and standards for social media, electronic health records (EHRs), reporting, and conferring. Chapter 21, Informatics and Health Care Technologies is responsive to what today's nurses need to know about how best to use new technologies and information to coordinate care and achieve desired outcomes. There is recognition that more health care facilities and organizations are combining virtual services with in-person care to ease hospital burden and provide better patient experiences and satisfaction. Central to this transition is telehealth, remote monitoring, and mobile care teams.

Unit IV, Developmentally Appropriate Care

Unit IV provides the basis for understanding growth and development across the lifespan and acknowledges nursing's differing requirements arising from the various developmental stages and abilities to meet developmental tasks. This content is framed to recognize the historical context and core tenets of developmental theories, while reinforcing that inclusivity and acceptance without bias are essential to good nursing care.

Unit V, Actions Basic to Nursing Care

Unit V introduces the foundational skills used by nurses: maintaining asepsis, measuring vital signs, assessing health, promoting safety, incorporating complementary and alternative therapies, administering medication, and caring for surgical patients. Chapter 29 was reorganized around the person-centered, systems-based, and population-based aspects of safety and security to intentionally integrate the spheres of practice and highlight three new domains in AACN's *Essentials*: person-centered care (domain 2), systems-based practice (domain 7), and population health (domain 3). Chapter 31 relies on guidance from professional nursing organizations with expertise in perioperative nursing.

Unit VI, Promoting Healthy Physiologic Responses

Unit VI explores the nurse's role in helping patients meet basic physiologic needs: hygiene; skin integrity and wound care; activity; rest and sleep; comfort and pain management; nutrition; urinary elimination; bowel elimination; oxygenation and perfusion; and fluid, electrolyte, and acid–base balance. Chapter 33 contains the latest guidance on pressure injury prevention, staging, and management. Chapter 36 addresses the opioid crisis and challenges students to consider different perspectives regarding legal ramifications and related structural disparities. Chapter 40 includes cardiovascular content as it pertains to its role in oxygenation. In each chapter, guidelines are included for assessing and diagnosing unhealthy responses and for planning, implementing, and evaluating appropriate care strategies.

Unit VII, Promoting Healthy Psychosocial Responses

Unit VII uses the same format as Unit VI to focus on the psychosocial needs of patients: self-concept; stress and adaptation; loss, grief, and dying; sensory functioning; sexuality; and spirituality.

THEMES

The following themes are interwoven throughout the text to provide a broad knowledge base of nursing essentials while emphasizing holistic care.

Thoughtful Person-Centered Care

Our subtitle reflects today's emphasis on person-centered care. Readers will now see an even stronger emphasis on clinical reasoning, clinical judgment, decision making, and reflective practice in every chapter. Central to this model are the nurse's personal attributes, knowledge base, and clinical experience; clinical reasoning, clinical judgment, and decision making; patient-centered nursing process; and reflective practice leading to personal learning.

Nursing as an Art and Science

Nursing as a science is characterized by a growing body of knowledge that links technical and interpersonal interventions to desired patient outcomes; as an art, nursing demands of its practitioners sufficient competency to creatively design individualized strategies to assist patients to reach personal health goals. A unique spirit of caring always must prevail.

Professional Formation of the Nurse

Responding to emphases in the AACN's *Essentials*, this edition weaves content about the professional formation of the nurse into every chapter. The goal is to form students who own the professional identity of the nurse and are intentional about developing the character and values of the nurse as well as the knowledge, skills, and attitudes. Every effort has been made to incorporate content from the ANA *Nursing: Scope and Standards of Practice* (4th ed.), AACN's *Essentials,* and the National Academy of Sciences, Engineering and Medicine's *The Future of Nursing 2020–2030.*

Integrated Nursing Process

After the nursing process is introduced in Unit III, it provides the organizational framework for successive chapters. The *2021 Nursing Scope and Standards of Practice* highlights the continuing importance of nursing process:

> Regardless of the theoretical knowledge base upon which nursing and its practice are derived, that knowledge fits within the multidimensional nursing process, the analytical, critical-thinking framework guiding professional thinking and activities.

Chapters in Units VI and VII, which deal with physiologic and psychosocial responses, begin with a succinct background discussion of the concept, followed by identification of factors that influence how different individuals respond to these needs. Phases in the nursing process are used to describe related nursing responsibilities. Throughout these chapters, students will find numerous practical examples of how to conduct focused assessments; develop and write problem statements; identify goals and outcomes; and select, implement, and evaluate appropriate nursing interventions. These examples will reinforce the student's mastery of nursing process skills. Some chapters in Units VI and VII conclude with a Nursing Care Plan that illustrates each phase of the nursing process and a sample documentation of nursing assessment or intervention. Others feature Evolving Case Studies based on NCSBN's model of evolving cases with directed questions at each level of the Clinical Judgment Measurement Model. The answers to these cases are included only in the instructor materials to allow nurse educators to use them as desired. In addition, Concept Maps demonstrating the nursing process are included in several chapters. The basic concept map structure for nursing students just starting to consider the nursing process incorporates: (1) beginning pathophysiologic principles, laboratory values, and medications; (2) actual and potential patient problems; and (3) related nursing interventions. Concept mapping provides the learner the opportunity to visually depict and explore connections between disease processes, problems identified by nurses, and individualized nursing interventions. Although concept maps can take many forms, the beginning maps in this text focus on identifying connections using a specific format that provides students a starting point for mapping. The concept map in Chapter 31, Perioperative Nursing, depicts a different structure, designed to show students a way to organize their thoughts as they begin to think like nurses.

Critical Thinking, Clinical Reasoning, and Clinical Judgment

This edition describes carefully curated options that are discussed separately and in tandem to build ways of knowing through the lens of clinical judgment. Clinical judgment is foundational to what we do as nurses. Building a shared understanding of the elements fundamentally shifts the focus of students to the processes they will need to learn and apply. Addressed are:

- Tanner's (2006) Model of Clinical Judgment
- Lasater's (2007) Clinical Judgment Rubric
- Nielson, Stragnell, and Jester (2007) Reflection Tool
- Gibb's Model of Reflection (1988)
- Nursing Process

The 10th edition continues to invite students to reflect on their ability to be the critical difference for recipients of their thoughtful practice. The revised *Self-Reflective Practice* boxes, *Focused Critical Thinking Guides*, and *Developing Clinical Reasoning and Clinical Judgment* material in each chapter challenge students to use new knowledge and experience to "think through" learning exercises designed to demonstrate how careful thinking can change outcomes. The ninth edition added Reflective Practice Leading to Personal Learning content to Chapters 8 and 9 in Unit I and each of the chapters in Units III, VI, and VII. In addition to a brand-new chapter on Clinical Judgment, the 10th edition added a new feature, Thoughtful Person-Centered Practice: Challenging Topics, which offers evolving scenarios of challenging and relevant issues based on Tanner's Clinical Judgment Model (2006) and the reflection tool developed by Nielson, Stragnell, and Jester (2007). These exercises challenge students to reflect upon and critique how they would respond to real practice situations—each designed to promote their professional formation and ability to think, value, and practice like a nurse.

Competency Models

Competency models outline very specific tasks or goals and are directly related to the measurement of nursing clinical judgment. These competency models are used in the development, implementation, and evaluation of nursing curricula and accredited programs nationwide. Framing clinical judgment as an expectation explains the significance to students the moment they begin a fundamentals course. This text was organized initially around what was called blended competencies (cognitive, technical, interpersonal, and ethical/legal) and these were later complemented with QSEN—this represents a history of embedding competencies, so this is not a new concept for this text.

- Competency Outcomes Performance Assessment Model (COPA, 1999/2009)
- QSEN influence: each chapter begins with "Reflective Practice: Cultivating QSEN Competencies"
- American Association of Colleges of Nursing (AACN, 2021): *The Essentials*
- National League for Nursing: *Competencies for Graduates of Nursing Programs* (2012) and *Hallmarks of Excellence in Nursing Education Model* (NLN, 2020)
- Competencies outlined in the revised ANA (2021) *Nursing Scope and Standards of Practice* 4th edition
- Interprofessional Education Collaborative (IPEC, 2016): *Core Competencies for Interprofessional Collaborative Practice*

Four Spheres of Care

The AACN 2021 *Essentials* noted that nursing education has historically emphasized clinical education in acute care. The first edition of our text did exactly that. But we quickly realized that students would be practicing in very diverse settings and that we needed to prepare them for these expanded roles, many in the community. We think you will see increased content in the 10th edition and examples of what *The Essentials* call the four spheres of care: (1) disease prevention/promotion of health and well-being, which includes the promotion of physical and mental health in all patients as well as management of minor acute and intermittent care needs of generally healthy patients; (2) chronic disease care; (3) regenerative or restorative care; and (4) hospice/palliative/supportive care.

Emphasis on Partnering With Patients, Families/Caregivers, and Professional Caregivers

Today, we have witnessed the health care "industry" transform patients to "customers," who buy health care (if they are able) as a commodity in the marketplace. We do not believe that a "customer orientation" serves patients or nurses well. One of our students shared her belief that she owes less to a "customer" and even to a "client" than she does to a "patient." We, therefore, use the term *patient*—in its most positive sense—to designate the recipient of nursing care, whether the patient is an individual, family group, or community. *Family* is defined by the patient and includes anyone they rely on for support, comfort, and care.

Careful attention is paid to directing students to identify, value, and develop the interpersonal skills that will allow them to effectively partner with patients, family, and professional caregivers. This edition highlights interprofessional collaborative practice and nursing strategies for actively engaging patients, family (as identified by the patient), guardians, caregivers, and the public in the development of health goals and strategies to achieve these goals.

Health, Justice, Equity, Diversity, and Inclusion

A health- rather than an illness-orientation provides a framework for presentation of content. This edition includes expanded content on the social determinants of health, health literacy, health disparities, and health equity. Special features such as *Promoting Health, Teaching Tips*, and *Health Literacy* boxes help to highlight this important content and new information on web-based resources for culturally respectful care is provided.

As nurses, we continue to practice in a health system plagued by disparities. As authors, we are committed to making health care work for everyone, especially the most vulnerable. While previous editions of this text highlighted the social determinants of health and offered practical resources for assessing special needs, for advocating for vulnerable individuals and groups, and for designing effective strategies to promote equity, the 10th edition heeds nursing leaders' call to prepare nurses who are anti-racist and highlights ANA's Standard on Respectful and Equitable Practice. New Vulnerable Populations Alerts are valuable additions to this edition.

Care has been taken to communicate that both nurses and patients may identify their gender and/or sexual orientation on a spectrum, and that they come from every racial and ethnic background and socioeconomic group. When not addressing a specific case, we have tried to avoid gender distinctions in personal pronouns. We also very intentionally differentiate the concepts of gender identity, gender expression, sexual identity, sexual orientation, and biological sex or sex assigned at birth—we focus on saying what we mean and only what is germane to providing nursing care. Every effort has been made to highlight diversity, equity, and inclusion themes and to use recommended language that honors each individual we describe. We understand that this language is changing rapidly and anticipate future modifications.

Health and Self-Care of the Nurse

If the pandemic taught us anything, it underscored the critical importance of the health and well-being of caregivers. In this edition, you will find a new Nurse Self-Care alert, enhanced content on wellness strategies and resilience.

Compassion Fatigue and Burnout

In our efforts to instill a commitment to service and excellence in our graduates, we have often failed as educators to address appropriate work/life balance challenges. Our ANA Code of Ethics continues to instruct nurses that their primary commitment is to patients, while at the same time reminding them they have duties to self. We directly address these challenges of commitment in the 10th edition with expanded content in Chapter 1, new Nurse Self-Care alerts throughout the text, and highlighted resources for self-care.

Climate Change and Environmental Health

ANA's *Nursing: Scope and Standards of Practice* (2021) includes Standard 17, Resource Stewardship and 18, Environmental Health. The 10th edition added new content on environmental health, and the United Nations Sustainable Development Goals offers students practical strategies and climate actions they can use to partner in their communities to help limit global warming and take care of our planet.

Attention to Care of the Older Person

Because the age of the population is increasing, nurses encounter growing numbers of older patients in all practice settings. Chapter 24: Middle and Older Adulthood, the *Focus on the Older Adult* boxes, and general considerations for the older patients that appear within the text aim to sensitize students to the special nursing needs of this population. Readers of the 10th edition will find expanded information related to health disparities; a discussion of cascade iatrogenics; technology-based and online resources for older adults; expanded information on developmental and disability considerations; and updated guidelines for health-related screenings, examinations, and immunizations for the aging adult.

Healthy Work Environments

This edition addresses current issues of disruptive interpersonal behavior (including incivility and bullying), cyber terror, lateral violence, aggressive behavior, and nurses' use of social media to help readers understand what it takes to have a healthy work environment.

Evidence-Based Practice

Content on research and evidence-based practice has been updated and is included in Unit I for increased emphasis early in the learning experience. See the John Hopkins Evidence-Based Practice Model and new hierarchy of evidence pyramid. The updated feature, *PICOT in Practice: Asking Clinical Questions*, encourages readers to delve into research to solve a clinical question using the PICOT format and guidelines. Updated *Research in Nursing: Bridging the Gap to Evidence-Based Practice* boxes, appearing throughout the book, promote the value of research, and apply its relevance to nursing practice. Students are challenged to become informed participants in, and consumers of, clinical research. To that end, students can explore additional research in nursing journal articles provided for each chapter on our website (http://thePoint.lww.com/Taylor10e).

Focus on Nursing Skills

Skills are presented in a concise, straightforward, and simplified format that is intended to facilitate competent performance of nursing skills. A scientific rationale accompanies each nursing action; many color photographs and illustrations further reinforce mastery. Students are encouraged to think critically about the skills they are performing. *Delegation Considerations* assist students and graduate nurses in developing the critical decision-making skills necessary to transfer responsibility for the performance of an activity to another individual and to ensure safe and effective nursing care. The *Developing Clinical Reasoning and Judgment* features support development of clinical reasoning and clinical judgment skills. *Unexpected Situations and Related Interventions* are included to help students think critically about the skills they are performing. *Special Considerations*, including modifications and age and community-based care considerations, are given where appropriate and guide students to implement person-centered interventions. Also included are *Documentation Guidelines* and *Sample Documentation* to help students learn what and how to document when performing skills.

Hand Hygiene icons alert students to this crucial step that is the best way to prevent the spread of microorganisms (see the *How to Use Fundamentals of Nursing* section on pp. xvi–xxv).

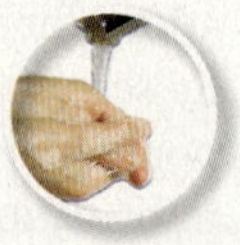

Patient Identification icons alert students to this critical step ensuring the right patient receives the intervention to help prevent errors (see the *How to Use Fundamentals of Nursing* section on pp. xvi–xxv).

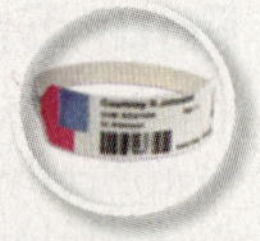

Focus on Community and Expanded Nursing Roles

Patients today spend fewer days in the hospital, are frequently transferred both within the hospital and between health care institutions and home, and need to rely on rapidly proliferating community-based health care resources. Content on accountable care organizations, medical homes, and medical neighborhoods, as well as content on the new roles for nurses (nurse coach, clinical nurse leader, nurse navigator, and nurse care coordinator) highlight both traditional and innovative care in institutional and community-based practice settings. New content includes the Robert Wood Johnson Foundations Healthy Communities resources and CDC's Division of Community Health (DCH), which created Partnerships to Improve Community Health (PICH).

Focus on Safety

New content highlights today's emphasis on patient safety, including expanded safety information related to children, adolescents, and older adults. The National Academy of Sciences, Engineering and Medicine safety content, 2020 Joint Commission National Patient Safety Goals, and Sentinel Event Statistics are highlighted, and new information is provided on health care–associated infections (HAIs). Safe Patient Handling and Mobility Practices are included in this edition as well as expanded content on patient "hand-offs."

In addition, QSEN boxes and Safety Alerts help students cultivate the Quality and Safety Education for Nurses (QSEN) and blended competencies they will need to serve patients and the public well.

Pandemic Precautions

It is difficult to determine where we will be as the learning package publishes. We obviously strongly recommend following the CDC and your institutional guidelines on use of personal protective equipment and the guidelines to reduce transmission. That said, you will not see masks worn in most photos unless generally indicated. We are hopeful that we will all soon be practicing in a postpandemic world.

Up-to-Date Clinical and Practice Information

Revisions in each clinical chapter will help educators and students remain current. Sample new content includes:

- Updated information from AACN's *Essentials*, the ANA *Nursing: Scope and Standards of Practice* (4th ed.), and National Academy of Sciences, Engineering and Medicine's *The Future of Nursing 2020–2030*
- NEW! Content on diversity, inclusion, and equity that addresses institutional and systemic racism
- AACN's Four Spheres of Care

- Updated content on the Formation of the Professional Identity of the Nurse
- NEW! Feature: Evolving Case Study that reflects the Next Generation NCLEX (NGN)
- NEW! Information on deaths of isolation and despair
- United Nations Sustainable Development Goals
- NEW! Content on climate change and environmental health
- NEW! Content on moral agency, moral distress, moral injury, incivility, and academic ethics
- Challenging topic on reproductive ethics
- Challenging topic on nurse death by suicide
- Leadership's role in preventing clinician burnout
- Pandemic consideration throughout—as applicable
- Community Health needs assessment
- Healthy People 2030
- Updated mental health content
- Comparison of clinical judgment models
- Quick priority assessments
- NEW! Content on triage and nurse triage role
- Updated content on documentation
- New! Information on telehealth, remote monitoring, and mobile care teams
- NEW! Content on disabilities and a vulnerable populations alert
- NEW! Content on adverse childhood experiences
- NEW! Content on treatment of transgender children and gender dysphoria
- Updated content on human suffering and compassionate presence
- Meeting the spiritual needs of millennials
- Expanded information on genetics, genomics, and epigenetics
- Information on SIDS and SUID (sudden unexplained infant death)
- Expanded discussion of childhood obesity
- Dangers associated with substance use disorder and opioid use disorder
- Expanded information on multiple drug–resistant organisms; use of care bundles or evidence-based protocols; the impact of staffing issues on HAIs
- ANA recommendations on reducing use of restraints
- Periop: "never events," new guidelines for preop fasting and skin prep, and operative positioning recommendations by AORN (Association of periOperative Registered Nurses)
- The Joint Commission universal protocol and "time-out"
- Noise prevention in acute care and ICU
- Expanded content on self-care including new information on mindfulness and a new Nurse Self-Care alert
- The Joint Commission Sentinel Alert on fatigue in health care workers
- Role of Pain Resource Nurse
- New content on biological sex, biological sex identification, and sexual orientation
- SBAR/SBARR/I-SBAR-R communication to improve patient "hand-offs" from one professional caregiver to another
- CUS communication tool to assist in effective communication related to patient safety concerns
- Updated ANA Principles of Delegation
- Updated content on maintaining privacy, confidentiality, and professionalism and the use of social media
- Content on Bedside Reports and Purposeful rounding
- Updated medication math calculations designed to highlight common errors
- Enhanced content on the opioid crisis including new standards by The Joint Commission such as the Prescription Drug Monitoring Program (PDMP), individualizing and performing a comprehensive pain assessment, and current pain management guidelines
- Inclusion of new terms and treatments associated with pressure injuries and wounds
- Cardiopulmonary resuscitation (CPR) for the mind: Facts About Mental Health First Aid

Self-Assessment Guides

Fundamentals of Nursing has always encouraged students to be independent learners. Checklists throughout the text (e.g., blended skills assessment, use of nursing process, health assessments) allow students to evaluate their personal strengths and limitations and develop related learning goals.

SPECIAL FEATURES

Many features appear throughout the text to help students grasp important content. Refer to the "How to Use *Fundamentals of Nursing*" section on pages xiii–xxii to learn more about them.

COMPREHENSIVE, INTEGRATED FUNDAMENTALS AND SKILLS SOLUTIONS

We are delighted to offer an expanded suite of digital solutions that offer instructors and students using the Taylor, Lynn, and Bartlett Fundamentals and Skills suite of content everything they need to conduct their fundamentals course and integrate clinical skills learning throughout the curriculum. To learn more about any solution with the Taylor suite, please contact your local Wolters Kluwer representative.

Lippincott CoursePoint+

Lippincott*® *CoursePoint+ is an integrated, digital curriculum solution for nursing education that provides a completely interactive experience geared to help students understand, retain, and apply their course knowledge and be prepared for practice. The time-tested, easy-to-use, and trusted solution includes engaging learning tools, evidence-based practice, case studies, and in-depth reporting to meet students where they are in their learning, combined with the most trusted nursing education content on the market to help prepare students for practice. This easy-to-use digital learning solution of *Lippincott*® *CoursePoint+*, combined with unmatched support, gives instructors and students everything they need for course and curriculum success!

Lippincott® *CoursePoint+* includes:

- An interactive eBook provides on-demand access to the full contents of this textbook.
- Leading content provides a variety of learning tools to engage students of all learning styles.

- A personalized learning approach gives students the content and tools they need at the moment they need it, giving them data for more focused remediation and helping to boost their confidence and competence.
- Powerful tools, including varying levels of case studies, interactive learning activities, and adaptive learning powered by PrepU, help students learn the critical thinking and clinical judgment skills to help them become practice-ready nurses.
- Preparation for Practice tools improve student competence, confidence, and success in transitioning to practice.
  - **vSim for Nursing:** Help students be practice-ready with the next generation of vSim for Nursing. The virtual simulation program that so many nursing educators and students rely on has been taken to the next level, providing the most realistic, true-to-life clinical experience. Co-developed by Laerdal Medical and Wolters Kluwer, vSim® for Nursing | Fundamentals provides real-world, evidence-based scenarios written by the National League for Nursing, with built-in point-of-care solutions for reference and remediation. With vSim for Nursing, students can develop their clinical judgment, competence, and confidence. The next generation of vSim for Nursing offers increased realism and fidelity, improved communication, and enhanced opportunities to develop clinical judgment.
  - **Lippincott Advisor for Education:** With over 8,500 entries covering the latest evidence-based content and drug information, Lippincott Advisor for Education provides students with the most up-to-date information possible, while giving them valuable experience with the same point-of-care content they will encounter in practice.
- Unparalleled reporting provides in-depth dashboards with several data points to track student progress and help identify strengths and weaknesses.
- Unmatched support includes training coaches, product trainers, and nursing education consultants to help educators and students implement CoursePoint+ with ease.

Lippincott Skills for Nursing Education

Developed with complete consistency with *Fundamentals of Nursing*, the companion skills title, *Taylor's Clinical Skills for Nursing Education*, 6th Edition, by Pamela Lynn is now available in a new digital solution.

Help student nurses develop skill competency and clinical judgment with ***Lippincott® Skills for Nursing Education***, an unparalleled nursing education skills solution.

Available anytime, anywhere, ***Lippincott Skills for Nursing Education*** is designed specifically to empower nursing faculty and students to support teaching, learning, and reporting on nursing skills across the curriculum. Expert-authored skill instructions, evidence-based rationales, numerous videos, and case studies help the novice nursing student master new skills and confidently prepare for skills lab and clinical settings.

Used alone or integrated with *Lippincott® CoursePoint*, ***Lippincott Skills for Nursing Education*** offers an efficient learning experience backed with tools to monitor and motivate student preparedness and skill competency.

Taylor's Clinical Nursing Skills Collection, authored by Pamela Lynn, EdD, MSN, RN, delivers a robust set of essential skills for the undergraduate nurse and meets the needs of students throughout the curriculum.

ADDITIONAL RESOURCES FOR TEACHING AND LEARNING

To further facilitate teaching and learning, a carefully designed teaching and learning package has been developed to assist faculty and students.

Instructor Resources

Tools to assist you with teaching your course are available in Lippincott CoursePoint+, with select tools available upon adoption of this text on thePoint® at http://thepoint.lww.com/Taylor10e.

- A thoroughly revised and augmented **Test Generator** contains more than 2900 NCLEX-style questions mapped to chapter learning outcomes.
- An extensive collection of materials is provided for each book chapter:
  - **Lesson Plans** outline learning outcomes and identify relevant resources from the robust instructor and student resource packages to help you prepare for your class.
  - **Pre-Lecture Quizzes** (and answers) allow you to check students' reading.
  - **PowerPoint Presentations** provide an easy way to integrate the textbook with your students' classroom experience; multiple-choice and true/false questions are included to promote class participation.
  - **Guided Lecture Notes** are organized by outcome and provide corresponding PowerPoint slide numbers to simplify preparation for lecture.
  - **Discussion Topics** (and suggested answers) can be used in the classroom or in online discussion boards to facilitate interaction with your students.
  - **Assignments** (and suggested answers) include group, written, clinical, and Web assignments to engage students in varied activities and assess their learning.
  - **Case Studies** with related questions (and suggested answers) give students an opportunity to apply their knowledge to a client case similar to one they might encounter in practice.
- Sample **Syllabi** are provided for one- and two-semester courses.
- **NEW! AACN Essentials Content Mapping**, which are competency-based and include expected competencies for entry-level nurses and advanced-level nurses.
- A **QSEN Competency Map** identifies content and special features in the book related to competencies identified by the QSEN Institute.
- An **Image Bank** lets you use the photographs and illustrations from this textbook in your course materials.
- Access to all **Student Resources** is provided so that you can understand the student experience and use these resources in your course as well.

Student Resources

An exciting set of learning resources is available to students using Lippincott CoursePoint+. Select resources are available on thePoint* at http://thepoint.lww.com/Taylor10e using the codes printed in the front of students' textbooks.

- Interactive learning resources appeal to a variety of learning styles.
  - **Concepts in Action Animations** bring physiologic and pathophysiologic concepts to life.
  - **Practice & Learn Case Studies** present case scenarios and offer interactive exercises and questions to help students apply what they have learned.
  - **Watch & Learn Videos** reinforce select skills from the textbook and appeal to visual and auditory learners.
- **Journal Articles** offer access to current articles relevant to each chapter and available in Wolters Kluwer journals to familiarize students with nursing literature.

Study Guide

A comprehensive study aid for reviewing key concepts, *Study Guide for Fundamentals of Nursing: The Art and Science of Person-Centered Care*, 10th Edition, has been thoroughly revised and presents a variety of exercises, including case studies and practice NCLEX-style questions, to reinforce textbook content and enhance learning.

Skill Checklists

Skill Checklists for Fundamentals of Nursing: The Art and Science of Person-Centered Care, 10th Edition (included in Lippincott CoursePoint+ or available in print) offers step-by-step forms to evaluate student competency for the skills included in this textbook. A more complete list of skills and associated skill checklists is available in *Lippincott Skills for Nursing Education*.

Lippincott DocuCare

Available for separate purchase, Lippincott® DocuCare combines Web-based academic EHR simulation software with clinical case scenarios, allowing students to learn how to use an EHR in a safe, true-to-life setting, while enabling instructors to measure their progress. Lippincott DocuCare's nonlinear solution works well in the classroom, simulation lab, and clinical practice.

HOW TO USE
FUNDAMENTALS OF NURSING

Dear Student,

Congratulations on choosing an exciting and rewarding profession! All of us who have been part of the writing of this text welcome you warmly to our profession and value our role as your guides to excellent practice. We have tried in this text to present in a readable and enjoyable format, the scientific and technical knowledge you will need to design safe and effective nursing care. But we want to do more than prepare you intellectually and technically. You will also find narratives that will teach you valuable interpersonal skills and content specifically designed to prepare you to meet the ethical and legal challenges in today's practice. So take a deep breath and dig in. Your patients are counting on you and so are we!

Carol Taylor, Pamela Lynn, and Jennifer L. Bartlett

HERE'S HOW TO GET STARTED!

FOLLOW THE STORY LINES!

Get to know your patients by reading the chapter opening **Case Scenarios**.

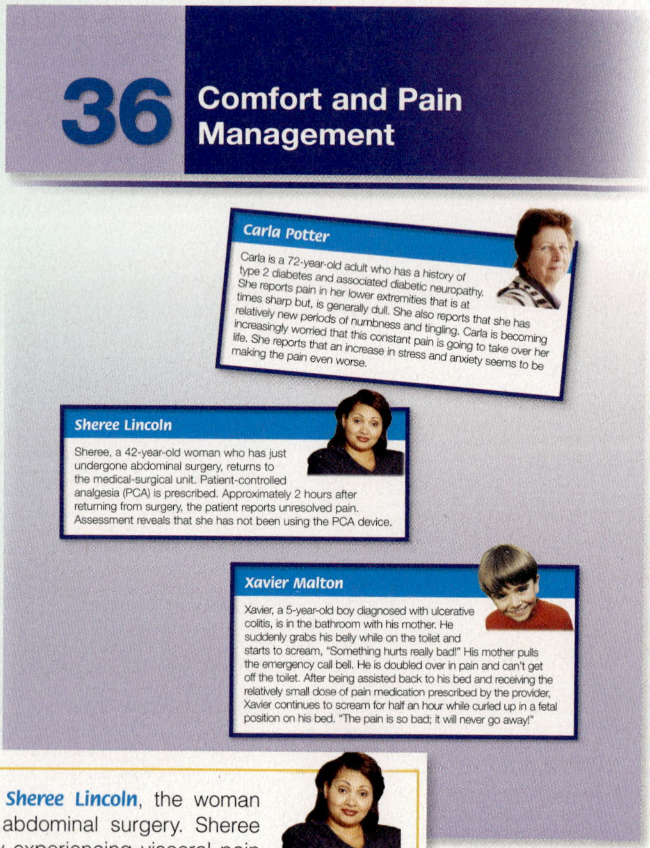

Narratives throughout the chapter refer to these scenarios, helping you to consider how the chapter content applies to care of real patients. For your convenience, a list of these case scenarios and threaded narratives, along with their location in the book, appears in the "Case Studies in This Book" section later in this front matter.

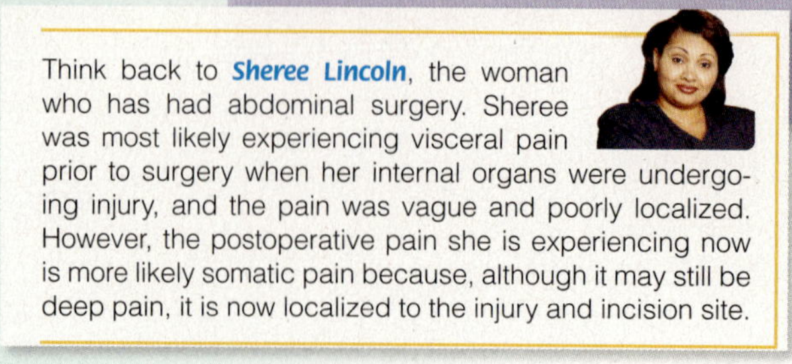

NEWLY UPDATED! Unfolding Patient Stories, written by the National League for Nursing, are an engaging way to begin meaningful conversations in the classroom. These vignettes, which unfold in two parts each and are interspersed throughout the text, feature patients from Wolters Kluwer's *vSim Fundamentals* (codeveloped by Laerdal Medical) and DocuCare products; however, each Unfolding Patient Story in the book stands alone, not requiring purchase of these products. For your convenience, a list of these case studies, along with their location in the book, appears in the "Case Studies in This Book" section later in this front matter.

Unfolding Patient Stories: Marvin Hayes • Part 1

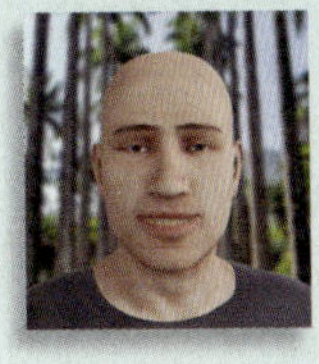

Marvin Hayes, a 43-year-old male, is being seen at the clinic. He has a family history of colorectal cancer. What questions can the nurse ask to identify disturbances in bowel elimination? What are the signs and symptoms of colon and rectal cancer? What patient education would the nurse provide when orders are written to obtain a stool sample and schedule a colonoscopy? (Marvin Hayes' story continues in Chapter 42.)

Care for Marvin and other patients in a realistic virtual environment: ***vSim*** *for Nursing* (thepoint.lww.com/vSimFunds). Practice documenting these patients' care in DocuCare (thepoint.lww.com/DocuCareEHR).

GET READY TO LEARN!

Before reading the chapter content, read the **Learning Outcomes**. These roadmaps help you understand what is important and why. Create your own learning outline or use them for self-testing.

Learning Outcomes

After completing the chapter, you will be able to accomplish the following:

1. Explain the components, purposes, and types of health assessments.
2. Prepare the patient and the environment for a health assessment.
3. Conduct a health history.
4. Use the techniques of inspection, palpation, and auscultation appropriately during a physical assessment.
5. Conduct a physical assessment in a systematic manner.
6. Document health assessment findings in a concise, descriptive, and legally appropriate manner.
7. Describe nursing responsibilities related to diagnostic and laboratory testing as part of health assessment.

NEW! Nursing Concepts list in the chapter opener highlight connections to nursing concepts for ease of identification.

Nursing Concepts

- Assessment
- Clinical Decision Making/Clinical Judgment
- Communication
- Therapeutic Communication

Key Terms are bolded throughout the narrative; explanations to help you become familiar with new vocabulary are presented online at https://thepoint.lww.com/taylor10e

STAY CURRENT ON SAFETY, TECHNOLOGY, AND LEGAL DEVELOPMENTS!

QSEN boxes highlight content related to QSEN competencies, which are key to ensuring students understand how to avoid harming patients and providers with best practice in individual performance and facility wide.

QSEN PATIENT-CENTERED CARE

The health practices and beliefs of patients and/or family members/caregivers related to fever and other symptoms may be influenced by cultural beliefs and practices. Culturally and ethnically sensitive strategies must be considered when providing interventions and patient education related to fever.

Technology Alerts feature new technology in development that will likely be in place by the time students are practicing. By understanding as students that technology is always changing, they will be better prepared to embrace change later.

Technology Alert

One system, ON-Q Pain Relief System, involves administration of local anesthetic medication directly at the affected surgical site. The benefit of this temporary system is earlier mobility and effective pain relief, with fewer side effects because of decreased opioid use postoperatively (Cinar et al., 2021; Porter et al., 2021).

Legal Alerts highlight important laws that affect nurses and are applicable to nursing practice.

Legal Alert

Patients have the right to be treated with dignity and to be involved in developing their pain management plan of care.

LEARN TO PRACTICE WELLNESS STRATEGIES AND SELF-CARE!

NEW! Nursing Self-Care Alerts remind us that we cannot be there for others if we do not take care of ourselves.

Nursing Self-Care Alert

Although the benefits of wearing a mask far outweighed the potential risks, nurses (and other members of the interprofessional health care team) had to take extra measures during the pandemic to protect their skin from breakdown due to prolonged use of masks and other necessary PPE.

Examine the **Nursing Care Plan** box (often derived from the chapter opener cases) to discover common health problems and the wide variety of independent and collaborative interventions that nurses manage.

Nursing Care Plan for Mr. Bitner 35-1

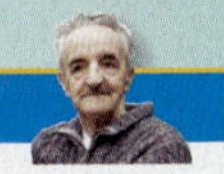

Mr. Bitner is an alert, widowed, 86-year-old man who was admitted to a long-term care facility 2 months ago. He is ambulatory and performs most of his own care. His admitting medical diagnoses include diabetes mellitus and hypertension. He adds to this list "a touch of arthritis." His daughter complains to the charge nurse that her father seems to be spending more and more time during the day napping and that he says he does not sleep well at night. A comprehensive sleep assessment of Mr. Bitner after his daughter's expression of concern reveals the following data:

- *Sleep–wakefulness pattern:* Patient goes to bed between 2000 and 2100 and gets out of bed between 0700 and 0800 because the staff are getting his roommate out of bed at this time. Patient states he never falls asleep before midnight because he always watched the late news at home. He usually wakes twice during the night to void and often cannot go back to sleep. During the day, patient is frequently observed dozing in his chair. If not discouraged, he returns to his room midmorning and afternoon for a 1-hour nap.
- *Effect of sleep pattern on everyday living:* Patient states: "I'm always tired. I don't seem to have much energy anymore." Patient has not socialized yet with other residents and, without strong encouragement, does not participate in group activities. From his point of view, the patient states that life holds little reason for him to be awake. "I worked for the railroad for almost 50 years and I never overslept once."
- *Sleep aids:* Patient denies ever using medication to fall asleep. States he often relaxed at home in the evening

View the **Concept Map** (from selected chapter opener cases) to see how the nursing process can be visually represented when planning care for a patient.

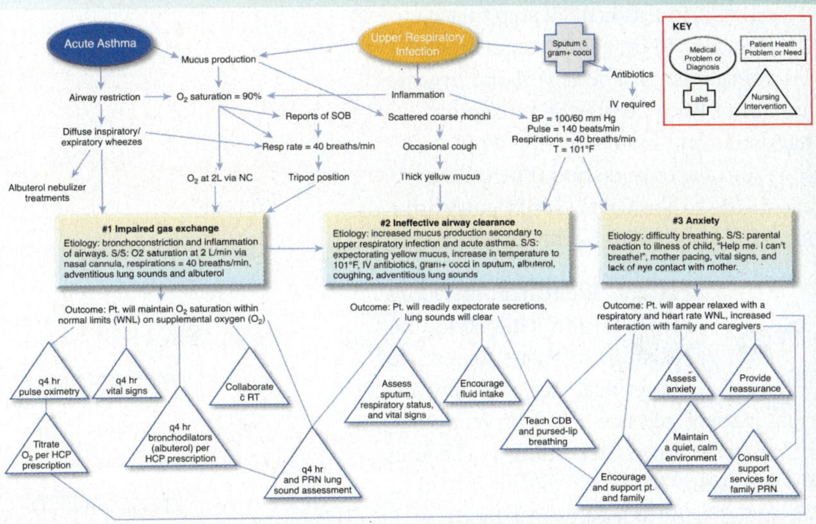

Evaluation

- **Diagnosis #1** Tyrone continues to have oxygen saturation below normal limits, tachypnea, and wheezing. Continue to monitor response to collaborative interventions. Notify physician for an increase in respiratory distress and a decrease in pulse oximetry.
- **Diagnosis #2** Tyrone continues to have audible adventitious sounds. He is readily expectorating secretions. Continue to monitor.
- **Diagnosis #3** Tyrone made eye contact with nurse as she explained the actions of his bronchodilators. Mother stopped pacing and sat beside son to provide comfort and reassurance. Continue interventions.

Concept map that displays the use of the nursing process in designing a care plan for Tyrone Jacobs. c̄ = with; IV = intravenous; pt. = patient; q = each/every (from L., *quaque*).

Then use these tools to further develop your nursing process skills:

Focused Assessment Guides with sample interview questions will help strengthen your assessment skills.

Focused Assessment Guide 27-1

HEALTH HISTORY

Factors to Assess	Questions and Approaches
Present health history	"When did you first begin having this problem?" "Did it happen suddenly or slowly?" "Show me exactly where you are having this problem." "What other symptoms have you had with this problem?" "How have you treated this problem?"
Past health history	"Tell me about the childhood illnesses, such as measles or mumps, that you had." "What are you allergic to?" "Describe any accidents, injuries, and surgeries you have had." "What prescribed or over-the-counter medications do you use?" "Do you take any herbal or dietary supplements?" "What is the date of your most recent immunization for tetanus; pertussis; polio; measles; rubella; mumps; influenza; hepatitis A, B, and C; and pneumococcus?"

Examples of Actual and Potential Patient Problems and Needs teach you how to identify and formulate patient problems, and identify needs based on etiologic factors and assessment data.

Examples of Actual or Potential Health Problems and Needs

FLUID, ELECTROLYTE, AND ACID–BASE BALANCE

Actual or Potential Health Problems and Needs	Possible Etiologic Factors	Potential Signs and Symptoms
Fluid overload	Renal failure, decreased cardiac output, excessive IV infusion/fluid intake, excessive sodium intake	• "I've noticed that my wedding ring is tight . . . also my clothes don't fit as well as they used to. I guess I've gained some weight." • Reports dyspnea with exertion, feeling weak and fatigued • Pitting edema in feet, ankles, lower legs, taut, shiny skin • Adventitious breath sounds and increased blood pressure • 10-lb (4.5-kg) weight gain over past month
Fluid imbalance	Inability to obtain or swallow	• Change in mental status

DEVELOP THE NECESSARY SKILLS!

Carefully follow the concise, straightforward, and simplified format of the nursing **Skills** that show both actions and rationales. Special considerations, delegation considerations, and documentation guidelines and samples are also included.

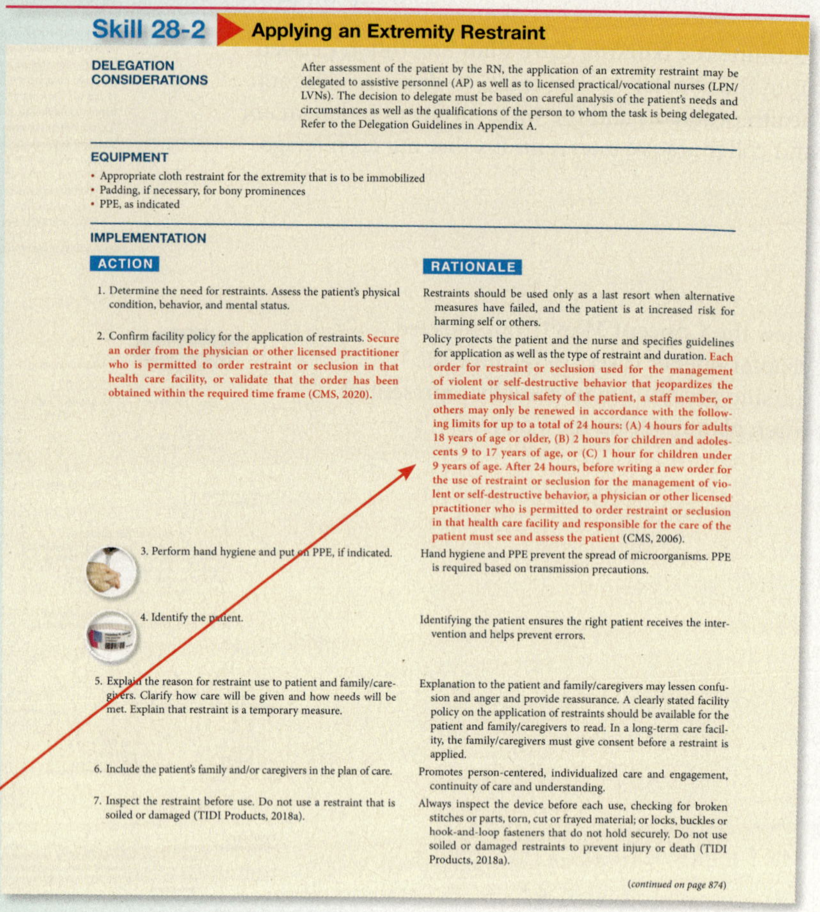

Skill 28-2 Applying an Extremity Restraint

DELEGATION CONSIDERATIONS

After assessment of the patient by the RN, the application of an extremity restraint may be delegated to assistive personnel (AP) as well as to licensed practical/vocational nurses (LPN/LVNs). The decision to delegate must be based on careful analysis of the patient's needs and circumstances as well as the qualifications of the person to whom the task is being delegated. Refer to the Delegation Guidelines in Appendix A.

EQUIPMENT

- Appropriate cloth restraint for the extremity that is to be immobilized
- Padding, if necessary, for bony prominences
- PPE, as indicated

IMPLEMENTATION

ACTION	RATIONALE
1. Determine the need for restraints. Assess the patient's physical condition, behavior, and mental status.	Restraints should be used only as a last resort when alternative measures have failed, and the patient is at increased risk for harming self or others.
2. Confirm facility policy for the application of restraints. Secure an order from the physician or other licensed practitioner who is permitted to order restraint or seclusion in that health care facility, or validate that the order has been obtained within the required time frame (CMS, 2020).	Policy protects the patient and the nurse and specifies guidelines for application as well as the type of restraint and duration. Each order for restraint or seclusion used for the management of violent or self-destructive behavior that jeopardizes the immediate physical safety of the patient, a staff member, or others may only be renewed in accordance with the following limits for up to a total of 24 hours: (A) 4 hours for adults 18 years of age or older, (B) 2 hours for children and adolescents 9 to 17 years of age, or (C) 1 hour for children under 9 years of age. After 24 hours, before writing a new order for the use of restraint or seclusion for the management of violent or self-destructive behavior, a physician or other licensed practitioner who is permitted to order restraint or seclusion in that health care facility and responsible for the care of the patient must see and assess the patient (CMS, 2006).
3. Perform hand hygiene and put on PPE, if indicated.	Hand hygiene and PPE prevent the spread of microorganisms. PPE is required based on transmission precautions.
4. Identify the patient.	Identifying the patient ensures the right patient receives the intervention and helps prevent errors.
5. Explain the reason for restraint use to patient and family/caregivers. Clarify how care will be given and how needs will be met. Explain that restraint is a temporary measure.	Explanation to the patient and family/caregivers may lessen confusion and anger and provide reassurance. A clearly stated facility policy on the application of restraints should be available for the patient and family/caregivers to read. In a long-term care facility, the family/caregivers must give consent before a restraint is applied.
6. Include the patient's family and/or caregivers in the plan of care.	Promotes person-centered, individualized care and engagement, continuity of care and understanding.
7. Inspect the restraint before use. Do not use a restraint that is soiled or damaged (TIDI Products, 2018a).	Always inspect the device before each use, checking for broken stitches or parts, torn, cut or frayed material; or locks, buckles or hook-and-loop fasteners that do not hold securely. Do not use soiled or damaged restraints to prevent injury or death (TIDI Products, 2018a).

(*continued on page 874*)

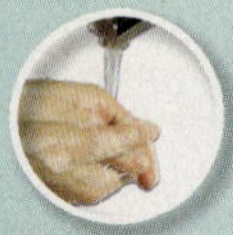

Hand Hygiene icons in Skills and Guidelines for Nursing Care alert students to this crucial step that is the best way to prevent the spread of microorganisms. The term *hand hygiene* applies to both the use of antiseptic handrubs and hand washing with soap and water and should be utilized according to the CDC (2002) guidelines for hand hygiene in health care settings.

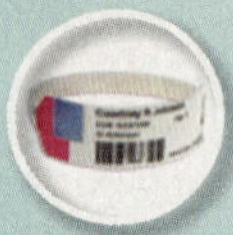

Patient Identification icons in Skills and Guidelines for Nursing Care alert students to this critical step ensuring the right patient receives the intervention to help prevent errors. According to The Joint Commission (2022), the patient should be identified using at least two methods.

Nursing Alerts in Skills and Guidelines for Nursing presented in red text draw attention to crucial information in the steps of the skills.

Guidelines for Nursing Care outline important points to remember in practice and will help you gain competence in performing nursing skills.

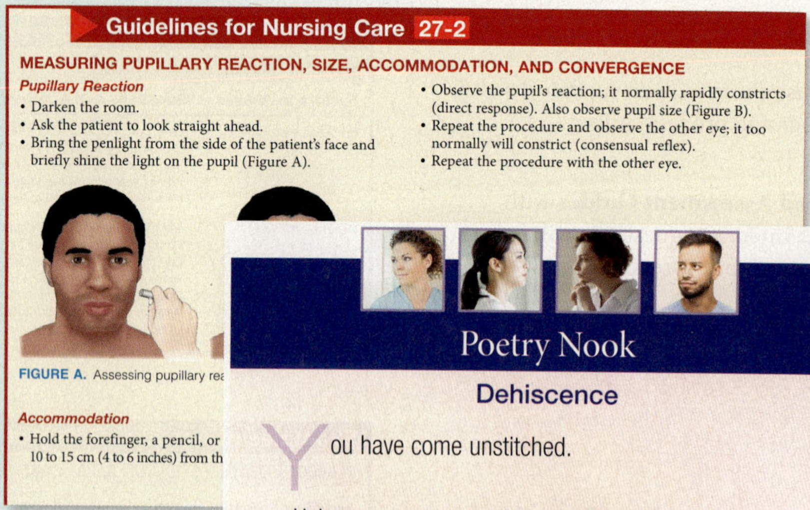

Guidelines for Nursing Care 27-2

MEASURING PUPILLARY REACTION, SIZE, ACCOMMODATION, AND CONVERGENCE

Pupillary Reaction

- Darken the room.
- Ask the patient to look straight ahead.
- Bring the penlight from the side of the patient's face and briefly shine the light on the pupil (Figure A).
- Observe the pupil's reaction; it normally rapidly constricts (direct response). Also observe pupil size (Figure B).
- Repeat the procedure and observe the other eye; it too normally will constrict (consensual reflex).
- Repeat the procedure with the other eye.

FIGURE A. Assessing pupillary rea

Accommodation

- Hold the forefinger, a pencil, or
10 to 15 cm (4 to 6 inches) from th

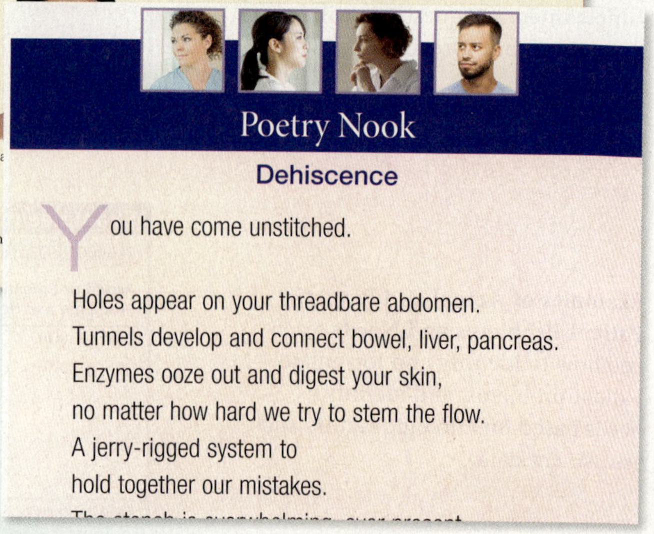

Poetry Nook

Dehiscence

You have come unstitched.

Holes appear on your threadbare abdomen.
Tunnels develop and connect bowel, liver, pancreas.
Enzymes ooze out and digest your skin,
no matter how hard we try to stem the flow.
A jerry-rigged system to
hold together our mistakes.

NEW! Poetry Nook designed to engage your emotional, spiritual, and artistic sides, provide you the opportunity to integrate learning from your liberal arts coursework in a meaningful, creative way.

PROMOTE HEALTH AND WELLNESS!

Learn not only to treat illness but also to promote the health and wellness of your patients.

Check out the **Promoting Health** boxes, which include assessment checkpoints for specific health and wellness topics and suggestions for designing a self-care prescription.

Use the **Promoting Health Literacy** boxes to help identify patients and families at risk for poor health outcomes and discover the key questions that all patients should ask their providers.

Develop appropriate nurse–patient communication using **Teaching Tips** boxes to help improve your patient's and family's outcomes.

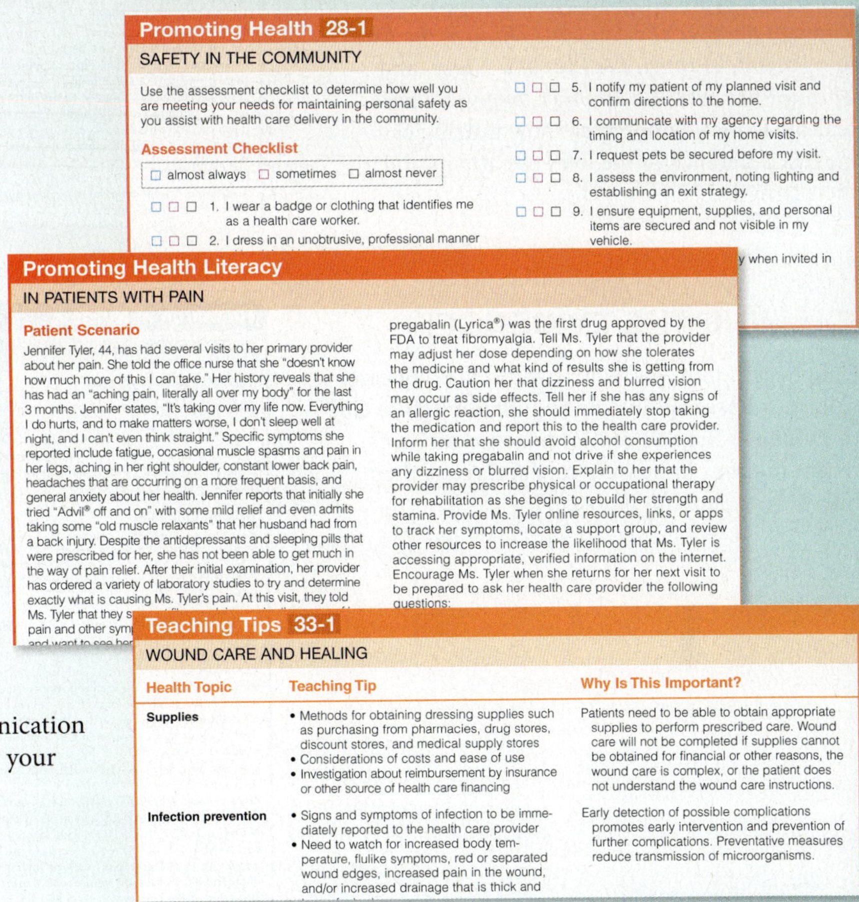

Promoting Health 28-1
SAFETY IN THE COMMUNITY

Use the assessment checklist to determine how well you are meeting your needs for maintaining personal safety as you assist with health care delivery in the community.

Assessment Checklist

☐ almost always ☐ sometimes ☐ almost never

☐ ☐ ☐ 1. I wear a badge or clothing that identifies me as a health care worker.
☐ ☐ ☐ 2. I dress in an unobtrusive, professional manner
☐ ☐ ☐ 5. I notify my patient of my planned visit and confirm directions to the home.
☐ ☐ ☐ 6. I communicate with my agency regarding the timing and location of my home visits.
☐ ☐ ☐ 7. I request pets be secured before my visit.
☐ ☐ ☐ 8. I assess the environment, noting lighting and establishing an exit strategy.
☐ ☐ ☐ 9. I ensure equipment, supplies, and personal items are secured and not visible in my vehicle.
...y when invited in

Promoting Health Literacy
IN PATIENTS WITH PAIN

Patient Scenario

Jennifer Tyler, 44, has had several visits to her primary provider about her pain. She told the office nurse that she "doesn't know how much more of this I can take." Her history reveals that she has had an "aching pain, literally all over my body" for the last 3 months. Jennifer states, "It's taking over my life now. Everything I do hurts, and to make matters worse, I don't sleep well at night, and I can't even think straight." Specific symptoms she reported include fatigue, occasional muscle spasms and pain in her legs, aching in her right shoulder, constant lower back pain, headaches that are occurring on a more frequent basis, and general anxiety about her health. Jennifer reports that initially she tried "Advil® off and on" with some mild relief and even admits taking some "old muscle relaxants" that her husband had from a back injury. Despite the antidepressants and sleeping pills that were prescribed for her, she has not been able to get much in the way of pain relief. After their initial examination, her provider has ordered a variety of laboratory studies to try and determine exactly what is causing Ms. Tyler's pain. At this visit, they told Ms. Tyler that they s... pain and other sym...

pregabalin (Lyrica®) was the first drug approved by the FDA to treat fibromyalgia. Tell Ms. Tyler that the provider may adjust her dose depending on how she tolerates the medicine and what kind of results she is getting from the drug. Caution her that dizziness and blurred vision may occur as side effects. Tell her if she has any signs of an allergic reaction, she should immediately stop taking the medication and report this to the health care provider. Inform her that she should avoid alcohol consumption while taking pregabalin and not drive if she experiences any dizziness or blurred vision. Explain to her that the provider may prescribe physical or occupational therapy for rehabilitation as she begins to rebuild her strength and stamina. Provide Ms. Tyler online resources, links, or apps to track her symptoms, locate a support group, and review other resources to increase the likelihood that Ms. Tyler is accessing appropriate, verified information on the internet. Encourage Ms. Tyler when she returns for her next visit to be prepared to ask her health care provider the following questions:

Teaching Tips 33-1
WOUND CARE AND HEALING

Health Topic	Teaching Tip	Why Is This Important?
Supplies	• Methods for obtaining dressing supplies such as purchasing from pharmacies, drug stores, discount stores, and medical supply stores • Considerations of costs and ease of use • Investigation about reimbursement by insurance or other source of health care financing	Patients need to be able to obtain appropriate supplies to perform prescribed care. Wound care will not be completed if supplies cannot be obtained for financial or other reasons, the wound care is complex, or the patient does not understand the wound care instructions.
Infection prevention	• Signs and symptoms of infection to be immediately reported to the health care provider • Need to watch for increased body temperature, flulike symptoms, red or separated wound edges, increased pain in the wound, and/or increased drainage that is thick and	Early detection of possible complications promotes early intervention and prevention of further complications. Preventative measures reduce transmission of microorganisms.

BE A PATIENT ADVOCATE!

Read the scenarios in the **Nursing Advocacy in Action** boxes and learn how you can advocate for vulnerable individuals.

NEW! Vulnerable Populations alerts will help you identify and individualize care for populations with actual or potential vulnerabilities.

Consider the special needs of the older adult with the **Focus on the Older Adult** boxes.

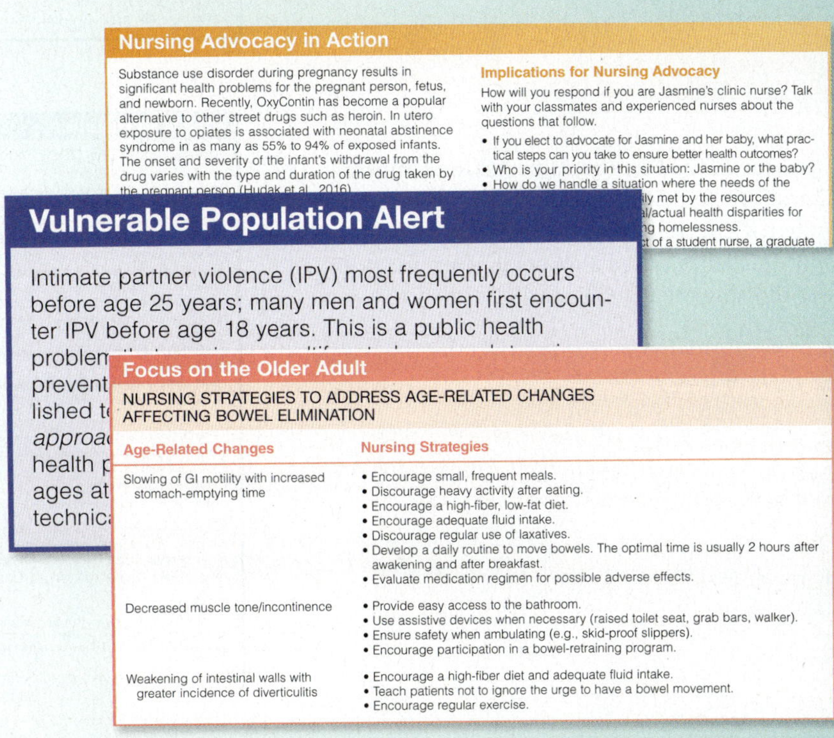

Nursing Advocacy in Action

Substance use disorder during pregnancy results in significant health problems for the pregnant person, fetus, and newborn. Recently, OxyContin has become a popular alternative to other street drugs such as heroin. In utero exposure to opiates is associated with neonatal abstinence syndrome in as many as 55% to 94% of exposed infants. The onset and severity of the infant's withdrawal from the drug varies with the type and duration of the drug taken by the pregnant person (Hudak et al., 2016).

Implications for Nursing Advocacy

How will you respond if you are Jasmine's clinic nurse? Talk with your classmates and experienced nurses about the questions that follow.

• If you elect to advocate for Jasmine and her baby, what practical steps can you take to ensure better health outcomes?
• Who is your priority in this situation: Jasmine or the baby?
• How do we handle a situation where the needs of the ...ily met by the resources ...l/actual health disparities for ...ng homelessness. ...t of a student nurse, a graduate

Vulnerable Population Alert

Intimate partner violence (IPV) most frequently occurs before age 25 years; many men and women first encounter IPV before age 18 years. This is a public health problem ... prevent... lished t... *approa*... health p... ages at... technic...

Focus on the Older Adult
NURSING STRATEGIES TO ADDRESS AGE-RELATED CHANGES AFFECTING BOWEL ELIMINATION

Age-Related Changes	Nursing Strategies
Slowing of GI motility with increased stomach-emptying time	• Encourage small, frequent meals. • Discourage heavy activity after eating. • Encourage a high-fiber, low-fat diet. • Encourage adequate fluid intake. • Discourage regular use of laxatives. • Develop a daily routine to move bowels. The optimal time is usually 2 hours after awakening and after breakfast. • Evaluate medication regimen for possible adverse effects.
Decreased muscle tone/incontinence	• Provide easy access to the bathroom. • Use assistive devices when necessary (raised toilet seat, grab bars, walker). • Ensure safety when ambulating (e.g., skid-proof slippers). • Encourage participation in a bowel-retraining program.
Weakening of intestinal walls with greater incidence of diverticulitis	• Encourage a high-fiber diet and adequate fluid intake. • Teach patients not to ignore the urge to have a bowel movement. • Encourage regular exercise.

GAIN NEW INSIGHTS!

Students, patients, nurses, and family caregivers share their experiences in boxes entitled *Through the Eyes of a Student, Through the Eyes of a Patient, Through the Eyes of a Nurse,* and *Through the Eyes of a Family Caregiver*. These real-life stories demonstrate how nursing can make a difference in the lives of patients and their families.

Through the Eyes of a Student

I entered my patient's room, knowing that she had had surgery less than 12 hours before my arrival, and introduced myself. I asked how she was feeling, to which she immediately responded, "I feel really sick. I think I'm going to throw up. I need something—now!" I told her that I would check the medication orders and be back as soon as possible. I walked quickly to the medication administration record, and there it was glaring at me in black and white on the eMAR: "Prochlorperazine, 10 mg IM q 6 hr PRN nausea or vomiting." My mind raced as I thought, "I have never given an IM injection. There has to be something else prescribed." I knew there wasn't. I found my clinical instructor and announced, "My patient needs an IM injection." Given the anxiety I was feeling, everything went surprisingly well as we prepared the medication. I went over the procedure one last time before entering the patient's room.

times, wiped the area with alcohol, and asked her if she was ready for the injection. *Big mistake!* She swiftly replied, "No, but get it over with." I took a minute to reassure her (and silently, me) again.

A little voice in my head repeated the words my *technologies* professor had said a million times, "Darting action is the key to a successful injection." So, I aimed at the bull's-eye that appeared in front of my eyes. My hand, which seemed to be moving in slow motion, propelled downward at a 90-degree angle. Secretly, I prayed that I would not hit my own hand. I looked down and it was a bull's-eye, thank goodness, but the needle had not penetrated the muscle! The patient successfully tensed her muscle tight enough to intercept the needle midflight. At that moment, she relaxed, probably because she thought the worst was over, and I pushed the needle into place. I stabilized the syringe at the end of the barrel,

EXAMINE THE EVIDENCE!

Gain insight into the "why" behind nursing care. Consider **Research in Nursing: Bridging the Gap to Evidence-Based Practice** boxes to discover recent findings in nursing care and relate their relevance to nursing practice.

Research in Nursing

BRIDGING THE GAP TO EVIDENCE-BASED PRACTICE

Stethoscope Hygiene

Stethoscopes, like other patient care equipment, should be cleaned between patients and undergo routine disinfection to prevent the spread of microorganisms. This simple intervention is rarely done despite guideline recommendations (Holleck et al., 2020). What can be done to improve compliance by health care professionals?

Related Evidence

Holleck, J. L., Campbell, S., Alrawili, H., Frank, C., Merchant, N., Rodwin, B., Perez, M. F., Gupta, S., Federman, D. G., Chang, J. J., Vientos, W., & Dembry, L. (2020). Stethoscope hygiene: Using cultures and real-time feedback with bioluminescence-based adenosine triphosphate technology to change behavior. *American Journal of Infection Control, 48*(4), 380–385. https://doi.org/10.1016/j.ajic.2019.10.005

The purpose of this quality improvement project was to determine whether demonstrating what is growing on the stethoscopes of providers via culture or bioluminescence technology alters perceptions and improves compliance with stethoscope hygiene. In addition, the researchers sought to gain a better understanding of the beliefs and the barriers to stethoscope hygiene. Participants included medical students, house staff, and attending physicians on the medical wards at a Department of Veterans Affairs (VA) tertiary care teaching hospital. Beginning with the first week of their medicine inpatient rotations at the VA, providers were given the opportunity to culture their stethoscopes and swab for bioluminescence-based adenosine triphosphate testing before and after disinfection with alcohol pads, alcohol-based hand rub, or hydrogen peroxide disinfectant wipes. Beginning with the second week of their rotations, actual photographic images of stethoscope culture plates before and after disinfection were presented for visual impact at a morning report. Bioluminescence scores of stethoscopes before and after disinfection were provided in real-time and again when presenting images of the stethoscope cultures. Pre-surveys exploring beliefs and barriers to stethoscope hygiene were administered initially prior to any intervention and post-surveys were administered 2 days after presentation of the results. Baseline observations of hand and stethoscope hygiene rates were discreetly recorded at the start of rotations, after presenting the culture images and bioluminescence scores during the second week and during the fourth week of provider rotations. The bacteria isolated, colony-forming units (CFUs), and bioluminescence scores were tracked. This 4-week period was repeated for a total of three cycles. A total of 1,245 observed hand hygiene opportunities showed that compliance improved from 72.5% to 82.3% ($p < .001$). Observed patient–provider encounters (590) revealed no significant change in stethoscope hygiene rates of 10% initially and 5% afterward ($p = .08$), although self-reported rates trended from 56% to 67% postintervention ($p = .06$). Perceptions regarding stethoscope hygiene importance improved 8.5/10 to 9.3/10; $p = .04$. Disinfection with alcohol pads, alcohol-based hand rub, and hydrogen peroxide disinfectant wipes were equivalent in CFU reduction ($p = .21$). The top three barriers to stethoscope hygiene were forgetfulness, time constraints, and limited access to supplies. The authors concluded that showing providers what is growing on their stethoscopes improved "buy in" regarding stethoscope hygiene importance. Objective observations failed to show improvement in stethoscope hygiene rates, but hand hygiene performance improved. The authors noted a significant gap between what providers think they are doing and what they are actually doing.

Relevance to Nursing Practice

Disinfection of patient care equipment, such as stethoscopes, reduces bacteria on the equipment, including the potential to reduce and limit transmission of pathogens. Stethoscopes, like other patient care equipment, should be cleaned between patients and undergo routine disinfection. Nurses and other health care providers need to be aware of the potential barriers to implementation and make a conscious effort to implement equipment hygiene as part of patient care. Facilities must ensure adequate access to disinfection supplies and consider interventions to support use of disinfectants to reduce barriers to implementation.

Read the **PICOT in Practice: Asking Clinical Questions** to think about how you can do a systematic search, formulate questions, and apply evidence-based answers in your practice by following the PICOT model.

PICOT in Practice

ASKING CLINICAL QUESTIONS: ACUPUNCTURE/ACUPRESSURE

Scenario: You are a nurse working with a large maxillofacial surgery group who attended a conference on integrative nursing. One presenter that stood out discussed the benefits of acupuncture/acupressure in managing the gag reflex in patients undergoing dental procedures. Gagging is a common problem encountered during dental treatment, making therapeutic procedures distressing and often difficult or even impossible to perform. One of the surgeons asks if you learned something new at the conference and you discuss the results of the presentation.

The office currently only uses sedatives to facilitate sedation in patient undergoing procedures. You wonder if acupuncture/acupressure compared to sedatives has any benefit in the care of patients "specifically pediatric patients" undergoing procedures.

- **Population:** Children receiving sedation
- **Intervention:** Use of acupuncture/acupressure
- **Comparison:** Use of sedatives
- **Outcome:** Decreased gag reflex
- **Time:** During dental procedures

PICOT Question: Does the use of acupuncture/acupressure by a nonanesthesiologist compared to administration of sedatives result in depression of gag reflex in children undergoing dental treatment and improved experience?

Findings:

1. Ashley, P. F., Chaudhary, M., Lourenço-Matharu, L. (2018). Sedation of children undergoing dental treatment. *Cochrane Database of Systematic Reviews,* (12), CD003877. https://doi.org/10.1002/14651858.CD003877.pub5

Included 50 studies with a total of 3,704 children up to age for further well-designed and well-reported clinical trials to evaluate other potential sedation agents.

2. Eachempati, P., Kumbargere Nagraj, S., Kiran Kumar Krishanappa, S., George, R. P., Soe, H. H. K., Karanth, L. (2019). Management of gag reflex for patients undergoing dental treatment. *Cochrane Database of Systematic Reviews,* (11), CD011116. https://doi.org/10.1002/14651858.CD011116.pub3

The interventions used to manage gagging include antinausea medicines, sedatives, local and general anesthetics, herbal remedies, behavior therapy and cognitive behavior therapy, acupressure, acupuncture, laser, and prosthetic devices. This systematic review included four trials with 328 people (263 adults and 65 children who were ages 4 years and older). Of the trials reviewed, one compared acupuncture and acupressure (with thumb, device, and sea band) at P6 (point located three finger breadths below the wrist on the inner forearm in between the two tendons) to sham acupuncture and acupressure with and without sedation. One trial compared acupuncture at the P6 point to sham acupuncture. These trials reported both completion of dental procedure and reduction in gagging as their outcomes.

Level of Evidence I: systematic review.

Recommendations: Conscious sedation or moderate sedation is the ability of the patient to independently maintain an open mouth and respond sensibly to verbal commands. In addition, the patient will retain adequate function of protective reflexes such as the gag reflex. There is a fine line between a sedated patient and an anesthetized patient. The ideal sedative agent would reduce anxiety and improve behavior. Oral midazolam probably improves the behavior of children during

PREPARE FOR NCLEX!

Start preparing for NCLEX right from the beginning of your nursing education. The **Practicing for NCLEX** section at the end of each chapter uses the multiple-choice question format to test your knowledge of basic through complex concepts. Answers with rationales are provided for immediate reinforcement.

PRACTICING FOR NCLEX

1. Thirty-six hours after having surgery, a patient has a slightly elevated body temperature and generalized malaise as well as pain with redness at the surgical site. Which action is most appropriate?

   MAR

   - Acetaminophen 650 mg every 6 hours prn fever
   - Cefazolin (antibiotic) 1 g 1 hour preoperatively
   - Cefazolin 1 g, every 6 hours 3 times, postoperatively

   a. Documenting the findings and continuing to monitor

You may also be interested in Lippincott PassPoint, our adaptive, online NCLEX-preparation tool. Through PassPoint, you can take quizzes accessing thousands of NCLEX-style questions and even take simulated NCLEX questions that adapt to your answers—just like the real exam. To learn more about PassPoint, visit thePoint.lww.com/PassPoint.

Concept Mastery Alerts highlight and clarify the most common misconceptions in nursing fundamentals, as identified by Lippincott's online adaptive learning platform. Our team reviewed data from thousands of fundamentals students across North America to identify the points of confusion for most students to help you learn more effectively.

Concept Mastery Alert

Of the many ways to avoid falls in the acute care setting, the best outcome for a patient at risk for falling is that the patient will not experience a fall and remains free of injury.

COORDINATE YOUR STUDY PLAN!

From traditional texts to video and interactive products, the Taylor Fundamentals Suite is tailored to fit every learning style. This integrated suite of products offers students a seamless learning experience you won't find anywhere else.

LIPPINCOTT COURSEPOINT

Powered by PrepU, Lippincott's adaptive learning engine, CoursePoint allows you to study more efficiently and access our digital course content precisely when you need it. With CoursePoint, you can access hundreds of quiz questions for each chapter, as well as a complete electronic version of the textbook and valuable reference and study resources.

ACKNOWLEDGMENTS

This revision is the work of many talented and committed people; we wish to gratefully acknowledge the assistance of all who have contributed in any way to the completion of this project. Our first debt of gratitude is to all the nurse educators and students who have adopted the text and shared with us their experiences in using the teaching and learning package. We are deeply grateful for their revision suggestions and trust they will enhance the learning experiences of others.

The work of this revision was capably facilitated by our Development Editor, Kelly Horvath. She worked tirelessly behind the scenes to make sure that a superb, state-of-the-art product was delivered on time! When emails are flying back and forth on Sundays and holidays, you know you have the best! Our very special thanks to our Senior Acquisitions Editor Jonathan Joyce, Senior Development Editor, Julie Vitale, and Editorial Coordinator Erin Hernandez for their hard work and guidance throughout the project. Thank you to Stephen Druding of the Design department, and Jennifer Clements, Art Director, who brought a fresh look to the entire Taylor Suite of products. The Instructional Services Consultants also deserve special thanks for their focus on our products to provide curriculum guidance, instructional design, technology support, and training. We also want to thank Andrea Mann, who worked creatively on many aspects of the teaching/learning package to ensure that faculty and students alike are getting the best resources to facilitate learning.

We thank all who generously gave their time, ideas, and resources, and we gratefully acknowledge the special contributions of the following:

- Rick Brady, Joe Mitchell, Ken Kasper, Barbara Proud, Gates Rhodes, and Kathy Sloane, photographers.
- Marie Clark, who developed the math problems and solutions in the "Medications" chapter.
- Kathleen Lucente, RN, MT, CIC, Infection Control Manager at Paoli Hospital, Paoli, Pennsylvania, for advising and updating us on changing infection-control protocols.

We gratefully acknowledge the influence of our mentors and teachers who have influenced our thoughts and writing; each person we have been privileged to care for as nurses; our students, who continually challenge us to find more effective means to teach nursing; our professional colleagues; and perhaps most important, our families and friends, whose love sustained us through the long hours of research and writing.

CONTENTS

UNIT II Health Care Delivery

UNIT III Processes of Thoughtful, Person-Centered Practice

Case Studies in this Book

TWO-PART CASES THAT UNFOLD ACROSS CHAPTERS

CASES THAT UNFOLD WITHIN CHAPTERS

CONCEPT MAPS

CARE PLANS

EVOLVING CASE STUDIES

Research in Nursing

BRIDGING THE GAP TO EVIDENCE-BASED PRACTICE

Guidelines for Nursing Care

Fundamentals of Nursing

The Art and Science of Person-Centered Care

UNIT I

Foundations of Thoughtful, Person-Centered Nursing Practice

Nursing is both an art and a science. It is a profession that uses specialized knowledge and skills to promote wellness and to provide care for people in both health and illness in a variety of practice settings. Unit I introduces concepts that provide the foundation for professional nursing practice. Chapters in this unit explore nursing and professional formation; theory, research, and evidence-based nursing practice; health, wellness, and health disparities; cultural diversity; basic needs and health of people, families, and the community; ethical and legal dimensions of nursing practice; communication; teaching and counseling; and leadership, managing, and delegating.

Historical perspectives, educational preparation, professional organizations, and guidelines for professional nursing practice serve as a basis for understanding what nursing is and how it is organized. Nursing theories and nursing research provide a foundation for evidence-based nursing practice, defining the rationale for nursing actions and offering a focus for nursing care. The diverse society in which nurses care for others mandates the ability to provide respectful care for all, especially the most vulnerable, and a commitment to antiracism. An understanding of basic human needs and the individualized definitions of wellness and illness prepare the nurse to integrate the human dimensions—the physical, intellectual, emotional, sociocultural, spiritual, and environmental aspects of each person—into nursing care to promote wellness, prevent illness, restore health, and facilitate coping with altered function or death. An understanding of the influence of values on human behavior and of the ethical dimensions of nursing practice is essential to responsible and accountable patient care. Sensitivity to the legal implications of professional nursing practice is imperative in today's culture. Finally, this unit describes competencies that are essential to every professional nurse: professional communication; teaching and counseling; and leadership, management, and delegation.

Unit I explores the foundations for thoughtful, person-centered nursing practice from both the perspective of the nurse and a person-centered holistic understanding of the patient. You will be introduced to a challenging and rewarding profession and be provided with a knowledge base to ground the development of caregiving skills and professional relationships and behaviors. You will also find a heightened emphasis on the nurse's self-care behaviors.

> **Basic to any philosophy of nursing seems to be these three concepts: (1) reverence for the gift of life; (2) respect for the dignity, worth, autonomy, and individuality of each human being; (3) resolution to act dynamically in relation to one's beliefs."**

Ernestine Wiedenbach (1900–1996), *a faculty member at Yale University School of Nursing, where she developed her model of nursing from years of experience in various nursing positions*

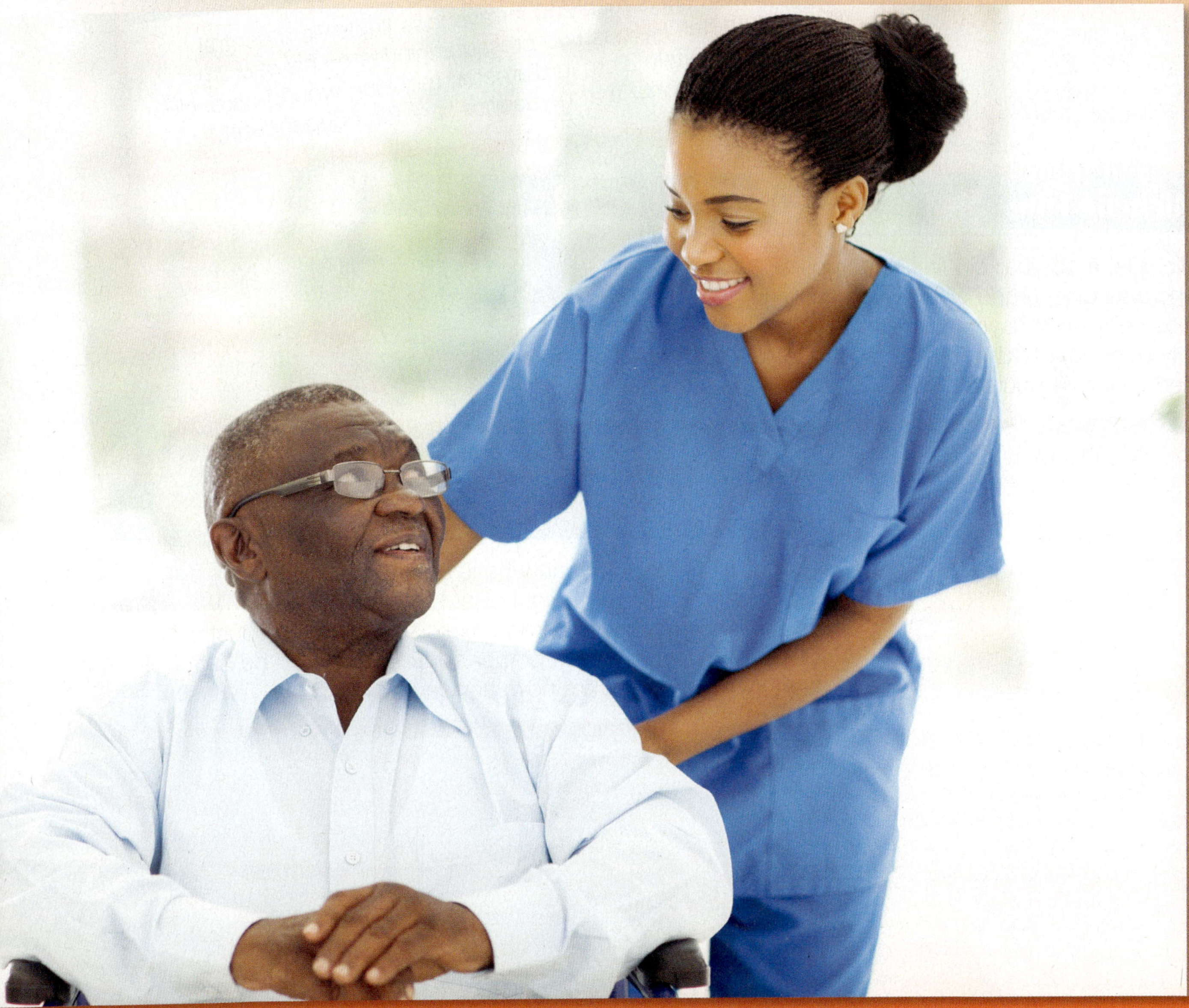

1 Introduction to Nursing and Professional Formation

Roberto Pecorini

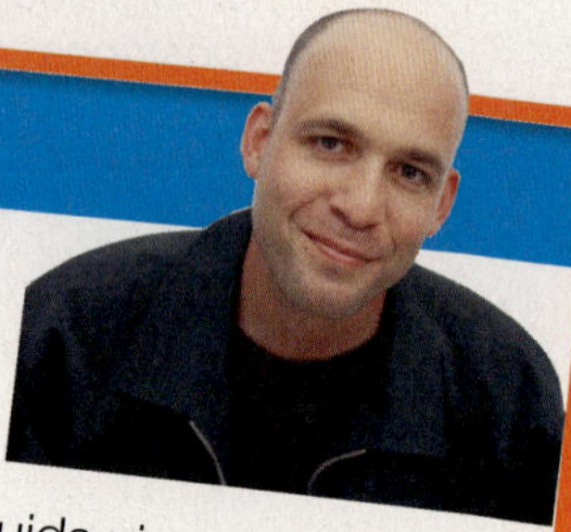

Roberto is a 38-year-old man diagnosed with metastatic colon cancer. Having undergone radiation treatments and chemotherapy, he is extremely weak and malnourished. He is receiving intravenous fluids via a central venous catheter. He has two pressure injuries on his sacrum, each approximately 2 cm in diameter, requiring wound care. He also has a colostomy that he cannot care for independently.

Michelle Fine

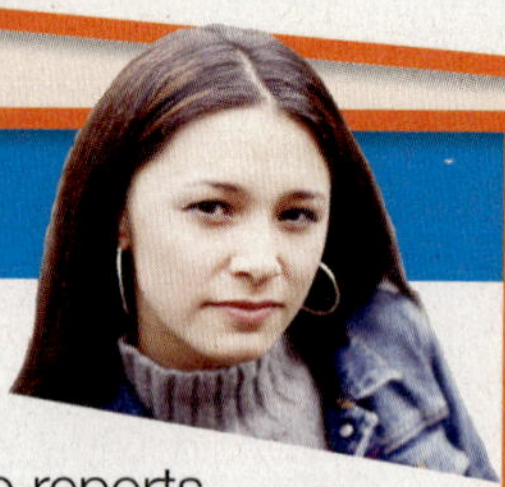

Michelle, a 19-year-old first-time mother who was discharged with her healthy 7-lb 8-oz baby girl 2 days ago, calls the nursery. She reports, "My baby isn't taking to my breast and she hasn't had any real feeding for 24 hours."

Ahmad Basshir

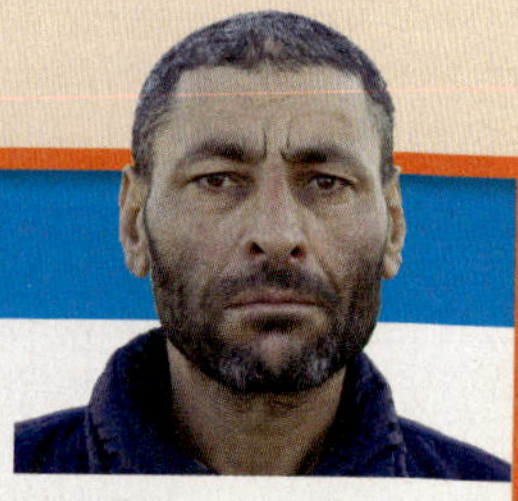

Ahmad, a 62-year-old man who is at risk for heart disease, is being taught about lifestyle modifications, such as diet and exercise. He states, "Just save your breath. Why should I bother about all that? I'd be better off dead than living like I am now, anyway!"

Learning Outcomes

After completing the chapter, you will be able to accomplish the following:

1. Describe the historical background of nursing, definitions of nursing, and the status of nursing as a profession and as a discipline.
2. Explain the aims of nursing as they interrelate to facilitate maximal health and quality of life for patients.
3. Explain how nursing qualifies as a profession.
4. Describe the various levels of educational preparation in nursing.
5. Discuss the effects on nursing practice of nursing organizations, standards of nursing practice, nurse practice acts, and the nursing process.
6. Identify current trends in nursing.
7. Discuss the importance of self-care in relation to the demands of the nursing profession and the duty to model healthy behaviors.

Nursing Concepts

- Professional behaviors
- Self

What is nursing? Consider the following examples of who nurses are and what they do:

- Delton Nix, RN, graduated from an associate degree nursing program 3 years ago. He is now working full-time as a staff nurse in a hospital medical unit while attending school part-time toward a baccalaureate degree in nursing; his goal is to become a nurse anesthetist.
- Jeiping Wu, RN, MSN, FNP, specializes as an advanced practice family nurse practitioner. She has an independent practice in a rural primary health clinic.
- Samuel Cohen, LPN, decided to follow his life's dream to become a nurse after 20 years as a postal worker. After examining all his options and goals, he completed a practical nursing program and is now a member of an emergency ambulance crew in a large city.
- Amy Orlando, RN, BSN, graduated 2 years ago and recently began a new job in an urban community health service.
- Ed Neill, RN, DNP, is the Chief Nursing Informatics Officer at a large health system.
- Roxanne McDaniel, RN, PhD, with a doctorate in nursing, teaches and conducts research on moral distress at a large university.

These examples show how difficult it is to describe nursing simply. If everyone in your class were asked to complete the sentence, "Nursing is . . . ," there would be many different responses, because each person would answer based on their own personal experience and knowledge of nursing. As you progress toward graduation and as you practice nursing after graduation, your own definition will reflect changes as you learn about and experience nursing.

Nursing is a profession focused on assisting people, families, and communities to attain, recover, and maintain optimum health and function from birth to old age. Nurses act as a bridge between an often extremely vulnerable public and the health care resources that can literally make the difference between life and death, health and disease or disability, and well-being and discomfort. Yale School of Nursing faculty member and philosopher Mark Lazenby, PhD, APRN, FAAN, describes nursing as a "profoundly radical profession that calls society to equality and justice, to trustworthiness, and to openness. The profession is also radically political: it imagines a world in which the conditions necessary for health are enjoyed by all people" (Lazenby, 2017). According to an annual Gallup survey, the public has rated nursing as the most honest and ethical profession in America for 18 years straight. The only exception was 2001 when firefighters following the attacks on September 11 were named the most honest and ethical.

In 2020, the world celebrated the International Year of the Nurse and Midwife on the 200th anniversary of the birth of Florence Nightingale. You will want to research Nursing Now (http://www.nursingnow.org/launch/), a 3-year (2018–2020) global campaign that aimed to improve health by raising the profile and status of nursing worldwide. Run in collaboration with the World Health Organization (WHO) and the International Council of Nurses, Nursing Now sought to empower nurses to take their place at the heart of tackling 21st-century health challenges and maximize their contribution to achieving Universal Health Coverage. The campaign focused on five core areas: (1) ensuring that nurses and midwives have a more prominent voice in health policy making; (2) encouraging greater investment in the nursing workforce; (3) recruiting more nurses into leadership positions; (4) conducting research that helps determine where nurses can have the greatest impact; and (5) sharing of best nursing practices.

While the world was celebrating nurses and midwives in 2020, the COVID-19 pandemic struck, placing nurses and other health care professionals on the frontlines, literally, of the battle to save lives. With most visitors restricted from hospitals and nursing homes, nurses were suddenly the last human faces seen by the dying and the family's only point of contact. For too many nurses, the appropriate personal protective equipment (PPE) was in short supply, and many had to make anguished decisions about how to balance their commitment to patients, their families, and themselves. Nurses suddenly became superheroes, and the public offered us free hotel rooms, free food, and nightly cheers. Some nurses understandably were less enthused about the public accolades and more concerned about not having the PPE and other resources needed to do their jobs well. Never was nursing more valued, more challenging, or more dangerous. Never was the public more appreciative of nurses.

QSEN Reflective Practice: Cultivating QSEN Competencies

CHALLENGE TO ETHICAL AND LEGAL SKILLS

During nursing school, I was working as a nurse's aide on a busy oncology unit. It was here that I met Roberto Pecorini, a 38-year-old man diagnosed with metastatic colon cancer. He had undergone radiation treatments and chemotherapy and was extremely weak and malnourished. He was receiving numerous intravenous fluids via a central venous catheter. In addition, he had developed two pressure injuries on his sacrum, each approximately 1½ in in diameter, that required wound care. He also had a colostomy that he could not care for independently.

Although the staff was very helpful, the orientation I received to the unit was brief because they were very short staffed. During one occasion, shortly after I had been oriented to the floor, I was working a night shift and was the only nurse's aide on the unit. The nurses I was working with asked me to care for Mr. Pecorini, including performing several tasks and skills with which I was unfamiliar. In addition to my lack of familiarity with skills such as changing central line dressings and performing blood draws and wound care, I was not licensed to perform these tasks. I felt uncomfortable performing these skills on my own. However, the nurses were extremely busy, and I wanted to help them as much as possible. If I performed these skills on my own, I could be putting the patient at risk. Moreover, I could be threatening the licenses of the nurses.

Thinking Outside the Box: Possible Courses of Action

- Perform the tasks requested despite the fact that I had little experience with them.
- Inform the nurses that I did not feel comfortable completing these skills on my own and ask that they assign me other tasks within my scope of duty.
- Ask the nurses to be present when I performed these tasks so that they could observe my skills and intervene if necessary.
- Refrain from performing these tasks and alert the nurse manager the following day that I was assigned to tasks outside my scope of duty.

Evaluating a Good Outcome: How Do I Define Success?

- The patient received safe, comprehensive care without being placed at risk.
- I performed tasks and skills within my scope of practice.
- The nurses understood my job duties and appropriately delegated the necessary tasks.
- The nurses' licensure was not put in jeopardy.
- I felt comfortable and competent in my job performance.

Personal Learning: Here's to the Future!

Since I felt uncomfortable in performing the duties assigned to me by the nurses, I confronted them and told them that I had recently been oriented to the floor and did not have experience with these skills. Although somewhat surprised that I didn't have the experience, they understood and did not want me to do anything I felt uncomfortable with. The nurses were used to having an LPN as a night aide, and the LPN's scope of practice was broader than mine. Throughout the night, I observed the nurses performing the skills and tasks, with the nurses walking me through several of the skills that I was allowed to perform but in which I did not feel proficient. In the morning, we spoke with the nurse manager, who realized the need for clarifying the job duties of the nurse's aides and the appropriate delegation of tasks. I feel that I made the right decision in speaking to the nurses because patient safety could have been compromised by my inexperience. The nurses' licensure also could have been put at risk. As a result of our conversation with the nurse manager, the orientation for new nurse's aides was reorganized, helping greatly to define the scope of duties for the aides.

Colleen Kilcullen, Georgetown University

QSEN SELF-REFLECTION ON QUALITY AND SAFETY COMPETENCIES DEVELOPING KNOWLEDGE, SKILLS, AND ATTITUDES FOR CONTINUOUS IMPROVEMENT

How do you think you would respond in a similar situation? Why? What does this tell you about yourself and about the adequacy of your skills for professional practice? How was the nursing student's action ethical? Legal? Please explain. What other *knowledge, attitudes,* and *skills* do you need to develop to continuously improve the quality and safety of care for patients like Mr. Pecorini?

Patient-Centered Care: What role did the different members of the nursing team play in creating a partnership with Mr. Pecorini to best coordinate his care? What special talents do you bring to creating this partnership?

Teamwork and Collaboration/Quality Improvement: What communication skills do you need to improve to ensure that you function as a competent, caring, and responsible member of the patient-care team and ensure that you obtain assistance when needed? How would you have responded if nursing leadership did not address your concerns? What special talents do you bring to promoting a well-functioning interdisciplinary team?

Safety/Evidence-Based Practice: What priority did Mr. Pecorini's care team accord to his health, well-being, and safety? What evidence in the nursing literature supports adhering to the scope of practice and roles?

Informatics: Can you identify the essential information that must be available in Mr. Pecorini's electronic record to support safe patient care and coordination of care? Can you think of other ways to respond to or approach the situation?

According to *Nursing: Scope and Standards of Practice* (American Nurses Association [ANA], 2021),

> "Nursing incorporates the art and science of caring and focuses on the protection, promotion, and optimization of health and abilities; prevention of illness and injury; facilitation of healing; and alleviation of suffering through compassionate presence. Nursing is the diagnosis and treatment of human response, and advocacy in the care of individuals, families, groups, communities, and populations in recognition of the connection of all humanity (p. 1)."

Nursing care involves a wide range of activities, from carrying out complicated technical procedures to something as seemingly simple as holding a hand. Nursing is a blend of science and art. The science of nursing is the knowledge base for the care that is given, and the art of nursing is the skilled application of that knowledge to help others achieve maximum health and quality of life. For a contemporary description of the scope of nursing practice (the "who," "what," "where," "when," "why," and "how" of nursing practice), be sure to read the complete *Nursing: Scope and Standards of Practice* (ANA, 2021). Today, 4 million nurses in the United States practice in over 200 different specialties, such as anesthesia, mental health, school nursing, cardiac care, pediatrics, surgery, oncology, obstetrics, and geriatrics. They are caregivers, administrators, researchers, innovators, and policy makers. The federal government projects that more than 200,000 new registered nurse positions will be created each year from 2016 to 2026 (AACN, 2019). Nursing is the largest of the health professions and the foundation of the nation's health care workforce (www.nursingworld.org). Read Mancuso and Davidson (2020) "Thirty million strong: What our profession needs to look like in the upcoming decade" to learn how nurses need to lead to meet the health needs of the world.

This chapter introduces you to professional nursing, including a brief history of nursing from its beginnings to the present, and provides the definitions and aims of professional nursing. The educational preparation for professional nursing, professional nursing organizations, and guidelines for professional nursing practice are discussed to help you better understand what nursing as a profession is and how it is organized. (For an example demonstrating the importance of licensure to nursing practice and responsibilities, see the Reflective Practice box on the previous page.) This edition of the text highlights the professional formation of the nurse and importance of self-care for all nurses. Because nursing is a part of an ever-changing society, current trends in nursing also are discussed.

HISTORICAL PERSPECTIVES ON NURSING

Caregivers for the ill and injured have always been a part of history. The roles, settings, and responsibilities, however, have changed over time, as is summarized in the following section.

Development of Nursing From Early Civilizations to the 16th Century

Most early civilizations believed that illness had supernatural causes. The theory of animism attempted to explain the cause of mysterious changes in bodily functions. This theory was based on the belief that everything in nature was alive with invisible forces and endowed with power. Good spirits brought health; evil spirits brought sickness and death. In providing treatment, the roles of the health care provider and the nurse were separate and distinct. The health care provider was the medicine man who treated disease by chanting, inspiring fear, or opening the skull to release evil spirits (Dolan et al., 1983). The nurse usually was the mother who cared for her family during sickness by providing physical care and herbal remedies. This nurturing and caring role of the nurse has continued to the present.

As ancient Greek civilizations grew, temples became the centers of medical care because of the belief that illness was caused by sin and the gods' displeasure (*disease* literally means "dis-ease"). During the same period, the ancient Hebrews developed rules through the Ten Commandments and the Mosaic Health Code for ethical human relationships, mental health, and disease control. Nurses cared for sick people in the home and the community and also practiced as nurse–midwives (Dolan et al., 1983).

In the early Christian period, nursing began to have a formal and more clearly defined role in society. Led by the idea that love and caring for others were important, women called "deaconesses" made the first organized visits to sick people, and members of male religious orders gave nursing care and buried the dead. Both male and female nursing orders were founded during the Crusades (11th to 13th centuries). Hospitals were built for the enormous number of pilgrims needing health care, and nursing became a respected vocation. Although the early Middle Ages ended in chaos, nursing had developed purpose, direction, and leadership.

At the beginning of the 16th century, many Western societies shifted from a religious orientation to an emphasis on warfare, exploration, and expansion of knowledge. Many monasteries and convents closed, leading to a tremendous shortage of people to care for the sick. To meet this need, women who were convicted of crimes were recruited into nursing in lieu of serving jail sentences. In addition to having a poor reputation, these nurses received low pay and worked long hours in unfavorable conditions.

Florence Nightingale and the Birth of Modern Nursing

From the middle of the 19th century to the 20th century, social reforms changed the roles of nurses and of women in general. It was during this time that nursing as we now know it began, based on many of the beliefs of Florence Nightingale. Born in 1820 to a wealthy family, she grew up in England, was well educated, and traveled extensively. Despite strong opposition from her family, Nightingale began training as a nurse at the age of 31. The outbreak of the Crimean

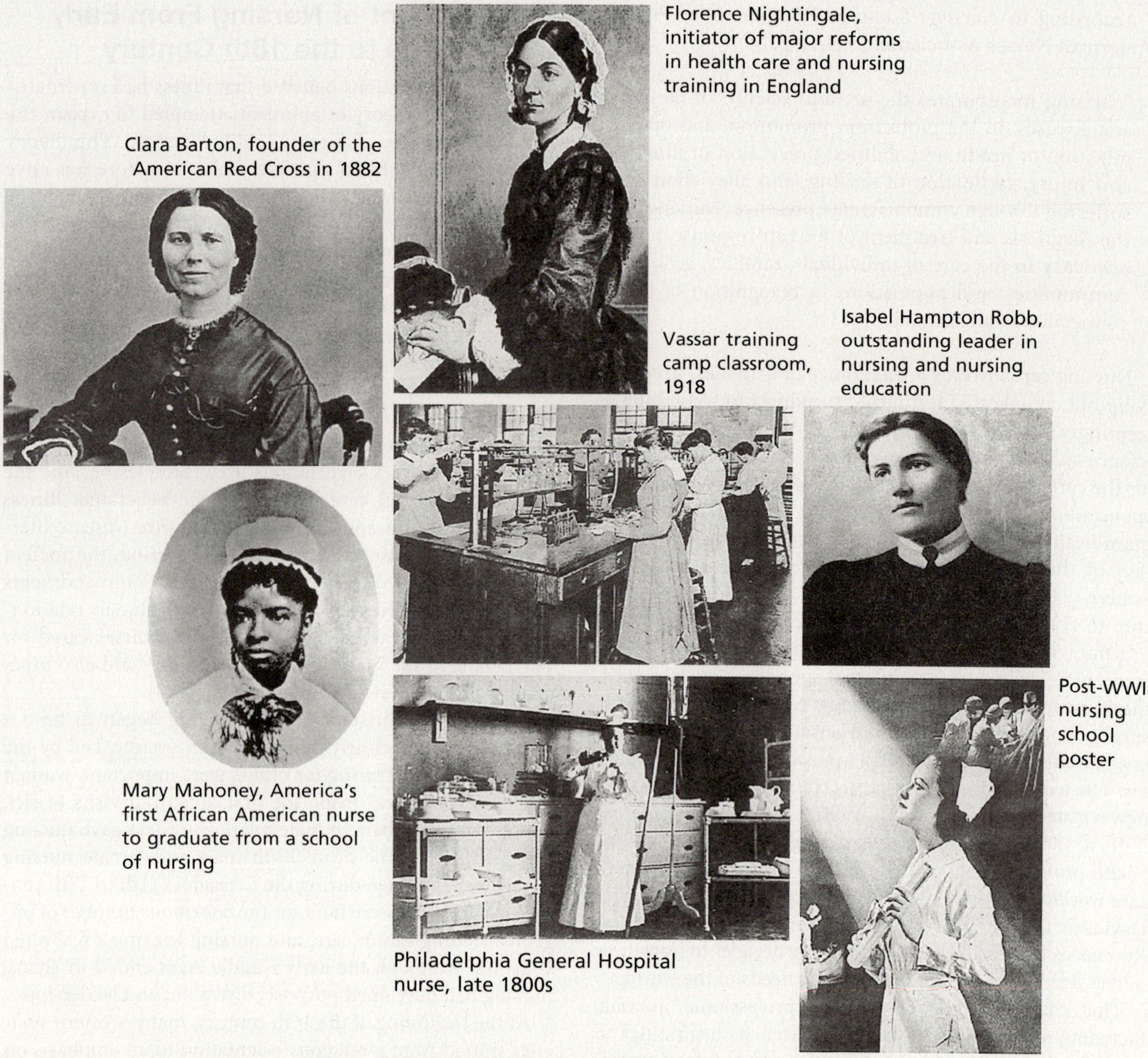

FIGURE 1-1. Images of nurses spanning more than 100 years of service. (Courtesy of the Center for the Study of the History of Nursing, University of Pennsylvania.)

War and a request by the British to organize nursing care for a military hospital in Turkey gave Nightingale an opportunity for achievement (Kalisch & Kalisch, 2004). As she successfully overcame enormous difficulties, Nightingale challenged prejudices against women and elevated the status of all nurses. After the war, she returned to England, where she established the first training school for nurses and wrote books about health care and nursing education. Today we celebrate Florence Nightingale as a disaster nurse, care provider, educator, manager, consultant, and statistician. Her contributions include:

- Identifying the personal needs of the patient and the role of the nurse in meeting those needs
- Establishing standards for hospital management
- Establishing a respected occupation for women
- Establishing nursing education
- Recognizing the two components of nursing: health and illness
- Believing that nursing is separate and distinct from medicine
- Recognizing that nutrition is important to health
- Instituting occupational and recreational therapy for sick people
- Stressing the need for continuing education for nurses
- Maintaining accurate records, recognized as the beginnings of nursing research

Florence Nightingale, other historically important nurses, and images of early nursing can be seen in Figure 1-1. Figure 1-2 illustrates "monumental moments" in nursing. People important to the early development of nursing are listed in Table 1-1 (on page 10). See Chapter 10 for a list of contemporary nurse leaders. A historical overview of

Monumental Moments in Nursing

1836
While recuperating in a British hospital, **Dorothea Dix** met prison reformers and mental health professionals who inspired her later work as an advocate for the humane treatment of the mentally ill. She founded or expanded more than **30** hospitals for mentally ill patients during her lifetime.

1860
Considered the founder of modern nursing, **Florence Nightingale** established the first secular nursing school in London. She was integral to elevating nursing training and the nursing profession. (See page 6 for a full timeline of her life.).

1862
Walt Whitman became a nurse after his brother was wounded during the Battle of Fredericksburg. His brother recovered, and Whitman went on to care for wounded soldiers throughout the Civil War. Many of his experiences at field hospitals were reflected in his poetry and prose.

1879
Mary Eliza Mahoney became the first Black female nurse in the United States. Throughout her 40-year career, Mahoney faced extreme discrimination, but she paved the way for other Black women in the field of nursing. Mahoney was inducted into the **National Women's Hall of Fame in 1993.**

1881
Clara Barton, a self-taught nurse who served on battlefields during the Civil War, established the **American Red Cross.**

1900
The first issue of the **American Journal of Nursing** was distributed.

1911
The American Nurses Association (ANA) was formally established. While the organization officially began in 1896, its name was changed in 1911, and it began representing nurses throughout the country.

1923
Yale Nursing School was founded, becoming the first independent nursing school in the United States. The school was unique among colleges and universities at that time because it accepted women.

1934
ANA's House of Delegates approved an **eight-hour day** for nurses and conducted a national campaign to promote better working hours.

1940
There were **369,287** nurses in the U.S., according to the U.S. Census. That included **361,215 women** and **8,072 men.**

1945
ANA intensified efforts to **recruit nurses** for military service as an alternative to President Roosevelt's proposal to draft nurses into military services.

1962
By the end of 1962, all state nurses associations accepted all qualified registered nurses (RNs) into membership, **regardless of race, color or creed.**

1964
ANA's House of Delegates approved a recommendation for making the **baccalaureate degree** the educational foundation for professional nursing.

1964
Congress passed the **Nurse Training Act,** the most comprehensive nursing legislation in American history. The act reflected the federal government's enlarged financial commitment to nursing education.

1974
The first hospice program was created in the United States by **Florence Wald,** who believed that individuals with incurable diseases should focus on connecting with their families instead of enduring endless treatments.

1982
The American Academy of Nursing identified **41** hospitals as **Magnet Hospitals.** Magnet Hospitals are workplaces that follow models of nursing practice and provide positive working environments for nurses.

1986
The National Institute of Nursing Research was established at the National Institutes of Health to support and conduct clinical and basic research on issues of health and illness across the lifespan.

1988
ANA promoted the use of nurses to plan and implement **psychological** and **psychosocial** nursing care for clients with AIDS-related health problems.

1988
The estimated number of RNs in the U.S. was **2,033,032**, and of those, **1,627,032** were employed in nursing, according to ANA.

1992
Eddie Bernice Johnson became the first RN elected to the United States Congress.

1993
The ANA Board of Directors designated **May 6 - 12** as permanent dates to observe National Nurses Week.

1995
ANA supported the **Fair Pay Act** to require employers to provide equal pay for jobs of comparable skill, effort, responsibility and working conditions.

2000
The National Sample Survey of Registered Nurses estimated there were **2,696,540** RNs in the U.S.

2008
There were an estimated **3,063,162** licensed RNs living in the United States, as of March 2008, according to a report from the U.S. Department of Health and Human Services.

2018
$71,730: the annual median salary for RNs, according to the U.S. Bureau of Labor Statistics.

2020
In celebration of the 200th anniversary of Florence Nightingale's birth, the World Health Organization designated 2020 as the **International Year of the Nurse and the Midwife.**

2020
The Washington Post partnered with ANA to present **Star Nurses,** a premiere event that recognized leading nurses in the Greater Washington area and named six Nightingale Award winners, on September 1, 2020.

2020
4 million: The Nation's RN population, according to ANA.

2020
Since the **global outbreak of covid-19,** ANA has advocated for clear, evidence-based guidelines and resources to keep RNs and health-care workers safe, so that they can effectively protect the public.

FIGURE 1-2. Monumental moments in nursing. (Used with permission, Star Nurses publication from *The Washington Post*.)

Table 1-1 People Important to the Early Development of Nursing in North America

PERSON	CONTRIBUTION
19th Century	
Florence Nightingale	Defined nursing as both an art and a science, differentiated nursing from medicine, created freestanding nursing education; published books about nursing and health care; is regarded as the founder of modern nursing (see text for further information)
Clara Barton	Volunteered to care for wounds and feed Union soldiers during the Civil War; served as the supervisor of nurses for the Army of the James, organizing hospitals and nurses; established the Red Cross in the United States in 1882
Dorothea Dix	Served as superintendent of the Female Nurses of the Army during the Civil War; was given the authority and the responsibility for recruiting and equipping a corps of army nurses; was a pioneering crusader for the reform of the treatment of the mentally ill
Mary Ann Bickerdyke	Organized diet kitchens, laundries, and an ambulance service, and supervised nursing staff during the Civil War
Louise Schuyler	A nurse during the Civil War; returned to New York and organized the New York Charities Aid Association to improve care of the sick in Bellevue Hospital; recommended standards for nursing education
Linda Richards	Graduated in 1873 from the New England Hospital for Women and Children in Boston, Massachusetts, as the first trained nurse in the United States; became the night superintendent of Bellevue Hospital in 1874 and began the practice of keeping records and writing orders
Jane Addams	Provided social services within a neighborhood setting; a leader for women's rights; recipient of the 1931 Nobel Peace prize
Lillian Wald	Established a neighborhood nursing service for the sick poor of the Lower East Side in New York City; the founder of public health nursing
Mary Elizabeth Mahoney	Graduated from the New England Hospital for Women and Children in 1879 as America's first Black nurse
Harriet Tubman	A nurse and an abolitionist; active in the underground railroad movement before joining the Union Army during the Civil War
Nora Gertrude Livingston	Established a training program for nurses at the Montreal General Hospital (the first 3-year program in North America)
Mary Agnes Snively	Director of the nursing school at Toronto General Hospital and one of the founders of the Canadian Nurses Association
Sojourner Truth	Provided nursing care to soldiers during the Civil War and worked for the women's movement
Isabel Hampton Robb	A leader in nursing and nursing education; organized the nursing school at Johns Hopkins Hospital; initiated policies that included limiting the number of hours in a day's work and wrote a textbook to help student learning; the first president of the Nurses Associated Alumnae of the United States and Canada (which later became the American Nurses Association)
20th Century	
Mary Adelaide Nutting	Became the first professor of nursing in the world as a faculty member of Teachers' College, Columbia University; with Lavinia Dock, published the four-volume *History of Nursing*
Elizabeth Smellie	A member of the original Victorian Order of Nurses for Canada (a group that provided public health nursing); organized the Canadian Women's Army Corps during World War II
Lavinia Dock	A nursing leader and women's rights activist; instrumental in the Constitutional amendment giving women the right to vote
Mary Breckenridge	Established the Frontier Nursing Service and one of the first midwifery schools in the United States

the foundational documents for nursing is presented in Box 1-1. You may also want to check the WHO's *State of the world's nursing 2020* report, which provides the latest, most up-to-date evidence on policy options for the global nursing workforce. It presents a compelling case for considerable yet feasible investment in nursing education, jobs, and leadership (https://www.who.int/publications/i/item/9789240003279).

Box 1-1 Timeline of the Development of Foundational Nursing Documents

1859	Florence Nightingale publishes Notes on Nursing: What It Is and What It Is Not.
1896	The Nurses' Associated Alumnae of the United States and Canada is founded. Later to become the American Nurses Association (ANA), its first purpose is to establish and maintain a code of ethics.
1940	A "Tentative Code" is published in the *American Journal of Nursing,* although never formally adopted.
1950	*Code for Professional Nurses,* in the form of 17 provisions that are a substantive revision of the "Tentative Code" of 1940, is unanimously accepted by the ANA House of Delegates.
1952	*Nursing Research* publishes its premiere issue.
1956	*Code for Professional Nurses* is amended.
1960	*Code for Professional Nurses* is revised.
1968	*Code for Professional Nurses* is substantively revised, condensing the 17 provisions of the code into 10 provisions.
1973	ANA publishes its first *Standards of Nursing Practice.*
1976	*Code for Nurses with Interpretive Statements,* a modification of the provision and interpretive statements, is published as 11 provisions.
1980	ANA publishes *Nursing: A Social Policy Statement.*
1985	The National Institutes of Health organizes the Center for Nursing Research.
	ANA publishes *Titling for Licensure.*
	Code for Nurses with Interpretive Statements retains the provisions of the 1976 version and includes revised interpretive statements.
	The ANA House of Delegates forms a task force to formally document the scope of practice for nursing.
1987	ANA publishes *The Scope of Nursing Practice.*
1990	The ANA House of Delegates forms a task force to revise the 1973 *Standards of Nursing Practice.*
1991	ANA publishes *Standards of Clinical Nursing Practice.*
1995	ANA publishes *Nursing's Social Policy Statement.*
	The Congress of Nursing Practice directs the Committee on Nursing Practice Standards and Guidelines to establish a process for periodic review and revision of nursing standards.
1996	ANA publishes *Scope and Standards of Advanced Practice Registered Nursing.*
1998	ANA publishes *Standards of Clinical Nursing Practice*, 2nd edition (also known as *Clinical Standards*).
2001	*Code of Ethics with Interpretive Statements* is accepted by the ANA House of Delegates.
	ANA publishes *Bill of Rights for Registered Nurses.*
2002	ANA publishes *Nursing's Agenda for the Future: A Call to the Nation.*
2003	ANA publishes *Nursing's Social Policy Statement*, 2nd edition.
2004	ANA publishes *Nursing: Scope and Standards of Practice.*
2008	*APRN Consensus Model* is published by the APRN Consensus Work Group and APRN Joint Dialogue Group.
	ANA publishes *Professional Role Competence Position Statement.*
	ANA publishes *Specialization and Credentialing in Nursing Revisited: Understanding the Issues, Advancing the Profession.*
2010	ANA publishes *Nursing's Social Policy Statement: The Essence of the Profession*
	ANA publishes *Nursing: Scope and Standards of Practice*, 2nd edition.
2015	ANA publishes *Code of Ethics for Nurses with Interpretive Statements.*
	ANA publishes *Nursing: Scope and Standards of Practice*, 3rd edition.
2021	ANA publishes Nursing: Scope and Standards of Practice, 4th edition.

Source: From American Nurses Association (ANA). (2021). *Nursing: Scope and standards of practice* (4th ed.).

Development of Nursing From the 19th to 21st Centuries

Both the work of Florence Nightingale and the care provided for battle casualties during the Civil War focused attention on the need for educated nurses in the United States. Schools of nursing, founded in connection with hospitals, were established on the beliefs of Nightingale, but the training they provided was based more on apprenticeship than on educational principles. Hospitals saw an economic advantage in having their own schools, and most hospital schools were organized to provide more easily controlled and less expensive staff for the hospital. This resulted in a lack of clear guidelines separating nursing service and nursing education. As students and as graduates, female nurses were under the control of male hospital administrators and health care providers. The lack of educational standards, the male dominance in health care, and the pervading Victorian belief that women were subordinate to men combined to contribute to several decades of slow progress toward professionalism in nursing (Kalisch & Kalisch, 2004).

World War II had an enormous effect on nursing. For the first time, as large numbers of women worked outside the home, they became more independent and assertive. These changes in women and in society led to an increased emphasis on education. The war itself had created a need for more nurses and resulted in a knowledge explosion in medicine and technology, which broadened the role of nurses. After World War II, efforts were directed at upgrading nursing education. Schools of nursing were based on educational objectives and were increasingly developed in university and college settings, leading to degrees in nursing for men, women, and minorities.

Nursing achievement has broadened in all areas, including practice in a wide variety of health care settings, the development of a specific body of knowledge, the conduct and publication of nursing research, and the recognition of the role of nursing in promoting access to affordable quality health care. Increased emphasis on nursing knowledge as the foundation for evidence-based practice (EBP) has led to the growth of nursing as a professional discipline. The American Association of Colleges of Nursing (AACN, 2019) is careful to point out that, although often working collaboratively, nursing does not "assist" medicine or other fields. Nursing operates independently of, not auxiliary to, medicine and other disciplines. Nurses' roles range from direct patient care and case management to establishing nursing practice standards, developing quality assurance procedures, and directing complex nursing care systems.

In the 2021 *The Essentials: Core Competencies for Professional Nursing Education* document, the AACN proposes a vision for the future of the nursing workforce, including ways educators can help graduates to be "work ready":

> Nursing education for the 21st century ought to reflect a number of contemporary trends and values and address several issues to shape the future workforce, including diversity, equity, and inclusion [see Chapter 3]; four spheres of care (including an enhanced focus on primary care); systems-based practice; informatics and technology [see Chapter 21]; academic partnerships; and career-long learning. (p. 5)

You will want to read this document carefully as you prepare for your career in today's professional nursing.

Noting that, historically, nursing education emphasized clinical education in acute care, authors of the *Essentials* document emphasized that the future of health care delivery will occur within four spheres of care: (1) disease prevention/promotion of health and well-being, which includes the promotion of physical and mental health in all patients as well as management of minor-acute and intermittent care needs of generally healthy patients; (2) chronic disease care, which includes management of chronic diseases and prevention of sequelae; (3) regenerative or restorative care, which includes critical/trauma care, complex acute care, acute exacerbations of chronic conditions, and treatment of physiologically unstable patients that generally requires care in a mega-acute institution; and (4) hospice/palliative/supportive care, which includes end-of-life care as well as palliative and supportive care for individuals requiring extended care, those with complex, chronic disease states, or those requiring rehabilitative care (2021, p. 6). See Box 1-2.

Box 1-2 Four Spheres of Nursing Care

Wellness, Disease Prevention	Promotion of physical and mental health in all patients as well as management of minor-acute and intermittent care needs of generally healthy patient
Chronic Disease Management	Management of chronic diseases and prevention of sequelae
Regenerative/ Restorative Care	Critical/trauma care, complex acute care, acute exacerbations of chronic conditions, and treatment of physiologically unstable patients that generally requires care in a mega-acute institution
Hospice/Palliative Care	Includes end-of-life care as well as palliative and supportive care for individuals requiring extended care, those with complex, chronic disease states, or those requiring rehabilitative care

Source: American Association of Colleges of Nursing. (2021). *The essentials: Core competencies for professional nursing education* (pp. 5–6). https://theaacn.org/.

To learn more about the history of nursing, visit the Penn Nursing Science Nursing, History, and Health Care website: https://www.nursing.upenn.edu/nhhc.

DEFINITIONS OF NURSING

The word *nurse* originated from the Latin word *nutrix*, meaning "to nourish." Most definitions of **nursing** describe the nurse as a person who nourishes, fosters, and protects and who is prepared to take care of sick, injured, older, and dying people. With the expanding roles and functions of the nurse in today's society, however, any one definition may be too limited.

The International Council of Nurses (ICN) captures much of what nursing means in its definition:

> Nursing encompasses autonomous and collaborative care of individuals of all ages, families, groups, and communities, sick or well and in all settings. Nursing includes the promotion of health, prevention of illness, and the care of ill, disabled, and dying people. Advocacy, promotion of a safe environment, research, participation in shaping health policy and in patient and health systems management, and education are also key nursing roles.

In addition to the definition of nursing shared at the beginning of the chapter, the ANA describes the social context of nursing, the knowledge base for nursing practice, the scope of nursing practice, standards of professional nursing practice, and the regulation of professional nursing in its *Nursing's Social Policy Statement* (2010). Within today's definitions of nursing, we find all the elements of professional nursing. Nurses focus on human experiences and responses to birth, health, illness, and death within the context of people, families, groups, and communities. The knowledge base for nursing practice includes diagnosis, interventions, and evaluation of outcomes from an established care plan. In addition, the nurse integrates objective data with knowledge gained from an understanding of the patient's or group's subjective experience, applies scientific knowledge in the nursing process and other clinical judgment models, and provides a caring relationship that facilitates health and healing.

The central focus in all definitions of nursing is the patient (the person receiving care), which includes the physical, emotional, social, and spiritual dimensions of that person. Nursing is no longer considered to be concerned primarily with illness care. Nursing's concepts and definitions have expanded to include the prevention of illness; the promotion and maintenance of health for people, families, groups, and communities; and care for seriously ill and dying people.

NURSING'S AIMS AND COMPETENCIES

Four broad aims of nursing practice can be identified in the definitions of nursing:

1. To promote health
2. To prevent illness
3. To restore health
4. To facilitate coping with disability or death

To meet these aims, the nurse uses four blended competencies: cognitive, technical, interpersonal, and ethical/legal. More recently these competencies have been further specified as the Quality and Safety Education for Nurses (QSEN) project competencies: patient-centered care, teamwork and collaboration, quality improvement, safety, EBP, and informatics (Sherwood & Barnsteiner, 2012). These competencies are described in Chapter 13. The Reflective Practice Boxes that begin each chapter of this book offer examples of practical challenges to these competencies that actual nursing students have encountered.

The primary role of the nurse as caregiver is given shape and substance by the interrelated roles of communicator, teacher, counselor, leader, researcher, advocate, and collaborator. These roles are described in Table 1-2 and throughout

Table 1-2 Nursing Roles in All Settings

ROLE	FUNCTION
Caregiver	The provision of care to patients that combines both the art and the science of nursing in meeting physical, emotional, intellectual, sociocultural, and spiritual needs. As a caregiver, the nurse integrates the roles of communicator, teacher, counselor, leader, researcher, advocate, and collaborator to promote wellness through activities that prevent illness, restore health, and facilitate coping with disability or death. The role of caregiver is the primary role of the nurse.
Communicator	The use of effective interpersonal and therapeutic communication skills to establish and maintain helping relationships with patients of all ages in a wide variety of health care settings
Teacher/educator	The use of communication skills to assess, implement, and evaluate individualized teaching plans to meet learning needs of patients and their families
Counselor	The use of therapeutic interpersonal communication skills to provide information, make appropriate referrals, and facilitate the patient's problem-solving and decision-making skills
Leader	The assertive, self-confident practice of nursing when providing care, effecting change, and functioning with groups
Researcher	The participation in or conduct of research to increase knowledge in nursing and improve patient care
Advocate	The protection of human or legal rights and the securing of care for all patients based on the belief that patients have the right to make informed decisions about their own health and lives
Collaborator	The effective use of skills in organization, communication, and advocacy to facilitate the functions of all members of the health care team as they provide patient care

the text. You will also discover that nurses play many specialized roles in today's evolving health care environment, such as case manager, navigator, informaticist, safety and quality officer, ethicist, to name just a few. As you progress through your clinical rotations, pay attention to the many diverse roles nurses play and begin to reflect on what might be the perfect fit for you. Nurses carry out their roles in many different settings, with care increasingly provided in the home and in the community. Examples of settings for care are fully described in Unit II.

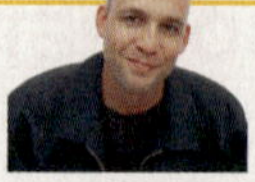

Recall **Roberto Pecorini**, the 38-year-old patient with metastatic cancer. When providing care for Mr. Pecorini, the nurse assumes the role of competent, caring, and responsible caregiver, creates a respectful partnership while identifying best practices, maintains the patient's safety throughout, and appropriately educates the patient and advocates for the patient's rights.

Promoting Health

Health is a state of optimal functioning or well-being. As defined by the WHO, a person's health includes physical, social, and mental components and is not merely the absence of disease or infirmity. Health is often a subjective state: people medically diagnosed with an illness may still consider themselves healthy. Wellness, a term that is often associated with health, is an active state of being healthy by living a lifestyle that promotes good physical, mental, emotional, and spiritual health. Models of health and wellness are described in Chapter 3.

Health is an essential part of each of the other aims of nursing. Nurses promote health by identifying, analyzing, and maximizing each patient's own individual strengths as components of preventing illness, restoring health, and facilitating coping with disability or death.

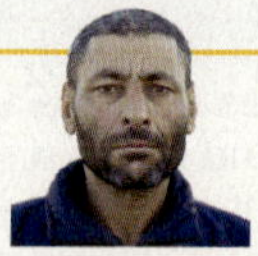

When teaching **Mr. Basshir**, the patient described at the beginning of the chapter with risk factors for heart disease, the nurse would focus the teaching plan to rely on the patient's strengths. Although his statements reflect a reluctance to learn and change, emphasizing the patient's strengths would help the patient feel more in control of his health, and thus, hopefully, spur him to make the necessary changes.

Health promotion is motivated by the desire to increase a person's well-being and health potential. A person's level of health is affected by many different interrelated factors that either promote health or increase the risk for illness. These factors include genetic inheritance, cognitive abilities, educational level, race and ethnicity, culture, age and biologic sex, developmental level, lifestyle, environment, and socioeconomic status. A level of health or wellness is also strongly influenced by what is termed "health literacy." Health literacy is the ability of people to obtain, process, and understand the basic information needed to make appropriate decisions about health. Examples of ways that nurses can promote health literacy are included throughout this text.

Healthy People 2030 also establishes health promotion guidelines for the nation as a whole. The guidelines are focused on meeting five overarching goals:

1. Attain healthy, thriving lives and well-being, free of preventable disease, disability, injury, and premature death.
2. Eliminate health disparities, achieve health equity, and attain health literacy to improve the health and well-being of all.
3. Create social, physical, and economic environments that promote attaining full potential for health and well-being for all.
4. Promote healthy development, healthy behaviors, and well-being across all life stages.
5. Engage leadership, key constituents, and the public across multiple sectors to take action and design policies that improve the health and well-being of all.

Box 1-3 lists the foundational principles that explain the thinking that guides decisions about Healthy People 2030.

Patient-centered health promotion is the framework for nursing activities. The nurse considers the patient's self-awareness, health awareness, and use of resources while providing care. Through knowledge and skill, the nurse:

- Facilitates patients' decisions about lifestyle that enhance the quality of life and encourage acceptance of responsibility for their own health

Box 1-3 Healthy People 2030: Foundational Principles

- Health and well-being of all people and communities are essential to a thriving, equitable society.
- Promoting health and well-being and preventing disease are linked efforts that encompass physical, mental, and social health dimensions.
- Investing to achieve the full potential for health and well-being for all provides valuable benefits to society.
- Achieving health and well-being requires eliminating health disparities, achieving health equity, and attaining health literacy.
- Healthy physical, social, and economic environments strengthen the potential to achieve health and well-being.
- Promoting and achieving the Nation's health and well-being is a shared responsibility that is distributed across the national, state, tribal, and community levels, including the public, private, and not-for-profit sectors.
- Working to attain the full potential for health and well-being of the population is a component of decision making and policy formulation across all sectors.

Source: Office of Disease Prevention and Health Promotion. *Healthy People 2030 Framework.* https://www.healthypeople.gov/2020/About-Healthy-People/Development-Healthy-People-2030/Framework.

- Increases patients' health awareness by assisting in the understanding that health is more than just not being ill, and by teaching that certain behaviors and factors can contribute to or diminish health
- Teaches self-care activities to maximize achievement of goals that are realistic and attainable
- Serves as a role model
- Encourages health promotion by providing information and referrals

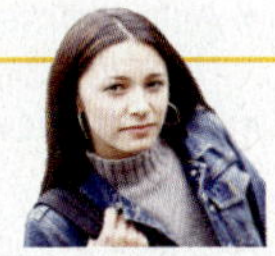

Recall **Michelle Fine**, the young mother with a new baby who calls the nursery for help with breastfeeding. Making a referral for home care follow-up before Michelle's discharge from the hospital would have been an appropriate intervention to offer support, guidance, and additional teaching.

Preventing Illness

The U.S. Department of Health and Human Services Office of Disease Prevention and Health Promotion (ODPHP) leads efforts to improve the health of all Americans. The objectives of disease prevention activities are to reduce the risk of illness, to promote good health habits, and to maintain optimal functioning. Nurses prevent illness primarily by teaching and by personal example. Examples include:

- Educational programs in areas such as prenatal care for pregnant people, smoking-cessation programs, and stress-reduction seminars
- Community programs and resources that encourage healthy lifestyles, such as aerobic exercise classes, "swimnastics," and physical fitness programs
- Literature, television, radio, or Internet information on a healthy diet, regular exercise, and the importance of good health habits
- Health assessments in institutions, clinics, and community settings that identify areas of strength and risks for illness

As you think back to the early days of the COVID-19 pandemic in 2020 and the critical importance of frequent handwashing, social distancing, and wearing masks, what efforts did you take to model appropriate behaviors? When we learned in the summer of 2020 that if 95% of Americans wore masks in public we could prevent 33,000 deaths by October 1, 2020, it was hard to understand why so many still refused to wear masks (http://www.healthdata.org/news-release/new-ihme-covid-19-model-projects-nearly-180000-us-deaths). At 4 million strong, U.S. nurses have the potential to be a real powerhouse if we each reach out in our personal spheres of influence to encourage healthy behaviors.

Take time to check out Health.gov, the ODPHP's website (https://health.gov) to familiarize yourself with many helpful resources that you can use for yourself, your family, and your patients.

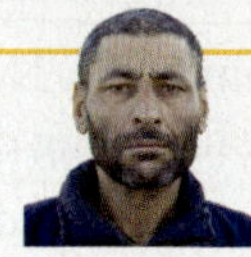

Think back to **Ahmad Basshir**, the 62-year-old man at risk for heart disease who was described at the beginning of the chapter. By addressing Mr. Basshir's resistance to change and teaching him the lifestyle modifications necessary to reduce his risk for developing heart disease, the nurse contributes to illness prevention by promoting healthier behavior.

Restoring Health

Activities to restore health encompass those historically considered to be the nurse's responsibility. These focus on the person with an illness and range from early detection of a disease to rehabilitation and teaching during recovery. Such activities include:

- Performing assessments that detect an illness (e.g., taking blood pressure, measuring blood sugars)
- Referring questions and abnormal findings to other health care providers as appropriate
- Providing direct care of the person who is ill by such measures as giving physical care, administering medications, and carrying out procedures and treatments
- Collaborating with other health care providers in providing care
- Planning, teaching, and carrying out rehabilitation for illnesses such as heart attacks, arthritis, and strokes
- Working in mental health and chemical-dependency programs

Facilitating Coping With Disability and Death

Although the major goals of health care are promoting, maintaining, and restoring health, these goals cannot always be met. Nurses also facilitate patient and family coping with altered function, life crisis, and death. Altered function decreases a person's ability to carry out activities of daily living (ADLs) and expected roles. Nurses facilitate an optimal level of function through maximizing the person's strengths and potentials, through teaching, and through referral to community support systems. Nurses provide care to both patients and families at the end of life, and they do so in hospitals, long-term care facilities, hospices, and homes. Nurses are active in hospice programs, which assist patients and their families in multiple settings in preparing for death and in living as comfortably as possible until death occurs.

NURSING AS A PROFESSIONAL DISCIPLINE

As definitions of nursing have expanded to describe more clearly the evolving roles and actions of nurses, increased attention has been given to nursing as a professional discipline. Nursing uses existing and new knowledge to solve problems creatively and meet human needs within ever-changing boundaries. Nursing is recognized as a **profession** based on the following defining criteria:

- Well-defined body of specific and unique knowledge
- Strong service orientation
- Recognized authority by a professional group
- Code of ethics
- Professional organization that sets standards
- Ongoing research
- Autonomy and self-regulation

Nursing involves specialized skills and application of knowledge based on an education that has both theoretical and clinical practice components. Nursing is guided by standards set by professional organizations and an established code of ethics. Nursing focuses on human responses to actual or potential health problems and is increasingly focused on wellness, an area of caring that encompasses nursing's unique knowledge and abilities. Nursing is increasingly recognized as scholarly, with academic qualifications, research, and publications specific to the profession that are widely accepted and respected. In addition, nursing interventions are focused on EBP, which is practice based on research and not intuition.

Nursing has evolved through history from a technical service to a thoughtful, person-centered process that maximizes potential in all human dimensions. This has been an active development process, using lessons from the past to gain knowledge for practice in the present and in the future.

PROFESSIONAL FORMATION

If nursing is a profession and not merely a job, nurse educators have a responsibility to form the professional identities of their students and graduates. You should be learning from every faculty member in every class and clinical encounter, not only how to *do* nursing but how to *be* a nurse. Maureen Shawn Kennedy (2018), editor of the *American Journal of Nursing*, charged nurse educators to transform nursing students into nurses who have a sense of themselves that is influenced by the characteristics, norms, and values of the nursing discipline, resulting in each individual thinking, acting, and feeling like a nurse. See Box 1-4.

If we educators are successful, you will graduate with a professional identity that creates a sense of belonging to a group that holds the same values. You will practice with respected colleagues with whom you can touch base when you need to make tough decisions in stressful situations. Most importantly, those who experience your care will know that they are being cared for in a professional manner by someone who adheres to a code of ethical conduct. The authors of this text take Kennedy's charge seriously, and, in every chapter, we aim to forge your professional identity and suggest not only how to do nursing but also how to be a nurse. Our goal is to help you become a competent, compassionate, responsible professional who can be trusted to be who the public you serve needs.

Box 1-4 Tips for Thinking, Acting, and Feeling Like a Nurse

Think like a nurse,

- Make sure that solid research/nursing science informs every aspect of your evidence-based practice.
- Always be prepared to answer the question, "Why are you doing it this way?"
- Value being able to think strategically and creatively about the plan of care for patients with complex needs.
- Ask yourself, if this was the person you loved most, "would I be happy about the care being delivered?"
- Be intellectually humble and never fail to ask for help when you are unsure of what counts as a best response.

Act like a nurse,

- Demonstrate over and over again that your primary concern is the patient, family, and community you serve.
- Prioritize patient safety and high-quality care.
- Inspire confidence and trust in your being a competent, compassionate, and responsible nurse.
- Learn how to advocate effectively for anyone not receiving optimal care or for colleagues being disrespected in the workplace.
- Create a culture that supports everyone's doing the right thing simply because it's the right thing to do.
- Live a healthy life so that you can be energized for each day's practice.

Feel like a nurse.

- Take deserved pride and joy in being the critical difference that makes health care "work" for even, or especially for, the most vulnerable.
- Renew your ability to empathize with patients, families, and communities in need and to respond compassionately; take a break when compassion fatigue or burnout threatens your care.
- Practice self-compassion when your best efforts fail to resolve patient problems or challenging practice situations.
- Recognize moral distress and seek help in responding.
- Value your growing resilience even in times of crisis . . . delight in the positive energy and strength you bring to your team.

EDUCATIONAL PREPARATION FOR NURSING PRACTICE

Educational preparation for nursing practice involves several different types of programs that lead to **licensure**, or the legal authority to practice as a nursing professional. Students may choose to enter a practical nursing program and become a licensed practical nurse (LPN) or they may enter a diploma, an associate degree, or a baccalaureate program to be licensed as a registered nurse (RN). State laws in the United States recognize both the LPN and the RN as credentials to practice nursing. Increasingly, various levels of nursing education are providing programs for educational advancement. For example, the LPN can complete an associate degree and become an RN, and the RN prepared at the diploma or associate degree level can attain a bachelor of science in nursing (BSN) degree. There are also programs that provide RN-to-master's degrees, as well as BSN-to-DNP or PhD, and master's degree-to-DNP or PhD. Graduate programs in nursing provide master's and doctoral degrees. For a guide to the many different types of nursing programs, read "Professional Registered Nurses Today: The Who of Nursing" (ANA, 2021) and check out the AACN website (https://www.aacnnursing.org/).

Educational preparation for the nurse has become a major issue in nursing; the multiple methods of preparation are confusing to employers, consumers of health care services, and nurses themselves. Nursing organizations are working hard to answer questions such as "What is technical nursing?" and "What is professional nursing?" as well as "Should graduates of different programs take the same licensing examination and have the same title?" These questions are likely to be resolved during your nursing career. The AACN believes that baccalaureate education should be the minimum level required for entry into professional nursing practice in today's complex health care environment. Most RNs today enter practice with a baccalaureate degree offered by a 4-year college or university or an associate degree offered by a community college. Employers are expressing a strong preference for new nurses with baccalaureate preparation. Findings from the AACN's latest survey on the Employment of New Nurse Graduates show that 46% of employers require new hires to have a bachelor's degree, while 88% strongly prefer baccalaureate-prepared nurses (AACN Nursing Fact Sheet).

The AACN's Essentials notes that nursing has been identified as having the potential for making the biggest impact on a transformation of health care delivery to a safer, higher quality, and more cost-effective system (AACN, 2008, 2021). The 2021 Essentials document describes the outcomes expected of graduates of baccalaureate programs and emphasizes ten domains: Knowledge for Nursing Practice, Person Centered Care, Population Health, Scholarship for the Nursing Discipline, Quality and Safety, Interprofessional Partnerships, Systems Based Practice, Informatics and Healthcare Technologies, Professionalism, and Personal, Professional, and Leadership Development. In addition to domains, there are featured concepts associated with professional nursing practice that are integrated within the Essentials. These include clinical judgment, communication, compassionate care, diversity, equity and inclusion, ethics, evidence-based practice, health policy, and social determinants of health.

The following sections discuss current education for LPNs and RNs as well as graduate nursing education, continuing education for nurses, and in-service education.

Practical and Vocational Nursing Education

Practical (also labeled vocational) nursing programs were established to teach graduates to give bedside nursing care to patients. Schools for practical nursing programs are located in varied settings, such as high schools, technical or vocational schools, community colleges, and independent facilities. Most programs are 1 year in length, divided into one third classroom hours and two thirds clinical laboratory hours. On completion of the program, graduates can take the National Council Licensure Examination–Practical Nurse (NCLEX–PN) for licensure as an LPN. LPNs work under the direction of a health care provider or RN to give direct care to patients, focusing on meeting health care needs in hospitals, long-term care facilities, and home health facilities.

Registered Nursing Education

Three types of educational programs traditionally lead to licensure as an RN: (1) diploma, (2) associate degree, and (3) baccalaureate programs. Graduates of all three programs take the NCLEX–RN examination. Although it is a national examination, it is administered by—and the nurse is licensed in—the state in which the examination is taken and passed. *It is illegal to practice nursing unless one has a license verifying completion of an accredited (by state) program in nursing and has passed the licensing examination.* Nurses gain legal rights to practice nursing in another state by applying to that state's board of nursing and receiving reciprocal licensure. Read more in Chapter 7.

The U.S. Department of Labor, Bureau of Labor Statistics (BLS), annually collects and publishes data on employment and earnings for more than 800 occupations. As of 2020, the BLS reports that employment of registered nurses is projected to grow 12% from 2018 to 2028, much faster than the average for all occupations. Reasons for this accelerated growth include an increased emphasis on preventive care, increasing rates of chronic conditions, and demand for health care services from the baby boomer generation as members of this group lead longer and more active lives.

Diploma in Nursing

Many nurses practicing in the United States today received their basic nursing education in a 3-year, hospital-based diploma school of nursing. The first schools of nursing established to educate nurses were diploma programs; until the 1960s, they were the major source of graduates. In recent years, the number of diploma programs has decreased greatly.

Graduates of diploma programs have a sound foundation in the biologic and social sciences, with a strong emphasis on clinical experience in direct patient care. Graduates work in acute, long-term, and ambulatory health care facilities.

Associate Degree in Nursing

Most associate degree in nursing (ADN) programs are offered by community or junior colleges. These 2-year educational programs often attract students with more diverse backgrounds than do the other types of programs. Associate degree education prepares nurses to give care to patients in various settings, including hospitals, long-term care facilities, and home health care and other community settings. Graduates are technically skilled and well prepared to carry out nursing roles and functions. As defined by the National League for Nursing (NLN), competencies of the ADN on entry into practice encompass the roles of provider of care, manager of care, and member of the discipline of nursing.

Baccalaureate in Nursing

The first baccalaureate nursing programs were established in the United States in the early 1900s. The number of programs and the number of enrolling students, however, did not increase markedly until the 1960s. Most graduates receive a BSN.

Recommendations by national nursing organizations that the entry level for professional practice be at the baccalaureate level have resulted in increased numbers of these programs. Although BSN nurses practice in a wide variety of settings, the 4-year degree is required for many administrative, managerial, and community health positions.

In BSN programs, the major in nursing is built on a general education base, with concentration on nursing at the upper level. Students acquire knowledge of theory and practice related to nursing and other disciplines, provide nursing care to individuals and groups, work with members of the health care team, use research to improve practice, and have a foundation for graduate study. Nurses who graduate from a diploma or associate degree program and wish to complete requirements for a BSN may choose to enroll in an on-campus, online, or external degree RN-to-BSN program. In addition, there are accelerated BSN programs for people who already have a degree in another area.

Emerging Entry Points

Beyond the mainstream entry routes to a career as an RN, a number of additional pathways are emerging and proving effective at attracting new audiences into the nursing profession. These alternative routes include entry-level master's programs, accelerated programs for graduates of nonnursing disciplines, community college–based baccalaureate programs, and RN completion programs for LPNs and other allied health providers.

Graduate Education in Nursing

The two levels of graduate education in nursing are the master's and doctoral degrees. A master's degree prepares advanced practice nurses (APRNs) to function in educational settings, in managerial roles, as clinical specialists, and in various advanced practice areas, such as nurse–midwives and nurse practitioners (Table 1-3). Many master's graduates gain national certification in their specialty area—for example, as family nurse practitioners (FNPs) or nurse midwives. The clinical nurse leader (CNL) is an emerging nursing role developed by the AACN (2012) in collaboration with an array of leaders from the practice environment. The CNL, an advanced clinician with education at the master's degree level, puts EBP into action to ensure that patients benefit from the latest innovations in care delivery. The CNL role is not one of administration or management. Nurses

Table 1-3 Expanded Educational and Career Roles of Nurses

TITLE	DESCRIPTION
Clinical nurse specialist Examples: enterostomal therapist, geriatrics, infection control, medical-surgical, maternal–child, oncology, quality assurance, nursing process	A nurse with an advanced degree, education, or experience who is considered to be an expert in a specialized area of nursing; carries out direct patient care; consultation; teaching of patients, families, and staff; and research
Nurse practitioner	A nurse with an advanced degree, certified for a special area or age of patient care; works in a variety of health care settings or in independent practice to make health assessments and deliver primary care
Nurse anesthetist	A nurse who completes a course of study in an anesthesia school; carries out preoperative visits and assessments; administers and monitors anesthesia during surgery; and evaluates postoperative status of patients
Nurse–midwife	A nurse who completes a program in midwifery; provides prenatal and postnatal care; and delivers babies for patients with uncomplicated pregnancies
Clinical nurse leader	A nurse prepared at the graduate level who oversees the lateral integration of care for a distinct group of patients and who may actively provide direct patient care in complex situations. The CNL role is not one of administration or management.
Nurse educator	A nurse, usually with an advanced degree, who teaches in educational or clinical settings; teaches theoretical knowledge and clinical skills; conducts research
Nurse administrator	A nurse who functions at various levels of management in health care settings; is responsible for the management and administration of resources and personnel involved in giving patient care
Nurse researcher	A nurse with an advanced degree who conducts research relevant to the definition and improvement of nursing practice and education
Nurse entrepreneur	A nurse, usually with an advanced degree, who may manage a clinic or health-related business, conduct research, provide education, or serve as an adviser or consultant to institutions, political facilities, or businesses

with doctoral degrees meet requirements for academic advancement and organizational management. They also are prepared to carry out research necessary to advance nursing theory and practice.

The newest graduate nursing degree is the doctor of nursing practice (DNP). In 2004, the AACN, in consultation with a variety of stakeholder groups, called for moving the current level of preparation necessary for advanced practice from the master's degree to the DNP by the year 2015. According to their position statement, the DNP is designed for nurses seeking a terminal degree in nursing practice and offers an alternative approach to research-focused doctoral programs. DNP-prepared nurses are well equipped to fully implement the science developed by nurse researchers prepared in PhD, DNSc, and other research-focused doctorates. For more information on the AACN's position, refer to the AACN Fact Sheet on the DNP, available at https://www.aacnnursing.org/News-Information/Fact-Sheets/DNP-Fact-Sheet.

As you begin clinical practice, it is a good idea to talk with as many nurses with graduate degrees as you can to see if one of their roles might become your next goal. In 2018, 17.1% of the nation's RNs held a master's degree and 1.9% a doctoral degree as their highest educational preparation. The current demand for master's- and doctorally prepared nurses for advanced practice, clinical specialties, teaching, and research roles far outstrips the supply (AACN, 2019).

Continuing Education

The ANA defines continuing education as those professional development experiences designed to enrich the nurse's contribution to health. Colleges, hospitals, voluntary facilities, nursing organizations, and private groups offer formal continuing education through courses, seminars, and workshops. In many states, continuing education is required for an RN to maintain licensure. You will quickly learn that successful nurses are lifelong learners!

In-Service Education

Many hospitals and health care facilities provide education and training for employees of their institution or organization, called in-service education. This is designed to increase the knowledge and skills of the nursing staff. Programs may involve learning, for example, a specific nursing skill or how to use new equipment.

PROFESSIONAL NURSING ORGANIZATIONS

One of the criteria of a profession is having a professional organization that sets standards for practice and education. Nursing's professional organizations are concerned with current issues in nursing and health care, and influence health care policy and legislation. The benefits of belonging to a professional nursing organization include networking with colleagues, having a voice in legislation affecting nursing, and keeping current with trends and issues in nursing.

International Nursing Organization

The ICN, founded in 1899, was the first international organization of professional women. By sharing a commitment to maintaining high standards of nursing service and nursing education and by promoting ethics, the ICN provides a way for national nursing organizations to work together.

National Nursing Organizations

Professional nursing organizations in the United States include the ANA, the NLN, the AACN, the American Academy of Nursing (AAN), and many other specialty organizations such as the American Association of Critical-Care Nurses (AACN). The National Student Nurses' Association (NSNA) prepares students to participate in professional nursing organizations.

American Nurses Association

The ANA is the professional organization for RNs in the United States. Founded in the late 1800s, its membership is comprised of the state nurses' associations to which individual nurses belong. Its primary mission is to advance the profession of nursing to improve health for all. It is the premier organization representing the interests of the 4 million RNs in the United States. It advances the nursing profession by fostering high standards of nursing practice, promoting a safe and ethical work environment, bolstering the health and wellness of nurses, and advocating on health care issues that affect nurses and the public. Publications of the ANA include the *Code of Ethics for Nurses, American Nurse Today, The American Nurse,* and *OJIN: The Online Journal of Issues in Nursing.* The website NurseBooks.org provides access to the publishing program of the ANA. ANA electronic newsletters include *ANA SmartBrief, Nursing Insider, ANA ImmuNews,* and *Capitol Update.*

National League for Nurses

The NLN is an organization open to all people interested in nursing, including nurses, nonnurses, and facilities. Established in 1952, its objective is to foster the development and improvement of all nursing services and nursing education. The NLN conducts one of the largest professional testing services in the United States, including pre-entrance testing for potential students and achievement testing to measure student progress. It also serves as the primary source of research data about nursing education, conducting annual surveys of schools and new RNs. The organization also provides voluntary accreditation for educational programs in nursing.

American Association of Colleges of Nursing

The AACN is the national voice for baccalaureate and higher-degree nursing education programs. The organization's goals focus on establishing quality educational standards, influencing the nursing profession to improve health care, and promoting public support of baccalaureate and graduate education, research, and nursing practice. National accreditation for collegiate nursing programs is provided (based on meeting standards) through the AACN by the Commission on Collegiate Nursing Education (CCNE).

American Academy of Nursing

The AAN serves the public and the nursing profession by advancing health policy and practice through the generation, synthesis, and dissemination of nursing knowledge. Its 2019–2020 policy priorities included Advancing Health Equity and Championing Wellness; Promoting Innovation and Sustainability; and Reducing Patient, Provider, and System Burden. Becoming a fellow of the Academy is a prized distinction. The AAN's approximately 2,700 fellows are nursing leaders in education, management, practice, and research (https://www.aannet.org/home).

National Student Nurses Association

Established in 1952 with the assistance of the ANA and the NLN, the NSNA is the national organization for students enrolled in nursing education programs. Through voluntary participation, students practice self-governance, advocate for student and patient rights, and take collective, responsible action on social and political issues.

Specialty Practice and Special-Interest Nursing Organizations

A wide variety of specialty practice and special-interest nursing organizations are available to nurses. These organizations provide information on specific areas of nursing, often have publications in the specialty area, and may be involved in certification activities. Examples of these organizations are listed in Box 1-5.

GUIDELINES FOR NURSING PRACTICE

Nursing controls and guarantees its practice through standards of practice, nurse practice acts and licensure, the ANA's *Code of Ethics for Nurses*, professional values, and the use of the nursing process. Each of these, which you will meet in later chapters, will guide your nursing education as a student and how you practice after graduation.

Box 1-5 Examples of U.S. Specialty Practice and Special Interest Nursing Organizations

American Academy of Nurse Practitioners
American Assembly for Men in Nursing
American Association for the History of Nursing
American Association of Nurse Attorneys
American Holistic Nurses Association
Association of Nurses in AIDS Care
American Association of Critical Care Nurses
Dermatology Nurses Association
Hospice Nurses Association
Oncology Nurses Society
Sigma Theta Tau International
Transcultural Nursing Society

Standards of Nursing Practice

The ANA's 2021 *Nursing: Scope and Standards of Practice* defines activities that are specific and unique to nursing. **Standards** allow nurses to carry out professional roles, serving as protection for the nurse, the patient, and the institution where health care is provided. The competencies articulated in the Standards describe expected levels of performance that integrate knowledge, skills, abilities, and judgments. Each nurse is accountable for their own quality of practice and is responsible for the use of these standards to ensure knowledgeable, safe, and comprehensive nursing care. Review the 2021 ANA standards that apply to the practice of professional nursing for all RNs, in all settings.

Concept Mastery Alert

Standards of Practice address the key steps involved in caring for patients; Standards of Professional Performance address the key concepts that the nurse integrates into their role as a professional nurse.

Nurse Practice Acts and Licensure

Nurse practice acts are laws established in each state in the United States to regulate the practice of nursing. They are broadly worded and vary among states, but all of them have certain elements in common, such as the following:

- Protect the public by defining the legal scope of nursing practice, excluding untrained or unlicensed people from practicing nursing.
- Create a state board of nursing or regulatory body having the authority to make and enforce rules and regulations concerning the nursing profession.
- Define important terms and activities in nursing, including legal requirements and titles for RNs and LPNs.
- Establish criteria for the education and licensure of nurses.

The board of nursing for each state has the legal authority to allow graduates of approved schools of nursing to take the licensing examination. Those who successfully meet the requirements for licensure are then given a license to practice nursing in the state. The license, which must be renewed at specified intervals, is valid during the life of the holder and is registered in the state. Many states have a requirement for a specified number of continuing education units to renew and maintain licensure. The license and the right to practice nursing can be denied, revoked, or suspended for professional misconduct (e.g., incompetence, negligence, chemical impairment, or criminal actions).

There are two ways in which nurses can practice in a state other than in the one they were originally licensed. One is by **reciprocity**, which allows a nurse to apply for and be endorsed as an RN by another state. Some states are members of the Nurse Licensure Compact (NLC), allowing a nurse who is licensed and permanently lives in one of the member states to practice in the other member states without additional licensure. The Enhanced Nurse Licensure Compact (eNLC) increases access to care while maintaining public protection at the state level. Nurses with an original NLC multistate license will be grandfathered into the new eNLC. New applicants residing in compact states will need to meet 11 uniform licensure requirements (National Council of State Boards of Nursing, 2017).

As nursing roles continue to expand and issues in nursing are resolved, revised nurse practice acts will reflect those changes. All nurses must be knowledgeable about the specific nurse practice act for the state in which they practice. Check out the National Council of State Boards of Nursing Nurse Practice Act Toolkit, available at https://www.ncsbn.org/npa-toolkit.htm, to:

- Learn about the law and regulations that guide and govern nursing practice
- Locate your state nurse practice act and regulations
- Access nurse practice act educational resources

Code of Ethics and Professional Values

Professional values provide the foundation for nursing practice and will guide your interactions with patients, colleagues and the public. In 1998, the AACN (2008) identified five values that epitomize the caring, professional nurse: altruism, autonomy, human dignity, integrity, and social justice. These values are further specified in the ANA Code of Ethics for Nurses (ANA, 2015). Both are described in Chapter 6.

It is never too early for students to be intentional about cultivating the character that comports with professional nursing. Begin by asking yourself:

- Am I able to commit myself wholeheartedly to securing the interest of my patients—even when this entails self-sacrifice?
- Recognizing that we live in a society with great diversity, am I committed to respecting my patients' right to make their own decisions about health care?
- Am I able to respect the inherent worth and uniqueness of each individual and population, even when this is difficult?
- Do I value my own integrity sufficiently to challenge workplace cultures that expect me to be less than my personal best?
- Am I committed to making health care work for everyone, especially the most vulnerable?

Nursing Process and Other Clinical Judgment Models

The **nursing process** is another of the major guidelines for nursing practice. The essential activities involved in the nursing process are assessing, diagnosing, planning, implementing, and evaluating (see Unit III). The ANA *Nursing: Scope and Standards of Nursing Practice* (ANA, 2021) states that regardless of the theoretical knowledge base upon which nursing practice is derived, the knowledge fits within the multidimensional nursing process, the analytical, critical-thinking framework guiding professional thinking and activities. Nurses implement their roles through the nursing process, which integrates both the art and the science of nursing—that is, the nursing process is nursing made visible.

The nursing process is used by the nurse to identify the patient's health care needs and strengths, to establish and carry out a care plan to meet those needs, and to evaluate the effectiveness of the plan to meet established outcomes. The nursing process allows nurses to use critical thinking and clinical reasoning when providing thoughtful, person-centered care that is individualized and holistic and to define those areas of care that are within the domain of nursing. Clinical reasoning and judgment and the nursing process are fully described in Unit III. This unit also explores newer models including the Tanner/Lasater model and the National Council of State Boards of Nursing Clinical Judgment model.

THOUGHTFUL, PERSON-CENTERED PRACTICE FRAMEWORK

This text uses as its framework thoughtful, person-centered practice, which is described in Chapter 13. As you read through the text, you will see multiple examples of each of its elements and begin to develop facility in each of these elements. Your formation in professional nurse practice will include:

- Personal attributes, knowledge base, and clinical experience, which culminates in your development of blended and QSEN competencies and growing confidence;
- Clinical reasoning, judgment, and decision-making skills;
- Patient-centered nurse process competencies in assessing, diagnosing/problem identification, planning, implementing, and evaluating; and
- Ability to routinely engage in reflective practice leading to personal learning and improvement.

With each clinical experience, you should become more confident in your ability to think, act, and feel like a professional nurse—one who earns your patients' and the public's trust.

CURRENT TRENDS IN HEALTH CARE AND NURSING

The National Advisory Council on Nurse Education and Practice (NACNEP) identifies critical challenges to nursing practice in the 21st century: a growing population of hospitalized patients who are older and more acutely ill, increasing health care costs, and the need to stay current with rapid advances in medical knowledge and technology. You are sure to experience all of these as you begin your clinical practice. Complicating these challenges are an existing shortage of nurses (more acute in some regions than others), an aging nurse workforce, and prospects of a worsening nurse shortage (NACNEP, 2010, p. 1). The ANA identified four health care trends that will affect American nurses:

- Nursing shortages will offer unique opportunities.
- Job opportunities are expanding outside the hospital, and nurses will play a much bigger role in communities.
- Technology will play a larger role in nursing practice.
- Nurses will collaborate more with other health care providers.

According to the Association of American Medical Colleges (AAMC), many Americans are "medically homeless" and find it difficult to navigate the health care system when they need care or advice. In addition, the existing health care system financially rewards "patchwork" care provided by assorted clinicians instead of encouraging continuity and care coordination. These problems are compounded by a lack of shared health information systems that could make critical health information available to both patients and providers (AAMC, 2008, p. 2). You will learn more about these realities in Unit II. This much is clear: the public needs professional nurses who are "prepared to work when they are hired, willing to continue to learn, and ready to adapt their skills to the needs of the working environment" (NACNEP, 2010). The most recent NACNEP report (2016) emphasizes needed changes in policy, legislation, and research to strengthen nursing's ability to lead and to practice population health management initiatives and more health care transitions out of hospitals into the community (Fig. 1-2 on page 9).

The NLN has identified 10 trends to watch for in nursing education (Heller et al., 2000):

- Changing demographics and increasing diversity
- The technologic explosion
- Globalization of the world's economy and society
- The era of the educated consumer, alternative therapies, and genomic and palliative care
- The shift to population-based care and the increasing complexity of patient care
- The cost of health care and the challenge of managed care
- The impact of health policy and regulation
- The growing need for interdisciplinary education and for collaborative practice
- The current nursing shortage, and opportunities for lifelong learning and workforce development
- Significant advances in nursing science and research

Each of these trends continues to influence what and how you are taught and the challenges you will daily encounter in practice.

In 2011, the Institute of Medicine (IOM), now the National Academy of Sciences, Engineering, and Medicine, released the results of a groundbreaking study on the role of nurses in realizing a transformed health care system. The report, *The Future of Nursing: Leading Change, Advancing Health*, is "a thorough examination of how nurses' roles, responsibilities and education should change to meet the needs of an aging, increasingly diverse population and to respond to a complex, evolving health care system." The four key messages underlying the IOM's recommendations for transforming the nursing profession (IOM, 2011, p. 4) are as follows:

1. Nurses should practice to the full extent of their education and training.
2. Nurses should achieve higher levels of education and training through an improved education system that promotes seamless academic progression.
3. Nurses should be full partners, with health care providers and other health professionals, in redesigning health care in the United States.
4. Effective workforce planning and policy making require better data collection and an improved information infrastructure.

To read more about these recommendations for the future of nursing, visit the IOM website: http://www.nationalacademies.org/hmd.

An exciting follow-up to the *Future of Nursing* report is the Campaign for Action, which aims to ensure that everyone in America can live a healthier life, supported by a system in which nurses are essential partners in providing care and promoting health (Figures 1-3 and 1-4). Campaign for Action is working in every state to mobilize nurses, health providers, consumers, educators, and businesses to strengthen nursing on multiple fronts, using the recommendations from the IOM's *Future of Nursing* report. The Campaign for Action works on seven major interrelated issues that together contribute to a healthier America through nursing: improving access to care, fostering interprofessional collaboration, promoting nursing leadership, transforming nursing education, increasing diversity in nursing, collecting workforce data, and building healthier communities. Visit the Campaign for Action website, https://campaignforaction.org.

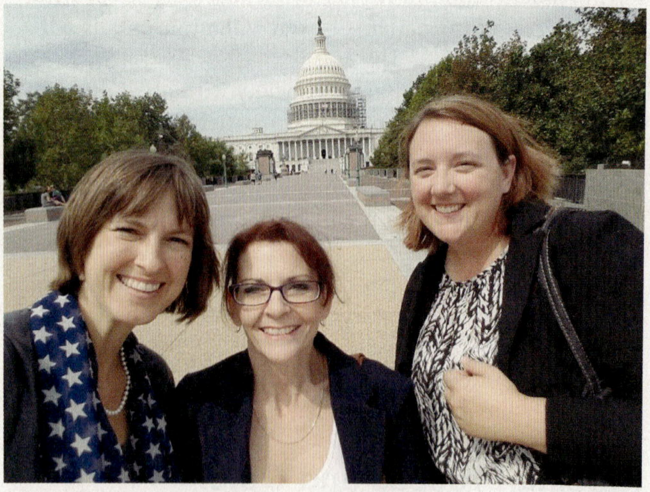

FIGURE 1-3. Faculty and student lobby on the hill. (*Source:* From left to right: Jennifer Jagger, CNM, MSN, FACNM, Georgetown University faculty and Midwives-PAC chair [OR]; Pamela Jellen, SNM [IL]; and Mandy Walters, SWHNP [WI] pose in front of the Capitol on their way to visit legislators.) Visit the Campaign for Action website, https://campaignforaction.org. See also Figures 1-3 and 1-4.

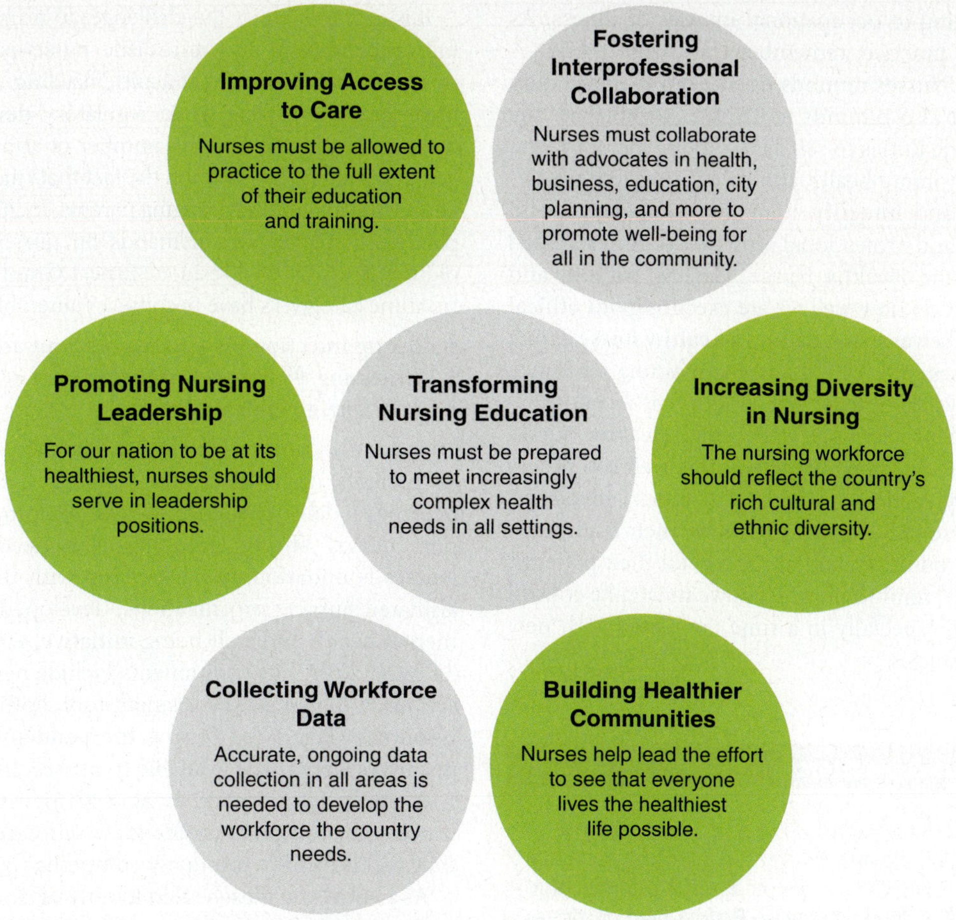
Improving Access to Care
Nurses must be allowed to practice to the full extent of their education and training.
Fostering Interprofessional Collaboration
Nurses must collaborate with advocates in health, business, education, city planning, and more to promote well-being for all in the community.
Promoting Nursing Leadership
For our nation to be at its healthiest, nurses should serve in leadership positions.
Transforming Nursing Education
Nurses must be prepared to meet increasingly complex health needs in all settings.
Increasing Diversity in Nursing
The nursing workforce should reflect the country's rich cultural and ethnic diversity.
Collecting Workforce Data
Accurate, ongoing data collection in all areas is needed to develop the workforce the country needs.
Building Healthier Communities
Nurses help lead the effort to see that everyone lives the healthiest life possible.

FIGURE 1-4. Campaign for Action. Building a healthier America through nursing. (*Source:* From Campaign for Action. https://campaignforaction.org/issues. Used with permission.)

Recognizing the key role nurses play in the health of Americans, the National Academies of Sciences, Engineering, and Medicine is currently working on a consensus report, *The Future of Nursing 2020–2031*, that charts a path for the nursing profession to help the United States create a culture of health, reduce health disparities, and improve the health and well-being of the U.S. population in the 21st century. The report explores how nurses can work to reduce health disparities and promote equity, while keeping costs at bay, utilizing technology, and maintaining patient and family-focused care into 2030. This committee is considering newly emerging evidence related to the COVID-19 pandemic, and the report includes recommendations regarding the role of nurses in responding to the crisis created by a pandemic (https://www.nationalacademies.org/our-work/the-future-of-nursing-2020-2030).

The January 2017 issue of the *American Journal of Nursing* identified the top health care policy news stories of 2016. Gun violence topped the list. There were over 14,000 deaths and almost 29,000 injuries related to gun violence in the United States in 2016. Access to care was the second theme. In 2016, sexual and biologic sex minorities, including lesbian, gay, bisexual, and transgender people, were officially designated by the National Institutes of Health as a "health disparity population," allowing for more research on improving health and health care access for this population. Other access-to-care stories involved mental health care (one in five Americans experience mental health challenges, and resources are frequently unavailable), the rising costs of prescription drugs, and rural health care access (Sofer, 2017). Identified as stories to watch in 2017 were new cancer initiatives and precision medicine; climate change and health; changing trends in the use, misuse, and cost of drugs; and obesity (Potera, 2017). All of these remain relevant.

To address these challenges, employers will continue to seek nurses who have knowledge, skills, and attitudes that are aligned with the requirements of their practice environments, those who can work effectively in interprofessional teams across a variety of health care settings and those who can provide traditional nursing services as well as other needed services such as case and practice leadership, case management, health promotion, and disease prevention.

SELF-CARE

Hopefully this chapter has made you excited about your chosen profession and eager to begin professional practice. There are so many rewards that nursing offers each of us. You will, however, quickly learn that nursing is also a demanding profession, one the U.S. Department of Labor identifies as a hazardous occupation because of the numbers of nurses who miss workdays owing to occupational injuries or illness. As you begin clinical practice, remember that while the ANA Code of Ethics for Nurses reminds us that our primary duty is to the patient, it also reminds us (ANA, 2015a) that "the nurse owes the same duties to self as to others, including the responsibility to promote health and safety, preserve wholeness of character and integrity, maintain competence, and continue personal and professional growth." ANA designated 2017 the year of the Healthy Nurse, Healthy Nation, and invited us to reflect on how well we are executing our ethical duty to care for ourselves. ANA defines a **healthy nurse** as one who actively focuses on creating and maintaining a balance and synergy of physical, intellectual, emotional, social, spiritual, personal and professional well-being. Healthy nurses live life to the fullest capacity, across the wellness/illness continuum, as they become stronger role models, advocates, and educators, personally, for their families, their communities and work environments, and ultimately for their patients. Wei and Wei (2020) remind nurses that we must take control of our own health, especially in a time populated with new challenges and obstacles.

Nurse Self-Care Alert

Self-care is vital. See Figure 1-5 for a practical illustration of how you can elevate six strategies into a self-care model using the ENERGY acronym: **E**nergy source, **N**urturing kindness, **E**motional hygiene, **R**efocusing purpose, **G**erminating positivity, and **Y**our uniqueness.

It is easy to identify the challenges to nurses' living life to the full: understaffing and unrealistic nurse–patient ratios; night rotations; increased patient acuity; needing to come in early or leave late to complete work; regulatory demands; mandatory overtime; and an increasing number of abusive patients, families, and staff, not to mention the fact that many nurses are older and caring for children or aging parents. In 2020, the COVID-19 pandemic created new demands on nurses and exacerbated old demands. ANA President Ernest Grant (2020) wrote that frontline caregivers have become a vulnerable population:

- Risking infection by working without adequate PPE
- Witnessing the ravages of the disease
- Experiencing ethical conflicts

Suddenly, nurses having to balance their obligations to patients, themselves, their families, and communities became a daily challenge. Grant announced that to support nurses' short- and long-term needs, the American Nurses Foundation, in partnership with the ANA and three affiliated nursing organizations, developed a comprehensive mental health and well-being initiative, which is available at bit.ly/2yLKuU2. Its components include peer-to-peer conversations, a digital self-assessment tool, hotlines, and provider resources (Fig. 1-6). During the pandemic, more self-care resources were made available to nurses than ever before.

A study by Thacker et al. (2016) revealed that many nurses may not practice adequate self-care, especially when they feel they have too many competing priorities.

As a nurse, you must be alert to early signs of fatigue, as well as:

- **Compassion fatigue**: Loss of satisfaction from providing good patient care

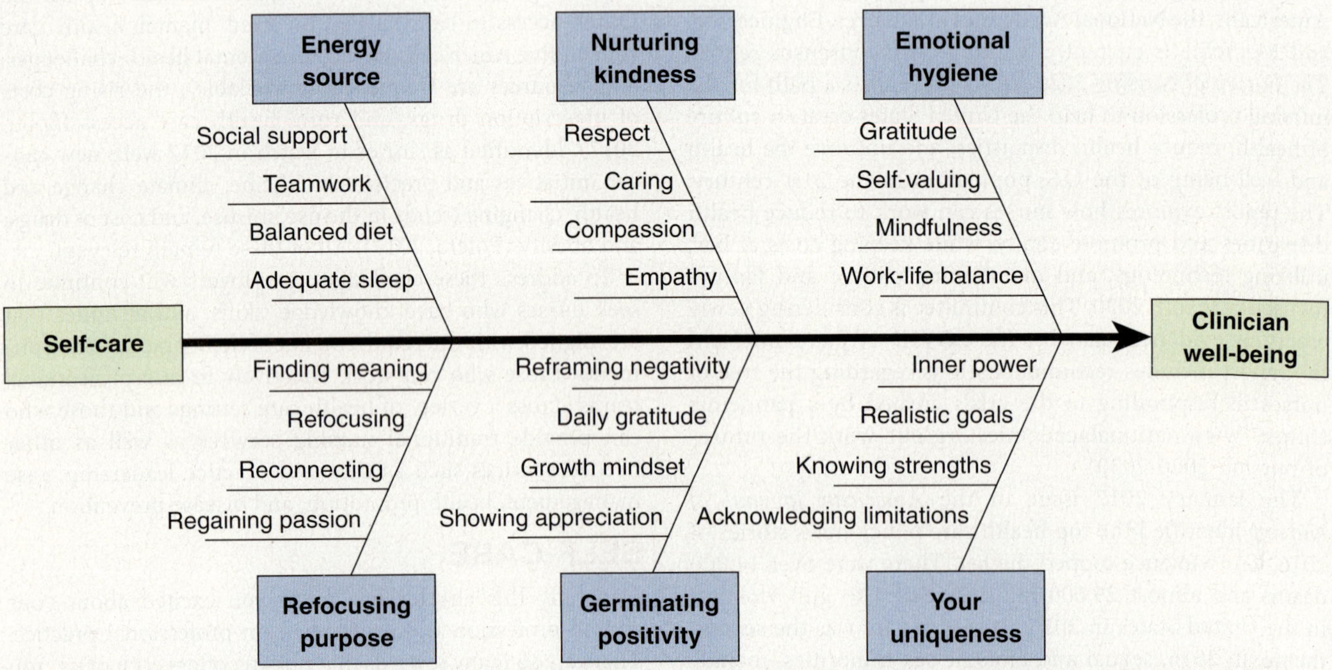

FIGURE 1-5. Use the ENERGY acronym for self-care: **E**nergy source, **N**urturing kindness, **E**motional hygiene, **R**efocusing purpose, **G**erminating positivity, and **Y**our uniqueness. (*Source:* Used with permission from Wei, H., & Wei, T. L. (2020). The power of self-care: An ENERGY model to combat clinician burnout. *American Nurse Journal*, *15*(10), 28–31. https://www.myamericannurse.com/wp-content/uploads/2020/09/an10-Energy-916.pdf)

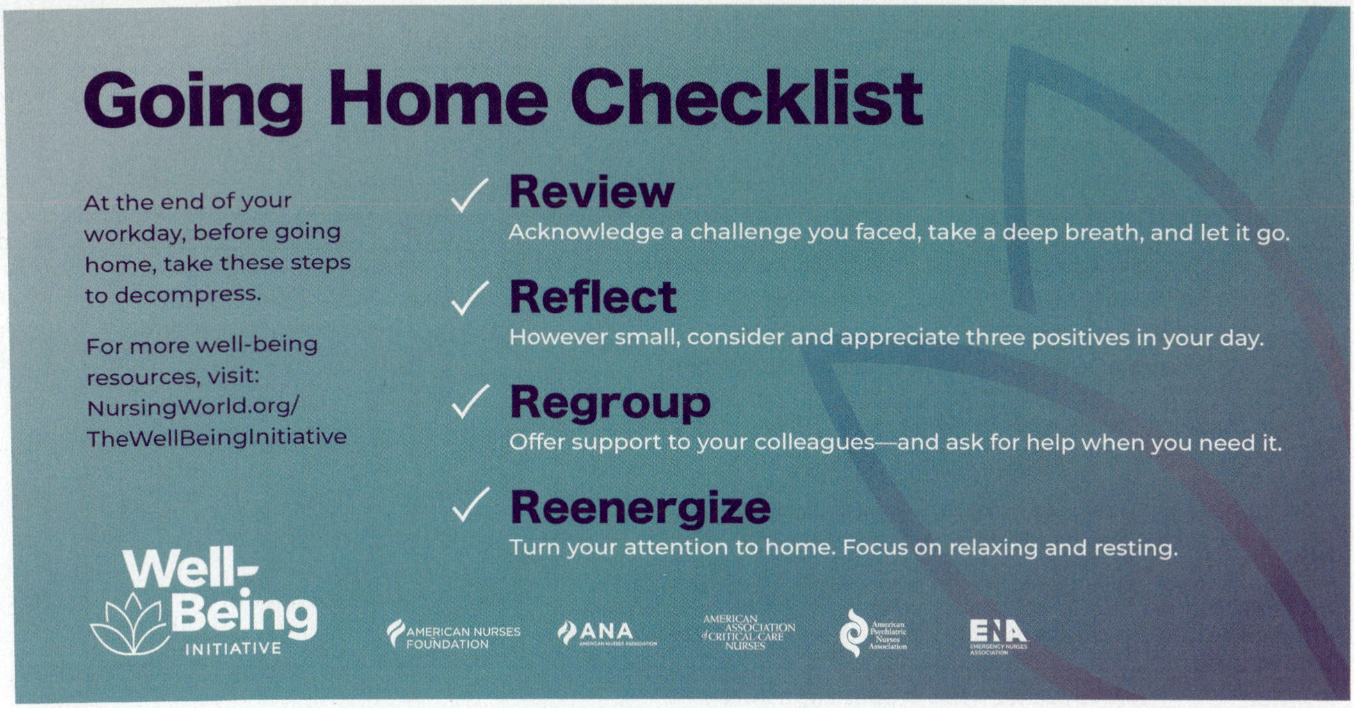

FIGURE 1-6. Going home checklist from the Well-Being Initiative. (*Source:* Used with permission from the American Nurses Foundation. https://www.nursingworld.org/_4a330c/globalassets/covid19/well-being-initiative-going-home-checklist-sharegraphic_06162020-final.png)

- **Burnout**: Cumulative state of frustration with the work environment that develops over a long time
- **Secondary traumatic stress**: A feeling of despair caused by the transfer of emotion distress from a victim to a caregiver, which often develops suddenly

Healthy self-care practices include stress reduction training, the use of relaxation techniques, time management, assertiveness training, work–life balance measures, and meditation or mindfulness-based practices. Many health care professionals are learning how to use mindfulness practices as daily elements of their self-care. Howland and Bauer-Wu (2015, p. 12) describe **mindfulness** as the "capacity to intentionally bring awareness to present-moment experience with an attitude of openness and curiosity." Mindfulness promotes healing as you pause, focus on the present, and listen. Stopping to focus on your breathing before walking into a patient encounter helps you to focus your mind and allows you to then be more centered and more fully present with the patient.

Nurse Self-Care Alert

Ponte and Koppel (2015) recommend using the STOP technique to reduce stress and be able to respond more skillfully during challenging times.

S—Stop and take a step back
T—Take a few breaths
O—Observe inside yourself
P—Proceed after you pause

Nurse Self-Care Alert

Nurse Sharon Tucker advocates a "Vital Signs Selfie Campaign" (Tucker, 2016). She urges nurses everywhere to take evidence-based action on an important set of vital signs for nurses using the BP–T–P–R technique:

- BP = Being Present (Have I cultivated the art of being truly present in each human encounter? Does my lifestyle support this?)
- T = Tracking (Am I tracking the numbers most important to my health: blood pressure, weight, blood sugar, lipid levels?)
- P = Practicing health and wellness behaviors (Am I a model of healthy behaviors?)
- R = Refueling (Do I get adequate sleep and find meaning, energy, and joy in many aspects of my life? When I am running on empty, how do I refuel?)

What do *your* vital signs say about *your* health and your ability to practice the art and science of thoughtful, person-centered care? And finally, check out the Professional Quality of Life Measure website (https://www.proqol.org) and keep its "Caring for Yourself in the Face of Difficult Work" pocket card handy (Fig. 1-7 on page 26). It just might turn out to be a life-saver as you start your clinical practice.

There is now a growing body of literature on **resilience**. Rajamohan et al. (2020) define resilience as an individual's aptitude for overcoming an adverse life circumstance with a hopeful attitude; utilizing healthy internal coping mechanisms; and utilizing external resources, such as supportive work

CARING FOR YOURSELF IN THE FACE OF DIFFICULT WORK

Our work can be overwhelming. Our challenge is to maintain our resilience so that we can keep doing the work with care, energy, and compassion.

10 things to do each day

1. Get enough sleep.
2. Get enough to eat.
3. Vary the work that you do.
4. Do some light exercise.
5. Do something pleasurable.
6. Focus on what you did well.
7. Learn from your mistakes.
8. Share a private joke.
9. Pray, meditate or relax.
10. Support a colleague.

For more information see your supervisor or visit www.istss.org, www.proqol.org and www.compassionfatigue.org

FOCUSING YOUR EMPATHY

Your empathy for others helps you do your job. It is important to take good care of your feelings and thoughts by monitoring how you use them. The most resilient workers are those that know how to turn their feelings to work mode when they go on duty, but off-work mode when they go off duty. This is not denial; it is a coping strategy. It is a way they get maximum protection while working (feelings switched to work model) and maximum support while resting (feelings switched off-work mode).

How to become better at switching between Work and Off-Work Modes

1. Make this a conscious process. Talk to yourself as you switch.
2. Use images that make you feel safe and protected (work-mode) or connected and cared for (non-work mode) to help you switch.
3. Develop rituals that help you switch as you start and stop work.
4. Breathe slowly and deeply to calm yourself when starting a tough job.

FIGURE 1-7. Caring for Yourself in the Face of Difficult Work" pocket card.

environments, mindfulness-based stress reduction training, and assertive communication skills training (p. 54). They devised the acronym REST to put these strategies into a practical format that you can use to categorize protective factors:

- **R**elationships with self and others
- **E**xercise (care of the mind, body, and spirit)
- **S**oul (compassionate emotional care)
- **T**ransformative thinking leading to thoughtful action

You will certainly experience stress as you struggle to meet your duties to self, to family, and to your patients and communities, as you meet all the demands of being a student. Be aware and reflective, pay attention to what your body is telling you, cultivate the type of supportive relationships that you can lean into for support, and learn about and utilize the resources you need. As you move through the chapters in this text, you will find appropriate self-care alerts and promoting health boxes. Remember, we cannot give what we don't have. If our own basic needs are not met, we will not be able to identify and meet the needs of the patients, families, and communities we serve.

DEVELOPING CLINICAL REASONING AND CLINICAL JUDGMENT

1. Consider the roles and functions of professional nursing (see Table 1-2). Interview several nurses in different settings to see how much value they attach to these roles and how much time they can devote to them. Two great questions to ask practicing nurses: What breaks your heart? What makes you come alive?
2. Describe how a nurse would meet the aims of nursing as described in this chapter—promoting health, preventing illness, restoring health, and facilitating coping with death or disability—when caring for the following patients:
   - A single mother who has just delivered her first child and is scheduled to be discharged 12 hours after delivery.
   - An 82-year-old woman who wants to begin an exercise program.
   - A 70-year-old woman newly diagnosed with atrial fibrillation who is admitted for a cardioversion and currently taking blood-thinning medication.
   - A fellow nursing student who is tired of COVID-19 restrictions who wants to "party" now that she is back in school, but your university is currently in a "hot spot" where COVID-19 numbers are rising.

   As you consider these situations, try to identify factors that either promote or inhibit the fulfilling of these aims.
3. How would you rate the adequacy of your self-care? On any given day would you describe yourself as "energized to heal" or "just about making it"? Ask nurses to talk about how they balance their duty to make patients their primary commitment with the duty to self-care.
4. Review Box 1-3, Tips for Thinking, Acting, and Feeling Like a Nurse. Talk with other students about how you

each would want to think, act, and feel in these situations:

- You realize when asked to discharge an 84-year-old male patient with chronic obstructive pulmonary disease (COPD) and other comorbidities that he lives alone and has no family or neighbor caregivers. His discharge orders include having to make follow-up appointments with other providers and to get new prescriptions filled. No one seems to have "caught" that his self-care activities are limited. You know the hospital is "full" and there is a crunch for beds.
- You are working labor and delivery and a woman, who speaks Spanish only, is frightened because the obstetrician just told her that she may need a cesarean delivery because her water broke hours ago and the baby doesn't seem to be in any hurry to come. You speak some Spanish, but not fluently, and no one yet has tried to secure translation services. You understand how frightened the mom must be and this obstetrician is not known for his bedside manner.
- You are a professional nurse working in a community nursing home. Among your other responsibilities are wound care. You always sign your new dressings and are dismayed when returning to work after a 3-day holiday to see that no one had changed what should be a daily dressing. When you report this, you are asked, "Why do you care so much? These residents don't know what is going on. They won't complain."

PRACTICING FOR NCLEX

1. A nurse is planning education for a patient who is scheduled for a diagnostic procedure to rule out a cerebral aneurysm. Which aspect of nursing does the nurse use as the basis for education?
   a. Art of nursing
   b. Science of nursing
   c. Caring aspect of nursing
   d. Holistic approach to nursing
2. A group of students in a community health course is discussing disaster management. Which nursing leader will the students identify as the founder of the Red Cross?
   a. Clara Barton
   b. Florence Nightingale
   c. Lillian Wald
   d. Lavinia Dock
3. A nurse is engaged in community health promotion activities. What activity best reflects this type of health promotion?
   a. Teaching about fall prevention and home safety at a senior center
   b. Holding a blood glucose screening for diabetes at a local church
   c. Educating hospice volunteers on therapeutic communication
   d. Providing education on crutch walking to a child with a fractured tibia
4. A nurse historian is researching changes in professional nursing and nursing education in the mid-20th century. What trend promoted advancement of the profession and of nursing education?
   a. Increased need for nurses and knowledge explosion led to emphasis on education.
   b. Focus on the war effort slowed development of knowledge in medicine and technology.
   c. Role of the nurse focused on acute technical skills used in hospital settings.
   d. Nursing care was dependent on the medical profession to define its priorities.
5. According to *Nursing: Scope and Standards of Practice* (ANA, 2021), "Nursing is the diagnosis and treatment of human response, and advocacy in the care of individuals, families, groups, communities, and populations in recognition of the connection of all humanity. Which actions are consistent with these nursing roles? Select all that apply.
   a. Offering emotional support to a patient overwhelmed by a new diagnosis of ovarian cancer
   b. Making a diagnosis of appendicitis when a patient reports right lower quadrant pain
   c. Providing classes on nutrition and physical activity at a senior center
   d. Administering an antibiotic to a patient with a documented infection
   e. Working with the health department to provide free influenza vaccinations to children
   f. Requesting the health care provider change prescription for the patient whose pain is still unrelieved
6. A nurse working in a rehabilitation facility focuses on the goal of restoring health for patients. Which nursing interventions could the nurse use to meet this goal? Select all that apply.
   a. Counseling adolescents in a drug rehabilitation program
   b. Performing range-of-motion exercises for a patient on bedrest
   c. Demonstrating insulin injection to a patient with diabetes
   d. Recommending a yoga class for a busy executive
   e. Providing hospice care for a patient with end-stage cancer
   f. Teaching a nutrition class at a local high school
7. Nursing students are learning about the criteria that establish nursing as a profession. Which statements by the students indicate they have correctly described characteristics of a profession? Select all that apply.
   a. Nursing is composed of a well-defined body of general knowledge.
   b. Nursing interventions are dependent upon medical practice.
   c. Nursing is a recognized authority by a professional group.
   d. Nursing practice is regulated by the medical profession.
   e. Nursing has a code of ethics.
   f. Nursing is influenced by ongoing research.

8. A nurse considers returning to school to obtain a master's degree in nursing. Which practice discipline requiring graduate level education could the nurse consider?
   a. Rehabilitation nurse
   b. Critical care nurse
   c. Oncology nurse
   d. Nurse practitioner
9. Nurses in the United States follow regulations outlined by each state's nurse practice act. A nurse moving to a different state anticipates finding which elements are common to all states' nurse practice acts?
   a. Definition of the legal scope of nursing practice for those registered
   b. Provision of continuing education programs to meet state requirements
   c. Determining the scope of content covered in the NCLEX examination
   d. Creating institutional policies for health care practices
10. Nurses of a statewide nursing organization come together to plan for the challenges to health care for the 21st century. What current trend in health care should be a focus of the plan?
   a. Decreasing numbers of hospitalized patients
   b. Increasing numbers of older and more acutely ill patients
   c. Decreasing health care costs owing to managed care
   d. Decreasing advances in medical knowledge and technology

ANSWERS WITH RATIONALES

1. **b.** The science of nursing is the knowledge base for care that is provided. In contrast, the skilled application of that knowledge is the art of nursing. Providing holistic care to patients based on the science of nursing is considered the art of nursing.
2. **a.** Clara Barton established the Red Cross in the United States in 1882. Florence Nightingale elevated the status of nursing to a respected occupation, improved the quality of nursing care, and founded modern nursing education. Lillian Wald was the founder of public health nursing. Lavinia Dock was a nursing leader and women's rights activist instrumental in establishing women's right to vote.
3. **a.** Nurses promote health and prevent illness primarily by teaching, through personal example and administering preventative vaccinations. Performing blood glucose screening for diabetes detects a disease after it has developed, rather than diabetes prevention. Therapeutic communication during hospice care and crutch walking are additional interventions used for diseases or health problems already present.
4. **a.** During World War II, large numbers of women worked outside the home. They became more independent and assertive, leading to an increased emphasis on education. The war itself created a need for more nurses and resulted in a knowledge explosion in medicine and technology.
5. **a, c, d, e, f.** Education, emotional support, nursing interventions such as administering medications, preventing influenza and infectious diseases, and advocating for improved pain management are roles of the nurse. Making a medical diagnosis is not within the scope of professional nursing practice.
6. **a, b, c.** Activities to restore health focus on the person with an illness and range from early detection of a disease to rehabilitation and teaching during recovery. These activities include drug counseling, teaching patients how to administer their medications, and performing range-of-motion exercises for bedridden patients. Recommending a yoga class for stress reduction helps prevent illness, and teaching a nutrition class helps promote health. A hospice nurse facilitates coping with disability and death.
7. **c, e, f.** Nursing is recognized increasingly as a profession based on the following defining criteria: well-defined body of specific and unique knowledge, strong service orientation, recognized authority by a professional group, code of ethics, professional organization that sets standards, ongoing research, and autonomy and self-regulation.
8. **d.** A master's degree (MSN) prepares advanced practice nurses, nurse practitioners (NPs), nurse midwives, clinical specialists, or clinical nurse leaders.
9. **a.** State nurse practice acts regulate practice by defining the legal scope of practice, creating a state board of nursing to make and enforce rules and regulations, define important terms and activities in nursing, and establish criteria for the education and licensure of nurses. The state's board of nursing has the legal authority define the education required to take NCLEX but does not provide that education or determine the content of the examination. The board has the legal authority to allow graduates of approved schools to take the licensing examination. Institutional policies are created by the institutions themselves.
10. **b.** The National Advisory Council on Nurse Education and Practice identifies the following critical challenges to nursing practice in the 21st century: A growing population of hospitalized patients who are older and more acutely ill, increasing health care costs, and the need to stay current with rapid advances in medical knowledge and technology.

Bibliography

American Association of Colleges of Nursing (AACN). (2008). *The essentials of baccalaureate education for professional nursing practice*. AACN.

American Association of Colleges of Nursing (AACN). (2012). *Clinical nurse leader: Frequently asked questions*. https://www.aacnnursing.org/CNL/About/FAQs

American Association of Colleges of Nursing (AACN). (2019a). *Nursing fact sheet*. https://www.aacnnursing.org/News-Information/Fact-Sheets/Nursing-Fact-Sheet

American Association of Colleges of Nursing (AACN). (2019b). *DNP fact sheet: The doctor of nursing practice (DNP)*. https://www.aacnnursing.org/News-Information/Fact-Sheets/DNP-Fact-Sheet

American Association of Colleges of Nursing. (2021). *The essentials: Core competencies for professional nursing education*. https://www.aacnnursing.org/Portals/42/AcademicNursing/pdf/Essentials-2021.pdf

American Nurses Association (ANA). (n.d.). *Healthy nurse, healthy nation*. http://www.nursingworld.org/MainMenuCategories/WorkplaceSafety/Healthy-Nurse

American Nurses Association (ANA). (2009). *What is nursing?* https://www.nursingworld.org/practice-policy/workforce/what-is-nursing/

American Nurses Association (ANA). (2010). *Nursing's social policy statement*. Author.

American Nurses Association (ANA). (2015a). *Code of ethics for nurses with interpretive statements*. http://www.nursingworld.org/MainMenuCategories/EthicsStandards/CodeofEthicsforNurses/Code-of-Ethics-For-Nurses.html

American Nurses Association (ANA). (2015b). *Four health care trends that will affect American nurses*. http://nursingworld.org/Content/Resources/4-Health-Care-Trends-That-Will-Affect-American-Nurses.html

American Nurses Association (ANA). (2015c). Nursing: Scope and standards of practice (3rd ed.). Author.

Association of American Medical Colleges (AAMC). (2008). *The medical home: AAMC position statement.* AAMC.

Benner, P., Sutphen, M., Leonard, V., & Day, L. (2010). *Educating nurses: A call for radical transformation.* Jossey-Bass.

Brown, S. R., Purviance, D., & Southard, E. P. (2020). Nurse fatigue: Short on sleep, short on safety. *American Nurse Journal, 15*(1), 24–26.

Buerhaus, P. (2007). Dealing with reality: Confronting the global nursing shortage. *Reflections on Nursing Leadership, 33*(4), 16.

Buerhaus, P., Staiger, D., & Auerbach, D. (2009). *The future of the nursing workforce in the United States: Data, trends and implications* (p. 210). Jones & Bartlett.

Campaign for Action. (n.d.). https://campaignforaction.org/about

Cochran, K. L., Moss, M., & Mealer, M. (2020). Prevalence of coping strategy training in nursing school curricula. *American Journal of Critical Care, 29*(2), 104–110.

D'Antonio, P. (2006). History for a practice profession. *Nursing Inquiry, 13*(4), 242–248.

Davidson, J. E., Accardi, R., Sanchez, C., &, Zisook, S. (2020). Nurse suicide: Prevention and grief management. *American Nurse Journal, 15*(1), 14–17.

Dolan, J. A., Fitzpatrick, M. L., & Herrmann, E. K. (1983). *Nursing in society: A historical perspective.* W. B. Saunders.

Ellis, J., & Hartley, C. (2019). *Nursing in today's world: Challenges, issues, trends* (11th ed.). Wolters Kluwer.

Fleming, K., Mazzatta, G. R., Matarese, K., & Eberle, J. (2020). Compassion fatigue and the ART model. *Nursing, 50*(3), 58–61.

Grabbe, L., Higgins, M. K., Baird, M., Craven, P. A., & San Fratello, S. (2020). The community resilience model to promote nurse well-being. *Nursing Outlook, 68*(3), 324–336.

Grant, R. (2016). The U.S. is running out of nurses. *The Atlantic.* https://www.theatlantic.com/health/archive/2016/02/nursing-shortage/459741.

Grant, E. J. (2020). Speaking out: A critical time for nurses and all vulnerable populations. *American Nurse Journal, 15*(6), 12.

Hammer, J. (2020, March 1). Thou shalt not underestimate Florence Nightingale. *Smithsonian*, 25–33, 78–79.

Healthy People 2030 Framework. https://health.gov/healthypeople

Heller, B. R., Oros, M. T., & Durney-Crowley, J. (2000). The future of nursing education: Ten trends to watch. *Nursing and Health Care Perspectives, 21*(1), 9–13.

Hill, K. (2010). Improving quality and patient safety by retaining nursing expertise. *OJIN: The Online Journal of Issues in Nursing, 15*(3). https://doi.org/10.3912/OJIN.Vol15No03PPT03

Hope, A. A., & Munro, C. L. (2020). Leading systems toward improving professional well-being. *American Journal of Critical Care, 29*(2), 84–86.

Howland, L. C., & Bauer-Wu, S. S. (2015). The mindful nurse. *American Nurse Today, 10*(9), 12–43.

Hundt, B. (2020). Reflections on Nightingale in the year of the nurse. *American Nurse Journal, 15*(5), 26–29.

Institute of Medicine of the National Academies. (2011). *The future of nursing: Leading change, advancing health.* The National Academies Press.

International Council of Nurses. (n.d.). *Definition of nursing.* https://www.icn.ch/nursing-policy/nursing-definitions

The Joint Commission. (2018). Sentinel Event Alert 59: Physical and Verbal Violence against health care workers.

Jordan, C. (2017). Recover energy, find balance, and reduce stress. *American Nurse Today, 12*(9), 41.

Kalisch, P. A., & Kalisch, B. J. (2004). *American nursing: A history.* Lippincott Williams & Wilkins.

Kelly, L. A., & Lefton, C. (2017). Effect of meaningful recognition on critical care nurses' compassion fatigue. *American Journal of Critical Care, 26*(6), 438–444.

Kennedy, M. S. (2018). To be a nurse. What does it really mean? *American Journal of Nursing, 118*(11), 7.

Lazenby, M. (2017). *Caring matters most.* Oxford University Press.

Lewenson, S. B., & Graham-Perel, A. (2020). "You don't have any business being this good": An oral history interview with Bernadine Lacey. *American Journal of Nursing, 120*(8), 40–47.

Mancuso, L., & Davidson, P. M. (2020). Thirty million strong. What our profession needs to look like in the upcoming decade. *American Journal of Nursing, 120*(5), 11.

Monroe, M., Morse, E., & Price, J.M. (2020). The relationship between critical care work environment and professional quality of life. *American Journal of Critical Care, 29*(2), 145–149.

Monumental Moments in Nursing. (2020, September 2). Star Nurses Publication. The Washington Post.

National Academy of Sciences, Engineering, and Medicine. (2019). *Taking action against clinician burnout: A systems approach to professional well-being.* The National Academies Press.

National Academies of Sciences, Engineering, and Medicine. (2021). *The future of nursing 2020–2030.* https://www.nationalacademies.org/our-work/the-future-of-nursing-2020-2030

National Advisory Council on Nurse Education and Practice (NACNEP). (2010). *Preparing nurses for new roles in population health management. Eighth Annual Report to the Secretary of the U.S.* Department of Health and Human Services and the U.S. Congress.

National Advisory Council on Nurse Education and Practice (NACNEP). (2016). *Addressing new challenges facing nursing education: Solutions for a transforming healthcare environment.* Health Resources and Services Administration (HRSA).

National Council of State Boards of Nursing. (n.d.). *Nurse practice act toolkit.* https://www.ncsbn.org/npa-toolkit.htm

National Council of State Boards of Nursing. (2017). *Enhanced Nurse Licensure Compact (eNLC) implementation.* https://www.ncsbn.org/enhanced-nlc-implementation.htm

Nightingale, F. (1992). *Notes on nursing: What it is and what it is not.* (Commemorative ed.). J. B. Lippincott.

Owens, I. T. (2020). Supporting nurses' mental health during the pandemic. *Nursing2020, 50*(10), 54.

Ponte, P. R., & Koppel, P. (2015). Cultivating mindfulness to enhance nursing practice. *American Journal of Nursing, 115*(6), 48–55.

Potera, C. (2017). Stories to watch in 2017. *American Journal of Nursing, 117*(1), 17.

Price-Spratlen, L., & Mahoney, M. (2006). February, black history month: A time to review nursing's past, present, and future. *Washington Nurse, 36*(1), 12–13.

ProQOL (Professional Quality of Life Measure). (2021). https://proqol.org/proqol-measure

Rajamohan, S., Davis, C. R., & Ader, M. (2020). REST: Breaking through to resilience. *Nursing, 50*(8), 53–56.

Reiser, V. L., & Gonzalez, J. F. Z. (2020). Confronting compassion fatigue in oncology nurses. *Nursing, 50*(5), 54–60.

Robert Wood Johnson Foundation. (2009). *The chronic care model.* http://www.improvingchroniccare.org/index.php?p=The_Chronic_Care_Model&s=2

Rosier, P. K., Dupont, M., & Crowell, J. (2019). Successful strategies for improving nurse certification rates. *American Nurse Today, 14*(7), 34–35.

Savel, R. H., & Munro, C. L. (2017). Quiet the mind: Mindfulness, meditation, and the search for inner peace. *American Journal of Critical Care, 26*(6), 433–435. https://doi.org/10.4037/ajcc2017914

Sheppard, K. (2016). Compassion fatigue: Are you at risk? *American Nurse Today, 11*(1), 53–55.

Sherwood, G., & Barnsteiner, J. (2012). *Quality and safety in nursing: A competency approach to improving outcomes.* Wiley-Blackwell.

Silverstein, W., & Kowalski, M. O. (2017). Adapting a professional practice model. *American Nurse Today, 12*(9), 78, 80–83.

Smith, T. (2009). A policy perspective on the entry into practice issue. *OJIN: The Online Journal of Issues in Nursing, 15*(1).

Sofer, D. (2017). The top health care policy news stories of 2016. *American Journal of Nursing, 117*(1), 14.

Thacker, K., Haas Stavarski, D., Brancato, V., Flay, C., & Greenawald, D. (2016). CE: Original Research: An investigation into the health-promoting lifestyle practices of RNs. *American Journal of Nursing, 116*(4), 24–31; quiz 31.

Trossman, S. (2019). Time to end nurse abuse. *American Nurse Today, 14*(10), 32–34. 1 in 4 nurses assaulted. #EndNurseAbuse

Tucker, S. J. (2016). The vital signs selfie campaign. *American Journal of Nursing, 116*(5), 11.

Turnock, B. J. (2016). *Public health: What it is and how it works* (6th ed.). Aspen Publishers.

University of Pennsylvania School of Nursing. (n.d.) *Penn nursing science: Nursing history and health care.* https://www.nursing.upenn.edu/nhhc

U.S. Department of Health and Human Services, Health Resources and Services Administration. (2010). *The registered nurse population: Findings from the 2008 National sample survey of registered nurses.* Author. https://bhw.hrsa.gov/sites/default/files/bhw/nchwa/rnsurveyfinal.pdf

U.S. Department of Health and Human Services Health, Resources and Services Administration, Bureau of Health Workforce. (2014). *The future of the nursing workforce: National- and State-level projections, 2012–2025.* Author. https://bhw.hrsa.gov/sites/default/files/bureau-health-workforce/data-research/nchwa-hrsa-nursing-report.pdf

U.S. Department of Health and Human Services, Office of Disease Prevention and Health Promotion. (n.d.) *Healthy People 2020.* https://www.healthypeople.gov

U.S. Department of Health and Human Services, Office of Disease Prevention and Health Promotion. (n.d.) *Healthy People 2030 Framework.* https://www.healthypeople.gov/2020/About-Healthy-People/Development-Healthy-People-2030/Framework

U.S. Bureau of Labor Statistics. (2020). *Occupational outlook handbook: Registered nurses.* https://www.bls.gov/ooh/healthcare/registered-nurses.htm#tab-1

Wall, B. M. (2008). Celebrating nursing history. *American Journal of Nursing, 108*(6), 26–29.

Wei, H., & Wei, T. L. (2020). The power of self-care: An ENERGY model to combat clinician burnout. *American Nurse Journal, 15*(10), 28–31.

Whitle, K. A., & Castaldi, C. L. (2017). Creating and developing a professional CV. *American Nurse Today, 12*(9), 58–60.

World Health Organization. (2020, April 6). *State of the World's Nursing Report—2020.* https://www.who.int/publications/i/item/9789240003279.

2 Theory, Research, and Evidence-Based Practice

Joe Wimmer

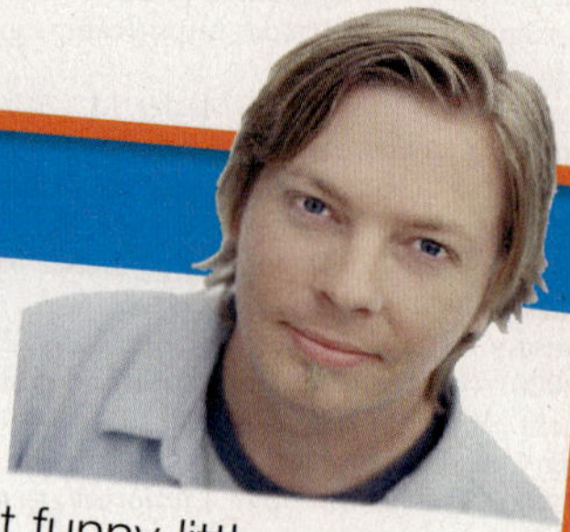

Joe, a first-time father of a healthy 8-lb baby girl delivered several hours ago, is visiting with his wife and new daughter. He asks, "Why is my daughter wearing that funny little cap on her head?"

Rachel Whang

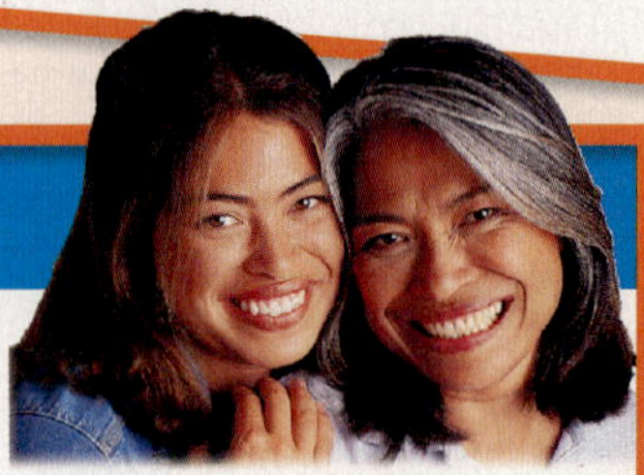

Rachel, the daughter of a 57-year-old patient being discharged with an order for intermittent nasogastric tube feedings, is being taught how to perform the procedure. During one of the teaching sessions, Rachel asks, "How will I know that the tube is in the right place?"

Maribella Santos

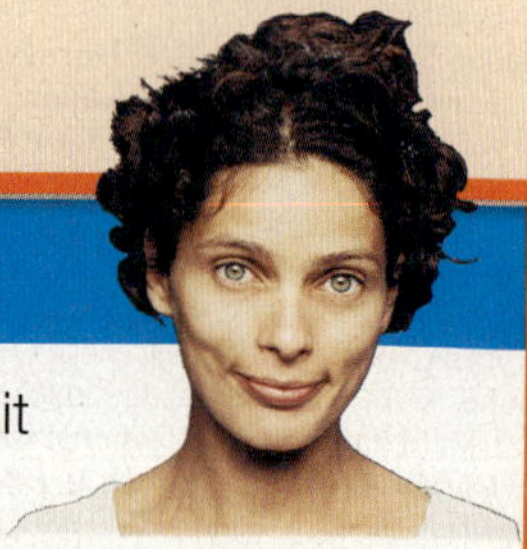

Maribella, who had just arrived back on the unit after undergoing abdominal surgery, is complaining of nausea. A while later she states, "My nausea is gone. The nurse did something with her hands and the feeling just went away."

Learning Outcomes

After completing the chapter, you will be able to accomplish the following:

1. Explain the sources of nursing knowledge and historical influences on nursing knowledge.
2. Compare and contrast systems theory, adaptation theory, and developmental theory.
3. Explain the significance of the four concepts common to all nursing theories.
4. Discuss the evolution of nursing research.
5. Compare and contrast quantitative and qualitative research methods.
6. Describe evidence-based practice in nursing, including the rationale for its use.
7. Outline the steps in implementing evidence-based practice.
8. Read and understand, on a beginning level, a published research article.
9. Use a framework to evaluate the salience of a research study.

Nursing Concepts

- Evidence-based practice
- Quality improvement

Nursing is a unique health care discipline in which nurses provide a service based on knowledge and skill. Nursing has two essential elements: a body of knowledge and the application of that knowledge in nursing care interventions. The body of knowledge provides the rationale for nursing interventions. There is a growing knowledge base developed specifically for nursing through theory development and research (see the accompanying Reflective Practice display for an example). Rationales for nursing interventions also come from many different disciplines, including anatomy, physiology, chemistry, nutrition, psychology, and sociology. This chapter discusses the concepts of nursing knowledge, nursing theory, nursing research, and evidence-based practice (EBP) as separate entities, but in fact, they are often intertwined in clinical practice.

NURSING KNOWLEDGE

Knowledge is an awareness of reality acquired through learning or investigation. Every person collects, organizes, and arranges facts to build a knowledge base relevant to one's personal reality. The knowledge base for professional nursing practice includes nursing science, philosophy, and ethics; biology and psychology; and the social, physical, economic, organizational, and technologic sciences. Nursing's Social Policy Statement (American Nurses Association [ANA], 2010, pp. 13–14; Fowler, 2015) lists the following as issues that nurses address in partnership with individuals, families, communities, and populations:

- Promotion of health and wellness
- Promotion of safety and quality of care
- Care, self-care processes, and care coordination
- Physical, emotional, and spiritual comfort, discomfort, and pain
- Adaptation to physiologic and pathophysiologic processes
- Emotions related to the experience of birth, growth and development, health, illness, disease, and death
- Meanings ascribed to health, illness, and other concepts
- Linguistic and cultural sensitivity
- Health literacy
- Decision making and the ability to make choices
- Relationships, role performance, and change processes within relationships
- Social policies and their effects on health
- Health care systems and their relationships to access, cost, and quality of health care
- The environment and the prevention of disease and injury

As you reflect on this list, you can see why your nursing education is so important and why professional nurses are lifelong learners.

Sources of Knowledge

Knowledge comes from a variety of sources and may be traditional, authoritative, or scientific.

Traditional Knowledge

Traditional knowledge is that part of nursing practice passed down from generation to generation. When questioned about the origin of such nursing practices, nurses might reply, "We've always done it this way." Changing bedclothes is an example of how traditional knowledge has affected nursing practice. It is customary in acute care settings to change a patient's bedclothes daily, whether soiled or not. There are no research data to support this, yet virtually millions of hospital beds are changed daily because this practice is accepted as a necessary component of quality patient care. Until this practice is challenged scientifically and its assumed value disproved, it will remain a traditional part of patient care. Table 2-1 (on page 33) illustrates practical examples of moving from traditions to EBP. Read Upvall, Bourgault, Pigon, and Swartzman (2019) to see exemplars illustrating de-implementation of tradition-based practices.

Authoritative Knowledge

Authoritative knowledge comes from an expert and is accepted as truth based on the person's perceived expertise—for example, when a senior staff nurse teaches a new graduate nurse a more efficient method of doing a technical procedure, such as inserting an intravenous catheter. The senior

QSEN Reflective Practice: Cultivating QSEN Competencies

CHALLENGE TO COGNITIVE SKILLS

One of the nurses, Danielle, on a surgical floor where I was assigned, took a course in therapeutic touch. When she returned to work, she was eager to use her new "intervention." My patient, Maribella Santos, had come back to the unit after undergoing abdominal surgery. Upon her return, she complained of nausea. Danielle used her "unruffling" technique to calm the patient, whose nausea then "disappeared." Excited, I reported this in postconference, only to learn from my instructor that therapeutic touch was "a lot of bunk" without scientific support.

Thinking Outside the Box: Possible Courses of Action

- Accept my instructor's dismissal of therapeutic touch.
- Learn more about therapeutic touch from my colleague Danielle and professional literature.
- Become an advocate for therapeutic touch if it *does* work!

Evaluating a Good Outcome: How Do I Define Success?

- Patient is not harmed by anyone using an unproven therapy.
- Patient benefits from my openness to new (potentially beneficial) therapies.
- I rely on research and EBP, not hearsay, as a basis for my clinical judgments and actions.

Personal Learning: Here's to the Future!

I was surprised to find the literature so inconclusive about the benefits of therapeutic touch. Obviously, its adherents claim that they can measure its efficacy. Others find these claims unsupported. Since this event happened at the beginning of my clinical rotation, I decided to observe Danielle throughout my rotation. What I saw made me a believer in this technique. Danielle was using therapeutic touch as an adjuvant to other therapies and it seemed to be working. I want to learn more about this technique. My goal is to attend a workshop on therapeutic touch to see if it is something I can incorporate into my practice.

Katherine Figliala, Georgetown University

QSEN SELF-REFLECTION ON QUALITY AND SAFETY COMPETENCIES DEVELOPING KNOWLEDGE, SKILLS, AND ATTITUDES FOR CONTINUOUS IMPROVEMENT

How do you think you would respond in a similar situation? Why? What does this tell you about yourself and about the adequacy of your competencies for professional practice? Can you think of other ways to respond? Do you agree with the criteria that the nursing student used to evaluate a successful outcome? Why or why not? What *knowledge, skills*, and *attitudes* do you need to develop to continuously improve the quality and safety of care?

Patient-Centered Care: What information should be communicated to Maribella Santos and other patients about the use of therapeutic touch to involve them as partners in the use of this technique?

Teamwork and Collaboration/Quality Improvement: Other members of the professional caregiving team can have positive and negative effects on us. In what ways do you practice so as to remain open to learning new interventions from colleagues and not allow negativity to inhibit your creativity?

Safety/Evidence-Based Practice: What sources of knowledge did the nursing student use? Did the nursing student use theory and research? If so, please explain how. Would you consider therapeutic touch to be EBP? Why or why not? How might the patient's personal values or beliefs have affected the response? Might patients be harmed through the use of a new intervention such as therapeutic touch? What safeguards exist in practice sites to prevent reckless experimentation on patients? When a review of the literature proves inconclusive, on what should we base our judgment about the efficacy of therapeutic touch or other interventions?

Informatics: What research strategy is likely to yield the best evidence about the efficacy of therapeutic touch? Can you identify the essential information that must be available in a patient's record about the use of therapeutic touch?

nurse has gained knowledge through experience, and the new graduate nurse accepts it as truth based on the perceived authority of the experienced nurse. Authoritative knowledge generally remains unchallenged as long as presumed authorities maintain their perceived expertise.

As you begin your clinical experience, you may observe experienced nurses doing procedures differently than you learned to do them in a fundamentals course or skills lab. You should always bring a questioning attitude to these discoveries. "I notice that your technique is different from what I learned. Can we talk about the differences and what informs your practice?" Your student status allows you to honestly question even the experts, and, in this way, we all learn to identify best practices. Today's safety emphasis on "see something, say something," mandates that we question differences in practice.

Table 2-1 Moving From Traditions to Evidence-Based Practice Interventions

CATEGORY	TRADITION	EVIDENCE-BASED INTERVENTION
Respiratory	Saline instillation for secretion removal	Normal saline should not be instilled as a routine step with endotracheal suctioning; instilling saline will not enhance removal of secretions.
	Excessive sedation; avoiding sedation and daily awakening practice	Interrupt sedation daily to assess patients' neurologic status and/or readiness for reduced ventilator support or extubation.
Psychosocial	Restricting intensive care unit visitation	Open visitation 24/7 enhances patient/family engagement and does not have adverse physiologic impact on patients' outcomes.
Hospital-acquired conditions	Early removal of urinary catheters to reduce catheter-associated urinary tract infections is not possible in the intensive care unit	Nurse-driven interventions to reduce catheter-associated infections focus on addressing the need for the catheter, sterile/aseptic catheter insertion, keeping drainage bag below the level of the bladder at all times, daily catheter care, and prompt removal of catheter.

Source: Select Examples used with permission of American Association of Critical Care Nurses, from Select examples from Makic, M. B. F., & Rauen, C. (2016). Maintaining your momentum: Moving evidence into practice. *Critical Care Nurse*, *36*(2), 13–18; permission conveyed through Copyright Clearance Center, Inc.

Scientific Knowledge

Scientific knowledge is knowledge obtained through the scientific method (implying thorough research). New ideas are tested and measured systematically using objective criteria.

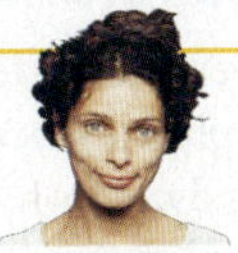

Think back to **Maribella Santos**, the woman complaining of nausea after undergoing abdominal surgery. The nurse would integrate scientific knowledge about the effects of surgery and anesthesia on the body and the side effects of pain medication to develop the postoperative care plan.

Significance of Knowledge Sources

All sources of knowledge are useful in the collective body of knowledge that constitutes the nursing profession. Although these three sources provide nursing with important contributions, each has inherent strengths and limitations. Both traditional and authoritative knowledge are practical to implement but are often based on subjective data, limiting their usefulness in a wide variety of practice settings. For this reason, nurses increasingly focus on scientific knowledge to provide care, commonly called EBP, a topic that will be thoroughly discussed later in this chapter. Table 2-1 illustrates the importance of scientific knowledge.

Historical Influences on Nursing Knowledge

The development of nursing knowledge has been influenced by the early work of Florence Nightingale, later nurse researchers and theorists, and societal changes.

Nightingale's Contributions

Nightingale influenced nursing knowledge and practice by demonstrating efficient and knowledgeable nursing care, defining nursing practice as separate and distinct from medical practice, and differentiating between health nursing and illness nursing (Hammer, 2020; Hundt, 2020). (See Chapter 1 for further information.)

The training of nurses was initially carried out under the direction and control of the medical profession. Because the conceptual and theoretical basis for nursing practice came from outside the profession, nursing struggled for years to establish its own identity and to receive recognition for its significant contributions to health care.

Societal Influences on Nursing Knowledge

Most early schools of nursing established in the United States were adapted from Nightingale's model. There was no planned educational curriculum; instead, knowledge was acquired from lectures by physicians and through practical experience by caring for sick people in hospitals. This service orientation for nursing education remained the strongest influence on nursing practice until the 1950s. Nursing care was carried out under the control and direction of the hospital administration and physicians practicing in that hospital. Nursing care was based on traditional ideas about following orders, as well as on common wisdom about caring for others based on either "common sense" or widely accepted scientific principles (Chinn & Kramer, 2019). As a result, nursing knowledge remained undeveloped and fragmented.

During the first half of the 20th century, a change in the structure of society resulted in changed roles for women and, in turn, for nursing. As a result of World Wars I and II, women increasingly entered the workforce, became more independent, and sought higher education. At the same time, nursing education began to focus more on education than hands-on training, and nursing research was conducted and published. As women became more independent and assertive, nursing's need for a clearly defined identity based on unique contributions to the health care system emerged. In the mid-20th century, the idea of nursing as a science became more generally accepted, and philosophic beliefs and a knowledge base for nursing practice began to evolve. Today the proliferation of graduate nursing programs, including the PhD in nursing, demonstrate society's acceptance of nursing science.

In the 21st century, the Institute of Medicine (IOM), now the National Academy of Sciences, Engineering, and Medicine (NASEM), issued its seminal report, *The Future of Nursing* (IOM, 2011), which identifies research priorities for transforming nursing practice, nursing education, and nursing leadership. "Taken together, the recommendations are meant to provide a strong foundation for the development of a nursing workforce whose members are well educated and well prepared to practice to the full extent of their education, to meet the current and future health needs of patients, and to act as full partners in leading change and advancing health" (IOM, 2011, p. 271). The IOM report and the 2015 update on progress are available at https://nam.edu. Recognizing the key role nurses play in the health of Americans, the NASEM is currently working on an updated consensus report, *The Future of Nursing 2020–2031*, that charts a path for the nursing profession to help the United States create a culture of health, reduce health disparities, and improve the health and well-being of the U.S. population in the 21st century.

NURSING THEORY

A **theory** is composed of a group of concepts that describe a pattern of reality. **Concepts**, such as ideas, are abstract impressions organized into symbols of reality. Concepts describe objects, properties, and events and relationships among them. A group of concepts that follow an understandable pattern makes up a **conceptual framework or model**. Concepts can be thought of as the individual bricks and boards used to build a house, with the conceptual framework being the blueprint that specifies where each brick and board should go. Theories can be tested, changed, or used to guide research or to provide a base for evaluation. They are derived through two principal methods: **deductive reasoning**, in which one examines a general idea and then considers specific actions or ideas, and **inductive reasoning**, in which the reverse process is used—one builds from specific ideas or actions to conclusions about general ideas.

Nursing theory is developed to describe nursing. Nursing theory differentiates nursing from other disciplines and activities in that it serves the purposes of describing, explaining, predicting, and controlling desired outcomes of nursing care practices. Thus, theories provide a means of testing knowledge through research and for expanding nursing's knowledge base to meet the health care needs of patients in an ever-changing society.

Interdisciplinary Base for Nursing Theories

Nursing theories are often based on, and influenced by, other broadly applicable processes and theories. The ideas and principles of the theories described briefly in the following sections are basic to many nursing concepts and are a part of the nursing literature. Nurses need to understand these theories and terminologies as they develop their own knowledge base in nursing.

Box 2-1 Key Points in General Systems Theory

- A system is a set of interacting elements, all contributing to the overall goal of the system. The whole system is always greater than the sum of its parts.
- Systems are hierarchical in nature and are composed of interrelated subsystems that work together in such a way that a change in one element could affect other subsystems, as well as the whole.
- Boundaries separate systems both from each other and from their environments.
- A system communicates with and reacts to its environment through factors that enter the system (input) or are transferred to the environment (output).
- An open system allows energy, matter, and information to move freely between systems and boundaries, whereas a closed system does not allow input from or output to the environment (no totally closed systems are known to exist in reality).
- To survive, open systems maintain balance through feedback.

General Systems Theory

General systems theory has been used in a wide range of disciplines since it emerged in the 1920s. Its primary theorist, Ludwig von Bertalanffy, developed the theory for universal application. This theory describes how to break whole things into parts and then to learn how the parts work together in "systems." It emphasizes relationships between the whole and the parts and describes how parts function and behave. These concepts may be applied to different kinds of systems, for example, molecules in chemistry, cultures in sociology, organs in anatomy, and health in nursing. The key points in general systems theory are outlined in Box 2-1.

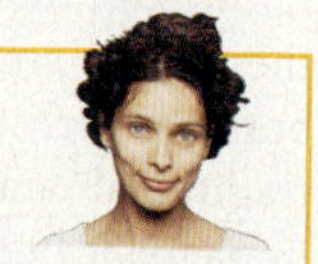

Recall ***Maribella Santos***, the woman described in the Reflective Practice box who received therapeutic touch? The nurse would need to integrate knowledge of systems theory, including system communication, open systems, and energy transfer to better understand the goal of this technique.

Adaptation Theory

Adaptation theory defines adaptation as the adjustment of living matter to other living things and to environmental conditions. Adaptation is a continuously occurring process that effects change and involves interaction and response. Human adaptation occurs on three levels: the internal (self), the social (others), and the physical (biochemical reactions). Chapter 43 describes adaptation in relation to stress.

Developmental Theory

Developmental theory outlines the process of growth and development of humans as orderly and predictable, beginning with conception and ending with death. Although the pattern has definite stages, the progress and behaviors of a person within each stage are unique. Heredity, temperament, emotional and physical environment, life experiences, and health status influence the growth and development of a person.

Several theorists have made important contributions to developmental theory, but only two are mentioned here because their work is often used to develop nursing theory and to organize nursing practice. Erik Erikson based his theory of psychosocial development on the process of socialization, emphasizing how people learn to interact with the world. Erikson recognized the role of social, biologic, and environmental factors in development, and defined specific tasks or conflicts that people accomplish or overcome during what he defined as the eight stages of life. Chapters 22 to 24 present more information on developmental theory.

Abraham Maslow developed his theory of human needs in terms of physical and psychosocial needs considered essential to human life, rather than by chronologic age as Erikson did. As described in Chapter 4, Maslow defined five levels of need in a hierarchy, with different needs existing simultaneously.

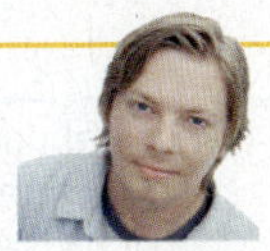

Think back to **Joe Wimmer**, the new father of a baby girl. When explaining about the use of the cap on the baby's head, the nurse would incorporate knowledge of Maslow's hierarchy of needs, specifically physiologic needs, and the need to minimize heat loss as a priority.

As you continue in your nursing education and practice, you will learn how systems, adaptation, and developmental theories are used in planning and giving holistic care to patients. The following sections on specific nursing theories will help you better understand the knowledge base used to develop the concepts unique to nursing.

Nursing Theories

Even though nurses have difficulty agreeing on precise definitions of nursing, theory-based nursing directs nurses toward a common goal, with the ultimate outcome being improved person-centered care. Nursing theory provides rational and knowledgeable reasons for nursing interventions, based on descriptions of what nursing is and what nurses do. In addition, nursing theory gives nurses the knowledge base necessary for acting and responding appropriately in nursing care situations, provides a base for discussion, and, ideally, helps resolve current nursing issues. Theory gives nurses who know and practice theory better problem-solving skills, so that nursing interventions are better organized, considered, and purposeful. Nursing theory also prepares nurses to question assumptions and values in nursing, thus further defining nursing and increasing the knowledge base.

Nursing theories identify and define interrelated concepts important in nursing and clearly state the relationships between and among these concepts. Nursing theories should be simple and general; simple terminology and broadly applicable concepts ensure their usefulness in a wide variety of nursing practice situations. Nursing theories should also increase the nursing profession's body of knowledge by generating research to guide and improve practice. Overall, nursing theory guides nursing practice by providing a knowledge base, organizing concepts, providing guidelines for practice, and identifying nursing care goals.

Nursing theories may be descriptive or prescriptive (Meleis, 2018). Descriptive theories describe a phenomenon, an event, a situation, or a relationship. They further identify the properties and components of each of these as well as the circumstances in which it occurs. Prescriptive theories address nursing interventions and the consequences of those interventions; they are designed to control, promote, and change clinical nursing practice.

The aims of nursing, described in Chapter 1, are the same for all nursing theorists, but the values, assumptions, and beliefs individualize each theory when it is applied to nursing care. Theoretical frameworks of nursing provide a focus for nursing care activities. The person receiving care is the central theme, but the way each theorist defines that person, the environment, health, and nursing gives a unique focus specific to a particular theory. The ultimate goal of each framework is holistic patient care, individualized to meet needs, promote health, and prevent or treat illness. Selected theories of nursing are outlined in Table 2-2 (on pages 36–37) and in an appendix in *Nursing: Scope and Standards of Practice*, 4th ed (ANA, 2021).

Common Concepts in Nursing Theories

Four concepts common in nursing theory that influence and determine nursing practice are (1) the person (patient), (2) the environment, (3) health, and (4) nursing. Each of these concepts is usually defined and described by a nursing theorist, and although these concepts are common to all nursing theories, both the definitions and the relations among them may differ from one theory to another. Of the four concepts, the most important is that of the person. The focus of nursing, regardless of definition or theory, is the person (Fig. 2-1).

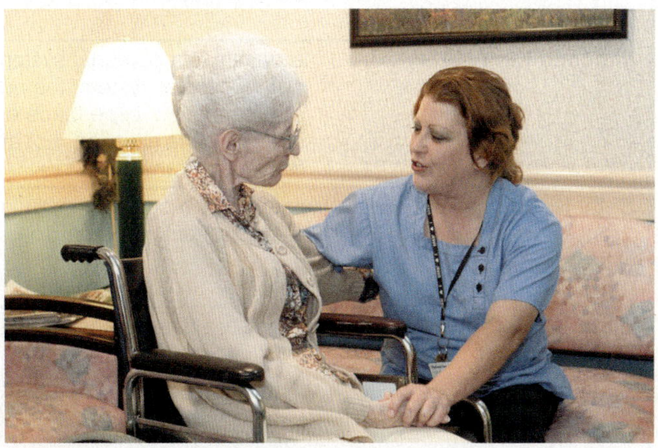

FIGURE 2-1. Four concepts common to all nursing theories are person, environment, health, and nursing. The most important concept, and the focus of nursing, is the person. (*Source:* From Eliopoulos, C. [2013]. *Gerontological nursing* [8th ed.]. Wolters Kluwer. *Photo by Rick Brady.*)

Table 2-2 Selected Theorists and Theories of Nursing

NURSING THEORIST AND DATE OF THEORY	CENTRAL THEME	APPLICATION TO CLINICAL PRACTICE
Florence Nightingale (1860)	Meeting the personal needs of the patient within the environment.	Concern for the environment of the patient, including cleanliness, ventilation, temperature, light, diet, and noise.
Hildegard Peplau (1952)	Nursing is a therapeutic, interpersonal, and goal-oriented process.	Nursing interventions are directed toward developing the patient's personality for productive personal and community living.
Virginia Henderson (1955)	The patient is a person who requires help to reach independence.	Nursing practice is independent; autonomous nursing functions are identified, and self-help concepts are described.
Faye Abdullah (1960)	Nursing is a problem-solving art and science used to identify the nursing problems of patients as they move toward health and cope with illness-related health needs.	The 21 nursing-care problems identified were based on research and can be used to determine patient needs and formulate nursing-focused care.
Ida Jean Orlando (1961)	The nurse reacts to the patient's verbal and nonverbal expression of needs both to understand the meaning of the distress and to know what is needed to alleviate it.	Uses the nursing process to provide solutions to problems as well as to prevent problems.
Ernestine Wiedenbach (1964)	Nursing as an art; nursing is providing nurturing care to patients.	Clinical nursing includes a philosophy, a purpose, the practice, and the art. Care is directed toward a specific purpose to meet the patient's perceived health care needs.
Lydia E. Hall (1966)	Focus is on rehabilitation, encompassing nursing's autonomy, the therapeutic use of self, treatment within the health care team (cure), and nurturing (care).	The major outcome of nursing care is rehabilitation and feelings of self-actualization by the patient.
Myra E. Levine (1967)	Emphasis is on the ill person in the health care setting; describes detailed nursing skills and actions.	The patient is the center of nursing activities, with nursing care provided based on four conservation principles to help patients adapt to their environment.
Martha Rogers (1970)	Emphasis is on the science and art of nursing, with the unitary human being central to the discipline of nursing.	Nursing interventions are directed toward repatterning human environment fields or assisting in mobilizing inner resources.
Dorothea Orem (1971)	Self-care is a human need; self-care deficits require nursing actions.	Nursing is a human service, and nurses design interventions to provide or to manage self-care actions for sustaining health or recovering from illness or injury.
Imogene King (1971)	The patient is a personal system within a social system; the nurse and the patient experience each other and the situation, act and react, and transact.	Nursing is a process of human interactions as nurses and patients communicate to mutually set goals, and explore and agree on the means to reach those goals.
Betty Newman (1972)	Humans are in constant relationship with stressors in the environment.	The major concern for nursing is keeping the patient's system stable through accurately assessing the effects of environmental stressors and assisting the patient with adjustments required for optimal wellness.
Sister Callista Roy (1974)	Humans are biopsychosocial beings existing within an environment. Needs are created within interrelated adaptive modes: physiologic self-concept, role function, and interdependence.	Nursing interventions are required when people demonstrate ineffective adaptive responses.
Madeleine Leininger (1978)	Caring is the central theme of nursing care, knowledge, and practice.	This provides the foundation of transcultural nursing care. Caring improves human conditions and life processes.

Table 2-2 Selected Theorists and Theories of Nursing *(continued)*

NURSING THEORIST AND DATE OF THEORY	CENTRAL THEME	APPLICATION TO CLINICAL PRACTICE
Jean Watson (1979)	Nursing is concerned with promoting and restoring health, preventing illness, and caring for the sick.	Clinical nursing care is holistic to promote humanism, health, and quality of living. Caring is universal and is practiced through interpersonal relationships.
Margaret A. Newman (1979)	Nursing interventions are purposeful, using a total-person approach to patient care to help people, families, and groups attain and maintain wellness.	Nursing care is directed toward reducing stress factors and adverse conditions that increase the risk for or actually affect optimal patient functions.
Dorothy E. Johnson (1980)	Nursing problems arise when there are disturbances in the system or subsystem, or the level of behavioral functioning is below an optimal level.	Nursing interventions are designed to support/maintain health, educate, counsel, and modify behavior.
Rosemarie Parse (1981)	The person continually interacts with the environment and participates in maintaining health.	Health is a continual, open process (rather than an absence of illness), with nursing care planned based on the patient's perspective of health and care.
Nola Pender (1982)	The goal of nursing is the optimal health of the person, with a focus on how people make health care decisions.	Factors significant to health-promoting behaviors include a person's beliefs about the importance of health and the perceived benefits of, and perceived barriers to, those behaviors. Participation in health-promoting behaviors is modified by one's demographic and biologic characteristics, interpersonal influences, and situational and behavioral factors.
Patricia Benner and Judith Wrubel (1989)	Nursing practice occurs within a context of caring and skill development. Caring is a common bond of people situated in a state of being that is essential to nursing.	They presented a systematic description of stages of nursing practice: novice, advanced beginner, competent, proficient, and expert.
Katherine Kolcaba (2003)	Patient comfort exists in three forms: relief, ease, and transcendence. If a patient is comfortable, they will feel emotionally and mentally better which will aid in recovery.	The role of the nurse is to assess a patient's comfort needs and create a nursing care plan to meet those needs.

Nursing Theory in Clinical Practice

As a discipline, nursing is increasingly defining its own independent functions and contributions to health care. The development and use of nursing theory provide autonomy (independence and self-governance) in the practice of nursing in many ways. Nursing theories are patterns that guide the thinking about, being, and doing of nursing (ANA, 2021). As nurses demonstrate that nursing care does indeed make a difference and that nursing services are valuable, the discipline becomes more independent. Having a body of knowledge specific to the discipline allows members to be viewed by others as experts; this, in turn, gives nurses authority to carry out actions. In addition, interventions carried out and based on sound rationales are trusted and respected.

Today, it has become even more necessary and important for nurses to demonstrate efficient, cost-effective, high-quality care within organized health care delivery systems. By practicing theory-based nursing combined with clinical reasoning and judgment skills, nurses are able not only to deliver care that meets those criteria but also to describe and document what it is they do. Professional nurses use theories from nursing and from the behavioral sciences to collect, organize, and classify patient data and to understand, analyze, and interpret patients' health situations. Theoretical concepts and theories guide all phases of the nursing process, including planning, implementing, and evaluating nursing care, while also describing and explaining desired responses to and outcomes of care.

The major concepts of a chosen model or theory guide each phase of the nursing process. The concepts serve as categories to guide the nurse in determining what information is relevant and should be collected to make assessments and to formulate nursing diagnoses. The concepts also suggest the appropriate types of nursing interventions and patient outcomes to be included in the care plan (refer back to Table 2-2 for the purpose and clinical application of selected nursing theories). It is important to realize that as the focus of nursing changes, so does the applicability of the concepts within a specific theory.

NURSING RESEARCH

Research most simply defined means to examine carefully or to search again. Research as scientific inquiry is a process that uses observable and verifiable information (**data**), collected in a systematic manner, to describe, explain, or predict events. Research is conducted to validate and refine current knowledge or to develop new knowledge. The goals of research are to develop explanations (in theories) and to find solutions to problems.

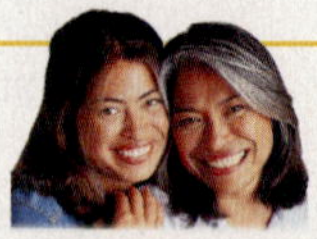

Consider ***Rachel Whang***, the daughter who is being taught how to give tube feedings and is asking about ensuring proper tube placement. The nurse would recommend the best method to use based on scientific evidence from research.

Nursing research, broadly defined, encompasses research to improve the care of people in the clinical setting as well as the broader study of people and the nursing profession, including studies of education, policy development, ethics, and nursing history. Research is included as an essential component of nursing by the ANA (2021), by the International Council of Nurses, and by nursing specialty organizations. Be sure to check ANA's *Nursing: Scope and Standards of Practice*, 4th ed (ANA, 2021) to become familiar with the expected competencies for scholarly inquiry.

> Research-focused nurses engage in the science of nursing and spirit of inquiry by designing, implementing, and evaluating research studies directed to the generation of new knowledge to improve and reform nursing practice and the systems in which nursing practice occurs. They conduct research directed to specific and salient nursing practice phenomena and serve as a leader in integrating research findings into the practice of nursing (ANA, 2021, p. 31).

The ANA Code of Ethics for Nurses (2015) counsels that all nurses must participate in the advancement of the profession through knowledge development, evaluation, dissemination, and application to practice. Nurses engage in **scholarly inquiry** in order to expand the body of knowledge that forms and advances the theory and practice of the discipline in all its spheres. One of the many ways to promote nursing's development of greater autonomy and strength is nursing research. Nurses, depending on their level of education, conduct or participate in research to improve their efforts to deliver high-quality, cost-efficient care. Nurses also increasingly use the findings of research to provide evidence-based nursing practice (discussed in the next section).

Nursing research is fundamental to the recognition of nursing as a profession. As an occupation, nursing has existed since the beginning of human history. One of the essential elements that differentiate a profession from an occupation is the existence of a unique and distinct knowledge base. The ultimate goal of expanding nursing's body of knowledge is to learn improved ways to promote and maintain health. As health care and illness patterns change, nursing interventions must change. Ongoing practice-based research reflects the nursing profession's commitment to meet the ever-changing demands of health care consumers.

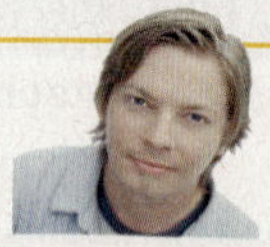

Remember ***Joe Wimmer***, the new father described at the beginning of the chapter. Before responding to Mr. Wimmer, the nurse would need knowledge of newborn heat loss and methods to minimize it. A review of the literature would provide theoretical information necessary to explain the scientific rationale for using caps on the heads of newborns to reduce heat loss.

Evolution of Nursing Research

While caring for victims of the Crimean War, Florence Nightingale kept careful and objective records. These records provided baseline data that she later used to determine which nursing interventions were most effective in treating her patients.

Although nurses have always provided care through nursing interventions and have evaluated the response of the patient, for a long time those interventions were primarily based on a philosophy of "It's always been done that way." As advances were made in technology and medical research during the 20th century, nursing leaders realized that research about the practice of nursing was necessary to meet the health needs of modern society. Increasing numbers of nurses began to conduct research and publish articles telling other nurses how to conduct nursing research.

During the 1950s and 1960s, nursing research was increasingly recognized as important. The first issue of *Nursing Research* was published in 1952. Early studies provided the basis for the development of nursing practice standards and the most effective educational preparation for registered nurses. The ANA sponsored a series of nursing research conferences. A focus on clinical studies to examine quality of care and the development of outcomes of care grew out of the newly developed intensive care units (ICUs).

The 1970s and 1980s focused on clinical research, with published studies of clinical interventions, such as vital signs and treatment procedures. Primary patient care was a popular method of nursing care, with research investigating outcomes and quality of care. The nursing process also was studied, with research into assessment and effective nursing diagnosis of patient responses to the effects of illness. Studies of nursing education were concerned with student learning experiences and clinical evaluation methods, as well as differentiation of practice by educational preparation. In addition, models, conceptual frameworks, and theories were developed to guide nursing practice. More nurses were prepared at the master's and doctoral levels, and federal funding for nursing research increased. Journals specific to nursing research (both generally and in specialty areas) were published.

Of major importance was the ANA's 1985 creation of the National Center for Nursing Research, which was subsequently

Box 2-2 National Institute of Nursing Research (NINR): Featured Research Highlights

Program That Can Provide Long-Term Physical and Mental Health Improvement Among Adolescents

- Being overweight or obese or having depressive symptoms can interfere with health and academic performance among young people, yet the number of overweight and obese young people has increased in recent years.
- To help find the best way to address weight and depression among teens, scientists tested the long-term effectiveness of the COPE (Creating Opportunities for Personal Empowerment) Healthy Lifestyles TEEN (Thinking, Emotions, Exercise, Nutrition) program.
- The COPE Healthy Lifestyles TEEN program, which involves teacher-led physical activity and positive behavioral skills training, was compared with an attention control program, Healthy Teens. The interventions were presented as part of required health classes in 11 high schools. In all, 779 students aged 14 to 16 participated in the study.

Researchers measured the two programs' effects on overweight and obesity, as well as depressive symptoms, at 12 months following the interventions. After these 12 months, students participating in the COPE Healthy Lifestyles TEEN program had lower body mass index than those participating in the Healthy Teens program. None of those in the COPE Healthy Lifestyles TEEN intervention became obese, and only about 5% moved from a healthy weight to overweight, whereas 10% of those in the Healthy Teens control group moved into overweight or obesity. Among the subgroup of participants with severely elevated depressive symptoms, participants in the COPE Healthy Lifestyles TEEN group improved after 12 months, while depressive symptoms in the Healthy Teens group remained elevated. The researchers concluded that the COPE Healthy Lifestyles TEEN program may help at-risk youth improve their physical and mental health. They also note that the program was delivered by teachers as part of their curriculum, making it easily available to students who may need it the most.

Citation

Melnyk, B. M., Jacobson, D., Kelly, S. A., Belyea, M. J., Shaibi, G. Q., Small, L., O'Haver, J. A., & Marsiglia, F. F. (2015). Twelve-month effects of the COPE Healthy Lifestyles TEEN Program on overweight and depressive symptoms in high school adolescents. *Journal of School Health, 85*(12), 861–870.

Source: From National Institute of Nursing Research. https://www.ninr.nih.gov/researchandfunding/researchhighlights#cope-teen. Used with permission.

promoted to the National Institute of Nursing Research (NINR) in 1993, thereby gaining equal status with the other 27 National Institutes of Health. The NINR website funds research that establishes the scientific basis for quality patient care. According to the NINR, the goals of nursing research are to:

- Build the scientific foundation for clinical practice
- Prevent disease and disability
- Manage and eliminate symptoms caused by illness
- Enhance end-of-life and palliative care

In September 2016, NINR released its new Strategic Plan: Advancing science, improving lives: A vision for nursing science. The new Strategic Plan describes four areas of scientific focus:

1. Symptom science: promoting personalized health strategies
2. Wellness: promoting health and preventing illness
3. Self-management: improving quality of life for people with chronic conditions
4. End-of-life and palliative care: the science of compassion

An additional two areas were deemed of high priority across all of NINR's scientific programs: (1) Promoting innovation: technology to improve health and (2) 21st-century nurse scientists: innovative strategies for research careers (Grady, 2017).

The NINR website offers a series of Featured Research Highlights, which summarize the recent work of NINR-supported researchers across the country. Box 2-2 provides an example of one of these Research Highlights. Be sure to visit the NINR website to explore featured resources: Palliative Care: Conversations Matter, NINR Director's Lecture Series, Stories of Discovery, Grant Programs Supported by NINR, NINR Strategic Plan and Research Highlights.

Methods of Conducting Nursing Research

Nursing research is conducted by quantitative and qualitative methodology. Each method is summarized here to help you understand published research so that findings may be used in your clinical practice.

Quantitative Research Methods

Quantitative research involves the concepts of basic and applied research. Box 2-3 provides definitions of important terms for quantitative research. **Basic research**, sometimes

Box 2-3 Important Terms in Quantitative Research

- **Variable:** Something that varies and has different values that can be measured
- **Dependent variable:** The variable being studied, determined as a result of a study
- **Independent variable:** Causes or conditions that are manipulated or identified to determine the effects on the dependent variable
- **Hypothesis:** Statement of relationships between the independent and dependent variables that the researcher expects to find
- **Data:** Information the researcher collects from subjects in the study (expressed in numbers)
- **Instruments:** Devices used to collect and record the data, such as rating scales, pencil-and-paper tests, and biologic measurements. Instruments should be both reliable (produce the same results [data] on repeated use) and valid (test what they are supposed to test)

Table 2-3 Types of Quantitative Research

TYPE	PURPOSE
Descriptive Research	To explore and describe events in real-life situations, describing concepts and identifying relationships between and among events; often used to generate new knowledge about topics with little or no prior research
Correlational Research	To examine the type and degree of relationships between two or more variables; the strength of the relationship varies from a −1 (perfect negative correlation, in which one increases as the other decreases) to a +1 (perfect positive correlation, with both variables increasing or decreasing together)
Quasi-experimental Research	To examine cause-and-effect relationships between selected variables; often conducted in clinical settings to examine the effects of nursing interventions on patient outcomes
Experimental Research	To examine cause-and-effect relationships between variables under highly controlled conditions; often conducted in a laboratory setting

called pure or laboratory research, is designed to generate and refine theory, and the findings are often not directly useful in practice. **Applied research**, also called practical research, is designed to directly influence or improve clinical practice.

The types of quantitative research depend on the level of current knowledge about a research problem (Table 2-3). The steps of quantitative research are followed carefully, although they may be designed in different ways. Table 2-4 presents an overview of the basic steps of the quantitative research process. If you are already familiar with the steps in the nursing process you should be able to recognize the similarities.

Qualitative Research Methods

Qualitative research is a method of research conducted to gain insight by discovering meanings. At its core is the idea that reality is based on perceptions, which differ for each person and change over time. The research design follows many of the same steps as quantitative research but differs in that the researcher primarily analyzes words or narratives rather than numbers. Table 2-5 outlines and briefly describes the methods of qualitative research. Chicca (2020) offers a helpful introduction to qualitative nursing research.

Protection of the Rights of Human Subjects

Many nurses work in health care institutions in which patients are invited to participate in clinical research. With their focus on the overall well-being of the patient, nurses play an important role in ensuring that patient interests are not sacrificed to research interests. Nursing priorities include determining that

Table 2-4 Steps of the Quantitative Research Process

STEP	DESCRIPTION
1. State the research problem	This is often stated as a question, which should be focused narrowly on the problem being studied. For example: "What is the optimal time for taking a rectal temperature with a digital thermometer?"
2. Define the purpose of the study	The purpose explains "why" the problem is important and what use the findings will be.
3. Review-related literature	The literature review provides information about what is already known, as well as providing information about concepts and how the concepts have been measured. It also identifies gaps in knowledge that will be studied.
4. Formulate hypotheses and variables	Hypotheses are statements about two or more variables. Scientific hypotheses must be testable using variables that can be measured, manipulated, or controlled in a study.
5. Select the research design	The design is a carefully determined, systematic, and controlled plan for finding answers to the question of the study. This provides a "road map" for all aspects of the study, including how to collect and analyze the data.
6. Select the population and sample	The population is the group to be studied. The sample refers to specific people or events in the population from which data will be collected.
7. Collect the data	Sources of data may include people, literature, documents, and findings (e.g., from sources such as laboratory data or measurements of vital signs). Data may be collected from interviews, questionnaires, direct measurement, or examinations (such as physical or psychological tests).
8. Analyze the data	Statistical procedures are used to analyze the data and provide answers to the research question.
9. Communicate findings and conclusions	Through publications and presentations, the researcher explains the results of the study and links them to the existing body of knowledge in the literature. The researcher also describes the implications of the study and suggests directions for further research.

Table 2-5 Qualitative Research Methods

METHOD	DESCRIPTION
Phenomenology	The purpose of phenomenology (both a philosophy and a research method) is to describe experiences as they are lived by the subjects being studied. Analysis of data provides information about the meaning of the experience within each person's own reality (e.g., the experience of health or of having a heart attack).
Grounded Theory	The basis of grounded theory methodology is the discovery of how people describe their own reality and how their beliefs are related to their actions in a social scene. The findings are grounded in the data from subjects and are used to formulate concepts and to generate a theory of the experience, supported by examples from the data (e.g., coping with a seriously ill child).
Ethnography	Developed by the discipline of anthropology, ethnographic research is used to examine issues of a culture that are of interest to nursing.
Historical	Historical research examines events of the past to increase understanding of the nursing profession today. Many historical studies focus on nursing leaders, but there is increasing interest in the historical patterns of nursing practice.

the studies have met appropriate scientific and ethical criteria before their implementation and protecting patient rights. Specific patient rights include **informed consent**, the patient's right to consent knowledgeably to participate in a study without coercion (knowing that this consent may be withdrawn at any time) or to refuse to participate without jeopardizing the care that they will receive, the right to confidentiality, and the right to be protected from harm. Nurse ethicist Christine Grady and her colleagues propose seven requirements that provide a coherent framework for evaluating the ethics of clinical research with human subjects (Emmanuel et al., 2000):

- Value: Enhancements of health or knowledge must be derived from the research.
- Scientific validity: The research must be methodologically rigorous.
- Fair subject selection: Scientific objectives, not vulnerability or privilege, and the potential for and distribution of risks and benefits, should determine communities selected as study sites and the inclusion criteria for individual subjects.
- Favorable risk–benefit ratio: Within the context of standard clinical practice and the research protocol, risks must be minimized and potential benefits enhanced, and the potential benefits to people and knowledge gained for society must outweigh the risks.
- Independent review: Unaffiliated people must review the research and approve, amend, or terminate it.
- Informed consent: People should be informed about the research and provide their voluntary consent.
- Respect for enrolled subjects: Subjects should have their privacy protected, the opportunity to withdraw, and their well-being monitored.

Federal regulations require that institutions receiving federal funding or conducting studies of drugs or medical devices regulated by the Food and Drug Administration establish institutional review boards (IRBs). The IRBs review all studies conducted in the institution to determine the risk status of all studies and to ensure that ethical principles are followed (Marzinsky & Smith-Miller, 2019). See Chapter 6 for a full discussion of values and ethics in nursing.

The National Cancer Institute (NCI) offers an online training tutorial (with a certificate) titled, "Protecting Human Research Participants." You can access the tutorial on NCI's website, https://phrp.nihtraining.com/users/login.php. You will also find helpful resources on the Office for Human Research Protections (OHRP) website, http://www.hhs.gov/ohrp.

Application of Research to Practice

Younas (2020) defines **research utilization (RU)** as a process of transforming research knowledge into practice, with knowledge referring to both conducting and analyzing research. It enables nurses to improve patient care by informing practice on interventions that may no longer be useful. Despite the clinical and practical importance of research, studies have indicated that nurses seldom use it to guide practice. Instead, they rely on personal experience, peer support, and trial and error (p. 63). The most common impediments to nursing research include restricted access to resources, limited time to participate in research-related activities, and lack of educational preparation needed by nurses for research. Research about nursing education, administration, and practice all affect patient care directly or indirectly. Too often, practicing nurses mistakenly think research is far removed from caring for patients at the bedside. This false impression has slowed the progress of practice-based nursing research. Yet much of what bedside nurses routinely do constitutes research. The nursing process (i.e., assessing, diagnosing/problem identification, planning, implementing, and evaluating) represents the basic framework of the research process.

Summarizing research about why the adoption of EBP in nursing has been sluggish, Ost et al. (2020) identify the most frequent barriers in EBP implementation as inadequate knowledge and skills, a lack of experienced mentors to facilitate the process, and the perception that implementing EBP is too time-consuming. "Overcoming these barriers is essential because the provision of support and resources to implement EBP has been reported to result in improved quality of care, lower costs, and better patient outcomes," (p. 59)—things we all value!

QSEN EVIDENCE-BASED PRACTICE (EBP)

Nurses who value the concept of EBP as integral to determining best clinical practice regularly read relevant professional journals to keep their practice up to date. They similarly value the need for continuous improvement in clinical practice based on new knowledge.

Unless the research findings of nurse researchers are used by practicing nurses to improve the quality of patient care, clinical nursing research is useless. Nursing students developing clinical skills must understand the scientific rationale that makes one course of action preferable to another. Throughout this text, Research in Nursing boxes highlight current studies that have the potential to make a positive difference in nursing practice and patient outcomes.

EVIDENCE-BASED PRACTICE

Nurses make decisions about many different aspects of patient care each day. For example, questions for consideration range from, "What site should I use to take an infant's temperature?" to "How can I move my patient in bed to decrease complications and promote safety?" Patient safety and health may be adversely affected unless the most current best evidence is used to answer questions and make clinical decisions. When frontline caregivers began to see critically ill patients with COVID-19 in their emergency rooms and critical care units, what initially complicated their treatment and care was the lack of knowledge about how to effectively treat these patients, their disease, and their symptoms. Patient outcomes improved as professionals quickly shared what they were learning, but everyone was eager for the research to support best practice.

Evidence-based practice (EBP) in nursing is a problem-solving approach to making clinical decisions, using the best evidence available (considered "best" because it is collected from sources such as published research, national standards and guidelines, and reviews of targeted literature). See Figure 2-2 for a hierarchy of evidence.

Makic and Rauen (2016) identify essential elements of EBP as (1) the integration of best research and other forms of evidence to guide practice; (2) viewing clinical expertise as a component in care effectiveness; and (3) considering patients' preferences, values, and engagement in care decisions as essential to providing optimal evidence-based care to patient and their families (Fig. 2-3).

The information that is collected is analyzed and used to answer questions (the science of nursing), taking into consideration patient preferences and values, as well as the clinical experiences of the nurse (the art of nursing). EBP may consist of specific nursing interventions or may use guidelines established for the care of patients with certain illnesses, treatments, or surgical procedures.

Implementing EBP in clinical practice can present multiple challenges. Resistance to using EBP may arise in the current health care setting as a result of the nursing shortage, the acuity level of patients, nurses' skill in reading and evaluating published research, and an organizational culture that does not support change. Other factors include insufficient time to implement new ideas; insufficient time to read research; lack of authority to change patient care procedures; lack of support from physicians, managers, and other staff members; and inadequate infrastructure support, such as libraries and ethics committees (Yoder et al., 2014). However, to achieve desired outcomes for quality patient care and to demonstrate clinical nursing effectiveness, it is critical that nurses gain the necessary knowledge and skills to provide the best possible nursing care. The practice settings in which nurses work must support changes made

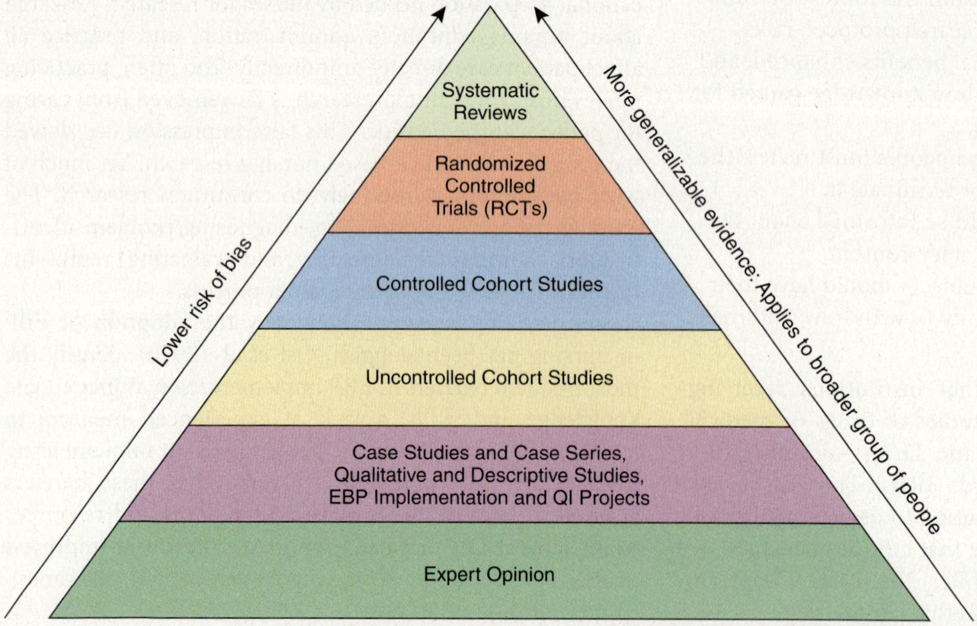

FIGURE 2-2. Hierarchy of evidence for intervention questions. (*Source:* Adapted from Melnyk, B. M., & Fineout-Overholt, E. [2015]. *Evidence-based practice in nursing: A guide to best practice* [3rd ed., p. 92]. Wolters Kluwer Health. Used with permission.)

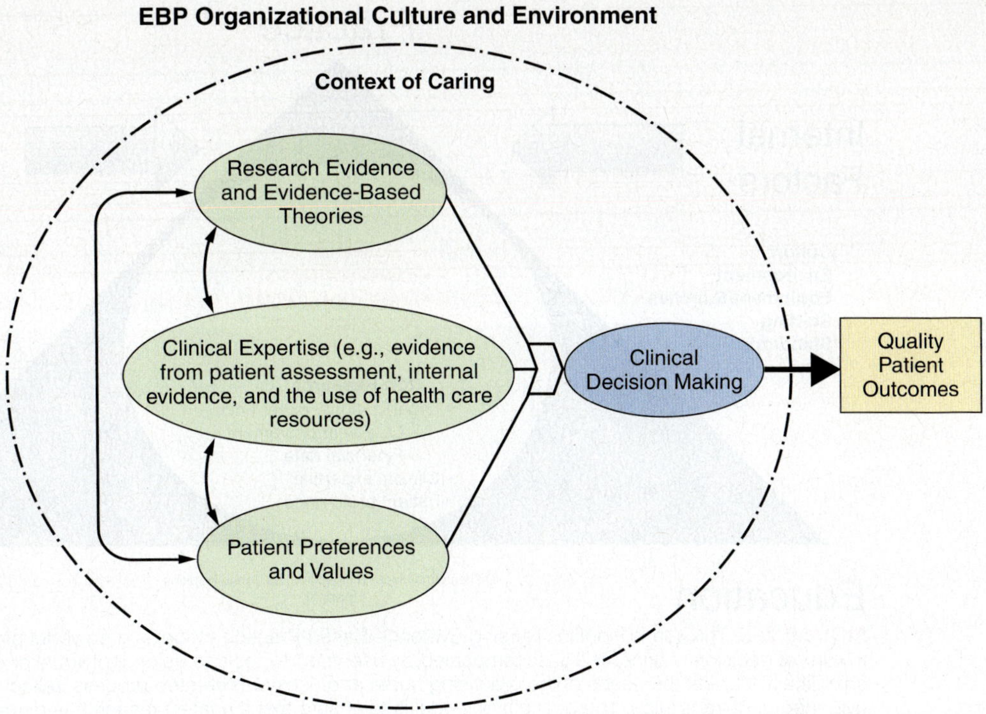

FIGURE 2-3. The merging of science and art: Evidence-based practice (EBP) within a context of caring and an EBP culture and environment results in the highest quality of health care and patient outcomes. (*Source:* From Melnyk, B. M., & Fineout-Overholt, E. [2015]. *Evidence-based practice in nursing: A guide to best practice* [3rd ed., p. 5]. Wolters Kluwer Health. Used with permission.)

based on EBP. The changes may be implemented by an individual nurse, by groups of nurses working together, or by interdisciplinary teams of health care providers.

Unfolding Patient Stories: Sara Lin • Part 1

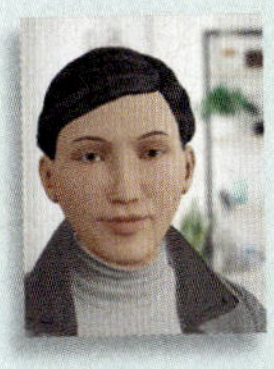

Sara Lin, an 18-year-old female, returned from the recovery room to the medical-surgical unit following an appendectomy. An intravenous (IV) line and indwelling urinary catheter were placed in the operating room. Sara is awake and can begin oral fluids and advance activity, as tolerated. The nurse reviews the provider's orders and confirms the continuation of the IV for fluids and antibiotics. How does evidence-based practice support the nurse's clinical decision to contact the provider for an order to discontinue the urinary catheter? (Sara Lin's story continues in Chapter 19.)

Care for Sara and other patients in a realistic virtual environment: ***vSim** for Nursing*. (thepoint.lww.com/vSimFunds). Practice documenting these patients' care in DocuCare (thepoint.lww.com/DocuCareEHR).

Johns Hopkins Nursing Evidence-Based Practice Model

The Johns Hopkins Nursing Evidence-Based Practice (JHNEBP) model is a powerful problem-solving approach to clinical decision making and is accompanied by user-friendly tools to guide individual or group use. It is designed specifically to meet the needs of the practicing nurse and uses a three-step process called PET: practice question, evidence, and translation (Fig. 2-4 on page 44). The goal of the model is to ensure that the latest research findings and best practices are quickly and appropriately incorporated into patient care. Check the Johns Hopkins Medicine website for helpful tools: http://www.hopkinsmedicine.org/evidence-based-practice/jhn_ebp.html.

Rationale for Using Evidence-Based Practice

The impetus for EBP is based on the IOM report (2001) *Crossing the Quality Chasm: A New Health System for the 21st Century*, which challenged health care professionals to provide care based on scientific evidence. In addition, those interested in quality and cost control want evidence that the services and interventions being funded or reimbursed are effective in securing valued goals.

Until the mid-1990s, many large hospitals had research utilization departments directed by doctoral-prepared nurse scientists. These departments conducted research within the hospital to answer clinical practice questions and used the research findings to dictate practice changes. Today, few hospitals use findings from their own research to direct clinical nursing practice. As a result of recent advances in information technology, findings from published literature can be found, analyzed, and applied to answer clinically relevant questions. Key databases and search engines may be easily accessed on most work computer stations as well as home computer systems. Many research articles in journals and guidelines developed by expert panels can be downloaded, read, evaluated, and shared with colleagues.

Therefore, the use of EBP mandates the analysis and systematic review of research findings. The first step for you as a student is to be able to read and understand a research article. To help you, the typical format of a research journal article

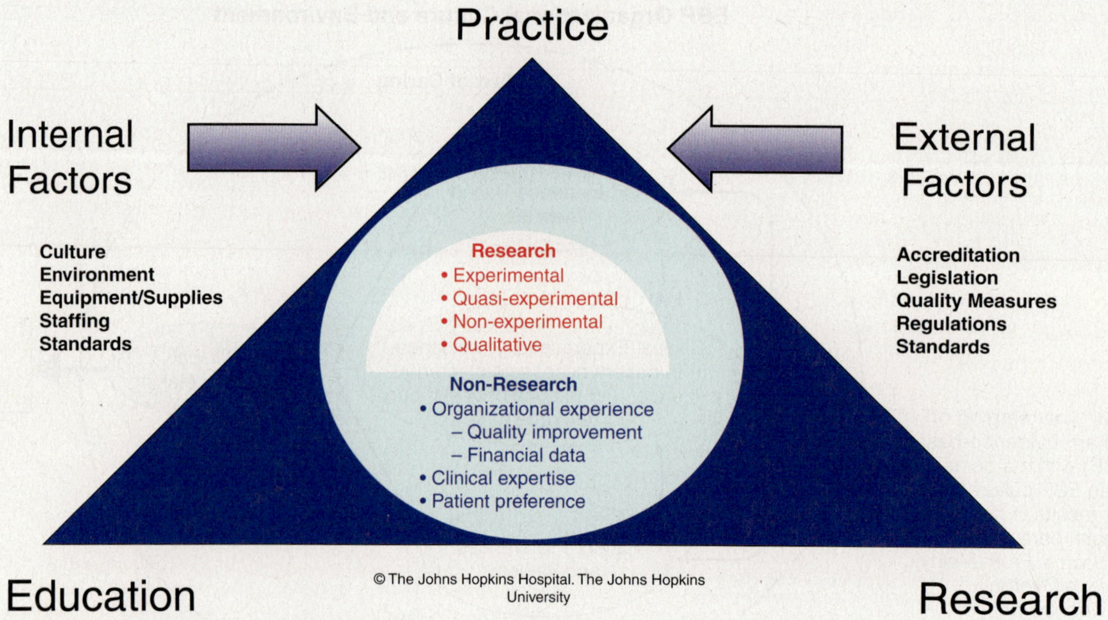

FIGURE 2-4. The Johns Hopkins Nursing Evidence-Based Practice model is a powerful problem-solving approach to clinical decision making and is accompanied by user-friendly tools to guide individual or group use. It is designed specifically to meet the needs of the practicing nurse and uses a three-step process called PET: practice question, evidence, and translation. The goal of the model is to ensure that the latest research findings and best practices are quickly and appropriately incorporated into patient care. (*Source:* From John Hopkins Medicine Center for Evidence-Based Practice. Used with permission. © The Johns Hopkins Hospital/The Johns Hopkins University.)

with a description of each part is outlined in Table 2-6. See also Box 2-4 for a helpful checklist to use when reading and critiquing a research article.

Steps of the Evidence-Based Practice Process

To practice EBP, nurses carry out the following six steps (Melnyk & Fineout-Overholt, 2019).

Step 1: Formulate the burning clinical question. There are several different methods that can be used to ask clinical questions. The most common method is the PICOT format, described in Table 2-7. See the accompanying PICOT in Practice, for a sample of the development of a clinical question using PICOT and the EBP decision-making process; additional samples are found in selected chapters of this book.

Table 2-6 Parts of a Research Journal Article

SECTIONS (IN USUAL ORDER)	DESCRIPTION
Abstract	The abstract is at the beginning of the article. It summarizes the entire article and usually provides the purpose of the study; a description of the subjects, data collection, and data analysis; and a summary of important findings.
Introduction • Review of the literature • Statement of the purpose	The literature review discusses relevant studies that have been conducted in the area of this study. A statement of the specific goals or purpose of the study often follows the review.
Method • Subjects • Design • Data collection • Data analysis	The methods section describes in detail how the study was conducted, including the type and number of subjects, the research design used, what data were collected and how, and the types of analysis done. There should be enough information so that the study could be replicated (repeated).
Results	The results (findings) are often presented both in words and in charts, tables, or graphs. It is important to understand what the results were and whether they are meaningful.
Discussion (Conclusions)	The discussion section reports what the results mean in regard to the purpose of the study and the literature review. It may also include suggestions for further research and application to nursing education or practice, as appropriate.
References	The references are at the end of the article and include a list of articles and books used by the researcher.

Box 2-4 Checklist for Reading and Critiquing a Research Article

1. Review the elements of the article.
   - Title describes the article.
   - Abstract summarizes the article.
   - Introduction makes the purpose clear.
   - Problem is properly introduced.
   - Purpose of the study is explained.
   - Research question(s) are clearly presented.
   - Theoretical framework informs the research.
   - Literature review is relevant and comprehensive and includes recent research.
   - Methods section details how the research questions were addressed or hypotheses were tested.
   - Analysis is consistent with the study questions and research design.
   - Results are clearly presented and statistics clearly explained.
   - Discussion explains the results in relation to the theoretical framework, research questions, and significance to nursing.
   - Limitations are presented and their implications discussed.
   - Conclusion includes recommendations for nursing practice, future research, and policymakers.
2. Determine the level and quality of the evidence using a scale (several can be found in ANA's Research Toolkit http://www.nursingworld.org/Research-Toolkit/Appraising-the-Evidence).
3. Decide if the study is applicable to your practice.

Source: From Kaplan, L. (2012). Reading and critiquing a research article. *American Nurse Today, 7*(10). Used with permission. *American Nurse Today*, October 2012.

Table 2-7 Asking Clinical Questions in PICOT Format

COMPONENTS	CONSIDERATIONS
P = Patient, population, or problem of interest	Need for explicit description; may include setting, limiting to subgroups (such as by age)
I = Intervention of interest	The more defined, the more focused the search of the literature will be; may include exposure, treatment, patient perception, diagnostic test, or predicting factor
C = Comparison of interest	Usually a comparison to another treatment or the usual standard of care
O = Outcome of interest	Specifically identifying the outcome to enable a literature search to find evidence that examined the same outcome, perhaps in different ways
T = Time	The time when the comparison of interest is completed and the outcome can be evaluated

Step 2: Search for the best evidence. It is important to collect information that is regarded as the strongest level of evidence. The level for strength of evidence is numerical, with level 1 being the strongest and level 7 the lowest. The strongest ("best") evidence is provided by findings from systematic reviews, EBP guidelines,

PICOT in Practice

ASKING CLINICAL QUESTIONS: PRESSURE INJURY

Scenario: You are a staff nurse in a specialty long-term care facility for adult patients with spinal cord injuries. Patients admitted to your unit usually are young and have had injuries that resulted in tetraplegia. The patients are at risk for pressure injuries.

In a monthly staff meeting, you report that the incidence of pressure injuries on the unit in each of the most recent quarters was higher than it had been for any of the previous 12 quarters. The nurse manager notes that monies have been allocated in the current budget for purchase of new equipment as needs are identified. The nurse manager gives the staff information on a new type of low air loss alternating pressure mattress that is reported to be "more effective in preventing pressure injuries than the alternating pressure mattress overlays now being used." The nurse manager requests that the staff make a recommendation about purchase of the new pressure injury prevention mattress.

- **Problem:** Adults at risk for pressure injuries
- **Intervention:** Low air loss alternating pressure mattress
- **Comparison:** Alternating pressure mattress overlays
- **Outcome:** Incidence of pressure injuries
- **Time:** During admission to a long-term care facility

PICOT Question: Is the use of a low air loss alternating pressure mattress more effective than an alternating pressure mattress overlay in preventing pressure injuries among a population of patients with tetraplegia during admission to a long-term care facility?

Findings

1. European Pressure Ulcer Advisory Panel, National Pressure Injury Advisory Panel and Pan Pacific Pressure Injury Alliance (2019). Prevention and Treatment of Pressure Ulcers/Injuries: Quick Reference Guide. http://www.internationalguideline.com/guideline

2. Nixon, J., Smith, I. L., Brown, S., McGinnis, E., Vargas-Palacios, A., Nelson, E. A., Coleman, S., Collier, H., Fernandez, C., Gilberts, R., Henderson, V., Muir, D., Stubbs, N., Walker, K., Wilson, L., & Hulme, C. (2019). Pressure Relieving Support Surfaces for Pressure Ulcer Prevention (PRESSURE 2): Clinical and Health Economic Results of a Randomized Controlled Trial. *EClinicalMedicine, 14*, 42–52.

(continued)

PICOT in Practice (*continued*)

ASKING CLINICAL QUESTIONS: PRESSURE INJURY

Results of four high-quality systematic reviews reveal insignificant evidence to conclude superiority of one type of support surface over another. Guidelines across multiple organizations support that the use of support surfaces is not a stand-alone intervention for the prevention of pressure injuries. A pressure injury prevention program should include a routine assessment of skin, risk for pressure injuries, weight and mobility of patient, nutritional status, skin moisture, pressure redistribution when in bed and chair, repositioning, and patient and caregiver education.

Level of Evidence C: A body of evidence with inconsistencies that cannot be explained, reflecting genuine uncertainty surrounding the topic.

Strength of Recommendation: Weak positive recommendation: Probably do it.

Recommendations: Based on the staff's review of the literature, a recommendation NOT to buy the new pressure prevention mattress was made to the nurse manager.

In addition, the staff recommend that the current nursing protocol for prevention of pressure injuries be reviewed to assure that current evidence-based recommendations for assessment risk and non-support surface interventions were included. The decision about which support surface intervention to use should be evidence based and individualized to meet the needs for pressure redistribution for the right patient at the right time. The staff made the following recommendation based on the *Prevention and Treatment of Pressure Ulcers/Injuries Guide:*

1. Use a high specification reactive single-layer foam mattress or overlay in preference to a foam mattress without high specification qualities for individuals at risk of developing pressure injuries.
2. Assess the relative benefits of using a medical grade sheepskin for individuals at risk of developing pressure injuries.
3. For individuals with obesity, select a support surface with enhanced pressure redistribution, shear reduction and microclimate features.

Box 2-5 American Association of Critical Care Nurses' Resources for Online Searches

Systematic Reviews

A systematic review is a review of available research studies focusing on a single question. The systematic review summarizes, appraises, and synthesizes large bodies of evidence relevant to a focused research question.

- Cochrane Collaboration: www.cochrane.org
- Database of Abstracts of Reviews of Effectiveness (DARE): www.brad.ac.uk/library/elecinfo/dare.php
- Clinical Evidence: www.clinicalevidence.bmj.com
- The Joanna Briggs Institute (Library of Systematic Reviews): https://jbi.global/
- PubMed: www.ncbi.nlm.nih.gov/entrez/query/static/clinical.shtml#reviews
- National Health Service (NHS) Evidence Health Information Resources—Specialist Collections: https://library.hud.ac.uk/freeresources/helpsheets/NLHsummary.pdf

Guideline Database

Guideline databases are searchable databases of evidence-based clinical practice guidelines.

- U.S. National Guideline Clearinghouse: www.guideline.gov
- U.S. Agency for Healthcare Research and Quality: www.ahrq.gov
- New Zealand Guidelines Group: www.nzgg.org.nz
- Trip Database: www.tripdatabase.com
- National Institute for Health Care Excellence (NICE): https://www.evidence.nhs.uk
- Institute for Healthcare Improvement: www.ihi.org/IHI/topics
- Centers for Disease Control: www.cdc.gov/hai
- Australian National Health and Medical Research Council: https://www.nhmrc.gov.au/guidelines
- Michigan Quality Improvement Consortium Guidelines: www.mqic.org/guidelines.htm

Professional Organizations

Professional organizations often offer position statements, guidelines, protocols, and other documents to promote evidence-based practice.

- American Association of Critical Care Nurses: www.aacn.org
- Society of Critical Care Medicine: www.learnicu.org/Pages/Guidelines.aspx
- American College of Chest Physicians: https://www.chestnet.org/topic-collections/critical-care

Online Clinical Databases

These databases allow literature searches for primary sources of evidence and research.

- The Cumulative Index of Nursing and Allied Health Literature (CINAHL) is a comprehensive resource for nursing and allied health literature; https://www.ebsco.com/products/research-databases/cinahl-database or access through www.aacn.org
- MEDLINE is the U.S. National Library of Medicine's (NLM) database that references journal articles focused on biomedicine. It can be searched for free through PubMed: www.ncbi.nlm.nih.gov/pubmed

Journals

Professional journals may contain abstracts with expert commentaries. Here are some suggestions; others exist beyond this listing.

- *Evidence-Based Nursing*: www.ebn.bmj.com
- *Evidence-Based Medicine*: www.ebm.bmj.com
- *British Medical Journal's Clinical Evidence*: www.clinicalevidence.com
- *American Journal of Critical Care,* Clinical Pearls Section: http://ajcc.aacnjournals.org
- *American College of Physicians Journal Club*: From AACN Searching for Evidence Toolkit. Resources for Online Search.

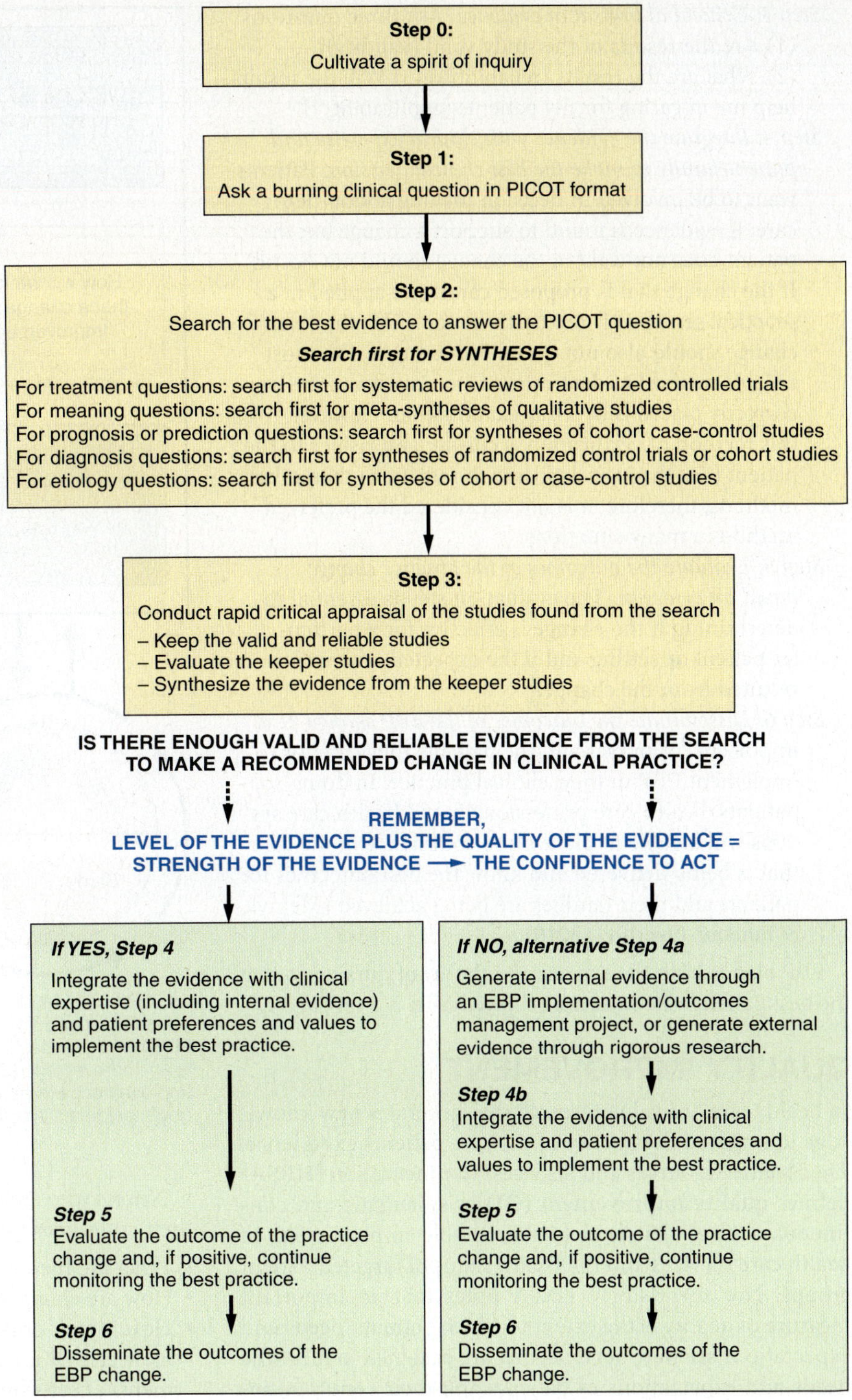

FIGURE 2-5. Steps of the evidence-based practice process leading to high-quality health care and best patient outcomes. (*Source:* From Melnyk, B. M., & Fineout-Overholt, E. [2015]. *Evidence-based practice in nursing: A guide to best practice* [3rd ed., p. 15]. Wolters Kluwer Health. Used with permission.)

and meta-analyses. **Systematic reviews** summarize findings from multiple studies of a specific clinical practice question or topic and recommend practice changes and future directions for research. **Evidence-based practice guidelines** synthesize information from multiple studies and recommend best practices to treat patients with a disease (e.g., hypertension), a symptom (e.g., chronic pain), or a disability (e.g., cognitive impairment). These guidelines are typically written by a panel of experts. A *meta-analysis* uses statistical analysis of the effect of a specific intervention across multiple studies, providing stronger evidence than results from a single study. If systematic reviews, EBP guidelines, and meta-analyses are not available, collect reviews of descriptive or qualitative studies or articles of original quantitative studies listed in databases such as MEDLINE and CINAHL (Cumulative Index to Nursing and Allied Health Literature). Box 2-5 provides a suggested list of resources for collecting evidence.

Step 3: Critical appraisal of evidence. Ask three questions: (1) Are the results of the study valid (validity)? (2) What are the results (reliability)? (3) Will the results help me in caring for my patients (applicability)?

Step 4: Integrate the evidence with clinical expertise and patient/family to make the best clinical decision. Patients want to be involved in decision making about their care; if evidence is found to support a change but the patient does not want it, the change should not occur. If the change that is proposed cannot be applied in a practical sense, or is too costly or too risky, then the change should also not occur. For example, the most reliable method to determine if a nasogastric tube is correctly placed is by x-ray examination. However, this method of verification is costlier and riskier to the patient (i.e., through exposure to radiation) than other methods; therefore, it is not considered the preferred method in many situations.

Step 5: Evaluate the outcomes of the practice change based on evidence. The evaluation step is essential to determining if the change is effective for a particular patient or setting and if the expected outcomes resulted from the change.

Step 6: Disseminate the outcomes of the EBP change. It is important for nurses and the patients they care for to implement EBP in their clinical practice. In doing so, patients, health care professionals, and health care systems will be able to place more confidence in the care that is being delivered and know the best outcomes for patients and their families are being achieved (Melnyk & Fineout-Overholt, 2019).

EBP blends both the science and the art of nursing so that the best patient outcomes are achieved (Fig. 2-5 on page 47).

QUALITY IMPROVEMENT

In health care, we value research that generates new knowledge to improve the quality of the care patients experience. The Health Resources and Services Administration (HRSA) defines **quality improvement (QI)** as systematic and continuous actions that lead to measurable improvement in health care services and the health status of targeted patient groups. Not surprisingly HRSA notes that an important measure of quality is the extent to which patients' needs and expectations are met. Services that are designed to meet the needs and expectations of patients and their communities include:

- Systems that affect patient access
- Care provision that is evidence based
- Patient safety
- Support for patient engagement
- Coordination of care with other parts of the larger health care system
- Cultural competence, including assessing health literacy of patients, patient-centered communication, and linguistically appropriate care

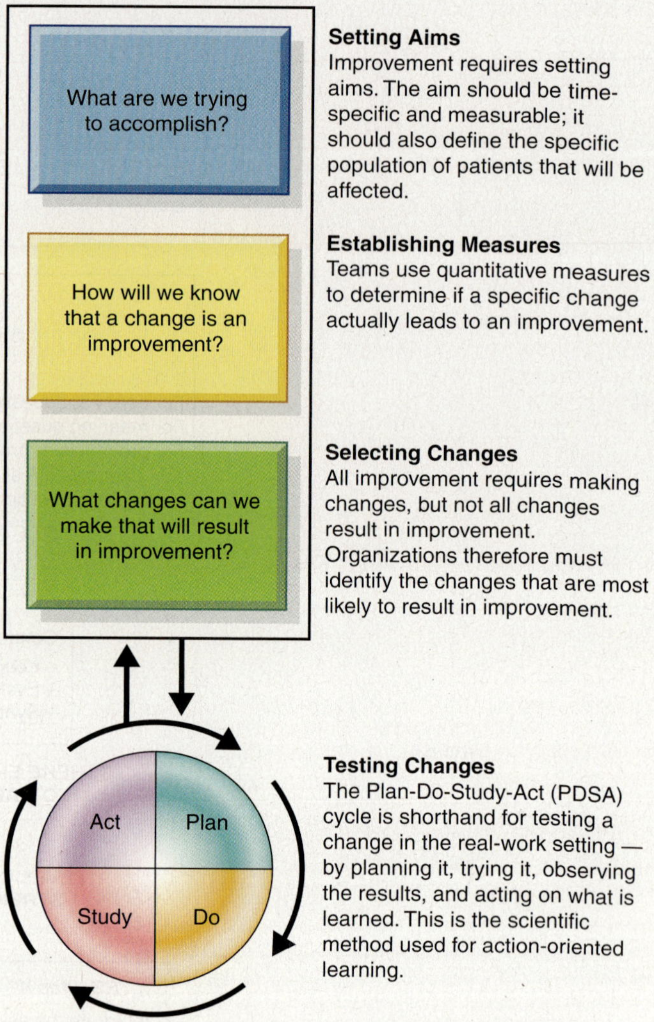

FIGURE 2-6. Model for improvement. Plan-Do-Study-Act (PDSA) cycle to test and implement changes in real-work settings. The PDSA cycle guides the test of change to determine if the change is an improvement. (*Source:* Adapted from Institute for Health Care Improvement. Health system and services research. https://www.hrsa.gov/sites/default/files/quality/toolbox/508pdfs/qualityimprovement.pdf)

Nurses who are part of QI teams work collaboratively with their colleagues asking the questions:

- What are the desired improvements?
- How are changes and improvements measured?
- How is staff organized to accomplish the work?
- How can QI models be leveraged to accomplish improvements effectively and efficiently?
- How is change managed?

There are many QI models in use. Figure 2-6 illustrates how the popular Plan-Do-Study-Act (PDSA) model is used to test and implement changes in real-work settings. Read more about QI and performance improvement in everyday clinical practice in Chapter 18 and check out the Institute for Healthcare Improvement website for more resources (http://www.ihi.org/). If you are committed to developing the skills to lead the way to health care quality and safety, you will also want to study Tucker and Melnyk's

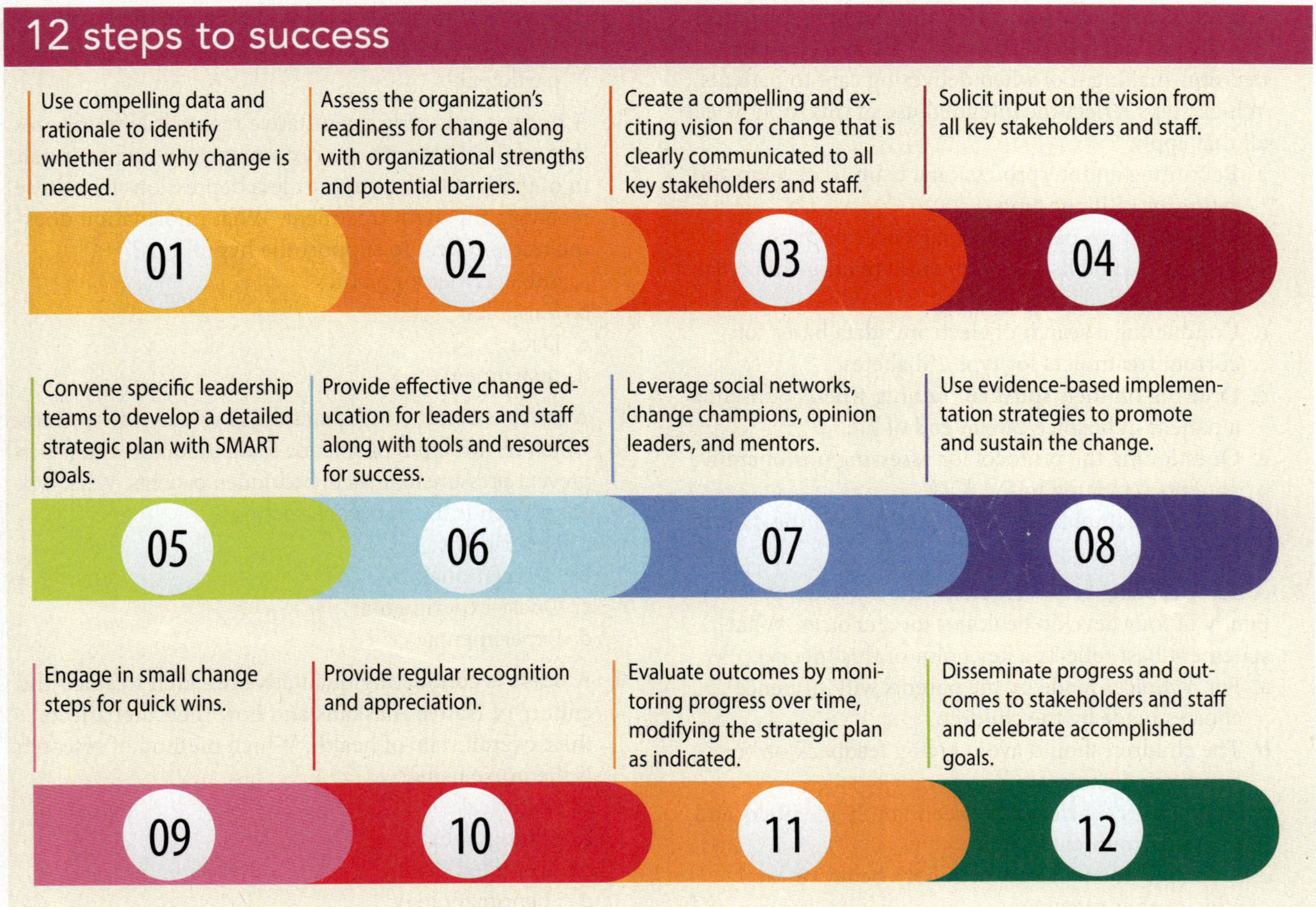
12 steps to success
01
Use compelling data and rationale to identify whether and why change is needed.
02
Assess the organization's readiness for change along with organizational strengths and potential barriers.
03
Create a compelling and exciting vision for change that is clearly communicated to all key stakeholders and staff.
04
Solicit input on the vision from all key stakeholders and staff.
05
Convene specific leadership teams to develop a detailed strategic plan with SMART goals.
06
Provide effective change education for leaders and staff along with tools and resources for success.
07
Leverage social networks, change champions, opinion leaders, and mentors.
08
Use evidence-based implementation strategies to promote and sustain the change.
09
Engage in small change steps for quick wins.
10
Provide regular recognition and appreciation.
11
Evaluate outcomes by monitoring progress over time, modifying the strategic plan as indicated.
12
Disseminate progress and outcomes to stakeholders and staff and celebrate accomplished goals.

FIGURE 2-7. Twelve steps to success. Tucker and Melnyk developed this 12-step model for leading and sustaining successful organizational change. (*Source:* Used with permission from Tucker, S., & Melnyk, B. M. [2019]. Leading organizational change and building wellness cultures for maximum ROI and VOI. In B. Melnyk & T. Raderstorf [Eds.], *Evidence-based leadership, innovation and entrepreneurship in nursing and healthcare: A practical guide.* (2019). Springer Publishing. https://www.myamericannurse.com/wp-content/uploads/2019/06/ant6-Evidence-based-practice-515.pdf)

12-step guide to implementing EBP, which is illustrated in Figure 2-7.

DEVELOPING CLINICAL REASONING AND CLINICAL JUDGMENT

1. Describe your own beliefs about the patient, the nurse, health, and what nursing is. Compare and contrast your answers with those of another student. How do they differ and how are they alike? How do you think such differences might influence nursing practice for each of you?
2. In preparation for your clinical assignment, you read three research articles about positioning and moving patients who are at risk for pressure injuries (bedsores). The staff nurse responsible for the patient tells you, "Oh, I don't pay any attention to that stuff." How should you respond?
3. Describe the research strategy you would use to identify evidence-based interventions to reduce sexual misconduct and assault on your campus; or to promote the use of handwashing, social distancing, and masks to reduce COVID-19 transmission; or to help people stop smoking.
4. Go the National Institute of Nursing Research website and click on Research Highlights. Choose one recently funded study and talk with another student about how the research findings might inform your clinical practice.

PRACTICING FOR NCLEX

1. A nursing student questions the primary nurse about instilling air into a nasogastric tube to confirm placement, when they learned that x-ray validation of the tube's tip in the stomach reflects best practice. The student is validating safe nursing practice with which type of knowledge?
   a. Instinctive knowledge
   b. Scientific knowledge
   c. Authoritative knowledge
   d. Traditional knowledge

2. A nurse is using the Johns Hopkins Nursing Evidence-Based Practice (JHNEBP) model PET as a clinical decision-making tool when delivering care to patients. Which steps reflect the intended use of this tool? Select all that apply.
   a. Recruiting an interprofessional team to develop and refine an EBP question
   b. Drawing from personal experiences of being a patient to establish a therapeutic relationship with a patient
   c. Conducting a search of electronic data bases for current treatments for type 2 diabetes
   d. Drawing on their spiritual training when counseling a patient in hospice care at end of life
   e. Questioning the protocol for assessing postoperative patients returning to the ICU
   f. Studying pathophysiology to understand the disease states of assigned patients
3. A nurse is using general systems theory to assist a family of four develop healthier food choices. What statement best reflects a key point of this theory?
   a. Food choices made by the parents will influence choices made by the children.
   b. The children should avoid giving feedback on the family food choices.
   c. Boundaries are closed between family members and their environments.
   d. A change in one family member's behavior rarely affects other members.
4. A charge nurse meets with staff to outline a plan to provide transcultural nursing care for patients in their health care facility. The charge nurse explains that transcultural care as the central theme of nursing care, knowledge, and practice was promoted by which theorist?
   a. Madeline Leininger
   b. Jean Watson
   c. Dorothy E. Johnson
   d. Betty Newman
5. After their clinical experience, nursing students are given a reflective assignment to discuss the concepts in nursing theory that influence and determine nursing practice. What part of this theory is most important when delivering thoughtful care?
   a. Environment
   b. Health
   c. Nursing
   d. Person
6. Nursing students have been assigned to discuss a section of a research article examining 24-hour visitation for patients in the intensive care unit (ICU). What topic will the student assigned to the applicability section plan to discuss?
   a. Description of the tool that was used to gather the data
   b. How the results could be used in the student's practice
   c. Statistical methods used to determine the results
   d. Whether informed consent was obtained from the participants
7. A nurse conducting quantitative research hypothesizes that adolescents with anorexia nervosa who participate in outpatient therapy report less depression than those receiving inpatient treatment. What information does the nurse collect to support the hypothesis?
   a. Subjects' demographics
   b. Variables
   c. Data
   d. Instruments
8. A nurse is conducting quantitative research to examine which of two types of silicone foam sacral dressings best prevent pressure injuries in bedridden patients. What type of research is the nurse conducting?
   a. Descriptive
   b. Correlational
   c. Quasi-experimental
   d. Experimental
9. A nurse is conducting qualitative research to study the culture of Native Alaskans and how their diet affects their overall state of health. Which method of research is the nurse using?
   a. Historical
   b. Ethnography
   c. Grounded theory
   d. Phenomenology
10. A nurse is formulating a clinical question using the PICOT format. The nurse begins with determining the "P," which focuses on which element?
   a. Comparison to another similar protocol
   b. Clearly defined, focused literature review of procedures
   c. Specific identification of the purpose of the study
   d. Explicit descriptions of the population of interest
11. A group of nurses in the postanesthesia care unit propose a study to determine which of two antiemetic medications from the same classification best relieve postoperative nausea. Before implementing the study, whose approval will the nurses need?
   a. Organization's surgical director
   b. Pharmacy director and staff
   c. Institutional review board
   d. Director of nursing

ANSWERS WITH RATIONALES

1. **b.** Scientific knowledge is obtained through the scientific method or research; this leads to evidence-based practice. Instinct, such as. "I feel this is correct," is not a source of knowledge. Traditional knowledge is the part of nursing practice passed down from generation to generation, often without research data to support it. Examples include daily bathing and changing bed linens each day. Authoritative knowledge comes from an expert and is accepted as truth based on the person's perceived expertise.

2. **a, c, e.** The JHNEBP model is a powerful problem-solving approach to clinical decision making, which uses a three-step process called PET: practice question, evidence, and translation. The goal of the model is to ensure that the latest research findings and best practices are quickly incorporated into patient care. Steps in PET include, but are not limited to, recruiting an interprofessional team, developing and refining the EBP question, and conducting internal and external searches for evidence.
3. **a.** General systems theory defines a system as a set of interacting elements contributing to the overall goal of the system. A change in one element could affect other subsystems, as well as the whole. To survive, open systems maintain balance through feedback, in this case, family members. An open system allows energy, matter, and information to move freely between systems and boundaries, such as with members of the health care team, whereas a closed system does not allow input from or output.
4. **a.** Madeline Leininger's theory provides the foundations of transcultural nursing care by making caring the central theme of nursing. Jean Watson stated that nursing is concerned with promoting and restoring health, preventing illness, and caring for the sick. The central theme of Dorothy E. Johnson's theory is that problems arise because of disturbances in the system or subsystem or functioning below optimal level. Betty Newman proposed that humans are in constant relationship with stressors in the environment and the major nursing focus is keeping the patient system stable through accurate assessment of these stressors.
5. **d.** Of the four concepts, the most important is the person. The focus of nursing, regardless of definition or theory, is the person.
6. **b.** Applicability refers to how study results could be used in practice. Method includes the design and data analysis. Informed consent affirms the patient's right to agree to participate in a study without coercion, to refuse to participate without jeopardizing their care, the right to confidentiality, the right to be protected from harm, and the ability to withdraw from the study at any time.
7. **c.** Data refer to information that the researcher collects from subjects in the study, generally expressed in words, numbers, graphs, and charts. A variable is something (such as conditions, equipment, interventions) that varies and has different values (outcomes) that can be measured. Instruments are devices used to collect and record the data, such as rating scales, pencil-and-paper tests, and biologic measurements.
8. **c.** Quasi-experimental research is often conducted in clinical settings to examine the effects of nursing interventions on patient outcomes. Descriptive research is often used to generate new knowledge about topics with little or no prior research. Correlational research examines the type and degree of relationships between two or more variables. Experimental research examines cause-and-effect relationships between variables under highly controlled conditions.
9. **b.** Ethnographic research was developed by the discipline of anthropology and is used to examine issues of culture of interest to nurses. Historical research examines events of the past to increase understanding of the nursing profession today. The basis of grounded theory methodology is the discovery of how people describe their own reality and how their beliefs are related to their actions in a social scene. The purpose of phenomenology (both a philosophy and a research method) is to describe experiences as they are lived by the subjects being studied.
10. **d.** The *P* in the PICOT format represents an explicit description of the patient population of interest. *I* represents the intervention, *C* represents the comparison, *O* stands for the outcome, and *T* stands for the time.
11. **c.** Federal regulations require that institutions receiving federal funding or conducting studies of drugs or medical devices regulated by the Food and Drug Administration establish institutional review boards (IRBs). The IRBs reviews studies conducted in the institution to determine the risk status of the studies and to ensure that ethical principles are followed. While organizations may have internal procedures for conducting research, such as including surgeons, the director of nursing, the pharmacy director, and staff, these are not government mandates. The type of study, such as randomized-controlled study, will be determined by the nurse in collaboration with the prescriber and approval of the IRB.

Bibliography

Alligood, M. (2014). *Nursing theory: Utilization and application* (5th ed.). Elsevier Mosby.

Alligood, M. (2018). *Nursing theorists and their work* (9th ed.). Elsevier/Mosby.

American Nurses Association (ANA). (2010). *Nursing's social policy statement*. Author.

American Nurses Association. (2015). *Code of ethics for nurses with interpretive statements*. http://www.nursingworld.org/MainMenuCategories/EthicsStandards/CodeofEthicsforNurses/Code-of-Ethics-For-Nurses.html

American Nurses Association (ANA). (2021). *Nursing: Scope and standards of practice* (4th ed.). Author.

Armola, R. R., Bourgault, A. M., Halm, M. A., Board, R. M., Bucher, L., Harrington, L., Heafey, C., Lee, R. K., Shellner, P. K., Medina, J., & 2008–2009 Evidence-Based Practice Resource Work Group of the American Association of Critical-Care Nurses. (2009). Upgrading the American Association of Critical Care Nurses' evidence-leveling hierarchy. *American Journal of Critical Care, 18*(5), 405–409.

Aromataris, E., & Pearson, A. (2014). The systematic review: An overview. *The American Journal of Nursing, 114*(3), 53–58.

Aromataris, E., & Ritano, D. (2014). Constructing a search strategy and searching for evidence. A guide to the literature search for a systematic review. *The American Journal of Nursing, 114*(5), 49–56.

Brennan-Cook, J. (2020). Implementation of evidence-based practice in long-term care. *American Nurse Journal, 15*(9), 45–48.

Bridges, E., McNeill, M., & Munro, N. (2016). Research in review: Driving critical care practice change. *American Journal of Critical Care, 25*(1), 76–84.

Capili, B. (2020). How does research start? *American Journal of Nursing, 120*(10), 41–44.

Capili, B. (2021). Selection of study participants. *American Journal of Nursing, 121*(1), 64–67.

Chicca, J. (2020). Introduction to qualitative nursing research. *American Nurse Journal, 15*(6), 28–32.

Chinn, P., & Kramer, M. (2019). *Knowledge development in nursing: Theory and process* (10th ed.). Elsevier/Mosby.

Crable, J., Highfield, M.E. F., & Patmon, F. (2021). Evidence-based practice knowledge, attitudes, practices and barriers. *Nursing, 51*(9), 58–65.

Cronenwett, L., Sherwood, G., Barnsteiner, J., Disch, J., Johnson, J., Mitchell, P., Sullivan, D. T., & Warren, J. (2007). Quality and safety education for nurses. *Nursing Outlook, 55*(3), 122–131.

Emmanuel, E. J., Wendler, D., & Grady, C. (2000). What makes clinical research ethical? *Journal of the American Medical Association, 283*(20), 2701–2711.

Fitne's Virtual Learning Resource Center. (n.d.). *Nurse theorists: Portraits of excellence, volumes I, II, and III; Excellence in action*. http://www.fitne.net/products.jsp

Fowler, M. (2015). *Guide to nursing's social policy statement*. American Nurses Association.

Gaffney, T. (2021). Mitigating the threat of lost knowledge. *American Nurse Journal, 16*(1), 8–9, 58.

Glasofer, A., & Townsend, A. B. (2021a). Determining the level of evidence: Experimental research appraisal. *Nursing, 51*(1), 60–63.

Glasofer, A., & Townsend, A. B. (2021b). Determining the level of evidence: Nonresearch evidence. *Nursing2021, 51*(3), 53–57.

Grady, P. A. (2017). Advancing science, improving lives. NINR's new strategic plan and the future of nursing science. *Journal of Nursing Scholarship, 49*(3), 247–248.

Grady, P. A., & Gough, L. L. (2015). Nursing science: Claiming the future. *Journal of Nursing Scholarship, 47*(6), 512–521.

Grove, S. K., & Gray, J. R. (2019). *Understanding nursing research: Building an evidence-based practice* (7th ed.). Elsevier.

Hammer, J. (2020, March 1). *Thou shalt not underestimate Florence Nightingale* (p. 32). Smithsonian Magazine.

Hood, L. (2014). *Leddy & Pepper's conceptual bases of professional nursing* (8th ed.). Lippincott Williams & Wilkins.

Hundt, B. (2020). Reflection on Nightingale in the Year of the Nurse. *American Nurse Journal, 15*(5), 26–29.

Institute of Medicine (IOM). (2001). *Crossing the quality chasm: A new health system for the 21st century.* National Academy of Sciences.

Institute of Medicine (IOM). (2011). *The future of nursing: Leading change, advancing health.* The National Academies Press.

Kolcaba, K. (2003). *Comfort theory and practice.* Springer Publishing Company.

Kreil, S. (2021). Operationalizing new knowledge, innovations, and improvement. *American Nurse Journal, 16*(3), 3438.

Linnen, D. (2016). The promise of big data. Improving patient safety and nursing practice. *Nursing, 46*(5), 28–34; quiz 34–35.

Makic, M. B. F., & Rauen, C. (2016). Maintaining your momentum: Moving evidence into practice. *Critical Care Nurse, 36*(2), 13–18.

Makic, M. B., Rauen, C., Watson, R., & Poteet, A. W. (2014). Examining the evidence to guide practice: Challenging practice habits. *Critical Care Nurse, 34*(2), 28–45; quiz 46.

Marzinsky, A., & Smith-Miller, C. A. (2019). Nurse research and the institutional review board. *American Nurse Today, 14*(10), 20–24.

McEwen, M., & Wills, E. (2019). *Theoretical basis for nursing* (5th ed.). Wolters Kluwer Health.

Meleis, A. I. (2018). *Theoretical nursing: Development and progress* (6th ed.). Wolters Kluwer.

Melnyk, B. M. (2018). Breaking down silos and making use of the evidence-based practice competencies in healthcare and academic programs: An urgent call to action. *Worldviews on Evidence-based Nursing, 15* (1), 3–4.

Melnyk, B. M., & Fineout-Overholt, E. (2002). Key steps in evidence-based practice. Asking compelling clinical questions and searching for the best evidence. *Pediatric Nursing, 28*(3), 262–263, 266.

Melnyk, B. M., & Fineout-Overholt, E. (2015). *Evidence-based practice in nursing: A guide to best practice* (3rd ed.). Wolters Kluwer Health.

Melnyk, B. M., & Fineout-Overholt, E. (2019). *Evidence-based practice in nursing: A guide to best practice* (4th ed.). Wolters Kluwer Health.

National Academies of Sciences, Engineering, and Medicine. (2015). *Assessing progress on the Institute of Medicine Report the Future of Nursing.* The National Academies Press.

National Academies of Sciences, Engineering, and Medicine. (2021). *The future of nursing 2020–2030.* https://www.nationalacademies.org/our-work/the-future-of-nursing-2020-2030

Ost, K., Blalock, C., Fagan, M., Sweeney, K. M., & Miller-Hoover, S. R. (2020). Aligning organizational culture and infrastructure to support evidence-based practice. *CriticalCare Nurse, 40*(3), 59–63.

Peterson, M. H., Barnason, S., Donnelly, B., Hill, K., Miley, H., Riggs, L., Whiteman, K. (2014). Choosing the best evidence to guide clinical practice: Application of AACN levels of evidence. *Critical Care Nurse, 34*(2), 58–68.

Pickler, R. H., Abshire, D. A., Chao, A. M., Chlan, L. L., Stanfill, A. G., Hacker, E. D., Kawar, L. N., McCarthy, A. M., & Talsma, A. (2020). Nursing science and COVID-19. *Nursing Outlook, 68*(5), 685–688.

Polit, D., & Beck, C. (2021). *Nursing research: Generating and assessing evidence for nursing practice* (11th ed.). Wolters Kluwer Health.

Reynolds, S. (2020). Using audit and feedback to improve compliance with evidence-based practices. *American Nurse Journal, 15*(10), 16–19.

Scala, E., Price, C., & Day, J. (2016). An integrative review of engaging clinical nurses in nursing research. *Journal of Nursing Scholarship, 48*(4), 423–430.

Titler, M. G., Kleiber, C., Steelman, V. J., Rakel, B. A., Budreau, G., Everett, L. Q., Buckwaiter, K. C., Tripp-Reimer, T., & Goode, C. J. (2001). The Iowa model of evidence-based practice to promote quality care. *Critical Care Nursing Clinics North American, 13*(4), 497–509.

Tucker, S., & Melnyk, M. (2019). A leader's guide to implementing evidence-based practice. *American Nurse Today, 14*(6), 6–9.

Upvall, M. J., Bourgault, A. M., Pigon, C., & Swartzman, C. A. (2019). Exemplars illustrating de-implementation of tradition-based practices. *Critical Care Nurse, 39*(6), 64–69.

Walker, L. O. (2020). Gifts of wise women: A reflection on enduring ideas in nursing that transcend time. *Nursing Outlook, 68*(3), 355–364.

Williams, B. (2015). Understanding qualitative research. *American Nurse Today, 10*(7), 40–42.

Yoder, L. H., Kirkley, D., McFall, D. C., Kirksey, K. M., StalBaum, A. L., & Sellers, D. (2014). CE: Original Research: Staff nurses' use of research to facilitate evidence-based practice. *The American Journal of Nursing, 114*(9), 26–37.

Younas, A. (2020). Identifying international barriers and facilitators to research utilization. *Nursing, 50*(7), 63–67.

3 Health, Wellness, and Health Disparities

Ruth Jacobi

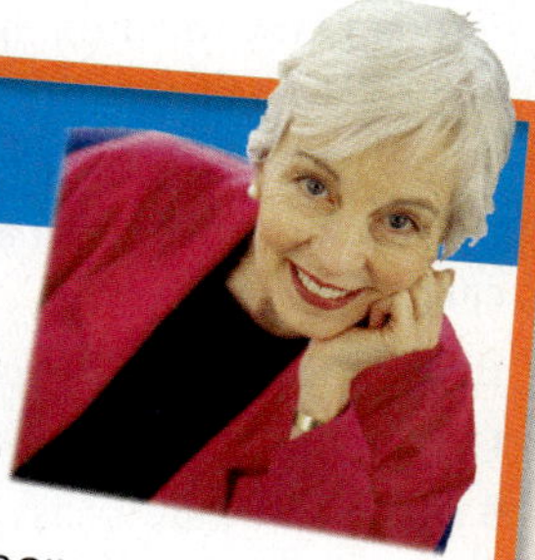

Ruth is a 62-year-old woman who was hospitalized after a "mini-stroke." She has now returned to her pre-event level of functioning and is being prepared for discharge. She states, "I know that I have an increased risk for a major stroke, so I want to do everything possible to stay as active and as healthy as I possibly can."

Sara Thurston

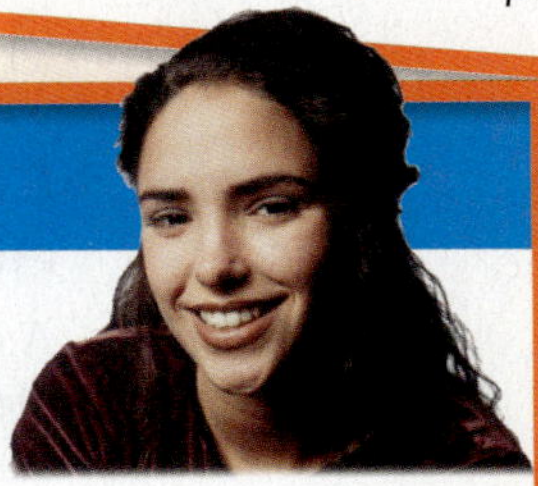

Sara, a college freshman, is encouraged to visit the student health center by her roommate because she rarely visits the dining hall for meals, runs 5 to 8 miles a day, and has recently lost a significant amount of weight. She is very thin now, and when she does eat a meal, she just seems to move the food around on her plate. Sara states, "I'm plenty healthy, just a bit 'nuts' about being fit!"

Daniel Sternman

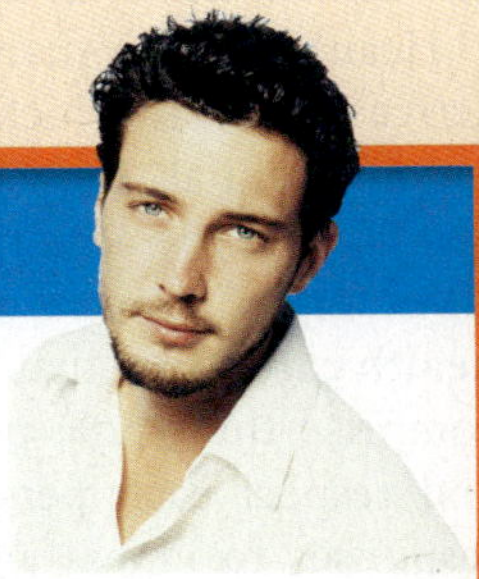

Daniel, a 27-year-old man with a history of schizophrenia, comes to the mental health clinic, loudly demanding relief from the voices that are telling him to hurt himself. Mr. Sternman is well known by the clinic staff. His medical record reveals that he has had numerous visits to the clinic and that he has difficulty interacting and dealing with various staff members.

Learning Outcomes

After completing the chapter, you will be able to accomplish the following:

1. Describe concepts and models of health, wellness, disease, and illness.
2. Compare and contrast acute illness and chronic illness.
3. Discuss the factors that play a role in health equity and health disparities including social determinants of health.
4. Explain how the human dimensions, basic human needs, and self-concept influence health and illness.
5. Summarize the role of the nurse in promoting health, preventing illness, and addressing disparities in health care.
6. Explain the levels of preventive care.
7. Define diversity, inclusion, and equity and explain what it means to be antiracist.

Nursing Concepts

- Health care disparities
- Health, wellness, and illness
- Diversity, equity, and inclusion

The primary objectives of the nurse as caregiver are to promote health; to prevent illness; to restore health; and to facilitate coping with illness, disability, or death. These objectives focus care on maximizing the health of people of all ages and in all populations, in all settings, and in both health and illness.

Health is more than just the absence of illness; it is an active process in which a person moves toward their maximum potential. Each person has a different definition of health. (See the accompanying Reflective Practice box for an example.) To give thoughtful, person-centered **holistic health care**—care that addresses the many dimensions that comprise the whole person—the nurse must understand and respect each person's own definition of health and responses to illness and should be familiar with models of health and illness. The nurse's knowledge of health and illness is even more important because of today's focus on health promotion and advocacy, the continuing trend toward care being provided in the home and community, the increasing numbers of older adults, the growing incidence of chronic illnesses and mental health problems, and the ongoing efforts to maximize health care outcomes for all populations (diversity, equity, inclusion).

The 2013 report by the Institute of Medicine (renamed the National Academy of Sciences, Engineering, and Medicine in 2015) and the National Research Council (*U.S. Health in International Perspective: Shorter Lives, Poorer Health*) provides additional impetus to foster positive health behaviors. Compared to 16 other affluent countries, the United States has a serious health disadvantage, despite the fact that the country spends twice as much per person on health care in comparison to the other nations in the survey. Americans fare worse in nine key health areas: infant mortality and low birth weight, injuries and homicides, teenage pregnancies and sexually transmitted infections, prevalence of HIV and AIDS, drug-related deaths, obesity and diabetes, heart disease, chronic lung disease, and disability. There is agreement that the United States must vigorously investigate potential explanations for this health disadvantage as well as intensify efforts to strengthen systems responsible for health and social services, education, and employment; promote healthy lifestyles; and design healthier environments. Some of these problems are longstanding concerns, and many evidence-based strategies have been implemented to address these challenges. The United States can no longer afford to ignore these compelling issues. Better health must be an achievable outcome for all Americans (Woolf & Aron, 2013). As this text goes to publication, Congress is again trying to decide how best to meet the health care needs of U.S. citizens. See Chapter 11, The Health Care Delivery System.

CONCEPTS OF HEALTH AND WELLNESS

A classic definition of health is that **health** is a state of complete physical, mental, and social well-being, not merely the absence of disease or infirmity (World Health Organization, 1974). The health of the public is measured globally by **morbidity** (how frequently a disease occurs) and **mortality** (the number of deaths resulting from a disease). On a personal level, however, most people define health according to how they feel ("I feel really sick"), the absence or presence of symptoms of illness ("I have a terrible pain in my stomach"), or their ability to carry out activities of daily living ("I felt so much better that I got up and cooked supper"). The accompanying feature, Through the Eyes of a Student (on page 56), presents a personal viewpoint of the meaning of health. How would you describe health?

Each person defines health in terms of their own values and beliefs. The person's family, culture, community, and society also influence this personal perception of health.

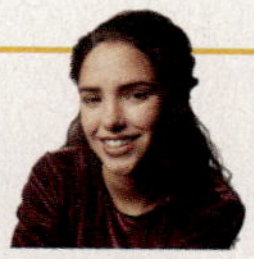

Think back to ***Sara Thurston***, the college freshman who rarely eats and runs several miles almost daily. According to her statement, she considers herself to be healthy. However, her roommate is concerned because of what she views as excessive exercise and Sara's poor nutrition. The nurse needs to investigate Sara's views further to determine exactly what Sara believes to be healthy. Doing so provides a foundation on which to develop an appropriate care plan.

QSEN Reflective Practice: Cultivating QSEN Competencies

CHALLENGE TO ETHICAL AND LEGAL SKILLS

My first college roommate, Sara Thurston, seemed the ideal roommate when I first met her. A good student, she was thoughtful, outgoing, and fun. By October, however, I was really worried about her. I noticed that she rarely wanted to come to the dining hall with our group of friends. When she did come, she just seemed to pick at her food. She also spent a lot of time at the athletic center, running 5 to 8 miles almost daily. I wasn't surprised when she started losing significant amounts of weight. What worried me was her lack of willingness to talk about her nutritional habits and health. She told me that she was plenty healthy, just a bit "nuts" about being fit! She also kidded that I'd be healthier if I worked out more often with her. While she was certainly right about that, I was worried that she had a serious eating disorder and wasn't sure what I could do to help. She politely told me to "mind my own business" when I asked her if she had ever spoken with anyone about her health and eating.

Thinking Outside the Box: Possible Courses of Action

- Respect Sara's wishes and simply try to be a good friend without continuing to confront her about her nutritional status.
- Tell Sara I am concerned that she has a serious eating disorder, and then plan the next steps with her, fully respecting her right to seek or refuse professional help.
- Tell Sara that if she fails to get professional help, I will contact her parents or a counselor at school.

Evaluating a Good Outcome: How Do I Define Success?

- Sara gets whatever help she needs to address her eating problems and regain health.
- Sara's right to make her own decisions is respected.
- My obligations as a friend are fulfilled.
- My beginning ability to identify and correctly respond to health problems affirms my choice for nursing.

Personal Learning: Here's to the Future!

Unfortunately, I did not intervene because (1) I failed to recognize how serious a problem this would become, and (2) I wasn't sure what I could do after Sara refused my initial offers of help. Sara dropped out of school at the end of our freshman year and she has not returned my calls, so I'm not sure how she is doing. I've read more about eating disorders, and I now know how important it is to get professional help early. I learned too late that Sara had been in treatment for anorexia during high school and that the pressures of college life had led to a relapse. I think I valued her friendship more than I valued getting her the help that she needed to address a serious health problem.

QSEN SELF-REFLECTION ON QUALITY AND SAFETY COMPETENCIES DEVELOPING KNOWLEDGE, SKILLS, AND ATTITUDES FOR CONTINUOUS IMPROVEMENT

How do you think you would respond in a similar situation? Why? What does this tell you about yourself and about the adequacy of your skills for professional practice? Can you think of other ways to respond? Do you agree with the criteria that the nursing student used to evaluate a successful outcome? Why or why not? What *knowledge, skills,* and *attitudes* do you need to develop to continuously improve quality and safety when caring for patients like Sara?

Patient-Centered Care: What is the best approach when Sara denies that she has an eating problem? If Sara refuses any help, is it better to focus on her positive attributes and avoid conflict regarding her current situation? How might the student's and Sara's developmental level have affected their responses? How should you, as her roommate and friend, proceed? What is the best way to communicate emotional support, concern, and caring to Sara?

Teamwork and Collaboration/Quality Improvement: What communication skills do you need in order to facilitate your role as a patient advocate for Sara? As a student nurse, what other skills do you need to respond appropriately in this situation? Should you offer to make an appointment for her with a professional (nutritionist, counselor, nurse) or offer to accompany her to an appointment?

Safety/Evidence-Based Practice: Can you secure any evidence in nursing literature that provides information related to eating disorders and the need for professional treatment? Should you share this information with Sara? What response best contributes to a safe environment for Sara?

Informatics: If you were completing a rotation in a clinical setting as a student nurse, what information should you document electronically regarding your assessment of a patient like Sara and her response to any interventions?

Through the Eyes of a Student

Carrie was a 17-year-old who attended my high school, dated my best friend Ricky, and participated in many of the same clubs and activities as I did. By looking at her, I never would have guessed anything was wrong. However, once I got to know her, I learned that she was diagnosed with cancer and that the disease had spread through her heart and lungs. The situation, as doctors continually told her, did not look promising. Yet, she never once let that slow her down, and she lived each day to the fullest. It was almost 1 year ago that I watched as this friend passed away from bone cancer. However, until the days before her last breath, in my eyes, she was a happy and healthy girl. She never once let the disease get the best of her, and she fought for life every second of every day. Her constant optimism and determined smile touched and moved so many others. So you ask me, was Carrie healthy?

Health to me is a state of mind, not the physical condition of a person's body. Carrie, in my opinion, was the definition of healthy: She was happy, she lived her life to the fullest, and she continually inspired others to embrace life. The dictionary may state that health is the absence of a disease; however, for me, it is the way a person thinks and reacts to life. A person's health consists of being able to work to the best of her capability, look out for herself, and her ability to respond to life enthusiastically. In my eyes, a person like Carrie can be physically unwell, but in terms of living, is healthy. Perhaps this is where health and wellness differ, in that, to me, health means the person's entire state of being and is decided by the person, whereas wellness refers more to the physical condition of a person and is determined more readily by society. The words *illness* and *disease* also correspond with these words. I believe that illness, such as health, is a matter of thinking, while disease is a medical term that relates to physical condition and wellness. All of these states are constantly changing, and I have probably experienced the best and worst of all of them. However, as I embark on this new and exciting journey of college, I consider myself extremely healthy. I am living each day to the fullest, trying to impact other people's lives, and am filled with optimism. This all may change shortly, but as I look back on Carrie's life and the effect she has had on me, I will always try to live my life in a healthy and grateful way.

—Molly Proskine, Georgetown University

Health integrates all the human dimensions—the physical, intellectual, emotional, sociocultural, spiritual, and environmental aspects of the whole person. The nurse giving holistic care must equally consider all these interrelated dimensions of the whole person (Fig. 3-1).

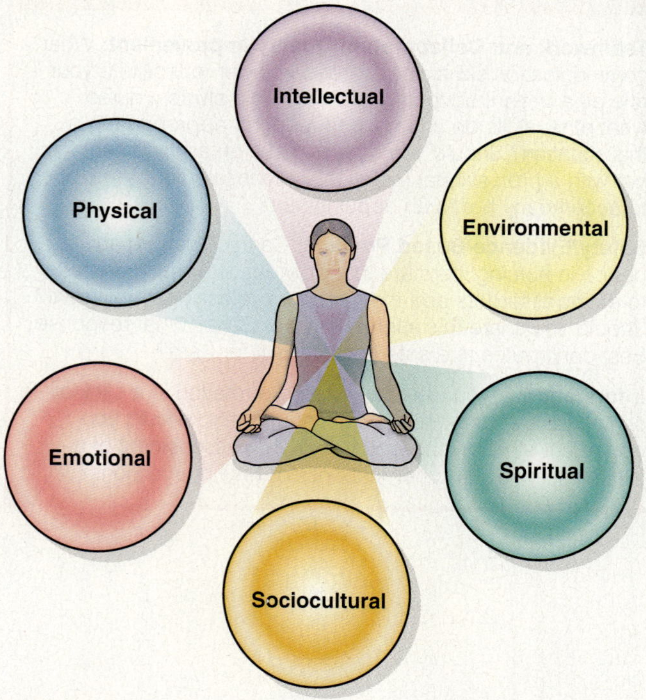

FIGURE 3-1. The human dimensions. All of these interdependent parts compose the whole person.

Unfolding Patient Stories: Kim Johnson • Part 1

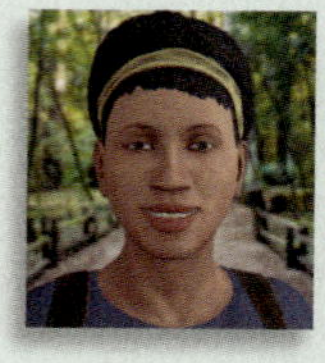

Kim Johnson—a 26-year-old police officer—is hospitalized with a thoracic spinal cord injury from a gunshot wound and is now paraplegic. What factors influencing health status and recovery should the nurse consider for each human dimension when developing an individualized, holistic care plan for Kim? (Kim Johnson's story continues in Chapter 11.)

Care for Kim and other patients in a realistic virtual environment: ***vSim** for Nursing* (thepoint.lww.com/vSimFunds). Practice documenting these patients' care in DocuCare (thepoint.lww.com/DocuCareEHR).

Wellness—a term often used interchangeably with health—is an active state of being healthy, including living a lifestyle that promotes good physical, mental, and emotional health. Dunn (1977) described his model of high-level wellness as functioning to one's maximum potential while maintaining balance and a purposeful direction in the environment. Dunn differentiated "wellness" from "good health," believing that good health is a passive state simply denoting that the person is not ill at this time. Wellness is a more active state, regardless of one's level of health. Dunn also defined processes that help people know who and what they are. These processes, which are a part of each person's perception of their own wellness state, are *being* (recognizing oneself as separate and individual), *belonging* (being part of a whole), *becoming* (growing and developing), and *befitting* (making personal choices that befit oneself for the future). Dunn's model encourages the nurse to care for the total person, with regard for all factors affecting the person's state of being while striving to reach maximum potential.

CONCEPTS OF ILLNESS AND DISEASE

Disease is a medical term, referring to pathologic changes in the structure or function of the body or mind. Box 3-1 lists common causes of disease. An **illness** is the response of the person to a disease; it is a process in which the person's level of functioning is changed when compared with a previous level. This response is unique for each person and is influenced by self-perceptions, others' perceptions, the effects of changes in body structure and function, the effects of those changes on roles and relationships, and cultural and spiritual values and beliefs. A disease is traditionally diagnosed and treatment is prescribed by a health care provider or advanced practice nurse, whereas nurses focus on the person with an illness. However, the terms *disease* and *illness* are often used interchangeably. It is important for nurses to remember that patients may have an illness or injury but still achieve maximum functioning and quality of life, and consider themselves to be healthy.

Classifications of Illness

Illnesses are classified as either acute or chronic. A person may have an acute illness, a chronic illness, or both at the same time; for example, an adult with diabetes (a chronic illness) may also have an acute episode of severely low blood sugar.

Acute Illness

An **acute illness** usually has a rapid onset of symptoms and lasts only a relatively short time. Although some acute illnesses are life threatening, simple acute illnesses, such as the common cold or diarrhea, do not usually require medical treatment. If medical care is required, a specific treatment with medication (e.g., an antibiotic for pneumonia), surgical procedures (e.g., an appendectomy for appendicitis), or another medical treatment usually return the person to normal functioning.

Box 3-1 Common Causes of Diseases

- Inherited genetic defects
- Developmental defects resulting from exposure to such factors as viruses or chemicals during pregnancy
- Biologic agents or toxins
- Physical agents such as temperature, chemicals, and radiation
- Generalized tissue responses to injury or irritation
- Physiologic and emotional reactions to stress
- Excessive or insufficient production of body secretions (hormones, enzymes, and so forth)

Chronic Illness

Chronic illness is a broad term that encompasses a number of different physical and mental alterations in health, each having one or more of the following characteristics:

- It is a permanent change.
- It causes, or is caused by, irreversible alterations in normal anatomy and physiology.
- It requires special patient education for rehabilitation.
- It requires a long period of care or support.

Chronic illnesses usually have a slow onset and many have periods of **remission** (the disease is present, but the person does not experience symptoms) and **exacerbation** (the symptoms of the disease reappear).

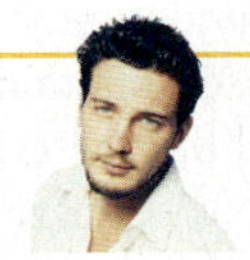

Recall **Daniel Sternman**, the young man with schizophrenia. The nurse would integrate knowledge of this disorder, understanding that it is a chronic illness that can be treated. The patient's arrival at the clinic with reports of hearing voices would indicate to the nurse that symptoms of the disorder have reappeared, necessitating treatment.

The Centers for Disease Control and Prevention (CDC) reports that chronic diseases and conditions—such as heart disease, stroke, cancer, type 2 diabetes, obesity, and arthritis—are among the most common, costly, disabling and preventable of all health problems (CDC, 2016a, 2016b). A 2014 CDC study found that, each year, nearly 900,000 Americans die prematurely from the 5 leading causes of death (heart disease, cancer, chronic lower respiratory disease, stroke, and unintentional injury), yet 20% to 40% of the deaths from each cause could have been prevented.

The chronic disease burden in the United States largely results from a short list of risk factors that can be effectively addressed for individuals and populations. These risk factors include tobacco use, poor diet and physical inactivity (both strongly associated with obesity), excessive alcohol consumption, uncontrolled high blood pressure, and hyperlipidemia (CDC, 2019).

To help to meet the chronic disease burden, the CDC uses four cross-cutting strategies: (1) epidemiology and surveillance to monitor trends and inform programs, (2) environmental approaches that promote health and support healthy behaviors, (3) health system interventions to improve the effective use of clinical and other preventive services, and (4) community resources linked to clinical services that sustain improved management of chronic conditions. This approach is based on the assumption that establishment of community conditions to support healthy behaviors and promote effective management of chronic conditions will deliver healthier students to schools, healthier workers to employers and businesses, and a healthier population to the health care system (Bauer et al., 2014, p. 45).

Because chronic illnesses are the leading health problem in the world, the health promotion and illness prevention activities discussed later in this chapter are vital to nursing care. Nurses will be caring for more patients with chronic illnesses in the future. Although not all people with a chronic illness require care, all who are chronically ill must accept certain conditions to be able to live with the illness on a day-to-day basis for the rest of their lives. People with a chronic illness often grieve over losses or changes in physical structure and function; worry about their finances, status, roles, and dignity; and face the possibility of an earlier death.

To successfully adapt to a chronic illness, the person must learn to live as normally as possible and maintain a positive self-concept and sense of hope, despite symptoms and treatments that may make the person feel different from others. Activities of daily living, relationships, and self-care activities must often be modified, and it is important that the person maintain a feeling of being in control of their own life and the prescribed treatments.

Nurses care for people of all ages with chronic illnesses, providing that care in all types of settings, including homes, hospitals, clinics, long-term care facilities, and other institutions. Regardless of the age of the patient or the effects and demands of the illness or the setting, the nurse must make every effort to promote health for patients with chronic illness, with a focus on care that emphasizes what is possible rather than what can no longer be.

Diseases and Deaths of Isolation and Despair

In this decade, both clinicians and researchers are studying two seemingly associated demographic trends: income stagnation and rising premature mortality from suicides, drug poisoning, and alcoholic liver disease among U.S. non-Hispanic Whites with low education. Some are now suggesting that these population-level trends indicate that despair induced by financial stressors is a shared pathway to these causes of disease and death. See Figure 3-2 for a schema illustrating this progression from economic stagnation to deaths of despair (Shanahan et al., 2019). What these trends, exacerbated during the pandemic, make clear, is the complexity of factors influencing the health of individuals and communities. You will want to be very alert to all the variables that influence health and well-being. Until recently, we paid scant attention to socioeconomic circumstances.

Illness Behaviors

When a person becomes ill, certain illness behaviors may occur in identifiable stages (Suchman, 1965). These behaviors are how people cope with altered functioning caused by the disease. They are unique to the person and are influenced by age, sex assigned at birth, family values, economic status, culture, educational level, and mental status.

There is no specific timetable for the stages-of-illness behaviors, which may occur rapidly or slowly. Nursing roles throughout the stages remain constant. In all stages, the nurse accepts the patient as an individual, gives nursing care based on prioritized needs, and facilitates recovery through physical care, emotional support, and health education.

Stage 1: Experiencing Symptoms

How do people define themselves as "sick"? The first indication of an illness usually is recognizing one or more symptoms that are incompatible with their personal definition of health. Although pain is the most common symptom indicating illness, other common symptoms include rash, fever, bleeding, or cough. If the symptoms last for a short time or are relieved by self-care, the person usually takes no further action. If the symptoms continue, however, the person enters the next stage.

Stage 2: Assuming the Sick Role

The person now self-defines as being sick, seeks validation of this experience from others, gives up normal activities, and assumes a "sick role." At this stage, most people focus on their symptoms and bodily functions. Depending on individual health beliefs and practices, the person may choose to do nothing, may research symptoms on Internet sources, may buy over-the-counter medications, may try alternative remedies to relieve symptoms, or may seek out a health care provider for diagnosis and treatment. In our society, an illness becomes "legitimate" when a health care provider

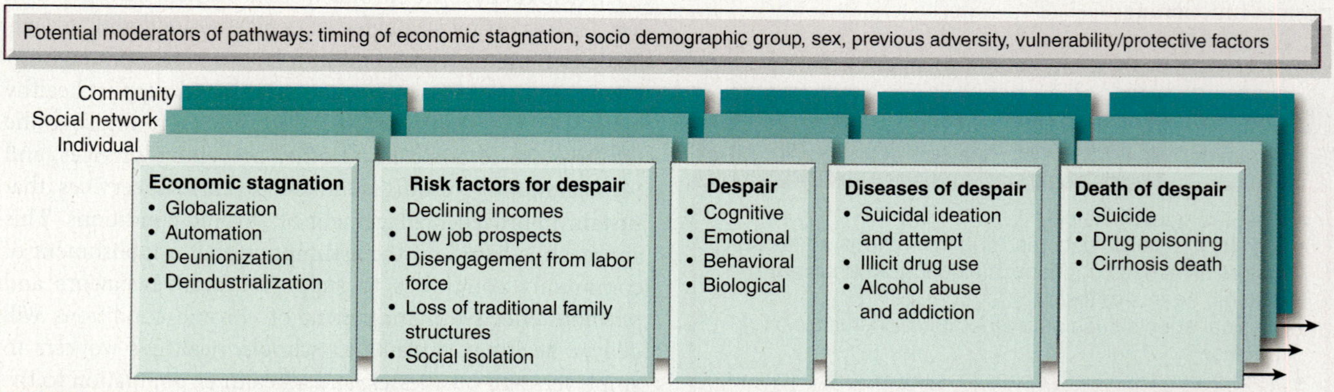

FIGURE 3-2. Potential moderators of pathways: timing of economic stagnation, sociodemographic group, sex, previous adversity, vulnerability/protective factors. (*Source:* Used with permission from Shanahan, L., Hill, S. N., Gaydosh, L. M., Steinhoff, A., Costello, E. J., Dodge, K. A., Harris, K. M., & Copeland, W. E. [2019]. Does despair really kill: A roadmap for an evidence-based answer. *American Journal of Public Health, 109*[6], 854–858.)

diagnoses it and prescribes treatment. After seeking help from the health care provider, the person becomes a patient and enters the next stage.

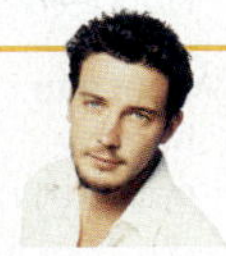

Recall **Daniel Sternman**, the young man with schizophrenia. His arrival at the mental health clinic indicates that he is seeking help from a health care provider. The nurse would interpret this behavior as signaling his assumption of the sick role.

Stage 3: Assuming a Dependent Role

This stage is characterized by the patient's decision to accept the diagnosis and follow the prescribed treatment plan. The person may initially have difficulty conforming to the recommendations of the health care provider and may decide to seek a second opinion or deny the diagnosis. The lack of independence is more troubling for some people who, based on their diagnosis, often require assistance in carrying out activities of daily living and need emotional support through acceptance, approval, physical closeness, and protection.

If the disease is serious (such as a heart attack or stroke), the patient may enter the hospital for treatment. If the symptoms can be managed by the patient or family alone or with the assistance of home care providers, the patient is cared for at home. To facilitate adherence to the treatment plan, the patient needs effective relationships with caregivers, knowledge about the illness, and an individualized care plan. The patient's responses to care depend on a variety of factors, including the seriousness of the illness, the patient's degree of fear about the disease, the loss of roles, the support of others, and previous experiences with illness care. The optimal outcome expected by both caregivers and family is to get well and resume normal roles.

Stage 4: Achieving Recovery and Rehabilitation

Recovery and rehabilitation might begin in the hospital and conclude at home, or may be totally concluded at a rehabilitation center or at home. Most patients complete this final stage of illness behavior at home. In this stage, the person gives up the dependent role and resumes normal activities and responsibilities. If the care plan includes health education, the person may return to health at a higher level of functioning and health than before the illness.

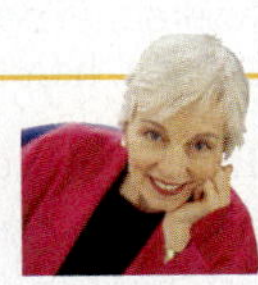

Remember **Ruth Jacobi**, the woman being prepared for discharge after a mini-stroke. The patient's stated desire to be as active and as healthy as she possibly can reflects her desire to give up the dependent role. The nurse would use this knowledge as a basis for the patient's teaching plan, thereby fostering a return to health, possibly at a level higher than before the patient's mini-stroke.

Effects of Illness on the Family

Most nursing care is given to patients with some form of support system, usually family members. When an illness occurs, daily life changes for both the patient and the family. For example, a chronic illness creates stress for the patient and family because of possible lifelong alterations in roles or lifestyle, frequent hospitalizations, economic problems, and decreased social interactions among family members. The responses of family members to an illness are also individualized. Some family members want to be with the patient all the time, while others might avoid visiting. Parents of a sick child often react with blame, overprotection, and severe anxiety, and family members of patients requiring intensive care often feel alone and frightened. In both cases, they might also feel guilty and imagine the worst possible outcome. See Chapter 4 for more information.

Care for Family Caregivers

Carpenter and Gould (2020) note that in the United States alone an, estimated 65.7 million unpaid family caregivers provide care to someone who is ill, has a disability, or is an older adult. "Even with strong support systems the caregiver may experience depression, social isolation, weight loss, irregular sleep patterns, lack of interest in activities that once brought joy, increased alcohol or drug use, or stress manifesting itself in physical ailments" (p. 53). Nurses working with family caregivers are wise to urge them to take responsibility for their own health and well-being. Suggestions include:

- Engage in self-compassion—be kind to yourself
- Practice gratitude
- Do something for yourself daily
- Ask for help
- Find a support group
- Seek professional help for yourself if needed
- Check out available resources
- Be realistic about expectations—know that you and your loved one may need to explore other options

How might you use this list to counsel a parent caring for a child with cerebral palsy or a spouse with early-onset dementia?

DISPARITIES IN HEALTH CARE

Healthy People 2030 defines **health equity** as the attainment of the highest level of health for all people. Although health care is increasingly focused on the promotion of health and the prevention of illness, there continue to be disparities that lead to different health outcomes among different populations of people. A **health disparity** is defined by Healthy People 2030 as a "particular type of health difference that is closely linked with social, economic, and/or environmental disadvantage" (Healthy People 2030, n.d.a).

Health disparities are influenced by many different factors, including race and ethnicity, poverty, sex assigned at birth, age, mental health, educational level, disabilities, sexual orientation, health insurance, and access to health care. Healthy People 2030 defines **social determinants of health** as the conditions in the

Economic Stability	Neighborhood and Physical Environment	Education	Food	Community and Social Context	Health Care System
Employment	Housing	Literacy	Hunger	Social integration	Health coverage
Income	Transportation	Language	Access to healthy options	Support systems	Provider availability
Expenses	Safety	Early childhood education		Community engagement	Provider
Debt	Parks	Vocational training		Discrimination	Linguistic and cultural competence
Medical bills	Playgrounds	Higher education			Quality of care
Support	Walkability				

Health Outcomes
Mortality, Morbidity, Life expectancy, Health care expenditures, Health status, Functional limitations

FIGURE 3-3. Social determinants of health. (*Source:* Used with permission: The Henry J. Kaiser Family Foundation.)

environments in which people are born, live, learn, work, play, worship, and age that affect a wide range of health, functioning, and quality-of-life outcomes and risks (Healthy People 2030), as shown in Figure 3-3. Kristof (2020) writes that "A newborn in a ZIP code of North Philadelphia with a largely poor and Black population has a life expectancy 20 years shorter than a newborn in mostly White central Philadelphia just four miles away; that's not because one infant has displayed 'weak character'." A Kaiser Family Foundation study found that only 19% of Black adults 65 years or older have documented their wishes at the end of life compared with 65% of White adults in the same age group. In addition, a perception exists in the health care community that the Black population avoids end-of-life discussions and underuses palliative and hospice services (ANA Center for Ethics and Human Rights, 2020). See also the discussion of social determinants of health in Chapter 4 and Healthy People 2020's list of social determinants across the life stages in Box 3-2.

Box 3-2 Social Determinants Across the Life Stages

From infancy through old age, the conditions in the social and physical environments in which people are born, live, work, and age can have a significant influence on health outcomes.

Children

- Early and middle childhood provide the physical, cognitive, and social-emotional foundation for lifelong health, learning, and well-being. A history of exposure to adverse experiences in childhood, including exposure to violence and maltreatment, is associated with health-risk behaviors such as smoking, alcohol and drug use, and risky sexual behavior, as well as health problems such as obesity, diabetes, heart disease, sexually transmitted diseases, and attempted suicide.
- Features of the built environment, such as exposure to lead-based paint hazards and pests, negatively affect the health and development of young children.

Adolescents

- Because they are in developmental transition, adolescents and young adults are particularly sensitive to environmental influences. Environmental factors, including family, peer group, school, neighborhood, policies, and societal cues, can either support or challenge young people's health and well-being. Addressing young people's positive development facilitates their adoption of healthy behaviors and helps to ensure a healthy and productive future adult population.
- Adolescents who grow up in neighborhoods characterized by poverty are more likely to be victims of violence; use tobacco, alcohol, and other substances; become obese; and engage in risky sexual behavior.

Adults

- Access to and availability of healthier foods can help adults follow healthful diets. For example, better access to retail venues that sell healthier options may have a positive impact on a person's diet. These venues may be less available in low-income or rural neighborhoods.
- Longer hours, compressed work weeks, shift work, reduced job security, and part-time and temporary work are realities of the modern workplace and are increasingly affecting the health and lives of U.S. adults. Research has shown that workers experiencing these stressors are at higher risk of injuries, heart disease, and digestive disorders.

Older Adults

- Availability of community-based resources and transportation options for older adults can positively affect health status. Studies have shown that increased levels of social support are associated with a lower risk for physical disease, mental illness, and death.

Source: HealthyPeople.gov. Social determinants across the life stages. https://www.healthypeople.gov/2020/leading-health-indicators/2020-lhi-topics/Social-Determinants/determinants.

Disparities in health outcomes are especially common in racial and ethnic minorities, in whom higher rates of obesity, cancer, diabetes mellitus, and AIDS are seen. See the U.S. Department of Health and Human Services Office of Minority Health for Specifics (USDHHS, 2016). The Health Equity Institute urges the following measures to eliminate avoidable health inequities and health disparities (Health Equity Institute):

- Attention to the root causes of health inequities and health disparities—specifically, health determinants, a principal focus of Healthy People 2020 and 2020–2030.
- Particular attention to groups that have experienced major obstacles to health associated with socioeconomic disadvantages and historical and contemporary injustices.
- Promotion of equal opportunities for all people to be healthy and to seek the highest level of health possible.
- Distribution of socioeconomic resources needed to be healthy in a manner that progressively reduces health disparities and improves health for all.
- Continuous efforts to maintain a desired state of equity after avoidable health inequities and health disparities are eliminated.

Note that health equity is different from equality. In order to ensure that individuals are provided with the resources they need to have access to the same opportunities, different types and degrees of support are needed. If both a 6-ft and a 4-ft person are hoping to see over a 7-ft wall, giving them each a 12-in stool helps one and frustrates the other. What will each of your patients need to optimize their health? One size fits all definitely does not apply here!

Fostering Diversity, Inclusion, and Equity

As nurses are being called to work actively to create health equity, it is important to reflect on why health disparities are so persistent, seemingly in spite of many collective efforts to address them. We know that **institutional or structural racism**, the systematic distribution of resources, power, and opportunity in our society to the benefit of people who are White and to the exclusion of people of color, plays a role, as does **unconscious or implicit bias**, prejudice in favor of or against one thing, person, or group as compared to another, in a way that is usually considered unfair. Unconscious bias occurs automatically, as the brain makes quick judgments based on past experiences and backgrounds. Until everyone in health care is committed to creating a culture of respectful diversity, inclusion, and equity, disparities will persist. The status quo of race-neutral, race-blind, or culturally competent care will only strengthen existing disparities. Know that the ANA *Code of Ethics for Nurses with Interpretive Statements* (Provision 8.3) obligates nurses to advance health and human rights and reduce disparities (ANA, 2015). The ANA also published a Position Statement in 2018 titled "The Nurse's Role in Addressing Discrimination: Protecting and Promoting Inclusive Strategies in Practice Settings, Policy, and Advocacy."

Koschmann et al. (2020) issued an urgent call for **antiracism** in nursing practice, which requires every nurse to engage in a daily practice of actively combating **racism**, including structures, institutions, and practices: "Rather than race-neutral or culturally competent care, antiracist practice actively stands against racism. We must face the epidemic of racism head on by applying rigorous changes to nursing practice, research and education, and, as is always true with our profession, do this with empathy and respect" (p. 540). See Figure 3-4 (on page 62), Becoming Anti-Racist, for practical strategies to help you move into the learning and growth zones.

Monica McLemore (2020) describes five tools and skills nurses can implement incrementally. She uses "SPLIT" to describe these: ***S***imulation, ***P***ublic health, ***L***eading, ***I***mmersion, and ***T***ension. For McLemore, SPLIT is a simple way to think about what we can do right now about the awareness people are starting to gain of the lived experiences of Black, Indigenous, and other people of color. "We [nurses] need to publicly address the fact that we are on the side of the people we serve . . . People are looking for us to lead—learners, the unit staff, all the places within our health care institutions where we have some racial and ethnic diversity . . . As nurses, we need to enlist the tools we have and adapt them to assist us as novices in racial justice and antiracism work. There are no CliffsNotes or shortcuts." (p. 70)

Diversity is about welcoming individuals of all races, religions, nationalities, cultures, ages, sexual orientations, and identities. **Inclusion** is about giving everyone a sense of purpose and belonging, a feeling of being valued. The example is often giving that diversity is about inviting different people to a dance. When we are dancing with one another that is inclusion. If you walk into a cafeteria where Whites sit at one table and Blacks and other people of color at different tables, you may have diversity but not inclusion. Similarly, **equity** is not about treating everyone the same, it is about ensuring that everyone has access to the conditions they need to thrive. What one person needs to manage diabetes may be very different than what another needs. It is never too early to begin assessing the cultures you will experience in different work settings and to question those cultures in which inclusion is the exception and equity an unrealized goal. See the Challenging Topics feature on page 62.

Vulnerable Populations

National trends in efforts to prevent health disparities focus on **vulnerable populations**, such as racial and ethnic minorities, those living in poverty, women, children, older adults, residents of rural areas and low-income areas of cities, and people with disabilities and special health care needs. Be sure to check out the Vulnerable Populations Alert in this and other chapters. Emphasis is given to disparities in access to care, quality of care, health insurance status, specific sources of ongoing care, and quality and access to care for people with limited English proficiency. It is critical that nurses recognize that disparities exist and plan specific and individualized interventions for patients who are most at risk.

(text continues on page 64)

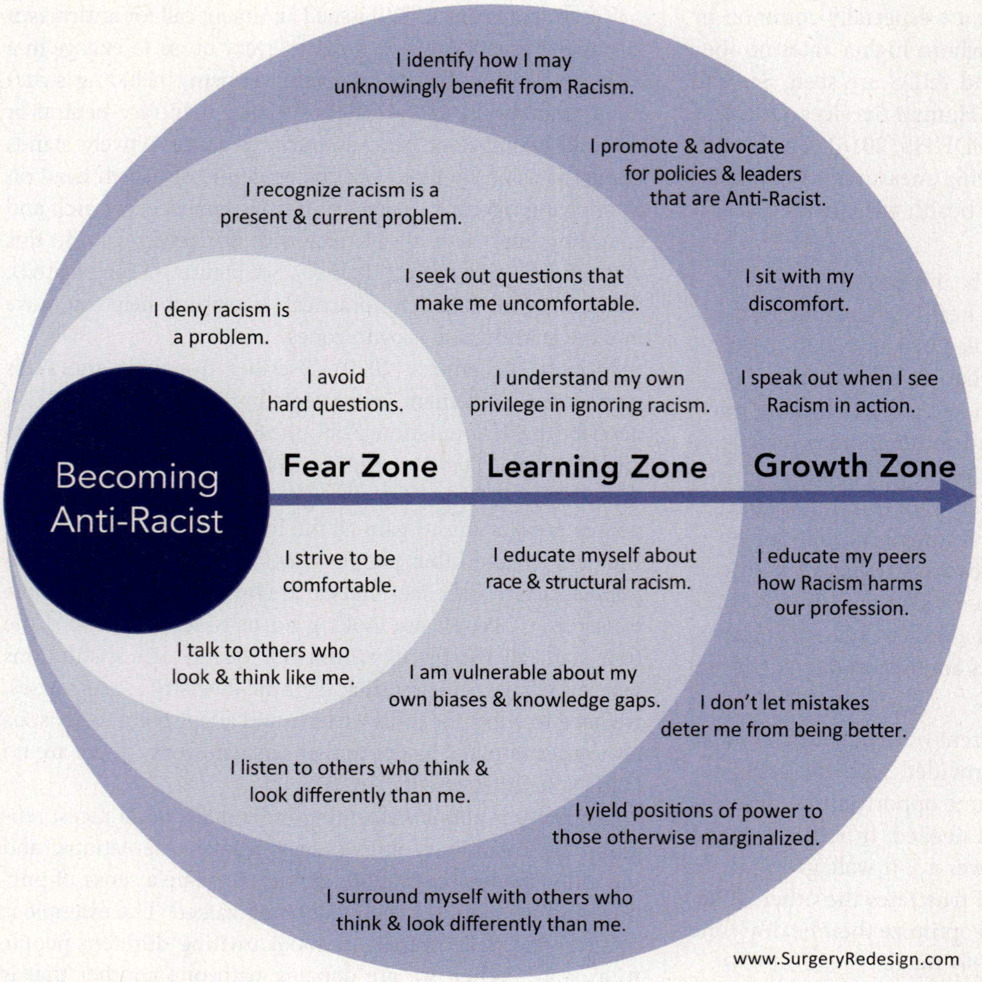

FIGURE 3-4. Becoming antiracist. (*Source:* Used with permission. https://www.surgeryredesign.com/.)

Thoughtful, Person-Centered Practice: Challenging Topics

Health Equity and Persistent Health Disparities

Many controversial issues make it challenging to know how to respond as a professional nurse in select scenarios. Often, the nurse's personal and/or professional values may conflict with options desired by patients, families, colleagues, employers and communities. Too often our practice environments prioritize generating revenues and saving money over excellent patient care. Where institutional racism and unconscious bias create a culture that exacerbates health disparities, nurses often struggle to meet the all too real needs of vulnerable patients.

Read the scenario below and see if you can articulate what you believe, why you believe this, and how these beliefs are likely to inform the decisions you make and your behavior, especially when you are confronted with competing obligations. Based on Tanner's Clinical Judgment Model (2006), consider reflection-in-action and reflection-on-action (Nielson et al., 2007):

Reflection-in-Action

As you read, consider what the new nurse is thinking in the moment—what happened? How did the patient, family, and/or health care provider respond? What did the nurse do next?

Scenario

I was excited to be doing a senior year clinical rotation in an emergency room in a major city. We got very busy one evening during a Black Lives Matter protest following the shooting of a local, unarmed young Black man. Allegedly, some of the protestors became violent and started looting, and the police began using tear gas, rubber bullets and force for crowd control. We received a number of patients with eye damage, bruising, some broken bones, and bleeding. When I brought my concerns about one patient who was still sitting in the waiting room in obvious discomfort, needing to be seen, to the attention of one of the physicians, I was told that many of these patients got what was coming to them and not to worry. "These thugs are tough, they'll survive." I was startled to hear an opinion like this coming from a physician whose expertise I admired.

Effective Noticing (Cues)

1. What did you notice about the situation initially? What information/observations are significant? What information deviates from what is expected/normal/usual?

Effective Interpreting

2. How would you prioritize this data? What other assessment data, evidence and/or information would you need to consider the situation? How would you obtain this additional information?
3. What do you think about this situation? Consider personal and previous nursing experiences that you have had and formal knowledge (physiology, psychology, sociology, communication skills) that may be of assistance in providing care in this situation.

Scenario

Shocked by the physician's comment, I stepped back and returned to my duties with another patient. How could this physician even know if this was a peaceful protester or someone turned violent—and should that even matter? How in heaven's name could I effect change as a student and a guest in this emergency room? In school, we learned a lot about health equity and health disparities, and I was aware that not all patients received exactly the same care—but this racist comment shocked me into silence. I remembered that my code of ethics taught me to practice with compassion and respect for the inherent dignity, worth, and unique attributes of every person. What did this mean that evening in our busy emergency department? I didn't feel comfortable continuing to advocate for this patient, but I also didn't feel comfortable leaving him alone. Did I have any obligation to challenge the status quo? Later that night I had difficulty trying to fall asleep. I kept wondering about that patient and the many others like him, still facing indifference or worse from health care professionals on a daily basis.

Effective Responding

4. How would you describe the obligations you have in this scenario to your patient, to yourself, and to your team? Do you agree with the statement that being antiracist is not political rhetoric but is rather a moral imperative.
5. If you cannot fulfill each of these obligations how will you prioritize them? What basis/rationale do you use for prioritization? Remember that the ANA *Code of Ethics for Nurses* reminds us that nurses "are responsible for contributing to a moral environment that demands respectful interactions among colleagues, mutual peer support, and open identification of difficult issues, which include ongoing professional development of staff in ethical problem solving."

Effective Reflecting

6. This was not the first racist comment or behavior that this student observed in this hospital, which made her question the institutional culture and ethical environment. As a student, she certainly wasn't in a position of power to effect change.
7. Do you agree with the choice the nurse made? Would you have made the same choice, why or why not? What would inform your decision? If the nurse had refused to back down and reported her concerns up the chain of command would you champion her cause?
8. Do you agree with the criteria the nurse used to evaluate her decision? How do you evaluate your clinical and moral judgments?
9. What resources can you access to better inform your decision?
10. Whether or not you would decide to challenge the physician, how might you use reflective practice to evaluate your decision so you can respond more confidently in the future? What criteria will you use to evaluate a good response?
11. What personal attributes and competencies are most likely to lead to a good response?

Reflection-on-Action

Then look back at the nurse's decisions and reflect on your learning—how did your knowledge and/or skills expand based on this scenario? What attitude, value, or belief shifts did you experience (if any) after reading this scenario? What would you do differently if you were in this situation? What more do you need to know to be able to manage this or a similar situation in the future?

Nielson, A., Stragnell, S., & Jester, P. (2007). Guide for reflection using the Clinical Judgment Model. *Journal of Nursing Education*, *46*(11), 513–516.

Tanner, C. A. (2006). Thinking like a nurse: a research-based model of clinical judgment in nursing. *Journal of Nursing Education*, *45*(6), 204–211.

Vulnerable Population Alert: Caring for Patients Who Are Homeless

Depending on where you live and practice, you may rarely or frequently encounter patients who are homeless. People who are homeless do not have a regular and appropriate place to sleep at night, may include adults and children, and may be sheltered or unsheltered.

If your patient is homeless, how will this influence the treatment plan:

- for a patient with a newly diagnosed cancer?
- for someone who has been exposed to COVID-19 and needs to self-quarantine for 14 days?
- for a patient who needs IV antibiotics and daily dressing changes?
- for a patient in renal failure who needs dialysis?
- for a child who needs a liver small bowel transplant?

Resources

Homeless Advocacy Project https://haplegal.org/

National Alliance to End Homelessness: How to get help if you are experiencing homelessness https://endhomelessness.org/how-to-get-help-experiencing-homelssness/

Substance Abuse and Mental Health Services Administration: Homelessness programs and resources www.samhsa.gov/homelessness-programs-resources

U.S. Department of Health and Human Services: Resources https://www.hhs.gov/programs/social-services/homelessness/index.html

Source: Adapted from Mcenroe-Petitte, D. M. (2020). Caring for patients who are homeless. *Nursing, 2020, 50*(3), 24–31.

Health Disparities and COVID-19

In 2020, we definitely witnessed the dramatic consequences of health disparities. Writing in July 2020 (https://www.healthaffairs.org/do/10.1377/hblog20200716.620294/full/), Wen and Sadeghi commented that, with nearly 3 million confirmed COVID-19 cases and more than 131,000 deaths, communities of color are bearing the brunt of the pandemic.

> New federal data reveals that African Americans and Latinos in the U.S. have been three time more likely to contract COVID-19 than white residents and nearly twice as likely to die from it. Some counties with a majority of African American residents have almost six times the death rate compared to counties that are predominantly white. In some states such as Illinois, Latinos have nearly seven times the rate of COVID-19 cases compared to white peoples, while African Americans have the highest death rate.

Wen and Sadeghi explain that health disparities during the COVID-19 pandemic reflect two important patterns of inequity: (1) underrepresented communities have a higher likelihood of contracting the virus by living in urban areas and disproportionately working in higher-risk environments, and (2) racial minorities also experience higher rates of chronic medical conditions, including obesity, diabetes, and kidney disease, which are risk factors for severe illness from COVID-19.

On August 4, 2020, the American Academy of Nursing and the American Nurses Association issued a call for social justice to address racism and health equity in communities of color (https://www.nursingworld.org/news/news-releases/2020/the-american-academy-of-nursing-and-the-american-nurses-association-call-for-social-justice-to-address-racism-and-health-equity-in-communities-of-color/). Noting that our Code of Ethics obligates nurses to be allies and to speak up against racism, discrimination, and injustice, the statement urges every nurse to:

> . . . remove areas of bias that perpetuate negative behaviors and reinforce harmful stereotypes and stigmas. This extends to those biases held by nurses and other health care providers. Working together, health professionals, public health officials, health care and industry leaders, system administrators, and policy makers, can confront and directly address these behaviors along with the unfair practices that lead to discrimination against Black and Brown individuals and communities of color. It is imperative in this time of incredible uncertainty and unrest, that we create and sustain cultures of understanding, belonging, open dialogue, and inclusion in workplaces, within our profession, and in communities. Commitment to addressing bias is a meaningful starting point to make lasting change.

Calling us to continued vigilance, the statement urges us to be change agents by responding to racism when we experience or see it occur, further our understanding of implicit and unconscious bias, and work within our own institutions to develop cultures of inclusivity. Moreover, we can advocate for policies at the local, state, and national level that address health equity, which will not only improve well-being now, but also continue to lay the foundation for better health in the future. See Box 3-3 for key resources on health disparities.

Nurse Self-Care Alert

The *Nursing: Scope and Standards of Practice* (ANA, 2021) reminds us that nurses must first respect themselves before being capable of respecting others. They must become clear on how equity, diversity, inclusion, and social justice inform them as people. This can be a difficult, painful exploration when meeting your own beliefs and biases. Box 3-4 outlines ANA Standard 9: Respectful and Equitable Practice. What work will you need to do to be able to practice with cultural humility and inclusiveness?

FACTORS AFFECTING HEALTH AND ILLNESS

As discussed, many factors influence a person's health status, health beliefs, and health practices. These factors may be internal or external and may or may not be under the person's conscious control. To plan and provide thoughtful, person-centered care, the nurse must understand how these factors influence behavior in both healthy and ill patients.

Basic Human Needs

A basic human need is something essential that must be met for emotional and physiologic health and survival. A person whose needs are met may be considered to be healthy, and a person who has one or more unmet needs is at an increased risk for illness. (Basic human needs are discussed in detail in Chapter 4.)

Human Dimensions

The factors influencing a person's health–illness status, health beliefs, and health practices relate to the person's human dimensions (see Fig. 3-1). Each dimension interrelates with each of the others and influences the person's behaviors in both health and illness. Nursing assessments of strengths and weaknesses in each dimension are used to develop a plan of care that is thoughtful, person-centered, and holistic. The nursing process, used to plan, implement, and evaluate plans of care, is discussed in Unit III.

Physical Dimension

The physical dimension includes genetic inheritance, age, developmental level, race, and sex assigned at birth. These components strongly influence the person's health status and health practices. For example, inherited genetic disorders

Box 3-3 Internet Resources on Health Disparities

Resource	URL
Kaiser Family Foundation: Communities of Color at Higher Risk for Health and Economic Challenges due to COVID-19	https://www.kff.org/coronavirus-covid-19/issue-brief/communities-of-color-at-higher-risk-for-health-and-economic-challenges-due-to-covid-19/
Johns Hopkins University: Racial Data Transparency: State COVID-19 Data by Race	https://coronavirus.jhu.edu/data/racial-data-transparency
Rural Health Information Hub	https://www.ruralhealthinfo.org/
National Academies of Sciences, Engineering, and Medicine—Birth Settings in America: Outcomes, Quality, Access, and Choice (2020)	https://www.nap.edu/catalog/25636/birth-settings-in-america-outcomes-quality-access-and-choice
Highlights	https://www.nap.edu/resource/25636/interactive/
Root Cause Coalition—2020 Status of Health Equity Report	https://www.rootcausecoalition.org/sherreport/
How to use the report	https://register.gotowebinar.com/recording/737019542241680897
County Health Ranking—2020 County Health Rankings State Reports	https://www.countyhealthrankings.org/reports/state-reports
The Century Foundation—Racism, Inequality, and Health Care for African Americans	https://production-tcf.imgix.net/app/uploads/2019/12/19172443/AfAmHealth_Jamila_PDF.pdf
Kaiser Family Foundation: Changes in Health Coverage by Race and Ethnicity since the ACA, 2010–2018	https://www.kff.org/racial-equity-and-health-policy/issue-brief/changes-in-health-coverage-by-race-and-ethnicity-since-the-aca-2010-2018/
Archived Podcast: American Hospital Association: Advancing Health, Part 1	https://www.aha.org/advancing-health-podcast/2020-02-18-using-collaboration-advance-health-equity
Part 2	https://www.aha.org/advancing-health-podcast/2020-03-05-value-using-collaboration-advance-health-equity

include Down syndrome, hemophilia, cystic fibrosis, and color blindness. Toddlers are at greater risk for drowning, and adolescents and young adult males are at greater risk for automobile crashes from excessive speed. There are specific racial traits for disease, including sickle cell anemia, hypertension, and stroke. A young, biologically female person whose mother and grandmother had breast cancer is more likely to have an annual clinical breast examination and mammogram.

Emotional Dimension

How the mind affects body functions and responds to body conditions also influences health. Long-term stress affects body systems, and anxiety affects health habits; conversely, calm acceptance and relaxation can actually change the body's responses to illness. As examples of the negative effects of emotions, a student may always have diarrhea before examinations, and an adolescent with poor

Box 3-4 ANA Standard 9. Respectful and Equitable Practice

The registered nurse practices with cultural humility and inclusiveness.

Competencies

The registered nurse:

- Demonstrates respect, equity, and empathy in actions and interactions with all health care consumers.
- Respects consumer decisions without bias.
- Participates in life-long learning to understand cultural preferences, worldviews, choices, and decision-making processes of diverse consumers.
- Reflects upon personal and cultural values, beliefs, biases, and heritage.
- Applies knowledge of differences in health beliefs, practices, and communication patterns without assigning values to the differences.
- Considers the effects and impact of discrimination and oppression on practice within and among diverse groups.
- Uses appropriate skills and tools for the culture, literacy, and language of the individuals and population served.
- Communicates with appropriate language and behaviors, including the use of qualified health care interpreters and translators in accordance with consumer needs and preferences.
- Serves as a role model and educator for cultural humility and the recognition and appreciation of diversity and inclusivity.
- Identifies the cultural-specific meaning of interactions, terms, and content.
- Advocates for policies that promote health and prevent harm among diverse health care consumers and groups.
- Promotes equity in all aspects of health and health care.
- Advances organizational policies, programs, services, and practice that reflect respect, equity, and values for diversity and inclusion.

Source: Used with permission. ANA. (2021). *Nursing: Scope and standards of practice* (4th ed., p. 93). Silver Spring, MD: Author.

self-esteem may begin to experiment with drugs. Many researchers today are linking the rising deaths by suicide to a sense of meaninglessness related to the shrinking of the family and our sense of connectedness as well as the diminishing role of religion. The positive effects of emotions include reducing surgical pain with relaxation techniques and reducing blood pressure with biofeedback skills.

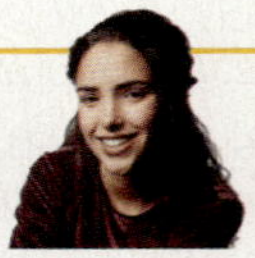

Knowledge of the emotional dimension would be important when planning care for ***Sara Thurston***, the college freshman described at the beginning of the chapter. The nurse needs to examine how she responds to stress and anxiety.

Intellectual Dimension

The intellectual dimension encompasses cognitive abilities, educational background, and past experiences. Whether or not someone can understand the causes of disease and the importance of healthy lifestyle behaviors can have a huge impact on health and wellness. These influence the person's responses to teaching about health and reactions to nursing care during illness. They also play a major role in health behaviors. Examples involving this dimension include a young college student with diabetes who follows a diabetic diet but drinks beer and eats pizza with friends several times a week, and a middle-aged man who quits taking his high blood pressure medication after developing unpleasant side effects.

Environmental Dimension

The environment has many influences on health and illness. Housing, sanitation, climate, and pollution of air, food, and water are elements in the environmental dimension. Examples of environmental causes of illness include deaths in older adults from inadequate heating and cooling; an increased incidence of asthma and respiratory problems in large cities with smog; and an increased incidence of skin cancer in people who live in hot, sunny areas of the world.

Sociocultural Dimension

Health practices and beliefs are strongly influenced by a person's economic level, lifestyle, family, and culture. In general, low-income groups, racial and ethnic minorities, and other underserved populations are less likely to seek medical care to prevent illness and have fewer treatment options, while high-income groups are more prone to stress-related habits and illness. The family and the culture to which a person belongs influence the person's patterns of living and values about health and illness; such patterns are often unalterable. All of these factors are involved in personal care, patterns of eating, lifestyle habits, and emotional stability. Examples of other sociocultural situations that influence health and illness are an adolescent who sees nothing wrong with smoking or drinking because their parents smoke and drink; and parents of a sick infant who do not seek medical care because they have no health insurance.

Spiritual Dimension

Spiritual beliefs and values are important components of a person's health and illness behaviors (see Chapter 47). It is important that nurses respect these values and understand their importance for the individual patient. Examples of the influences of the spiritual dimension on health care include the Roman Catholic requirement of baptism for both live births and stillborn babies; kosher dietary laws, prohibiting the intake of pork and shellfish, practiced by Orthodox and Conservative Jews; and opposition to blood transfusion, common to Jehovah's Witnesses. Perhaps most importantly, as noted above, religion allows people to feel as if they are a part of something larger than themselves and more meaningful than their individual lives, which promotes resilience.

Self-Concept

Another variable influencing health and illness is a person's self-concept (see Chapter 42), which incorporates both how they feel about themselves (self-esteem) and the way they perceive their physical self (body image). Self-concept has both physical and emotional aspects and is an important factor in the way a person reacts to stress and illness, follows self-care health practices, and relates to others.

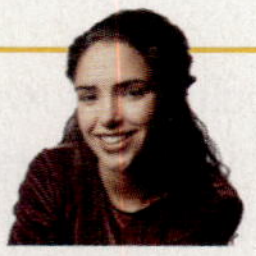

Consider ***Sara Thurston***, the college freshman with a suspected eating disorder. Although she has lost a significant amount of weight, she states that she is healthy but just "nuts" about being fit. Her self-concept is most likely one of being overweight. Consequently, she rarely eats. In contrast, people who are overweight may feel that nothing will change the way they look and refuse to follow a diet and exercise program.

A person's self-concept results from a variety of past experiences, interpersonal interactions, physical and cultural influences, and education. It includes perceptions of one's own strengths and weaknesses. Illness can alter a person's self-concept, as it affects roles, independence, and relationships with important others.

Risk Factors for Illness or Injury

A **risk factor** is something that increases a person's chances for illness or injury. Like other components of health and illness, risk factors are often interrelated. Risk factors may be further defined as modifiable (things a person can change, such as quitting smoking) or nonmodifiable (things that cannot be changed, such as a family history of cancer). As a person's number of risk factors increases, so does the possibility of illness. For example, an executive who is overweight and is under pressure to increase sales may smoke and drink alcohol in excess. These factors, combined with a family history of heart disease, place this person at higher risk for illness.

Table 3-1 Major Areas of Risk Factors

RISK FACTOR	EXAMPLES
Age	School-aged children are at high risk for communicable diseases. After menopause, females are more likely to develop cardiovascular disease.
Genetic factors	A family history of cancer or diabetes predisposes a person to developing the disease.
Physiologic factors	Obesity increases the possibility of heart disease. Pregnancy places increased risk on both the pregnant person and the developing fetus.
Health habits	Smoking increases the probability of lung cancer. Poor nutrition can lead to a variety of health problems.
Lifestyle	Multiple sexual relationships increase the risk for sexually transmitted infections (e.g., gonorrhea or AIDS). Events that increase stress (e.g., divorce, retirement, work-related pressure) may precipitate accidents or illness.
Environment	Working and living environments (such as those where hazardous materials and poor sanitation are present) may contribute to disease.

Table 3-2 Examples of Nursing Activities by Level of Health Promotion and Preventive Care

LEVEL	TOPIC
Primary	Weight loss Diet Exercise Smoking cessation Reduced alcohol consumption Avoidance of illicit drugs Farm safety Seat belts and child safety seats Immunizations Water treatment Safer sex practices Effective parenting
Secondary	Screenings (blood pressure, cholesterol, glaucoma, HIV, skin cancer) Pap smears Mammograms Testicular examinations Family counseling
Tertiary	Medication Medical therapy Surgical treatment Rehabilitation Physical therapy Occupational therapy Job training

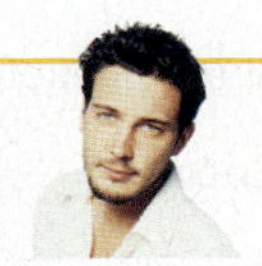

Remember **Daniel Sternman**, the man with schizophrenia. The Mayo Clinic (2019) had identified the following as risk factors for developing mental problems: having a blood relative with a mental illness; stressful life situations, such as financial problems or a loved one's death or divorce; an ongoing chronic medical condition; brain damage as a result of serious injury; traumatic experiences; use of alcohol or recreational drugs; being abused or neglected as a child; having few friends or few healthy relationships; and a previous mental illness.

The six general types of risk factors are described in Table 3-1. Risk factors for each developmental level across the lifespan are included in Unit IV, and cultural influences on risk factors are discussed in Chapter 5.

HEALTH PROMOTION AND ILLNESS PREVENTION

Health promotion is the behavior of a person who is motivated by a personal desire to increase well-being and health potential. In contrast, illness/disease prevention, also called health protection, is behavior motivated by a desire to avoid or detect disease or to maintain functioning within the constraints of an illness or disability (Murdaugh et al., 2019). Health promotion and illness prevention activities are traditionally described as occurring on primary, secondary, and tertiary levels (Leavell & Clark, 1965). Definitions and examples of nursing activities for each level are discussed in the next section and are detailed in Table 3-2.

Primary Health Promotion and Illness Prevention

Primary health promotion and illness prevention are directed toward promoting health and preventing the development of disease processes or injury. Nursing activities at the primary level may focus on people or groups. Examples of primary-level activities are immunization clinics, family-planning services, providing poison-control information, and accident-prevention education. Other nursing interventions include teaching about a healthy diet, the importance of regular exercise, safety in industry and farms, using seat belts, using social distancing and face masks during the pandemic, and safer sex practices.

Health-risk assessments are an important part of primary health promotion and preventive care. A health-risk assessment is an assessment of the total person. The resulting "picture" of the person indicates areas of risk for disease or injury as well as areas that support health. A variety of formats are used to perform this assessment, but all take a broad approach to health, focusing on lifestyle and behaviors. Box 3-5 (on pages 68–69) contains an

Box 3-5 Health-Style Self-Test

All of us want good health, but many of us do not know how to be as healthy as possible. Health experts now describe *lifestyle* as one of the most important factors affecting health. In fact, it is estimated that as many as 7 of the 10 leading causes of death could be reduced through common-sense changes in lifestyle. That's what this brief test, developed by the Public Health Service, is all about. Its purpose is simply to tell you how well you are doing to stay healthy. The behaviors covered in the test are recommended for most Americans. Some of them may not apply to people with certain chronic diseases or disabilities, or to pregnant people. Such people may require special instructions from their health care providers.

Cigarette Smoking

If you *never smoke* enter a score of 10 for this section and go to the next section on Alcohol and Drugs.

almost always	sometimes	almost never	
2	1	0	1. I avoid smoking cigarettes.
2	1	0	2. I smoke only low-tar and nicotine cigarettes *or* I smoke a pipe or cigars.

Smoking score: ________

Alcohol and Drugs

almost always	sometimes	almost never	
2	1	0	1. I avoid drinking alcoholic beverages *or* I drink no more than one or two drinks a day.
2	1	0	2. I avoid using alcohol or other drugs (especially illegal drugs) as a way of handling stressful situations or the problems in my life.
2	1	0	3. I am careful not to drink alcohol when taking certain medicines (e.g., medicine for sleeping, pain, colds, and allergies), or when pregnant.
2	1	0	4. I read and follow the label directions when using prescribed and over-the-counter drugs.

Alcohol and drugs score: ________

Eating Habits

almost always	sometimes	almost never	
2	1	0	1. I eat a variety of foods each day, such as fruits and vegetables, whole-grain breads and cereals, lean meats, dairy products, dry peas and beans, and nuts and seeds.
2	1	0	2. I limit the amount of fat, saturated fat, and cholesterol I eat (including fat on meats, eggs, butter, cream, shortenings, and organ meats such as liver).
2	1	0	3. I limit the amount of salt I eat by cooking with only small amounts, not adding salt at the table, and avoiding salty snacks.
2	1	0	4. I avoid eating too much sugar (especially frequent snacks of sticky candy or soft drinks).

Eating habits score: ________

Exercise and Fitness

almost always	sometimes	almost never	
2	1	0	1. I maintain a desired weight, avoiding overweight and underweight.
2	1	0	2. I do vigorous exercises for 15 to 30 minutes at least three times a week (examples include running, swimming, brisk walking).
2	1	0	3. I do exercises that enhance my muscle tone for 15 to 30 minutes at least three times a week (examples include yoga and calisthenics).
2	1	0	4. I use part of my leisure time participating in individual, family, or team activities that increase my level of fitness (such as gardening, bowling, golf, and baseball).

Exercise/fitness score: ________

Stress Control

almost always	sometimes	almost never	
2	1	0	1. I have a job or do other work that I enjoy.
2	1	0	2. I find it easy to relax and express my feelings freely.
2	1	0	3. I recognize early, and prepare for, events or situations likely to be stressful for me.
2	1	0	4. I have close friends, relatives, or others whom I can talk to about personal matters and call on for help when needed.
2	1	0	5. I participate in group activities (such as church and community organizations) or hobbies that I enjoy.

Stress control score: ________

Safety

almost always	sometimes	almost never	
2	1	0	1. I wear a seat belt while riding in a car.
2	1	0	2. I avoid driving while under the influence of alcohol and other drugs.
2	1	0	3. I obey traffic rules and the speed limit when driving.
2	1	0	4. I am careful when using potentially harmful products or substances (such as household cleaners, poisons, and electrical devices).
2	1	0	5. I avoid smoking in bed.

Safety score: ________

What Your Scores Mean to You

Scores of 9 and 10

Excellent! Your answers show that you are aware of the importance of this area to your health. More important, you are putting your knowledge to work for you by practicing good health habits. As long as you continue to do so, this area should not pose a serious health risk. It's likely that you are setting an example for your family and friends to follow. Because you got a very high test score on this part of the test, you may want to consider other areas where your scores indicate room for improvement.

Box 3-5 Health-Style Self-Test *(continued)*

Scores of 6 to 8

Your health practices in this area are good, but there is room for improvement. Look again at the items you answered with "Sometimes" or "Almost never." What changes can you make to improve your score? Even a small change can often help you achieve better health.

Scores of 3 to 5

Your health risks are showing! Would you like more information about the risks you are facing and about why it is important for you to change these behaviors? Perhaps you need help in deciding how to make the changes you desire. In either case, help is available.

Scores of 0 to 2

Obviously, you were concerned enough about your health to take the test, but your answers show that you may be taking serious and unnecessary risks with your health. Perhaps you are unaware of the risks and what to do about them. You can easily get the information and help you need to improve, if you wish. The next step is up to you.

Suggested Self-Care Behaviors

Start by asking yourself a few frank questions: *Am I really doing all I can to be as healthy as possible? What steps can I take to feel better? Am I willing to begin now?* If you scored low in one or more sections of the test, decide what changes you want to make for improvement. You might pick that aspect of your lifestyle where you feel you have the best chance for success and tackle that one first. Once you have improved your score there, go on to other areas.

Lifestyle practices that promote health include:

- Sleeping regularly, 7 to 8 hours per night
- Eating regular meals, which include recommended food groups
- Maintaining ideal body weight
- Having a regular schedule of exercise
- Using alcohol in moderation, if at all
- Not smoking
- Maintaining positive mental health and self-concept
- Practicing safer sex
- Wearing seatbelts, using car seats for children, and wearing bicycle helmets
- Having recommended screenings and checkups by your medical and dental health care providers

If you already have tried to change your health habits (e.g., to stop smoking or exercise regularly), don't be discouraged if you haven't yet succeeded. The difficulty you have encountered may be due to influences you've never really thought about—such as advertising—or to a lack of support and encouragement. Understanding these influences is an important step toward changing the way they affect you.

There's help available. In addition to personal actions you can take on your own, there are community programs and groups (such as the YMCA or the local chapter of the American Heart Association) that can assist you and your family to make the changes you want to make. If you want to know more about these groups or about health risks, contact the National Health Information Center (https://health.gov/our-work/health-literacy/resources/national-health-information-center).

There's a lot you can do to stay healthy or to improve your health, and there are organizations that can help you. Start a new "health style" today!

example of a health-style self-test the patient completes. As you work with patients in both hospital and community settings to provide care, use this self-test to help your patients assess their state of health and health risks and learn a new health style through recommended lifestyle practices that support health. But first use it to assess your own state of health and health risks.

The patient-centered assessment method (PCAM) is a tool nurses can use to assess patient complexity using the social determinants of health that often explain why some patients engage and respond well in managing their health, while others with similar health conditions do not experience the same outcomes (see the PCAM tool in Chapter 15, Fig. 15-4). You are best able to recognize factors affecting peoples' ability to manage their health care if you pay attention to their health and well-being (lifestyle behaviors, impact of their physical health on their mental health, and their ability to enjoy daily activities), their social environment (status of employment, housing, transportation, and social networks), and their health literacy and communication skills (understanding of their symptoms and risk factors, language and cultural differences, and learning difficulties).

Concept Mastery Alert

During primary prevention, teaching is an important activity. However, before teaching can be initiated, it is essential that the nurse engage the patient in a discussion about their health risks and the implications of these risks. Then, once the risks are identified, the nurse can develop a patient-specific teaching strategy to help the patient address the risks.

Secondary Health Promotion and Illness Prevention

Secondary health promotion and illness prevention focus on screening for early detection of disease with prompt diagnosis and treatment of any found. The goals of secondary preventive care are to identify an illness, reverse or reduce its severity or provide a cure, and thereby return the person to maximum health as quickly as possible. The Patient Protection and Affordable Care Act (ACA) of 2010, which broadens the scope of preventive care, also helps reduce health disparities so that underserved groups can reach their full health potential. Examples of nursing activities at this level are assessing children for normal growth and development and encouraging regular medical, dental, and vision examinations. Proposals to repeal the ACA are placing these preventive care options in jeopardy. Other activities include screenings (e.g., blood pressure, cholesterol, skin cancer), recommending gynecologic examinations and mammograms for females at appropriate ages, and teaching testicular self-examination to males. Direct nursing care interventions at the secondary level include administering medications and caring for wounds.

Concept Mastery Alert

Screenings are a major activity involved in secondary health promotion.

Tertiary Health Promotion and Illness Prevention

Tertiary health promotion and illness prevention begins after an illness is diagnosed and treated, with the goal of reducing disability and helping rehabilitate patients to a maximum level of functioning. Nursing activities on a tertiary level include teaching a patient with diabetes how to recognize and prevent complications, using physical therapy to prevent contractures in a patient who has had a stroke or spinal cord injury, and referring a patient to a support group after removal of a breast because of cancer. Nurses play an important role in monitoring the responses of the patient to the prescribed therapy and in providing services to facilitate the patient's recovery or improve quality of life while living with the effects of an illness or injury.

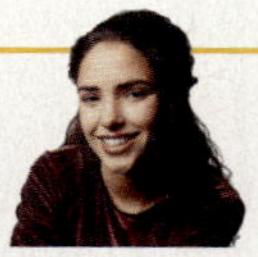

Think back to ***Sara Thurston***, the college freshman. If she is diagnosed with an eating disorder, the nurse would use tertiary preventive care by referring the patient to an eating disorders support group. For Ruth Jacobi, the woman being discharged after a mini-stroke, tertiary preventive care would include educating her about the warning signs and symptoms of a major stroke and about measures to reduce her risk.

MODELS OF HEALTH PROMOTION AND ILLNESS PREVENTION

Models of why and how people behave in ways to promote health and prevent illness help health care providers understand health-related behaviors and adapt care to people from diverse economic and cultural backgrounds. This knowledge can be used to overcome barriers to health from disparities in care resulting from such factors as the increasing number of people without health insurance, a predicted increase in underrepresented populations, and a lack of accessible and essential health care services for low-income and rural populations.

Health Belief Model

Free or low-cost screens and health information are available in most areas to help detect disease early and to educate people about healthy living. Why, then, don't more people take advantage of these services or change their lifestyles? This question can be answered with the widely used health belief model, which describes health behaviors.

The health belief model (Rosenstock, 1974) focuses on what people perceive or believe to be true about themselves in relation to their health. This model is based on three components of individual perceptions of threat of a disease: (1) perceived susceptibility to a disease, (2) perceived seriousness of a disease, and (3) perceived benefits of action.

Perceived susceptibility to a disease is the belief that one either will or will not contract a disease. It ranges from being afraid of developing a disease to completely denying that certain behaviors may cause illness. For example, one person who smokes cigarettes may believe they are at risk for lung cancer and may stop smoking, while another person may believe smoking poses no serious threat and continues to smoke.

Perceived seriousness of a disease concerns the person's perception of the threat that disease poses to health and its effects on the person's lifestyle. Perceived seriousness depends on how much the person knows about the disease and can result in a change in health behavior. If a person who smokes knows that lung cancer can cause physical disability or death and therefore affect their ability to work and care for the family, the person is more likely to stop smoking.

The perceived benefits of action are the person's beliefs about how effectively measures will prevent illness. This factor is influenced by the person's conviction that carrying out a recommended action will prevent or modify the disease and by the person's perception of the cost and unpleasant effects of performing the health behavior (compared with not taking any action). For example, the person may believe that stopping smoking will prevent future breathing problems and that the initial withdrawal symptoms can be overcome; therefore, they may stop smoking.

In addition to these three components, a person's health beliefs are affected by modifying factors including demographic variables (such as age and sex assigned at birth), sociopsychologic variables (such as personality and peer group pressure), and structural variables (such as knowledge and prior contact with the disease). These factors interact to influence the perceived benefits of preventive action minus the perceived barriers to preventive action. Another modifying factor is a cue to action, including activities such as others' advice, mass-media campaigns, literature, appointment-reminder telephone calls or postcards, and the illness of a significant other. The likelihood of taking a recommended preventive health action is thus a composite of individual perceptions and modifying factors. We saw this dramatically when research revealed that teens and young adults who vaped were five to seven times more likely to be infected with COVID-19 than those who did not use e-cigarettes (Gaiha et al., 2020). A belief that their youth will protect them or that their symptoms will not be severe (both of which are not true) reduces their likelihood of stopping vaping. Recent research indicates that self-efficacy should be added as another component of the health belief model. Self-efficacy, one's own belief in the ability to reach goals and complete tasks, is a strong influence on a person's choices, particularly regarding health behaviors (Murdaugh et al., 2019).

The health belief model is useful when teaching about health and illness. You can assess the patient's related beliefs and together structure goals to help realistically meet health needs. Teaching and health promotion activities are ineffective, however, unless the patient believes that they are important and necessary. How would you use the health belief model to change teen vaping behaviors?

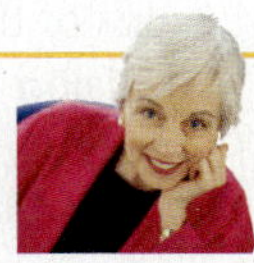

Consider **Ruth Jacobi**, the woman being discharged after a mini-stroke. The patient indicates that she is positively motivated to achieve health, providing the nurse with valuable information about her health beliefs. Together, the nurse and patient can determine realistic goals. The nurse, then, could use this model to develop the patient's teaching plan, including information about the underlying disease process, risk factors for stroke, and ways to reduce the patient's risk for a major stroke.

Health Promotion Model

The health promotion model (Murdaugh et al., 2019) was developed to illustrate how people interact with their environment as they pursue health. The model incorporates individual characteristics and experiences, as well as behavior-specific knowledge and beliefs, to motivate health-promoting behavior. Nurses can use the components of the model to design and provide interventions to promote health for people, families, and communities.

Individual characteristics and experiences can be useful to predict if a person will incorporate and use health-related behaviors. If a behavior has been used before and becomes a habit, it is more likely to be used again. Personal biologic, psychological, and sociocultural factors—including age, sex assigned at birth, strength, self-esteem, perceived health status, definition of health, acculturation, and socioeconomic status—all help predict a given health-related habit. For example, the person who has high self-esteem, defines self as healthy, and has an adequate income is less likely to use alcohol or tobacco and more likely to follow a healthy diet and take part in regular exercise. Conversely, a person with low self-esteem, a fatalistic attitude toward health, and low socioeconomic status is more likely to have poor nutrition, not exercise, and use addictive substances.

Behavior-specific knowledge, beliefs, and relationships are considered major motivators for health-promoting behaviors. These include the knowledge that that there will be a positive outcome from a specific health behavior, the belief that one has the skill and competence to engage in health behaviors, and the influences of others (especially family, peers, and health care providers). Situational influences, such as no-smoking policies, also influence health behaviors. Barriers to action, which include perceptions of unavailability, inconvenience, expense, difficulty, or time, usually result in avoidance of a behavior.

A revised health promotion model includes three additional variables: activity-related affect, a commitment to a plan of action, and immediate competing demands and preferences. Behaviors may induce either a positive or negative subjective response or affect. If the activity initiates a positive reaction, the behavior will likely be repeated; if the emotional reaction is negative, the person will likely avoid that behavior. A person initiates a health-related behavior by committing to a plan of action, accompanied by developing associated strategies to perform the valued behavior. Failure to sustain the behavior may result from competing demands. For example, a person may begin a low-fat diet but "give in" to the convenience of fast foods. Health-related behavior is the outcome of the model and is directed toward attaining positive health outcomes and experiences throughout the lifespan (Murdaugh et al., 2019).

Health–Illness Continuum

The health–illness continuum is one way to conceptualize a person's level of health. This model views health as a constantly changing state, with high-level wellness and death at opposite ends of a graduated scale, or continuum (Fig. 3-5). This continuum illustrates the ever-changing state of health as a person adapts to changes in internal and external environments to maintain a state of well-being. For example,

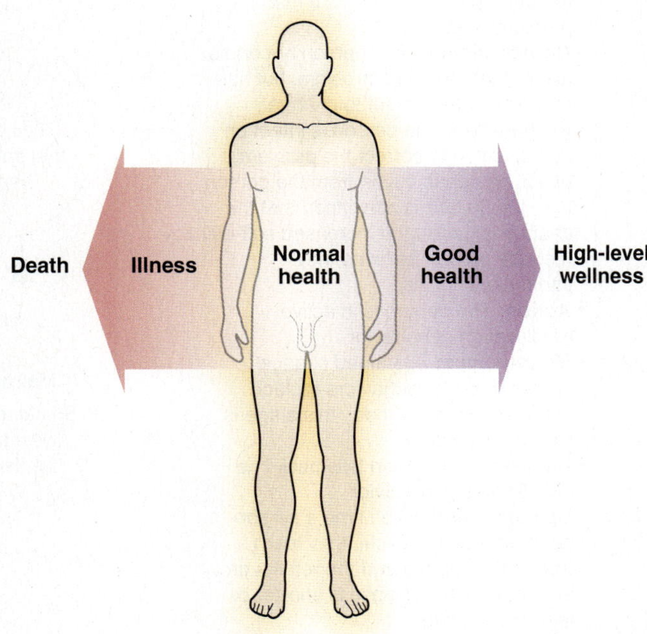

FIGURE 3-5. The health–illness continuum.

patients with cancer may view themselves at different points on the continuum at any given time, depending on how well they believe they are functioning with the illness.

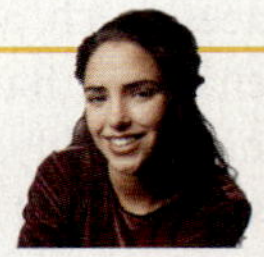

Think back to ***Sara Thurston***, the college freshman described in the Reflective Practice display. The nurse could apply the health–illness continuum model when assessing this patient, recognizing that the stressors of college life have resulted in a shift along the continuum for this patient away from high-level wellness.

Agent–Host–Environment Model

The agent–host–environment model of health and illness, developed by Leavell and Clark (1965), views the interaction between an external agent, a susceptible host, and the environment as causes of disease in a person. It is a traditional model that explains how certain factors place some people at risk for an infectious disease—a model that is currently helpful in addressing COVID-19. These factors are constantly interacting, and a combination of factors may increase the risk of illness. The use of this model is limited when dealing with noninfectious diseases, and other models have proved more useful.

Stages of Change Model

Prochaska and DiClemente developed the Stages of Change Model in the late 1970s and early 1980s while trying to help people with addictions. The model is widely used today by counselors addressing a broad range of behaviors including injury prevention, overcoming drug and alcohol addictions, and weight loss. Figure 3-6 illustrates stages in the model. As you read brief descriptions of the stages below, think about the communication and interventions nurses might use in each stage to help someone change problematic behaviors.

Precontemplation. In this stage, people are not even thinking about trying to change their behavior. DiClemente lists as reasons the four Rs: reluctance, rebellion, resignation, and rationalization. Counselors can validate the lack of readiness to change and encourage self-exploration.

Contemplation. People ambivalently consider the need to change the problematic behavior. Counselors can help by focusing on educating about the pros and cons of the behavior and change, and clarify that the decision to change is one that only the individual can make.

Determination: Commitment to Action. Now the decision is made to move forward and preparation ensues. Counselors are most helpful in this stage by helping people make realistic plans, with small steps that anticipate difficulties, and by identifying creative strategies to address the difficulties. It is helpful to affirm that the individual has the ability to change behaviors.

Action: Implementing the Plan. When someone publicly begins to implement the plan and begins to achieve success, it reinforces the decision to change behavior. If family, friends, and coworkers understand

- **Precontemplation:** A logical starting point for the model, where there is no intention of changing behavior; the person may be unaware that a problem exists
- **Contemplation:** The person becomes aware that there is a problem, but has made no commitment to change
- **Preparation:** The person is intent on taking action to correct the problem; usually requires buy-in from the person (i.e., the person is convinced that the change is good) and increased self-efficacy (i.e., the person believes they can make change)
- **Action:** The person is in active modification of behavior
- **Maintenance:** Sustained change occurs and new behaviors replace old ones; per this model, this stage is also transitional
- **Relapse:** The person falls back into old patterns of behavior
- **Upward spiral:** Each time a person goes through the cycle, they learn from each relapse and (hopefully) grow stronger so that relapse is shorter or less devastating

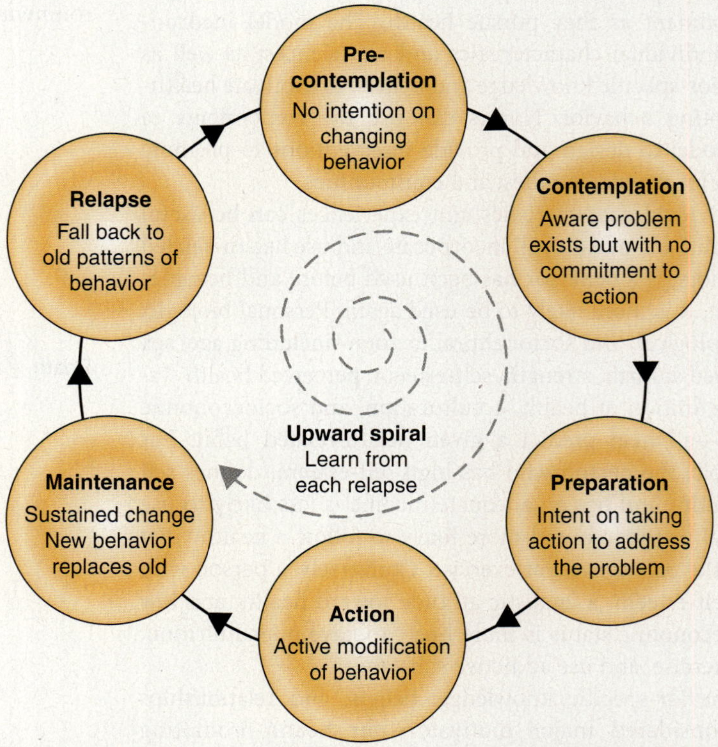

FIGURE 3-6. Prochaska and DiClemente's stages of change model. (*Source:* Adapted from Prochaska, J. O., & DiClemente, C. C. [1983]. Stages and processes of self-change of smoking: toward an integrative model of change. *Journal of Consulting and Clinical Psychology*, *51*[3], 390–395.)

that the person has decided to eat differently or stop drinking, they can become supporters. Counselors can bolster the person's ability to change by reiterating long-term benefits.

Maintenance, Relapse, and Recycling. During this stage, people focus on sustaining the new behavior in a stage that can last from 6 months to 5 years. Counselors can be helpful by exploring strategies to support the new behaviors and by continuing support during relapse.

NURSING CARE TO PROMOTE HEALTH AND PREVENT ILLNESS

The current focus on health promotion and illness prevention at local, state, national, and global levels is important to nursing. Chapter 1 provides information about Healthy People 2030, a national agenda to promote health. The "Healthy People Tools and Resources" page on the Healthy People 2020 website (https://www.healthypeople.gov/2020/tools-resources) identifies tools and evidence-based resources nurses can use to improve the health of their community. See Chapters 4 and 12 for other suggestions. Chapters 23 and 24 discuss recommended screenings, immunizations, and safety practices across the lifespan.

Nurse Self-Care Alert

As emphasized in Chapter 1, nurses must take care of their own health to be able to give effective nursing care to others. Good personal health enables nurses not only to practice more efficiently but also to serve as role models for patients and families. Nurses can help patients acquire new health behaviors by modeling the very behaviors they are trying to promote. It is difficult for nurses to be sincerely attentive to the needs of patients when their own needs are not being met. Because no one is perfectly healthy all of the time, nurses who are preparing for professional practice should spend time getting to know themselves. From this self-knowledge should come a commitment to actively pursue holistic health. See healthynurse@ana.org and respond to the Healthy Nurse, Healthy Nation Grand Challenge (Dawson, 2017). To help you increase your self-knowledge, complete the health-style self-test in Box 3-5 on pages 68–69.

Concept Mastery Alert

Primary role is not the same as primary prevention. Primary role is individually directed, whereas primary prevention focuses on activities that foster health for individuals, groups, and communities.

The Promoting Health boxes highlighted throughout this text may also be useful to you as well as to your patients. Use these guides to assess and identify both your strengths and risks for alterations in health. The guides can also serve as a basis for teaching self-care to patients.

As we move further into the 21st century, resources for health care practices for self and others, along with knowledge of health care trends, can help promote health and advocacy for patients and families of all ages and in all settings. Eliminating disparities in health care improves the quality of life for all people. Examples of nurse-led interventions that reduce disparities and provide access to quality health care include:

- A nurse-led clinic in an urban area in Milwaukee, Wisconsin, was established to treat low-income uninsured patients with hypertension and diabetes. Interventions include laboratory tests, low-cost medications, free patient education, and consultations as needed. This program was specifically designed "to reduce excessive wait times, inconvenient locations, and a lack of cultural awareness by health care providers" (Melville, 2011).
- A postdischarge, nurse-led clinic in San Francisco, California, helps patients transition from the inpatient to outpatient setting. This bridge clinic serves vulnerable populations including new immigrants, substance abusers, people experiencing homelessness, and mentally ill patients. Outreach activities include review of medications, assessment of new symptoms, health promotion and education, and referrals as needed. Surveys of these patients have demonstrated significant improvement in self-management for these vulnerable populations (Newbold et al., 2012).
- Residents of impoverished communities in Philadelphia, Pennsylvania, can receive a variety of services at one location. The Family Practice and Counseling Network (FPCN) includes three nurse-led health centers that provide immediate and long-term health care coordinated by a team of nurses including registered and advance practice registered nurses. This care coordination facilitates communication and produces quality patient outcomes (Trossman, 2012).

DEVELOPING CLINICAL REASONING AND CLINICAL JUDGMENT

1. Identify a family in which someone has a chronic illness. Interview as many of the other family members as possible, and discuss the effect of the illness on them. What do you observe about the effects of the illness in relation to the patient's age, type of illness (e.g., AIDS vs. cancer), sex assigned at birth, and family role?
2. List the six human dimensions described in this chapter, and identify your personal strengths and weaknesses in each area. For example, you may have inherited a genetic tendency toward being overweight (a weakness), but have controlled your weight through nutrition and exercise (a strength). After considering your strengths and weaknesses, develop a personal plan for health promotion.
3. In what ways can poverty, race or ethnic group, lack of education, and poor social support influence health outcomes? Does current information about the biologic and

genetic characteristics of underrepresented and underserved populations explain the health disparities experienced by these groups? For example is race or racism a risk for many different types of health problems? Can you identify additional barriers that interfere with quality health care?

4. Not infrequently, nurses become the target of disrespect, racist beliefs, and biases. How would you respond if a White new father asked you to post a sign in the nursery stating that no Black nurses were to touch his baby? What if a patient told you that they didn't want you to be their nurse because of your race, ethnicity, gender, or any other aspect of your identity?
5. Review your institution's policies on sexual misconduct and assault. One in 5 women and 1 in 16 men will face sexual assault while in college, according to a government report. What is your perception of your risk for sexual assault or misconduct? Describe the model of health professional nurses might use to reduce sexual misconduct on campus. What is it about this model that makes it ideal for addressing this challenge?

PRACTICING FOR NCLEX

1. A nurse working in an ambulatory care center provides care for patients experiencing varying levels of health and illness. The nurse bases care on which concepts of health and illness? Select all that apply.
   a. Health and illness are the same for all people.
   b. Health and illness are individually defined by each person.
   c. People with acute illnesses may consider themselves healthy.
   d. People with chronic illnesses have poor health beliefs.
   e. Health is more than the absence of illness.
   f. Illness is the response of a person to a disease.
2. A community health nurse is developing a support group for patients coping with chronic health problems. What chronic health conditions does the nurse anticipate group members might want to discuss? Select all that apply.
   a. Diabetes mellitus
   b. Bronchial pneumonia
   c. Rheumatoid arthritis
   d. Ulcerative colitis
   e. Fractured hip
   f. Otitis media
3. Nurses from hospital in a low-income area of the city are developing educational materials and programs focused on health care for vulnerable populations. When planning community outreach, which members of the community will the nurses include? Select all that apply.
   a. White male diagnosed with HIV
   b. Black teenager who is 6 months pregnant
   c. Hispanic male who has type 2 diabetes
   d. Low-income family living in rural America
   e. Middle-class teacher living in a large city
   f. White infant born with cerebral palsy
4. A nurse has volunteered to give influenza immunizations at a local health clinic. In which level of health promotion and illness prevention is the nurse participating?
   a. Tertiary
   b. Secondary
   c. Primary
   d. Promotive
5. A community health nurse cares for vulnerable populations. What problem will the nurse prioritize for a patient who is homeless?
   a. Love and belonging
   b. Safety
   c. Self-esteem
   d. Self-actualization
6. A clinic nurse works with a population experiencing health disparities. Which patient does the nurse identify as having the highest risk for postponing annual breast examinations and mammograms?
   a. Patient whose best friend had a benign breast lump removed
   b. Patient who lives in a low-income neighborhood
   c. Patient who has a family history of breast cancer
   d. Patient whose family encourages regular physical examinations
7. A nursing student is writing a paper about nurses performing health promotion activities at the tertiary level. Which nursing actions will the student include? Select all that apply.
   a. Running an immunization clinic in a lower-income area of a city
   b. Teaching a patient with an amputation how to care for the residual limb
   c. Providing range-of-motion exercises for a patient who is paralyzed
   d. Teaching parents of toddlers how to childproof their homes
   e. Providing screening for scoliosis for school students
   f. Teaching new parents how to choose and use an infant car seat
8. A nurse is caring for a patient who has been managing their chronic spasticity well for 10 years. The patient states having had increasing spasticity and few falls due to unremitting muscle spasms. The nurse, patient, and health care provider discuss the possibility the patient may be experiencing which phase of illness?
   a. Acute onset of illness
   b. Permanent complication
   c. Need for hospice care
   d. Exacerbation of disease

9. A nurse incorporates concepts from current models of health when providing health promotion classes for patients. What is a key concept of both the health–illness continuum and the high-level wellness models?
   a. Illness as a fixed point in time
   b. The importance of family
   c. Wellness as a passive state
   d. Health as a dynamic state

10. A public health nurse is planning interventions for a community and plans to determine the frequency of diseases in the area. What information will best guide the nurse?
   a. Morbidity table
   b. Disease eradication statistics
   c. Mortality rates
   d. Annual hospital admissions

ANSWERS WITH RATIONALES

1. **b, c, e, f.** Each person defines health and illness individually, based on a number of factors. Health is more than just the absence of illness; it is an active process in which a person moves toward their maximum potential. An illness is the response of the person to a disease.
2. **a, c, d.** Diabetes, arthritis, and ulcerative colitis are chronic diseases causing permanent, irreversible alterations in normal anatomy and/or physiology. They require a lengthy period of care, support, and patient education. Pneumonia, fractures, and otitis media are acute illnesses, characterized by a rapid onset and typically short duration.
3. **b, c, d, f.** National trends in the prevention of health disparities are focused on vulnerable populations, such as racial and ethnic minorities, those living in poverty, women, children, older adults, residents of rural areas and lower-income areas of cities, and people with disabilities and special health care needs.
4. **c.** Giving influenza injections is an example of primary health promotion and illness prevention. Secondary prevention includes early detection of disease with prompt diagnosis and treatment. Tertiary prevention focuses on reducing disability and providing rehabilitation to a maximum level of functioning.
5. **b.** Safety is the most appropriate focus as adults and children experiencing homelessness do not have a regular and appropriate place to sleep; they may be sheltered or unsheltered. After meeting safety needs, the nurse can focus on love and belonging, self-esteem, or self-actualization.
6. **b.** Healthy People 2020 defines health disparity as a "particular type of health difference that is closely linked with social, economic, and/or environmental disadvantage." Disparities are influenced by race and ethnicity, poverty, sex assigned at birth, age, mental health, educational level, disabilities, sexual orientation, health insurance, and access to health care.
7. **b, c.** Tertiary health promotion and disease prevention begins after an illness is diagnosed and treated to reduce disability and to help rehabilitate patients to a maximum level of functioning. Tertiary interventions include providing ROM exercises and patient teaching for residual limb care. Providing immunizations and teaching parents how to childproof their homes and use an appropriate car seat are primary health promotion activities. Providing screenings is a secondary health promotion activity.
8. **d.** Exacerbation of a chronic illness occurs when the symptoms of a disease reappear after having been absent for a time.
9. **d.** Both these models view health as a dynamic (constantly changing state).
10. **a.** Morbidity refers to how frequently a disease occurs; mortality is the number of deaths resulting from a disease. These statistics may be placed in tables as a reference for others.

Bibliography

Agency for Healthcare Research and Quality. (2020). *National healthcare quality and disparities reports.* https://www.ahrq.gov/research/findings/nhqrdr/index.html

American Nurses Association. (2015). *Code of ethics for nurses with interpretive statements.* Author.

American Nurses Association. (2018). *The nurse's role in addressing discrimination: Protecting and promoting inclusive strategies in practice settings, policy, and advocacy.* https://www.nursingworld.org/_4ab207/globalassets/practiceandpolicy/nursing-excellence/ana-position-statements/social-causes-and-health-care/the-nurses-role-in-addressing-discrimination.pdf

American Nurses Association. (2021). *Nursing, scope and standards of practice,* 4th ed. Author.

ANA Center for Ethics and Human Rights. (2020). Health disparities and end-of-life. *American Nurse Journal, 15*(10), 41.

Arcaya, M. C., & Figueroa, J. F. (2017). Emerging trends could exacerbate health inequities in the United States. *Health Affairs (Millwood), 36*(6), 992–998.

Artiga, S., Orgera, K., & Pham, O. (2020). *Disparities in health and health care: Five key questions and answers.* https://www.kff.org/disparities-policy/issue-brief/disparities-in-health-and-health-care-five-key-questions-and-answers/

Bauer, U. E., Briss, P. A., Goodman, R. A., & Bowman, B. A. (2014). Prevention of chronic disease in the 21st century: Elimination of the leading preventable causes of premature death and disability in the USA. *The Lancet, 384*(9937), 45–52.

Butler, A., Covington, K., & Parxh, B. (2021). Identifying and tackling racial disparities in health care. *Nursing 2021, 51*(9), 40–43.

Carpenter, H., & Gould, L. (2020). Care for family caregivers. *American Nurse Journal, 15*(9), 53.

Case, A., & Deaton, A. (2020). *Deaths of despair and the future of capitalism.* Princeton University Press.

Centers for Disease Control and Prevention (CDC). (n.d.). *Ten essential public health services and how they can include addressing social determinants of health inequities.* https://www.cdc.gov/publichealthgateway/publichealthservices/pdf/ten_essential_services_and_sdoh.pdf

Centers for Disease Control and Prevention. (2014, May 1). *Up to 40 percent of annual deaths from each of five leading US causes are preventable.* http://www.cdc.gov/media/releases/2014/p0501-preventable-deaths.html

Centers for Disease Control and Prevention (CDC). (2016a). *How you can prevent chronic diseases.* http://www.cdc.gov/chronicdisease/about/prevent/index.htm

Centers for Disease Control and Prevention (CDC). (2016b). *Chronic diseases and health promotion.* http://www.cdc.gov/chronicdisease/overview/index.htm

Centers for Disease Control and Prevention (CDC). (2019). *Chronic diseases in America.* https://www.cdc.gov/chronicdisease/resources/infographic/chronic-diseases.htm

Chadha, N., Lim, B., Kane, M., & Rowland, B. (2020). *Toward the abolition of biological race in medicine.* Transforming clinical education, research, and practice. https://belonging.berkeley.edu/race-medicine

Dawson, J. M. (2017). The healthy nurse, healthy nation grand challenge—join now. *American Nurse Today, 12*(5), 27.

DiJulio, B., Hamel, L., Wu, B., & Brodie, M. (2017, November 2). *Serious illness in late life: The public's views and experiences.* Kaiser Family Foundation. https://www.kff.org/other/report/serious-illness-in-late-life-the-publics-views-and-experiences/

Disparities in healthcare quality among racial and ethnic minority groups. Selected findings from the AHRQ 2010 NHQR and NHDR. (2011). *Agency for healthcare research and quality.* http://www.ahrq.gov/qual/nhqrdr10/nhqrdrminority10.htm

Dunn, H. L. (1977). *High-level wellness.* Slack, Inc.

Ernst, M. E., Wiliams, J. R., & McCabe, B. E. (2021). Racial/ethnic differences in stress, coping, and distress among mothers with a child in the ICU. *American Journal of Critical Care, 30*(4), 275–284.

Fauteux, N. (2021). What lies ahead for nursing? *American Journal of Nursing, 121*(4), 57–60.

Gaiha, S. M., Cheng, J., & Halpern-Felsher, B. (2020). Association between youth smoking, electronic cigarette use, and coronavirus disease 2019. *Journal of Adolescent Health, 67*(4), 519–523. https://doi.org/10.1016/j.jadohealth.2020.07.002.

Halsted, C., & Hart, V. T. (2021). Mental health in nursing: A student perspective. *Nursing 2021, 51*(1), 52–55.

Health Equity Institute. (n.d.) *Defining health equity*. http://healthequity.sfsu.edu/content/defining-health-equity

HealthyPeople.gov. *Development of the national health promotion and disease prevention objectives for 2030*. https://www.healthypeople.gov/2020/About-Healthy-People/Development-Healthy-People-2030

Healthy People 2020. (n.d.a). *Disparities*. http://www.healthypeople.gov/2020/about/DisparitiesAbout.aspx

Healthy People 2020. (n.d.b). *Healthy people tools and resources*. https://www.healthypeople.gov/2020/tools-resources

Koschmann, K. S., Jeffers, N. K., & Heidari, O. (2020). "I can't breathe": A call for antiracist nursing practice. *Nursing Outlook, 68*(5), 539–541.

Kristof, N. (2020, January 18). *Are my friends' deaths their fault or ours?* The New York Times. https://www.nytimes.com/2020/01/18/opinion/sunday/deaths-despair-personal-responsibility.html

Kristor, N. D., & WuDunn, S. (2020). *Tightrope: American reaching for hope*. New York: Alfred A. Knopf.

Leavell, H. R., & Clark, E. G. (1965). *Preventive medicine for the doctor in the community* (3rd ed.). McGraw Hill.

Lewinson, S. B., & Graham-Perel, A. (2020). "You don't have any business being this good": An oral history interview with Bernadine Lacey. *American Journal of Nursing, 120*(8), 40–47.

McSpedon, C. (2020). A conversation with Monica R. McLemore. *American Journal of Nursing, 120*(9), 68–70.

Mayo Clinic. (2019). *Mental illness: Risk factors*. https://www.mayoclinic.org/diseases-conditions/mental-illness/symptoms-causes/syc-20374968

Melnyk, B. M., et al. (2021). Promoting nurse mental health. *American Nurse Journal, 16*(1), 20–22, 59.

Melville, N. A. (2011). *Nurse-led clinics show success in chronic disease management*. http://www.medscape.com/viewarticle/753418

Murdaugh, C. L., Parsons, M. A., & Pender, N. J. (2019). *Health promotion in nursing practice* (8th ed.). Pearson Education, Inc.

Newbold, E., Schneidermann, M., & Horton, C. (2012). The bridge clinic: A nurse-led postdischarge clinic improves care transitions in a public hospital. *American Journal of Nursing, 112*(7), 56–59.

Oerther, S. E., & Rosa, W. E. (2020). Advocating for equality: The backbone of the sustainable development goals. *American Journal of Nursing, 120*(12), 60–62.

Okun, T. White Supremacy Culture. *dRworks*. www.dismantlingracism.org https://www.dismantlingracism.org/uploads/4/3/5/7/43579015/okun_-_white_sup_culture.pdf

Park, M., Alston, A. D., & Washington-Brown, L. (2021). Toward national conversation about race, health risk, and nursing. *American Nurse Journal, 16*(1), 5–7, 58.

Prochaska, J. O., & DiClemente, C. C. (1983). Stages and processes of self-change of smoking: Toward an integrative model of change. *Journal of Consulting and Clinical Psychology, 51*(3), 390–395.

Project Implicit. https://implicit.harvard.edu/implicit/takeatest.html

Roberts, D. (2020). The elephant in the room. *Nursing 2020, 50*(2), 42–46.

Rosenstock, I. M. (1974). Historical origins of the health belief model. *Health Education Monographs, 2(4)*, 328–335.

Shanahan, L., Hill, S. N., Gaydosh, L. M., Steinhoff, A., Costello, E. J., Dodge, K. A., Harris, K. M., & Copeland, W. E. (2019). Does despair really kill: A roadmap for an evidence-based answer. *American Journal of Public Health, 109*(6), 854–858.

Sherwood, G., & Barnsteiner, J. (2012). *Quality and safety in nursing: A competency approach to improving outcomes*. Wiley-Blackwell.

Suchman, E. A. (1965). Stages of illness and medical care. *Journal of Health and Human Behavior, 6*(3), 114–128.

Trossman, S. (2012). Issues up close: Model of care coordination. *American Nurse Today, 7*(1), 38–39.

University of Washington Department of Epidemiology Equity, Diversity, and Inclusion Committee. (2019). Glossary of Equity, Diversity, and Inclusion Terms. [September 26, 2020]

U.S. Department of Health and Human Services (USDHHS) Office of Minority Health. (2016). *Policy and data*. http://www.minorityhealth.hhs.gov/omh/browse.aspx?lvl=1&lvlid=4

Wen, L. S., & Sadeghi, N. B. (2020, July 20). Addressing racial health disparities in the COVID-19 pandemic: Immediate and long-term policy solutions. *Health Affairs Blog*.

Woolf, S. H., & Aron, S. (Eds.). (2013). *U.S. health in international perspective: Shorter lives, poorer health*. National Research Council and Institute of Medicine. National Academies Press.

Woolf, S. H. (2017). Progress in achieving equity requires attention to root causes. *Health Affairs (Millwood), 36*(6), 984–991.

World Health Organization. (1974). https://www.who.int/about/governance/constitution

World Health Organization. (2014). In *Basic documents*. 48th ed. Author.

4 Health of the Individual, Family, Community, and Environment

Rolanda Simpkins

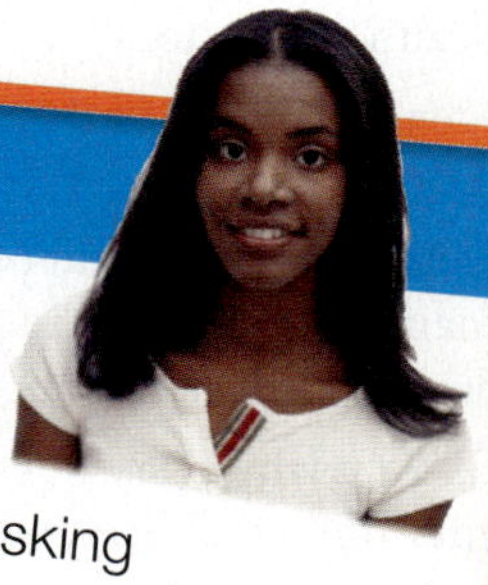

Rolanda, a 16-year-old adolescent who is sexually active, comes to the clinic seeking information about contraception. She states, "My mother would 'kill me' if she knew I was asking about this."

Samuel Kaplan

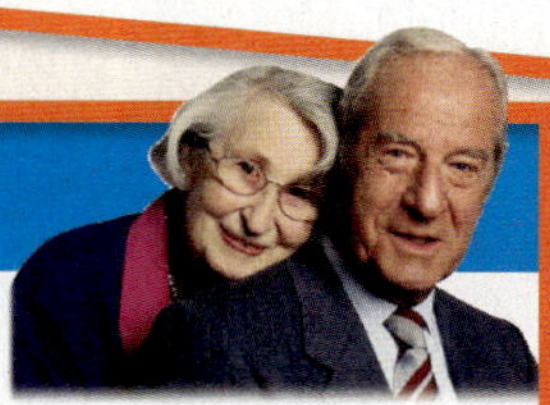

Samuel is the 80-year-old husband of a 76-year-old woman who was diagnosed with Alzheimer disease 1 year ago. Visibly tearful, he states, "I don't think that I can continue to care for my wife at home anymore. But how can I even consider putting her in a nursing home?"

Carlotta Rios

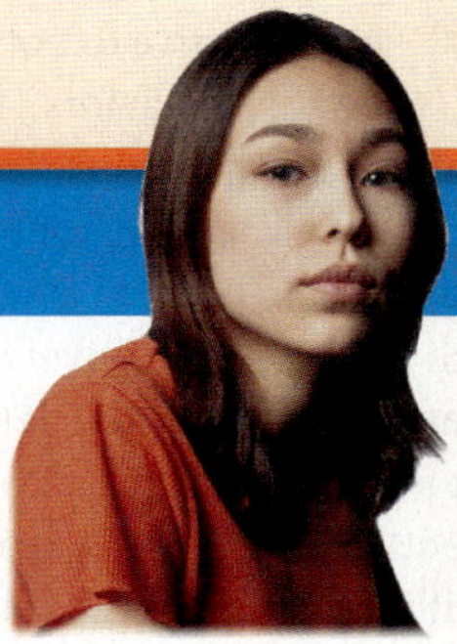

Carlotta is a 17-year-old girl who was brought to the mental health–psychiatric unit because of attempted suicide. She is not fluent in English and lives with her sister because of the recent death of her mother. Carlotta expresses a desire to "disappear" and not return to her sister's home. Further assessment reveals possible verbal abuse by her sister.

Learning Outcomes

After completing the chapter, you will be able to accomplish the following:

1. Describe each level of Maslow's hierarchy of basic human needs.
2. Explain nursing care necessary to meet needs in each level of Maslow's hierarchy.
3. Discuss family concepts, including family roles, structures, functions, developmental stages, tasks, and health risk factors.
4. Identify aspects of the community that affect individual and family health.
5. Describe nursing interventions to promote and maintain health of the individual as a member of a family and as a member of a community.
6. Explain why every nurse should be committed to environmental health, building a culture of health, and promoting the United Nations Sustainable Development Goals.

Nursing Concepts

- Health, wellness, and illness
- Family

Humans are complex organisms, influenced by and responsive to both internal and external environments. Our behaviors, feelings about ourselves and others, values, and the priorities we set for ourselves all relate to our physiologic and psychosocial needs. These needs are common to all people, and meeting these needs is essential for the health and survival of all people; therefore, they are called **basic human needs**. Basic human needs can be met or unmet in a variety of ways. A person can meet some needs independently, but most needs require relationships and interactions with others for partial or complete fulfillment. Satisfying one's needs often depends on the physical and social environment, especially one's family and community.

Holistic nursing care, which is based on considering all human dimensions affecting how the patient's basic human needs are met in health and in illness, allows the nurse to provide thoughtful, person-centered, health-oriented care. This chapter discusses how basic human needs, the family, the community, and the environment affect the health of every individual. (For an example, see the accompanying Reflective Practice box.)

Concept Mastery Alert

A holistic framework of care involves not just the individual patient but all those around the patient, most importantly the family and their active participation in promoting health.

THE INDIVIDUAL

In nursing, we consider the physical, safety, psychosocial, and spiritual needs of each individual patient. Abraham Maslow (1968) developed a hierarchy of basic human needs that describes which needs of a person are the most important at any given time (Fig. 4-1). Certain needs are more basic or essential than others and must be at least minimally met before other needs can be considered.

Maslow's hierarchy is useful for understanding relationships among basic human needs and for establishing priorities of care. The hierarchy is based on the theory that something is a basic need if it has the following characteristics:

- Its lack of fulfillment results in illness.
- Its fulfillment helps prevent illness or signals health.
- Meeting it restores health.
- It takes priority over other desires and needs when unmet.
- The person feels something is missing when the need is unmet.
- The person feels satisfaction when the need is met.

Nursing care is often directed toward meeting unmet or threatened needs. Maslow's hierarchy provides a framework for nursing assessment and for understanding the needs of patients at all levels, so that interventions to meet priority needs become a part of the care plan. Many nursing interventions are aimed at meeting patients' basic human needs. The following sections describe each level of need in more detail.

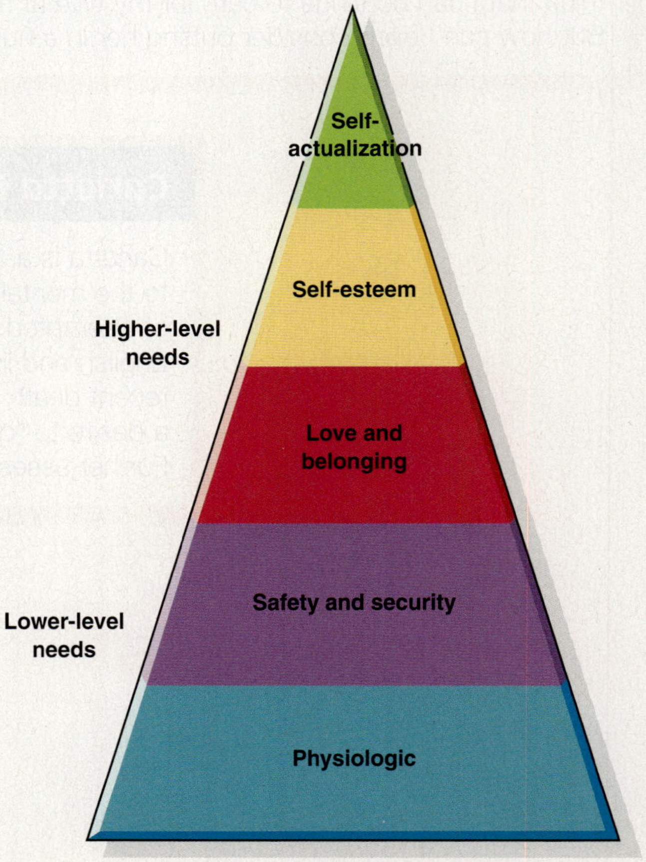

FIGURE 4-1. Maslow's hierarchy of basic human needs.

QSEN Reflective Practice: Cultivating QSEN Competencies

CHALLENGE TO ETHICAL AND LEGAL SKILLS

Junior year was full of excitement and new experiences. I was both nervous and excited about our mental health clinical rotation. Although the staff was very helpful and cooperative to provide as great an experience as they could, I found this clinical rotation to be difficult. I was going to be speaking with patients who had mental health problems and developing nurse–patient relationships that were different from the ones that I'd had in the past. To tell the truth, I was fearful. I was afraid I would say the wrong thing, causing the person to react, possibly injuring himself or others.

One patient really made an impression on me—Carlotta Rios, a 17-year-old girl who was brought to the unit because of attempted suicide. Her first language was Spanish and she was not fluent in English, and she lived with her sister because her mother had recently passed away. The nurses asked me to speak with her because I spoke Spanish.

When talking with her, I found out that Carlotta did not like living with her sister because the sister verbally abused her, always putting her down and constantly reminding Carlotta that the only reason she was here was because of her sister. Carlotta reported that her sister constantly told her about all of the sacrifices that she was making just so that Carlotta could be with her. According to Carlotta, her sister said that Carlotta did not appreciate everything that her sister was doing. The sister constantly reminded Carlotta of everything she bought for her, keeping a record so that Carlotta would pay her back. Carlotta said that she was not happy and figured that the only way she would stop feeling bad and that her sister would be happy again would be if Carlotta disappeared. Carlotta no longer wanted to exist.

Talking with Carlotta further, I found out that she did not want to return to her sister's home. Unfortunately, this was a problem because legally she was not considered an adult. Therefore, Carlotta's sister would have to be contacted. Yet, it seemed that Carlotta's current family and living situation was not the safest. It also seemed to be the cause of Carlotta's desperate attempt to take her life. If she chose not to return to her sister's house, Carlotta would be taken to court in handcuffs and placed in a foster home. Although this placement would only be until she turned 18 years old, which was at the end of the month, it also meant that once she was 18 years old, she would be on her own. It was apparent that she was not ready for such a drastic change.

Thinking Outside the Box: Possible Courses of Action

- Call Carlotta's sister and have her pick Carlotta up, because she is legally responsible for the patient.
- Gain the trust of the patient by speaking to her as an adult and informing her of all the options, ultimately assisting her with carrying them out.
- Call someone with whom she felt comfortable to provide support and also to hear the options available; in this way, the patient would have the opinion of someone she knew and trusted before she made a decision on which course of action to take.

Evaluating a Good Outcome: How Do I Define Success?

- Patient's safety is ensured.
- Patient benefits from the course of action decided on.
- The patient's human dignity is respected.
- No violations of the American Nurses Association's Code of Ethics occur.
- Patient makes the most appropriate decision, resulting in the best outcome for her.
- My ethical and legal obligations and those of the hospital are met.

Personal Learning: Here's to the Future!

I figured the best way to approach this situation was to develop a trusting relationship. So, after getting Carlotta up, we went to a brighter, better-lit room, where we had breakfast. I started by asking simple questions, eventually progressing to those that pertained to why she was in the hospital. Throughout our talks, I reinforced that her sister was considered the person legally responsible for Carlotta, explaining that if Carlotta decided not to call home, she would be taken in handcuffs to court and then would be placed in a foster home. I told her that this would only be until she turned 18 years old; upon turning 18, she then would be on her own. After listening to all of her options, she decided that she would call her sister to let her know where she was. She also told her sister that she would be staying with a best friend until she had figured things out. For Carlotta, this was the best decision to make because she felt safest. As a result of informing her sister, Carlotta would not have to go to court. Subsequently, any upset or disruption for her sister would be minimized, further adding to Carlotta's feelings of being safe. The priority for Carlotta was a safe environment. We were able to establish a trusting relationship and work together toward this end.

Stephanie Cuellar, Georgetown University

QSEN SELF-REFLECTION ON QUALITY AND SAFETY COMPETENCIES DEVELOPING KNOWLEDGE, SKILLS, AND ATTITUDES FOR CONTINUOUS IMPROVEMENT

How do you think you would respond in a similar situation? Why? What does this tell you about yourself and about the adequacy of your skills for professional practice? Can you think of other ways to respond? What *knowledge, skills,* and *attitudes* do you need to develop to continuously improve quality and safety when caring for patients like Carlotta?

(*continued*)

QSEN Reflective Practice: Cultivating QSEN Competencies *(continued)*

CHALLENGE TO ETHICAL AND LEGAL SKILLS

Patient-Centered Care: What additional information would be important for the nursing student to obtain from Carlotta to provide a more complete picture of the family situation? What family risk factors were evident here? Have these factors been addressed? What is the best way to communicate emotional support to Carlotta?

Teamwork and Collaboration/Quality Improvement: What communication skills do you need to continue to function as a resource and advocate for Carlotta? Would collaboration with your instructor or her nurse have resulted in additional alternatives or another approach with Carlotta? Are there community resources that might prove helpful to Carlotta? Do you think some form of family therapy might prove helpful to Carlotta and her sister?

Safety/Evidence-Based Practice: Is there anything more you could have done to acknowledge that you understood Carlotta's concern about the future? How do you think your response contributed to a safe environment for Carlotta? What evidence in nursing literature provides guidance for decision making regarding ensuring a safe environment and giving Carlotta the support that she needs?

Informatics: Can you identify essential information that must be documented in Carlotta's electronic record regarding communication that you had with her? Is it important to document your assessment of Carlotta's current mental status? Can you identify any additional information that supports safe patient care and coordination of care?

Physiologic Needs

Physiologic needs—for oxygen, water, food, elimination, temperature, sexuality, physical activity, and rest—must be met at least minimally to maintain life. These needs are the most basic in the hierarchy of needs and the most essential to life, and therefore have the highest priority. Most healthy children and adults meet their physiologic needs through self-care, but meeting physiologic needs is often a major part of the nursing care plan for young, old, disabled, and ill people who require assistance in meeting them.

Oxygen is the most essential of all needs because all body cells require oxygen for survival. Oxygenation of body cells is carried out primarily by the respiratory and cardiovascular systems; any alteration in the structure or function of these systems can result in an increased need for oxygen. This need may be acute (such as when cardiopulmonary resuscitation is needed) or chronic (requiring special positioning, treatments, and teaching). Nurses evaluate patients' oxygen needs by assessing skin color, vital signs, anxiety levels, responses to activity, restlessness, and mental responsiveness.

A balance between the intake and elimination of fluids is also essential to life. Healthy people drink fluids to satisfy thirst, and they maintain fluid balance through various physiologic processes. Disruption in the water balance of the body results in either dehydration or edema (the collection of fluid in body tissues). Dehydration results from conditions such as severe diarrhea or vomiting, whereas edema is caused by diseases of the cardiovascular or renal system, trauma, and other factors. Measuring intake and output, testing the resiliency of the skin, checking the condition of the skin and mucous membranes, and weighing the patient help assess a patient's water balance.

Food and elimination are related physiologic needs, with a balance maintained through digestive and metabolic processes. The need for food is manifested through hunger. Insufficient nutrient intake results in nutrient and electrolyte imbalances and weight loss. Waste products are eliminated from the body through the skin, lungs, kidneys, and intestines. A patient's nutritional status is assessed with a variety of indicators, including weight, muscle mass, strength, and laboratory values.

The human body functions best within a narrow temperature range, usually considered as plus or minus 98.6°F (37°C). Homeostatic mechanisms and adaptive responses, such as sweating or shivering, help maintain this temperature. Nurses assess body temperature as a vital sign (see Chapter 26).

Sexuality is an integral component of each person and may be affected by physical and emotional illnesses. Sexual practices depend on a variety of factors, such as a person's age, sociocultural background, self-esteem, and level of health. Health care providers are increasingly aware that consideration of sexuality is a vital part of holistic care.

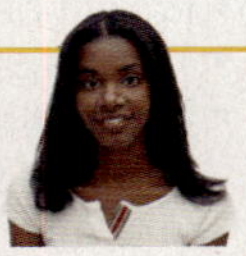

Recall **Rolanda Simpkins**, the 16-year-old girl described at the beginning of the chapter requesting information about contraception. The nurse can use knowledge about Rolanda's sexuality and sexual practices to help determine the most appropriate method of contraception for her.

Physical activity and rest are also basic physiologic needs. Physical activity depends on intact and functioning neuromuscular and skeletal systems. Rest and sleep allow time for the body to rejuvenate and be free of stress. Individual requirements for rest and sleep vary widely, but the adverse health effects of deprivation have been well documented. Factors that influence sleep include age, environment, exercise, stress, and drug use.

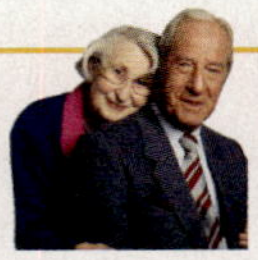

Think back to **Samuel Kaplan**, the 80-year-old man caring for his wife with Alzheimer disease at home. The nurse assesses the effect of providing this care on Mr. Kaplan's activity, rest, and sleep patterns, thereby developing an appropriate care plan for him to ensure that his needs are met as well.

Safety and Security Needs

Safety and security needs come next in priority after physiologic needs, and have both physical and emotional components. Physical safety and security means being protected from potential or actual harm. Nurses carry out a wide variety of activities to meet patients' physical safety needs, such as the following:

- Using proper hand hygiene and sterile techniques to prevent infection
- Using electrical equipment properly
- Administering medications knowledgeably
- Skillfully moving and ambulating patients
- Teaching parents about household chemicals that are dangerous to children

Specific safety interventions are discussed in Chapter 28.

Emotional safety and security involves trusting others and being free of fear, anxiety, and apprehension. Patients entering the health care system often fear the unknown and may have significant emotional security needs. Nurses can help meet such needs by encouraging spiritual practices that provide strength and support, by allowing as much independent decision making and control as possible, and by carefully explaining new and unfamiliar procedures and treatments.

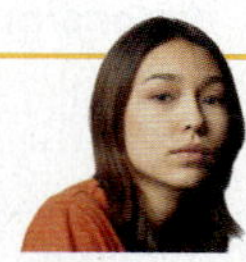

Remember **Carlotta Rios**, the adolescent described in the Reflective Practice display. The nurse fosters the development of a trusting relationship to promote emotional safety and security. Doing so assists Carlotta in her decision-making process about going home.

Love and Belonging Needs

All humans have a basic need for love and belonging. After physiologic and safety and security needs, this is the next priority, and is often called a higher-level need. **Love and belonging needs** include the understanding and acceptance of others in both giving and receiving love, and the feeling of belonging to groups such as families, peers, friends, a neighborhood, and a community.

People who believe that their love and belonging needs are unmet often feel lonely and isolated. They may withdraw physically and emotionally, or they may become overly demanding and critical. Often, these behaviors signal that the person has unmet love and belonging needs. Nurses should always consider love and belonging needs (Fig. 4-2) when developing a care plan, including nursing interventions such as:

- Including family and friends in the care of the patient
- Establishing a nurse–patient relationship based on mutual understanding and trust (by demonstrating care, encouraging communication, and respecting privacy)
- Referring patients to specific support groups (such as a cancer support group or Alcoholics Anonymous)

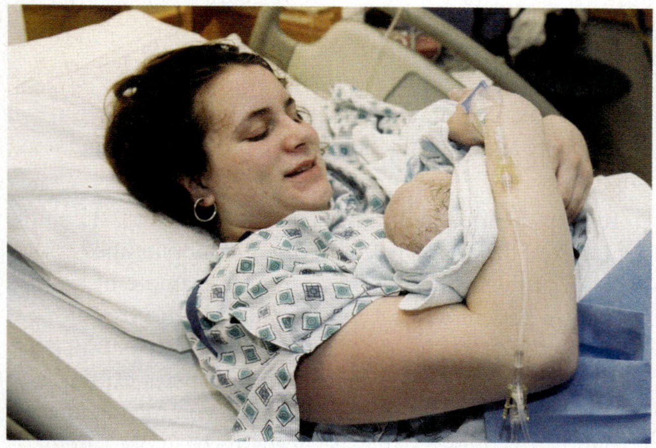

FIGURE 4-2. By providing time for the mother and newborn to bond, the nurse is helping to fulfill the need for love and belonging of both mother and child.

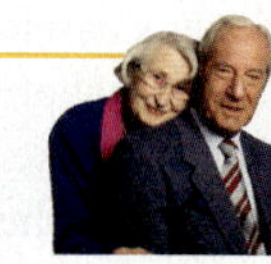

Think back to **Samuel Kaplan**, the man caring for his wife with Alzheimer disease. The nurse could refer Mr. Kaplan to a support group for caregivers of people with Alzheimer disease to help meet Mr. Kaplan's needs for love and belonging.

Self-Esteem Needs

The next highest priority on the hierarchy is **self-esteem needs**, which include the need for a person to feel good about themselves, to feel pride and a sense of accomplishment, and to believe that others also respect and appreciate those accomplishments. Positive self-esteem facilitates the person's confidence and independence.

Many factors affect self-esteem. When a person's role changes (e.g., through illness or the death of a spouse), self-esteem can be seriously altered because the person's responsibilities and relationships also change. A change in body image, such as the loss of a breast, an injury, or a growth spurt during puberty, may also affect self-esteem. Nurses must remember that the person's perception of the change—rather than the actual change itself—is what affects that person's self-esteem. Nurses can help meet patients' self-esteem needs by respecting their values and beliefs, encouraging patients to set attainable goals, and facilitating support from family, friends, or significant others. These actions promote a sense of worth and self-acceptance.

Self-Actualization Needs

The highest level on the hierarchy of needs is **self-actualization needs**, which include the need for people to reach their full potential through development of their unique capabilities. In general, each lower level of need must be met to some degree before this need can be satisfied. The process of self-actualization continues throughout life. Maslow lists the following qualities that indicate achievement of individual potential:

- Acceptance of self and others as they are
- Focus of interest on problems outside oneself

- Ability to be objective
- Feelings of happiness and affection for others
- Respect for all people
- Ability to discriminate between good and evil
- Creativity as a guideline for solving problems and pursuing interests

To help meet patients' self-actualization needs, the nurse focuses on the person's strengths and possibilities rather than on problems. The following is an example of a nurse assisting a patient to meet self-actualization needs:

> During a clinic visit, a patient with diabetes expresses difficulty with his prescribed dietary recommendations, but also recognizes that he needs to be more careful or "I'll end up losing a leg or having trouble seeing because of this disease." A nurse coach recognizes that the patient is the best expert about his own health, and listens carefully as he reviews his eating habits and discusses what he thinks he needs to do differently. Based on assessment data and the patient's desire to change his behavior, the nurse and patient together create an action plan to begin the process of change and move toward the optimal way for him to achieve his goals.

Nursing interventions are aimed at providing a sense of direction and hope and providing teaching that is aimed at maximizing potentials.

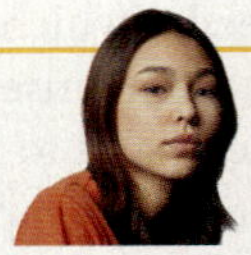

Recall ***Carlotta Rios***, the 17-year-old who had attempted suicide. By focusing on her strengths as well as helping her explore alternatives to her current lifestyle, the nurse helps to meet Carlotta's self-actualization needs by fostering personal growth and assisting her to find meaning to her life.

Table 4-1 The Human Dimensions and Basic Human Needs

	BASIC HUMAN NEED	EXAMPLES
Physical dimension	Physiologic needs	Breathing Circulation Temperature Intake of food and fluids Elimination of wastes Movement
Environmental dimension	Safety and security needs	Housing Community/neighborhood Climate
Sociocultural dimension	Love and belonging needs	Relationships with others Communications with others Support systems Being part of a community Feeling loved by others
Emotional dimension	Self-esteem needs	Fear Sadness Loneliness Happiness Accepting self
Intellectual and spiritual dimensions	Self-actualization needs	Thinking Learning Decision making Values Beliefs Fulfillment Helping others

Applying Maslow's Theory

Nurses can apply Maslow's hierarchy of basic needs in the assessing, diagnosing, planning, implementation, and evaluation phases of patient care. The hierarchy can be used with patients at any age, in all settings where care is provided, and in both health and illness. It helps the nurse identify unmet needs as they become health care needs. The hierarchy of basic needs allows the nurse to locate the patient on the health–illness continuum and to incorporate the human dimensions and health models into meeting needs (Table 4-1).

As the nurse identifies and carries out interventions to help meet patients' needs, it is important to remember that Maslow's hierarchy is only a framework or guideline, and that, in actuality, each person sets their own priorities for needs. In addition, basic human needs are interrelated, and may require nursing actions at more than one level at a given time. For example, in caring for a person coming into the emergency department with a heart attack, the nurse's immediate concern is the patient's physiologic needs (e.g., oxygen and pain relief). At the same time, safety needs (e.g., for oxygen use precautions and for ensuring that the person does not fall off the examining table) and love and belonging needs (e.g., for having a family member nearby if possible) are still major considerations. You will learn how nurses meet basic human needs throughout the rest of this book.

THE FAMILY

Almost every person is a member of a number of groups, such as family, friends, professional colleagues, a church congregation, or a school class. Each of these groups involves a specific part of the person's life and is important to the person. However, only one group—the family—is typically concerned with all parts of a person's life and with meeting the individual's basic human needs to promote health.

A **family** can be defined simply as any group of people who live together and depend on one another for physical, emotional, and financial support. Families are essential to the health and survival of the individual family members, as well as to society as a whole. The family is a buffer between the needs of the individual member and the demands and expectations of society. The role of the family is to help meet the basic human needs of its members while also meeting the needs of society (Pender et al., 2019).

Family Structures

A family may consist of two or more people who may be related or unrelated either biologically or legally; members may be of the same assigned sex or different assigned sex, and members may be of the same or various generations. A family may include unmarried people with a meaningful commitment to each other (Pender et al., 2019). Nurses must remember that there are no absolute "rights" or "wrongs" about what makes a family, and one person's values must not be imposed on another person. Respect for all kinds of family members and relationships is essential to person-centered, individualized patient care.

Nuclear Family

The **nuclear family**, also called the traditional family, is composed of two parents and their children. Contemporary descriptions of a nuclear family vary. Pender et al. (2019) define a nuclear family as "two or more persons who depend on one another for emotional, physical, or financial support."

There is great variability in nuclear family structure in today's "postmodern families." The parents may be of any sexual orientation and are usually either married or in a committed relationship; family members live together until the children leave home as young adults. The nuclear family may be composed of biologic parents and children, adoptive parents and children, surrogate parents and children, or step-parents and children. Multiple research studies have concluded that family processes, such as the quality of parenting and harmony between parents, rather than family structures, contribute to a child's well-being (American Academy of Pediatrics).

In the past, the traditional nuclear family typically consisted of a breadwinner husband and caregiver wife. In contemporary nuclear families, both parents may work for pay while sharing roles in providing physical and emotional safety and security. The two major causes of this change are increased education and career opportunities for women, and changes in our economy resulting in a need for additional income to maintain a desired standard of living. The contemporary nuclear family often lives in close geographic proximity to relatives, such as aunts, uncles, and grandparents, who are a part of the **extended family**. Couples without children and couples with grown children who no longer live at home are considered nuclear families as well. The **blended family** is another form of a nuclear family, formed when parents bring unrelated children from previous relationships together to form a new family.

Single-Parent Family

For decades, the share of U.S. children living with a single parent has been rising, accompanied by a decline in marriage rates and a rise in births outside of marriage. A new Pew Research Center study of 130 countries and territories shows that the United States has the world's highest rate of children living in single-parent households (Kramer, 2019).

Many single-parent families are headed by women. Single parents often have special problems and needs, including financial concerns and role shifts (i.e., having the roles of both parents), and they may remarry or enter into new relationships. The situation and needs of the single-parent family are important considerations when planning and implementing nursing care.

Other Family Structures

In addition to traditional and single-parent families, cohabiting adults and single adults are other family structures. Cohabiting families are people who choose to live together for a variety of reasons, including relationships, financial need, or changing values. Cohabiting families include unmarried adults living together (they may be of any age, including retired people who choose not to marry because it would impose financial hardship) and communal or group marriages. Other family structures include binuclear (where divorced parents assume joint custody of children) and dyadic nuclear (in which the couple chooses not to have children).

Single adults may not be living with others, but they are part of a family of origin, may have a social network with significant others, or may even regard a pet as family. Most single adults living alone are either young adults who achieve independence and enter the workforce or older adults who never married or are left alone after the death of a spouse.

With changes in family structure have come other influences on the basic human needs of family members. Considerations for the family, and for nursing care, include support systems (in our mobile society, family members may live hundreds or thousands of miles away), availability of childcare, time for leisure and recreation, struggles to meet financial commitments, and changing role models. During the COVID-19 pandemic, numerous family stressors taxed families, including the need for working parents to assume responsibility for their children's online learning and the need to socially distance to protect high-risk family members—which included grandparents no longer having visits from their children and grandchildren and some frontline nurses sleeping in hotels to avoid transmitting COVID-19 to a dependent family member. Not all was negative about the pandemic; this author's niece, an attorney with three children ages 7 and younger, wrote: "Yes, the pandemic has been a challenge. Huge challenge! But facing and overcoming challenges with dignity and grace is what life is all about! From a work/life balance, this has turned out to be a blessing to spend more quality time with the kids."

Family Functions

Families have important functions that affect how individual family members meet their basic human needs and maintain their health. The family provides the individual with an environment for development and social interactions. Families also are important to society as a whole because they provide new and socialized members for society.

Family functions occur in five major areas. Physically, the family provides a safe, comfortable environment necessary for growth, development, and rest or recuperation. Economically, the family provides financial aid to family members and also helps meet society's needs. The reproductive function of many families is to have and raise children. The affective and coping functions of the family provide emotional comfort to family members and help members establish their identity and maintain it in times of stress. Finally, through socialization, the family teaches; transmits beliefs, values, attitudes, and coping mechanisms; provides feedback; and guides problem solving (Friedman et al., 2003).

Developmental Tasks of Families

Duvall and Miller (1984) identified critical family developmental tasks and stages in a family life cycle. Duvall's theory, based on Erikson's theory of psychosocial development (described in Chapter 23), states that all families have certain basic tasks for survival and continuity, as well as specific tasks related to developmental stages throughout the life of the family. These stages and developmental tasks are outlined in Table 4-2. If the family does not meet certain developmental tasks, societal disapproval may lead to intervention by children's services, social services, police departments, welfare facilities, or health departments. The successful mastery of each developmental stage is important to the family's adaptation and growth through successive stages. See the accompanying Vulnerable Population Alert.

Table 4-2 Family Stages, Tasks, Health Risk Factors, and Nursing Interventions to Promote Health

FAMILY STAGE[a]	TASKS	STAGE-SPECIFIC RISK FACTORS	STAGE-SPECIFIC NURSING INTERVENTIONS/ REFERRALS
Couple and family with young children	Establish a mutually satisfying marriage/relationship Plan to have or not to have children Have and adjust to infant Support needs of all family members Adjust to cost of family life Adapt to needs and activity of children Cope with loss of energy and privacy Encourage and support growth and development and educational achievements	Inadequate knowledge of contraception and family planning Inadequate knowledge of sexual and marital roles Lack of knowledge about child safety and health Child abuse and neglect First pregnancy before age 16	Family planning clinics Prenatal classes Well-child clinics Vision and hearing screenings Dental health information Parent support groups Safety in the home, daycare, school, neighborhood, and community
Family with adolescents and young adults	Maintain open communications Support moral and ethical family values Balance teenagers' freedom with responsibility Maintain supportive home base Strengthen marital relationships	Family of origin Family value of aggressiveness Inadequate problem-solving abilities Conflict between family members Physical or sexual abuse Sexually transmitted diseases	Accident prevention programs Sex education Mental health programs Screening for chronic illness
Family with middle-aged adults	Maintain ties with younger and older generations Prepare for retirement	Depression Exposure to environmental or work-related health risks, such as sunlight, asbestos, radiation, coal dust, and air or water pollution	Blood pressure screenings Screening for chronic illness
Family with older adults	Adjust to retirement Adjust to loss of spouse May move from family home	Increasing age with loss of physical function Chronic illness Depression Death of spouse	Screening for chronic illness Home safety information Retirement information Pharmacology information

[a]Family includes all forms: nuclear, extended, single-parent, etc.
Source: Data from Duvall, E., & Miller, B. (1984). *Marriage and family development* (6th ed.). Harper Collins; Aldous, J. (1975). *The developmental approach to family analysis.* University of Minnesota Press.

Vulnerable Population Alert: Children During the Pandemic

How aware are you of all the ways children in the communities you serve are being affected by the pandemic? Talk with your classmates about how this knowledge might impact your ability to diagnose actual and potential health problems and needs and target your interventions to better health outcomes for children.

Households with children continue to be hit harder by the financial pressures caused by the COVID-19 pandemic, according to the latest results of the U.S. Census Bureau's experimental Household Pulse Survey. Nationally, 24.7 million adults in mortgaged or rented households reported a later or deferred housing payment in May, 2020. Children especially affected by the negative economic impacts of the pandemic are facing both living in households where the rent or mortgage payments were late and where there was not enough food (https://www.census.gov/library/stories/2020/06/the-risks-children-face-during-pandemic.html).

Lockdown measures intended to keep people safe from COVID-19 in the United States may have some school children in danger says Margo Lindauer, director of the Domestic Violence Institute at Northeastern. Seven months into the pandemic, Lindauer worries that the closure of schools, along with the added stress of balancing work, child care, and distance learning, has led to a rise in child abuse. And it's little wonder: People have spent more time insides their homes, some have lost jobs, and some have contracted the virus. All of these factors together are causing a perfect storm of increased rates of violence and decreased reporting of child abuse. The detrimental impacts of isolation and potential exposure to abuse, neglect, and food insecurity in many instances is worse than figuring out safe ways to get kids, at least temporarily or periodically, back in the classroom. The longer the pandemic goes on, the worse it's going to get (https://news.northeastern.edu/2020/10/13/closed-schools-could-be-putting-children-at-risk-during-the-covid-19-pandemic/).

With many schools still closed during the pandemic, educators worry that students without access to technology and no way to access online instruction will fall behind. The digital divide disproportionately impacts students of color, according to an analysis from USAFacts, which shows that 37% of American Indian and Alaska Native children, 19% of Black children, and 17% of Hispanic children lack access to the internet compared to 12% of White and Asian children (https://www.usnews.com/news/education-news/articles/2020-04-01/schools-rush-to-get-students-internet-access-during-coronavirus-pandemic).

The Family in Health and Illness

People learn health care activities, health beliefs, and health values in the family. When patients enter the health care system, they bring their own personal behaviors and needs, but they also bring (in a sense) their family too.

Friedman and associates (2003) identified the importance of family-centered nursing care in four ways. First, the family is composed of interdependent members who affect one another. If some form of illness occurs in one member, all other members become involved in the illness. Second, because there is a strong relationship between the family and the health status of its members, the role of the family is essential in every level of nursing care. Third, the level of health of the family and in turn each of its members can be significantly improved through health promotion activities. Finally, illness of one family member may suggest the possibility of the same problem in other members. Through assessment and intervention, the nurse can assist in improving the health status of all family members.

Illness may precipitate a health crisis in a family. If an illness is relatively minor, such as a viral infection in a child, changes in family tasks may be minor and brief. But if a family member's injury or illness is serious, the roles and responsibilities, as well as functions, of other family members change. This is especially true if the illness is chronic and long term, results in disability, or decreases the person's time to live. Some families find it difficult to adapt to the stress of changes in financial, social, and caregiving resources, whereas other families experience renewed family closeness and stability. Regardless of how the family adapts, members of the family must constantly adjust roles and responsibilities to manage the needs of the ill family member and the family.

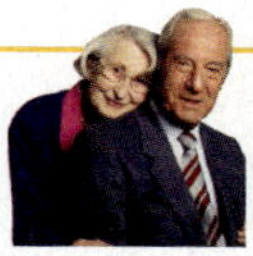

Remember **Mr. Kaplan**, the 80-year-old man caring for his wife with Alzheimer disease. Now the primary caregiver, Mr. Kaplan's role has changed. The disease and family role changes may affect the family's ability to function. The nurse would incorporate knowledge of this when developing the most appropriate plan for Mr. Kaplan and his wife.

Nursing interventions for a family in a health crisis include providing teaching that is honest, open, and respectful; using therapeutic communication skills; applying knowledge of family dynamics; and making referrals to community health care and financial resources to support realistic hope. In addition, it is important to involve family members in planning and implementing care. Review the content on caring for family caregivers in Chapter 3.

Family Risk Factors

Family patterns of behavior, the environment in which the family lives, and genetic factors can all place family members at risk for health problems. Nurses should assess these factors before developing nursing care plans. Typical questions in a family assessment include the following (Pender et al., 2019):

- What is the family's structure?
- What is the family's socioeconomic status?
- What are family members' cultural background and religious affiliation?
- Who cares for children if both parents work?

- What are the family's health practices (e.g., types of foods eaten, meal times, immunizations, bedtime, exercise)?
- How does the family define health?
- What habits are present in the family (e.g., do any family members smoke, drink to excess, or use drugs)?
- How does the family cope with stress?
- Is any family member the primary caregiver for another family member?
- Do close friends or family members live nearby and can they help if necessary?

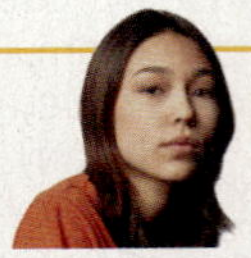

These questions are extremely important to ask when assessing **Carlotta Rios**, the adolescent described in the Reflective Practice display; Rolanda Simpkins, the 16-year-old wanting contraceptive counseling; and Samuel Kaplan, the older adult caring for his ill wife at home. Each person's answers provide the nurse with valuable information to help determine the best way to meet their needs. For Rolanda, understanding more about her relationship with her mother will guide the education and counseling. For Carlotta, this includes information about viable options for her living arrangements, including physical and emotional safety. For Mr. Kaplan, this assessment provides information about available sources of help so that he can continue to care for his wife at home or, if necessary, to ease the transition and adjustment to moving his wife to a long-term care facility.

The health assessment for a family should also consider the risk factors for altered health described in Box 4-1.

Nursing Interventions to Promote Family Health

The nurse can help reduce risk factors with activities that promote health for all family members at any level of development. Recall that each person has their own definition of health, based in part on family beliefs and values about health and illness. The nurse assists both the person and the family to meet basic human needs. Examples of stage-specific risk factors and nursing interventions to promote health in the family are shown in Table 4-2 (on page 84). Nurses may carry out such activities themselves or may refer the individual or family to other health care providers. Health promotion activities and nursing actions can reduce the risk for illness and facilitate healthy behaviors at any age within the family life cycle.

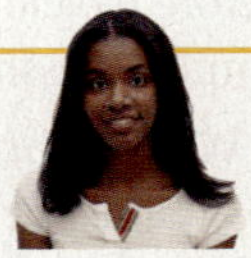

Consider **Rolanda Simpkins**, the adolescent seeking contraceptive information. The nurse needs to evaluate further her statement that her mother would "kill her," questioning Rolanda further to determine the family's health beliefs and practices.

Box 4-1 Risk Factors for Altered Family Health

Lifestyle Risk Factors

- Lack of knowledge about sexual and marital roles, leading to teenage marriage and pregnancy; divorce; sexually transmitted infections; child, spouse, or elder abuse; and lack of prenatal or child care
- Alterations in nutrition—either more or less than body requirements at any age
- Chemical dependency, including the use of alcohol, drugs, and nicotine
- Inadequate dental care and hygiene
- Unsafe or unstimulating home environment

Psychosocial Risk Factors

- Inadequate childcare resources, when both parents work, for preschool and school-aged children
- Inadequate income to provide safe housing, food, clothing, and health care
- Conflict between family members

Environmental Risk Factors

- Lack of knowledge or finances to provide safe and clean living conditions
- Work or social pressures that cause stress
- Air, water, or food pollution

Developmental Risk Factors

- Families who have new babies, especially if support systems are unavailable
- Older adults, especially those living alone or on a fixed income
- Unmarried adolescent parents who lack personal, economic, and educational resources

Biologic Risk Factors

- Birth defects
- Intellectual disability
- Genetic predisposition to certain diseases, including cardiovascular diseases and cancer

THE COMMUNITY

A person, as an individual and as a member of a family, is also a member of a community. The most basic definition of a **community** is a specific population or group of people living in the same geographic area under similar regulations and having common values, interests, and needs. A community may be a small neighborhood within a city or a large rural area, including a small town. Communities are based on shared characteristics of people, the area, social interaction, and familial, cultural, or ethnic heritage and ties. Within a community, people interact and share resources. The community environment affects the ability of the person to meet basic human needs. This section discusses the relationship of the community to basic human needs, including influences on health and illness. Be sure to check out the content on social determinants of health in Chapter 3.

The physical and social environments of communities have been implicated by the Institute of Medicine (renamed the

National Academy of Sciences, Engineering, and Medicine as of 2015) and the National Research Council as possible contributing factors to health disadvantages in the United States as compared to other high-income countries (Woolf & Aron, 2013). Americans die younger and have a consistent pattern of poor health and death and suffering from illness and injuries compared to the other wealthiest nations in the world. Designing healthier community environments is one of the recommended strategies to promote more favorable health outcomes in the United States. See Chapter 3 for additional explanations of and implications for this U.S. health disadvantage.

Many community factors affect the health of residents. A healthy community enables people to maintain a high quality of life and productivity. For example, a healthy community:

- offers access to health care services for all members of the community, which provide both treatment for illnesses and activities to promote health.
- has roads, schools, playgrounds, and other services to meet needs of the people in the community.
- maintains a safe and healthy environment.

The Robert Wood Johnson Foundation (n.d.) has identified healthy communities as one of its four focus areas. See the foundation's website (http://www.rwjf.org/en/our-focus-areas/focus-areas/healthy-communities.html) for examples of programs to build healthy communities. Similarly, the Division of Community Health (DCH) and Partnerships to Improve Community Health (PICH) support the implementation of evidence-based strategies to improve the health of communities and reduce the prevalence of chronic disease. The DCH focus areas are tobacco use and exposure, poor nutrition, physical inactivity and lack of access to opportunities for chronic disease prevention, risk reduction, and disease management.

The health of a community's residents is affected by the social support systems, the community health structure, environmental factors, and facilities providing assistance for those in need of shelter, housing, and food. Examples of community factors affecting health are listed in Box 4-2 and are discussed further in the following sections.

Box 4-2 Examples of Community Factors Affecting Health

- Number and availability of health care institutions and services
- Housing codes
- Police and fire departments
- Nutritional services for low-income infants, parents, school-aged children (e.g., lunch programs), and older adults
- Zoning regulations separating residential and industrial areas
- Waste disposal services and locations
- Air and water pollution
- Food sanitation
- Health education services and dissemination
- Employment opportunities
- Recreational opportunities
- Violent crimes or drug use

Social Support Systems

A person's social support systems are made up of all the people who help meet financial, personal, physical, and emotional needs. In most instances, family, friends, and neighbors provide the best social support within a community. To understand the social support systems of a community, it is important to know who provides support (such as family, neighbors, friends, church, and organizations).

Community Health Care Structure

The health care structure of a community directly affects the health of the people living within it. The size and location of the community often determine what services are available. For example, urban residents may have public transportation to a variety of health care providers, whereas rural residents may need to travel long distances on their own for care. County and state funding for community health care services also determines the type and number of available health care institutions and facilities.

Economic Resources

Personal finances and health care insurance coverage affect a person's access to health care services within a community. As private health insurance costs continue to escalate, fewer citizens have optimal insurance. Many part-time and service-industry jobs provide no insurance benefits at all, resulting in a substantial number of citizens without any financial assistance for health care screenings or care for illnesses.

Signed in March 2010, the Patient Protection and Affordable Care Act (PPACA), often referred to simply as the Affordable Care Act, aims to provide improved health security and access to health care for all Americans through comprehensive health insurance reforms being implemented in stages over several years. Major provisions of the act provide a right to coverage for Americans with preexisting conditions, allow young adults up to 26 years of age to continue to be covered under their parents' plan, and end lifetime limits on coverage. In addition, the act expands Medicaid coverage to millions of low-income Americans and makes numerous improvements to the Children's Health Insurance Program, or CHIP (Affordable Care Act, n.d.; HealthCare.gov). The PPACA has many more provisions to facilitate health insurance coverage and help care for underserved populations and eliminate disparities in health care. As this text goes to publication, efforts are underway to repeal the PPACA, which could result in many more citizens losing their insurance and access to basic health care services. Chapter 11 further discusses the costs of health care.

Effect on Individuals and Families

The community has a strong influence on health promotion and illness-prevention activities of individuals and families in the community (Fig. 4-3 on page 88). Just as there are family risk factors for the health of individual members, so are there community risk factors involving resources, economics, and services. For nursing assessments and interventions to be

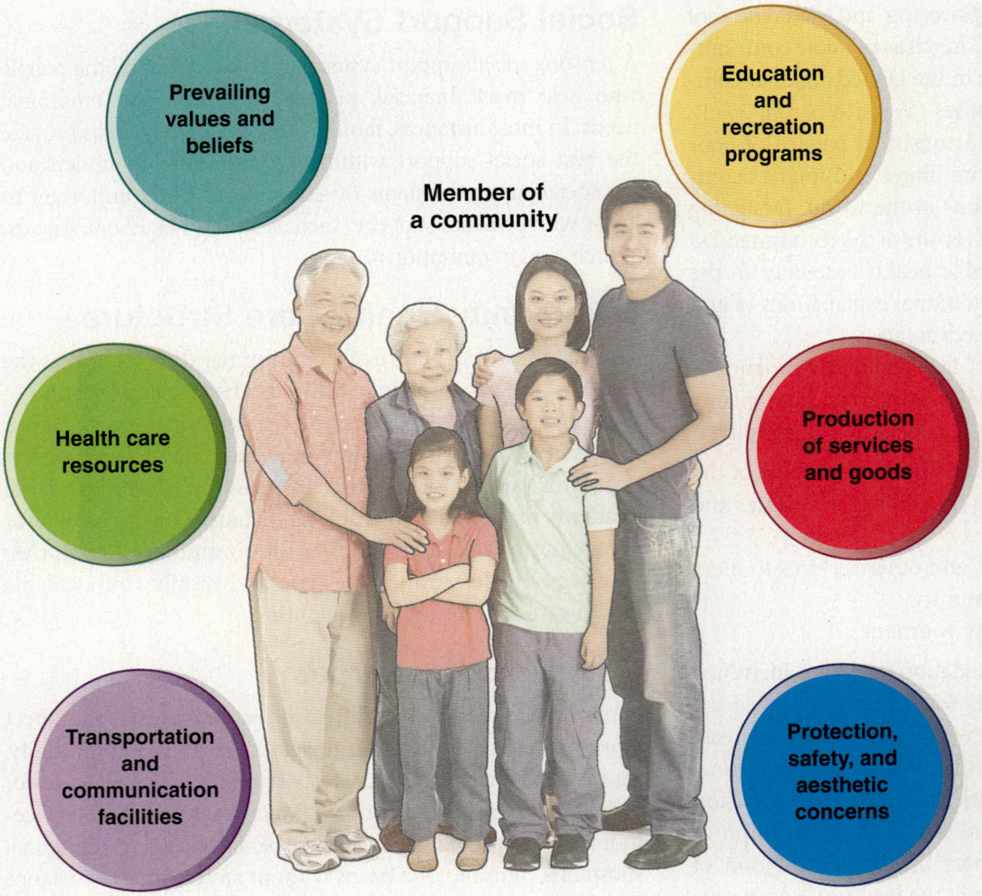
Prevailing values and beliefs
Education and recreation programs
Member of a community
Health care resources
Production of services and goods
Transportation and communication facilities
Protection, safety, and aesthetic concerns

FIGURE 4-3. Many characteristics of a community influence the health of its members. This diagram shows six categories of characteristics that influence the health of a member of a community.

comprehensive and individualized, the nurse must consider the community's influence.

Consider the following examples of how the community can affect the individual's and family's needs:

> ***Tara, 20 years old,*** lives in a two-room apartment with her 6-month-old daughter in a lower-income area of a major city. The apartment lacks adequate heat and plumbing. Tara has no family living nearby, and she and her husband are separated and no longer live together. Tara rarely leaves her apartment because she fears for her safety due to the neighborhood's high crime rate. She is on a public assistance program but has never taken her baby to a local clinic for checkups because of her concerns that the neighborhood is not safe.

> ***Anne, 22 years old,*** lives in a small house in a rural area. Her 4-year-old son is in a community preschool program with afterschool care. She is a single mother and works as an assistant at an insurance facility. Anne often sees her family members, who live nearby. Anne and her son have regular health assessments.

These two different examples illustrate that the community plays a major role in the health of people who live there. Tara and her baby are at much greater risk for illness than are Anne and her son. Even if the two women had identical health care needs, their care plans would include different interventions because of their different community environments.

Nursing in the Community

In contrast to community health nursing, which focuses on whole populations within a community, community-based nursing is centered on the health care needs of individuals and families. Nurses practicing community-based nursing provide interventions to manage acute or chronic health problems, promote health, and facilitate self-care. Nursing care provided within a community must be culturally competent and family centered.

Concept Mastery Alert

Community health nursing focuses on whole populations; *community-based nursing* focuses on the members of the population, specifically the individuals and families within the population.

Nurses providing community-based care must know about the location and specialties of health care providers, the availability and accessibility of services and supplies, and other public health services. Additional considerations include facilities (such as daycare or long-term care), housing, and the number and type of facilities providing services.

QSEN PATIENT-CENTERED CARE

QSEN urges nurses to understand how diverse cultural, ethnic, and social backgrounds function as sources of patient, family, and community values. Nurses working in the community are ideally positioned to collect data on traditions that affect different members of the community and to communicate patient values, preferences, and expressed needs to other members of the health care team.

The Future of Nursing, an Institute of Medicine report, emphasizes nursing as a vital component in all efforts to reform the health care system (Institute of Medicine, 2011; National Academies of Sciences, Engineering, and Medicine, 2021). The Affordable Care Act further reaffirms that nurse-managed centers in communities offer high-quality care to underserved populations in a cost-effective manner (Domrose, 2012). More than 250 nurse-managed health centers in the United States are improving health outcomes in communities because they understand community needs (Collins, 2012). Nurses in these centers carry out a variety of activities that focus on wellness and prevention, including immunizations, prenatal care, health education, and medication supervision. Nurses promote health as individuals, as caregivers within institutional settings, and as community-based health care providers. Nurses also provide community services as volunteers in health-related activities (e.g., screenings, educational programs, and blood drives) and as role models for health practices and lifestyles.

Nurses working in a variety of health care settings consider community influences when developing individualized nursing care plans and when making referrals to community facilities and support groups. Community-based nurses are employed in many different kinds of practice settings, including home care (Fig. 4-4), community health centers, school nursing, occupational nursing, and independent nursing practice. Community-based care is discussed in more detail in Chapter 12.

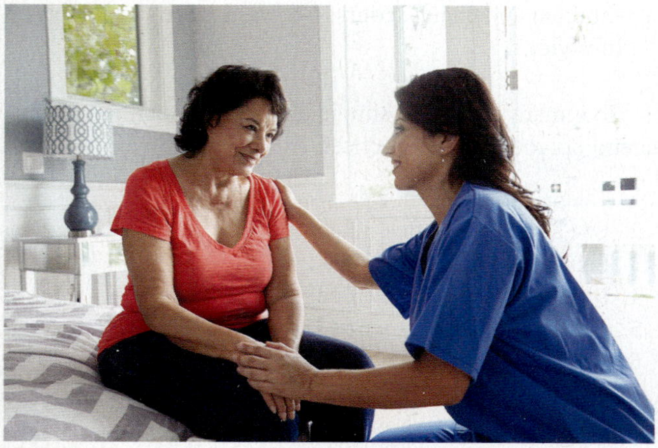

FIGURE 4-4. A nurse at work in a home health care setting. (*Source: Photo by Monkey Business Images/Shutterstock.*)

THE ENVIRONMENT

All nurses are to be aware of the principles of environmental health for nursing (American Nurses' Association, 2007). Provision 9.4 of the ANA Code of Ethics for Nurses with Interpretive Statement (2015) counsels that social justice extends beyond human health and well-being to the health and well-being of the natural world:

> Consistent with Florence Nightingale's historic concerns for environmental influences on health, . . . the profession's advocacy for social justice extends to ecojustice. Environmental degradation, aridification, earth resources exploitation, ecosystem destruction, waste, and other environmental assaults disproportionately affect the health of the poor and ultimately affect the health of all humanity. As nursing seeks to promote and restore health, prevent illness and injury, and alleviate pain and suffering, it does so within the holistic context of healing the world (p. 37).

See Box 4-3 for the top 10 reasons why nurses and environmental health go together. ANA's *Nursing: Scope and Standards of Practice* (2021) includes Standards 17, Resource Stewardship and 18, Environmental Health.

The community environment in which a person lives and works can have either helpful or harmful effects on health. **Environmental health** may be defined as that aspect of human health determined by physical, chemical, biologic, and psychosocial factors in the environment. Environmental barriers to accessing health care within a community may include lack of transportation, distance to services, and location of the services.

Box 4-3 Top 10 Reasons Why Nurses and Environmental Health Go Together

1. Nurses provide healing and safe environments for people.
2. Nurses are trusted sources of information.
3. Nurses are the largest health care occupation.
4. Nurses work with persons from a variety of cultures.
5. Nurses effect decisions in their own homes, work settings, and communities.
6. Nurses are good sources of information for policy makers.
7. Nurses translate scientific health literature to make it understandable.
8. Nurses with advanced degrees are engaged in research about the environment and health.
9. Health organizations recognize nurses' roles in environmental health.
10. Nursing education and standards of nursing practice require that nurses know how to reduce exposures to environmental health hazards.

Source: Reprinted with permission from Smith, C. M. (2016). Why nurses are involved with environmental health. In J. Leffers C. M. Smith, K. Huffling, R. McDermott-Levy, & B. Sattler (Eds.), *Environmental health in nursing, Alliance of nurses for healthy environments* (pp. 2–5).

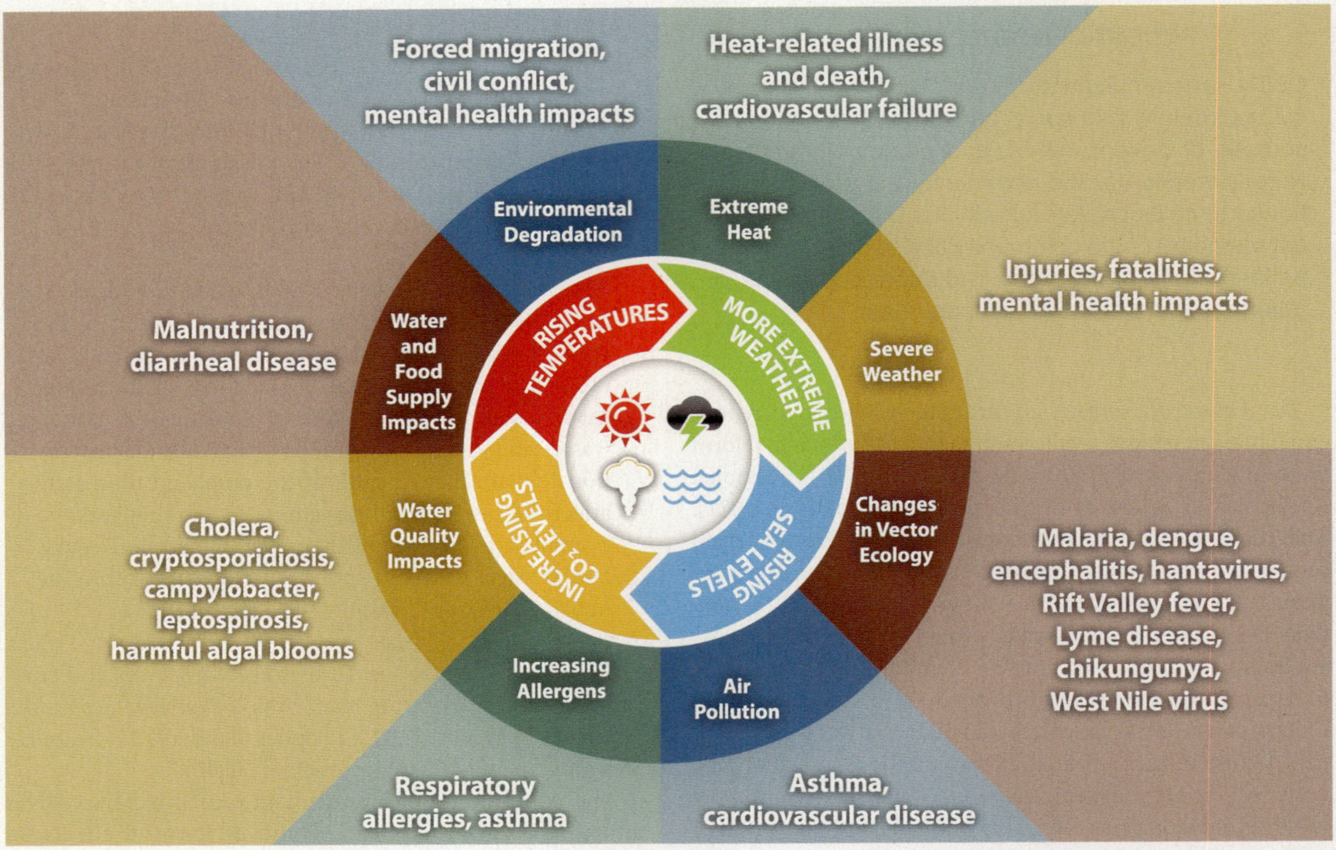

FIGURE 4-5. Impact of climate change on human health. (*Source:* Used with permission from Centers for Disease Control and Prevention. Climate effects on health. https://www.cdc.gov/climateandhealth/effects/default.htm.)

The quality of air and water differs across communities. Large urban areas are often affected by air pollution, whereas many smaller communities are at risk for water pollution from run-off of chemical or livestock wastes. Aging infrastructure also exacerbates these challenges. Read about the water crisis in Flint Michigan and its long-term effects. There is also increasing concern about how global warming and a growing potential for natural disasters affect health. As this chapter is being written, fires are raging in California, Oregon, and Colorado, and parts of Louisiana and Texas are suffering the devastating effects of hurricanes. The United Nations reports that no corner of the globe is immune from the devastating consequences of **climate change/crisis**:

> Rising temperatures are fueling environmental degradation, natural disasters, weather extremes, food and water insecurity, economic disruption, conflict and terrorism. Sea levels are rising, the Artic is melting, coral reefs are dying, oceans are acidifying, and forests are burning. It is clear that business as usual is not enough. As the finite costs of climate change reaches irreversible highs, now is the time for bold collective action (https://www.un.org/en/un75/climate-crisis-race-we-can-win).

See Figure 4-5 for an illustration of the impact of climate change on human health.

Climate Actions

ACT NOW is the United Nations campaign for individual action on climate change and sustainability. ACT NOW issued a call with particular urgency for nurses:

> Every one of us can help limit global warming and take care of our planet. By changing our habits and making choices that have less harmful effect on the environment, we have the power to confront the climate challenge and build a more sustainable world. Our lives depend on a healthy planet. Let's seize the moment and change course—toward more sustainable lifestyles.

How many of the 10 simple climate actions they recommend do you already practice?

1. Take a 5-minute shower
2. Use a reusable coffee mug
3. Eat a plant-based meal
4. BYOB—bring your own bag
5. Turn off your lights when leaving the room
6. Recycle your plastic waste
7. Drive less
8. Try zero-waste fashion
9. Unplug your appliances
10. Buy local

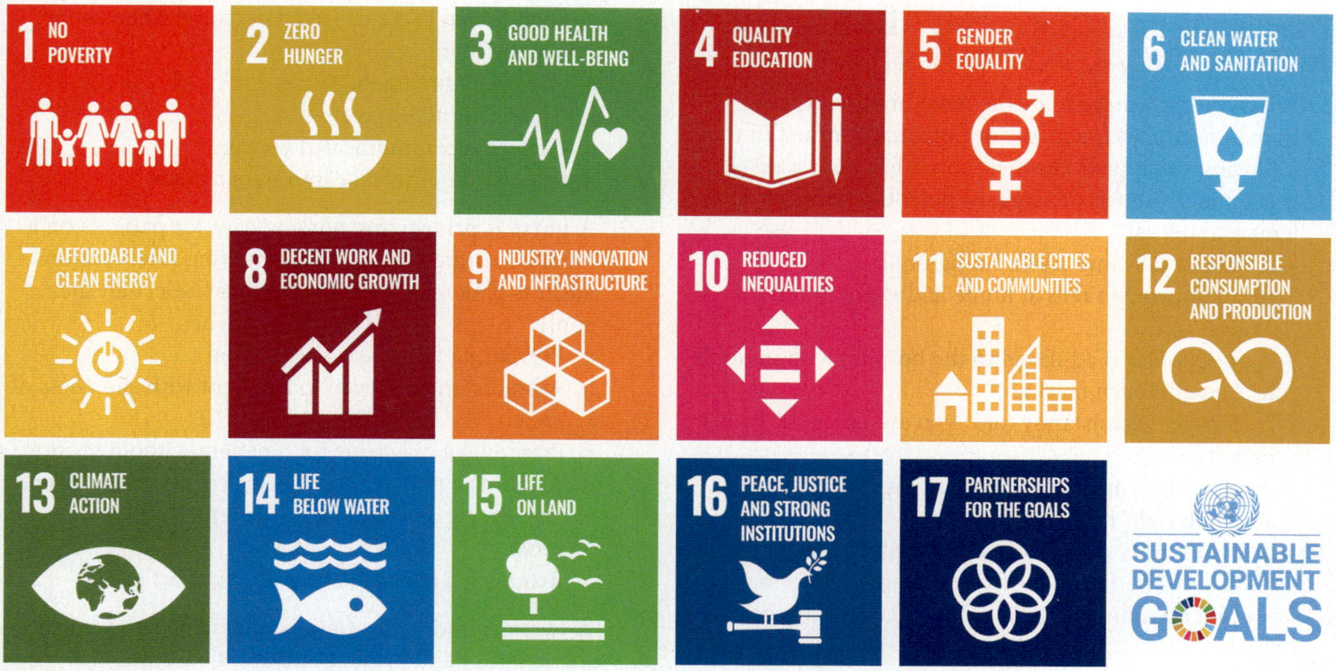
1 NO POVERTY
2 ZERO HUNGER
3 GOOD HEALTH AND WELL-BEING
4 QUALITY EDUCATION
5 GENDER EQUALITY
6 CLEAN WATER AND SANITATION
7 AFFORDABLE AND CLEAN ENERGY
8 DECENT WORK AND ECONOMIC GROWTH
9 INDUSTRY, INNOVATION AND INFRASTRUCTURE
10 REDUCED INEQUALITIES
11 SUSTAINABLE CITIES AND COMMUNITIES
12 RESPONSIBLE CONSUMPTION AND PRODUCTION
13 CLIMATE ACTION
14 LIFE BELOW WATER
15 LIFE ON LAND
16 PEACE, JUSTICE AND STRONG INSTITUTIONS
17 PARTNERSHIPS FOR THE GOALS
SUSTAINABLE DEVELOPMENT GOALS

FIGURE 4-6. The United Nations Sustainable Development Goals. (*Source:* Reprinted with permission from the United Nations Sustainable Development Goals. https://www.un.org/sustainabledevelopment/student-resources/.)

Check the ACT NOW website and download their app to measure your impact at actnow.aworld.org. Your class may want to download their poster to educate your classmates.

Reducing Waste in Clinical Settings

Read the article in your bibliography about reducing waste in the clinical setting and be sure to assess what is happening in your practice sites (Saber, 2020; Wohlford et al., 2020). How committed are the frontline caregivers you observe to improving environmental sustainability and to realizing cost savings? Be sure to check out the Alliance of Nurses for Healthy Environments (https://envirn.org/) and Sustainable Solutions for Health Care (https://www.practicegreenhealth.org/). Would you use the label "environmentally 'woke' nurse" to describe yourself?

SUSTAINABLE DEVELOPMENT GOALS

"Since the inception of modern nursing, our leaders have continuously recognized social and environmental determinants as substantive forces in creating and sustaining health. . . . The [United Nations] Sustainable Development Goals represent an inspired transnational humanitarian agenda" (Rosa & Hasmiller, 2020, p. 69). See Figure 4-6. Rosa and Hasmiller offer a distinctive invitation for the nursing profession to innovate, collaborate, and lead in making improvements toward collective health and well-being while capitalizing on the gains of the past century. After carefully reviewing the 17 Sustainable Development Goals and the Robert Wood Johnson Foundation's principles to build a culture of health in Box 4-4, talk with your classmates about a class project you can do locally to achieve one of the goals that will link your project to global health efforts and contribute to the legacy of our profession. You may want to check out Sustainable Solutions for Health Care (https://www.practicegreenhealth.org/).

We know the contributions Florence Nightingale and other nurse leaders made to global health. What will your contributions be?

Box 4-4 10 Principles for a Culture of Health

1. Good health flourishes across geographic, demographic, and social sectors.
2. Attaining the best health possible is valued by our entire society.
3. Individuals and families have the means and the opportunity to make choices that lead to the healthiest lives possible.
4. Business, government, individuals, and organizations work together to build healthy communities and lifestyles.
5. No one is excluded.
6. Everyone has access to affordable, quality health care because it is essential to maintain, or reclaim, health.
7. Health care is efficient and equitable.
8. The economy is less burdened by excessive and unwarranted health care spending.
9. Keeping everyone as healthy as possible guides public and private decision making.
10. Americans understand that we are all in this together.

Source: Used with permission, Robert Wood Johnson Foundation. (2019). *Building a culture of health: How we got here.* https://www.rwjf.org/en/cultureofhealth/about/how-we-got-here.html.

DEVELOPING CLINICAL REASONING AND CLINICAL JUDGMENT

1. What do you believe to be the most important basic human need that is actually or potentially unmet in the following situations? How will this affect your assessment and diagnosis of actual or potential health problems and needs?
   - A toddler falls into a swimming pool.
   - An older woman falls at home and is not found for 3 days.
   - A preschooler is admitted to the hospital with multiple bruises and burn marks.
   - A teenager is constantly told "you are no good" by his parents.
   - A long-term care facility resident says, "I never did anything right in my life."
2. Our own family experiences often affect the way we relate to the families of our patients. Describe at least two possible responses to the families described below.
   - Suspecting child abuse, a nurse asks a mother about her child's bruises. The woman says, "In our family, we believe in 'spare the rod and spoil the child.'"
   - A single woman wants to have a child and comes to a fertility clinic for information on artificial insemination.
   - Several members of a patient's large extended family are in the patient's long-term care facility room and are trying to do everything for the patient.
3. If a natural disaster were to strike your town (e.g., tornado, earthquake, flood, fire), leaving many homeless, what priorities would guide your rescue efforts? What needs should take priority, and how could these best be met?
4. Use the Pender, Murdaugh, and Parsons questions in the text to facilitate assessing a family's risk factors for health problems. Ideally, you will assess families in two or more sections of your town or city. How do you explain the differences you discover? How will you use these to plan care for these families?
5. Reading your local newspaper, you learn that local rivers and creeks are not infrequently full of raw sewage, given the high-intensity rain storms affecting your neighborhood. What is surprising is that few seem to know this, and on any given day, you are likely to see numerous people jogging, biking, fishing, and walking kids and dogs along the waterways, not to mention boating, kayaking, and paddleboarding within them. You read that while volunteers have found dangerous levels of *Escherichia coli* in local waterways, the city has no plans for formal testing or notifying the public. How might you work to address this challenge as a proponent for environmental health?

PRACTICING FOR NCLEX

1. Nurses in a long-term care facility use Maslow's hierarchy of basic human needs to plan care for their patients. What is the expected outcome when using this hierarchy?
   a. Accurate nursing diagnoses
   b. Clear priorities of care
   c. Concerns communicated concisely
   d. Integration of science into nursing care
2. A nurse is prioritizing nursing care for patients on a medical-surgical unit. Which nursing interventions address patients' physiologic needs? Select all that apply.
   a. Preventing falls during admission
   b. Administering oxygen to a patient with shortness of breath
   c. Providing a magazine for a patient without visitors
   d. Assisting a patient who had a stroke eat their dinner
   e. Facilitating a visit from the patient's significant other
   f. Referring a patient to a cancer support group
3. A nurse provides care for postoperative patients using meticulous hand hygiene and aseptic technique. Which of Maslow's basic human needs is the nurse addressing?
   a. Physiologic
   b. Safety and security
   c. Self-esteem
   d. Love and belonging
4. A nurse caring for patients in a long-term care facility develops strategies to help patients achieve Maslow's highest level of needs: self-actualization. Which concepts will the nurse incorporate when planning care? Select all that apply.
   a. Humans are born with a fully developed sense of self-actualization.
   b. Self-actualization needs are met by depending on family, friends, and others for help.
   c. No matter the patient's age, the self-actualization process continues throughout life.
   d. Loneliness and isolation occur when self-actualization needs are unmet.
   e. A person achieves self-actualization by focusing on problems outside self.
   f. Self-actualization needs may be met by creatively solving problems.
5. A nurse in a family-centered health clinic is assessing a new family composed of two parents and three preschool children. Which value does the nurse include in a family-centered approach to health care?
   a. Each person in the family will be evaluated and treated independently of the others.
   b. Time will be saved as there is only one clinic to contact for health problems.
   c. All members of the family can be part of health-related decisions.
   d. Interdependence of family members affects them in illness and health.

6. A nurse performs an assessment of a family consisting of a single parent, a grandparent, and two children. What interview questions will the nurse direct toward the mother to best determine the family's affective and coping functions? Select all that apply.
   a. Who is the person you depend on for emotional support?
   b. Who is the person you depend on for financial support in your family?
   c. Do you plan on having any more children?
   d. Who keeps your family together in times of stress?
   e. What family traditions do you pass on to your children?
7. A nurse caring for families in a free health care clinic assesses for psychosocial risk factors for altered family health. Which example best describes one of these risk factors?
   a. The family does not have dental care insurance or resources to pay for it.
   b. Both parents work and leave a 12-year-old child to care for his younger brother.
   c. Both parents and their children are considerably overweight.
   d. The youngest member of the family has cerebral palsy and needs assistance from community services.
8. A nurse working in an "Aging in Place" facility interviews a married couple in their late 70s. Based on Duvall's Developmental Tasks of Families, what developmental task is most appropriate for the nurse to assess?
   a. Maintenance of a supportive home base
   b. Strength of the marital relationship
   c. Ability to cope with loss of energy and privacy
   d. Adjustment to retirement years
9. A nurse working in a new community performs an assessment to determine the health of the community. What finding indicates a healthy community?
   a. Meets all the needs of its inhabitants
   b. Mixes residential and industrial areas
   c. Offers access to health care services
   d. Consists of modern housing and condominiums
10. A nurse is practicing community-based nursing in a mobile health clinic. Which example best demonstrates community-based nursing?
    a. Caring for a mother and her child who have diabetes
    b. Providing shelter for vulnerable populations within the community
    c. Providing local same-day surgery facilities
    d. Assisting families in crisis and overseeing the crisis hotline
11. After receiving a change-of-shift report, the nurse on a medical-surgical unit sets initial priorities for care. According to Maslow's hierarchy of needs, which patient requires immediate assessment?
    a. Patient requesting help to phone family to ask them to visit
    b. Patient who needs education on changing their wound dressing prior to discharge
    c. Patient who calls for assistance because they are breathing fast and feel faint
    d. Patient who needs assistance to walk to the bathroom to void

ANSWERS WITH RATIONALES

1. **b.** Maslow's hierarchy of basic human needs is useful for establishing priorities of care.
2. **b, d.** Physiologic needs—oxygen, water, food, elimination, temperature, sexuality, physical activity, and rest—must be met at least minimally to maintain life. Providing food and oxygen are examples of interventions to meet these needs. Preventing falls helps meet safety and security needs; providing art supplies may help meet self-actualization needs; facilitating visits from loved ones helps meet self-esteem needs; and referring a patient to a support group helps meet love and belonging needs.
3. **b.** By using meticulous hand hygiene and aseptic technique, nurses prevent infection, which falls under safety. An example of a physiologic need is clearing a patient's airway. Self-esteem needs may be met by allowing an older adult to talk about a past career. An example of helping meet a love and belonging need is contacting a hospitalized patient's family to arrange a visit.
4. **c, e, f.** Self-actualization, or reaching your full potential, is a process that continues throughout life. A person achieves self-actualization by focusing on their unique capabilities, being creative, and demonstrating the capacity for happiness and affection for others. Humans are not born with a fully developed sense of self-actualization, and self-actualization needs are not met specifically by depending on others for help. Loneliness and isolation are not always the result of unmet self-actualization needs.
5. **d.** Families likely share beliefs and values about health and illness. The nurse can help reduce risk for all family members at any level of development and recognizes interdependence of families affect one another in illness and health promotion.
6. **a, d.** The five major areas of family function are physical, economic, reproductive, affective and coping, and socialization. Affective areas of function include feelings and coping, assessed by determining who provides emotional support in times of stress. Assessing the financially responsible individual focuses on the economic function. Inquiring about having more children assesses the reproductive function, asking about family traditions assesses the socialization function, and checking the environment assesses the physical function.
7. **b.** Inadequate childcare resources are a psychosocial risk factor. Not having access to dental care and obese family members are lifestyle risk factors. Having a family member with birth defects is a biologic factor.
8. **d.** The developmental tasks of the family with older adults are to adjust to retirement and possibly to adjust to the loss of a spouse and loss of independent living. Maintaining a supportive home base and strengthening marital relationships are tasks of the family with adolescents and young adults. Coping with loss of energy and privacy is a task of the family with children.

9. **c.** A healthy community offers access to health care services to treat illness and to promote health. A healthy community cannot usually meet all the needs of its residents, but should be able to help with health issues such as nutrition, education, recreation, safety, and zoning regulations to separate residential sections from industrial areas. The age of housing is irrelevant as long as residences are maintained according to code.
10. **a.** Community health nursing focuses on whole populations within a community, and community-based nursing is centered on the health care needs of individuals and families. Nurses practicing community-based nursing provide interventions to manage acute or chronic health problems, promote health, and facilitate self-care.
11. **c.** The nurse prioritizes the patient with rapid breathing who feels faint, who may need oxygen or additional assistance with physiologic needs. Family visits help meet love and belonging needs, while assisting the patient to prevent falls and proper dressing change technique meets safety and security needs.

Bibliography

ACT NOW. Ten simple climate actions. https://www.un.org/sustainabledevelopment/wp-content/uploads/2021/02/ActNow-action-guide.pdf

Affordable Care Act (ACA). (n.d.). https://www.medicaid.gov/affordable-care-act/index.html

Aldous, J. (1975). *The developmental approach to family analysis*. University of Minnesota Press.

American Academy of Pediatrics. (n.d.a). *Types of families*. https://www.healthychildren.org/English/family-life/family-dynamics/types-of-families/Pages/default.aspx

American Academy of Pediatrics. (n.d.b). *Family life: Single parent families*. http://www.healthychildren.org/English/family-life/family-dynamics/types-of-families/pages/Single-Parent-Families.aspx

American Academy of Pediatrics. (2015a). *Family life: Gay and lesbian parents*. http://www.healthychildren.org/English/family-life/family-dynamics/types-of-families/Pages/Gay-and-Lesbian-Parents.aspx

American Academy of Pediatrics. (2015b). *Family life: Stresses of single parenting*. http://www.healthychildren.org/English/family-life/family-dynamics/types-of-families/pages/Single-Parent-Families.aspx

American Nurses Association. (2007). *ANA's principles of environmental health for nursing practice with implementation strategies*. Author.

American Nurses Association. (2015). *Code of Ethics for Nurses with Interpretive Statements*. Author.

American Nurses Association. (2021). *Nursing: Scope and standards of practice* (4th ed.). Author.

Caouette, S., Boss, L., & Lynn, M. (2020). Original Research: The relationship between food insecurity and cost-related medication nonadnerence in older adults: A systemic review. *American Journal of Nursing, 120*(6), 24–36.

Centers for Disease Control and Prevention (CDC). *Climate effects on health*. https://www.cdc.gov/climateandhealth/effects/default.htm

Centers for Disease Control and Prevention (CDC), Division of Community Health (DCH). (2017). *Partnerships to improve community health (PICH)*. http://www.cdc.gov/nccdphp/dch/programs/partnershipstoimprovecommunityhealth/index.html

Collins, A. M. (2012). Promoting community health. *American Journal of Nursing, 112*(6), 65–66.

Development of the National Health Promotion and Disease Prevention Objectives for 2030. https://www.healthypeople.gov/2020/About-Healthy-People/Development-Healthy-People-2030

Domrose, C. (2012). A healthy day in the neighborhood. *Nurse, 21*(8), 16–17.

Dossey, B. M., Rosa, W. E., & Beck, D. M. (2019). Nightingale and the sustainable development goals: From Nightingale to now. *American Journal of Nursing, 119*(5), 44–49.

Duvall, E. M., & Miller, B. C. (1984). *Marriage and family development* (6th ed.). HarperCollins.

Edelman, C., Kudzma, E. C., & Mandle, C. (2014). *Health promotion throughout the lifespan* (8th ed.). Mosby Elsevier.

Ellis, J., & Hartley, C. (2012). *Nursing in today's world: Trends, issues, and management* (10th ed.). Wolters Kluwer Health/Lippincott Williams & Wilkins.

Fateux, N. (2020). Embracing a role from nursing's past. *American Journal of Nursing, 120*(5), 65–68.

Friedman, M. M., Bowden, V. R., & Jones, E. G. (2003). *Family nursing: Research, theory, and practice* (5th ed.). Prentice Hall.

HealthCare.gov. (n.d.). *The children's health insurance program (CHIP)*. https://www.healthcare.gov/medicaid-chip/childrens-health-insurance-program/

Healthy People 2020. (2016). *Education and community-based programs*. http://www.healthypeople.gov/2020/topicsobjectives2020/overview.aspx?topicid=11

Institute of Medicine of the National Academies. (2011). *The future of nursing: Leading change, advancing health*. Washington, DC: The National Academies Press.

Kramer, S. (2019). *U.S. has the world's highest rate of children living in single-parent households*. Pew Research Center. https://www.pewresearch.org/fact-tank/2019/12/12/u-s-children-more-likely-than-children-in-other-countries-to-live-with-just-one-parent/

Maslow, A. (1968). *Toward a psychology of being* (2nd ed.). Van Nostrand–Reinhold.

National Academies of Sciences, Engineering, and Medicine, Health and Medicine Division. (2011). *The future of nursing: Focus on education*. http://www.nationalacademies.org/hmd/Reports/2010/The-Future-of-Nursing-Leading-Change-Advancing-Health/Report-Brief-Education.aspx

National Academies of Sciences, Engineering, and Medicine. The future of nursing 2020–2030. (2021). https://www.nationalacademies.org/our-work/the-future-of-nursing-2020-2030

Nicholas, P. K., Breakey, S., Tagliareni, M. E., Simmonds, K., & Sabo, K. K. (2021). Climate change and population health: Incorporating stages of nursing's political development. *Nursing Outlook, 69*(1), 65–73.

Pender, N. J., Murdaugh, C. L., & Parsons, M. A. (2019). *Health promotion in nursing practice* (8th ed.). Pearson Education, Inc.

Robert Wood Johnson Foundation. (n.d.). *Healthy communities*. http://www.rwjf.org/en/our-focus-areas/focus-areas/healthy-communities.html

Robert Wood Johnson Foundation. (2019). *Building a culture of health: How we got here*. https://www.rwjf.org/en/cultureofhealth/about/how-we-got-here.html

Rosa, W. E., Burnett, C., Butler, C., Rolle, P., Salvage, J., Wignall, A., & Mason, D. J. (2021). The ICN global nursing leadership institute: Integrating the SDGs into leadership and policy development. *American Journal of Nursing, 121*(12), 54–58.

Rosa, W. E., & Hassmiller, S. B. (2020). The sustainable development goals and building a culture of health. *American Journal of Nursing, 120*(6), 69–71.

Rosa, W. E., Kurth, A. E., Sullivan-Marx, E., Shamian, J., Shaw, H. K., Wilson, L. L., & Crisp, N. (2019). Nursing and midwifery advocacy to lead the United Nations sustainable development agenda. *Nursing Outlook, 67*(6), 628–641.

Saber, D. A. (2020). Healthcare's role in environmental sustainability. *American Nurse Journal, 15*(10), 50–53.

Schenk, E. C., Potter, T. M., Cook, C., Huffling, K., & Rosa, W. E. (2021). Nurses promoting inclusive, safe, resilient, and sustainable cities and communities: Taking action on COVID-19, systemic racism, and climate change. *American Journal of Nursing, 121*(7), 66–69.

Sherwood, G., & Barnsteiner, J. (2012). *Quality and safety in nursing*. Wiley-Blackwell.

Smith, C. M. (2016). Why nurses are involved with environmental health. In J. Leffers, C. M. Smith, K. Huffling, R. McDermott-Levy, & B. Sattler (Eds.), *Environmental health in nursing, Alliance of nurses for healthy environments* (pp. 2–5).

Stanhope, M., & Lancaster, J. (2019). *Foundations for population health in community/public health nursing* (5th ed.). Elsevier.

Terry, L., Bowman, K., & West, R. (2019). Becoming an environmentally 'woke' nurse: A phenomenological study. *Nursing Outlook, 67*(6), 725–733.

Titelman, P. (Ed.). (2014). *Differentiation of self: Bowen family systems theory perspectives*. Routledge.

United Nations. *Shaping our future together. The climate crisis—A race we can win*. https://www.un.org/en/un75/climate-crisis-race-we-can-win

USGCRP. (2016). The impacts of climate change on human health in the United States: A scientific assessment. In A. Crimmins, J. Balbus, J. L. Gamble, C. B. Beard, J. E. Bell, D. Dodgen, R. J. Eisen, N. Fann, M. D. Hawkins, S. C. Herring, L. Jantarasami, D. M. Mills, S. Saha, M. C. Sarofim, J. Trtanj, & L. Ziska (Eds.), *U.S. Global Change Research Program*. 312 pp. http://dx.doi.org/10.7930/J0R49NQX

Wohlford, S., Esteves-Fuentes, N., & Carter, K. F. (2020). Reducing waste in the clinical setting. *American Journal of Nursing, 120*(6), 48–55.

Woolf, S. H., & Aron, L. (Eds.). (2013). *U.S. health in international perspective: Shorter lives, poorer health*. The National Academies Press.

5 Culturally Respectful Care

Danielle Dorvall

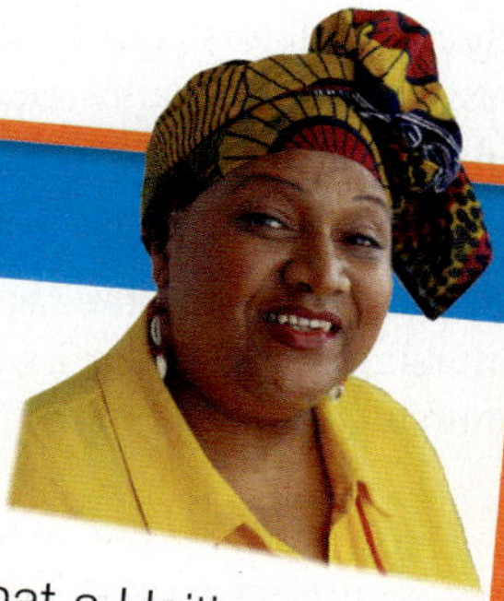

Danielle is an immigrant from Haiti who has been in the United States for approximately 8 months. She recently had surgical repair of a fractured femur and is now confined to a hospital bed in skeletal traction. She asks that a Haitian folk healer from her neighborhood be allowed to come to the hospital to help heal her broken leg.

Khalifa Abdul Hakim

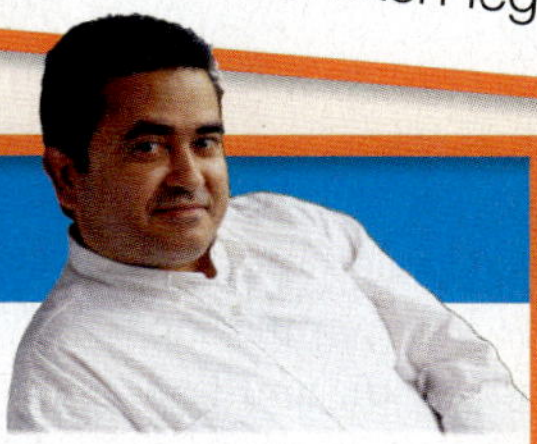

Khalifa, the husband of a Muslim patient, requests that only female health care providers care for his wife. In the Muslim culture, it is deemed immodest for a married woman's body to be seen by any male other than her husband.

Janice Goldberg

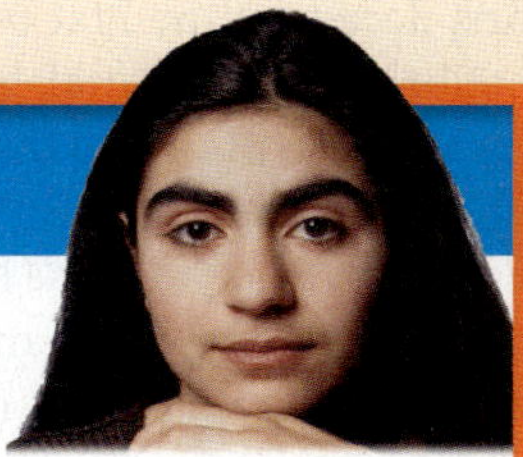

Janice, a 23-year-old woman of Jewish ancestry, comes to the women's health clinic for a routine examination. During the visit, she asks, "I've been dating this man who also is Jewish, and we're thinking about getting married and having children. But I've heard about a hereditary disorder called Tay-Sachs disease that occurs in Jewish people. Should I be concerned?"

Learning Outcomes

After completing the chapter, you will be able to accomplish the following:

1. Explain concepts of cultural diversity and respect.
2. Describe influences that affect culturally respectful health care.
3. Discuss examples of how diversity affects health and illness care, including culturally based traditional care.
4. Identify factors commonly included in a transcultural assessment of health-related beliefs and practices.
5. Practice cultural respect when assessing and providing nursing care for patients from diverse cultural groups.
6. Discuss factors in the health care system and in nursing that facilitate or impede culturally competent nursing care.

Nursing Concepts

- Identity (including culture/diversity)

Analysis of the 2010 U.S. census data reveals sweeping changes over the last 20 years. The U.S. population is bigger, older, more Hispanic and Asian, and less inclined toward marriage and traditional families than in 1990. Other trends reveal that the United States is more embracing of several generations living under one roof, more inclusive of same-sex couples, more aware of multiracial identities, more suburban, and less rural. "The end of the first decade of the 21st century marks a turning point in the nation's social, cultural, geographic, racial and ethnic fabric. It's a shift so profound that it reveals an America that seemed unlikely a mere 20 years ago—one that will influence the nation for years to come in everything from who is elected to run the country, states and cities to what types of household will be built and where" (El Nassar & Overberg, 2011).

An essay in *The Economist* in 2020 noted that baby boomers (born between 1946 and 1964) have dominated American politics since the 1990s, when they became the largest living generation and started to cast the largest number of votes. The year 2020, however, might be called the year of the young, in which protesters against racial injustice have mostly been in their 20s. The young have also been hardest hit by the consequences of the COVID-19 virus (losing jobs or taking a significant pay cut). "America is moving from largely white, baby-boomer-dominated politics and culture in the second half of the 20th century to a more racially diverse country fuelled by younger generations: millennials [born between 1981 and 1996], Gen Z-ers and their juniors." This report continues:

> Younger generations differ from their elders in attitudes, ethnicity, and education.... millennials and Gen Z-ers are most likely to say governments should do more to solve problems, that same-sex marriage is good for society, that climate change is caused by human activity and that blacks are treated less fairly than whites (*The Economist*, 2020).

The essential knowledge and skills for understanding cultural diversity and providing thoughtful, person-centered culturally respectful care have become essential components of nursing practice. For an example, see the accompanying Reflective Practice display. This chapter focuses on concepts of cultural diversity and cultural respect and discusses their influence on nursing care.

CONCEPTS OF CULTURAL DIVERSITY AND RESPECT

Cultural diversity is the coexistence of different ethnic, sex assigned at birth, racial, and socioeconomic groups within one social unit. These groups include, but are not limited to, people of varying religion, language, physical size, sexual orientation, age, disability, occupational status, and geographic location. Culture is an integral component of both health and illness because of the cultural values and beliefs that we learn in our families and communities. Nurses and other health care providers must be familiar with the concepts of cultural diversity in order to understand characteristics common to certain populations.

Nurses must also be sensitive to cultural factors in order to provide culturally respectful care to people from diverse backgrounds. The concept of **cultural respect** enables nurses to deliver services that are respectful of and responsive to the health beliefs, practices, and cultural and linguistic needs of diverse patients. Moreover, cultural respect is critical to reducing health disparities and improving access to high-quality health care (National Institutes of Health [NIH], 2017).

It is also vital to remember that each person may be a member of multiple cultural, ethnic, and racial groups at one time. Therefore, different cultural values may guide a person in different situations based on what is most important to that person at the time. In addition, any person should be viewed foremost as an individual, not as a representative of a cultural group. **Intersectionality** refers to the simultaneous experience of categorical and hierarchical classifications including, but not limited to, race, class, gender, sexuality, and nationality. It also refers to the fact that what is often perceived as disparate forms of oppression, such as racism, classism, sexism, and xenophobia, are actually mutually dependent and intersecting in nature, and together they compose a unified system of oppression. Thus, the privileges we enjoy and the discrimination we face are a product of our unique positioning in society as determined by these social classifiers (https://www.thoughtco.com/intersectionality-definition-3026353).

Culture

Culture is a shared system of beliefs, values, and behavioral expectations that provides social structure for daily living. The NIH defines culture as the combination of a

QSEN Reflective Practice: Cultivating QSEN Competencies

CHALLENGE TO INTELLECTUAL SKILLS

I had thought that I was pretty much used to all sorts of questions from patients about why a guy like me would go into nursing. Today, however, I was surprised when Khalifa Abdul Hakim, the husband of a newly admitted patient, demanded that I leave his wife's room immediately. Stepping into the corridor with me, he explained that he and his family were Muslim and that in their culture it was deemed immodest for the body of a married woman to be seen by any male other than her husband. He asked me to make sure it was clear in his wife's chart that there should be no male nurses. He also asked about female physicians. Since we were short-staffed and all trying to cover for one another to get through the day, I wasn't sure that I could make that promise, especially since our unit has three or four male nurses. I wasn't clear if this was just a personal preference or a religious or cultural matter or both, or if it really mattered at all. I had absolutely no clue how to respond. I understood the importance of culturally appropriate care, but couldn't remember learning how to respond to a request like this. I also wasn't sure if the hospital had a policy about something like this.

Thinking Outside the Box: Possible Courses of Action

- Find someone to swap patients with me and just not have to deal with the situation (probably the simplest response).
- Use the opportunity to research Muslim culture and talk with the patient's male family members about what is important to them. Since we are seeing more Muslim patients, suggest an in-service program on this topic for everyone.
- Explain to Mr. Hakim that his wife is in a U.S. hospital, and that while here, they should observe U.S. customs, meaning she may have male nurses or other male health care providers.
- Check the hospital's policy about this request and then follow it.

Evaluating a Good Outcome: How Do I Define Success?

- I know enough to do whatever is necessary to ensure the patient's health and well-being as well as respect the integrity of all participants involved.
- The patient and her family feel sufficiently comfortable in our environment (culturally appropriate care) for healing to be maximized.
- I know more at the end of the experience than when I started.

Personal Learning: Here's to the Future!

I was pretty surprised when two of the older, more experienced nurses said they had never encountered such a request and they didn't know if the hospital had a policy about it. Luckily, one of them referred me to our patient-advocate person, and she came right up to the unit. I had never met her before, but I was impressed with her knowledge and her strong commitment to patient advocacy. She showed me the hospital policy that obligates all workers to respect the beliefs and values of patients unless this entails compromising their own integrity or the safety of other persons. She said that we will be seeing more Muslim patients in the future and recommended a website to get more information. I haven't checked it out yet, but I did talk some with the patient's family and have a better understanding why this matters to them. So now I'm trying to cultivate the attitude that each patient and family could be an important learning opportunity for me if I'm open to what they have to teach!

QSEN SELF-REFLECTION ON QUALITY AND SAFETY COMPETENCIES DEVELOPING KNOWLEDGE, SKILLS, AND ATTITUDES FOR CONTINUOUS IMPROVEMENT

How do you think you would respond in a similar situation? Why? Do you agree with the criteria this nursing student used to evaluate a successful outcome? Why or why not? What *knowledge, skills,* and *attitudes* do you need to develop to improve the quality and safety of care for families like the Hakims?

Patient-Centered Care: What role does the nurse's cultural sensitivity, respect, and accommodation play in creating a successful person-centered partnership with the Hakims? What lessons did the student learn about the importance of cultural humility and competence?

Teamwork and Collaboration/Quality Improvement: What communication skills do you need to improve to ensure that you function as a valuable member of the patient-care team and to obtain assistance when needed? What did you learn about the importance of a referral—in this case to the patient advocate? How could this experience be used to improve care for other Muslim families?

Safety/Evidence-Based Practice: What role should safety considerations play in evaluating whether or not there was adequate staff to meet Mr. Hakim's request? Are there research studies about how best to accommodate cultural beliefs and preferences?

Informatics: Can you identify the essential information that must be available in Ms. Hakim's electronic record to support safe patient care and coordination of care? Can you think of other ways to respond to or approach the situation?

body of knowledge, a body of belief, and a body of behavior. Elements include personal identification, language, thoughts, communications, actions, customs, beliefs, values, and institutions that are specific to ethnic, racial, religious, geographic, or social groups. For nurses who practice thoughtful, person-centered care, these elements influence beliefs and belief systems surrounding health, healing, wellness, illness, disease, and delivery of health services.

Culture influences roles and interactions with others as well as within families and communities and is apparent in the attitudes and institutions unique to particular groups (Andrew et al., 2020). The characteristics of culture include the following:

- Culture helps shape what is acceptable behavior for people in a specific group. It is shared by, and provides an identity for, members of the same cultural group.
- Culture is learned by each new generation through both formal and informal life experiences. Language is the primary means of transmitting culture.
- The practices of a particular culture often arise because of the group's social and physical environment.
- Cultural practices and beliefs may evolve over time, but they mainly remain constant as long as they satisfy a group's needs.
- Culture influences the way people of a group view themselves, have expectations, and behave in response to certain situations. Because a culture is made up of people, there are differences both within cultures and among cultures.

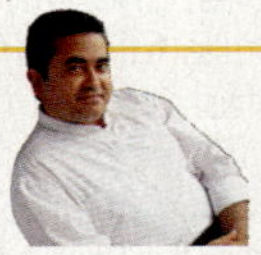

Recall **Mr. Hakim**, the Muslim man described in the Reflective Practice display. The nurse's knowledge of his culture and beliefs are important for ensuring culturally respectful care as well as staffing needs. The nurse needs to understand actions and behaviors that would be acceptable to Mr. Hakim and his wife.

Within most cultures are **subcultures**. A subculture is a large group of people who are members of the larger cultural group but who have certain ethnic, occupational, or physical characteristics that are not common to the larger culture. For example, nursing is a subculture of the larger health care system culture, and teenagers and older adults are often regarded as subcultures of the general population in the United States.

Most societies include both dominant culture groups and minority culture groups. The dominant group has the most ability to control the values and sanctions of the society. It usually is (but does not have to be) the largest group in the society. Minority groups usually have some physical or cultural characteristic (such as race, religious beliefs, or occupation) different from those of the dominant group.

When a minority group lives within a dominant group, many members may lose the cultural characteristics that once made them different, and they may take on the values of the dominant culture. This process is called **cultural assimilation** or acculturation. For example, when people immigrate and encounter a new dominant culture as they work, go to school, and learn the dominant language, they often move closer to the dominant culture. The process and the rate of assimilation are individualized.

Mutual cultural assimilation also occurs, with both groups taking on some characteristics of the other. For example, many Hispanic immigrants to the United States learn to speak English, and many Americans learn to cook and enjoy traditional Hispanic foods. We all gain from the many cultures with which we live. Although we seldom think about it, the clothes we wear, the foods we eat, the music we enjoy, many of the words we use, and the leisure activities we practice are all influenced by acculturation.

A person may experience **culture shock** when placed in a different culture they perceive as strange. Culture shock may result in psychological discomfort or disturbances, because the patterns of behavior a person found acceptable and effective in their own culture may not be adequate or even acceptable in the new culture. The person may then feel foolish, fearful, incompetent, inadequate, or humiliated. These feelings can eventually lead to frustration, anxiety, and loss of self-esteem.

Ethnicity

Ethnicity is a sense of identification with a collective cultural group, largely based on the group members' common heritage. One belongs to a specific ethnic group or groups either through birth or through adoption of characteristics of that group. People within an ethnic group generally share unique cultural and social beliefs and behavior patterns, including language and dialect, religious practices, literature, folklore, music, political interests, food preferences, and employment patterns. Ethnicity largely develops through day-to-day life with family and friends within the community.

Race

Although the term *ethnicity* is often used interchangeably with race, these terms are not the same. Racial categories are typically based on specific physical characteristics such as skin pigmentation, body stature, facial features, and hair texture. Because of the significant blending of physical characteristics through the centuries, however, race is becoming harder to define using simple classifications, and physical characteristics are not considered a reliable way to determine a person's race. Federal standards for race classification provide five categories, Native American or Alaska Native, Asian, Black or African American, Native Hawaiian or Other Pacific Islander, and White, and provide the opportunity for people to identify themselves in multiple categories.

In recent years, the concept of "race" has become increasingly controversial (Park et al., 2021). The authors contrast the historical thinking that racial categories reflect our genetic composition, making it a *biologic* concept with the more recent thinking of race as a *socially constructed* concept. If the more recent thinking is correct, "using a racial category as an attributing factor for undesirable health conditions may reinforce racism and that such attribution may not be scientifically warranted because association isn't causation" (p. 5). See also Chadha et al. "Toward the abolition of biological race in medicine" (2020).

Factors Inhibiting Sensitivity to Diversity

A variety of factors may affect a person's sensitivity to others. When one assumes that all members of a culture, ethnic group, or race act alike, **stereotyping** is at work. Stereotyping may be positive or negative. Negative stereotyping includes racism, ageism, and sexism. These are mistaken beliefs that certain races, an age group, or one biologic sex is inherently superior to others, leading to discrimination against those considered inferior. Take a moment to look carefully at the images in Figure 5-1. What assumptions might you bring to your encounters with these people? Are you aware of any personal biases that could influence the way you respond to them? Many of us aren't even aware of biases that influence our ability to create respectful, trusting relationships. When we hold attitudes toward people or associate stereotypes with them without our conscious knowledge it is called **implicit bias**. If you have never taken the implicit bias test, check it out: https://implicit.harvard.edu/implicit/takeatest.html. What did you learn about any personal biases that you may not have recognized that you hold?

Also affecting cultural sensitivity are **cultural imposition**, which is the belief that everyone else should conform to your own belief system, and **cultural blindness**, which occurs when one ignores differences and proceeds as though they do not exist. Cultural imposition and cultural blindness can be observed within the health care system, especially in regard to nonmainstream methods of care. **Culture conflict** occurs when people become aware of cultural differences, feel threatened, and respond by ridiculing the beliefs and traditions of others to make themselves feel more secure about their own values (Andrews et al., 2020).

CULTURAL INFLUENCES ON HEALTH CARE

The United States is multicultural, multiethnic, and multiracial. The U.S. Census Bureau (2019a) projected that net international migration is expected to add one person to the U.S. population every 34 seconds. Therefore, nurses must be aware of, and sensitive to, the needs of a diverse patient population. Most people interpret the behaviors of others in terms of their own familiar culture. This process usually works both ways; for example, in a health care setting, the patient evaluates the attitudes and actions of the health care provider at the same time the health care provider interprets the behavior of the patient. What may seem reasonable and important to a patient may seem ridiculous and irrelevant to an insensitive nurse. The reverse is also true: practices a nurse perceives as logical and effective may seem senseless or even dangerous to a patient.

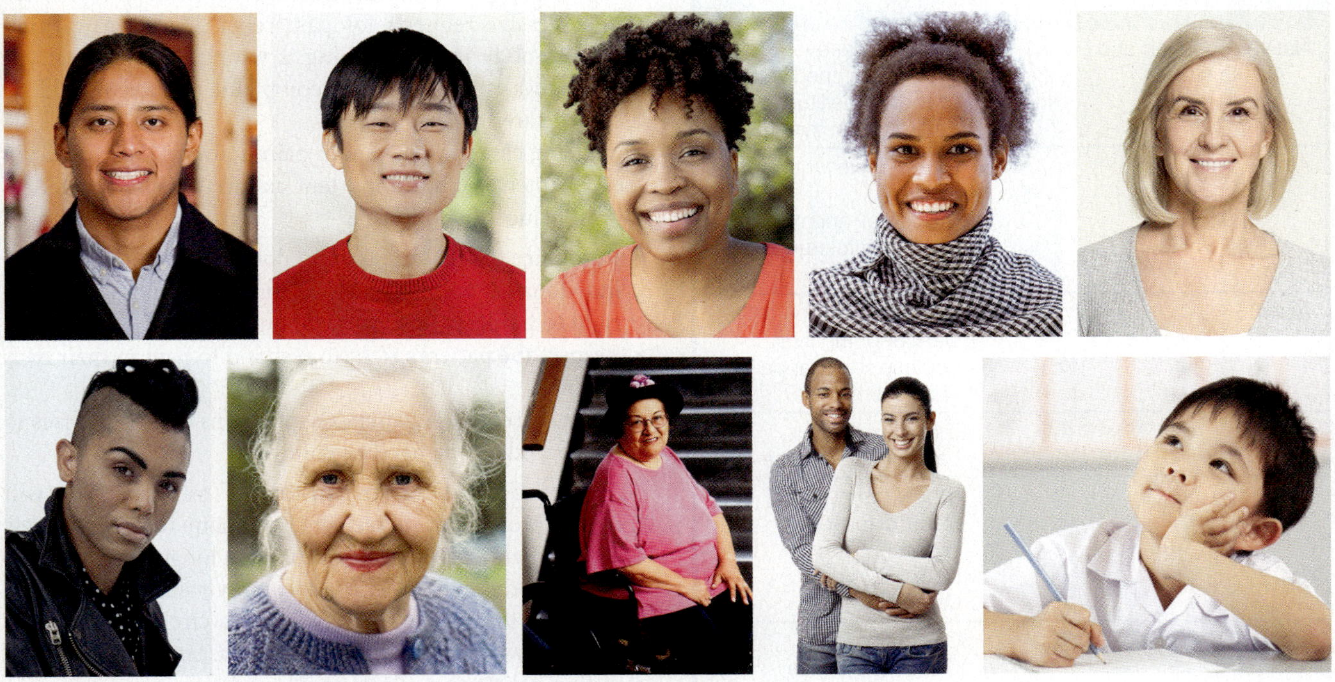

FIGURE 5-1. Identifying our own prejudices is the first step toward eliminating them. Think about the assumptions you make regarding the people in these images. (*Source:* Used with permission from Shutterstock. Top row, from left to right: *Photos by Fotos593, FabrikaSimf, pixelheadphoto digitalskillet, Hagen Production, fizkes.* Bottom row, far right: *Photo by wavebreakmedia.*)

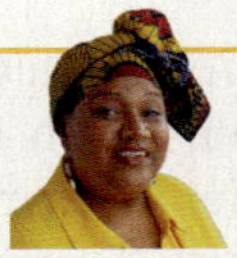

Consider **Danielle Dorvall**, described at the beginning of the chapter. She might view skeletal traction as worthless, while the nurse may view her request for a folk healer in the same way. The nurse needs to be aware of these possible attitudes and beliefs to ensure maximum effective care while still meeting the patient's cultural needs.

The following sections describe general considerations in providing **culturally competent care**.

Physiologic Variations

Studies have shown that certain racial and ethnic groups are more prone to being diagnosed with certain diseases and conditions. For example, a hereditary disorder, Tay-Sachs disease, is associated with people of Eastern European Jewish descent. Although the incidence of this disorder has declined over the years owing to improved and earlier testing, it is still a concern. Use knowledge of such risk factors when interviewing a patient to complete a health history. Table 5-1 provides examples of diseases that are more often diagnosed in specific populations. This is not a comprehensive list.

Remember, according to the newer understanding of race as a socially constructed concept, the fact that cirrhosis of the liver and fetal alcohol syndrome are found more frequently in Native Americans and Alaska Natives does not mean that these individuals have a genetic propensity for these diseases, but rather that structural racism in the United States and elsewhere has produced living circumstances that promote these disorders more frequently in these communities—a critical distinction.

Table 5-1 Examples of Common Health Problems in Specific Populations

POPULATION	COMMON HEALTH PROBLEMS
Native American and Alaska Native	Heart disease Cirrhosis of the liver Diabetes mellitus Fetal alcohol syndrome
African American	Hypertension Stroke Sickle cell anemia Lactose intolerance Keloids
Asian	Hypertension Cancer of the liver Lactose intolerance Thalassemia
Hispanic	Diabetes mellitus Lactose intolerance
White	Breast cancer Heart disease Hypertension Diabetes mellitus Obesity
Eastern European Jewish	Cystic fibrosis Gaucher disease Spinal muscular atrophy Tay-Sachs disease

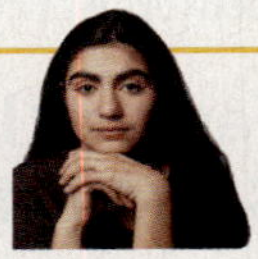

Recall **Janice Goldberg**, the young woman described at the beginning of the chapter. Knowledge of the Tay-Sachs disorder and screening and early detection methods would be important for the nurse to use as a foundation when counseling and teaching Janice.

Reactions to Pain

Health care researchers have discovered that many of the expressions and behaviors exhibited by people in pain are culturally prescribed. Some cultures allow or even encourage the open expression of emotions related to pain, whereas other cultures encourage suppression of such emotions.

You should not assume that a patient who does not complain of pain is not having pain. If you make this assumption, you may overlook the pain-reduction needs of a patient who deals with pain quietly and stoically. To avoid this error, be sensitive to nonverbal signals of discomfort, such as holding or applying pressure to the painful area, avoiding activities that intensify the pain, and uncontrollable, spontaneous expressions of discomfort, such as facial grimacing and moaning. You also should not consider patients who freely express their discomfort as constant complainers with excessive requests for pain relief. Pain is a warning from the body that something is wrong. Pain is what the patient says it is, and every complaint of pain should be assessed carefully.

Nursing care for a patient in pain is always individualized (see Chapter 36), but important culture-sensitive considerations include the following:

- Recognize that culture is an important component of individuality, and that each person holds (and has the right to hold) various beliefs about pain.
- Respect the patient's right to respond to pain in their own manner.
- Never stereotype a patient's perceptions of or responses to pain based on the person's culture.

Finally, if you study the history of medicine, you will find that professional caregivers held many incorrect beliefs about the pain patients perceived. For a long time, the belief that infants did not feel pain led to many painful procedures, such as the insertion of chest tubes or a circumcision being performed without any type of analgesia. Similarly, the longstanding beliefs that Black people did not experience pain like White people, routinely led to the undermanagement of their pain during painful procedures.

Mental Health

Most mental health data originated in research and observations made of White, middle-class people. But many ethnic groups have their own respectable patterns of behavior for psychological well-being as well as different psychological reactions to certain situations. For example, many Hispanic people deal with problems within the family and consider it inappropriate to tell problems to a stranger. Some Chinese people consider mental illness a stigma and seeking psychiatric help a disgrace to the family. In times of high stress or anxiety, some Puerto Rican individuals may demonstrate a hyperkinetic seizurelike activity known as *ataques*; this behavior is a culturally accepted reaction. Be aware of these variations and accept them as culturally appropriate (Giger & Davidhizer, 2020).

Assigned Sex Roles

In some cultures, the man is the dominant figure and generally makes decisions for all family members. For example, if approval for medical care is needed, the man may give it regardless of which family member is involved. In male-dominant cultures, women are often passive. On the other hand, in some cultures, women are dominant.

Knowing who is dominant in the family is important when planning nursing care. For example, if the dominant member is ill and can no longer make decisions, the whole family may be anxious and confused. If a nondominant family member is ill, the person may need help in verbalizing needs, particularly if the needs differ from those the dominant member perceives as being important.

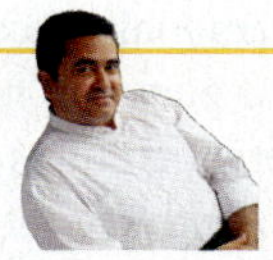

Think back to **Mr. Hakim**, the Muslim man concerned about his wife's care providers being male. Because Mr. Hakim—not his wife—made the request about no male care providers, the nurse would interpret this as indicating that Mr. Hakim is the dominant family member. This assumption, however, would need to be tested.

Language and Communication

When people from another part of the world where English is not the dominant language move to the United States, they may speak their own language fluently but have difficulty speaking English. This is especially true for people in the family who do not work outside the home and for people who live in proximity to others who speak their primary language. Assimilation is likewise slower for people who stay at home, especially if they live in communities of their ethnic and cultural background. Children usually assimilate more rapidly and learn the language of the dominant culture quickly if they leave home each day to go to school and make new friends in the dominant culture. Wage earners also tend to learn a new language more quickly through the work setting. Language acquisition is thus tied to necessity and assimilation rather than to degree of difficulty.

Because the United States has such a diverse population, with many languages spoken, communication problems can arise during health care activities. This problem is not unique to non–English-speaking patients; even in different regions of the country, certain dialects or word meanings can cause differences in understanding. Consider how difficult it must be to describe symptoms or give a personal health history when you do not understand the questions being asked. In addition, patients may forget English words or revert to their more familiar language when experiencing the stress of an injury, illness, or pain. Imagine for a moment finding yourself in an emergency room with crushing chest pain in a foreign country where no one speaks your language. **Linguistic competence** refers to the ability of caregivers and organizations to understand and effectively respond to the linguistic needs of patients and their families in a health care encounter.

Nurses who work in a geographic area with a high population of residents who speak a language other than English should learn pertinent words and phrases in that language. (See the accompanying Through the Eyes of a Student account on page 102.) Many facilities also have a qualified interpreter, or one can be found in the community. To avoid misinterpretation of questions and answers, it is important to use an interpreter who understands the health care system. Sometimes a family member or friend can translate for the nurse, but such a person may be protective and not the most reliable means of transferring information; thus, guidelines discourage using family members or friends as translators.

QSEN PATIENT-CENTERED CARE

Be sure you are familiar with the resources available in your agency and policies for interacting with people who do not speak English. You should know that not infrequently professional caregivers are reluctant to secure the assistance of trusted interpreters because this involves more time than usual.

Keep in mind that talking more loudly to someone who does not understand what you are saying is not helpful. Remember that language difference is a communication problem, not a hearing problem. Make sure you are familiar with the linguistic resources available in your practice settings and pertinent policies.

The U.S. Department of Health and Human Services Office of Minority Health created a health care language services implementation guide to help health care organizations implement effective language access services to meet the needs of their patients with limited English proficiency, thereby increasing their access to health care. You will find this guide, along with many other helpful resources at the website http://www.minorityhealth.hhs.gov. Also see Marcus, MacMillan, Ketchie, and Clark (2020) for a study of how nurses perceive technology used in language interpretation for patients with limited English proficiency.

Through the Eyes of a Student

I was doing my maternity rotation and was assigned to labor and delivery. I was caring for a woman who spoke no English—she and her husband were from Central America and had been in the United States for only 2 months.

When I arrived at 7 AM, the night nurse was giving a report about my patient to the day nurse. The night nurse was frantic—no one understood the couple, all efforts to locate a translator had come up empty, and, quite frankly, she had no idea exactly what condition this woman was in.

I quickly began to think back on my 2 years of Spanish. Could I be of any help to this couple? I wondered. Would I remember enough to communicate with them about giving birth? Then I decided that any little bit of communication at this point was better than none, so I spoke up. I told both nurses that I spoke some Spanish and asked if I could be of any help. The night nurse literally hugged me!

I began by telling the expectant couple that I was a nursing student and that I spoke some Spanish. We exchanged introductions and then I asked the woman some assessment questions. Nothing I said was complicated—all of my sentences were short and simple, but who needed more than that?

Then the couple asked me some questions. They had heard about "cutting open the stomach" to deliver a baby. I naturally assumed that they meant a cesarean delivery. They looked so afraid but I had to be honest. They wanted to know how it was done and why. The words I could not remember or did not know I acted out. They looked so relieved when I was finished.

The man said that they thought all babies were born this way in our country. He said that they had never heard of this procedure until coming to the United States. No wonder they were so frightened!

The doctor came in, examined the woman, and said she was fully dilated. The doctor asked if I could teach a crash course in Lamaze breathing to the woman. She also asked me if I would stay throughout the delivery because she would need assistance in translating directions to the woman. Of course, I said yes.

The woman was terrified. I told her that it was normal to be afraid and that I would be with her during the delivery. She took my hand and whispered, "Muchas gracias." I never felt more useful than I did at that moment.

—A. Kelly Gaylor, Holy Family College, Philadelphia

One of the most culturally variable forms of nonverbal communication is eye contact. The American-dominant culture emphasizes eye contact while speaking, but many other cultures regard this behavior in different ways. For example, direct eye contact may be considered impolite or aggressive by many people who are Asian, Native American, Indochinese, Middle Eastern and North African (MENA), and Appalachian; people from these groups may avert their eyes while speaking. Hispanic people may look downward in deference to age, assigned sex, social position, economic status, or authority. Muslim–Arab women often indicate modesty by avoiding eye contact with men, and Hasidic Jewish men may avoid direct eye contact with women (Andrews et al., 2020). Although the above examples are not true of all members of a group, they provide some general guidelines.

When caring for a patient from a cultural or ethnic group different from your own, it is important to perform a transcultural assessment of communication (Andrews et al., 2020):

- What language does the patient speak during usual activities of daily living?
- How well does the patient speak and write in English?
- Does the patient need an interpreter? Are there people the patient would not want to serve as an interpreter?
- How does the patient prefer to be addressed?
- What cultural values and beliefs of the patient (such as eye contact, personal space, or social taboos) may change your techniques of communication and care?
- How does the patient's nonverbal behavior affect the responses of members of the health care team?
- What are the cultural characteristics of the patient's communications with others?

Chapter 8 provides additional information on communicating with non–English-speaking patients. Box 5-1 illustrates two mnemonics which may be helpful if you are intent on developing culturally sensitive medical interviewing skills.

Orientation to Space and Time

Personal space is the area around a person regarded as part of the person. This area, individualized to each person and to different cultures and ethnic groups, is the area into which others should not intrude during personal interactions. If others do

Box 5-1 Culturally Sensitive Medical Interviewing Tools

Ethnic

E. Explanation (How do you explain your illness?)
T. Treatment (What treatment have you tried?)
H. Healers (Have you sought any advice from folk healers?)
N. Negotiate (mutually acceptable options)
I. (Agree on) intervention
C. Collaboration (with patient, family, and healers)

Learn Model

L. Listen to the patient's perspective
E. Explain and share your own perspective
A. Acknowledge differences and similarities between these two perspectives
R. Recommend a treatment plan
N. Negotiate a mutually agreed-on treatment plan

Source: Cultural Competency, College of Medicine, Medical University of South Carolina, http://etl2.library.musc.edu/cultural/communication/communication_4.php

not consider a person's personal space, that person may become uncomfortable or even angry. When providing nursing care that involves physical contact, you should know the patient's cultural personal space preferences. For example, people from some Middle Eastern and African cultures commonly sit and stand close to one another when talking, whereas people of from some Asian and European cultures may be more comfortable with more distance between themselves and others.

Many people and almost all institutions in the United States value promptness and punctuality. When arriving for an appointment, doing a job, or carrying out an activity, being on time and getting the job done promptly are viewed as important. This is not true in some other cultures. For example, in some South Asian cultures, being late is considered a sign of respect. In addition, while some cultures are future oriented (including activities that promote future good health), other cultures are more concerned with the present or the past. Understanding the patient's orientation to time is important as you communicate, for example, the need to be on time for appointments for health care procedures and when taking medications.

Food and Nutrition

Food preferences and preparation methods often are culturally influenced. Certain food groups serve as staples of the diet based on culture and remain so even when members of that culture are living in a different country.

Patients in a hospital or long-term care setting often do not have much choice of foods. This means that people with cultural food preferences may not be able to select appealing foods and thus may be at risk for inadequate nutrition. When assessing the possible causes of a patient's decreased appetite, try to determine whether the problem may be related to culture. It may be possible for family or friends to bring in foods that satisfy the patient's nutritional needs while still meeting dietary restrictions. Dietary teaching must be individualized according to cultural values about the social significance and sharing of food.

Family Support

In many cultural and ethnic groups, people have large, extended families and consider the needs of any family member to be equal to or greater than their own. They may be unwilling to share private information about family members with those outside the family (including health care providers). Other cultural groups have great respect for the elders in the family and would never consider institutional care for them. Including the family in planning care for any patient is a major component in nursing care to meet individualized needs, especially if those needs can be met only through consideration of all members of the family.

Socioeconomic Factors

Low income is a major problem in the United States and is often described as having created a culture of poverty. A report from the U.S. Census Bureau (2019b) noted that an estimated 11.8% of the U.S. population had an income below the poverty threshold. Of that population, the lowest income was found in African Americans, Native Americans, and Alaska Natives. In 2018, 16.2% of all children lived in poverty—that's about one in every five children. On a single night in January 2016:

- An estimated 194,716 people in families, or 61,265 family households were identified as homeless. See Macenroe-Petitte (2020) for a comprehensive article on care for patients who are homeless.
- More than 19,000 were living on the street, in a car, or in another place not meant for human habitation.
- 120,819 were children under the age of 6 (National Alliance to End Homelessness, n.d.).

At the time of writing this chapter, data are not available to see how the pandemic has affected poverty rates in the United States and homelessness. We do know that children and adults face poverty and hunger in every county across the United States. Feeding America reported in 2021 that:

- In 2019, 34 million people lived in poverty in America. For a family of four, that means earning just $25,000 per year.
- Before the coronavirus pandemic, more than 35 million people struggled with hunger in the United States, including more than 10 million children.
- A household that is food insecure has limited or uncertain access to enough food to support a healthy life.
- Children are more likely to face food insecurity than any other group in the United States.
- The coronavirus pandemic has left millions of families without stable employment. More than 50 million people, including 17 million children, may experience food insecurity (https://www.feedingamerica.org/hunger-in-america/facts).

There has been much debate about how to define poverty. In terms of economics, a person or family whose income falls below an established threshold is considered to be experiencing poverty. The U.S. Census Bureau defines poverty according to money or income guidelines that vary by family size and composition. If the family's total income is less than a set threshold, all members of the family are considered to be experiencing poverty. Others have stated that poverty is a relative term that reflects a judgment based on community standards. Such standards vary at different times and in different places; what is judged to be poverty in one community might be regarded as wealth in another (Spector, 2017). No matter how poverty is defined, it is an increasingly devastating epidemic, fueled by real estate foreclosures and credit debt that has evolved into a culture of its own. At highest risk are children, older people, families headed by single mothers, and the future generations of those now living in poverty. Access to financial resources affects how individuals and families meet their basic needs and maintain their health. Poverty often leads to problems such as lack of health insurance, inadequate care of infants and children, lack of access to basic health care services, and homelessness. All these are of concern to nursing.

The feminization of poverty threatens to increase the number of people who are living at poverty level. The number of female-headed households is increasing as a result of divorce, abandonment, unmarried motherhood, and changes in abortion laws. Because it is now common that two incomes are required in a household for economic survival, a single woman supporting a household is at a financial disadvantage. The number of single-parent families headed by women is associated closely with the increasing number of children living in poverty and the number of homeless families with children.

The increasing population of older people has also raised problems associated with poverty. Many older people live on fixed incomes that often do not keep up with inflation, and many (particularly widows) are on the borderline of poverty or have already slipped below the poverty level. Socioeconomic status often differs by the cultural group of the older adult. For example, Pacific/Asian, African American, Native American, and Hispanic elders generally have lower incomes than elders in the majority population. The work history of the cultural group, especially those who have labored all their lives as agricultural workers, often means that a person has no Social Security or Medicare benefits.

In some cases, the culture of poverty is passed from generation to generation. This appears to be especially true in such groups as migrant farm workers, families living on public assistance, and people who live in isolated areas such as Appalachia. Poverty cultures often have the following characteristics:

- Feelings of despair, resignation, and fatalism
- "Day-to-day" attitude toward life, with no hope for the future
- Unemployment and need for financial or government aid
- Unstable family structure, possibly characterized by abusiveness and abandonment
- Decline in self-respect and retreat from community involvement

Poverty has long been a barrier to adequate health care. It prevents many people from consistently meeting their basic human needs. The lack of affordable or adequate housing is a problem experienced frequently by those in poverty. When low-income housing is available, it sometimes lacks such necessities as running water, heat, and electricity. To stretch their available money and to pool resources, many people live in crowded conditions, with several families living together in one household.

Research has demonstrated that crowded living conditions foster depersonalization, correlate with higher crime rates, and lead to psychological problems such as schizophrenia, alienation, and feelings of worthlessness (Spector, 2017). Such conditions also contribute to an increased incidence and severity of disease and illness because of the closer proximity of people, the sharing of utensils and belongings, poor sanitation, and poor health habits.

Accessing health care facilities frequently requires transportation, which often is neither affordable nor available to people experiencing poverty. Their access to health insurance also is frequently limited, and they often must choose between purchasing food and obtaining health care. Those in upper-income groups tend to live longer and to experience less disability than those in lower-income groups. Other barriers to health care include isolation, language or communication difficulties, seasonal occupations, migration patterns, depersonalization, and institutional prejudice (Spector, 2017).

Concept Mastery Alert

The increase in the number of single-parent female families (also known as the feminization of poverty), has had the greatest potential for increasing the number of people living in poverty.

Health Disparities

The term *health disparities* refers to health differences between groups of people; they can affect how frequently a disease affects a group, how many people get sick, or how often the disease causes death. You can read more about disparities in Chapters 3 and 4. Many different populations are affected by disparities, including racial and ethnic minorities; residents of rural areas; women, children, and older adults; and persons with disabilities.

CULTURAL INFLUENCES ON HEALTH AND ILLNESS

People's values and beliefs about health, illness, and health care are influenced by cultural, ethnic, or religious groups. For example, in some groups, illnesses are classified as either natural or unnatural. "Natural illnesses" are caused by dangerous agents, such as cold air or impurities in the air, water, or food. "Unnatural illnesses" are punishments for failing to follow God's rules, resulting in evil forces or witchcraft causing physical or mental health problems.

In some cultures, the power to heal is thought to be a gift from God bestowed on certain people. People in these cultures believe that these folk or traditional healers know what is wrong with them through divine intervention and experience. A patient accustomed to traditional healers may think that health care providers are incompetent because they have to ask many questions before they can treat an illness. Traditional healers speak the patient's primary language, often are more accessible, and are usually more understanding of the patient's cultural and personal needs.

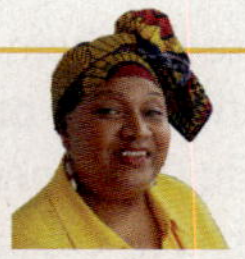

Think back to **Danielle Dorvall**, the immigrant from Haiti asking for a folk healer. Respecting her use of a folk healer, as appropriate, would demonstrate an understanding of her cultural beliefs.

People from different cultures may also have different beliefs about the best way to treat an illness or disease.

For example, herbs are a common method of treatment in many cultures. In fact, many medications used today have a basis in herbs or other plant sources that have been used for centuries to cure illnesses. If a patient traditionally drinks an herbal tea to alleviate symptoms of an illness, there is no reason that both the herbal tea and prescribed medications cannot be used, as long as the tea is safe to drink and the ingredients do not interfere with or exaggerate the action of the medication.

Other traditional therapies include the use of cutaneous stimulation, therapeutic touch, acupuncture, and acupressure. Cutaneous stimulation by massage, vibration, heat, cold, or nerve stimulation reduces the intensity of the sensation of pain. Therapeutic touch is an intentional act that involves an energy transfer from the healer to the patient to stimulate the patient's own healing potential. Acupuncture, long used in China, is a method of preventing, diagnosing, and treating pain and disease by inserting special needles into the body at specified locations. Acupressure involves a deep-pressure massage of appropriate points of the body. Read more about these therapies in Chapter 29.

CULTURALLY RESPECTFUL NURSING CARE

Providing culturally respectful nursing care means that care is planned and implemented in a way that is sensitive to the needs of individuals, families, and groups from diverse populations within society. Among the elements of **cultural competence** (Purnell, 2014) are the following:

- Developing an awareness of your own existence, sensations, thoughts, and environment to prevent them from having an undue influence on those from other backgrounds
- Demonstrating knowledge and understanding of the patient's culture, health-related needs, and culturally specific meanings of health and illness
- Accepting and respecting cultural differences in a manner that facilitates the patient's and family's abilities to make decisions to meet their needs and beliefs
- Not assuming that the health care provider's beliefs and values are the same as the patient's
- Resisting judgmental attitudes such as "different is not as good"
- Being open to and comfortable with cultural encounters
- Accepting responsibility for your own education in cultural competence by attending conferences, reading professional literature, and observing cultural practices

These elements suggest that becoming culturally competent is a life-long challenge, and that nurses should strive to be culturally humble—recognizing what we don't yet know about those entrusted to our care and being willing to learn what we need to know. The Office of Minority Health of the U.S. Department of Human Services created "Think Cultural Health" (https://www.thinkculturalhealth.hhs.gov), an online service whose goal is to advance health equity at every point of contact through the development and promotion of culturally and linguistically appropriate services. Nurses who recognize and respect cultural diversity are better equipped to exhibit cultural sensitivity and provide nursing care that accepts the significance of cultural factors in health and illness. See Box 5-2 for other helpful web resources.

The health care system is itself a culture with customs, rules, values, and a language of its own, with nursing as its largest subculture. As you progress through your education, you will be acculturated into the culture of the health care system and will develop values related to health and health care. Box 5-3 (on page 106) lists some common cultural norms of the health care system.

Although nursing as a whole is actively recruiting more diverse members, many nurses are members of, and have

Box 5-2 Multicultural Web Resources

Diseases and Conditions, Centers for Disease Control and Prevention

www.cdc.gov/DiseasesConditions

Provides information on all diseases but concentrates on infectious disease topics. Available in English and Spanish.

EthnoMed

www.ethnomed.org

Provides information on cultural beliefs, medical issues, and related topics pertinent to the health care of immigrants in Seattle and throughout the United States. It focuses on Cambodian, Ethiopian, Hispanic, Oromo, Somali, Tigrean, and Vietnamese cultures.

Health Information Translations

www.healthinfotranslations.org

Health education resources in multiple languages for diverse populations. Searchable by keyword, topic, and language.

Healthy Roads Media

www.healthyroadsmedia.org

A source of health information on over 100 topics and patient education materials in many formats. Search by topic or language.

MedlinePlus

https://medlineplus.gov/languages/languages.html

Allows users to browse for authoritative health information in over 50 languages.

U.S. Committee for Refugees and Immigrants

http://refugees.org/research-reports

Culturally appropriate material for consumers and health care professionals. Search by topic or language.

Source: Adapted from Schnall, J. G., & Fowler, S. (2014). Multicultural web resources. *The American Journal of Nursing, 114*(6), 63–64.

Box 5-3 Cultural Norms of the Health Care System

Beliefs
- Standardized definitions of health and illness
- Omnipotence of technology
- Critical importance of safety and quality measures

Practices
- Maintenance of health and prevention of illness
- Annual physical examinations and diagnostic procedures

Habits
- Documentation
- Frequent use of jargon
- Use of a systematic approach and problem-solving methodology

Likes
- Promptness
- Neatness and organization
- Compliance

Dislikes
- Tardiness
- Disorderliness and disorganization

Customs
- Professional deference and adherence to the pecking order found in autocratic and bureaucratic systems
- Use of certain procedures attending birth and death

the same value systems as, the dominant U.S. middle-class culture. When a nurse with a particular set of cultural values about health interacts with a patient with a different set of cultural values about health, the following factors affect this interaction (Andrews et al., 2020):

- The cultural background of each participant
- The expectations and beliefs of each about health care
- The cultural context of the encounter (e.g., hospital, clinic, home)
- The extent of agreement between the two persons' sets of beliefs and values

The ESFT model (**E**xplanatory model of health and illness, **S**ocial and environmental factors, **F**ears and concerns, **T**herapeutic contracting) is a cross-cultural communication tool that helps health care professionals strengthen communication and identify potential threats to treatment adherence (Box 5-4). Nurses can use this model to improve health care outcomes and address health disparities.

Nursing care can become complicated when the patient and the nurse have distinctly different cultural norms. Cultural imposition in health care is the tendency for health personnel to impose their beliefs, practices, and values on people of other cultures. Closely related to cultural imposition is **ethnocentrism**, the belief that the ideas, beliefs, and practices of one's own culture are superior to those of another's culture. When health professionals assume that they have the right to make choices and decisions for patients of

Box 5-4 The ESFT Model

The ESFT model guides providers in understanding a patient's explanatory model (a patient's conception of their illness), social and environmental factors, and fears and concerns, and also guides providers in contracting for therapeutic approaches.

E—Explanatory Model of Health and Illness
- What do you think caused your problem?
- Why do you think it started when it did?
- How does it affect you?
- What worries you most?
- What kind of treatment do you think you should receive?

S—Social and Environmental Factors
- How do you get your medications?
- Are they difficult to afford?
- Do you have time to pick them up?
- How quickly do you get them?
- Do you have help getting them if you need it?

F—Fears and Concerns
- Does the medication sound okay to you?
- Are you concerned about the dosage?
- Have you heard anything about this medication?
- Are you worried about the adverse effects?

T—Therapeutic Contracting
- Do you understand how to take the medication?
- Can you tell me how you will take it?

Source: The U.S. Department of Health and Human Services, Office of Minority Health. A physician's practical guide to culturally competent care. https://cccm.thinkculturalhealth.hhs.gov

another culture, patients may respond in the same way that minority cultures often respond to such an attitude by the dominant culture: by becoming passive, resistive, angry, or resistant to treatment.

Unless nurses are willing to examine carefully and clarify their own attitudes and values and to be sensitive to others who are "different," their use of cultural concepts when providing care will be unsuccessful. The nurse's role is to understand the patient's needs and to adapt care to respectfully meet those needs. A careful merging of modern and traditional cultural beliefs is a necessary prerequisite for safe, considerate, and successful nursing care of all patients.

National standards issued by the Office of Minority Health (2001) were developed to ensure that all people entering the health care system be provided equitable and effective treatment in a culturally and linguistically appropriate manner. Examples of these standards are provided in Box 5-5. The Office of Minority Health (2016) has now released The National Standards for Culturally and Linguistically Appropriate Services in Health and Health Care.

Theory of Cultural Humility

Foronda (2021) defines **cultural humility** as "the recognition of diversity and power imbalances among individuals, groups or communities, with the action of being open, self-aware, egoless, flexible, exuding respect and supportive

Box 5-5 Assuring Cultural Competence in Health Care

- Ensure that all patients/families receive from all staff members effective, understandable, and respectful care that is provided in a manner compatible with their cultural health beliefs and practices and preferred language.
- Implement strategies to recruit, retain, and promote at all levels of the organization a diverse staff and leadership that are representative of the demographic characteristics of the service area.
- Ensure that staff at all levels and across all disciplines receive ongoing education and training in culturally and linguistically appropriate service delivery.
- Offer and provide language assistance services, including bilingual staff and interpreter services, at no cost to each patient/family with limited English proficiency at all points of contact, in a timely manner during all hours of operation.
- Make available easily understood patient-related materials and post signs in the language of the commonly encountered groups and/or groups represented in the service area.
- Ensure that data on the individual patient's/family's race, ethnicity, and spoken and written language are collected in health records, integrated into the organization's management information systems, and periodically updated.
- Maintain a current demographic, cultural, and epidemiologic profile of the community, as well as a needs assessment, to accurately plan for and implement services that respond to the cultural and linguistic characteristics of the service area.

Source: The Office of Minority Health, Public Health Service, U.S. Department of Health and Human Services. (2001). Assuring cultural competence in health care: Recommendations for national standards and an outcomes-focused research agenda. *Federal Register*, *65*(247), 80865–80879.

interactions, focusing on both self and other to formulate a tailored response. Cultural humility is a process of critical self-reflection and lifelong learning, resulting in mutually positive outcomes" (p. 9). The accompanying "Through the Eyes of a Nurse: I am the Jewish Nurse" which is found on p. 110, is an excellent example of cultural humility. You may also want to check out Foronda's Rainbow Model of Cultural Humility (2020). Foronda (2021) also offers a guide to debriefing for cultural humility created to help learners critically reflect on past events with the lens of better recognizing and understanding diversity and cultural humility.

Cultural Assessment

The National Center for Cultural Competence urges health care professionals who value cultural competence to enhance their understanding of the following:

- Beliefs, values, traditions, and practices of a culture
- Culturally defined, health-related needs of individuals, families, and communities
- Culturally based belief systems of the etiology of illness and disease and those related to health and healing
- Attitudes toward seeking help from health care providers

When caring for patients from a different culture, it is important to first ask how they want to be treated based on their values and beliefs. An effective way to identify specific factors that influence a patient's behavior is to perform a cultural assessment. The primary informant should be the patient, if possible. If the patient is not able to respond to the questions, a family member or a friend can be consulted. A useful tool for this is the Andrews et al. (2020), part of which is included in Box 5-6. See also the Giger and Davidhizar (2013) and Purnell models for transcultural competence

Box 5-6 Transcultural Assessment: Health-Related Beliefs and Practices

- To what cause(s) does the patient attribute illness and disease (e.g., divine wrath, imbalance in hot/cold or yin/yang, punishment for moral transgressions, hex, soul loss, pathogenic organism)?
- What are the patient's cultural beliefs about the ideal body size and shape? What is the patient's self-image compared to the ideal?
- What name does the patient give to their health-related condition?
- What does the patient believe promotes health (e.g., eating certain foods; wearing amulets to bring good luck; sleep; rest; good nutrition; reducing stress; exercise; prayer; rituals to ancestors, saints, or intermediate deities)?
- What is the patient's religious affiliation (e.g., Judaism, Islam, Pentecostalism, West African voodooism, Seventh-Day Adventism, Catholicism, Mormonism)? How actively involved in the practice of this religion is the patient?
- Does the patient rely on cultural healers (e.g., *curandero*, shaman, spiritualist, priest, minister, monk)? Who determines when the patient is sick and when the patient is healthy? Who influences the choice/type of healer and treatment that should be sought?
- In what types of cultural healing practices does the patient engage (e.g., use of herbal remedies, potions, massage; wearing of talismans, copper bracelets, or charms to discourage evil spirits; healing rituals, incantations, prayers)?
- How are biomedical/scientific health care providers perceived? How do the patient and the patient's family perceive nurses? What are the expectations of nurses and nursing care?
- What comprises appropriate "sick role" behavior? Who determines what symptoms constitute disease/illness? Who decides when the patient is no longer sick? Who cares for the patient at home?
- How does the patient's cultural group view mental disorders? Are there differences in acceptable behaviors for physical versus psychological illnesses?

Source: Adapted from Andrews, M., Boyle, J., & Collins Transcultural Nursing Assessment Guide. (2020). *Transcultural concepts in nursing care* (8th ed.). Wolters Kluwer.

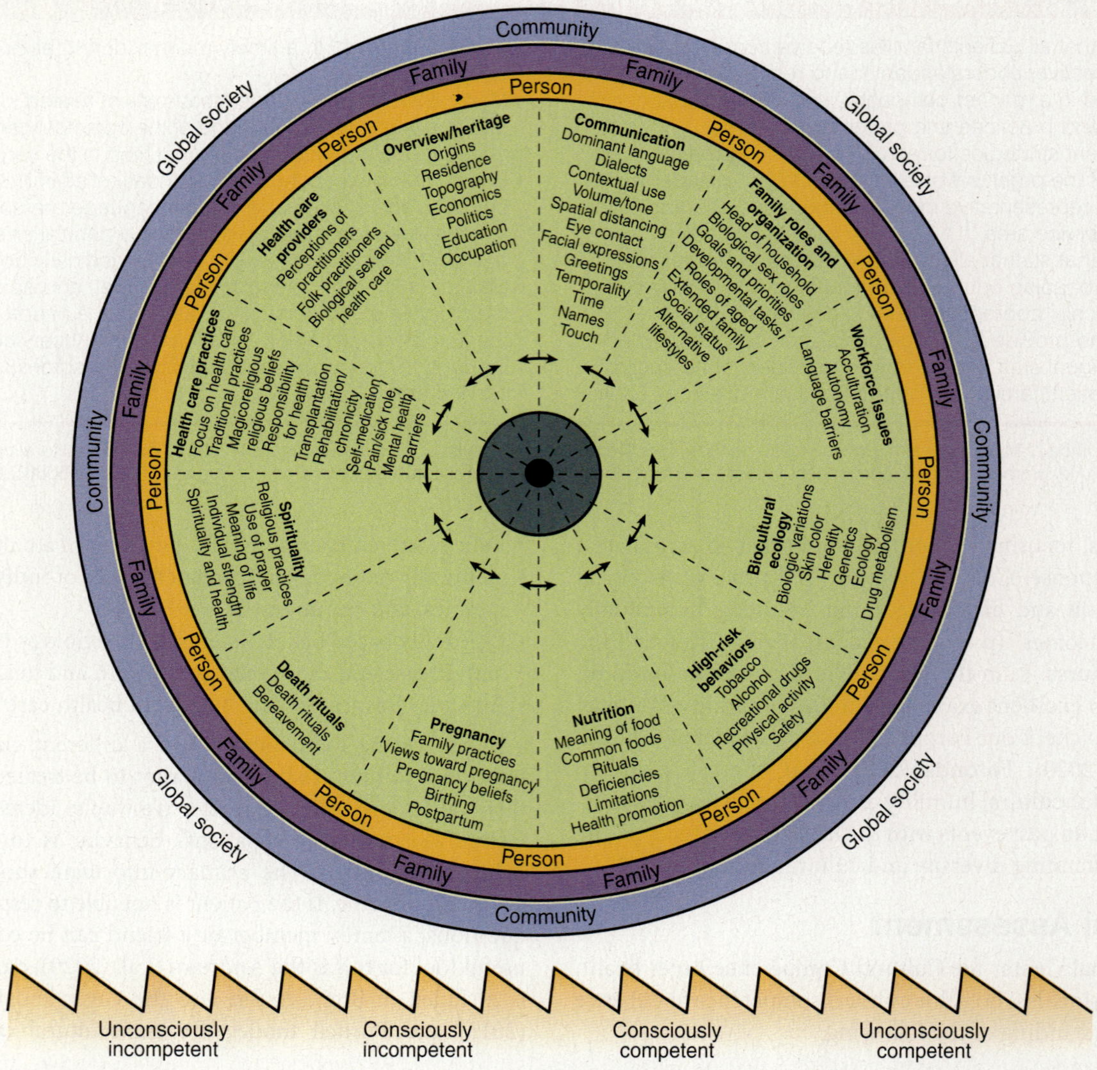

FIGURE 5-2. The Purnell Model for Cultural Competence. This schematic depicting the model is a circle with an outlying rim representing global society, a second rim representing community, a third rim representing family, and an inner rim representing the person. The interior of the concentric circles is divided into 12 pie-shaped wedges depicting cultural domains (constructs) and their concepts. The center of the model is empty, which represents unknown aspects about the cultural group. Along the bottom of the model is a saw-toothed line representing the concept of cultural consciousness. This line relates primarily to the health care provider, although organizations may also be represented on this nonlinear line according to their stage of cultural competence as an organization. (*Source:* Reprinted by permission of SAGE Publications. From Purnell, L. [2002]. The Purnell model for cultural competence. *Journal of Transcultural Nursing*, *13*[3], 193–196; discussion 200–201.)

(Figs. 5-2 and 5-3). The Giger and Davidhizar model takes into account six cultural phenomena: communication, space, social orientation, time, environmental control, and biologic variations. The Campinha-Bacote Model of Cultural Competence (2011) emphasizes becoming culturally competent and integrating cultural awareness, cultural knowledge, cultural skill, cultural encounters, and cultural desire.

You can also anticipate a patient's cultural needs by obtaining this information through research before initiating contact with the patient. Remember, however, that *information about any culture is general, and that it must be individualized for the specific patient once the actual interaction begins.*

Guidelines for Nursing Care

Transcultural nursing, now both a specialty and a formal area of practice, originated from work by Dr. Leininger (1991), a nurse–anthropologist. Her Theory of Cultural Care Diversity and Universality provides the foundation for providing culturally respectful care for patients of all ages, as well as families, groups, and communities. A nurse who is culturally respectful has the knowledge and skills to adapt nursing care to cultural similarities and differences. Cultural competence takes time. It involves developing awareness, acquiring knowledge, and practicing skills. Each patient must be considered a unique person. What is true of one person

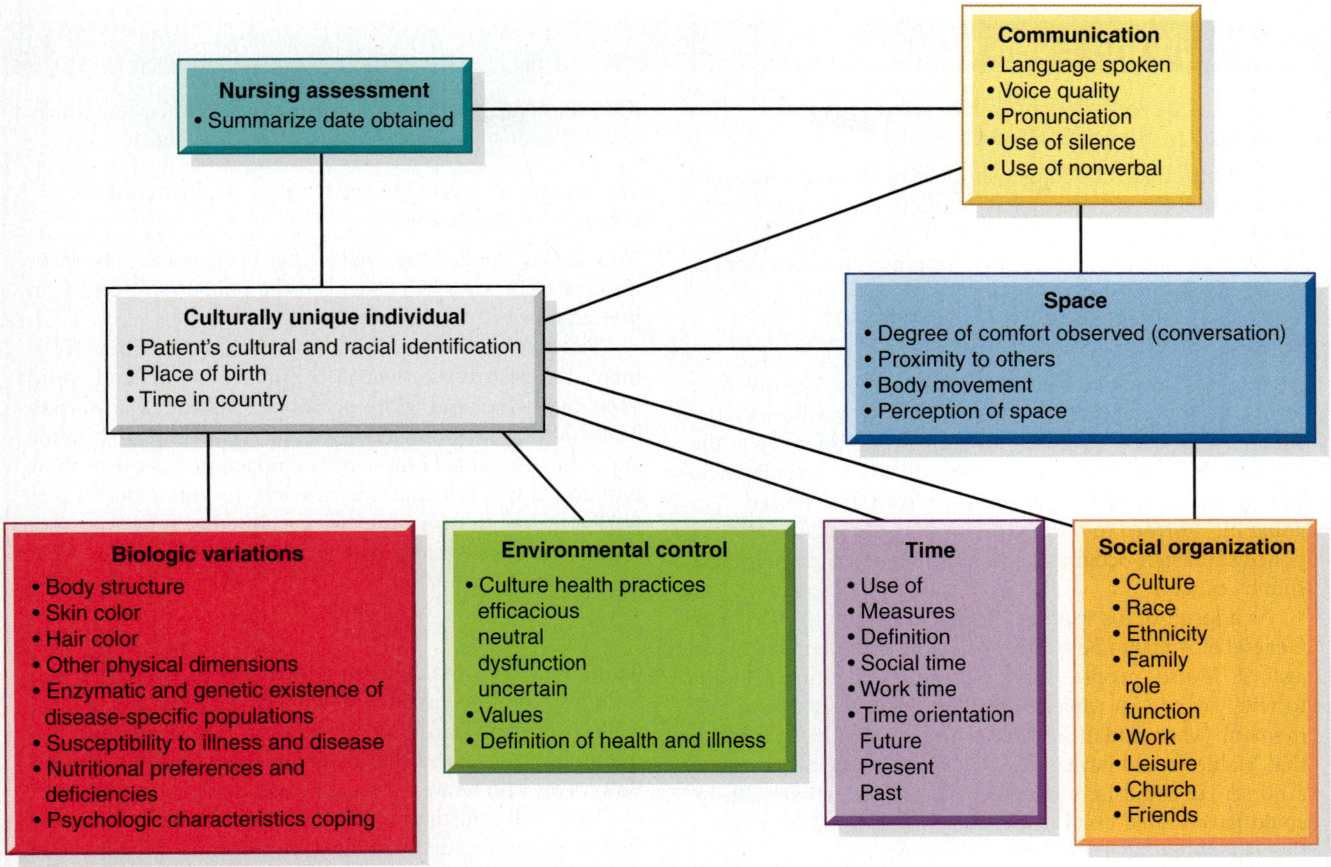

FIGURE 5-3. Schematic of Giger and Davidhizar's Transcultural Assessment Model. (*Source:* From Giger, J. N., & Davidhizar, R. [2013]. *Transcultural nursing: Assessment and intervention* [6th ed., p. 7]. Elsevier/Mosby.)

may not be true of another, even if they are from the same cultural background.

Concept Mastery Alert

Regardless of the culture background of the patient, nurses need to assess each patient individually to provide culturally respectful care. Asking open-ended questions provides an opportunity to obtain specific information from the patient about their beliefs related to health care.

When providing care to a person from a culture that is different from your own or the dominant culture, you may use past experiences with members of that culture as a guide but never as the answer to all cultural issues. Learn from your mistakes and do not repeat them. All nurses make mistakes at some time when caring for patients from different cultures. Inadvertent mistakes are just that, but repeated mistakes are careless and disrespectful; they will adversely affect your interaction with patients and coworkers. The following sections provide additional guidelines for providing culturally appropriate nursing care.

Develop Cultural Self-Awareness

Before you can provide culturally competent care to patients from diverse backgrounds, you'll need to become aware of the role of cultural influences in your own life. Objectively examine your own beliefs, values, practices, and family experiences. As you become more sensitive to the importance of these factors, you'll also become more sensitive to cultural influences in others' lives. Identify your biases. How do they affect your feelings about others? How could they affect your nursing care of others? For a powerful example of how one nurse transcended possible cultural biases, read the accompanying Through the Eyes of a Nurse on page 110.

Develop Cultural Knowledge

Learn as much as possible about the belief system and practices of people in your community and of patients in the area in which you work. Practice techniques of observation and listening to acquire knowledge of the beliefs and values of patients for whom you provide care. Some people, especially those of minority cultures, may have been belittled or ridiculed and may be hesitant to discuss their beliefs and practices. Approach this topic with patients carefully. If you are motivated by sincerity, respect, and concern, your attitude will convey this, and most patients will respond positively. On the other hand, if you are motivated merely by curiosity and have a condescending attitude, most patients will respond negatively.

(text continues on page 112)

Through the Eyes of a Nurse

"I am the Jewish Nurse": RN Who Treated Synagogue Shooter Shares Story

In a country that is no longer shocked by mass murders and random shootings at places that should feel safe, from schools to synagogues to yoga studios, there is one act that has risen out from among the violence that is perhaps the most shocking act of all:

Kindness and Compassion

Ari Mahler, an ER nurse from Pittsburg, was one of three Jewish doctors and nurses who cared for Robert Bowers, the shooter who killed 11 Jewish worshipers and injured 6 at the Tree of Life Congregation on October 27, 2018. After Bowers, who had a long history of anti-Semitism and posted "I'm going in," stormed into the synagogue and began shooting, a police shoot-out occurred, and it's thought that Bowers was shot by officers.

As a result of his wounds, Bower was taken to Allegheny General Hospital to be treated, where he continued his tirade against Jewish people, even reportedly shouting, "Death to Jews" as he was wheeled into the hospital. It was at that moment, when a man so filled with hate that he murdered, that Mahler could have chosen so many paths in his role as a nurse. He could have declined the patient assignment, he could have hurled cruel words back, or he could have taken the patient but failed to care for him properly.

Instead, Mahler chose to rise above hate and instead, cared for Bowers, in his own words, with "empathy."

In a revealing Facebook post, Mahler described how he was the Jewish nurse who cared for one of the country's most hate-filled shooters and how the interaction with Bowers was a deliberate one meant to honor the lives that had been lost, not add to the hate that took them.

"I am The Jewish Nurse," Mahler began his post. "Yes, that Jewish Nurse. The same one that people are talking about in the Pittsburgh shooting that left 11 dead. The trauma nurse in the ER that cared for Robert Bowers who yelled, 'Death to all Jews,' as he was wheeled into the hospital. The Jewish nurse who ran into a room to save his life."

Mahler went on to describe how he was nervous for writing up a post on what happened with Bowers, noting his past growing up Jewish, with a father who was a Rabbi, and experiencing anti-Semitism.

"I found drawings on desks of my family being marched into gas chambers, swastikas drawn on my locker, and notes shoved inside of it saying, 'Die Jew. Love, Hitler.'" Mahler explained. "It was a different time back then, where bullying was not monitored like it is now. I was weak, too. Rather than tell anyone, I hid behind fear. Telling on the people who did this would only lead to consequences far worse."

He then stated that sadly, he was not shocked by the fact that this shooting took place, mentioning today's climate as one that "doesn't foster nurturing, tolerance, or civility … I don't know why people hate us so much, but the underbelly of anti-Semitism seems to be thriving," he added.

"I wanted him to feel compassion. I chose to show him empathy."

And despite the fact that Mahler has been lauded a hero for his care of Bowers, he challenged the public sentiment who praised him because he is Jewish.

"I'm sure he had no idea I was Jewish," he wrote. "Why thank a Jewish nurse, when 15 minutes beforehand, you'd shoot me in the head with no remorse? I didn't say a word to him about my religion. I chose not to say anything to him the entire time. I wanted him to feel compassion. I chose to show him empathy. I felt that the best way to honor his victims was for a Jew to prove him wrong. Besides, if he finds out I'm Jewish, does it really matter? The better question is, what does it mean to you?"

He Didn't See "Evil"

Citing [HIPAA], Mahler also added that he couldn't reveal the specifics of his interaction with Bowers, but did say that when he looked into his eyes, he didn't see "evil," and, like the professional nurse that he is, he didn't base his care for Bowers on who he was or what he had done.

"I can tell you that as his nurse, or anyone's nurse, my care is given through kindness, my actions are measured with empathy, and regardless of the person you may be when you're not in my care, each breath you take is more beautiful than the last when you're lying on my stretcher," he went on to say.

Love

In the comment section of his post, Mahler received an outpouring of love and support for his actions and his care of the mass murderer, including from his fellow Jewish nurses. "As a Jewish nurse I applaud you for doing the right thing," wrote Janet. "It is what we do. We may crumble later but we do our job and do it well."

For those who are wondering just why Mahler acted the way he did and chose to go public with his decision to treat a murderer with any shred of kindness at all, the nurse minced no words in explaining exactly why he did what he did:

"Love," he said. "That's why I did it."

"Love as an action is more powerful than words, and love in the face of evil gives others hope. It demonstrates humanity. It reaffirms why we're all here. The meaning of life is to give meaning to life, and love is the ultimate force that connects all living beings. I [couldn't] care less what Robert Bowers thinks, but you, the person reading this, love is the only message I wish to instill in you. If my actions mean anything, love means everything."

Source: https://nurse.org/articles/jewish-nurse-treated-synagogue-shooter/

Thoughtful, Person-Centered Practice: Challenging Topics

Respecting Cultural and Religious Beliefs

As students, we quickly learn to respect the cultural and religious beliefs of our patients and their families. While cultural "competence" is an elusive goal, we learn the benefits of cultural humility and respect. That said, our primary commitment to patients entails working with them and their surrogates to identify and choose the treatment goals and plans of care best able to secure their physical health and well-being, which at times, becomes good dying. In the following scenario, the nurse must decide whether to support or challenge the beliefs of the patient's oldest daughter.

Read the scenario and see if you can articulate what you believe, why you believe it, and how these beliefs are likely to inform the decisions you make and your behavior, especially when you are confronted with competing obligations. Based on Tanner's Clinical Judgment Model (2006), consider reflection-in-action and reflection-on-action (Nielson et al., 2007):

Reflection-in-Action

As you read, consider what the nurse is thinking in the moment—what is happening? Why do the patient's two daughters want different things? How should the nurse respond? What is nursing's role?

Scenario

You are caring for a 78-year-old male patient from West Africa who came to the United States to visit his youngest daughter, who is studying at the state university. He is accompanied by his oldest daughter who lives with him in West Africa. His wife is deceased. There are four other sons, all living in West Africa. He presents to the emergency department after 8 days of suffering from fever, chills, nausea, and vomiting. His daughter reports that he's been unable to hold fluids. A computed tomography (CT) scan of the abdomen shows a small bowel obstruction with a dilated bowel. He has a history of other comorbidities (hypertension, type 2 diabetes, and kidney disease stage III). Deemed not to be a good candidate for surgery, he is in the intensive care unit with multiorgan failure. He is now unresponsive with a worsening prognosis. Both daughters are acting as his spokesperson. The critical care intensivist believes it is time to transition to purely palliative goals and to stop the "life-sustaining" interventions that now seem to be "death-prolonging." His oldest daughter is horrified and insists that we do not stop any treatments. She is denying his condition and bleak prospects. She explains that the family's role in their culture is to try everything or "he will know that we didn't do all we could and he will follow us after death." She continues, "It is important to live a fulfilling life and to die of natural causes. The goal of life is to become an ancestor after death. After death, an individual lives in a spirit world, receiving a new body that is identical to the earthly body, with the capacity to move about as an ancestor. Having life cut short through an accident or by an unnatural death may prevent this from occurring."

Effective Noticing (Cues)

1. What did you notice about the situation initially? What information/observations are significant? What information deviates from what is expected/normal/usual?

Effective Interpreting

2. How would you prioritize this data? What other assessment data, evidence, and/or information would you need to consider the situation? How would you obtain this additional information?
3. What do you think about this situation? Consider personal and previous nursing experiences that you have had and formal knowledge (physiology, psychology, communication skills) that may be of assistance in providing care in this situation.
4. Once the nurse finds herself caught in the three-way dilemma of respecting the family's culture, helping the family help the patient die well, and supporting the recommendation of the critical care intensivist, she is less certain of how to proceed because she has never been in a situation like this before. What sort of "fact finding" would you recommend and what resources can you tap? How could you best learn what you need to know about this family's culture? Are there hospital policies or other resources you can consult?
5. Now see if you can articulate what you believe, why you believe this, and how these beliefs are likely to inform the decisions you make and your behavior, especially when you are confronted with competing obligations.

Effective Responding

6. How would you describe and prioritize the obligations you have in this scenario to advocate for your patient being allowed to die well—which, in the team's analysis, means transitioning to purely palliative goals, versus your obligation to respect this family's cultural beliefs and continue to do everything medically possible?
7. If you cannot fulfill each of these obligations, how will you prioritize them? What basis/rationale do you use for prioritization? What counsel does the ANA *Code of Ethics for Nurses* offer?
8. If you want to learn more about West African culture, what resources would you use? If you want to educate the oldest daughter about how end-of-life decisions are made in the United States, what resources would you use?

Scenario

The patient's youngest daughter, who has been living in the United States for 2 years, understands the advice the critical care team is offering and is willing to change the treatment goals to prepare her father for a comfortable and dignified death. The nurse decides it is important to support this daughter while trying to be respectful of the older daughter's wishes.

(continued)

Thoughtful, Person-Centered Practice: Challenging Topics *(continued)*

Effective Reflecting

9. Which statement below best captures your beliefs?
   a. Respecting the patient's culture trumps imposing our U.S. medical culture—even when this is oriented to securing a respectful and peaceful death for the patient.
   b. Helping this patient die well is more important than respecting the family's culture. Think Maslow's hierarchy.
10. Do you agree with the choice the nurse made? Would you have made the same choice? Why or why not? What would inform your decision?
11. Whether you decide to advocate for the critical care intensivist or the oldest daughter—both of whom want to do right for the patient—how might you use reflective practice to evaluate your decision so you can respond more confidently in similar situations in the future? What criteria will you use to evaluate a good response?
12. What personal attributes and competencies are most likely to lead to a good response?

Reflection-on-Action

Then look back at the nurse's decisions and reflect on your learning—how did your knowledge and/or skills expand based on this scenario? What attitude, value, or belief shifts did you experience (if any) after reading this scenario? What would you do differently if you were in this situation? What more do you need to know to be able to manage this or a similar situation in the future?

Nielson, A., Stragnell, S., & Jester, P. (2007). Guide for reflection using the Clinical Judgment Model. *Journal of Nursing Education, 46*(11), 513–516.

Tanner, C. A. (2006). Thinking like a nurse: A research-based model of clinical judgment in nursing. *Journal of Nursing Education, 45*(6), 204–211.

Omenka, O. I., Watson, D. P., & Hendrie, H. C. (2020). Understanding the healthcare experiences and needs of African immigrants in the United States: A scoping review. *BMC public health, 20*(1), 27. https://doi.org/10.1186/s12889-019-8127-9

Accommodate Cultural Practices in Health Care

Incorporate factors from the patient's cultural background into health care whenever possible if the practices would not be harmful to the patient's health. To ignore or contradict the patient's background may result in the patient refusing care or failing to follow prescribed therapy. Modify care to include traditional practices and practitioners as much as possible, and be an advocate for patients from diverse cultural groups.

Accommodate the cultural dietary practices of patients as much as possible. Dietary departments in many hospitals and long-term care facilities can provide meals that are consistent with special dietary practices. Families may be encouraged to bring food from home for patients with particular preferences when this practice does not violate policy. Teaching patients and families about therapeutic diets may also be appropriate within the framework of particular cultural practices.

Respect Culturally Based Family Roles

Consider the cultural role of the family member who makes most of the important decisions. In some cultures, it is the husband or father, whereas in others it may be a grandmother or another respected elder. To disregard this person's role or to proceed with nursing care that is not approved by this person can result in conflict or in disregard for the patient's and family's values. Be careful to involve this person in the nursing care planning. See the accompanying Challenging Topics (on pages 111–112) feature to read about the struggles of one family to make decisions that honored their father.

Avoid Mandating Change

Keep in mind that health practices are part of the overall culture and that changing them may have widespread implications for the person. Provide support and reinforcement for the patient if it is necessary to change a health practice with a cultural basis.

Do not force patients to participate in care that conflicts with their values. If a patient is forced to accept such care, resulting feelings of guilt and alienation from a religious or cultural group are likely to threaten that patient's well-being.

Seek Cultural Assistance

Seek assistance from a respected family member, member of the clergy, or traditional healer, as appropriate, so that the patient is more likely to accept health care services. Acknowledging the role of the person's traditional healer can be an important way of building trust. Folk medicine practitioners can work closely with professional health practitioners in the interest of the patient and family. Such efforts promote mutual understanding, respect, and cooperation.

DEVELOPING CLINICAL REASONING AND CLINICAL JUDGMENT

1. Analyze the following situations, identifying potential sources of cultural imposition:
   - A young Ethiopian woman with terminal breast cancer requests that her uncle, who is the family elder, make all treatment decisions. Her primary nurse is an active feminist.
   - A Native American woman refuses a life-saving amputation of her leg because she believes it is essential to enter the next world "whole." Her attending believes she is being foolish because he can "save her life."
2. Interview family members or friends who have recently received health care, such as for a health screening, diagnostic testing, emergency care, routine checkup, office or clinic visit, or hospitalization. What aspects of the health care culture were most distressing to them? What factors

were most helpful? Do their answers vary according to the setting for care or the attitudes of the health care providers involved? If so, why do you think they felt as they did?
3. College students have their own culture. What in your school's culture is influencing your health positively and negatively? If you don't want to be the passive recipient of negative cultural forces, what choices do you have?
4. Visit the Georgetown University National Center for Cultural Competence website (http://nccc.georgetown.edu). Pay special attention to the self-assessment resources. Share with your classmates what you learned about your own cultural competence/humility.
5. On a given evening while you are doing a clinical rotation in a busy emergency department you meet the following patients: A "drunk driver" who killed a mother and her twin sons in another car; a man with chronic back pain whom the experienced staff characterize as "drug-seeking"; a 79-year-old man transferred from a nursing home, who fell in the bathroom and broke his hip; and a person who is homeless and is reporting stomach pain. Are you aware of any *personal* biases that might interfere with these patients receiving your best care? What *institutional* biases might contribute to their receiving less optimal care?
6. When we think about culture we often jump quickly to religious or ethnic cultures. How might belonging to a university football or lacrosse team influence a student's health and well-being?

PRACTICING FOR NCLEX

1. A nurse is caring for patients of diverse cultures in a community health clinic. Which concepts will the nurse incorporate to guide the plan of care? Select all that apply.
   a. The United States has become less inclusive of same-sex couples.
   b. Cultural diversity is limited to people of varying cultures and races.
   c. Cultural diversity is separate and distinct from health and illness.
   d. People may be members of multiple cultural groups at one time.
   e. Culture guides what is acceptable behavior for people in a specific group.
   f. Cultural practices may evolve over time but mainly remain constant.
2. At the last staff meeting, the nurse manager discussed the organizational initiative to improve provision of culturally competent care. During rounds, which behaviors inconsistent with this goal require the manager to intervene? Select all that apply.
   a. A staff nurse tells the AP that patients should not be given a choice, but should shower or bathe daily.
   b. A nurse asks the family of a patient who has died if they would like to wash their loved one's body.
   c. A nurse tells another nurse that Jewish dietary restrictions are just a way for them to get special foods.
   d. A Catholic nurse insists that a patient diagnosed with terminal bladder cancer see the chaplain in residence.
   e. A nurse obtains a translator to speak to the patient in their native language.
   f. A nurse refuses to care for a married gay patient who is HIV positive because the nurse is against same-sex marriage.
3. An ambulatory care nurse serving a large, culturally diverse population is planning a free blood pressure screening clinic. Based on the nurse's understanding of racial differences in health and illness, which groups will the nurse target for screening? Select all that apply.
   a. Native American people
   b. African American people
   c. Alaska Native people
   d. Asian people
   e. White people
   f. Hispanic people
4. A nurse is using the Explanatory Model of Health and Illness (ESFT) model to assess how a patient from another culture views their diagnosis of chronic obstructive pulmonary disease (COPD). What interview question is most appropriate to assess the E aspect of this model?
   a. How do you get your medications?
   b. How does having COPD affect your lifestyle?
   c. Are you concerned about the side effects of your medications?
   d. Can you describe how you will take your medications?
5. A nurse tells a patient, "tonight's menu selection is pork. I understand many people in your culture do not eat pork; may I order something else for you?" When the patient states they no longer observe this dietary practice, the nurse understands that the patient has experienced what transition?
   a. Cultural assimilation
   b. Cultural imposition
   c. Culture shock
   d. Ethnocentrism
6. The charge nurse overhears a nurse state, "That patient is 78 years old—too old to learn how to change a dressing." How should the charge nurse respond?
   a. "Please don't impose your view of the patient's culture on them."
   b. "I wish you would try to demonstrate more cultural sensitivity."
   c. "Try to be open to your patient's culture, to make the biggest impact."
   d. "Grouping all older adults as having trouble learning is a form of stereotyping."

7. A young Hispanic mother comes to the local clinic because her baby is sick. She speaks only Spanish, and the nurse speaks only English. Which action should the nurse take next?
   a. Use short words and speak loudly
   b. Obtain a medical interpreter
   c. Explain why care cannot be provided
   d. Provide instructions in writing
8. A nurse is interviewing a newly admitted patient from another culture. What question best displays cultural sensitivity?
   a. "Do you think you'll be able to eat the food we have here?"
   b. "You do understand that we can't prepare special meals?"
   c. "What types of food do you typically prepare for meals?"
   d. "Could you make an exception on what food you eat while you are here?"
9. A nurse tells a new mother from Africa that she should not carry her infant in a sling because bassinets are safer. The charge nurse suggests the nurse is displaying which behavior?
   a. Cultural imposition
   b. Clustering
   c. Cultural competency
   d. Stereotyping
10. A community organization includes provision of culturally competent care in their mission. Which action has the organization set as a priority?
   a. Learning the predominant language of the community
   b. Obtaining significant information about the community
   c. Treating each patient at the clinic as an individual
   d. Recognizing the importance of the patient's family
11. A surgeon will not attempt a life-saving repair of a ruptured aneurysm unless the patient agrees to receive blood transfusions. Although receiving blood products is against the patient's religious beliefs, the surgeon ordered four units of packed red blood cells. What action will the nurse take first?
   a. Administer the blood transfusion
   b. Call the patient's family and ask them to reason with the patient
   c. Discuss obtaining a court order to save the patient's life
   d. Maintain the patient's comfort and support their decision

ANSWERS WITH RATIONALES

1. **d, e, f.** A person may belong to multiple cultural, ethnic, and racial groups at one time. Culture guides what is acceptable behavior for people in a specific group. Cultural practices and beliefs may evolve over time, mainly remaining constant as long as they satisfy a group's needs. The United States has become more inclusive of same-sex couples. The definition of cultural diversity includes, but is not limited to, people of varying cultures, racial and ethnic origin, religion, language, physical size, biologic sex, sexual orientation, age, disability, socioeconomic status, occupational status, and geographic location. Cultural diversity, an integral component of health and illness, includes culture, ethnicity, and race.
2. **a, d.** Cultural imposition occurs when someone believes others should conform to their beliefs, such as whether or not to shower or bathe daily, when a Catholic nurse insists that a terminally ill patient see a chaplain. Cultural blindness occurs when a nurse treats all patients the same regardless of culture. Culture conflict occurs when a nurse judges a patient's dietary restrictions as a way to get their favorite foods. When a nurse refuses to respect an older adult's ability to speak for themselves, or refuses to treat a patient based on their sexual orientation, stereotyping has occurred.
3. **b, d, e.** African American people, Asian people, and White people are more prone to developing hypertension. Alaska Native individuals and Native American individuals are prone to heart disease, diabetes, cirrhosis, and fetal alcohol syndrome.
4. **b.** The ESFT model, a cross-cultural communication tool, guides providers in understanding a patient's explanatory model (a patient's conception of their illness), social and environmental factors, and fears and concerns and also guides providers in contracting for therapeutic approaches. Asking the questions: "How does having COPD affect your lifestyle?" explores the explanatory model, "How do you get your medications?" refers to the social and environmental factor, "Are you concerned about the side effects of your medications?" addresses fears and concerns, and "Can you describe how you will take your medications?" involves therapeutic contracting.
5. **a.** Assimilation occurs when minority groups living within a dominant group lose the cultural characteristics that make them different. Cultural imposition occurs when one person believes that everyone should conform to their own belief system. Culture shock occurs when a person is placed in a different culture perceived as strange, and ethnocentrism is the belief that the ideas, beliefs, and practices of one's own cultural group are best, superior, or most preferred to those of other groups.
6. **d.** Stereotyping is assuming that all members of a group are alike. This is not an example of cultural competence nor is the nurse imposing her culture on the patient. The information in this scenario does not suggest the nurse is not open to her patient's culture.
7. **b.** Requesting an interpreter reflects best practice. Qualified interpreters, available in many facilities or via video or phone, have knowledge of health care and can provide assistance. Using short words, talking loudly, and providing instructions in writing will not aid communication. Explaining why care cannot be provided will not meet the patient's health needs; the nurse is required to provide care. Since the patient doesn't speak English, this will not be understood.
8. **c.** Asking patients what types of foods they eat for meals is culturally sensitive. The other questions are culturally insensitive.

9. **a.** The nurse is trying to impose her belief that bassinets are preferable to baby slings on the African mother—in spite of the fact that African women have safely carried babies in these slings for years.

10. **c.** In all aspects of nursing, patients should be treated as individuals; this remains true when providing culturally competent care. Additional ways to provide culturally competent care include learning the predominant language in the community, researching the patient's culture, and recognizing the influence of family on the patient's life.

11. **d.** The nurse does not force patients to participate in care that conflicts with their values. Imposing such care may engender feelings of guilt and alienation from a religious or cultural group and create a threat to the patient's well-being.

Bibliography

Alspach, J. G. (2018). Implicit bias in patient care: An endemic blight on quality care. *Critical Care Nurse, 38*(4), 12–16.

Andrews, M. M., Boyle, J. S., & Collins Transcultural Nursing Assessment Guide. (2020). *Transcultural concepts in nursing care* (8th ed.). Wolters Kluwer.

Atkins, R. (2014). Instruments measuring perceived racism/racial discrimination: Review and critique of factor analytic techniques. *International Journal of Health Service, 44*(4), 711–734.

Beard, K. V., Gwanmesia, E., & Miranda-Diaz, G. (2015). Culturally competent care: Using the ESFT model in nursing. *The American Journal of Nursing, 115*(6), 58–62.

The boomers' last stand. (2020). *The Economist*, 22–23.

Campinha-Bacote, J. (2011). The process of cultural competence in the delivery of health care services. In M. K. Douglas & D. F. Pacquiao (Eds.), *Core curriculum for transcultural nursing and health care.* Sage Publications.

Chadha, N., Lim, B., Kane, M., & Rowland, B. (2020). Toward the abolition of biological race in medicine. Transforming clinical education, research, and practice. https://belonging.berkeley.edu/race-medicine

El Nassar, H., & Overberg, P. (2011). Census tracks 20 years of sweeping change. USA Today.

Expert Panel on Global Nursing and Health, American Academy of Nursing. (2010). *Standards of practice for culturally competent nursing care executive summary.* https://tcns.org/wp-content/uploads/2018/03/Standards_of_Practice_for_Culturally_Compt_Nsg_Care-Revised_.pdf

Fadiman, A. (2012). *The spirit catches you and you fall down: A Hmong child, her American doctors, and the collision of two cultures.* Farrar, Straus and Giroux.

Fitzgerald, E. M., Cronin, S. N., & Boccella, S. H. (2016). Anguish, yearning and identity: Toward a better understanding of the pregnant Hispanic woman's prenatal care experience. *Journal of Transcultural Nursing, 27*(5), 464–470.

Foronda C. (2020). A Theory of cultural humility. *Journal of Transcultural Nursing. 31*(1), 7–12. https://doi.org/10.1177/1043659619875184.

Foronda, C. (2021). Debriefing for cultural humility. *Nurse Educator, 46*(5), 268–270. https://doi.org/10.1097/NNE.0000000000000957.

Foronda, C., Baptiste, D. L., Reinholdt, M. M., Ousman, K. (2016). Cultural humility: A concept analysis. *Journal of Transcultural Nursing, 27*(3), 210–217. https://doi.org/10.1177/1043659615592677.

Giger, J. N. (2016). *Transcultural nursing* (7th ed.). Elsevier/Mosby.

Giger, J. N., & Davidhizar, R. (2002). The Giger and Davidhizar transcultural assessment model. *Journal of Transcultural Nursing, 13*(3), 185–188; discussion 200–201.

Giger, J. N., & Davidhizaar, R. (2020). *Transcultural nursing: Assessment and intervention* (8th ed). St. Louis, MO: Elsevier.

Kersey-Matusiak, G. (2019). *Delivering culturally competent nursing care: Working with divers and vulnerable populations.* G. Springer Publishing.

Leininger, M. M. (1991). *Culture care diversity and universality: A theory of nursing.* John Wiley & Sons.

Limbo Sagar, P. (2012). *Transcultural nursing theory and models. Application in nursing education, practice and administration.* Springer Publishing Company.

Macenroe-Petitte, D. M. (2020). Caring for patients who are homeless. *Nursing, 50*(3), 24–30.

Mahler, A. (2018). I am the Jewish Nurse. https://nurse.org/articles/jewish-nurse-treated-synagogue-shooter/

Marcus, J., MacMillan, D., Ketchie, M., & Clark, P. C. (2020). Nurses perceptions of technology used in language interpretation for patients with limited English proficiency. *American Journal of Nursing, 120*(9), 48–58. doi: 10.1097/01.NAJ.0000697652.73975.37.

Muronda, V. C. (2016). The culturally diverse nursing student: A review of the literature. *Journal of Transcultural Nursing, 27*(4), 400–412.

National Alliance to End Homelessness. (n.d.). https://endhomelessness.org/homelessness-in-america/who-experiences-homelessness/children-and-families/

National Institutes of Health (NIH). (2017). *Clear communication: Cultural respect.* https://www.nih.gov/institutes-nih/nih-office-director/office-communications-public-liaison/clear-communication/cultural-respect

Office of Minority Health, Public Health Service, U.S. Department of Health and Human Services.(n.d.). *The National CLAS Standards.* Office of Minority Health. https://minorityhealth.hhs.gov/omh/browse.aspx?lvl=2&lvlid=53

Office of Minority Health, Public Health Service, U.S. Department of Health and Human Services. (2001). Assuring cultural competence in health care: Recommendations for national standards and an outcomes-focused research agenda. *Federal Register, 65*(247), 80865–80879.

Okun, T. White Supremacy Culture. dRworks. www.dismantlingracism.org https://www.dismantlingracism.org/uploads/4/3/5/7/43579015/okun_-_white_sup_culture.pdf

Park, M., Alston, A. D., & Washington-Brown, L. (2021). Toward national conversation about race, health risk, and nursing. *American Nurse Journal, 16*(1), 5–7, 58.

Pew Research Center. (2016). *On views of race and inequality, blacks and whites are worlds apart.* http://www.pewsocialtrends.org/2016/06/27/on-views-of-race-and-inequality-blacks-and-whites-are-worlds-apart

Project Implicit. (2011). https://implicit.harvard.edu/implicit/education.html

Purnell, L. D. (2014). *Guide to culturally competent health care* (3rd ed.). F.A. Davis Company.

Roberts, D. C. (2020). The elephant in the room. *Nursing, 50*(12), 42–46.

Schnall, J. G., & Fowler, S. (2014). Multicultural web resources. *The American Journal of Nursing, 114*(6), 63–64.

Shen, Z. (2015). Cultural competence models and cultural competence assessment instruments in nursing: A literature review. *Journal of Transcultural Nursing, 26*(3), 308–321.

Shrestha, L. B., & Heisler, E. J. (2011). *The changing demographic profile of the United States. CRS Report for Congress: RL32701.* Congressional Research Service.

Smith, L. S. (2017a). Cultural competence: A guide for nursing students. *Nursing, 47*(10), 18–20.

Smith, L. S. (2017b). Cultural competence: A nurse educator's guide. *Nursing, 47*(9), 18–21.

Spector, R. (2017). *Cultural diversity in health and illness* (9th ed.). Prentice Hall.

Squires, A. (2017). Evidence-based approaches to breaking down language barriers. *Nursing, 47*(9), 34–40.

Think Cultural Health. (2013). *The National Standards for Culturally and Linguistically Appropriate Services in Health and Health Care: A Blueprint for Advancing and Sustaining CLAS Policy and Practice (The Blueprint).* http://www.integration.samhsa.gov/EnhancedCLASStandardsBlueprint.pdf

U.S. Census Bureau. (2019a). *Income and poverty in the United States.* https://www.census.gov/library/publications/2019/demo/p60-266.html

U.S. Census Bureau. (2019b). Census bureau projects U.S. and world populations on new year's day. https://www.census.gov/newsroom/press-releases/2019/new-years-2020.html

U.S. Department of Health and Human Services Office of Minority Health. (n.d.a). *Think cultural health.* https://thinkculturalhealth.hhs.gov/

U.S. Department of Health and Human Services Office of Minority Health. (n.d.b). *Center for linguistic and cultural competency in health care.* http://www.minorityhealth.hhs.gov/omh/browse.aspx?lvl=2&lvlid=34

Wichinski, K. A. (2015). Providing culturally proficient care for transgender patients. *Nursing, 45*(2), 58–63.

Yosef, A. R. (2008). Health beliefs, practice, and priorities for health care of Arab Muslims in the United States: Implications for care. *Journal of Transcultural Nursing, 19*(3), 284–291.

6 Values, Ethics, and Advocacy

Chengyu Zhang

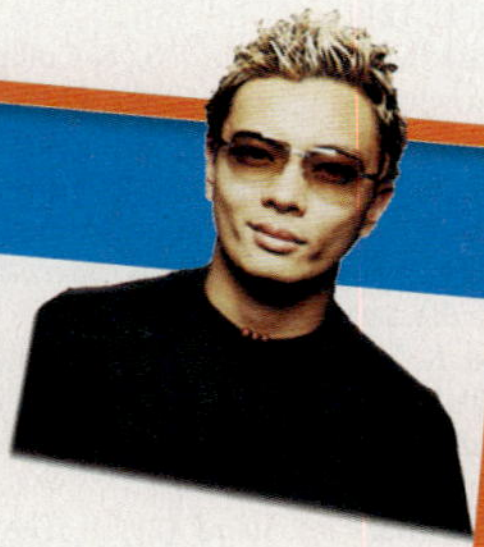

Chengyu is an alert 32-year-old man in the intensive care unit who is begging to be removed from the ventilator. He understands that it is highly unlikely that he will be able to breathe on his own without the ventilator. He writes on the communication board, "If I die, I die. I can't keep living like this."

Marissa Sandoval

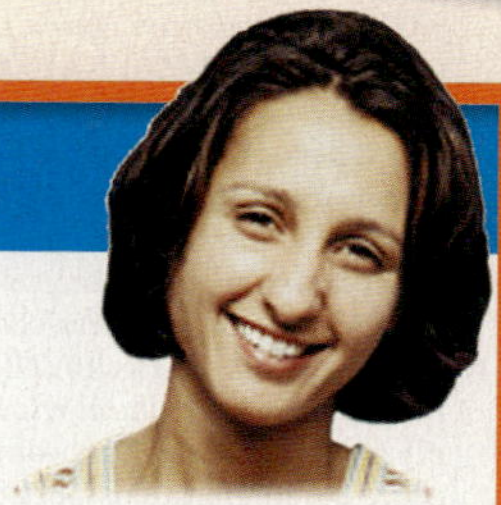

Marissa, a 44-year-old woman who has just recently undergone extensive surgery to treat uterine cancer, is experiencing several serious postoperative complications. She states, "I don't know why all of these things are happening. I ask the doctors. So does my family. But we get no answers. We just want to know what is happening." The nurse is surprised to observe that the oncology nurse practitioner not only does not answer Marissa's questions but also dismisses her fears without any explanation.

William Raines

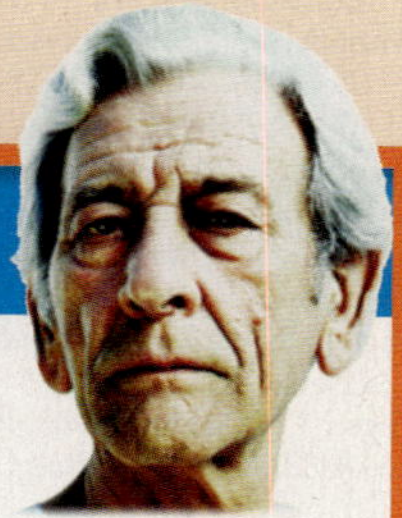

Mr. Raines, a 68-year-old man experiencing homelessness, is diagnosed with schizophrenia, developmental delays, and uncontrolled hypertension. He was admitted for control of moderately severe elevated blood pressure. A review of his medical record reveals that Mr. Raines was getting samples of medications for blood pressure treatment from the pharmaceutical representatives at the clinic, but recent policy changes stopped this practice approximately 4 weeks ago. Mr. Raines is about to be discharged with several prescriptions for medications but no way to fill them.

Learning Outcomes

After completing the chapter, you will be able to accomplish the following:

1. List five common modes of value transmission.
2. Describe three steps in the valuing process.
3. Use values clarification strategies in clinical practice.
4. Compare and contrast the principle-based and care-based approaches to bioethics.
5. Describe nursing practice that is consistent with the code of ethics for nursing.
6. Describe moral distress and ways to promote moral resilience.
7. Recognize ethical issues as they arise in nursing practice.
8. Use an ethical framework and decision-making process to resolve ethical problems.
9. Identify four functions of institutional ethics committees.
10. Describe three typical concerns of the nurse advocate.

Nursing Concepts

- Ethics

The unique nature of nursing places nurses both at the bedside and in groups of professionals where critical decisions are made about the best way to treat injury and disease and to solve health care problems. Often, the question confronting the nurse is not "How do I do this?" but, rather, "Should I do this?" or even, "How can we *not* do this?" The more that science and technology increase the options available to patients and health care professionals, the more frequently nurses will find themselves asking "We can do this, but should we, here and now, for this patient?" An example of this would be: "Should the professionals in the intensive care unit keep Mr. Zhang on ventilatory support?"

Nurses also are increasingly distressed by the failure of society to provide adequate care for its most vulnerable members. Nothing is more disturbing for professional nurses than seeing firsthand the consequences of unmet health care needs (Olsen & Keilman, 2020). When nurses care for patients like Mr. Raines, who lack the financial resources to obtain the medications and treatment they need, they have special advocacy obligations. A shortage of nurses further complicates the nursing work environment, creating the necessity for nurses to be skilled advocates for safety and quality care as well as for their own needs. Never has it been more important for nurses to grasp the ethical dimensions of professional practice and to be confident in "doing the ethically right thing simply because it's the right thing to do!" With their moral integrity on the line every day, nurses understand the need to be as skilled ethically as they are intellectually, interpersonally, and technically. Nurses who understand how patients' values and their own values shape nurse–patient interactions, and who continually develop sensitivity to the ethical dimensions of nursing practice, are best able to provide thoughtful, person-centered quality care and advocate effectively for their patients. For an example, see the accompanying display, Reflective Practice: Challenge to Ethical and Legal Skills (on page 118) that includes self-reflective questions.

VALUES

Values are beliefs about the worth of something, about what matters, that act as a standard to guide one's behavior. If you think back to how you spent your last weekend, you may observe something about your own values. The amount of time, passion, and money you devote to relationships, work, study, fitness activities, leisure, and other experiences reveals something about the importance (value) you attach to these endeavors. As nurses, we need to routinely monitor whether our values support excellent practice.

A **value system** is an organization of values in which each is ranked along a continuum of importance, often leading to a personal code of conduct. A person's values influence beliefs about human needs, health, and illness; the practice of health behaviors; and human responses to illness. For example, people who place a high value on health and personal responsibility often work hard to reach their fitness goals. People who value high-risk leisure activities may attach less value to life and health. Nurses who work effectively with patients are sensitive to how a patient's values and their own values influence their interactions. How might you use values to analyze people's very different approaches to using measures like handwashing, social distancing, and mask wearing to reduce the transmission of COVID-19 during the pandemic? Similarly, what values prompted many to eagerly find a way to get vaccinated once the vaccines were available when others chose not to be vaccinated?

Development of Values

A person is not born with values; rather, values are formed during a lifetime involving influences from the environment, family, and culture.

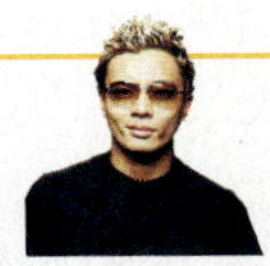

Recall **Chengyu Zhang**, the 32-year-old man in the intensive care unit asking to be removed from the ventilator, even if it means that he will die. The nurse can integrate knowledge of the patient's culture and family and their influence on the patient's value of independence as a key aspect in planning his care.

As children observe the actions of their parents and siblings, they quickly learn what has high and low value for family members. If the parents spend a good portion of each day cooking, for example, and the family spends a long time eating and talking at the table, the children learn to value

QSEN Reflective Practice: Cultivating QSEN Competencies

CHALLENGE TO ETHICAL AND LEGAL SKILLS

I have faced a common ethical dilemma both as a student in the clinical area and as a summer nurse extern. My lack of confidence prevents me from being a patient advocate. My lack of status in the unit makes it very difficult for me to stand up to more senior, experienced staff to act as a patient advocate. However, patient advocacy is a crucial duty for any nurse. I feel that when I neglect this duty, I am being unethical because I am not fulfilling one of the most important nursing roles. An example of this dilemma occurred during one of my first weeks on the gynecologic surgical floor, where I was an extern this summer.

Mrs. Marissa Sandoval was a 44-year-old woman who had just recently undergone extensive surgery for treatment of newly diagnosed uterine cancer. She also developed several postoperative complications. Mrs. Sandoval and her family were unhappy about the lack of answers they were getting from the attending surgeon and her oncology nurse practitioner about the complications she was experiencing from the surgery. After observing the nurse practitioner interacting with the patient and her family in her room, I could easily understand the patient's distress. In addition to not answering any of the family's questions, he dismissed all of her legitimate fears without an explanation. I felt this was a terrible way to treat a patient and that as patient advocate, I had an ethical and professional duty to make sure the patient and her family received adequate answers.

Thinking Outside the Box: Possible Courses of Action

- Confront the nurse practitioner, explaining the patient's anxiety and asking him to return to her room to answer the questions.
- Try to answer the patient's questions to the best of my ability.
- Pretend that the nurse practitioner was acting appropriately. Tell the patient that he will return tomorrow during rounds, and that she will have the opportunity to ask questions then.
- Ask another, more experienced nurse to answer my patient's questions.
- Tell the patient not to worry so much because the doctors and nurses will take good care of her.

Evaluating a Good Outcome: How Do I Define Success?

- The patient receives satisfactory answers to her questions.
- The situation is handled in a respectful manner for all parties involved.
- The American Nurses Association (ANA)'s Bill of Rights for Registered Nurses is followed: "Nurses have the right to freely and openly advocate for themselves and their patients, without fear of retribution."
- No one involved in the situation suffers from a violation of integrity.
- The ANA Code of Ethics is followed: "The nurse promotes, advocates for, and strives to protect the health, safety, and rights of the patient."

Personal Learning: Here's to the Future!

In retrospect, when I examine the situation, I don't think that I handled the situation in the most ethical manner. Rather than dealing with the situation myself, I sought out the help of a more experienced nurse to answer the patient's questions to the best of her ability. Unfortunately, because of the complexity of the case, the more experienced nurse was not able to answer all of the questions adequately. I should have spoken with the surgeon and oncology nurse practitioner and expressed my concern regarding the patient's questions going unanswered. However, I was greatly intimidated by this surgeon and nurse practitioner, and I did not want to confront them. My actions demonstrate that I was compromising my role as a patient advocate. I compromised this role because of personal anxiety and lack of confidence associated with confronting other members of the team.

I am trying to base my personal practice on a strong ethical foundation, and act accordingly, as I hold my own actions to a high ethical standard. However, I am not a very confrontational person. This, coupled with my great insecurities about working in the hospital, makes it difficult for me to confront other health care providers when I think they are acting in an unethical manner. Therefore, while I think my personal actions have a strong ethical foundation, I have a lot of room for growth when acting ethically to confront coworkers. I hope that as I grow more comfortable in the hospital, I will not compromise my role as a patient advocate because of my personal fears.

Elizabeth Nalli, Georgetown University

QSEN SELF-REFLECTION ON QUALITY AND SAFETY COMPETENCIES DEVELOPING KNOWLEDGE, SKILLS, AND ATTITUDES FOR CONTINUOUS IMPROVEMENT

How do you think you would respond in a similar situation? Why? What does this tell you about yourself and about the adequacy of your values and skills for professional practice? How was the nursing student's action ethical? Legal? Please explain. What other *knowledge, attitudes,* and *skills* do you need to develop to continuously improve the quality and safety of care for patients like Mrs. Sandoval?

Patient-Centered Care: What role did each member of the nursing team play in creating a partnership with Mrs. Sandoval to best coordinate her care? What special talents would you bring to this partnership?

Teamwork and Collaboration/Quality Improvement: What communication skills do you need to improve to ensure that you function as a competent, caring, and responsible

QSEN Reflective Practice: Cultivating QSEN Competencies *(continued)*

CHALLENGE TO ETHICAL AND LEGAL SKILLS

member of the patient-care team and that you obtain assistance when needed? How would you have responded if experienced nurses, nursing leadership, and the patient's surgeon and nurse practitioner were not responsive to your concerns? What special talents would you bring to promoting a well-functioning interdisciplinary team?

Safety/Evidence-Based Practice: What priority did everyone involved in Mrs. Sandoval's care accord to her health, well-being, and safety? What evidence in the nursing literature supports practicing within the scope of practice and roles?

Informatics: Can you identify the essential information that must be available in Mrs. Sandoval's electronic record to support safe patient care and coordination of care? Can you think of other ways to respond to or approach the situation?

food and the good times it represents. Similarly, children learn that helpfulness is a good and respected quality if praised when helping parents, grandparents, and siblings. Common modes of value transmission include modeling, moralizing, laissez-faire, rewarding and punishing, and responsible choice.

Through *modeling,* children learn what is of high or low value by observing parents, peers, and significant others. Thus, modeling may lead to socially acceptable or unacceptable behaviors. Children whose caregivers use the *moralizing* mode of value transmission are taught a complete value system by parents or an institution (e.g., church or school) that allows little opportunity for them to weigh different values.

Those who use the *laissez-faire* approach to value transmission leave children to explore values on their own (no single set of values is presented as best for all) and to develop a personal value system. This approach often involves little or no guidance and may lead to confusion and conflict.

Through *rewards* and *punishments,* children are rewarded for demonstrating values held by parents and punished for demonstrating unacceptable values. Finally, caregivers who follow the *responsible choice* mode of value transmission encourage children to explore competing values and to weigh their consequences. Support and guidance are offered as children develop a personal value system.

Reflect for a moment on values you hold and see if you can identify how you developed these values. Will your values serve your patients well?

Values Essential to the Professional Nurse

Professional values provide the foundation for nursing practice and guide the nurse's interactions with patients, colleagues, and the public. In 1998, the American Association of Colleges of Nursing (AACN) identified five values that epitomize the caring professional nurse. Table 6-1 (on page 120) lists these values and sample behaviors illustrating each of them. See also the revised *Essentials* (AACN, 2021) for a description of the domains for nursing. Person-centered care is described as holistic, individualized, just, respectful, compassionate, coordinated, evidence-based, and developmentally appropriate (p. 11).

What other values epitomize the thoughtful, caring professional nurse? Every nurse should critically examine their personal values to see if they match these essential professional values. For example, if you value self-promotion to the extent that you won't make the sacrifices demanded by a genuine commitment to the welfare of the patients entrusted to your care, you will never be successful as a nurse. Similarly, if you attach low value to respecting people who are different from you, you may interact with patients and colleagues in a way that is demeaning and unprofessional. It is helpful to identify nurses in your practice setting who epitomize nursing's essential values and to learn from observing their behavior. It is never too late to develop the values that epitomize the caring professional nurse. Ask yourself now how you would respond if you saw an experienced nurse or health care provider in your clinical rotation acting in a way that was harmful to patients. Would you intervene? What if it was as simple as someone not washing hands before a clinical encounter? What if a nurse instructing you contaminated a urinary catheter before getting ready to insert it?

To encourage health care professionals to respect and accept the individuality of patients, some educators have advised that professionals be "value neutral" and "nonjudgmental" in their professional roles. Professional nurses do not assume that their personal values are more correct than those of their patients. This encourages effective care for patients with values different from the nurse's. For example, a nurse who strongly believes that any premarital or extramarital sex is wrong can still offer competent and compassionate nursing care to a young sex worker with active herpes lesions. On the other hand, when it comes to health, safety, and well-being, nurses do make judgments. If the same patient, after receiving education, indicates that they are unconcerned about whom they might infect in future sexual encounters, the nurse has an ethical obligation to try to protect the patient and others from the harm the patient's values may cause.

In August 2014, 50 nursing leaders came together in Baltimore, Maryland, for a summit meeting on nursing ethics in the 21st century. The goals of the summit were to "identify the strategic nursing ethics priorities for the profession and create a blueprint for the future that key individuals and professional organizations will adopt and implement to

Table 6-1 Professional Values

PROFESSIONAL VALUES	SAMPLE PROFESSIONAL BEHAVIORS	SELF-REFLECTION
Altruism		
Altruism is a concern for the welfare and well-being of others. In professional practice, altruism is reflected by the nurse's concern for the welfare of patients, other nurses, and other health care providers.	• Demonstrating understanding of the cultures, beliefs, and perspectives of others • Advocating for patients, particularly the most vulnerable • Taking risks on behalf of patients and colleagues • Mentoring other professionals	• Am I willing to move out of my comfort zone to advocate for my patients? • Would my instructor and classmates say that "my primary commitment is to my patient(s)?"
Autonomy		
Autonomy is the right to self-determination. Professional practice reflects autonomy when the nurse respects patients' rights to make decisions about their health care.	• Honoring the right of patients and families to make decisions about health care • Planning care in partnership with patients • Providing information so that patients can make informed choices	• Do I routinely find the time to provide the information and support patients need to make truly autonomous decisions to advance their well-being and interests?
Human Dignity		
Human dignity is respect for the inherent worth and uniqueness of individuals and populations. In professional practice, human dignity is reflected when the nurse values and respects all patients and colleagues.	• Providing culturally respectful and sensitive care • Protecting the patient's privacy • Preserving the confidentiality of patients and health care providers • Designing care in partnership with the patient and with sensitivity to individual patient needs	• Do I demonstrate the same respect and compassion for *every* human I meet—even when this is challenging? • Am I willing to "go the extra mile" for each and every patient?
Integrity		
Integrity is acting in accordance with an appropriate code of ethics and accepted standards of practice. Integrity is reflected in professional practice when the nurse is honest and provides care based on an ethical framework that is accepted within the profession.	• Providing honest information to patients and the public • Documenting care accurately and honestly • Seeking to remedy errors made by self or others • Demonstrating accountability for own actions	• At the end of the day, can I lay my head on my pillow and feel peaceful and fall asleep because I lived the day according to my values and ethics.
Social Justice		
Social justice is upholding moral, legal, and humanistic principles. This value is reflected in professional practice when the nurse works to assure equal treatment under the law and equal access to quality health care.	• Supporting fairness and nondiscrimination in the delivery of care • Promoting universal access to health care • Encouraging legislation and policy consistent with the advancement of nursing care and health care	• Am I acutely aware when people are not being treated fairly, when they lack access to quality care? Does my awareness lead to advocacy? Do I share professional nursing's commitment to securing access to affordable quality care for *all*?

Source: Data from American Association of Colleges of Nursing (AACN). (2008). *The essentials of baccalaureate education for professional nursing practice.* Author. See also AACN's revised *Essentials* (2021) and *ANA's Scope and Standards of Practice.* 4th ed. (2021).

build capacity within nursing; create and support ethically principled, healthy, sustainable work environments; and contribute to the best possible patient, family and community outcomes" (http://www.bioethicsinstitute.org/nursing-ethics-summit-report). Nurses participating in the summit made promises to carry on this work—to themselves, to each other, and to the profession. It is interesting to read the promises nurses continue to make on the summit's website when they sign the pledge.

Values Clarification

Values clarification is a process by which people come to understand their own values and value system. It is a process of discovery, allowing the person to discover through feelings and analysis of behavior what choices to make when alternatives are presented. Values clarification is beneficial for nurses. When nurses understand the values that motivate patients' decisions and behaviors, they can tap these values when teaching and counseling patients. For example, a man who does not value his own health and well-being may be motivated by the value he attaches to being a good father for his children to make needed lifestyle changes.

Values theorists most often describe the process of valuing as focusing on three main activities (Raths et al., 1978):

1. Choosing
2. Prizing (treasuring)
3. Acting

When you decide to value something, you choose freely from alternatives after careful consideration of the consequences of each alternative. Prizing something you value involves pride, happiness, and public affirmation. Finally, the person who values something acts on the value by combining choice and behavior with consistency and regularity.

Example of Values Clarification by the Nurse

If you value inherent human dignity in your nursing practice, you choose freely to believe in the worth and uniqueness of each person, to realize that you have other options (e.g., you could treat with dignity only those people who are most like you), and to believe that respecting each person's human dignity yields the best consequences for you and for all of society.

You also will prize your choice. For example, you especially enjoy when patients let you know they appreciate your care and when nursing colleagues and supervisors compliment you on interpersonal skills. You also prize your ability to defend this value when someone's human dignity is being ignored.

Clarifying this value of respect for human dignity will motivate you to incorporate this value into your practice. You strive to respect human dignity consistently in your personal as well as professional life.

As you become more conscious of this value, you will be sensitive to actions that are inconsistent with it. For example, you may feel uncomfortable hearing other nurses gossiping during break about a patient they do not like, realizing that this behavior contradicts a basic respect for human dignity.

Clinical Applications

Nurses who understand the valuing process can use this knowledge when counseling patients whose values fail to support healthy choices.

PATIENT PLACES LOW VALUE ON HEALTH AND HEALTH BEHAVIORS

You become frustrated when repeated attempts to teach or counsel a 26-year-old pharmaceutical salesperson meet with failure. Although hospitalized with a serious duodenal ulcer, all he can talk about is his job and meeting his sales quota.

To facilitate values clarification for this patient, first help him identify his basic values. Ask him, "What three things are most important to you in life?" or have him rank the following behaviors for how he would most likely spend an unexpected free day:

_____ Enjoy some quiet time alone (e.g., thinking, reading, listening to music)
_____ Spend time with family, friends
_____ Do something active (e.g., hiking, playing ball, swimming)
_____ Watch television
_____ Volunteer time and energy to help someone else
_____ Use time for my job
_____ Other

Discuss with the patient what his rankings suggest about his values. Ask whether his rankings would be different if asked how he *wished* he could spend the free day versus how he would *most likely* spend it.

VALUES OF PATIENT AND FAMILY MEMBERS CONFLICT

You sense a growing tension while counseling the young parents of a child with asthma. Questioning them ("You seem uncomfortable with what I'm saying now. Is there something wrong?") reveals that the wife smokes, has a pet cat, and has told her husband that even if these behaviors are hurting their child, she is unwilling to give them up.

To facilitate values clarification, suggest that both parents complete the following exercise, then talk with them about their different responses:

Where do you stand on the following issues? (Mark each as SA, strongly agree; A, agree; D, disagree; SD, strongly disagree; U, undecided.)

_____ A parent's primary obligation is to meet the needs of their children.
_____ Each member of a family is entitled to pursue personal pleasures, even if these are not in the best interest of all.
_____ Pleasure is more important than health.
_____ The choices one family member makes can dramatically affect other family members (positively or negatively).

This exercise will help the parents evaluate their basic values, explore areas of conflict, and perhaps move toward joint choosing, prizing, and acting on several health-promoting values.

ETHICS

Ethics is a systematic study of principles of right and wrong conduct, virtue and vice, and good and evil as they relate to conduct and human flourishing. The ability to be ethical, to make decisions and act in an ethical manner, begins in childhood and develops gradually. See Chapter 22 for two popular theories of moral development, Kohlberg's justice-based account and Gilligan's care-based account.

Many people use the term *ethics* when describing the systematic ethics incorporated within a code of professional conduct, such as nursing codes of ethics. The term **morals**, although similar in meaning, usually refers to personal or communal standards of right and wrong. It is important to distinguish ethics from religion, law, custom, and institutional practices. The fact that an action is legal or customary does not in itself make the action ethically or morally right. For example, many people believe that abortion and physician-assisted suicide are unethical in spite of their being legal options in some states and countries.

Since our values reflect what we believe is important, they are intimately related to and direct our ethical conduct. If I place a high value on patient safety and well-being, I am more likely to inconvenience myself to secure the patient's safety and well-being—even when this entails sacrifice—than a nurse who places less value on securing the patient's interests.

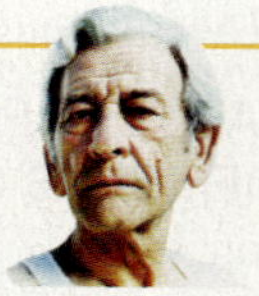

Recall ***Mr. Raines***, the 68-year-old man experiencing homelessness and poverty who is being discharged with several medication prescriptions. Due to policy changes, this patient can no longer receive his medications at the clinic free of charge. Whether health care is a commodity that can be bought and sold in the marketplace ("Too bad, Mr. Raines, if you don't have insurance to cover your meds or money in your pocket…"), or a social good owed everyone, is a basic question in ethics.

Nursing Ethics

The *Encyclopedia of Bioethics* describes the scope of **bioethics** as a number of fields and disciplines grouped broadly under the rubric "the life sciences." At the heart of bioethics are three paramount human questions (Callahan, 1995):

- What kind of person should I be in order to live a moral life and make good ethical decisions?
- What are my duties and obligations to other people whose life and well-being may be affected by my actions?
- What do I owe the common good or the public interest in my life as a member of society?

Nursing ethics, which is a subset of bioethics, is the formal study of ethical issues that arise in the practice of nursing and of the analysis used by nurses to make and evaluate ethical judgments.

As nurses assume increasing responsibility for managing care, we must be prepared to recognize the ethical dimensions of our practice and to participate competently in ethical decision making. The newly revised American Nurses Association's (ANA) Scope and Standards of Practice (2021) has enhanced content to prepare every nurse to be better able to respond to the ethical challenges in everyday practice. Recommended are:

- Continuous appraisal of personal and professional values and how they may impact interpretation of an issues and decision making
- Awareness of the ethical obligations mandated in ANA's Code of Ethics for Nurses with Interpretive Statements (ANA, 2015)
- Knowledge of ethical principles and their application in the decision-making process, and
- Having the motivation and skills to implement a chosen decision.

Common ethical issues encountered by nurses in daily practice include cost-containment issues that jeopardize patient welfare; beginning and end-of-life decisions; breaches of patient confidentiality; and incompetent, unethical, or illegal practices by colleagues.

Theories of Ethics

Ethical theories or frameworks are systems of thought that attempt to explain how we ought to live and why. These theories may be broadly categorized as action-guiding theories that address the question "What should I do?" or character-guiding theories that address the question "What kind of person should I be?" Action-guiding theories fall into two main categories:

- Utilitarian. The rightness or wrongness of an action depends on the consequences of the action.
- Deontologic. An action is right or wrong based on a rule, independent of its consequences.

This distinction is important because it is involved in many ethical conflicts we experience in practice. For example, one nurse may believe that abortion is ethically justified in situations that result in the best consequences for the woman, child, and society (utilitarian argument). Another nurse may believe that abortion is wrong based on a rule that an innocent life should never be taken (deontologic argument).

Concept Mastery Alert

The utilitarian focus is based on "usefulness"—that is, actions are right when they promote the greater good and wrong when they do not. The deontologic focus views actions as right or wrong, regardless of the consequences.

Nurse ethicists frequently use two popular theoretical and practical approaches to "doing ethics": the principle-based approach and the care-based approach.

Principle-Based Approach

The **principle-based approach** to ethics combines elements of both utilitarian and deontologic theories and offers specific action guides for practice. The Beauchamp and Childress principle-based approach to bioethics (2012) identifies four key principles: **autonomy**, **nonmaleficence**, **beneficence**, and **justice** (Table 6-2). Many nurses add **fidelity**, veracity, accountability, privacy, and confidentiality to this list because they play a central role in the tradition of nursing (and medical) ethics and guide the behavior of health care professionals toward patients and their families.

Table 6-2 Principles of Bioethics

PRINCIPLE	MORAL RULE	IMPLICATIONS FOR NURSING PRACTICE
Autonomy (self-determination)	Respect the rights of patients or their surrogates to make health care decisions.	Provide the information and support patients and families need to make the decision that is right for them, including collaborating with other members of the health care team to advocate for the patient.
Nonmaleficence	Avoid causing harm.	Seek not to inflict harm; seek to prevent harm or risk of harm whenever possible.
Beneficence	Benefit the patient, and balance benefits against risks and harms.	Commit yourself to actively promoting the patient's benefit (health and well-being or good dying). Be sensitive to the fact that individuals (patients, family members, and professional caregivers) may identify benefits and harms differently. A benefit to one may be a burden to another.
Justice	Give each their due; act fairly.	Always seek to distribute the benefits, risks, and costs of nursing care justly. This may involve recognizing subtle instances of bias and discrimination.
Fidelity	Keep promises.	Be faithful to the promise you made to the public to be competent and to be willing to use your competence to benefit the patients entrusted to your care. Never abandon a patient entrusted to your care without first providing for the patient's needs.

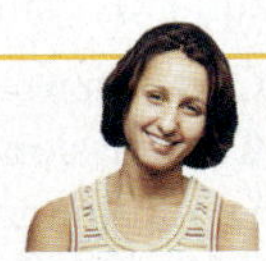

Recall **Marissa Sandoval**, the 44-year-old woman who developed complications following extensive surgery for uterine cancer. The nurse would likely feel that the surgeon and residents are not being faithful (principle of fidelity) to their responsibility to address the patient's questions and fears. Unless the nurse can effectively advocate for Marissa with the medical team, the nurse's own ability to be faithful to Marissa and accountable for her well-being will be compromised.

The principles offer general guides to action. All things being equal, we ought to act at all times in a manner that respects the autonomy of others, benefits others, does not harm, treats others fairly, and is faithful to the promises we make to others. Rarely is this as simple as it sounds. Be sensitive to the fact that individuals (patients, family members, and professional caregivers) may identify benefits and harms differently. A benefit to one may be a burden to another.

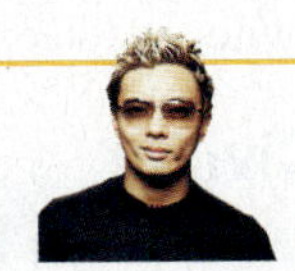

Review the request by **Mr. Zhang**, the 32-year-old man described at the beginning of the chapter. Although the nurse may view the request for removal from the ventilator as harmful, most likely leading to the patient's death, the patient's view differs—that is, he does not want to be dependent on a ventilator to live. When conflict about how to apply these principles cannot be resolved, the nurse can request an ethics consult, which is described at the end of this chapter.

Ethical dilemmas arise when attempted adherence to basic ethical principles results in two conflicting courses of action. There is no foolproof method for identifying which principle is most important when there is conflict between competing principles. Popularized versions of the principle-based approach to bioethics have too frequently resulted in a type of "quandary ethics" that diminishes in importance the everyday ethical concerns of nurses (Taylor, 1997) and misleadingly suggests that how ethical dilemmas are resolved is unimportant, as long as a person can justify their recommendation with recourse to a principle. Thus, many health care professionals equate ethics with decisions about whether to "pull the plug," ignoring the ethical challenges involved in daily decisions about what constitutes an honest day's work, how respectful we are to others, how truthful, how responsible, and how compassionate.

Care-Based Approach

Dissatisfaction with the principle-based approach to bioethics has led many nurses to look to care as the foundation for nursing's ethical obligations. The nurse–patient relationship is central to the **care-based approach**, which directs attention to the specific situations of individual patients viewed within the context of their life narrative. The care-based approach is essential to person-centered care. The care perspective directs that how you choose to "be" and act each time you encounter a patient or colleague is a matter of ethical significance. Ethics is not reduced to a decision to withhold or withdraw life-sustaining treatment. Characteristics of the care perspective include the following (Taylor, 1993):

- Centrality of the caring relationship
- Promotion of the dignity and respect of patients as people
- Attention to the particulars of individual patients
- Cultivation of responsiveness to others and professional responsibility
- A redefinition of fundamental moral skills to include virtues like kindness, attentiveness, empathy, compassion, reliability

Feminist Ethics

Feminist ethics is a particular type of ethical approach popular among nurses of all genders. It critiques existing patterns of oppression and domination in society, especially as these affect women and those experiencing poverty. The many forms of feminist ethics range in focus from assigned sex–related inequities to concern for the least well off. Nurses working within a feminist framework promote social policy that reflects a fundamental trust in women and those on the margins. This trust is recognition that all people deserve the opportunity to make legitimate choices about conditions that affect their lives and are deserving of respect whenever they exercise such facility. This approach reflects a full commitment to full personhood for marginalized people, and provides for basic human needs that are consistent with a person's capacity to flourish and that honors human dignity and relationality (Holland, 2001, pp. 74–75).

ETHICAL CONDUCT

Nurses committed to high-quality care base their practice on professional standards of ethical conduct as well as professional values. The study of professional ethical behavior begins in nursing school, continues in formal and informal discussions with colleagues and peers, and culminates when nurses "try on" and adopt the behaviors of role models who practice professional nursing consistent with high ethical standards. How do nurses learn the standards for professional ethical behavior? At the very least, nurses should cultivate the virtues of nursing, understand ethical theories that dictate and justify professional conduct, and be familiar with codes of ethics for nurses and standards for professional nursing conduct.

Moral Agency

Once professional nurses understand what is reasonable for the public to expect of them, the next step is to determine if you have the capacity to meet these expectations (i.e., "Am I trustworthy?"). What makes a nurse trustworthy is not holding a credential that is publicly recognized or bestowed by the requisite credentialing body. Rather, trustworthiness is proved in every clinical encounter when the nurse demonstrates that they are able to be trusted, in the moment, with the challenge at hand. This may be as simple (relatively speaking) as a change in the plan of care, such as transitioning from curative to purely palliative goals. Or it could as complex as rethinking obligations to critically ill patients in a pandemic when a shortage of personal protective equipment (PPE) forces choosing between the patient's need for cardiopulmonary resuscitation and the health of frontline caregivers. It is never a given.

Moral agency is quite simply the ability to be what is professed: a moral human, a moral parent, a moral professional nurse. **Moral agency** may be defined as the capacity to be ethical and to do the ethically right thing for the right reasons. For the professional nurse, moral agency is the capacity to be trusted to meet the reasonable expectations of the publics we serve, as articulated in the American Nurses' Association's Social Policy statement and Code of Ethics.

The fact that we want to be ethical nurses does not automatically mean we have some natural ability to always do the ethically right thing because we know it is the right thing to do. This ability, moral agency, must be cultivated in the same way that nurses cultivate the ability to do the scientifically right thing when providing care. To see an illustration of how the elements of moral agency "work" in an actual situation, see Box 6-1. You will quickly see that agency requires the development of who we *are* as nurses that goes well beyond scope of practice, assigned roles, and a laundry list of tasks. Agency also requires internal and demonstrated motivation, professional support rooted in nursing's norms and values, and an environment where action is possible. Agency requires tenacity, courage, resilience, and perseverance.

Nurse Virtues

Virtues are human excellences, cultivated dispositions of character and conduct that motivate and enable us to be good human beings. Clinical virtues enable nurses to provide good care to patients. While there is no official list of essential virtues of nurses, the following virtues are frequently named:

- Competence
- Compassionate caring
- Subordination of self-interest to patient interest
- Self-effacement
- Trustworthiness
- Conscientiousness
- Intelligence
- Practical wisdom
- Humility
- Courage
- Integrity

Since these human qualities cannot be "put on" the way one puts on a set of scrubs or identity badge, it is important that they are part of the nurse's character, part of who the nurse is. As you read the above list, reflect on which virtues are already strengths and which you will need to practice until they become part of who you are. Once again, nurses must work hard to cultivate the dispositions of character that invite, and keep earning, the public's trust.

Civility

Civility might be one of the virtues we would include in a list of nursing virtues but it seems to merit its own focus in today's health care world. You will read more about this critical element in each nurse's ethical comportment in Chapter 8 on communication, but this chapter would be remiss not to call it to your attention as you begin to reflect on your personal "fit" for nursing. It is a strange world where topics like workplace bullying and lateral violence are commonplace. What can you promise yourself now that will ensure your presence in practice settings will be treasured? Ebberts and Sollars (2020) surveyed float nurses and asked them on a Likert scale of 1 to 5 the score they thought their unit would merit, with 1 being "strongly disagree" and 5 being "strongly

Box 6-1 Elements of Moral Agency in Action

Situation: *A 75-year-old patient with end-stage lung cancer suffers a respiratory arrest and is coded, ventilated, and admitted to the intensive care unit (ICU). When the receiving nurse reviews his chart, she discovers that upon admission, his nurse documented that he "did not want to be resuscitated" and that he wanted to prepare an advance directive specifying "no heroics." There is no do-not-resuscitate order on the chart, and the nurse can find no advance directive.*

Moral Sensibility

The ICU nurse notes the discrepancy between the patient's documented preferences and the treatment and care that he has received. She senses personal discomfort/distress about this disregard for his wishes.

Moral Responsiveness

The nurse can decide to ignore her discomfort and simply provide excellent technologic care or acknowledge her discomfort and respond. She decides to talk with the attending physician about his knowledge concerning the patient's preferences and learns that the attending was unaware of the patient's documented preferences and has no personal knowledge of these. She contacts the nurse who originally admitted the patient and learns that although the patient was quite clear about his preference, no one followed up and translated this conversation into orders on his chart. She calls an ethics consult when the attending says that there is "nothing to be done now that treatment is initiated."

Moral Reasoning and Discernment

During the ethics consult, family members agree that the patient would not be happy to find himself on a ventilator and request that he be weaned—even if this results in his death. The ethicist explains that weaning him from an ineffective treatment (the ventilator will not cure his lung cancer) that is disproportionately burdensome is an ethically justified action.

Moral Accountability

The nurse initiated the ethics consult because she believed that she could not be an advocate for this patient and merely provide good physical care. Once she knew (or suspected) that his preferences had been ignored, she felt accountable for determining how the system had failed him and for remedying the problem. The nurse prides herself on being responsible and accountable and therefore could not "stick her head in the sand" and pretend that this was not her problem. After the ethics consult, she participates in plans to find an optimal time and conditions to wean the patient from the ventilator and makes sure that his family is present. The patient does not survive the weaning, and although they are grieving, his family members are grateful to the nurse for her care for the patient and for them.

Moral Character

Because she had cultivated the virtues of responsibility and fidelity, the nurse's course of action was natural.

Moral Motivation

As a health professional, the nurse's primary motivation needs to be secure the interests of the patient—even if this entails moving beyond her comfort zone. "Not rocking the boat" or not wanting to displease the patient's attending are not acceptable motivations.

Moral Valuing

Because she places a high value on patient well-being and being an effective patient advocate, the nurse was willing to confront the attending physician and initiate an ethics consult, even though these actions caused her some discomfort and the expense of time and inconvenience.

Transformative Ethical Leadership

When her colleagues asked her where she got the "guts" to follow through with this course of action, the nurse knew that the culture within the hospital had to change so that more nurses would choose to do the same thing she did without fearing negative consequences. She asks the nurse educator on her unit to explore the possibility of pursuing this theme in a future Nursing Grand Rounds and is willing to work to make this happen.

agree." How would you respond to these statements if currently doing a clinical rotation?

- I felt welcome on the unit.
- Someone offered me help when I needed it.
- If floated again, I would enjoy coming back to this unit.
- I had the resources I needed to complete my assignment.
- I witnessed someone expressing appreciation to another for good work.
- Staff showed concern for my well-being.
- I received appreciation for my work.

Gandhi is often quoted, "Be the change you want to see." How will you make your workplace a welcoming and supportive environment?

Nursing Codes of Ethics

Codes of ethics for nursing include the International Council of Nurses' (ICN) *ICN Code of Ethics for Nurses* (https://www.icn.ch/system/files/2021-10/ICN_Code-of-Ethics_EN_Web_0.pdf), the *ANA Code for Nurses With Interpretive Statements* (http://www.nursingworld.org/codeofethics), and the Canadian Nurses Association (CNA) *Code of Ethics for Registered Nurses* (https://www.cna-aiic.ca/en/on-the-issues/best-nursing/nursing-ethics). Students will also want to be familiar with the National Student Nurses' Association (NSNA) *Code of Academic and Clinical Conduct*, which can be found on the NSNA website (www.nsna.org). Epstein and Turner (2015) write that to practice competently and with integrity, today's nurses must have in place several key elements that guide the profession, such as an accreditation process for education and a rigorous system for licensure and certification (see Chapter 1) as well as a relevant code of ethics.

According to the ANA (2015), people who become nurses are expected not only to adhere to the moral norms of the profession but also to embrace them as part of what it means to be a nurse. The ethical tradition of nursing is self-reflective, enduring, and distinctive. A **code of ethics** is a set of principles that reflect the primary goals, values, and obligations of the profession.

Box 6-2 American Nurses Association Code for Nurses

1. The nurse practices with compassion and respect for the inherent dignity, worth, and unique attributes of every person.
2. The nurse's primary commitment is to the patient, whether an individual, family, group, community, or population.
3. The nurse promotes, advocates for, and protects the rights, health, and safety of the patient.
4. The nurse has authority, accountability, and responsibility for nursing practice; makes decisions; and takes action consistent with the obligation to promote health and to provide optimal care.
5. The nurse owes the same duties to self as to others, including the responsibility to promote health and safety, preserve wholeness of character and integrity, maintain competence, and continue personal and professional growth.
6. The nurse through individual and collective effort, establishes, maintains, and improves the ethical environment of the work setting and conditions of employment that are conducive to safe, quality health care.
7. The nurse, in all roles and settings, advances the profession through research and scholarly inquiry, professional standards development, and the generation of both nursing and health policy.
8. The nurse collaborates with other health professionals and the public to protect human rights, promote health diplomacy, and reduce health disparities.
9. The profession of nursing, collectively through its professional organizations, must articulate nursing values, maintain the integrity of the profession, and integrate principles of social justice into nursing and health policy.

The ANA Code of Ethics for Nurses serves the following purposes:

- It is a succinct statement of the ethical obligations and duties of every person who enters the nursing profession.
- It is the profession's nonnegotiable ethical standard.
- It is an expression of nursing's own understanding of its commitment to society. See Box 6-2.

The ICN writes that, to achieve its purpose, the Code of Ethics for Nurses must be available to students and nurses throughout their study and work lives. They recommend that nursing students do the following:

- Study the standards under each element of the Code.
- Reflect on what each standard means to them. Think about how they can apply ethics in their own nursing domain: practice, education, research, and management.
- Discuss the Code with coworkers and others.
- Use a specific example from experience to identify ethical dilemmas and standards of conduct as outlined in the Code. Identify how they would resolve the dilemma.
- Work in groups to clarify ethical decision making and reach a consensus on standards or ethical conflict.
- Collaborate with their national nurses' association, coworkers, and others in continuous application of ethical standards in nursing practice, education, management, and research.
- Codes help nurses accomplish these goals only to the extent that nurses uphold them.

Code requirements may exceed legal requirements. While violations of the law subject a nurse to civil or criminal liability (see Chapter 7), violations of the code of ethics may result in a reprimand, censure, suspension, or expulsion from the profession.

Standards of Professional Nursing Practice

Standard 7 of the ANA's Scope and Standards of Practice describes the nurse's ethical obligations. The Competencies in this standard begin with the statement that the "registered nurse uses the Code of Ethics for Nurses with Interpretive Statements (ANA, 2015) as a moral foundation to guide nursing practice and decision-making." The criteria that follow are derived from the Provisions of the Code of Ethics, reinforcing the importance of every nurse being familiar with the Code. Standard 8 outlines the competencies that enable the registered nurse to demonstrate advocacy in all roles and settings. Note that this is a brand-new standard, appearing for the first time in the 2021 *ANA Scope and Standards of Practice*. In the past, in spite of all the attention our Code of Ethics give to advocacy, many nurses viewed advocacy as an ethical ideal, not a nonnegotiable moral obligation. Our profession now wants every nurse to view advocacy as a duty and to prioritize advocating for any patient whose needs are unmet. As you begin your clinical practice, make sure to ask yourself if any of your patients have special advocacy needs and then determine what must happen for you to be an effective advocate. Make sure you are familiar with both standards! Also note that the 2021 revision of ANA's *Scope and Standards of Professional Practice* includes new content on models of ethical decision making and an appendix on ethics, morals, and ethical theories and approaches.

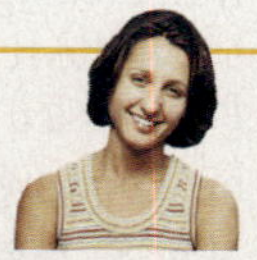

Remember ***Marissa Sandoval***, the 44-year-old woman who wants answers but is not getting them? Integration of these standards would be essential for the nurse to act professionally and ethically when obtaining the needed answers.

Bill of Rights for Registered Nurses

Two of the chief reasons nurses cite for the declining quality of nursing care at their facilities are inadequate staffing and decreased nurse satisfaction. Advocacy on behalf of nurses and the profession has resulted in a tangible tool, the Bill of Rights for Registered Nurses, to aid in improving

Box 6-3 Ethics Inventory

Think about a recent ethical challenge you encountered in practice.

- What signals you to an ethical challenge? Intellectual disconnect? Queasy feeling in the pit of your stomach? Discomfort or disappointment in the way you or your team are responding? Yuck factor?
- Pay attention to how you reason as you think about how you should and would respond.
  - What informs your judgment? Rephrased, how do you calibrate your moral compass?
  - Are there moral "rules" that apply?
  - Do you have a responsibility to respond? Are you personally able and willing to respond? Which elements of moral agency will be most critical?
  - If you have conflicting duties or obligations, how will you determine which take priority?
- Are there any universal (nonnegotiable) moral obligations that obligate all health care professionals? What guidance does the ANA Code of Ethics offer for this situation?
- Does the agency/institution have an ethics environment or culture that promotes ethical decision making and behavior? Are there institutional or other external variables making it difficult or impossible to respond?
- Are you confident in your ability to respond ethically?
  - What counts as a good response? What criteria/principles do you use to inform and justify your response?
    - Promotes human dignity and the common good
    - Maximizes good and minimizes harm
    - Justly distributes goods and harms
    - Respects rights
    - Is responsive to vulnerabilities
    - Promotes virtue
    - Other
  - What criteria/principles do you use to critique/evaluate your response?
    - I stayed out of trouble—not greatly inconvenienced.
    - My/our reputation is intact.
    - "I could tell my children what I/we did and feel proud." (Washington Post test)
    - I'm able to put my head on my pillow and fall asleep peacefully.
    - I am transparent in my deliberations, decisions, and behavior.
    - Other
- To whom would you turn if you were uncertain about how to proceed?
- What agency resources exist to help you think through and secure a good response? How confident are you that these resources would facilitate a good resolution of your concern?
- What barriers are nurses likely to encounter when trying to resolve these types of challenges? What would make intervening most challenging in this practice setting? Would you expect nurses wanting to intervene to experience moral distress?
- If you believe that institutional or other variables are making it impossible to do what you believe is the ethically right thing to do, what are your options?

workplaces and ensuring nurses' ability to provide safe, quality patient care. The Bill of Rights is intended to empower nurses by making clear what is absolutely nonnegotiable in the workplace.

The seven basic tenets of the Bill of Rights for Registered Nurses are:

1. Nurses have the right to practice in a manner that fulfills their obligations to society and to those who receive nursing care.
2. Nurses have the right to practice in environments that allow them to act in accordance with professional standards and legally authorized scopes of practice.
3. Nurses have the right to a work environment that supports and facilitates ethical practice, in accordance with the Code of Ethics for Nurses and its interpretive statements.
4. Nurses have the right to freely and openly advocate for themselves and their patients, without fear of retribution.
5. Nurses have the right to fair compensation for their work, consistent with their knowledge, experience, and professional responsibilities.
6. Nurses have the right to a work environment that is safe for themselves and their patients.
7. Nurses have the right to negotiate the conditions of their employment, either as individuals or collectively, in all practice settings (http://nursingworld.org/NursesBillofRights, used with permission).

ETHICAL EXPERIENCE AND DECISION MAKING

Ethical experience comes in many varieties for professional nurses. See the accompanying Box 6-3, Ethics Inventory. Two types of ethical problems commonly faced by nurses are ethical dilemmas and moral distress. In an ethical dilemma, as described earlier, two (or more) clear moral principles apply but support mutually inconsistent courses of action. **Moral distress** occurs when you know the right thing to do, but either personal or institutional factors make it difficult to follow the correct course of action.

Moral Distress and Resiliency

When nurses are unable to translate their ethical judgments into action, their integrity is compromised. Nurses need sound analytic skills and the ability to engage in ethical reasoning to resolve ethical dilemmas and moral distress. The American Association of Critical-Care Nurses has developed a helpful model to "Recognize and Address Moral Distress," (https://www.aacn.org/~/media/aacn-website/clincial-resources/moral-distress/recognizing-addressing-moral-distress-quick-reference-guide.pdf) part of which is illustrated in Figure 6-1 (on page 128). Rushton and Kurtz (2015) and Rushton et al. (2016) offer helpful hints for developing the necessary capacities to deal with moral distress, including recognizing the symptoms of moral

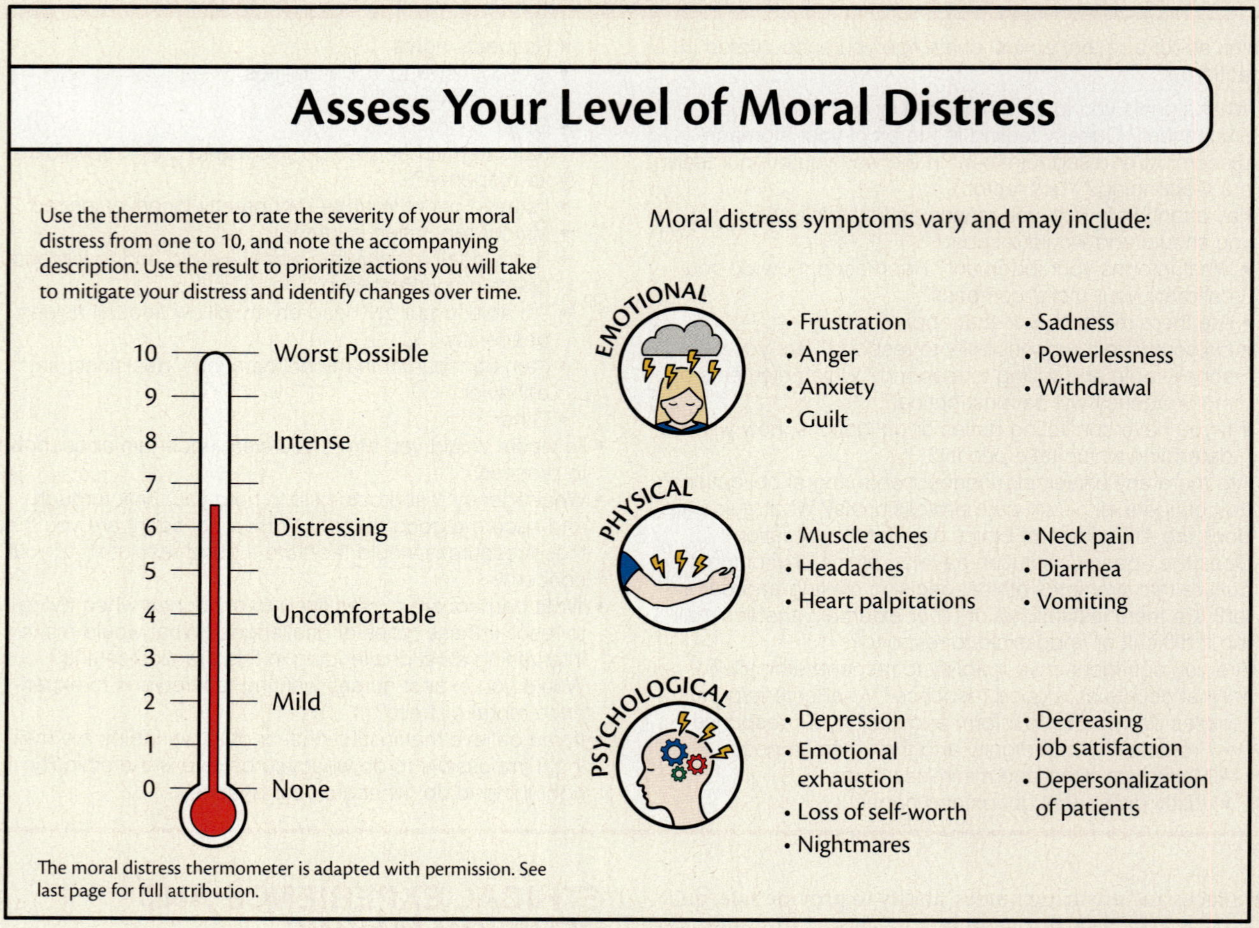

FIGURE 6-1. Assess your level of moral distress. (*Source:* Used with permission. American Association of Critical Care Nurses. [2020]. Recognize and Address Moral Distress. The moral distress thermometer is the result of research works authored by Lucia Wocial, PhD., RN and Dr. Michael Weaver at the Indiana University School of Nursing, with graphics and associated software developed by Robert "Skip" Comer, research associate at the Indiana University-Purdue University Indianapolis School of Informatics and Computing.)

distress and speaking up about your ethical concerns. Rushton et al. (2016) urge all nurses to become agents in creating a workplace environment that minimizes moral distress. In keeping with Provision 6 of the ANA's Code of Ethics, "recognize and honor your responsibility to work collectively toward a culture in which ethical practice is expected, valued and supported."

Today a number of resources are being developed to address moral distress in health care. Epstein et al. (2019) published a validated tool to measure moral distress, the measure of moral distress for health care professionals (MMD-HP). Rosenthal and Clay (2015) launched The Moral Distress Education Project. The aim of the project is to educate, inform, and destigmatize moral distress. The program includes a "welcome video" in which core multidisciplinary experts on moral distress were interviewed, and multiple resources. The video can be viewed at http://moraldistressproject.med.uky.edu/moral-distress-home. More recently nurse leaders met to explore strategies to develop moral resilience and support ethics practice. Their executive summary resulted in group consensus on recommendations for addressing moral distress and building moral resilience in four areas: practice, education, research, and policy (Rushton et al., 2017). An increasing number of practice sites now have moral distress consult services available to health care professionals.

The capacity to recover, adapt, and even thrive in the face of threats, misfortune, or challenging times is termed *resilience*. **Moral resilience** is the developed capacity to respond well to morally distressing experiences and to emerge strong. While there are numerous guides about developing resilience, the American Psychological Association's 10 ways to build resilience are often cited. Included in the association's list are the importance of cultivating good relationships, accepting that change is a part of living, refusing to view crises as insurmountable, nurturing a positive view of self and taking care of self, and keeping things in perspective.

Giving Voice to Values

Giving Voice to Values (GVV) is an innovative approach to values-driven leadership development in business education and the workplace, pioneered by Dr. Mary C. Gentile. GVV is not about persuading people to be more ethical. Rather GVV starts from the premise that most of us already want to act on our values, but that we also want to feel that we have a reasonable chance of doing so effectively and successfully. Rather than a focus on ethical analysis, the GVV curriculum focuses on ethical implementation and asks the question: "What if I were going to act on my values? What would I say and do? How could I be most effective?" GVV is all about shifting the discussion in ethics from the cognitive realm—"What is the right thing to do?"—to the practical realm: "When I know the right thing to do, how can I act effectively in a way that honors my values?" Perhaps most interesting, Gentile draws on what she learned about muscle memory in a self-defense class. The GVV approach is all about developing a "*moral* muscle memory." If we practice finding ways to be comfortable and skillful doing the things that mean the most to us, that accord with our highest aspirations, we will do this routinely. Then we can bring our whole identity to work with us and not feel alienated from our truest, most authentic self. The converse leads to burnout and moral distress (http://www.givingvoicetovaluesthebook.com/).

Moral Injury

A popular definition describes **moral injury** as occurring when there has been: (1) a betrayal of what is right, (2) by someone who holds legitimate authority or by oneself (Litz et al., 2009), (3) in a high-stakes situation (Shay, 1991, 2014). Consequences of moral injury can manifest as unique components of the psychological symptoms of posttraumatic stress disorder when the deeply held moral and ethical values of a person are transgressed. Putting it simply, moral injury is "a deep soul wound that pierces a person's identity, sense of morality, and relationship to society" (Silver, 2011, https://bit.ly/2YGfbTt).

Research attempting to better qualify and quantify moral injury and morally injurious experiences (MIEs) are increasingly being developed, refined, tested, and conceptually extended to populations such as in teachers exposed to violence, traumatized refugees, people who have experienced sexual violence, police officers, social workers, and nurses.

The term *moral injury* has been adopted to describe the emotional, spiritual, and psychological wounds affecting individuals that result from exposure to a potentially cruel or unjust environment's ethical and moral dilemmas. Moral injury has also been a consequence after perpetrating, failing to prevent, or bearing witness to acts that transgress deeply held moral beliefs and individual expectations (MIEs) (Litz et al., 2009).

Nurse Self-Care Alert

Violations of moral values and beliefs can put an individual at risk for burnout, posttraumatic stress disorder (PTSD), and other trauma-related problems. Exposure to morally injurious experiences (MIEs), or even potential MIEs, are associated with poor mental health outcomes (e.g., depression, anxiety, PTSD, suicidal thinking) and also seem to influence behaviors such as hostility (Williamson et al., 2018). Be sure to seek help from trusted sources if you find yourself experiencing this.

While moral injury has most commonly been associated with war veterans, there is empirical evidence of moral injury occurring in nurses. See Figure 6-2. One moral injury study of nurses who had been involved with a patient safety incident (historically called *second victims*) found that they experience moral injury symptoms of guilt, shame, spiritual/existential crisis, and loss of trust after such involvement (Stovall et al., 2020). Other symptoms experienced by the nurses involved with a patient safety incident included depression, anxiety, anger, self-harm, and social problems. These nurses also had difficulty with making meaning of the incident, had a change in worldview, suffered hyperarousal and other physical symptoms, and even considered leaving their job or the nursing profession altogether.

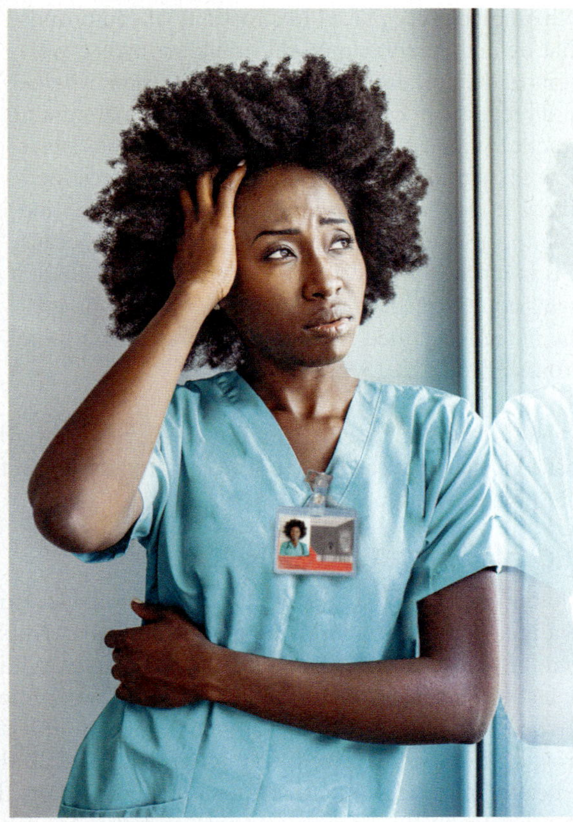

FIGURE 6-2. Moral injury, described as "a deep soul wound that pierces a person's identity, sense of morality, and relationship to society," also affects nurses. (*Source:* Used with permission from Shutterstock. *Photo by Dragana Gordic.*)

One group has developed a Moral Injury Symptom Scale-Healthcare Provider edition in an effort to capture the constellation of moral injury symptoms experienced by physicians, nurses, and other health care providers (Mantri et al., 2020). With the challenges of providing care with limited resources during the COVID-19 pandemic, experts in this field have begun to wonder whether undiagnosed moral injuries among health care providers may underlie burnout and other emotional conditions so often reported by those on the front lines of clinical care (Kopacz et al., 2019). Research in these areas is forthcoming.

Conscientious Objection

The ANA Code of Ethics for Nurses recognizes that some nurses are asked to tolerate practice conditions that seriously violate their personal and professional standards and integrity and supports nurses who refuse to accept these conditions. **Conscientious objection** is the refusal to participate in certain types of treatment and care based on the fact that these activities violate the nurse's personal and professional ethical beliefs and standards. Lachman (2014) writes that having moral integrity means being faithful to deeply held religious or moral conviction and that the willingness to live and act according to an internally consistent set of basic moral ideas is considered a desirable character trait (p. 196).

> Where nurses are placed in situations of compromise that exceed acceptable moral limits or involve violations of the moral standards of the profession, whether in direct patient care or in any other forms of nursing practice, they may express their conscientious objection to participation. Where a particular treatment, intervention, activity, or practice is morally objectionable to the nurse, whether intrinsically so or because it is inappropriate for the specific patient, or where it may jeopardize both patients and nursing practice, the nurse is justified in refusing to practice on moral grounds (ANA, 2015, p. 21).

If you find yourself feeling compromised by activities you are asked to perform, be sure to speak with your instructor or a respected colleague.

Making Ethical Decisions

The Joint Commission mandates that all accredited facilities have a mechanism for addressing ethical problems. Nurses should be familiar with (and use) the resources within their institutions. Most institutions have ethics committees (discussed on page 135), and many employ staff ethicists. A growing number have nurse ethicists. Nurses will also find helpful resources for ethical decision making on the ANA website (www.nursingworld.org) and the American Association of Critical-Care Nurses website (www.aacn.org). Also see the section on creating and sustaining healthy work environments in Chapter 19.

In order for the nurse to be confident in ethical decision making, the steps of the nursing process may be used to help guide ethical decisions:

Step 1: Assess the Situation (Gather Data). Recognize and then describe the situation and contextual factors that give rise to the ethical problem. This involves the main people involved (their views and interests); the patient's overall nursing, medical, and social situation; and relevant legal, administrative, and staff considerations.

Step 2: Diagnose (Identify) the Ethical Problem. Clarify that the issue is ethical in nature: (1) Is there a conflict at the personal, interpersonal, institutional, or societal level? Is there a question that arises at the level of thought or feeling? (2) Does the question have a moral or ethical component? Why? For example, does it raise issues of rights, moral character? State the problem clearly. Identify your relationship to the decision. Identify time parameters. Make sure that the problem is an ethical problem rather than a communication or legal problem. Some suggest that whenever human dignity is being threatened, you have an ethical problem.

Step 3: Plan (Identify and Weigh Alternatives). Identify options and explore the probable short-term and long-term consequences of each for each stakeholder. Use ethical reasoning to decide on a course of action that you can justify ethically:

- Identify your personal and professional moral positions and values and those of other involved people.
- Apply pertinent ethical theories and principles.
- Apply codes of conduct and ethics, professional position statements or guides, and institutional policies as applicable.
- Consider consulting with a respected and wise colleague or an institutional ethics committee or consultant.
- Decide on the course of action that you are best able to support.

Step 4: Implement Your Decision. Implement your decision and begin to compare the outcome of your action with what you considered and hoped for in advance.

Step 5: Evaluate Your Decision. What have you learned from this process that will help you in the future? How can you improve your reasoning and decision making in the future? In what ways does your institutional culture need to change to prevent similar conflicts in the future?

The accompanying patient care study (Box 6-4) illustrates this five-step model of ethical decision making. Other models of decision making are described in *Nursing: Scope and standards of practice*, 4th ed. (ANA, 2021).

Box 6-4 Patient Care Study Using a Five-Step Process for Resolving Ethical Conflict

Jean Watts is a labor and delivery room nurse in a small community hospital that serves both private and clinic patients. Jean has always felt that certain members of the obstetrics–gynecology medical staff have treated these two groups of patients differently. On this particular morning, Jean is caring for a woman who is scheduled for an elective cesarean delivery. The woman (who is a clinic patient) has made it very clear that she wants to be awake for the delivery and has requested epidural or spinal anesthesia. Jean is dismayed when the anesthesiologist enters the delivery room because the anesthesiologist's success rate with epidural anesthesia is poor. The anesthesiologist unsuccessfully attempts to perform an epidural block. After waiting 20 minutes for results, the obstetrician is growing impatient and instructs the anesthesiologist to put the patient to sleep. Jean feels the rights of this patient are being violated but is unsure how she should respond.

Step 1: Assess the Situation (Gather Data)

The patient is in stable medical condition (elective cesarean delivery, not an emergency) and has made it very clear that she wishes to be awake for the delivery. The patient is not a private paying patient of the obstetrician. The nurse believes that her role is to promote and protect the patient's interests; she knows of no reason in this case why the patient's preferences should be disregarded.

The anesthesiologist has a poor success record with epidural anesthesia.

The obstetrician seems to want to complete the delivery quickly. In the past, he has seemed to give more weight to following wishes of private patients than those of clinic patients. He is the head of the obstetrics–gynecology department; he believes that nurses should obey health care providers unquestioningly.

Nurses have in the past expressed dissatisfaction with the different levels of care being provided to private and clinic patients, but no one to date has formally addressed the concern.

Step 2: Diagnose (Identify) the Ethical Problem

Jean objects to the obstetrician's intent to disregard the patient's wish to be awake for her delivery; she is aware of no good reasons justifying this course of action.

The nurse will be a participant in carrying out the decision.

The decision for this case must be made immediately; it would also be helpful to plan to avoid situations like this in the future.

Step 3: Plan

a. *Identify Options*

The nurse can say nothing to the obstetrician and help with the delivery. If asked by the patient later why she needed to be put to sleep, the nurse can (1) tell the truth, (2) refer her to the obstetrician, (3) express sympathy that she could not be awake, or (4) say nothing. *Outcome:* The patient's wishes are disregarded; delivery occurs quickly, and the obstetrician is happy; the nurse fulfills obligation to the health care provider and hospital but feels she has betrayed the patient's trust. *Long-term outcome:* There is a good probability the same problem will happen again.

OR

The nurse can remind the obstetrician that the patient was adamant about wanting to be awake and suggest that a different anesthesiologist be called in. If the obstetrician agrees, the patient may get her wish and everyone is satisfied with the outcome (the nurse must still decide how to prevent recurrence of this dilemma). If the obstetrician refuses and insists that the patient be put to sleep, the nurse can (1) refuse to participate (but if another nurse is unavailable or unwilling to replace her, the nurse will have abandoned the patient and harm may ensue); or (2) participate and proceed as described or resolve to speak to the obstetrician in a "cool moment" after the delivery to see how to avoid this problem in the future. If the nurse is not satisfied with the obstetrician's response, then she must decide whether to move through the proper administrative channels. Depending on the institution and people involved, the nurse may be affirmed or censured for this move. *Long-term outcome:* Future patients may be helped by the nurse following through with her concerns.

OR

The nurse can say nothing and assist with this delivery, believing it to be the wisest course of action for the time being, but resolve to take the steps described to correct the perceived injustice. *Outcome:* There is no benefit for the present patient but there is potential benefit to future patients.

b. *Think the Ethical Problem Through*

Basic moral principles: The good of patients (beneficence) should be the nurse's primary concern (ANA Code of Ethics for Nurses); this strongly suggests that the nurse should act, but it does not address the nurse's obligation to do so if she feels it would jeopardize her own good (job security).

Respect for persons would suggest that the patient's autonomy (right to self-determination) should be respected unless there is strong justification for not doing so.

Justice would suggest that whether a patient pays the obstetrician privately should have no bearing on the quality of care received.

Care-based ethics would obligate Jean to serve as an effective advocate for her patient, respecting the nurse's commitment to be faithful to the nurse–patient relationship.

c. *Make a Decision*

Jean feels from past interactions with this obstetrician that her speaking up will not influence his decision to have the patient put to sleep. She decides to speak with the obstetrician after the delivery and follow-up with whatever approach is necessary to avoid recurrence.

Steps 4–5: Implement and Evaluate Your Decision

Jean will never know whether speaking up might have resulted in the patient's wishes being respected. Although she is dissatisfied with the outcome of this case, she hopes to prevent this from happening to other clinic patients in the future. In this instance, a hospital committee was formed to study the problem and make recommendations. If Jean had been told to "mind her own business" unless she wanted trouble, she would have had to make a decision weighing patient benefit on one hand with potential personal risk or harm on the other.

Ethically Relevant Considerations

Fletcher et al. (2005) recommend attention to eight ethical considerations that have the greatest weight and relevance in the care of patients, which bridge between ethical principles, an ethics of caring, and the clinical situation (p. 12).

1. **The Balance between Benefits and Harms in the Care of Patients.** Nurses are superbly positioned to contribute to reasoning about the benefits or burdens of treatment and the related harms, since their relationships with patients enable them to see more than physiologic effects.
2. **Disclosure, Informed Consent, and Shared Decision Making.** There are three basic models of health care decision making. In the *paternalistic model*, clinicians decide what ought to be done to benefit the patient and inform the patient, and the patient's role is to comply. In the *patient sovereignty model*, patients or their surrogates, expressing their right to be autonomous, tell the clinician what they want, and the clinician's role is to comply. Most ethicists reject these models in their extremes and recommend a model of *shared decision making*, which respects and uses the preferences of the patient and the expertise and judgment of the clinician. *The object of all clinical decision making is decisions that secure the health, well-being, or good dying of the patient and that honor and respect the integrity of all participants in the decision-making process.* Nurses can play an important role in ensuring that patients and their surrogates receive the information and support that they need to make health care decisions that secure their interests.
3. **Norms of Family Life.** Most patients are not isolated individuals. Nurses who are sensitive to how a patient's injury or illness affects family members and significant others can better appreciate how this influences decisions about care, and can bring this information to the interdisciplinary team.
4. **The Relationship between Clinicians and Patients.** The healing encounter is central to nursing ethics. As nurses reason ethically about what should be done, it is always in the context of our relationships with and duties to patients and their families as well as with other professional caregivers. Much ethical distress for nurses results from the strong conviction that we owe individual patients more than our work environments allow us to deliver.
5. **The Professional Integrity of Clinicians.** While the 2015 ANA Code of Ethics for Nurses clearly states that the primary commitment of the nurse is the patient, it also states that the nurse owes the same duties to self as to others—including the responsibility to preserve integrity, to maintain competence, and to continue personal and professional growth. Nurses should think long and hard when they find themselves asked to sacrifice personal integrity to meet the needs of another.
6. **Cost Effectiveness and Allocation.** The increasing awareness of how difficult it is to make valued and scarce health resources available to all in need has resulted in new appreciation for the moral relevance of cost effectiveness. Nurses who are committed to patient advocacy bridge the sometimes overwhelming needs of patients and their families and the limited resources available to professional caregivers. Justice is the principle of bioethics that speaks to distributing the benefits and burdens of health care delivery fairly. Nurses are uniquely positioned within the interdisciplinary team to speak to what it means to give patients or patient cohorts "their due."
7. **Issues of Cultural and/or Religious Variation.** Since many conflicts about what should be done are rooted in different cultural or religious beliefs and values, nurses who are sensitive to the cultural and religious identity of patients and caregivers can help mediate these conflicts. Read more about culturally respectful care in Chapters 5 and 47.
8. **Considerations of Power.** Differences in power underlie many of the ethical challenges encountered in clinical practice. Injury and illness make even sophisticated consumers of health care vulnerable. Nurses and other caregivers should be vigilant to challenge any abuses of power by clinicians. Clinicians who believe that they lack power to influence care settings and delivery may also experience ethical conflict and distress.

Examples of Ethical Problems

Ethical problems commonly arise between nurses and patients, nurses and health care providers, nurses and other nurses, and nurses and their employing institutions. Moreover, nurses are often most conflicted when good practice seems to require acting against their personal moral convictions. As you read through the following mini-cases, try to determine how you would respond. The process of ethical decision making described previously should prove helpful. Note that many ethical challenges will be addressed in other chapters, especially Chapters 44 and 46. Read through the accompanying Thoughtful, Person-Centered Practice: Challenging Topics Reproductive Decisions.

Paternalism

An alert older resident who lives in a long-term care facility and who is now at high risk for falls refuses to call the nurse for assistance when getting out of bed. The nurse must decide whether to obtain an order to restrain the patient. Does preventing potential harm justify violating the patient's right to autonomy and make it acceptable for the nurse to act as a "parent," choosing an action the patient does not want because the nurse believes it to be in the patient's best interest?

Deception

A postoperative patient asks the student nurse, who is about to administer an intramuscular injection for pain, "Is this your first shot?" It does happen to be the student's first

Thoughtful, Person-Centered Practice: Challenging Topics

Reproductive Decisions

Many controversial issues make it challenging to know how to respond as a professional nurse in select scenarios. Often, the nurse's personal and/or professional values may conflict with options desired by patients, families, employers, and communities. Not infrequently, nurses have to make clinical judgments that balance promoting and safeguarding personal integrity and respecting the values and preferences of patient. The Baccalaureate *Essentials* for nurses includes the ability to communicate to the health care team your personal bias on difficult health care decisions that impact your ability to provide care (AACN, 2008, Essential VIII: Professionalism and Professional Values; also see AACN, *The essentials: Core competencies for professional nursing education* (2021).

Read the scenario below and see if you can articulate what you believe, why you believe this, and how these beliefs are likely to inform the decisions you make and your behavior, especially when you are confronted with competing obligations. Based on Tanner's Clinical Judgment Model (2006), consider reflection-in-action and reflection-on-action (Nielson et al., 2007):

Reflection-in-Action

As you read, consider what the new nurse is thinking in the moment—what happened? How did the patient, family, and/or health care provider respond? What did the nurse do next?

Scenario

As a new graduate nurse on a high-risk labor and delivery unit, I was floating around the floor without a specific assignment. I was asked to assist fellow staff members and, in general, "lighten the load" around the unit. As things got busy, the charge nurse asked me to take over a patient who was in the early stages of an induced abortion. I had heard the patient's back story in huddle but had not had direct contact with the patient yet that day. She was middle aged and a recent immigrant from Ethiopia. Her husband was the sole breadwinner of the family, and her water broke at 20 weeks. She was forced to choose between: (1) staying on bed rest to possibly maintain her unsafe pregnancy to viability; or (2) terminating her pregnancy, which would allow her to continue taking her 3-year-old son to his weekly brain cancer treatments. She chose to terminate. She was in pain, and she was alone. In that moment, I was faced with the decision of whether to help the suffering patient, her unborn baby, my charge nurse, and my fellow staff *or* stand by my cultural, religious, and ethical beliefs, which have always told me that abortion is never the answer, and refuse to care for this patient.

Effective Noticing (Cues)

1. What did you notice about the situation initially? What information/observations are significant? What information deviates from what is expected/normal/usual?

Effective Interpreting

2. How would you prioritize this data? What other assessment data, evidence, and/or information would you need to consider the situation? How would you obtain this additional information?
3. What do you think about this situation? Consider personal and previous nursing experiences that you have had and formal knowledge (physiology, psychology, communication skills) that may be of assistance in providing care in this situation.

Scenario

I chose to attend the delivery and support the patient and my team. In this scenario, I believe I made the correct decision based on the outcomes I expected prior to entering the room. I supported the laboring mother, cherished the dying fetus and helped my distressed fellow staff. Though I was in moral distress following the delivery, the outcomes for those involved (patient, fetus, and staff) outweighed my feelings and personal stance. I recognized the abortion was happening regardless of my beliefs or personal values. The fetus would die regardless of what my parents taught me or what upbringing instilled in me. The negative effects on the mom and family outweighed the statistical and physiologic improbability of the fetus's survival. The way for me to create the best outcomes would be by supporting and caring for those involved in this difficult situation. I felt a little like I was doing damage control—there was no way to affect the outcome. Last, I realized, though I think something is wrong, it may not be. Certainly, it was not perceived as wrong to the others involved in the delivery. Now, I consider outcomes as selflessly as possible, and I do not treat patients how I want to be treated. Instead, I treat them how they want to be treated.

Effective Responding

4. How would you describe the obligations you have in this scenario to your patient, to yourself, and to your team?
5. If you cannot fulfill each of these obligations, how will you prioritize them? What basis/rationale do you use for prioritization? Remember that the ANA *Code of Ethics for Nurses* reminds us that "the nurse's primary commitment is to the patient," while at the same time states that "the nurse owes the same duties to self as to others, including the responsibility to promote health and safety, preserve wholeness of character and integrity, maintain competence, and continue personal and professional growth.

Effective Reflecting

This hospital does perform abortions and also respects a health care professional's decision not to participate. In this instance, the nurse has a long-held belief in the sanctity of life and has always believed that abortion is wrong. However, she also finds herself wanting to be an advocate for her patient and is concerned about all the talk in the unit from nurses who are judging the patient to be a "bad" mother. No one wants to accept responsibility for this assignment.

(continued)

Thoughtful, Person-Centered Practice: Challenging Topics *(continued)*

Reproductive Decisions

6. Do you agree with the choice the nurse made? Would you have made the same choice? Why or why not? What would inform your decision? If the nurse had refused to participate, would you respect this choice?
7. Do you agree with the criteria the nurse used to evaluate her decision? How do you evaluate your clinical and moral judgments?
8. What resources can you access to better inform your decision?
9. Whether you decide to accept or refuse the assignment, how might you use reflective practice to evaluate your decision so you can respond more confidently in the future? What criteria will you use to evaluate a good response?
10. What personal attributes and competencies are most likely to lead to a good response?

Reflection-on-Action

Then look back at the nurse's decisions and reflect on your learning—how did your knowledge and/or skills expand based on this scenario? What attitude, value, or belief shifts did you experience (if any) after reading this scenario? What would you do differently if you were in this situation? What more do you need to know to be able to manage this or a similar situation in the future?

Nielson, A., Stragnell, S., & Jester, P. (2007). Guide for reflection using the Clinical Judgment Model. *Journal of Nursing Education, 46*(11), 513–516.

Tanner, C. A. (2006). Thinking like a nurse: a research-based model of clinical judgment in nursing. *Journal of Nursing Education, 45*(6), 204–211.

injection, and the student is anxious. Would the student's intent to decrease the patient's anxiety justify telling the patient, "No, I've given several before"?

Privacy and Social Media

A nursing student in your class shows you her recent Facebook posting that includes a photo of a patient with a large sacral pressure injury. She says that since the patient is lying face down, this is not an invasion of privacy. What patient information can you post ethically on social media sites? How would you respond? Be familiar with guidelines for use of social media issued by the NSNA, ANA, and the National Council State Boards of Nursing. See more on social media in Chapters 7 and 21.

Confidentiality

A nurse asks a middle-aged woman who is crying quietly, "Would you like to share what's troubling you?" The woman tells the nurse that she has no idea how she will pay for this clinic visit because she entered the country illegally 2 months ago and is trying to earn enough money to help her family back home. She begs the nurse not to tell anyone. If the nurse believes that this anxiety is interfering with the patient's ability to obtain needed health care, would it be ethical to break the woman's confidence to obtain help for her?

Allocation of Scarce Nursing Resources

A nurse has just been pulled from your unit, leaving it understaffed. Among your patients is a 33-year-old man recovering from a heart attack who is being discharged in the morning (he tells you that he still has many questions); an older adult who is close to death; and a woman with cancer who has been vomiting all day and who is in severe pain. You know that you cannot meet everyone's needs well. How do you "distribute" your nursing care? (You really like the patient who is going home in the morning.)

Valid Consent or Refusal

A resident is attempting to perform a spinal tap on an adolescent whom you know dislikes the resident. After one failed attempt, the adolescent tells the resident to stop. The resident asks you to administer an antianxiety medication to the patient to enable the resident to get the spinal tap done quickly. Should you administer the medication knowing that the patient no longer consents to the procedure?

Conflicts Concerning New Technologies

A woman who is infertile asks you what you think about in vitro fertilization. She tells you that she is "desperate to produce a child for her husband and in-laws" but also has grave reservations about the whole process. "I've read about couples who end up with seven frozen embryos, and I think that would kill me, thinking I've got seven potential kids 'on ice.'" How do you respond? What informs your response?

Unprofessional, Incompetent, Unethical, or Illegal Physician Practice

A nurse who works in the operating room notices that a pediatric surgeon who has been on the staff for several years and has done excellent work suddenly seems not to be concentrating during surgery and to be making more mistakes than usual. Rumors have been circulating about the surgeon having a problem with cocaine abuse after his recent divorce. The parents of one pediatric patient are dissatisfied with the progress the patient is making and ask the nurse for an opinion about the surgeon. Should the nurse voice personal concerns? Is the nurse ethically obligated to report the physician to the proper hospital authority for investigation?

Unprofessional, Incompetent, Unethical, or Illegal Nurse Practice

When you make your morning rounds, a patient tells you that one of the nurses fondled her body and made suggestive remarks during the previous night shift. You suspect that the patient may simply be trying to cause trouble, and because you like the nurse in question, you find it hard to believe the patient. What should you do?

Short Staffing Issues

Restructuring has resulted in chronic understaffing on the unit where you work. You believe that patients are now at risk because there simply are not enough nurses to provide quality care. Some nurses are talking about forming a union and going on strike. Because yours is the only major hospital in a rural area, you are unsure whether striking is a morally legitimate option. Because efforts to get management to address the issues have repeatedly failed, you are also contemplating "going public" with your concerns. Your brother works for the local newspaper, and he would be willing to do a story about the situation at the hospital. What do you do?

Beginning-of-Life Issues

You are a psychiatric mental health nurse working in a Catholic hospital whose ethical and religious directives forbid abortion and abortion counseling. You are talking with a single woman recently hospitalized with bipolar disorder who is in the first trimester of an unplanned pregnancy and who is expressing great ambivalence about continuing the pregnancy. You personally believe that your ethical obligation is to assist this woman in exploring abortion as an option and to refer her to outside resources if she elects to abort. The charge nurse tells you that these are not appropriate conversations within this hospital. How do you reconcile your clinical obligations with your employee responsibilities?

End-of-Life Issues

You are the nurse case manager for a woman with a history of cancer whose cancer has recurred after many years and is now seriously advanced. She frequently tells you when you come to visit her at home that she is unwilling to fight anymore and wants to die with some dignity while she is still in control. She begs you to get her something that will "put me gently to sleep once and for all before my pain gets worse." You believe that this is the woman's sincere wish, not just depression speaking, and you honestly believe that she would be better off spared the last stage of her fatal illness. According to your religious beliefs, however, assisted suicide is wrong under any circumstances. How do you reconcile your desire to help this woman with your profession's ethical code and your religious conviction that what she is asking for is wrong? (For a fuller discussion of ethical issues at the end of life, see Chapter 44.)

Nurses and Ethics Committees

An increasing number of health care institutions have developed ethics committees whose chief functions include education, policy making, case review and consultation, quality, and in some cases research. Some committees focus on clinical ethics and some on organizational ethics. These committees are well equipped to deal with the complexities of modern health care because they are multidisciplinary and provide a forum for different views to be aired without fear of repercussion.

Increasingly, hospitals are hiring ethics consultants to address the ethical issues that arise in the care of patients. Nurses bring an important voice to the ethics committee or consultant. When clinical issues are being reviewed, nurses can help to ensure that the technical facts are understood, that the appropriate decision makers have been identified, that the patient's medical and overall best interests have been identified, and that the course of action selected from the alternatives is justified by sound ethical principles. Nurses' strong backgrounds in interpersonal communications allow us to contribute unique knowledge about the patient and family to the discussion and to facilitate the ethics committee's group dynamics. Nurses also play an important role in policy making. We are frequently able to identify what policies are needed to address recurring ethical concerns and to suggest needed modifications of existing policies.

CONFLICTS OF COMMITMENT

While the ANA Code of Ethics offers practical guidance on many of the ethical challenges nurses face, it also creates a conflict for nurses with two of its provisions:

Provision 2: The nurse's primary commitment is to the patient, whether an individual, family, group, or community.

Provision 5: The nurse owes the same duties to self as to others, including the responsibility to preserve integrity, to maintain competence, and to continue personal and professional growth.

The profession of nursing calls all nurses to be self-sacrificing in order to meet the needs of the patients, families, and communities we serve. But we must always remember that no one can give what they don't have. If your basic needs aren't met, you will not be able to be there for your patients.

Nurses aren't always good about reflecting on whether or not they have an optimal work–life balance. As a student, this can be as simple as making sure you are prepared and well rested before you arrive for clinical practice. This dilemma gets a bit more complicated if you are responsible for dependent children or adults. What if you are asked or mandated repeatedly to work an extra shift and your family is feeling short-changed? What happens in the rare event of a calamity? Envision an active shooter in your unit: Is your first responsibility to try to save your patients, or is it to take care of yourself? The pandemic made all these questions more than theoretical as every nurse working with patients with COVID-19 had to balance duties to these and other patients, family, and self.

A helpful exercise is to try to identify all the parties to whom you are responsible and then prioritize the parties. As a professional nurse, your patients and employer will definitely make it on to this list. But who gets your top priority? Patients? Your employer or team? Yourself? Your family?

Through the Eyes of a Nurse

Writing about a surgeon coercing a patient's wife to consent to a procedure she knew her husband didn't want; a nurse shared this narrative.

While it's easy to identify and place blame on the unethical actions of the cardiac surgeon, you cannot ignore those of the nurse—me. According to the ANA Code of Ethics Provision 3.5 in 2015, "[Nurses] must take appropriate action in all instances of incompetent, unethical, illegal, or impaired practice that place the best interests of the patient in jeopardy." I had that gut feeling in my stomach that what was occurring was unethical and a disservice to my patient. However, I did not fulfill one of my most important roles as a nurse, and that was to be an advocate to my patient. I should have expressed my concern to the surgeon about what had occurred as well as management. While it may have been uncomfortable and intimidating to stand up to those authority figures, without acknowledging and bringing to light this scenario, a similar injustice could happen to many others. Initiating an ethics consult would have been a great way to bring everybody together to focus on what the patient's wishes were and to support his wife as the surrogate decision maker so she could authorize a valid decision. It is now years later, my moral agency is enhanced, and were this incident to occur today, I believe there would be a totally different outcome.

–Megan Konopacke, RN

ADVOCACY IN NURSING PRACTICE

As bridges between vulnerable patients and the resources they need to secure health outcomes, nurses have always been strong patient advocates. **Advocacy** is the protection and support of another's rights. This role is increasingly important because of patients' changing expectations and demands, and because in our increasingly market-driven health care economy there are no guarantees that the health care system will work to secure patient safety and health. Provision 3 of the ANA Code of Ethics for Nurses with Interpretive Statements reads, "The nurse promotes, advocates for, and protects the rights, health and safety of the patient." Provision 8 obliges nurses to collaborate with other health professionals and the public to protect human rights, promote health diplomacy, and reduce health disparities (ANA, 2015). See the accompanying Through the Eyes of a Nurse.

The ANA declared 2018 the Year of Advocacy and featured examples of members advocating for patients and the profession in various roles and settings, highlighted at www.RNAction.org and distributed through various ANA digital and social media channels. The RNACtion is a website where you can sign up for latest updates and for opportunities to be involved in advocacy campaigns. The current advocacy campaigns include: Health care reform, nursing workforce development, gun violence, safe staffing, home health, workplace violence, and the opioid epidemic. What other advocacy issues would you like to see addressed? See the Nursing Advocacy in Action box in this and other chapters.

Nurses who value patient advocacy:

- Make sure that their loyalty to their employing institution or colleagues does not compromise their primary commitment to the patient
- Give priority to the good of the individual patient rather than to the good of society in general
- Carefully evaluate the competing claims of the patient's autonomy (self-determination) and the patient's well-being

When respecting autonomy, the nurse supports the patient's right to make decisions with informed consent (Chapter 7). When promoting the patient's well-being, the nurse acts in the best interests of the patient. Ideally, both autonomy and patient well-being are promoted in every nurse–patient interaction; however, conflicts sometimes arise.

Nursing Advocacy in Action

Patient Scenario

Mrs. Abigail Winthur is repeatedly asking the staff in your nursing home *not* to encourage her husband to eat. Mr. Winthur, age 88, has advanced Alzheimer disease. He seems to enjoy eating and has no difficulty swallowing, but an aide has to sit by Mr. Winthur and lift the spoon to his mouth and place his cup in his hand. If you merely put the tray in front of him, he will most likely not eat.

Mrs. Winthur reports that her husband would never want to live the way he is now and she is sure that he would refuse to eat if capable of doing so. She also states that society is going to have to decide what to do about all the people we are currently "warehousing." She seems to love her husband, but she is very open about the difficulty of having been his caregiver for 3 years. He had always been a gentle man, but then suddenly he became aggressive and would just as soon hit or punch her as take her hand. Your nurse colleagues are split: some believe Mrs. Winthur's request should be honored, but others are adamant that they and other nurses should at least try to feed a patient who can swallow and who seems to enjoy eating when someone is helping him.

Implications for Nursing Advocacy

How would you respond if you were Mr. Winthur's nurse? Talk with your classmates and experienced nurses about these questions:

- If you elect to advocate for Mr. and Mrs. Winthur, what practical steps can you take to ensure better health outcomes?
- What is it reasonable to expect of a student nurse, a graduate nurse, and an experienced nurse in this situation?
- What advocacy skills are needed to effectively respond to this challenge?

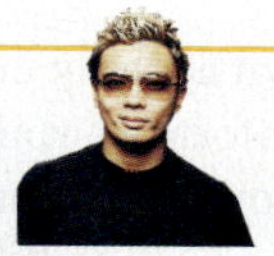

When **Mr. Zhang**, the 32-year-old man described at the beginning of the chapter, requests to be removed from the ventilator, the principle of autonomy demands respect for his treatment preferences at the same time that the principle of nonmaleficence obligates preventing the harm of his likely death. Nurses sensitive to the need to promote both patient autonomy and well-being may often experience conflict, but they are nonetheless more likely to succeed in securing the patient's genuine best interests.

Representing Patients

Most nurses would agree that much nursing time is spent representing patients' interests or guiding patients in protecting their own rights. The nurse is often involved as an intermediary between the patient and the family, especially when the patient and family have conflicting ideas about the management of health care situations. For example, a patient with terminal cancer tells his nurse that he wants to go home to die. The patient's family, however, tells the nurse that they cannot care for him at home. As an advocate, the nurse recognizes the rights of both the patient and his family. The nurse then works to help find a solution that benefits both the patient and the family. By informing the family of the availability of home care and hospice care, the nurse gives them information that may help satisfy the patient's desire for a dignified death (Fig. 6-3). Working alone, most people could not get the financial help needed for such care. Nurses have the resources available to help, and can arrange referrals from other health care workers, such as social workers, to achieve the desired outcomes.

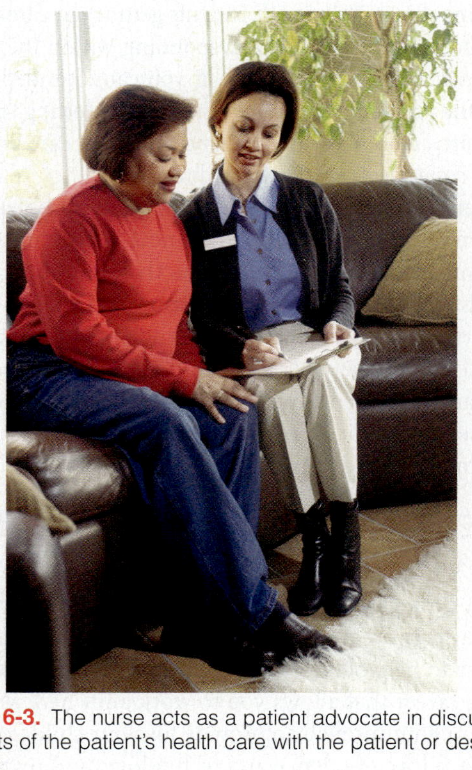

FIGURE 6-3. The nurse acts as a patient advocate in discussing all aspects of the patient's health care with the patient or designated surrogate.

Nurses may also serve as intermediaries between patients and the medical profession. Nurse ethicist Patricia Murphy (1990) documented a moving account of how nurses interceded for a 43-year-old woman with amyotrophic lateral sclerosis who was on a ventilator but wished to die. The patient's primary health care providers refused to help remove her from the ventilator, and more than 20 other health care providers declined to accept her as a patient when they learned what she wanted to do. After unsuccessful appeals for help to the county medical society and her own attorney, the patient's visiting nurse, working with a supportive social worker, contacted her state nurses' association and finally secured the assistance needed to help the patient achieve her goal of a dignified death.

Patients with special advocacy needs include those who are uninformed about their rights and opportunities, those with sensory impairment, those who do not speak the dominant language fluently or at all, the very young and the older adult, those who are seriously ill, those who are mentally or emotionally impaired, those with physical disabilities, and those who lack adequate financial or human resources.

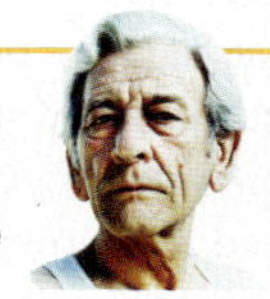

Consider **Mr. Raines**, the 68-year-old man described at the beginning of the chapter. Advocacy for his special needs would be critical in developing his discharge care plan.

Promoting Self-Determination

Advocacy is linked to the belief that making choices about health is a fundamental human right that promotes the person's dignity and well-being. Ethical dilemmas may arise when people are unable or unwilling to make choices or when they are not given the opportunity to do so. Faulty communication among patients, family members, and caregivers frequently contributes to these dilemmas. Nurses have an important advocacy role in educating the public about the value of written advance directives (described in Chapter 44).

Nurses as advocates must realize that they do not make ethical decisions for their patients. Instead, they facilitate their patients' own decision making. Nurses interpret findings for their patients, provide information to be considered, help them verbalize and organize their feelings, call in those people who should be involved in the decision making (e.g., family, primary nurse, health care provider, or clergy), and help patients assess all of their options. In this way, nurses advocate for the right of patients to make their own decisions concerning their health.

Not all individuals want to make their own treatment decisions, and nurses should not violate the spirit of autonomy (self-determination) by forcing the decision-making role on anyone. Nurses sometimes advocate for patients by helping them delegate decisions to a preferred decision maker whom they trust. In addition, when acting as a patient advocate, nurses must be careful to clarify exactly what it is that they mean by advocacy because, in most instances, this does not simply mean supporting patients in all of their preferences.

For example, if a patient in the early stages of Alzheimer disease, with the support of her husband, asks a nurse for help in terminating her life, the nurse would have strong ethical grounds for refusing to advocate for that particular request.

Concept Mastery Alert

Advocacy supports decision making, but it does not involve making the decision for the patient.

Whistle-Blowing

Every nurse who witnesses unsafe care has a duty to patients to report it. However, for too long, nurses may have failed to speak up out of fear of retribution.

In 2009, Anne Mitchell and Vicki Galle, two long-time registered nurses at Winkler County Memorial Hospital in Kermit, Texas, were charged with violating the law by sending an anonymous letter to the state medical board that expressed concern about Dr. Arafiles, who practiced at the hospital. After receiving a complaint of harassment from the physician, the Winkler County Sheriff's Department investigated and filed criminal charges against both nurses that carried potential penalties of 10 years imprisonment and a fine of up to $10,000. Mitchell and Galle, who had a combined 47 years of employment at the hospital, were also fired from their positions.

Charges of misuse of official information against Galle were dropped. Mitchell endured a 4-day jury trial and was found not guilty. The nurses then filed a federal civil suit against their accusers alleging violation of civil rights, among other violations, and won a $750,000 settlement. The Texas attorney general's office ultimately indicted the hospital and the government officials who had originally accused the nurses of wrongdoing.

In 2011, Dr. Arafiles pleaded guilty and was sentenced to 60 days in jail and 5 years' probation, a $5,000 fine, and surrendering his medical license. The Winkler County sheriff, county attorney, and hospital administrator received jail sentences for their roles in trying to silence the two nurses who complained to the Texas Medical Board about Arafiles. As expressed by the ANA, "The criminal convictions of all those involved in prosecuting the nurses sends a powerful message: Those who retaliate against nurses who speak up in the interests of patients will be held accountable" (ANA, 2011).

Being Politically Active

Nursing has had a continuing voice in the political arena on behalf of those least well served by the health care system, including people who are homeless, minorities, women, and children. As the government becomes more involved in the delivery and funding of health care services, and as those designing rationing plans speak seriously of age and other variables as criteria for limiting care, nurses must continue to advocate for the health care needs of those least empowered to do so for themselves. Nurses are a powerful bloc of voters—3 million strong—whose potential for influencing health care legislation is growing. Recall that 2020 was a particularly contentious election year. Did you vote? What informed your vote? See Chapter 7 for helpful guides to contacting your legislative representatives.

Ethics and Academic Integrity

Before leaving this chapter, it's important to think carefully about your role as a student in an academic environment. It should go without saying that any school of nursing expects honesty; integrity; ethical behavior; and civility of all of its members, faculty, students, and staff. Charged with preparing the next generation of professional nurses who will inherit the mantle of being the most trusted professionals, nursing programs and educators are mandated to model and uphold rigorous standards of integrity. A recent Outlook and Perspective in *Nursing Outlook* (July/August 2020) noted that students cite the high pressure to succeed, an intensely competitive culture, and anxiety about the postgraduation job market as factors that push high-performers to cheat, plagiarize, or commit other dishonesty. Most telling is the evidence that those who act dishonestly as students may well carry over this behavior into their lives as working clinicians. So, if you find yourself tempted to cheat in order to get better grades, remember what is at stake: your own integrity, but also that of the profession and the well-being of those you profess to serve.

Final Note About Trustworthiness

Common to all of the standards discussed previously is the obligation for nurses to be competent and willing to use their competence to secure the health and well-being or good dying of the patient. Who you choose to be on any day you arrive for practice literally has the power to influence how people are born, live, age, suffer, and die. When you become aware that something is interfering with patients getting the care that they need, you are responsible for responding within the scope of your practice and responsibility. If you cannot independently resolve the problem, you are responsible for alerting the appropriate party, who may be the attending health care provider, a nursing supervisor, or a medical director.

Although some nurses believe that "the problem is out of my hands" once they notify the next person in the chain of command, the problem remains theirs until appropriate action is taken. Thus, you should know and use the chain of command and continue to refer a problem upward until it is resolved and the patient's needs are met. Good professional nurses are competent, compassionate, collaborate advocates for patients, families, and communities. They are remembered for being and making the critical difference.

DEVELOPING CLINICAL REASONING AND CLINICAL JUDGMENT

1. Each student who chooses nursing as a career does so for different reasons and based on different values. A desire to help others, a desire for a steady income, wanting a career that allows you to work anywhere at any time, a commitment to provide for your children's well-being, a love of science and technology, and respect for

your parents' wishes are all values that may lead to you to choose nursing as a career.

- Interview your classmates and identify the values that brought everyone to nursing. When a classmate lists more than one value, ask that classmate to rank them in order of their importance. Compare your lists.
- Discuss which values, if any, provide the best motivation for professional nursing. Do you think that there are certain values that are incompatible with professional nursing and should be grounds for rejecting candidates for professional nursing?
- Make a judgment about how well your personal values equip you for professional nursing. Would your patients affirm your values? Are any modifications needed?

2. Make a list of values that might positively or negatively influence someone's ability to lose weight. Think about how you could use this knowledge when counseling patients who are overweight.
3. Another student tells you, "Who I am outside of school is no one's business and has no effect on my nursing." Do you agree? Why or why not?
4. Using any current ethical issue (e.g., assisted suicide, how to allocate scarce organs for transplantation, everyone's right to health care), poll your classmates to identify a range of opinions among them. Reflect on what it is that causes people to reach different conclusions about what is the ethically right thing to do. How might you use this knowledge as you experience ethical conflict in your professional practice?
5. You are observing a birth and hear the mother cry out in pain when the obstetrician starts suturing a tear after the delivery. You ask the obstetrician if she would like more lidocaine to numb the area, but she says the repair will not take long. The mother is now screaming each time she feels the needle puncture. How do you advocate for the patient? You have heard other nurses complain that this obstetrician frequently ignores the pain of Black patients.
6. During an observation experience in the operating room, you see the scrub nurse break the sterile field and continue as if nothing happened. Your clinical instructor is not in the hospital, and you don't know where your OR preceptor is at this moment. What should you do? What will you do?

PRACTICING FOR NCLEX

1. A nurse caring for patients in the intensive care unit develops values from their experiences when forming a personal code of ethics. Which statements correctly guide this process? Select all that apply.
   a. People are born with values.
   b. Values act as standards to guide behavior.
   c. Values are ranked on a continuum of importance.
   d. Values influence beliefs about health and illness.
   e. Value systems are not related to personal codes of conduct.
   f. Nurses should not let their values influence patient care.

2. The parent of a young school-age child wants them to learn about healthy dietary choices related to diabetes. Which method of value transmission would be most helpful?
   a. Depriving the child of their favorite toy when they consume foods not on their diet
   b. Lecturing the child on the merits of healthy and unhealthy food choices
   c. Allowing the child to experiment and discuss the outcomes on their blood glucose
   d. Offering healthy meals and snacks and acting as a role model for healthful eating

3. A nurse who is working in a hospital setting uses value clarification to help patients understand the values that motivate patient behavior. What patient actions help the nurse determine if they demonstrate "prizing" during this process? Select all that apply.
   a. They stop smoking after a diagnosis of lung cancer.
   b. They show off a new outfit that after losing 20 lb.
   c. They choose to work fewer hours following a myocardial infarction.
   d. They adopt a low-cholesterol diet.
   e. They join a gym and schedule classes throughout the year.
   f. They proudly display a certificate for completing a marathon.

4. A nurse incorporates the "five values that epitomize the caring professional nurse" (identified by the American Association of Colleges of Nursing) into their home health care practice. Which attribute best reflects agreement with the code of ethics and accepted standards of practice?
   a. Altruism
   b. Autonomy
   c. Human dignity
   d. Integrity

5. A nurse caring for patients in the city-run health clinic expresses a commitment to social justice. Working toward which action best exemplifies this attribute?
   a. Providing honest information to patients and the public
   b. Promoting universal access to health care
   c. Planning care in partnership with patients
   d. Documenting care accurately and honestly

6. Nursing students are discussing the care-based approach to ethical practice. What actions will the students ensure are included in the discussion? Select all that apply.
   a. Understanding that the needs of the many prevail versus the needs of the few
   b. Promoting the dignity and respect of patients as people
   c. Attending to the individual attributes of each patient
   d. Cultivating responsiveness to others and professional responsibility
   e. Understanding that moral skills include kindness, attentiveness, compassion, and reliability

7. A patient with brain cancer questions whether they should agree to palliative radiation treatments despite possible memory loss, or enjoy their remaining time with friends and family. What is the most appropriate response by the nurse?
   a. "I can't advise you. This is such an individual decision."
   b. "If you receive the radiation, might you live a bit longer?"
   c. "What does your family think you should do?"
   d. "What is most important to you with the time you have left?"
8. A hospice nurse is caring for a patient with end-stage cancer. Which action demonstrates the nurse's commitment to promoting the patient's autonomy?
   a. Competently administering pain medication
   b. Giving undivided attention when listening to patient concerns
   c. Keeping a promise to obtain a counselor
   d. Supporting the patient in obtaining a durable power of attorney
9. A patient with an advanced directive and do-not-resuscitate order is sobbing and reporting severe pain. The nurse contacts the provider, who refuses to increase the medication dose due to the patient's hypotension. What actions would the nurse take next? Select all that apply.
   a. Lodge a complaint with the state board of nursing
   b. Consult with the ethics committee
   c. Contact a different health care provider
   d. Speak with the nurse manager
   e. Request a palliative care consultation
10. A nursing student is on clinical rotation in a long-term care facility. Which action best reflects the student acting as advocate?
   a. Telling the health care team that a patient clearly stated they do not want to be transported to the hospital
   b. Avoiding input in care conferences, as patient advocacy is primarily performed by the health care provider
   c. Assisting the primary nurse in making good health care decisions for patients and residents
   d. Deferring to whatever decisions patients and residents want
11. At an interprofessional meeting, nurses discuss appropriate uses for an organizational ethics committee. Which referral do the nurses identify as appropriate?
   a. Giving input into policies affecting work life balance
   b. Providing interprofessional input on clinical care
   c. Determining if the patient's cultural beliefs are valid
   d. Advising the board of nursing on policy for licensure
12. A patient with dysphagia has been admitted with a third episode of aspiration pneumonia in less than a year. The health care provider insists that for safety, the patient must have a feeding tube placed. The patient declines the tube and later asks the nurse if they should reconsider. What is the most appropriate nursing response?
   a. "The feeding tube will prevent aspiration and is the safest option for you."
   b. "You could swallow thickened liquids and puréed foods more easily."
   c. "Tell me your understanding of what may happen without the feeding tube."
   d. "You said cooking and dining with your family is important, and I understand your decision."

ANSWERS WITH RATIONALES

1. **b, c, d.** A value is a belief about the worth of something, about what matters, that acts as a standard to guide our behavior. A value system is an organization of values in which each is ranked along a continuum of importance, often leading to a personal code of conduct. A person's values influence beliefs about human needs, health, and illness; the practice of health behaviors; and human responses to illness. Values guide the practice of nursing care. An individual is not born with values; rather, values are formed during a lifetime from information from the environment, family, and culture.
2. **d.** Through modeling by observing parents, peers, and significant others, children learn what is of high or low value. When punishment is used to transmit values, children create negative associations with those values. Using lecturing and moralizing modes of value transmission, usually taught by parents or an institution (e.g., church or school), offers little opportunity for the child to weigh different values. Using a laissez-faire approach to value transmission, where no single set of values is presented as best, is not appropriate for a young child; this approach could permit permanent consequences of diabetes to develop.
3. **b, f.** Prizing something you value involves pride, happiness, and public affirmation, such as losing weight or running a marathon. When choosing, you choose freely from alternatives after careful consideration of the consequences of each alternative, such as quitting smoking and working fewer hours. Finally, the person who values something *acts* on the value by combining choice and behavior with consistency and regularity, such as joining a gym for the year and following a low-cholesterol diet faithfully.
4. **d.** The American Association of Colleges of Nursing defines integrity as acting in accordance with an appropriate code of ethics and accepted standards of practice. Altruism is a concern for the welfare and well-being of others. Autonomy is the right to self-determination, and human dignity is respect for the inherent worth and uniqueness of individuals and populations.
5. **b.** The American Association of Colleges of Nursing lists promoting universal access to health care as an example of *social justice*. Providing honest information and documenting care accurately and honestly are examples of *integrity*, and planning care in partnership with patients is an example of *autonomy*.

6. **b, c, d, e.** A care-based approach, essential to thoughtful, person-centered care, directs attention to the specific patient situation, viewed within the context of their life narrative. The care-based approach includes the following characteristics: centrality of the caring relationship; promotion of patient dignity and respect; attention to patient particulars; cultivation of responsiveness to others; professional responsibility; and redefinition of fundamental moral skills like kindness, attentiveness, empathy, compassion, and reliability. An action is right or wrong based on a rule, independent of its consequences, such as "the needs of the many outweigh the needs of the few."
7. **d.** Advocacy is the protection and support of another's rights. The nurse assesses the patient's goals and advocates to support their wishes. Nurses do not make ethical decisions for patients; rather; the nurse facilitates patient decision making by interpreting and providing information, encouraging verbalization of feelings, and facilitating communication with family, primary nurse, health care provider, or clergy.
8. **d.** The principle of autonomy obligates nurses to provide information and support patients' and their surrogates' need to make decisions that advance their interests. Acting with *justice* means giving each person their due, acting with fidelity involves keeping promises to patients, and acting with nonmaleficence means avoiding doing harm to patients.
9. **b, d, e.** Ethical distress results from knowing the right thing to do but finding it almost impossible to execute due to institutional or other constraints (in this case, the nurse fears inability to collaborate with the provider). The nurse uses available resources such as seeking guidance from the nurse manager, attempting to secure a palliative care consult, and consulting the ethics committee. The state board of nursing does not regulate medical practice. The nurse does not circumvent the patient's health care provider.
10. **a.** Advocacy is the protection and support of another's rights. Among the patients with special advocacy needs are the very young and the very old, those who are seriously ill, and those with disabilities. Patient advocacy is the responsibility of every member of the professional caregiving team—not just nurses. Nurse advocates do not make health care decisions for their patients and residents; rather, they facilitate patient decision making. Advocacy does not entail supporting patients in all their preferences.
11. **b.** The Joint Commission mandates that accredited facilities have a mechanism for addressing ethical problems. Health care institutions often have multidisciplinary ethics committees who provide case review and consultation and participate in education, policy making, quality, and (in some cases) research. Nurses contribute unique knowledge about the patient and family, interpret technical facts, identify appropriate decision makers, represent the patient's best interests, and help ensure the course of action is justified by sound ethical principles. Nurses play an important role in policy making, identifying needed policies to address ethical concerns or suggest needed modifications of existing policies. The human resource department focuses on employee policy; the health care team cannot judge or force a patient to reevaluate their cultural beliefs and observances.
12. **c.** The nurse assesses the patient's understanding of the cause and consequences of aspiration and pneumonia. The nurse can provide further information on pneumonia and sepsis if needed, while supporting the patient's decision. The patient has already declined treatment; therefore, the nurse assesses whether the patient understands the decision before discussing the intervention. The nurse may suggest safer swallowing options or consultation with a speech therapist after assessing the patient's knowledge.

Bibliography

Alspach, J. G. (2018). Implicit bias in patient care: An endemic blight on quality care. *Critical Care Nurse, 38*(4), 12–16.

American Association of Colleges of Nursing (AACN). (2008). *The essentials of baccalaureate education for professional nursing practice.* Author.

American Association of Colleges of Nursing (AACN). (2021). *The essentials: Core competencies for professional nursing education.* Author.

American Association of Critical-Care Nurses. (n.d.). *4 A's to rise above moral distress.* http://www.aacn.org/WD/Practice/Docs/4As_to_Rise_Above_Moral_Distress.pdf

American Association of Critical-Care Nurses. (2016). *AACN standards for establishing and sustaining healthy work environments: A journey to excellence* (2nd ed.). http://www.aacn.org/wd/hwe/docs/hwestandards.pdf

American Nurses Association (ANA). (n.d.). *ANA position statements on ethics and human rights.* http://www.nursingworld.org/MainMenuCategories/EthicsStandards/Resources/Ethics-Position-Statements

American Nurses Association (ANA). (2010). *Nursing's social policy statement: The essence of the profession.* Author.

American Nurses Association (ANA). (2011). *Principles for social networking and the nurse.* https://www.nursingworld.org/~4af4f2/globalassets/docs/ana/ethics/social-networking.pdf

American Nurses Association (ANA). (2015). *Code of ethics for nurses with interpretive statements.* Author. http://nursingworld.org/DocumentVault/Ethics-1/Code-of-Ethics-for-Nurses.html

American Nurses Association (ANA). (2021). *Nursing: Scope and standards of practice* (4th ed.). Author.

American Psychological Association. (2015). *The road to resilience.* http://www.apa.org/helpcenter/road-resilience.aspx

Anders, L. (2020). How a lesson in patient advocacy changed my career. *Nursing, 50*(7), 40–41.

Beauchamp, T. L., & Childress, J. F. (2019). *Principles of biomedical ethics* (8th ed.). Oxford University Press.

Berlinger, N. (2017). Workarounds are routinely used by nurses—but are they ethical? *American Journal of Nursing, 117*(10), 53–55.

Callahan, D. (1995). Bioethics. In W. T. Reich (Ed.). *Encyclopedia of bioethics* (Rev. ed., pp. 247–256). Macmillan.

Canadian Nurses Association. (2017). *Code of ethics for registered nurses.* Author.

Clark, C. M. (2019). Combining cognitive rehearsal, simulation, and evidence-based scripting to address incivility. *Nurse Educator, 44*(2), 64–68.

Currier, J. M., Holland, J. M., Drescher, K., & Foy, D. (2015). Initial psychometric evaluation of the Moral Injury Questionnaire—Military version. *Clinical Psychology & Psychotherapy, 22*(1), 54–63. https://doi.org/10.1002/cpp.1866

Currier, J. M., Holland, J. M., Rojas-Flores, L., Herrera, S., & Foy, D. (2015). Morally injurious experiences and meaning in Salvadorian teachers exposed to violence. *Psychological Trauma: Theory, Research, Practice, and Policy, 7*(1), 24–33. https://doi.org/10.1037/a0034092

DeGrazia, M., Porter, C., Sheehan, S., Whitamore, S., White, D., Nuttall, P.W., Blanchard, T., Davis, N., Steadman, J., & Hickey, P. (2021). Building moral resiliency through the nursing education and support team initiative. *American Journal of Critical Care, 30*(2), 95–102.

DiGangi Condon, K. A., Berger, J. T., & Shurpin, K. M. (2021). I've got the power: Nurses moral distress and perceptions of empowerment. *American Journal of Critical Care, 30*(6), 461–465.

Ebberts, M., & Sollars, K. (2020). Educating nurses about incivility. *Nursing, 50*(10), 64–68.

Epstein, B., & Turner, M. (2015). The nursing code of ethics: Its value, its history. *Online Journal of Issues in Nursing, 20*(2), 4. https://doi.org/10.3912/OJIN.Vol20No02Man04

Epstein, E. G., Whitehead, P. B., Prompahakul, C., Thacker, L. R., & Hamric, A. B. (2019). Enhancing understanding of moral distress: The measure of moral distress for health care professionals. *AJOB Empirical Bioethics, 10*(2), 113–124. https://doi.org/10.1080/23294515.2019.1586008

Fitzgerald, H., Knackstedt, A., & Trotochaud, K. (2018). Novel ethics champion programs. *American Nurse Today, 13*(3), 52–54.

Fletcher, J. C., Spencer, E. M., & Lombardo, P. A. (Eds.). (2005). *Fletcher's introduction to clinical ethics* (3rd ed.). University Publishing Group.

Fowler, M. D. M. (Ed.). (2010 Reissue). *Guide to the code of ethics for nurses: Interpretation and application.* American Nurses Association.

Fowler, M. D. M. (2015). *Guide to nursing's social policy statement: Understanding the profession from social contract to social covenant.* American Nurses Association.

Fry, S. T., Veatch, R. M., & Taylor, C. (2011). *Case studies in nursing ethics* (4th ed.). Jones and Bartlett Publishers.

Gentile, M.C. (2010). *Giving voice to values*. Yale University Press.

Gibson, J. A. (2021). Ethical considerations when patients initiate their own discharge. *Nursing, 51*(9), 12–14.

Hamric, A. B., & Epstein, E. G. (2017). A health system wide moral distress consultation service: Development and evaluation. *HEC Forum, 29*(2), 127–143. https://doi.org/10.1007/s10730-016-9315-y

Hewitt, J. (2019). Just healthcare and human flourishing: Why resource allocation is not just enough. *Nursing Ethics, 26*(2), 405–417.

Hiler, C. A., Hickman, R. L. Jr., Reimer, A. P., & Wilson, K. (2018). Predictors of moral distress in a US sample of critical care nurses. *American Journal of Critical Care, 27*(1), 59–66.

Holland, S. (2001). Beyond the embryo: A feminist appraisal of the embryonic stem cell debate. In S. Holland, K. Lebacqz, & L. Zoloth. (Eds.). *The human embryonic stem cell debate* (pp. 73–86). A Bradford Book.

Humphrey-Carothers, F., Kalia, N., Lam, C. K., Minor, S. A., Bernacki, E. J., & Tao, X. G. (2021). Standardizing the accommodations process for health care workers during COVID-19. *American Journal of Nursing, 121*(4), 50–55.

International Council of Nurses. (2012). *ICN code of ethics for nurses: Ethical concepts applied to nursing*. Imprimeries Populaires.

Kopacz, M. S., Ames, D., & Koenig, H. G. (2019). It's time to talk about physician burnout and moral injury. *Lancet Psychiatry, 6*(11), e28.

Koskenvuori, J., Stolt, M., Suhonen, R., & Leinto-Kilp, H. (2018). Healthcare professionals' ethical competence: A scoping review. *Nursing Open, 6*(1), 5–17.

Lachman, V. D. (2014). Conscientious objection in nursing: Definition and criteria for acceptance. *MedSurg Nursing, 23*(3), 196–198.

Lechasseur, K., Caux, C., Dollé, S., & Legault, A. (2018). Ethical competence: An integrative review. *Nursing Ethics, 25*(6), 694–706.

Litz, B. T., Stein, N., Delaney, E., Lebowitz, L., Nash, W. P., Silva, C., & Maguen, S. (2009). Moral injury and moral repair in war veterans: A preliminary model and intervention strategy. *Clinical Psychology Review, 29*(8), 695–706. https://doi.org/10.1016/j.cpr.2009.07.003

Mantri, S., Lawson, J. M., Wang, Z., & Koenig, H. G. (2020). Identifying moral injury in healthcare professionals: The Moral Injury Symptom Scale-HP. *Journal of Religion and Health, 59*(5), 2323–2340. https://doi.org/10.1007/s10943-020-01065-w

Murphy, P. (1990). Helping Joanne die with dignity: A nursing profile in courage. *Nursing, 20*(9), 44–49.

National Council of State Boards of Nursing (NCSBN). (2011). *White paper: A nurse's guide to the use of social media*. https://www.ncsbn.org/Social_Media.pdf

National Student Nurses' Association. (n.d.). *Recommendations for: Social media usage and maintaining privacy, confidentiality and professionalism*. https://www.ncsbn.org/NSNA_Social_Media_Recommendations.pdf

National Student Nurses' Association. (2009). *Code of ethics: Part II. Code of academic and clinical conduct and interpretive statements*. www.nsna.org

Olsen, D. P. (2017). What nurses talk about when they are talking about ethics. *American Journal of Nursing, 117*(11), 63–67.

Olsen, D. P. (2021). Care and ethics: Inseparable and relational. *American Journal of Nursing, 121*(8), 57–62.

Olsen, D. P., & Keilman, L. J. (2020). The moral distress of nurses when patients forgo treatment because of cost. *American Journal of Nursing, 120*(9), 61–66.

Olson, L. L. (2021). Envisioning an ethical climate in nursing education programs. *OJIN: The Online Journal of Issues in Nursing, 26*(1), Manuscript 7. DOI: 10.3912/OJIN.Vol26No01Man07 https://doi.org/10.3912/OJIN.Vol26No01Man07

Pavlish, C., Brown-Saltzman, K., Hersh, M., Shirk, M., & Nudelman, O. (2011). Early indicators and risk factors for ethical issues in clinical practice. *Journal of Nursing Scholarship, 43*(1), 13–21.

Pavlish, C., Brown-Saltzman, K., Hersh, M., Shirk, M., & Rounkle, A. M. (2011). Nursing priorities, actions, and regrets for ethical situations in clinical practice. *Journal of Nursing Scholarship, 43*(4), 385–395.

Prestoa, A. S., Sherman, R. O., & Demezier, C. (2017). Chief nursing officers' experience with moral distress. *The Journal of Nursing Administration, 47*(2), 101–107.

Raths, L. E., Harmin, M., & Simon, S. B. (1978). *Values and teaching* (2nd ed.). Charles E. Merrill.

Rosenthal, M. S., & Clay, M. C. (2015). *The moral distress education project*. http://moraldistressproject.med.uky.edu/moral-distress-home

Rushton, C. H. (2021). Preserving integrity and staying power as a nurse in a pandemic. *American Journal of Nursing, 121*(3), 68–69.

Rushton, C. H., Broome, M., & The Nursing Ethics for the 21st Century Summit Group. (2014). *A blueprint for 21st century nursing ethics: Report of the national nursing summit*. http://www.bioethicsinstitute.org/nursing-ethics-summit-report

Rushton, C. H., Caldwell, M., & Kurtz, M. (2016). CE: Moral distress: A catalyst in building moral resilience. *American Journal of Nursing, 116*(7), 40–49.

Rushton, C. H., & Kurtz, M. J. (2015). *Moral distress and you: Supporting ethical practice and moral resilience in nursing*. American Nurses Association.

Rushton, C. H., Schoonover-Shoffner, K., & Kennedy, M. S. (2017). Executive summary: Transforming moral distress into moral resilience in nursing. *American Journal of Nursing, 117*(2), 52–56.

Shay, J. (1991). Learning about combat stress from Homer's Iliad. *Journal of Traumatic Stress, 4*(4), 561–579.

Shay, J. (2014). Moral injury. *Psychoanalytic Psychology, 31*(2), 182–191. https://doi.org/10.1037/a0036090

Sherman, R. O., & Cohn, T. M. (2018). Discovering your true north. *American Nurse Today, 13*(7), 14–15.

Stephens, T. M. (2017). Situational awareness and the Nursing Code of Ethics. *American Nurse Today, 12*(11), 56–58.

Steers, M. N., & Gallups, S. F. (2020). Ethical tipping point: Nurses' presence on social media. *Nursing, 50*(12), 52–54.

Storch, J. L., Rodney, P., & Starzomski, R. (Eds.). (2013). *Toward a moral horizon: Nursing ethics for leadership and practice*. Pearson/Prentice Hall.

Stovall, M., Hansen, L., & van Ryn, M. (2020). A critical review: Moral injury in nurses in the aftermath of a patient safety incident. *Journal of Nursing Scholarship, 52*(3), 320–328. https://doi.org/10.1111/jnu.12551

Taylor, C. (1993). Nursing ethics: The role of caring. *AWHONN's Clinical Issues in Perinatal and Women's Health Nursing, 4*(4), 552–560.

Taylor, C. R. (1997). Everyday nursing concerns: Unique? Trivial? Or essential to healthcare ethics? *HEC Forum, 9*(1), 68–84.

Ulrich, C. M., & Grady, C. (2019). *Moral distress and moral strength among clinicians in health care systems: A call for research. NAM Perspectives*. Commentary, National Academy of Medicine. https://doi.org/10/31478/20/1909c

Warmer, S. L. (2017). Getting political about advocacy. *Nursing, 47*(11), 47–49.

Webster, L., & Wocial, L. D. (2020). Ethics in a pandemic. *American Nurse Journal, 15*(9), 18–23.

Williamson, V., Stevelink, S. A. M., & Greenberg, N. (2018). Occupational moral injury and mental health: Systematic review and meta-analysis. *The British Journal of Psychiatry, 212*(6), 339–346. https://doi.org/10.1192/bjp.2018.55

Wocial, L. D. (2020). Resilience as an incomplete strategy for coping with moral distress in critical care nurses. *Critical Care Nurse, 40*(6), 62–66.

Yonkaitis, C. F. (2021). The elevator pitch: A 60-second advocacy tool for nurses. *American Nurse Journal, 16*(1), 54–55.

For a nice introduction to ethical theories and thought experiments, check out The Ethics Center: https://ethics.org.au/knowledge/ethics-explainers/

7 Legal Dimensions of Nursing Practice

Ramone Scott

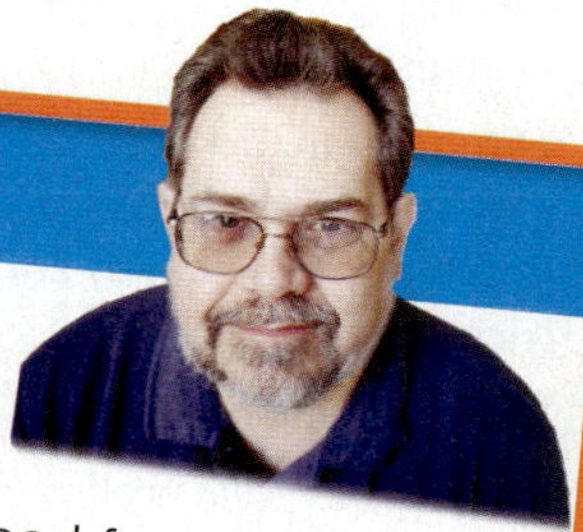

Ramone, a 66-year-old man, had surgery to repair a fractured hip earlier in the day. His nurse just administered a dose of an intravenous antibiotic that had been prescribed for a different patient.

Meredith Bedford

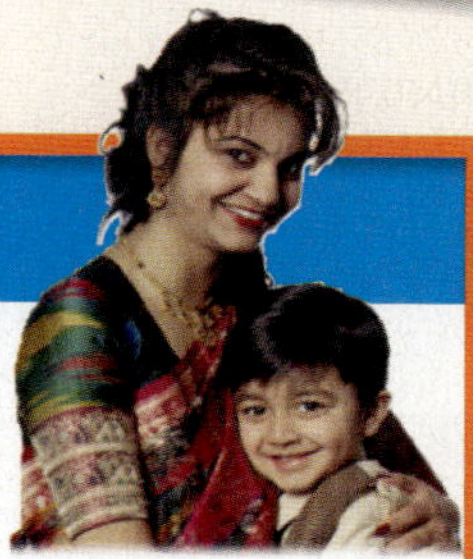

Meredith is the mother of a terminally ill child with a brain tumor who is admitted to a residential hospice for better pain and symptom management. One morning she tells the nurse, "I'm very unhappy with the care my son is receiving. I'm going to talk with my attorney as soon as possible to press charges against the hospice."

Ella Rodriguez

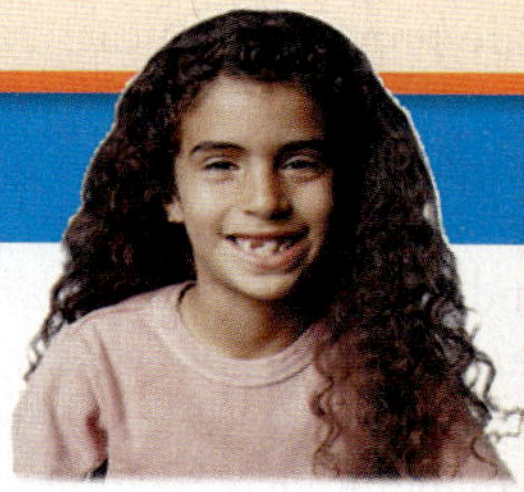

Ella, an 8-year-old girl, comes to the emergency department (ED) with a right forearm fracture. She requires diazepam sedation for a closed reduction procedure. The ED's protocol for administration to a child states that a health care provider must be present throughout the entire sedation procedure. One of the health care providers has been working his 14th hour, and the ED is overflowing. He orders the nurse to begin the sedation protocol, stating that he will be back in the room in 10 minutes.

Learning Outcomes

After completing the chapter, you will be able to accomplish the following:

1. Define "law" and describe four sources of laws.
2. Describe the professional and legal regulation of nursing practice.
3. Identify the purpose of credentialing, using as examples accreditation, licensure or registration, and certification.
4. Identify grounds for suspending or revoking a license or registration.
5. Differentiate between intentional torts (assault and battery, defamation, invasion of privacy, false imprisonment, fraud) and unintentional torts (negligence).
6. Evaluate personal areas of potential liability in nursing.
7. Describe the legal procedure that occurs when a plaintiff files a complaint against a nurse for negligence.
8. Describe the roles of the nurse as defendant, fact witness, and expert witness.
9. Use appropriate legal safeguards in nursing practice.
10. Explain the purpose of incident reports.
11. Describe laws affecting nursing practice.

Nursing Concepts

- Legal issues

As the roles and duties of nurses have expanded, so has our legal accountability. In the past, many nurses worked under the supervision of a health care provider, few carried liability insurance, and even if a nurse's actions directly caused harm to a patient, the primary liability for the nursing action fell on the employing facility or health care provider. In modern practice, nurses assess and diagnose patients and plan, implement, and evaluate nursing care. Full legal responsibility and accountability for these nursing actions rest with the nurse. (See the accompanying Reflective Practice box for an example.) Nurses are increasingly the subjects of both civil and criminal negligence cases and are being brought to court to defend their practice. While nurses shouldn't practice in constant fear of being sued, it would be foolish not to learn how to be legally prudent. Similarly, many nurses do not appreciate the true extent of authority the nursing boards maintain and the issues they may address and consequently fail to take steps to maintain their license in good standing.

Although many nurses continue to work in traditional settings such as hospitals and long-term care facilities, more nurses are working in nontraditional community settings such as home care facilities, clinics, daycare centers, and nurse-managed health centers. Advanced practice nurses may have independent practices. It is critical for nurses to document their actions carefully and act in ways to prevent malpractice accusations. Nurses who wish to avoid legal conflicts need to develop trusting nurse–patient relationships (satisfied patients rarely sue), practice within the scope of their competence, and identify potential liabilities in their practice and work to prevent them. Nurses are less likely to be sued than other health care professional because they spend more time with patients and take time to answer their questions.

LEGAL CONCEPTS

As you begin professional practice, it is essential to understand how the law defines the nurse's legal responsibilities and duties.

Definition of Law

A **law** is a standard or rule of conduct established and enforced by the government that is intended chiefly to protect the rights of the public. Public law is law in which the government is involved directly. It regulates relationships between people and the government—for example, describing the powers of the government. Private law, also called civil law, regulates relationships among people. Civil law includes laws relating to contracts; ownership of property; and the practice of nursing, medicine, pharmacy, and dentistry. Criminal law, a type of public law, concerns state and federal criminal statutes, which define criminal actions such as murder, manslaughter, criminal negligence, theft, and illegal possession of drugs.

Sources of Laws

Four sources of laws exist at both the federal and state level: constitutions, statutory law, administrative law, and common law.

Constitutions

Federal and state constitutions indicate how the federal and state governments are created, and they give authority and state the principles and provisions for establishing specific laws. Although they contain relatively few laws (called constitutional laws), constitutions serve as guides to legislative bodies.

Statutory Law

A legislative body enacts **statutory law**. Statutory laws must be in keeping with both the federal constitution and the state constitution. Nurse practice acts are an example of statutory laws. These are discussed fully in the later section entitled "Professional and Legal Regulation of Nursing Practice."

Administrative Law

Executive officers (e.g., the President of the United States, state governors, and city mayors) administer facilities that, among other functions, are responsible for law enforcement. These facilities have the power to make administrative rules and regulations, in conformity with enacted law, that act as

QSEN Reflective Practice: Cultivating QSEN Competencies

CHALLENGE TO ETHICAL AND LEGAL SKILLS

This past summer, I worked in the emergency department (ED) of a very reputable hospital. Overall, I felt that the department was a desirable working environment and that the relationships between health care providers and nurses were very open. However, one incident occurred that I felt put the patient's safety at risk.

Ella Rodriguez, an 8-year-old girl, had come to the ED with a right forearm fracture. She required diazepam sedation for a closed reduction procedure. The ED's protocol for administration to a child states that a health care provider must be present throughout the entire sedation procedure. One of the health care providers had been working for 14 hours, and the ED was overflowing. He ordered the nurse to begin the sedation protocol, stating that he would be back in the room in 10 minutes. The nurse taking care of the patient was a new graduate and did not feel comfortable giving the drug alone, but also did not feel comfortable speaking up to the doctor. She proceeded to go into the room and inject the first dose of diazepam, against protocol.

This nursing action completely undermined the patient's safety because the nurse not only stated previously that she did not feel comfortable with the sedation procedure, but she also went against protocol. Since both the health care provider and the nurse had a duty to follow the protocol, if harm resulted from their failure to do so, there would be grounds for negligence. Although the health care provider was also responsible for giving the nurse orders against protocol, her obligation to herself and the patient should have been the priority, and thus, she should have refused to give the drug until the health care provider was in the room.

Thinking Outside the Box: Possible Courses of Action

- Hope that nothing happens to the patient until the health care provider comes back into the room.
- Get the health care provider back into the room; if he refuses an invitation to be present, report this to someone in a leadership position.
- Ask the nurse why she is violating protocol.
- Seek the help of my preceptor immediately.

Evaluating a Good Outcome: How Do I Define Success?

- Patient is benefited or at the very least not harmed.
- The health care provider, nurse, and unit leaders accept responsibility for safely implementing protocols.
- All health care team members demonstrate accountability for failures to adhere to protocols.
- Patient safety is put first, even when this means challenging other members of the team.

Personal Learning: Here's to the Future!

My preceptor, the charge nurse, realized that the nurse was in the room administering the medication. Once he realized this, he immediately got the health care provider to go into the patient's room. After the procedure was completed successfully, he discussed the implications of both the nurse's and the doctor's actions with each of them together and separately. I did not have time to respond to this incident because the charge nurse had acted so quickly and appropriately.

Obviously, I think that the nurse should have spoken to the health care provider and refused to give the medication, but I can understand her feelings, especially being a new graduate. The entire situation can be very intimidating, but as nurses, our responsibility is to the patient. By not standing up for the patient and herself, the nurse put the patient in danger and herself in danger, and did nothing to change the climate of the ED. The experienced and exceptionally capable charge nurse was not afraid to stand up to the doctor. Not only did his actions put the patient's safety first, but he also demonstrated to the nurse, myself, and other nurses that it is imperative that nurses stand up for themselves and patients.

I believe that no matter what the circumstance is, nurses need to stand up for themselves and their patients, especially now, when our health care climate yields to nurses' voices being heard. The only way that nurses' roles and reputations will change is if we, the nurses, speak up, and speak loudly. Right now, we have a unique opportunity to change the way medicine is practiced to benefit both patients and nurses. If all nurses grab this opportunity and make something of it, we can really make a difference, but it needs to be a collective effort to be successful. Regardless of how small the problem is, it must be addressed.

Julia Strobel, Georgetown University

QSEN SELF-REFLECTION ON QUALITY AND SAFETY COMPETENCIES DEVELOPING KNOWLEDGE, SKILLS, AND ATTITUDES FOR CONTINUOUS IMPROVEMENT

How do you think you would respond in a similar situation? Why? What does this tell you about yourself and about the adequacy of your skills for professional practice? How was the nurse's action ethical? Legal? Please explain. What other *knowledge, attitudes,* and *skills* do you need to develop to continuously improve the quality and safety of care for patients like Ella Rodriguez?

Patient-Centered Care: What role did each member of the nursing team play in creating a partnership with Ella's parents to best coordinate her care? What special talents do you bring to creating this partnership?

Teamwork and Collaboration/Quality Improvement: What communication skills do you need to improve to ensure that you function as a competent, caring, and responsible

(*continued*)

QSEN Reflective Practice: Cultivating QSEN Competencies *(continued)*

CHALLENGE TO ETHICAL AND LEGAL SKILLS

member of the patient-care team and that you obtain assistance when needed? How would you have responded if ordered by a health care provider to break protocol? What special talents do you bring to promoting a well-functioning interdisciplinary team?

Safety/Evidence-Based Practice: What priority did all involved in Ella's care accord to her health, well-being, and safety? What evidence in the nursing literature supports practicing as directed by this protocol? What in the safety literature dictates how nurses should respond in similar situations?

Informatics: Can you identify the essential information that must be available in Ella Rodriguez's electronic record to support safe patient care and coordination of care? Can you think of other ways to respond to or approach the situation?

laws and are enforceable. Boards of nursing are administrative facilities at the state level. The rules and regulations that they adopt are administrative laws. An example of a municipal administrative facility is the city board of health.

Common Law

The government provides for a judiciary system, which is responsible for resolving controversies. It interprets legislation at the local, state, and national levels as it has been applied in specific instances and makes decisions concerning law enforcement. A body of law known as **common law** has evolved from these accumulated judiciary decisions. Common law is thus court-made law. Most law involving malpractice is common law.

Common law is based on the principle of *stare decisis,* or "let the decision stand." After a decision has been made in a court of law, the principle in that decision becomes the rule to follow in other similar cases. The case that first sets down the rule by decision is called a precedent. Court decisions can be changed, but only with strong justification. Common law helps prevent one set of rules from being used to judge one person and another set to judge another person in similar circumstances.

Court System

A lawsuit is a civil action brought in a court of law. **Litigation** is the process of bringing and trying a lawsuit. The person or government who claims to have incurred losses as the result of an action by a defendant is called the **plaintiff**. The **defendant** is presumed innocent until proved guilty of a crime or tort. Criminal law is concerned with actions that are harmful to society as a whole. A prosecutor or district attorney brings charges against a person, persons, or corporate entity believed to have committed a crime.

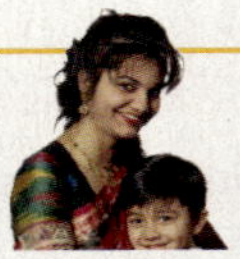

Recall ***Meredith Bedford***, the mother of the terminally ill child threatening to bring charges against the hospice. The mother would be considered the plaintiff, while those named in the lawsuit would be considered the defendants.

The two levels of courts in the United States are trial courts and appellate courts. The trial court, the first-level court, hears all the evidence in a case and makes decisions based on facts, usually through a jury. The appellate court hears only cases questioning a point of law decided by the trial court. No witnesses testify at the appellate court level. The opinions of appellate judges are published and become common law.

PROFESSIONAL AND LEGAL REGULATION OF NURSING PRACTICE

Nurses who practice safely respect both the voluntary and legal controls of nursing practice. Both controls are designed to ensure quality health care and to protect society from unsafe actions. Take time to study the ANA Model Representing Regulation of Professional Nursing Practice, which depicts the components and relationships of the key regulatory influencers governing nursing practice:

- Evidence
- Nursing Practice
- Key Regulatory Influencers
  - Code of Ethics, Nursing Professional Scope and Standards, and Specialty Certification
  - Practice Setting, Organizational Policies, and Procedures
  - Nurse Practice Acts, Rules and Regulations, Population Focus, Consensus Model
- Safety
- Quality (ANA, 2021, pp. 38–42)

Nurse Practice Acts

Your state's nurse practice act is the most important law affecting your nursing practice. Each state has a **nurse practice act** that protects the public by broadly defining the legal scope of nursing practice. Remember from Chapter 1 that the scope of nursing practice describes the "who," "what," "when," "where," "why," and "how" of nursing practice. You should obtain a copy of this act from your State Board of Nursing and study it carefully. Visit the website of the National Council of State Boards of Nursing (NCSBN) for more information about nurse practice acts and how to contact your State Board of Nursing (https://www.ncsbn.org/boards.htm). Each nurse is expected to care for patients within defined practice

Table 7-1 Who Makes Nursing Practice Rules?

SOURCE OF PRACTICE RULES	EXAMPLES OF ISSUES COVERED	WHERE RULES ARE DOCUMENTED	HOW TO INITIATE CHANGE
Federal legislation	• Medicare and Medicaid provisions related to reimbursement for nursing services	• Federal statutes	• Review documents • Draft desired legislative changes • Obtain support of colleagues, nursing organizations, other health care providers, and the public, if appropriate • Obtain support and sponsorship from a U.S. congressperson or senator, who will introduce the bill • Lobby for the bill's passage
State legislation	• Scope of practice for RNs, LPNs, advanced practice nurses • Nursing educational requirements • Composition and disciplinary authority of board of nursing	• Nurse practice act • Medical practice act • Other statutes	• Review documents • Draft desired legislative changes • Obtain support of colleagues, nursing organizations, other health care providers, and the public, if appropriate • Obtain support and sponsorship from a state legislator, who will introduce the bill • Lobby for the bill's passage
Board of nursing	• Delegation • Medication administration • Unprofessional conduct • Licensing	• Rules and regulations • Position statements • Declaratory rulings (as found in meeting minutes or newsletters), which may be specific to a particular setting or institution	• Review documents • Initiate a formal query to the licensing board • Obtain board support for change • The board may issue a position statement or declaratory ruling or hold a formal public hearing before voting to promulgate new rules or change existing ones
Health care institution	• Clinical procedures, such as wound dressing changes • Policies specific to the institution, specialty, or practice setting • Personnel and employment policies	• Unit-based policies • Institutional policies • Institutional credentialing policies	• Review institutional policies • Follow institutional policies or the chain of command to make inquiries or propose change

limits. Practicing beyond those limits (e.g., performing an appendectomy) makes you vulnerable to charges of violating the state nurse practice act.

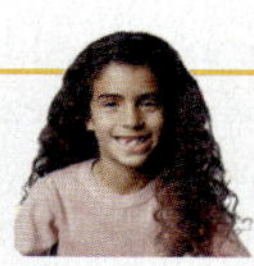

Consider **Ella Rodriguez**, the 8-year-old with the fractured arm requiring administration of sedation based on a protocol. The nurse should integrate knowledge of the state's nurse practice act when administering the medication, understanding the need to adhere to the ED's protocol that requires a health care provider to be present throughout the administration.

Nurse practice acts list the violations that can result in disciplinary actions against a nurse and also intend to prevent untrained or unlicensed people from practicing nursing. Table 7-1 illustrates different sources of rules affecting nursing practice, examples of issues covered, where these rules are documented, and suggestions for initiating change. More than 3.9 million U.S. nurses have great potential to influence health care if we would only contact our representatives and "raise our voices." To get what we want, we must make sure our legislators hear us loud and clear. What easier way to do this than with a letter or e-mail? An example of an e-mail to a member of Congress to support funding for the Nurse Reinvestment Act (NRA) is shown in Box 7-1 (on page 148), and a student describes a lobbying experience in Through the Eyes of a Student (on page 148).

Standards

Voluntary standards, developed and implemented by the nursing profession itself, are not mandatory but are used as guidelines for peer review. Professional nursing organizations continually reassess the functions, standards, and qualifications of their members. These organizations are guided by their own assessment of society's need for nursing and by the public's expectations of nursing. Examples of voluntary standards include the American Nurses

Box 7-1 Example of an E-Mail to Congress to Support Funding for the Nurse Reinvestment Act (NRA)

Explanation of Numbered Points

1. Use your Congress member's e-mail address, which can be found at http://www.house.gov and http://www.senate.gov. Send an individual e-mail to each member of Congress separately, with only one e-mail address in the "To:" line. You may want to send an e-mail to the member who represents voters from the place where you work, if you live in a different state or district from where you work. If you do this, be sure to write the e-mail to describe the impact that the legislation will have on your patients, who are the legislator's constituents.
2. You can copy this e-mail to a professional nursing organization or leave this blank. Do not copy it to another member of Congress.
3. State as clearly as possible the legislation you are addressing (e.g., nursing shortage). Although not necessary, you can use the bill number, if known.
4. If you want to attach a letter you have written that is longer and more fully explains your position, you may do so here.
5. An e-mail needs to be shorter and more succinct than a letter. The person reading it should be able to view your entire message on one screen without scrolling down. If you want to write more, attach a letter.
6. Put your name and address at the top to show the legislator that you are a voter in their district or state.
7. The legislator's title—either "Representative" or "Senator"—and last name make up the salutation.
8. Body of the e-mail:
   - State what you want the legislator to do in the first sentence.
   - Identify yourself as a concerned nurse.
   - Tell why the legislator should do what you are asking.
   - Ask the legislator to vote for/support what you are asking.

Finally, use spell-check and reread the e-mail to make sure the message you want to get across is clear and concise.

Source: Used with permission. Sharp, N. (2003). The "write stuff." *Nursing Spectrum, 13*(2), 12–13.

Association (ANA) standards of practice (see Chapter 1; ANA, 2021), professional standards for the accreditation of education programs and service organizations, and standards for the certification of individual nurses in general and specialty areas of practice. The ANA (2021) describes the Standards of Professional Nursing Practice as authoritative statements of the duties that all registered nurses, regardless of role, population, specialty, setting or Advanced Practice Registered Nurse foci, are expected to competently perform.

Legal standards, on the other hand, are developed by a legislature and are implemented by authority granted by the state to determine minimum standards for the education of nurses, to set requirements for licensure or registration, and to decide when a nurse's license may be suspended or revoked. Examples of legal standards include state nurse practice acts and rules and regulations of nursing.

Credentialing

Nursing has taken several steps to ensure the competence of its health care providers, including the credentialing process. **Credentialing** refers to ways in which professional competence is ensured and maintained.

Three processes are used for credentialing in nursing. The first is **accreditation**, which is the process by which an educational program is evaluated and recognized as having met certain standards. The second is **licensure**, which is the process by which a state determines that a candidate meets certain minimum requirements to practice in the profession and grants a license to do so. The third is **certification**,

Through the Eyes of a Student

I was extremely nervous to go to Capitol Hill and meet with my congressional representative; I had begun to feel so comfortable in my scrubs at the hospital that I felt out of place in a suit. I was very fortunate that Representative Christopher Shays agreed to meet with me to discuss my views on medical malpractice liability. Although the meeting was very short, Mr. Shays gave me his attention and respect and listened to my point of view and that of the ANA with political tact. He said that he appreciated my taking time to meet with him and share my views on the subject as a voter and student nurse. He found the issue to be especially important in Connecticut because our state is currently facing crises in regard to high medical malpractice insurance rates and a large number of health care providers having to end their practice because of these rates. Mr. Shays shared his belief that it is critical to reform medical malpractice to provide quality, affordable health care. He explained his view that excessive jury awards have driven the cost of health care up for everyone, and that he believes a noneconomic damage cap of $250,000 will help in containing health care costs and make insurance more affordable to Americans. I was able to reiterate the ANA's view of postponing judgment on the institution of a medical malpractice cap until an impartial commission could complete and release a report on the effect of the controversial topic, helping him to make an informed decision. I thanked Mr. Shays for his time, and he thanked me for sharing my views on the subject and wished me luck in my study of such a "noble profession." It was thrilling to talk to Mr. Shays, if only briefly, and to feel like such an important part of the legislative process. Nurses definitely have the power to impact our nation's health care legislation.

—Maureen McFadden, Georgetown University

which is the process by which a person who has met certain criteria established by a nongovernmental association is granted recognition in a specified practice area.

Accreditation

State constitutions give states a responsibility for the public welfare. State legislative bodies have used this principle to enact laws controlling occupational and professional groups. One function of these laws is to see that schools preparing health care providers maintain minimum standards of education. Nursing, like most other health care professions, operates under state laws that promote the general welfare by determining minimum standards of education through accreditation of schools of nursing. State-approved, or accredited, educational programs in nursing include practical or vocational, associate degree, diploma, baccalaureate, and graduate programs in nursing (see Chapter 1).

Legal accreditation of a school preparing nursing personnel by the State Board of Nursing is different from voluntary accreditation. The National League for Nursing Accrediting Commission (NLNAC) and the American Association of Colleges of Nursing (AACN) are voluntary facilities that accredit schools when they meet certain criteria. Most schools choose to seek this voluntary accreditation, and many prospective students prefer selecting accredited schools. Accreditation by NLNAC or AACN is not a legal requirement for a school to exist; state accreditation is a legal requirement.

Licensure

Licensure is a specialized form of credentialing based on laws passed by a state legislature. A license is a legal document that permits a person to offer to the public skills and knowledge in a particular jurisdiction, where such practice would otherwise be unlawful without a license. Licensure is discussed in Chapter 1. In addition to successfully completing an accredited nursing program of study and passing the National Council Licensure Examination (NCLEX), to maintain a license in good standing a nurse must meet other requirements as determined by the state or territory. These requirements typically include good moral character, continuing clinical competence or continuing education, the absence of a criminal record, English proficiency, and compliance with specific provisions of the state's nursing laws. Some states require criminal background checks. It is critical to remember that licensure is not a constitutional right, it is a revocable privilege. As many nurse attorneys are quick to point out the licensing board is there to protect the public not to be an advocate for you. See the National Council of State Boards (NCSBN) website (https://www.ncsbn.org) for answers to your questions about licensure. The NCSBN also offers a video for new nurses about licensure, available at https://www.ncsbn.org/8243.htm.

According to the NCSBN, a mutual recognition model of nurse licensure allows a nurse to have one license in their state of residency and to practice in other states (both physically and electronically) as well, subject to each state's practice law and regulation, unless otherwise restricted. This multistate nurse licensure model is governed by the Nurse Licensure Compact (NLC). All states that currently belong to the NLC also operate the single-state licensure model for those nurses who reside legally in an NLC state but do not qualify for multistate licensure. *You must legally reside in an NLC state to be eligible for a multistate license.* For questions related to the multistate license or privilege to practice, contact the Board of Nursing in your state of residence (https://www.ncsbn.org/nlc.htm).

Once earned, a license to practice is a property right and may not be revoked without due process. This includes notice of an investigation, a fair and impartial hearing, and a proper decision based on substantial evidence. Crucial to a nurse's successful defense are early legal counsel, character, and expert witnesses and thorough preparation for all proceedings. Since legal counsel can be expensive, it is important to have your own liability insurance, as your employer's coverage does not address this.

State Boards of Nursing may revoke or suspend a nurse's license or registration for various reasons. Drug or alcohol use or misuse is currently the most frequent reason. You may be surprised to learn that sleep deprivation may result in disciplinary action. Other reasons for revocation or suspension of a license or registration include fraud, deceptive practices, criminal acts, previous disciplinary action by other state boards, gross or ordinary negligence, and physical or mental impairments, including those resulting from aging.

Certification

Whereas licensure measures entry-level competence, certification validates specialty knowledge, experience, and clinical judgment. Nursing certification is offered by many U.S. professional organizations, including two primary organizations: the American Association of Critical-Care Nurses, which represents the specialty with the largest number of certified nurses, and the American Nurses Credentialing Center (https://www.nursingworld.org/ancc/), a subsidiary of ANA, which began certifying nurses in 1974. The latter is the largest and most prestigious nurse credentialing organization in the United States and has certified more than a quarter million nurses since 1990. Although certification, which involves special testing, is voluntary, nurse specialists are increasingly becoming certified.

Certification is one means to demonstrate advanced proficiency and a commitment to ensuring competence in the context of the current U.S. health care crisis, evidenced by daily reports of unsafe care, rising litigation, escalating costs, and a worsening nursing shortage.

Concept Mastery Alert

Nursing deals with the public. Thus, the ultimate goal of all laws and professional regulations involved with nursing practice is public safety.

CRIMES AND TORTS

A wrong committed against a person or that person's property may be categorized as a crime or a tort, or sometimes both. A **crime** is a violation punishable by the state, whereas a **tort** is subject to action in a civil court with damages usually being settled with money. By its very nature, a wrong tried as a crime is considered a more serious offense, with more legal implications, than a tort.

Crime

Though there may only be one victim of a crime, criminal acts are considered to be against the public as well. In a criminal case, the government, called "the people," prosecutes the offender. When a crime is committed, the factor of intent to commit wrong is present in most cases. Nonetheless, people who break certain laws are guilty of a crime regardless of whether they intended it. For example, failure to observe the Federal Food, Drug, and Cosmetic Act may constitute a crime.

Criminal law is in most cases statutory law (e.g., Federal Controlled Substance Acts and kidnapping laws or state criminal codes that define murder, manslaughter, criminal negligence, rape, fraud, illegal possession of drugs, theft, assault, and battery); only infrequently is it common law. Examples of common law are informed consent and the right to refuse treatment. Crimes are further classified as misdemeanors or felonies. A **misdemeanor** is a less serious crime, commonly punishable with a fine, imprisonment for less than 1 year, or both, or with parole. A **felony** (e.g., rape, murder) is punishable by imprisonment in a state or federal penitentiary for more than 1 year.

Torts

Torts may be intentional or unintentional acts of wrongdoing. Some of the intentional torts for which nurses may be held liable include assault and battery, defamation of character, invasion of privacy, false imprisonment, and fraud. A person committing an intentional tort is considered to have knowledge of the permitted legal limits of their words or acts. Violating these limits is grounds for prosecution. For example, although a policy specifies that a nurse may use restraints to protect an incompetent patient, restraining a competent patient to administer medications forcefully while the patient is refusing is assault and battery. Unintentional torts are referred to as negligence. A nurse who fails to initiate proper precautions to prevent patient harm (e.g., falls, skin breakdown) is subject to the charge of negligence. The nurse may not intend to cause harm; nevertheless, harm results.

An act that is a tort may also be a crime. For example, gross negligence demonstrating that the offender is guilty of complete disregard for another's life may be tried as both a civil and criminal action. It is then prosecuted under both civil and criminal law.

Intentional Torts

ASSAULT AND BATTERY

Assault is a threat or an attempt to make bodily contact with another person without that person's consent. **Battery** is an assault that is carried out and includes willful, angry, and violent or negligent touching of another person's body or clothes or anything attached to or held by that other person. Forcibly removing a patient's clothing, administering an injection after the patient has refused it, and pushing a patient into a chair are all examples of battery. Threatening to do any of these actions if the patient does not cooperate is assault. If an aggressive patient threatens harm, only actions necessary for self-protection or the aid of another are permitted.

Every person has the right to be free from invasion of their person, and adult patients who are alert and oriented have the right to refuse any treatment. The fact that treatment is desirable does not allow the nurse or health care provider to proceed without the consent of the patient or to go beyond the limits to which the patient has consented (see "Informed Consent or Refusal" within "Legal Safeguards for the Nurse").

DEFAMATION

Defamation of character is an intentional tort in which one party makes derogatory remarks about another that diminish the other party's reputation. *Slander* is spoken defamation of character; *libel* is written defamation. Defamation of character is grounds for an award of civil damages. Damages are awarded to the plaintiff based on the amount of harm done to the plaintiff. Nurses who make false or exaggerated statements about their patients or coworkers run the risk of being sued for slander or libel. A person charged with slander or libel may be found not liable if it can be proved that the statement was made not to injure another but was made for a nonmalicious, justifiable purpose.

INVASION OF PRIVACY

The U.S. Supreme Court has interpreted the right against invasion of privacy as a constitutional right. The Fourth Amendment gives citizens the right of privacy and the right to be left alone. State courts have also strongly protected a patient's right to have information kept confidential. What is *confidential*? All information about patients is considered private or confidential, whether written on paper, saved on a computer, or spoken aloud. This includes patient name and all identifiers, such as address, telephone number, e-mail address, Social Security number, and any other personal information. It also includes the reason that the patient is sick or in the hospital, office, or clinic, the treatments the patient receives, and information about past health conditions. Protected health information may be found in the patient medical record, computer systems, telephone calls and voice mails, fax transmissions, e-mails that contain patient information, and conversations about patients between clinical staff.

The Health Insurance Portability and Accountability Act (HIPAA) was finalized in 2002. Most facilities now require workers to undergo HIPAA training and to review and sign a confidentiality agreement when hired and at each performance review. As a student in a health care setting, you should discuss privacy guidelines with your instructor and nurse mentors. HIPAA ensures that patients have the following rights:

- To see and copy their health record
- To update their health record
- To request correction of any mistakes
- To get a list of the disclosures a health care institution has made independent of disclosures made for the purposes of treatment, payment, and health care operations

- To request a restriction on certain uses or disclosures
- To choose how to receive health information

If a health institution wants to release a patient's health information for purposes other than treatment, payment, and routine health care operations, the patient must sign an authorization. Box 20-2 in Chapter 20 gives a list of permitted disclosures of patient health information and incidental disclosures. Other disclosure of confidential information, such as inappropriately discussing a patient's problem with a third party, may be construed as invasion of privacy and may subject the nurse to liability. The nurse's intimate knowledge of the patient increases legal risk in this regard.

The doctrine of privileged communication specifies that people in a protected relationship, such as a doctor and patient, cannot be forced, even during legal proceedings, to reveal communication between them unless the person who benefits from the protection agrees to it. State laws determine which relationships are protected by the privilege doctrine, and not all states privilege nurse–patient communication.

HIPAA includes punishments for anyone caught violating patient privacy: Those who do so for financial gain can be fined as much as $250,000 or be jailed for up to 10 years. Even accidentally breaking the rules can result in penalties—and embarrassment—for you and your organization.

Certain acts by nurses could constitute invasion of privacy, as the following examples illustrate:

- Unnecessary exposure of patients while moving them through a corridor or while caring for them in rooms they share with others
- Talking with patients in rooms that are not soundproof
- Discussing patient information with people not entitled to the information (e.g., with the patient's employer or the press, or even the patient's family if not authorized to do so)
- Pressing the patient for information not necessary for care planning
- Interacting with the patient's family in ways not authorized by the patient
- Using tape recorders, dictating machines, computers, and the like without taking precautions to ensure the patient's confidentiality (see Chapter 20 and Box 7-2)
- Preparing written or oral class assignments about patients without concealing their identity
- Carrying out research without taking proper precautions to ensure the anonymity of patients

Cybersecurity has become a top priority for all health care systems. Finn and Dion (2017a) recently wrote, "Just as nurses have been on the front lines of fighting disease and illness, they are now combatting cybercriminals trying to rob our patients of privacy, personal information, and identities. More than ever, nurses are required to perform a task—provide information security—that falls well outside their job description and for which they receive little training." Finn and Dion quote past ANA president Pamela Cipriano, "Nurses' ethical practice commands the safeguarding of a patient's right to privacy and confidentiality including their data and information. By being vigilant and using best practices to secure devices and the flow of information, nurses protect patients and maintain their trust." Jordan (2020) urges nurses to be aware of the most common types of attacks to improve our ability to recognize, avoid, and respond to them to protect ourselves, our coworkers, the organization, and—of course—our patients.

Box 7-2 Privacy and Confidentiality of Health Care Records

Security measures that a nurse should be aware of, particularly when using computerized health care records, include the following:

- Authorized users of an automated information system should have individual passwords and identification codes that are changed frequently. Nurses should never allow anyone else to use their log-on ID, nor should they perform any function using another person's log-on ID.
- Terminals, including those at the point of care, should have key locks as an additional measure to prevent unauthorized access to data.
- The computer system should "time out" when not in use for a specific period. The authorized user then needs to reenter the password and identification code to regain access.
- Nurses should log off the system when they leave a workstation and take other reasonable measures to ensure that unauthorized users cannot view or access confidential information.
- Temporary employees, such as traveling nurses, should have temporary passwords assigned.
- Employees who leave the organization should have their passwords and IDs terminated.
- The system should be able to track which users viewed, deleted, or updated patient information.
- Some information, such as results of acquired immunodeficiency syndrome testing, should not be stored on a computer.
- Computer printouts must be discarded appropriately because they may contain sensitive data about a patient.
- Nurses should not copy or provide data, either in printed or machine-readable form, for themselves or anyone else except as required to fulfill the responsibilities of their jobs.
- Most nurses sign agreements that they will use Internet access only to perform the responsibilities of their job. Internet access is not to be used for non–job-related business.
- The organization should have a policy regarding the use of patient data in research. Patient identifiers should be removed before the data are analyzed.
- Every nurse must be aware of the laws and statutes that protect the confidentiality of medical records. Most states have guidelines on the sharing of medical information. Your State Board of Nursing may revoke your license for serious breaches of patient confidentiality.

Protecting the privacy and confidentiality of health care records is the duty of every nurse. Any nurse who is aware of an actual or suspected breach of confidentiality must report it.

At times, a person's right to privacy may conflict with other rights, such as the public's right to information. When in doubt about disclosing confidential information, consult the nursing supervisor, ethics committee, or public relations department of the institution.

FALSE IMPRISONMENT

Unjustified retention or prevention of the movement of another person without proper consent can constitute false imprisonment. For example, only a reasonable amount of restraint should be used in circumstances that warrant it. The indiscriminate and thoughtless use of restraints on a patient can constitute false imprisonment. Springer (2015) cautions that restraints must not be used for coercion, punishment, discipline, or staff convenience. Serious sanctions by the state health department, The Joint Commission, or both, may result from improper restraint use. Be sure to check your institution's restraint policy before attempting to restrain any patient.

A person cannot be legally forced to remain in a health facility, such as a hospital, if that person is of sound mind, even when health care providers believe that the person should remain for additional care. Health facilities have special forms to use when a patient insists on being discharged against medical orders. The patient signs to indicate not holding the facility responsible for any harm that may result from leaving. People who are mentally ill may be committed to a psychiatric institution for treatment without their consent (involuntary commitment) only when it can be proved that they may be harmful to themselves or others.

FRAUD

Fraud is willful and purposeful misrepresentation that could cause, or has caused, loss or harm to a person or property. Misrepresentation of a product is a common fraudulent act. A person fraudulently misrepresenting themself to obtain a license to practice nursing may be prosecuted under the state's nurse practice act. Also, misrepresenting the outcome of a procedure or treatment may constitute fraud. Nurses who report vital signs or other assessment data that they have not obtained are acting fraudulently.

Unintentional Torts

NEGLIGENCE AND MALPRACTICE

Negligence is defined as performing an act that a reasonably prudent person under similar circumstances would not do or, conversely, failing to perform an act that a reasonably prudent person under similar circumstances would do. As the definition implies, an act of negligence may be an act of omission or commission. **Malpractice** is the term generally used to describe negligence by professional personnel. Reising (2012) identifies the following common categories of malpractice claims:

- *Failure to follow standards of care.* EXAMPLE: You fail to follow the standards for administering insulin or other injectable medications.
- *Failure to use equipment in a responsible manner.* EXAMPLE: You attempt to use a bariatric patient lift for the first time without getting help, and the patient falls.
- *Failure to assess and monitor.* EXAMPLE: You fail to follow your hospital's standards for postoperative assessments after receiving a patient from the operating room, and response to a ruptured suture line is delayed.
- *Failure to communicate.* EXAMPLE: You fail to communicate your concerns about an older adult patient being discharged home; this patient lives alone. The patient is soon rehospitalized because no provisions were made to secure the nursing care needed after discharge.
- *Failure to document.* EXAMPLE: You believe a patient is in danger of arresting, but your repeated calls to a health care provider to see the patient are ignored, so you work up the chain of command. Before any health care provider sees the patient, he arrests and, despite a code, dies. You document the arrest, code, and death; however, you failed to document all the steps you took to get the patient the medical attention he needed. Sixteen months later, the family sues, and you try to remember what action you took that evening—most of which was never recorded.
- *Failure to act as a patient advocate or to follow the chain of command.* EXAMPLE: You are in the operating room and watch a surgeon break the sterile field twice. No one else seems to notice. You are intimidated by this surgeon and fail to bring this to anyone's attention. You learn that the patient developed a serious infection postoperatively.

ELEMENTS OF LIABILITY

Liability involves four elements that must be established to prove that malpractice or negligence has occurred: duty, breach of duty, causation, and damages. *Duty* refers to an obligation to use due care (what a reasonably prudent nurse would do) and is defined by the standard of care appropriate for the nurse–patient relationship. *Breach of duty* is the failure to meet the standard of care. *Causation*, the most difficult element of liability to prove, shows that the failure to meet the standard of care (breach) actually caused the injury. *Damages* are the actual harm or injury resulting to the patient. Examples of these four elements are presented in Table 7-2.

STANDARDS OF CARE

Whether negligence has occurred depends on a standard of care: what a reasonably prudent person would or would not have done under similar circumstances. All nurses are responsible for following the standards of care for their particular areas of practice. For example, labor and delivery nurses must understand how standards for nursing practice differ from those for medical obstetric practice (according to the state's nurse practice act); must be familiar with specific standards for obstetric nursing (e.g., Association of Women's Health, Obstetrics, and Neonatal Nursing [AWHONN]); and must carry out the nursing responsibilities detailed in the hospital's policies and procedures and in their job description. If hospital policy dictates an assessment of each patient in the early stages of labor every 30 minutes, for

Table 7-2 Proof of Malpractice

An example of how a plaintiff (person bringing the lawsuit) proves that the nurse defendants are guilty of malpractice.

ELEMENT	EXAMPLE
Duty	Hospital staff nurses are responsible for: • Accurate assessment of patients assigned to their care • Alerting responsible health care professionals to changes in a patient's condition • Competent execution of safety measures for patients
Breach of duty	• Failure to note and report that an older adult patient assessed as alert on admission is exhibiting periods of confusion • Failure to execute and document use of appropriate safety measures (e.g., upper and lower bedside rails, use of restraints if necessary, assisted ambulation)
Causation	• Failure to use appropriate safety measures; this failure causes the patient to fall while attempting to get out of bed, resulting in a fractured left hip
Damages	• Fractured left hip, pain and suffering, lengthened hospital stay, and need for rehabilitation

example, nurses must adhere to this standard unless they document a reason for doing otherwise.

Table 7-3 (on page 154) lists areas of potential liability associated with each of the ANA standards of clinical nursing practice. Nursing errors can result in serious outcomes for the patient, as these examples show. To read more about standards, see Chapters 13 and 18.

Malpractice Litigation

When a patient believes they have been injured because of the negligence of a nurse or other health care professional and pursues legal action, one of three outcomes usually occurs:

- All parties work toward a fair settlement.
- The case is presented to a malpractice arbitration panel (in the United States).
- The case is brought to trial court.

The steps involved in malpractice litigation are as follows:

1. The basis for the claim is determined to be appropriate and timely; all elements of liability are present (duty, breach of duty, causation, and serious damages).
2. All parties named as defendants (nurses, health care providers, health care facility), as well as insurance companies and attorneys, work toward a fair settlement.
3. The case is presented to a malpractice arbitration panel. The panel's decision is either accepted or rejected, in which case a complaint is filed in trial court.
4. The defendants contest allegations (argue that there is no basis for alleging deviation from the appropriate standard of care or for proving causation and damages).
5. Pretrial discovery activities occur: review of medical records and depositions of plaintiff, defendants, and witnesses.
6. Trial takes place; both sides present their evidence and arguments.
7. Decision or verdict is reached by the judge or jury.
8. If the verdict is not accepted by both sides, it may be appealed to an appellate court.

The nurse may be involved in legal proceedings as a defendant, a fact witness, or an expert witness. For a tangible illustration of how the legal process operates, you and your class may want to implement the malpractice lawsuit simulation developed by Jenkins and Lemak (2009). See also Starr (2020), "You've been sued" and Brous articles on the elements of a nursing malpractice case (2019b, 2019c, 2020).

NURSE AS DEFENDANT

A nurse who is named a defendant should work closely with an attorney while preparing the defense. The attorney representing the nurse's interests is secured by either the nurse (if carrying personal liability insurance) or the employing facility. Recommendations for the nurse defendant include the following:

- Do not discuss the case with anyone at your facility (exception for the risk manager), with the plaintiff, with the plaintiff's lawyer, with anyone testifying for the plaintiff, or with reporters.
- Do not alter the patient's records. Tampering with a chart is the worst mistake you can make; you may well ruin your defense.
- Cooperate fully with your attorney. Do not hide any information from the attorney. Make sure you are fully prepared before you go on the witness stand.
- Be courteous on the witness stand. Do not volunteer any information.

NURSE AS FACT WITNESS

Either the defense or the prosecuting attorney may call a nurse who has knowledge of the actual incident prompting the legal case to testify as a **fact witness**. Fact witnesses, who are placed under oath, must base their testimony on only firsthand knowledge of the incident and not on assumptions. The nurse will be asked if the testimony is based on independent recollection of the incident or on documentation in the patient record. The nurse may testify, "I do not remember Ms. Jones, but I see from review of her record that I cared for her on the evenings of June 10, 13, 14, and 17." When in doubt about facts, the nurse should simply testify, "I do not remember that." New research into memory is showing that people often remember things differently from the way they were; this challenges the value of eyewitness memory. Thus, accurate documentation remains the nurse's best defense.

Table 7-3 Areas of Potential Liability for Nurses

AREAS OF POTENTIAL LIABILITY	EXAMPLES
Standard I: Assessment The registered nurse collects pertinent data and information relative to the health care consumer's health or the situation. • Incomplete database obtained (occurs frequently when patient is too ill at admission to respond to questions) • Significant omissions or errors in recorded database • Failure to note in the patient's care plan (and to execute) the need for more frequent nursing assessments • Failure to recognize and to report significant changes in the patient's condition	• Child too weak to be weighed on admission; chart contains no record of patient's weight; dosage of postoperative antibiotic therapy (which should be calculated on child's weight) too small to prevent infection; abscess develops • Nurse fails to detect and report observable signs that an older adult patient is at risk for abuse in her home from her granddaughter • Previously alert patient was exhibiting periods of confusion; found beating roommate with a hairbrush • Mother's labor is failing to progress, nurses unaware of signs of fetal distress; obstetrician not informed; irreversible cerebral damage to fetus • Healthy patient making slower than usual postanesthesia recovery; signs of developing cerebrovascular accident (slurred speech, difficulty moving extremities, falling to one side) present and unnoted
Standard II: Diagnosis The registered nurse analyzes the assessment data to determine actual or potential diagnoses, problems, and issues. • Failure to identify priority nursing diagnosis critical to the patient's care • Nursing diagnosis incorrectly developed and "labels" the patient negatively	• Nowhere in the resident's care plan it was noted that the patient had a history of choking on food ("impaired swallowing") and that close supervision was indicated during meals; patient aspirated Brussels sprout and died • Homosexual male patient without acquired immunodeficiency syndrome (AIDS) admitted for gallbladder surgery questions the few interactions he has with staff; nursing diagnosis on Cardex reads "High Risk for Violence: Directed at Others (AIDS), related to homosexuality"
Standards III and IV: Outcome Identification and Planning The registered nurse identifies expected outcomes for a plan individualized to the health care consumer or the situation and develops a plan that prescribes strategies to attain expected, measurable outcomes. • No indication in nursing care plan that nurses were aware of and sensitive to the patient's health care priorities	• Obese patient with a history of impaired circulation continually refuses to ambulate after major abdominal surgery; patient dies after a massive pulmonary embolism; care plan showed no concern or attempt to compensate for patient's lack of mobility; family states that no nurse consulted them to encourage mobility
Standard V: Implementation The registered nurse implements the identified plan. • Patient's record contains no documentation of attempts to teach appropriate self-care measures to patient and family • Nursing interventions deviate from usual standard of care (understaffing, indifference on part of nurse, inexperience of nurse, faulty or scarce equipment or resources)	• Male patient discharged from short-procedure unit on crutches; falls first day home, refracturing leg; alleges his not receiving instructions for crutch walking caused fall; patient record contains no documentation of patient education • Skin breakdown on frail, older, homebound patient worsens with eventual muscle deterioration; sepsis; nurses seem confused about treatment regimen for pressure injuries; treatment is inconsistent
Standard VI: Evaluation The registered nurse evaluates progress toward attainment of goals and outcomes. • No evidence in care plan and nursing notes that nurses evaluated whether the patient achieved target goals • Patient discharged before key goals are met and without follow-up instruction	• Male patient, newly started on insulin therapy, discharged after giving himself the insulin only once, and without understanding the relationship among food, exercise, and insulin. No referral made to visiting nurse; patient readmitted after 2 weeks with dangerously low blood sugar after overdose with insulin

Source: American Nurses Association (ANA). (2021). *Nursing Scope and Standards of Practice* (4th ed.). Author.

NURSE AS EXPERT WITNESS

A nurse may be called by either attorney to testify as an **expert witness** to explain to the judge and jury what happened based on the patient's record and to offer an opinion about whether the nursing care met acceptable standards. Nurse expert witnesses need a solid educational background and strong clinical experience comparable with those of the nurse defendant. The expert witness also needs an understanding of the legal aspects of nursing and malpractice liability as well as knowledge of the state nurse practice act and the standard of nursing care where the incident occurred.

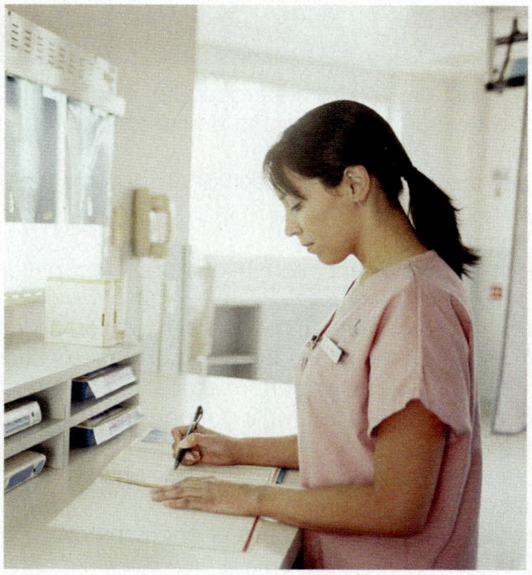

FIGURE 7-1. Competent practice is the nurse's most important legal safeguard. Careful documentation ensures a record of competent practice.

LEGAL SAFEGUARDS FOR THE NURSE

The U.S. health care system has a variety of safeguards to protect nurses from exposure to legal risks while performing the duties of their role and to ensure that the practice environment is geared toward enhancing patient and personal safety. As you read the following sections, consider the scenario featured in the Nursing Advocacy in Action display and the implications for nursing practice.

Competent Practice

Competent practice remains the nurse's most important and best legal safeguard (Fig. 7-1). Each nurse is responsible for making sure that their educational background and clinical experience are adequate to fulfill the nursing responsibilities delineated in the job description.

Legal safeguards include the following:

- Developing and maintaining interpersonal communication skills
- Respecting legal boundaries of practice
- Knowing and following institutional procedures and policies
- "Owning" personal strengths and weaknesses; seeking means of growth, education, and supervised experience to ensure continued competence for new and evolving responsibilities
- Evaluating proposed assignments; refusing to accept responsibilities for which you are unprepared
- Keeping current in nursing knowledge and skills
- Respecting patient rights and developing rapport with patients
- Working within the facility to develop and support management policies
- Keeping careful documentation

Remember that the medical record is the best, and sometimes the only, available evidence if you must defend your actions. Nurse attorney Edie Brous (2014, p. 60) recommends the following:

- Document all clinical observations and critical diagnostics.
- Document conversations with other providers regarding patient issues.
- Document which specific health care provider was notified of which specific concerns at what specific time.
- Document that the chain of command has been engaged when necessary.
- Make sure that the medical record reflects that you pursued your concerns to resolution.

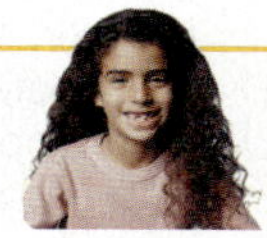

Think back to **Ella Rodriguez**, the girl with a fractured arm requiring the administration of sedation according to the facility's protocol. The nurse should incorporate knowledge of the legal safeguards for competent practice when preparing to administer the medication as well as knowledge of the unit's protocol. In addition, the nurse should identify personal limitations and confront the health care provider, stressing the need for his presence to ensure the patient's safety.

Nursing Advocacy in Action

Patient Scenario

Mr. Spahn is a 49-year-old attorney who suffered a cerebral bleed. After his brain surgery, his surgeon informed the family that Mr. Spahn has massive, irreversible neurologic damage. In short, barring an act of God or nature he will have no meaningful recovery. His wife is already suing the first hospital that treated her husband because they delayed performing the appropriate diagnostic tests. She and her daughter complain frequently about the nursing care Mr. Spahn is receiving now, and no one wants to take care of him because they are afraid of being named in a lawsuit. Mrs. Spahn keeps a notebook in which she writes down the name of every caregiver who helps her husband. She has placed numerous calls to complain to administration about everything from the cleanliness of the room to a torn sheet. You believe that he is receiving less than optimal care because everyone is afraid of his family bringing a lawsuit.

Implications for Nursing Advocacy

How will you act if you are Mr. Spahn's nurse? Talk with your classmates and experienced nurses about the questions that follow.

- If you elect to advocate for Mr. Spahn, what practical steps can you take to ensure better health outcomes?
- What is it reasonable to expect of a student nurse, a graduate nurse, and an experienced nurse in this situation?
- What advocacy skills are needed to effectively respond to this challenge?

Box 7-3 Nursing Malpractice Prevention

Most Frequent Allegations Against Nurses and Related Prevention Tips

1. **Failure to ensure patient safety**
   - Monitor patients in a timely manner consistent with facility policy and the changing needs of the patient. Assess and document potential for injury. Incorporate safety needs into the care plan.
   - Clearly define criteria for use of restrictive devices. Ensure that the use of restrictive devices is consistent with facility policy. Use the least restrictive devices that will be effective in preventing injury.
   - Update your knowledge involving patient safety and new interventions to prevent and reduce injury.
   - Evaluate whether patients at high risk for injury are routinely identified before injury results.
2. **Improper treatment or performance of treatment**
   - Question treatments that you believe are improper. Know your facility's policy for questioning a problematic order.
   - Use proper techniques when performing procedures, and follow facility procedures.
   - Seek assistance when unsure of a new procedure. Never perform an intervention until you know what you are doing, why you are doing it, and your ongoing assessment and teaching responsibilities.
   - Update your clinical skills through continuing education classes, conferences, and workshops.
3. **Failure to monitor and report**
   - Follow health care provider orders regarding monitoring of patients unless changes in the patient's condition necessitate a change in the frequency of monitoring; report the need for change to the health care provider.
   - Report any requested information or significant changes in a patient's condition. If unsure of the significance of an observed change, consult with an experienced colleague.
   - Perform appropriate and timely nursing assessments.
   - Ensure that the nurse–patient ratio is adequate.
4. **Medication errors and reactions**
   - Verify any questionable medical orders.
   - Verify patient's name and date of birth before administering medication and use appropriate facility-specific identifiers such as bar coding.
   - Listen to any patient questions or objections regarding a medication, and investigate the patient's concerns before administering the medication.
   - Refer to a drug reference for any questions about appropriate dosages, side effects, and reactions.
   - Know your facility's policies on verbal and written medication orders and on medication administration.
   - Update your knowledge of medications and new medication administration protocols.
5. **Failure to follow facility procedure**
   - Know your facility's procedures. Ensure that your orientation to new responsibilities familiarizes you with pertinent policies and procedures.
   - If you must deviate from a procedure, discuss the incident with your supervisor and decide on appropriate action.
   - Advise the appropriate person of procedures that need to be revised.
6. **Documentation**
   - Document significant information about your patients objectively and factually.
   - Know and follow the facility's documentation policies.
   - Document specific times that you performed actions, made observations, or performed patient assessments.
   - Document legibly when writing, spell correctly, and use only facility-approved abbreviations.
   - Be sensitive to privacy considerations when documenting on a computer.
   - Routinely evaluate the quality of documentation and update your knowledge of new documentation methodologies.
7. **Equipment use**
   - Learn how to operate equipment in a safe and appropriate manner. Never operate equipment with which you are unfamiliar.
   - Use predetermined procedures when teaching patients how to use equipment, and ensure that all nurses involved in patient education are teaching the same procedures.
   - Provide home care patients with the telephone number of a 24-hour backup hospital or home care service available in case of emergency.
   - Have patients demonstrate their competence with equipment before allowing them to use it.
   - Attend orientations and in-services on the use of new or modified equipment.
8. **Adverse incidents**
   - If an adverse incident occurs, complete the appropriate documentation and report the incident to the designated person following facility policy.
   - Do not assume, voice, or record any blame for the incident.
   - Know the institutional chain of command for reporting instances when patient care is at issue.
   - Support facility loss prevention programs that identify potential liabilities, guard against patient injuries, and maximize the defense of the facility and its employee nurses.
9. **Patients with human immunodeficiency virus (HIV)**
   - Be conscious of actions that could result in a lawsuit:
     - Discrimination in treatment
     - Nosocomial (in-hospital) transmission of virus
     - Breach of confidentiality
     - Participation in testing a patient for HIV without first obtaining informed consent
   - Know and follow facility policies and procedures for the care of patients with infectious diseases.
   - Update your knowledge of HIV infection; be familiar with national standards (such as those established by the Centers for Disease Control and Prevention) and pertinent state/province laws.

Competent practice includes developing sensitivity to common sources of patient injury, such as falls, restraints, and malfunctioning equipment, and then taking specific measures to prevent patient injury. Box 7-3 lists the most frequent allegations against nurses and related prevention tips.

Issues That Affect Competent Practice

Staying competent for our practice in today's rapidly changing health care world will always be a challenge. New technologies, medications, protocols, and policies will always challenge our ability to learn and adapt. What also challenges competence is nurse fatigue (no surprise) and the potential for developing substance use disorders. Sherman (2017) makes it a point to ask nurses in each of her presentations on building resilience to "stand up" if they practice particular resilience-building strategies. In each session, sleeping 7 hours was the *least* practiced resiliency strategy. "It is not uncommon for nurses not to take breaks, to eat on the run and to rarely use the restroom—almost a badge of honor in some settings. And now, our lack of self-care is starting to catch up with us as the work environment becomes more stressful."

Nurse Fatigue

We now know that fatigued and sleep-deprived nurses place their patients and themselves at serious risk for harm. The ANA issued a position statement addressing nurse fatigue in 2014. They urged registered nurses (RNs) and employers in all care settings to collaborate to reduce the risks of nurse fatigue and sleepiness associated with shift work and long work hours. Fatigued nurses are more likely to express concern that they made a wrong decision about a patient's care (Scott et al., 2014). During the COVID-19 pandemic the amazing salaries and benefits some employers were offering to attract nurses, especially those skilled in critical care, made it very tempting for nurses to assume more shifts than any nurse should reasonably carry. It is a good practice as students to make it a habit to be rested before appearing for clinical responsibilities and to continue this practice throughout your career.

The Impaired Nurse

About 1 in 10, or 10% to 15% of all nurses, may be impaired or in recovery from alcohol or drug use disorder. The stresses involved in nursing and health care, combined with the availability of controlled substances, make nurses prime candidates for alcohol and drug use disorders. Startlingly, more than half of all impaired nurses began using substances during their nursing education days.

In the past, nurses with substance use disorders usually were promptly punished by firing and license suspension. Today, substance use is recognized as a treatable disorder; the objective is to detect problems early and get nurses into treatment. The ANA strongly supports "alternative to discipline" or "peer assistance" programs.

Students should recognize their level of risk and know to seek help promptly if they suspect a personal problem or a problem on the part of a classmate or colleague. Students can talk with a trusted faculty member. Practicing nurses should consult management. O'Neill (2015, p. 9) suggests that nurses who suspect that a colleague may have a substance use disorder ask themselves the following questions:

- What do I observe?
- How does this affect patient care or teamwork?
- What should I do when I have a concern?
- Would my colleague benefit from assistance?

Box 7-4 Indications That a Nurse May Have a Substance Use Disorder (SUD)

As nurses, we care for our patients, but we don't always care for our coworkers or ourselves. As you read the list below, you may discover that you are working with or have worked with a nurse who displays signs, symptoms, and behavioral changes that may indicate substance use.

Behavioral Changes

- Changes or shifts in job performance
- Absences from the unit for extended periods
- Frequent trips to the bathroom
- Arriving late or leaving early
- Making an excessive number of mistakes, including medication errors

Behavioral changes may have physical manifestations:

- Subtle changes in appearance that may escalate over time
- Increasing isolation from colleagues
- Inappropriate verbal or emotional responses
- Diminished alertness, confusion, or memory lapses

Narcotics Discrepancies

- Incorrect narcotic counts
- Large amounts of narcotic wastage
- Numerous corrections of medication records
- Frequent reports of ineffective pain relief from patients
- Offers to medicate coworkers' patients for pain
- Altered verbal or phone medication orders
- Variations in controlled substance discrepancies among shifts or days of the week

Source: Adapted from National Council of State Boards of Nursing (NCSBN). (2018). *A nurse manager's guide to substance use disorder in nursing.* Author. https://www.ncsbn.org/Mgr_SUDiN_Brochure_2014.pdf

Box 7-4 describes signs and symptoms to watch for. The public's trust and well-being and the well-being of the nurse are both at stake. See the NCSBN video on substance use disorder in nursing: https://www.ncsbn.org/333.htm.

Informed Consent or Refusal

Every person is granted freedom from bodily contact by another person unless consent is granted. In most states, you must be 18 to legally provide medical consent. States vary in the types of medical treatment they allow minors to authorize without their parents' consent; be sure to check your state law.

In all health care facilities, informed and voluntary consent is needed for admission, for each specialized diagnostic or treatment procedure, and for any experimental treatments or procedures. The consent must be written, designated for the procedure to be performed, and signed by the patient or person legally responsible for the patient. A signed consent is not needed in an emergency if there is an immediate threat to life or health, if experts would agree that it is an emergency, and if the patient is unable to consent and a legally authorized person cannot be reached.

Box 7-5 Checklist to Ensure Informed Consent

Disclosure

Patient/surrogate has been informed of the (1) nature of the procedure, (2) risks (nature of the risk, magnitude, probability that the risk will materialize) and benefits, (3) alternatives (including the option of nontreatment), and (4) fact that no outcomes can be guaranteed.

Comprehension

Patient/surrogate can correctly repeat in their own words that for which the patient/surrogate is giving consent.

Competence

The patient understands the information needed to make *this* decision, is able to reason in accord with a relatively consistent set of values and can communicate a preference.

The surrogate (if needed) meets the above criteria, knows the patient's wishes to the extent that this is possible, and is free from undue emotional stress and conflict of interests.

Voluntariness

The patient is voluntarily consenting or refusing. Care has been taken to avoid manipulative and coercive influences.

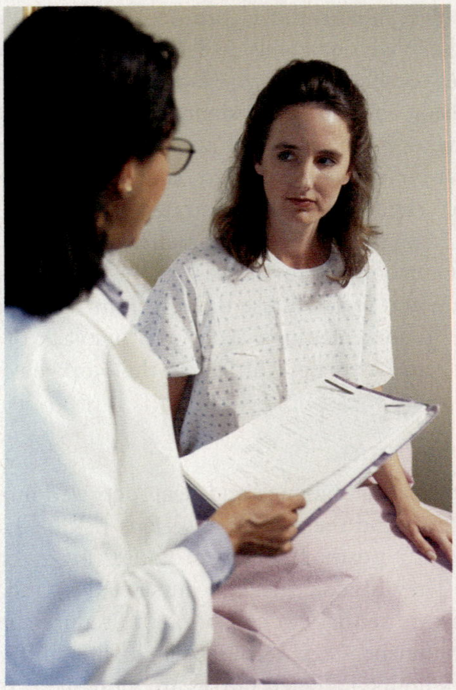

FIGURE 7-2. Informed consent is a process. A mere signature does not guarantee each of the elements of consent: disclosure, comprehension, competence, and voluntariness.

While informed consent is a protection against lawsuits, the central values underlying informed consent include promoting the patient's well-being and respecting the patient's self-determination (President's Commission for the Study of Ethical Problems in Medicine and Biomedical and Behavioral Research, 1982). For this reason, you should make sure that patients have all the information they need, and that they understand the information, to validly consent to or refuse what is being proposed. Patients who do not speak English require the services of a translator; be sure to check your facility's policies about translation and be familiar with resources. Using a family member to translate is rarely acceptable. Similarly, patients with low literacy may be unable to read what they are signing and require extra help. Elements of informed consent include *disclosure*, *comprehension*, *competence*, and *voluntariness* (Box 7-5). Feeg et al. (2021) describe the distress students experienced when they observed failures to respect the rights of patients in their clinical practice sites.

Obtaining informed consent is the responsibility of the person who will perform the diagnostic or treatment procedure or the research study. Your role as a nurse is to confirm that a signed consent form is present in the patient's chart and to answer any patient questions about the consent. Unless you are obtaining consent for a nurse-prescribed and nurse-initiated intervention, as a nurse you sign the consent form as a witness to the patient signing the form, not as having obtained the consent yourself (Fig. 7-2). In some instances, you may be responsible for having a patient sign the consent form after a clinician has explained the procedure, its risks and benefits, and alternative treatments to the patient. Increasingly, nurses are performing procedures requiring consent, or are part of interdisciplinary teams that meet with the patient to obtain consent for complex interventions (e.g., bone marrow transplantation).

Documenting the consent process with a printed consent form should not be confused with the actual explanation given to the patient and the informed consent itself. When documenting consent, assess whether patients understand what they are signing and are acting voluntarily, and report any problems to the clinician doing the procedure. Having patients describe in their own words what they understand they are consenting to is the best way to make sure that they understand. Nurses often question the patient's understanding of the proposed procedure and its risks or the patient's ability to consent voluntarily to the procedure. Impediments include the effects of anxiety, pain, medication, depression, language barriers, and temporary or permanent states of disorientation and confusion.

Consequences of not obtaining a valid consent include the possibility of charges of battery against the nurse, the doctor, and the health care facility, which has a duty to protect patients and is responsible for its employees' actions.

Concept Mastery Alert

Although, at times, a nurse may be responsible for having a patient sign the consent form, in **all** instances, the nurse is responsible for answering any questions the patient may have and for making sure that the signed consent form is on the patient's chart. If the nurse determines that the patient is unsure or has questionable understanding, the nurse is responsible for notifying the person who had obtained the consent about the situation so that person can clarify or reexplain the information.

A patient's refusal to sign a consent form should be documented, and the patient should be informed of the possible consequences of the refusal. The patient should sign a release form indicating their refusal to consent and releasing the nurse, health care provider, and facility from responsibility for outcomes of this act. This statement should be witnessed.

Unfolding Patient Stories: Jared Griffin • Part 1

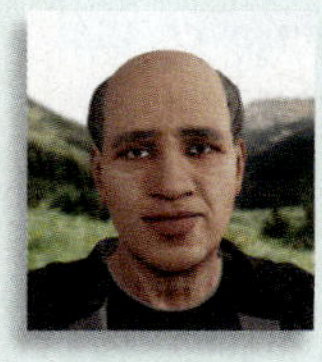

Jared Griffin, a 63-year-old male, is being admitted to the hospital for knee surgery. What is the purpose of informed consent, what circumstances require it, and who is responsible for obtaining informed consent? What is the nurse's role with informed consent for Jared's surgery? (Jared Griffin's story continues in Chapter 46.)

Care for Jared and other patients in a realistic virtual environment: ***vSim** for Nursing* (thepoint.lww.com/vSimFunds). Practice documenting these patients' care in DocuCare (thepoint.lww.com/DocuCareEHR).

Contracts

A contract is an exchange of promises between two parties. The agreement may be in writing or oral, although oral contracts may be more difficult to prove. The law of contracts provides a remedy for a breach of contract so that the person who suffers from a broken contract may be compensated for any resulting loss. For a contract to be legally enforceable, it must involve real consent of the parties, a valid consideration, a lawful purpose, competent parties, and the format required by law.

Practicing nurses enter into legally valid and binding contracts with both their employers and their patients. Thus, it is important to understand and be able to fulfill the terms of a nursing agreement before agreeing to a contract. Your employment contract should specify what it is reasonable for you to expect of your employer and what the employer can expect of you. An employer that repeatedly expects you to assume supervisory responsibilities without benefit or who fires you without just cause is likely to be guilty of contract violations. Similarly, you may be guilty of contract violations if you refuse to accept reasonable assignments, repeatedly fail to arrive on time for work, or are habitually unable to complete reasonable work assignments. Any action by your employer that violates a federal or state law is the basis of a grievance, even if the employment contract permits the action. Examples include a female nurse receiving less pay for performing the same work as a male nurse, or a supervisor's failure to promote an employee based on race. When discrimination is suspected, complaints should be filed with the Equal Employment Opportunity Commission (EEOC).

Contracts with patients are often implied. There may not be a written contract specifying what is reasonable for patients to expect of nurses, but courts will uphold an implied contract obligating the nurse to be competent and to provide responsible care.

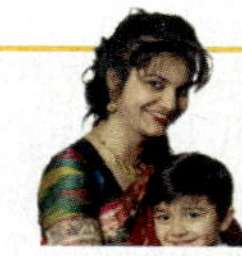

Remember **Meredith Bedford**, the mother of the terminally ill child, who is threatening to sue the hospice. The nurse needs to understand the implied contract between the patient (and his family) and the health care team.

Collective Bargaining

The 2015 ANA Code of Ethics for Nurses states that the nurse, "through individual and collective effort, establishes, maintains and improves the ethical environment of the work setting and conditions of employment that are conducive to safe, quality health care."

Although individual contracts serve many nurses adequately, many nurses have joined other groups of workers whose interests are better protected when contracts are negotiated for them as a group. Collective bargaining is a legal process in which representatives of organized employees negotiate with employers about such matters as wages, hours, and conditions. Arbitration, strikes, and threats of strikes may be used to enhance the terms of employment and to enforce contracts.

Many nurses choose their state nurses' association, rather than a trade organization, as their collective bargaining representative. Other nurses question whether collective bargaining is an appropriate role for a professional organization. When deciding whether to participate in collective bargaining, ask yourself the following questions:

- Will collective bargaining help my professional and economic status?
- Can I address my professional concerns through collective bargaining?
- Can I devote the time and effort that such organized activity demands?
- Can I change my working conditions as a person, or do I need to organize with other nurses to bring about the desired change?

Patient Education

U.S. courts affirm the patient's right to know what is necessary to manage their health, and view patient education as a legal duty of the nurse. Standards for patient education are derived from national professional standards and from state nurse practice acts as well as the local standards described in facility policies, procedure manuals, and job descriptions. Special forms for documenting the nurse's assessment of the patient's learning needs and for subsequent teaching are available in some facilities. Failure to conduct or document an assessment of a patient's learning needs and teaching may later be construed as negligence.

Determine in your practice setting what specific aspects of patient education are the responsibility of nursing. Consult your job description, and be familiar with facility policies regarding patient education and its documentation. Remember that an important aim of nursing is to assist patients in managing their own care. Discuss the nursing care plan with patients and family members, and identify their learning needs and learning readiness. Document the teaching plan as part of the nursing care plan. Document all nursing efforts to educate the patient and family about health care management, and also document the patient's response. If a patient refuses health education or refers you to a family member (e.g., "Talk to my wife about my pills; she'll be giving them to me at home"), document this in the patient's record. If patient education greatly increases the patient's anxiety and the patient requests not to be given any more information, document the patient's initial response to teaching, the patient's request that it be stopped, and, if you complied, your reason for doing so.

Because a lack of time is frequently offered as the reason for failing to document patient education, assess what type of patient documentation is performed routinely in your setting. If possible, develop forms or checklists that will facilitate rapid documentation. For example, preoperative checklists make it easy to record preoperative teaching and are often introduced as evidence in court that preoperative teaching was done. Similarly, other forms have been developed for documenting teaching for patients who have diabetes, teaching after a myocardial infarction, and teaching postpartum and baby care to parents. The teaching role of the nurse is discussed in Chapter 9.

Executing Provider Orders

Nurses are legally responsible for carrying out the orders of a legitimate provider in charge of a patient unless a reasonable person would anticipate the order would lead to injury. Follow these guidelines:

1. Be familiar with the parties designated in your state's nurse practice act who can legally write orders for the nurse to execute (e.g., in many states, a physician assistant cannot legally write orders for the nurse).
2. Be familiar with your institution's or facility's policy regarding provider orders.
3. Attempt to get all provider orders in writing. Verbal orders (VOs) and telephone orders (TOs) should be countersigned within 24 hours. Take the following steps to prevent errors caused by TOs:
   a. Limit TOs to true emergency situations when there is no alternative.
   b. Designate which nurses may take TOs (e.g., those who have more education and experience).
   c. Repeat the TO back to the provider for confirmation.
   d. Document the order, its time and date, the situation necessitating the order, the provider prescribing and reconfirming the order as it is read back, and your name. Indicate if the order is a VO or TO.
   e. When possible, have two nurses listen to a questionable TO, with both nurses countersigning the order. See Chapter 19 for additional guidelines on executing verbal, telephone, and fax orders.
4. The Joint Commission (2016b) now permits licensed independent health care providers to send orders via text messaging "as long as a secure text messaging platform is used, and the required components of an order are included." To read more about The Joint Commission's position on sending orders by text message, visit www.jointcommission.org/assets/1/6/Update_Texting_Orders.pdf.
5. Question any health care provider order that is:
   a. Ambiguous
   b. Contraindicated by normal practice (e.g., an abnormally high dose of medication)
   c. Contraindicated by the patient's present condition (e.g., as a patient's present condition improves, the patient may no longer need aggressive forms of treatment)

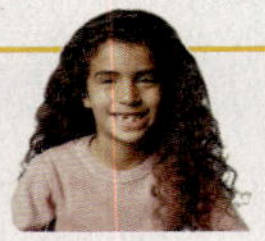

Remember **Ella Rodriguez**, the young girl requiring a sedation protocol for closed reduction of her fracture. The nurse should understand that the child is at risk for complications if the health care provider is not present during the drug administration. Therefore, the nurse should question the health care provider's order to "start without him" to ensure the patient's safety.

It is a good practice to double-check any order that a patient questions. See Chapter 20 for another discussion of orders.

Delegating Nursing Care

Professional nurses are responsible for delegating nursing activities, but, although RNs may delegate elements of care, they do not delegate the nursing process itself. As a nurse, you remain accountable for any actions you delegate. The ANA/NCSBN joint statement on national guidelines for nursing delegation can be found at https://www.nursingworld.org/_4962ca/globalassets/practiceandpolicy/nursing-excellence/ana-position-statements/nursing-practice/ana-ncsbn-joint-statement-on-delegation.pdf. Chapter 10 addresses nursing's delegation responsibilities.

Documentation

Documentation is discussed in detail in Chapter 20. Although most nurses prefer to spend their time interacting with patients rather than documenting in a patient's record, careful documentation is a crucial legal safeguard for the nurse. Documentation must be factual, accurate, complete, and entered in a timely fashion. The law presumes that if something was not documented, it was not done. This includes even routine acts, such as taking vital signs, repositioning patients, and ensuring the patient's safety. In 2004, The Joint Commission created a list of "Do Not Use" abbreviations that should not be included in documentation. Be sure to check your facility's policies on what and how to document. This is now updated (2019).

Be sure that the nursing care plan is part of the patient's permanent record. Facilities should have flow sheets or a documentation form that enables you to check off routine aspects of care rapidly and completely. You should also write a comprehensive nursing note for each patient problem you address. This note should include the current nature of the problem, how you intervened, the patient's response, and, when appropriate, future priorities for care. After a problem is noted, nursing documentation should demonstrate continuity of care until the problem is resolved.

A common problem reported by nurses is not knowing how to document a situation in which the nurse believes a patient needs medical attention, but the responsible health care providers are not responding to calls for assistance. In this case, the best legal safeguard is to document the facts of the incident, being careful not to make incriminatory statements, such as "Anyone could see we were losing this patient rapidly" or "Once again, Dr. Jones was unavailable when her patient needed her." The note should document the time the health care provider was called, the time of response or lack of response, and the subsequent nursing response (e.g., nursing supervisor notified). Such a note documents that you are carefully assessing the patient, recognizing significant cues, and reporting them appropriately. The nursing supervisor should write the next note after reviewing the case and choosing a course of action. A patient's nonadherence to a treatment also should be documented, along with your attempts to increase adherence.

Appropriate Use of Social Media

Social media platforms have created new opportunities for defamation and violation of a patient's privacy and confidentiality rights. Fortier (2019) offers eight rules of social media etiquette:

- Be aware of your facility's social media policy, review your state nurse practice act, and read "A Nurse's Guide to the Use of Social Media" for tips on best practices.
- Follow organizational policies about checking e-mail and social media profiles while at work. Don't conduct personal business or expect privacy on work computers.
- Don't take photos or videos of patients at work, even if there are not identifiers.
- Never share patient information in a public forum, including social media.
- Avoid disparaging posts. If you speak badly about patients, families, colleagues, or employers online, it could constitute cyberbullying or professional misconduct.
- Don't post if you're angry or need to vent.
- Anything you post remains accessible even if you delete it later. The time, place, and content of a social media post can be tracked and retrieved.
- Serve as a positive representative of the profession online.

Be familiar with guidelines for use of social media issued by the National Student Nurses' Association, ANA, and the National Council State Boards of Nursing (2018). Inappropriate use of social and electronic media may be reported to a State Board of Nursing. If the board finds the allegations to be true, the nurse may face disciplinary action by the board, including a reprimand or sanction, assessment of a monetary fine, or temporary or permanent loss of licensure. If a nurse's improper use of social media violates state and federal laws established to protect patient privacy, the violations may result in both civil and criminal penalties, including fines and possible jail time. Nurses may also face employment consequences, including termination (https://www.ncsbn.org/Social_Media.pdf).

Adequate Staffing

Understaffing, sometimes called short staffing, is a problem that results in reduced quality of nursing care and may jeopardize patient safety. Temporary management solutions to understaffing, such as floating nurses from one unit to another, or asking (or mandating) nurses to work overtime or double (back-to-back) shifts, are ineffective because they can further jeopardize patient safety. A nurse in an understaffed facility will be held to a professional standard of judgment for accepting responsibility for work and for delegating nursing responsibilities to others. Thus, if a patient claims negligent care, a nurse claiming to have been overworked that evening because of an unrealistic assignment does not have adequate grounds for a legal defense. If patient injury results, the facility and nurse employee will most likely be named as codefendants. Some state nursing associations are using "protest of assignment forms" to track employer practices of routine understaffing.

Whistle-Blowing

Many nurses who are frustrated with unsafe practice environments are speaking up. **Whistle-blowing** is a warning from a present or past member of an organization to the public concerning a serious wrongdoing or danger created or masked by the organization. The decision to whistle-blow can be difficult since some nurses have been threatened with the loss of their jobs and licenses. Whistle-blower laws are intended to prevent employers from taking retaliatory action against nurses, such as suspension, demotion, harassment, or discharge, for reporting improper patient care or business practices. As part of the ANA Nationwide State Legislative Agenda, the ANA and State Nurses Associations are promoting strong whistle-blower laws on the state level that provide legal protections for nurses advocating for patients without fear of reprisal. Many states now have protections in other legislation such as safe staffing and mandatory overtime prohibition. See information about whistle-blower protection at http://www.nursingworld.org to learn more, and see the whistle-blowing section in Chapter 6 on page 138.

Professional Liability Insurance

Although a nurse's best legal safeguard is always competent practice, the increasing number of malpractice claims naming nurses as defendants makes it wise for nurses to carry their own liability insurance. Liability insurance will also support nurses facing licensure disciplinary actions. Nurses may obtain this insurance through the ANA and other nursing associations, as well as from other sources.

Reasons for purchasing a personal professional liability insurance policy include:

- *Protection of the nurse's best interests.* If the nurse is named as a defendant in a malpractice action along with the facility, a conflict of interest could arise between the nurse and the facility. Nurses have no assurance that their best interest will be represented unless they have their own coverage, which provides their own attorney.
- *Limitations of employer's coverage.* Most health care facilities carry "claims-made" insurance, which means that if the nurse is no longer working there or the facility closes, the nurse is not covered when a claim is filed.
- *Care or advice given outside of work.* An employer's policy covers the nurse only within the confines of the work setting.

Nurse attorney White (2011) explores the personal, professional, and historical influences on why nurses should or should not have their own malpractice insurance. As well, White urges nurses to regularly evaluate their circumstances and decide not only whether to carry their own malpractice insurance but what kind and how much. Pohlman (2015) notes that an individual policy provides benefits not usually covered in employer policies, such as coverage for assault, first aid expenses, violations of the HIPAA, libel or slander, depositions, property damage, and license protection benefits. Nurse attorney Brous (2012c, 2016a) is adamant that every nurse should carry liability insurance to defend themselves from licensure disciplining.

Risk-Management Programs

Hoping to reduce malpractice claims, many health care facilities have initiated risk-management programs designed to identify, analyze, and treat risks. Elements of a comprehensive risk management program include the following:

- *Safety program.* The aim is to provide a safe environment in which the basic safety needs of patients, employees, and visitors are met.
- *Product safety program.* The aim is to ensure safe and adequate equipment; this involves ongoing equipment evaluation and maintenance.
- *Quality assurance program.* The aim is to provide quality health care to patients; this involves ongoing evaluation of all systems used in the care of patients.

Nurses with legal questions often find risk managers a helpful resource. Many risk managers encourage nurses and other clinicians to report "near misses" to better identify factors contributing to errors. A "near miss" is an error that would have happened except for someone's alertness and ability to identify and prevent the error.

Just Culture

A "just culture" encourages open reporting of errors, recognizes that errors may be systemic rather than personal failures, and focuses on determining the root of the problem when events such as errors and near misses occur. According to the theory of just culture, three types of behaviors contribute to errors:

- *Human error,* which occurs unintentionally and without malicious intent
- *At-risk behavior,* which encompasses acts designed to cut corners and save time despite the known but seemingly justified behavior
- *Reckless behavior,* which consists of acts that disregard all safety measures

Tocco and Blum (2013, p. 17) describe actions every nurse can take to promote a just culture:

- Report errors, near misses, and other events to your manager and colleagues.
- Encourage colleagues to report their own events.
- Discuss with colleagues what can be done to prevent future events.
- Partner with your manager in communicating your unit's experiences to the nursing practice council or quality council. This promotes learning from these events, which translates to safer care.
- Help colleagues "connect the dots" by linking changes in practice to learning from events.

The NCSBN of Nursing developed a Taxonomy of Error, Root Cause Analysis and Practice-responsibility (TERCAP) tool to track elements of nursing practice breakdown (https://www.ncsbn.org/websites.htm). The most recent TERCAP analysis of 4,000 cases of practice breakdown (2011–2016) revealed:

• Lack of professional responsibility	73% (2,903)
• Lack of clinical reasoning	49% (1,964)
• Lack of intervention	47% (1,867)
• Documentation error	42% (1,662)
• Misinterpretation	37% (1,490)
• Medication error	33% (1,299)
• Lack of attentiveness	25% (1,048)
• Lack of prevention	27% (1,082)

NCSBN has a national web-based network for anonymous reporting of student errors and near misses: Safe Students Reports (SSRs). Nothing like this exists in any other health profession, nor outside the United States. This network allows programs to analyze data related to student errors and near misses and to compare themselves to other programs. See the other web-based resources at NCSBN.

Incident, Variance, or Occurrence Reports

An **incident report**, also called a variance or occurrence report, is used by health care facilities to document the occurrence of anything out of the ordinary that results in, or has the potential to result in, harm to a patient, employee, or visitor (Fig. 7-3). These reports are used for quality improvement and should not be used for disciplinary action against staff members. They are a means of identifying risks. More harm than good results from ignoring mistakes. Incident reports improve the management and treatment of patients by identifying high-risk patterns and initiating in-service

Medication Occurrence Information Report/PI **ADDRESSOGRAPH**
Send completed form to Risk Management
This document is part of a quality improvement process
CONFIDENTIAL: Do Not PHOTOCOPY
Do Not File in Patient Record
All Sections Must Be Completed

Patient age:______

Definition of occurrence: *Any preventable event that may cause or lead to inappropriate medication use or patient harm while the medication is in the control of the health care professional, patient, or consumer. Such events may be related to professional practice, health care products, procedures, and systems, including prescribing, order communication, product labeling, packaging, and nomenclature; compounding; dispensing; distribution; administration; education; monitoring; and use.*

Section A: Report filed by (please print): ____________ Title: ____________ Date/Time: ____________
Location of event
Floor/Unit: ________ Date of event: ________ Time of event (24 hour): ________ ☐ Inpatient ☐ Outpatient

Error discovered: ☐ Within same shift ☐ Within 24 hours ☐ Greater than 24 hours

Staff involved in initial error: ☐ Staff RN ☐ Facility RN ☐ Pharmacist ☐ NP ☐ House staff ☐ Attending MD Name: ________
Other staff also involved (i.e., perpetuated the error): ☐ Staff RN ☐ Facility RN ☐ Pharmacist ☐ Health care provider

Staff that discovered error: ☐ Staff RN ☐ Facility RN ☐ Pharmacist ☐ Health care provider

Health care provider notified? ☐ No ☐ Yes Date: ____________ Time: ____________ Attending: ____________

Section B: Medication type: ☐ IV ☐ Non-IV
Medication(s) involved: A. ____________ B. ____________
Incident documented in medical record? ☐ Yes ☐ No
Patient/family aware of incident? ☐ Yes ☐ No
(If yes, please comment below)

TYPE OF ERROR *(See reverse for definitions)*	**BREAKDOWN POINT** *(Where in process did the initial error occur?)*	**BREAKDOWN POINT** *(Where in process did the initial error occur?)* *(continued from the previous column)*
☐ Prescribing ☐ Omission—Total # ______ Schedule: ______ ☐ Monitoring error ☐ Wrong patient ☐ Wrong time ☐ Wrong route ☐ Wrong dose/quantity/extra dose • dose ordered ______ • dose given ______ ☐ Medication D/C'd, given • extra doses: ______ ☐ Wrong drug • med ordered ______ • med given ______ ☐ Medication not ordered • med given ______ • dose ______ ☐ Wrong drug preparation ☐ Wrong rate of administration ☐ Given to patient with known allergy ☐ Investigational protocol not followed ☐ Other ______	☐ Prescribing *circle:* • illegible handwriting • wrong chart/order sheet • incorrect order • incomplete order • other, please describe below ☐ Order processing *circle:* • carbon not pulled/pulled late • order not transcribed • transcribed incorrectly • other, please describe below ☐ Dispensing *circle:* • incorrectly entered into computer by pharmacist/not entered at all • wrong strength sent • wrong med sent • label incorrect/unclear • delay in delivery of medication • other, please describe below *(continued next column)*	☐ Administration *circle:* • med given, but not charted • med charted, but not given • held med given • incorrect medication taken from floor stock/Pyxis and given • incorrect dose/rate calculation • pump error –tubing clamped –incorrect rate setting –pump malfunction –pump turned off ☐ Other, please describe below **ERROR SEVERITY/OUTCOME** ☐ **Category A:** Circumstances or events that have the capacity to cause error ☐ **Category B:** Error occurred; medication not given ☐ **Category C:** Medication given but did not cause patient harm ☐ **Category D:** Resulted in the need for increased patient monitoring but no harm ☐ **Category E:** Resulted in the need for treatment or intervention and caused temporary patient harm ☐ **Category F:** Resulted in initial or prolonged hospitalization and caused temporary patient harm ☐ **Category G:** Resulted in permanent patient harm ☐ **Category H:** Resulted in a near-death event (e.g., anaphylaxis, cardiac arrest) ☐ **Category I:** Resulted in patient death

COMMENTS/DESCRIBE EVENT (include any intervention/treatment given and outcome):
____
____
____

Section C: ANALYSIS/RECOMMENDATIONS/ACTION PLAN *(Manager to complete):*
Possible causes: ☐ abbreviation ☐ calculation error ☐ communication confusing/intimidating/lacking ☐ computer order entry ☐ decimal point/leading zero missing/trailing zero ☐ equipment design ☐ facsimile order ☐ handwriting illegible ☐ inexperienced staff ☐ staffing level ☐ labeling (GUMC) confusing/incomplete/inaccurate ☐ labeling (manufacturer) confusing/incomplete/inaccurate ☐ similar name ☐ patient identification ☐ shift change ☐ floating staff ☐ poor lighting ☐ performance deficit ☐ preparation error ☐ procedure/protocol not followed ☐ reference manual confusing/inaccurate/unclear/outdated ☐ verbal order confusing/incomplete/misunderstood ☐ written order confusing/incomplete/misunderstood ☐ other ______
____
____

Signature of Manager: ____________ Date: ____________

FIGURE 7-3. Sample medication occurrence information report.

programs to prevent future problems. These forms also make all the facts about an incident available to the facility in case of litigation. Increasingly, facilities use paperless computer-based reporting systems that are secure, timely, efficient, and effective. These may also offer online help and formal education and serve as a valuable tool for data analysis.

The nurse responsible for a potential or actual harmful incident or who witnesses an injury is the one who completes the incident form. This form should contain the complete name of the person or people involved and the names of all witnesses; a complete factual account of the incident; the date, time, and place of the incident; pertinent characteristics of the person or people involved (e.g., alert, ambulatory, asleep) and of any equipment or resources being used; and any other variables believed to be important to the incident.

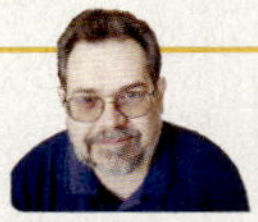

Think back to **Ramone Scott**, the patient who received the wrong medication. The nurse should document the incident, including the actions taken upon finding the error such as immediately stopping the medication, assessing the patient, and notifying the health care provider. In addition, the nurse should document continued follow-up assessments and interventions taken to ensure the patient's safety.

A health care provider completes one section of the incident form with documentation of the medical examination of the patient, employee, or visitor with an actual or potential injury.

In some states, incident reports may be used in court as evidence. When documenting a patient incident, be sure to include a complete account of what happened in the patient's record as well as in the incident report. *Documentation in the patient record, however, should not include the fact that an incident report was filed.*

Sentinel Events

The Joint Commission's Sentinel Event Policy defines a **sentinel event** as an unexpected occurrence involving death or serious physical or psychological injury, or the risk thereof. Serious injury specifically includes loss of limb or function. The phrase "or the risk thereof" includes any process variation for which a recurrence would carry a significant chance of a serious adverse outcome. Such events are called "sentinel" because they signal the need for immediate investigation and response. Some examples of sentinel events are wrong-side surgery, suicide, and operative and postoperative complications.

QSEN SAFETY

Safety is one of the core Quality and Safety Nursing Competencies. Every nurse is expected to be alert to anything in a clinical culture that can compromise patient safety and well-being. Be sure to speak up if you see something and be willing to participate in an analysis of the causes contributing to a sentinel event.

Accredited organizations are expected to identify and respond appropriately to all sentinel events occurring in the organization or associated with services that the organization provides or provides for. Appropriate response includes a thorough and credible root cause analysis, implementation of improvements to reduce risk, and monitoring of the effectiveness of those improvements. **Root cause analysis** involves digging progressively deeper into the event, repeatedly asking why the event occurred, and exploring the circumstances that led to it to determine where improvements can be made. Nurses play a critical role in responding to sentinel events.

Never Events

In 2011, the National Quality Forum released a newly revised list of 29 events that they termed "serious reportable events": extremely rare medical errors that should never happen to a patient. Often termed "never events," these include errors such as surgery performed on the wrong body part or on the wrong patient, leaving a foreign object inside a patient after surgery, or discharging an infant to the wrong person. By reporting and following suggested guidelines when a never event occurs, the likelihood of such an error happening again is greatly decreased.

There is growing consensus that hospitals should not be reimbursed for the treatment of the consequences of never events. The Leapfrog Group, a voluntary program aimed at recognizing and rewarding big leaps in health care safety, quality, and customer value, gives public recognition to hospitals if they agree to the following when a never event occurs within their facility:

- Apologize to the patient and family
- Waive all costs related to the event and follow-up care
- Report the event to an external facility
- Conduct a root cause analysis of how and why the event occurred

See The Leapfrog Group website, https://ratings.leapfroggroup.org/measure/hospital/responding-never-events.

Patients' Rights

The American Hospital Association developed "A Patient's Bill of Rights" in 1972 (revised in 1992 and 2003). Renamed "The Patient Care Partnership" (Box 7-6), it addresses the expectations, rights, and responsibilities of the patient while receiving care in the hospital, and ranges from "high-quality hospital care" to "helping prepare you and your family for when you leave the hospital." With care moving increasingly from the hospital to the community, legally prudent nurses must be familiar with how different institutions and professional groups define patient rights and responsibilities.

Other bills of rights include the Pregnant Patient's Bill of Rights, the Indian Patient's Bill of Rights, a Nursing Home Bill of Rights, and the Veterans Administration Code of Patient Concern. Each emphasizes a specific aspect of patient rights within a particular health facility and implies a code of ethics that the nurse observes professionally.

Box 7-6 The Patient Care Partnership: Understanding Expectations, Rights, and Responsibilities

When you need hospital care, your doctor and the nurses and other professionals at our hospital are committed to working with you and your family to meet your health care needs. Our dedicated doctors and staff serve the community in all its ethnic, religious, and economic diversity. Our goal is for you and your family to have the same care and attention we would want for our families and ourselves.

The sections below explain some of the basics about how you can expect to be treated during your hospital stay. They also cover what we will need from you to care for you better. If you have questions at any time, please ask them. Unasked or unanswered questions can add to the stress of being in the hospital. Your comfort and confidence in your care are very important to us.

What to Expect During Your Hospital Stay

- **High-quality hospital care.** Our first priority is to provide you the care you need, when you need it, with skill, compassion, and respect. Tell your caregivers if you have concerns about your care or if you have pain. You have the right to know the identity of doctors, nurses, and others involved in your care, as well as when they are students, residents, or other trainees.
- **A clean and safe environment.** Our hospital works hard to keep you safe. We use special policies and procedures to avoid mistakes in your care and keep you free from abuse or neglect. If anything unexpected and significant happens during your hospital stay, you will be told what happened and any resulting changes in your care will be discussed with you.
- **Involvement in your care.** You and your doctor often make decisions about your care before you go to the hospital. Other times, especially in emergencies, those decisions are made during your hospital stay. When they take place, making decisions should include:
  - *Discussing your medical condition and information about medically appropriate treatment choices.* To make informed decisions with your doctor, you need to understand several things:
    - The benefits and risks of each treatment
    - Whether it is experimental or part of a research study
    - What you can reasonably expect from your treatment and any long-term effects it might have on your quality of life
    - What you and your family will need to do after you leave the hospital
    - The financial consequences of using uncovered services or out-of-network providers

  Please tell your caregivers if you need more information about treatment choices.
  - *Discussing your treatment plan.* When you enter the hospital, you sign a general consent to treatment. In some cases, such as surgery or experimental treatment, you may be asked to confirm in writing that you understand what is planned and agree to it. This process protects your right to consent to or refuse a treatment. Your doctor will explain the medical consequences of refusing recommended treatment. It also protects your right to decide if you want to participate in a research study.
  - *Getting information from you.* Your caregivers need complete and correct information about your health and coverage so that they can make good decisions about your care. That includes:
    - Past illnesses, surgeries, or hospital stays
    - Past allergic reactions
    - Any medicines or diet supplements (such as vitamins and herbs) that you are taking
    - Any network or admission requirements under your health plan
  - *Understanding your health care goals and values.* You may have health care goals and values or spiritual beliefs that are important to your well-being. They will be taken into account as much as possible throughout your hospital stay. Make sure your doctor, your family, and your care team know your wishes.
  - *Understanding who should make decisions when you cannot.* If you have signed a health care power of attorney stating who should speak for you if you become unable to make health care decisions for yourself, or a "living will" or "advance directive" that states your wishes about end-of-life care, give copies to your doctor, your family, and your care team. If you or your family needs help making difficult decisions, counselors, chaplains, and others are available to help.
- **Protection of your privacy.** We respect the confidentiality of your relationship with your doctor and other caregivers, and the sensitive information about your health and health care that are part of that relationship. State and federal laws and hospital operative policies protect the privacy of your medical information. You will receive a Notice of Privacy Practices that describes the ways that we use, disclose, and safeguard patient information and that explains how you can obtain a copy of information for our records about your care.
- **Help preparing you and your family for when you leave the hospital.** Your doctor works with hospital staff and professionals in your community. You and your family also play an important role. The success of your treatment often depends on your efforts to follow medication, diet, and therapy plans. Your family may need to help care for you at home.

You can expect us to help you identify sources of follow-up care and to let you know if our hospital has a financial interest in any referrals. As long as you agree we can share information about your care with them, we will coordinate our activities with your caregivers outside the hospital. You can also expect to receive information and, where possible, training about the self-care you will need when you go home.

- **Help with your bill and filing insurance claims.** Our staff will file claims for you with health care insurers or other programs, such as Medicare and Medicaid. They will also help your doctor with needed documentation. Hospital bills and insurance coverage are often confusing. If you have questions about your bill, contact our business office. If you need help understanding your insurance coverage or health plan, start with your insurance company or health benefits manager. If you do not have health coverage, we will try to help you and your family find financial help or make other arrangements. We need your help with collecting needed information and other requirements to obtain coverage or assistance.

While you are here, you will receive more detailed notices about some of the rights you have as a hospital patient and how to exercise them. We are always interested in improving. If you have questions, comments, or concerns, please contact ________________.

Source: © Used with permission by American Hospital Association. (2003). *Patient care partnership [extract].* https://www.aha.org,/system/files/2018-01/aha-patient-carepartnership.pdf

Good Samaritan Laws

Good Samaritan laws are designed to protect health care providers when they give aid to people in emergency situations. For example, a nurse at the scene of an automobile accident may give emergency care without fear of a legal suit if such care appears necessary, unless care is given in a grossly negligent manner.

Every state in the United States and the District of Columbia has Good Samaritan laws, although the laws vary considerably. Nurses are covered in some states but not in others; in some states, only certain acts are covered. While in many states no person has a legal obligation to help another (except in employment situations), and a health care provider, like any other person, may choose to help or to leave the scene of an emergency, other states consider it mandatory for anyone to give help. Refer to the specific laws in your state. Regardless, in many situations, nurses may have an ethical responsibility to assist. In the event that health care providers assist a person in an emergency situation when it is impossible to obtain consent for the care, they are expected to use good judgment to determine that an emergency exists and to give care that a reasonably prudent person with a similar background and in similar circumstances would provide.

Student Liability

As a student nurse, you are responsible for your own acts, including any negligence that may result in patient injury. Moreover, you are held to the same standard of care as an RN. You are also responsible for being familiar with facility policies and procedures.

Legal Alert

Your legal responsibilities include careful preparation for each new clinical experience and a duty to notify your clinical instructor if you feel in any way unprepared to carry out a nursing procedure. *For no reason should you attempt a clinical procedure if you are unsure of the correct steps involved.*

A hospital may also be held liable for the negligence of a student nurse enrolled in a hospital-controlled program because the student is considered an employee. The status of students enrolled in college and university programs is less clear, as is the liability of the educational institution in which they are enrolled and the health care facility offering a site for clinical practice.

Nursing instructors may share responsibility for damages in the event of patient injury if an assignment called for clinical skills beyond a student's competency or the instructor failed to provide reasonable and prudent clinical supervision. Because the status of patients can change rapidly, especially in an acute care setting, notify your instructor or a staff member of any significant changes in the patient's condition, even if you are unsure of the meaning of these changes.

Most nursing programs require students to carry personal professional liability insurance. *School policies provide coverage only for clinical nursing done for educational purposes at the direction of the school.* Moreover, student nurses who work as nursing assistants or in some other health care role are legally permitted to offer only those services included in their job description. Even if you feel confident about medication administration, catheter insertion, or another professional nursing act, you risk disciplinary action if you perform such a procedure outside the supervised clinical practice setting.

LAWS AFFECTING NURSING PRACTICE

Just as many safeguards help protect nurses from the risk of legal action, many laws govern the practice of nursing to protect both nurses and patients from harm.

Occupational Safety and Health

The Occupational Safety and Health Act of 1970 set legal standards in the United States to ensure safe and healthful working conditions. The act, intended to reduce work-related injuries and illnesses, has affected health care facilities and increased certain responsibilities for many nurses. In 1991, the Occupational Safety and Health Administration (OSHA) established safety standards for workers who may be exposed to bloodborne pathogens in their employment. Following are examples of situations that could violate standards if care is not taken, because of the potential threat to worker safety:

- Use of electrical equipment
- Use of isolation techniques for patients with infectious diseases and the management of contaminated equipment and supplies
- Use of radiation, such as infrared or ultraviolet radiation, sound or radio waves, and laser beams
- Use of chemicals, such as those that are toxic or flammable

OSHA's regulations, frequently updated, have specific applications, and fines can be severe for infractions. Nurses can help implement this law by promoting health and safety precautions wherever they work. Nurses employed in industrial settings have a particularly important role. A new Office of Occupational Health Nursing was created at OSHA to underscore the major role that such nurses play in striving for safe and healthful workplaces.

In 2020, unions representing hundreds of thousands of nurses and health care workers filed a lawsuit against OSHA, alleging that the agency is violating its duties to keep workers safe by failing to issue an infectious-disease standard to protect them during the pandemic.

National Practitioner Data Bank

The Health Care Quality Improvement Act of 1986 encourages identification and discipline of health care providers who engage in unprofessional conduct and restricts their ability to move from state to state without a disclosure of their previous performance. When a state licenses, certifies, or registers practitioners, they become subject to the National Practitioner Data Bank requirements. The Act provides immunity from civil damages for peer review and establishes the National Practitioner Data Bank as an information clearinghouse. Nurses may be reported to the National Practitioner Data Bank for medical malpractice payments, adverse licensure actions, or adverse professional actions. In a 2020 webinar, nurse attorney Edie Brous stated that an analysis of National Practitioner Data Bank allegations against nurses revealed that only 2% were for negligence/malpractice. The other 98% were for adverse licensure actions.

Reporting Obligations

Because of the unique nature of nurse–patient interactions, the nurse frequently has knowledge that a state requires to be reported, such as of child abuse, rape, or a communicable disease. Legislation varies; thus, nurses must know what needs to be reported in their local area and to what authority.

Nurses are frequently the first members of the public to detect abuse. Abuse includes a physical, verbal, sexual, or emotional attack; neglect; and abandonment. Targets of abuse include infants, children, and adults of all ages. Abusers are people of all genders, ages, races, socioeconomic groups, and religious backgrounds. Nurses are obligated both ethically and legally to report abuse. In many states, the failure to report actual or suspected abuse is itself a crime. Nurses are protected by law against suits from alleged abusers if they file a report of suspected abuse in good faith that turns out to be erroneous.

Controlled Substances

The United States has special laws governing the distribution and use of controlled substances (drugs with misuse potential) such as narcotics, depressants, stimulants, and hallucinogens. Drug use and misuse laws are specific, and violations are considered criminal acts. Nursing responsibilities for controlled substances include storing them in special locked compartments and adhering to specific documentation responsibilities.

Discrimination and Sexual Harassment

Title VII of the Civil Rights Act of 1964 protects employees from discrimination based on race, color, religion, sex, or national origin, and provides that pregnant women receive the same protection as other employees and applicants. The EEOC, which enforces Title VII, defines sexual harassment as "unwelcome sexual advances, requests for sexual favors, and other verbal or physical conduct of a sexual nature" occurring in the following circumstances (EEOC, 1980, sections 3950.10 to 3950.11):

- Submission to sexual advances is implicitly or explicitly considered a condition of employment.
- Submission to sexual advances is used as a basis for employment decisions.
- Sexual harassment interferes with job performance even if it only creates an intimidating, offensive, or hostile atmosphere.

See Chapter 46 for a more detailed discussion of sexual harassment and hostile environment.

Health Insurance Portability and Accountability Act

See the discussion of "Invasion of Privacy" on page 150.

Restraints

The Nursing Home Reform Act of 1987 states that long-term care facility residents have the right to be free from physical or chemical restraints imposed for purposes of discipline or convenience and that are not required to treat medical symptoms. When caring for a patient who requires restraints, be sure that you are familiar with your institution's policies and the guidelines set forth by The Joint Commission. Safe use of restraints is discussed in Chapter 28. Also see the discussion of restraints earlier in this chapter under the heading "False Imprisonment." Articles by Lawson et al. (2020) and by Kisacik et al. (2020) explore nurses' knowledge, attitudes, and practices about using restraints in critical care.

People With Disabilities

At least 43 million Americans have physical or mental disabilities. Discrimination against such people persists in such crucial areas as employment, housing, public accommodations, education, transportation, communication, and health services. The 1990 Americans With Disabilities Act (ADA), amended in 2008, provides a broad definition of "disability" to cover any person who has a physical or mental impairment that substantially limits one or more major life activities or who has a record of such impairment. In addition to impairments that have traditionally been perceived as disabilities, the ADA also specifically protects people who have communicable diseases such as AIDS or HIV infection; people who are recovering from drug or alcohol use disorders; and people who are regarded as being disabled, whether they are disabled or not. The ADA imposes two requirements on businesses covered by the Act: It prohibits such entities from discriminating against people with disabilities and requires covered entities to "reasonably accommodate" people who are protected by the Act.

Wills

State and provincial laws regulate requirements for wills. The person who makes a will is called the testator. A will describes the intentions of a testator (for who will manage the estate and how property is to be disposed) to be carried out upon their death. A person who receives money or property from a will is called a beneficiary.

Depending on state law, nurses may be asked occasionally to witness a testator's signing of their will and should be familiar with the following guidelines:

- The witness should feel sure that the testator is of sound mind—that is, that the testator knows what they are doing and is free of the influence of drugs that could distort thinking.
- The witness should feel sure that the testator is acting voluntarily and is not being coerced in any way concerning the terms of their will.
- Witnesses should watch the testator sign the will, and they should sign in the presence of each other. State law indicates how many witnesses must acknowledge the testator's signature on a will; two or three witnesses are most commonly required.
- Witnesses to the signature on a will do not need to read it, but they should be sure that the document being signed is a will and not some other type of document.
- In most states, a person who is a beneficiary in a will is disqualified from being a witness to the testator's signature.

Legal Issues Related to Dying and Death

Legal responsibilities for the dying or deceased patient are discussed in Chapter 44. Legal issues include advance directives, Patient Self-Determination Act (PSDA), do-not-resuscitate/allow natural death orders, assisted suicide/medically assisted dying, direct voluntary euthanasia, determination of death, organ donation, autopsy, and inquest.

DEVELOPING CLINICAL REASONING AND CLINICAL JUDGMENT

1. Nursing's collaborative responsibilities include helping other health care providers obtain informed and voluntary consent for treatment in difficult situations. How might a nurse facilitate the process of obtaining informed consent in the following situations?
   - A 15-year-old boy with cancer who is tired of therapy needs a new course of chemotherapy.
   - Parents who speak little English are being asked to consent to surgery for their newborn.
   - An older adult who has had pain with eating for 6 months is being offered an exploratory laparotomy. She tells the surgeon, "I don't care what you do, just get rid of this pain."
   - Rehabilitation options are being considered for an older adult who is intermittently confused.
2. You are caring for a recently hospitalized patient who had been living in a retirement community. When his daughters, who tend to be critical, come to visit, they tell you that they hope their father's care here will be better than it was in the retirement community, which they are in the process of suing. How would you respond to the daughters, and what, if anything, would you share with other nurses about this incident?
3. The erratic behavior of a teenage patient on your unit is causing nurses to suspect that he is getting illegal drugs from his friends who visit. You are asked to keep a watchful eye. When changing his bed linens later in the day, you discover a cache of drugs. What are your next steps?
4. Recent layoffs have reduced the number of professional nurses on your unit, and you are increasingly concerned about patient safety as well as quality-of-care issues. What would you do about your concern for your personal liability for inadequate care?
5. A patient posts a video about you on social media that you had no idea was being filmed. By the time you see it, more than 500 people have viewed it. How do you respond? A colleague posts an image of sacral pressure injury with the words, "we don't get paid enough to do this work." When you question her, she tells you there is no way to identify the patient involved. How do you respond?
6. When you bring an antipsychotic medication to your alert long-term care facility resident, she refuses to take it, saying, "I don't like the way it makes me feel." When you report this to one of the nurses, she tells you that they always crush the medication and administer it in food so that the resident doesn't know what she is getting. How do you respond?

PRACTICING FOR NCLEX

1. A nursing professor pulls a student aside to discuss documenting a patient's blood pressure of 202/122 but not reporting this to the primary nurse. When discovered, the patient was transferred to the intensive care unit for treatment and monitoring. How does the faculty best explain to the student that their inaction reflects negligence?
   a. "You did not re-assess your patient."
   b. "There was poor interprofessional communication with the health care team."
   c. You failed to act as a reasonably prudent nurse would under similar circumstances."
   d. "This action is consistent with a felony criminal action."
2. Nursing students approaching graduation and licensure are required to read the state nurse practice act. Which topics in the law will they identity as guides to professional practice? Select all that apply.
   a. Actions resulting in discipline
   b. Clinical procedures
   c. Medication administration
   d. Scope of practice
   e. Delegation policies
   f. Medicare reimbursement
3. A nurse on a surgical unit is concerned about a colleague's possible substance use disorder. Which signs and symptoms could support the nurse's suspicion? Select all that apply.
   a. Exhibiting diminished alertness and somnolence while working
   b. Attending multiple continuing education conferences
   c. Offering to medicate coworkers' patients for pain

d. Making incorrect narcotics counts and creating wastage
e. Leaving the unit frequently

4. A new graduate nurse tells the preceptor they want to obtain recognition in wound care, a specialty area of nursing. What credential will this nurse need to seek?
a. Accreditation
b. Licensure
c. Certification
d. Board approval

5. The nurse reports to their manager that informed consent was not obtained from a patient for whom HIV testing was already performed. The nurse suggests which intentional tort may have been committed?
a. Assault
b. Battery
c. Invasion of privacy
d. False imprisonment

6. A patient died during routine outpatient surgery, and the nurse was accused of having failed to monitor and interpret vital signs. Which fact must be established to prove them guilty of malpractice or negligence?
a. The surgeon testifies the nurse's action was pure negligence, saying that the patient could have been saved.
b. This patient should not have died since they were healthy, physically active, and involved in the community.
c. The nurse intended to harm the patient and was willfully negligent, as evidenced by the tragic outcome.
d. The nurse had a duty to monitor the patient, and due to the nurse's failure to perform this duty, the patient died.

7. An attorney representing a patient's family who is suing for wrongful death calls the nurse to obtain a better understanding of the nurse's actions. How will the nurse respond?
a. "I can't talk with you; you will have to contact my attorney."
b. "I will answer your questions, so you'll understand how the situation occurred.
c. "I hope I won't be blamed for the death because it was so busy that day."
d. "First tell me why you are doing this to me. This could ruin my career!"

8. A nurse follows a prescription written by the health care provider to administer a medication to which the patient is allergic. How does the nurse interpret their liability for administering this medication?
a. The nurse is not responsible because they were following the provider's orders.
b. The nurse is responsible because they administered the medication.
c. The health care provider is responsible because they ordered the drug.
d. The nurse, health care provider, and pharmacist bear responsibility for their actions.

9. A nurse answers a call light and finds the patient on the floor. After the health care provider examines the patient and finds no injury, the nurse returns the patient to bed and fills out an incident report. What statements are true about incident reports? Select all that apply.
a. They can be used as disciplinary action against staff members.
b. They can be used as a means of identifying risks.
c. They can be used for quality control.
d. They must be completed by the facility manager.
e. They make facts available in litigation cases.
f. They should be documented in the patient record.

10. A nursing student is preparing to administer medications and asks the clinical instructor about legal liability in clinical practice. What is the most appropriate response?
a. "Students are not responsible for their acts of negligence resulting in patient injury."
b. "Student nurses are held to the same standard of care that would be used to evaluate the actions of a registered nurse."
c. "Hospitals are exempt from liability for student negligence if the student nurse is properly supervised by an instructor."
d. "Most nursing programs carry group professional liability making student personal professional liability insurance unnecessary."

11. The nurse manager reviews the medical record of a patient who has accused a nurse of negligence after requiring a "needless" admission to the intensive care unit postoperatively. Which entry in the electronic health record requires follow-up by the manager?
Exhibit: Electronic health record (EHR)
Nursing Notes: Postoperative follow-up
12:20 pm: patient still reporting incisional pain of 10/10, provider contacted, increased morphine from 1 mg to 2 mg every hour
2: 15 pm: dime-sized, dark red–brown blood stain on dressing; area circled
2:30 pm: patient reports incisional pain, 7/10, 2 mg morphine administered
2:45 pm: vital signs T 99.2°, P 120, RR 20, BP 84/48; will continue to monitor
a. Inappropriately recorded vital signs
b. Pain treated without appropriate assessment
c. Failure to follow up on tachycardia and hypotension
d. Lack of interpretation of vital signs and follow-up

12. A patient admitted through the emergency department for a severe infection is receiving intravenous (IV) antibiotics. The patient, who has been oriented, demands the nurse remove the IV because the patient is leaving now. What action will the nurse take?
a. Apply soft wrist restraints
b. Perform a neurologic assessment
c. Explain that after signing an "against medical order form," the patient may leave
d. Call the patient's family to encourage the patient to stay

ANSWERS WITH RATIONALES

1. **c.** Negligence is defined as performing an action that the reasonably prudent nurse would not perform or failing to act as a reasonably prudent nurse would in similar circumstances. Negligence may be an act of omission or commission. Criminal law concerning state and federal criminal statutes includes murder, manslaughter, criminal negligence, theft, and illegal possession of drugs. Public law regulates relationships between people and the government. Private or civil law includes laws relating to contracts, ownership of property, and the practice of nursing, medicine, pharmacy, and dentistry.
2. **a, d.** Each state has a nurse practice act that protects the public by broadly defining the legal scope of nursing practice. Practicing beyond those limits makes nurses vulnerable to charges of violating the state nurse practice act. Nurse practice acts also list the violations that can result in disciplinary actions against nurses. Clinical procedures are covered by the health care institutions themselves. Medication administration and delegation are topics covered by the board of nursing. Laws governing Medicare reimbursement are enacted through federal legislation.
3. **a, c, d, e.** Signs of substance use in nurses may include diminished alertness or somnolence, leaving the unit frequently, incorrect narcotic counts, wastage, offers to medicate colleagues' patients, or changes in job performance, among others. Attending professional conferences is an example of a nurse who is fully engaged with their work.
4. **c.** Certification is the process by which a person who has met certain criteria established by a nongovernmental association is granted recognition in a specified practice area. Nursing is one of the groups operating under state laws that promote the general welfare by determining minimum standards of education through accreditation of schools of nursing. Licensure is a legal document that permits a person to offer to the public skills and knowledge in a particular jurisdiction, where such practice would otherwise be unlawful without a license. State board of approval ensures that nurses have received the proper training to practice nursing.
5. **b.** Assault is a threat or an attempt to make bodily contact with another person without that person's consent. Battery is an assault that is carried out. Every person is granted freedom from bodily contact by another person unless consent is granted. The Fourth Amendment gives citizens the right of privacy and the right to be left alone; a nurse who disregards these rights is guilty of invasion of privacy. Unjustified retention or prevention of the movement of another person without proper consent can constitute false imprisonment.
6. **d.** Liability involves four elements that must be established to prove that malpractice or negligence has occurred: duty, breach of duty, causation, and damages. Duty refers to an obligation to use due care (what a reasonably prudent nurse would do) and is defined by the standard of care appropriate for the nurse–patient relationship. Breach of duty is the failure to meet the standard of care. Causation, the most difficult element of liability to prove, shows that the failure to meet the standard of care (breach) caused the injury. Damages are the actual harm or injury resulting to the patient.
7. **a.** The nurse should not discuss the case with anyone at the facility (except the risk manager), with the plaintiff, with the plaintiff's lawyer, with anyone testifying for the plaintiff, or with reporters. This is one of the cardinal rules for nurse defendants.
8. **d.** Nurses are legally responsible for carrying out the orders of the health care provider in charge of a patient unless an order would lead a reasonable person to anticipate injury if it was carried out. If the nurse should have anticipated injury and did not, both the prescribing health care provider and the administering nurse are responsible for the harms to which they contributed.
9. **b, c, e.** Incident reports are used for quality improvement and should not be used for disciplinary action against staff members. They are a means of identifying risks and are filled out by the nurse responsible for the injured party. An incident report makes facts available in case litigation occurs; in some states, incident reports may be used in court as evidence. A health care provider completes the incident form with documentation of the medical examination of the patient, employee, or visitor with an actual or potential injury. Documentation in the patient record should not include the fact that an incident report was filed.
10. **b.** Student nurses are held to the same standard of care that would be used to evaluate the actions of a registered nurse. Student nurses are responsible for their own acts of negligence if these result in patient injury. A hospital may also be held liable for the negligence of a student nurse enrolled in a hospital-controlled program because the student is considered an employee of the hospital. Nursing instructors may share responsibility for damages in the event of patient injury if an assignment called for clinical skills beyond a student's competency or the instructor failed to provide reasonable and prudent clinical supervision. Most nursing programs require students to carry personal professional liability insurance.
11. **d.** Nurses are responsible for gathering assessment data including vital signs and interpreting them considering the patient's condition and trends. The nurse did not document interventions from the health care provider for typical symptoms of shock, including tachycardia and hypotension.
12. **c.** A person cannot be legally forced to remain in a health facility, such as a hospital, if that person is of sound mind. The patient signs an "against medical orders" form when insisting on being discharged, to indicate not holding the facility responsible for harm from leaving. Applying soft wrist restraints when the patient has expressed wanting to leave constitutes battery, which includes willful, angry, and violent or negligent touching of another person's body or clothes or anything attached to or held by that other person. The patient has been oriented, so another assessment is not indicated. The patient, not the family, has autonomy.

Bibliography

Abreu, T. (2021). Adverse event reporting and root cause analysis. *American Nurse Journal, 16*(6), 44–47.

American Association of Critical-Care Nurses and AACN Certification Corporation. (2002). *Safeguarding the patient and the profession: Executive summary*. Author.

American Nurses Association. (2014). *Addressing nurse fatigue to promote safety and health: Joint responsibilities of registered nurses and employers to reduce risks*. https://www.nursingworld.org/practice-policy/nursing-excellence/official-position-statements/id/addressing-nurse-fatigue-to-promote-safety-and-health/

American Nurses Association. (2015). *Code for nurses with interpretive statements*. Author.

American Nurses Association. (2019). National guidelines for nursing delegation. https://www.nursingworld.org/_4962ca/globalassets/practiceandpolicy/nursing-excellence/ana-position-statements/nursing-practice/ana-ncsbn-joint-statement-on-delegation.pdf

American Nurses Association. (2020). *Principles for nurse staffing* (3rd ed.) https://www.nursingworld.org/practice-policy/nurse-staffing/staffing-principles/

American Nurses Association. (2021). *Nursing: Scope and standards of practice* (4th ed.). Author.

American Nurses Association. (2021a). What is the role of the state board of nursing. https://nursejournal.org/resources/what-is-the-role-of-the-state-board-of-nursing/

Ashton, L. M. (2016). Compact state licensure: Take the "fast lane" to nursing practice. *Nursing, 46*(12), 50–54.

Balestra, M. L. (2018). Social media missteps could put your nursing license at risk. *American Nurse Today, 13*(3), 20–21, 63.

Barnsteiner, J., & Disch, J. (2017). Creating a fair and just culture in schools of nursing. *American Journal of Nursing, 117*(11), 42–48.

Brent, N. J. (2019). When a BON disciplinary process is based on substance misuse disorder. *American Nurse Today, 14*(3), 14–16.

Brous, E. A. (2012a). Common misconceptions about professional licensure. *American Journal of Nursing, 112*(10), 55–59.

Brous, E. A. (2012b). Professional licensure protection strategies. Part 3. *American Journal of Nursing, 112*(12), 43–47.

Brous, E. A. (2012c). Professional licensure: Investigation and disciplinary action. Part 2. *American Journal of Nursing, 112*(11), 53–60.

Brous, E. (2014). Lessons learned from litigation. *American Journal of Nursing, 114*(2), 58–60.

Brous, E. (2016a). Lessons learned from litigation: Discrimination against nurses. *American Journal of Nursing, 116*(2), 60–63.

Brous, E. (2016b). Legal considerations in telehealth and telemedicine. *American Journal of Nursing, 116*(9), 64–67.

Brous, E. (2021). Immunity from civil liability, Part 1. *American Journal of Nursing, 121*(4), 61–64.

Brous, E. A. (2019a). The BON discipline cascade. *American Nurse Today, 14*(11), 26–28.

Brous, E. A. (2019b). The elements of a nursing malpractice case, Part 3A: Causation. *American Journal of Nursing, 119*(11), 54–59.

Brous, E. A. (2019c). The elements of a nursing malpractice case, Part 1: Duty. *American Journal of Nursing, 119*(7), 64–67.

Brous, E. A. (2020). The elements of a nursing malpractice case, Part 4: Harm. *American Journal of Nursing, 120*(3), 61–64.

Brous, E. A., & Olsen, D. P. (2017). Lessons learned from litigation: Legal and ethical consequences of social media. *American Journal of Nursing, 117*(9), 50–54.

Claffey, C. (2018). Near-miss medication errors provide a wake-up call. *Nursing, 48*(1), 53–55.

Doherty, C. L., Pawlow, P., & Becker, D. (2018). The consensus model: What current and future NPs need to know. *American Nurse Today, 13*(1), 65–67.

Dolan, J., & Dolan Looby, S. E. (2017). Determinants of nurses' use of physical restraints in surgical intensive care unit patients. *American Journal of Critical Care, 26*(5), 373–379.

Equal Employment Opportunity Commission (EEOC). (1989). Sex discrimination guidelines. In *EEOC rules and regulations.* Commerce Clearing House.

Feeg, V. D., Mancino, D. J., Rushton, C. H., Menndez, K. J. W., & Baierlein, J. (2021). Ethical dilemmas for nursing students and faculty: In their own voices. *Nursing Education Perspectives, 42*(1), 29–35.

Finn, S. S., & Dion, K. W. (2017a). Security tips for using personal technology. Reflections on Nursing Leadership. http://www.reflectionsonnursingleadership.org/features/more-features/Vol43_1_security-tips-for-using-personal-technology

Finn, S. S., & Dion, K. W. (2017b). Security tips for using personal technology at your employer's site. Reflections on Nursing Leadership. http://www.reflectionsonnursingleadership.org/features/more-features/Vol43_2_security-tips-for-using-personal-technology-at-your-employer-s-site

Finn, S. S., & Dion, K. W. (2017c). Security tips for using your employer's technology. Reflections on Nursing Leadership. http://www.reflectionsonnursingleadership.org/features/more-features/Vol43_2_security-tips-for-using-personal-technology-at-your-employer-s-site

Fortier, M. E. (2019). Social media: New communication platform but old rules still apply. *American Nurse Today, 14*(5).

Fotsch, R. (2020). Frequently asked questions about the nurse licensure compact. *American Nurse Journal, 15*(3), 44–46.

Glannon, J. W. (2010). *The law of torts: Examples and explanations* (4th ed.). Aspen Publishers.

Green, D. (2019). Becoming a nurse investigator. *American Nurse Today, 14*(4), 66–67.

Jenkins, R. C., & Lemak, C. H. (2009). A malpractice lawsuit simulation: Critical care providers learn as participants in a mock trial. *Critical Care Nurse, 29*(4), 52–60.

The Joint Commission. (2016a). *Sentinel event policy and procedures.* http://www.jointcommission.org/Sentinel_Event_Policy_and_Procedures

The Joint Commission. (2016b). *Update: Texting orders.* http://www.jointcommission.org/assets/1/6/Update_Texting_Orders.pdf

The Joint Commission. (2019). Facts about the official "do not use" list of abbreviations. https://www.jointcommission.org/-/media/tjc/documents/fact-sheets/do-not-use-list-8-3-20.pdf?db=web&hash=2489CB1616A30CFFBDAAD1FB3F8021A5

Jordan, M. (2020). Cybersecurity awareness. *American Journal of Nursing, 15*(2), 10–13.

Kavalar, F., & Alexander, R. S. (2014). *Risk management in healthcare institutions* (3rd ed.). Jones & Bartlett Learning.

Kisacik, Ö. G., Sönmez, M., & Coşgun, T. (2020). Use of physical restraints in critical care units: Nurses' knowledge, attitudes, and practices. *Critical Care Nurse, 40*(3), 37–47.

Laskowshi-Jones, L. (1998). Reaching beyond the rules. Understanding—and influencing—your scope of practice. *Nursing, 28*(9), 42–47.

Lawson, T. L., Tan, A., Thrane, S. E., Happ M, B., Mion, L. C., Tate, J., & Balas, M. C. (2020). Predictors of new-onset physical restraint use in critically ill adults. *American Journal of Critical Care, 29*(2), 92–102.

McGill, M., Loveless, B., & McGill, M. (2019). Social media in healthcare: A 360-degree view. 25–26.

Miller, L. A. (2011). The National Practitioner Data Bank: A primer for clinicians. *Journal of Perinatal and Neonatal Nursing, 25*(3), 224–225.

Myers, L., Heard, L., & Mort, E. (2020). Lessons learned from medical malpractice claims involving critical care nurses. *American Journal of Critical Care, 29*(3), 174–180.

National Council of State Boards of Nursing (NCSBN). (n.d.). *New nurses: Your license to practice video.* https://www.ncsbn.org/8243.htm

National Council of State Boards of Nursing (NCSBN). (2014). *What you need to know about substance use disorder in nursing.* https://www.ncsbn.org/SUD_Brochure_2014.pdf

National Council of State Boards of Nursing (NCSBN). (2018). White paper: A nurse's guide to the use of social media. https://www.ncsbn.org/NCSBN_SocialMedia.pdf

National Practitioner Data Bank. https://www.npdb.hrsa.gov/index.jsp

National Quality Forum. (n.d.). List of serious reportable events (SREs). http://www.qualityforum.org/Topics/SREs/List_of_SREs.aspx

National Quality Forum. (2011). *Serious reportable event in healthcare—2011 update: A consensus report.* Author.

National Student Nurses' Association. (n.d.). Recommendations for social media usage and maintaining privacy, confidentiality and professionalism. http://www.nsna.org/Portals/0/Skins/NSNA/pdf/NSNA_Social_Media_Recommendations.pdf

Newman, A. B., & Kjervik, D. K. (2016). Critical care nurses' knowledge of confidentiality legislation. *American Journal of Critical Care, 25*(3), 222–227.

Nurses Service Organization (NSO) and CAN HealthPro. (2011). Understanding nurse liability, 2006–2010: A three-part approach.

Nyhus, J. (2021). Drug diversion in healthcare. Prevention and detection for nurses. *American Nurse Journal, 15*(5), 24–27.

Olsen, D. P., & Brous, E. (2018). The ethical and legal implications of a nurse's arrest in Utah. *American Journal of Nursing, 118*(3), 47–53.

Olsen, L. (2018). When a nurse's privacy is breached by social media. *American Nurse Today, 13*(1), 40.

O'Neill, C. (2015). When a nurse returns to work after substance abuse treatment. *American Nurse Today, 10*(7), 8–12.

O'Neill, S. P. (2021). Individual nurse liability insurance. Understand your options. *American Nurse Journal, 16*(5), 54–56, 58.

Paradiso, L., & Sweeney, N. (2019). Just culture: It's more than policy. *Nursing Management, 50*(6), 38–45. https://doi.org/10.1097/01.NUMA.0000558482.07815.ae

Pohlman, H. (2015). Why you need your own malpractice insurance. *American Nurse Today, 10*(11), 28–30.

President's Commission for the Study of Ethical Problems in Medicine and Biomedical and Behavioral Research. (1982). *Making healthcare decisions: A report (Vol. 1).* U.S. Government Printing Office.

Puente, J. (2017). The enhanced nurse licensure compact. *American Nurse Today, 12*(10), 50–53.

Reising, D. L. (2012). Make your nursing care malpractice-proof. *American Nurse Today, 7*(1), 24–28.

Rose, C. (2015). Choosing the right restraint. *American Nurse Today, 10*(1).

Scott, L. D., Arslanian-Engoren, C., & Engoren, M. C. (2014). Association of sleep and fatigue with decision regret among critical care nurses. *American Journal of Critical Care, 23*(1), 13–23.

Sharp, N. (2003). The "write stuff." *Nursing Spectrum, 13*(2), 12–13.

Sherman, R. (2017). Building leadership resiliency. EmergingRNLeader. http://www.emergingrnleader.com/building-leadership-resiliency

Springer, G. (2015). When and how to use restraints. *American Nurse Today, 10*(1).

Starr, K. T. (2014). Whistleblower liability: Are you ready to put your job on the line? *Nursing, 44*(2), 16–17.

Starr, K. T. (2017). Background checks: Do you have something to report? *Nursing, 47*(10), 11–12.

Starr, K. T. (2020). You've been sued, part 1. *Nursing, 50*(6), 13–14.

Stone, L., Rice, J., & Garcia, R. (2021). Addressing substance use disorder and diversion in the health care environment. *American Nurse Journal, 16*(2), 27–30.

Thede, L. (2010). Informatics: Electronic health records: A boon or privacy nightmare? *OJIN: The Online Journal of Issues in Nursing, 15*(2). https://doi.org/10.3912/OJIN.Vol15No02InfoCol01

Tocco, S., & Blum, A. (2013). Just culture promotes a partnership for patient safety. *American Nurse Today, 8*(5), 16–17.

Trossman, S. (2019a). Preventing harm. Reporting, recognition, and just culture can make a difference. *American Nurse Today, 14*(2), 30–32.

Trossman, S. (2019b). Time to end nurse abuse. *American Nurse Today, 14*(10), 32–34.

U.S. Equal Employment Opportunity Commission. (n.d.). *Sex-based discrimination.* https://www.eeoc.gov/laws/types/sex.cfm

Walker, R. (2011). Elements of negligence and malpractice. *The Nurse Practitioner, 36*(5), 9–11.

White, C. L. (2011). Do I need my own malpractice insurance? *Plastic Surgical Nursing, 31*(4), 185–187.

8 Communication

Susie Musashi

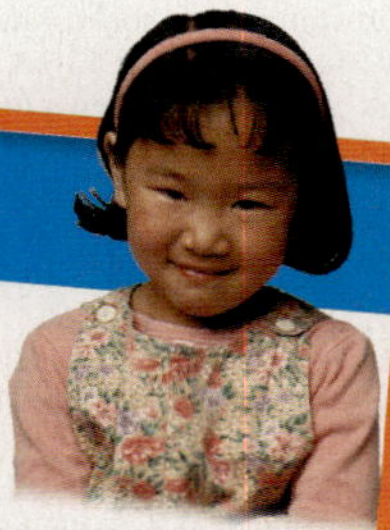

Susie is a 3-year-old patient with second-degree burns on both legs. Every time a health care provider enters her room, she begins to cry, turning her body toward the wall and curling up with her knees to her chest. Her family lives approximately 1½ hours away and can visit her only about once or twice a week.

Irwina Russellinski

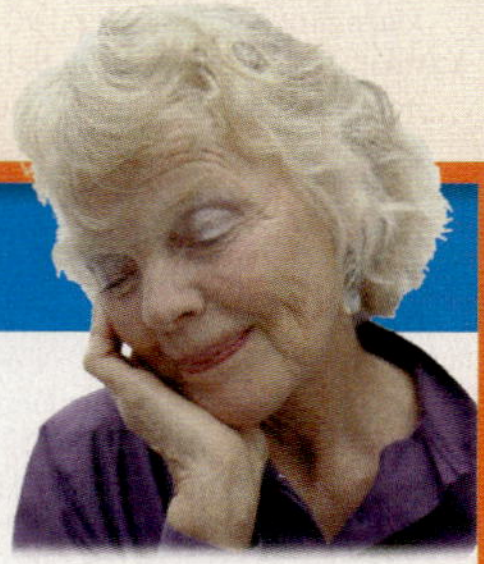

Irwina, a 75-year-old woman, has been transferred to a long-term care facility from the hospital after being diagnosed and treated for pneumonia. Her health record reveals that she is hard of hearing, "pleasantly confused" at times, and speaks "broken English." An initial nursing assessment is needed.

Randolph Gordon

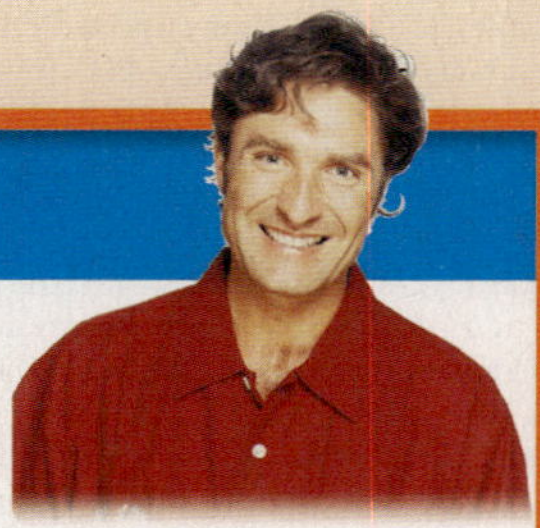

Randolph, a middle-aged man diagnosed with end-stage liver failure, is being cared for in the intensive care unit (ICU). He has been comatose for several weeks. He has numerous tubes and drainage devices in place and is receiving multiple therapies that require continuous electronic monitoring.

Learning Outcomes

After completing the chapter, you will be able to accomplish the following:

1. Describe the communication process and identify factors that influence communication.
2. Describe ways in which people communicate nonverbally.
3. Discuss professional responsibilities when using electronic communication and other communication technologies.
4. Describe the interrelation between communication and the nursing process.
5. Identify patient goals for each phase of the therapeutic nurse–patient relationship.
6. Use appropriate communication techniques when interacting with patients from different cultures.
7. Use a standardized communication technique (e.g., SBAR) to communicate with other nurses and health care providers.
8. Evaluate yourself in terms of the interpersonal competencies needed in nursing.
9. Describe how each type of ineffective communication hinders communication.
10. Describe strategies that counteract disruptive professional communication and behaviors.
11. Establish therapeutic relationships with patients assigned to your care.
12. Describe effective interventions for patients with impaired communication.

Nursing Concepts

- Clinical Decision Making/Clinical Judgment
- Communication
- Therapeutic communication
- Collaboration/teamwork
- Professionalism

A nurse who wishes to be an effective caregiver must first learn how to be an effective communicator. Good communication skills enable nurses to get to know their patients and, ultimately, to diagnose and meet their needs for nursing care. Nursing students who sit face to face with patients to obtain a comprehensive nursing history intuitively grasp the importance of the nurse's communicator role. To adequately document the patient's health history, the nursing student must understand and implement proper communication techniques. Communication skills are the building blocks of professional relationships between nurse and patient, nurse and nurse, and nurse and other health care team members. Refer to the accompanying Reflective Practice box on page 174.

Many experienced nurses identify the quality of their interpersonal relationships as the single most significant element in determining their helper effectiveness. On nursing units where nurses freely exchange ideas and information, solve problems together when something goes wrong rather than assigning blame, compliment one another, and use humor creatively, staff morale is high and there is a higher level of attainment of patient outcomes. On the other hand, when harassment or disruptive communication and/or behaviors occur in the workplace between health care professionals, the consequences can affect the emotional and physical well-being of those involved, the functioning of the organization, and the safety of patient care. The American Association of Critical-Care Nurses (AACN) provides standards for establishing and sustaining healthy work environments, and states the quality of the work environment is linked to excellent nursing practice and patient care outcomes (AACN, 2016). These standards include skilled communication: "Nurses must be as proficient in communication skills as they are in clinical skills" (AACN, 2016, p. 2). Effective communication supports collaborative relationships and continuous improvement in patient safety and quality of care (AACN; ANA & AONE, n.d.; Settani et al., 2019).

QSEN TEAMWORK AND COLLABORATION

Nurses must communicate with team members in a manner that promotes open communication and mutual respect. Communication and collaboration between the nurse, patient, and other health care professionals results in quality person-centered care.

PROCESS OF COMMUNICATION

Communication is the process of exchanging information and generating and transmitting meanings between two or more people. It is the foundation of society and the most primary aspect of a nurse–patient interaction. Without communication, it would be impossible to share family experiences, gain knowledge, establish and maintain practice protocols, and enhance caregiving. By nature, humans are social beings, and human needs are met in collaboration with other humans. Human relationships enable us to meet our physical and safety needs. Communication also assists in meeting our psychosocial needs of love, belonging, and self-esteem. The ability to communicate is basic to human functioning and well-being.

David K. Berlo (1960) is credited with the classic description of the communication process, which involves a source (encoder), message, channel, and receiver (decoder). This communication process is initiated based on a stimulus, in this case, a patient need that must be addressed. The need might be due to a patient's discomfort or desire for information or to address any uncertainty the patient might be experiencing. The sender or source (encoder) of the message is a person or group who initiates or begins the communication process.

QSEN Reflective Practice: Cultivating QSEN Competencies

CHALLENGE TO ETHICAL AND LEGAL SKILLS

Recently, I was accompanying a nurse in the ICU when I encountered some behaviors that I found to be unprofessional and lacking in interpersonal communication skills. We were caring for Mr. Randolph Gordon, a middle-aged patient who was in end-stage liver failure and had been comatose for several weeks. The extent of drains, tubes, and technologies being used to care for Mr. Gordon was overwhelming. It was almost difficult to recognize him as a human being. I was taken aback when the nurse and some residents entered the patient's room and immediately began to assess the technologic equipment, without any regard for or recognition of the patient. They proceeded to have a conversation about the patient's poor condition, unsightly appearance, and foul smell at the bedside, in the direct presence of the patient. They did not speak to the patient and they made no attempt to interact with the patient, not even the slightest touch of a hand.

Thinking Outside the Box: Possible Courses of Action

- Ignore the conversation between the nurse and residents and acknowledge the patient through words or touch.
- Calmly ask the nurse and residents to leave the room before discussing the patient's condition.
- Confront the nurse and residents, stating that they need to pay attention to the patient and his psychosocial and emotional well-being.

Evaluating a Good Outcome: How Do I Define Success?

- The patient's health care team will act with professionalism.
- The health care team will demonstrate respect for the patient's human dignity.
- The health care team will have regard for the whole patient, with attention to spiritual, emotional, and social issues.
- The health care team will set a good example for others in our expression of caring.

Personal Learning: Here's to the Future!

I was somewhat disappointed by my actions in this situation because I did not confront the nurse and the residents when they were acting unethically and unprofessionally. I did, however, ask the nurse if this was common behavior in the ICU—that is, demonstrating little regard for the patient's holistic well-being. The nurse stated that unfortunately this was the case. The patients in the ICU are critically ill, and many health care professionals become extremely focused on the physical and technologic aspects of care. I was hesitant to interrupt the nurse and the residents because of my status as a nursing student. I feared that my opinion would not be respected. I know that I will not be able to change the actions of everyone. However, in the future, I will demonstrate my concern for the patient, hoping that those around me will follow my example. I think that I should have immediately gone to the patient and said hello or touched his hand, even if he was comatose. Maybe my actions would have reminded the nurse and residents that there was a person in that bed. Then, possibly, they might have followed my lead.

Colleen Kilcullen, Georgetown University

QSEN SELF-REFLECTION ON QUALITY AND SAFETY COMPETENCIES DEVELOPING KNOWLEDGE, SKILLS, AND ATTITUDES FOR CONTINUOUS IMPROVEMENT

How do you think you would respond in a similar situation? Why? What does this tell you about yourself and about the adequacy of your skills for professional practice? What knowledge, skills, and attitudes do you need to develop to continuously improve quality and safety in a situation like the one experienced by this student nurse?

Patient-Centered Care: How could the nursing student's communication skills have demonstrated empathy and emotional support for this patient? Did her handling of this situation facilitate her ability to deliver effective care and treatment in other environments? What reasons can you propose to suggest the rationale for the nurse's and residents' behavior?

Teamwork and Collaboration/Quality Improvement: How do you think the residents would have reacted if the nursing student had approached them about their behavior? Can you think of other ways to respond? Describe a plan that the nursing student could use to go about changing the staff's behavior. What communication skills might effectively communicate empathy and caring by all the professional staff caring for this patient?

Safety/Evidence-Based Practice: Do you agree with the criteria to evaluate a positive outcome in this situation? Did the nursing student meet the criteria? Please explain why or why not. Should one of the priorities of care for Mr. Gordon have included a review at the bedside of his current condition and treatment therapies with respect for the possibility that the patient might be able to hear the discussion, even though he is not able to communicate with the staff? What evidence in nursing literature provides guidance for evidence-based practice for the student when caring for an unresponsive patient?

Informatics: Can you identify essential information that should be documented in Mr. Gordon's electronic record regarding physical assessments and electronic monitoring in addition to efforts to communicate with this patient? Do you think the understanding you gained from this situation improves your ability to care effectively for other comatose patients and communicate respect and emotional support?

The **message** is the actual communication product from the source. It might be a speech, interview, conversation, chart, gesture, memorandum, or nursing note. The **channel** of communication is the medium the sender has selected to send the message. The channel might target any of the receiver's senses. The message can be sent to the receiver through the following channels:

- Auditory—spoken words and cues
- Visual—sight, observations, and perception
- Kinesthetic—touch

Nurses use all three of these channels to communicate with patients and other health care providers.

The receiver (decoder) must translate and interpret the message sent and received. Through the translation of the message, the receiver must then make a decision about an accurate response. To be an effective communicator, the nurse needs to be considerate of the receiver, and select a message that appeals to the patient's interests and that requires minimal effort and time to decode.

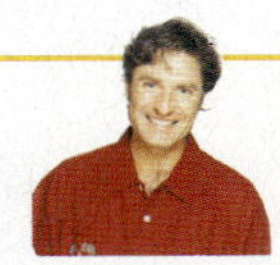

Recall **Randolph Gordon**, the middle-aged man who is comatose. When planning Mr. Gordon's care, the nurse would need to incorporate knowledge about changes in mental status and their effect on communication. The patient's current mental status mandates that the messages sent to the patient by the nurse and other health care providers be simple, clear, and easy to understand.

Confirmation of the message provides **feedback** (i.e., evidence) that the receiver has understood the intended message. **Noise**—factors that distort the quality of a message—can interfere with communication at any point in the process. These distractors might be from the television, or from pain or discomfort experienced by the patient.

Communication is a reciprocal process in which both the sender and the receiver of messages participate simultaneously. The communication process is illustrated in Figure 8-1. Messages might be influenced on either end by the person's previous knowledge, past experiences, feelings, or sociocultural level.

Read the situation in Box 8-1 (on page 176) and test your knowledge and use of communication.

FORMS OF COMMUNICATION

The sending and receiving of messages is accomplished through verbal and nonverbal communication techniques. These can occur separately or simultaneously. Nurses must consider both verbal and nonverbal communication when sending and interpreting communicated messages.

Verbal Communication

Verbal communication is an exchange of information using words, including both the spoken and written word. Verbal communication depends on **language**, or a prescribed way of using words so that people can share information

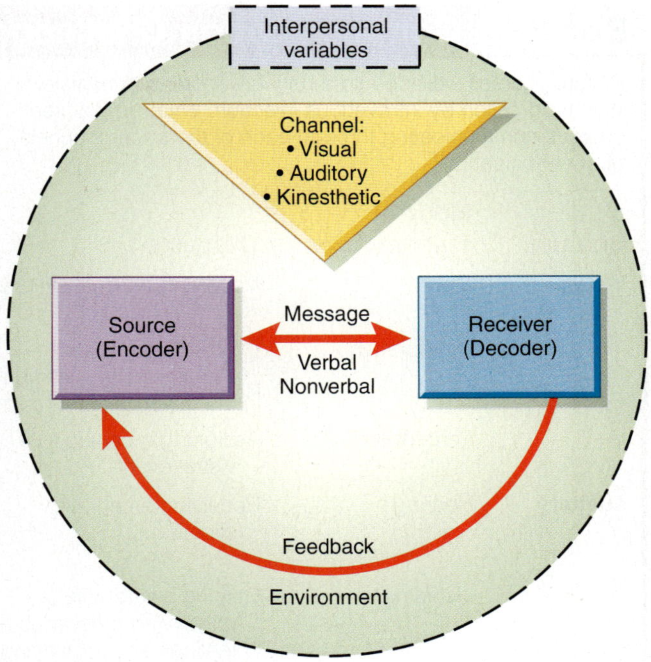

FIGURE 8-1. The various components in the process of communication.

effectively. Language includes a common definition of words and a method of arranging the words in a certain order.

A person's use of written and spoken language forms reveals aspects of the person's intellectual development, educational level, and geographic and cultural origin. Nurses must also consider whether English is a second language for the patient. Language helps nurses assess what the patient knows and feels. In turn, nurses must develop their own language skills to assist in reciprocal responses in the communication process.

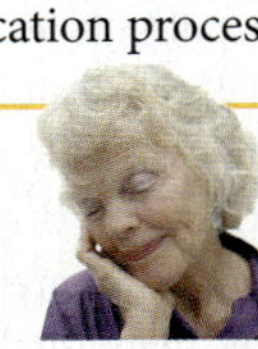

Think back to **Irwina Russellinski**, the older adult woman transferred to a long-term care facility after treatment for pneumonia. According to her health record, the patient speaks "broken English." Therefore, the nurse must incorporate knowledge of this when attempting to communicate verbally with the patient, making adaptations during the interaction to ensure that messages are clear.

Nurses use verbal communication extensively when providing patient care, including verbal interactions with patients and family, collaborating with the health care team, developing plans of care, and evaluating patient progress. Other examples of verbal communication include public speaking, collaboration for publication, and dissemination of health information. Words and language in the previous examples communicate messages to others.

Nonverbal Communication

The transmission of information without the use of words is termed **nonverbal communication**. Nonverbal communication includes facial expressions, eye contact, space, time, boundaries, and body movements (Videbeck, 2020). Nonverbal

Box 8-1 Communication Challenges

Picture yourself walking into a patient's room to administer a pain medication by intravenous injection. What do you see yourself communicating through each of the three channels of communication?

Then, read the following and think about all the ways nurses might unintentionally communicate that they are not concerned about the patient or his pain. Use this exercise to guide both your verbal and nonverbal messages to patients.

Channel	Mode of Transmission	Outcome	Nursing Behavior
Visual	Sight	Receiving a visual stimulus	Patient sees nurse walking into the room holding desired medication.
	Observation	Interpreting a visual stimulation by making note of nonverbal enhancement	Patient makes note of the nurse's sense of competence, confidence, and sympathetic expression.
	Perception	Assigning meaning to a visual event	Patient concludes that the nurse is willing and able to help him and feels comforted.
Auditory	Hearing	Receiving an auditory stimulus	Patient hears the nurse say, "I understand your hip is hurting. This medication should help you to start feeling better within minutes."
	Listening	Gaining awareness of underlying messages and feelings accompanying auditory events	Patient senses that the nurse said he should start feeling better soon and really wants this to happen because she cares about him.
Kinesthetic	Procedural touch	Performing nursing procedures and techniques	Patient feels the nurse touching him while preparing to inject the medication into the IV access.
	Caring touch	Conveying emotional support	Patient feels that the nurse cares about him as a person when she touches his shoulder upon first entering the room while asking about his pain.

communication is as important as verbal communication, if not more so (Videbeck, 2020). Nonverbal communication often helps to understand subtle and hidden meanings in what the patients or others are saying verbally (Keltner & Steele, 2019). For example, a nurse asks the patient, "How do you feel today?" The patient responds, "I feel all right." However, the nurse notes that the patient does not maintain eye contact and his facial expression is tense. This should prompt the nurse to investigate further because of the incongruence of the patient's verbal and nonverbal communication (Fig. 8-2).

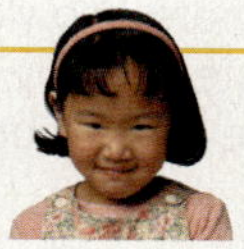

Consider ***Susie Musashi***, the 3-year-old described at the beginning of the chapter. Interpretation of her nonverbal behavior is essential to implementing an effective plan of care. For example, the nurse needs to interpret what the child's crying indicates, such as fear, pain, or loneliness. In addition, the nurse needs to examine the meaning of the child's turning away from the door. Does she want to be left alone? Is she frightened? Once this information is obtained and analyzed, the nurse is better equipped to develop a plan of care to meet Susie's needs.

Information is exchanged through nonverbal communication in various ways. Body language may mirror or enhance what is verbally communicated (Keltner & Steele, 2019). When verbal and nonverbal communication do not match, nonverbal communication often conveys the speaker's actual meaning (Videbeck, 2020). Consequently, if verbal and nonverbal messages conflict, behaviors can negate a verbal message and the listener will believe the nonverbal message (Boyd, 2018; Keltner & Steele, 2019). Therefore, nurses must be aware of both the nonverbal messages they send and the nonverbal messages they receive from patients. Nurses working with patients from diverse cultural backgrounds should attempt to understand cultural variations to avoid misunderstanding nonverbal communication. The various forms of nonverbal communication follow.

Touch

Touch (a person's tactile sense) is a very personal behavior and means different things to different people. Familial, regional, class, and cultural influences largely shape tactile experiences. Factors such as age and sex also play a key role in meanings associated with touch. Despite its individuality, touch is viewed as one of the most effective nonverbal ways to express feelings of comfort, love, affection, security, anger, frustration, aggression, excitement, and many others.

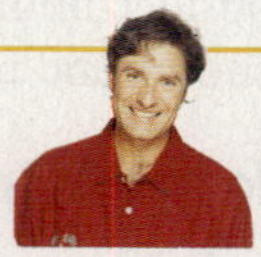

Recall ***Mr. Gordon***, the patient with end-stage liver disease who is in a coma. Although the patient may not respond verbally or be able to comprehend, the nurse could use touch to indicate concern and respect for the patient, thus sending a message that someone is there for him.

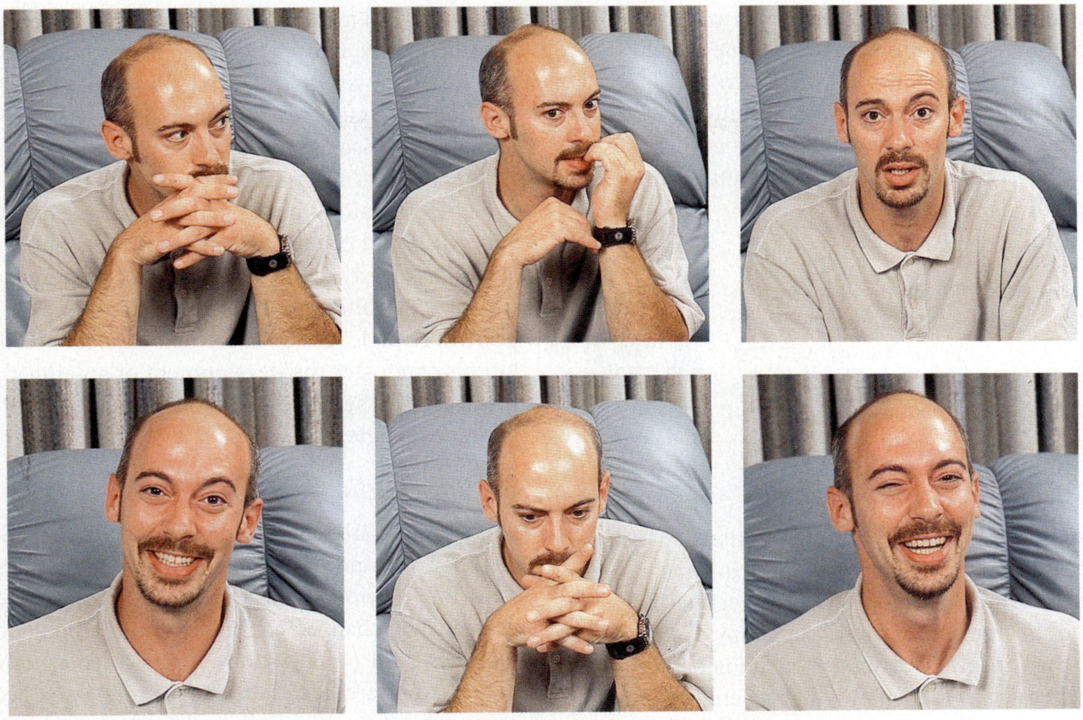

FIGURE 8-2. Eye contact, the lack of it, facial expression, posture, gesture, and silence send nonverbal messages to the receiver. What messages do you receive from each of these photographs?

Eye Contact

Communication often begins with eye contact, looking into the other person's eyes. A glance, for example, is often an attention-getting method to open conversation. In many cultures, eye contact suggests respect and a willingness to listen and to keep communication open. Its absence often indicates anxiety or defenselessness, or avoidance of communication. Some view eye contact as the nonverbal communication that reveals a person's true nature. However, some Native American and Asian cultures view eye contact as an invasion of a person's privacy or as confrontational. In other cultures, people are taught to avoid eye contact or, out of respect, not to make eye contact with a superior.

In addition to the messages sent by eye contact, the eyes carry other nonverbal messages. For example, the eyes fix in a stare during anger, tend to narrow in disgust, and ordinarily open wide in fear. Some people who experience fear might be unable to speak and only their eyes will send the message of anxiety. A blank stare can indicate daydreaming or inattentiveness.

Facial Expressions

The face is the most expressive part of the body. Examples of the various messages facial expressions convey are anger, joy, suspicion, sadness, fear, and contempt. Some people have extremely expressive faces, whereas others mask their feelings, making it more difficult to determine what the person is really thinking. Nurses need to learn to control their own facial expressions.

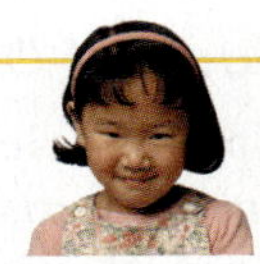

Consider **Susie Musashi**, the 3-year-old with burns. Preschoolers are naturally curious. So, she might watch the nurse's reaction when the nurse changes the burn dressings for the first time. Any sign of repulsion or disgust could greatly impact the child's self-image and recovery.

Posture

The way a person holds the body carries nonverbal messages. People in good health and with a positive attitude usually hold their bodies in good alignment. Depressed or tired people are more likely to slouch. Posture also often provides nonverbal clues concerning pain and physical limitations, for instance, a rigid, stiff appearance might be a good indicator of tension and pain.

Gait

A bouncy, purposeful walk usually carries a message of well-being. A less purposeful, shuffling gait often means the person is sad or discouraged. Certain gaits are associated with illness. For example, patients recovering from recent abdominal surgery usually walk slightly bent over and slowly and might need the assistance of handrails or a helping person.

Gestures

Gestures using various parts of the body can carry numerous messages—for example, thumbs up may mean victory, kicking an object often expresses anger, wringing the hands or tapping a foot usually indicates anxiety or anger, and a waving hand serves to beckon someone to come on, or if waved in another way, signifies that someone should leave. Gestures are often used extensively when two people speaking in different languages attempt to communicate with each other. Gestures may have different meanings in different cultures, and nurses must consider how culture influences the meaning (Tuohy, 2018).

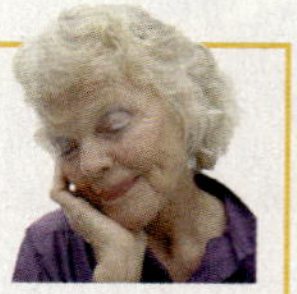

Remember **Mrs. Russellinski**, the 75-year-old recovering from pneumonia. Gestures would be very helpful in communicating with the patient, especially in light of the patient's hearing and language deficits.

General Physical Appearance

Many illnesses cause at least some alterations in general physical appearance. Observing for changes in appearance is an important nursing responsibility for detecting illness or evaluating the effectiveness of care and therapy. For example, a person with an insufficient intake of fluids has dry skin that wrinkles easily, eyes that might be sunken and dull in appearance, and poor muscle tone. On the other hand, the person in good health tends to radiate a healthy status through general appearance.

Mode of Dress and Grooming

A person's clothing and grooming practices carry significant nonverbal messages. For example, healthy people tend to pay attention to details of dress and grooming, whereas people feeling ill often demonstrate little interest in personal appearance. It is often a sign of returning health when interest in their physical appearance and mode of dress returns.

Sounds

Crying, moaning, gasping, and sighing are oral but nonverbal forms of communication. Such sounds can be interpreted in numerous ways. For example, a person might cry because of sadness or joy. Gasping often indicates fear, pain, or surprise. A sigh might be a sign of reluctant agreement to do something or of relief.

Silence

Periods of silence during a conversation often carry important nonverbal messages. A silence between two people might indicate complete understanding of each other, that both are thinking, or that they are angry with each other. Silence and its possible uses and meanings are discussed later in this chapter.

Communication Technologies

Electronic Communication

The Internet and a variety of social websites provide new and challenging opportunities for nurses to communicate and collaborate with other health care providers. The challenges of using social media include protecting patient privacy and confidentiality and preventing unintended consequences for the employer or the nurse. Protocols for using e-mail, sending text messages, and accessing the social media sites are vital for wise use of these forms of electronic communication. Student nurses also must know these guidelines for use of electronic communication venues. Educational institutions should orient students to professional expectations as well as clearly defined policies and procedures regarding use of electronic communication and social networking policies (Daigle, 2020). Increased exposure to these expectations can foster the development of an ethical conscience that begins when one is a student and carries into future practice (Daigle, 2020).

Social Media

Social media are web-based technologies that allow users to create, share, and participate in dialogue in virtual communities and networks. The availability of social media sites has dramatically changed communications among people, communities, and organizations. Social media networks allow nurses to share ideas, develop professional connections, access educational offerings and forums, receive support, and investigate evidence-based practices (Chan & Leung, 2018). Facebook, WhatsApp Messenger, Twitter, and LinkedIn are common social media sites used by nurses and other health care professionals (Chan & Leung, 2018). Concerns about social media occur when nurses inadvertently reveal information about patients that compromise the patients' privacy. Nurses must adhere to Health Insurance Portability and Accountability Act (HIPAA) regulations that protect patient confidentiality and privacy and be aware of their employers' policies about using social media. Health care facilities may specifically address personal use of computers in the facility and types of websites that may be accessed during working hours from employer computers. Health care facility policies often do not address employee use of social media when not at work, but disclosing information that violates the privacy and confidentiality of patients or professional standards and posting defamatory remarks about an employer, supervisor, coworker, or patient have serious consequences for nurses (National Council of State Boards of Nursing [NCSBN], 2018). Nurses are accountable for their use of social media and can be reported to a regulatory authority for an allegation of inappropriate use of social media, reflective of deviation from required professional competencies and standards for practice (Scruth et al., 2015).

Both the American Nurses Association (ANA) and the NCSBN have issued guidelines for RNs regarding use of social media. These organizations agree that professional boundaries must be followed in the social media environment. Refer to Box 8-2 for a discussion of the six principles for social networking relevant to registered nurses and nursing students endorsed by the ANA.

Often, inappropriate disclosures of information are unintentional. Nurses may expect that information they post is private, but, in reality, it can be shared with multiple other

Box 8-2 American Nurses Association's Principles for Social Networking

1. Nurses must not transmit or place online individually identifiable patient information.
2. Nurses must observe ethically prescribed professional patient–nurse boundaries.
3. Nurses should understand that patients, colleagues, institutions, and employers may view postings.
4. Nurses should take advantage of privacy settings and seek to separate personal and professional information online.
5. Nurses should bring content that could harm a patient's privacy, rights, or welfare to the attention of appropriate authorities.
6. Nurses should participate in developing institutional policies governing online conduct.

Source: Reprinted with permission from American Nurses Association (ANA). (2011). *ANA's Principles for social networking and the nurse.* Author.

recipients. It is also incorrect to assume that once information has been deleted from a site, it is no longer available. Describing a patient by using a room number or diagnosis rather than a name is still considered a breach of confidentiality and a violation of patient privacy.

Potential consequences for inappropriate use of social and electronic media by nurses vary, depending, in part, on the particular nature of the nurse's conduct (NCSBN, 2018). Inappropriate use of social and electronic media may be reported to the nurse's state board of nursing; reports of inappropriate disclosure by a nurse may be investigated on the grounds of unprofessional conduct, unethical conduct, moral turpitude, mismanagement of patient records, and/or breach of confidentiality (NCSBN, 2018). Disciplinary action by the board of nursing could include a reprimand or sanction, monetary fine, or temporary or permanent loss of licensure (NCSBN, 2018). In addition, improper use of social media by a nurse may violate state and federal laws related to patient privacy and confidentiality, with the potential for civil and criminal penalties, including monetary fines and possible incarceration (NCSBN, 2018). Employers may use social media to screen potential employees as long as they do not violate discrimination laws. Any information you have provided about yourself on a social media website may influence a hiring decision. In addition, you could also face employment consequences, including loss of employment, if content or conduct on a social media site violates the policies of an employer (NCSBN, 2018; Scruth et al., 2015).

The responsibility for understanding the use of social media to maintain professional standards lies with the practitioner. The ease with which information can be posted on a social media site allows minimal time to consider the implications and the effect a posting can have on a nurse's personal and professional life (NCSBN, 2018). Clear professional boundaries should be established by educational institutions for nursing students upon entry into nursing programs to support safe use of social media and to promote a positive image for the nursing profession (Daigle, 2020).

E-Mail and Text Messages

E-mail and text messages are efficient means to communicate with staff members and, in some cases, patients. The risk for violating patient privacy and confidentiality exists any time a message is sent electronically. Health care facilities usually have security measures in place to safeguard e-mail and text communications. E-mail and text messages should be concise and avoid text abbreviations. Nurses should be aware of facility policies and guidelines regarding the use of electronic communication with patients. The patient may have to sign an authorization permitting e-mail communication from the health care facility. Any e-mails sent to a patient must be duplicated and become part of the health record for that patient. While e-mail and text messages are additional communication tools, it is always necessary to follow facility policies and adhere to your professional code of conduct. Individualizing patient care requires nurses to determine which form of communication is most beneficial for each patient.

Telehealth and Telemedicine

Health and mobile health technologies make use of telecommunications and virtual technology to deliver health care services and health-related information outside of traditional health care facilities (Koivunen & Saranto). These technologies are used to support and promote long-distance clinical health care, patient and professional health-related education, public health, and health administration (The Office of the National Coordinator for Health Information Technology, 2017). Telehealth nursing uses technology to deliver nursing care and conduct nursing practice remotely to improve efficiency and patient access to health care (Adzhigirey et al., 2019). The use of connected health technologies does not alter the standards of professional practice (American Nurses Association, 2019). Effective communication between the patient and nurses is a significant part of provision of effective nursing care. The use of effective communication skills is essential to ensure successful telehealth encounters, positive patient experiences, and successful interprofessional collaboration (Sweeney Gustin et al., 2020). Both verbal and nonverbal communication skills impact and contribute to successful telehealth visits and collaboration (Sweeney Gustin et al., 2020). When engaging in telehealth activities, nurses should dress professionally; decrease distractors, such as environmental noise and clutter; ensure privacy and lack of interruptions; and make use of key nonverbal cues, including leaning in, nodding, and making eye contact, to communicate interest, empathy, and engagement with the patient or professional (Sweeney Gustin et al., 2020). Being a good listener is also essential (Mataxen & Webb, 2019). Telehealth nurses make use of clinical knowledge, technical skills, and communication skills to prioritize, initiate, and evaluate patient care.

LEVELS OF COMMUNICATION

Throughout our lives and the lives of our patients, communication occurs at varying levels. Nurses engage in four levels of communication during practice: intrapersonal communication, interpersonal communication, small-group communication, and organizational communication.

Intrapersonal Communication

Intrapersonal communication, or self-talk, is communication within a person. This communication is crucial because it affects the nurse's behavior and can enhance or detract from positive interactions with the patient and family. Imagine two different nursing students preparing for the first experience with a critically ill patient. Both are frightened. One tells herself, "Calm down, you've been in challenging situations before and always survived. You can handle this." The other repeatedly tells himself, "There's no way you can survive this experience. The instructor will be all over you, and you might as well admit defeat before you start." Obviously, the first student's positive self-talk is more helpful than that of the second student.

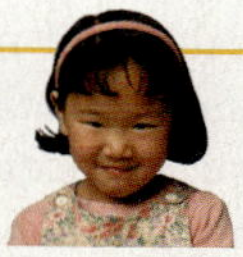

Consider **Susie Musashi**, the 3-year-old receiving treatment for her burns. The nurse may use self-talk when preparing to interact with the child, thereby helping her to focus on the child and her behaviors. In doing so, the nurse may be better able to interpret the child's messages. The nurse might say to herself, "I will use broad opening statements to help the patient and family express their feelings. I will talk to the patient on her level. I must maintain eye contact with the patient and family and answer their questions. I will not make light of the situation or appear unconcerned."

Understanding the importance of intrapersonal communication can also help you to work with patients and families whose negative self-talk affects their health and self-care abilities.

Interpersonal Communication

Interpersonal communication occurs between two or more people with a goal to exchange messages. Most of the nurse's day is spent communicating with patients, family members, and members of the health care team. The ability to communicate effectively at this level influences your sharing, problem solving, goal attainment, team building, and effectiveness in critical nursing roles (e.g., caregiver, teacher, counselor, leader, manager, patient advocate).

Group Communication

Group communication includes small-group and organizational group communication. To determine the effectiveness or ineffectiveness of a group, one studies the group dynamics.

Small-Group Communication

Small-group communication occurs when nurses interact with two or more people. To be functional, members of the small group must communicate to achieve their goal. Examples of small-group communication include staff meetings, patient care conferences, teaching sessions, and support groups. The more people involved in the communication process, the more complex it becomes.

Organizational Communication

Organizational communication occurs when people and groups within an organization communicate to achieve established goals. Nurses on a practice council working to review unit policies or nurses working with interdisciplinary groups on strategic planning or quality assurance use organizational communication to achieve their aims.

Group Dynamics

When determining the effectiveness or ineffectiveness of a group, one studies the group dynamics. **Group dynamics** involve how individual group members relate to one another during the process of working toward group goals.

Although effective leadership facilitates a group's achievement of its goals, success or failure largely results from members' behavior and associated communication. Ideally, all group members use their talents and interpersonal strengths to help the group to accomplish its goals. The group's ability to function at a high level depends on each member's sensitivity to the needs of the group and its individual members. Effective groups have members who are mutually respectful. If a group member dominates or thwarts the group process, then the leader or other group members must confront that member to promote the needed collegial relationship. Effective and ineffective groups are contrasted in Table 8-1.

FACTORS INFLUENCING COMMUNICATION

Factors influencing communication include level of development; sociocultural differences; roles and responsibilities; space and territoriality; physical, mental, and emotional state; and environment.

Developmental Level

The rate of language development is directly correlated with the patient's neurologic competence and cognitive development. Thus, it is helpful to understand the process of language development and the stages of intellectual and psychosocial development. This helps you communicate effectively with patients and family of all age ranges.

Table 8-1 Characteristics of Effective and Ineffective Groups

VARIABLE	EFFECTIVE GROUP	INEFFECTIVE GROUP
Group identity	Members value and "own" the aims of the group; aims are clearly articulated.	Group's aims are not of major importance to members. Members accept imposed goals.
Cohesiveness	Members generally trust and like one another and are loyal to the group; high commitment; high degree of cooperation.	Members often feel alienated from the group and from one another; low commitment; members tend to work better alone than with the group.
Patterns of interaction	Honest, direct communication flows freely and is two-way; members support, praise, and critique one another.	Communication is sparing and/or one-way; little self-disclosure; self-serving roles (i.e., dominator, blocker, or aggressor) may be unchecked.
Decision making	Problems are identified, appropriate method of decision making is used (i.e., individual, minority, majority, consensus, or unanimous); decision is implemented and followed through; group commitment to decision is high.	Problems are allowed to build without resolution; little responsibility is shown for problem solving; group commitment to decision is low.
Responsibility	Members feel strong sense of responsibility for group outcomes.	Little responsibility for group felt by group members.
Leadership	Effective style of leadership meets desired aims. Participation and leadership are distributed among all members.	Ineffective leadership styles are used. Leadership is delegated and based on authority.
Power	Sources of power are recognized and used appropriately; needs or interests of those with little power are considered.	Power is used and abused to "fix" immediate problems; little attention to needs of powerless.

Source: Johnson, D. W., & Johnson, F. P. (2017). *Joining together: Group theory and group skills.* (The counselling series) (12th ed.). Pearson; Townsend, M., & Morgan, K. I. (2018). *Psychiatric mental health nursing: Concepts of care in evidence-based practice* (9th ed.). F.A. Davis Company; and Videbeck, S. L. (2020). *Psychiatric mental health nursing* (8th ed.). Wolters Kluwer.

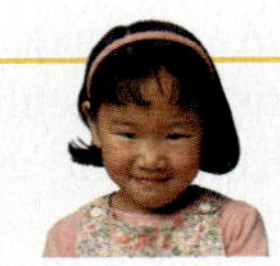

Remember **Susie Musashi**, the 3-year-old child with burns. The nurse would incorporate knowledge of the typical preschooler fears (such as fear of new places and fear of the dark) when developing the child's plan of care. Preschoolers gain self-esteem by receiving compliments about their appearance. The presence of the burns directly affects the child's appearance, possibly threatening self-esteem. Therefore, the nurse also needs to consider the child's current fears related to her burns and burn treatment and their effect on the child's self-esteem.

The stages of development are presented in Chapters 22, 23, and 24. Knowing how each age group commonly perceives health, illness, and body functions should guide your interactions with patients. For instance, a 10-year-old child has limited understanding of what an infection is; therefore, explain things in simple terms so that the child cooperates with the treatment without being frightened. Because adolescents are developing abstract thinking, more detailed and accurate explanations can be given to them. Being familiar with commonly used slang usually helps when communicating with adolescents. Communicating with adults can be affected by their past positive or negative health-related experiences and by inaccurate information. When communicating with older adults, assess for any problems with hearing or sight (discussed later in this chapter, on pages 202–203), confusion, or depression, any of which could affect nurse–patient interaction.

Sociocultural Differences

Nurses need to recognize ways in which culture and social determinants of health, such as economic condition, education and literacy (including health literacy), and overall lifestyle influence a patient's functioning and preferred mode of communicating. This will help you understand what the patient understands. Detailed discussion of considerations related to social determinants of health and health care are provided in Chapters 3 and 4.

Culture refers to the common lifestyles, languages, behavior patterns, traditions, and beliefs that are learned and passed from one generation to the next. Development of cultural competence requires becoming aware of your own personal cultural beliefs and identifying prejudices or attitudes that could affect interactions with persons different from you or be a barrier to good communication (Kersey-Matusiak, 2019). Likewise, understanding a patient's culture helps you understand nonverbal communication and deliver appropriate nursing care to the patient and family. For example, women in some cultures may speak of personal concerns only to their spouses; in such instances, a maternal care nurse might talk with the patient's husband about the woman's postdelivery care. Additional discussion of culture and provision of person-centered culturally respectful care is provided in Chapter 5.

According to Census Bureau data from the 2017 American Community Survey, the number of U.S. residents who speak a language other than English at home has reached an all-time high: one in five (Zeigler & Camarota, 2018). Patients with limited proficiency in English have difficulty understanding health care instructions, understanding test results and diagnoses, and participating in treatment decisions (Chung et al., 2020). Low health literacy and, difficulty understanding and using health information compound these issues (The Joint Commission, 2020a). In addition, the health care system is a culture with its own customs, values, and language. Try to remain aware of these cultural variations and be careful to use lay terminology when speaking with patients, unless you know that the patient is a health care professional. Use of medical terminology (e.g., myocardial infarction for heart attack, cerebrovascular accident for stroke [brain attack], or cholecystectomy for gallbladder operation) or abbreviations usually alienates patients and can inhibit further communication. Detailed discussion of considerations related to health literacy is provided in Chapter 9.

A patient's language proficiency, support system, cultural preferences, and socioeconomic circumstances should be evaluated upon contact with health care services and admission to health care facilities to facilitate communication and improve the quality of care (Moscrop et al., 2019). The Joint Commission (2020a) recommends an approach to communicating health information that encompasses language needs, individual understanding, and cultural and other communication issues. Nurses and other health care providers should be adaptive and culturally sensitive to patient needs to ensure effective communication; thoughtful, person-centered care; and improved patient outcomes (Chung et al., 2020; Tuohy, 2019).

Roles and Responsibilities

Patients function through various roles and responsibilities; the number and types of roles vary but may include family (child, spouse, partner), occupation (student, employer), and activities (club member, choir member) (Videbeck, 2020). Identification of the role or roles a person occupies may give the nurse some insight into the person's identity. Stereotyping a person according to a role or roles, however, can be misleading and should be avoided. This can be hazardous, for instance, when nurses assume that patients who are health care professionals know everything about their condition and need little nursing assistance, teaching, and counseling.

The challenge in the provision of care is to respect the patient's roles and responsibilities, especially because these roles influence their preferred manner of communicating, without denying the patient needed care. For example, a successful attorney might have a "take-charge" demeanor and seem utterly self-sufficient; a skilled nurse will note this but still provide an opening for the patient to verbalize their needs. "You seem well prepared for this procedure and in control, but I know that patients often have questions that never get answered or fears that remain unvoiced. Is there anything I can help you with while I'm here?" Similarly, be careful not to ignore an uncomplaining patient (occupying the role of patient) who never asks for anything, because the power differences in the health care professional–patient relationship may make communication intimidating.

Space and Territoriality

People are most comfortable in areas they consider their own. We generally feel relief when we come home, take our shoes and professional clothes off, and relax. This urge to maintain an exclusive right to certain space is termed territoriality. You might have already noticed that patients behave differently when being interviewed in their homes, at a health fair in the mall, or in an institutional setting. Similarly, health care professionals might behave differently when they are "on their own turf" in a health care setting compared to when they enter a patient's home as a guest caregiver. It is important to understand how territoriality influences the nurse–patient relationship.

The actual physical difference between the nurse and patient during interaction is also important. *Proxemics* is the study of distance zones between people during communication (Videbeck, 2020). Each person has a sense of how much personal or private space is needed and what distance between people is optimum. Figure 8-3 demonstrates the four communication zones. Activities that are likely to occur during each of these zones include:

- Intimate zone: interaction between parents and children or people who desire close personal contact
- Personal zone: distance when interacting with close friends
- Social zone: space when interacting with acquaintances such as in a work or social setting
- Public zone: communication when speaking to an audience or small groups

An understanding of personal space and distancing characteristics can enhance the quality of communication (Videbeck, 2020). Some aspects of communication zones are dictated

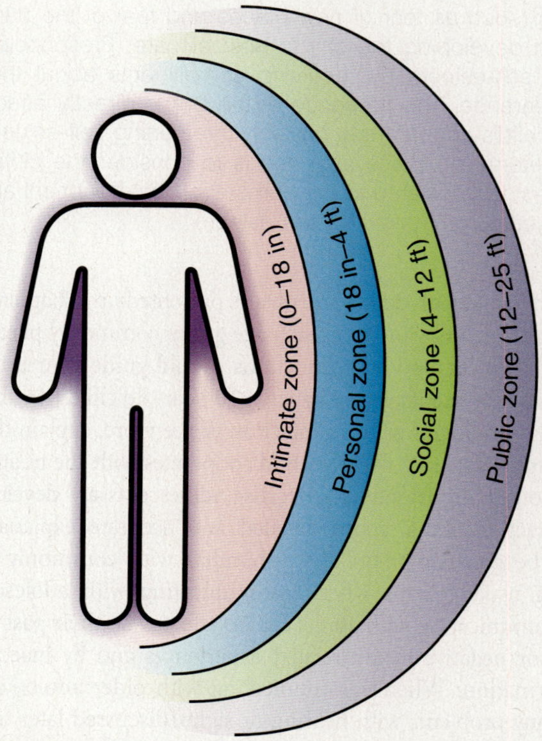

FIGURE 8-3. These four distance zones around the body are recognized as communication zones.

through culture, and some are idiosyncratic. Anywhere from 18 in to 4 ft might be optimal distance to sit from a patient during an intake interview. For example, some European Americans and African Americans might require more personal space between two people who are speaking than some people in other cultures (Mediterranean, Hispanic, Asian, Middle Eastern, East Indian) who might be comfortable at a closer distance when speaking (Videbeck, 2020). It is best to take cues from patients, noting whether they are moving backward from you if you are too near or leaning forward to get closer to you. Because many nursing interventions place one in proximity to a patient and entail forced intimacy, be sensitive to how offensive this might be to certain patients who are accustomed to large areas of private space. Develop the habit of seeking the patient's permission before entering the intimate or personal zone (Videbeck, 2020). Although most people consider their hands, arms, shoulders, and back within a social zone, increased levels of privacy are accorded to (1) mouth and feet; (2) face, neck, and front of body; and (3) genitalia.

Physical, Mental, and Emotional State

The degree to which people are physically comfortable and mentally and emotionally free to engage in interactions also influences communication. A full bladder, a dull headache, crushing chest pain, anxiety about a pending diagnosis or concern about what is happening at home or at work, and fear can all negatively influence communication. For example, patients who think that a nurse wants to hurt them will be difficult to interview. Be sensitive to the patient's physical, mental, and emotional barriers to effective communication.

Cognitively impaired patients and patients with other communication difficulties present special communication challenges. For example, an older adult who has dementia and is agitated due to pain from an abscessed tooth might be unable to communicate with the nurse. Nurses and other health care providers must consider augmentative and alternative communication (AAC) strategies to adjust conversation when providing care to "communication vulnerable" patients (Stans et al., 2018). AAC strategies include formal assistive communication systems (e.g., voice communication aids), handwriting, pictograms, and gesturing (Stans et al., 2018).

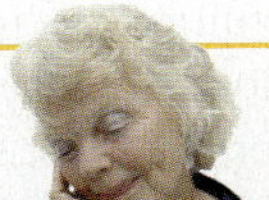

Remember **Irwina Russellinski**, the 75-year-old woman who was described as "being pleasantly confused" at times and requiring an initial nursing assessment. The patient's level of confusion presents challenges for the nurse when eliciting information for the nursing history. This challenge could be further complicated by the patient's limited use and understanding of English. The nurse needs to speak clearly, distinctly, and in terms that the patient understands, asking for clarification as needed. The nurse should make use of translation resources provided by the long-term facility. In addition, the nurse needs to allow ample time for the patient to respond and explore other sources for needed information. It is important for the nurse to convey patience and caring through nonverbal measures.

Values

Communication is influenced by the way people value themselves, one another, and the purpose of any human interaction. For example, nurses who believe that teaching is an important aspect of nursing and who value empowering patients will communicate this to patients. Conversely, a nurse who believes teaching is an unimportant chore is unlikely to be an effective teacher. Similarly, the patient's motivation (or lack of motivation) to develop new self-care behaviors cannot help but influence nurse–patient communication.

Environment

Communication happens best when the environment facilitates an easy exchange of needed information. The environment most conducive to communication is one that is calm and nonthreatening. The goal is to minimize distractions and ensure privacy. The use of music, art, and interior decorations might help put the patient at ease. A patient with newly diagnosed human immunodeficiency virus (HIV) infection may find it difficult to discuss sexual history or genital warts in an area that lacks privacy. A toddler might find it easier to communicate if a parent, favorite stuffed animal, or blanket is nearby.

USING PROFESSIONAL COMMUNICATION IN THE NURSING PROCESS

The ability to communicate with patients, other nurses, and other health care professionals is essential for effective use of the nursing process. Knowledge of the communication process and effective communication techniques is fundamental to all steps of the nursing process. At the same time, the nursing process provides the guidance and direction needed to communicate in a professional manner clearly, effectively, and compassionately.

Assessing

The major focus of assessment is to gather information in both verbal and nonverbal communication forms. Before the assessment, the nurse should determine if the patient needs any assistive devices in order to communicate effectively and understand conversations (e.g., hearing aid, glasses, etc.). Identify the patient's preferred language and secure an interpreter if one is needed, or plan for use of other AAC strategies to address patient communication needs (Stans et al., 2018).

The written word is used to obtain patient data and when reading patients' records or charts before meeting them. The spoken word is used to give and to receive reports to and from other health personnel. This is commonplace when admitting a patient to a hospital unit or before visiting the patient at home. One-to-one communication is used with patients to obtain thorough nursing histories, physical examinations, and other assessments. Effective communication techniques, as well as observational skills, are used extensively during

Examples of Actual or Potential Health Problems and Needs

COMMUNICATION

Actual or Potential Health Problems and Needs	Possible Etiologic Factors	Potential Signs and Symptoms
Impaired Verbal Communication	• Insufficient stimuli • Cultural incongruence • Physiologic condition • Alteration in perception • Emotional disturbance	• Difficulty speaking • Slurred speech • Inappropriate verbalization • Disoriented to person, place, or time • Inability to speak language of caregiver
Hearing Impairment	• Congenital condition • Physiologic condition • Consequence of aging • Chronic exposure to loud noises	• Lack of response to verbal queries/directions • Inappropriate verbalization • Difficulty understanding verbal communication • Frequently asking to have conversation repeated

Source: International Council of Nurses (ICN). (2019). *Nursing diagnosis and outcome statements.* https://www.icn.ch/sites/default/files/inline-files/ICNP2019-DC.pdf; Wolters Kluwer. (2020). Problem-based care plans. In *Lippincott Advisor.* Wolters Kluwer.

this phase. The data collected verbally and nonverbally are analyzed, documented, and shared with appropriate people through oral and written communication.

Diagnosing Actual or Potential Health Problems and Needs

An assessment of the patient may lead to the identification of one or more actual or potential health problems and needs related to communication. Following the formulation of the actual or potential health problems and needs, the nurse communicates findings to other nursing and health care professionals through the use of the written and spoken word. The written actual or potential health problem or need becomes a permanent part of the patient's health record. Examples of health problems and needs with related etiology and signs and symptoms can be found in the box titled Examples of Actual or Potential Health Problems and Needs: Communication.

Outcome Identification and Planning

The planning step requires communication among the patient, nurse, and other team members as mutually agreed-upon outcomes are developed and interventions are determined. Because a nurse is rarely able to implement all parts of a plan alone, oral and written communication is needed to inform others of what needs to be done to meet the set objectives or goals. The formal written plan of care is a form of communication. Without communication, the plan of care could not be implemented and continuity in care would not be possible.

Implementing

Nurses assume many roles when they implement the plan of care. Verbal and nonverbal communication methods enhance basic caregiving measures and are used to teach, counsel, and support patients and their families during the implementation phase. Even a simple nursing intervention, such as "encourage patient to drink 100 mL of fluid every hour while awake," requires countless messages to be sent and received between the nurse and the patient and the nurse and other nurses and health care providers. The nurse explains the importance of an adequate fluid intake, along with the amount and frequency of intake. The nurse communicates the plan to others involved in the care of the patient. The patient, in turn, speaks of their preference for fluids and ability or inability to meet targeted objectives. The patient's verbal and nonverbal messages are assessed during each nurse–patient interaction. The implementation of the nursing care plan is then documented in the patient's record.

Evaluating

Nurses often rely on verbal and nonverbal cues from patients to verify whether patient objectives or goals have been achieved. Communication, through the exchange of positive and negative messages between the nurse and the patient, also facilitates the revision of parts of the plan of care.

DOCUMENTING COMMUNICATION

Continual assessment of the patient's needs and conditions requires accurate documentation in the appropriate location. Because one nurse cannot provide 24-hour coverage for patients, significant information must be passed on to others; effective communication among health care professionals is essential to the coordination and continuity of thoughtful, person-centered care. The use of various forms of documenting and reporting, including nursing progress notes and plans of care, are important parts of effective communication. Documentation, reporting, and the use of electronic communication are discussed in detail in Chapter 20.

EFFECTIVE PROFESSIONAL COMMUNICATION

Cooperation, coordination, and collaboration in interactions between nurses and other health care professionals are a vital part of the provision of safe, effective, high-quality, and thoughtful person-centered care. Effective professional communication is an integral aspect of these interactions, supporting the continuum of teamwork necessary to deliver patient care (Bochatay, 2019; Tingle, 2018). Nurses and other health care professionals utilize various communication processes, including hand-off communication and other structured communication techniques, to support effective exchange of information.

Hand-off Communication: SBAR

A "hand-off" occurs when the responsibility for care is transferred from one care provider to another (PSNet, 2019). Hand-off communication involves the process of accurate presentation and acceptance of patient-related information from one caregiver or team to another caregiver or team. Hand-off communication occurs between nurses and other departments in the facility, during nurse-to-nurse report, or in nurse-to-other health care professional discussions and occurs numerous times per day. However, miscommunication between health care providers during hand-off communication and inadequate hand-off communication are significant contributing factors to adverse patient events, such as wrong-site surgery, delay in treatment, falls, and medication errors (The Joint Commission, 2017; PSNet, 2019).

In an effort to eliminate breakdowns in communication and potential adverse events, the Joint Commission has included a goal to improve the effectiveness of communication among caregivers as a National Patient Safety Goal (The Joint Commission, 2021). Structured communication techniques can help health care team members ensure accuracy and make decisions (Pettit & Duffy, 2015). Implementation of a standardized communication tool has been shown to reduce the risk of transmitting inaccurate and incomplete information (Galatzan & Carrington, 2018). However, standardized hand-off tools "must be flexible to meet various needs of each nurse, nursing unit, health-care environment, and patient situation" (Galatzan & Carrington, p. 485).

The Joint Commission, Joint Commission International, and the Institute for Healthcare Improvement (IHI) have all recommended using the SBAR method to improve hand-off communication (IHI, 2017; The Joint Commission, 2017; Joint Commission International [JCI], 2018). **SBAR**, which stands for **S**ituation, **B**ackground, **A**ssessment, and **R**ecommendations, provides a consistent method for hand-off communication that is clear, structured, and easy to use. This technique was originally developed by the U.S. Navy to accurately transmit critical information, and later adapted by Kaiser Permanente of Colorado to facilitate communication in health care (JCI, 2018). The **S** (Situation) and **B** (Background) provide objective data, whereas the **A** (Assessment) and **R** (Recommendations) allow for presentation of subjective information. The SBAR method has been used to enhance the clarity and efficiency of communication between health care team members (Padgett, 2018). The SBAR format is widely used in health care and can be modified to meet the specific situations related to shift reports, conversations with physicians and other health care providers, and transfer of patients. SBAR has been successfully used to improve hand-off communication, bedside shift report, teamwork, and the perception of patient safety culture (Bonds, 2018; Clark et al., 2020). An electronic SBAR template has been used to improve documentation and communication between nurses and other health care providers (Panesar et al., 2016; Sermersheim et al., 2020). Figure 8-4 (on page 186) provides an example of a basic SBAR communication tool used between a nurse and another health care provider. SBAR is also discussed in Chapters 12, 17, and 20.

Technology Alert

An SBAR template has been implemented as part of electronic documentation. The use of an electronic SBAR hand-off has been associated with improved communication, as well as more complete documentation and increased frequency of documentation of communication among nurses and health care providers (Panesar et al., 2016; Sermersheim et al., 2020).

I-SBAR-R and the QSEN Institute

The Quality and Safety Education for Nurses (QSEN) Institute identifies quality and safety competencies for nursing, with the goal of preparing future nurses with the knowledge, skills, and attitudes necessary to improve the quality and safety of the health care systems within which they work (QSEN, n.d.). QSEN also provides teaching strategies and resources to assist nurse educators to meet the QSEN goals. One such teaching resource suggests a revised SBAR for use with nursing students to improve communication and support safe practice. This adapted form includes the initial identification of "yourself and your patient (**I**)" and the opportunity to ask and respond to questions, or "readback (**R**)," at the close of the communication (Quality and Safety Education for Nurses [QSEN] Institute, 2008). This reformulated **I-SBAR-R** supports clear identification of the nurse and the patient when communicating patient care information or concerns with another health care provider.

SBAR and The Joint Commission: The Hand-Off TST

The Joint Commission Center for Transforming Healthcare developed the Hand-off Communication Targeted Solutions Tool (TST), which examines hand-off communication problems and identifies causes for failures and barriers to improvement (The Joint Commission Center for Transforming Healthcare, n.d.). This tool also provides evidence-based solutions to improve hand-off communication targeted to specific causes of inadequate hand-off at an individual organization (The Joint Commission Center for Transforming Healthcare, n.d.).

Rising Level of Concern Communication: CUS

Structured communication techniques can help health care team members communicate effectively and accurately;

S

SITUATION

I am calling about ______________________________

The patient's Code status is: ______________

The problem I am calling about is: ______________________

(e.g., I AM CONCERNED THE PATIENT IS GOING TO ARREST)

I have just assessed the patient personally:

Vital signs are: Blood pressure ________/________, Pulse ________, Respiration ____________, and temperature ________

I am concerned about the:

Blood pressure because it is	over 200 or	less than 100 or	30 mm Hg below usual
Pulse because it is	over 130 or	less than 40 and symptomatic	
Respiration because it is	less than 8 or	over 30	
Temperature because it is	less than 96 or	over 104	
Urine output because it is	less than 25 mL/hr or 200 mL/8 hr		
O_2 saturation because it is	less than 88% on 6/L nasal cannula		

Other: ______________________________

B

BACKGROUND

The patient's mental status is:

Alert and oriented to person, place, and time

Confused and cooperative or non-cooperative

Agitated or combative

Lethargic but conversant and able to swallow

Stuporous and not talking clearly and possibly not able to swallow

Comatose Eyes closed Not responding to stimulation.

The skin is:

Warm and dry

Pale

Mottled

Diaphoretic

Extremities are cold

Extremities are warm

The patient is not or is on oxygen.

The patient has been on __________ (L/min) or (5) oxygen for __________ minutes (hours)

The oximeter is reading __________ %

The oximeter does not detect a good pulse and is giving erratic readings.

A

ASSESSMENT

This is what I think the problem is: ______________________

"SAY WHAT YOU THINK IS THE PROBLEM"

The problem seems to be cardiac infection neurologic respiratory

I am not sure what the problem is but the patient is deteriorating.

The patient seems to be unstable and may get worse, we need to do something.

R

RECOMMENDATION

From Physician ______________________________

Transfer the patient to Critical Care.

Come to see the patient at this time.

Talk to the patient or family about Code status.

Ask a consultant to see patient now.

Are any tests needed:

Do you need any tests like CXR ABG EKG CBC BMP

Others: ______________________________

If a change in treatment is ordered then ask:

How often do you want vital signs?

How long do you expect this problem will last?

If the patient does not get better when would you want us to call again?

FIGURE 8-4. Sample SBAR Communication Tool. (*Source:* Reprinted with permission from the Institute for Healthcare Improvement. http://www.ihi.org/knowledge/Pages/Tools/SampleSBARCommunicationTool.aspx)

these patient advocacy tools can also help team members take action to escalate concerns (Clapper, 2018). CUS is another communication tool, recommended for use to assist in effective communication related to patient safety concerns. **CUS**, which stands for I'm **C**oncerned, I'm **U**ncomfortable, This is un**S**afe (This is a **S**afety issue), was developed from an airline safety program and provides mutually agreed-upon critical language for communication (Tocco, 2014). CUS offers a consistent method for health care team members to speak up about patient safety concerns in an assertive manner that is clear, structured, and easy to use (Agency for Healthcare Research and Quality, 2020). CUS can be used when the nurse feels there is an unsafe situation and needs to effectively communicate this concern to other health care providers.

Additional information related to effective reporting and professional and interprofessional communication is discussed in Chapter 20.

USING PROFESSIONAL COMMUNICATION IN THE THERAPEUTIC RELATIONSHIP

Nurses and other health care personnel enter health care in order to help people. Relationships between health care providers and patients develop in part through use of purposeful communication. A caring, **therapeutic relationship** exists among people who provide and receive assistance in meeting human needs. It sets the climate for the participants to move toward common goals. Therefore, the patient's needs are met as the result of a successful therapeutic relationship.

When a nurse and patient are involved in a caring, therapeutic relationship, known as the **nurse–patient relationship**, the nurse is the carer and the patient is the person being cared for, in the context of mutual respect and value. The relationship between the nurse and patient is focused on promoting or restoring the health and well-being of the patient; the quality of the relationship between these people is the most significant element in determining its effectiveness. "Of all the problems that can arise in nursing care, perhaps the most common is failure to establish rapport and a helping–trust relationship with the other person" (Watson, 1985, p. 24). Communication is the means used to establish rapport and trusting, therapeutic relationships. In this book, the terms therapeutic relationship and nurse–patient relationship are used interchangeably to refer to such relationships between nurses and patients (Fig. 8-5).

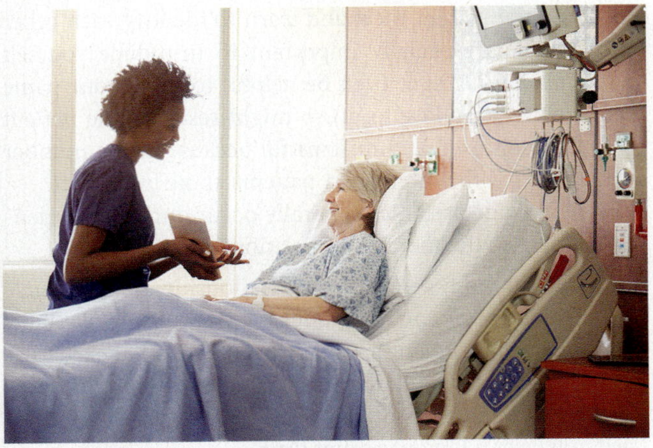

FIGURE 8-5. A therapeutic relationship between the nurse and patient sets the climate for participants to move toward common goals. (*Source: Photo by Monkey Business Images/Shutterstock.*)

Therapeutic Versus Social Relationships

The difference between a therapeutic relationship and a friendship is important. Therapeutic relationships contain many of the qualities of a social relationship—they have in common the components of care, concern, trust, and growth. They are also very different:

- The therapeutic relationship does not occur spontaneously, as do most social relationships. It occurs for a specific purpose with a specific person.
- The therapeutic relationship is characterized by an unequal sharing of information. The patient shares information related to personal health problems, whereas the nurse shares information in terms of a professional role. In a friendship, information sharing is more likely to be similar in quantity and type.
- The therapeutic relationship is built on the patient's needs, not on those of the nurse. In a friendship, needs of both participants are generally considered. A friendship might grow out of a therapeutic relationship, but this is separate from the purposeful, time-limited interaction described as a nurse–patient relationship.

It is important to remember that therapeutic relationships are professional relationships. It can be helpful to identify nurse models who, through their appearance, demeanor, and behavior, communicate a clear sense of professionalism or confidence and expertise in their practice. Patients and the public are more likely to trust and value nurses who appear competent and confident and who are focused on the patients entrusted to their care. Rudeness, sloppiness, inattention to person, sexually inappropriate behavior, and other breaches of professionalism undermine nursing's professional image and the effectiveness of individual nurses. Nursing and professionalism is discussed in detail in Chapter 1. Caring; therapeutic relationships; and thoughtful, person-centered care are also discussed in Chapter 13.

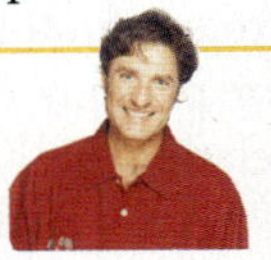

Think back to **Mr. Gordon**, the patient described in the Reflective Practice display, and consider the behavior of the nurse and residents caring for the patient. Unfortunately, their focus was not on the patient as a whole but, rather, on the patient's devices and technologic equipment. The nurse needs to keep in mind the highly technical nature of the ICU and work to implement a plan of care that focuses on the "whole" patient.

Characteristics of the Therapeutic Nurse–Patient Relationship

The therapeutic (nurse–patient) relationship is intangible, and therefore difficult to describe. It is thought that it has at least the following basic characteristics:

- It is a caring, person-centered relationship.
- It is dynamic. Both the person providing the assistance and the person being helped are active participants to the extent each is able.

- It is purposeful and time limited. This means there are specific goals that are intended to be met within a certain period.
- Although both parties in the therapeutic relationship have responsibilities, the person providing the assistance is professionally accountable for the outcomes of the relationship and the means used to attain them. Nurses should present their helping abilities as honestly as possible and not promise to provide more assistance than they can offer.

Goals of the Therapeutic Relationship

The goals of a therapeutic relationship (nurse–patient relationship) are determined cooperatively and are defined in terms of the patient's needs. Broadly speaking, common goals might include increased independence for the patient, greater feelings of worth, and improved health and well-being. Selected nursing interventions will help the person move toward the goal. As the patient's needs and goals change, so do the nursing care interventions implemented to attain the patient's goals. You might also have many needs to be met, but in the therapeutic relationship between the nurse and the patient, those are temporarily set aside—the focus is on the patient's needs (Videbeck, 2020).

Phases of the Therapeutic Relationship

The therapeutic (nurse–patient) relationship is often described as having three phases: (1) the orientation phase, (2) the identification and exploration (or working) phase, and (3) the resolution (or termination) phase (Peplau, 1952; Registered Nurses' Association of Ontario [RNAO], n.d.). In clinical practice, the phases are not that clear-cut, with varying overlap and interlock (Videbeck, 2020). In the therapeutic relationship, the communication process follows the sequence of the nursing process. Both processes are continuous and reciprocal. Box 8-3 summarizes goals for patients during the phases of an effective therapeutic relationship.

Nurse–patient relationships vary in depth, length, and focus. In some situations, one nurse initiates the therapeutic relationship and works with the patient and family through to termination. More often (e.g., in acute care settings), different nurses at different times are implementing different phases of the relationship. In addition, a brief therapeutic encounter might last only a few minutes, focusing on the patient's immediate needs; a longer hospitalization might result in a relationship that lasts weeks (Keltner & Steele, 2019). The current environment of health care includes brief hospitalization and time-limited care (Keltner & Steele). In this context, Keltner and Steele suggest the phases of the therapeutic (nurse–patient) relationship are often not a sequence of processes, but different emphases or goals. The nurse concentrates on nursing approaches in a particular phase, depending on the status and needs of the individual patient (Keltner & Steele, p. 85).

Box 8-3 Summary of Patient Goals for the Three Phases of the Therapeutic Nurse–Patient Relationship

Orientation Phase

- The patient will call the nurse by name.
- The patient will accurately describe the roles of the participants in the relationship.
- The patient and nurse will establish an agreement about:
  - Goals of the relationship
  - Location, frequency, and length of the contacts
  - Duration of the relationship

Working Phase

- The patient will actively participate in the relationship.
- The patient will cooperate in activities that work toward achieving mutually acceptable goals.
- The patient will express feelings and concerns to the nurse.

Termination

- The patient will participate in identifying the goals accomplished or the progress made toward goals.
- The patient will verbalize feelings about the termination of the relationship.

Source: Adapted from Townsend, M., & Morgan, K. I. (2018). *Psychiatric mental health nursing: Concepts of care in evidence-based practice* (9th ed.). F.A. Davis Company; Videbeck, S. L. (2020). *Psychiatric mental health nursing* (8th ed.). Wolters Kluwer.

In preparation for the orientation phase, nurses might use interpersonal communication to prepare for the data-gathering phase of the interaction with the patient.

Orientation Phase

The nurse–patient relationship ideally begins between the nurse and patient during the data-gathering part of the nursing process. It can also be initiated at other times during the nurse–patient relationship. In the orientation phase, the tone and guidelines for the relationship are established. The nurse and the patient meet and learn to identify each other by name. It is especially important to introduce yourself to the patient; it might even be helpful to write your name for the patient. Failure to do so might result in the patient becoming confused and mistrustful because of the number of caregivers with whom most patients come in contact.

The following activities generally occur during the orientation phase of the therapeutic relationship:

- The roles of both people in the relationship are clarified.
- An agreement or contract about the relationship is established. The agreement is usually a simple verbal exchange related to goals and the means of achieving them or occasionally a written document, especially if the relationship extends over a long period of time.
- The patient is provided with an orientation to the health care facility, its services, admission routines, and any

pertinent information the patient requires to decrease anxiety. This orientation should be identified as one of the goals in the nurse–patient relationship.

The development of a trusting relationship is critical to the development of the nurse–patient relationship. Exhibiting openness and interest in the concerns of the patient paves the way for developing trust and communicating care and respect.

Working Phase

The working phase is usually the longest phase of the nurse–patient relationship. During this phase, the nurse works together with the patient to meet the patient's physical and psychosocial needs. Interaction is the essence of the working phase. Nurse–patient interactions that occur at this time are purposeful in that they are designed to ensure achievement of health goals or objectives that were mutually agreed upon.

In addition, the nurse as caregiver provides the patient with whatever assistance might be needed to perform activities of daily living. For example, if a patient with impaired mobility is unable to get out of bed except to use a bedside commode, the nurse or caregiver needs to help with daily hygiene.

The nursing roles of teacher and counselor (see Chapter 9) are performed primarily during this phase. These roles involve motivating the patient to learn and to implement health-promotion activities, to facilitate the patient's ability to execute the plan of care, and to express feelings about health problems, nursing care, any progress or setbacks, and any other areas of concern. This is where your interpersonal skills are used to their fullest. A breakdown of the nurse–patient relationship on one of these levels could result in serious consequences. Satisfactory interaction preserves people's integrity while promoting an atmosphere characterized by minimal fear, anxiety, distrust, and tension. People feel harmonious and contented with each other as they work cooperatively to reach common goals.

Termination Phase

The termination phase occurs when the conclusion of the initial agreement is acknowledged. This might happen at change-of-shift time, when the patient is discharged, or when a nurse takes vacation or employment elsewhere. At this point, you'll examine with the patient the goals of the therapeutic relationship for indications of their attainment or for evidence of progress toward them. If the goals/outcomes have been reached, this fact should be acknowledged. Such acknowledgment generally results in a feeling of satisfaction for the patient and nurse. If the goals/outcomes have not been reached, the progress can be acknowledged and either the patient or you might make suggestions for future efforts.

Ordinarily, emotions are associated with the termination of a nurse–patient relationship. If the goals have been met, there is often regret about ending a satisfying relationship, even though a sense of accomplishment persists. If the goals have not been achieved, the patient might experience anxiety and fear about the future. Whatever the feelings, patients should be encouraged to express their emotions about the termination.

You can prepare for the termination of the nurse–patient relationship in various ways. It is thoughtful to set the stage for the patient to establish a therapeutic relationship with another nurse, if appropriate. You can also assist the patient transferring from one facility to another or from one unit in a facility to another by offering explanations concerning the transfer. In some instances, you might introduce the patient to personnel who will be giving care.

Interpersonal relations are discussed in greater detail in the classic works of nursing theorists Orlando (1961), Paterson and Zderad (1976), Peplau (1952), Travelbee (1971), and Watson (1985).

Factors Promoting Effective Communication Within the Therapeutic Relationship

Despite the fact that patient stays in health care facilities are shorter than in the past and there is now an increased reliance on technology, skilled professional communication with patients and their families is essential and remains a vital part of the therapeutic (nurse–patient) relationship. Nurses who are competent, honest, skilled communicators are viewed as effective and compassionate caregivers. This focus on therapeutic relationships is a critical component of what nurses do and plays a vital role in promoting healing, enhancing safety, and improving clinical outcomes.

Dispositional Traits

A dispositional trait is a characteristic or customary way of behaving. Nurses who consistently demonstrate warmth and friendliness; openness and rapport; empathy, honesty, authenticity, and trust; caring; and competence are well disposed to communicate effectively.

WARMTH AND FRIENDLINESS

Initiation of a therapeutic (nurse–patient) relationship depends on the nurse's ability to begin the orientation phase successfully. A pleasant greeting and friendly smile can facilitate this phase and place the patient at ease. By maintaining qualities of warmth and friendliness throughout the nurse–patient relationship, you will convey continuous acceptance of the patient and interest in discussing the patient's feelings and concern.

OPENNESS AND RESPECT

One key factor to effective communication is to be open, accepting, frank, respectful, and without prejudice. Patients who feel that a nurse is being judgmental might withhold significant information. You need to develop sensitivity to the unique challenges presented by each patient. Attention to patient variables that might influence the process of communicating (e.g., biologic sex, expressed gender role identification, developmental level, culture, life experience)

Box 8-4 Relating to Patients from Different Cultures

Assess your personal beliefs surrounding people from different cultures

- Review your personal beliefs and past experiences.
- Set aside any values, biases, ideas, and attitudes that are judgmental and may negatively affect care.

Assess communication variables from a cultural perspective

- Determine the ethnic identity of the patient, including generation in the United States.
- Use the patient as a source of information when possible.
- Assess cultural factors that may affect your relationship with the patient and respond appropriately.

Plan care based on the communicated needs and cultural background

- Learn as much as possible about the patient's cultural customs and beliefs.
- Encourage the patient to reveal cultural interpretation of health, illness, and health care.
- Be sensitive to the uniqueness of the patient.
- Identify sources of discrepancy between the patient's and your own concepts of health and illness.
- Communicate at the patient's personal level of functioning.
- Evaluate effectiveness of nursing actions and modify plan of care when necessary.

Modify communication approaches to meet cultural needs

- Be attentive to signs of fear, anxiety, and confusion in the patient.
- Respond in a reassuring manner in keeping with the patient's cultural orientation.
- Be aware that in some cultural groups, discussion concerning the patient with others may be offensive and may impede the nursing process.

Understand that respect for the patient and communicated needs is central to the therapeutic relationship

- Communicate respect by using a kind and attentive approach.
- Learn how listening is communicated in the patient's culture.
- Use appropriate active listening techniques.
- Adopt an attitude of flexibility, respect, and interest to help bridge barriers imposed by culture.

Communicate in a nonthreatening manner

- Conduct the interview in an unhurried manner.
- Follow acceptable social and cultural amenities.
- Ask general questions during the information-gathering stage.
- Be patient with a respondent who gives information that may seem unrelated to the patient's health problem.
- Develop a trusting relationship by listening carefully, allowing time, and giving the patient your full attention.

Use validating techniques in communication

- Be alert for feedback that the patient does not understand.
- Do not assume meaning is interpreted without distortion.

Be considerate of reluctance to talk when the subject involves sexual matters

- Be aware that in some cultures, sexual matters are not discussed freely with members of the opposite sex.

Adopt special approaches when the patient speaks a different language

- Use a caring tone of voice and facial expression to help alleviate the patient's fears.
- Speak slowly and distinctly, but not loudly.
- Use gestures, pictures, and play acting to help the patient understand.
- Repeat the message in different ways if necessary.
- Be alert to words the patient seems to understand and use them frequently.
- Keep messages simple and repeat them frequently.
- Avoid using medical terms and abbreviations that the patient may not understand.
- Use an appropriate language dictionary.

Use interpreters to improve communication

- Ask the interpreter to translate the message, not just the individual words.
- Obtain feedback to confirm understanding.
- Use an interpreter who is culturally sensitive.

Source: Used with permission from Giger, J. N., & Haddad, L. G. (2021). *Transcultural nursing. Assessment and intervention* (8th ed.). Elsevier.

can make the difference between effective and ineffective interactions. For example, respectful communication includes acknowledging and respecting a person's identity through use of the terms the individual uses to describe themselves (GLAAD, 2016). If necessary, respectfully and privately ask what terms they use to describe themselves (e.g., pronouns "he" and "she," or gender-neutral pronouns, such as "they"), then use those terms (GLAAD, 2016). Box 8-4 provides another example of respectful ways to relate to patients, in this case, patients from different cultures (see also Chapter 5).

EMPATHY

Empathy is an objective understanding of the way in which a patient sees their situation, identifying with the way another person feels, putting yourself in another person's circumstances, imagining what it would be like to share that person's feelings and communicating this understanding to the patient (Keltner & Steele, 2019; Videbeck, 2020). In contrast, sympathy is the expression of sorrow for someone's situation, involving compassion and kindness. Sympathy shifts the emphasis from the patient to the nurse as the nurse shares feelings and personal concerns and projects them onto the patient. Employing sympathy rather than empathy limits the nurse's ability to focus objectively on the patient's needs (Videbeck, 2020).

Empathy is one of the approaches that nurses use to communicate emotional support in their relationships with patients (Keltner & Stele, 2019). An empathic nurse is sensitive to the patient's feelings and problems but remains objective enough to help the patient work to attain positive outcomes. You can establish successful therapeutic relationships without appearing cold or stern by retaining the quality of empathy. For example, although it is understandable for team members to become impatient with family members who never seem satisfied with the care their loved one is receiving, it helps to empathize with the family, who may be feeling frightened and helpless. Appropriate responses employing empathy may include:

"This must be a hard time for you; how are you coping?"
"Is there any way I can be of help?"

When the patient and family sense that you have some idea of what they are experiencing, and that you are committed to helping, the basis is set for a trusting nurse–patient relationship.

HONESTY, AUTHENTICITY, AND TRUST

Patients should be able to trust that nurses are who they say they are (professional care givers). Patients should also be able to believe that nurses can be trusted to do everything within their level of expertise to secure the resources and to help meet the patient needs.

CARING

Patients quickly sense whether they are merely a "task to be performed" (task-centered caring), or a person of worth who is both cared about and cared for (relation-centered caring). Expert nurses know how to communicate genuine caring the minute they step into a patient's space by how they look at and touch the patient and what they say and do. Patients who feel cared for will feel accepted.

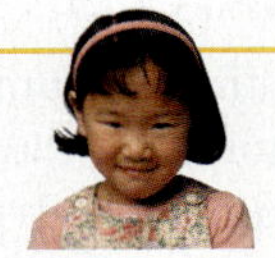

Think back to **Susie Musashi**, the 3-year-old child with burns. How the nurse approaches the child will set the stage for the interaction. Consider how the child would respond to a nurse who enters the room and scolds the child for crying as compared to the nurse who enters the room and approaches the child's bed, touching the child's shoulder or hand gently and softly. The message conveyed by the second action would be much more caring.

COMPETENCE

Competent nurses are skilled in all aspects of basic nursing and can meet their patients' health care needs through their technical, cognitive, interpersonal, and ethical/legal skills. Take responsibility for evaluating your own strengths and weaknesses so that your patients will receive optimal care. Consequently, your patients will develop trust in and respect for you as their nurse, facilitating therapeutic relationships and good communication.

Rapport Builders

Rapport, a feeling of mutual trust experienced by people in a satisfactory relationship (Fig. 8-6), facilitates open communication. Good rapport can be achieved by paying attention to the following variables.

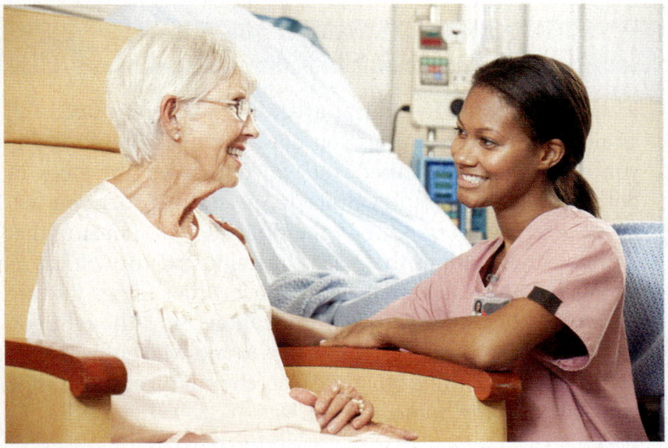

FIGURE 8-6. Rapport between the nurse and the patient or family is a necessary first step in planning care.

SPECIFIC OBJECTIVES

Having a purpose for an interaction provides guidance toward achieving a meaningful encounter with the patient. One objective might be to perform a head-to-toe physical assessment when greeting the patient and at the beginning of each shift. Another objective might be the discussion of a patient's feelings about being newly diagnosed with diabetes. The shortest encounter with a patient can have an objective, even if it is as simple as conveying a feeling of friendliness. Be flexible at all times, and follow the patient's cues to work toward meeting all needs.

COMFORTABLE ENVIRONMENT

A comfortable environment, in which both the patient and the nurse are at ease, helps to promote interactions. Suitable furniture, proper lighting, and a moderate temperature are important. Also, effective relationships are enhanced when the atmosphere is relaxed and unhurried. If you seem preoccupied and on the run, or if the patient is ill at ease for fear of missing visitors or because of another commitment, communication is impaired.

PRIVACY

It might not always be possible to carry on conversations alone with the patient in a room, but every effort should be made to provide privacy and to prevent conversations from being overheard by others. Sometimes merely drawing the curtains around the bed in a hospital or long-term care facility or sitting in a corner of the waiting room or lounge can provide the sense of privacy that is so important in most interactions. Home visits might need to be timed to ensure the privacy the patient desires and needs.

CONFIDENTIALITY

The confidentiality with which patient information is to be treated should be established with the patient. Indicate with whom the information that the patient gives will be shared. The patient should know about the right to specify who might have access to the information. Failure to consider this factor can be considered a breach of the patient's right to privacy. See Chapter 20 for guidelines concerning patient confidentiality.

Through the Eyes of a Patient

I know you come to clinical every day with your head full of all the important things you need to do for me. Probably you worry about whether you will remember the steps to both simple and complex procedures and fear that you will never get everything done in the time allotted. I'm sure that there are many things that your clinical instructor will use as a basis for your evaluation, and perhaps other things that are important to you for your self-evaluation. But I thought you might like to know what's important to me. Most of what I've listed are simple things that you can communicate each time you walk into my home or room.[a]

- Really listen to me.
- Ask me what I think.
- Don't dismiss my concerns.
- Don't treat me like a disease, treat me like a person.
- Talk *to* me, not *at* me.
- Respect my privacy.
- Don't keep me waiting.
- Don't tell me what to do without telling me how to do it.
- Keep me informed.
- Remember who I used to be.
- Let me know you care.

Thanks for giving me this chance to share with you what matters to me.

[a]The list of nursing interventions that are valued highly by patients was compiled by Roberta Messner after a review of many patient satisfaction studies. These are cited in Messner, R. L. (1993). What patients really want from their nurses. *American Journal of Nursing, 93*(8), 38–41.

PATIENT VERSUS TASK FOCUS

Communication in the nurse–patient relationship should focus on the patient and patient needs, not on the nurse or an activity in which the nurse is engaged. Refer to the accompanying box, Through the Eyes of a Patient. Consider the following example, in which the nurse's comment focuses on the patient and the patient needs:

Patient: I don't know why these injections scare me, but they do.
Nurse: You are afraid of these injections?

In contrast, consider this example, in which the nurse's comment focuses instead on the nursing activity:

Patient: I don't know why these injections scare me, but they do.
Nurse: I give hundreds of injections. Don't be so immature.

USING NURSING OBSERVATIONS

Observations, which involve both effective noticing and interpreting, are especially useful for validating information. For example, a nurse suspects that a patient is afraid to hear the results of certain blood tests, but the patient insists that the results are unimportant. The nurse then observes the patient pacing in the corridor, apparently deep in thought. Observing the patient's behavior helps validate the nurse's suspicion that the patient is fearful and the patient's assertion of being unconcerned appears to be a cover-up for truer feelings.

Observation serves several important purposes:

- It helps increase the awareness of a patient's nonverbal messages.
- It is the primary source of information when a patient is unwilling or unable to communicate verbally.
- It demonstrates caring and interest in the patient. (Patients often recognize when a nurse is unobservant and, rightly or wrongly, commonly conclude that the nurse does not care about them.)
- It is an important component of clinical reasoning and clinical judgment (see Chapters 13 and 19).

OPTIMAL PACING

Consider the pace of any conversation or encounter with a patient. For instance, it would be ineffective to rush through a list of questions when obtaining a nursing history; it is more effective to let the patient set the pace. Let the patient know at the beginning of the interaction if time is limited so that the patient does not feel that you are rushing because of a lack of concern or personal interest.

DEVELOPING PROFESSIONAL THERAPEUTIC COMMUNICATION SKILLS

Although humans communicate during virtually all waking moments, the therapeutic use of communication requires training and practice. Box 8-5 contrasts therapeutic and nontherapeutic communication. Nursing students might feel awkward when first trying to develop therapeutic relationships. Practice makes perfect, however, and you will soon feel at ease if you work on developing the following communication skills.

Conversation Skills

Conversation, or the exchange of verbal communication, is a social interaction. As social beings, humans learn as children how to converse with others; nursing students, therefore, have already had years of experience communicating verbally. However, you can improve your communications with patients and achieve a more effective relationship in the following ways:

- Control the tone of your voice so that you are conveying exactly what you mean to say and not a hidden message. Your tone should indicate interest rather than boredom, patience rather than anger, acceptance rather than hostility, and so forth.
- Be knowledgeable about the topic of conversation and have accurate information. When possible, be familiar with the subject of conversation before discussing it with

Box 8-5 Therapeutic versus Nontherapeutic Communication

Patient Scenario

Mr. Commens is a 65-year-old divorced man who lives alone. His grown children are married and live out of town. He was recently diagnosed with cancer of the colon and underwent a colon resection. He is now home recuperating and has received a new diagnosis. The home health care nurse is scheduled to visit Mr. Commens.

Nontherapeutic Communication

Nurse: Hello, Mr. Commens! I'm glad you're home. I only have 30 minutes to visit with you. It's been a very busy day.

Mr. Commens: I'm sorry you are having a bad day. I have been to the doctor and I'm very concerned about the report I received.

Nurse: Yes, I've had a busy day but not a bad day. I guess your day has been busy too. What report are you talking about?

Mr. Commens: Well, I need more tests because they think the cancer has spread.

Nurse: Now, who told you that? Maybe the test was wrong, or you misunderstood the health care provider. Mr. Commens, I'll call your health care provider. Is there anything else bothering you?

Mr. Commens: No.

Nurse: I'll call your doctor and then call you tomorrow.

In this scenario, the nurse seems unconcerned about Mr. Commens' test results and gives him the idea the nurse does not believe the information he has relayed. The nurse is more concerned about their own busy day and less concerned about the patient.

Therapeutic Communication

Nurse: Hello, Mr. Commens! I'm sorry I am running a little behind schedule. Now that I'm here, we will have as much time as we need to discuss how you're feeling and your visit to the health care provider. How are you feeling?

Mr. Commens: (His eyes are cast down to the floor and he is wringing his hands.) Well, I feel all right. I've had some pain in my right side.

Nurse: Mr. Commens, how would you describe and rate your pain on a scale of 1 to 10?

Mr. Commens: Aching and about an 8.

Nurse: Mr. Commens, you seem concerned and a little preoccupied. Is there something bothering you?

Mr. Commens: Yes, I suppose there is. My doctor said my cancer has spread to my hip. I guess that's why I have pain in my right side. I have so many decisions to make and I'm very confused. The doctor said I need to start chemotherapy. I don't even know how I'll get there. My family is out of town.

Nurse: Mr. Commens, would it help if I spoke to your health care provider to obtain specific details about your treatment plan? This would then assist me in obtaining some help when you begin your chemotherapy.

Mr. Commens: That would be wonderful! If you call the doctor, then you can explain everything to me, and maybe it will help me to understand what I'll be going through. Also, it might help me in making decisions about my treatments.

Nurse: Mr. Commens, would you then like me to be here when you call your children about your diagnosis and treatment plan? I might be able to answer some of the questions they might have about your treatments.

Mr. Commens: That would be wonderful. I feel so much more relaxed knowing you are going to help me. Thank you so much.

Nurse: Mr. Commens, I'll call your health care provider and clarify the information you have received, and I'll be back at 5 PM. Maybe at that time, we can call your family.

Mr. Commens: That sounds like a good plan, but we might need to call my children at 6 PM.

Nurse: That's just fine. I will be back at 5 PM to discuss the information I have, and we will call your children at 6 PM.

Interpretation

The first example of communication focuses on the nurse's needs, not the patient's needs. Most of the interaction in the first scenario blocks the communication process. The second example allows the patient to verbalize his concerns and his lack of decision making. The nurse provides the patient with broad opening statements and patient goals to assist in his planning and decision making.

the patient. If the topic is unfamiliar to you (e.g., the availability of community resources for family caregivers of patients with special needs), admit that to the patient and family and direct them to other resources. Convey confidence and honesty to the patient.

- Be flexible. You might want to discuss a certain subject but learn that the patient wishes to discuss something else. It is better to follow the patient's lead whenever possible; in due time, you can return to the subject. For example, you arrive at the patient's bedside to administer a medication, but the patient begins to talk about diet issues. It is better to take a little time to talk about the patient's interest than to insist on talking about only the procedure at hand, as long as there is enough time for the conversation.
- Be clear and concise, and make statements as simple as possible. Patients are often anxious and fail to understand the message unless the patient understands the language used. Stay on one subject at a time. This helps prevent confusion.
- Avoid words that might have different interpretations. The study of the meaning of words is called **semantics**. Even when two people speak the same language, some words—such as love, hate, freedom, and health—might have different meanings to different people.
- Be truthful. A patient who is given false information will soon distrust the nurse. If you're not sure about something, admit you don't know and seek an answer rather than make a comment that may be an error.
- Keep an open mind. An attitude of "I know better than the patient" is quickly discerned by the patient. Patients can make valuable contributions to their own health care.
- Take advantage of available opportunities. During most caregiving situations, you can facilitate conversation that makes even the most routine task meaningful. For instance, when giving a bed bath to a patient, ask about

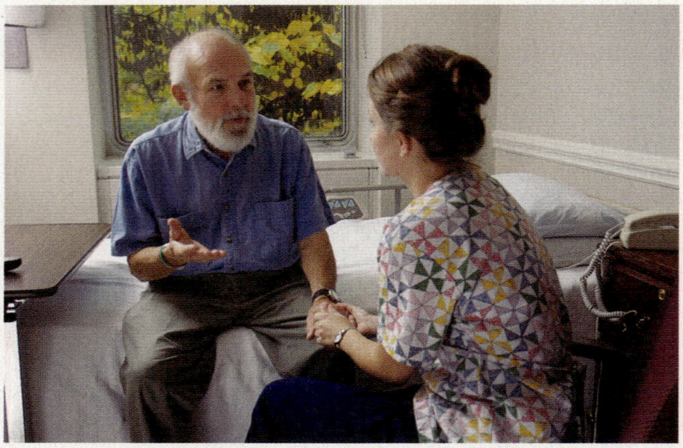

FIGURE 8-7. Listening attentively, with concentration and genuine concern, is key to productive communication.

the patient's employment. This would allow the patient to verbalize any positive or negative feelings about the job and being temporarily absent from it, reducing the anxiety that often occurs with the loss of work. It is often comforting to know that someone understands and cares.

Listening Skills

Listening is a skill that involves both hearing and interpreting what the other says. It requires attention and concentration to sort out, evaluate, and validate clues to better understand the true meaning of what is being said (Fig. 8-7). The accompanying box, Through the Eyes of a Student, relates one student's experience with attentive listening. The following techniques are recommended to improve listening skills:

- When possible, sit when communicating with a patient (George et al., 2018; Videbeck, 2020). Do not cross your arms or legs because that body language conveys a message of being closed to the patient's comments (Videbeck, 2020).
- Be alert and relaxed and take sufficient time so that the patient feels at ease during the conversation.
- Keep the conversation as natural as possible, and avoid sounding overly eager.
- If culturally appropriate, maintain eye contact with the patient, without staring, in a face-to-face pose. This technique conveys interest in the conversation and willingness to listen.
- Indicate that you are paying attention to what the patient is saying by using appropriate facial expressions and body gestures. Be attentive to both your own and the patient's verbal and nonverbal communication.
- Think before responding to the patient. Responding impulsively tends to disrupt communication and listening.
- Do not pretend to listen. Most patients are sensitive to an attitude of feigned attention or to boredom and apathy.
- Listen for themes in the patient's comments. What are the repeated themes in the person's speech and behavior? What topics does the patient tend to avoid? What subjects tend to make the patient shift the conversation to other subjects? What inconsistencies and gaps appear in the patient's conversations?

Silence

You can use silence appropriately, allowing the patient to gather their thoughts and to proceed at their own pace to initiate a conversation or to continue speaking (Videbeck, 2020). During periods of silence, you can reflect on what has already been shared and observe the patient without having to concentrate simultaneously on the spoken word.

Through the Eyes of a Student

It was my first day of clinical rotation and I was assigned to Mr. Anderson, who was in his early 90s. He was in the hospital because he had a second heart attack. Mr. Anderson had lived alone for 5 years after the death of his wife. He wanted to remain independent, but his daughter, who was herself in her late 60s, and his doctor believed that he would not be able to function well on his own any longer. Mr. Anderson was distressed about this belief.

Because it was my first day and, unlike some of my classmates, I had never worked in a hospital before, I felt insecure and nervous. There really wasn't a lot of work for us to do. We weren't allowed to give medication yet, and my patient was pretty self-sufficient. Because my skills were shaky, I took my time taking vital signs, assisted Mr. Anderson with his bath and toileting, and made his bed. After checking his chart, I began my nursing interview with him. I was overjoyed to discover that he was a real talker! His memory was tremendous—either that or he was a great improviser! He recalled stories about his childhood and his wife with great detail and emotion. He smiled and laughed when he spoke of his daughter and grandchildren. He told me about his daughter's childhood illnesses, as well as his own. We talked about the Depression and world wars and about music, art, and education. He asked me about my family, and I felt like I had made a friend.

The next day, Mr. Anderson told me about his fears. He talked about losing his wife, about his health and body deteriorating, and about losing his independence and home. He despised having to be sent to a long-term care facility and having to depend on others. It hurt him a lot and made me sad. Mr. Anderson left on my second day, and as I said goodbye, I wished I could do something for him.

I've thought about him a lot since then, and I've come to realize that in those 2 days that I knew Mr. Anderson, I did do something for him besides washing him and changing his sheets. I listened to him. Although his family had little time for him and the doctors quickly flew in and out of the room, I let him talk and heard all he said, both in words and in his eyes. He will always be a good memory for me—and I think I'll be a good memory for him.

—Kristina Hofmeister
Holy Family College, Philadelphia, PA

Periods of silence during communication can carry a variety of meanings:

- The patient might be comfortable and content in the nurse–patient relationship. Continuous talking is unnecessary.
- The patient might be trying to demonstrate stoicism and the ability to cope without help.
- The patient might be exploring inner thoughts or feelings, and a conversation would disrupt this. In effect, the patient is really saying, "I need some time to think."
- The patient might be fearful and use silence as an escape from a threat.
- The patient might be angry and use silence to display this emotion.
- The patient's culture may require longer pauses between verbal communication.

In time, you might discuss the silence with the patient, especially if you wish to understand its meaning. Fear of silence sometimes leads to too much talking by the nurse. Also, excessive talking tends to place the focus on the nurse rather than on the patient.

Touch

Touch is a powerful means of communication with multiple meanings. It can connect people; provide affirmation, reassurance, and stimulation; decrease loneliness; increase self-esteem; and share warmth, intimacy, approval, and emotional support. It can also communicate frustration, anger, aggression, and punishment, and invade personal space and privacy.

Touch is the most highly developed sense at birth. Tactile experiences of infants and young children appear to be essential for the normal development of self and awareness of others. It has also been found that many older people long for touch, especially when isolated from loved ones because of hospitalization or being in a long-term care facility. Many older people have no living family to provide them with the caring touch so necessary for the sense of well-being. In such an instance, you can provide some special care by holding the patient's hand (Fig. 8-8).

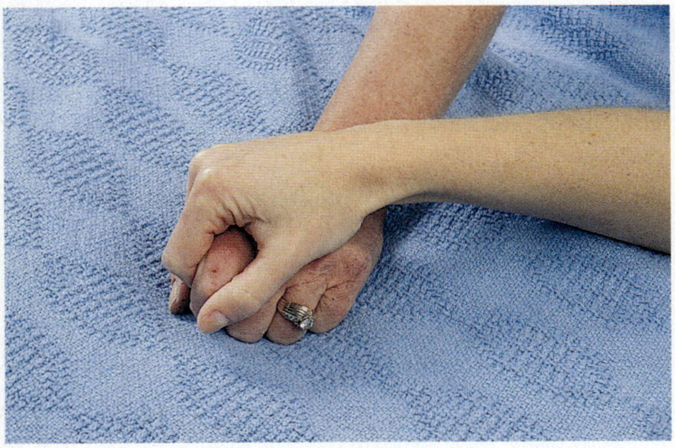

FIGURE 8-8. A reassuring handclasp uses touch to convey a message. Sometimes touch can be a more effective way of expressing concern and interest than verbal communication. (*Source:* Used with permission from Shutterstock. *Photo by B. Proud.*)

Many situations require touching the patient while implementing nursing care. Physical closeness between the patient and the nurse is essential and inevitable. Therefore, every nurse needs to become comfortable with the judicious use of this nonverbal communication technique so that a sense of security, rather than anxiety, results. As well, dexterity and sureness in the use of the hands help to assure the patient of your expertise when measuring blood pressure or giving an injection. Touch can be a powerful therapeutic tool when used at the right time. Anxiety or discomfort might result, however, when a patient does not understand the meaning of a tactile gesture or when the patient simply dislikes being touched. Because of the personal nature of touching, be sure to weigh the benefit of touch against the detrimental use of touch for each patient. The nurse should observe the patient for cues that show whether touch is desired or indicated, and ask the patient about touching prior to implementation (Videbeck, 2020).

Interest has continued to grow in the phenomenon known as therapeutic touch. A nurse trained in therapeutic touch may use it to promote comfort, relaxation, healing, and a sense of well-being. Many nurses are studying therapeutic touch in nursing educational programs and through special courses or workshops. It is becoming a widely accepted form of therapy, as well as a subject for nursing research. Refer to Chapters 29 and 36 for additional discussion of therapeutic touch.

Humor

Humor is increasingly valued as both an interpersonal skill for the nurse and a healing strategy for patients. Nurses can use humor effectively to maintain a balanced perspective in their work and to encourage patients to do the same. Nurses with a sense of humor are able to laugh at themselves and accept their failures, confront the absurdities of everyday practice without falling apart, and challenge patients to situate their current dilemma within the context of their larger life experiences. Laughter releases excess physical and psychological energy and reduces stress, anxiety, worry, and frustration. Humor, like other interpersonal competencies, is a learned skill. When used inappropriately, however, it can be destructive. You'll need an awareness of how various cultures perceive the use of humor in the presence of an illness. You might also find it helpful to identify nurses who use humor well and to "try on" observed behaviors. The use of humor is also discussed in Chapter 36.

Interviewing Techniques

The purpose of the patient interview is to obtain accurate and thorough information. In nursing, the interview is a major tool for collecting data during the assessment step of the nursing process and is an important component of clinical reasoning and clinical judgment (see Chapters 13, 14, and 15). Consequently, every nurse needs to become proficient in the use of the communication techniques described previously as well as interviewing techniques designed to gather and validate information.

All interviews should begin with an explanation of the purpose of the interview. During the interview, you'll use interviewing techniques to obtain needed information while remaining flexible in approach. The interview itself is a therapeutic interaction and might be an essential part of the orientation phase of the therapeutic relationship. At the end of the interview, plans for further interactions can be made. The following interviewing techniques are useful in nearly all nurse–patient interactions, especially the interview.

Open-Ended Question or Comment

When collecting patient information, such as during a nursing history, use the open-ended question technique to allow the patient a wide range of possible responses. Use of open-ended questions allows patients to express what they understand to be true, yet is specific enough to prevent digressing from the issue at hand. It encourages free verbalization and more descriptive information (Videbeck, 2020). The greatest advantage of this technique is that it prevents the patient from giving a simple yes or no answer that has the effect of limiting the patient's response. The following is an example of an open-ended question and the response:

Nurse: What did your health care provider tell you about your need for this hospitalization?

Patient: He told me that my blood pressure is dangerously high and that I need some special tests done while I am here.

Closed Question or Comment

The closed (focused) question or comment provides the receiver with limited choices of possible responses and might often be answered by one or two words, "yes" or "no." Closed questions are used to gather specific information from a patient and to allow the nurse and patient to focus on a particular area. Closed questions are often a barrier to effective communication. The following is an example of an appropriate use of a closed question:

Nurse: What medicines have you been taking at home?

Patient: Let me see, my doctor gave me a water pill and a blood pressure pill to take every day.

Validating Question or Comment

This type of question or comment serves to validate what the nurse believes they have heard or observed. Overusing validating questions and comments might lead the patient to think the nurse is not listening, however. To continue the example used in the previous technique, the nurse could validate the patient's reply as follows:

Nurse: At home, you have been taking both a water pill and a blood pressure pill every day. Did you take them today?

Patient: Yes, I took one of each with my breakfast.

Clarifying Question or Comment

At times, a patient's thoughts and/or communication may be unclear. The nurse should never assume understanding of the patient's meaning; the nurse should ask for clarification if there is doubt (Videbeck, 2020). The use of the clarifying question or comment allows the nurse to gain an understanding of a patient's comment. When used properly, this technique can prevent possible misconceptions that could lead to identification of an inappropriate diagnosis or patient problem. However, overuse of clarifying questions or comments can lead the patient to believe that the nurse is not listening or lacks appropriate knowledge. The following is an example of effective use of this technique:

Patient: I have never needed to take medicine before in my life.

Nurse: Is this the first health problem you have had?

Patient: Yes, I've always been healthy.

Reflective Question or Comment

The reflective question technique involves repeating what the person has said or describing the person's feelings. It encourages patients to elaborate on their thoughts and feelings. An example of this technique follows:

Patient: I've been really upset about my blood pressure and have to take these pills.

Nurse: You've been upset …

Patient: I guess I'm worried about what could happen if my blood pressure gets too bad.

Sequencing Question or Comment

Sequencing is used to place events in a chronologic order or to investigate a possible cause-and-effect relationship between events. Nursing assessment is facilitated when events leading to a problem are placed in sequence. This technique is evident in the following example:

Patient: I don't feel like myself anymore since I've been taking my blood pressure medicine. I'm tired and don't have any energy.

Nurse: Your tiredness began after you started taking your medicine?

Directing Question or Comment

It might become necessary at times to obtain more information about a topic brought up earlier in the interview or to introduce a new aspect of the current topic. In this way, the nurse can gain additional valuable information to consider in assessing the patient's health status and educational or counseling needs. The following is an example of this technique:

Nurse: You mentioned your dad earlier. Did he develop complications related to high blood pressure?

Patient: Yes.

Nurse: What sort of complications?

Patient: Kidney failure. He was on dialysis for years before getting a transplant.

Nurse: Are you afraid this might happen to you?

Assertive versus Aggressive Behaviors and Communication

When interacting with patients, family members, other nurses, health care providers, and other members of the

Table 8-2 Examples of Assertive, Nonassertive, and Aggressive Speech

	ASSERTIVE	NONASSERTIVE	AGGRESSIVE
Nurse to Nurse	"I know we all lose track of time occasionally, but I'm finding it harder and harder to cover for you when you take extra time for lunch. I don't think it's fair for your patient and me to have to wait an extra 30 minutes every day for you to come back from lunch. Can we talk about this?"	"Huh? No, I didn't really mind. Luckily I wasn't too busy today." Thought: "What a sucker I am. Now I'll have to grab a quick bite so that I can get back to the unit in time to do the 1,400 treatments."	"I'm sick and tired of covering for you. You are lazy and unreliable and I'm going to talk to the unit leader about you and let her know how irresponsible you are! What kind of nurse are you! I hope you lose your job!"
Nurse to Health Care Provider	"I know we talked about Mr. Esposito's pain medication before, but I've collected some new data. Even with the change in dosage, he is only getting 1–1½ hours of relief. I believe a different analgesic agent may work better for him."	"Um … yes I know you already changed the dosage. It's just that I thought it still wasn't working. Maybe I didn't give it enough time. Thanks for listening to me anyway. I'm sorry to bother you with this."	"What is it going to take to convince you that Mr. Esposito is not exaggerating his pain level so he can get more meds? I thought nurses and doctors were going to be more respectful of each other and collaborate, but this whole attempt to talk to you is a disaster. I need to report you to someone and maybe none of us will have to deal with you anymore. You give doctors a bad name."
Student Nurse to Preceptor	"Miss Cheng has a new order to be straight catheterized. I reviewed the procedure, but I'd sure appreciate your talking me through this because I've never done it before and I'm terrified."	"Uh...I'm sorry to be such a pain again. I have to do this catheterization and don't know where to begin. I know you must be busy, but, uh, is there any way you might have time for me?"	"If this is an example of how helpful experienced nurses on this unit are to student nurses, then the profession is in a lot of trouble. Are you one of the believers in that saying that 'nurses eat their young'? Remind me to try and avoid you in the future."

health care team, nurses should communicate in a way that demonstrates respect for all parties. **Assertive behavior** is the ability to stand up for yourself and others using open, honest, and direct communication. The focus is on the issue and not the person. Assertive behaviors, which are one hallmark of professional nursing relationships, are very different from aggressive (i.e., harsh, injurious, or destructive) behaviors. They also differ greatly from avoidance or acquiescent behaviors. Assertiveness involves making a choice about how to behave in order to gain a desired outcome, not just about being firm in order to get what is wanted (Ellis, 2018). The key to assertiveness is expressing feelings and beliefs in a nondefensive manner. "I" statements—"I feel..." and "I think..."—play an important role in assertive statements (Videbeck, 2020). The use of assertive behaviors and communication respectfully expresses views, opinions, and concerns regarding patient care without judgment, belittlement, or blaming another person and without aggression (Ellis, 2018). Table 8-2 provides examples of assertive, nonassertive, and aggressive speech.

Characteristics of the assertive nurse's self-presentation include a confident, open body posture; eye contact; use of clear, concise "I" statements; and the ability to effectively share their thoughts, feelings, and emotions. The assertive nurse's attitude toward work is characterized by working to capacity with or without supervision, the ability to remain calm under supervision, the freedom to ask for help when necessary, the ability to give and accept compliments, and honesty in admitting mistakes and taking responsibility for them. Refer also to the previous discussion of the "CUS" communication technique—another example of a method for health care team members to assertively speak up about patient safety concerns, located on pages 185–187.

Aggressive behavior, on the other hand, involves asserting one's rights in a negative manner that violates the rights of others. Aggression can be verbal or physical. It is communication that is marked by tension and anger and inhibits the formation of good relationships and collaboration. Characteristics of aggressive verbal behavior include using an angry tone of voice and being condescending, and threatening (Marquis & Huston, 2021). Aggressive behavior is rude and intimidating. The focus is usually on "winning at all costs" or demonstrating personal excellence (Marquis & Huston, 2021). Comments such as "do it my way" or "that's just enough out of you" are examples of aggressive verbal statements. People speaking in an aggressive manner may invade another's personal space, speak loudly, and use gestures that are very emphatic or threatening. Aggressive people enhance their self-esteem and prove their superiority through destructive comments directed at others.

BARRIERS TO COMMUNICATION

Nurses who have a good understanding of their own feelings and responses are better able to communicate and respond to others. The failure to verbalize clearly and compassionately, however, blocks effective communication. Recognition of the patient as a human being, listening carefully, and avoiding nontherapeutic statements help the nurse to provide optimal, compassionate patient care. Respectful behavior and communication between nurses and other members of the health care team promotes a safer patient environment with positive outcomes and improved job satisfaction.

Failure to Perceive the Patient as a Human Being

Nurses must focus on the whole patient and not merely the patient's diagnosis. Patients report that nothing is more discomforting than to be treated as merely an object of care rather than a patient. Patients should be addressed in the manner of their preference; ask a patient how they prefer to be addressed or what they prefer to be called. Err on the side of formality over informality (Mr., Mrs., Ms., Mx.); use neutral and inclusive language when speaking with all patients (The Joint Commission, 2011). Do not use slang terminology such as "honey" or "sweetie." What distinguishes nursing from other health professions is its focus on the whole person, not simply the illness or dysfunction.

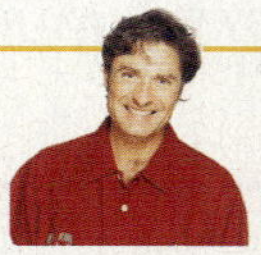

Think back to **Mr. Gordon**, the patient with end-stage liver disease. In the scenario, the nursing student voiced concerns about the staff nurse and residents focusing only on the technical aspects of the patient's care. To effectively communicate this concern to these people, the student should use open, honest, and direct (assertive) communication when speaking with them, stressing the need for providing care to the whole patient.

Failure to Listen

Failure to listen to cues in the patient's responses and conversation can occur from a lack of concentration on what the patient says—an absence of use of active listening skills (refer to previous discussion of Listening Skills on page 194). Patients might or might not feel to be able to speak freely to the nurse. Often, the signals indicating their readiness to talk are subtle. Do not miss valuable opportunities for important communication by approaching patients with a closed mind or focusing on your own needs rather than on the patient's needs. Nurses who lack confidence in their own ability to meet the challenges a patient presents might become defensive in response to a patient's comments. Nurse defensiveness is a huge barrier to open and trusting communication.

Nontherapeutic Comments and Questions

Certain types of comments and questions should be avoided in most situations because they tend to impede effective communications. A description of each type follows.

Clichés

A **cliché** is a stereotyped, trite, or pat answer. Most health care clichés suggest that there is no cause for anxiety or concern, or they offer false assurance. Patients tend to interpret them as a lack of real interest in what they have said. For example, even though the common question "How are you?" could start a conversation, it can cause a problem if patients hearing this suspect that the nurse is not sincerely interested in how they feel. Avoid the following common clichés because they tend to impede effective communication:

"Everything will be all right."
"Don't worry. You will be just fine in another day or two."
"Your doctor knows best."
"Cheer up. Tomorrow is another day."

Another type of cliché makes a sweeping generalization that does not necessarily apply to a specific patient. It also tends to cut off communications and makes people feel as though they are insignificant. Consider the following examples:

"Men tolerate pain poorly. That must be why you are complaining of severe pain."
"Everybody is afraid of surgery. Why should you be any different?"
"You teenagers are all alike. You aren't cooperative because you deny authority."

Such comments rarely promote communication with the patient to whom they are addressed.

Questions Requiring Only a Yes or No Answer

Questions that can be answered by simply saying yes or no tend to cut off discussion, even when the person might wish to continue. Consider the following question:

Nurse: Did you have a good day?

The question begs for a noncommittal answer, which tells the nurse little. This is a better question:

Nurse: Tell me about your sessions in therapy. How did you feel they went today?

Another pitfall is to pose a question to which the patient can say no when that answer could present a problem. Consider the following question that a nurse asks a postoperative patient:

Nurse: Are you ready to get out of bed?

By offering the patient the chance to say no, the nurse might have created difficulties if the patient should be getting out of bed.

At times, of course, questions that can be answered with yes or no are appropriate, such as in these examples:

Nurse: Did you take your insulin before breakfast this morning?
Nurse: Do you have pain when I move your arm this way?

The problem with yes or no questions arises when seeking more detailed information or when the question might create difficulty.

Questions Containing the Words Why and How

Questions using the words *why* and *how* may be intimidating to many patients. Consider the following questions:

Nurse: Why were you not tired enough to sleep?

Nurse: How did you ever decide to go on a crash diet?

These two questions would be better stated as follows:

Nurse: What were you doing while you were unable to sleep?

Nurse: What things prompted you to decide to go on a crash diet?

Questions that Probe for Information

Questions that too obviously probe for information might cut off communication. Patients who are made to feel as though they are receiving the "third degree" become resentful, usually stop talking, and try to avoid further conversation. Although more information might be needed, it is better to follow the patient's lead. Letting the patient take the initiative allows you to delve more deeply at a time when the patient is ready. A nurse who says, "Let's get to the bottom of this" is likely to destroy conversation, unless the patient is ready to face the real cause of the problem.

Leading Questions

A leading question suggests what response the speaker wishes to hear. Leading questions tend to produce answers that might please the nurse but are unlikely to encourage the patient to respond honestly without feeling intimidated. Consider the following examples:

Nurse: You aren't going to smoke that cigarette, are you?

Nurse: You have been well cared for by your nurses, haven't you?

These questions direct patients to give an answer that pleases the nurse rather than to express their own thoughts.

Comments that Give Advice

Giving advice often implies that the nurse knows what is best for patients and denies them the right to make decisions and have feelings. It also tends to increase the patient's dependence on caregivers. However, advice does have a rightful place when it is requested and when the person giving the advice has expert knowledge that the patient does not.

Judgmental Comments

Judgmental comments tend to impose the nurse's standards on the patient. Consider the comment of a nurse who notes that a young woman is crying:

Nurse: You aren't acting very grown up. How do you think your husband would feel if he saw you crying like this?

The nurse judges the patient as being immature, and the nurse's apparent hostility could end effective communication. A better comment in this situation might be as follows:

Nurse: I would like to help. Tell me, what is making you cry?

Consider the following exchange between a nurse and a patient about to have surgery:

Patient: I think I have a right to be afraid of this operation.

Nurse: Tell me what makes you feel afraid.

This patient is likely to feel safe when allowed to express feelings without being judged.

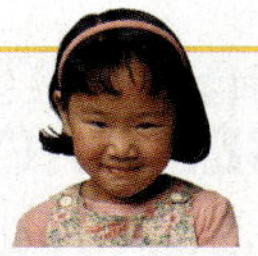

Remember **Susie Musashi**, the 3-year-old with burns who is crying. A response such as "You're acting like a baby. You're a big girl now" would be intimidating, especially to a young child who is striving for acceptance. Instead, a response such as "Can you tell me what is making you cry or feel so sad?" would allow the child to verbalize her concerns without feeling intimidated or scolded. This response also would help in establishing a trusting nurse–patient relationship.

Changing the Subject

A quick way to stop conversation is to change the subject. Rejection of a topic by the nurse closes it off from exploration (Hays & Larson, 1963, as cited in Videbeck, 2020, p. 100). The patient might be at a point of readiness to discuss something and will likely feel frustrated if put off by a change in the topic of conversation. Or, the patient may feel personally rejected along with expressed ideas or topic (Hays & Larson, 1963, as cited in Videbeck, 2020, p. 100). Consider this example:

Patient: When can I expect to be told about my insulin?

Nurse: Let's discuss your diet now so that you will know what to eat when you get home. We can discuss your insulin some other time.

A nurse might also change the subject when feeling uncomfortable about the topic of conversation (Videbeck, 2020). For example, the patient's needs are being met when the nurse allows the patient to speak of impending death, thoughts of suicide, or contemplated abortion. The nurse is ignoring the patient, however, if the nurse changes the subject because of feeling uncomfortable talking about it.

Giving False Assurance

Because it is easier and more pleasant to deal with positive outcomes than negative outcomes, nurses might try to convince the patient that things are going to turn out well even when knowing the chances are not good. False assurance might give patients the impression that the nurse is not interested in their problems. The use of clichés gives a patient false assurance. Communication might be impeded when providing the patient and family with false assurance. If you inadvertently do use false assurance, then you should explain with an apology and implement effective communication techniques.

Gossip and Rumor

Gossip and rumor are common forms of communication, particularly in health care settings, sometimes referred to as "the grapevine." Gossip and rumor can produce detrimental effects on relationships and group building. Gossiping might be used to inform, influence others, entertain, or ventilate. It can be harmless but could also damage the reputation of others. Rumors serve similar functions but become more widespread. Both rumors and gossip might cause blocks to team building and damage the reputations of the people who are the subject of the information.

DISRUPTIVE INTERPERSONAL BEHAVIOR AND COMMUNICATION

Disruptive behavior has a negative effect on clinical outcomes and interpersonal relationships, and includes incivility, bullying, and aggressive patient and family behavior. Adverse events occur when communication between health care professionals is ineffective, abusive, or negative. The Joint Commission established a leadership standard that requires hospitals and other accredited institutions to establish a code of conduct defining acceptable, disruptive, and unacceptable behavior (The Joint Commission, 2016). This standard also mandates facility leaders to create and implement a process for managing unprofessional and inappropriate behaviors when they occur (The Joint Commission, 2016). In addition, the Joint Commission advises hospitals to educate all staff about the code of conduct, develop reporting systems, use mediators when necessary, and document all efforts to address unacceptable behavior (The Joint Commission, 2016). Disruptive interpersonal behavior compromises patient safety, influences satisfaction with care, decreases productivity, and contributes to health care errors and poor patient and staff outcomes (Clark, 2019; Layne et al., 2018).

Incivility and Bullying

Incivility is rude, disruptive, intimidating, and undesirable verbal and nonverbal communication and behaviors directed at another person (Clark, 2019). Incivility also includes failing to act when action is warranted, such as refusing to assist a coworker or share important information about a patient's care, or remaining silent while others are treated with disrespect (ANA, 2015). Incivility is considered by some as a precursor to bullying behavior or lateral violence, and by others as a form of bullying (Armstrong, 2018).

Anger and aggressive behavior between nurses, or nurse-to-nurse hostility, has been labeled **horizontal violence**. This negative behavior is also referred to as **bullying**, **lateral violence**, and professional incivility. All are breaches in the workplace norms of respect and courtesy and forms of psychological and social harassment and involve covert or overt behaviors (McPherson & Buxton, 2019; Millis, 2018). Bullying occurs when a person is subjected to intimidating behaviors that have a negative effect on them; the conduct is persistent and may involve direct physical or verbal behaviors or indirect behaviors (Meires, 2018a; Millis, 2018).

Covert bullying includes withholding information from a colleague, gossiping and spreading rumors, using nonverbal communication such as eye-rolling and other body language, and social isolation. Overt bullying behaviors include accusing a nurse of errors made by someone else (scapegoating) or humiliating a person in the presence of others.

Bullying behaviors and communication occur in all health care environments and affect nurses at all levels of practice, including new graduates and nursing. The potential source of the disruptive behavior, the bully, may be a coworker, a supervisor, or another health care provider. Many nurses choose to leave the workplace or unit to find a "bully-free" place to work (Bambi et al., 2019; Sauer & McCoy, 2018).

The physical and emotional toll on those employed in a toxic work environment can be significant. Commonly reported physical consequences include frequent headaches, sleep disturbances, gastrointestinal symptoms, and decreased energy (Lever et al., 2019). Psychological manifestations, such as an increased level of stress, anxiety, fear, frustration, and loss of self-esteem, can result in burnout, emotional exhaustion, depression, and suicidal ideation or attempt (Bambi et al., 2019; Lever et al., 2019). Bullying is associated with nursing practice errors and affects patient safety and patient outcomes; in addition, teamwork is negatively influenced, resulting in deterioration in the quality of care and a greater potential for error (Johnson & Benham-Huchins, 2020; Meires, 2018a).

Verbally and Physically Aggressive Patients

Adverse events also occur when nurses and other health care professionals care for verbally and/or physically abusive patients. Aggression in health care settings can take many forms and occurs for numerous reasons (Baby et al., 2019). Workplace violence is defined as violent acts, including physical assaults and threats of assault, directed toward persons at work on duty (NIOSH, 2014). Patient and/or family violence ranges from verbal harassing, threatening, yelling, bullying, and hostile sarcasm to physical slapping, punching, biting, and throwing of objects (Locke et al., 2018). Refer to the Vulnerable Population Alert 8-1: Nurses Caring for Verbally and Physically Abusive Patients for additional information and resources related to this issue.

Decreased quality of communication may be interpreted as a lack of caring and support, with resulting decreased satisfaction with the level of nursing care. Poor-quality communication between the nurse and the patient and/or family and decreased patient/family satisfaction may make people more likely to justify aggressive behavior toward the nurse (Yagil & Dayan, 2020). The U.S. Department of Labor Occupational Safety and Health Administration (OSHA) (2016) has established guidelines for preventing workplace violence for health care and social service workers. Health care institutions are encouraged to develop workplace violence prevention programs, document reports of violence, investigate reported events in a timely manner, and provide training on workplace violence for all workers (Benyon, 2019; OSHA, 2016; Zuzelo,

Vulnerable Population Alert 8-1: Nurses Caring for Verbally and Physically Abusive Patients

An Occupational Health and Safety Report states that violence and assault against health care workers, especially nurses, is on the rise—and some studies suggest it has spiked nearly 110% (Occupational Health & Safety, 2020).

A number of surveys (OSHA, 2015c) highlight the prevalence of violence among different health care professions and found that:

- 21% of registered nurses and nursing students reported being physically assaulted—and 50% verbally abused—in a 12-month period
- 12% of emergency department nurses experienced physical violence—and 59% experienced verbal abuse—during a 7-day period
- 13% of employees in Veterans Health Administration hospitals reported being assaulted in a year

Health care worker safety affects companies and businesses too. OSHA (2015) reports that between 2002 and 2013, incidents of serious workplace violence (those requiring days off for the injured worker to recuperate) were four times more common in health care than in private industry on average. The costs to help a worker who has suffered violence or hire a new nurse can be immensely high—sometimes as much as $103,000.

Workplace Violence Prevention Resources

- American Nurses Association (ANA, 2019b) provides information about different levels of violence and laws and regulations. Access the ANA position statement on incivility, bullying, and workplace violence. See https://www.nursingworld.org/practice-policy/advocacy/state/workplace-violence2/.
- Centers for Disease Control and Prevention (CDC) and National Institute for Occupational Safety and Health (2019) online course "Workplace violence prevention for nurses" helps nurses better understand workplace violence and how to prevent it. See cdc.gov/niosh/topics/violence/training_nurses.html.
- OSHA's (2016) Guidelines for Preventing Workplace Violence for Healthcare and Social Service Workers describe the five components of an effective workplace violence prevention program, with extensive examples. See www.osha.gov/Publications/osha3148.pdf.
- Preventing Workplace Violence: A Road Map for Healthcare Facilities expands on OSHA's (2015a) guidelines by presenting case studies and successful strategies from a variety of health care facilities. See www.osha.gov/Publications/OSHA3827.pdf.
- OSHA's (2015b) Workplace Violence Prevention and Related Goals: The Big Picture explains how you can achieve synergies between workplace violence prevention, broader safety and health objectives, accreditation, and a "culture of safety." See www.osha.gov/Publications/OSHA3828.pdf.

Additional Sources

Occupational Health & Safety (OH&S). (2020). *Nurses are suffering more violence in the workplace.* https://ohsonline.com/articles/2020/02/10/nurses-are-suffering-more-violence-in-the-workplace.aspx; Occupational Safety and Health Administration (OSHA). (2015c). *Workplace violence in healthcare. Understanding the challenge.* https://www.osha.gov/sites/default/files/OSHA3826.pdf

2020). Clearly developed policies and procedures must be in place and include a policy of zero tolerance (American Association of Critical-Care Nurses, 2019; American Nurses Association, 2015; Zuzelo, 2020). A nurse subject to verbal and/or physical aggression is a victim of violence, regardless of the etiology of the attack; such attacks cannot be considered an expected part of nursing (Zuzelo, 2020).

Communication is the first line of defense against patient violence (Locke et al., 2018). Nurses should use effective, therapeutic communication techniques (discussed earlier in the chapter) to build trust, establish a rapport, meet patient and family expectations, and validate feelings as well as respond to patient needs (Baby et al., 2019; Locke et al., 2018). Nurses should also be prepared to use appropriate responses to disruptive and/or aggressive behavior as outlined in the next section.

Responses to Disruptive Behaviors and Communication

When disruptive behavior occurs, it is best to maintain a professional demeanor, respond assertively and address the issue directly with those involved (Meires, 2018b). If this is not possible, ask to speak to the person in private and address any disrespectful remarks or behaviors. Nurses may also see guidance and support through nurse-managers and/or other appropriate channel, as outlined by the institution (American Nurses Association, 2015). Nurses should factually document the occurrence of any bullying behaviors. Facility administrative policies and procedures should be implemented to deal with individual situations in a constructive manner.

Addressing disruptive behaviors requires the determination that bullying and other behaviors and inappropriate communication will no longer be tolerated in order to promote a healthy work environment. The previously discussed standard from The Joint Commission (2016) regarding preventing disruptive behaviors in health care facilities includes the following key recommendations:

- Education must be provided for all staff regarding respectful, professional behavior and communication. (See the accompanying Research in Nursing box on page 202.)
- All staff members must be held accountable for their behavior and use of communication techniques.
- Zero-tolerance policies must be implemented regarding disruptive behaviors, and protection must be provided for those who report these behaviors and communication.
- Those in leadership positions must attend training regarding professional standards of behavior and communication techniques and function as a positive role model.
- Surveillance and reporting systems must be available to identify unprofessional behaviors and communication.
- Emphasis must be placed on the importance of documenting bullying behaviors and disruptive communication.

Research in Nursing

BRIDGING THE GAP TO EVIDENCE-BASED PRACTICE

Workplace Incivility

Incivility and bullying behaviors in the workplace contribute to toxic work environments. These disruptive behaviors negatively affect health care providers and can lead to nurse turnover and impact retention of nurses. Communication issues are a component of bullying and workplace incivility. Can increased awareness of incivility and communication strategies reduce incivility?

Related Research

Howard, M. S., & Embree, J. L. (2020). Educational intervention improves communication abilities of nurses encountering workplace incivility. *The Journal of Continuing Education in Nursing, 51*(3), 138–144. https://doi:10.3928/00220124-20200216-09

This quasi-experimental mixed-method study examined the use of an educational intervention to increase the awareness and knowledge of incivility and bullying and enhance the communication skills of novice nurses. Twenty-eight nurses who had completed general nursing orientation within the past year were assigned to the control group. Twenty-one nurses who were in general nursing orientation programs at the time of the study were assigned to the experimental group. The majority (67.3%) of participants had less than 3 years of experience as a nurse. All participants completed the Workplace Civility Index (WCI), an evidence-based questionnaire used to assess nurses' sense of civility and to increase awareness related to personal actions and intensions. Lower WCI scores signify very uncivil behavior; higher scores indicate very civil behavior. The nurses in the experimental group then completed an asynchronous, learner-paced e-learning educational activity designed to encourage productive communication and dialogue, increase awareness and knowledge of incivility and bullying, and increase participants' ability to engage in difficult conversations successfully. The control group did not receive any intervention. All participants completed the post-WCI. WCI scores improved significantly for the experimental group post intervention ($p < .00001$). The WCI scores decreased significantly for the control group ($p = .000227$). The researchers suggested this decrease was a result of increased self-awareness and self-reflection of uncivil behavior on the part of the control group participants. All participants in the experimental group noted the successful use of a positive conflict-management strategy in the workplace to address an issue after the educational intervention. The researchers concluded that an asynchronous, learner-paced e-learning educational activity is an effective intervention to decrease incivility and increase perceived comfort levels during critical conversations between nurses and other health care providers.

Relevance to Nursing Practice

Workplace mistreatment negatively affects the well-being of nurses and can have detrimental effects. Nurses must act in a manner that demonstrates that bullying and other negative behaviors will not be tolerated in order to promote a healthy work environment. Nurses must develop skills to respond assertively and address this issue directly with those involved. One way to address incivility is through educational activities to encourage use of productive and critical communication skills and increase awareness of incivility. A proactive approach has the potential to increase job satisfaction, foster personal growth, and positively affect the retention of registered nurses.

The ANA states that nurses and employers in all settings have an ethical, moral, and legal responsibility to create a healthy and safe work environment for nurses and all members of the health care team, health care consumers, families, and communities (ANA, 2015). Nurses and their employers must collaborate to create a culture of respect that is free of incivility, bullying, and workplace violence (ANA, 2015).

Nurses who refuse to be victims can help break the cycle of violence. Once bullying and other disruptive behavior and communication are recognized as problems, the need for a culture change is evident. Education is crucial. Nurses need to learn effective communication strategies to combat bullying and react to aggressive behaviors (Baby et al., 2019; Locke et al., 2018; Meires, 2018a). Assertiveness and aggression training are effective in addressing these issues. Threats or violent behavior require a calm attitude before interacting with the aggressor; being upset will escalate the situation (Curtin, 2019). Proactive response includes learning how to react professionally and protectively "in the moment"; documenting and reporting the incident; welcoming new nurses; using conflict-management strategies when responding to aggressive behavior; and insisting that the disruptive behavior and communication are addressed. Nurses who have always cared for others need to also care for themselves and their peers.

An organizational response coupled with individual nurses' efforts to address disruptive behaviors and communication at all levels can create a healthy work environment, positively affect job satisfaction, improve the retention of nurses, and result in more positive patient outcomes.

IMPAIRED VERBAL COMMUNICATION

The ability to communicate is our most human characteristic. Human communication is essential for learning, working, and social interaction. Impaired communication can affect every aspect of a person's life. Impaired verbal communication is a decreased, delayed, or absent ability to use speech.

Specific communication strategies may be necessary for patients with impaired verbal communication. There are many reasons for verbal communication impairments. For example, older adults may have speech, language, and hearing disorders. Nurses and other caregivers should avoid "elderspeak" when communicating with older adults. Elderspeak involves using diminutive words, exaggerated voice intonation, high pitch, and exaggerated punctuation that imply that the older adult is not competent. Elderspeak is non–person-centered communication based on stereotypes of older adults and is a form of ageism (Williams et al., 2018). Children and adults may have neurodevelopmental issues, such as autism spectrum disorder, traumatic brain injury, and dementia, which may contribute to impairment in communication. Strategies to address impairments in verbal communication include use of a calm and reassuring approach, use of nonverbal gestures to aid the patient in understanding what is being communicated, and seeking clarification and validation to ensure that the intended messages have been conveyed (Townsend & Morgan, 2018). Communication adjustments may be necessary but must be respectful, positive, and individualized. Chapter 24 also addresses communication with older adults.

The causes of hearing loss include chronic ear infections, heredity, birth defects, health problems at home, certain drugs, head injury, viral or bacterial infection, exposure to loud noise, aging, and tumors. Causes of speech and language disorders are related to hearing loss, cerebral palsy, and other nerve and muscle disorders; severe head injury; stroke (brain attack); viral diseases; cognitive, intellectual, or developmental disabilities; certain drugs; physical impairments, such as cleft lip or palate; vocal abuse or misuse; and inadequate speech and language. Box 8-6 offers guidelines for communicating with patients with special needs.

Box 8-6 Communicating With Patients Who Have Special Needs

Patients Who Are Visually Impaired

- Acknowledge your presence in the patient's room.
- Identify yourself by name.
- Remember that the visually impaired patient will be unable to pick up most nonverbal cues during communication. Speak in a normal tone of voice.
- Explain the reason for touching the patient before doing so.
- Indicate to the patient when the conversation has ended and when you are leaving the room.
- Keep a call light or bell within easy reach of the patient.
- Orient the patient to the sounds in the environment and to the arrangement of the room and its furnishings.
- Be sure the patient's eyeglasses are clean and intact or that contacts are in place.

Patients Who Are Deaf or Hard of Hearing

- Orient the patient to your presence before initiating conversation. This may be done by gently touching the patient or moving so that you can be seen.
- Talk directly to the patient while facing them. If the patient is able to lip read, use simple sentences and speak in a quiet, natural manner and pace. Be aware of nonverbal communication.
- Do not chew gum or cover your mouth when talking with the patient.
- Demonstrate or pantomime ideas you wish to express, as appropriate.
- Use sign language or finger spelling, as appropriate.
- Write any ideas that you cannot convey to the patient in another manner.
- Be sure that hearing aids are clean, functioning, and inserted properly.

Patients With a Physical Barrier (Laryngectomy or Endotracheal Tube)

- Select one or more simple means of communication that the patient is physically able to use. Options include eye blinks or hand squeezes to communicate yes or no; writing pads or magic slates; communication boards with words, letters, or pictures; flash cards; sign language.
- Be sure that everyone communicating with the patient—family, friends, and caregivers—understands and is able to use the communication devices selected.
- Demonstrate patience with the time needed to communicate effectively, and reinforce the patient's efforts.
- Ensure that the patient has an effective means of signaling need for assistance, such as a call bell or alarm.

Patients Who Are Cognitively Impaired

- Establish and maintain eye contact with the patient to hold attention.
- Communicate important information in a quiet environment where there is little to distract the patient's attention.
- Keep communication simple and concrete. Break down instructions into simple tasks and avoid lengthy explanations. Do not use pronouns or abstract terms. Use pictures or drawings when appropriate.
- Whenever possible, avoid open-ended questions. Ask "Would you like to wear the brown pants or the gray pants?" instead of "What would you like to wear?"
- Be patient and give the patient time to respond. If the patient does not respond after 2 minutes, repeat what you said. If there is still no response, take a break before continuing the conversation so that neither you nor the patient becomes frustrated.

Patients Who Are Unconscious

- Be careful of what is said in the patient's presence. Hearing is believed to be the last sense lost; therefore, the unconscious patient is often likely to hear even though there is no apparent response.
- Assume that the patient can hear you. Talk in a normal tone of voice about things you would ordinarily discuss.
- Speak with the patient before touching. Remember that touch can be an effective means of communication with the unconscious patient.
- Keep environment noises at as low a level as possible. This helps the patient focus on the communication.

Patients Who Do Not Speak English

- Use an interpreter whenever possible.
- Use a dictionary that translates words from one language to another so that you can speak at least some words in the patient's language.
- Speak in simple sentences and in a normal tone of voice.
- Demonstrate or pantomime ideas you wish to convey, as appropriate.
- Be aware of nonverbal communication. Remember that many nonverbal communication cues are universal.

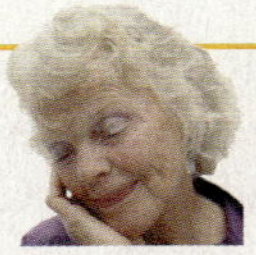

When caring for **Irwina Russellinski**, the older adult woman transferred after being treated for pneumonia, the nurse needs to investigate the cause and degree of the patient's hearing loss and what, if any, treatments or measures have been used to manage the problem. The nurse also needs to gather additional data about the patient's confusion and her cultural background. Based on this information, the nurse would be able to develop a plan of care that addresses Mrs. Russellinski's needs.

A nurse who suspects a speech, language, or hearing problem should refer the patient to a speech–language pathologist or audiologist. A speech–language pathologist is a professional educated in the study of human communication, its development, and its disorders. An audiologist is a professional educated in the study of normal and impaired hearing.

REFLECTIVE PRACTICE LEADING TO PERSONAL LEARNING

Remember that the goal of reflective practice is to look at an experience, understand it, and learn from it. As you begin to develop the use of and expertise in professional therapeutic communication, reflect on your experiences—successes and failures—in order to improve your practice. How can you do it better the next time? What did you learn today that can help you tomorrow? Begin your reflection by paying close attention to the following while providing nursing care:

- Did your preparation and practice related to the use of verbal and nonverbal communication techniques result in your feeling confident in your ability to communicate with your patient and their family? Did your competence and confidence inspire the patient's and family's trust?
- How did you prioritize the data you collected? What patterns in the data did you identify? What knowledge from your learning, personal experience, and intuition did you use to make decisions and develop your plan of care?
- How confident are you that you have successfully communicated information to other members of the health care team?
- Were you aware of any cultural or ethnic beliefs or practices that may have influenced your communication or development of a relationship with patients or family members? Were you aware of any stereotypes or prejudices that may have negatively influenced an encounter? If so, how did you address these?
- Was the patient's or family's participation in the process at an optimal level? How may you have better engaged the patient and family? Did the patient sense that you are respectful, caring, and competent?

Perhaps the most important questions to reflect on are: Are your patients and their families/caregivers better for having had *you* share in the critical responsibility of being a part of their health care team? Are your patients now receiving thoughtful, person-centered, prioritized, holistic, evidence-based treatment and care because of your efforts?

DEVELOPING CLINICAL REASONING AND CLINICAL JUDGMENT

1. Working with another student, attempt to express the following using nonverbal communication only:
   - I am in pain.
   - I am genuinely concerned about your well-being.
   - I couldn't care less that you are my patient, and I wish I were anywhere else but here caring for you.
   - I am afraid that you will hurt me.

   Describe what this exercise can teach you about the importance of nonverbal communication. Explain how this understanding will influence your nursing practice.
2. Conversation is both an art and an essential nursing tool. If you had 30 minutes to spend with each of the following patients while doing a procedure that allows you to communicate, what would you talk about (communicate) and why? Compare your answers with another student's, and explore what your conversations would communicate to the patients involved.
   - An older adult recently admitted to a long-term care facility
   - A 6-year-old boy newly admitted to a hospital for asthma
   - An HIV-positive, 33-year-old man who has just been given the news that he has acquired immunodeficiency syndrome (AIDS)
   - A 45-year-old amputee who has been in a rehabilitation hospital for 3 weeks after a motorcycle accident
   - A 19-year-old woman who has just had an elective abortion and is in the recovery unit
   - An unconscious patient in a critical care unit
3. An experienced nurse observes your distress after leaving the room of a patient who has just told her family that her cancer has recurred and is in an advanced state. She tells you that you better "toughen up" if you want to survive in nursing. She counsels not getting emotionally involved with patients and families: "Become a rock." How do you respond to this nurse and why? Of what value, if any, is empathy?

PRACTICING FOR NCLEX

1. The charge nurse overhears an AP yelling loudly to a patient who is hard of hearing, while transferring them from the bed to a chair. Upon entering the

room, which response by the charge nurse is most appropriate?
   a. "Please speak more quietly so you don't disturb the other patients."
   b. "Let me help you with your transfer technique."
   c. "When you are finished, be sure to apologize for shouting."
   d. "When your patient is safe and comfortable, meet me at the desk."
2. A public health nurse is leaving the home of a young mother who has an infant with special needs. The neighbor states, "How is she doing, since the baby's father is no help?" What is the nurse's best response?
   a. "New mothers need support."
   b. "The lack of a father is difficult."
   c. "How are you today?"
   d. "It is a very sad situation."
3. A toddler with vomiting, diarrhea, and dehydration is being seen at an acute care center. During the admission interview, what question will the nurse ask the parents to elicit the most useful information?
   a. "Watching your child vomiting and in discomfort must have been scary."
   b. "This started yesterday, correct?"
   c. "Has this child has had anything to drink?"
   d. Could you tell me the color and approximate amount of the vomiting?
4. A nurse enters a patient's room and examines the patient's intravenous (IV) fluids and cardiac monitor. When asked, "who are you?", which response by the nurse is most appropriate?
   a. "I'm just the IV therapist checking your IV."
   b. "I've been transferred to this division and will be caring for you."
   c. "I'm sorry, my name is John Smith and I am your nurse."
   d. "I am John Smith, your nurse, and I'll be caring for you until 11 PM."
5. A nurse enters the room of a patient with cancer. The patient is crying and states, "I feel so alone." How will the nurse best communicate a therapeutic response?
   a. The nurse stands at the patient's bedside and states, "I understand how you feel. My mother said the same thing when she was ill."
   b. The nurse places a hand on the patient's arm and states, "You feel so alone."
   c. The nurse stands in the patient's room and asks, "Why do you feel so alone? Your wife has been here every day."
   d. The nurse holds the patient's hand and asks, "Tell me what feeling so alone is like for you?"
6. A primary nurse is preparing a discharge plan for a patient who has been hospitalized following a double mastectomy. Which statement is most appropriate for the nurse to use in the termination phase of the therapeutic relationship?
   a. "Let's review the progress you've made in meeting your goals."
   b. "I'd like to review your medication schedule with you."
   c. "I need to document today's teaching session in the electronic health record."
   d. "Should we include your family in today's session?"
7. A nursing student is nervous and concerned about working at a clinical facility. Which action would best decrease anxiety and help ensure successful delivery of patient care?
   a. Determining the established goals of the institution
   b. Ensuring that verbal and nonverbal communication is congruent
   c. Engaging in self-talk to plan the day and decrease fear
   d. Speaking with fellow colleagues about how they feel
8. A nurse says to their nurse manager, "I need the day off, and you didn't give it to me!" The manager replies, "I wasn't aware you needed the day off, and it isn't possible since staffing is inadequate." How could the nurse best modify the communication for a more positive interaction?
   a. "I placed a request to have 8th of August off for a doctor's appointment, but I'm scheduled to work."
   b. "Could I make an appointment to discuss my schedule with you? I requested the 8th of August off for a doctor's appointment."
   c. "I will need to call in on the 8th of August because I have a doctor's appointment."
   d. "Since you didn't give me the 8th of August off, will I need to find someone to work for me?"
9. During a nursing staff meeting to discuss delayed documentation, the nurses unanimously agree that they will ensure all vital signs are reported and charted within 15 minutes following assessments. This decision is consistent with which characteristics of effective communication? Select all that apply.
   a. Group decision making
   b. Group leadership
   c. Group power
   d. Group identity
   e. Group patterns of interaction
   f. Group cohesiveness
10. A nurse notices a patient is walking to the bathroom with a stooped gait, facial grimacing, and grunting sounds. Based on these nonverbal cues, what action will the nurse take next?
   a. Assess for pain and the need for analgesia.
   b. Ask the patient if they feel anxious.
   c. Offer to sit with the patient and listen to their feelings.
   d. Suggest the patient increase their fluid intake to prevent constipation.

11. A nursing student is preparing to administer morning care to a patient. What question by the student is most important to ask?
    a. "Would you prefer a bath or a shower?"
    b. "May I help you with a bed bath now or later this morning?"
    c. "I will be giving you your bath. Do you use soap or shower gel?"
    d. "I prefer a shower in the evening. When would you like your bath?"
12. A nurse enters a patient's room and finds them vomiting bright red blood. After taking vital signs, the nurse communicates the event to the health care provider using the SBAR format. Which information will the nurse include in the "A" portion of the SBAR communication?

    Exhibit: Electronic health record (EHR)

Past medical history	Vital Signs
Peptic ulcer	T 98.8°F, P 111, RR 20, BP 98/50
Bleeding disorder	Pulse oximetry 96%

    a. Admitted with peptic ulcer and bleeding disorder
    b. Found vomiting in bathroom
    c. Anti-ulcer medication recommendation
    d. Vital signs, oxygen saturation, bright red emesis
13. The nurse preceptor and a new graduate nurse on the surgical unit are performing preoperative assessments on a group of patients. What statement by the graduate nurse requires the preceptor to intervene?
    a. "I am sure everything will be fine; you have nothing to worry about."
    b. "When you return from surgery, you'll need to cough and deep breathe."
    c. "Many people on this unit have had that procedure with good success."
    d. "You seem fearful, can I answer any questions about the procedure?"
14. A patient states, "I have been experiencing complications of diabetes." What question will the nurse use to elicit additional information?
    a. "Do you take two injections of insulin to prevent complications?"
    b. "Are you using diet and exercise to help regulate your blood sugar?"
    c. "Have you been experiencing the complications of neuropathy?"
    d. "Can you tell me about the complications you've experienced?"
15. During an interaction with a patient diagnosed with epilepsy, a nurse notes that the patient is silent after hearing the plan of care. How does the nurse best respond? Select all that apply.
    a. Fill the silence with lighter conversation directed at the patient.
    b. Use the time to perform the care that is needed uninterrupted.
    c. Discuss the silence with the patient to ascertain its meaning.
    d. Allow the patient time to think and explore inner thoughts.
    e. Determine if the patient's culture requires pauses between conversation.
    f. Arrange for a counselor to help the patient cope with emotional issues.

ANSWERS WITH RATIONALES

1. **d.** The charge nurse should direct the AP to see to the patient's safety, then address any concerns privately. The nurse then can discuss appropriate use of therapeutic communication.
2. **a.** The nurse must maintain confidentiality when providing care. The statement "New mothers need support" is a general statement that all new parents need help. The statement is not judgmental of the family's roles. "How are you today?" is dismissive of the neighbor's question.
3. **d.** Using a clarifying question or comment allows the nurse to gain an understanding of the parents' observations, avoiding misunderstandings that could lead to an inappropriate nursing diagnosis. A reflective question technique involves repeating what the person has said or describes the person's feelings. Assertive questions are direct, demonstrating the ability to stand up for self or others, using open and honest communication. Open-ended questions encourage free verbalization and expression of what the parents believe to be true.
4. **d.** The nurse should identify themselves, ensure the patient knows what will be happening, and the duration of their relationship.
5. **d.** The use of touch conveys acceptance, and the implementation of an open-ended question allows the patient time to verbalize freely.
6. **a.** The termination phase occurs when the conclusion of the initial agreement is acknowledged. Discharge planning correlates with the termination phase of a therapeutic relationship and the progress toward the patient's goals are reviewed.
7. **c.** By engaging in positive self-talk, or intrapersonal communication, the nursing student can plan the day, decrease fear and anxiety, and enhance clinical performance.
8. **b.** Effective communication involves sending clear, nonthreatening, and respectful information to the receiver. The nurse identifies the subject of the meeting and determines a mutually agreed upon time.
9. **a, d, e, f.** Solving problems involves group decision making; ascertaining the task is important and agreeing to complete the task on time is characteristic of group identity. Group patterns of interaction involve honest communication and member support; cohesiveness occurs when members generally trust each other, have a high commitment to the group, and a high degree of cooperation. Group leadership occurs when groups use effective styles of leadership to meet goals; with group power, sources of power are recognized and appropriately used to accomplish group outcomes.
10. **a.** A patient who presents with nonverbal communication of a stooped gait, facial grimacing, and grunting sounds is most likely communicating pain. The nurse should clarify this nonverbal behavior.

11. **b.** The nurse should ask permission to assist the patient with a bath. This allows for patient preferences and consent for care that involves entering the patient's personal space.

12. **d.** The SBAR method is used to improve hand-off communication. SBAR, which stands for Situation, Background, Assessment, and Recommendations, provides a clear, structured, and easy to use framework. Vital signs, oxygen saturation, and the presence of emesis and its color are assessments.

13. **a.** Telling a patient that everything will be fine is a cliché. This statement gives false assurance and may give the patient the impression that the nurse is dismissive of a patient's concerns or condition.

14. **d.** Requesting information regarding the patient's specific complications of diabetes will guide the nurse to further questioning and related assessments.

15. **c, d, e.** Appropriate use of silence allows the patient to initiate or to continue speaking; the nurse can reflect on what has been shared while observing the patient without having to concentrate simultaneously on conversation. In due time, the nurse might discuss the meaning of silence with the patient. The nurse considers whether the patient's culture may require longer pauses between verbal communication. Fear of silence sometimes leads to excessive talking by the nurse, displacing focus from the patient. The nurse should not assume silence requires a consult with a counselor.

Bibliography

Adzhigirey, L., Berg, J., Bickford, C. J., Broadnax, T., Denton, C., Leistner, G., McMenamin, J., Nims, P., & Smedley, L. (2019). *Telehealth nursing. A position statement.* Telehealth Nursing Special Interest Group. American Telemedicine Association.

Agency for Healthcare Research and Quality (AHRQ). (2020, January). *Pocket guide: TeamSTEPPS.* https://www.ahrq.gov/teamstepps/instructor/essentials/pocketguide.html#cus

American Association of Critical-Care Nurses (AACN). (2016). *AACN standards for establishing and sustaining healthy work environments. A journey to excellence* (2nd ed.). https://www.aacn.org/nursing-excellence/standards/aacn-standards-for-establishing-and-sustaining-healthy-work-environments

American Association of Critical-Care Nurses (AACN). (2019, May 1). *AACN position statement: Preventing violence against healthcare workers.* https://www.aacn.org/policy-and-advocacy/aacn-position-statement-preventing-violence

American Nurses Association (ANA). (2011). *ANA's Principles for social networking and the nurse.* https://www.nursingworld.org/practice-policy/nursing-excellence/official-position-statements/ana-principles/

American Nurses Association (ANA). (2015, July 22). *Position statement. Incivility, bullying and workplace violence.* https://www.nursingworld.org/practice-policy/nursing-excellence/official-position-statements/id/incivility-bullying-and-workplace-violence/

American Nurses Association (ANA). (2019a). *ANA Core principles on connected health.* https://www.nursingworld.org/practice-policy/nursing-excellence/official-position-statements/ana-principles/

American Nurses Association (ANA). (2019b). *Workplace violence.* https://www.nursingworld.org/practice-policy/advocacy/state/workplace-violence2/

American Nurses Association (ANA) and AONE. (n.d.). *ANA/AONE Principles for collaborative relationships between clinical nurses and managers.* Author. https://www.nursingworld.org/practice-policy/nursing-excellence/official-position-statements/ana-principles/

Andrews, M., Boyle, J. S., & Collins, J. (2020). *Transcultural concepts in nursing care* (8th ed.). Wolters Kluwer.

Armstrong, N. (2018). Management of nursing workplace incivility in the health care settings. A systematic review. *Workplace Health & Safety, 66*(8), 403–410. https://doi.org/10.1177/2165079918771106

Baby, M., Gale, C., & Swain, N. (2019). A communication skills intervention to minimise patient perpetrated aggression for healthcare support workers in New Zealand: A cluster randomised controlled trial. *Health and Social Care in the Community, 27*(1), 170–181. https://doi.org/10.1111/hsc.12636

Bambi, S., Guazzini, A., Piredda, M., Lucchini, A., Grazia DeMarinis, M., & Rasero, L. (2019). Negative interactions among nurses: An explorative study on lateral violence and bullying in nursing work settings. *Journal of Nursing Management, 27*(4), 749–757. https://doi.org/10.1111/jonm.12738

Bartley, A., & Jacobs, T. (2013). IHI expedition. Engaging frontline teams to create a culture of safety. Institute for Healthcare Improvement. [PowerPoint presentation]. http://www.ihi.org/Engage/Memberships/Passport/Documents/IHI%20Expedition%20Engaging%20Frontline%20Teams%20to%20Create%20a%20Culture%20of%20Safety%20Session%203.pdf

Beiler, J., Opper, K., & Weiss, M. (2019). Integrating research and quality improvement using TeamSTEPPS. A health team communication project to improve hospital discharge. *Clinical Nurse Specialist, 33*(1), 22–32. https://doi.org/10.1097/NUR.0000000000000417

Benyon, B. (2019). Violence against nurses: A major issue in healthcare. *Oncology Nursing News.* https://www.oncnursingnews.com/web-exclusives/violence-against-nurses-a-major-issue-in-healthcare

Berlo, D. (1960). *The process of communication: An introduction to theory and practice.* Holt, Rinehart and Winston.

Bochatay, N. (2019). Discussing teamwork in health care: From interprofessional collaboration to coordination and cooperation. *Health Information and Libraries Journal, 36*(4), 367–371. https://doi.org/10.1111/hir.12282

Bonds, R. L. (2018). SBAR Tool implementation to advance communication, teamwork, and the perception of patient safety culture. *Creative Nursing, 24*(2), 116–123. https://doi.org/10.1891/1078-4535.24.2.116

Boyd, M. A. (2018). *Psychiatric nursing. Contemporary practice* (6th ed.). Wolters Kluwer.

Centers for Disease Control and Prevention and the National Institute for Occupational Safety and Health (NIOSH). (2019). *Workplace violence prevention for nurses.* CDC Course No. WB2908-NIOSH Pub. No. 2013-2155. https://www.cdc.gov/niosh/topics/violence/training_nurses.html

Chan, W. S., & Leung, A. Y. (2018). Use of social network sites for communication among health professionals: Systematic review. *Journal of Medical Internet Research, 20*(3), e117. https://doi.org/10.2196/jmir.8382

Chung, S., Huang, Q., LaMori, J., Doshi, D., & Romanelli, R. J. (2020). Patient-reported experiences in discussing prescribed medications with a health care provider: Evidence for racial/ethnic disparities in a large health care delivery system. *Population Health Management, 23*(1), 78–84. https://doi.org/10.1089/pop.2018.0206

Clapper, T. C. (2018). TeamSTEPPS® is an effective tool to level the hierarchy in healthcare communication by empowering all stakeholders. *Journal of Communication in Healthcare, 11*(4), 241–244. https://doi.org/10.1080/17538068.2018.1561806

Clark, A., Wolgast, K. A., Mazur, N., & Mekis, A. (2020). Leading change in nurse bedside shift report. *Nursing Clinics in North America, 55*(1), 21–28. https://doi.org/10.1016/j.cnur.2019.10.002

Clark, C. M. (2019). Fostering a culture of civility and respect in nursing. *Journal of Nursing Regulation, 10*(1), 44–50.

Curtin, L. (2019). Workplace violence: Don't risk it, de-escalate it. *American Nurse Today, 14*(5), 72. https://www.myamericannurse.com/wp-content/uploads/2019/03/ant5-Curtin-417.pdf

Daigle, A. (2020). Social media and professional boundaries in undergraduate nursing students. *Journal of Professional Nursing, 36*(2), 20–23. https://doi.org/10.1016/j.profnurs.2019.08.007

Eliopoulos, C. (2018). *Gerontological nursing* (9th ed.). Wolters Kluwer.

Ellis, P. (2018). What it means to be an assertive leader. *Wounds UK, 14*(3), 52–54.

Galatzan, B. J., & Carrington, J. M. (2018). Exploring the state of science of the nursing hand-off communication. *CIN: Computers, Informatics, Nursing, 36*(10), 484–493. https://doi.org/10.1097/CIN.0000000000000461

George, S., Rahmatinick, S., & Ramos, J. (2018). Commit to sit to improve nurse communication. *Critical Care Nurse, 38*(2), 83–85. https://doi.org/10.4037/ccn2018846

Giger, J. N., & Hadsdad, L. G. (2017). *Transcultural nursing. Assessment and intervention* (8th ed.). Elsevier.

GLAAD. (2016). *GLAAD media reference guide* (10th ed.). https://www.glaad.org/reference

Howard, M. S., & Embree, J. L. (2020). Educational intervention improves communication abilities of nurses encountering workplace incivility. *The Journal of Continuing Education in Nursing, 51*(3), 138–144. https://doi.org/10.3928/00220124-20200216-09

Institute for Healthcare Improvement (IHI). (n.d.). *Develop a culture of safety.* http://www.ihi.org/resources/Pages/Changes/DevelopaCultureofSafety.aspx

Institute for Healthcare Improvement. (2017). *SBAR Tool: Situation-background-assessment-recommendation.* http://www.ihi.org/resources/Pages/Tools/SBARToolkit.aspx

Johnson, A. H., & Benham-Hutchins, M. (2020). The influence of bullying on nursing practice errors: A systematic review. *AORN Journal, 111*(2), 199–210. https://doi.org/10.1002/aorn.12923

Johnson, D. W., & Johnson, F. P. (2017). *Joining together: Group theory and group skills. (The counselling series)* (12th ed.). Pearson.

The Joint Commission Center for Transforming Healthcare. (n.d.). *Hand-off communications targeted solutions tool.* https://www.centerfortransforminghealthcare.org/what-we-offer/targeted-solutions-tool/hand-off-communications-tst/

The Joint Commission. (2011). *Advancing effective communication, cultural competence, and patient-and-family-centered care for the lesbian, gay, bisexual, and transgender (LGBT) community: A field guide.* https://www.jointcommission.org/-/media/tjc/documents/resources/patient-safety-topics/health-equity/lgbtfieldguide_web_linked_verpdf.pdf?db=web&hash=FD725DC02CFE6E4F21A35EBD839BBE97&hash=FD725DC02CFE6E4F21A35EBD839BBE97

The Joint Commission. (2016). *Sentinel Event Alert 40. Behaviors that undermine a culture of safety.* https://www.jointcommission.org/resources/patient-safety-topics/sentinel-event/sentinel-event-alert-newsletters/sentinel-event-alert-issue-40-behaviors-that-undermine-a-culture-of-safety/

The Joint Commission. (2017). *Sentinel Event Alert 58. Inadequate hand-off communication.* https://www.jointcommission.org/resources/patient-safety-topics/sentinel-event/sentinel-event-alert-newsletters/sentinel-event-alert-58-inadequate-hand-off-communication/

The Joint Commission. (2018). *Sentinel Event Alert 59. Physical and verbal violence against health care workers.* https://www.jointcommission.org/resources/patient-safety-topics/sentinel-event/sentinel-event-alert-newsletters/sentinel-event-alert-59-physical-and-verbal-violence-against-health-care-workers/

The Joint Commission. (2020a). *Patient-centered communications* [Fact sheet]. https://www.jointcommission.org/resources/news-and-multimedia/fact-sheets/

The Joint Commission. (2021). *2021 National patient safety goals.* https://www.jointcommission.org/standards/national-patient-safety-goals/

Joint Commission International (JCI). (2018). *Communicating clearly and effectively to patients. How to overcome common communication challenges in health care.* A White Paper by Joint Commission International. https://store.jointcommissioninternational.org/assets/3/7/jci-wp-communicating-clearly-final_(1).pdf

Keltner, N. L., & Steele, D. (2019). *Psychiatric nursing* (8th ed.). Elsevier.

Kersey-Matusiak, G. (2019). *Delivering culturally competent nursing care. Working with diverse and vulnerable populations* (2nd ed.). Springer Publishing Company.

Koivunen, M., & Saranto, K. (2018). Nursing professionals' experiences of the facilitators and barriers to the use of telehealth applications: A systematic review of qualitative studies. *Scandinavian Journal of Caring Sciences, 32*(1), 24–44. https://doi.org/10.1111/scs.12445

Layne, D. M., Nemeth, L. S., Mueller, M., Schaffner, M. J., Stanley, K. M., Martin, M. M., & Wallston, K. A. (2018). Negative behaviours in health care: Prevalence and strategies. *Journal of Nursing Management, 27*(1), 154–160. https://doi.org/10.1111/jonm.12660

Lever, I., Dyball, D., Greenberg, N., & Stevelink, S. A. M. (2019). Health consequences of bullying in the healthcare workplace: A systematic review. *Journal of Advanced Nursing, 75*(12), 3195–3209. https://doi.org/10.1111/jan.13986

Locke, L., Bromley, G., & Federspiel, K. A. (2018). Patient violence: It's not all in a day's work. *American Nurse Today, 13*(5), 10–13.

Marquis, B. L., & Huston, C. J. (2021). *Leadership roles and management functions in nursing. Theory and application* (10th ed.). Wolters Kluwer Health.

Mataxen, P. A., & Webb, L. D. (2019). Telehealth nursing: More than just a phone call. *Nursing, 49*(4), 11–13. https://doi.org/10.1097/01.NURSE.0000553272.16933.4b

McPherson, P., & Buxton, T. (2019). In their own words: Nurses countering workplace incivility. *Nursing Forum, 54*(3), 455–460. https://doi.org/10.1111/nuf.12354

Meires, J. (2018a). The essentials: Here's what you need to know about bullying in nursing. *Urologic Nursing, 38*(2), 95–102. https://doi.org/10.7257/1053-816X.2018.38.2

Meires, J. (2018b). The essentials: Using emotional intelligence to curtail bullying in the workplace. *Urologic Nursing, 38*(3), 150–153. https://doi.org/10.7257/1053-816X.2018.38.3.150

Messner, R. L. (1993). What patients really want from their nurses. *American Journal of Nursing, 93*(8), 38–41.

Millis, S. (2018). Changing workplace culture. What would it take to speak up? *The Dissector, 46*(2), 14–17.

Moscrop, A., Ziebland, S., Roberts, N., & Papanikitas, A. (2019). A systematic review of reasons for and against asking patients about their socioeconomic contexts. *International Journal for Equity in Health, 18*(1), 112. https://doi.org/10.1186/s12939-019-1014-2

National Council of State Boards of Nursing (NCSBN). (2018). *A nurse's guide to the use of social media.* [Brochure]. Author. https://www.ncsbn.org/3739.htm

National Institute for Occupational Safety and Health (NIOSH). (2014). *Violence in the workplace.* Current intelligence bulletin 57. DHHS (NIOSH) Publication Number 96–100. https://www.cdc.gov/niosh/docs/96-100/default.html

Occupational Health & Safety (OH&S). (2020). *Nurses are suffering more violence in the workplace.* https://ohsonline.com/articles/2020/02/10/nurses-are-suffering-more-violence-in-the-workplace.aspx

Occupational Safety and Health Administration (OSHA). (2015a). *Preventing workplace violence: A road map for healthcare facilities.* Publication OSHA 3827. https://www.osha.gov/sites/default/files/OSHA3827.pdf

Occupational Safety and Health Administration (OSHA). (2015b). *Workplace violence prevention and related goals. The big picture.* Publication OSHA 3828. https://www.osha.gov/sites/default/files/OSHA3828.pdf

Occupational Safety and Health Administration (OSHA). (2015c). *Workplace violence in healthcare. Understanding the challenge.* Publication OSHA 3826. https://www.osha.gov/sites/default/files/OSHA3826.pdf

Occupational Safety and Health Administration (OSHA). (2016). *Guidelines for preventing workplace violence for healthcare and social service workers.* U. S. Department of Labor. https://www.osha.gov/Publications/osha3148.pdf

The Office of the National Coordinator for Health Information Technology (ONC). (2017). *Telemedicine and telehealth.* HealthIT.gov. https://www.healthit.gov/topic/health-it-initiatives/telemedicine-and-telehealth

Orlando, I. J. (1961). *The dynamic nurse–patient relationship.* G. P. Putnam's Sons.

Padgett, T. M. (2018). Improving nurses' communication during patient transfer: A pilot study. *The Journal of Continuing Education in Nursing, 49*(8), 378–384.

Panesar, R. S., Albert, B., Messina, C., & Parker, M. (2016). The effect of an electronic SBAR communication tool on documentation of acute events in the pediatric intensive care unit. *American Journal of Medical Quality, 31*(1), 64–68.

Paterson, J., & Zderad, L. (1976). *Humanistic nursing.* Wiley.

Patient Safety Network (PSNet). (2019). *Handoffs and signouts.* Agency for Healthcare Research and Quality (AHRQ). https://psnet.ahrq.gov/primer/handoffs-and-signouts

Peplau, H. (1952). *Interpersonal relations in nursing.* Putnam.

Pettit, A. M., & Duffy, J. J. (2015). Patient safety: Creating a culture change to support communication and teamwork. *The Journal of Legal Nurse Consulting, 26*(4), 23–26.

Quality and Safety Education for Nurses (QSEN) Institute. (n.d.). *QSEN competencies.* https://qsen.org/competencies/pre-licensure-ksas/

Quality and Safety Education for Nurses (QSEN) Institute. (2008). *Reformulating SBAR to "I-SBAR-R."* http://qsen.org/reformulating-sbar-to-i-sbar-r

Quality Improvement Organizations. Centers for Medicare & Medicaid Services. (2020). *TeamSTEPPS® in LTC: Communication strategies to promote quality and safety.* https://qioprogram.org/teamstepps%C2%AE-ltc-communication-strategies-promote-quality-and-safety

Registered Nurses' Association of Ontario (RNAO). (n.d.). *Nursing best practice guidelines. Phases of the therapeutic relationship.* https://bpgmobile.rnao.ca/node/1038

Sauer, P. A., & McCoy, T. P. (2018). Nurse bullying and intent to leave. *Nursing Economic, 36*(5), 219–245.

Scruth, E. A., Pugh, D. M., Adams, C. L., & Foss-Durant, A. M. (2015). Electronic and social media: The legal and ethical issues for healthcare. *Clinical Nurse Specialist, 29*(1), 8–11.

Sermersheim, E. R., Moon, M. C., Streelman, M., McCullum-Smith, D., Fromm, J., Yohannan, S., & Powell, R. (2020). Improving patient throughput with an electronic nursing handoff process in an academic medical center. *Journal of Nursing Administration, 50*(3), 174–181. https://doi.org/10.1097/NNA.0000000000000862

Settani, S. S., Silva, G. B. S., Julião, I. H. T., da Silva, M. C. F., da Silva, J. C. B., Oliveira, D. A. L., Barbosa, L. M. S., & Silva, C. C. (2019). Integrative literature review article. Nursing communication and its impact on patient safety. *Journal of Nursing, 13*, 327–333. https://doi.org/10.5205/1981-8963.2019.239573

Stans, S. E. A., Dalemans, R. J. P., Roentgen, U. R., Smeets, H. W. H., & Beurskens, A. J. H. M. (2018). Who said dialogue conversations are easy? The communication between communication vulnerable people and health-care professionals: A qualitative study. *Health Expectations, 21*(5), 848–857. https://doi.org/10.1111/hex.12679

Sweeney Gustin, T., Kott, K., & Rutledge, C. (2020). Telehealth etiquette training. A guideline for preparing interprofessional teams for successful encounters. *Nurse Educator, 45*(2), 88–92. https://doi.org/10.1097/NNE.0000000000000680

Tingle, J. (2018). Communication breakdown in healthcare settings. *British Journal of Nursing, 27*(20), 1204–1205.

Tocco, S. (2014). Managing our fears to improve patient safety. *American Nurse Today, 9*(5), 34–38. http://www.medscape.com/viewarticle/825934_5

Townsend, M., & Morgan, K. I. (2018). *Psychiatric mental health nursing: Concepts of care in evidence-based practice* (9th ed.). F.A. Davis Company.

Travelbee, J. (1971). *Interpersonal aspects of nursing* (2nd ed.). F. A. Davis.

Tuohy, D. (2018). Effective intercultural communication in nursing. *Nursing Standard, 34*(2), 45–50.

Tuohy, D. (2019). Effective intercultural communication in nursing. *Nursing Standard, 34*(2), 45–50. doi: 10.7748/ns.2019.e11244

Videbeck, S. L. (2020). *Psychiatric mental health nursing* (8th ed.). Wolters Kluwer.

Watson, J. (1985). *Nursing: The philosophy and science of caring.* Colorado Associated University Press.

Williams, K. N., Perkhounkova, Y., Jao, Y. L., Bossen, A., Hein, M., Jihey, S., Chung, J., Starykowicz, A., & Turk, M. (2018). Person-centered communication for nursing home residents with dementia: Four communication analysis methods. *Western Journal of Nursing Research, 40*(7), 1012–1031. https://doi.org/10.1177/0193945917697226

Wolters Kluwer. (2022). Problem-based care plans. In *Lippincott Advisor.* Wolters Kluwer.

Yagil, D., & Dayan, H. (2020). Justification of aggression against nurses: The effect of aggressor distress and nurse communication quality. *Journal of Advanced Nursing, 76*(2), 611–620. https://doi.org/10.1111/jan.14269

Zeigler, K., & Camarota, S. A. (2018). *Almost half speak a foreign language in America's largest cities. Nationally, one in five spoke a language other than English in 2017.* Center for Immigration Studies. https://cis.org/Report/Almost-Half-Speak-Foreign-Language-Americas-Largest-Cities

Zuzelo, P. R. (2020). Workplace violence. Opportunities to improve the context of health care. *Holistic Nursing Practice, 34*(1), 68–70. https://doi.org/10.1097/HNP.0000000000000366

9 Teaching and Counseling

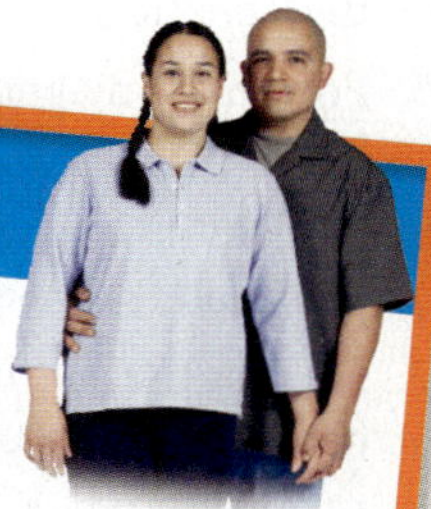

Marco García Ramírez

Marco accompanies his wife, Claudia, to the antepartal clinic for a routine visit. They are expecting their first child in 5 months. He reports that they are happy and excited but also scared and very nervous. They are planning for a home birth, asking lots of questions about childbirth and their new responsibilities as parents: "We're both wondering if we'll be good parents."

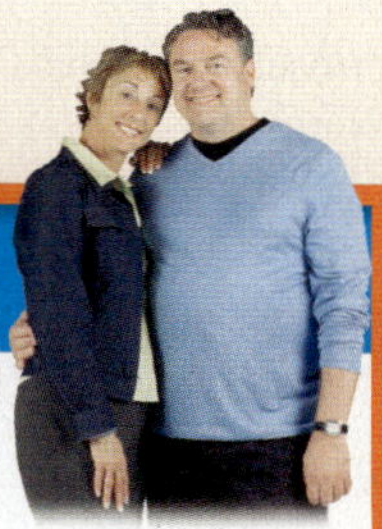

Rachel Blumenthal

Rachel, age 40, is the second wife of a 57-year-old man who has suffered a serious myocardial infarction. They have been married for only 1 year. She says, "I'm a little embarrassed to talk with the cardiologist, but I have lots of questions about what my husband will be able to do after he gets home. I'm also wondering about resuming sexual activity."

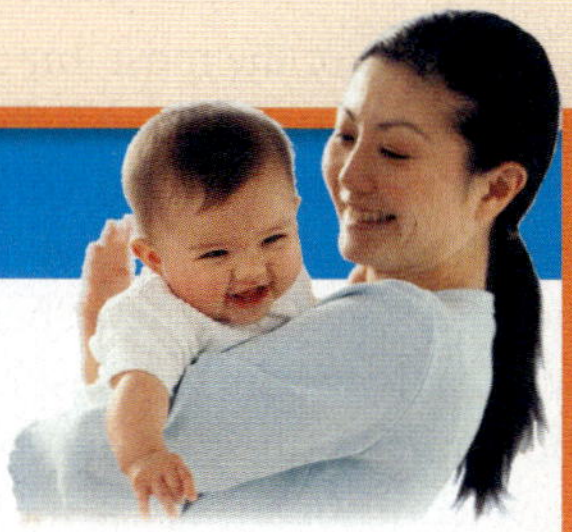

Alicia Bonet

Alicia is the young mother of a baby boy; the baby's health care provider is recommending that he start long-term aspirin therapy. Ms. Bonet is quite concerned about agreeing to long-term aspirin therapy and asks, "I've heard so much about Reye syndrome and aspirin. What should I do? What would you recommend?"

Learning Outcomes

After completing the chapter, you will be able to accomplish the following:

1. Describe the teaching–learning process.
2. Describe factors that are assessed in the learning process.
3. Discuss strategies to improve health literacy and promote patient safety.
4. Describe factors that influence adherence with the therapeutic plan.
5. Formulate diagnoses/patient problems for identified learning needs.
6. Explain how to create and implement a culturally considerate, age-specific teaching plan for a patient.
7. Discuss the role of a nurse coach in promoting behavior change.
8. Identify methods for evaluating learning.
9. Explain what should be included in the documentation of the teaching–learning process.
10. Discuss the nurse's role as a counselor.
11. Describe how the nursing process is used to help patients solve problems.
12. Explain how patient education and counseling is used to motivate a patient toward health promotion.

Nursing Concepts

- Assessment
- Clinical Decision Making/Clinical Judgment
- Communication
- Health promotion
- Teaching and learning/patient education

One of the most important nursing roles involves helping patients and their families learn how to respond to their health care problems and how to promote health. Many patients lack the knowledge and self-care abilities they need to achieve their health goals. To work effectively with patients, nurses must be skilled teachers and counselors. Both roles require strong communication skills. Many factors have contributed to an intensified need for effective patient teaching and counseling: current trends toward shorter hospital stays and decreased time for interactions between health care professionals and patients, dependence on complex technologies, an increased emphasis on health promotion, consumer empowerment, cost containment, and an increase in chronic illness. Nurses are challenged with the task of creating an environment conducive to learning that motivates individuals to want to learn and makes it possible for them to learn—a learner-centered approach (Bastable, 2019; Sykes et al., 2013, as cited in Bastable, 2019, p. 16). Nurses are facilitators (Bastable, 2019), engaging patients and their family/caregivers as partners in the learning process and challenged by limited time and resources and patients who may or may not be ready, willing, or able to learn. Refer to the accompanying Reflective Practice box for one student's experience in responding to a request from a patient's family member for information to help in making an informed health care decision.

Never has the demand for quality education and counseling been greater. Nurses who are skilled educators and counselors can improve patients' health and well-being and reduce the demand for professional services. Current trends in health care are making it essential that patients are prepared to assume responsibility for self-care management (Bastable, 2019). Nurses must ensure that patients, families, and caregivers receive the information they need and demonstrate learning essential knowledge and skills to maintain optimal health. The Institute of Medicine (IOM, 2001) identified the importance of education in patient- and family-centered care in their report *Crossing the Quality Chasm,* proposing that access to understandable health information is essential to empower patients to participate in their care, and patient-centered organizations take responsibility for providing access to that information. (Note: The IOM titling has changed in recent years and is now referred to more broadly as The National Academies of Sciences, Engineering, and Medicine.) It is critical for health care professionals to inform and engage patients in their own health care through education (IOM, 2013). The Joint Commission (n.d.a) reinforced the importance of and supported this crucial need for educating patients by sponsoring the Speak Up initiative. This patient safety program aims to empower and educate patients and make them a partner in their care. The Speak Up campaign features infographics, animated videos, and brochures, and use has expanded to more than 70 countries (The Joint Commission, n.d.b). All Speak Up materials are available in English and Spanish and can be translated into other languages; they are available for use without copyright or reprinting permissions.

AIMS OF TEACHING AND COUNSELING

Patient education is the "process of assisting people to learn health-related behaviors that they can incorporate into everyday life with the goal of achieving optimal health and independence in self-care" (Bastable, 2019, p. 15), influencing the patient's behavior to effect changes in knowledge, attitudes, and skills needed to maintain and improve health. Research supports the fact that educated patients experience better health and have fewer complications. This results in fewer hospitalizations and emergency department, clinic, and health care provider visits. To be successful, patient education must be ongoing and interactive. It must also take into account the patient's plan of care, educational level, need for care no matter what the setting or environment, and other **social determinants of health**. Patient education plans should be developed with the patient in collaboration with the entire health care team, including, for example, physicians, dietitians, respiratory therapists, social workers,

QSEN Reflective Practice: Cultivating QSEN Competencies

CHALLENGE TO ETHICAL AND LEGAL SKILLS

It was during my senior practicum in pediatrics last spring that I met Alicia Bonet, the young mother of a baby boy for whom I was caring. The baby's health care provider was recommending long-term aspirin therapy (unfortunately, I cannot remember what condition the child had for which long-term aspirin therapy was being recommended). Ms. Bonet was quite concerned about agreeing to aspirin therapy, asking me if I knew much about Reye syndrome. Then she asked me what I would recommend about whether or not to agree to long-term aspirin therapy. Not really understanding the risks versus the benefits of aspirin therapy or how it actually ties into Reye syndrome, I did not feel competent to answer Ms. Bonet's questions, let alone make an educated recommendation to her.

Thinking Outside the Box: Possible Courses of Action

- Tell the mother that I could not be of help to her in making this decision because of my lack of knowledge about either topic.
- Inform her that I would have to ask other nurses and members of the health care team to explain both topics to me (due to my lack of knowledge) before I could give her my opinion.
- Be honest with the mother about my lack of knowledge about either aspirin therapy or Reye syndrome and offer to gather information from reputable sources for both of us so that we could discuss the topics.
- Provide her with information from the hospital library or the internet so that she could educate herself (but not for my education so that I could assist her in making her decision).
- Lie to the mother (or withhold the fact that I did not know much about aspirin therapy or Reye syndrome) and make an uneducated recommendation simply because I had the "authority" to do so.
- Ignore the mother's request, pretending not to have time to discuss her questions, rather than admitting my own ignorance or taking the time to educate myself.

Evaluating a Good Outcome: How Do I Define Success?

- The mother's needs are met. Not only does she receive a professional, educated, and competent recommendation, but she also is given the opportunity to make her own educated decisions by being given the information she needs.
- My intellectual competence is challenged and improved. I am able to admit a deficit in my knowledge and embrace the opportunity to improve it.
- The mother and patient benefit from my actions (or at least are not harmed) by the mother's informed choice.
- The mother's autonomy is encouraged—by providing her with all the necessary information, I enable her to make a healthy, educated decision.
- Quality care is provided to the patient and their family by competent professionals.
- The mother expresses an understanding of the information presented to her, feels comfortable asking additional questions, and makes an educated decision with which she is comfortable.

Personal Learning: Here's to the Future!

After explaining to the mother that I was not very familiar with aspirin therapy or Reye syndrome, I first attempted to gather research information from the internet for her. However, because I did not have a password to access the internet from the nurse's station, I could not obtain the research I needed on my own. My next step was to ask my preceptor how to gather data for the mother if I could not get it from the internet. She suggested calling down to the hospital library and asking them to put together an information packet that could be easily understood by a patient. I did this, and several hours later, the packet arrived on the floor. After flipping through it briefly, I was satisfied with its contents and delivered it to Ms. Bonet. While I wished I had had the time to read all the information myself so that I could sit down with the mother and discuss it in detail, the day had been particularly busy. The best I could do was to pass the information on to the mother and hope she would read it herself. She was very grateful that I went to the trouble of gathering so much information for her, and she did not seem at all annoyed or disappointed that I did not have time to sit down with her to review the material. I did let her know that she could feel free to ask me any questions after she read the material, but she never got a chance to read the packet before my shift ended (because her son had visitors). As a result, we never got around to discussing her concerns.

One of the things that I learned from this experience is that it is okay to admit to a patient that you do not have all the answers. Moreover, admitting this helps to allay any doubt that they may have about my intellect or abilities as a nurse. Admitting a lack of knowledge is not a weakness, but a strength, for half the battle is knowing what you do not know. If anything, my willingness to admit my lack of knowledge and eagerness to educate both myself and my patient (by doing research) helped inspire trust and faith in me by my patient. I also learned that sometimes doing the best we can is better than doing nothing at all, even if the best we can do is not very much. Although I really needed to be able to sit down with Ms. Bonet and review the research with her, simply providing her with the material was enough to enable her to make an informed decision on her own. That simple act most likely empowered her to be much more comfortable with her decision in the end.

Although this occurred only a few months ago, I feel safe saying that my professional intellectual skills are quite adequate now—actually, they were quite adequate back then, too. Not knowing everything in nursing is not a reflection of inadequate professional intellectual skills, because it is impossible to know everything in this field. The fact that I knew that my knowledge was lacking, but that I knew where to go to find an answer, tells me my professional intellectual skills are more than adequate.

Tracey Sara Miller, Georgetown University

(*continued*)

QSEN Reflective Practice: Cultivating QSEN Competencies *(continued)*

CHALLENGE TO ETHICAL AND LEGAL SKILLS

QSEN SELF-REFLECTION ON QUALITY AND SAFETY COMPETENCIES DEVELOPING KNOWLEDGE, SKILLS, AND ATTITUDES FOR CONTINUOUS IMPROVEMENT

How do you think you would respond in a similar situation? Why? What does this tell you about yourself and about the adequacy of your skills for professional practice? What *knowledge, skills,* and *attitudes* do you need to develop to continuously improve quality and safety in a situation like the one experienced by this student nurse?

Patient-Centered Care: How did the nursing student's communication skills improve the nurse–patient relationship? Did her handling of this situation facilitate her ability to deliver effective care and treatment in other environments? What, if any, teaching and learning principles did the nursing student use?

Teamwork and Collaboration/Quality Improvement: How important are effective communication skills when collaborating with other team members and hospital staff? Are there other referrals or community resources that might prove helpful to Ms. Bonet regarding her questions about long-term aspirin use for her child?

Safety/Evidence-Based Practice: Is there anything else the nursing student could have done to facilitate a positive outcome? Do you agree with the criteria to evaluate a successful outcome? Did the nursing student meet the criteria? What evidence in nursing evidence for practice provides guidance to assist Ms. Bonet with effective decision making in this situation? If time had not been a factor and you were able to discuss the materials in the packet with the baby's mother, would that have been an opportunity to assess Ms. Bonet's understanding of the information provided?

Informatics: Can you identify essential information that should be documented in the child's electronic record regarding your efforts to communicate with the mother about the specific concerns she expressed? Do you think the self-confidence gained from dealing effectively with this situation improves your ability to respond to patient's questions and accurately document their concerns?

pharmacists, community-based care providers, wellness facilities, and long-term care facilities.

The basic purpose of teaching and counseling is to help patients and families develop the self-care abilities (knowledge, attitude, skills) they need to maximize their functioning and quality of life (or to have a dignified death). For example, a patient newly diagnosed with diabetes must (1) acquire knowledge about diabetes as a disease process and related medical management and self-care; (2) value health sufficiently to make certain lifestyle modifications (attitude); and (3) master certain skills, such as medication administration. When done effectively, teaching and counseling are powerful tools for helping patients achieve health goals. Teaching provides the knowledge that patients need to make informed health care decisions and to implement a plan of care. **Counseling** provides the resources and support that patients need to participate actively in self-care and to facilitate their coping with their circumstances.

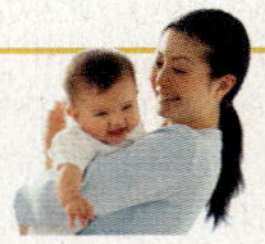

Recall **Alicia Bonet**, the young mother worried about long-term aspirin therapy and Reye syndrome. By providing Ms. Bonet with information, the nurse enables her to reach a decision that is based on sound knowledge and one with which she is comfortable.

Maintaining and Promoting Health

Nurses can help patients value health and develop specific health practices that promote wellness. Health teaching related to health promotion is varied, and ranges from teaching passive exercises to a patient with left-sided paralysis, to designing a safe exercise program for a young athlete, to teaching cooking for good nutrition to a group of middle-school children.

Preventing Illness

Educational intervention related to illness prevention, a major theme in health teaching and counseling, takes many forms. You can counsel women of childbearing age about health practices that promote optimal fetal development, teach parents how to make their home safe for a toddler, counsel people at high risk for heart disease, cancer, or communicable diseases, or explain preventive health screening to adults.

Restoring Health

Once a patient is ill, teaching and counseling focus on developing self-care practices that promote recovery. Pre- and postoperative teaching, sexual counseling for a patient recovering from a myocardial infarction, and lifestyle counseling for a patient with an ostomy are all examples of teaching and counseling directed at restoring health.

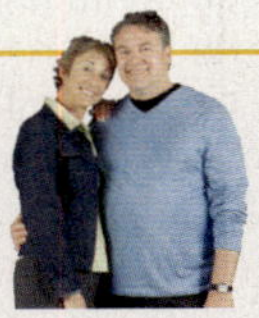

Consider **Rachel Blumenthal**, the wife of the patient who had suffered a myocardial infarction. She is concerned about his activity level. When developing an appropriate teaching plan, the nurse would need to assess Mr. and Mrs. Blumenthal's knowledge base before determining their actual learning needs. In addition, the nurse would need to consult with the patient's cardiologist to determine the patient's status and levels of activity that are safe in relation to his health status. These actions help to ensure that the teaching plan includes accurate information and is individualized to Mr. and Mrs. Blumenthal's needs.

Facilitating Coping

Developmental lifestyle changes and acute, chronic, and terminal illness all place demands on patients and families that may become overwhelming. As a nurse, you will work not only with patients but also with their families and friends to help them adjust to changes in health status and whatever lifestyle modifications may be required. Not all patients fully recover from their illness or injury; many patients will need to learn to adapt and cope with short-term, long-term, or permanent health alterations.

Promoting Outcomes

Nurses who are skilled teachers and counselors work to promote the following outcomes:

- An optimal level of wellness and related self-care practices
- Disease prevention or early detection
- Quick recovery from trauma or illness with minimal or no complications
- Enhanced ability to cope with developmental lifestyle changes and acute and chronic health conditions, and/or terminal illness

Potential topics for health teaching and counseling are identified in Box 9-1.

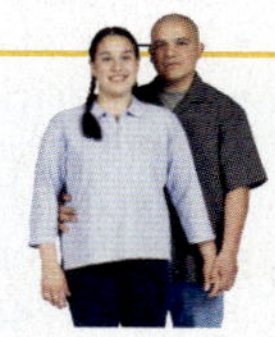

Remember ***Marco García Ramírez***, the father-to-be described in the beginning of the chapter. Pregnancy and childbirth are associated with developmental lifestyle changes. The nurse needs to incorporate knowledge of these changes when working with the couple to develop an appropriate teaching plan for Mr. García Ramírez and his wife. The goal of teaching would be a positive adaptation to their new role as parents.

NURSE AS TEACHER

Teaching is a planned method or series of methods used to help someone learn. The person using these methods is the teacher. **Learning** is the process by which a person acquires or increases knowledge or changes behavior in a measurable way as a result of the experience. You assume the role of teacher and your patient assumes the role of learner when there are identified learning needs. This teacher–learner relationship is enhanced by the therapeutic nurse–patient relationship, in which mutual respect and trust are established (see Chapter 8). You build on this trust by sharing information that you and your patient mutually identify as important.

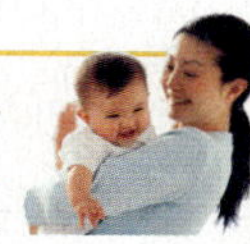

Think back to ***Alicia Bonet***, the young mother with questions about long-term aspirin therapy. The nurse developed trust with Ms. Bonet by honestly identifying that she lacked the necessary knowledge about the therapy. The nurse promoted an ongoing therapeutic relationship by seeking the information, thereby solidifying trust.

The patient may ask for information, or you may initiate teaching after assessing and diagnosing/identifying a learning need. Key concepts that are important to consider in regard to patient education include the following (Lowenstein et al., 2009):

- Listen to your patients and their families
- Every interaction is an opportunity to teach
- Keep education patient (person) centered
- Begin teaching at the first patient encounter
- Engage and motivate

Like other clinical interventions, effective patient teaching demands analytic and problem-solving skills. To maximize

Box 9-1 Topics for Health Teaching and Counseling

Promoting Health

- Developmental and maturational issues
- Normal childbearing
- Hygiene
- Nutrition
- Exercise
- Mental health
- Spiritual health

Preventing Illness

- First aid
- Safety
- Immunizations
- Screening
- Identification and management of risk factors

Restoring Health

- Orientation to treatment center and staff
- Patients' and nurses' expectations of one another
- The illness and physical condition: anatomy and physiology, etiology of problem, significance of symptoms, prognosis
- The nursing and other health care regimens and how the patient can participate in care
- Self-care practices the patient and family/caregivers need to manage the patient's condition independently

Facilitating Coping

- How the patient's physical and mental condition affects other areas of functioning; lifestyle counseling
- Measures that maximize independence and enhance self-concept
- Stress management
- Environmental alterations
- Community resources
- Appropriate referrals (e.g., physical therapy, occupational therapy, self-help groups, psychiatric–mental health counselor)
- Grief and bereavement counseling

Box 9-2 Steps of the Teaching–Learning Process

Assess Learning Needs and Learning Readiness

1. Use all appropriate sources of information. Collaborate with the patient and family/caregivers.
2. Identify the knowledge, attitudes, or skills needed by the patient and family/caregivers.
3. Assess the patient's emotional and experiential readiness to learn.
4. Assess factors affecting the patient's ability to learn, including age and development level, family/caregiver support networks and financial resources, cultural influences, literacy, and language barriers.
5. Develop critical pathways or teaching plans that span care delivery settings from hospital to home to take advantage of optimal learning readiness.
6. Identify the patient's strengths.
7. Use anticipatory guidance.

Identify the Patient's Learning Needs

1. Be realistic.
2. Collaborate and validate with patient or family/caregivers through conversations, questionnaires, and checklists.

Develop Learning Outcomes

1. Identify specific, attainable, measurable, short-term and/or long-term outcomes for patient learning.
2. Make sure that proposed behavioral changes are realistic and explored in the context of the patient's resources and lifestyle.
3. Decide which domain of learning is involved (cognitive, psychomotor, affective).
4. Prioritize.
5. Collaborate with the patient and family/caregivers. Valuing of the outcomes increases likelihood of learning success.

Develop a Teaching Plan

1. Select content, content sequencing, and appropriate teaching strategies/activities.
2. Relate the teaching content to the patient's learning style, interests, resources, and patterns of everyday living.
3. Pay careful attention to time constraints, scheduling, and the physical environment.
4. Decide on group versus individual teaching and formal versus informal methodologies.
5. Formulate a verbal or written contract with the patient.

Implement Teaching Plan and Strategies

1. Prepare the physical or online environment, with attention to comfort and privacy.
2. Communicate effectively with individuals; small groups; and, in some instances, large groups.
3. Gather all materials and equipment.
4. Deliver the content in an organized manner using the selected teaching strategies.
5. Be flexible.
6. Keep teaching sessions short.
7. Vary strategies for sensory stimulation, which promotes learning.
8. Relate the material to the patients' life experiences, which will help them assimilate new knowledge.
9. Plan how you will evaluate learning.
10. Assess verbal and nonverbal feedback.

Evaluate Learning

1. Evaluate whether the learner outcomes were met:
   - Observe a return demonstration
   - Ask the patient to restate the instructions
   - Ask the patient questions to determine whether teaching reinforcement is needed
   - Use written test or questionnaires
   - Consult with the patient's family/caregivers
   - Consider patient feedback and comments
2. Reinforce and celebrate learning.
3. Evaluate teaching:
   - Self-evaluation
   - Patient questionnaires
4. Revise the plan if the learner outcome is not met:
   - Alter content and teaching strategies
   - Use motivational counseling
   - Reschedule teaching sessions
5. Document the teaching–learning process:
   - Patient and family learning needs and identified barriers to learning
   - Mechanisms used to overcome learning barriers
   - Patient and family/caregiver readiness to learn
   - Current knowledge regarding the patient's condition and health status
   - Learning outcomes agreed on by the nurse, patient, and family/caregiver
   - Identification of learning outcomes
   - Information and skills taught
   - Teaching methods used
   - Patient and family/caregiver response
   - Evaluation of what patient and family/caregivers learned and need for follow-up

the effectiveness of patient teaching, remember the acronym TEACH:

T: Tune into the patient
E: Edit patient information
A: Act on every teaching moment
C: Clarify often
H: Honor the patient as a partner in the education process

Learning to be an effective teacher is a critical component of professional development. A basic understanding of the teaching–learning process helps you develop your own teaching and learning skills. The process of patient teaching, which resembles the nursing process, consists of several steps that are necessary to provide teaching and to measure learning (refer to Box 9-2). This process is often condensed because of limited time or resources, but the basic principles apply each time the teaching–learning process occurs. Being a successful teacher requires excellent communication skills and sensitivity to all the factors that affect the patient's ability to learn (Fig. 9-1).

Factors Affecting Patient Learning

By taking into consideration the patient's age and developmental level, and the impact of social determinants of health,

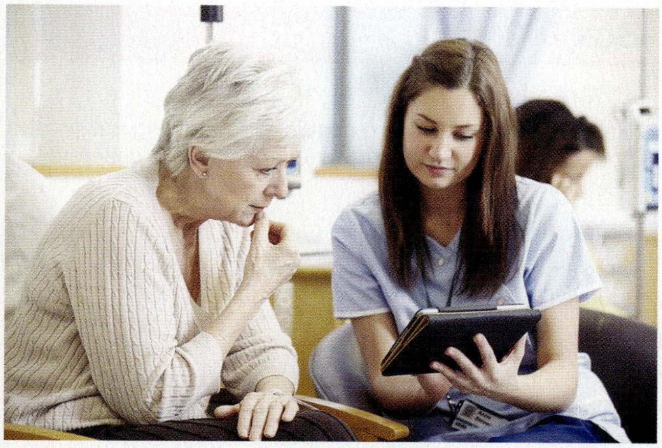

FIGURE 9-1. Effective communication is essential to the teaching–learning process. (*Source: Photo by Monkey Business Images/Shutterstock.*)

including family support networks and financial resources, cultural influences and language limitations, and health literacy level, you can individualize the teaching plan and maximize learning. This will support the nursing goal of helping the patient to manage their own health care needs.

Age and Developmental Level

People learn throughout life, although what they learn and how learning occurs change according to developmental stages. Three critical developmental areas to consider when developing a teaching plan are the patient's physical maturation and abilities, psychosocial development, and cognitive capacity. Other concerns related to the teaching–learning process include the patient's emotional maturity and moral and spiritual development.

CHILD AND ADOLESCENT LEARNERS

Piaget's theory of intellectual development is a major learning theory (see Chapter 22). If you understand how children and adolescents develop learning abilities, you can use this knowledge when teaching patients.

When the patient is an infant, teaching is directed toward the parents. Toddlers and preschoolers may have some degree of understanding about medical tests or procedures, but health teaching continues to be directed toward the parents. For patients in this age range, it helps for one nurse to establish a relationship with the patient and family/caregivers and to be consistently involved in patient-teaching activities.

An example of teaching considerations for young children would be the case of a 4-year-old girl diagnosed with diabetes: The child must begin to take insulin every day, and the nurse should recognize the child's limitations in understanding diabetes. Information should be simplified to include only the most basic facts, with concrete examples or demonstrations; a detailed discussion of the pathophysiology of diabetes would not be appropriate. The girl could be told that she needs a shot every day to keep her from getting sick or feeling "funny." She could be allowed to play with the syringes and to give shots to a doll.

Children today, even at very young ages, have likely been exposed to online games with colorful animations that teach basic information. Their manual dexterity skills may be more advanced, and they may be more comfortable with tasks previously viewed as challenging for this age group. Preschool children are often eager to demonstrate a skill they have been taught and may ask many questions. Explanations should be short and composed of simple words. Compared to adults, children have shorter attention spans and a greater need for nurturing, support, and creative participation in learning activities.

School-aged children are capable of logical reasoning and should be included in the teaching–learning process whenever possible. Teaching strategies that include clear explanations and reasons for procedures, stated in a simple and logical manner, are most successful. These children are open to new learning experiences but need learning to be reinforced by either a parent or health care personnel as they become more involved with their friends and school activities.

The cognitive processes of adolescents are similar to those of adults; thus, the content and strategies of patient teaching for this age group resemble those used for teaching adults. There are some important considerations to keep in mind, however. For example, when teaching a sexually active 16-year-old girl about contraceptive methods, you would assess whether the young patient has reached the stage Piaget refers to as formal operations (the ability to use logical reasoning to solve hypothetical problems). If the patient's intellectual development is delayed and she is still in the period of concrete operations (use of logical reasoning to solve concrete problems), she may be less skilled in thinking abstractly—that is, she may not perceive pregnancy as a real possibility, and therefore may not fully understand the need for contraception. If so, you can alter the teaching plan to include online teaching aids that are easily accessible and explain the topic in concrete terms. Peer group acceptance is critical for most adolescents. Teaching strategies designed for an adolescent patient should recognize the adolescent's need for independence and the need to establish a trusting relationship that demonstrates respect for the adolescent's opinions.

Motor development is also a concern in the teaching–learning process. A 4-year-old girl diagnosed with diabetes may not be able to administer her own insulin shots if she lacks the fine motor skills needed to manipulate the equipment, but a 13-year-old patient could probably master the technique quickly.

ADULT LEARNERS

As people age, their personalities and learning abilities change. Most psychologists who have studied the teaching–learning process base their work on children and adolescents, because a large amount of learning occurs early in life. The science of teaching (**pedagogy**) generally refers to the teaching of children and adolescents. In recent years, the study of teaching adults (**andragogy**), beginning at young adulthood, 20 to 40 years of age, has gained more attention (Knowles, 1990).

Adults need to be taught differently than children. Knowles (1990) listed the following four assumptions about adult learners:

1. As people mature, their self-concept is likely to move from dependence to independence.
2. The previous experience of the adult is a rich resource for learning.
3. An adult's readiness to learn is often related to a developmental task or a social role.
4. Most adults' orientation to learning is that material should be useful immediately, rather than at some time in the future.

Thus, andragogy focuses on a specific problem or need and on the immediate application of new material. In general, adult learners must believe that they need to learn before they become willing to learn. Nurses often must use their counseling skills (discussed later) to motivate patients to participate in the teaching–learning process. Adults may need to be shown the importance of learning new information, health practices, or skills.

Because health promotion and injury avoidance are important activities throughout the lifespan, teaching methods need to be further modified when working with older adults. When developing a teaching plan for older adults, first identify any learning barriers such as sensory loss, limited physical mobility, or inability to comply with the recommended therapeutic regimen. Sensory deficits that can affect learning in older adults include the presence of cataracts that can cloud vision and a decrease in lens accommodation that necessitates adequate lighting and high contrast, larger font printed materials; a decrease in peripheral vision that requires that teaching materials be kept immediately in front of the learner; or a hearing loss that make it imperative for the teacher to speak slowly and clearly (CDC, 2019; Eliopoulos, 2018). Successful teaching plans for older adults incorporate extra time, short teaching sessions, accommodation for sensory deficits, and reduction of environmental distractions. Older adults also benefit from instruction that relates new information to familiar activities or information.

Family/Caregiver Support Networks and Financial Resources

No matter what the patient's age, working with the patient's family/caregivers can be a great help in patient teaching. Assess the family's/caregiver's role and style by talking with them and observing how the patient and family interact. This assessment will yield information about family/caregiver function, stress, transitions, and expectations. Informal conversations with both the patient and family/caregivers can provide data that will help in developing the teaching plan. The COPE model (Houts et al., 1996) described in Box 9-3 is one method of helping family members/caregivers become effective problem solvers and support your teaching efforts.

Family caregiving—providing care for a family member, partner, or friend with a chronic, disabling, or serious health condition—is nearly universal today (National Alliance for Caregiving [NAC] & American Association of Retired Persons [AARP], 2020). In 2020, it was estimated that about 53 million family caregivers in the United States provided unpaid care to an adult family member or friend, or child with limitations due to health or functional needs (NAC & AARP, p. 4). In addition, compared to data from 2015, a greater proportion of caregivers of adults are providing care to multiple people, with 24% caring for two or more recipients (up from 18%) (NAC & AARP, p. 4). This family caregiver also often provides support when the patient is hospitalized. It is important to identify and provide education related to the learning needs of caregivers and provide meaningful supports for family caregivers. Family caregivers should be involved in collaboration with health care team members regarding care planning. Family caregivers should be viewed as partners in providing care, and you should view yourself as a health educator who teaches patients and their families/caregivers how to solve problems rather than as an expert meant to solve problems for them. Refer to the accompanying Research in Nursing box for a review of a quality improvement project that provides evidence for practice to improve patient outcomes through improved education of caregivers of patients with cognitive impairment.

The patient's and family's/caregiver's financial resources should be evaluated. The patient and/or their family/caregivers may be unable to afford to follow a new treatment regimen or other parts of the proposed plan of care. The patient's and family's/caregiver's financial resources must be taken into consideration by the health care team when planning care. If needed, refer patients and families to community-based support groups and funding sources.

Box 9-3 COPE Model

C: Creativity

Help the family overcome obstacles to carrying out health care management and learning how to generate alternatives.

O: Optimism

Help the family caregivers learn how to view the caregiving situation with confidence.

P: Planning

Help the family learn how to plan for future problems and how to develop contingency plans that reduce uncertainty.

E: Expert Information

Help the family learn how to obtain expert information from health care providers about what to do in specific situations. This information empowers caregivers by encouraging them to develop plans for solving caregiving problems.

Source: Adapted from American Psychological Association (APA). (2011). *Creativity, optimism, planning and expert information (COPE).* https://www.apa.org/pi/about/publications/caregivers/practice-settings/intervention/cope; Houts, P. S., Nezu, A. M., Nezu, C. M., & Bucher, J. A. (1996). The prepared family caregiver: A problem-solving approach to family caregiver education. *Patient Education & Counseling, 27*(1), 63–73.

Research in Nursing

BRIDGING THE GAP TO EVIDENCE-BASED PRACTICE

Educational Needs of Family Caregivers

Family caregivers are partners in the provision of patient care and require appropriate education and meaningful support. Nurses need to identify the educational needs of patients and family caregivers to provide effective health education, supporting informed decisions about health care. Well-informed caregivers are a critical component of the care for many patients.

Related Research

Agarwal, K. S., Bhimarij, A., Xu, J., Bionat, S., Pudlo, M., Miranda, D., Campbell, C., & Taffet, G. E. (2020). Decreasing heart failure readmissions among older patients with cognitive impairment by engaging caregivers. *The Journal of Cardiovascular Nursing, 35*(3), 253–261. https://doi.org/10.1097/JCN.0000000000000670

This quality improvement project examined the impact of caregiver inclusion in nursing discharge patient education on readmission in older adults with cognitive impairment and heart failure. Patients age 70 years or older discharged from hospital heart failure (HF) units with a primary diagnosis of HF were screened for cognitive impairment using Mini-Cog testing. If the patient's Mini-Cog score was less than 4 (indicating cognitive impairment), the patient's caregivers were included in an enhanced nursing discharge education and planning program. Readmission within 30 days to any of the hospital-system facilities was tracked. In patients with cognitive impairment, involving caregivers in nursing discharge teaching was associated with decreased 30-day readmission ($P = .01$). The researchers concluded involving caregivers in discharge education is an important intervention to reduce readmission rates for older patients with cognitive impairment and HF.

Relevance to Nursing Practice

Many family caregivers lack experience in carrying out this role and need the best possible assistance to maintain their role and provide support to their family member. Nurses have the ability to empower caregivers by providing instruction and counseling to assist them to identify and implement strategies to provide care, learn the practical skills required for their particular situation, what to expect related to progression of illness and prevent complications.

Cultural Influences and Language Differences

As our society becomes more ethnically diverse, you will be providing care and education to patients from many different cultural and ethnic backgrounds. Different cultural backgrounds create different attitudes and reactions to changes in health and can influence how people express themselves (Bastable, 2019). A thorough assessment is essential prior to establishing a plan of action and educational outcomes (Bastable, 2017; Schaffler et al., 2019).

It is important to keep in mind that culture can also influence how people express themselves verbally and nonverbally (Bastable, 2017). In addition, be sure to identify language differences or barriers and develop strategies to address them, clearly communicating this in the plan of care. Do not assume that a family member/caregiver is adequately translating information critical to the patient's learning. The Joint Commission standards and accreditation requirements include an expectation for hospitals to accommodate the oral and written communication needs of all patients (The Joint Commission, 2011). This includes translated, clearly stated patient education information.

To successfully provide care, you may need to seek information from a variety of sources, such as the nursing literature and evidence for practice and books that describe the health practices and values of other cultures. Numerous resources provide assistance in meeting patient education needs for culturally and ethnically diverse populations. Professionally trained interpreters should be used for assessment, teaching, and other important interactions (Bastable, 2019; Gutman et al., 2018). Telephone interpreting services and translation software apps are possible services to be used if an interpreter is not available in-person. Patient education specialists from four health systems in central Ohio offer free, easy-to-read, copyrighted health information on more than 300 topics in multiple languages on the Health Information Translations (n.d.) website (healthinfotranslations.org). The National Library of Medicine, through the website Medline Plus, provides patient education materials in multiple languages that include tutorials with animated graphic materials and accompanying handouts (U.S. National Library of Medicine, 2020). The National Library of Medicine provides additional patient materials through HealthReach, a national collaborative partnership that has created a resource of quality multilingual, multicultural public health information (U.S. National Library of Medicine, n.d.). Box 9-4 outlines

Box 9-4 Culturally Considerate Patient Teaching

- Develop an understanding of the patient's culture.
- Work with a multicultural team in developing educational programs.
- Be aware of personal assumptions, biases, and prejudices.
- Understand the core cultural values of the patient or group. Listen to the patient and family/caregivers. Explore customs or taboos (Bastable, 2019).
- Understand the patient's religious practices and determine how their beliefs influence perceptions of health and health care (Bastable, 2019).
- Develop written materials in the patient's preferred language.

strategies for providing patient education in a culturally considerate manner.

Health Literacy

Health literacy is the ability to access, read, understand, evaluate, communicate, and act on health information to promote, maintain, and improve health; health literacy is associated with the capacity and self-efficacy to manage health and well-being (Okan, 2019). More than a quarter of U.S. adults (approximately 80 million people) have limited health literacy and thus would have difficulty with common health tasks (AHRQ, 2011). Health literacy has been found to strongly correlate with many of the social determinants of health, contributing to disparities in health (Mantwill & Divani, 2019). Health literacy requires a complex group of reading, listening, and analytical and decision-making skills and the ability to apply these skills to health situations (Network of the National Library of Medicine [NNLM], n.d.a). These skills include, for example, accessing health care services, interpreting test results, analyzing relative risks and benefits, locating health information, reading health prevention pamphlets, measuring medication doses, and understanding and complying with verbal or written health care instructions (NNLM, n.d.a). Limited health literacy affects adults in all racial, ethnic, age, education, and income groups; however, the older adult and immigrant populations, those with limited education, those with low incomes, minority populations, and non-native speakers of English are most likely to experience low health literacy (NNLM, n.d.a; USDHHS, 2010).

Federal initiatives such as the Affordable Care Act of 2010 and the National Action Plan to Improve Health Literacy from USDHHS (2010) have made health literacy a national priority to improve the health of all Americans. Awareness of the health literacy issue gives health care professionals the opportunity to support patients and families in overcoming barriers to health, including addressing social determinants of health, and empowering patients to take control of their health care needs (Office of Disease Prevention and Health Promotion, 2020b; USDHHS, 2010).

Nurses need to identify patients and family caregivers with limited health literacy for health education to be effective (Eadie, 2014). The Newest Vital Sign (NVS) is a screening tool to identify patients at risk for low health literacy. It was developed by Pfizer to improve communications between patients and providers and can be administered during initial assessments to assess the patient's literacy skills involving both numbers and words (Pfizer, n.d.). The NVS has been reported to perform moderately well in identifying limited literacy (Brangan et al., 2018; Pfizer, n.d.; Powers et al., 2010). The NVS uses a nutrition label from an ice cream container (Fig. 9-2) and a score sheet for recording the patient's answers to six oral questions that refer to the label (Fig. 9-3 on page 220). Based on the number of correct responses, the health care provider can then further assess the patient's health literacy level as indicated. The time spent administering this tool more than compensates for the time providers might need clarifying a diagnosis, treatment, or medications if they had not recognized a patient's limited health literacy.

The *Ask Me 3*® is another intervention to address health literacy by promoting understanding and improving communication between patients and their providers (Institute for Healthcare Improvement [IHI], n.d.). It is an educational program that encourages patients and families to ask three specific questions of their providers to better understand their health conditions and what they need to do to stay healthy (IHI, n.d.). Providers are encouraged to answer these questions in a clear, forthright manner. The *Ask Me 3*® questions are:

- What is my main problem?
- What do I need to do?
- Why is it important for me to do this?

The health care provider's response should include plain language without medical jargon, may incorporate the use of visual models to explain a disease or procedure, and should include a teach-back demonstration that verifies their understanding of the information. The Teach-Back Method assesses health literacy, seeking to confirm that the learner understands the health information received from the health professional (Agency for Healthcare Research and Quality [AHRQ], 2017). It is a particularly important intervention when a person has difficulty reading and comprehending written materials or has limited English proficiency. Patients and family/caregivers have the opportunity to repeat back to the health care provider the key points they understand from a teaching session. The health care provider should speak slowly and clearly and focus on the most important concepts, stopping at intervals to check the patient's and family's/caregiver's understanding by asking the patient or family member/caregiver to teach it back—asking them to explain in their own words what they need to know or do (AHRQ, n.d.). Clarification and repetition of information is provided as needed. The Teach-Back Method has been proven to be effective in a wide variety of patient care settings (Dinh et al., 2016; Nickles et al., 2020; Prochnow et al., 2018; Ryan-Madonna et al., 2019). See the accompanying Promoting Health Literacy display in this and other chapters throughout this book for examples of implementation of this program in action.

Collaboration between health care providers and patients to achieve effective health education is dependent upon accurate communication. Both the nurse and patient need to be part of setting goals and objectives to support success (Bastable, 2017). Strategies to enhance health literacy should be learner centered (Bastable, 2017). All patients, regardless of literacy level, need and should receive accessible and actionable health information to make informed decisions about their health (Duncan, 2020). Nurses must be knowledgeable about the prevalence of low health literacy and its impact on patients and make a concentrated effort to be well informed about effective strategies for health care communication (Scott, 2016).

Nutrition Facts

Serving size			½ cup
Servings per container			4
Amount per serving			
Calories	250	Fat Cal	120
			%DV
Total Fat 13 g			20%
Sat fat 9 g			40%
Cholesterol 28 mg			12%
Sodium 55 mg			2%
Total Carbohydrate 30 g			12%
Dietary fiber 2 g			
Sugars 23 g			
Protein 4 g			8%

*Percentage Daily Values (DV) are based on a 2,000 calorie diet. Your daily values may be higher or lower depending on your calorie needs.

Ingredients: Cream, Skim milk, Liquid sugar, Water, Egg yolks, Brown sugar, Milk fat, Peanut oil, Sugar, Butter, Salt, Carrageenan, Vanilla extract.

FIGURE 9-2. Sample ice cream label from the Newest Vital Sign (NVS) health literacy assessment tool. (*Source:* From Pfizer Inc. [n.d.]. *Health literacy. Public policy researchers. The Newest Vital Sign [NVS].* https://www.pfizer.com/health/literacy/public-policy-researchers/nvs-toolkit. Reprinted with permission from Pfizer Inc.)

Promoting Health Literacy

IN PATIENTS WHO SMOKE

Patient Scenario

Jack Boyer is 37 years old and has been smoking since he was 17 years of age. During a routine health visit, he admits to a one pack per day habit. In response to a question from his health care provider, Jack admits that several previous attempts to stop smoking failed after a day or two. He states on his history form that he is married and has two sons, 7 and 3 years of age, and also lists that his father died following a heart attack at the age of 60. Jack tells his health care provider that he is essentially healthy but is under a lot of stress. Because of the downturn in the economy, his job in automotive sales is at risk. His wife works full-time as an administrative assistant. The health care provider expresses concern to Jack about the effects of second-hand smoke on his family. Jack states, "I know all about that and when I smoke in the car, I keep the window down and blow the smoke outside. At home, I try to smoke outside most of the time except when the weather is bad." The physical examination reveals that Jack has hypertension (BP 164/92), is 15 lb overweight, and is currently having difficulty sleeping. The health care provider explains that he would like to monitor Jack's blood pressure for 1 month before prescribing antihypertensive medication. He recommends that Jack make a serious effort to stop smoking and reviews the harmful effects of nicotine use and the long-term benefits for Jack as well as his family, if he stops smoking. The health care provider explains that the nurse will discuss information about quitting smoking when he makes an appointment for his next visit. As Jack is speaking with the nurse, he comments that maybe he'll switch to chewing tobacco since there's no smoke involved with that.

Nursing Considerations: *Tips for Improving Health Literacy*

Provide Jack with information about ways to help him quit smoking. Mention that counseling and behavior cessation therapies have proven effective and that often it takes repeated attempts to quit. Jack needs to understand the harmful effects of second-hand smoke on his family, as well as the fact that people who stop smoking greatly reduce their risk of lung cancer, heart disease, and respiratory symptoms. Explain to him that smokeless tobacco is also a significant health risk and not a safe substitute for smoking cigarettes. Give him information about nicotine replacement products (gum, inhalers, patches) found effective in treating tobacco dependence. Several non-nicotine medications are also available but need to be prescribed by his health care provider. For extra help, suggest he call 1-800-QUIT-NOW, which connects callers with counselors who are trained specifically to help smokers quit (National Cancer Institute, n.d.). When Jack returns for his follow-up appointment, he needs to be prepared to ask his health care provider the following questions to help him understand that tobacco addiction is a chronic condition and what the positive outcomes of quitting will be:

- What is my main problem?
- What do I need to do?
- Why is it important for me to do this?

What additional measures can you take to help increase health literacy in this patient? What other measures would be helpful if Jack did not speak English, could not read, or had other factors that could affect his health literacy?

The Newest Vital Sign

Score Sheet for the Newest Vital Sign Questions and Answers

READ TO SUBJECT:
This information is on the back of a container of a pint of ice cream.

ANSWER CORRECT? Yes / No

1. If you eat the entire container, how many calories will you eat?
   Answer: 1,000 is the only correct answer

2. If you are allowed to eat 60 g of carbohydrates as a snack, how much ice cream could you have?
   Answer: Any of the following is correct: 1 cup (or any amount up to 1 cup), half the container. Note: If patient answers "two servings," ask "How much ice cream would that be if you were to measure it into a bowl?"

3. Your doctor advises you to reduce the amount of saturated fat in your diet. You usually have 42 g of saturated fat each day, which includes one serving of ice cream. If you stop eating ice cream, how many grams of saturated fat would you be consuming each day?
   Answer: 33 is the only correct answer

4. If you usually eat 2,500 calories in a day, what percentage of your daily value of calories will you be eating if you eat one serving?
   Answer: 10% is the only correct answer

READ TO SUBJECT:
Pretend that you are allergic to the following substances: penicillin, peanuts, latex gloves, and bee stings.

5. Is it safe for you to eat this ice cream?
   Answer: No

6. Ask only if the patient responds "no" to question 5: Why not?
   Answer: Because it has peanut oil

Number of correct answers:

Interpretation

Score of 0–1 suggests high likelihood (50% or more) of limited literacy.
Score of 2–3 indicates the possibility of limited literacy.
Score of 4–6 almost always indicates adequate literacy.

FIGURE 9-3. Score sheet for the Newest Vital Sign (NVS) includes questions and answers that refer to the label. (*Source:* From Pfizer Inc. [n.d.]. *Health literacy. Public policy researchers. The Newest Vital Sign [NVS].* https://www.pfizer.com/health/literacy/public-policy-researchers/nvs-toolkit. Reprinted with permission from Pfizer Inc.)

Learning Domains

People learn in three domains: cognitive, psychomotor, and affective (Bloom, 1956). The ability of patients to manage their daily lives and maintain or resume their former roles depends on the extent to which their cognitive, psychomotor, and affective learning result in behavioral changes. These domains influence the nurse's selection of teaching and evaluation strategies. Effective teaching often involves the promotion of behaviors in all three domains.

Cognitive learning involves the storing and recalling of new knowledge in the brain (e.g., the patient describes how salt intake affects blood pressure). Cognitive learning includes intellectual behaviors such as the acquisition of knowledge, comprehension, application (using abstract ideas in concrete situations), analysis (relating ideas in an organized way), synthesis (assimilating parts of information as a whole), and evaluation (judging the worth of a body of information). Learning a physical skill involving the integration of mental and muscular activity is called **psychomotor learning** (e.g., the patient demonstrates how to change dressings using clean technique). **Affective learning** includes changes in attitudes, values, and feelings (e.g., the patient expresses renewed self-confidence after physical therapy).

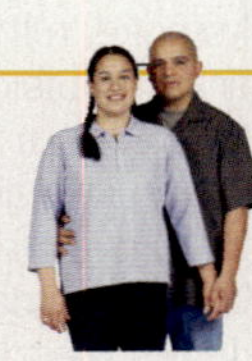

Recall ***Marco García Ramírez***, the father-to-be with concerns about his new role. The nurse would develop a teaching plan that focuses on the three domains of learning. The nurse would address the cognitive domain by teaching Mr. García Ramírez and his wife about labor and delivery, including the labor process and what events will occur. Teaching the couple about newborn care and breathing techniques to use during labor would address the psychomotor domain. Learning in the affective domain would be demonstrated if Mr. García Ramírez reports that he and his wife do not fear labor and feel comfortable handling a newborn.

Effective Communication Techniques

A critical component of effective patient education is the nurse's ability to be an effective communicator. Professional communication is discussed in detail in Chapter 8. Key points of effective communication associated with patient teaching include the following:

- Be sincere and honest; show genuine interest and respect.
- Avoid giving too much detail; stick to the basics.
- Ask if the patient has any questions.
- Be a "cheerleader" for the patient. Avoid lecturing.
- Use simple words.
- Vary your tone of voice.
- Keep the content clear and concise.
- Listen and do not interrupt when the patient speaks.
- Ensure that the environment is conducive to learning and free of interruptions.
- Be sensitive to the timing of teaching sessions. A shorter session is best for a younger child, and an adult may need to choose an opportune time to learn new information.

NURSING PROCESS FOR PATIENT AND FAMILY/CAREGIVER TEACHING

Patient teaching is approached most effectively using the steps of the nursing process. The teaching–learning process and the nursing process are interdependent. Health care providers have a responsibility to identify the patient's learning needs and determine their readiness to learn (Bastable, 2017).

Assessing

Usually, patients themselves are the best source of assessment information. Patients are considered primary sources of information. By using effective interviewing techniques (see Chapter 8), you can obtain the data needed to identify learning needs. An important component is assessing what the patient wants to learn; motivation to learn is increased by focusing on what the patient feels is most important to know or to be able to do (Bastable, 2017). In addition, relevant information may be obtained before actually meeting the patient by reviewing the patient's past and current health records. These records are considered secondary sources of information and can provide a history of health problems as well as documentation of the nursing assessments, diagnoses/patient problems, nursing physical examinations, and nursing interventions that have been performed.

QSEN PATIENT-CENTERED CARE

Partner with the patient and family/caregivers to determine what they consider to be important and what they identify as the best educational outcomes. Ask the patient and family/caregivers what they need and care most about.

The patient's family/caregivers and significant others are also valuable sources of assessment data. They are sometimes needed to provide assessment data when the patient cannot communicate because of health problems, language barriers, or impaired sensory functions. At other times, family members/caregivers or significant others may be the most appropriate source of certain information; for example, if seeking information about how much salt is used in the family's cooking, you could speak with the person who prepares the meals at home and include that person in any teaching about food preparation. The patient's permission is needed before family members/caregivers are involved in the teaching–learning process.

In addition to identifying the patient's learning needs, you should assess your own knowledge base and teaching skills. Nurses cannot teach information and skills to patients if they themselves lack the information and skills to be taught. Often, knowing where to find information or an appropriate resource person is the first step in correcting your knowledge deficits.

Assessment of the Learner

Assessment of the learner is the first and most important step in the teaching–learning process (Bastable, 2019). Four elements should be considered in each assessment of the learner. First, identify **learning needs**, gaps in knowledge that exist between what the person knows and what someone needs or wants to know (Bastable, 2019). Gaps may be a result of a lack of knowledge, attitude, or skill (Holli & Beto, 2018). Assessment through structured interviews, informal conversations, questionnaires and/or observation, for example, will reveal what the patient considers of importance to learn. The nurse then considers new knowledge, attitudes, or skills necessary for patients and families to learn in order to manage their health care, based on the individual patient's health problems.

Assess **learning readiness**. The patient's anxiety, motivation for learning, willingness to engage in the teaching–learning process, and support system contribute to readiness to learn. Readiness is distinguished from the patient's actual ability to learn, which is the third element. Assess the patient's **learning style(s)**. A person's learning style is the individual preferences for and abilities to process content of various instructional messages (Holli & Beto, 2018). These preferences influence how easy or difficult learning is for the individual and impact teaching and learning interventions. The fourth element of assessment is of the patient's **learning strengths**. Strengths are the personal resources that can be harnessed to facilitate the teaching–learning process. Box 9-5 (on page 222) provides additional information related to these assessment parameters. Additional factors to consider in assessment of the learner include motivation and adherence.

Motivation

When assessing a patient's learning readiness, consider the patient's motivation. Patients who are ready to learn are able and motivated to process new information, develop new skills, and explore new attitudes and behaviors. Motivation is an internal impulse (such as emotion or physical pain) that encourages the patient to take action or change behavior.

Box 9-5 Assessment Parameters

1. **Learning Needs**
   - Knowledge, skills, and attitudes that are of priority to the patient
   - New knowledge, skills, or attitudes that are necessary for patients and families to learn in order to manage their health care
2. **Learning Readiness**
   - Physical readiness
   - Complexity of task
   - Health status
   - Physical abilities
3. **Emotional Readiness**
   - Emotional health
   - Motivation for learning
   - Self-concept and body image
   - Sense of responsibility for self
   - Support system
   - Developmental considerations
4. **Experiential Readiness**
   - Social and economic stability
   - Past coping mechanisms
   - Attitude toward learning
   - Cultural background
   - Literacy
   - Communication skills
5. **Learning Style**
   - Preferences in thinking and problem solving
   - Differences in processing information
   - Personality
   - Past experiences with learning
   - Comprehension, reasoning, memory, or psychomotor skills
   - Visual, tactile (kinesthetic), auditory learners
6. **Learning Strengths**
   - Past experiences with learning
   - High motivation
   - Strong network
   - Adequate financing

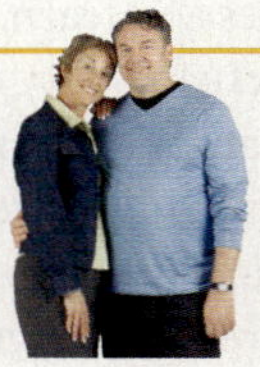

Think back to **Rachel Blumenthal**, the wife of the patient who had a myocardial infarction. Although further assessment is necessary, analysis of Mrs. Blumenthal's questions would lead the nurse to suspect that she is interested in finding out information, because she is showing motivation and a beginning readiness to learn.

A patient's health beliefs can have great influence on motivation. The health belief model identifies several health beliefs as critical for patient motivation (Rosenstock, 1974). Motivation is enhanced when:

- Patients view themselves as susceptible to the health problem in question
- Patients view the health problem as a serious threat
- Patients believe there are actions they can take to reduce the probability of acquiring the health problem
- Patients believe the threat related to taking these actions is not as great as the health problem itself

The health belief model was designed to explain why people are willing to take actions to support their health, but it evolved into a strategy for predicting the likelihood that patients would adhere to therapies. Motivation plays a key role in the health belief model because it spurs the patient to behave in ways for health promotion and health protection. Examples of motivational triggers include personal crisis and loss of social role due to disease symptoms. You can use the health belief model when developing teaching plans, evaluating the ideas or beliefs that motivate a patient, and applying these to the teaching plan. For example, if you are able to modify a patient's perception of disease susceptibility, the patient might become more receptive to learning.

Adherence

The terms adherence and compliance are often used interchangeably to refer to a patient's efforts to follow health care advice (Robinson et al., 2008, as cited in Bastable, 2017, p. 158). Both terms refer to the ability to maintain health-promoting regimens determined by or in conjunction with the health care provider, respectively (Bastable, 2017). Compliance refers to the extent to which a patient's behavior coincides with the clinical advice, implying the health care provider is viewed as the authority and the patient passively follows recommendations, a paternalistic attitude toward patients (Bastable, 2017; Hugtenburg et al., 2013). **Adherence** refers to the extent to which a person's behavior corresponds with the agreed-upon recommendations from a health care provider as a result of a team approach to the treatment plan, in which the patient and health care provider are part of the team (Gardner, 2015; Sabaté, 2003, as cited in Bastable, 2017, p. 158). The term *adherence* supports a more inclusive and active patient role, emphasizing agreement between the patient and health care provider, and is seen as more patient (person) centered than compliance (Hurlow & Hensley, 2015; Vlasnik et al., 2005, as cited in Bastable, 2017, p. 159). Use of the term *adherence* reflects the patient's right to choose whether or not to follow treatment recommendations (Hurlow & Hensley, 2015). Therefore, the term adherence will be used in this discussion.

Nursing assessment of the patient's learning needs is vital to developing a plan of care with which the patient can adhere. Patients are considered to adhere when they follow the agreed-upon treatment plan and use the information they have learned. Accurate and thorough assessment of a patient's learning needs, motivation (as outlined above), and current knowledge, behaviors, skills, and self-care activities provide insight into the patient's adherence to previous plans of care as well as information to help to develop new teaching plans that support adherence and address any nonadherence (Hugtenburg et al., 2013).

Nonadherence occurs when patients do not follow treatment recommendations that are mutually agreed upon (Resnick, 2005, as cited in Bastable, 2019). The terms nonadherence and noncompliance are also often used interchangeably; the term nonadherence is used in this discussion for continuity. Patients may ignore instructions or not follow them appropriately; nonadherence may also occur unintentionally

(Bastable, 2017). Nonadherence may contribute to situations that threaten the patient's health. Nonadherence can be associated with a lack of learning readiness and motivation, confusion, disappointment, misunderstanding, fear, or inability to learn. Treatment factors such as side effects, lifestyle issues such as transportation, and sociodemographic factors such as inadequate finances may also contribute to nonadherence.

Patients control the choices they make about following the plan of care and using what they have been taught, but it is your responsibility as a nurse to help patients improve their health by sharing knowledge, solving problems, and providing support while the patient integrates the new knowledge and practices the new skills. When patients understand their health problem, treatment rationale, medication regimen, recommended plan of care, and the benefits of adherence, they are more likely to keep to the plan. Accurate understanding of the patient's situation, effective patient teaching, and tailoring of the plan to the patient contribute greatly to increasing the probability for patient adherence (Aronson, 2007; Mathew & Thukha, 2018). Health care providers should assist patients to be proactive and take an active part in their treatment to encourage positive behaviors and adherence (Makiling & Smart, 2020; Richie, 2016). Box 9-6 identifies ways to support patients and families in adhering to the plan of care.

Box 9-6 Promoting Patient and Family/Caregiver Adherence

- Be certain that health care instructions are understandable and designed to support patient goals.
- Include the patient and family/caregivers as partners in the teaching–learning process.
- Use interactive teaching strategies.
- Remember that teaching and learning are processes that rely on strong interpersonal relationships with patients and their families.

Diagnosing Actual or Potential Health Problems and Needs

An assessment of the patient and family/caregivers may lead to the identification of one or more diagnoses or patient problems related to patient education—the knowledge, attitudes, or skills needed to support health promotion. Following the formulation of the diagnoses or patient problems, the nurse communicates findings to other nursing and health care professionals through the use of the written and spoken word. The written actual or potential health problem or need becomes a permanent part of the patient's health record. Examples of health problems and needs with related etiology and signs and symptoms can be found in the box titled Examples of Actual or Potential Health Problems and Needs: Patient Education.

Outcome Identification and Planning

Planning for learning involves the development of a teaching plan. Teaching plans follow the steps of the teaching–learning and nurses' processes. One type of teaching plan is presented in Box 9-7 (on page 224). It is directed toward teaching appropriate nipple care to reduce the likelihood of nipple cracking and redness in breastfeeding women.

Examples of Actual or Potential Health Problems and Needs

PATIENT EDUCATION

Actual or Potential Health Problems and Needs	Possible Etiologic Factors	Potential Signs and Symptoms
Dressing ADL Deficit	Extreme fatigue and weakness	• Unable to choose clothing • Impaired ability to put on and remove clothing • Unable to use assistive devices • Decreased strength in right upper and lower extremities • Flaccid left upper extremity
Impaired Health Maintenance	Insufficient understanding of diabetes treatment regimen	• Unable to identify procedure for insulin administration • Inadequate identification of signs and symptoms of hypo- and hyperglycemia • Blood-glucose levels labile, ranging from 210 to 400 over past weeks • Dietary recall reveals excessive carbohydrate and sugar consumption
Knowledge Deficiency	Inaccurate follow-through related to fiber-rich diet for diverticular disease	"I thought I should never eat fiber again." "I've been avoiding beans and vegetables." Inaccurate identification of dietary regimen Unable to identify appropriate food choices Unable to verbalize rationale for fiber-rich diet. Dietary recall reveals lack of fiber-rich foods. Reports some "problems" with constipation; last stool 3 days ago.

Source: International Council of Nurses (ICN). (2019). *Nursing diagnosis and outcome statements.* https://www.icn.ch/sites/default/files/inline-files/ICNP2019-DC.pdf permission statement; Wolters Kluwer. (2020). *Problem-based care plans.* (2020). In *Lippincott advisor.* Wolters Kluwer. https://advisor.lww.com/lna/home.

Box 9-7 Sample Teaching Plan

Actual or Potential Health Problems and Needs: Ineffective breastfeeding

Possible Etiologic Factors: Insufficient knowledge of nipple care

Potential Signs and Symptoms: Reports sore nipples, redness, cracking, pain when baby latches on; unable to verbalize appropriate nipple care

Long-Term Outcome: Patient will be able to breastfeed as long as desired without nipple problems

(Short-Term) Learner Outcome	Date Met	Content	Method/Material	Learner Activity
Patient describes measures to prevent nipple cracking (cognitive).	8/10/25 L.I.	Protective measures: • Avoid soap/alcohol/drying agents on nipples. • Pat nipples dry after bathing and keep dry.	Discussion Audiovisual: Flip chart on breastfeeding	Read handout: Nipple care. Review "Breastfeeding—skin and nipple changes." National Library of Medicine. (2018) http://www.nlm.nih.gov/medlineplus/ency/patientinstructions/000632.htm
Patient begins protective measures immediately (psychomotor).	8/10/25 L.I.	• Apply a thin layer of 100% highly purified anhydrous (HPA) lanolin on nipple. • Avoid use of nursing pads or bras that contain plastic.		Read handout: Sore nipples
Patient describes the correct procedure for breastfeeding (cognitive).	8/10/25 L.I.	• Discuss possible positions to use to hold and support the baby during breastfeeding. • Review available breastfeeding aids. • Start baby on less sore side.	Discussion Audiovisual: Flip chart on breastfeeding	Read handout: Positioning baby for breastfeeding. View "Breastfeeding and breast milk." National Institute of Child Health and Human Development (2017). https://www.nichd.nih.gov/health/topics/breastfeeding
Patient demonstrates correct procedure for breastfeeding (psychomotor).	8/10/25 L.I.	• Get baby onto areola area. • Position baby properly. • Change position for each feeding. • Remove baby from breast.	Discovery: Guide through each step; assist as necessary Return demonstration	
Patient displays increasing confidence in breastfeeding skills and self-care (affective).	8/10/25 L.I.	After feeding: • Air dry the nipples. • Inspect for open or cracked areas. • Apply lanolin.	Discovery	
Patient values good nutrition and hydration and rest at home (affective).	8/10/25 L.I.	Home considerations: • Maintain "demand feedings."	Lecture with discussion Audiovisual: Poster	Refer to handouts at home as needed; call maternity department's information number for any questions
Patient can list the signs of thrush (cognitive).	8/10/25 L.I.	• Ensure good nutrition. • Get adequate rest. • Know the signs and symptoms of thrush.		

Standardized teaching plans are available for major topics of health teaching. Such plans must be tailored to the patient's learning needs and abilities. Remember that factors such as age, developmental level, family/caregiver support networks, financial resources, cultural influences, language proficiency, and health literacy affect the patient's ability to learn and take them into consideration when individualizing the teaching plan. Incorporation of teaching plans into critical path documentation systems is discussed in Chapters 17 and 20.

Thoughtful planning of patient teaching maximizes the patient's learning while ensuring the most efficient use of your time and skills. Learner outcomes are developed for each diagnosis of or patient problem related to a learning need. The nursing actions become the content, teaching strategy, and learner activity columns of the written plan. This phase requires thought and creativity. Your efforts are rewarded when the patient meets the outcomes at the end of the implementation phase.

Box 9-8 Verbs That Can Be Used When Writing Learner Outcomes

Cognitive Domain

compares	identifies
defines	names
describes	prepares
designs	plans
differentiates	solves
explains	states
gives examples	summarizes

Affective Domain

chooses	justifies
defends	relates
displays	revises
forms	selects
gives	shares
helps	uses
initiates	values

Psychomotor Domain

adapts	manipulates
arranges	moves
assembles	organizes
begins	rearranges
changes	shows
constructs	starts
creates	works
demonstrates	

When planning for learning, decide with the patient who should be included in the learning sessions. When the patient is a young child, one or both parents or a caregiver may be the primary learners. For an adult patient, a spouse, partner, caregiver, or close friend who will be giving the care that is to be learned may be included. For instance, the person who does the household's cooking is usually asked to be present for nutritional teaching. Teaching plans are developed according to the needs of the people being taught.

One or several nurses can prepare and use a teaching plan. When two or more nurses plan and coordinate the implementation of the plan, this is called team teaching. An advantage of team teaching is that it takes advantage of the talents of more than one nurse.

Duplicating teaching that has already been completed by other members of the health care team wastes time and causes frustration. Accurate and thorough documentation of all patient teaching, along with review of the health record before teaching sessions and effective communication with members of the interdisciplinary team, can prevent this problem.

Several factors should be considered while formulating any teaching plan, as discussed in the next sections.

Patient Learning Outcomes

Learner outcomes are written in the same manner as the patient outcomes in the nursing process (see Chapter 17). When planning for the patient's learning, first determine which of the three learning domains (cognitive, psychomotor, or affective) is the focus of teaching. Then write learning outcomes that reflect what learning is to occur. Learning outcomes should be stated as desired or expected patient behaviors, rather than as nursing interventions. For a patient having difficulty sleeping, for example, an appropriate learning outcome is "Avoid foods, beverages, and over-the-counter medications in the evening that contain caffeine" rather than "Teach the patient about foods and beverages that contain caffeine," which states a nursing behavior. A well-constructed learning outcome is measurable and serves as a guide for planning evaluation methods.

Choosing the verb for a learning outcome is probably the most difficult part of writing outcomes (Box 9-8). But a careful choice based on the learning domain that is the focus of the teaching makes it easier to plan the content, teaching strategies, learner activities, and evaluation.

Concept Mastery Alert

The domains of learning guide the learning outcomes. It is helpful to remember the following: "cognitive" is "knowledge"; "psychomotor" is "action"; "affective" is "feelings."

The number of outcomes needed for each diagnosis/patient problem varies. It's better to have several specific outcomes than to try to cover everything with only one or two broad outcomes. Many nurses write one long-term, general outcome for each diagnosis/patient problem, followed by several short-term, specific outcomes. For example, a long-term outcome for the sample teaching plan could be: "The patient will be able to breastfeed her infant as long as desired without sore nipples." This outcome could be met in 2 weeks or 2 years, depending on how long the woman decides to breastfeed. Long-term outcomes are general statements. On the other hand, the short-term outcomes written in the learner outcome column of the sample teaching plan (see Box 9-7) are specific behaviors to be accomplished within a specified time (e.g., "The patient immediately begins protective measures to prevent nipple cracking").

Patients and appropriate family members or caregivers should be included in planning the outcomes. When patients value the learning outcomes, their readiness to learn is enhanced, increasing the likelihood that they will achieve the goals.

Teaching Content

After writing the learner outcomes, decide what information the patient needs to complete them. This is the content of the teaching plan. The most effective teaching plans address the most important topics relevant to the patient's care. New nurses usually need to research the subject to be taught to determine what information exists about the topic. Extensive information is easily accessible online, along with handouts, books, and journal articles available in many nursing units. Content supported by nursing research is called evidence-based and reflects the most accurate and clinically supported information (see Chapter 2).

Nurses are often concerned about just how much patients should learn about topics such as illness, procedures, medications, and surgeries. Patients benefit, for example, from explanations of the physical sensations they will experience during a procedure. They appreciate knowing in advance what they will feel, taste, hear, see, and smell.

Content explaining why certain treatments and medications are needed is included in the teaching plan. Information on the prevention of illness or its complications should also be covered. Again, patients are more likely to implement a plan that they understand and value.

Teaching Methods and Instructional Materials

The techniques used by a teacher to promote learning are called teaching methods. A **teaching method** is the way information is taught that brings the learner into contact with what is to be learned (role play, group discussion, demonstration, simulation) (Bastable, 2017, 2019). **Instructional materials** are the objects or vehicles (such as printed handouts, videos, podcasts) used to communicate information (Bastable, 2017, 2019).

TEACHING METHODS

No one method is right for teaching all learners in all settings, nor is one method more effective for changing behavior in any of the three domains (Bastable, 2017). Combine methods or use one method with one or more instructional materials to meet the needs of the learner. Bastable (2017) emphasizes the importance of selecting appropriate methods for the individual learner and those that will actively involve the learner to achieve positive outcomes. Choose methods depending on your familiarity with the method, the availability of educational resources and teaching materials, and the characteristics of the individual patient or audience. Select the technique that requires the most active participation of the learner to increase the chance for learning success (Holli & Beto, 2018). It is also important to use age/developmental level-appropriate methods; for example, a 10-year-old child will be more receptive to gaming or role play, whereas an adult could learn similar material through a self-instruction module.

Use a variety of teaching strategies to enhance learning. Box 9-9 provides suggested teaching strategies for the three learning domains. The sample teaching plan (see Box 9-7 on page 224) shows how teaching strategies vary according to the learner outcomes and content of that particular plan. Again, be creative in choosing your methods. When providing teaching and learning opportunities and interventions, try to stimulate as many of the patient's senses as possible. Seeing, hearing, and touching reinforce what is read or heard. Continuously assess and validate how learning was accepted and understood, and provide repetition as necessary. Descriptions of common teaching strategies follow.

Role Modeling

The old saying "actions speak louder than words" explains why role modeling is effective. Patients watch their nurses closely; use this as an opportunity to improve a patient's behavior. Nurses have many opportunities to be personal examples of competency in skill performance, enthusiasm, and interest about an issue, and appropriate interactions with others (Bastable, 2017). For example, nurses who formerly smoked can be role models for patients who are trying to quit smoking. Nurses who diligently wash their hands before any patient encounter or procedure demonstrate the value and importance of handwashing.

Box 9-9 Suggested Teaching Strategies for the Three Learning Domains

Cognitive Domain
- Lecture or discussion
- Panel discussion
- Discovery
- Audiovisual materials
- Printed materials
- Programmed instruction
- Computer-assisted instruction programs

Affective Domain
- Role modeling
- Discussion
- Panel discussion
- Audiovisual materials
- Role playing
- Printed materials

Psychomotor Domain
- Demonstration
- Discovery
- Audiovisual materials
- Printed materials

Consider ***Marco García Ramírez***, the father-to-be concerned about his role as a parent. The nurse acts as a role model to the couple when demonstrating newborn care.

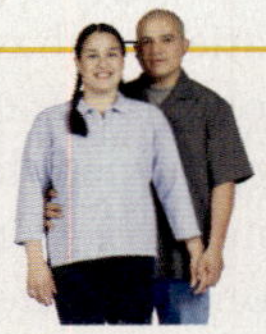

Lecture

In education, lecture refers to a presentation of information by a teacher to a learner. It is a passive method of informing and transferring knowledge and relies on the listening skills of the learner (Holli & Beto, 2018). To be more effective, lectures should include question-and-answer periods and collaboration with the learner. This strategy can be used to deliver information to a large group of patients but is more effective when the session is interactive; it is rarely used for individual instruction, except in combination with other strategies.

Discussion

Discussion involves a two-way exchange of information, ideas, and feelings between the teacher and learners. Discussion promotes active participation by learners (Holli & Beto, 2018). It is an effective method when used by a nurse who is comfortable with leading a group and knowledgeable about group processes (see Chapter 8). It can also be an effective method for one-on-one instruction. The Teach-Back Method can be an integral part of a discussion (refer to page 218).

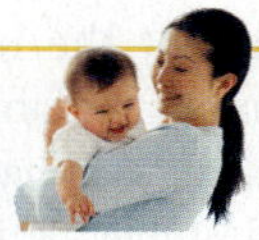

Remember **Alicia Bonet**, the young mother who had to make a decision about long-term aspirin therapy for her baby. The nurse could use a discussion to present information to Ms. Bonet about aspirin therapy, its risks and benefits, and Reye syndrome. The nurse would also provide time for Ms. Bonet to ask questions and think about the information presented.

Panel Discussion

A panel discussion involves a presentation of information by two or more people. Panel discussions can be used to impart factual material but are also effective for sharing experiences and emotions. Debates are a form of panel discussion that includes multiple sides of a controversial topic. These methods are often used as educational interventions for a large group, although, as with lecture, very few learners may actually get a chance to actively participate in the discussion (Holli & Beto, 2018).

Demonstration and Return Demonstration

Demonstration of techniques, procedures, exercises, and the use of special equipment, combined with a lecture and discussion, is an effective strategy. You can evaluate the patient's learning using a return demonstration, as with the Teach-Back Method technique described earlier (refer to page 218). Practice sessions are often included for the learner. Models of body parts or practice models, such as a resuscitation model, are frequently used. Childbirth educators usually demonstrate the birth of a baby by using a pelvic model, knitted uterus, and baby doll.

Discovery

In discovery learning, a problem or situation is presented to the patient or group of patients, who are then guided to discover the solution or approach. Discussion of other possible approaches and solutions can follow the patient's own solutions. This active participation in the learning process results in improved problem solving, creativity, responsibility, and independent thinking (Bruner, 1961). For instance, you could give a group of diabetic patients a short description of a situation that includes signs and symptoms, asking them to decide whether they indicate hypoglycemia (low blood sugar) or hyperglycemia (high blood sugar) and what measures to take. Then discuss the group's decision as a further learning experience. Even if the patients choose a poor solution, it can be turned into an effective learning experience. Other learning models that are based upon discovery learning include problem-based learning, simulation-based learning, and case-based learning.

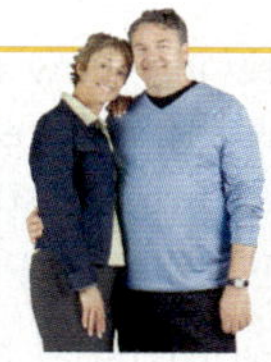

Recall **Rachel Blumenthal**, the wife of the patient who had a myocardial infarction. The nurse could present the couple with a "what-if" situation, such as, "What if your husband started to have chest pain while you were cuddling and kissing? How would you handle the situation?" From her answer, the nurse would be able to tell how well Mr. and Mrs. Blumenthal understand information provided related to home care. The nurse would also have an opportunity for reinstruction, reinforcement, and validation of learning.

Role Playing

Role playing gives the learner a chance to experience, relive, or anticipate an event. You explain a scenario and allow the patient to play out the scene with you or with one or more other learners. It is intended to arouse feelings and elicit emotional responses in the learners and is used primarily to achieve objectives in the affective domain (Bastable, 2019). Role playing can be used to work through emotional traumas or to plan for possible traumas; gain an understanding of others and why they behave the way they do; and practice new behaviors in a relatively safe environment (Holli & Beto, 2018). For example, role playing could help a teenage girl prepare to tell her parent about her pregnancy by letting the girl play herself while you play the girl's parent. This would help the patient rehearse what she wanted to say and anticipate the emotional atmosphere that she will experience. Role playing is a good strategy for children as well as adults. Puppets and dolls can be used as part of the process to help young children express negative feelings about hospitalization and traumatic procedures (Fig. 9-4).

INSTRUCTIONAL MATERIALS AND LEARNING ACTIVITIES

While planning teaching methods, also decide what instructional materials will be used to communicate the information, and any learning activities the patient should do independently. There are many ways that the patient can

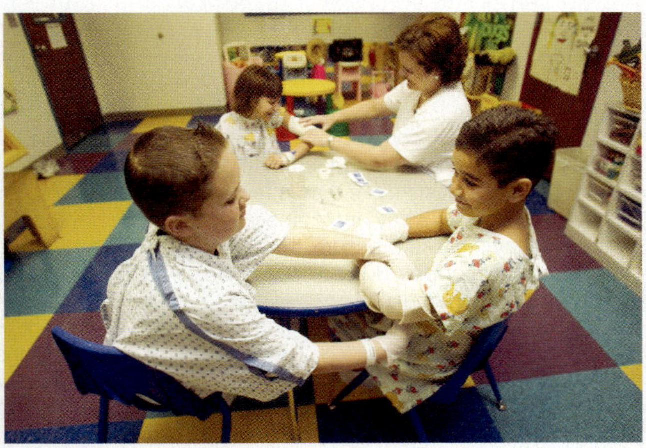

FIGURE 9-4. Role playing can help children learn and express negative feelings resulting from hospitalization and traumatic procedures. (*Source:* Used with permission from Shutterstock. *Photo by Joe Mitchell.*)

preview new material or reinforce what has already been taught. Printed materials, audiovisual materials, and programmed instruction materials are often assigned as part of the teaching plan.

Audiovisual Materials

Audiovisual materials such as computer programs, online courses, technology-driven learning tools, presentations using presentation tools such as PowerPoint or Prezi, films, television programs, flip charts, posters, and diagrams are popular and effective teaching strategies when combined with a lecture or discussion. Chosen materials must be in the preferred language of the learner and be at an appropriate level for the learner. As discussed earlier, never assume that the patient is literate. Also, never use AV materials as the sole source of learning for a patient. The patient may view the material independently, but it should be preceded and followed with a discussion or evaluation of comprehension of the material, with opportunity for questions, clarification, and validation.

Written Materials

The first consideration with printed material is availability. Many brochures, fact sheets, and pamphlets are available at no cost from online sources. Many nurses have also written materials for distribution to patients. Writing instruction sheets, books, and comic books for health teaching can be rewarding as well as useful. Like audiovisual materials, printed materials are generally used in conjunction with other strategies. It is also relatively easy to make games, which are a popular and fun way for patients to learn. For instance, cards with pictures of foods can be used to create a nutritional instruction game.

Select printed materials carefully based on how well they present the needed content in a format that is attractive, understandable, and helpful. Graphics and pictures can be used to enhance explanation and promote understanding (Bastable, 2017). The use of pictures can be an effective method of education for populations with limited health literacy (Winokur et al., 2019). Printed materials must be in the preferred language of the learner and be at an appropriate level for the learner. This may be challenging, in part because health care information and directions have traditionally been written at a 10th-grade level or higher; guidelines suggest health education material should be written at a 4th- to 6th-grade level, using short sentences and simple words, and incorporate pictures (Patient Safety Network, 2019). A sample of patient education material appears in Box 9-10.

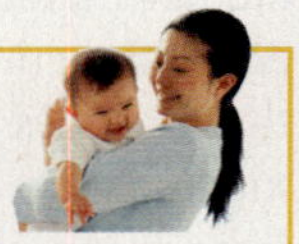

Consider how the nurse handled the situation of **Alicia Bonet**, the young mother described in the Reflective Practice box. The nurse provided Ms. Bonet with written materials that were at a level she could understand, thereby helping her make her decision.

Box 9-10 Heart Attack: Know the Symptoms. Take Action

Important Information

Fill out the next two sections and put this card in your wallet with your ID.

It will help emergency medical staff treat you after you call 9-1-1.

Medicines you are taking:

____

____

____

Medicines you are allergic to:

____

____

____

Health Care Provider

Name: ______________________________

Office phone: ______________________________

After-hours phone: ______________________________

Person You Would Like Contacted If You Go to the Hospital.

Name: ______________________________

Home phone: ______________________________

Work phone: ______________________________

- Chest Pain or Discomfort
  Discomfort in the center or left side of the chest that lasts more than a few minutes or goes away and comes back. May feel like pressure, squeezing, fullness, or pain. May also feel like heartburn or indigestion.
- Other Upper Body Pain or Discomfort
  May be felt in one or both arms, the back, shoulders, neck, jaw, or upper part of the stomach (above the belly button).
- Shortness of Breath
  May be the only symptom, or it may occur before or along with chest pain or discomfort. May occur when resting or during easy activities.
- Other Possible Symptoms
  May include breaking out in a cold sweat, feeling unusually tired, nausea, or lightheadedness. Any sudden new symptom or change in usual symptoms also should be a concern.

If you think you might be having heart attack symptoms or a heart attack, call 9-1-1 immediately. Do not ignore your pain or discomfort. Every minute matters when it comes to getting treatment for heart attacks.

Never delay calling 9-1-1 to take aspirin or do anything else you think might help.

If you are unable to reach 9-1-1, have someone else drive you to the hospital right away. Don't drive yourself to the hospital. You may cause a car accident.

Source: National Heart, Lung, and Blood Institute. (2011). *Heart attack: Know the symptoms. Take action.* U.S. Department of Health and Human Services. https://www.nhlbi.nih.gov/files/docs/public/heart/heart_attack_fs_en.pdf

Demonstration Materials

Demonstration materials stimulate a learner's senses as well as add variety, realism, and enjoyment to the teaching–learning experience (Bastable, 2017). Models and real equipment and displays, such as posters, flip charts, and bulletin boards are examples of demonstration materials. Demonstration materials bring the learner closer to reality and actively engage the patient in learning (Bastable, 2017).

Programmed Instruction

Most programmed instruction books or booklets are prepared so that learners can use them independently of a teacher. However, educators generally agree on the need to spend time with the learner before and after the program to clarify the information, answer questions, and provide the personal touch necessary for a learner's motivation. Because this is a self-paced strategy, it can be beneficial for many learners. Printed materials must be in the preferred language of the learner and be at an appropriate level for the learner.

Web-Based Instruction and Technology

Websites appropriate to the patient's disease process, wellness interests, or health promotion focus can be valuable teaching and learning resources. There are various free or affordable applications (apps) that provide choices for nurses and patients to identify what works best in individual circumstances (Shustack, 2019). There are many websites and/or apps can support instruction. These sites and tools provide consumer information that is formatted for easy reading and access. Programmed instruction or web-based instruction and apps can be particularly useful for patients in isolated areas, especially when it is interspersed with opportunities to see the nurse or other health care provider in person. Be sure to evaluate the website or app chosen by the patient and advise the patient on its suitability and accuracy because some information found on the internet is not grounded in scientific, medical, or nursing research. Opportunities for the use of technology integrated into patient education are endless. For example, mobile phone–based social networking has been used to support self-management education and behaviors for patients with hypertension (Ghezeljeh et al., 2018).

Technology Alert

Technology platforms are being developed and used to help patients and their families engage in the care process. One example of such a network uses the intensive care unit patient's bedside television to deliver patient education using a combination of direct instruction and model patient re-enactments of situations in order to display situations that could be encountered during the hospital stay. The use of this technology resulted in patient and caregiver reports of perceived decreased anxiety and that television was a useful tool for providing health literacy education (Thompson Bastin et al., 2019).

Box 9-11 Example of a Contractual Agreement Between a Nurse and a Patient

I will participate in the learning activities needed to help me learn about my low-sodium diet. During my hospital stay, I will attend the class on low-sodium diets, read the materials given to me, and ask questions as I need to. I will work with S. Moore, RN, to plan my meals and food preparation at home. If I need help when I get home, I will contact S. Moore.

Jim Mall

I will provide Jim Mall with the experiences needed for him to follow his low-sodium diet accurately.

S. Moore, RN

Contractual Agreements

A **contractual agreement** is a pact between two people setting out mutually agreed-on goals. Contracts between nurses and patients are common in many health care settings. The contracts are usually informal and not legally binding. When teaching a patient, such an agreement can serve to motivate both the patient and you as the teacher to do what is necessary to meet the patient's learning outcomes. The agreement notes the responsibilities of both the teacher and the learner, emphasizing the importance of the mutual commitment, as well as provides a measurement of how close the patient is to reaching the goals (Holli & Beto, 2018) (Box 9-11). If the contracted outcomes are achieved, you can boost the patient's self-esteem with rewards; if the outcomes are not achieved, you can try different teaching techniques.

Implementing

Implementing the teaching plan requires interpersonal skills and effective communication techniques, as well as organizational and time management skills. Teaching the patient can be a major part of the working phase of the helping relationship (refer to Chapter 8).

Time Constraints

Nurses often encounter challenges in finding time to meet patients' needs, so consideration of time constraints is important when implementing teaching and learning activities. Lack of time to teach is cited by nurses as the greatest barrier to being able to carry out their role effectively (Bastable, 2017, p. 14). Set priorities in order to teach essential content thoroughly. Less important content can be taught last so that the more important learner outcomes can be met within the time available. If time permits, the remaining content can be addressed.

To meet time constraints, nurses often plan together. Teamwork and cooperation allow nurses to meet deadlines. Patient education is provided during hospitalization, home visits, and clinic visits, and in scheduled learning opportunities through outpatient programs or referrals to community-based programs. Home health care nurses often receive referrals from hospital nurses to continue the teaching begun

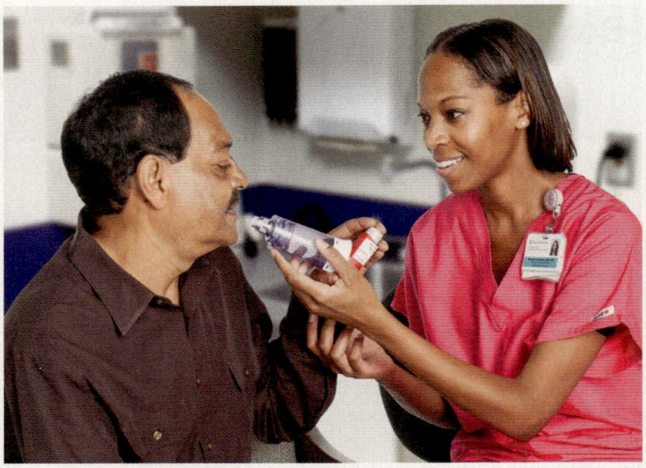

FIGURE 9-5. One-to-one teaching is used in many nurse–patient situations.

during a patient's hospitalization. Discharge planning from a facility must be started early to ensure continuity of teaching.

Scheduling

It is better to plan shorter, more frequent teaching sessions than one or two longer sessions. Short sessions allow patients to digest the new material and prevent them from becoming too tired or uncomfortable because of a health problem. Sessions of 15 to 30 minutes are generally well tolerated. Usually, more formal classroom programs last for more than 1 hour; in such cases, provide a break after every 50 minutes of class time. Include the patient when planning the time and frequency of lessons. Scheduling teaching sessions when the patient is least stressed will enhance teaching.

Group Versus Individual Teaching

Learner outcomes influence the use of group versus individual, one-on-one instruction. Some learner outcomes are met more readily in a one-to-one encounter, which provides a nonthreatening environment to meet individual needs and goals (Bastable, 2017) (Fig. 9-5). Other learner outcomes are achieved more easily in a group, which can foster social skills and maintain contact with others through shared experiences (Bastable, 2017). For example, the outcome "The patient will change the dressing using clean technique" is best taught and evaluated in a private session. The outcome "The patient will discuss feelings about diabetes self-management" might be met more easily in a group discussion with other patients.

Formal Versus Informal Teaching

Many nurse–patient interactions can include **informal teaching**. These unplanned teaching sessions are often effective because they deal with the patient's immediate learning needs and concerns. Discussion as simple as reinforcing the correct technique for postoperative deep breathing exercises or explaining or clarifying information about a scheduled procedure is actually teaching. Informal teaching may also lead to additional planned, formal sessions. **Formal teaching** is planned, scheduled teaching done to address specific identified learner outcomes. Both forms are effective when used appropriately.

Additional Implementation Considerations

Nurses must continually observe the patient for additional assessment data that could alter the original teaching plan. This requires skill in adapting and reorganizing the teaching plan. Following are important considerations when implementing a teaching plan:

- *Promote patient learning by using a warm and accepting approach.* Your attitude has more effect on the patient than any other factor (Fig. 9-6). Avoid taking a condescending attitude and using technical and medical terms (unless the patient has a background in this area). A nonthreatening teaching–learning atmosphere allows learning to occur.
- *Consider the physical environment when implementing the teaching plan.* Some planning may be needed to ensure adequate space and lighting, comfortable chairs, and good ventilation. Privacy is also important, as is freedom from distractions and interruptions.
- *Review the patient's expectations and role functions as a learner.* To avoid any misunderstandings, review the contractual agreement before implementing the teaching plan. The patient is expected to listen, observe, engage, and attempt to understand what is being taught.
- *Assess the patient's comfort level.* Some people are uncomfortable in the role of learner. You need to recognize this problem in order to assist the patient to assume the role more easily. If the patient must learn special techniques or procedures (e.g., colostomy care, self-injections, eye medication instillation), assure the patient that it takes time and practice before anyone can perform new skills confidently.
- *Be prepared and organized before implementing the teaching plan.* Gather and organize all teaching aids (e.g., posters, films, printed materials) before the teaching session. A disorganized teacher distracts the learner and hinders learning. Also, a procedure or skill must be taught in the correct sequence so that the patient does not become confused.

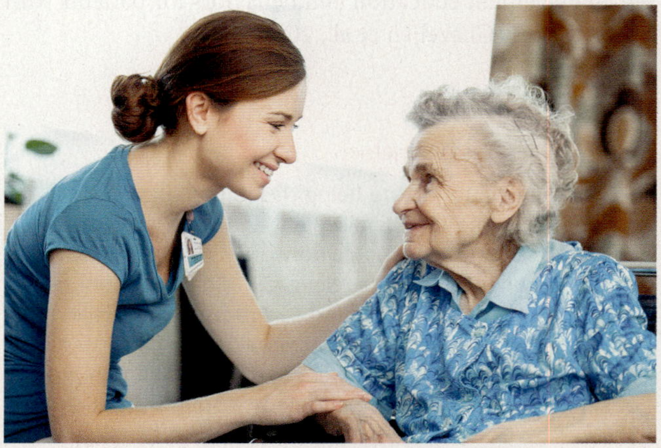

FIGURE 9-6. The nurse's warm approach is an important factor in interpersonal relationships. (*Source: Photo by Monkey Business Images/Shutterstock.*)

- *Make each learning session interesting and enjoyable for the patient.* Have an enthusiastic and positive attitude, and make learning fun by creative use of planned teaching strategies. When you approach teaching positively, the patient is more likely to approach learning in a similar way.

Role of the Nurse as Coach

With the implementation of the 2010 Affordable Care Act and the goals outlined in the *Healthy People 2030* initiative, there is a clear need to address the direction of health care in the future (Office of Disease Prevention and Health Promotion, 2020; USDHHS, 2019). Health challenges are more complex these days, and nurses need to be prepared to move from a disease-based model of care toward a health and wellness promotion model. The IOM's (2011) report, *The Future of Nursing: Leading Change, Advancing Health*, emphasizes the need for nurses to assume a leadership role that includes collaborating and coordinating care across teams of health professionals. The nurse coach role is an integral component of this partnership and assists patients and families to make changes that promote healthier lifestyles.

Nurses who incorporate coaching into their professional practice can improve the quality and effectiveness of care. A **nurse coach** integrates coaching competencies to facilitate a process of change or development that assists individuals or groups to realize their potential and ability to cope with health challenges (Delaney et al., 2020; Hess et al., 2013). Nurse coaches utilize a whole-person, relationship-centered approach to educate and empower patients (Delaney et al., 2020). A nurse coach establishes a partnership with a patient and uses discovery to identify the patient's personal goals and agenda in a way that will result in change rather than using teaching and education strategies directed by the nurse as the expert. Nurse coaches may practice in any setting or specialty area, such as diabetes education or cardiac rehabilitation, and may be staff nurses, advanced-practice nurses, educators, and administrators. The nurse coach role is supported by coaching education, training, and experience and is influenced by the population served.

The nurse coaching process includes the following (Delaney et al., 2020; Hess et al., 2013):

- Establishing relationships and identifying readiness for change
- Identifying opportunities, issues, and concerns
- Establishing patient (person)-centered goals
- Creating the structure of the coaching interaction
- Empowering and motivating patients activate lasting wellness behaviors to reach goals
- Assisting the patient to determine progress toward goals

The role of nurse coach is evolving and should not be confused with that of a preceptor or mentor. A nurse coach explores the patient's readiness for change, plans and structures the coaching interactions, supports the achievement of the patient's desired goals, and with the patient determines how to evaluate the attainment of patient goals (American Holistic Nurses Association, n.d.). Health maintenance organizations and various health and wellness programs have nurse coaches to assist patients to improve health outcomes. Professional nursing organizations recognize the need to further define the definition of a nurse coach and develop a nurse coach certification program and process.

Evaluating

The nurse and the patient and family/caregivers work together to measure how well the outcomes specified in the plan of care have been achieved.

Evaluating Learning

Nurses cannot be sure that patients have actually learned the content without some type of proof or feedback. The key to evaluation is the learner outcomes in the teaching plan that describe the behaviors to be measured. The results of evaluation provided evidence to guide future action in planning and carrying out educational interventions (Bastable, 2019). Methods for obtaining feedback about learning are discussed in the following section.

METHODS OF EVALUATION

There are several methods of evaluation of learning. For instance, cognitive domain learning may be evaluated through oral questioning, affective domain learning through the patient's response, and psychomotor domain learning by a return demonstration. Consider this learner outcome in the cognitive domain: "The patient will be able to describe what a blood pressure reading represents." To evaluate this, you could ask the patient, "Tell me what this blood pressure reading means to you." The patient then has a chance to talk about the reading while you evaluate the patient's understanding of it.

Asking direct questions is often an efficient method of evaluating learner outcomes. Simply ask the patient a question, and the answer reflects the patient's level of knowledge about a topic. Direct questions can also be used to evaluate the patient's affective learning.

Another way to decide whether learner outcomes have been met is to analyze the patient's own comments. Patients may state that they understand the information while avoiding further discussion of the topic. In such instances, using effective communication techniques when reintroducing the topic at a later time might provide the evaluation data needed.

Sometimes observational skills can help determine whether the patient is using the material learned. For example, observing what the patient has ordered for lunch shows whether dietary lessons are being put into practice. A nurse also uses observation when evaluating the patient's psychomotor skills. A return demonstration is an excellent way of evaluating psychomotor domain learning (Fig. 9-7 on page 232). Providing an opportunity for and encouraging patients to change their own dressing, for example, provides concrete evidence of satisfactory or unsatisfactory performance of the procedure. However, you must take care to promote a nonstressful environment when the time comes for the patient's return demonstration.

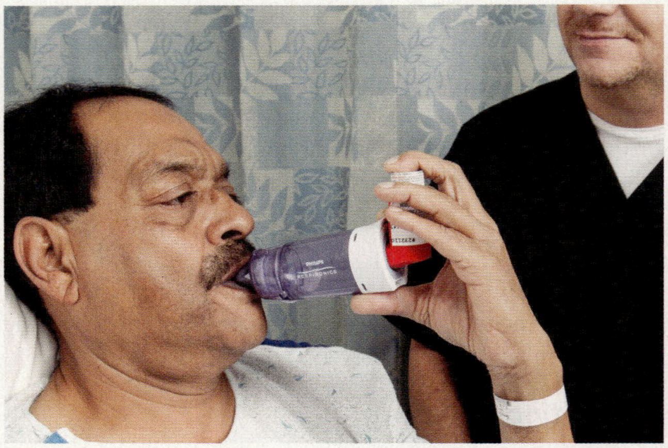

FIGURE 9-7. Patient correctly demonstrates what has been taught, validating learning has occurred.

TIMING OF EVALUATION

Evaluation of learning is ongoing. If learning is only evaluated as soon as teaching is completed, the results may be misleading. Nurses may evaluate what the patient has learned from educational sessions the previous day. Home health care nurses may evaluate what the patient learned in the hospital, as well as what is being taught during home visits. Hospital nurses often check with family members/caregivers or significant others after discharge to evaluate whether learner outcomes have been met.

Reinforcing and Celebrating Learning

Most people feel encouraged and supported when their efforts are acknowledged by another person, especially when they trust and value the other person. This is especially true in health care, where patients often feel overwhelmed by their illness. To make the most of this dynamic, use **positive reinforcement** to affirm the efforts of patients who have mastered new knowledge, attitudes, or skills. Reinforcement may be as simple as a few words of acknowledgment ("You've mastered this diet quickly"), as spontaneous as a warm hug, or as planned as the entire staff joining to celebrate a patient's independent ambulation. **Negative reinforcement**—criticism or punishment—is generally ineffective; undesirable behavior is usually best ignored. Behavior modification programs that reward desired behaviors and ignore undesired behaviors can be designed for some patients.

Evaluating Teaching

Evaluation of teaching must occur so that you can capitalize on your strengths and work on improving weaknesses. Like all nursing roles, effective teaching requires practice and experience. Even nurse educators agree that they are always discovering better ways to promote learning. It is important not to feel discouraged when evaluations of your teaching are less than perfect.

It is best to evaluate your own teaching effectiveness immediately after a teaching session. This involves a quick review of how well you feel you implemented the plan. Mentally noting both the strengths and weaknesses of the teaching session helps you plan better for subsequent sessions.

Box 9-12 Factors Affecting Teaching Effectiveness

- Ignoring the restrictions of the patient's environment
- Failing to accept that patients have the right to change their mind
- Using medical jargon
- Failing to negotiate goals
- Duplicating teaching that other team members have done
- Overloading the patient with information
- Choosing the wrong time for teaching
- Not evaluating what the patient has learned
- Not reviewing educational media, or relying exclusively on media
- Failing to document patient teaching and plan for follow-up or teaching reinforcement

You can also seek feedback from patients. You can use a simple questionnaire at the end of a teaching session or after discharge to gain the patient's perception of your teaching effectiveness. Use a standardized questionnaire from the facility or prepare your own. When using an outcome format that requires only circles or checkmarks as answers, provide space for comments.

Revising the Plan

During evaluation, you or your patient might decide that revisions are needed in the teaching plan. When revising the plan, you should identify teaching factors that might have reduced teaching effectiveness (Box 9-12). A reassessment might indicate that some patient factors were not considered in the original plan, and adjustments might be made accordingly to meet the patient's needs. Often, the use of a different teaching strategy is all that is needed for a patient to achieve the learner outcomes.

Revision is a natural part of the teaching–learning process and should not be viewed negatively. Neither you nor the patient has "failed" when an outcome is not met. Most outcomes can be met with a change in approach, although sometimes the learner outcomes may be unrealistic. Further assessment might reveal that the content might be too complex or the time too short for successful achievement.

Unfolding Patient Stories: Rashid Ahmed • Part 1

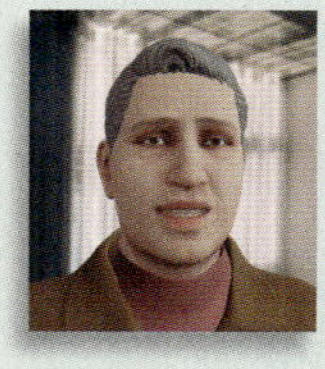

Rashid Ahmed is a 50-year-old male admitted to the medical unit with a diagnosis of dehydration from severe nausea, vomiting, and diarrhea. The nurse receives provider's orders containing abbreviations that are unclear and not accepted by the hospital. What steps would the nurse take to clarify the orders and deter the provider's use of error-prone documentation? Why is it important for all health care professionals to follow agency policies on documentation? (Rashid Ahmed's story continues in Chapter 20.)

Care for Rashid and other patients in a realistic virtual environment: ***vSim** for Nursing* (**thepoint.lww.com/vSimFunds**). Practice documenting these patients' care in DocuCare (thepoint.lww.com/DocuCareEHR).

Documenting

The nurse is legally responsible for documenting teaching in the patient's health record. Documentation of the teaching–learning process includes a summary of the learning need, the plan, the implementation of the plan, and the evaluation results. The evaluative statement is crucial and *must show concrete evidence that demonstrates that learning has occurred.* If the desired learning has not occurred, the patient's health record should indicate updated plans to address the problem or how the problem was resolved. It is not enough to document only what you taught; your charting *must show evidence that the patient or family member/caregiver has actually learned* the material taught.

NURSE AS COUNSELOR

Counseling is the "art of providing listening, advice, guidance, or direction regarding an action or decision to help a person change" (Holli & Beto, 2018, p. 137). Nurses counsel patients through this interpersonal process to assist patients in adapting to difficulties or changes in life experiences (Peplau, 1991) and help patients make decisions that promote their overall well-being. Counseling focuses on improving coping abilities, reinforcing healthy behaviors, fostering positive interactions, or preventing illness and disability (Boyd, 2018). Family members/caregivers or significant others are often included in counseling sessions. Everyone participating must feel comfortable in the situation and surroundings. Like teaching, counseling may be formal or informal.

The interpersonal skills of warmth, friendliness, openness, and empathy—skills required to develop therapeutic nurse–patient relationships—are necessary for successful counseling. Refer to Chapter 8 for discussion of therapeutic nurse–patient relationships. An effective counselor needs to be a caring person. Caring is based on a humanistic philosophy and caring is foundational to the nursing profession (Watson, 2008). A humanistic approach to counseling rooted in professional caring helps the patient strive toward the greatest health potential. Caring is important in all nursing roles but is fundamental in the counseling role.

Some advanced-practice psychiatric mental health nurses specialize in counseling, and this form of counseling has an important professional role. The focus in this chapter, however, is on the everyday counseling that is a basic component of all nurses' practice. This counseling involves listening carefully to the patient's or family's/caregivers questions, concerns, demands, and grievances and then responding in an effective manner.

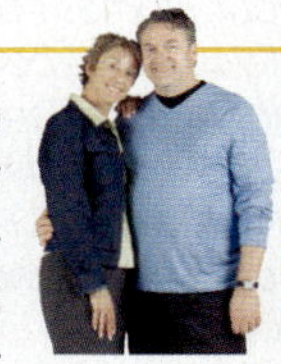

Consider **Rachel Blumenthal**, the wife of the patient who had a myocardial infarction. By carefully listening to Mrs. Blumenthal's concerns, including her comment about being embarrassed to talk with her husband's cardiologist, the nurse helps to establish a trusting relationship that forms the basis for counseling.

Knowing appropriate responses to what a patient says might be difficult at first, but practice helps develop this skill (refer to Chapter 8 for discussion of communication techniques). Each nurse–patient (or nurse–family/caregiver) interaction is unique; a nurse's response that works well with one patient might intimidate or anger another. Sensitivity to the unique needs of each patient and a willingness to get involved and make a difference are essential for effective counseling. Because counseling skills take time to cultivate, nursing students and new nurses should be aware of their limits and not rush to counsel without first considering consultation with more experienced nurses. Table 9-1 (on page 234) presents typical counseling situations you might experience and analyzes both effective and ineffective nursing responses. You might want to role play these situations with a friend.

In counseling situations, you do not tell patients what to do to solve the problem but instead assist and guide them to solve problems and make decisions. If the patient lacks the knowledge and skills to approach a problem systematically, you can combine the teaching and counseling roles to help the patient solve the dilemma successfully.

The nursing process is an essential tool when guiding/counseling patients. The nursing process is used to organize the nurse–patient counseling situation described in Box 9-13 (on page 235). Additional examples of health problems centered on counseling needs with related etiology and signs and symptoms can be found in the box titled Examples of Actual or Potential Health Problems and Needs: Counseling Needs (on page 235).

Types of Counseling

Counseling may be short or long term or motivational and may occur as the result of a situation or event or a developmental crisis.

Short-Term Counseling

Short-term counseling focuses on the immediate problem or concern of the patient or family/caregiver. It can be a relatively minor concern or a major crisis, but in any case, it requires immediate attention (Fig. 9-8). Short-term counseling might

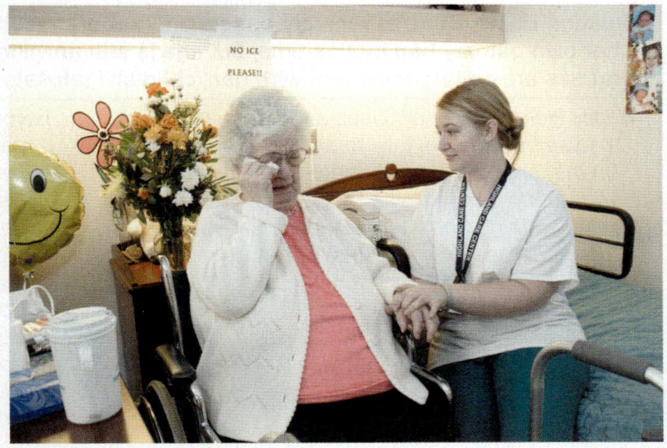

FIGURE 9-8. Counseling may involve a concern that needs immediate attention. (*Source:* Used with permission from Shutterstock. *Photo by Rick Brady.*)

Table 9-1 Analysis of Nursing Responses in Common Counseling Situations

INEFFECTIVE RESPONSE	ANALYSIS	EFFECTIVE RESPONSE	ANALYSIS
Situation A: You walk into the room of Ms. Goldstein, who learned earlier in the day that her tumor is malignant. She is crying.			
"Oh cheer up! Tomorrow's got to be a brighter day."	Provides false reassurance; communicates insensitivity to patient's feelings.	Touch forearm and sit next to her quietly. After several minutes, say, *"I can't even begin to imagine how difficult this must be for you. Please let me know if there is anything I can do to help."*	Uses touch, silence, and caring appropriately.
Situation B: You have been teaching 60-year-old Mr. Hyong diabetic self-care for 4 days, and he is still asking the same questions and refusing to administer his own insulin or check his blood sugar.			
"Well, I guess we are getting nowhere here. Is there anyone else who might be able to do this for you?"	Rejects patient without first evaluating the teaching plan and exploring patient variables that might be hindering learning.	*"We may have a bit of a problem here.… I hear you asking the same questions every day. Let's see if together we can figure out why this isn't making sense to you."*	Enlists patient in problem solving.
Situation C: One morning, you walk into the room of an older resident who had withdrawn and become totally dependent on the nurses for basic care on her transfer into the long-term care facility. You are surprised to discover that she has washed and dressed herself—for the first time.			
"Well, I'm happy to see that you have rejoined the ranks of the living. Did you wash off your glasses?"	Misses opportunity to celebrate the resident's achievement of an important goal.	Hugs resident warmly, looks her in the eye, and exclaims, *"Don't you look wonderful today? What are you celebrating?"* Defers an assessment of how thorough the morning care has been until later.	Rejoices spontaneously in the resident's achievement and reinforces this behavior. Gives the resident a reason to continue to make progress. Uses touch appropriately.
Situation D: You are helping Mr. Stein out of bed; he has been on bed rest for 2 weeks because of a painful and debilitating illness. A fiercely independent man, he is embarrassed to need your support and looks disgusted with himself when he steps on your foot.			
"What's the problem, Honey? Haven't been eating your Wheaties?"	Uses terms of endearment, which often denote disrespect and condescension to patients, no matter in what spirit they are uttered.	"No problem, Mr. Stein, my husband steps on my toes all the time when we go dancing!" After a few minutes . . . *"It must be hard when you are used to doing everything for yourself to all of a sudden find yourself needing others for simple things.…"*	Uses humor and empathy appropriately; invites the patient to share his feelings.
Situation E: Ms. Berretta recently underwent surgery resulting in a urinary diversion. She should be able to change her own ostomy bag by this time, but she is still unwilling to look at the stoma and participate alone in her care. The nurses are getting impatient with her "childish" refusals to learn.			
"Really Helen, I'll do it myself but you'll be the loser once you get home with this thing and there's no one around to help."	Uses a threat in an attempt to coerce learning (negative reinforcement). Displays unwillingness to explore what is blocking Ms. Berretta's readiness to learn.	Before beginning Ms. Berretta's care: *"I think we need to talk before your care today. You will be discharged soon, and I want you to feel confident about caring for your stoma. I understand that until you can accept it, you don't want to learn anything about it. Would you like to talk about this with me, or would you prefer me to make a referral to someone else?"*	Communicates respect for patient and sensitivity to her needs, without ignoring what is the real problem. Offers the possibility of a referral to another health care professional if the patient so wishes.

Box 9-13 Example of Counseling for Problem Solving Using the Nursing Process

Situation

Monday, 1930, Amy Purcell has been admitted to the children's unit with dehydration resulting from diarrhea. Amy is responding well to intravenous (IV) fluids. Her mother is visibly distraught.

Assessing

- Amy is doing well but will need 24 hours of IV therapy.
- Amy and her twin sister Susan have never been separated from their parents or each other. They are 2 years old.
- Mrs. Purcell has no idea who will care for Susan when Mr. Purcell goes to work in the morning.
- The Purcells have no regular childcare arrangements and have no family members in the area.
- Mrs. Purcell wants to stay with Amy during her hospitalization.
- The Purcells' neighbor is home during the day. Sometimes Amy and Susan play at her house.
- There is a day care center near their home, but Susan might be upset about going there. It's also expensive.
- Mr. Purcell cannot afford to take Tuesday off but will take Wednesday morning off.
- Insurance does not cover a private room, which would allow Susan to come to stay in the hospital too.

Diagnosing

Actual Health Problems and Need: Anxiety
Etiologic Factors: Stress of daughter's hospitalization, need for childcare for Susan, and uncertain resources
Signs and Symptoms: Refer to Assessment data above.

Planning Goal

Mrs. Purcell will demonstrate decreased anxiety over the care of Susan during Amy's hospitalization.

Together, Mrs. Purcell and the nurse have planned the following:

- The neighbor will come to the Purcell home to care for Susan when Mr. Purcell leaves for work on Tuesday morning.
- The neighbor will bring Susan to the hospital for the afternoon visiting hours to be with Mrs. Purcell and Amy.
- Mr. Purcell will come to the hospital after work to have dinner with the family.
- Mr. Purcell will take Susan home for bedtime.
- On Wednesday morning, Mr. Purcell will take off work in the morning. He and Susan will go to the hospital to pick up Mrs. Purcell and Amy.

Implementing

Plan implemented by the Purcells with support of the nursing staff.

Evaluating

Mrs. Purcell told the nurse that she feels that both Amy and Susan did well with the care they received from their parents. The family's stress was minimized, and she is relieved that everything went so well. The nurse decides that the goals were met.

be used during a situational crisis, which occurs when a patient faces an event or situation that causes a disruption in life. For example, a patient in the hospital finds out that his wife has been involved in a car accident; she received only a few scratches, but their only car was demolished. As a nurse, you are in an excellent position to help the patient decide what can be done to solve this situational crisis. You can guide the patient to resources to help solve the travel, financial, and emotional difficulties that arise as a result of the accident. This holistic approach is especially important because the crisis could hinder the patient's recovery.

Long-Term Counseling

Long-term counseling extends over a prolonged period. A patient might need the counsel of the nurse at daily, weekly, or monthly intervals. A patient experiencing a

Examples of Actual or Potential Health Problems and Needs

COUNSELING NEEDS

Actual or Potential Health Problems and Needs	Possible Etiologic Factors	Potential Signs and Symptoms
Decisional Conflict	• Conflict with moral obligation • Insufficient support system	• "I don't know what to do!" • Delay in decision making • Inability to authorize withdrawal of life-sustaining treatment despite believing this to be in the patient's best interests
Hopelessness	Prolonged social isolation and belief that "even God has abandoned me"	• Progression of debilitating symptoms • Poor eye contact • Flat affect
Situational Low Self-Esteem	Recent lay-off and divorce	• Indecisive • "I can't do what you are asking me to do." • "I am worthless."

Source: ICNP® is owned and copyrighted by the International Council of Nurses (ICN). Reproduced with permission of the copyright holder. (2019). *Nursing diagnosis and outcome statements.* https://www.icn.ch/sites/default/files/inline-files/ICNP2019-DC.pdf; Wolters Kluwer. (2022). Problem-based care plans. In *Lippincott Advisor.* Wolters Kluwer.

developmental crisis, for example, might need long-term counseling. A developmental crisis can occur when a person is going through a developmental stage or passage. For example, many women going through menopause need help adjusting to the changes they experience. Long-term counseling may occur in nurse-led support groups.

Motivational Interviewing

Motivational interviewing is an evidence-based counseling approach to evoke and strengthen a patient's motivation and commitment to change (Miller & Rollnick, 2013). This method of guidance promotes behavior change by guiding patients to explore their own values and motivation for change and the advantages and disadvantages of their decisions (Caccavale et al., 2020; Morgan & Townsend, 2021). Motivational interviewing incorporates active listening and verbal therapeutic communications techniques, focusing on what the patient wants rather than on what the nurse thinks should be the next steps in behavior change (Morgan & Townsend, 2021). Four main principles guide this technique: expressing empathy, supporting self-efficacy, developing discrepancy, and rolling with resistance (Dart, 2011). These principles allow the patient to share their perspectives; ensure the nurse does not impose their own beliefs onto the patient; assist the patient to gain insight into the difference between where they are and where they want to be; and allows the patient to share their negative thoughts without challenge from the nurse (Dart, 2011).

Gance-Cleveland (2013) proposed that the traditional model of counseling may not prove effective for an issue such as the childhood obesity epidemic. Instead, a collaborative, family-centered model that includes motivational interviewing may help the family identify health goals. Instead of focusing on solutions to the obesity issue, the nurse attempts to gain a better understanding of the barriers that exist to changing family behaviors. With this technique, families gain the self-confidence needed to promote better health outcomes. This is not the traditional approach, and it requires time to establish relationships and explore family perspectives, but motivational interviewing can be an effective alternative to deal with a severe health problem.

When assessing a motivational problem, always consider the patient's cultural values. Often the way a person feels about something is strongly influenced by that person's cultural background. For instance, if a person has grown up in a family in which illness is perceived as an inevitable result of aging, it may be difficult to motivate that person to practice preventive measures for health (see Chapter 5). Such a problem may seem insurmountable, yet a caring nurse can work toward helping patients with this mindset become interested in promoting their own health.

Referrals

Sometimes a patient needs specialized counseling from a nurse with advanced training or from other health care professionals. In these cases, offer to refer the patient to the appropriate professional (e.g., psychiatric or mental health nurse, psychologist or psychiatrist, social worker, clergy, financial counselor, sex therapist, or occupational therapist). In other cases, a simple referral to a community resource, such as a neighborhood support group, may be appropriate to address the patient's needs. When making a referral, be sure to address any barriers that might prevent the patient from acting on the referral. Patients might fail to follow-up with a referral for financial reasons, because they do not understand the reason for or value of the referral, because they lack transportation, because the facility is not open at times convenient for them or there are other access issues.

REFLECTIVE PRACTICE LEADING TO PERSONAL LEARNING

Remember that the goal of reflective practice is to look at an experience, understand it, and learn from it. As you begin to use and develop expertise as a teacher and counselor, reflect on your experiences—both successes and failures—in order to improve your practice. How can you do it better next time? What did you learn today that can help you tomorrow? Begin your reflection by paying close attention to the following while providing nursing care:

- Did your preparation and practice related to the use of verbal and nonverbal communication techniques result in your feeling confident in your ability to provide care to meet the identified educational and counseling needs? Did your competence and confidence inspire the patient's and family's/caregiver's trust?
  - How did you prioritize the data you collected? What patterns in the data did you identify? What knowledge from your learning, personal experience and intuition did you use to make decisions and develop your plan of care?
- How confident are you that the data you reported and recorded accurately communicate the status of the patient? How successfully have you communicated who this patient and family/caregivers are to the interdisciplinary team?
- Were you aware of any cultural or ethnic beliefs or practices that may have influenced your communication or development of a helping relationship with patients or family members/caregivers? Were you aware of any stereotypes or prejudices that may have negatively influenced the encounter? If so, how did you address these?
- Did the patient and family/caregivers participate in the process at an optimal level? How might you have better engaged the patient and family/caregivers? Did the patient sense that you are respectful, caring, and competent?

Perhaps the most important questions to reflect on are: Are your patients and their families/caregivers better for having had *you* share in the critical responsibility of being a part of their health care team? Are your patients now receiving thoughtful, person-centered, prioritized, holistic, evidence-based treatment and care because of your efforts?

DEVELOPING CLINICAL REASONING AND CLINICAL JUDGMENT

1. Explain what the following statement means: "It is as important for patients to understand and value the proposed treatment regimen as it is for them to understand how to implement the proposed regimen." What are the implications of this for teaching and counseling?
2. A patient your age has just learned that she has tested positive for the human immunodeficiency virus (HIV). Make a list of some of the learning (cognitive, psychomotor, affective) that you think should take place. What sorts of things might affect their readiness to learn? How would you tailor your nursing in response to these variables?
3. Mrs. Riley is being readmitted to your hospital unit with complications related to her diabetes. A coworker voices her frustrations and says, "We've taught her everything she needs to know to do a better job of managing her diabetes. I don't know what more we can do." How do you respond?

PRACTICING FOR NCLEX

1. A nurse is teaching first aid to counselors of a summer camp for children with asthma. This is an example of what aim of health teaching?
   a. Promoting health
   b. Preventing illness
   c. Restoring health
   d. Facilitating coping
2. A nurse is teaching patients of all ages in a hospital setting. Which teaching examples are appropriate for the patient's developmental level? Select all that apply.
   a. The nurse plans long teaching sessions to discuss diet modifications for an older adult diagnosed with type 2 diabetes.
   b. The nurse recognizes that a female adolescent diagnosed with anorexia is still dependent on her parents and includes them in all teaching sessions.
   c. The nurse designs an exercise program for a sedentary older adult male patient based on the activities he prefers.
   d. The nurse includes an 8-year-old patient in the teaching plan for managing cystic fibrosis.
   e. The nurse demonstrates how to use an inhaler to an 11-year-old male patient and includes his mother in the session to reinforce the teaching.
   f. The nurse continues a teaching session on STIs for a sexually active male adolescent despite his protest that "I've heard enough already!"
3. A nurse is teaching an adult patient how to care for their new ostomy appliance. Which evaluation method is most appropriate to confirm that the patient has learned the information?
   a. Ask Me 3
   b. Newest Vital Sign (NVS)
   c. Teach-Back Method
   d. TEACH acronym
4. A nurse is planning teaching strategies in the affective domain of learning for patients with alcohol use disorders. Which teaching–learning activities will the nurse use? Select all that apply.
   a. Preparing a lecture on the harmful long-term effects of alcohol on the body
   b. Asking the patient to discuss reasons people with alcohol use disorders drink and exploring other methods of coping with problems
   c. Requesting that patients perform a return demonstration for using relaxation exercises to relieve stress
   d. Helping patients to reaffirm their feelings of self-worth and relate this to their alcohol use disorder
   e. Using a pamphlet to discuss the tenets of the Alcoholics Anonymous program with patients
   f. Reinforcing the mental benefits of gaining self-control over a substance use disorder
5. A nurse is preparing a teaching plan for a patient with asthma on the use of an inhaler. What teaching method is most appropriate for this patient?
   a. Demonstration
   b. Lecture
   c. Discovery
   d. Panel session
6. The nurse has taught a patient with diabetes how to administer subcutaneous insulin injections. Which is the best strategy to evaluate if the teaching goal has been met?
   a. Ask the patient the insulin dose and times of day they will administer insulin.
   b. Observe the patient's technique in drawing up and administering insulin.
   c. Have the patient explain the skill they have just learned.
   d. Document the teaching session in the patient's electronic health record.
7. A registered nurse acts as nurse coach to provide teaching to patients who are recovering from a stroke. Which statement directs the nurse in performing this role?
   a. The nurse uses discovery to identify the patients' personal goals and create a plan that will result in change.
   b. The nurse is the expert in providing teaching and education strategies to provide dietary and activity modifications.
   c. The nurse becomes a mentor to the patients and encourages them to create their own fitness programs.
   d. The nurse assumes an authoritative role to design the structure of the coaching session and support the achievement of patient goals.

8. A nurse on the rehabilitation unit is counseling a young adult athlete who sustained a traumatic below-the-knee amputation following a motorcycle accident. The patient refuses to eat or ambulate, stating, "What's the point? My life is over. I'll never be the football player I dreamed of becoming." What is the nurse counselor's best response?
   a. "You're young and have your whole life ahead of you. You should focus on your rehabilitation and make something of your life."
   b. "I understand how you must feel. I wanted to be a famous singer, but I wasn't born with the talent to be successful at it."
   c. "You should concentrate on other sports that you could play even with prosthesis."
   d. "I understand this is difficult for you. Would you like to talk about it now or would you prefer me to make a referral to someone else?"
9. A nurse is caring for a patient who is admitted to the hospital with traumatic injuries sustained in a motor vehicle accident. While hospitalized, the patient's spouse tells the patient that their house flooded, damaging their belongings. When the nurse notes that the patient is visibly upset by this news, the nurse suggests which type of counseling?
   a. Long-term developmental
   b. Short-term situational
   c. Short-term motivational
   d. Long-term motivational
10. A nurse develops a contractual agreement with a morbidly obese patient to achieve optimal weight goals. Which statement best describes the nature of this agreement?
    a. "This agreement forms a legal bond between the two of us to achieve your weight goals."
    b. "This agreement will motivate the two of us to do what is necessary to meet your weight goals."
    c. "This agreement will help us determine what learning outcomes are necessary to achieve your weight goals."
    d. "This agreement will limit the scope of the teaching session and make stated weight goals more attainable."
11. A nurse in the diabetes clinic initiates education for a patient with a new diagnosis of diabetes. The nurse notes the patient has completed 2 years of college. What action does the nurse select for the initial teaching session?
    a. Providing the patient with handouts related to blood-glucose management
    b. Demonstrating the use of the blood-glucose monitor and tool to record blood-glucose readings
    c. Assessing the patient's knowledge of diabetes and their ability to interpret the health information
    d. Explaining the dietary restrictions including foods that are prohibited
12. The nurse coach at a cardiac rehabilitation office is meeting with a patient who has learned they have heart failure. Which nursing actions might the nurse coach include in coaching sessions for this patient? (Select all that apply.)
    a. Provide education based on the patient's personal goals.
    b. Explore the patient's readiness for change.
    c. Assist the patient to determine progress toward goals.
    d. Direct the patient to exercise daily.
    e. Identify goals for the patient.

ANSWERS WITH RATIONALES

1. **b.** Teaching first aid is a function of the goal to prevent illness. Promoting health involves helping patients to value health and develop specific health practices that promote and maintain wellness. Restoring health occurs once a patient is ill, and teaching focuses on developing self-care practices that promote recovery. When facilitating coping, nurses help patients come to terms with whatever lifestyle modification is needed for their recovery or to enable them to cope with permanent health alterations.

2. **c, d, e.** Successful teaching plans for older adults incorporate extra time, short teaching sessions, accommodation for sensory deficits, and reduction of environmental distractions. Older adults also benefit from instruction that relates new information to familiar activities or information. School-aged children are capable of logical reasoning and should be included in the teaching–learning process whenever possible; they are also open to new learning experiences but need learning to be reinforced by either a parent or health care provider as they become more involved with their friends and school activities. Teaching strategies designed for an adolescent patient should recognize the adolescent's need for independence, as well as the need to establish a trusting relationship that demonstrates respect for the adolescent's opinions.

3. **c.** The Teach-Back Method tool is a method of assessing literacy and confirming that the learner understands health information received from a health professional. The Ask Me 3 is a brief tool intended to promote understanding and improve communication between patients and their providers. The NVS is a reliable screening tool to assess low health literacy, developed to improve communications between patients and providers. The TEACH acronym is used to maximize the effectiveness of patient teaching by *t*uning into the patient, *e*diting patient information, *a*cting on every teaching moment, *c*larifying often, and *h*onoring the patient as a partner in the process.

4. **b, d, f.** Affective learning includes changes in attitudes, values, and feelings (e.g., the patient expresses renewed self-confidence to be able to give up drinking). Cognitive learning involves the storing and recalling of new knowledge in the brain, such as the learning that occurs during a lecture or by using a pamphlet for teaching. Learning a physical skill involving the integration of mental and muscular activity is called psychomotor learning, which may involve a return demonstration of a skill.

5. **a.** Demonstration of techniques, procedures, exercises, and the use of special equipment is an effective patient-teaching strategy for a skill. Lecture can be used to deliver information to a large group of patients but is more effective when the session is interactive; it is rarely used for individual instruction, except in combination with other strategies. Discovery is a good method for teaching problem-solving techniques and independent thinking. Panel discussions can be used to impart factual material but are also effective for sharing experiences and emotions.
6. **b.** The nurse cannot assume that the patient has actually learned the content unless there is some type of proof of learning. The key to evaluation is ensuring the learner meets the outcomes stated in the teaching plan, in this case, by demonstrating the psychomotor skill.
7. **a.** A nurse coach establishes a partnership with a patient and, using discovery, facilitates the identification of the patient's personal goals and agenda to lead to change rather than using teaching and education strategies with the nurse as the expert. A nurse coach explores the patient's readiness for coaching, designs the structure of a coaching session, supports the achievement of the patient's desired goals, and with the patient determines how to evaluate the attainment of patient goals.
8. **d.** This answer communicates respect and sensitivity to the patient's needs and offers an opportunity to discuss their feelings with the nurse or another health care professional. The other answers do not allow the patient to express their feelings and receive the counseling they need.
9. **b.** Short-term counseling might be used during a situational crisis, which occurs when a patient faces an event or situation that causes a disruption in life, such as a flood. Long-term counseling extends over a prolonged period; a patient experiencing a developmental crisis, for example, might need long-term counseling. Motivational interviewing is an evidence-based counseling approach that involves discussing feelings and incentives with the patient. A caring nurse can motivate patients to become interested in promoting their own health.
10. **b.** A contractual agreement is a pact two people make, setting out mutually agreed-on goals. Contracts are usually informal and not legally binding. When teaching a patient, such an agreement can help motivate both the patient and the teacher to do what is necessary to meet the patient's learning outcomes. The agreement notes the responsibilities of both the teacher and the learner, emphasizing the importance of the mutual commitment.
11. **c.** While the nurse takes the patient's level of education into account when providing teaching, the first step is assessing the patient's knowledge and readiness to learn. The nurse would not provide handouts or AV material without reviewing the information and assessing the patient's understanding. Discussing or demonstrating psychomotor skills, an intervention, is performed after assessment.
12. **a, b, c.** The nurse coach facilitates change or development that assists the individual to cope with health challenges. The nurse coach establishes a partnership with the patient to support the patient to identify and work toward the patient's personal agenda and goals; nurse coaches do not use teaching and other strategies directed by the nurse as an expert. A, b, and c are patient-driven, person-centered interventions to educate and empower the patient. D and e are interventions identified and directed by the nurse, not by the patient, which is not part of the coaching process.

Bibliography

Agarwal, K. S., Bhimaraj, A., Xu, J., Bionat, S., Pudlo, M., Miranda, D., Campbell, C., & Taffet, G. E. (2020). Decreasing heart failure readmissions among older patients with cognitive impairment by engaging caregivers. *Journal of Cardiovascular Nursing, 35*(3), 253–261. https://doi.org/10.1097/JCN.0000000000000670

Agency for Healthcare Research and Quality (AHRQ). (n.d.). *Implementation quick start guide. Teach-Back. The guide to improving patient safety in primary care settings by engaging patients and families.* Retrieved July 8, 2020 from https://www.ahrq.gov/sites/default/files/wysiwyg/professionals/quality-patient-safety/patient-family-engagement/pfeprimarycare/teach-back_quickstart_full.pdf

Agency for Healthcare Research and Quality (AHRQ). (2011, March). *Health literacy interventions and outcomes: an updated systematic review. Evidence report/technology assessment. Number 199.* AHRQ Publication No. 11-E006. https://www.ahrq.gov/downloads/pub/evidence/pdf/literacy/literacyup.pdf

Agency for Healthcare Research and Quality (AHRQ). (2017, December). *Teach-Back: Intervention.* https://www.ahrq.gov/patient-safety/reports/engage/interventions/teachback.html

Agency for Healthcare Research and Quality (AHRQ). (2020, March). *Health literacy universal precautions toolkit* (2nd ed.). Use the teach-back method: Tool #5. https://www.ahrq.gov/professionals/quality-patient-safety/quality-resources/tools/literacy-toolkit/healthlittoolkit2-tool5.html

American Holistic Nurses Association. (n.d.). *Coaching, health coaching & nurse coaching.* Retrieved July 8, 2020 from https://www.ahna.org/Home/Resources/Nurse-Coaching

American Psychological Association (APA). (2011). *Creativity, optimism, planning and expert information (COPE).* https://www.apa.org/pi/about/publications/caregivers/practice-settings/intervention/cope

Andrews, M., Boyle, J. S., & Collins, J. (2020). *Transcultural concepts in nursing care* (8th ed.). Wolters Kluwer.

Aronson, J. K. (2007). Compliance, concordance, adherence. *British Journal of Clinical Pharmacology, 63*(4), 383–384.

Ayaz-Alkaya, S., Terzi, H., Işik, B., & Sönmez, E. (2020). A healthy lifestyle education programme for health literacy and health-promoting behaviours: A pre-implementation and post-implementation study. *International Journal of Nursing Practice, 26*(2), e12793. https://doi.org/10.1111/ijn.12793

Bastable, S. B. (2017). *Essentials of patient education* (2nd ed.). Jones & Bartlett Learning.

Bastable, S. B. (2019). *Nurse as educator. Principles of teaching and learning for nursing practice* (5th ed.). Jones & Bartlett Learning.

Bentley, D., & Potts, J. W. (2019, July 31). *Medication adherence and compliance.* Fresenius Medical Care. https://fmcna.com/insights/education/medication-adherence-and-compliance-/

Bloom, B. S. (1956). *Taxonomy of educational objectives: The classification of educational goals.* David McKay.

Boyd, M. A. (2018). *Psychiatric nursing. Contemporary practice* (6th ed.). Wolters Kluwer.

Brangan, S., Ivanišić, M., Rafaj, G., & Rowlands, G. (2018). Health literacy of hospital patients using a linguistically validated Croationa version of the Newest Vital Sign screening test (NVS-HR). *PLoS ONE, 13*(2), e0193079. https://doi.org/10.1371/journal.pone.0193079

Bruner, J. S. (1961). The act of discovery. *Harvard Educational Review, 31*, 21–32.

Caccavale, L. J., Gokee LaRose, J., Mazzeo, S. E., & Bean, M. K. (2020). An examination of adolescents' values in a motivational interviewing-based obesity intervention. *American Journal of Health Behaviour, 44*(4), 526–533. https://doi.org/10.5993/AJHB.44.4.13

Centers for Disease Control and Prevention (CDC). (2019, October 17). *Health literacy. Older adults. Challenges.* https://www.cdc.gov/healthliteracy/developmaterials/audiences/olderadults/understanding-challenges.html

Clarke, C., Whitmore, L., & Webb, A. (2020). Patient education pictorial boards: Improving patients' understanding of venous leg ulcer and compression therapy. *Wounds UK, 16*(2), 54–60.

Dart, M. (2011). *Motivational interviewing in nursing practice. Empowering the patient.* Jones and Bartlett.

Delaney, C., Barrere, C., & Bark, L. (2020). A metaphor analysis of patients with chronic conditions experiences with holistic nurse coaching. *Holistic Nursing Practice, 34*(1), 24–34. https://doi.org/10.1097/HNP.0000000000000359

Dinh, T. T. H., Bonner, A., Clark, R., Ramsbotham, J., & Hines, S. (2016). The effectiveness of the Teach-Back Method on adherence and self-management in health education for people with chronic disease: A systematic review. *JBI Database of Systematic Reviews and Implementation Reports, 14*(1), 210–247. https://doi.org/10.11124/jbisrir-2016-2296

Duangchan, C., & Matthews, A. K. (2020). The effects of nurse-led smoking cessation interventions for patients with cancer: A systematic review. *Pacific Rim International Journal of Nursing Research, 24*(1), 118–139.

Duncan, Y. (2020). Resources for patient health literacy skills: Information in orientation and continuing professional development programs. *The Journal of Continuing Education in Nursing, 51*(4), 155–157.

Eadie, C. (2014). Health literacy: A conceptual review. *Academy of Medical-Surgical Nurses, 23*(1), 1–13.

Eliopoulos, C. (2018). *Gerontological nursing* (9th ed.). Wolters Kluwer Health.

Fraser, S. J., Brown, W. J., Whiteford, H. A., & Burton, N. W. (2018). Impact of nurse-led behavioural counselling to improve metabolic health and physical activity among adults with mental illness. *International Journal of Mental Health Nursing, 27*(2), 619–630. https://doi.org/10.1111/inm.12343

Gance-Cleveland, B. (2013). Motivational interviewing for adolescent obesity. *American Journal of Nursing, 113*(1), 11.

Gardner, C. L. (2015). Adherence: A concept analysis. *International Journal of Nursing Knowledge, 26*(2), 96–101.

Ghezeljeh, T. N., Sharifian, S., Isfahani, M. S., & Haghani, H. (2018). Comparing the effects of education using telephone follow-up and smartphone-based social networking follow-up on self-management behaviors among patients with hypertension. *Contemporary Nurse, 54*(4-5), 362–373. https://doi.org/10.1080/10376178.2018.1441730

Gutman, C. K., Cousins, L., Gritton, J., Klein, E. J., Brown, J. C., Scannell, J., & Lion, K. C. (2018). Professional interpreter use and discharge communication in the pediatric emergency department. *Academic Pediatrics, 18*(8), 935–943.

Hart, J., & Nutt, R. (2020). Improving inpatient education and follow-up in patients with heart failure: A hospital-based quality improvement project. *Nursing Economic$, 38*(2), 74–85.

Hasan, A. A., & Jaber, A. A. (2019). The effect of a family intervention on primary caregivers' psychological outcomes: Finding from the integrative literature review. *Perspectives in Psychiatric Care, 55*(2), 277–290. https://doi.org/10.1111/ppc.12339

Health Information Translations. (n.d.). *Quality health education resources for diverse populations.* Retrieved July 7, 2020 from healthinfotranslations.org

Helvaci, A., Gok Metin, Z., Ozdemir, L., & Ergun, P. (2019). The effects of a nurse-led education and counselling program on dyspnea, health status, and care dependency in patients with chronic obstructive pulmonary disease: A feasibility study. *Home Health Care Management & Practice, 31*(4), 249–256. https://doi.org/10.1177/1084822319850819

Hess, D., Dossey, B., Southard, M., Luck, S., Gulino-Schaub, B., & Bark, L. (2013). *The art and science of nurse coaching: The provider's guide to coaching scope and competencies.* American Nurses Association.

Holli, B. B., & Beto, J. A. (2018). *Nutrition counseling and education skills. A guide for professionals* (7th ed.). Wolters Kluwer.

Houts, P. S., Nezu, A. M., Nezu, C. M., & Bucher, J. A. (1996). The prepared family caregiver: A problem-solving approach to family caregiver education. *Patient Education & Counseling, 27*(1), 63–73.

Hudson, S., Rikard, R. V., Staiculescu, I., & Edison, K. (2018). Appendix C. Improving health and the bottom line: The case for health literacy. In *National Academies of Sciences, Engineering, and Medicine; Health and Medicine Division; Board on Population Health and Public Health Practice; Roundtable on Health Literacy. Building the case for health literacy: Proceedings of a workshop.* National Academies Press (US). https://www.ncbi.nlm.nih.gov/books/NBK518850/

Hugtenburg, J. G., Timmers, L., Elders, P. J. M., Vervloet, M., & van Dijk, L. (2013). Definitions, variants, and causes of nonadherence with medication: A challenge for tailored interventions. *Patient Preference and Adherence, 7*, 675–682.

Hurlow, J., & Hensley, L. (2015). Achieving patient adherence in the wound care clinic. *Today's Wound Clinic, 9*(9).

Institute for Healthcare Improvement (IHI). (n.d.). *Ask Me 3®: Good questions for your good health.* Retrieved July 10, 2020 from http://www.ihi.org/resources/Pages/Tools/Ask-Me-3-Good-Questions-for-Your-Good-Health.aspx

Institute of Medicine (IOM). (2001). *Crossing the quality chasm: A new health system for the 21st century.* National Academies Press.

Institute of Medicine (IOM). (2011). *The future of nursing: Leading change, advancing health.* National Academies Press. https://www.nap.edu/read/12956/chapter/1

Institute of Medicine (IOM). Committee on the Learning Health Care System in America. (2013). Chapter 7: Engaging patients, families, and communities. In M. Smith, R. Saunders, L. Stuckhardt, & J. M. McGinnis (Eds.), *Best care at lower cost: The path to continuously learning health care in America.* National Academies Press. https://www.ncbi.nlm.nih.gov/books/NBK207234

International Council of Nurses (ICN). (2019). *Nursing diagnosis and outcome statements.* https://www.icn.ch/sites/default/files/inline-files/ICNP2019-DC.pdf

The Joint Commission. (2011, February 9). *R³Report Issue 1: Patient-centered communication.* https://www.jointcommission.org/standards/r3-report/r3-report-issue-1—patient-centered-communication/

The Joint Commission. (2020). *National patient safety goals.* https://www.jointcommission.org/standards/national-patient-safety-goals/

The Joint Commission. (n.d.a). *Speak Up Campaigns.* Retrieved August 1, 2020 from https://www.jointcommission.org/en/resources/for-consumers/speak-up-campaigns/

The Joint Commission. (n.d.b). *Facts about Speak Up™.* Retrieved August 2, 2020 from https://www.jointcommission.org/resources/for-consumers/speak-up-campaigns/facts-about-speak-up/

Keener, K. A., & Winokur, E. J. (2018). Digitally recorded education. Effects on anxiety and knowledge recall in patients receiving first-time chemotherapy. *Clinical Journal of Oncology Nursing, 22*(4), 444–449. https://doi.org/10.1188/18.CJON.444-449

Kim, S., Song, Y., Park, J., & Utz, S. (2020). Patients' experiences of diabetes self-management education according to health-literacy levels. *Clinical Nursing Research, 29*(5), 285–292. https://doi.org/10.1177/1054773819865879

Knowles, M. S. (1990). *The adult learner: A neglected species* (4th ed.). Gulf Publishing.

Lee, J., Choi, M., Yoo, Y., Ahn, S., Jeon, J. Y., Kim, J. Y., & Byun, J. Y. (2019). Impacts of an exercise program and motivational telephone counselling on health-related quality of life in people with Parkinson's disease. *Rehabilitation Nursing, 44*(3), 161–170. https://doi.org/10.1097/rnj.0000000000000106

Lowenstein, A. J., Foord-May, L., & Romano, J. C. (2009). *Teaching strategies for health education and health promotion. Working with patients, families, and communities.* Jones and Bartlett.

Makiling, M., & Smart, H. (2020). Patient-centered health education intervention to empower preventive diabetic foot self-care. *Advances in Skin & Wound Care, 33*(7), 360–365. https://doi.org/10.1097/01.ASW.0000666896.46860.d7

Mantwill, S., & Diviani, N. (2019). Health literacy and health disparities: A global perspective. In O. Okan, U. Bauer, D. Levin-Zamir, P. Pinheiro, & K. Sørensen (Eds.), *International handbook of health literacy. Research, practice and policy across the lifespan* (pp. 139–152). Policy Press. https://library.oapen.org/handle/20.500.12657/24879

Mathew, S., & Thukha, H. (2018). Pilot testing of the effectiveness of nurse-guided, patient-centered heart failure education for older adults. *Geriatric Nursing, 39*(4), 376–381. https://doi.org/10.1016/j.gerinurse.2017.11.006

McDonall, J., Hutchinson, A. F., Redley, B., Livingston, P. M., & Botti, M. (2019). Usability and feasibility of multimedia interventions for engaging patients in their care in the context of acute recovery: A narrative review. *Health Expectations, 22*(6), 1187–1198. https://doi.org/10.1111/hex.12957

Miller, W. R., & Rollnick, S. (2013). *Motivational interviewing: Helping people change* (3rd ed.). The Guilford Press.

Morgan, K. I., & Townsend, M. C. (2021). *Psychiatric mental health nursing.* (10th ed.). F. A. Davis Company.

National Alliance for Caregiving (NAC) and American Association of Retired Persons (AARP). (2020). *Caregiving in the U.S.* https://www.aarp.org/content/dam/aarp/ppi/2020/05/full-report-caregiving-in-the-united-states.doi.10.26419-2Fppi.00103.001.pdf

National Cancer Institute. (n.d.). *Smokefree.gov.* U. S. Department of Health and Human Services. Retrieved July 9, 2020 from https://smokefree.gov/

National Center for Education Statistics. (n.d.). *National Assessment of Adult Literacy (NAAL).* Retrieved July 20, 2020 from https://nces.ed.gov/naal/index.asp

National Heart, Lung, and Blood Institute. (2011, January). *Heart attack: Know the symptoms. Take action.* U.S. Department of Health and Human Services. https://www.nhlbi.nih.gov/files/docs/public/heart/heart_attack_fs_en.pdf

National Institute of Child Health and Human Development. (2017, January 31). *Breastfeeding and breast milk.* National Institute of Health. https://www.nichd.nih.gov/health/topics/breastfeeding

National Library of Medicine. (2018, September 25). *Breastfeeding-skin and nipple changes.* Medline Plus. https://medlineplus.gov/ency/patientinstructions/000632.htm

Network of the National Library of Medicine (NNLM). (n.d.a). *Health literacy.* National Library of Medicine. National Institute of Health. Retrieved July 20, 2020 from https://nnlm.gov/initiatives/topics/health-literacy

Network of the National Library of Medicine (NNLM). (n.d.b). *Clinical conversations training program. Health literacy.* National Library of Medicine. National Institute of Health. Retrieved July 20, 2020 from https://nnlm.gov/mar/guides/clinical-conversations-training-program/health-literacy

Nickles, D., Dolansky, M., Marek, J., & Burke, K. (2020). Nursing students use of Teach-Back to improve patients' knowledge and satisfaction: A quality improvement project. *Journal of Professional Nursing, 36*(2), 70–76.

Office of Disease Prevention and Health Promotion (ODPHP). (n.d). *Health communication and health information technology.* Retrieved July 10, 2020 from https://www.healthypeople.gov/2020/topics-objectives/topic/health-communication-and-health-information-technologyhttps://www.healthypeople.gov/2020/topics-objectives/topic/health-communication-and-health-information-technology

Office of Disease Prevention and Health Promotion (ODPHP). (2020a). *HealthyPeople 2030.* U.S. Department of Health and Human Services. https://health.gov/healthypeople

Office of Disease Prevention and Health Promotion (ODPHP). (2020b). *Social determinants of health.* U.S. Department of Health and Human Services. https://www.healthypeople.gov/2020/topics-objectives/topic/social-determinants-of-health

Okan, O. (2019). From Saranac Lake to Shanghai: A brief history of health literacy. In O. Okan, U. Bauer, D. Levin-Zamir, P. Pinheiro, & K. Sørensen (Eds.), *International handbook of health literacy. Research, practice and policy across the lifespan* (pp. 21–38). Policy Press. https://library.oapen.org/handle/20.500.12657/24879

Patient Safety Network (PSNet). (2019, September). *Health literacy.* Agency for Healthcare Research and Quality (AHRQ). https://psnet.ahrq.gov/primer/health-literacy

Peplau, H. E. (1991). *Interpersonal relations in nursing.* Springer.

Pfizer Inc. (n.d.). *Health literacy. Public policy researchers. The Newest Vital Sign (NVS).* Retrieved July 10, 2020 from https://www.pfizer.com/health/literacy/public-policy-researchers/nvs-toolkit

Powers, B. J., Trinh, J. V., & Bosworth, H. B. (2010). Can this patient read and understand written health information? *Journal of the American Medical Association, 304*(1), 76–84.

Prochnow, J. A., Meiers, S. J., & Scheckel, M. M. (2019). Improving patient and caregiver new medication education using an innovative Teach-Back toolkit. *Journal of Nursing Care Quality, 34*(2), 101–106. https://doi.org/10.1097/NCQ.0000000000000342

Richardson Ingram, R., & Kautz, D. D. (2018). Creating 'Win-Win' outcomes for patients with low health literacy: A nursing case study. *MEDSURG Nursing, 27*(2), 132–134.
Richie, D. (2016). *What is the difference between adherence versus compliance in patient behavior? Podiatry Today*. http://www.podiatrytoday.com/blogged/what-difference-between-adherence-versus-compliance-patient-behavior
Robert Wood Johnson Foundation. (2011, October 13). *Health literacy: Reducing the burden of a complex healthcare system*. http://www.rwjf.org/en/culture-of-health/2011/10/health-literacy-reducing-the-burden-of-a-complex-healthcare-system.html
Rosenstock, I. (1974). Historical origins of the health belief model. *Health Education Monographs, 2*(4), 328–335.
Ryan-Madonna, M., Lauder, B., & Levin, R. F. (2019). Effectiveness of the Teach-Back Method for improving caregivers' confidence in caring for hospice patients and decreasing hospitalizations. *Journal of Hospice & Palliative Nursing, 21*(1), 61–70. https://doi.org/10.1097/NJH.0000000000000492
Schaffler, J. L., Tremblay, S., Laizner, A. M., & Lambert, S. (2019). Developing education materials for caregivers of culturally and linguistically diverse patients: Insights from a qualitative analysis of caregivers' needs, access and understanding of information. *Health Expectations, 22*(3), 444–456. https://doi.org/10.1111/hex.12867
Scott, S. A. (2016). Health literacy education in baccalaureate nursing programs in the United States. *Nursing Education Perspectives, 37*(3), 153–158.
Shustack, L. (2019). Going digital with patient teaching. *Nursing, 49*(1), 65–66. https://doi.org/10.1097/01.NURSE.0000549742.35131.e4
Tay, L. H., Ong, A.K. W., & Lang, D. S. P. (2018). Experiences of adult cancer patients receiving counselling from nurses: A qualitative systematic review. *JBI Database Systematic Review Implement Report, 16*(10), 1965–2012. https://doi.org/10.11124/JBISRIR-2017-003606
Thompson Bastin, M. L., Short, G. T., Cook, A. M., Rust, K., & Flannery, A. H. (2019). Patients' and care providers' perceptions of television-based education in the intensive care unit. *American Journal of Critical Care, 28*(4), 307–315. https://doi.org/10.4037/ajcc2019156
U.S. Department of Health and Human Services (USDHHS). Office of Disease Prevention and Health Promotion. (2010). *Health literacy. National action plan to improve health literacy*. https://health.gov/our-work/health-literacy/national-action-plan-improve-health-literacy
U.S. Department of Health and Human Services (USDHHS). (2019, October 23). *About the Affordable Care Act*. https://www.hhs.gov/healthcare/about-the-aca/index.html
U.S. Department of Health and Human Services (USDHHS). Office of Disease Prevention and Health Promotion. (n.d.). *Health literacy*. Retrieved July 1, 2020 from https://health.gov/our-work/health-literacy
U.S. National Library of Medicine. (2020, July 10). *MedlinePlus. Health information in multiple languages*. https://medlineplus.gov/languages/languages.html
U.S. National Library of Medicine. (n.d.). *HealthReach. Health information in many languages*. Retrieved July 15, 2020 from https://healthreach.nlm.nih.gov/
Watson, J. (2008). *Nursing: The philosophy and science of caring* (Revised edition). University Press of Colorado.
Winokur, E. J., Rutledge, D. N., & McGowan, J. J. (2019). A picture is worth a thousand words: Pictographs to improve understanding of discharge instructions. *Journal of Emergency Nursing, 45*(5), 531–537. https://doi.org/10.1016/j.jen.2019.01.007
Wittenberg, E., Ferrell, B., Kanter, E., & Buller, H. (2018). Health literacy. Exploring nursing challenges to providing support and understanding. *Clinical Journal of Oncology Nursing, 22*(1), 53–61. https://doi.org/10.1188/18.CJON.53-61
Wolters Kluwer. (2022). Problem-based care plans. In *Lippincott Advisor*. Wolters Kluwer.

10 Leading, Managing, and Delegating

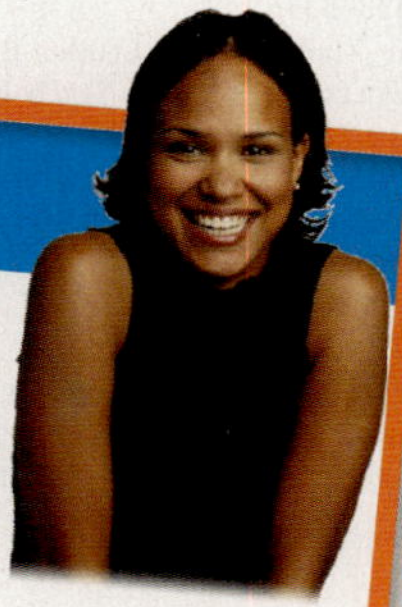

Rehema Kohls

Rehema is a college sophomore who comes to the health care center requesting information about sexually transmitted infections (STIs). During the visit, she says, "So many of my friends are concerned about STIs. They all say we should start a group on campus to discuss this problem, and they want me to set it up and be the leader. But I wouldn't know where to start or what to do!"

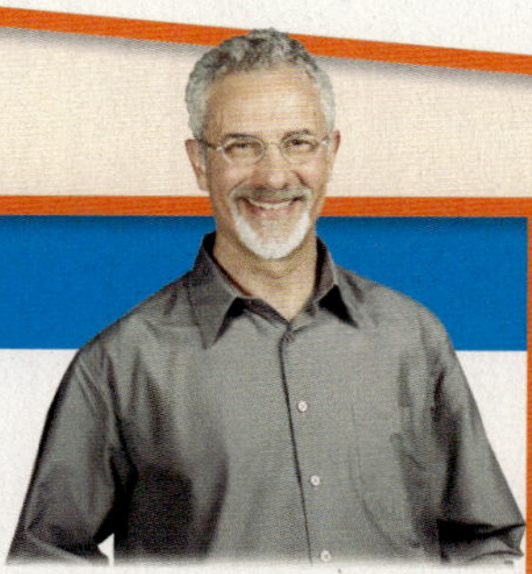

Stephen Wall

Stephen, a 65-year-old widower who lives alone, is admitted to the intensive care unit after an automobile accident in which he sustained trauma to the head, chest, abdomen, and lower extremities. He is being monitored continuously via numerous invasive devices and requires complex care. His closest family member, a 40-year-old son, lives approximately 75 miles away.

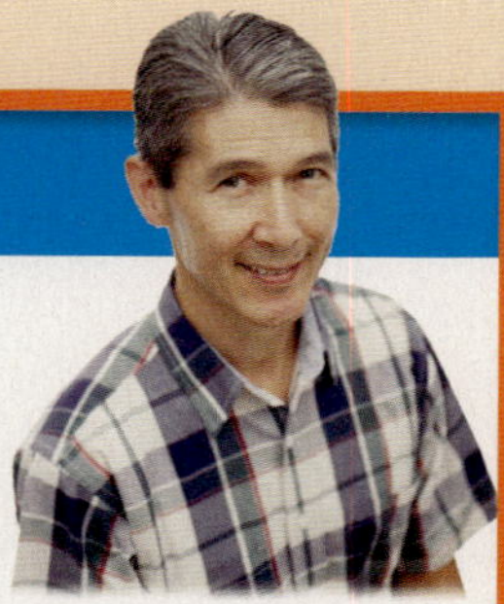

Jack Camp

Jack, a middle-aged single man with a history of diabetes mellitus, is receiving care for a compound fracture of his left lower extremity being treated with an external fixator. His adherence to his diabetic therapy regimen is questionable; he states, "I really love my sweets!" The patient frequently voices loud complaints about his room, the food, and the hospital routine. He also uses his call light very frequently, stating, "I just want to see if it's working and if the nurses will come check on me."

Learning Outcomes

After completing the chapter, you will be able to accomplish the following:

1. Identify the qualities, four skills, and differing styles of leaders.
2. List the five managerial functions.
3. Discuss the difference between leadership and management.
4. Discuss the significance of Magnet recognition for a health care organization.
5. Summarize the steps in the process of change.
6. Describe areas in which beginning nurses can develop leadership skills.
7. Recognize the responsibilities associated with the delegation of nursing care.
8. Describe the role of a mentor.

Nursing Concepts

- Leadership and management

Today's health care providers are experiencing challenges such as fiscal constraints, workforce shortages, increased sophistication of health care consumers, and technologic and pharmacologic advances. Never before has there been such a need for nurses to work competently and collaboratively with other health care professionals to deliver accessible, cost-effective, high-quality health care to all. Although nurses may assume leadership roles by virtue of their positions, they only become effective leaders over time by understanding the complexities of coordinating care, remaining open to differing points of view, and understanding the interdependency of the entire health care team (see Chapter 12 for more on Interprofessional Collaboration and the Reflective Practice box on page 244).

Leadership and management are intertwined, but leadership roles differ from management tasks or functions. In *The Seven Habits of Highly Effective People,* Covey (1999) clarified the difference, citing a quote from Peter Drucker: "Management is doing things right; leadership is doing the right things." This suggests that leadership involves philosophy, perception, and judgment, whereas management tasks are the core of the management role (Stachowiak & Bugel, 2013). A supportive leader uses strategies that facilitate the delivery of safe, high-quality patient care in a positive environment.

Now, more than ever, it is important for nursing as a profession to be self-directed as it charts its future. The American Nurses Association (ANA) recommends recognition and reimbursement for the role that nurses play in providing effective **care coordination**. This core competency for registered nurses (RNs) has a positive impact on patient outcomes and the quality of care and reduces health care costs through more efficient use of resources. Then ANA president, Cipriano (2017), reflecting on the challenging political situation in the United States, suggested that we nurses will persevere by keeping our values, principles, and ethical practice at the forefront; staying true to our mission; and being strong advocates. "I have confidence in our moral compass and ANA's vision and new strategic plan to strengthen our profession, our voice, and our ability to advocate for all health care consumers as well as the 3.6 [now 3.9] million nurses who rely on us in this, and in any, time of change" (www.nursingworld.com).

LEADERSHIP

The concept of leadership is one of the most researched, studied, and debated fields of inquiry. **Leadership** has been described as the ability to direct or motivate a person or group to achieve set goals. Effective leaders in groups or systems do this by encouraging others to be their best selves as they work collaboratively in the pursuit of common organizational or unit goals. Brene Brown states that a leader is anyone who takes responsibility for finding the potential in people and processes and who has the courage to develop that potential. "Leadership is not about titles or the corner office. It's about the willingness to step up, put yourself out there, and lean into courage. The world is desperate for braver leaders. It's time for all of us to step up" (https://daretolead.brenebrown.com/).

Leaders have power, whether explicit or implied. For example, elected class leaders have **explicit power** by virtue of their position. However, students in the class with no designated leadership position may, by force of their personality, have more power to influence the class than designated leaders; this is **implied power**.

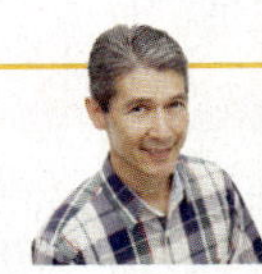

Consider **Jack Camp**, the patient described in the Reflective Practice scenario. The patient assumed a position of "running things in his business," thus having the explicit power of his position. In addition, the patient used "implied power" while hospitalized to exert control over his situation. The nurse's understanding of power would be important in developing a plan to deal with the patient's behavior.

Power to influence a group depends on the person's leadership style and how the person fulfills leadership responsibilities. The dynamics of leadership involve applying that power for personal or organizational growth or change. Nurses who use leadership skills can become proficient in effecting desired changes in many areas, including their patients' health patterns, the health care facility, the community, the nursing profession, and the health care system in general.

Leadership Qualities

Most people admire a charismatic, dynamic, enthusiastic, visionary leader who is poised, confident, and self-directed. When you read these characteristics, who comes to your

QSEN Reflective Practice: Cultivating QSEN Competencies

CHALLENGE TO ETHICAL AND LEGAL SKILLS

While in a clinical rotation in my junior year, I was assigned the dreaded Jack Camp (I still remember his name). He was a middle-aged single man receiving care for a compound fracture of his left lower extremity being treated with an external fixator. He had a bad case of diabetes, and an even worse sweet tooth. Before I even met him, the nurses on the floor were saying things like "good luck," which made this junior nursing student extra paranoid (although I was grateful for the warning). The patient was known for voicing loud complaints about his room, the food, and the hospital routine. He also was using his call light very frequently. The nurses called him names and discussed their dislike of him in the nurses' station, which was in the center of the unit.

As the day progressed, I found out that all this patient wanted was some attention, because he was used to running things in his business. I actually found him entertaining.

Thinking Outside the Box: Possible Courses of Action

- Ignore the comments of the other nurses on the floor, hoping that no one else hears them.
- Report the nurses to my clinical instructor, possibly causing tension on the floor.
- Politely tell the nurses to keep it down and refrain from talking about the patient, risking my own comfort level; after all, I am only a visiting student—what do I know?

Evaluating a Good Outcome: How Do I Define Success?

- Act as a patient advocate despite my limited power, which means correcting unethical behaviors as cordially as possible.
- Have the courage to go to the next level if the nurses' behavior is not corrected.
- Inform the patient politely to modify his behavior.

Personal Learning: Here's to the Future!

My response was to ignore the nurses' comments and hope no one else heard them either. I was not courageous enough to be the patient advocate that we had been taught to be. I knew my response should have been to ask them to keep it down, which would allow them to maintain their personal opinions while at the same time keeping the comments from jeopardizing patient confidentiality. From this experience, I learned that you have to be a leader, speak up, and take the risk. Part of that means being able to go against the group, risking being ostracized. In doing so, others may follow your lead, but if they choose not to follow, at least you know you advocated for your patient. Since this experience, I have not been in a situation that has challenged my personal ethics, but I have the self-confidence to believe that I can be the leader that I spoke so passionately about.

Kim Gray, Georgetown University

QSEN SELF-REFLECTION ON QUALITY AND SAFETY COMPETENCIES DEVELOPING KNOWLEDGE, SKILLS, AND ATTITUDES FOR CONTINUOUS IMPROVEMENT

How do you think you would respond in a similar situation? Why? What does this tell you about yourself and about the adequacy of your skills for professional practice? What *knowledge, skills,* and attitudes do you need to develop to continuously improve quality and safety in a situation like the one experienced by this student nurse?

Patient-Centered Care: How could the nursing student initiate improved communication between Mr. Camp and the nurses working on his unit? Did her handling of this situation facilitate her ability to advocate for patients in similar situations? Would it be helpful to elicit Mr. Camp's preferences and expressed needs and ensure that they are included as part of the care plan?

Teamwork and Collaboration/Quality Improvement: How do you think the nursing staff would have reacted had the nursing student approached them regarding their comments about Mr. Camp? Can you think of other ways to respond? Describe a plan the nursing student could use to go about changing the staff's behavior. Which type of leadership style might have been most effective with this group?

Safety/Evidence-Based Practice: Is there anything more the nursing student could have done to contribute to a safe patient care environment, confront her fears, and promote a positive outcome in this situation? What evidence in nursing literature provides guidance for the leadership qualities necessary to enlist support and cooperation with the nursing staff in this environment?

Informatics: What information should be included in the patient handoff at the close of the student nurse's shift? Can you identify the essential information that must be available in Mr. Camp's electronic record to support safe patient care, coordination of care, and communication with staff?

mind? Not everyone can be as dynamic and inspirational as such individuals, yet leaders do need to be comfortable with themselves (i.e., have a positive self-image) and present themselves as role models for followers. Ideally, they also have a vision that energizes the group and brings forth the best efforts of members. Critical thinkers and responsible decision makers commit high energy to achieving goals and are skilled in enlisting support and cooperation.

Leaders value learning and must be knowledgeable. Contemporary nurse managers draw upon their own staff for clinical and organizational knowledge. Understanding the culture in your practice environment is necessary to be successful. Flexibility is a must for all nursing leaders. All nursing functions and roles require flexibility. The needs of patients, families, and the nursing team can change from minute to minute. For example, a nurse coordinator may plan to involve staff in a discussion about how best to distribute new work responsibilities, but if there are three unexpected new admissions to the unit, the discussion may need to be postponed to a quieter time.

Leadership potential is present in all nurses. With education and practice, these qualities can be developed to the point at which a nurse is skilled in the many behaviors necessary for leadership. In 2021, the ANA in *Nursing: Scope and Standards of Nursing Practice,* 4th edition, defined specific professional performance guidelines for leadership. Be sure to become familiar with the leadership competencies expected of all registered nurses. Professional nurses are accountable for these standards.

Box 10-1 offers a checklist with numerous suggestions for how you might approach the challenge of becoming a

Box 10-1 Checklist for the Beginning Nurse Who Wishes to Develop Leadership Skills

Basic Attitudes and Skills

Read the statements on the right and circle the appropriate response: (1) rarely characterizes me, (2) sometimes characterizes me, and (3) often characterizes me. Then choose the behaviors and activities you would like to develop as you prepare to assume nurse leadership roles.

1	2	3	1. I am self-directed. I know what I want and take the necessary steps to get it.
1	2	3	2. I know my strengths and limitations and feel confident with who I am and who I am becoming.
1	2	3	3. I get an idea ("vision") and energize others to help me "make it happen."
1	2	3	4. I coordinate or direct the activities of others, matching their abilities to the necessary task
1	2	3	5. I think critically about a situation without letting my feelings or those of others bias my analysis
1	2	3	6. Once I have identified a problem, I work at it until I resolve it—to the extent that this is within my power.
1	2	3	7. When I need help, I know where to find it and ask for it.
1	2	3	8. I recognize and encourage the talents of others and offer sincere compliments.
1	2	3	9. I accept responsibility for my decisions and behavior.
1	2	3	10. I accept compliments and enjoy my success.
1	2	3	11. I confront individuals who are abusing my rights or those of others in my group.
1	2	3	12. I use assertiveness techniques when defending rights.
1	2	3	13. I am flexible and can change direction once I see the value of another course of action.
1	2	3	14. I follow an appropriate chain of command when problem solving.
1	2	3	15. I question how nursing interventions might be improved.

The higher your score the better. Reread the statements where you checked "1" and see how you might plan to improve in these areas.

Beginning Execution of Leadership Role Responsibilities

Read the list of behaviors on the right and check the appropriate box met or not met.

Met	Not Met	
☐	☐	1. Recognize some personal need you have been ignoring and take steps to ensure that it is met.
☐	☐	2. Think of some group you belong to (e.g., school, work, church, or social) whose members' needs are not being met, and plan with other members to tackle the problem.
☐	☐	3. Recognize the special advocacy needs of a patient you believe is being underserved by the health care system. Become an advocate for this patient.
☐	☐	4. Find a nursing research study that recommends a specific type of care for one of your patients. Implement the recommendation and compare your findings with those of the researchers. Work collaboratively with the interdisciplinary team to implement needed changes.
☐	☐	5. Join a professional nursing organization and become an active member; Play a leadership role in your student nursing organization or other college association or group.
☐	☐	6. Analyze the media's portrayal of nurses in a specific television program, film, or book. Talk with a friend about how this portrayal of nursing influences your profession. Share your comments with the producer or author.
☐	☐	7. Contact your legislator to share your views about pending legislation. See Chapter 7.
☐	☐	8. Think about leaders you admire and respect; interview current nursing leaders; develop a plan for personal professional growth and development.
☐	☐	9. Develop a mentoring relationship with a nursing leader.

nurse leader. You can monitor your progress by periodically reviewing the checklist.

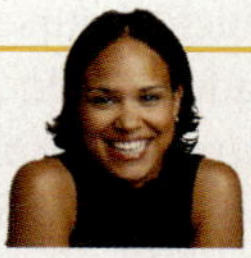

Recall **Rehema Kohls**, the college sophomore considering starting a campus group on STIs. The nurse would apply knowledge of leadership qualities when helping Rehema to decide about leading the group. In addition, the nurse would demonstrate these qualities when interacting with Rehema.

Personal Leadership Skills

Nurses recognize key qualities that are vital for a successful leader. The following list includes basic skills needed for nursing leadership and is not meant to be all inclusive, but instead to serve as a basis for development (Sherman, 2012b):

- Commitment to excellence
- Problem-solving skills, including a clear vision and strategic focus, that allow movement forward toward a creative solution (see the Nursing Advocacy in Action display)
- Commitment to and passion for your work
- Trustworthiness and integrity
- Respectfulness
- Accessibility
- Empathy and caring
- Desire to be of service
- Responsibility to enhance the personal growth of all staff

The ability to know yourself is the cornerstone of success in either implicit or explicit leadership roles. In a *Harvard Business Review* article, Drucker (1999), a scholar of leadership, wrote that to be successful in our current knowledge culture (of which nursing is a part), one must possess self-knowledge. With self-knowledge, we can place ourselves in positions in which we can make the greatest contribution. In terms of nursing leadership roles, this translates into formal authority of position, such as a unit coordinator or director, or a clinical leader without a formal title (Box 10-2).

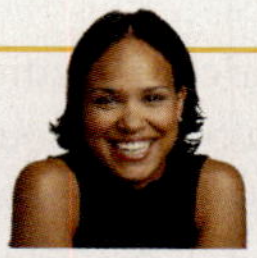

Think back to **Rehema Kohls**, the college sophomore who is thinking about starting a campus discussion group on STIs. The nurse would incorporate knowledge of Drucker's identified need for self-knowledge and personal inquiries when helping Rehema decide about starting and leading the group.

Emotional Intelligence

Goleman (2005) defines **emotional intelligence** in its simplest terms as the ability or skill to be intelligent about emotions, our own and those of others. If you want to be successful as a leader, you will want to reflect on your ability to use your emotional intelligence to help yourself and others achieve valued goals. As you read about the four attributes below, use your self-assessment skills to determine which you can claim as strengths and which need more work.

1. **Self-management:** You're able to control impulsive feelings and behaviors, manage your emotions in healthy ways, take initiative, follow through on commitments, and adapt to changing circumstances.
2. **Self-awareness:** You recognize your own emotions and how they affect your thoughts and behavior. You know your strengths and weaknesses and have self-confidence.
3. **Social awareness**: You have empathy. You can understand the emotions, needs, and concerns of other people; pick up on emotional cues; feel comfortable socially; and recognize the power dynamics in a group or organization.
4. **Relationship management:** You know how to develop and maintain good relationships, communicate clearly, inspire and influence others, work well in a team, and manage conflict.

Leadership Styles

Many different styles of leadership are present in contemporary health care settings. The complexity and persistent, rapid change in health care drive many of the leadership styles that you will observe. It is helpful to think of leadership as a behavior, as something one person does to influence another. This influence takes many forms and requires much creativity, intellect, and savvy. Different styles are

Box 10-2 Personal Inquiries for Determining Complementary Leadership Roles and Working Environments

- **Identify your strengths:** Continually improve the things you do best. Discover your "intellectual arrogance" (being bright is no substitute for knowledge). Work on acquiring the skills and knowledge you need to fully realize your strengths. Remedy your bad habits.
- **Evaluate how you accomplish work:** We all work in ways that yield the best results for us. Are you a visual or auditory learner? Do you learn best by reading or writing? Do you work more productively in teams or alone? Are you more productive as a decision maker or as an advisor?
- **Clarify your values:** Working in an organization or on a unit whose value system is unacceptable or incompatible with yours will lead to frustration and poor performance. Identify your values and seek a work environment that is complementary, not adversarial.
- **Determine where you belong and what you can contribute:** In small or large organizations, as a decision maker or as an advisor, prepare for opportunities that emerge in response to these queries. In this dynamic industry, set reasonable short- to medium-range goals.
- **Assume responsibility for relationships:** Cultivate relationships and analyze the differences you may have with others. Know and understand the strengths, performance modes, and values of your coworkers and managers.

Nursing Advocacy in Action

Patient Scenario

Everybody loves Sarah. Mature for her 9 years, Sarah has advanced leukemia, and her only medical hope now is to transfer to a hospital 3,000 miles from home that has the bone marrow that she needs. There are, however, several problems.

1. Sarah's family is homeless and visits rarely. She makes excuses for them—saying how hard it is to be on the street and always trying to find shelter—but she couldn't hide her disappointment when no one visited on Christmas and her birthday. You have met the parents and were struck by their immaturity.
2. Sarah's health care provider is working passionately to get Sarah to the transplant center; the latest hurdle is ensuring that they will accept her given the fact that the family has no insurance or finances.
3. Many of Sarah's professional caregivers aren't sure that the bone marrow transplant is a good idea. It is doubtful the funds would be found to send any of her family with her, and the possibility exists that, if unsuccessful, she could die at the transplant center surrounded by strangers.

You mention these concerns to Sarah's doctor, who replies, "But this is her only hope for cure!"

Implications for Nursing Advocacy

How will you respond if you are Sarah's nurse? Talk with your classmates and experienced nurses about the questions that follow.

- If you elect to advocate for Sarah, what practical steps can you take to ensure better health outcomes?
- What is it reasonable to expect of a student nurse, a graduate nurse, and an experienced nurse in this situation?
- What advocacy skills are needed to effectively respond to this challenge?

applicable in different contexts and with different levels of employees. Some of these styles are explained in the next section. New graduates should carefully choose organizations that match their preferred leadership style.

Autocratic Leadership

Autocratic leadership, also called directive leadership or authoritarian leadership, involves the leader assuming control over the decisions and activities of the group. It is often an efficient process, yet many people may resent this leadership approach when it is used regularly. Staff and team members have limited opportunity to contribute suggestions and participate in organizational decisions. High staff turnover and burnout are more common with this style of leadership.

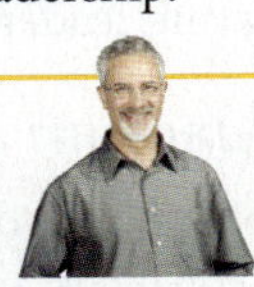

Consider **Stephen Wall**, the 65-year-old patient in the intensive care unit. The nurse would demonstrate autocratic leadership to perform specific care activities and to delegate responsibilities to appropriate personnel.

Many experienced nurses are used to working under autocratic leaders because this approach was used in most hospitals in earlier years. It may have evolved from nursing's historical military and religious past, or from the industrial model of command and control prevalent in many organizations. Although some health care workers still respond best to the directive approach, this style of leadership is gradually being replaced by the democratic style of leadership as nurses demand and receive more say in decision making.

Some situations may require an autocratic leadership style. For example, Nurse A discovers that one of her patients is bleeding excessively from his surgical incision. She knows that he needs immediate attention, so she gives specific orders to another team member to attend to the other patients. She tells the RN on her team to call the surgical resident to come as soon as possible. She implements a nursing care plan to prevent further blood loss or complications. Nurse A assumed the autocratic style of leadership in this situation so that all necessary tasks would be accomplished immediately. Although she rarely uses this style, she implemented it effectively in this emergency situation. This example illustrates that leadership is context dependent.

Democratic Leadership

Democratic leadership, also called participative leadership, is characterized by a sense of equality among the leader and other participants. Decisions and activities are shared. Participants are encouraged to develop their skills and strengths within the group. The group and leader work together to accomplish mutually set goals and outcomes. As professionals, nurses generally respond well to this style of leadership when they are the followers and feel more comfortable when they are the leaders of democratic groups. Group satisfaction and motivation are excellent benefits of this style. In situations in which a rapid response is essential, however, a democratic approach to leadership that requires gathering the input of team members may slow decision making.

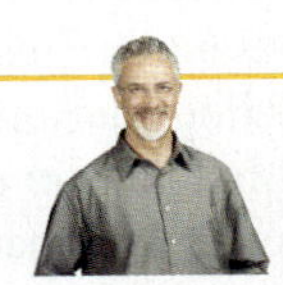

Recall **Stephen Wall**, the patient in the intensive care unit. The nurse would use democratic leadership to work collaboratively with other health care disciplines to plan the most effective care for the patient. For example, the nurse may need to work with the surgical and neurologic staff, respiratory therapy, physical therapy, and social services in developing the patient's care plan.

An example of democratic leadership follows. Nurse B, a head nurse, observes that staff members have not been documenting patient teaching and learning in their progress notes. Nurse B is not sure why this is occurring but believes that this problem must be solved. He calls a staff meeting and leads a discussion to seek information on possible causes and solutions. Nurse B decides that staff members need to be included in the problem-solving approach. He thinks the staff will be more motivated to document their teaching and the patients' learning if they have a say in what changes in practice are necessary and how they will be implemented. Nurse B has used the democratic style of leadership and **decentralized decision-making process** to resolve this issue.

Laissez-Faire Leadership

In **laissez-faire leadership**, also called nondirective leadership, the leader relinquishes power to the group, such that an outsider could not identify the leader in the group. This approach encourages independent activity by group members. This style depends on the strengths of followers to direct the group activities. It is most effective when all staff are clinical experts with a deep understanding of both clinical and administrative processes. This style is rarely useful because task achievement is difficult when each nurse is working independently, and the staff on most units and departments have varying levels of clinical maturity. However, it can be used effectively when the leader wants a problem to be solved completely by expert staff group members.

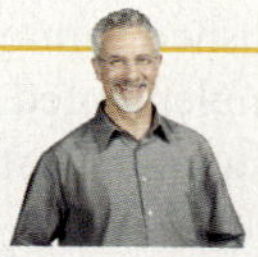

Consider **Stephen Wall**, the patient with multiple trauma who is in the intensive care unit. The patient has multiple priority needs, requiring interdependent actions of many people. Use of laissez-faire leadership would not be effective in this situation.

Similarly, one of the greatest failings of nursing leadership is leaving every nurse, every shift, to figure out how best to respond to Jack Camp's behaviors, rather than planning together and facilitating what a team based "best" response looks like.

Servant Leadership

The Robert K. Greenleaf Center for Servant Leadership (https://www.greenleaf.org) defines **servant leadership** as a philosophy and set of practices that enriches the lives of individuals, builds better organizations, and ultimately creates a more just and caring world. It begins with the natural feeling that one wants to serve. Greenleaf recognized that, although some prize leadership because of their love for power and material possessions, others aspire to leadership because of wanting to serve:

> The difference manifests itself in the care taken by the servant first to make sure that other people's highest priority needs are being served. The best test, and most difficult to administer, is: Do those served grow as people? Do they, while being served, become healthier, wiser, freer, more autonomous, more likely themselves to become servants? And what is the effect on the least privileged in society? Will they benefit or at least not be further deprived?

Box 10-3 Five Key Practices for Servant Leaders

1. **Develop your vision.** What do you see in the future, related to a current or anticipated need? A leader's vision inspires and motivates others to follow and to engage.
2. **Listen and learn before speaking and acting.** Be mindfully present with others, learning and assessing their concerns, values, and priorities. Have an open mind and leave all judgment and assumptions behind.
3. **Envision and invest in others' greatness.** What do you see in others? How can you help them grow?
4. **Give away your power.** Allow others to have a voice, to exercise control, and to practice leading themselves, reassured by the knowledge that you have their backs.
5. **Build community by developing strategic relationships.** Invest in those who support the organization's values, show passion, can play to their strengths, and demonstrate a positive attitude. Provide ongoing opportunities for collaborations, sharing, reflection, encouragement, and celebration, as well as hard work

Source: Inspired by Fahlberg, B., & Toomey, R. (2016). Servant leadership: A model for emerging nurse leaders. *Nursing, 46*(10), 49–52; adapted from Boone, L. W., & Makhani, S. (2012). Five necessary attitudes of a servant leader. *Review of Business, 33*(1), 83–96. Used with permission.

Relationships are the key to successful servant leadership. It is easy to see why many nurses find servant leadership a great fit with nursing values, roles, and responsibilities. Fahlberg and Toomey (2016) believe that many of the best nursing leaders practice servant leadership. "We lead, speak up, volunteer, and advocate because it is the right thing to do. We want to make something better. We see a wrong and we want to make it right, so we do something. Soon, others join in, becoming leaders as they learn and grow through their service" (p. 50). Box 10-3 presents five key practices for servant leaders.

Quantum Leadership

Porter-O'Grady and Malloch (2003), in *Quantum Leadership: A Textbook of New Leadership*, argued that leaders must move beyond the traditional modes used by all levels of workers. They, like Drucker (1999) and others, focused on the impact of the information age, identified at the turn of the century, on work and workers. The vertical command and control structures that generated the leadership styles previously mentioned are no longer useful for managers and workers, nor do they yield productivity for organizations. The explosion of information and technology in health care, as in other industries, has spawned, by necessity, the "knowledge worker." This social transformation is affecting aspects of all our lives, including, perhaps most importantly, how we lead and manage our organizations.

We are in a difficult transition period between the old and the new. In the old, change was viewed as an entity to be planned, carefully managed, and accepted. In the new "quantum age," change is conceived as dynamic, ever present, and continually unfolding. We are forced to experience change at the same time we perceive it, with little or no opportunity to definitively and laboriously plan and manage it. **Quantum leadership** theory views an organization and its members as interconnected and collaborative—a helpful approach when unpredictable events and changing environments present themselves (Curtin, 2013). Nursing leaders can model these new behaviors by combining these new attributes with the requisite technical skills. Never was this more needed than when the 2020 pandemic stretched all our resources thin.

Transactional Leadership

Transactional leadership style is based on a task-and-reward orientation. Team members agree to a satisfactory salary and working conditions in exchange for commitment and compliance to their leader. Health care organizations have often used transactional leadership strategies to provide direction and recognize employees' progress in meeting pre-established goals and work deadlines. Transactional leaders maintain control by rewarding good behavior and punishing behavior they perceive as detrimental or negative. Employees have minimal opportunities for creative thinking and involvement in organizational decisions, and employer and employee may not share a common vision. Transactional leaders provide little inspiration for nurses to participate in reforming health care, problem solving, or engaging in practices and research that promote nursing excellence (Habel & Sherman, 2012).

Transformational Leadership

Transformational leadership can create revolutionary change. Often described as charismatic, transformational leaders are unique in their ability to inspire and motivate others. They create intellectually stimulating practice environments and challenge themselves and others to grow personally and professionally, and to learn. Gifted in creating a common vision, they demonstrate passion for their vision and keep others similarly focused. One of the unique qualities of transformational leaders is their vulnerability. They communicate honestly and openly and can express emotions as well as ideas as they share themselves with others. They show concern and care for others and are willing to take risks. They pay attention to process as well as outcomes.

An example of transformational leadership is as follows. Nurse C is troubled by the plight of women and children in the city where she lives. She unites with other nurses and health care professionals to design and implement strategies to meet their needs. Within 18 months, a nursing center is funded and running, improving maternal–child outcomes in the area. The founding group of health care professionals continues to meet monthly to dream about future strategies and to support each other in their work. They are proudest of the improved self-esteem and independence in many of the women they serve.

Transformational leaders have a positive and compelling vision, fostering a new culture for nursing practice and patient care. This style of leadership is a key component of organizations that achieve Magnet status.

DEVELOPMENT OF THE MAGNET RECOGNITION PROGRAM

More than two decades ago, the Task Force on Nursing Practice in Hospitals of the American Academy of Nursing (AAN) conducted a study of 41 hospitals to identify and describe variables that created an environment that attracted and retained well-qualified nurses who promoted quality patient care through providing excellence in nursing services. These institutions were called "Magnet" hospitals because they attracted and retained professional nurses who experienced a high degree of professional and personal satisfaction through their practice. These institutions used a decentralized decision-making process, self-governance at the unit level, and respect for and acknowledgment of professional autonomy.

In 1990, the American Nurses Credentialing Center (ANCC), a subsidiary of ANA, developed a formal process to recognize excellence in nursing service and to confer "Magnet" status. Magnet status is awarded for 4 years, after which organizations must reapply. Originally, 14 characteristics, called the Forces of Magnetism, were recognized that identified quality patient care, excellent nursing care, and innovations in professional nursing practice. A statistical analysis and review of evaluators' reports has resulted in the configuration of the original 14 attributes into five model components, effective in 2009:

- Transformational leadership
- Structural empowerment
- Exemplary professional practice
- New knowledge, innovation, and improvements
- Empirical quality results

This new model includes the original 14 forces but reflects a greater focus on measuring outcomes and eliminates redundancy in documentation.

SIGNIFICANCE OF MAGNET RECOGNITION

Achieving Magnet status serves patients, nurses, and health care organizations. It empowers organizations to:

- Attract and retain top talent
- Improve care, safety, and satisfaction
- Foster a collaborative culture
- Advance nursing standards and practice
- Grow business and financial success

Research and surveys provide evidence that Magnet hospitals have better patient outcomes, shorter lengths of stay, higher patient satisfaction, and higher nurse job satisfaction and nurse retention than hospitals without this governance style of leadership (ANCC, 2013; Habel & Sherman, 2012; Hawkins & Shell, 2012). The achievement of Magnet status has a profound impact on the quality of patient care and nursing practice. According to Bashaw (2011), Magnet recognition has become the "apex of achievement for nursing professionals and health care organizations." More than 400 hospitals have achieved Magnet status. Additional information regarding the Magnet Recognition Program is available at the ANCC at https://www.nursingworld.org/organizational-programs/magnet/.

IMPLEMENTATION OF A "JUST CULTURE"

Health care organizations that achieve Magnet status have created a focus on positive patient care outcomes, collaboration, shared decision making, and a climate in which patient safety is a priority. Creation of a **just culture** indicates an organizational commitment to accountability and universal safety in health care. Nurses are encouraged to disclose clinical errors and potential error situations without the fear of punitive actions. This accountability then allows other nurses to learn from this experience. The open communication resulting from development of a just culture allows health care workers to discuss concerns and challenges related to patient care and turn them into opportunities for improvement. The combination of Magnet principles and a just culture can produce a health care vision focused on transparency, accountability, communication, collaboration, and the pursuit of health care excellence (Bashaw, 2011; Bashaw et al., 2012; Shepard, 2011). Read more about just culture in Chapter 7.

MANAGEMENT

All nurses, to the extent that they work with others and influence others to be their best, can become leaders. However, some nurses hold positions in the health care system that also make them managers. The role of **management** is to plan, organize, direct, and control available human, material, and financial resources to deliver quality care to patients and families.

The managerial role is frequently conceptualized as the technical dimension of formal leadership roles. These technical areas of expertise, particularly in the financial or clinical resource management dimension, are mandatory for contemporary nurse managers. A few of their direct responsibilities, identified in a previous section, can be viewed in these traditionally broad areas (Marquis & Huston, 2017):

- *Planning:* identifying problems and developing goals, objectives, and related strategies to meet the demands of the clinical arena
- *Organizing:* acquiring, managing, and mobilizing resources to meet both clinical and financial objectives
- *Staffing:* hiring, orienting, scheduling to facilitate team building; also includes staff development
- *Directing:* leading others in achieving goals within the constraints of the current fiscal and workforce shortage scenarios, a demanding task for managers and staff alike
- *Controlling:* implementing mechanisms for ongoing evaluation, particularly in areas of clinical quality and financial accountability

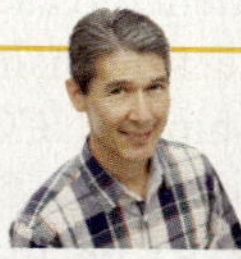

Remember ***Jack Camp***, the patient with diabetes and an external fixator. The nurse manager for this unit could address the problem of the staff's overt criticism of the patient. Using planning, organizing, directing, and controlling, the nurse manager could ultimately create an environment that is conducive to the patient's recovery and health and satisfying to staff caring for this patient.

It is increasingly challenging for the nurse manager to be both a clinical and a managerial expert; the explosion of clinical knowledge and expectations for managerial expertise place unrealistic demands on this role (Shingler-Nace & Gonzalez, 2017). Typical nurse managers are expected to manage their unit budget within prescribed constraints, deliver a high level of quality care to patients on the unit, develop and serve as mentors for junior staff, comply with regulatory requirements, and be experts at human resource management. Although the role might seem overwhelming, it can also be quite satisfying to the manager, the staff, and the organization. Collaboration and appropriate support from both superiors and subordinates can empower and motivate staff, facilitating a highly functioning team and best practice clinical environment.

Marquis and Huston (2017) caution that management and leadership should be intertwined for each to be effective. Some view leadership as an expected function of management, while others consider leadership as more complex, with an emphasis on improving productivity and empowering the workforce rather than just controlling specific organizational details. However, a leader without management skills can cause chaos in an organization, while a manager who fails to lead is equally ineffective. Nurse managers must be effective leaders to be successful. Nurse managers who cannot create a healthy group environment; who fail to resolve interpersonal issues that lower morale and result in numerous complaints from patients, nurses, and health care providers; and who cannot develop a plan to resolve detrimental interpersonal issues lack leadership skills. See Table 10-1 for a comparison of the roles and characteristics of nurse leaders and managers. What is certainly true is that both nursing leadership and management roles require passion to make health care work for those who need it, a commitment to advance the well-being of their staff, and in-depth knowledge of the field and successful strategies to achieve these aims.

Centralized and Decentralized Management Structures

In a centralized management structure, senior managers generally make decisions. Those further down in the hierarchy of the organization are often responsible for implementing decisions into which they had little input. In a decentralized management structure, on the other hand, decisions are made by those who are most knowledgeable about the issues being decided. Nurses are thus intimately involved in decisions concerning patient care. Nurse managers are accountable for what happens on their nursing unit, including patient census, staffing, supplies, and budget. A decentralized system invites greater accountability and responsibility because most nurses feel more responsible for decisions they have made themselves. Magnet facilities promote **shared governance** practices that give nurses more input and influence over their jobs and how

Table 10-1 Nursing Leadership and Management: A Breakdown of the Roles

ROLE	DEFINITION	KEY RESPONSIBILITIES	QUALITIES/ CHARACTERISTICS
Nurse Leader	A nurse leader oversees a team of nurses and other health care professionals, making decisions and directing patient care initiatives. They have advanced clinical knowledge and are focused on improving patient health outcomes.	• Staying up to date on the latest health care research • Working to shorten the average length of patient hospital stays and reduce readmission rates • Aiming to reduce health care costs by improving efficiency • Providing team members with the knowledge and tools they need to deliver safe, top-quality care • Ordering and reviewing diagnostic tests • Developing treatment plans to improve care and patient outcomes • Providing care directly to patients • Advocating for and educating patients and family caregivers • Reducing the turnover rate of registered nurses	*Nurse leaders need to communicate well with team members and efficiently delegate tasks. Empathy and compassion are a must, since they work directly with patients. Effective nurse leaders also need to have strong problem-solving and critical thinking skills.*
Nurse Manager	Nurse managers are not typically involved in direct patient care; rather, they are focused on managing daily operations and supervising staff. The position requires an understanding of business management, as nurse managers are often in charge of budgeting.	• Overseeing day-to-day operations • Supervising and providing training to team members • Working with various stakeholders to optimize care and meet budget requirements • Handling escalating situations between patients and health care providers • Designing and managing a budget • Overseeing insurance and other reimbursements • Overseeing electronic health record systems • Hiring and evaluating nursing staff • Collaborating with other managers to achieve optimal patient outcomes	*Nurse managers must be able to juggle multiple priorities, communicate effectively, and work well with various stakeholders. They should be task-oriented individuals who are also able to advocate and serve as mentors for the staff members who report to them.*

the organization makes decisions that affect them. Every nurse brings their own wisdom, expertise, and experience that are not leveraged enough if not tapped into. Shared governance models ensure that every nurse has a voice. Especially as nursing fatigue rates rise, employers struggle to retain nurses, and nursing performance has a more direct impact on the financial bottom line of hospitals. The shared governance model is essential to ensuring that nurses are empowered to have as much influence over their work environment as possible (https://www.nursingworld.org/search/?q=shared+governance+in+nursing).

You will most likely experience both modes of decision making—centralized and decentralized—in nursing units. Financial targets and other broad strategic directions are frequently established at executive levels of the organization. Clinical issues, processes of care delivery, clinical outcomes, and unit governance are usually resolved at the unit or department level.

Conflict Management and Engagement

Nurse managers frequently encounter conflict between employees and between themselves and employees. Unresolved conflict can lower morale and threaten quality care. **Conflict management** is a process to work through conflicts in a way that minimizes negative effects and promotes positive consequences. **Conflict engagement** teaches skills to help nurses perform well in the face of conflict instead of finding a workaround to avoid conflict.

Creating connection with others is a powerful tool in conflict engagement. Gerardi (2015b) recommends the PEARLA approach. PEARLA stands for **P**resence, **E**mpathy, **A**cknowledgment, **R**eflect (or **R**eframe), **L**isten openly, and **A**sk questions. When someone is agitated, taking the time to create a connection can deescalate the situation and lessen feelings of threat. The better we understand another's concerns, wants, and needs, the more likely we are to build trust as a foundation for problem solving (Gerardi, 2015b, p. 61).

It is important for each of us to recognize our "hot buttons" and patterns under stress. Gerardi (2015a, p. 61) recommends:

- Recognizing the physical sensations we experience when triggered by a situation (flushing, increased heart rate, shallow breathing)
- Taking a step back and breathing deeply three times

- Noticing and delaying our initial response in order to stop the habit of "fixing" or "solving" a situation too quickly
- Becoming curious about what we don't know, including discerning what the other person needs

Marquis and Huston (2017) described six styles for dealing with conflict—avoiding, accommodating, competing, compromising, collaborating, and smoothing—and noted that "the situation itself, the urgency of the decision, the power and status of the players, the importance of the issue, and the maturity of the people involved in the conflict" determine which strategy is most appropriate. Box 10-4 further defines these conflict resolution strategies.

Johansen (2012) describes a nursing management situation that demonstrates these conflict resolution strategies. Nurse C, who works in an emergency department, receives her assignment and notices that Nurse J has a much lighter assignment. Nurse J has a reputation for being difficult and always getting her way. Because of the number of her assigned patients and the severity of their conditions, Nurse C approaches the charge nurse, Nurse S, and asks her to modify her assignment. Nurse S declines to change it, does not want to address this with Nurse J, and reminds Nurse C how difficult Nurse J can be if confronted with an unpleasant situation. Nurse C decides to discuss this situation with Nurse P, the nurse manager. To manage this conflict, Nurse P can use one of the following strategies:

- *Avoid* the situation, with the result that both Nurse C and Nurse P feel frustrated and powerless.
- Respond in a dominating or *competing* manner and tell Nurse S that the assignments are unacceptable. She intimidates Nurse S and also is upset because the nurses on the unit are not resolving their own problems.
- Ask Nurse C to accept the assignment in order to *accommodate* the charge nurse. Nurse P understands the inequity of this assignment but lets Nurse C know that she appreciates her team commitment and will remember this in the future.
- Attempt a *compromise* by providing Nurse S with a rationale for modifying the assignment. Both Nurse C and Nurse S should discuss the assignment with Nurse J and see if they can find a mutually agreeable solution.
- *Collaborate* with all parties to resolve the assignment issue and promote a safer work situation.
- Use a *smoothing* approach that involves complimenting all parties in an attempt to prevent emotional outbursts and focus on agreement.

Box 10-4 Conflict Resolution Strategies

Avoiding: There is awareness of the conflict situation, but the parties involved decide to either ignore the conflict, or avoid, or postpone its resolution. The conflict has not been resolved and may resurface later in an exaggerated form.

Collaborating: This is a joint effort to resolve the conflict with a win–win solution. All parties set aside previously determined goals, determine a priority common goal, and accept mutual responsibility for achieving this goal. This focus on problem solving is based on mutual respect, honest communication, and shared decision making.

Competing: This approach results in a win for one party at the expense of the other group. This win–lose confrontation can leave the loser frustrated, with a desire to "get even" in the future. This strategy may be used when one party has more knowledge regarding the situation, or when resistance is appropriate because of ethical concerns or unsafe patient care practices.

Compromising: For this technique to be effective, both parties must be willing to relinquish something of equal value. If that does not occur, either or both parties may feel that they have lost the conflict and given up more than the other group.

Cooperating/Accommodating: One party makes a conscious decision to let the other group win and may collect an "IOU" for use in the future. This party's original loss may result in a more positive outcome in the future.

Smoothing: Smoothing is an effort to compliment the other party and focus on agreement rather than disagreement, thus reducing the emotion in the conflict. The original conflict is rarely resolved with this technique.

Source: Adapted from Marquis, B., & Huston, C. (2017). *Leadership roles and management functions in nursing* (9th ed., pp. 558–559). Wolters Kluwer Health.

Managing Change

Change is the process of transforming or modifying something. It might be a planned change, an unplanned change, a developmental change, or, as Porter-O'Grady and Malloch (2003) suggested, a quantum change and ever present. Nursing and the health care system are continually changing and evolving—that momentum will only escalate in the years to come. Factors such as the increasing number of chronically ill and older people, the increasing role of government and industry in health care, the rising cost of health care, and the changing patterns of health care delivery have produced a need for innovation and change in health care. Patient care safety and quality issues play a vital role in the transformation occurring in the health care system. Nurse managers, once they have assessed the need for change, function as visionary, assertive, and supportive role models in the implementation of the planned change.

Change Theory

There are many theories of change, most based on the classic theory of change proposed by Lewin (1951). Lewin identified three stages of change:

1. *Unfreezing:* The need for change is recognized.
2. *Moving:* Change is initiated after a careful process of planning.
3. *Refreezing:* Change becomes operational.

These three rather simplistic stages do not fully reveal the very dynamic and personal nature of change of any kind. In health care, we can find numerous examples of using change theory to transform practice. Not so long ago, childbirth in the United States was routinely "medicalized." Women came to the hospital to deliver their babies; pain medications that interfered with the natural process of labor were routinely administered, necessitating forceps and assisted deliveries; and husbands, partners, and siblings were banished from the delivery room. Nurse midwives and others recognized the need for change (*unfreezing*) and set about researching childbirth and ways to improve infant and family outcomes. After a careful process of planning (*moving*), multiple natural childbirth options in health care facilities and in the home were made available to women and couples; today they represent mainstream care (*refreezing*).

Similarly, someone who takes good health for granted may fail to develop healthy lifestyle practices until illness results in recognition of the need for change (*unfreezing*). A careful process of consultation and study may lead to the development of a well-developed fitness plan (*moving*), which ideally becomes part of the person's everyday life (*refreezing*). Effective nurses pay attention to their ability to influence the person's thinking and behavior in each stage of change.

Planned Change

Planned change is a purposeful, systematic effort to bring about change. Nurse managers most often implement planned change. The eight steps in the process of change, which are somewhat similar to the steps of the nursing process, are shown in Box 10-5. Kotter (1996) emphasized that for change to be successful, it is important to progress in sequence through each of the eight stages. Skipping any of the steps can result in the vision being sabotaged, momentum faltering, and frustration increasing for all involved in the process.

Before planning to make a change, a nurse manager should consider the following:

- What is amenable to change? Considering this question may reveal a behavior not amenable to change.
- How does the group function as a unit? Certain forces within a group may favor change, whereas other forces may resist it.
- Is the person or group ready for change and, if so, at what rate can that change be expected to be accepted? The pace of change must be consistent with the person's or group's readiness to assimilate change. Readiness involves both the ability and willingness to change. In contemporary health care organizations, change is dynamic, persistent, and very challenging. The concept of flexibility previously mentioned is put to a real test in any clinical or managerial arena.
- Are the changes major or minor? A series of small changes may be more easily accomplished than one large, dramatic change. The nursing leader/manager must support the staff during the difficult task of acquiring new skills and, frequently, new professional identities.

In today's dynamic health care environment, nurses play a pivotal role in the change process. They must be prepared to initiate and implement quality change projects. The Robert Wood Johnson Foundation and the Institute for Healthcare Improvement originated a program called Transforming Care at the Bedside (TCAB) that focuses on instituting changes to improve patient care on medical-surgical units. Nurses are empowered to address inefficiencies and changes in workflow in an effort to improve the quality of patient care. An additional change effort, the Care Innovation and Transformation (CIT) initiative, was developed by the American Organization of Nurse Executives (AONE). This program supports nurse managers and provides training and tools to ensure a successful change environment.

Box 10-5 Planned Change: An Eight-Step Process

Planned change is a purposeful, systematic effort to alter or bring about change through the intervention of a change agent. The same steps apply whether dealing with individuals or groups.

1. *Recognize symptoms that indicate a change is needed and collect data.*
2. *Identify a problem to be solved through change.* Analyze the symptoms and reach a conclusion. Note resistance or barriers to change and factors that promote the desired change.
3. *Determine and analyze alternative solutions to the problem.* Consider the advantages, disadvantages, and consequences of each alternative. An analysis of various proposed solutions to a problem may result in using a combination of alternatives.
4. *Select a course of action from possible alternatives.* Avoid initiating too many courses of action and thereby dissipating resources and energy.
5. *Plan for making the change.* This step is crucial to effect change successfully. Start by stating specific objectives, designing a plan for change, developing timetables, selecting people to assist with making the change, and anticipating how to stabilize change and deal with resistance to change. Unless a plan is clearly designed, effecting change is likely to be a chaotic experience.
6. *Implement the selected course of action to effect change.* Put the plan for change into effect. During this period, flexibility is important to adapt to unforeseen problems.
7. *Evaluate the effects of change by comparing them with objectives stated in the plan for change.* Adjustments can be made in the plan as necessary after evaluation. If the results of evaluation indicate that the course of action selected to solve a problem has been unsuccessful, an adjustment should be made or another course of action selected.
8. *Stabilize the change.* When a solution has been found, take measures to make the change permanent. Continue follow-up until the change is firmly established.

Resistance to Change

If you find yourself in a clinical setting undergoing small or big change, it can be helpful to ask yourself the following questions:

- How patient am I with myself and with others?
- Am I open to new experiences and to growth?
- Do I believe that good will come of the change? Hope is that human excellence that allows us to envision a positive future and work to bring it into being.
- Am I a positive influence on others and on our institution?

People may resist change for various reasons. You may find it helpful to locate yourself on the Fisher change curve in Figure 10-1. One nurse in the early days of orienting to a new electronic medical record shared that she found herself in all of the places on any given day! The nurse manager/leader must identify if any resistance is present in order to determine which techniques are needed to overcome it. Change alters the balance of a group, and resistance is an expected accompaniment to change.

People resist change for a number of reasons, as noted below.

THREAT TO SELF

People generally view change in terms of how they are affected personally. Personal threats may include a loss of self-esteem, a belief that more work will be required, or a belief that social relationships will be disrupted. For example, when hospitals began to use more assistive personnel (AP) for routine nursing care, many nurses resisted, not only because of quality concerns but also because they found themselves legally and professionally responsible for supervising the care given by these aides. There was also concern that some professional nurses would be replaced by AP.

LACK OF UNDERSTANDING

Someone who does not understand the nature of change is likely to resist. The people who will be affected by the change must become involved and educated if their resistance is to be overcome. For example, nurses who do not realize the effectiveness of using care plans tend to resist preparing them because they believe they are not beneficial for providing patient care.

LIMITED TOLERANCE FOR CHANGE

Some people simply do not like to function in a state of flux or disequilibrium. A person may understand the need for change but may be unable to cope with it emotionally. For example, a nurse may resist change because of the temporary confusion the change is likely to cause.

DISAGREEMENTS ABOUT THE BENEFITS OF CHANGE

Resistance may occur when the change agent and those resisting change have different information. If the information known by the people resisting change is more accurate and relevant than the change agent's information,

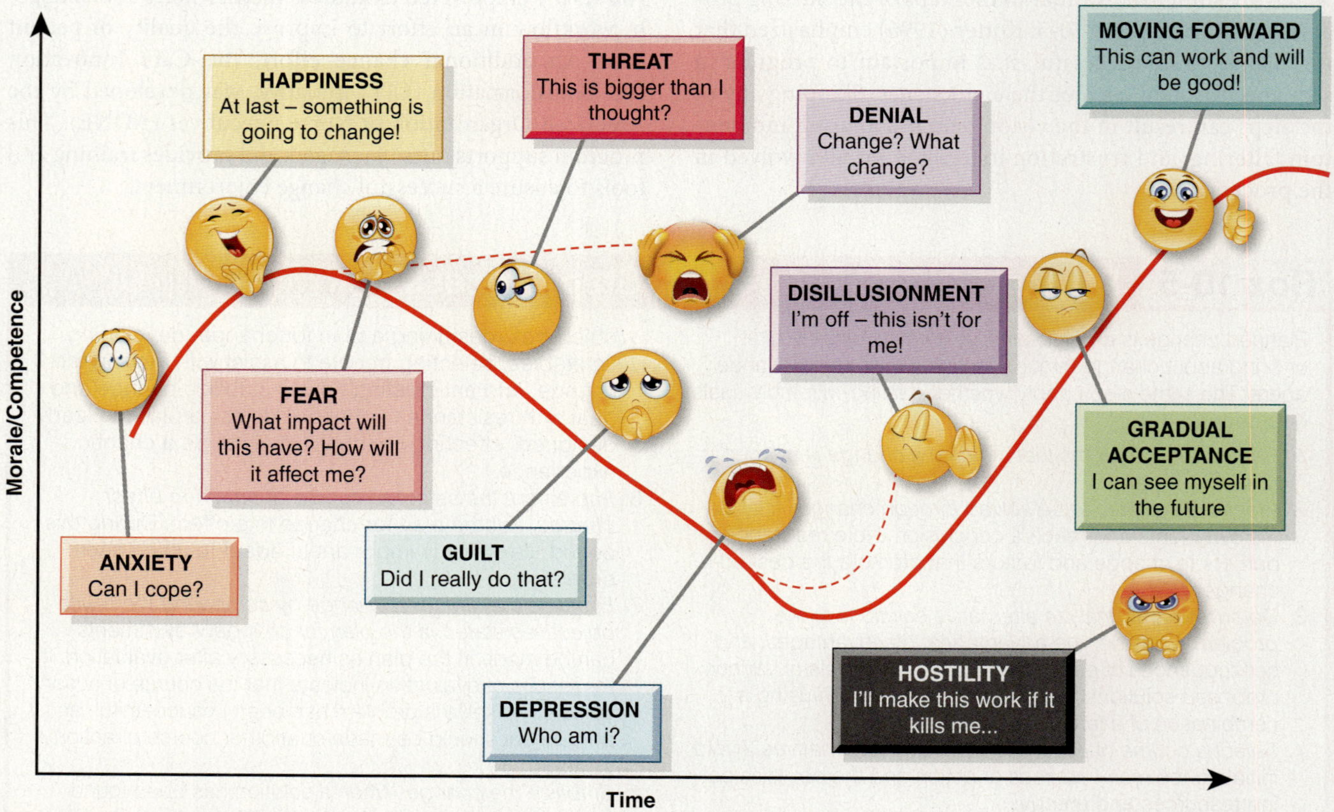

FIGURE 10-1. Fisher Change Curve. (© BusinessBalls Ltd [and J. M. Fisher] [1999/2012]. Not to be sold or published. The author(s)/ Businessballs Ltd. accepts no liability for any issues arising https://www.businessballs.com/change-management/personal-change-stages-john-fisher/.)

resistance may be beneficial. For example, the supervisor of community health services proposes to implement, in a low-income neighborhood, a home health care plan that has been effective in a middle-class section of the city. The nurse in charge of the health program in the low-income area resists, believing that the same plan would not be successful in a financially and educationally disadvantaged neighborhood.

FEAR OF INCREASED RESPONSIBILITY

Many people are worried about having to take on more complex responsibilities, especially if they feel unprepared for the planned changes. The changes may seem overwhelming, so they naturally resist them.

Overcoming Resistance to Change

Resistance can be subtle or distinct, gentle or aggressive. Responding to resistance is both a leadership responsibility and a challenge in which the leader uses leadership qualities, leadership style, and knowledge of group dynamics to influence others toward a desired outcome. Nurses acting as change agents find the following guidelines helpful for overcoming resistance to change:

- Explain the proposed change to all affected people in simple, concise language.
- List the advantages of the proposed change, both for the individual and for members of the group.
- Relate the proposed change to the person's or group's existing beliefs and values.
- Help overcome resistance by providing opportunities for open communication and feedback.
- Indicate clearly how the change will be evaluated.
- If possible, introduce change gradually. Involve everyone affected by the change in the design and implementation of the process.
- Provide incentives for commitment to change, such as money, status, time off, or a better working environment.

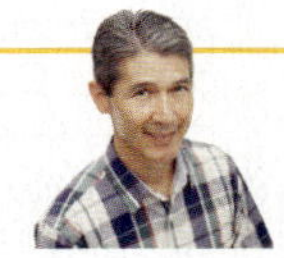

Think back to **Jack Camp**, the patient described in the Reflective Practice display. The nurse could apply these guidelines when attempting to change staff behavior and the patient's behavior. Ultimately, a positive outcome for both could be achieved.

Management Strategies

Two management strategies often used in health care and in many businesses are the SWOT analysis and SOAR strategic planning. Imagine for a moment that you are part of a team developed to ensure that as many employees as possible will get the COVID-19 vaccine as soon as it becomes available. You have heard many of the employees voice concerns about the vaccine's safety and want to begin to address these fears early on. If you use a SWOT analysis, you will work with your team to identify Strengths within the organizations to facilitate a good plan, Weaknesses that will make adopting any plan to realize your goals challenging, Opportunities, and Threats (Stavros & Cole, 2013).

SOAR analysis (Strengths, Opportunities, Aspirations, and Results) is a strategic planning technique that helps organizations focus on their current strengths and opportunities and create a vision of future aspirations and the result they can bring (Fig. 10-2). SOAR focuses on what is known

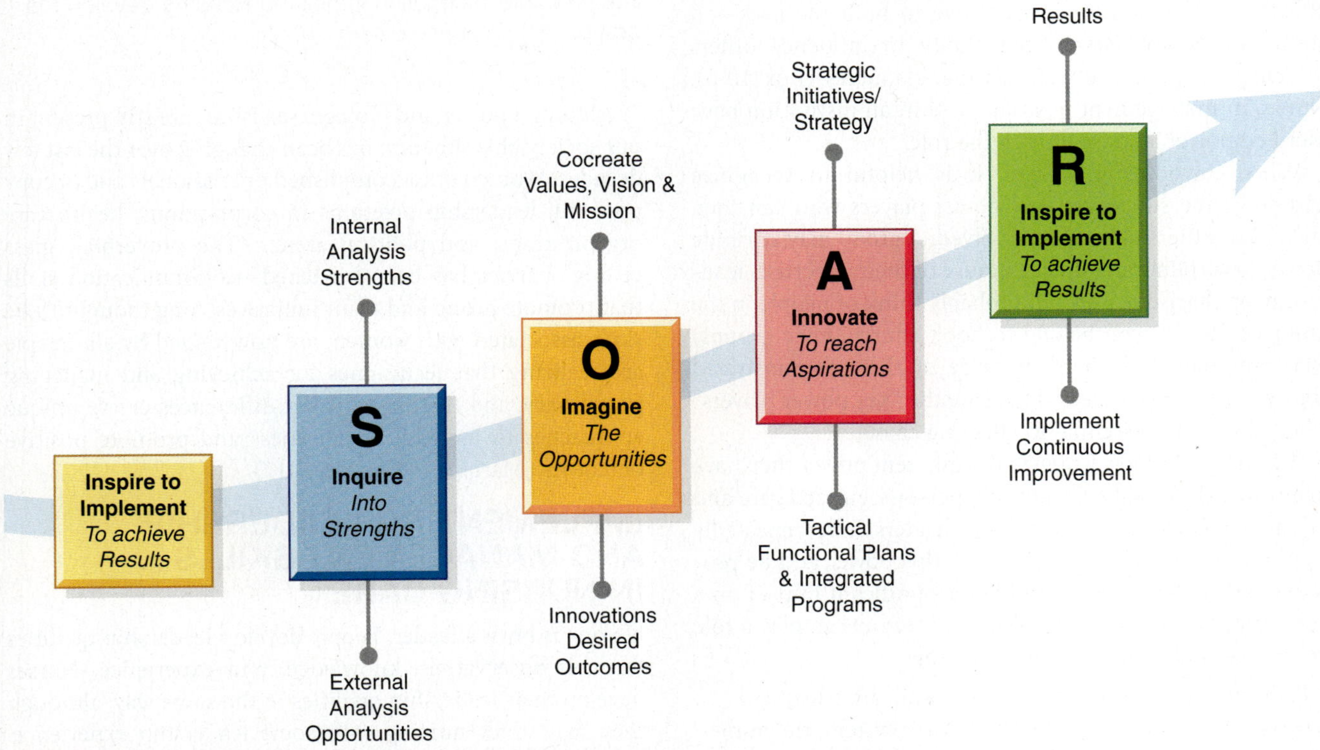

FIGURE 10-2. SOAR framework. (*Source:* Used with permission from www.soar-strategy.com)

Box 10-6 Five Power Sources

Leaders have five major sources of power in their power grid.

1. Coercive power is the "stick" of leadership where staff are sanctioned for failing to comply with the leader's desires. Coercive power relies on fear but rarely inspires nurses to work with a leader for the long term.
2. Legitimate power emanates from a position or title. It can be short-lived if the leader is ineffective because to be influential, leaders must have followers.
3. Reward power is based on a leader's ability to give something of value in return for performance. Nurse leaders have reward and recognition power that needs to be used in a meaningful, sustainable, and practical way.
4. Expert power is built on the individual's specialized knowledge and access to information. Many nurse leaders struggle with giving up their expert power as clinicians when moving into a leadership role.
5. Referent or relationship power is built on a leader's personal brand. Leaders with referent power are respected and have what is sometimes called "social capital" because people chose to follow them.

Source: Used with permission. Sherman, R. O., & Cohn, T. M. (2019). Using leadership power wisely. *American Nurse Today, 14*(9), 18–19.

to work in order to create a shared vision for the future, rather than on internal weaknesses or perceived threats that may not eventuate (Stavros & Cole, 2013). Can you think of ways you might use elements of these strategies to begin to hone your leadership and management competencies?

Power

Nurses in leadership and managerial roles who wish to be effective change agents are sensitive to both the uses and abuses of power. **Power**, the ability to influence others to achieve a desired effect, has many sources (Box 10-6). Nurses in management positions within an institution have ascribed power associated with the role.

When introducing change, it is helpful to recognize and enlist the support of key power players who can then encourage others to become involved. A group may attribute power to certain individuals because of their expertise, leadership, or charisma. You can probably think of people in the groups to which you belong (school, church, civic groups) who are "natural leaders" because of their demonstrated ability to influence others. These are the "key power players" whose support is essential to effecting change.

All nurses should recognize the inherent power they have to ensure safe, quality, thoughtful, person-centered care and to cause change. Various nursing leaders have repeatedly emphasized that nurses need to use this power and be proactive rather than reactive to have a significant impact on a new vision for nursing. The following factors can play a role in increasing the power base of nursing:

- *Right timing:* Consumers and legislators are frustrated with errors reported in the health care system, the number of uninsured people, and overall problems with the health care system in the United States. Nurses, as the most respected health care providers, are poised to help improve health care and implement health care reform.
- *Size of the nursing profession:* This is one of nursing's greatest assets, with at least 3.9 million RNs in the United States. Nurses are an impressive voting bloc.
- *Nursing's referent power:* The public has expressed a high degree of trust and credibility in the nursing profession.
- *Increasing knowledge base and education for nurses:* More nurses are assuming advanced practice roles, and nursing graduates are strongly encouraged to achieve higher levels of education.
- *Nursing's unique perspective:* The caring component of nursing coupled with evidence-based practice and critical thinking has positioned nurses to deliver complex care to a variety of patients and positively affect quality of care.
- *Desire of consumers and providers for change:* Consumers are increasingly aware of the need for accessible, affordable, and safe quality care (Marquis & Huston, 2017).

Transformational leaders empower their staff by communicating and encouraging learning as well as promoting and verifying a sense of value about the powerful, life-saving work that nurses perform. Nurses who feel they have no control over their environment are more likely to express frustration toward a coworker and to leave their position or even the profession.

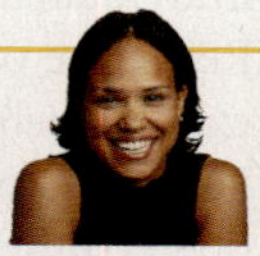

Recall **Rehema Kohls**, the college sophomore considering starting a campus discussion group about STIs. The nurse at the health care center sees that Rehema is considered by her peers to have power and to be a leader. The nurse would integrate this information in helping Rehema develop the group.

Although power and biologic sex issues are still present in our society, this situation has been changing over the last few decades. Women are accomplished professionals and occupy powerful leadership positions in corporations, health care organizations, and political arenas. The proverbial "glass ceiling" barrier has been broached—communication skills that promote group and team initiatives, long thought to be skills associated with women, are now valued by all. People are realizing that techniques for achieving and managing power vary, and that biologic sex differences create unique approaches to increase effectiveness and promote positive outcomes (Marquis & Huston, 2017).

IMPLEMENTING LEADERSHIP AND MANAGEMENT SKILLS IN NURSING CARE

No one is born a leader. People develop leadership qualities through observation, knowledge, and experience. Nurses develop their leadership qualities in the same way, although they may enter nursing with some leadership experience. Nursing students and beginning practicing nurses have some leadership responsibilities but are usually still working at developing leadership skills and learning where and how to apply them. Fortunately, they have support systems for guidance.

Approach leadership like any other new role or skill: slowly and carefully. Nursing students and beginning nurses should be prepared with all the necessary tools or skills before attempting a new leadership role. Initially, nurses develop leadership skills in well-defined clinical situations. With each experience, growth occurs and leadership is strengthened. Have you ever volunteered to lead a group project? Remember that all nurse managers, nurse administrators, and nursing leaders began as inexperienced nurses. If you return to Box 10-1, you will find very concrete suggestions for developing your leadership potential. Read also the accompanying Thoughtful Person-Centered Practice: Challenging Topics (on pages 258–259), to learn about an unexpected leadership challenge that confronted a new graduate nurse.

Nurses who become effective leaders can play a major role in influencing future changes in the health care system.

Patient Care Coordination

Even new graduate nurses have leadership and coordination responsibilities when they begin nursing. Nursing leadership begins with nursing care of the individual patient. Although patients are partners in their care planning, most do not have the knowledge base and skills to direct the plan. Through interpersonal skills and effective communication techniques, nurses lead their patients to acquire new knowledge, solve problems, and change behaviors.

Managing care for even one patient can be an overwhelming responsibility for those new to nursing and its challenges. The student guide to organizing clinical responsibilities in Chapter 18 offers practical help.

An ongoing leadership challenge for all nurses is time management (Leis & Andersen, 2020). The following are helpful steps for using your time effectively:

- Establish goals and priorities for each day. Identify what you need to accomplish each day, differentiating "need to do" from "nice to do" tasks. Be sure to include the patient and the patient's family in establishing these priorities. Ask, "What is it important for you to accomplish today?"
- Evaluate your goals in terms of their ability to meet the needs of the patients entrusted to your care as well as your duties to yourself and your colleagues (other students and members of the team). If one student has a patient whose care requires assistance, other students can plan their day to be able to help at a particular time. This sort of teamwork is an important element of care coordination.
- Establish a timeline. Allocate priorities to hours in your workday so that you will recognize when you are falling behind schedule in time to correct it before the day is lost.
- Evaluate your success or failure in managing time. If you fail to accomplish your goals in the time available, determine whether your goals were overambitious, whether things happened beyond your control (e.g., your patient's condition worsened, requiring more care, or another student required your assistance), or whether you wasted time that could have been better spent (Fig. 10-3).
- Use the results of this evaluation to direct your next day's priorities and timeline.

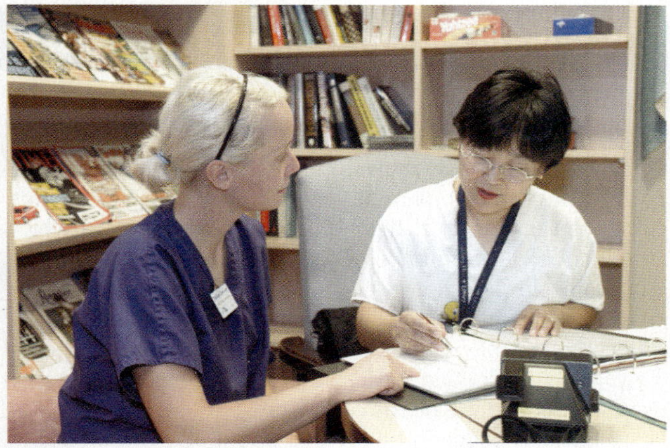

FIGURE 10-3. A student reviews her success in managing time with her clinical instructor. (*Source:* Used with permission from Shutterstock. *Photo by Joe Mitchell.*)

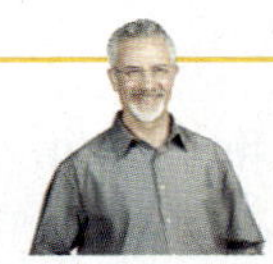

Remember ***Stephen Wall***, the 65-year-old patient in the intensive care unit with multiple injuries. Because of his multiple and complex needs, time management for the nurse is crucial. Applying the steps just identified in this situation would be very helpful when planning and providing care.

Clinical Nurse Leader Role

To have a positive effect on fragmented health care and promote improved collaboration within the entire health care team, the American Association of Colleges of Nursing (AACN) created the nursing professional role of clinical nurse leader (CNL). This master's-prepared nurse who has earned the certified CNL credential works collaboratively with the health care team to facilitate, coordinate, and oversee care provided to patients (Sheets et al., 2012; Stachowiak & Bugel, 2013). This role is not considered an administrative or management role, but rather one of leadership in all health care settings. The CNL should be able to clearly communicate with other health care professionals, integrate evidence-based practices into patient care, and evaluate risks and outcomes that may require change in care plans for patients (AACN, 2012). The person-centered focus of the CNL role includes functioning as a patient advocate, educator, and provider of patient care in complex situations.

Questions have arisen about a perceived overlap or duplication between the roles of the CNL and those of the clinical nurse specialist and case manager. Some nursing professionals also question the need for the CNL at this time. Clinical nurse specialists are advanced practice nurses with specialist education in a defined area of practice; case managers are

Thoughtful Person-Centered Practice: Challenging Topics

Nurse Suicide

Many controversial issues make it challenging to know how to respond as a professional nurse in select scenarios. When our obligations or duties are conflicting, this creates a particular type of challenge. How can we be sure which duty or obligation trumps? Often, the nurse's personal and/or professional values may conflict with options desired by patients, families, employers/colleagues, and communities. Not infrequently, nurses have to make clinical judgments balancing promoting and safeguarding personal integrity and respecting the needs of others.

Read the scenario below and see if you can articulate what you believe, why you believe this, and how these beliefs are likely to inform the decisions you make and your behavior, especially when you are confronted with competing obligations. Based on Tanner's Clinical Judgment Model (2006), consider reflection-in-action and reflection-on-action (Nielson, Stragnell, & Jester, 2007).

Reflection-in-Action

As you read, consider what the new nurse is thinking in the moment—what happened? How did the patient, family, and/or health care provider respond? What did the nurse do next?

Scenario

As a brand-new graduate nurse, I was just beginning my orientation to a step-down medical unit. I was excited about being hired to this unit and was eager to prove my worth to my nurse colleagues. On this particular day, the unit was short-staffed, and I had pulled a full patient load. One of my patients was especially complex and needed several procedures that I had never done before. I was understandably nervous but grateful that I had a preceptor to help me. As the morning evolved, I was becoming increasingly distressed because my preceptor was sitting at the nursing station and seemed indifferent to my appeals for help. She referred me to others for help and I couldn't understand her indifference to my growing distress. When I summoned my courage and sat next to her on my lunch break to ask why she wasn't being more helpful, she admitted that she's been suffering from depression and just narrowly avoided overdosing the prior evening. Her husband walked out 2 weeks ago, leaving her with a 2-year-old son. She said she's finding it more and more difficult to find a reason to want to live. She begged me not to share what she confided in me because at least for the present she needs this job.

Effective Noticing (Cues)

1. What did you notice about the situation initially? What information/observations are significant? What information deviates from what is expected/normal/usual?

Effective Interpreting

2. How would you describe and prioritize the obligations you have in this scenario to respect your preceptor's request to not divulge what she told you "confidentially" with your obligation to get her help? Do you have an obligation to inform the charge nurse of the unit? Are your preceptor's depression and thoughts of suicide affecting patient care? Do you have obligations to yourself and your own well-being?
3. If you cannot fulfill each of these obligations, how will you prioritize them? What basis/rationale do you use for prioritization? Remember that the ANA *Code of Ethics for Nurses* reminds us that "the nurse's primary commitment is to the patient," while at the same time states that "the nurse owes the same duties to self as to others, including the responsibility to promote health and safety, preserve wholeness of character and integrity, maintain competence, and continue personal and professional growth."
4. What do you know about the suicide rate among nurses? What are the warning signs, and how can nurse colleagues be most helpful? What are the modifiable workplace issues that can be addressed to reduce suicide risk?

Scenario

Now I am really feeling overwhelmed, and I have patients to take care of. I decided that dealing with her suicidal thoughts was "above my pay grade" and went to the charge nurse. I was not sure if violating her request to keep this private was the right thing to do. I sure didn't want to feel responsible for her suicide should this happen.

Effective Responding

5. My nurse manager told me about a previous workplace where physicians within his organization had partnered with the American Foundation of Suicide Prevention (AFSP.org) to develop the first physician suicide prevention program in 2009 following similar circumstances. The Healer Education Assessment and Referral (HEAR) program educated clinicians about mental health issues and professional risks and assessed colleagues to detect those in need of help (Moutier et al., 2012; Norcross et al., 2018). They partnered to extend the program to nurses. Now, 4 years later, they identify approximately 40 nurses a year who are high risk and actively expressing suicidality and refer them into treatment. This program also has the potential to identify nurses with substance use disorder and refer them anonymously into treatment while maintaining their license, job, and professional identity. What other resources can you access to better inform your decision?
6. Whether or not you decide to inform the charge nurse, how might you use reflective practice to evaluate your decision so you can respond more confidently in the future? What criteria will you use to evaluate a good response?
7. What personal attributes and competencies are most likely to lead to a good response?

Effective Reflecting

8. Do you agree with the choice the nurse made? Would you have made the same choice? Why or why not? What would inform your decision?
9. How do you evaluate your professional and moral judgments?

Thoughtful Person-Centered Practice: Challenging Topics *(Continued)*

Reflection-on-Action

Then look back at the nurse's decisions and reflect on your learning—how did your knowledge and/or skills expand based on this scenario? What attitude, value, or belief shifts did you experience (if any) after reading this scenario? What would you do differently if you were in this situation? What more do you need to know to be able to manage this or a similar situation in the future?

Nielson, A., Stragnell, S., & Jester, P. (2007). Guide for reflection using the Clinical Judgment Model. *Journal of Nursing Education, 46*(11), 513–516.

Tanner, C. A. (2006). Thinking like a nurse: a research-based model of clinical judgment in nursing. *Journal of Nursing Education, 45*(6), 204–211.

Suicide Resources

Davidson, J. E. (2/20/2020). *Suicide in nursing: We are at risk. Sigma Reflection on Nursing Leadership.* https://www.reflectionsonnursingleadership.org/features/more-features/suicide-in-nursing

Davidson, J. E., Accardi, R., Sanchez, C., & Zisook, S. (2020). Nurse suicide: Prevention and grief management. *American Nurse Today, 15*(1), 1–6.

Davidson, J. E., Choflet, A., Earley, M. M., Clark, P., Dilks, S., Morrow, L., Tucker, S., & Mims, T. (2021). Nurse suicide prevention starts with crisis intervention. *American Nurse Journal, 16*(2), 14–18.

Howard, M. S., Buck, M., Carpenter, H., & McMillan, K. (2021). Navigating the loss and grief of a nurse suicide. *American Nurse Journal, 16*(3), 14–16.

Montalvo, W. (2020). Caring counts. Preventing suicide among nurses. *American Nurse Journal, 15*(2), 3227.

Moutier, C., Norcross, W., Jong, P., Norman, M., Kirby, B., McGuire, T., & Zisook, S. (2012). The suicide prevention and depression awareness program at the University of California, San Diego School of Medicine. *Academic Medicine, 87*(3), 320–326.

Norcross, W. A., Moutier, C., Tiamson-Kassab, M., Jong, P., Davidson, J. E., Lee, K., & Zisook, S. (2018). Update on the UC San Diego Healer Education Assessment and Referral (HEAR) Program. *Journal of Medical Regulation, 104*(2), 17–26.

Patrician, P. A., Petersen, C., & McGuinness, T. M. (2020). Suicide among RNs: An analysis of 2015 data from the National Violent Death Reporting System. *American Journal of Nursing, 120*(10), 24–28.

closely involved with discharge plans, length-of-stay issues, and insurance constraints (Stachowiak & Bugel, 2013). Refer to Chapters 11 and 12 for additional discussions regarding case management.

Delegating Nursing Care

New graduate nurses use leadership techniques when they direct the work of nonprofessional staff and volunteers and when they delegate tasks to nonprofessional staff. These people, who are unlicensed and function in an assistive role to RNs, are referred to as AP by the ANA, replacing the former term, nursing assistive personnel (NAP). AP may include nurses' aides, certified nursing assistants, or other unlicensed caregivers within the health care environment.

In 2019, ANA issued a Joint Statement on Delegation with the National Council of State Boards of Nursing (https://www.ncsbn.org/Delegation_joint_statement_NCSBN-ANA.pdf). **Delegation** involves the transfer of responsibility for the performance of an activity to another person while retaining accountability for the outcome. It is a critical competency and essential skill for an RN in today's health care environment. RNs may never delegate any elements of the nursing process itself.

QSEN SAFETY

Nurses are responsible for minimizing the risk of harm to patients and providers through both system effectiveness and individual performance. You want to be sure when delegating nursing responsibilities to AP that they are prepared to safely assume this function and that your state nursing practice act and facility policies approve this delegation.

The ANA, which is committed to monitoring the regulation, education, and use of AP, recommends adherence to 10 broad principles guiding RNs prior to delegating care. In addition to the RN's responsibility, several principles focus on the accountability of the health care organization. Organizational accountability for delegation relates to providing sufficient resources, including:

- Sufficient staffing with an appropriate staff mix
- Documenting competencies for all staff providing direct patient care and for ensuring that the RN has access to competence information for the staff to whom the RN is delegating care
- Organizational policies on delegation are developed with the active participation of all nurses and acknowledge that delegation is a professional right and responsibility.

Initially, the RN must be fully aware of the parameters for delegation as outlined in their state's Nurse Practice Act as well as the employing organization's policies and procedures regarding delegation (Daley, 2013). As a general rule, you should not delegate the assessment, planning, and evolution steps of the nursing process. AP can collect patient data but only the nurse can interpret this data. This means that professional nurses are responsible for the initial patient assessment, discharge planning, health education, care planning, triage, interpretation of patient data, care of invasive lines, administering parenteral medications. What you can delegate are assistance with basic care activities (bathing, grooming, ambulation, feeding) and things like taking vital signs, measuring intake and output, weighing, simple dressing changes, transfers, and postmortem care. Facilities are responsible for ensuring that AP are qualified and capable of performing nursing tasks that RNs may delegate to them. RNs should have involvement in the development of facility policies regarding delegation and also have access to any information regarding competency of the AP on their team.

Before the RN delegates any nursing intervention, a number of additional factors, including the qualifications and capabilities of the AP, should be considered: (1) the stability of the patient's condition, (2) the complexity of the activity to be delegated, (3) the potential for harm, (4) the predictability of the outcome, and (5) the overall context of other patient needs. The RN remains accountable for any delegated nursing care or outcomes and is responsible for the supervision of the AP to whom tasks are delegated. AP need an awareness of any patient precautions, when to seek assistance, and what should immediately be reported to the RN. Inappropriate delegation decisions can jeopardize the safety of patients and endanger a nurse's professional practice.

Concept Mastery Alert

Even if a task is delegatable, AP are not permitted to perform it independently. Your hospital may allow AP to ambulate patients, but only you can decide if your AP should ambulate a particular patient at a particular time.

Delegation skills must be developed, practiced, and strengthened. Nurse educators are encouraged by the ANA to integrate principles for delegation into the curriculum and ensure that nursing students have opportunities to practice delegation skills. Chapter 18 has additional information on delegation and the student nurse. Professional development offerings assist RNs to develop critical thinking skills that promote good judgment and provide strategies to delegate effectively. Experienced and reliable AP who perform delegated skills competently allow RNs to focus more on assessment and development or revision of the nursing care plan and learn skills that improve their nursing practice. The Decision Tree for Delegation by Registered Nurses distributed by the ANA and NCSBN is a helpful guide for nurses who are learning to delegate (Fig. 10-4). Refer to Chapter 18 for additional information on nursing delegation, including the five rights of delegation. Gradually, new nurses assume increased leadership responsibilities as they become primary nurses, case managers, or unit coordinators. An understanding of the function and organization of both the nursing department and health care organization is required to be an effective leader.

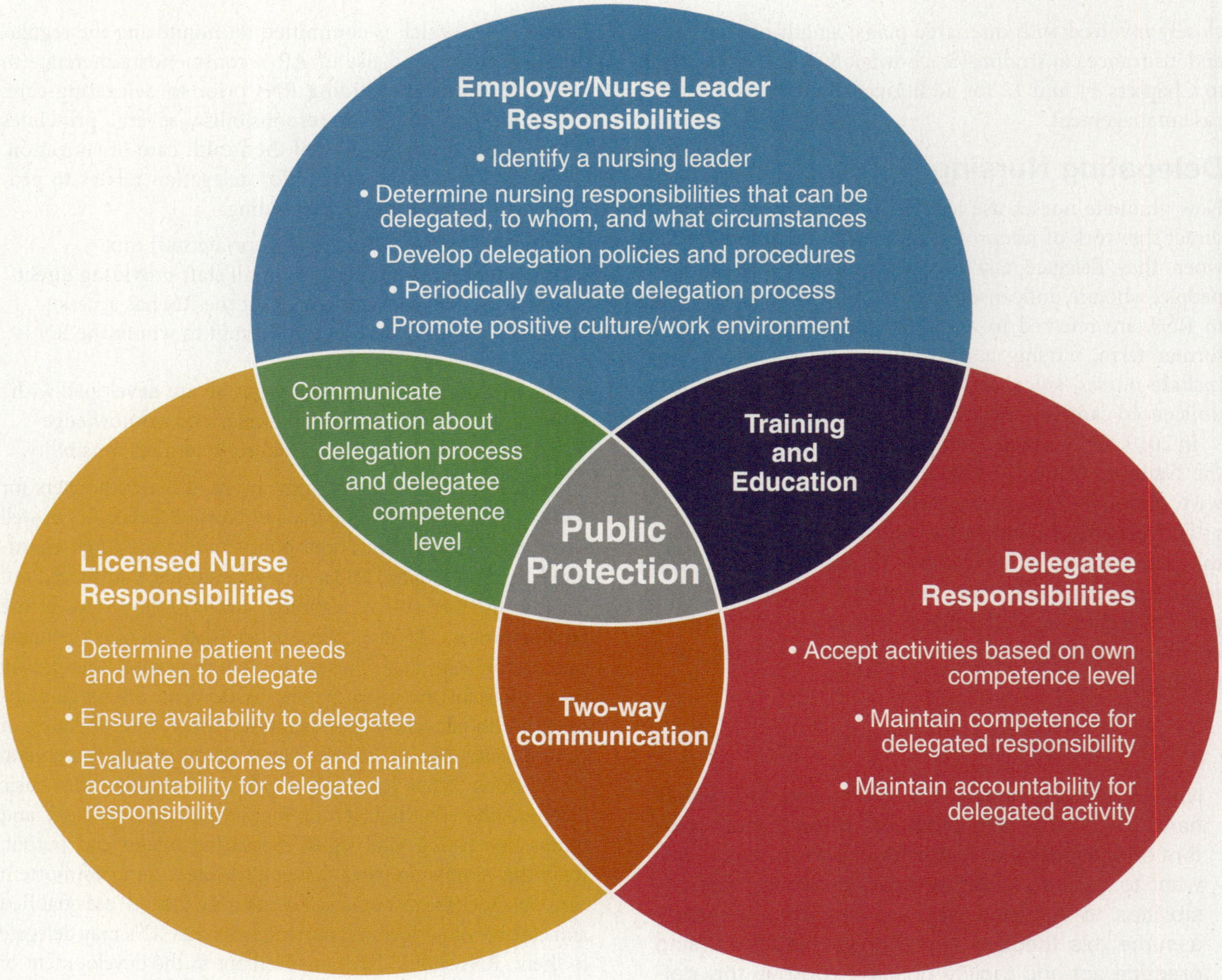
Employer/Nurse Leader Responsibilities
• Identify a nursing leader
• Determine nursing responsibilities that can be delegated, to whom, and what circumstances
• Develop delegation policies and procedures
• Periodically evaluate delegation process
• Promote positive culture/work environment
Communicate information about delegation process and delegatee competence level
Training and Education
Public Protection
Licensed Nurse Responsibilities
• Determine patient needs and when to delegate
• Ensure availability to delegatee
• Evaluate outcomes of and maintain accountability for delegated responsibility
Two-way communication
Delegatee Responsibilities
• Accept activities based on own competence level
• Maintain competence for delegated responsibility
• Maintain accountability for delegated activity

FIGURE 10-4. Joint Statement on Delegation. (*Source:* Used with permission. NCSBN Board of Directors/ANA Board of Directors. 2019. National guidelines for Nursing Delegation. To read the entire statement, go to https://www.ncsbn.org/NGND-PosPaper_06.pdf)

Knowledge of the Administrative Structure

Nursing Department

The nursing team can also be viewed in the broader context of the entire nursing department of a health care institution or facility. Nurses should have an interest in the functioning of the department. Using this knowledge, nurses can seek information or change through appropriate channels. The more nurses understand how the nursing department runs, the better able they are to work constructively to meet the department's objectives.

Employing Institution or Facility

Nurses at all levels need to be knowledgeable about the administrative structure and functions of their employing institution or facility. When problems arise concerning professional, unit, departmental, or institutional or facility objectives, nurses must be able to use the proper channels of communication and refer problems up the chain of command. For example, if a nurse believes that work assignments are routinely incompatible with basic patient safety and quality but gets no response after discussing this with an immediate nursing supervisor, the nurse should take those complaints to the director of nursing. If the director of nursing fails to respond adequately, the nurse should determine to whom the director of nursing reports and should approach that person. Similarly, a nurse concerned about medical care should first approach the attending physician. If the attending physician fails to respond, the nurse must then contact the nursing coordinator and, in consultation with the nursing coordinator, approach the medical director. The structure of these channels is shown in the facility's organization chart, which details the relationships among the various administrative positions, departments, and job titles. Sometimes, the nurse is referred to committees that deal with specific issues.

Support for Leadership Training

Nurses intent on developing their leadership ability have multiple resources available to them—mentorship, preceptorship, participation in professional organizations, and continuing education.

Mentorship

Mentorship is a relationship in which an experienced person (the mentor) advises and assists a less experienced person (protégé). This is an effective way of easing a new nurse into leadership responsibilities. Mentors link with protégés by common interest and provide support, information, and network links. The relationship does not include financial reward.

Mentors should be excellent role models. If you find a nurse with expertise in practice or topics that interest you, you can ask if they would be interested in becoming your mentor. The advantages of having an effective mentor are many. Ideally, good mentors can suggest options for your growth and development and identify helpful resources. Good mentors will welcome your questions and provide honest feedback on your progress. Many nurses who are passionate about nursing and the profession's future are happy to share what brings meaning and purpose to their lives.

Mentorship is valuable in all types of nursing positions. As a nurse climbs the ladder of leadership responsibility, a mentor who is experienced in management and administrative functions may be of great assistance. A mentor can be key in helping a less experienced nurse assume added responsibilities and position changes. Many mentorship relationships also become lasting friendships.

Preceptorship

An alternative model for leadership training is preceptorship. The preceptor (experienced nurse) is selected (and generally paid) to introduce an employee to new responsibilities through teaching and guidance. This orientation ensures that the new RN gains the appropriate knowledge, skills, and support to care for patients safely and efficiently. Preceptors also assist new RNs to learn the policies and procedures of a new facility and can serve as a mentor by modeling excellent nursing practice. The relationship is limited by the new employee's needs. When you are ready to select your first professional nursing position you will want to carefully evaluate how different institutions orient new nurses. You may also find it helpful to explore student internships in a setting or specialty of interest (Fig. 10-5).

Participation in Nursing and Other Professional Organizations

The many nursing organizations at the international, national, state, district, and local levels are discussed in Chapter 1. They are major forces for nursing leadership and have active groups throughout the United States and abroad. The more than 100 professional organizations address specialty interests, goals, and purposes, as well as advocate for

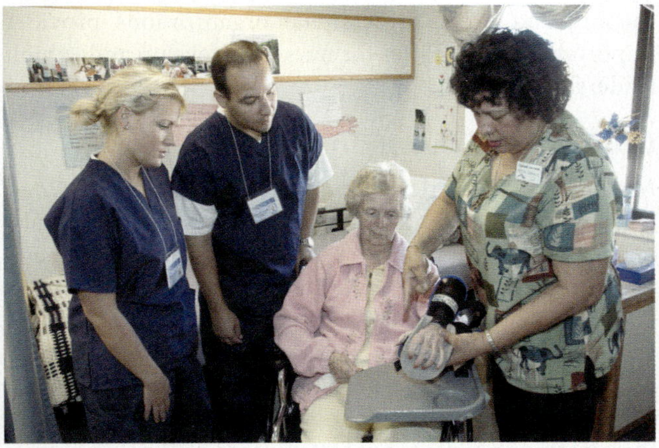

FIGURE 10-5. The nurse preceptor advises and teaches nursing students by example. (*Source:* Used with permission from Shutterstock. Photo by Joe Mitchell.)

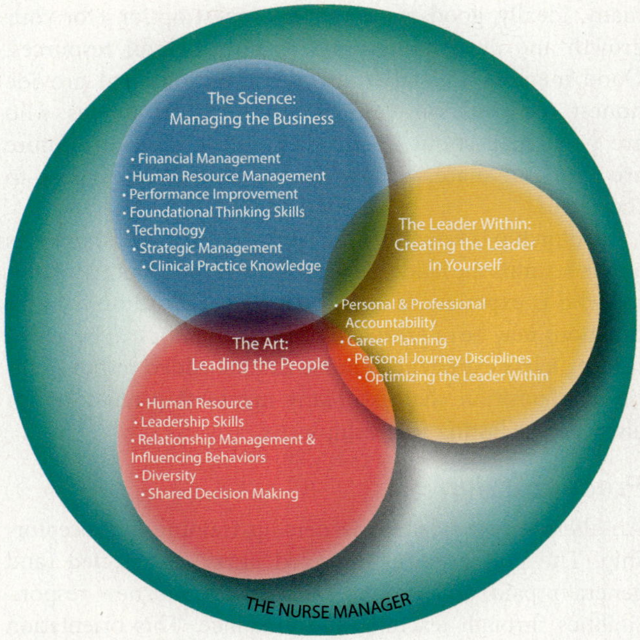

FIGURE 10-6. Nurse manager learning domain framework. (© 2006 Nurse Manager Leadership Partnership. By the American Organization for Nursing Leadership [AONL]. [2015]. Executives [AONE]. All rights reserved.)

nurses and nursing. Representatives of these nursing organizations also work with ANA lobbyists in Congress and state legislatures regarding nursing concerns, health care issues, and quality care.

The AONE, now the American Organization for Nursing Leadership (AONL), recognizing the need for leadership development for nurse managers, united with the American Association of Critical-Care Nurses (AACN) and the Association of periOperative Registered Nurses (AORN) to develop a model that includes content on the science and art of management for nurses, and creation of the leader within yourself (Fig. 10-6) (AONE, 2012). This model is intended to engage nurses in exploring potential solutions to achieve their management goals.

Nursing leadership can define what the future should look like and help make it happen. Participation in nursing and other professional organizations provides important opportunities for nurses to develop and exhibit leadership.

Continuing Education

Many programs for developing leadership, managerial, and administrative skills are available to nurses. Courses can be taken by correspondence or over the Internet. Periodicals and books also provide continuing education for emerging leaders. Many continuing education programs are available to prepare nurses before they assume higher levels of leadership; some are geared to nurses already in such positions. Nurses should choose a program that matches their learning needs. Many State Boards of Nursing require evidence of continuing education credits prior to renewal of RN licenses.

Developing Resilience

Every nurse needs to be a leader to make health care work for those who need it. Nursing is often hard work, and at times the challenges can be daunting. Never has it been more important for nurses who are passionate about patients, families, and communities, as well as their own health, to be intentional about developing resilience—the capacity to thrive not only in spite of, but because of, challenges. Here are a few hints for developing resilience:

- Begin and end the day with gratitude.
- Practice mindfulness: What is the most important thing right now? See Chapter 1.
- Appreciate that all humans are limited; some things can't be "fixed."
- Appreciate the power of connectedness and presence.
- Stop frequently to stretch and take deep diaphragmatic breaths.
- Reflect frequently on what brings you joy, makes you smile.
- Keep a positive, hopeful outlook. Hope allows us to envision a positive future and work to bring this into being.

A piece in *The New York Times* during the pandemic (Zimmerman, 2020) lists optimism (that is also realistic), a moral compass, religious or spiritual beliefs, cognitive and emotional flexibility, and social connectedness as the tools common to resilient people. Most important among these are the quality of our close personal relationships, especially with parents and primary caregivers.

Nurse Self-Care Alert

During the pandemic, we learned anew how important resilience is for all health care professionals. How many of the practices that promote resilience have you incorporated into your life? Do you have a positive vision for the future that you are working to achieve, and are you making time to nourish supportive close personal relationships?

Leadership and Advancing Clinician Well-Being

As the National Academy of Sciences, Engineering, and Medicine make clear, patient-centered, high-quality care relies on the well-being, health, and safety of health care clinicians. Its 2019 report, *Taking action against clinical burnout*, makes clinicians' well-being a priority for every health care professional leader, citing how the alarmingly high rates of **clinician burnout** in the United States, including that of nurses, are detrimental to the quality of care being provided, harmful to individuals in the workforce, and costly. Key messages from the report include:

- Clinician burnout—a workplace syndrome resulting from chronic job stress—is a major problem across the nation. Substantial symptoms are present in 35% to 54% of nurses and physicians, and 45% to 60% of medical students and residents. Current understanding suggests that burnout is a growing public health concern among all types of clinicians and learners.

- Burnout has high personal costs for individual clinicians and learners as well as high social and economic costs for their organizations and society as a whole. Burnout threatens the successful achievement of important health care quality goals: better care, improved population health, and lower health care costs. Mitigating clinician burnout and supporting professional well-being is essential to providing high-quality patient care.
- Emotional exhaustion, depersonalization, and loss of sense of professional efficacy—the three dimensions of burnout—are a barrier to professional well-being. Although the absence of burnout does not equate to a state of professional well-being, addressing the factors contributing to burnout and the barriers to well-being is critical to reaching the goal of professional well-being among clinicians. This will ultimately help health systems improve patients', families', and clinicians' experiences and outcomes.

Nurse leaders are fortunate to have excellent resources to address how we can create supportive work environments to prevent clinician burnout and distress. Read more about the American Association of Critical Care Nurses *Standards for Establishing and Sustaining Healthy Work Environments* in Chapter 19 and check the AONL's Elements of a Healthy Practice Environment at: https://www.aonl.org/elements-healthy-practice-environment. You will also want to be familiar with the ANCC's Pathways to Excellence. This program acknowledges that nurses operate on the frontlines of health care, dedicating their working lives to protecting promoting, and improving health care for all. To do this to the best of their ability, they need to operate in an environment that supports their own needs and promotes high standards (https://www.nursingworld.org/organizational-programs/pathway/overview/). Read Pabico (2020) for a discussion titled "Dispelling common myths about ANCC's Pathway to Excellence."

The authors of this text celebrate the leadership potential in every nurse and our profession's ability to be the critical difference for those in need.

DEVELOPING CLINICAL REASONING AND CLINICAL JUDGMENT

1. Interview several experienced nurses and ask them what qualities make for the best nursing leaders. Reflect on your personal experience in groups (e.g., within your family, church, school, community). Identify the roles you characteristically assume and what qualities you bring to the group (e.g., enthusiasm, positive thinking, vision, self-direction). Consider whether those qualities will serve you well in professional nursing groups and situations. Are there new qualities you need to develop if you want to become an effective nurse leader? Why?
2. Identify a situation in your class or school that "cried out for change." Discuss with your classmates which students emerged as leaders to address the need for change. Review and critique the steps they engaged in to bring about change. See if your group can reach consensus about the adequacy of their leadership behaviors.
3. Identify a health challenge where you live. Examples include things like increases in the suicide rate and opioid addiction, inadequate mental health services, and disparities in access to needed health services. Brainstorm with your classmates how nurse leaders might effectively address these challenges and become a catalyst for needed change.

PRACTICING FOR NCLEX

1. A charge nurse on the step-down unit will likely use which leadership style during resuscitation efforts for a cardiac arrest?
   a. Democratic
   b. Laissez-faire
   c. Servant
   d. Autocratic
2. A chief nursing officer with a transformational leadership style is developing a plan for success to obtain Magnet status. What are the most appropriate strategies for the leader to use? Select all that apply.
   a. Sharing their vision of excellence in patient care and high-level education
   b. Encouraging nurses to incorporate evidence-based practice through hospital committees and to join nursing organizations
   c. Promoting compliance by reminding subordinates that they have a good salary and working conditions
   d. Ensuring employees are kept abreast of new developments in their department and the larger organization
   e. Writing the Magnet application and supporting documentation with limited input from the nursing staff
   f. Encouraging nurse managers and nurses to self-schedule as long as proper coverage is maintained
3. After observing conflicts between nurses about scheduling, a nurse manager compliments the nurses for achieving the monthly goal of no patient falls. What strategy for conflict resolution did the manager display?
   a. Collaborating
   b. Competing
   c. Compromising
   d. Smoothing

4. A nurse who is considered a servant leader is working in an economically depressed community setting up a free mobile health clinic. Which actions best exemplify a servant leader? Select all that apply.
   a. Motivating coworkers to solicit funding to set up the clinic
   b. Setting only realistic goals that are present oriented and easily achieved
   c. Forming an autocratic governing body to keep the project on track
   d. Spending time with supporters to help them grow in their roles
   e. Ensuring that other's lowest priority needs are served
   f. Prizing leadership because of the need to serve others
5. A nurse manager is planning to update a health care provider's office from paper to electronic health records (EHR) by using the eight-step process for planned change. Place the following actions in the order in which they should be initiated:
   a. The nurse devises a plan to switch to EHR.
   b. The nurse records the time spent on written records versus EHR.
   c. The nurse attains approval from management for new computers.
   d. The nurse analyzes all options for converting to EHR.
   e. The nurse installs new computers and provides an in-service for the staff.
   f. The nurse explores possible barriers to changing to EHR.
   g. The nurse follows up with the staff to check compliance with the new system.
   h. The nurse evaluates the effects of changing to EHR.
6. A nurse manager who is working to institute the SBAR communication process for all health care providers is meeting resistance to the change. How does the manager best approach the resistance?
   a. Containing the anxiety in a small group and moving forward with the initiative
   b. Explaining the change and listing the advantages to the person and the organization
   c. Reprimanding those who oppose the new initiative and praising those who willingly accept the change
   d. Quickly introducing the change and involving staff in implementation of the change
7. A nurse is asked to act as a mentor to a new nurse. What action will the mentor expect to perform?
   a. Accepting payment to introduce the new nurse to their responsibilities
   b. Hiring the new nurse and assigning duties related to the position
   c. Enabling the new nurse to participate in professional organizations
   d. Advising and assisting the new nurse to adjust to the work environment of a busy emergency department
8. An RN on a telemetry unit is falling behind while performing assessments and administering medications. Which task can the nurse safely delegate to the AP?
   a. Assessing a patient who has just arrived on the unit
   b. Teaching a patient with newly diagnosed diabetes about foot care
   c. Documenting a patient's I & O in the electronic health record
   d. Helping a postoperative patient out of bed for the first time
9. Nursing students enrolled in a leadership and management course attend clinical on a surgical unit. As they are planning their day, they note one student has a complex patient with multiple medications and the need for frequent turning, pressure injury wound care, and tube feedings. Which action by the group best reflects effective teamwork and coordination?
   a. Asking patients to prioritize what they want to accomplish each day
   b. Including a "nice to do" for every "need to do" task on the list
   c. "Front loading" their schedules with "must do" priorities
   d. Scheduling times to assist the student with the complex patient
10. The nurses at an acute care hospital participate in a committee focused on achieving Magnet status. Which action do the nurses suggest to help achieve this goal?
    a. Centralizing the decision-making and scheduling process
    b. Promoting self-governance at the unit level
    c. Deterring professional autonomy to promote teamwork
    d. Promoting evidence-based practice over innovative nursing practice
11. A nursing student is actively working toward strengthening their leadership skills. What action will best assist the student to meet this goal?
    a. Being self-reliant in solving problems
    b. Being self-directed and asking for assistance when needed
    c. Using written communication instead of face-to-face communication
    d. Reporting nurses who do not follow policies to the nurse manager
12. A nurse erroneously administered two tablets of acetaminophen totaling 650 mg to their patient. When reporting this to the nurse manager, the nurse states, "there are two tablets in a package labeled '325 mg. acetaminophen.' The prescription reads 'administer

325 mg of acetaminophen;' therefore, I administered what was in the package." Based on a philosophy of just culture, what should happen next?
a. The nurse should be found at fault for not clarifying the order.
b. The package labeling should be reviewed with the pharmacy.
c. The nurse should be disciplined.
d. No follow-up is needed as the medication is over the counter.

13. Nursing students enrolled in a leadership and management course discuss the roles of the nurse manager during post conference. What roles should the students include in the discussion? Select all that apply.
a. Developing and overseeing a unit budget for staff and patient care
b. Hiring, evaluating, and promoting staff growth
c. Performing patient care
d. Developing treatment plans to improve care and patient outcomes
e. Handling escalating situations between caregivers and patients

ANSWERS WITH RATIONALES

1. **d.** Autocratic leadership assumes control over the decisions and activities of the group, such as taking charge of emergencies, dictating schedules and work responsibilities, and scheduling mandatory in-service training. Polling other nurses is an example of democratic leadership, which is characterized by a sense of equality among the leader and other participants, with decisions and activities being shared. In laissez-faire leadership, the leader relinquishes power to the group and encourages independent activity by group members. Examples of laissez-faire leadership style are allowing the nurses to divide up the tasks and encouraging them to work independently.

2. **a, b.** Transformational leaders inspire, motivate, create intellectually stimulating practice environments, and challenge themselves and others to grow personally and professionally. They demonstrate caring and vulnerability, communicating honestly and openly. They are risk takers and pay attention to process as well as outcomes. Instituting a reward program and reminding workers that they have a good salary and working conditions are examples of transactional leadership, which is based on a task-and-reward orientation. Ensuring that employees keep abreast of new developments in nursing care is a characteristic of quantum leadership. The group and leader work together to accomplish mutually set goals and outcomes with the democratic leadership style, and the laissez-faire style encourages independent activity by group members, such as setting their own schedules and work activities.

3. **d.** The manager who avoids conflict by complimenting the parties and avoids disagreements is using smoothing to reduce the emotion of the conflict. The original conflict is rarely resolved with this technique. Collaborating is a joint effort to resolve the conflict with a win–win solution. All parties set aside previously determined goals, determine a priority common goal, and accept mutual responsibility for achieving this goal. Competing results is a win for one party at the expense of the other group. Compromising occurs when both parties relinquish something of equal value.

4. **a, d, f.** To serve as servant leaders, nurses need to invest in those who support the organization's values, show passion, can play to their strengths, and demonstrate a positive attitude. They should develop their vision to see the future related to a current anticipated need and motivate others to follow and engage. They also need to provide ongoing opportunities for collaborations, sharing, reflection, encouragement, and celebration as well as hard work. The servant leader allows others to have a voice, to exercise control, and to practice leading themselves. The servant first makes sure that other people's highest priority needs are being served. The best test, and most difficult to administer, is: Do those served grow as people? Do they, while being served, become healthier, wiser, freer, more autonomous, more likely themselves to become servants?

5. **b, f, d, c, a, e, h, g.** Planned change involves the following steps: (1) recognize symptoms that indicate a change is needed and collect data, (2) identify a problem to be solved through change, (3) determine and analyze alternative solutions, (4) select a course of action from possible solutions, (5) plan for making the change, (6) implement the change, (7) evaluate the change, and (8) stabilize the change.

6. **b.** Change is ubiquitous, as is resistance to change. The manager should explain the proposed change to all affected, list the advantages of the proposed change for all parties, introduce the change gradually, and involve everyone affected by the change in the design and implementation of the process. The manager should not use the reward/punishment style to overcome resistance to change.

7. **d.** Mentorship is a relationship in which an experienced person (the mentor) advises and assists a less experienced person (protégé). This is an effective way of easing a new nurse into leadership responsibilities. An experienced nurse who is paid to introduce an employee to new responsibilities through teaching and guidance describes a preceptor, not a mentor. The nurse mentor does not hire or schedule new nurses. Nurses do not need mentors to join professional organizations.

8. **c.** Documenting a patient's I & O on a flow chart does not require professional judgment and can be delegated to AP. Professional nurses are responsible for the initial patient assessment, discharge planning, health education, care planning, triage, interpretation of patient data, care of invasive lines, administering parenteral medications. What they can delegate are assistance with basic care activities (bathing, grooming, ambulation, feeding) and things like taking vital signs, measuring intake and output, weighing, simple dressing changes, transfers, and postmortem care.

9. **d.** The students use teamwork and collaboration to appropriately coordinate patient care; this is the best response. By asking the patient to prioritize what they want to accomplish each day, the nurse is demonstrating an effective time management technique. To manage time, the nurse should establish goals and priorities for each day, differentiating "need

to do" from "nice to do" tasks; the nurse should include the patient in this process. The nurse should also establish a time line, allocating priorities to hours in the workday in to keep track of falling behind and correct the problem before the day is lost.

10. **b**. Magnet hospitals use a decentralized decision-making process, self-governance at the unit level, and respect for and acknowledgment of professional autonomy. In Magnet hospitals, 14 characteristics, the Forces of Magnetism, have been recognized that identify quality patient care, excellent nursing care, and innovations in professional nursing practice.

11. **b.** Leader behavior includes being self-directed and knowing your limitations; demonstrating a commitment to excellence; having a clear vision and strategic focus that allow movement forward toward a creative solution; showing commitment to and passion for your work; and displaying problem-solving skills, trustworthiness and integrity, respectfulness, accessibility, empathy and caring, desire to be of service, and responsibility to enhance the personal growth of all staff.

12. **b.** A just culture is committed to accountability and safety. Nurses are encouraged to disclose clinical errors and potential error situations without the fear of punitive actions, allowing others to learn from this experience. Health care workers within the organization discuss concerns and challenges related to patient care, turning them into opportunities for improvement.

13. **a, b, e.** Responsibilities of the nurse manager include overseeing day-to-day operations, designing and managing a budget, supervising and providing training to team members, hiring and evaluating nursing staff, handling escalating situations between patients and health care providers, and collaborating to attain optimal patient outcomes. Nurse managers' roles do not typically include performing patient care or developing treatment plans.

Bibliography

Alvoet, P. E. (2019). Should you pursue leadership? 10 questions to help you decide. *American Nurse Today, 14*(1), 51–53.

American Association of Colleges of Nursing (AACN). (2012). *Leading initiatives: Frequently asked questions.* https://www.aacnnursing.org/cnl/about/faqs

American Nurses Association (ANA). (n.d.). *Care coordination and the essential role of nurses.* http://www.nursingworld.org/care-coordination

American Nurses Association (ANA). (2012). *News release: American Nurses Association urges recognition and funding for nurses' essential role in patient care coordination.* https://www.nursingworld.org/practice-policy/nursing-excellence/official-position-statements/id/care-coordination-and-registered-nurses-essential-role/

American Nurses Association (ANA). (2021). *Nursing: Scope and standards of practice: Nursing* (4th ed.). Author.

American Nurses Association (ANA) and the National Council on of State Boards of Nursing (NCSBN). (n.d.). *Joint statement on delegation.* https://www.ncsbn.org/Delegation_joint_statement_NCSBN-ANA.pdf

American Nurses Credentialing Center (ANCC). (2013). *Magnet model.* https://www.nursingworld.org/organizational-programs/magnet/

American Organization of Nurse Executives (AONE). (2012). *NMLP learning domain framework.* http://www.aone.org/resources/nurse-manager-leadership-partnership

American Organization for Nursing Leadership (AONL). (2019). *Elements of a healthy practice environment.* https://www.aonl.org/system/files/media/file/2020/02/elements-healthy-practice-environment_1.pdf

American Organization of Nurse Executives. (2015). *AONE nurse manager competencies.* Author. http://www.aone.org/resources/nurse-leader-competencies.shtml

Bashaw, E. (2011). Fusing Magnet® and just culture. *American Nurse Today, 6*(9), 42–45.

Bashaw, E., Rosenstein, A., & Lounsbury, K. (2012). Culture trifecta: Building the infrastructure for Magnet® and just culture. *American Nurse Today, 7*(9), 36–41.

Bond, M. J., & Birkholz, L. J. (2020). What if the bully is the manager? *Nursing, 50*(3), 48–52.

Brown, B. (2018). *Dare to lead.* Random House.

Cipriano, P. F. (2017). How do we manage in uncertain times? *American Nurse Today, 12*(2), 33.

Clavell, J. T., & Prado-Inzerillo, M. (2018). Inspire others through transformational leadership. *American Nurse Today, 13*(11), 39–41.

Covey, S. (1999). *The seven habits of highly effective people.* Simon and Schuster.

Curtin, L. (2013). Quantum leadership: Upside down. *American Nurse Today, 8*(3), 56.

Daley, K. (2013). Helping nurses strengthen their delegation skills. *American Nurse Today, 8*(3), 18.

Dark, T., & Ellis, W. M. (2020). Level loading nurse assignments based on the work intensity. *American Nurse Journal, 15*(1), 46–49.

Davidson, J. E., Choflet, A., Earley, M. M., Clark, P., Dilks, S., Morrow, L., Tucker, S., & Mims, T. (2021). Nurse suicide prevention starts with crisis intervention. *American Nurse Journal, 16*(2), 14–18.

Demming, J. D., & O'Neill, L. (2020). Leaders' role in stopping workplace violence. *American Nurse Journal, 15*(9), 66–68.

Drucker, P. F. (1999). Managing oneself. *Harvard Business Review, 77*(2), 64–74, 185.

Edmonson, C., & Weberg, D. (2019). Leadership styles that promote innovation. *American Nurse Today, 14*(7), 21–23.

Fahlberg, B., & Toomey, R. (2016). Servant leadership: A model for emerging nurse leaders. *Nursing, 46*(10), 49–52.

Ferguson, R. (2018). Care coordination at the end of life: The nurse's role. *Nursing, 48*(2), 11–13.

Gelinas, L. (2020). Mentors: Learning from experts and expert teams. *American Nurse Journal, 15*(4), 4.

Gerardi, D. (2015a). Conflict engagement: Emotional and social intelligence. *The American Journal of Nursing, 115*(8), 60–65.

Gerardi, D. (2015b). Conflict engagement: Creating connection and cultivating curiosity. *The American Journal of Nursing, 115*(9), 60–65.

Goleman, D. (2005). *Emotional intelligence. The 10th Anniversary Edition.* Bantam Books.

Greenleaf, R. K. (2002). *Servant leadership: A journey into the nature of legitimate power and greatness.* Paulist Press.

Hawkins, J. E., & Shell, A. (2012). Magnet® hospitals are attracted to the BSN but what's in it for nurses? *Nursing, 42*(3), 50–52.

Hicks, T. P., Sullivan, M., Sexton, J. B., & Adair, K. C. (2019). Transforming culture through resilience and teamwork. *American Nurse Today, 14*(2), 41–43.

Howard, M. S., Buck, M., Carpenter, H., & McMillan, K. (2021). Navigating the loss and grief of a nurse suicide. *American Nurse Journal, 16*(3), 14–16.

Institute of Medicine (IOM). (2010). *The future of nursing:Leading change, advancing health.* http://www.nationalacademies.org/hmd/Reports/2010/The-Future-of-Nursing-Leading-Change-Advancing-Health.aspx

Johansen, M. (2012). Keeping the peace: Conflict management strategies for nurse managers. *Nursing Management, 43*(2), 50–54.

Keasler, T. (2013). Nurse residency program empowers new grads. *The American Nurse, 45*(4), 13.

Kerfoot, K. (2020). Patient-centered staffing as the path forward. *American Nurse Today, 14*(9), 87–90.

Kotter, J. (1996). *Leading change.* Harvard Business School Press.

Leis, S. J., & Anderson, A. (2020). Time management strategies for new nurses. *American Journal of Nursing, 120*(12), 63–66.

Lewin, K. (1951). *Field theory in social science.* Harper & Row.

Marquis, B. L., & Huston, C. J. (2017). *Leadership roles and management functions in nursing: theory and application* (9th ed., pp. 558–559). Wolters Kluwer.

Monroe, M., Morse, E., & Price, J. M. (2020) The relationship between critical care work environment and professional quality of life. *American Journal of Critical Care, 29*(2), 145–149.

National Academies of Sciences, Engineering, and Medicine. (2019). *Taking action against clinician burnout: A systems approach to professional well-being. The National Academies Press.* https://doi.org/10.17226/25521.

National Council of State Boards of Nursing. (2016). National guidelines for nursing delegation. *Journal of Nursing Regulation, 7*(1), 5–14.

Northouse, P. G. (2019). *Leadership and practice*, 8th ed. Sage.

Pabico, C., & Graystone, R. (2018). Comparing Pathway to Excellence® and Magnet Recognition® Programs. *American Nurse Today, 13*(3), 46–48.

Pabico, C. (2020). Dispelling common myths about ANCC's Pathway to Excellence. *American Nurse.* https://www.myamericannurse.com/dispelling-common-myths-about-anccs-pathway-to-excellence/

Patrician, P. A., Petersen, C., & McGuinness, T. M. (2020). Suicide among RNs: An analysis of 2015 data from the national violent death reporting system. *American Journal of Nursing, 120*(10), 24–28.

Porter-O'Grady, T., & Malloch, K. (2003). *Quantum leadership: A textbook of new leadership.* Jones & Bartlett.

Rodriguez-Garcia, C., Marquez-Hernandez, M. V., Belmonte-Garcia, T., Gutierrez-Puertas, L, & Granadas-Gamez, G. (2020). How Magnet hospital status affects nurses, patients, and organizations: A

systemic review. *American Journal of Nursing, 120*(7), 28–39.
Savel, R. H., & Munro, C. L. (2017). Servant leadership: The primacy of service. *American Journal of Critical Care, 26*(2), 97–99.
Sheets, M., Bonnah, B., Kareivis, J., Abraham, P., Sweeney, M., & Strauss, J. (2012). CNLs make a difference. *Nursing, 42*(8), 54–58.
Shepard, L. H. (2011). Creating a foundation for a just culture workplace. *Nursing, 41*(8), 46–48.
Sherman, R., & Habel, M. (2012). Transformational leadership: A growing promise for nursing. *Nurse.com, 21*(15), 24–29.
Sherman, R. (2012a). Evidence-based effective nursing leadership. *Nurse com, 21*(9), 50–55.
Sherman, R. (2012b). What followers want in their nurse leaders. *American Nurse Today, 7*(9), 62–64.
Sherman, R. (2017). Building trust in your leadership. *American Nurse Today, 12*(6), 24–26.
Sherman, R. O. (2017). Transcending your comfort zone. *American Nurse Today, 12*(9), 22–23.
Sherman, R. O., & Cohn, T. M. (2019). Using leadership power wisely. *American Nurse Today, 14*(9), 18–19.
Sherwood, G., & Barnsteiner, J. (2012). *Quality and safety in nursing*. Wiley-Blackwell.
Shingler-Nace, A., & Gonzalez, J. Z. (2017). EBM: A pathway to evidence-based nursing management. *Nursing, 47*(2), 43–46.
Stachowiak, M. E., & Bugel, M. J. (2013). The clinical nurse leader and the case manager: Are both roles needed? *American Journal of Nursing, 113*(1), 59–63.
Stavros, J. M., & Cole, M. L. (2013). SOARing towards positive transformation and change. The ABAC ODI Visions. *Action Outcome, 1*(1), 10–34.
Strickler, J., Bohling, S., Kneis, C., O'Connor, M., & Yee, P. L. (2016). Developing nurse leaders from within. *Nursing, 46*(5), 49–51.
Thompson, R. (2019). What if you're the bully? *American Nurse Today, 14*(1), 22–25.
Zimmerman, E. (2020, June 18). What makes some people more resilient than others. *The New York Times*. https://www.nytimes.com/2020/06/18/health/resilience-relationships-trauma.html

UNIT II

Health Care Delivery

Nurses care for patients in a wide variety of settings. Knowledge of the varied methods of care delivery is necessary in today's complex health care system. As the health care environments change, nurses are increasingly providing care to promote wellness and restore health outside traditional hospital settings. Patients may receive health care services as inpatients or ambulatory outpatients in a hospital, through voluntary or public health facilities, in daycare centers and schools, in offices and clinics, in their home, or through crisis intervention centers. A health care team often provides care to meet a full range of physical, psychological, sociocultural, economic, and spiritual needs. Health care services may be financed through federal funding, health maintenance organizations, or private insurance. All these factors, combined with increasing concern about health care provision and costs, have raised questions about cost containment, consumer rights, fragmentation of care, vulnerable populations, and changing patient populations and needs.

As patients move among health care settings, the nurse is most often the member of the health care team responsible for coordinating care and teaching so that continuity of care is maintained. Unit II provides information about the various settings in which nursing care is provided and the resources for that care. Chapter 11 discusses the health care system as a whole, highlighting access, quality and safety, and affordability concerns. Newer models of organizing health care, such as patient-centered medical homes and accountable care organizations, are presented. Chapter 12 focuses on how nurses work with the interprofessional health care team and considers nursing care provided in the home and other community-based settings. Care coordination and continuity during handoffs are important as patients are admitted, transferred, and discharged from health care settings. Because health care is increasingly provided to patients in their own homes, Chapter 12 describes the characteristics and roles of the home health care nurse as well as the components of a home visit. The information in this unit enables the nurse to work within the health care system to meet individualized patient needs and provide holistic, thoughtful, person-centered care.

“... a realization that the call to the nurse is not only for the bedside care of the sick, but to help in seeking out the deep-lying basic causes of illness and misery, that in the future there may be less sickness to nurse and to cure.”

Lillian Wald (1867–1940), *a visionary humanitarian who initiated child-labor law revision, improved housing conditions in tenements, supported education for people with mental disabilities, originated public health nursing, and founded the Visiting Nurse Service at the Henry Street Settlement House, in New York City.*

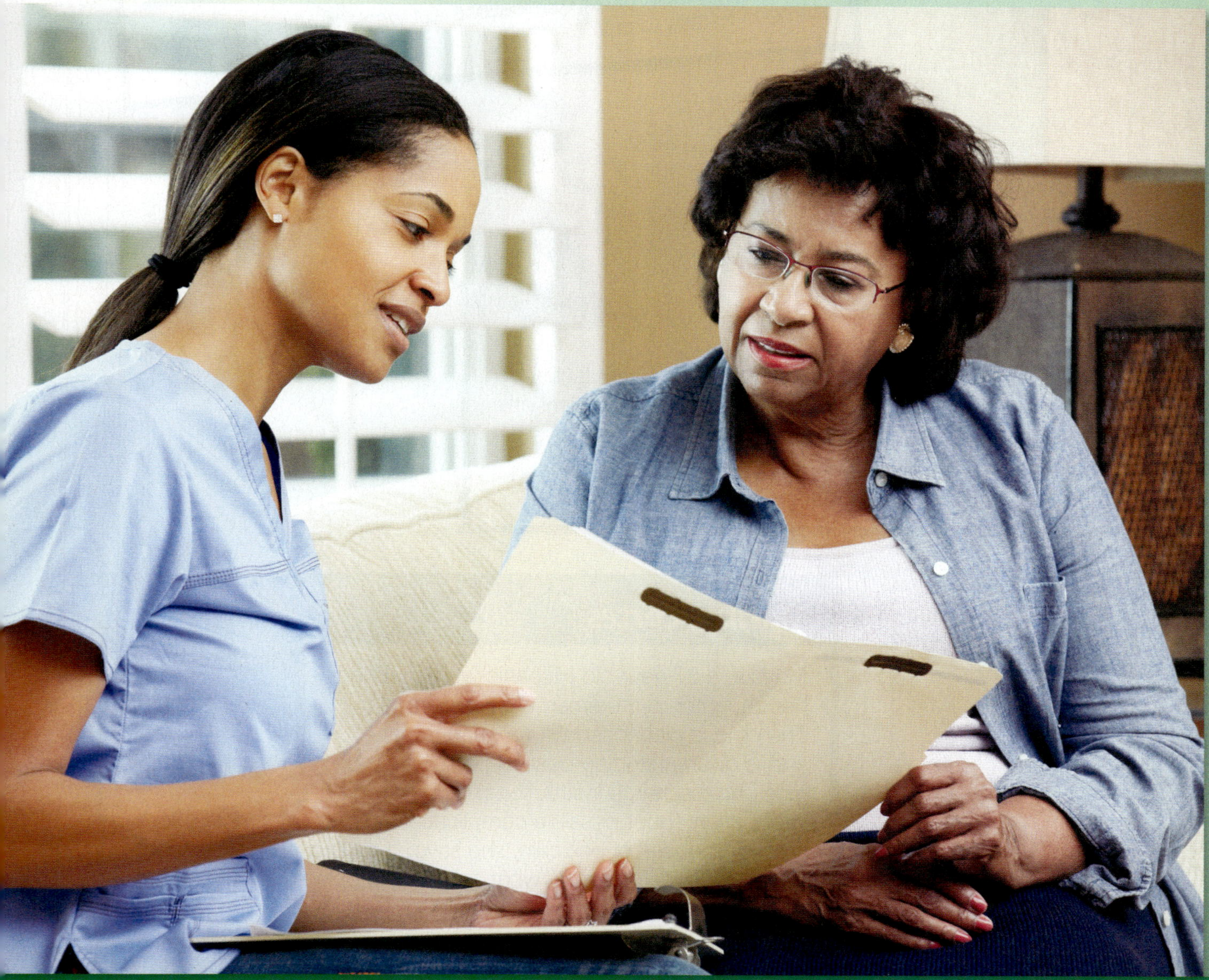

11 Health Care Delivery System

Paul Cochran

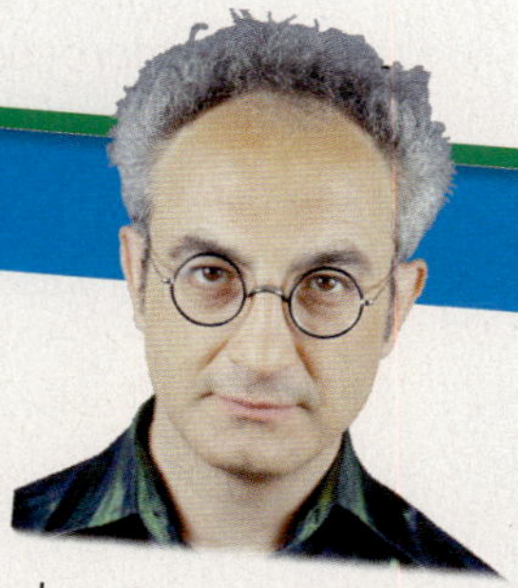

Paul is a 55-year-old man with a history of mental illness and numerous visits to mental health inpatient and outpatient facilities; he comes to the mental health clinic for follow-up. He says, "I ran out of my medications last week, but I feel fine. Do I still need to take them?"

Margaret Ritchie

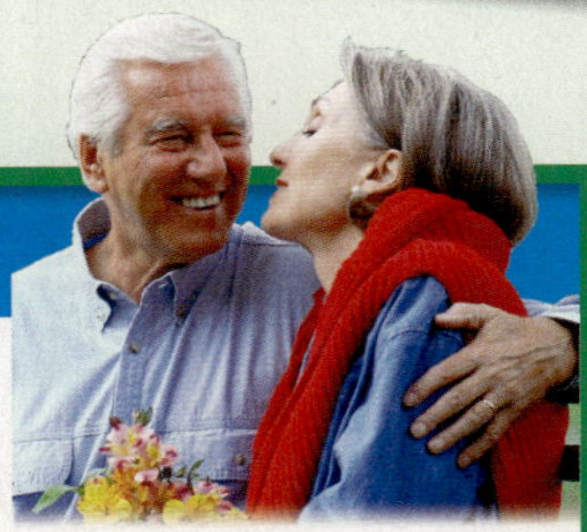

Margaret, a 63-year-old woman, is caring at home for her 67-year-old husband who has been diagnosed with amyotrophic lateral sclerosis (ALS, or Lou Gehrig disease). She states, "All of the help from the home care facility has been a blessing. But I need more help and some equipment now that our insurance won't cover. Plus, now the doctor says that his condition has really worsened, and he probably has 6 months or less to live."

Maritza Cortes

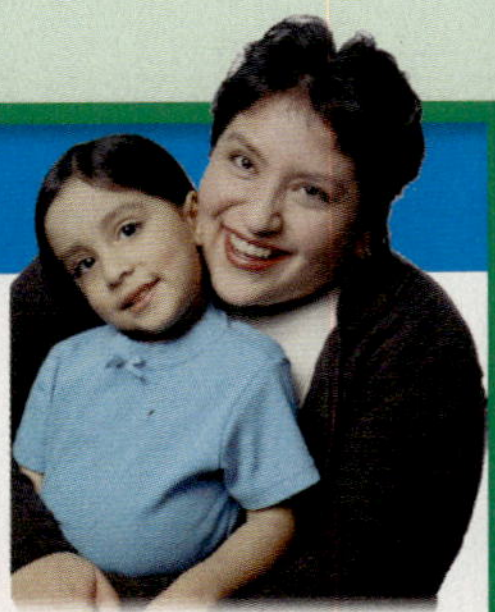

Maritza, a 37-year-old Hispanic woman, brings her daughter to the emergency department. The child is diagnosed with a strep throat and is given a starting dose of penicillin. After receiving discharge instructions, including information about possible complications, and a prescription for additional doses of penicillin, she says, "I can't afford to get the prescription filled. Exactly what are these problems, and what are my son's chances for having them, too?"

Learning Outcomes

After completing the chapter, you will be able to accomplish the following:

1. Identify elements of a well-functioning health care delivery system.
2. Describe strategies to increase access to affordable, high-quality care.
3. Compare and contrast these health care delivery systems: health care providers and hospitals, multispecialty practice groups, community health centers, prepaid group practices, accountable care organizations, medical homes, and medical neighborhoods.
4. Evaluate four basic ways to pay for health care.
5. Compare and contrast settings and facilities that provide health care.
6. Describe the members of the interprofessional health care team.
7. Discuss selected trends and issues affecting health care delivery.
8. Describe the role of nursing in meeting the challenges of health care reform.

Nursing Concepts

- Health care systems
- Health policy
- Quality improvement

Designing a system for and delivering health care that adequately meets the needs of a diverse public is a complex challenge. Health care planners have always worried about access, quality, and cost. Who should have access to what quality of care at what cost? What you think about health care in the United States largely depends on your past experiences. If you are well insured or independently wealthy, you can access the best health care in the world. If you lack insurance and have limited financial resources, you may die of a disease that might have been prevented or treated in an early stage if you had access to quality care. The COVID-19 pandemic in 2020 quickly alerted the public to the disproportionate incidence of COVID-19 among communities of color. As treatments and vaccines became available, just and equitable distribution plans were the topic of much study.

The U.S. system has been criticized for providing too little care to some and too much of the wrong type of care to others. Many now believe that a moral society owes health care to its citizens—that health care is like clean water, sanitation, and basic education. Others, however, believe that health care is a commodity, like automobiles, to be sold and purchased in the marketplace. If you lack the funds to buy a car, that may be sad, but society has no obligation to purchase a car for you.

As you read this chapter, ask yourself what you believe about health care. Is it simply unfortunate if people cannot afford the health care that they and their families need? Learning about how health care works may not seem as exciting as learning how to administer medications safely, but your nursing practice every day will be affected by decisions made by governments, insurers, and health care institutions. Nursing's challenge as profits and politics increasingly dictate health priorities is to keep health care strongly focused on the needs of patients and the public. Health care in the United States is a business; revenues need to be generated to make care possible. But health care can never be *only* a business. First and primarily, it is a service a moral society provides for its vulnerable members. Nurses play a critical role in keeping health care centered on the patient and family. See the accompanying Reflective Practice display on pages 272–273.

HEALTH CARE: THE BIG PICTURE

In 2001, describing a "new health system for the 21st century," the Institute of Medicine (IOM) called for six outcomes, envisioning a system that is safe, effective, efficient, patient-centered, timely, and equitable. (Note: The IOM titling has changed in recent years and is now referred to more broadly as The National Academies of Sciences, Engineering, and Medicine.) In 2007, the Institute for Healthcare Improvement (IHI) in Cambridge, Massachusetts, developed the IHI Triple Aim framework (Fig. 11-1) to improve the patient care

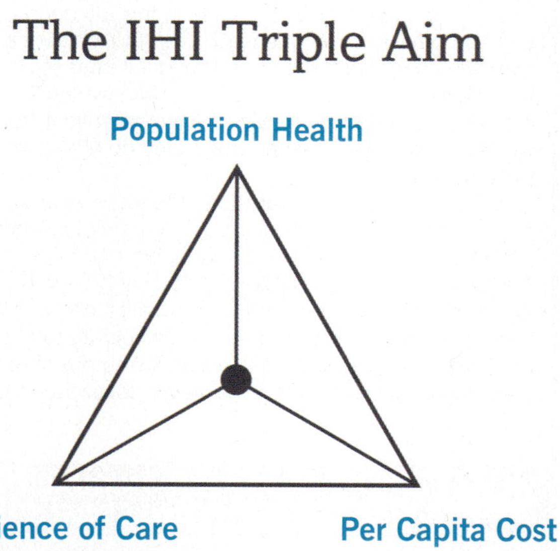

FIGURE 11-1. The IHI Triple Aim is a framework developed by the Institute for Healthcare Improvement that describes an approach to optimizing health system performance. It is IHI's belief that new designs must be developed to simultaneously pursue three dimensions, which we call the "Triple Aim": (1) Improving the patient experience of care (including quality and satisfaction); (2) improving the health of populations; and (3) reducing the per capita cost of health care. (*Source:* From Berwick, D. M., Nolan, T. W., & Whittington, J. [2008]. The Triple Aim: care, health, and cost. *Health Affairs [Millwood]*, *27*[3], 759–769. The IHI Triple Aim framework was developed by the Institute for Healthcare Improvement in Boston, Massachusetts [www.ihi.org].)

QSEN Reflective Practice: Cultivating QSEN Competencies

CHALLENGE TO COGNITIVE SKILLS

Maritza Cortes, a 37-year-old Hispanic woman, came into the emergency department (ED) this summer with her daughter who was diagnosed with strep throat using a rapid strep test. The child was given an initial dose of penicillin and was getting ready for discharge. When I entered the patient's room to give her mother the discharge instructions and the prescription for 10 more doses of penicillin, Ms. Cortes said that she could not afford the medication and probably would not be able to have the prescription filled. I told her that it is essential to fill the medication because strep throat can lead to rheumatic fever and glomerulonephritis. She then asked me to elaborate, requesting exact information about the chances of her son also developing these complications. She wanted exact numbers and did not settle for my answer of "No matter what the percentage is, the medication is still necessary." She also wanted me to elaborate on the disease processes of rheumatic fever and glomerulonephritis. Although I do know basic information about these conditions, I did not feel comfortable being the primary and sole informer.

Thinking Outside the Box: Possible Courses of Action

- Make up a percentage to tell the mother and give a partial explanation of the diseases so that she would sign the discharge papers.
- Look up the answer in books available in the ED or search the internet.
- Try to persuade her that numbers don't matter and that the possible diseases are very severe.
- Ask the nurse to inform me or explain the information to me while we are with the patient.
- Ask the health care provider to inform me or provide the information to me while we are with the patient.

Evaluating a Good Outcome: How Do I Define Success?

- Ms. Cortes receives adequate information regarding the medication and the conditions that may follow strep throat.
- Ms. Cortes obtains medication and gives it to her daughter, as prescribed.
- The standards of nursing care and protocols of the hospital are maintained.
- I am able to acknowledge that I need the help of others, seeking out their help; in return, those people help me.

Personal Learning: Here's to the Future!

Because I was working under my preceptor's license and he had to cosign my signature, I decided that he would be the best person to go to first. My preceptor said that this situation is a common occurrence in this ED because many people come in to get checked, even though they know that they cannot afford the medication, if necessary. As a justification to themselves, patients often want to know what are the exact chances for developing complications, which will likely influence whether or not they go ahead and fill the prescription.

My preceptor and I returned to the room, where he was able to explain rheumatic fever and glomerulonephritis in detail in Spanish. Because he was able to do this at the education level of the patient's mother and be very direct and persuasive, she was no longer concerned about exact numbers. She stated that she would try to get the medication filled, and then she signed the discharge document. Unfortunately, there is no way to follow-up in these situations. I still wonder if the patient was able to get her medications.

Medical information is always changing, and what people held as standards of practice years ago differ from what we practice today. Similarly, what we hold today may be obsolete and even wrong in the years ahead. As a student, I find overwhelming the vast information that is necessary to be a competent nurse, especially in pharmacology. In this example, I probably should have been able to give the patient a comprehensive explanation of rheumatic fever and glomerulonephritis. However, I didn't feel comfortable. I do feel that I have learned a lot in the past years as a student, but I know that the knowledge I need to act as a professional nurse is much greater! While it is overwhelming and very challenging at times, I think continued learning is one reason why nursing is such a wonderful profession. I think it will never get boring.

Julia Strobel, Georgetown University

QSEN SELF-REFLECTION ON QUALITY AND SAFETY COMPETENCIES DEVELOPING KNOWLEDGE, SKILLS, AND ATTITUDES FOR CONTINUOUS IMPROVEMENT

How do you think you would respond in a similar situation? Why? What does this tell you about yourself and about the adequacy of your skills for professional practice? Can you think of other ways to respond? What other knowledge, attitudes, and skills do you need to develop to continuously improve the quality and safety of care for patients like Ms. Cortes's daughter?

Patient-Centered Care: What made creating a partnership with Ms. Cortes and her daughter so challenging? What abilities did the student's preceptor possess and use to achieve a good outcome? What special talents do you bring to creating successful partnerships? Reread the preceptor's statement about this type of situation being common in the ED. Do such statements reflect culturally competent nursing? Or are such statements judgmental? Support your response.

Teamwork and Collaboration/Quality Improvement: What communication skills do you need to improve to

QSEN Reflective Practice: Cultivating QSEN Competencies *(continued)*

CHALLENGE TO COGNITIVE SKILLS

ensure that you function as a competent, caring, and responsible member of the patient care team and that you obtain appropriate assistance when needed? What special talents do you bring to promoting a well-functioning team?

Safety/Evidence-Based Practice: What priority did all involved with Ms. Cortes accord to her daughter's health, well-being, and safety? What resources should be available to those who lack the financial resources to purchase prescribed medications or treatment? Were the team members successful advocates for this family? Did the nursing student seek out the most appropriate resources for information? Why or why not? What other resources could have been helpful? Do you agree with the criteria to evaluate a successful outcome? Did the nursing student meet the criteria? Explain your answers.

experience, improve the health of a population, and reduce per capita health care costs *at the same time* (www.ihi.org; Berwick et al., 2008). Considered radical in 2007, the Triple Aim is now used throughout health care and was more recently revised to the Quadruple Aim to include workers and job satisfaction. This fourth aim recognizes the difficulties frontline caregivers experience while trying to simultaneously improve the patient experience and the health of a population while reducing costs, and directs attention to providing the knowledge, resources, and partnerships frontline caregivers need. Never was this truer than during the pandemic when caregiver burnout rates increased to alarming levels.

The IOM report, *Best Care at Lower Cost*, concluded that Americans would be better served by a nimbler health care system that is consistently reliable and that constantly, systematically, and seamlessly improves (Smith et al., 2012). It states its vision as follows: "… achieving a learning healthcare system—one in which science and informatics, patient–clinician partnerships, incentives, and culture are aligned to promote and enable continuous and real-time improvement, in both the effectiveness and efficiency of care—is both necessary and possible for the nation." The IOM (2015) report, *Transforming Health Care Scheduling and Access: Getting to Now*, reviews what is currently known and experienced with respect to health care access, scheduling, and wait times nationally, and offers preliminary observations about emerging best practices and promising strategies. In 2017 the National Academy of Medicine released its report, *Vital Directions for Health and Health Care*, which identifies fundamental challenges (persistent inequities in health, rapidly aging population, new and emerging health threats, persisting care fragmentation and discontinuity, health expenditure costs and waste, and constrained innovation due to outmoded approaches). The report's good news is that "the nation is equipped to tackle these formidable challenges from a position of unprecedented knowledge and substantial capacity." Described as realistic tools are:

- A new paradigm of health care delivery and financing
- Fully embracing the centrality of population and community health
- Increased focus on individual and family engagement
- Biomedical innovation, precision medicine, and new diagnostic capabilities
- Advances in digital technology and telemedicine
- Promise of "big data" to drive scientific progress.

See Figure 11-2. Sadly, the pandemic of 2020 revealed widespread weaknesses in the ability of the U.S. health care delivery system to respond to unprecedented challenges.

Access to Health Care

People have access to health care if they are able to obtain health care when they need it. Access depends on the ability to pay and the availability of services. Nearly 48 million nonelderly Americans were uninsured in 2011. Decreasing the number of uninsured is a key goal of the 2010 **Patient Protection and Affordable Care Act (PPACA)**, which provides Medicaid or subsidized coverage to qualifying people with incomes up to 400% of poverty, beginning in 2014. A

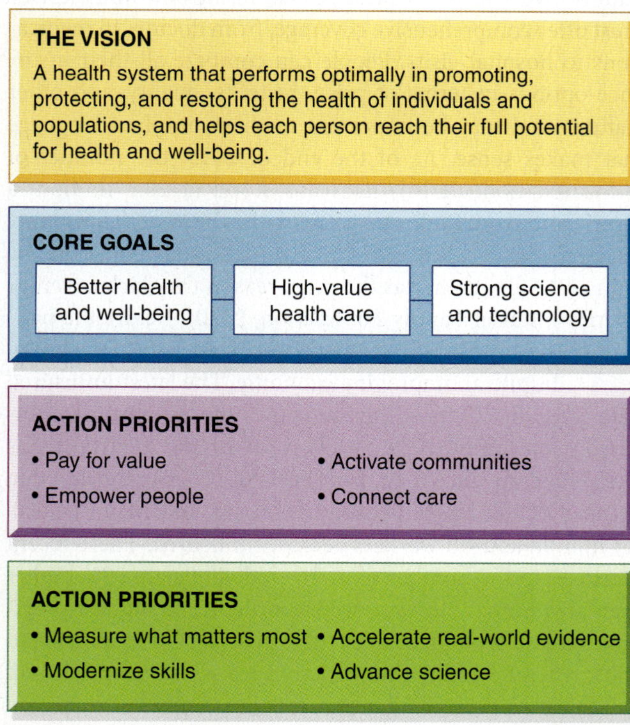

FIGURE 11-2. Vital directions for health and health care framework. (*Source:* Dzau, V. J., McClellan, M. B., McGinnis, J. M., & Finkelman, E. M. (Eds.). [2017]. Vital directions for health & health care: An initiative of the National Academy of Medicine. Reproduced with permission from the National Academy of Sciences, Courtesy of the National Academies Press, Washington, D.C.)

Box 11-1 Summary: Key Facts about the Uninsured Population

How many people are uninsured?
For the third year in a row, the number of uninsured increased in 2019. In 2019, 28.9 million nonelderly individuals were uninsured, an increase of more than one million from 2018. Coverage losses were driven by declines in Medicaid and non-group coverage and were particularly large among Hispanic people and for children. Despite these recent increases, the uninsured rate in 2019 was substantially lower than it was in 2010, when the first ACA provisions went into effect and prior to the full implementation of Medicaid expansion and the establishment of Health Insurance Marketplaces.

Who are the uninsured?
Most uninsured people have at least one worker in the family. Families with low incomes are more likely to be uninsured. Reflecting the more limited availability of public coverage in some states, adults are more likely to be uninsured than children. People of color are at higher risk of being uninsured than non-Hispanic White people.

Why are people uninsured?
Even under the ACA, many uninsured people cite the high cost of insurance as the main reason they lack coverage. In 2019, 73.7% of uninsured adults said that they were uninsured because the cost of coverage was too high. Many people do not have access to coverage through a job, and some people, particularly poor adults in states that did not expand Medicaid, remain ineligible for financial assistance for coverage. In addition, undocumented immigrants are ineligible for Medicaid or Marketplace coverage.

How does not having coverage affect health care access?
People without insurance coverage have worse access to care than people who are insured. Three in ten uninsured adults in 2019 went without needed medical care due to cost. Studies repeatedly demonstrate that uninsured people are less likely than those with insurance to receive preventive care and services for major health conditions and chronic diseases.

What are the financial implications of being uninsured?
The uninsured often face unaffordable medical bills when they do seek care. In 2019, uninsured nonelderly adults were over twice as likely as those with private coverage to have had problems paying medical bills in the past 12 months. These bills can quickly translate into medical debt since most of the uninsured have low or moderate incomes and have little, if any, savings.

Source: Tolbert, J., Orgera, K., & Damico, A. (2020, November 6). *Key facts about uninsured population.* Kaiser Family Foundation. https://www.kff.org/uninsured/issue-brief/key-facts-about-the-uninsured-population/

key element of the health care law that took effect in 2014 provided a new way to get health insurance: The **Health Insurance Marketplace**. The Marketplace was designed to help people more easily find health insurance that fits their budget. Every health insurance plan in the new Marketplace must offer comprehensive coverage, from doctors to medications to hospital visits. People can compare all their insurance options in terms of price, benefits, quality, and other features that may be important to them, in plain language that makes sense. As of the end of 2015, the number of uninsured nonelderly Americans stood at 28.5 million, a significant reduction. Even under the PPACA (commonly referred to as just the ACA), many uninsured people site the high cost of insurance as the main reason they lack coverage (Henry J. Kaiser Family Foundation, 2020). Before the pandemic, the uninsured rate had been increasing for several years—despite an improving economy. The latest uninsured data from the Census Bureau shows the number of uninsured people grew to 29.2 million (or 10.8%) in 2019. It has likely gone up since then. FamiliesUSA (2020) reported that because of job losses between February and May of 2020, 5.4 million laid-off workers became uninsured. These recent increases in the number of uninsured adults are 39% higher than any annual increase ever recorded. The highest previous increase took place over the 1-year period from 2008 to 2009, when 3.9 million nonelderly adults became uninsured.

These record-breaking increases in the number of uninsured have taken place during the country's worst public health crisis in more than a century and the sharpest and deepest economic downturn since World War II. Nevertheless, no federal COVID-19 legislation signed into law has attempted to restore or preserve comprehensive health insurance. Continual efforts to eliminate the ACA threaten the well-being of the 23 million who get health insurance through the ACA.

See Box 11-1, Figure 11-3, and HealthCare.gov for more up-to-date information as you are reading this chapter. Also see the Vulnerable Population Alert.

Shortage of Providers

A 2013 U.S. Subcommittee on Primary Health and Aging reported that nearly 57 million people in the United States—one in five Americans—live in areas without adequate access to primary health care due to a shortage of providers in their communities. The facts in this report are sobering:

- Fifty years ago, half of the doctors in the United States practiced primary care, but today fewer than one in three do.
- As many as 45,000 people die each year because they do not have health insurance and do not get to a doctor on time.
- The average primary care physician in the United States is 47 years old, and one quarter are nearing retirement.
- In 2011, about 17,000 doctors graduated from U.S. medical schools. Despite the fact that over half of patient visits are for primary care, only 7% of the nation's medical school graduates now choose a primary care career (Sanders, 2013).

The report cites nurse Linda Aiken noting that nurse practitioners are a good solution for the shortage of primary care predicted to worsen as millions of currently uninsured Americans get health insurance as a result of the ACA. "Research shows that care by nurse practitioners is excellent, highly satisfactory to patients, accessible, and affordable."

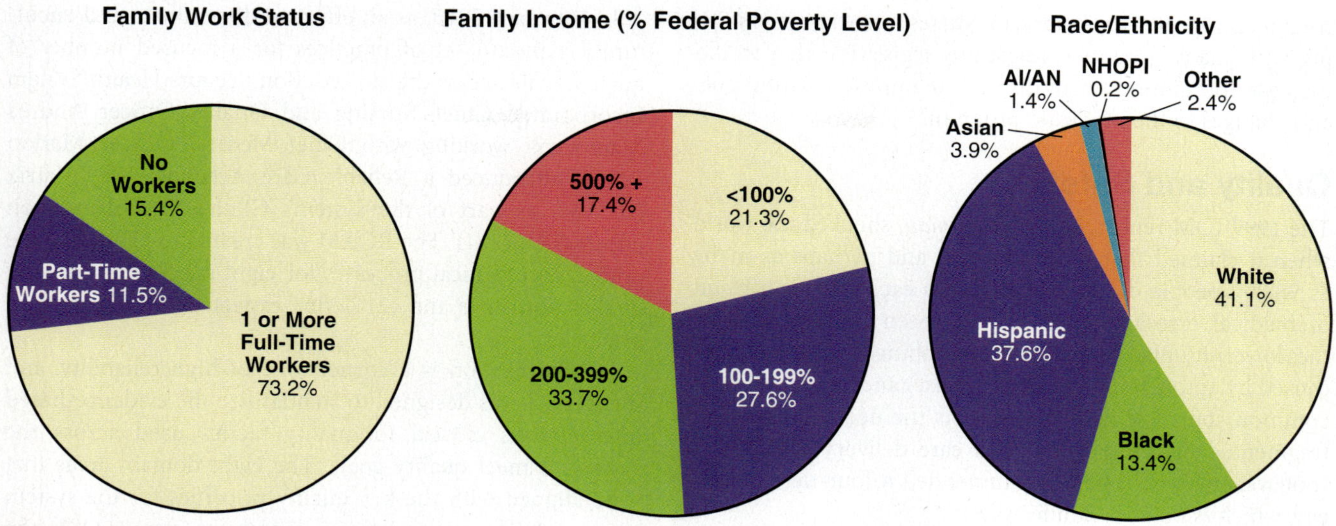

FIGURE 11-3. Characteristics of the nonelderly uninsured, 2019. Includes nonelderly individuals ages 0 to 64 years. AIAN, American Indian/Alaska Native; NHOPI, Native Hawaiians and Other Pacific Islanders. Hispanic people may be of any race but are categorized as Hispanic; other groups are all non-Hispanic. The 2019 Census Bureau poverty threshold for a family of three was $20,578. (*Source:* KFF analysis of 2019 American Community Survey, 1-Year Estimates.)

Although nursing is currently one of the fastest growing occupations in the country, demand is rapidly outpacing supply. An expected 1.2 million vacancies will emerge for registered nurses between 2014 and 2022. By 2025, the shortfall is expected to be more than twice as large as any nurse shortage since the mid-1960s. A major reason for the projected shortages is the aging of the baby boomer generation and their demand for health care services (Grant, 2016).

Legislation Addressing Health Care Access

Although the ACA greatly reduced the number of uninsured in the United States, it was bitterly opposed by many who

Vulnerable Population Alert: Caring for Persons Who Are Undocumented

Shifting immigration policies under the Trump administration are leading to substantially increased fears among the immigrant community. Many public health nurses report that families are no longer keeping clinic appointments, vaccinating children, or showing up at food banks or even church. What do you need to know to best care for undocumented immigrants in your clinical sites and communities?

Gostin, L. O. (2019, September 5). Is affording undocumented immigrants health coverage a radical proposal? *Journal of the American Medical Association*, *322*(15), 1438–1439. https://doi.org/10.1001/jama.2019.15806. https://newsatjama.jama.com/2019/09/05/jama-forum-is-affording-undocumented-immigrants-health-coverage-a-radical-proposal/

More than 10 million undocumented immigrants in the United States are systematically excluded from federal health insurance programs: Medicaid, Medicare, the Affordable Care Act (ACA) marketplaces, and the Children's Health Insurance Program (CHIP). Lawful immigrants can participate in these programs, with limitations, which vary by program.

Refugees are generally eligible for Medicaid but only for the first 7 years of residence. Asylum seekers qualify for ACA exchanges starting 180 days after applying for asylum. Several states extend Medicaid and CHIP to lawfully present children and pregnant women without the 5-year wait. Currently, Medicaid payments for emergency services are the only federal funds allowed for undocumented immigrants; federal law requires hospitals to stabilize patients with life-threatening conditions, irrespective of immigration status.

Consequently, almost half of undocumented nonelderly adults and one third of undocumented children are uninsured. For basic medical care, immigrants often turn to 1,400 federally funded health care centers providing services on a sliding-scale based on ability to pay, irrespective of residency status.

There are, however, strong reasons to afford health coverage for this population: modest economic costs, safeguarding the public's health by curbing the spread of infectious diseases, and complying with international law that requires health coverage for migrants. Many countries fail to afford migrants equitable access to health coverage, so adopting a policy of providing undocumented immigrants on par with other residents—integrated into existing federal health insurance programs—would help the United States regain moral leadership, in line with World Health Organization (WHO) and United Nations (UN) guidelines, and potentially save money (discussed below).

Treating Fear: Sanctuary Doctoring

This web page contains presentation materials, video, patient flyers, and lapel pins designed to be simple and useful in helping physicians and health-care professionals meet the needs of their patients who may be undocumented or suffering stresses related to close family or community members being undocumented. https://hsd.luc.edu/bioethics/content/sanctuary-doctor/

Artiga, S., & Diaz, M. (July 15, 2019). Health coverage and care of undocumented immigrants. KFF Disparities Policy. https://www.kff.org/disparities-policy/issue-brief/health-coverage-and-care-of-undocumented-immigrants/

Health coverage for immigrants. HealthCare.gov. https://www.healthcare.gov/immigrants/coverage/

sought its repeal. The American Nurses Association is joining with many groups to reject any legislation that would increase the number of uninsured or impose harmful cuts and changes to the Medicaid program.

Quality and Safety

The 1999 IOM report, *To Err Is Human,* shocked the world when it claimed that at least 44,000 and perhaps as many as 98,000 people die in U.S. hospitals each year as a result of medical errors that could have been prevented. Even the lower number exceeds the combined annual deaths caused by automobile accidents, breast cancer, and AIDS. A common source of medical errors is the decentralized and fragmented nature of the health care delivery system—or "nonsystem." The report recommended a four-tiered strategy, which is now well underway:

- Establishing a national focus to create leadership, research, tools, and protocols to enhance our knowledge about safety
- Identifying and learning from errors by developing a nationwide public mandatory reporting system and by encouraging health care organizations and practitioners to develop and participate in voluntary reporting systems
- Raising performance standards and expectations for improvements in safety through the actions of oversight organizations, professional groups, and group purchasers of health care
- Implementing safety systems in health care organizations to ensure safe practices

In 2001, the IOM defined **quality** as the degree to which health services for people and populations increase the likelihood of desired health outcomes and are consistent with professional knowledge. More simply, quality is the right care for the right person at the right time. Every year, the Agency for Health Care Research and Quality (AHRQ) issues national reports on quality and disparities. To learn more about health care quality, visit the websites listed in the Internet Resources for this chapter, which can be found on.

Increasingly, quality of care is being measured and used to evaluate hospitals and other providers and to award reimbursement.

Reliable Care Accountability Matrix

High reliability organizations are organizations that operate in complex, high-hazard domains for extended periods without serious accidents or catastrophic failures. Characteristics of high reliability organizations include preoccupation with failure, reluctance to simplify, sensitivity to operations, deference to expertise, and commitment to resilience (AHRQ, 2016). To deliver care in a highly reliable way and achieve quality—the right care for the right person at the right time—consistent and evidence-based practices must be translated and communicated to the front-line staff. Nurses represent the majority of health care workers and are on the front line to assure the provision of safe and reliable care. An example of nurse leadership making a critical difference follows.

In February 2015, as an effort to disseminate and enculture a standard set of practices for a focused number of quality goals across the system, Bon Secours Health System Incorporated Chief Nursing and Quality Officer Andrea Mazzoccoli working with Chief Medical Officer Marlon Priest, introduced a Reliable Care Accountability Matrix (RCAM) as part of the system's Clinical Transformation efforts (Fig. 11-4). The RCAM was created to (1) define the critical core clinical processes for eight specific domains of quality outcomes and (2) define expectations for standard practices.

Standardization is a cornerstone of high reliability, and the RCAM was designed to standardize the evidence-based interventions critical to quality tactics used across the system to meet quality goals. The eight domain areas that were aligned with the key quality priorities for the system are: mortality; readmissions; length of stay (LOS); the Hospital Consumer Assessment of Healthcare Providers and Systems (HCAHPS); hand hygiene; and the prevention of *Clostridioides difficile*, surgical site infections, and catheter-associated urinary tract infections. Each domain contained no more than five standards of practice derived from the system Learning Communities and national standards believed to be critical in achieving goals.

The RCAM define expectations of performance of the tactics, for example:

- Validating that a Foley catheter is removed via the nurse-driven Foley catheter removal protocol at the time the catheter is no longer necessary via a chart audit
- Validating that sepsis order sets are used through an audit of usage

RCAM validators use face-to-face validation techniques that combine outcome data, observations, chart reviews, and interviews to assess compliance with the RCAM components and provide feedback to Bon Secours hospitals on any identified gaps in process. Alongside the work to create a reliable culture, this standard became a focal point of conversations to hold one another accountable. The RCAM is leading to significant improvement in desired outcomes on key measures.

Pay for Performance/Value-Based Purchasing

Pay for performance is a strategy using financial incentives to reward providers for the achievement of a range of payer objectives, including delivery efficiencies, submission of data and measures to the payer, and improved quality and patient safety. Using the concept of **value-based purchasing**, the Hospital Value-based Purchasing (VBP) Program requires the Centers for Medicare and Medicaid Services (CMS) to redistribute a portion of the Medicare payments to hospitals for inpatient services based on performance on quality measures. The National Committee for Quality Assurance (NCQA) developed the Healthcare Effectiveness Data and Information Set (HEDIS), a tool used by more than 90% of U.S. health plans to measure performance in important

RELIABLE CARE ACCOUNTABILITY MATRIX (2.0)

Ensuring Reliable, Evidence-Based Compassionate Care for *Every Patient, Every Time*

CLOSTRIDIOIDES DIFFICILE PREVENTION

Goal: 0 Clostridioides Difficile Infections

- Demonstrate compliance with BSHSI policy on cleaning of C. diff rooms with OxyCide
- Demonstrate compliance in the use of BSHSI C. diff algorithm for testing (including the ED).
- Establish and implement process to review the use of proton pump inhibitors (PPI).

CATHETER ASSOCIATED URINARY TRACT INFECTION PREVENTION

Goal: 0 Catheter Associated Urinary Tract Infections

- Conduct daily Foley necessity review.
- Demonstrate compliance with BSHSI nurse-driven removal protocol.
- Demonstrate use of Foley alternatives.
- Demonstrate compliance with Lippincott standard of care for perineal care.

SURGICAL SITE INFECTION PREVENTION

Goal: 0 Surgical Site Infections

- Chlorhexidine gluconate (CHG) bathing before surgery.
- Demonstrate compliance on SCIP measures.
- Maintain normothermia perioperatively, unless otherwise clinically indicated.
- Establish and follow perioperative and postoperative glucose control protocols.
- Use wound protectors for open colorectal surgeries.

HAND HYGIENE

Goal: 100% Compliance

- Demonstrate compliance with BSHSI hand hygiene policy.
- Evidence of daily unit level hand hygiene compliance monitoring.
- Evidence of monthly audit completed.

LENGTH OF STAY MANAGEMENT

Goal: Facility Specific

- Demonstrate use of BSHSI's interdisciplinary rounding (IDR) model.
- Communicate with patients and display estimated discharge date on whiteboards.
- Establish protocol based workflow for the use of EPIC Monitors.
- Compliance for review and evaluation of observation status every 12 hours.
- Evidence for clinical pathway use for highest LOS DRGs.

READMISSION PREVENTION

Goal: 0 Avoidable Readmissions

- Demonstrate compliance with the readmission risk assessment tool (RRAT) completion, on admission, with care management plans targeted by risk score.
- Document evidence of PCP identification on admission.
- Evidence of appropriate follow up appointment made, prior to discharge.
- Demonstrate medication reconciliation and medication education.

MORTALITY REDUCTION

Goal: 0 Preventable Deaths

- Demonstrate compliance with system ventilator bundles.
- Demonstrate a minimum of 75% use of the BSHSI sepsis order set.
- Evidence of compliance with Modified Early Warning Score (MEWS) standard.
- Evidence of advanced care planning and appropriate palliative care consult within 24 hours.
- Document weekly review of deaths and the SSER classification for all deaths and safety events.

EXPERIENCE OF CARE

Goal: Top Decile

- Demonstrate compliance with shift change report at the bedside.
- Demonstrate compliance of purposeful interval/hourly rounding and leader rounding on all units.
- Post Hospital Consumer Assessment of Healthcare Providers and System (HCAHPS) scores and verbatims with PDCA action plans at the nursing unit.
- Demonstrate compliance with the BSHSI standard daily safety huddles.
- Evidence of leader rounding to influence.

FIGURE 11-4. Reliable Care Accountability Matrix (RCAM). The Reliable Care Accountability Matrix identifies the critical core clinical processes for eight specific domains of quality outcomes. (*Source:* Updated from Bon Secours Health System, 2016. https://www.chausa.org/publications/catholic-health-world/archives/issues/july-1-2016/set-clear-goals-measures-to-achieve-results-from-c-suite-to-bedside) dimensions of care and service. Altogether, HEDIS consists of 80 measures across five domains of care. Because so many plans collect HEDIS data, and because the measures are so specifically defined, HEDIS makes it possible to compare the performance of health plans on an "apples-to-apples" basis. Health plans also use HEDIS results themselves to see where they need to focus their improvement efforts.

HEDIS measures address a broad range of important health issues. Among them are asthma medication use, persistence of beta-blocker treatment after a heart attack, controlling high blood pressure, comprehensive diabetes care, breast cancer screening, antidepressant medication management, childhood and adolescent immunization status, and childhood and adult weight/body mass index (BMI) assessment.

In 2011, Medicare finalized a plan to alter reimbursements based on the quality-of-care hospitals provide and patients' satisfaction during their stays. This was a dramatic step toward paying for better care, not just more care. Seventy percent of the bonuses initially were based on how often hospitals followed guidelines on 12 clinical care measures. The other 30% were determined by how patients rated hospitals on their experiences (Rau, 2011).

The HCAHPS Survey is the first national, standardized, publicly reported survey of patients' perspectives of hospital care. HCAHPS (pronounced "H-caps"), also known as the CAHPS Hospital Survey, is a 21-item survey instrument and data collection methodology for measuring patients' perceptions of their hospital experience. While many hospitals have collected information on patient satisfaction for their own internal use, until HCAHPS there were no common metrics and no national standards for collecting and publicly reporting information about patients' experience of care. Since 2008, HCAHPS has allowed valid comparisons to be made across hospitals locally, regionally, and nationally. The HCAHPS Survey asks recently discharged patients about aspects of their hospital experience that they are uniquely suited to address. The core survey items ask "how often" or whether patients experienced a critical aspect of hospital care, rather than whether they were "satisfied" with the care.

Eleven HCAHPS measures (seven summary measures, two individual items, and two global items) are publicly reported on the Medicare.gov Hospital Compare website (http://www.medicare.gov/hospitalcompare) for each participating hospital. The six composites summarize how well nurses and doctors communicate with patients, how responsive hospital staff are to patients' needs, how well hospital staff help patients manage pain, how well staff communicate with patients about medicines, and whether key information is provided at discharge. The two individual items address the cleanliness and quietness of patients' rooms, while the two global items report patients' overall rating of the hospital and whether they would recommend the hospital to family and friends (HCAHPS Fact Sheet, 2021).

In April 2015, CMS added HCAHPS Star Ratings to the Hospital Compare website. HCAHPS Star Ratings summarize the results for each HCAHPS measure and present it in a format that is increasingly familiar to consumers, making it easier to use the information and spotlight excellence in health care quality. Scores are calculated using seven groups of measures: mortality, safety of care, readmission, patient experience, effectiveness of care, timeliness of care, and efficient use of medical imaging (Medicare.gov, 2017). As of December 2016, only 83, or 1.8%, of participating hospitals had earned the highest five-star rating.

Penalties for Excess Readmissions

In October 2012, more than 2,000 hospitals were penalized by the government because many of their patients were readmitted soon after discharge. These hospitals forfeited more than $280 million in Medicare funds because the government considers readmissions a prime symptom of an overly expensive and uncoordinated health system. Until now, hospitals had little financial incentive to ensure that patients get the care they need once they leave the hospital (Rau, 2012).

Affordability

How Health Care Is Financed

Health care financing involves two streams of money: the collection of money for health care (money going in) and reimbursement of health care providers for health care (money going out). The United States is a **multipayer system**: its "payers" include both private insurance companies and the government. Distinctive to the United States is the dominance of the private element over the public. The United States spends 17% to 18% of its gross domestic product (GDP) on health care—more than any other country in the world. The government estimates that an aging population, improving economy, and the health care overhaul will push spending on medical services to almost 20% of the U.S. gross domestic product by 2021 (CMS.gov, 2021). While some argue that nothing is more important than health and no price is too high to pay, the increasing percentage of the GDP being allocated to health care means less money for education, defense, homeland security, public parks, the arts, and other priorities. See Table 11-1 for a description of strategies to reduce health care costs.

Many believe that the solution to rising U.S. health care costs is a **single-payer system**—that is, have one entity such as a government run the organization, collect all health care fees, and pay out all health care costs. In the current U.S. free market system, there are tens of thousands of different health care organizations and huge administrative waste. The Physicians for a National Health Program (PNHP) promote a single-payer system in which all hospitals, doctors, and other health care providers would bill one entity for their services. "This alone would reduce administrative waste greatly and save money, which could be used to provide care and insurance to those who currently don't have it" (PNHP, 2016). During President Obama's efforts to reform health care, the Senate did not allow discussion of a single-payer system.

Table 11-1 Strategies to Reduce Health Care Costs

Strategy	Description	Comments
CHANGES IN REIMBURSEMENT AND REGULATORY ENVIRONMENT		
Prospective payment system: Diagnosis-Related Groups (DRGs) and Resource Utilization Groups (RUGs)	Inpatient hospital services for Medicare patients are grouped into DRGs with a fixed reimbursement amount with adjustments based on case severity, rural/urban/regional costs, and teaching costs; RUGs in long-term care.	This changes the financial incentives linked to doing more in order to gain more reimbursement.
Capitation and managed care	**Capitation** gives providers a fixed amount per enrollee of health plan. In managed care, the provider or system receives a capitated payment for each patient enrolled in the program and assumes financial risk.	This aims to build a payment plan for select diagnoses or procedures that consist of best standards of care at the lowest cost. Quality of care may suffer if there is too much emphasis on cost.
Bundled payments	Provider receives a fixed sum of money to provide a range of services.	Again, the fixed sum aims to decrease costs of health care by changing the financial incentives.
Rate setting	Government could set targets or caps for spending on health care services. Government could establish prices for services or even payment approaches that public and private payers would use.	Could equalize prices across payers and focus competition on health management and customer service. Diagnoses can be modified to game the system. Some see this as heavy-handed.
Comparative effectiveness analysis	Explicitly assess and weigh the benefits and costs of new technologies, and make decisions about whether a medical benefit is worth the cost and whether it should be covered by a public or private insurance program.	This forces providers to factor in costs when making decisions about new technologies and challenges the "more is always better" thinking.
Increasing patient cost sharing	This leads to higher deductibles.	Higher cost sharing reduces demand (and some people with few resources may not seek indicated services), which over the longer run will dampen incentives for research and investment. Can raise barriers to even necessary and appropriate care.
CHANGES IN CARE DELIVERY		
Strategy	*Description*	*Comments*
Utilizing quality improvement tools (such as Lean Six Sigma, PDSA) to reduce waste and improve safety	These efforts link interventions to valued outcomes.	Today's greater focus on quality makes it less likely that patients will suffer unnecessary or harmful treatment.
Improving transitions across settings (to decrease 30-day readmissions)	Make sure that all vital information essential to care coordination gets transferred with the patient.	Better patient handoffs will improve outcomes and the patient and family experience.
Making the delivery of medical services more efficient and less costly	October 1, 2014 is the compliance date for use of new codes that classify diseases and health problems; estimated to save $6 billion over 10 years. These code sets, known as the *International Classification of Diseases, 10th Edition* diagnosis and procedure codes, or ICD-10, will include codes for new procedures and diagnoses that improve the quality of information available for quality improvement and payment purposes.	Efforts to increase efficiency and cost without sacrificing quality are welcome.
Eliminating unnecessary costs such as those resulting from fraud and abuse	For too long, measures to identify and address fraud and abuse have been inadequate, which have greatly contributed to rising health care costs.	Nurses can play an important role in reporting suspected fraud and abuse.
Improving population health	These efforts change the focus from individual patients to targeted populations.	Efforts to improve population health could have a long-term effect on disease prevalence and help reduce health care spending.

PDSA, plan, do, study, act.
Source: Partially adapted from The Henry J. Kaiser Family Foundation. Health Care Costs: https://www.kff.org/health-costs/

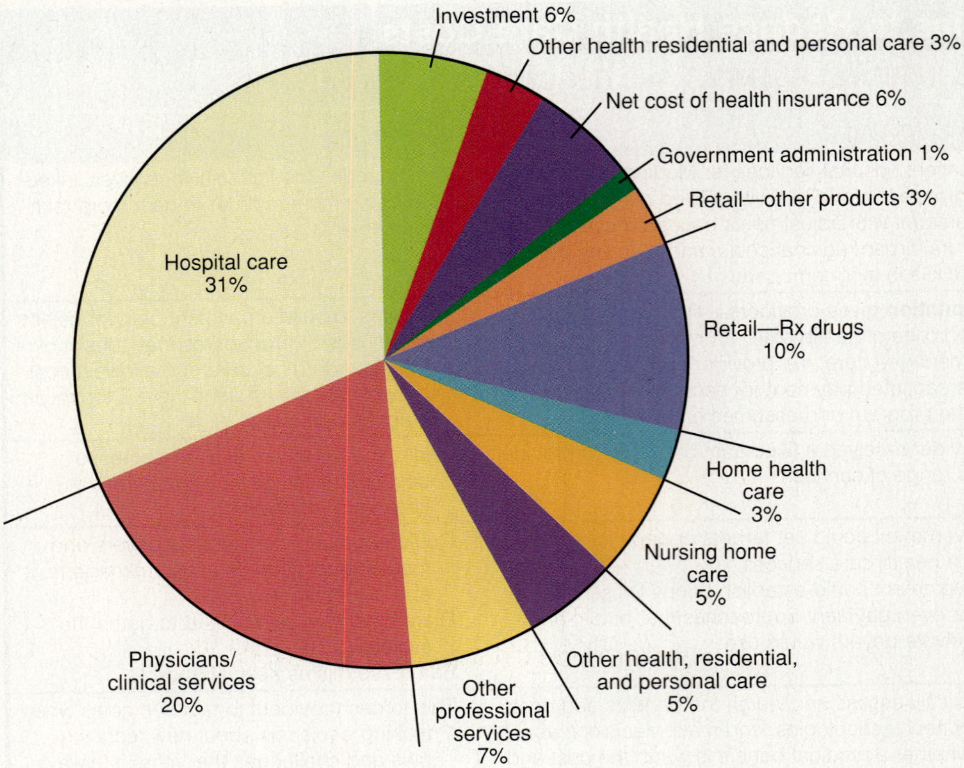

FIGURE 11-5. How the U.S. health care dollar is spent.

How the U.S. Health Care Dollar Is Spent

Hospital care and health care provider/clinical services together account for 51% of the nation's health care expenditures. With greater understanding of the social determinants of health (see Chapter 3 and Fig. 11-10 later in this chapter), everyone is trying to figure out how to get more health care dollars out of the hospital and into the community to promote health and prevent illness. This is an ongoing challenge. Figure 11-5 shows a pre–COVID-19 breakdown of how the U.S. health care dollar was spent. During the pandemic hospital revenues were reduced dramatically as the public skipped annual health screenings and delayed elective surgeries and treatment. The IOM report, *Best Care at Lower Cost* concluded that a substantial proportion of U.S. health care expenditures is wasted, leading to little improvement in health or the quality of care. The IOM workshop summary, *The Health Care Imperative: Lowering Costs and Improving Outcomes,* estimates excess costs in six domains: unnecessary services, services inefficiently delivered, prices that are too high, excess administrative costs, missed prevention opportunities, and medical fraud (Yong et al., 2010). Figure 11-6 illustrates how commercial health plans spend each of your premium health care dollars.

How the U.S. Health Care System Compares Internationally

The 2010 Commonwealth Fund International comparison of the U.S. health care system concluded that despite having the costliest health system in the world, the United States consistently underperforms in most dimensions of performance relative to other countries. "Compared with six other nations—Australia, Canada, Germany, the Netherlands, New Zealand, and the United Kingdom—the U.S. health care system ranks last or next-to-last in five dimensions of a high-performance health system: quality, access, efficiency, equity, and healthy lives" (Davis et al., 2010). The report was hopeful that newly enacted health reform legislation in the United States would address these problems by extending coverage to those without and helping to close gaps in coverage, leading to improved disease management, care coordination, and better outcomes over time. A 2015 Commonwealth Fund brief showed that—before the major provisions of the ACA were introduced—the United States had worse outcomes and spent more on health care, largely because of greater use of medical technology and higher prices, compared to other high-income countries. By benchmarking the performance of the U.S. health care system against other countries—and by updating with new data as they become available—we could gain important insights into our strengths and weaknesses and help policymakers and delivery system leaders identify areas for improvement. Sobering highlights of the report include:

- The United States spends more on health care as a share of the economy—nearly twice as much as the average Organisation for Economic Co-operation and Development (OECD) country—yet has the lowest life expectancy and highest suicide rates among the 11 nations.
- The United States has the highest chronic disease burden and an obesity rate that is two times higher than the OECD average.

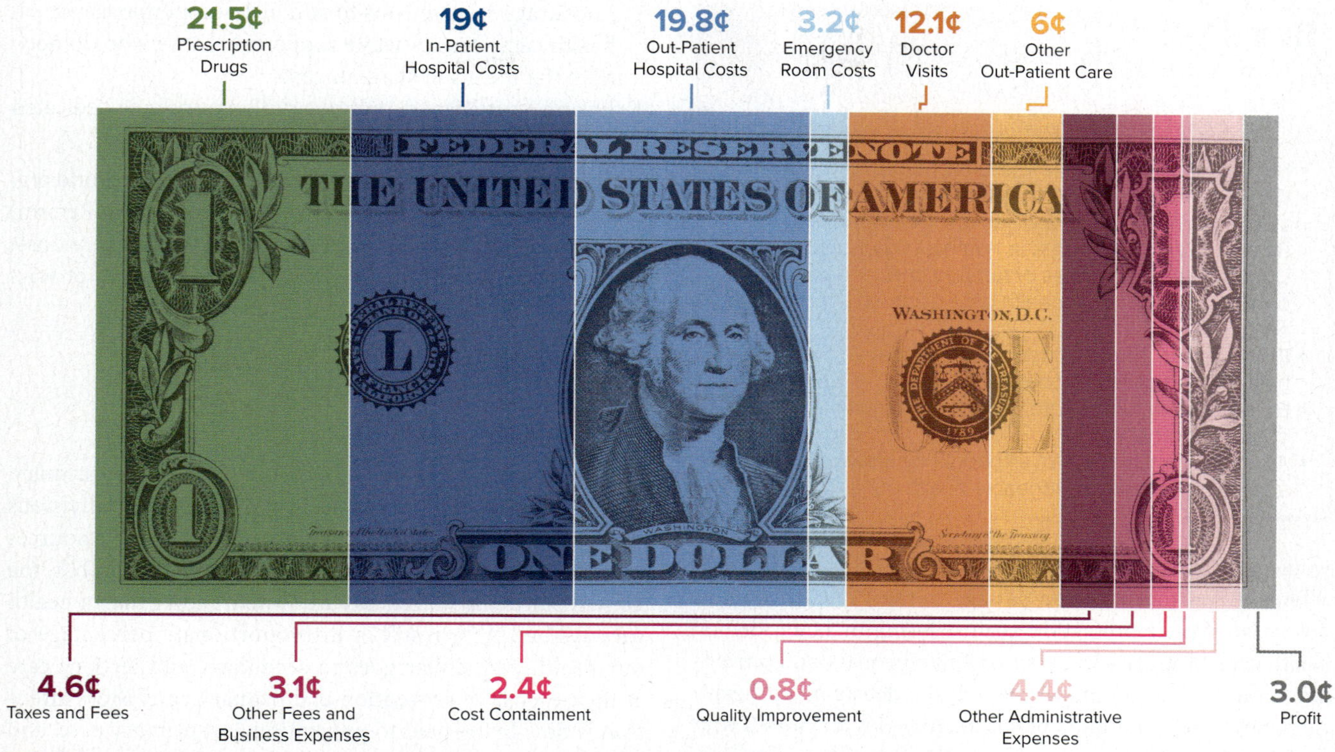

FIGURE 11-6. How commercial health plans spend each of your premium health care dollars. (*Source*: This data represent how commercial health plans spend your premiums. Used with permission, AHIP. https://www.ahip.org/health-care-dollar/)

- Americans had fewer physician visits than peers in most countries, which may be related to a low supply of physicians in the United States.
- Americans use expensive technologies, such as MRIs, and specialized procedures, such as hip replacements, more often than our peers.
- The United States outperforms its peers in terms of preventive measures—it has one of the highest rates of breast cancer screening among women ages 50 to 69 years and the second-highest rate (after the United Kingdom) of flu vaccinations among people age 65 and older.
- Compared to peer nations, the United States has among the highest number of hospitalizations from preventable causes and the highest rate of avoidable deaths.

A similarly discouraging 2013 IOM report, *U.S. Health in International Perspective: Shorter Lives, Poorer Health,* concludes that while the United States is among the wealthiest nations in the world, it is far from the healthiest. Despite spending far more per person on health care than any other nation, the United States has more people dying at younger ages than people in almost all other high-income countries. Among 16 peer nations, all affluent democracies, the United States is at or near the bottom in nine key areas of health: infant mortality and low birth weight, injuries and homicides, teenage pregnancies and sexually transmitted infections (STIs), prevalence of HIV and AIDS, drug-related deaths, obesity and diabetes, heart disease, chronic lung disease, and disability. Included as factors linked to the U.S. disadvantage are inadequate health care, unhealthy behaviors, and adverse economic and social conditions. "The tragedy is not that the U.S. is losing a contest with other countries, but that Americans are dying and suffering from illness and injury at rates that are demonstrably unnecessary" (Woolf & Aron, 2013).

An important study from the 2020 social progress index shows that the quality of life in the United States has dropped over the last decade (2020 Social Progress Index: https://www.socialprogress.org/?tab=2&code=USA). Out of 163 countries assessed worldwide, the United States, Brazil, and Hungary are the only ones in which people are worse off than when the index began in 2011. The United States ranks No. 1 in the world in quality of universities but No. 91 in access to quality basic education. The United States leads the world in medical technology, but we are No. 97 in access to quality health care. The data for the 2020 index predates COVID-19, which has had a disproportionate impact on the United States and seems likely to exacerbate the slide in America's standing.

HEALTH CARE REFORM

On March 23, 2010, President Obama signed comprehensive health reform legislation, the Patient Protection and Affordable Care Act (PPACA), into law. The intent of the law was to expand coverage, control health care costs, and improve the health care delivery system. While the law is complex, nurses should be familiar with how the law affects their practice, health care delivery, and the choices available to the public. Excellent information about the law can be found at www.healthcare.gov and www.nursingworld.org.

The American Nurses Association website chronicles nurses' decades-long efforts to advocate for health care reforms that

Box 11-2 Nurses Can Make a Difference in Health Care Policy and Reform

- Stay informed about current issues and pending legislation.
- Write or e-mail members of Congress to support legislation to improve nursing and patient care. See Chapter 7.
- Belong to and participate in nursing organizations.
- Document the outcomes of nursing care and develop a database to influence health care costs and quality of care.
- Participate in efforts to design and implement innovative health care delivery models.
- Be a leader in local, state, and national nursing and consumer groups.
- Advocate for the rights of all people for equal, affordable, accessible, and knowledgeable health care.

would guarantee access to high-quality health care for all. It acknowledges that with the passage of the PPACA, millions now have greater protection against losing or being denied health care coverage and better access to primary and preventive services. It also reminds us that the debate about health care is not over and offers practical strategies for nurses who choose to be politically active for continuing reform. The 2016 ANA Principles for Health System Transformation include the following:

1. Ensure universal access to a standard package of essential services for all citizens and residents.
2. Optimize primary, community-based, and preventive services while supporting the cost-effective use of innovative, technology-driven, acute, hospital-based services.
3. Encourage mechanisms to stimulate economic use of health care services while supporting those who do not have the means to share in costs.
4. Ensure a sufficient supply of a skilled workforce dedicated to providing high-quality health care services.

Check out the ANA website (http://www.nursingworld.org/MainMenuCategories/Policy-Advocacy/HealthSystemReform) to see the many resources ANA provides for nurses passionate about health care reform. See Box 11-2 for examples of ways that nurses can promote health care reform.

ORGANIZING HEALTH CARE: PRIMARY, SECONDARY, AND TERTIARY CARE

Health care can be broken down into three levels: primary, secondary, and tertiary (Table 11-2). While these divisions seem simple, it is challenging to decide what resources should be allocated to each level. Many claim that the United States has an illness care system rather than a health care system. As a result, a disproportionate percentage of our health care dollar goes to secondary and tertiary care at the expense of prevention and primary care. More attention is now being paid to prevention and primary care, and new opportunities are opening up for nurses at all levels of practice. If care coordination entails not only the right care for the right patient at the right time but also the right provider, decisions about how to organize care must also address which providers are best able to deliver affordable, safe, high-quality care.

The IOM study report, *The Future of Nursing, Leading Change, Advancing Health* (2011), calls on private and

Table 11-2 Primary, Secondary, and Tertiary Health Care

CARE LEVEL	GOAL	PRACTITIONER	PRACTICE SITE	ACTIVITIES
Primary Health Care	Common health problems (sore throats, diabetes, arthritis, depression, or hypertension) and preventive measures (vaccinations, mammograms) that account for 80–90% of visits to clinicians	Family practice physicians Nurse practitioners Midwives	Family planning centers Primary care centers Urgent care centers Employment health centers	Family planning Prenatal and well-baby care Immunization against specific diseases Health risk screenings Diagnostic tests Health education Medications
Secondary Health Care	Problems that require more specialized clinical expertise, such as hospital care for a patient with a myocardial infarction or stroke	Physicians in specialties such as internal medicine, pediatrics, neurology, psychiatry Advance practice nurses	Hospital-based clinics Emergency departments Hospitals Psychiatric institutes Same-day surgery units	Disease identification and management
Tertiary Health Care	Management of rare and complex disorders such as pituitary tumors and congenital malformations	Subspecialist physicians such as cardiovascular surgeons, pediatric hematologists Advance practice nurses	Tertiary care medical centers	Rare and complex disease management

Source: Adapted from Bodenheimer, T., & Grumbach, K. (2016). *Understanding health policy: A clinical approach* (7th ed.). McGraw-Hill.

Through the Eyes of a Nurse

Asked to describe what keeps me up at night, I spoke about an upcoming summit . . . one in which health care innovation would be featured prominently as part of a conversation about health care reform. I spoke about my concern, as the sole nurse leader in attendance, whether the space would be created in such an important forum for a larger conversation to take place—about how, in the face of emerging technologies and provider shortages, we can better utilize our health care workforce for potentially tens of millions who, under the Affordable Care Act, will likely soon find themselves with improved access to care.

. . . I believe the greatest challenge for nurse leaders is to influence the culture of care so that patients are able to optimally benefit from the knowledge, competencies, and skills of nurses. Nurses bring unique cost-saving value to health care and have the capacity to be system innovators. I believe nurses must be empowered to participate as leaders in care delivery redesign to assure changes will be meaningful for patients. And yet, nurses remain on the periphery of many policy and reform conversations.

- Care coordination managed by nurses decreases costs. One IOM-commissioned study published in 2011 showed uncoordinated care raises costs by 75%, compared to similar cases with coordinated care.
- There is a strong link between patient satisfaction, nurse staffing, and revenue. Thirty percent of Medicare value-based performance scores are based on patient satisfaction scores (HCAHPS)—the single most important aspect of which is patient perceptions of excellent nursing care. In addition, increasing the proportion of RNs providing care within the team improves patient outcomes (decreased falls, reduced rates of complications, and lower mortality) and costs.
- Expanding access to advance practice registered nurses (APRNs) will provide additional primary coverage to people who otherwise find it difficult or impossible to have timely access to primary care.
- Women who deliver with midwives have fewer C-sections and higher breastfeeding rates, pointing to the cost effectiveness of midwifery services. A 2011 Agency for Healthcare Research and Quality brief found that the cost of a cesarean delivery was almost $2,000 higher than for a vaginal delivery. Considering there are approximately four million births per year in this country and 32% are delivered by C-section, that is a total of $2.5 billion per year. Reducing this number by even 5% by increasing access to midwifery care for low-risk pregnancies would result in about $128 million in savings on hospitalizations alone.

These are just a few of the compelling arguments with respect to the value of nurses.

—Karen A. Daley, PhD, RN, FAAN, President, American Nurses Association

Source: Reprinted with permission from Daley, K. A. (2013). President's perspective: What keeps me up at night? *The American Nurse, 45*(1), 3.

public funders, health care organizations, nursing education programs, and nursing associations to expand opportunities for nurses to lead and manage collective efforts with health care providers and other members of the health care team to conduct research as well as redesign and improve practice environments and health systems. Recognizing the key role nurses play in the health of Americans, the National Academies of Sciences, Engineering, and Medicine is currently working on a consensus report, *The Future of Nursing 2020–2031*, that charts a path for the nursing profession to help the United States create a culture of health, reduce health disparities, and improve the health and well-being of the U.S. population in the 21st century. This committee is considering newly emerging evidence related to the COVID-19 pandemic, and the report includes recommendations regarding the role of nurses in responding to the crisis created by a pandemic (https://www.nationalacademies.org/our-work/the-future-of-nursing-2020-2030). This is an exciting time to be a nurse. See the accompanying display, Through the Eyes of a Nurse.

ORGANIZING HEALTH CARE: HEALTH CARE DELIVERY SYSTEMS AND CARE COORDINATION

For a long time, health care delivery in the United States has been characterized by fragmentation at the national, state, community, and practice levels. A 2008 Commonwealth Fund study (Shih et al., 2008) found that:

- Patients and families navigate unassisted across different providers and care settings, fostering frustrating and dangerous patient experiences.
- Poor communication and lack of clear accountability for a patient among multiple providers lead to medical errors, waste, and duplication.
- The absence of peer accountability, quality improvement infrastructure, and clinical information systems foster poor overall quality of care.
- High-cost, intensive medical intervention is rewarded over higher-value primary care, including preventive medicine and the management of chronic illness.

As you read about the following delivery systems, note that great progress is being made to address this fragmentation, and nurses are playing ever more important roles in care coordination. See Chapter 12 for a discussion of the nurse navigator role. As noted in Chapter 1, the IOM report on nursing (IOM, 2011, p. ix) states that "accessible, high quality care cannot be achieved without exceptional nursing care and leadership."

Health Care Providers and Hospitals

Until recently in the United States, most medical care was delivered by fee-for-service private health care providers in solo or small group practices. Most hospitals were not-for-profit community hospitals. Health care providers, who were rarely employees of the hospital, wielded great power because hospitals depended on the patients whom health care providers admitted or referred for treatment. Under a **fee-for-service** arrangement (in which everything a provider "does" for a patient leads to a bill generated and a fee paid), financial incentives reward doing more care, not necessarily better care.

Multispecialty Group Practice

As new drugs and technologies proliferated, it became increasingly difficult for general practitioners of medicine to provide all the services their patients needed. In the late 1800s, when the Mayo Clinic was founded in Rochester, Minnesota, health care providers from different specialties united to share income, expenses, facilities, equipment, and support staff. The **multispecialty group practice** that resulted was better able to provide comprehensive care. While the Mayo Clinic generally served as a referral center, other multispecialty centers developed to serve specific communities.

Community Health Centers

Community health centers are regionalized services for vulnerable geographic populations with an emphasis on primary care and education. Their primary objective is to ensure that everyone who needs care has access regardless of the ability to pay. Most of these services rely on nurses to provide primary care. Mary Breckinridge's Frontier Nursing Service, which successfully served a poor rural area in Kentucky that lacked basic medical and obstetric care, was a pioneer organization at its inception in the 1920s.

Today the National Association of Community Health Centers (www.nachc.com) reports that community health centers serve the primary health care needs of more than 22 million patients in over 9,000 locations across the United States. According to NACHC, these health centers play a crucial role during tough economic times, providing affordable health services for millions of uninsured and newly jobless Americans. Community health centers save money every time an uninsured patient opts for an examination and treatment at the first sign of a health issue instead of waiting until a costly emergency room visit is the only option. These centers also save money for Americans looking for work whose families could otherwise face poor health without care or large medical debts.

Prepaid Group Practice

Health maintenance organizations (HMOs) are prepaid, group-managed care plans that allow subscribers to receive all the medical services they require through a group of affiliated providers. There may be no additional out-of-pocket costs, or subscribers may pay only a small fee, called a copayment. An HMO may employ all its providers (including health care providers), or it may be a group of clinicians in alliance who provide care as independent practitioners. In most HMOs, the patient does not have a choice about health care providers but receives all services from clinicians who are associated with or part of the HMO. HMOs often have a goal of primary care to reduce costs by preventing illness. HMOs are popular with large employers who support the concept of **managed care**, and they are also associated with Medicare in some states.

Preferred provider organizations (PPOs) allow a third-party payer (facilities that pay health care providers for services provided to people, such as a health insurance company) to contract with a group of health care providers to provide services at a lower fee in return for prompt payment and a guaranteed volume of patients and services. Although patients are encouraged to use specific providers, they may also seek care outside the panel without referral by paying additional out-of-pocket expenses. One type of PPO is called a preferred provider arrangement, in which a contract is made with an individual health care provider rather than with a group of providers. Similarly, a point-of-service plan encourages the use of specified health care providers and services but pays a portion of expenses for referrals made to health care providers outside the organization by the patient's primary care health care provider.

Accountable Care Organizations

One of the more innovative models of care delivery to emerge from the PPACA is the **accountable care organization (ACO)**. This new organizational structure is a departure from the traditional fee-for-service model of reimbursement. In the fee-for-service model, providers are incentivized to do more and more, but not necessarily in a coordinated manner. ACOs turn this model around by offering incentives to provide integrated, well-coordinated care to patients.

ACOs are made up of several types of organizations that deliver care: hospitals, primary care settings, and specialty care practices. Together, the organizations in an ACO come together to deliver the most efficient and high-quality care for the population served; only one bill is generated that covers *all* the care delivered across the various settings (e.g., before the hospitalization, during the inpatient stay, and after discharge from the hospital). In addition, when providers (hospitals and outpatient practice settings) deliver higher quality and more efficient care, they share in the savings from delivering well-integrated care.

Because nurses have the skill set to coordinate care across settings, they are especially well suited to make a real contribution to improved population health within ACOs.

Medical Homes to Medical Neighborhoods

A **medical home** is an enhanced model of primary care that provides whole-person, accessible, comprehensive, ongoing, and coordinated patient-centered care. Figure 11-7 illustrates a conceptual model for a medical home oriented to the Institute for Health Improvement's Quadruple Aim.

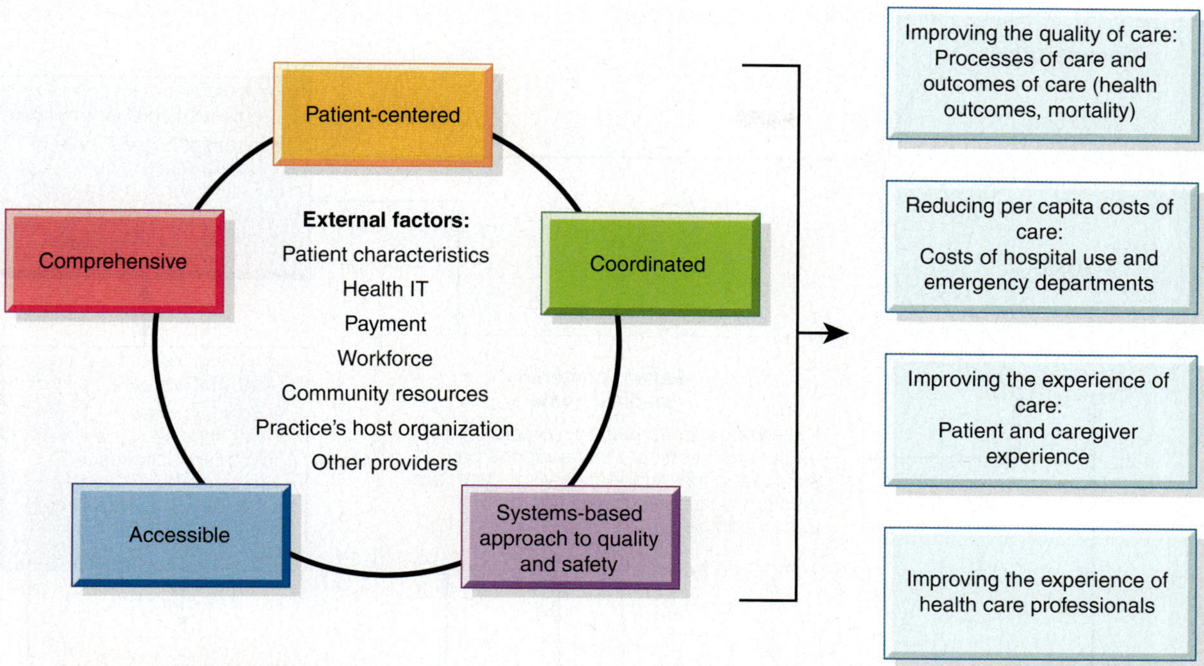

FIGURE 11-7. Conceptual framework for the effectiveness of the medical home. (*Source:* Used with permission. Agency for Healthcare Research and Quality. [2013]. The medical home: What do we know, what do we need to know? A review of the earliest evidence on the effectiveness of the patient-centered medical home model. AHRQ Publication No. 12-0020-1-EF.)

First advanced by the American Academy of Pediatrics in the 1960s, the medical home concept gained momentum in 2007 when four major physician groups agreed to a common view of the patient-centered medical home (PCMH) model (AHRQ, 2013). The 2012 Patient-Centered Primary Care Collaborative research project demonstrated that the data about PCMHs are clear, consistent, and compelling: "The PCMH improves health outcomes, enhances the patient experience of care and reduces expensive, unnecessary hospital and ED care" (Nielsen et al., 2012).

A 2011 Agency for Healthcare Research and Quality (AHRQ) white paper defines a **medical neighborhood** as a PCMH and the constellation of other clinicians providing health care services to patients within it, along with community and social service organizations as well as state and local public health facilities (Fig. 11-8 on page 286). Defined in this way, the PCMH and the surrounding medical neighborhood can focus on meeting the needs of the individual patient but also incorporate aspects of population health and overall community health needs in its objectives (Taylor et al., 2011, p. 5). But despite all our efforts to improve health care, the report starkly concludes:

> The medical neighborhood in its current form is highly fragmented, with little coordination among the myriad clinicians and institutions . . . primary care—and increasingly a PCMH as the provider of that primary care—should be at the core of the neighborhood, but for many patients it is not. Without a medical home, patients and their families often are left to navigate the system on their own. The current functioning of the neighborhood largely reflects the fee for service environment—in which few or no incentives exist for care coordination activities—and a historical emphasis on specialty-based medical practice in independent small groups or solo practice. Other factors, however, including existing professional norms and a lack of tools to share information across clinicians, also play a role in the way the medical neighborhood currently functions.

Care Coordination

The AHRQ Care Coordination Measures Atlas acknowledges that there is no consensus definition for care coordination but offers the following (McDonald et al., 2010):

> **Care coordination** is the deliberate organization of patient care activities between two or more participants (including the patient) involved in a patient's care to facilitate the appropriate delivery of health care services. Organizing care involves the marshaling of personnel and other resources needed to carry out all required patient care activities and is often managed by the exchange of information among participants responsible for different aspects of care.

Nurses are critical to the success of any care coordination strategy. Chapter 12 explores this topic more fully.

PAYING FOR HEALTH CARE

Few citizens can afford to pay for health care from their own resources. The costs of most people's health care are covered by public or private health insurance. The four basic

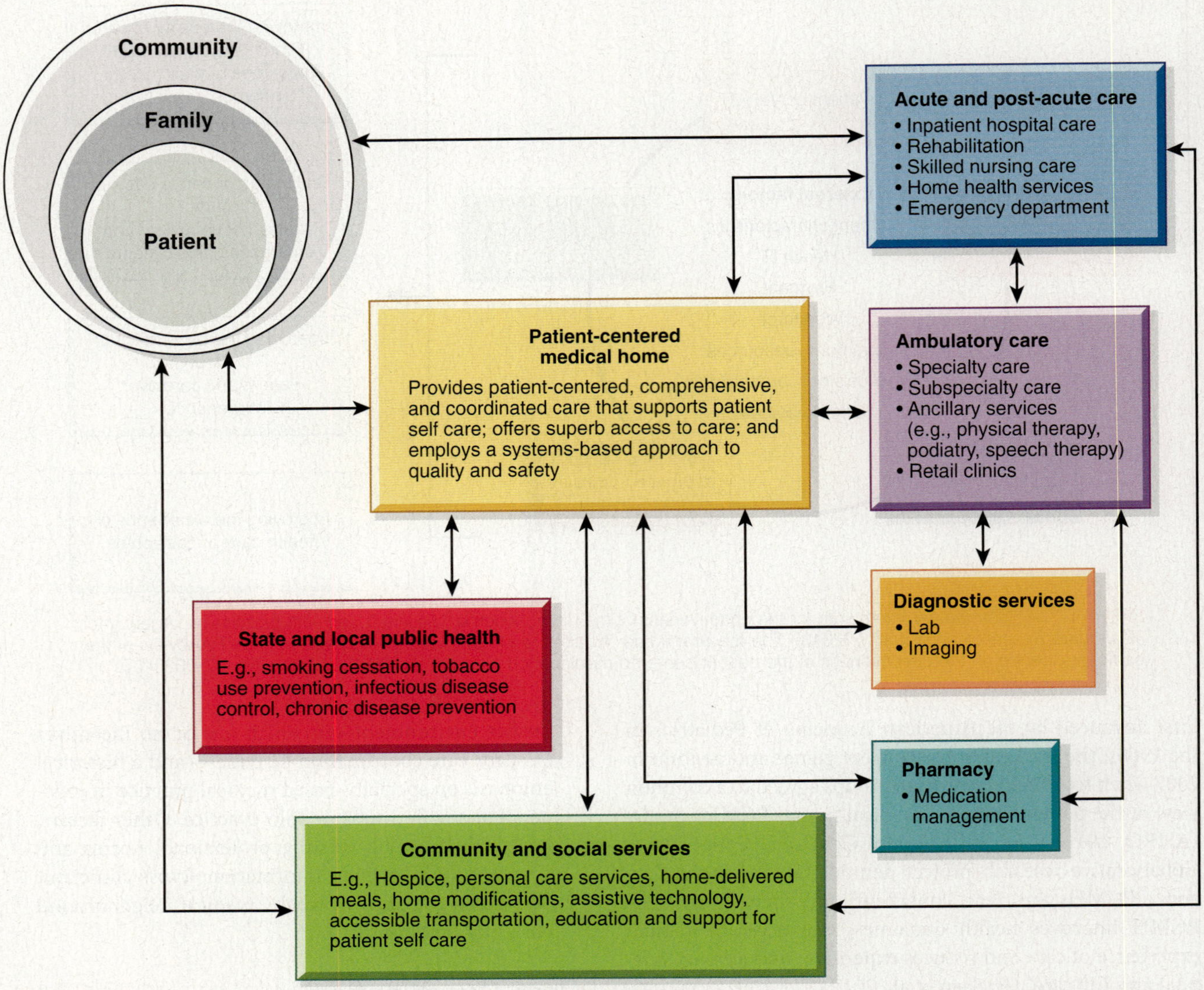

FIGURE 11-8. Medical neighborhood. (*Source:* Reprinted with permission from Taylor, E. F., Lake, T., Nysenbaum, J., Peterson, G., & Meyers, D. [2011]. *Coordinating care in the medical neighborhood: critical components and available mechanisms. White Paper [Prepared by Mathematica Policy Research under Contract No. HHSA290200900019I TO2]. AHRQ Publication No. 11–0064.* Agency for Healthcare Research and Quality.)

modes of paying for health care are out-of-pocket payment, individual private insurance, employer-based group private insurance, and government financing.

Out-of-Pocket Payment

During the first half of the 20th century, most Americans paid for health care with cash payments. This simple method of financing is increasingly rare because today most families cannot afford the high costs of health care. Most Americans continue to believe that the basic health care needs of all should be met regardless of ability to pay.

Individual Private Insurance

Personal health care can be financed by private insurance through large, nonprofit, tax-exempt organizations or through smaller, private, for-profit insurance companies. To be insured, members pay monthly premiums either by themselves or in combination with employer payments. These plans are called third-party payers because the insurance company pays all or most of the cost of care. The premiums on private insurance plans tend to be higher than those for managed care plans, but members can choose their own health care providers and services desired.

Employer-Based Private Insurance

Employer-sponsored coverage remains the most common source of health care coverage in the United States. In 2014, 66% of nonelderly workers received an offer of coverage from their employer—less than the 71% rate in 1999. Employees who worked part time were less likely to be offered coverage from their employer than were employees working full time. The percentage of workers covered has declined over the last 15 years, and the decline is greatest among families with low and modest incomes (Long et al., 2016).

Government Financing

The largest federally funded health care programs are Medicare and Medicaid. Other federally funded programs include the Children's Health Insurance Program (CHIP) and the Veteran's Health Administration (VHA).

Medicare

The 1965 **Medicare** amendments to the Social Security Act established national and state health insurance programs for older adults under Title XVIII. Within a decade, almost all citizens over 65 years of age held Medicare insurance for hospital care, extended care, and home health care. Medicare coverage was increased in 1972 to include permanently disabled workers and their dependents, if they also qualified for Social Security benefits.

In 1983, Medicare converted to a prospective payment plan based on patient classification categories, called **diagnosis-related groups (DRGs)**. The federal government implemented DRGs in an effort to control rising health care costs. The plan pays the hospital a fixed amount that is predetermined by the medical diagnosis or specific procedure rather than by the actual cost of hospitalization and care. Medicare was expanded in 1988 to include catastrophic care costs and expensive medications.

In 2007, based on changes in DRGs made by the CMS, the criteria for reimbursement to hospitals became severity of illness and projected cost of care. The plan pays only the amount of money preassigned to a treatment for the diagnosis (e.g., an appendectomy); if the cost of hospitalization is greater than that assigned, the hospital must absorb the additional cost. If the cost is less than that assigned, the hospital makes a profit. In addition, Medicare no longer reimburses hospitals for conditions that result from preventable errors and lead to increased costs. Such conditions include pressure injuries, injuries caused by falls, infections associated with indwelling urinary catheters, vascular catheter–associated infections, infections of the mediastinum after coronary artery bypass graft, air embolisms, adverse reactions to incompatible blood infusions, and sponges or instruments left inside a patient during surgery.

People who receive Medicare pay both a deductible cost and a monthly premium for full insurance coverage. Part A of Medicare, which pays most inpatient hospital costs, is paid by the federal government. Part B of Medicare, which is voluntary, is paid by a monthly premium; it covers most outpatient costs for physician visits, medications, and home health services. Because the full cost of some services is not covered by Medicare, a supplemental insurance policy offered by a private insurance company is recommended. Also, because Medicare is federally funded, benefits may change annually according to Congressional decisions related to the federal budget. There continues to be talk about "phasing out" Medicare. In the second decade of the 21st century there continues to be a national debate about whether the United States can continue to operate Medicare in the same form along with other government programs and still control spiraling health care costs. In the United States, as in other countries, **entitlement reform** is being considered for benefits paid by the government to citizens in order to improve the national budget and reduce debt. See Medicare and You (2016), available at https://www.medicare.gov/Pubs/pdf/10050.pdf.

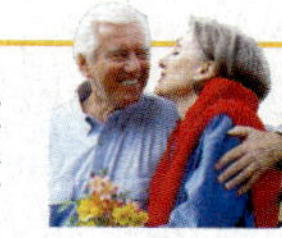

Remember **Margaret Ritchie**, the older adult woman caring for her husband at home. Most likely, she and her husband have Medicare. Medicare does pay for home health care services if the patient meets specific criteria. However, Medicare does not cover all equipment that may be necessary. Medicare does not pay for nursing home care.

Medicaid

Medicaid was established in 1965 under Title XIX of the Social Security Act. Medicaid is a federally funded public assistance program for people of any age who have low incomes; for blind, older adult, and disabled people covered by supplemental security benefits; and for beneficiaries of Aid to Families with Dependent Children. This coverage depends on individual state regulations. Visit www.medicaid.gov to learn more about this program.

Current budgetary considerations are leading state and federal facilities to trim Medicaid expenditures. The rapid growth of an aging population and an increased number of people experiencing poverty, many of whom are women and children, are draining the Medicaid budget. In an attempt to survive, Medicaid programs are implementing changes such as reducing benefits or placing patients into managed care programs.

Children's Health Insurance Program

The CHIP, formerly the State Children's Health Insurance Program (SCHIP), was created by the Balanced Budget Act of 1997, was enacted as Title XXI of the Social Security Act, and has allocated about $20 billion over 10 years to help states insure low-income children who are ineligible for Medicaid but cannot afford private insurance. States receive an enhanced federal match (greater than the state's Medicaid match) to provide this coverage. In 2007 the program was extended, and in 2009 was reauthorized by Congress and signed by President Obama. Together, Medicaid and CHIP serve more than 42 million children who would otherwise not have access to regular medical care. While Medicaid and CHIP have helped bring the rate of uninsured children to the lowest level in more than two decades, many more children are eligible but not covered as of yet.

Veterans Health Administration

The Veterans Health Administration is home to the United States' largest integrated health care system, consisting of 152 medical centers, nearly 1,400 community-based outpatient clinics, community living centers, veterans' centers, and domiciliaries. Together these health care facilities and the more than 53,000 independent licensed health care practitioners who work within them provide comprehensive care to more than 8.3 million veterans each year. The VHA has an annual medical care appropriation of more than $47 billion.

HEALTH CARE SETTINGS AND SERVICES

Health care is provided within many different types of facilities to meet the varying needs of people. When one considers that only patients who require complex surgery, those who are acutely ill or seriously injured, and some who are having babies are hospitalized—and then only for a minimum period of time—it is apparent that most health care services are provided in settings outside the hospital. These settings include clinics, homes, schools, prisons, daycare centers for children and older adults, crisis-intervention centers, mental health centers, drug and alcohol rehabilitation programs, storefront clinics, and churches.

Hospitals

There are approximately 5,000 community hospitals in the United States. Community hospitals are short-term, general, nonfederal, and special (e.g., orthopedic, cancer, and academic medical center) hospitals. Each year, community hospitals admit more than 35 million people, treat nearly 118 million people in their emergency departments, and deliver over 4 million babies (American Hospital Association, 2020). Most hospital stays are short, although longer stays occur in patients who have serious infections, major trauma, mental illnesses, and cardiovascular diseases. Today's shorter hospital stays have resulted from many factors, including improved treatment of diseases, an increased emphasis on preventive care, federal regulations, and other health care reimbursement policies. The shorter stay means that most hospital care is focused on the acute care needs of the patient. Nurses play a critical role in ensuring that patients and their family caregivers are prepared to meet their health care needs by the time of discharge.

Classification

Hospitals are classified as public or private, and as for profit or nonprofit. Public hospitals, which are nonprofit institutions, are financed and operated by local, state, or national facilities. Patients admitted to a public hospital may not have health insurance, and services are provided at little or no cost to the patient. Tax revenue or public funds cover the cost. Private hospitals may be for profit or nonprofit and are operated by communities, churches, corporations, and charitable organizations. The Catholic health ministry is the largest group of nonprofit health care providers in the nation. Every day one in six patients in the United States is cared for in a Catholic hospital. Many patients cared for in private hospitals have some type of personal health insurance or health care plan.

Size and Services

Hospitals range in size from as few as 20 beds to large medical centers with hundreds of beds. Various services are provided, depending on the size and location of the hospital. Most hospitals provide emergency care, inpatient care, surgery, diagnostic tests, and patient education. Other hospital services may include intensive care, obstetric care, palliative care, social services, outpatient clinics and surgery, educational programs, and long-term skilled nursing care facilities. Hospitals may provide care for all types of illnesses and trauma or may specialize in the treatment of certain types of illness. Specialty hospitals, or special units in general hospitals, meet the varied needs of certain patient groups such as children and patients of all ages needing rehabilitation, cancer care, psychiatric or drug-dependency care, or patients with severe burns.

Inpatient and Outpatient Services

Hospitals provide both inpatient and outpatient services. An **inpatient** is a person who enters a hospital and stays overnight for an indeterminate time (from days to months). Hospitals also have many services for **outpatients**—those who are not hospitalized overnight but who require diagnosis or treatment. Patients who do not require inpatient care can receive treatment, care, and education on an outpatient basis. Examples of outpatient services include surgical procedures, diagnostic tests, medications, physical therapy, counseling, and health education. A form of hospital outpatient care occurs in short-stay units, where patients having diagnostic tests or surgery enter the hospital, have the procedure, and then return to the hospital room for a brief (1 to 6 hours) recovery period before going home. Patients may also be categorized as outpatients when they are admitted, treated, and discharged within 23 hours.

Nurses' Role in Hospitals

Although the trend is changing, hospitals still employ more nurses than any other type of facility. The percentage of RNs working in hospitals is declining, but about 61% of RNs are still employed in hospitals (Bureau of Labor Statistics, U.S. Department of Labor, 2017). The U.S. Department of Labor projects that the number of RNs employed in hospitals will decrease while those employed in outpatient settings, home health, and long-term care will increase. Nurses employed in hospitals have many roles. Although many nurses are direct care providers, other roles include manager of other members of the health care team providing patient care, administrator, nurse practitioner, clinical nurse specialist, patient educator, in-service educator, and researcher.

The Magnet Recognition Program for Excellence in Nursing and the Pathway to Excellence Program are administered by the American Nurses Credentialing Center (ANCC), a subsidiary of the American Nurses Association. Magnet hospitals must meet strict requirements and standards that define the highest quality of nursing practice and patient care. A designation as a magnet hospital recognizes quality patient care, nursing excellence, and innovations in professional nursing practice (American Nurses Credentialing Center, 2020). See Chapter 10 for more about Magnet Hospitals.

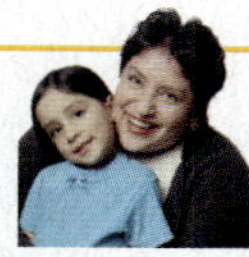

Think back to ***Maritza Cortes***, the mother who brings her daughter to the emergency department for care. The nurse in this situation acts primarily in the caregiver role. However, the nurse also plays a major role as educator, using knowledge about the infection to teach the mother about possible complications and the need for continued antibiotic treatment.

Primary Care Centers

Health care providers and advanced practice nurses provide primary health care services in offices and clinics. Services include the diagnosis and treatment of minor illnesses; performing minor surgical procedures; and providing obstetric care, well-child care, counseling, and referrals (Fig. 11-9). Federally qualified health centers (FQHCs), also known as community health centers, are nonprofit primary care clinics located in high-need areas across the country. Community health centers must serve everyone in the community, regardless of their health insurance and ability to pay, and often offer on-site mental health and dental services. An RN working in a health care provider's office makes health assessments, performs technical procedures, assists the health care provider, and provides health education and counseling.

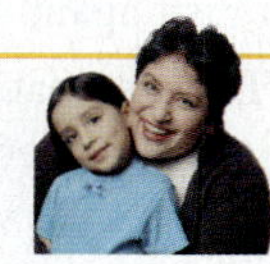

Recall ***Maritza Cortes***, the mother of the child with a strep throat. One might commonly think of primary health care services for typical childhood illnesses, but in this case, Ms. Cortes used the emergency department. Possibly, the mother thought that her child was too ill and needed to be seen immediately. In this case, the nurse would develop a teaching plan for Ms. Cortes about typical childhood illnesses. Maybe she did not know of anywhere else to obtain services. In this case, the nurse could contact social services to obtain information about community clinics for Ms. Cortes. Her finances may also have led to her decision to use the emergency department. In this case, the nurse also could contact social services to arrange for financial assistance.

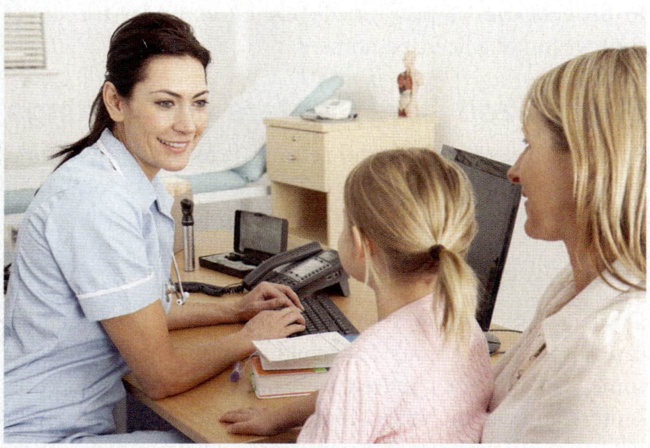

FIGURE 11-9. A nurse assesses a patient during a well-child visit at a primary care center. (*Source:* Used with permission from Shutterstock. *Photo by Monkey Business Images.*)

Advanced practice registered nurses (APRNs) are registered nurses educated at the master's or post-master's level in a specific role and for a specific population; examples include nurse practitioners, midwives, and clinical nurse specialists. APRNs work independently or collaboratively with health care providers to make assessments and care for patients who require health maintenance or health promotion activities. Depending on state regulations, APRNs may have their own offices and clinics to provide primary care and treatment to patients and refer only complex health problems to a health care provider.

Ambulatory Care Centers and Clinics

Ambulatory care centers and clinics (facilities that deliver outpatient medical care) may be located in hospitals or they may be freestanding services provided by a group of health care providers who work together. Ambulatory care centers and clinics are often located in convenient areas such as shopping malls or other community facilities. Many ambulatory care centers and clinics offer walk-in services so that appointments are unnecessary, and many are also open at times other than traditional office hours. They may be managed by an APRN. Small clinics staffed by APRNs are increasingly being established in nontraditional sites, such as drugstores and grocery stores. These clinics have dramatically improved access to care for the uninsured and those with other barriers to health care.

Nurses in ambulatory care centers and clinics provide technical services (e.g., administering medications), determine the priority of care needs, and provide teaching about all aspects of care. The urgent care center is a special type of ambulatory care center that provides walk-in care for illnesses and minor trauma. Outpatient or same-day surgical centers, discussed in Chapter 31, are another form of ambulatory care center.

Home Health Care

Home health care is one of the most rapidly growing areas of the health care system. Home health care may be provided through community health departments, visiting nurses' associations, hospital-based case managers, and home health facilities. These facilities provide many different health-related services, including skilled nursing assessment, teaching and support of patients and family members, and direct care for patients.

Home health care is important for many reasons. The prospective payment system of reimbursement encourages early discharge from the hospital, and has created a new, acutely ill population that needs skilled care at home. More older people are living longer and have multiple chronic illnesses, and with sophisticated technology people can live relatively comfortably in their own homes. Health care consumers demand that services be humane and that provisions be made for a dignified death at home. Read more about home care in Chapter 12.

Nurses who provide care in the home make assessments and provide physical care, administer medications, teach, and support family members. They also collaborate with other health care providers, such as physicians, physical therapists (PTs), occupational therapists, respiratory therapists (RTs), and social workers to plan and provide patient care. See Chapter 12.

Extended-Care Services

Extended-care services provide medical and nonmedical care for people with chronic illnesses or disabilities. Through a variety of facilities, and in conjunction with family members and other caregivers, extended-care services assist with activities of daily living for people of any age who are physically or mentally unable to care for themselves independently. In 2012, about 9 million people over the age of 65 used long-term care services; that number is projected to increase to 12 million by 2020.

Most extended care is provided to people by family or friends; for example, 70% of older adults requiring extended care are not in any type of facility. It is always helpful for nurses to be sensitive to the needs of family caregivers, who often labor at great health and financial costs to themselves. Visit the Family Caregiver Alliance National Center on Caregiving website (www.caregiver.org) to learn more about the experiences of caregivers.

Extended care may last for periods ranging from days to years. Facilities that provide this care are often independent but may be associated with a hospital. Extended-care facilities include transitional subacute care, assisted-living facilities, intermediate- and long-term care facilities, homes for medically fragile children, retirement centers, and residential institutions for mentally and developmentally or physically disabled patients of all ages. One of the newest concepts in extended care is called "aging in place." In this type of care, patients remain in their homes or move to a living space, such as an apartment, while they are still physically able to care for themselves, and then have access to services that are a part of the health care community as needed as long as they live. What is essential for this health care paradigm is a community committed to meeting one another's needs. Also popular today are senior retirement communities. These residential care homes offer many options to older people. Some offer a range of services from independent apartment living to skilled nursing care, to match the needs of older adults as they age. Many also include memory care units for people with dementia who require specialized care.

Extended-care facilities have proliferated in recent years for two reasons. First, as many patients are discharged from the hospital earlier in their recovery period, they require care that is beyond the scope of home care. These patients receive transitional, subacute care in an extended-care facility. Second, as the population ages, many older adults will not have caregivers available and would be unable to carry out activities of daily living independently. Although extended-care facilities, especially long-term care facilities, have had a negative image in the past, much has changed. Most long-term care facilities focus on maintaining residents' function and independence, with concern for the living environment as well as the health care provided. A focus on maximizing the quality of life for residents has led to surroundings that include plants and animals as well as numerous intergenerational programs. Many of the overall improvements in long-term care resulted from the 1987 Omnibus Budget Reconciliation Act (OBRA), which included legislation to maintain standards of quality assurance in the long-term care industry.

Nurses can share the American Association of Retired Persons' (AARP) nine things to do before choosing a nursing home with families seeking a nursing home placement:

1. Check the grounds. Perhaps most important—do you get a sense of security and safety? And, if your loved one enjoys being outdoors, are there nice sitting areas?
2. Schmooze the residents and ask about living conditions and interactions with other residents.
3. Talk with family members if they are willing to give their unvarnished opinions.
4. Ask tough questions so you can get a real sense of the place and feeling for the culture.
5. Check the staff turnover rates.
6. Have a meal.
7. Give a smell and sound test.
8. Make a safety check.
9. Visit again during off hours (Strauss, 2017).

Because patients entering extended-care facilities require so many different levels of care, it is difficult to generalize about the services provided. Those entering convalescent centers remain only until they have recovered. In some instances, an older adult may choose to move into a retirement or assisted-living facility that provides health care services only when needed. Other people who enter a long-term care facility may require complete care as long as they live. The nurse's roles in extended-care facilities may include being a provider of direct care, supervisor, administrator, safety or quality nurse, or teacher. Because most patients are older, increasing numbers of gerontology nurse specialists are contributing their knowledge and expertise to the care of these patients. Almost all extended-care facilities require that skilled nursing care be available at all times. The care given to patients can be performed only by or under the direct supervision of a licensed nurse.

Specialized Care Centers and Settings

Specialized care centers and settings provide services for a specific population or group. They are usually located in easily accessible locations within a community.

Daycare Centers

Daycare centers have a variety of purposes. Some centers care for healthy infants and children whose parents work; some also care for children with minor illnesses. Eldercare centers and senior citizen centers provide a place for older adults to socialize and to receive care while family members work. Some daycare centers provide health-related services and care to people who do not need to be in a health care institution but cannot be at home alone. Such centers provide services to older adults for physical rehabilitation, for people with functional needs (e.g., cerebral palsy), and for chemical dependency and mental health.

Nurses who work in daycare centers administer medications and treatments, conduct health screenings, teach, and counsel.

Mental Health/Behavioral Centers

A mental health center may be associated with a hospital or may provide services as an independent facility. The services provided may be crisis-centered or may involve long-term counseling. Patients receive outpatient care through a variety of interventions, including individual and group counseling, medications, and assistance with independent living. Crisis intervention centers are also mental health centers. They typically provide 24-hour services and hotlines for people who are suicidal, using drugs or alcohol, or in abusive situations. These centers also provide information and services for victims of rape and abuse. In most communities, needed mental health services are inadequately funded, and you may experience difficulty in matching existing resources with a patient's or family's needs.

Nurses who work in mental health centers must have strong communication and counseling skills and must be thoroughly familiar with community resources specific to the needs of patients being served in order to make appropriate referrals.

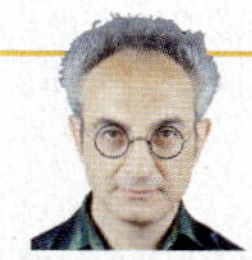

Remember **Paul Cochran**, the patient with a mental illness who ran out of his medications. The nurse needs knowledge of local mental health centers to ensure continuity of care, including follow-up with medication regimen.

Rural Health Centers

Rural health centers are often located in geographically remote areas that have few health care providers. Many rural health centers are run by APRNs who serve as the patient's primary health provider for the care of minor acute illnesses as well as chronic illnesses. Patients who are seriously ill or injured are given emergency care and then transported to the nearest large hospital. Nurses who practice independently may do so in collaboration with a health care provider. Many rural health care settings and providers now have immediate access to information about diagnosis and treatment of illness through telecommunication and computers. Health disparities facing Americans living in rural areas have recently been compounded by closures of rural hospitals. Two types of facilities have increased in recent years to meet the needs of rural patients:

- Critical access hospitals must have fewer than 25 acute inpatient beds, be located more than 35 miles from another hospital, provide around-the-clock emergency care services, and maintain an average length-of-stay of 96 hours or less for acute care patients.
- Freestanding emergency departments may be affiliated with a larger facility or operate independently.

The screening and education provided by nurses and nurse practitioners in rural communities continues to help patients live healthier lives (Peterson, 2020, p. 18).

Schools

School nurses are often the major source of health assessment, health education, and emergency care for the nation's children. The role of the school nurse reflects changes in society itself: children in schools today are from many different racial and ethnic groups, have varying socioeconomic backgrounds, and have more complex disabilities that require expert knowledge and skills for management during school hours. School nurses provide many different services, including maintaining immunization records, providing emergency care for physical and mental illnesses, administering prescribed medications, conducting routine health screenings (e.g., vision, hearing, scoliosis), and providing health information and education.

Industry

Many large industries have their own ambulatory care clinic, staffed primarily by nurses. Occupational health nurses in industrial clinics focus on preventing work-related injury and illness by conducting health assessments, teaching for health promotion (e.g., stopping smoking, eating sensibly, using safety equipment, exercising regularly), caring for minor accidents and illnesses, and making referrals for more serious health problems.

Homeless Shelters

Homeless shelters are usually living units, such as an apartment building or home, that provide housing for people who do not have regular shelter. People experiencing homelessness are at increased risk for illness or injury because of factors such as exposure to the elements, exposure to violence, drug and alcohol use disorders, poor nutrition, poor hygiene, and overcrowding. Services provided by nurses in homeless shelters include immunizing children, teaching pregnant women, treating infections and illnesses, referring for diagnosis and treatment of STIs, and providing information about maintaining health. See the Vulnerable Populations Alert: Patients who are Homeless in Chapter 3.

Rehabilitation Centers

Rehabilitation centers specialize in services for patients requiring physical or emotional rehabilitation and for treatment of chemical dependency. These centers may be freestanding or associated with a hospital. The goal is to return patients to optimal health and to the community as independent members of society. Rehabilitation centers often use a multidisciplinary team composed of health care providers, nurses, PTs, occupational therapists, and counselors. The role of the nurse includes direct care, teaching, and counseling. The practice of rehabilitation nursing is based on a philosophy of encouraging independent self-care within the patient's capabilities.

Unfolding Patient Stories: Kim Johnson • Part 2

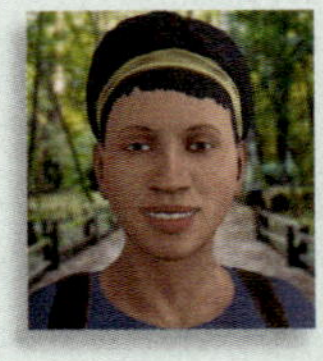

Recall **Kim Johnson** from Chapter 3, the 26-year-old police officer with paraplegia from a thoracic spinal cord injury. She is being transferred from the hospital to a rehabilitation facility. What education would the nurse provide on the purpose of a rehabilitation center? How can the nurse facilitate a smooth transition to the new facility for Kim and her parents? How may determinants of health play a role in her rehabilitation?

Care for Kim and other patients in a realistic virtual environment: ***vSim** for Nursing* (thepoint.lww.com/vSimFunds). Practice documenting these patients' care in DocuCare (thepoint.lww.com/DocuCareEHR).

Parish Nursing

Parish nursing is an expanding area of specialty nursing practice that emphasizes holistic health care, health promotion, and disease-prevention activities. It combines professional nursing practice with health ministry, emphasizing health and healing within a faith community. Parish nurses function as health educators, resource and referral aids, and facilitators of lay volunteer and support groups. Parish nurses reach out to those most vulnerable, such as older adults, those who have suffered a loss or change, single parents, and children. For more about parish nursing, see Chapter 47.

Health Care Services for the Seriously Ill and Dying

Health care services for the seriously ill and dying and for their families and caregivers include respite care, hospice, and palliative care. (End-of-life care is discussed further in Chapter 44.)

Respite Care

Respite care is a type of care provided for caregivers of homebound ill, disabled, or older adults. The main purpose is to give the primary caregiver some time away from the responsibilities of day-to-day care. Professionals or volunteers may provide care in an adult daycare center or in the patient's home. In most instances, the care is provided by qualified nursing assistants or volunteers. Professional nurses provide information about how to access respite care and may make referrals. Medicaid and most insurance providers do not cover the costs of respite care.

Hospice Services

Hospice is a program of palliative and supportive care services providing physical, psychological, social, and spiritual care for dying people, their families, and other loved ones. The interdisciplinary hospice team:

- Manages the patient's pain and symptoms
- Assists the patient with emotional, psychosocial, and spiritual aspects of dying
- Provides needed drugs, medical supplies, and equipment
- Instructs the family on how to care for the patient
- Delivers special services such as speech and physical therapy when needed
- Makes short-term inpatient care available when pain or symptoms become too difficult to treat at home, or the caregiver needs respite
- Provides bereavement care and counseling to surviving family and friends (National Hospice and Palliative Care Organization [NHPCO], 2020).

In 2017, an estimated 1.49 million Medicare beneficiaries received hospice services for 1 day or more (NHPCO, 2020). Approximately 44.6% of all deaths in the United States in 2011 were under the care of a hospice program. The number of hospice programs nationwide has increased since the first program in 1974 to over 4,300 programs today. The Medicare hospice benefit, enacted by Congress in 1982, is the predominant source of payment for hospice care. To be eligible for hospice benefits from Medicare or Medicaid, the patient must have a serious, progressive illness with a life expectancy of 6 months or less.

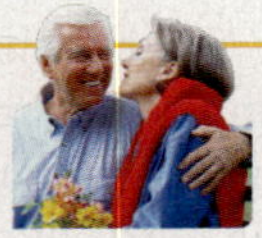

Think back to **Margaret Ritchie**, who is caring for her husband at home. The health care provider recently informed her of her husband's prognosis. The nurse might anticipate that hospice care would be appropriate for Mrs. Ritchie and her husband.

The hospice nurse combines the skills of the home care nurse with the ability to provide daily emotional support to dying patients and their families. Hospice nurses are especially skilled in pain and symptom management. Their focus is on improving the quality of life rather than merely prolonging its length, and on preserving dignity for the patient in death. After the death, the nurse continues to care for the patient's family during the bereavement period for up to 1 year. Nurses use this time to help families work through the grief process after their loss. (See Chapter 44 for more information.)

Palliative Care

Palliative care evolved from the hospice experience but also exists outside of hospice programs. It is not restricted to the end of life and can be used from the point of initial diagnosis. Palliative care, which may be given in conjunction with medical treatment and in all types of health care settings, is patient- and family-centered care that optimizes the quality of life by anticipating, preventing, and treating suffering.

The NHPCO identifies the following features that characterize palliative care philosophy and delivery:

- Care is provided and services are coordinated by an interdisciplinary team.

- Patients, families, palliative and nonpalliative health care providers collaborate and communicate about care needs.
- Services are available concurrently with or independent of curative or life-prolonging care.
- Patient and family hopes for peace and dignity are supported throughout the course of illness, during the dying process, and after death (NHPCO, 2020).

HEALTH CARE FACILITIES

Many different types of facilities provide health care services. This section discusses voluntary facilities, religious facilities, and government facilities.

Voluntary Facilities

Community facilities are often nonprofit voluntary facilities. They are financed by private donations, grants, or fundraisers (although some may charge minimal fees). Examples of volunteer facilities are Meals on Wheels, which supplies meals to older and homebound people; transportation services for older and physically disabled people; and shopping or house-cleaning services. Other nonprofit voluntary community facilities include the American Heart Association and the American Lung Association. Health care providers and nurses are often active members of these organizations, providing health screenings and educational programs.

Voluntary facilities may also provide a setting for support groups. These groups provide an education and support system for patients who are adjusting to their health problems. Members of these support groups have experienced the same type of problem. By sharing their experiences, members learn to solve problems when dealing with a stressful or crisis situation. Professional nurses most often provide information about and make referrals to these facilities to patients and family members. The following are examples of support groups:

- *Alcoholics Anonymous*—an international organization for people recovering from alcohol use disorders.
  The purpose is to help people stop drinking and remain sober. Meetings are held in accessible community locations, such as churches and hospitals.
- *Cancer support groups*—focus on support and solving problems experienced by people diagnosed with cancer. Most cancer support group meetings are held at hospitals.
- *Reach to Recovery*—for women who have had a breast removed for cancer or have had breast reconstruction surgery. Among other activities, members visit women before surgery, teach exercises to prevent muscle atrophy, and provide information about prostheses and clothing.

Other Government Facilities

In addition to Medicare, Medicaid, and the Veteran's Association, described earlier, there are other government health facilities.

Public Health Service

The Public Health Service (PHS) is a federal health facility under the direction of the U.S. Department of Health and Human Services. The PHS is a multifaceted program with a wide range of services. It is the medical branch of the U.S. Coast Guard and the principal source of Native American health care through the Indian Health Services. The PHS supplies funds to health centers that provide care to migrant workers and to community facilities that supply health care to the poor and uninsured. The principal budget of the PHS goes to grant programs for poor and uninsured people.

The Centers for Disease Control and Prevention (CDC) in Atlanta and the National Institutes of Health (NIH) are both part of the PHS. The CDC focuses on the epidemiology, prevention, control, and treatment of communicable diseases, such as STIs. The NIH is engaged in both funding and conducting various health research activities.

The PHS also supplies health care professionals (e.g., nurses, health care providers, dentists, pharmacists) to the U.S. Department of Justice to provide care in federal prisons. The service is also involved in some state-administered drug and alcohol use and mental health programs. PHS activities focus on community needs whenever possible. Nurses practicing in these settings provide direct care, provide information, and serve as patient advocates within the community. See Figure 11-10 (on pages 294–295) for an illustration of 10 essential public health services and how they can address social determinants of health (SDOH) inequities.

Public Health Facilities

Public health facilities are local, state, and federal facilities that provide PHS at the local, county, state, or federal level. They are usually funded by taxes and run by elected or appointed administrators. Local facilities provide services and programs to promote health and prevent illness, such as providing immunizations and screening for tuberculosis and STIs. Public health facilities work with state and local departments to ensure public health through activities such as inspections of restaurants and water supplies. They also provide educational programs and may provide direct care services for low-income people or people living in rural, isolated areas. Nurses who practice in public health facilities focus on prenatal care, well-child care, screening programs, education, and outreach into the community (Fig. 11-11 on page 295).

COLLABORATIVE CARE: THE INTERPROFESSIONAL HEALTH CARE TEAM

In any type of facility, setting, or framework, nurses work with other members of the interprofessional health care team to plan, provide, and evaluate patient care (Box 11-3 on page 296). The likelihood of achieving valued patient outcomes is greatly enhanced when nurses are skilled in collaborating with other members of the professional caregiving team.

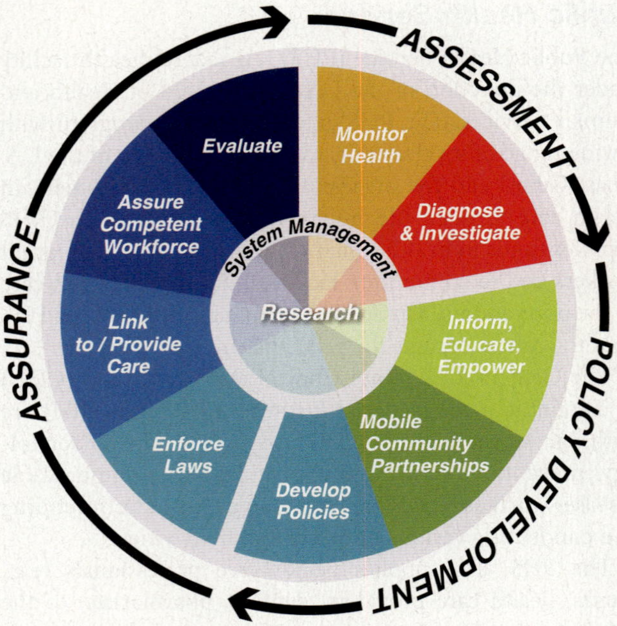

10 Essential Public Health Services

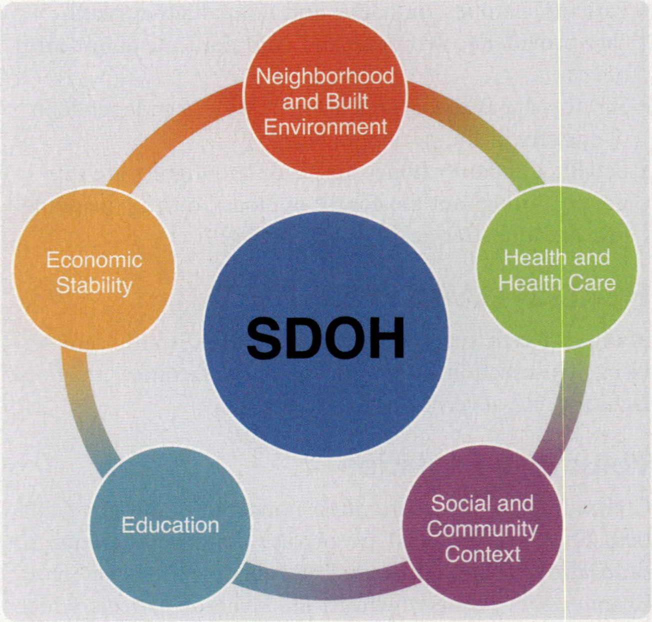

Five Key Areas of SDOH (HP 2020)

	Roles of Public Health Agency (Based on 10 Essential Public Health Services)	Examples of How Essential Public Health Services Can Address
1.	Monitor health status to identify and solve community health problems	Include SDOH measures as basis for addressing community health problems and inequities Ensure community health assessments (CHA) include SDOH measures and engage communities and multi-sectoral partners in CHA efforts
2.	Diagnose and investigate health problems and health hazards in the community	Include community-level determinants of health in investigations, as well as policies and practices that involve other sectors to support them. For example • Ensure water sources meet required standards • Ensure brownfield sites Identify hazardous waste that might contaminate a community • Address deteriorating housing conditions to prevent lead poisoning and other hazards to health
3.	Inform, educate, and empower people about health issues	Ensure outreach and education efforts address social and structural determinants of health inequities Ensure access to culturally and linguistically appropriate approaches to community health (e.g., REACH) to help address SDOH. Approaches should take into account such challenges as structural racism and stigma against immigrants, both of which can decrease likelihood of seeking needed health care.
4.	Mobilize community partnerships and action to identify and solve health problems	Engage and collaborate with community members and non-traditional partners associated with SDOHs, such as • Housing authorities • Law enforcement • Schools • Community organizations

FIGURE 11-10. Ten essential public health services and how they can include addressing social determinants of health inequities. Public health departments and their partners need to consider how conditions in the places where people live, learn, work, and play affect a wide range of health risks and outcomes. These social determinants of health (SDOH), and actions to address the resulting health inequities, can be incorporated throughout all aspects of public health work. Through broader awareness of how the key public health practices can better incorporate consideration of SDOH, public health practitioners can transform and strengthen their capacity and impact to advance health equity. (*Source:* U.S. Department of Health and Human Services, Centers for Disease Control and Prevention. https://www.cdc.gov/publichealthgateway/publichealthservices/pdf/ten_essential_services_and_sdoh.pdf)

5.	Develop policies and plans that support individual and community health efforts	Leverage evidence-based policies in non-health sectors that affect SDOH and health outcomes, such as • Safe and affordable housing that can reduce risk for asthma, lead poisoning, homelessness • Full-day kindergarten that can reduce adverse health prospects such as teenage pregnancy Develop and implement state/community health improvement plans that include and address the SDOH in collaboration with community partners
6.	Enforce laws and regulations that protect health and ensure safety	Develop strategies to ensure enforcement of existing regulations and laws that affect health, such as • Housing and health codes to prevent childhood lead poisoning. • Batterer intervention program laws to prevent violence against women and children
7.	Link people to needed personal health services and ensure the provision of health care when otherwise unavailable	Educate community members about their eligibility for and access to entitlement programs • Medicaid, including its medical, mental health, and housing benefits • TANF • SNAP Ensure that essential health benefits and the free preventive services provisions of the Affordable Care Act are correctly and equitably implemented
8.	Assure competent public and personal health care workforce	Support staff training and development efforts that help workforce incorporate social determinants of health inequity into their job responsibilities Promote hiring of workforce that reflects population being served
9.	Evaluate effectiveness, accessibility, and quality of personal and population-based health services	Ensure evaluation and research designs include interventions that address SDOH inequity Use performance management and quality improvement methods to explore and address more effectively the root causes of issues, which often include SDOH
10.	Research for new insights and innovative solutions to health problems	Expand research agendas to include SDOH and related health outcomes, especially in evaluation of natural experiments where a project is already addressing SDOH but is not studying health effects (e.g., implementation of the Essentials for Childhood Framework) Use community-based participatory research designs Apply evidence-based practices (e.g., *The Community Guide*) to address health inequity and demonstrate improved health outcomes

FIGURE 11-10. *(Continued)*

QSEN TEAMWORK AND COLLABORATION

In order to function effectively within nursing and interprofessional teams, fostering open communication, mutual respect, and shared decision making to achieve quality patient care, each nurse must demonstrate awareness of personal strengths and limitations as a team member and initiate plans for self-development.

In 2012, the U.S. Department of Health and Human Services awarded $4 million over 5 years to fund a new coordinating center to promote interprofessional education and collaborative practice in health care at the University of Minnesota Academic Health Center. The goal is to foster efforts to create a U.S. health care system that engages patients, families, and communities in collaborative, team-based care.

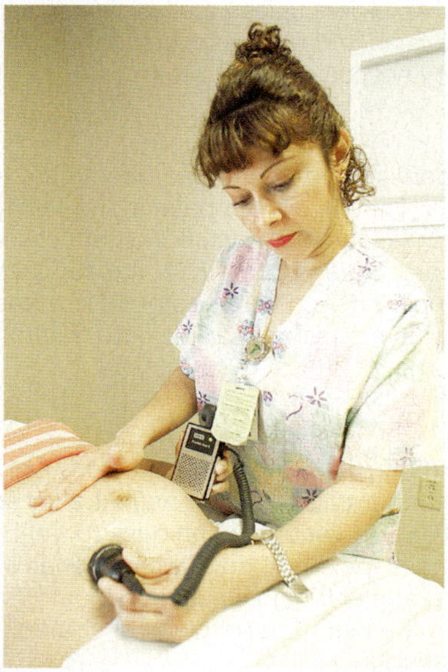

FIGURE 11-11. A nurse provides prenatal care at a public health clinic. (*Source:* Used with permission from Shutterstock. *Photo by Joe Mitchell.*)

Box 11-3 Collaborative Roles of Members of the Interprofessional Health Care Team

Physician

The physician is primarily responsible for the diagnosis of illness and the medical or surgical treatment of that illness. Physicians are granted the authority to admit patients to a health care facility by the health care facility or institution itself and to practice care within that setting through such actions as prescribing medications, interpreting the results of laboratory and diagnostic tests, and performing procedures and surgery. A person becomes a physician after extensive education and clinical practice and a licensing examination. Physicians may choose to be general practitioners or to specialize in the treatment of one type of illness or body system (such as a cardiologist) or a specific type of surgery (such as an orthopedic surgeon).

Hospitalists are health care providers who provide care to patients when they visit the emergency department or are admitted to the hospital. They communicate with the patient's primary care health care provider but provide care while the patient is in the hospital. They also may take after-hour, weekend, and holiday calls and services for one or more health care providers.

Advanced Practice Registered Nurse

The Advanced Practice Registered Nurse (APRN) is a registered nurse educated at the master's or post-master's level in a specific role and for a specific population. Whether they are nurse practitioners, clinical nurse specialists, nurse anesthetists, or nurse midwives, APRNs play a pivotal role in the future of health care. APRNs are often primary care providers and are at the forefront of providing preventive care to the public.

Physician Assistant

A physician assistant (PA) has completed a specific course of study and a licensing examination in preparation for providing support to the physician. The PA's responsibilities usually depend on the supervising physician and might include conducting physical examinations and suturing lacerations. In most states, nurses are not legally bound to follow a PA's orders unless a physician cosigns the orders. This is an important aspect to investigate if PAs are employed by hospitals in your area.

Nurse

Nurses supervise and coordinate direct care to patients and families. They teach the patient and family self-care and conduct research to ensure cost effectiveness and quality of care. Nurses coordinate the services of other health care providers. See Chapter 1 for a description of the many roles nurses play and their different levels of education.

Physical Therapist

A physical therapist (PT) seeks to restore function or to prevent further disability in a patient after an injury or illness. PTs use various techniques to treat patients, including massage, heat, cold, water, sonar waves, exercises, and electrical stimulation. Most PTs are also educated in the use of psychological strategies to motivate patients.

Occupational Therapist

Occupational therapists evaluate the patient's functional level and teaching activities to promote self-care in activities of daily living. They assess the home for safety and provide adaptive equipment as necessary.

Speech Therapist

A speech therapist is trained to help patients who are deaf or hard of hearing speak more clearly, to assist patients who have had a stroke to relearn how to speak, and to correct or modify a variety of speech disturbances in children and adults. Speech therapists also diagnose and treat swallowing problems in patients who have had a head injury or a stroke.

Social Worker

Social workers assist patients and families in dealing with the social, emotional, and environmental factors that affect their well-being. They make referrals to appropriate community resources and provide assistance with securing equipment and supplies, as well as with health care finances. In recent years, their role in discharge planning has been highlighted.

Pharmacist

A pharmacist, prepared at the doctoral level, is licensed to formulate and dispense medications. The pharmacist is also responsible for keeping a file of all patient medications and for informing the health care provider when a potential or actual medication error in prescribing has occurred or when prescribed drugs may interact adversely. The pharmacist is an excellent resource for information related to medications for both patients and nurses.

Respiratory Therapist

A respiratory therapist (RT) is trained in techniques that improve pulmonary function and oxygenation. RTs may also be responsible for administering a variety of tests that measure lung function and for educating the patient about the use of various devices and machines prescribed by the health care provider.

Dietitian

A registered dietitian (RD) manages and plans for the dietary needs of patients, based on knowledge about all aspects of nutrition. RDs can adapt specialized diets for the individual needs of patients, counsel and educate individual patients, and supervise the dietary services of an entire facility.

Chaplain/Spiritual Care Provider

Spiritual care providers identify and respond to the spiritual needs of patients, families, and other members of the interdisciplinary team. They may be members of the clergy, pastoral care workers with graduate degrees, or lay volunteers.

Assistive Personnel

Assistive personnel (AP) help nurses provide direct care to patients. As defined by individual state boards of nursing, AP may have the title of certified nursing assistants, orderlies, attendants, or technicians.

Take advantage of every opportunity to get to know the members of the interprofessional teams you will join as a student and learn what each member can contribute. Practice working collaboratively to make health care "work" for your patients and families. Read more about the care coordination role nurses play in Chapter 12.

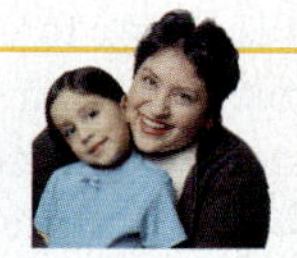

Think about ***Maritza Cortes***, the woman who brought her daughter to the emergency department. Her statement about not having the money needed to have the prescription filled would alert the nurse to the need for consulting social service. The social worker could provide Ms. Cortes with information about available financial assistance and community resources. Which members of the health care team are best equipped to meet the health care needs of Maritza and her daughter, Margaret Ritchie and her husband, and Paul Cochran? How would you collaborate with these members of the team?

TRENDS AND ISSUES IN HEALTH CARE DELIVERY

This section discusses some current issues and trends in health care. In your career as a nurse, you may find that as some issues are resolved, other new challenges arise. It is important for you both personally and professionally to be knowledgeable about all health care trends affecting the health care delivery system (Box 11-4).

Focus on Preventive Care

People's health awareness and desire to be involved in their own health care have strongly influenced the delivery of health care services in our society. Stress management programs, nutritional awareness, exercise and fitness programs, and antismoking and antidrug campaigns are all examples of this trend. These programs have never been more important in the United States as violence escalates and deaths from opioid misuse are increasing dramatically. Equally important to health are measures such as legislating the use of seat belts, promoting automobile and airplane safety, controlling smog, gun control, and eliminating hazardous wastes.

Box 11-4 Trends to Watch in Health Care Delivery

- Changing demographics
- Increasing diversity
- Technology explosion
- Globalization of economy and society
- Educated and engaged consumers
- Increasing complexity of patient care
- Costs of health care
- Effect of health policy and regulation
- Shortages of key health care professionals and educators

Knowledgeable and Engaged Consumers

A **consumer** is someone who uses a commodity or service. Health care consumers (patients or clients) are increasingly knowledgeable about health, prefer to control and make decisions about their own health, and want to be active participants in planning and implementing their health care. It is therefore critical for nurses to develop skills for creating successful partnerships with patients and their families. Consumers of health care services are better educated about the services they require and the services that are available, largely because so much health information is available on the internet. A downside is that many patients learn erroneous information from internet sites. It is critical for nurses to discover what patients know about their health challenges and to respectfully correct false or inappropriate information. Patients are also concerned about access to services, the cost of those services, and the quality of the care received. Consumers are questioning escalating costs and the proliferation and duplication of services. Consumers have become actively involved in the administration of health care facilities and have helped develop standards for care, patient rights, and cost-containment measures as protection for patients when they enter a health care setting.

The CMS now requires providers to meet several patient engagement benchmarks. More than 50% of the patients that clinicians see must now get timely access to their health information, including diagnostic test results, medication lists, and a clinical summary of their office visit, within one business day. While this is an important effort by the U.S. government to engage the public in self-care, respectful, trusting, and compassionate health care professional–patient relationships remain the most effective strategy to achieve these goals.

Mobile Health

The millennial generation enthusiastically embraced health apps, smartphones, and tablets, and savvy health care professionals and entrepreneurs are responding quickly to their demands. Patients can now access their medical records online, schedule appointments, and communicate with professional caregivers online. Tablets give access to electronic health record data, drug reference materials, and other valuable data that in the past was available only in the office or hospital. Patients, especially those with chronic illnesses, are similarly using apps and smartphone devices that let them measure weight, blood pressure, blood glucose, and more.

During the 2020 pandemic, there was an unprecedented increase in telehealth medical visits, which many expect to continue. Many nurses are filming teachable moments, such as how to dress a port, and then e-mailing the video to the patient or family caregiver. This trend will only increase and provide more opportunities for nurses to provide effective, quality care. Read more about informatics in Chapter 21.

Racial Justice and Equity

The year 2020 will forever be remembered in the United States not only because of the pandemic, but also because new instances of racial violence commanded the attention of the world and popularized the Black Lives Matter movement. In health care, there are now recurrent calls for all members of the interprofessional team to become antiracist, and we move toward zero tolerance for racism. We, of course, need to become newly aware of our personal beliefs and attitudes that reveal what might have been unconscious biases and predjudices. But we must also be ready to speak out as we encounter any institutional structures that perpetuate harmful and hurtful inequity and inequality. Remaining silent is no longer an option (Roberts, 2020). Read more about this in Chapter 3.

HEALTH CARE: A RIGHT, A PRIVILEGE, OR AN OBLIGATION OF A MORAL SOCIETY?

Two major factors influencing the provision of health care in the United States are the ability to pay for care and the location of facilities. Poor or uninsured people, minorities, residents of rural areas, and older adults often have inadequate access to health care services. In the United States, there are still too many who have inadequate health insurance or none at all. As this book goes to press, we are still waiting to see the effects a new political administration will have on health reform.

Although many people assume that everyone has a right to health care, consider these questions that pose ethical dilemmas for nurses who provide care, as well as for consumers of health care services:

- Do people who engage in risky behaviors or who do not make necessary lifestyle changes deserve the same health care as people who live healthy lives?
- Who should pay for health care needed by the unemployed and homeless?
- Is someone who pays for national television coverage to ask for an organ donation for his child any more deserving than someone who has been waiting months for just such a transplant?
- Should citizens pay higher insurance premiums or taxes so that someone addicted to drugs who overdoses can have intensive care?
- Should undocumented workers in the United States have the same access to health care as U.S. citizens?
- What priorities should we use when deciding how to distribute COVID-19 vaccines: ability to pay, age, prisoners, nursing home residents and those who work there, health care workers, other essential workers, etc.?
- Should vaccination status be used as a criterion for allocating critical care beds, ventilators, or other therapies that are in short supply?
- If 20 people need a heart transplant and only one heart is available, who decides who gets another chance at life and how should these decisions be made?

These are only a few of the questions being raised, and there are no easy answers. Carefully review the *Code of Ethics for Nurses* (Chapter 6) and the American Nurses Association website resources on health care reform to guide your responses.

NURSES' ROLE IN HEALTH CARE REFORM

Since the delivery of health care continues to change rapidly, it is fitting to conclude with a note about nurses' continuing role in health care reform. Changes taking place in health care give nurses the opportunity to help shape health care for the future. Projections about competencies of future health care practitioners, coupled with the national health promotion and disease prevention objectives outlined in the *Healthy People 2030* project (www.healthypeople.gov), underscore the importance of nursing's role in improving access to care, quality of care, and cost of care.

The U.S. health care system is facing many challenges, including rapidly increasing numbers of older adults, changing expectations of health care consumers, rapidly expanding technologies, increasing disparities, and an emphasis on improved quality and safety of care. The goals of health care reform focus on cost containment, improved access, and increased quality of services for all citizens. Where do nurses fit into the reform movement? First, nurses are becoming a stronger voice in protesting health-related problems in our nation and proposing solutions. Second, nurses in greater numbers are increasing their education and becoming APRNs and Doctors of Nursing Practice (DNPs) or PhDs. As such, more nurses now provide primary health care services in areas and to people long neglected: older adults, women, infants, people living in poverty, and those living in rural areas.

Nurses are seated at the tables where decisions are being made about how best to design, deliver, finance, and evaluate health care. In addition, the focus of nursing care provided by all nurses is holistic care essential to promoting health and preventing illness. The issues of who gets health care and who pays the bills continue to have major importance for society in the 21st century. These issues will present both challenges and opportunities for nurses of the future.

DEVELOPING CLINICAL REASONING AND CLINICAL JUDGMENT

1. How might prenatal and well-child care differ for two women: one without health insurance and the other with a good health insurance plan? Why do you think this happens? What can nurses do to ensure respectful, compassionate care of high quality for all?
2. Talk with your classmates about what should be in an essential health services package available for all. Would you include dental care, mental health services, complementary and alternative treatment modalities, women's health services including birth control and abortion, long-term care? Why is it so difficult for health planners to agree on what services are essential?
3. Think back to Paul Cochran, Margaret Ritchie and her husband, and Maritza and her children. What biases might professional caregivers hold even unconsciously that could

interfere with their providing optimal care? Reflect on any personal biases that might impair your ability to make health care "work" for all, especially the most vulnerable.

4. Interview as many people as you can about what the government's role should be in providing health care. Why in the United States are so many distrustful of "big" government playing an expanded role in health care?

PRACTICING FOR NCLEX

1. Nursing students are reviewing information about health care delivery systems in post conference. Which statements describing current U.S. health care delivery practices should be included in the discussion? Select all that apply.
   a. Access to care depends only on the ability to pay, not the availability of services.
   b. The Patient Protection and Affordable Care Act provides private health care insurance to underserved populations.
   c. Every health insurance plan in the Health Insurance Marketplace offers comprehensive coverage, from doctors to medications to hospital visits.
   d. The uninsured pay for more than one third of their care out of pocket and are usually charged lower amounts for their care than the insured pay.
   e. Fifty years ago, half of the doctors in the United States practiced primary care, but today fewer than one in three do.
   f. Quality of care can be defined as the right care for the right person at the right time.
2. Nurses provide care to patients in secondary health care facilities. Which patients do the nurses anticipate will receive this type of care? Select all that apply.
   a. Patient seeking treatment at a community clinic for possible strep throat
   b. Patient treated in the hospital following a myocardial infarction
   c. Child brought to the emergency department following a seizure
   d. Individual with osteogenesis imperfecta being treated in a medical center
   e. Child visiting a specialist to correct a congenital heart defect
   f. Patient who has a hernia repair in an ambulatory care center
3. A nurse working in a primary care facility prepares insurance forms in which the provider is given a fixed monetary amount per enrollee in the health plan. What term do the nurses apply to this type of reimbursement?
   a. Capitation
   b. Prospective payment system
   c. Bundled payment
   d. Rate setting
4. A nurse working in a pediatric clinic provides codes for a patient's services to a third-party payer who pays all or most of the care. How does the nurse refer to this method of payment?
   a. Out-of-pocket payment
   b. Individual private insurance
   c. Employer-based group private insurance
   d. Government financing
5. A nurse researcher follows current trends in health care delivery. Which present-day trends does the nurse observe? Select all that apply.
   a. Globalization of the economy and society
   b. Slowdown in technology development
   c. Decreasing diversity
   d. Increasing complexity of patient care
   e. Changing demographics
   f. Shortages of key health care professionals and educators
6. A nursing student is assisting with nursing care for patients in a primary care center. Based on the setting, what activities will the student expect to perform?
   a. Assisting with major surgery
   b. Performing health assessments
   c. Maintaining patients' function and independence
   d. Maintaining immunization records
7. The caregiver for a patient who is immobile and requires tube feedings asks the nurse to explain respite care. How does the nurse best explain this type of care?
   a. "It's a type of service that allows time away for caregivers."
   b. "It provides comfort and end-of-life services for the terminally ill and their families."
   c. "It is skilled care provided to older adults in a long-term care facility."
   d. "It provides living units available to people without regular shelter."
8. A nurse caring for patients in a primary care setting submits paperwork for reimbursement from managed care plans for services provided. What best describes managed care?
   a. System designed to control cost of care while maintaining quality
   b. Care coordination to maximize positive outcomes to contain costs
   c. Delivery of services from initial contact through ongoing care
   d. Based on a philosophy of ensuring death in comfort and dignity
9. As part of a clinical paper, a nursing student interviews a hospice nurse about their role. How will the student describe the type of care the nurse provides?
   a. Physical, psychological, social, and spiritual care for dying patients, their families, and loved ones
   b. Preventive, primary care, focusing on diabetes education, immunizations, and prenatal care
   c. Care focusing on rare diseases and specialty care
   d. Care to meet the patient's health care needs while giving a break to the patient's caregiver

10. Nursing students learn advance practice nurses can write medication prescriptions. Which roles may be performed by an advanced practice registered nurse? Select all that apply.
    a. Primary care provider
    b. Hospitalist
    c. Physical therapist
    d. Anesthetist
    e. Midwife
    f. Pharmacist
11. The nurses at a large community hospital with several campuses are members of a committee working toward obtaining Magnet status. What activity will best meet their goal?
    a. Recruiting excellent surgeons and medical doctors
    b. Offering health prevention activities in the community
    c. Providing high-quality patient care, using innovative practices
    d. Seeking culturally diverse clergy to meet patient's spiritual concerns
12. During a meeting with nurses at all levels in an acute care hospital, the Director of Nursing discusses lost revenue due to Medicare penalties. The nurses plan improvements in practice designed to prevent penalties from which events? Select all that apply.
    a. Urinary catheter–related infections
    b. Blood infections from central venous catheters
    c. Excessive readmissions
    d. Pressure injuries
    e. High blood pressure
13. Nursing students are asked to provide interprofessional care during their clinical experience. Which member of the health care team will the student contact for an uninsured patient?
    a. Nurse practitioner
    b. Admissions coordinator
    c. Social worker
    d. Hospital chaplain

ANSWERS WITH RATIONALES

1. **c, e, f.** The Health Insurance Marketplace is designed to help people more easily find health insurance that fits their budget. All plans in the Marketplace offers comprehensive coverage, from doctors to medications to hospital visits. There are many less primary care providers in the United States than there were 50 years ago. Quality is the right care for the right person at the right time. Access to care depends on both the ability to pay and the availability of services. The Patient Protection and Affordable Care Act provides Medicaid or subsidized coverage to qualifying people with incomes up to 400% of poverty. The uninsured pay for more than one third of their care out of pocket and are often charged higher amounts for their care than the insured pay.
2. **b, c, f.** Secondary health care treats problems that require specialized clinical expertise, such as an MI, a seizure, and a hernia repair. Treating strep throat is primary health care. Tertiary health care involves management of rare and complex disorders, such as osteogenesis imperfecta and congenital heart malformations.
3. **a.** Capitation plans give providers a fixed amount per enrollee in the health plan to build a payment plan that consists of the best standards of care at the lowest cost. The prospective payment system groups inpatient hospital services for Medicare patients into DRGs. With bundled payments, providers receive a fixed sum of money to provide a range of services. Rate setting means that the government could set targets or caps for spending on health care services.
4. **b.** The four basic modes of paying for health care are out-of-pocket payment, individual private insurance, employer-based group private insurance, and government financing. The *International Classification of Diseases, 10th Edition* and procedure codes, or ICD-10, includes codes for new procedures and diagnoses that improve the quality of information available for quality improvement and payment purposes. With individual private insurance, members pay monthly premiums either by themselves or in combination with employer payments. These plans are called third-party payers because the insurance company pays all or most of the cost of care. Out-of-pocket payment is paying for health care with cash payments. Employer-based private insurance is employer-sponsored coverage and government financing is provided through Medicare and Medicaid, and other federally funded programs.
5. **a, d, e, f.** Trends to watch in health care delivery include globalization of the economy and society, increasing complexity of patient care, changing demographics, shortages of key health care professionals and educators, technology explosion, and increasing diversity.
6. **b.** Performing health assessments is a common role of the nurse in a primary care center. Assisting with major surgery is a role of the nurse in the hospital setting. Maintaining patients' function and independence is a role of the nurse in a rehabilitation or extended-care facility, and keeping student immunization records up to date is a role of the school nurse.
7. **a.** Respite care is provided to enable a primary caregiver time away from the day-to-day responsibilities of homebound patients.
8. **a.** Managed care is a way of providing care designed to control costs while maintaining the quality of care.
9. **a.** The hospice nurse combines the skills of the home care nurse with the ability to provide daily emotional support to dying patients and their families. Respite care caregivers of homebound ill, disabled, or older adults. Palliative care, which can be used in conjunction with medical treatment and in all types of health care settings, is focused on the relief of physical, mental, and spiritual distress. Extended-care facilities include transitional subacute care, assisted-living facilities, intermediate and long-term care, homes for medically fragile children, retirement centers, and residential institutions for mentally and developmentally or physically disabled patients of all ages.
10. **a, d, e.** The Advanced Practice Registered Nurse (APRN) is a registered nurse educated at the master's or post-master's level in a specific role and for a specific population. Whether they are nurse practitioners, clinical nurse specialists, nurse anesthetists, or nurse midwives, APRNs play a pivotal role in

the future of health care. APRNs are often primary care providers and are at the forefront of providing preventive care to the public. Hospitalists are health care providers who provide care to patients when they visit the emergency department or are admitted to the hospital. A physical therapist completes a specific training program to learn to help patients restore function or to prevent further disability in a patient after an injury or illness. A pharmacist, prepared at the doctoral level, is licensed to formulate and dispense medications.

11. c. Magnet hospitals meet strict requirements and standards representing the highest quality of professional nursing practice and patient care, nursing excellence, and innovations in practice. Physicians are recruited by the medical department, health prevention activities in the community could be conducted by nursing staff but are not required activities; chaplains, nurses, and others may provide spiritual care, but it is not the focus of a Magnet designation.

12. a, b, c, d. Medicare penalties are given to hospitals when patients are readmitted soon after discharge; this is designed to ensure patients receive needed coordinated care after discharge. In addition, Medicare no longer reimburses hospitals for conditions that result from preventable errors and lead to increased costs. These include pressure injuries, injuries caused by falls, infections associated with indwelling urinary catheters, vascular catheter–associated infections, infections of the mediastinum after coronary artery bypass graft, air embolisms, adverse reactions to incompatible blood infusions, and retained sponges or instruments during surgery.

13. c. Social workers assist patients and families in dealing with the social, emotional, and environmental factors that affect their well-being. They make referrals to appropriate community resources, participate in discharge planning to obtain equipment and supplies, and assist with health care finances. Nurse practitioners assist in managing the medical and nursing needs of a patient, the admissions coordinator performs administrative intakes and may assign beds, and the hospital chaplain attends to patients' spiritual needs.

Bibliography

Agency for Healthcare Research and Quality (AHRQ). (2013). The medical home: What do we know, what do we need to know? A review of the earliest evidence on the effectiveness of the patient-centered medical home model. AHRQ Publication No. 12(14)-0020-1-EF.

Agency for Healthcare Research and Quality (AHRQ). (2016). *High reliability*. https://psnet.ahrq.gov/primers/primer/31/high-reliability

AHIP. (2020). *Where does your health care dollar go?* https://www.ahip.org/wp-content/uploads/AHIP_HealthCareDollar-2020.pdf

American Hospital Association (AHA). (2020). *About the AHA*. http://www.aha.org/about/index.shtml

American Journal of Nursing. (2017). Supporting family caregivers. No longer home alone. Supplement to May 2017. *American Journal of Nursing, 117*(5), S1–S24.

American Nurses Association. (2016). *ANA's principles for health system transformation 2016*. https://www.nursingworld.org/~4afd6b/globalassets/practiceandpolicy/health-policy/principles-healthsystemtransformation.pdf

American Nurses Association. (n.d.). *Health system reform resources*. https://www.nursingworld.org/practice-policy/health-policy/health-system-reform/resources/

American Nurses Credentialing Center (ANCC). (2020). *ANCC magnet recognition program. ANCC pathway to excellence*. https://www.nursingworld.org/organizational-programs/magnet/

Berwick, D. M., Nolan, T. W., & Whittington, J. (2008). The triple aim: Care, health, and cost. *Health Affairs (Millwood), 27*(3), 759–769. https://doi.org/10.1377/hlthaff.27.3.759

Bodenheimer, T., & Grumbach, K. (2016). *Understanding health policy: A clinical approach* (7th ed.). McGraw-Hill.

Brooks, J. A. (2016). Understanding hospital value-based purchasing. *American Journal of Nursing, 116*(5), 63–66.

Bureau of Labor Statistics, U.S. Department of Labor. (2017). *Occupational outlook handbook, Registered nurses*. https://www.bls.gov/ooh/healthcare/registered-nurses.htm

Catholic Health Association. (2020). *Facts-statistics. Catholic health care in the United States*. https://www.chausa.org/about/about/facts-statistics

Centers for Disease Control and Prevention (CDC). (n.d.). *Hospital utilization (in non-Federal short stay hospitals)*. https://www.cdc.gov/nchs/fastats/hospital.htm

Centers for Medicare and Medicaid Services, Office of the Actuary, National Health Statistics Group. (2019). National health care expenditures data. https://www.cms.gov/Research-Statistics-Data-and-Systems/Statistics-Trends-and-Reports/NationalHealthExpendData/index.html

Centers for Medicare and Medicaid Services. (2022). Medicare and you. https://www.medicare.gov/Pubs/pdf/10050-medicare-and-you.pdf

Chua, K. P. (2006). Overview of the U.S. health care system. http://www.stritch.luc.edu/lumen/MedEd/IPM/ipm3/BPandJ/HealthCareSystemOverview-AMSA%2020062_25_09.pdf

CMS.gov. NHE Fact Sheet. (2021). https://www.cms.gov/Research-Statistics-Data-and-Systems/Statistics-Trends-and-Reports/NationalHealthExpendData/NHE-Fact-Sheet

Craig, C., Eby, D., & Whittington, J. (2011). *Care coordination model: Better care at lower cost for people with multiple health and social needs. IHI Innovation Series white paper*. Institute for Healthcare Improvement. http://www.ihi.org/knowledge/Pages/IHIWhitePapers/IHICareCoordinationModelWhitePaper.aspx

Daley, K. A. (2013). President's perspective: What keeps me up at night? *The American Nurse, 45*(1), 3.

Davis, K., Schoen, C., & Stremikis, K. (2010). *Mirror, mirror on the wall: How the performance of the U.S. health care system compares internationally—2010 Update*. The Commonwealth Fund. http://www.commonwealthfund.org/Publications/Fund-Reports/2010/Jun/Mirror-Mirror-Update.aspx?page=all

Family Caregiver Alliance. *National center on caregiving*. https://www.caregiver.org

Frankel, A., Haraden, C., Federico, F., & Lenoci-Edwards, J. (2017). *A framework for safe, reliable, and effective care. White paper*. Institute for Healthcare Improvement and Safe & Reliable Healthcare.

Grant, R. (2016). *The U.S. is running out of nurses. The Atlantic*. https://www.theatlantic.com/health/archive/2016/02/nursing-shortage/459741

HCAHPS Fact Sheet. (2021). *Centers for Medicare & Medicaid Services (CMS)*. https://hcahpsonline.org/globalassets/hcahps/facts/hcahps_fact_sheet_march_2021.pdf

Healthcare.gov. https://www.healthcare.gov

Henry J. Kaiser Family Foundation. *Program on Medicaid and the uninsured*. https://www.kff.org/about-program-on-medicaid-and-the-uninsured/

Henry J. Kaiser Family Foundation. *Health care costs*. https://www.kff.org/health-costs/

Henry J. Kaiser Family Foundation. *Health reform*. https://www.kff.org/health-reform/

Institute for Healthcare Improvement (IHI). (2017). *The IHI triple aim initiative*. http://www.ihi.org/offerings/Initiatives/TripleAIM/Pages/default.aspx

Institute of Medicine (IOM). (1999). *To err is human: Building a safer health system*. The National Academies Press.

Institute of Medicine (IOM). (2001). *Crossing the quality chasm: A new health system for the 21st century*. The National Academies Press.

Institute of Medicine (IOM). (2011). *The future of nursing: Leading change, advancing health*. The National Academies Press.

Institute of Medicine and National Research Council. (2013). *U.S. health in international perspective: Shorter lives, poorer health*. The National Academies Press.

Institute of Medicine (IOM). (2015). *Transforming health care scheduling and access: Getting to now*. The National Academies Press.

Kurtzman, E. T., & Buerhaus, P. I. (2008). New Medicare payment rules: Danger or opportunity for nursing? *American Journal of Nursing, 108*(6), 30–35.

Long, M., Rae, M., & Claxton, A. (2016). *Trends in employer-sponsored insurance offer and coverage rates, 1999–2014*. The Henry J. Kaiser Family Foundation. http://www.kff.org/private-insurance/issue-brief/trends-in-employer-sponsored-insurance-offer-and-coverage-rates-1999-2014

Martin, A. B., Lassman, D., Washington, B., Catlin, A., & National Health Expenditure Accounts Team. (2012). Growth in US health spending remained slow in 2010; Health share of gross domestic product was unchanged from 2009. *Health Affairs (Millwood), 31*(1), 208–219.

Matthews, J. (2017). Overview and summary: Healthcare reform: Nurses impact policy. *The Online Journal of Issues in Nursing, 22*(2). https://doi.org/10.3912/OJIN.Vol22No02ManOS.

McClellan, M., McKethan, A. N., Lewis, J. L., Roski, J., & Fisher, E. S. (2010). A national strategy to put accountable care into practice. *Health Affairs (Millwood), 29*(5), 982–990. http://content.healthaffairs.org/cgi/content/abstract/hlthaff.28.2.w219

McDonald, K. M., Schultz, E., & Albin, L. (2010). *Care Coordination Atlas Version 3 (Prepared by Stanford University under subcontract to Battelle on Contract No. 290-04-0020). AHRQ Publication No. 11-0023-EF*. Agency for Healthcare Research and Quality.

Medicare.gov. (2017). *Hospital compare*. https://www.medicare.gov/care-compare/?providerType=Hospital&redirect=true

National Academy for State Health Policy. (2013). www.nashp.org

National Academy of Medicine. (2017). *Vital directions for health and health care: Priorities from a national academy of medicine initiative*. https://nam.edu/vital-directions-for-health-health-care-priorities-from-a-national-academy-of-medicine-initiative

National Academy of Sciences. (2003). *Executive summary: Health professions education. A bridge to quality.* http://www.nap.edu/openbook.php?record_id=10681&page=R1

National Academies of Sciences, Engineering, and Medicine. (2021). *The future of nursing 2020–2030.* https://www.nationalacademies.org/our-work/the-future-of-nursing-2020-2030

National Association of Community Health Centers (NACHC). (2013). *About our health centers.* http://www.nachc.org/about-our-health-centers

The National Center for Coverage Innovation at Families USA. (2020). The COVID-19 Pandemic and Resulting Economic Crash Have Caused the Greatest Health Insurance Losses in American History. Publication ID: COV2020-254. https://www.familiesusa.org/wp-content/uploads/2020/07/COV-254_Coverage-Loss_Report_7-17-20.pdf

National Hospice and Palliative Care Organization. (2020). *Hospice Facts and Figures.* https://www.nhpco.org/hospice-facts-figures/

Nielsen, M., Langner, B., Zema, C., Hacker, T., & Grundy, P. (2012). *Benefits of implementing the primary care patient-centered medical home: cost and quality Results.* Patient-Centered Primary Care Collaborative. www.pcpcc.org/sites/default/files/media/benefits_of_implementing_the_primary_care_pcmh.pdf

Petersen, K. (2020). Meeting healthcare needs in rural America. *Nursing, 50*(8), 16–18.

Physicians for a National Health Program (PNHP). (2016). What is single payer? http://www.pnhp.org/facts/what-is-single-payer

Rambur, B., & Pulcini, J. (2022). Understanding the language of health reform. *American Journal of Nursing, 122*(1), 48–53.

Rau, J. (2011). *Medicare announces rules for quality bonuses to hospitals.* Kaiser Health News.

Rau, J. (2012). *Medicare to penalize 2,217 hospitals for excess readmissions.* Kaiser Health News.

Roberts, D. (2020). The elephant in the room. *Nursing, 50*(2), 42–46.

Rudowitz, R., Artiga, S., & Young, K. (2016). *What coverage and financing is at risk under a repeal of the ACA Medicaid expansion?* The Henry J. Kaiser Family Foundation. http://www.kff.org/medicaid/issue-brief/what-coverage-and-financing-at-risk-under-repeal-of-aca-medicaid-expansion

Sanders, B. (2013). *Subcommittee on primary health and aging.* Primary Care Access. http://www.sanders.senate.gov/imo/media/doc/PrimaryCareAccessReport.pdf

Shih, A., Davis, K., Schoenbaum, S. C., Gauthier, A., Nuzum, R., & McCarthy, D. (2008). Organizing the U.S. health care delivery system for high performance. S.S. Commonwealth Fund Study.

Smith, M., Saunders, R., Stuckhardt, L., & McGinnis, J. M. (Eds.). (2012). *Best care at lower cost: The path to continuously learning health care in America.* The National Academies Press.

Sofaer, S., & Schumann, M. J. (2013). *Fostering successful patient and family engagement: Nursing's critical role.* http://www.naqc.org/WhitePaper-PatientEngagement

Strauss, G. (2017). Inspect like a pro: 9 things to consider before choosing a nursing home. *AARP Bulletin, 58*(9), 18–19.

Taylor, E. F., Lake, T., Nysenbaum, J., Peterson, G., & Meyers, D. (2011). *Coordinating care in the medical neighborhood: critical components and available mechanisms. White Paper (Prepared by Mathematica Policy Research under Contract No. HHSA290200900019I TO2). AHRQ Publication No. 11-0064.* Agency for Healthcare Research and Quality. http://pcmh.ahrq.gov/sites/default/files/attachments/Coordinating%20Care%20in%20the%20Medical%20Neighborhood.pdf

Tolbert, J., Orgera, K., & Damico, A. (2020, November 6). *Key facts about uninsured population.* Kaiser Family Foundation. https://www.kff.org/uninsured/issue-brief/key-facts-about-the-uninsured-population/

U.S. Department of Health and Human Services, Centers for Disease Control and Prevention. (2019). https://doi.org/10.1001/jama.2019.15806

Woolf, S. H., & Aron, L. (Eds.). (2013). *U.S. health in international perspective: Shorter lives, poorer health, National Research Council and Institute of Medicine. 2012 Patient-Centered Primary Care Collaborative/Millbank Memorial Fund.* The National Academies Press.

Yong, P. L., Saunders, R. S., & Olsen, L. (Eds.). (2010). *The healthcare imperative: Lowering costs and improving outcomes. Workshop Series Summary.* The National Academies Press.

12 Interprofessional Collaborative Practice and Care Coordination Across Settings

Jeff Hart

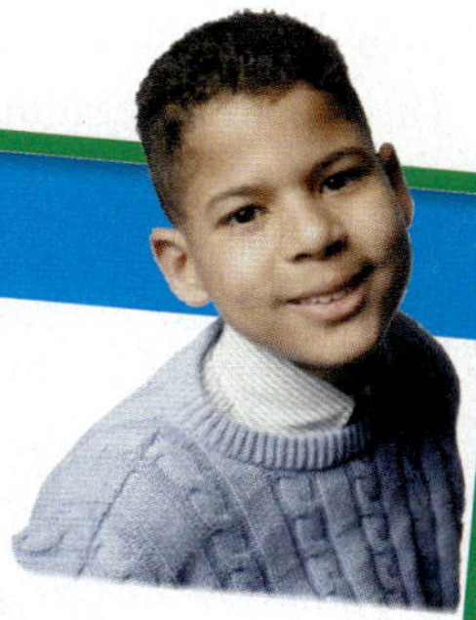

Jeff is a 9-year-old boy with a genetic disease that includes severe intellectual disability. He is transferred from the state home for children to the hospital for respiratory complications.

Laura Degas

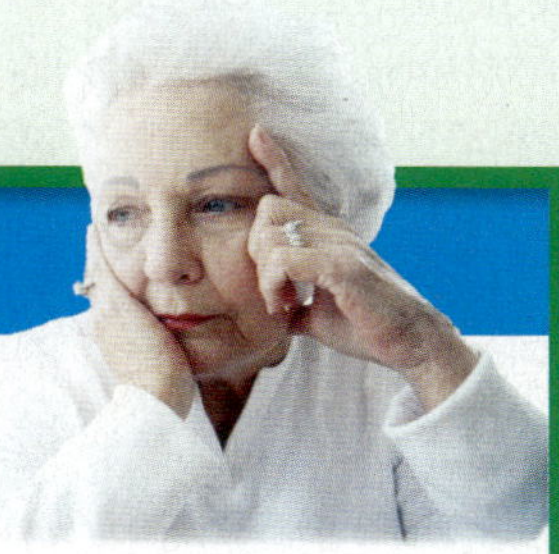

Laura, a 78-year-old woman, has been caring for her sister Ellen at home. She says, "She was diagnosed with Alzheimer's disease 2 years ago. This surgery to fix her broken hip has really been tough. I want to take her home, but I'm not sure if I can give her the care that she needs now."

Joey Marshall

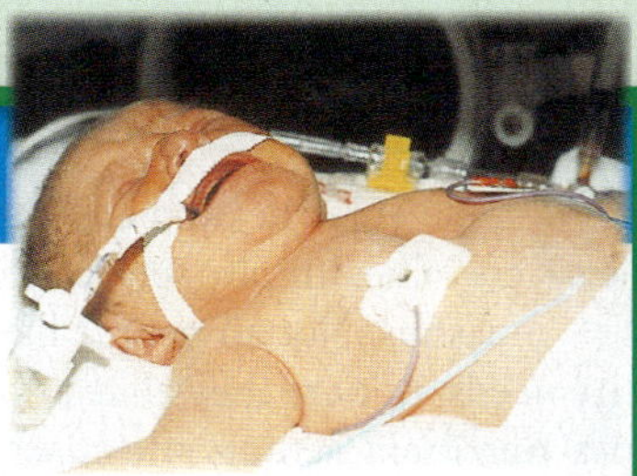

Joey, an extremely low–birth-weight baby (1,100 g), spent 7 months in the hospital before being discharged home. His mother is caring for him, his twin (who is healthier), and their 3-year-old sister. Joey is still being fed artificially, is on a ventilator, and needs care around the clock.

Learning Outcomes

After completing the chapter, you will be able to accomplish the following:

1. Identify key elements of community health.
2. Describe the qualities and roles of the community-based nurse.
3. Describe the role of the nurse in ensuring continuity of care and coordinating care between and among health care settings and the home.
4. Describe collaborative practice.
5. Discuss the importance of care coordination, including admissions, transfers, and discharges.
6. Discuss considerations for establishing an effective nurse–patient relationship when admitting a patient to a health care setting.
7. Compare and contrast admission of a patient to an ambulatory care setting and a hospital setting.
8. Discuss transfer of patients within and among health care settings.
9. Explain how nurses use the components of discharge planning to provide continuity of care.
10. Describe the components of the home health care system, including facilities, patients, referrals, primary caregivers, reimbursement sources, and legal considerations.
11. Explain the essential components of the pre-entry and entry phases of the home visit.
12. Explain the importance of documentation in home care.

Nursing Concepts

- Interprofessional practice
- Collaborative practice
- Community-based care
- Care coordination

People enter health care settings and become consumers of health care services (patients) for many different reasons. Not all people have the same types of health care needs, nor are they alike as patients. Some are admitted to a treatment setting and discharged the same day, some remain in an acute care setting for months, and some require extended care at home or in another community setting. Increasingly, people are seeking health care services in the communities where they live, study, work, pray, and play.

Entering and leaving a health care setting, as well as receiving care at home, are experiences that produce anxiety for both patients and family members. The nurse is often the health care provider who helps the patient and family make a smooth transition from one care setting to another. (See the accompanying Reflective Practice display for an example.) Planning for and providing individualized nursing interventions that promote health and wellness, prevent illness, and support coping with disability are critical in today's culturally diverse society. It is no longer enough only to consider the patient's needs within the hospital setting; nurses must also consider how those needs will be met as the patient makes the transition from the acute care setting to some type of long-term care or to care at home with support and services from the patient's community.

Five concepts essential to nursing care of patients within and across health care settings, discussed in this chapter, are community health, community-based nursing care, continuity of care, collaborative practice, and care coordination.

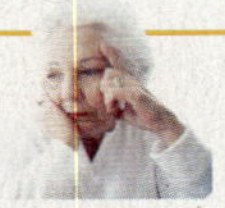

Consider **Laura Degas**, whose sister Ellen has Alzheimer disease. Because of her sister's increased complexity of care after undergoing a hip repair, Ms. Degas is unsure if she can continue to care for Ellen at home. The nurse would work with Ms. Degas to determine her needs and possibly enlist the aid of social services for assistance with a referral to home care and appropriate resources and community services.

COMMUNITY HEALTH

It's important for every nurse to recognize that healthy communities are not just about physical health. The Robert Wood Johnson Foundation writes:

> Where we live shouldn't determine how long or how well we live. In our communities we should all be surrounded by conditions that enable us to live the healthiest life possible, such as access to healthy food, quality schools, stable housing, good jobs with fair pay, and safe places to exercise and play. Unfortunately, in many communities, there are persistent barriers to health and opportunity to thrive (https://www.rwjf.org/en/our-focus-areas/focus-areas/healthy-communities.html).

See the accompanying Through the Eyes of a Pediatrician box on page 306.

The Centers for Disease Control and Prevention (CDC) defines a community as typically defined by a geographic area but notes that they can also be based on shared interests or characteristics such as religion, race, age, or occupation. People within a community come from different backgrounds and have unique cultures, customs, and values. The CDC report on community needs assessment writes that utilizing this wide range of ideas and wisdom is critical to assessing the community needs and strategizing areas for improvement (2013).

Healthy People 2030 defines Leading Health Indicators (LHIs) as a small subset of high-priority *Healthy People 2030* objectives selected to drive action toward improving health and well-being. Most LHIs address important factors that impact major causes of death and disease in the United States,

QSEN Reflective Practice: Cultivating QSEN Competencies

CHALLENGE TO TECHNICAL SKILLS

Joey Marshall, an extremely low–birth-weight baby (1,100 g), spent 7 months in the hospital before being discharged home. His mother is now at home full time caring for him, his twin (who is healthier), and their 3-year-old sister. Joey is still being fed via tube feedings, is on a ventilator, and needs care around the clock. When I first visited Joey on the day he was discharged home, I was frightened at the sight of such a small baby surrounded by beeping machines and tubes. While this was not a new sight for Joey's mom, she seemed very uncomfortable being his primary caregiver. She said she had lots of practice taking care of him in the hospital, but nothing had prepared her for the reality of his coming home and needing help around the clock.

Thinking Outside the Box: Possible Courses of Action

- Take a "pass" on this family and tell my instructor that this family's needs exceed my capacity to care; an adult with a lot of tubes is one thing, but a BABY!
- Ask for an experienced mentor to guide me through a comprehensive family assessment and plan to meet everyone's needs; use this as a challenge but ask for help until I feel competent and confident.
- Act like I know what I'm doing and pray I don't make mistakes!

Evaluating a Good Outcome: How Do I Define Success?

- Joey's mother develops the competence and confidence she needs to provide Joey's care at home.
- I am honest about my ability and seek help when I need it.
- I learn something from each situation that will prepare me to meet the next clinical challenge.
- I don't let my fear interfere with my learning.

Personal Learning: Here's to the Future!

I decided that options #1 (taking a pass) and #3 (acting like I knew what I was doing) weren't really options, although they seemed tempting. An experienced home health care nurse who once worked in the neonatal intensive care unit (NICU) agreed to visit this family with me, and she talked me through a comprehensive assessment. I was able to use my fear to identify with how Joey's mom was feeling, and I believe I was able to make her feel comfortable. I told her that we would learn how to do everything together! By the end of this rotation, we were both comfortable with Joey's care. I learned a valuable lesson: to seek help when I am in over my head and to relish a challenge. I hope I will remember this experience as I grow more confident so that I never forget how overwhelmed many families feel when they first bring a loved one home!

QSEN SELF-REFLECTION ON QUALITY AND SAFETY COMPETENCIES DEVELOPING KNOWLEDGE, SKILLS, AND ATTITUDES FOR CONTINUOUS IMPROVEMENT

How do you think you would respond in a similar situation? Why? What does this tell you about yourself and about the adequacy of your skills for professional practice? Can you think of other ways to respond? What other knowledge, attitudes, and skills do you need to develop to continuously improve the quality and safety of care for patients like Joey?

Patient-Centered Care: What made creating a partnership with Ms. Marshall so challenging? What abilities did the experienced home health care nurse and student use to achieve a good outcome? What special talents do you bring to creating successful partnerships?

Teamwork and Collaboration/Quality Improvement: What communication skills do you need to improve to ensure that you function as a competent, caring, and responsible member of the patient care team and that you obtain appropriate assistance when needed? How is collaborative practice and teamwork different for home health care nurses? What special talents do you bring to promoting a well-functioning team? How did the student's commitment to quality care influence her response?

Safety/Evidence-Based Practice: What priority did the student give to Joey's health, well-being, and safety? What does research demonstrate about the safety of providing care in the home that once happened in the hospital? Did the nursing student seek out the most appropriate resources for help in responding to Joey and his mother's complex needs? What other resources could have been helpful? Do you agree with the criteria to evaluate a successful outcome? Did the nursing student meet the criteria? Explain your answer.

and they help organizations, communities, and states across the nation focus their resources and efforts to improve the health and well-being of all people. *Healthy People 2030* includes 23 LHIs. To learn how LHIs are connected to other Healthy People objectives and the *Healthy People 2030* vision, check out the graphic in Figure 12-1 (on page 306). You can also visualize the graphic and tap on select boxes to review the overall health and well-being measures, LHIs, and developmental and research objectives at: https://health.gov/healthypeople/objectives-and-data/about-objectives/healthy-people-2030-objectives-and-measures.

The IRS requires not-for-profit hospitals to conduct community health needs assessments to demonstrate how they are meeting these needs. For an excellent example of

Through the Eyes of a Pediatrician

A baby born in Flint, where I am a pediatrician, is likely to live almost 20 fewer years than a child born elsewhere in the same county. She's a baby like any other, with wide eyes, a growing brain and a vast, bottomless innocence—too innocent to understand the injustices that without her knowing or choosing have put her at risk.

Throughout the United States, geography defines and describes inequities in health, wealth, mobility, and longevity. The reasons for this are both visible and hidden. Life in a distressed neighborhood means limited access to health care and healthy food. It means living with violence, racism, poverty, and uncertainty. It means bearing the brunt of environmental injustice—not having safe and affordable water, as Flint knows too well, or living in the shadow of a polluting factory. More air pollution increases the rate of respiratory disease and reduces student achievement. We are also beginning to understand the interplay of water access and air quality with COVID-19 severity.

Science tells us that children exposed to multiple adversities, both in their home and neighborhood, have a far greater likelihood of challenges later in life. From addiction to eviction, those pressures change children on a molecular, cellular, and behavioral level—and make them sick. The effects of toxic stress can be as disruptive as environmental pollution on their bodies, increasing risk for chronic diseases like asthma and hypertension, and lowering life expectancy. [Read more about adverse childhood events (ACEs) in Chapter 43.]

Source: Used with permission. Hanna-Attisha, M. (2020, May 17). Babies don't choose where they are born. *The New York Times*, p. 10.

how this works you may want to see the San Diego 2019 Community Health Needs Assessment (https://hasdic.org/wp-content/uploads/2019-CHNA-Executive-Summary.pdf). Figures 12-2 through 12-4 illustrate their process map, engagement participants, and findings: Top 10 community health needs. You will find many examples of community health needs assessments in the literature. The Johns Hopkins Hospital & Johns Hopkins Bayview Medical Center 2018 Community Health Needs Assessment identified the following socioeconomic and direct health care needs in decreasing order of priority:

Socioeconomic Needs
- Employment
- Crime/neighborhood safety
- Housing/homelessness
- Education
- Food environment

Direct Health Needs
- Behavioral health/substance use
- Behavioral health/mental health
- Chronic diseases
- Uninsured/underinsured
- Dental services

The Guide to Community Preventive Services (www.thecommunityguide.org) is an online collection of evidence-based recommendations from the Community Preventive Services Task Force that identifies promising, cost-effective ways to improve community and population health. "Robust

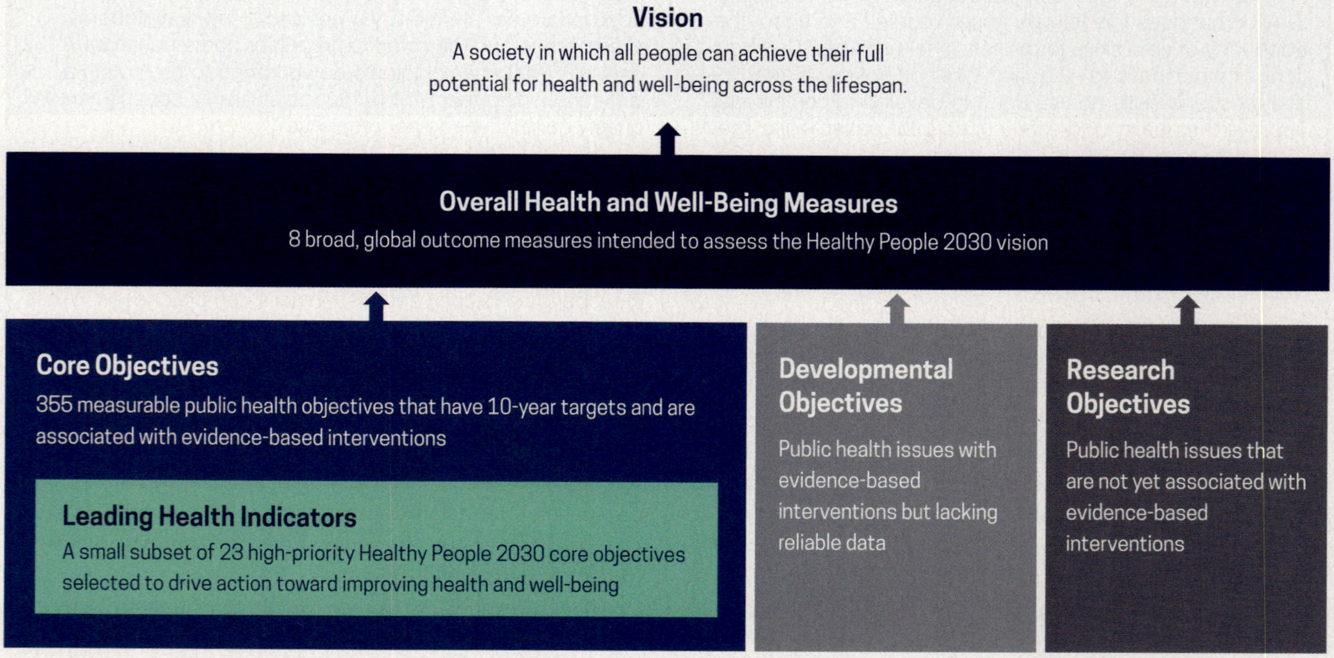

FIGURE 12-1. *Healthy People 2030* Objectives and Measures. (Healthy People 2030 Objectives and Measures.)

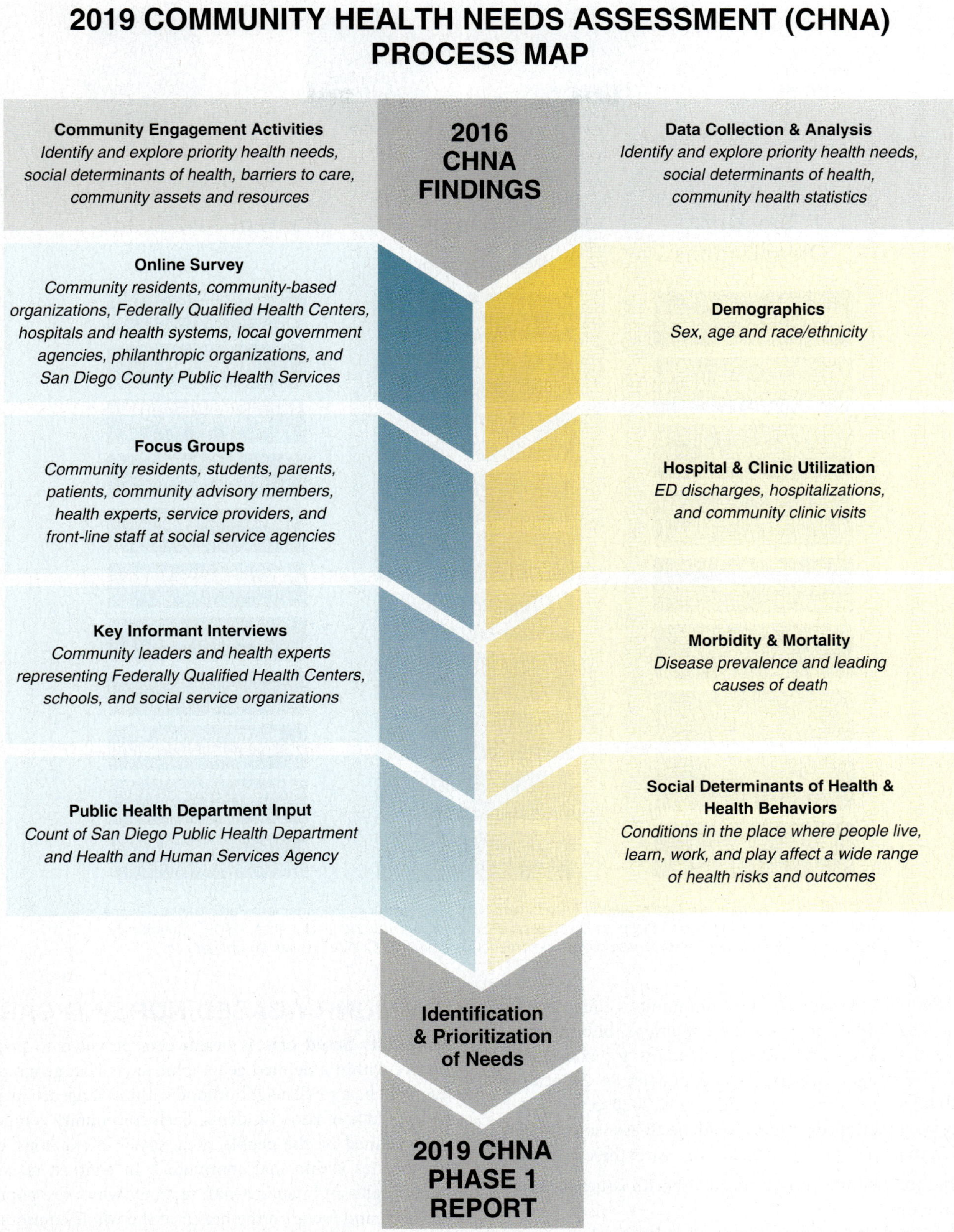

FIGURE 12-2. Community Health Needs Assessment (CHNA) Process Map. (*Source:* San Diego State University and Hospital Association of San Diego and Imperial Counties. [2019]. *Community health needs assessment.* https://hasdic.org/wp-content/uploads/2019-CHNA-Executive-Summary.pdf)

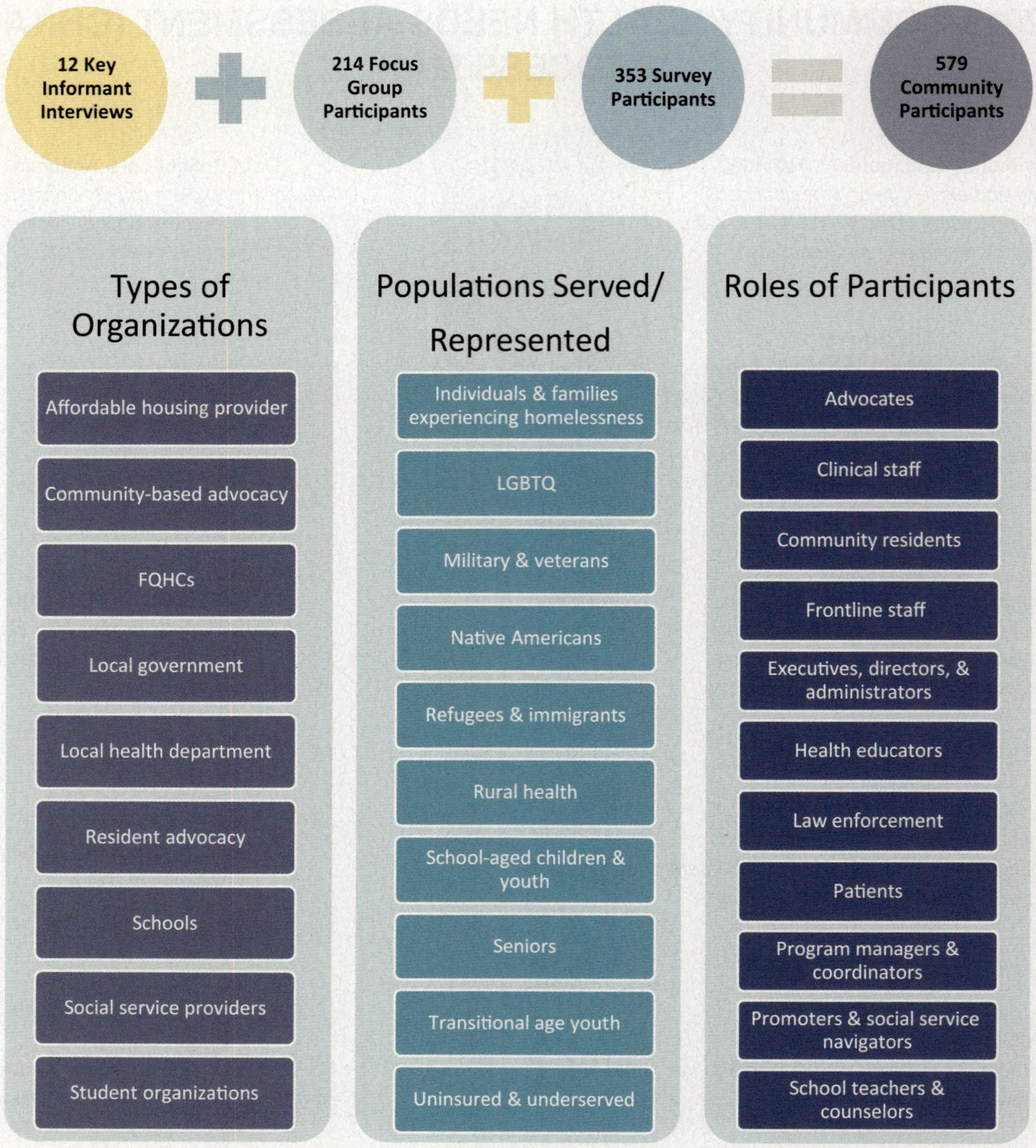

FIGURE 12-3. Community Health Needs Assessment (CHNA) Community Engagement Participants. (*Source:* San Diego State University and Hospital Association of San Diego and Imperial Counties. [2019]. *Community health needs assessment.* https://hasdic.org/wp-content/uploads/2019-CHNA-Executive-Summary.pdf)

and continuously updated, the Community Guide covers a broad range of health topics and conditions, offering more than 240 findings and recommendations for community preventive programs, services and policies in 21 priority health topics areas" (Suzuki & Edmonds, 2020, p. 55).

Are you aware of community health needs assessments being done in your area? Are you prepared to answer these questions?

- What are the three most important health issues in your community?
- What are the three most important unhealthy behaviors in your community?
- What are the three most important factors that impact your well-being in your community?

Also check out Figure 12-5, which illustrates the national dialogue to build awareness of mental health issues in communities.

COMMUNITY-BASED NURSING CARE

Community-based care is health care provided to people who live within a defined geographic area. That geographic area might be a small neighborhood within a large urban area or a large area of rural residents. Each community is unique and is defined by the people, area, social interactions, and common ties within that community. In contrast to community health and public health nursing (which are population based and focus on the health of the whole community by targeting community interventions like immunizations, infection prevention, environmental health, and opioid crisis response), community-based care centers on individual and family health care needs. It emphasizes the provision of comprehensive, coordinated, and continuous services for patients with acute or chronic health problems. Within a framework of community-based care, nurses help people wherever they

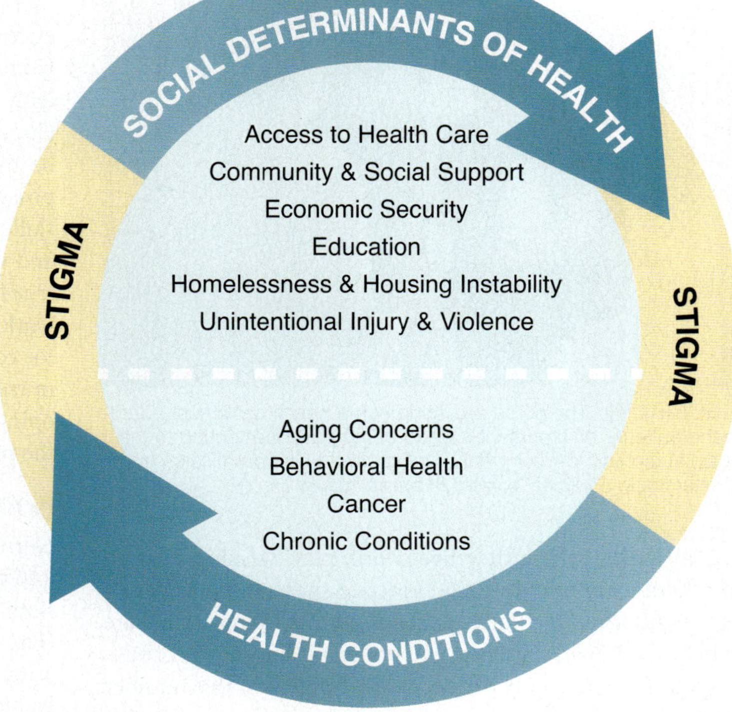

FIGURE 12-4. Community Health Needs Assessment (CHNA) Top 10 Community Health Needs. This figure illustrates the interactive nature of social determinants of health (SDOH) and health conditions, each impacting the other period in addition, an underlying theme of stigma and the barriers it creates arose across community engagement. For instance, stigma impacts the way in which people access needed services that address SDOH, which consequently impacts their ability to maintain and manage health conditions. Due to the complexity of this underlying theme, the CHNA Committee plans to explore and understand ways in which hospitals and health systems could better address stigma in patient care during phase two of the CHNA process. (*Source:* San Diego State University and Hospital Association of San Diego and Imperial Counties. [2019]. *Community health needs assessment.* https://hasdic.org/wp-content/uploads/2019-CHNA-Executive-Summary.pdf)

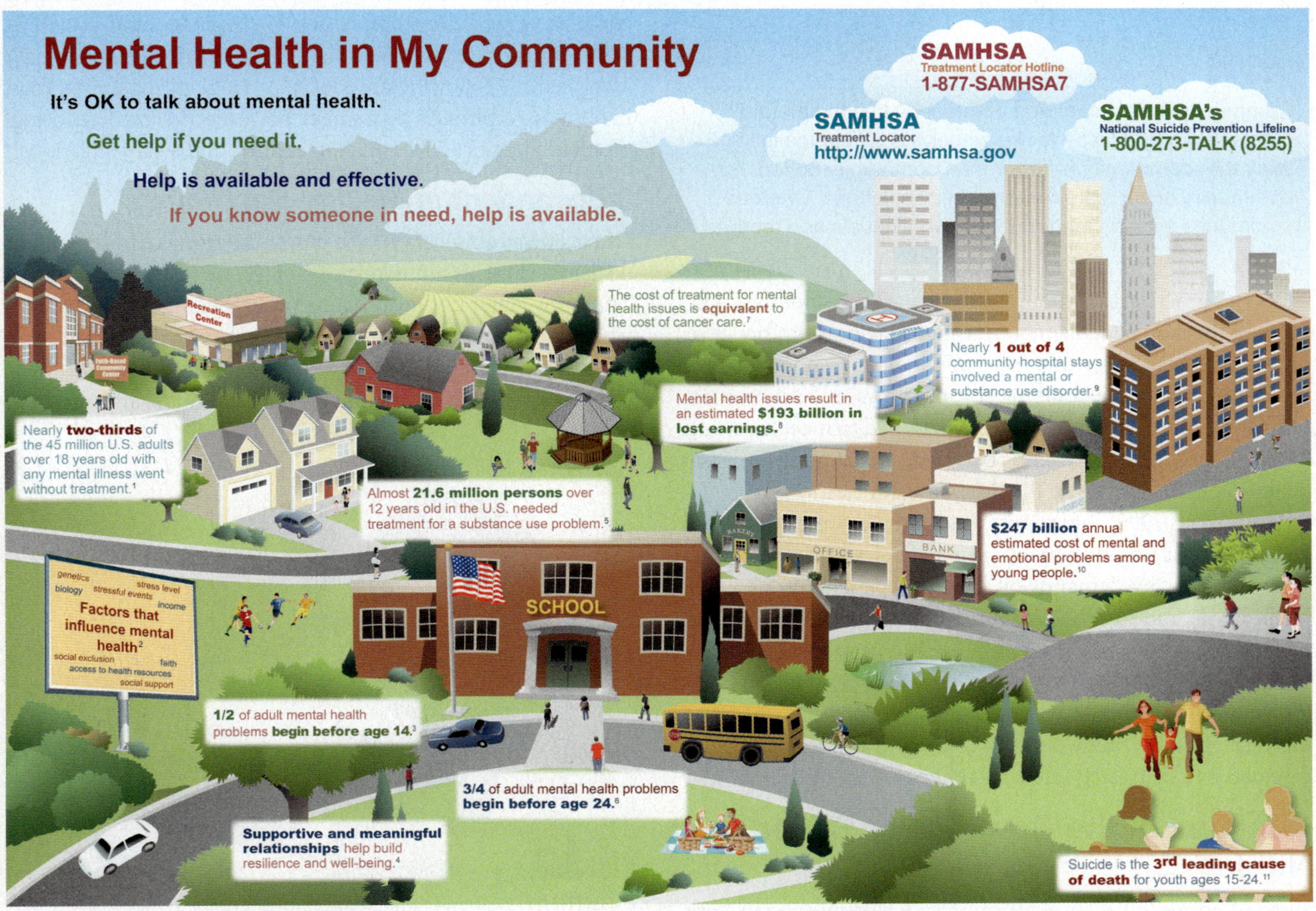

FIGURE 12-5. Mental Health in My Community. (*Source:* Substance Abuse and Mental Health Services Administration (SAMHSA). *Mental health in my community: Information graphic.* https://store.samhsa.gov/product/Mental-Health-in-My-Community-Information-Graphic/SMA13-4725)

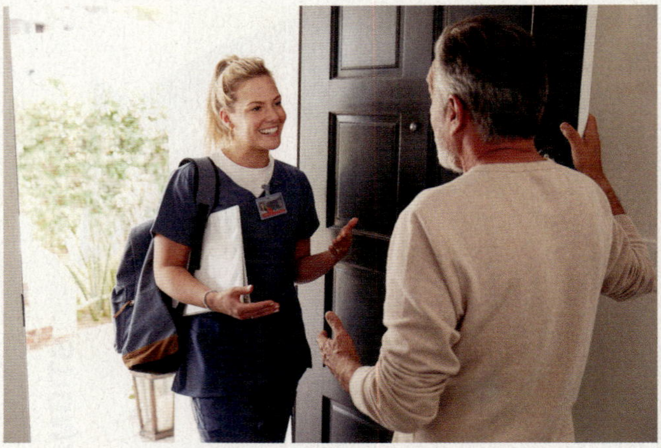

FIGURE 12-6. The nurse providing home health care must adapt to the patient's environment instead of the patient adapting to the hospital or clinic environment. (*Source:* Used with permission from Shutterstock. *Photo by Monkey Business Images.*)

are, including where they live, work, play, worship, and go to school. Community-based practice sites can be as varied as neighborhood clinics, patients' homes, long-term care facilities, schools, churches, and prisons. Almost 30% of RNs work in such nonacute patient care settings, and this number is growing. When health care is provided in the community, the nurse must adapt to the patient's environment and blend clinical skills with flexibility (Fig. 12-6).

Concept Mastery Alert

Community-based care and community health care are different. A helpful way to remember the difference is to think that community is larger than community based. So, community health care focuses on populations, whereas community-based care focuses on individuals and families.

Nurses practicing community-based care consider the continuity of the care patients require when moving from one level or setting of care to another; they provide interventions to promote health, manage acute or chronic illnesses, and promote self-care. Community-based care is designed to meet the needs of people as they move into, between, and among different health care settings within the overall health care system.

Until about 1990, community-based nurses were considered generalists, but recently many have gained advanced skills to meet the growing demands of acutely ill patients being cared for at home and in other community settings. These specialties include enterostomal therapy, cardiac care, mental health, maternal and child health, and palliative care. Specialized nursing knowledge and skills coupled with sophisticated technology increasingly allow many patients with acute and chronic health care needs to be treated safely and effectively in the home.

Qualities of the Community-Based Nurse

Nurses choose to practice community-based nursing in both urban and rural settings for various reasons. Many nurses enjoy practicing in an autonomous setting where they can use their expertise in an expanded role. Others enjoy managing their time independently and like the satisfaction experienced when patients welcome them into their home and life. Community-based nurses find satisfaction in networking with community facilities to provide individualized care. Community settings also provide an opportunity for nurses to be creative in delivering care. Community-based nurses must possess several key qualities: they must be knowledgeable and skilled in their practice, able to make decisions independently, and willing to remain accountable. While these qualities hold true for all nurses, the fact that many nurses in the community work independently makes these qualities even more critical for community-based nurses. For example, if a home hospice nurse fails to appropriately assess a patient and report a developing complication to the team, the patient may never receive the needed proactive care.

Knowledgeable and Skilled

Nurses who provide care in the community must have the knowledge and skills needed to provide appropriate care. Both effective communication and clinical skills are essential (Fig. 12-7). In fact, many community-based facilities require a minimum of 1 year of clinical practice as a prerequisite for employment. Physical assessment skills are necessary to identify positive and negative changes in a patient's health status. Procedures such as administering intravenous fluids, changing complex wound dressings, caring for ostomies, and providing ventilator care are often required. Home health care nurses have identified the following areas of knowledge as most important in home care: physical assessment, body mechanics, diagnosing/problem identification, infection control, and legal regulations.

Independent in Making Decisions

Nurses providing care in the community make independent decisions and assume responsibility for decision making. They are generally away from other health care providers when providing care and must be able to make patient care decisions independently. The combination of a sound theoretical foundation, proficiency in clinical skills, and ability to

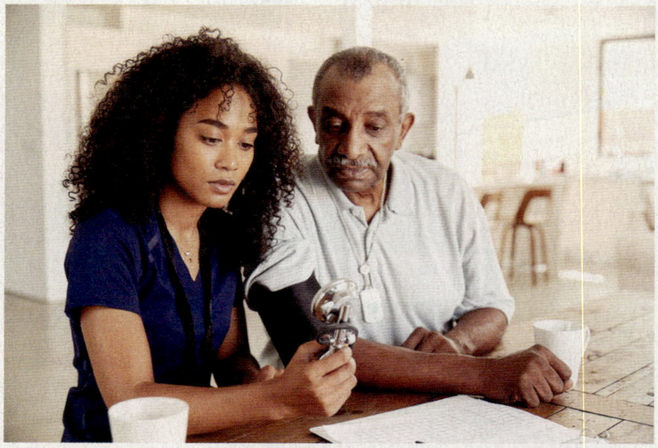

FIGURE 12-7. Home health care nurses combine effective communication skills with a sound clinical knowledge base when caring for patients and their families. (*Source:* Used with permission from Shutterstock. *Photo by Monkey Business Images.*)

solve problems creatively enables the nurse to make appropriate patient care decisions.

Accountable

Accountability is another important characteristic of community-based nurses. In a hospital, the nurse generally works a shift and then reports to the next shift nurse, who continues to care for the patient. Nurses seeing patients in their homes generally are not followed by a next shift but instead rely on family or other caregivers to continue the care. If there is no caregiver in the home, the nurse returns to face the same issues at the next visit. The nurse is accountable to the patient, the family, and the primary health care provider. Community-based nurses must consider questions such as the following:

- Whom do I call if the patient's physician or nurse practitioner is not available?
- What should I do if a family member becomes acutely ill?
- How do I learn to perform advanced procedures?
- How do I document the patient's decisions about treatment?
- How do I work collaboratively and ensure that other providers know about and document the care plan?

Roles of the Community-Based Nurse

In addition to having excellent caregiving skills, the community nurse is a patient advocate, coordinator of services, and patient and family educator/counselor.

Patient Advocate

Advocacy—the protection and support of another's rights—is an important role of community nurses. Patients often need help understanding the complex health care system, handling insurance problems, or dealing with state and federal regulations affecting their care and their environment. For example, the nurse may have to convince the patient's insurance carrier of the need for continued home health services. Patients may need help understanding complex billing issues related to their care. Home health care nurses can often mobilize services needed to improve the patient's environment.

QSEN THOUGHTFUL, PATIENT-CENTERED PRACTICE

Emotional support and alleviation of fear and anxiety along with involvement of family and friends are two principles of thoughtful patient-centered practice. When hospitals and nursing homes prevented families from visiting loved ones with COVID-19, including those who were in critical care units and dying, nurses turned to technology to support these patients and residents. Suddenly nurses were becoming skilled in using electronic tablets and smartphones to facilitate communication with families. Nurses became a welcome bridge for loved ones desperate to see a family member, often in the last minutes before death. And ultimately, nurses themselves became the last human to touch a patient or resident before death.

Community nurses who are committed to advocating for vulnerable patients and families work long hours and face many challenges. It is sometimes difficult to establish and maintain professional boundaries and to sever ties when appropriate with families the nurse has come to know and love. It is helpful to be aware of these challenges and to be able to discuss them with respected team leaders and colleagues. Read more about advocacy in Chapter 6.

Coordinator of Services

The community-based nurse generally coordinates all other health care providers visiting the patient and is the primary source of communication and coordination of the patient's care with the primary health care provider. The nurse uses effective communication skills with other health care providers while coordinating services for the patient.

A community-based nurse is also responsible for coordinating community resources needed by the patient. A sound knowledge of community resources enables the nurse to provide comprehensive services to the patient. For example, the nurse must understand the role of a social worker or physical therapist to determine a need for these services. The nurse should know about available community resources, such as Meals on Wheels, the American Cancer Society's services, services for patients who are visually impaired or deaf/hard of hearing, and local services for the aging. As the coordinator of care, the nurse directs the various services toward a common goal of improving the patient's health and promoting independence. How will you learn which community resources are available for Jeff Hart, Laura Degas, and Joey Marshall's families (described at the beginning of the chapter) and for all the patients for whom you will provide care?

Patient and Family Educator/Counselor

Nurses providing community-based care in a clinic or home teach patients and families about all aspects of care, including disease processes and treatments, nutrition, medications, and treatment and care of wounds. The nurse identifies learning needs; then the nurse, patient, and family mutually develop goals for teaching information necessary to promote health. Family members or other caregivers may be taught any skill that they are able and willing to perform.

The nurse provides the information necessary to keep the patient safe until the next visit, using methods that work best in the home or other community setting. The goal is to increase the patient's ability to provide self-care and the caregiver's ability to care for the patient. The teaching and learning process is fully described in Chapter 9 as well as the counseling responsibilities of the nurse.

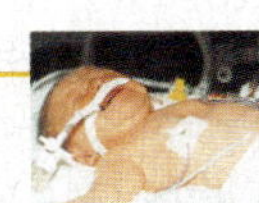

Remember **Joey Marshall**, the high-risk infant coming home after 7 months in the NICU. In this situation, the home health care nurse fills many roles; one of the major roles will be that of educator, with the goal of teaching Joey's mother so that she can ultimately care for Joey independently.

CONTINUITY OF CARE

Over their lifetimes, most people require many different health services offered in a variety of health care settings. Although a patient's health care may involve many different providers and settings (discussed in Chapter 11), the nurse is often the primary person responsible for communicating the patient's needs, teaching self-care, and, in many instances, providing care. As a result, one of the primary responsibilities of the nurse as caregiver is ensuring continuity of care.

Continuity of care is a process by which health care providers give appropriate, uninterrupted care and facilitate the patient's transition between different settings and levels of care. Continuity of care ensures a smooth transition between ambulatory or acute care and **home health care**, or other types of health care in community settings. Continuity depends on excellent communication as patients move from one caregiver or health care site to another. Too often, communication breakdowns among caregivers result in medical errors or deficient plans of care. In recent years, **patient handoffs**—transferring responsibility for a patient from one caregiver to another with the goal of providing timely, accurate information about a patient's care plan, treatment, current condition, and anticipated changes (Runy, 2013)—have been carefully researched. In 2006, The Joint Commission National Patient Safety Goals required hospitals to implement a standardized approach to handoff communications that includes:

- The handoff situation
- Who is, or should be, involved in the handoff communication
- Opportunities for people involved in handoffs to ask and respond to questions
- An outline for when to use certain communication techniques, such as repeat-back or read-back or the SBAR technique
- What print or electronic information should be available during the handoff (The Joint Commission, 2017)

In 2010, the requirement became a standard. On September 12, 2017 the Joint Commission issued a Sentinel Alert Event 58 providing advice to senders and receivers of handoff communication (https://www.jointcommission.org/-/media/tjc/documents/resources/patient-safety-topics/sentinel-event/sea_58_hand_off_comms_9_6_17_final_(1).pdf).

One popular approach to handoffs is the **situation–background–assessment–recommendation (SBAR)** strategy mentioned above and described in Chapter 8. According to the Institute for Healthcare Improvement (2017), SBAR provides a framework for communication between members of the health care team about a patient's condition. It is an easy and focused way to set expectations for what will be communicated and how between members of the team, which is essential for developing teamwork and fostering a culture of patient safety. See Box 12-1 for examples of simple SBAR communications. **ISBARQ** is a revised approach, adding introduction and question and answer components to SBAR (Runy, 2013):

I—Introduction: People involved in the handoff identify themselves, their roles, and their jobs

S—Situation: Complaint, diagnosis, treatment plan, and patient's wants and needs

B—Background: Vital signs, mental and code status, list of medications, and lab results

A—Assessment: Current provider's assessment of the situation

R—Recommendation: Identify pending lab results and what needs to be done over the next few hours and other recommendations for care

Q—Question and answer: An opportunity for questions and answers

Figure 12-8 (on page 314) illustrates a format for a more complex handoff. Following are 10 tips for effective handoffs (Runy, 2013):

1. Allow for face-to-face handoffs whenever possible.
2. Ensure two-way communication during the handoff process.
3. Allow as much time as necessary for handoffs.
4. Use both verbal and written means of communication.
5. Conduct handoffs at the patient bedside whenever possible. Involve patients and families in the handoff process. Provide clear information at discharge.
6. Involve staff in the development of handoff standards.
7. Incorporate communication techniques, such as SBAR, in the handoff process. Require a verification process to ensure that information is both received and understood.
8. In addition to information exchange, handoffs should clearly outline the transfer of patient responsibility from one provider to another.
9. Use available technology, such as the electronic medical record, to streamline the exchange of timely, accurate information.
10. Monitor use and effectiveness of the handoff. Seek feedback from staff.

Read more about patient handoffs in Chapter 20.

TeamSTEPPS is an evidence-based teamwork system designed for health care professionals to improve patient safety and improve communication and teamwork skills among health care professionals. The system is rooted in more than 20 years of research and lessons from the application of teamwork principle (Agency for Healthcare Research and Quality [AHRQ], 2017). TeamSTEPPS uses a variety of team strategies and tools to enhance performance and patient safety, including the SBAR tool for shift-to-shift handoffs and for situations that require immediate attention and action.

Another tool, increasingly used by nurses to get a supervisor's attention when it's really needed, is CUS: I am **C**oncerned, I am **U**ncomfortable, I believe **S**afety is at risk. *Example*: "I'm concerned that Ms. C is not her usual self. I'm uncomfortable that she is behaving so oddly. I believe she is not safe; she may have something serious going on that we are missing."

The Joint Commission Center for Transforming Healthcare (2012) describes targeted solutions for five specific causes of communication failures, as shown in Figure 12-9 (on page 315).

Box 12-1 Sample SBAR (Situation–Background–Assessment–Recommendation) Communications

SBAR Scenario #1

RN calling provider regarding patient's elevated temperature, breathing difficulties, and deteriorating condition

S—"Jeff's temperature this evening shot up to 103°C, and his respirations are labored; RR of 40, HR of 95 BPM, and O_2 Sat of 82% on room air. He is pale and also drooling."
B—"Jeff was transferred 2 days ago from the state home for children with respiratory difficulties. Jeff is a 9-year-old with a genetic disease that includes severe intellectual disability."
A—"I am concerned about Jeff's deteriorating condition."
R—"Another nurse is staying with Jeff, offering O_2 and positioning and suctioning, but I need you to come to the bedside and assess this patient."

SBAR Scenario #2

RN calling team manager regarding home hospice patient's inadequate pain management

S—"Ms. Tadesse is grimacing and moaning—she appears uncomfortable."
B—"She is in end-stage breast cancer and her family has been told that death is imminent—expected sometime this week."
A—"Her daughter has been administering the PRN morphine sulfate as ordered, but it no longer seems to be keeping her mother comfortable."
R—"Should we have the palliative care provider reevaluate Ms. Tadesse's analgesics and recommend a better pain management regimen?"

SBAR Scenario #3

RN calling provider about inadequate social support services for a patient scheduled for a discharge from a hospital rehab unit to home

S—"Mr. Ames is scheduled for discharge today. His wife appeared to "take him home" and arrived via taxi. She is a frail, 89-year-old woman who seems overwhelmed by the care she will need to provide in the home. She states that there are no families or friends capable of helping her care for her husband."
B—"Mr. Ames has spent the last week in a hospital rehabilitation unit following a right-sided total knee replacement. He weighs 320 lb. He has signed the discharge papers. There is no home care follow-up ordered."
A—"I am concerned about the Ameses because Mr. Ames still needs help ambulating. Prior to his surgery, Mr. Ames, who is 75 years old, was the primary caretaker for the couple. Without good home care services, I am concerned about their ability to manage."
R—"Should we invite the social worker and the case manager to reevaluate this family prior to his discharge and set up visiting nurses to assist?"

INTERPROFESSIONAL COLLABORATIVE PRACTICE

The "old" definition of teamwork in health care was working side by side with other health care professionals while performing your own skills. The Quality and Safety Education for Nursing (QSEN) project now defines teamwork as functioning effectively within your professional and interprofessional teams, fostering open communication, mutual respect, and shared decision making to achieve quality patient care (qsen.org). In 2011, the American Association of Colleges of Nursing partnered with other professional groups to establish core competencies for interprofessional collaborative practice. The World Health Organization (WHO) defines interprofessional **collaborative practice** as what happens when multiple health workers from different professional backgrounds work together with patients, families, carers, and communities to deliver the highest quality of care (WHO, 2010). The goal is to deliberatively work together to build a safer and better patient-centered and community/population-oriented U.S. health care system.

Components of Effective Team Structure

According to Salas et al. (2008), a team is composed of two or more people who:

- Interact interdependently and adaptively
- Have complementary skills
- Have effective leadership
- Work toward a common goal (*This is the MOST important component of team structure. Knowledge of the common goal accounted for 14% of the difference in team function.*)
- Have clear roles and responsibilities (*This is the second most important component of team structure; it accounted for 12% of the difference in team function.*)
- Hold themselves mutually accountable for achieving the goal

Core Competencies for Interprofessional Collaborative Practice

The IPEC core competencies were first adopted in 2011 and then updated in 2016. The 2016 update reflects two significant changes in the health care system, the increasing focus on the Triple Aim (improving the experience of care, improving the health of populations, and reducing the per capita cost of health care) and the implementation of the Patient Protection and Affordable Care Act; see Chapter 11. You can read more about these competencies in Chapter 14. Also note that *The Essentials: Core Competencies for Professional Nursing Education* now includes a sixth competency: Interprofessional partnerships. Its sub competencies align with these Interprofessional Education Collaborative competencies:

- Values and ethics
- Roles and responsibilities
- Communication
- Teams and teamwork

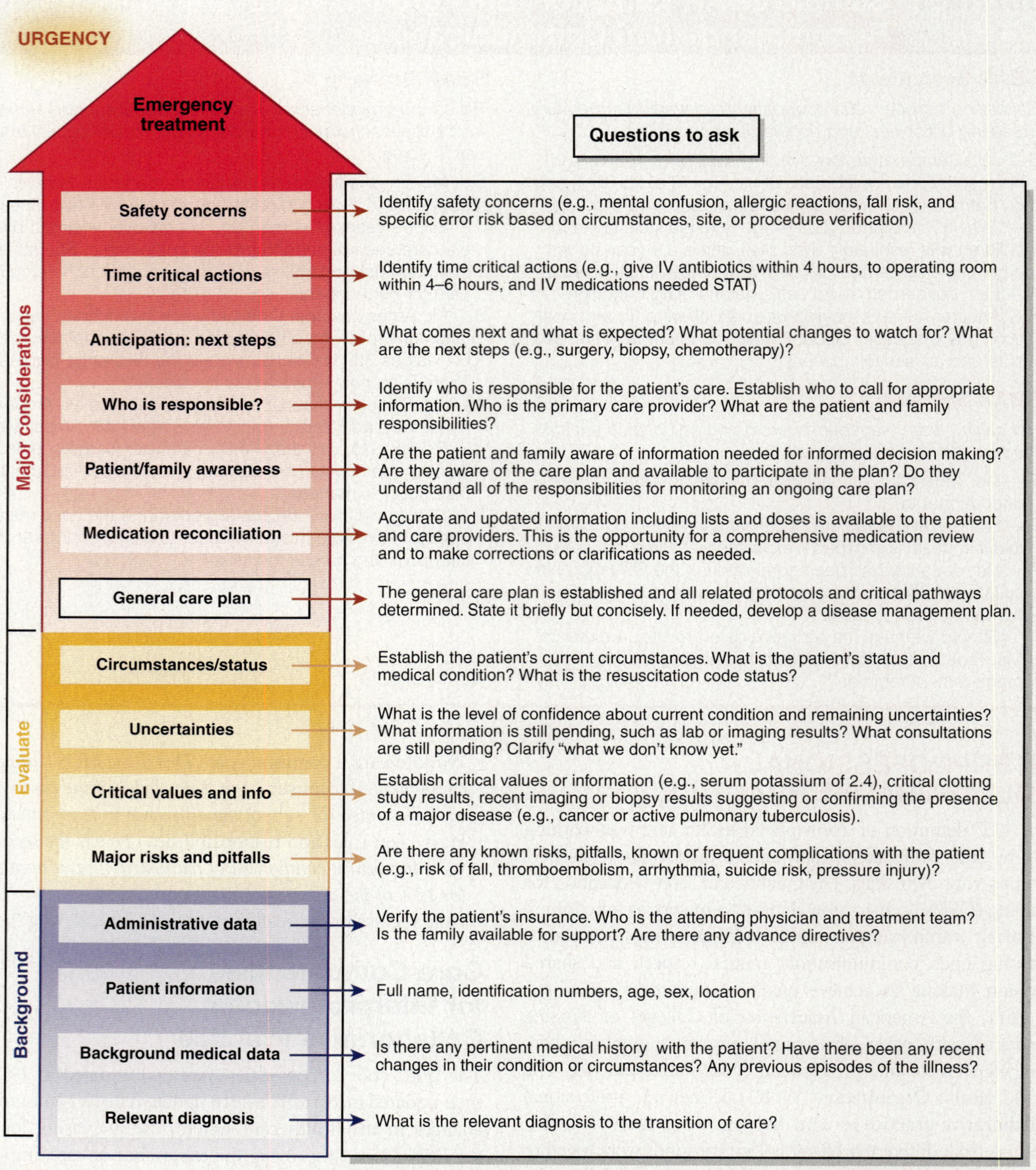

FIGURE 12-8. The U.S. Department of Defense Handoff Model. (*Source:* Reprinted from Healthcare Team Coordination Program. [2005]. *Department of Defense Patient Safety Program: Healthcare communications toolkit to improve transitions in care.* Department of Defense Patient Safety Program.)

Competency 1

Work with individuals of other professions to maintain a climate of mutual respect and shared values. (Values/Ethics for Interprofessional Practice)

Competency 2

Use the knowledge of one's own role and those of other professions to appropriately assess and address the health care needs of patients and to promote and advance the health of populations. (Roles/Responsibilities)

Competency 3

Communicate with patients, families, communities, and professionals in health and other fields in a responsive and responsible manner that supports a team approach to the promotion and maintenance of health and the

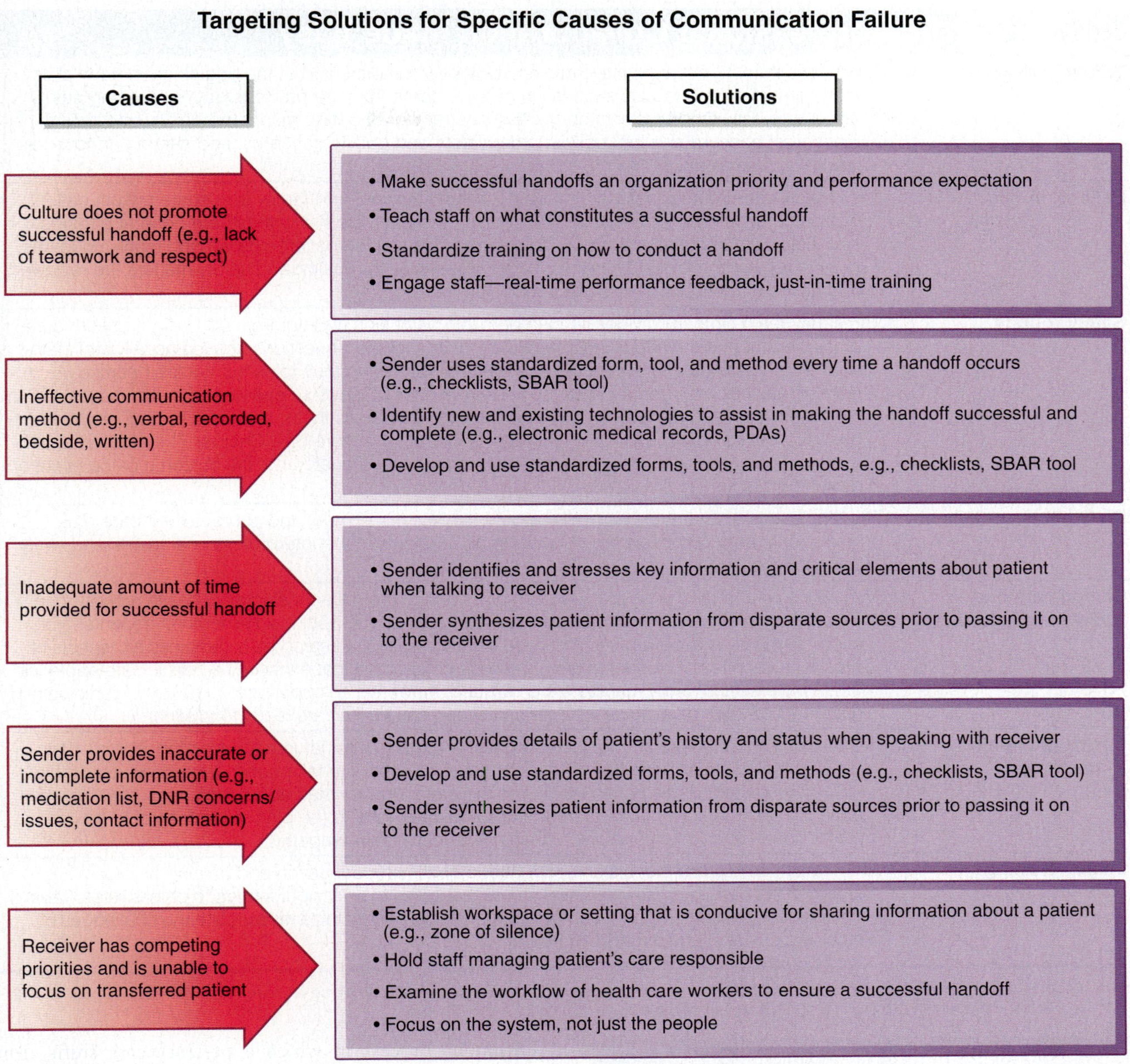

FIGURE 12-9. Targeted solutions for specific causes of communication failures. (*Source:* Reprinted with permission. Agency for Healthcare Research and Quality [AHRQ]. [2012]. *Improving transitions of care: Hand-off communications.* Joint Commission Center for Transforming Healthcare. https://psnet.ahrq.gov/)

prevention and treatment of disease. (Interprofessional Communication)

Competency 4

Apply relationship-building values and the principles of team dynamics to perform effectively in different team roles to plan, deliver, and evaluate patient/population-centered care and population health programs and policies that are safe, timely, efficient, effective, and equitable. (Teams and Teamwork)

As you begin to develop the knowledge, attitudes, and skills for interprofessional collaborative practice, you'll want to ask yourself these questions:

- What will I bring as strengths to collaborative practice?
- What about me might be problematic for my team?
- How will this self-knowledge direct my goals for self-development?

Chapter 11 describes the responsibilities of different members of the interprofessional health care team. Try to learn about the roles and responsibilities of your team colleagues as you begin practice. Sigmon (2020) notes that interprofessional collaborative teams that include nurses, physicians, social workers, pharmacists, and physical and occupational therapists can help health care organizations improve patient and family experiences, ensure good outcomes, and reduce costs while simultaneously enhancing the workplace. She is quick to point out that even when teamwork and collaboration are a job requirement, effective collaboration can be challenging. See Table 12-1 (on page 316) for strategies you can use to improve collaboration and see how many are in place during your clinical rotations.

Table 12-1 Interprofessional Collaboration Made Easy

Safety huddles	Short (less than 10 minutes) interprofessional safety huddles held at the beginning of each shift focus on safety and quality successes and concerns from the previous day, discussing safety and quality issues for patients on the day's schedule, updating mandated quality and safety measures, encouraging input about other safety and quality concerns, and sharing announcements or information.
Patient rounds	The goal of interprofessional team rounding with the patient and family is to share critical patient care information and develop a collaborative care plan. Optimally these are done at bedside and include the patient and family. The team discusses the patient's health and family concerns, daily care, treatment goals, and discharge plans. Health, quality, and safety matters are reviewed, and all team members participate in decision making.
Safety rounds	The safety team typically divides its members into pairs who walk through up to eight patient care areas and meet with various staff members. Using scripted questions, the teams talk with staff from all professions and record their comments, identifying their roles but not their names. At debriefings the safety team evaluates near miss causes, adverse events and safety issues. When concerns are noted, an action plan is developed to address them, and specific staff members are assigned for follow up. The aim is to promote a just culture (see Chapter 7) that focuses on evaluating choices and processes that impact safety and quality, not the outcome of the event or assigning blame.
Daily goals worksheet	The aim is to identify one or two daily targets for patients to meet and improve their care. The worksheets help communicate patient needs and risks to the interprofessional teams and verify goal completion.
Shared care and discharge plans	A shared care and discharge plan—written or as part of the patient's electronic health record—can be used for interprofessional team collaboration in all clinical settings. Rather than depending on separate medical, behavioral, and nursing treatment plans, a shared plan combines all aspects of care, with each team member offering a unique perspective that enhances a holistic care approach. When patients and family members are included, they have an opportunity to develop, participate in, and negotiate their care, voice their concerns, and ensure they are ready for discharge.
Structured family meetings	The meeting should have a leader who creates an agenda, structures the meeting, summarizes the discussion for all participants, assigns team members to take action, and conducts follow-up. Active patient participation (talking to the patient rather than about them) can help increase patients' sense of independence and improve adherence to the plan of care. Structured interprofessional family meetings also can increase care team empathy.
Shared training	When health care professionals and staff attend continuing education and training sessions together, they are in a risk-free environment that gives them insight into each other's roles. Talking freely about a common goal can help team members empathize, appreciate the challenges of other professions, and strengthen bonds.

Source: Adapted with permission, Sigmon, LB. (2020). Interprofessional collaboration made easy. *American Nurse Journal, 15*(11), 36–38. Copyright © 2021. HealthCom Media. Used with permission. All rights reserved. MyAmericanNurse.com

Unfolding Patient Stories: Vernon Russell • Part 1

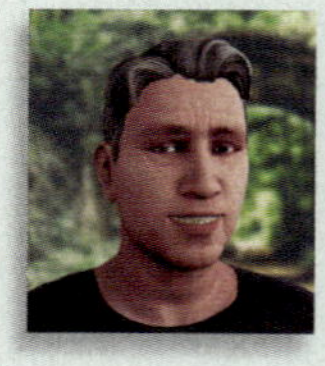

Vernon Russell—a 55-year-old who presents with left hemiplegia, garbled speech, and confusion—is admitted to the hospital with a stroke. He is divorced and lives with his son. What concepts would the nurse need to integrate to establish an effective, professional relationship with Vernon and his son? How does the nurse promote coordination of care between the interprofessional team members for stroke management? (Vernon Russell's story continues in Chapter 43.)

Care for Vernon and other patients in a realistic virtual environment: ***vSim** for Nursing* (thepoint.lww.com/vSimFunds). Practice documenting these patients' care in DocuCare (thepoint.lww.com/DocuCareEHR).

CARE COORDINATION

A 2012 Health Policy Brief produced by *Health Affairs*, a journal on health policy, describes **care transition** as a continuous process in which a patient's care shifts from being provided in one setting of care to another, such as from a hospital to a patient's home or to a skilled nursing facility and sometimes back to the hospital. It reports: "Poorly managed transitions can diminish health and increase costs. Researchers have estimated that inadequate care coordination, including inadequate management of care transitions, was responsible for $25 to $45 billion in wasteful spending in 2011 through avoidable complications and unnecessary hospital readmissions" (Burton, 2012). Because of all the complexities in delivering safe and affordable health care of good quality (see Chapter 11), care coordination has emerged as a central responsibility of all health care professionals, and especially nurses. In simple terms, care coordination is a mechanism to make sure that patients get the right care at the right time in the most efficient and cost-effective manner, by the right person in the right setting. The aim is to link patients with resources in the community to enhance their well-being, improve information exchange, and reduce fragmentation and duplication of services.

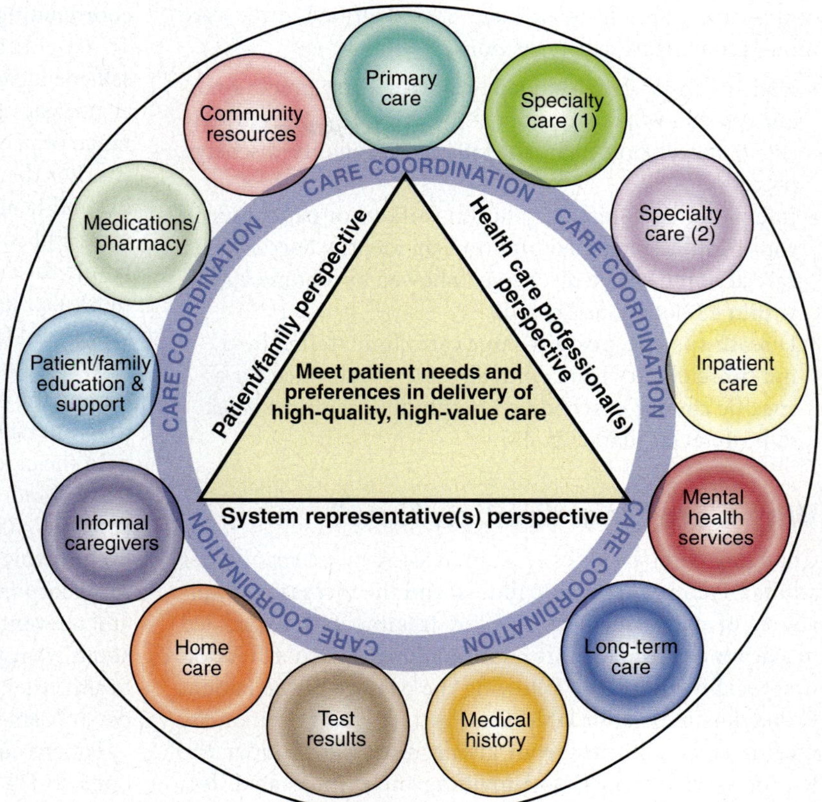

FIGURE 12-10. Care Coordination Ring. The central goal of care coordination is shown in the middle of the diagram. The *colored circles* represent some of the possible participants, settings, and information important to the care pathway and workflow. The *blue ring* connecting the *colored circles* is Care Coordination—namely, anything that bridges gaps (*white spaces*) along the care pathway. (*Source:* Reprinted with permission from McDonald, K. M., Schultz, E., Albin, L., Pineda, N., Lonhart, J., Sundaram, V., Smith-Spangler, C., Brustrom, J., & Malcolm, E. [2010]. *Care Coordination Atlas Version 3 [prepared by Stanford University under subcontract to Battelle on Contract No. 290–04–0020]. AHRQ publication No. 11–0023-EF.* Agency for Healthcare Research and Quality.)

A recent systematic review (AHRQ, 2014a) identified over 40 definitions for **care coordination**. The reviewers proposed the following broad definition: "Care coordination is the deliberate organization of patient care activities between two or more participants (including the patient) involved in a patient's care to facilitate the appropriate delivery of health care services. Organizing care involves the marshaling of personnel and other resources needed to carry out all required patient care activities and is often managed by the exchange of information among participants responsible for different aspects of care." Figure 12-10 illustrates care coordination.

Successes and failures in care coordination will be perceived in different ways by patients and families, health care professionals, and system representatives. Patients and families are pleased when care coordination helps ensure that the patient's needs and preferences for health services and information sharing across people, functions, and sites are met over time. Patients are unhappy during transitions to different providers and settings when communication regarding their history and health care needs requires more effort. According to the AHRQ review, health care professionals notice failures in coordination particularly when the patient is directed to the wrong place in the health care system or has a poor health outcome as a result of poor handoffs or inadequate information exchanges. They also perceive failures when they are obliged to exert an unreasonable effort to accomplish coordination during transitions to other health care entities. System representatives focus more on coordination failures when patients experience a clinically significant mishap from fragmentation of care or when system finances are adversely affected, such as when a preventable hospital readmission occurs.

Validation of Nursing Care Coordination Activities

Nurses have long been involved in care coordination activities, but only recently have these efforts been recognized as an integral contribution to effective and efficient use of health care resources and quality patient outcomes. Nurses have long developed care plans that account for patients' needs and preferences, conducted health teaching for patients and their families prior to discharge, and coordinated care across a variety of settings following discharge from a health care facility. It is who nurses are and what they do. The ANA launched an effort to validate the care coordination activities of RNs and seek funding for these essential components of patient care. Its position statement affirms the vital role that nurses play in the care coordination process, either as members of a multidisciplinary health care team or independently within the scope of their nursing practice. These efforts result in improved patient outcomes, increased efficiency in health care systems, and lower health care costs (American Nurses Association [ANA], 2014).

Bracken (2016) an acute care nurse practitioner, described how nurse practitioners can use a provisional bundle of predischarge, postdischarge, and bridging interventions to decrease costly readmissions for patients with chronic obstructive pulmonary disease. She identified three care models to increase safe transitions:

- High-intensity care team led by both a nurse practitioner and a social worker to support the primary care provider (PCP) and support high-risk patients through the discharge process
- Integration of community health workers or patient navigators into the inpatient unit to help identify barriers to care at home before discharge, followed by a home visit within 48 hours of discharge
- Disease-specific, postdischarge care clinic staffed by a multidisciplinary team, with all patients admitted for a specific condition scheduled in the clinic within 1 week of hospital discharge (p. 25).

Why Care Coordination Now?

Changing demographics (e.g., increasing numbers of older adults), increasing chronic illness, and the increasing availability of costly medications and treatments have all led to a heavy demand for care coordination. Care coordination is especially important following the passage of the Patient Protection and Affordable Care Act (PPACA). Financial incentives are shifting from giving more care (under the fee-for-service model) to providing more integrated, less costly care. The move toward "bundled payment" with shared savings provides incentives for care coordination and avoids fragmentation or duplication of services. Costs decrease when better information exchanges reduce the need for repeat procedures, which often happen when one provider doesn't know what others have ordered. Quality of care is enhanced when better handoffs result in treatment plans being aligned across settings. Chapter 11 describes some of the models of care coordination: providers and hospitals, multispecialty group practice, community health centers, prepaid group practice, accountable care organizations, and medical homes/medical neighborhood. Care coordination in discharge planning is addressed later in this chapter.

Nurse Self-Care Alert

One of the greatest sources of moral distress for nurses (see Chapter 6) is not being able to make health care work for those who need it. Limited access to necessary services coupled with limited resources for those without health insurance or independent means to pay for needed care means many families suffer without appropriate care to keep them healthy or to promote recovery (Olsen & Keilman, 2020). Look for moral distress resources in your clinical practice sites and talk with nurses about how they cope.

Care Coordinator

The **care coordinator** is the care provider (nurse case manager, social worker, community health worker, or lay person) who is responsible for identifying a patient's health goals and coordinating services and providers to meet those goals. To be effective, care coordinators must have expertise in self-management and patient advocacy, and must be adept at navigating complex systems and communicating with a range of people, from family members to PCPs and specialists. It is the responsibility of the care coordinator to identify life and health goals with the patient and to coordinate services and community supports to work with the patient and family toward better health outcomes. The care coordinator must also understand the strengths and gifts that the individual and family bring (their "assets").

This begins with conversations between the care coordinator and the patient about life goals and health goals, and how they interact. These conversations must be nonjudgmental, with the care coordinator taking an open, learning stance to understand the person's life context, challenges, struggles, and gifts. The care coordinator has ultimate responsibility for ensuring that the care plan is delivered as described, and for incorporating new knowledge to keep the care plan fresh and relevant. As the care coordinator and patient learn more about what promotes and what gets in the way of improved health, they are able to modify the care plan to meet the person's emerging strengths and needs.

Patient navigation is just one of the new roles being developed to fill a void in care coordination. The Academy of Oncology Nurse & Patient Navigators clarifies the difference between a nurse navigator and a patient navigator in the context of the patient with a cancer diagnosis:

Nurse navigator: This term describes a clinically trained nurse responsible for the identification and removal of barriers to timely and appropriate cancer treatment. The nurse navigator guides the patient through the cancer care continuum from diagnosis through survivorship. More specifically, the nurse navigator acts as a central point of contact for a patient and coordinates all components involved in cancer care, including surgical, medical, and radiation oncologists; social workers; patient education; community support; and financial and insurance assistance. The nurse navigator has the clinical background to perform this role and is a critical member of the multidisciplinary cancer team.

Patient navigator: This term describes all types of navigators; the patient navigator may be a nurse, a social worker, or a lay person. The primary distinction is that the patient navigator (1) does not necessarily have a clinical background and (2) focuses on the support aspects of care. Thus, a lay person or a social worker can be a patient navigator. Depending on the patient navigator's background and training, their function can vary. In general, the patient navigator provides assistance with scheduling, financial assistance, psychosocial support, and community support.

See Figure 12-11 for an example of how an oncology nurse navigator might assist a patient newly diagnosed with cancer.

One Patient's Story

Ellen McLoughlin, an oncology nurse navigator, helps Ms. Remos who is newly diagnosed with colon cancer.

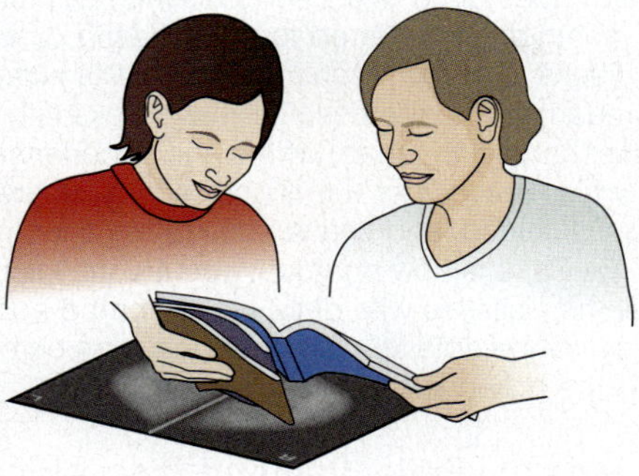

Explanation

Ms. Remos has many questions about her cancer after she gets home from her visit with her oncologist—questions she didn't think to ask. Her nurse navigator brings numerous resources and patience as she sits with Ms. Remos and answers Ms. Remos' questions. At this point she is building a trusting partnership with Ms. Remos and her husband.

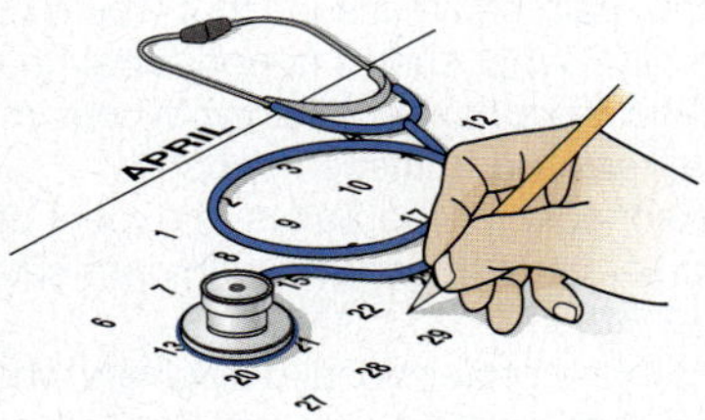

Scheduling

The thought of scheduling surgery and follow-up appointments that worked with the Remos' busy life was overwhelming Ms. Remos. The nurse navigator was able to schedule appointments for Ms. Remos that didn't interfere with when she needed to be home with her children or at work.

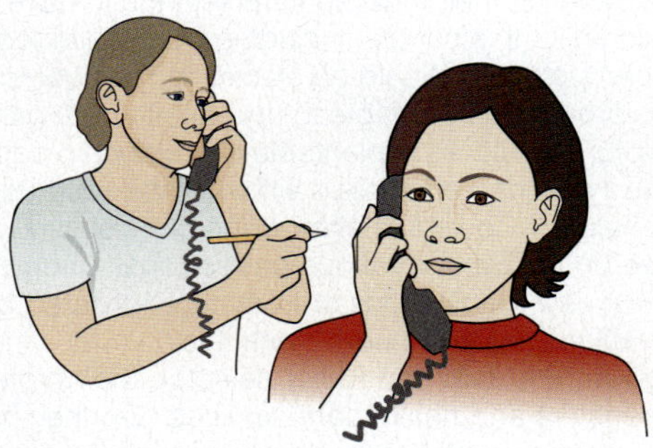

Information/Advice

Although Ms. Remos' surgeon talked with her about pre- and postoperative care, Ms. Loughlin was able to explain how Ms. Remos could best prepare for surgery and what she could do afterward to maximize her recovery. She was also able to help Mr. Remos plan to have family assist with childcare both during the hospitalization and after when Ms. Remos got home.

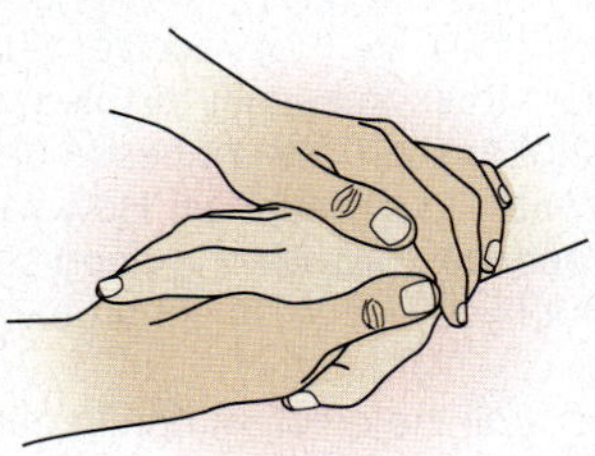

Support

The nurse navigator met with Ms. Remos the evening before her surgery and waited for her in the recovery room. Ms. Remos was grateful she could talk about her fears. The nurse navigator was also able to support Ms. Remos' husband and children.

FIGURE 12-11. An example of an oncology nurse navigator. (*Source:* Adapted with permission of *The Wall Street Journal* from Landro, L. [2011, August 16]. When a doctor isn't enough. Nurse Navigators help patients through maze of cancer-treatment decisions, fears. *The Wall Street Journal.* http://online.wsj.com/article/SB1000142405 3111904253204576510472828240848.html. Copyright © 2011 Dow Jones & Company, Inc. All Rights Reserved Worldwide. License number 4294870825526.)

Populations With Special Care Coordination Needs

Vulnerable populations are groups that are not well integrated into the health care system because of ethnic, cultural, economic, geographic, or health characteristics. Their isolation can result in these groups not obtaining necessary health care. Examples of vulnerable populations include:

- people with disabilities or multiple chronic conditions. (Think of Jeff Hart, the 9-year-old boy with severe intellectual disability, and review the case study of the Saxas presented in Box 12-2 on page 320.)
- people with mental illnesses or substance use disorders. See Figure 12-4, for facts about "Mental Health in My Community."
- cultural, racial, and ethnic minorities.
- people experiencing poverty in rural and urban areas, including those who are homeless.
- undocumented immigrants.

Nurses are often on the front lines of advocating for these groups, but advocacy requires special knowledge, attitudes, and skills. We all have to ask ourselves, first, if we may have biases that interfere with our willingness to create respectful patient-centered partnerships with vulnerable people.

Box 12-2 Care Coordination and Continuity Case Study

Read this scenario and discuss your answers to the questions that follow with your fellow students.

Mr. and Mrs. Saxa are an older couple (both in their mid-70s) who live independently. They live in the same house they raised their family in and are active members of their church. They have two grown children who live across the country but who are attentive and visit regularly, and they have four young grandchildren. Mr. Saxa is still driving, but his children are increasingly concerned about his safety behind the wheel.

Mrs. Saxa has type 1 diabetes and hypertension but has been able to manage her diet well and maintains good control of her hypertension with her medications. She takes six medications.

Mr. Saxa is also hypertensive, and recently underwent hip replacement surgery. While hospitalized for this surgery, he developed some difficulty urinating, and now sees a urologist. He also began anticoagulation therapy while hospitalized. Despite these issues, he has done quite well postoperatively, progressing from a walker to a cane that he now uses for stability. He currently takes seven medications.

The Saxas have a primary care provider (PCP) who has been their "family doctor" for decades. He is in a solo practice and does not have an electronic medical record system. In addition to their PCP, Mrs. Saxa sees an endocrinologist and a cardiologist, and Mr. Saxa sees a cardiologist, a urologist, and an orthopedic surgeon.

Mr. Saxa is a plumber. Mrs. Saxa did some secretarial work years ago but has primarily been a homemaker. Since Mr. Saxa retired and his employer does not offer retiree benefits, they rely on Medicare. They have a small nest egg of about $45,000.

In September, Mrs. Saxa has an episode of chest discomfort and shortness of breath and is taken to the emergency department (ED) of the local hospital. A hospitalist evaluates her in the ED and sends her to the lab for blood work and to the radiology department for a chest film. He calls in a cardiology consult and subsequently admits her to the critical care unit with a diagnosis of congestive heart failure, ruling out myocardial infarction, renal insufficiency, and rheumatoid arthritis. The cardiologist on call orders a cardiac catheterization to rule out coronary artery disease. She is found to have significant occlusion of the left anterior descending artery and the right coronary artery. A cardiovascular surgeon is consulted and a coronary artery bypass graft (CABG) is scheduled and later performed.

Mrs. Saxa recovers from the surgery and is discharged to a rehabilitation facility. While she is in rehabilitation, there is an outbreak of seasonal flu, and although Mrs. Saxa doesn't actually get the flu, she is significantly affected by staffing shortages. Meanwhile, Mr. Saxa is urged by his daughter to get a flu shot. Since his PCP is on vacation, he goes to an urgent care center in his local strip mall, where the nurse practitioner administers the flu shot. Mrs. Saxa receives physical and occupational therapy three times a week in rehab and does quite well. She is discharged from rehab after 1 month and is referred to home health care.

Two weeks after her discharge, Mrs. Saxa suffers a stroke and is readmitted to the hospital. Two weeks later she is again discharged to rehab, where she experiences another stroke, which leaves her with significant hemiparesis. Her progress is limited, and she is admitted to a long-term care facility. Mr. Saxa is now adamant about continuing to drive because he visits his wife daily. He is worried about how long they will be able to afford the long-term care facility, which is the only one close to their home.

Questions for Reflection and Discussion

1. What are the main health issues that would concern you with this family? What sort of nonphysical health care needs are the Saxas experiencing? Who is most likely to identify and respond to these needs?
2. What is reasonable for the Saxas to expect of the nurses they encounter in each of the health care settings they experience?
3. How likely are the professional caregivers who encounter the Saxas in their multiple care settings to have complete histories of this couple, including both their medical and social histories? Would an electronic medical history that could be made available to new health care providers be helpful? Would an implantable microbiochip capable of being scanned and linked with medical records access be helpful? Could this information be misused?
4. How do the Saxas' various professional caregivers learn about new medications or treatments ordered by each other? Are there concerns with this?
5. How do you think the Saxas selected their professional caregivers and health care services? Do they have any way of knowing what quality to expect? If they are dissatisfied with the care they receive, what avenues are open to them to express their displeasure?
6. Make a list of all the different health care settings the Saxas are likely to experience. How well do you understand the services provided in each setting? What criteria would you use to select an excellent facility or service?
7. Make a list of all the different health care providers the Saxas are likely to experience. How well do you understand their respective roles? What criteria would you use to evaluate their care?
8. How will the Saxas' provider visits and hospitalizations be paid for? Will the Saxas bear any financial burden? What health care costs are they likely to incur? Medications? Medical supplies?
9. Think about how the Saxas' experience would differ if they were members of a vulnerable population, for example, experiencing poverty in an urban area, recent immigrants, non–English-speaking, rural, etc.
10. Who, if anyone, is best qualified to coordinate the care the Saxas are receiving? How likely are they to experience satisfactory care coordination and continuity?

Source: Adapted from Dr. Patricia Cloonan, Georgetown University School of Nursing and Health Studies.

Do we believe that people with substance use disorders, people who are homeless, older adults, or people who do not speak English deserve the same respectful, compassionate, person-centered care that we would want for those we love most? Are we moved by the plight of those most in need? You will find vulnerable population alerts scattered throughout the text.

In 2013, a columnist for *The Washington Post* wrote about a "scary, abandoned hospital" in Washington, DC (the city had a $417 million budget surplus at the time) that was serving as a makeshift family homeless shelter; no one seemed to care about 600 kids crammed inside. "Stop and think about that. Six hundred kids with chubby cheeks and Spider-Man sneakers and Dora hats are beginning their journey in life on an army cot in a cafeteria or an old hospital bed in a city shelter. And that's an improvement from the time they spent sleeping in cars, bus shelters, Metro stations, apartment–house lobbies or on a different couch every night" (Dvorak, 2013). Nurses have a proud tradition of seeking to meet the needs of the most vulnerable; will the next generation of nurses continue this?

Nurses also need specialized knowledge and skills to serve these people. It takes a special effort to "walk in the shoes" of a teenage single mother with three children under the age of four, or a homeless man with a history of chronic drug and alcohol abuse, to learn about who they are, what they need, and how best to help them. Think about a vulnerable population where you live, and try to interview some of its members. See if your class can devise a strategy to learn about them and then begin to meet their needs. Think about how community-based care coordination efforts can improve the health and well-being of the most vulnerable in your region.

Admissions, Transfers, and Discharges

As a result of increasing costs and of health care cost reimbursement programs that are prospective rather than retrospective (meaning that costs are predetermined for specific illnesses or treatments, including severity of illness and cost of care), hospital admissions and lengths of hospital stay have decreased. More patients are having surgery, diagnostic tests, and emergency care in ambulatory care settings or on a hospital outpatient basis. The 2020 pandemic further reduced visits to the hospitals. Even patients who are admitted often stay for less than 24 hours, are admitted the morning of the surgery, or go home during an interim period between diagnosis and care. All this makes care coordination particularly challenging.

All people who enter a health care setting take on a new role. They must add to their already established roles (e.g., spouse, parent, sibling, student) the role of patient. They also enter an environment in which strangers surround them and in which they encounter different sounds, sights, and smells. A competent, responsible, and caring nurse can make all the difference to an anxious, frightened, or confused patient and family.

To meet patients' health care needs during the admission process, nurses provide holistic care and establish the basis for how patients will respond to and evaluate the remainder of their stay. Box 12-3 describes guidelines for establishing an effective nurse–patient relationship to ensure that each patient is considered as a unique person who merits respect in any setting.

During admission, the nurse acts not only as a health care provider but also as an advocate concerned about the welfare of the patient and the family. The admission period corresponds to the orientation phase of the helping relationship described in Chapter 15. In addition, regulatory guidelines direct both the continuity and the quality of care. For example, The Joint Commission standards for admission to a hospital assert that each patient's need for nursing care should be assessed by a registered nurse (RN). This assessment includes consideration of biophysical, psychosocial, environmental, self-care, educational, and discharge planning factors. In addition, nurses collaborate, as appropriate, with health care providers and members of other clinical disciplines to make decisions regarding the patient's need for nursing care.

Box 12-3 Establishing an Effective Nurse–Patient Relationship During Hospital Admission

- Recognize and take steps to reduce the patient's anxiety. Anxiety is a natural reaction to the unknown, but it can be reduced by therapeutic communication, teaching, and acceptance. Some common concerns that cause anxiety are: *Will I have pain? Who will take care of my family if I die? Will strangers be looking at my body? How much will this cost? What if I can't keep my job?*
- Encourage the patient and family to participate in and make decisions about all aspects of care.
- Remember that the medical or surgical condition for which the patient is being treated is only one part of the patient's life. Other concerns include family needs, financial status, and the future.
- Communicate with patients as individuals so that they can maintain their own identity. Ask patients how you should address them; some people prefer Mr., Mrs., Miss, or Ms. (last name), whereas others would rather be called by their first name. Do not call all older adults "Grandma" or "Grandpa." Do not refer to Mr. Jones, admitted to room 2218 for treatment of a ruptured appendix, as "the appendix in 2218."
- Take time to learn who the patient being admitted is, including that patient's cultural and religious background. Respect the patient's values and beliefs even though they may differ from yours.

Admission to an Ambulatory Care Facility

In ambulatory care facilities, described in Chapter 11, the patient receives health care services but does not remain overnight. Ambulatory facilities include physician and nurse practitioner offices, clinics, hospital outpatient services, emergency departments (EDs), and same-day surgery centers. The goal of these facilities is to provide health care services to patients who are able to provide self-care at home. People go to ambulatory settings for health promotion, health maintenance, or medical or surgical treatment.

In most office and clinic facilities, patients enter a reception area where they are asked to complete a short health history (unless they have already done so during a previous visit) and sign a statement acknowledging the HIPAA privacy rule (see Chapters 7, 20, and 21). They then receive a physical assessment (often specific to the reason for the visit) in an examination room. Depending on their needs, patients may be given, for example, diagnostic tests, immunizations, or prescriptions for medications, or may undergo minor surgery. All patients require teaching, which should include written instructions about care at home, health promotion activities, and how to contact someone for further questions. Referrals to community facilities, support groups, or other types of health care settings may also be necessary.

Admission to ambulatory or same-day surgery facilities is somewhat different. Screening tests, teaching, and admission procedures are usually completed previously. Patients arrive at the setting, have the procedure, and go home when recovery is satisfactory. If patients have outpatient or short-stay surgery in the hospital setting, the regular admission procedures are completed on arrival; in most instances, screening tests and teaching are done before the day of surgery. It is the nurse's responsibility to assess what has been done and tailor the care plan to the patient's needs.

Concept Mastery Alert

Patients are admitted to all different types of ambulatory care facilities for many different reasons. Regardless of the setting or reason, teaching is a priority.

Admission to the Hospital

A scheduled admission to the hospital usually begins in the admitting office. Admitting office staff obtain information about the patient and input that information into the computer. The admission data become part of the patient's permanent record.

The identification number (often included as a barcode), as well as the patient's name, admitting provider's name, and any other information required by the particular institution, is printed on an identification wristband that is placed on the patient's wrist. This wristband is an important safety component during the patient's stay because it is one of two identifiers, required by the Joint Commission national safety standards, used to accurately identify a patient during activities such as medication administration, blood and fluid administration, diagnostic tests, and surgery. A wristband is worn by all patients. The patient's date of birth is commonly used as the second identifier.

During the initial interview, the admitting staff provide other information about legal and ethical components of care. The patient is asked to sign forms that give consent to treatment and allow the hospital to contact health care insurance companies or public facilities (e.g., Medicare) for reimbursement of services. Patients are asked if they have established advance directives, such as a living will or durable power of attorney, to indicate their treatment preferences about prolonging life. If they have established advance directives, a copy becomes a part of their hospital record. If they have not, the purpose is explained and they are given a form to complete if they wish to do so. (Chapter 44 discusses advance directives and provides a sample form.) Providers must give patients a clear written explanation of how health information will be used and disclosed, and the patient must sign a privacy statement. Patients may also be asked to provide the names of family or friends to whom health status information may be given. Finally, almost all hospitals give some form of a Patient Care Partnership (formerly titled a Patient Bill of Rights) to patients to inform them about what to expect while in the hospital. This document, usually available in several languages, includes the rights to high-quality hospital care, a clean and safe environment, involvement in care, protection of privacy, help when leaving the hospital, and help with insurance claims (American Hospital Association, 2003).

After the necessary forms have been completed in the admitting office, a nurse who works in that area may complete the admission health history and physical assessment, or the patient may be taken to an assigned room for these admission procedures. Laboratory studies and x-rays, as well as the admitting office procedures, are usually completed on an outpatient basis before the day of admission. If the patient has an unscheduled admission or will have only a limited stay (e.g., a patient admitted the morning of a diagnostic examination who is intending to return home later that day), admission procedures and assessments may be completed on the unit.

PREPARING THE ROOM FOR ADMISSION

The admitting office notifies the unit to which the patient is to be admitted before the patient arrives so that the room can be prepared. Although the nurse may delegate most of the activities in preparing the room for an admission, it is a nursing responsibility to ensure that other personnel do them. Guidelines for Nursing Care 12-1 outlines the activities carried out in anticipation of the patient's arrival.

ADMITTING THE PATIENT TO THE UNIT

Although other members of the health care team may assist in the admitting procedure, the nurse is responsible for ensuring the patient's safety, comfort, and well-being upon arrival in the unit. The admitting nursing history and assessment are described in Chapter 15, where you will find examples of paper and electronic assessment records. The admission assessment is used to develop the nursing care plan for the patient and is also used as a database for discharge planning and home care. In addition, an inventory of personal belongings and valuables is completed to ensure their return to the patient on discharge or their transfer with the patient to another unit or facility. A **medication reconciliation** form is completed on admission. The form is checked and filled out again with each transfer and on discharge to ensure that all medications have been correctly ordered or discontinued as the patient moves through the system.

The nurse should welcome the patient to the unit in the same courteous manner as when welcoming a guest into their own home. In most instances, the patient will be accompanied by family members who may either remain with the patient to provide support and information or who may wait in the waiting room during the admission procedure. The nurse assesses the needs of the patient and family, and they should mutually agree about whether family should be present during admission.

Guidelines for Nursing Care 12-1

PREPARING THE ROOM FOR PATIENT ADMISSION

- Position the bed. For ambulatory patients, the bed should be in its lowest position. Place the bed in its highest position if the patient will arrive on a stretcher. Ensure that the furniture in the room is arranged to allow easy access to the bed.
- Open the bed by folding back the top bed linens (see photo).
- Assemble routine equipment and supplies. Place a hospital admission pack (which contains such items as a hygiene supplies, water pitcher, drinking glass, tissues, soap, and lotion) in the room. A hospital gown or pajamas should be in the room, although the patient may choose to wear their own pajamas or gown. Equipment for taking vital signs (i.e., stethoscope, sphygmomanometer, thermometer) and height and weight should be in the room or readily available. If laboratory work has not been done previously, a container for a clean urine specimen should be available.
- Make sure that the call light and TV remote control are readily available for the patient.
- Assemble special equipment and supplies. The patient may require oxygen therapy, cardiac monitoring, or suction equipment. Ensure that the equipment is functioning properly and is ready for the patient's use on arrival.
- Adjust the physical environment of the room; this may include turning on lights and setting the room temperature.

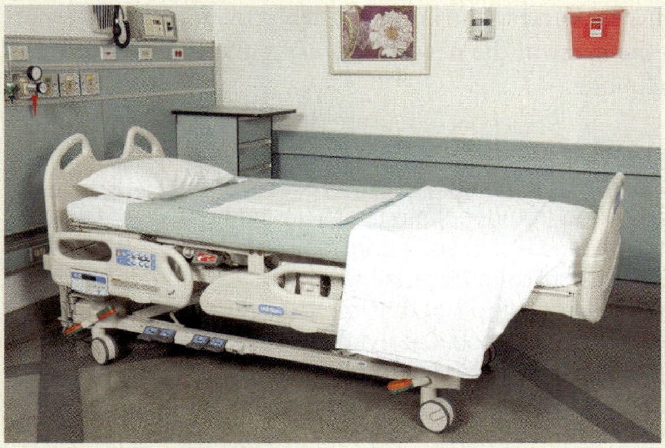
An "open" bed, ready for the patient's arrival.

Transferring Within and Between Health Care Settings

Patients often move within a setting as well as between settings, as in these examples:

- Within the hospital, such as from the ED to a hospital room, from an intensive care unit (ICU) to a hospital room (and vice versa), from one unit to another, or from one room to another room on the same unit
- To and from acute care settings and long-term settings
- From acute care settings to the patient's home
- From ambulatory care settings to acute care settings

When a transfer occurs, the patient must readjust to new surroundings, a new roommate, new routines, and new people providing care. If the transfer is to a higher level of care, as in a move to the ICU, the patient and family often experience unfamiliar sights and sounds. A transfer to a long-term care facility may not be desired by the patient or family but may be necessary if family members cannot provide care at home or if no other support people are available. All of these factors cause stress and anxiety.

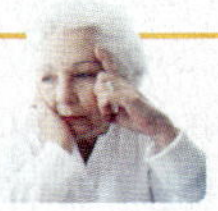

Recall **Laura Degas**, the woman who is not sure if she will be able to care for her sister at home. If it is determined that Ms. Degas cannot care for her sister at home, she may decide to have her sister transferred to a long-term care facility. In this case, the nurse must provide Ms. Degas with support and guidance to ease the transition and help minimize the stress and anxiety of this move.

The nurse may not be responsible for the actual physical move but is responsible for ensuring that the comfort, safety, and teaching needs of the patient and family are met. Although documentation and procedures differ depending on the institution and type of transfer, patient needs are always a priority in ensuring a smooth transition and continuity of care.

TRANSFER WITHIN THE HOSPITAL

When a patient is transferred within the hospital, personal belongings must be moved to the new room. Every effort must be made to ensure that belongings are not misplaced or lost. The patient's records are moved to the new unit or made available electronically. Other hospital departments (e.g., dietary, pharmacy, physical therapy) must be notified of the transfer.

When a patient is transferred to another unit, the nurse in the original area gives a verbal report about the patient to the nurse in the new area using the approved handoff technique. The report should include the patient's name, age, providers, admitting diagnosis, surgical procedure (if applicable), current condition and manifestations, allergies, medications and treatments, laboratory data, and any special equipment that will be needed to provide care. Patient goals and nursing care priorities are identified, and the existence of advance directives is noted. Accurate, concise, and complete verbal communication is essential.

TRANSFER TO AN EXTENDED CARE FACILITY

When a patient is transferred from the hospital to an extended care facility or other community setting, the patient is discharged from the hospital and a copy of the medical record may be sent to the extended care facility (depending on the provider's preference and the facility's protocol). The original record, which is a legal document, remains at the hospital. All of the patient's belongings are sent to the facility with the patient. Prescriptions and appointment cards for return visits to the provider's office may also be sent.

In most instances, a detailed assessment and care plan is sent from the hospital to the extended care facility. In addition, the nurse at the hospital often provides a verbal report to the nurse at the new facility using the approved handoff technique.

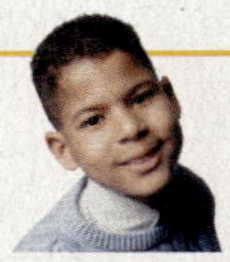

Remember **Jeff Hart**, the 9-year-old boy transferred from the state facility to the hospital because of respiratory complications. Once the child's problems have been resolved, the nurse will prepare Jeff to be transferred back to the state facility. Information about the events of the hospitalization will be documented and reported. Communication between health care team members at the hospital and those at the state facility helps ensure continuity of care for Jeff.

Discharge from a Health Care Setting

Patients are discharged from a health care facility when the expected outcomes of care are met and the patient or caregiver has the necessary knowledge and skills to provide any additional care still needed. In meeting the needs of the patient being discharged from a health care setting, the nurse considers that the person may be expecting a change from a dependent role to a more independent (self-care) role. Although discharge is almost always a welcome event, it also can be stressful.

DISCHARGE PLANNING

The purpose of planning for continuity of care, commonly referred to in hospitals and community facilities as **discharge planning**, is to ensure that patient and family needs are consistently met as the patient moves from a care setting to home. Essential components of discharge planning include assessing the strengths and limitations of the patient, the family or support person, and the environment; implementing and coordinating the care plan; considering individual, family, and community resources; and evaluating the effectiveness of care. Done well, discharge planning and teaching go a long way to reducing hospital readmissions.

Planning for discharge actually begins on admission, when information about the patient is collected and documented. The key to successful discharge planning is an exchange of information among the patient, the caregivers, and those responsible for care while the patient is in a care setting and after the patient returns home. This coordination of care is usually the nurse's responsibility.

With earlier hospital discharges, patients often are still acutely ill when they go home, and many require complicated treatment and care by family members. It is no longer unusual for family members to change sterile dressings, administer tube feedings, monitor intravenous medications, manage high-technology equipment, give complete physical care, and prepare special diets. If they are unprepared or unable to carry out these interventions correctly, the patient may experience an exacerbation of the illness or complications that could require readmission or additional treatment. The nurse must ensure that family members are taught the necessary knowledge and skills, and that referrals are made to facilities such as home health care or social services to provide support and assistance during the recovery period.

The hospital discharge process includes identifying which patients need which level of discharge planning. All patients need discharge planning in general, but certain patients have more comprehensive needs for specific services. The nurse who conducts the initial nursing assessment is in the best position to determine these special needs.

Patients who meet any of the following criteria need a formal discharge plan and referral to another facility:

- Lack of knowledge of the treatment plan
- Social isolation
- Recently diagnosed chronic disease
- Major surgery
- Prolonged recuperation from major surgery or illness
- Emotional or mental instability
- Complex home care regimen
- Financial difficulties
- Lack of available or appropriate referral sources
- Terminal illness

GUIDELINES FOR DISCHARGE PLANNING

For a patient hospitalized with a serious illness or injury, discharge planning may be done over time; for a patient treated in an ambulatory facility, it may be completed relatively quickly. A nursing case manager or discharge planner is often responsible for discharge planning for patients in acute care settings and may follow a care plan or a critical path established for the patient. Regardless of the plan used, the nurse assesses the patient's needs and identifies problems, develops goals with the patient, carries out teaching, and makes referrals. An example of discharge planning is provided in Box 12-4.

Assessing and Identifying Health Care Needs

The first step in discharge planning involves collecting and organizing data about the patient. When assessing the patient for discharge, the nurse includes the family, if possible, because both the patient and family must be actively involved for an effective transition from the health care setting to home. Factors to assess in discharge planning are listed in the accompanying Focused Assessment Guide 12-1 (on page 326). Other assessment formats may be used, depending on institutional procedures, to evaluate the patient's ability to carry out activities of daily living (e.g., bathing, dressing, toileting, transferring, continence, feeding) and instrumental activities of daily living (using the telephone, shopping, preparing food, doing housekeeping

Box 12-4 Discharge Planning Example

Scenario

Mr. Smith is a 55-year-old married man, admitted to the hospital with a diagnosis of stroke. He now has left-side weakness and difficulty communicating verbally. He has had a history of high blood pressure for 10 years. If his blood pressure remains stable, Mr. Smith is to be discharged from the hospital in 3 days. He will be going home with four new medications. A low-sodium diet is prescribed.

After reviewing the medical record, the nurse interviews Mr. and Mrs. Smith. The assessment reveals that Mr. Smith has a limited ability to transfer from bed to chair. Both Mr. and Mrs. Smith are fearful of discharge. Mr. Smith believes that he will be able to return to work as an accountant in 3 weeks and hates the thought of becoming disabled at his age, but Mrs. Smith thinks he will never work again. They have never faced a life-threatening or disabling illness in the past. They have no strong cultural preferences for diet. They have two adult children who live out of state with their own families. Mrs. Smith has a younger sister who lives nearby. The Smiths are both college educated. They live in a suburban area in a two-story home with narrow stairs leading to the second floor's two bathrooms and three bedrooms. Their doctor's office is about 1 mile away, and shopping is nearby.

Mrs. Smith is worried about moving Mr. Smith in and out of bed. She needs instruction in the new medications and diet regimen. She is terrified that she may be unable to handle an emergency in the middle of the night. Financially, this two-income family has abruptly become a one-income family. Mr. Smith is not 65 years old and thus is not yet eligible for Medicare, although he does have disability insurance that will cover a portion of his salary.

Planning

How would the nurse coordinate this discharge plan? The health care provider or advance practice nurse must be consulted for diet, medication, other treatments, and home health care orders. The dietitian needs to counsel the Smiths on a low-sodium diet and on creative ways to prepare low-salt meals. Physical therapy has already been initiated at the hospital and will continue through home health care. An occupational therapist will visit to help the Smiths find the best way to tend to personal hygiene, grooming, and other meaningful life activities. The social worker has been called for financial assessment to determine exactly what services the Smiths can expect to have reimbursed by their insurance plan and how they will manage their out-of-pocket expenses.

The nurse discusses Mr. and Mrs. Smith's health care needs with the home health care facility. A teaching plan for medications is implemented. The physical therapist teaches Mrs. Smith how to transfer Mr. Smith into and out of the bed and assures her that he will help her practice at home. Written information about high blood pressure, stroke, low-sodium diet, and prescribed medications is given to the Smiths, along with the telephone number of a local support group for people who have had strokes. Although Mrs. Smith still verbalizes concern about providing care at home, she says that she feels more in control now. Mr. Smith is beginning to realize that recovery may take longer than he anticipated. At the time of discharge, the nurse tells the Smiths that someone from the hospital will call them the next day and that the home health care nurse will visit them that afternoon.

and laundry, taking medications, accessing transportation). The medical record and health care provider orders are also consulted for the exact medication and treatment plan before the nursing care plan is developed.

Health problems, developed from the discharge planning assessment, identify the needs of both the patient and the family. The nurse determines whether problems are present now or are potential problems. For example, a patient with chronic respiratory problems may have assistance from a member of the family who has come to stay for 1 month, but after that, the patient will be alone at home. In this case, the situation is not an actual problem now but could become one unless planning is done to meet needs when there is no longer a family caregiver.

Setting Goals With the Patient

The expected goals of the discharge plan are set mutually and must be realistic. If the patient is involved in establishing goals, the expected outcomes of the care plan are more likely to be met. The patient may fail to follow the plan if the goals are not mutually agreed on or are not based on a complete assessment of the patient's needs. For example, the nurse or another health care provider may do a thorough job of teaching a patient about a special diet, but the patient may not actually follow the diet after discharge because of being unable to afford the special food, being unable to get to the grocery store, or not having a refrigerator at home for food storage.

Teaching

The AHRQ (www.ahrq.gov) offers the following suggestions for establishing and maintaining rapport with patients during education sessions:

- Offer a warm greeting
- Establish eye contact
- Slow down
- Use plain, nonmedical words
- Limit content
- Use the teach-back technique
- Report key points
- Involve the patient, family, and significant others (with the patient's permission)
- Use visual displays to reinforce information

Important teaching topics about self-care at home must be covered before discharge. These topics include medications, procedures and treatments, diet, referrals, and health status.

The patient needs to understand the drug name, dosage, purpose, effects, times to be taken, and possible side effects. Information about medications should be given both verbally and in writing. Copies of the medication administration record are often given to the patient to use as a pattern for times and amounts of medications administered in the hospital. Patients often find it helpful when the nurse draws a clock face and writes the names of the medications in the correct time slots.

Focused Assessment Guide 12-1

DISCHARGE PLANNING

Factors to Assess	Questions and Approaches
Health data	Establish a database that includes age, biologic sex, height and weight, medical diagnoses, past medical history, current health problems, surgery, and functional limitations (e.g., impaired sight or hearing, amputation, use of wheelchair or walker).
Personal data	Ask the patient: "What language do you prefer to use?" "How do you feel about being discharged? Do you have any special fears or concerns?" "What are your expectations for recovery?" "What do you do to help you cope with stress? Are these things helpful?"
Caregivers	Establish the caregiver's age, biologic sex, relationship to the patient, past experiences with this illness or treatment, values and beliefs, and cultural practices that might affect prescribed care. Ask the caregiver: "Do you live with the patient?" "What are your expectations about providing care at home?" "What are your fears about providing care at home?"
Environment	Assess the home, noting if there will be barriers to using prescribed assistive devices (e.g., wheelchairs or walkers); if the patient will be able to use bathroom facilities safely; and if hot water, heat, and room for supplies are available. See the home safety checklist in Chapter 28, Box 28-1. Assess the community, noting location (such as rural or urban), whether health care is available and accessible, whether transportation is available, and any known environmental hazards.
Financial and support resources	Discuss expenses of prescribed care, including dressing supplies, medications, equipment, and special foods. Discuss available resources, including Medicare and Medicaid, parish nursing, and meal services to the home. Discuss—especially if the patient will be living alone—support services and resources and how they can be accessed. Include friends, church groups, and support groups specific to the patient's age and health care needs.

All steps of a procedure (e.g., dressing changes) should be demonstrated, practiced, and provided in writing. Some nurses make short videos to demonstrate complex procedures to patients for the patient to take home. The patient or caregiver should then perform the procedure or treatment in the presence of the nurse to demonstrate the ability to carry out the procedure. The caregiver should know the purpose of what is being done and how to get supplies.

Teaching about diet should clearly describe the purpose of the diet and its expected outcomes. Patients find examples of written diet plans and meals helpful. If the patient has been in the hospital, it is helpful to save menu or meal forms to use as a reference at home.

Appointments for the first visit to a health care provider or facility are often made before discharge. In addition, the patient and family members should know how to contact the providers of follow-up care and should know whom to call if they have questions or problems. Nurses can help patients by making sure that they have the phone numbers of the primary care doctor and the names and phone numbers of community resources. Patients should also know the signs and symptoms of potential complications and when to contact emergency care. This referral information takes into account the patient's economic situation, access to transportation, support systems, and home environment.

All aspects of the illness or effects of treatment should be clearly described, both verbally and in written materials. Many forms of written information are available for patients, ranging from printed literature (e.g., from the American Heart Association) to teaching materials developed by the health care facility. Written instructions are given to the patient. Please note that handing the patient written instructions is NOT the same as teaching. The patient should be able to talk about the anticipated physical and emotional effects of the illness and also describe what will be done to achieve the highest level of health possible. All teaching should be documented in the patient's record and the discharge summary. The patient's or family member's demonstrations of care procedures must be satisfactory, and the patient and caregiver must have exposure to and practice with the equipment that they will be using at home.

Painter (2021) noted that managing home dialysis can be one of the most complex and challenging tasks family caregivers face. In her article on preventing home dialysis complications she offers a very practical guide to help nurses provide caregivers with the tools they need to manage their family member's health care at home.

Meeting Eligibility Requirements for Community-Based Settings

The physician or nurse practitioner must write an order for all home care services, and the patient must meet eligibility criteria for reimbursement for home health care visits. As much patient information as possible should be given to the home health facility, including the kind of surgery or injury, medications, the patient's physical and mental status, significant social factors (e.g., frail caregiver with health problems, or no caregiver), and the family's expected needs.

EVALUATING DISCHARGE PLANNING EFFECTIVENESS

Evaluating the discharge plan is crucial to ensure that the discharge planning works. Planning and referrals must be scrutinized to ensure the quality and appropriateness of services. Evaluation is ongoing, and care plans may need to be changed. A few weeks after the patient goes home, further evaluation of the discharge process is usually conducted by a telephone call, a questionnaire, or a home visit.

"Baby Steps to Discharge"

Nurses at Methodist Children's Hospital neonatal intensive care unit identified their unit's discharge as problematic for the nursing staff and patients' families. Research revealed that nurses were unsatisfied with the overall discharge process, the amount of time they had to teach parents, the number of times staff members stayed beyond their scheduled shifts to meet discharge needs, and whether discharge documentation was charted in the Baby Discharge Checklist section of the electronic health record. To address these problems, they developed a checklist to facilitate discharge better meeting the needs of their patients, families, and staff (Davidson, Roberts et al., 2020). See Figure 12-12 (on page 328), and be sure to check out the Baby Steps to Home website at babystepstohome.com.

Leaving the Hospital Against Medical Advice

A patient sometimes decides to leave the hospital or other care setting against medical advice (AMA). Although the patient is legally free to do so, this choice carries a risk for increased illness or complications. Torrey (2020) offers the following advice to patients who choose to leave AMA:

- **If you want to leave, you most likely can**. The only exception may be mental health patients for whom a discharge may place them or others at risk of harm.
- **AMA discharges do not void the terms of your insurance**. Doing so will not result in a refusal of payments or trigger an increase in premium. Be aware, however, that you will incur additional medical expenses if you have to be readmitted as a result of the premature discharge.
- **You will be asked to sign discharge papers**. This document is separate from any SRE complaint you may have filed. The discharge papers state that you have decided to leave against your doctor's advice. Have an advocate on hand to review the document and help you understand the terms.
- **You do not have to sign the papers**. You have the legal right to leave and there is no law requiring you to sign discharge documents. With that being said, you should prepare a letter explaining why you have decided to leave. Keep a copy of the letter for yourself and give a copy to the hospital administrator.

Telehealth

Telehealth.hhs.gov defines **telehealth**, sometimes called telemedicine, as:

> the use of electronic information and telecommunication technologies to provide care when you and the doctor aren't in the same place at the same time. If you have a phone or a device with internet access, you already have everything you need to get medical care or services through telehealth—you may be able to:
>
> - Talk to your doctor live over the phone or video chat.
> - Send and receive messages from your doctor using chat messaging, email, secure messaging, and secure file exchange.
> - Use remote patient monitoring so your doctor can check on you at home. For example, you might use a device to gather ECG or other vitals to help your doctor stay informed on your progress.

Types of care you can get using telehealth include general health care like wellness visits; prescriptions for medicine; dermatologic; eye exams; nutrition counseling; mental health counseling; and urgent care conditions such as sinusitis, back pain, urinary tract conditions, common rashes, etc. Some of the reasons why virtual visits are growing in popularity include:

- Limiting physical contact reduces everyone's exposure to COVID-19.
- Visiting virtually can address health issues wherever patients are, even from the comfort of home.
- Staying put cuts down on commuting, travel in bad weather, time off from work, and the need for child care.
- Using virtual health care tools can shorten wait times to see a provider and expand the range of access to specialists who live further away. (See https://telehealth.hhs.gov/patients/understanding-telehealth/#what-does-telehealth-mean.)

During the COVID-19 pandemic, many individuals chose to use telehealth visits rather than in-person doctor appointments for routine visits. Marsa (2020) reported that virtual doctor visits skyrocketed by 300% among Medicare-eligible seniors since the start of the pandemic and that nearly half of those surveyed were comfortable using telemedicine in the future. Some of the barriers that previously impeded the widespread adoption of home-based diagnostics and telemedicine in the past were removed by emergency rules during the pandemic. Physicians were allowed to practice across state lines; be reimbursed for in-home telemedicine

BABY STEPS TO DISCHARGE

Milestone	Done	Action	Criteria	Date/Initial	Entered into Baby Discharge Checklist (under Assessments) in EMR
24 Hrs of life (>2kg at Birth)	☐	Hep B	Signed consent form, info sheet given Infant >2 kg at birth Infants born <2 kg at birth get Hep B at 30 days of life		☐
24–48 Hrs of life	☐	Newborn Screen #1 (PKU) Form#:	All neonates 24–48 hours of life		☐
	☐	CCHD Screening (≥34 weeks, regardless of respiratory support)	For infants ≥34 weeks, perform CCHD screen at 24–48 hrs of life (regardless of respiratory support) Unless an ECHO is performed)		☐
1–2 wks of life	☐	Newborn Screen #2 (PKU) Form#:	All neonates 1–2 weeks of life		☐
>1800 grams	☐	Wean to open crib	Progressive weight gain Stable temps on air control made at 28°C for 24 hours		N/A
PO Feed "A/B" at 50% for 24 hrs	☐	Infant Guided Feeding	≥ 32 weeks ≤ 2 LMP HFNC respiratory support On full enteral gavage feedings		N/A
>32 weeks CGA and thereafter	☐	Hearing Screen (Regardless of NGT)	Weaned to an open crib 32 weeks post conception One room air unless plan to D/C on O2 Off phototherapy May be prior to last 2 doses of abx or diuretics OR within the last 24 hrs of abx		☐
≥34 weeks, off respiratory support	☐	CCHD Screening (≥34 weeks, off respiratory support)	For infants ≥34 weeks, repeat screening when off respiratory support. Unless an ECHO was performed		☐
Immunizations	☐	2 month	Signed consent obtained		☐
	☐	4 month			☐
	☐	6 month			☐
	☐	Synagis	TOC.Synagis.com OR SynagisTOC.com		☐
			34 Think, "Out the Door"		
Circumcision Requested **Y** or **N**	☐	Provider identified:	Signed consent form (in-house) Must void within 8 hrs post procedure Provide instruction regarding circ care		☐
Safe Sleep	☐	Safe Sleep Link Watched	≥34 weeks >1500 grams No respiratory distress No contraindications to sleeping supine https://nichd.nih.gov/sts/news/videos/Pages/default.aspx		☐
CPR	☐	CPR Kit Given	<34 weeks gestation at birth Infants d/c'd on apnea monitors AND/OR Cardiac/blood pressure meds/trachs OR MD Order		N/A
	☐	CPR Kit Watched			☐
Car Seat	☐	Car Seat Position Tolerance Test	<37 weeks gestation Specified high-risk criteria as defined by MD/NNP		☐
RX	☐	Medication Teaching	Medication teaching with return demo Rx copied by RN Filled Rx verified by 2 RNs		Record in Nursing Note Place in Maroon Chart
ROP	☐	ROP Follow-Up Screening	RN (with caregivers) schedules follow-up appointment		Record in NICU Discharge Instructions
Special Diets	☐	Dietary Teaching	All caregivers going home with EBM fortification or formulas		Record in NICU Discharge Instructions
WIC Recipients	☐	WIC form	Providers must sign WIC forms prior to D/C		☐
Follow-Up Appointments		Phone Number	Provider Name/Appointment		Record in NICU Discharge Instructions
Pediatrician	☐	( )			☐
Developmentalist	☐	( )			☐
	☐	( )			☐
	☐	( )			☐
	☐	( )			☐
	☐	( )			☐
Night before D/C	☐	Obtain Weight, Length & FOC	All infants must be discharged with recent Weight, Length and FOC measurements		Record in NICU Discharge Instructions
Footprint Sheet	☐	Verify Footprints page	If infant was born in-house, attach infant ID bracelet to Footprint Sheet, verify parental bracelet, and obtain mother's signature. If infant was a transfer, confirm parental identification with valid government ID.		Place a copy in Maroon chart, record driver's license number in Discharge instructions (if applicable).
Discharge Order Received	☐	Financial clearance obtained	All infants must be cleared by a financial counselor After hours admitting		

Notes: ______________________________

Abbreviations: A/B, feeding score A or B; Abx, antibiotics; CCHD, critical congenital heart disease; CGA, corrected gestational age; CPR, cardiopulmonary resuscitation; D/C, discharge; EBM, expressed breast milk; ECHO, echocardiogram; EMR, electronic medical record; FOC, frontal occipital circumference; Hep B, hepatitis B; HFNC, high-flow nasal cannula; LPM, L/min; MD, physician, N/A, not available; NGT, nasogastric tube; NICU, neonatal intensive care unit; NNP, neonatal nurse practitioner; O2, oxygen; PKU, phenylketonuria; PO, by mouth; RN, registered nurse, ROP, retinopathy of prematurity; RX, prescription; WIC, special supplemental nutrition program for women, infants, and children.

Reprinted with permission from Methodist Children's Hospital.

FIGURE 12-12. Baby Steps to Discharge.

and audio (phone) visits; and use FaceTime, Skype, or Zoom to communicate with their patients, which had long been considered taboo because of privacy issues. Check out the AARP website for a discussion of the pros and cons of telemedicine (Marsa, 2020) and Olsen (2020) for tips about how to use a smartphone, tablet, or computer for telehealth appointments. Be sure you are prepared to answer your patients' questions about telehealth knowledgeably.

HOME HEALTH CARE NURSING

This chapter would not be complete without addressing some of the particulars of home health care nursing, which is rapidly expanding for many reasons. The need for home health care services is increasing as the population ages. Because fewer people live in the same community as their parents, home health care providers may be needed to care for ill parents when children live far away. Because patients are discharged from hospitals earlier in their recovery, many need skilled professional care after they return home. In addition, people are more often choosing to die with comfort and dignity in their own homes. Also, third-party payers (such as insurance companies and managed care organizations) try to reduce the escalating costs of health care through the use of managed care programs that include home health care.

Nurses provide home health care within a system that includes home health facilities, patients, referral sources, health care providers or other primary caregivers, reimbursement sources, and legal considerations. The system functions best when its members communicate, cooperate, and collaborate with each other.

Types of Home Health Care Facilities

There are several different types of public and private home health care facilities. All home health care facilities must meet uniform standards for licensing, certification, and accreditation by state facilities or federal programs (such as Medicare). Home care facilities differ in how they are organized and administered. Box 12-5 describes different types of home health care facilities.

Home health care facilities are either certified or not certified by Medicare. A facility must be certified by Medicare to receive reimbursement from Medicare for services. Facilities may not be certified by Medicare for many reasons: for example, home care facilities that do not provide skilled nursing care (e.g., services provided by an RN) cannot receive Medicare reimbursement. Medicare is the largest single payer of home care services. It provides payment for services through a prospective payment plan based on an "episode of care" (usually considered a 60-day period). All patients receiving home health care services must have an order from their primary health care provider.

Home health care services include high-technology pharmacy services, skilled professional services, custodial care, medical equipment services, hospice and respite services (discussed in Chapter 11), and community support services. Box 12-6 lists examples of these services.

Depending on the facility and its geographic location, professional providers may include RNs, licensed practical/vocational

Box 12-5 Types of Home Health Care Facilities

Official or public facilities: These facilities are operated by state or local governments and primarily financed by tax funds. Most offer home care and disease-prevention programs in the community.

Voluntary or private not-for-profit facilities: These facilities are supported by donations, endowments, charities (such as the United Way), and insurance reimbursements. They are governed by a board of directors, usually representing the community they serve.

Private, proprietary facilities: Most private, proprietary facilities are for-profit organizations governed by individual owners or national corporations. Their services are paid for through health care insurance or individual self-pay.

Institution-based facilities: These facilities operate under a parent organization, such as a hospital. The home care facility is governed by the institution, and most referrals for care come from within the institution.

Box 12-6 Examples of Home Health Care Services

High Technology Services

- Intravenous therapy
- Home uterine monitoring
- Ventilator management
- Chemotherapy

Skilled Professional and Paraprofessional Services

- Nursing care (provided by a licensed practical nurse, a registered nurse, a clinical nurse specialist, or a nurse practitioner)
- Home health care aides
- Personal care
- Physical therapy
- Occupational therapy
- Speech therapy
- Medical social work
- Respiratory therapy

Custodial Services

- Homemaking and housekeeping
- Hourly or shift coverage
- Live-in services
- Companionship

Home Medical Services

- Providing durable medical equipment such as beds, braces, canes, crutches, wheelchairs, commodes, and oxygen

Hospice Services

- Pain management
- Physician and nurse practitioner services
- Spiritual support
- Respite care
- Bereavement counseling

Community Support Services

- Meals on Wheels
- Transportation
- Friendly visitors
- Delivery services
- Emergency answering services

nurses, nurse practitioners and clinical nurse specialists, home care aides, enterostomal therapists, mental health specialists, speech therapists, respiratory therapists, physical therapists, occupational therapists, social workers, dietitians, and a chaplain or spiritual care provider. Regardless of how many providers are involved, the responsibility for care coordination (also called case management) remains with the RN.

Patients and Family Caregivers

The patient in home health care is both the person receiving care and the person's family, who often are also the caregivers. When a patient enters the hospital, the family most often plays a minor role in actual care. Families and friends visit with the patient and sometimes stay overnight, but they are generally not involved in direct patient care. Hospital staff provide personal care for the patient and administer medications and treatments. After the patient is discharged, the responsibility for care is shifted to family caregivers, who may or may not be physically or mentally able to handle this responsibility.

Today's emphasis on home health care means that family caregivers have increased responsibilities. Patients are discharged "quicker and sicker." Chronically ill patients may need long-term care at home that may not be covered by Medicare, and changes in Medicare funding may mean that fewer home visits are covered. The financial burden of care is more than many families can afford, and home health care nurses must be alert for signs of such financial problems (e.g., no food in the refrigerator or kitchen cupboards). A referral for services such as Meals on Wheels may be necessary to provide adequate nutrition for the patient.

In addition to the financial burden, family members face the challenges of handling equipment, providing new types of care to loved ones, and dealing with unfamiliar and often terrifying sounds, odors, and substances. Most caregivers are women, and many of them are over age 65. Older women may themselves have health problems or may not have the physical strength or energy to care for their family members. The Family Caregiver Alliance: National Center on Caregiving "supports and sustains the important work of families nationwide caring for adult loved ones with chronic disabling health conditions." Make time to visit their website to become familiar with their resources so you can refer them to family caregivers (https://www.caregiver.org/). The Alliance offers a national telephone hotline, online resources, and printed publications which serve as a central source of information and assistance to family caregivers in every state. Even family members who are themselves nurses may find that providing care at home is very different from providing care in the hospital. The accompanying Through the Eyes of the Family Caregiver display describes one such experience. Carpenter and Gould (2020) offer a sample of what nurses can share with caregivers of family or others:

- Engage in self-compassion
- Practice gratitude
- Do something for yourself daily
- Ask for help
- Find a support group
- Seek professional help for yourself if needed
- Check out available resources
- Be realistic about expectations (p. 53)

The home health care nurse must identify the needs of the family and caregiver. The nurse assesses whether the patient and family understand and agree with the care plan and determines if the caregivers understand the instructions provided and are capable of providing care. The nurse can help the patient and family identify and use community resources to meet their needs. If a caregiver feels overwhelmed, the nurse can provide resources to relieve the stress. The nurse also supports family decisions about complex treatments or end-of-life care. The following questions may be used for discussion:

- What is most important to you?
- What do you want for your life and your family's?
- How do you want to spend the rest of your life?
- How is this technology supporting or not supporting what you want?

Referrals for Home Care

A referral source is a person who recommends home care services and supplies the home health care facility with details about the patient's needs. The referral source may be a nurse, health care provider, social worker, therapist, or discharge planner. The referral may be to a home health facility, a hospice, or a community resource. Families sometimes generate their own referrals by contacting a home care facility. If the facility believes the patient qualifies for services, the facility contacts the patient's provider and requests a referral for the patient.

Orders for Home Care

Home health care cannot begin without an order from a primary provider, nor can it proceed without the primary caregiver's approved treatment plan. This is a legal and reimbursement requirement. A nursing assessment visit to identify a patient's needs can be scheduled only after a referral is made and an initial set of primary caregiver's orders are received. At the nursing assessment visit, the nurse begins to formulate the care plan and sends it to the primary caregiver for review and approval. Box 12-7 identifies the data needed to create an effective home care plan. The primary

Box 12-7 Data Required for an Effective Home Care Plan

- Mental status
- Types of services and equipment required
- Prognosis and rehabilitation potential
- Functional limitations
- Activities permitted
- Nutritional requirements
- Medications and treatments
- Safety measures to protect against injury
- Instructions for timely discharge

Through the Eyes of the Family Caregiver

"I'm so glad to have you home, but what do I do now?" (and this is just the first day….)

I am a nurse and have been a nurse for 30 years. I have a diploma in nursing, a baccalaureate in nursing, a master's in counseling, and a doctorate in nursing. I have taught others how to be nurses for more than 25 years. Nothing in all my educational and practice experiences prepared me to care for the complex needs of my husband, Jacque, when he had surgery 2 years ago. Following diagnosis of metastatic thyroid cancer, a large lower thoracic spinal cord tumor (which put pressure on the spinal nerves, causing leg weakness and bladder malfunction) and the thyroid gland were removed surgically, and steel rods were implanted almost the entire length of the spine. After 30 days in the hospital for diagnosis, surgery, and recovery, Jacque came home—unable to do more than move from the bed to a chair, and with a catheter in his bladder that was attached to a drainage bag.

Before he came home, I got a hospital bed with electric controls, a bedside commode, and a bedside table. I cleared out the family room furniture, got a friend to put the television up on a table (so it could be seen from the hospital bed), and thought I was all ready to give my husband expert care. The first challenge came when he got up in a chair to eat his dinner—we had no chairs with a high enough seat or a straight enough back to allow use of the bedside table. I ran up and down stairs to look at chairs, and finally decided the antique armchair in the living room would work, and it did. Now another problem—where to hang the catheter drainage bag? And how best to move so it didn't pull when he moved? And remember to empty the bag before he gets up!

I fixed a wonderful homecoming meal for this man I love, and he could only eat a few bites. Now back to bed and a new problem. He got out of the bed and into the chair just fine, but now he can't get out of the chair and into the bed because his legs are still so weak. What did I do wrong—it worked in the hospital. It took me 2 days to realize that I forgot to lower the bed height so Jacque wouldn't have to push up so hard to get his bottom on the bed.

Then, after finally literally hauling him back in bed, I realized that I did not know how to move him up in bed. The physical therapist had taught him how to get up in a chair, but not how to move himself up in bed (they always did it for him in the hospital). This is a 250-lb man we are talking about. I could turn him from side to side, but I couldn't physically move him up in bed and he couldn't stay where he was. After a lot of trials, we figured out that he could wiggle one side of his body at a time and slowly inch up in bed. Now, he was exhausted and in pain, and I felt totally incompetent. Thank goodness, the home health care nurse is coming to visit tomorrow.

If I felt this way, how must family members feel who know nothing about caring for someone who is sick or in pain? I have such respect for all those family members who provide such wonderful care and for the nurses who provide home care that calms the fears and answers the questions.

—Priscilla LeMone

caregiver's signature on the care plan authorizes the home care facility to provide services. The plan is reviewed as necessary, but at least once every 60 days.

Safety Considerations

As a nurse making the first home visit, you should evaluate safety issues beforehand and once in the home; this includes the safety of the patient and of family and professional caregivers (Marrelli & Rennell, 2020). Once you arrive in the patient's home, you will want to do a home safety assessment since hazards in the home are a major contributor to falls, poisonings, violence, fire, and other accidents. A fall resulting in a fractured hip, for example, is often the beginning of serious debilitation in a person with dementia who until then was otherwise healthy. Chapter 28 offers a detailed home safety checklist, which you can adapt to any home setting.

QSEN SAFETY

It is essential for nurses making home visits to cultivate the knowledge, skills, and attitudes that will enable them to minimize the risk of harm to patients and providers through both system effectiveness and individual performance.

Try to assess the safety of the neighborhood where the patient lives before your first visit. You may need to arrange the visit at a time when it is safe to be in the area, and you should always know the exact destination before arriving for the visit. In some unsafe areas, police or security officers may accompany nurses. Make sure your car is in good working order, and call ahead to let the patient know when to expect you. You should only carry a small amount of money, and you should not bring medications with you. Never leave electronics, a purse or wallet, cell phone, laptop, or other valuables out in the open. Other guidelines for safety include carrying a cell phone programmed with emergency numbers, making sure that someone from the facility knows your itinerary, and being continuously alert to the environment (Elliot, 2014). In rare situations where your best efforts to address unsafe environments are unsuccessful (patient who is receiving oxygen therapy persists in smoking, a family member is verbally abusive and threatening), be sure to seek guidance from you supervisor and know your facility protocols for refusing to put yourself in a hazardous situation. It is wise to review the *NIOSH hazard review: Occupational hazards in home healthcare* before starting home visits (https://www.cdc.gov/niosh/docs/2010-125/pdfs/2010-125.pdf?id=10.26616/NIOSHPUB2010125).

Infection Prevention

Trying to keep homebound patients, their family caregivers, and the community infection free is a central responsibility for home health nurses. Cleanliness in the home and handwashing are key to infection prevention. If you remember how challenging it was for you to master the principles of asepsis and infection control described in Chapter 25, you will be able to empathize with family caregivers who need to learn complicated procedures and how to handle wastes. Hand hygiene, personal protective equipment, and environmental cleaning are critical to breaking the chain of transmission in the home. Handwashing with soap and water or an alcohol-based handrub is the most important measure for preventing transmission. Teach family caregivers how to effectively wash their hands:

Before:

- Direct contact with a patient
- Performing invasive procedures
- Handling dressings or touching open wounds
- Preparing and administering medications
- Feeding a patient

After:

- Contact with blood, body fluids, broken skin or mucous membranes
- Contact with items known or considered to be contaminated
- Removal of gloves
- Use of toilet or wiping nose

Between:

- Performing procedures on the same patient in which soiling of the hands is likely (Embil et al., 2009).

The CDC offers numerous resources to stop the spread of germs at home, work, and school.

Reimbursement Sources

A reimbursement source pays for home health care services. Although Medicare is the largest single source of reimbursement, services are also reimbursed by Medicaid, private insurance, patients or their families, and other public funding. The reimbursement source evaluates each care plan, and only interventions identified on the plan are approved for reimbursement.

Medicare pays the cost of the first 100 home visits following a hospital stay (Centers for Medicare & Medicaid Services, 2016). Medicare does not reimburse visits to support general health, health promotion, or socioeconomic needs. To be approved for Medicare reimbursement, the patient must meet the criteria listed in Box 12-8.

In addition, Medicare provides reimbursement only if the nurse teaches about a new or acute situation, assesses an acute change in the patient's condition, or performs a skilled procedure requiring the professional skill, knowledge, ability, and judgment of a licensed nurse. It is imperative to thoroughly document all nursing interventions with each home visit for reimbursement to occur.

Legal Considerations

Legal considerations in home care involve a variety of factors, including issues of privacy and confidentiality, the patient's access to health information, the patient's freedom from reasonable restraint, informed consent, and matters of negligence and malpractice. The same codes and standards that guide all other nurses also guide nurses providing care in the home. The ANA's *Home Health Nursing: Scope and Standards of Practice* (2014) is the basis for practice in the home. The standards address the nursing process, interdisciplinary collaboration, quality assurance, professional development, and research. Another source of guidance is the section on Patient Rights and Responsibilities in the

Box 12-8 Eligibility Requirements for Medicare Reimbursement for Home Health Care Services

All people with Medicare Part A and/or Part B who meet all of these conditions are covered:

- You must be under the care of a doctor, and you must be getting services under a care plan established and reviewed regularly by a doctor.
- You must need, and a doctor must certify that you need, one or more of these:
  - Intermittent skilled nursing care (other than just drawing blood)
  - Physical therapy, speech-language pathology, or continued occupational therapy services. These services are covered only when the services are specific, safe, and an effective treatment for your condition. The amount, frequency, and time period of the services need to be reasonable, and they need to be complex or only qualified therapists can do them safely and effectively. To be eligible, either: (1) your condition must be expected to improve in a reasonable and generally predictable period of time, or (2) you need a skilled therapist to safely and effectively make a maintenance program for your condition, or (3) you need a skilled therapist to safely and effectively do maintenance therapy for your condition
- The home health facility caring for you must be Medicare certified.
- You must be homebound, and a doctor must certify that you're homebound.

You're not eligible for the home health benefit if you need more than part-time or "intermittent" skilled nursing care.

You may leave home for medical treatment or short, infrequent absences for nonmedical reasons, like attending religious services. You can still get home health care if you attend adult day care.

Source: Medicare.gov. (n.d.). *Your medicare coverage: Home health services.* https://www.medicare.gov/coverage/home-health-services.html

Box 12-9 Examples of Home Health Care Patient Rights

Home health care patients have the right to:

- Be fully informed of all patient rights and responsibilities
- Appropriate and professional care relating to provider orders
- Choice of care providers
- Receive information necessary to give informed consent prior to the start of any procedure or treatment
- Refuse treatment within the confines of the law and to be informed of the consequences of their action
- Privacy
- Receive a timely response from the facility to their requests for service
- Reasonable continuity of care
- Be informed within reasonable time of anticipated termination of service or plans for transfer to another facility
- Voice grievances and suggest changes in service or staff without fear of restraint or discrimination

Source: These are part of a longer list of patient rights and responsibilities published by the National Association for Home Care & Hospice. *Code of ethics. Patient rights and responsibilities.* http://www.nahc.org/about/code-of-ethics

National Association for Home Care & Hospice (NAHC) Code of Ethics. Home care facilities are required by federal law to address the concepts in the Bill of Rights with all home care patients in the initial visit. Box 12-9 provides a few examples from the Bill of Rights. Nurses can best avoid lawsuits by knowing standards of practice, providing care that is consistent with facility policies, and documenting all carefully and accurately.

HOME VISITS

Home health care patients often feel frightened, in pain, and abandoned, and family members often feel nervous about their new roles as caregivers. The home health care nurse must keep these concerns and needs in mind when planning and carrying out care.

Pre-entry Phase of the Home Visit

In the referral process, the provider or discharge planner of a hospital contacts the home care facility and provides a brief medical history, along with indications for home health services. During this pre-entry phase, the referral nurse at the home care facility collects as much information as possible about the patient's diagnoses, surgical experience, socioeconomic status, and treatments ordered. This is called the pre-entry phase. Once assigned the case, the nurse reviews the information and calls the patient to schedule a visit. During this phone conversation, the nurse can determine whether the patient's caregiver can answer questions related to the patient's and family's needs and also learn about the patient's cognitive abilities, orientation, and caregiver status. This information is important to the nurse planning the first visit.

Concept Mastery Alert

In home health care services, a great deal is usually known about the patient prior to the first visit. The nurse begins the initial patient assessment by collecting patient data in the pre-entry phase.

Entry Phase of the Home Visit

The second phase of the visit is the entry phase. In the entry phase, the nurse develops rapport with the patient and family, makes assessments, determines health problems, establishes desired outcomes (along with the patient and family), plans and implements prescribed care, and provides teaching. The nurse must remember that they are a guest in the patient's home and are offering services that the patient may accept or reject. Important considerations include negotiating and honoring visit times, establishing a rapport with the patient and family, defining what nursing care will be provided, and teaching to promote independence in self-care.

The nurse must gain the trust of the patient and family, and must recognize and respect their values. Accepting the patient's living conditions is necessary, even when they differ from those of the nurse. The nurse must ask permission before using the patient's home for activities such as handwashing. The nurse might believe that the furniture in the patient's home or sick room needs to be rearranged to allow the use of equipment and to remove safety hazards, but the patient should give permission before any changes are made.

Nurses who provide home health care interventions do so based on an individualized care plan for each patient, based initially on identifying individualized health care needs. In identifying the patient's needs and determining the interventions, the nurse fulfills the roles discussed earlier in the chapter.

Identifying Needs and Determining Interventions

The ability to assess patients accurately is an important skill for home health care nurses. Most of the initial assessment takes place during the first home visit, although ongoing focused assessment occurs during subsequent visits. The nurse must be skilled not only in physical assessment but also in psychological, socioeconomic, environmental, spiritual, and cultural assessment. Skilled assessment allows the nurse to make appropriate diagnoses. In addition, the nurse must determine and provide culturally respectful care (see Chapter 5); although important for inpatients, this is even more important in the patient's home. Family caregivers must also be considered, taking into account the various roles that each family member plays and how they contribute to the patient's health status. Specific interventions are based on the patient's needs, but controlling infection and teaching the patient and caregiver are part of all home visits.

Teaching the Patient and Caregivers

Because home health care is meant to be short term and intermittent, the nurse includes the family and friends in the teaching process so that they can learn how to care for the patient after the nurse's home care is no longer needed. The nurse designs and implements the teaching plan based on the patient's and caregiver's readiness to learn. It must be adapted to the patient's and caregiver's physical and emotional status, and it must be understandable and "doable."

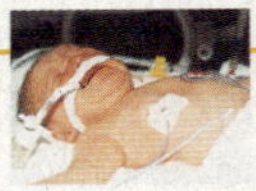

Consider **Joey Marshall**, the infant discharged home after 7 months. Because of the complex technology associated with his care, and because his mother feels anxious and afraid, the nurse needs to provide the necessary teaching about his care, but in small sessions to avoid overwhelming the mother.

Teaching should identify both the positive outcomes of following instruction and the serious consequences of failing to do so. The nurse points out the major problem areas specific to care in the home, focusing on the information needed to keep the patient safe until the nurse's next home visit.

Documenting Care Given in the Home

Documenting care given in the home is mandated by regulatory and federal facilities (see Chapter 20). The nurse may document the visit on preprinted forms or checklists or may use a computer.

The documented care plan, the visit plan, and progress notes are routinely used by regulatory facilities and payer sources (e.g., private insurance or Medicare) to determine whether various state and federal regulations are being met and if payment is warranted. Figure 12-13 illustrates goals for a patient newly admitted to home hospice with related nursing measures and actions. The care plan establishes specific measurable goals and specifies a time frame for reaching the goals. The care plan accurately reflects the condition of the patient, the patient's functional limitations and safety needs, the need for skilled care, specific provider orders, anticipated progress, criteria for discharge, supplies needed, a visit schedule for all health care providers, and a list of support systems available.

The nurse writes (or types) progress notes to document each visit to the patient's home. These notes must accurately describe the patient's condition, the skilled care provided, the patient's response, the patient's progress toward discharge, and an ongoing plan for continued care. They also include the nurse's plan for the next visit. To meet reimbursement requirements, each progress note must indicate that the care provided requires the knowledge and skills of a professional nurse.

DEVELOPING CLINICAL REASONING AND CLINICAL JUDGMENT

1. Interview a nurse employed in a hospital and a nurse employed by a home health care facility. How are their roles and responsibilities alike? How do they differ? Ask both what they believe about the fragmentation of care in their setting. How well are nurses working with their colleagues to coordinate care?
2. Compare and contrast the needs of the following patients and their families:
   - A 2-year-old admitted to an ambulatory surgery center for minor surgery
   - A 34-year-old woman discharged home after treatment for a fractured arm in the ED
   - A 50-year-old woman returning to a clinic to learn the results of her mammogram
   - A 78-year-old man being transferred from the hospital to a long-term care facility

   What care priorities are these patients and families likely to have? How can you best establish a partnership with these patients and families? How likely are today's health care providers to meet the holistic needs (physical, psychological, social, and spiritual) of these patients?
3. Discuss with your fellow students what you would do in the following home health care situations:
   - An 85-year-old patient cannot move by himself and refuses to eat. His 83-year-old wife tries to care for him, but she is under a great deal of stress and begins to cry when you enter their apartment.
   - A 43-year-old woman is receiving home care after surgery to repair a herniated vertebral disc ("slipped disc"). When you arrive for the scheduled visit, you find that her speech is slurred, and she does not remember how much pain medication she has taken.
   - A 2-year-old has a malignant brain tumor. He is not expected to live more than 1 week and is receiving hospice care.

   What knowledge, attitudes, and skills are required to successfully address these patients' needs?
4. A 55-year-old man with end-stage lung cancer is discharged home with a referral to a visiting nurse facility. He is receiving oxygen therapy. When the first visiting nurse enters his home, she finds the patient smoking, oblivious to the dangers with the oxygen in the room. When the nurse explains her safety concerns, he states that he may as well just die now if he isn't able to smoke because smoking is the only pleasure he has left.
5. How can continuity and care coordination be achieved for Jeff Hart, Laura Degas, and Joey Marshall? What community resources should competent community-based nurses be able to recommend? Are there any barriers to these families accessing these resources?

Visit Actions	Goal Description:
☐ Mileage/Drive Time* ☐ Demographics ☐ Vital Signs* ☐ Physical Assessment* ☐ View/Edit POC ☐ Interventions/Goals* ☐ New Order ☐ Order Supplies ☐ Supplies Delivered ☐ Aide Care Plan	Patient/Caregiver verbalizes understanding of anorexia/dehydration in terminal patient and caregiver demonstrates offering, but not forcing food/fluids to patient. Pain will be managed at a level acceptable to the patient. A nursing care plan will be established. Patient/Caregiver will verbalize/demonstrate appropriate pain management. Patient exhibits signs of symptom reduction or relief. Medications will be managed appropriately as evidenced by steady symptom control. Patient/Caregiver will verbalize/demonstrate compliance with medication regimen. Patient/Caregiver will verbalize knowledge of signs and symptoms/ preventative measures/ response in the event of bleeding/hemorrhage. **Send to Physician** YES **Read to Physician** YES **Send to Facility** NO

Nurse to assess medication response and instruct on schedule actions, purpose, side effects, compliance, and need to report side effects to staff.

Nurse to assess for bleeding/hemorrhage and take measures to control/manage.

Instruct on preventative measures/response.

1) Admit to hospice
2) HOV may accept orders from primary care physician/practitioner partners and/or on call group when needed
3) May add/adjust visit order frequency for the interdisciplinary team
4) Patient, primary caregiver, and/or facility staff may administer medications
5) Patient may transfer level of care and/or location as necessary and determined by team. Notify the attending practitioner of changes. If admitted to inpatient unit (IPU), may initiate IPU orders
6) May obtain chest x-ray or PPD (tuberculosis [TB] skin test) as indicated for TB screening
7) Follow wound care guidelines for red unbroken skin (stage 1) and/or minor wound care
8) Ventricular access device maintenance: follow Arizona home care policies for catheter type
9) May initiate O_2 at 2–4 L via NC continuously or PRN as indicated
10) Durable medical equipment (DME) as indicated for patient condition
11) May insert urinary catheter up to 18 Fr for relief of urinary retention or incontinence. May use lidocaine gel (2%) topical for discomfort during insertion. May replace for malfunction PRN
12) Urinary catheter care: irrigate with 30–50 cc sterile 0.9% NaCl PRN
13) May use facility bowel care regimen if applicable and if not, then use standard HOV home care bowel orders

FIGURE 12-13. Goals for a patient newly admitted to home hospice with related nursing measures and actions (*mandatory actions). (*Source:* Used with permission. Hospice of the Valley, Phoenix, AZ.)

PRACTICING FOR NCLEX

1. A discharge nurse manager is preparing the plan for a patient returning home after receiving a kidney transplant. What actions will the nurse perform to ensure continuity of care? Select all that apply.
   a. Conduct an admission health assessment
   b. Evaluate the effectiveness of the current nursing care plan
   c. Participate in transferring the patient to the postoperative care unit
   d. Make referrals to appropriate facilities
   e. Maintain records of patient satisfaction with services received
   f. Assess the strengths and limitations of the patient and family
2. A discharge nurse is evaluating patients and their families to determine the need referrals to other facilities after hospitalization. Which patients will the nurse recommend for these services? Select all that apply.
   a. Older adult diagnosed with dementia in the hospital
   b. Adult diagnosed with Parkinson disease
   c. Adult woman receiving chemotherapy for breast cancer
   d. Adolescent being discharged with a cast on his leg
   e. New mother who delivered a healthy infant via a cesarean birth
   f. Adult man diagnosed with end-stage cancer
3. A home health nurse is scheduled to visit a patient recently discharged from the hospital with a new colostomy. During the entry phase of the home visit, what actions will the nurse perform? Select all that apply.
   a. Collect information about the patient's diagnosis, surgery, and treatments
   b. Call the patient to make initial contact and schedule a visit
   c. Develop rapport with the patient and their family
   d. Assess the patient to identify their needs
   e. Assess the physical environment of the home
   f. Evaluate safety issues including the neighborhood in which the patient lives
4. A nurse and AP are planning to receive a patient who sustained a traumatic head injury in a motor vehicle accident. Which activity can the nurse safely delegate to the AP?
   a. Collecting information for a health history
   b. Performing a physical assessment
   c. Contacting the health care provider for medical orders
   d. Preparing the bed and collecting needed supplies
5. A home care nurse is observing the patient's family member perform a wound irrigation and dressing change for a postoperative wound dehiscence containing purulent drainage. In which situation will the nurse provide additional education?
   a. The family member places the old dressing in a separate bag at the bedside.
   b. The patient takes an analgesic a half-hour prior to the dressing change.
   c. The family member states they washed their hands an hour ago.
   d. The patient returns to bed during the dressing change.
6. A patient is being transferred from the intensive care unit (ICU) to a medical-surgical unit. What is the responsibility of the ICU nurse during the transfer of care?
   a. Providing a verbal report to the nurse on the new unit
   b. Giving a detailed written report to the unit secretary
   c. Delegating the responsibility for providing information
   d. Making a copy of the patient's medical record
7. A nurse is reviewing the discharge plan with a patient who had major abdominal surgery. Which statement by the nurse is most appropriate?
   a. "I'll bet you will be so glad to be home and sleep in your own bed."
   b. "Tell me about your understanding of your recovery needs after discharge."
   c. "Be sure to take your pain medications and change your dressing."
   d. "You will just be fine! Please stop worrying."
8. A nurse is caring for a patient who has been hospitalized for dehydration secondary to a urinary tract infection. The patient states, "I'm leaving. There are too many germs here, and I'll probably get sicker than when I came in." As this patient has capacity for decision making, which response is most consistent with the nurse's legal accountability?
   a. "Only the primary health care provider can authorize your discharge from a hospital."
   b. "Let me gather your belongings and prepare the discharge paperwork."
   c. "I will inform the health care provider that you want to leave and request a psychiatric consult."
   d. "Your choice carries risks for complications, so I must ask you to sign a release form."
9. A nurse is considering moving from the hospital setting to home health care. In speaking with other professionals, what qualities does the nurse find they should possess to be successful? Select all that apply.
   a. Making accurate assessments
   b. Researching new treatments for chronic diseases
   c. Communicating effectively
   d. Delegating tasks appropriately
   e. Performing clinical skills effectively
   f. Making independent decisions

10. A nurse asks the AP to prepare the hospital room for a new ambulatory patient. Which aspect of the room will the nurse ask the AP to correct?
    a. The bed linens are folded back.
    b. A hospital gown is on the bed.
    c. Equipment for taking vital signs is in the room.
    d. The bed is in the highest position.
11. A nurse on a medical-surgical unit is teaching a patient's family about hospice care. How does the nurse best explain the focus of this care?
    a. Hospice care focuses on symptom and pain relief.
    b. Nutrition is provided orally or by tube to maintain intake.
    c. Surgical procedures are performed when medically necessary.
    d. Services are provided until the patient's death.
12. A visiting nurse is performing the initial assessment and plan for a patient who receives Medicare and was recently discharged from the acute care hospital. Before implementing the plan of care, what follow-up is required by the nurse?
    a. Validating the patient's consent for care
    b. Obtaining the health care provider's signature and approval
    c. Determining how the patient will pay for services
    d. Ensuring that a family member or friend can assist with implementation
13. When transferring a patient from the operating room to the medical-surgical unit, a nurse uses the SBAR format for handoff communication. Place the components of the SBAR communication (Situation, Background, Assessment, and Recommendations) in their proper order.
    a. This 20-year-old patient presented to the ER with right lower quadrant pain, fever, and an elevated WBC count.
    b. The patient is postlaparoscopic appendectomy.
    c. The patient may need pain medication in 30 minutes.
    d. The patient is sleepy, but responsive; five small bandages on the abdomen are clean and dry.

ANSWERS WITH RATIONALES

1. **b, d, f.** The primary roles of the discharge planner as patients move from acute to home care are evaluating the nursing plan for effectiveness of care, making referrals for patients, and assessing the strengths of patients and their families. The staff typically performs an admission health assessment and assists with patient transfers from the OR. In most facilities, maintaining records of patient satisfaction is the role of the public relations manager or office manager.
2. **a, b, f.** The patients who are most likely to need a formal discharge plan or referral to another facility are those who are emotionally or mentally unstable (e.g., those with dementia), those who have recently diagnosed chronic disease (e.g., Parkinson disease), and those who have a terminal illness (e.g., end-stage cancer). Other candidates include patients who do not understand the treatment plan, are socially isolated, have had major surgery or illness, need a complex home care regimen, or lack financial services or referral sources.
3. **c, d, e.** In the entry phase of the home visit, the nurse develops rapport with the patient and family, makes assessments, determines nursing diagnoses, establishes desired outcomes, plans and implements prescribed care, and provides teaching. In the pre-entry phase of the home visit, the nurse collects information about the patient's diagnoses, surgical experience, socioeconomic status, and treatment orders. In the pre-entry phase, the nurse also gathers supplies needed, makes an initial phone contact with the patient to arrange for a visit, and assesses the patient's neighborhood for safety issues.
4. **d.** The nurse may delegate preparation of the bed and collection of needed supplies to assistive personnel but performs the other activities listed.
5. **c.** The nurse teaches the patient and family to effectively wash their hands before and after having direct contact with the patient, before performing invasive procedures, when handling dressing or touching open wounds, and when administering medications or feeding the patient. All other options are correct.
6. **a.** The transferring (ICU) nurse gives a verbal report on the patient's condition and nursing care needs to the receiving nurse. This information should not be given to a unit secretary, nor can this be delegated to others. The medical record is transferred with the patient; a copy is not made for transfers within the agency.
7. **b.** The purpose of discharge planning is to ensure for continuity of care for the patient and family needs. The nurse uses open-ended assessment questions to begin a planning session. Essential components of discharge planning include assessing the strengths and limitations of the patient, the family or support person, and the environment; implementing and coordinating the care plan; considering individual, family, and community resources; and evaluating the effectiveness of care. Answers a and c are examples of communication or interventions, which may be included after an assessment. The statement "You will just be fine! Please stop worrying." is a cliché and is avoided.
8. **d.** The patient is legally free to leave the hospital against medical advice (AMA); however, patients who leave AMA must sign a form releasing the health care provider and hospital from legal responsibility for their health status. This signed form becomes part of the medical record.
9. **a, c, e, f.** Nurses working in the community must have the knowledge and skills to make accurate assessments, work independently, communicate effectively, and perform clinical skills accurately. Community-based nurses may be researchers and occasionally delegate care, but these are not key qualities for this type of nursing.
10. **d.** A properly prepared hospital room includes a bed in the lowest position for an ambulatory patient, an open bed with top linens folded back, routine and special equipment and supplies assembled, and the physical environment of the room adjusted.

11. **a.** Hospice services include pain management, physician and nurse practitioner services, spiritual support, respite services, and bereavement counseling.

12. **b.** The nurse assesses the patient eligible for home services and presents the plan to the health care provider for approval. This approval allows for provision of care and reimbursement of services.

13. **b, a, c, d.** The SBAR communication for this patient should be: The patient is post laparoscopic appendectomy. This 20-year-old patient presented to the ER with right lower quadrant pain, fever, and an elevated WBC count. The patient may need pain medication in 30 minutes. The patient is sleepy, but responsive; there are five small bandages on the abdomen that are clean and dry.

Bibliography

Academy of Oncology Nurse & Patient Navigators. *Frequently asked questions*. https://www.aonnonline.org/faq/

Agency for Healthcare Research and Quality (AHRQ). (2012). *Improving transitions of care: Hand-off communications*. Joint Commission Center for Transforming Healthcare. http://psnet.ahrq.gov/resource.aspx?resourceID=24737

Agency for Healthcare Research and Quality (AHRQ). (2013). Re-engineered discharge (RED) toolkit. https://www.ahrq.gov/professionals/systems/hospital/red/toolkit/index.html

Agency for Healthcare Research and Quality (AHRQ). (2014a). *Care coordination measures atlas update*. https://www.ahrq.gov/ncepcr/care/coordination/atlas.html

Agency for Healthcare Research and Quality (AHRQ). (2014b). Module 2: Communicating change in a resident's condition. Appendix: Example of the SBAR and CUS tools. http://www.ahrq.gov/professionals/systems/long-term-care/resources/facilities/ptsafety/ltcmod2ap.html

Agency for Healthcare Research and Quality (AHRQ). (2017). *About TeamSTEPPS®*. https://www.ahrq.gov/teamstepps/about-teamstepps/index.html

Allard, B. L. (2018). Transitional care—The pathway to integrated care delivery. *American Nurse Today, 13*(1), 54, 56–60.

American Association of Colleges of Nursing. (2021). *The Essentials: Core competencies for professional nursing education*. https://www.aacnnursing.org/AACN-Essentials

American Hospital Association (AHA). (2003). *The patient care partnership*. https://www.aha.org/system/files/2018-01/aha-patient-care-partnership.pdf

American Journal of Nursing. (2017). *Supporting family caregivers: No longer home alone*. http://journals.lww.com/ajnonline/pages/collectiondetails.aspx?TopicalCollectionId=38

American Nurses Association (ANA). *Public health nursing*. https://www.nursingworld.org/practice-policy/workforce/public-health-nursing/

American Nurses Association (ANA). (2013). *Care coordination quality measures panel*. https://www.nursingworld.org/get-involved/share-your-expertise/pro-issues-panel/care-coordination-quality-measures-panel/

American Nurses Association (ANA). (2014). *Home health nursing: Scope and standards of practice* (2nd ed.). ANA.

Arora, V. M., Greenstein, E. A., Woodruff, J. N., Staisiunas, P. G., & Farnan, J. M. (2013). Implementing peer evaluation of handoffs: Associations with experience and workload. *Journal of Hospital Medicine, 8*(3), 132–136.

Bracken, N. (2016). Reducing readmissions in COPD patients. *American Nurse Today, 11*(7), 24–29.

Buhler-Wilkerson, K. (2007). No place like home: A history of nursing and home care in the U.S. *Home Healthcare Nurse, 25*(4), 253–259.

Burton, R. (2012). *Health policy brief: Improving care transitions*. Health Affairs. http://www.healthaffairs.org/healthpolicybriefs/brief.php?brief_id=76

Carpenter, H., & Gould, L. (2020). Care for family caregivers. *American Nurse Journal, 15*(9), 53.

Centers for Disease Control and Prevention (CDC). (n.d.). *Stop the spread of germs*. https://www.cdc.gov/coronavirus/2019-ncov/downloads/stop-the-spread-of-germs.pdf

Centers for Disease Control and Prevention (CDC). Infection control. https://www.cdc.gov/infectioncontrol/index.html

Centers for Disease Control and Prevention (CDC). (2010). *NIOSH hazard review. Occupational hazards in home healthcare*. https://www.cdc.gov/niosh/docs/2010-125/pdfs/2010-125.pdf?id=10.26616/NIOSHPUB2010125

Centers for Medicare & Medicaid Services. (2016). *Home health PPS*. https://www.cms.gov/Medicare/Medicare-Fee-for-Service-Payment/HomeHealthPPS/index?redirect=/HomeHealthPPS

Craig, C., Eby, D., & Whittington, J. (2011). *Care coordination model: Better care at lower cost for people with multiple health and social needs*. Institute for Healthcare Improvement. http://brainxchange.ca/Public/Files/Primary-Care/HQPC/Coordinated-Care-Model-IHIC.aspx

Curle, B. W., & Maduro, R. (2020). Discharge unit efficiency. *American Nurse Journal, 15*(9), 85–88.

Davidson, N., Roberts, B., Potts, C., Rieger, A., Herrera, A., & Altman, M. (2020). "Baby steps to discharge": An interprofessional, developmental milestone-based checklist for the neonatal intensive care unit. *Critical Care Nurse, 40*(5), 75–78. https://doi.org/10.4037/ccn2020911

DeMarco, R. F., & Healey-Walsh, J. (2020). *Community and public health nursing* (3rd ed.). Wolters Kluwer.

Dvorak, P. (2013). 600 homeless children in DC, and no one seems to care. *The Washington Post*. https://www.washingtonpost.com/local/600-homeless-children-in-dc-and-no-one-seems-to-care/2013/02/08/a728a0ea-722b-11e2-8b8d-e0b59a1b8e2a_story.html?utm_term=.5e0edaa53b7d

Elliot, B. (2014). Considering home healthcare nursing? *Nursing, 44*(12), 57–59.

Embil, J. M., Dyck, B., & Plourde, P. (2009). Prevention and control of infections in the home. *Canadian Medical Association Journal, 180*(11), E82–E86.

Friedrich, C., Sick, B., & North, S. (2021). Building experiential interprofessional education. *American Nurse Journal, 16*(11), 45–49.

Hanna-Attisha, M. (2020, May 17), Babies don't choose where they are born. *The New York Times*, p. 10.

Institute for Healthcare Improvement. (2017). *SBAR toolkit*. http://www.ihi.org/resources/Pages/Tools/sbartoolkit.aspx

Interprofessional Education Collaborative (IPEC). (2016). *Core competencies for Interprofessional collaborative practice: 2016 Update*. https://ipec.memberclicks.net/assets/2016-Update.pdf

Irani, E., Hirschman, K. B., Cacchione, P. Z., & Bowles, K. H. (2020). The role of social, economic, and physical environmental factors in care planning for home health care recipients. *Research in Gerontological Nursing, 13*(3), 130–137. https://doi.org/10.3928/19404921-20191210-01

Johnson, M., Cowin, L. S. (2013). Nurses discuss bedside handover and using written handover sheets. *Journal of Nursing Management, 21*(1), 121–129.

The Joint Commission. (2012). *Joint commission center for transforming healthcare releases tool to tackle miscommunication among caregivers*. http://www.jointcommission.org/center_transforming_healthcare_tst_hoc

The Joint Commission. (2017). *Sentinel Event Alert*. https://www.jointcommission.org/-/media/tjc/documents/resources/patient-safety-topics/sentinel-event/sea_58_hand_off_comms_9_6_17_final_(1).pdf?db=web&hash=5642D63C1A5017BD2147015 14DA00139&hash=5642D63C1A5017BD21470151 4DA00139

The Joint Commission. (2018). *2018 National patient safety goals®*. https://www.jointcommission.org/standards_information/npsgs.aspx

Landro, L. (2011). When a doctor isn't enough: Nurse navigators help patients through maze of cancer-treatment decisions, fears. *The Wall Street Journal*. http://online.wsj.com/article/SB100014240531119042532045765104728282408848.html

Marrelli, T. (2015). How to succeed as a home care nurse. *American Nurse Today, 10*(1), 43–44.

Marrelli, T. M., & Rennell, N. (2020). Home care safety. *American Nurse Journal, 15*(5), 8–12.

Marsa, L. (2020, August 31). The future of telehealth and what it means for older adults. https://www.aarp.org/health/conditions-treatments/info-2020/telehealth-goes-mainstream.html

McDonald, K. M., Schultz, E., Albin, L., Pineda, N., Lonhart, J., Sundaram, V., Smith-Spangler, C., Brustrom, J., & Malcolm, E. (2010). *Care coordination Atlas Version 3 (prepared by Stanford University under subcontract to Battelle on Contract No. 290-04-0020) AHRQ publication No. 11-0023-EF*. Agency for Healthcare Research and Quality.

Medicare.gov. (n.d.). *Your medicare coverage. Home health services*. https://www.medicare.gov/coverage/home-health-services.html

Middleton, B., Bloomrosen, M., Dente, M. A., Hashmat, B., Koppel, R., Overhage, J. M., Payne, T. H., Rosenbloom, S. T., Weaver, C., Zhang, J., & American Medical Informatics Association. (2013). Enhancing patient safety and quality of care by improving the usability of electronic health record systems: Recommendations from AMIA. *Journal of the American Medical Informatics Association, 20*(e1), e2–e8.

Miles, R. (2016). Boost your career with community outreach involvement. *American Nurse Today, 11*(7), 34–36.

National Association for Home Care & Hospice. *Code of ethics: Patient rights and responsibilities*. http://www.nahc.org/about/code-of-ethics

National Transitions of Care Coalition. (n.d.). *Care transition bundle: Seven essential intervention categories*. https://www.ntocc.org/

Olsen, D. P., & Keilman, L. J. (2020). The moral distress of nurses when patients forgo treatment because of cost. *American Journal of Nursing, 120*(9), 61–66.

Olsen, D. P. (2020, August 31). How to connect with your doctor virtually. AARP. https://www.aarp.org/health/conditions-treatments/info-2020/connecting-virtual-doctor-visits.html

Painter, D. (2021). Preventing home dialysis complications. *American Journal of Nursing, 121*(1), 57–63.

Peikes, D., Chen, A., Schore, J., & Brown, R. (2009). Effects of care coordination on hospitalization, quality of care, and health care expenditures among Medicare beneficiaries: 15 randomized trials. *Journal of the American Medical Association, 301*(6), 603–618.

Petersen, K. (2020). Meeting healthcare needs in rural America. *Nursing, 50*(8), 16–18.

Polster, D. (2015). Patient discharge information: Tools for success. *Nursing, 45*(5), 42–49; quiz 49–50.

Rachwal, C. M., Langer, T., Trainor, B. P., Bell, M. A., Browning, D. M., & Meyer, E. C. (2018). Navigating communication challenges in clinical practice: A new approach to team education. *Critical Care Nurse, 38*(6), 15–22.

Rantz, M. J., Skubic, M., Alexander, G., Popescu, M., Aud, M. A., Wakefield, B. J., Koopman, R. J., & Miller, S. J. (2010). Developing a comprehensive electronic health record to enhance nursing care coordination, use of technology, and research. *Journal of Gerontological Nursing, 36*(1), 13–17.

Rhodes, J. R., Stowe, T., & Williams, L. (2020). Discharge lounges for optimal outcomes: A quality improvement project. *Nursing, 50*(12), 65–68

Runy, L. A. (2013). Patient handoffs: The pitfalls and solutions *of transferring patients safely from one caregiver to another.* http://216.92.22.76/discus/messages/21/Patient_Handoffs_-_2008_Article-2338.pdf

Salas, E., DiazGranados, D., Weaver, S. J., & King, H. (2008). Does team training work? Principles for health care. *Academic Emergency Medicine, 15*(11), 1002–1009.

Sigmon, L. B. (2020). Interprofessional collaboration made easy. *American Nurse Journal, 15*(11), 36–38.

Steppie, S., & Kirchner, J. (2020). Office-based nursing in practice. *Nursing, 50*(6), 41–44.

Sullivan, M., Kiovsky, R. D., Mason, D. J., Hill, C. D., & Dukes, C. (2015). Interprofessional collaboration and education. *The American Journal of Nursing, 115*(3), 47–54.

Suzuki, L. K., & Edmonds, J. K. (2020). The community guide: A living resource for nursing practice. *American Journal of Nursing, 120*(3), 55–57.

Telehealth.HHS.Gov. (2021, January 13). *What is telehealth.* https://telehealth.hhs.gov/patients/understanding-telehealth/

Torrey, T. (2020). *Leaving the hospital against medical advice. Verywell health.* https://www.verywellhealth.com/choosing-to-leave-the-hospital-against-medical-advice-2614871

U.S. Department of Defense. (2005). Department of defense patient safety program: Healthcare communications toolkit to improve transitions in care.

U.S. Department of Health & Human Services. (2017). *Your rights under HIPAA.* https://www.hhs.gov/hipaa/for-individuals/guidance-materials-for-consumers/index.html

Urban Institute: Health Policy Center. (n.d.). https://www.urban.org/search?search_api_views_fulltext=vulnerable%20populations

World Health Organization (WHO). (2010). *Framework for action on interprofessional education & collaborative practice.* World Health Organization. http://whqlibdoc.who.int/hq/2010/WHO_HRH_HPN_10.3_eng.pdf

UNIT III

Processes of Thoughtful, Person-Centered Practice

Unit III begins with an exploration of each element of thoughtful, person-centered practice. Chapter 13 invites you to reflect on your readiness for professional practice. Is your motivation love of humanity and the sincere desire to help people who need nursing care? Do you have the personal attributes, knowledge base, and competencies to begin safe practice? Are you committed to learn how to reason clinically, to make clinical judgments and decisions about treatment and care? This chapter introduces the three major clinical judgment models: Nursing Process (ADPIE), Tanner/Lasatar, and the National Council of State Boards of Nursing (NCSBN) Clinical Judgment Action Model. It also describes the blended and QSEN competencies nurses need to use the process for promoting patient well-being. Chapter 14, a brand-new chapter in this edition, demonstrates how the NCSBN Clinical Judgment Action Model informs and enhances professional practice. Chapters 15 to 19 explore each step of the nursing process (Assessing, Diagnosing/Problem Identification, Outcome Identification and Planning, Implementing, and Evaluating). Chapter 20 introduces you to the critical skill of documenting your nursing work and reporting to other members of the team. The unit concludes with Chapter 21, which focuses on informatics and technology.

The phases of clinical judgment models are not separate items but rather parts of a whole, used to identify patient problems and needs, establish priorities of care, maximize strengths, and resolve actual or potential alterations in human responses to health and illness, thereby promoting health to the highest level possible for each patient. The phases are iterative, which means they are interrelated and repetitive.

Assessment, the systematic and continuous collection and communication of data, allows analysis of data to identify patient problems and strengths. During outcome identification and planning, the nurse and patient mutually identify expected outcomes and agree on nursing interventions necessary to meet these outcomes. The nurse implements the plan of care, adapting it to each person, documenting nursing actions and patient responses. After implementation, the nurse and patient evaluate the effectiveness of the plan based on achievement of outcomes and determine if the plan should be continued, modified, or terminated.

The nursing process is nursing practice in action. Unit III provides the information necessary to begin to apply the nursing process. As blended competencies are learned and practiced, the process becomes an integral component of each nurse–patient interaction. The outcome is thoughtful, person-centered practice.

QSEN Reflective Practice Cultivating QSEN Competencies *(continued)*

CHALLENGE TO ETHICAL AND LEGAL SKILLS

and I believe that the patient felt my primary commitment was to her. Unfortunately, this only highlighted the fact that no one else's primary commitment had been to her. I certainly promoted, advocated for, and strove to protect this patient's health, safety, and rights. However, it seemed that the nurses went out of their way not to do that for this patient.

Tracey Sara Miller, Georgetown University

QSEN SELF-REFLECTION ON QUALITY AND SAFETY COMPETENCIES DEVELOPING KNOWLEDGE, SKILLS, AND ATTITUDES FOR CONTINUOUS IMPROVEMENT

How do you think you would respond in a similar situation? Why? What does this tell you about yourself and about the adequacy of your skills for professional practice? What *knowledge, attitudes,* and *skills* do you need to develop to continuously improve the quality and safety of care for patients like Ms. Warner?

Person-Centered Care: Why do you believe that the nursing staff was so critical of this patient? What was it about the student's attitudes and responses to Ms. Warner that created such a successful partnership?

Teamwork and Collaboration: Do you think that the nursing student should have approached the nursing staff about what she found? How might a student or professional nurse effectively change negative staff behavior that is disrespectful of a patient's inherent dignity?

Safety/Evidence-Based Practice: What safety challenges resulted from the nursing staff's indifference and condescension, and how did the student correct these? What might the nursing research suggest as best practice in similar situations?

Informatics: Can you identify the essential information that must be available in Ms. Warner's electronic record to support safe patient care and coordination of care? Can you think of other ways to respond to or approach the situation?

clinical reasoning and judgments that they evaluate and review through reflective practice, so that they continually learn from practice for the benefit of future patients (Hill et al., 2017, p. 240).

Before reading further, take a minute to read the Reflective Practice display, review the concepts in Box 13-1, and consider the essential elements of thoughtful, person-centered care shown in Figure 13-1 on page 346.

Box 13-1 Thoughtful, Person-Centered Practice

Person

Each person is unique and has their own set of beliefs, values, memories, hopes, and history. People are holistic beings with emotional, physical, social, and spiritual dimensions and needs that all meld together to create the whole individual person. The fact that a person has a disease is only one aspect of the whole in the same way as having red hair is only one aspect of the whole person. Therefore, each person's health journey and personal care are individual. Clinical care is an interaction between the carer and the cared for. Each of the people within this relationship is unique, so the respect and valuing of the person applies to both. Relationships based on this principle can become therapeutic.

Professional Nurse

Professional nursing requires cultivated personal attributes, mastery of the science of nursing, and reflective clinical experience in which nurses develop the blended competencies and QSEN competencies that promote thoughtful and effective person-centered practice.

Reflective Practice Leading to Personal Learning

Reflective practice occurs when the carer has a profound awareness of self; awareness of one's own biases, prejudgments, prejudices, and assumptions; and understands how these may affect the therapeutic relationship. This awareness is developed through the process of reflection, thinking back on what has occurred for the purpose of learning in order to improve.

Clinical Reasoning, Judgment, and Decision Making

Clinical reasoning is the process for analyzing a situation, making a judgment, deciding on possible alternative reasons, and choosing an action to be taken. It is built on a foundation of knowledge, experience, and the personal attributes of the person doing the reasoning. Critical thinking is fundamental in the process of clinical reasoning. Care can become ritualistic and depersonalized when nurses fail in clinical reasoning and judgment.

Person-Centered Nursing Process

The nursing process describes the way in which care is organized through a series of actions undertaken in response to the individual needs of the patient. The components of the nursing process are assessing, diagnosing/problem identification, planning, implementing, and evaluating.

Nurse's Action in Response to Individual Clinical Need

The healing action that occurs in response to individual need completes the cycle of thoughtful practice when it is considered, personalized, appropriate, valued, and effective.

Source: Adapted from Hill, R., Hall, H., & P. Glew. (2017). *Fundamentals of nursing and midwifery: A person-centered approach to care* (3rd ed.). Wolters Kluwer/Lippincott Williams & Wilkins.

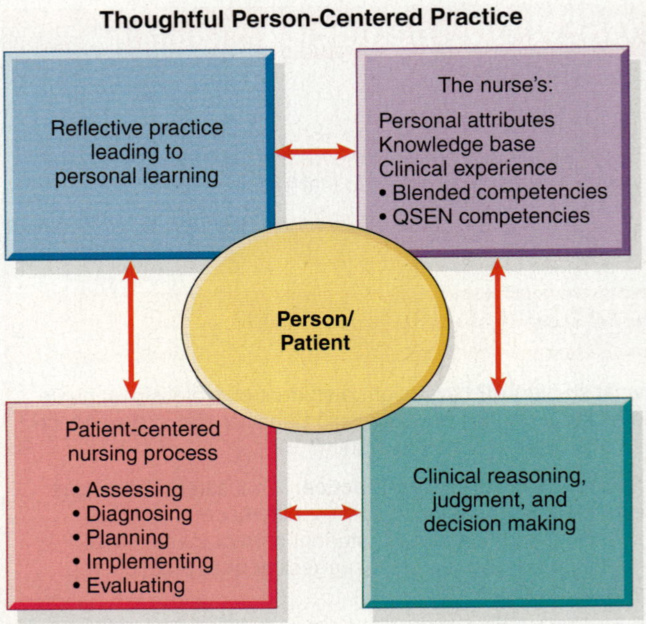

FIGURE 13-1. The components of thoughtful practice are all interrelated and function together to create thoughtful, person-centered care. (*Source:* Adapted from Hill, R., Hall, H., & Glew P. [2017]. *Fundamentals of nursing and midwifery: A person-centered approach to care* [3rd ed.]. Wolters Kluwer/Lippincott Williams & Wilkins. p. 240.)

THOUGHTFUL, PERSON-CENTERED PRACTICE

If you are new to health care, you probably can't imagine what health care would be like if it wasn't person centered. Sadly, U.S. health care in the 20th century focused more often on disease and on generating revenues than on patients. Despite major efforts to refocus the delivery of health care based on the needs of the patient, we are in danger of failing again. Physician Abraham Verghese (2011) coined the term *iPatient:*

> I've gotten into some trouble in Silicon Valley for saying that the patient in the bed has almost become an icon for the real patient who is in the computer. I've actually coined a term for that entity in the computer. I call it the *iPatient*. The iPatient is getting wonderful care all across America. The real patient often wonders, where is everyone? When are they going to come by and explain things to me? Who's in charge? There's a real disjunction between the patient's perception and our own perceptions . . . of the best medical care.

Nurses have always been on the frontlines of keeping care delivery focused on the needs of real patients in real time. But today's demanding work environments are forcing some nurses to focus more on accomplishing a set of tasks than on helping patients. From the very beginning of your professional practice, remember that nursing is about creating therapeutic relationships with actual patients, about making health care work for all who need it, especially the most vulnerable. Being a good nurse isn't just a matter of being "busy" doing "tasks"—it is about being and making the critical difference for patients and families with health care needs. Reflect for a moment on how you will respond when another nurse informs you that your patient is requesting medication for pain. How will your response differ if you have a *person* versus a *task* orientation? Hint: The nurse with a task orientation merely wants to safely administer and document the prescribed medication. The nurse with a person orientation uses every clinical encounter to assess how the person is doing and to communicate respect, compassion, and care.

The idea of **person-centered care** emerged about 30 years ago as a return to the holistic roots of health care. Promoters of this model of care included the Picker Institute, the Planetree membership network, and the 2001 Institute of Medicine's seminal report *Crossing the Quality Chasm.* (The Institute of Medicine has since been renamed the National Academy of Sciences, Engineering, and Medicine.) With the introduction of the Hospital Consumer Assessment of Healthcare Providers and Systems (HCAHPS) patient experience of care survey, there now exists a standardized tool to evaluate the way care is provided from the patient's perspective. Although there are different definitions of person-centered care, the 10 vital person-centered care principles listed in Box 13-2 offer a comprehensive illustration.

Theories of Caring

Nurses who practice thoughtful, person-centered care are committed to developing caring professional relationships based on respect and mutual trust. This holistic approach, which is consistent with theories based on human caring, seeks to promote humanism, health, and quality of living. Caring is viewed as universal and is practiced through interpersonal relationships. When the relationship between the caregiver and the person who is being cared for is focused on promoting or restoring the health and well-being of the person being cared for in the relationship or facilitating their dying with respect and comfort, it becomes a **therapeutic relationship** (Hill et al., 2017). Dossey and Dossey (1998) write:

> Our majestic predecessors in nursing, such as Florence Nightingale, spoke boldly about the need to honor the psychological and spiritual aspects of our patients. For her and many others, it was unthinkable to consider sick humans as mere bodies who could be treated in isolation from their minds and spirits. In Nightingale's holistic approach, the role of love and empathy was considered paramount. . . . But with the rise of scientific, materialistic medicine in the nineteenth and twentieth centuries, these lessons in love . . . were set aside and virtually lost. . . . In study after study, social contact, the richness of one's interactions with others, is correlated with positive health outcomes. . . . We're being asked to integrate a holistic approach and extend love, compassion, and empathy" (pp. 35–38).

Box 13-2 Reflective Practice: Thoughtful, Person-Centered Practice

1. All team members are considered caregivers.	• Identify the team members you worked with while implementing the plan of care. Everyone in the workforce from housekeeping staff to the CEO is part of the patient's care team. • Next to each describe what they contributed to person-centered care for your patient. • Star or highlight those with whom you had meaningful conversations and briefly describe what you learned.
2. Care is based on continuous healing relationships.	• Describe what you did to make your interactions with the patient/family qualify as a healing relationship versus a mere business transaction or provision of a service. • This principle reinforces a focus on the continuum of care. In what ways did your care anticipate and prepare your patient and family for the days ahead?
3. Care is customized and reflects patient needs, values, and choices.	• Describe what you learned about this patient/family as unique individuals (strengths, needs, values, and preferences) that allowed you to creatively individualize the care plan. • What strategies did you use to elicit the patient's needs, values, and choices? • In what specific ways is your care plan different from any standardized care plan?
4. Knowledge and information are freely shared between and among patients, care partners, health care providers, and caregivers.	• Describe one way you shared information with the patient/family and one way you shared information with the health care team that enhanced the partnership and the care plan. • What did you learn from other members of the team that enhanced your ability to care for this patient/family?
5. Care is provided in a healing environment of comfort, peace, and support.	• When we think of healing environment we usually think of music, healing gardens, soothing colors. Assess your patient's healing environment and describe what you did to facilitate the creation of such an environment. How can you adapt these principles in critical care settings, emergency rooms, clinics, etc.? • In what ways are you able to address variables that negatively influence healing: Poverty, noise, time pressures, etc. • What percentage of the care plan and *your* care plan addresses patient needs other than physiologic needs? • To what degree are the psycho-social-spiritual needs of the patients identified and addressed? To what degree do they appear in your care plan? • Describe the measures you used to promote the patient's/family's comfort and peace and to provide support.
6. Families and friends of the patient are considered an essential part of the care team.	• Has the patient identified family members or others they wish to be part of the care team? If the patient is not able to articulate preferences, is there a legally valid surrogate making decisions? In what ways have you communicated with these people and provided the information and support they need to help the patient?
7. Patient safety is a visible priority.	• What is the institutional commitment to safety measures such as hand hygiene and other protocols to prevent hospital-acquired infections, medication and other errors, falls, etc.? • In what ways is this particular patient at risk for safety concerns, falls, infection, violence, etc. and what have you done to address these risks?
8. Transparency is the rule in the care of the patient.	• True person-centered care requires transparency between providers and patients and among providers. Patients or their designees need information so they can make informed decisions. Does your patient have the information they need to make informed decisions? If not, in what ways are you addressing this?
9. All caregivers cooperate with one another through a common focus on the best interests and personal goals of the patient.	• In what ways are clinical decisions or institutional policies motivated by goals other than the best interests and personal goals of the patient and how is this constraining the care plan? What have you done to address these variables? • What institutional resources exist to help you address these variables?
10. The patient is the source of control for their care.	• Assess the degree to which your patient or their designee is the source of control for the care plan. • What factors are constraining this and what are you doing to address these factors?

Source: Principles from Rodak, S. (2012). *10 Guiding Principles for Patient-Centered Care.* https://www.beckershospitalreview.com/quality/10-guiding-principles-for-patient-centered-care.html. Reprinted with permission from Becker's Hospital Review.

Numerous nurse theorists have struggled to describe the caring central to the work of nursing. Travelbee (1971), an early nurse theorist, developed the Human-to-Human Relationship Model, which defined nursing as an interpersonal process whereby the professional nurse practitioner assists an individual, family, or community to prevent or cope with the experience of illness and suffering and, if necessary, to find meaning in these experiences. Benner and Wrubel (1989) wrote that caring is a basic way of being in the world, and that caring is central to human expertise, curing, and healing. "Nursing is viewed as a caring practice whose science is guided by the moral art and ethics of care and responsibility. . . . Nurses provide care for people in the midst of health, pain, loss, fear, disfigurement, death, grieving, challenge, growth, birth, and transition on an intimate front-line basis. Expert nurses call this the *privileged place of nursing*" (p. xi). Watson's (2008) theory of transpersonal caring begins with the conviction that humans are to be valued, cared for, respected, nurtured, understood, and assisted. She believes that caring can be demonstrated and practiced, and that nurses should create caring environments in which patients are accepted as they are and are invited to grow and realize their full potential. She reminds nurses that this model is transformative in that the nurse–patient relationship influences both the nurse and the patient for better or for worse. Finally, Swanson (1991) identified five caring processes and defined caring as "a nurturing way of relating to a valued other toward whom one feels a personal sense of commitment and responsibility" (p. 165).

There is no universally accepted definition of caring. You should become familiar with the care models described in Table 13-1 and see if you agree with the convictions held by nurse members of the International Association of Human Caring (IAHC). Members of the IAHC believe:

- **Caring** is the human mode of being.
- Caring is the essence of nursing and the moral imperative that guides nursing praxis (education, practice, and research).
- Caring is both spiritual and human consciousness that connects and transforms everything in the universe.
- Caring in nursing is action and competencies that aim toward the good and welfare of others.
- Caring in nursing is a special way of being, knowing, and doing with the goal of protection, enhancement, and preservation of human dignity.
- Care is culturally diverse and universal and provides the broadest and most important means to study and explain nursing knowledge and nursing care practices (www.humancaring.org).

Before reading further, reflect on how these convictions will influence your future practice. If you agree that caring is essential to being human and is the way nurses promote healing, what are your personal strengths and growth opportunities for caring? How can you plan to focus your attention on human caring as you struggle to master tasks such as safely transferring patients, assisting with bathing, or administering medications? How likely are the recipients of your care to describe you as a competent, compassionate, caring nurse? In what ways might nurses relate to patients who may evoke negative feelings? How will you prevent this in your practice? You can read more about care ethics in Chapter 6 and about how to become a healing presence in Chapter 47.

Table 13-1 Comparison of Benner's *The Helping Role of the Nurse* with Swanson's *Caring Process* and Watson's *Carative Factors*

BENNER: THE HELPING ROLE OF THE NURSES	SWANSON'S CARING PROCESS	WATSON'S CARATIVE FACTORS
• Creating a climate for establishing a commitment to healing • Providing comfort measures and preserving personhood in the face of pain and extreme breakdown • Presencing • Maximizing the patient's participation and control in the patient's recovery • Interpreting kinds of pain and selecting appropriate strategies for pain management and control • Providing comfort and communication through touch • Providing emotional and informational support to patients and families • Guiding patients through emotional and developmental changes	• Knowing: avoiding assumptions, centering on the one cared for, assessing thoroughly, seeking cues, engaging the self of both • Being with: being there, conveying ability, sharing feelings, not burdening • Doing for: comforting, anticipating, performing competently/skillfully, protecting, preserving dignity • Enabling: informing/explaining, supporting/allowing, focusing, generating alternatives/thinking it through, validating/giving feedback • Maintaining belief: believing in/holding in esteem, maintaining a hope-filled attitude, offering realistic optimism, "going the distance"	• Humanistic altruistic system of values • Instillation of faith/hope • Sensitivity to self and others • Helping/trusting human care relationship • Expressing positive and negative feelings • Creating problem-solving caring process • Transpersonal teaching/learning • Supportive, protective, and/or corrective mental, physical, societal, and spiritual environment • Human needs assistance • Existential–phenomenologic–spiritual forces

Source: Adapted from Benner, P., & Wrubel, J. (1989). *The primacy of caring in health and illness* (p. 50). Addison-Wesley; Swanson, K. M. (1991). Empirical development of a middle range theory of caring. *Nursing Research*, *40*(3), 161–166; and Watson, J. (2008). *Nursing: The Philosophy and Science of Caring* (rev. ed.). University Press of Colorado.

PROFESSIONAL NURSE

Nurses committed to thoughtful, person-centered practice are careful to assess whether they possess the prerequisite personal attributes along with learned knowledge, blended competencies, and QSEN competencies.

Personal Attributes

Not everyone "has what it takes" to be a professional nurse. As you read the following list of attributes, reflect on how well they characterize you at this stage of your human and professional development.

Open-mindedness. This may also be termed *humility.* Are you open to learn what your patients, families, and colleagues have to teach you?

A profound sense of the value of the person. Do you believe that everyone, literally everyone, matters? Can you think of anyone who deserves less than your best care effort? Are you willing to go to bat for the most vulnerable in our midst? Are you committed to learning how to advocate for those not well served by today's health care system?

Self-awareness and knowledge of your own beliefs and values. Do you know what you believe, why you believe it, and the consequences of your beliefs? Are you sensitive to how your beliefs and values influence your professional relationships?

A sense of personal responsibility for your actions. At the end of the day, will people (your patients and team) be better because of their experiences with you? Are you committed to using your personal expertise, time, and power to coordinate all the care patients and families need?

Motivation to do what you do to the best of your ability because you care about the well-being of those entrusted to your care. Does love get you up and motivate your study and practice? Do you want to be your personal best for those who will count on you? In what ways does your practice (and life) reflect a love of humanity?

Leadership skills. Have you tried to use your influence to help others attain valued goals? Are you committed to using your leadership strengths with patients, families, and colleagues to achieve valued health goals? Learn more about developing your leadership skills in Chapter 10.

Bravery to question the "system." When the plan of care isn't working for a patient or your work environment is interfering with your ability to give good care, are you willing to challenge the status quo, and can you do this effectively? Denise Thornby, previous president of the American Association of Critical Care Nurses, was famous for challenging nurses to "make waves" when change was needed—even when this demanded personal courage. She reminded all of us that the day we don't wake up we will have already created our legacy:

> Every day, every moment, you make choices on how to act or respond. Through these acts, you have the power to positively influence. As John Quincy Adams sagely said, 'The influence of each human being on others in this life is a kind of immortality.' So, I ask you: What will be your act of courage? How will you influence your environment? What will be your legacy? When the day arrives that you are no longer able to show up for practice, what do you want colleagues to say about you? What will be *your* legacy?

Knowledge Base

In order to reason through a clinical situation, you must be able to draw upon a body of nursing knowledge that comes from the sources of knowledge described in Chapter 2. Added to this must be research evidence. Box 13-4 outlines the knowledge required for competent clinical reasoning and judgment in nursing. The specific knowledge required in a given care interaction depends on the actual clinical situation. For example, if the situation calls for reasoning about the manifestation of a clinical problem, the nurse will need to understand the disease or condition, its epidemiology, the mechanisms of its pathophysiology, its physical and psychological manifestations, signs and symptoms, and the probabilities of its progression or outcome.

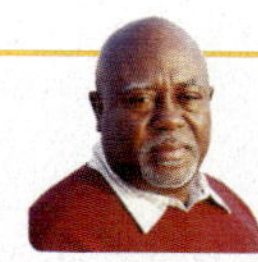

Think back to the nurse who could not locate **Jermaine's** tibial pulse. The nurse needs to know the complications of vascular surgery on the femoral artery and the significance of not being able to palpate the tibial pulse.

If the clinical situation involves a problematic hospital discharge of a patient with disabilities, for example, the nurse's knowledge base must include knowledge of support services available in the local community or knowledge of how and when to contact other team members with this expertise. These knowledge requirements are essential for the development of clinical reasoning and judgment, discussed later in this chapter.

Blended Competencies

Nurses aim to design and manage each patient's care scientifically, holistically, and creatively. To do this successfully, nurses need many cognitive, technical, interpersonal, and ethical/legal competencies, along with the willingness to use them creatively and critically when working with patients to promote or restore health, to prevent disease or illness, and to facilitate coping with altered functioning. Understanding the importance of these competencies helps you work consciously to develop them while beginning to master the nursing process. Cognitive and technical competencies equip nurses to manage clinical problems stemming from the patient's changing health or illness state. Interpersonal and ethical skills are essential, moreover, for nurses concerned about the patient's broader well-being.

This text uses the term **blended competencies** because, in most instances, nursing actions require all four competencies. A nurse who sets out to suction a patient, for example, must understand the evidence that supports this action, be

Box 13-3 Take the Challenge

Read the following professional behaviors, and circle the number that best reflects the proficiency you now have in each of these essential nursing competencies.

1 = no skills
2 = somewhat skilled
3 = moderately skilled
4 = well skilled
5 = excellent skills

Cognitive Competencies

1	2	3	4	5	• Offer a scientific rationale for the plan of care.
1	2	3	4	5	• Select those nursing interventions that are most likely to yield desired outcomes.
1	2	3	4	5	• Use clinical reasoning and judgment to problem solve creatively.

Technical Competencies

1	2	3	4	5	• Use technical equipment with sufficient competence and ease to achieve goal with a minimum of distress to involved participants.
1	2	3	4	5	• Creatively adapt equipment and technical procedures to the needs of particular patients in diverse circumstances.

Interpersonal Competencies

1	2	3	4	5	• Creative use of looks, speech, and touch to communicate respect and to enhance sense of worth
1	2	3	4	5	• Skilled use of compassionate presence and conversation to demonstrate empathy and to obtain sufficient knowledge about the patient to personalize care and serve as an effective advocate
1	2	3	4	5	• Responsible, competent attentiveness to the holistic needs of patients such that trust is built and patients experience comfort of security
1	2	3	4	5	• Value mutual enrichment of both participants in the nurse–patient relationship

Ethical/Legal Competencies

1	2	3	4	5	• Self-motivated to act in ways that advance the interests of patients (consistently trustworthy)
1	2	3	4	5	• Accountable for practice to self, patients served, the caregiving team, and society
1	2	3	4	5	• Consistently serve as effective patient advocate
1	2	3	4	5	• Skilled in mediating ethical conflict among the patient, significant others, health care team, and other interested parties
1	2	3	4	5	• Practice nursing faithful to the tenets of professional codes of ethics
1	2	3	4	5	• Use legal safeguards that reduce the risk of litigation

skilled in handling the required equipment, use the encounter to promote the patient's sense of well-being, and practice in an ethically and legally defensible manner. Few nurses excel naturally in all four of these competencies, and even experienced nurses continue working on becoming more proficient in the knowledge, attitudes, and skills that lead to excellence. These competencies were first introduced and defined in Chapter 1. Box 13-3 will help you to assess your proficiency in these competencies.

Developing Cognitive Competencies

Cognitively skilled nurses are critical thinkers. **Critical thinking** is defined as "a systematic way to form and shape one's thinking. It functions purposefully and exactingly. It is thought that is disciplined, comprehensive, based on intellectual standards, and, as a result, well-reasoned" (Paul, 1993, p. 20).

DEVELOPING THE METHOD OF CRITICAL THINKING

To develop the critical thinking skills essential to quality nursing practice, nurses find it helpful when posed with a challenge to work methodically through a set of five types of considerations: the purpose of thinking, adequacy of knowledge, potential problems, helpful resources, and critique of judgment/decision.

Purpose of Thinking

The first step when thinking critically about a situation is to identify the purpose or goal of your thinking. This helps to discipline your thinking by directing your thoughts toward the goal. The purpose of critical thinking might be to make a judgment about a particular patient or situation or to make a decision about how best to intervene.

Adequacy of Knowledge

At the outset of critical thinking, you need to judge whether the knowledge you have is accurate, complete, factual, timely, and relevant. If you reason with false information or a lack of important data, it is impossible to draw a sound conclusion. You also want to be sure that you understand all the details relevant to the issue. What is at stake? How much time do you have to make a decision? How much room is there for error?

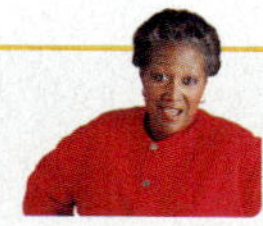

Consider **Addie Warner**, the patient described as "demanding" by some staff. Rather than accept that description, the nurse answers the patient's call light, thereby obtaining information from which to make an informed decision.

Potential Problems

As you become skilled in critical thinking, you will learn to "flag" and remedy pitfalls to sound reasoning. Common problems include working with untested or faulty assumptions, accepting an unproven claim or line of argument, allowing bias to color your thinking, and reasoning illogically, such as making a generalization on the basis of a single experience or case or allowing emotion to rule reason. The more familiar you are with these common blocks to critical thinking, the easier it is to detect them in your own thinking.

Helpful Resources

Wise professionals are quick to recognize their limits and seek help to remedy their deficiencies. Experienced clinicians know that learning is continuous and expect their practice to involve challenges that demand new knowledge. Critical thinkers know what help they need to assist their reasoning and what resources to tap. Key resources include experienced clinicians, texts and journals, institutional policies and procedures, and professional groups and writings.

Critique of Judgment/Decision

Ultimately, you must identify alternative judgments or decisions, weigh the merits of each, and reach a conclusion. It helps to try to predict the consequences of your major options before concluding your reasoning. You will also want to evaluate the alternative you selected as your decision begins to influence your actions.

After using this method to work through an intellectually challenging situation, critique your use of the method in light of the **standards for critical thinking**: clear, precise, specific, accurate, relevant, plausible, consistent, logical, deep, broad, complete, significant, adequate (for the purpose), and fair.

Focused Critical Thinking Guides

Focused Critical Thinking Guide 13-1 (on page 352) illustrates the use of these five considerations to facilitate critical thinking about a care dilemma experienced by a nursing student. The merits of thinking critically about which of the options is most likely to meet that patient's needs are easily seen. Because nurses are accountable for the well-being of their patients, sloppy reasoning is both dangerous and inexcusable—even for someone new to nursing and clinical practice. Other Focused Critical Thinking Guides are found throughout the book.

DEVELOPING THE PERSONAL ATTRIBUTES TO THINK CRITICALLY

Reasoning has a logical or cognitive (thinking) component as well as an emotional or affective (feeling) component, both of which are affected by the personal attributes of the thinker. Critical thinking is also affected by a person's beliefs and values. Nurses must be independent thinkers—that is, they must be careful not to allow the status quo or a persuasive person to control their thinking.

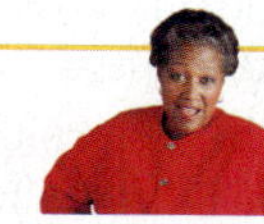

Remember **Addie Warner**, the older woman who was considered demanding by some staff? The student describing her experience with Mrs. Warner in the Reflective Practice box demonstrated independent thinking by not accepting staff members' emotional description of the patient. Rather, the student confronted the situation, obtained information, and then acted based on this information.

When confronted with an intellectual challenge, such as "Why does this patient resist change?" the nurse should proceed cautiously, consulting with the patient and respected colleagues and reviewing the literature. Only then can the nurse reach a true clinical judgment. Compare this with a nurse who makes a snap judgment that a patient is "unreasonable" based only on hearing the comments of another nurse—even if that nurse is the nurse manager.

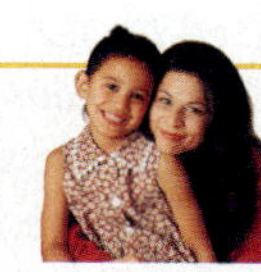

Recall **Charlotte Horvath**, the single mother needing wound care teaching. A nurse who is not an independent thinker might quickly assume that Ms. Horvath just wasn't interested in caring for her child at home. But a nurse who is an independent thinker would investigate the situation further before making a decision. Contrast these approaches:

"A good mother who loves her child would find a way to come to a teaching session." [implies judgment]
"Can you tell me what is making it difficult for you to come to a teaching session?"

Alfaro-LeFevre (2002–2020) has carefully developed a list of **critical-thinking indicators** (CTIs), which are evidence-based descriptions of behaviors that demonstrate the knowledge, characteristics, and skills that promote critical thinking in clinical practice (Boxes 13-4 on page 353 and 13-5 on page 354). If you are serious about developing the critical thinking skills needed for professional practice, now would be a good time to sit down with several people who know you well to see which critical thinking characteristics you possess and which need work. One way to do this is to ask these questions about each characteristic in Box 13-5:

1. Ask the people who know you well: "On a scale of 1 to 7 (with 1 being almost never and 7 always), to what degree do I demonstrate this characteristic that promotes critical thinking?"
2. Think of examples of times when you demonstrated and failed to demonstrate these characteristics. Ask yourself: "What were the consequences in these situations?"

13-1 Focused Critical-Thinking Guide

MAINSTREAM VERSUS ALTERNATIVE MEDICINE

You are a nursing student. Your friend, Amy Chang, confides to you that she is very worried about her grandmother. When you meet Mrs. Chang, she demonstrates many of the assessment findings related to heart failure. Although her family has entreated her to seek medical attention, Mrs. Chang insists on relying on herbal teas and traditional Chinese remedies. Now 88 years old, Mrs. Chang came to America from mainland China when she was 14. Although she raised a family that is now thoroughly "Americanized," Mrs. Chang has resisted embracing her new culture and now wants nothing to do with "American medicine." Amy, who is also a nursing student, loves her grandmother dearly and is frustrated by her stubborn refusal to see an internist. Both of you have reason to believe that she could be helped by medical attention. What do you do?

1. Identify goal of thinking

Clarify your thinking about alternative medicine so that you can decide how you ought to respond to Mrs. Chang's worsening physical condition.

2. Assess adequacy of knowledge

Pertinent circumstances: Although you have strong reason to believe that Mrs. Chang is suffering from congestive heart failure, she has not been medically diagnosed, and you lack definitive knowledge about her medical condition and the likelihood that she would respond to treatment. You do know that she places a high value on traditional Chinese culture and strongly believes that if she is to be healed, the healing will result from herbal teas and traditional Chinese remedies. She has no confidence in American medicine. Her family describes her as being extremely strong willed and very lovable. You do not know if she has the benefit of seeing a competent practitioner of Chinese medicine.

Prerequisite knowledge: To decide how you should respond in this situation, you need to know that mainstream American medicine is not the only beneficial system of medicine. It would be helpful for you and Mrs. Chang's family to learn more about Chinese medicine and the probability of its benefiting her (as well as the possibility of its harming her) in her present condition. You will also need to learn more about what is essential to Mrs. Chang's well-being. How much value does she place on physical health? How important is it for her to live (and possibly die) within the familiar and comforting boundaries of her culture? You will want to assess what teaching, counseling, and support Mrs. Chang needs to reach an informed and voluntary decision that is right for her.

Room for error: Because Mrs. Chang's life may literally be at stake, there is not much room for error in the manner you and her family choose to respond. Even if her condition is not life threatening, her sense of well-being may be severely threatened if she feels forced to pursue treatment that is alien and frightening.

Time constraints: Although you are uncertain about the seriousness of her condition, you understand that the sooner Mrs. Chang receives effective therapy, the better. Unless her condition suddenly deteriorates, this is not a decision that needs to be made within the next 24 hours.

3. Address potential problems

The most serious obstacle to critical thinking in this situation would be an inability to weigh the respective merits of alternative healing systems. Cultural bias may result in the untested assumption that American medicine is necessarily superior to all other systems of healing and that it would be morally wrong to support a choice of anything else. The love of Mrs. Chang's family and their desire to do everything possible to keep her well may interfere with their ability to allow her the freedom to make the choice that is right for her.

4. Consult helpful resources

Your first challenge will be to learn more about traditional Chinese medicine by consulting with local authorities and available literature. The National Institutes of Health have now established an Office of Alternative Medicine, which may provide helpful information and which is easily accessed through their website. Your most important resource may be Mrs. Chang herself; it will be important to try to learn from her as much as you can about what she values and what her goals are at this point in her life. You will also want to be sure that Mrs. Chang has the benefits of a competent practitioner of Chinese medicine.

5. Critique judgment/decision

After getting to know Mrs. Chang better, you realize that she is firmly committed to her ways and adamant about not going to an American doctor or into a hospital at this point of her life. Thus, you (with her family) have several options: to force her to see an internist against her will, possibly deceiving her to get her to the internist's office, or to support her choice to rely on familiar remedies, which may or may not successfully resolve her problems. The first alternative may save her life, and her family can see no other choice. You realize that by making this choice, the family is imposing its values on Mrs. Chang and violating her autonomy, her right to determine the course of her life. You decide to support her and to try to explain to her family the importance of doing this. You understand that if her condition is serious and her traditional remedies prove ineffective, her death may be hastened, but she accepts this consequence and prefers it to embracing an alien and frightening culture. An alternative strategy that might result in a win–win result would be to find an American Chinese physician who practices both Chinese and American medicine. If Mrs. Chang could be persuaded to visit this practitioner, she would experience the best of both medical traditions.

Box 13-4 Knowledge and Intellectual Skills Critical-Thinking Indicators (CTIs)

Knowledge

Requirements vary, depending on the context (e.g., specialty practice).

Relates Knowledge of

- ☐ Nursing and medical terminology
- ☐ Nursing versus medical and other models, roles, and responsibilities
- ☐ Scope of nursing practice (qualifications; applicable standards, laws, and rules and regulations)
- ☐ Related anatomy, physiology, and pathophysiology
- ☐ Spiritual, social, and cultural concepts
- ☐ Normal and abnormal growth and development (pediatric, adult, and gerontologic implications)
- ☐ Normal and abnormal function (bio-psycho-social-cultural-spiritual)
- ☐ Factors affecting normal function (bio-psycho-social-cultural-spiritual)
- ☐ Nutrition and pharmacology principles
- ☐ Behavioral health and disease management
- ☐ Signs and symptoms of common problems and complications
- ☐ Nursing process, nursing theories, research, and evidence-based practice
- ☐ Reasons behind policies, procedures, and interventions; diagnostic studies implications
- ☐ Ethical and legal principles
- ☐ Risk management and infection control
- ☐ Safety standards, healthy workplace standards, and principles of learning and safety cultures
- ☐ Inter-relationship of health care disciplines and systems
- ☐ Reliable information resources

Demonstrates

- ☐ Focused nursing assessment skills (e.g., breath sounds or IV site assessment)
- ☐ Mathematical problem solving for drug calculations
- ☐ Related technical skills (e.g., n/g tube or other equipment management)

Clarifies

- ☐ Personal biases, values, beliefs, needs
- ☐ How own culture, thinking, personality, and learning style preferences differ from others'
- ☐ Level of commitment to organizational mission and values

Intellectual Skills/Competencies

Demonstrates Nursing Process and Decision-Making Skills

- ☐ Communicates effectively orally and in writing
- ☐ Identifies practice scope: applies standards, principles, laws, and ethics codes
- ☐ Makes safety and infection control a priority; prevents and deals with mistakes constructively
- ☐ Includes patient, family, and key stakeholders in decision making; teaches patient, self, and others
- ☐ Identifies purpose and focus of assessment
- ☐ Assesses systematically and comprehensively
- ☐ Distinguishes normal from abnormal; identifies risks for abnormal
- ☐ Distinguishes relevant from irrelevant; clusters relevant data together
- ☐ Identifies assumptions and inconsistencies; checks accuracy and reliability (validates data)
- ☐ Recognizes missing information; gains more data as needed.
- ☐ Concludes what's known and unknown; draws reasonable conclusions—gives evidence to support them
- ☐ Identifies both problems and their underlying cause(s) and related factors; includes patient and family perspectives
- ☐ Recognizes changes in patient status; takes appropriate action
- ☐ Considers multiple ideas, explanations, and solutions
- ☐ Determines individualized outcomes and uses them to plan and give care
- ☐ Manages risks, predicts complications
- ☐ Weighs risks and benefits; anticipates consequences and implications—individualizes interventions accordingly
- ☐ Sets priorities and makes decisions in a timely way
- ☐ Reassesses to monitor outcomes (responses)
- ☐ Promotes health, function, comfort, and well-being
- ☐ Identifies ethical issues and takes appropriate action
- ☐ Uses human and information resources; detects bias

Additional Related Skills

- ☐ Advocates for patients, self, and others
- ☐ Engages and empowers patients, families, peers, and coworkers
- ☐ Fosters positive interpersonal relationships; addresses conflicts fairly; promotes healthy workplace and learning cultures
- ☐ Promotes teamwork (focuses on common goals, respects diversity; encourages others to contribute in their own way)
- ☐ Facilitates and navigates change
- ☐ Organizes and manages time and environment
- ☐ Gives and takes constructive criticism
- ☐ Delegates appropriately (matches patient needs with worker competencies; determines worker learning needs, supervises and teaches as indicated; monitors results personally)
- ☐ Leads, inspires, and helps others move toward common goals
- ☐ Demonstrates systems thinking (shows awareness of relationships existing within and across health care systems)

Source: Reprinted with permission from Alfaro-LeFevre, R. (2002–2020). *Critical thinking indicators (CTIs)*. www.AlfaroTeachSmart.com.

It can be helpful to see if you and others you invite to evaluate your characteristics reach the same conclusions about your strengths and areas for improvement.

Another way to use this list is to try to determine as a class which characteristics in Box 13-5 accurately describe your class! Alternatively, you can compare groups. For example, as a rule, which characteristics do nurses as a group and other health care providers as a group demonstrate?

As you begin clinical practice, you can also use the lists in Box 13-4 to critique your competence for professional practice.

Box 13-5 Personal Critical-Thinking Indicators (CTIs)

PERSONAL CTIs are brief descriptions of behaviors, attitudes, and characteristics often seen in critical thinkers. These are the behaviors that promote development of critical thinking habits. The below is the ideal—no one's perfect. Characteristics vary depending on circumstances such as comfort and familiarity with the people and situations at hand. What matters is *patterns* of behavior over time (is the behavior usually evident?). If you're a critical thinker, you probably can pick some characteristics you'd like to improve (critical thinkers are innately focused on improvement).

- ☐ **Self-aware:** Identifies own learning, personality, and communication style preferences; clarifies biases, strengths, and limitations; acknowledges when thinking may be influenced by emotions or self-interest.
- ☐ **Genuine/authentic:** Shows true self; demonstrates behaviors that indicate stated values.
- ☐ **Effective communicator:** Listens well (shows deep understanding of others' thoughts, feelings, and circumstances); speaks and writes with clarity (gets key points across to others).
- ☐ **Curious and inquisitive:** Asks questions; looks for reasons, explanations, and meaning; seeks new information to broaden understanding.
- ☐ **Alert to context:** Looks for changes in circumstances that warrant a need to modify approaches; investigates thoroughly when situations warrant precise, in depth thinking.
- ☐ **Reflective and self-corrective:** Carefully considers meaning of data and interpersonal interactions, asks for feedback; corrects own thinking, alert to potential errors by self and others, finds ways to avoid future mistakes.
- ☐ **Analytical and insightful:** Identifies relationships; expresses deep understanding.
- ☐ **Logical and intuitive:** Draws reasonable conclusions (if this is so, then it follows that because…); uses intuition as a guide; acts on intuition only with knowledge of risks involved.
- ☐ **Confident and resilient:** Expresses faith in ability to reason and learn; overcomes problems and disappointments.
- ☐ **Honest and upright:** Looks for the truth, even if it sheds unwanted light; demonstrates integrity (adheres to moral and ethical standards; admits flaws in thinking).
- ☐ **Autonomous/responsible:** Self-directed, self-disciplined, and accepts accountability.
- ☐ **Careful and prudent:** Seeks help as needed; suspends or revises judgment as indicated by new or incomplete data.
- ☐ **Open and fair-minded:** Shows tolerance for different viewpoints; questions how own viewpoints are influencing thinking.
- ☐ **Sensitive to diversity:** Expresses appreciation of human differences related to values, culture, personality, or learning style preferences; adapts to preferences when feasible.
- ☐ **Creative:** Offers alternative solutions and approaches; comes up with useful ideas.
- ☐ **Realistic and practical:** Admits when things aren't feasible; looks for useful solutions.
- ☐ **Proactive:** Anticipates consequences, plans ahead, acts on opportunities.
- ☐ **Courageous:** Stands up for beliefs, advocates for others, doesn't hide from challenges
- ☐ **Patient and persistent:** Waits for right moment; perseveres to achieve best results.
- ☐ **Flexible:** Changes approaches as needed to get the best results.
- ☐ **Health-oriented:** Promotes a healthy lifestyle; uses healthy behaviors to manage stress.
- ☐ **Improvement-oriented (self, patients, systems): Self**—identifies learning needs; finds ways to overcome limitations, seeks out new knowledge. **Patients**—promotes health; maximizes function, comfort, and convenience. **Systems**—identifies risks and problems with health care systems; promotes safety, quality, satisfaction, and cost containment.

Source: Reprinted with permission from Alfaro-LeFevre, R. (2019). *Critical thinking indicators (CTIs).* www.AlfaroTeachSmart.com.

Developing Technical Competencies

Some people are naturally "good with their hands" and quickly master intricate procedures that involve working with technical equipment. Others have to practice procedures many times before they feel competent handling the equipment and performing clinical activities independently. Whatever your natural level of technical skill, developing the following habits can help you master the manual skills essential in the nursing process:

- When a procedure demands manual dexterity or a complex series of steps, practice the necessary skill until you feel confident in your ability before attempting to perform it with a patient. Simulation exercises are a great help in developing both your competence and confidence.
- Take time to familiarize yourself with new equipment before using it in a clinical procedure. Understand how it works and what supplies are needed to ensure optimal functioning. If possible, anticipate problems and know how to remedy them.
- Identify nurses who are technical experts and ask them to share their secrets. Many experienced clinicians have developed quality, time-saving techniques they are willing to share.
- Never be ashamed to ask for help when feeling unsure of how to perform a procedure or manage equipment. Don't overlook the patient or family caregiver as a source of helpful hints for care they routinely provide. Never forget that the patient's well-being—and sometimes the patient's life—depend on your technical competence.

Many nursing procedures are described in the clinical chapters in this text. Performance checklists break each procedure down into its component parts, allowing you to evaluate your performance of each step of the procedure. This type of self-testing enables you to quickly identify and remedy any deficiencies in technical skills.

Developing Interpersonal Competencies

Interpersonal skills are essential to thoughtful, person-centered practice. Interpersonal caring involves promoting the dignity and respect of patients as people and establishing a caring relationship. As a result, both the nurse and patient experience mutual enrichment.

QSEN PATIENT-CENTERED CARE

Beginning with your first clinical encounters, learn to value seeing health care situations "through the patient's eyes." You will want to willingly support patient-centered care for individuals and groups whose values differ from your own.

PROMOTING HUMAN DIGNITY AND RESPECT

If you are committed to respecting patients' human dignity, you will find it helpful to reflect on these questions:

- What obligates me to respect patients' human dignity? Why should I respect all patients equally? Are some patients more deserving of respect than others? Can a patient ever forfeit the right to be respected?
- What does it mean to respect the dignity of patients? What are five concrete ways I can demonstrate respect?
- What are my strengths and deficiencies when it comes to respecting patients?
- In what ways (if any) must I change to be faithful to the duty of respecting the dignity of each patient, family member, and colleague?
- What patients most challenge my ability to give care respectfully? How do I respond to this challenge? What does this teach me for the future?

Nurses often underestimate their power to help a patient heal simply through their respectful and caring presence. Each time a nurse walks into a room, the nurse communicates one of two messages: (1) "You are a job to be done—you mean nothing to me" or (2) "You are a person of worth, and I care about you." Even a 60-second nurse–patient interaction can enhance or jeopardize human well-being. Therefore, nurses must be sensitive about what their looks, speech, and touch communicate to patients and colleagues. The more vulnerable the patient and the more threatened the patient's sense of self, the more powerful effect the nurse's message has on the person's sense of worth and well-being.

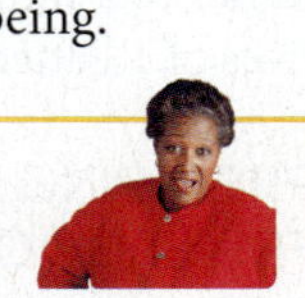

Consider **Addie Warner**, the patient described in the Reflective Practice display. Imagine the message that she received from staff who consider her difficult when she used her call light to ask for help. Most likely, the message conveyed was negative. Compare this to the message communicated by the nursing student who helped get her out of bed and get washed: a more positive message supporting the patient's self-worth.

The learning activity in Box 13-6 (on page 356) was developed for nurses caring for older adults in a long-term care facility. To help develop interpersonal skills, try these activities with a friend. Take turns being both the nurse and the older adult and talk about how different types of nursing presence makes you feel.

ESTABLISHING CARING RELATIONSHIPS

Increasingly, nurses report that new systems of care and the demand to work "harder, faster, and smarter" to keep up in today's competitive health care arena are making traditional nurse–patient relationships difficult to attain. Note that when the ANA revised the definition of nursing in *Nursing: Scope and Standards of Practice*, it highlighted nurse caring:

> This revised definition presents a reordering of the content from the 2015 version, including the art and science of caring, replacing abilities with human functioning, and incorporating references to compassionate presence and recognition of the connection of all humanity. Such refinements reflect an evolution of thinking over the past five years and present enhancements intended to lead into the future (2021, p. 1).

As you begin your nursing practice, ask yourself what priority you assign to caring. Nurses who accept that there can be no excellence in nursing in the absence of this relationship commit themselves to finding creative means to establish compassionately caring relationships. Obviously, many variables influence the quality of relationships that are possible, not the least of which is how sick the patient is and the patient's length of stay. Helpful reflection questions include the following:

- Do I know my patients well enough to promote anything more than their physical well-being?
- If asked to describe a patient, would I be able to report on anything other than the patient's physical condition?
- Is the care I routinely provide really holistic, individualized, prioritized according to medical need and the patient's valued interests and goals, and continuous? Do my care plans reflect this?
- What does the content of the patient report and nursing documentation communicate about nursing priorities in my practice setting?
- What are my strengths and deficiencies in creating caring relationships?
- In what ways (if any) must I change/grow to establish better caring relationships?

Nurses committed to caring relationships routinely use opportunities for conversation to communicate genuine interest in who the patient is and what the patient is experiencing to provide meaningful nursing assistance. For example, rather than just chatting aimlessly with a talkative patient, a nurse skilled in developing caring relationships will direct the conversation. Here are some leading statements or questions that are often successful in eliciting useful information from older adults:

- "Tell me something about your life at home. What do you miss most now that you are here?"

Box 13-6 Developing Interpersonal Skills

Human Dignity: How Who I Am as a Caregiver Affects Others

Description

The purpose of this exercise is to explore the notion of "therapeutic use of self." You will be challenged to reflect on the effect your looks, speech, and touch have on other people. Role-play and guided discovery will be used to enable you to experience the affirming and negating influences of different means of human relating.

Objectives

Upon conclusion of this exercise, you will be able to:

1. Demonstrate how looks, words, and touch can be used to harm or benefit others.
2. Describe how the way you approach others enhances or diminishes their well-being.
3. Identify one care behavior you plan to modify to improve your nursing practice.

Learning Activities

Invite an experienced nurse to demonstrate how looks, words, and touch can be used to communicate two different messages to others: "You are a job to be done—you mean nothing to me" and "You are precious, and I care about you." After the demonstration, team up with another student, and experience giving and receiving these messages. Share the feelings that you both experienced. After these preliminary exercises, role-play the following suggested nursing situations (or others of your choosing), and once again process the experience. Talk about the relevance of this experience to human interaction in general, and conclude the exercise by writing a goal for your practice.

Worksheet

A. Practice looking at a colleague two different ways:
   1. "You are a job to be done—you mean nothing to me."
   2. "You are precious, and I care about you."

B. Practice speaking to a colleague in two different ways:
   1. Indifferent: "Your patient, your light."
   2. Helpful: "I think Mrs. Jones's light is on again. Do you need help?"

C. Practice touching a colleague in two different ways:
   1. Indifferent: Pick up your colleague's wrist and feel for a pulse.
   2. Using warm lotion, massage your colleague's hands.

D. Talk about how each of these looks, words, and touches made you feel. Talk about how you think they make patients feel.

E. Role-play each of the following situations in two different ways, trying to incorporate looks, words, and touches that communicate:

   First time: You are a job to be done—you mean nothing to me.

   Second time: You are precious, and I care about you.

   1. Student feels overwhelmed by patient care assignment and approaches clinical instructor to discuss her options.
   2. Student walks into patient's room to begin morning care.
   3. Student assists older adult to stand and ambulate around room.
   4. Student brings medication to patient.
   5. Student approaches another student and asks for help changing the bed linens of an obese patient who is on complete bed rest.

F. Name one thing you have decided to try to do differently when you take care of your patients as a result of this session.

G. Does what you experienced today have any implications for who you are when you are not nursing?

- "What family members and friends do you see most often? Who do you think knows you best and would you trust to speak for you if you were ever unable to speak for yourself?"
- "Most of us have some goal or dream that keeps us going. It might be owning our own home, seeing some relationship patched up, or being able to celebrate the birth of a grandchild. What is your dream?"
- "When you've had troubles in the past, what did you draw on for strength? What keeps you going?"
- "It looks like you've got a lot of time for thinking these days . . . would you like to share what's been on your mind?"
- "It looks like we'll be spending some time together . . . what would you like to do with this time? How may I help you?"
- "What would you like us to know that will help us to better meet your needs?"
- "Hospitals can be scary places [Alternatively, "illness can be scary," "bringing a loved one home from the hospital and shouldering the burden of caregiving alone can be scary"] . . . how can I help you?"

Nurses who are sensitive to the well-being of their patients can find many ways to communicate caring. Happily, most caring is mutually enriching, and nurses who care find themselves reenergized for the more demanding aspects of their practice. Read one patient's account of the importance to her of a nurse's caring in the accompanying Through the Eyes of a Patient display.

PREPARING YOUR ATTENTION AND INTENTION FOR EACH CLINICAL ENCOUNTER

A physician colleague who became a chaplain shared with me that he now appreciates that the most important thing he brings to each bedside encounter is himself, and how his presence comforts and heals. Before visiting a patient, he stops to prepare two things in order to create greater connection and meaning: his *attention* and *intention*. You may find his practice of using the experience of handwashing helpful.

There are many ways different people prepare their attention and intention. I have developed a simple

Through the Eyes of a Patient

I recently spent 2 months in a university teaching hospital while doctors tried to find a way to regulate my heartbeats. Many of the days were filled with tests, some of which were frightening. I was given many drugs—most of which turned out not to be helpful. I was a 2-hour car ride away from my home, family, and friends—which meant there wasn't always a familiar face at my bedside.

I quickly learned I could judge what kind of day I was going to have as soon as I saw my nurse each morning. All of them brought my medicines and helped with the treatment plan. With some nurses, however, I also experienced the comfort and security of knowing that my expressed needs would be promptly and respectfully tended to. If I needed help getting up to the bathroom or asked for something for pain, I could count on help coming quickly. And finally there were those few with whom I knew I was going to have a great day because they would "make it happen" no matter how sick I was feeling. These were the nurses who offered a hug with their medicines, who had a moment to sit and listen, who teased about the "fashion statements" I was making with my nightgowns, and who "walked me through" new tests so that at least I felt better prepared to face the unknown. Most often, it wasn't what they did but how they did it.

I wish all nurses understood the power they have to influence a patient's basic sense of well-being. A hospital can be a pretty scary, lonely place. Nurses can make all the difference! Will you?

—Mildred Taylor, Pottsville, PA

ritual for myself. Before I enter my patient's room, I stop. While washing (or gelling) my hands, I prepare my attention. I bring my awareness to my feet on the ground, then to my breath, and to the flow of water (or gel) over my hands, as if they are washing aside (evaporating away) my preoccupations, leaving only my best intentions. I make a blessing before I dry my hands (or as my hands are drying): I lift up my hands. May I be of service? Then I take a full breath and remind myself: "What matters for you, my patient, is what matters for me. May I meet you in your world as it is for you and accompany you from there. Whatever time I have with you, may I be fully present. May I serve you with all of my life experience as well as my expertise. May I listen fully with a generous heart, without judgment, and without having to fix what cannot be fixed. May my presence allow you to connect with your source of comfort, strength, and guidance as it is for you. May I be well used" (Feldstein, 2011).

ENJOYING THE REWARDS OF MUTUAL EXCHANGE

In any helping profession, but especially in nursing, countless opportunities exist to interact with others. Those committed to interpersonal caring enrich everyday interactions by investing them with something of themselves and, in return, receiving something from the other (Fig. 13-2). Think of your last encounter with a patient. Whether you were administering a medication, checking vital signs, or preparing the patient for discharge, you had the choice of merely accomplishing the given task or accomplishing the task while simultaneously communicating a personal gift of support, caring, strength, and peacefulness. Frequently overlooked, these interpersonal gifts might contribute to a patient's healing as significantly as medical interventions. Rather than deplete their giver, these interpersonal gifts invite similar gifts from the recipient, which in return enrich the caregiver. Nothing causes burnout faster than a practice that is reduced to the performance of multiple tasks stripped of their human significance. When a patient is given care in a way that "makes a difference" in terms of their well-being, the patient's gratitude, even when unspoken, helps renew the nurse's energy.

Too seldom do we stop our busy practices long enough to reflect on how who we are that day is influencing the well-being of those receiving our care. It is helpful to question:

- How conscious am I of how my mood influences the well-being of others?
- Have I ever consciously tried to transmit strength, peace, support, or joy to another? What were the results?
- Am I aware of any situation in which my fatigue, anxiety, frustration, or negativity was communicated to a patient in a manner that negatively influenced the patient's well-being?
- Am I conscious of ways in which patients enrich me personally or enrich my practice?
- In what ways is my practice different when I am attuned to the interpersonal dimensions of nurse–patient interactions?
- In what ways must my practice change if I am to facilitate healing in every patient encounter?

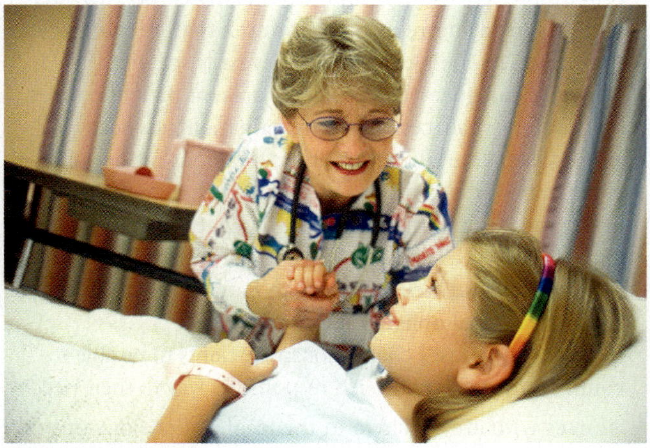

FIGURE 13-2. Interpersonal caring enriches the lives of everyone participating, providing a mutual exchange of giving and receiving.

Developing Ethical and Legal Competencies

Nurses who prize their role in securing patient well-being are sensitive to the ethical and legal implications of nursing practice. Chapters 6 and 7 describe essential components of ethical and legal competence for nurses. Although it can take years to master effective patient advocacy skills and to become proficient in mediating ethical conflict, even beginning nurses are responsible for certain basic ethical skills. For example, one of the greatest challenges nursing students face is balancing the competing demands of home life, school, and the hospital or practice setting.

Nurse Self-Care Alert

Learning to be true to yourself, to the patients for whom you are responsible, to the caregiving team, and to the profession and society is an ongoing struggle for nurses. At no time was this struggle more acute than during the COVID-19 pandemic.

Examining your sense of accountability is crucial as you assume professional responsibilities.

Nurses committed to interpersonal caring hold themselves accountable for the human well-being of patients entrusted to their care. Being accountable means being attentive and responsive to the health care needs of individual patients. It means that your concern for the patient transcends whatever happens during your shift, and that you ensure continuity of care when you leave a patient. In today's system of increasingly fragmented care, patients often find themselves unable to point to any single caregiver who knows their overall situation and is capable and willing to coordinate the efforts of the health care team. Being responsive and responsible earns a patient's trust that "all will be well" as health care needs are addressed. Nurses committed to responsible, compassionate caring reflect on the following:

- To what extent does my commitment to securing the human well-being of those in my care dictate my work priorities?
- How comfortable am I voicing unmet patient needs to other members of the health care team? Is meeting the patient's needs more important to me than remaining in my comfort zone? Am I an effective advocate?
- Do other caregivers listen when I present patient concerns because of my successful record of patient advocacy?
- What system variables (e.g., nurse–patient ratios, skill mix, availability of resources) need to change for us to better meet the human needs of our patients?
- Have I read ANA's *Code of Ethics for Nurses with Interpretive Statements* (2015), and am I ready to meet nursing's ethical obligations?
- In what ways must I change for my patients to be able to count on me to respond in a responsible way to their needs?

Nurses who are sensitive to the legal dimensions of practice are careful to develop a strong sense of both ethical and legal accountability. Competent practice is a nurse's best legal safeguard. Nurses seeking to develop legal competence may find it helpful to ask these questions:

- Do I know the legal boundaries of my practice? Have I read my state nurse practice act?
- Am I familiar with ANA's *Nursing: Scope and Standards of Practice* (2021)?
- Am I familiar with pertinent institutional procedures and policies?
- Do I "own" my personal strengths and weaknesses and seek assistance as needed?
- Am I careful never to accept responsibility for an assignment for which I am unprepared?
- Am I knowledgeable about, and respectful of, patient rights?
- Does my documentation provide a legally defensible account of my practice?

When working to develop ethical and legal accountability, nurses must recognize that both deficiencies and excesses of responsible caring are problematic. Although it is reasonable to hold oneself accountable for promoting the human well-being of patients, nurses can err by setting unrealistic standards of responsiveness and responsibility for themselves. Prudence is always necessary to balance responsible self-care with care of others. Inexperienced nurses may feel totally responsible for effecting patient outcomes beyond their control and may become frustrated and sad when unable to produce the desired outcome. Conversations with other nurses about what is reasonable to hold ourselves and others accountable for are always helpful.

QSEN Competencies

The overall goal of the **QSEN (Quality and Safety Education for Nurses)** project is to meet the challenge of preparing future nurses who will have the knowledge, skills, and attitudes (KSAs) necessary to continuously improve the quality and safety of the health care systems within which they work.

Using the Institute of Medicine (now the National Academy of Sciences, Engineering, and Medicine) competencies, QSEN faculty and a National Advisory Board defined quality and safety competencies for nursing and proposed targets for the KSAs to be developed in nursing pre-licensure programs for each competency. See the QSEN website (www.qsen.org) and Box 13-7 for a description of these competencies. To highlight the importance of these competencies, each chapter in this text has a feature entitled *Reflective Practice: Developing QSEN Competencies.* These special features are written by nursing students and will help you to assess your developing mastery of these competencies.

Clinical Reasoning, Decision Making, and Clinical Judgment

The terms *critical thinking, clinical reasoning,* and *clinical judgment* are often used interchangeably. Alfaro-LeFevre (2020, p. 7) offers these helpful distinctions:

- Critical thinking—a broad term—includes reasoning *both* inside and outside the clinical setting.

Box 13-7 New Fundamentals in Nursing: Introducing Beginning Quality and Safety Education for Nurses (QSEN) Competencies

Patient-Centered Care

The traditional concept involves listening to the patient and demonstrating respect and compassion. The QSEN competency emphasizes recognition of the patient or designee as the source of control and full partner in providing compassionate and coordinated care based on respect for patients' preferences, values, and needs. The KSAs include:

- K—Integrate understanding of multiple dimensions of person-centered care: patient, family, and community preferences and values; coordination and integration of care; information, communication, and education; physical comfort and emotional support; involvement of family and friends; and transition and continuity.
- S—Elicit patient values, preferences, and expressed needs as part of the clinical interview, implementation of care plan, and evaluation of care.
- A—Value seeing health care situations "through patients' eyes."

Teamwork and Collaboration

The traditional view of teamwork may involve working side by side with other health care professionals while forming nursing skills. The updated QSEN definition calls for functioning effectively within nursing and interprofessional teams, fostering open communication, mutual respect, and shared decision making to achieve quality patient care. Important beginning KSAs include:

- K—Describe scope of practice and roles of health care team members.
- S—Follow communication practices that minimize risk associated with handoff among providers and across transition in care.
- A—Acknowledge own potential to contribute to effective team functioning.

Evidence-Based Practice

Traditional practices involve adhering to internal policies to standardize skills execution. The QSEN definition specifies the integration of best current evidence with clinical expertise and patient and family preferences and values for delivery of optimal health care. Important, beginning KSAs reveal significant changes in fundamentals of nursing:

- K—Describe evidence-based practice to include components of research evidence, clinical expertise, and patient and family values.
- S—Base individualized care plan on patient values, clinical expertise, and evidence.
- A—Value the concept of evidence-based practice as integral to determining best clinical practice.

Quality Improvement

A long-standing approach to quality involves routinely updating nursing policies and procedures. The QSEN updated concept of quality improvement recommends use of data to monitor the outcomes of care processes and use of improvement methods to design and test changes to continuously improve the quality and safety of health care systems. The KSAs recommended for early introduction include:

- K—Recognition that nursing and other health professions students are parts of systems of care and care processes that affect outcomes for patients and families.
- S—The Delphi ratings did not identify a beginning skill in quality improvement but rather recommended introduction and emphasis in intermediate or advanced experiences.
- A—Appreciate continuous quality improvement as essential in the daily work of all health care professionals.

Safety

A simplistic, traditional definition of safety is to use bed rails properly to ensure "that my patient does not fall during my shift." The QSEN update assures recognition of a culture of safety and minimization of risk of harm to patients through both system effectiveness and individual performance. Safety KSAs rated as important to introduce early include:

- K—Examine human factors and other basic safety design principles as well as commonly used unsafe practices (e.g., workarounds, dangerous abbreviations).
- S—Demonstrate effective use of strategies to reduce risk of harm to self or others.
- A—Value the contributions of standardization and reliability to safety.

Informatics

Traditionally, documentation consists of timely and accurate charting. However, the QSEN-updated definition is expanded and calls for using information and technology to communicate, manage knowledge, mitigate error, and support decision making. The KSAs identified as important for early introduction include:

- K—Explain why information and technology skills are essential for safe patient care.
- S—Apply technology and information management tools to support safe processes of care.
- A—Value technologies supporting decision making, error prevention, and care coordination.

Source: Reprinted with permission of Slack Incorporated from Preheim, G., Armstrong, G. E., & Barton, A. J. (2009). The NEW fundamentals in nursing: Introducing beginning quality and safety education for nurses (QSEN) competencies. *Journal of Nursing Education, 48*(12), 694–697; permission conveyed through Copyright Clearance Center, Inc.

- **Clinical reasoning** and **decision making**—specific terms—refer to the process you use to think about patient problems in the clinical setting—for example, deciding how to prevent and manage mobility issues. For reasoning about other clinical issues (e.g., teamwork, collaboration, and streamlining workflow), nurses usually use critical thinking.
- **Clinical judgment** refers to the result (outcome) of critical thinking, clinical reasoning, and decision-making—the conclusion, decision, or opinion you make after analyzing information (Fig. 13-3).

People use critical-thinking skills whenever they want to use clear, focused thinking to achieve a result. You can think critically about how to survive the day's challenges, to find a

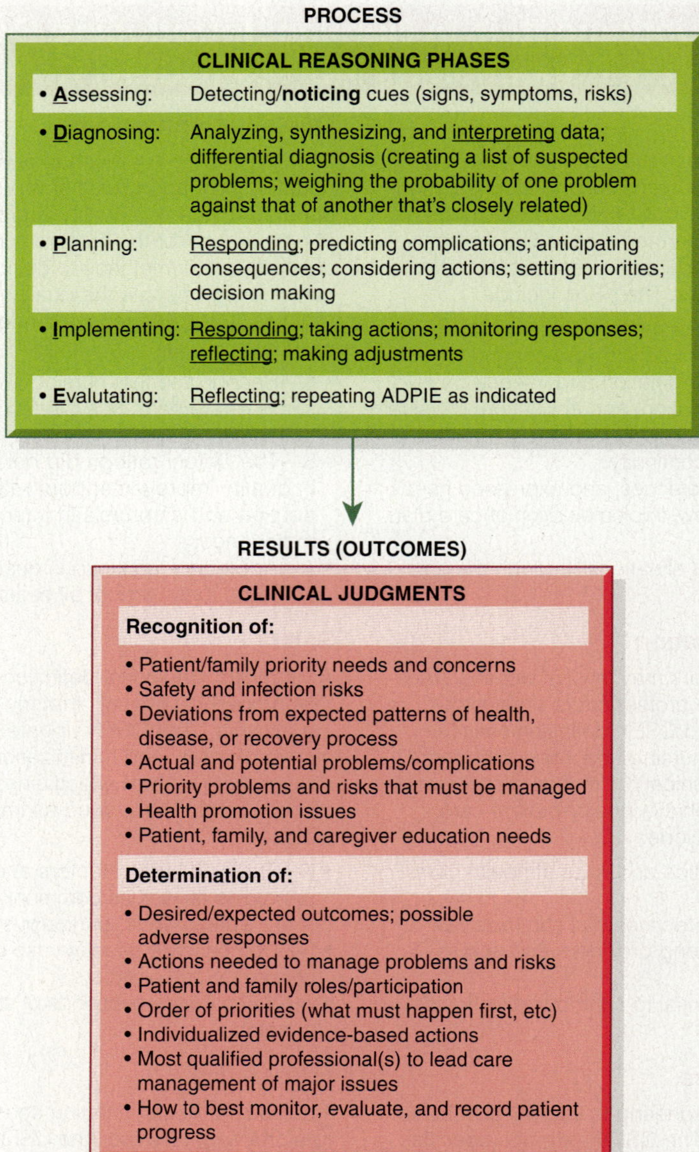

FIGURE 13-3. The process and outcomes of clinical reasoning using ADPIE. Underlined terms indicate Tanner's clinical judgment model (noticing, interpreting, responding, reflecting). (*Source:* Adapted with permission from © 2019 Alfaro-LeFevre. www.AlfaroTeachSmart.com.)

partner for life, to pass a licensing exam, or to become president! Critical thinking in nursing—which includes clinical reasoning, decision making, and clinical judgment—is purposeful, informed, outcome-focused thinking that:

- Is guided by standards, policies, ethics codes, and laws (individual state practice acts and state boards of nursing regulations).
- Is driven by patient, family, and community needs, as well as nurses' needs to give competent and efficient care (e.g., streamlining charting to free up nurses for patient care).
- Is based on principles of the nursing process, problem solving, and the scientific method (which requires forming opinions and making decisions based on evidence).
- Focuses on safety and quality, constantly reevaluating, self-correcting, and striving to improve personal, professional, and system practices.
- Carefully identifies the key problems, issues, and risks involved and includes patients, families, and key stakeholders in decision making early in the process.
- Uses logic, intuition, and creativity and is grounded in specific knowledge, skills, and experience.
- Calls for strategies that make the most of human potential and compensate for problems created by human nature (e.g., finding ways to prevent errors, using information technology, and overcoming the powerful influence of personal views). (Alfaro-LeFevre, 2020, p. 8)

Levett-Jones et al. (2010) prepared the clinical reasoning (CR) model depicted in Figure 13-4 after studying the work of Hoffman, Alfaro-LeFevre, and Andersen. They describe eight main steps or phases in the clinical reasoning cycle. However, in reality, the distinctions between these phases are not so clear. While clinical reasoning can be broken down into steps—look, collect, process, decide, plan, act, evaluate,

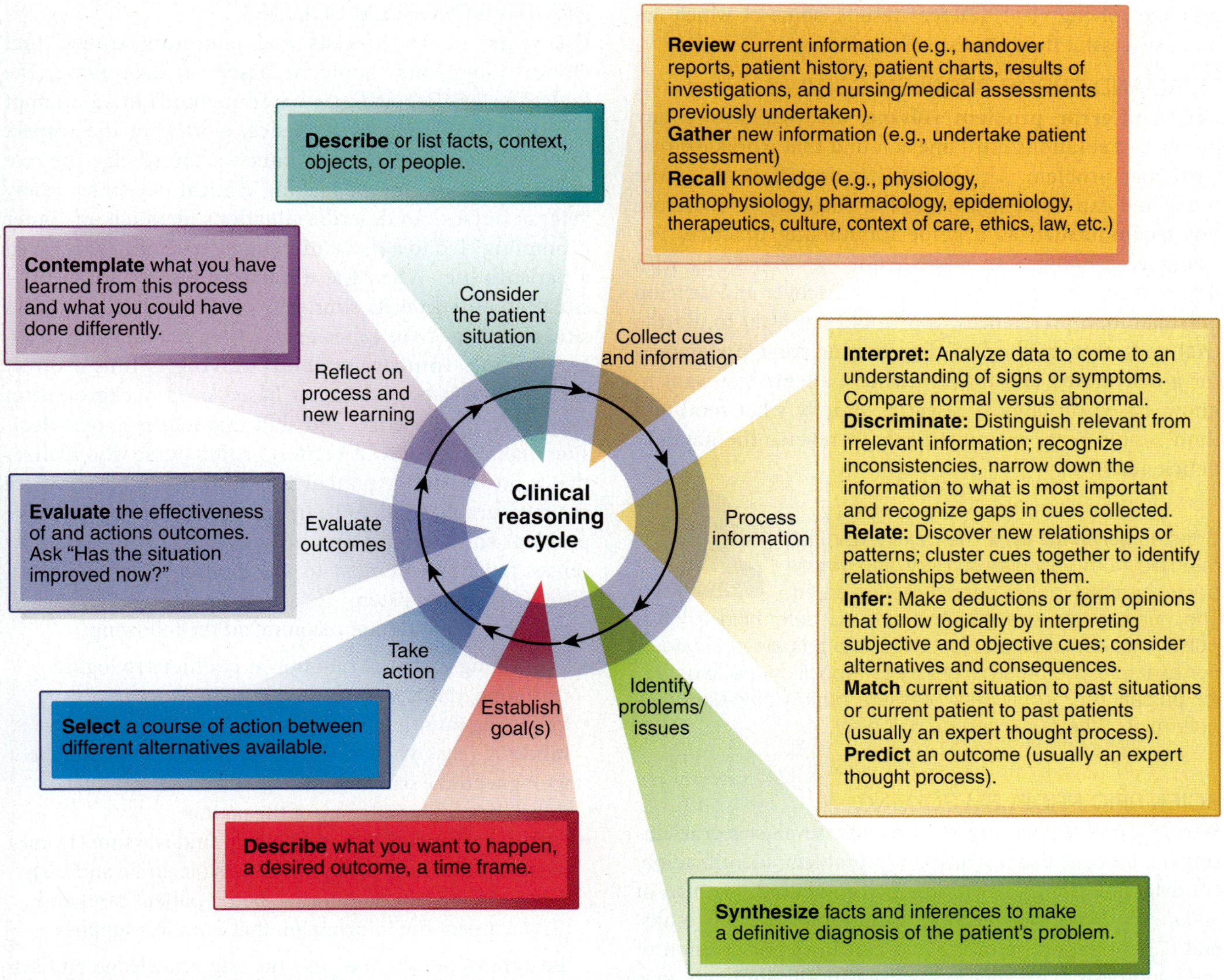

FIGURE 13-4. The clinical reasoning cycle. (*Source:* Reprinted from Elsevier, from Levett-Jones, T., Hoffman, K., Dempsey, J., Jeong, S. Y., Noble, D., Norton, C. A., Roche, J., & Hickey, N. [2010]. The "five rights" of clinical reasoning: An educational model to enhance nursing students' ability to identify and manage clinically "at risk" patients. *Nurse Education Today, 30*[6], 515–520, with permission from Elsevier.)

and reflect—these phases often merge and the boundaries between them become blurred. Remember to learn to recognize, understand, and work through each phase, rather than making assumptions about patient problems and initiating interventions that have not been adequately considered.

Effective use of the CR model by nursing students and its application in practice by novice nurses are directly linked to the five rights of clinical reasoning: the ability to collect the right cues and take the right action for the right patient at the right time and for the right reason (Levett-Jones et al., 2010). The demand on nurses to execute higher-order reasoning skills is increasing as clinical environments become more complex. This complexity requires nurses to be capable of clear, ordered thinking; identifying problems accurately; and effective decision making that demonstrates good clinical judgment (Hill et al., 2017, p. 262). Clinical reasoning includes the ability to recognize clinical problems and to solve them using the cognitive skills of critical thinking, creative thinking, and intuitive thinking. Using all of these skills, the clinician in the nursing context is capable of "thinking like a nurse" (Tanner, 2006, p. 204) in order to make a clinical judgment and come to a decision that results in a nursing action. You may find it helpful to ask these three questions:

1. What did you observe?
2. What do you make of what you saw?
3. What course of action will you take? (Koharchik et al., 2015)

Each of the nursing process chapters that follow has a section highlighting the type of clinical reasoning necessary to successfully implement that step of the nursing process.

Problem Solving

One of the strengths of clinical reasoning is that it is based on a methodology that is familiar to most nursing students: problem solving. Problem solving is a basic life skill; identifying a problem and then taking steps to resolve it are a matter of common sense. However, different approaches to problem solving yield different results, some of which are more successful than others.

TRIAL-AND-ERROR PROBLEM SOLVING

Trial-and-error problem solving involves testing any number of solutions until one is found that works for that particular problem. This method is not efficient for the nurse and can be dangerous to the patient; it is therefore not recommended as a guide for nursing practice. For example, although you might enjoy experimenting with different types of ethnic food as you discover and develop personal food preferences, you would not want to use the trial-and-error method of determining food preferences for a dehydrated and malnourished patient. You want to know, based on clinical research, exactly what food and fluid supplements are most likely to reverse the patient's deficiencies.

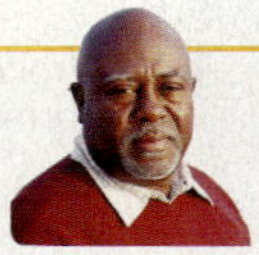

Consider ***Jermaine Byrd***, the patient who has returned from vascular surgery and whose posterior tibial pulse cannot be palpated. The nurse might use trial-and-error to determine if the pulse is indeed absent or just difficult to palpate or locate. For example, the nurse might try to reposition the fingers for palpation or apply less pressure during palpation to determine if the pulse can be palpated.

SCIENTIFIC PROBLEM SOLVING

Scientific problem solving is a systematic, seven-step problem-solving process that involves: (1) problem identification, (2) data collection, (3) hypothesis formulation, (4) plan of action, (5) hypothesis testing, (6) interpretation of results, and (7) evaluation, resulting in a conclusion or revision of the hypothesis. This method is used most commonly in a controlled laboratory setting but is closely related to the more general problem-solving processes commonly used by health care professionals as they work with patients. The nursing process is an example of this type of problem-solving process.

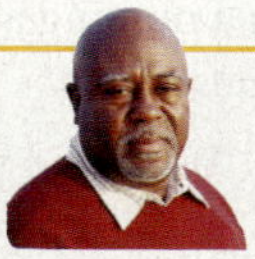

Again, think back to ***Jermaine Byrd***, the postoperative patient with a nonpalpable pulse. The nurse uses scientific problem solving to investigate the situation. For example, after attempts at repositioning yield no change, the nurse would collect more data, such as the temperature and the color of Mr. Byrd's extremity when compared with the opposite leg, existence of pulses above and below the posterior tibial pulse, complaints of pain, numbness, or tingling in the extremity, and Mr. Byrd's overall condition. These findings would lead the nurse to identify whether Mr. Byrd is experiencing vascular compromise, if his pulse was difficult to palpate, or if the nurse needs more skill in palpation. In addition, the nurse could summon the assistance of another nurse to negate or validate the findings. Once the problem is identified, the nurse can then plan care appropriately to meet Mr. Byrd's need.

INTUITIVE PROBLEM SOLVING

For years, nurse theorists and educators argued that clinical judgments should be based on data alone (the logical, scientific, evidence-based method) in an attempt to establish nursing as a science, worthy of the respect of other professions. Today, nurses acknowledge the role of intuitive thinking in making clinical decisions. Many veteran nurses can describe situations in which an "inner prompting" led to a quick nursing intervention that saved a patient's life. When these nurses directly apprehend a situation based on its similarity or dissimilarity to other situations they have experienced, they use intuitive problem solving. **Intuitive problem solving** is thus a direct understanding of a situation based on a background of experience, knowledge, and skill that makes expert decision making possible. A recovery room nurse who realizes that a postoperative patient is deteriorating before there are measurable signs to suggest trouble is using intuitive problem solving, as is an oncology nurse who somehow senses the right moment to teach, offer encouragement, affirm, or simply listen.

Advocates of intuition recommend the following:

- Welcoming flashes of intuition as additions to logical reasoning, rather than as disruptions
- Validating intuitions, and when an intuition cannot be validated (e.g., when the nurse senses that something is wrong with the patient, although there are no clinical signs), careful monitoring of the patient
- Furthering nursing research to help find ways to: (1) cultivate intuition and its typical results (accurate and early diagnosis, vigilant monitoring, better patient care) and (2) document the information that intuition supplies

Beginning nurses must use nursing knowledge and scientific problem solving as the basis for the care they give; intuitive problem solving comes with years of practice and observation. If the beginning nurse has an intuition about a patient, that information should be discussed with the faculty member, preceptor, or supervisor.

CRITICAL THINKING: INTUITIVE, LOGICAL, OR BOTH?

While this text makes a strong case for clinical reasoning that is logical, scientific, and evidence based, it also promotes clinical reasoning that is creative and intuitive. Alfaro-LeFevre, an expert in critical thinking, is quick to note that critical thinking is contextual and changes depending on the circumstances. As an example, she cites brainstorming sessions as a good method for nurturing intuition, because logical thinking may constrain and block ideas. On the other hand, developing policies, procedures, and plans of care requires more logical, evidence-based thought. In summary, when intuition is used alone, there are increased risks and fewer benefits. Intuition often moves problem solving forward quickly, but it may result in a lot of trial-and-error approaches. Logic is the safest approach, but it doesn't foster out-of-the-box ideas and may inhibit right-brain thinkers from getting started. Pairing intuitive and logical thinkers who have learned specific strategies to promote reasoning (e.g., mind mapping) can bring great results (Alfaro-LeFevre, 2020).

Concept Mastery Alert

Critical thinking often involves scientific problem solving, but it also involves intuition, logic, and creative thinking. A person integrates and adapts the use of all these strategies to address the situation.

Creative Thinking

Critical thinking and clinical reasoning also involve reflection and creative thinking. **Creative thinking** involves imagination, intuition, and spontaneity, factors that underpin the art of nursing. Creative thinking is brought into play when you ask "why" or "what if" questions and is most useful when conventional solutions have not resolved a situation. Creative nurse thinkers are able to "think outside the box" and imagine possible consequences, generate original approaches, and identify alternative perspectives. The solution to a challenge may involve resources as yet untapped, effective, and cost saving and may lead to interventions as yet undiscovered and untried. The process of brainstorming may bring out, along with unworkable options, one or two realistic suggestions that would not have surfaced otherwise. Each Reflective Practice box that opens a chapter invites readers to think outside the box as they contemplate possible courses of action.

CLINICAL JUDGMENT MODEL

For decades in nursing and nursing education, clinical judgment was taught using the nursing process. According to ANA (2021):

> Regardless of the theoretical knowledge base upon which nursing practice is derived, the knowledge fits within the multidimensioinal nursing process, the analytical, critical thinking framework guiding professional thinking and activities. The nursing process is conceptualized as a cyclic, iterative, and dynamic process, including assessment, diagnosis, outcomes identification, planning, implementation, and evaluation. The nursing process supports evidence-based practice and relies heavily on the bidirectional feedback loops between components (pp. 11–12).

Students learned the intricacies of assessing patients, diagnosing actual and potential health problems and needs, developing patient outcomes and related plans of care, and implementing and finally evaluating the plans of care. These processes are essential to learning how to think and practice like a nurse and are central to mastering the fundamentals of nursing. This unit describes each phase in the nursing process and your responsibilities. More recently, nurse educators are critiquing the nursing process as being too simple to adequately capture the processes of clinical judgment both beginning and experienced nurses use to ground their practice. A seminal article written by Tanner in 2006 offered a research-based model of clinical judgment highlighting four aspects:

- Noticing, a perceptual grasp of the situation at hand
- Interpreting, developing a sufficient understanding of the situation to respond
- Responding, deciding on a course of action deemed appropriate for the situation
- Reflecting, attending to patients' responses to the nursing action while in the process of acting.

Tanner aimed to offer a model to faculty to help students diagnose breakdowns, identify areas for needed growth, and focus attention on those areas. In 2007, Lasatar used the four phases of Tanner's clinical judgment model to provide the basis for a clinical judgment rubric. Her aim was to offer a bigger picture of clinical judgment development, which would allow students to grasp what clinical judgment involves, evaluate their growth in this area, and identify goals. In the Lasatar (2007) rubric, each of Tanner's four phases is further described by two or three dimensions that elucidate what is meant by each phase (see Table 14-1 on pages 386–387).

In 2009, the National Council of State Boards of Nursing (NCSBN) began to study the importance of clinical judgment in the nursing profession. Of note, their report found that 50% of entry level nurses were involved in practice errors (Smith & Crawford, 2003) and that 65% of entry level nurse errors were related to poor clinical decision making (Brennan et al., 2004). Not surprisingly, only 20% of employers were satisfied with the decision-making abilities of entry level nurses. Further NCSBN study revealed that clinical judgment was one of the top five required skills needed upon entry into the field of nursing. Two other high priority skills in the top five were problem solving and critical thinking. These studies led to the development of the NCSBN Clinical Judgment Measurement and Action Models, which are described in Chapter 14 (NCSBN, 2020). Chapter 14 also shows you how to use recurrent features in this text to help you become proficient in the different phases of the most common clinical judgment models. See Table 13-2 (on page 364) for a comparison of the uses and reasoning phases of each of three major clinical judgment models (CJMs) now influencing nursing education. Note that Alfaro is quick to point out that although CJMs are usually presented as linear models showing step-by-step progression, CJMs are iterative, meaning that the phases are interrelated and repetitive. They require paying attention to changing circumstances and continually reflecting and adjusting until the best results are achieved (Alfaro, 2020).

NURSING PROCESS

As the practice of nursing became more complex in the second half of the 20th century, nurses began to study the process of nursing to both understand and improve the means that nurses use to accomplish their aims.

Table 13-2 Three Major Clinical Judgment Models[a]

CLINICAL JUDGMENT MODEL AND COMMON USES	REASONING PHASES				
Nursing Process (ADPIE[b]) (NCLEX; Education; Simulation; Clinical practice; Interprofessional communication; Documentation)	Assess	Diagnose or Analyze[c]	Plan	Implement	Evaluate
Tanner/Lasater (Education; Simulation; Minimal clinical practice use)		Noticing/Interpreting	Responding		Reflecting
NCSBN CJAM[c] (NGN; No education or practice use as of 2019)		Recognize cues Analyze cues Prioritize hypotheses	Generate solutions	Take action	Evaluate outcomes

[a]Notice that using "phases" instead of "steps" implies that clinical reasoning is a fluid process rather than step by step.

[b]Assess, Diagnose, Plan, Implement, Evaluate.

[c]Clinical judgment requires more than analyzing—it requires bringing data together to come to conclusions (e.g., make decisions; determine priority risks and problems). Therefore, "Diagnose/Decide" may be a more appropriate term. Too many nurses spend too much time analyzing when there are *time pressures* to make decisions (some call this "analysis paralysis").

Source: Reprinted with permission from Alfaro-LeFevre, R. (2020). Comparison of Nursing Process, Tanner/Lasatar, and NGN Clinical Judgment Models. https://www.alfaroteachsmart.com/textbooktools.html.

Historical Perspective

Since Hall first used the term "nursing process" in 1955, many nurses have struggled to define exactly what constitutes the "work of nursing" and what makes nurses successful. In the 1960s, nursing theorists began to describe nursing as a distinct entity among the health care professions and also to delineate specific steps in a process approach to nursing practice. In 1967, Yura and Walsh published the first comprehensive book on nursing process, in which they described four steps in the nursing process: assessment, planning, intervention, and evaluation. They viewed the nursing diagnosis as the logical conclusion of the assessment phase, whereas Gebbie and Lavin (1974) later made nursing diagnosis a separate step in the process. These and other studies led to the development of the five-step nursing process commonly used today: assessment, diagnosis, outcome identification and planning, implementation, and evaluation. Although most nurses call this simply the nursing process, some use the acronym **ADPIE**, assessing, diagnosing, planning, implementing, and evaluating, or **AAPIE**, assessing, analyzing, planning, implementing, and evaluating.

The steps of the nursing process were legitimized in 1973, when the ANA Congress for Nursing Practice developed standards of practice to guide nursing performance. The scope defines the range and boundaries of nursing practice (see Chapter 1 for more information). The standards are authoritative statements by which the nursing profession describes responsibilities for which its practitioners are accountable. These standards were revised in 1991, 1998, 2004, 2010, 2015, and 2021. The six standards of practice (assessment, diagnosis, outcome identification, planning, implementation, and evaluation) describe a competent level of nursing care as demonstrated by the critical-thinking model of the nursing process. The nursing process encompasses all significant actions taken by registered nurses and forms the foundation of the nurse's decision making.

Although the ANA refers to a six-step nursing process, many practitioners still commonly refer to a five-step nursing process that combines outcome identification and planning into one step. The five-step nursing process is presented throughout this textbook.

The Joint Commission requires that care be documented according to the nursing process, and the National League for Nursing has recommended that educational programs incorporate the nursing process as their intellectual process. In 1982, the state board examinations for professional nursing practice underwent major revisions and began to use the nursing process as an organizing concept. The revised examinations are structured to test the practitioner's ability to assess patients, to diagnose health problems amenable to nursing therapy, and to plan, implement, and evaluate nursing care. The examinations had previously organized content on a medical model, structured according to medical specialties—medicine, surgery, maternity, pediatrics, and psychiatry. In 2023 or 2024, the state board examinations for professional nursing practice are scheduled to be based on the National Council of State Boards of Nursing's clinical judgment measurement model.

Description of the Nursing Process

The **nursing process** is a systematic method that directs the nurse, with the patient's participation, to accomplish the following: (1) assess the patient to determine the need for nursing care, (2) determine nursing diagnoses for actual and potential health problems and needs, (3) identify expected outcomes and plan care, (4) implement the care, and (5) evaluate the results. The phases in this person-centered, outcome-oriented process are interrelated; each phase depends on the accuracy of the steps preceding it. The process provides a framework that enables the nurse, along with the patient, to accomplish the following:

- Systematically collect patient data (assessing)
- Clearly identify patient strengths and actual and potential health problems and needs (diagnosing)

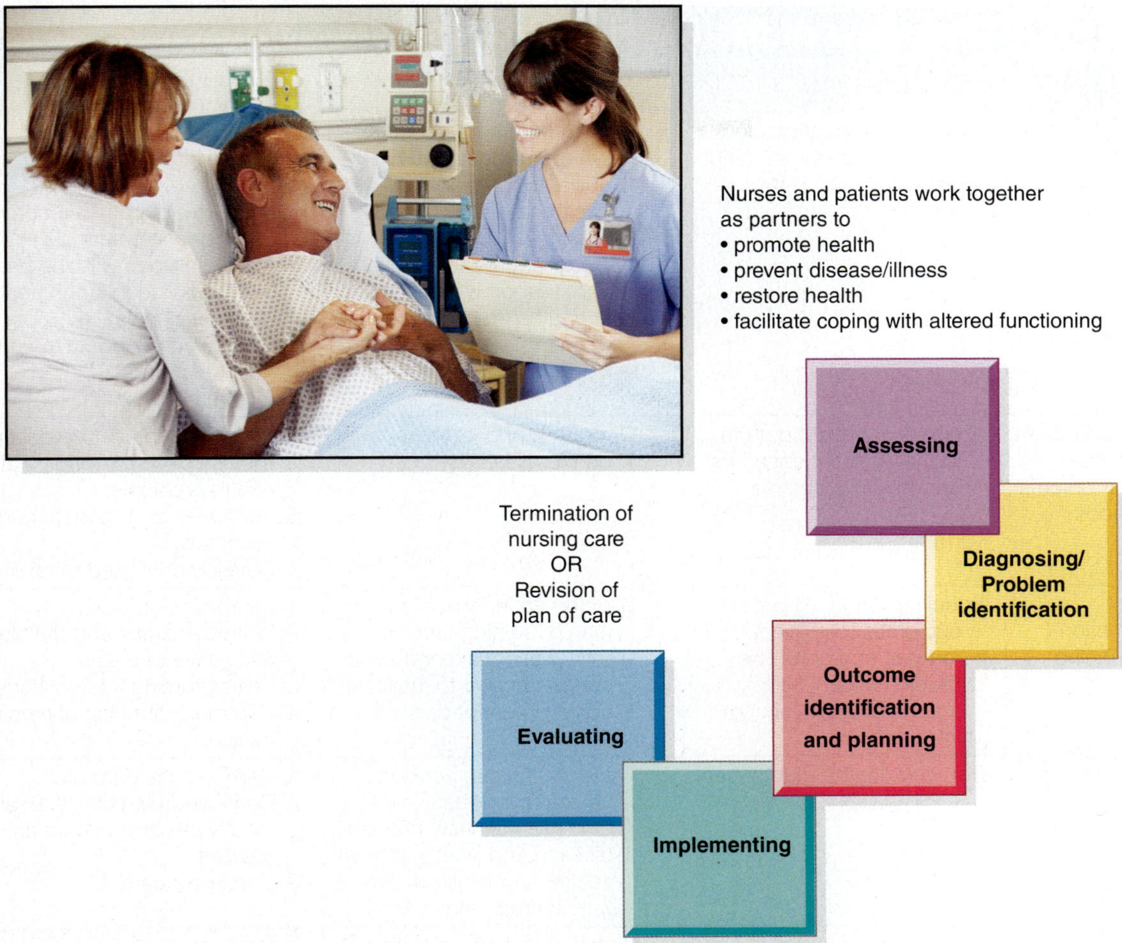

FIGURE 13-5. The iterative phases in the thoughtful, person-centered, outcome-oriented nursing process are dynamic and interrelated. Each of the five phases depends on the accuracy of the preceding step. (*Source:* Photo used with permission from Shutterstock. *Photo by Monkey Business Images.*)

- Develop a holistic plan of individualized care that specifies the desired patient goals and related outcomes and the nursing interventions most likely to assist the patient to meet those expected outcomes (planning)
- Execute the plan of care (implementing)
- Evaluate the effectiveness of the plan of care in terms of patient goal achievement (evaluating)

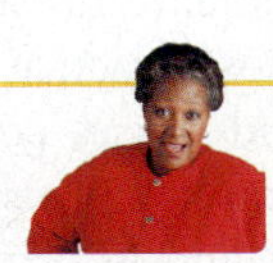

Consider **Addie Warner**, the older adult who had suffered a CVA and is considered "demanding" by some staff. The nurse uses the nursing process framework to determine the Mrs. Warner's presenting problem—that is, her reason for using the call light. By systematically collecting information, determining the Mrs. Warner's strengths and needs, quickly developing a plan for these needs, executing it, and then determining the effectiveness of the plan, the nurse provides Mrs. Warner with safe, quality, effective care.

The five phases of the nursing process are shown in Figure 13-5 and described in Table 13-3 (on page 366). In each phase of the process, the nurse and patient work together as partners (Fig. 13-6); the patient's health state and resources influence the patient's level of participation. When the patient is an infant or is unconscious or uncooperative, the nurse works through the steps of the process with the help of a family member or support person whenever possible.

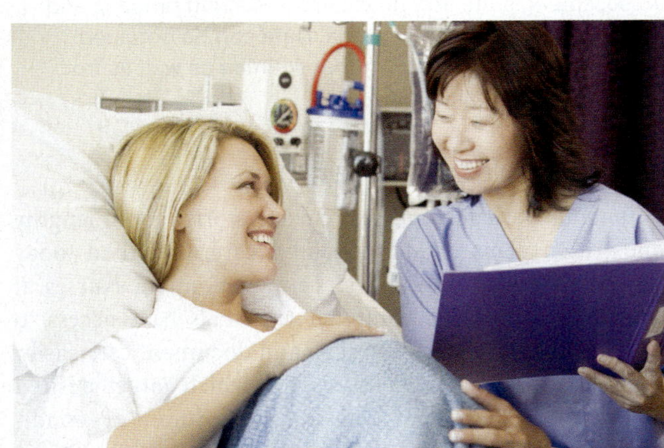

FIGURE 13-6. Nurses develop powerful partnerships with patients when using the nursing process to plan and deliver care.

Table 13-3 Overview of the Nursing Process

COMPONENT	DESCRIPTION	PURPOSE	ACTIVITIES
Assessing	Collection, validation, and communication of patient data	Make a judgment about the patient's health status, ability to manage their own health care, and need for nursing. Plan individualized holistic care that draws on patient strengths and is responsive to changes in the patient's conditions.	1. Establish the database: • Nursing history • Physical assessment • Review of patient record and nursing literature • Consultation with the patient's support people and health care professionals 2. Continuously update the database. 3. Validate data. 4. Communicate data.
Diagnosing Actual or Potential Health Problems and Needs	Analysis of patient data to identify patient strengths and health problems	Develop a prioritized list of problems/needs.	1. Interpret and analyze patient data. 2. Identify patient strengths and health problems. 3. Formulate and validate nursing problems. 4. Develop prioritized list of problems.
Outcome identification and planning	Specification of (1) patient outcomes to prevent, reduce, or resolve the problems identified; and (2) related nursing interventions	Develop an individualized plan of nursing care. Identify patient strengths that can be tapped to facilitate achievement of desired outcomes.	1. Establish priorities. 2. Write outcomes and develop an evaluative strategy. 3. Select nursing interventions. 4. Communicate plan of nursing care.
Implementing	Carrying out the plan of care	Assist patients to achieve desired outcomes—promote wellness, prevent disease and illness, restore health, and facilitate coping with altered functioning.	1. Carry out the care plan. 2. Continue data collection, and modify the plan of care as needed. 3. Document care.
Evaluating	Measuring the extent to which the patient has achieved the outcomes specified in the plan of care; identifying factors that positively or negatively influenced outcome achievement; revising the plan of care if necessary	Continue, modify, or terminate nursing care.	1. Measure how well the patient has achieved desired outcomes. 2. Identify factors that contribute to the patient's success or failure. 3. Modify the plan of care (if indicated).

Concept Mastery Alert

Assessment is the first phase in the nursing process and always involves gathering data. Data can be obtained from the patient, family, or other sources as well as from the physical examination.

Nursing Process Trends

Although experienced nurses may tell stories about lengthy handwritten plans of individualized care, the trend today is toward standardization and computerization. Nurses at centralized or bedside computer terminals have access to databases that allow them to plan and document care easily. Critical pathways (see Chapter 17)—which target desired outcomes for particular illnesses, procedures, or conditions—and accompanying multidisciplinary staff actions along a timeline provide the standard guidelines for care in many institutions. Although there were national efforts to develop the state of nursing knowledge and science and a standard nursing language (described in Table 13-4), today most practice sites do not use standard nursing language and nurses contribute to common problem and intervention lists. This work is described in subsequent chapters on diagnosis, planning, and implementation.

Characteristics of the Nursing Process

Various words and phrases have been used to describe the nursing process. Key descriptors include *systematic*, *dynamic*, *interpersonal*, *outcome oriented*, and *universally applicable*.

Systematic

Each nursing activity is part of an ordered sequence of activities. Moreover, each activity depends on the accuracy

Table 13-4 Examples of Groups Developing Standard Languages (Vocabularies)

GROUP NAME	FOCUS	PURPOSE
North American Nursing Diagnosis Association (NANDA) International	Diagnoses	Increase the visibility of nursing's contribution to patient care by continuing to develop, refine, and classify phenomena of concern to nurses (see Nursing Diagnosis Quick Reference section). *Website:* www.nanda.org
Nursing Interventions Classification (NIC)	Interventions	Identify, label, validate, and classify actions nurses perform, including direct and indirect care interventions (interventions done directly with patients, e.g., teaching; those done indirectly, e.g., obtaining laboratory studies). *Website:* https://nursing.uiowa.edu/cncce/nursing-interventions-classification-overview
Nursing-Sensitive Outcomes Classification (NOC)	Outcomes	Identify, label, validate, and classify nursing-sensitive patient outcomes and indicators to evaluate the validity and usefulness of the classification, and define and test measurement procedures for the outcomes and indicators. *Website:* https://nursing.uiowa.edu/cncce/nursing-outcomes-classification-overview
Home Health Care Classification (HHCC)	Diagnoses, interventions, and outcomes	Provide a structure for documenting and classifying home health and ambulatory care. Consists of two interrelated taxonomies: HHCC of Nursing Diagnoses and HHCC of Nursing Interventions. *Website:* http://www.sabacare.com
International Classification for Nursing Practice (ICNP)	Diagnoses, interventions, and outcomes	Capture nursing's contributions to health and provide a framework into which existing vocabularies and classifications can be cross-mapped, enabling comparison of nursing data from various countries throughout the world. *Website:* https://www.icn.ch/what-we-do/projects/ehealth-icnp/about-icnp
Systematized Nomenclature of Medicine—Clinical Terms (SNOMED CT)	Comprehensive clinical terminology	Integrate, link, and map terms from various disciplines such as medicine, nursing, and occupational therapy. *Website:* https://www.nlm.nih.gov/healthit/snomedct/index.html

Source: Adapted with permission from Alfaro-LeFevre, R. (2014). *Applying nursing process: A tool for critical thinking* (8th ed., p. 100). Wolters Kluwer/Lippincott Williams & Wilkins.

of the activity that precedes it and influences the actions that follow it. Without a complete and accurate database, the nurse cannot identify patient strengths and problems. Lacking knowledge of these, the nurse and patient cannot develop a plan of care based on realistic and valued patient goals. Unless the goals and outcomes are well written, nursing actions and evaluation lack focus and might be ineffective. The nursing process directs each step of nursing care in a sequential, ordered manner.

Concept Mastery Alert

During the evaluation phase, the nurse reviews the patient's outcome attainment and determines if outcomes have been met, partially met, or not met. Evidence interpretation is more associated with the diagnosing/problem identification phase.

Dynamic

Although the nursing process is presented as an orderly progression of phases, in reality, there is great interaction and overlapping among the five phases. No single phase in the nursing process is a one-time phenomenon; each phase flows into the next. In some nursing situations, all five phases occur almost simultaneously.

Interpersonal

Always at the heart of nursing is the human being. Read one student's account of this truth in the accompanying Through the Eyes of a Student feature (on page 368). The nursing process ensures that nurses are person centered rather than task centered (Fig. 13-7). Rather than simply approaching a patient to take vital signs, the nurse might ask, "How are you today, Mr. Byrd? Are we helping you to achieve your

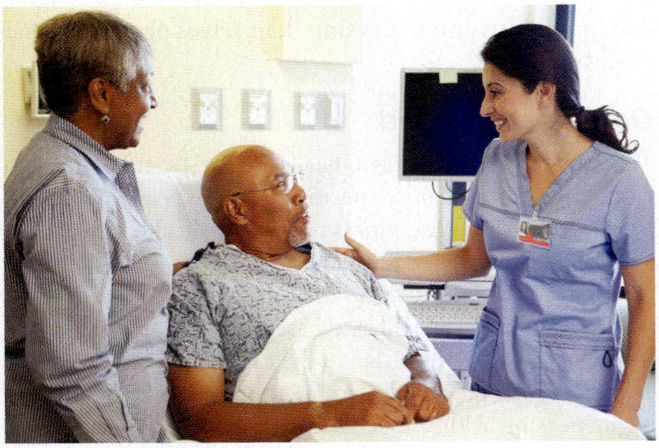

FIGURE 13-7. Nurses focus on people, not problems or tasks. The nursing process is thoughtful and person centered, not task centered.

Through the Eyes of a Student

My first experience with an open wound was with a woman who had a stage IV sacral decubitus. I needed to do a dressing change with packing. I was fearful of what the wound would look like. I thought for sure I was going to be "grossed out," and I was—not by the appearance of the wound, but by the odor. The stench was awful! I started to feel queasy and began to sweat, and I thought I was going to pass out and fall right over on the patient. While I was packing the wound, I kept thinking that I was never going to get out of that room. I looked over at my clinical instructor and searched her face for approval of my technique, and I wondered if she also smelled anything and if it was making her feel sick too!

After the procedure was over and I left the room, I asked my instructor if all wounds smell that awful and would the smell always make me feel sick. Her response was that sometimes an odor will be really bad, and it might make me feel sick. With this kind of reassurance, I thought this is it—I never want to smell that again, and no way do I want to be a nurse.

Later, I realized that I had forgotten there was someone else in that room: the patient. She had to stay in there with that wound and its odor. It was for this reason I changed my mind about leaving nursing. I remembered that it was wanting to help patients to deal with their wounds that made me decide to be a nurse in the first place.

—Barbara L. Dlugosz
Holy Family University, Philadelphia, PA

goals? What are the most important things you would like to accomplish today? [or] What are the most important things you would like us to work on today?" The nurse might also consider any new data that indicate a need to modify the patient's plan of care.

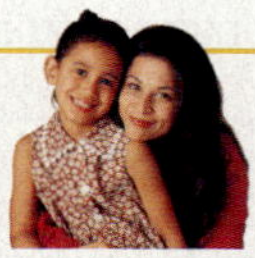

Consider **Charlotte Horvath**, the single mother who requires wound care teaching but has failed to attend any scheduled teaching sessions. A nurse who values the interpersonal dimensions of nursing would investigate with Ms. Horvath the reasons underlying her inability to make the teaching sessions. This investigation may reveal many reasons, such as an inability to get away from work, fear, feelings of being overwhelmed, or lack of awareness about the importance of the wound care.

The nursing process encourages nurses to work together to help patients use their strengths to meet all their human health needs. This is different from viewing the patient as a "problem to be solved" and interacting mechanically to provide the solution. Working intimately with patients helps nurses to explore their own strengths and limitations and to develop themselves personally and professionally.

Outcome Oriented

The nursing process offers a means for nurses and patients to work together to identify specific outcomes related to health promotion, disease and illness prevention, health restoration, and coping with altered functioning; to determine which outcomes are most important to the patient; and to match them with the appropriate evidence-based nursing actions. When these outcomes are recorded in the care plan and prioritized, each nurse can quickly determine the patient's priorities and begin nursing with a clear sense of how to proceed. The patient benefits from continuity of care, and each nurse's care moves the patient closer to outcome achievement.

Universally Applicable in Nursing Situations

The one constant in health care is change. When nurses have a working knowledge of the nursing process, they find that they can practice nursing with well or ill people, young or old, in any type of practice setting. Mastering the nursing process gives you a valuable tool you can use with ease in any nursing situation.

It should be clear from this discussion that the nursing process provides a framework for all the nurse's activities. In each nurse–patient interaction, it is important to assess the patient, note any significant alterations in health status, determine whether the nursing action is helping the patient achieve their goals, and modify the care plan as necessary. Thus, the nurse who feeds a child through a special tube as ordered by a health care provider continually assesses how the child is responding to the feeding and whether the child or family will be able to manage the feedings independently when the child is discharged. Depending on the results of the nursing assessment, new diagnoses or problems may be indicated, along with related additions to the plan of care. The nursing process offers direction for all the activities carried out by the nurse when caring for patients.

Documenting the Nursing Process

The ability to communicate clearly is a critical nursing skill. Accurate, concise, timely, and relevant documentation provides all the members of the caregiving team with a picture of the patient. The patient record is the chief means of communication among members of the interdisciplinary team. Legally speaking, a nursing action that was not documented was not performed. If accused of negligent care, a nurse might tell the court of having faithfully assessed the patient's needs, diagnosed problems, and implemented and evaluated an effective care plan. However, unless the patient's health records contain documentation supporting these claims, the court has no reason to accept the nurse's word rather than that of the patient or family who are claiming that such care was not given.

Each chapter in this unit offers specific documentation guidelines for nursing process activities; Chapter 20 discusses

Box 13-8 Example of the Nursing Process in Action

Assessing

You are checking on a patient who had abdominal surgery yesterday and hear that the patient has considerable pain: "It kept me up all night." The patient has been reluctant to ask for any pain medication, fearing effects of the drug. "I don't want to become a junkie." The patient's blood pressure and pulse rate are slightly elevated.

Diagnosing/Problem Identification

You analyze the data just described and identify pain/discomfort as a problem. The patient agrees that this is becoming a problem.

Outcome Identification and Planning

You decide to work with the patient to achieve the outcome: *By 1500, patient reports sufficient relief of pain to enable him to rest and to get out of bed to go to the bathroom.* The patient wants to accomplish the outcome. You identify teaching as the primary evidence-based nursing intervention.

Implementing

After asking the patient about his experiences with pain-relieving medications, you explain that although many of these drugs are addictive when misused, there is no harm if they are taken as prescribed postoperatively. You also explain that it is important for him to experience enough pain relief to be able to cough and deep breathe, ambulate, and do other things important to his recovery. You suggest that the medication will be most effective if taken before his pain peaks and becomes intense. You administer the prescribed medication for pain when the patient indicates that he is willing to give it a try.

Evaluating

After enough time has elapsed for the medication to take effect, you check back with the patient to evaluate whether he has obtained relief and met his outcome. If the patient is satisfied and you both feel that comfort is no longer a problem, you terminate the care plan for this diagnosis. If the patient still feels pain or is dissatisfied with the medication, each of the preceding steps of the nursing process is reevaluated, and necessary changes are made in the care plan.

documentation in general. It is helpful to practice documentation while learning any given nursing activity; like any other nursing skill, documentation improves with practice. Examples of nursing documentation, nursing assessments, plans of care, and notes are provided throughout this text.

Benefits of the Nursing Process

When used well, the nursing process achieves for the patient scientifically based, holistic, individualized care; the opportunity to work collaboratively with nurses and other team members; and continuity of care. Nurses who use the nursing process in a thoughtful and systematic way achieve a clear, efficient, and cost-effective plan of action by which the entire nursing team can achieve the best results for patients; the satisfaction that they are making an important difference in the lives of their patients; and the opportunity to grow professionally as they evaluate the effectiveness of interventions and variables that contribute positively or negatively to the patient's achievement of valued outcomes. See Box 13-8 for an example of the nursing process in action. The accompanying Promoting Health Literacy box is another example of how nurses can make a difference.

Evaluating the Use of the Nursing Process

The primary purpose of the nursing process is to help nurses committed to thoughtful, person-centered practice manage each patient's care scientifically, holistically, and creatively.

Promoting Health Literacy

IN PATIENTS AND FAMILIES WITH ASTHMA

Patient Scenario

Your mom calls to tell you that your neighbor back home spent the night in the emergency department with her 3-year-old son Bobby, whom you used to baby-sit. When Bobby experienced chest tightness and shortness of breath, his pediatrician recommended a quick trip to the local emergency department. For the present, Bobby's parents are comforted that he was able to be discharged and is now breathing easier. They were terrified, however, to learn that he may have asthma and wanted your opinion on what they should do. They have an appointment scheduled with their pediatrician.

Nursing Considerations: *Tips for Improving Health Literacy*

Call Bobby's mom and give her an information sheet about childhood asthma and tips on finding out more information about the disease online from a credible source. Explain that it is a potentially serious disorder if not treated properly, but with good management children are able to sleep, learn, and play. Encourage her to follow the pediatrician's recommendations and to be prepared to ask her pediatrician three questions:

- What is Bobby's main problem?
- What do they need to do?
- Why is it important for them to do this?

What additional measures can you take to help increase health literacy in this patient/family? What other measures would be helpful if Bobby's parents do not speak English, cannot read, or have learning difficulties?

Box 13-9 Checklist for Evaluating Your Use of the Nursing Process

Assessing

- ☐ The initial database is obtained by means of a nursing history and nursing examination.
- ☐ Assessment data are documented:
  - ☐ Accurately—Questionable data are validated.
  - ☐ Completely—Use of a systematic guide ensures that recorded data describe (1) the patient's functional ability to meet each basic human need, and (2) responses to health and illness.
  - ☐ Concisely—Irrelevant data and meaningless generalizations are avoided.
  - ☐ Factually—Patient behaviors are recorded rather than the nurse's interpretation of these behaviors.
  - ☐ Timely—Current data are recorded for the team.
- ☐ The initial database communicates a "real sense" of the patient that makes possible individualized care.
- ☐ Focused assessment data are recorded for each patient problem.
- ☐ Data collection and documentation are ongoing and responsive to changes in the patient's condition.

Diagnosing/Problem Identification

- ☐ A prioritized list of actual or potential health problems and needs is in the care plan.
- ☐ Each problem statement:
  - ☐ Is derived from an accurate and validated interpretation of a cluster of significant patient data or "cues"
  - ☐ Contains a precise problem statement describing what is unhealthy about the patient and what needs to change—suggests patient goals
  - ☐ Identifies factors that contribute to the problem (etiology)—these suggest nursing interventions
  - ☐ Uses nonjudgmental language and is written using legally advisable terms
- ☐ Each problem is compatible with institution/agency guidelines.
- ☐ Old problems are deleted from the care plan once resolved, and new problems are added as soon as identified.

Outcome Identification and Planning

- ☐ A comprehensive, individualized, and up-to-date care plan that specifies patient outcomes and nursing orders for each diagnosis/problem is developed with the assistance of the patient and family.
- ☐ Planning is comprehensive:
  - ☐ Initial
  - ☐ Ongoing
  - ☐ Discharge
- ☐ Long-term goals alert the entire nursing team to realistic patient expectations after discharge.
- ☐ Short-term outcomes:
  - ☐ When achieved, demonstrate a resolution of the patient problem
  - ☐ Describe a single, observable, and measurable patient behavior
  - ☐ Are valued by the patient and family
  - ☐ Are realistic in terms of the resources of the patient and the nurse
- ☐ Nursing orders:
  - ☐ Clearly and concisely describe the nursing intervention to be performed (ongoing assessment; nursing treatments and procedures; teaching, counseling, advocacy)
  - ☐ Are individualized to the patient
  - ☐ Are consistent with standards of care and supportive of other therapies/evidence-based practice
  - ☐ Are effective in accomplishing the desired patient outcomes
- ☐ The care plan encourages patient and family participation.

Implementing

- ☐ The patient record contains daily documentation of the nursing measures used to (1) assist the patient to meet basic human needs, (2) resolve health problems, and (3) implement select aspects of the medical care plan.
- ☐ The care plan is implemented:
  - ☐ Competently
  - ☐ Confidently
  - ☐ Responsibly
  - ☐ Caringly
  - ☐ Creatively

Evaluating

- ☐ Evaluative statements are recorded on the care plan to document the patient's level of outcome achievement at targeted times.
- ☐ Ongoing evaluation of the patient's responses to the care plan is used to make decisions about terminating, continuing, or modifying nursing care.

To do this successfully, the nurse needs the correct personal attributes, a sound knowledge base, and many competencies, along with the willingness to use them creatively and critically when working with patients to promote or restore health, prevent disease or illness, and facilitate coping with altered functioning.

The chapters that follow in this unit describe each step of the nursing process in detail. As a student nurse beginning to use the nursing process, you should evaluate your growing skill in using the nursing process correctly. The assessment tool in Box 13-9 will help you assess your proficiency in the skills essential for competent use of the nursing process. After completing the exercise, share your self-evaluation with a trusted colleague or clinical instructor and see whether your assessment of your abilities agrees with your colleague's or instructor's assessment. Celebrate your natural and developed strengths. Begin now to plan a strategy to boost those skills in which you are deficient. It may sound trite, but it is true: Your patients will be grateful you cared enough to be your best. Nurses sensitive to mastering both the art and the science of thoughtful, person-centered practice evaluate whether they have the prerequisite skills for each nurse–patient encounter, as well as the skills needed to perceive, respond to, and appreciate the uniqueness of each patient. Quality care is each nurse's responsibility.

Concept Mapping

Concept mapping is an instructional strategy in which learners identify, graphically display in a diagram or drawing, and identify interrelationships between core concepts.

Concept maps—also called cognitive maps, mind maps, and metacognitive tools for learning—are a proven means to promote critical thinking and self-directed learning. They allow for a visual picture of the internal processes nurses use in critical thinking and relationship analysis. Be alert . . . your concept maps offer your instructor a key visual about how your brain is working and your developing ability to link related concepts.

Schmehl (2014, p. 3) articulates that "concept mapping, as it is used in nursing, serves as a pathway to the intersection of critical thinking and theory-to-practice application." Concepts maps assist nursing students in designing a care plan based on the individual patient concerns and problems. Using a concept map promotes critical thinking, the ability to recognize relationships and connection between data, and the ability to apply this knowledge to patient care (Schmehl, 2014).

There are many excellent resources that discuss different ways to approach concept mapping. Schuster (2016) uses boxes to cluster, organize, and link information.

According to Schmehl (2014), the basic steps in concept map care planning are as follows:

1. *Collect patient problems and concerns on a list.* Remember that this list can include a symptom, a lab value, a diagnostic test result, a treatment, or collaborative care concerns. These data can be obtained by you from the assessment, from the patient directly, from the medical record, and from interactions with the interprofessional team.
2. *Connect and analyze the relationships*, differentiating between groupings of main and related problems. Take time to question, compare, contrast, and group your data.
3. *Create a diagram* demonstrating problem recognition, critical thinking, and nursing actions. Use shapes, connecting lines, descriptive phrases, and learning styles to emphasize nursing actions related to the care plan. As your concept maps become more complex, use a key with your diagram to keep track of what each box, link, shape, or color represents. Keep in mind that creativity is encouraged; no two maps will look the same!
4. *Keep in mind key concepts*: the nursing process, holism, safety, and advocacy.

Figure 13-8 (on pages 372–376) presents examples of concept maps prepared by a student with the related patient database problem list forms. Simple concept maps demonstrating the nursing process for featured patients can be found in Chapters 31, 33, 34, 40, 41, and 45.

REFLECTIVE PRACTICE

Reflection is a normal human activity. We frequently think about what has just happened and how it has affected us, but often this reflection is superficial. **Reflective practice** is a purposeful activity that leads to action, improvement of practice, and better patient outcomes. It is about looking at an event, understanding it, and learning from it. Learning from reflection is not automatic; it requires a deeper understanding of how and why reflection contributes to the competence of the effective nurse. Schön (1983) has identified three types of reflection.

1. *Reflection in action* happens in the here and now of the activity and is also known as "thinking on your feet."
2. *Reflection on action* occurs after the fact and involves thinking through a situation that has occurred in the past. It is used as a means of evaluating the experience and deciding what could have been done differently.
3. *Reflection for action* is the desired outcome of the first two types of reflection: it helps the person to think about how future actions might change as a result of the reflection.

Gibbs's model of reflective practice (1988) is used by many nurses to learn from and improve their practice (Table 13-5 on page 377).

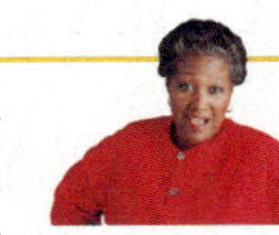

Suppose the nursing student caring for **Addie Warner** mistakenly gives her the medications she was supposed to give to another patient. She can use the critical reflection in action through the critical incident analysis described in Table 13-6 (on page 377) to learn from this experience.

Try to identify a recent situation that left you feeling disappointed in yourself. Then use Gibbs's reflective cycle questions to analyze what happened so that you can use what you learned about yourself to guide future experiences.

Nurses who are sincerely committed to thoughtful, person-centered care learn early to make reflection and self-evaluation an integral part of their nursing practice. Self-evaluation skills promote professional development, enhance self-esteem, and help you develop self-awareness. The Reflective Practice exercises in each chapter illustrate this practice. Each exercise describes a particular challenge to the student's competence, a range of possible responses, the criteria the student used to evaluate a good response, and a brief statement about what the student learned from this experience. A nurse who is just beginning to develop in the caregiver role may find it helpful to conclude each caregiving experience with a brief moment of reflection that identifies and celebrates the nursing skills used and targets skills that still need to be developed. This practice can keep you from feeling overwhelmed by everything that remains to be mastered and yet strongly motivated to learn new skills.

DEVELOPING CLINICAL REASONING AND CLINICAL JUDGMENT

1. A nursing student realizes that her college roommate's behavior has changed dramatically during the past month. Once outgoing and funny, the roommate is now withdrawn and moody, rebuffing efforts to discuss her behavior changes. Compare and contrast the processes and likely outcomes of using different methods

(text continues on page 377)

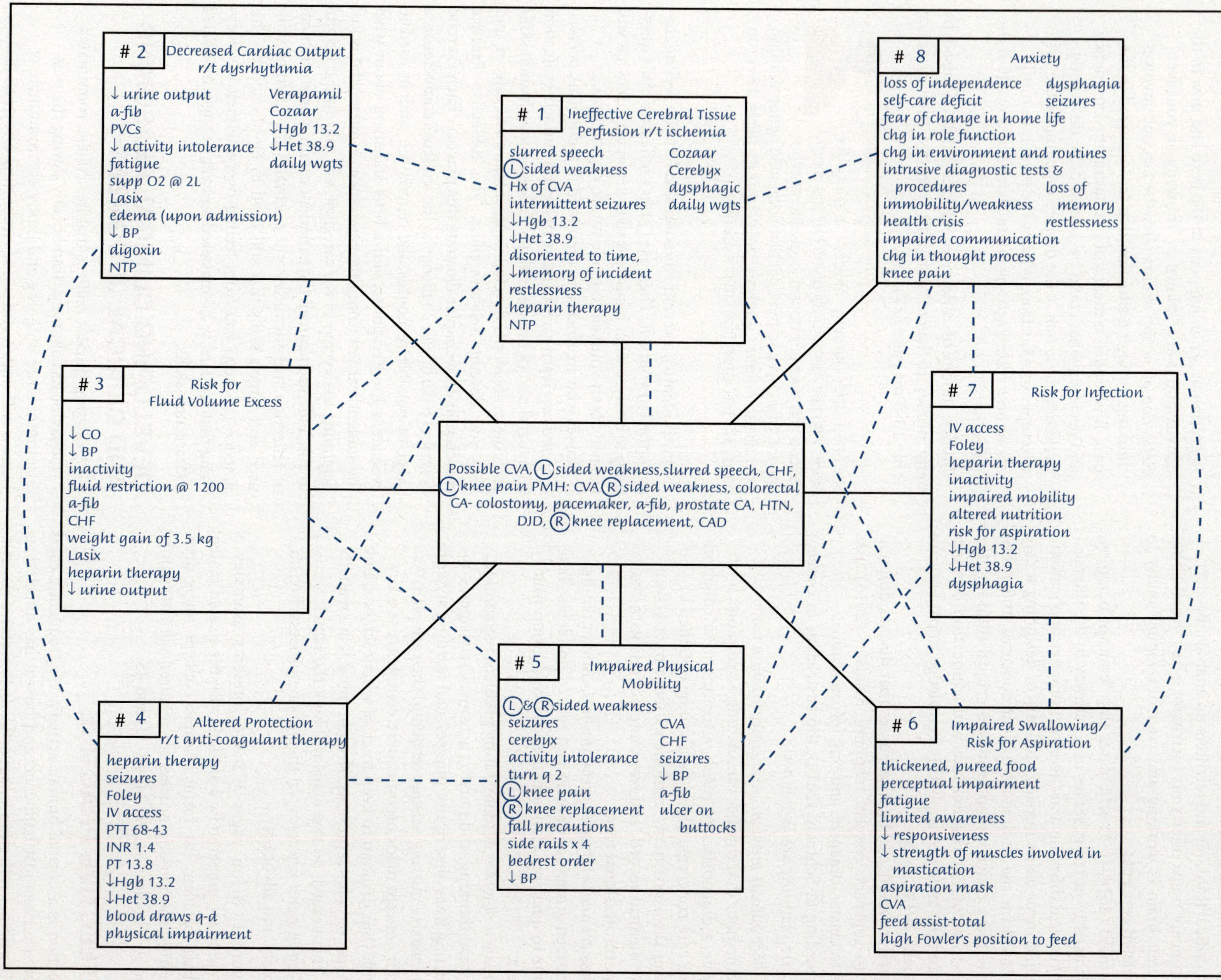

FIGURE 13-8. Sample beginning concept map focused on data clustering. (*Source:* Adapted from Schuster, P. M. [2002]. *Concept mapping: A critical-thinking approach to care planning.* F.A. Davis. Completed forms used with permission from Janet Heck, Delaware County Community College.) (*continued*)

Patient Database

Admission Information			**Student Name:** JANET HECK		
Date of Care 2—27—24	**Patient Initials** DR	**Age** 79	**Growth & Development** Ego Integrity vs Despair	**Sex** M	**Adm date** 2—24—24

Medical Diagnosis/Surgical Procedure:
Possible CVA, (L) sided weakness, slurred speech, CHF, (L) knee pain

Past Medical History: CVA (R) sided weakness, colorectal CA—colostomy, pacemaker, A-fib, prostate CA, HTN, DJD, (R) knee replacement, CAD

Psychosocial History	**Smoking** yes (no)	**Alcohol** yes (no)
Religious Preference: Protestant	**Marital Status:** Widower	
Health Care Insurance: Keystone 65	**Occupation:** Retired	
Advanced Directives	**Living Will** yes (no)	**Do Not Rescucitate** yes (no)

Medications:	**Allergies:** NKA
Name of Medication	**Why is patient taking this medication?**
IV Heparin 24 cc/hr /raised to 28 cc/hr per PTT protocol	anti-coagulant -prevention of thrombi (a-fib)
K-DUR 20 meQ qd	potassium supplement (K 3.5)
Lasix 40 mg po qd	diuretic - treat CHF/edema upon admission
Digoxin 0.25 mg po qd	to treat a-fib, ↑ CO
Verapamil SR 120 mg qd	calcium channel blocker, treat dysrhythmia (a-fib)
NTP 1" q 6 to chest wall	coronary dilator, ↑ blood flow, treat CHF ↓ BP
Protonix 40 mg qd	suppress gastric acid
Cozaar 50 mg & Het 212.5 mg qd	blocks angiotension II, acts to vasodilate & ↓ BP
Cerebyx 1000 mg IV @ 10 cc/hr	anti-convulsant; treat seizures

Laboratory Data

Lab Value	On adm	Current	Why abnormal	Lab Value	On adm	Current	Why abnormal
WBS	8.6	9.2	WNL	Na	128	NOT DONE	WNL
Hemoglobin	14.1	13.2↓	heparin; ↓nutrition	K	3.5	"	WNL (but K supp administered)
Hematocrit	42.2	38.9↓	heparin; ↓nutrition	Cr	1.2	"	WNL
Platelets	233	232	WNL	BUN	11	"	WNL
PT	13.8	—	WNL	Blood Glucose	114	"	WNL
INR	1.4	—		ABG	NOT DONE		
PTT	68	43↓	heparin therapy	Other Mg	1.9	"	WNL
Troponin	<0.5	—	WNL	Other CA	8.5	"	WNL
CPK	47	—	WNL	Other Dig	1.4	"	WNL

Diagnostic Tests

CXR ✓shows CHF	**EKG** ✓A-fib	**Echocardiogram** —
Other CT-scan (−) No Δ; bleed (x2)	**Other**	

FIGURE 13-8. *(continued)*

Treatments:	Daily wgts
	Pulse Ox q shift – > 90% (on 2L NC)
	No neuro checks ordered
	Turn q 2•

Diet

Type: Pureed, ↓NA 2 gm	**Restrictions:** thickened only 1200 cc po fluid	**Appetite:** Good
Difficulty Swallowing: (yes) no		**Assist with Feeds:** (yes) no

Fluid Status

IV solution & rate:	Heparin 28 cc/hr	**Type of IV access:**	Peri	**Site condition:**	Ø swelling, Ø redness
24 hr intake:	1460	**24 hr output:**	1000	**Balance:**	+460
5 hr intake:	480	**5 hr output:**	250	**Balance:**	+230
Weight:	86.2 kg admin; 89.7 kg		**Amount of gain or loss:**		+3.5 kg

Elimination

Continent:	**Bladder:** (yes) no	**Bowel:** (yes) no
Foley: (yes) no	**Urine color:** dark amber	**Last BM:** 2/27/24

Activity

Activity Order: Bedrest	**Gait:** N/A	**Use of Assistive Devices:** N/A
Risk for Falls: (yes) no	**Weakness:** (yes) no	**Restraints:** yes (no)

Vital Signs 8 am	**BP** 112/60	**P** 66	**R** 16	**T** 97 SAO2 99%
Any additional vs 1200	94/60	70	18	97 (AX) SAO2 99%

Narrative Assessment Notes for Clinical Day:

2/27/24 0800. Rec'd pt sleeping– responsive to verbal stimuli. Pt is oriented to person, place only. Responds slowly c̄ one word answers or head motion. Heparin infusion running at 24 cc/hr s̄ incident IV site #11 shows ↓ swelling and ↓ redness. Pt denies pain. VS BP 112/60, T 97+(0); P66, R16, Pt on 2L O_2 via nc, SAO_2 @ 99%. Pt has colostomy bag - no BM present. Foley draining c̄ dark amber urine. Pt's lungs are clear but decreased in bases. BS(+), Radial and DI pulses palpable +2. Skin warm and dry. Rash evident on face– pt picks and scratches at face especially nose and mouth frequently. Inspected nose and mouth, both clear c̄ no evidence of inflammation or sores. Pt weak in both LE and upper extremities, limited mvmt. Pt grimaces upon manipulation or mvmt of (L) knee. (R) arm spasms frequently– subsides c̄ touch. Pt dozes on & off but responsive to verbal stimuli. Pt has duoderm on (L) buttock - unable to inspect wound. Complete bed bath given c̄ mouthcare, pt tolerated well. Capillary refill brisk. ↓ edema present. PEARL; heart sounds S, S_2 c̄ murmur ———— JM DCCCSN

FIGURE 13-8. (*continued*)

Problem #1 Ineffective Cerebral Tissue Perfusion r/t ischemia (thrombosis)
Short-term Goal: Cerebral perfusion pressure will be maintained during hospital stay.
Long-term Goal: Pt will participate in rehabilitation exercises to regain optimal strength in (L) extremities.

Nursing Interventions:	Patient's Response:
1. Monitor VS q 4, check pupils	1. BP 112/60, T97, P66, RR16, PEARL @ 0800
2. Monitor I & O strict q shift.	2. BP 94/60, T97, P70, RR18, PEARL @ 1200
3. Monitor pulse Ox q shift	3. Pt on restricted 1200 cc fluids po, 5 hr intake=480, SAO_2 99% on 2L NC.
4. Keep head of bed 30 or lower (except when feeding)	4. Pt responsive to verbal stimuli, oriented to person & place.
5. Cluster activities to ↓ ICP.	5. Pt tolerated assessment, bath and feeding before tiring.
6. Administer heparin infusion.	6. Pts PTT 68 to 43.

Summarize your impressions of patient progress towards goals: Pt displays Ø worsening of symptoms of reduced of cerebral perfusion. Continue interventions.

Problem #2 Decreased Cardiac Output r/t dysrhythmia
Short-term Goal: Pt will maintain optimally compensated cardiac output evidenced by clear lung sounds, Ø SOB, increased urine output on ↑activity tolerance while hospitalized.
Long-term Goal: Pt will comply c̄ medication regimen to maintain optimal cardiac output after discharge.

Nursing Interventions:	Patient's Response:
1. Assess rate & quality of apical & peripheral pulses.	1. Pulses palpable +2, apical rate S_1S_2 c murmur; Ø pulse deficit.
2. Assess BP q 4	2. BP 112/60 @ 0800, 94/80 @ 1200.
3. Assess lung sounds q 2	3. Lungs clear but decreased in bases bilaterally.
4. Assess urine output.	4. Urine output 50 cc/hr (250 in 5 hrs)
5. Assess SAO_2.	5. Pt SAO_2 99% c 2L O_2 via nc.
6. Weigh pt daily.	6. Pt has gained 3.5 kg from 2/24 to 2/27.

Summarize your impressions of patient progress towards goals: Pt is maintaining good cardiac output as evidenced by ↑ urine output, clear lung sounds and ↓ edema. Continue interventions.

Problem #3 Risk for Fluid Volume Excess
Short-term Goal: Pt will maintain optimal fluid balance as evidenced by stable wgt, clear lung sounds, Ø edema and adequate urine output.
Long-term Goal: Pt will maintain fluid balance upon discharge by compliance c̄ medication regimen and fluid intake.

Nursing Interventions:	Patient's Response:
1. Weigh pt daily.	1. Pt gained 3.5 kg since admission.
2. Monitor strict I & O (1200 cc/24 hr)	2. Pt's intake was 480, output 250 in 5 hrs.
3. Evaluate urine output.	3. Urine output is 50 cc/hr for 5 hrs (0800—1300)
4. Administer Lasix as ordered.	4. Lasix given @ 1000 40 mg po.
5. Monitor electrolytes (side effect of diuretic)	5. All electrolytes WNL.
6. Assess for edema.	6. Ø edema present.

Summarize your impressions of patient progress towards goals: Pt is maintaining optimum fluid balance presently c̄ exception of wgt gain. Continue interventions.

Problem #4 Altered Protection r/t anticoagulant therapy
Short-term Goal: Pt will maintain therapeutic blood level of anticoagulant as evidenced by PTT, PT and INR WNL.
Long-term Goal: Pt will set up schedule for bloodwork to be drawn after discharge to maintain therapeutic levels.

Nursing Interventions:	Patient's Response:
1. Monitor pt for adverse effects to anti-coagulant.	1. Pt shows Ø signs of unexplained bleeding– Ø bruising, Ø petechic.
2. Monitor vs q 4.	2. Pts BP 112/60, T978, P66, RR16 @ 0800, 94/60, T974, P20, RR18@1200.
3. Ensure IV infusion & site is uninterrupted.	3. Heparin infusing s̄ incident, IV site shows Ø signs of inflammation or bleeding.
4. Monitor lab results of PTT, PT, INR and intact.	4. Pts PTT 68 to 43, PT 13.8, INR 1.4.
5. Monitor Hgb & Het for internal bleeding.	5. Hgb ↓ 13.2, Het 38.9 ↓

Summarize your impressions of patient progress towards goals: Pt currently shows Ø signs of bleeding caused by anti-coagulant therapy. Continue to monitor –check H&H to see if continues downward trend. Continue interventions.

FIGURE 13-8. *(continued)*

Problem #5 Impaired Physical Mobility
Short-term Goal: Pt will maintain maximum level of function and risk of complications will be reduced while hospitalized.
Long-term Goal: Pt will regain optimal level of functioning as dictated by severity of CVA.

Nursing Interventions:	Patient's Response:
1. Assess pt's degree of weakness in both upper & lower extremities.	1. Pt's (L) side shows ↑ weakness to (R) side.
2. Determine active & passive ROM capabilities.	2. Pt can move (R) arm independently, other extremities require passive ROM.
3. Monitor skin integrity for potential breakdown.	3. Pt's skin intact c̄ exception of (L) buttock -opaque dsg- cannot assess.
4. Change pt's position q 2.	4. Pt appears comfortable, Ø breakdown present.
5. Use pressure relieving devices to ↓ stress.	5. Placed pillows under legs to elevate heels, pillow under (R) or (L) side to ↓ pressure on sacrum.
6. Implement fall precautions for pt safety.	6. Side rails x 4, bed in low, locked position.

Summarize your impressions of patient progress towards goals: Pt has Ø falls. Pt shows Ø skin breakdown and passive ROM performed on lower extremities & (L) arm. Continue interventions.

Problem #6 Impaired Swallowing/Risk for Aspiration
Short-term Goal: Pt will not experience aspiration while hospitalized.
Long-term Goal: Pt will maintain adequate nutrition, as evidenced by stable wgt and albumin WNL.

Nursing Interventions:	Patient's Response:
1. Before mealtime, provide adequate rest periods.	1. Pt was able to stay alert through meal.
2. Provide oral care before feeding.	2. Pt's mouth moistened, displayed good appetite.
3. Place pt in high Fowler's position for feeding.	3. Pt swallowed and chewed well.
4. Prompt pt to chew/swallow.	4. Pt responsive to prompts.
5. Identity food given to pt before each mouthful.	5. Pt nodded recognition- frowned to display distaste.
6. Crush pills and place in pureed food.	6. Pt took all medications s̄ incident

Summarize your impressions of patient progress towards goals: Pt did not aspirate and completed 75% of meals. Continue interventions.

Problem #7 Risk for Infection
Short-term Goal: Pt will remain free of infection as evidenced by VS WNL, Ø purulent drainage from tubes.
Long-term Goal: Pt will remain free of infection post discharge.

Nursing Interventions:	Patient's Response:
1. Monitor VS q 4.	1. VS WNL: Temp 97, HR66
2. Monitor WBC.	2. WBC WNL - 9.2.
3. Monitor pt for S & S of infection.	3. Pt shows Ø S & S of inflammation, swelling, drainage at any IV site.
4. Practice aseptic technique at all times.	4. Pt remains free of infection.
5. Monitor appearance of urine.	5. Pt's urine is dark, amber color. MD notified. Culture ordered.
6. Encourage intake of protein & calorie rich foods.	6. Pt completes app. 75% of food offered.

Summarize your impressions of patient progress towards goals: Pt has remained free of S/S of infection—awaiting results of urine culture. Continue interventions.

Problem #8 Anxiety
Short-term Goal: Pt will demonstrate a reduced level of anxiety evidenced by ↓ seizures, ↓ restlessness.
Long-term Goal: Pt will demonstrate positive coping mechanisms.

Nursing Interventions:	Patient's Response:
1. Acknowledge awareness of pt's anxiety.	1. Pt appeared grateful, nodded affirmatively.
2. Maintain a calm manner c̄ pt.	2. Pt appears calm and responsive.
3. Maintain frequent contact c̄ pt.	3. Pt demonstrates recognition when I appear.
4. Use simple language & brief statements to explain procedures & tasks.	4. Pt followed commands appropriately.
5. Reduce sensory stimuli.	5. Pt appears calm and resting comfortably.

Summarize your impressions of patient progress towards goals: Pt is experiencing less restlessness and appears more comfortable c̄ environment. Continue interventions.

FIGURE 13-8. *(continued)*

Table 13-5 Gibbs's Model of Reflection

Description	What happened? Don't make judgments yet or try to draw conclusions; simply describe.
Feelings	What were your reactions and feelings? Again, don't move to analyzing these yet.
Evaluation	What was bad or good about the experience? Make value judgments.
Analysis	What sense can you make of the situation? Bring in ideas from outside the experience to help you. What was really going on? Were different people's experiences similar or different in important ways?
Conclusions (general)	What can be concluded, in a general sense, from these experiences and the analyses you have undertaken?
Conclusions (specific)	What can be concluded about your own specific, unique, personal situation or way of working?
Personal Action Plan	What are you going to do differently in this type of situation next time? What steps are you going to take on the basis of what you have learned?

Source: Reprinted with permission from Gibbs, G. (1988). *Learning by doing: A guide to teaching and learning methods.* Further Education Unit, Oxford Polytechnic. http://www.brookes.ac.uk/services/upgrade/study-skills/reflective-gibbs.html.

of problem solving (trial-and-error, scientific, intuitive) and the nursing process to address the roommate's needs.

2. The nursing process is an interpersonal process that is always person centered rather than task centered. Discuss with other students the meaning of this claim. Think through and discuss the implications of approaching patients as "problems to be solved" rather than as unique human beings with inherent dignity.
3. Describe how you would structure an assessment of the following situation, using critical-thinking considerations: purpose of thinking, adequacy of knowledge, potential problems, helpful resources, and critique of judgment/decision.

   A 28-year-old woman is admitted to a hospital for multiple contusions and a hairline fracture of the skull. She claims that she "fell down the steps," but on examination, several of the injuries seem inconsistent with a fall. The woman sticks to her story that her fall was an accident. You are her nurse.

   Assess whether your attitudes and dispositions would help or hinder the task of critical thinking if you were the nurse in this situation. Share your self-evaluation with another student and compare your responses.
4. Using the just-described scenario, identify the cognitive, technical, interpersonal, and ethical and legal skills you would need to meet the nursing needs of this woman. If possible, compare your list with that of an experienced nurse and discuss differences.

Table 13-6 Critical Reflection in Action Through Critical Incident Analysis

REFLECTIVE PRACTICE	REFLECTIVE QUESTIONS	LEARNING
Self-awareness These questions are aimed at helping the nursing student to become more aware of self.	What was my role in the incident?	I gave the drug to the wrong patient. The drug was meant for my second patient—not Addie Warner. I was in a rush and did not check the eleven rights of drug administration.
	What did I learn about myself?	When I am in a rush I take shortcuts.
Reflection These questions are aimed at helping the student to identify deficits in knowledge and the actions or inactions that contributed to the situation.	What circumstances may have contributed to my error?	The unit was very busy and I was already behind on my work and trying to do three things at once. I asked someone to check the drug with me, but I knew they were also busy and not focused on the task at hand.
	Were there any knowledge deficits that contributed to my error? If so, how might I overcome these?	I already knew the eleven rights but did not check them, so the deficit relates to acting on my knowledge rather than a lack of knowledge.
	Were there any environmental issues that may have contributed to the error occurring?	This patient had been so demanding all morning that she certainly had me "on edge" and worried about finishing all I had to do before needing to leave the floor for post-conference.
	What did I learn from the incident?	This reinforced the importance of checking and also of my role in safe administration of medication. I also learned why I can't let demanding patients "rattle" me. Luckily the patient did not suffer an adverse reaction, but it did make me stop and think about my practice.
	How might I act differently in the future?	I will think about the patient first and ensure I am not rushed during drug administration. I will ask for help.

Source: Reprinted with permission from Hill, R., Hall, H., & Glew, P. (2017). *Fundamentals of nursing and midwifery: A person-centered approach to care* (3rd ed.). Wolters Kluwer/Lippincott Williams & Wilkins.

PRACTICING FOR NCLEX

1. A nursing student is committed to providing thoughtful, person-centered care. Which nursing actions demonstrate this type of care? Select all that apply.
   a. Assisting patients to select meals based on their cultural observances
   b. Providing nursing care based on patients' needs and preferences
   c. Documenting nursing interventions in the electronic health record
   d. Reviewing fingerstick blood glucose levels with the primary nurse
   e. Listening to a patient's concern for their ill significant other
2. A patient who is receiving cancer chemotherapy tells the nurse, "The treatment for this cancer is worse than the disease itself. I'm stopping treatment." Which nursing action best promotes a patient-centered, therapeutic relationship?
   a. Determining if the patient database is adequate to address the problem
   b. Considering whether to suggest a counseling session for the patient
   c. Reassessing the patient and determining how to best support them
   d. Identifying possible interventions and critiquing the merit of each option
3. The nursing philosophy in an acute care hospital includes a commitment to deliver thoughtful, person-centered care. Which description of the nursing process best supports this commitment?
   a. Systematic
   b. Interpersonal
   c. Dynamic
   d. Universally applicable in nursing situations
4. A staff nurse tells a new graduate nurse not to bother studying too hard, since most clinical reasoning becomes second nature and intuitive once they begin practicing. Which response by the student is appropriate?
   a. Intuitive problem solving comes with years of practice and observation based on nursing knowledge and science.
   b. For nursing to remain a science, nurses must continue to be vigilant about avoiding intuitive reasoning.
   c. The emphasis on logical, scientific, evidence-based reasoning has held nursing back; we need intuitive, creative thinkers.
   d. The nurse's preference dictates whether they are logical, scientific thinkers or intuitive, creative thinkers.
5. The nurse uses blended competencies when caring for patients in a rehabilitation facility. Which interventions reflect the use of cognitive skills? Select all that apply.
   a. Monitoring for side effects of medications
   b. Safely administering an injectable medication
   c. Teaching a patient about diabetes and its management
   d. Acting as witness by signing a surgical consent form
   e. Helping a patient identify their progress in physical therapy
   f. Comforting a patient who has received bad news
6. A nurse uses critical-thinking skills to develop the care plan for an older adult with dementia awaiting placement in a long-term care facility. Which statements describe characteristics of the critical thinking used by nurses engaged in clinical reasoning? Select all that apply.
   a. Functions independently of nursing standards, ethics, and state practice acts
   b. Based on the principles of the nursing process, problem solving, and the scientific method
   c. Driven by patient, family, and community needs as well as nurses' needs to give competent, efficient care
   d. Avoids designs to compensate for problems created by human nature, such as medication errors
   e. Constantly reevaluating, self-correcting, and striving for improvement
   f. Focuses on the big picture rather than identifying the key problems, issues, and risks involved with patient care
7. A nurse is caring for a patient with type 2 diabetes who has an infected foot ulcer requiring dressing changes. Which nursing action best demonstrates the QSEN competency of patient-centered care?
   a. Asking the patient if they would like their spouse to be present for a teaching session
   b. Researching new procedures to care for foot ulcers when developing a care plan for this patient
   c. Leading a grand rounds or unit-based discussion on complications of diabetes
   d. Using the electronic medical record to review trends of the patient's blood glucose levels
8. The nursing assessment of a patient with a diagnosis of anorexia nervosa reveals the patient consumes a vegan diet of 700 calories daily and has lost 30 lb in 4 months. The nurse's recommendation to meet with a nutritionist is the outcome of which process?
   a. Clinical judgment
   b. Nursing process
   c. Clinical reasoning
   d. Critical thinking
9. A nurse working in a long-term care facility reviews the electronic health records of patients who have fallen in the last month to determine if there is a common risk factor. Which QSEN competency is the nurse demonstrating?
   a. Patient-centered care
   b. Evidence-based practice
   c. Teamwork and collaboration
   d. Informatics

10. A new graduate nurse phones the surgeon to report their patient is having severe incisional pain. The surgeon asks about vital signs and appearance of the wound, causing the nurse to return to the bedside for additional assessments. Upon reflection with the preceptor, which characteristic of the nursing process should the nurse have remembered?
    a. Centric
    b. Dynamic
    c. Interpersonal
    d. Systematic

11. The nurse is formulating a care plan for a patient in a long-term care facility who has lost 12 lb in the last 2 months. To arrive at a patient-centered nursing judgment, what will the nurse do first?
    a. Ensure the patient is receiving foods they like, including favorites.
    b. Make sure the patient's dentures are clean and inserted at mealtimes.
    c. Assess the patient's food intake and hydration over the last 1 to 3 days.
    d. Request that the nursing assistant feed the client at mealtime.

12. When implementing a thoughtful, patient-centered care plan, which action does the nurse prioritize?
    a. The patient's loved ones are considered part of the team.
    b. A caring relationship with mutual trust is established.
    c. Measures for safety are visibly incorporated.
    d. Transparent communication is observed.

13. An oncology nurse is analyzing a patient's strengths and finds the patient is well educated, learns quickly, and is resilient. In which phase of the nursing process will the nurse use this information?
    a. Diagnosing
    b. Evaluating
    c. Planning
    d. Implementing

ANSWERS WITH RATIONALES

1. **a, b, e.** The nursing process ensures that nurses are person centered rather than task centered. Attending to cultural preferences and needs and listening to a patient's concerns are patient-centered actions. Documentation and communication with other members of the health care team are not specifically patient centered.

2. **c.** Reassessing the patient allows the nurse and patient to clarify the patient's goal(s) and develop interventions to best meet them. Once the problem is addressed, it is important for the nurse to judge the adequacy of the knowledge, identify potential problems, use helpful resources, and critique the decision.

3. **b.** Interpersonal. All other options are characteristics of the nursing process but focus on the patient best illustrates the interpersonal dimension of the nursing process.

4. **a.** When intuition is used alone, increased risks and fewer benefits may occur. Beginning nurses must use nursing knowledge and scientific problem solving as the basis of care; intuitive problem solving comes with years of practice and observation. If the beginning nurse has an intuition about a patient, that information should be discussed with the faculty member, preceptor, or supervisor. There is a place for intuitive reasoning in nursing, but it will augment, not replace logical, scientific reasoning. Critical thinking is contextual and changes depending on the circumstances, not on personal preference.

5. **a, c.** Using critical thinking to teach a patient about a disease process and management and monitoring for side effects of medications are cognitive competencies. Performing an injection correctly is a technical skill; witnessing/signing an informed consent form is a legal/ethical action, and comforting a patient is an interpersonal skill.

6. **b, c, e.** Critical thinking applied to clinical reasoning and clinical judgment is guided by standards, policies and procedures, and ethics. When applying principles of nursing process, problem solving, and the scientific method, clinical reasoning identifies the key problems, issues, and risks. This is driven by patient, family, and community needs as well as nurses' needs to give competent, efficient care. It also calls for strategies that make the most of human potential and compensate for problems created by human nature. It is constantly reevaluating, self-correcting, and striving to improve the quality and safety of health care systems (Alfaro-LeFevre, 2014).

7. **a.** Patient-centered care commits to developing caring relationships based on mutual trust to communicate and deliver care based on patient preferences and values. Evidence-based practice integrates the best current evidence for safe practice with clinical expertise. Teamwork and collaboration shares patient information or opportunities for learning with others. Informatics manages patient information, mitigates error, and supports decision making using the electronic medical record and other databases.

8. **a.** Clinical judgment is the outcome of critical thinking and clinical reasoning, using the nursing process as a framework. Clinical reasoning refers to ways of thinking about patient care issues including weighing and validating options (determining, preventing, and managing patient problems). Critical thinking includes reasoning both outside and inside of the clinical setting.

9. **d.** Informatics uses information and technology to communicate, manage knowledge, mitigate error, and support decision making. Thoughtful, patient-centered care emphasizes recognition of the patient or designee as the source of control and full partner in compassionate and coordinated care, based on respect for patients' preferences, values, and needs. Evidence-based practice integrates the best current evidence with clinical expertise and patient and family preferences and values to deliver optimal health care. Teamwork and collaboration refer to effective functioning within nursing and interprofessional teams, fostering open communication, mutual respect, and shared decision making to achieve quality patient care.

10. **d.** The nursing process is systematic, iterative, and overlapping. By reporting an isolated symptom, the nurse has overlooked the benefit of systematic and inclusive assessment. While the nursing process is presented as an orderly progression of phases, there is a dynamic interaction and flow of phases into one another.

11. **c.** The nurse uses the nursing process to arrive at a clinical judgment. After analyzing the assessment data, the nurse determines, through clinical reasoning, whether the related factors in the patient's weight loss, such as dislike of menu options, lack of dentition, or inability to perform activities of daily living such as feeding, should be the focus of interventions.
12. **c.** Although developing a thoughtful, patient-centered approach is focused on caring and mutual trust, the nurse uses the nursing process and Maslow's hierarchy of needs to prioritize care. Safety is a higher-level need than love and belonging, and therefore the priority.
13. **a.** Assessing for strengths and weaknesses is the first step of the nursing process, which has been completed. Next, the nurse clusters cues and develops diagnoses that give rise to interventions. Evaluating the plan is followed by completing or modifying the plan.

Bibliography

Alfaro-LeFevre, R. (2014). *Applying nursing process: The foundation for clinical reasoning* (8th ed.). Wolters Kluwer/Lippincott Williams & Wilkins.

Alfaro-LeFevre, R. (2020). *Critical thinking, clinical reasoning, and clinical judgment: A practical approach* (7th ed.). Elsevier.

Alfaro-LeFevre, R. (2002–2020). *Teaching smart/learning easy*. http://www.AlfaroTeachSmart.com

American Association of Colleges of Nursing (AACN). (2008). *The essentials of baccalaureate education for professional nursing practice*. Author.

American Nurses Association (ANA). (2010). *Nursing's social policy statement* (2010 ed.). Author.

American Nurses Association (ANA). (2015). *Code for nurses with interpretive statements*. Author.

American Nurses Association (ANA). (2021). *Nursing: Scope and standards of practice* (3rd ed.). Author.

Benner, P. (2001). *From novice to expert*. Addison-Wesley.

Benner, P. (2005). Extending the dialogue about classification systems and the work of professional nurses. *American Journal of Critical Care, 14*(3), 242–243, 272.

Benner, P., & Wrubel, J. (1989). *The primacy of caring in health and illness*. Addison-Wesley.

Brennan, T. A., Leape, L. L., Laird, N. M., Hebert, L., Localio, A. R., Lawthers, A. G., Newhouse, J. P., Weiler, P. C., Hiatt, H. H., & Harvard Medical Practice Study I. (2004). Incidence of adverse events and negligence in hospitalized patients: Results of the Harvard Medical Practice study I. 1991. *Quality and Safety in Health Care, 13*(2), 145–151; discussion 151–152.

Bulechek, G. M., Butcher, H. K., & Dochterman, J. (Eds.). (2013). *Nursing interventions classification [NIC]* (6th ed.). Elsevier.

Craft-Rosenberg, M., & Delaney M. (1997). Nursing diagnosis extension and classification (NDEC). In Rantz, M. J., & LeMone, D. (Eds.), *Classification of nursing diagnoses: Proceedings of the Twelfth Conference, North American Nursing Diagnosis* (pp. 26–31). CINAHL Information Services.

Cronenwett, L., Sherwood, G., Barnsteiner J., Disch, J., Johnson, J., Mitchell, P., Sullivan, D. T., & Warren, J. (2007). Quality and safety education for nurses. *Nursing Outlook, 55*(3), 122–131.

Daley, B. J. (1996). Concept maps: Linking nursing theory to clinical nursing practice. *Journal of Continuing Education in Nursing, 27*(1), 17–27.

Davies, E. (1995). Reflective practice: A focus for caring. *Journal of Nursing Education, 34*(4), 167–174.

Dickison, P., Haerling K. A., & Lasater K. (2019). Integrating the National Council of State Boards of Nursing Clinical Judgment Model into Nursing Educational Frameworks. *Journal of Nursing Education, 58*(2) 72–78. https://doi.org/10.3928/01484834-20190122-03.

Dochterman, J. M., & Jones, D. A. (2003). *Unifying nursing languages: The harmonization of NANDA, NIC, NOC*. American Nurses Association.

Dossey, B. M., & Dossey, L. (1998). Body, mind, spirit. Attending to holistic care. *American Journal of Nursing, 98*(8), 35–38.

Feldstein, B. D. (2011). Bridging with the sacred: reflections of a physician Chaplain. *Journal of Pain and Symptom Management, 42*(1), 155–161.

Fitzpatrick, M. A. (2015). The essence of nursing. *Supplement to American Nurse Today, 10*(5).

Gebbie, K., & Lavin, M. A. (1974). Classifying nursing Diagnoses. *American Journal of Nursing, 74*(2), 250–253.

Gibbs, G. (1988). *Learning by doing: A guide to teaching and learning methods. Further Education Unit*. Polytechnic. http://www.brookes.ac.uk/services/upgrade/study-skills/reflective-gibbs.html

Hall, L. E. (1955). *Quality of nursing care. Address given at the Department of Baccalaureate and Higher Degree Programs of the New Jersey League for Nursing. Public Health News (June)*. New Jersey State Department of Health.

Hill, R., Hall, H., & Glew, P. (2017). *Fundamentals of nursing and midwifery: A person-centered approach to care* (3rd ed.). Wolters Kluwer/Lippincott Williams & Wilkins.

Herdman, T. H., & Kamitsuru, S. (Eds.). (2018). *Nursing diagnoses: Definitions and classification, 2018–2020* (11th ed.). Thieme.

Horton-Deutsch, S., & Sherwood, G. D. (2017). *Reflective practice: Transforming education and improving outcomes* (2nd ed.). Sigma Theta Tau.

Institute of Medicine (IOM). (2001). *Crossing the quality chasm*. The National Academies Press.

Institute of Medicine (IOM). (2003). *Health professions education: A bridge to quality*. The National Academies Press.

Iowa Intervention Project. (1997). Nursing interventions classification (NIC): An overview. In M. J. Rantz & P. LeMone (Eds.), *Classification of nursing diagnoses: Proceedings of the Twelfth Conference, North American Nursing Diagnosis* (pp. 32–39). CINAHL Information Systems.

Jacobs, S. (2016). Reflective learning, reflective practice. *Nursing, 46*(5), 62–64.

Koharchik, L., Caputi, L., Robb, M., & Culleiton, A. L. (2015). Fostering clinical reasoning in nursing students. *American Journal of Nursing, 115*(1), 58–61.

Kuiper, R., O'Donnell, S., Pesut, D., & Turrise, S. (2017). *The essentials of clinical reasoning for nurses*. Sigma Theta Tau.

Lasatar, K. (2007). Clinical judgment development: Using simulation to create an assessment rubric. *Journal of Nursing Education, 46*(11), 496–503.

Levett-Jones, T., Hoffman, K., Dempsey, J., Jeong, S. Y., Noble, D., Norton, C. A., Roche, J., & Hickey, N. (2010). The 'five rights' of clinical reasoning: An educational model to enhance nursing students' ability to identify and manage clinically 'at risk' patients. *Nurse Education Today, 30*(6), 515–520.

Mangubat, M. D. B. (2017). Emotional intelligence: Five pieces to the puzzle. *Nursing, 47*(7), 51–53.

Moorhead, S., Johnson, M., Maas, M. L., & Swanson, E. (2013). *Nursing outcomes classification (NOC)* (5th ed.). Elsevier.

Mueller, A., Johnston, M., & Bligh, D. (2002). Joining mind and mapping care planning to enhance student critical thinking and achieve holistic nursing care. *Nursing Diagnosis, 13*(1), 24–27.

National Council of State Boards of Nursing (NCSBN). (2020). NGN FAQs for Educators. https://www.ncsbn.org/11447.htm

Paul, R. W. (1993). *Critical thinking: How to prepare students for a rapidly changing world*. Foundation for Critical Thinking.

Preheim, G. J., Armstrong, G. E., & Barton, A. J. (2009). The NEW fundamentals in nursing: Introducing beginning quality and safety education for nurses (QSEN) competencies. *Journal of Nursing Education, 48*(12), 694–697.

Rodak, S. (2012). *10 Guiding principles for patient-centered care*. ASC Communications.

Scheffer, B. K., & Rubenfeld, M. G. (2000). A consensus statement on critical thinking in nursing. *Journal of Nursing Education, 39*(8), 352–359.

Schmehl, P. (2014). *Introduction to concept mapping in nursing: Critical thinking in action*. Jones & Bartlett Learning.

Schön, D. (1983). *The reflective practitioner: How professionals think in action*. Basic Books.

Schuster, P. M. (2016). *Concept mapping: A critical-thinking approach to care planning* (4th ed.). F.A. Davis.

Smith, J., & Crawford, L. (2003). Medication errors and difficulty in first patient assignments of newly licensed nurses. *JONAS Healthcare Law, Ethics and Regulation, 5*(3), 65–67.

Sommer, S. K. (2020). Relationships between decision-making processes in developing clinical judgment skills. *Nurse Educator, 45*(4), 184. https://doi.org/10.1097/NNE. 0000000000000776

Swanson, K. M. (1991). Empirical development of a middle range theory of caring. *Nursing Research, 40*(3), 161–166.

Tanner, C. A. (2006). Thinking like a nurse: A research-based model of clinical judgment in nursing. *Journal of Nursing Education, 45*(6), 204–211.

Taylor, C. (1995). Rethinking nursing's basic competencies. *Journal of Nursing Care Quality, 9*(4), 1–13.

Travelbee, J. (1971). *Interpersonal aspects of nursing* (2nd ed.). F.A. Davis.

Verghese, A. (2011). A doctor's touch. TED talk. http://www.ted.com/talks/abraham_verghese_a_doctor_s_touch.html

Watson, J. (2008). *Nursing: The philosophy and science of caring* (rev. ed.). University Press of Colorado.

Watson, J. (2016). Human caring literacy. In S. Lee, P. Palmieri, & J. Watson (Eds.), *Global advances in human caring literacy* (pp. 3–20). Springer Publishing Company.

Weyant, R. A., Clukey, L., Roberts, M., & Henderson, A. (2017). Show your stuff and watch your tone: Nurses' caring behaviors. *American Journal of Critical Care, 26*(2), 111–117.

Yura, H., & Walsh, M. B. (1988). *The nursing process: Assessing, planning, implementing, evaluating* (5th ed.). Appleton-Century-Crofts.

Zonsius, M. S., Cothran, F. A., & Miller, J. M. (2020). Acute care for patients with dementia. A review of best practices for integrating person-centered care throughout the hospital stay. *American Journal of Nursing, 120*(4), 34–42.

14 Clinical Judgment

Ashley Dotski

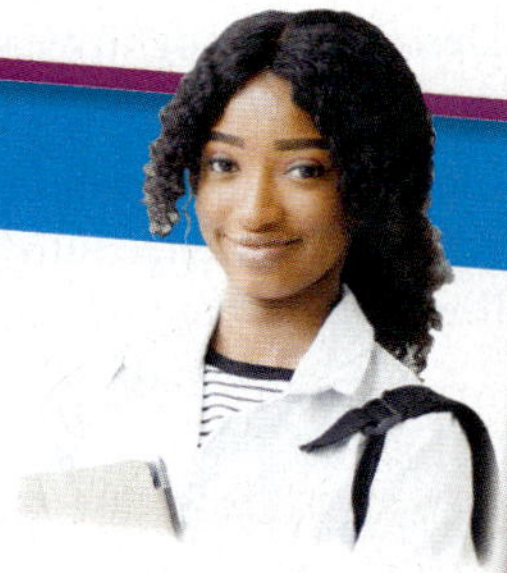

Ashley is a student nurse with no clinical experience and no legacy of nursing in her family or circle of friends. She wants to be a nurse and is interested in pediatrics but is open to exploring different possibilities in nursing. Ashley is focused on developing her critical thinking skills before she begins her first clinical rotation.

Daniel Ramirez

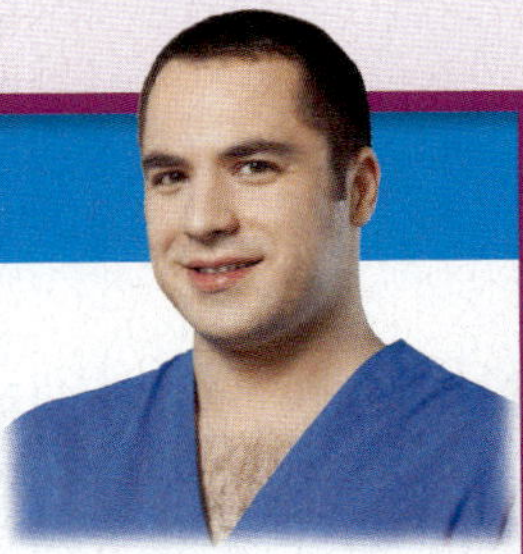

Daniel, a student nurse, has divulged to an academic advisor that he suffers from some test anxiety and is nervous about the licensure test. He states, "I tend to do worse on the first exam in a course because I need to get a feel for the teaching and the teacher's testing style before I figure out how to study."

Kallie McDonald

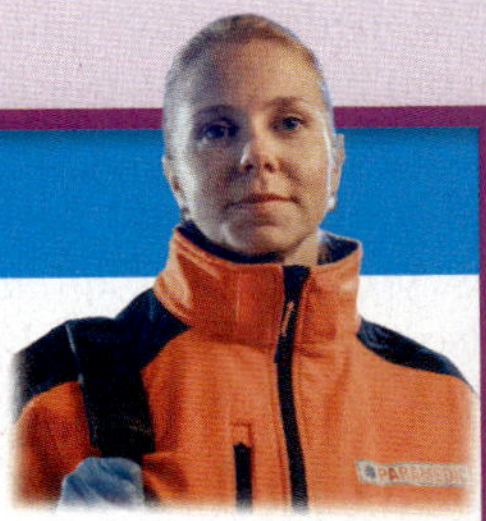

Kallie is a paramedic returning to school to be a nurse. They are trying to not divulge that they have some health care background for fear they will be held to a higher standard than the other student nurses.

Learning Outcomes

After completing the chapter, you will be able to accomplish the following:

1. Describe the concepts of critical thinking, clinical reasoning, and clinical judgment.
2. Compare and contrast models, frameworks, and theories related to the development of clinical judgment.
3. Explain how competency models are used in nursing education.
4. Describe the cognitive theories that underpin clinical decision making.
5. Identify your plan to integrate previous and newly gained knowledge into your nursing practice to drive the development of clinical judgment.

Nursing Concepts

- Advocacy
- Clinical decision making/clinical judgment
- Collaboration/teamwork and collaboration
- Ethics
- Professional identity
- Managing care

Your exploration and development of clinical judgment will continue well past your formal undergraduate education. Clinical judgment, informed by experience, develops over the course of your professional nursing career. The brief descriptions of educational principles presented will help you appreciate foundational concepts and theories as they relate to your personal and professional development. Education is based on fairly predictable pedagogical and andragogical principles. We will explore some of these principles and theoretical models as we provide you context for the development of clinical judgment and highlight concrete steps you can take to cultivate an adaptive decision-making process. We will also spend time highlighting specific tools and resources used throughout this text to provide exemplars of how to engage in this developmental work. This chapter is designed to foster your clinical judgment by including you in the process of education through an exploration of the common threads that guide nurse educators who foster, facilitate, and guide you through your exploration of the profession of nursing.

See the Reflective Practice box on the next page and consider your role in maximizing your personal professional development and the professional development of your peers.

CONCEPTS RELATED TO CLINICAL JUDGMENT

Critical thinking, clinical reasoning, and clinical judgment occur in the quiet moments. For example, framing your approach to a patient using their identified pronouns requires a measure of clinical judgment. Identifying and then using an algorithm or protocol based on your clinical findings requires clinical judgment. Reviewing the evidence and contributing to the development or revision of that algorithm or protocol requires clinical judgment. We use clinical judgment to determine whether we must immediately call the provider, or if there are additional assessments that we should perform to formulate a recommendation. Deciding whether something you know about the patient, such as their HIV+ status, is germane to the SBAR report you give to the oncoming nurse requires clinical judgment. To frame clinical judgment and ensure we are all using the same working definitions, we should review some key terms. Although there are subtle differences in how nurse educators define these terms, we are going to explore the core tenets of critical thinking, clinical reasoning, and clinical judgment.

Critical Thinking

Alfaro-LeFevre (2020a) posits that we should replace the word *critical* in *critical thinking* with *important* because the thinking that is done with respect to nursing care is important! The term critical thinking applies to thinking that occurs within the clinical and education settings but also applies in everyday life. What is important to remember is that critical thinking is a skill that can be developed—it often requires intentional focus and work, but the ability to think, reason, consider options, and problem solve can be learned. Snyder's (1993) definition of critical thinking references problem solving that is "both creative/intuitive and logical/analytic" (p. 207). Alfaro-LeFevre's (2020a) definition describes critical thinking as "knowing how to focus your thinking to get the results you need (includes applying logic, intuition, standards, and evidence-based practice)" (p. 8). Take a moment and put the term critical thinking into your own words. When you think about critical thinking, do you include elements of an orderly process that is reasonable, possible, and logical?

Consider this definition of **critical thinking** from Scriven and Paul (1987): "Critical thinking is the intellectually disciplined process of actively and skillfully conceptualizing, applying, analyzing, synthesizing, and/or evaluating information gathered from, or generated by, observation, experience, reflection, reasoning, or communication, as a guide to belief and action" (p. 1). Other thought leaders have recognized critical thinking as a *concept* that does not have one universally accepted definition. Ennis (2016) offers an abbreviated, parallel definition: "reasonable reflective thinking focused on deciding what to believe or do" (p. 166). Student nurses often use critical thinking with test processing, when navigating new systems such as an electronic health record (EHR) or learning management systems (LMS), when learning in

QSEN Reflective Practice: Cultivating QSEN Competencies

CHALLENGE TO ETHICAL AND LEGAL SKILLS

I'm in my second adult medical-surgical clinical rotation this semester and am finally able to apply some of the skills I learned as a paramedic. Simulations are my favorite part of the course because we get to actually do everything. The team-based simulations are used to reinforce our learning and are not graded. I've found that my team of three student nurses tends to move quickly through every simulation and does most things correctly because I provide guidance and instruction throughout the entire scenario. During the debriefing yesterday, one of my peers pretty much called me bossy and asked me to "stop telling tell them what to do all the time." The other student nodded in agreement, and the faculty facilitating the debrief chastised me for jumping in and "not giving them a chance to think and prioritize for themselves."

Thinking Outside the Box: Possible Courses of Action

- I could nod in agreement and admit that I was bossy.
- I could explain my background and counter that I should not have to slow down to match their (too slow) speed.
- I could refrain from saying anything at all and talk to my two peers after the debriefing.

Evaluating a Good Outcome: How Do I Define Success?

- The simulated patient benefited from my actions—there was timely, correct intervention for this health problem.
- My peers and I all need to apply the information we've learned in class in specific situations, using the appropriate resources.
- Presentation matters, so perhaps my tone and assumption of the dominant role is something I could reconsider.
- If I am doing the right thing at the right time, my peers should benefit from watching me even if their preference is to make their own decisions and do it themselves.
- In this situation, I need to separate my personal feelings from my professional interactions.

Personal Learning: Here's to the Future!

I opted to explain my background as a paramedic and provide evidence-based rationale for my decision making in the simulation. My faculty facilitator did a really good job in separating the simulation actions from my professionalism and intraprofessional collaboration abilities. As we walked through the simulation itself and reviewed our thinking and decisions at various points, I realized that I had missed a few things that would have slightly altered the order of our actions. It was interesting because one of my peers interjected that he didn't feel heard by the team during the simulation, and he had tried to mention the change in respirations twice. I learned that my team had valuable insight and that I (and the simulated patient) would have benefited from more intentionally including my peers in the process. We each approached the situation a little differently and had access to different information at various points, which means collaboration was actually necessary. During the debrief, the faculty facilitator guided us to talking about team process. It was clear I was not the appointed formal leader and that leadership does not always mean being the loudest or the first person to speak. I also listened to their words more closely and realized they had not used the word *bossy* at all; in fact, they were careful to talk about the situation objectively because they like and respect me. I probably need to work on my emotional intelligence and make time to focus on building relationships with my peers. I met with the faculty facilitator after the group debrief to gain more insight into the perceptions of others and discuss specific goals.

QSEN SELF-REFLECTION ON QUALITY AND SAFETY COMPETENCIES DEVELOPING KNOWLEDGE, SKILLS, AND ATTITUDES FOR CONTINUOUS IMPROVEMENT

How do you think you would respond in a similar situation? Why? What does this tell you about yourself and about the adequacy of your skills for professional practice? Can you think of other ways to respond or approach the situation? What *knowledge, skills,* and *attitudes* do you need to develop to continuously improve quality and safety when caring for simulated patients in a team-based learning model?

Patient-Centered Care: How could missing key data points change the course of action? Did the patent feel confident in all members of your team? Did the patient view you as in charge or as bossy? How do team dynamics impact on patient confidence, rapport, satisfaction, and outcomes?

Teamwork and Collaboration/Quality Improvement: What is emotional intelligence? How does self-reflection foster development of interpersonal, intraprofessional, and interprofessional communication skills? What roles and responsibilities can you identify for members of the health care team? What do you know about TeamSTEPPS® (https://www.ahrq.gov/teamstepps/index.html), and how would training in these strategies and tools improve team performance? How does teamwork link to quality care? Would an analysis of team function in the clinical setting be beneficial as a quality improvement study?

Safety/Evidence-Based Practice: How is safety actually and potentially impacted by team performance? Doesn't having team members with varied personal, educational, and experiential backgrounds provide an opportunity for individualizing care using the best-known evidence? When considering beginning clinical knowledge, what is the value of brainstorming knowledge and agreeing on a plan of care before acting?

Informatics: How do we integrate informatics when delivering patient care? How does the technology available increase our access to varied and valuable information? How do we make space during a crisis to gather information from the person observing the monitor, looking in the EHR, completing a medication calculation, or pulling up a protocol? How do we leverage communication and technology information to provide safe, quality care (even to a simulated patient)?

teams, and when balancing daily activities with the pressures of school. As student nurses, not being provided *one* definition can be challenging, but sifting through the varied perspectives and formulating your own understanding and application of the concept of critical thinking to nursing practice requires . . . critical thinking!

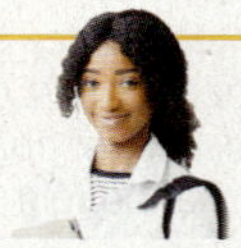

Recall **Ashley Dotski**, the student nurse who is looking to hone her critical thinking skills. Ashley could consider completing a PrepU assignment on the concept of Critical Thinking to identify strengths and gaps in her understanding of the definitions and applications of critical thinking in nursing.

Clinical Reasoning

Like critical thinking, clinical reasoning has multiple layers and context-based descriptions. Reasoning, in general, is not unique to nursing. Hypothetico-deductive reasoning is a component of Piaget's cognitive development theory and relates to the formal operational stage in adolescence (Piaget & Inhelder, 1969). Transitioning from concrete thinking to abstract thinking allows for hypothesis testing and considering elements outside of what is immediately perceived. Deductive reasoning relies on applying widely accepted knowledge and principles to a model or a combination of models to solve problems—this is referred to as *backward reasoning*. Proving your point by testing identified theories or hypotheses and predicting consequences utilizes deduction. Inductive reasoning requires observing, then drawing conclusions—this is referred to as *forward reasoning*. Inductive reasoning processes require the ability to recognize patterns and connections and form hypotheses and theories. Inductive reasoning requires experience, knowledge, a holistic view, intuition, and organized thinking. Although deductive and inductive both have value, inductive reasoning is more often used by expert practitioners (Shin, 2019).

The American Association of Colleges of Nursing (AACN, 2021) positions clinical reasoning as a precursor to clinical judgment, and considers critical thinking, knowledge from nursing and other disciplines, and clinical reasoning as foundational to clinical judgment and the associated clinical decision making (CDM). Specifically, **clinical reasoning** is defined as "thought processes that allow healthcare providers to arrive at a conclusion" (AACN, 2021, p. 62). Alfaro-LeFevre (2020a) defines clinical reasoning and decision making as "the process you use to think about patient problems in the clinical setting" (p. 8). This idea of viewing clinical reasoning as the *process* of thinking that results in a clinical judgment is fairly accepted in nursing. Although critical thinking is relevant in everyday life (although in a different form than what we consider critical thinking in health care), clinical reasoning occurs in the clinical setting. For example, clinical reasoning is required when providing thoughtful, person-centered care; when engaging in quality improvement projects; when integrating evidence-based practice; when providing teaching; and in many other instances (Alfaro-LeFevre, 2020a and 2020b). Think about it this way: critical thinking may be used to access the EHR and to learn to navigate through the screens, but clinical reasoning is used to decide what you should review, when to review it, and how each piece of data relates to the others to create a clinical picture.

Clinical Judgment

Clinical judgment is the result or observed outcome of critical thinking and decision making (NCSBN, 2019a). AACN (2021) defines clinical judgment as "the skill of recognizing cues regarding a clinical situation, generating and weighing hypotheses, taking action, and evaluating outcomes for the purpose of arriving at a satisfactory clinical outcome" (p. 62). Hopefully you noticed that this definition mirrors the nursing process, which is discussed later in this chapter. As you move through the rest of this chapter, consider the overlap and use of the terms critical thinking, clinical reasoning, clinical decision making, and clinical judgment. Memorizing definitions is not the goal. Rather, your first goal is to understand how the concepts relate to your learning, the teaching strategies, your assignments, the exams, and other course-related activities. Then apply the concepts in the clinical setting and consider how they are fundamental to nursing practice. Finally, it is important that you acknowledge the impact your clinical judgment has on patient outcomes.

Situational Awareness

Situational awareness (SA), also referred to as *situation awareness*, is "the perception of the elements in the environment in a volume of time and space, the comprehension of their meaning and the projection of their status in the near future" (Endsley, 1995, p. 36). Originally used in training crews of military aircraft and in other tactical and strategic systems, SA is known to increase in difficulty as the complexity and dynamic nature of an environment increases (Endsley, 1995). Picking up on the (sometimes subtle) cues that indicate a patient is deteriorating, recognizing the implications of these assessments, and notifying the team to implement a protocol demonstrates how the idea of SA is applied in health care. Nurses face significant challenges when managing the delivery of thoughtful, person-centered care with the complexities in the health care environment, increased workload and associated cognitive load, frequent interruptions, and ongoing distractions (Walshe et al., 2021). Novice nurses tend to have a narrower focus than their more experienced counterparts and focus on tasks and cues immediately available. Experienced nurses, who have developed intuition, are continually scanning the environment to prioritize their nursing actions (Sitterding et al., 2014).

Protocols, early warning systems embedded in the EHR, and standardized hand-off tools all serve to facilitate the situational awareness of health care teams and address safety issues in the clinical environment. Nurses need to be involved in the development and implementation of these systems to ensure they are feasible and address the needs of nurses. For example, there is debate over whether the

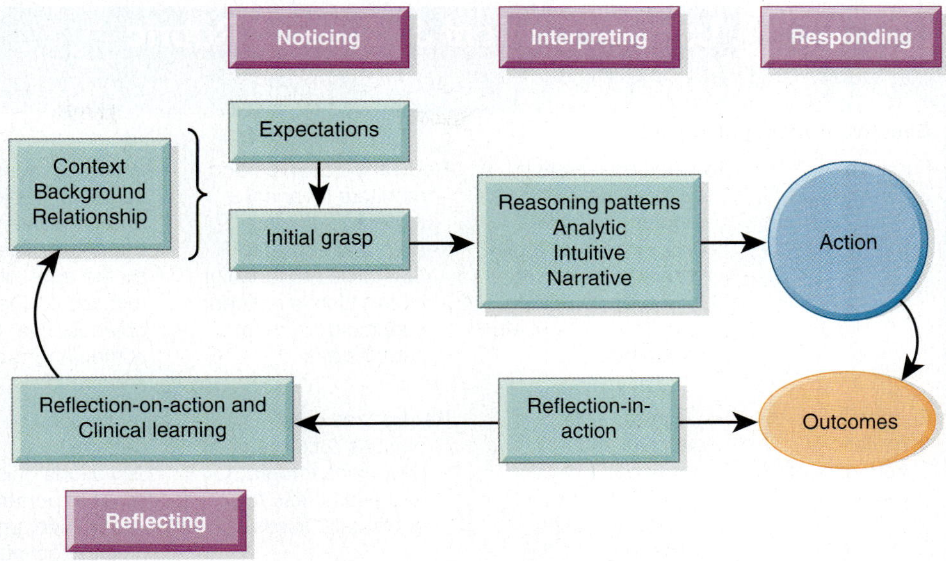

FIGURE 14-1. Clinical Judgment Model. (*Source:* Adapted with permission from Tanner, C. A. [2006]. Thinking like a nurse: a research-based model of clinical judgment in nursing. *Journal of Nursing Education*, *45*[6], 204–211. https://doi.org/10.3928/01484834-20060601-04)

amount of documentation in the computer required to trigger a warning in the EHR interferes with the nurse's ability to spend time with the patient and instinctively use their nursing skills to recognize important cues. It takes time to learn to balance nursing clinical judgment with our reliance on information technology and communication tools that provide safety checklists and protocols. **Cognitive load** is a term used to reference the amount of information a person can hold in their memory at one time. Although related to multitasking, the reprioritization and refocusing nurses do on an ongoing basis is unique and mentally taxing, which is why factors such as patient acuity and staffing levels are important to consider. Developing schema and strategies to manage the cognitive load is essential for maintaining SA.

Generally speaking, SA is required prior to decision making and clinical judgment (Fore & Sculli, 2013), which is why the term is relevant to health care professionals. As you review the clinical judgment models described in this chapter, look for elements of SA, specifically the concepts of perception, comprehension, and projection.

MODELS RELATED TO CLINICAL JUDGMENT

Nursing draws on developments from other disciplines and generates our own models to facilitate the development of clinical judgment. Although what follows is not an exhaustive discussion, we will highlight a few key models and frameworks that will support you in your development of clinical judgment.

Tanner's Clinical Judgment Model

When nurse educators think about developing clinical judgment, one of the first models referenced is Tanner's (2006) Clinical Judgment Model. This research-based model accounts for the impact the nurse's knowledge, experience, and values have on assessment and action in a situation; the importance of knowing our patients and considering their perspectives; the influence of context and culture on a situation; the recognition that nurses typically use more than one reasoning pattern; and the importance of reflection to foster the development of clinical knowledge and improving clinical reasoning (Tanner). Clinical judgment for this model is defined as "an interpretation or conclusion about a patient's needs, concerns, or health problems, and/or the decision to take action (or not), use or modify standard approaches, or improvise new ones as deemed appropriate by the patient's response" (Tanner, 2006, p. 204). The model is provided in Figure 14-1.

The core elements of the model include:

- Noticing: initial grasp and perceptions of the situation that are impacted by context, the nurse's practical experience, knowledge of expected versus unexpected data, ethical perspectives, and the nurse–patient relationship
- Interpreting: attributing meaning to the data through multiple reasoning patterns
- Responding: deciding on an action (or inaction) and monitoring outcomes
- Reflecting: in-action and on-action

What makes this model the go-to for many student nurses and nurse educators is that the first three components of the model are supported by reflection. *Reflection in-action* occurs when actively engaged in the situation and during ongoing monitoring and assessment; *reflection on-action*, which mirrors a debrief or post-conference, occurs after the situation and drives clinical learning. Note that this model is cyclical, like the experiential learning model (further described on p. 394), which indicates that the learning that occurs informs future experiences. Although there are certainly times when nurses do not consciously move through each step of this model, it reflects the way nurses arrive at decisions and, more importantly, the way student nurses develop clinical judgment.

Based on Tanner's Clinical Judgment Model, Lasater (2007) developed and tested a rubric to describe the development of clinical judgment, the Lasater Clinical Judgment Rubric (LCJR; Table 14-1 on page 386).

Table 14-1 Lasater Clinical Judgment Rubric

	EXEMPLARY	ACCOMPLISHED	DEVELOPING	BEGINNING
Effective noticing involves:				
Focused observation	Focuses observation appropriately; regularly observes and monitors a wide variety of objective and subjective data to uncover any useful information	Regularly observes and monitors a variety of data, including both subjective and objective; most useful information is noticed; may miss the most subtle signs	Attempts to monitor a variety of subjective and objective data but is overwhelmed by the array of data; focuses on the most obvious data, missing some important information	Confused by the clinical situation and the amount and kind of data; observation is not organized and important data are missed, and/or assessment errors are made
Recognizing deviations from expected patterns	Recognizes subtle patterns and deviations from expected patterns in data and uses these to guide the assessment	Recognizes most obvious patterns and deviations in data and uses these to continually assess	Identifies obvious patterns and deviations, missing some important information; unsure how to continue the assessment	Focuses on one thing at a time and misses most patterns and deviations from expectations; misses opportunities to refine the assessment
Information seeking	Assertively seeks information to plan intervention; carefully collects useful subjective data from observing and interacting with the patient and family	Actively seeks subjective information about the patient's situation from the patient and family to support planning interventions; occasionally does not pursue important leads	Makes limited efforts to seek additional information from the patient and family; often seems not to know what information to seek and/or pursues unrelated information	Is ineffective in seeking information; relies mostly on objective data; has difficulty interacting with the patient and family and fails to collect important subjective data
Effective interpreting involves:				
Prioritizing data	Focuses on the most relevant and important data useful for explaining the patient's condition	Generally focuses on the most important data and seeks further relevant information but also may try to attend to less pertinent data	Makes an effort to prioritize data and focus on the most important, but also attends to less relevant or useful data	Has difficulty focusing and appears not to know which data are most important to the diagnosis; attempts to attend to all available data
Making sense of data	Even when facing complex, conflicting, or confusing data, is able to (a) note and make sense of patterns in the patient's data, (b) compare these with known patterns (from the nursing knowledge base, research, personal experience, and intuition), and (c) develop plans for interventions that can be justified in terms of their likelihood of success	In most situations, interprets the patient's data patterns and compares with known patterns to develop an intervention plan and accompanying rationale; the exceptions are rare or in complicated cases where it is appropriate to seek the guidance of a specialist or a more experienced nurse	In simple, common, or familiar situations, is able to compare the patient's data patterns with those known and to develop or explain intervention plans; has difficulty, however, with even moderately difficult data or situations that are within the expectations of students; inappropriately requires advice or assistance	Even in simple, common, or familiar situations, has difficulty interpreting or making sense of data; has trouble distinguishing among competing explanations and appropriate interventions, requiring assistance both in diagnosing the problem and developing an intervention
Effective responding involves:				
Calm, confident manner	Assumes responsibility; delegates team assignments; assesses patients and reassures them and their families	Generally displays leadership and confidence and is able to control or calm most situations; may show stress in particularly difficult or complex situations	Is tentative in the leader role; reassures patients and families in routine and relatively simple situations, but becomes stressed and disorganized easily	Except in simple and routine situations, is stressed and disorganized, lacks control, makes patients and families anxious or less able to cooperate

Table 14-1 Lasater Clinical Judgment Rubric *(continued)*

	EXEMPLARY	ACCOMPLISHED	DEVELOPING	BEGINNING
Clear communication	Communicates effectively; explains interventions; calms and reassures patients and families; directs and involves team members, explaining and giving directions; checks for understanding	Generally communicates well; explains carefully to patients; gives clear directions to team; could be more effective in establishing rapport	Shows some communication ability (e.g., giving directions); communication with patients, families, and team members is only partly successful; displays caring but not competence	Has difficulty communicating; explanations are confusing; directions are unclear or contradictory; patients and families are made confused or anxious and are not reassured
Well-planned intervention/flexibility	Interventions are tailored for the individual patient; monitors patient progress closely and is able to adjust treatment as indicated by patient response	Develops interventions on the basis of relevant patient data; monitors progress regularly but does not expect to have to change treatments	Develops interventions on the basis of the most obvious data; monitors progress but is unable to make adjustments as indicated by the patient's	Focuses on developing a single intervention, addressing a likely solution, but it may be vague, confusing, and/or incomplete; some monitoring may occur
Being skillful	Shows mastery of necessary nursing skills	Displays proficiency in the use of most nursing skills; could improve speed or accuracy	Is hesitant or ineffective in using nursing skills	Is unable to select and/or perform nursing skills

As you can see in Lasater's rubric, the four components of Tanner's model each have three to four dimensions that further explicate each of the four components. These 11 total dimensions are similar to competencies insomuch as they are very direct, clear, and action-oriented (see the far-left column of the rubric). Like any rubric you may have used in previous coursework to guide your development of an assignment and your teacher's grading of the assignment, a scale defines and describes level of accomplishment, which may be associated with points or a grade. In the LCJR, four levels of performance are possible: *exemplary*, *accomplished*, *developing*, or *beginning* (top row of the rubric). Detailed descriptions of actions taken by a student nurse who is deemed exemplary, accomplished, developing, or beginning for each of the 11 dimensions are included to guide use of the rubric. Although originally designed for the evaluation of a single simulation scenario, the rubric outlines the expectations of student nurses and provides a concrete way to show progression in the development of clinical judgment. A rubric like this is very valuable when used over the duration of a nursing program. Your program likely has a clinical evaluation tool that may reflect some of the ideas outlined in the LCJR. Your faculty will also evaluate your performance in the skills laboratory or simulation setting according to predefined standards that reflect expected development, expected performance, and the culture and values of your program. As an aside, learning to use a rubric early in your career will assist you not just in school; rubrics are often associated with grants, publishing scholarly works, a clinical ladder or evaluation tool at work, and many other instances where standardized evaluation is required.

Developing Nurses' Thinking Model

The Developing Nurses' Thinking (DNT) model has undergone several revisions and has been tested in several studies (Jensen et al., 2014; Tesoro, 2012; Tesoro et al., 2021). The initial model considered four evidence-based concepts: domain knowledge that includes the nursing process, discrete critical thinking processes, safety issues, and repeated practice of the model to develop habits (Tesoro, 2012). The latest iteration used by Tesoro et al. (2021) contains the same concepts but emphasizes the level of actual or potential danger and demonstrates the cyclic nature of the nursing process. The model identifies 17 critical thinking processes including information seeking, contextual perspective, predicting, discriminating, intuition/pattern recognition, and creativity. The DNT model was used to develop clinical reasoning prompts designed to assist student nurses in making clinical judgments on a case study. Although the prompts primarily increased confidence, one of the things brought to light by research using the DNT model is the value and necessity of threading clinical judgment models and frameworks into curricula to provide students repeated opportunities to develop critical thinking, clinical reasoning, and clinical judgment (Tesoro et al., 2021). Your school may integrate a clinical judgment model (or a combination of models) into their lessons, reflections, and evaluation tools to allow for repeated exposure to these concepts, to provide a framework for you, and to track your growth.

California Critical Thinking Disposition Inventory

The California Critical Thinking Disposition Inventory (CCTDI) measures the willingness of an adult learner to think critically. Based on an expert consensus in the American Philosophical Association (APA) Delphi Report on critical thinking (Facione, 1990), the CCTDI describes the characteristics of an ideal critical thinker and measures seven attributes:

> the disposition toward truth-seeking or bias, toward open-mindedness or intolerance, toward anticipating possible consequences or being heedless of them, toward proceeding in a systematic or unsystematic way, toward being confident in the powers of reasoning or mistrustful of thinking, toward being inquisitive or resistant to learning, and toward mature and nuanced judgment or toward rigid simplistic thinking (Insight Assessment, 2021).

The CCTDI provides insight into the tendency of a person to engage in life-long or career-long learning, which is good information for a student nurse who, based on the ever-changing, complex health care environment, is never done learning.

National Council of State Boards of Nursing

"National Council of State Boards of Nursing (NCSBN) is an independent, not-for-profit organization through which nursing regulatory bodies act and counsel together on matters of common interest and concern affecting public health, safety and welfare, including the development of nursing licensure examinations" (NCSBN, 2022, p. 1). Most nurse educators and nursing students associate NCSBN with the standardized tests required for nursing licensure, NCLEX-PN and NCLEX-RN. With any update of the exam, an associated test plan is posted online for nurse educators to use to ensure concepts are addressed in the curriculum. For example, in addition to outlining key concepts, the test plans highlight specific diagnostics and laboratory values that students need to know for the exam (as opposed to laboratory values expected to be referenced). You can access the most up-to-date test plans at https://www.ncsbn.org/testplans.htm; this is a good resource to access when crafting a study plan for the exam. NCSBN released clinical judgment and action models that are directly related to NCLEX.

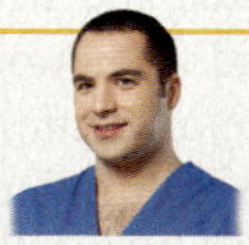

Recall ***Daniel Ramirez***, the student nurse who benefits from information about the teacher and exam when preparing a study plan. Daniel can start integrating NCLEX-style practice questions into his study plan early in the nursing program to increase his comfort with the types of questions he will be asked on the licensure exam.

Clinical Judgment Measurement Model

Although not a clinical judgment model, NCSBN's Clinical Judgment Measurement Model (CJMM) works behind the scenes of the standardized test required for nursing licensure upcoming new version of the NCLEX, the Next Generation NCLEX (NGN), set to release in 2023 to evaluate the development of clinical judgment (see Fig. 14-2 for the NCSBN Clinical Judgment Measurement Model). Layers 0–2 of the model emphasize how clinical judgment informs the clinical decisions made to address the client's needs. Evaluation of those decisions determines if the processes in layers 3 and 4 should be completed again. Layers 3 and 4 are focused on expected behaviors of a student in a specific clinical or case scenario. These behaviors are directly related to what NCSBN deems an appropriate clinical decision on the NGN (NCSBN, 2019a). Although this action model (described more fully in the next section) and measurement model are relatively new, they are related to the core elements of the nursing process, which have guided nursing education and practice for decades. See Figure 14-3 for the NCSBN Clinical Judgment Overview that overlays the five steps of the nursing process with the six NCSBN cognitive skills.

Clinical Judgment Action Model

The Clinical Judgment Action Model (CJAM) developed by NCSBN is used in the context of the 2023 release of the NGN. The action model aligns the six cognitive operations from layer 3 of the CJMM (recognize cues, analyze cues, prioritize hypotheses, generate solutions, take actions, and evaluation outcomes) with specific situational factors from layer 4 including environmental, client observation, medical record, and time pressure cues (NCSBN, 2019a). The NCSBN model is based on the humanistic–intuitive, information-processing, and cognitive continuum cognitive theories and models (Betts et al., 2019; see p. 394). This textbook, your faculty, and the NGN utilize evolving case studies to walk through these six steps in a clinical scenario that includes specific cues. Make sure you spend time on the evolving cases embedded at the end of eight chapters in this book (see p. 1081 for an example).

Forming, refining, and evaluating hypotheses in the context of clinical judgment challenges student nurses because they are learning how to simultaneously follow a systematic thought process to assess, prioritize, and diagnose, while allowing for creativity and individualization to meet the needs of the patient. Consider what is meant and how to describe specific elements of the CJAM. For example, when we talk about generating solutions, what you are actually doing is determining the desired outcomes, exploring the evidence to determine the best solution(s), identifying what resources are needed (Billings, 2019; Hensel & Billings, 2020), thinking about social determinants of health (SDoH) that may limit potential solutions, acknowledging your bias when considering options, and balancing creative solutions with realistic options.

Keep in mind that although the 2023 NGN requires your faculty to restructure some test items in your curriculum,

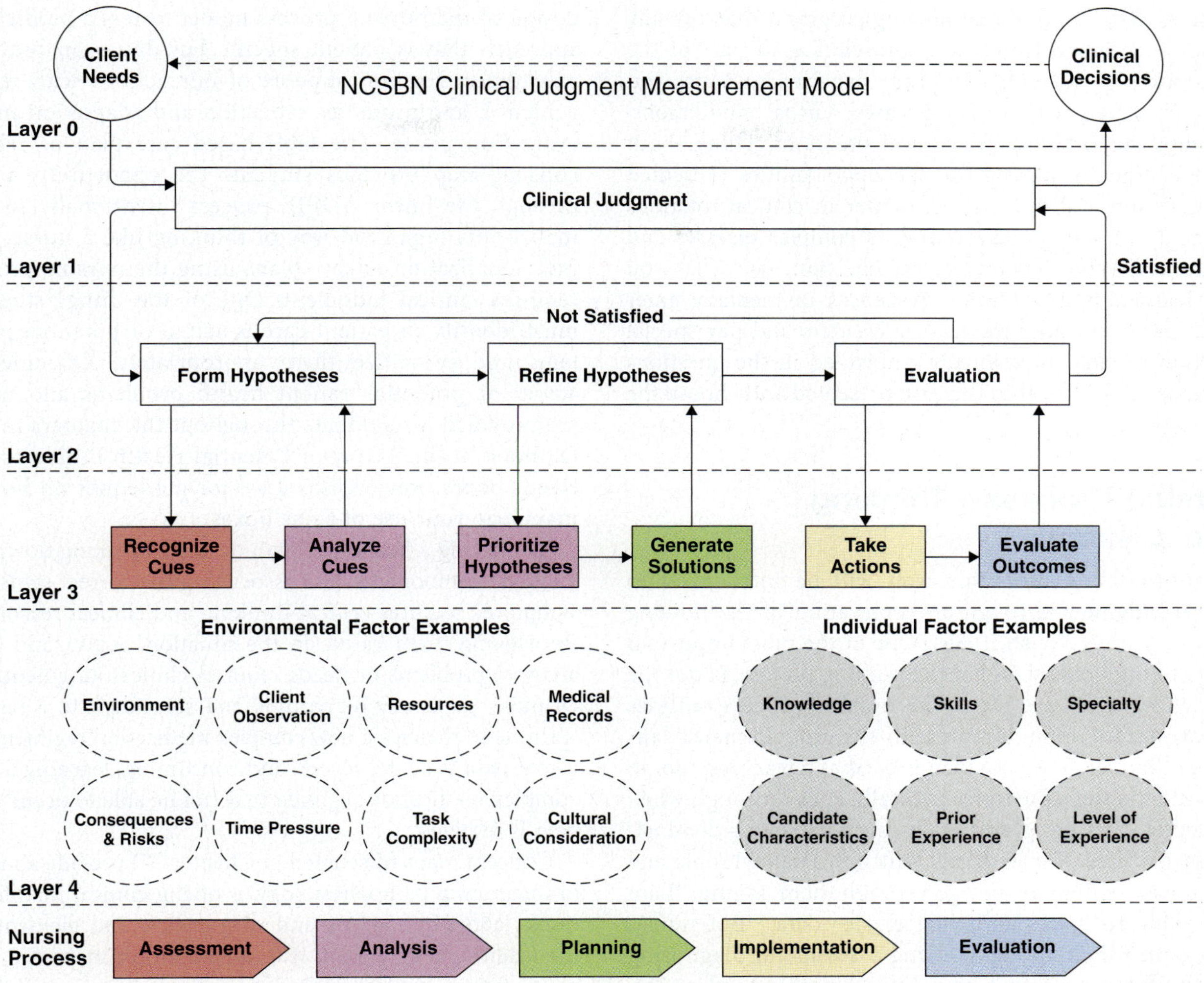

FIGURE 14-2. The NCSBN Clinical Judgment Measurement Model. (*Source:* Reprinted with permission from the National Council of State Boards of Nursing [NCSBN®]. [2021]. NCSBN clinical judgment measurement model. www.ncsbn.org/14798.htm)

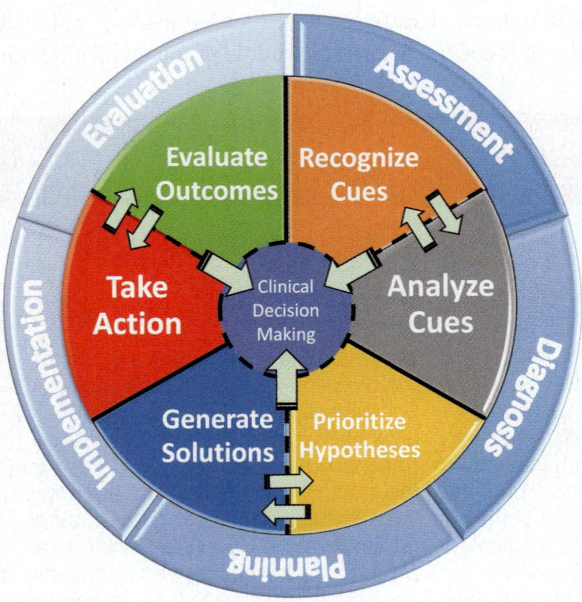

FIGURE 14-3. NCSBN Clinical Judgment Overview. (*Source:* Reprinted with permission from Brenton, A., & Petersen, E. K. [2019]. *Next generation NCLEX® [NGN] Educator Webinar Part I.* National Council of State Boards of Nursing [NCSBN®].)

you benefit from their transparency, instruction, and opportunities for practice because you must pass the NCLEX for licensure. However, nursing education addresses more than the NCLEX—nurse educators are working with you to facilitate your development as a practicing nurse who thrives in the complex health care environment. The development of clinical judgment is foundational and draws on your understanding and application of best evidence, situational awareness, advances in technology and communication, person-centered care (that includes SDoH, a holistic perspective, the impact of health policy, families and others close to the patient), and your ability to access and use your resources. Think beyond the NCLEX and classroom instruction. Integrate what you learn from your interactions with a live EHR in the clinical practice setting or the simulated EHR (such as DocuCare) used for simulation, laboratory, and other assignments. Integration of this technology is essential for clinical practice, which is why navigation of resources such as this may be embedded in the NGN and should become part of your study plan. Access and use various elements associated with your textbook to consider what you are studying from different perspectives, applications, and foci. Keep in mind that nursing programs intentionally include laboratory, simulation, and clinical as part of the preparation of students—let these experiences assist you when presented with evolving cases; virtual simulations; and, most importantly, live clinical situations. Think about this the other way, too—use the opportunities presented in simulation and that you encounter in clinical rotations to round out your understanding of complex diseases and syndromes. When reading a test question, use what you have learned from clinical experiences to mentally enter the scenario, consider the facts as written, and pay special attention to cues intentionally embedded in the questions to situate yourself within the case presented and choose the best answer.

Nursing Process—Thinking Like a Nurse

In most nursing programs, you will be introduced to clinical judgment through an exploration of the nursing process (Yura & Walsh, 1988). One of the most important things to understand is that the nursing process is not the same thing as a care plan. The nursing process outlines the way nurses think; it represents the unique, shared language of nurses. The care plan is used as a teaching tool to explicate the steps the nurse mentally goes thorough when developing, delivering, and evaluating a patient's individualized plan of care. Nurses do not walk into a patient room and announce the steps as they go through them, saying, "I am now going to assess and then cluster data!" But nurses *do* organize their thoughts using assessment, diagnosing or identifying an actual or potential problem, planning, identifying interventions with rationale, and evaluation (ADPIE). This nursing process represents a mental model (an organized way of thinking that shapes our worldview and helps us to understand complex aspects of a situation) that guides our assessments and behaviors. The formal design of the nursing process model fosters a predictable approach that is patient specific but draws on previous experience, requires support of our actions with recent evidence, and promotes reflection and adaptation in the evaluation phase. The table-based care plan or related concept map provides students the opportunity to go through the linear ADPIE process intentionally to formalize this organized way of thinking like a nurse. The individualization of care plans using the nursing process requires clinical judgment. One of the things students must identify in patient care is actual or potential problems and prioritize them appropriately. Examples of actual or potential patient health problems and needs are provided for students throughout the chapters in this textbook in the Actual or Potential Health Problems and Needs boxes. Review Box 14-1 for guidelines on how to maximize your use of these boxes.

Identifying a health problem or need, breaking down the etiologic components, and associating the correct signs and symptoms requires critical thinking and clinical reasoning. Prioritizing them based on the situation, acuity, and hierarchy of problems or needs requires clinical judgment. For example, pain may be chronic and secondary to a patient learning to manage a new complex medication regimen; but if that pain is acute, severe, and consuming, learning a new complex medication regimen may not be able to occur until pain is resolved.

Concept maps (discussed in Chapter 17) provide a means of integrating pathophysiology, evolving clinical manifestations, laboratory values and diagnostics, and elements of the traditional care plan. Although concept maps can take many forms, they should show progression (i.e., *X leads to Y*) and demonstrate relationships. In a free-form map, think about placing risk factors, pathophysiology, and disease processes at the top of the map; connecting to clinical manifestations, disease sequelae (consequences), and related problem identification in the middle of the map; and ending

Box 14-1 How to Use Actual or Potential Health Problems and Needs Boxes

Identifying a Problem or Need

Actual or Potential Health Problem or Need	Possible Etiologic Factors	Potential Signs and Symptoms
For this text, these health problems or needs come from one of the two sources below the table. However, in the clinical setting, most electronic health records (EHRs) include an auto-populated list that an interprofessional team member can draw upon to craft a plan of care that reflects best practice, takes standard reimbursement into account, and can be individualized for each patient.	Etiology requires determining the underlying cause—what is the root of the problem or need. Try not to use another problem or medical diagnosis here. Ask yourself what is going on with the patient to cause this problem or need. For example, we would not use chronic obstructive airway disease (COPD; a medical diagnosis) here. We could, however, state chronic mucus production, air trapping, and increased airway reactivity.	These are the signs and symptoms of the problem or need (not the etiology). For example, if you are going to identify a problem related to airway clearance (mechanical issue), be sure to describe the mucus and cough; if you are prioritizing a problem related to gas exchange (chemical issue), be sure to include a pulse oximetry reading and arterial blood gas results. Be sure to include objective and subjective data.

Source: International Council of Nurses (ICN). (2019). *Nursing diagnosis and outcome statements.* https://www.icn.ch/sites/default/files/inline-files/ICNP2019-DC.pdf; Wolters Kluwer. (2020). *Problem-based care plans.* In Lippincott Advisor. Wolters Kluwer. https://advisor.lww.com/lna/home.do

with interventions and outcomes at the bottom of the map. Concept maps are very valuable when considering the care of a patient with complex disease processes that are interrelated (see the concept map on p. 1045).

DEVELOPING COMPETENCY IN NURSING PRACTICE

Clinical judgment is foundational to every action taken by a nurse from identifying a problem and associated interventions to advocating for a patient whose voice needs to be heard. These actions, which are supported by clinical judgment, often fall into a competency model. Framing educational outcomes as competencies makes them measurable. In nursing, we are very outcome-focused with our patients and in our process of nursing education. These outcomes often focus on behaviors and attainment of certain thresholds. The American Nurses Association (ANA) *Nursing: Scope and Standards of Practice* (2021) defines a **competency** as "an expected level of performance that integrates knowledge, skills, abilities, and judgment" (p. 52). In many cases, competencies are complex and are not simply met once and checked off on a checklist—they require intentional reassessment by the educators and repeated exploration from different perspectives on the part of the student. Understanding education through the competency lens provides you perspective into checklists, rubrics, evaluation tools, rubrics, and even your program outcomes.

Competency Outcomes Performance Assessment Model

The Competency Outcomes and Performance Assessment Model (COPA; Lenburg et al., 2009) integrates essential practice competencies, outcomes and outcome statements, interactive learning strategies, and objective competency evaluation to validate competence in an effort to promote patient safety. This model was adapted in 2011 to prepare learners for effective role performance in the clinical practice environment by specifying specific, core behaviors in the affective, cognitive, and psychomotor realms that reflect competence (Lenburg et al., 2011; see Box 14-2 for an overview of these competencies). This concept of assessing students' knowledge, skills, and attitudes (KSAs) is a fundamental practice in nursing education. Asking what model is used for your competency evaluation informs your preparation and performance in simulation and skills laboratory settings. Knowing that educational rationale underpins the decisions made by faculty provides you context and will help you leverage resources provided to be successful in competency evaluation.

Professional Guidance

Nurse educators rely on standards of education and practice published by national leaders to guide their development of your curriculum and the associated methods of teaching. This development is intentional, collaborative, and often linked with accreditation of a nursing program.

Box 14-2 The Eight Core COPA Practice Competencies With Examples of Related Affective, Cognitive, and Psychomotor Skills

1. **Assessment and Intervention Skills**
   a. Safety and protection
   b. Assessment and monitoring
   c. Therapeutic treatments and procedures
2. **Communication Skills**
   a. Oral skills
      1. Talking, listening, with individuals
      2. Interviewing; history taking
      3. Group discussion, interacting
      4. Telling, showing, reporting
   b. Writing skills
      1. Clinical reports, care plans, charting
      2. Agency reports, forms, memos
      3. Articles, manuals
   c. Computing skills (information processing; using computers)
      1. Related to clients, agencies, other authorities
      2. Related to information search and inquiry
      3. Related to professional responsibilities
3. **Critical Thinking Skills**
   a. Evaluation; integrating pertinent data from multiple sources
   b. Problem solving; diagnostic reasoning; creating alternatives
   c. Decision making; prioritizing
   d. Scientific inquiry; research process
4. **Human Caring and Relationship Skills**
   a. Morality, ethics, legality
   b. Cultural respect; cooperative interpersonal relationships
   c. Client advocacy
5. **Management Skills**
   a. Administration, organization, coordination
   b. Planning, delegation, supervision of others
   c. Human and material resource utilization
   d. Accountability and responsibility; performance appraisals and QI
6. **Leadership Skills**
   a. Collaboration; assertiveness, risk taking
   b. Creativity, vision to formulate alternatives
   c. Planning, anticipating, supporting with evidence
   d. Professional accountability, role behaviors, appearance
7. **Teaching Skills**
   a. Individuals and groups; clients, coworkers, others
   b. Health promotion; health restoration
8. **Knowledge Integration Skills**
   a. Nursing, health care, and related disciplines
   b. Liberal arts, natural and social sciences, and related disciplines

Source: Lenburg, C. B., Klein, C., Abdur-Rahman, V., Spencer, T., & Boyer, S. (2009). The COPA model: A comprehensive framework designed to promote quality care and competence for patient safety. *Nursing Education Perspectives, 30*(5), 312–317; Lenburg, C. B., Abdur-Rahman, V. Z., Spencer, T. S., Boyer, S. A., & Klein, C. J. (2011). Implementing the COPA model in nursing education and practice settings: Promoting competence, quality care, and patient safety. *Nursing Education Perspectives, 32*(5), 290–296. https://doi.org/10.5480/1536-5026-32.5.290

American Association of Colleges of Nursing

In 2021, the American Association of Colleges of Nursing (AACN) re-envisioned their *Essentials* (2021), a document that guides nurse educators in the United States and internationally. This is important to you as a student because the core tenets described in the *Essentials* surface in your course and program/student learning outcomes, especially if your program is accredited by the Commission on Collegiate Nursing Education (CCNE). "*The Essentials: Core Competencies for Professional Nursing Education* has been built on the strong foundation of nursing as a discipline, the foundation of a liberal education, and principles of competency-based education" (AACN, 2021, p. 2). Using a competency model originally designed for physicians (Englander et al., 2013), the *Essentials* outlines 10 domains with associated competencies and sub-competencies. These competencies and sub-competencies specify behaviors that students must demonstrate in their entry-level or graduate-level programs and are designed to translate to the practice of nursing today. This goal-focused perspective requires measurable attainment of competencies in distinct spheres of care. The domains are listed in Box 14-3.

In addition to the other *featured concepts* (communication; compassionate care; evidence-based practice; health policy; SDoH; ethics; and diversity, equity, and inclusion), the *Essentials* specifically addresses the integration of clinical judgment. AACN's definition of clinical judgment recognizes clinical judgment as one of nursing's core attributes and foundational to the practice of nursing. There is an identifiable link between nursing knowledge that is rooted in evidence from myriad sources, nursing theory, and ways of knowing; knowledge gained from other disciplines and liberal education; critical thinking and reasoning; and CDM. This CDM, which is based on clinical judgment, directly impacts patient outcomes (AACN, 2021). AACN intentionally designed their competencies and sub-competencies to require consistent reiteration and consideration over the course of a nursing program, which means you will likely revisit the complex concepts outlined in the domains from many perspectives several times over your course of study. This guiding document articulates who we are and what we do as nurses, and provides a competencies-based map for both educators and students.

Box 14-3 AACN *Essentials* Competency Domains

- Domain 1: Knowledge for Nursing Practice
- Domain 2: Person-Centered Care
- Domain 3: Population Health
- Domain 4: Scholarship for Nursing Practice
- Domain 5: Quality and Safety
- Domain 6: Interprofessional Partnerships
- Domain 7: Systems-Based Practice
- Domain 8: Information and Healthcare Technologies
- Domain 9: Professionalism
- Domain 10: Personal, Professional, and Leadership Development

National League for Nursing

The competencies identified by the National League for Nursing (NLN, 2012, 2022) include human flourishing, nursing judgment, professional identity, and spirit of inquiry. Other key concepts integrated into the competencies-based education model address "context and environment; knowledge and science; personal and professional development; quality and safety; relationship-centered care; and teamwork" (NLN, 2021). The NLN Commission for Nursing Education Accreditation (CNEA) standards of accreditation build on the core values of NLN and these core competencies. Accreditation requires, in addition to other things, integration of experiential learning opportunities that "foster the acquisition of professional nursing values, encompassing, but not limited to, leadership skills, clinical reasoning and judgment, reflective thought, and ethically responsive care to diverse populations" (NLN CNEA, 2021, p. 37). The description of these professional values underscores the relevance of clinical judgment to good nursing care.

American Nurses Association

It is impossible to discuss competency in nursing education and not refer to the ANA for the *Nursing: Scope and Standards of Practice* (2021). The scope and standards publication articulates the necessity for nurses to use clinical judgment when identifying an actual or potential problem or need; when engaging in ethical decision making; and in conjunction with creative and critical thinking to evaluate the safety, quality, and effectiveness of nursing care (ANA, 2021). The scope and standards publication integrates several competency models including IPEC and QSEN, and specifically introduces the concept of structural competence. The 18 standards address each component of the nursing process (ADPIE, with outcome identification and planning addressed separately), ethics, advocacy, respectful and equitable practice, communication, collaboration, leadership, education, scholarly inquiry, quality of practice, professional practice evaluation, resource stewardship, and environmental health. Although not an exhaustive list, the guidance document also includes core competencies for each standard in relation to the scope of practice for registered nurses and graduate-level prepared registered nurses (ANA, 2021).

Quality and Safety Education for Nurses

Nursing education addresses collaborative, interprofessional-based initiatives that demonstrate responsiveness to national trends. Funded by the Robert Wood Johnson Foundation and developed by thought leaders in nursing, the competencies associated with Quality and Safety Education for Nurses (QSEN) outline the KSAs essential for prelicensure (and graduate) nurses. Using the Institute of Medicine (now the National Academy of Sciences, Engineering, and

Medicine) competencies from 2003, the seminal QSEN work (Cronenwett et al., 2007) focused on six areas: patient-centered care, teamwork and collaboration, evidence-based practice, quality improvement, safety, and informatics. The QSEN Institute website contains information on publications, conferences, and students resources you may find helpful: https://qsen.org/category/qs/.

You have likely noticed that this text intentionally includes threaded cases that focus on cultivating QSEN competencies. The QSEN boxes, such as the Reflective Practice display on p. 383 in this chapter, highlight the six main competencies to build your knowledge and ability to apply the competencies to a challenging clinical situation. We do this by asking you to consider possible courses of action, evaluate possible outcomes, and relate this reflection to your development as a student nurse. The questions posed facilitate multiple ways of thinking, thus expanding your frame of reference. Use these boxes embedded throughout this text to orient yourself to the QSEN competencies that directly relate to the integration of concepts foundational to the development of clinical judgment.

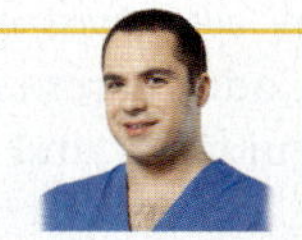

Recall **Daniel Ramirez**, the student nurse who has expressed some anxiety with test-taking. Learning to integrate and apply the core QSEN concepts provides an opportunity for Daniel to think about clinical situations from several angles. This is a helpful skill when asked to prioritize actions.

Interprofessional Education Collaborative

The Interprofessional Education Collaborative (IPEC) core competencies were developed by a team of interprofessional health care collaborators who published their initial competencies in 2001 and updated them in 2016. Interprofessional competencies are defined by IPEC as: "Integrated enactment of knowledge, skills, values, and attitudes that define working together across the professions, with other health care workers, and with patients, along with families and communities, as appropriate to improve health outcomes in specific care contexts" (IPEC, 2016, p. 8). In addition to receiving support from myriad national professional organizations, their work informs curriculum and accreditation standards through a Health Professions Accreditors Collaborative (HPAC) that includes professional organizations from nursing, pharmacy, dentistry, osteopathy, public health, and medical education. Their competency-based interprofessional education framework includes the following four competencies (IPEC, 2016, p. 10):

1. Work with individuals of other professions to maintain a climate of mutual respect and shared values. (Values/Ethics for Interprofessional Practice)
2. Use the knowledge of one's own role and those of other professions to appropriately assess and address the health care needs of patients and to promote and advance the health of populations. (Roles/Responsibilities)
3. Communicate with patients, families, communities, and professionals in health and other fields in a responsive and responsible manner that supports a team approach to the promotion and maintenance of health and the prevention and treatment of disease. (Interprofessional Communication)
4. Apply relationship-building values and the principles of team dynamics to perform effectively in different team roles to plan, deliver, and evaluate patient/population-centered care and population health programs and policies that are safe, timely, efficient, effective, and equitable. (Teams and Teamwork)

Sub-competencies flesh out the specific, measurable competencies that comprise interprofessional collaboration as a standalone domain in curricula for health care professionals.

As you consider the competences from COPA, AACN, NLN, ANA, QSEN, and IPEC, you will likely notice some common threads and terms. Compare the competencies you have learned about with what you see in your course and program/student learning outcomes. Taking the time to understand the roots of your curriculum helps you to appropriately appreciate concepts and competencies designed to foster the development of your clinical judgment as a nurse, member of a profession, and collaborator.

CLINICAL DECISION-MAKING THEORIES, MODELS, AND FRAMEWORKS

Nursing is not alone in the endeavor to develop clinical judgment, although critical thinking and judgment take different forms and have different foci depending on the end goal. CDM is often based on a defined process or framework that provides a rational structure for student nurses. In nursing, our understanding and application of clinical judgment in CDM is rooted in several cognitive theories. The following examples represent just a few of the cognitive theories related to processing, reasoning, and decision making.

Humanistic–Intuitive Approach

The humanistic–intuitive approach is referenced by nurses with respect to Benner's (1982) novice to expert model of development. Novice nurses make clinical judgments that do not consider all of the contextual elements and rely on concrete, analytic methods and planning to inform their decision making. Most new graduates function at the novice level. In practicing nurses, that thinking expands with attainment of the next four levels (advanced beginner, competent, proficient, and expert) and culminates in intuitive responses that seamlessly sort data and consider a holistic approach. Think about your experiences in clinical: do you ever wonder how the expert nurse seems to just instinctively know how to respond to unpredictable situations? Clinical judgment and decision-making models move from facts and rules to dynamic decision making with clinical experience (Benner, 1982; Betts et al., 2019).

Information-Processing Model

Another cognitive model that informs decision making mirrors the way we think of a computer processor. The information-processing model requires memory that is classified as sensory (collects and transforms), short term (temporary), and long term (more permanently stored). The information-processing model proposes a sequential way of thinking that involves encoding/input, storage, and retrieval/output. This cognitive theory proposes a straightforward way of considering human response to a stimulus that results in a response. Although a helpful model, we recognize that humans do not often process only one stimulus at a time, and we have emotions, histories, motivations, and other factors that can complicate this process.

Cognitive Continuum Theory

Originally posited by Hammond, a psychologist, in 1978 in relation to policy formation, the cognitive continuum theory (CCT) acknowledges and integrates both intuitive and analytical cognitive characteristics. The recognition that intuition influences CDM supports the delivery of creative, individualized, holistic, person-centered care. This intuitive aspect requires acknowledgment of potential biases and thoughtful use in conjunction with analysis to mitigate risk and errors (Standing, 2008). Standing (2008) built upon Hammond's original work and the work of Hamm (in medicine) to customize the cognitive continuum of clinical judgment and CDM for nursing that integrates intuition and analysis. What is significant about this model that will benefit student nurses is the consideration of the myriad activities performed by nurses from direct patient care to engaging in research and developing policy. It integrates accountability, ethical and professional comportment, competence, soundness of decisions, and consideration of other variables such as viability and time (Standing, 2008). Interprofessional team clinical judgment and CDM may be strengthened by the use of CCT by providing a shared language for CDM, mitigating potential bias, opening the door to a discussion of ideas based on experience, facilitating collaborative engagement in brainstorming solutions, and filling gaps in communication (Parker-Tomlin et al., 2017).

Rest Framework

Ethics underpins the cognitive theories and approaches, and there are many focused ethical decision-making models available to students and practitioners. Some models are rooted in deontology (duty-based), utilitarianism (greatest good for the greatest number), rights (Kant's categorical imperative), virtues (character based), or the feminist approach; these theories and associated approaches inform ethical decision-making frameworks that are often focused on consequences, duties, or virtue. Other models specifically draw on the beliefs, values, and obligations outlined in the professional code of ethics for that profession to craft a decision-making model tailored to their accepted professional roles and responsibilities (see Chapter 6 for more on ethics).

Based on the variation in nursing education and the complex health care environment, there is a recommendation to embed Rest's four-component model of moral reasoning into nursing curricula because it captures the cognitive processes that precede moral action and emphasizes the development of a person as a moral agent (Robichaux et al., 2022). The four components of the model include (Rest, 1982):

1. Moral sensitivity: development of an awareness that there is an ethical issue; requires empathy and perspective-taking
2. Moral judgment/reasoning: consideration of several courses of action to account for the potential impact on those involved (person-centered); occurs along with CDM and informs clinical judgment
3. Moral motivation/focus: cognitive process of decision making that involves prioritizing (often) competing values
4. Moral character: implementing a plan of action; related to professional identity formation

This last phase reflects integration of your professional and personal values and attributes, which is referred to as *wholeness of character* in our Code (ANA, 2015). The Code represents who we are as nurses, providing ethical guidance and supporting the profession of nursing. See Chapter 6 for a fuller discussion of the Code of Ethics for Nurses (ANA, 2015). As you progress in nursing school, keep in mind that decision-making schemata that you develop reflect your personal and professional role and identity formation.

INTEGRATING PREVIOUS KNOWLEDGE

Experiential learning reflects elements of competency models and clinical judgment models. In experiential learning, the cyclic nature of learning is driven by concrete experience, termed *prehension*, followed by *reflective observation*, which leads to the formation of abstract concepts that are then tested in new situations through experimentation, the integration of which is termed *transformation*. The process then begins anew with the active experimentation affecting the next experience (Kolb, 1984). Leveraging previously acquired knowledge in meaningful ways is essential for student nurses.

Educational Experience

Learning is cumulative. Lessons learned in your prerequisite courses inform your thinking, your perspectives, and your learning ethos. Ethos in this instance refers to the guiding beliefs, or ethics, of a group, person, or organization (Ethos, 2021). It is also a term used in rhetoric to reference Aristotle's description of ethos, which contains *phronesis* (wisdom or intelligence), *arete* (general moral virtue of your argument), and *eunoia* (the trust and rapport you establish with your audience), all of which are germane to establishing a writer's credibility, knowledge, and moral character (Gaiman, 2021). Although we are not going to dive into a philosophical debate on the value of rhetoric, nursing programs require students to build on previously acquired knowledge from the humanities, social science, and natural sciences (AACN, 2021). "The study of history, critical race theories, critical theories of nursing, critical digital studies, planetary health and climate science, politics, public policies, policy formation, fine arts, literature, languages, and the behavioral, biological, and natural sciences are key to the understanding of one's self and others, civil readiness, and engagement and forms the basis for clinical reasoning and subsequent clinical judgments" (AACN, 2021, p. 4). Developing empathy, a tolerance for ambiguity, the ability to take the perspective of others, and advocacy are all rooted in the liberal arts. One of the elements included in this textbook is a Poetry Nook—these poems were all written by a poet and nurse, Amy Haddid. They have been included to activate your creative side, to engage you in a different way, to change your thinking, and to provide personal insight in a way only poetry can.

As you read each poem, consider the following reflection questions:

- How did this poem make you feel?
- Who is speaking in the poem? Why is their perspective important?
- What meaning do you attribute to the words in each stanza or section?

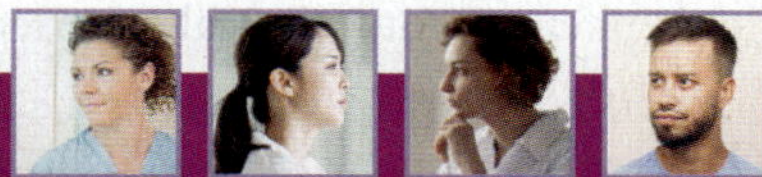

Poetry Nook

Imaging Prep

You sigh, irritated with my veins.
A furtive glance at my other arm
spells uncertainty, or worse,
inexperience.

You run

your fingers down my arm,
resting in the pale antecubital
space, moving on above my wrist.
Veins roll and hide at
your touch. You commit

to the arm with the tourniquet,
poke the needle in and shimmy
the sheath, sliding the
sharp
back out. We wait for the
blood
to fill the tubing. When none

comes, you push the tubing
ahead a bit and hit a wall
in my vein. I gasp. You pause,
sigh again.

The flush flaming your neck
speaks of shame and pigheaded
resolve to stick with this site.

Each try burns as you jiggle
the tubing in and out. If you
keep at it,
I will wear your
handiwork
for weeks. I hiss
to let you know
it hurts.
Weighing the cost
of
crying out, *Stop.*

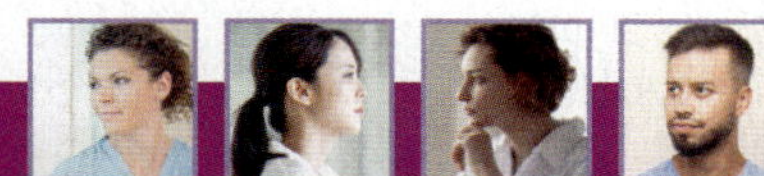

Poetry Nook

Making Camp

The hall to intensive care is always
lit. At night, families and others,
unprepared, no gear or supplies,
make camp
in the waiting rooms, retreat
to corners, arrange makeshift
pillow forts. Lay claim to sofas,
drape and shape with sheets
to draw property lines. Downstream,
the more private consultation room,
sleeps two but reeks of bad news.
The tinny heave of the coffee machine
marks time over the family burrowed
under the information desk. They stay
close in case something changes,
hover at the end of the bed ten minutes
every hour. At dawn, they bend,
stiff and rumpled at the sinks, splash
water on their faces, avoiding any
glimpses of their mirrored lives, then
pat dry with harsh paper towels.
They lean against walls
to get the best signal,
texting, talking and casing
out who might still be there.

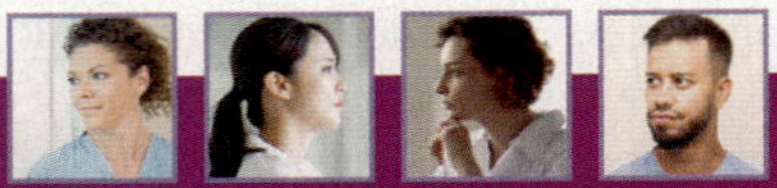

Poetry Nook

Blame Placing

Holding the scalpel in his gloved hand
like a baton, poised above the black crust
that was once her big toe—
tap, tap, tap, ready, begin.
The already hardened
medical students and residents
flank the maestro.
I stand by the head of the bed,
reach for the patient's hand,
hold it in both of mine.

The surgeon cuts away
at the decay
with constant clinical patter.
At first the patient does not flinch,
her hand held in mine.
She grips me, bites
her bottom lip, holds her breath
against the pain.

Now we're getting somewhere.
See how it bleeds. That's a good sign.
I whisper close to her ear,
Take a deep breath.
It will help ease the pain.
The smallest cry escapes
as she exhales. She turns crimson.

The performance interrupted,
he addresses me, *Nurse, let go of her hand.*
She grabs me tighter.
He drops the scalpel,
snaps off both sterile gloves.
I want to see you in the hall, now!
Extracting my hands,
I follow him out of the room.

He punctuates each word with a jab
to my chest, just above my name tag,
When I tell you to let go
of my patient, do it.

He pivots to leave. Not quite finished
he turns back, face so close to mine
I feel his breath, *You made things worse*
by babying her. Students in tow
who watched their mentor's show
follow.

I return to dress her bloody foot,
hope that there is something ordered
for her pain. *I'm sorry,*
I got you in trouble, she says.

- Where is the nurse in the poem? Describe the attributes of the nurse (and other health care professionals) in the poem.
- How does the technical structure of the poem impact on your appreciation of the poem and on the clarity of the message of the poem?
- Write your own poem about a clinical experience.

Your view of education and your role as a student nurse evolves over the course of your education. Although you may have completed a learning style inventory and are well aware of your preferred education delivery mode, you will learn increased adaptability as you flex to assimilate new content from many different sources. For example, simulation requires flexing within a predictable and replicable model; clinical requires responding to individual and situational constraints; and didactic content may include small group work, specific technology-based applications that require more mental work from you up front, or more traditional lecture peppered with narratives, videos, and evolving case studies.

This blending of delivery models may not always suit your auditory, visual, or kinesthetic preference(s), but varied teaching and learning modalities help you consider different perspectives and strategies and allow for the development of multiple ways of knowing. Clinical judgment is informed by balancing empirical, aesthetic, personal, ethical (Carper, 1978), and sociopolitical (White, 1995) ways or patterns of knowing. Unknowing represents the nurse's ability to appreciate that they cannot and do not know the patient before their first encounter—the patient's perspective and their unique needs take precedence over our clinical habits and assumptions (Heath, 1998; Munhall, 1993). Depending on the specific situation, nurses integrate the ways or patterns of knowing, sometimes emphasizing one component over another to improve patient outcomes.

Life Experience

We need diversity in nursing—our intention in health care is to mirror the populations we serve. Your unique experiences have shaped who you are as a person, and they are important. The goal is to help you develop your professional and personal identity within the confines of professional practice. This means that we foster decision making by enforcing school policies regarding late work, addressing areas that require attention through formal action plans, and partnering with you to define goals for your education. Any critical thinking and reasoning skills you already have in your repertoire will serve you well as we work together to adapt these skills for the clinical environment where our clinical judgment informs important clinical decisions that impact on the populations we serve.

Health Care Experience

Striking the balance between integrating your previous experience in health care to provide context for your burgeoning nursing practice and allowing your preconceived notions and role-specific knowledge to interfere with your development as a nurse requires intentionality. Instead of thinking, "that's not the way we do it in the real world," reframe your thinking to consider the underlying principles. Here is an example to consider: a nurse inserting an indwelling catheter does not follow the procedure you were shown when you onboarded as a patient care technician or does not strictly adhere to the carefully constructed checklist you memorized for check-off that week in lab. What you have to consider is whether the nurse adhered to the principles of sterility, the situational constraints (e.g., room set-up, available equipment, patient anatomy, nurse's dominant hand), and patient physical and psychological safety. Reframing your thinking to account for things you may not have considered at first glance builds your trust of the interprofessional team and fosters a collaborative approach. Nursing students benefit the health care environment by bringing positivity and elevating routine practice because of their questions regarding policy and procedure and constant observance. Ask questions, but keep in mind that your tone and words matter. Recognize that learning the steps is essential when practicing the urinary catheterization skill for the first time, but the ability to adapt while adhering to the underlying infection-control principles demonstrates clinical judgment.

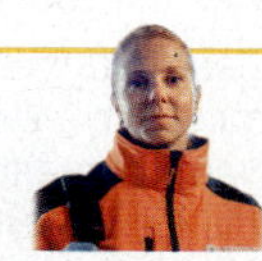

Recall **Kallie McDonald**, the paramedic transitioning to nursing. As a paramedic, Kallie completed an associate degree and is familiar with a defined scope of practice related to licensure. Because of the comprehensive response expected of the paramedic, Kallie has developed clinical judgment skills and routinely engages in complex decision making. Kallie's focus should be on honing those skills and integrating them into their evolving professional identity as a nurse.

IMPORTANCE OF REFLECTION

While in nursing school, you are going to be asked to formally reflect, often in writing, more than you expect. The practice of reflection is different than journaling—it is intentional, focused, directed, and purposeful. Guided reflection templates or guidelines may reflect your program/student learning outcomes, course outcomes, competencies or sub-competencies, or other measurable elements. For example, Nielsen et al. (2007) developed a Guide for Reflection that is based on Tanner's Clinical Judgment Model (Box 14-4 on page 398).

This Reflection Guide provides prompts in the form of both questions and directives that guide the thinking of the student nurse. Take a look under the Interpreting header. Do you see how this guide forces the student to arrive at a conclusion? There is also an expectation that rationales are provided, which integrates evidence-based practice. Now look under the Responding header. Do you see how this includes prompts that guide your thinking of thoughtful, person-centered interventions? Pay special attention to the second question regarding the identification of stressors: this question provides the space and grace for the student nurse to reflect on their feelings. The last four questions on the guide drive home the necessity of reflecting on learning. You will see these headers in the Thoughtful, Person-Centered Practice: Challenging Topics boxes (for example, on pages 398–399) included throughout this textbook. Take the time to consider the challenge presented and walk through the questions to reflect deeply and with purpose.

Simulation debriefing (or debrief) is another touch point for reflection. Reflection during a debrief is often done verbally with groups of participants. A simulation debrief facilitator typically uses a semi-structured debriefing guide that prompts pointed questions to engage participants and allow them to dialogue, vent, critique, celebrate, and tie learning back to the clinical practice setting. If serving as a participant observer in a simulation (not directly involved with the scenario), your perspective provides additional information for the team to consider, especially during the debrief. Facilitators often require specific training to integrate team dynamics into a debriefing session. An individual written reflection may also be included with a simulation experience. This may be used before the group debrief to allow individual participants time to process and organize their thoughts and feelings, or after the debrief to reinforce learning. Knowing the information is very different from applying it in the moment in response to a specific scenario designed to elicit a response from you. The debrief and/or reflection provides the space and mechanism for focusing on the process of clinical reasoning ("What did you do next? What were you thinking when you made that decision?") to guide you in your ability to make sound clinical decisions based on clinical judgment ("How are you going to apply what you learned to your clinical practice?").

DEVELOPING CLINICAL REASONING AND CLINICAL JUDGMENT

This section is found in each chapter of this textbook to foster intentional reflection and foster clinical reasoning and clinical judgment related to the specific content of the chapter. The questions are designed to help you reflect and apply critical thinking skills to develop your abilities related to clinical judgment. Since this entire chapter was focused on clinical judgment, instead of providing prompts, we will explore why the questions are included in each chapter.

1. The first question in the clinical chapters refers you to the concept map, care plan, or evolving case study. The evolving case studies are modeled after a template provided by NCSBN, in which a scenario is interrupted by questions designed to hone your ability to recognize cues, prioritize cues, prioritize hypotheses, generate solutions, take action, and evaluate outcomes.
2. The remaining questions are designed to deepen your critical thinking, explore your process of clinical reasoning, and employ CDM based on clinical judgment.

Box 14-4 Guide for Reflection Using Tanner's Clinical Judgment Model

Instructions

This Guide for Reflection is intended to help you think about a given clinical situation you have encountered during the past week and your nursing response to that situation. The situation can be a specific physiologic patient problem, such as an elevation in temperature, respiratory difficulty, or electrolyte imbalance. You may choose to describe a situation involving a patient's family. The situation can be a description of your role in interdisciplinary problem solving. The reflection situation may describe an ethical issue you encountered in practice. Use the guide for reflection as a way to tell the story of the situation you encountered.

The guide provides you with a way of thinking about care that supports the development of your clinical judgment. Although there are many ways of organizing your thinking about patient care and professional nursing practice, Tanner's (2006) Clinical Judgment Model provides the framework for the questions in this guide.

Introduction

Describe a nursing situation you encountered this week (see the instructions above).

Background

- Describe your relationship to the patient at the time you noticed the situation (e.g., previous contact with patient and/or family, the quality of your relationship).
- Consider experiences you have had that helped you provide nursing care in the situation. Describe your formal knowledge (e.g., physiology, psychology, communication skills), previous nursing experiences with a similar problem, and/or personal experiences that helped guide you as you worked with the patient.
- Describe your beliefs about your role as the nurse in working on the situation.
- Describe any emotions you had about the situation.

Noticing

- What did you notice about the situation initially?
- Describe what you noticed as you spent more time with the patient and/or family.

Interpreting

- Describe what you thought about the situation (e.g., its cause, potential resolutions, patterns you noticed).
- Describe any similar situations you have encountered in practice before. Describe any similarities and differences you observed when compared with the current situation.
- What other information (e.g., assessment data, evidence) did you decide you needed as you considered the situation? How did you obtain this information? What help with the problem did you get from your preceptor?

Your conclusion: What did your observations and data interpretation lead you to believe? How did they support your response to the situation? Include pertinent pathophysiology and/or psychopathology.

Responding

- After considering the situation, what was your goal for the patient, family, and/or staff? What was your nursing response, or what interventions did you do? List all actions that you took.
- Describe stresses you experienced as you responded to the patient or others involved in the situation.

Reflection-in-Action

- What happened? How did the patient, family, and/or staff respond? What did you do next?

Reflection-on-Action and Clinical Learning

- Describe three ways your nursing care skills expanded during this experience.
- Name three things you might do differently if you encounter this kind of situation again.
- What additional knowledge, information, and skills do you need when encountering this kind of similar situation in the future?
- Describe any changes in your values or feelings as a result of this experience.

Source: Nielsen, A., Stragnell, S., & Jester, P. (2007). Guide for Reflection Using the Clinical Judgment Model. *Journal of Nursing Education*, *46*(11), 513–516. https://doi.org/10.3928/01484834-20071101-06

Thoughtful, Person-Centered Practice: Challenging Topics

Artificial Intelligence (AI) and Informatics in Health Care

Many controversial issues make it challenging to know how to respond as a professional nurse in select scenarios. Often, the nurse's personal and/or professional values may conflict with options desired by patients, families, employers, and communities. Not infrequently, nurses have to make clinical judgments balancing promoting and safeguarding personal integrity and respecting the values and preferences of patient. The *Essentials* for nursing education includes that nurses need to acknowledge their own personal and professional values, and demonstrate an awareness of their conscious and unconscious biases (AACN, 2021).

Read the scenario below and see if you can articulate what you believe, why you believe this, and how these beliefs are likely to inform the decisions you make and your behavior, especially when you are confronted with competing obligations. Based on Tanner's Clinical Judgment Model (2006), consider reflection-in-action and reflection-on-action (Nielsen et al., 2007):

Reflection-in-Action

As you read, consider what the new nurse is thinking in the moment—what happened? How did the patient and health care team respond? What did the nurse do next?

Thoughtful, Person-Centered Practice: Challenging Topics *(continued)*

Artificial Intelligence (AI) and Informatics in Health Care

Scenario

As a new graduate nurse, I was trained in the use of an electronic health record (EHR) and have worked to seamlessly complete my documentation in the moment while I am still in the patient's room. Medication administration now moves pretty quickly and I've learned how to navigate the screens to look up my medications and administer the medications following the general tenets of the rights of medication administration and three checks that were drilled into me while in nursing school. But I admit that I've streamlined the process a bit and rarely think about the actual steps. The triggers and notifications that pop up on the screen are sometimes a nuisance, but I've figured out a way to bypass things that do not seem to apply to my patient. Sometimes I think this system was designed to annoy me while making it impossible to compete straightforward tasks quickly. For example, the last time I entered my patient's vitals in the EHR, something popped up about sepsis, which is ridiculous . . . my patient does not have a potentially life-threatening infection.

Effective Noticing (Cues)

1. What did you notice about the situation initially? What information/observations are significant? What information deviates from what you have been taught is best practice?

Effective Interpreting

2. How could the information provided in the pop-up be useful? What other assessment data, evidence and/or information would you need to consider in the situation?
3. What do you think about this situation? Does the nurse's clinical judgment ever take precedence over standards of care, protocols, or instruments intentionally included in the EHR? Is this one of those times?

Scenario

On rounds an hour later, the primary provider met with the team and indicated that the patient, admitted with a basic urinary tract infection (UTI) was demonstrating early signs of sepsis. The temperature, respirations, and heart rate were all slightly elevated, which prompted the provider to order a stat blood draw for a lactate, which was also elevated. The team was instructed to initiate the sepsis protocol.

Now, consider the nurse's decision to implement shortcuts and reflect on your learning. See if you can articulate what you believe, why you believe this, and how these beliefs are likely to inform the decisions you make and your behavior, especially when you confronted with competing obligations.

Effective Responding

4. How would you describe the obligations you have in this scenario to your patient, to yourself, and to your team? Where do speed and efficiency rank in relation to effective clinical judgment?
5. How did the team approach benefit the patient in this scenario? What if the primary provider had not followed up on the prompt triggered in the EHR by the data you entered?
6. How will you locate the sepsis protocol? Who will you identify to assist you with the implementation of the protocol? What can you delegate and what requires your immediate attention? How will you prioritize your actions?

Effective Reflecting

As you reflect on this case, consider your role and the role of other members of the health care team.

7. Do you need to report that you ignored the trigger in the EHR? Do you think the provider is aware that you did not react? Could this affect your working relationship?
8. What do you really know about the indicators of sepsis? What could be going on behind the scenes in the EHR that prompted this message? What resources can you access to better inform your decision making in the future?
9. What do you know about artificial intelligence, machine learning, and informatics, in general? How do they impact patient outcomes? Are your shortcuts possibly undermining the benefits of integrating machine learning into clinical environments?

Reflection-on-Action

Then look back at the scenario—how might this have been different if the provider had also ignored the message in the EHR? How did your knowledge and/or skills expand based on this scenario? How will you continue to explore informatics and how it can potentially impact on patient outcomes, both positively and negatively? What are the risks and benefits of integrating technology? What attitude, value, or belief shifts did you experience (if any) after reading this scenario? How will you maintain core practice standards once you graduate?

Lasater, K. (2007). Clinical judgment development: Using simulation to create an assessment rubric. *Journal of Nursing Education, 46*(11), 496–503. https://case.edu/nursing/sites/case.edu.nursing/files/2018-06/Clinical-Judgement-Development.pdf

Nielson, A., Stragnell, S., & Jester, P. (2007). Guide for reflection using the Clinical Judgment Model. *Journal of Nursing Education, 46*(11), 513–516. https://doi.org/10.3928/01484834-20071101-06

Tanner, C. A. (2006). Thinking like a nurse: A research-based model of clinical judgment in nursing. *Journal of Nursing Education, 45*(6), 204–211. https://doi.org/10.3928/01484834-20060601-04

Box 14-5 Tips for NCLEX Success

- If all things are equal in a question, choose the answer that relates to airway, breathing, or circulation (ABC)—focus on the things that are life threatening first.
- If all the data presented in a question are focused on the renal system (for example), look for an answer related to renal function, not any of the other systems.
- If the answers represent unexpected and expected events or data points, the unexpected item is typically the most concerning.
- Mentally enter the patient-care setting described and form an image of the scene to rank-order interventions—walk through the steps of what you would do if you were standing in the described setting.
- If you have enough information in a question to formulate a differential diagnosis, move to an intervention (not assessment) in your answer—in other words, *when in distress, do not assess.*
- Read the question, review all the possible answers, eliminate answers immediately deemed wrong, and then read the question again—this helps you answer the question you are being asked and forces you to take an extra moment to consider the specific system/priority/strategy/area being tested.
- All cues in a question are important—if age, sex, assessment data, or other elements are included, they are provided to give you situational context that matters when determining the best course of action; when reviewing a chart or other data for a question, watch for patterns and make connections to determine which information is relevant or irrelevant.
- Focus on hallmark presenting signs and symptoms; consider resolution or improvement of these signs and symptoms as a cue that the intervention/treatment/medication has been effective.
- Even if you are not in a program that emphasizes a concept-based curriculum, pay attention to concepts that are related—for example, although very different etiologies, classic (cast-based) compartment syndrome, circumferential burns, cardiac tamponade, and increased intracranial pressure all share core tenets of assessment and intervention.
- When answering a question that a patient asks the nurse (on an NCLEX-style question), answer the patient's question directly and then consider the most therapeutic option.
- Think about what is *reasonable* based on the patient, available resources, your role, and the setting—for example, if the setting is the community, the patient will not have a peripheral intravenous catheter in place for medication administration.
- Only choose to call the provider as the priority answer if you need an intervention that is outside your scope of practice (such as surgery), only once you have enough data to make a reasonable SBAR report, and only when the required intervention is not listed in one of the other answers.

PRACTICING FOR NCLEX

Although the NCLEX-formatted questions included in every chapter will help you solidify your understanding of the content within the chapter, make sure you spend time reviewing the rationale. Learning *why* an answer is wrong is just as important as verifying your answer is correct—test processing is a skill you will need to develop. Also consider the rationale provided for prioritizing. Test processing is not a trick or a game, it is a skill that can be learned. There are several mental schemas that can be used to assist you in choosing the correct answer. Box 14-5 provides a few tips.

If your nursing program allows you to return to questions before submitting your exam, never leave an answer blank—mark your initial instinct before moving on to the next question; when you return to review the question, unless you notice something new in the question that you did not catch on the first read or suddenly remember a hallmark or other key element that provides irrefutable rationale, keep your original answer. These five questions are focused on the content from this chapter. Please keep in mind that *all* NCLEX-style questions require clinical judgment. Reflect on your development of content expertise and test processing as you work your way through the NCLEX-style questions at the end of each chapter in this textbook. Review the most recent NCSBN test plan for insight into the types of questions to expect on NGN, including multiple response, hot-spot, drop-down, drag-and-drop, and matrix/grid (NCSBN, 2019b).

1. A student nurse walks into a patient room, introduces themselves, and begins to complete a full head-to-toe assessment. The clinical faculty member enters the room, introduces themselves, and asks the student to step out of the room for a moment. The student meets the faculty member in the hallway and is asked to identify 15 cues or observations they noted during their initial contact with the patient and the patient's environment. Although the student is unable to reach 15 observations, the faculty guides the student to recognize the linen on the floor, old dinner tray on the windowsill, empty water pitcher, twisted oxygen tubing, the patient's pallor, and several other things requiring action. What is the value of engaging in this kind of activity with students in the clinical setting?
   a. Developing situational awareness is important to risk prevention, timely implementation of interventions, and prioritizing actions
   b. Managing cognitive load begins with systematically sorting mental images and immediately addressing pressing concerns
   c. Nursing best practice requires that an environmental scan be completed and documented in the electronic health record (EHR)
   d. Designing interventions that increase patient satisfaction is an essential focus for nurses when completing their initial assessments

2. A nursing program uses Tanner's Clinical Judgment Model, a research-based model that accounts for

differences in the patient, environment, and individual student nurse. What makes Tanner's reflection step unique?

a. The emphasis is on noticing, interpreting, and responding; reflection is less important.
b. Reflection occurs both in-action (in the moment) and on-action (after the situation).
c. Reflection occurs first in the model that is focused on rapid decision making and patient outcomes.
d. Reflection is the last step in a linear model and is designed to minimize bias in the student nurse.

3. Nursing programs prepare students for safe clinical practice. As a student nurse, why is a basic understanding of NCSBN's Clinical Judgment Measurement Model (CJMM) important? Select all that apply.
   a. Successful completion of the NCLEX is required for professional licensure in the United States.
   b. Nurse educators use the CJMM and NCLEX test plans to develop exam questions.
   c. Students should be intimately familiar with theoretical models of education to answer questions.
   d. Appreciation of the core principles assists students in understanding the structure and intent of nursing exams.
   e. There is overlap in the core components of clinical judgment models, measurement models, and the nursing process.
4. Nursing students and those studying other health sciences (medicine, pharmacy, physical therapy, etc.) are often engaged in competency-based education. What is the value of competency-based education?
   a. It provides comprehensive skills checklists for students to check their progress and move on to other elements.
   b. It allows for student individualization based on their unique experience and preferences.
   c. It provides specific guidance on the expected level of performance that integrates knowledge, skills, abilities, and judgment.
   d. Like most other education models, it is a high-level way of thinking that is not related to clinical judgment.
5. The development of clinical judgment requires intentional focus and a willingness to grow and change both personally and professionally. How can a nursing student best foster the development of clinical judgment?
   a. Engaging in learning that only appeals to their preferred learning style
   b. Focusing on knowledge acquisition that is straightforward and clear
   c. Developing a model for learning that integrates feedback and reflection
   d. Focusing inward to develop emotional intelligence and communication skills

ANSWERS WITH RATIONALES

1. **a.** The case represents a concrete example of how students develop situational awareness and how that awareness develops with experience. Cognitive load management occurs in many ways; the use of mental images may not facilitate cognitive load management. Although an environmental scan is important, it is generally not documented in the EHR. Patient satisfaction is not the priority when completing the initial assessment; rapport formation, solid assessments, and good patient outcomes are associated with patient satisfaction.
2. **b.** Reflection drives the clinical judgment cycle and allows for the integration of new knowledge that will inform future situations. Reflection is as important in Tanner's model as the other elements of noticing, interpreting, and responding. The focus of the model is the development of clinical judgment, rather than rapid decision making; as clinical judgment is developed, decision making improves and may lead to better patient outcomes. Tanner's model is cyclic, not linear; although bias may be addressed as part of the development of clinical judgment, it is not the focus.
3. **a, b, d, e.** Nurses in the United States must pass NCLEX prior to being issued a license to practice as a professional nurse. To help students achieve this goal, nurse educators model course exams on the NCSBN's NCLEX test plan in terms of content and style. Understanding the *why (rationale for actions)* is often helpful when students are engaged in studying, working to apply the information they have learned, and developing test-taking strategies. There is overlap between the models and processes identified as foundational to nursing education, which demonstrates the importance of fundamental concepts. A deep understanding of theoretical and philosophical models is not necessary for student nurses.
4. **c.** The definition of a competency included in the *Nursing: Scope and Standards of Practice* (ANA, 2021) identified includes knowledge, skills, abilities, and judgment. Competency-based education is more than a checklist and often requires repeated exposure to concepts for mastery in a variety of contexts. Although the delivery of education can flex to meet the needs of students, testing is standardized to address core competencies. Competency-based education is very direct and concrete; the development of competence requires clinical judgment.
5. **c.** Each nursing student is in charge of their learning, including integrating feedback from exams, clinical experiences, simulations, and other assignments—reflecting on what has been learned and integrating new learning. Adaptability is key. Classroom and clinical learning presents information in myriad ways and in different settings. Students should learn what they can from each situation and adapt their studying style as needed. Nursing knowledge, like patient care, is rarely straightforward and clear. Picking up on cues, emphasizing the correct element, answering the question being asked, and maintaining a person-centered focus that is individualized and nuanced requires practice and time. Students must give themselves the space and grace needed to learn and apply information in various situations. There is a reciprocity in learning that requires an inward and outward combination. Engagement with others and the environment is essential for shaping thinking and development of clinical judgment.

Bibliography

Alfaro-LeFevre, R. (2020a). *Critical thinking, clinical reasoning, and clinical judgment: A practical approach* (7th ed.). Elsevier.

Alfaro-LeFevre, R. (2020b, March). *Comparison of NGN, nursing process, and Tanner/Lasater clinical judgment models (CJMs)*. http://www.alfaroteachsmart.com/docs/NGN-CJMsComparisonTool.pdf

American Association of Colleges of Nursing (AACN). (2021, April 6). *The essentials: Core competencies for professional nursing education*. https://www.aacnnursing.org/Portals/42/AcademicNursing/pdf/Essentials-2021.pdf

American Nurses Association. (2015). *Code of ethics for nurses with interpretive statements*. Nursebooks.

American Nurses Association (ANA). (2021). *Nursing: Scope and standards of practice* (4th ed.). Nursebooks.

Bartlett, J. L. (2015). A simulation template for a new simulation program. *Clinical Simulation in Nursing, 11*(11), 479–481. https://doi.org/10.1016/j.ecns.2015.09.003

Benner, P. (1982). From novice to expert. *The American Journal of Nursing, 82*(3), 402–407. https://doi.org/10.1097/00000446-198282030-00004

Betts, J., Muntean, W., Kim, D., Jorion, N., & Dickison, P. (2019). Building a methods for writing clinical judgment items for entry-level nursing exams. *Journal of Applied Testing Technology, 20*(S2), 21–36. https://ncsbn.org/Building_a_Method_for_Writing_Clinical_Judgment_It.pdf

Billings, D. M. (2019). Teaching nurses to make clinical judgments that ensure patient safety. *Journal of Continuing Education in Nursing, 50*(7), 300–302. https://doi.org/10.3928/00220124-20190612-04

Carper, B. (1978). Fundamental patterns of knowing in nursing. *Advances in Nursing Science, 1*(1), 13–23. https://doi.org/10.1097/00012272-197810000-00004

Cronenwett, L., Sherwood, G., Barnsteiner, J., Disch, J., Johnson, J., Mitchell, P., Sullivan, D. T., & Warren, J. (2007). Quality and safety education for nurses. *Nursing Outlook, 55*(3), 122–131. https://doi.org/10.1016/j.outlook.2007.02.006

Endsley, M. R. (1995). Toward a theory of situational awareness in dynamic systems. *Human Factors, 37*(1), 32–64. https://doi.org/10.1518/001872095779049543

Englander, R., Cameron, T., Ballard, A. J., Dodge, J., Bull, J., & Aschenbrener, C. A. (2013). Toward a common taxonomy of competency domains for the health professions and competencies for physicians. *Academic Medicine, 88*(8), 1088–1094.

Ennis, R. (2018). Critical thinking across the curriculum: A vision. *Topoi, 37*(1), 165–184. https://philpapers.org/rec/ENNCTA-2

Ethos. (2021). Merriam-Webster.com Dictionary. Merriam-Webster. Retrieved December 12, 2021, from https://www.merriam-webster.com/dictionary/ethos

Facione, P. A. (1990). *Critical thinking: A statement of expert consensus for purposes of educational assessment and instruction—The Delphi report*. California Academic Press. https://www.insightassessment.com/article/expert-consensus-on-critical-thinking

Fore, A. M., & Sculli, G. L. (2013). A concept analysis of situational awareness in nursing. *Journal of Advanced Nursing, 69*(12), 2613–2621. https://doi.org/10.1111/jan.12130

Gaiman, N. (2021, September 9). What is ethos? Definition of ethos with examples. https://www.masterclass.com/articles/what-is-ethos-definition-of-ethos-with-examples#what-are-the-origins-of-ethos

Heath, H. (1998). Reflection and patterns of knowing in nursing. *Journal of Advanced Nursing, 27*(5), 1054–1059. https://doi.org/10.1046/j.1365-2648.1998.00593.x

Hensel, D., & Billings, D. M. (2020). Strategies to teach the National Council of State Boards of Nursing Clinical Judgment Model. *Nurse Educator, 45*(3), 128–132. https://doi.org/10.1097/NNE.0000000000000773

Insight Assessment. (2021). California Critical Thinking Disposition Inventory (CCTDI). Retrieved December 15, 2021, from https://www.insightassessment.com/article/california-critical-thinking-disposition-inventory-cctdi-2

Institute of Medicine. (2003). *Health professions education: A bridge to quality*. National Academies Press. https://www.nap.edu/login.php?record_id=10681&page=https%3A%2F%2Fwww.nap.edu%2Fdownload%2F10681

Interprofessional Education Collaborative. (2016). Core competencies for interprofessional collaborative practice: 2016 update. https://ipec.memberclicks.net/assets/2016-Update.pdf

Jensen, R., da Cruz Dde, A., Tesoro, M. G., & Lopes, M. H. (2014). Translation and cultural adaptation for Brazil of the Developing Nurses' Thinking model. *Revista Latino-Americana de Enfermagem, 22*(2), 197–203. https://doi.org/10.1590/0104-1169.3232.2402

Kolb, D. A. (1984). *Experiential learning: Experience as the source of learning and development*. Prentice Hall.

Lenburg, C. B., Abdur-Rahman, V. Z., Spencer, T. S., Boyer, S. A., & Klein, C. J. (2011). Implementing the COPA model in nursing education and practice settings: Promoting competence, quality care, and patient safety. *Nursing Education Perspectives, 32*(5), 290–296.

Lenburg, C. B., Klein, C., Abdur-Rahman, V., Spencer, T., & Boyer, S. (2009). The COPA model: A comprehensive framework designed to promote quality care and competence for patient safety. *Nursing Education Perspectives, 30*(5), 312–317.

Munhall, P. L. (1993). Unknowing: Toward another pattern of knowing in nursing. *Nursing Outlook, 41*(3), 125–128.

National League for Nursing (NLN). (2012). Objectives and competencies for graduates of practical/vocational, diploma, baccalaureate, master's practice doctorate, and research doctorate programs in nursing. http://www.nln.org/professional-development-programs/competencies-for-nursing-education/nln-competencies-for-graduates-of-nursing-programs

National League for Nursing (NLN). (2022). NLN Competencies for graduates of nursing programs. Retrieved January 30, 2022, from http://www.nln.org/professional-development-programs/competencies-for-nursing-education/nln-competencies-for-graduates-of-nursing-programs

National League for Nursing Commission for Nursing Education Accreditation (NLN CNEA). (2021, October). Accreditation standards for nursing education programs. https://irp.cdn-website.com/cc12ee87/files/uploaded/CNEA%20Standards%20October%202021.pdf

NCSBN. (2019a). NGN talks: The clinical judgment model and action model video transcript. Retrieved December 12, 2021, from https://www.ncsbn.org/Transcript_NGNTalk_Episode07.pdf

NCSBN. (2019b, April). NCLEX-RN Examination: Test plan for the National Council Licensure Examination for Registered Nurses. Retrieved December 12, 2021, from https://www.ncsbn.org/2019_RN_TestPlan-English.pdf

NCSBN. (2022). NCSBN: Leading regulatory excellence. Retrieved March 5, 2022, from https://www.ncsbn.org/index.htm

Nielsen, A., Stragnell, S., & Jester, P. (2007). Guide for reflection using the clinical judgment model. *The Journal of Nursing Education, 46*(11), 513–516. https://doi.org/10.3928/01484834-20071101-06

Parker-Tomlin, M., Boschen, M., Morrissey, S., & Glendon, I. (2017). Cognitive continuum theory in interprofessional healthcare: A critical analysis. *Journal of Interprofessional Care, 31*(4), 446–454. https://doi.org/10.1080/13561820.2017.1301899

Piaget, J., & Inhelder, B. (1969). *The psychology of the child*. Basic Books.

Rest, J. R. (1982). A psychologist looks at the teaching of ethics. *Hastings Center Report, 12*(1), 29–36.

Robichaux, C., Grace, P., Bartlett, J., Stokes, F., Lewis, M. S., & Turner, M. (2022). Ethics education for nurses: Foundations for an integrated curriculum. *Journal of Nursing Education, 61*(3), 123–130. https://doi.org/10.3928/01484834-20220109-02

Scriven, M., & Paul, R. (1987). Critical thinking. National Council for Excellence in Critical Thinking, 8th Annual International Conference on Critical Thinking and Education Reform. Retrieved December 15, 2021, from http://www.criticalthinking.org/pages/defining-critical-thinking/766

Shin, H. S. (2019). Reasoning processes in clinical reasoning: from the perspective of cognitive psychology. *Korean Journal of Medical Education, 31*(4), 299–308. https://doi.org/10.3946/kjme.2019.140

Sitterding, M. C., Ebright, P., Broome, M., Patterson, E. S., & Wuchner, S. (2014). Situation awareness and interruption handling during medication administration. *Western Journal of Nursing Research, 36*(7), 891–916. https://doi.org/10.1177/0193945914533426

Smith, M. K. (2013, June 20). David A. Kolb on experiential learning. http://www.infed.org/biblio/b-explrn.htm

Snyder, M. (1993). Critical thinking: A foundation for consumer-focused care. *Journal of Continuing Education in Nursing, 24*(5), 206–210.

Standing, M. (2008). Clinical judgement and decision-making in nursing – nine modes of practice in a revised cognitive continuum. *Journal of Advanced Nursing, 62*(1), 124–134. https://doi.org/10.1111/j.1365-2648.2007.04583.x

Tanner, C. A. (2006). Thinking like a nurse: A research-based model of clinical judgment in nursing. *The Journal of Nursing Education, 45*(6), 204–211. https://doi.org/10.3928/01484834-20060601-04

Tesoro, M. G. (2012). Effects of using the developing nurses' thinking model on nursing students' diagnostic accuracy. *Journal of Nursing Education, 51*(8), 436–443. http://dx.doi.org/10.3928/01484834-20120615-01

Tesoro, M. G., Simmons, A. M., de Barros, A. L. B. L., Lopes, C. T., Guandalini, L. S., Cruz, E. D. A., & Maurício, A. B. (2021). Effects of clinical reasoning prompts on nursing students' clinical judgment for a patient experiencing respiratory distress. *International Journal of Nursing Knowledge, 32*(1), 37–43. https://doi.org/10.1111/2047-3095.12286

Walshe, N., Ryng, S., Drennan, J., O'Connor, P., O'Brien, S., Crowley, C., & Hegarty, J. (2021). Situation awareness and the mitigation of risk associated with patient deterioration: A meta-narrative review of theories and models and their relevance to nursing practice. *International Journal of Nursing Studies, 124*, 104086. https://doi.org/10.1016/j.ijnurstu.2021.104086

White, J. (1995). Patterns of knowing: Review, critique, and update. *Advances in Nursing Science, 17*(4), 73–86. https://doi.org/10.1097/00012272-199506000-00007

Yura, H., & Walsh, M B. (1988). *The nursing process: Assessing, planning, implementing, and evaluating* (5th ed.). Appleton & Lange.

15 Assessing

Susan Morgan

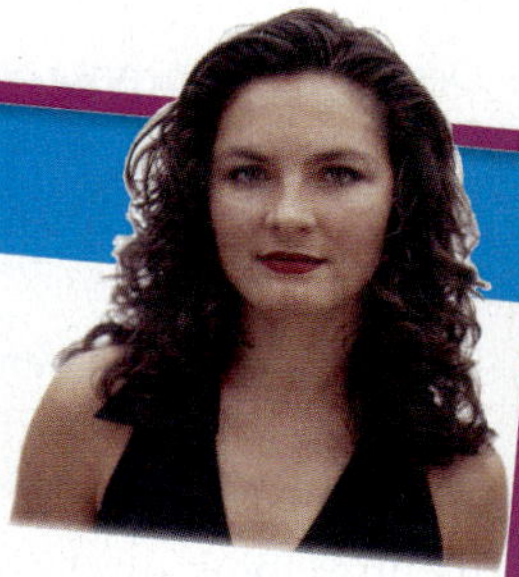

Susan is a 34-year-old woman newly diagnosed with multiple sclerosis (MS). She says, "How am I going to tell my husband? We were just married last year and planned to do lots of hiking and outdoor sports. It's not fair for him to be tied down to me if I can't be the wife and partner that he thought he had married."

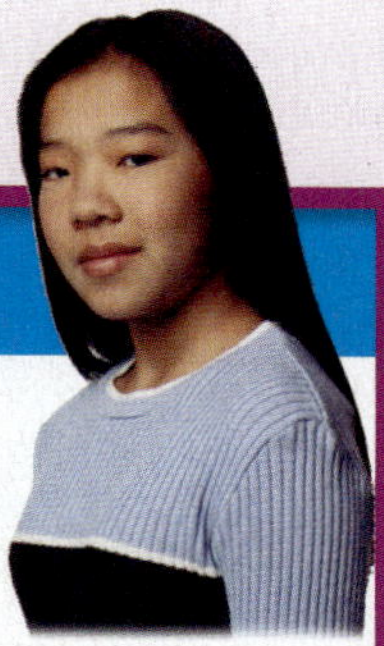

Sylvia Wu

Sylvia, a 17-year-old adolescent, has just arrived back in the United States after a visit to her family in mainland China. She comes to the emergency department because she woke up that morning with flulike symptoms (cough, sore throat, fever, muscle aches, fatigue). "I'm scared because of everything I've seen on television and read in the newspapers about that new virus."

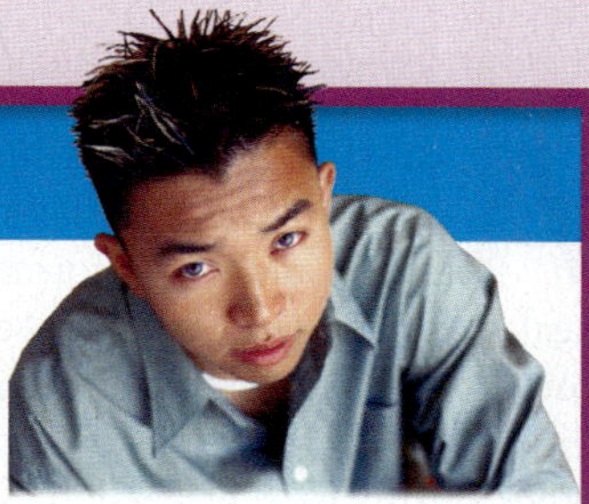

James Farren

James is a college junior who comes to the student health center complaining of difficulty sleeping, eating, and studying. He reveals that his mother died when he was 8 years old, and last semester his father died suddenly in a car crash. "Ever since my dad died, nothing seems to mean anything anymore. All I see is gray."

Learning Outcomes

After completing the chapter, you will be able to accomplish the following:

1. Define and describe the purpose of six types of nursing assessments.
2. Explain the relationship between nursing assessment and medical assessment.
3. Differentiate between objective and subjective data.
4. Identify five sources of patient data useful to the nurse.
5. Describe the purpose of nursing observation, interview, and physical assessment.
6. Obtain a nursing history using effective interviewing techniques.
7. Plan patient assessments by identifying assessment priorities and structuring the data to be collected systematically.
8. Identify common problems encountered in data collection, noting their possible causes.
9. Explain when data need to be validated and several ways to accomplish this.
10. Describe privacy, confidentiality, and professionalism issues related to patient assessment and data storage.
11. Describe the importance of knowing when to report significant patient data and of proper documentation.
12. Obtain and document purposeful, prioritized, complete, systematic, accurate, and relevant patient data in a standard format.

Nursing Concepts

- Assessment
- Communication
- Clinical reasoning
- Clinical judgment
- Nursing

Assessing is the systematic and continuous collection, analysis, validation, and communication of patient **data**, or information. These data reflect how health functioning is enhanced by health promotion or compromised by illness and injury. A **database** includes all the pertinent patient information collected by the nurse and other health care professionals. The database enables you to partner with patients to develop a comprehensive and effective care plan. Assessment, the first phase of the nursing process, is the first of six American Nurses Association (ANA) Standards of Practice: The registered nurse collects pertinent data and information relative to the healthcare consumer's health or the situation (ANA, 2021). Be sure to visit the website to read each of the competencies in this standard. Collecting patient data is a vital step in the nursing process because the remaining steps depend on purposeful, prioritized, complete, systematic, accurate, and relevant data. Assessment is critical for safety, accuracy, and efficiency (Alfaro-LeFevre, 2014, p. 46).

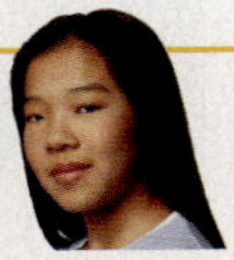

Refer to the Reflective Practice box regarding **Sylvia Wu**, a patient who fears that she has a virus. The nurse's assessment would reveal possible risk factors. In addition, the patient's statements about her fears provide further data on which to develop a care plan.

The initial comprehensive nursing assessment results in baseline data that enable the nurse to:

- make a judgment about a person's health status, ability to manage their own need for self-care, and the need for nursing care.
- plan and deliver thoughtful, person-centered nursing care that draws on the person's strengths and promotes optimum functioning, independence, and well-being.
- refer the patient to a provider or other health care professional, if indicated.

In addition to an initial assessment of the patient, the nurse makes ongoing assessments. These assessments alert the nurse to changes in the patient's responses to health and illness and suggest necessary changes in the plan of nursing care or care offered by other health care professionals.

During the assessment step of the nursing process, the nurse establishes the database by interviewing the patient to obtain a **nursing history**. The nursing history identifies the patient's health status, strengths, actual and potential health problems, health risks, and need for nursing care. The nurse may also perform a nursing physical examination to collect data. Other sources of patient information used by the nurse include the patient's family and significant others, the patient record, other health care professionals, and nursing and other health care literature.

After the nurse has established the database, data about the patient are collected continuously because the patient's health status can change quickly. Questionable data are verified (validated) as part of the assessment step of the nursing process. All pertinent data are recorded and communicated to other health care professionals so that the data can best benefit the patient (Fig. 15-1 on page 406). In addition to collecting data, nurses might use intuition to assess patients (see Chapter 13).

UNIQUE FOCUS OF NURSING ASSESSMENT

When nurses make nursing assessments, they do not duplicate medical assessments. Medical assessments target data pointing to pathologic conditions, whereas nursing assessments focus on the patient's responses to health problems. For example, is there interference with the patient's ability to meet basic human needs? Can the patient perform the activities of daily living? Although the findings from a nursing assessment may contribute to the identification of a

QSEN Reflective Practice: Cultivating QSEN Competencies

CHALLENGE TO INTELLECTUAL SKILLS

While on a clinical rotation in the emergency department, I met Sylvia Wu, a 17-year-old adolescent who had just arrived back in the United States after a visit to her family in mainland China. She came to the emergency department because she woke up that morning with flulike symptoms (cough, sore throat, fever, muscle aches, fatigue) and was terrified because of everything she had seen on television and read in the newspapers about the latest virus. Of the 64 people who have died already, she knows that most of the cases are in Asia. She came to the emergency department begging to be told that she doesn't have the virus but just fatigue or a cold. I want to calm her, but I honestly don't know what she has. Besides, I am starting to feel a bit anxious myself because the one thing everyone knows about this virus is the fact that it is extremely "contagious." I could feel myself recoil when Sylvia sneezed.

Thinking Outside the Box: Possible Courses of Action

- Reassure Sylvia and tell her not to worry because the overwhelming probability is that her symptoms aren't anything serious.
- Quickly get someone with more experience to care for Sylvia because I don't want to be anywhere near her if she does have this virus.
- Document and report her concerns, trying to keep her isolated and away from other patients, while trying to find more information about this new virus quickly, since I'm not sure about its signs and symptoms.

Evaluating a Good Outcome: How Do I Define Success?

- Sylvia gets the medical treatment she needs, and her fears are appropriately addressed.
- In the event that Sylvia does have a highly communicable disease, the risk for disease transmission to others is reduced.
- I manage to control my fears, being able to respond to Sylvia's concerns appropriately.
- I learn something about my immediate response to feeling at risk and my commitment to professionalism.

Personal Learning: Here's to the Future!

Although I am not proud of my response, I falsely reassured Sylvia that this was probably nothing. As a result, I did not report or document her fears. Unfortunately, Sylvia was diagnosed with the virus, and several others in our emergency department at that time became infected. For some reason, I escaped. In the future, I hope I'll never be so insensitive to a patient's concerns or insights again.

QSEN SELF-REFLECTION ON QUALITY AND SAFETY COMPETENCIES DEVELOPING KNOWLEDGE, SKILLS, AND ATTITUDES FOR CONTINUOUS IMPROVEMENT

How do you think you would respond in a similar situation? Why? What does this tell you about yourself and about the adequacy of your skills for professional practice? What factors might have influenced this nursing student's actions? What types of data could have led the nursing student to a different course of action? How might the nursing student have assessed the patient differently? Do you agree with the criteria that the nursing student used to evaluate a successful outcome? Why or why not? What *knowledge, skills,* and *attitudes* do you need to develop to continuously improve the quality and safety of care for patients like Ms. Wu?

Patient-Centered Care: How would you develop a partnership with Ms. Wu, knowing her fears? If steps are needed to keep others safe, how can you communicate to Ms. Wu that she is your care priority?

Teamwork and Collaboration/Quality Improvement: What communication skills do you need to improve to ensure that you function as a member of the patient care team and to obtain assistance when needed? How might the transmission of this infection have been prevented?

Safety/Evidence-Based Practice: What does the evidence point to as "best practice" in situations like this to keep everyone safe and to treat Ms. Wu effectively? Are you familiar with the latest Centers for Disease Control and Prevention (CDC) guidelines for isolation precautions?

Informatics: Can you identify the essential information that must be available in Ms. Wu's electronic record to support safe patient care and coordination of care? Can you think of other ways to respond to or approach the situation? What else might the nursing student have done to ensure a successful outcome?

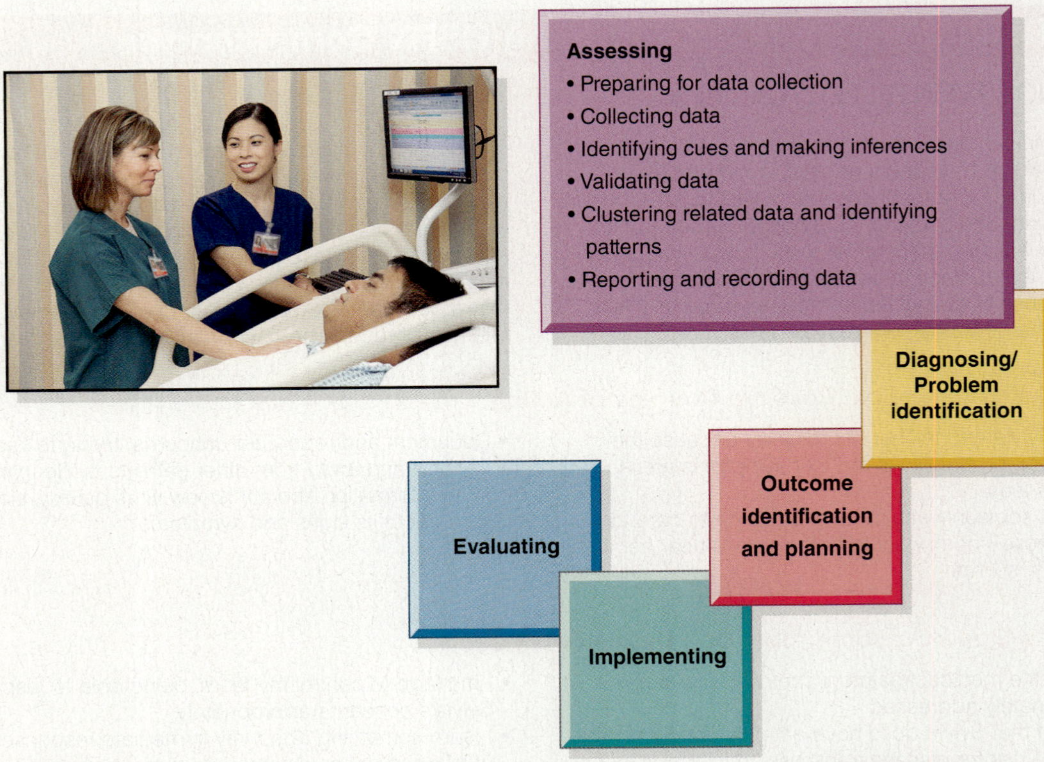

FIGURE 15-1. Assessing. The primary source of patient information is the patient. Other resources include the patient's support people, the patient record, information from other health care professionals, and information from nursing and health care literature.

medical diagnosis, the unique focus of nursing assessments is on the patient's responses to actual or potential health problems and needs.

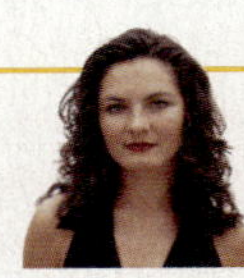

Remember ***Susan Morgan***, a patient recently diagnosed with MS? By looking at the data supplied by the patient, the nurse would be able to determine that the patient's new diagnosis of MS is affecting her body image and self-esteem. The nurse then would use this information to focus assessment questions to obtain additional information to be included in the database, from which a care plan specific to Susan's needs can be developed.

ASSESSMENT, CLINICAL REASONING, AND CLINICAL JUDGMENT

Since the entire nursing process rests on the initial and ongoing assessment of the patient, it is imperative to use excellent critical thinking and clinical reasoning and judgment skills when gathering, analyzing, validating, and communicating data. According to Alfaro-LeFevre (2010, p. 49), among the critical thinking activities linked to assessment are:

- Assessing systematically and comprehensively, using a nursing framework to identify nursing concerns and a body systems framework to identify medical concerns
- Detecting bias and determining the credibility of information sources
- Distinguishing normal from abnormal findings and identifying the risks for abnormal findings
- Making judgments about the significance of data, distinguishing relevant from irrelevant
- Identifying assumptions and inconsistencies, checking accuracy and reliability, and recognizing missing information

To promote sound clinical reasoning and judgment, your nursing assessments should be:

Purposeful. When preparing for data collection, identify the purpose of the nursing assessment (comprehensive, focused, emergency, time-lapsed) and then gather the appropriate data. The circumstances of the patient's situation may also dictate the nature and amount of data you collect.

Prioritized. It is essential to get the most important information first. We address how to do this later in this chapter.

Complete. As much as possible, identify all the patient data needed to understand a patient health problem and develop a care plan to maximize the patient's health and well-being. For example, knowing that a patient has lost weight is not fully meaningful until you discover (1) if the weight loss was intentional or unintentional, (2) if it was related to a change in eating or exercise patterns or to some underlying pathologic condition, and (3) how the patient views and is responding to the weight loss.

Systematic. Using a systematic way to gather data, you will always know if you've missed something important.

Factual and accurate. Both you and the patient, as well as family members and other caregivers, may intentionally or unintentionally misrepresent or distort patient information. For example, a patient who values being thin may describe a weight gain of several pounds as the onset of obesity. If you are concerned with accuracy and factual reality, you will continually verify what you hear with what you observe, using other senses and validating all questionable data. At the outset of data collection, it is crucial that you determine whether the patient or caregiver who is supplying the data is reliable. If you suspect that your own personal bias or stereotyping may be influencing your data collection, you should consult with another nurse. You should also describe observed behavior rather than interpreting the behavior. For example: "Patient frequently is observed lying with his face to the wall. Attempts to engage him in conversation fail. He refused lunch today and ate only soup for dinner." In contrast, the statement "Patient is depressed" is an interpretation of the patient's behavior, not a factual statement. Recording the patient's behaviors factually allows other health care professionals to explore causes of the behavior with the patient.

Relevant. Because recording comprehensive data can be very time consuming, one challenge facing you as a nurse is to determine what types of and how much data to collect for each patient. As described throughout this chapter, the aim is to record concisely all pertinent data. Often, only experience will teach you what data are needed in specific cases.

Recorded in a standard manner. Data cannot be efficiently used unless you record the information according to the facility's policy so that all caregivers can easily access what you learned.

Learning how to collect, validate, and communicate data that are purposeful, prioritized, complete, systematic, accurate, and relevant is the focus of the remainder of this chapter. Many assessment activities are challenging for those new to nursing, who often lack the types of clinical experiences that facilitate expert clinical reasoning. Thus, students are urged to ask questions frequently about data and to test their inferences and judgments.

ASSESSMENT AND INTERPERSONAL COMPETENCE

The nurse's interpersonal competence is critical beginning with the very first assessment by the nurse. The patient's initial impression of the nurse is crucial, especially with patients who are new to the health care environment or who have had bad experiences. *The patient may judge all nurses encountered in the future in light of this first impression.* When the nurse communicates respect and genuine concern for the patient, the patient is encouraged to discuss health concerns and problems freely. The nurse's competence and professionalism, as well as the interpersonal qualities of being respectful and caring, invite the patient's confidence and assure the patient that help is available. Successful assessments begin with the trust and confidence an interpersonally competent nurse inspires. See the Guidelines for Nursing Care: Promoting a Caring Interview 15-1 on page 420.

Alfaro-LeFevre (2014, p. 66) recommends avoiding these communication errors:

- Using first names without permission, which is disrespectful
- Using honey, dear, sweetie, pop, or grandma
- "Talking down" (e.g., "so you have a pain in your tummy?")
- Using medical terminology with lay people
- Ignoring patients' nonverbal communication

TYPES OF NURSING ASSESSMENTS

Traditional nursing assessments include the comprehensive initial assessment, the focused assessment, the emergency assessment, quick priority assessments, triage assessments, and the time-lapsed assessment. This chapter focuses on assessing the health status of an individual patient, but as you develop expertise in nursing assessments you will also be able to assess communities and special populations, such as schoolchildren, members of the LGBTQIA$^+$ communities, the homeless, and people with infectious diseases.

Initial Assessment

The **initial assessment** is performed shortly after the patient is admitted to a health care facility or service. Most institutions have policies specifying the time interval within which this assessment must be completed. The purpose of this assessment is to establish a complete database for problem identification and care planning. The nurse collects data concerning all aspects of the patient's health, establishing priorities for ongoing focused assessments and creating a reference baseline for future comparison. See Figure 15-2 (on page 408) for a sample of an initial assessment in an electronic medical record. For an example of a handwritten admission database, see Figure 15-3 (on pages 409–410).

Focused Assessment

In a **focused assessment**, the nurse gathers data about a specific problem that has already been identified. Helpful questions include:

- What are your signs and symptoms?
- When did they start?
- Were you doing anything different than usual when they started?
- What makes your symptoms better? Worse?
- Are you taking any remedies (medical or natural) for your symptoms?

A focused assessment may be done during the initial assessment if the patient's health problems surface, but it is routinely part of ongoing data collection. Another

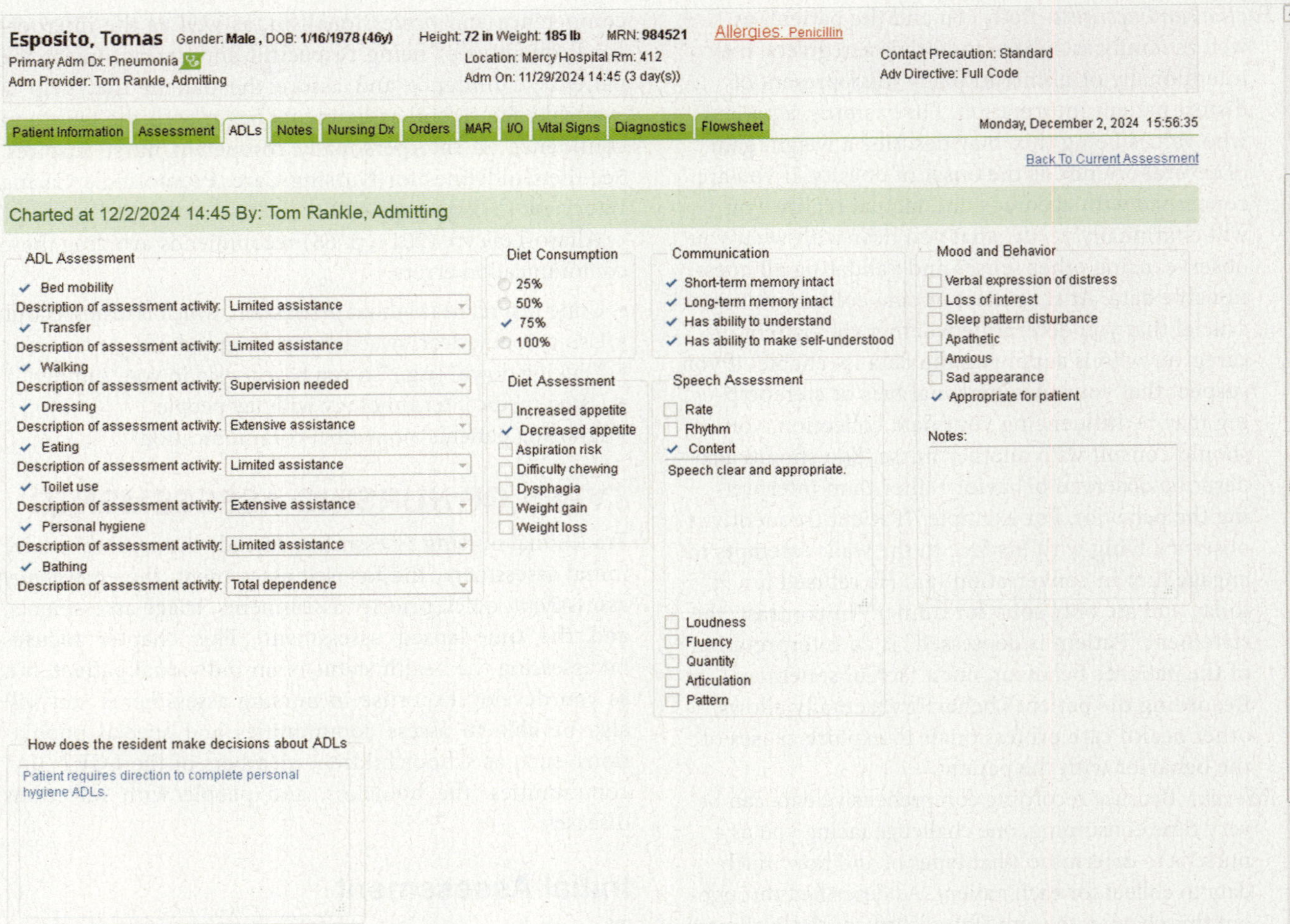
Esposito, Tomas Gender: Male, DOB: 1/16/1978 (46y) Height: 72 in Weight: 185 lb MRN: 984521 Allergies: Penicillin
Primary Adm Dx: Pneumonia
Adm Provider: Tom Rankle, Admitting
Location: Mercy Hospital Rm: 412
Adm On: 11/29/2024 14:45 (3 day(s))
Contact Precaution: Standard
Adv Directive: Full Code

Patient Information | Assessment | ADLs | Notes | Nursing Dx | Orders | MAR | I/O | Vital Signs | Diagnostics | Flowsheet

Monday, December 2, 2024 15:56:35

Back To Current Assessment

Charted at 12/2/2024 14:45 By: Tom Rankle, Admitting

ADL Assessment
✓ Bed mobility
Description of assessment activity: Limited assistance
✓ Transfer
Description of assessment activity: Limited assistance
✓ Walking
Description of assessment activity: Supervision needed
✓ Dressing
Description of assessment activity: Extensive assistance
✓ Eating
Description of assessment activity: Limited assistance
✓ Toilet use
Description of assessment activity: Extensive assistance
✓ Personal hygiene
Description of assessment activity: Limited assistance
✓ Bathing
Description of assessment activity: Total dependence

Diet Consumption
25%
50%
✓ 75%
100%

Diet Assessment
☐ Increased appetite
✓ Decreased appetite
☐ Aspiration risk
☐ Difficulty chewing
☐ Dysphagia
☐ Weight gain
☐ Weight loss

Communication
✓ Short-term memory intact
✓ Long-term memory intact
✓ Has ability to understand
✓ Has ability to make self-understood

Speech Assessment
☐ Rate
☐ Rhythm
✓ Content
Speech clear and appropriate.
☐ Loudness
☐ Fluency
☐ Quantity
☐ Articulation
☐ Pattern

Mood and Behavior
☐ Verbal expression of distress
☐ Loss of interest
☐ Sleep pattern disturbance
☐ Apathetic
☐ Anxious
☐ Sad appearance
✓ Appropriate for patient

Notes:

How does the resident make decisions about ADLs
Patient requires direction to complete personal hygiene ADLs.

FIGURE 15-2. Section of sample electronic nursing admission assessment form. (Used with permission. Fictitious data.)

purpose of the focused assessment is to identify new or overlooked problems. Each of the clinical chapters in this text offers focused assessment guides describing factors to assess and related questions and approaches for common problems.

Quick Priority Assessments

Quick priority assessments (QPAs) are short, focused, prioritized assessments you do to gain the most important information you need to have first. They are important because they can "flag" existing problems and risks (Alfaro-LeFevre, 2014, p. 50).

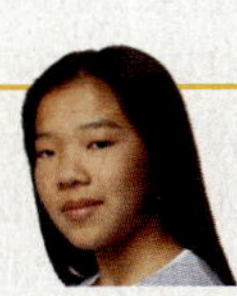

Recall **Sylvia Wu**, the 17-year-old who comes to the emergency department because she thinks that she might have a virus. The nurse would use a focused assessment to evaluate her complaints that relate specifically to her respiratory status. If the nurse suspects a communicable disease, they would also need to consider what precautions to take before continuing with the assessment. This information would be supplemented by additional data about the patient's recent travel to mainland China.

Emergency Assessment

When a patient presents with a physiologic or psychological crisis, the nurse performs an **emergency assessment** to identify life-threatening problems. A long-term care facility resident who begins choking in the dining room, a bleeding patient brought to the emergency department with a stab wound, an unresponsive patient in the rehabilitation unit, and a factory worker threatening violence are all candidates for an emergency assessment. In the first example, the source of the choking is assessed; in the second, the blood loss and wound characteristics; in the third, airway, breathing, and circulation; and in the fourth, the potential for immediate harm.

Time-Lapsed Assessment

The **time-lapsed assessment** is scheduled to compare a patient's current status to the baseline data obtained earlier. Most patients in residential settings and those receiving nursing care over longer periods of time, such as homebound patients with visiting nurses, are scheduled for periodic time-lapsed assessments to reassess their health status and to make necessary revisions in the care plan. This assessment can be comprehensive or focused.

MR# 56923

Acct# 06947328

Name Martha Rosenfeld

DOB 04/17/1952

* 0 0 1 5 0 4 . 1 0 0 9 *

Nursing Admission History

COMPLETE OR IMPRINT WITH ADDRESS-O-PLATE

IMPORTANT: DO NOT WRITE IN MARGINS

Admission Data

Date 8/19/2024	Time 2100	
T 38.5	P 92	R 18
BP 108/76	Ht	Wt

☒ **ID Bracelet ON Patient**

Allergies ☐ **Allergy Bracelet On**

☐ No Known Allergies

☒ Medication

Medication	Reaction
Morphine	Rash
Penicillin	Rash

☐ Food

☐ Latex ☐ IV Contrast (Dye)/Iodine

☐ Uncertain

☐ Other

Advance Directives

1. Advance Directive Information was provided to the patient.
   ☒ Yes ☐ No
2. Does the patient have an Advance Directive?
   ☒ Yes ☐ No
3. If patient has an Advance Directive, is it on the chart?
   ☒ Yes ☐ No
4. If patient has an Advance Directive and it is not on chart, was a request made to provide a copy of Advance Directive for chart?
   ☐ Yes ☐ No N/A
5. If patient has an Advance Directive, do they want to review or revise it?
   ☐ Yes ☒ No
6. If patient does not have an Advance Directive, would they like assistance in developing one?
   ☐ Yes ☐ No N/A
7. If patient does not have an Advance Directive and would like assistance in developing or if patient would like assistance in revising an Advance Directive, was Social Work consulted?
   ☐ Yes ☐ No ☒ N/A

Orientation to Room/Unit

☒ Light/Emerg Call ☒ Patient Handbook

☒ Bed Controls/Siderails ☒ Safety

☒ Visiting Hours ☒ TV/Pt Ed Channels

☒ Oriented to JDU ☒ Hourly Rounds

☐ Inability to Understand Instructions

Explained to: ☐ Family ☒ Patient

Health History (see review of systems on back)

Information Source

☒ Patient ☐ Other (name/relationship):

Stated Reason for Hospitalization

Uncontrolled pain & nausea r/t cancer

☐ Unable to Obtain Hx at Present
Reason:

☒ History of falls at home/prior hospitalizations
☒ Yes ☐ No

☒ Patient is afraid of falling?
☒ Yes ☐ No

☒ Chemotherapy ☐ Radiation Therapy

☐ Transplant (type)

☒ Cancer (type) Stomach

☒ Past Surgeries J-tube placement, Mediport

☐ Isolation Care Precaution Other than Standard

Type

Other Pertinent Info

Medications ☐ None

Current medications being taken:
(include over-the-counter medications, herbals, and non-traditional medications)

Name/Dose/Frequency	Last Taken
Oxycontin 60mg BID	0800
Reglan 10mg TID	0800
Protonix 40mg daily	0800
Peri-colase 2 tabs BID	0800

Are you taking investigational study drugs? ☐ Yes ☒ No

(specify)

Are you currently using any mode of alternative therapy? ☒ Yes ☐ No

(specify) Medical Cannabis

Spiritual/Cultural/Social Information

Are there any religious traditions, ethnic practices or cultural practices that need to be part of your care

☒ No ☐ Yes (explain):

☐ Unable to Obtain Social/Discharge info due to:

Lives: ☐ Alone ☒ Spouse ☐ Children ☐ Parents
☐ Other (specify)

☐ Smokes

How Long? ______ Packs/Day ______

Time of first cigarette.

☐ Informed of Hospital Smoking Policy

☐ Interested in Smoking Cessation Education

Would you like to have nicotine replacement therapy while here in the hospital?

☐ Yes ☐ No

☐ Alcohol

How Long? ______ Amount? ______

☐ Last Drink (time/amount)

☐ Previous treatment and response.

☒ Recreational Drugs (type/amount/last used)

Medical Cannabis daily 8/18

☐ Previous treatment and response.

Contact/Support Person Present: ☒ Yes ☐ No

Name David Rosenfeld

Relationship Spouse

Home Phone

Work Phone

Valuable/Personal Property

Prosthetic Devices ☐ None

With Pt:	Yes	No
☐ Dentures	☐	☐
☐ Type:		
☒ Glasses	☒	☐
☐ Contact Lenses	☐	☐
☒ Hearing Aid (R/L)	☒	☐
☐ Limb Prosthesis	☐	☐
☐ Glass Eye	☐	☐

Assistive Devices ☐ None

With Pt:	Yes	No
☐	☐	☐

Valuable/Personal Items/Medications

Item	Home	W/Pt	Secured
	☐	☐	☐
	☐	☐	☐

☒ Sent Home with (relationship) Spouse

☐ Secured Location

Non-RN Signature	Unit	Date/Time

FORM 0015-04 (REV. 10/09) JG 11-1551

PAGE 1 OF 2

FIGURE 15-3. Nursing admission database. (*continued*)

Nursing Admission History

Patient Name: *Rosenfeld, Martha* | DOB: *04/17/1952* | MR#: *56923*

Social Work/Case Management Screen
Enter consult in Jeff Chart or call SW/CM Consult line at 5-2587 if any condition is present.
- ☐ Trauma or New SCI
- ☐ Difficulty Coping with Diagnosis/Traumatic Incident
- ☐ Mental Health Impairment (eating disorder/suicide)
- ☐ Unknown Identity/Unknown Next of Kin
- ☐ No Parent on Admission for a Minor Under 18
- ☐ Boarding Home/Nursing Home Return
- ☐ Unable to Return Home
- ☐ Financial Difficulties (lack of gas, electric, water, medication coverage, etc.)
- ☐ Lack of Transportation for Discharge
- ☐ Assistance with Advance Directive
- ☐ Abuse/Neglect (child/older adult/domestic violence)
- ☐ Drug/Alcohol/Substance Abuse
- ☐ Positive Drug Screen of Newborn/Parent of Newborn/Child
- ☐ No Prenatal Care
- ☐ Pregnant Woman Under 16
- ☐ Fetal Demise
- ☐ Adoption/Foster Care Placement
- ☐ Other Concerns that would impede Discharge
- ☐ Other Concerns Impeding Psychosocial Functioning (non-compliance, end of life issues)
- ☐ Other ______

☒ **No Conditions Identified**

Screening Criteria for Nutrition
Enter consult in Jeff Chart or contact Department of Nutrition and Dietetics at ext. 5-7144 if any condition is present.
- ☐ Food Allergy
- ☒ Unintentional Weight Loss > 15lbs in past 3 months
- ☒ On Tube Feeding or anticipate Tube Feeding
- ☐ On TPN or anticipate TPN
- ☐ Stage 2 or greater Decubitus Ulcer or Non-healing Wound
- ☐ Jaw/Mandibular Fx/Wired Jaw
- ☐ Anorexia Nervosa or Bulemia
- ☐ Difficulty swallowing or other problems that prevent eating
- ☐ Continuous vomiting > 5 days
- ☐ Esophagectomy
- ☐ Enterocutaneous Fistula or Repair
- ☐ Radical Neck Surgery
- ☐ Whipple Procedure
- ☐ Other ______

☐ **No Conditions Identified**

Pregnant Woman (above criteria plus the following)
- ☐ Gestational Diabetic
- ☐ Hyperemesis
- ☐ Lactating (assessment by RN/Lactation specialist at Center City)
- ☐ Other ______

☒ **No Conditions Identified**

Rehab Screen
Physician order in Jeff Chart for new onset of deficits in:

Occupational Therapy
- ☐ Bathing ☐ Dressing/Grooming
- ☐ Feeding ☐ Toileting
- ☐ Range of Motion ☐ Home Management
- ☐ Judgement/Safety ☐ Vision
- ☐ Cognition and Perception

☒ **No Conditions Identified**

Physical Therapy
- ☐ Strength, Balance Coordination, Range of Motion
- ☐ Transfers ☐ Stairs ☐ Bed Mobility
- ☐ Wheel Chair Mobility ☐ Ambulation
- ☐ Other ______

☒ **No Conditions Identified**

Speech Language Pathology
- ☐ Communication ☐ Speech/Language
- ☐ Swallowing
- ☐ Other ______

☒ **No Conditions Identified**

MRSA Screen
Has patient been diagnosed with MRSA? ☐ Yes ☒ No
If yes, document facility and date and order MDRO Precautions.

Were you admitted from an outside facility?
If yes, order MRSA screen.
Were you hospitalized within the past 30 days?
If yes, order MRSA screen.

EENT ☐ **No Hx/Conditions Identified**
- ☐ Glaucoma/ Cataracts ☐ Sinus Problems
- ☐ Loose Teeth ☐ Difficulty Hearing ☐ TMJ
- ☐ Airway Device ______
- ☐ Hoarseness ☐ Mouth Sores
- ☐ Dental Problems ☐ Stiff Neck
- ☐ Bleeding Gums ☐ Epistaxis

Hearing Deficit: ☐ Right ☒ Left *wears hearing aid*
Vision Deficit: ☐ Right ☐ Left
Comments:

Resp ☐ **No Hx/Conditions Identified**
- ☐ Tuberculosis ☒ Asthma ☐ Pneumonia
- ☐ COPD ☐ Emphysema ☐ Home O_2

Cough: ☐ Productive ☐ Non-Productive
Dyspnea: ☐ At Rest ☐ With Exertion
☐ Sleep Apnea (at home use of): ☐ BiPap ☐ CPAP
Comments: *No exacerbation >5 years, no meds*

Cardiac ☒ **No Hx/Conditions Identified**
- ☐ High Blood Pressure ☐ Irregular Heartbeat
- ☐ Palpitations ☐ Murmur ☐ Chest Pain/Angina
- ☐ Heart Attack ☐ Phlebitis/Varicose Veins
- ☐ Bleeding Disorder ☐ Angioplasty/Stents
- ☐ Pacemaker ☐ Implanted Defibrillator/AICD
- ☐ Venous Access Device (e.g. PICC, Infusaport)

Comments:

GI ☐ **No Hx/Conditions Identified**
- ☒ Nausea ☐ Vomiting ☐ Diarrhea
- ☐ Ulcers ☐ Blood in Stool ☒ Constipation
- ☐ Liver Disease ☐ Jaundice
- ☐ Gallbladder Prob. ☐ Hepatitis
- ☐ Inflammatory Bowel Disease ☐ Pancreatitis
- ☒ Hiatal Hernia (Heartburn/Acid Reflux) (circled)
- ☐ Incontinence ☐ GI Diversion

Weight: ☐ Recent Gain ☒ Recent Loss
Last BM *8/16*
Comments: *Diagnosed stomach cancer 5/2020*

GU/Repro ☒ **No Hx/Conditions Identified**
- ☐ Kidney Disease ☐ Kidney Stones
- ☐ Blood in Urine ☐ Difficulty Urinating
- ☐ Prostate Problems ☐ Hesitancy ☐ Urgency
- ☐ Dribbling ☐ Incontinence ☐ Frequency
- ☐ Nocturia

Urinary Diversion ______
Indwelling Foley ______
When/Where inserted? ______
- ☐ Dialysis Access Location ______
- ☐ Vaginal/Penile Discharge
- ☐ Breast Problems ☐ Hysterectomy
- ☐ Vaginal Bleeding
- ☐ LMP ______ ☐ Pregnant (____ weeks)

Comments: *post-menopause*
(Call pharmacy at 5-7147 if pregnant or lactating)
☐ Pharmacy called

Neuromuscular ☒ **No Hx/Conditions Identified**
- ☐ Back Pain ☐ Arthritis/Gout
- ☐ Joint Pain/Swelling
- ☐ Amputation ______
- ☐ Contracture ______
- ☐ Fractures ______
- ☐ Unsteady Gait
- ☐ Requires Assistance to Ambulate
- ☐ Limited ROM
- ☐ Unable to Bear Weight (RLE / LLE)
- ☐ Blurred Vision ☐ Migraines ☐ Headaches
- ☐ Seizures ☐ Dizziness ☐ Stroke
- ☐ Numbness/Tingling
- ☐ Paralysis: location ______
- ☐ Inappropriate Behavior
- ☐ Slurred Speech ☐ Aphasia ☐ Dysphagia

Muscle: ☐ Weakness ☐ Flaccid ☐ Spastic
Location ______
Comments:

Endocrine ☐ **No Hx/Conditions Identified**
- ☐ Thyroid Disease/Goiter
- ☐ Heat or Cold Intolerance
- ☐ Long Term Steroids
- ☐ Fever ☐ Night Sweats
- ☐ Diabetes Type 1 ☒ Diabetes Type 2
- ☐ Diabetes Other

Comments: *Diet controlled*

Comfort ☐ **No Hx/Conditions Identified**
Patient Goal *improve pain & nausea*
Where is Pain Now?

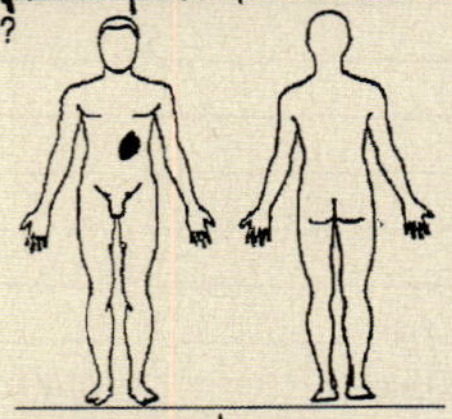

Describe the pain *Aching, dull*
How long have you had this pain? *4 months*
What relieves the pain? *nothing*
What makes it worse? *nothing*
List pain meds *Oxycontin*
Are they effective? *NO*
Does pain interfere with daily activities? *Yes*
With sleep? *yes*
Which number best describes your pain?
(no pain) 0 1 2 3 4 5 6 7 (8 circled) 9 10 (worst pain)

Psych ☐ **No Hx/Conditions Identified**
- ☐ Alcohol/Drug Abuse ☐ Other Addictions
- ☐ Psychiatric Disorder ☐ Suicidal Ideations
- ☐ Grieving ☐ Chronic Anxiety
- ☒ Depressed Affect ☐ Hallucinations
- ☐ Confusion ☐ Aggressive behavior
- ☐ Restraint use ______

Comments: *has appointment with psychiatrist*

Skin ☒ **No Hx/Conditions Identified**
- ☐ Skin Problems ☐ Rashes ☐ Ulcers
- ☐ Infection: site ______

Comments:

IMPORTANT: DO NOT WRITE IN MARGINS

RN Signature	Unit	Date/Time	Updated By	Unit	Date/Time
Katherine Blalock, RN	*C53*	*8/19/2024*			

FORM 0015-04 (REV. 10/09) JG 11-1551 **PAGE 2 OF 2**

FIGURE 15-3. *(continued from previous page)*

Triage Assessment

Many nurses serve as **triage** professionals who screen patients to determine the extent and severity of the their problems and then recommend appropriate follow-up. A triage nurse working for an internal medicine practice in a university hospital will take phone calls from patients without appointments experiencing distressing symptoms such as shortness of breath, pressure or tightness in the chest, or increases in temperature. The importance of triage nurses during the COVID-19 pandemic was quickly apparent. The Oncology Nursing Society (2020) offered special guidance to their telephone triage nurses, citing the fear and uncertainties persons with cancer were experiencing about coming for their regular clinic appointments, knowing they were at higher risk of acquiring COVID-19. Triage nurses fielding phone calls were instructed to (1) assess the need for an in-person appointment, (2) assess risk of developing serious complications from COVID-19, (3) assess for symptoms of COVID-19, and (4) educate on risk reduction (https://voice.ons.org/news-and-views/covid-19-telephone-triage-for-patients-with-cancer).

Triage nurses need highly specialized nursing knowledge and clinical reasoning and judgment skills since the life and well-being of their patients are literally in their hands.

Patient-Centered Assessment Method

The **Patient-Centered Assessment Method (PCAM)** is a tool health care practitioners can use to assess patient complexity using the social determinants of health (see Chapter 3); these determinants may explain why some patients engage and respond well in managing their health while others with the same or similar health conditions do not experience the same outcomes. The PCAM assessment tool helps you ask questions to gain understanding about the patient's:

- health and well-being—lifestyle behaviors, impact of physical health on mental health, ability to enjoy daily activities
- social environment—status of employment, housing, transportation, and social networks
- health literacy and communication skills—understanding of symptoms and risk factors, language and cultural differences, learning difficulties

Questions about these health determinants may help you discover other factors that are affecting the person's ability to manage their health.

The PCAM method recognizes that patient response to health issues may be related to multiple chronic medical conditions as well as social and environmental factors, and it is very likely a combination of both. Factors that interfere with a patient's usual care and decision making can make providing health care more difficult and complex, and can affect the patient's health and recovery. If you are committed to learning about these factors and addressing them as part of your patients' medical care, you can have a positive effect on their health and improve your partnership with patients and their families.

The PCAM assessment tool (Fig. 15-4 on pages 412–413) is action oriented, with the final section focused on the actions that can be taken to address the needs and issues identified in the assessment. The tool is available at https://med.umn.edu/familymedicine/research/faculty-research/pcam. Other helpful online tools to assess patient assets and risks, in light of what we know about the social determinants of health, are available from the CDC and the National Association of Community Health Centers (NACHC):

Ten Essential Public Health Services and How They Can Include Addressing Social Determinants of Health Inequities, retrieved from https://www.cdc.gov/stltpublichealth/publichealthservices/pdf/ten_essential_services_and_sdoh.pdf

PRAPARE: Protocol for Responding to and Assessing Patient Assets, Risks, and Experiences, retrieved from http://www.nachc.org/wp-content/uploads/2016/09/PRAPARE_One_Pager_Sept_2016.pdf

PREPARING FOR DATA COLLECTION

Establishing assessment priorities and systematically structuring data collection are two important considerations when preparing for data collection.

Establishing Assessment Priorities

Before beginning to collect data on any patient, think carefully about the type of data needed to develop a satisfactory care plan. This also includes identifying data of a lower priority that you should not repeatedly collect. For example, data already collected from the patient and in the patient record should not be repeatedly sought unless there is a need for validation. Repetitious questioning can be annoying to a patient and may cause the patient to wonder about a lack of communication among health care professionals. A careful review of the patient record before interviewing the patient helps prevent this problem.

Nurses spend more or less time on different assessment components depending on the patient's reason for needing nursing care.

> **QSEN PATIENT-CENTERED CARE**
>
> **Pediatric nurses are careful to establish the developmental age and milestones obtained by children admitted to a pediatric unit so that they can respect and promote the child's achievements. A school nurse who suspects child abuse pays careful attention to the child's statements about living conditions at home and relationships with family members and caregivers. A nurse preparing to discharge a patient from same-day surgery makes sure that the patient has the human and physical resources needed for appropriate postoperative care.**

The purpose for which the assessment is being performed offers the best guidance for what type and how much data to

Patient Centered Assessment Method (PCAM)

ID ____________________ Date: __ __/__ __ __/2 0 __ __

Nurse/Clinician:

Instructions: Use this assessment as a guide, ask questions in your own words during the consultation to help you answer each question. Circle one option in each section to reflect the level of complexity relating to this patient. To be completed either during or after the consultation.

Health and Well-being			
1. Thinking about your patient's **physical health needs**, are there any symptoms or problems (risk indicators) you are unsure about that require further **investigation**?			
No identified areas of uncertainty or problems already being investigated	Mild vague physical symptoms or problems; but do not impact on daily life or are not of concern to patient	Mod to severe symptoms or problems that impact on daily life	Severe symptoms or problems that cause significant impact on daily life
2. Are the patient's **physical health problems** impacting on their **mental well-being**?			
No identified areas of concern	Mild impact on mental well-being, e.g., "feeling fed-up," "reduced enjoyment"	Mod to severe impact upon mental well-being and preventing enjoyment of usual activities	Severe impact upon mental well-being and preventing engagement with usual activities
3. Are there any problems with your patient's **lifestyle behaviors** (alcohol, drugs, diet, exercise) that are impacting on **physical** or **mental well-being**?			
No identified areas of concern	Some mild concern of potential negative impact on well-being	Mod to severe impact on patient's well-being, preventing enjoyment of usual activities	Severe impact on patient's well-being with additional potential impact on others
4. Do you have any **other concerns** about your patient's **mental well-being**? How would you rate their severity and impact on the patient?			
No identified areas of concern	Mild problems—don't interfere with function	Mod to severe problems that interfere with function	Severe problems impairing most daily functions
Social Environment			
1. How would you rate their **home environment** in terms of **safety and stability** (including domestic violence, insecure housing, neighbor harassment)?			
Consistently safe, supportive, stable, no identified problems	Safe, stable, but with some inconsistency	Safety/stability questionable	Unsafe and unstable
2. How do **daily activities** impact on the patient's well-being? (include current or anticipated unemployment, work, caregiving, access to transportation or other)			
No identified problems or perceived positive benefits	Some general dissatisfaction but no concern	Contributes to low mood or stress at times	Severe impact on poor mental well-being
3. How would you rate their **social network** (family, work, friends)?			
Good participation with social networks	Adequate participation with social networks	Restricted participation with some degree of social isolation	Little participation, lonely and socially isolated

FIGURE 15-4. Patient-Centered Assessment Method (PCAM). (*Source:* Used with permission. © Maxwell, Hibberd, Pratt, Peek and Baird 2013. PCAM may not be copied or shared with any third party without inclusion of this copyright declaration. There are no license costs for the use of PCAM and the developers are committed to PCAM being freely available to use.)

4. How would you rate their **financial resources** (including ability to afford all required medical care)?			
Financially secure, resources adequate, no identified problems	Financially secure, some resource challenges	Financially insecure, some resource challenges	Financially insecure, very few resources, immediate challenges
Health Literacy and Communication			
1. How well does the patient **now understand** their health and well-being (symptoms, signs, or risk factors) and what they need to do to manage their health?			
Reasonable to good understanding and already engages in managing health or is willing to undertake better management	Reasonable to good understanding <u>but</u> do not feel able to engage with advice at this time	Little understanding which impacts on their ability to undertake better management	Poor understanding with significant impact on ability to manage health
2. How well do you think your patient can **engage** in health care discussions? (Barriers include language, deafness, aphasia, alcohol or drug problems, learning difficulties, concentration)			
Clear and open communication, no identified barriers	Adequate communication, with or without minor barriers	Some difficulties in communication with or without moderate barriers	Serious difficulties in barriers
Service Coordination			
1. Do **other services** need to be involved to help this patient?			
Other care/services not required at this time	Other care/services in place and adequate	Other care/services in place but not sufficient	Other care/services not in place and required
2. Are current services involved with this patient **well coordinated**? (Include coordination with other services you are now recommending)			
All required care/services in place and well coordinated	Required care/services in place and adequately coordinated	Required care/services in place with some coordination barriers	Required care/services missing and/or fragmented
Routine Care	**Active monitoring**	**Plan Action**	**Act Now**

What action is required?	**Who needs to be involved?**	**Barriers to action?**	**What action will be taken?**
Notes:			

FIGURE 15-4. (*continued*)

collect. Assessment priorities are influenced by the patient's health orientation, developmental stage, culture, and need for nursing. Following the comprehensive nursing assessment, the patient's health problems dictate assessment priorities for future nurse–patient interactions.

Health Orientation

Nurses may use health assessments, such as the Health-Style Self-Test in Chapter 3 and the Promoting Health displays in each clinical chapter, to help patients identify potential and actual health risks and to explore the habits, behaviors, beliefs, attitudes, and values that influence their wellness. The literature abounds in specialized assessment tools that focus on relationships; psychological, environmental, and physical self-care; relaxation; spirituality; humor and play; movement and exercise; sleep and dreams; nutrition; and sexuality. These assessments generally gather a different type of patient data compared to the assessments of patients being treated for disease-related treatment.

Developmental Stage

Nursing assessments vary according to the patient's developmental needs. For example, when assessing an infant, special attention is given to weight gain and physical growth, feeding and elimination problems, sleep–activity cycles, and the parenting skills of caregivers. When a child is hospitalized, it is important to note how independent the child is with basic care measures (toileting, hygiene, dressing, eating), what words the child uses to indicate the need to void and defecate, play preferences, and so on.

Culture

When assessing patients, remember the influence of cultural factors such as race, ethnicity, religious beliefs, and socioeconomic factors. Consideration of the patient's culture begins with how you approach the patient and whether or not you make direct eye contact or shake the person's hand. Chapter 5 offers practical guidelines for incorporating cultural considerations into nursing assessments. Also assess the need for an interpreter. In what language does the patient wish to communicate? If an interpreter is necessary, be sure to follow your facility's policy about using a professional interpreter, since it is inappropriate to rely on the patient's family members for this service.

Need for Nursing

The likely duration of the nurse's interaction with the patient (e.g., same-day surgery vs. surgery requiring a long recovery in an intensive care unit) and the nature of nursing care needed by the patient (e.g., assistance with the birth of a baby vs. support and home care throughout a terminal illness) are both factors that powerfully influence the type of data the nurse collects. A general assessment guideline is to gather only data that are helpful when planning and delivering care. It would be inappropriate, for example, to collect a detailed sexual history of a patient admitted to the hospital overnight after a slight concussion. Conversely, if your patient is a pregnant woman admitted to the hospital for observation because of bleeding during their first trimester, you should not fail to ask whether they has any questions about resuming sexual activity after returning home.

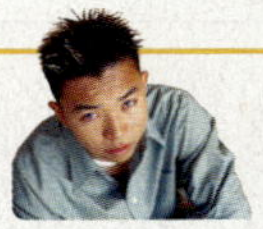

Think back to ***James Farren***, the college junior described at the beginning of the chapter. The nurse would assess his sleeping, eating, and activity habits as well as his emotional status to gain further insight into his possible problems. However, a detailed assessment of his elimination habits would probably be inappropriate at the present time.

Structuring the Assessment

Because many different types of data are collected about patients, data collection must be structured systematically. Systematic guidelines specifically developed for a nursing assessment help ensure that comprehensive, holistic data are collected for each patient and lead easily to formulating nursing diagnoses. When the nurse internalizes such assessment guidelines, it is easier to focus on the patient during the assessment rather than worrying about what to assess next.

Most schools of nursing and health care institutions have a **minimum data set** that specifies the information that must be collected from every patient and uses a structured assessment form to organize or cluster this data. Many nursing assessment guides are based on holistic models rather than medical models. Gordon's (1994) framework identifies 11 functional health patterns and organizes patient data within these patterns. Maslow's hierarchy of five levels of human needs may also be used to organize data. A medical model often organizes data collection according to body systems. Although the medical model is helpful for formulating diagnoses related to physiologic problems, it neglects patient problems and strengths in psychosocial and spiritual dimensions of health and well-being.

Some students use the HELP mnemonic shown in Box 15-1 to ensure systematic person-centered observation.

Whichever approach you use for structuring your nursing assessment, always conclude by asking the patient if there is anything else they would like you to know so that you will be better able to provide care. This allows the patient to address anything critical that you may have missed.

Table 15-1 describes models for organizing assessment data.

COLLECTING DATA

There are two types of data: subjective and objective. **Subjective data** are information perceived only by the affected person; these data cannot be perceived or verified by another person. Examples of subjective data are feeling nervous, nauseated, or chilly, and experiencing pain. Subjective data also are called symptoms or covert data.

Objective data are observable and measurable data that can be seen, heard, felt, or measured by someone other than the person experiencing them. Objective data observed by one person can be verified by another person observing the same patient. Examples of objective data are an elevated

Box 15-1 HELP Mnemonic for Patient Observation

Help: Observe the first signs patient may need help. Look for signs of distress (pallor, pain, labored breathing).
Environmental equipment: Look for safety hazards; ensure that all equipment is working (IVs, oxygen, catheter).
Look: Examine the patient thoroughly.
People: Who are the people in the room? What are they doing?

Table 15-1 Models for Organizing or Clustering Data

HOLISTIC			MEDICAL
Human Needs (Maslow)	**Functional Health Patterns (Gordon)**	**Human Response Patterns (Unitary Person)**	**Body System Model**
Physiologic (Survival) Needs: Food, fluids, oxygen, elimination, warmth, physical comfort *Safety and Security Needs:* Things necessary for physical safety (e.g., a cane) and psychological security (e.g., a child's favorite toy) *Love and Belonging Needs:* Family and significant others *Self-Esteem Needs:* Things that make people feel good about themselves and confident in their abilities (e.g., being well groomed, having accomplishments recognized) *Self-Actualization Needs:* Need to grow, change, and accomplish goals	*Health Perception/Health Management:* Perception of general health status and well-being; adherence to preventive health practices *Nutritional–Metabolic:* Patterns of food and fluid intake, fluid and electrolyte balance, general ability to heal *Elimination:* Patterns of excretory function (bowel, bladder, skin) and patient's perception *Activity/Exercise:* Pattern of exercise, activity, leisure, recreation, and ADLs; factors that interfere with desired to expected individual pattern *Cognitive–Perceptual:* Adequacy of sensory modes such as vision, hearing, taste, touch, smell, pain perception, cognitive functional abilities *Sleep/Rest:* Patterns of sleep and rest–relaxation periods during a 24-hour day, as well as quality and quantity *Self-Perception/Self-Concept:* Attitudes about self, perception of abilities, body image, identity, general sense of worth, and emotional patterns *Role/Relationship:* Perception of major roles and responsibilities in current life situation *Sexuality and Reproductive:* Perceived satisfaction or dissatisfaction with sexuality, reproductive state, and pattern *Coping/Stress Tolerance:* General coping pattern, stress tolerance, support systems, perceived ability to control and manage situations *Value Belief:* Values, goals, or beliefs that guide choices or decisions	*Exchanging:* Nutritional status, temperature, elimination, oxygenation, circulation, fluid balance, skin, and mucous membranes, risk for injury *Communicating:* Ability to express thoughts verbally; orientation, speech impairments, language barriers *Relating:* Establishing bonds, social interaction, support systems, role performance (including parenting, occupation, and sexual role) *Valuing:* Religious and cultural preference and practices, relationship with deity, perception of suffering; acceptance of illness *Choosing:* Ability to accept help and make decisions, adjustment to health status, desire for independence/dependence, denial of problem, adherence to therapies *Moving:* Activity tolerance, ability for self-care, sleep patterns, diversional activities, disability history, safety needs, breastfeeding *Perceiving:* Body image, self-esteem, ability to use all five senses, amount of hopefulness, perception of ability to control current situation *Knowing:* Knowledge about current illness or therapies; previous illnesses; risk factors, expectations of therapy, cognitive abilities; readiness to learn, orientation, memory *Feeling:* Pain, grieving, risk for violence, anxiety level, emotional integrity	Neurologic Cardiovascular Respiratory Gastrointestinal Musculoskeletal Genitourinary Psychosocial

Source: Data from Alfaro-LeFevre, R. (2014). *Applying nursing process. The foundation for clinical reasoning* (8th ed.). Wolters Kluwer Health/Lippincott Williams & Wilkins.

temperature reading (e.g., 101°F), skin that is moist, and refusal to look at or eat food. Objective data also are called signs or overt data. Table 15-2 (on page 416) compares subjective and objective data.

Paying attention to both subjective and objective data promotes clinical reasoning and judgment because often the two types of data complement and clarify one another. Many providers were taught to use the OLD CARTS mnemonic to structure their assessment of patient symptoms:

- **O**nset: When did your symptom(s) begin?
- **L**ocation: Where is the symptom?
- **D**uration: Is it episodic? How long does it last?
- **C**haracteristics: How would you describe it?
- **A**lleviating and **A**ggravating factors: What makes it worse?
- **R**elieving factors: What makes it better?
- **T**reatments: Have you tried anything to make it better?
- **S**everity: On a scale of 1–10, with 1 being the lower number, how serious is the symptom?

Table 15-2 Comparison of Objective and Subjective Data

OBJECTIVE DATA	SUBJECTIVE DATA
32-year-old man Height: 5′8″ Weight: 9/18/24—224 lb 2/4/24—202 lb	"I'm beginning to feel better about myself now that I'm losing weight and I seem to have more energy."
Posterior, left midcalf is warm and red.	"My leg hurts when I walk."
Patient observed fidgeting with bed covers; facial features are tightly drawn.	"I'm so afraid of what they might find when they cut me open tomorrow."

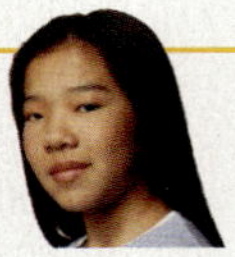

Review the data provided in the scenario for **Sylvia Wu** in the Reflective Practice display. Her reports of flulike symptoms provide the nurse with subjective data. Hearing her cough, noting any sputum produced, inspecting her throat for redness and irritation, and checking her temperature would provide the nurse with objective data that help to clarify and substantiate the patient's reported symptoms.

Sources of Data

Patient

The patient is the primary and usually the best source of information. Unless specified otherwise, the data recorded in the nursing history are assumed to have been collected from the patient. Most patients are willing to share information when they know it is helpful for planning their care. (See the accompanying feature box, Through the Eyes of a Student.) Although subjective data collected from the patient are usually accurate, you should be alert for certain difficulties. For example, a patient who is acutely ill may not be able to communicate adequately if the pain is severe or if consciousness is altered. An emotionally upset patient may distort information; for example, patients who are fearful because they think their illness may threaten their work or life may deny certain symptoms or deliberately give misleading facts. If you become aware that a patient's report of symptoms differs from physical findings or data obtained from other sources, note this and explore the cause of the discrepancy.

Data from patients with limited mental or communication capacity, such as young children and older adults with dementia, cannot be relied on as accurate. However, learn early to avoid the mistake of too quickly judging that a family member is a better source of information than the patient. Children and people with decreased mental capacity or impaired verbal ability should be encouraged to respond to interview questions as best as they can. Automatically turning to a family member, friend, or caregiver for information communicates powerfully that you either have no time for the patient to express their needs or mistakenly doubt the patient's ability to communicate these needs.

Family and Significant Others

Family members, friends, and caregivers are especially helpful sources of data when the patient is a child or has limited capacity to share information with the nurse. Partners can supply information concerning their spouses. Friends often accompany a patient to a health facility and can supply

Through the Eyes of a Student

During my chronic medical–surgical rotation, my clinical group was placed on an oncology floor. My first thought was "Oh no, not the cancer floor!" The word *fear* didn't even begin to describe how I felt. These patients had enough problems without some "green" nursing student aggravating them all day. I kept thinking these people are extremely ill and won't want to be bothered by my intruding questions.

Nonetheless, I knew I had to do it. Not only did I have to take care of this patient all day, but I also had to develop a database and care plan. I knew I would have to do a lot more than give him his morning care and leave him alone. I would have to carry on an extended conversation with this patient to get all the information I needed.

As if all of this wasn't enough to make me throw in the white flag, when my patient assignment was given, I discovered my patient was a man only 1 year older than me. A 28-year-old man with terminal cancer—this was too scary!

Clinical day came, as I knew it would, and I was shaking. I walked in that room and together the patient and I planned his care. I explained to him the things I needed to talk about with him and I couldn't believe it—he didn't tell me to go away! We talked at length about his disease process and how it had affected his plans and goals. He opened up to me about his spirituality, his relationships with friends and family, and other personal subjects. Periodically, he would cringe, and I could tell it was time for a break. He was hurting too badly to go on at that time.

At the end of that day, my viewpoint was totally different than it had been that morning. I walked away from that room and off that floor feeling like I had made a difference for this person. We had shared a lot and he seemed so appreciative for the time I took to talk with him. The information he shared helped me to develop a better care plan that was more responsive to his particular needs. The amazing part was that all I had to do was just be myself and allow him to do the same and our day flowed smoothly. The lesson I learned here was important for me: Cultivate competence, keep calm and hold on to compassion, and nursing offers many rewards!

—Nancy E. Driskill, Southeast Missouri State University
Cape Girardeau, Missouri

useful information. Take care to determine that the patient does not object to you gathering data from family and friends, and also that family and friends want to participate. Also, everyone involved should clearly understand the confidentiality of this data. Whenever data are gathered from support people, indicate this in the nursing history.

Patient Record

Records prepared by different members of the health care team provide information essential to comprehensive nursing care. You should review records early when gathering data—in some instances, before the first contact with the patient. This review helps to focus the nursing assessment and to confirm and amplify information obtained from other sources.

The patient's health record or chart, which lists such information as age, sex, occupation, religious preference, next of kin, and financial status, is one type of record. The health record includes information entered by various health care professionals such as physicians, social workers, dietitians, physiotherapists, and laboratory technicians.

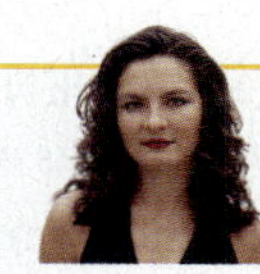

For **Susan Morgan**, the 34-year-old patient recently diagnosed with MS, the nurse would review her medical record for information related to her diagnosis and treatment plans, including specialized consultations and therapy, as well as her current home situation. This information would help the nurse determine the approach to performing the nursing history and physical examination, as well as planning her care.

If you want your care to be supportive of the patient while responding to changes in health status, you must be familiar with the many sections of the patient record in addition to the documentation of the nursing care plan and nursing notes. The following parts of the patient record are important sources of data.

MEDICAL HISTORY, PHYSICAL EXAMINATION, AND PROGRESS NOTES

These parts of the record include the findings of physicians and nurse practitioners as they assess and treat the patient; they focus on identifying pathologic conditions and their causes and on determining the medical regimen for treatment.

CONSULTATIONS

The patient's health care providers may invite specialists to assess and treat the patient. The focus of these parts of the record is additional findings related to the patient's medical diagnosis and treatment.

REPORTS OF LABORATORY AND OTHER DIAGNOSTIC STUDIES

Reports of laboratory studies and other diagnostic tests, such as radiographs, include objective data that can either confirm or conflict with data collected during the nursing history or examination. Diagnostic studies help clinicians establish a diagnosis and monitor the patient's response to treatment. The results of these studies may also help nurses evaluate the success of nursing interventions.

REPORTS OF THERAPIES BY OTHER HEALTH CARE PROFESSIONALS

Other health care professionals who interact with the patient also record their findings and note what progress the patient is making in their specific areas—for example, nutrition, physical therapy, spiritual health, or speech therapy. These reports also help the nurse assess the patient's progress and help determine the patient's ability to return home and manage care independently. For example, a nurse would carefully check a speech therapist's evaluation of a patient's ability to swallow while working with a dietitian to develop and administer the care plan for nutrition via a feeding tube.

Records of previous admissions for health care and records from other health facilities, such as a social service facility or a home health care facility, are also valuable sources of data. They contain information about the patient's previous medical or surgical problems and response patterns, which may be important determinants of the current care plan. See Chapters 8, 11, and 20 for a description of the critical information that should be shared when patients are "handed off" or transitioned from one caregiver or team to another.

Assessment Technology

Nurses can also gain valuable data about patients from technologies such as cardiac and respiratory monitors. For example, a patient's bedside monitoring can provide round-the-clock information on blood pressure, heart rate, respirations, and cardiac activity.

Other Health Care Professionals

Nurses can learn a great deal about a patient's normal health habits and patterns and response to illness by talking with other nurses, physicians, social workers, and others on the health care team (Fig. 15-5 on page 418). Although such communication is always important, it is especially critical when patients are transferred from home to an institution or from one hospital or institution to another. The only way to ensure continuity of care is to make special efforts to share pertinent information.

Nursing and Other Health Care Literature

To obtain a comprehensive patient database, it may be necessary to consult the nursing and related literature on specific health problems. For example, a nurse who has not cared for a patient with Paget disease before should read about the clinical manifestations of the disease and its usual progression to know what to look for when assessing the patient. In addition to information about medical diagnoses, treatment, and prognosis, a literature review offers nurses important information about nursing diagnoses, developmental norms, and psychosocial and spiritual practices that is helpful when assessing and caring for patients.

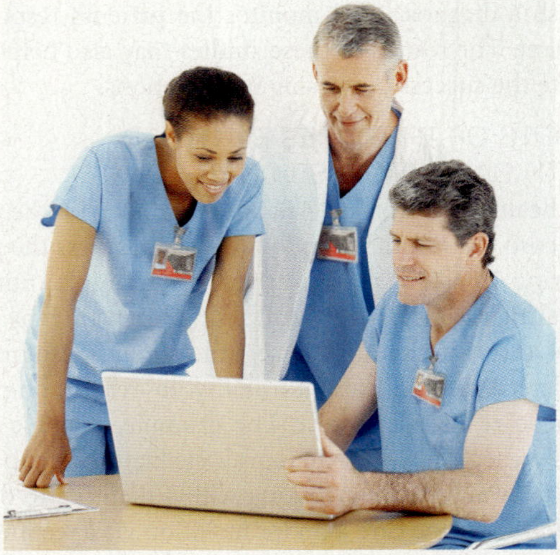

FIGURE 15-5. Nurses can learn a great deal about a patient's health habits, patterns, and responses to illness by talking with other nurses, physicians, social workers, and other members of the health care team. This exchange of information is particularly important when patients transfer from one health care setting to another, or to home.

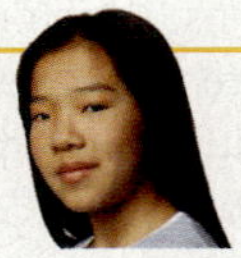

For **Sylvia Wu**, the possible diagnosis of a virus that is potentially lethal is very frightening. To provide the most appropriate care, the nurse would need to know as much as possible about the disease. Then the nurse would be better able to act as an advocate for the patient.

Methods of Data Collection

The nursing history and physical assessment are primary components of data collection (see Chapter 27). These data may be documented on separate assessment tools or incorporated into a combined database assessment form, as shown in Figure 15-2 on page 408.

Observation is a key nursing skill when performing both the nursing history and the physical examination. **Observation** is the conscious and deliberate use of the five senses to gather data. Skilled nurses observe and interpret meaningful stimuli (data) in each nurse–patient interaction. You can develop such observation skills by training yourself to carefully observe the following each time you encounter a patient:

- What are the patient's current responses (physical and emotional) to their situation? Be alert to signs of distress—difficulty breathing, bleeding, pain, heightened anxiety—as well as anything out of the ordinary, such as sudden eruption of rash or a change in level of consciousness.
- What is the patient's current ability to manage their care (need for additional information or nursing assistance)?
- What factors are relevant in the immediate environment? Consider the safety of the environment as well as the functioning of equipment (e.g., intravenous therapy, oxygen, drains). Who are the people in the room and at home? What are the temperature and odor of the room?
- What other factors are relevant in the larger environment (hospital or community)?

Nursing History

Ideally, the nursing history captures and records the uniqueness of the patient so that care may be planned to meet the patient's individual needs. You should obtain the nursing history as soon as possible after a patient presents for care and then follow with the nursing physical assessment. You should clearly identify the patient's strengths and weaknesses; health risks, such as hereditary and environmental factors; and potential and existing health problems. While obtaining the nursing history, you focus on getting to know the person.

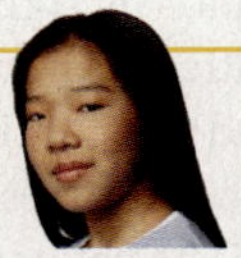

When obtaining the nursing history from **Sylvia Wu**, the nurse would ascertain when the patient had traveled in China, how long she had been there, how long she had been home, with whom she may have been in contact, and whether these people exhibited any signs and symptoms. This information is important for determining the patient's actual risk for developing a particular virus.

COMPONENTS OF A NURSING HISTORY

Components of a nursing history include:

- Profile: name, age, sex, race/ethnicity, marital status, religion, occupation, education
- Reason for seeking health care
- Health literacy and communication skills
- Usual health habits and patterns and related needs for nursing assistance
- Cultural considerations in relation to diet, decision making, and activities
- Current state of physical and mental health, functioning of body systems, degree of pain, and past medical and surgical history
- Current medications, allergies, and record of immunizations and exposure to communicable diseases
- Perception of health status and what health and illness mean to the patient, as well as usual responses or coping patterns
- Developmental history, family history, environmental history, and psychosocial history
- Patient's and family's expectations of nursing and of the health care team
- Patient's and family's educational needs and ability and willingness to learn
- Patient's and family's ability and willingness to participate in the care plan
- Whether an advance directive exists or if the patient wants help to prepare an advance directive
- Patient's personal resources (strengths) and deficits
- Patient's potential for injury

PATIENT INTERVIEW

You obtain the nursing history by interviewing the patient. An **interview** is a planned communication. You need strong interviewing skills to establish a successful working partnership

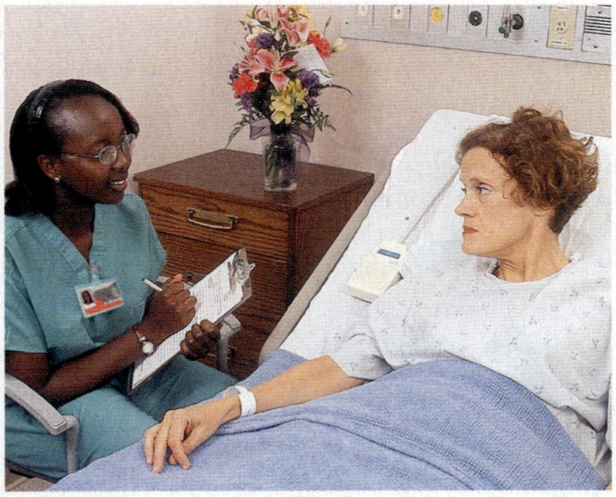

FIGURE 15-6. In the interview, both the seating arrangement and the distance from the patient are important in establishing a relaxed and comfortable environment for data collection. (*Source:* Used with permission from Shutterstock. *Photo by B. Proud.*)

with the patient, to communicate care and concern for the patient, and to obtain the necessary patient data. Many students find it helpful to role-play the nurse–patient interview before attempting this in a clinical setting. It is also helpful to watch how experienced nurses interview patients, create partnerships, and earn their trust. Figure 15-6 depicts a seating arrangement and distance from the patient appropriate for the interview. See the accompanying Guidelines for Nursing Care 15-1: Promoting a Caring Interview (on page 420) for tips on conducting an effective interview. The interview occurs in four phases: the preparatory phase, introduction, working phase, and termination. More detailed information on interviewing techniques is provided in Chapter 8.

Physical Assessment

Physical assessment is the examination of the patient for objective data that may better define the patient's condition and help the nurse plan care. The physical assessment normally follows the nursing history and interview and may verify data gathered during the history or yield new data. Health care providers traditionally have performed the intake physical assessment, which commonly is the mechanism of entry into the health care delivery system as well as the basis for medical treatment. Some nurses in advanced practice roles perform comprehensive intake physical assessments similar to those of their physician colleagues, which identify health and illness states, and then recommend or prescribe appropriate care. In any case, all nurses conduct selected aspects of physical assessment for nursing purposes.

Unlike the physical assessment performed by the clinician to identify pathologic conditions and their causes, the nursing physical assessment focuses primarily on the patient's functional abilities. If a neurologic deficit is present, the nurse identifies how it affects the patient's reasoning and sensorimotor abilities. For example, a patient who has had a cerebrovascular accident (brain attack or stroke) is examined to determine ability to comprehend and communicate information and perform the tasks of everyday life.

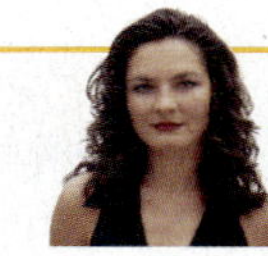

The physical assessment for **Susan Morgan**, the young woman newly diagnosed with MS described at the beginning of the chapter, would include investigation of the patient's muscle strength and endurance level and the effects of MS on the patient's ability to perform daily activities. In the physical examination the nurse would be alert for indications of fatigue or inability to complete specific activities. This information would help the nurse respond appropriately to the patient's concerns about her marriage.

The purposes of the nursing physical assessment include the appraisal of health status, the identification of health problems, and the establishment of a database for nursing interventions (Fig. 15-7).

Nurses practicing in different settings may use different physical assessment techniques for different purposes. Nurses in the medical intensive care unit use sophisticated, high-technology assessment techniques, whereas nurses in a rehabilitation center use a wide range of physical assessment skills that focus on identifying functional and nonfunctional response patterns to disabilities.

The nursing physical assessment involves the examination of all body systems in a systematic manner, commonly using a head-to-toe format; this is called the **review of systems (ROS)**. Four methods are used to collect data during the physical assessment:

- *Inspection*: the process of performing deliberate, purposeful observations in a systematic manner
- *Palpation*: use of the sense of touch to assess skin temperature, turgor, texture, and moisture as well as vibrations within the body

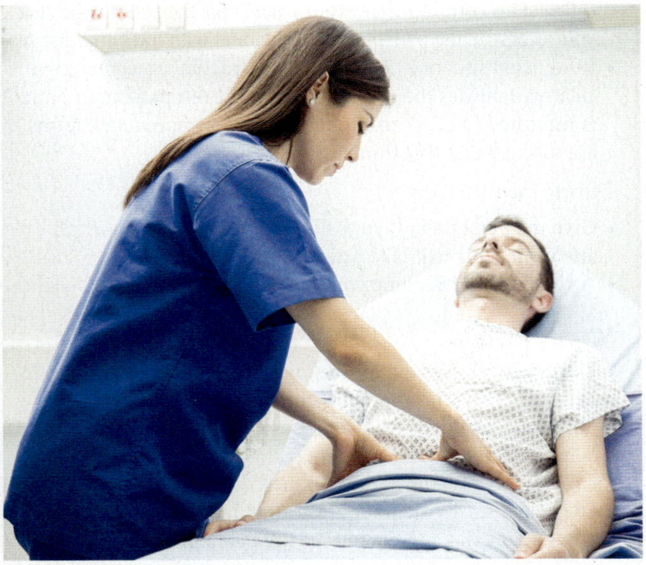

FIGURE 15-7. The nurse conducts a physical examination. No matter what the setting or the age of the patient, the physical examination should include appraisal of health status, identification of health problems, and establishment of a database for nursing intervention. (*Source:* Used with permission from Shutterstock. *Photo by Antoniodiaz.*)

Guidelines for Nursing Care 15-1

PROMOTING A CARING INTERVIEW

These guidelines can help you to establish trust, create a positive attitude, and reduce anxiety—both yours and the patient's!

How to Establish Rapport

Before you go into the interview

- Get organized: Be sure that you have everything you need to have with you.
- Prepare for the interview by reading current and past records and reports.
- Don't rely on memory: Have a printed or electronic assessment tool to guide the questions you will ask.
- Plan enough time: The admission interview usually takes 30 to 60 minutes.
- Ensure privacy: Make sure that you have a quiet, private setting, free from interruptions or distractions.
- Get focused: Clear your mind of other concerns. Say to yourself, "Getting to know this person is the most important thing I have to do right now."
- Visualize yourself as being confident, warm, and helpful: This helps you to be confident, warm, and helpful—your genuine interest comes through.
- Approach the patient with an open mind and be aware of any stereotypes or prejudices that might affect this encounter.

When you begin the interview

- Begin by sitting at eye level with the patient (Fig. 15-6 on page 419). Chairs placed at right angles to each other and about 3 to 4 ft (0.9 to 1.2 m) apart facilitate an easy exchange of information. If the patient is in bed, placing the chair at a 45-degree angle to the bed is helpful.
- Introduce yourself and give your name and position. This sends the message that you accept responsibility and are willing to be accountable for your actions. This is especially important if you are a student.
- Verify the person's name and ask what they would like to be called. This communicates your respect for the patient and that you recognize the patient as an individual with likes and dislikes.
- In unusual situations in which a contractual agreement that clearly identifies the responsibilities of both patient and nurse is indicated (e.g., a gerontologic nurse entrepreneur), terms are discussed at this time.

During the interview

- Give the person—not your notes or computer—your full attention. This will take practice.
- Avoid rushing. Become comfortable with the patient's silence.

How to Listen

- Listen actively—listen for feelings as well as words.
- Let the person know in a diplomatic manner when you see body language that sends a message that conflicts with what is being said, for example, "You say that you aren't having pain, but you look uncomfortable to me."
- Use short, supplemental phrases that let the person know you understand and encourage the person to continue, for example, "I see," "Mmhm," and "Then what?"
- Be patient if the person has a memory block.
- Avoid the impulse to interrupt.
- Allow for pauses in conversation. Silence gives both you and the person time to gather thoughts, and allows you to reflect on the accuracy of the information the patient has provided.

How to Ask Questions

- Ask questions about the person's main problems first, for example, "What are the main reasons you are here today?" and "What do you hope happens today (or during your visit/time here)?"
- Focus your questions to gain specific information about signs and symptoms, for example, "Show me where the problem is" and "Can you describe how this feels more specifically?"
- Don't use leading questions, for example, "You don't smoke, do you?"
- Do use exploratory statements, for example, "Tell me more about your sleeping patterns."
- Use communication techniques that enhance your ability to think critically and get the facts:
  1. Use phrases that help you see the other person's perspective, for example, "What are the problems as you see them?"
  2. Restate the person's own words, for example, "Let me repeat what you said to make sure I understand."
  3. Ask open-ended questions, for example, "How are you feeling?" rather than "Are you feeling well?"
  4. Avoid close-ended questions—those requiring a one-word answer—unless the person is too ill to elaborate or you are trying to clarify a response by getting a yes or no.

What to Observe

- Carefully assess areas connected to verbal complaints.
- Use your senses.
- Note general appearance.
- Observe body language. Does the person appear comfortable? Nervous? Withdrawn? Apprehensive? What behaviors do you see?
- Notice interaction patterns. Be aware of the person's responses to your interviewing style (e.g., sometimes cultural and personal differences create communication barriers).

How to Terminate the Interview

- Give a warning, for example, "We have 5 minutes to finish up . . . let's be sure we have covered the most important things you want us to know."
- Ask people to summarize their most important concerns and then summarize the most important concerns as you see them.
- Ask, "What else?," for example, "Is there anything else you want us to know to better plan your care?"
- Offer yourself as a resource, for example, "Let me know if anything changes or you have any questions."
- Explain care routines and provide information about who is accountable for nursing care decisions. Patients are often confused about who is responsible for what.
- Explain where the data being recorded are stored, how they will be used, and who has access to them.
- End on a positive note and encourage the person to become an active participant, for example, "We have a good start here. We want you to be actively involved in making decisions about your care."

Source: Adapted from Alfaro-LeFevre, R. (2014). *Applying nursing process. The foundation for clinical reasoning* (8th ed., pp. 62–65). Wolters Kluwer Health/Lippincott Williams & Wilkins.

Table 15-3 Patient Variables That Can Negatively Influence an Interview and Suggested Nursing Responses

PATIENT VARIABLES	EFFECT ON INTERVIEW	NURSING RESPONSE
High anxiety	Patient may speak rapidly or incoherently and may jump from one topic to another; patient may deny or misrepresent what they are experiencing.	Normalize anxiety: "Many people find it difficult to talk about their health and become anxious"; approach patient gently, speak slowly and softly; underscore importance of the patient sharing what they are experiencing so that nurses can help.
Pain	Patient offers clipped responses and "yes" or "no" answers whenever possible; overriding concern is pain relief.	Do everything possible to make patient comfortable before the interview, try nonpharmacologic remedies and if necessary obtain an order for and administer pain medication; if pain persists, obtain only vital data and defer remainder of interview until patient is more comfortable.
Language difficulty (patient not fluent in nurse's language because patient speaks a different language, has a limited education, or fears saying the "wrong thing")	Vital patient data will not be communicated; patient may mistakenly be labeled "indifferent" or "noncommunicative."	Speak clearly (do not raise voice) using simple language; whenever possible, obtain the assistance of an interpreter and follow facility guidelines.
Previous negative experience with nurses or health care delivery system	Patient is aloof, unwilling to participate in interview; general attitude: "Why should I waste my time telling you anything . . . it won't do me any good."	"I know other people who have had a tough time with nurses or the system . . . life isn't perfect . . . but how about giving us a chance this time to show you what nurses can do?" Communicate respect for the patient and competence.
Unrealistic expectations of health care professionals	Patient expects nurses and other health care professionals magically to know everything about the patient and to "take care" of the patient; "surrenders" self to the system—"you know best" attitude.	Communicate clearly that no one knows or understands the patient like the patient does, and invite the patient to become involved in their care; "No two people are alike, and unless you tell me a little more about yourself and how you are feeling, there is no way we'll be able to plan good care."

- *Percussion*: the act of striking one object against another to produce sound
- *Auscultation*: the act of listening with a stethoscope to sounds produced within the body

Nurses may also use physical assessment skills to evaluate selected body systems. These techniques and the basic skills for physical assessment are described in Chapter 27.

Problems Related to Data Collection

Common problems that occur in data collection include inappropriate organization of the database, omission of pertinent data, inclusion of irrelevant or duplicate data, erroneous or misinterpreted data, failure to establish rapport and partnership with the patient, recording an interpretation of data rather than observed behavior, and failure to update the database. Tables 15-3 and 15-4 describe possible causes and remedies for such problems.

IDENTIFYING CUES AND MAKING INFERENCES

Nurses now use the language of cues and inferences to describe the early analysis of data. The subjective and objective data you identify ("the patient does not respond when I speak to him on his left side") is a **cue** that something may be wrong. The judgment you reach about the cue (the patient's hearing may be impaired on his left side) is an **inference**. See Figure 15-8 to see a nurse responding to nonverbal cues.

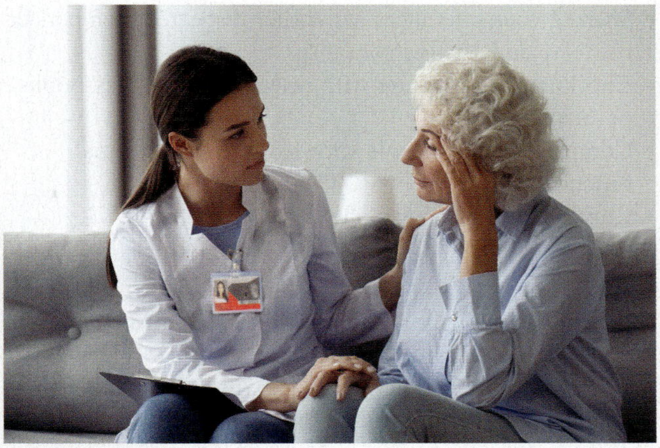

FIGURE 15-8. A nurse responds to a patient's nonverbal cues during a home visit. (*Source:* Used with permission from Shutterstock. *Photo by fizkes.*)

Table 15-4 Common Problems of Data Collection, Possible Causes, and Suggested Remedies

PROBLEM	POSSIBLE CAUSES	SUGGESTED REMEDIES
Database inappropriately organized	Failure to plan for the assessment by identifying needed data; use of inappropriate tools for data collection	Review the guidelines for specifying pertinent data. Consider modifying tool for data collection or select an alternative tool.
Pertinent data omitted	Not following up on cues during data collection; inappropriate guidelines	Identify potentially relevant factors in advance of collection. Practice interview strategies.
Irrelevant or duplicate data collected	Failure to identify specific purpose of data collection; failure to review available patient records; use of inappropriate tools for data collection	Determine specific purpose of data collection for each patient. Consider existing data before initiating collection. Consider modifying data collection tool or selecting alternative.
Erroneous or misinterpreted data collection	Failure to observe carefully or validate during data collection; interviewer prejudices or stereotypes	Sharpen observation skills by independently observing the same situation with a peer and comparing notes afterward. Role-play several validation techniques.
Failure to establish rapport	Failure to establish sufficient rapport or use appropriate communication techniques with patient; failure to know what information is wanted	Review and practice communication techniques discussed in Chapter 8. Role-play several explanations of purpose of data collection. Identify general data desired before collection.
Interpretation of data is recorded rather than the observed behavior	Nurse jumps to hasty conclusion about patient's behavior and deprives others of exploring with patient possible causes of the behavior; deficient validation	Review the distinction between data and interpretation of data. Practice documenting observed patient behavior concisely.
Failure to update the database	Erroneous belief that assessment is concluded after the initial database is recorded; low priority attached to ongoing data collection	Recollect that it is impossible to give quality, individualized care without knowledge of changes in the patient's status. Ongoing data collection is critical to the deletion or modification of old problems and the identification of new problems.

Until you check the patient's hearing, you cannot be sure that your inference is correct. Inferences may be validated in multiple ways:

- Physical examination, using the proper equipment and procedure (you may need to have an expert confirm your findings)
- Clarifying statements ("You said this is not a problem, but I sense you may still be worried.")
- Sharing your inferences with other respected members of the team and seeking consensus
- Checking your findings with research reports, textbooks, or journals
- Comparing cues to your knowledge base of normal function
- Checking consistency of cues

Figure 15-9 illustrates the process for validating inferences.

The nurse may validate data during collection or at the end of the data-gathering process. When it is clear that the data are correct, the nurse is ready to analyze the data and formulate nursing diagnoses/health problems—the next phase of the nursing process. Figure 15-10 (on page 424) illustrates the role clinical reasoning and judgment plays in moving from assessment to diagnosis/problem identification.

VALIDATING DATA

Validation is the act of confirming or verifying. The purpose of validating is to keep data as free from error, bias, and misinterpretation as possible. Validation is an important part of assessment because invalid information can lead to inappropriate nursing care. Because it is neither possible nor necessary to validate all data, nurses need to decide which items need verification. For example, data need to be verified when there are discrepancies: a patient tells you he is fine and has no concerns, but you note that he demonstrates tense body musculature and seems curt in his responses. When there is a discrepancy between what the person is saying and what you are observing, validation is necessary to determine accuracy. Validation in this instance may take the form of your saying, "You tell me you feel fine, but right now your body and behaviors are telling me something else. Tell me more about this."

Data also need verification when they lack objectivity. For example, you suspect that the patient hears in one ear but does not seem to hear well in the other. You should validate the data before proceeding and should determine whether the patient does indeed have a hearing problem. Suspicions are not objective. In this instance, you need to test the patient's hearing in both ears. Speaking toward the

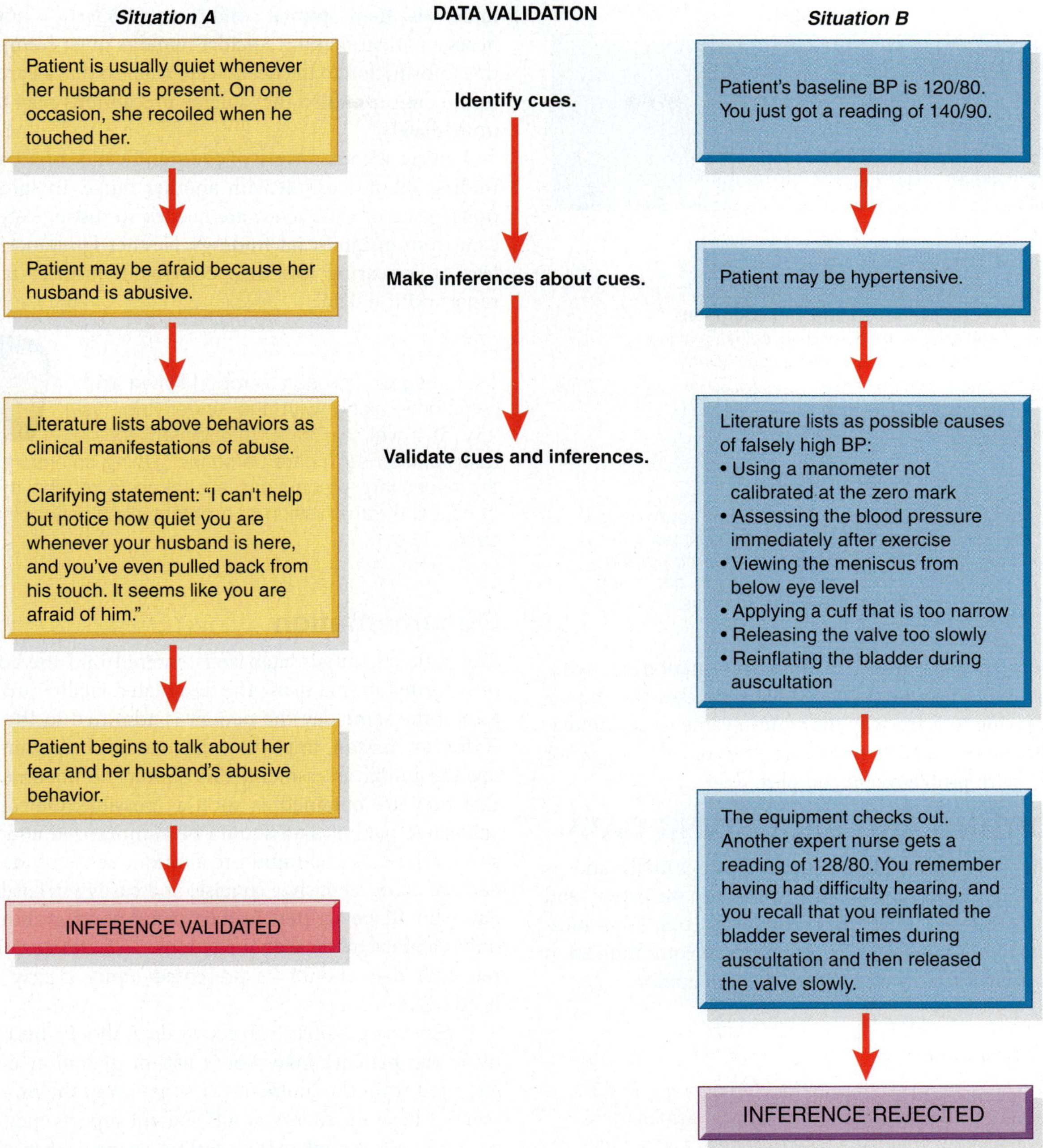

FIGURE 15-9. The process used to validate cues and inferences.

suspected better ear, you explain, "It seems to me that you hear better out of one ear than the other. I would like to test this. I'll bring a watch slowly toward your right ear first and then toward your left. Please look straight ahead and tell me when you first hear the watch ticking." You can then record how far the watch was from each ear when the patient first heard it ticking.

Concept Mastery Alert

Whenever there is any data discrepancy or conflict, the nurse must investigate further, gathering focused information to support, confirm, or negate the suspicions.

CLUSTERING RELATED DATA AND IDENTIFYING PATTERNS

As described earlier, as you prepare to collect your data you also decide how to organize or cluster the data. Table 15-1 on page 415 illustrates three holistic models (Maslow's human needs, Gordon's functional health patterns, and human response patterns) along with the body system medical model. Once you have organized your data according to the purpose of your assessment, you begin to look for and test your initial impressions about patterns of human functioning. Alfaro-LeFevre (2014) recommends testing your first impressions to decide what's relevant, making tentative decisions about what the data suggest, and focusing your

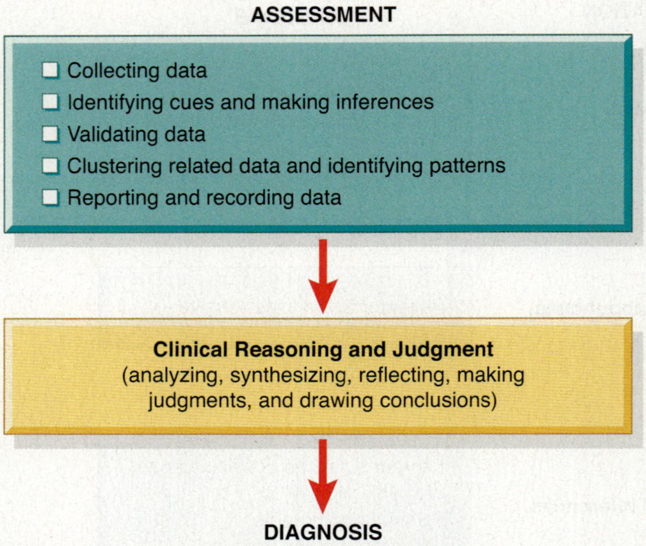

FIGURE 15-10. How the phases of assessment set the stage for diagnosis/problem identification. (*Source:* Reprinted with permission from Alfaro-LeFevre, R. [2014]. *Applying nursing process. The foundation for clinical reasoning* [8th ed., p. 49]. Wolters Kluwer Health/Lippincott Williams & Wilkins.)

assessment to gain more in-depth information to better understand the patient's situation. She stresses the importance of trying to learn why the pattern came to be, emphasizing that there is usually more than one contributing factor because health problems are complex.

REPORTING AND RECORDING DATA

The patient data the nurse collects, both initially and as patient contact continues, are of no benefit to the patient and the health care team unless they are appropriately communicated. See the Legal Alert box. Appropriate communication involves correct timing and proper documentation.

Legal Alert

Nurses are responsible for alerting the appropriate health care professional whenever assessment data differ significantly from the patient's baseline, indicating a potentially serious problem. Interventions for which the nurse may be legally responsible include increasing the frequency of assessments and initiating necessary changes in the treatment regimen.

Timing

Data should be reported verbally immediately whenever assessment findings reveal a critical change in the patient's health status that necessitates the involvement of other nurses or health care professionals. A nurse who observes an elevated temperature of 103.2°F (39.5°C) in a patient scheduled for surgery that morning must report this to the charge nurse and to the surgeon, who might then cancel surgery. Failure to communicate this finding could result in the patient's receiving preoperative sedation, being taken to the operating room, and even having the surgery performed under less than optimal conditions. Similarly, a nurse who hears a patient making suicidal remarks must communicate this information to the health care team so that all are alerted to the danger and so that suicide precautions may be taken immediately.

A nurse who is unsure of the significance of a particular finding should consult with another nurse. In some situations, years of experience are needed to distinguish significant from insignificant findings. Neither ignorance nor the fear of appearing less than competent justifies failure to report critical data.

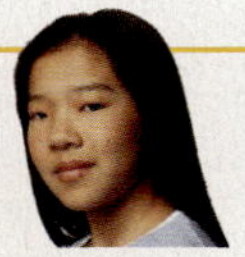

The nurse would need to report **Sylvia Wu's** symptoms along with the underlying history of travel to China immediately to the appropriate health care personnel. Doing so ensures that the necessary precautions are taken to reduce the risk of infection transmission of a potentially highly communicable virus.

Documentation

The patient's initial database is entered into the computer or recorded in ink, using the designated facility protocol or forms, the same day the patient is admitted to the facility. If, for any reason, important data cannot be obtained during the initial assessment, this should be documented so that they are obtained as soon as possible. Objective and subjective patient data should be summarized and written so that the data communicate a unique sense of the patient and are comprehensive, concise, and easily retrievable. The data should be written legibly, using good grammar and only standard medical abbreviations. To facilitate quick data retrieval, data should be presented under clearly marked headings.

Whenever possible, subjective data should be recorded using the patient's own words within quotation marks: "I feel tired from the moment I first get up in the morning. It seems I have no energy at all." Patient reports may also be paraphrased: Patient reports feeling dyspneic, has difficulty catching breath when walking one flight of stairs.

Avoid the tendency to record data using nonspecific terms with different meanings or interpretations—words such as *adequate, good, average, normal, poor, small, large.* One nurse's idea of what "average" fluid intake is may be very different from that of another nurse. Always be specific. Chapter 20 offers general documentation guidelines.

Privacy, Confidentiality, and Professionalism

One of your primary ethical responsibilities is safeguarding the privacy of your patients. When gathering patient data, you will learn much about patients that they wish to keep private, and patients have every right to expect that you will maintain their privacy. If family members are with a patient you plan to assess you need to ask them to step outside or get the patient's consent for them to be present. Please review the privacy information in Chapter 7 and be sure you are familiar with your institution's policies on privacy and on the requirements of the Health Insurance Portability and Accountability Act (HIPAA). Recently, the ANA (www.nursingworld.org) and the National Council of State Boards of Nursing (https://www.ncsbn.org) united to provide guidelines on social media for nurses. Check their websites for organization guidelines upholding professional boundaries in a social networking environment. You will also find a statement on social media usage and maintaining privacy, confidentiality, and professionalism on the National Student Nurses' Association website, www.nsna.org.

REFLECTIVE PRACTICE LEADING TO PERSONAL LEARNING

Remember that the goal of reflective practice is to look at an experience, understand it, and learn from it. As you begin to develop expertise in assessing patients' health status and well-being, reflect on your experiences—successes and failures—in order to improve your practice. How can you do it better next time? What did you learn today that can help you tomorrow? Begin your reflection by paying close attention to the following during the assessing phase of the nursing process:

- Did your preparation for the assessing experience bring you to the interview and physical examination feeling confident in your ability to gather reliable, accurate, and complete data while inspiring the patient's confidence and trust?
- How confident are you that the data you reported and recorded accurately communicates the health problems, issues, risks, and strengths of the patient? How successfully have you communicated who this patient/family are to your interdisciplinary colleagues?
- If you were unsure of any of your findings, perhaps had difficulty feeling a pulse, did you ask readily for help?
- Were you aware of any stereotypes or prejudices that might have negatively influenced the clinical encounter? If yes, how did you address these?
- Was patient/family participation in the process at an optimal level? How might you have better engaged the patient and family? As you concluded your assessment, did the patient know your name, know what to expect of you and of nursing, sense that you are competent, respectful, and caring, and know what is expected in terms of developing the care plan and participating in its execution?

Perhaps the most important questions to reflect on are: Are your patients and their families/caregivers better for having had *you* share in the critical responsibility of assessing their health problems and identifying and tapping their strengths? Are your patients now receiving thoughtful, person-centered, prioritized, holistic, evidence-based treatment and care because of your efforts?

DEVELOPING CLINICAL REASONING AND CLINICAL JUDGMENT

1. Working with another student, interview patients in both their home and institutional settings, and record your findings separately. Make a list of the objective and subjective data you gather about each patient interviewed and the inferences you make from these cues. Compare your data lists and inferences. Describe to each other how you plan to validate your inferences. Explore possible reasons for the differences you discover.
2. Allow another student to perform a comprehensive nursing assessment (interview and physical assessment) on you. Reflect on what you experienced. Offer the student feedback about which of their behaviors were helpful, comforting, or distressing. Change roles and talk about what you learned from this experience.
3. Collect several different forms for recording the initial comprehensive nursing assessment (hospital, long-term care facility, home care, school of nursing forms). Identify differences and explain them. Experiment with using the different forms, and make a list of features that help you get all the data you need in the easiest way possible. Review Table 15-3 on page 421. What other patient variables might negatively influence an interview? Nursing variables? How should you address these?
4. You are helping another student with a dressing change when he pulls out his cell phone and takes a picture of the stage IV pressure injury exposing bone and muscle on the patient's sacrum and says, "This is really gross." How do you respond and why?

PRACTICING FOR NCLEX

1. A nursing student tells the clinical instructor that their patient is fine and has "no complaints." Which question by the faculty coaches the student to provide evidence that supports their assessments?
   a. "Could you tell me how you validated this?"
   b. "Do you think your patient feels free to share their concerns?"
   c. "That's good to hear. Tell me about the care you provided."
   d. "Please reassess the patient; they were admitted with a serious problem."
2. A nursery nurse notifies the nurse practitioner (NP) that a newborn has signs of jaundice. The NP performs a brief skin assessment, then orders a blood test for bilirubin levels. Which type of assessment has the NP performed?
   a. Comprehensive
   b. Initial
   c. Time-lapsed
   d. Quick priority

3. The nurse is admitting a pregnant patient to the hospital for treatment of pregnancy-induced hypertension. The patient asks the nurse, "Why are you doing a history and physical exam when the doctor just did one?" What statements will the nurse use to explain the primary purpose of the nursing assessment? Select all that apply.
   a. "The nursing assessment will allow us to plan and deliver individualized, holistic nursing care that draws on your strengths."
   b. "It's hospital policy. I know we ask a lot of questions, but I will try to make this quick."
   c. "As a nursing student, I need to develop assessment skills about your health status and need for nursing care."
   d. "This validates that your responses with the medical exam are consistent and that all our data are accurate."
   e. "I will check your health status and see what kind of nursing care you may need."
   f. "This is to determine the necessity for referring your nursing care needs to a health care provider."
4. During shift report, a nurse says that a patient has no integumentary changes or skin care needs. During assessment, the nurse observes reddened areas over bony prominences. What action will the nurse take?
   a. Correct the initial assessment form
   b. Redo the initial assessment and document current findings
   c. Conduct and document an emergency assessment
   d. Perform and document a focused assessment of skin integrity
5. A nursing student is performing a nursing history for the first time. The student asks the primary nurse how anyone learns all the questions needed to get complete baseline data. What would be the nurse's best reply?
   a. "There's a lot to learn at first, but once it becomes part of you, you just ask the same questions over and over in each situation until you can do it in your sleep!"
   b. "You make the basic questions a part of you and apply critical thinking to modify them, to help you plan quality care."
   c. "It is really hard to learn how to do this well, as each history is different. I often feel like I'm starting fresh with each new patient."
   d. "Don't worry about learning all of the questions to ask. Every facility has its own assessment form you must use."
6. The nurse collects subjective and objective data during a patient assessment. When documenting, which data points will the nurse include as subjective data? Select all that apply.
   a. Feeling nauseated
   b. Edematous ankles
   c. Feeling anxious about test results
   d. Report of left arm tingling
   e. Pain rated 7 on a scale of 1 to 10
   f. Oral temperature of 101°F
7. When a nurse enters the patient's room to begin a nursing history, the nurse notes the patient's spouse is present. After greeting them, what action will the nurse take?
   a. Thank the spouse for being present
   b. Ask the spouse if they want to remain
   c. Ask the spouse to leave
   d. Ask the patient if they would like the spouse to stay
8. A nurse is performing an initial comprehensive assessment of a patient admitted to a long-term care facility. The nurse begins the assessment by asking the patient, "How would you describe your health status and well-being?" and, "What do you do to keep yourself healthy?" These questions reflect what model for organizing data?
   a. Maslow's hierarchy of needs
   b. Gordon's functional health patterns
   c. Human response patterns
   d. Body system model
9. The nurse notes a temperature of 102°F in a patient scheduled for surgery in 30 minutes. As the patient has been afebrile and asymptomatic until now, what action will the nurse take next?
   a. Inform the charge nurse
   b. Notify the surgeon
   c. Reassess the temperature
   d. Document the finding in the electronic health record
10. During a change-of-shift report, a nurse receives information that a patient admitted with hypertensive emergency has prescriptions for antihypertensive medications given at 8 AM and due at 8 PM. During the 8:00 PM assessment, the patient's blood pressure is 90/60, and they report slight dizziness upon standing. After returning the patient to bed, what action will the nurse take?
    Exhibit: Electronic health record, vital signs
    8:00 AM 182/100
    12:00 PM 168/98
    4:00 PM 160/88
    a. Record the BP in the electronic health record
    b. Notify the health care provider
    c. Administer the 8:00 PM medications
    d. Place the patient flat in bed
11. During an assessment, the nurse on a neurologic unit finds the patient confused to time and place but able to state their name. How will the nurse best record this in the electronic health record?
    a. Is more confused than yesterday
    b. States the year is 1975 and they are at a wedding
    c. Disoriented to person, time, and place
    d. Patient's speech is garbled
12. A nursing student is assigned to the emergency department (ED) to shadow the triage nurse. What activity will the student expect to perform?
    a. Acute and emergency interventions
    b. Daily care and assistance with ADLs
    c. Assessment and prioritization of care
    d. Care planning for return to home

13. The nurse is assigned to care for a group of patients. Which patient will the nurse assess first?
   a. Postoperative patient reporting pain 4/10
   b. Individual with pneumonia whose WBCs are now 7,000
   c. Adolescent with a burn to the face who is going home tomorrow
   d. Patient's pulse oximetry reading 89%, as reported by AP
14. The nurse assessing a patient plans to use the OLD CARTS mnemonic to organize their questions. What questions will the nurse include in the assessment? Select all that apply.
   a. "Can you tell me when the problem began"?
   b. "Where were you sitting when this started?"
   c. "Have your symptoms stopped and/or started again?"
   d. "Would you describe your pain as sharp, dull or burning?"
   e. "What do you believe has caused this problem?"
15. A nurse in the emergency department is assessing a young adult who has cognitive disability and is reporting severe abdominal pain. The patient is accompanied by the director of the group home where they live. When collecting data from this patient, which action reflects best practice?
   a. Ask the assessment questions of the director.
   b. Wait for the young adult's parents to arrive before performing the assessment.
   c. Ask the young adult questions and validate with the adult present.
   d. Perform the physical assessment, then the intake interview when the family arrives.
16. A nursing student on the surgical unit is assigned to perform a review of systems using the head-to-toe format on a patient admitted for a fractured femur. Using this format, what system will the student assess first?
   a. Genitourinary
   b. Neurologic
   c. Respiratory
   d. Musculoskeletal

ANSWERS WITH RATIONALES

1. **a.** The instructor is reminding the student that all data must be validated. Questioning the use of the word "fine" allows the nurse to determine if this is a social and reflexive response, and there may be another need the nurse can meet. Concluding that the patient does not trust the student is premature and is based on an invalidated inference. Saying "That's good to hear" and asking the student to describe the care provided is incorrect because it accepts the invalidated inference. Telling the student to reassess the patient because they were admitted with a serious problem is incorrect because it is possible that the condition is resolving.
2. **d.** A quick priority assessment (QPA) is a short, focused assessment to obtain the most important information first. A comprehensive initial assessment is performed shortly after admission. The time-lapsed assessment is used to compare a patient's current status to baseline data obtained earlier.
3. **a, e, f.** Medical assessments target data pointing to pathologic conditions, whereas nursing assessments focus on the patient's responses to actual and potential health problems. The initial comprehensive nursing assessment results in baseline data that enable the nurse to make a judgment about a patient's health status, the ability to manage their own health care and the need for nursing. It also helps nurses plan and deliver individualized, holistic nursing care that draws on the patient's strengths and promotes optimum functioning, independence, and well-being, and enables the nurse to refer the finding(s) to the health care provider or collaborate with other health care professionals where indicated. Citing hospital policy or student learning is a secondary reason, and although it may be true that a nurse may need to develop assessment skills, it is not the main reason for a nursing history and assessment. The assessment augments the medical examination but is not performed to check its accuracy.
4. **d.** Perform a focused skin assessment for the new problem, documenting the current date. The initial assessment was entered in the permanent health record, correct at the time, and cannot legally be rewritten. An emergency assessment is performed for a life-threatening problem.
5. **b.** Once a nurse learns what constitutes the minimum data set, it can be adapted to each patient situation. It is not true that each assessment is the same even when using the same minimum data set, nor is it true that each assessment is uniquely different. Nurses committed to thoughtful, person-centered practice individualize their questions to each patient and situation. When using a standard facility assessment tool the nurse must still use critical thinking to individualize questions or follow up on patient information.
6. **a, c, d, e.** Subjective data are information perceived only by the affected person. Examples of subjective data are feeling nauseated, anxious, tingling, and experiencing pain. Objective data are observable and measurable data that can be seen, heard, felt, or measured by someone other than the person experiencing them. Examples of objective data are fever or 101°F or edema.
7. **d.** The patient has the right to privacy and to determine who will be present during the nursing history and exam. The nurse does not presume the patient's preference, as the decision belongs to the patient, not their spouse.
8. **b.** Gordon's functional health patterns begin with the patient's perception of health and well-being and progress to data about nutritional–metabolic patterns, elimination patterns, activity, sleep/rest, self-perception, role relationship, sexuality, coping, and values/beliefs. Maslow's model is based on the human needs hierarchy. Human responses include exchanging, communicating, relating, valuing, choosing, moving, perceiving, knowing, and feeling. The body system model is based on the functioning of the major body systems.
9. **c.** The nurse validates assessment findings that deviate from normal patterns or are unsupported by other data. Should the initial measurement be in error, it would have been premature to notify the charge nurse or the surgeon. The nurse must be sure that all data are accurate prior to documenting and reporting. If there is a question about accuracy, the data should be validated before documenting.

10. **b.** When assessment findings reveal a critical change in the patient's health status, the nurse reports the data (verbally) immediately. The nurse verifies the BP and notifies the health care provider, who may prescribe withholding blood pressure medications, assessment of orthostatic vital signs, among other actions. There is no indication the patient needs to lie flat at this time.

11. **b.** While the patient is confused, it is most important to clearly describe the behavior for comparison to past and future behavior. Citing the actual year and events (orientation to time and place) provides context; "patient confused" is open to misinterpretation. Garbled speech refers to speech that is unclear; the patient may have difficulty with pronunciation or speak slowly, which is not necessarily reflective of confusion.

12. **c.** The triage nurse screens patients to determine the extent and severity of their problems. They use highly specialized nursing knowledge and clinical reasoning and make clinical judgments to prioritize who must be seen immediately and who can wait. Patients in the ED are stabilized and transferred to the appropriate level of care; therefore, daily care, assistance with ADLs, planning for return home, and providing interventions are not part of the triage nurse's role. Should the patient need emergency interventions, the triage nurse moves the patient to the appropriate area in the ED.

13. **d.** The nurse uses Maslow's hierarchy of needs to prioritize assessing the patient with hypoxemia, manifested by a pulse oximetry reading of 89%. The postoperative patient is reporting moderate pain; the patient with pneumonia has normal WBCs; the adolescent patient with a burn to the face is stable for discharge. These patients can be seen as soon as possible.

14. **a, c, d.** The OLD CARTS mnemonic refers to **O**nset: "When did your symptom(s) begin"?. **L**ocation: "Where is the symptom"?. **D**uration: "Is it episodic or constant?" or "How long does it last"?. **C**haracteristics: "How would you describe it?." **A**lleviating and **A**ggravating factors: "What makes it better or worse?." **R**elieving factors: "What makes it better?." **T**reatments: "Have you tried anything to make it better?." **S**everity: "On a scale of 1–10, with 1 being the lower number, how serious is the symptom?."

15. **c.** Children and people with decreased mental capacity or impaired verbal ability should be encouraged to respond to interview questions as best as they can. This communicates support of the patient's autonomy, expression of their needs, and respect for their abilities. The information is then validated with family members or guardians as appropriate.

16. **b.** The nursing physical assessment involves the examination of all body systems in a systematic manner, commonly using a head-to-toe format called the review of systems (ROS). This assessment begins at the top of the body with the neurologic system and moves downward.

Bibliography

Alfaro-LeFevre, R. (2010). *Applying nursing process: A tool for critical thinking* (7th ed.). Wolters Kluwer Health/Lippincott Williams & Wilkins.

Alfaro-LeFevre, R. (2014). *Applying nursing process. The foundation for clinical reasoning* (8th ed.). Wolters Kluwer Health/Lippincott Williams & Wilkins.

Alfaro-LeFevre, R. (2020). *Critical thinking, clinical reasoning, and clinical judgment* (7th ed.). Elsevier.

American Nurses Association (ANA). (2010). *Nursing's social policy statement: The essence of the profession.* Author.

American Nurses Association (ANA). (2021). *Nursing: Scope and standards of practice* (4th ed.). Author.

Bickley, L. S. (2017). *Bates' guide to physical examination and history taking* (12th ed.). Wolters Kluwer Health.

Gordon, M. (1994). *Nursing diagnosis: Process and application* (3rd ed.). Mosby.

Herman, A. E. (n.d.). *How visually intelligent are you? Here's how to test yourself.* https://www.inc.com/leigh-buchanan/visual-intelligence-exercises.html

Herman, A. E. (2016). *Visual intelligence: Sharpen your perception, change your life.* An Eamon Dolan Book. See also www.artfulperception.com.

Jensen, S. (2019). *Nursing health assessment: A best practice approach* (3rd ed.). Wolters Kluwer Health.

Johnson, M., Jefferies, D., & Nicholls, D. (2012). Developing a minimum data set for electronic nursing handover. *Journal of Clinical Nursing, 21*(3–4), 331–343.

Toney-Butler, T. J., & Unison-Pace, W. J. (Updated 2019 July 30). Nursing admission assessment and examination. In: *StatPearls [Internet]*. StatPearls Publishing; 2020. https://www.ncbi.nlm.nih.gov/books/NBK493211/

Viser, L. S., & Montejano, A. (2019). *Fast facts for the triage nurse* (2nd ed.). Springer.

16 Diagnosis/Problem Identification

Martin Prescott

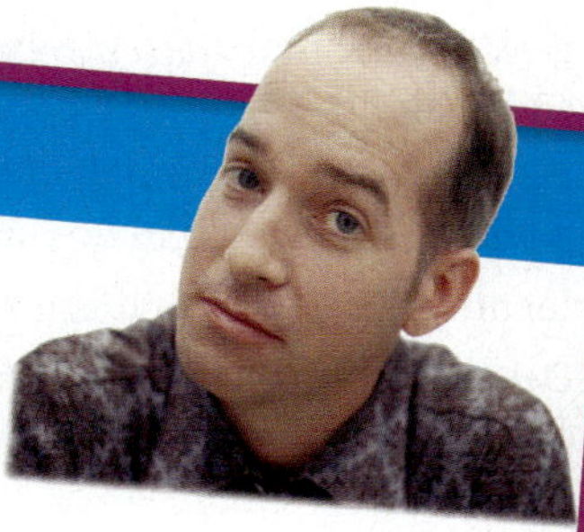

Martin, a 46-year-old man, comes to the health clinic for a routine physical examination. During the assessment, he states, "I've had problems with constipation and have seen some blood when I wipe myself after a bowel movement. It's just hemorrhoids, right? Nothing to worry about?"

Antonia Zuccarelli

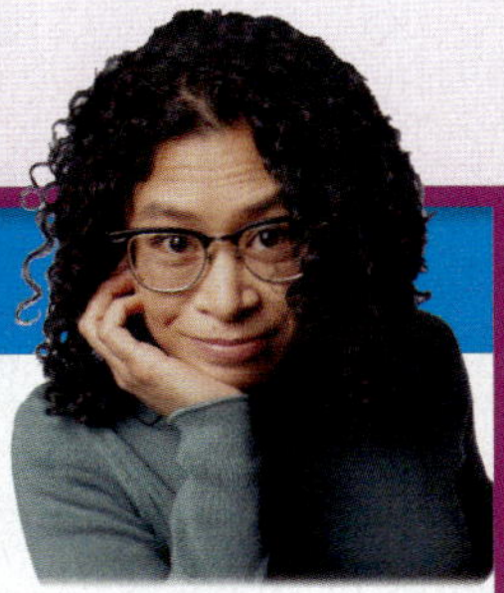

Antonia is a middle-aged woman newly diagnosed with cancer that is treatable. However, she continually fails to show up for follow-up appointments for both continuing diagnosis and treatment.

Angie Clarkson

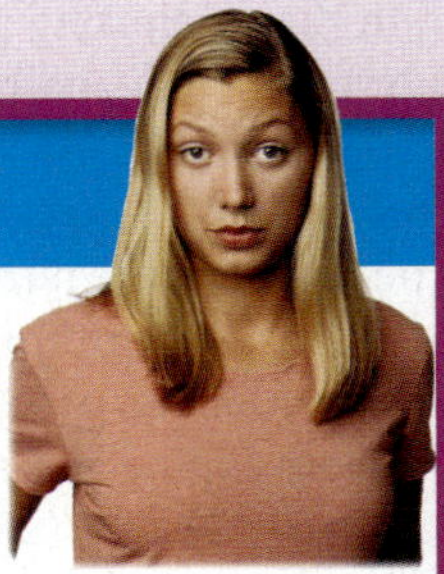

Angie, a college sophomore, tearfully reports to her student nurse colleague that she believes she is a survivor of date rape. She had too much to drink at a party and can only remember waking up in a strange room with a guy she just met, unsure if she passed out because of the alcohol or date-rape drugs. A virgin, Angie was sure there was penetration because of blood and semen stains she discovered upon waking. It is now a month later and she has not been able to "get her life together" and move on.

Learning Outcomes

After completing the chapter, you will be able to accomplish the following:

1. Apply basic principles of diagnostic reasoning to identify actual and potential diagnoses, problems, and issues.
2. Explain why it is critical to partner with the patient and family to identify priority actual and potential diagnoses, problems, and issues and strengths.
3. Describe two historical uses of the term diagnosis.
4. Describe the four steps involved in data interpretation and analysis.
5. Develop diagnostic/problem statements using the guidelines presented in this chapter.
6. Identify three types of diagnoses.
7. Describe means to validate actual and potential diagnoses, problems, and issues.

Nursing Concepts

- Nursing process
- Clinical decision making

Diagnosing Problem identification—the second step/phase in the nursing process—begins after the nurse has collected and recorded the patient data. The purposes of **diagnosing/analyzing** are to (1) identify how a person, group, or community responds to actual or potential health and life processes; (2) identify factors that contribute to or cause health problems (etiologies); and (3) identify resources or strengths that the person, group, or community can draw on to prevent or resolve problems. See the accompanying Reflective Practice display for an example.

In the diagnosing phase of the nursing process, the nurse interprets and analyzes data gathered from the nursing assessment (Fig. 16-1). Some refer to this phase of the process as analysis. Recall Figure 15-9 in the preceding chapter. The data help the nurse identify patient strengths and health problems. A **health problem** is a condition that necessitates intervention to prevent or resolve disease or illness or to promote coping and wellness.

Alfaro-LeFevre (2014, p. 92) counsels nurses to understand the types of problems they should focus on to better understand their responsibilities relating to the diagnosis and management of health problems. She lists the following as concerns that are central to your role as a nurse:

- Recognizing safety and infection transmission risks and addressing these immediately
- Identifying human responses—how problems, signs and symptoms, and treatment regimens *affect patients' lives*—and promoting optimum function, independence, and quality of life

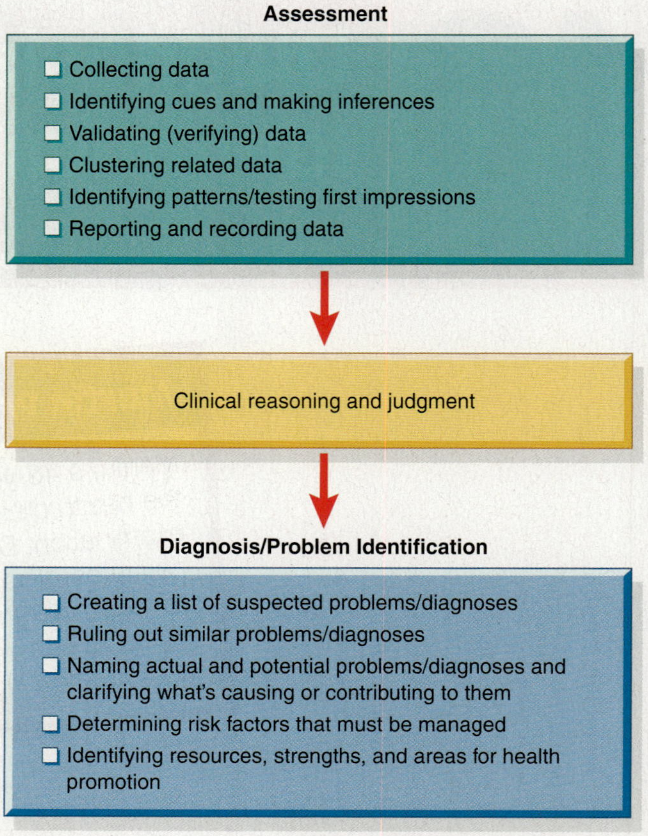

FIGURE 16-1. This diagram shows how the activities of assessment lead to a pivotal point in the nursing process: diagnosis. Diagnosis is a pivotal point for the following reasons: (1) The purpose of diagnosis is to clarify the exact nature of the problems and risks that must be addressed to achieve the overall expected outcomes of care. If you do not completely understand the problems and what factors are contributing to them, how do you know what to do about them? If you don't pay attention to risks, how are you going to prevent problems? (2) The conclusions you make during this phase affect the entire care plan. If your conclusions are correct, your plan is likely to be on target. If they are not—for example, if you are operating on assumptions rather than sound reasoning that is based on evidence—your plan is likely to be flawed, maybe even dangerous. (*Source:* Used with permission from Alfaro-LeFevre, R. [2014]. *Applying nursing process: The foundation for clinical reasoning* [8th ed.]. Wolters Kluwer Health/Lippincott Williams & Wilkins.)

- Anticipating possible complications and taking steps to prevent them
- Initiating urgent interventions—you do not want to wait to make a final diagnosis if there are signs and symptoms indicating the need for immediate treatment

When a health problem is identified, the nurse must decide which health care professional can best address the problem. Actual or potential health problems that can be prevented or resolved by independent nursing intervention have historically been termed **nursing diagnoses**. The nurse formulates, validates, and lists actual or potential problems for each patient (Fig. 16-2 on page 432). These problem statements provide the basis for selecting nursing interventions that will achieve valued patient outcomes for which the nurse is responsible. See the Legal Alert box for Alfaro's rule about the legal implications of diagnoses (Alfaro-LeFevre, 2014, p. 92).

QSEN Reflective Practice: Cultivating QSEN Competencies

CHALLENGE TO COGNITIVE AND INTERPERSONAL SKILLS

Angie Clarkson, a college sophomore, told me, her college friend, tearfully that she believes she is a survivor of date rape her first week in school. She knows she had too much to drink at a party and can only remember waking up in a strange room with a guy she met at the party. She is not sure if she passed out because of the alcohol or if one of the date-rape drugs was involved. A virgin, Angie was sure there had been penetration because of the blood and semen stains she discovered upon waking. It is now a month later and she has not been able to "get her life together" and move on. Angie told me that I am the first person she has told because she feels "so ashamed" and can't believe she let this happen to her. This is my first encounter with an experience like this. I don't do drugs or alcohol and am not sexually active.

Thinking Outside the Box: Possible Courses of Action

- Try to be a good friend and simply suggest she get professional help.
- Advocate for Angie by finding out what resources exist on campus.
- Inform Angie that everything she is describing sounds like a significant health problem and explain how to get professional help and why getting help is so important.

Evaluating a Good Outcome: How Do I Define Success?

- Angie gets the professional help she needs to survive this well.
- I prove worthy of her trust in me.
- I use this experience to learn more about a common problem on campus and the adequacy of existing resources.
- I learn something about my ability to diagnose a health problem and plan accordingly.

Personal Learning: Here's to the Future!

Responding to Angie's clear cry for help certainly moved me out of my comfort zone and made me aware of how my newly developing clinical skills will at times complicate something as simple as being a friend. I felt somewhat responsible for helping Angie cope with being raped and believed that I had to do more than simply provide a listening ear. I was pleasantly surprised to discover all the resources that exist on campus. I guess I wasn't surprised that it took quite a bit of coaxing to get Angie to seek professional help. When I showed her some of what is written about the challenges of moving beyond date rape, she seemed to find her experience validated and finally agreed to try the student health service counseling center. I felt positive about my role in helping to make this happen.

QSEN SELF-REFLECTION ON QUALITY AND SAFETY COMPETENCIES DEVELOPING KNOWLEDGE, SKILLS, AND ATTITUDES FOR CONTINUOUS IMPROVEMENT

How do you think you would respond in a similar situation? Why? What does this tell you about yourself and about the adequacy of your personal attributes and competencies for professional practice? Do you agree with the criteria that the nursing student used to evaluate a successful outcome? Why or why not? What *knowledge, skills,* and *attitudes* do you need to develop to continuously improve the quality and safety of care for patients like Ms. Clarkson?

Patient-Centered Care: How would you develop a partnership with Ms. Clarkson, knowing her fears? How can you communicate to her that she is your care priority and that she can trust you?

Teamwork and Collaboration/Quality Improvement: *In this case, your teamwork will involve campus resources.* What communication skills do you need to improve to ensure that you can access these resources and make them work for Ms. Clarkson? If your research revealed inadequate campus resources, what could you do to advocate for improved quality?

Safety/Evidence-Based Practice: What does the evidence point to as "best practice" in a situation like this? Can you think of campus activities that would promote enhanced safety for all students?

Informatics: Can you identify electronic resources that might help Ms. Clarkson or you? Can you think of other ways to respond to or approach the situation? What else might the nursing student have done to ensure a successful outcome?

Legal Alert

The term *diagnosis* implies that there's a situation or problem requiring appropriate, qualified treatment. This means that if you identify a problem, you must decide if you are *qualified* to treat it and willing to *accept responsibility* for treating it. If you are not, you are responsible for getting help.

Alfaro recommends using both a nursing model and a body systems approach (see Chapter 15) to organize assessment data to detect both nursing and medical problems.

Today you can find literature on both nursing diagnosis care plans and problem-based care plans. In this chapter, we will continue to teach you what a nursing diagnosis is and how to write these statements, which many nursing programs

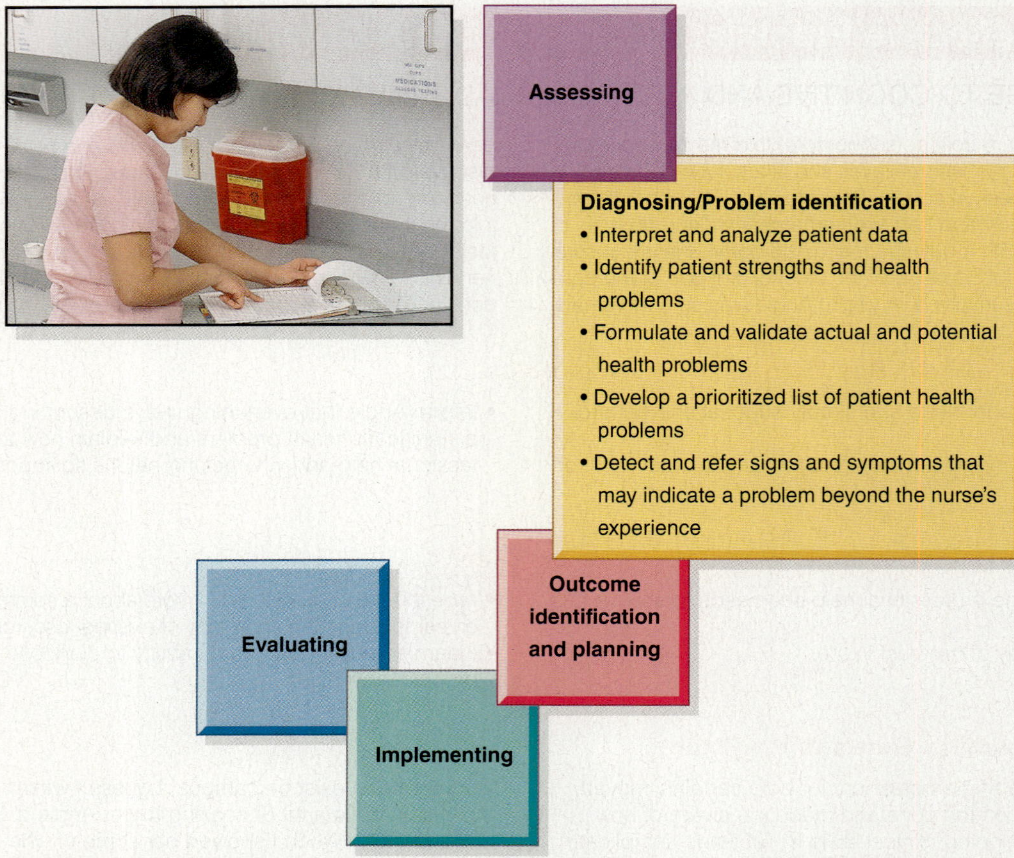

FIGURE 16-2. Diagnosing is the interpretation and analysis of patient data to identify patient strengths and health problems that nursing intervention can prevent or resolve. Patient problems may change from day to day as the patient's responses to health and illness change. (*Source:* Used with permission from Shutterstock. *Photo by B. Proud.*)

require. We will also teach you how to identify and write actual and potential problem statements, which you will increasingly use in your practice sites. This text selects examples of patient problems from Lippincott Advisor (2020) and the International Council of Nurses International Classification for Nursing Practice (ICNP) Nursing Diagnosis and Outcome Statements (2019) lists.

EVOLUTION OF NURSING DIAGNOSIS

The term *nursing diagnosis* first appeared in the literature in the 1950s. As early as 1966, Hammond wrote that nurses need to be competent in information-seeking strategies and should have a good background of theoretical knowledge to search for cues and evaluate evidence. These skills and knowledge result in accurate diagnosing.

Key milestones in the evolution of nursing diagnosis as an integral component of the nursing process include the following:

- **1953:** The term *nursing diagnosis* was introduced by Fry (1953) to describe a step necessary in developing a care plan.
- **1972:** The New York State Nurse Practice Act identified diagnosing as part of the legal domain of professional nursing; practice acts in many other states have been revised similarly since then.
- **1973:** The American Nurses Association's Standards of Practice included diagnosing as a function of professional nursing.
- **1973:** Kristine Gebbie and Mary Ann Lavin, of St. Louis University, called the First National Conference on the Classification of Nursing Diagnoses, beginning a national effort to identify, standardize, and classify health problems treated by nurses. At this first meeting, the National Group, since renamed the North American Nursing Diagnosis Association (NANDA) and subsequently renamed NANDA International (NANDA-I), appointed a task force to accomplish the following goals:
  - Gather information and disseminate it through the Clearinghouse for Nursing Diagnosis.
  - Encourage educational activities at regional and state levels to promote the implementation of nursing diagnoses. These activities include conferences to organize nurses to identify additional diagnostic labels and workshops to teach nurses about nursing diagnoses.
  - Promote and organize activities to continue the development, classification, and scientific testing of nursing diagnoses. These activities include planning national conferences, identifying criteria for accepting diagnoses, surveying current research activities, and exploring varied methods for classification.

- **1980:** The American Nurses Association (ANA) Social Policy Statement defined nursing as "the diagnosis and treatment of human response to actual or potential health problems" (ANA, 1980).
- **March 1990:** At the Ninth Conference of NANDA, the General Assembly approved an official definition of nursing diagnosis:

  > Nursing diagnosis is a clinical judgment about individual, family, or community responses to actual or potential health problems/life processes. Nursing diagnosis provides the basis for selection of nursing interventions to achieve outcomes for which the nurse is accountable (NANDA, 1990).

- **March 1990:** The first issue of *Nursing Diagnosis*, NANDA's official journal, was published.
- **2004:** The ANA Standards of Nursing Practice revised the Standard 2 Diagnosis, to include the word *issues:* "The registered nurse analyzes the assessment data to determine the diagnoses or issues." In 2015, the ANA Standards of Practice read: "The registered nurse analyzes assessment data to determine actual or potential diagnoses, problems, or issues" (p. 55) (Box 16-1). Adding "issues" to the standard reflects the realities of today's health care setting. Today's nurses deal with specific problems (diagnoses) and ill-defined problems (issues).
- **2015:** The National Academy of Medicine (NAM)'s report (2015), *Improving Diagnosis Healthcare*, highlighted the catastrophic impact of diagnostic errors and designated eight specific goals to address the problem. The first two goals are relevant to nursing education (Gleason et al., 2021):

Box 16-1 Checklist for Identifying Actual and Potential Problems

1. List current medications (include over-the-counter and herbal drugs). Ask yourself whether any of the patients or problems could be related to any of the medications (remember SODA).
   Side effect?
   Overdose?
   Drug interaction?
   Allergy or adverse reaction?
2. List current and past allergies, diseases, surgeries, or trauma.
3. Consider whether any of the patient's current problems are related to questions 1 or 2 above.
4. Complete the following checklist:
   (Circle those that apply)

Is there a problem with breathing?	Yes	No	AR[1]	Pos[2]
Is there a problem with circulation?	Yes	No	AR	Pos
Is there a problem with comfort?	Yes	No	AR	Pos
Is there a problem with nutrition?	Yes	No	AR	Pos
Is there a problem with urinary or bowel illumination?	Yes	No	AR	Pos
Is there a problem with fluid or electrolyte balance?	Yes	No	AR	Pos
Is there a problem with ability to think or perceive environment?	Yes	No	AR	Pos
Is there a problem with communication?	Yes	No	AR	Pos
Is there a problem with safety (risk for injury or falls)?	Yes	No	AR	Pos
Is there a problem with sleeping or exercising?	Yes	No	AR	Pos
Is there a risk for infection (self or transition to others)?	Yes	No	AR	Pos
Is there a risk for impaired skin integrity?	Yes	No	AR	Pos
Is there a psychological development of self-esteem problem?	Yes	No	AR	Pos
Is there a sociocultural problem?	Yes	No	AR	Pos
Is there a problem with roles, relationships, or sexuality?	Yes	No	AR	Pos
Does the person have a problem with taking medications?	Yes	No	AR	Pos
Does the patient require teaching?	Yes	No	AR	Pos
Is there a problem with health maintenance at home?	Yes	No	AR	Pos
Is this admission going to cause difficulties at home?	Yes	No	AR	Pos
Is there a problem with personal or religious beliefs?	Yes	No	AR	Pos
Is there a problem with coping or managing stress?	Yes	No	AR	Pos
Could this person be pregnant?	Yes	No	AR	Pos

[1]AR = At risk for problem (no signs and symptoms present, but risk factors are evident).
[2]Pos = Possible problem (insufficient data, but you suspect a problem).
Source: © 2018 R. Alfaro-LeFevre. www.AlfaroTeachSmart.com

- Goal 1: Facilitate more effective teamwork in the diagnostic process among health care professionals, patients, and their families.
- Goal 2: Enhance health care professional education and training in the diagnostic process.

- 2021: *The Essentials: Core competencies for professional nursing education* articulates as a basic competency for entry-level professional nursing education: "Diagnose actual or potential health problems and needs." This is further specified as:
  - Synthesize assessment data in the context of the individual's current preferences, situation, and experience.
  - Create a list of problems/health concerns.
  - Prioritize problems/health concerns.
  - Understand and apply the results of social screening, psychological testing, laboratory data, imaging studies, and other diagnostic tests in actions and plans of care.
  - Contribute as a team member to the formation and improvement of diagnoses (p. 32).
- 2021: The *ANA Scope and Standards of Practice* (4th ed.) includes the competency, "Uses assessment data, standardized classification systems, technology, and clinical decision support tools to articulate actual or potential diagnoses, problems, and issues." Note that ANA defines the outcomes of diagnosing as "diagnoses, problems, and issues." This language will be used throughout this chapter.

Now an accepted and essential phase in the nursing process, nursing diagnosis was initially confused with medical diagnosis, sparking controversy. *Medical* diagnosis refers to a provider's assignment of a syndrome or disease label to a set of signs, symptoms, and other findings. In contrast, *nursing* diagnosis is a "clinical judgment concerning a human response to health conditions and/or life processes, or a vulnerability for that response, by an individual, family, group, or community. A nursing diagnosis provides the basis for selection of nursing interventions to achieve outcomes for which the nurse has accountability" (Herdman & Kamitsuru, 2018).

Although the confusion between medical and nursing diagnoses has been resolved, many nurses have been slow to understand and to accept the "work" of diagnosing. Gleason et al. (2021) underscore the critical importance of nurses being part of the diagnostic team if we are to aggressively confront the problem of diagnostic error:

> . . . we believe nurses are essential members of the diagnostic team and should enter practice with the expectation to participate actively and meaningfully in the diagnostic process, and that nursing education should prepare them to assume this responsibility and accountability (p. 363).

UNIQUE FOCUS OF DIAGNOSING

In the diagnosing phase of the nursing process, the nurse expresses nursing's unique concern for a patient by analyzing patient data to identify each patient's unique actual and potential health problems and needs. This may lead to diagnosing a problem that nurses can independently treat or a problem best treated collaboratively by the interprofessional team.

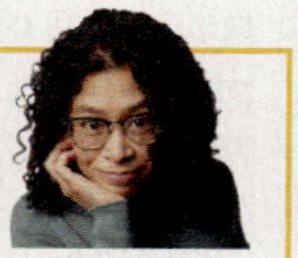

Consider **Antonia Zuccarelli**, the middle-aged woman recently diagnosed with cancer but failing to maintain follow-up. Although the patient's diagnosis of cancer is important, the nurse would focus on the patient's lack of follow-up and the possible underlying reasons. For example, the patient may not realize the importance of the follow-up, thereby indicating a lack of knowledge. Or the patient may be too overwhelmed with the diagnosis, possibly denying its existence and being unable to cope.

Alfaro-LeFevre (2014, pp. 93–94) describes the shift from diagnose and treat (DT) to predict, prevent, manage, and promote (PPMP). The latter approach focuses on early evidence-based intervention to prevent and manage problems and their potential complications. It requires three activities for nurses:

1. In the presence of known problems, predict the most common and most dangerous complications and take immediate action to (a) prevent them, and (b) manage them in case they cannot be prevented.
2. Whether problems are present or not, look for evidence of risk factors (things that evidence suggests contribute to health problems). If you identify risk factors, you aim to reduce or control them, thereby preventing the problems themselves.
3. In all situations, ensure that safety and learning needs are met, and promote optimum function and independence.

As nurses interpret and analyze patient data, they may identify health problems that are better treated by physicians (medical diagnoses) or by nurses working with other health care professionals (collaborative problems). In such a case, the nurse reports the findings to the physician or other appropriate health care professionals and works collaboratively with them to resolve the problem. Gleason et al. (2021) are quick to note that nurses working in highly medicalized environments are expected to identify and intervene in a wide range of medical diagnoses, including life-threatening conditions such as stroke, pulmonary embolism, and sepsis.

Patient Problems Versus Medical Diagnoses

Medical diagnoses identify diseases, whereas problem statements focus on unhealthy responses to health and illness. Medical diagnoses describe problems for which the physician or advanced practice nurse directs the primary treatment. A medical diagnosis remains the same for as long as the disease is present, whereas patient problems may change from day to day as the patient's responses change. These distinctions reflect key differences in medical and nursing practices.

Myocardial infarction (heart attack) is a medical diagnosis. Examples of patient problems for a person with myocardial

Table 16-1 A Comparison: Nursing Diagnosis and Medical Diagnosis

	NURSING DIAGNOSIS	MEDICAL DIAGNOSIS
Definition	A nursing diagnosis is a clinical judgment about individual, family, or community responses to actual or potential health problems or life processes. Nursing diagnosis provides the basis for selection of nursing interventions to achieve outcomes for which the nurse is accountable (NANDA-I).	Traumatic or disease condition or syndrome validated by medical diagnostic studies
Focus	Monitoring human responses to actual and potential health problems	Correcting or preventing pathology of specific organs or body systems
Sample data cluster	56-year-old mother of seven; 5 ft 4 in, 167 lb; "Whenever I sneeze lately, I dribble urine. This is embarrassing."	22-year-old woman; "Whenever I have to urinate, it burns terribly. I also feel like I have to go all the time—real bad." Small, frequent voidings, cloudy urine; T—100.8°F
Problem statement	Stress Incontinence of Urine; etiology, degenerative changes in pelvic muscles and structural supports associated with advanced age, obesity, gravid uterus	Cystitis
Select nursing responses	Teach Kegel exercises to increase muscle tone; explore patient's willingness and motivation to pursue weight reduction and exercise program; evaluate need for bladder-training program.	Report signs and symptoms to physician; obtain urine culture; report results to physician; administer appropriate physician-prescribed antibiotic.

infarction may include Acute anxiety, Activity intolerance, Knowledge deficiency, Acute pain, Altered tissue perfusion, Coping impairment, and Death anxiety (Lippincott Advisor, 2020).

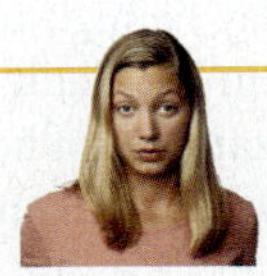

Think back to **Angie Clarkson**, the college sophomore who was a victim of date rape. Possible nursing diagnoses might include Rape Trauma Response (ICNP, 2019), Coping impairment, Situational low self-esteem, and Infection risk (Lippincott Advisor, 2020).

Table 16-1 shows how health care professionals successfully interpret different clusters of data to identify a patient problem and a medical diagnosis. In the first example, a patient problem is identified and successfully treated. In the second example, the nurse's early detection and reporting of the problem to the health care provider led to the health care provider's prompt medical diagnosis of cystitis and successful antibiotic therapy.

DIAGNOSTIC REASONING, CLINICAL REASONING, AND CLINICAL JUDGMENT

Successful implementation of each phase of the nursing process requires high-level skills in clinical reasoning and judgment. To correctly diagnose health problems:

- Be familiar with lists of actual and potential health problems and needs (see Lippincott Advisor and ICNP, 2020 and 2019), read professional literature, and keep reference guides handy.
- Trust clinical experience and judgment but be willing to ask for help when the situation demands more than your qualifications and experience can provide.
- Respect your clinical intuition, but before writing a problem statement without evidence, increase the frequency of your observations and continue to search for cues to verify your intuition.
- Recognize personal biases and keep an open mind.

Questions to facilitate clinical reasoning and judgment during diagnostic reasoning include the following:

- Are my data accurate and complete? Do the objective data support the subjective data? How do I know that this information is reliable?
- Have I correctly distinguished normal from abnormal findings for this patient and decided if abnormal data may be signs and symptoms of a specific health problem?
- Have I made and validated deductions or opinions that follow logically from patient cues?
- Has the patient or the patient's surrogates validated (if able to do so) that these are important problems?
- Have I given the patient or the patient's surrogate an opportunity to identify problems that I may have missed?
- Is each problem statement supported by evidence? Might these cues signify a different problem?
- Have I tried to identify what is causing the actual or potential problem, and what strengths/resources (including but not limited to support systems, health literacy, and engagement in self-care) the patient might use to avoid or resolve the problem?
- Have I followed facility guidelines to correctly document problem statements in a way that clearly communicates patient problems to other health care professionals?

- Have I documented diagnoses, problems, strengths, and issues in a manner that facilitates the development of the expected outcomes and collaborative plan (ANA, 2021, p. 78)?

Gleason et al. (2017) counsel nurses, if what you are observing in a patient does not align with an assigned diagnosis, or if observed changes appear to indicate a new or different diagnosis, this creates an opportunity and an obligation to intervene and mitigate diagnostic errors before there is harm. From your earliest days in clinical practice, you want to cultivate the art of thinking like a nurse, which requires a "flexible and nuanced ability to recognize salient aspects of an undefined clinical situation, interpret their meanings, and respond appropriately" (Tanner, 2006).

DIAGNOSTIC REASONING AND INTERPERSONAL COMPETENCE

Diagnostic statements are best made and used by nurses who have strong interpersonal and communication skills. These skills make it more likely that a patient will be able to trust you sufficiently to talk about their responses to health problems and life processes. You must be able to demonstrate your desire to listen to the patient's narrative to gain trust: "Tell me your story."

The best use of diagnosis/analysis is in partnership with patients, families, groups, and communities. To work in partnership, nurses need to speak to people with respect and care, listen effectively, respect the opinions and views of others, and know how to validate perceptions with patients and families (Skelley et al., 2020); see Figure 16-3. Learning these skills is a challenge, so the interpersonal aspects of nursing need to be an integral part of learning to use the diagnosis/problem identification phase of the nursing process.

DATA INTERPRETATION AND ANALYSIS

Most experienced nurses begin the work of interpreting and analyzing data while they are still collecting (assessing) the data. The term **cue** is often used to denote significant data or data that influence this analysis. Significant data should "raise a red flag" for the nurse, who then looks for patterns or clusters of data that signal an actual or possible health problem.

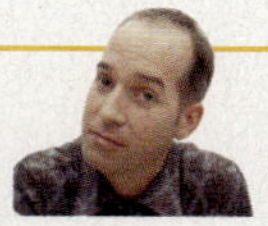

Recall ***Martin Prescott***, the 46-year-old man with bleeding associated with bowel movements. The report of bleeding accompanied by the patient's complaint of constipation should alert the nurse to a potential problem involving the patient's bowel elimination.

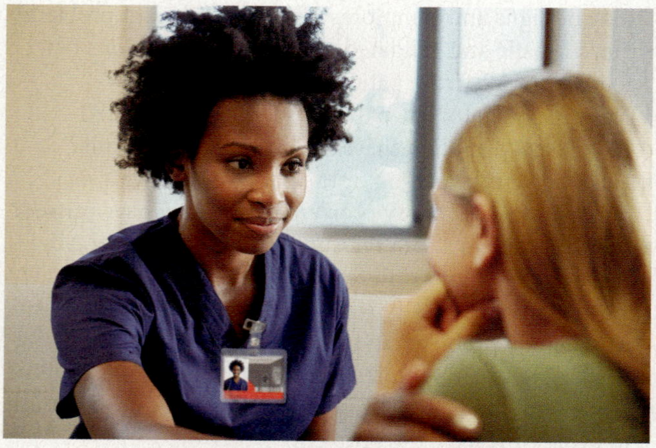

FIGURE 16-3. This nurse is using respectful listening to elicit the patient's trust and promote a partnership to identify and prioritize patient problems. (*Source:* Used with permission from Shutterstock. *Photo by Monkey Business Images.*)

Recognizing Significant Data

Sorting out healthy patient responses from those that are not healthy is not as clear-cut as it may seem. To avoid erroneously labeling selected patient health patterns as unhealthy (**diagnostic error**) while failing to detect an actual unhealthy behavior, nurses must be familiar with comparative standards to be used in data interpretation and analysis.

A **standard**, or a norm, is a generally accepted rule, measure, pattern, or model to which data can be compared in the same class or category. For example, when determining the significance of a patient's blood pressure reading, appropriate standards include normative values for the patient's age group, race, and illness category. The patient's own normal range, if known, is an important standard. A pressure of 150/90 mm Hg may be high for someone whose pressure normally is 120/70 mm Hg, but it may be normal for a person with hypertension. Examples of how standards can be used to identify significant cues include the following (Gordon, 1994):

- Changes in a patient's usual health patterns that are unexplained by expected norms for growth and development: *Example: An infant who took to breastfeeding easily as a newborn suddenly stops sucking when put to the breast and begins to lose weight.*
- Deviation from an appropriate population norm: *Example: A first-year college student begins to accelerate her exercise habits dramatically and starts inducing vomiting after binge eating. She rapidly loses weight.*
- Behavior that is nonproductive in the whole-person context: *Example: A college student breaks up with her boyfriend and begins to believe that she is "unfit" for any other relationship, withdrawing from her friends and social activities.*
- Behavior that indicates a developmental lag or evolving dysfunctional pattern: *Example: A 16-year-old single mother with a 6-month-old infant continues to "party hard" with her friends, hangs out at the mall, and shows no interest in caring for her son, who is repeatedly left with concerned family members.*

Recognizing Patterns or Clusters

A **data cluster** is a grouping of patient data or cues that point to the existence of a health problem. Diagnostic statements should always be derived from clusters of significant data rather than from a single cue. The danger of deriving a nursing diagnosis from a single cue is illustrated in the following example. Diagnosing a woman recovering from gallbladder surgery with a coping impairment solely on the basis of tears may misinterpret the patient's crying, which may be a healthy release of emotion. If the same patient begins to exhibit a cluster of significant cues, such as refusing to eat, preferring bed rest to scheduled ambulation, and reporting increasing discomfort, an unhealthy pattern is emerging.

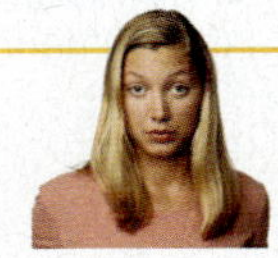

Think back to **Angie Clarkson**, the college sophomore. Her verbalization of the rape trauma is significant. However, even more significant is Angie's report that the event happened more than 1 month ago, and she is having difficulty "getting her life together" and moving on.

Table 16-2 (on page 438) offers examples of how clusters of significant data lead to formulation of accurate diagnostic statements.

Identifying Strengths and Problems

The next step in analyzing data is to determine the patient's strengths and problems. It also helps to determine whether the patient agrees with the nurse's identification of strengths and problems and is motivated to work toward problem resolution. If you recall the situation described in the Reflective Practice box on p. 431, you'll understand how important it is to create a partnership with the patient and family in order to respect the patient's priorities.

Determining Patient and Family Strengths

If a patient appears to meet a standard, the nurse concludes that the patient has strength in that particular area, and that this strength contributes to the patient's level of wellness. For example, a person with a history of maintaining a well-balanced diet is usually better able to cope with illness than a person who has a history of unhealthy eating.

Patient strengths might include healthy physiologic functioning, emotional health, cognitive abilities, coping skills, interpersonal strengths, and spiritual strengths. Resources such as the presence of support people, adequate finances, and a healthy environment may all contribute to patient strengths. Many people take their strengths for granted and may not know how to use them effectively when responding to illness. Discussing observed strengths with patients and counseling patients about ways to develop and use their strengths are important nursing measures.

Determining the Patient's Problem Areas

A person who does not meet a certain health standard probably has a limitation in that area and may benefit from professional care. For example, a person with a long history of constipation probably needs care to help overcome this problem. If you are preparing to discharge an 80-year-old patient with chronic pulmonary obstructive disease home and realize that they live alone with no one to help them manage their diet, medicines, and new therapies, you need to report their problem areas, or you can be sure you will quickly see them readmitted to the hospital in crisis. Ideally, you will be able to identify community resources that can be accessed to help them successfully transition home. It is always helpful to remember the social determinants of health discussed in Chapter 3. The Patient-Centered Assessment tool in Chapter 15 uses the social determinants of health to explain why some patients engage and respond well in managing their health, while others with the same or similar health condition do not experience the same outcomes and success.

Determining Problems the Patient Is Likely to Experience

Nurses also identify potential health problems. For example, a nurse notes that a patient has signs of a wound infection, but laboratory test results show that the patient's white blood cell count has not increased, as is usual when such an infection is present. The nurse concludes that the body apparently is not building up normal defenses to combat the infection. The nurse then predicts the problems this patient is likely to encounter, such as a longer-than-normal healing period. Potential problems alert other caregivers to problems the patient may experience if certain trends in the patient's condition continue unreversed. This prediction has implications for nursing care, such as the need for measures related to the patient's diet, fluid intake, urine output, and mobility. You will want to be familiar with the common lists of problems endorsed by your school or program. Box 16-1 on page 433 offers a practical checklist for identifying actual and potential problems. You may find it helpful to use this checklist when you first meet your assigned patients. If your practice site uses an electronic medical record, problem lists will be preloaded for your convenience. Figure 16-4 (on page 439) provides a systematic problem analysis worksheet that you may find helpful, especially when doing concept mapping. Alfaro reminds us that diagnosis is incomplete until we identify not only the problems but also the underlying causes and contributing factors of the problems.

Identifying Potential Complications

Patients may experience many complications related to their diagnoses, medications or treatment regimens, or invasive diagnostic studies. While new to nursing, you can more easily prevent potential complications—or at least make sure that they are detected early and managed well—if you research the potential complications associated with your patient's diagnoses, diagnostics, and treatment, and if you report all abnormal data. For example, slurred speech, changes in skin color or moistness, inability to move an extremity or abnormal movement, and changes in levels of consciousness may all be indications of serious and life-threatening complications. Remember, if you are unsure about the significance of data, always confer with someone more experienced.

Table 16-2 Formulating an Accurate Diagnostic Statement Based on Data Clusters

DATA INTERPRETATION AND ANALYSIS		FORMULATION OF TENTATIVE PROBLEM STATEMENT	VALIDATION
Significant Cues	*Sample Data Clusters*		
Patient 1			
Change in a patient's usual health patterns that is unexplained by expected norms for growth and development	• "I guess I lost about 20–30 lb over the last 6 months—I think I've just been too busy to eat." • Height: 5 ft 8 inches • Weight: 102 lb • 35-year-old mother of twin boys; returned to work (executive secretary) for first time since delivery of twins 7 months ago	Malnutrition risk; possible etiologic factors: stress of new job; role conflict and demands	Accurate problem statement: Patient validates this problem, agreeing with contributing factors
Patient 2			
Deviation from an appropriate population norm	• Teacher notices and reports frequency of bruises on third-grade boy who is repeatedly observed alone during recess periods and who is withdrawn in classroom. • In conversation with the school nurse, one of the boy's parents remarks: "That boy brings out the worst in me! I don't know why, but I often have to smack him hard to make him listen."	Risk To Be Victim of Child Abuse	Incomplete problem statement: Additional data collection yields new information: • Father out of work for past 18 months • Father was abused as a child Problem restated: Risk to be a victim of child abuse; possible etiologic factors: increased family stress and father's history of being abused
Patient 3			
Behavior that is nonproductive in the whole-person context	• Fiancé abruptly terminated relationship 3 months before established wedding date • Noticeable change in physical appearance; frequently wears same clothes; makeup, jewelry, hairstyling are absent; strong body odors present • No desire to be with others; goes home (lives alone) immediately after work • Stopped attending aerobics classes	Situational low self-esteem; possible etiologic factor: feeling rejected by fiancé	Premature problem statement resulting from incomplete data collection. Patient has a long history of major depressive states, one of which may have resulted in the breakup of this relationship. Medical diagnosis and treatment indicated. Changes in appearance are indicative of depressive state. Need to explore related problems
Patient 4			
Behavior indicating developmental lags or evolving dysfunctional patterns	• Admitted to long-term care facility 2 months ago • "I have nothing to live for anymore . . . why don't I die?" • Wishes to remain in room seated in chair; will only ambulate with great urging • Anything requiring movement has become "too much bother" • Decreased muscle mass, tone, and strength; reduced joint mobility	Deconditioning; possible etiologic factor: difficult transition to long-term care facility	Accurate but routinized problem statement that may result in staff's acceptance of status quo unless a more specific cause is identified

SYSTEMATIC PROBLEM ANALYSIS WORKSHEET

Instructions:

1. List the focus problem, diagnosis, or issue in the box below.
2. Put a check mark in all boxes on the right that correspond to factors that contribute to the problem, diagnosis, or issue you identified.
3. Decide what factors must be managed and who will manage them.
4. Use back of page or figure of man as needed.

Actual/potential diagnosis, problem, or issue

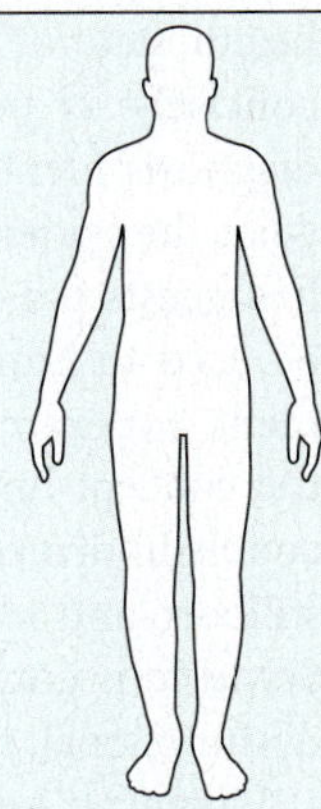

CONTRIBUTING OR RELATED (RISK) FACTORS

1. Main reason for admission or contact?

2. Vulnerability—constitutional or age-related factors?
❑ Age ____ Weight ____ Height ____ Mental Status? ____
❑ Communication ability? ❑ Smoker? ❑ Drinker (alcohol)?
❑ Skin status? ❑ Nutrition-hydration status?
❑ Mobility or self-care problems?
❑ Bowel elimination or urine elimination problems?
❑ Immune system status? ❑ Overall health status/resilience?
❑ Other?

3. Allergy, medication, or treatment-related factors?
❑ Allergies? ❑ Considered all meds (Rx, OTC, herbal)?
❑ Treatments?

4. Co-existing medical problems, injuries, or pathophysiology
❑ Neuro? ❑ Resp? ❑ Cardiac-circulatory? ❑ GI? ❑ GU?
❑ Diabetes? ❑ Hypertension? ❑ Depression? ❑ Other?

5. Environmental factors? Patient identified factors?
❑ Current environment (include work)? ❑ Role-related?
❑ Other factors?

6. Comfort factors? Mobility problems? Self-care problems?
❑ Pain level? ❑ Pain management? ❑ Self-mobile? ❑ Other?

7. Socioeconomic, spiritual, cultural factors?
❑ Family issues? ❑ Coping problems? ❑ Support systems limited?
❑ Other?

FIGURE 16-4. Systematic problem analysis worksheet. (*Source:* Used with permission. Alfaro-LeFevre, R. [2020]. *Critical thinking, clinical reasoning, and clinical judgment* [7th ed.]. Elsevier, p. 162.)

Reaching Conclusions

The nurse reaches one of three basic conclusions after interpreting and analyzing the patient data. Different nursing responses result from each conclusion:

No Problem

- No nursing response is indicated.
- Reinforce the patient's health habits and patterns.
- Initiate health promotion activities to prevent disease or illness or to promote a higher level of wellness.
- Wellness diagnosis might be indicated.

Possible Problem

- Collect more data to confirm or disprove a suspected problem.

Actual or Potential Diagnosis, Problem, or Issue

- Document the diagnosis, problem, or issue.
- Begin planning, implementing, and evaluating care designed to prevent, reduce, or resolve the problem.
- Consult with the appropriate health care professionals and work collaboratively on the problem as indicated.
- If unable to treat the problem because the patient denies the problem and refuses treatment, make sure that the patient understands the possible outcomes of this stance.

Partnering With the Patient and Family

Remember that your best source of information usually is an aware patient. Although some patients still enter the health care system expecting physicians and nurses to tell them what is "wrong" and to "fix it," increasingly patients want to play a leading role in identifying and treating their health problems.

Concept Mastery Alert

Be sure to ask patients what they believe their most important problems or issues are and have them confirm what your assessment reveals and helps you prioritize the resulting list of diagnoses/problems.

FORMULATING AND VALIDATING NURSING DIAGNOSES AND PROBLEM STATEMENTS

Terminology for Writing NANDA-I Approved *Nursing* Diagnoses

When the nurse recognizes a cluster of significant patient data indicating a health problem that can be treated by independent nursing interventions, a *nursing* diagnosis should be written.

If you are just beginning to understand and write nursing diagnoses, consult the list of health problems accepted by NANDA-I for testing and study (https://www.nanda.org/). The NANDA-I list is a beginning list of suggested terms for health problems that might be identified and treated by nurses. Each of the diagnoses in *NANDA International Nursing Diagnoses: Definitions and Classification, 2018–2020* is presented in taxonomic order and includes the basic components of a nursing diagnosis: definition and defining characteristics.

There are distinct advantages to nurses' use of common terminology when formulating nursing diagnoses. These range from communication advantages (everyone uses the same words to describe common problems) to promoting the development of nursing science by facilitating research and the dissemination of research findings to establishing the foundation for any cost–benefit analysis for nursing practice. Pocket-sized handbooks of NANDA-I–approved nursing diagnoses are available and should help students unfamiliar with this grouping of health problems.

Types of *Nursing* Diagnoses

There are basically three types of nursing diagnoses: problem focused, risk, and health promotion.

A **problem-focused nursing diagnosis** is a clinical judgment concerning an undesirable human response to a health condition/life process that exists in an individual, family, group, or community. A **risk nursing diagnosis** is a clinical judgment concerning the vulnerability of an individual, family, group, or community for developing an undesirable human response to health conditions/life processes. A **health promotion nursing diagnosis** is a clinical judgment concerning motivation and desire to increase well-being and to actualize human health potential. These responses are expressed by a readiness to enhance specific health behaviors and can be used in any health state. Health promotion responses may exist in an individual, family, group, or community.

Terminology for Writing Problem Statements

Most diagnostic statements are written either as two-part statements listing the patient's problem and its cause (etiology) or as three-part statements that also include the problem's signs and symptoms (Table 16-3). You will find examples of three-part diagnoses/patient problems in every clinical chapter.

Concept Mastery Alert

The acronyms PE and PES can be helpful in remembering how to write a nursing diagnosis. PE stands for "problem" and "etiology"; PES stands for "problem," "etiology," and "signs and symptoms."

Problem

The purpose of the problem statement is to describe the health state or health problem of the patient as clearly and concisely as possible. Because this section of the nursing diagnosis identifies what is unhealthy about the patient and what the patient would like to change in their health status, it suggests patient outcomes. Quantifiers or descriptors may be used to limit or specify the meaning of a problem statement. For example, the descriptor "anticipatory" placed before the concept "grieving" clarifies the diagnosis for a pregnant couple informed prenatally that their child will most likely be stillborn and who are already grieving the death of their child. Some common descriptors include terms such as decreased, dysfunctional, impaired, ineffective, or situational.

Lippincott Advisor (https://advisor.lww.com/lna/turnaway.do) uses the following headings under problem-based care plans:

Activity and Rest
Behavioral Health
Cognition
Comfort

Table 16-3 Formulating Problem Statements

	DEFINITION	PURPOSE	EXAMPLE
Problem	Identifies what is unhealthy about the patient, indicating the need for change (clear, concise statement of the patient's health problem)	Suggests the patient outcomes (expectations for change)	Activities of daily living (ADL) deficit ↓
Etiology	Identifies the factors that are maintaining the unhealthy state or response (contributing or causative factors)	Suggests the appropriate nursing measures	Fear of falling in the tub and obesity ↓ ↓
Signs and Symptoms	Identify the subjective and objective data that signal the existence of the problem (cues that reflect the existence of a problem)	Suggest evaluative criteria	Strong body and urine odor, unclean hair: "I'm afraid I'll fall in the tub and break something." (5 ft 4 inches, 170 lb)

Examples:
Two-part diagnostic statement: ADL deficit; possible etiologic factors: fear of falling in tub and obesity
Three-part diagnostic statement: ADL deficit; possible etiologic factors: fear of falling in tub and obesity; signs and symptoms: strong body and urine odor, unclean hair, statement of fearing fall in tub, and height and weight: 5 ft 4 inches, 170 lb

Elimination
Health Promotion
Nutrition
Patient Safety
Roles and Relationships
Skin and Wounds
Ventilation and Perfusion

When expanded, each heading identifies related problems; for example, under Activity and Rest, common problems are: Activity intolerance

ADL deficit
Bathing/hygiene ADL deficit
Deconditioning
Discharge planning
Dressing ADL deficit
Fatigue
Sleep deprivation

ETIOLOGY

The etiology identifies the physiologic, psychological, sociologic, spiritual, and environmental factors believed to be related to the problem as either a cause or a contributing factor. Because the etiology identifies the factors that maintain the unhealthy patient state and prevent the desired change, the etiology directs nursing intervention. Unless the etiology is correctly identified, nursing actions might be inefficient and ineffective. For example, a patient with diabetes who is frequently admitted to the hospital with hyperglycemia and who has a poor history of dietary and pharmacologic management is diagnosed to be nonadherent. Mistakenly assuming that the nonadherence is related to a knowledge deficit, the nurse channels all nursing activities and energies into teaching the patient how to manage the diabetes. However, this would be useless if the nonadherence were actually a result of the patient's decreased will to live, an etiology that would necessitate a different group of nursing interventions.

SIGNS AND SYMPTOMS

The subjective and objective data that signal the existence of the actual or potential health problem are the third component of the nursing diagnosis. It is important to remember that the signs and symptoms are part of assessment. Although they are written last in the formal problem statement, they are considered first. Table 16-3 defines the components of a diagnosis/problem statement and shows how they affect patient outcomes, nursing measures, and evaluation.

Guidelines for Writing Diagnostic Statements

Remember these guidelines to ensure that your diagnostic statements are correctly written.

1. Phrase the diagnostic statement as an actual or potential diagnosis, problem, or issue.
2. Check to make sure that the patient problem precedes the etiology.
3. Consider when at-risk populations or associated conditions should be identified.
4. Signs and symptoms, when included in the nursing diagnosis, should follow the etiology.
5. Write in legally advisable terms.
6. Use nonjudgmental language.
7. Be sure the problem statement indicates what is unhealthy about the patient or what the patient wants to change (enhance).
8. Avoid using defining characteristics, medical diagnoses, or something that cannot be changed in the problem statement.
9. Reread the diagnosis to make sure that the problem statement suggests patient outcomes and that the etiology will direct the selection of nursing measures.

Common errors in writing diagnostic statements are shown in Table 16-4 (on p. 442), along with suggestions for correcting them.

When recording problems in electronic health records (EHRs), remember that different EHRs organize data differently, and that the documentation for nursing assessments and for nursing diagnoses/problems/issues may vary. Be sure to check your facility's policies. You should be able to select your diagnostic statement within the system's problem list, and the problem list may trigger a message to place an order for an intervention or care set of orders for the patient if this is not already present.

What Is *Not* a Diagnostic Statement

The diagnostic statement is written in terms of a patient problem, alteration in health state, or patient strength, which guides nurses and others to select interventions to achieve valued outcomes. Table 16-5 (on page 443) uses a patient with diabetes mellitus to illustrate what nursing diagnostic statements are not.

Validating Diagnostic Statements

After a tentative diagnostic statement is formulated, it should be validated. An affirmative response to each of the following questions validates a tentative diagnostic statement:

- Is my patient database (assessment data) sufficient, accurate, and supported by nursing research?
- Does my synthesis of data (significant cues) demonstrate the existence of a pattern?
- Are the subjective and objective data I used for determining the existence of a pattern characteristic of the health problem I defined?
- Is my tentative problem statement based on scientific nursing knowledge and clinical expertise?
- Is my degree of confidence above 50%, that other qualified practitioners would formulate the same statement based on my data?

Remember that you are responsible for validating the problem statements you write, even when using computer-assisted problem lists. The use of standardized language and EHRs may make diagnosis writing easier by suggesting possible diagnoses/problems to match your recorded assessment findings. However, computers cannot replace humans and critical thinking, especially when it comes to complex

Table 16-4 Common Errors in Writing Nursing Diagnoses and Recommended Corrections

ERROR	EXAMPLE	CORRECTION	EXAMPLE
Writing the diagnosis in terms of needs and not response	Needs assistance with bathing related to bed rest	Write the diagnosis in terms of response rather than need.	Bathing self-care deficit related to immobility
Making legally inadvisable statements	Nonadherence due to hostility toward nursing staff (the words *due to* imply a direct cause-and-effect relationship) Spouse abuse related to husband's immaturity and violent temper Impaired skin integrity related to patient's lying on back all night	Use "related to" rather than "due to" or "caused by" to link the etiology to the problem statement. Write diagnosis in legally advisable terms: statements that may be interpreted as libel or that imply nursing negligence are legally hazardous to all the nurses caring for the patient.	Nonadherence related to hostility toward nursing staff (denotes a relation between the problem and etiology but not necessarily a causal relation) Risk for Violence: Spouse abuse; signs and symptoms: husband's reported inability to control behavior Impaired Skin Integrity related to mobility deficit
Identifying as a problem a patient response that is not necessarily unhealthy	Mild anxiety related to impending surgery	Include in the problem statement of the nursing diagnosis only patient responses that are unhealthy or that the patient wants to change.	No need for nursing diagnosis: mild anxiety before surgery is a healthy response that motivates preoperative self-care behavior
Identifying as a problem signs and symptoms of illness	Cough related to long history of smoking	Avoid including signs and symptoms of illness in the problem statement of the nursing diagnosis.	Ineffective airway clearance related to 20-year history of smoking
Identifying as a patient problem or etiology what cannot be changed	Alterations in bowel elimination: Permanent colostomy related to cancer of bowel Grieving related to death of spouse	Express the problem statement and etiologic factors in terms that can be changed; otherwise, nursing energies are being directed to a hopeless task.	Self-Care Deficit: Care of colostomy, related to severe anxiety about cancer and feelings of powerlessness Dysfunctional Grief related to inability to accept death of spouse
Identifying environmental factors rather than patient factors as a problem	Cluttered home related to inability to discard anything	Express the problem statement in terms of unhealthy patient responses rather than environmental conditions.	Injury risk; signs and symptoms: cluttered home (inability to discard anything)
Reversing clauses	Deficient knowledge related to alteration in parenting	Avoid reversing the problem statement and etiologic statement.	Impaired Parenting related to knowledge deficit: child growth and development, discipline
Having both clauses say the same thing	Impaired comfort related to pain (pain is the comfort alteration; what is contributing to the pain?)	Be sure that the two parts of the diagnosis do not mean the same thing.	Unrelieved incisional pain; etiology: fear of addiction
Including value judgments in the nursing diagnosis	Poor home maintenance related to laziness	Write the diagnosis without value judgments; avoid words such as *poor, inadequate, abnormal, unhealthy.*	Impaired Homemaking related to low value ascribed to home safety and cleanliness
Including the medical diagnosis in the diagnostic statement	Impaired home maintenance related to arthritis	Do not include the medical diagnosis in the nursing diagnosis statement.	Impaired Homemaking related to mobility, endurance, and comfort alterations

Common errors adapted from Mundinger, M. O., & Jauron, G. D. (1975). *Developing a nursing diagnosis. Nursing Outlook, 23*(2), 94–98. Guidelines for writing nursing diagnoses adapted from Iyer, P., Taptich, B., & Bernocchi-Losey, D. (1991). *Nursing process and nursing diagnoses* (2nd ed.). W. B. Saunders.

Table 16-5 What a Nursing Diagnostic Statement Is *Not*, and Why

WHAT A NURSING DIAGNOSTIC STATEMENT IS *NOT*	EXAMPLE	RATIONALE
Medical diagnosis	Diabetes mellitus	Although there is nursing care associated with medical illnesses, the illness is not primarily amenable to nursing intervention. Nursing's concern is the *person* who has the illness and the effect of the illness on human functioning.
Medical pathology	Hypoglycemia	Nurses need to understand the pathology underlying disease states to plan appropriate nursing care, but once again, nursing's focus is the person, not the pathology. The person's response to hypoglycemia, how hypoglycemia affects human functioning—these are the domain of *nursing*.
Diagnostic tests, treatments, equipment	Fasting blood glucose Insulin therapy Insulin syringe Infusion pump	Nursing's concern is the person's response to the diagnostic study, treatment, or equipment. If the need for insulin therapy reveals a deficient knowledge or self-care deficit, this becomes the diagnostic, not insulin therapy in and of itself.
Therapeutic patient needs	Needs to learn the relation among diet, exercise, and insulin	The problem should be written as a patient health problem rather than a patient need. *Example:* Altered health maintenance (diabetic care); possible etiologic factor: lack of knowledge of relation among diet, exercise, and insulin.
Therapeutic nursing goals	To develop therapeutic diabetic self-care behaviors	The problem should be written from the patient perspective rather than the nursing perspective and phrased as a patient health problem. *Example:* Activities of daily living deficit: diabetic self-care behaviors; etiologic factors: decreased value on life and decreased motivation to learn.
A single sign or symptom	After successfully administering own insulin for 3 days, patient tells nurse, "You give me my shot today."	A problem statement is not developed until a pattern or cluster of significant cues is detected. The signs and symptoms lead to the identification of the problem statement but are not the problem statement. In this situation, no problem statement is indicated until further data collection, interpretation, and analysis take place.
An *invalidated* nursing inference	Above incident leads to the nursing inference: Nonadherence related to depression	This is a premature problem statement that may not accurately reflect a patient problem. More data and the validation of the tentative problem (nursing inference) are needed before the problem statement can be recorded.

diagnostic reasoning. While the computer can process data faster than you can, it will not be aware of what is happening to your patient at this moment in time. You need to validate your diagnostic statements and recognize when your computer is making an obvious error.

In addition, patients who are able to participate in decision making should be encouraged to validate the problem. "It seems to me that bathing has become a problem now that you are afraid of falling in the tub. What's your sense of this?" Refer to Table 16-2 on page 438 for a list of possible outcomes of validating tentative nursing diagnoses.

Next Steps

In Chapter 17, you will learn how to plan nursing care to address the patient health problems and issues you have identified. One of your first tasks will be to prioritize your diagnostic statements, and Chapter 17 will teach you how to allow patient preference, Maslow's hierarchy of human needs, and your anticipation of future problems to guide your clinical reasoning about nursing priorities. You will also be able to use your knowledge of concept mapping (Chapters 13 and 14) to diagram the relationships between your diagnoses/problems and evidence-based interventions.

DOCUMENTING NURSING DIAGNOSES AND PATIENT PROBLEMS

The nurse documents validated nursing diagnoses and actual and potential patient problems in the patient record. Depending on the documentation system in use, nursing diagnoses and problems might be recorded in the nursing care plan and on the multidisciplinary problem list at the front of the patient record. Table 16-3 on page 440 illustrates how to document nursing diagnoses/patient problems using both two- and three-part diagnostic statements.

At one time, nurses were urged to only use NANDA-I accepted terms to state nursing diagnoses. Today, accepted terms vary. Nurses should use the terms recommended by their school, employer, or specialty organization (e.g., Association of periOperative Nurses [AORN] or Association of Rehabilitation Nurses [ARN]). The terms most commonly used will be the terms chosen for standard plans and computerized systems.

Importance of Patient Problems in Electronic Health Records

The goal of the EHR is to enable the interdisciplinary team caring for the patient to more easily view the patient's risks, health promotion possibilities, and actual current and long-term care problems. Documenting patient problems in the EHR is important for the patient and others providing care. You should use the EHR to:

- view the patient's ongoing risks (e.g., Risk for Dysfunctional Grief, Risk for Falls) and problems (e.g., Impaired Gastrointestinal System Function: Constipation, Burn Wound) that others have identified and documented.
- decide on and document new patient problems based on the patient assessment findings.
- facilitate communication of the patient's actual problems with nurses and others on the care team.
- use the list of patient problems to make decisions about what mutual goals the patient desires (patient outcomes) and what can be done (nursing interventions).
- determine and document when the patient problems are resolved.

NURSING DIAGNOSIS: A CRITIQUE

Current nursing diagnosis literature contains many examples of nurses writing about how using nursing diagnoses has improved their clinical practice; articles also detail the many benefits nursing diagnosis brings to the profession. Conversely, other articles point out the limitations of nursing diagnosis and urge nurses to be cautious so that an uncritical use of nursing diagnosis does not restrict their practices.

The primary benefit of nursing diagnosis for the patient is the individualization of patient care—this is true whether nurses are identifying what are called nursing diagnoses or actual or potential problems. For example, nurses might be caring simultaneously for three women who have had a modified radical mastectomy because of breast cancer. Although the postoperative nursing management of these women is similar, priorities of care may differ. A prioritized list of nursing diagnoses/problems enables nurses to direct their energies toward these differing patient priorities. Here are some examples of nursing diagnoses/problems for three different women with modified radical mastectomy:

Patient A
- Disturbed Body Image
- Coping impairment

Patient B
- Acute Pain
- Bathing/hygiene ADL deficit

Patient C
- Impaired Sexual Functioning
- Risk for Powerlessness

The use of nursing diagnoses/problems also allows patients to be informed and willing participants in their care, as they validate their diagnoses/problems and assist in prioritizing them. The process of prioritizing nursing diagnoses/patient problems is the first step in planning care, addressed in Chapter 17.

Improved communication between nurses and other health care professionals is probably the most important benefit of accurate, up-to-date diagnostic statements—expressed in well-defined and standardized terminology—for nurses. This communication aids in planning, charting, patient data retrieval, health team conferences, change-of-shift reports, and health care follow-up. It also promotes nursing accountability for the problems that nurses diagnose.

If the diagnostic process is used incorrectly, however, a patient might be "misdiagnosed." Common sources of error include the following:

- *Premature diagnoses based on an incomplete database:* For example, a diagnosis of Coping impairment is made after the patient verbally attacks one nurse who was attempting to teach him self-care for his wound.
- *Erroneous diagnoses resulting from an inaccurate database or a faulty data analysis:* For example, a diagnosis of Dysfunctional Grief is made in a patient observed crying after learning that her cancer had returned, before anyone had time to evaluate whether this was simply an appropriate response to bad news.
- *Routine diagnoses resulting from the nurse's failure to tailor data collection and analysis to the unique needs of the patient:* For example, a diagnosis of Knowledge deficiency is made in a patient with diabetes who is frequently hospitalized with diabetes-related complications, when she actually has excellent knowledge of diabetes and related self-care demands but has lacked the motivation to care for herself appropriately.
- *Errors of omission:* Failure to modify diagnoses and to identify new diagnoses as the patient's status changes may also be problematic. Failures in diagnosis lead to failures in nursing care.

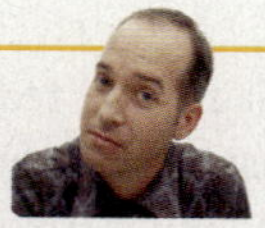

Recall **Martin Prescott**, the 46-year-old man with rectal bleeding and constipation. Although an initial nursing problem statement may involve Knowledge deficiency of possible causes of rectal bleeding, further assessment may reveal that the patient's constipation resulting from a diet inadequate in fiber and fluids is the underlying cause of the bleeding. Thus, the nurse would need to revise the problem statement to focus on Constipation; etiology: inadequate intake of high-fiber foods and fluids; signs/symptoms: hard stool and rectal bleeding.

The above examples of misdiagnosis don't show the limitations of nursing diagnosis; rather, they are problems of nurses diagnosing incorrectly. More serious criticisms of nursing diagnoses are raised by nurses who claim that a classification of standardized diagnoses limits nursing, curbing nurses' originality and ability to think things through.

Although some nurses believe that diagnosis offers a valued shortcut to practice, critics find this attitude offensive, and respond that rather than invest nursing's energies in perfecting a shortcut, nurses need to change working conditions that interfere with in-depth problem solving and thoughtful nursing care.

Early critics of diagnostic labeling point out that instead of identifying what is unique and positive about nursing, nursing diagnoses make a clear statement that nurses are concerned about what is deviant, wrong, or pathologic (Hagey & McDonough, 1984). These critics claim that the ever-changing and dynamic human person with a need for nursing care becomes objectified. The practice of many experienced nurses who find nursing diagnoses helpful in targeting care for patients with diverse needs counters these concerns.

Nurses who are sensitive to transcultural issues raise important concerns about the cultural limitations of some diagnoses. Foremost among these concerns is that some diagnoses and behaviors assume that the patient is "wrong," and the provider is "right" and deny the validity of cultural and health care beliefs and practices that are different from those of the nurse (Geissler, 1991). Examples of nursing diagnoses that often are misused in labeling such cultural deviations as abnormal include Impaired Verbal Communication, Impaired Socialisation, and Nonadherence. Nurses who provide culturally sensitive care (see Chapter 5) and who work collaboratively with the patient as a partner avoid these problems.

In conclusion, diagnosis/analyzing has become a valued and essential phase in the nursing process. Used correctly, it is a powerful tool for individualizing patient care and ensures that nurses' energies are being used in the most efficient way to meet prioritized and holistic patients' needs. Nurses who are as concerned about the art and spirit of nursing as they are about its science are careful to avoid labeling patients in a way that objectifies them or limits the potential range of nurse–patient interactions.

REFLECTIVE PRACTICE LEADING TO PERSONAL LEARNING

Remember that the object of reflective practice is to look at an experience, understand it, and learn from it. As you begin to develop your expertise in diagnosing health problems and identifying patient strengths, reflect on your experiences—both successes and failures—in order to improve your practice. How can you do it better next time? What did you learn today that can help you tomorrow? Alfaro-LeFevre (2014) recommends paying close attention to the following during the diagnosing phase of the nursing process:

- Has patient and family participation in the process been at an optimal level? How might you have better engaged the patient and family?
- Are your data reliable, accurate, and complete? How do you know this?
- Have you identified the assumptions you made about patient cues?
- Are your conclusions based on facts (evidence) rather than guesswork?
- Have you considered alternate conclusions, ideas, and solutions?

Perhaps the most important questions to reflect on are: Are your patients and their families/caregivers better for having had *you* share in the critical responsibility of diagnosing their health problems and identifying and tapping their strengths? Are your patients now receiving thoughtful, person-centered, prioritized, holistic, evidence-based treatment and care because of your efforts?

DEVELOPING CLINICAL REASONING AND CLINICAL JUDGMENT

1. Find a patient with a well-established medical condition. List potential medical diagnoses and actual and potential diagnoses, problems, and issues that a nurse can treat. Explain the differing purposes of medical diagnoses and the diagnoses, problems, and issues that nurses and the collaborative team can treat. What is nursing's diagnostic contribution to the interdisciplinary team's effort to care for this patient?
2. Try to assess a patient with another student and independently identify their strengths. Compare the lists you generated. What explains your differences?
3. Interview two patients with the same medical diagnosis. Develop a prioritized list of diagnoses/problems/issues for both, and reflect on the differences. Compare and contrast the strengths of both patients. If you can do this exercise with another student, it would be helpful to explore why there are differences in your lists of nursing diagnoses and patient strengths.
4. Reflective nurses realize that they bring their personal attributes, knowledge, and competencies to the process of diagnosing. What personal strengths and limitations do you expect to influence your ability to diagnose health problems and identify and tap strengths?

PRACTICING FOR NCLEX

1. A registered nurse is formulating nursing diagnoses for a patient with multiple fractures. Which actions does the nurse take during this step of the nursing process? Select all that apply.
   a. Conducting a nursing interview to collect patient data
   b. Analyzing data collected in the nursing assessment
   c. Developing a care plan for the patient
   d. Pointing out the patient's strengths
   e. Assessing the patient's mental status
   f. Identifying community resources to help the family cope
2. A nurse is caring for a patient who presents with dyspnea, tachypnea, productive cough, fever, and low oxygen saturation. When developing the nursing care plan, which health problems might the nurse identify for this patient? Select all that apply.
   a. Bronchial pneumonia
   b. Impaired gas exchange
   c. Impaired Respiratory System Function
   d. Altered breathing pattern
   e. Impaired Thermoregulation

3. After assessing a patient recovering from a stroke in a rehabilitation facility, the nurse's initial analysis suggests a potential health problem of situational low self-esteem. How will the nurse record the problem when they believe more data are needed?
   a. No problem
   b. Possible problem
   c. Actual nursing diagnosis
   d. Clinical problem other than nursing
4. When caring for a patient who sustained a spinal cord injury, the nurse formulates the health problem:
   Impaired Tissue Integrity
   Etiology: sensory and motor deficit
   Signs and symptoms: difficulty turning, reddened areas on heels and sacrum

   Which phrase gives direction to the underlying cause of the problem?
   a. Impaired Tissue Integrity
   b. Sensory and motor deficit
   c. Signs and symptoms
   d. Reddened areas of skin on the heels and back
5. A nurse is caring for a patient who refuses to look at or care for a new colostomy. The patient states, "I don't care what I look like anymore. I'm not washing up, let alone touching or changing this bag!" The nurse formulates the health problem: Difficulty Coping: Impaired Acceptance of Health Status, reflecting which type of health problem?
   a. Collaborative
   b. Interdisciplinary
   c. Medical
   d. Nursing
6. A nursing student obtains a blood pressure reading of 148/100. To determine the significance of this reading, what action will the nurse take first?
   a. Comparing this reading to standards and trends in the medical record
   b. Checking the taxonomy of nursing diagnoses for a pertinent label
   c. Checking a medical text for the signs and symptoms of high blood pressure
   d. Consulting with experienced nurse colleagues
7. A nursing student tells the primary nurse that their patient has not had a bowel movement for 2 days and suggests adding the health problem "Constipation" to the care plan. How would the nurse best respond?
   a. "Did you assess the patient's usual bowel patterns and appearance of the last stool?"
   b. "This early diagnosis will help us manage the problem before it becomes severe."
   c. "Have you determined if this is an actual or a possible diagnosis?"
   d. "This condition requires a medical diagnosis."
8. A nurse is caring for a patient who has been admitted the second time this month for hypertensive emergency. The care plan contains the health problem:
   Nonadherence
   Etiology: lack of knowledge of purpose of medications
   Signs and symptoms: BP, 220/112; readmitted for hypertensive crisis after 2 weeks

   When meeting the patient, which action will the nurse take first?
   a. Teach the patient that nonadherence may lead to stroke and heart disease
   b. Discuss what will motivate the patient to adhere to the medication regimen
   c. Explain that these medications are essential to their health and illness prevention
   d. Determine the patient's knowledge about the medications and their side effects
9. A nurse in the psychiatric clinic is developing a problem list for a patient. What statement best reflects a correctly written, two-part problem?
   a. Difficulty Coping: Impaired Family Coping
      Etiology: inability to maintain marriage
   b. Difficulty Coping: Impaired Acceptance of Health Status
      Etiology: anger management issues
   c. Impaired Cognition: Distorted Thought Process
      Etiology: psychosis as evidence by hallucinations
   d. Impaired Cognition: Decisional Conflict
      Etiology: placement of parent in a long-term care facility
10. A nurse is developing a problem list for a care plan. Which reflects a correctly written three-part problem statement? Select all that apply.
   a. Difficulty Coping: Impaired Family Coping:
      Etiology: lack of knowledge about tube feeding
      Signs and symptoms: child needing tube feeding discharged to home
   b. Impaired Nutritional Status: Impaired Nutritional Intake
      Etiology: striving for perfect weight, wishes to excel in gymnastics
      Signs and symptoms: 20-lb weight loss in 1 month
   c. Need to learn how to care for child on ventilator at home
      Etiology: discharge of child after 3-month hospital stay
      Signs and symptoms: repeated comments, "I know I'll harm her because I'm not a nurse." and "I can't do medical things."
   d. Impaired Spiritual Status
      Etiology: inability to accept diagnosis of terminal illness
      Signs and symptoms: comments such as, "I don't deserve this"; "I've tried to live my life well"; and "How could God make me suffer this way?"
   e. Impaired Tissue Integrity: Impaired Skin Integrity
      Etiology: failure of home health aides to turn patient every 2 hours
      Signs and symptoms: stage 3 pressure wound on sacrum.

11. A nurse is caring for a patient recovering from a stroke that paralyzed the dominant arm. The nursing assistant reports that the patient was unable to bathe, comb their hair, or brush their teeth. Which health problem should the nurse add to the care plan?
   a. Lack of motivation to complete self-care activities
   b. Risk for: Activities of Daily Living Deficit
   c. ADL deficit: impaired dressing and grooming
   d. Impaired musculoskeletal system function: paralysis
12. A nurse is caring for a patient who had abdominal surgery yesterday. The nurse observes the patient guarding the area with hands and a pillow, refusing to move, and grimacing. What information does the nurse use to formulate the health problem statement?
   a. Symptoms
   b. Diagnostic statement
   c. Etiology
   d. Cue
13. When developing the admission care plan for a patient with multiple sclerosis and quadriplegia, the nurse formulates the patient problem: Impaired Tissue Integrity: Impaired Skin Integrity. What action will the nurse take next?
   a. Elevate the patient's heels off the bed using a pillow
   b. Develop a goal that the patient will consume protein at each meal
   c. Delegate assessment of the skin on the patient's back to the AP
   d. Teach the patient to turn themselves in bed every hour
14. A nurse has performed an admission assessment on a patient. What step does the nurse perform after clustering the data?
   a. Developing interventions
   b. Nursing judgments
   c. Diagnosing and analyzing
   d. Concept mapping
15. A nurse notices a patient crying after meeting with the health care provider. Prior to formulating a health problem of difficulty coping, the nurse seeks to further support the problem by gathering which data?
   a. Abnormal vital signs
   b. Underlying cause of the tears
   c. Admitting diagnosis
   d. Patient's support system

ANSWERS WITH RATIONALES

1. **b, d, f.** Diagnosing includes identifying actual or potential health problems for individuals, groups, or communities; identifying factors that contribute to or cause health problems (etiologies); and identifying resources or strengths the individual, group, or community can draw on to prevent or resolve problems. The nurse assesses and collects patient data in the assessment step and develops the care plan during the planning phase of the nursing process.
2. **b, c, d, e.** Nursing diagnoses are actual or potential health problems that can be prevented or resolved by independent or interdependent nursing interventions. These include Impaired gas exchange, supported by low oxygen saturation; Impaired Respiratory System Function; Altered breathing pattern, supported by dyspnea and tachypnea; and Impaired Thermoregulation. Pneumonia is a medical diagnosis.
3. **b.** When a possible problem exists, the nurse must collect more data to confirm or disprove the suspected problem. The conclusion, "no problem," indicates no nursing response is required. When an actual problem is identified, the nurse continues using the steps of the nursing process by planning, goal setting, implementing, and evaluating care to resolve the problem. A clinical problem other than nursing diagnosis requires a collaborative approach with the appropriate health care professionals.
4. **b.** The etiology, sensory and motor deficits, identifies the contributing or causative factors of the problem. The problem, "Impaired Tissue Integrity: Impaired Skin Integrity," states the undesirable health condition, life processes, or human response. The phrase, "Signs and symptoms: non-blanchable reddened areas on heels and back," contains the defining characteristics of the problem.
5. **d.** Difficulty Coping: Impaired Acceptance of Health Status is a nursing problem, falling within the scope of independent nursing practice. Collaborative and interdisciplinary problems are resolved through a teamwork approach with other health care professionals. A medical problem is a traumatic or disease condition validated by medical diagnostic studies.
6. **a.** A standard, or a norm, is a generally accepted rule, measure, pattern, or model to which data can be compared within the same class or category. When interpreting the significance of a patient's blood pressure reading, the nurse uses normative values for the patient's age group, race, and illness category and compares these to the patient's recent results. Identifying the reason for deviation from a norm gives direction to the etiology of a health problem (e.g., insufficient knowledge, nutrition, stress, and coping, or other).
7. **a.** Patient health problems are derived from clusters of related data and patterns, rather than a single cue. The nurse determines if this is the patient's usual bowel pattern, or whether an underlying reason exists for the lack of a bowel movement. Constipation is a health problem the nurse can resolve with independent or interdependent nursing actions.
8. **d.** Using the nursing process, the nurse first assesses the patient's knowledge base; this also confirms the accuracy of the problem statement. Problem statements with unclear etiologies may lead to inappropriate, erroneous, or unhelpful interventions. If the patient has difficulty affording medications or is experiencing side effects, a collaborative problem can be resolved jointly by the nurse, social worker, and health care provider.
9. **d.** A correctly written two-part problem statement includes the health problem and the etiology or cause. The problem statement and etiology should avoid signs and symptoms, medical diagnoses, and something that cannot be changed. Inability to maintain marriage and anger issues do not identify the underlying cause of the problem and may themselves reflect the true problem. Psychosis is a medical diagnosis, which should not be used to support a patient problem.

10. **d.** Correctly written problem statements contain a problem the nurse can treat with independent or interdependent interventions, a clearly stated etiology or cause of the problem, and supporting signs and symptoms. Option (a) may be more easily resolved with the problem statement, knowledge deficiency. Option (a) further states the tube feeding is the underlying cause of the problem; it is a factor that cannot be changed. Option (c) is written in terms of needs and not an unhealthy response. Option (e), while written in three parts, places blame or implies negligence, which is legally inadvisable and should be avoided. A clear etiology is not stated in option (e), impeding direction for appropriate interventions or outcomes.
11. **c.** The nurse clusters the data that demonstrates the patient's (actual) inability to perform bathing and grooming. For that reason, a "potential problem" or "risk" is not appropriate. There is no evidence the patient lacks motivation, and paralysis is not a problem the nurse can resolve.
12. **d.** A cue denotes significant data or "red flags," that, when occurring in a pattern or cluster, point to the existence of a health problem.
13. **b.** After the health problem is developed, the nurse begins the planning phase of the nursing process, which includes goal development. Elevating the heels and teaching the patient to turn are interventions used during the implementation phase. Delegating an assessment to the AP is an incorrect activity; assessment falls within the role and scope of practice of the professional nurse. In addition, the nurse must perform the skin assessment to develop the problem and plan care.
14. **c.** After clustering the data, the nurse analyzes the data and formulates a nursing diagnosis. Interventions are based on and developed after goal setting. Nursing judgments are outcomes based on critical thinking and clinical reasoning. A concept map is a diagram or pictorial representation of the (student) nurse's understanding of the interactions and relationships of the patient's problems and plan of care.
15. **b.** The nurse continues gathering data, determining the presence of a problem of grief, impaired coping, etc., by determining the underlying cause of the tears. If the patient received news that a biopsy was free from cancer, perhaps no problem exists. If the patient was told they have a terminal illness, the nurse can continue to gather data and plan to support the patient's physical and emotional needs.

Bibliography

Alfaro-LeFevre, R. (2014). *Applying nursing process: The foundation for clinical reasoning* (8th ed.). Wolters Kluwer Health/Lippincott Williams & Wilkins.

Alfaro-LeFevre, R. (2020). *Critical thinking, clinical reasoning, and clinical judgment* (7th ed.). Elsevier.

American Association of Colleges of Nursing (AACN). (2008). *The essentials of baccalaureate education for professional nursing practice.* Author.

American Association of Colleges of Nursing (AACN). (2021). *The essentials: Core competencies for professional nursing education.* Author.

American Nurses Association (ANA). (1980, 2010). *Nursing's social policy statement.* Author.

American Nurses Association (ANA). (2004, 2010, 2015, 2021). *Nursing: Scope and standards of practice.* Author.

American Nurses Association (ANA). (2015). *Code for nurses with interpretive statements.* Author.

Aspinall, M. J. (1976). Nursing diagnosis: The weak link. *Nursing Outlook, 24*(7), 433–437.

Carpenito, L. J. (2017). *Nursing diagnosis: Application to clinical practice* (15th ed.). Wolters Kluwer.

Carroll-Johnson, R. M. (Ed.). (1991). Classification in nursing diagnosis: Proceedings of the ninth national conference. J. B. Lippincott.

Fry, V. S. (1953). The creative approach to nursing. *American Journal of Nursing, 53*(3), 301–302.

Gebbie, K. M., & Lavin, M. A. (1973). Summary of the first national conference. C. V. Mosby.

Geissler, E. M. (1991). Transcultural nursing and diagnosis. *Nursing and Health Care, 12*(4), 190–192, 203.

Gleason, K. T., Davidson, P. M., Tanner, E. K., Baptiste, D., Rushton, C., Day, J., & Newman-Toker, D. E. (2017). Defining the critical role of nurses in diagnostic error prevention: A conceptual framework and a call to action. *Diagnosis, 4*(4), 201–210. https://doi:10.1515/dx-2017-0015.

Gleason, K., Harkless, G., Stanley, J., Olson, A. P. J., & Graber, M. L. (2021). The critical need for nursing education to address the diagnostic process. *Nursing Outlook, 69*(3), 362–369.

Gordon, M. (1976). Nursing diagnosis and the diagnostic process. *American Journal of Nursing, 76*(8), 1298–1300.

Gordon, M. (1994). *Nursing diagnosis: Process and application* (3rd ed.). C. V. Mosby.

Gordon, M. (1998). Nursing nomenclature and classification system development. *Online Journal of Issues in Nursing, 3*(2).

Hagey, R. S., & McDonough, P. (1984). The problem of professional labeling. *Nursing Outlook, 33*(3), 151–157.

Hammond, K. R. (1966). Clinical inference in nursing: A psychologist's viewpoint. *Nursing Research, 15*(1), 27–38.

Herdman, T. H. (2008). Nursing diagnosis: Is it time for a new definition? *International Journal of Nursing Terminologies & Classifications, 19*(1), 2–13.

Herdman, T. H., & Kamisuru, S. (Eds.). (2018). North American Nursing Diagnosis Association International (NANDA-I). *NANDA international nursing diagnoses: Definitions and classification, 2018–2020* (11th ed.). Theime.

International Council of Nurses. (2019). International Classification for Nursing Practice (ICNP) Catalogue. https://www.icn.ch/sites/default/files/inline-files/ICNP2019-DC.pdf

Kritek, P. B. (1985). Nursing diagnosis in perspective: Response to a critique. *Image—The Journal of Nursing Scholarship, 17*(1), 3–8.

Lindsey, A. M. (1990). Identification and labeling of human responses. *Journal of Professional Nursing, 6*(3), 143–150.

Lippincott Advisor. (2020). Problem-based care plans. https://advisor.lww.com/lna/home.do?m=selection&selectedBookId=43

Mundinger, M. O., & Jauron, G. D. (1975). Developing a nursing diagnosis. *Nursing Outlook, 23*(2), 94–98.

National Academies of Medicine. (2015). *Improving diagnosis in health care.* National Academies Press, https://doi:10.17226/21794.

North American Nursing Diagnosis Association (NANDA). (1990). *Taxonomy I revised with official diagnostic categories.* Author.

North American Nursing Diagnosis Association International (NANDA-I). https://www.nanda.org

Skelly, C. L., Hall, C. A., & Risher, C. R. (2020). Shared decision making and patient-centered care. *American Nurse Journal, 15*(2), 45–47.

Tanner, C. A. (2006). Thinking like a nurse: A research-based model of clinical judgment in nursing. *Journal of Nursing Education, 45*(6), 204–211. https://doi:10.3928/01484834-20060601-04.

17 Outcome Identification and Planning

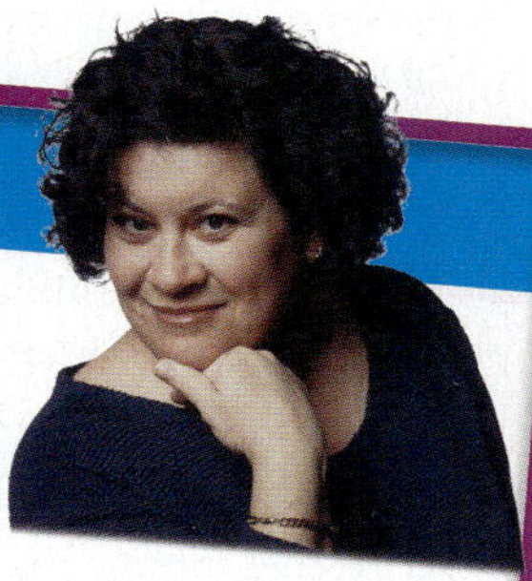

Glenda Kronk

Glenda, a 35-year-old woman, comes to the health center for a routine checkup. During the visit, she expresses a strong motivation and desire to become physically fit, lose weight, increase her muscle tone, and improve her cardiorespiratory capacity. "I know it will involve some major lifestyle changes, including diet. What's with all these diets and diet supplements now?" she asks.

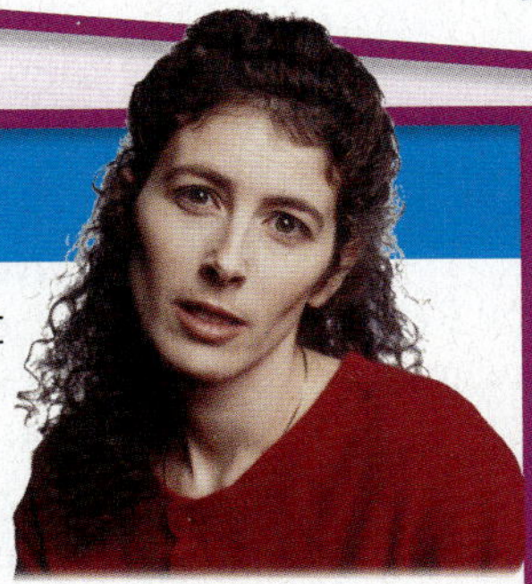

Darla Jefferson

Darla, a 29-year-old single woman, is about 14 weeks pregnant. She describes herself as a "hopeless addict" who has tried to stop "more times than I can remember." Although currently drug-free, she is not hopeful of preventing relapse. She does not know the baby's father and has mixed feelings about keeping the baby, saying, "On the one hand I want someone to love me, but I'm not sure I'd want me for a mother."

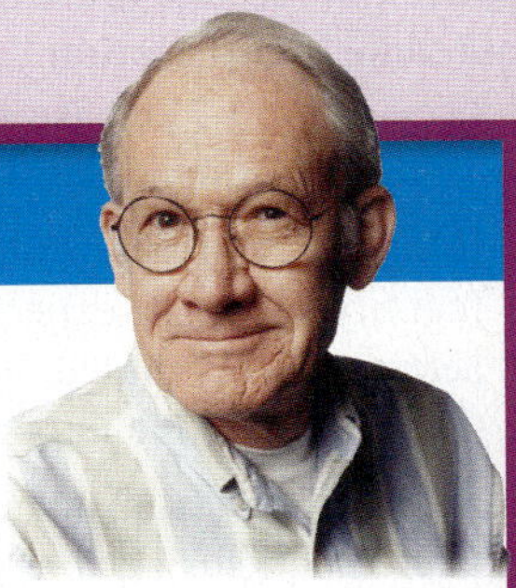

Elijah Wolinski

Elijah is a thin, frail, 85-year-old man who is bedbound due to severe degenerative joint disease. He is being cared for by his 56-year-old nephew at his home. Assessment on a home visit reveals Elijah lying on soiled linens with a large pressure injury on his sacrum, approximately 5 cm in diameter and about 2 cm deep with purulent drainage.

Learning Outcomes

After completing the chapter, you will be able to accomplish the following:

1. Describe the purpose and benefits of outcome identification and planning.
2. Identify three elements of comprehensive planning.
3. Prioritize patient health problems and nursing responses.
4. Describe how patient goals/expected outcomes and nursing orders are derived from diagnoses/patient problems.
5. Develop a nursing care plan with properly constructed outcomes and related nursing interventions.
6. Differentiate nurse-initiated interventions, physician-initiated interventions, and collaborative interventions.
7. Use criteria to evaluate planning skills.
8. Describe five common problems related to planning, their possible causes, and remedies.
9. Describe the rationale for standardized outcomes (NOC) and interventions (NIC) for nursing.

Nursing Concepts

- Nursing Process
- Managing Care
- Clinical Decision Making
- Clinical Reasoning and Judgment

After the nurse collects and interprets patient data, identifying patient strengths and health problems, it is time to plan for nursing actions (see the accompanying Reflective Practice box for an example). During the **outcome identification** and **planning** phase of the nursing process (Fig. 17-1 on page 452), the nurse works in partnership with the patient and family to:

- Establish priorities
- Identify and write expected patient outcomes
- Select evidence-based nursing interventions
- Communicate the nursing plan of care

A **goal** is an aim or an end. A **patient outcome** is an expected conclusion to a patient health problem, or in the event of a wellness diagnosis, an expected conclusion to a patient's health expectation. The words *goal, objective,* and *outcome* are often used interchangeably. In some practice settings, the term *goal* or *objective* is used to describe what is wanted, and the term *outcome* is used to describe the results achieved. In nursing, the phrase **expected outcomes** is used to refer to the more specific, measurable **criteria** used to evaluate the extent to which a goal has been met. This chapter uses *outcome* to refer to expected patient outcomes.

The nurse, patient, and family should work together as much as possible in the outcome identification and planning stage. If the outcomes specified in the care plan are not valued by the patient or do not contribute to the prevention, resolution, or reduction of the patient's problems or the achievement of the patient's health expectations, the care plan may be ineffective. Similarly, if social determinants of health create barriers that prevent the patient from realizing the outcomes, these need to be explored. Outcome determination is, therefore, a critical skill for successfully intervening with patients.

This chapter describes outcome identification and planning as a formal process, a deliberate phase in the nursing process. A formal plan of care allows nurses to:

- Individualize care that maximizes outcome achievement
- Set priorities
- Facilitate communication among nursing personnel and their colleagues
- Promote continuity of high-quality, cost-effective care
- Coordinate care
- Evaluate the patient's responses to nursing care
- Create a record that can be used for evaluation, research, reimbursement, and legal purposes
- Promote the nurse's professional development

Nurses also engage in informal planning in practice. This is the link between identifying a patient's strength or problem and providing an appropriate nursing response.

A nurse on a busy surgical unit learns that a postoperative patient is complaining of incisional pain; they quickly reshuffles priorities to allow time to assess the course and qualities of the pain, and to determine nursing measures to reduce discomfort. Planning has occurred. A postpartum nurse realizes the evening before the mother's discharge that they has not seen the father hold his new daughter; they make a mental note to observe the father–daughter interactions that evening and facilitate their bonding. Planning has occurred. A nurse in a geriatric daycare center hears a patient choking and rushes to their side to perform the Heimlich maneuver if necessary. Planning has occurred.

Informal planning on a more deliberate level is illustrated by a hospice nurse who drives home pondering how best to support a patient with terminal cancer who is gradually relinquishing her hold on life. The hospice nurse may elect to initiate a more formal process of planning the next day when consulting with colleagues who have cared for patients with similar health needs.

In each of these examples, the process of informal planning allowed an individual nurse to think about how best to help a particular patient—ideally, with good results. What is lacking is a coordinated plan known by everyone caring for the patient.

QSEN Reflective Practice: Cultivating QSEN Competencies

CHALLENGE TO ETHICAL AND LEGAL SKILLS

While working in a women's shelter, I met Darla Jefferson, a 29-year-old single woman who was about 14 weeks pregnant. Darla described herself as a "hopeless addict" who had tried to stop "more times than I can remember." She was drug-free at the moment but not hopeful of preventing relapse. She did not know her baby's father and had mixed feelings about keeping the baby. She said, "On the one hand I want someone to love me, but I'm not sure I'd want me for a mother." I knew I needed to explore her commitment to this pregnancy, but I am strongly opposed to abortion and did not think I could talk with her objectively about her decision. I needed to develop a plan for dealing with this issue.

Thinking Outside the Box: Possible Courses of Action

- Tell Darla that I believe it is her responsibility to have this baby and to then make a decision about whether to offer the baby for adoption based on her assessment of her parenting readiness.
- Help Darla assess her readiness to become a parent and, in light of this, explore all her options regarding continuing or terminating the pregnancy.
- Get someone else to talk with Darla so that she gets the counseling she needs and I am not morally compromised.

Evaluating a Good Outcome: How Do I Define Success?

- Darla gets the help she needs to make the decision that is right for her and her unborn baby.
- I am faithful to both my nursing responsibilities to counsel this patient and my duty to maintain my moral integrity.

Personal Learning: Here's to the Future!

Unfortunately, I overestimated my ability to counsel Darla without compromising myself, and as a result, I don't think I was as helpful to her as I should have been. Ideally, I planned to objectively explore her readiness to be a mother and then have an open and unbiased discussion about her options. When she began to talk about getting an abortion, I found myself urging her to have the baby and then place the baby up for adoption if she still felt she couldn't care for the infant after delivery. Regrettably, I let my personal opinions come through in the discussion. Through my actions, I think she lost trust in me. I'm going to talk with other nurses to see how they handle this challenge.

QSEN SELF-REFLECTION ON QUALITY AND SAFETY COMPETENCIES DEVELOPING KNOWLEDGE, SKILLS, AND ATTITUDES FOR CONTINUOUS IMPROVEMENT

How would you respond in a similar situation? Why? What does this tell you about yourself and about the adequacy of your competencies for professional practice? Can you think of other ways to respond? What actions might have proved more effective? What actions might be helpful for the nursing student so that when faced with similar situations in the future, the outcome would be more positive? Do you agree with the criteria that the nursing student used to evaluate a successful outcome? Why or why not? What *knowledge, skills,* and *attitudes* do you need to develop to continuously improve the quality and safety of care for patients like Ms. Jefferson?

Patient-Centered Care: How would you develop a successful partnership with Ms. Jefferson, knowing that she may choose an alternative that is unethical for you? Are nurses obligated to be ethically neutral when issues like this come up? How can you best communicate empathy and that you respect her even when you disagree with choices she makes?

Teamwork and Collaboration/Quality Improvement: What communication and interpersonal skills do you need to improve to ensure that you function as a member of the patient care team and to obtain assistance when needed? What does quality care for Ms. Jefferson look like?

Safety/Evidence-Based Practice: What does the evidence point to as "best practice" for Ms. Jefferson? What safety needs do she and her unborn baby have and how can you meet them?

Informatics: Can you identify the essential information that must be available in Ms. Jefferson's electronic record to support safe patient care and coordination of care? Can you think of other ways to respond to or approach the situation? What else might the nursing student have done to ensure a successful outcome?

UNIQUE FOCUS OF NURSING OUTCOME IDENTIFICATION AND PLANNING

The primary purpose of the outcome identification and planning step of the nursing process is to design a plan of care with and for the patient that, once implemented, results in the prevention, reduction, or resolution of patient health problems and the attainment of the patient's health expectations, as identified in the patient outcomes.

Become familiar with the registered nurse competencies for Standards 3 (Outcomes Identification) and 4 (Planning) in ANA's *Nursing: Scope and Standards of Practice* (2021). A comprehensive care plan additionally specifies any routine

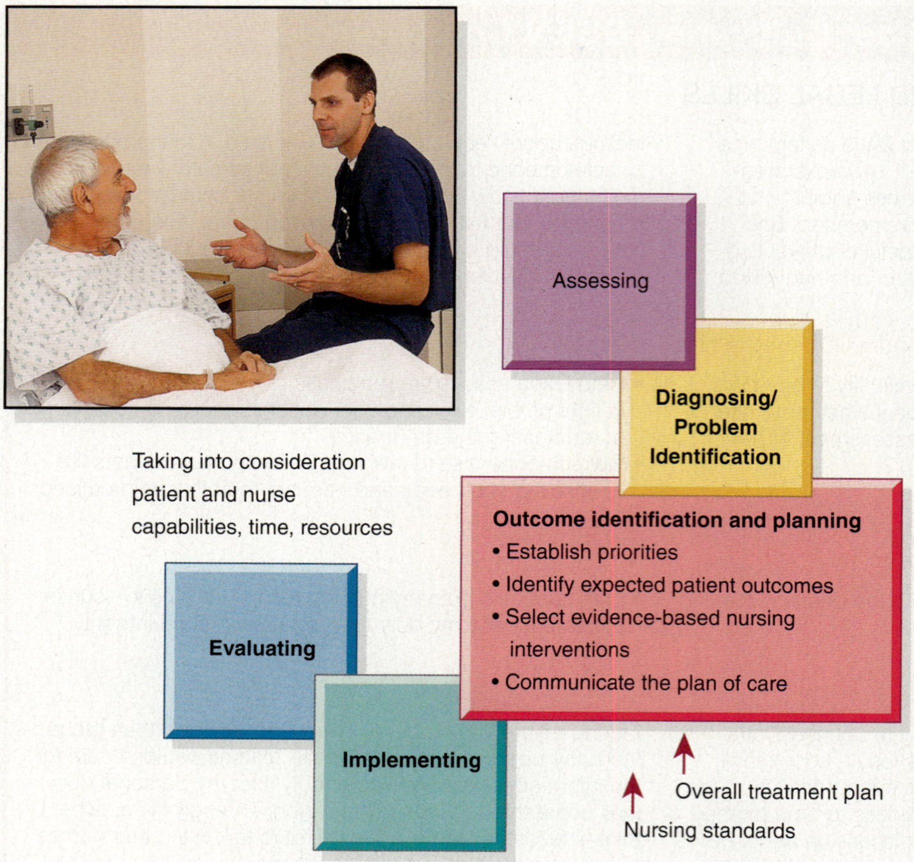

FIGURE 17-1. Outcome identification and planning. The nurse and patient work together to establish priorities, identify expected patient outcomes, and select evidence-based nursing interventions. The care plan should be consistent with nursing standards, congruent with other planned therapies, and realistic in terms of the patient's and nurse's abilities or resources. Ensuring that the care plan is recorded is also an important nursing responsibility. (Used with permission from Shutterstock. *Photo by B. Proud.*)

nursing assistance the patient needs to meet basic human needs (e.g., assistance with hygiene or nutrition) and describes appropriate nursing responsibilities for fulfilling the collaborative and medical care plan. For example, health care providers may delegate to nurses caring for a surgical patient the redressing of the surgical incision, the administration of prescribed medications and intravenous therapy, and the responsibility for scheduling laboratory studies. Nurses design care plans that incorporate their independent, dependent, and collaborative responsibilities. See the clinical decision making process illustrated in Figure 17-2 to help determine when you can act independently within your scope of practice. Because nursing is concerned with the patient's responses to health and illness, the plan of care is supportive of nursing's broad aims: to promote wellness, prevent disease and illness, promote recovery, and facilitate coping with altered functioning (see Chapter 1).

Critical Thinking/Clinical Reasoning and Judgment in Outcome Identification and Planning

Successful implementation of each phase of the nursing process requires high-level skills in critical thinking and specifically in clinical reasoning and judgment. To plan health care correctly, in your role as nurse, you must:

- Be familiar with standards and facility policies for setting priorities, identifying and recording expected patient outcomes, selecting evidence-based nursing interventions, and recording the care plan (Box 17-1).
- Remember that the goal of thoughtful, person-centered practice is to keep the patient and the patient's interests and preferences central in every aspect of planning and outcome identification.
- Keep the "big picture" in focus: What are the discharge goals for this patient, and how should this direct each nurse's interventions?
- Trust clinical experience and judgment but be willing to ask for help when the situation demands more than your qualifications and experience can provide; value collaborative practice.
- Respect your clinical intuitions, but before establishing priorities, identifying outcomes, and selecting nursing interventions, be sure that research supports your plan.
- Recognize your personal biases and keep an open mind.

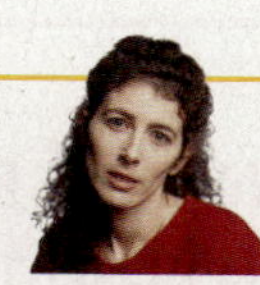

Remember **Darla Jefferson**, the pregnant woman with a history of drug abuse described in the Reflective Practice box on page 451. Although the nursing student planned to engage the patient in an unbiased discussion of her alternatives, the student was unable to adhere to the plan, inserting personal opinions in the discussion. As a result, the care plan was thwarted and the patient lost trust in the student.

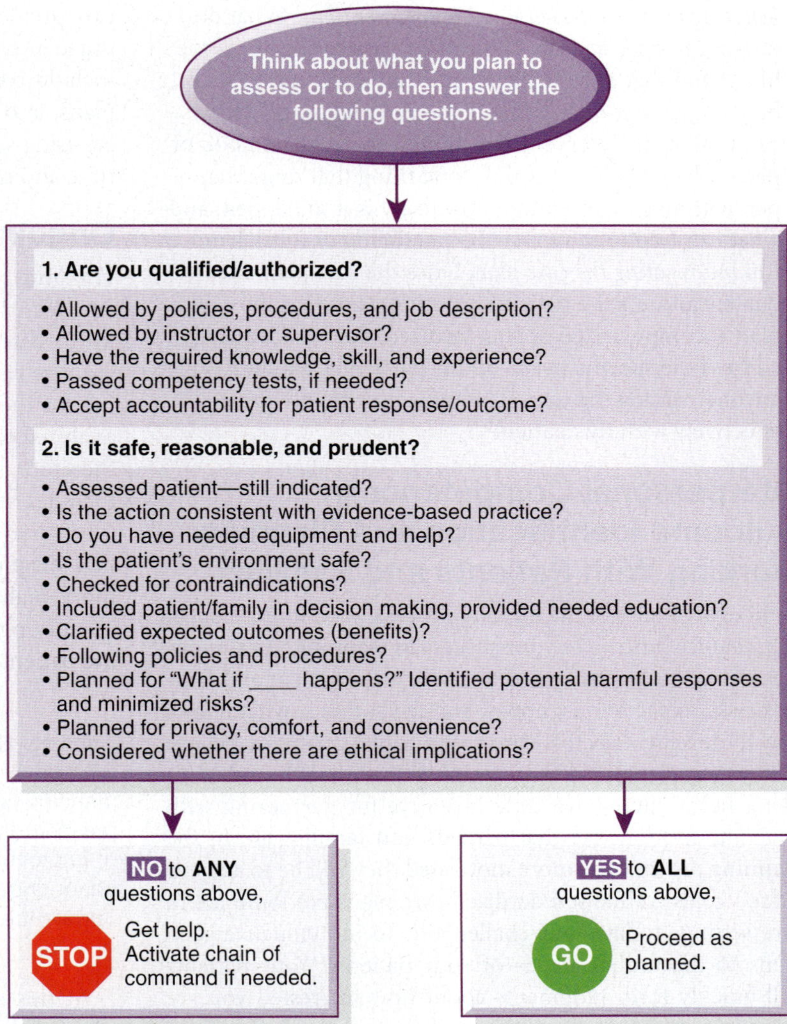

FIGURE 17-2. Clinical decision making and scope of practice. (*Source*: © 2019 R. Alfaro-LeFevre. http://www.AlfaroTeachSmart.com.)

Questions to facilitate clinical reasoning and judgment during planning and outcome identification include:

- *Setting priorities:* Which problems require my immediate attention or that of the team? Which problems are my responsibilities, and which should I refer to someone else? Which problems are most important to the patient?
- *Identifying outcomes:* What must I observe in the patient to demonstrate the resolution of the problems identified by the nursing diagnoses and general problem list? What is the time frame for accomplishing these outcomes? Do the outcomes need to be modified in light of the patient's response (or lack of response) to the planned interventions?

Box 17-1 Applying Standards to Plan Nursing Care

The standards you must apply when identifying outcomes and related nursing interventions are determined by:

- *The law.* Your state's nurse practice act outlines the scope of nursing practice. Your State Board of Nursing also outlines what you are and are not allowed to do.
- *Specialty professional organizations,* such as the American Association of Critical Care Nurses or Emergency Nurses Association, which develop standards for specialty practice.
- *The Joint Commission.* This powerful accrediting body has developed detailed standards that must be followed to keep accreditation.
- *The Agency for Healthcare Research and Quality (AHRQ).* This organization develops, reviews, and updates clinical guidelines to aid health care providers to prevent, diagnose, and manage clinical conditions.
- *Your employer.* Each facility usually develops its own unique set of standards (standards of care, guidelines, policies, procedures, critical pathways, standard care plans, and so forth) that reflect how nursing care should be given in specific situations.

Source: Reprinted with permission from Alfaro-LeFevre, R. (2010). Applying nursing process: A tool for critical thinking (7th ed., pp. 144–145). Wolters Kluwer Health/Lippincott Williams & Wilkins.

- *Selecting evidence-based nursing interventions:* What do nursing science and my clinical experience suggest is the likelihood that this particular nursing intervention will help the patient realize their expected outcomes? How can I tailor my interventions to increase the likelihood of patient benefit? What is the worst thing that might happen with this intervention, how likely is it to happen, and what can I do to minimize the possibility of this harm?
- *Communicating the care plan:* Does the care plan adequately address the patient's priorities today? If the care plan is computerized or standardized, does it adequately address the specific needs of this particular patient? Will anyone reading the care plan know how to intervene effectively with this patient?

Interpersonal Competence in Outcome Identification and Planning: Working With Patients and Families

As in every phase of the nursing process, your interpersonal competence influences your success in planning. As a nurse, you are uniquely positioned to understand patient and family needs, expectations, hopes, and fears; this is what allows you to develop effective care plans. Unless patients believe that you are committed to meeting their health and well-being needs, they have little incentive for partnering with you. The more active that patients and families are in the planning process, the more motivated they will be to achieve valued goals. While standardized care plans predominate in care settings today, your challenge is to individualize such plans to the unique needs of your patients. Your patients will quickly form judgments about how interested you are in learning enough about them to help them realistically set and meet valued outcomes.

COMPREHENSIVE PLANNING

In acute care settings, three basic stages of planning are critical to comprehensive nursing care: initial, ongoing, and discharge. In other settings such as long-term care, hospice care, or a community clinic, initial and ongoing planning may be the primary types of planning. If a nurse develops a comprehensive plan of care on the patient's first day but fails to update the plan, the plan will not be effective or efficient. Failure to update the plan of care as needed is a common problem in all health care settings.

Initial Planning

Initial planning is performed by the nurse with the admission nursing history and the physical assessment. This comprehensive plan addresses each problem listed in the prioritized nursing diagnoses and identifies appropriate patient goals and the related nursing care. **Standardized care plans** are prepared care plans that identify the nursing diagnoses, outcomes, and related nursing interventions common to a specific population or health problem. (An example of a standardized care plan is shown later in the chapter.) They can provide an excellent basis for the initial plan if the nurse individualizes them. Resources for standardized plans include computerized plans, textbooks with prepared care plans, and facility-developed plans/maps/critical pathways. By using such standardized plans, the nurse is free to direct time and expertise to individualizing the plan.

Ongoing Planning

Ongoing planning is carried out by any nurse who interacts with the patient. Its chief purpose is to keep the plan up to date to facilitate the resolution of health problems, manage risk factors, and promote function. The nurse caring for the patient uses new data as they are collected and analyzed to make the plan more specific and accurate and, therefore, more effective. The work of ongoing planning includes stating nursing diagnoses/problems more clearly (both the problem statement and the cause), developing new diagnoses/problems, adjusting patient outcomes to be more realistic, developing new outcomes as needed, and identifying nursing interventions that will best accomplish the patient goals.

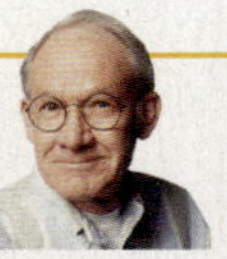

Consider **Elijah Wolinski**, the frail, older adult who developed a pressure injury. Ongoing planning is necessary because the patient's pressure injury would most likely take some time to heal or improve. In addition, other needs may become apparent during subsequent home visits, requiring the nurse to update the care plan.

At this stage of planning, standardized plans based on medical conditions or procedures may be useful in developing new nursing diagnoses/problems and related nursing interventions, but individualizing the plan is necessary to meet unique patient needs. For example, the standard nursing order "force fluids" might be rewritten as "offer 60-mL cranberry or orange juice between meals, and keep fresh water at bedside." A preliminary order such as "explore with the patient existing supports" might be replaced with "keep daughter Barbara informed of mother's progress and coach her in effective support strategies: Barbara Clems, (h) (703) 448–3211, (w) (202) 654–8999."

Discharge Planning

Discharge planning is best carried out by the nurse who has worked most closely with the patient and family, possibly in conjunction with a nurse or social worker with a broad knowledge of existing community resources. In acute care settings, comprehensive discharge planning begins when the patient is admitted for treatment—or even before admission. Careful planning ensures that the nurse uses teaching and counseling skills effectively to help the patient and family develop sufficient knowledge of the health problem and the therapeutic regimen to carry out necessary self-care behaviors at home competently. Discharge planning is further discussed in Chapter 12.

ESTABLISHING PRIORITIES

To develop a prioritized list of nursing diagnoses/problems, the nurse needs guidelines for ranking diagnoses as high, medium, or low priority. High-priority diagnoses pose the greatest threat to the patient's health and well-being. Diagnoses/problems that are not life threatening are ranked as medium priorities, and diagnoses/problems that are not specifically related to the current level of health or well-being are of low priority. In all levels, psychosocial needs must be considered as well as physiologic needs.

In addition to developing a prioritized list of nursing diagnoses/problems, nurses working within an interdisciplinary team need to set priorities for nursing care that take account of all the patient's health needs, as recorded on the general problem list. This involves looking at all problems to determine the relationships among the problems (what's causing or contributing to what). Thus, it generally makes sense to deal with medical (or suspected medical) problems first. If these can be resolved, many human response problems are gone. If a nurse sees the classic signs and symptoms of appendicitis and tries to identify and manage a nursing diagnosis of pain without consulting a physician or nurse practitioner, the patient's appendix might rupture before a nursing plan to relieve pain is even developed!

Three helpful guides to facilitate clinical reasoning when prioritizing patient problems include Maslow's hierarchy of human needs, patient preference, and anticipation of future problems.

Maslow's Hierarchy of Human Needs

Because basic needs must be met before a person can focus on higher ones, patient needs may be prioritized according to the following hierarchy:

1. Physiologic needs
2. Safety needs
3. Love and belonging needs
4. Self-esteem needs
5. Self-actualization needs

For example, a geriatric patient who is incontinent of urine and sitting in a wet disposable brief (physiologic need) will be unable to participate fully in a music therapy diversional activity (self-esteem need) until the more basic need is met. (Chapter 4 more fully discusses basic human needs.)

Patient Preference

Thoughtful, person-centered practice directs you to first meet the needs that the patient thinks are most important, as long as this order does not interfere with other vital therapies. For example, a woman is admitted to an orthopedic unit with a fractured pelvis and multiple lacerations after an automobile accident. The morning after the accident, she complains of pain and needs assistance with bathing and attention to her lacerations, but she refuses to do anything until she calls home to find out who is caring for her 15-month-old twins. The nurse should help her to call home before beginning other care as long as it does not interfere with life-saving emergency care.

Anticipation of Patient Needs

Nurses must tap their knowledge base to consider the potential effects of different nursing actions. Assigning low priority to a diagnosis that the patient wants to ignore but can result in harmful future consequences for the patient might be nursing negligence. For example, a patient experiencing obesity patient with multiple sclerosis and greatly decreased limb strength who spends most of their day in bed may see no value in diet modification and position changes. A nurse who is alert to the potentially serious problem of pressure injuries would assign high priority to this diagnosis, nonetheless, and incorporate weight management and position changes into the care plan despite the patient's reluctance.

Critical Thinking/Clinical Reasoning and Judgment and Establishing Priorities

The work of setting priorities demands careful clinical reasoning. Alfaro-LeFevre (2014, p. 132) suggests that nurses ask themselves these four questions:

1. What problems need immediate attention and what could happen if I wait to attend to them? Nurses can then initiate actions to solve problems with simple solutions, such as repositioning a patient to improve her breathing or calling a family member in.
2. Which problems are my responsibilities and which do I need to refer to someone else?
3. Which problems can be dealt with by using standard plans (e.g., critical paths, standards of care)?
4. Which problems aren't covered by protocols or standard plans but must be addressed to ensure a safe hospital stay and timely discharge (or simply safe care of high quality)?

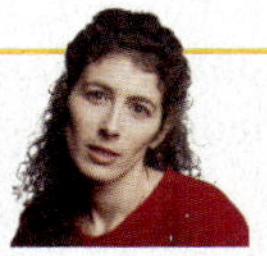

Think back to **Darla Jefferson**, the pregnant woman with a history of drug abuse. The nurse would incorporate clinical reasoning by asking these four questions, thereby ultimately arriving at the patient problems requiring the most immediate attention.

When planning nursing care for each day, consider the following:

- Have changes in the patient's health status influenced the priority of nursing diagnoses/problems? For example, when a routine home visit to an older adult reveals evidence of possible elder abuse, a new diagnosis may result in a new set of care priorities.
- Have changes in the way the patient is responding to health and illness or the care plan affected those nursing diagnoses/problems that can be realistically addressed? For example, a nurse might have identified coping as a

high-priority problem for the patient after the patient learned the medical diagnosis and planned to initiate counseling. If the patient adamantly requests to be left alone for a day to think things through, however, the nurse has to modify priorities of care for that day.

- Are there relationships among diagnoses/problems that require that one be worked on before another can be resolved?
- Can several patient problems be dealt with together?

After answering these questions, the nurse ranks the diagnoses/problems in the order in which they should be addressed. Setting priorities enables the nurse to make sure that time and energy are being directed first to the patient's most important problems.

IDENTIFYING AND WRITING OUTCOMES

Learning to identify and write appropriate outcomes takes practice. The following sections will help you to identify outcomes that will maximize your effectiveness when working with patients.

Deriving Outcomes From Nursing Diagnoses/Problems

Outcomes are derived from the problem statement. For each problem in the care plan, at least one outcome should be written that, if achieved, demonstrates a direct resolution of the problem statement (Table 17-1).

Other outcomes that contribute to the resolution of the problem may be written as well. For example, for the diagnosis *Body weight problem: Overweight; etiologic factors: excessive snacking and inactivity*, in addition to the outcome "Within 12 weeks (by 12/6/25), the patient will lose 20 lb and reach target weight (122 lb)," the following goals are appropriate: "Within 3 days of teaching, the patient will identify 10 low-calorie snack foods he is willing to try; the patient will have 3-day diet recall consistent with nutritionally balanced 1,500-calorie diet; the patient will report incorporating three half-hour periods of walking at 5 miles per hour into each week." If the patient can identify low-calorie snack foods and adopt a more active lifestyle, there is a greater likelihood that he will reach his target weight, but it is entirely possible for a patient to achieve these secondary outcomes without resolving the chief problem. Remember, at least one outcome per problem statement must directly resolve the problem.

Table 17-1 Examples of Goals/Outcomes to Relieve Problems

PROBLEM STATEMENT OF THE NURSING DIAGNOSIS	RELATED PATIENT GOAL/OUTCOME
Pain	Within 8 hours, patient will report pain is absent or diminished
Nutrition Problem: More Than Body Requirements	Within 2 weeks (by 12/6/25), patient will reach target weight of 122 lb
Impaired Physical Mobility	Before discharge, patient will ambulate length of hallway independently

The **Nursing Outcomes Classification (NOC)** developed by the Iowa Outcomes Project presents the first comprehensive standardized language used to describe the patient outcomes that are responsive to nursing intervention (Moorhead et al., 2013). The current classification lists 490 outcomes with definitions, indicators, measurement scales, and supporting references. The outcomes may be used for individuals, families, or communities. Explicit linkages between the North American Nursing Diagnosis Association-International (NANDA-I) diagnoses and the NOC facilitate a comprehensive approach to care planning. Remember whenever you use standardized language to ensure that it adequately captures the uniqueness of your patients and families.

Establishing Long-Term Versus Short-Term Outcomes

Outcomes may be either long term or short term. Long-term outcomes require a longer period (usually more than a week) to be achieved than do short-term outcomes. They also may be used as discharge goals, in which case they are more broadly written and communicate to the entire nursing team the desired end results of nursing care for a particular patient. For example, two women, both 77 years of age, are on a nursing unit after undergoing similar operations for fractured left hips. One woman has spent the past 2 years in bed in a long-term care facility; the other woman fractured her hip at the YMCA, where she swims daily. Their nursing care should not be the same because it is directed toward different long-term goals, even though their short-term goals may be similar (Box 17-2).

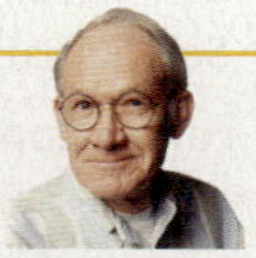

Consider ***Elijah Wolinski***, the frail, older adult with a pressure injury. The nurse might establish a long-term outcome such as, "The patient's sacral area will exhibit no evidence of a pressure injury." Short-term outcomes might include, "The patient's sacral pressure injury demonstrates an absence of purulent drainage within 1 week of initiating wound care. By week 2, the patient's pressure injury has decreased in size by 1 cm. By week 2, the patient's caregiver demonstrates measures to relieve pressure on the skin while the patient is in bed."

Determining Patient-Centered Outcomes

Alfaro-LeFevre (2020, p. 164) recommends that nurses first ask patients to describe two or three major goals they would like to achieve. Nurses then should be realistic and consider:

Box 17-2 Examples of Long- and Short-Term Outcomes

Patient on Bed Rest From Long-Term Care Facility

Long-Term Outcome

Mrs. Goldstein returns to the long-term care facility pain free with her incision healed and her left leg in good alignment.

Short-Term Outcomes

- Whenever observed, patient will be lying in bed with legs in correct alignment (abductor pillow in place, if ordered).
- Before discharge, Mrs. Goldstein's hip incision will show signs of healing (skin surfaces approximate, free from signs of infection—redness, swelling, heat, purulent drainage).
- Whenever observed, patient will report that comfort measures and medication are satisfactorily managing pain.

Active Patient From Private Home

Long-Term Outcome

Mrs. Silverstein returns home to her husband pain free with incision healed, fully mobile (full weight bearing on left leg), and capable of independent activities of daily living.

Short-Term Outcomes

- By 1/28/25, the patient will verbalize willingness to participate in physical therapy program.
- By 2/4/24, the patient will ambulate (with nursing assistance and walker) to bathroom (full weight bearing).
- By 2/11/24, the patient will ambulate with nursing assistance only (no walker) in her room.
- Goals for incision and pain relief same as for Mrs. Goldstein.

- Patient's health state and overall prognosis
- Expected length of stay
- Growth and development
- Patient values and cultural considerations
- Other planned therapies for the patient
- Available human, material, and financial resources
- Risks, benefits, and current scientific evidence
- Changes in status that indicate the need to modify usual expected outcomes

Moorhead et al. (2013, p. 32) recommend considering the following factors when selecting outcomes: (1) the type of health concern, (2) the nursing or medical diagnoses, (3) patient characteristics, (4) available resources, (5) patient preferences, and (6) treatment potential.

Family Involvement

One of the most important considerations in writing outcomes is to encourage the patient and family to be as involved in goal development as their abilities and interest permit. When developing patient outcomes, the nurse, patient, and family look at the problem statement of the nursing diagnosis/problem and ask, "What patient changes or outcomes will result in the prevention or resolution of this problem?" The answer, when carefully worded, becomes the patient outcome.

Using Cognitive, Psychomotor, and Affective Outcomes

Outcomes may be categorized according to the type of change needed by a patient. Cognitive outcomes describe increases in patient knowledge or intellectual behaviors—for example: "Within 1 day after teaching, the patient will list three benefits of continuing to apply moist compresses to leg ulcer after discharge." Psychomotor outcomes describe the patient's achievement of new skills—for example, "By 6/12/25, the patient will correctly demonstrate application of wet-to-dry dressing on leg ulcer." Affective outcomes describe changes in patient values, beliefs, and attitudes. Difficult both to write and to evaluate, affective outcomes could be critical to the resolution of a complex patient problem—for example, "By 6/12/25, the patient will verbalize valuing health sufficiently to practice new health behaviors to prevent recurrence of leg ulcer." In this example, even if the patient intellectually grasps the reasons for taking care of her leg and can competently redress her ulcer, unless she is motivated to take care of herself, her knowledge and skills will not result in healthy outcomes. See Chapter 19 for other examples of these outcomes.

Identifying Clinical, Functional, and Quality-of-Life Outcomes

Another way to think about the types of outcomes to identify is to categorize them as clinical, functional, or quality of life. Alfaro-LeFevre (2014, p. 137) presents them as follows:

Clinical outcomes describe the expected status of health issues at certain points in time, after treatment is complete. They address whether the problems are resolved or to what degree they are improved.

Functional outcomes describe the person's ability to function in relation to the desired usual activities.

Quality-of-life outcomes focus on key factors that affect someone's ability to enjoy life and achieve personal goals.

Identifying Culturally Appropriate Outcomes

The American Nurses Association (ANA) Scope and Standards of Practice (2021) direct nurses to practice in a manner that is *congruent with cultural diversity and inclusion principles.* See Chapter 5 for a discussion of culturally appropriate care.

Identifying Outcomes Supportive of the Total Treatment Plan

When identifying outcomes, always remember that nurses nurse *people*, not problems. This means that every outcome you write should support the overall treatment plan and "make sense" in terms of the overall goals for the patient. For example, identifying nutritional outcomes may be appropriate for a patient who is losing weight, but if this patient is in a hospice and dying, this may not be an appropriate outcome if it is incompatible with the overall goal of a peaceful death with dignity.

Writing Patient-Centered Measurable Outcomes

To be measurable, outcomes should have the following:

- *Subject:* the patient or some part of the patient.
- *Verb:* the action the patient will perform.

  Verbs helpful in writing measurable outcomes include:

Define	List	Explain
Prepare	Verbalize	Select
Identify	Describe	Apply
Design	Choose	Demonstrate

- *Conditions:* the particular circumstances in or by which the outcome is to be achieved. Not every outcome specifies conditions.
- *Performance criteria:* the expected patient behavior or other manifestation described in observable, measurable terms.
- *Target time:* when the patient is expected to be able to achieve the outcome. The target time or time criterion may be a realistic, actual date or other statement indicating time, such as "before discharge," "after viewing film," or "whenever observed."

  Here are two examples of properly constructed measurable outcomes:

  "During the next 24-hour period, the patient's fluid intake will total at least 2,000 mL."

  "At the next visit, 12/23/25, the patient will correctly demonstrate relaxation exercises."

It often helps to include special conditions when writing an outcome if this information is important for other nurses—for example, "Before discharge, the patient will ambulate independently the length of hallway and back, using a Philadelphia collar to support cervical vertebrae."

A memory jog for writing goals and outcomes is the word SMART (Doran, 1981):

S—specific
M—measurable
A—attainable
R—realistic
T—time-bound

Avoiding Common Errors in Outcomes

Common errors when writing patient outcomes include the following:

Expressing the patient outcome as a nursing intervention

Incorrect: "Offer Mr. Myer 60-mL fluid every 2 hours while awake."

Correct: "Mr. Myer will drink 60-mL fluid every 2 hours while awake, beginning 2/24/25."

Using verbs that are not observable and measurable

Incorrect: "Mrs. Gaston will know how to bathe her newborn." Verbs to be avoided when writing goals include "know," "understand," "learn," and "become aware." These verbs are too general and cannot be measured. Verbs for writing outcomes should be observable and measurable (as listed previously).

Correct: "After attending the infant care class, Mrs. Gaston will correctly demonstrate the procedure for bathing her newborn."

Including more than one patient behavior/manifestation in short-term outcomes

Incorrect: "Patient will list dangers of smoking and stop smoking."

Correct: "By next meeting, 3/11/25, the patient will (1) identify three dangers of smoking and (2) describe a plan he is willing to try to stop smoking. By 6/20/25, the patient will report that he no longer smokes."

Writing outcomes that are so vague that other nurses are unsure of the goal of nursing care

Incorrect: "Patient will cope better."

Correct: "After teaching, 10/20/25, the patient will (1) describe two new coping strategies he is willing to try and (2) demonstrate decreased incidence of previously observed ineffective coping behaviors (chain smoking, withdrawal behavior, heavy alcohol consumption)."

Ensuring Quality Outcomes

The Committee on Quality Health Care in America of the Institute of Medicine, now the National Academy of Sciences, Engineering, and Medicine (2001), in its report *Crossing the Quality Chasm*, highlights six aims to be met by health care systems with regard to the quality of care:

1. *Safe:* avoiding injury
2. *Effective:* avoiding overuse and underuse
3. *Patient centered:* responding to patient preferences, needs, and values
4. *Timely:* reducing waits and delays
5. *Efficient:* avoiding waste
6. *Equitable:* providing care that does not vary in quality to all recipients

Institutions measuring their achievement of these aims will welcome nursing's efforts to determine its effectiveness (Moorhead et al., 2013, p. 32).

Joint Commission National Patient Safety Goals

The Joint Commission publishes standards and requirements for Joint Commission accreditation and certification programs. Be sure to check their website (www.jointcommission.org) and pay special attention to the National Patient Safety Goals. The purpose of the National Patient Safety Goals is to improve patient safety, focusing on problems in health care safety and how to solve them. The 2020 Hospital National Patient Safety goals included (https://www.jointcommission.org/en/standards/national-patient-safety-goals/):

- Identify patients correctly
- Improve staff communication

- Use medicines safely
- Use alarms safely
- Prevent infection
- Identify patient safety risks
- Prevent mistakes in surgery

Chapter 19 describes other examples to ensure quality outcomes.

Healthy People Goals

Healthy People identifies our nation's health improvement priorities. For more than 30 years, Healthy People has established evidence-based national health objectives with clear targets that allow us to monitor progress, motivate action, and guide efforts to improve health across the country.

With a focus on ambitious, yet achievable, 10-year goals and targets, the Healthy People 2020 initiative. Healthy People 2030 sets data driven national objectives to achieve health and well-being over the next decade. Healthy People 2030 includes 355 core- or measurable-objectives as well as developmental and research objectives. Leading health indicators (LHIs) are a small subset of high priority objectives selected to drive action toward improving health and well-being (https://health.gov/healthypeople).

- Establishes 26 Leading Health Indicators selected from high-priority objectives—the majority of which are making positive progress toward achieving their targets
- Gathers and displays the best-available evidence and data to improve public health practices and strengthen existing health policies
- Provides user-centered tools for health professionals to improve the health of their communities
- Develops a platform for the public to give input and suggest additional objectives to ensure current public health priorities are represented

IDENTIFYING NURSING INTERVENTIONS

The **Nursing Interventions Classification (NIC)** project defines a **nursing intervention** as "any treatment based upon clinical judgment and knowledge that a nurse performs to enhance patient/client outcomes" (Bulechek et al., 2013, p. 2). The NIC project further goes on to describe the types of interventions:

> The Classification includes interventions that nurses do on behalf of patients, both independent and collaborative interventions, both direct and indirect care. NIC interventions include both the physiologic (e.g., Acid–Base Management) and the psychosocial (e.g., Anxiety Reduction)…. Interventions are included for illness treatment (e.g., Hyperglycemia Management), illness prevention (e.g., Fall Prevention), and health promotion (e.g., Exercise Promotion). Most of the interventions are for use with individuals, but many are for use with families (e.g., Family Integrity Promotion) and some for entire communities (e.g., Environmental Management: Community). Indirect care interventions (e.g., Supply Management) are also included.

Carpenito-Moyet (2017a, pp. 37–38) describes how the major focus of intervention differs according to the type of nursing diagnoses or collaborative problem being addressed. For actual nursing diagnoses, interventions seek to:

- Reduce or eliminate contributing factors of the diagnosis/problem
- Promote higher-level wellness
- Monitor and evaluate status

For risk nursing diagnoses, interventions seek to:

- Reduce or eliminate risk factors
- Prevent the problem
- Monitor and evaluate status

For possible nursing diagnoses, interventions seek to:

- Collect additional data to rule out or confirm the diagnosis

For collaborative problems, interventions seek to:

- Monitor for changes in status
- Manage changes in status with nurse- and physician-prescribed interventions
- Evaluate response

Your challenge in the planning phase of the nursing process is to identify the nursing interventions most likely to achieve the outcomes. There are nurse-initiated, physician-initiated, and collaborative interventions.

Nurse-Initiated Interventions

A **nurse-initiated intervention** is an autonomous action based on scientific rationale that a nurse executes to benefit the patient in a predictable way related to the nursing diagnosis and projected outcomes. According to Alfaro-LeFevre (2014, pp. 142–143), nursing interventions are actions performed by the nurse to:

1. Monitor patient health status and response to treatment
2. Reduce risks
3. Resolve, prevent, or manage a problem
4. Promote independence with activities of daily living
5. Promote optimum sense of physical, psychological, and spiritual well-being
6. Give patients the information they need to make informed decisions and be independent

Nurse-initiated interventions do not require a health care provider's (or other team member's) order. Nurse-initiated interventions, such as patient goals, are derived from the nursing diagnosis/patient problem. But whereas the problem statement of the diagnosis suggests the patient goals, it is the cause of the problem (etiology) that suggests the nursing interventions (Fig. 17-3 on page 460). Effective nurses select nursing interventions that specifically address factors that cause or contribute to the patient's problems. For example, many factors may contribute to obesity, such as deficient

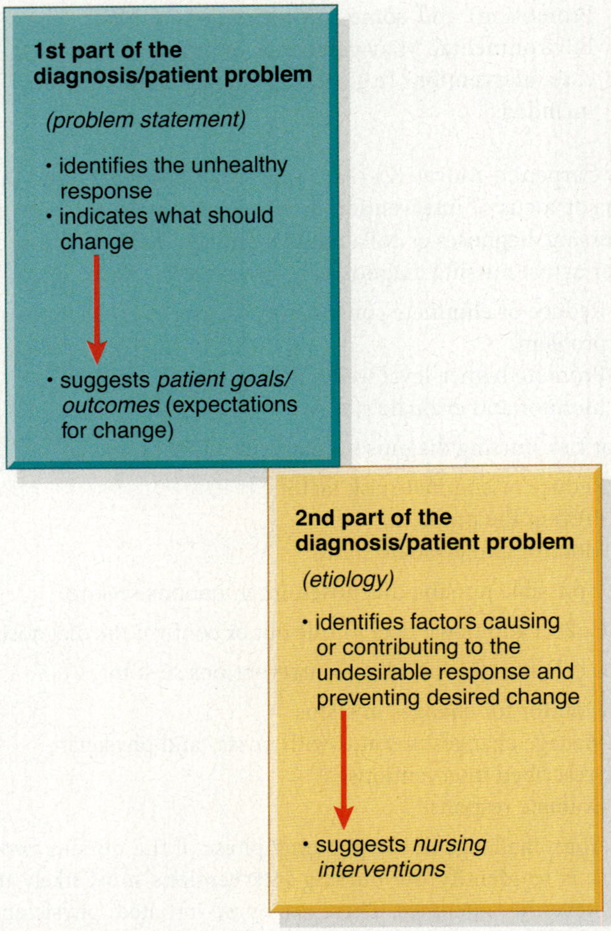

FIGURE 17-3. Deriving patient goals/outcomes and nursing orders from nursing diagnoses/problems.

nutritional knowledge, convenience of high-calorie fast foods, lifetime snacking habits, limited food budget, little exercise, food desert, and low self-esteem. The nurse working with a patient who wants to lose weight could attempt to deal with all these factors, but this approach would be inefficient. When a carefully developed nursing diagnosis identifies the specific factors that contribute to a particular patient's weight problem, nursing interventions can be selected to deal directly with these factors.

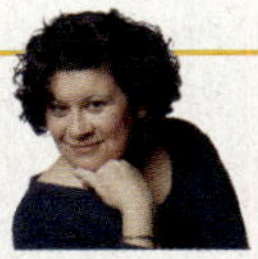

Remember **Glenda Kronk**, the woman desiring to improve her fitness. Based on assessment, the nurse determines the factors that have played a role in the patient's current status, developing appropriate nursing diagnoses and outcomes from which to establish appropriate interventions. For example, if the patient has been sedentary over the past several years, interventions should focus on measures to increase the patient's activity level, thereby promoting improvement in her overall health and fitness.

Similarly, nursing interventions for a patient with the diagnostic statement *Body weight problem: Overweight; etiologic factors: lifetime snacking habits and heavy reliance on high-calorie fast foods* might include education about the fat content and calories in fast foods and exploration of ways the patient could change eating habits to eat more nutritionally balanced meals with fewer calories. Thus, the nursing approach is not the same for every patient with a weight problem. The art of thoughtful, person-centered nursing practice involves the careful identification of the specific nursing interventions needed by particular patients to meet their individual needs.

Identifying and Selecting Appropriate Nurse-Initiated Interventions

After writing the patient outcomes, the nurse identifies various nursing interventions to help the patient achieve the outcomes. The Nursing Interventions Classification (NIC), the first comprehensive, validated list of nursing interventions applicable to all settings that can be used by nurses in multiple specialties, greatly facilitates the work of identifying appropriate interventions. Go to this website to see the NIC taxonomy: https://nursing.uiowa.edu/cncce/nursing-interventions-classification-overview. Bulechek et al. (2013, p. 13) write that the selection of a nursing intervention for a particular patient is part of the clinical judgment of the nurse. They identify six factors that should be considered when choosing an intervention: (1) desired patient outcomes, (2) characteristics of the nursing diagnosis, (3) research base for the intervention, (4) feasibility for doing the intervention, (5) acceptability to the patient, and (6) capability of the nurse.

The effectiveness of the nurse is directly proportional to the nurse's knowledge of varied nursing strategies. Consider the following different nursing care options identified by three nurses when they are asked to describe nursing care for a woman 2 days after cesarean delivery who is complaining of pain in the incisional area.

Nurse A

- Check to see what type of pain medication is ordered, and give it if the time interval is sufficient.

Nurse B

- Assess the quality of the pain, and use this time to communicate support by means of expression and squeeze of hand.
- Administer analgesic if indicated.
- Assess effectiveness of the analgesic ordered.

Nurse C

- Assess quality of the pain, and explore the possibility of contributing factors such as the effects of increased gas in the abdominal area or concern about the newborn, herself, or other family members.
- Use empathic listening (possibly touch) to communicate support and to encourage the mother to share her concerns.
- Change the patient's position in bed.
- Offer a backrub.
- If appropriate, suggest activity that will distract attention from the pain (e.g., watching a film about newborn care or listening to music).

Box 17-3 Guidelines for Selecting Nursing Interventions

Nursing interventions should be:

- Valued, whenever possible, by the patient and family
- Appropriate in terms of the diagnosis/patient problem and related patient outcomes, safe, and efficient
- Consistent with research findings and standards of care
- Realistic in terms of the abilities, time, and resources available to the nurse and patient
- Compatible with the patient's values, beliefs, and cultural and psychosocial background
- Compatible with other planned therapies

- Give the prescribed medication for pain and observe its effect.
- When administering the medication, use the power of positive suggestion to enhance its effectiveness: "This will start taking the pain away in about 10 minutes and will help you relax."

It is possible that the patient simply needs her prescribed analgesic to achieve the outcome: "Patient will report minimal to no pain at assessment every 2 hours." In that case, all three nurses would be effective in meeting the patient's need for nursing care. It is highly possible, however, that the prescribed medication is not sufficient or the pain is compounded by the mother's fears about caring for her new baby or by her worries that the baby will ruin her relationship with her husband. Therefore, Nurse C, whose knowledge level is more comprehensive, is likely to be most effective in resolving the patient's problem.

The more varied the options available to the nurse, the more effective the nursing response. In different situations, a skilled nursing procedure, the appropriate use of silence, respectful listening, humor, teaching, counseling, and touch can all be effective nursing strategies. Nurses who are merely task oriented and satisfied to meet every patient problem with a mechanical procedure are limiting their effectiveness.

When selecting nursing interventions for individual patients, use the guidelines in Box 17-3. These guidelines help ensure that the patient will achieve the outcome. Ongoing evaluation enables the nurse to determine the effectiveness of the selected interventions.

Reducing Variation

If there is one thing that systemness and the 2020 pandemic taught us, it is that we all need to quickly adopt best practices. In a 2020 viewpoint on "Choices for the 'new normal,'" Donald Berwick, president emeritus of the Institute for Health Care Improvement states that clinicians in the new normal may be less tolerant of unwarranted variation in health care practice. What COVID-19 did was make all frontline caregivers seek guidance from trusted sources. "This is the way we do it here" gave way very quickly to "What are experts saying is the best course of action for all of us?" Never before has there been a greater emphasis on all professional caregivers researching and sharing best practices. Nurses have a critical role to play in researching and communicating best practices. Berwick's question is one we all need to ponder: "Will the new normal embrace global learning, shared knowledge, and trusted authority as foundations for reducing harmful, wasteful, and unscientific variation in care?" (Berwick, 2020).

If you are interested in learning about best practices, you may want to check out the American Association of Critical Care Nurses website (https://www.aacn.org/clinical-resources). There you will find:

- Practice Alerts, directives to guide evidence-based nursing practice within the context of a healthy work environment;
- CSI Innovation Projects, strategies, interventions, tools, and outcomes from successful nurse-led change initiatives; and
- Clinical Pearls and other resources.

Individualizing Evidence-Based Interventions

Nurse researchers are attempting to establish a statistical pattern for predicting the probability of success for select nursing interventions. Using the student care plan at the end of this chapter, review the scientific rationale for the selected nursing orders. You should always be prepared to explain why you are doing intervention "a" as opposed to intervention "b" or "c." You should know how likely it is that the proposed intervention will achieve the desired outcomes and what the associated risks are. Nurses should answer four key questions when determining individualized evidence-based interventions:

1. What can be done to prevent or minimize the risks or causes of this problem?
2. What can be done to manage the problem?
3. How can I tailor interventions to meet expected outcomes?
4. How likely are we to get desired versus adverse responses to the interventions, and what can we do to reduce the risks and increase the likelihood of beneficial responses?

Alfaro-LeFevre (2014, p. 148) cautions nurses using standard and electronic plans to always do this with a critical mind. Remember that you are responsible for:

- detecting changes in patient status that may contraindicate using the plan.
- using good judgment about which parts of the plan apply and which do not.
- recognizing when problems are not covered by the plan and finding other ways to address them. (Some facilities, e.g., have an additional page that can be placed on the record to address "out-of-the-box" situations.)
- adding unique patient requirements (e.g., walker) in appropriate places.

You can learn more about evidence-based practice in Chapter 2 and in the Research in Nursing and PICOT in Practice recurring displays in the clinical chapters (Units VI and VII). Competent nurses use research findings (science of nursing), experience, and knowledge of the patient (art of nursing) to help select effective nursing interventions. Consultation with nurse colleagues and continuing education also assist nurses to develop effective nursing approaches to patients' problems.

Recording Nurse-Initiated Interventions in the Patient Record

Nursing interventions describe, and thus communicate to the entire nursing staff and health care team, the specific nursing care to be implemented for the patient. Each nursing intervention should include:

- Date
- Verb: Action to be performed
- Subject: Who is to do it
- Descriptive phrase: How, when, where, how often, how long, or how much
- Signature

Well-written nursing interventions accomplish the following:

- Assist the patient to meet specific outcomes that are related directly to one outcome.
- Clearly and concisely describe the nursing action to be performed (i.e., answer the questions who, what, where, when, and how).
- Are dated when written and when the care plan is reviewed.
- Are signed by the nurse prescribing the order or intervention.
- Use only those abbreviations accepted in the institution. (These are usually found in the facility's policy manual; a list of commonly accepted abbreviations appears in Chapter 20.)
- Refer the nurse to the facility's procedure manual or other literature for the steps of routine, lengthy procedures.

Here are some examples of well-stated nursing interventions:

- Offer patient 60-mL water or juice (prefers orange or cranberry juice) every 2 hours while awake for a total minimum PO intake of 500 mL.
- Teach patient the necessity of carefully monitoring fluid intake and output; remind patient each shift to mark off fluid intake on record at bedside.
- Walk with patient to bathroom for toileting every 2 hours (on even hours) while patient is awake.

Concept Mastery Alert

Outcome statements reflect the result or what to achieve; interventions state how the nurse will go about trying to achieve the result.

The set of nursing interventions written to assist a patient to meet an outcome must be comprehensive. Comprehensive nursing interventions specify what *observations* (assessments) need to be made and how often; what nursing *interventions* need to be done and when they must be done; and what *teaching, counseling,* and *advocacy* needs patients and families have.

Many sets of nursing interventions are inadequate because they fail to indicate the ongoing assessment priority needs for a specific problem or goal. Clearly stating assessment priorities helps all nurses to be more sensitive to important patient data.

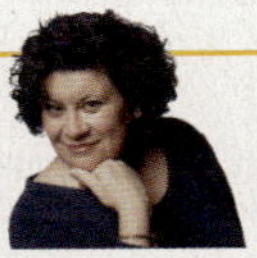

Review the scenario for **Glenda Kronk** at the beginning of the chapter. The nurse would need to establish assessment priorities. In assisting Glenda to reach her target weight, appropriate nursing interventions might include the following: "6/17/25: Continue to assess (1) patient's motivation to participate in weight-loss program and (2) factors that positively or negatively influence weight loss."

Similarly, nurses should not assume that all patients have the same teaching needs. Many patients have an excellent knowledge base, which in some cases may be greater than that of the nurse for a particular disease. Patients who are learning to live with a chronic illness may need counseling instead of teaching. However, it is important to obtain proof of the patient's knowledge or competency before proceeding with the care plan. For example, a diabetic patient would need to state the signs and symptoms of hypo- and hyperglycemia or give a return demonstration of doing a fingerstick blood glucose test. In summary, comprehensive nursing interventions relate to individual patient needs.

Physician-Initiated and Collaborative Interventions

An intervention is initiated by a physician in response to a medical diagnosis but is carried out by a nurse in response to a doctor's order. For example, a physician examining a patient brought into the emergency department after a motor vehicle accident might ask the nurse to administer a medication to relieve pain and to schedule the patient for radiographs and other diagnostic tests. The nurse who performs these interventions is implementing **physician-initiated interventions**. Both the physician and nurse are legally responsible for these interventions, and nurses are expected to be knowledgeable about how to execute these interventions safely and effectively. Nurses who question the appropriateness of physician-initiated interventions are legally responsible to seek clarification of the order with responsible parties. Under no circumstances should a nurse implement a questionable intervention, even at the urging of a physician or other professional. Chapter 7 addresses nurses' legal responsibility for their actions.

Nurses also carry out treatments initiated by other providers such as pharmacists, respiratory therapists, or physician assistants; these are **collaborative interventions**. For example, nurses caring for a patient after a motor vehicle accident may eventually implement interventions written by a physical therapist, occupational therapist, or other member of the health care team.

Structured Care Methodologies

Efforts to standardize nursing care have taken different forms. Popular past approaches have included procedures (1960s), standards of care (1970s), algorithms (1980s), and clinical practice guidelines (1990s). Each of these approaches aimed to help the nurse identify and select interventions that produce optimal care, reduce legal risks, and lower health care costs.

Procedure: A set of how-to action steps for performing a clinical activity or task

Standard of care: A description of an acceptable level of patient care or professional practice

Algorithm: A set of steps that approximates the decision process of an expert clinician and is used to make a decision; these clinical rules are typically embedded in a branching flow chart

Clinical practice guideline: A statement or series of statements outlining appropriate practice for a clinical condition or procedure

National guidelines such as those published by the U.S. Agency for Health Care Research and Quality (AHRQ; http://www.ahrq.gov) and the Cochrane Library (http://www.cochranelibrary.com) are generally based on the latest, most comprehensive scientific evidence and expert analysis. They provide standards for delivering and evaluating care for patients with the same diagnosis. Box 17-4 compares structured care methodologies. Additional examples are provided in Chapter 19.

Box 17-4 Structured Care Methodologies

Algorithm

- Useful in management of high-risk subgroups within the cohort; may be "layered" on top of a pathway to control care practices that are used to manage a specific problem
- Binary decision trees that guide stepwise assessment and intervention
- Intense specificity; no provider flexibility
- May use analytical research methods to ensure cause and effect

Critical Pathway

- Represents a sequential, interdisciplinary, minimal practice standard for a specific patient population
- Provides flexibility to alter care to meet individualized patient needs
- Abbreviated format, broad perspective
- Phase or episode driven
- Ability to measure cause-and-effect relationship between pathway and patient outcomes prohibited by lack of control; changes in patient outcomes directly attributable to the efforts of the collaborative practice team

Guideline

- Broad, research-based practice recommendations
- May or may not have been tested in clinical practice
- Practice resources helpful in construction of structured care methodologies
- No mechanism for ensuring practice implementation

Order Set

- Preprinted provider orders used to expedite the order process after a practice standard has been validated through analytical research
- Complements and increases compliance with existing practice standards
- Can be used to represent the algorithm or protocol in order format

Protocol

- Prescribes specific therapeutic interventions for a clinical problem unique to a subgroup of patients within the cohort
- Multifaceted; may be used to drive practice for more than one discipline
- Broader specificity than an algorithm; allows for minimal provider flexibility by way of treatment options
- May be "layered" on top of a pathway

Source: Agency for Health Care Policy and Research's (now Agency for Healthcare Research and Quality) Clinical Practice Guideline Development, AHCPR program note in Publication 93-0023, 1993.

Classification Systems

One of the first things you will need to do when beginning a new practice site is to learn about the classification system used in that setting.

Omaha System

The Omaha System (OS) is one of the oldest of the ANA-recognized standardized terminologies describing and measuring the impact of health care services. It is a research-based, comprehensive, standardized taxonomy or classification that exists in the public domain. It is designed to enhance practice, documentation, and information management. It is intended for use across the continuum of care for individuals, families, and communities who represent all ages, geographic locations, medical diagnoses, socioeconomic ranges, spiritual beliefs, ethnicity, and cultural values. It was developed in the 1970s by the Visiting Nurse Association of Omaha to document and manage home care services, but it is now widely applied across health care disciplines and settings. The OS has three aspects:

1. Structure: characteristics of the care providers, their tools and resources, and the physical/organizational setting)

2. Process: both interpersonal and technical aspects of the treatment process
3. Outcome: change in the patient's symptoms and functioning

The OS also has three steps: problem, intervention, and outcome. The four intervention categories are health teaching, guidance, and counseling; treatments and procedures; case management; and surveillance. Current users and their sites now include the continuum of care: home care, public health, and school health practice settings; nurse-managed center staff; hospital-based and managed care case managers; educators and students; occupational health nurses; faith community staff; acute care and rehabilitation hospital/long-term care staff; researchers; members of various disciplines; and computer software vendors. The majority of OS users are located in the United States (http://www.omahasystem.org/overview.html).

Clinical Care Classification System

The Clinical Care Classification (CCC) System was founded by Dr. Virginia K. Saba who has pioneered and spearheaded Nursing Informatics nationally and internationally (see Chapter 21). The CCC System (V-2.5) offers a new approach to documenting nursing practice in an electronic health record (EHR). It consists of a standardized framework representing three unique levels:

1. 176 Nursing Diagnoses
2. 804 Nursing Intervention/Actions
3. 528 Nursing Outcomes, each of which are classified by 21 Care Components representing four Healthcare Patterns to form one system—the CCC System (https://www.sabacare.com/framework/).

Consulting

A nurse designing the care plan may discover that more information is needed about the nature of the problems underlying the need for nursing or about specific interventions. **Consultation**, a process in which two or more people with varying degrees of experience and expertise discuss a problem and its solution, often proves helpful. Nurses might consult with nurse specialists and other members of the health care team, including health care providers, nutritionists, social workers, therapists, pastoral caregivers, and ethicists (Fig. 17-4). Consultations are a valuable means for nurses to expand their nursing knowledge and repertoire of effective strategies.

QSEN TEAMWORK AND COLLABORATION

It is always important for nurses to know their own strengths, limitations, and values when identifying the best interventions to address patient problems and to value the perspectives and expertise of all health team members. Knowing when to consult and doing so is essential to excellent practice. It is never too early to begin learning who and what your best resources are.

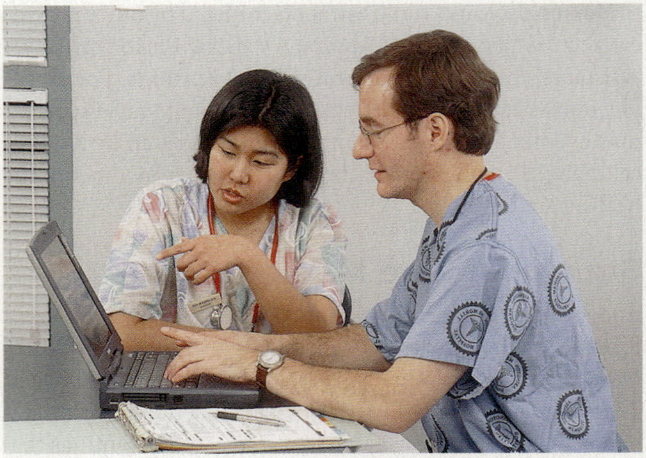

FIGURE 17-4. Consulting with a nursing colleague or other member of the health care team can help the nurse develop an effective nursing care plan. (Used with permission from Shutterstock. *Photo by B. Proud.*)

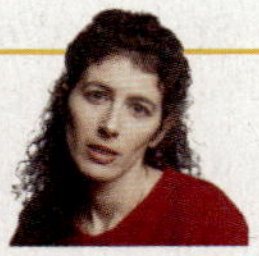

Review the Reflective Practice box (on page 451) describing **Darla Jefferson**. The nurse would consult other health care team members for assistance. For example, the nurse might consult social services for assistance with drug treatment and rehabilitation. Should the patient decide to keep her baby, social services also would be helpful, such as with obtaining food stamps and infant formula through government programs, appropriate housing, and follow-up in the community. A consultation with a nutritionist would be helpful prenatally to help Darla meet the requirements for herself and her fetus, and also postpartum to ensure that the infant is receiving adequate nutrition to grow and develop.

DEVELOPING EVALUATIVE STRATEGIES

Well-written outcomes define evaluative strategies to be used by the nurse. Patient outcomes are meaningless unless nurses evaluate the patient's progress toward their achievement. The nurse records the date the outcome was written and the date it is achieved. An evaluative statement (Box 17-5) includes a statement about achievement of the desired outcome (met, partially met, not met) and lists actual patient behavior as evidence supporting the statement. If the plan is not achieved, recommendations for revising the care plan are included in the evaluative statement. Chapter 19 deals specifically with the evaluative component of the nursing process.

COMMUNICATING AND RECORDING THE NURSING CARE PLAN

The **nursing care plan** (patient care plan) is the written guide that directs the efforts of the nursing team working with the patient to meet their health goals. It specifies nursing diagnoses/problems, outcomes, and associated nursing interventions. Well-written care plans offer many benefits to

Box 17-5 Evaluative Statement

Documents that patient has met, partially met, or not met the goal/outcome.

Goal/Outcome Statement

Beginning 6/8/25, the patient will ambulate half the length of hallway with assistance three times daily.

Evaluative Statement

6/8/25—Goal partially met; patient refused to ambulate in the morning but did walk to the bathroom once in the afternoon with the assistance of one nurse.

Recommendation: Review reason for progressive ambulation with patient; assess motivation to increase independence.

—M. Stenulis, RN

the patient, nurse, nursing unit, nursing administration, and nursing profession. Primarily, nursing care plans ensure that the nursing team works efficiently to deliver holistic, goal-oriented, person-centered care to patients.

A well-written nursing care plan:

- Represents an effective philosophy of nursing and advances nursing's four aims: promoting health, preventing disease and illness, promoting recovery, and facilitating coping with altered functioning
- Is prepared by the nurse who best knows the patient and is recorded on the day the patient presents for treatment and care, according to facility policy, with modifications to the initial plan signed and dated
- Is responsive to the individual characteristics, values and needs of the patient, and is culturally appropriate
- Clearly identifies the nursing assistance the patient needs and nursing's collaborative responsibilities for fulfilling the medical and interdisciplinary care plan (clearly specifies nursing diagnoses/problems, patient outcomes, nursing interventions, and evaluative strategies)
- Directs the nurse's assessment priorities, caregiving behaviors, and teaching, counseling, and advocacy behaviors
- Is based on scientific principles and incorporates findings of nursing research
- Meets the developmental, psychosocial, and spiritual needs of the patient, as well as the patient's physiologic needs
- Is updated to reflect changes in the patient's status and related needs for nursing care
- Addresses the discharge needs of the patient and family
- Provides for as much patient and family participation as possible
- When appropriate, is compatible with the medical care plan and that of the interdisciplinary team
- Creates a record that can be used for evaluation, research, reimbursement, and legal purposes

Many suggestions for care plans appear in the nursing literature. Each school of nursing and each health care institution and facility has its own format, which may reflect a particular nursing theory. Common to all formats is a minimum of three columns for documenting nursing diagnoses, patient outcomes, and nursing interventions. Formats vary in the ways assessment data and the nursing evaluation are addressed. Many facilities now post an abbreviated care plan on the wall in the patient's room highlighting priority outcomes.

Institutional and Facility Care Plans

The Joint Commission requires health care institutions and facilities to formulate, maintain, and support a patient-specific plan for care, treatment, and rehabilitation.

Types of Nursing Care

In most institutions and facilities, care plans, regardless of their format, communicate directions for three different types of nursing care: nursing care related to basic human needs, nursing care related to nursing diagnoses/problems, and nursing care related to the medical and interdisciplinary care plan.

NURSING CARE RELATED TO BASIC HUMAN NEEDS

The plan should concisely communicate to caregivers the data about the patient's usual health habits and patterns, obtained during the nursing history, that are needed to direct daily care. For example, it is important to know whether a toddler is toilet trained and what words the child uses to indicate the need to void or defecate. Directives about the patient's usual health habits and patterns might be modified by current treatment orders, such as an order to fast for a diagnostic procedure or to limit or increase activity. This information is useful to caregivers only if it is kept current as the patient's condition changes. Any nurse should be able to find in the care plan the instructions needed to provide competent care.

NURSING CARE RELATED TO NURSING DIAGNOSES/PROBLEMS

The plan contains outcomes and nursing interventions for every nursing diagnosis/problem, as well as a place to note the patient's responses to care. This section is the heart of the nursing care plan because it represents the independent component of nursing practice. When well developed, it demonstrates the nurse's clinical competence (knowledge of the science of nursing), sensitivity to the individual needs of the patient, and creativity in mobilizing the resources of the patient and the caregiving team to meet the patient's health needs.

NURSING CARE RELATED TO THE MEDICAL AND INTERDISCIPLINARY CARE PLAN

The care plan also records current medical orders for diagnostic studies and treatment and specified related nursing care.

Formats for Care Plans

A great variety of formats are used to communicate care plans. In addition to traditional written care plans, you should be familiar with the following.

COMPUTERIZED CARE PLANS

Nurses now often use **computerized nursing care plans** as part of the electronic medical record. The benefits of computerized plans include ready access to a large knowledge base; improved record keeping and a resulting improvement in audits and quality assurance; documentation by all members of the health care team with printouts for the patient's record and for change-of-shift reports; and less time spent on paperwork. One nurse researcher, however, has studied a potential negative impact of computerized plans on the professionalization of staff nurses. Harris (1990) cautions that computerized systems for patient care planning and the larger systems in which they are embedded contribute to the loss of autonomy, loss of individualization of care, and loss of nursing expertise. Individual nurses, as well as researchers, need to respond to this challenge from Harris (1990, p. 73): "Does a lot of nursing time spent in procedural, rule-governed, step-by-step thinking processes destroy part of the nurse's ability to care, to empathize, to intuit, to gain insight, to function in the expert mode?"

CONCEPT MAP CARE PLANS

A concept map care plan is a diagram of patient problems and interventions. Your ideas about patient problems and treatments are the "concepts" that are diagrammed. These maps are used to organize patient data, analyze relationships in the data, and enable you to take a holistic view of the patient's situation (Schuster, 2016). Examples of concept map care plans are shown in Chapters 13 and 14 and throughout the text.

CHANGE-OF-SHIFT REPORTS

Chapter 12 describes the importance of critical patient information being communicated with each patient transfer or "hand-off." This includes what happens each time nurses finish their shift and hand off patients to other nurses. Many facilities have developed forms to facilitate this exchange of information, including the Situation-Background-Assessment-Recommendation/Introduction-Situation-Background-Assessment-Recommendation-Question and Answer (SBAR/ISBARQ) formats described in Chapters 8, 12, and 20. Three advantages of using a standardized hand-off tool are:

1. Helps you get organized
2. Prevents omissions of key information that must be communicated
3. Promotes dialogue and critical thinking between caregivers

See Figure 17-5 for a standardized hand-off tool different from the SBAR. As you rotate through different clinical facilities, pay attention to their policies and procedures for hand-offs, and follow them carefully.

MULTIDISCIPLINARY (COLLABORATIVE) CARE PLANS

Clinical pathways (critical pathways, CareMaps) are tools used in case management to communicate the standardized, interdisciplinary care plan for patients. Case management is a health care delivery system intended to provide high-quality, cost-effective care for individuals, families, and groups. The emphasis is on clearly stating expected patient outcomes and the specific times within which it is reasonable to achieve these outcomes. Chapter 20 provides examples of how critical pathways are used with select documentation tools in a computerized system.

Student Care Plans

The care plans that students are required to develop are often more detailed than those used in practice settings. The aim is to assist you to assimilate each of the five phases of the nursing process. Although care plan formats vary among different nursing programs, most are designed so that the student systematically proceeds through the interrelated steps of the nursing process. Many use a five-column format. See the accompanying poem, Her First Nursing Care Plan.

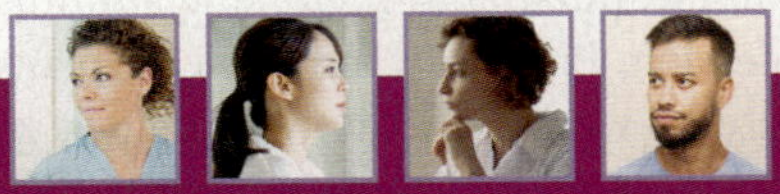

Poetry Nook

Her First Nursing Care Plan

Amy Haddad, PhD, RN

She plans her care, cares about her plan
that speaks in imperatives with an authority
she does not own. She plans to watch, count, ease,
flush, remove, monitor, offer, relieve, be
there, listen, encourage, pray, prevent, provide
care to every system in the human body.
She is hungry for the treat of praise, "Good work!"
that follows the trick of a perfect care plan.
The patient is the notepaper on which she writes.
He is young, a husband, a father,
wiped out (not a nursing term)
from surgery for stomach cancer. The word,
metastatic in the doctor's notes is Greek
to her. She misspells it—*metastes*—cannot
grasp the implications, instead she includes
all the organs the cancer touched on its clockwise
march around his abdomen. The strange terms—
omentum, celic gutter, hepatic flexure—
entrance her. She looks in her anatomy
book to find where the organs rest in case
her teacher asks. Her plan is filled with problems
the cancer creates during her shift.
She worries a bit no one has told
the patient what *metastes* means. Certain
it is not her place to tell such a truth,
she sticks to her plan.

Date/Time:

ISHAPED Patient Centered Bedside Report Tool

I — Introduction

Patient Label:
Room #: ______ Code Status ______ Do Not Announce? ______
Attending: ______ Consults: ______
Primary/Family Contact Information:

S — Story

CC: ______ Diagnosis: ______
Communication Issues: Interpreter Needed?: □ Yes □ No Language: ______ Deaf □ HOH □ Auxiliary Aids: ______ □ Blind
Admission Process: □ Admission HX □ Med Rec □ Vaccine Screening □ MRSA Screening □ Pt Belongings List □ Fall Safety Contract

H — History

Past Medical History: ______
Allergies: Home O_2 □ Yes □ No Smoker □ Yes □ No □ Other: ______

A — Assessment

Last Vital Signs: Time: ____ BP: ____ HR: ____ R: ____ Temp: ____ O_2 Sat: ____ Freq: ____
Pain: □ Yes □ No Location: ______ Level/Scale: ______ Last Pain Med/Time: ______ Type: ______
IV access: Type: PIV/CVL/PICC Site: ______ Fluid: ______
PIV/CVL/PICC Site: ______ Fluid: ______
Drips: ______
Abnormal Labs: ______
AccuChecks: Schedule and Coverage: ______
Neurological Status: A and O x ______ □ Other: ______
Musculoskel./Activity: □ OOB Ad Lib □ OOB Assist □ Total Care □ Bed Rest □ PT/OT Consult (date): ______ □ Other: ______
Cardiovascular: □ Regular □ Irregular □ Edema □ Pacemaker □ Remote Telemetry □ Dialysis: schedule ______
Respiratory Status: □ WNL □ Exceptions: ______ SpO_2 ______ % on ______ L/min ______ (mode) □ Chest Tube
Oxygen: O_2 Order Verified □ Yes □ NA Weaning O_2 □ Yes □ No □ Bipap/ Cpap Pulse-Ox Monitoring Cont □ Other ______
GI: Diet: ______ □ Feeder □ Assist □ Independent □ Tube Feed via ______ (mode)
Last BM: ______ □ NGT: Suction ______ □ Ostomy: ______ □ Other: ______
GU: □ Voids □ Foley: Insertion Date: ______ Indication: ______ □ D/C'd: ______ Due to Void: ______
Skin: Pressure Ulcer: □ Yes □ No □ At-Risk Location(s) ______ □ Documented Pt Last Turned: ______
□ WOCN Consult (date): ______ Incisions/Drains: □ Yes □ No Location(s) ______
Wound Care/Dressing Changes: □ Yes □ No Site(s): ______ □ Frequency: ______ Last Changed ______
Psychosocial/Family:

P — Plan

Today's Goal(s): ______
Oxygen Wean Goal: ______
Tests/Procedures/Labs: ______
PRN Meds/Last Dose ______
Discharge Plan/Teaching ______
CM / SW Needs ______
Core Measures: □ Checklist □ CHF □ Pneumonia □ AMI □ SCIP

E — Error-Prevention

Isolation: □ No □ Yes Type: ______ Organism/Site: ______
Fall Risk: □ Low □ Moderate □ High Score: ____ Bed Alarm On: □ No □ Yes □ Interventions/Orders Initiated ______ □ Safety Plan
High-Risk Medications:

RISKS:	Sepsis	Aspiration	Elopement	Suicide	Restraints	Seizure	ETOH Withdraw
	□ Yes □ No	□ Yes □ No Precautions Initiated: □ Yes □ No	□ Yes □ No	□ Yes □ No	□ Yes □ No □ Behavior □ Medical	□ Yes □ No □ Bed Padded	□ Yes □ No CIWA: ______

D — Dialogue

Question and answer occurred: □ Yes □ No Patient/family had opportunity to participate: □ Yes □ No If no, why:

Not part of the Permanent Medical Record: 2018-2019

FIGURE 17-5. Nurse-to-nurse shift reports are essential elements of care coordination. (Reprinted with permission, Inova Health System Foundation, Falls Church, VA.)

The sample student care plan shown in Box 17-6 (on pages 468–469) demonstrates a plan developed for a 72-year-old woman admitted to the hospital after experiencing a ministroke (i.e., brain attack, transient ischemic attack) at home. Her condition is stable, and the three prioritized diagnoses written in the plan address her inability to deal with this new medical diagnosis and to prevent a major stroke (high priority), ineffective coping (medium priority), and constipation (low priority).

(text continues on page 470)

Box 17-6 Sample Student Care Plan N.B.

Assessment/Diagnosis	Goal/Outcome	Nursing Orders
Subjective data: "Will I get a stroke now? I don't think I could handle that." "How can I help myself prevent it?" *Objective data:* Admitting diagnosis: TIA BP: 184/120 *Strengths:* Past pattern of adhering to prescribed health behaviors.	Before discharge, the patient will: • Describe the terms *TIA* and *stroke,* identifying the underlying disease process, causes, symptoms, and treatment	Assess what the patient knows about TIA and stroke (correct any misinformation). Assess learning needs, readiness to learn, and factors that will influence learning. Plan teaching and learning sessions to involve family members designated by patient. Include in the teaching plan a description of TIA and stroke and the underlying disease process, causes, symptoms, and treatment plan.

Health Problem: Impaired Health Maintenance Response to TIA and Stroke Prevention
Etiologic factor: knowledge deficit.
	After discussion with the health care provider and nurse, the patient will:
	• Correctly describe the treatment plan:
	  • Medications (drugs, intended effect, dose, time, route)
	  • Dietary modifications
	  • Exercise prescription
	  • Signs and symptoms to report
	  • Follow-up appointment date
		After the treatment plan has been developed, make sure the patient and family can restate it (teaching) and value the prescribed lifestyle modification (counseling).

Subjective data: Husband died 8 months ago; moved in with daughter 6 months ago after selling family home. Daughter reports mother had been a very independent, strong woman in the past—seemed to "crumple" after husband's death. History of headaches. *Objective data:* Clutches daughter's hand. *Strengths:* History of handling life stressors well. *Limitations:* In the past, her husband was her primary support.	Beginning 9/7/25, the patient will: • Verbalize her feelings related to the loss of her husband, loss of family home, loss of health • Identify coping patterns that have helped her in the past • Identify three personal strengths and three outside supports that will help her now	Once during each shift, primary nurse should sit at patient's bedside for at least several minutes to communicate caring and to explore with the patient her current stressors and the adequacy of her coping response. • Assess factors compounding her losses. • Reinforce her personal strengths and support systems; counsel her to tap into these now. • Suggest local support groups, if indicated. Primary nurse to explore with daughter, Lisa, how her mother's moving in with her has affected the family. Recommend support systems.
Health Problem: Coping Impairment ***Etiologic factors:*** illness, recent death of husband, and relocation with daughter.	Before discharge, the patient will: • Verbalize that she feels "okay" (sufficiently in charge of her life) about returning home	

Subjective data: "I move my bowels every 2 or 3 days; get constipated at least once a week. Often Ducolax or Metamucil helps."
"I drink plenty of fluids and eat fruits and vegetables."
History of hemorrhoids secondary to straining.
Objective data: No bowel movement in past 4 days.
On bed rest since hospitalized.
Health Problem: Constipation
Etiologic factors: decreased physical activity and long-term laxative use (Ducolax, Metamucil).
	Beginning 9/7/25, the patient will:
	• Pass soft, formed stool every 1 to 3 days without use of laxatives
	By 9/10/25, the patient will:
	• Verbalize the importance of the following natural aids to bowel elimination:
	  • Daily intake of foods high in bulk
	  • Daily fluid intake of 8 to 10 glasses
	  • Regular time for elimination
	  • Daily physical exercise: walking
		Monitor bowel elimination patterns; identify causative factors of constipation and successful corrective measures.
		Explain the importance of adhering to a regular time for defecation (patient suggests after breakfast)—adhere to this in the hospital.
		When given medical clearance, assist patient with progressive ambulation.
		Recommend that she include brisk walking into daily health habits (build strength to 20- to 30-minute brisk walk daily).
		Explain the long-term effects of laxative abuse on the bowel, and discourage use of laxatives.
		Reinforce the patient's fluid intake and ingestion of high-bulk foods, such as fresh fruits and salad.

Scientific Rationale	Evaluation
Each person's learning needs are different; each person learns in their own unique way; learning is dependent on readiness.	9/10/25—Outcome not met. Patient says her head is "too old" to learn all this stuff. Equates stroke with death. *Revision:* Reteach content in simpler terms. Reassess learning readiness. —*M. Foley, SN*
The more support people knowledgeably committed to the care plan, the greater the probability the patient will achieve goals.	
New self-care behaviors are dependent on knowledge.	
New self-care behaviors are dependent on motivation. Unless the patient is committed to stroke prevention and values this outcome, she will not follow the treatment plan.	9/10/25 Too early to evaluate. —*M. Foley, SN*
The nurse's unhurried, attentive, and caring presence communicates to the patient that she is important to the nurse and that the nurse values her well-being. It is an invitation to the patient to become actively involved in recovery. Also, it is logical to explore adequacy of past and current coping mechanisms before suggesting new approaches.	9/10/25 Outcome partially met. Patient speaks freely about how much she misses her husband and how fearful this hospitalization makes her. When asked about living with her daughter, she becomes uncharacteristically quiet. —*M. Foley, SN* 9/10/25 Outcome met. Patient talks about how everything seemed better in the past after she talked it over with her husband and God. —*M. Foley, SN* 9/10/25 Outcome not met. Patient couldn't think of anything about herself that is healthy or strong. Says "maybe" her family can help her now. *Revision:* Counsel regarding personal strengths. Help her to experience them. —*M. Foley, SN*
Adult children of aging parents frequently experience overwhelming stress as they try to deal with their own and their parents' problems. Supporting this family is supporting the patient indirectly.	9/11/25 Too early to evaluate. —*M. Foley, SN*
This patient's elimination problems will not be resolved until all the specific causes of her constipation and successful corrective measures are identified. Needs to be an ongoing assessment priority. This encourages positive use of circadian rhythms.	9/10/25 Outcome partially met. Soft, formed stool passed every 2 to 3 days with aid of docusate. —*M. Foley, SN* 9/10/25 Outcome met. Patient correctly related value of four natural aids to elimination. Questions whether she will be strong enough to walk. *Revision:* Encourage assisted ambulation. —*M. Foley, SN*
Peristalsis is stimulated by physical exercise.	
Laxative abuse leads to decreased peristaltic response to food and loss of intestinal tone.	
Commenting on these positive self-care behaviors reinforces them.	

Assessing

The student records the assessment data that led to the determination of each diagnosis in the Assessment/Diagnosis column. Recording these data helps to link specific defining characteristics with diagnostic problem statements.

Diagnosing/Problem Identification

Nursing diagnoses/problems are recorded in the Assessment/Diagnosis column in a prioritized list beginning with the top-priority problem. For each diagnosis/problem, a clear and concise problem statement is followed by an etiology statement that identifies specific contributing factors.

Outcome Identification and Planning

The outcome identification and planning column (Goal/Outcome column) contains the expected changes in patient health status or in patient behaviors (i.e., patient outcomes). If achieved, these changes resolve the problem statement in the nursing diagnosis.

Implementing

Sets of nursing orders that describe specific nursing interventions are written for each patient outcome. (Refer to the Nursing Orders column in Box 17-6 on pages 468–469.) These orders specify what nursing interventions are to be performed, how they are to be performed, when they are to be performed, and who is to perform them. In many nursing programs, students are asked to document the source of their proposed nursing interventions. Although students may be able to "pull from their head" some nursing strategies, developing the practice of consulting the nursing literature is a sure means to increase nursing knowledge. Some programs also require students to provide a scientific rationale for the interventions they propose, as shown in Box 17-6 (on pages 468–469). A succinct rationale statement demonstrates that the student is deliberately choosing the nursing intervention because of its high probability to effect the desired change.

Evaluating

Incorporating evaluative statements in the care plan clearly communicates the message that nursing care is never complete until achievement of patient outcomes is evaluated. For examples, see the Evaluation column in Box 17-6 (on pages 468–469). Just as some say that teaching does not occur if learning does not take place, so nursing care is incomplete if the desired patient goals are not achieved.

PROBLEMS RELATED TO OUTCOME IDENTIFICATION AND PLANNING

Problems commonly encountered while developing nursing care plans include failure to involve the patient in the planning process, insufficient data collection, use of inaccurate or insufficient data to develop nursing diagnoses/problems, outcomes that are stated too broadly, outcomes that are derived from poorly developed nursing diagnoses, failure to write nursing orders clearly, written nursing orders that do not resolve the problem, and failure to update the care plan.

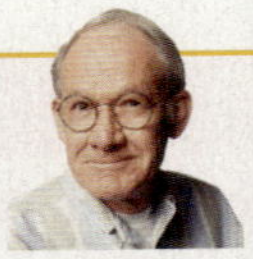

Recall **Elijah Wolinski**, the frail, older adult with a pressure injury. Since the nurse is providing care in the patient's home, a written care plan is extremely important because more than one caregiver may be involved in the patient's care. In addition, the nurses caring for Mr. Wolinski must update the plan regularly to ensure that, regardless of who is providing the care, the correct care is given consistently.

A FINAL WORD ABOUT STANDARDIZED LANGUAGES AND HOLISTIC, PERSON-CENTERED CARE

Moorhead et al. (2013, p. 3) lament that while nurses' clinical-reasoning and decision making skills are integral to quality health care and account for much of the health care system "safety net," little attention has been focused on the outcomes of nursing interventions. They write that, as part of improving health care quality and safety, "it is imperative that nursing define its interventions and outcomes and that these standardized nomenclatures be included in clinical nursing information systems and in large data sets used for systematic analysis."

The use of NIC (Bulechek et al., 2013, p. vi):

- helps demonstrate the impact that nurses have on the system of health care delivery
- standardizes and defines the knowledge base for nursing curricula and practice
- facilitates the appropriate selection of a nursing intervention
- facilitates communication of nursing treatments to other nurses and other providers
- enables researchers to examine the effectiveness and cost of nursing care
- assists educators to develop curricula that better articulate with clinical practice
- facilitates the teaching of clinical decision making to novice nurses
- assists administrators in planning more effectively for staff and equipment needs
- promotes the development of a reimbursement system for nursing services
- promotes the development and use of nursing information systems
- communicates the nature of nursing to the public

As you can see, there are numerous reasons to use standardized language. As nurses, however, we must always remember that our primary commitment is to patients, not to standardized language. Our focus must always be on ensuring that the nursing care plan accurately captures the diagnoses and problems of the very real patient with whom we are planning care and those interventions most likely to resolve those problems. If you have established a successful partnership with the patient and family, they should be able to read the care plan and say, "Wow, you really captured our priorities!"

REFLECTIVE PRACTICE LEADING TO PERSONAL LEARNING

Remember that the object of reflective practice is to look at an experience, understand it, and learn from it. As you begin to develop your expertise in outcome identification and planning, reflect on your experiences—both successes and failures—in order to improve your practice. How can you do it better next time? What did you learn today that can help you tomorrow? Begin your reflection by paying close attention to the following during the planning phase of the nursing process:

- Did your preparation for partnering with the patient and family to identify outcomes and plan care enable you to feel confident in your ability to identify pertinent outcomes, select evidence-based interventions, and communicate the care plan? Did you inspire the patient's confidence and trust? Did you seek help if you were unsure about how to identify pertinent outcomes or select evidence-based interventions?
- How confident are you that, once implemented, this plan will address the clinical, functional, and quality-of-life concerns of the patient? How can you become more familiar with the many outcomes and interventions that may be applicable for future patients?
- Were you aware of any personal stereotypes or prejudices that may have negatively influenced this clinical encounter? If yes, how did you address them?
- Was the patient's and family's participation in the process at an optimal level? How might you have better engaged the patient and family? Does the care plan accurately reflect patient priorities and preferences? To what degree do you think the patient's participation in planning will influence the achievement of outcomes?

Perhaps the most important question to reflect on is: Are your patients/caregivers better for having had *you* share in the critical responsibility of partnering with them to identify outcomes and plan the care that will result in them achieving these outcomes? Are your patients now receiving thoughtful, person-centered, prioritized, holistic, evidence-based treatment and care because of your efforts?

DEVELOPING CLINICAL REASONING AND CLINICAL JUDGMENT

1. Write diagnostic statements for three patients experiencing obesity, and make sure that the etiologies for the problem statement differ. Describe how these different etiologies result in different care plans.
2. Use one of the nursing diagnoses/problems from Exercise 1 and write related cognitive, psychomotor, and affective goals for this patient. Explain the different purposes of each type of goal and why it may be necessary to include all three to resolve a patient problem successfully.
3. An alert 82-year-old widow who has a history of unsafe behaviors has recently been discharged from the hospital to her home. Caregivers attempted to secure her consent to be transferred to a long-term care facility, but she flatly refused. Responsible for her home care, you list Risk for Injury as a priority diagnosis/problem. First, list the nursing measures that you believe are most likely to achieve the outcome of preventing injury. Then talk with several other students to compare your lists of interventions and the evidence that supports each, and discuss how practicing nurses can be sure they select the best nursing interventions for each expected patient outcome.
4. You learn that the patient you will be caring for tomorrow has lymphedema in both legs and is newly admitted to the hospital. You don't know anything about lymphedema. What resources will you consult to prepare yourself to identify actual and potential diagnoses/problems, outcomes, and interventions? Share this exercise with another student and compare the lists you generate.

PRACTICING FOR NCLEX

1. A nurse is planning care for a patient admitted to the hospital for treatment of a drug overdose. What actions will the nurse take during the outcome identification and planning step of the nursing process? Select all that apply.
   a. Formulating nursing diagnoses
   b. Identifying expected patient outcomes
   c. Selecting evidence-based nursing interventions
   d. Explaining the nursing care plan to the patient
   e. Assessing the patient's mental status
   f. Evaluating the patient's outcome achievement
2. Nurses on a hospital unit work to improve staff communication, as outlined in The Joint Commission's National Patient Safety Goals. What process will best provide for continuity of the plan of care?
   a. Checking two patient identifiers, such as name and date of birth, prior to administering medications
   b. Ensuring two nurses check doses of high-risk medications such as anticoagulants or insulin
   c. Giving handoff report in the patients' rooms to update the next nurse on the plan of care
   d. Obtain a patient sitter for a confused individual who has fallen trying to get out of bed
3. A nurse on a mother–baby unit engages in informal planning while providing ongoing nursing care. What actions are included in this type of planning? Select all that apply.
   a. Sitting down with a patient and prioritizing existing diagnoses
   b. Assessing a woman for postpartum depression during patient education
   c. Planning interventions for a patient with a risk for bleeding
   d. Taking time to speak with a new mother who just received bad news
   e. Reassessing a patient who reports their pain medication is not working
   f. Coordinating home care for a patient being discharged later today

4. To plan the day, a nurse is prioritizing patient diagnoses according to Maslow's hierarchy of human needs. What patient problem will the nurse address first?
   a. Altered body image perception
   b. Impaired gas exchange
   c. Grief
   d. Situational low self-esteem
5. Nurses on an oncology unit plan to adopt use of critical pathways for patients receiving chemotherapy. What positive features of this system will the nurses anticipate? Select all that apply.
   a. Accessible computerized practice standards, easily individualized for patients
   b. Binary decision tree for stepwise assessment and intervention
   c. Ability to measures the cause-and-effect relationship between pathway and patient outcomes
   d. Research-based practice recommendations that may or may not have been tested in clinical practice
   e. Preprinted provider prescriptions, using standards validated through research, to streamline care
   f. Outcomes with suggested time frames for achievement
6. A nurse is developing outcomes in the affective domain for a patient with a foot ulcer related to diabetes. Which outcome best addresses this domain?
   a. Within 1 day after teaching, the patient will list three benefits of continuing to apply moist compresses to foot ulcer after discharge.
   b. By 6/12/25, the patient will correctly demonstrate application of wet-to-dry dressing on the foot ulcer.
   c. By 6/19/25, the patient's pressure ulcer will decrease in size from 3 to 2.5 inches.
   d. By 6/12/25, the patient will verbalize they value their health sufficiently to control diabetes and prevent recurrence of diabetic ulcers.
7. A nurse is developing a clinical outcome for a patient who is an avid runner and is recovering from a stroke resulting in right-sided paresis. Which clinical outcome is most appropriate to include in the care plan?
   a. After receiving 3 weeks of physical therapy, patient will demonstrate improved movement on the right side of her body.
   b. By 8/15/25, patient will be able to use right arm to dress, comb hair, and feed herself.
   c. Following physical therapy, patient will begin to gradually participate in walking/running events.
   d. By 8/15/25, patient will verbalize feeling sufficiently prepared to participate in running events.
8. A nurse is caring for a patient with dehydration who has a prescription to encourage oral fluids. Which outcome statement will best direct nursing interventions?
   a. Offer patient 60 mL of fluid every 2 hours while awake.
   b. During the next 24-hour period, patient's fluid intake will total at least 2,000 mL.
   c. Teach the patient the importance of drinking enough fluids to prevent dehydration by 1/15/25.
   d. At the next visit on 12/23/24, patient will know to drink at least 3 L of water per day.
9. A nurse is writing outcomes for a patient admitted with a cardiac condition causing fluid overload and edema. Which reflects an appropriately worded outcome?
   a. Offer to elevate the patient's legs on a stool while out of bed
   b. Patient will restrict fluids to 1,500 mL per 24-hour period
   c. Monitor the patient's intake and output
   d. Weigh the patient each morning prior to breakfast
10. A nursing student is presenting their concept map care plan for a patient with sickle cell anemia in post-conference. How does the student best describe the "concepts" that are being diagrammed in the plan?
    a. Protocols for treating the patient's medical problem
    b. Evidence-based treatment guidelines
    c. Synthesis of the patient's problems and treatment
    d. Clinical pathways reflecting evidence-based treatment for sickle cell anemia
11. A nurse is updating the plan of care with nurse-initiated interventions. Which intervention is appropriate to include?
    a. Administering acetaminophen for a headache
    b. Offering emotional support to a patient
    c. Consulting with a physical therapist
    d. Attending a team meeting for care planning

ANSWERS WITH RATIONALES

1. **b, c, d.** During the outcome identification and planning step of the nursing process, the nurse, patient, and family collaborate to establish priorities and identify and write expected patient outcomes. The nurse selects evidence-based nursing interventions, and communicates the care plan. These steps may overlap; however, formulating and validating nursing diagnoses are typically performed during the diagnosing step. Assessing mental status is part of the assessment step, and evaluating patient outcomes occurs during the evaluation step of the nursing process.
2. **c.** One of the published standards and requirements for accreditation and certification required by The Joint Commission is to "improve staff communication." Communicating the plan of care with the patient and oncoming and off going nurses meets this goal. Using patient identifiers relates to the goal of safely identifying patients, checking high-risk medications relates to decreasing medication errors, and obtaining a patient sitter relates to general safety and fall reduction.
3. **b, d, e.** Informal planning is a link between identifying a patient's strength or problem and providing an appropriate nursing response, often while rearranging priorities. Examples of this include the nurse integrating assessment for postpartum depression during patient care, providing a therapeutic presence for a patient who received bad news, or reassessing a patient for pain during rounding. Formal planning involves prioritizing diagnoses, formally planning

interventions, and coordinating the home care of a patient being discharged.

4. **b.** Because basic needs must be met before a person can focus on higher ones, Maslow's hierarchy of needs sets the priorities as: (1) physiologic needs, (2) safety needs, (3) love and belonging needs, (4) self-esteem needs, and (5) self-actualization needs. Answer (b) is an example of a physiologic need, (a and d) are examples of a self-esteem need, and (c) is an example of a love and belonging need.

5. **a, c, f.** Critical pathways represent a sequential, interdisciplinary, minimal practice standard for a specific patient population, that provide flexibility to alter care to meet individualized patient needs. They provide the ability to measure a cause-and-effect relationship between pathway and patient outcomes. An algorithm is a binary decision tree that guides stepwise assessment and intervention with intense specificity and no provider flexibility. Guidelines are broad, research-based practice recommendations that may or may not have been tested in clinical practice, and an order set is a preprinted provider order used to expedite the order process after a practice standard has been validated through analytical research.

6. **d.** Affective outcomes describe changes in patient values, beliefs, and attitudes. Cognitive outcomes (a) describe increases in patient knowledge or intellectual behaviors; psychomotor outcomes (b) describe the patient's achievement of new skills; and (c) is an outcome describing a physical change in the patient.

7. **b.** Clinical outcomes describe the expected status of health issues at certain points in time, after treatment is complete. Functional outcomes (b) describe the person's ability to function in relation to the desired usual activities. Quality-of-life outcomes (c) focus on key factors that affect someone's ability to enjoy life and achieve personal goals. Affective outcomes (d) describe changes in patient values, beliefs, and attitudes.

8. **b.** The outcomes in (a) and (c) make the error of expressing the patient goal as a nursing intervention. Incorrect: "Offer the patient 60 mL fluid every 2 hours while awake." Correct: "The patient will drink 60 mL fluid every 2 hours while awake, beginning 1/3/25." The outcome in (d) makes the error of using verbs that are not observable and measurable. Verbs to be avoided when writing outcomes include "know," "understand," "learn," and "become aware."

9. **b.** The terms goal, objective, and outcome are often used interchangeably to refer to the expected conclusion to the patient's health problem or expectation. Nurses use the phrase expected outcomes to refer to the more specific, observable, and measurable changes. Options a, c, and d are stated as interventions, rather than outcomes.

10. **c.** A concept map care plan is a diagram synthesizing patient problems and interventions. The nurse's ideas about patient problems and treatments are the "concepts" that are diagrammed. These maps are used to organize patient data, analyze relationships in the data, and provide a holistic view of the patient's situation. Answers (a) and (b) are incomplete because the concepts being diagrammed may include protocols and standardized treatment guidelines but the patient problems are also diagrammed concepts. Clinical pathways are tools used in case management to communicate the standardized, interdisciplinary care plan for patients.

11. **b.** A nurse-initiated intervention is related to the nursing diagnosis and projected outcome. It is an autonomous action based on scientific rationale. The physician or health care provider uses a physician-initiated interventions or order in response to the medical diagnosis: nurses execute these interventions safely and effectively. Collaborative interventions are initiated by other providers including pharmacists, respiratory therapists, or physician assistants.

Bibliography

Alfaro-LeFevre, R. (2010). *Applying nursing process: A tool for critical thinking* (7th ed.). Wolters Kluwer Health/Lippincott Williams & Wilkins.

Alfaro-LeFevre, R. (2014). *Applying nursing process. The foundation for clinical reasoning* (8th ed.). Wolters Kluwer Health/Lippincott Williams & Wilkins.

Alfaro-LeFevre, R. (2020). *Critical thinking, clinical reasoning, and clinical judgment: A practical approach* (7th ed.). Elsevier.

American Nurses Association (ANA). (2010). *Nursing's social policy statement*. Author.

American Nurses Association (ANA). (2015). *Standards of clinical nursing practice* (3rd ed.). Author.

Atay, S., & Karabacak, U. (2012). Care plans using concept maps and their effects on the critical thinking dispositions of nursing students. *International Journal of Nursing Practice, 18*, 233–239.

Berwick, D. M. (2020). Choices for the "New Normal." *JAMA, 323*(21), 2125–2126. https://doi.org/10.1001/jama.2020.6949

Bulechek, G. M., Butcher, H. K., Dochterman, J., & Wagner, C. M. (Eds.). (2013). *Nursing interventions classification (NIC)* (6th ed.). Elsevier.

Carpenito-Moyet, L. J. (2017a). *Nursing diagnosis: Application to clinical practice* (15th ed.). Wolters Kluwer Health/Lippincott Williams & Wilkins.

Carpenito-Moyet, L. J. (2017b). *Nursing care plans. Transitional patient and family centered care* (7th ed.). Wolters Kluwer.

Committee on Quality Health Care in America, Institute of Medicine (IOM). (2001). *Crossing the quality chasm: A new health system for the 21st century*. National Academy Press.

Doran, G. T. (1981). There's a S.M.A.R.T. way to write management's goals and objectives. *Management Review, 70*(11), 35–36.

Harris, B. L. (1990). Becoming deprofessionalized: One aspect of the staff nurse's perspective on computer-mediated nursing care plans. *Advances in Nursing Science, 13*(2), 63–74.

International Council of Nurses. (2019). Nursing Diagnosis and Outcome Statements. International Classification for Nursing Practice (ICNP) Catalogue. https://www.icn.ch/sites/default/files/inline-files/ICNP2019-DC.pdf

Iowa Intervention Project. (1997). Nursing interventions classification (NIC): An overview. In M. J. Rantz & P. LeMone (Eds.), *Classification of nursing diagnoses: Proceedings of the twelfth conference, North American nursing diagnosis* (pp. 32–39). CINAHL Information Systems.

Johnson, M., Bulechek, G., McCloskey Dochterman, J., Maas, M., & Moorhead, S. (Eds.). (2001). *Nursing diagnoses, outcomes and interventions: NANDA, NIC, NOC, linkages*. Mosby.

The Joint Commission. (2020). https://www.jointcommission.org/en/standards/national-patient-safety-goals/

Moorhead, S., Johnson, M., Maas, M. L., & Swanson, E. (Eds.). (2013). *Nursing outcomes classification (NOC)* (5th ed.). Elsevier.

Mueller, A., Johnston, M., & Bigh, D. (2002). Joining mind mapping and care mapping to enhance student critical thinking and achieve holistic nursing care. *Nursing Diagnosis, 13*(1), 24–27.

Saathoff, A. (2019). Predictive analytics, clinical decision support, and the future of sepsis treatment. Use data to make predictions, recommend interventions and improve outcomes. *American Nurse Today, 14*(3), 36–40.

Schnehl, P. (2014). *Introduction to concept mapping in nursing*. Jones & Bartlett.

Schuster, D. M. (2016). *Concept mapping: A critical thinking approach to care planning* (4th ed.). F. A. Davis.

Skelly, C. L., Hall, C. A., & Risher, C. R. (2020). Shared decision making and patient-centered care. *American Nurse Journal, 15*(2), 45–47.

Wolters Kluwer. (2022). Problem-based care plans. In *Lippincott Advisor*. Wolters Kluwer.

18 Implementing

Antoinette Browne

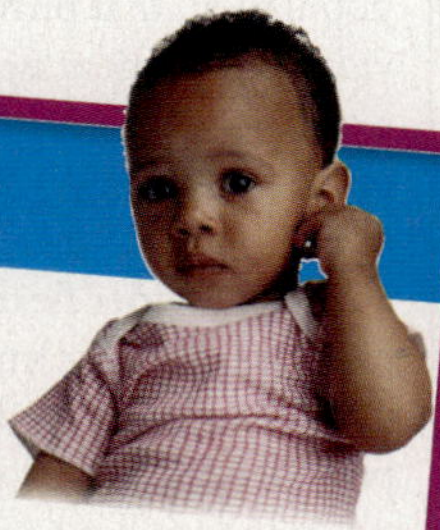

Antoinette, a toddler, is brought to the well-child community clinic by her grandmother. The health history reveals recurrent nausea, vomiting, and diarrhea. Her physical examination reveals a negligible gain in height and weight, lethargy, and a delay in achieving developmental milestones.

Estelle Morrissey

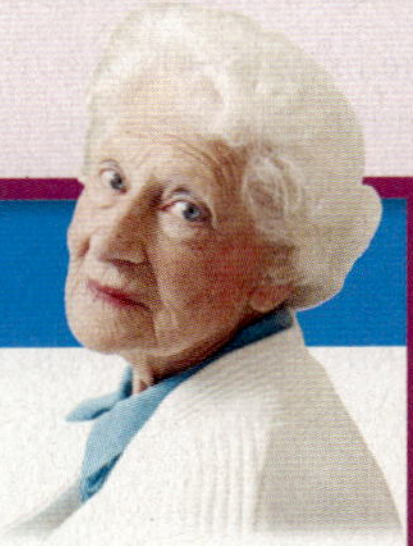

Estelle is an 86-year-old woman who is in a long-term care facility because of multiple chronic health problems. She is alert and oriented to person, place, and time. She states, "I'm all alone. There's no one left and I want to die. Can you help me?"

James McMahon

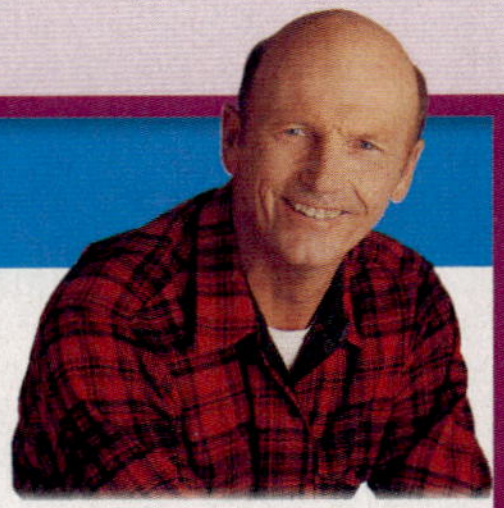

James, a 62-year-old man, is admitted to the intensive care unit in hepatic failure. He is critically ill, being monitored continuously, and receiving intravenous fluids and medications via central and peripheral IV catheters.

Learning Outcomes

After completing this chapter, you will be able to accomplish the following:

1. List examples of how nursing interventions and nursing outcomes classifications can be used to implement care.
2. Use cognitive, interpersonal, technical, ethical/legal, and QSEN competencies to implement a plan of nursing care.
3. Use the eight implementation guidelines provided in the chapter.
4. Describe six variables that influence the way a plan of care is implemented.
5. Use ongoing data collection to determine how to safely and effectively implement a plan of care.
6. Explain why reassessment after nursing intervention is important.
7. Discuss what to do if a patient does not cooperate with the plan of care.
8. Describe the risks and responsibilities of delegating nursing interventions.

Nursing Concepts

- Managing care
- Nursing process

During the **implementing** phase of the nursing process, the evidence-based nursing actions planned in the previous step are carried out. The purpose of implementation is to help the patient achieve valued health outcomes: promote health, prevent disease and illness, restore health, and facilitate coping with altered functioning. The plan of care is best implemented when patients who are able and willing to participate have maximum opportunities to engage in self-care. Family members and other support people, as well as other health care professionals, may also be involved in successfully implementing the plan of care (Table 18-1 on page 477). During the implementation phase, the nurse continues to collect data and to modify the plan of care as needed (Fig. 18-1 on page 478). All activities are documented in the format used by the nurse's institution or facility. For an example of implementation, see the accompanying Reflective Practice box on page 476.

UNIQUE FOCUS OF NURSING IMPLEMENTATION

In all nurse–patient interactions, the nurse is concerned with the patient's response to health and illness and the patient's ability to meet basic human needs. Whereas other health care professionals focus on selected aspects of the patient's treatment regimen, nurses are concerned with how the patient is responding to the plan of care in general. Be sure to review the competencies in Standard 5. Implementation in the American Nurses Association's (ANA's) *Nursing: Scope and Standards of Practice* (2021).

Nursing's Scope of Practice

Scope of practice describes the services that a qualified health professional is deemed competent to perform and permitted to undertake—in keeping with the terms of their professional license. The ANA states that the *Nursing: Scope and Standards of Practice* describes the "who," "what," "where," "when," "why," and "how" of nursing practice:

- **Who:** Registered Nurses (RN) and Advanced Practice Registered Nurses (APRN) comprise the "who" constituency and have been educated, titled, and maintain active licensure to practice nursing.
- **What:** Nursing is the protection, promotion, and optimization of health and abilities; prevention of illness and injury; facilitation of healing; alleviation of suffering through the diagnosis and treatment of human response; and advocacy in the care of individuals, families, groups, communities, and populations.
- **Where:** Where there is a patient in need of care.
- **When:** Whenever there is a need for nursing knowledge, compassion, and expertise.
- **Why:** The profession exists to achieve the most positive patient outcome in keeping with nursing's social contract and obligation to society (www.nursingworld.org/practice-policy/scope of practice/).

See Figure 17-2 in the preceding chapter (p. 453), which illustrates clinical decision making and scope of practice. The greater familiarity nurses have with their scope of practice, the better able they are to practice thoughtful, person-centered nursing. Benner (1984) classifies the ways nurses intervene with their patients as the domains of nursing practice:

- Helping role
- Teaching–coaching function
- Diagnostic and patient-monitoring function
- Effective management of rapidly changing situations
- Administering and monitoring therapeutic interventions and regimens
- Monitoring and ensuring the quality of health care practices
- Organizational and work-role competencies

The Nursing Interventions Taxonomy Structure

In 1992, McCloskey, Dochterman, and Bulechek published *Nursing Interventions Classification (NIC),* a report of research to construct a taxonomy of nursing interventions. New editions appeared in 1996, 2000, 2004, 2008, and 2013. Each of the interventions listed has a label, a definition, a set

QSEN Reflective Practice: Cultivating QSEN Competencies

CHALLENGE TO TECHNICAL SKILLS

James McMahon, a 62-year-old man, is admitted to the intensive care unit (ICU) in hepatic failure. He is critically ill, being monitored continuously, and receiving intravenous (IV) fluids and medications via central and peripheral IV catheters. During a recent clinical rotation in the ICU, I followed an extremely busy nurse who was caring for Mr. McMahon. He had several IV infusion lines and required numerous technologic devices for monitoring and care. The nurse asked me to hang a new bag of IV medication. I found myself completely overwhelmed and confused by the myriad tangle of IV lines and knew that I wouldn't be able to determine how to run the medication without the guidance of the nurse. I became frustrated because I should have been able to perform this task quickly and correctly if I had been working independently. I didn't want to risk hanging the IV medication and infusing it into a line with another fluid that was possibly incompatible. Nor did I want to risk running the medication through the incorrect port. The nurse was extremely busy, and I felt pressured to perform this task immediately.

Thinking Outside the Box: Possible Courses of Action

- Request that the nurse hang the medication once she was through with her other tasks.
- Hang the medication, hoping that it was compatible with the other fluids that were already infusing.
- Ask another nurse on the unit to hang the medication.
- Wait until the nurse was through with what she had to do, admit to her that I felt uncomfortable hanging the medication on my own, and then ask that she walk me through the process.

Evaluating a Successful Outcome: How Do I Define Success?

- The patient remains free from harm while receiving the necessary medication.
- The nurse recognizes the need to provide me with more guidance.
- I feel comfortable and competent in my skills.
- The patient receives efficient, safe care.

Personal Learning: Here's to the Future!

Luckily, there was a positive ending to this situation. I explained to the nurse that I was confused by the maze of IV lines and that I was uncomfortable administering the IV medication on my own. The nurse immediately recognized that the patient's lines were tangled and disorganized and some were unlabeled. With me at her side, she took the time to reorganize and label all of the lines, making it easier to visualize all of the medications and fluids the patient was receiving. We referenced a drug book to ensure that the medication was compatible with the other fluids that were running. She also walked me through the process of hanging the medication and connecting it to the appropriate port. The nurse appreciated the fact that I waited to ask her for help. As a result, the patient remained safe from injury. In addition, the nurse realized that she shouldn't have asked me to perform this task independently. I benefited from the experience because I became more familiar with this particular skill. As of now, I still find myself feeling somewhat anxious and uncomfortable with certain technical skills. However, I am finding that with each new clinical experience, I become more comfortable and more independent in my practice.

Colleen Kilcullen, Georgetown University

QSEN SELF-REFLECTION ON QUALITY AND SAFETY COMPETENCIES DEVELOPING KNOWLEDGE, SKILLS, AND ATTITUDES FOR CONTINUOUS IMPROVEMENT

How do you think you would respond in a similar situation? Why? What does this tell you about yourself and about the adequacy of your competencies for professional practice? Do you agree with the criteria that the nursing student used to evaluate a successful outcome? Why or why not? What *knowledge, skills,* and *attitudes* do you need to develop to continuously improve the quality and safety of care for patients like Mr. McMahon? What factors might have influenced the nurse in assigning this task to the student? Did the nurse effectively delegate this intervention? Why or why not? Did the student adhere to ethical and legal guidelines with the response? If so, explain how. If not, what issues were present?

Patient-Centered Care: How can you keep your focus on providing respectful and compassionate care for Mr. McMahon—even when feeling overwhelmed?

Teamwork and Collaboration/Quality Improvement: What communication and interpersonal skills do you need to be able to approach other nurses and team members when you need help? What does quality care for Mr. McMahon "look like?" What did the experienced nurse teach the student by taking the time to label the lines and medications?

Safety/Evidence-Based Practice: What does the evidence point to as "best practice" for administering Mr. McMahon's medications? What safety needs does he have and how can you meet them? What have you learned about the dangers of "busyness"?

Informatics: Can you identify the essential information that must be available in Mr. McMahon's drug record to support safe patient care and coordination of care? Can you think of other ways to respond to or approach the situation? What else might the nursing student have done to ensure a successful outcome?

Table 18-1 Professional Nursing Relationships: Role Responsibilities and Related Competencies

RELATIONSHIP	ROLE RESPONSIBILITIES	RELATED COMPETENCIES
Nurse–patient	• Communicate to patients that someone is concerned about them (as well as the disease) and is interested in how change in health state will affect their overall well-being. • Create an environment in which patients can commit their energies to health promotion or restoration or peaceful dying, confident that basic human needs are being addressed. • Challenge patients to develop self-care abilities that promote holistic health.	• Repertoire of therapeutic interpersonal behaviors: attending, listening, interviewing, nonverbal communication, touching, facilitating, coaching • Ability to establish trusting nurse–patient–family relationships • Demonstrated competence in the nursing roles of caregiver, teacher, counselor, advocate
Nurse–patient–family	• Develop in the patient and family the knowledge, attitude, and skills that will enable them to respond to the self-care challenges of their health or illness state. • Intervene as appropriate to promote healthy family functioning. • Educate the family to be wise and assertive health care consumers.	
Nurse–nurse	• Support one another's efforts to deliver quality nursing care; work collaboratively with nursing administration to improve quality care. • Provide creative leadership—formally or informally—to make the nursing unit a satisfying and challenging place to work. • Supervise the nursing care given by other nursing personnel; affirm the nursing strengths of others, and constructively address the nursing deficiencies encountered. • Enhance the professional development of self and other nurses through active participation in professional organizations.	• Communication • Teaching/counseling/advocacy • Assertiveness • Collaboration • Coordination • Group process • Organization • Leadership • Delegation • Change strategies • Problem solving • Decision making • Conflict resolution
Nurse–health care team	• Communicate clearly nursing's perspective regarding the patient and family to the health care team. • Coordinate the inputs of the multidisciplinary team into a comprehensive care plan. • Serve as a liaison between the patient and family and the health care team, as necessary.	

of activities that a nurse performs to carry out the intervention, and a short list of background readings. Advantages of having a standard classification of nursing interventions are discussed in Chapter 17.

The researchers involved in the development of NICs are also committed to developing a classification of patient outcomes for nursing interventions, called Nursing Outcomes Classifications (NOCs). This research aims to:

1. Identify, label, validate, and classify nursing-sensitive patient outcomes and indicators
2. Evaluate the validity and usefulness of the classification in clinical field testing
3. Define and test measurement procedures for the outcomes and indicators

This research continues in an effort to develop a common nursing language to optimize the design and delivery of safe, high-quality, and cost-effective care.

Care Coordination, Continuity, and the Nurse

One of nursing's major contributions to the interprofessional health care team is the role of coordinator (discussed in Chapter 12). Care can easily become fragmented when patients are seen by numerous specialists—each interested in a different aspect of the patient—and in different settings. At best, patients express feeling that no one single person really knows them and can talk with them about what is going on and how it all may affect them in the future. At worst, the orders of different specialists may conflict with one another and be counterproductive. Therefore, it is important for you as the nurse to make rounds with other health care professionals and to read the results of consultations that patients have had with specialists. You can then interpret the specialists' findings for patients and family members, prepare patients to participate maximally in the care plan in both institutional

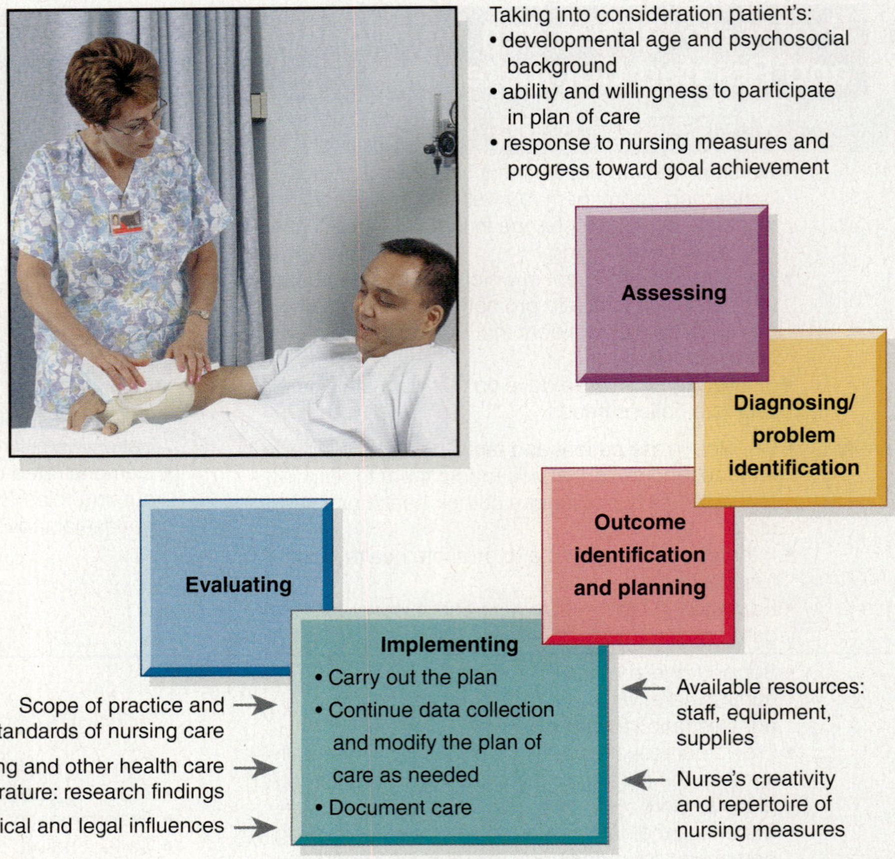

FIGURE 18-1. Implementing involves carrying out the plan of care, which is modified in response to patient changes. Numerous variables influence the way the care plan is implemented (see *arrows*). (*Source:* Used with permission from Shutterstock. *Photo by B. Proud.*)

and community settings, and serve as a liaison among the members of the health care team. Nurse case managers and navigators are specialists in the role of care coordinator and work in both inpatient and community settings.

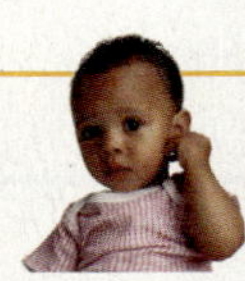

Think back to **Antoinette Browne**, the toddler described at the beginning of the chapter. As a result of the child's delays, multiple disciplines would likely be involved in caring for her. The nurse would play a major role as coordinator for the child's care, ensuring communication among all team members. In addition, the nurse would act as the liaison between the other members of the team to ensure that the child's grandmother understands the care plan.

CRITICAL THINKING/CLINICAL REASONING AND JUDGMENT, AND IMPLEMENTING

As you implement the plan of care, you are constantly engaging in clinical reasoning and judgment about what you are doing. Since patient conditions can change dramatically in minutes, you must reassess the patient for changes in status that may dictate a different set of interventions. You also want to be sure that research supports the interventions you have selected and be open to better ways of addressing patient problems and issues. **Clinical inquiry** is defined as the ongoing process of questioning and evaluating practice and advancing informed practice (Mick, 2017, p. 39). In every clinical setting, we should hear nurses and other members of the team actively questioning whether there are better ways to achieve desired patient outcomes. "Am I offering everything that is currently available to achieve the best outcome?" Finally, you are always monitoring the patient's responses to your interventions so that you can modify the care plan if needed. Remember Alfaro's rule (Alfaro-LeFevre, 2014, p. 161):

Assess, reassess, revise, record:

- *Assess* patients before performing nursing actions.
- *Reassess* them to determine their responses after you perform nursing actions.
- *Revise* your approach as indicated.
- *Record* patient responses and any changes you made in the care plan.

As a student, you should always ask if you are competent to implement the plan of care. If you doubt that your cognitive, interpersonal, or technical competencies are adequate to successfully implement the care plan, it is your responsibility to ask for help. Getting help when you need it demonstrates your primary commitment to the patient. Expert nurses understand that learning is a lifelong practice and that we need one another to continue to master clinical skills.

IMPLEMENTING AND INTERPERSONAL COMPETENCE

Nursing is rarely a solo activity. Nurses are always working with patients, families, communities, and other nurses and health care professionals (see Table 18-1 on page 477). While nurses need knowledge of best practice interventions and technical skills to implement the care plan, it is also true that the nurse's interpersonal competence to a large degree determines how successfully the plan is implemented. If your patients and team do not trust you, it will be difficult to motivate everyone's best effort toward achieving goals. Alfaro-LeFevre (2014, p. 161) writes that "your ability to communicate (listen, speak, and write effectively) with patients, families, assistive personnel (APs), and other professionals makes the difference between competent, efficient care and care that is sloppy, unprofessional, and prone to errors." You may want to talk with patients about what qualities and attributes they value in a nurse. You are sure to discover that your respect, empathy, compassion, accountability, and trustworthiness are highly valued.

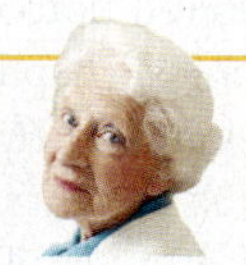

Remember **Estelle Morrissey** telling her nurse, "I'm all alone. There's no one left and I want to die. Can you help me?" A skilled nurse would try to find out what Estelle really wants. Is she simply lonely and longing for companionship, or is this an authentic request for assistance in suicide if this is a legal option in your state? The nurse who responds to Ms. Morrissey might document the following intervention.

> Found Ms. Morrissey alone in her room when the other residents were in the dining room. She told me, "There's no one left and I want to die. Can you help me?" I sat down beside her and asked her what she really wants and she replied that she misses her husband (who died 5 years ago) and her friends from church. I asked her if she wanted me to see if anyone from her church would be able to visit and she visibly brightened. Upon leaving her room, I called her minister to arrange a visit, and we hope to set up a visitation schedule.
>
> 9/22/25, 1000, Carol Taylor, RN

This example demonstrates the importance of documenting what you do so that anyone else hearing Ms. Morrissey's concerns would know what is planned and be able to evaluate its effectiveness.

One tip for practice is to cultivate the habit of reflecting on your clinical encounters each day. As you walk out of a human encounter, mentally look back at what you are leaving in your "wake." Were you one more anonymous person who did something "to" the patient? Were you toxic? Or were you the one who will be remembered as making or being the critical difference for the patient? The choice is yours in every encounter. At the end of your shift, ask, "Are my patients better for having had me today?" "Is my team better for my being in it today?"

TYPES OF NURSING INTERVENTIONS

Nursing Interventions Classification

The NIC project defines a **nursing intervention** as "any treatment based upon clinical judgment and knowledge that a nurse performs to enhance patient/client outcomes" (Bulechek et al., 2008, p. xxi). The NIC project goes on to describe types of interventions:

> Nursing interventions include both direct and indirect care; those aimed at individuals, families and community; and those for nurse-initiated and other provider-initiated treatments.

A **direct care intervention** is a treatment performed through interaction with the patient(s). Direct care interventions include both physiologic and psychosocial nursing actions and include both the "laying on of hands" actions and those that are more supportive and counseling in nature.

An **indirect care intervention** is a treatment performed away from the patient but on behalf of a patient or group of patients. Indirect care interventions include nursing actions aimed at management of the patient care environment and interdisciplinary collaboration. These actions support the effectiveness of direct care interventions.

A community (or public health) intervention is targeted to promote and preserve the health of populations. Community interventions emphasize the health promotion, health maintenance, and disease prevention of populations and include strategies to address the social and political climate in which the population resides.

Independent and Collaborative Interventions

When you carry out the interventions identified in the care plan, you are implementing the care plan. When implementing the care plan, you function independently and collaboratively. See Chapter 17 for descriptions of nurse-initiated, health care provider–initiated, and collaborative interventions.

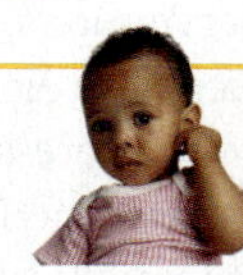

The three types of nursing interventions can be illustrated by the example of **Antoinette Browne**, the toddler with gastrointestinal symptoms and delayed growth and development. If the health care provider orders a series of gastrointestinal studies, it is the nurse's responsibility to prepare the patient by executing the health care provider's order for cleansing the bowel. This nursing action is a health care provider–initiated intervention. When the nurse senses that the grandmother seems unusually fearful of the outcome of the studies, and explores the grandmother's fears and then follows up with appropriate teaching and counseling, the nurse is using nurse-initiated interventions. When a multidisciplinary team conference is held to discuss the patient's failure to progress, the nurse works collaboratively with the psychiatrist, gastroenterologist, social worker, and child development specialist to develop a comprehensive care plan; this involves collaborative nursing interventions.

Carpenito-Moyet (2017, pp. 37–38) describes how the major focus of intervention differs according to the type of nursing diagnoses or problem being addressed.

For actual nursing diagnoses/problems, interventions seek to:

- Reduce or eliminate contributing factors of the diagnosis or problem
- Promote higher-level wellness
- Monitor and evaluate status

For risk nursing diagnoses/problems, interventions seek to:

- Reduce or eliminate risk factors
- Prevent the problem
- Monitor and evaluate status

For possible nursing diagnoses/problems, interventions seek to:

- Collect additional data to rule out or confirm the diagnosis

For collaborative problems, interventions seek to:

- Monitor for changes in status
- Manage changes in status with nurse-prescribed and health care provider–prescribed interventions
- Evaluate response

Protocols and Standing Orders

Protocols and standing orders expand the scope of nursing practice in certain clearly defined situations. **Protocols** are written plans that detail the nursing activities to be executed in specific situations. Although some protocols specify routine aspects of nursing care (e.g., protocols that describe nursing responsibilities when a patient is admitted to or discharged from the institution), other protocols include **standing orders** that empower the nurse to initiate actions that ordinarily require the order or supervision of a health care provider. Examples include admission protocols for obstetrics and gynecology patients, protocols for bowel programs that allow the nurse to select and administer necessary bowel interventions, standard orders for narcotic overdoses that specify the agents the nurse is to administer to reverse respiratory depression in an emergency, and standard orders for pain management that enable the nurse to select the strength of the medication to be given within preset ranges.

Care Bundles

The Institute for Health Improvement (IHI) defines **care bundle** as a structured way of improving processes of care and patient outcomes: A small straightforward set of evidence-based practices—generally three to five—that, when performed collectively and reliably, have been proven to improve patient outcomes. The power of a bundle "comes from the body of science behind it and the method of execution, with complete consistency . . . A bundle ties the practices together into a package of interventions that people know must be followed for every patient, every single time" (http://www.ihi.org/resources/Pages/ImprovementStories/WhatIsaBundle.aspx).

The IHI website has examples of care bundles that have dramatically improved patient outcomes including the central line bundle and ventilator bundle.

IMPLEMENTING THE PLAN OF CARE

When carrying out the plan of care, nurses use specialized abilities to (1) determine the patient's new or continuing need for nursing assistance, (2) promote self-care, and (3) assist the patient to achieve valued health outcomes. Nurses must also organize necessary resources and anticipate unexpected outcomes and situations. Novice nurses need to be sure they possess the nursing competencies necessary to carry out the plan of care, and to consult with their instructor or preceptor if unsure of their knowledge or ability.

Reassessing the Patient and Reviewing the Plan of Care

As you begin your professional practice, you will be expected at any time to provide a rationale for your actions. Does research demonstrate that this is the best intervention to achieve a desired outcome? The student care plans at the end of many clinical chapters provide a rationale for each intervention, and it may be helpful to check out some of these care plans now.

A patient's condition can change dramatically in a matter of minutes. Therefore, it is critical to assess the patient carefully before initiating any nursing intervention to make sure that the care plan is still responsive to the patient's needs and prioritized to the most pressing of those needs.

Each nurse implementing the plan should:

- Be sure that each nursing intervention is supported by a sound scientific rationale, as demanded by **evidence-based practice** (see Chapter 2)
- Be sure that each nursing intervention is consistent with your scope of practice and professional standards of care and consistent with the protocols, policies, and procedures of the institution or facility
- Be sure that the nursing actions are safe for this particular patient and individualized to their preferences
- Clarify any questionable orders

Using Patient Boards or Dry-Erase Boards

Increasingly, a variety of practice sites are using dry erase dry-erase boards as a convenient two-way communication system between patients and their professional caregivers. They allow nurses to communicate with the patient and the patient's family and to let patients know that their voices are being heard. They are an excellent way to involve patients in their care plan and have been shown to increase patient satisfaction. They typically include the patient's priority goals and comfort/pain scales as well as reminders to providers to wash their hands and reminders to patients to "Please call don't fall."

The content on these boards will change according to the unit and its priorities. Figures 18-2 and 18-3 illustrate patient dry-erase boards for a hospital inpatient adult unit and a pediatric emergency room.

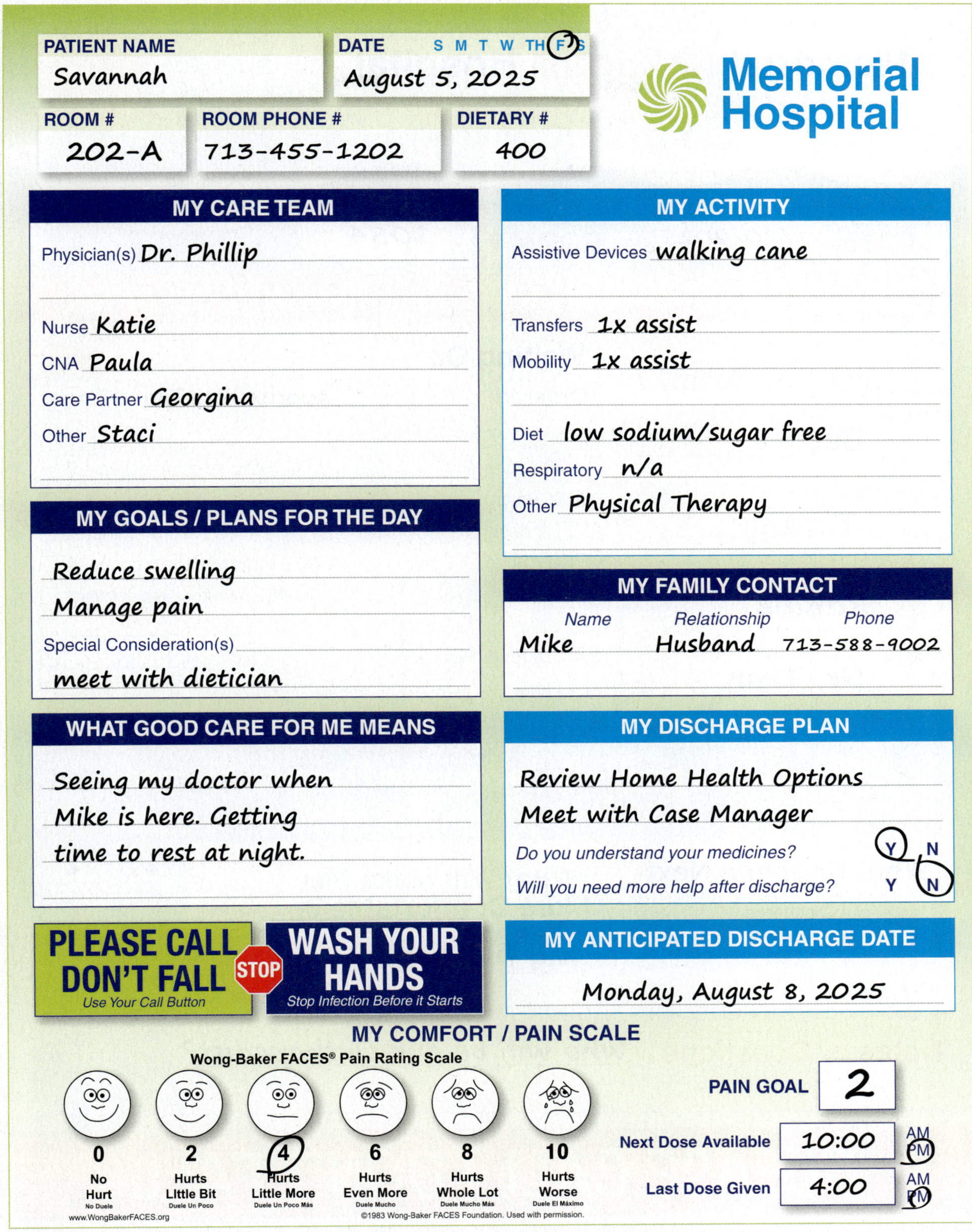

FIGURE 18-2. Adult inpatient dry-erase board. (*Source:* Used with permission, VisiCare™ 2017. For Information/inquires click http://www.VisiCare.com. VisiCare™ is a DBA of Insignia Marketing, Inc. Patent pending. 281-465-0040 Info@VisiCare.com.)

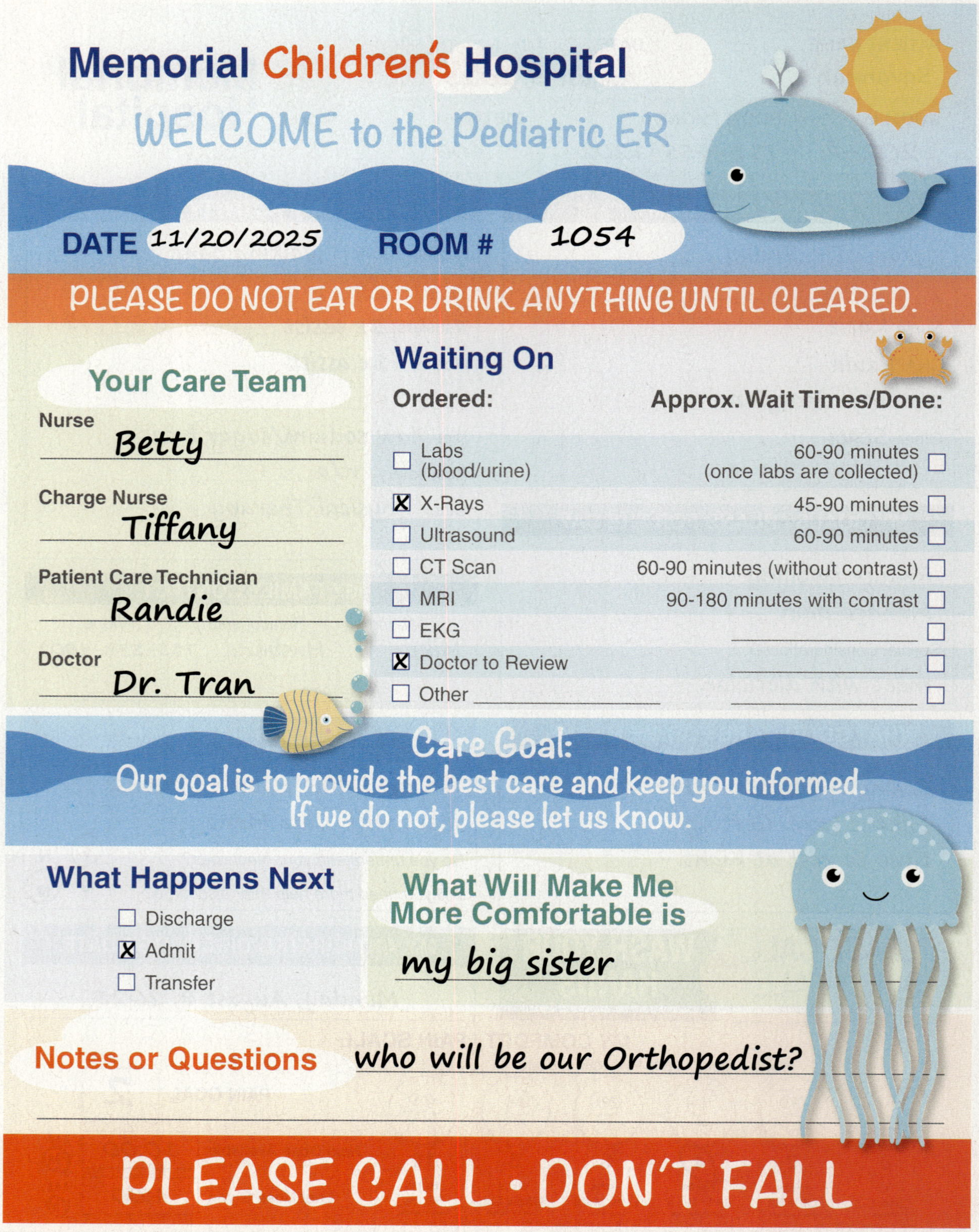

Memorial Children's Hospital

WELCOME to the Pediatric ER

DATE 11/20/2025 ROOM # 1054

PLEASE DO NOT EAT OR DRINK ANYTHING UNTIL CLEARED.

Your Care Team

Nurse
Betty

Charge Nurse
Tiffany

Patient Care Technician
Randie

Doctor
Dr. Tran

Waiting On

Ordered:	Approx. Wait Times/Done:
☐ Labs (blood/urine)	60-90 minutes (once labs are collected) ☐
☒ X-Rays	45-90 minutes ☐
☐ Ultrasound	60-90 minutes ☐
☐ CT Scan	60-90 minutes (without contrast) ☐
☐ MRI	90-180 minutes with contrast ☐
☐ EKG	☐
☒ Doctor to Review	☐
☐ Other	☐

Care Goal:
Our goal is to provide the best care and keep you informed.
If we do not, please let us know.

What Happens Next
☐ Discharge
☒ Admit
☐ Transfer

What Will Make Me More Comfortable is
my big sister

Notes or Questions who will be our Orthopedist?

PLEASE CALL • DON'T FALL

FIGURE 18-3. Pediatric emergency room dry-erase board. (*Source:* Used with permission, VisiCare™ 2017. For Information/inquires click http://www.VisiCare.com. VisiCare™ is a DBA of Insignia Marketing, Inc. Patent pending. 281-465-0040 Info@VisiCare.com.)

Make sure you learn about how dry-erase boards are being used on your clinical units, what information you can expect to find there, and what your responsibilities are to update content. These boards become meaningless if not updated frequently in response to patient changes.

Clarifying Prerequisite Nursing Competencies

To implement the plan of nursing care, nurses need blended intellectual, interpersonal, technical, and ethical/legal competencies as well as mastery of the Quality and Safety Education for Nurses (QSEN) Competencies that are described in Chapter 13 and illustrated in the Reflective Practice displays that introduce each chapter. Each nurse has a unique blend of these competencies and can act effectively to the extent that their abilities match the patient's need for nursing care.

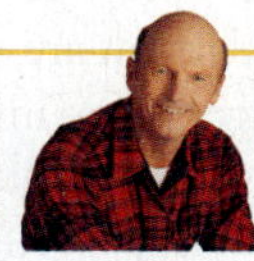

Remember **James McMahon**, the critically ill patient in the ICU. Although technologic skills are key in this area, the nurse also needs to implement care that integrates intellectual, interpersonal, and ethical and legal competencies because of the patient's complex needs. QSEN competencies—patient-centered care, teamwork and collaboration, evidence-based practice, quality improvement, safety, and informatics—also promote a good outcome.

Always notify your nursing instructor or nurse mentor if you believe that you lack any competencies needed to safely implement the care plan.

QSEN SAFETY

Nurses committed to safety and minimizing the risk of harm to patients and providers will examine human factors and other basic safety design principles as well as commonly used unsafe practices such as work-arounds and dangerous abbreviations. These nurses value their own role in preventing errors.

Planning Ahead and Organizing Resources

In today's hectic health care environments, successful implementation of the plan of care requires a high degree of organization and efficiency.

Patient and Patient Visitors

Make sure that the patient is physically and psychologically prepared for what you are going to do. Give the nursing intervention the best chance for success by ensuring that the patient is not in too much pain to cooperate, understands what is being attempted and why they should cooperate, and is not distracted (e.g., by wanting to talk with visitors or watch TV). If visitors are in the room, check with the patient to see if they want the visitors to stay during the procedure. If a family caregiver needs to learn new caregiving skills, try to schedule your interventions at a time appropriate for the patient and convenient for the family caregiver.

Equipment

Anticipate all the equipment you will need to successfully carry out the intervention, and arrange it so that it is easily accessible. Be sure to order sufficient supplies at the beginning of the shift for the care you expect to provide, and be thoughtful of the nurse who will follow you by leaving adequate supplies. Follow facility policy when ordering supplies to ensure proper charges.

Nurse Self Care Alert

To avoid injury on the job, take the time to use proper assistive devices, such as lifts for heavy patients or transfer boards for patients with limited mobility.

Environment

Think through the proper environment for each intervention. Thoughtful, person-centered practice means paying special attention to respecting the patient's dignity, privacy, and safety needs. Remember routine measures as simple as closing a door or pulling drapes. These considerations are of special importance when patients or residents share rooms. For example, administering an enema can be embarrassing for the patient and unpleasant for the patient's roommate. With some planning, the intervention can be scheduled in a private bathroom or at a time when the roommate is absent.

Personnel

Identify whether you can carry out the planned intervention alone or if you need assistance. To avoid injury to both patients and professional caregivers, be sure that interventions are attempted by the right person or by a sufficient number of people. Because it is easy to underestimate the strength it takes to lift or support a large patient, it is always safer to err on the side of having too much help rather than not enough. Teams of student nurses can begin each rotation by asking, "Who thinks they might need help today?" The team can then plan to coordinate care so that help is available when needed.

Time Management

One of the most essential skills you will develop in your clinical experiences is time management. Almost any experienced nurse will tell you that in today's health care environments where efficiency reigns, prioritizing face time with patients is an everyday challenge. Too often, the demand to utilize the electronic medical record to chart every bit of assessment data and intervention further limits time spent with patients. Remember that Benner includes both the nurse's helping role and organizational and work-role competencies in the domains of nursing. Be sure as you plan care for the patients in your caseload that you anticipate the time needed for the interventions you intend to carry out and prioritize these from most to least important.

Anticipating Unexpected Outcomes and Situations

When you learn about new nursing procedures and interventions, you often see a list of possible adverse effects. An **adverse reaction** is an unwanted or harmful reaction experienced following the administration of a drug, diagnostic test, or therapeutic intervention under normal conditions of use.

Although everyone hopes never to encounter these complications, they do occur with some frequency. The skilled nurse knows what might happen if an intervention "goes wrong" and is prepared to deal with the new challenge. This may be as simple as accurately assessing how much support a patient may need to avoid a fall when ambulating for the first time after surgery or being prepared to respond to complaints of burning at a new intravenous (IV) site. For further consideration of unexpected outcomes and situations, refer to *Taylor's Clinical Nursing Skills* by Pamela Lynn and *Taylor's Video Guide to Clinical Nursing Skills* by Wolters Kluwer.

Unfolding Patient Stories: Mona Hernandez • Part 1

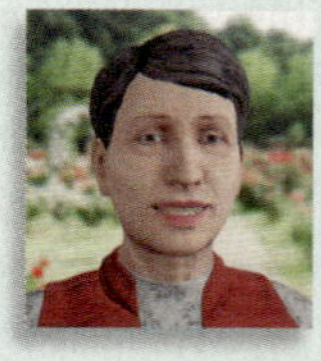

Mona Hernandez, a 72-year-old female admitted to an acute care unit with pneumonia, is receiving oxygen via nasal cannula and intravenous fluids. An activity order is written for "out of bed to chair and ambulate three times a day." How would the nurse plan activity for Mona? What unexpected outcomes should the nurse anticipate when getting her out of bed for the first time? What steps can the nurse take to ensure patient safety with activity? (Mona Hernandez's story continues in Chapter 30.)

Care for Mona and other patients in a realistic virtual environment: ***vSim** for Nursing* (thepoint.lww.com/vSimFunds). Practice documenting these patients' care in DocuCare (thepoint.lww.com/DocuCareEHR).

Ensuring Quality and Patient Safety: Preventing Errors and Omissions

Keeping patients safe and delivering high-quality care require a vigilance today that was unknown as recently as 10 years ago. Anytime you feel tempted not to wash your hands or clean them with gel or foam before a patient encounter, ask yourself if you are willing to complicate your patient's recovery by introducing infection, increasing the length of stay and related costs. Every nurse should be familiar with the easily accessible resources available at the following websites and web pages:

- Agency for Healthcare Research and Quality (AHRQ), Quality and Patient Safety website: https://www.ahrq.gov/professionals/quality-patient-safety/index.html
- The Institute for Health Care Improvement's Patient Safety web page: http://www.ihi.org/Topics/PatientSafety/Pages/default.aspx
- The Joint Commission's Patient Safety web page: https://www.jointcommission.org/topics/patient_safety.aspx

Alfaro-LeFevre (2014) counsels nurses to keep patients safe during implementation by preventing errors and omissions and building safety nets (Fig. 18-4). Starting with your first clinical experience, develop the habit of monitoring closely for error-prone situations. The goal is to "catch" possible errors and omissions early. Remember that anyone can make a mistake and everyone, including the most senior health care provider or nurse, needs surveillance.

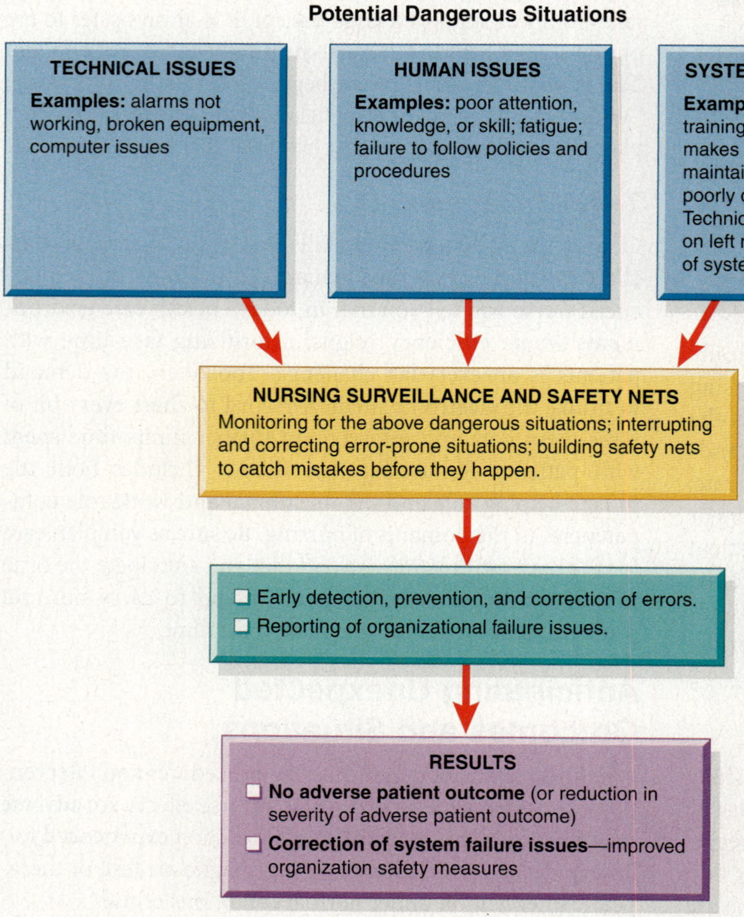

FIGURE 18-4. How monitoring for dangerous situations promotes early correction of problems and keeps patients safe. (© 2010 www.AlfaroTeachSmart.com. Used with permission.)

Nursing Advocacy in Action

Patient Scenario

The emergency department (ED) is very rushed and overcrowded. Mrs. Penuela, who speaks little English, grabs you when you walk into the waiting area and begs someone to look at her husband, who is holding his head and moaning. When you finally get him in the unit to be assessed, he has a blood pressure of 240/150 mm Hg. He speaks a little more English than his wife, but is not fluent. However, you are able to learn that he stopped taking his blood pressure medication because he couldn't afford the prescription. He also lost his job and the family lost their house because of an inability to make mortgage payments. They are now living with her brother. Mr. Penuela is in the ED for several hours while intravenous medications are administered. You are shocked to discover that the only discharge orders for Mr. Penuela are a prescription for the same medication he was on previously, which he couldn't afford. His doctor tells you that the ED isn't a charity or social service—"our job is to fix medical problems."

Implications for Nursing Advocacy

How will you respond if you are Mr. Penuela's nurse? Talk with your classmates and experienced nurses about the questions that follow.

- If you elect to advocate for the Penuelas, what practical steps can you take to ensure better health outcomes?
- What is it reasonable to expect of a student nurse, a graduate nurse, and an experienced nurse in this situation?
- What advocacy skills are needed to effectively respond to this challenge?

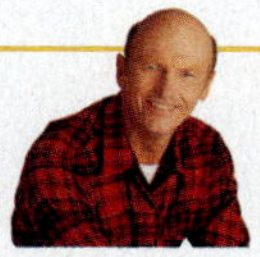

Remember **James McMahon**, the critically ill patient in the ICU. When the nurses caring for Mr. McMahon spent times relabeling and organizing his lines they were preventing a possible error.

Henneman et al. (2010) recommend the following strategies to identify, interrupt, and correct errors:

- *Error identification strategies:* knowing the patient, knowing the "players," knowing the plan of care, surveillance, knowing policy and procedure, double-checking, using systematic processes, and questioning.
- *Error interruption strategies:* offering help, clarifying, and verbally interrupting.
- *Error correction strategies:* persevering, being physically present, reviewing or confirming the plan of care, offering options, referencing standards or experts, and involving another nurse or health care provider.

The Joint Commission encourages patients to become active, involved, and informed participants on the health care team. Figure 18-5 illustrates The Joint Commission's initiative to get patients to more actively participate in their care by speaking up. The website offers numerous videos and infographics in English and Spanish that you can use with your patients.

Promoting Self-Care: Teaching, Counseling, and Advocacy

Although most people can meet their basic human needs independently, illness and the stress of diagnostic and therapeutic measures may interfere with a person's usual practice of self-care. Nurses assess patients' abilities to meet their human needs independently. Nurses can fail patients by doing too much for them and by encouraging negative, sick-role behaviors, such as inappropriate dependence. Conversely, there is a time and a place for the "tender loving care" that says to a patient, "I know you may be able to do this for yourself, but just this once, how about if I do it, and we'll talk!" Balancing the need to encourage a patient's best self-care effort with the effort to make each patient feel cared for is an important component of the art of nursing.

If patients and their families want to participate actively in seeking wellness, preventing disease and illness, recovering health, and learning to cope with altered functioning, they need effective self-care behaviors. Nurses sensitive to the importance of patients learning to direct and manage their own care use nurse–patient interactions for both planned and spontaneous teaching, counseling, and advocacy. These nursing roles are described in Chapters 6 and 9. See also the accompanying Nursing Advocacy in Action box. Referring families to a community support group or other resources further enhances the self-care behaviors being developed. See Through the Eyes of a Family Caregiver (on page 487) for a description of one wife's experiences when her husband was discharged home.

Remember: the only way you can be sure that patients or family caregivers have mastered a skill is watching them perform it. Once you observe them doing a procedure correctly you can be confident that learning—as well as teaching—has occurred.

Assisting Patients to Meet Health Outcomes

In this phase of the implementation process, the nursing team carries out the nursing orders detailed in the nursing care plan. If the care plan is well constructed, carrying out its orders is the nurse's most important task and should receive top priority. The nursing actions planned to promote patient goal or outcome achievement and the resolution of health problems should be carefully executed. Implementation guidelines are listed in Box 18-1 on page 487.

Because understaffing is a problem in many practice settings, nurses must learn to use their time wisely and to maximize each patient encounter. Inserting an IV can be simply that, or it can be an opportunity to gather additional focused data, to communicate concern for what the patient

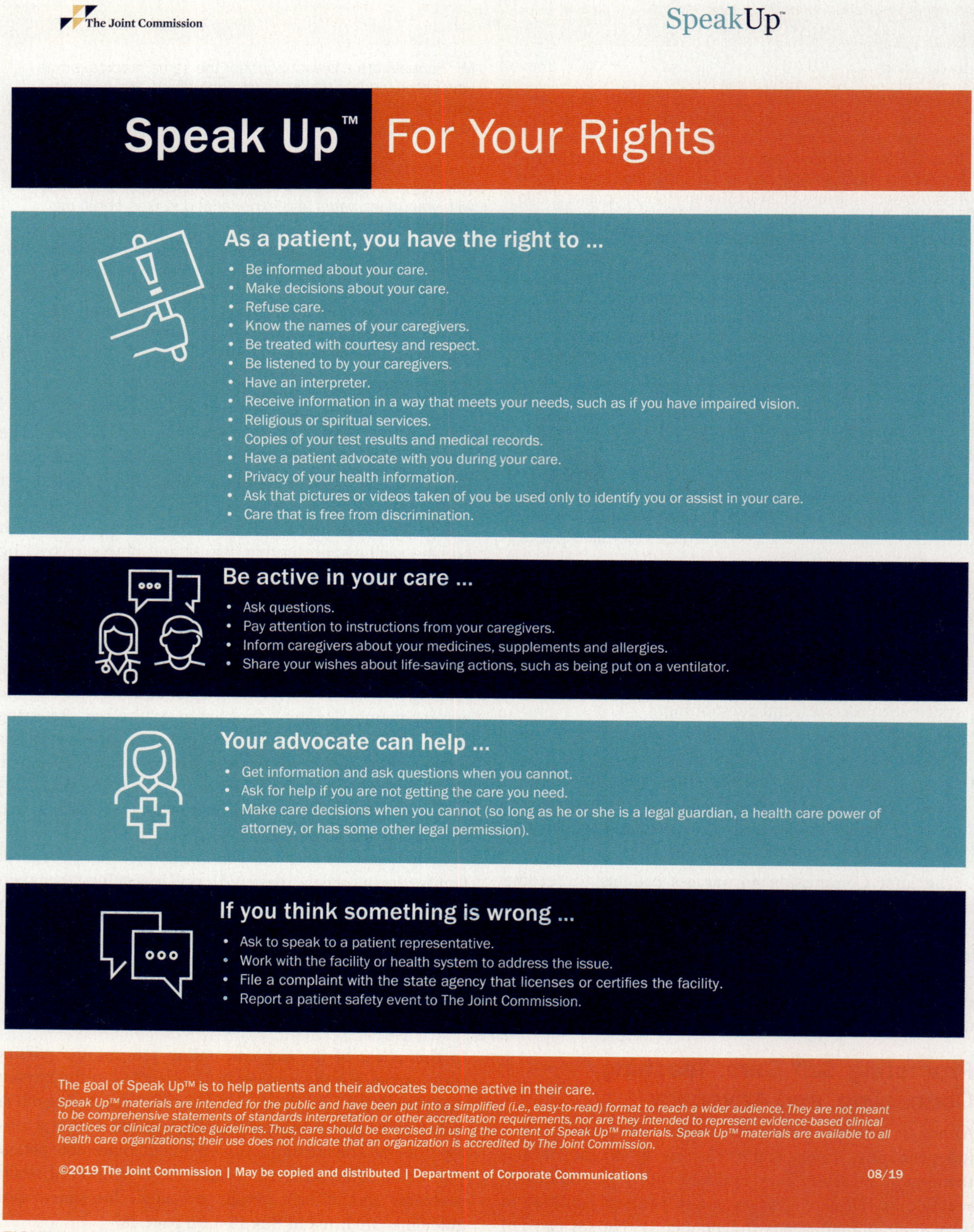

The Joint Commission

SpeakUp™

Speak Up™ For Your Rights

As a patient, you have the right to ...

- Be informed about your care.
- Make decisions about your care.
- Refuse care.
- Know the names of your caregivers.
- Be treated with courtesy and respect.
- Be listened to by your caregivers.
- Have an interpreter.
- Receive information in a way that meets your needs, such as if you have impaired vision.
- Religious or spiritual services.
- Copies of your test results and medical records.
- Have a patient advocate with you during your care.
- Privacy of your health information.
- Ask that pictures or videos taken of you be used only to identify you or assist in your care.
- Care that is free from discrimination.

Be active in your care ...

- Ask questions.
- Pay attention to instructions from your caregivers.
- Inform caregivers about your medicines, supplements and allergies.
- Share your wishes about life-saving actions, such as being put on a ventilator.

Your advocate can help ...

- Get information and ask questions when you cannot.
- Ask for help if you are not getting the care you need.
- Make care decisions when you cannot (so long as he or she is a legal guardian, a health care power of attorney, or has some other legal permission).

If you think something is wrong ...

- Ask to speak to a patient representative.
- Work with the facility or health system to address the issue.
- File a complaint with the state agency that licenses or certifies the facility.
- Report a patient safety event to The Joint Commission.

The goal of Speak Up™ is to help patients and their advocates become active in their care.

Speak Up™ materials are intended for the public and have been put into a simplified (i.e., easy-to-read) format to reach a wider audience. They are not meant to be comprehensive statements of standards interpretation or other accreditation requirements, nor are they intended to represent evidence-based clinical practices or clinical practice guidelines. Thus, care should be exercised in using the content of Speak Up™ materials. Speak Up™ materials are available to all health care organizations; their use does not indicate that an organization is accredited by The Joint Commission.

©2019 The Joint Commission | May be copied and distributed | Department of Corporate Communications 08/19

FIGURE 18-5. Improve safety: Urge your patients to speak up. (*Source:* Used with permission. © 2019 The Joint Commission.)

Through the Eyes of a Family Caregiver

"The nurses never told me there'd be days like this."

I wasn't prepared for a roller coaster ride when my husband became ill. My husband was admitted to the hospital in an emergency condition, became confused when his electrolytes were off balance, went into cardiac arrest and had CPR, was placed on a ventilator, and was sedated because he was too apprehensive about the ventilator. I had reached the lowest point as I sat by his bedside for days, talking to him and wondering if he heard me.

My spirits soared the day they brought him out of his sleep state and he recognized me and was hungry for real food. The next day when I went to the hospital, I plummeted to the low point again when he was crumpled in bed like a confused rag doll with his hospital gown up to his chest and the sheet to his ankles. I started to cry, and the nurse came and put her arm around me. She said, "Don't think he's taken a turn for the worse. There will be good days and bad days as he recovers." No one had prepared me for that—and her arm around me and her words were so consoling.

When I brought him home after 6 weeks in the hospital, I was not prepared for his anger at being confined to the house (in a heat wave) and not being allowed to drive. His reasoning that he had to get a haircut because he hadn't had one in 2 months made sense to him. My saying that no one would care about the length of his hair did not soothe his anger.

He couldn't accept the fact that he was too weak to go up and down the steps more than once a day, so he insisted on going to the basement. Going down was simple; coming up wasn't. We forgot there was no railing (which he needed to haul himself up) on the last four steps. He solved the problem by sitting on the steps and lifting himself up a step at a time. Then he got to the floor at the top and couldn't stand up. I couldn't lift him. We were stuck. Again, I took a nose dive.

I thought I understood how difficult it would be for him to readjust. I knew he would be depressed and expected him to lean on me. But I was not prepared for his frustration to come out as anger at me. It would have been helpful to have someone prepare me. Or, it would be nice to have a nurse put her arm around me now when my roller coaster plummets.

—Eleanor Faven, Philadelphia, Pennsylvania

Box 18-1 Implementing Guidelines

- When implementing nursing care, remember to act in partnership with the patient/family.
- Before implementing any nursing action, reassess the patient to determine whether the action is still needed.
- Approach the patient competently. Know how to perform the nursing action, why the action is being performed, and potential adverse responses. Have all equipment and supplies ready.
- Approach the patient caringly. Explain the nursing action using language the patient understands. Communicate genuine concern for what the patient is experiencing.
- Modify nursing interventions according to the patient's (1) developmental and psychosocial background, (2) ability and willingness to participate in the care plan, and (3) responses to previous nursing measures and progress toward goal/outcome achievement.
- Check to make sure that the nursing interventions selected are consistent with your scope of practice and standards of care and within legal and ethical guides to practice.
- Always question that the nursing intervention selected is the best of all possible alternatives. Consult colleagues and the nursing and related literature to see if other approaches might be more successful. Evaluate the effectiveness of the intervention selected, noting any factors that positively or negatively influenced the outcome.
- Develop a repertoire of skilled nursing interventions. The more options one can choose from, the greater the likelihood of success.

is experiencing and offer support, and to teach and counsel as appropriate. How the nurse uses the time for inserting the IV determines how effective the nurse is in helping the patient to achieve the patient's goals and outcomes. See the accompanying Through the Eyes of a Student display (on page 488) for one student's account of an important bath.

When working with patients to achieve the outcomes specified in the care plan, remember that nothing about the care plan is fixed. Some of the most important variables that influence how the care plan is implemented follow.

Patient Variables

Ideally, the patient is primary in determining how nursing interventions are implemented. Successful nurses modify their nursing actions according to the patient's (1) changing ability and willingness to participate in the care plan and (2) previous responses to nursing interventions and progress toward achieving goals or outcomes. Other important variables are the patient's developmental stage, psychosocial background, and culture.

DEVELOPMENTAL STAGE

Addressing the developmental needs of a patient involves identifying the patient's developmental stage, as well as the developmental tasks related to this stage and their relationship to nursing care. However, be careful not to let stereotypes about developmental stages and tasks influence patient care. To implement a comprehensive and holistic care plan, nurses must find creative ways to meet developmental needs. This is of greatest importance when patients are separated from their families and home environments for long periods.

Through the Eyes of a Student

One of my first patients was a woman with a history of Alzheimer's disease. When I was assigned this patient, I knew that I was not going to have a good day. I had been introduced to her the week before, when I had orientation. She was sitting in a geriatric chair in the hallway, where she sang at the top of her lungs and threw tissues on the floor. Occasionally, she would curse at a person passing by.

I took a deep breath and entered her room. At her bedside, I introduced myself. With a few choice words, she told me to get out of her room. I tried to ignore her response and prepared her breakfast tray. She proceeded to throw her scrambled eggs around the room. After I took the tray away from her and finished cleaning up the mess, it was time for preconference. At preconference, my instructor told me that we were going to "tub" my patient. I had visions of a grand fiasco in the tub room, and I dreaded giving her the bath.

My instructor and I took her to the tub room by wheelchair. Once we convinced her to get in the tub, she did nothing but yell that it was cold. We started the water and she yelled even louder. I knew everyone could hear her in the hallway as she cursed and yelled, but as the bath proceeded, she quieted down and stopped fighting me. We completed the bath and wheeled her back down the hall to her room. I bundled her up in blankets and put her in the Geri chair in the hallway. She was so relaxed from the bath that she let me brush her hair and put it in a ponytail. While I was brushing her hair, she fell asleep. I did my chart until her lunch arrived. When I set her up for her lunch and told her I would be leaving, she thanked me, and it made my day. All the struggling I went through all day with her and she thanked me. When I went home, I felt really good about helping her. During all my worrying about the day being a fiasco and the embarrassment of having a patient yell at me, I had lost sight of the patient herself and what she needed me to do for her. By her thanking me at the end of the day, I realized that when my clinical instructor forced me to do something for my patient that the regular staff of the hospital wouldn't do, I was meeting her basic needs, and my patient recognized that.

—Jeanene C. Smith

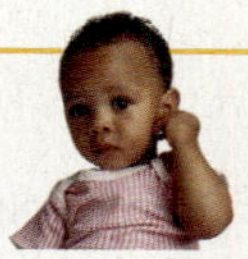

Think back to **Antoinette Browne**, the toddler with physical and developmental delays. The nurse would creatively adapt interventions to meet the needs of this toddler.

PSYCHOSOCIAL BACKGROUND AND CULTURE

When choosing nursing interventions, the nurse should consider and respect the patient's socioeconomic background and culture. Confronted with a malnourished patient on a limited income who rents a single room in a boarding home, a nurse cannot simply teach the importance of including more protein in the diet. To be effective, the nurse must explore the realistic issue of whether the patient can afford and obtain foods rich in protein. Moreover, the nurse needs to assess whether the patient values this intervention and is willing to make the necessary changes. Similarly, if the diet you recommend is unfamiliar to the patient who eats different foods for economic or cultural reasons, your intervention is unlikely to be successful. A nurse midwife recently shared that a colleague once took her aside and said, "You can't do that." Their practice was mainly for high-risk adolescent teens in a low-income area of the city, and she had just suggested that the patient buy organic kale to make smoothies. The colleague reminded her that the young woman lived in a food desert, might not own a blender, and was probably not the one who cooked in her family.

Nurse Variables

Nurse variables that influence the implementation of the care plan include levels of expertise, creativity (ability to match patient needs with specific nursing strategies), willingness to provide care, and available time. Focused Critical Thinking Guide 18-1 illustrates the importance of a nurse's ability to think critically about intervention strategies.

Resources

The most elaborately designed care plan cannot be fully effective without adequate staff, equipment, and supplies. These resources are all important determinants of patient care. The patient's financial resources and the adequacy of community-based resources also influence the care plan.

Scope of Practice and Current Standards of Care

All nursing actions for implementing the care plan must be consistent with the nurse's scope of practice and standards of care. See Chapter 19 for a discussion of these standards. All nurses are responsible for learning the standards that dictate practice in their specialty. Failure to practice according to these standards may result in a charge of negligence.

Research Findings

Nurses concerned about improving the quality of nursing care use research findings to enhance their nursing practice. Reading professional nursing journals and attending continuing education workshops and conferences are excellent ways to learn about new nursing strategies that have proved effective. Evidence-based practice resources online include the following:

- The Agency for Healthcare Research and Quality (AHRQ): http://ahrq.gov
- The Cochrane Effective Practice Organization of Care's reviews on effective quality improvement and implementation: http://epoc.cochrane.org

18-1 Focused Critical Thinking Guide

INTERVENTION STRATEGIES

One of the nurses on the oncology unit where you have been working for 6 months since graduation wants to develop a "humor room" where patients, their families, and staff can "take a break" from the serious business of illness. Designed to lift the spirits, amuse, distract, and thus speed the healing process, humor rooms are gaining popularity as new therapeutic tools. Funny books, comic movies on a large-screen TV, games, and puzzles—and ideally, even clowns, magicians, musicians, and stand-up comedians—are being envisaged. Several nurses have vocally expressed their lack of support for the project and think the idea is "stupid" at best, and potentially a great waste of money, time, and energy that could be devoted to "tried and true" methods of healing. You have been asked to support the project and must decide how to respond.

1. Identify goal of thinking

Clarify your thinking about humor as a therapeutic measure so that you can decide whether to support this project.

2. Assess adequacy of knowledge

Pertinent circumstances: The nurse who wants to develop the humor room is more popular with patients than she is with her colleagues. Her nurse friends are quick to point out that while it's true that she is "a bit flaky" and unorthodox, she is an efficient nurse who is well loved by her patients and their families. The hospital is in the midst of cutting expenses and has laid off both professional and nonprofessional employees.

Prerequisite knowledge: To decide how you should respond in this situation, you need to research the healing benefits of humor. Are there clinical studies demonstrating its effectiveness as a therapeutic measure? If studies point to humor's effectiveness, you will need to determine: (1) what priority it should have among other treatment modalities and (2) the feasibility of creating a humor room in the current climate of cutting expenses. Is there a creative way to finance this venture?

Room for error: Since life and death do not hinge on how you elect to respond to this plea for support, there is a relatively wide margin for error. Because personal energy and finances are limited, however, you do not want to involve your unit in a futile project.

Time constraints: There is no rush for an immediate decision on your part, which gives you adequate time to develop the knowledge base you need to make an informed decision.

3. Address potential problems

The most serious obstacle to critical thinking in this situation would be the lack of an open mind and refusal to weigh the merits of a new treatment modality. Complicating factors include divided loyalties among the nurses and the tendency to support or refuse support for the project on the basis of whether one likes the nurse advocating the project, rather than on the merits of the project. Finally, the lowered morale caused by layoffs may squash all creativity and willingness to "dream new dreams."

4. Consult helpful resources

Your first challenge will be to learn more about humor as a healing measure. Ideally, you may be able to consult a local expert and invite the expert to meet with the staff. Alternatively, you can research the literature, looking for clinical studies and reports of the first-person experiences of others.

5. Critical judgment/decision

After a search of the literature that convinced you and some of the other nurses of the clinical benefits of humor, you decide to explore the feasibility of developing a humor room. Your options are to "play it safe" and not rock the boat during a difficult period in the hospital by trying something new, or to become an advocate for the project and commit your energies to making it happen. You decide that a creative project may be exactly what the staff needs to rediscover the "joy of nursing" and begin to explore means to fund the project. You plan to "start small" and to reassess the project every 6 months. Since your research educated you about the potential benefits *and harms* humor can create, you decide that your first objective must be to educate the staff.

- *Toolkit: Implementation of Clinical Practice Guidelines*, available at the Registered Nurses' Association website, http://www.rnao.org
- Intervention Mapping, Step 5: Program Implementation Plan, available at the Intervention Mapping website, http://interventionmapping.com
- American Association of Critical-Care Nurses (AACN) Practice Alerts: https://www.aacn.org/clinical-resources/view-all-issues#page/1?%7B75C75579-1BCC-4DD7-9044-A01AB54B2FAD%7D%5B%5D=%7BFE23A6BE-FE7F-4E2D-B539-A6F2BA208E88%7D

The evidence-based practice literature continues to identify the high demands of providing patient care and limits on available time, resources, and structures as barriers to evidence-based practice. It is important as you begin planning and implementing care for patients to perceive evidence-based practice as a consistent approach to providing safe, quality patient care, rather than an "extra duty" or student care plan demand (Mick, 2017). Read Bridges, McNeill, and Munro (2016) for an exhilarating description of how research published in the preceding year will lead to practice change in critical care, address challenges at the bedside, and introduce new care strategies.

Research in Nursing boxes throughout this text demonstrate the difference nursing research can make in improving patient outcomes. Proponents of nursing implementation science are beginning to address the challenges of implementing research findings into practice.

Ethical and Legal Guides to Practice

To practice good nursing, you need to be knowledgeable about the laws and regulations that affect health care and the ethical dimensions of clinical practice. Without this understanding, a sincere motivation to benefit the patient and a conscientious attempt to implement nursing orders will not be sufficient. Each nurse is responsible for becoming sensitive to the ethical and legal dimensions of practice, and moral and legal accountability are inherent in the practice of professional nursing.

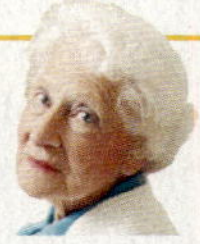

Look back on the scenario presented at the beginning of the chapter for **Estelle Morrissey**. Ethical and legal guidelines are crucial in determining how the nurse intervenes. In addition, the nurse needs to evaluate the ethical and legal ramifications of their actions in light of the patient's request to die.

Chapters 6 and 7 discuss the ethical and legal dimensions of practice. Hospital risk managers and ethics committees are increasingly available as institutional resources for nurses.

CONTINUING DATA COLLECTION AND RISK MANAGEMENT

Sensitivity to how the patient is responding to nursing interventions and to the patient's progress toward outcome achievement allows the nurse to modify nursing interventions appropriately.

A vital nursing intervention is ongoing risk management. While monitoring the patient's responses to the care plan, nurses are also alert to the development of new problems that may result in the identification of new diagnoses or collaborative problems. As nurses get to know patients and recognize clusters of significant data, they can identify problems for which the patient is at risk and intervene appropriately to promote health and to prevent disease.

DOCUMENTING NURSING CARE

Remembering the legal truth, "It wasn't done if it wasn't documented," each nurse carefully documents all nursing interventions. See Chapter 20 for guidelines for written documentation, and see the nursing care plans at the end of clinical chapters for samples of documented nursing interventions.

WHEN A PATIENT DOES NOT COOPERATE WITH THE PLAN OF CARE

When a patient does not follow the plan of care despite your best efforts, it is time to reassess strategy. The first objective is to identify why the patient is not following the therapy. One possibility is that the care plan may not be right for this patient. In this event, what is needed is not a change in the patient but rather a change in the plan of care. If you determine, however, that the care plan is adequate, you must identify and remedy the factors contributing to the patient's nonadherence. Common reasons for nonadherence include:

- Lack of family support
- Lack of understanding about the benefits of adherence
- Low value attached to outcomes or related interventions
- Adverse physical or emotional effects of treatment (such as pain and fatigue)
- Inability to afford treatment
- Limited access to treatment

Remember the difference between labeling patients "nonadherent" and judging them as "bad people" versus being open to understand the reasons for someone's failing to act on the care plan. Think about the effect on the patient both of these nursing responses to learning that a patient hasn't been taking his blood pressure medicines will have. "What's wrong with you? Don't you know that high blood pressure can kill you?" versus "Can you tell me why taking your medications as scheduled is so difficult for you? I would like to understand."

DELEGATING NURSING CARE

Because of the pressure to reduce health care costs and the increasing demand for nursing services in the midst of a critical shortage of professional nurses, many employers of nurses have increased their use of **assistive personnel (APs)**, sometimes referred to informally as "nurse extenders" or "techs." APs are people trained to function in an assistive role to the licensed registered nurse (RN) in the provision of patient activities as delegated by and under the supervision of the registered professional nurse. **Delegation** is the transfer of responsibility for the performance of an activity to another person while retaining accountability for the outcome. In some cases, the new mix of professional and nonprofessional staff is threatening patient safety. Never has it been more important for nurses to critically identify which nursing interventions require professional nurses and which can be safely delegated; this can be especially challenging for new nurses. See the Five Rights of Delegation in Box 18-2. Chapter 10 includes additional discussion of delegation, including the ANA's *Principles for Delegation.*

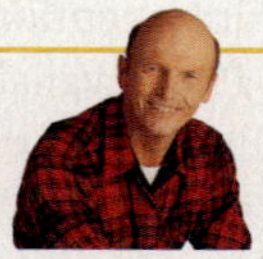

Review the patient scenario for **James McMahon**, the critically ill patient described at the beginning of the chapter and in "Reflective Practice: Challenge to Technical Skills." The nurse's ability to delegate effectively is important for providing safe, efficient care.

Box 18-2 Five Rights of Delegation

Right Task

- The activity falls within the delegatee's job description or is included as part of the established written policies and procedures of the nursing practice setting. The facility needs to ensure that the policies and procedures describe the expectations and limits of the activity and provide any necessary competency training.

Right Circumstance

- The health condition of the patient must be stable. If the patient's condition changes, the delegatee must communicate this to the licensed nurse, and the licensed nurse must reassess the situation and the appropriateness of the delegation.

Right Person

- The licensed nurse along with the employer and the delegatee is responsible for ensuring that the delegatee possesses the appropriate skills and knowledge to perform the activity.

Right Directions and Communication

- Each delegation situation should be specific to the patient, the licensed nurse, and the delegatee.
- The licensed nurse is expected to communicate specific instructions for the delegated activity to the delegatee; the delegatee, as part of two-way communication, should ask any clarifying questions. This communication includes any data that need to be collected, the method for collecting the data, the time frame for reporting the results to the licensed nurse, and additional information pertinent to the situation.
- The delegatee must understand the terms of the delegation and must agree to accept the delegated activity.
- The licensed nurse should ensure that the delegatee understands that they cannot make any decisions or modifications in carrying out the activity without first consulting the licensed nurse.

Right Supervision and Evaluation

- The licensed nurse is responsible for monitoring the delegated activity, following up with the delegatee at the completion of the activity, and evaluating patient outcomes. The delegatee is responsible for communicating patient information to the licensed nurse during the delegation situation. The licensed nurse should be ready and available to intervene as necessary.
- The licensed nurse should ensure appropriate documentation of the activity is completed.

Source: Used with permission. National Council of State Boards of Nursing/American Nurses Association. (2019, April 1). National guidelines for nursing delegation. https://www.nursingworld.org/~4962ca/globalassets/practiceandpolicy/nursing-excellence/ana-position-statements/nursing-practice/ana-ncsbn-joint-statement-on-delegation.pdf

Delegation and the Student Nurse

Student nurses may find that they have been delegated to provide care they cannot safely perform. Whenever you are asked by a staff nurse to perform an intervention for which you lack training, consult with your instructor to see if you can safely perform the intervention with supervision. Never attempt to perform interventions beyond your capacity without supervision, even if instructed to do so by a staff nurse. Review the Reflective Practice feature at the beginning of this chapter. Students who work as nursing assistants while enrolled in professional programs are especially likely to be asked to perform interventions beyond their mastery. You may be able to turn these requests into learning opportunities. For example, you might say, "I've never practiced that procedure but I'd love the opportunity to observe one of the experienced nurses do this."

GUIDE FOR STUDENTS

Organizing Care

Student nurses organizing their nursing care in advance for a particular clinical day can use the guidelines for student clinical responsibilities in Box 18-3 to help identify nursing measures for which they will be responsible. In addition to these guidelines, working out a time schedule may provide clear direction for the clinical day and ensure that the patient's needs are met. Some faculty require students to prepare clinical logs, which are also an excellent guide to organization. Figure 18-6 (on page 492) illustrates guidelines for a clinical log.

Box 18-3 Organizing Student Clinical Responsibilities

To organize clinical responsibilities, check:

1. Patient profile
2. Name by which patient wishes to be addressed
3. Patient's chief complaint and reason for admission
4. Patient's current health status: Note any physical or emotional changes indicating the need to modify the care plan.
5. Routine assistance patient needs to meet basic human needs
6. Priorities for nursing care:
   a. Priorities identified by the patient as "most important." The nurse might state, "I'll be your nurse until 3 PM, and I'm interested in learning what you would most like to accomplish today."
   b. Prioritized nursing diagnoses/problems, patient outcomes, and related nursing interventions
   c. Medical orders that need to be implemented
   d. Interdependent or collaborative nursing responsibilities
7. Special "events" of the day that may require special observation of the patient, teaching, preparation, or aftercare:
   a. Diagnostic tests
   b. Consultations with specialists
   c. New therapies (physical therapy, medications, surgery, radiotherapy, and the like)
8. Special safety or risk management needs
9. Special teaching, counseling, or advocacy needs
10. Special needs of the family

Evaluation Criteria for Clinical Logs

Student	Date

Element/Criteria	Points possible	Score
Epidemiology of Primary Diagnosis • Incidence • Prevalence • Risk factors • Case-fatality rate	10	
Pathophysiology • Presented in understandable patient education terms • Brief explanation is congruent with actual physiologic processes of disease	10	
Tests/Procedures • Brief explanation of why indicated • Analysis of findings accurate • Pre-post patient education developmentally appropriate • Pre-post nursing interventions appropriate	10	
Medications • Provide a list of all medications that the patient is receiving • Brief explanation of the indication in terms that a patient would understand	10	
Physiologic/Psychosocial Assessment Summary • Assessment findings accurate • Includes physiologic, psychosocial, and spiritual findings (as identified)	10	
Nursing Diagnosis • 5 appropriate nursing diagnoses identified • Diagnoses presented in appropriate format • Priority nursing diagnosis selected is appropriate	10	
Nursing Process: Interventions/Rationale/Evaluation. (Determined by clinical faculty weekly) • Measurable goals established/short-term goal supports achievement of long-term goal but are not the same goal • Interventions are clear and concise and include frequency of action • Three appropriate interventions provided for each LT and ST goal • Rationales clearly support intervention in plan of care and are referenced • Evaluation statements for short-term goal are clear and concise (LTG not evaluated) • Unmet goals include action plan	20	
Self-Identified Strengths and Opportunities for Self Improvement • Congruent with Strengths Identified by Instructor	2	
National Patient Safety Goals: Identify one of the National Patient Safety Goals and how you addressed it during your shift (use a different one for each log).	4	
Cultural Considerations Appropriately Incorporated in Your Care with an Example	2	
Values: Describe an example of how your nursing care emulates the principles of Social Justice, Human Flourishing, OR Commitment to the Common Good that we stand for in the Department of Nursing at Georgetown University	4	
Professional Roles • Self-identities roles utilized in providing care	2	
Reflective Practice: Thought Question of the Week • Question posed by student upon reflecting on the day of care. May be based on patient care or condition, nursing, staff issues, etc.	2	
Format: Typed, spelling, grammar, APA for references	4	
Note: Papers are due within 48 hours. Please submit to your clinical faculty member via e-mail or Blackboard as per their preference. Rules for grading apply as with all NHS papers.	100	

FIGURE 18-6. Evaluation tool for clinical logs. (*Source:* Used with permission. Georgetown University School of Nursing and Health Studies.)

Nursing Oneself

It is difficult for nurses to be sincerely attentive to patient needs if their own human needs are not met. Make sure you come to your clinical rotation well rested and having had a nutritious meal. Because no one is perfectly healthy or "whole" all the time, nurses preparing for professional practice should spend time getting to know themselves. Activities that promote psychological health when practiced regularly include self-awareness, communication, time management, preparation for crisis and loss, developing and maintaining support systems, and practicing self-care in all areas. The characteristics of emotional health include self-esteem, self-knowledge, satisfying interpersonal relationships, environmental mastery, stress management, a positive body image, a sense of humor, and the ability to experience pleasure. See related content in Chapter 1.

Nurses who want to be competent practitioners learn early to nurse themselves and other nurses before attempting to nurse patients. Good personal health enables nurses not only to practice more efficiently, but also to be a health model for patients and their families. Nurses can help patients to imitate good health behaviors and eventually integrate them into their daily life through the process of identification. Use the Promoting Health displays in each clinical chapter (Units VI and VII) for yourself as well as for your patients. You will also find Nurse Self-Care Alerts like the one below throughout the text.

Nurse Self-Care Alert

The Occupational Safety and Health Administration (OSHA) cites three factors that make hospitals such hazardous workplaces:

Unique risks: Hospital workers lift, reposition, and transfer patients who have limited mobility. Other unique risks include needlesticks and violence.

Unique culture: Caregivers feel an ethical duty to "do no harm" to patients. Some will put their own safety and health at risk to help a patient.

They are not assembly lines: Employees must react to unpredictable events with split-second decisions.

Read more at: https://www.osha.gov/dsg/hospitals/documents/1.1_Data_highlights_508.pdf.

REFLECTIVE PRACTICE LEADING TO PERSONAL LEARNING

Remember that the object of reflective practice is to look at an experience, understand it, and learn from it. As you begin to develop your expertise in implementing the care plan, reflect on your experiences—successes and failures—in order to improve your practice. How can you do it better next time? What did you learn today that can help you tomorrow? Begin your reflection by paying close attention to the following during the implementing phase of the nursing process:

- Did your commitment to engage your patients and families and to collaborate with your fellow students, instructor, and other members of the team as you implemented the care plan result in successful partnerships?
- Did your preparation result in your feeling confident about the nursing interventions you performed? Did your competence and confidence inspire the patient's and team's trust?
- Were you able to offer a scientific rationale for each intervention you employed (evidence-based practice)?
- Did your patients make real progress toward realizing expected outcomes as a result of your interventions?
- Did you need to modify the care plan as a result of ongoing assessments? Did you think of better interventions to produce the expected outcomes?
- Did your vigilance and awareness of potential error and omissions prevent error?

Perhaps the most important question to reflect on is: Are your patients and their families/caregivers better for having had *you* share in the critical responsibility of partnering with them to implement the care plan?

DEVELOPING CLINICAL REASONING AND CLINICAL JUDGMENT

1. Team up with another student and take turns role-playing a nurse visiting an older man who is homebound and needs his vital signs and nutritional status assessed. Discuss with each other the truth or falsity of this claim: "*Who the nurse is*, is as important as, and sometimes more important than, *what the nurse does*."
2. Receive the same clinical assignment as another student and independently outline your care priorities, specifying what you plan to accomplish during each of your clinical hours. Talk with the other student about the differences in what you both hope to accomplish and how you would do this. Try to imagine what these differences would mean to the patient.
3. You are the only RN on a 50-bed wing in a long-term care facility. You have one LPN working with you and two personal care assistants. Each of the 50 residents requires assistance with activities of daily living, all take at least some medications, and most require monitoring for multiple chronic (and sometimes acute) illnesses. When the home is short-staffed, you are sometimes the only RN covering two 50-bed units. How will you decide which interventions to delegate?
4. Describe how you would probably respond, and how you would like to respond (if these are different), to hearing another nurse in the shift report say that one of the patients you are assigned to was a real "PIB" ("pain in the butt") all day and "just impossible" to care for. Reflect on the importance of the language we use to report on a patient to one another.

PRACTICING FOR NCLEX

1. A school nurse determines that a student who has lost weight is at risk for an eating disorder and would benefit from a nutritional assessment. What action will the nurse take?
   a. Perform a focused nutritional assessment
   b. Seek direction from the student's health care provider
   c. Suggest the student visit the nurse-run clinic
   d. Request a consultation with a nutritionist
2. A nurse is caring for a group of patients. Which actions are appropriate to include in the implementation phase of care? Select all that apply.
   a. Changing the dressings on a burn victim's arm
   b. Assessing a patient's nutritional intake
   c. Formulating a nursing diagnosis for a patient with epilepsy
   d. Turning a patient in bed every 2 hours to prevent pressure injuries
   e. Checking a patient's insurance coverage at the initial interview
   f. Determining availability of community resources for a patient with dementia
3. Nurses use the Nursing Interventions Classification (NIC) Taxonomy structure as a resource to plan nursing care for patients. What information is found in this structure?
   a. Case studies illustrating a complete set of activities that a nurse performs to carry out nursing interventions
   b. Nursing interventions, each with a label, a definition, and a set of activities that a nurse performs to carry it out, with a short list of background readings
   c. Complete list of nursing diagnoses, outcomes, and related nursing activities for each nursing intervention
   d. Complete list of reimbursable charges for each nursing intervention
4. A nurse works in a long-term care facility where standing orders are in place for influenza vaccines for all residents. What is the nurse's priority, when carrying out the prescriptions?
   a. Assessing whether the patient previously received the vaccine
   b. Refusing to give the vaccine without a written prescription
   c. Determining if the standing orders are inappropriate for their unit
   d. Calling the nursing supervisor to determine if this is a permitted action
5. A nurse performs nurse-initiated nursing actions when caring for patients in a skilled nursing facility. Which reflect these types of actions? Select all that apply.
   a. Administering an antibiotic to a patient with pneumonia
   b. Consulting with a psychiatrist for a patient who misuses opiates
   c. Checking the skin of bedridden patients for skin breakdown
   d. Ordering a kosher meal for an orthodox Jewish patient
   e. Recording a patient's intake and output
   f. Preparing a patient for surgery according to facility protocol
6. A nurse enters the patient's room to perform pin-site care for a patient wearing a halo vest to stabilize the cervical spine. What action will the nurse take first?
   a. Administer pain medication
   b. Reassess the patient
   c. Prepare the equipment
   d. Explain the procedure to the patient
7. The charge nurse tells a nursing student to change a surgical dressing while they take care of other patients. The student has not changed dressings before and does not feel confident performing the procedure. What action should the student take?
   a. Tell the charge nurse that they lack the technical competencies to change the dressing independently
   b. Assemble the equipment for the procedure and follow the steps in the procedure manual
   c. Ask another student nurse to work collaboratively with them to change the dressing
   d. Tell the clinical instructor they have not had experience with the delegated task
8. A nurse develops a care plan for an adolescent patient who gave birth to a premature infant. When presented with the collaborative care plan, including home health care visits, the patient states, "We will be fine on our own. I don't need any more care." What is the nurse's best response?
   a. "You know your personal situation better than I do; I will respect your wishes."
   b. "If you don't accept these services, your baby's health will suffer."
   c. "Let's take a look at the plan again and see if we can adjust it to fit your needs."
   d. "I'm going to assign your case to a social worker who can explain the services better."
9. An RN working on a hospital unit frequently delegates patient care to assistive personnel (AP). Which activities are appropriate for the nurse to safely delegate? Select all that apply.
   a. Performing patient assessments
   b. Making patient beds
   c. Giving patients bed baths
   d. Administering oral medications
   e. Ambulating patients
   f. Assisting patients with meals

10. A nursing student is prioritizing interventions for a patient with diabetes who needs diagnostic testing, dressing changes, meal planning and counseling, and assistance with hygiene. The patient states, "I must have my hair washed before I can do anything else; I'm ashamed of the way I look." How will the student best prioritize this patient's care?
    a. Explain to the patient that there is not enough time to wash their hair today because of the busy schedule
    b. Schedule the testing and meal planning first and complete hygiene as time permits
    c. Perform the dressing changes first, schedule the testing and counseling, and complete hygiene last
    d. Wash the patient's hair and perform hygiene, schedule testing and counseling, then change the dressing
11. A nurse is caring for a patient with a painful, non-healing surgical wound. The patient does not request pain medication because they do not want to be a burden. What actions will the nurse implement to improve pain relief? Select all that apply.
    a. Reestablishing the pain level the patient finds acceptable as the pain management goal
    b. Obtaining a dry-erase board to remind the patient of the plan of care
    c. Assessing the patient's pain and offering analgesia during hourly rounding
    d. Placing the analgesic underneath other medications and quickly handing it to the patient
    e. Asking the family members to speak to the patient about pain relief
12. A nursing unit has adopted use of a care bundle for insertion of central venous catheters. During the procedure, which action by a nurse requires the charge nurse to intervene?
    a. They discard the sterile drapes in the insertion kit.
    b. The primary nurse reminds everyone in the room to wear a mask.
    c. The team includes every item in the bundle during the procedure.
    d. The nursing student states using the bundle improves patient outcomes.

ANSWERS WITH RATIONALES

1. **a.** Performing a focused assessment is an independent nurse-initiated intervention, not requiring a prescription from or intervention by the health care provider, advanced practice nurse, or nutritionist.
2. **a, d, f.** During the implementing step of the nursing process, nursing actions that were formulated during the planning process are carried out. The purpose of the implementation phase is to assist the patient in achieving valued health outcomes, for example promote health, prevent disease and illness, restore health, and facilitate coping with altered functioning. Assessing a patient's nutritional status or insurance coverage occurs in the assessment step, and formulating nursing diagnoses occurs in the diagnosing/analyzing step.
3. **b.** The Nursing Interventions Classification (NIC) Taxonomy lists nursing interventions, each with a label, a definition, a set of activities that a nurse performs to carry it out, and a short list of background readings. It does not contain case studies, diagnoses, or charges.
4. **a.** Standard orders empower the nurse to initiate actions ordinarily requiring the order, prescription or supervision of a health care provider. The nurse first assesses whether the patient has already received the vaccine. The standing order is a valid prescription given to cover common, recurring actions the nurse can use when indicated.
5. **c, d, f.** Nurse-initiated interventions, or independent nursing actions, include nurse-prescribed interventions resulting from their assessment of patient's actual or potential health problems. Protocols and standard orders empower the nurse to initiate actions that ordinarily require the order or supervision of a health care provider. Consulting with a psychiatrist is a collaborative intervention.
6. **b.** Before implementing any nursing action, the nurse returns to the first step of the nursing process, reassessing whether the action is still needed. Then the nurse may collect the equipment, explain the procedure, and, if necessary, administer pain medications.
7. **a.** Student nurses should notify their nursing instructor or nurse preceptor if they believe they lack any competencies needed to safely implement the care plan. Once educated and technically prepared, the nursing student may perform a dressing change.
8. **c.** When a patient rejects the care plan, the nurse works to identify the underlying barriers. If the nurse determines that the care plan is adequate, the nurse works with the patient to formulate mutually developed goals and interventions.
9. **b, c, e, f.** AP assist the RN to provide care as delegated by and under their supervision. Typical tasks delegated include actions for stable patients (e.g., vital signs hygiene, bed-making, ambulating patients, and helping to feed patients). Performing the initial patient assessment and administering medications are the responsibility of the RN.
10. **d.** When time constraints and safety permit, priorities identified by the patient as most important are completed first. Washing the patient's hair and assisting with hygiene put the patient first, setting the tone for an effective nurse–patient partnership.
11. **a, b, c.** The nurse reassesses the patient's knowledge and acceptance of the plan of care, including the level of pain the patient finds acceptable. Using a dry-erase board and hourly rounding further communicate and reinforce the care plan. The nurse develops a compassionate and trusting relationship with the patient; the nurse and patient mutually determine the plan for pain management, not their family.
12. **a.** Care bundles are sets of evidence-based interventions that, when performed together and consistently, improve the process of care and patient outcomes. Discarding sterile drapes from the insertion kit circumvents this process.

Bibliography

Agency for Healthcare Research and Quality (AHRQ). Quality and patient safety. https://www.ahrq.gov/professionals/quality-patient-safety/index.html

Alfaro-LeFevre, R. (2010). *Applying nursing process: A tool for critical thinking* (7th ed.). Wolters Kluwer Health/Lippincott Williams & Wilkins.

Alfaro-LeFevre, R. (2014). *Applying nursing process: The foundation for clinical reasoning* (8th ed.). Wolters Kluwer Health/Lippincott Williams & Wilkins.

Alfaro-LeFevre, R. (2020). *Critical thinking, clinical reasoning, and clinical judgment: A practical approach* (7th ed.). Elsevier.

Alspach, J. G. (2017). The checklist: Recognize limits, but harness its power. *Critical Care Nurse, 37*(5), 12–18.

American Nurses Association (ANA). (2010). *Nursing's social policy statement* (2010 ed.). Author.

American Nurses Association. (2015). *Code of ethics for nurses*. Author.

American Nurses Association (ANA). (2021). *Nursing: Scope and standards of practice* (4th ed.). Author.

American Nurses Association (ANA) and the National Council on of State Boards of Nursing (NCSBN). (n.d.). *Joint statement on delegation*. https://www.ncsbn.org/Delegation_joint_statement_NCSBN-ANA.pdf

Begley, R., Cipriano, P. F., & Nelson, R. (2020). *The business of caring: Promoting optimal allocation of nursing resources*. Healthcare Financial Management Association. https://www.hfma.org/content/dam/hfma/Documents/industry-initiatives/business-of-caring-promoting-optimal-allocation-nursing-resources.pdf

Benner, P. (1984). *From novice to expert: Excellence and power in clinical nursing practice*. Addison-Wesley.

Benner, P., & Wrubel, J. (1989). *The primacy of caring: Stress and coping in health and illness*. Addison-Wesley.

Bridges, E., McNeill, M., & Munro, N. (2016). Research in review: Driving critical care practice change. *American Journal of Critical Care, 25*(1), 76–84.

Brown, J., & Braden, C. J. (2020). Nursing turbulence in critical care: Relationships with nursing workload and patient safety. *American Journal of Critical Care, 29*(3), 182–191.

Bulechek, G. M., Butcher, H. K., & Dochterman, J. C. (Eds.). (2008). *Nursing interventions classification (NIC)* (5th ed.). Elsevier/Mosby.

Bulechek, G. M., Butcher, H. K., Dochterman, J. C., & Wagner, C. M. (Eds.). (2013). *Nursing interventions classification (NIC)* (6th ed.). Elsevier.

Carpenito, L. J. (2017). *Nursing diagnosis: Application to clinical practice* (15th ed.). Philadelphia, PA: Wolters Kluwer.

Dark, T., & Ellis, W. M. (2020). Level loading nurse assignments based on the work intensity. *American Nurse Journal, 15*(1), 46–49.

Dickerson, J., & Latina, A. (2017). Team nursing: A collaborative approach improves patient care. *Nursing, 47*(10), 16–17.

Freel, J., & Fleharty, B. (2021). Standardizing handoff communication. *American Nurse Journal, 16*(3), 30–33.

Hackett. T., & Bigott, V. (2021). New graduate nurse time management. *American Nurse Journal, 16*(5), 30–32.

Henneman, E., Gaawlinski, A., Blank, F., Henneman, P., Jordan, D., & McKenzie, J. (2010). Strategies to identify, interrupt, and correct medical errors: Theoretical framework. *American Journal of Critical Care, 19*(6), 500–509.

Herman, A. E. (2016). *Visual intelligence*. An Eamon Dolan Book. Mariner Books.

Institute for Health Care Improvement. *Patient safety*. http://www.ihi.org/resources/Pages/ImprovementStories/WhatIsaBundle.aspx

Institute of Medicine. (2010). *The future of nursing: Leading change, advancing health*. The National Academies Press.

Iowa Intervention Project. (1993). The NIC taxonomy structure. *Image—The Journal of Nursing Scholarship, 25*(3), 187–192.

Iowa Intervention Project. (1997). Nursing interventions classification (NIC): An overview. In M. J. Rantz & P. LeMone (Eds.), *Classification of nursing diagnoses: Proceedings of the Twelfth Conference, North American Nursing Diagnosis* (pp. 32–39). CINAHL Information Systems.

The Joint Commission. *Patient safety*. https://www.jointcommission.org/en/resources/patient-safety-topics/patient-safety/

The Joint Commission. *Speak up for your rights*. https://www.jointcommission.org/resources/for-consumers/speak-up-campaigns/for-your-rights

Kerfoot, K. (2019). Patient-centered staffing as the path forward. *American Nurse Today, 14*(9), 87–90.

Leis, S. J., & Anderson, A. (2020). Time management strategies for new nurses. *American Journal of Nursing, 120*(12), 63–66.

Locklear, K. (2021). The BOSS method: Using simulation to teach management and organizational skills. *Nursing, 51*(7), 15–18.

Macdonald, B. J., & Dickinson, J. K. (2021). Breaking out of the system and moving to strengths-based care. *Nursing, 51*(8), 39–42.

McCauley, K. M. (2005). A message from the American Association of Critical-Care Nurses. *American Journal of Critical Care, 14*(3), 186.

McCloskey, J. C., & Bulechek, G. M. (Eds.). (1992). *Nursing interventions classification (NIC)*. Mosby-Year Book.

McCloskey, J. C., & Bulechek, G. M. (Eds.). (1995). Validating and coding of the NIC taxonomy structure. *Image—The Journal of Nursing Scholarship, 27*(1), 43–49.

Mick, J. (2017). Call to action: How to implement evidence-based nursing practice. *Nursing, 47*(4), 36–43.

Moorhead, S., Johnson, M., Maas, M. L., & Swanson, E. (Eds.). (2013). *Nursing outcomes classification (NOC)* (5th ed.). Elsevier.

National Council of State Boards of Nursing/American Nurses Association. (2019, April 1). National guidelines for nursing delegation. https://www.nursingworld.org/~4962ca/globalassets/practiceandpolicy/nursing-excellence/ana-position-statements/nursing-practice/ana-ncsbn-joint-statement-on-delegation.pdf

Porter, J. S., & Strout, K. A. (2016). Developing a framework to help bedside nurses bring about change. *The American Journal of Nursing, 116*(12), 61–65.

Skelly, C. L., Hall, C. A., & Risher, C. R. (2020). Shared decision making and patient-centered care. *American Nurse Journal, 15*(2), 45–47.

Stephens, T. M. (2020). Build resilient teams to tackle nursing burnout. *American Nurse Journal, 15*(3), 10–14.

Tedone, D. A. (2020). Eliminating horizontal violence from the workplace. *Nursing, 50*(8), 57–60.

Tucker, S. (2019). Implementation: The linchpin of evidence-based practice changes. *American Nurse Today, 14*(3), 8–12.

Ulrich, B., Barden, C., Cassidy, L., & Varn-Davis, N. (2019). Critical care nurse work environments 2018: Findings and implications. *Critical Care Nurse, 39*(2), 67–84.

19 Evaluating

Tyler Jameson

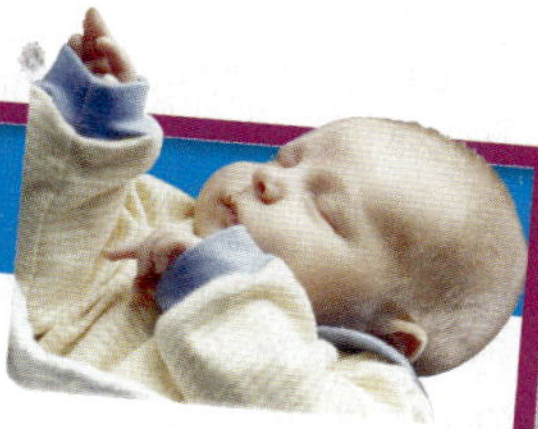

Tyler, a term neonate born 30 hours ago, has yet to pass stool. Follow-up assessment reveals that he does not have a patent anus, a finding that was not detected in the neonate's initial assessment.

Mioshi Otsuki

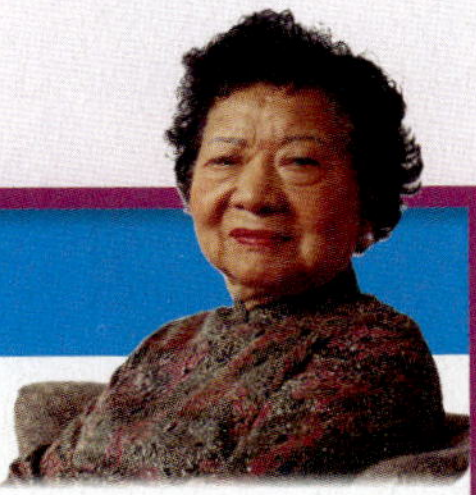

Mioshi, an older adult woman with a history of heart failure being treated with diuretics, is receiving home care. Questioned about her prescribed drug-therapy regimen, Ms. Otsuki states, "I take this one labeled 'furosemide' every day in the morning along with this other one labeled 'Lasix.'"

Nicholas Soros

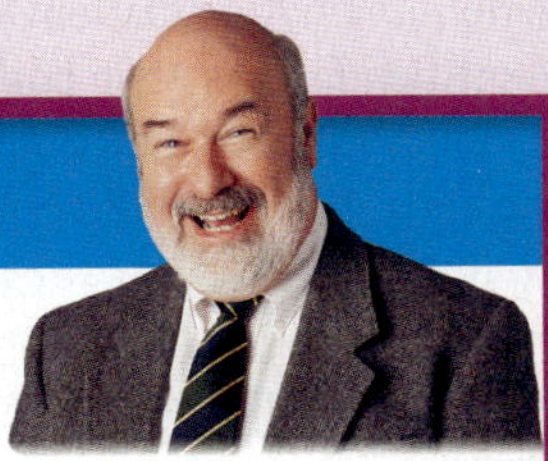

Nicholas is a 68-year-old patient newly diagnosed with diabetes. His initial assessment revealed that he was about 50 lb overweight due to poor diet and lack of exercise. A plan was developed to help Mr. Soros better manage his diabetes through planned weight reduction and regular exercise. At a follow-up visit, assessment reveals a weight gain of 5 lb. He stated, "I'm too old to worry about diet and exercise. You can control my diabetes with medication, right?"

Learning Outcomes

After completing the chapter, you will be able to accomplish the following:

1. Describe evaluation, its purpose, and its relation to the other steps in the nursing process.
2. Evaluate the patient's achievement of four types of outcomes specified in the care plan.
3. Manipulate factors that contribute to success or failure in outcome achievement.
4. Use the patient's response to the care plan to modify the plan as needed.
5. Explain the relation between quality-assurance/quality-improvement programs and excellence in health care.
6. Describe the AACN's six essential standards for establishing and sustaining healthy work environments and the seven crucial conversations in health care.
7. Value self-evaluation as a critical element in developing the ability to deliver quality thoughtful, person-centered nursing care.

Nursing Concepts

- Nursing process
- Evaluation
- Quality improvement

In the fifth phase of the nursing process, **evaluating**, the nurse and patient together measure how well the patient has achieved the outcomes specified in the care plan. When evaluating patient outcome achievement, the nurse identifies factors that contribute to the patient's ability to achieve expected outcomes and, when necessary, modifies the plan of care (Fig. 19-1 on page 500). The purpose of evaluation is to allow the patient's achievement of expected outcomes to direct future nurse–patient interactions. Based on the patient's responses to the plan of care, the nurse decides to:

- Terminate the plan of care when each expected outcome is achieved
- Modify the plan of care if there are difficulties achieving the outcomes
- Continue the plan of care if more time is needed to achieve the outcomes

When evaluation points to the need to modify nursing care, the nurse reviews each preceding phase of the nursing process (assessing, diagnosing, planning, and implementing). Successful evaluation helps ensure that valued patient outcomes are attained. It also enhances the public's image of nursing and promotes continued selection and funding of nursing services in the competitive health care market.

UNIQUE FOCUS OF NURSING EVALUATION

As members of the health care team, nurses are involved in many types of evaluation. Nurses measure patient outcome achievement, how effectively nurses help targeted groups of patients to achieve their specific outcomes, the competence of individual nurses, and the degree to which external factors—such as different types of health care services, specialized equipment or procedures, or socioeconomic factors—influence health and wellness. *The patient, however, is always the nurse's primary concern.* A nurse may perform a nursing procedure competently, creatively, and with care, but if this nursing intervention does not help the patient reach desired outcomes, it is not fully meaningful. Either directly or indirectly, the aim of all nursing evaluation is quality nursing care that aids patient outcome achievement. Therefore, the most important act of evaluation performed by nurses is evaluating outcome achievement with the patient (see the Reflective Practice box for an example).

The Institute of Medicine (IOM)'s Committee on Quality of Health Care in America is educating the public about what patients can reasonably expect from their health care (Box 19-1 on page 500). (Note the IOM was renamed the National Academy of Sciences, Engineering, and Medicine in 2015.) Even beginning nurses can use these guidelines to evaluate the care they are providing.

CLINICAL REASONING AND JUDGMENT AND EVALUATING

The five classic elements of evaluation are:

1. Identifying evaluative criteria and standards (what you are looking for when you evaluate—i.e., expected patient outcomes)
2. Collecting data to determine whether these criteria and standards are met
3. Interpreting and summarizing findings
4. Documenting your judgment
5. Terminating, continuing, or modifying the plan

Each element requires the nurse to use critical thinking and clinical reasoning and judgment about how best to evaluate the patient's progress toward valued health outcomes. In the nursing process, evaluative criteria are the patient outcomes developed during the planning phase. Because patient outcomes reflect desired changes in patient status, and because nursing actions are directed toward these outcomes, they are the core of evaluation in thoughtful, person-centered nursing practice. Determining whether patient outcomes have been or are being met and then identifying the appropriate nursing response are the functions of evaluation.

QSEN Reflective Practice: Cultivating QSEN Competencies

CHALLENGE TO INTERPERSONAL SKILLS

I first met Mr. Nicholas Soros, a 68-year-old patient newly diagnosed with diabetes, in the clinic. He was about 50 lb overweight, and his health history revealed the need for major dietary changes and an exercise program. The interdisciplinary team devised a plan to help Mr. Soros better manage his diabetes through planned weight reduction and regular exercise, for which I did much of the initial teaching. Unfortunately, when Mr. Soros returned for his next checkup, he had gained 5 additional pounds and reported being "too old" to worry about diet and exercise. "You can control my diabetes with medication, right?" When I reported this to the nurse practitioner, he told me that Mr. Soros knows what to do and now it is his responsibility. I wasn't perfectly comfortable with this response and thought that Mr. Soros needed more than someone wagging a finger in his face.

Thinking Outside the Box: Alternate Courses of Action

- Remind Mr. Soros of what he needs to do and tell him that responsibility for this is his!
- After I make sure that he does indeed know what to do, spend time making sure that he values his health sufficiently to try these new behaviors.
- Make sure that Mr. Soros trusts us sufficiently to value working with us to achieve his health goals.

Evaluating a Good Outcome: How Do i Define Success?

- Mr. Soros achieves his target weight and is faithful to a program of regular exercise.
- Mr. Soros feels that his independence and ability to determine his own life plan are respected, at the same time feeling that we care about his health status.
- I learn more about developing a trusting nurse–patient relationship, exploring the relationship's role in helping patients to achieve valued health outcomes.

Personal Learning: Here's to the Future!

I learned something about myself and an important distinction between teaching and counseling. Clearly, just teaching Mr. Soros about diet and exercise wasn't sufficient. Mr. Soros was in no way going to change his lifestyle until he valued his health enough to make needed changes, including understanding why these changes were important. I also learned how important nurse–patient relationships are. When Mr. Soros came for his third visit, he asked the nurse who greeted him where I was, telling her "I want to see that nurse who cared about me!"—positive reinforcement for the relationship's importance.

Megan Kyle, Georgetown University

QSEN SELF-REFLECTION ON QUALITY AND SAFETY COMPETENCIES DEVELOPING KNOWLEDGE, SKILLS, AND ATTITUDES FOR CONTINUOUS IMPROVEMENT

How do you think you would respond in a similar situation? Why? What does this tell you about yourself and about the adequacy of your competencies for professional practice? Do you agree with the criteria that the nursing student used to evaluate a successful outcome? Describe the type of teaching plan that the nursing student may have used at the initial teaching session. How might that teaching plan have changed based on the patient's response at the next visit? Would the outcomes identified initially need to be revised based on any changes in the teaching plan? Explain why or why not. What *knowledge, skills,* and *attitudes (KSAs)* do you need to develop to continuously improve the quality and safety of care for patients like Mr. Soros?

Patient-Centered Care: How can you establish a successful partnership with a patient who lacks the motivation to make critical lifestyle changes?

Teamwork and Collaboration/Quality Improvement (QI): When colleagues aren't willing to go that "extra mile" to work with vulnerable patients, how can you intervene successfully? What needs to change to improve quality in this setting? What does quality care for Mr. Soros "look like"?

Safety/Evidence-Based Practice: What does the evidence point to as "best practice" for Mr. Soros? What safety needs does he have and how can you meet them?

Informatics: Can you identify the essential information that must be available in Mr. Soros's record to support safe patient care and coordination of care? Are there any apps that might be useful in coaching Mr. Soros? Can you think of other ways to respond to or approach the situation? What else might the nursing student have done to ensure a successful outcome?

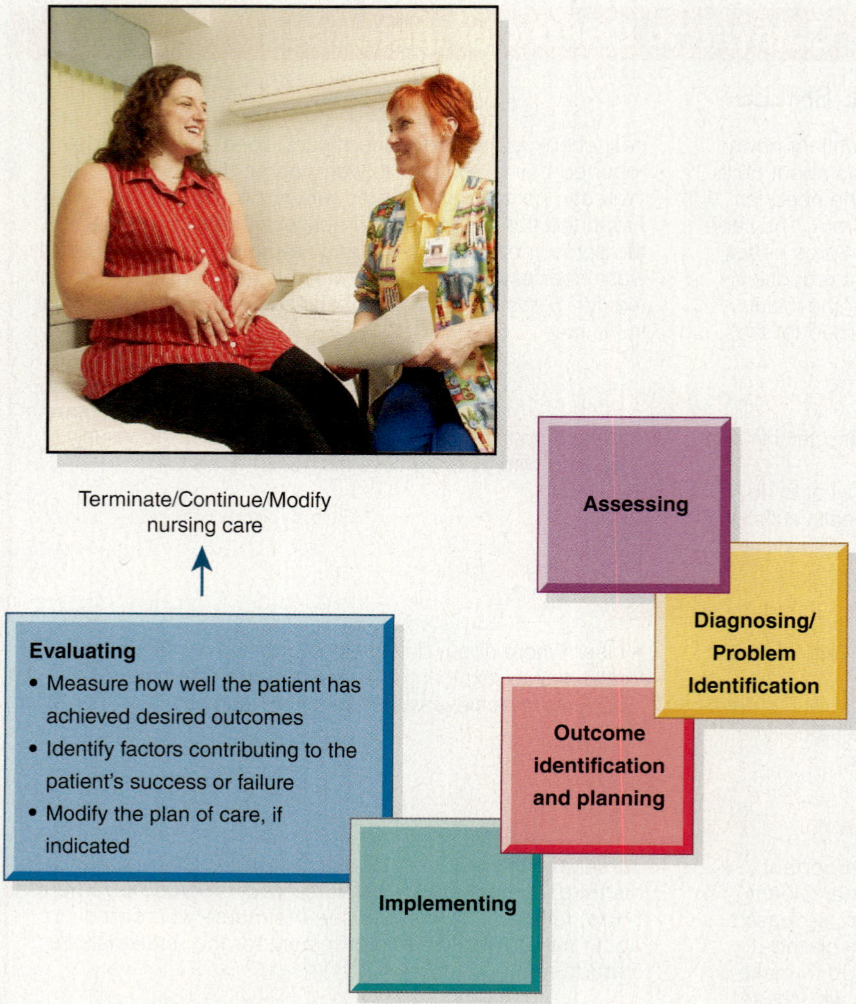

FIGURE 19-1. Evaluating. The nurse and patient together measure how well the patient has achieved the outcomes specified in the plan of care. Factors that contribute to the patient's success or failure are identified, and the plan of care is modified if necessary. Patient responses to the plan of care determine whether nursing care is to be continued as is, modified, or terminated. (*Source:* Used with permission from Shutterstock. *Photo by Joe Mitchell.*)

Box 19-1 What Patients Should Expect From Their Health Care

1. **Beyond patient visits:** You will have the care you need when you need it . . . *whenever* you need it. You will find help in many forms, not just in face-to-face visits. You will find help on the Internet, on the telephone, from many sources, by many routes, in the form you want it.
2. **Individualization:** You will be known and respected as an individual. Your choices and preferences will be sought and honored. The usual system of care will meet most of your needs. When your needs are special, the care will adapt to meet you on your own terms.
3. **Control:** The care system will take control only if and when you freely give permission.
4. **Information:** You can know what you wish to know, when you wish to know it. Your medical record is yours to keep, to read, and to understand. The rule is: "Nothing about you without you."
5. **Science:** You will have care based on the best available scientific knowledge. The system promises you excellence as its standard. Your care will not vary illogically from doctor to doctor or from place to place. The system will promise you all the care that can help you, and will help you avoid care that cannot help you.
6. **Safety:** Errors in care will not harm you. You will be safe in the care system.
7. **Transparency:** Your care will be confidential, but the care system will not keep secrets from you. You can know whatever you wish to know about the care that affects you and your loved ones.
8. **Anticipation:** Your care will anticipate your needs and will help you find the help you need. You will experience proactive help, not just reactions, to help you restore and maintain your health.
9. **Value:** Your care will not waste your time or money. You will benefit from constant innovations, which will increase the value of care to you.
10. **Cooperation:** Those who provide care will cooperate and coordinate their work fully with each other and with you. The walls between professions and institutions will crumble, so that your experiences will become seamless. You will never feel lost.

Source: Republished with permission of National Academies Press from The Institute of Medicine's Committee on Quality Health Care in America. (1999). *Crossing the quality chasm: A new health system for the 21st century, by the National Academy of Sciences.* National Academies Press; permission conveyed through Copyright Clearance Center, Inc.

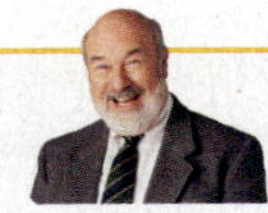

Think back to **Nicholas Soros**, the 68-year-old man diagnosed with diabetes who needs to lose weight and to exercise. The outcomes identified initially most likely focused on weight loss and adherence to an exercise program. Teaching at this initial visit also focused on ways to achieve these outcomes. However, the patient's statements and weight gain on his next clinic visit would lead the nurse to the conclusion that the outcomes identified were not being achieved. Therefore, some changes in the patient's care plan are necessary.

Identifying Evaluative Criteria and Standards

Although the terms *criteria* and *standards* are often used interchangeably in reference to the evaluation step, they have distinct definitions. **Criteria** are measurable qualities, attributes, or characteristics that identify skills, knowledge, or health states. They describe acceptable levels of performance by stating what is expected of the nurse or the patient. Chapter 17 describes how patient criteria are identified and formulated as patient outcomes.

Standards are the levels of performance accepted by and expected of nursing staff or other health team members. They are established by authority, custom, or consent. A good example of standards is the American Nurses Association's (ANA's) *Nursing: Scope and Standards of Practice* (2021), which you read about in Chapter 1. Be sure to be familiar with the evaluation competencies for registered nurses outlined in Standard 6, Evaluation. Chapters 17 and 18 describe *clinical practice guidelines,* a term used interchangeably with standards and protocols, all of which describe how care should be managed in certain situations. The goal is to design and deliver nursing care that evidence supports as likely to produce the expected patient outcomes (i.e., **evidence-based practice**).

Collecting Evaluative Data

The nurse collects evaluative data to determine whether or not the patient has met the desired outcomes. While the nurse collects data in the nursing assessment to identify patient health problems, the data collected in the evaluation step are used to determine whether the identified health problems have been or are being resolved through outcome achievement.

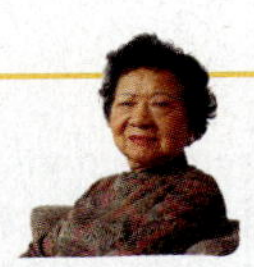

Consider **Mrs. Otsuki**, the older adult who is inadvertently taking double the dose of prescribed diuretic. This initial assessment indicates a need for teaching. Thus, when evaluating outcome achievement for this patient, the nurse would determine whether the patient demonstrates understanding of her drug-therapy regimen and is no longer taking two doses of the same drug.

This section discusses (1) the different types of data collected to evaluate the achievement of different types of patient outcomes and (2) time criteria for data collection.

Types of Outcomes

Nurses write outcomes during the planning phase of the nursing process. Chapter 17 describes four types of outcomes: cognitive, psychomotor, affective, and physiologic. The type of patient data collected to support the evaluation of outcome achievement depends on the nature of the outcome. The data collected to determine the degree of outcome achievement are recorded in the corresponding evaluative statements (Box 19-2 on page 502).

Time Criteria

In addition to knowing *what type* of data to collect to determine outcome achievement, the nurse needs to know *when* to collect the data. When the patient outcomes were developed, a time frame was established for determining whether the specified changes have been achieved. At the designated time, the nurse, in collaboration with the patient, the family, and other members of the nursing team, evaluates the patient's attainment of the outcome. If outcomes are developed in observable and measurable terms, the task of collecting data for evaluation is clear-cut. Examples of three types of time criteria follow:

- By 7/8/25, the patient will walk the length of the hallway with support of a walker.
- Beginning 7/8/25, the patient will demonstrate a weight loss of 3 lb per month until target weight (135 lb) is achieved (6/8/25, weight: 151 lb).
- Before discharge, parents will correctly demonstrate chest physiotherapy procedures for patient.

Nurses should evaluate patient outcome achievement as early as possible. Celebrating outcome attainment with the patient usually helps encourage the patient and leads to further outcome achievement. When failure to meet designated outcomes is detected early, the care plan can be modified to remedy the failure.

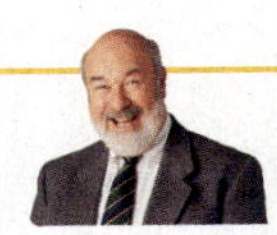

Think back to **Nicholas Soros**, the 68-year-old patient with diabetes. By recognizing the lack of outcome achievement on the next visit, the nurse can gather additional data to revise the care plan. For example, perhaps Mr. Soros did not completely understand the nurse's teaching. Or, he may have had difficulty accepting his diagnosis, thereby interfering with his ability to comply with the plan, ultimately leading to weight gain instead of a weight loss.

The most common mistake nurses make when evaluating in acute care settings is waiting until the day the patient is to be discharged before evaluating outcome achievement. At that point, it is too late to revise the care plan.

Box 19-2 Evaluating Four Types of Outcomes in the Plan of Nursing Care

Diagnosis/Problem

Readiness for effective parenting; etiologic factor: no previous experience in childrearing (fear)

Assessment Data

Subjective: "My husband and I are both afraid we won't know what to do when we get the baby home"

Objective: Both parents are single children, report no childrearing experience; healthy newborn son delivered 2/4/25; first born

Strengths

VIB (very important baby): parents are both 38; history of infertility with one miscarriage; strong motivation to learn and use good parenting skills; strong support network

Expected Outcomes	Nursing Interventions	Evaluative Statement (Actual Outcomes)
Psychomotor Outcomes Before discharge, parents will demonstrate confidence in: • Holding baby • Diapering, dressing baby • Bathing baby • Feeding baby	Assess both parents' knowledge of childrearing practices; identify and reinforce motivation to learn; correct any misinformation. Develop and implement at a time convenient for both parents a teaching plan to include: • The primary nurse role-modeling techniques for comfortably and safely holding, talking to, and dressing baby • Parents independently viewing videos on: baby care, baby bath, and breastfeeding, followed by one-on-one discussion • Class for new parents: nurse to demonstrate baby bath and discuss general principles of care • Primary nurse observing mother and infant during initial feeding sessions and offering teaching and support as necessary	2/6/25 Outcome partially met. Both parents have correctly demonstrated safe techniques for holding, dressing, and bathing baby. Mother is still concerned baby is not getting enough milk. *Revision:* Continue to spend time with mother and infant during feeding—provide positive reinforcement. *F. Morales, RN*
Cognitive Outcomes By 2/6/25, parents will report appropriate action to be taken if questions or problems arise after discharge: • Name and number of primary nurse • Name and number of pediatrician • La Leche League contact and number	Answer parents' questions and address related concerns. Assess parents' knowledge of infant problems frequently encountered by new parents. Inform parents of available community resources and describe appropriate action to take if questions or problems arise.	2/6/25 Outcome met. Parents discussed some infant problems related to feeding, elimination, and illness and reported appropriate community resource to contact. *F. Morales, RN*
Affective Outcome Before discharge, parents will verbalize decreased anxiety in regard to caring for son.	Assess parents' level of anxiety and potential negative effects on childrearing. Discuss this with parents. Explore adequacy of parents' coping strategies—increased knowledge, practice in supportive environment, community resources. Counsel as necessary. Compliment parents on new parenting skills. Allow for ventilation of anxiety or specific fears. Respond with teaching or emotional support, as necessary.	2/6/25 Outcome partially met. Except for concern about breastfeeding, *both* parents expressed feeling comfortable and eager to care for their son at home. *F. Morales, RN*
Physiologic Outcomes At 1-month postpartal telephone interview, 3/4/25 (by parents' report), the baby will demonstrate adequate: • Weight gain (birth weight, 7 lb 6 oz) • Sleep–wakefulness patterns • Comfort level indicating adequate parenting	Use a 1-month postdelivery telephone interview to assess the adequacy of parenting skills. With positive report of growth and development, compliment (reinforce) the parents. With negative report, teach or counsel and refer as appropriate.	3/4/25 Outcome met. Parents' report of baby's weight gain and behavior indicates good parenting skills. *F. Morales, RN*

Interpreting and Summarizing Findings

Before the nurse can make a judgment about the patient's achievement of outcomes, it is necessary to study and interpret the data collected. Just as clusters of data are interpreted before the nurse identifies and validates a nursing diagnosis/problem, so too do evaluative data need to be interpreted. For example, a patient who is expected to walk the length of the hallway with support of a walker asks to be taken back to her room because she feels weak. The nurse must gather more data to determine if this is a one-time incident linked to medications or a temporary metabolic imbalance, or whether it signals a consistent inability to achieve this goal. Interpreting evaluative data requires clinical reasoning and judgment and is a skill that must be practiced.

When interpreting and summarizing findings, consider factors that influence outcome achievement. Numerous patient, nurse, and health care system variables contribute positively or negatively to patient outcome achievement. Identifying these variables allows the nurse to reinforce positive factors by drawing on them in the future, as well as to deal with other variables that are creating problems. The more sensitive and responsive nurses are to these variables, the more rewarding their practices will be.

Examples of positive factors include a patient's strong motivation to learn new health behaviors, a nurse who comes to work well rested and with a new care idea learned from a nursing journal, and a health care institution or facility that offers incentives for quality nursing and has an optimal nurse-to-patient ratio.

A nurse who understands what factors are helpful to the patient who is trying to reach desired outcomes can often manipulate these factors. For example, if a patient is learning to ambulate independently after hip surgery and you notice that he seems to make his best effort when his wife is present, mention this to her and plan to ambulate the patient at least once a day when she is present. Conversely, if a patient seems more fearful when his wife is present, note in the care plan that ambulation is best attempted when the patient's wife is not on the unit. Ideally, this fear would be explored with the patient before discharge so that he can continue to make progress when he is discharged home with his wife.

Table 19-1 (on page 504) presents variables that may negatively influence patient outcome achievement. Nurses need to think critically about the effects of these variables and respond creatively to them.

Documenting Your Judgment

After the data have been collected and interpreted to determine patient outcome achievement, the nurse makes and documents a judgment summarizing the findings. This is termed the **evaluative statement**. The two-part evaluative statement includes a decision about how well the outcome was met, along with patient data or behaviors that support this decision. Outcomes may have been met, partially met, or not met:

- 1/21/25—Outcome met. Patient reports 1 week of no tobacco use. C. Taylor, RN
- 1/21/25—Outcome partially met. Patient reports decreasing tobacco use from one pack per day to 4 to 6 cigarettes per day. Continue to implement and monitor plan. C. Taylor, RN
- 1/21/25—Outcome not met. Patient reports no change in tobacco use. Revision: Reexplore patient's commitment to try tobacco-use control strategies and adequacy of personal support systems to eliminate tobacco use. C. Taylor, RN

The nurse signs and dates the evaluative statement (see Box 19-2) or follows the documentation guidelines specified in the institution's computerized documentation systems.

Unfolding Patient Stories: Sara Lin • Part 2

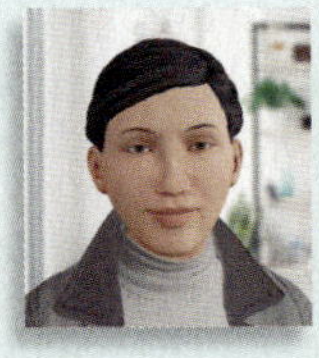

Recall **Sara Lin**, from Chapter 2, who is on the medical-surgical unit following an appendectomy. Her indwelling urinary catheter was discontinued, and she can begin oral fluids and advance activity, as tolerated. How would the nurse evaluate that Sara is tolerating oral fluids? How would the nurse evaluate that her activity, fluid intake, and urine output are adequate?

Care for Sara and other patients in a realistic virtual environment: ***vSim** for Nursing* (thepoint.lww.com/vSimFunds). Practice documenting these patients' care in DocuCare (thepoint.lww.com/DocuCareEHR).

Modifying the Care Plan

When evaluation reveals that the patient has made little or no progress toward outcome achievement, the nurse needs to reevaluate each preceding step of the nursing process to try to identify the contributing factors causing problems with the care plan. New assessment data may need to be collected, diagnoses may be added or altered, outcomes may need to be modified or rewritten, nursing orders may be changed, or evaluation may be targeted more frequently.

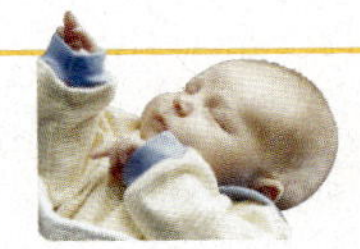

Remember **Tyler Jameson**, the neonate who has not passed any stool after 30 hours. The initial outcome may have stated that the neonate would pass stool within 18 to 24 hours after birth. However, this outcome was developed based on data that was inaccurate. Therefore, the nurse, learning of the new data, would revise the outcome to correlate with the neonate's condition, dependent on the treatment to correct the anomaly.

Review the checklist in Box 13-9 (on page 370) for help in evaluating your use of the nursing process. Table 19-2 (on pages 505–506) suggests appropriate nursing responses to common problems encountered during evaluation of each step in the nursing process.

(text continues on page 506)

Table 19-1 Patient, Nurse, and Health Care System Variables That May Detract From Quality Nursing Care

VARIABLES	POSSIBLE SOLUTIONS
Patient Variables	
Patient who is physically and cognitively capable of self-care gives up, refuses to cooperate with therapeutic regimen, or thwarts the regimen	Identify one nurse who is able to develop a trusting relationship with the patient and determine the reason underlying the observed behavior: • No longer finds meaning and purpose in life • Overwhelming sense of powerlessness • Previous history of being "hurt," "exploited," "cheated" by the health care system • Inability to accept illness and related lifestyle changes Counsel appropriately. Use a team conference to develop a consistent plan of nursing care.
Patient who quietly accepts whatever is done or not done for him or her; seldom communicates needs or dissatisfaction	Note on the care plan the need to assess this patient thoroughly because the patient will probably not advocate for self. Educate the patient to become a more assertive health care consumer.
Nurse Variables	
Nurse who sincerely desires to give 150% all the time and who becomes quickly frustrated when observing substandard care; may feel alienated from other staff; excellent candidate for burnout	Learn to give quality care during designated work period; leave on time; avoid the temptation to do the work of others; leave work concerns at work. After establishing a reputation for delivering quality nursing care, seek creative solutions for nursing problems (strategies to increase nursing resources, motivation, morale) and try them—hopefully with a support network. View concerns as challenges rather than overwhelming obstacles. Develop a realistic sense of how much nursing care and of what quality can be delivered with existing resources. If resources do not permit quality care, explore change strategies within the institution. If administration is not supportive, explore other practice settings.
Nurse with overwhelming outside concerns: • Preparation for marriage, childbirth, divorce • Illness (self or family members) • Role conflict (familial roles, school, work, and the like) • New apartment, house	During periods of peak demand, may need to accept less than optimal performance at work. If this becomes the norm rather than the exception, carefully evaluate priorities. May need to cut work hours rather than "cheat" patients.
Nurse who is bored	After reflection, write down *personal* objectives related to work. Explore avenues within work setting for professional growth and development: initiate changes in nursing unit to improve patient care and to stimulate peer development; join institutional committees; participate actively in staff development programs; develop patient and family support groups. Look for new position that offers new challenges within or outside the institution. Join professional organizations and participate actively. Evaluate educational goals and explore possibilities—continuing education programs and degree work.
Health Care System Variables	
Inadequate staffing	Develop and use a patient classification system that incorporates an identification of the kind and amount of nursing services required. Record staffing patterns and relate to needs for nursing care and patient outcomes. Clearly demonstrate and document that adequate staffing makes a difference. Present these data to nursing administration with the request for additional staff. If necessary, use professional bargaining unit.
Nursing administration has sold out nursing; insensitivity to nursing demands within the institution	It may be impossible to practice quality, progressive nursing in this environment. If there seems to be no hope for change after appropriate channels have been explored, look for a new practice setting. Evaluate the new setting on the basis of what experience has taught you.

Table 19-2 Common Problems Noted During Evaluation of the Nursing Process

PROBLEM	NURSING RESPONSE
Assessing	
1. Inaccurate database → inaccurate nursing diagnoses/problems and a distorted care plan	1. a. Identify the patient or nurse variables responsible for inaccuracy. b. Revise the recorded database.
2. Database does not reflect changes in patient condition	2. Review with the entire nursing staff the importance of making assessment a priority in every patient interaction as well as the recording of the new data obtained.
3. Database is superficial: • Fails to communicate uniqueness of patient • Lacks sufficient detail on major problems or developments	3. a. Rethink the critical relation between an adequate database and quality care. b. Develop interviewing and physical assessment skills. c. Begin to identify the key data that need to be collected for specific nursing and medical diagnoses and problems and assess patient response to therapeutic regimen.
Diagnosing/Problem Identification	
1. General sense that nursing diagnoses/problems are "common sense" and, therefore, do not need to be put in writing → failure to address patient's real problems	1. Carefully develop and record priority nursing diagnoses/problems for several patients and fairly evaluate whether this makes a difference in terms of the continuity of quality care.
2. General sense that nurses are too busy doing treatments, "passing meds," and documenting care to develop nursing diagnoses/problems carefully → independent dimension of nursing remains underdeveloped	2. Examine practice and see whether independent nursing has a place; what percentage of every day is devoted to independent nursing functions? If this percentage is nonexistent or small, there understandably may be no felt need for nursing diagnoses/problems—but a desperate need to revise practice priorities.
3. Nursing diagnoses/problems are too vague to be helpful → routinized patient care	3. a. Revise the problem statement to describe more accurately what is unhealthy about the patient (the behavior that needs to be changed). b. Revise the etiology to more accurately identify what is making the problem a problem—this should be a guide to nursing intervention.
4. Nursing diagnoses/problems are not up to date → no one uses the care plan	4. Have a process for periodically reviewing the care plan to delete diagnoses/problems when problems have been resolved and to add a new diagnosis/problem as needed.
Planning	
1. The care plan contains only the standard knowledge most nurses would know without a written plan	1. Make use of standardized (computerized) plans as a basis for care planning. Devote nursing energies to individualizing this plan.
2. The long-term goal is vague, standard; fails to make clear the discharge goal for this patient	2. Practice writing specific long-term goals that clarify for all nurses the aim toward which all nursing care is directed (e.g., patient returns home ambulatory with walker, right hip incision healing, able to manage activities of daily living with minimal assistance from spouse).
3. The nursing outcomes, even if met, do not necessarily guarantee a resolution of the patient problem	3. When writing goals, it often helps to develop outcomes related to etiologic factors. Because the stated etiology may be incomplete or inaccurate, at least one outcome must be written so that if it is achieved, the problem in the nursing diagnosis is resolved.
4. The outcomes are incorrectly developed; progress toward goal achievement is difficult to evaluate	4. After writing outcomes, check them against the following criteria: • Subject is the patient or some part of the patient. • The patient behavior is stated in observable, measurable terms. • Criteria of acceptable performance are specified. • Time criteria are included in notes.
5. Nursing orders are superficial → patient receives routinized care	5. Review nursing orders to ensure that they indicate the specific nursing strategies or interventions most likely to result in successful outcome achievement for this patient (e.g., particular comfort measures that are successful adjuncts to analgesic administration for a particular patient). In specifying the "who, what, when, where, how, and how much" of nursing interventions, be sure to list the type of equipment and supplies needed in various treatments. As new patient data are obtained, update nursing orders. Delete inappropriate or unnecessary orders.
6. The initial care plan fails to be updated → care plan will not be consulted by nurses—if used, it will be to patient's detriment	6. If personal accountability for updating plan fails, develop a process on the nursing unit to ensure care plan review and revision.
7. The care plan addresses the immediate needs of the patient but fails to anticipate discharge needs → patient returns home unable to manage self-care activities	7. Work hard at developing the ability to project yourself into the patient's home after discharge. Learn to anticipate problems and concerns and prepare the patient and family for these. Use all discharge resources in the institution. Learn from patients what their needs were after previous discharge.

(*continued*)

Table 19-2 Common Problems Noted During Evaluation of the Nursing Process *(continued)*

PROBLEM	NURSING RESPONSE
Implementing	
1. Nurses are not aware of patient priorities and the care plan; lack of continuity; inefficient use of nursing resources → patient fails to achieve goals/outcomes	1. a. Use shift report to update staff on status of priority nursing diagnosis and concomitant nursing care. b. Review care plan and nursing notes before beginning care.
2. Nursing care becomes routine and mechanized → patient never has the sense of being personally known by nurses	2. Explore creative strategies to make quality nursing care on this particular unit a challenge rather than a burden; use ongoing education, problem-solving strategies by the nursing team, gaming, and other incentives.
3. Documentation is inadequate → because there is no complete written record of nursing care, legally this care was never provided	3. a. Develop the philosophy that quality nursing care deserves to be documented. Review legal reasons for careful documentation. b. Become familiar with the flow sheets and note format used within the work setting so that charting can be done quickly and comprehensively.
Evaluating	
1. It is not done → mastery of nursing process is stunted; severely limits accomplishment of nursing aims	1. Develop the belief that quality nursing care does not happen automatically and that only ongoing evaluation will identify needed areas of revision. Devise an evaluative strategy and carry it out. Study its effect on quality of care after 6 months' implementation.

After identifying the factors contributing to the outcomes not being achieved, use the evaluative statement to suggest necessary revisions in the care plan. Revisions may include (1) deleting or modifying the nursing diagnosis/problem, (2) making the outcome statement more realistic, (3) increasing the complexity of the outcome statement, (4) adjusting time criteria in the outcome statement, or (5) changing the nursing intervention(s). Increasing the complexity of an outcome after it has been achieved facilitates optimal function. For example, the initial outcome for a patient with the diagnosis Impaired Mobility might be "patient transfers from the bed to the chair." After this is achieved, however, the outcome needs to be stepped up in complexity to "patient walks around room with support of walker."

The following is an example of a specified outcome for a resident in long-term care: "Resident will participate in a minimum of two planned social activities per week beginning 9/16/25." If the resident did not meet that outcome, this evaluative statement may be written: "9/27/25—Outcome not met. Resident chose not to participate in any group activities this week." Many courses of action are then available to the nurse. Possible revisions to any care plan include the following:

- *Delete or modify the diagnosis/problem.* In the example, lack of participation in social activities may not be a problem or concern for the resident. The nurse should evaluate and validate data pointing to the diagnosis/problem.
- *Make the outcome statement more realistic.* The nurse would carefully determine the resident's need for activities and ability or desire to participate in activities.
- *Adjust time criteria in outcome statement.* The nurse might reevaluate after 3 weeks. The resident may need more time to adjust to living in an institution, as well as more encouragement.
- *Change nursing interventions.* The nurse could make a special effort to become familiar with the resident's interests, and match these with available programs and activities.

Once the nurse—ideally, in partnership with the patient—makes a decision about how to respond, this must be communicated to the patient or the patient's surrogate and to other members of the professional caregiving team, via the patient's record.

Think back to **Mioshi Otsuki**, the older adult taking too much diuretic medication. The home care nurse would work with the patient to develop a teaching plan about her heart failure, specifically related to her drug-therapy regimen. This plan then would be documented in the patient's record and communicated to all people involved in the patient's care, such as other home care facility nurses who may be on call or filling in to visit the patient, or home health aides involved in providing personal care and hygiene for the patient.

EVALUATING QUALITY CARE

In addition to each nurse's evaluation of patient outcome achievement and subsequent modifications to the care plan, many informal and formal mechanisms are used to ensure quality nursing care.

Performance Improvement in Everyday Clinical Practice

Nurses sometimes discover problems with the delivery of nursing care in their practice setting. The IOM's Committee on Quality of Health Care in America suggests 10 rules to redesign and improve care:

1. Care based on continuous healing relationships
2. Customization based on patient needs and values
3. The patient as the source of control
4. Shared knowledge and the free flow of information
5. Evidence-based decision making
6. Safety as a system priority
7. The need for transparency
8. Anticipation of patient's needs
9. Continuous decrease in waste
10. Cooperation among clinicians

Each nurse must decide how to respond when compromised patient care has been identified. Nurses committed to healthier patients, quality care, reduced costs, and the personal satisfaction of knowing that they are *actually making a difference* versus merely *wishing things were different* value **performance improvement**. The following four steps are crucial in improving performance:

1. Discover a problem
2. Plan a strategy using indicators
3. Implement a change
4. Assess the change; if the outcome is not met, plan a new strategy

See Box 19-3 for an example of a performance-improvement strategy. In this example, oncology nurses believe that advance directives are not being used optimally to improve end-of-life care for the seriously ill and dying. Remember, the central focus of these efforts is always improving the patient's experience and outcomes. The Institute for Healthcare Improvement (2018) has created a model for a Quality Improvement Charter, the guiding document that helps a team structure its improvement project and develop and communicate a shared vision. The charter begins to answer the three essential questions of the Model for Improvement:

- What are we trying to accomplish?
- How will we know that a change is an improvement?
- What change can we make that will result in improvement?

See their website for a helpful template (http://www.ihi.org/resources/Pages/Tools/QI-Project-Charter.aspx).

An important resource for nurses committed to performance improvement is the Quality and Safety Education for Nurses (QSEN) project. The overall goal of the QSEN Institute initiatives is to prepare nurses with the knowledge, skills and attitudes (KSAs) necessary to continuously improve the quality and safety of their health care systems. Visit the QSEN website, www.qsen.org, to view a variety of educational materials.

Peer review, the evaluation of one staff member by another staff member on the same level in the hierarchy of the organization, is an important mechanism nurses can use to improve their professional performance. This can be done formally or informally by inviting a peer you respect to give you feedback on nursing skills you are trying to develop—for example, "How do you think that session went with the patient's daughter? She's been so critical of us and I'm trying to understand the situation from her point of view and respond appropriately."

Establishing and Sustaining Healthy Work Environments

According to the study *Silence Kills: The Seven Crucial Conversations for Healthcare* (Maxfield et al., 2005), the prevalent culture of poor communication and collaboration among health professionals is significantly related to continued medical errors and staff turnover. Additionally,

Box 19-3 Example of Steps in Performance Improvement

The following four steps are crucial in improving performance:

1. **Discover a problem.** Advance directives are a powerful legal tool for people to indicate their end-of-life care preferences. Nurses on an oncology unit are becoming frustrated because many of the patients on their unit lack advance directives. By the time decisions need to be made about ventilators, coding, dialysis, and so forth, patients are often no longer able to communicate their preferences. The hospital has a policy about advance directives, but no one seems to be taking responsibility for initiating discussions with patients when they are first admitted—or in the outpatient setting.
2. **Plan a strategy using indicators.** The nurses call an interdisciplinary meeting with the oncologists, social workers, and spiritual caregivers, who decide that the nurse case manager will be responsible for working with patients on admission to see if they want help in preparing an advance directive. Each case manager will be responsible for documenting within 48 hours of admission the patient's decision regarding an advance directive. Staff nurses will be able to direct patient and family requests to do advance planning to the case manager and appropriate team members. The ethics committee was asked to do an in-service on advance directives for the team.
3. **Implement a change.** Case managers begin assuming this responsibility, and one nurse volunteers to monitor progress at 3-month intervals by checking charts for advance directive content and by speaking with the staff nurses who voiced the initial frustration about decision making.
4. **Assess the change.** If the goal is not met, plan a new strategy. At the end of 6 months, everyone seems satisfied that the new plan is working, but a decision is made to schedule a 6-month follow-up evaluation to prevent backsliding.

Source: Reprinted with permission from Haase, R., & Miller, K. (1999). Performance improvement in everyday clinical practice. *American Journal of Nursing, 99*(5), 52, 54.

a lack of adequate support systems, skills, and personal accountability results in communication gaps that can cause harm to patients. Results of this national study of more than 1,700 health professionals, conducted by the American Association of Critical-Care Nurses (AACN) and VitalSmarts, include these facts:

- Up to 84% of health care providers and 62% of nurses and other clinical care providers have seen coworkers taking shortcuts that could be dangerous to patients.
- Up to 88% of health care providers and 48% of nurses and other providers work with people who show poor clinical judgment.
- Fewer than 10% of health care providers, nurses, and other clinical staff directly confront their colleagues about their concerns, and one in five health care providers said they have seen harm come to patients as a result.
- The 10% of health care workers who raise these crucial concerns observe better patient outcomes, work harder, and are more satisfied and more committed to staying in their jobs.

The study pinpoints seven categories of common communication problems that are rarely addressed. See Table 19-3 for examples of the seven crucial conversations in health care that nurses and other professionals must learn to master. If you find yourself in one of these situations, ask an experienced and trusted colleague how best to respond, and don't accept an answer such as "Spare yourself some grief and do nothing."

Table 19-3 The Seven Crucial Conversations in Health Care

CATEGORY OF CONVERSATION	EXAMPLES	RECOMMENDATIONS
1. Broken rules	Colleague fails to wash hands.	Confront your colleague and tell her that you noticed that she failed to wash her hands and that this could be harmful to herself, the patient, or other patients. If the behavior continues, report your concerns to the nurse manager and work up the chain of command.
2. Mistakes	Nurse administers medication to the wrong patient and asks you to keep an eye on the patient for adverse reactions. She does not plan to report the error.	Tell your colleague that you'll be happy to help watch the patient but that a full report needs to be made. If appropriate, help your colleague identify what contributed to her giving the medication to the wrong patient.
3. Lack of support	Nurse refuses to help a colleague move an obese patient although she has time to do so.	Explain to this nurse that teamwork is essential to good outcomes and that her behavior is simply unacceptable. "When we have patients with special needs and need all hands on deck, everyone who's free is obligated to help out!" Develop and enforce zero tolerance for selfish behavior.
4. Incompetence	Nurse fails to correctly administer dialysis. She wasn't finished with her orientation to the unit and attempted a procedure before she was prepared to do it solo.	In addition to reporting the error, help the nurse identify that overconfidence in their abilities can have deadly results for patients. The nurse manager will need to address the incompetence.
5. Poor teamwork	A particularly difficult family is splitting the team by choosing (and rewarding) favorites among the staff and complaining to them about other workers. The staff is encouraging this behavior.	Someone needs to call the team together and name the divisive behavior and get everyone working together again. If there is staff who are problematic, appropriate channels need to be used to address these behaviors.
6. Disrespect	When a student nurse asks a physician if she has time to answer a few questions for her patient, the physician screams at her and tells her that she has more important things to do than babysit her patient and tells the student to find someone else to answer the questions.	The student should calmly tell the physician that her response is inappropriate and that she is entitled to respectful conversation, then seek the counsel of an experienced nurse. The physician's behavior should be reported.
7. Micromanagement	A student asks her clinical preceptor, "Will you walk me through this procedure before I do it, since it's my first time?" The preceptor then takes over, doing the procedure for the student, and starts watching her every move.	The student should inform her preceptor that she merely wanted to review the steps of the procedure to make sure that she would perform it correctly and that it is essential for the student to gain experience by trying new procedures. If the preceptor's behavior does not change, the student should seek the counsel of her instructor.

Source: Adapted from Maxfield, D., Grenny, J., Patterson, K., McMillan, R., & Switzler, A. (2005). *Silence kills.* https://psnet.ahrq.gov/issue/silence-kills-seven-crucial-conversations-healthcare

Box 19-4 The American Association of Critical-Care Nurses Standards for Establishing and Sustaining Healthy Work Environments

- **Skilled communication.** Nurses must be as proficient in communication skills as they are in clinical skills.
- **True collaboration.** Nurses must be relentless in pursuing and fostering true collaboration.
- **Effective decision making.** Nurses must be valued and committed partners in making policy, directing and evaluating clinical care, and leading organizational operations.
- **Appropriate staffing.** Staffing must ensure the effective match between patient needs and nurse competencies.
- **Meaningful recognition.** Nurses must be recognized and must recognize others for the value each brings to the work of the organization.
- **Authentic leadership.** Nurse leaders must fully embrace the imperativeness of a healthy work environment, authentically live it, and engage others in its achievement.

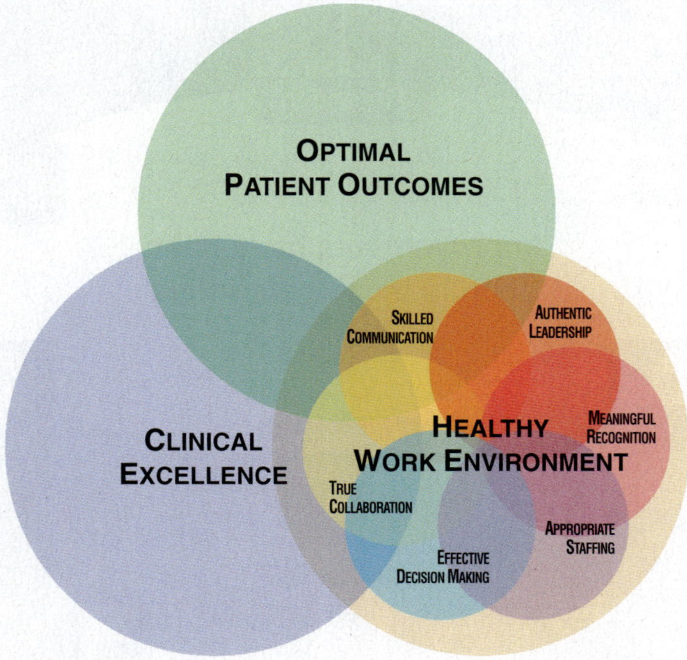

Interdependence of a healthy work environment, clinical excellence, and optimal patient outcomes.

Source: Used with permission from American Association of Critical-Care Nurses (AACN). (2005). AACN standards for Establishing and Sustaining Healthy Work Environments: A Journey to Excellence. *American Journal of Critical Care, 14*(3), 187–197. Author.

A follow-up to this study, conducted by VitalSmarts, AACN, and the Association of periOperative Registered Nurses (AORN), revealed that safety tools fail to address a second category of communication breakdowns: "undiscussables." These are risks that are widely known but not discussed: dangerous shortcuts, incompetence, and disrespect (Maxfield et al., 2010). This study revealed that too many nurses are in situations in which they feel it is unsafe to speak up about problems or are unable to get others to listen.

AACN's commitment *to actively promote the creation of healthy work environments that support and foster excellence in patient care* is a superb example of nursing leadership. See Box 19-4 for AACN's six essential standards for establishing and sustaining healthy work environments. The standards represent *evidence-based* and *relationship-centered* principles of professional performance. Each standard is considered essential, because studies show that effective and sustainable outcomes do not emerge when any standard is considered optional. For copies of the *Silence Kills* report and the AACN Standards for Establishing and Sustaining Healthy Work Environments, visit https://www.aacn.org/nursing-excellence/healthy-work-environments/~/media/aacn-website/nursing-excellence/healthy-work-environment/silencekills.pdf?la=en or https://www.aacn.org/nursing-excellence/standards/aacn-standards-for-establishing-and-sustaining-healthy-work-environments.

In 2015, AACN conducted a public forum campaign to identify aspects of nurses' work environments inhibiting optimal patient care.

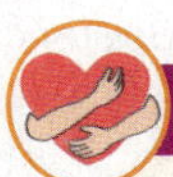

Nurse Self-Care Alert

The barriers to practice assessment identified five main themes contributing to workplace stressors: (1) staff shortages and higher workloads; (2) government regulations and hospital requirements; (3) disrespectful behaviors and unrealistic expectations of patients and their families; (4) lack of authentic leadership within practice environments; and (5) hostile workplace culture. These stressors are known to compromise nurses' job satisfaction and engagement, increase role conflict, lead to friction with leadership, and promote poor relationships between coworkers (Grant et al., 2020).

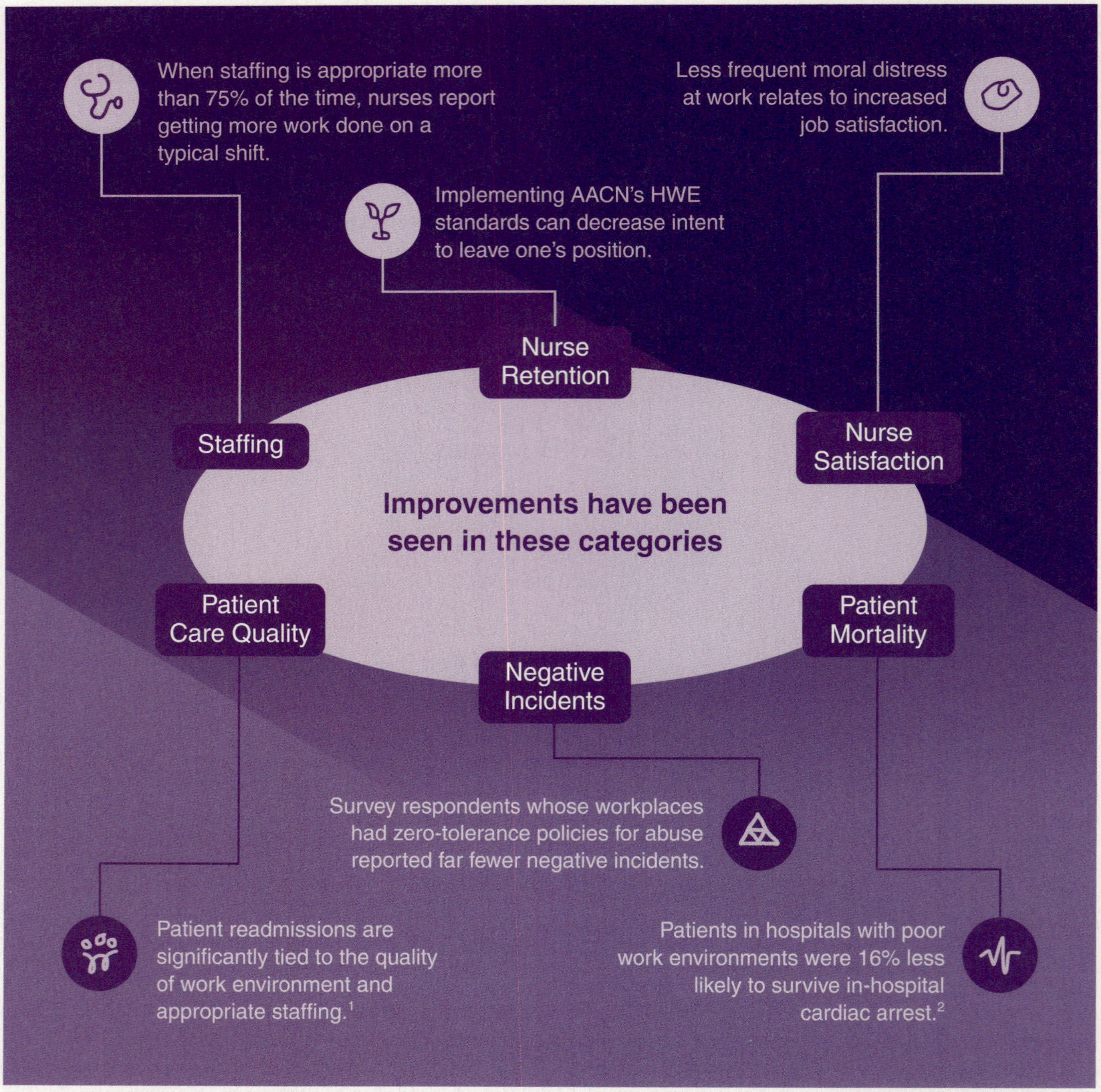

FIGURE 19-2. Implementing standards works. A healthy work environment (HWE) can affect everything in your unit, from nurse engagement and retention to patient outcomes. AACN's Critical Care Nurse Work Environment shows that nurse work environments have improved, but there's still a lot of work to be done. (*Source:* Used with permission from American Association of Critical-Care Nurses [AACN] [2020]. *AACN healthy work environments*. https://www.aacn.org/nursing-excellence/healthy-work-environments)
[1]Ma C, McHugh, M. D., Aiken, L. (2015). Organization of hospital nursing and 30-day readmissions in Medicare patient undergoing surgery. *Med Care, 53*(1), 65–70.
[2]McHugh, M. D., Rochman, M. F., Sloan, D. M., et al. (2016). Better nurse staffing and nurse work environments associated with increased survival if in-hospital cardiac arrest patients. *Med Care*, *54*(1), 74–80.

Nurses who are committed to thoughtful, patient-centered care will want to pay careful attention to these known barriers to quality care.

In February 2019, AACN released the results of "Critical Care Nurse Work Environments 2018: Findings and implications (Ulrich et al., 2019). Figure 19-2 clearly demonstrates the difference implementing the health work environments makes. You will want to pay attention in your different clinical rotations to the presence or absence of these standards in your different work cultures.

Evaluative Programs

In the United States, regulatory facilities such as State Boards of Nursing, the Joint Commission, and the Professional Standards Review Organization, along with the National Health Planning and Resources Development Act of 1975, require nurses to document that nursing standards are being implemented and maintained. Each of these facilities is concerned with quality care and quality control. The decreased availability of resources to treat patients in hospitals and the unavailability of sufficient alternative treatment settings pose a strong challenge to the nursing profession to find ways to avoid compromising quality of care. Numerous professional organizations are working to meet this challenge. Selected web resources for patients and families can be found on their websites.

Quality Assurance

Quality-assurance programs are special programs that promote excellence in nursing. These range from small programs conducted by nurses on a nursing unit to those developed for an entire institution, state, or country.

Quality-assurance programs enable nursing to be accountable to society for the quality of nursing care. Such programs also respond to the public mandate for professional accountability. They help ensure survival of the profession, encourage nursing's fidelity to its moral and ethical responsibilities, and assist nursing to comply with other external pressures.

There are two different approaches to ensuring quality. *Quality by inspection* focuses on finding deficient workers and removing them. However, nurses and others working in a setting using this approach may be afraid to admit a mistake or error and wrongly attempt to hide a problem. Such behavior is never acceptable and may result in serious harm to patients. *Quality as opportunity,* on the other hand, focuses on finding opportunities for improvement and fosters an environment that thrives on teamwork, with people sharing the skills and lessons they have learned. Mistakes are viewed as a result of a problem in the system rather than due to a lack of motivation or lack of effort by a particular worker. In work environments using this approach, nurses respond with openness and a desire to learn because their integrity and self-worth are not threatened. Our outcome should be to work in an environment in which quality measurements encourage our best efforts.

In 1975, the ANA developed a model quality-assurance program consisting of seven steps:

1. Identify values.
2. Identify structure, process, and outcome standards and criteria.
3. Measure the degree of attainment of criteria and standards.
4. Make interpretations about strengths and weaknesses based on such measurements.
5. Identify possible courses of action.
6. Choose a course of action.
7. Take action.

The ANA hoped the model would be used to develop and implement quality-assurance programs within institutions.

The ANA model directs attention to three essential components of quality care: structure, process, and outcome. Other types of quality-assurance programs may focus only on one of these components or on a mixture of components.

- A **structure evaluation** or audit focuses on the environment in which care is provided. Standards describe physical facilities and equipment; organizational characteristics, policies, and procedures; fiscal resources; and personnel resources.
- The focus of a **process evaluation** is the nature and sequence of activities carried out by nurses implementing the nursing process. Criteria make explicit acceptable levels of performance for nursing actions related to patient assessment, diagnosis, planning, implementation, and evaluation.
- **Outcome evaluation** focuses on measurable changes in the health status of the patient, or the end results of nursing care. While the proper environment for care and the right nursing actions are important aspects of quality care, the critical element in evaluating care is demonstrable changes in patient health status.

Concept Mastery Alert

It is important to distinguish the different types of evaluation in quality assurance. A helpful way to remember the different types is to focus on the meaning of the word. For example, *structure* implies buildings or facilities; *process* implies action or activities; *outcome* implies changes in health.

From Quality Assurance to Quality Improvement

Concerns about the spiraling costs of health care, coupled with the success of industrial models for QI, led to a strong commitment to QI in the 1990s. **Quality improvement (QI)**—also known as continuous quality improvement (CQI) or total quality management (TQM)—consists of systematic and continuous actions that lead to measurable improvement in health care services and the health status of targeted patient groups. The U.S. Department of Health and Human Service, Health Resources and Services Administration (HRSA), identifies the four key principles of QI (HRSA, 2011):

- Focus on systems and processes
- Focus on patients
- Focus on being part of the team
- Focus on use of the data (Read about Quality Improvement in Chapter 2.)

From the patient's point of view, one of the most important outcomes of QI is the recognition that patient satisfaction in health care is as important as customer satisfaction in retail business. With increased competition for the health care dollar, providers are learning that it is important to offer services that patients value and to offer them in a way that is valued by patients. By reemphasizing the critical nature of nursing's *person* versus *task* orientation, QI underscores the need for nurses to blend cognitive, technical, interpersonal, and ethical/legal competencies successfully.

Patient Satisfaction

An evaluative program that focuses on patient satisfaction is a powerful tool for patients and families who want to know what care will be like before choosing a health care facility.

Hospital Consumer Assessment of Healthcare Providers and Systems (HCAHPS), the Centers for Medicare and Medicaid Services' patient satisfaction program, is the first national, standardized, publicly reported survey of patients' perspectives of hospital care. The program provides consumers with information about a hospital's performance in key areas of communication, pain control, timeliness of care, discharge instructions, hospital cleanliness, and treatment with courtesy and respect. The survey was designed to produce data about patients' perspectives of care that allow objective and meaningful comparisons of hospitals on topics that are important to consumers. Public reporting of the survey results creates new incentives for hospitals to improve quality of care. Public reporting also serves to enhance public accountability in health care by increasing the transparency of the quality of hospital care provided in return for the public investment.

Are you helping or hurting your hospital? With your first clinical rotation, you can ask yourself how you think your patients would respond if asked the following questions:

- During this hospital stay, how often did nurses treat you with courtesy and respect, listen carefully to you, and explain things in a way you could understand?
- During this hospital stay, after you pressed the call button, how often did you get help as soon as you wanted it?

You can see how your local hospitals compare by searching the website https://www.medicare.gov/hospitalcompare/search.html.

Nursing's Patient Safety and Quality Initiative

In March of 1994, the ANA Board of Directors launched a major multiphase initiative to investigate the impact of health care restructuring on the safety and quality of patient care as well as on nursing. Through its Patient Safety and Quality Initiative, the ANA highlighted the strong linkages between nursing actions and patient outcomes.

In 1998, the ANA funded the development of a national database to house **nursing-sensitive quality indicators**, which are indicators specific to nursing that identify structures of care and care processes that influence care outcome. Examples of nursing-sensitive quality indicators for acute care settings are the mix of RNs, LPNs, and unlicensed staff caring for patients, the total number of nursing care hours provided per patient day, and the rates of pressure injuries and patient falls. The goals of the **National Database of Nursing Quality Indicators (NDNQI)** are to promote and facilitate the standardization of information submitted by hospitals across the United States on nursing quality and patient outcomes.

The ANA Patient Safety and Quality Initiative has focused on educating RNs about quality measurement; informing the public and purchasing/regulating constituencies about safe, quality health care; and investigating research methods and data sources to empirically evaluate the safety and quality of patient care.

QSEN QUALITY IMPROVEMENT

Use data to monitor the outcomes of care processes and use improvement methods to design and test changes to continuously improve the quality and safety of health care systems. If you find something in your work setting that "isn't working," design a small test of change in daily work (using an experiential learning method such as Plan-Do-Study-Act) and use measures to evaluate the effect of change. Read more about Plan-Do-Study-Act in Chapter 2.

Concurrent versus Retrospective Evaluation

Nursing care and patient outcomes may be evaluated while the patient is receiving care (i.e., a concurrent evaluation) or after the patient has been discharged (i.e., a retrospective evaluation). **Concurrent evaluation** is conducted by using direct observation of nursing care, patient interviews, and chart review to determine whether the specified evaluative criteria are met. **Retrospective evaluation** may use postdischarge questionnaires, patient interviews (by telephone or face to face), or chart review (nursing audit) to collect data.

The type of retrospective audit most familiar to nurses working in hospitals is the Joint Commission retrospective chart review. This accrediting body initially required hospitals to conduct a certain number of audits per year.

REFLECTIVE PRACTICE LEADING TO PERSONAL LEARNING

Remember that the object of reflective practice is to look at an experience, understand it, and learn from it. As you begin to develop your expertise in evaluating the plan of care, reflect on your experiences—successes and failures—in order to improve your practice. How can you do it better next time? What did you learn today that can help you tomorrow? Begin your reflection by paying close attention to the following:

- How effectively did you engage your patients and families in evaluating the plan of care? To what degree does patient/family satisfaction motivate your efforts to provide high-quality, safe care?
- What value do you attach to monitoring the patient's achievement of expected outcomes? In what ways did this monitoring result in valuable changes to the plan of care?
- Did your experience with evaluation reveal the need for changes in yourself or in your practice setting? How might these be accomplished?

The cultivation of evaluation as a critical component of the nursing process helps ensure nursing's continued success in achieving desired changes in patient health status. Nursing actions are far too valuable and costly to be haphazardly implemented. Evaluation that is carefully planned and executed can direct and redirect these actions to maximize the patient's benefit. This is the outcome and challenge of nursing evaluation.

Perhaps the most important questions to reflect on are: Are your patients and families/caregivers better for having had *you* share in the critical responsibility of partnering with them to evaluate the development and implementation of the plan of care? Are your patients now receiving thoughtful, person-centered, prioritized, holistic, evidence-based treatment and care because of your efforts?

DEVELOPING CLINICAL REASONING AND CLINICAL JUDGMENT

1. Interview five students who have personal fitness goals. Ask them to describe what personal factors have helped or hindered them in achieving their goals. Note commonalities and differences. Reflect on how you can help patients tap their own personal strengths to achieve their outcomes more successfully.
2. Interview several patients and ask them what qualities in a nurse are most helpful as they try to achieve their health outcomes. Similarly, ask what nurse qualities are most problematic. Reflect on how you measure up in terms of both positive and negative nurse qualities.
3. Interview three or more experienced nurses in the same practice setting. Ask them what system variables (such as philosophy of care, nurse-to-patient ratio, professional and nonprofessional staff mix, nursing management, adequacy of resources) most influence their ability to deliver quality care. Identify variables you want to look for when you interview for a job.
4. Specify how nurses might use the AACN standards and crucial conversation recommendations to change the outcomes in the following situations:
   - A nurse knows that a patient's pain medication isn't working but decides not to call his attending health care provider, because the health care provider was verbally abusive to her in the past and believes his patients "don't need analgesics."
   - A new policy was developed to make sure that obese patients are transferred safely without harm to themselves or staff. The nurse manager places the new policy in the policy manual but fails to educate staff in the new bariatric unit. Moreover, some nurses have been quite vocal about not putting themselves at risk with these patients and have refused to participate in collaborative efforts to move these patients safely.
   - Two nurses call in sick, and staffing is at an all-time low. Additional patients are added to each nurse's assignment, increasing the probability that errors will be made. The nurses are frustrated and angry.

PRACTICING FOR NCLEX

1. A university student works with the student health nurse to develop a weight loss plan that includes increasing activity and avoiding empty calories. At the next session, the student has lost 1 lb instead of the projected 5 lb. What action will the nurse take next?
   a. Congratulate the student and continue the care plan
   b. Terminate the care plan since it is not working
   c. Give the student more time to reach the targeted outcome
   d. Modify the plan after discussing possible reasons for partial success
2. A visiting nurse is following up with a patient who was given a prescription for a diuretic and told to chart her weight daily. The patient's weight has increased 5 lb since the nurse's last visit. What actions will the nurse take first?
   a. Explain to the patient that it is clear she is not adhering to her prescription and the health care provider will be notified
   b. Document the 5-lb weight gain and ask the patient about sodium intake and medication side effects
   c. Terminate the plan of care while determining the cause for the weight gain
   d. Encourage the patient to continue the prescription and return in 1 week
3. During orientation to the critical care unit, a nurse learns that staff follow existing clinical practice guidelines, also called standards, for patient care. Which activities does the nurse expect to be included in these guidelines? Select all that apply.
   a. Monitoring vital signs and pulse oximetry every hour
   b. Using intuition to troubleshoot patient problems
   c. Repositioning a patient on bed rest every 2 hours
   d. Becoming a nurse mentor to a student nurse
   e. Administering pain medication prescribed by the health care provider
   f. Becoming involved in community nursing events
4. After reviewing the admission SBAR and plan of care, the nurse begins to evaluate patient outcomes. Which statement reflects a clear evaluation of the patient's primary problem?

   Electronic health record (EHR)

   8:00 AM Admission note

   S. Patient with profound wheezing, tachycardia, and anxiety

   B. Patient has history of asthma, for which she regularly uses inhalers and carries a rescue inhaler

   A. Pulse oximetry 89%, cyanosis of lips, dyspnea with increased work of breathing

   R. Admit to telemetry unit, add IV corticosteroids and mini-nebulizer treatments

   a. The patient states they were terrified when they were fighting to breathe and the wheezing would not stop.
   b. The nurse determines the patient's strengths include adherence to their medication regimen.
   c. The care plan includes the health problem of impaired gas exchange, etiology, bronchospasm.
   d. At 10:00 AM, no wheezing on auscultation, pulse oximetry is 94%, the patient reports no anxiety; the outcome has been met.

5. A nurse is writing nursing outcomes in the affective domain for a patient who is trying to stop smoking. Which outcome statement will the nurse include in the care plan?
   a. "The patient will state the relationship between smoking and coronary artery disease."
   b. "After the teaching session, the patient will redemonstrate the proper application of a nicotine patch."
   c. "The patient will state they value a healthy body sufficiently to stop smoking prior to discharge."
   d. "The patient will state that any changes in cough should be reported to the health care provider"
6. A nurse writes the outcome for a patient who is trying to lose weight: "The patient will explain the relationship between weight loss, increased exercise, and decreased calorie intake." This outcome reflects which domain of learning?
   a. Cognitive
   b. Psychomotor
   c. Affective
   d. Physical changes
7. A nurse is writing an evaluative statement for a patient who is trying to lower cholesterol through diet and exercise. Which evaluative statement is most correctly written?
   a. "Outcome met."
   b. "1/21/25—Patient reports no change in diet."
   c. "Outcome not met. Patient reports no change in diet or activity level."
   d. "1/21/25—Outcome met. Cholesterol level has decreased 10 mg."
8. A nurse is attempting to improve care on the pediatric unit of a hospital. Which improvements might the nurse employ when following the recommendations of the Institute of Medicine's Committee on Quality of Health Care in America? Select all that apply.
   a. Basing patient care on continuous healing relationships
   b. Customizing care to reflect the competencies of the staff
   c. Using evidence-based decision making
   d. Having a charge nurse as the source of control
   e. Using safety as a system priority
   f. Recognizing the need for secrecy to protect patient privacy
9. As part of a hospital-wide quality-assurance program, an electronic medical record review for the last 6 months reveals a higher incidence of falls on a specific unit. The nurse authoring the study refers to the review as what type of evaluation?
   a. Quality by inspection
   b. Retrospective evaluation
   c. Concurrent study
   d. Quality by indicator
10. The nurse manager of a unit with an excellent safety record meets with staff to present the findings of a recent audit. The manager states, "We're doing well, but I believe we can do better. Who's got an idea to foster increased patient well-being and satisfaction?" This leader has demonstrated they value which process?
    a. Quality assurance
    b. Quality improvement
    c. Process evaluation
    d. Outcome evaluation
11. Nurses note that allowing patients to choose the time of their breakfast to improve patient satisfaction has resulted in medication delays for patients who have prescriptions for medications taken on an empty stomach. Which action will direct the nurses to the best outcome?
    a. Asking the pharmacy to dispense the medication at bedtime
    b. Suggesting a quality improvement project piloting a 6:00 AM administration
    c. Requesting that the health care provider prescribe the medication for midnight
    d. Telling the nurse manager that patients are getting their medications late
12. The nurse on a medical-surgical unit attends a class on the seven crucial conversations in health care. After observing a colleague administer an incorrect dose of medication without reporting it, which action will the nurse take?
    a. Speak to the nurse privately and tell her if she does not complete an event report, you will report her to the unit manager
    b. Tell the nurse you overheard her discussing giving too much medication, and she must complete an event report or you will
    c. Explain that you are aware of the medication incident, and you can assist her in notifying the health care provider for patient safety
    d. Give the nurse a copy of the handout from the class and explain that this class in crucial conversations was very helpful
13. A nurse is using the classic elements of evaluation when caring for patients. Place the steps of evaluation in the proper order they are carried out.
    a. Interpreting and summarizing findings
    b. Collecting data to determine whether evaluative criteria and standards are met
    c. Documenting your judgment
    d. Terminating, continuing, or modifying the plan
    e. Identifying evaluative criteria and standards (i.e., expected patient outcomes)
14. The care plan for a patient just diagnosed with diabetes contains the expected outcome: "the patient will correctly measure the insulin dose and self-administer the injection, using correct technique by 12/12/24."

The nurse observes the client fumbled with the syringe and drew up less insulin than prescribed. What action will the nurse take first?

a. Document that the plan of care was unsuccessful
b. State continuation of the care plan is indicated
c. Assess the patient's vision and dexterity and revise the plan
d. Designate a family member to administer the insulin

ANSWERS WITH RATIONALES

1. **d.** Since the student has only partially met her outcome, the nurse should first explore the factors making it difficult for her to reach her outcome and then modify the care plan. As the plan is not completely working as written, continuing without further assessment is contraindicated. It is premature to terminate the care plan before the outcome is met. The student may need additional support and time to reach the outcome.
2. **b.** The nurse documents the goal has not yet been achieved and also suspects the patient has not adhered to the prescription, perhaps due to frequent urination or other side effects. The nurse further assesses the patient's understanding of the medication's purpose and effects, understanding of the disease process and complications.
3. **a, c, e.** Standards are the levels of performance accepted and expected by the nursing staff or other health care team members. They are established by authority, custom, or consent. Standards would include monitoring patient status every hour, repositioning a patient on bed rest every 2 hours, and administering pain medication prescribed by the health care provider. Using intuition to troubleshoot patient problems, becoming a nurse mentor to a student nurse, and becoming involved in community nursing events are not included in patient care standards.
4. **d.** The two-part evaluative statement includes a decision about how well the outcome was met, along with patient data or behaviors that support this decision. Outcomes may have been met, partially met, or not met. The nurse collects evaluative data to measure outcome achievement. While this may justify terminating the care plan, that is not necessarily so. Data to assess health problems and patient variables are collected during the first step of the nursing process.
5. **c.** Affective outcomes pertain to changes in patient values, beliefs, and attitudes. Cognitive outcomes involve increases in patient knowledge; psychomotor outcomes describe the patient's achievement of new skills; physical changes are actual bodily changes in the patient (e.g., weight loss, increased muscle tone).
6. **a.** Cognitive outcomes involve increases in patient knowledge; psychomotor outcomes describe the patient's achievement of new skills; affective outcomes pertain to changes in patient values, beliefs, and attitudes; and physical changes are actual bodily changes in the patient (e.g., weight loss, increased muscle tone).
7. **d.** The evaluative statement should contain a date; the words "outcome met," "outcome partially met," or "outcome not met"; and the patient data or behaviors that support this decision. The other answer choices are incomplete statements.
8. **a, c, e.** Care should be based on continuous healing relationships and evidence-based decision making. Customization should be based on patient needs and values with the patient as the source of control. Safety should be used as a system priority, and the need for confidentiality of care with transparency for the patient and designated individuals, rather than secrecy is used.
9. **b.** Quality by inspection focuses on finding deficient workers and removing them. Concurrent evaluation uses direct observation of nursing care, patient interviews, and chart review to determine whether the specified evaluative criteria are met. Retrospective evaluation may use post discharge questionnaires, patient interviews (by telephone or face to face), or chart review (nursing audit) to collect data. Quality as opportunity focuses on finding opportunities for improvement and fosters an environment thriving on teamwork, with people sharing the skills and lessons they have learned.
10. **b.** Unlike quality assurance, quality improvement (QI) is internally driven. QI focuses on patient care rather than organizational structure and processes rather than people, and has no end points. Its goal is improving quality rather than assuring quality. Process evaluation and outcome evaluation are types of quality-assurance programs.
11. **b.** Quality improvement or continuous quality improvement involves systematic, continuous actions that lead to measurable improvement in health care services and the health status of targeted patient groups. Quality-assurance programs enable nursing to be accountable for the quality of nursing care. Making changes without gathering needed data may prove unsafe or a waste of time. Reporting to the nurse manager does not reflect professional commitment to improving processes.
12. **c.** *Crucial Conversations for Healthcare,* addresses "undiscussable" communication breakdowns and gaps that can result in patient harm, medical errors, and staff turnover. When nurses feel unsafe to report problems or are not heard, dangerous shortcuts, incompetence, and disrespect may ensue. Threatening the nurse with reporting them is unprofessional and inconsistent with the crucial conversations. Providing a handout is passive aggressive and does not clearly relate the medication error to this concept.
13. **e, b, a, c, d.** The five classic elements of evaluation in order are (1) identifying evaluative criteria and standards (what the nurse looks for during evaluation, that is, expected patient outcomes); (2) collecting data to determine whether these criteria and standards are met; (3) interpreting and summarizing findings; (4) documenting your judgment; and (5) terminating, continuing, or modifying the plan.
14. **c.** When an outcome is not achieved, the nurse can (1) delete or modify a diagnosis; (2) revise the diagnosis, making it more realistic; (3) adjust the time criteria, or (4) modify the nursing interventions. This outcome was not successfully met; further assessment and revision is indicated. It is inappropriate for the nurse to designate a family member to take over insulin administration without additional assessment and patient permission.

Bibliography

Agency for Healthcare Quality and Research (AHQR). (2019). *Culture of safety*. https://psnet.ahrq.gov/primer/culture-safety

Albanese, M. P., Evans, D. A., Schantz, C. A., Bowen, M., Disbot, M., Moffa, J. S., Piesieski, P., & Polomano, R. C. (2010). Engaging clinical nurses in quality and performance improvement activities. *Nursing Administration Quarterly, 34*(3), 226–245.

Alfaro-LeFevre, R. (2014). *Applying nursing process. The foundation for clinical reasoning* (8th ed.). Wolters Kluwer Health/Lippincott Williams & Wilkins.

Alfaro-LeFevre, R. (2020). *Critical thinking, clinical reasoning, and clinical judgment: A practical approach* (7th ed.). Elsevier.

American Association of Critical-Care Nurses (AACN). (2016). *AACN standards for establishing and sustaining healthy work environments: A journey to excellence* (2nd ed.). Author. https://www.aacn.org/WD/HWE/Docs/HWEStandards.pdf

American Nurses Association (ANA). (1976). *ANA quality assurance workbook*. Author.

American Nurses Association (ANA). (1999). *Nursing quality indicators: Guide for implementation* (2nd ed.). Author.

American Nurses Association (ANA). (2010). *Nursing's social policy statement*. Author.

American Nurses Association (ANA). (2021). *Nursing: Scope and standards of practice* (4th ed.). Author.

Barnsteiner, J., & Disch, J. (2017). Creating a fair and just culture in schools of nursing. *American Journal of Nursing, 117*(11), 42–48.

Bloch, D. (1975). Evaluation of nursing care in terms of process and outcome: Issues in research and quality assurance. *Nursing Research, 24*(4), 256–263.

Buhlman, N. (2016). How nurses' work environment influences key performance indicators. *American Nurse Today, 11*(3), 54–58.

Connor, J. A. (2016). Measurement of quality of nursing practice in congenital cardiac care. *American Journal of Critical Care, 25*(2), 128–135.

Connor, J. A., Ziniel, S. I., Porter, C., Doherty, D., Moonan, M., Dwyer, P., Wood, L., & Hickey, P. A. (2018). Interprofessional use and validation of the AACN Healthy Work Environment Assessment Tool. *American Journal of Critical Care, 27*(5), 363–371.

Donabedian, A. (1980). *The definition of quality and its approaches*. Health Administration Press.

Donabedian, A. (1982). *The criteria and standards of quality: Explorations in quality assessment and monitoring*. Health Administration Press.

Easter, K., & Tamburini, L. M. (2018). Understanding patient safety and quality outcome data. *Critical Care Nurse, 38*(6), 58–66.

Grant, S., Davidson, J., Manges, K., Dervenchyan, A., Wilson, E., & Dowdell, E. (2020). Creating healthful work environments to deliver on the quadruple aim. A call to action. *Journal of Nursing Administration, 50*(6), 314–321.

Haase, R., & Miller, K. (1999). Performance improvement in everyday clinical practice. *American Journal of Nursing, 99*(5), 52, 54.

Health Resources and Services Administration (HRSA), U.S. Department of Health and Human Services. (2011). *Quality improvement*. HRSA. https://www.hrsa.gov/quality/toolbox/508pdfs/qualityimprovement.pdf

Hughes, R. G. (2008). Chapter 44: Tools and strategies for quality improvement and patient safety. In R. G. Hughes (Ed.). *Patient safety and quality: An evidence-based handbook for nurses*. Agency for Healthcare Research and Quality (US). https://www.ncbi.nlm.nih.gov/books/NBK2682

Institute for Healthcare Improvement. (2018). *Quality improvement charter*. http://www.ihi.org/resources/Pages/Tools/QI-Project-Charter.aspx

Institute of Medicine (IOM). (1999). *Measuring the quality of health care*. National Academy Press.

Institute of Medicine (IOM). (2001). *Crossing the quality chasm: A new health system for the 21st century*. National Academy Press.

Institute of Medicine (IOM). (2007). *Advancing QI research: Challenges and opportunities*. National Academies Press.

Institute of Medicine (IOM). (2008). *Knowing what works in healthcare: A roadmap for the nation*. National Academies Press.

The Joint Commission. (2012). Improving patient and worker safety. https://www.jointcommission.org/-/media/tjc/documents/resources/patient-safety-topics/patient-safety/tjc-improvingpatientandworker-safety-monograph.pdf

The Joint Commission. (2017). *Sentinel event policy and procedures*. https://www.jointcommission.org/sentinel_event_policy_and_procedures

Jones, P. A., Parliman, A., Groneman, M., & Schneider, J. (2018). Quality improvement: A structured daily checklist. *American Nurse Today, 13*(11), 58–60.

Kohn, L. T., Corrigan, J. M., & Donaldson, M. S. (Eds.). Committee on Quality of Health Care in America. Institute of Medicine (IOM). (2000). *To err is human: Building a safer health system*. National Academy Press.

Maxfield, D., Grenny, J., Lavandero, R., & Groah, L. (2010). *The silent treatment: Why safety tools and checklists aren't enough to save lives*. https://www.aacn.org/nursing-excellence/healthy-work-environments/~/media/aacn-website/nursing-excellence/healthy-work-environment/silencekills.pdf?la=en

Maxfield, D., Grenny, J., McMillan, R., Patterson, K., & Switzler, A. (2005). *Silence kills: The seven crucial conversations for healthcare*. http://www.aacn.org/WD/Practice/Docs/PublicPolicy/SilenceKillsExecSum.pdf

Montalvo, I. (2007). The national database of nursing quality indicators (NDNQI). *The Online Journal of Issues in Nursing, 12*(3). http://www.nursingworld.org/MainMenuCategories/ANAMarketplace/ANAPeriodicals/OJIN/TableofContents/Volume122007/No3Sept07/NursingQualityIndicators.html

Pabico, C. (2020). Dispelling common myths about ANCC's pathway to excellence. *American Nurse Journal, 15*(5), 34–37.

Pabico, C., & Graystone, R. (2018). Comparing Pathway to Excellence and Magnet Recognition® Programs. *American Nurse Today, 13*(3), 46–48.

Pelletier, M. (2019). High reliability in healthcare: The chief nursing officer's critical role. *American Nurse Today, 14*(4), 41–43.

Phaneuf, M. (1976a). *The nursing audit: Self-regulation in nursing practice*. Appleton-Century-Crofts.

Phaneuf, M. (1976b). Quality assurance: A nursing view. *New Zealand Nursing Journal, 69*(2), 9–11.

Stausmire, J. M., & Ulrich, C. (2015). Making it meaningful: Finding quality improvement projects worthy of your time, effort and expertise. *Critical Care Nurse, 35*(6), 57–61.

Ulrich, B., Barden, C., Cassidy, L., & Varn-Davis, N. (2019). Critical care nurse work environments 2018: Findings and implications. *Critical Care Nurse, 39*(2), 67–84.

20 Documenting and Reporting

Phillippe Baron

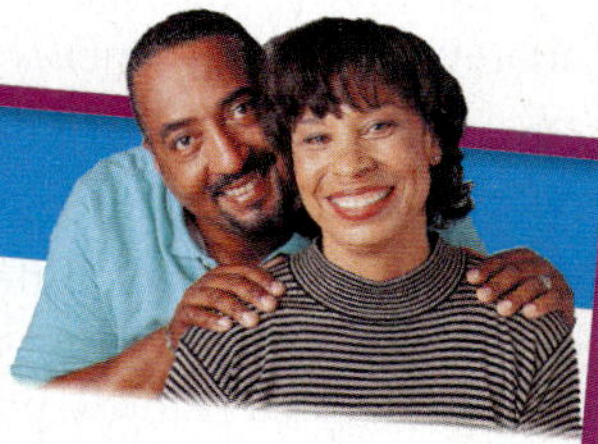

Phillippe is a 52-year-old man being discharged from the outpatient surgery department after undergoing a colonoscopy for removal of three polyps. He will be going home with his wife, who is a nurse, and they both require discharge teaching.

Millie Delong

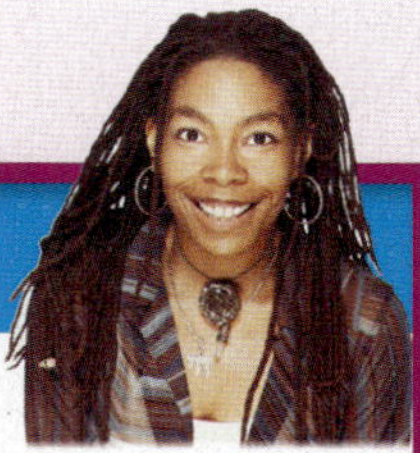

Millie, a 44-year-old woman, develops a wound infection following abdominal surgery. Wound care with normal saline irrigations is ordered four times a day.

Jason Chandler

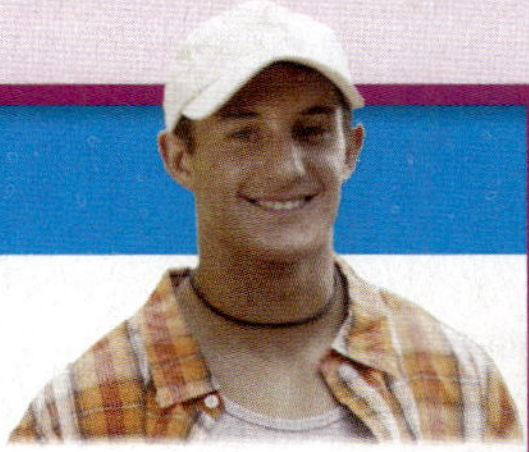

Jason, 15 years old and in police custody, is brought to the emergency department for treatment because he allegedly consumed a latex bag containing a handful of pieces of crack cocaine to avoid arrest. Treatment with insertion of nasogastric tube and bowel preparation solution is ordered. Jason is refusing treatment because he denies possession of drugs entirely.

Learning Outcomes

After completing the chapter, you will be able to accomplish the following:

1. Use standard professional guidelines for effective nursing documentation.
2. Identify measures to protect confidential patient information.
3. Identify approved abbreviations and symbols used for documentation and distinguish these from error-prone abbreviations and symbols.
4. Describe the purposes of different types of patient health records.
5. Compare and contrast different methods of documentation, including electronic health records, source-oriented records, problem-oriented medical records, PIE charting, focus charting, charting by exception, and the case management model.
6. Describe the purpose and correct use of each of the following formats for nursing documentation: nursing assessment, nursing care plan, critical/collaborative pathways, progress notes, flow sheets, discharge summary, and home care documentation.
7. Recognize that documentation by the nurse should be complete, accurate, current, and concise because the patient health record is a legal document.
8. Describe the nurse's role in communicating with other health care professionals by reporting.

Nursing Concepts

- Collaboration
- Documentation

Effective communication among health care professionals is essential to the coordination and continuity of thoughtful person-centered care. Communicating effectively enables personnel to support and complement one another's services and to avoid duplications and omissions in care. This chapter describes two methods of communication central to nurses' professional role: documenting and reporting. The first day you care for patients, you will find yourself conferring with colleagues, recording your interventions, and reporting on your patient's progress toward valued goals and outcomes. As you develop these skills, you will see a link between communicating information and clinical reasoning and clinical judgment. As you document data, you are looking for relationships and patterns—things that might otherwise be overlooked. As you confer with the patient and the patient's family and professional caregivers, you may learn something about the patient or situation that enhances your data set and clarifies the patient's health problem and related need for care (see the Reflective Practice box for an example). This chapter will help you assume communication responsibilities with confidence and skill. The communication process itself and specific communication techniques are discussed in Chapter 8.

DOCUMENTING CARE

Documentation is the written or electronic legal record of all pertinent interactions with the patient: assessing, diagnosing, planning, implementing, and evaluating. You can expect to repeatedly hear "If it wasn't charted, it wasn't done" from your clinical instructors. Today, increasingly sophisticated management information systems help manage patient-specific data and information. These records contain data used to facilitate quality, evidence-based patient care, serve as financial and legal records, help in clinical research, and support decision analysis. Information specialists aim to create an environment that supports timely, accurate, secure, and confidential recording and use of patient-specific information.

The **patient record** is a compilation of a patient's health information (PHI). Each health care institution or facility has policies that specify the nurse's documentation responsibilities. The Joint Commission specifies that nursing care data related to patient assessments, nursing diagnoses or patient needs, nursing interventions, and patient outcomes are permanently integrated into the patient record. Each nurse is expected to practice according to local policies and professional standards.

Guidelines for Effective Documentation

The patient record is the only permanent legal document that details the nurse's interactions with the patient. It is the nurse's best defense if a patient or patient surrogate alleges nursing negligence. Unfortunately, there are often omissions in the nursing documentation, along with repetitious or inaccurate entries. Although these errors might go undetected and have no effect on the patient, they might also seriously affect the care the patient receives, undermine nursing's credibility as a professional discipline, and cause legal problems for the nurses involved. Adherence to the documentation guidelines shown in Box 20-1 (on page 521) helps to prevent errors. Be sure to also check the guidelines later in this chapter for electronic documentation.

Responding to the widespread nursing concern that the time spent documenting nursing care comes at the expense of providing safe, quality patient care, the American Nurses Association (ANA) introduced a tool to streamline the nursing documentation process in 2003 and revised the tool in 2010. Available as a brochure entitled ANA's Principles for Nursing Documentation: Guidance for Registered Nurses, this guide includes policy statements, principles, and recommendations to assist nurses with documentation and to comply with institutional and regulatory requirements.

The policy statements and principles outlined in the guide are based on the ANA Code of Ethics for Nurses with Interpretive

QSEN Reflective Practice: Cultivating QSEN Competencies

CHALLENGE TO ETHICAL AND LEGAL SKILLS

Working in the emergency department (ED) this summer never ceased to amaze me. Police brought Jason Chandler to the ED, a 15-year-old male who was in custody for drug charges. Apparently, as police approached Jason, he consumed a latex bag containing a handful of pieces of crack cocaine to avoid arrest. He was brought to the ED as a precaution. If the bag broke inside his gastrointestinal tract, it would have toxic consequences. Jason was refusing treatment because he denied the possession of drugs entirely. The ED attending health care provider was unsure of his legal rights for treating the boy and called the hospital attorney. The attorney said the physician could force treatment if there were probable signs that ingestion had occurred. However, the boy was not showing any clinical manifestations of chemical ingestion. This was a dilemma because if the drugs leached into the boy's gastrointestinal tract, the health care provider stated that he most likely would not survive. The legal issue was whether the officer's statement of witnessing the ingestion was enough to constitute the need for treatment. The physician was about to begin treating the patient when his mother arrived, threatening to sue anyone and everyone who "touched her little boy."

My preceptor and I were assigned to this patient and were given orders to insert a nasogastric (NG) tube so that a bowel preparation solution (GoLYTELY) could be used to flush out the drugs. The hospital attorney concluded that there was probable cause to justify forced treatment. However, the mother was furious and said she would bring legal action under these circumstances, despite what the doctor or attorney said. As we entered the room to insert the NG tube and begin treatment, the boy, who was handcuffed to the bed, was screaming at us not to touch him.

Thinking Outside the Box: Possible Courses of Action

- Go with my preceptor and assist with the NG tube insertion.
- Refuse to treat the patient for fear of becoming part of a lawsuit.
- Allow my preceptor to sedate the patient against his will, to make the NG tube insertion easier.
- Inform the health care provider that I do not feel comfortable proceeding with treatment on a patient who refuses it and shows no clinical manifestations of drug toxicity.

Evaluating a Good Outcome: How Do I Define Success?

- The patient is benefited or, at the very least, not harmed by our actions.
- The hospital and its employees act in a legally defensible manner and are not sued by the patient's family.
- The patient accepts treatment.
- The mother is able to realize the need for medical intervention.
- Hospital policy is maintained.
- I learn more about our legal and ethical responsibilities.

Personal Learning: Here's to the Future!

My preceptor and I went into the room and explained to the patient and his mother the procedure of NG tube insertion and what the bowel preparation solution was expected to do. I think the mother appreciated that we were not talking to them in a condescending fashion and, therefore, began to see us as trying to help her son, not harm him. She asked a couple of questions about side effects of the medication and how the NG tube worked. She began to show signs of calming down until the health care provider walked into the room. Then she started to show her frustration again. Therefore, my preceptor politely asked the provider to leave. Subsequently, we were able to insert the NG tube, despite some resistance from the patient. Several hours later, the patient passed a package of crack rocks intact.

Obviously, this situation was very new to me. I had never dealt with a patient who was threatening to sue and who was clearly upset by what was happening. I was able to see the collaboration between the attending health care provider, the toxicologist, the hospital attorney, and the nurses and myself. This was an interesting case because the treatments were clearly necessary for the patient's well-being, but everyone wanted to make sure they were legally able to impose treatment. I learned that a hospital attorney is a good resource when legal questions or ambiguous situations arise.

I think that my professional legal skills need a fair amount of work. Unfortunately, I also believe that nurses violate the law more often than is recognized—for example, subtle breaches of the law such as failure to ensure patient safety and failure to follow facility policy. Although I feel that I understand many of the obvious legal violations, I think I have a lot to learn regarding legal issues in the nursing practice.

Julia Strobel, Georgetown University

QSEN SELF-REFLECTION ON QUALITY AND SAFETY COMPETENCIES DEVELOPING KNOWLEDGE, SKILLS, AND ATTITUDES FOR CONTINUOUS IMPROVEMENT

How do you think you would respond in a similar situation? Why? What does this tell you about yourself and about the adequacy of your competencies for professional practice? Can you think of other ways to respond? What legal and ethical principles were involved in this situation? Which ones had the potential to be violated? Why was the clinical instructor more successful than the health care provider? Did the preceptor and nursing student ensure the patient's rights? How might this situation have been different if the patient were over 18 years of age? What knowledge, skills, and attitudes do you need to develop to continuously improve the quality and safety of care for patients like Jason?

(continued)

QSEN Reflective Practice: Cultivating QSEN Competencies *(continued)*

CHALLENGE TO ETHICAL AND LEGAL SKILLS

Patient-Centered Care: How can you establish a successful partnership with a patient and family refusing treatment?

Teamwork and Collaboration/Quality Improvement: What role did the hospital attorney play? What other team members would be helpful? What needs to change to improve quality in this setting?

Safety/Evidence-Based Practice: What does the evidence point to as "best practice" for Jason? What safety needs does he have and how can you meet them?

Informatics: Can you identify the essential information that must be available in Jason's record to support safe patient care and coordination of care? Can you think of other ways to respond to or approach the situation? What else might the nursing student have done to ensure a successful outcome?

Statements (ANA, 2015a) and Scope and Standards of Practice (ANA, 2021). In addition, the formulated principles in many instances are based on standards set forth by state and federal regulatory facilities and the Centers for Medicare & Medicaid Services (CMS), and through accrediting organizations, such as the Joint Commission and the National Committee for Quality Assurance (NCQA). The 2010 ANA Standards identify the following characteristics of effective documentation: accessible; accurate, relevant, and consistent; auditable; clear, concise, and complete; legible/readable (particularly in terms of the resolution and related qualities of EHR content as it is displayed on the screens of various devices); thoughtful; timely, contemporaneous, and sequential; reflective of the nursing process; and retrievable on a permanent basis in a nursing-specific manner (ANA, 2010, p. 12). Note that revised standards may be available after this text goes to publication.

Privacy and Confidentiality

Nurses and other professional caregivers learn and communicate private information about patients and their families every day.

What Information Is Confidential?

All information about patients is considered private or confidential, whether written on a paper, saved on a computer, or spoken aloud. This includes patient names and all identifiers such as address, telephone and fax number, Social Security number, and any other personal information. It also includes the reason the patient is sick or in the hospital, office, or clinic; the assessments and treatments the patient receives; and information about past health conditions. Protected health information might be found in the patient medical record, computer systems, telephone calls, voice mails, fax transmissions, e-mails that contain patient information, and conversations about patients among clinical staff.

While most nurses are staunch advocates of a patient's right to privacy and confidentiality, it is possible to violate these rights. For example, one nurse gives patient information over the phone to a patient's alleged spouse without knowing whether the patient wants the spouse to know; another talks about a difficult patient in the elevator; and another gives patient information to a professional caregiver who "knows" the patient but is not involved in the patient's care. Additional examples of breaches of confidentiality and security include the following:

- Discussing patient information in any public area
- Leaving patient medical information in a public area
- Leaving a computer unattended in an accessible area with medical record information unsecured
- Failing to log off a computer terminal
- Sharing or exposing passwords
- Copying or providing data, for yourself, coworkers, or any other party, except as required to fulfill job responsibilities
- Improperly accessing, reviewing, or releasing the record of a patient for whom one has no responsibility out of concern or curiosity, or requesting another person to do so
- Improperly accessing, reviewing, or releasing a patient record to use information in a personal relationship
- Improperly accessing, reviewing, or releasing the patient record of a public personality for the intent of giving or selling information to the media
- Improperly accessing, reviewing, or releasing confidential information of another member of the workforce who is also a patient
- Improperly accessing, reviewing, or releasing confidential information that may bring harm to the organization or people associated with it

Table 20-1 (on page 522) provides specific measures to use to ensure that information about your patients remains confidential.

Professional codes of ethics, facility policies, and state and federal privacy legislation dictate how patient information can be communicated (spoken verbally and in writing), where and how it can be stored, the appropriate people and entities to whom it may be divulged, and the purposes for which it may be divulged. Nurses must be familiar with these guidelines.

Legal Alert

Take note! There have been reports of school suspensions for nursing and medical students who unprofessionally share patient experiences on social media platforms such as Facebook, Instagram, blogs, and YouTube. What may be an inadvertent or unintentional report of patient information may lead to your suspension or dismissal. Take the time to review the social media guidelines for nurses developed by the ANA National Student Nurses' Association and the National Council of State Boards of Nursing.

Box 20-1 Documentation Guidelines

Aim: Complete, accurate, concise, current, factual, and organized data communicated in a timely and confidential manner to facilitate care coordination and serve as a legal document.

Content

- Enter information in a complete, accurate, concise, current, and factual manner.
- Make sure your documentation reflects the nursing process and your professional responsibilities.
- Record patient findings (observations of behavior) rather than your interpretation of these findings.
- Avoid words such as "good," "average," "normal," or "sufficient," which may mean different things to different readers. It is best to document measurable, verifiable objective data.
- Avoid generalizations such as "seems comfortable today." A better entry would be "on a scale of 1 to 10, patient rates back pain 2 to 3 today as compared with 7 to 9 yesterday; vital signs returned to baseline."
- Note problems as they occur in an orderly, sequential manner; record the nursing intervention and the patient's response; update problems or delete as appropriate.
- Record precautions or preventive measures used.
- Document in a legally prudent manner. Know and adhere to professional standards and facility/institutional policy for documentation.
- Document the nursing response to questionable medical orders or treatment (or failure to treat). Factually record the date and time and the name of the health care provider who was notified of the concern and the exact health care provider response. If this occurs by phone, have a second nurse listen to the conversation and cosign the note. Verbal orders should always be documented as VO with the date, time, and name and credentials of the health care provider who gave the orders. If a nurse administrator was contacted, document the name of the administrator and date and time of contact. Documentation should give legal protection to the nurse, other caregivers, the health care facility or institution, and the patient.
- Document objectively. Avoid slang terms, stereotypes, or derogatory terms when charting. Document quotes from the patient and behaviors. Do not document your opinions or subjective feelings about a patient situation.
- Refrain from copying and pasting notes in an EHR, because the data may be outdated or inaccurate.

Timing

- Document in a timely manner. Follow facility policy regarding the frequency of documentation and modify this if changes in the patient's status warrant more frequent documentation.
- If you forget to document something, record it as soon as you can, following the procedures for making late entries. Example: Late entry: Patient reported passing gas at 8:00 AM this morning but no stool yet. Notified the surgical resident, Dr. Cotter—C. Taylor, RN.
- Indicate in each entry the date and both the time the entry was written and the time of pertinent observations and interventions. This is crucial when a case is being reconstructed for legal purposes.
- Most facilities use military time, one 24-hour time cycle, to avoid confusion between am and pm times (see accompanying figure).
- Document nursing interventions as closely as possible to the time of their execution. The more seriously ill the patient, the greater the need to keep documentation current. Never leave the unit for a break when caring for a seriously ill patient until all significant data are recorded.
- Never document interventions before carrying them out.
- Write a progress note for each of these instances:
  - Upon admission, transfer to another unit, and discharge
  - When a procedure is performed
  - Upon receiving a patient postoperatively or postprocedure
  - Upon communicating with health care providers regarding critical patient information (e.g., abnormal lab value result)
  - For any change in patient status

Format

- Check to make sure you have the correct chart before writing.
- Record on the proper form or screen as designated by facility policy.
- With paper charts, print or write legibly in dark ink to ensure permanence. Use correct grammar and spelling. Use standard terminology, only commonly accepted terms and abbreviations, and symbols (see Box 20-3 on page 524). Alternatively, follow computer documentation guidelines.
- Date and time each entry.
- Record nursing interventions chronologically on consecutive lines. Never skip lines. Draw a single line through blank spaces.

Accountability

- Sign your first initial, last name, and title to each entry. Do not sign notes describing interventions not performed by you that you have no way of verifying.
- Do not use dittos, erasures, or correcting fluids. Draw a single line through an incorrect entry, and write the words "mistaken entry" or "error in charting" above or beside the entry and sign. Then rewrite the entry correctly.
- Identify each page of the record with the patient's name and identification number.
- Recognize that the patient record is permanent. Follow facility policy pertaining to the color of ink and the type of pen or ink to be used. Ensure that the patient record is complete before sending it to medical records.

Confidentiality

- Patients have a moral and legal right to expect that the information contained in their patient health record will be kept private. Students should be familiar with facility policy and pertinent legislation about who has access to patient records other than the immediate caregiving team, and the process used to obtain access (see HIPAA guidelines).
- Most facilities allow students access to patient records for educational purposes. Students using patient records are bound professionally and ethically to keep in strict confidence all the information they learn by reading patient records. Actual patient names and other identifiers should not be used in written or oral student reports.
  - Students should never use their cellphone in the clinical setting.
  - Students should never use any computer in the clinical setting for personal communication.
  - Students should never take photos of any patient or clinical setting.
  - Students should never use any patient information on any social media platform.

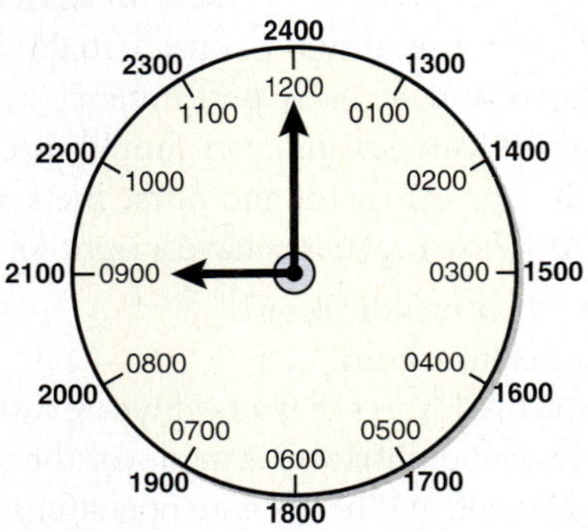

The military clock uses one 24-hour time cycle instead of two 12-hour cycles (e.g., 9:00 AM is 0900 and 9:00 PM is 2100).

Table 20-1 Tips for Preventing Breaches in Patient Confidentiality

TYPE OF BREACH	HOW TO PREVENT IT
Computers	
Displaying information on a screen (especially handheld computers) that is viewed by unauthorized users	Make sure display screens do not face public areas. For portable devices, install encryption software that makes information unreadable or inaccessible.
Sending confidential e-mail messages via public networks such as the Internet, where they can be read by unauthorized users	Use encryption software when sending e-mail over public networks.
Sharing printers among units with differing functions and information (unauthorized users can read printouts)	Request that your unit have a separate printer not shared with another unit.
Copiers	
Discarded copies of patient health information in trash cans adjacent to copiers	Use secure disposal containers (similar to mailboxes) adjacent to copiers.
Cordless and Cellular Phones	
Holding conversations vulnerable to eavesdropping outsiders with scanning equipment	Use phones with built-in encryption technology.
Fax Machines	
Faxing confidential information to unauthorized persons	Before transmission, verify the fax number and that the recipient is authorized to receive confidential information.
Voice Pagers	
Sending confidential messages that can be overheard on the pager	Restrict use of voice pagers to nonconfidential messages.

Source: Reprinted with permission from Holmes, H. N. (Ed.). (2006). *Documentation in action.* Wolters Kluwer Health/Lippincott Williams & Wilkins.

Health Information Privacy

The U.S. Office for Civil Rights enforces the Health Insurance Portability and Accountability Act (HIPAA) Privacy Rule, which protects the privacy of individually identifiable health information; the HIPAA Security Rule, which sets national standards for the security of electronic protected health information; the HIPAA Breach Notification Rule, which requires covered entities and business associates to provide notification following a breach of unsecured protected health information; and the confidentiality provisions of the Patient Safety Rule, which protect identifiable information being used to analyze patient safety events and improve patient safety (https://www.hhs.gov/hipaa/for-professionals/index.html). Congress passed HIPAA in 1996. The HIPAA has been updated to include regulations about electronic patient information with the addition of the 2003 Security Rule and 2013 Omnibus rule.

Most facilities now require workers to undergo HIPAA training and to review and sign a confidentiality agreement, both when hired and at each performance review. As a student in a health care setting, you should discuss privacy guidelines with your instructor and nurse mentors.

According to HIPAA, patients have a right to:

- see and copy their health record.
- update their health record.
- get a list of the disclosures that a health care institution has made independent of disclosures made for the purposes of treatment, payment, and health care operations.
- request a restriction on certain uses or disclosures.
- choose how to receive health information.

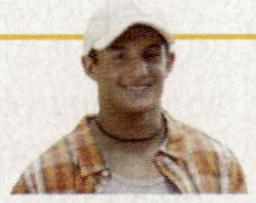

Consider **Jason Chandler**, the adolescent brought to the ED by the police. The nurse needs to be knowledgeable about HIPAA regulations to ensure that Jason's confidentiality is maintained. In addition, the nurse should keep in mind that Jason is a minor, and any authorizations would probably require a parent's consent.

If a health institution wants to release patient health information (PHI) for purposes other than treatment, payment, or routine health care operations, the patient must be asked to sign an authorization. Box 20-2 provides a list of permitted disclosures of PHI and incidental disclosures.

Legal Alert

Take note! **HIPAA legislation includes punishments for anyone caught violating patient privacy. Those who do so can be fined, face imprisonment, and/or revoked licensure. Even accidentally breaking the rules can result in penalties—and embarrassment—for you and your organization.**

Facility Policies

Most facilities have specific policies regarding patient records. Everyone with access to the record (i.e., direct caregivers) is expected to maintain its confidentiality (see the earlier discussion about privacy). Most facilities grant student nurses access to patient records for educational purposes. In this

Box 20-2 The Health Insurance Portability and Accountability Act of 1996 Authorization Rule

If a health institution wants to release a patient's health information (PHI) for purposes other than treatment, payment, and routine health care operations, the patient must be asked to sign an authorization.

Permitted Disclosure of PHI

While the authorization rule covers most situations in which patient information is released for purposes other than treatment, payment, and routine health care operations, there are some exceptions to the authorization rule for the good of the general population.

These three exceptions show situations in which authorization is not required prior to releasing the patient's information:

Public Health Activities

- Tracking and notification of disease outbreaks
- Infection control
- Statistics related to dangerous problems with drugs or medical equipment

Law Enforcement and Judicial Proceedings

- Medical records crucial to the investigation and prosecution of a crime
- Medical records to identify victims of crime or disasters
- Medical personnel reporting incidents of child abuse, neglect, or domestic violence
- Medical records released according to a valid subpoena

Deceased People

- PHI needed by coroners, medical examiners, and funeral directors
- PHI needed to facilitate organ donations
- PHI provided to law enforcement in the case of a death from a potential crime

Incidental Disclosure of PHI

Incidental disclosure of PHI is defined as a secondary disclosure that cannot reasonably be prevented, is limited in nature, and occurs as a by-product of an otherwise permitted use or disclosure of PHI.

Examples of Permitted Incidental Disclosures

Use of sign-in sheets: Provided that the sign-in sheet does not contain information on the reason for the patient's visit

The possibility of a confidential conversation being overheard: Provided that the surroundings are appropriate for a confidential conversation and voices are kept down

Placing patient charts outside exam rooms: Provided that unauthorized public traffic is not permitted in the area of the exam rooms and face sheets are turned toward the wall

Use of white boards: Provided that only the minimum information needed for the purpose of the white board is used

X-ray light boards that can be seen by passers-by: Provided that patient x-rays are not left unattended on the light board

Calling out names in the waiting room: Provided that the reason for the patient's visit is not mentioned

Leaving appointment reminder voicemail messages: Provided that the minimum amount of information is disclosed

instance, *the student assumes responsibility to hold patient information in confidence*. Never use a patient's name when preparing written or oral reports for school.

Facility policies also indicate which personnel are responsible for recording on each form in the record; such policies may also describe the order in which the forms are to appear in the record. Additional policies may concern the frequency with which entries are to be made, whether routine care is recorded, how health personnel identify themselves after making an entry, which abbreviations are acceptable, and how recording errors are handled. Box 20-3 (on page 524) provides a list of commonly used abbreviations. Table 20-2 (on pages 525–527) identifies the Institute for Safe Medication Practices (ISMP) list of error-prone abbreviations, symbols, and dose designations. One of the strategies the Joint Commission is using to achieve National Patient Safety Goals is a list of "Do Not Use" abbreviations, acronyms, and symbols (Table 20-3 on page 528). Be sure to know the latest Joint Commission and facility policies regarding the use of abbreviations, acronyms, and symbols in your practice setting. It is now recommended that students minimize the use of abbreviations, and instead write or type out the full terms and other words to create a clear record for the caregivers who follow. Develop the habit of practicing whatever type of documentation you will be using in your clinical rotations.

Unfolding Patient Stories: Rashid Ahmed • Part 2

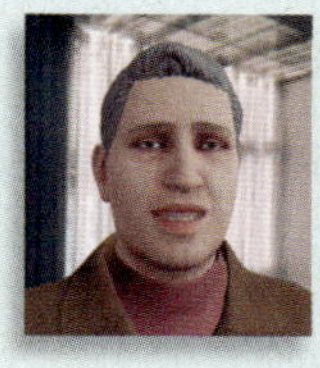

Recall from Chapter 9, **Rashid Ahmed**, a 50-year-old male admitted to the medical unit with a diagnosis of dehydration from severe nausea, vomiting, and diarrhea. What factors should the nurse consider when planning patient education for Rashid? How can the nurse create an environment conducive to learning? What teaching methods can be used to enhance the clarity and retention of information? Why is it important for the nurse to evaluate learning after education is provided, and what evaluation methods can be used?

Care for Rashid and other patients in a realistic virtual environment: ***vSim** for Nursing* (thepoint.lww.com/vSimFunds). Practice documenting these patients' care in DocuCare (thepoint.lww.com/DocuCareEHR).

The storage of patient records after treatment is a function of the health facility's record department. Many patient records are microfilmed for compact storage or are entered into a computer to expedite accessibility of information.

(text continues on page 528)

Box 20-3 Abbreviations and Symbols Commonly Used by Health Practitioners[a]

Activities

AMB	ambulatory
BRP	bathroom privileges
CBR	complete bed rest
OOB	out of bed
up ad lib	up as desired

Assessment Data

abd	abdomen
BP	blood pressure
bx	biopsy
C	Celsius (centigrade)
c/o	complains of
CTA	clear to auscultation
dx	diagnosis
F	Fahrenheit
FUO	fever of unknown origin
GI	gastrointestinal
GU	genitourinary
H/A	headache
h/o	history of
HPI	history of present illness
Imp	impressions
lt or l	left
MAE	moves all extremities
NAD	no apparent distress
NKA	no known allergies
N/V	nausea and vomiting
neg	negative
P	pulse
PE	physical examination
PMH	past medical history
R	respirations
R/O	rule out
ROS	review of systems
rt or ®	right
SOB	short of breath
Sx	symptoms
T	Temperature
Tx	Treatment
⊕	positive
Θ	negative

Diseases

ASCVD	arteriosclerotic cardiovascular disease
ASHD	arteriosclerotic heart disease
BPH	benign prostatic hypertrophy
CA	cancer
CAD	coronary artery disease
CHF	congestive heart failure
COPD	chronic obstructive pulmonary disease
CVA	cerebrovascular accident
DM	diabetes mellitus
HTN (↑ BP)	hypertension
MI	myocardial infarction
PE	pulmonary emboli
PVD	peripheral vascular disease
STD	sexually transmitted disease
STI	sexually transmitted infection
URI	upper respiratory infection
UTI	urinary tract infection

Diagnostic Studies

ABG	arterial blood gases
BE	barium enema
CBC	complete blood count
CO2	carbon dioxide
C&S	culture and sensitivity
CXR	chest x-ray
ECG (EKG)	cardiogram
lytes	electrolytes
RBC	red blood cells
UA	urinalysis
UGI	upper GI
WBC	white blood cells

Symbols

↑	increase
↗	increasing
↓	decrease
↙	decreasing
2°	secondary to
=	equal to
≠	unequal
♀	female
♂	male
°	degree
▲	change
x̄	except

Miscellaneous

ā	before
ad lib	as desired
AMA	against medical advice
ASAP	as soon as possible
BM	bowel movement
BSD	bedside drainage
c̄ (C)	with
CABG	coronary artery bypass graft
CPR	cardiopulmonary resuscitation
DNR (no code)	do not resuscitate
Dsg	dressing
dx	diagnosis
FOB	foot of bed
Fx	fracture
GHWT	good handwashing technique
HOB	head of bed
Hx	history
I&O	intake and output
IM	intramuscular
IV	intravenous
KVO	keep vein open
NG	nasogastric
noc	night
NPO (npo)	nothing by mouth
NS (NIS) (N/S)	normal saline
O_2	oxygen
OT	occupational therapy
p̄	after
postop	postoperative
preop	preoperative
prep	preparation
PRN (p.r.n.)	as needed
PT	physical therapy
pt	patient
ROM	range of motion
RX	treatment
s̄(S)	without
SOB	side of bed
S/P	status post
STAT	immediately
SubQ or SQ	subcutaneous
TF	tube feeding
TPR	temperature, pulse, respirations
TX	treatment
VS	vital signs
WA	while awake
×	times

[a]Use only those abbreviations and symbols accepted by your institution.

Table 20-2 ISMP Error-Prone Abbreviations

The abbreviations, symbols, and dose designations found in this table have been reported to ISMP through the ISMP National Medication Errors Reporting Program (ISMP MERP) as being frequently misinterpreted and involved in harmful medication errors. They should NEVER be used when communicating medical information. This includes internal communications, telephone/verbal prescriptions, computer generated labels, labels for drug storage bins, medication administration records, as well as pharmacy and prescriber computer order entry screens.

ABBREVIATIONS	INTENDED MEANING	MISINTERPRETATION	CORRECTION
µg	Microgram	Mistaken as "mg"	Use "mcg"
AD, AS, AU	Right ear, left ear, each ear	Mistaken as OD, OS, OU (right eye, left eye, each eye)	Use "right ear," "left ear," or "each ear"
OD, OS, OU	Right eye, left eye, each eye	Mistaken as AD, AS, AU (right ear, left ear, each ear)	Use "right eye," "left eye," or "each eye"
BT	Bedtime	Mistaken as "BID" (twice daily)	Use "bedtime"
cc	Cubic centimeters	Mistaken as "u" (units)	Use "mL"
D/C	Discharge or discontinue	Premature discontinuation of medications if D/C (intended to mean "discharge") has been misinterpreted as "discontinued" when followed by a list of discharge medications	Use "discharge" and "discontinue"
IJ	Injection	Mistaken as "IV" or "intrajugular"	Use "injection"
IN	Intranasal	Mistaken as "IM" or "IV"	Use "intranasal" or "NAS"
HS hs	Half-strength At bedtime, hours of sleep	Mistaken as bedtime Mistaken as half-strength	Use "half-strength" or "bedtime"
IU[a]	International unit	Mistaken as IV (intravenous) or 10 (ten)	Use "units"
o.d. or OD	Once daily	Mistaken as "right eye" (OD-oculus dexter), leading to oral liquid medications administered in the eye	Use "daily"
OJ	Orange juice	Mistaken as OD or OS (right or left eye); drugs meant to be diluted in orange juice may be given in the eye	Use "orange juice"
Per os	By mouth, orally	The "os" can be mistaken as "left eye" (OS—oculus sinister)	Use "PO," "by mouth," or "orally"
q.d. or QD[a]	Every day	Mistaken as q.i.d., especially if the period after the "q" or the tail of the "q" is misunderstood as an "i"	Use "daily"
qhs	Nightly at bedtime	Mistaken as "qhr" or every hour	Use "nightly"
qn	Nightly or at bedtime	Mistaken as "qh" (every hour)	Use "nightly" or "at bedtime"
q.o.d. or QOD[a]	Every other day	Mistaken as "q.d." (daily) or "q.i.d. (four times daily) if the "o" is poorly written	Use "every other day"
q1d	Daily	Mistaken as q.i.d. (four times daily)	Use "daily"
q6pm, etc.	Every evening at 6 pm	Mistaken as every 6 hours	Use "daily at 6 PM" or "6 PM" o daily"
SC, SQ, sub q	Subcutaneous	SC mistaken as SL (sublingual); SQ mistaken as "5 every;" the "q" in "sub q" has been mistaken as "every" (e.g., a heparin dose ordered "sub q 2 hours before surgery" misunderstood as every 2 hours before surgery)	Use "subcut" or "subcutaneously"
ss	Sliding scale (insulin) or ½ (apothecary)	Mistaken as "55"	Spell out "sliding scale;" use "one half" or "½"

(continued)

Table 20-2 ISMP Error-Prone Abbreviations *(continued)*

ABBREVIATIONS	INTENDED MEANING	MISINTERPRETATION	CORRECTION
SSRI	Sliding scale regular insulin	Mistaken as selective serotonin reuptake inhibitor	Spell out "sliding scale (insulin)"
SSI	Sliding scale insulin	Mistaken as Strong Solution of Iodine (Lugol's)	
i/d	One daily	Mistaken as "tid"	Use "1 daily"
TIW or tiw	3 times a week	Mistaken as "3 times a day" or "twice in a week"	Use "3 times weekly"
U or u[a]	Unit	Mistaken as the number 0 or 4, causing a 10-fold overdose or greater (e.g., 4U seen as "40" or 4u seen as "44"); mistaken as "cc" so dose given in volume instead of units (e.g., 4u seen as 4cc)	Use "unit"
UD	As directed ("ut dictum")	Mistaken as unit dose (e.g., diltiazem 125 mg IV infusion "UD" misinterpreted as meaning to give the entire infusion as a unit [bolus] dose)	Use "as directed"
DOSE DESIGNATIONS AND OTHER INFORMATION	**INTENDED MEANING**	**MISINTERPRETATION**	**CORRECTION**
Trailing zero after decimal point (e.g., 1.0 mg)[a]	1 mg	Mistaken as 10 mg if the decimal point is not seen	Do not use trailing zeros for doses expressed in whole numbers
"Naked" decimal point (e.g., .5 mg)[a]	0.5 mg	Mistaken as 5 mg if the decimal point is not seen	Use zero before a decimal point when the dose is less than a whole unit
Abbreviations such as mg. or mL. with a period following the abbreviation	mg mL	The period is unnecessary and could be mistaken as the number 1 if written poorly	Use mg, mL, etc. without a terminal period
Drug name and dose run together (especially problematic for drug names that end in "l" such as Inderal 40 mg; Tegretol 300 mg)	Inderal 40 mg Tegretol 300 mg	Mistaken as Inderal 140 mg Mistaken as Tegretol 1,300 mg	Place adequate space between the drug name, dose, and unit of measure
Numerical dose and unit of measure run together (e.g., 10 mg, 100 mL)	10 mg 100 mL	The "m" is sometimes mistaken as a zero or two zeros, risking a 10- to 100-fold overdose	Place adequate space between the dose and unit of measure
Large doses without properly placed commas (e.g., 100000 units; 1000000 units)	100,000 units 1,000,000 units	100000 has been mistaken as 10,000 or 1,000,000; 1000000 has been mistaken as 100,000	Use commas for dosing units at or above 1,000, or use words such as 100 "thousand" or 1 "million" to improve readability
DRUG NAME ABBREVIATIONS	**INTENDED MEANING**	**MISINTERPRETATION**	**CORRECTION**
To avoid confusion, do not abbreviate drug names when communicating medical information. Examples of drug name abbreviations involved in medication errors include:			
APAP	acetaminophen	Not recognized as acetaminophen	Use complete drug name
ARA A	vidarabine	Mistaken as cytarabine (ARA C)	Use complete drug name
AZT	zidovudine (Retrovir)	Mistaken as azathioprine or aztreonam	Use complete drug name
CPZ	Compazine (prochlorperazine)	Mistaken as chlorpromazine	Use complete drug name
DPT	Demerol-Phenergan-Thorazine	Mistaken as diphtheria-pertussis-tetanus (vaccine)	Use complete drug name

Table 20-2 ISMP Error-Prone Abbreviations *(continued)*

DRUG NAME ABBREVIATIONS	INTENDED MEANING	MISINTERPRETATION	CORRECTION
DTO	diluted tincture of opium, or deodorized tincture of opium (Paregoric)	Mistaken as tincture of opium	Use complete drug name
HCl	hydrochloric acid or hydrochloride	Mistaken as potassium chloride (The "H" is misinterpreted as "K")	Use complete drug name unless expressed as a salt of a drug
HCT	hydrocortisone	Mistaken as hydrochlorothiazide	Use complete drug name
HCTZ	hydrochlorothiazide	Mistaken as hydrocortisone (seen as HCT250 mg)	Use complete drug name
$MgSO_4$[a]	magnesium sulfate	Mistaken as morphine sulfate	Use complete drug name
MS, MSO_4[a]	morphine sulfate	Mistaken as magnesium sulfate	Use complete drug name
MTX	Methotrexate	Mistaken as mitoxantrone	Use complete drug name
NoAC	Novel/new anticoagulant	Mistaken as "no anticoagulant"	Use complete drug name
PCA	procainamide	Mistaken as patient-controlled analgesia	Use complete drug name
PTU	propylthiouracil	Mistaken as mercaptopurine	Use complete drug name
T3	Tylenol with codeine No. 3	Mistaken as liothyronine	Use complete drug name
TAC	triamcinolone	Mistaken as tetracaine, Adrenalin, cocaine	Use complete drug name
TNK	TNKase	Mistaken as "TPA"	Use complete drug name
TPA or tPA	tissue plasminogen activator, Activase, (alteplase)	mistaken as TNKase (tenectaplase) or as another tissue plasminogen activator, Retavase (retaplase)	Use complete drug name
$ZnSO_4$	zinc sulfate	Mistaken as morphine sulfate	Use complete drug name
STEMMED DRUG NAMES	**INTENDED MEANING**	**MISINTERPRETATION**	**CORRECTION**
"Nitro" drip	nitroglycerin infusion	Mistaken as sodium nitroprusside infusion	Use complete drug name
"Norflox"	norfloxacin	Mistaken as Norflex	Use complete drug name
"IV Vanc"	intravenous vancomycin	Mistaken as Invanz	Use complete drug name
SYMBOLS	**INTENDED MEANING**	**MISINTERPRETATION**	**CORRECTION**
ʒ	Dram	Symbol for dram mistaken as "3"	Use the metric system
♏	Minim	Symbol for minim mistaken as "mL"	
x3d	For three days	Mistaken as "3 doses"	Use "for three days"
> and <	Greater than and less than	Mistaken as opposite of intended; mistakenly use incorrect symbol; "<10" mistaken as "40"	Use "greater than" or "less than"
/(slash mark)	Separates two doses or indicates "per"	Mistaken as the number 1 (e.g., "25 units/10 units" misread as "25 units and 110" units)	Use "per" rather than a slash mark to separate doses
@	At	Mistaken as "2"	Use "at"
&	And	Mistaken as "2"	Use "and"
+	Plus or and	Mistaken as "4"	Use "and"
°	Hour	Mistaken as a zero (e.g., q2° seen as q20)	Use "hr," "h," or "hour"
Φ or	Zero, null sign	Mistaken as numerals 4, 6, 8, and 9	Use 0 or zero, or describe intent using whole words

[a]These abbreviations are included on The Joint Commission's "minimum list" of dangerous abbreviations, acronyms, and symbols that must be included on an organization's "Do Not Use" list, effective January 1, 2004. Visit www.jointcommission.org for more information about this Joint Commission requirement.

Source: © Institute for Safe Medication Practices. (2021). List of Error Prone Abbreviations. https://www.ismp.org/recommendations/error-prone-abbreviations-list

Table 20-3 The Joint Commission Official "Do Not Use" List[a]

DO NOT USE	POTENTIAL PROBLEM	USE INSTEAD
U, u (for unit)	Mistaken for "0" (zero), the number "4" (four), or "cc"	Write "unit"
IU (International Unit)	Mistaken for IV (intravenous) or the number 10 (ten)	Write "International Unit"
Q.D., QD, q.d., qd (daily)	Mistaken for each other	Write "daily"
Q.O.D., QOD, q.o.d, qod (every other day)	Period after the Q mistaken for "I" and the "O" mistaken for "I"	Write "every other day"
Trailing zero (X.0 mg)[b]	Decimal point is missed	Write X mg
Lack of leading zero (.X mg)		Write 0.X mg
MS	Can mean morphine sulfate or magnesium sulfate	Write "morphine sulfate"
MSO_4 and $MgSO_4$	Confused for one another	Write "magnesium sulfate"

[a]Applies to all orders and all medication-related documentation that are handwritten (including free-text computer entry) or on preprinted forms.

[b]Exception: A "trailing zero" may be used only when required to demonstrate the level of precision of the value being reported, such as for laboratory results, imaging studies that report the size of lesions, or catheter/tube sizes. It may not be used in medication orders or other medication-related documentation.

Source: © The Joint Commission. (2018). Official "Do Not Use" List. FACT SHEET. https://www.jointcommission.org/-/media/tjc/documents/resources/patient-safety-topics/patient-safety/do_not_use_list_9_14_18.pdf.

You should also know your facility's policies regarding the patient's right to access records. Be sure to check the policy where you work to find out answers to the following common questions from patients:

- Can I take my patient record home?
- Can I access my patient record electronically?
- How long do you retain records?
- How long will it take to get a copy of my record?
- How much does it cost?
- I do not want some parts of my record (e.g., psychiatric information) released to anyone. What do I do?
- What can I do to get errors in my record corrected?
- May I look at my family's medical record?
- Who can look at my record?
- Who do I tell if my name has changed?

Your facility should have an information officer or clinical informaticist who can help you answer these questions.

Delegating Documentation

An issue of growing importance concerns documentation made by assistive personnel. Because professional nurses frequently supervise the care that assistive personnel give, it must be clear which assessments and interventions may be charted by assistive personnel and which require documentation by a professional nurse. Make sure you know and follow your facility's protocols. As a general rule, you should only document the assessments and interventions you perform.

Purposes of Patient Records

Patient records serve many purposes. The ANA states that the most important of these is "communicating within the health care team and providing information for other professionals, primarily for individuals and groups involved with accreditation, credentialing, legal, regulatory and legislative, reimbursement, research, and quality activities" (ANA, 2010, p. 5).

Communication

The primary purpose of the patient record is to help health care professionals from different disciplines (who interact with the patient at different times) communicate with one another. Communication fosters continuity of care. For example, a critically ill patient in an academic health center may be seen by an attending health care provider, several consulting physicians, different teams of medical residents, an assigned social worker or case manager, assorted therapists, a hospital chaplain, and many nurses. Because these people are never all in the same room at the same time, the patient record is the primary means of communication. A nurse may check the patient record to see if the health care provider has spoken with the patient or the patient's surrogate about a do-not-resuscitate order (DNR) or an allow natural death order (AND). The health care provider may read the nurse's note to see how the family is responding to the recommendation to withhold or withdraw life-sustaining treatment.

Note also that other health care professionals make judgments about nurses and nursing's contributions to the health care team partially on the basis of what is documented in the patient record.

Diagnostic and Therapeutic Orders

Patient records include diagnostic and therapeutic orders. Anyone reviewing the chart can find all the diagnostic studies ordered for the patient since admission, the results of these studies, and related orders for care. Illegible handwritten notes have been the source of many inaccuracies in patient health records. Whenever you are unsure of what has been written or entered in an electronic record, check the original order. Never guess about what is written. A patient's life and your license are literally at risk if you incorrectly transcribe or execute an order.

VERBAL ORDERS

Verbal orders (VOs) must be given directly by the physician or nurse practitioner to a registered professional nurse or registered professional pharmacist, who receives, reads back, documents and executes the order. In "**read-back**," the recipient reads back the message as they heard and interpreted it. The person giving the order then confirms that such recording and interpretation of the order is correct.

Health care institutions limit use of verbal orders and have individual facility policies for their use. Here is a sample institutional policy for VOs:

A. The registered professional nurse or registered professional pharmacist who receives the VO will:
   a. record the orders in the patient's medical record with the letters VO (verbal order).
   b. read back the order to verify accuracy of the order.
   c. date and note the time the orders were issued
   d. record VOs, the name of the physician or nurse practitioner who issued the orders, followed by the nurse's own name and title.

B. At the soonest possible time, the physician or nurse practitioner who issued the VOs must:
   a. review the orders to ascertain whether they are correct.
   b. sign the orders with name, title, and pager number.
   c. date and note the time they sign the orders.

C. The registered professional nurse must see that the orders are transcribed according to the facility's procedure.

D. Verbal orders should be limited to urgent situations where immediate written or electronic communication is not feasible (National Coordinating Council for Medication Error Reporting and Prevention, 2020).

E. According to the Institute for Safe Medication Practices, 2017, the potential for verbal orders to be misunderstood, misheard, or transcribed incorrectly make them error prone. Health care facilities should have policies and procedures specifying when verbal orders are acceptable, defining the prohibitions and limitations on verbal orders, and establishing requirements for clear communication of verbal orders, including a read-back process (Cohen, 2017).

F. According to Wakefield et al. (2012, p. 11), "recommendations to ameliorate potential dangers associated with verbally communicated orders include 'read-backs' and other strategies to improve the safety of VOs and/or limit their use, and to ensure that the verbal communication was understood and accurately transcribed into the hospitals' ordering systems."

Care Planning

Each health care professional working with the patient has access to the patient's baseline and ongoing data and can see how the patient is responding to the treatment plan from day to day. For example, if recorded data indicate that a patient is gradually becoming weaker and cannot now tolerate ambulation, orders for physical therapy and other nurse-initiated ambulation need to be modified. Modifications of the care plan are based on these data.

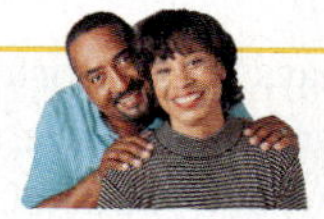

Think back to **Phillippe Baron**, the patient who had undergone a colonoscopy. The nurse uses the patient's chart to obtain information about the patient, including events of the colonoscopy and how the patient responded, to develop an individualized discharge teaching plan.

Quality Process and Performance Improvement

"Documentation is the primary source of evidence used to continuously measure performance outcomes against predetermined standards" (ANA, 2010, p. 7). Records may be reviewed to evaluate the quality of care patients have received and the competence of the nurses providing that care. For example, in a nursing audit, a committee decides in advance the standards of care it wants to evaluate (e.g., pertaining to nursing assessment, nursing documentation, or safety measures). A number of records are then randomly selected and reviewed for evidence that the nurses met the selected standards of care. If deficiencies are found, in-service training may be used to remedy the problem and improve the quality of care. Accrediting facilities, such as the Joint Commission on Accreditation of Healthcare Organizations (JCAHO), may also use record review to determine whether a particular facility or health care institution is meeting its standards.

Research

Researchers may study patient records, hoping to learn how best to recognize or treat identified health problems from the study of similar cases. The aim is to promote evidence-based practice in nursing and quality health care.

Decision Analysis

Information from record review often provides the data needed by administrative strategic planners to identify needs as well as the means and strategies most likely to address these needs. Record review may reveal both underused and overused services, patients with prolonged stays who require special assistance, and financial information about which services generate revenue compared with those that cost the institution or facility money.

Education

Health care professionals and students reading a patient's record can learn a great deal about the clinical manifestations of particular health problems, effective treatment modalities, and factors that affect patient goal achievement.

Credentialing, Regulation, and Legislation

Documentation allows reviewers to monitor health care practitioners' and the health care facility's compliance with standards governing the profession and provision of care.

Legal Documentation

Patient records are legal documents that might be used as evidence in court proceedings. One in four malpractice suits are decided on the basis of the patient's record. Documentation plays an important role in implicating or absolving health care practitioners charged with improper care. The record can also be used in accident or injury claims made by the patient. All nurses need to be well informed about facility policies and professional standards for documentation.

Reimbursement

Patient records are used to demonstrate to payers (e.g., insurance companies) that patients received the intensity and quality of care for which reimbursement is being sought.

Historical Documentation

Because all entries on records are dated, the record has value as a historical document. Years later, information concerning a patient's past health care may be pertinent.

Methods of Documentation

Different methods of documentation are used by different health care facilities to achieve certain aims. Understanding a variety of systems helps nurses adapt quickly in new practice settings.

Computerized Documentation and Electronic Health Records

Increasingly, computer systems are used for nursing documentation in the patient record. In such systems the nurse may:

1. call up the admission assessment tool on the computer screen and key in patient data (see Chapter 15 for illustrations).
2. develop the care plan using computerized care plans available for each diagnosis or problem.
3. add to the patient database as new data are identified and modify the care plan accordingly.
4. receive a work list showing the treatments, procedures, and medications necessary for each patient throughout the care of the patient.
5. document care immediately, using the computer terminal at the patient's bedside.

According to HealthIT.gov (n.d.), "Electronic health records (EHRs) and the ability to exchange health information electronically can help you provide higher quality and safer care for patients while creating tangible enhancements for your organization." EHRs help providers better manage care for patients and provide better health care by:

- Providing accurate, up-to-date, and complete information about patients at the point of care
- Enabling quick access to patient records for more coordinated, efficient care
- Securely sharing electronic information with patients and other clinicians
- Helping providers more effectively diagnose patients, reduce medical errors, and provide safer care
- Improving patient and provider interaction and communication, as well as health care convenience (Fig. 20-1)
- Enabling safer, more reliable prescribing
- Helping promote legible, complete documentation and accurate, streamlined coding and billing

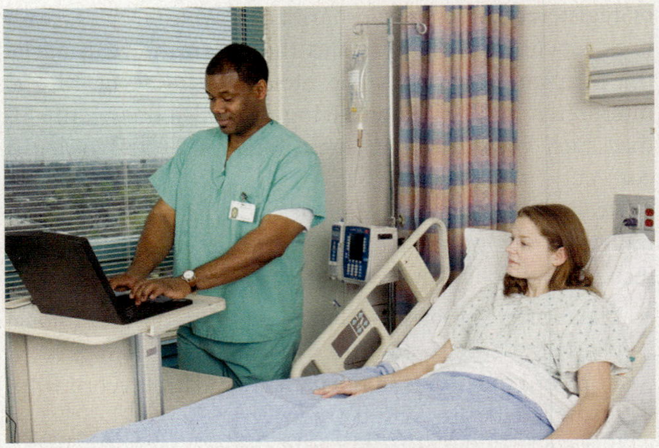

FIGURE 20-1. Computerized bedside charting allows the nurse to remain in contact with the patient while electronically documenting patient information. (*Source:* Used with permission from Shutterstock. *Photo by B. Proud.*)

- Enhancing privacy and security of patient data
- Helping providers improve productivity and work–life balance
- Enabling providers to improve efficiency and meet their business goals
- Reducing costs through decreased paperwork, improved safety, reduced duplication of testing, and improved health (https://www.healthit.gov/faq/what-are-advantages-electronic-health-records)

With computer-based records, or **electronic health records (EHRs)**, data can be distributed among many caregivers in a standardized format, allowing them to compare and uniformly evaluate patient progress easily. Besides tracking the progress of individual patients, computerized outcome information can aid in comparing the progress of groups of patients with similar diagnoses. These results will contribute to research; education; and, ultimately, better and more efficient nursing practice. Box 20-4 defines terms used to discuss electronic records in health care.

The Agency for Healthcare Research and Quality (AHRQ, 2018) reports EHRs can improve the quality and safety of health care in the following ways:

- Help reduce medical errors and adverse events
- Enable better documentation and file organization
- Provide patients with information that assists their adherence to medication regimens and scheduled appointments
- Assist health care providers track their treatment protocols
- Allow patient information to flow between and within health care facilities and practices can enhance primary care provider decision making and improve care coordination (Cross et al., 2015)
- Allow faster and more complete access to the patient record and may improve communication among members of the health care team (some evidence exists that electronic documentation may be associated with improved patient outcomes and decreased costs [Hripcsak & Albers, 2013])
- Improve the communication and management of laboratory information in patient care, particularly results reporting and test order management (Henricks, 2011)

Box 20-4 Terms Used to Discuss Electronic Records in Health Care

Computerized Provider Order Entry (CPOE): This section of the EHR is for the orders written by the health care provider that are deemed necessary for the patient such as required lab tests, procedures, medications, and treatments. This section was formerly known as the section of the paper medical record known as "physician orders."

Clinical Decision Support (CDS): CDS includes academic information, medical logic, and analytic programs built into the EHR that can assist the health care provider make diagnoses and clinical decisions about patient care. Examples of CDS data include patient genetic information, past patient health history data that influences current health problem, potential drug–drug interactions, pharmacogenomic information applicable to the patient, interpretation of abnormal lab test results, data received from the medical devices used in patient care such as infusion pumps, ventilators, and bedside monitors. CDS applications continue to be promoted as one of the key features of EHRs. CDS applications are constantly being upgraded within EHRs. CDS systems give the health care provider ability to synthesize fragments of evidence documented in the entire record to understand the etiology of a disease and its clinical manifestation in individual patients. A comprehensive discussion of current CDS capabilities can be found in Greenes' "Clinical Decision Support" (Greenes, 2014).

Electronic health record (EHR): The EHR is the patient care record created when facilities under different ownership share their data. The goal is for this sharing to be nationwide, creating a situation in which a person's health care record is accessible by designated health care providers anywhere in the nation. The patient will decide which portions of a record will be available to whom.

Electronic medical record (EMR): An EMR is an electronic patient care record created by a facility or facilities having common ownership. Although these EMRs today are often called EHRs, they are not true EHRs because the data are not shared between providers in facilities under different ownership.

Health information exchange (HIE): An HIE is an organization that provides services to enable the electronic sharing of health-related information.

Electronic database: An electronic database is a collection of data that allows easy searching and easy retrieval of similar pieces of data from many records.

Medication Administration Record (MAR): The electronic Medication Administration Record (MAR or eMAR) is used to electronically track and record administration of patient medications. At a minimum the MAR includes the patient's name, and each medication's name, dose, frequency, and route. The MAR is commonly linked to bar code medication administration systems. For example, when a nurse scans a bar code on their identification badge, on the patient's wristband, and on the medication to be administered, the data are delivered to a computer software system where algorithms check various databases and generate real-time warnings or approvals. Most systems then automatically document, in real time, the administration of the medication in an eMAR (Shah et al., 2016).

Personal Health Records (PHRs): These are patient records of their own medical data and health history. PHRs can be interfaced with applications within EHRs and are used by most large facilities. PHRs are allowing patients to take a more active role in managing their health care by documenting their past health history and current health care goals. This communication feature has enhanced patient-centered care provided by health care providers.

Source: Evans, R. S. (2016). Electronic health records: Then, now, and in the future. *Yearbook of Medical Informatics, 25*(Suppl 1), S48–S61. https://www.ncbi.nlm.nih.gov/pmc/articles/PMC5171496/pdf/ymi-11-0s48.pdf

- EHR clinical decision support (CDS) systems, provide appropriate, timely, patient-specific reminders and information and are essential to cope with the growth in medical knowledge; when implemented effectively, CDS has been shown to improve quality and can be particularly effective for increasing appropriate use of evidence-based preventive services (Wright et al., 2015)
- EHR computer provider order entry (CPOE) is associated with a 13% to 99% reduction in medication errors and a 30% to 84% reduction in adverse drug events (ADEs) (Ammenwerth et al., 2008)

In spite of the touted benefits of EHRs, many providers, including nurses, report high dissatisfaction. According to Balestra (2017), "Although these systems promised to improve the quality of patient care, increase efficiency, and reduce costs, health care providers are finding that current EHRs instead require time-consuming data entry, can interfere with patient interactions, and cause medical errors." Nurse Stephanie Drobny shared her dismay when a patient grumbled about nurses always talking behind his back—and she realized it happened when they were charting in his room. "The idea that charting about a patient in his presence would be perceived as secretive had never occurred to me" (Balestra, 2017, p. 11). Drobny responded by flipping her position so that she now sits side by side with the patient, and they both focus on the computer and enter the responses together. While the initial assessment now takes 20 to 30 minutes, she discovered that patients have become partners, their health literacy is improved, and she more rapidly gains their trust: a big payoff for a simple change.

Pfeifer (2020), reporting on a Kaiser Health News and Fortune Magazine study on EHRs (Schulte & Fry, 2019), describes serious consequences that can befall patients with the use of EHRs. Rather than the promised higher quality care, lower costs, and an overall healthier population, the authors describe "systemic failures in transmission of physician orders, mix-ups in patient profiles that could lead to catastrophic medication errors, and issues with 'interface,' where online systems used by pharmacies and laboratories might fail to communicate with each other." See the Office of the National Coordinator for Health Information Technology nine SAFER Guides (https://www.healthit.gov/topic/safety/safer-guides).

With the increasing use of computerized patient information systems to store and analyze patient data have come policies and procedures to ensure the privacy and confidentiality of patient information. Policies should specify what types of patient information can be retrieved, by whom, and for what purpose. Patient consent is necessary for the use and release of any stored information that can be linked to the patient.

The ANA, the American Medical Record Association, and the Canadian Nurses Association offer the following guidelines and strategies for safe computer charting:

- Never give your personal password or username to anyone, including any other health care provider.
- Don't leave a computer terminal unattended after you have logged on.
- Know and follow the recommended protocol for correcting errors. To correct an error after it has been entered, mark the entry "mistaken entry," add the correct information, and date and initial the entry. If you record information in the wrong chart, write "mistaken entry—wrong chart" and sign off. Follow similar guidelines in electronic records.
- Never create, change, or delete records unless you have specific authority to do so.
- If you inadvertently delete part of the permanent record, type an explanation into the computer file with the date, time, and your initials, and submit an explanation in writing to your manager.
- Do not leave information about a patient displayed on a monitor where others may see it. Keep a log that accounts for every printout of a computerized file that you've generated from the system.
- Never use email to send protected health information unless it has been encrypted to protect it from unauthorized access.
- Follow the facility's confidentiality procedures for documenting sensitive material, such as a diagnosis of acquired immunodeficiency syndrome (AIDS) or human immunodeficiency virus (HIV) infection.

Legal Alert

Remember, each time you log in to an electronic health record (EHR) with your password, you create a trail that can be traced, and you are liable for everything you document—or fail to document.

PERSONAL HEALTH RECORDS

Many people today are preparing online personal health records (PHRs) to manage their health care via computer. These records contain the person's medical history, including diagnoses, symptoms, and medications. Some patients scan in doctors' notes, test results, CT images, and insurance information. They may give health care professionals their password so that they can log on and may give permission to share the record with other family members. The chief reason for a PHR is to provide easy access to up-to-date, complete health information to assist in self-care and communication with providers.

Tethered/connected PHRs are the most common kind of personal health record. A tethered, or connected, PHR is linked to a specific health care organization's EHR system or to a health plan's information system. With a tethered PHR, patients can access their own records through a secure portal and see, for example, the trend of their lab results over the last year, their immunization history, or due dates for screenings.

When talking with patients who are considering using a PHR, advise them to check the service's privacy policy carefully to see how much control they will have over their information and whether the service can share or exchange their data, and ask their health care providers if they are willing to read their PHR. Helpful information may be found at https://www.healthit.gov/faq/what-are-benefits-personal-health-records and https://www.healthit.gov/sites/default/files/about-phrs-for-providers-011311.pdf.

HEALTH INFORMATION EXCHANGE

An electronic **health information exchange (HIE)** allows physicians, nurse practitioners, physician assistants, nurses, pharmacists, other health care providers, and patients to appropriately access and securely share a patient's vital medical information electronically, improving the speed, quality, safety, and cost of patient care. Appropriate, timely sharing of vital patient information can better inform decision making at the point of care and allow providers to avoid readmission and medication errors, improve diagnoses, and decrease duplicate testing (Health Information Exchange, n.d.). Benefits of an HIE include the following:

- Provides a vehicle for improving quality and safety of patient care.
- Provides a basic level of interoperability among EHRs maintained by individual health care providers and organizations.
- Stimulates consumer education and patients' involvement in their own health care.
- Helps public health officials meet their commitment to the community.
- Creates a potential loop for feedback between health-related research and actual practice.
- Facilitates efficient deployment of emerging technology and health care services.
- Provides the backbone of technical infrastructure for leverage by national and state-level initiatives (Health Information Exchange, n.d.).

The following resources provide more information about electronic health and medical records and HIE:

- American Nursing Informatics Association: www.ania.org
- HealthIT.gov: www.healthit.gov
- Healthcare IT News: www.healthcareitnews.com
- Healthcare Information and Management Systems Society (HIMSS): www.himss.org
- American Health Information Management Association (AHIMA): https://www.ahima.org/

Source-Oriented Records

Many nurses, especially in rural and underserved areas, continue to practice in settings that do not use EHRs. Traditional paper records are still used in such settings, in a variety of formats. A **source-oriented record** is a paper format in which

Box 20-5 Examples of Forms and Information in Source-Oriented Patient Records

Admission Record
Legal name, identification number
Age, birth date, biologic sex/gender
Marital status
Occupation and employer
Religious preference
Next of kin and person to notify in case of emergency
Date, time, reason for admission
Name of the attending health care provider
Insurance information
Discharge data

Admission Nursing Assessment (see Chapter 15)
Results of nursing history and physical assessment

Graphic Record
Daily temperatures, pulse and respiratory rates, blood pressure (vital signs), pain level
Daily weight
Special measurements, such as the patient's fluid intake and output

Flow Sheet to Record Routine Care (see Fig. 20-5)

Respiratory	IV therapy	Sleep
Cardiac	Wound	Safety
Pain	Tubes	Equipment
Nutrition	Hygiene	Teaching
Elimination	Activity	Progress sheet

Narrative Nurse's Notes
Descriptions of pertinent observations of patient
Statements that specify the nursing care, including teaching, received by patient and patient's responses to nursing care
Statements that describe patient's condition and progress, or lack of progress, toward recovery and goal achievement
Descriptions of patient's complaints and how patient is coping or failing to cope with them, and nursing's response

Medication Record (see Chapter 30)
Name of prescribed medications administered on a regular or PRN basis
Dosage of medication administered
Route by which medication was administered, unless given orally
Time medication was administered
Name or initials of person administering the medication

Medical History and Examination Record
Results of physical examination performed by health care provider
Current medical condition
Health history, including previous illnesses
Family medical history
Confirmed or tentative diagnosis
Plan of medical therapy

Health Care Provider's Order Record
Orders for medications
Orders for treatments
Other directives pertinent to a particular patient's care

Health Care Provider's Progress Notes
Interpretations of patient's pathology
Responses of patient to medical therapy

Miscellaneous Forms
Laboratory reports
X-ray film reports
Consultation reports
Dietary requirements
Results of social service consultations
Types and results of physical, respiratory, and x-ray therapy

each health care group keeps data on its own separate form. Sections of the record are designated for nurses, health care providers, laboratory, x-ray personnel, and so on. Notations are entered chronologically, with the most recent entry being nearest the front of the record. An advantage of the source-oriented record is that each discipline can easily find and chart pertinent data. The main disadvantage is that data are fragmented, making it difficult to track problems chronologically with input from different groups of professionals.

Although the specifics vary among health facilities, the general characteristics of source-oriented records are essentially the same. Types of forms typically used in a source-oriented patient record are shown in Box 20-5. Notes written to inform caregivers of the progress a patient is making toward achieving expected outcomes are called **progress notes**. Progress notes written by nurses in a source-oriented record are **narrative notes** and address routine care, patient data, and patient problems identified in the care plan. They include a description of the status of the problem, related nursing interventions, patient responses to interventions, and needed revisions to the care plan.

Alfaro-LeFevre (2014, p. 183) identifies the following charting memory jogs when writing narrative notes:

- Assessment, Intervention, Response, Action (AIRA). Chart the assessment data you observed, the interventions you performed, the patient's response to interventions, and any actions you took based on the response.
- Date, Action, Response, Action (DARA). This has the same meaning as above.

Problem-Oriented Medical Records

Another type of paper record used in some health facilities is the **problem-oriented medical record (POMR)**, or problem-oriented record. The POMR is organized around a patient's problems rather than around sources of information. With POMRs, all health care professionals record information on the same forms. The advantages of this type of record are that the entire health care team works together in identifying a master list of patient problems and contributes collaboratively to the care plan. Progress notes clearly focus on patient problems. The POMR includes the defined database, problem list, care plans, and progress notes.

The **SOAP format** (Subjective data, Objective data, Assessment [the caregiver's judgment about the situation], Plan) is used to organize entries in the progress notes of the POMR. Variants of the SOAP format include SOAPE, SOAPIE, and SOAPIER (Intervention, Evaluation, and Response). Caregivers select numbered problems from the master list on the front of the patient record and then work up the problem or "SOAP it" on the progress sheet. Some nurses believe that the SOAP method of charting focuses too narrowly on problems and advocate instead a return to the traditional narrative format.

PIE Charting: Problem, Intervention, Evaluation

The **PIE charting** system is unique in that it does not develop a separate care plan. The care plan is incorporated into the progress notes, which identify problems by number (in the order they are identified). In this documentation system, a patient assessment is performed and documented at the beginning of each shift using preprinted fill-in-the-blank assessment forms (flow sheets). Patient problems identified in these assessments are numbered, documented in the progress notes, worked up using the Problem, Intervention, Evaluation (**PIE**) format—or Problem, Intervention, Evaluation, Revision (**PIER**), and evaluated each shift. Resolved problems are dropped from daily documentation following the nurse's review. Continuing problems are documented and numbered each day. One advantage of this system is that it promotes continuity of care. It also saves time because there is no separate care plan. The disadvantage of not having a formal care plan is that nurses need to read all the nursing notes to determine problems and planned interventions before initiating care. Unlike the SOAP method, which originated from the medical record, the PIE format has a nursing origin.

Focus Charting

The purpose of **focus charting** is to bring the focus of care back to the patient and the patient's concerns. Instead of a problem list or list of nursing or medical diagnoses, a focus column is used that incorporates many aspects of a patient and patient care. The focus may be a patient strength, problem, or need. Topics that may appear in the focus column include patient concerns and behaviors, therapies and responses, changes of condition, and significant events such as teaching, consultation, monitoring, management of activities of daily living, or assessment of functional health patterns. The narrative portion of focus charting uses the Data–Action–Response (DAR) format (Fig. 20-2). The principal advantage of focus charting is the holistic emphasis on the patient and the patient's priorities. Ease of charting is also cited as an advantage of focus charting because each note does not need to incorporate data, action, and response. Some nurses report, however, that the DAR categories are artificial and not helpful when documenting care.

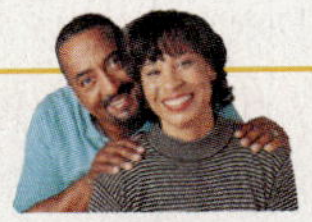

For Mr. **Baron**, the nurse may use focus charting to document specific aspects of teaching related to the colonoscopy and postprocedural care. In addition, because of the effects of anesthesia from the colonoscopy procedure, Mr. Baron may not completely remember all that is taught. Therefore, the nurse documents to include the patient's wife in the discharge teaching to ensure that the information taught was indeed understood. Remember that Mrs. Baron is a nurse. Her clinical knowledge and any necessary reinforcement of information would also be documented.

Charting by Exception

Charting by exception (CBE) is a shorthand method of documenting normal findings, based on standardized normals, standards of practice, and predetermined criteria for assessments and interventions. Significant findings or **exceptions** to the predefined norms are only documented in detail. CBE is common on EHRs. Many patient examination findings are completed by health care providers using checklists and checkboxes on EHRs, instead of fully written descriptions. When a health care provider charts by exception, it means that only exceptions to normal findings are documented. If nothing is documented the patient's status is assumed to match the normal findings established for the data.

For example, on a pulmonary exam, the normal finding may be clear breath sounds at 12 to 20 breaths per minute. Providers

Date/Time	Focus	Patient Care Notes
7/11/25 0915	High risk for trauma	**DATA:** Patient crying when I entered room; confided that she is afraid to go home because her injuries are the result of her husband's battery, which she had not previously wanted anyone to know. **ACTION:** Attending notified and discharge cancelled; Abuse network called with patient's permission and they are sending a counselor this afternoon to talk with her. — C. Taylor, RN
1000	Pain	**DATA:** Patient complaining of pain in right rib area **ACTION:** Tylenol 3 administered as ordered. — C. Taylor, RN
1030	Pain	**RESPONSE:** Patient reports relief from rib pain, still anxious about aftermath of discharge. — C. Taylor, RN

FIGURE 20-2. Sample focus patient care notes.

who find this on examination of the patient do not need to chart this in CBE. However, if the patient had a respiratory rate above or below the normal or had clear lung sounds with occasional wheezes, the provider would need to clearly document this. However, these lung sounds can go undocumented in CBE, since the majority of breath sounds were clear. Nuances and subtleties found on examination can easily go undocumented.

Benefits of CBE have been noted to be less time needed for charting (freeing more time for direct patient care), a greater emphasis on significant data, easy retrieval of significant data, timely bedside charting, standardized assessment, greater interdisciplinary communication, better tracking of important patient responses, and lower costs (King et al., 2014; Nguyen et al., 2014).

However, there are drawbacks to CBE. Distinctive findings on examination of the patient can go undocumented. In CBE, the clinical portrayal of the patient is based on a standardized checklist of normal findings rather than full descriptions of examination findings. A lack of detail in documentation can compromise patient safety and place the health care provider in legal jeopardy. A patient's medical record is expected to accurately reflect the complete description of distinctive findings and details discovered on patient examination. A chart that is missing pertinent information could fail to draw attention to potential problems. In addition, nurses' notes with few explanations, little description of key findings, or no mention of periodic patient checks could be construed as negligence by a plaintiff's attorney guided by the premise, not charted, not done (Brown, 2016; Nursing Service Organization [NSO], 2020).

Case Management Model

Managed care's emphasis on quality, cost-effective care delivered within a limited time frame has led to the development of interdisciplinary documentation tools that clearly identify those outcomes that select groups of patients are expected to achieve on each day of care. The case management model promotes collaboration, communication, and teamwork among caregivers; makes efficient use of time; and increases quality by focusing care on carefully developed outcomes. One limitation of this model, however, is that it works best for "typical" patients with few individualized needs. At present, there is little consensus about which documentation tools are best for recording routine aspects of care and avoiding repetition.

COLLABORATIVE PATHWAYS

Collaborative pathways—also called **critical pathways** or care maps—are used in the case management model. The collaborative pathway specifies the care plan linked to expected outcomes along a timeline. In some documentation systems, the collaborative pathway is part of a computerized documentation system that integrates the collaborative pathway and documentation flow sheets designed to match each day's expected outcomes. CBE is frequently used with collaborative pathway documentation systems.

OCCURRENCE CHARTING

When a patient fails to meet an expected outcome or a planned intervention is not implemented in the case management model, this variance from the plan is documented. The usual format for **occurrence charting** or **variance charting** is the unexpected event, the cause of the event, actions taken in response to the event, and discharge planning, when appropriate. The variances most likely to be documented are those that affect quality, cost, or length of stay.

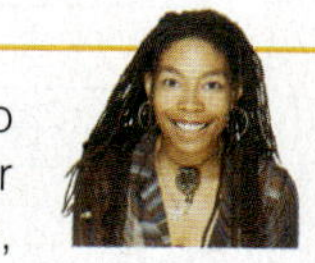

Consider **Millie Delong**, the woman who developed a wound infection. Typically, after abdominal surgery, infection is a complication, not a normal or expected occurrence. Therefore, using the case management model, the nurse needs to document this unexpected outcome with variance charting.

Formats for Nursing Documentation

When the nursing process is fully implemented, nursing documentation in the patient's permanent record includes the following formats.

Initial Nursing Assessment

A typical electronic form used to record the initial database obtained from the nursing history and physical assessment is illustrated in Chapter 15. Accurate documentation of these data is important to provide a baseline for later comparisons as the patient's condition changes.

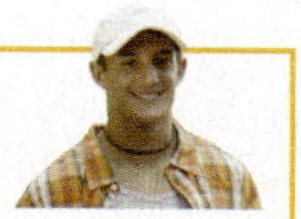

Think back to **Jason Chandler**, the adolescent brought to the ED in police custody. Owing to the nature of the admission, a complete nursing assessment would be inappropriate. However, the nurse needs to thoroughly assess the patient for signs and symptoms indicating problems associated with swallowing the package of drugs. Later, once the initial situation is resolved, an initial history and physical examination would be performed.

Care Plan

Patient records must communicate the patient's problems or diagnoses; related goals, outcomes, and interventions; and progress or resolution of the problems. The nursing care plan may be written separately or incorporated into a multidisciplinary plan. In a traditional nursing care plan, nursing diagnoses, goals and expected outcomes, and nursing interventions are written for each patient (see the sample student plan in Chapter 17 and the care plans at the end of each clinical chapter). Standardized care plans may also be used that identify common problems and related care for select patient groups. These generally incorporate standards of high-quality care, but unless such care plans are individualized, they may not sufficiently address individual patient needs. Formats for care plans vary greatly.

Patient Care Summary

The patient care summary contains an overview of valuable patient information such as documentation, lab and test results, orders, and medications. Figure 20-3 shows one such example.

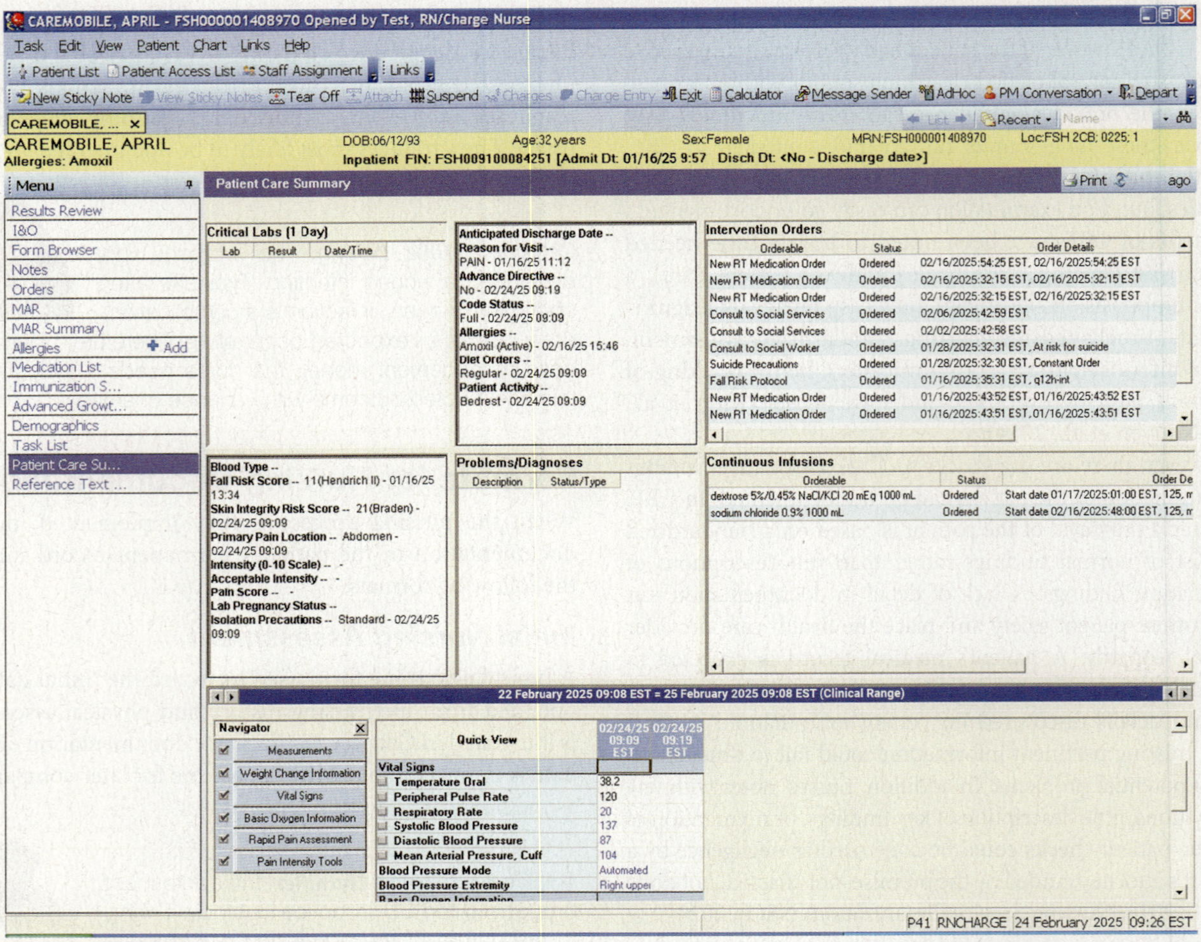

FIGURE 20-3. Electronic patient care summary.

Critical/Collaborative Pathways

The case management plan is a detailed, standardized care plan that is developed for a patient population with a designated diagnosis or procedure. It includes expected outcomes, a list of interventions to be performed, and the sequence and timing of those interventions. The critical/collaborative pathway is an abbreviated summary of key information taken from the more detailed case management plan.

Progress Notes

The purpose of progress notes is to inform caregivers of the progress a patient is making toward achieving expected outcomes. The method used to record the patient's progress depends on the documentation system being used. Common examples include narrative nursing notes, SOAP notes, PIE notes, focus charting, CBE, and the case management model. Figure 20-4 shows an example of a home hospice nurse's charting following a home visit.

Flow Sheets and Graphic Records

Flow sheets are documentation tools used to efficiently record routine aspects of nursing care (Fig. 20-5). Well-designed flow sheets enable nurses to quickly document the routine aspects of care that promote patient goal achievement, safety, and well-being. The **graphic record** is a form used to record specific patient variables such as pulse, respiratory rate, blood pressure readings, body temperature, weight, fluid intake and output, bowel movements, and other patient characteristics.

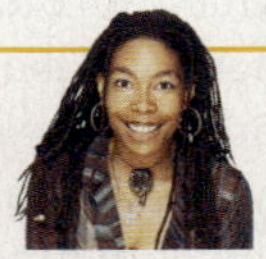

A graphic record would be used for both **Millie Delong** and Phillippe Baron, described at the beginning of the chapter. Specifically for Ms. Delong, documentation of vital signs is significant because she has a wound infection. Because Mr. Baron is post colonoscopy, his vital signs also need to be assessed frequently. In addition, fluid intake and output are key postoperative assessment findings to be documented.

Medication Administration Records

The patient's medication record must include documentation of all the medications administered to the patient (drug, dose, route, time), the nurse administering the drug, and, for some medications (e.g., analgesics), the reason the drug was administered and its effectiveness. Some electronic medication administration records (eMARs) allow providers to look up detailed information about a medication's indications, contraindications, expected and adverse effects, and safe dosage ranges. Sample medication records are shown in Chapter 30.

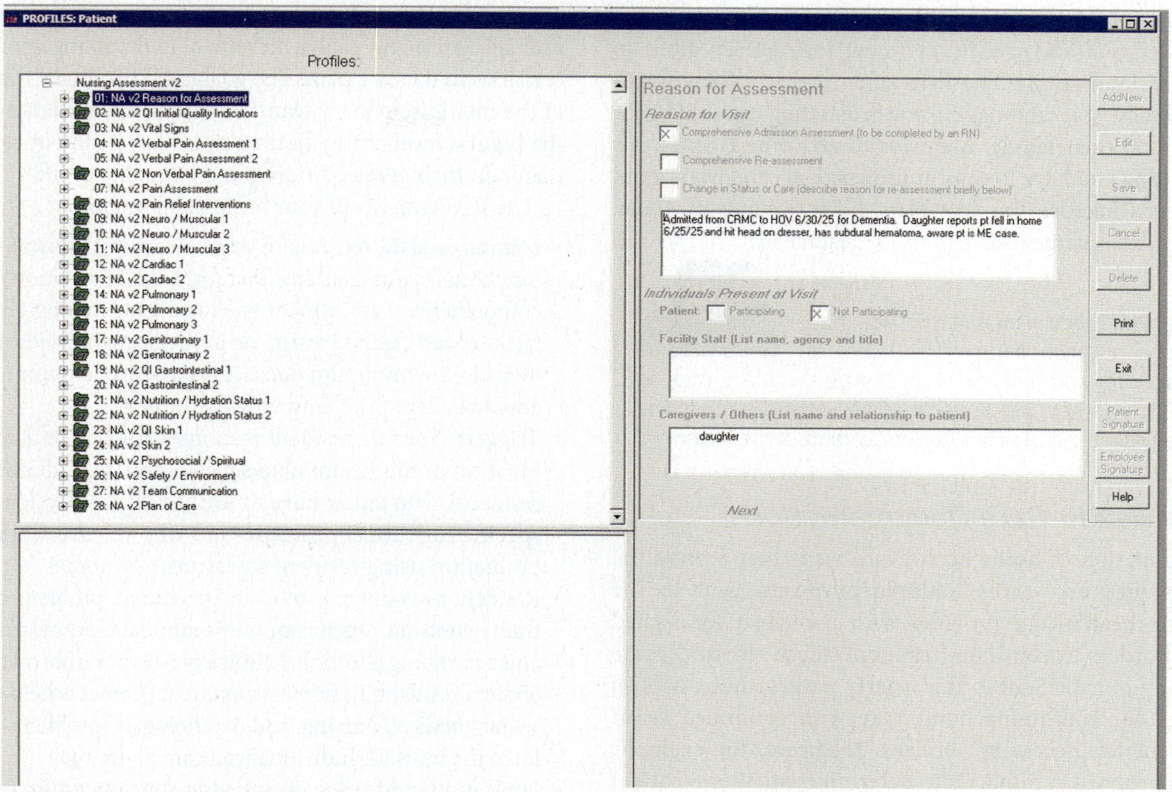

FIGURE 20-4. Electronic nursing documentation following a home hospice visit. (Used with permission. Forms completed with fictitious data.)

Acuity Records

Twenty-four–hour reports are increasingly used in conjunction with acuity reports, with which nurses rank patients as high-to-low acuity in relation to both the patient's condition and need for nursing assistance or intervention. A trauma patient whose condition is changing rapidly and who requires intensive nurse monitoring and intervention merits a higher acuity rank than a patient whose condition is stable. Acuity rankings are often used to determine staffing requirements. A nursing unit with patients with higher acuity rankings requires more professional nurses than a unit with the same number of patients who have lower acuity ranks.

Discharge and Transfer Summary

When a patient is discharged from care or transferred from one unit, institution, or facility to another, a **discharge summary** should be written that concisely summarizes the reason for treatment, significant findings, the procedures performed

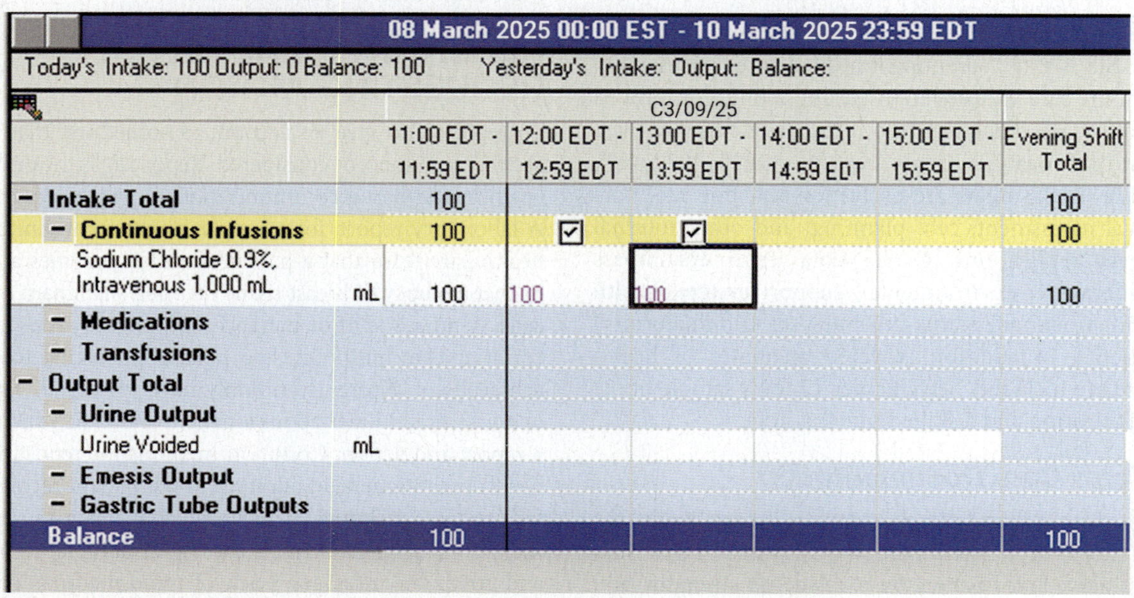

08 March 2025 00:00 EST - 10 March 2025 23:59 EDT

Today's Intake: 100 Output: 0 Balance: 100 Yesterday's Intake: Output: Balance:

		C3/09/25					
		11:00 EDT - 11:59 EDT	12:00 EDT - 12:59 EDT	13:00 EDT - 13:59 EDT	14:00 EDT - 14:59 EDT	15:00 EDT - 15:59 EDT	Evening Shift Total
− Intake Total		100					100
− Continuous Infusions		100	☑	☑			100
Sodium Chloride 0.9%, Intravenous 1,000 mL	mL	100	100	100			100
− Medications							
− Transfusions							
− Output Total							
− Urine Output							
Urine Voided	mL						
− Emesis Output							
− Gastric Tube Outputs							
Balance		100					100

FIGURE 20-5. Intake and output flow sheet. Used with permission. Forms completed with fictitious data.

and treatment rendered, the patient's condition on discharge or transfer, and any specific pertinent instructions given to the patient and family. The EHR often prepares these forms electronically. You can imagine how frustrating it would be for patients and their family caregivers to arrive in a new treatment setting and have to inform professional caregivers about their needs because the care plan didn't accompany them. Review the discharge instructions in Chapter 12.

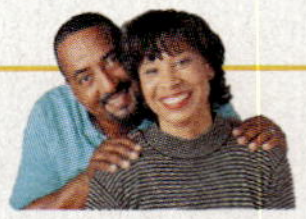

Consider **Phillippe Baron**, the man who had undergone a colonoscopy. The nurse is responsible for completing the discharge summary, making sure to include specific aspects of self-care teaching and both the patient's and wife's understanding of the teaching.

Home Health Care Documentation

Documentation of home health care visits that reports the patient's progress serves multiple purposes. Sent to the attending health care provider with a request for signed medical orders to continue treatment, these records ensure continuity of care. Sent to third-party payers, they establish the need for continuing home care with continued reimbursement for necessary services. Medicare, for example, reviews progress summaries to determine whether a patient meets one of these Medicare requirements:

- The patient is homebound and still needs skilled nursing care.
- Rehabilitation potential is good.
- The patient's status is not stabilized.
- The patient is dying.
- The patient is making progress in expected outcomes of care.

The **Outcome and Assessment Information Set (OASIS)** is a group of data elements that:

- represent core items of a comprehensive assessment for an adult home care patient.
- form the basis for measuring patient outcomes for purposes of outcome-based quality improvement (OBQI).

The OASIS is a key component of Medicare's partnership with the home care industry to foster and monitor improved home health care outcomes (see https://edit.cms.gov/files/document/draft-oasiseall-items-instrument-02012022.pdf). Overall, the OASIS items are useful for outcome monitoring, clinical assessment, care planning, and other internal facility-level applications. OASIS data items encompass sociodemographic, environmental, support system, health status, and functional status attributes of (nonmaternity) adult patients. In addition, selected attributes of health service use are included. See Chapter 12 for a sample home health certification and a skilled nursing note.

Long-Term Care Documentation

Documentation in long-term care settings is specified by the Resident Assessment Instrument (RAI), which helps staff gather definitive information on a resident's strengths and needs and addresses these in an individualized care plan. The RAI helps staff track changes in a resident's status by evaluating resident goal achievement and making appropriate revisions in the care plan. The goal is to coordinate the efforts of the multidisciplinary team to ensure that residents achieve the highest level of functioning possible (quality of care) and maintain their sense of individuality (quality of life).

The RAI consists of four basic components:

- **Minimum data set**: A core set of screening, clinical, and functional status elements that form the foundation of the comprehensive assessment of all residents in long-term care facilities certified to participate in Medicare or Medicaid. The items in the minimum data set standardize communication about resident problems and condition.
- Triggers: Specific resident responses for one or a combination of minimum data set elements that identify residents who either have or are at risk for developing specific functional problems and who require further evaluation using resident assessment protocols.
- Resident assessment protocols: Structured, problem-oriented frameworks for organizing minimum data set information and examining additional clinically relevant information about a resident. Resident assessment protocols help identify social, medical, nursing, and psychological problems and form the basis for individualized care planning.
- Utilization guidelines: Specified in state operation manuals that direct when and how to use the RAI.

Statutory law, federal regulations, and the Health Care Financing Administration specify how the RAI is implemented. A RAI must be completed for residents of Medicare skilled nursing facilities or Medicaid nursing facilities, hospice residents, and short-term stay or respite residents who reside in a facility for longer than 14 days.

Benefits of using the RAI process include the following:

- Residents respond to individualized care.
- Staff communication becomes more effective.
- Resident and family involvement increases.
- Documentation becomes clearer.

REPORTING CARE OR REQUESTING ACTION

To report is to give an account of something that has been seen, heard, done, or considered. Reporting is the oral, written, or computer-based communication of patient data to others. A laboratory report, for example, might communicate to the health care team that a patient's cardiac enzymes are normal or that a biopsy of breast tissue revealed malignant or atypical cells. A nurse's shift or handoff report or nursing note might communicate the progress a patient is making toward goal achievement. Nurses commonly have to consult a physician or nurse practitioner about a patient situation which requires a report and action. Common methods for reporting among health practitioners, in addition to the patient record, include face-to-face meetings, telephone conversations, fax documents, messengers, written messages, audiotaped messages, and computer messages. Each of these methods has certain benefits and limitations, as detailed in Table 20-4.

Table 20-4 Common Methods of Communication Among Health Care Professionals

METHOD	ADVANTAGES	DISADVANTAGES
Face-to-face meeting	• Message can be delivered immediately. • Nonverbal messages are readily conveyed. • Message can be clarified; receiver's questions can be raised and answered.	• Both the communicating and the receiving people must be available at the same time, in the same place. • Ordinarily, there is no permanent record for later use.
Faxed documents	• Message can be delivered in short time. • Graphic images can be sent. • Paper record is available. • Validation by sender possible.	• Requires fax telephone number and fax machine by both sender and receiver. • Requires time to transmit across telephone system which can be busy and not immediately transmitted. • Complete confidentiality not possible.
Telephone or video conferencing	• Message can be delivered immediately. • Message can be clarified; receiver's questions can be raised and answered. • Two parties need not be present in same place.	• Only the tone of voice and voice inflections can be communicated—no nonverbal messages unless video conferencing method or some other real-time conferencing means are used.
Written message	• Message can be exchanged at times convenient for the people involved. • Record is available. • Time efficient if message is understood.	• Message usually cannot be validated with the sender.
Audiotaped message	• Message can be exchanged at times convenient for the people involved. • Record is available. • Time efficient if information communicated is complete.	• Message usually cannot be validated with the sender.
Computer message	• Message can be delivered immediately—even to those at a great distance. • Parties need not be present in same place. • Two-way communication is possible by e-mail. • Record is available. • Many people can participate in exchange.	• No nonverbal messages can be communicated. • Privacy concerns remain an issue.

To ensure patient safety, the Institute for Healthcare Improvement (www.ihi.org) 2021 promotes the SBAR (or ISBAR) communication technique as a framework for communication between members of the health care team about a patient's condition (see http://www.ihi.org/resources/Pages/Tools/SBARToolkit.aspx):

- **I**dentity/**I**ntroduction: Communicate who you are, your credentials, your relationship to the patient, where you are, and why you are communicating.
- **S**ituation: Communicate concisely what is occurring in the patient situation and why you are consulting the health care provider—what is happening.
- **B**ackground: Explain significant details of the patient's history related to the current situation—brief patient information.
- **A**ssessment: Give your analysis of the current situation—what you think.
- **R**ecommendation: Explain the action requested or the health care provider's recommendation regarding the current situation—what you want.

Note that there are different ISBAR formats: earlier versions used simply SBAR, and some newer versions use ISBARR, with the last R being a read-back of orders/response. See Chapters 8 and 12 for more on ISBAR and other frameworks for patient handoffs. ISBAR or SBAR is an easy-to-remember, concrete mechanism useful for framing any conversation between two health care providers regarding a patient situation. It is useful when one clinician is requesting another clinician's immediate attention and action. It allows for an easy and focused way to set expectations for what will be communicated, and how, between members of the team, which is essential for developing teamwork and fostering a culture of patient safety. For example, it is a communication framework that should be used when a nurse is requesting the consultation and action of a physician regarding a patient situation.

QSEN TEAMWORK AND COLLABORATION

Open communication, mutual respect, and shared decision making are all essential to achieving quality patient care. Practice using an approved patient handoff until you become proficient in reporting off to a colleague.

Many students find collaborative communication with health care providers about patient conditions challenging and intimidating. See Box 20-6 (on page 540) for suggestions about

Box 20-6 ISBARR Report to a Health Care Provider

Before calling the health care provider:

1. Assess the patient.
2. Review the record for the appropriate health care provider to call.
3. Know the admitting diagnosis.
4. Read the most recent physician and nursing notes.
5. Have the record at hand and be ready to report allergies, medications, IV fluids, and lab and test results.
6. Every **ISBARR** report is different. Focus on the problem. Be concise. Not everything in the following outline needs to be reported—just what is needed for the situation.

I Identity/Introduction	State NAME, TITLE, and UNIT	"I am Ellen McLoughlin, a nursing instructor from Georgetown University precepting a nursing student, working on 3 Main."
S Situation	I am calling about: (Patient Name and Room Number) The PROBLEM I am calling about is:	"I am calling about Ms. Miriam Klein, room 9. She is scheduled this morning for a prophylactic bilateral mastectomy to prevent breast cancer but she is now having second thoughts."
B Background	State Admission Diagnosis and Admission Date State Pertinent Medical History Brief synopsis of Treatment if pertinent Most recent Vital Signs Changes in VS or Assessment from prior assessment	"Ms. Klein was admitted yesterday. She has a strong family history of breast and ovarian cancer. She tested positive earlier this year for BRCA1 (breast cancer gene). She signed the informed consent for the mastectomy in your office and had all her preop testing done, but she has been up all night expressing second thoughts."
A Assessment	Give your analysis and conclusions about the present situation. Words like "might be" or "could be" are helpful. A diagnosis is not necessary. If the situation is unclear, at least try to indicate what body system might be involved. State how severe the problem seems to be. If appropriate, state that the problem could be life threatening.	"This seems to be more than the usual presurgery anxiety. She has clearly stated that she regrets signing the informed consent and wishes to withdraw her consent."
R Recommendation	Say what you think would be helpful or needs to be done (medications, treatment, tests, x-rays, EKG, CT, transfer to critical care, health care provider evaluation, consultant evaluation). Ask about any Changes in Orders	"Shall I hold the preop orders and notify the OR that we need to place the surgery on hold until you can see her and determine if she wants this done?" "Is there anything else I can do at this time?"
R Read-back	Restate orders you have been given. Clarify how often to do vital signs. Under what circumstances to call back.	"I understand you want me to hold the preop medications and call the OR to place the surgery on hold. Thank you. I will tell her that you should be here within the hour."

Note: Be sure to document the change in condition and the health care provider notification.

Source: Adapted from ISBARR (Critical Situation) Report, © Joint Commission Resources; Enlow, M., Shanks, L., Guhde, J., & Perkins, M. (2010). Incorporating interprofessional communication skills (ISBARR) into an undergraduate nursing curriculum. *Nurse Educator*, *35*(4), 176–180.

how to do this well. Be professional whenever making a report about care or requesting a consultation. Ensure that you have all the pertinent data, and be concise. Most importantly, keep the report focused on the patient. The communication should be objective and brief. It should never involve gossip, floor politics, or any social commentary. It is never professional to speak disrespectfully about a patient or family; such comments reflect negatively on you and may negatively impact patient care.

Change-of-Shift/Handoff Reports

A **change-of-shift report** or **handoff** is given by a primary nurse to the nurse replacing them, or by the charge nurse to the nurse who assumes responsibility for continuing care of the patient. The change-of-shift report may be given in written form or orally in a meeting (Fig. 20-6), or it may be

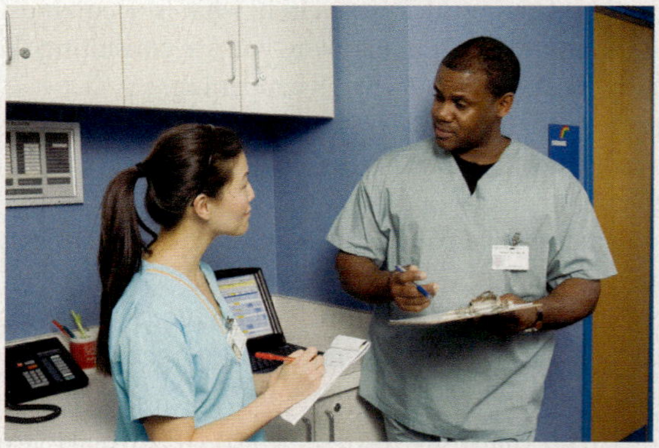

FIGURE 20-6. During a change-of-shift report, a nurse from the ending shift provides a summary of the patient's condition and current status of care to the nurse coming on duty. (*Source:* Used with permission from Shutterstock. *Photo by B. Proud.*)

Bedside Shift Report Checklist

- ❑ Introduce the nursing staff to the patient and family. Invite the patient and family to take part in the bedside shift report.
- ❑ Open the medical record or access the electronic work station in the patient's room.
- ❑ Conduct a verbal SBAR report with the patient and family. Use words that the patient and family can understand.
    - **S** = **Situation.** What is going on with the patient? What are the current vital signs?
    - **B** = **Background.** What is the pertinent patient history?
    - **A** = **Assessment.** What is the patient's problem now?
    - **R** = **Recommendation.** What does the patient need?
- ❑ Conduct a focused assessment of the patient and a safety assessment of the room.
    - Visually inspect all wounds, incisions, drains, IV sites, IV tubings, catheters, etc.
    - Visually sweep the room for any physical safety concerns.
- ❑ Review tasks that need to be done, such as:
    - Labs or tests needed
    - Medications administered
    - Forms that need to be completed (e.g., admission, patient intake, vaccination allergy review, etc.)
    - Other tasks: ______________________
- ❑ Identify the patient's and family's needs or concerns.
    - Ask the patient and family:
        - *"What could have gone better during the last 12 hours?"*
        - *"Tell us how your pain is."*
        - *"Tell us how much you walked today."*
        - *"Do you have any concerns about safety?"*
        - *"Do you have any worries you would like to share?"*
    - Ask the patient and family what the goal is for the next shift. This is the patient's goal — not the nursing staff's goal for the patient.
        - *"What do you want to happen during the next 12 hours?"*
        - Follow up to see if the goal was met during the verbal SBAR at the next bedside shift report.

FIGURE 20-7. Bedside shift report checklist. (*Source:* From Agency for Healthcare Research and Quality. https://www.ahrq.gov/sites/default/files/wysiwyg/professionals/systems/hospital/engagingfamilies/strategy3/Strat3_Tool_2_Nurse_Chklst_508.pdf)

audio- or videotaped. The trend today is toward a standardized, streamlined shift report system at the bedside—the **bedside report** (see Chapter 8). Vital elements of the bedside report include the oncoming and outgoing nurse assessing the patient together, reviewing medication records and the health care provider's and nursing orders, and establishing patient goals for the shift. The AHRQ identifies the goal of the nurse bedside report strategy as helping to ensure the safe handoff of care between nurses by involving the patient and family. It is the patient who defines who is family and who can participate in the report. Evidence demonstrates that the bedside shift report can improve patient safety and quality, the patient experience of care, nursing staff satisfaction, and time management and accountability between nurses (Fig. 20-7). Some nurses prefer to restrict the handoff to two nurses in a private environment free from distraction and interference.

Typical information shared among nurses, patients, and families in a change-of-shift report includes the following:

- Basic identifying information about each patient: name, room number, bed designation, diagnosis, and attending and consulting health care providers

- Current appraisal of each patient's health status:
  - Changes in patient's status during your shift and the patient's response to nursing and medical therapy
  - Pertinent monitoring, lab, and radiology data; data that are irregular or data that have been noted to be irregular in the past and have now been resolved
  - Abnormal findings in your physical or head-to-toe assessment
  - Patient progress in regard to diagnoses/health problems and goal achievement
  - Pain level and pain management needs
- Current orders (especially any newly changed orders):
  - Changes in medications, intravenous fluids, diet, toileting, and activity level
  - Upcoming or ongoing tests and procedures, and specific instructions for these such as NPO after midnight
- Abnormal occurrences during your shift
- Any unfilled orders that need to be continued onto the next shift
- Patient and family questions, concerns, and needs
- Reports on patients who have been transferred or discharged

Telephone/Telemedicine Reports

Telephones and telemedicine equipment can link health care professionals immediately and enable nurses to receive and give critical information about patients in a timely fashion. For example, the hematology lab may call to report a dangerously low platelet count, and the nurse may in turn call the attending health care provider to obtain new medical orders. When reporting significant changes in a patient's condition to health care providers and other health care professionals, be prepared to do the following:

- Identify yourself and the patient, and state your relationship to the patient. (Example: "Dr. Gomez-Lobo, this is Laura Bishop, case manager with St. Mary's Home Health Care. I'm calling about Mr. John Clouser, a patient of yours who was just discharged home following a workup for recurrent chest pain.)
- Report concisely and accurately the change in the patient's condition that is of concern and what has already been done in response to this condition. (Example: "When I first arrived in his home, he was complaining of feeling dizzy, and his blood pressure was 190/110. Yesterday morning in the hospital, it was 150/90. His wife appears anxious and says she doesn't know how she is going to take care of him. I had him rest for 30 minutes, and when I checked his pressure again it was 186/110.")
- Report the patient's current vital signs and clinical manifestations.
- Have the patient's record at hand to make knowledgeable responses to any health care provider's inquiries. In examples given above, the health care provider would probably want to know all the vital signs and might ask questions about the treatment regimen, both in the hospital and upon discharge.
- Concisely record the time and date of the call, what was communicated to the health care provider, and the health care provider's response. Read back any changes to the orders.

Transfer and Discharge Reports

Nurses report a summary of a patient's condition and care when transferring patients from one unit, institution, or facility to another (e.g., from the postanesthesia care unit to a surgical floor) and when discharging patients. The nurse making the report should concisely summarize all the patient data that caregivers need to provide immediate care. See Chapter 12 for transfer and discharge reporting guidelines.

Reports to Family Members and Significant Others

Nurses play a crucial role in keeping the patient's family and significant others updated about the patient's condition and progress toward goal achievement. Always clarify with the patient which visitors, if any, are entitled to progress reports—for example: "Mrs. Neale, do you object to our disclosing your health information to family or friends?" It is necessary to ask the patient which specific family members and/or significant others have permission to receive information, and this should be documented. Similarly, clarify what types of information may be communicated, and be familiar with facility policy about such communications. Some facilities provide family members approved by the patient a "code" to use when calling the facility to ask about the patient's condition. If the patient objects to disclosure, nurses are not permitted to discuss the patient's health condition with family or friends.

If a patient is not able to communicate objections, such as in an emergency situation or when unconscious, professional caregivers must use their best professional judgment to decide whether to talk to family and friends. Procedural outcomes should be reported to the patient by the health care provider who performed the procedure. For example, the nurse is generally not the caregiver who informs family members that a patient's biopsy has revealed a malignancy. The nurse does, however, often explain what this will mean for the patient after the family has this information. Information should be shared in a manner that is honest, compassionate, and respectful of the person's ability to understand medical concepts.

Incident Reports

An **incident report**, also termed a **variance report** or occurrence report, is a tool used by health care facilities to document unexpected events that result in, or have the potential to result in, harm to a patient or person or damage property. An incident report should be filed whenever an unexpected event occurs. These reports are used for risk management and quality improvement and are not intended to be used for disciplinary action against staff members. Incident reports improve the management and treatment of patients by identifying high-risk patterns so that staff development programs can be initiated to prevent future problems. These forms also make all the facts about an incident available to the facility in case of litigation.

You should be familiar with facility policy about your responsibilities and obligations if involved personally in an incident that results in, or has the potential to result in, harm to a patient, employee, or visitor, or if you witness such an incident. An example of an incident report form and a fuller discussion of this topic appear in Chapter 7.

CONFERRING ABOUT CARE

To **confer** is to consult with someone to exchange ideas or to seek information, advice, or instructions. A nurse may confer with another nurse, such as when a primary care nurse consults with a nurse clinical specialist about a particular patient's care. A nurse may consult a physician or nurse practitioner about treatment plans for a hospitalized patient. A school nurse may confer with a child's teacher or a psychologist about a behavior problem. A community health nurse and a health care provider may confer about a patient's activity regimen. Health practitioners also confer with each other to validate information. Health care professionals increasingly use electronic support groups to consult with clinicians who share similar interests or who have expertise in other specialty areas. See Box 20-7 for an illustration of how one health care system is using creative conferrals to motivate change in contemporary nursing practice and nursing care delivery.

Box 20-7 Delivering Optimal Care to Patients and Their Families

Nursing leadership at MedStar Health is committed to leading the organization along a path to a clearly defined goal: the delivery of optimal care to patients and their families. To guide these efforts, the MedStar Way, a set of activities, has been devised to motivate change in contemporary nursing practice and nursing care delivery.

1. Senior Leader Rounding—to promote communication and access within the nursing team
2. Multidisciplinary Team Rounding—to ensure consistent documentation and timely communication, and discuss the care plan
3. Nurse Leader Rounding—to support a culture of service, assess patient and staff needs, and promote the patient/family experience
4. Nursing Staff Hourly Rounds—to anticipate and evaluate patient needs, and improve safety and satisfaction
5. Nurse-to-Nurse Bedside Shift Reports—to ensure safe handoffs, and keep the patient and family involved in the care plan
6. Huddles at the Beginning of Each Shift—to improve teamwork and communication, and ensure timely response to issues and concerns
7. White Boards in Patient Rooms—to encourage communication, teamwork, and efficiency, and to assure the patient that the team is working together to provide optimal care
8. Post-discharge Phone Calls—to ensure quality clinical outcomes and increase patient satisfaction

Source: Reprinted with permission. (2013, June). The MedStar Way: Delivering optimal care to patients and their families. *MedStar Nursing Insights and Innovations*, *1*(2), 7.

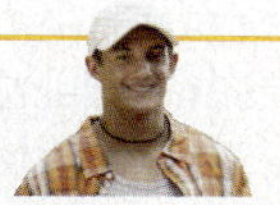

Think back to **Jason Chandler**, the adolescent who was brought into the ED by the police. He was refusing treatment. To determine the legal implications of administering treatment to the patient, the health care provider consulted the hospital's attorney for legal guidance. Doing so helped to clarify which actions were and were not acceptable.

Consultations and Referrals

When nurses detect problems they cannot resolve because the problems are outside the scope of independent nursing practice or the nurses' expertise, they consult with or make referrals to other professionals. The process of inviting another professional to evaluate the patient and make recommendations to you about the patient's treatment is called a **consultation**. The EHR may be designed to automatically initiate nursing consults to selected services based on what you document. For example, if you click on the "yes" box when answering the question, "Does the patient have financial concerns regarding hospitalization?" a nursing consult may be automatically sent to the social work department.

The process of sending or guiding the patient to another source for assistance is called a **referral**. A patient may be referred by a hospital to a community health nursing service for assistance with home care. A school nurse may refer a student to a hospital ED. A community health nurse who learns that a patient with multiple sexual contacts is HIV positive will refer to the Department of Health for tracking of these contacts.

Most health facilities have policies for referrals. A facility may use a special form for making referrals. Referral policies usually indicate who may initiate a referral, how it is to be done, and so on. Referrals are especially important for providing continuity of care for people who need a variety of services. The health practitioners to whom a patient is referred must receive the information that is most useful to the continuity of care. The key question is, "What would I want to know about this patient if I were the person who would be continuing their care?" The patient must know and approve of a referral to another facility or to other health personnel.

Before requesting a consultation or making a referral, determine which profession has the needed expertise and which of its practitioners is appropriate for consultation or referral. A great disservice is done to patients when referrals are poorly made. Patients and family members also appreciate a phone number and practical tips about how to easily reach the referred practitioner.

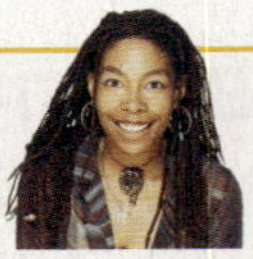

Recall **Millie Delong**, the woman with the wound infection. Obtaining a consultation from a wound, ostomy, and continence nurse may be appropriate to assist with measures for wound care. Additionally, consultation with an infection-control nurse may be necessary if the patient's wound remains infected or fails to heal.

Nursing and Interdisciplinary Team Care Conferences

Nurses and other health care professionals frequently confer in groups to plan and coordinate patient care. Such conferences are also used for instructing students and practitioners. A nursing care conference is a meeting of nurses to discuss some aspect of a patient's care. For example, several nurses who are caring for a generally uncooperative patient may initiate a conference. This would allow each nurse an opportunity to offer their opinion about the patient's problem and its cause, and then together they could discuss possible solutions to the problem.

Nurses may invite other health care practitioners to a nursing care conference concerning a patient's care. For example, in the Jason Chandler scenario, a clinical psychologist may be invited to address the possibility that a mental disorder is influencing this patient's behavior.

Nursing Care Rounds

Nursing care rounds are procedures in which a group of nurses visit selected patients individually, at each patient's bedside. The primary purposes of nursing care rounds are to gather information to help plan nursing care, to evaluate the nursing care patients have received, and to provide patients with an opportunity to discuss their care with those administering it. As each patient is visited, the nurse assigned provides a short summary of the patient's nursing diagnoses and goals and the care being given. Nurses may also make rounds with health care providers to share nursing's perspective with them.

Nursing care rounds have two principal advantages over discussions in a meeting room: Nursing personnel can actually see the patient as a report of care is given, and the patient and family can participate in discussions of patient-centered care. Nurses should use language the patient can understand when holding discussions at the bedside. Otherwise, the patient is likely to feel excluded and cannot intelligently participate in the discussion.

Purposeful Rounding

Purposeful rounding is a proactive, systematic, nurse-driven, evidence-based intervention that helps nurses anticipate and address patient needs (McLeod & Tetzlaff, 2015). Although nurses may struggle to reorganize their day to permit hourly rounding, it is difficult to dismiss the growing body of research that suggests effective, purposeful rounding can promote patient safety, encourage team communication, and improve staff ability to provide efficient patient care. Nurses at Stanford Health Care identified eight behaviors of purposeful rounding, which are listed in Table 20-5. Be sure to note their recommendation to use the recommended key phrase before leaving a patient room, "Is there anything else I can do for you before I go? I have time."

Research on hourly rounding in 14 hospitals revealed dramatic improvements:

- 12% increase in patient satisfaction scores
- 52% reduction in patient falls
- 37% reduction in call light use
- 14% decline in skin breakdowns

In addition, one hospital measured a 20% reduction in the distance walked each day by the nursing staff (Stanford Health Care, n.d.).

Table 20-5 Eight Behaviors of Purposeful Rounding

BEHAVIOR	EXPECTED RESULTS
Use Opening Key Words: Greet the patient and review the plan of care for the day.	Reduces anxiety, contributes to efficiency
Accomplish scheduled tasks.	Contributes to efficiency
Address four Ps: pain, personal needs (toileting), positioning, fall prevention.	Quality indicators, pain management, decubitus, and fall prevention
Address additional personal needs, questions.	Nurse-sensitive indicators: care and respect, listening
Conduct environmental assessment: bed alarms, IV pumps, hats, urinals.	Contributes to efficiency, safety, teamwork and addresses patient satisfaction
Ask "Is there anything else I can do for you before I go? I have time."	Increases efficiency, improves communication and teamwork (respect, caring, listening)
Tell each patient when you will be back.	Contributes to efficiency, provides reassurance
Document the round.	Quality and accountability

Source: Adapted from Nursing: Quality and safety: Purposeful rounding, Stanford Health Care website. Used with permission, Stanford Health Care. https://stanfordhealthcare.org/health-care-professionals/nursing/quality-safety/purposeful-rounding.html

REFLECTIVE PRACTICE LEADING TO PERSONAL LEARNING

Remember that the object of reflective practice is to look at an experience, understand it, and learn from it. As you begin to develop your expertise in documenting your nursing care and reporting to colleagues, reflect on your experiences—successes and failures—in order to improve your practice. How can you do it better next time? What did you learn today that can help you tomorrow? Begin your reflection by paying close attention to the following:

- Does your documentation today leave a complete, accurate, concise, current, timely, factual, and organized record of your nursing care?
- How easy was it for you to know what to chart, when to chart, and where? Are you confident that you followed your facility's protocols?
- Are you becoming sufficiently comfortable working with medical terminology? Are your words spelled correctly? Did you use only acceptable abbreviations?
- Are you able to find the information you need to know about your patient in the paper or electronic health record?
- Are you comfortable and confident both giving and receiving reports about your patient? Are you proficient in bedside reports and patient handoffs?
- Are you becoming skilled in purposeful rounding?

The cultivation of skill in documenting nursing care and reporting to colleagues is a critical component of professional nursing. Perhaps the most important questions to reflect on are: Are your patients and their families/caregivers better for having had *you* share in the critical responsibility of partnering with them to address their activity needs? Are your patients now receiving thoughtful, person-centered, prioritized, holistic, evidence-based treatment and care because of your efforts?

DEVELOPING CLINICAL REASONING AND CLINICAL JUDGMENT

1. Interview three practicing nurses and ask them to describe the documentation methods they have used in their practice. Which methods did they prefer? Which method was most effective, time efficient, and easiest to use?
2. A nurse overhears you complaining about writing narrative nursing notes and says to you, "Don't sweat it. I never worry about documentation—it's a waste of time. I'd rather spend my time doing things for patients than writing up what I did." Think about what you would like to say to this nurse and your rationale for this. Ask other students for their response, and compare your answers.
3. Imagine that you are a nurse in a long-term care facility, and that you and the facility are being sued for negligence by the family of an older resident who fell and fractured her hip last year. You know the resident but do not remember much about the day she fell. What data do you hope to find recorded in her health record? Which documentation system would most likely provide the type of information you think you need to reconstruct the events surrounding her fall?
4. How would you respond to each of the following requests for patient information? Compare your responses with those of another student and talk about any differences.
   - The mayor of your town, who is up for reelection, was just admitted to your unit after an acute myocardial infarction. You receive a phone call from his office requesting information about his condition.
   - A woman you have never seen approaches you in the hallway, identifies herself as a close friend of a married male patient on your unit, and requests information about his condition.
   - A case manager from a managed care organization calls you to ask about the progress an older surgical patient is making postoperatively. You have heard that the organization is eager to discharge her quickly, and you feel uncomfortable reporting any information over the phone.
   - A family member asks your advice about developing a PHR. She says she has heard that there are privacy concerns. How do you respond?

PRACTICING FOR NCLEX

1. A nurse is caring for a postoperative patient who has a prescription for morphine 2 mg IV every 3 hours. Which examples documenting pain management best reflect recommended guidelines? Select all that apply.
   a. 6/12/25 0945 Morphine 2 mg administered IV. Patient's response to pain appears to be exaggerated. M. Patrick, RN.
   b. 6/12/25 0950 Morphine 2 mg administered IV. Patient appears to be comfortable. M. Patrick, RN.
   c. 6/12/25 1015 Administered morphine 2 mg IV at 0945, patient reporting pain as 2 on a scale of 1 to 10. M. Patrick, RN.
   d. 6/12/25 0945 Patient reports severe pain in right lower quadrant. M. Patrick, RN
   e. 6/12/25 0945 Morphine IV 2 mg will be administered to patient every 3 hours. M. Patrick, RN
   f. 6/12/25 0945 Patient states they do not want pain medication despite return of pain. After discussion, patient agrees to try morphine 2 mg IV. M. Patrick, RN

2. When documenting a dressing change to a residual right limb, the nurse erroneously documents that the dressing change was performed on the left leg. How will the nurse most appropriately correct the documentation?
   a. Use white correction fluid to cover the error and neatly write over the correction
   b. Draw a single line through the error, write "mistaken entry," add correct information, and date and initial
   c. Blacken out the error with permanent marker and rewrite the note in the next available space
   d. Leave the entry in place, create a correctly written entry below, and cite the charting error above

3. A patient being discharged from the hospital asks to receive a copy of their medical record. What information will the nurse give the patient?
   a. "I'm sorry, but patients are not allowed to copy their medical records."
   b. "I can make a copy of your record for you right now."
   c. "You can read your record while you are still a patient, but copying records is not permitted according to HIPAA rules."
   d. "I'll check with the medical records department to determine how you request a copy."
4. A graduate nurse and preceptor are discussing protected health information (PHI) and HIPAA laws. The preceptor explains that PHI can be released without the patient's signed authorization in which situations? Select all that apply.
   a. News media are preparing to report on a patient who is a public figure.
   b. Data are needed for the tracking and notification of disease outbreaks.
   c. Protected health information is needed by a coroner.
   d. Child abuse and neglect are suspected.
   e. Protected health information is needed to facilitate organ donation.
   f. The sister of a patient with Alzheimer's disease wants to help provide care.
5. A nurse receives a call from a friend requesting information on her mother-in-law who was just admitted to the hospital. How does the nurse best respond?
   a. "You shouldn't be asking me to do this. I could be fined or lose my job for disclosing this information."
   b. "I'm sorry; per privacy laws, I can't give out patient information—even to my best friend or a family member."
   c. "Because of HIPAA, you could get in trouble for asking for this information unless you are authorized by the patient to receive it."
   d. "Why are you asking? Are you extremely worried?"
6. A nurse receives a prescription for an analgesic for a patient who has compound fractures of the tibia and fibula. What schedule will the nurse use to administer the medication?
   Electronic health record (EHR)
   Health care provider order sheet
   8:00 AM: Hydromorphone 1 mg IV every 2 hours PRN severe pain. –S. Jones, MD
   a. When the patient requests it
   b. Every 2 hours on the even hours
   c. Daily, every 2 hours
   d. As requested, 2 hours or more after the last dose
7. A health care provider has been urgently paged to another unit and asks a nurse to enter a pain medication prescription for their patient in the electronic medical record. Which response by the nurse is most appropriate?
   a. "Thank you for taking care of this; I'll be happy to enter a verbal order into the electronic health record."
   b. Get a second nurse to listen to the order, write the order on the health care provider order sheet, and ensure both nurses sign it.
   c. "I'm sorry; verbal orders can only be accepted in an emergency. Please enter this quickly before leaving this unit."
   d. Try calling another resident for the order or wait until the next shift.
8. A nurse is looking for trends in a postoperative patient's vital signs. In which part of the electronic health record will the nurse find this information?
   a. Admission sheet
   b. Admission nursing assessment
   c. Progress notes
   d. Graphic record
9. A nurse is using the PIE format to document care of a patient who is diagnosed with type 2 diabetes. What information does the nurse need to complete documentation in this format?
   a. Patient problem list
   b. Narrative notes describing the patient's condition
   c. Overall trends in patient status
   d. Planned interventions and patient outcomes
10. A nurse uses the ISBARR format to report the deteriorating mental status of a patient using morphine via a patient-controlled analgesia pump (PCA) for postoperative pain. Place the following nursing statements related to this call in the correct ISBARR order.
   a. "I am calling about Mr. Sanchez in Room 202 who is receiving morphine via a PCA pump for pancreatic cancer."
   b. "Mr. Sanchez has been difficult to arouse, and his mental status has declined over the past 12 hours."
   c. "You want me to discontinue the PCA pump until you see him tonight at patient rounds."
   d. "I am Rosa Clark, an RN working on the second floor of South Street Hospital."
   e. "Mr. Sanchez was admitted 2 days ago following a diagnosis of pancreatic cancer."
   f. "I suggest a decrease in the dose of morphine."
11. A new home health nurse and preceptor are reviewing charting for a patient with advanced lung cancer who receives Medicare benefits. When reviewing a draft of the new nurse's documentation, which statement will the preceptor correct?
   a. Explained to family that irregular respirations or agitation may occur when the patient is actively dying
   b. Patient seemed in better spirits and reported going out for ice cream with his family yesterday
   c. Stage 3 pressure ulcer dressing on sacral area is dry and intact; due to be changed tomorrow
   d. Performed medication reconciliation with focus on pain management and anticoagulation

12. The nurse on an oncology unit is caring for a patient admitted for dyspnea and wheezing. What is most important for the nurse to include in the change-of-shift report to the oncoming nurse?
   a. Partial bath was given
   b. Patient received physical therapy
   c. CT scan revealed a mass in the right lung
   d. Patient did not eat lunch today

ANSWERS WITH RATIONALES

1. **c, d, f.** The nurse should enter information in a complete, accurate, concise, current, and factual manner, indicating the date and both the time the entry was written and the time of pertinent observations and interventions. When charting, the nurse should avoid the use of stereotypes, derogatory terms, and judgments such as "response to pain appears to be exaggerated" or "seems to be comfortable." Stating that medication will be given does not document care given; this prescription/intervention belongs in the plan of care.
2. **b.** The nurse should not black out, use erasers or correcting fluids to correct documentation, or remove a page with an error and rewrite the data on a new page. To correct an error after it has been entered, the nurse should mark the entry "mistaken entry," add the correct information, and date and initial the entry. If the nurse records information in the wrong chart, the nurse should write "mistaken entry—wrong chart" and sign off. The nurse should follow similar guidelines in electronic records.
3. **d.** According to HIPAA, patients have a right to view and receive a copy of their health record; update their health record; get a list of the disclosures a health care institution has made, independent of disclosures made for the purposes of treatment, payment, and health care operations; request a restriction on certain uses or disclosures; and choose how to receive health information. The nurse should be aware of facility policies regarding the patient's right to access and copy records.
4. **b, c, d, e.** According to HIPAA, a health institution may share PHI without written patient authorization for tracking disease outbreaks, infection control, statistics related to dangerous problems with drugs or medical equipment, investigation and prosecution of a crime, identification of victims of crimes or disaster, reporting incidents of child abuse, neglect or domestic violence, responding to a valid subpoena, and providing information needed by coroners, medical examiners, funeral directors, and law enforcement in the case of a death from a potential crime and for facilitating organ donations. The nurse does not provide information to a news reporter without the patient's express authorization; typically, a hospital representative communicates with the media. A patient who has Alzheimer's disease will still need a release to share information; this may be given by the power of attorney.
5. **b.** The nurse should immediately clarify they must adhere to HIPAA laws to protect patient privacy and confidentiality. Mentioning penalties for breaches of privacy sidesteps the need to clearly introduce or reinforce the policy. It may be appropriate to ask the friend about her concerns, only after clarifying privacy laws.
6. **d.** PRN means "as needed." The nurse teaches the patient that the medication may be requested every 2 hours to treat pain. If pain occurs before 2 hours elapses, the nurse provides comfort measures and collaborates with the health care provider for a change in prescription.
7. **c.** In most facilities, health care providers may only issue verbal orders in an emergency. The provider is present but finds it impossible, due to the situation, to write or enter the order in the electronic health record. Calling another health care provider or waiting until the next shift would be inappropriate; the patient should not have to wait for the pain medication, and a provider is available who can quickly write/enter the order.
8. **d.** While one set of vital signs may appear on the admission nursing assessment, the best place to find sequential recordings demonstrating a pattern or trend is the graphic record. The admission sheet and flow sheet do not include ongoing vital sign documentation.
9. **a.** In the PIE format, patient problems are numbered; documented in the progress notes; worked up using the Problem, Intervention, Evaluation (PIE) format; and evaluated each shift. Resolved problems are dropped following the nurse's review. Narrative notes allow nurses to describe a condition, situation, or response in their own terms. Overall trends in patient status can be seen immediately when using charting by exception (CBE). Planned interventions and patient-expected outcomes are the focus of the case management model.
10. **d, a, e, b, f, c.** The order for ISBARR is: Identity/Introduction, Situation, Background, Assessment, Recommendation, and Read-back.
11. **b.** To receive Medicare services, the patient must be homebound, still needs skilled nursing care, or that the patient is dying, among others. Leaving the home for ice cream may interfere with home care benefits.
12. **c.** The nurse's shift or handoff report includes basic identifying information about the patient. The outgoing nurse includes the patient's current health status and changes during their shift, response to nursing and medical therapy, pertinent monitoring and assessment findings (e.g., lab and radiology data), pain management, changes in orders (medications, intravenous fluids, diet, and rationale), upcoming/ongoing tests and procedures, and instructions for these, such as NPO after midnight, unfilled prescriptions for the next shift to follow up on, and patient and family questions, concerns, and needs.

Bibliography

Agency for Healthcare Research and Quality (AHRQ), U.S. Department of Health & Human Services. (n.d.). *Bedside shift report checklist.* Author. https://www.ahrq.gov/sites/default/files/wysiwyg/professionals/systems/hospital/engagingfamilies/strategy3/Strat3_Tool_2_Nurse_Chklst_508.pdf

Agency for Healthcare Research and Quality (AHRQ), U.S. Department of Health & Human Services. (n.d.). *Nurse bedside shift report: Implementation handbook.* Author. https://www.ahrq.gov/professionals/systems/hospital/engagingfamilies/strategy3/index.html

Agency for Healthcare Research and Quality (AHRQ), U.S. Department of Health & Human Services. (2012). *Electronic health records improve nursing care, coordination, and patient safety: Research Activities, 381, 10.* Author. https://archive.ahrq.gov/news/newsletters/research-activities/may12/0512RA.pdf

Agency for Healthcare Research and Quality (AHRQ), U.S. Department of Health & Human Services. (2018). *Chartbook on care coordination. Use of electronic health records.* https://www.ahrq.gov/research/findings/nhqrdr/chartbooks/carecoordination/measure5.html

Alfaro-LeFevre, R. (2014). *Applying nursing process: The foundation for clinical reasoning* (8th ed.). Wolters Kluwer/Lippincott Williams & Wilkins.

American Nurses Association (ANA). (2015a). *Code of ethics for nurses with interpretive statements.* Author.

American Nurses Association (ANA). (2015b). *Scope and standards of practice* (3rd ed.). Author.

Ammenwerth, E., Schnell-Inderst, P., Machan, C., & Siebert, U. (2008). The effect of electronic prescribing on medication errors and adverse drug events: A systematic review. *Journal of the American Medical Informatics Association, 15*(5), 585–600.

ANA Principles of Nursing Documentation. (ANA) (2010). https://www.nursingworld.org/~4af4f2/globalassets/docs/ana/ethics/principles-of-nursing-documentation.pdf

Anderson, R. J., Sparbel, K., Barr, R. N., Doerschug, K., & Corbridge, S. (2018). Electronic health record tool to promote team communication and early patient mobility in the intensive care unit. *Critical Care Nurse, 38*(6), 23–35.

Baker, K., Rasmussen, K., & Shimp, K. (2018). The imperative for an electronic nurse scheduling system. *American Nurse Today, 13*(9), 90–92.

Balestra, M. L. (2017). Electronic health records: Patient care and ethical and legal implications for nurse practitioners. *Journal for Nurse Practitioners, 13*(2), 105–111.

Brown, G. (2016). Averting malpractice issues in today's nursing practice. *ABNF Journal, 27*(2), 25–27.

Buckley-Womack, C., & Gidney, B. (1987). A new dimension in documentation: The PIE method. *Journal of Neuroscience Nursing, 19*(5), 256–260.

Burke, L., & Murphy, J. (1988). *Charting by exception: A cost-effective quality approach.* Delmar.

Centers for Medicare & Medicaid Services. (2015). *Nursing home quality initiative.* http://www.cms.gov/Medicare/Quality-Initiatives-Patient-Assessment-Instruments/NursingHomeQualityInits/index.html?redirect=/NursingHomeQualityInits/45_NHQIMDS30TrainingMaterials.asp

Cohen, M. (2017). Medication errors. *Nursing2017, 47*(12), 72.

Conaty-Buck, S. (2017). Cybersecurity and healthcare records. *American Nurse Today, 12*(9), 62–65.

Cross, D. A., Cohen, G. R., Nong, P., Day, A. V., Vibbert, D., Naraharisetti, R., & Adler-Milstein, J. (2015). Improving EHR capabilities to facilitate stage 3 meaningful use care coordination criteria. *AMIA Annual Symposium Proceedings, 2015*, 448–455. eCollection 2015.

Drobny, S. D. (2017). Making patients partners in real-time electronic charting. *American Journal of Nursing, 117*(4), 11.

Enlow, M., Shanks, L., Guhde, J., & Perkins, M. (2010). Incorporating interprofessional communication skills (ISBARR) into an undergraduate nursing curriculum. *Nurse Educator, 35*(4), 176–180.

Evans, R. S. (2016). Electronic health records: Then, now, and in the future. *Yearbook of Medical Informatics, 25*(Suppl 1), S48–S61. https://www.ncbi.nlm.nih.gov/pmc/articles/PMC5171496/pdf/ymi-11-0s48.pdf

Flood, T. (2018). Promoting patient- and family-centered care with virtual rounding. *American Nurse Today, 13*(9), 84–85.

Greenes, R. A. (2014). *Clinical decision support: The road to broad adoption.* Elsevier.

HHS.gov. Health Information Privacy. (2022). *HIPAA for Professionals.* https://www.hhs.gov/hipaa/for-professionals/index.html

Health Information Exchange (HIE). (n.d.). *What is HIE?* http://www.healthit.gov/providers-professionals/health-information-exchange/what-hie

Health Insurance Portability and Accountability Act (HIPAA). (1996). *Public law. 104–191.* https://www.hhs.gov/hipaa/for-professionals/index.html

HealthIT.gov. (n.d.). *What are the advantages of electronic health records?* https://www.healthit.gov/providers-professionals/faqs/what-are-advantages-electronic-health-records

Henricks, W. H. (2011). "Meaningful use" of electronic health records and its relevance to laboratories and pathologists. *Journal of Pathology Informatics, 2*, 7. https://www.ncbi.nlm.nih.gov/pmc/articles/PMC3049251/

Hripcsak, G., & Albers, D. J. (2013). Correlating electronic health record concepts with healthcare process events. *Journal of the American Medical Informatics Association, 20*(e2), e311–318.

Holmes, H. N. (Ed.). (2006). *Documentation in action.* Wolters Kluwer Health/Lippincott Williams & Wilkins.

Hoover, R. (2017). Benefits of using an electronic health record. *Nursing Critical Care, 12*(1), 9–10.

Institute for Healthcare Improvement. (n.d.). *SBAR technique for communication: A situational briefing model.* http://www.ihi.org/resources/Pages/Tools/SBARTechniqueforCommunicationASituationalBriefingModel.aspx

The Joint Commission. (2017a). *Comprehensive accreditation manual.* Author.

The Joint Commission. (2017b). *Facts about the official "Do Not Use" list of abbreviations.* https://www.jointcommission.org/facts_about_do_not_use_list

Kahn, J. S., Aulak, V., & Bosworth, A. (2009). What it takes: Characteristics of the ideal personal health record. *Health Affairs (Millwood), 28*(2), 369–376.

King J., Patel V., Jamoom E. W., & Furukawa M. F. (2014). Clinical benefits of electronic health record use: national findings. *Health Services Research, 49*(1 Pt 2), 392–404.

Kutney-Lee, A., & Kelly, D. (2011). The effect of hospital electronic health record adoption on nurse-assessed quality of care and patient safety. *Journal of Nursing Administration, 41*(11), 466–472.

Lavin, M. A., Harper, E., & Barr, N. (2015). Health information technology, patient safety, and professional nursing care documentation in acute care settings. *OJIN: The Online Journal of Issues in Nursing, 20*(2), 6.

McGraw, D., Dempsey, J. X., Harris, L., & Goldman, J. (2009). Privacy as an enabler, not an impediment: Building trust into health information exchange. *Health Affairs (Millwood), 28*(2), 416–427.

McLeod, J., & Tetzlaff, S. (2015). The value of purposeful rounding. *American Nurse Today, 10*(11), 6–7.

Murphy, E. K. (2003). Charting by exception. *AORN Journal, 78*(5), 821–823.

National Coordinating Council for Medication Error Reporting and Prevention (NCCMERP) (2015). Recommendations to reduce medication errors associated with verbal medication orders and prescriptions. https://www.nccmerp.org/recommendations-reduce-medication-errors-associated-verbal-medication-orders-and-prescription

Nelson, R. (2016). Nurses' dissatisfaction with electronic health records remains high. *American Journal of Nursing, 116*(11), 18–19.

Nguyen, L., Bellucci, E., & Nguyen, L. T. (2014). Electronic health records implementation: an evaluation of information system impact and contingency factors. *International Journal of Medical Informatics, 83*(11), 779–796.

Nursing Service Organization (NSO). (2020). *Charting by exception: The legal risks.* https://www.nso.com/Learning/Artifacts/Articles/Charting-by-exception-the-legal-risks

The Office of the National Coordinator for Health Care Technology. Personal Health Records. What Health Care Providers Need to Know. https://www.healthit.gov/sites/default/files/factsheets/about-phrs-for-providers.pdf. Accessed on March 3, 2022.

The Office of the National Coordinator for Health Information Technology. *SAFER guides.* https://www.healthit.gov/topic/safety/safer-guides

Pagulayan, J., Eltair, S., & Faber, K. (2018). Nurse documentation and the electronic health record. *American Nurse Today, 13*(9), 48–54.

Pfeifer, G. M. (2020). How often do EHRs result in patient harm? *American Journal of Nursing, 120*(3), 16. doi: 10.1097/01.NAJ.0000656280.25749.1b

Santa, D., & Roach, E. E. (2017). Using mobile technology during patient handoffs. *American Nurse Today, 12*(9), 86–87.

Saranto, K., & Kinnunen, U. M. (2009). Evaluation nursing documentation—research designs and methods: Systematic review. *Journal of Advanced Nursing, 65*(3), 464–476.

Schulte, F., & Fry, E. (2019, March 18). Death by 1,000 clicks: Where electronic health records went wrong. *Kaiser Health News and Fortune Magazine.* https://khn.org/news/death-by-a-thousand-clicks/

Shah, K., Lo, C., Babich, M., Tsao, N. W., & Bansback, N. J. (2016). Bar code medication administration technology: A systematic review of impact on patient safety when used with computerized prescriber order entry and automated dispensing devices. *The Canadian Journal of Hospital Pharmacy, 69*(5), 394–402. https://doi.org/10.4212/cjhp.v69i5.1594

Shastay, A. (2019). Despite technology, verbal orders persist, read back is not widespread, and errors continue. *Home Healthcare Now, 37*(4), 230–233.

Siegrist, L. M., Stocks, B., & Dettor, R. E. (1985). The PIE system: Complete planning and documentation of nursing care. *Quality Review Bulletin, 11*(6), 186–189.

Stanford Health Care. (n.d.). *Nursing: Quality and safety: Purposeful rounding.* https://stanfordhealthcare.org/health-care-professionals/nursing/quality-safety/purposeful-rounding.html

Stelson, E. A., Carr, B. G., Golden, K. E., Martin, N., Richmond, T. S., Delgado, M. K., & Holena, D. N. (2016). Perceptions of family participation in intensive care unit rounds and telemedicine: A qualitative assessment. *American Journal of Critical Care, 25*(5), 440–447.

Thede, L. (December 12, 2008). "Informatics: Electronic Personal Health Records: Nursing's Role" *OJIN: The Online Journal of Issues in Nursing*, Vol. 14 No. 1. DOI: 10.3912/OJIN.Vol14No1InfoCol01 https://doi.org/10.3912/OJIN.Vol14No1InfoCol01

U.S. Department of Health & Human Services. (n.d.). *Health information privacy.* https://www.hhs.gov/hipaa/index.html

von Krogh, G., & Nåden, D. (2008). A nursing-specific model of EPR documentation: Organizational and professional requirements. *Journal of Nursing Scholarship, 40*(1), 68–75.

Wakefield, D. S., Wakefield, B. J., Despins, L., Brandt, J., Davis, W., Clements, K., & Steinmann, W. (2012). A review of verbal order policies in acute care hospitals. *The Joint Commission Journal on Quality and Patient Safety, 38*(1), 24–33.

Williams, C., Mostashari, E., Mertz, K., Hogin, E., & Atwal, P. (2012). From the office of the national coordinator: The strategy for advancing the exchange of health information. *Health Affairs (Millwood), 31*(3), 527–536.

Windle, P. E. (1994). Critical pathways: An integrated documentation tool. *Nursing Management, 25*(9), 80F–80L, 80P.

Wright, A., Sittig, D. F., Ash, J. S., Erickson, J. L., Hickman, T. T., Paterno, M., Gebhardt, E., McMullen, C., Tsurikova, R., Dixon, B. E., Fraser, G., Simonaitis, L., Sonnenberg, F. A., & Middleton, B. (2015). Lessons learned from implementing service-oriented clinical decision support at four sites: A qualitative study. *International Journal of Medical Informatics, 84*(11), 901–911.

21 Informatics and Health Care Technologies

Frank Albrecht

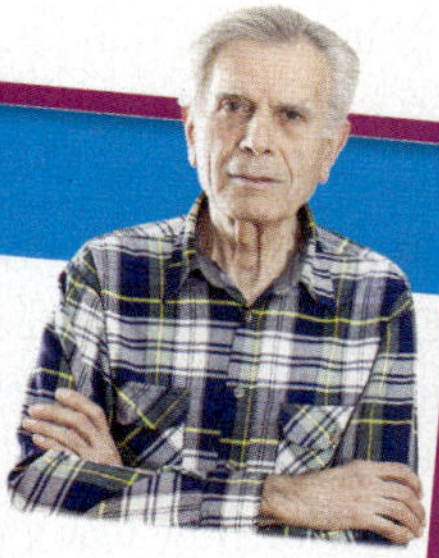

Frank is a 72-year-old patient who has chronic obstructive pulmonary disease. His wife, who has been his primary caregiver since his diagnosis 5 years ago, died last year and he now lives alone in their original two-level family home. He has been sleeping on the couch in the living room because he can no longer go upstairs. He has a daughter who lives across country who tries to get home once a month to be sure he has food and medications. Not surprisingly, Frank has had four hospital readmissions in the past year.

Jorge Bobadilla

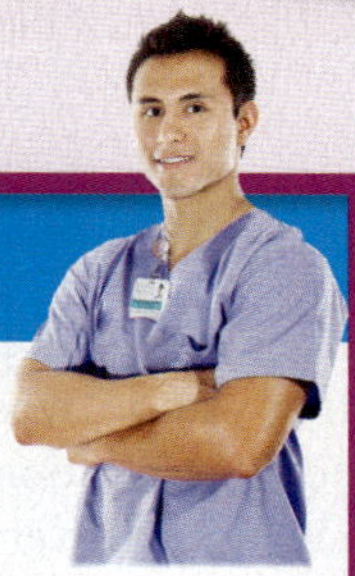

Jorge is the nurse manager on an orthopedic unit where the majority of patients are older and have had knee or hip replacements. Some have difficulty urinating after surgery and many have urinary catheters placed. Some are admitted to the hospital from nursing homes and have had indwelling urinary catheters for weeks. Jorge's unit is being watched closely for its high incidence of catheter-associated urinary tract infections (CAUTIs). Jorge wants help to monitor this problem.

Danielle Smith

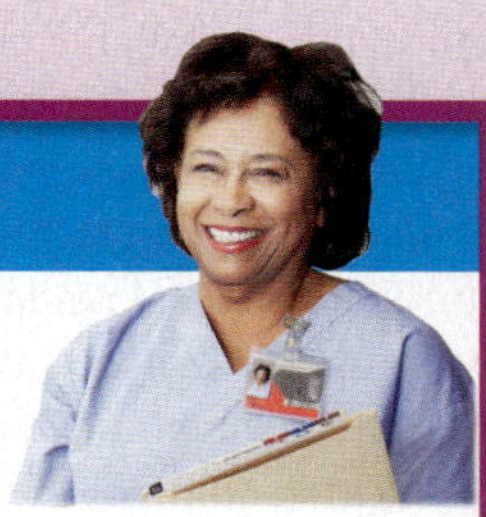

Danielle is a new nurse manager on a neurology intensive care unit. She has a passion for palliative care and knows that many intensive care unit patients and families would benefit greatly from timely referrals to palliative care so that appropriate treatment goals could be identified, and distressing symptoms addressed.

Learning Outcomes

After completing the chapter, you will be able to accomplish the following:

1. Describe nursing informatics and its contributions to nursing and quality health care.
2. Describe how the system development lifecycle (SDLC) process can be used to ensure the successful implementation of a new electronic health record (EHR).
3. Define terms basic to informatics: system usability, system optimization, standard technologies, interoperability, and security and privacy of electronic data.
4. Describe the two types of nurse informaticists and the responsibilities of each.
5. Describe how telehealth, telemedicine, and telecare are helping people achieve their health goals. What are the advantages of each?
6. Describe how using telehealth, remote monitoring, and mobile care teams, hospital-at-home programs can deliver quality inpatient care in the comfort of one's home.

Nursing Concepts

- Informatics

Technology in health care is now pervasive. Nurses in all types of care settings are interacting with increasing numbers of information and communications technologies and medical devices to aid in care delivery. The need for nurses trained in informatics to ensure optimized and evidence-based use of these devices and clinical information systems continues to grow. Nurses understand clinical workflows and how care is delivered, giving them the knowledge needed to help design technologic tools and **clinical information systems** that will support and transform health care. A clinical information system is a computer-based system designed for collecting, storing, manipulating, and making available clinical information important to the health care delivery process.

With an estimated 3.9 million nurses in the United States, all interacting with technology, it is important to ensure that all nurses possess a foundational understanding of how systems work and the concepts that allow for knowledgeable questioning and ongoing innovation. This chapter will help you develop an understanding of the concepts that are essential to nursing informatics (NI) practice; knowledge of these concepts will provide a sound framework to improve health care technologies with input from nurses who actually use the device or system. This chapter also covers emerging informatics trends that will need nursing input as they evolve into quality tools that drive clinical, administrative, and even financial outcomes.

HISTORY OF NURSING INFORMATICS

The science of **informatics** drives innovation that is defining future approaches to information and knowledge management in biomedical research, clinical care, and public health. Although seemingly of recent origin, at its core, informatics has been around for centuries. Many have asserted that the first informatics nurse (IN) was Florence Nightingale, who compiled and processed data to improve sanitation conditions in military hospitals during the Crimean War in the 1850s (Betts & Wright, 2006).

Informatics has come to represent a growing field with a focus on the use of technology and data to improve patient care. The American Nurses Association (ANA) recognized NI as a specialty and developed board certification in 1992. Several disciplines (nursing, medicine, pharmacology, nutrition, and dentistry) have developed informatics expertise within their respective domains, each adding their skills and knowledge to a dynamic field.

The importance of informatics nursing has been highlighted with the widespread implementation of the electronic health record (EHR), a digital version of a patient's chart or medical history. Informatics is not just about the EHR, though. Many areas within the scope of informatics deal with areas such as telehealth, mobile devices, patient portals, data analytics, and technologies for educating nurses in academic settings and for conducting research.

The need for expertise in the field of informatics has undoubtedly increased since the signing of the American Reinvestment and Recovery Act (ARRA) in 2009. The ARRA included the authorization of the Health Information Technology for Economic and Clinical Health (HITECH) Act, which allocated billions of dollars to stimulate the adoption of quality **health information technology (IT)** systems or EHRs that demonstrate **meaningful use** (ONC, 2009). HealthIT.gov defines meaningful as using certified EHR technology to:

- Improve quality, safety, efficiency, and reduce health disparities
- Engage patients and family
- Improve care coordination and population and public health
- Maintain privacy and security of patient health information

Ultimately, it is hoped that the meaningful use compliance will result in:

- Better clinical outcomes
- Improved population health outcomes
- Increased transparency and efficiency
- Empowered people
- More robust research data on health systems

Meaningful use regulations set specific objectives that eligible professionals (EPs) and hospitals must achieve to qualify for Centers for Medicare & Medicaid Services (CMS) Incentive Programs.

The percentage of hospitals with certified EHR technology increased from 72% to 97% between 2011 and 2014. In 2015, nearly 9 in 10 of office-based physicians (87%) had

QSEN Reflective Practice: Cultivating QSEN Competencies

CHALLENGE TO INTELLECTUAL AND ETHICAL SKILLS

I am a Critical Care Nurse Practitioner on a neuro intensive care unit in a university medical center. Because of an interest in palliative care and personal experience of the benefits that accompany early palliative care consults in intensive care units, I am growing more and more concerned with the failure of our staff to initiate consults to palliative care for our critically ill neuro patients with problematic symptoms. Neurocritical illness creates an unpredictable hospital course and many different opinions on a patient's prognosis. Many of our patients suffer permanent disability and with some diagnoses morality rates are above 50%. Palliative care could dramatically increase the well-being of our patients and their families. Sadly, too few of our physicians and nurses are familiar with palliative care and many confuse a referral to palliative care with "giving up" on a patient. Many of our surgeons believe they have an obligation to "rescue" our patients and even when the prognosis is grim, they may continue to order inappropriate life-sustaining/death-prolonging interventions. The medical director of our unit is not a fan of palliative care.

Thinking Outside the Box: Possible Courses of Action

- Accept the status quo and realize that I may just be ahead of my time. In no way do I want to be a martyr for the cause.
- Start trying to win over my colleagues one by one to value palliative care and hope that palliative care referrals increase.
- Educate my colleagues on how to use a validated screening tool to identify patients appropriate for palliative care consults and begin to measure how appropriate palliative care consults relate to length of stay, patient satisfaction/engagement scores, and in-hospital costs.

Evaluating a Good Outcome: How Do I Define Success?

- Our neuro patients and their families get the highest-quality care including timely referrals to appropriate palliative care.
- My ethical integrity is intact, and I am an effective advocate for our patients.
- I don't rock the boat and get our surgeons angry with me.
- I learn how to use data to bring about needed change.
- Staff learn how to use, and are comfortable using, a standardized screening tool to identify patients who would benefit from a palliative care referral. Our informaticists make this tool available electronically.

Personal Learning: Here's to the Future!

Luckily at the same time I was experiencing this challenge I enrolled in a Doctor of Nursing Practice (DNP) program where I learned how to use research to bring about system-wide change. It wasn't an easy journey and there were many obstacles, but I am happy to report that our unit will be examining ways to customize a screening tool that can be standardized for palliative care screenings with each patient admitted to the neuro ICU. Ideally our palliative care consults will increase threefold. I am definitely feeling good about my ability to improve the quality of care for our patients and families.

Danielle McCamey Smith, MS, CRNP, ACNP-BC
Georgetown University

QSEN SELF-REFLECTION ON QUALITY AND SAFETY COMPETENCIES DEVELOPING KNOWLEDGE, SKILLS, AND ATTITUDES FOR CONTINUOUS IMPROVEMENT

How do you think you would respond in a similar situation? Why? What does this tell you about yourself and about the adequacy of your competencies for professional practice? Can you think of other ways to respond? What *knowledge, skills,* and *attitudes* do you need to develop to continuously improve the quality and safety of care for patients?

Patient-Centered Care: How can you motivate your physician and nurse colleagues to sufficiently value person-centered care to learn more about palliative care and its benefits for your patient population? Similarly, how can you get your colleagues to invest in learning how to use a standardized palliative care screening tool and your institution to use the EHR to facilitate appropriate consults to palliative care?

Teamwork and Collaboration/Quality Improvement: How did you identify potential allies for the change you wished to create and work with barriers to changing the status quo?

Safety/Evidence-Based Practice: What research was most persuasive in getting staff "on board" for change? How did your research project findings support the need for change and convince administration that your proposal was sound and worth the investment of people and resources?

Informatics: What role might a nurse informaticist have played in bringing about needed change? What else might the nurse have done to ensure a successful outcome?

adopted an EHR system, up from 42% in 2008 (Charles et al., 2015; ONC, 2015a). Much of the focus of informatics work between 2003 and 2013 revolved around the EHR in the inpatient setting, but with changing payment models and care delivery systems consolidating and converging, informatics practice has begun to migrate outside the walls of the hospital and infiltrate new areas of practice.

NURSING INFORMATICS DEFINED

The ANA published the Nursing Informatics Scope of Practice in 1994, followed by Standards of Practice in 1995. Combined and updated versions were published in 2001, revised in 2008 and again in 2015 (ANA, 2015). This document contains standards of professional practice and competencies for INs in 16 categories of informatics practice, each including criteria that describe the expected knowledge, skills, and abilities necessary to meet each standard. Each of these categories supports nursing care delivery and evaluation of care using technology and associated analytics. These 16 areas are summarized in Table 21-1 (on pages 553–554).

The ANA defines **nursing informatics (NI)** as "the specialty that integrates nursing science with multiple information management and analytical sciences to identify, define, manage, and communicate data, information, knowledge, and wisdom in nursing practice. NI supports nurses, consumers, patients, the interprofessional health care team, and other stakeholders in their decision making in all roles and settings to achieve desired outcomes. This support is accomplished through the use of information structures, information processes, and information technology" (ANA, 2015, p. 1). See Figure 21-1. The American Medical Informatics Association (AMIA), which represents multiple disciplines in the field of informatics, defines NI as "the science and practice that integrates nursing, its information and knowledge, with information and communication technologies to promote the health of people, families, and communities worldwide" (AMIA, 2009). To put it simply and broadly, NI ensures that information used by nurses supports improvement in patient care delivery.

In addition to these definitions, nursing theorists introduced a classic NI framework. In the 1980s, Graves and

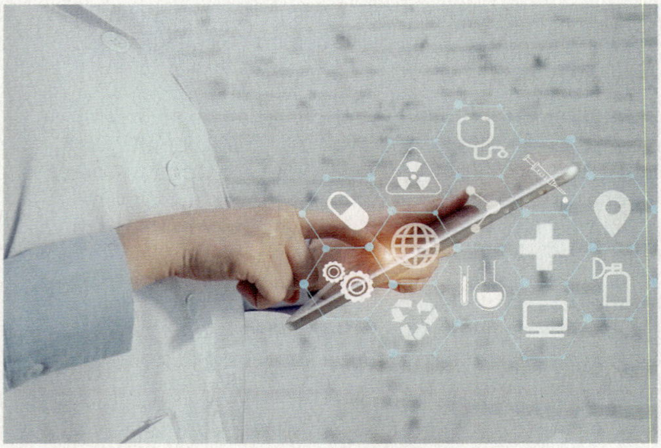

FIGURE 21-1. Nurse using tablet with medical interface icons. (*Source:* Used with permission from Shutterstock. *Photo by SOMKID THONGDEE.*)

Box 21-1 Informatics Scope and Standards Definitions: "DIKW"

Data: Discrete entities that are described without interpretation
Information: Data that have been interpreted, organized, or structured
Knowledge: Information that is synthesized so that relationships are identified
Wisdom: Appropriate use of knowledge to manage and solve human problems

Source: Data from American Nursing Association. (2015). *Nursing Informatics: Scope and Standards of Practice* (2nd ed.). © 2014 By American Nurses Association. Reprinted with permission. All rights reserved; Matney, S., Brewster, P. J., Sward, K. A., Cloyes, K. G., & Staggers, N. (2011). Philosophical approaches to the nursing informatics data-information-knowledge-wisdom framework. *Advances in Nursing Science*, *34*(1), 6–18.

Corcoran described the concepts of data, information, and knowledge as key components of NI practice. These components, each building on the next, lay the foundation for informatics in terms of how technology and clinical systems are used to continually advance care delivery and improve clinical outcomes. Taking individual data elements and combining them to provide meaningful information that leads to knowledge and enhanced patient care delivery is the essential premise of this framework. In the 2008 revision of the Informatics Scope and Standards, an additional concept, "wisdom," was added to reflect the appropriate use of knowledge (ANA, 2015; Topaz, 2013). Box 21-1 describes each of the components that provide the underpinnings for informatics practice. To read more about nursing informatics check out the American Nurses Informatics Association website (https://www.ania.org/) and the Healthcare Information and Management Systems Society, Inc. (HIMSS) website (https://www.himss.org/resources/what-nursing-informatics).

NURSING INFORMATICS EDUCATION

The ANA differentiates two types of nurse informaticists: the information nurse (IN) and the informatics nurse specialist (INS). The IN is a registered nurse with an interest or experience in an informatics field. This may be a nurse who has assisted with the implementation of an EHR and is considered a "superuser," with training being primarily on the job. Superuser is a term frequently used when describing someone who has become a system expert and can navigate the EHR with ease as they enter and review patient data. An INS is a registered nurse with formal graduate-level education in the field of informatics. The INS is often responsible for strategy development, implementation, and maintenance and evaluation of clinical systems requiring collaboration with multiple disciplines (ANA, 2015).

To educate these nurse specialists, universities began offering graduate education in NI, first at the University of Maryland and the University of Utah beginning in the 1980s. More than 40 NI graduate programs are now available across

Table 21-1 ANA Informatics Competencies

STANDARDS OF PRACTICE AREA	STANDARD	EXAMPLES OF COMPETENCIES
1. Assessment	The informatics nurse collects comprehensive data, information, and emerging evidence pertinent to the situation.	Uses evidence-based assessment technologies, instruments, tools, and effective communication strategies in collecting pertinent data to define the issue or problem Uses workflow analysis to examine current practice, workflow, and the potential impact of an informatics solution on that workflow
2. Diagnosis, problems, and issues identification	The informatics nurse analyzes assessment data to identify diagnoses, problems, issues, and opportunities for improvement.	Uses standardized clinical terminologies, taxonomies, and decision support tools, when available, to identify problems, needs, issues, and opportunities for improvement
3. Outcomes identification	The informatics nurse identifies expected outcomes for a plan individualized to the health care consumer or the situation.	Defines expected outcomes in terms of the health care consumer, health care worker, and other stakeholders, and their values, ethical considerations, and environmental, organizational, or situational considerations
4. Planning	The informatics nurse develops a plan that prescribes strategies, alternatives, and recommendations to attain expected outcomes.	Develops a customized plan considering clinical and business characteristics of the environment and situation Integrates current scientific evidence, trends, and research into the planning process
5. Implementation	The informatics nurse implements the identified plan.	Partners with the health care consumer, health care team, and others, as appropriate, to implement the plan on time, within budget, and within the plan requirements
5a. Coordination of activities	The informatics nurse coordinates planned activities.	Organizes components of the plan Provides leadership in the coordination of the information technology and health care activities for integrated delivery of efficient and cost-effective health care services
5b. Health teaching and health promotion	The informatics nurse employs informatics solutions and strategies for education and teaching to promote health and a safe environment.	Integrates informatics solutions, resources, ergonomics, and disability adaptations into clinical practice workflow and patient care routines
5c. Consultation	The informatics nurse provides consultation to influence the identified plan, enhance the abilities of others, and effect change.	Synthesizes data, information, knowledge, theoretical frameworks, and evidence when providing consultation
6. Evaluation	The informatics nurse evaluates progress toward attainment of outcomes.	Conducts a systematic, ongoing, and criterion-based evaluation of the outcomes in relation to the structures and processes prescribed by the project plan and indicated timeline
7. Ethics	The informatics nurse practices ethically.	Uses Code of Ethics for Nurses with Interpretive Statements (ANA, 2015) Employs informatics principles, standards, and methodologies to establish and maintain health care consumer confidentiality within legal and regulatory parameters
8. Education	The informatics nurse attains knowledge and competence that reflect current nursing and informatics practice.	Participates in ongoing education to advance their knowledge base and professional practice Shares educational findings, experiences, and ideas with peers
9. Evidence-based practice and research	The informatics nurse integrates evidence and research findings into practice.	Uses data to communicate evidence to promote effective care processes and decisions Uses the skills and tools available to the informatics nurse for research studies

(*continued*)

Table 21-1 ANA Informatics Competencies *(continued)*

STANDARDS OF PRACTICE AREA	STANDARD	EXAMPLES OF COMPETENCIES
10. Quality of practice	The informatics nurse contributes to quality and effectiveness of nursing and informatics practice.	Demonstrates quality by documenting the application of the nursing process in a responsible, accountable, and ethical manner, and by facilitating a unified or defined level of documentation by nurses in clinical practice Analyzes quality data to identify opportunities to improve nursing and informatics practice or outcomes
11. Communication	The informatics nurse communicates effectively in a variety of formats in all areas of practice.	Supports communication preferences of health care consumers, families, and colleagues Communicates strategies to improve and enhance the value of documentation
12. Leadership	The informatics nurse demonstrates leadership in the professional practice setting and the profession.	Promotes the organization's vision, the associated goals, and the strategic plan Mentors colleagues for the advancement of nursing informatics practice, the profession, and quality health care
13. Collaboration	The informatics nurse collaborates with the health care consumer, family, and others in the conduct of nursing and informatics practice.	Partners with others to effect change and produce positive outcomes through the sharing of data, information, and knowledge of the health care consumer or situation
14. Professional practice evaluation	The informatics nurse evaluates their own nursing practices in relation to professional practice standards and guidelines, relevant statutes, rules, and regulations.	Supports delivery of appropriate care and services in a culturally, ethically, and developmentally sensitive manner Interacts with peers and colleagues to enhance their own professional nursing practice or role performance
15. Resource utilization	The informatics nurse employs appropriate resources to plan and implement informatics and associated services that are safe, effective, and fiscally responsible.	Monitors the health care information needs of individual consumers and communities, as well as the available operational and technical enterprise resources to achieve desired outcomes
16. Environmental health	The informatics nurse supports practice in a safe and healthy environment.	Promotes a practice environment that reduces ergonomic and environmental health risks for workers and health care consumers Assists in the development of health and safety alerts within the clinical documentation and technology solutions

Source: American Nurses Association (ANA). (2015). *Nursing: Scope and standards of practice* (3rd ed.). American Nurses Association. Reprinted with permission. See also American Nurses Association (ANA). (2021). *Nursing: Scope and Standards of Practice* (4th ed.).

the United States, including several that are available completely online. NI education typically consists of a master's degree program, although some universities offer a post-master's program for those who already possess another graduate nursing degree.

NURSING INFORMATICS PRACTICE

The field of nursing has a wide variety of specialties, one of which is informatics. Even within the field of informatics there are multiple areas of practice where nurses can focus their work. Typically, an IN will have primary responsibilities in one of the areas described in the following sections but may be knowledgeable in many.

Nurses practicing in direct care roles should have general knowledge of these areas of informatics practice at a conceptual level to ensure efficient, effective, and safe use of clinical information systems and other technologies. A basic understanding of these concepts will also help nurses participate and collaborate in the required and ever-evolving interdisciplinary work of embedding technology into care delivery to drive improvement. The following sections describe several nurse informatics practice concepts and areas of practice, all essential for the effective use of technologic tools.

SYSTEM DEVELOPMENT LIFECYCLE

A fundamental framework for nurse informaticists in any care setting is the **system development lifecycle (SDLC)**. The concepts or phases of the SDLC are very similar to the concepts of the nursing process but with an informatics or technology focus. While for a practicing nurse, the areas of Assess, Plan, Implement, and Evaluate make up the foundational concepts of care, the SDLC requires focus in the areas of Analyze and Plan, Design and Build, Test, Train, Implement, Maintain, and Evaluate. A brief description of each phase of the SDLC follows.

QSEN INFORMATICS

Nurses who will be using a clinical information system should be involved in all phases of the SDLC to ensure the best chance that the system will meet its intended need.

Analyze and Plan

Before considering the employment of any type of new technology or an update to a system already in place, analysis and planning must take place. Questions need to be answered, such as:

- What is the purpose of this new technology or change to the current technology?
- What problem do we hope to solve?
- What data do we have to indicate the current state of the issue (how bad is the problem)?
- How will its use be incorporated into the current workflow of the nurse?
- Will it streamline nursing documentation, or will it increase the burden of documentation?
- Will it improve the overall usability and experience with the EHR?
- What technologic options are available if there are more than one?

Often this step is not given the necessary attention; well-intentioned people may go straight to the technologic solution without a thorough analysis of the actual need. In this phase of the SDLC, it is imperative to understand the organizational need and provide the supporting baseline data to justify the effort (Sengstack, 2016). Tools and resources used during this phase may include need assessment tools, data analytics programs, or workflow diagrams (Ozkaynak et al., 2016). During this phase, nurses can help to clarify the need and provide expertise in the current workflow.

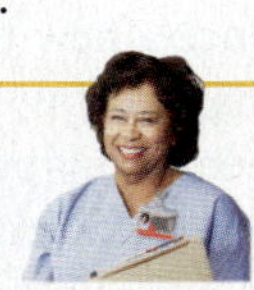

Recall the example above, in which **Danielle**, the new nurse manager was concerned about patient's receiving appropriate and timely palliative care. During this phase, Danielle would be instrumental in working with the informatics team to help understand the problem and explore potential solutions.

Design and Develop

Once thorough planning and analysis has resulted in an identified need for a new technology or an enhancement to a current system, the more granular work of designing begins. A basic tenet for informatics success is that nurses and other care providers using the clinical information system must be involved in the design for successful outcomes to be achieved (St. John, 2015).

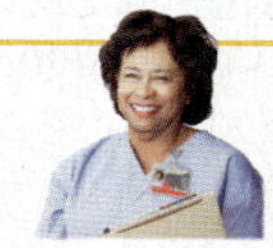

Danielle would be integral in helping the interdisciplinary team to design the best technical solution to support an improved process. With Danielle on the design team, all aspects of appropriate patient identification and subsequent follow-up actions could be addressed.

Questions asked during this phase may include:

- What should the screen display look like? How should it be laid out to be consistent with other screen layouts?
- Can the design support or improve the nurse's workflow as mapped out during the analysis and planning phase?
- Is there evidence supporting the effectiveness of the new technology and, if so, does it provide recommendations for the design?
- Can we use standard nursing terminology in the electronic system to better capture nursing's contribution to care delivery and patient outcomes?

Test

Testing of technology has several phases.

Technology Alert

Thorough testing helps to avoid unexpected issues (some of which can affect patient safety), since technology is complex with multiple interrelated components. A change or update to one part of a clinical information system, such as an EHR, can have effects on other areas not initially identified.

As part of the implementation for any new technology, or even a small change to a current EHR, an overall testing plan is developed that includes the use of testing scripts. These test scripts, ideally developed in collaboration with nurses who will be using the technology, ensure that all components of the system are working as designed and will support workflow during interaction with the system (Carlson, 2015). While testing is typically carried out by informatics specialists experienced in the testing of systems, the nurses using the system should provide input into the testing scripts and participate in user acceptance testing.

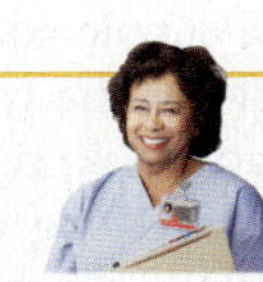

In our scenario, **Danielle** would be able to provide the essential components of test scripts to ensure that the new system updates are working as designed before they are built into the live system.

The phases of testing with brief descriptions are listed in Table 21-2.

Table 21-2 Technology Testing Phases

TESTING PHASE	WHEN PERFORMED	DESCRIPTION
Unit testing	During design and development	This is basic testing that occurs initially. • Do the screens contain the right information? • Was anything left out? • Is everything in the right place on the screen? • Are there any typos?
Function testing	After unit testing is complete	Uses test scripts to validate that a system is working as designed for *one* particular function. For example: • The EHR system sends a lab order to the lab system on the day they are scheduled 6 hours in advance. • The EHR system sets any order that has been active for over 365 days to a status of "auto-complete."
Integration testing	After function testing is complete	Uses test script to validate that a system is working as designed for an entire workflow that integrates multiple components of the system. For example: All steps in an EHR work as designed from order entry to administration of a medication (including the proper functioning and communication between order entry screens, the pharmacy system and the medication administration record).
Performance testing	After integration testing	Performance testing is more technical and ensures proper functioning of the system when there are high volumes of end users or care providers using the system at the same time. Can it handle the load?
User acceptance testing	After all testing above	An important final phase of testing where the nurse (or other system end user) test drives the new system or new functions of the EHR to ensure it's working as designed.

Source: From Carlson, S. (2015). Testing in the healthcare informatics environment. In P. Sengstack & C. Boicey (Eds.). *Mastering informatics: A healthcare handbook for success.* Sigma Theta Tau International Honor Society of Nursing (Sigma). Adapted and reprinted with permission of Sigma Theta Tau International Honor Society of Nursing (Sigma).

Train

Effective end-user training is a key element to an implementation's success. EHRs are complex and multifaceted. They have linkages that require end users to negotiate between different areas of the chart that can be confusing. While training end users effectively often takes a backseat to more visible activities like system configuration, it can make or break an implementation. Poor training can produce decreased efficiency, staff turnover, patient care errors, and poor-quality documentation followed by decreased billing revenue (Kulhanek, 2015).

The type of training required depends on the implementation project. For the installation of a new EHR, a classroom model of education will most likely be needed. If you are adding only a new module to a current system, web-based or online training may be adequate. If the change is a simple addition to current functionality, a tip sheet or just-in-time training may suffice. An organization's informatics training team should use principles of adult learning theory along with a framework, such as the five steps of ADDIE—analysis, design, development, implementation, and evaluation—in the training development process. The development of training materials needs nursing input to ensure that the technology supports nursing processes and workflows that will enable nurses to navigate the system as easily as possible (Kulhanek, 2015).

Implement

Implementation refers to the activities surrounding the activation of the new technology, or "flipping the switch" to begin using the new functionality in the EHR. The planning for this phase includes ensuring all testing has been completed, end users have been educated, and support resources are ready for any questions that arise (Houston, 2015). Nurse superusers are often employed during this implementation phase to assist if help is needed.

Maintain

Once a new technology is up and running, the maintenance phase begins. Many think that the most difficult work is behind them at this point; however, this next phase can be just as, if not more challenging than, previous phases. Keeping a system up and running requires ongoing allocation of resources and attention to detail (Settergren, 2015). A few of the tasks that occur during the maintenance phase for an EHR include:

- Ongoing updates to hospital and ambulatory order preference lists
- Ongoing updates to hospital and ambulatory medication preference lists
- Ongoing updates to provider patient lists
- Ongoing updates to scheduling blocks (ambulatory, radiology, and procedure areas)

- Monthly loads (new medications, medication pricing, and clinical alerts)
- Error work queue maintenance (e.g., billing errors, sure script errors, many types of interface errors)
- Pricing updates
- Quality measures updates
- Clinical decision support tools/rules
- Monthly updates from EHR vendor

Evaluate

The acquisition and management of EHRs represent a significant portion of an organization's financial bottom line. Millions of dollars are invested in these systems, not just to meet meaningful use objectives for the financial incentive, but to provide a higher quality of care than paper and pencil probably could. Once implemented, administrators across the nation are asking, "Is our EHR helping us realize our organizational goals? Is it reducing medication errors? Is it eliminating duplicate ordering of diagnostic testing? Is it allowing more time for our care providers to spend with the patients? Is it improving the overall health of our patients?" With expertise, guidelines, and tools still emerging in this area, organizations are beginning to address the evaluation of health IT. Evaluation may be the last phase of the SDLC, but it represents an essential step for nurses to be involved in before circling back to Assess and Plan based on the results of the evaluation (Sengstack, 2015).

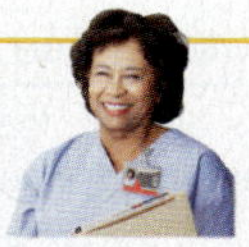

This would also be one of the most important phases for **Danielle** in our continued example. Are patients now receiving appropriate and timely palliative care? With the significant investment of the team's time to develop the new system functionality, it would seem that this is something Danielle should ensure happens.

See Table 21-3 (on page 558) for an example of the steps that should be taken when evaluating the effectiveness of the technology.

INFORMATICS CONCEPTS

The field of informatics possesses a unique body of knowledge and often uses terms that are not commonly part of typical health care interactions or communication. These terms—*usability, optimization, standard terminologies, interoperability*, and *security and privacy*—represent core concepts in the implementation and maintenance of clinical information systems. The discussion of these terms and concepts that follows is intended to heighten awareness among practicing nurses so that they can ask questions and use systems safely, and so that improvements can continue to be made to all technologies.

System Usability

The National Institute of Standards and Technology defines **usability** as "the extent to which a product can be used by specified users to achieve specified goals with effectiveness, efficiency, and satisfaction in a specified context of use" (NIST, 2017). EHRs and order entry systems are complex. Sometimes the way screens are formatted can be confusing, making it a real challenge to perform nursing tasks in a way that makes sense. The Healthcare Information and Management Systems Society (HIMSS) Electronic Health Record Usability Task Force report cited that usability was perhaps the most important factor that hindered the widespread adoption of EHRs prior to the signing of the HITECH Act in 2009 (Belden et al., 2009). Making clinical systems easy to use, intuitive, and supportive of nurses' workflow is what usability is all about. A system with effective usability can save time, reduce errors, and improve end user satisfaction (St. John, 2015). That is why it is so important to include nurses who will be using the technology in the planning and design phases of the SDLC.

Comprehensive tools for usability evaluation can be found through a number of sources both internal and external to the health care IT industry. The HIMSS EHR Usability Task Force (2009) supports the usability principles described in Box 21-2 (on page 559). These principles may seem foundational or simply common sense, but they are essential in the effective designing of safe, high-quality clinical information systems.

System Optimization

Once an EHR or other clinical information system is in use, and as nurses and other care providers become more proficient with the system, the need for improvements to better support and improve care delivery will usually become evident. Definitions of EHR **optimization** vary, but commonly include strategies to improve processes, maximize effective use, reduce errors, reduce costs, eliminate workflow inefficiencies, improve clinical decision support, and improve end-user skills and satisfaction with the system. Nurses in all settings can participate in organization-wide committees that discuss and make recommendations for improvements to the system. As EHR users, nurses quickly become the system experts and provide the richest source of ideas for strategies to improve system usability that can help to reduce potential errors and add value to patient care delivery. Optimization is all too often lumped into post-live maintenance and support, but it should be treated separately from routine maintenance (Settergren, 2015). Examples of EHR optimization include:

- Updating a nursing care plan to support an update to a procedure based on new evidence
- Reordering the sequence of screens that initially required nurses to go to three different places in the EHR to document a procedure
- Creating an alert to a nurse when a patient's urinary catheter has been in place for longer than 48 hours
- Adding a patient's code status and allergies to the header of the patient's main screen

Table 21-3 Examples of Technology Evaluation Steps

STEPS IN INFORMATICS EVALUATION	DESCRIPTION
1. Determine what will be evaluated.	Determine what to evaluate. Examples: • Adoption and use of the patient portal • Safety of using copy/paste function in the EHR • Effectiveness of modified early warning system on reducing codes called outside of the ICU • Effectiveness of allergy alerting
2. Determine the question.	A clear, focused question helps the team determine what data will need to be collected and how the data ultimately should be reported. Examples: • Has the implementation of the nurse-driven urinary catheter protocol reduced the number of catheter days for patients? • Have the new admission assessment screens resulted in timesaving and improved support of workflow for nurses? • What is the estimated amount of financial savings if automated report printouts were reduced by 50%?
3. Conduct a literature search.	Searches should be conducted in peer-reviewed journals by searching available databases such as Cumulative Index to Nursing and Allied Health Literature (CINAHL), PubMed, and Cochrane Reviews. • Has this topic been studied before? • What data was collected? • What were the findings? • Can we replicate the methods of the study?
4. Determine the needed data.	In this step, the specific data elements to be collected need to be determined. • What data is needed to answer the question? • Is it available? Can the data be easily queried and pulled into a report or spreadsheet for data manipulation? • Who will collect it? • What data collection tool will be used?
5. Determine the study type.	When determining your study design, first take into account the question you are asking, and the data you are collecting to answer the question. • Pre- or postevaluation of an intervention • Retrospective study • Observational study • Time/motion study • Case study • Randomized control trial • Descriptive evaluation of current state
6. Determine the data collection method and sample size.	Clarify exactly how the data will be collected. • Is the data already available in the EHR database (or other database), and you will need the assistance of someone skilled in running a query or developing a report? • Will you need to conduct a manual chart review? • Will you need to observe end users as they interact with the system? • Will you need to conduct a survey? • Will you need a focus group to gather data? • Check sample size and date ranges in previous studies on the same topic • Secure the help of a statistician.
7. Collect, analyze, and display data.	Whether using a table, bar chart, pie chart, or other method, ensure data displays include: • Title with date range and sample size as appropriate • Legends that clearly explain the content and colors • Labels on the x and y axis so the numerical value can be understood • Other descriptors necessary for interpretation
8. Document your outcome evaluation.	Without comprehensive documentation of your evaluation, the chance that any practice improvements occur becomes unlikely. Can use STARE-HI guidelines: http://www.imia-medinfo.org/new2/Stare-HI_as_published.pdf

Source: From Sengstack, P. (2015). Conducting quality healthcare IT outcome evaluations: Guidelines and resources. In P. Sengstack & C. Boicey (Eds.). *Mastering informatics: A healthcare handbook for success.* Sigma Theta Tau International Honor Society of Nursing (Sigma). Adapted and reprinted with permission of Sigma Theta Tau International Honor Society of Nursing (Sigma).

Box 21-2 Usability Concepts in System Design

Simplicity: Simplicity in design refers to everything from lack of visual clutter and concise information display to inclusion of only functionality that is needed to effectively accomplish tasks. A "less is more" philosophy is appropriate, with emphasis being given to information needed for decision making.

Naturalness: Naturalness refers to how automatically "familiar" and easy to use (intuitive) the application feels to the user.

Consistency: The more users can apply prior experience to a new system, the lower the learning curve, the more effective their usage, and the fewer their errors.

Minimizing cognitive load: Presenting all the information needed for the task at hand reduces cognitive load. For example, when reviewing results of a lipid profile, the provider will want to see the patient's latest and prior results, the medication list, the problem list, and the allergy list all in the same visual field so that decisions and subsequent actions may be performed without changing screens. Displaying information organized by meaningful relationships is one method of providing cognitive support to the user.

Efficient interactions: One of the most direct ways to facilitate efficient user interactions is to minimize the number of steps it takes to complete tasks and to provide shortcuts for use by frequent and/or experienced users.

Forgiveness and feedback: Forgiveness means that a design allows the user to discover it through exploration without fear of disastrous results. This approach accelerates learning while building in protections against unintended consequences.

Effective use of language: All language used in an EMR should be concise and unambiguous. Terminology used also must be that which is familiar and meaningful to the end users in the context of their work; no terms related to computers, technology, HL7, databases, and so forth should appear in the user interface.

Effective Information Presentation

Appropriate density when designing EMR screens: In clinical applications, there can be so much relevant information to display it can be tempting to pack as much as possible onto a screen. However, visual search times and user errors increase in proportion to density.

Meaningful use of color: Color should be used to convey meaning to the user.

Readability: Screen readability also is a key factor in objectives of efficiency and safety. Clinical users must be able to scan information quickly with high comprehension.

Preservation of context: Screen changes and visual interruptions should be kept to a minimum during completion of a particular task. Visual interruptions include anything that forces users to shift visual focus away from the area on the screen where they are currently reading or working to address something else, and then reestablish focus afterward.

Source: Data from St. John, C. (2015). Designing a usable healthcare information system. In P. Sengstack & C. Boicey (Eds.). *Mastering informatics: A healthcare handbook for success.* Sigma Theta Tau International.

- Configuring the system so that data entered by nurses in the pre-admission testing area then flows into the admission section of the chart so the admitting nurse does not need to duplicate the data entry

Standard Terminologies

When entering data into an EHR, nurses typically select items from drop-down lists or check boxes that represent an assessment parameter, an intervention, or a patient outcome. Behind the scenes, the data are stored in tables similar to spreadsheets. Each column in the table represents one concept—for example, activity level. The "activity level" column has data in rows that represent each time the data was entered by the nurse for a patient. It can also pull together many patients' activity levels that can be used in a report or analysis.

Whenever possible, data should be entered into the system using **standard terminology** instead of free text. For example, in Table 21-4 on page 560, the column A activity level was allowed to be entered as free text; nurses could type in anything. In column B, nurses were required to pick from a drop-down menu; responses were standardized. Imagine trying to find all the patients over the age of 65, who are on Medicare, whose activity level is "requires assistive device" from column A, where free text data entry was used; it would be impossible. Also, when assessing the acuity of patients to determine case mix and nurse shift assignments, it's important to know patient activity level. Using standard terms allows the development of reports and data that can help to make assignments based on patient care needs.

Without the ability to aggregate and analyze data entered into the EHR, it is a challenge to represent nursing's contribution to patient outcomes and to the organization's bottom line (Whittenburg & Jacobs, 2015). Data entered that represents patient assessment, interventions, and resultant outcomes need to be consistent so the care delivered by nurses can be quantified and nursing's contributions represented. Within this context, the nursing profession, with an estimated 3.4 million members, can contribute an enormous amount of valuable data related to the care of the patient.

Technology Alert

With data stored in a standardized electronic format, the value and contributions of nursing to patient outcomes can be measurable or retrievable (Welton & Harper, 2016). Using standard terminologies is just as important as the ability to use increasingly sophisticated tools to pull data from databases that can unlock an unlimited supply of data just waiting to be tapped into.

Nursing terminologies identify, define, and code care delivery concepts in an organized structure to represent nursing knowledge. The ANA recognizes 12 standard terminologies, which are listed in Table 21-5 on page 560; many of

Table 21-4 Activity Level Descriptions: Free Text versus Standard Terminology

	COLUMN A	COLUMN B
	Free Text	*Standard Terminology (Drop-Down Menu Used)*
Patient A	Stable—doesn't need help with walking	Walks without assistance
Patient B	Walks without problems	Walks without assistance
Patient C	Can't ambulate	Nonambulatory
Patient D	Needs a cane	Requires assistive device
Patient E	Can walk fine	Walks without assistance
Patient F	Okay—but sometimes uses a walker	Requires assistive device

these systems and classifications are described elsewhere in this text (see Chapters 16, 17, and 18).

In addition to sharing data among the various entities of a single organization, we are on a journey to share data across the nation, no matter where the data originates or where the patient is seen. Using standard terminology is a foundational step in this journey to ensure patient care can be delivered across the care continuum, and care providers have the right patient data, at the right time, to make safe clinical decisions.

Sharing data and information across nonaffiliated organizations has been an initiative of the Office of the National Coordinator for Health Information Technology, or ONC, part of the U.S. Department of Health and Human Services. In April 2015, Congress declared "a national objective to achieve widespread exchange of health information through interoperable certified EHR technology nationwide by December 31, 2018" (ONC, 2015b). The use of standard terminologies representing nursing care is a first step.

Interoperability

The term used to describe the ability to share patient data across health care systems is **interoperability**. The ONC (2015b) defines interoperability as:

> the ability of a system to exchange electronic health information with and use electronic health information from other systems without special effort on the part of the user. This means that all individuals, their families and health care providers should be able to send, receive, find and use electronic health information in a manner that is appropriate, secure, timely and reliable to support the health and wellness of individuals through informed, shared decision-making. With the right information available at the right time, individuals and caregivers can be active partners and participants in their health and care.

Table 21-5 Nursing Terminologies Recognized by the ANA

ANA-RECOGNIZED TERMINOLOGY/DATA SET	YEAR DEVELOPED	NURSING CONTENT
NANDA-Nursing Diagnoses, Definitions, and Classification	1973	Diagnoses
Omaha System	1975	Diagnoses, interventions, outcome ratings
Nursing Minimum Data Set (NMDS)	1985	Clinical data elements
Nursing Interventions Classification (NIC)	1987	Interventions
Perioperative Nursing Data Set (PNDS)	1988	Diagnoses, interventions, outcome
Clinical Care Classification (CCC) System	1988	Diagnoses, interventions, outcome ratings
Nursing Management Minimum Data Set (NMMDS)	1989	Management data elements
International Classification for Nursing Practice (ICNP)	1989	Diagnoses, interventions, outcome
Nursing Outcomes Classification (NOC)	1991	Outcomes
Logical Observation Identifiers Names and Codes (LOINC)	1994	Assessments, outcomes
ABC Codes	1996	Billing codes
SNOMED CT	2000	Diagnoses, interventions, outcomes, findings

Source: From Office of the National Coordinator for Health IT (ONC). (2017). *Standard nursing terminologies: A landscape analysis.* https://www.healthit.gov/sites/default/files/snt_final_05302017.pdf

In 2015, the ONC published *Connecting Health and Care for the Nation: A Shared Nationwide Interoperability Roadmap* (https://www.healthit.gov/sites/default/files/hie-interoperability/nationwide-interoperability-roadmap-final-version-1.0.pdf), which described a long-term goal to "build a strong foundation of health IT in our health care system, equipping every person with a long-term, digital picture of their health over their lifespan" (ONC, 2015b, p. iv). Whether a patient is cared for in a hospital, an ambulatory practice, an outpatient surgery center, or a skilled nursing facility, either in their home state or elsewhere in the country, the patient's data should be easily available to caregivers. Many EHR vendors are now beginning to provide the functionality to pull in patient data from other hospitals where the patient has received care in the past.

This journey toward interoperability will continue, and it will include advances in technologies that support the appropriate sharing of data and the use of standard terminologies. Not surprisingly, to support this effort, federal policies will need to address privacy and security issues surrounding data sharing for patient care and research, and nurses will need to educate themselves and their patients on the importance of understanding how their data is stored and used.

Security and Privacy of Electronic Data

The transition from paper charting to electronic documentation leads to an increased focus on security and privacy. In the paper-and-pen era, the chart was in only one physical location; a limited number of people had access to the chart, and you typically needed to fill out a request form to access it from Medical Records for review. Today, with data residing in electronic systems connected to networks, available from virtually anywhere with an Internet connection, the patient's data now becomes much easier to access by many more people—some without a justified need. Pertinent to this is the Health Insurance Portability and Accountability Act (HIPAA) and the Privacy Rule (see Chapter 20) as well as strategies to ensure the privacy and confidentiality of patient data (see Chapter 7).

Blockchain

Blockchain is digital information (the "block") stored in a public database (the "chain"). Carroll (2020) notes that blockchain can significantly increase data security within health care and the nursing profession due to its superior data accessibility, privacy, auditability, and efficiency. Some of the ways nurses can use blockchain to safeguard patient and personal data as well as purvey knowledge, adding value to the nursing profession include:

- Optimizing patient data management and portability
- Managing professional nurse credentialing and education
- Safeguarding clinical trials and expediting nursing research (pp. 62–63).

QSEN SAFETY

Nurses are responsible to minimize the risk of harm to patients and providers through both system effectiveness and individual performance. Ensuring secure and appropriate access to clinical systems starts with good management of passwords. Guidelines for keeping electronic systems secure with strong passwords can be found in Box 21-3.

Box 21-3 Keeping Data Safe Using Strong Passwords

Never share your password. Don't put it on a sticky note on the front of your computer or any other place that could be identified.

No well-managed site or business asks for your password. Be wary of e-mails, sites, or even callers who request your password—for any reason.

Don't reuse passwords. The password you use for social media should not be the same as the one for your bank account. You can use a common root for the password and make minor changes to reflect the system it's used for.

Use passwords that are easy to remember but hard to guess. You can use a mnemonic device that works for you but is unlikely to work for someone else. For example, create a phrase or sentence such as "I got my RN in 2010 from University of Miami" and then use the initial of each word to create a password, like this: IgmRNin2010fUM. To extend a password's usefulness to multiple sites, make variants by adding or deleting a couple of unique characters for each one. For some sites, you may want to use the entire phrase. You can also use a pass phrase as well, such as: "I like Wisconsin cheese" or "I will graduate in 2020."

Use at least eight characters for your password. Some sources recommend up to 15 characters at a minimum.

Consider using strong authentication or multifactor authentication. To prevent unauthorized users from accessing your account via a device not belonging to you, many companies or websites now offer users the option of verifying their identity. The typical method is to send a code via text or other message format to a mobile device registered to you. You then type in that code to verify that the person seeking access is really you.

Consider using a password manager. There are several programs or web services that let you create a different, very strong password for each of your sites. But you only have to remember that one password to access the program or secure site that stores all of your other passwords. Logons for sites you've selected can even populate the logon automatically when you "land" on those pages.

Source: Adapted from Finn, D., & Dion, W. (2017). *Security tips for using personal technology. Reflections on nursing leadership*. Sigma Theta Tau International Honor Society of Nursing (Sigma). http://www.reflectionsonnursingleadership.org/features/more-features/Vol43_1_security-tips-for-using-personal-technology

EMERGING AREAS IN THE FIELD OF INFORMATICS

As technology becomes increasingly sophisticated, and as care providers, patients, and consumers become more comfortable and proficient with the technologies, we will continue to see advances in health IT and informatics. Reportedly, computers double their capabilities every 12 to 18 months, as do the information technologies and software that use them (Emerging Future, 2012). Health care IT is seeing the emergence of numerous innovations that nurses will need to be familiar with as the pervasiveness of health care technologies grows. The following areas are evolving rapidly, and a basic understanding will help nurses prepare for, adapt to, and participate in the development, implementation, innovation, and evaluation of these tools.

Patient Portals

Engaging patients in their care and working together to improve health with supportive technology is an area that continues to advance. A primary patient engagement tool is the **patient portal**. This web-based tool can be securely accessed and provides functions to increase engagement. Portals are rapidly becoming the platform that links people to telehealth services, remote monitoring, and sometimes are a way to bring patient generated data to the health team. Portals can be accessible via a home computer or a smartphone, making engagement even easier. Depending on the vendor, patient portals can enable the patient to:

- Access medical history and other health information
- Complete various forms and questionnaires online
- Communicate securely and conveniently with providers
- Request prescription refills
- Pay bills
- Review lab results
- Schedule appointments
- Receive reminders for appropriate screenings (e.g., mammograms, flu shots, colonoscopy)
- Enter clinical data, such as blood pressure, glucose levels, weight, Fitbit data, and other activity tracking data
- Review progress notes
- Access educational materials based on diagnosis or procedure

Nurses are beginning to weave the functions of the portal into care delivery workflows in all settings, as patients are now beginning to expect their providers to be able to communicate using the functions and convenience that a portal provides. Supporting strong patient engagement using a tool such as the patient portal has shown to have multiple benefits (ONC, 2016), including:

- **Better health outcomes.** Encouraging patients to participate in their own health care can result in better preventive care and improve medication adherence.
- **Chronic condition management.** Patient access to information and direct communication with providers can increase the quality of life for patients with chronic disease. Patients can enter their own data on a daily basis for the provider to assess the need for intervention.
- **Timely access to care.** Engagement can result in a level of education that empowers patients to seek the right care at the right time.
- **Patient retention.** Patients who use the portal are nearly 2.6 times more likely to stay patients.
- **Patient-Centered Medical Home recognition.** Patient engagement is a basic element for all levels of Patient-Centered Medical Homes (PCMH) certification.

Encouraging patient engagement using the patient portal is a new competency for nurses that can occur during many different touchpoints in the care delivery process. Whether the patient is in the hospital, visiting a provider in the ambulatory clinic, or in the home health setting, use of the patient portal can be demonstrated and taught. Proxy access for children or for aging adults can also be a great benefit for those caring for loved ones. The convenience of being able to manage a loved one's care plan and communicate with providers via a portal can be an essential tool for healthy outcomes and reduced stress.

Health Care Analytics

Since the implementation of the first EHRs in the 1970s, organizations have been capturing and storing data in an electronic format. You can imagine that the data in those databases has grown exponentially over the years as nurses are continually contributing patient information. The tools to extract the data in order to identify trends and opportunities for improvement are becoming more mainstream and easier to use. Questions can be asked of the data to help drive clinical transformation and assess organizational program effectiveness. Data are now available to address problems in multiple areas. Here are some examples:

- **Clinical:** How many patients with congestive heart failure admitted over the last 3 months have been discharged to home with more than five medications? How many patients currently have had an indwelling urinary catheter in place for longer than 24 hours?
- **Populations:** Can we get a listing of all patients in our organization's Accountable Care Organization (ACO) who are diabetic and have not had a hemoglobin A1c drawn in the last year? (Note: The hemoglobin A1c test tells you the average level of blood sugar over the past 2 to 3 months. It's also called HbA1c, glycated hemoglobin test, and glycohemoglobin. People who have diabetes need this test regularly to see if their levels are staying within range. It can tell if you need to adjust your diabetes medicines.)
- **Administrative:** What nurse staffing ratios are recommended based on patient acuity? What is the hospital's daily census broken down by unit along with occupancy rate?
- **Financial:** Has revenue increased since implementing a new electronic bill pay system?

One way to think about **analytics** is this: If it is entered or stored in a database, then it can be pulled into a report.

With increasing sophistication of analytical tools, the ability now exists for data from disparate databases to be pulled into a single report. Organizations are taking data from Medicare claims and melding it with patient satisfaction data and clinical data. The questions that can be asked are virtually limitless with the right tools and expertise. As the tools become increasingly user friendly, nurses will have more opportunities to "self-serve" and "data mine" to find answers to questions that are posing a challenge to care delivery.

Three areas of analytics for which nurses should have a high level of understanding are *data visualization*, *predictive analytics*, and *big data* (Boicey, 2015). Each of these terms is used to describe aspects of analytics work that continues to evolve and is gaining traction in nursing and NI.

Data Visualization

Data visualization is the presentation of data in a pictorial or graphical format (Fig. 21-2). It enables decision makers to see analytics presented visually, so they can grasp difficult concepts or identify new patterns. Because of the way the human brain processes information, using charts or graphs to visualize large amounts of complex data is easier than poring over textual or numerical spreadsheets or reports (Boicey, 2015). Data visualization is a quick, easy way to convey concepts in a universal manner. These graphical formats can be bar charts, pie charts, maps (which can be interactive), bubble graphics, or infographics, and many other formats as well.

Predictive Analytics

Predictive analytics encompasses a variety of statistical techniques that analyze current and historical facts to make predictions about future or otherwise unknown events. In health care, we see this used as organizations attempt to identify patients who are at risk for readmission so case managers can intervene.

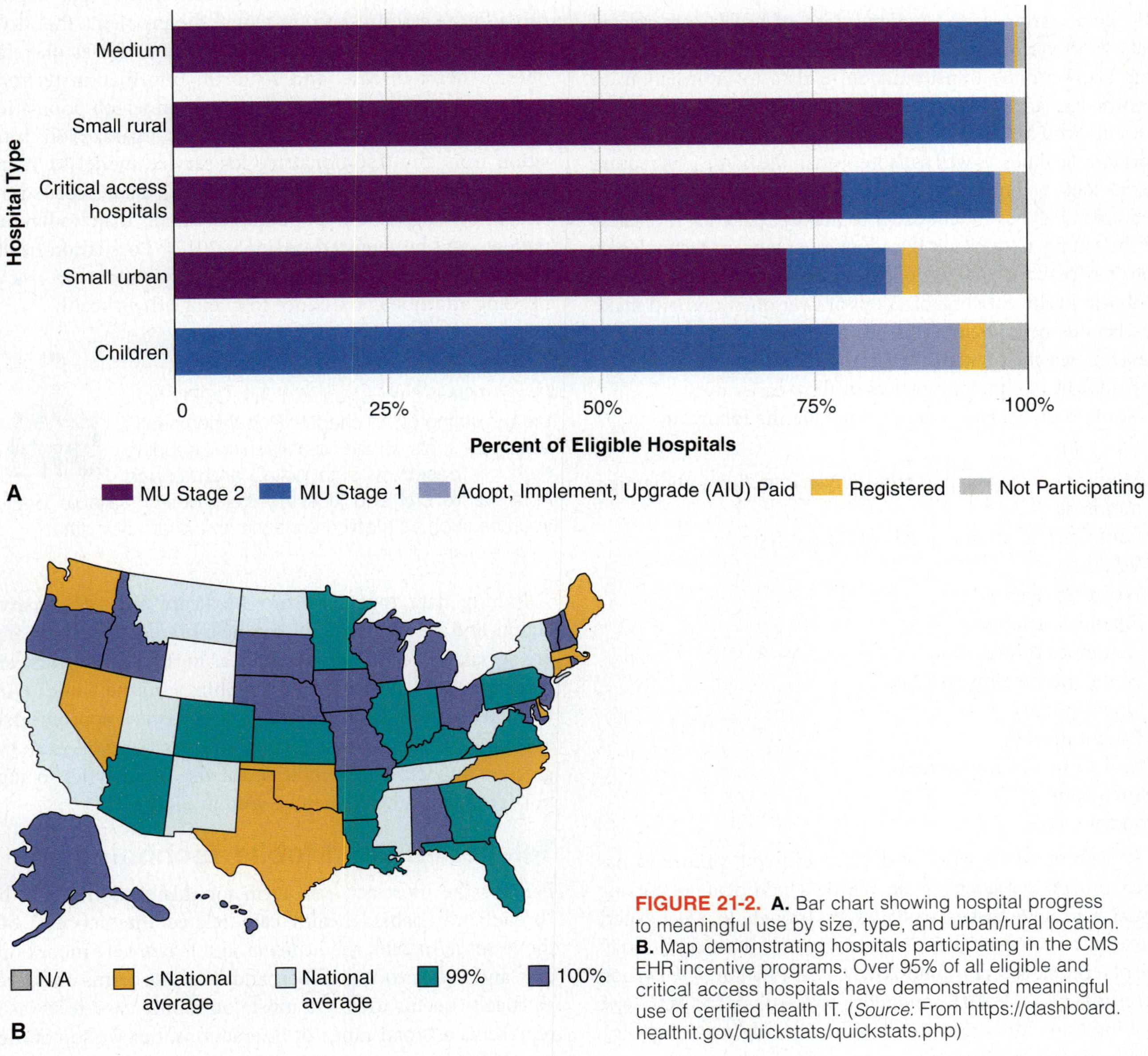

FIGURE 21-2. **A.** Bar chart showing hospital progress to meaningful use by size, type, and urban/rural location. **B.** Map demonstrating hospitals participating in the CMS EHR incentive programs. Over 95% of all eligible and critical access hospitals have demonstrated meaningful use of certified health IT. (*Source:* From https://dashboard.healthit.gov/quickstats/quickstats.php)

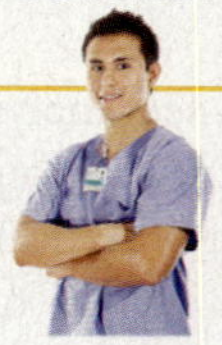

In the case of predicting which patients may develop catheter CAUTIs, recall **Jorge**, who needed a way to identify those patients at risk. Most EHRs now have the ability to display real-time analytic dashboards that indicate which patients on a given unit have had a catheter in place for more than 24 hours, putting them at a higher risk of developing a CAUTI. Many also have the ability to then trigger an alert to the nurse or to the manager to alert them to take action. With a real-time dashboard such as this, Jorge can easily identify any patient that may be at risk and intervene appropriately.

We also see predictive screening for patients who may be at risk for deterioration based on a number of clinical factors so that a preemptive rapid response can be called. Alerts and warnings built into clinical systems based on predictive models continue to evolve as evidence on their effectiveness grows.

Big Data

Big data comprises the accumulation of health care–related data from various sources, combined with new technologies that allow for the transformation of data to information, to knowledge, and ultimately to wisdom. The management of patients who are hospitalized, seen in clinics, or transferred to specialty facilities, as well as those seen in the home, will require us to look at analytics through a new lens. Delivering the required analytics functionality to manage patients, regardless of the setting, necessitates the adoption of big data technologies into our practice. Pulling together data from multiple sources will help health care organizations answer questions and make predictions never before possible as clinical systems advance, data entered into systems becomes increasingly interoperable, and analytics technology evolves to allow easier use.

Sources of available data can include the following:

- The EHR
- Medical devices such as from physiologic/hemodynamic monitors
- Radiology, laboratory, and pathology systems
- Ventilators
- Wearable devices
- Financial databases
- Genomics information
- Home monitoring systems
- Open sources
- Patient portals
- Real-time location systems
- Smart pumps
- Social media

A team of nurses based at the University of Minnesota has been providing leadership on big data pertinent to nursing practice. In 2016, these nursing leaders brought together expert nurse informaticists to ensure that nursing practice, through use of technology, contributes to a healthier nation. Their vision is described in the 2016 conference proceedings (https://www.nursing.umn.edu/sites/nursing.umn.edu/files/nursing_big_data_proceedings_2016.pdf) and excerpted below:

> We share a vision of better health outcomes resulting from the standardization and integration of the information nurses gather in electronic health records and other information systems, which is increasingly the source of insights and evidence used to prevent, diagnose, treat and evaluate health conditions. The addition of contextual data about patients, including environmental, geographical, behavioral, imaging, and more, will lead to breakthroughs for the health of individuals, families, communities and populations.

This is now an annual conference and includes nurse leaders from around the country.

Example: Using Analytics and Big Data to Support Population Health

Population health addresses the health status and health issues of aggregate populations. It brings significant health concerns into focus and addresses ways in which communities, health care providers, and public health organizations can allocate resources to overcome the problems that drive poor health conditions in the population, such as diabetes, obesity, heart disease, and so forth. Information technology is a part of the core infrastructure on which population health can be assessed and addressed. As organizations transition from the traditional fee-for-service model to value-based payment models (including ACOs), data, information, and knowledge about populations rather than individual patients will be required (HIMSS, 2017). Population health analytics can help organizations identify patients at risk of needing additional assistance to manage their health.

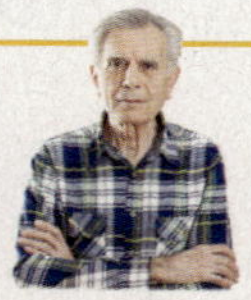

Recall **Frank**, the 72-year-old with COPD from the beginning of the chapter. Population health analytical tools would identify him as being high risk based on data pulled and trended from his record and possibly from other available data sources such as Medicare claims and pharmacy data.

Pulling data together from Medicare and other payor claims and data in the EHR can help predict which patients are at risk for readmission as well as locate patients who are receiving care outside of an organization's network. With this information, care managers can intervene appropriately and target those patients for whom resources will have the greatest impact. An example of the use of analytics to support population health can be seen in Figure 21-3.

Telehealth and Mobile Technologies

Perhaps the most accurate term for this section would be "broadband-enabled health care–related interactions," but the terms *telehealth*, *telemedicine*, and *telecare* are more popular and easier to remember, and all three terms are used. Telehealth seems to be the most commonly used term, as it represents a broad range of interactions, but we sometimes hear all three terms used interchangeably (Fig. 21-4).

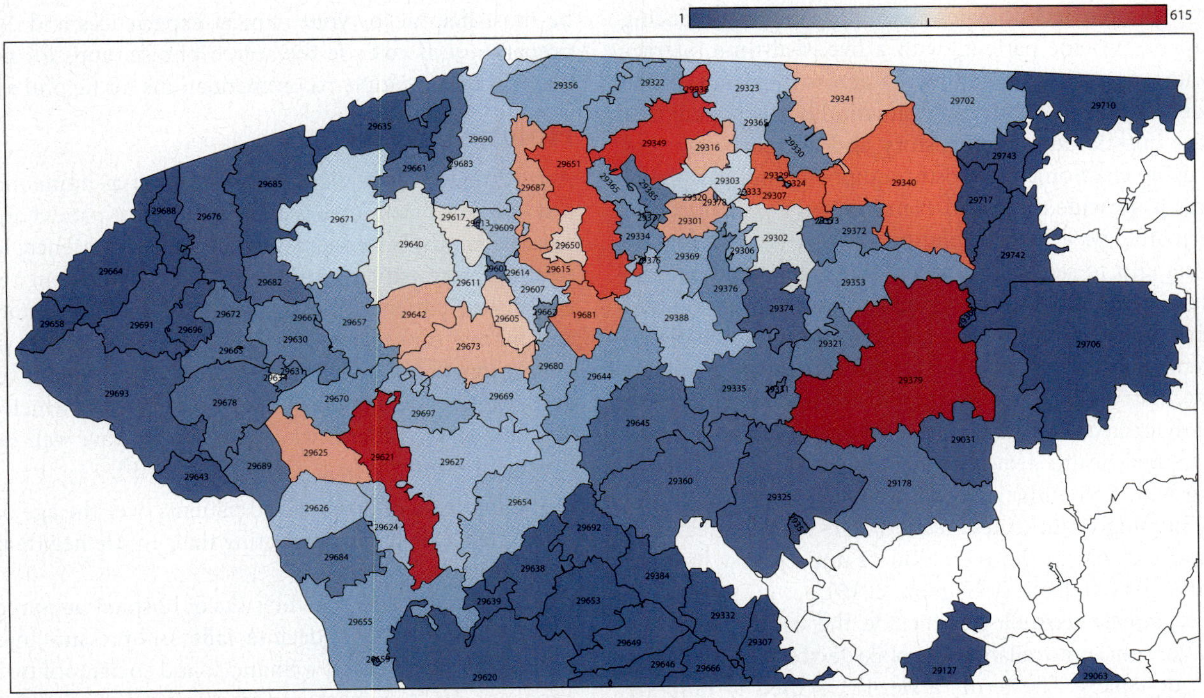

FIGURE 21-3. This example of data visualization illustrates the geographic location (zip codes in South Carolina) for all the patients from an accountable care organization (ACO) who have visited an emergency department (ED) because of the lack of availability of clinics or urgent care centers. The darker red areas indicate the greatest numbers of ED visits and help to provide the information needed by organizations to determine optimal placement of community outreach and establishment of care facilities. (*Source:* Adapted from Bon Secours Health System and Akbar Khan, 2017.)

The Health Resources and Services Administration (HRSA) of the U.S. Department of Health and Human Services defines **telehealth** as "the use of electronic information and telecommunications technologies to support and promote long-distance clinical health care, patient and professional health-related education, public health, and health administration. Technologies include videoconferencing, long distance imaging review, streaming media, and terrestrial and wireless communications" (HRSA & Federal Office of Rural Health Policy, 2015). Telehealth can involve more than just clinical services; it can also include remote nonclinical services such as provider training, administrative meetings, and continuing medical education.

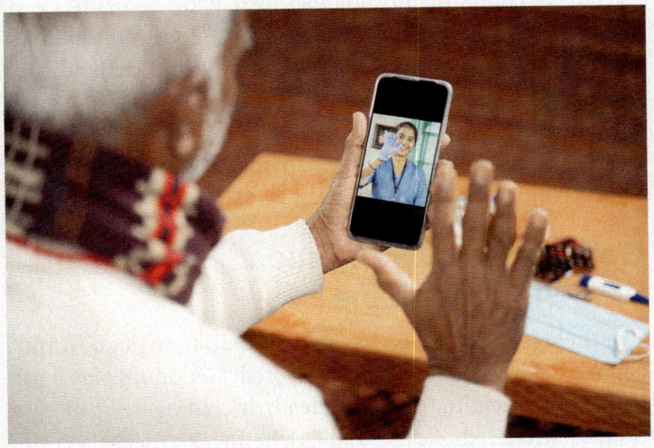

FIGURE 21-4. This nurse is using a telehealth visit to check up on a patient in his home. During the COVID-19 pandemic, he was reluctant to come to the clinic in the hospital. (*Source:* Used with permission form Shutterstock. *Photo by lakshmiprasada S.*)

The Federal Communications Commission defines **telemedicine** as the use of telecommunications technologies to support the delivery of all types of medical, diagnostic, and treatment-related services, usually by physicians or nurse practitioners. Examples include conducting diagnostic tests, monitoring a patient's progress after treatment or therapy, and facilitating access to specialists that are not located in the same place as the patient. Telemedicine involves only remote *clinical* services (FCC, n.d.).

Telecare generally refers to technology that allows consumers to stay safe and independent in their own homes. It may include consumer-oriented health and fitness apps, sensors and tools that connect consumers with family members or other caregivers, exercise tracking tools, digital medication reminder systems, and early warning and detection technologies (FCC, n.d.).

Telehealth does not necessarily promote new health care services, but simply provides a new way to deliver existing health care services. One of the key advantages of telehealth is allowing patients to remain in their communities while being seen by a health care provider at a remote site. Telehealth saves time and money for patients and reduces the time that patients are away from work. It also plays a more important role as we move away from the traditional fee-for-service system and toward new models of care, including Accountable Care Organizations (ACOs), PCMHs, and other strategies that focus on outcomes. Telehealth technologies are becoming more widely available in the marketplace, much easier to use and implement, and much more affordable (Arellano & Gagnon, 2015).

There are many examples of innovative ways that telehealth is being used to improve care within all health care settings. Simple technologies, such as videoconferencing equipment, provide patients with a live, real-time interaction with a specialist across town or across the country. The provider is able to conduct an evaluation of the patient that includes questioning about history and current symptoms while using electronic diagnostic equipment and peripheral cameras to provide the visual examination. For example, in teledermatology, a high-resolution camera is used for the dermatologist to see a close-up view of the patient's wound or skin condition. Remote monitoring equipment used in home health care allows a nurse to monitor a patient's adherence to medications or vital sign and weight readings. Telepsychiatry is also being explored within skilled nursing facilities located in communities where psychiatrists and other mental health providers are limited. By visually connecting with a provider early to evaluate the patient in the skilled nursing facility, these technologies show a great deal of promise to aid in the reduction of unnecessary hospital readmissions (Arellano & Gagnon, 2015).

Other mobile technologies include the use of "apps" or applications that are available on mobile devices such as smartphones or tablets. The term "mHealth" is used to describe the rapidly evolving use of mobile technologies to track and improve health outcomes. Nurses, physicians, other care providers, and patients are using apps that enable quick and easy access to screens that provide information and can track progress. They often provide a communication platform that allows discussion among key stakeholders including between peers, patients with similar conditions, or care providers. These apps can be interactive and engage users in ways that a typical website cannot. In 2012, 85% of adults in the United States owned a mobile phone, with 53% of these phones categorized as smartphones with the ability to install apps. In addition, nearly 19% of U.S. adults who owned a smartphone had at least one health care–related application on their phone. The majority of these apps focus on tracking diet and/or physical activity (Boudreaux et al., 2014). The number of mobile phone users with a health-related app installed will continue to increase at a rapid pace. With over 40,000 health-related apps available, it is important to evaluate the credibility and reliability of the app prior to use. While there is no one standard methodology or tool to assess the quality of an app, there are some emerging tools and frameworks that can be used including:

1. Health On the Net Foundation (HON) (https://www.healthonnet.org)
2. Healthcare Information and Management System Society: Selecting a Mobile App: Evaluating the Usability of Medical Applications (http://www.himss.org/selecting-mobile-app-evaluating-usability-medical-applications-0)
3. Commonwealth Fund: Developing a Framework for Evaluating the Patient Engagement, Quality, and Safety of Mobile Health Applications (http://www.commonwealthfund.org/~/media/files/publications/issue-brief/2016/feb/1863_singh_framework_evaluating_mobile_health_apps_ib_v2.pdf)

As nursing apps are constantly changing, we recommend that you consult with your faculty about what apps will be most helpful for your clinical experiences and NCLEX preparation. If you use the search phrase "apps for nurses," you will find multiple recommendations for helpful apps.

Hospital at Home

According to Khoury (2021), the hospital-at-home model is just one way health care is evolving to meet patient and cultural demands, better access, equity, and experience. Ideally, treating more patients at home will save inpatient care for the sickest patients. Using telehealth, remote monitoring, and mobile care teams, hospital-at-home programs deliver quality inpatient care in the comfort of one's home. There are numerous benefits to hospital-at-home models which target medium acuity patients whose conditions have well-defined treatment protocols (e.g., COPD and CHF):

- About a third of hospitalized patients over the age of 65 experience delirium, impacting their future health and functioning.
- Older patients also run the risks of hospital-acquired infections, functional decline, falls, and pressure injuries.
- Hospitalization exacts a financial and social tool by keeping patients from work and family responsibilities.

While hospital at home is claimed to benefit patients, providers, and hospitals, there is no question that a major driver is the financial benefit to hospitals and systems who continue to struggle to staff their hospitals, especially the emergency rooms and acute care units. While there is a great opportunity for nurses to provide leadership in what can be an enhanced experience to thousands of patients across the country, nurses must always use their lens of human dignity and well-being to make sure that patients benefit from this shift in delivery models. What experience do you have with patients and families who have experienced hospital at home? Is this available in your area? Would you recommend this experience if asked?

Unique Nurse Identifiers

Nursing has always struggled to identify and quantify nursing contributions to quality patient outcomes since nurse-sensitive outcomes have been difficult to quantify. "Implementing a unique nurse identifier (UNI) to leverage across systems and technologies will provide evidence of nursing's value to patient care delivery from multiple data sources" (Beale et al., 2021, p. 21). A UNI is a defined code or series of characters that represent an individual nurse within healthcare technology systems and across health care organizations. See the accompanying Table 21-6 to better understand the benefits of UNIs.

Genetics and Genomics: Precision Medicine

The field of genomics has the potential to significantly change the way health care is delivered. Genomics play a role in 9 of the 10 leading causes of death, including heart disease, cancer, stroke, diabetes, and Alzheimer's disease (WHO, 2004). Because genomic health care is heavily dependent on data storage and interpretation, no other area is better suited than informatics to support this evolving work.

Table 21-6 Unique Nurse Identifiers

TERM	DEFINITION	EXAMPLE
Audit trail	Records show who accessed a computer system, when it was accessed, and what actions or operations were performed.	Data are found and displayed in a report about barcode medication administration use derived from the technology and documentation within the electronic health record (EHR).
Interoperability	Different systems, devices, applications, and technologies access, exchange, and use health information for seamless portability.	Interoperability between an IV smart pump and the EHR creates a seamless and closed loop for medication ordering, dispensing, administration, and documentation.
Master data	Consistent and uniform set of identifiers describes core entities (patients, nurses, doctors, hospitals, units) that comprise a health system.	A list of patients in the health system master patient index can be referenced within all technologies and systems.
Meta data	Technology user footprint is created behind the scenes, showing what changes were made in an EHR, who made them and when, as well as what parts of a record were reviewed, for how long, how often, and by whom.	When a user marks a new lab value in a system as "reviewed," the system captures who the user was along with the date and time the reviewed button was selected. Similarly, when an order is marked as signed in the EHR, the user who signed the order is captured, along with the date and time the order was placed.
System integration	Design or construction of an application or technology to incorporate with new or existing hardware or software.	Clinical content from a vendor, such as clinical references or patient education material, are integrated into the EHR.

Source: Used with permission from Beale, N., Carroll, W., Aldrich, K., Alexander, S., Baernholdt, M., & Fields, W. (2021). What a unique nurse identifier means for the future. *American Nurse Journal, 16*(9), 21–24.

Genomics, or genomic medicine, is defined by the National Human Genome Research Institute (NHGRI) as "an emerging discipline that involves using genomic information about a person as part of their clinical care (e.g., for diagnostic or therapeutic decision making) and the other implications of that clinical use" (NHGRI, 2012). The World Health Organization differentiates the study of genetics and genomics in that genetics scrutinizes the functioning and composition of the single gene whereas genomics addresses all genes and their interrelationships in order to identify their combined influence on the growth and development of the organism.

Genomics can be used to make a diagnosis to assist in treatment decisions or to screen for risks for the development of certain diseases. This screening, or carrier testing, is a type of genetic testing performed on people who display no symptoms for a genetic disorder but may be at risk for passing it on to their children. A carrier for a genetic disorder has inherited one normal and one abnormal allele for a gene associated with the disorder. A child must inherit two abnormal alleles, one copy from each parent, in order for symptoms to appear (FDA, 2015).

Pharmacogenomics uses information about a person's genetic makeup, or genome, to choose the drugs and drug doses that are likely to work best for that particular person. This new field combines the science of how drugs work, called pharmacology, with the science of the human genome. Until recently, drugs have been developed with the idea that each drug works essentially the same at the prescribed dose for everyone. But genomic research has changed the "one-size-fits-all" approach and has opened the door to more personalized approaches to using and developing drugs. Some drugs may work differently in one person than in another, depending on a person's genetic makeup. Likewise, some drugs may produce more or fewer side effects depending on a person's gene expression. As the body of evidence grows, practitioners will be able to routinely use information about a patient's genetic makeup to choose the most effective and safe drugs (FDA, 2015).

EHR vendors are developing the ability to capture a patient's genetic information in the medical record. Standard terminologies to represent genetic information and gene variants in an electronic system will be imperative to ensure consistency across all care settings and throughout the patient's lifetime. Similar to alerts and reminders for allergies that appear when ordering medications, alerts can be configured in an EHR to notify providers that a genetic test indicates a need to tailor a dosage.

The field of genomics is in its infancy, but we are starting to see examples of its spread to larger populations. For example, the proportion of women with a family health history of breast or ovarian cancer who received genetic counseling increased from 34.6% to 52.9% from 2005 to 2010 (ODPHP, 2017). Also, the Affordable Care Act covers genetic counseling as a preventive service with no out-of-pocket costs for women who have a family health history consistent with increased risk for *BRCA* mutations. And, in 2015, the U.S. Food and Drug Administration (FDA) authorized and approved marketing for a carrier test from genetics testing and analysis company 23andMe. Their Bloom syndrome carrier test is a direct-to-consumer genetic test that can determine whether a healthy person has a variant in a gene that could lead to their offspring inheriting the serious disorder (FDA, 2015). As genomics becomes gradually more mainstream, nurses will see more functionality built into clinical information systems to address personalized care based on a patient's genetic makeup. Exciting times!

Box 21-4 Examples of Pharmacogenomics in Action

- Before prescribing the antiviral drug abacavir for human immunodeficiency virus, doctors now routinely test HIV-infected patients for a genetic variant that makes them more likely to have a bad reaction to the drug.
- The breast cancer drug trastuzumab works only for women whose tumors have a particular genetic profile that leads to overproduction of a protein called HER2.
- The FDA is considering genetic testing for another blood thinner, clopidogrel bisulfate, used to prevent dangerous blood clots. Researchers have found that clopidogrel bisulfate may not work well in people with a certain genetic variant.
- Cancer is a very active area of pharmacogenomic research. Studies have found that the chemotherapy drugs gefitinib and erlotinib work much better in lung cancer patients whose tumors have a certain genetic change. On the other hand, research has shown that the chemotherapy drugs cetuximab and panitumumab do not work very well in the 40% of colon cancer patients whose tumors have a particular genetic change.

Source: From National Human Genome Research Institute (NHGRI). (2016). *Frequently asked questions about pharmacogenomics.* https://www.genome.gov/27530645

Box 21-4 lists some examples of pharmacogenomics in action.

REFLECTIVE PRACTICE LEADING TO PERSONAL LEARNING

Remember that the object of reflective practice is to look at an experience, understand it, and learn from it. As you begin to develop your expertise in informatics, reflect on your experiences—successes and failures—in order to improve your practice. How can you do it better next time? What did you learn today that can help you tomorrow? Begin your reflection by paying close attention to the following:

The cultivation of skill in informatics is a critical component of professional nursing. Perhaps the most important questions to reflect on are: Are your patients and their families/caregivers better for having had *you* share in the critical responsibility of planning, delivering, and evaluating quality care? Are your patients now receiving thoughtful, person-centered, prioritized, holistic, evidence-based treatment and care because of your efforts?

DEVELOPING CLINICAL REASONING AND CLINICAL JUDGMENT

1. Does your organization use an EHR? If yes, does it use a standard terminology?
   Talk with professional nurses about their experiences with both paper and electronic health records and see what they believe are the advantages and disadvantages of both.
2. Your unit is encouraging you to discuss the use of patient portals with your patients and families during discharge planning. You understand that portals can deliver personal health information, online appointment scheduling, and personalized, condition-focused alerts and reminders in the form of e-mails, automated telephone calls, or text messages. You have never personally used a patient portal and aren't sure what to discuss in your discharge planning. What do you do?
3. You understand that your hospital and unit is far from reaching targeted rates on compliance with handwashing, which is resulting in an unacceptable number of hospital-acquired infections. Someone suggests that your nurse informaticist may be able to help you design and implement a solution. How might you be part of making this happen?

PRACTICING FOR NCLEX

1. A nurse informaticist is using the steps of the SDLC to design a new system for home health care documentation. The nurse analyzes the old system and develops plans for the new system. What step of this process will the nurse take next?
   a. Testing
   b. Designing
   c. Implementing
   d. Evaluating
2. After instituting a new system for recording patient data, a nurse evaluates the "usability" of the system. Which actions will the nurse include in this step? Select all that apply.
   a. Checking that the screens are formatted to allow for ease of data entry
   b. Reordering the screen sequencing to maximize effective use of the system
   c. Ensuring that the computers can be used by specified users effectively
   d. Checking that the system is intuitive and supportive of nurses
   e. Improving end-user skills and satisfaction with the new system
   f. Ensuring patient data is shareable across health care systems
3. A nurse is using informatics technology to determine which patients may be at risk for readmission. What term best describes this type of analytic?
   a. Data visualization
   b. Predictive analytics
   c. Big data
   d. Data recall

4. Nursing students enrolled in an informatics course question the purpose of "big data." Which statement do the students find best describes use of big data?
   a. Gathering data from multiple sources to help organizations answer questions and make predictions in multiple settings
   b. Predicting patients likely to be readmitted, allowing early intervention
   c. Promoting the most efficient staffing model for the organization
   d. Developing charts or graphs to visualize large amounts of complex data
5. A nurse incorporates use of the patient portal in the discharge teaching for a patient who received a kidney transplant. What services does the nurse explain are available with this technology? Select all that apply.
   a. Reviewing diagnostic and lab test results
   b. Making follow-up appointments
   c. Using health and fitness apps
   d. Entering clinical data, such as blood pressure
   e. Providing digital medication reminders
   f. Requesting prescription refills
6. A nurse is testing a new computer program designed to store patient data. During which phase of testing does the nurse determine whether the system can handle high volumes of end users and care providers using the system at the same time?
   a. Unit
   b. Function
   c. Integration
   d. Performance
7. Nurses test new technology in phases. When will the nurses plan to "test drive" the new system?
   a. Unit
   b. Function
   c. User acceptance
   d. Integration
8. A nurse is using the steps in informatics evaluation to assess a patient portal. Which activities might occur in the "determining the question" step? Select all that apply.
   a. Developing a clear, focused question to determine the data to be collected
   b. Determining what to evaluate
   c. Determining how the data ultimately should be reported
   d. Deciding what specific data elements need to be collected
   e. Clarifying exactly how the data will be collected
   f. Performing comprehensive documentation of the data collected
9. When signing in to the electronic medical record, a nurse is prompted to change their password. Which best-practice guideline does the nurse use to formulate the new password?
   a. Password should be at least 8 characters long and unique.
   b. Passwords should be memorable and used in other applications.
   c. Date of birth makes an ideal password.
   d. Nurses should share their passwords with their nurse managers.
10. A nurse designing a new EHR system for a pediatric office follows usability concepts in system design. Which concepts are recommended in system design? Select all that apply.
    a. Users should not explore with forgiveness for unintended consequences.
    b. Shortcuts for frequent users should not be incorporated into the system.
    c. Content emphasis should be on information needed for decision making.
    d. The less times users need to apply prior experience to a new system the better.
    e. All the information needed should be presented to reduce cognitive load.
    f. The number of steps it takes to complete tasks should be minimized.
11. A nurse wants to be an ethical practitioner. When using informatics, which action best represents ethical practice?
    a. Selecting appropriate standardized care plans to meet the patient's needs
    b. Gathering data for research studies using the electronic health record of multiple patients
    c. Maintaining confidentiality of patient records within legal and regulatory parameters
    d. Carrying out all electronic orders entered by the health care provider
12. During a feedback session on the updates to the electronic health record, nurses complain that they must use standard terminology rather than enter "free text" data in their own words. How will the nurses developing the system explain the purpose of standardization?
    a. It leads to fewer spelling errors and less misrepresentation of data.
    b. It provides for easier retrieval of data for use.
    c. The program was designed this way, and we cannot change it.
    d. Standardization uses preselected terminology, reducing lawsuits.
13. A nursing student who is planning their career trajectory tells the nurse preceptor how much they enjoy working with the electronic health record and informatics. What type of graduate program could the preceptor suggest?
    a. Clinical nurse specialist
    b. Nurse leader
    c. Superuser
    d. Informatics nurse specialist (INS)

ANSWERS WITH RATIONALES

1. **b**. The SDLC focuses on the areas of Analyze and Plan, Design and Build, Test, Train, Implement, Maintain, and Evaluate. After analyzing and planning the new system, the nurse would move on to the design step in which the basic design of the new system is developed. The nurse would then test the system, train employees, and implement, maintain, and evaluate the new system in that order.
2. **a, c, d.** Usability refers to the extent to which a product can be used by specified users to achieve specified goals with effectiveness, efficiency, and satisfaction in a specified context of use. Checking that screens are formatted to allow ease of data entry, ensuring that computers can be used by specified users effectively, and checking that the system is intuitive and supportive of nurses are all tasks related to the "usability" of the system. Maximizing screen sequencing and improving end-user skills and satisfaction with the new system refer to optimization. The ability to share patient data across health care systems is termed interoperability.
3. **b.** Predictive analytics uses statistical techniques to analyze current and historical facts to make predictions about future or otherwise unknown events. This is used by health care organizations to identify patients who are at risk for readmission, allowing case managers to intervene. Data visualization presents data in a pictorial or graphical format for analysis. Big data comprises the accumulation of health care–related data from various sources, transforming the data to information, to knowledge, and ultimately to wisdom. Data recall is not a technical term for analytics.
4. **a.** As organizations transition from traditional fee-for-service models to value-based payment models, information about populations rather than individuals is needed. Big data comprises the accumulation of health care–related data from multiple sources, combined with new technologies that allow for the transformation of data to information for patient care regardless of setting. Sources of available data can include the EHR; medical devices such as monitors, ventilators, and smart pumps; radiology, laboratory, and pathology systems; wearable devices and home monitoring systems; financial databases; genomics; open sources; patient portals; and real-time location systems. Predictive analytics uses statistical techniques to make predictions about future or unknown events, such as patients who are at risk for readmission. Data visualization presents data in a pictorial or graphical format for analysis. The growing population of older adults with complex health needs and a potential understaffing are important but are not the driving force for the development of this technology.
5. **a, b, c, d, f.** The patient portal can streamline services by allowing access to medical history and other health information; facilitating completion of online forms and questionnaires; offering secure and convenient communication with providers; and having the ability to place request prescription refills, pay bills, review lab results, schedule appointments, receive reminders for screenings and immunizations, enter clinical data such as blood pressure, glucose levels, weight, and other activity tracking data, review progress notes, and access educational materials based on diagnosis or procedure.
6. **d.** Performance testing is technical and ensures proper functioning of the system and its ability to handle high volumes of care providers using the system at the same time. Unit testing is basic testing that occurs initially. Function testing uses test scripts to validate that a system is working as designed for one particular function. Integration testing uses test script to validate that a system is working as designed for a workflow that integrates multiple components of the system.
7. **c.** During the phase "user acceptance," the nurse would "test drive" the new system to ensure it's working as designed. Unit testing is basic testing that occurs initially. Function testing uses test scripts to validate that a system is working as designed for one particular function. Integration testing uses test script to validate that a system is working as designed for an entire workflow that integrates multiple components of the system.
8. **a, c.** The nurse develops a clear, focused question to determine the data to be collected and the nurse determines how the data ultimately should be reported during the "determine the question" step. The nurse determines what to evaluate during the step "determine what will be evaluated." The nurse decides what specific data elements need to be collected during the "determine the needed data" step. The nurse clarifies exactly how the data will be collected during the "determine the data collection method and sample size" step. The nurse performs comprehensive documentation of the data collected during the "document your outcome evaluation" step.
9. **a.** Passwords should contain 8 to 15 characters, never be shared or re-used, and be easy to remember but hard to guess. Using multifactor authentication and a password manager can help organize and protect information. The password should not be shared with the nurse manager or others.
10. **c, e, f.** When designing a system, content emphasis should be on information needed for decision making. All the information needed should be presented to reduce cognitive load. The number of steps it takes to complete tasks should be minimized. The more users can apply prior experience to a new system, the lower the learning curve, the more effective their usage, and the fewer their errors. Forgiveness means that a design allows the user to discover it through exploration without fear of disastrous results or unintended consequences. Minimizing the number of steps needed to complete tasks and to provide shortcuts for use by frequent and/or experienced users facilitates efficient user interactions.
11. **c.** The ANA asserts ethical use of informatics principles, standards, and methodologies to establish and maintain health care consumer confidentiality be used within legal and regulatory parameters.
12. **b**. Using standard terminology in the electronic health record allows data to be easily retrieved and better captures nursing's contribution to care delivery and patient outcomes. For example, to capture all patients using canes, quad canes, and walkers, a common phrase such as "uses assistive device" allow data for all these mobility issues to be captured.
13. **d.** The INS is a registered nurse with formal graduate-level education in informatics. This nurse participates in strategy development, implementation, and maintenance and evaluation of clinical systems, in collaboration with multiple disciplines. The information nurse (IN) is a registered nurse with an interest or experience in informatics, who can assist with the implementation of the EHR or other types of informatics. "Superusers," often trained on the job, assist others to navigate the EHR. The clinical nurse specialist and nurse leader are patient care focused leadership roles.

Bibliography

American Medical Informatics Association (AMIA). (2009). *Nursing informatics work group: Nursing informatics defined.* https://www.amia.org/programs/working-groups/nursing-informatics

American Nurses Association (ANA). (2015). *Nursing informatics: Scope and standards of practice* (2nd ed.). Author.

Arellano, M., & Gagnon, R. (2015). Informatics in non-acute care settings. In P. Sengstack & C. Boicey (Eds.). *Mastering informatics: A healthcare handbook for success.* Sigma Theta Tau International.

Beale, N., Carroll, W., Aldrich, K., Alexander, S., Baernholdt, M., & Fields, W. (2021). What a unique nurse identifier means for the future. *American Nurse Journal, 16*(9), 21–24.

Belden, J. L., Grayson, R., & Barnes, J. (2009). *Defining and testing EMR usability: Principles and proposed methods of EMR usability evaluation and rating.* Healthcare Information and Management Systems Society.

Betts, H. J., & Wright, G. (2006). Lessons on evidence-based practice from Florence Nightingale. In C. A. Weaver, C. W. Delaney, P. Weber, & R. L. Carr (Eds.). *Nursing informatics for the 21st century: An international look at practice, trends and the future* (pp. 285–289). HIMSS.

Boicey, C. (2015). Healthcare analytics. In P. Sengstack & C. Boicey (Eds.). *Mastering informatics: A healthcare handbook for success.* Sigma Theta Tau International.

Boudreaux, E. D., Waring, M. E., Hayes, R. B., Sadasivam, R. S., Mullen, S., & Pagoto, S. (2014). Evaluating and selecting mobile health apps: strategies for healthcare providers and healthcare organizations. *Translational Behavioral Medicine, 4*(4), 363–371.

Carlson, S. (2015). Testing in the healthcare informatics environment. In P. Sengstack & C. Boicey (Eds.). *Mastering informatics: A healthcare handbook for success.* Sigma Theta Tau International.

Carroll, W. M. (2020). How blockchain can improve nursing. *Nursing, 50*(8), 62–63.

Carroll, W. M. (2021). *Emerging technologies for nurses: Implications for practice.* New York: Springer.

Charles, D., Gabriel, M., & Searcy, T. (2015). *ONC: Adoption of electronic health record systems among U.S. non-federal acute care hospitals: 2008–2014.* https://www.healthit.gov/sites/default/files/data-brief/2014HospitalAdoptionDataBrief.pdf

Dykes, P. C., Rozenblum, R., Dala, A., Massaro, A., Chang, F., Clements, M., Collins, S., Donze, J., Fagan, M., Gazarian, P., Hanna, J., Lehmann, L., Leone, K., Lipsitz, S., McNally, K., Morrison, C., Samal, L., Mlaver, E., Schnock, K., … Bates, D. W. (2017). Prospective evaluation of a multifaceted intervention to improve outcomes in intensive care: The Promoting respect and ongoing safety through patient engagement communication and technology study. *Critical Care Medicine, 45*(8), e806–e813.

Emerging Future, LLC. (2012). *Estimating the speed of exponential technological advancement in five years, ten years, twenty years, thirty years, forty years, fifty years.* http://theemergingfuture.com/docs/Speed-Technological-Advancement.pdf

Erickson, L., Hunt, C., & Blizzard, P. (2017). Leveraging technology to improve care and patient outcomes. *American Nurse Today, 12*(9), 71–72.

Federal Communications Commission (FCC). (n.d.). *Telehealth, telemedicine and telecare: What's what?* https://www.fcc.gov/general/telehealth-telemedicine-and-telecare-whats-what

Finn, D. S., & Dion, K. W. (2017). *Security tips for using personal technology.* From Reflections on Nursing Leadership. Sigma Theta Tau International website. http://www.reflectionsonnursingleadership.org/features/more-features/Vol43_1_security-tips-for-using-personal-technology

Food and Drug Administration (FDA). (2015). *FDA permits marketing of first direct-to-consumer genetic carrier test for Bloom syndrome.* https://www.fda.gov/news-events/press-announcements/fda-allows-marketing-first-direct-consumer-tests-provide-genetic-risk-information-certain-conditions

Gaisser, D. J., David, T., Rath, L., Clancy, G., Lawrence, C., Munoz-Rojas, D., Jones, U., & Smalls, J. (2021). International networking guidelines. *Nursing, 51*(7), 25–33.

Glassman, K. S. (2017). Using data in nursing practice. *American Nurse Today, 12*(11), 45–47.

Graves, J., & Corcoran S. (1989). The study of nursing informatics. *Journal of Nursing Scholarship, 21*, 227–231.

Hannans, J., & Olivio, Y. (2017). Craft a positive nursing digital identity with ePortfolio. *American Nurse Today, 12*(11), 48–49.

Healthcare Information and Management System Society (HIMSS) Usability Task Force. (2009). *Defining and testing EMR usability: Principles and proposed methods of EMR usability evaluation and rating.* https://www.researchgate.net/publication/277829258_Defining_and_Testing_EMR_Usability_Principles_and_Proposed_Methods_of_EMR_Usability_Evaluation_and_Rating

Healthcare Information and Management System Society (HIMSS). (2017). *Population health.* https://www.himss.org/

HealthIT.gov. (2015). *Meaningful use definition and objectives.* https://www.healthit.gov/providers-professionals/meaningful-use-definition-objectives

Health Resources and Services Administration (HRSA), Federal Office of Rural Health Policy. (2015). *Telehealth programs.* https://www.hrsa.gov/ruralhealth/telehealth/index.html

Houston, S. (2015). Healthcare system implementation. In P. Sengstack & C. Boicey (Eds.). *Mastering informatics: A healthcare handbook for success.* Sigma Theta Tau International.

Jordan, M. (2020). Cybersecurity awareness. *American Nurse Journal, 15*(2), 10–13.

Khoury, T. (2021). Hospital at home takes patient experience to new levels. https://www.vituity.com/blog/hospital-at-home-takes-patient-experience-to-new-levels/?%20utm_source=SBRIEF&utm_medium=BDOAD&utm_campaign=BD_2022_Q1_OAD%3ASBRIEF_eNewsletter_0208&utm_content=Blog-Hospitalat-Home-Koury

Khoury, T. (12/20/21). Hospital at home takes patient experience to new levels. https://www.vituity.com/blog/hospital-at-home-takes-patient-experience-to-new-levels/?%20utm_source=SBRIEF&utm_medium=BDOAD&utm_campaign=BD_2022_Q1_OAD%3ASBRIEF_eNewsletter_0208&utm_content=Blog-Hospitalat-Home-Koury

Kim, L. (2020). Cybercrime, ransomware, and the role of the informatics nurse. *Nursing, 50*(3), 63–65.

Kulhanek, B. (2015). Delivering healthcare informatics training. In P. Sengstack & C. Boicey (Eds.). *Mastering informatics: A healthcare handbook for success.* Sigma Theta Tau International.

Matney, S., Brewster, P. J., Sward, K. A., Cloyes, K. G., & Staggers, N. (2011). Philosophical approaches to the nursing informatics data-information-knowledge-wisdom framework. *Advances in Nursing Science, 34*(1), 6–18.

National Human Genome Research Institute (NHGRI). (2012). *NHGRI definition of 'genomic medicine.'* https://www.ncbi.nlm.nih.gov/pmc/articles/PMC5064852/#:~:text=As%20defined%20by%20the%20National,and%20rare%20and%20undiagnosed%20diseases.

National Institute of Standards and Technology (NIST). (2017). *Health IT usability.* https://www.nist.gov/programs-projects/health-it-usability

Nursing Knowledge. (2016). Big data science. *Conference Proceedings, June 1–3, 2016. Sponsored by the University of Minnesota.* https://www.nursingbigdata.org/sites/default/files/2021-04/nkbds-proceedings-2016.pdf

O'Brien, R. L., & O'Brien, M. W. (2021). Nursing orientation to data science and machine learning. *American Journal of Nursing, 121*(4), 32–39.

Office of Disease Prevention and Health Promotion (ODPHP). (2017). *Healthy People 2020: Genomics.* https://www.healthypeople.gov/2020/topics-objectives/topic/genomics

Office of the National Coordinator for Health Information Technology (ONC). (2009). *Policy making, regulation & strategy. Health IT legislation and regulations.* http://www.healthit.gov/policy-researchers-implementers/health-it-legislation-and-regulations

Office of the National Coordinator for Health Information Technology (ONC). (2015a). *Office based physician electronic health record adoption.* https://dashboard.healthit.gov/quickstats/pages/physician-ehr-adoption-trends.php

Office of the National Coordinator for Health IT (ONC). (2015b). *Connecting health and care for the nation: A shared nationwide interoperability roadmap.* https://www.healthit.gov/sites/default/files/hie-interoperability/nationwide-interoperability-roadmap-final-version-1.0.pdf

Office of the National Coordinator for Health IT (ONC). (2016). *Strategies for improving patient engagement through health IT.* https://www.healthit.gov/playbook/pdf/improving-patient-engagement-through-health-it.pdf

Office of the National Coordinator for Health IT (ONC). (2017). *Standard nursing terminologies: A landscape analysis.* https://www.healthit.gov/sites/default/files/snt_final_05302017.pdf

Ozkaynak, M., Unertl, K., Johnson, S., Brixeyk, J., & Haque, S. (2016). Clinical workflow analysis, process redesign and quality improvements. In J. Finnell & B. Dixon. *Clinical informatics study guide.* Springer International Publishing.

Santa, D., & Roach, E. E. (2017). Using mobile technology during patient handoffs. *American Nurse Today, 12*(9), 84, 86–87.

Sengstack, P. (2015). Conducting quality healthcare IT outcome evaluations: Guidelines and resources. In P. Sengstack & C. Boicey (Eds.). *Mastering informatics: A healthcare handbook for success.* Sigma Theta Tau International.

Sengstack, P. (2016). Information system lifecycles in health care. In J. Finnell & B. Dixon (Eds.). *Clinical informatics study guide.* Springer International Publishing.

Settergren, T. (2015). Maintaining and optimizing a healthcare information system. In P. Sengstack & C. Boicey (Eds.). *Mastering informatics: A healthcare handbook for success.* Sigma Theta Tau International.

Singh, K., Drouin, K., Newmark, L. P., Rozenblum, R., Lee, J., Landman, A., Pabo, E., Klinger, E. V., & Bates, D. W. (2016). Developing a framework for evaluating the patient engagement, quality, and safety of mobile health applications. *Issue Brief (Commonwealth Fund), 5*, 1–11.

St. John, C. (2015). Designing a usable healthcare information system. In P. Sengstack & C. Boicey (Eds.). *Mastering informatics: A healthcare handbook for success.* Sigma Theta Tau International.

Topaz, M. (2013). Invited editorial: The Hitchhiker's Guide to nursing informatics theory: Using the Data-Knowledge-Information-Wisdom framework to guide informatics research. *Online Journal of Nursing Informatics (OJNI), 17*(3). http://ojni.org/issues/?p=2852

Welton, J. M., & Harper, E. M. (2016). Measuring nursing care value. *Nursing Economics, 34*(1), 7–14; quiz 15.

Whittenburg, L., & Jacobs, A. (2015). Use of standard terminologies in healthcare IT. In P. Sengstack & C. Boicey (Eds.). *Mastering informatics: A healthcare handbook for success.* Sigma Theta Tau International.

Wilson, M. L. (2017). Understanding the technology that supports population health programs. *American Nurse Today, 12*(10), 28–30.

World Health Organization. (2004). *WHO definitions of genetics and genomics.* https://www.who.int/news-room/questions-and-answers/item/genomics

UNIT IV

Developmentally Appropriate Care

The chapters in Unit IV focus on growth and development through the life cycle. By considering all aspects of the person, nurses provide health care oriented toward wellness and maximize each patient's strengths to reach their potential. (The influences of the family on growth and development are discussed fully in Chapter 4.)

Chapter 22 gives an overview of developmental concepts and theories necessary to understanding growth and development across the lifespan. Major theorists and their contributions to the understanding of psychosocial, physical, cognitive, moral, and spiritual development are described.

Chapter 23 considers the individual from conception through young adulthood. Influences on biological growth and development, as well as physiologic, cognitive, psychosocial, moral, and spiritual development, are discussed. Common health problems of each age group and the role of the nurse in health promotion and illness prevention for each age group are considered.

Chapter 24 discusses the adult years in early, middle, and older-adult stages. The benefits, challenges, and problems associated with normal and abnormal aging are considered. The nurse's role in health care for the adult continues to be important through older adulthood. The chapter ends with a look at the paradigm of aging and stereotypes of older adults. Gerontology and the health care system related to this field are discussed.

"Basic to any philosophy of nursing seems to be these three concepts: (1) reverence for the gift of life; (2) respect for the dignity, worth, autonomy, and individuality of each human being; (3) resolution to act dynamically in relation to one's beliefs."

Ernestine Wiedenbach (1900–1996), *a faculty member at Yale University School of Nursing, who developed her model of nursing from years of experience in various nursing positions.*

"The concern of nursing is with man in his entirety, his wholeness. Nursing's body of scientific knowledge seeks to describe, explain, and predict about human beings."

Martha Rogers (1914–1994), *a nationally renowned nurse theoretician, author, lecturer, and consultant, whose "theory of man" inspired tremendous creativity, research activity, and intellectual growth in the nursing profession.*

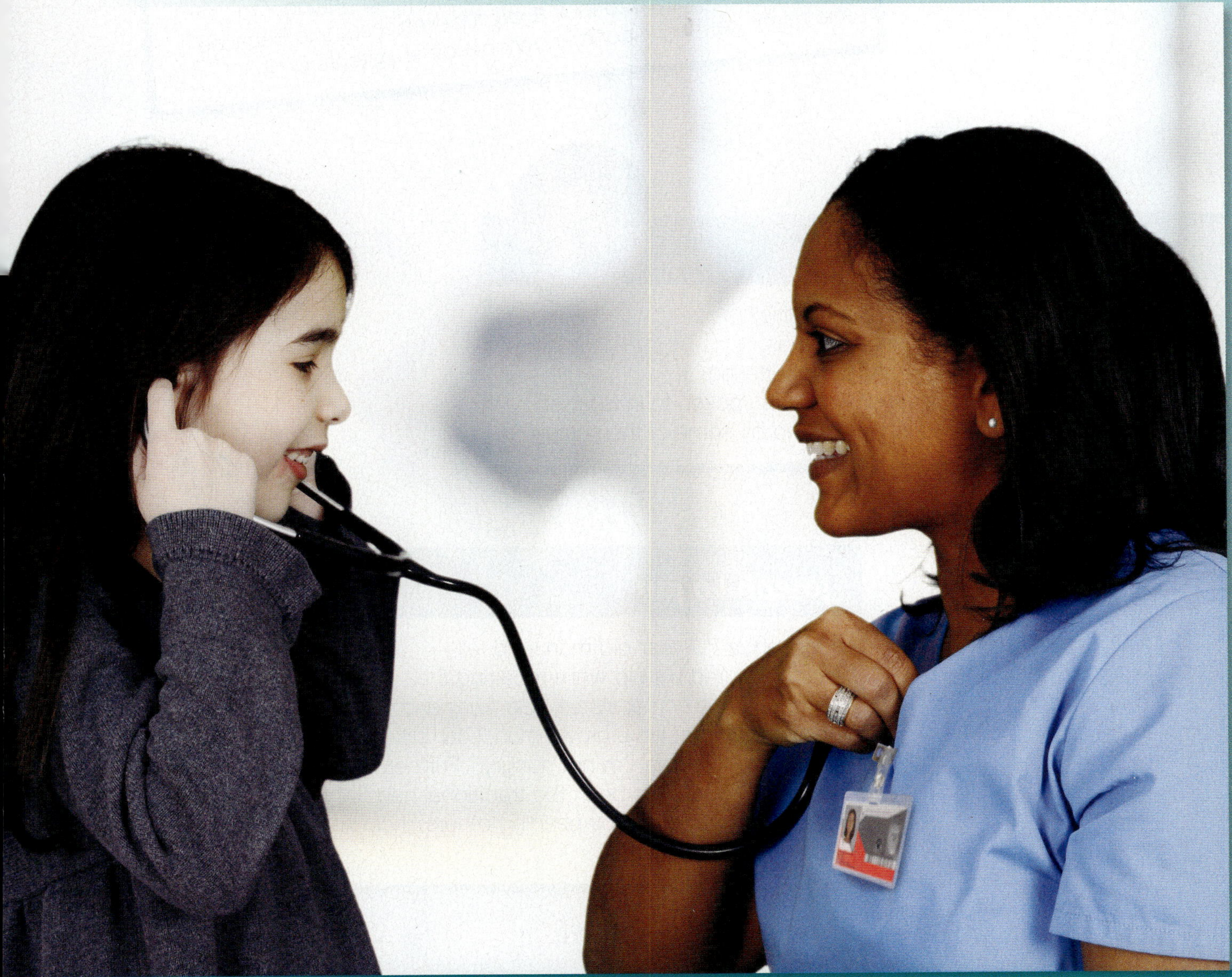

22 Developmental Concepts

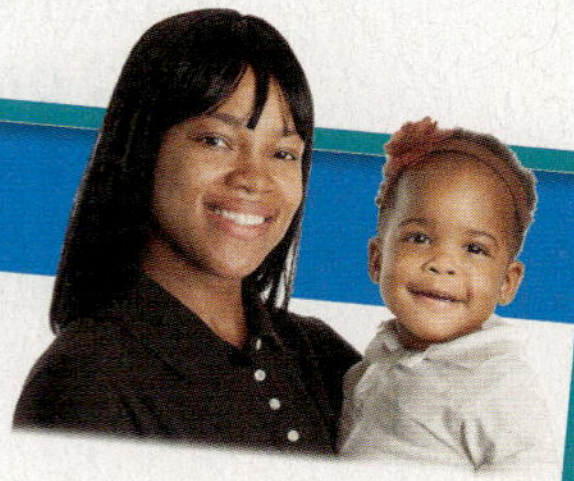

Melanie Kimber

Melanie, a 24-year-old single mother, voices concerns about rearing her 12-month-old daughter by herself. "She is just so active, putting toys in her mouth and getting into everything. I'm afraid to look away for even a second because she might get hurt. I don't know how other parents do it."

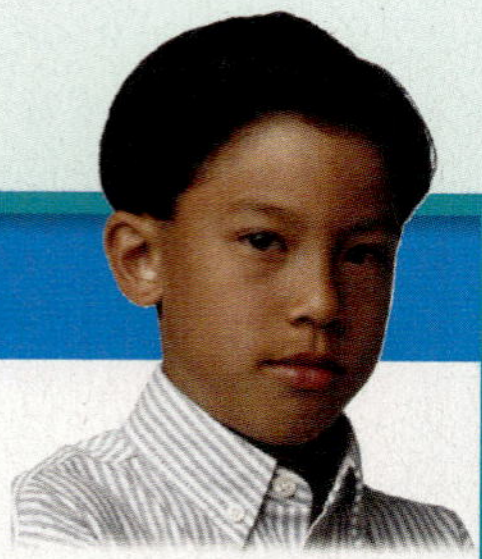

Juan Alvarez

Juan, an 8-year-old boy with encephalitis, becomes violent and combative at times, throwing himself against the bed and muttering words. He immediately calms down when spoken to in Spanish by both an interpreter who visits him and by some of the nurses.

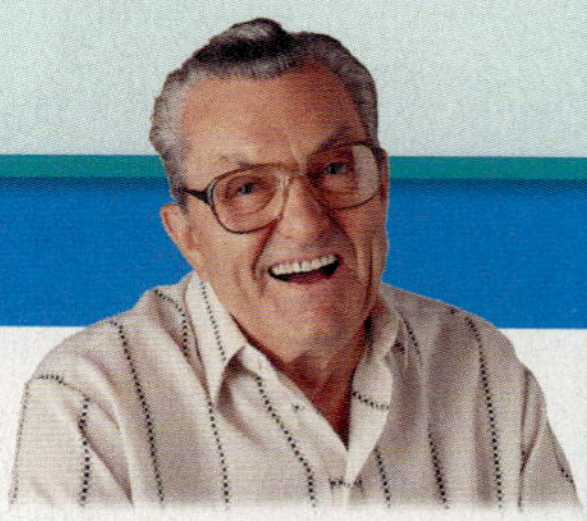

Joseph Logan

Joseph, a 70-year-old man who fell and fractured his hip while repairing the exterior of his home, states, "Go away and leave me alone. I'm a grown man, I can take care of myself … and get rid of this tray. I'm not hungry." Further investigation reveals that Mr. Logan has been the traditional head of his household and is now troubled by needing others, including his wife, to care for him.

Learning Outcomes

After completing the chapter, you will be able to accomplish the following:

1. Summarize basic principles of growth and development.
2. Identify the impact of genetics, genomics, and epigenetics/epigenomics on growth and development.
3. Discuss the theories of Freud, Erikson, Havighurst, Gould, Levinson, Piaget, Kohlberg, Gilligan, and Fowler.
4. Describe the importance of incorporating theories of growth and development in assessing and planning nursing care for individuals.
5. Explain implications for nursing practice based on an understanding of growth and development.

Nursing Concepts

- Development/human development
- Ethics
- Family
- Health promotion

Humans grow and develop throughout life. **Growth** is an increase in body size or changes in body cell structure, function, and complexity. **Development** is an orderly pattern of changes in structure, thoughts, feelings, or behaviors resulting from maturation, experiences, and learning. Development is a dynamic and continuous process as the individual progresses through life, characterized by a series of ascents, plateaus, and declines. The human processes of growth and development result from the interrelated effects of heredity and environment. Humans simultaneously grow and develop in physical, cognitive, psychosocial, moral, and spiritual dimensions. Each dimension represents an essential part of the whole person.

Nurses promote health in people from birth to death. All people, regardless of age, have unique health care needs that result from their physical, intellectual, emotional, sociocultural, spiritual, and environmental dimensions, which are influenced by their developmental level. To plan and give holistic and individualized care, the nurse must understand typical growth and development characteristics, tasks, and needs of patients of all ages. (See the accompanying Reflective Practice box on pages 576–577.)

This chapter presents theories and principles of growth and development across the lifespan that help us understand both healthy and ill people at various life stages. The major theories examining cognitive, psychosocial, spiritual, and moral development are discussed.

PRINCIPLES OF GROWTH AND DEVELOPMENT

Everyone's physical development has a predetermined genetic base because of inheritance patterns carried on the chromosomes. Thus, an unborn child begins life with specific physical attributes. Environmental factors from birth through the early years of growth provide initial psychological and social contact through positive or negative experiences with caregivers. As environmental influences expand beyond the immediate caregivers or family, development is influenced by a wide variety of psychosocial experiences as well as circumstances in the physical environment. Cognitive, moral, and spiritual developments are fostered through interactions within the family (as defined by the individual), school, and community.

The nurse can better understand these interrelated variables at specific life stages through theories of human growth and development. Growth and development are orderly and sequential as well as continuous and complex. All humans experience the same general growth patterns and developmental levels, but, because these patterns and levels are individualized, a wide variation in biological and behavioral changes is normal. Within each developmental level, certain milestones can be identified, such as the first time the infant rolls over, crawls, walks, or says their first words. Although growth and development occur in individual ways for different people, certain generalizations can be made about the nature of human development. These generalizations, outlined in Box 22-1 (on page 577), form the principles that help us understand growth and development.

FACTORS INFLUENCING GROWTH AND DEVELOPMENT

Many factors influence both growth and development. A person's growth and development may be facilitated or delayed by genetics; prenatal, individual, and caregiver factors; and environment and nutrition. Other factors influencing growth and development are health–illness state (discussed in Chapters 3, 4, 23, and 24) and culture (discussed in Chapter 5).

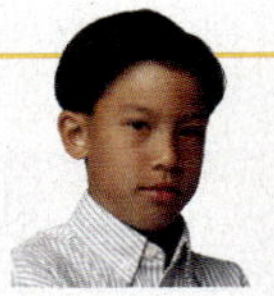

Think back to ***Juan***, the 8-year-old boy with encephalitis described at the beginning of the chapter. Although his behavior could be attributed to his infection, we have to consider social determinants of health when considering a child's lived experience.

Because of these often interrelated and interdependent factors, each person's growth and development is individualized. Scientists also continue to debate the idea of nature versus nurture, which considers the relative importance of the combined genes and environment that affect the development of a person.

Genetics, Genomics, and Epigenetics/Epigenomics

At conception, every human receives an equal number of chromosomes from each biological parent. The characteristics inherited from each parent are carried in gene pairs on

QSEN Reflective Practice: Cultivating QSEN Competencies

CHALLENGE TO ETHICAL AND LEGAL SKILLS

Two summers ago, while working in a nurse externship program, I worked with Juan, a Spanish-speaking 8-year-old boy diagnosed with encephalitis inflammation of the brain often secondary to viral or bacterial infection). The boy would become violent and combative at times, throwing himself against the bed and muttering words. Although the brain infection and inflammation could explain Juan's behavior, he became calm when a Spanish interpreter was with him. Juan also would appear calmer when nurses recognized his preferred language and attempted to speak Spanish. Unfortunately, most nurses and physicians would ignore Juan's screams in a language they did not understand, complain about his behavior, and rely on medication to calm him.

On one particular day, I was in the room with a physician who was writing an assessment note for Juan while I was getting Juan's bath water ready for morning care. As usual, Juan was muttering words and thrashing in the bed. I knew some measures to calm him; for example, I would try to use the few Spanish words I knew. The physician remained in her chair, looking at me and complaining about Juan's behavior, not making any effort to calm him. She said that she could not do anything to calm him down except prescribe sedative medications. I felt bad for the patient and knew he was frustrated. I knew that I could possibly help in this situation but did not want to show disrespect to the physician.

Thinking Outside the Box: Possible Courses of Action

- I could nod in agreement with the physician. After all, I was only a nursing student and appreciated that she certainly knew more than I did.
- I could tell her what measures I had used to help calm Juan.
- I could refrain from saying anything at all, wait until the physician had left, and then try to calm Juan.

Evaluating a Good Outcome: How Do I Define Success?

- The patient benefited from my actions.
- I did not disrespect the physician, and worked to develop a collaborative relationship with her.
- I was able to use my intuition, authority, and common sense to the best of my ability.
- Did I have the authority to jump in and give the physician advice on how to care for the patient?
- In this situation, my intuition and common sense told me to jump up and take action to provide compassionate care to Juan, who was frustrated and upset.

Personal Learning: Here's to the Future!

Unfortunately, in this situation, I did not respond as I would have liked to. I did not say anything, but watched Juan become upset and mutter Spanish words. During this whole time, the physician shook her head, looked down on him, and told me she just "couldn't do anything about him" except to give him medications. I waited until the physician left, and then tried to calm Juan myself. In this situation, I should have let the physician know about the methods used to calm Juan previously, which may have minimized the perceived or actual need for sedatives. However, as a junior level nursing student, I did not feel comfortable enough to use this type of authority. I now see how important it is for nurses and all staff members to communicate their opinions, beliefs, and observations about patients for the benefit of the patient. These suggestions and opinions need to be heard so that patients receive the best possible care. In the future, as a practicing nurse, I will respect my fellow staff members, but always make sure that my voice is heard concerning a patient's needs.

QSEN SELF-REFLECTION ON QUALITY AND SAFETY COMPETENCIES DEVELOPING KNOWLEDGE, SKILLS, AND ATTITUDES FOR CONTINUOUS IMPROVEMENT

How do you think you would respond in a similar situation? Why? What does this tell you about yourself and about the adequacy of your skills for professional practice? Can you think of other ways to respond or approach the situation? What *knowledge, skills,* and *attitudes* do you need to develop to continuously improve quality and safety when caring for patients like Juan?

Patient-Centered Care: Why was a third-party medical interpreter/translator not considered for Juan? What do you think Juan might have been experiencing and why? What if the nursing student had approached the physician about using other methods to calm Juan? Would you consider that action to be disrespectful? How do you think the physician would have responded to the nursing student's feedback about the use of the Spanish language to calm Juan? Would simply modeling the interventions and behavior that previously had worked with Juan provide cues for the physician?

Teamwork and Collaboration/Quality Improvement: Did the physician's age or gender impact on your decision making? What communication skills do you need to improve to ensure that you function as a member of the patient care team and minimize risk of harm to Juan? Would collaboration with your instructor or Juan's nurse have resulted in additional alternatives or another approach to communicate calmly and safely with Juan?

Safety/Evidence-Based Practice: Would Juan's stage of growth and development influence your nursing care? Do you think that the nursing student's stage of growth and development may have played a role in the student's response? Why or why not? Would an effort to identify common Spanish words and phrases and have them available to all caregivers make a difference? Are we missing cultural or other factors due to the language barrier? What evidence in nursing literature provides guidance for decision making

QSEN Reflective Practice: Cultivating QSEN Competencies *(continued)*

CHALLENGE TO ETHICAL AND LEGAL SKILLS

about methods to ensure a safe environment for a young child who does not understand English? How do we begin to assess and address social determinants of health related to Juan and his family and caregivers?

Informatics: Can you identify the essential information that needs to be included and documented in Juan's electronic record regarding efforts to communicate with him and give nursing care? Is it important to document your assessments and interventions? Can you identify any additional information that supports safe patient care and coordination of care? What technology can be used to ensure Juan has the medical interpreter/translator he may need? How can we ensure holistic care for Juan that takes into consideration individual and environmental factors?

the 23 pairs of chromosomes, which carry the genetic information that determines the person's cellular differentiation, growth, and function. As a result, physical characteristics such as height, bone size, and eye and hair color are inherited from our family of origin. Other characteristics, such as personality, are not as clearly identified with genetics, but research is ongoing in this area. Genetics also influences the development of many diseases, such as cancer and diabetes. **Heredity** is a term that is sometimes used interchangeably with genetics, but it more directly addresses the transmission of genetics, or what is passed down and inherited from generation to generation.

The Human Genome Project (HGP), completed in 2003, was an international 13-year collaborative research program whose goal was to map the genes in human DNA, determined to number approximately 20,500 by the HGP (National Human Genome Research Institute, 2020b). A **genome** is the complete set of DNA in an organism, including all its genes. You can appreciate the challenging complexity of the HGP when you consider that human DNA, developed from four different chemical building blocks called *bases*, involves approximately 3 billion bases arranged along the chromosomes in a particular order that is unique for each person (U.S. National Library of Medicine, 2021). The HGP deciphered the human genome by: (1) determining the order or sequence of all the bases in human DNA, (2) making maps that show the locations of genes on chromosomes, and (3) making linkage maps that track inherited traits over generations (National Human Genome Research Institute, 2020b). Another initiative, the 1000 Genomes Project (International Genome Sample Resource [IGSR], 2021), which ran between 2008 and 2015, provided the largest public catalog of human genome data available to date, while focusing on identifying genetic variances with frequencies of 1% or greater in the populations studied. These projects have led to the discovery of genetic sequencing and variants that provide valuable information regarding genomics.

Box 22-1 Principles of Growth and Development

Growth and development are orderly and sequential, as well as continuous and complex. All humans experience predictable growth patterns and developmental levels. Because these patterns and levels are complex and individualized, a wide variation in biological and behavioral changes is considered normal. Within each developmental level, certain milestones can be identified. For example, the timing of when the infant rolls over, crawls, walks, or talks is fairly predictable.

Growth and development follow regular and predictable trends. Cephalocaudal (proceeding from head to tail) development is the first trend, with the head and brain developing first, followed by the trunk, legs, and feet. The second trend is proximodistal development, which means that growth progresses from gross motor movements (such as learning to lift the head) to fine motor movements (such as learning to pick up a toy with the fingers). The last trend is symmetric development of the body, with both sides of the body developing equally.

Growth and development are both differentiated and integrated. As nerve pathways develop, they become more specialized, allowing the growing child to respond to different stimuli. Throughout the lifespan, each new learned ability builds on previously learned abilities so that increasingly complex tasks can be accomplished. For example, the toddler learning to use a spoon combines motor skills, hand–eye coordination, cognitive patterning, and social imitation from watching others. As children grow and develop, the task of learning to use a spoon becomes basic, forming the foundation for learning skills requiring more manual dexterity.

Different aspects of growth and development occur at different stages and at different rates and can be modified. For example, muscles and bones both grow most rapidly during the first year of life. During the toddler and preschool years, bone growth slows, but muscle fibers increase in size and strength. The most intense period of speech development is between 3 and 5 years of age. Sexual maturity begins during the preadolescent years and progresses into the adult years but is based on gender and sex role identity established from birth. Many factors can modify growth and development, including social determinants of health, love and affection from caregivers, and illnesses.

The pace of growth and development is specific for each person. Both physical and psychological skills and maturation vary among people. For example, while learning to walk, a child may concentrate energies on that task and temporarily lag in language development. In addition, a person's genetics places restrictions on the upper limits that can be achieved in growth.

QSEN INTERNATIONAL GENOME SAMPLE RESOURCE

The 1000 Genomes Project led to the creation of the IGSR to ensure access to the 1000 Genomes reference data, to track and incorporate additional published data on the existing populations, and to expand the project to populations not included in the original 1000 Genomes Project. This online database gives scientists access to data on genomes for research projects and is an excellent example of a high-quality electronic source that provides insight into the human genome.

Genomics is the study of the structure and interactions of all the genes in the human body, including their interactions with each other and the environment. Health care providers all over the world integrate genomics into their research, education, and practice (Office of Disease Prevention and Health Promotion, 2021). Genetic tests, coupled with family history tools, have the potential to identify people at risk for diseases. There are several emerging challenges related to genomic discoveries:

- Evidence-based review panels are needed to thoroughly evaluate the possible benefits and harms related to the expanding number of genetic tests and family health history tools.
- Valid and reliable national data are needed to establish baseline measures and track progress for populations while identifying disparities in their use and outcomes.
- Translating research recommendations into practice and policy requires specific knowledge of the topic and consideration of efficacy, equity, and transparency.
- Privacy and confidentiality must be considered when integrating genomic information into electronic health records (EHRs), clinical decision models, and education curricula (Office of Disease Prevention and Health Promotion, 2021).

Epigenetics is an emerging field of study that is still undergoing definition and refinement. First appearing in the 1940s, **epigenetics** is generally defined as the study of the changes that occur in organisms due to modification of gene expression and hereditability, not a change in the DNA sequence (Deans & Maggert, 2015; National Cancer Institute, 2020). One of the primary challenges when considering epigenetics is determining whether changes in gene expression are due to the inheritance of an expression state or another stimulus (Deans & Maggert, 2015). For example, **epigenomics**—epigenetic changes that occur in many genes or the entire organism—considers whether smoking, which affects how genomes are expressed in the person who smokes, also affects offspring of the person who smokes (National Cancer Institute, 2020; National Human Genome Research Institute, 2020a). Social epigenomics considers social determinants of health, specifically adverse social and environmental experiences in childhood and their relationship to the development of dysfunctional physiologic changes later in life (National Cancer Institute, 2020). See Chapter 3 for more on the social determinants of health.

Nurses must be prepared to answer questions and discuss the impact of genetic findings on health and illness. Advances in genetics and genomics affect everyday nursing practice in areas such as screening, diagnoses, treatment plans, and pharmacogenomics, as well as lifestyle choices and associated ethical challenges (American Nurses Association [ANA], n.d.). Resources for genetic technology and information are included in Box 22-2.

Box 22-2 Genetic Technology and Information Resources

American Academy of Pediatrics (AAP)

Council on Genetics (COG), https://www.aap.org/en/community/aap-councils/genetics/. Provides information about genetic testing and counseling for providers and patients.

American Nurses Association (ANA)

Ethics topics and articles, genetics, and personalized medicine, https://www.nursingworld.org/practice-policy/nursing-excellence/ethics/genetics/. Provides current publications and resources focused on genetics and genomics, with a focus on education and ethical issues.

International Society of Nurses in Genetics (ISONG)

https://www.isong.org/. Focused on supporting the professional growth of nurses with respect to human genetics and genomics in practice, education, and research; global perspective; precision medicine.

United States Surgeon General

My Family Health Portrait: https://www.cdc.gov/genomics/famhistory/knowing_not_enough.htm, from the Surgeon General. Aids in construction of a family health history, including risks for conditions that run in the family.

National Human Genome Research Institute (NHGRI)

www.genome.gov. Provides continued access to data obtained from the HGP, information about genetic services, and access to relevant research.

National Institutes of Health (NIH)

Genetic Testing Registry (GTR): http://www.ncbi.nlm.nih.gov/gtr. Serves as a repository for patient-submitted data on genetic conditions, genes, and labs; provides resources.

National Society of Genetic Counselors (NSGC)

Find a Genetic Counselor: http://www.nsgc.org/page/find-a-gc-search. Locates genetic nurse counseling services according to zip code location, and provides patient information, policies, and publications.

Prenatal, Individual, and Caregiver Factors

Fetal development can be affected by maternal age (with greater risk in pregnant persons younger than 15 years of age and those older than 35 years of age), inadequate prenatal care, inadequate maternal nutrition, and maternal substance use disorder. Individual factors that can affect development from birth through adolescence include congenital or genetic disorders, brain damage from accidents or abuse, vision and hearing impairments, chronic illness, inadequate nutrition, chemotherapy or radiation therapy, lead poisoning, poverty, and substance abuse. Caregiver factors that negatively affect development include neglect and abuse, mental illness, intellectual disabilities, and severe learning disabilities.

Environment and Nutrition

Environment and nutrition influence all stages of development. Environmental factors that may alter development include social determinants of health such as poverty, violence, unsafe living conditions, the presence of lead or mold in the home, and the quality of air and water in the surrounding environment. Environmental and nutritional effects can occur independently, but they are more likely to be interrelated, as seen in these examples:

- Infants who are malnourished in utero develop fewer brain cells than infants who have had adequate prenatal nutrition.
- Substance use disorder by a pregnant person increases the risk for congenital anomalies, low birth weight, and prematurity in the developing fetus.
- Failure to thrive, a condition of early infancy, has been linked to both nutritional and emotional deprivation.
- Environmental challenges, such as substandard housing and inadequate medical care, can compound the effects of poor nutrition.
- Child abuse, which is an extreme example of physical and emotional harm or deprivation, leads to deficits in physical or psychosocial development, or both.
- Substance use disorder by adolescents and young adults is associated with an increased incidence of teenage pregnancy, violence, accidents, and suicide. Abuse of alcohol and drugs is more prevalent in teenagers who have poor family relationships, low self-esteem, and poor social skills.
- Nutritional influences such as overeating and inactivity as well as genetic factors are directly related to obesity.

OVERVIEW OF CLASSIC DEVELOPMENTAL THEORIES

Human development and behavior have been studied since the beginning of the 20th century. Many theories seek to explain typical human responses at specific ages and stages of life. Although a psychological approach is common to most developmental theories, each theory has a different focus. The theories discussed in the following sections examine cognitive, social, and instinctual influences on human growth and development, with key points summarized in Table 22-1 (on page 580).

Theory of Psychoanalytic Development

Sigmund Freud

Freud's theory emphasizes the effect of instinctual human drives on behavior. Freud identified the underlying stimulus for human behavior as sexuality, which he called *libido.* Libido is defined as general pleasure-seeking instincts rather than purely genital gratification.

The four major components of the mind according to Freud's theory are the unconscious mind, the id, the ego, and the superego:

- The *unconscious mind* contains memories, motives, fantasies, and fears that are not easily recalled but that directly affect behavior.
- The *id* is the part of the mind concerned with self-gratification by the easiest and quickest available means. *Defense mechanisms* are a means of unconscious coping to reduce stress in the conscious mind when the id's impulses cannot be satisfied. (Defense mechanisms are discussed in Chapter 43.)
- The *ego* is the conscious part of the mind that serves as a mediator between the desires of the id and the constraints of reality so that a person can live effectively within their social, physical, and psychological environment. The ego includes intelligence, memory, problem solving, separation of reality from fantasy, and incorporation of experiences and learning into future behavior. Freud noted that the death of a loved one can result in the loss of a person's sense of identity, but once the loss is accepted, the ego is able to reconcile the loss and search for new attachments. Development of the ego allows the infant, by age 6 months, to view self as separate from others and to begin to alter behaviors in response to cues. Ego development continues throughout life.
- The *superego* is the part of the mind commonly called the conscience. It develops from the ego during the first year of life, as the child learns praise versus punishment for actions. The superego represents the internalization of rules and values so that socially acceptable behavior is practiced.

Each of the following developmental stages typically involves certain issues; any unresolved issues can persist into adulthood. Freud's work describes sexuality (including sex, gender, and sexual orientation) through a heteronormative lens.

ORAL STAGE (AGES BIRTH TO 18 MONTHS)

During the oral stage, the infant uses the mouth as the major source of gratification and exploration. Pleasure is experienced from eating, biting, chewing, and sucking. The infant's primary need is for security. A major conflict occurs with weaning.

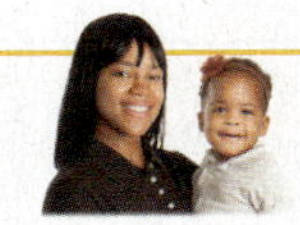

Recall **Ms. Kimber**, the young, single, frustrated mother of a 12-month-old child. The nurse might apply the concepts of Freud's theory in the nursing care of Ms. Kimber and her child by explaining the oral behaviors typical of the stage of her child's development.

Table 22-1 Key Points of Developmental Theories: Instinctual, Cognitive, and Social

	FREUD PSYCHOSEXUAL	PIAGET COGNITIVE	ERIKSON PSYCHOSOCIAL[a]	HAVIGHURST DEVELOPMENTAL
Infancy to toddlerhood	*Oral stage:* Focus on sucking, biting, chewing, and swallowing *Anal stage:* Focus on bowel and bladder control; anus becomes the center of gratification	*Sensorimotor stage:* Basic reflexes; coordinates more than one thought at a time; begins to reason and anticipate events	*Trust versus mistrust (infant):* Uncertainty; development of hope *Autonomy versus shame and doubt (toddler):* Exploration of the limits of abilities; development of will	Learning to walk; learning to talk; learning to control body waste elimination
Preschool to early school years	*Phallic stage:* Resolving Oedipal/Electra complex	*Preoperational stage:* Increased language; increased understanding of life events and relationships	*Initiative versus guilt:* Development of interpersonal skills through activities with others; development of purpose	Learning sex differences; forming concepts; getting ready to read
School years	*Latent stage:* No meaningful focus	*Concrete operational stage:* Develops logical thinking; incorporates others' perspectives *Formal operational stage:* Adopts life-guiding values or religious practices; uses abstract thinking and deductive reasoning; tests beliefs to establish values	*Industry versus inferiority:* Self-esteem based on feedback from others; development of competence	Learning physical skills; learning to get along with others; developing conscience and morality; developing fundamental skills in reading, writing, and math; developing concepts related to everyday living; achieving personal independence; developing attitudes toward social groups, institutions, and toward oneself
Adolescent to adult years	*Genital stage:* Reaching full sexual maturity		*Identity versus role confusion (adolescence):* Exploration for personal identity and a sense of self; development of fidelity *Intimacy versus isolation (young adulthood):* Development of happy relationships and a sense of commitment, safety, and caring; development of love	Achieving a gender role; achieving emotional independence; acquiring a set of values and an ethical system to guide socially responsible behavior; preparing for marriage, a family life, and a career
Middle adult years			*Generativity versus stagnation:* Establishment of career, relationships, family, and societal engagement; development of care	Achieving social and civic responsibility; accepting and adjusting to physical changes
Later adult years			*Ego integrity versus despair:* Change in productivity goals and evaluation of success; development of wisdom	Adjusting to decreasing physical status and health; adjusting to retirement

[a]Developmental goals identified by McLeod (2018).

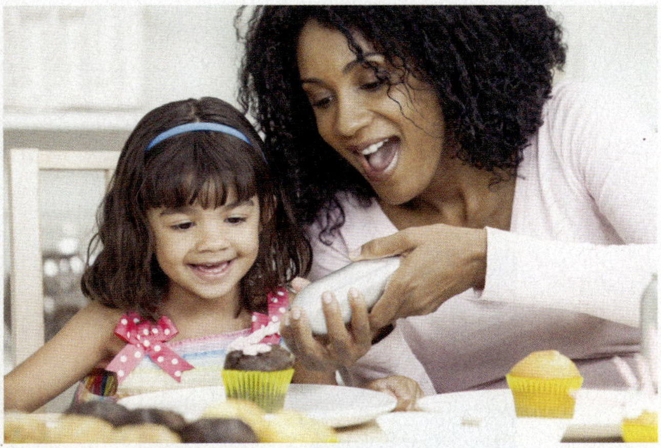

FIGURE 22-1. Sharing baking experiences allows this preschool girl to imitate activities that she often sees her mother enjoy.

ANAL STAGE (AGES 8 MONTHS TO 3 YEARS)

This stage begins with the development of neuromuscular control to allow control of the anal sphincter. Toilet training is a crucial issue that requires delayed gratification as the child compromises between enjoyment of bowel function and limits set by social expectations.

PHALLIC STAGE (AGES 3 TO 7 YEARS)

The child has increased interest in sex differences and in their own sex (Fig. 22-1). The child experiences conflict and resolution of that conflict with the parent of the same sex (named the *Oedipus complex* in boys and the *Electra complex* in girls, based on feelings of intimate sexual possessiveness for the opposite-sex parent). Curiosity about the genitals and masturbation increases during this stage.

LATENCY STAGE (AGES 7 TO 12 YEARS)

This stage marks the transition to the genital stage during adolescence. Increasing sex-role identification with the parent of the same sex prepares the child for adult roles and relationships.

GENITAL STAGE (AGES 12 TO 20 YEARS)

At this stage, sexual interest can be expressed in overt sexual relationships. Sexual pressures and conflicts typically cause turmoil as the adolescent makes adjustments in relationships.

Theory of Cognitive Development

Jean Piaget

Piaget and Inhelder (1969) developed a theory of **cognitive development** from infancy through adolescence. Piaget believed that learning occurs as a result of the internal organization of an event in which a mental schema (plan) is formed and serves as a base for further schemata as one grows and develops. Intellectual growth is a continual restructuring of knowledge to progress to higher levels of problem solving and critical thinking. Two continual processes of restructuring knowledge—assimilation and accommodation—stimulate intellectual growth in the child. **Assimilation** is the process of integrating new experiences into existing schemata. **Accommodation** is an alteration of existing thought processes to manage more complex information.

Piaget and Inhelder described four stages of cognitive development (although Piaget sometimes referred to three periods and combined the preoperational and concrete operational stages).

SENSORIMOTOR STAGE (BIRTH TO AGE 2 OR 3 YEARS)

This stage is marked by progression through a series of six substages with specific developmental tasks:

- Birth to 1 month: Demonstrates basic reflexes, such as sucking
- 1 to 4 months: Discovers enjoyment of random behaviors (such as smiling or sucking thumb) and repeats them
- 4 to 8 months: Relates own behavior to a change in environment, such as shaking a rattle to hear the sound or manipulating a spoon to eat
- 8 to 12 months: Coordinates more than one thought pattern at a time to reach a goal, such as repeatedly throwing an object on the floor; only objects in sight are considered permanent
- 12 to 18 months: Recognizes the permanence of objects, even if out of sight; can understand simple commands
- 18 to 24 months: Begins to develop reasoning and can anticipate events

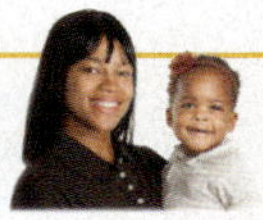

Recall **Ms. Kimber**, the single mother of a 12-month-old infant. Applying Piaget's theory, the nurse could develop a teaching plan for the mother that addresses appropriate anticipatory guidance to prevent injury while fostering the child's cognitive development.

PREOPERATIONAL STAGE (AGES 2 OR 3 TO 6 OR 7 YEARS)

This stage is characterized by the beginning use of symbols, through increased language skills and pictures, to represent the preschooler's world (Fig. 22-2 on page 582). This stage is divided into two parts: the preconceptual stage (ages 2 to 4 years) and the intuitive stage (ages 4 to 7 years). Play activities during this time help the child understand life events and relationships.

CONCRETE OPERATIONAL STAGE (AGES 6 OR 7 TO 11 OR 12 YEARS)

During this stage, children learn by manipulating concrete or tangible objects and can classify articles according to two or more characteristics. Logical thinking is developing, with an understanding of reversibility, relations between numbers, and loss of egocentricity that develops into the ability to incorporate another's perspective. Children become increasingly aware of external events and realize that their feelings and thoughts are unique and may not be the same as those of other children of their age. They have the ability to focus on multiple parts of a problem at the same time.

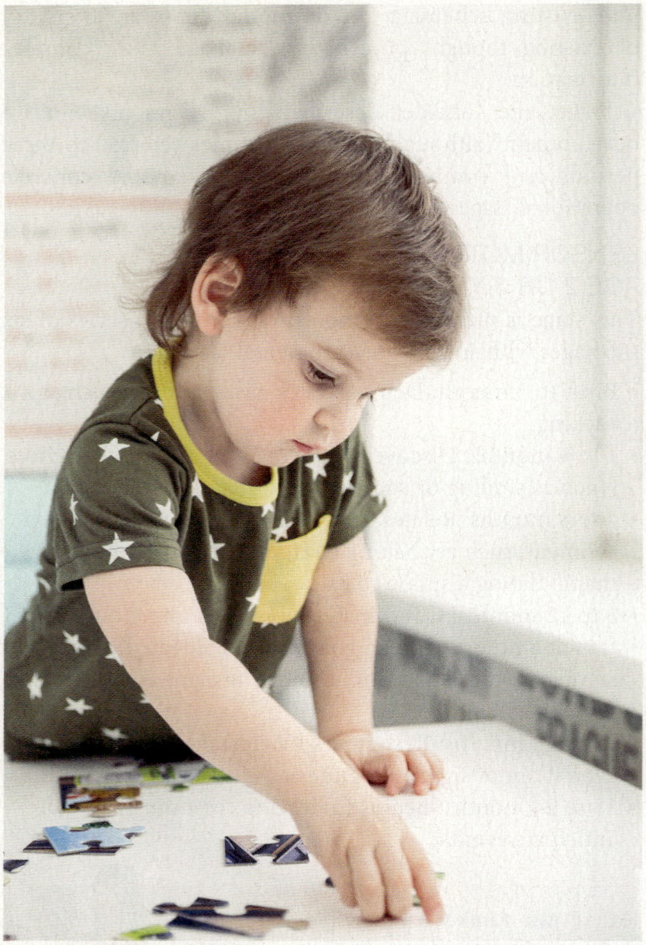

FIGURE 22-2. This child's cognitive development is characterized by the ability to learn simple sequences and relationships. (*Source: Photo by Yulia_B./Shutterstock.*)

FORMAL OPERATIONAL STAGE (AGES 11 OR 12 TO 14 OR 15 YEARS)

This stage is characterized by the use of abstract thinking and deductive reasoning. General concepts are related to specific situations and alternatives are considered. The world is evaluated by testing beliefs in an attempt to establish values and meaning in life.

Theories of Psychosocial Development

Erik Erikson

Erikson's (1963) developmental theory expanded on Freud's work to include cultural and social influences in addition to biological processes. His psychosocial theory is based on four major organizing concepts:

- Stages of development
- Developmental goals or tasks
- Psychosocial crises
- Process of coping

Erikson believed that development is a continuous process with distinct stages, characterized by the achievement of developmental goals that are affected by the social environment and significant others. He identified eight stages that progress from birth to old age and death. Each stage is characterized by a developmental crisis to be mastered, with possible successful or unsuccessful resolution of the crisis. Unsuccessful resolution at any one stage may delay progress through the next stage, but mastery can occur later.

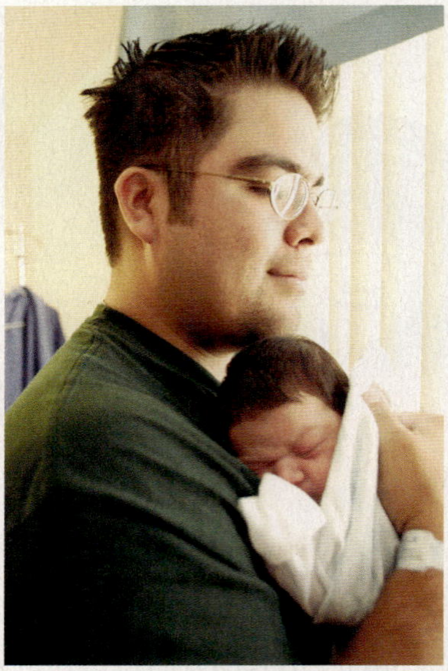

FIGURE 22-3. This caregiver provides comfort and affection to his daughter, teaching her to trust in others. (*Source:* Used with permission from Shutterstock. *Photo by Joe Mitchell.*)

TRUST VERSUS MISTRUST (INFANT)

The infant learns to rely on caregivers to meet basic needs of warmth, food, comfort, and forming trust in others. Mistrust can result from inconsistent, inadequate, or unsafe care (Fig. 22-3).

AUTONOMY VERSUS SHAME AND DOUBT (TODDLER)

As motor and language skills develop, the toddler (ages 1 to 3 years) learns from the environment and gains independence through encouragement from caregivers to feed, dress, and toilet themselves. If the caregivers are overprotective or have expectations that are too high, shame, doubt, and feelings of inadequacy may develop in the child.

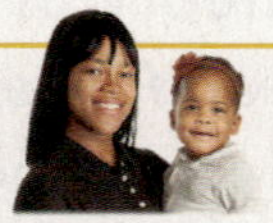

Think back to **Ms. Kimber**, the mother raising her child on her own. The nurse could apply Erikson's theory to explain her daughter's "getting into everything" as her need for learning about the environment and gaining independence. Additionally, the mother's anxiety level and the child's attempts to investigate the environment through locomotion and oral exploration, place the child at risk for injury from a fall or aspiration of a small object. With astute observation and knowledge of child development, the nurse plays a primary role in prevention by educating the mother.

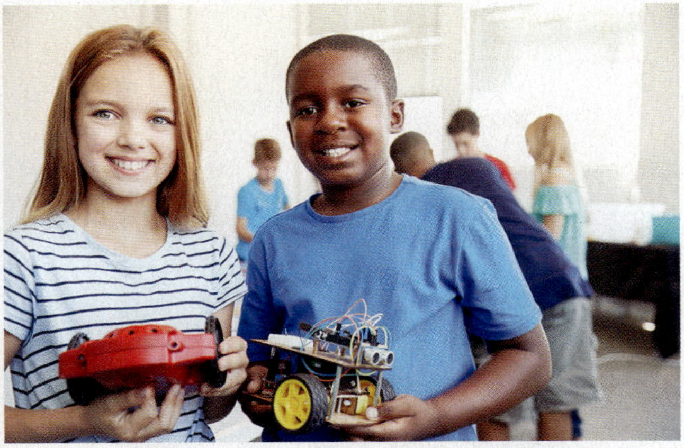

FIGURE 22-4. School-aged children focus on the end results of accomplishments—recognition and praise from family, teachers, and peers—in their development of a sense of competition and industry.

INITIATIVE VERSUS GUILT (PRESCHOOL)

Confidence gained as a toddler allows the preschooler (ages 4 to 6 years) to take the initiative in learning so that the child actively seeks out new experiences and explores the how and why of activities. If the child experiences restrictions or reprimands for seeking new experiences and learning, guilt results, and the child hesitates to attempt more challenging skills in motor or language development.

INDUSTRY VERSUS INFERIORITY (SCHOOL-AGED CHILDREN)

Focusing on the end result of achievements, the school-aged child gains pleasure from finishing projects and receiving recognition for accomplishments (Fig. 22-4). If the child is not accepted by peers or cannot meet parental expectations, a feeling of inferiority and lack of self-worth may develop.

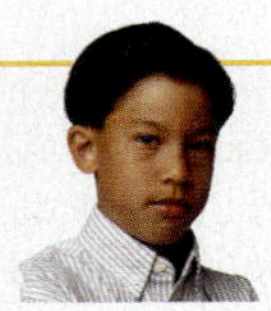

Think back to **Juan**, the 8-year-old boy described at the beginning of the chapter. The nurse could help to foster Juan's industry by offering positive reinforcement when he responds appropriately to efforts to calm him. The nurse also could incorporate activities that interest Juan into his plan of care to provide him with opportunities to succeed.

IDENTITY VERSUS ROLE CONFUSION (ADOLESCENCE)

With many physical changes occurring, the adolescent is in transition from childhood to adulthood. Hormonal changes produce secondary sex characteristics and mood swings. Trying on roles and even rebellion can be normal behaviors as the adolescent acquires a sense of self and decides what direction to take in life. Role confusion occurs if the adolescent is unable to establish identity and a sense of direction.

INTIMACY VERSUS ISOLATION (YOUNG ADULTHOOD)

The tasks for the young adult are to establish close, honest, loving relationships and make commitments to others. Fear of such commitments results in isolation and loneliness.

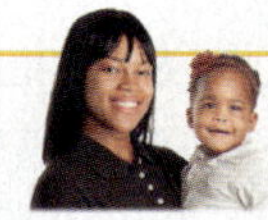

Recall **Ms. Kimber**, the mother described at the beginning of the chapter. She has identified a limited support system. Recognizing this, the nurse can assess further to identify the mother's potential problems with intimacy and subsequently, her progression toward generativity.

GENERATIVITY VERSUS STAGNATION (MIDDLE ADULTHOOD)

The middle adult years are marked by involvement with family, friends, and community. There is also a tendency to become concerned for the next generation and desire to make a contribution to the world. If this task is not met, stagnation occurs, and the person becomes self-absorbed and obsessed with their own needs, or regresses to an earlier level of coping.

EGO INTEGRITY VERSUS DESPAIR (LATER ADULTHOOD)

As a person enters the older years, reminiscence about life events provides a sense of fulfillment and purpose. Some older adults may not be fearful of dying if they feel they have achieved integrity. If a person believes their life has been a series of failures or missed opportunities, a sense of despair may prevail.

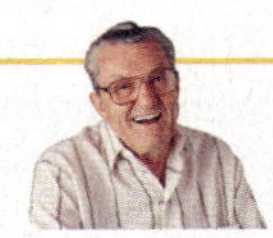

Think back to **Mr. Logan**, the 70-year-old man who broke his hip. Applying Erikson's theory, the nurse could assess Mr. Logan for indications of despair due to his feelings of dependency on others, and plan appropriate interventions that foster a sense of fulfillment and purpose.

Robert J. Havighurst

Havighurst (1972) believed that living and growing are based on learning, and that a person must continuously learn to adjust to changing conditions. He described learned behaviors as **developmental tasks** that occur at certain periods in life. Successful achievement leads to happiness and success in later tasks, whereas unsuccessful achievement leads to unhappiness, societal disapproval, and difficulty in later tasks. The developmental tasks arise from maturation, personal motives, and values that determine occupational and family choices and civic responsibility.

INFANCY AND EARLY CHILDHOOD

Developmental tasks for infancy and early childhood include:

- Achieving physiologic stability
- Learning to eat solid foods
- Learning to walk and talk
- Forming simple concepts of social and physical reality
- Learning to relate emotionally to parents or caregivers, siblings, and other people
- Learning to control the elimination of body wastes
- Learning to distinguish between right and wrong
- Learning sex differences and sexual modesty

MIDDLE CHILDHOOD

Developmental tasks for middle childhood include:

- Learning physical skills necessary for games
- Learning to get along with peers
- Developing fundamental skills in reading, writing, and mathematics
- Developing a conscience, morality, and a set of values
- Achieving personal independence

ADOLESCENCE

Developmental tasks for adolescence include:

- Accepting their body and using it effectively
- Achieving a masculine or feminine gender role (this binary reflects the time of Havighurst)
- Achieving emotional independence from parents and other adults
- Preparing for a career
- Preparing for marriage and family life
- Desiring and achieving socially responsible behavior
- Acquiring an ethical system as a guide to behavior

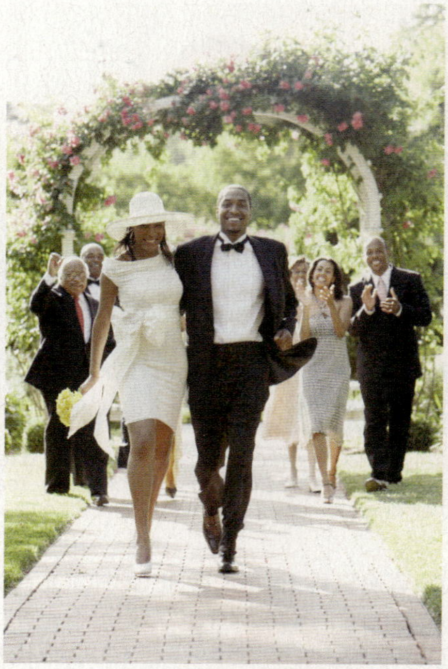

FIGURE 22-5. Choosing a life partner is often an important developmental task for young adults.

YOUNG ADULTHOOD

Developmental tasks for young adulthood include:

- Selecting a mate (Fig. 22-5)
- Learning to live with a (marriage) partner
- Starting a family and rearing children
- Managing a home
- Getting started in an occupation (see the accompanying Research in Nursing box)
- Taking on civic responsibility
- Finding a congenial social group

Research in Nursing

BRIDGING THE GAP TO EVIDENCE-BASED PRACTICE

The Impact of Job Loss on Maternal Sensitivity

Maternal sensitivity, the ability of a mother to be attuned and responsive to their child in nondistressed contexts, affects developmental outcomes in the child. The relationship between mother and child, especially the first 3 years of life, impacts social, cognitive, and emotional development. Job instability and unexpected job loss affect more than income; changing roles, emotional reactions, work–family conflict, change in caregiving dynamics, and education-related job mobility all potentially impact the mother–child bond.

Related Research

Prickett, K. C. (2020). Mothers' job loss and their sensitivity to young children's development. *Child Development*, *91*(6), 1970–1987. https://doi.org/10.1111/cdev.13398

Using the National Institute of Child Health and Human Development (NICHD) longitudinal Study of Early Child Care and Youth Development (SECCYD) dataset, which was started in 1991 with 1,364 infants from 10 locations across the United States, the researcher used autoregressive cross-lagged structural equation models to analyze data from the 1,211 mothers who engaged in the 36-month interview cycle. Four mediators were considered simultaneously: family income, work satisfaction, childcare transitions, and maternal depression. Although the analysis does not explain or control for all of the potential internal and external variables, findings from this analysis were threefold: (1) unexpected job loss, especially during the child's first year of life, was negatively associated with maternal sensitivity; (2) decreases in total family income and maternal depression are factors that explain the association between job loss and maternal sensitivity; and (3) maternal education level matters, with the strongest negative association between job loss and sensitivity seen in mothers who graduated high school or completed a GED but did not complete a bachelor's degree.

Relevance to Nursing Practice

Responsive parenting rooted in maternal sensitivity is a consistent predictor of short- and long-term child well-being. Considering the impact of myriad internal and external factors on maternal sensitivity is challenging. Targeting policy changes, specifically involving providing support for working mothers and reconsidering unemployment/maternal leave benefits, provides increased job stability. Intentional consideration and support of women and children at these vulnerable times decreases the negative impact of instability on maternal sensitivity and responsiveness.

MIDDLE ADULTHOOD

Developmental tasks for middle adulthood include:

- Accepting and adjusting to physical changes
- Attaining and maintaining a satisfactory occupational performance
- Assisting children to become responsible adults
- Relating to the spouse as a person
- Adjusting to aging parents
- Achieving adult social and civic responsibility

LATER MATURITY

Developmental tasks for later maturity include:

- Adjusting to decreasing physical strength and health
- Adjusting to retirement and reduced income
- Adjusting to death of a spouse
- Establishing an explicit affiliation with the person's age group
- Adjusting and adapting social roles in a flexible way
- Establishing satisfactory physical living arrangements

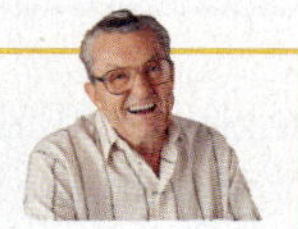

Recall **Mr. Logan**, the older man with the fractured hip described at the beginning of the chapter. Based on Mr. Logan's comments, the nurse could apply Havighurst's theory to conclude that Mr. Logan may be fluctuating between feelings of nonadjustment and feelings of acceptance of his declining health.

Roger Gould

Gould (1978), a psychiatrist trained in a psychoanalytic perspective, studied people between the ages of 16 and 60 years. He labeled the central theme for adults transformation and identified specific beliefs and developmental phases.

AGES 18 TO 22 YEARS: LEAVING THE PARENTS' WORLD

During the young adult years, individuals typically struggle with leaving their parents' world and challenging false assumptions from their childlike consciousness (e.g., "Only my parents can guarantee my safety."). However, these assumptions may be replaced with new false assumptions, such as, "Rewards will come automatically if I do what I am supposed to do."

AGES 22 TO 28 YEARS: GETTING INTO THE ADULT WORLD

Individuals in their 20s feel established as adults and separate from their families but believe they must still prove to their parents or guardians that they are competent, independent adults. They want to enjoy the present but build for the future.

AGES 29 TO 34 YEARS: QUESTIONING AND REEXAMINATION

Self-acceptance increases as the person's need to prove their competence disappears. Marriage and careers are generally well established, and young parents want to accept their own children for what they are becoming without imposing unnecessary rules. Questions about life in general are still present.

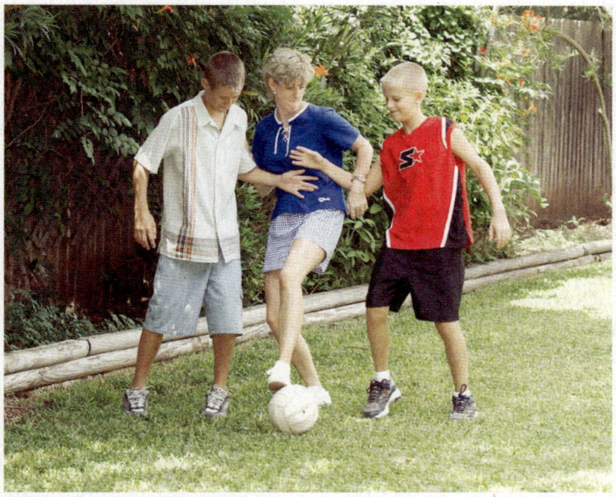

FIGURE 22-6. As her sons grow into young adults, this mom adapts to remain a positive influence in their lives. (*Source:* Used with permission from Shutterstock. *Photo by Joe Mitchell.*)

AGES 35 TO 43 YEARS: MIDLIFE DECADE

Adults in this age group tend to continually look inward and question themselves, their values, and their life. They see time as having an end and believe they have little time left to shape the behavior of their adolescent children (Fig. 22-6). They may be critical of their own parents, blaming them for many of their own problems.

AGES 43 TO 50 YEARS: RECONCILIATION AND MELLOWING

At this phase, adults accept the reality of boundaries for the lifespan and believe that personalities are set. They are interested in an active social life, community service, friends, and spouse. Life is viewed as neither simple nor controllable, which may result in periods of passivity, rage, depression, and despair.

AGES 50 AND OLDER: STABILITY AND ACCEPTANCE

Previous patterns of reflection and contemplation generally result in increased self-approval and self-acceptance. Increased marital happiness and contentment are associated with seeing the spouse as a valued companion.

Daniel Levinson and Associates

Levinson et al. (1978) based their theory on the organizing concept of "the evolution of individual life structure" (p. 40). The theory centers on the belief that the cycle of life at any point in time is formed by the interaction of three components: the self (values, motives), the social and cultural aspects of the person's life (family, career, religion, racial/ethnic background), and the person's particular set of roles (husband, father, friend, student). When anything changes in one component, the whole life structure must then reorganize. According to Levinson and associates, there are three major phases in young and middle adult life: novice, settling down, and midlife transition.

NOVICE PHASE

Early Adult Transition

The major concerns of the young adult (ages 17 to 22 years) are to break away from their parents or guardians, make

Box 22-3 Key Points of Moral and Faith Developmental Theories

Kohlberg: Moral Development

Preconventional, stage 1: Punishment and obedience—Oriented to obedience and punishment; right and wrong defined by punishments

Preconventional, stage 2: Instrumental relativist—Defines acts satisfying to self (and some satisfying to others) as right

Conventional, stage 3: Interpersonal concordance—Morality of maintaining good relations and approval of others; right and wrong are determined by the majority

Conventional, stage 4: Law and order—Being good extends to a person's duty to society; aware of need to respect authority

Postconventional, stage 5: Social contract—Right and wrong determined by personal values; laws are considered, but may be ignored or discounted

Postconventional, stage 6: Universal ethical principle—Deeply held moral principles are in accordance with a sense of self and are more important than laws; few adults ever reach this stage of development

Fowler: Faith Development

Fowler's six stages may occur over the course of a person's adult life.

Prestage: Undifferentiated faith—Centers on relationship with primary caregiver and the safety of the environment

Stage 1: Intuitive-predictive faith—Imitates religious behaviors of others; learning also occurs through stories and images

Stage 2: Mythic-literal faith—Accepts existence of deity; strong belief in justice; metaphors and symbolism often taken literally

Stage 3: Synthetic-conventional faith—Selection of principles to follow; development of a personal identity; concern for the rights and needs of others

Stage 4: Individuative-reflective faith—Angst possible; personal accountability for beliefs and feelings; awareness of conflicts in the complexities of faith

Stage 5: Conjunctive faith—Conflicts resolved; identification of truth

Stage 6: Universalizing faith—Enlightenment; universality of faith and principles

initial career choices, and establish intimate relationships. Many separations, losses, and transformations are necessary to terminate old relationships. This is also a time to begin to select personal values and establish goals, as the young adult's life structure begins to be more integrated.

Entering the Adult World

The years of the middle to late 20s (ages 22 to 28 years) are a time to build on previous decisions and choices, and to try different careers and lifestyles. By the late 20s, the young adult enters the age-30 transition period. The person often feels uneasy that something is missing. During this transition, decisions are made either to find a new direction in life or to make a stronger commitment to previous choices.

Age-30 Transition

This represents a transition time (ending around age 33 years) during which the overriding task of the novice phase—to establish a place in the world and create a viable, suitable life structure—is evaluated. This time of reflection allows for reconsideration of choices and the opportunity to make changes.

SETTLING DOWN: BUILDING A SECOND ADULT LIFE STRUCTURE

In the settling-down phase (ages 33 to 40 years), the adult invests energy into the areas of life that are most personally important. The areas of investment are primarily family, work, and community. The person strives to gain respect, status, and a sense of authority.

MIDLIFE TRANSITION AND ENTERING MIDDLE ADULTHOOD

Midlife Transition

Midlife transition (ages 40 to 45 years) involves a reappraisal of goals and values. The person's established lifestyle may continue, or they may choose to reorganize and change careers. This is an unsettled time, with the person often anxious and fearful. There is a focus on leaving a legacy and how short life is.

Entering Middle Adulthood

By this time (ages 45 to 50 years), the person has made choices and formed a new life structure. This allows for time to commit to new tasks.

Theories of Moral Development

Lawrence Kohlberg

Kohlberg (1969) developed a theory of **moral development** using levels that closely follow Piaget's theory of cognitive development (Box 22-3). Kohlberg recognized that a person's moral development is influenced by culture. Culture and sociocultural obligations affect the person's perceptions of justice in interpersonal relationships. A child's beginnings of moral development result from caregiver–child communications during the early childhood years, as the young child tries to please their parents and other caregivers (Fig. 22-7). The concept of morality emerges as a subset of a person's beliefs or values and governs choices made throughout life. Kohlberg's stages of moral development begin in childhood but may develop well into adolescence and adulthood. Rules and regulations established by society are eventually challenged and evaluated as a person either accepts societal rules into their own internal set of values or rejects them.

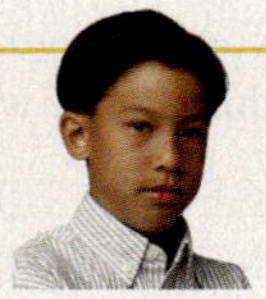

Remember **Juan**, the 8-year-old with encephalitis. Juan's language barrier and cultural heritage may be adding to the child's already heightened fears and anxieties related to hospitalization. The nurse's astute observation and application of Kohlberg's theory can further an understanding of the child's perceptions, beliefs, and, ultimately, his choices and actions.

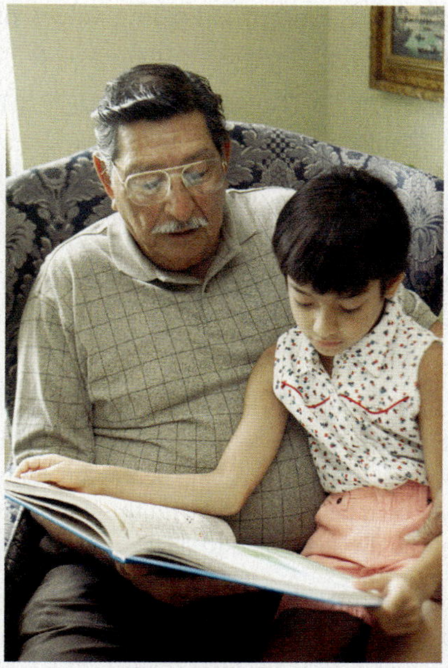

FIGURE 22-7. This grandfather reads traditional stories to their young granddaughter, teaching her important cultural values and beliefs, thereby influencing her moral development. (*Source:* Used with permission from Shutterstock. *Photo by Joe Mitchell.*)

PRECONVENTIONAL LEVEL

Kohlberg's preconventional level of moral development is based on external control, as the child learns to conform to rules imposed by authority figures. At stage 1, *punishment and obedience orientation*, the motivation for choices of action is the fear of physical consequences of authority's disapproval. As a result of the consequences, a perception of goodness or badness develops. At stage 2, *instrumental relativist orientation*, the thought of receiving a reward overcomes fear of punishment, and thus actions that satisfy this desire are selected.

CONVENTIONAL LEVEL

The conventional level of moral development involves identifying with significant others and conforming to their expectations. The person respects the values and ideals of family and friends, regardless of consequences. In stage 3, *"good boy–good girl" orientation*, the person strives for approval in an attempt to be viewed as good. At stage 4, *law and order orientation*, behavior follows social or religious rules from a respect for authority. In his later work, Kohlberg maintained that many adults are at this stage because they think abstractly and view themselves as members of society.

POSTCONVENTIONAL LEVEL

The postconventional level of moral development involves moral judgment that is rational and internalized as standards or values. At stage 5, *social contract and utilitarian orientation*, correct behavior is defined in terms of society's laws. These laws can be changed to meet society's needs, as long as they support respect for self and others. Stage 6, *universal ethical principle orientation*, represents the person's concern for equality for all human beings, guided by personal values and standards, regardless of those set by society or laws. Justice maybe internalized at an even higher level than society's level. Few adults ever reach this stage of development.

Carol Gilligan

Gilligan (1977, 1982) originally worked with Kohlberg. As she listened to women discuss their own real-life moral conflicts, she recognized that there was a conception of morality from the female viewpoint that was not represented in Kohlberg's work. Gilligan's theory views girls and women as developing a morality of response and care, and boys and men as developing a morality of justice. Gilligan's work must be considered within the context of gender roles and feminism of the 1970s and 1980s.

In Gilligan's theory, men and women have different ways of looking at the world. Men are more likely to associate morality with obligations, rights, and justice, whereas women are more likely to see moral requirements emerging from the needs of others within the context of a relationship. This moral orientation of women is called the *ethic of care*, which develops through three levels. Each level ends with a transitional period, a time when the girl or woman considers new approaches to moral considerations and moves to a new level.

LEVEL 1—PRECONVENTIONAL: SELFISHNESS

In level 1, the focus is on the girl's or woman's own needs. *Should* and *would* are the same. Morality is seen in terms of sanctions by society. Relationships are often disappointing, and as a result, a woman may isolate herself to avoid getting hurt. The transition that follows this level is characterized by the move from selfishness to responsibility—a move that integrates the responsibility to care for oneself with the desire to care for others.

LEVEL 2—CONVENTIONAL: GOODNESS

In level 2, moral judgment is based on shared norms and expectations, and societal values are adopted. Acceptance by others becomes critical, and the ability to protect and care for others becomes the defining characteristic of female goodness. This goodness involves self-sacrifice and bearing responsibility for others. As a woman examines her self-sacrifice, the second transition occurs, with the woman asking if her own needs are not also important. A shift from *goodness* to *truth* (as well as a new conception of goodness) takes place.

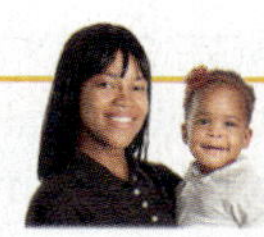

Think back to **Ms. Kimber**, the single mother. The nurse could apply Gilligan's theory to assist Ms. Kimber in adjusting to her role as both a single parent caring for a child and as a woman with her own set of needs.

LEVEL 3—POSTCONVENTIONAL: NONVIOLENCE

In level 3, a changed understanding of self and a redefinition of morality allow reconciliation of selfishness and responsibility. Nonviolence (the injunction against hurting) governs all moral judgments and actions. Care becomes a universal obligation toward self and others. Moral problems are usually considered within the contexts of maintaining relationships and promoting the welfare or preventing the harm of others.

Theory of Faith Development

James Fowler

Fowler (1981, p. 4) postulated a developmental theory of the spiritual identity of humans, based on work by Piaget, Kohlberg, and Erikson. Fowler describes **faith** as follows:

> Faith is not always religious in its content or context… Faith is a person's or group's way of moving into the force field of life. It is our way of finding coherence in and giving meaning to the multiple forces and relations that make up our lives. Faith is a person's way of seeing him or herself in relation to others against a background of shared meaning and purpose. Faith, therefore, is not necessarily religious, but it comprises the reasons one finds life worth living.

Fowler's theory is composed of a prestage and six stages of faith development (see Box 22-3 on page 586). The age when a certain stage occurs varies, but the sequence does not. Fowler explained that a relationship among self, shared causes or values, and others is the unifying factor in all stages, and that relationship is based on trust. Equilibrium, or a plateau in faith development, can occur at any stage from stage 2 and beyond.

PRESTAGE: UNDIFFERENTIATED FAITH

During the prestage, trust, courage, hope, and love compete with threats of abandonment and inconsistencies in the infant's environment. The strength of faith in this stage is based on the infant's relationship with the primary caregiver.

STAGE 1: INTUITIVE–PROJECTIVE FAITH

Intuitive–projective faith is most typical of the 3- to 7-year-old child. Children imitate religious gestures and behaviors of others, primarily their parents or guardians. They take on their elders' attitudes toward religious or moral beliefs without a thorough understanding of them. Imagination in this stage leads to long-lived images and feelings that they must question and reintegrate in later stages.

STAGE 2: MYTHICAL–LITERAL FAITH

Mythical–literal faith predominates in the school-aged child, who is having more social interaction. Stories represent religious and moral beliefs, and the child accepts the existence of a deity. The child can appreciate the perspectives of others as well as the concept of reciprocal fairness.

STAGE 3: SYNTHETIC–CONVENTIONAL FAITH

Synthetic–conventional faith is the characteristic stage of many adolescents. As the person experiences increasing demands from work, school, family, and peers, the basis for identity becomes more complex. The person has an emerging ideology but has not closely examined it until now. The person begins to question life-guiding values or religious practices in an attempt to stabilize their own identity.

STAGE 4: INDIVIDUATIVE–REFLECTIVE FAITH

Individuative–reflective faith is crucial for older adolescents and young adults because they become responsible for their own commitments, beliefs, and attitudes. Many adults do not develop to this stage, and for some people, it does not emerge until they are in their 30s or 40s. Searching for self-identity that is no longer defined by the faith of significant others, is a primary concern.

STAGE 5: CONJUNCTIVE FAITH

Conjunctive faith integrates other viewpoints about faith into a person's understanding of truth. The person can see the real nature of their own beliefs. Along with this realization, the person observes the divisions of faith development among people.

STAGE 6: UNIVERSALIZING FAITH

Universalizing faith involves making tangible the values of absolute love and justice for humankind. The faith relationship is characterized by total trust in the principle of actively *being in relation* to others in whom we invest commitment, belief, love, risk, and hope, and in the existence of the future, regardless of what religion or image of faith is involved.

APPLYING THEORIES OF GROWTH AND DEVELOPMENT TO NURSING CARE

The complex and interrelated elements that contribute to human growth and development involve not only biophysical factors, but also factors of personality development. The theories summarized in this chapter help us understand cognitive, psychosocial, moral, and spiritual development. To understand the whole person, nurses need to evaluate all the components of growth and development to appreciate certain life events or concerns (Fig. 22-8).

Although these theories offer a great deal of insight into the processes of human growth and development, they do have some limitations. You need to consider these developmental theories within the context of when they were developed. Although they have sustained relevance, some concepts are based on assumptions and beliefs that may not hold true in today's world. We also have a more-nuanced understanding of disparities, vulnerabilities, and social determinants of health that impact on growth and development. When planning holistic nursing care for patients with diverse needs, backgrounds, and ages, nurses should assess the patient as an individual and use interventions based on rationales from multiple developmental theories to provide comprehensive health care. Watch for the Vulnerable Population Alerts and Challenging Topics throughout this text—take time to reflect and acknowledge your role in addressing issues that impact health equity. Guidelines for incorporating the principles and theories of growth and development in nursing care are listed in Box 22-4.

Health care needs change quickly as a person grows and passes through life. These needs are unique for each person

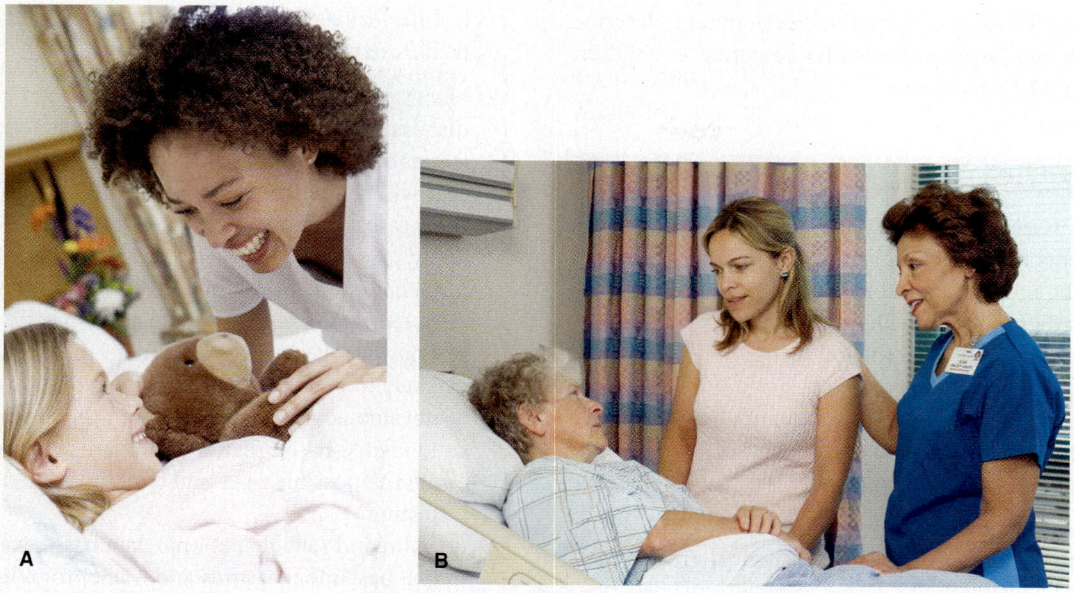

FIGURE 22-8. **A.** To provide holistic and individualized care, the nurse applies theories of growth and development when she displays compassion and provides emotional support to a young, hospitalized child. **B.** The nurse caring for an older adult includes the daughter, with whom the patient now lives, in discharge teaching. (*Source:* B: Used with permission from Shutterstock. *Photo by B. Proud.*)

but have certain similarities in specific developmental stages. The nurse must plan care based on the patient's general and unique health needs and must continually revise aspects of care as the growth process evolves or alterations in health status occur.

The nurse is also uniquely positioned to address the sensitive emotional, psychological, and educational issues related to genetic, genomic, and epigenetic discoveries. This focus on health rather than disease has the potential to result in significantly positive outcomes for the growth and development of all people.

DEVELOPING CLINICAL REASONING AND CLINICAL JUDGMENT

1. Identify developmental challenges for five of your family members or friends at different ages across the lifespan. Explain why meeting developmental needs is an essential role of nursing.
2. Compare and contrast the psychosocial theories of Erikson and Gould. Are the concepts in these theories relevant today? If yes, explain why. If no, what would you delete and what would you add?

Box 22-4 Incorporating Principles and Theories of Growth and Development

General guidelines for incorporating principles and theories of growth and development and family dynamics into daily practice of nursing care are listed here. They are provided as suggestions for working with patients of all ages.

- Be knowledgeable about the various stages of cognitive, psychosocial, moral, and spiritual development and prepared to support developmental stages typical of certain ages.
- Maintain flexibility in assessing patients and respect the uniqueness of each person. Although the literature describes development typical of a particular age, not everyone fits into an exact mold.
- Anticipate possible regression during difficult periods or times of crisis, then accept and support a person's return to a forward progression in development.
- Understand that environmental and cultural influences have a strong effect on development, especially psychosocial development. A deprived environment can be detrimental, whereas an enriched environment enhances development.
- Assess each person with an awareness that within each stage of development, a person may retain some behaviors of a previous stage, attain goals of the current stage, and begin to exhibit behaviors of the next stage. There is a time of transition to the next stage with no definitive beginning or ending.
- Remember that patients are members of families, and that the family can have both positive and negative influences on the development of individual members. Keep in mind that *family* is whomever the person identifies as family. Attempt to support good family relationships and healthy environments that assist members to reach their greatest potential for growth. Provide patient teaching to individuals and their families to aid in their understanding of periods of development.
- Be ready to provide health care to patients who are ill or who fail to meet developmental goals. Collaborate with other members of the health care team in providing care to prevent or minimize disruption of development and to promote optimal health throughout life.
- Provide environments and experiences that are developmentally challenging.

3. Using Piaget's theory of cognitive development, describe how you would explain the death of a parent to children ages 4, 9, and 13 years.

PRACTICING FOR NCLEX

1. A nurse assessing a toddler in a pediatric office tells the parents that the child is in the 90th percentile for height and weight and has blue eyes. The nurse explains these physical characteristics are primarily determined by which of the following?
   a. Socialization with caregivers
   b. Maternal nutrition during pregnancy
   c. Genetic information on chromosomes
   d. Meeting developmental tasks
2. A nurse caring for newborns understands that babies grow and develop according to individual growth patterns and developmental levels. Which terms describe these patterns? Select all that apply.
   a. Orderly
   b. Simple
   c. Sequential
   d. Unpredictable
   e. Differentiated
   f. Integrated
3. A 2-year-old grabs a handful of cake from the table and stuffs it in their mouth. According to Freud, what part of the mind is the child satisfying?
   a. Id
   b. Superego
   c. Ego
   d. Unconscious mind
4. A nurse is teaching parents of preschoolers the types of behavior to expect from their children based on developmental theories. Which statements describe this stage of development? Select all that apply.
   a. According to Freud, the child is in the phallic stage.
   b. According to Erikson, the child is in the trust versus mistrust stage.
   c. According to Havighurst, the child is learning to get along with others.
   d. According to Fowler, the child imitates religious behavior of others.
   e. According to Kohlberg, the child defines satisfying acts as right.
   f. According to Havighurst, the child is achieving gender-specific roles.
5. When caring for older adults in a long-term care facility, a nurse encourages an older adult to talk about past life events. One patient tells the nurse they were an angry person, lost many jobs, and ended up alone. According to Erikson, this patient is in what developmental stage?
   a. Despair
   b. Stagnation
   c. Inferiority
   d. Industry
6. Nursing students attending a class on genomics are discussing its use in current nursing practice. Which statements by the students identify genetic principles that will challenge nurses to integrate genomics in their research, education, and practice? Select all that apply.
   a. Genetic tests plus family history tools have the potential to identify people at risk for diseases.
   b. Pharmacogenetic tests can determine if a patient is likely to positive therapeutic response to a drug or develop adverse reactions from the medication.
   c. Evidence-based review panels are in place to evaluate the possible risks and benefits related to genetic testing.
   d. Valid and reliable national data bases exist to establish baseline measures and track progress toward targets.
   e. Genetic variation can either accelerate or slow the metabolism of many drugs.
   f. It is beyond a nurse's scope of practice to discuss the impact of genetic findings and impact on health and illness.
7. A nurse who is working with women in a drop-in shelter studies Carol Gilligan's theory of morality in women to use when planning care. According to Gilligan, what is the motivation for female morality?
   a. Law and justice
   b. Obligations and rights
   c. Response and care
   d. Order and selfishness
8. A school nurse uses Kohlberg's theory of moral development as a basis for a roundtable discussion with parents on bullying. According to Kohlberg, what factor initially influences the moral development of children?
   a. Parent/caregiver–child communications
   b. Societal rules and regulations
   c. Social and religious rules
   d. A person's beliefs and values
9. A school nurse uses Havighurst's principles and theories of growth and development when planning programs for high school students. With this information, the nurse can assist students to correlate their behavior and decisions to which age-appropriate developmental task?
   a. Finding a congenial social group
   b. Developing a conscience, morality, and a scale of values
   c. Achieving personal independence
   d. Achieving a masculine or feminine gender role
10. While assessing a patient in the medical clinic, the patient tells the nurse: "I'm currently a sales associate, but I'm considering a career move, which makes

me somewhat anxious." According to Levinson, what phase of adult life is this patient experiencing?
a. Entering the adult world
b. Settling down
c. Midlife transition
d. Entering middle-adulthood

11. When teaching parents about achievements in children, the nurse explains that, according to Piaget, children in which age group are able to grasp abstract ideas?
a. Toddler
b. Adolescence
c. Preschool age
d. School age

12. A parent shares with the nurse in the pediatric clinic that their 12-month-old cries when they leave the room or hide a favorite stuffed animal. The nurse explains that object permanence typically occurs in which group?
a. 0 to 6 months
b. 12 to 18 months
c. 24 to 36 months
d. 36 months to 4 years

13. A nurse working in a hospice setting uses reminiscence to help patients determine whether their life had meaning or if they wish to make amends. What stage of Erickson's development is the nurse applying with this approach?
a. Industry versus inferiority
b. Initiative versus guilt
c. Generativity versus stagnation
d. Ego integrity versus despair

ANSWERS WITH RATIONALES

1. **c.** Physical appearance and growth have a predetermined genetic base in inheritance patterns carried on the chromosomes.

2. **a, c, e, f.** Growth and development are orderly and sequential as well as continuous and complex. Growth and development follow regular and predictable trends and are both differentiated and integrated.

3. **a.** Freud defined the id as the part of the mind concerned with self-gratification by the easiest and quickest available means.

4. **a, d, e.** According to Freud, the child is in the phallic stage. According to Fowler, the child imitates religious behavior of others. According to Kohlberg, the child defines satisfying acts as right. According to Erikson, the child is in the initiative versus guilt stage. According to Havighurst, the child is learning sex differences, forming concepts, and getting ready to read. According to Havighurst, the adolescent, not the preschooler, is achieving gender-specific social roles.

5. **a.** Reminiscence during the older years of a person's life provides a sense of fulfillment and purpose (ego integrity). Generativity versus stagnation is a developmental stage of the middle adult years. Industry versus inferiority states that if a child is not accepted by peers or cannot meet parental expectations, feelings of lack of self-worth may develop.

6. **a, b, e.** Health care providers are being challenged to integrate genomics into their research, education, and practice. Genetic tests plus family history tools have the potential to identify people at risk for diseases. Pharmacogenetics studies how genetic variation affects a person's response to drugs, helping to determine if a patient is likely to have a strong therapeutic response or develop adverse effects to a drug. Genetic variation can either accelerate or slow the metabolism of many drugs (see Chapter 30). The need for (1) evidence-based review panels to thoroughly evaluate the possible benefits and harms related to the expanding number of genetic tests and family health history tools; and (2) valid and reliable national data to establish baseline measures and track progress toward targets (Office of Disease Prevention and Health Promotion, 2021) are emerging challenges in genomics. Nurses must be prepared to answer questions and discuss the impact of genetic findings on health and illness.

7. **c.** In Gilligan's theory, men and women have different ways of looking at the world. Women typically see moral requirements emerging from the needs of others within the context of a relationship. This moral orientation of women is called the *ethic of care*, which develops through three levels: Level 1—Preconventional: Selfishness, Level 2—Conventional: Goodness, Level 3—Postconventional: Nonviolence. Men typically associate morality with obligations, rights, and justice.

8. **a.** The beginnings of moral development result from parent/caregiver–child communications during early childhood, as the young child tries to please parents and caregivers. Kohlberg's stages of moral development begin in childhood but may continue developing into adolescence and adulthood. Rules and regulations established by society are eventually challenged and evaluated as a person either accepts societal rules into his or her own internal set of values or rejects them.

9. **d.** According to Havighurst, the role of the adolescent is to achieve a masculine or feminine gender role. Developing a conscience, morality, and a scale of values and achieving personal independence are roles of middle childhood. Finding a congenial social group is a role of young adulthood.

10. **c.** Midlife transition (ages 40 to 45 years) involves a reappraisal of goals and values. The established lifestyle may continue, or the person may choose to reorganize and change careers, creating anxiety or fear. In the middle to late 20s (ages 22 to 28 years) young adults build on previous decisions and choices and to try different careers and lifestyles. In the settling-down phase (ages 33 to 40 years), the adult invests energy into the areas of life that are most personally important. The years of entering middle adulthood (ages 45 to 50 years) revolve around having made choices and having formed a new life structure, and committing to new tasks.

11. **c.** According to Piaget's preoperational stage, increased language, increased understanding of life events, and relationships occur with language greatly increasing from ages 3 to 5 years.

12. **b.** Object permanence typically develops at age 12 to 18 months.

13. **d.** Reminiscence for the older adult provides a sense of fulfillment and purpose (integrity), perhaps removing the fear of dying. A sense of despair may ensue if a person believes that their life has been a series of failures or missed directions. Preschoolers (ages 4 to 6 years) take the initiative in learning and seeking out new experiences; when experiencing restrictions or reprimands, they typically hesitate to attempt more challenging (initiative vs. guilt). The school-aged child enjoys finishing projects and receiving recognition for accomplishments; children who are not accepted by peers or cannot meet parental expectations develop feelings of inferiority and lack of self-worth may develop (industry vs. inferiority). Middle adult years are marked by involvement with family, friends, community, and concern for the next generation; if this task is not met, stagnation occurs, and the person becomes self-absorbed or regresses to an earlier level of coping (generativity vs. stagnation).

Bibliography

American Nurses Association (ANA). (n.d.). *Genetics and personalized medicine.* Retrieved June 1, 2021, from https://www.nursingworld.org/practice-policy/nursing-excellence/ethics/genetics/

Deans, C., & Maggert, K. A. (2015). What do you mean, "epigenetic"? *Genetics, 199*(4), 887–896. https://doi.org/10.1534/genetics.114.173492

Erikson, E. H. (1963). *Childhood and society* (2nd ed.). W. W. Norton.

Fowler, J. W. (1981). *Stages of faith: The psychology of human development and the quest for meaning.* HarperCollins Publishers.

Freud, S. (1960). *The ego and the id: The standard edition of the complete psychological works of Sigmund Freud.* In J. Strachey (Ed.). W. W. Norton & Company, Inc.

Gilligan, C. (1977). In a different voice: Women's conceptions of the self and of morality. *Harvard Educational Review, 47*(4), 481–517.

Gilligan, C. (1982). *In a different voice: Psychological theory and women's development.* Harvard University Press.

Gould, R. L. (1978). *Transformations: Growth and change in adult life.* Simon & Schuster.

Havighurst, R. J. (1972). *Developmental tasks and education* (3rd ed.). David McKay.

International Genome Sample Resource [IGSR]. (2021). *The International Genome Sample Resource (IGSR) and the 1000 Genomes Project.* https://www.internationalgenome.org/about

Kohlberg, L. (1969). Stage and sequence: The cognitive–developmental approach to socialization. In D. A. Gaslin (Ed.). *Handbook of socialization: Theory and research* (pp. 347–380). Rand McNally.

Levinson, D. J., Darrow, C. N., Klein, E. B., Levinson, M. H., & McKee, B. (1978). *The seasons of a man's life.* The Random House Publishing Group.

McLeod, S. (2018, May 3). *Erik Erikson's stages of psychosocial development.* https://www.simplypsychology.org/Erik-Erikson.html

National Cancer Institute. (2020, July 24). *Epidemiology and genomics research program: Epigenomics and epigenetics research.* https://epi.grants.cancer.gov/epigen/

National Human Genome Research Institute. (2020a, August 16). *Epigenomics fact sheet.* https://www.genome.gov/about-genomics/fact-sheets/Epigenomics-Fact-Sheet

National Human Genome Research Institute. (2020b, December 22). *The human genome project.* https://www.genome.gov/human-genome-project

Office of Disease Prevention and Health Promotion. (2021, May 27). *Healthy People 2020: Genomics.* ttps://www.healthypeople.gov/2020/topics-objectives/topic/genomics#top

Piaget, J., & Inhelder, B. (1969). *The psychology of the child.* Basic Books.

Prickett, K. C. (2020). Mothers' job loss and their sensitivity to young children's development. *Child Development, 91*(6), 1970–1987. https://doi.org/10.1111/cdev.13398

U.S. National Library of Medicine. (2021, April 13). *Help me understand genetics.* https://medlineplus.gov/genetics/understanding/#hgp

23 Conception Through Young Adulthood

Nate Pelton

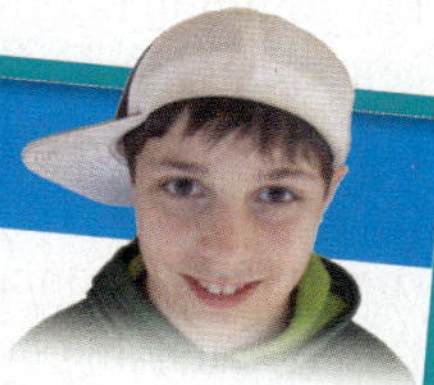

Nate, who is 11 years old, collided with another player while running in the outfield during a Little League baseball game. He was removed from the game after the collision because he reported a headache and, according to his coaches, appeared slightly dazed. His parents took him to the emergency department at the local hospital where Nate told the ED nurse, "I felt a little dizzy after the collision, but I feel fine now."

Darlene Schneider

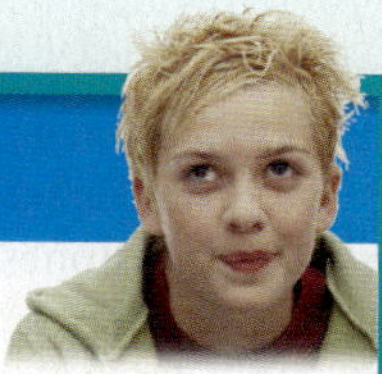

Darlene, a pregnant 14-year-old in her third trimester, comes to the prenatal clinic for the first time. Her history reveals sexual activity with multiple partners, smoking two packs of cigarettes per day, beer "four or five nights a week," and eating mostly "fast foods." She has received no prenatal care and hasn't been taking any prenatal vitamins. She is experiencing homelessness but occasionally stays with an older girlfriend since her parents "threw me out of the house."

Hillarie Browning

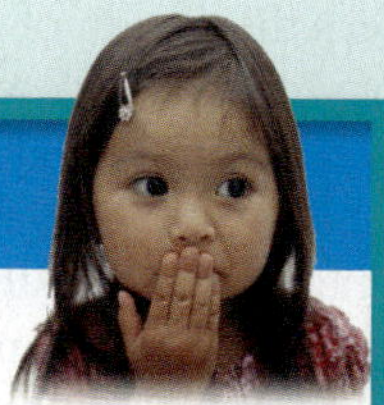

Hillarie, who is 2 years old, is brought to the emergency department by her father, James Browning. She is unresponsive. Mr. Browning says that she "took a tumble" down the stairs, but assessment reveals that her injuries are inconsistent with this type of fall.

Learning Outcomes

After completing the chapter, you will be able to accomplish the following:

1. Summarize major physiologic, cognitive, psychosocial, moral, and spiritual developments from conception through young adulthood.
2. Apply specific theoretical models and theories to each developmental period from conception to young adulthood.
3. List common health problems of each age period from conception through young adulthood.
4. Describe developmental and situational stressors common in each developmental period from conception to young adulthood.
5. Describe nursing interventions to promote health in patients from conception through young adulthood.

Nursing Concepts

- Development
- Family
- Identity
- Reproduction

Growth and development start at conception and continue over the course of a person's life. The nurse's knowledge of growth and developmental milestones provides a base for planning and implementing holistic, individualized nursing care. This chapter continues the discussion of developmental theories introduced in Chapter 22, with specific information related to the sequential stages of growth and development from conception through young adulthood.

Childhood encompasses the entire period before young adulthood and is divided into different stages. Included within this time span are the fetus, neonate, infant, toddler, preschooler, school-aged child, and adolescent. This chapter's discussion of each of these stages, as well as the period of young adulthood, includes physiologic, cognitive, psychosocial, and moral and spiritual development, as appropriate. We will also explore the nurse's role in promoting and maintaining health with each group of children and young adults. For an example that addresses the adolescent, see the Reflective Practice box.

CONCEPTION AND PRENATAL DEVELOPMENT

Human growth and development begin the moment the ovum is fertilized by the sperm. The fertilized ovum (zygote) contains the full complement of genetic information provided by each parent that determines biologic sex and influences personality, intellect, physical traits, and psychological traits. The growth and development stages of the fetus are orderly and continuous.

Pre-embryonic Stage

The pre-embryonic stage lasts for about 3 weeks. The zygote, which implants in the uterine wall, has three distinct cell layers. The endoderm (inner layer) becomes the respiratory system, the digestive system, the liver, and the pancreas. The mesoderm (middle layer) becomes the skeleton; connective tissue; cartilage; muscles; and the circulatory, lymphoid, reproductive, and urinary systems. The ectoderm (outer layer) becomes the brain, spinal cord, nervous system, and outer body parts (skin, hair, and nails).

Embryonic Stage

The embryonic stage occurs from the 4th through the 8th week. Rapid growth and differentiation of the cell layers take place. By the end of this stage, all basic organs have been established, the bones have begun to ossify, and some human features are recognizable. Because this is a period of such rapid growth and change, the embryo is especially vulnerable to any factor that might cause congenital anomalies (such as maternal use of alcohol, nicotine, over-the-counter [OTC] medications, or other drugs).

Fetal Stage

The fetal stage lasts from 9 weeks to birth. All body organs and systems continue to grow and develop. At the end of the first trimester (12 weeks' gestation), some reflexes are present, kidney secretion begins, the heartbeat can be heard by Doppler, and the sex of the fetus is distinguishable by outward appearance. At the end of the second trimester (24 weeks' gestation), fetal heart tones are able to be auscultated, the liver and pancreas are functioning, hair forms, sleep–wake patterns are established, lung surfactant is produced, and the eyelids open. At the end of the third trimester (40 weeks' gestation), the testes have descended, lung alveoli are formed, subcutaneous fat is deposited, and the fetus actively kicks. By birth, the average neonate weighs 7.5 lb (3.4 kg) and is 20 inches (50.8 cm) long.

During pregnancy, adequate maternal nutrition is essential for normal growth and development of the embryo and fetus. A fetus not receiving adequate nutrition may be small for gestational age, fail to have normal brain development, have learning disabilities as a child, and be at increased risk for chronic illnesses as an adult. Vitamin and mineral deficiencies can result in fetal megaloblastic anemia and neural tube defects (folic acid deficiency), inadequate bone calcification (vitamin D and calcium deficits), and hypothyroidism (iodine deficiency).

The number of premature births (those occurring before 37 weeks' gestation; also referred to as preterm births) decreased from 2007 to 2014 due in part to a decrease in the number of adolescents and young women giving birth. However, there was a slight increase in preterm births 5 years in a row between 2014 and 2019 (Centers for Disease Control [CDC], 2020c). Low birth weight is one of the leading causes of infant mortality and the leading cause of infant death during the first month of life. In 2018, 17% of

QSEN Reflective Practice: Cultivating QSEN Competencies

CHALLENGE TO ETHICAL AND LEGAL SKILLS

I was admitting Darlene Schneider, a pregnant, unmarried 14-year-old, to the prenatal clinic. This was her first visit, and she was already in her third trimester. A quick history revealed multiple factors putting both her and her fetus at risk for health problems: lack of family support (experiencing homelessness, occasionally staying with an older friend), father of the baby unknown, multiple sexual partners, diet consisting mainly of fast food, no prenatal vitamins, little to no exercise, and history of smoking (two packs of cigarettes per day) and alcohol consumption ("beer four to five times a week"). When she was seen by the medical resident, he asked her quite curtly if she was trying to kill her baby, telling her that it was probably too late for her to get the care she needed. "Why should we waste our time on you when other women here really want to be helped?" Although Darlene was trying to hide her emotions, I could tell from her expression that she was both angry and hurt. While I shared some of the resident's frustration, I knew we had to give Darlene a reason to trust us if we wanted her to start taking better care of herself and her fetus. I was also upset by the resident's lack of professionalism and wondered if I should say something to him.

Thinking Outside the Box: Possible Courses of Action

- Take advantage of the resident having been so harsh: after the resident finished his visit, I could try to be especially caring and explain why we were all concerned about her and her fetus. Then I could talk to her about what she needed to do to maximize good outcomes.
- Challenge the resident in the patient's presence, thereby showing her that at least I honestly cared about her.
- Confront the resident later in a moment when my emotions are not running so high, and directly address the issue. I would also indicate that although I am hopeful change will occur, I am prepared to report my concerns to a supervisor should this behavior occur again.
- Approach the resident outside the patient's presence and explain my concerns. Persuade the resident to apologize to Darlene in the interests of winning the patient's trust and compliance with the prenatal care program.

Evaluating a Good Outcome: How Do I Define Success?

- The respect for each person's human dignity (Darlene, the resident, myself) is affirmed.
- Each person feels empowered to make personal decisions that advance their interests and goals.
- The patient makes the needed lifestyle changes, with good outcomes for herself and her fetus.
- Personal integrity is maintained; no one has to sacrifice beliefs and values.
- Professional integrity is maintained.

Personal Learning: Here's to the Future!

In this situation, I don't think that I chose the best alternative because I tried to comfort Darlene and make excuses for the resident's behavior. I tried to explain that the resident was very busy and simply "out of sorts." I have to admit that, initially, I was probably just as shocked by the resident's response as Darlene. I did speak to the resident alone later and learned that this tactic was intentional. The resident had previous success with what he referred to as a form of "tough love" that involves shocking a patient into compliance. However, in this encounter, Darlene had no way of knowing that his response was well intended, and it was wholly unsuccessful. The resident ignored communication cues and did not take Darlene's specific circumstance into consideration. While talking further with Darlene, I became convinced that she wouldn't start hearing us until she could trust us. I wish I had had the courage to ask the resident to apologize to Darlene. His apology might have been exactly what was needed to get her to trust us, but that was not going to happen. I knew that I needed to work even harder to establish a trusting relationship with Darlene. Although this encounter did negatively affect this process, I needed to move forward and do my best to give Darlene and her fetus their best chance at a positive outcome. I'm learning that when patient welfare is at stake, I may have to sacrifice my own comfort level to challenge other professional caregivers and take the lead when the patient's relationship with the health care team is at risk. Hopefully, I'll learn how to do this in a way that promotes respectful, collaborative relationships.

QSEN SELF-REFLECTION ON QUALITY AND SAFETY COMPETENCIES
DEVELOPING KNOWLEDGE, SKILLS, AND ATTITUDES FOR CONTINUOUS IMPROVEMENT

How do you think you would respond in a similar situation? Why? What does this tell you about yourself and the adequacy of your skills for professional practice? Can you think of other ways to respond? What *knowledge, skills,* and *attitudes* do you need to develop to continuously improve quality and safety when caring for patients like Darlene?

Patient-Centered Care: What information should be communicated to Darlene regarding concerns about her pregnancy and the developing fetus? How could you involve the patient as a partner in coordinating her care to promote trust? How might you talk with Darlene about the various risk factors contributing to her health and that of her fetus? What is the best way to communicate emotional support to Darlene?

(*continued*)

QSEN Reflective Practice: Cultivating QSEN Competencies (continued)

CHALLENGE TO ETHICAL AND LEGAL SKILLS

Teamwork and Collaboration/Quality Improvement: What communication skills do you need to continue to function as a resource and advocate for Darlene? What if the nurse confronted the resident in front of the patient? Would you consider this professional behavior? Do you feel that the resident functioned in a professional manner? What is your role in facilitating the ongoing professional development and education of the resident? How will your constructive feedback make a difference? Do you agree with the nurse in the thinking that an apology from the resident would help encourage Darlene to trust health care professionals? Why or why not? Are there other community resources that may help Darlene in the care of her baby following the baby's birth?

Safety/Evidence-Based Practice: Is there anything more you could have done to acknowledge you understand Darlene's reasons for lack of trust and possible unwillingness to make changes to promote a positive outcome? How might a nurse's developmental stage have affected the actions taken toward the resident and the patient? What evidence in nursing literature provides guidance for decision making regarding ensuring a safe environment and giving Darlene the support that she needs?

Informatics: Can you identify essential information that must be documented in Darlene's electronic record about efforts to communicate with her and the specific concerns that she expressed? What other information must be available to support safe care for Darlene and her fetus and coordination of her care? Can you think of other ways to respond or approach the situation?

infant deaths were related to preterm birth and low birth weight. Infants born preterm are at increased risk for disorders such as respiratory problems, feeding and digestive difficulties, cerebral palsy, developmental delay, and sensory problems such as vision or hearing impairment (CDC, 2020c). Racial and ethnic disparities persist in relation to preterm birth. In 2019, the rate of preterm births among non-Hispanic Black women (14.4%) was higher than the rate among non-Hispanic White women (9.3%) or Hispanic women (10%; CDC, 2020c). Many people, including health care workers, are unaware of the magnitude of the potential and actual problems associated with preterm birth.

Other health risks for the developing fetus are discussed later in this chapter.

NEONATES: BIRTH TO 28 DAYS

At birth, the **neonate** must adapt to extrauterine life through several significant physiologic adjustments. The most important adjustments occur in the respiratory and circulatory systems as the neonate begins breathing and maintains circulation independent of the umbilical cord. The neonate is assessed immediately after birth. Of several existing measurement scales, the Apgar (1953) rating scale is the most commonly used tool for standardized assessment. This scale is used to assess neonates 1 and 5 minutes after birth (Table 23-1). An expanded Apgar score reporting form that includes ongoing assessment at 10, 15, and 20 minutes is recommended (as needed) to document resuscitative interventions (American College of Obstetricians and Gynecologists, 2015/2021).

Physiologic Development

The physical characteristics and behaviors of normal neonates are as follows:

- Reflexes include the Moro reflex, the stepping reflex, grasp reflex, hand-to-mouth activity, sucking, swallowing, blinking, sneezing, and yawning (Fig. 23-1).
- Body temperature responds quickly to the environmental temperature.
- Senses are used to respond to the environment; see color and form; hear and turn toward sound, smell, and taste; and feel touch and pain.
- Stool and urine are eliminated.
- Both an active crying state and a quiet alert state are exhibited (see Fig. 23-1).

The neonate inherits a transient immunity from infections as a result of maternal immunoglobulins that cross the placenta. Breastfeeding provides further protection

Table 23-1 Apgar Scoring Chart

CATEGORY[a]	0	1	2
Heart rate	Absent	<100 beats/min	>100 beats/min
Respiratory effort	Absent	Slow, irregular	Good, crying
Muscle tone	Flaccid	Some flexion of extremities	Active motion
Reflex irritability	No response	Weak cry or grimace	Vigorous cry
Color	Blue, pale	Body pink, extremities blue	Completely pink

[a]Each category is rated as 0, 1, or 2. The rating for each category is then totaled to a maximum score of 10. Normal neonates score between 7 and 10. Neonates who score between 4 and 6 require special assistance; those who score below 4 are in need of immediate life-saving support.

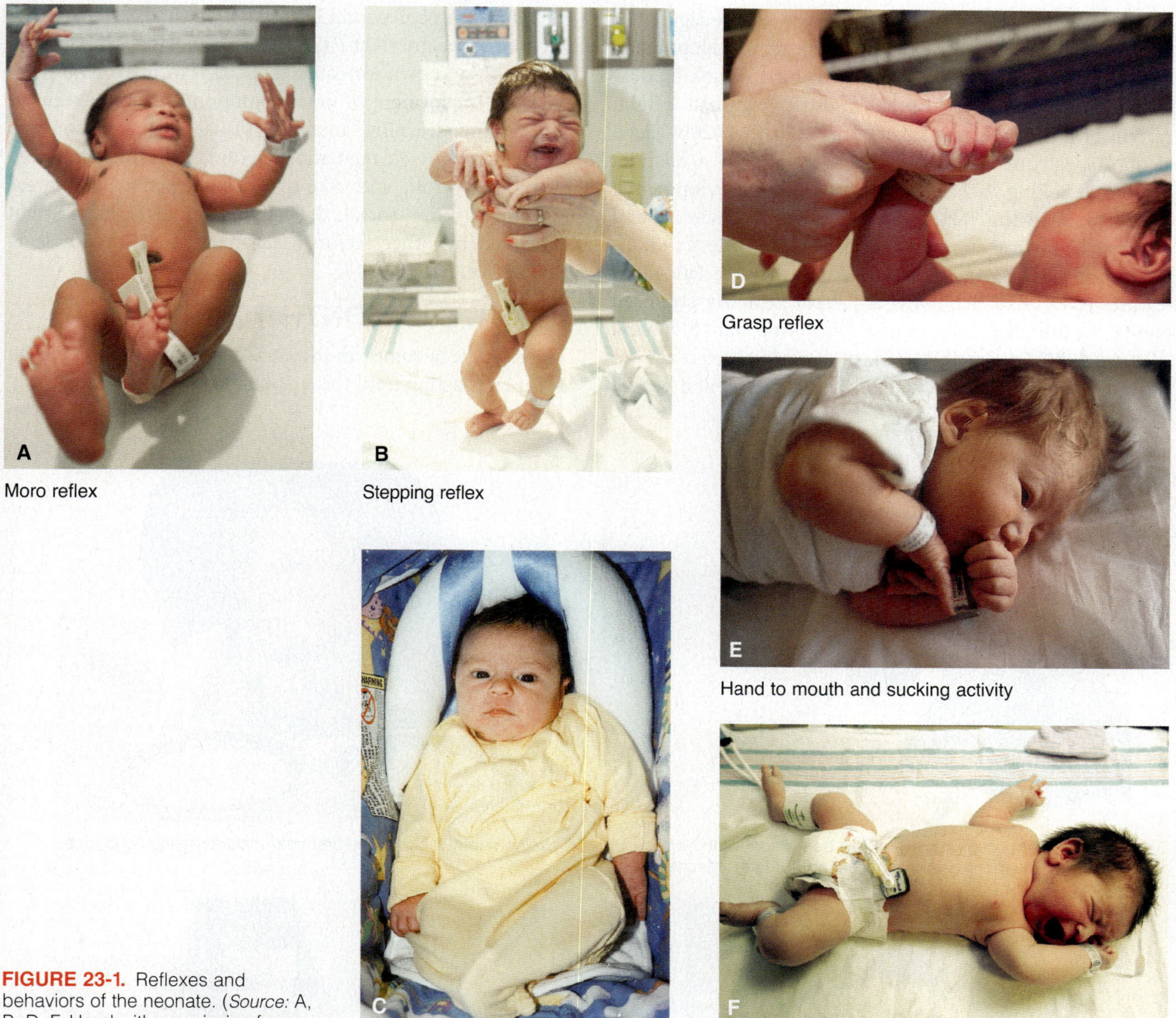

A Moro reflex

B Stepping reflex

C Quiet alert state

D Grasp reflex

E Hand to mouth and sucking activity

F Active crying state

FIGURE 23-1. Reflexes and behaviors of the neonate. (*Source:* A, B, D, F. Used with permission from Shutterstock. *Photos by Joe Mitchell.*)

against bacterial and viral infections through antibodies, immunoglobulins, and leukocytes in breast milk. The high lactose content in breast milk, combined with limited protein, promotes an acid environment that is unsuitable for bacterial growth. The American College of Obstetricians and Gynecologists (ACOG, 2018) recommends exclusive breastfeeding for the first 6 months of life, with continued breastfeeding, complemented by the introduction of solid foods, through the first year of life or for as long as mutually desired by the person breastfeeding and the infant.

Health of the Neonate

Difficulties related to the birth process, the transition to extrauterine life, or congenital anomalies may require intervention by health care personnel.

Respiratory difficulties may occur, especially if drugs given to the birthing person during labor and delivery have sedated the neonate. Premature neonates are vulnerable to respiratory distress syndrome because of their relatively immature lung function. Neonates delivered by cesarean birth are at risk for respiratory difficulties because of excess mucus in the lungs and may require frequent suctioning.

Incompatibility between the neonate's and birthing person's blood groups (Rh factor) requires prompt care at birth. Congenital malformations, such as cleft palate and cleft lip or neural tube defects (such as spina bifida) and hydrocephalus, may result in long-term health problems. When there are birth traumas that cause temporary symptoms—for example, caput succedaneum (localized edema of the scalp), molding (elongation of the skull as the baby passes through the birth canal), and subconjunctival hemorrhage—the parents and caregivers need to be reassured that the symptoms will disappear. The nonthreatening nature of physiologic jaundice, which commonly occurs in the neonate's first days, should also be explained to the parents and caregivers.

Neonates born to birthing persons who smoke cigarettes, drink alcohol, or use drugs are at risk for developmental deficits as well as complications during birth. Smoking during pregnancy can lead to preterm birth, low birth weight, certain birth defects, and infant death (CDC, 2020b). Fetal alcohol spectrum disorders (FASDs) caused by a birthing person's drinking include a range of neurodevelopmental disorders involving neurocognitive, neurobehavioral, and neuropsychological components; learning disorders and difficulties at school; growth disorders; and characteristic facial features (Oei, 2020; Schölin et al., 2021). A newly proposed mental health diagnosis in the *Diagnostic and Statistical Manual, Fifth Edition* (DSM-5), the standard reference for clinical diagnosis and practice for the field of mental health, includes Neurobehavioral Disorder associated with Prenatal Alcohol Exposure (ND-PAE). This diagnosis applies to children with a known exposure to alcohol in utero who present with impairment in neurocognition (general, executive functioning, learning, memory, visual–spatial reasoning), impairment in self-regulation (mood, behavior, attention, impulse control), and adaptive dysfunction in two areas (communication, social, daily living, motor), that are not explained by other factors (Hagan et al., 2016; Kable & Mukherjee, 2017).

INFANTS: 1 MONTH TO 1 YEAR

The neonate becomes an **infant** at 1 month, with the period of infancy lasting until the first birthday (Fig. 23-2).

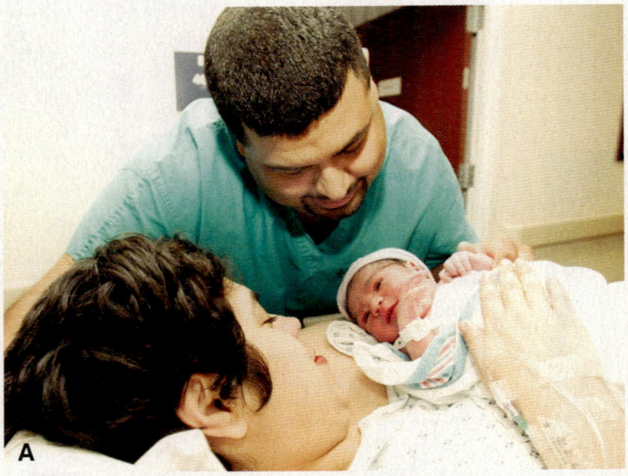

Bonding might occur in the first few hours after birth or later in the first few months and is necessary for later attachment.

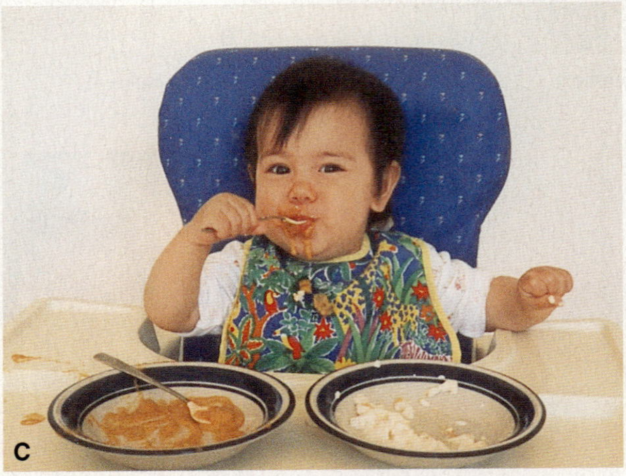

Developmental tasks of the first year include eating solid food.

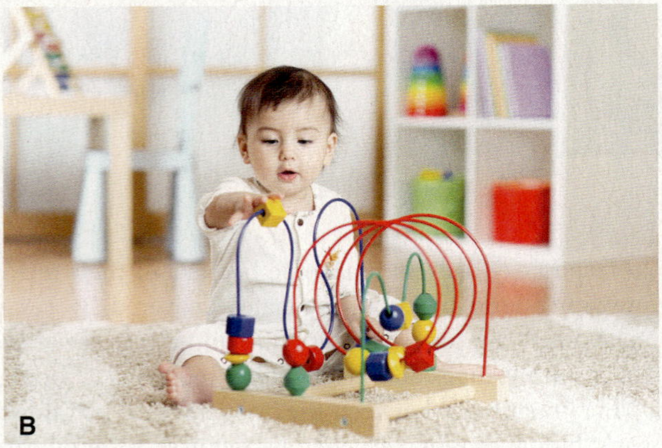

As the infant enters the second half of her first year, play will begin to involve manipulation of objects and the environment.

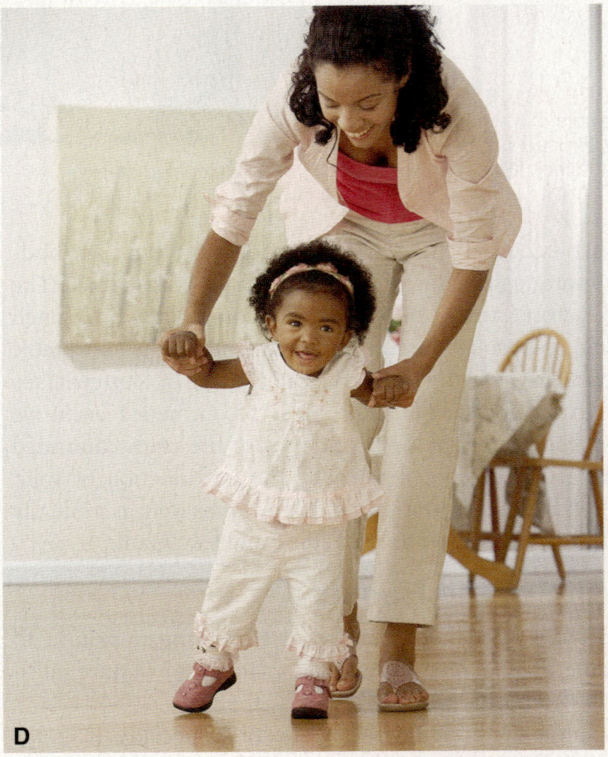

Later infancy is characterized by the ability to pull-to-stand, cruise, and often walk.

FIGURE 23-2. Development in the infant. (*Source:* A. Used with permission from Shutterstock. *Photo by Joe Mitchell.* B. Used with permission from Shutterstock. *Photo by Oksana Kuzmina.* D. Used with permission from Shutterstock. *Photo by Blend Images.*)

Physiologic Development

The physical characteristics of the infant include the following:

- The brain grows to about half the adult size.
- Body temperature stabilizes.
- Motor abilities develop, allowing the infant to use building blocks, to attempt to feed themselves, and eventually to crawl and walk.
- The eyes begin to focus and fixate.
- The heart doubles in weight, the heart rate slows, and blood pressure rises.
- Deciduous teeth begin to erupt at 4 to 6 months.
- Birth weight usually triples by 1 year, when the average male infant weighs 22 lb (10 kg) and the average female infant weighs 21 lb (9.5 kg); length increases by 50%.

Cognitive Development

Infants from birth to 1 year are in the sensorimotor stage of development described by Piaget (Piaget & Inhelder, 1969). Language development is in the prelinguistic phase. Babies begin to coo and make sounds soon after birth, and by age 12 months, they can convey their wishes through a few key words. Language development in infants has several consistent characteristics that occur with all languages:

- Use of syllable repetition (such as ma-ma, da-da, bye-bye)
- Universal early phonetic expressions (babbling sounds)
- Imitation of sounds and intonations spoken by caregivers

Psychosocial Development

Developmental Theories

The developmental theories discussed in Chapter 22 describe the infant as having the following characteristics:

- *Freud's theory* (1960): The infant is in the oral stage, striving for immediate gratification of needs and having a strong sucking need.
- *Erikson's theory* (1963): The infant develops trust if the caregiver can be counted on to provide food when the infant is hungry; trust is also facilitated by diaper changing, warmth, and comforting.
- *Havinghurst's theory* (1972): The infant meets developmental tasks by learning to eat solid food, walk, and talk.

Special Considerations

Other components of psychosocial development in the neonate and infant include attachment, bonding, play, and temperament.

ATTACHMENT AND BONDING

Attachment is an active, affectionate, reciprocal relationship between two people, which is somewhat different from bonding. **Bonding**, described by Klaus and Kennell (1982), occurs during a sensitive period in the first few hours after birth (although bonding also may occur later in the first few months) and is necessary for later attachment. Bonding may be considered the emotional linkage of two people, while attachment is considered the long-term maintenance and strengthening of that linked state. Physical (skin-to-skin) contact is a component of attachment research. Maternal proximity may influence the socioemotional development of the infant, and have positive effects on the infant's sleep patterns, internal body regulation, behavioral responses, development of colic (crying), speech development, trauma resilience, and their physical health as adults (Norholt, 2020).

PLAY

Infants and children discover their environment and begin to learn how to control it through play. Beginning as soon as the baby is aware of sensations and the enjoyment they produce, play progresses from entertaining oneself to interaction with others. The two dimensions of play are social play and cognitive play. Social play, such as rolling a ball back and forth between two children, is motivated by a desire for fun, pleasure, and engagement with others. Cognitive play, like when a child puts a puzzle together, is motivated by the desire to learn.

TEMPERAMENT

Temperament is primarily inborn, although it is influenced by environment. A baby or child may be said to be "easy," "slow to warm," or "difficult" (Thomas et al., 1968). The *easy* infant sleeps, eats, and eliminates easily; smiles spontaneously; and cries in response to significant needs. The *slow-to-warm* infant is more passive and distant. The *difficult* infant has volatile and labile responses, often is a restless sleeper, is highly sensitive to noises, and eats poorly. These traits often remain fairly consistent throughout the person's life. The behavior of caregivers as they care for the baby can positively or negatively influence the degree to which temperament dictates behavioral style.

Health of the Infant

Various health problems in infancy may require the intervention of health care personnel. Gastroenteritis and food allergies are common. Skin disorders, such as diaper dermatitis (diaper rash), seborrheic dermatitis (infant dandruff), prickly heat rash, acute infantile eczema, and oral thrush (infection of the oral mucous membrane by the fungus *Candida albicans*), are also common. Infant colic, failure to thrive, accidents, sudden infant death syndrome (SIDS), and child maltreatment are of particular concern during infancy.

Infant Colic

Colic is often described using *Wessel's rule of threes* that involves inconsolable crying or fussing in an infant that lasts more than 3 hours, occurs more than 3 days per week, and lasts for more than 3 weeks, although the duration was changed to 7 days in the modified Wessel's criteria (Hjern et al., 2020; Wolke et al., 2017). A recent update to the Rome IV criteria (established by gastroenterology experts) counters that the 3-hour designation may be arbitrary and culturally dependent, and that the inability to console or soothe the infant was a key element (Hjern et al., 2020; Zeevenhooven et al., 2017). Periods of colic are more frequent the first

Through the Eyes of a Caregiver

When my son Luke was first born, he was an easy-going, pleasant baby. Then, when he was about 3 weeks old, it started. He cried inconsolably every night from 5 PM until 12 AM. We could do nothing to comfort him. We took him to the pediatrician. The doctor said the word we already expected to hear: "colic." He gave us a prescription for an antacid and a muscle relaxant. He gave us some advice on how to comfort him . . . wrap him snugly, hold him like a football, eliminate milk and dairy from my diet (I was breastfeeding), and put pressure on his belly. None of these things worked. Eventually, we discovered that rocking him in our arms as we ran the shower seemed to calm him. Pink Floyd and *Dark Side of the Moon* also comforted him. We found this out quite accidentally when we played the vinyl record in an attempt to drown out his crying. These methods somewhat helped with the crying but did little to help my anxiety. I was concerned for my little son, who was clearly upset or maybe even in pain. At the same time, I found it very difficult to bond with him. I'd find myself dreading the evening, dreading being with my baby. When I'd come home from work, I'd take a deep breath and stand paralyzed at the front door, wondering if I had to go in. I could hear his crying from the doorstep. I felt horrible about these feelings. I questioned my parenting skills. At one point, I spoke with a nurse whose daughter had colic. She said, "My daughter's colic lasted 100 days, but it has taken me 14 years to forgive her!" This made me laugh for the first time in weeks. Then she asked how I was doing and if I wanted to talk about how I was feeling. I hadn't told anyone how I was feeling toward my son. How could I? I confided in her, though. I knew she wouldn't judge me. I knew she'd understand. After speaking with the nurse, I felt a lot better knowing that it was OK to feel the way I did. As time went on, Luke's crying spells got shorter and shorter, until the 99th day; then, miraculously, it ended. We had a party the next day, with a cake that said "Day 100. We made it." Today, he is a sweet, healthy child. He is no fussier than any other 3-year-old child. We have bonded exceptionally well. My husband and family were supportive and helped care for Luke when he had colic, but it was the nurse who helped care for me!

—Dana Jameson, Philadelphia, PA

6 weeks of life (17% to 25%) and then decrease between 6 and 12 weeks of life (11%, then down to 0.6% at 10 to 12 weeks; Wolke et al., 2017). This continuous crying can occur at any time but usually worsens in the evening. The infant cries loudly and draws the legs up to the abdomen. Despite the symptoms, the infant gains weight, and a change in feeding type or process does not improve colic. Although *Lactobacillus reuteri* DSM 17938, a probiotic, shows promise in the treatment of colic, acupuncture has not proven to be effective (Hjern et al., 2020). Parents, caregivers, and other family members may experience stress and anxiety due to the constant crying (de Kruijff et al., 2021; see Through the Eyes of a Caregiver).

Failure to Thrive

Failure to thrive (FTT) is a condition of inadequate growth in height and weight resulting from the infant's inability to obtain or use calories needed for growth. Collection of serial height, weight, and head circumference measurements on a reference scale such as a growth chart are helpful in determining this clinical finding (Homan, 2016). Infants with prolonged severe malnutrition may show signs of compromised cognitive and immune function, and may not meet developmental milestones (Franceschi et al., 2021). Causes and contributing factors most commonly include malnutrition or inadequate caloric intake but may also include organic causes such as gastrointestinal and genetic diagnoses. Contributing factors may include neglect or abuse, maternal education level, poverty, poor parenting skills, psychosocial family issues, and unusual health or nutritional beliefs (Franceschi et al., 2021; Homan, 2016). In most cases of FTT not caused by a physiologic problem, a team of health care providers is needed to meet the complex needs of the infant and caregivers.

Accidental Injuries

Among the safety issues that must be discussed with the infant's parents or guardians are the dangers related to aspiration and choking. The swallowing reflex matures progressively from birth, but until it is fully developed, aspiration is a risk. Also, because infants often put small objects in their mouths, choking is a risk. Choking may also result from small pieces of food, nuts, and popcorn. Parents and caregivers need instruction on what to do if the infant is choking. If the airway is obstructed and the infant is not coughing forcefully or does not have a strong cry, the parent or caregiver should give five quick back blows between the infant's shoulders while holding the infant prone over one arm. If this does not dislodge the object, the infant should be placed in a supine position over the rescuer's thighs with the infant's head supported, and five chest compressions to the lower third of the sternum should be given quickly. The cycle of five back blows, followed by five chest compressions should continue until the object is expelled or the infant becomes unresponsive. If the infant becomes unresponsive, CPR needs to be initiated (Topjian et al., 2020).

As the infant becomes more mobile, the risk for falls or for being caught in a dangling cord (such as in mini-blinds) increases. Preventive measures against such safety hazards must be taught to new parents or guardians. In addition, the law requires using special car safety seats and restraints for infants. See the accompanying display, Examples of Actual or Potential Health Problems and Needs: Infancy Through School Age.

Examples of Actual or Potential Health Problems and Needs

INFANCY THROUGH SCHOOL AGE

Actual or Potential Health Problem or Need	Possible Etiologic Factors	Potential Signs and Symptoms
Feeding ADL deficit	• Insufficient food or fluid intake • Barrier(s) to accessing fluid or water • Caregiver's insufficient knowledge about age-specific nutritional needs • Excessive fluid loss (vomiting and diarrhea)	• Change in disposition, crying, or activity • Decrease in urine output • Dry mucous membranes • Increase in heart rate • Failure to grow and meet developmental milestones
Injury risk	• Insufficient knowledge and adherence to safety standards with skates, bicycles, roller blades, and trampolines • Immunization level within community • Exposure to toxic chemical; unsafe water or food sources • Unsafe mode of transportation or inappropriate use of car seat restraints	

Source: Wolters Kluwer. (2020). *Problem-based care plans.* In Lippincott Advisor. Wolters Kluwer. https://advisor.lww.com/lna/home.do

Sudden Infant Death Syndrome and Sudden Unexpected Infant Death

Sudden infant death syndrome (SIDS) refers to the sudden death of an infant younger than age 1 year when consideration of the infant's history, a postmortem examination, and investigation of the scene where the death occurred fails to reveal a cause of death.

Approximately 1,250 infants died of SIDS in 2019, making SIDS the leading cause of death in infants 1 to 12 months old (CDC, 2021e). **Sudden unexpected infant death (SUID)** is an all-encompassing term used for sudden, unexplained infant deaths where the cause of death cannot readily be identified prior to an investigation (CDC, 2021e). SUID includes SIDS, accidental deaths (suffocation or strangulation), natural deaths (infections and cardiac, neurologic, or metabolic disorders), and homicides (American SIDS Institute, 2022); SUID accounted for about 3,400 deaths in the United States in 2019 (CDC, 2021e).

Approximately 900 children younger than age 1 year die annually from unintentional suffocation (or strangulation) in bed (CDC, 2021e). Suffocation deaths can occur when infants co-sleep with adults, other children, or animals (Task Force on Sudden Infant Death Syndrome, 2016). These accidental deaths occur most commonly when infants share a bed with adults (co-sleeping) and are inadvertently wedged beneath another person, trapped in a dangerous position, such as between the bed and the wall, and suffocated by bedding or an unapproved infant sleep positioner (ISP). In an effort to improve diagnostic and reporting practices, the CDC supports the SUID case registry and Sudden Death in the Young case registry to monitor national trends, identify risk factors, and focus on interventions to prevent these infant deaths (CDC, 2021a).

The rate of infant deaths attributed to SIDS has declined significantly since the early 1990s when the *Safe to Sleep* campaign promoted placing infants on their backs to sleep rather than in the prone position. The American Academy of Pediatrics (Task Force on Sudden Infant Death Syndrome, 2016) issued updated safe sleep guidelines for infants that include the following A-level recommendations:

- Place infant on back to sleep for every sleep.
- Use a firm sleep surface.
- Breastfeed.
- Place the infant on a separate sleep surface for room-sharing.
- Keep soft objects and loose bedding away from the infant's sleep area.
- Consider offering a pacifier at naptime and bedtime.
- Avoid smoke exposure, alcohol, and illicit drug use during pregnancy and after birth.
- Avoid overheating.
- Seek and obtain regular prenatal care.
- Immunize infants in accordance with AAP and CDC recommendations.
- Do not use home cardiorespiratory monitors as a strategy to reduce the risk of SIDS.
- Health care providers, staff in newborn nurseries and NICUs, and childcare providers should endorse and model the SIDS risk-reduction recommendations from birth.
- Media and manufacturers should follow safe sleep guidelines in their messaging and advertising.
- Continue the *Safe to Sleep* campaign, focusing on ways to reduce the risk of all sleep-related infant deaths, including SIDS, suffocation, and other unintentional deaths; pediatricians and other primary care providers should actively participate in this campaign.

Child Maltreatment

In the United States in 2020, 1 in 7 children experienced child abuse and neglect, with approximately 1,840 children dying due to abuse or neglect (CDC, 2021c). The Federal Child Abuse Prevention and Treatment Act (CAPTA), as amended and reauthorized by the CAPTA Reauthorization Act of 2010, defines child abuse and neglect as, at minimum, "Any recent act or failure to act on the part of a parent or caretaker which results in death, serious physical or emotional harm, sexual abuse or exploitation; or an act or failure to act which presents an imminent risk of serious harm" (Child Welfare Information Gateway, 2019b, p. 2). Although **child maltreatment** may occur at any age, most victims are from birth to age 4 years. Most states recognize four types of child maltreatment: physical abuse (nonaccidental physical injury), sexual abuse (visual depiction, rape, molestation, prostitution, incest, or other exploitation), emotional or psychological abuse (pattern of behavior), and neglect (failure to provide for physical, medical, educational, or emotional needs). Abandonment, parental/guardian substance use, and human trafficking are also classified as abuse or neglect in many states (Child Welfare Information Gateway, 2019b).

Childhood abuse and neglect have long-term physical, emotional or psychological, behavioral, and societal consequences for health—these traumatic experiences and the related negative effects are referred to as ***adverse childhood experiences*** (ACEs) (Child Welfare Information Gateway, 2019a). Individual outcomes vary widely and are affected by the age and developmental stage when the abuse or neglect occurred; the type of maltreatment; the frequency, duration, and severity of the maltreatment; and the relationship between the child and perpetrator. Long-term physical effects can include chronic health conditions such as cardiovascular disease, lung and bowel disease, cancer, and diabetes. Abuse or neglect can result in immediate neurologic consequences, such as brain damage from head trauma (shaking), but is also associated with long-term consequences such as reduced brain volume (size) and functional deficits in emotional regulation, learning, memory, motor function, and executive functioning (Child Welfare Information Gateway, 2019a). Additional psychological consequences of abuse or neglect can include an inability to regulate emotions, issues with executive functioning and cognitive skill development, attachment and social difficulties, mental health issues, and posttraumatic stress disorder with the associated symptoms. Unfortunately, these can lead to behavioral consequences including substance abuse, criminality, continuation of the abuse and neglect cycle, and sexual risk-taking. These consequences affect society and lead to significant direct and indirect costs (Child Welfare Information Gateway, 2019a).

Although child abuse occurs in all racial and ethnic groups and at all levels of society, certain factors increase the risk, including the following (Child Welfare Information Gateway, 2019a; Psychology Today, 2019):

- Caregivers' substance abuse; this includes manufacturing, distribution or selling, using, and prenatal exposure
- Caregivers experiencing stress from poverty or unemployment
- Caregivers' mental illness or other health problems
- History of violence in the family or community
- Physical or mental disabilities in the child or children that may increase caregiver burden
- Caregivers' lack of knowledge about parenting and the normal behaviors and development of children
- Lack of family and social support for caregivers, social isolation of families, lack of family cohesion, single caregiver, young caregivers

The fact that many cases of child abuse are not reported to police or social services is a national concern. Health care providers and facilities, teachers, daycare providers, and social workers are in an excellent position to recognize families at risk and offer interventions. In all 50 states, these professionals have a legal obligation to report suspected maltreatment (see Chapter 7). Organizations that serve as resources for child abuse concerns are listed in Table 23-2. The long-term treatment of children who are abused and their families is complex and requires input from the entire interprofessional team. Fostering the development of protective factors for victims of maltreatment at the individual, relationship, and community levels can prevent and mitigate some of the effects of abuse or neglect (Child Welfare Information Gateway, 2019a). Although children may overcome the ACEs and manage or recover from residual effects, they benefit from prevention, early recognition, and appropriate intervention.

Table 23-2 Child Abuse and Neglect Resources

ORGANIZATION	ACTIVITIES
Childhelp National Child Abuse Hotline http://www.childhelp.org Phone: 1-800-4-A-CHILD (1-800-422-4453)	Hotline counselors are available and can provide phone numbers for reporting abuse situations.
Child Welfare Information Gateway http://www.childwelfare.gov Phone: 1-800-394-3366	Provides access to information and resources to help protect children and strengthen families.
Prevent Child Abuse America http://www.preventchildabuse.org Phone: 1-800-244-5373 or 312-663-3520	National organization that provides access to hotlines, self-help groups, publications, and volunteer opportunities.
U.S. Department of Health and Human Services Children's Bureau https://www.acf.hhs.gov	Assists states in the delivery of child welfare services.

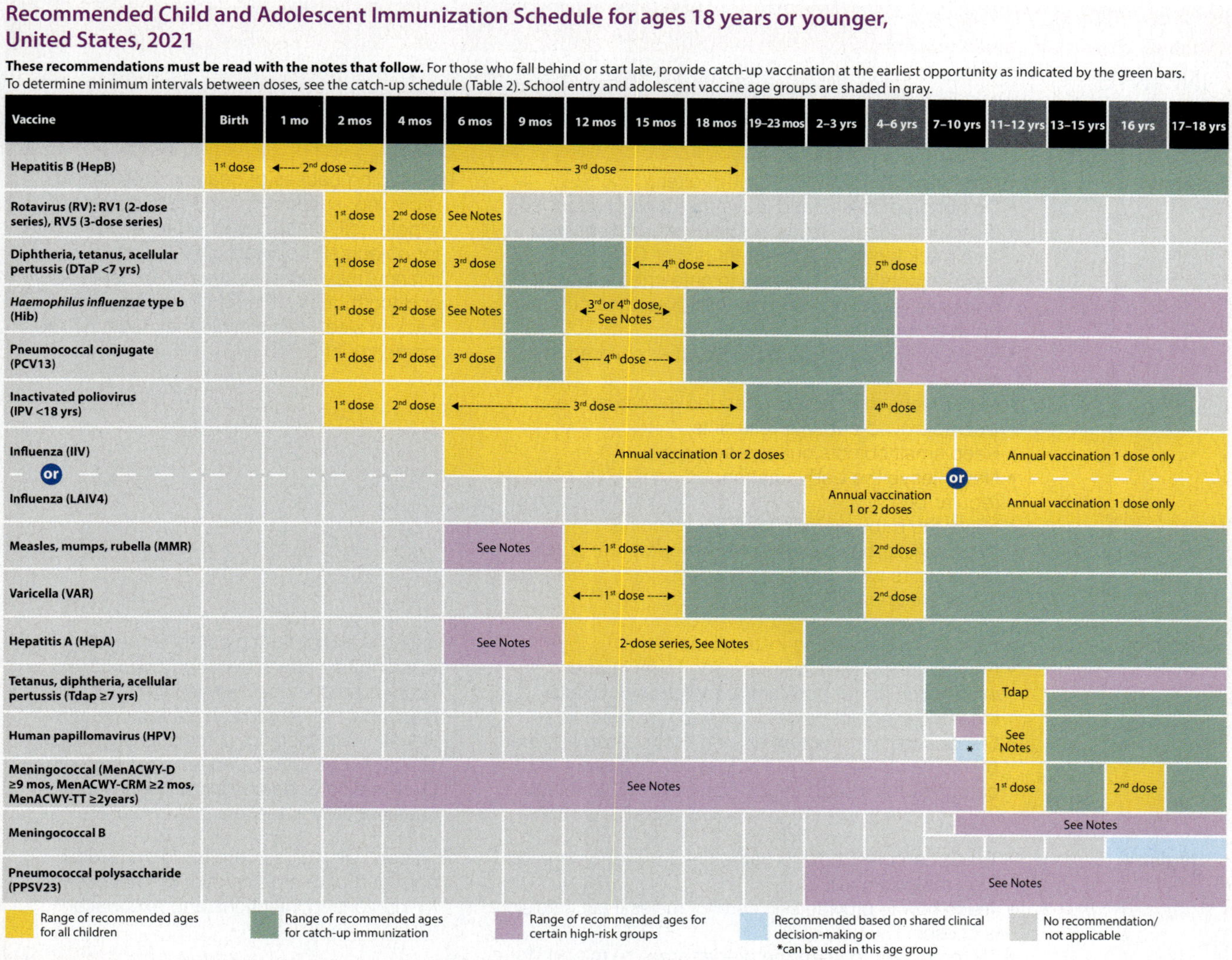

FIGURE 23-3. Recommended immunization schedule for children and adolescents aged 18 years or younger—United States, 2022. Footnote information available online. (*Source:* Reprinted from Centers for Disease Control and Prevention. https://www.cdc.gov/vaccines/schedules/downloads/child/0-18yrs-child-combined-schedule.pdf)

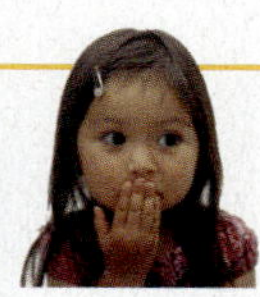

Recall 2-year-old **Hillarie Browning**. Her injuries are suspicious and may be a sign of child abuse. The nurse and other health care team members are required to report Hillarie's case to begin an investigation. Although Hillarie may not be a victim of child abuse, the safety and well-being of this child is of paramount importance. All efforts will be made to treat and protect this child.

Immunization against contagious diseases begins during the first year of life and should follow a regular schedule, as outlined in Figure 23-3. Health care providers need to listen to parents' or guardians' concerns about immunization and guide them to resources with current immunization information and schedules (CDC, 2021b). Guidelines for new or evolving vaccines, such as the COVID-19 or Ebola vaccine, are based on recommendations from the Advisory Committee on Immunizations Practices (AICP) and are frequently updated (https://www.cdc.gov/vaccines/hcp/acip-recs/index.html).

Role of the Nurse in Promoting Health and Preventing Illness

The most essential role of the nurse in promoting health of the infant is teaching family members or guardians and caregivers. Teaching ranges from providing basic information about prevention of diaper rash to facilitating grieving in parents who have lost a baby to SIDS. Examples of specific areas of preventive teaching for parents or guardians of infants are given in Teaching Tips 23-1 on page 604.

Technology Alert

The Centers for Disease Control and Prevention offers a CDC Vaccines Schedules App for clinicians and other health care professionals. This application provides free online access to the latest immunization schedules, associated footnotes, and immunization resources. Download the app here: https://www.cdc.gov/vaccines/schedules/hcp/schedule-app.html#download

Teaching Tips 23-1

INFANTS

Health Topic	Teaching Tip	Why Is This Important?
Safety	• Feed the baby slowly and burp often. • Do not prop bottles and leave the baby unattended. • If choking occurs, follow appropriate procedure to give back blows and chest thrusts or CPR. • Place infants on their backs in safe cribs with no crib bumpers, loose bedding, or toys. Keep the crib rails up at all times. • Avoid co-sleeping with parents, other children, and animals. • Never leave the baby unattended in or near water. • Use approved car seat restraints. • Keep small objects out of reach. • Never leave the baby unattended on a table, chair, or regular bed. • Place the baby on their back for sleeping. • Keep plastic bags and mini-blind cords out of reach. • Block stairs with gates. • Cover electrical outlets.	The leading causes of death in infants are drowning, suffocation, and falls. Infants wiggle, roll, creep, crawl, walk, and reach for objects. Propping bottles, even in later infancy, may increase the risk of aspiration and tooth decay. Placing babies on their back to sleep has significantly reduced the incidence of SIDS.
Nutrition	• Provide breastfeeding instructions. • Provide instructions on preparing formula and information about positioning for feeding. Stress the importance of holding the baby for feeding. • Discuss the introduction of solid foods, as prescribed by the health care provider. Instruct the parent or caregiver not to add sugar, salt, or honey to foods.	Feeding is a time for the caregiver and baby to strengthen attachment and bonding. There is no one best time to introduce solid foods, but they should be started one at a time. If breastfeeding, complimentary foods should not be introduced until age 6 months. Overfeeding or adding extra calories may cause obesity in the infant or in later life.
Hygiene	• Teach caregiver how to bathe the baby and care for the umbilical cord. • Teach how to provide skin care for males if circumcision is chosen. • Tell caregiver to keep the diaper area clean and dry.	Skin care, as well as care for the umbilical cord and circumcision site, are necessary for preventing infections and excoriations.
Elimination	• By age 2 months, babies usually have two stools a day. • Breastfed babies vary more in bowel consistency, color, and times than babies fed formula.	Renal and intestinal physiology develop throughout the first year of life.
Growth and Development	• Provide consistent care and love. • Growth and development differ for each infant, but there are some predictable milestones. • Provide educational toys appropriate to the age of the infant. • Talk and read to the baby. • Allow the baby to explore different shapes, sizes, tastes, and experiences.	The infant must be consistently loved and cared for in order to thrive, learn to trust, and achieve developmental tasks. Stimulation with age-appropriate toys and the freedom to explore influence intellectual development.
Promoting Health and Preventing Illness	• If a danger of lead ingestion exists, take appropriate measures and have the baby screened. • Maintain schedule of immunizations. • Contact health care provider for care of respiratory infections. • Wean baby off pacifier in the second 6 months of life. • Stress importance of supplemental fluoride if water is not fluoridated. • Continue well-baby checkups as recommended. • Do not smoke in the house or car with the baby. • Keep infants younger than 6 months out of direct sunlight and covered with protective clothing and hats.	Infants who ingest lead, such as from eating peeling lead-based paint, are at risk for brain damage, behavioral problems, and mental deficiency. Immunizations are an essential part of health care. Upper respiratory infections may spread to involve the middle ear or lungs. Fluoride is necessary for tooth structure. Cigarette smoke of any type (active or passive) is dangerous and may increase the risk of respiratory illnesses, asthma, and ear infections. Infants in daycare have increased exposure to respiratory and skin infections and infestations.

It is also important to assess the infant's growth and development. Growth rate is assessed in comparison with standardized growth charts developed for males and females, whose growth rates differ. Be careful when comparing an individual child's growth to standards on a chart for the following reasons:

- Every child has individual variations and short-term spurts and lags in growth.
- Atypical infants, such as those who are premature or have low birth weight, are not accounted for in such charts.
- At around age 3 months, weight gain is generally lower for breastfed infants. World Health Organization (WHO) growth charts were normed based on infants who are breastfed; therefore, current recommendations are to use the international WHO growth charts for children ages birth to younger than 2 years, and then transition to the CDC growth reference charts ages 2 through 20 years to monitor growth (CDC, 2015).

The inexpensive Denver Developmental Screening Test (DDST II) is commonly used to quickly assess for atypical developmental patterns in infants and children. The crucial areas of development assessed in the DDST II are gross motor behavior and skills, fine motor behavior and skills, language acquisition, and personal and social interaction. The test identifies problem areas that require more precise assessments. The DDST II is described in more detail in most pediatric nursing texts.

When an infant in late infancy is hospitalized, separation anxiety behaviors are common. **Separation anxiety** normally occurs when a child is separated from loved ones who offer security. It usually begins at about age 6 months and continues through the preschool period. At a later age, the young child is able to predict this happening and feels anxiety even before the separation occurs. The infant may initially cry and scream in the phase of protest, but then stop crying and appear depressed, which is the despair phase (Hockenberry et al., 2022). Nurses should facilitate parents or guardians staying with the hospitalized infant; when that is not possible, consistent health care providers are important to promote the infant's trust in others.

TODDLERS: 1 TO 3 YEARS

From ages 1 to 3 years, the child is considered a **toddler** (Fig. 23-4).

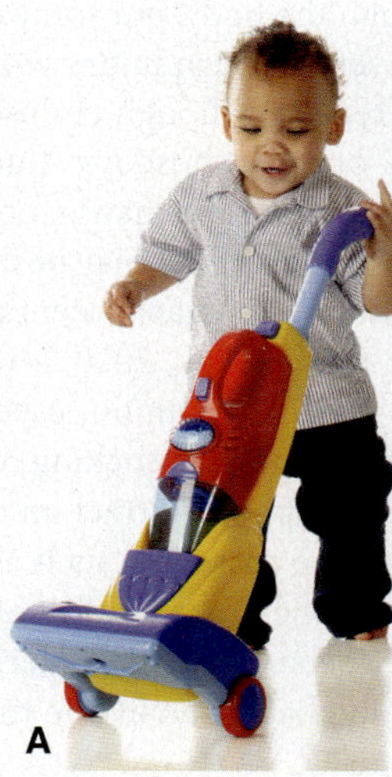

A Toddlers enter a stage of autonomy, promoting exploration.

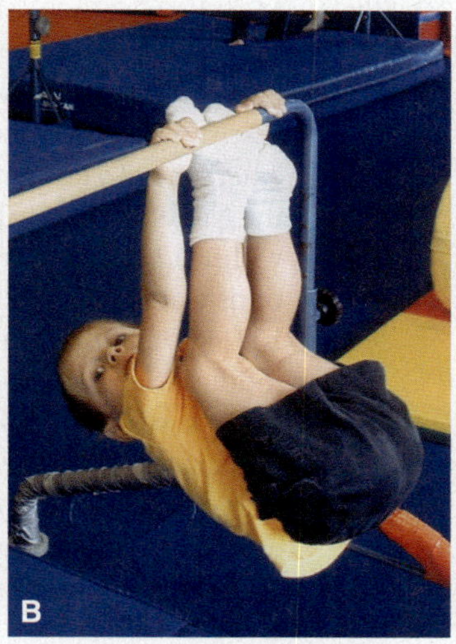

B The curious and independent toddler often has a desire to do things by himself.

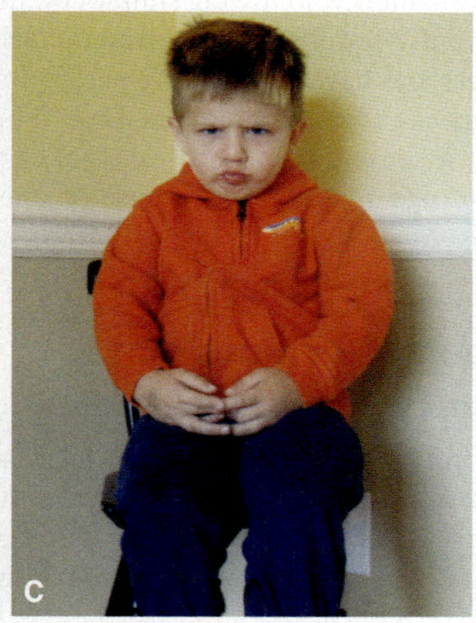

C Discipline helps toddlers learn inner control and understand limits.

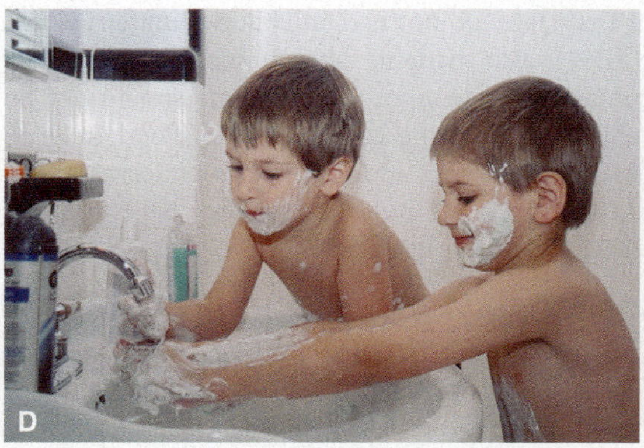

D Cognitive development can be promoted by allowing the toddler the opportunity to observe and imitate. Younger siblings particularly enjoy mimicking older siblings.

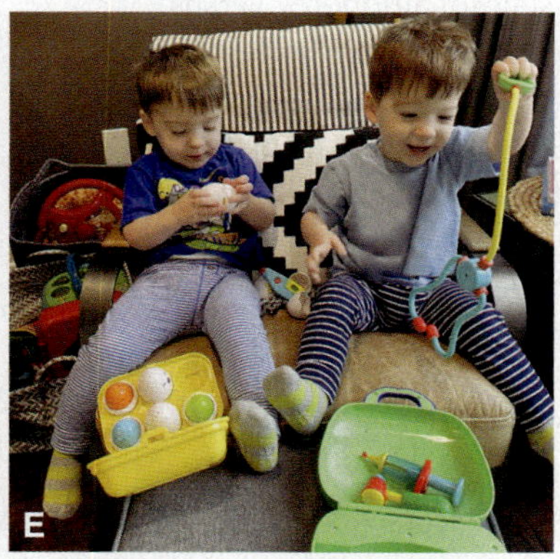

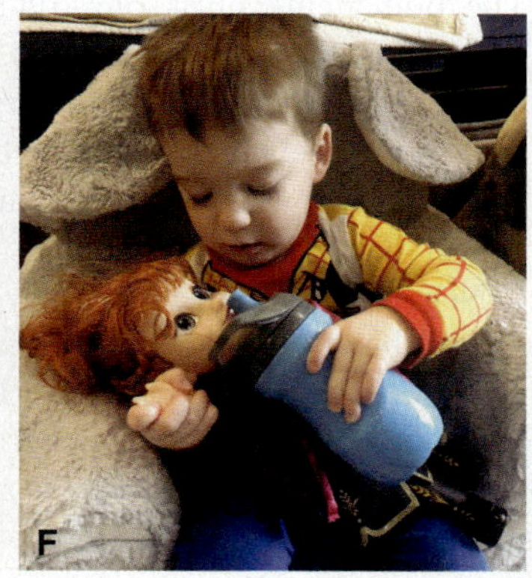

E, F Play in toddlerhood might be solitary or parallel.

FIGURE 23-4. Development in the toddler. (Courtesy of Amy Roach.)

Physiologic Development

Physiologic development continues steadily through the toddler years, but the pace is considerably slower than in infancy. In terms of growth and development, the toddler:

- Has rapid brain growth, increase in length of long bones of the arms and legs, and growth of muscles
- Uses fingers to pick up small objects
- Walks forward and backward, runs, kicks, climbs stairs, and rides a tricycle
- Drinks from a cup and uses a spoon
- Is typically four times the birth weight at age 2 years, averaging 30 to 35 lb (13.6 to 15.9 kg) and 23 to 37 inches (58.4 to 94 cm) in height.
- Has bladder control during the day and sometimes during the night (ages 2.5 to 3 years)
- Turns pages in a book and, by age 3 years, draws stick people

Cognitive Development

Toddlers are in Piaget's (Piaget & Inhelder, 1969) last two stages of sensorimotor development: beginning to understand object permanence, following simple commands, and anticipating events. Toddlers can understand self as separate from others and have a beginning perception of body image. Toddlers can identify and name several body parts, and they have a sense of biologic sex identity. Language begins at about age 1 year, with the use of one- or two-syllable sounds. At about age 2 years, children begin to use short sentences.

Psychosocial Development

Freud's Theory

The toddler is in Freud's (1960) anal stage. Increased muscle development and sphincter control encourage the child to focus on the pleasure of sphincter contraction and relaxation. Toilet training becomes a major focus during this period.

Erikson's Theory

The toddler enters Erikson's (1963) stage of autonomy versus shame and doubt. Autonomy is developing from independence in feeding, walking, dressing, and toileting, as well as the ability to express wishes verbally. Children who do not feel autonomous may be reluctant to explore and may be fearful of activities and people.

Negativism (characteristically expressed by saying, "no") and outbursts of temper result from the toddler's efforts at control over the environment. **Regression**, demonstrating behavior that is more characteristic of a younger age, can occur at any time in response to stressful circumstances. The most common regressive behaviors are excessive clinging to caregivers, loss of control over elimination, and the use of more infantile speech patterns.

Separation anxiety in response to separation from the mother figure intensifies at about age 18 to 24 months and can be as intense for the toddler as it was for the infant. The child may have feelings of anger, fear, grief, and revenge during this period, but, by age 24 months, the toddler begins to demonstrate increased independence from the mother or other primary caregiver (Hockenberry et al., 2022).

Havighurst's Theory

The toddler has the developmental task of learning to control the elimination of urine and feces and begins to learn sex differences, form concepts, learn language, and distinguish right from wrong (Havighurst, 1972).

Health of the Toddler

Accidents—such as motor vehicle crashes, poisonings, burns, drowning, choking and aspirations, and falls—are the major cause of death in toddlers. The number of young children visiting the ED due to ingestion of small button batteries has significantly increased. These batteries, typically 20 mm in diameter, are readily accessible and used in many toys and household products including remote controls, cell phones, and cameras. Ingestion and the associated injuries occur in children younger than age 6 years 70% of the time. Most batteries pass through the body, but some can lodge in the esophagus and cause serious burn injury within 2 hours. Battery removal may be required though endoscopy (upper gastrointestinal system) or bronchoscopy (lungs). Other emergency treatment (guided by information obtained from the National Battery Ingestion Hotline) may be implemented within 12 hours of ingestion to mitigate potential complications (Jatana et al., 2017; Khalaf et al., 2020; Mubarak et al., 2021). Dental problems are also common, especially if the toddler is allowed to go to sleep while sucking on a bottle of milk or sweetened liquid. Respiratory tract and middle-ear infections are common. Some surgeries, such as repair of a cleft lip and palate, may be done in the toddler years. Autistic disorder—with abnormal behavior, social interactions, and communication—is usually diagnosed by the time the child is 3 years old.

OTC cold medications can have serious adverse effects in infants and toddlers. The U.S. Food and Drug Administration (FDA) supports product labels on OTC cough and cold medicines that state "do not use" in children under the age of 2. The FDA is also changing labels to indicate that medications containing codeine or hydrocodone should not be used by children under the age of 18 (U.S. Food & Drug Administration, 2018). In addition to the concerns about misuse of the drugs, data indicate that they have minimal therapeutic value for this age group.

Role of the Nurse in Promoting Health and Preventing Illness

The role of the nurse in promoting health in the toddler continues to be primarily teaching, as shown by the examples in Teaching Tips 23-2. An important part of teaching is helping caregivers encourage their toddler's independence while setting firm limits.

Teaching Tips 23-2

TODDLERS

Health Topic	Teaching Tip	Why Is This Important?
Safety	• Lock medicines, cleaning supplies, and yard-care products out of reach. • Use safety plugs in electrical outlets. • Block stairs with gates. • Use approved car seat. • Never leave toddler unattended near water. Have toddler wear Coast Guard–approved life jackets around pools. • Do not give toddler small hard foods, small toys or toy parts, or balloons. • Keep plastic bags and mini-blind cords out of reach. • Teach danger in simple terms ("stove hot"). • Do not toss toddler in the air or swing by the arms.	Accidents are a leading cause of injuries and death in toddlers. It is necessary to childproof the home to prevent injury, as the toddler moves quickly, lacks judgment, and explores the world by seeing, touching, and tasting. Small objects or balloons may be aspirated and cause suffocation. Joints may be dislocated by swinging the child.
Nutrition	• Do not scold for messiness while eating. • Provide finger foods. • Short periods of loss of appetite are normal. • Avoid foods that are high in fat, sugar, and salt (often found in fast foods). • Watch for signs of food allergies. Reactions to milk, egg, peanuts, tree nuts, fish, shellfish, soy, and wheat are the most common.	The toddler is growing less rapidly than the infant and does not require as many calories. Feeding self, even if messy, promotes independence. Giving too much food or food that is high in calories may result in obesity. Children with food allergies are more likely to develop asthma or other allergies.
Hygiene	• Teach hand washing after eating and toileting. • Teach how to brush teeth. • Schedule dentist visit.	It is important to establish good hygiene and to serve as a role model. The first dentist visit may be just to become familiar with the office and provider.
Elimination	• Physical development is necessary for toilet training. • Begin training with bowel elimination. • Watch for signs of readiness (realizing wetness, staying dry for 2 or more hours). • Night dryness occurs later than day dryness.	The neuromuscular control necessary for elimination occurs between ages 1 and 3 years. Bowel training is a less complex task than bladder training.
Growth and Development	• Encourage independence in eating, dressing, and toileting. • Provide toys that emphasize gross motor skills and creativity. • Parallel play with other children is normal. • The concept of sharing is not yet developed. • Saying "no" to almost everything is normal.	The toddler gains a sense of security and control by being able to eat, dress, toilet self, and say "no."
Promoting Health and Preventing Illness	• If a danger of lead ingestion exists, take appropriate measures and have the toddler screened. • Complete immunizations. • See health care professionals for treatment of respiratory infections. • Do not smoke in the house or car with the child. • Limit sun exposure or use sun protection practices. • Learn CPR for emergencies.	Toddlers who ingest lead, such as from eating peeling lead-based paint, are at risk for brain damage, behavioral issues, and intellectual disability. Immunizations are an essential part of health care. Respiratory infections may lead to ear infections. Avoid smoking to reduce risk of respiratory illness, asthma, and ear infections. Passive smoke is dangerous. Infants in daycare have increased exposure to respiratory and skin infections and infestations. Children at high risk for development of skin cancer include those with light skin, freckling, or a family history.

Toddlers who require hospital care experience stress and separation anxiety when parents are not present. To decrease stress from unfamiliar surroundings and caregivers, nurses should facilitate parents or guardians staying with the hospitalized toddler as much as possible. Every effort should be made to have consistency of health care providers and to maintain familiar routines and rituals. When ill or in pain, toddlers often regress to earlier behaviors, such as wanting a bottle or thumb-sucking.

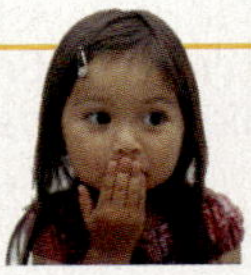

Recall 2-year-old **Hillarie Browning**. As Hillarie regains consciousness, the nurse should apply knowledge about the feelings of stress and separation for a hospitalized toddler when developing the care plan for this child, especially in light of possible child abuse. Consistency in staff members caring for the child and maintaining rituals would help foster trust and minimize upset.

PRESCHOOLERS: 3 TO 6 YEARS

At around age 3 years, toddlers begin to move into the next stage: **preschooler**. Although growth and development are slower than in infancy and toddlerhood, they are still steady (Fig. 23-5).

Physiologic Development

The physical characteristics of the preschooler include the following:

- The head is close to adult size by age 6 years.
- The body is less chubby and becomes leaner and more coordinated.
- Motor abilities include skipping, throwing and catching a ball, copying figures, and printing letters and numbers.
- A full set of 20 deciduous teeth is present; baby teeth begin to fall out and are replaced by permanent teeth.
- Average weight at ages 5 to 6 years is 45 lb (20.4 kg), with males being slightly heavier than females.

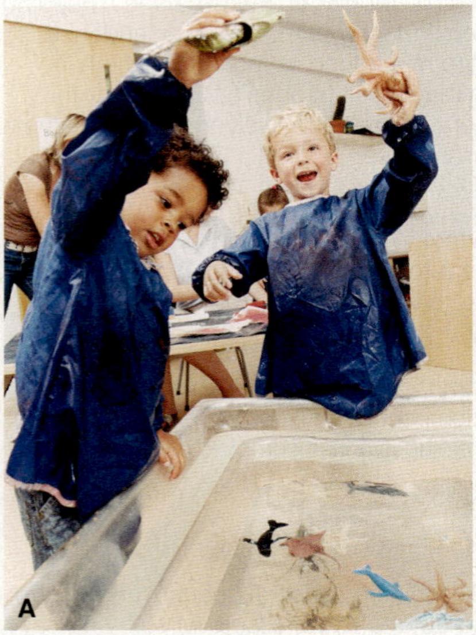

A

Preschooler play is associative and cooperative in its social dimension, and cognitive development is demonstrated in constructive and pretend play.

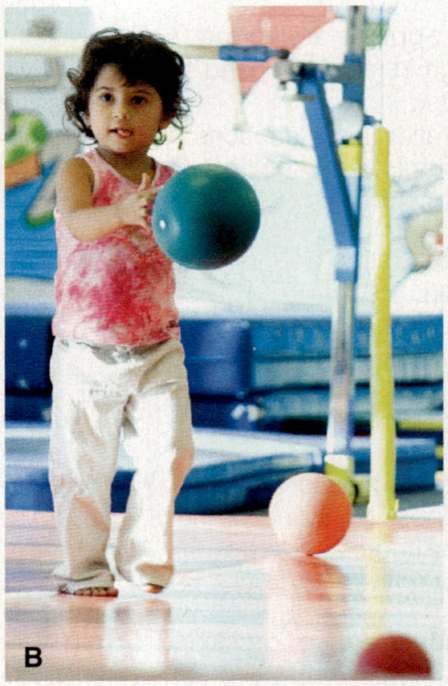

B

Motor abilities include throwing and catching a ball.

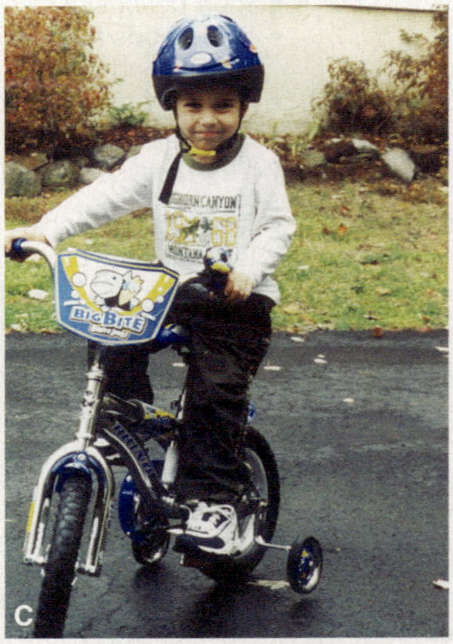

C

Safety is a common concern for caregivers.

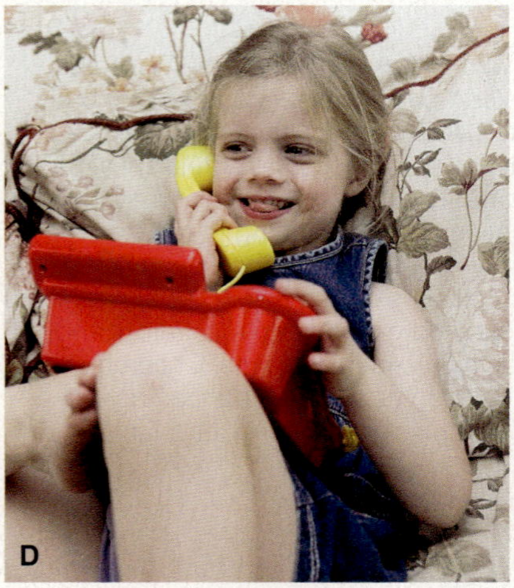

D

Preschoolers enjoy imitative play.

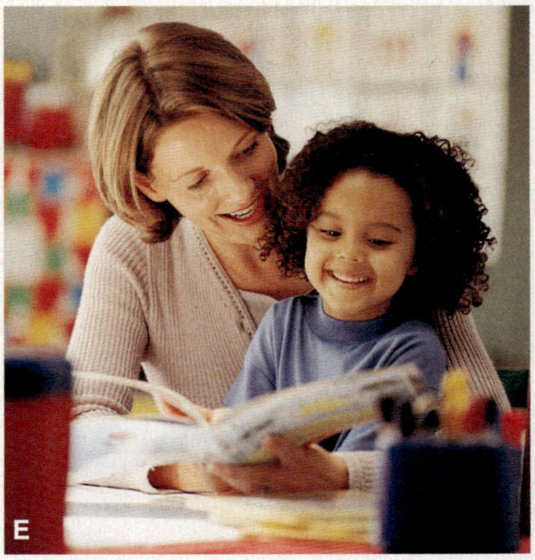

E

Cognitive development produces improved reasoning ability and readiness to read.

FIGURE 23-5. Development in the preschooler.

Cognitive Development

Preschoolers are in Piaget's (Piaget & Inhelder, 1969) preoperational stage of development. Passing through the preconceptual and intuitive phases, preschoolers demonstrate the following transitional changes:

- Egocentrism decreases as socialization with other children increases, and the ability to express self verbally improves.
- Play is more related to real-life events (rather than fantasy).
- Basic curiosity results in constant questions and improved reasoning ability.

Language development is seen in more elaborate and grammatically correct sentences, with 6- to 18-word sentences becoming common by age 6 years. Incessantly asking "Why?" increases the child's knowledge, encourages further conversations, and helps develop language abilities.

Preschoolers clearly identify themselves as male or female, start to develop a sexual orientation, can understand basic body functions, and have a curiosity about biologic sex differences. This curiosity often leads to "playing doctor," which is normal behavior at this stage. Many children in this age group want to look special or *dressed up* and gain increased self-esteem from compliments about their appearance.

Psychosocial Development

Freud's Theory

The preschooler is in Freud's (1960) phalic stage, with the biologic focus primarily genital. This is frequently associated with the Oedipal and Electra complexes (See Chapter 22). This affinity for a parent has since been discussed in relation to sexual identity formation, cultural and current political influences, and the complexities inherent in self-discovery (Dabbous, 2021; Flanders et al., 2016). As a result of this development and differentiation of self, the superego and conscience begin to develop.

Erikson's Theory

The preschooler is in Erikson's (1963) stage of initiative versus guilt. Inner turmoil occurs when natural curiosity is pitted against a constant examination of the propriety of one's actions by a rigid conscience. Realistic self-limits are learned through social interactions.

Havighurst's Theory

According to Havighurst (1972), the preschooler has four developmental tasks to accomplish: to learn biologic sex differences and modesty, to describe social and physical reality through concept formation and language development, to get ready to read, and to learn to distinguish right from wrong.

Special Considerations

Preschoolers often have fears—most commonly fear of new places, fear of the dark, and fear during nightmares. These fears are often made worse by the child's own fertile imagination and ability to fantasize. Support and validation of the preschooler's feelings by caregivers are essential.

Moral and Spiritual Development

Kohlberg's preconventional phase of moral reasoning dominates at this age. The focus of this stage is obeying rules to avoid punishment or receive a reward. The cognitive, psychosocial, and moral developments of the preschooler provide a base for spiritual development, as described by Fowler (1981). The preschooler may attend activities at church or synagogue with the family but does not understand religious concepts. The concept of a deity is literal, with God usually being viewed as a male human. Concepts such as heaven, hell, and holy spirits are incomprehensible and often frightening.

Health of the Preschooler

Preschoolers continue to have the health problems that are seen in toddlerhood. Communicable diseases and respiratory tract infections are common, especially with increased interaction with other children at nursery schools and daycare. Preschoolers are prone to accidents because of their increased curiosity about the world. Some congenital disorders—such as hypospadias, inguinal hernias, and cardiac anomalies—require surgery at this time. Dental caries become common if teeth are neglected. As language becomes more sophisticated, speech disorders may become apparent.

In the United States as well as worldwide, obesity is a significant threat to the health of children. The incidence of children with obesity has more than tripled since the 1970s. Although only one component of an obesity assessment, BMI measurement, discussed in detail in Chapter 37, is a standard used to determine obesity and correlating predictors. A national representative study of children and adolescents ages 2 to 19 years (Fryar et al., 2021) found that between 2017 and 2018, 19.3% fit into the category of obesity (body mass index [BMI] at or greater than the age- and sex-specific 95th percentile on the CDC growth charts), with 6.1% fitting into the category of extreme obesity (at or greater than 120% of the age- and sex-specific 95th percentile on the CDC growth charts). Young children (younger than 5 years old) who are overweight or obese are more likely to be obese as adolescents and adults, and have chronic health problems such as heart disease, high blood pressure, type 2 diabetes, stroke, cancer, asthma, and osteoarthritis. Racial and ethnic disparities persist, but there are also disparities rooted in income level. Based on published data, in 2019-2020, obesity rates ranged from 8.6% among youth in the highest income bracket to 23.1% among youth in the lowest income bracket (Robert Wood Johnson Foundation, 2021). Federally funded programs

Research in Nursing

BRIDGING THE GAP TO EVIDENCE-BASED PRACTICE

Considering Childhood Obesity in Light of COVID-19

Most people are aware that obesity has become an epidemic. In the United States by 2030, nearly 50% of Americans are projected to be obese, with women, non-Hispanic Black adults, and low-income adults most commonly predicted to fall into the severe obesity category (Ward et al., 2019). Experts contend that this is a complicated situation, which was negatively impacted by the COVID-19 pandemic. Communities need to consider multifaceted ways to provide support for children to make healthy decisions beginning at an early age, even with the additional stressor of a global pandemic.

Related Research

Alves, J. M., Yunker, A. G., DeFendis, A., Xiang, A. H., & Page, K. A. (2021). BMI status and associations between affect, physical activity, and anxiety among U.S. children during COVID-19. *Pediatric Obesity, 16*(9), e12786. https://doi.org/10.1111/ijpo.12786

The study considered 64 children ages 9 to 15 years from April 22 to July 29, 2020, the summer COVID-19 was at its height, and national (and global) shutdowns and stay-at-home measures were in full effect. The children kept logs regarding their physical activity, completed the state portion of the *State-Trait Anxiety Inventory* and the 10-item *Positive and Negative Affect Schedule for Children*. Results considered extraneous variables and are valid for the children in the study irrespective of age, sex, socioeconomic level, or maternal gestational diabetes diagnosis. Unsurprisingly, anxiety scores were over five standard deviations higher than pre-pandemic norms for children in this age range. Children classified as overweight or obese who reported more time engaged in physical activity, reported less anxiety. This supports the idea that physical activity is beneficial for children during periods of high stress. Leisure screen time, which averaged 6 hours per day, was associated with a negative effect in all children (healthy weight, overweight, and obese). A positive effect was significantly related to anxiety levels in all children. Although this study was performed at the height of the COVID-19 pandemic and highlights the potential negative implications for children with an elevated BMI at times of crisis.

Relevance to Nursing Practice

The long- and short-term effects of living through a global pandemic are still unknown. Stressors can have negative effects on the psychological and physical well-being and health of children—these effects can extend into adulthood. Considering potential ramifications of the pandemic provides the opportunity to develop mitigating strategies and inform future responses to large-scale, global issues that affect people of all ages.

including the Supplemental Nutrition Assistance Program (SNAP), the Women, Infants, and Children (WIC) program, the Child and Adult Care Food Program (CACFP), and Head Start provide much needed support for families. Reimagining school-based programs became a necessity during COVID-19, when meals normally obtained at school needed to be accessed by children and families in their homes. Work is ongoing to provide support and structure for dietary requirements and physical activity recommendations (Robert Wood Johnson Foundation, 2021). (See Research in Nursing box.)

Role of the Nurse in Promoting Health and Preventing Illness

Teaching Tips 23-3 provides examples of teaching to promote health in preschoolers. Nurses play a vital role in identifying children at risk for obesity, teaching families about the health consequences, providing information and health teaching, and promoting wellness in this vulnerable population. Assessments of dietary patterns and physical activity level of family members guide nursing interventions.

When caring for a preschool-aged child who is scheduled for surgery or requires hospitalization, nurses must recognize the importance of the child's fear of pain as well as separation anxiety. The nurse can help decrease fears by explaining procedures in language the child can understand and by being honest about how much pain a procedure will cause. Many health care institutions and facilities have pre-procedure visits so that the child having surgery becomes familiar with the setting and the activities that will be done. Allowing the child to practice procedures on a doll and encouraging the child to express their feelings openly are also beneficial (Fig. 23-6 on page 612). Encouraging caregivers to take an active role in the child's care helps to reduce fear and separation anxiety.

SCHOOL-AGED CHILDREN: 6 TO 12 YEARS

The **school-aged child**, ages 6 to 12 years, is typically sturdy and strong. Physical growth during this time is relatively slow but continues steadily, with both refinement and subtle changes taking place (Fig. 23-7 on page 612).

Physiologic Development

Physiologic development of school-aged children includes the following:

- The brain reaches 90% to 95% of adult size; by age 12 years, the nervous system is almost completely matured, resulting in coordinated body movements.
- Motor abilities progress from the ability to hold a pencil and print words at age 6 years to the ability to write in

Teaching Tips 23-3

PRESCHOOLERS

Health Topic	Teaching Tip	Why Is This Important?
Safety	• Lock medicines and cleaning and gardening supplies out of reach. • Use safety plugs in electrical outlets. • Teach child how to go up and down stairs. • Do not give small hard foods, small toys, or balloons. • Tape shut battery compartments of toys and household objects to limit access to button batteries. • Use approved car seats and bicycle helmets. • Teach simple traffic safety. • Teach to never talk to or get in the car with a stranger. Include information about inappropriate touching. • Never leave the child alone in public or unattended in a car. • Begin swimming lessons and teach water safety. • Teach danger of fire and have a home fire safety plan. • Limit use of bouncers or moonwalks and trampolines. Limit the number of children using them at one time and always have a parent present.	Accidents are the leading cause of injury and death in preschoolers, most often from motor vehicles, drowning, burns, and poisoning. Even minor head trauma may cause hematoma formation. Children are at risk for harm from physical and sexual abuse and must be taught how to recognize situations that may increase that risk. Broken bones and sprains are the most common type of bounce-related injuries; the number of children in the United States with this type of injury is 15 times higher now than 15 years ago.
Nutrition	• A gradual increase in calories, with nutritious snacks, is necessary. • Children who follow their own appetite patterns are less likely to be overweight. • Avoid foods that are high in fat, sugar, and salt (found in most fast foods). • Preschoolers like to eat one food at a time and prefer those that are mildly flavored and lukewarm.	The preschool child needs the same food group nutrition as the adult, but in smaller amounts. Lifelong eating patterns begin during this time frame, so healthy nutrition that promotes a normal BMI should be taught and modeled.
Hygiene	• Stress importance of hand washing before meals and after toileting. • Assist with brushing and flossing teeth after eating. • Teach disposal of used tissues. • Maintain regular dental checkups and care.	Preschoolers are able to carry out basic hygiene but continue to need assistance and reminders. Dental caries often begins during this age.
Elimination	• Toilet training is completed, but night wetting may persist.	Recognizing the need to empty the bladder during sleep takes a longer time in some children. They should not be punished for wetting the bed.
Growth and Development	• Night fears and bad dreams are common. • Make-believe play and imaginary friends are normal. • Although each child grows and develops differently, there are ranges of normal. • Play occupies most of the child's time; the child can play with others for periods of time. • Provide play materials that encourage physical activity, dramatic play, quiet play, and creativity. • Provide consistent, fair, and kind limits for behavior. • Masturbation is normal, although the child should learn that it is not acceptable in public.	Sleep problems usually resolve on their own; calm reassurance by parents is appropriate when they occur. Play is the work of the child; adults should provide time, space, equipment, and safety, but should not structure the child's play.
Promoting Health and Preventing Illness	• If a danger of lead ingestion or poisoning exists, take appropriate measures and have the child screened. • Maintain immunizations. • Have vision tested. • Have hearing tested if necessary (e.g., child does not seem to listen). • Maintain regular well-child checkups. • Preschoolers often fear dental and medical treatments. Avoid hospitalizations when possible; if necessary, prepare the child before the procedure.	Lead poisoning in preschoolers causes brain dysfunction. Immunizations and health-related checkups are essential in promoting health. Preschoolers often see dental or medical procedures as a punishment and fear damage to their bodies. Parents should set a good example and be honest with the child. Preparation for procedures and hospitalization can help decrease fear and separation anxiety.

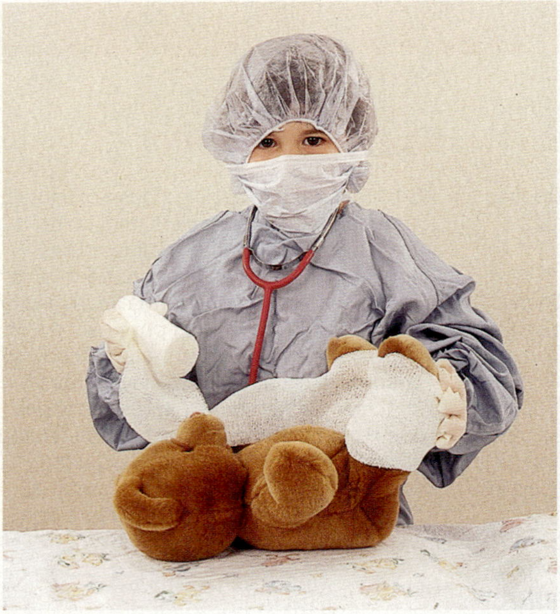

FIGURE 23-6. Abstract reasoning is necessary for children to understand that painful medical treatments given now will make them feel better later. Dramatic play may help the preschool child, who is not old enough to have developed abstract reasoning, to understand the uncomfortable experiences of the hospital stay. (*Source:* Used with permission from Shutterstock. *Photo by B. Proud.*)

script (if cursive is taught), type complete thoughts, and compose full sentences by age 12 years.

- Digital natives are able to interface with computer programs, learning management systems, and games with minimal instruction or supervision.
- Sexual organs grow, but are dormant until late in this period, when hormonal changes begin.
- All permanent teeth are present, except for the second and third molars, by age 12 years.
- Height increases 2 to 3 inches (5.1 to 7.6 cm) and weight increases 3 to 6 lb (1.4 to 2.7 kg) a year.

Cognitive Development

The school-aged child is in Piaget's (Piaget & Inhelder, 1969) concrete operational stage of development, organizing facts about the environment to use for problem solving. In this period, the child has the following characteristics:

- Thinks logically and develops concepts of mass, volume, weight, and measurement
- Deals best with actual objects and people, but can relate concepts and compare events
- Uses inductive reasoning to solve new problems
- Generalizes about people, places, and things
- Develops classification systems

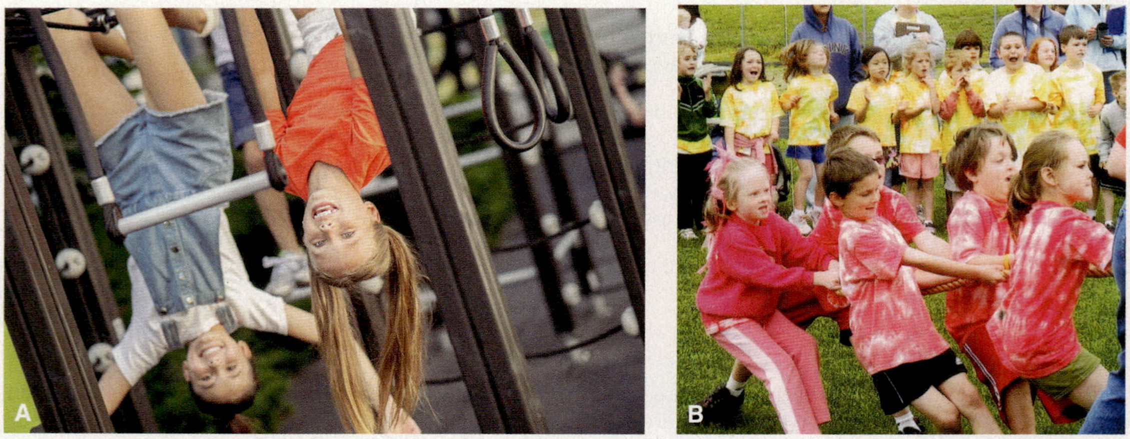

Play involves development of skill, games with rules, and competitive activities.

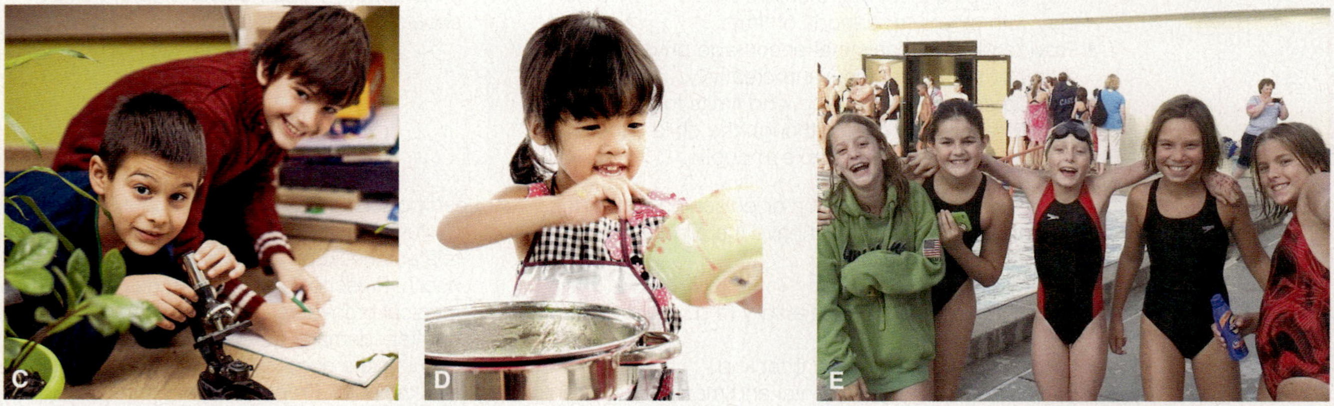

The school-aged child is aware of and understands a sequence of events. Making friends is important to the school-aged child.

FIGURE 23-7. Development in the school-aged child. (*Source:* A. Used with permission from Shutterstock. *Photo by Dmytro Zinkevych.* C. Used with permission from Shutterstock. *Photo by Una Shimpraga.*)

- Develops an awareness and understanding of other people's feelings and points of view
- Understands reversal of events

School-aged children have well-developed language skills and use language in a more sophisticated manner. Their ability to store information in long-term memory and retrieve it in the remembering (recall) process is more efficient. Texting and other social media platforms require knowledge of shorthand and social norms that begin to be understood and assimilated within this time frame.

Psychosocial Development

Freud's Theory

The school-aged child is in the latency stage, according to Freud (1960), with psychosocial energies being channeled toward strong identification with their own biologic sex and biologic sex–oriented creative activities. Privacy and understanding of their own body are important at this age.

Erikson's Theory

The school-aged child is in the industry-versus-inferiority stage, according to Erikson (1963), with the child focused on learning useful skills and thereby developing positive self-esteem. A sense of identity begins to emerge, and values are integrated. The emphasis is on doing, succeeding, and accomplishing.

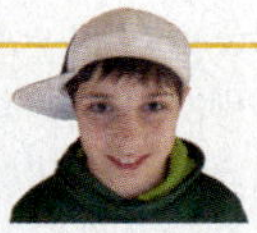

Think back to **Nate Pelton**, the 11-year-old baseball player. The nurse could apply Erikson's theory to understand that joining a sports team offers Nate the opportunity to develop physical skills, to learn to play as a member of a team, and to improve self-esteem. When children participate in sports, their parents/guardians or caregivers need to be actively involved to ensure safety while understanding that support and positive reinforcement help to promote a positive experience that will shape values and behaviors for adult life.

Havighurst's Theory

According to Havighurst (1972), the school-aged child has the following developmental tasks:

- Learning physical game skills
- Learning appropriate social roles
- Developing fundamental skills in reading, writing, and calculating
- Developing concepts necessary for everyday living
- Achieving personal independence
- Developing conscience, morality, and a scale of values

Special Considerations

Peer relationships become the major influence. They shape the child's view of their status or popularity, preferred or desirable skills and activities, and ability to be liked and accepted in diverse peer groups. Peer groups in middle childhood help prepare the child for getting along in the larger world. They help the child practice role-transition behaviors that will be needed when the child transitions from looking to the parent or guardian for guidance, to adult independence. Sexual orientation, gender identification, and sexual activity discussions among the peer group often begin at this stage. Unfortunately, as children become members of social groups, they may experience some form of bullying. Data indicate that bullying behavior becomes more common at school during unstructured moments such as recess and may be related to biologic sex or gender identity, physical appearance, disability or ability, and intellect. Bullying behavior intends to embarrass or harm the victim and creates a perceived imbalance of power between the aggressor (or aggressors) and the victim (Hockenberry et al., 2022).

Body image, self-concept, and sexuality are interrelated. Sexual development results in a strong need to understand body function and to have accurate information about sexuality.

Moral Development

Most of middle childhood is spent in the conventional phase of moral development. Behavior is based on familial and peer group beliefs, and conformity to the norm is common. Following school regulations, respecting teachers, and viewing justice as a means of fair play are all important.

Spiritual Development

In Fowler's (1981) theory, school-aged children view religious faith as a relationship that involves reciprocal fairness. They take part in rituals of their faith, with a basic understanding of the ritual's significance. The importance of spiritual beliefs and the possibility of life after death is accepted, even if not totally understood.

Health of the School-Aged Child

Accidents continue to be common in school-aged children. With increased interactions with other children in school, communicable conditions such as scabies, impetigo, and head lice are more prevalent. The CDC recommends vaccination with a two-dose series of the human papillomavirus (HPV) vaccine before age 15 years, with the first dose recommended at ages 11 or 12 years (can be given starting at age 9), to prevent the types of HPV that can cause cervical cancer and genital warts (CDC, 2021b). (See the accompanying PICOT in Practice display on page 614.)

Other common health-related problems of the school-aged child include obesity, attention-deficit hyperactivity disorder (ADHD), learning disability (LD), and enuresis (bed-wetting). In addition, chronic conditions such as sickle cell anemia, hyperactivity, seizure disorders, hypertension, type 1 diabetes mellitus, and obesity may affect the school-aged child. Scoliosis, an abnormal curvature of the spine, occurs most often in females between ages 10 and 13 years.

PICOT in Practice

ASKING CLINICAL QUESTIONS

Scenario: You are a nurse who works in a primary care clinic. A 13-year-old adolescent is being seen for a wellness visit prior to starting a new school year. You review the patient's electronic health record (EHR) and note that she has not had the human papillomavirus (HPV) vaccine. The patient says that no one told her that she needed the HPV vaccine.

You know that the adherence rates in your clinic are low for initiation and completion of the HPV series compared to national averages (CDC[a] estimates 66% initiation and 51% completion rates among adolescents in the United States). You wonder if automated calls and reminders for health care providers to offer the vaccine would increase the initiation and completion of the two-dose schedule for the HPV vaccine for females by age 19 years.

- **Population:** Adolescent females and males ages 11 to 19 years
- **Intervention:** Participation in centralized reminder and recall from state immunization information systems to increase HPV vaccination rates
- **Comparison:** No use of cues for health care providers
- **Outcome:** Initiation and completion of HPV vaccine
- **Time:** By age 19 years

PICOT Question: Among adolescents 11 to 19 years old, does the participation in centralized, automated calls and reminders from the state immunization information systems increase the initiation and completion rates of the two-dose HPV vaccine?

Findings:

Szilagyi, P., Albertin, C., Gurfinkel, D., Beaty, B., Zhou, X., Vangala, S., Rice, J., Campbell, J. D., Whittington, M. D., Valderrama, R., Breck, A., Roth, H., Meldrum, M., Tseng, C. H., Rand, C., Humiston, S. G., Schaffer, S., Kempe, A. (2020). Effect of state immunization information system centralized reminder and recall on hpv vaccination rates. *Pediatrics, 145*(5), e20192689. https://doi.org/10.1542/peds.2019–2689.

Szilagyi et al. (2020) conducted a four-arm pragmatic (effectiveness) randomized controlled trial across two states (New York and Colorado) between February 2017 and January 2019. The study focused on the impact of 1, 2, or 3 autodialer phone reminders per dose of the HPV vaccine sent to parents on behalf of the immunization information systems (IIS) and primary care practices about HPV vaccination. Practices where children received care (i.e., pediatrics, family medicine, and health center) were randomly selected. Within each practice, patients ages 11 to 17.9 years old who had not completed their HPV vaccine series (NY: n = 30,616 in 123 practices; CO: n = 31,502 in 80 practices) were randomly assigned to receive 0, 1, 2, or 3 autodialer messages per vaccine dose. The primary study outcome was initiation and/or completion of the HPV two- or three-dose vaccine series among adolescents ages 11 to younger than 19 years.

Although centralized reminder and recall by phone (autodialer) has been shown to improve childhood vaccination rates, immunization information systems–based centralized reminder and recall for the HPV vaccine did not raise HPV vaccination rates. In New York, HPV vaccine initiation rates ranged from 37.0% to 37.4%, and completion rates were between 29.1% and 30.1%, with no significant differences across study arms. In Colorado, HPV vaccine initiation rates ranged from 31.2% to 33.5% and were slightly higher for one reminder compared with none, but vaccine completion rates, ranging from 27.0% to 27.8%, were similar.

Level of Evidence: Randomized controlled trial

Recommendations: Studies have revealed that a strong provider recommendation is important in uptake of the HPV vaccine. You present a Plan-Do-Study-Act proposal to the interprofessional team responsible for clinic management. The goal of your project is to improve HPV vaccination rates using a multifaceted approach. Your proposal includes:

1. Adding a prompt in the clinic EHR to cue health care providers to discuss the HPV vaccine at all clinic visits with adolescents between ages 11 and 19 years and their parents.
2. Providing each health care provider and staff with the Centers for Disease Control and Prevention's *5 Ways to Boost Your HPV Vaccination Rates.*[b]
3. Adding a personalized patient reminder and recall system to notify patients who have completed the first dose to return to the clinic for the second dose of the vaccination at 5 to 6 months post the first dose.

[a]Centers for Disease Control and Prevention (CDC). (2017). *Understanding HPV coverage.* https://www.cdc.gov/hpv/partners/outreach-hcp/hpv-coverage.html

[b]Centers for Disease Control and Prevention (CDC). (2021). *5 Ways to boost your HPV vaccination rates.* https://www.cdc.gov/hpv/hcp/boosting-vacc-rates.html

Obesity

A sedentary lifestyle contributes to obesity in children who spend many hours using electronic devices, playing video games, and watching TV rather than actively playing. Many obese school-aged children also have diets that are high in saturated fats, do not meet fruit and vegetable daily requirements, and are low in fiber and calcium. As with adults, obesity in children results from consuming more calories than are expended. Genetics, health factors, and other social determinants of health may be contributing factors. (See Research in Nursing box on page 610.)

Specific Learning Disorders/Disabilities and Related Disorders

Learning disorders are conditions that affect how a person learns to read, write, speak, and perform calculations. Although the term *learning disability* is more commonly used in the legal and education systems, *specific learning disorder* is the medical term used in the DSM-5; *learning difference* may be informally used, but a medical diagnosis of a specific learning disorder often directly leads to recognition of a disability and the associated accommodations and specific school-based services (American Psychiatric Association [APA], 2021). Learning disorders tend to be discovered in school-aged children when they have difficulties in the classroom. Although many learning disorders persist over the course of a lifetime, educational support can provide essential tools and strategies that help to mitigate the challenges of a learning disorder. Three of the most common learning disabilities include the following (APA, 2021; National Institutes of Health [NIH], 2018):

- *Dyslexia:* difficulty in language skills, reading, and spelling
- *Dysgraphia:* writing disability; difficulty putting thoughts on paper
- *Dyscalculia:* difficulty with numbers and arithmetic (symbols)

Disorders associated with learning disabilities include dyspraxia (sensory integration disorder involving motor coordination) and attention-deficit/hyperactivity disorder (ADHD). ADHD is the most common chronic neurodevelopmental condition in U.S. children. It affects 8.4% of U.S. children (more than five million children) ages 2 through 17 years (Chang et al., 2020). Parents or guardians tend to seek intervention when they note behavioral, social, or academic performance issues rooted in a pattern of inattention and/or hyperactivity and impulsivity. A thorough history and physical, coupled with the use of valid and reliable instruments assist the health care provider in ruling out other conditions and diagnosing ADHD. Early diagnosis and intervention focus on symptom reduction, improved cognitive and social function, diagnosis and management of common comorbid conditions, and the mitigation of potential long-term effects of ADHD (Chang et al., 2020). Although interventions need to be individualized for each child, psychosocial interventions that include parent/guardian training and classroom interventions focused on behavior management are the standard of care. These psychosocial interventions are a first-line treatment for preschoolers and should continue as an adjunct therapy for children ages 6 to 17 years. Providing opportunities for regular exercise and promoting adequate sleep have been shown to have a positive effect on children with ADHD. Stimulant medications (methylphenidate, dexmethylphenidate/amphetamine, dextroamphetamine) provide effective treatment and are often prescribed first line for elementary school-aged children and adolescents (Chang et al., 2020).

Guidelines from the American Academy of Pediatrics (Wolraich et al., 2019) that were reaffirmed in 2019 outline the role of the health care provider in assisting children with special education needs. These recommendations include identifying children in need of early intervention or special education services; sharing information sharing with early intervention specialists, school personnel, or clinics, and involving parents or guardians in team meetings; identifying barriers to care; addressing school involvement in documented health care treatment plans; and working with school administrators to address the needs of children with disabilities/disorders at a system level.

Enuresis

Enuresis is diagnosed when a child is at least 5 years old and is still having involuntary urination, usually at night. Although this problem is significant to the child and their parents, it is a benign and self-limiting disorder, usually ending between ages 6 and 8 years.

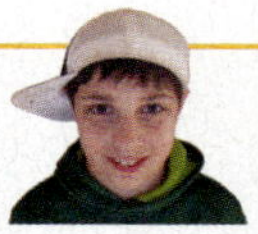

Recall 11-year-old **Nate Pelton**, who suffered a possible concussion during a baseball game as a result of a blow to his head in a collision with another teammate. Nurses working in the ED, schools, and public health settings should use the nursing process to provide education about the recognition and treatment of concussions and to collaborate with parents, young athletes, coaches, and school faculty to prevent and treat these injuries.

Role of the Nurse in Promoting Health and Preventing Illness

The nurse's role in promoting health for the school-aged child involves individual and family teaching, often conducted by school nurses. Multiple strategies can be implemented in schools to address the obesity epidemic, promote mental focus, and support general well-being. Recommended approaches include increasing opportunities for students to become involved in informal and formal physical activities and ensuring that students have access to affordable or free healthy food and beverage choices while at school.

Because school violence has become more common, school nurses must be prepared for a potential crisis. They need to be alert for warning signs of bullying and other dangerous behaviors and be involved in efforts to promote a safe environment in playgrounds, buses, and schools. This often includes collaboration between the school nurse, parents, and educators to determine creative strategies that promote healthier lifestyles and environments for school-aged children. The Teaching Tips 23-4 display (on page 616) provides examples of nursing activities specific for this age group. In addition, nurses often function as advocates for vulnerable populations (see the Nursing Advocacy in Action display on page 617).

QSEN BULLYING

Staying alert for bullying includes paying attention to social media, where cyberbullying is increasingly common. Cyberbullying can also occur through text, instant messaging apps, e-mail, or gaming platforms. Providing education and a method for reporting opens the door to conversation and debriefing on this important topic.

Teaching Tips 23-4

SCHOOL-AGED CHILDREN

Health Topic	Teaching Tip	Why Is This Important?
Safety	• Teach and require pedestrian traffic safety. • Wear seat belts and bicycle helmets. • Emphasize bicycle, scooter, skate, and skateboard safety. • Provide swimming lessons and water safety rules. • Rural children should be taught farm safety. • Teach how to "stop, drop, and roll" to extinguish clothing fire. • Teach the dangers of dangerous products and chemicals. • Keep guns locked up. Teach gun safety rules. • Teach use of proper equipment for contact sports. • Be alert for concussion sports injuries, use proper equipment, and follow treatment recommendations for concussions.	Accidents are the leading cause of death in school-aged children, most often caused by motor vehicle crashes, fires, falls, drowning, and poisonings. Gun injuries to the child firing the gun or to others occur in school-aged children. Accident prevention and safety education should be taught and reinforced both at home and at school. Concussions that are not treated properly increase the risk for long-term problems.
Nutrition	• School-aged children need adequate calories and may also require increased amounts of vitamin D and calcium. • Provide foods that meet nutritional needs and do not supply empty calories (as found in junk food and fast food). • Make mealtimes a positive, predictable, regular event.	Increased vitamin D and calcium are needed as bones enlarge and for females to prevent later osteoporosis. American children eat too much salt, sugar, and fats; nearly 25% of all school-aged children have an elevated cholesterol level. Eating patterns for school-aged children will improve over time. Both undernutrition and overnutrition are seen in this age group.
Hygiene	• Teach females how to wipe from front to back after urination. • Teach children not to share hats or combs.	Females are prone to urinary infections because of their short urethra. Head lice and ringworm are common in school-aged children and are easily spread to others.
Sexual Development	• Both females and males have characteristics of sexual maturity, including a growth spurt, growth of body hair, changes in body proportion, and the beginning of secondary physical sex changes. • Provide accurate information and answer questions honestly about sex, including anatomy, physiology, birth control, and STIs (including HIV). • Monitor TV watching and computer use.	Females have breast development, grow axillary and pubic hair, and may begin to menstruate. Males have testicular growth and grow axillary and pubic hair, and the penis enlarges. Males may also have temporary breast enlargement. School-aged children are curious, and if unsupervised, may watch pornographic content on television or online. Consider the level of violence they are exposed to in television shows or video games.
Growth and Development	• Best friends and groups of peer friends are important to the school-aged child. • Rules are rigidly followed during games with peers. • Encourage both quiet and active play activities. • Provide guidance and set limits for behavior, focusing on only one incident at a time. • Encourage feelings of industry by having realistic expectations and recognizing unique abilities and talents. • Provide positive statements demonstrating that the child is valued, loved, and important.	From ages 7 to 9 years, close friends are usually the same biologic sex and age. This is not as important from ages 10 to 12 years. Unrealistic expectations or excessive discipline may result in stress and feelings of inferiority.
Promoting Health and Preventing Illness	• Maintain records of immunizations, and have boosters as recommended. • Promote regular physical activity and exercise. • Script with children how to say no to smoking, alcohol, and drugs in common situations. • Maintain dental examinations. • Maintain well-child checkups, and have screenings (if at risk or indicated by symptoms) and treatment for chronic conditions such as asthma, diabetes mellitus, sickle cell anemia, hypertension, seizure disorder, hyperactivity, and obesity. • Have vision tested if school problems with reading, coordination, or inability to see the screen or monitor in front of the room occur.	Maintaining immunizations is essential to health; records are required for enrollment in school. Children need to know how to handle peer pressure to smoke, drink, and take drugs. Many school-aged children are at risk for and exhibit symptoms of chronic illnesses.

Nursing Advocacy in Action

Patient Scenario

You are working as a school nurse in a district where there are many poor families who have come to the United States (many illegally) to find work. At present, there is a lively debate in the country about whether these families should be identified and sent "home" or supported where they currently live in the United States. Many of the parents are afraid of being deported, and you learn that some have taken their children out of school. You know that the children benefit from being in school. In addition to the education, the free school lunch program is, for many children, the one meal of the day they can count on.

Implications for Nursing Advocacy

How will you respond if you are the school nurse approached by teachers who want to help the children? Talk with your classmates and experienced nurses about these questions:

- If you elect to advocate for these children, what practical steps can you take to ensure better health outcomes?
- What is it reasonable to expect of a student nurse, a graduate nurse, and an experienced nurse in this situation?
- What advocacy skills are needed to effectively respond to this challenge?
- What are the potential risks to being a moral agent in this situation? Professional, sociopolitical, or legal considerations?

Because school-aged children are striving for independence and control, hospitalization may mean a loss of freedom of choice (e.g., types of food, clothing, activities). Children of this age should be allowed to have some measure of control over allowable activities and should be encouraged to do what they can, such as playing competitive games and making their own beds (Fig. 23-8).

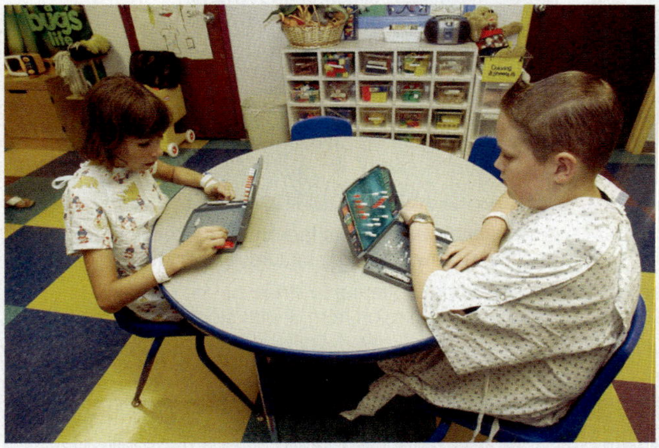

FIGURE 23-8. Allowing school-aged children to play competitive games promotes a positive hospital experience. (*Source:* Used with permission from Shutterstock. *Photo by Joe Mitchell.*)

ADOLESCENTS AND YOUNG ADULTS

The adolescent and young adult years are a time of both change and stability. **Adolescence** begins with puberty and extends from about age 12 to about age 18 years; the **young adult** period is considered to be ages 18 through 39 years. However, these time periods are highly individualized, and reflect a critical window of development and occasions for nursing intervention.

After experiencing rapid growth and development during adolescence, the young adult completes physical growth and develops internal and external controls and values acceptable to society. There are no specific measurements of maturity; each person is an individual and a wide range of normal values and behaviors are considered healthy (Fig. 23-9 on page 618). The world in which young adults live has changed dramatically, with globalization and a networked world contributing to increased knowledge and information availability, heightened risks due to unhealthy and risky behaviors, relatively low social mobility, and greater economic inequality than seen in previous generations (Institute of Medicine [IOM] & National Research Council [NRC], 2015).

Physiologic Development

Changes in the adolescent's body transform the adolescent from a child to an adult in appearance. Physiologic development includes the following:

- The feet, hands, and long bones grow rapidly, accompanied by an increase in muscle mass, especially in males.
- Primary and secondary sexual development occurs, with maturation of the genitalia; presence of body hair; breast development and menstruation in females; and facial hair growth, voice changes, and spermatogenesis in males.
- Sebaceous and axillary sweat glands become active.
- Full adult size is reached, although some young males may continue to grow in their 20s.

Puberty—the time when the ability to reproduce begins—starts at age 9 to 13 years in females (with menstruation usually beginning between ages 10 and 14 years) and at ages 11 to 14 years in males. Puberty can be divided into the following three stages (Table 23-3 on page 618):

- *Prepubescence:* Secondary sex characteristics begin to develop, but the reproductive organs do not yet function.
- *Pubescence:* Secondary sex characteristics continue to develop, and ova and sperm begin to be produced by the reproductive organs.
- *Postpubescence:* Reproductive functioning and the development of secondary sex characteristics reach adult maturity.

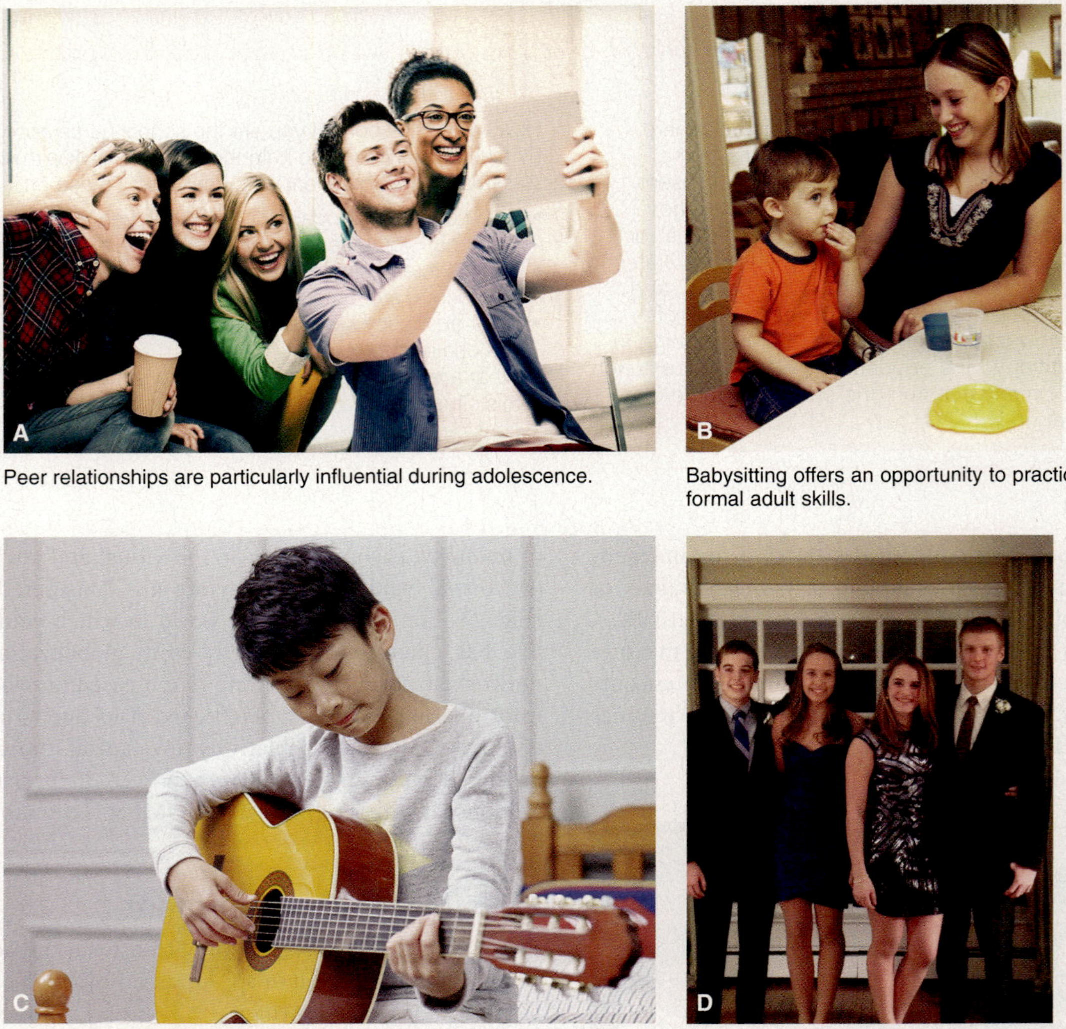

A. Peer relationships are particularly influential during adolescence.

B. Babysitting offers an opportunity to practice formal adult skills.

C. The development of self-identity in adolescence involves discovering talents and becoming emotionally independent.

D. A primary developmental task of adolescence is to achieve new and more mature relationships.

FIGURE 23-9. Development in the adolescent. (*Source:* B. Used with permission from Shutterstock. *Photo by Joe Mitchell.* C. Used with permission from Shutterstock. *Photo by Syda Productions.* D. Used with permission from Shutterstock. *Photo by allensima.*)

Table 23-3 Adolescent Sexual Development

STAGE	MALES	FEMALES
Prepubescence	• Progressive enlargement of testicles, seminal ducts, prostate gland • Enlargement and reddening of the scrotal sac • Increase in length and circumference of penis • Appearance of downy pubic hair	• Progressive enlargement of the ovaries • Ripening of Graafian follicles • Rounding of the hips • Appearance of breast buds • Enlargement of the fallopian tubes, vagina, and uterus • Appearance of downy pubic hair
Pubescence	• Increase in amount, pigmentation, and curling of pubic hair • Growth spurt involving height and weight increase • Deepening of the voice due to growth of larynx • Enlargement of testicles • Increased pigmentation and growth of scrotum • Growth of penis in length and circumference • Beginning of spermatogenesis	• Increase in amount, pigmentation, and curling of pubic hair • Growth spurt involving height and weight increase • Menarche • Appearance of axillary hair • Enlargement of vulva and clitoris • Development of breast tissue • Ovulation
Postpubescence	• Completion of sexual growth and development • Fertility	• Completion of sexual growth and development • Fertility

Cognitive Development

According to Piaget (Piaget & Inhelder, 1969), adolescence is the stage when the cognitive development of formal operations takes place. Deductive, reflective, and hypothetical reasoning are possible, and abstract concepts can be understood. Long-term goals can be set as the concept of time, its passage, and the future become real. Challenging the decision making of adults is common. Egocentrism returns, and imaginary audiences and daydreaming are common.

Young adults, in comparison to the adolescent, are more creative in thought, are objective and realistic, and are less self-centered. Their learning is enhanced through educational and life experiences.

Psychosocial Development

Freud's Theory

The adolescent and young adults are in Freud's (1960) genital stage. The libido re-emerges in a mature, adult form, and the person is capable of full sexual function. There is a sense of self and others. Creativity and pleasure are found in love and in work.

Erikson's Theory

According to Erikson's (1963) theory, the adolescent tries out different roles, personal choices, and beliefs in the stage called identity versus role confusion. Self-concept is being stabilized, with the peer group acting as the greatest influence.

The young adult, in the intimacy-versus-isolation stage, needs to complete tasks such as achieving independence from parents, establishing intimate relationships, and choosing an occupation or career. If such developmental tasks are not accomplished, the young adult may become isolated and self-absorbed.

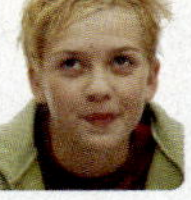

Think back to **Darlene Schneider,** the 14-year-old pregnant teenager. The nurse could apply knowledge of Erikson's theory to foster a sense of identity in Darlene by engaging her in essential self-care measures and providing her necessary information to facilitate decision making. In addition, establishing a trusting relationship with Darlene, and subsequently between her and other members of the health care staff, would help to further promote her self-exploration and identity formation.

Havighurst's Theory

According to Havighurst (1972), during adolescence, more mature relationships with peers is achieved, a gender-influenced social role is developed, personal appearance is accepted, and a set of values and ethical system as a guide to behavior are internalized.

Levinson's Theory

In Levinson's theory of individual life structure, the years from ages 18 to 22 are characterized by early adult transition (Levinson et al., 1978). This is a time of making initial career choices, establishing personal relationships, and selecting personal values and lifestyles. During the years from ages 22 to 28, the young adult builds on previous choices, but there may be a transient quality to occupational choices and friendships.

Gould's Theory

Gould's (1978) theory of transformation views young adults as having established their own control as adults separate from the family. They want to enjoy the present but also build for the future.

Special Considerations

CHOOSING AN OCCUPATION OR CAREER

A major psychosocial developmental requirement for the young adult is choosing a vocation. The young person's decision to enter the world of work is strongly influenced initially by the need to become independent of their family and to be self-sufficient. The choice of an occupation or a career is also guided by factors such as the desire to get married, raise a family, and become part of the community (Fig. 23-10 on page 620).

Occupational and career choices are largely tied to educational choices. Many careers require a college education. Adults learn from both informal and formal experiences and are largely goal-directed learners. If the person's identified goals are to increase career opportunities, maintain financial stability, and pursue upward mobility, the adult will be motivated to learn and change. The major factor in achieving satisfaction with a vocational choice is a person's belief that they are functioning to capacity and contributing to society.

ESTABLISHING A FAMILY

As discussed in Chapter 4, there are many different types and configurations of families. For many people, family is not determined by blood relation—families are chosen. Nurses have to keep in mind that the concept of *family* holds different meaning for different people—sometimes this is as simple as asking a patient to identify their *family*, *folks*, or *people*. Families provide a safe zone and a buffer between the needs of people and the expectations of society. Each family has the potential to provide a caring, supportive environment. For some couples, having children requires assistive reproductive technology, surrogacy, or adoption—these can be necessary but cost-prohibitive options. Although the process for establishing a family may vary, the entire family unit tends to be involved with the addition of a new family member.

Pregnancy is a period of adjustment requiring family members to be flexible enough to adapt to the changes that pregnancy and a new family member will bring. The cognitive, psychosocial, cultural, and educational dimensions of the prospective parents influence completion of the tasks. The verification of pregnancy may raise conflicting emotions in the pregnant person and partner, influenced by such factors as whether the pregnancy was planned or unplanned and how the baby may affect career goals. As

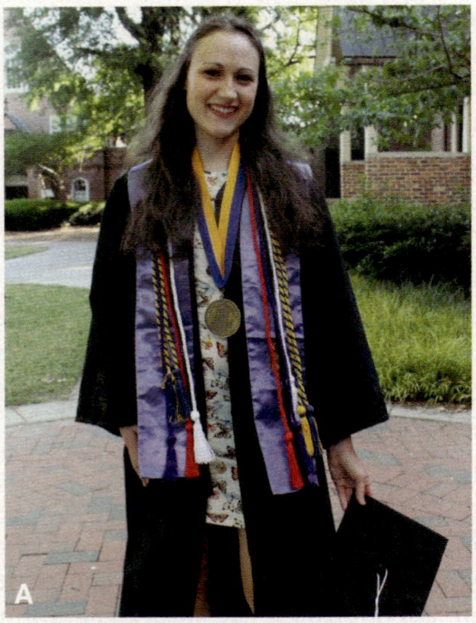

Graduating college or trade school is an important developmental milestone.

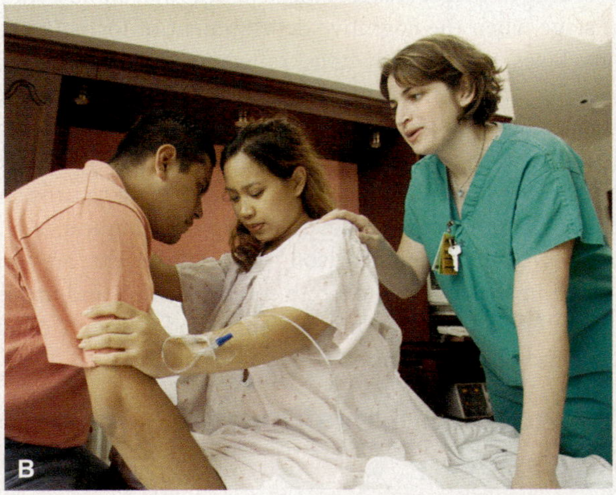

Choosing an occupation and starting a career are also important developmental milestones.

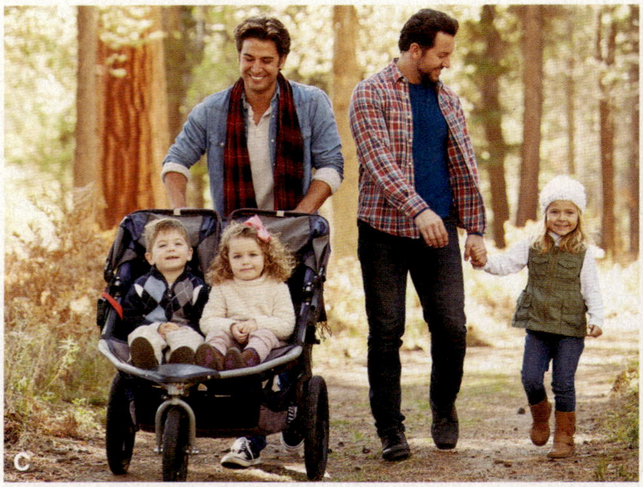

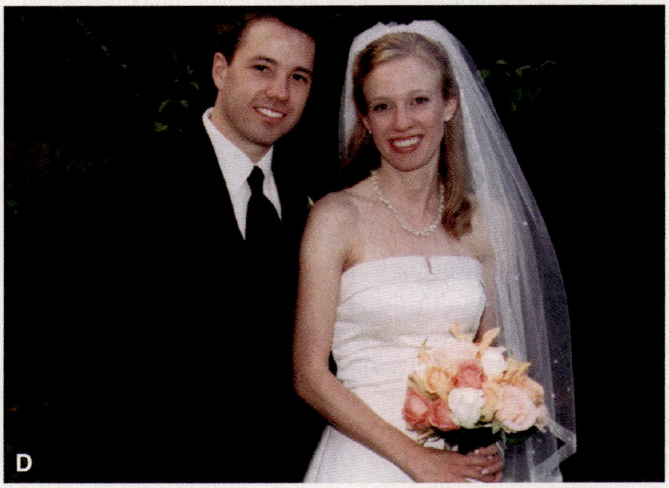

Developmental tasks of the young adult center on establishing intimate relationships, a home, and a family.

FIGURE 23-10. Development in the young adult. (A. Courtesy of K. Bartlett. C. Used with permission from Shutterstock. *Photo by Monkey Business Images.*)

physiologic changes occur and fetal movement is felt, the pregnant person begins to visualize themselves as a mother/parent and typically assumes responsibility for the health of the growing fetus. As the time for delivery becomes closer, there is a focus on maternal/parental tasks (such as preparing the baby's room and having clothing ready) and preparing for labor and delivery. During the pregnancy, the expectant partner needs to learn the normal physiologic and psychological changes of pregnancy, accept their supportive role in meeting the birthing person's needs, and explore their feelings about the developing fetus and the birth of the baby.

Moral Development

The child enters adolescence with a law-and-order orientation and may never progress beyond that point. Young adults who have mastered previous levels of moral development reach the conventional level and are concerned with maintaining expectations. They also value conformity, loyalty, and social order. Some people may enter the postconventional stage, in which they make moral judgments on the basis of universal beliefs.

Spiritual Development

Adolescents and young adults can think in the abstract and may question beliefs and practices that no longer serve to stabilize their identity or purpose. The individuating-reflective period in the young adult (defined by Fowler, 1981) brings discovery of the meaning of values as they relate to the achievement of social purposes and the acceptance of the value systems of others. Often, adolescents or young adults temporarily abandon traditional religious practices.

Health of the Adolescent and Young Adult

Although adolescence and young adulthood are times of maximum physiologic development and health, a wide variety of health problems can occur. Health promotion focuses on nutrition, relationships with self and others, and safety. The Advisory Committee on Immunization Practices now recommends routine vaccination with a quadrivalent meningococcal conjugate for children ages 11 to 12 years, with a booster of a serogroup B meningococcal vaccine provided at age 16 years (up to age 23 years, but preferably before age 18 years) when the risk for contracting meningococcal disease is highest (CDC, 2019). College freshmen living in dormitories and young adults living in military barracks are at risk for meningococcal disease and require the vaccine for protection from it. Young adults who received the Tdap vaccine at ages 11 to 12 years should have a tetanus and diphtheria (Td) booster every 10 years. Since 2000, there has been a recurrence of pertussis (whooping cough). Tdap vaccine may be given as one of these boosters if the Tdap was not previously received (CDC, 2020a). The CDC also recommends the vaccination of females ages 15 years and older who did not receive the two-dose series of the HPV vaccine when they were younger. The HPV vaccine for those ages 15 years and older is a three-dose series that prevents the types of HPV that most commonly cause cervical cancer and genital warts (CDC, 2021b). See the accompanying box, Examples of Actual or Potential Health Problems and Needs: Adolescence, for health issues in adolescents.

Injuries

Injuries are the leading cause of death for adolescents and young adults. Motor vehicle crashes are the most common cause of mortality, often associated with the use of alcohol or other drugs. In 2019, a total of 2,375 teenagers ages 13 to 19 years died in a motor vehicle accident. Drivers ages 16 to 19 years are three times more likely to be involved in a fatal crash than drivers ages 20 years and older (Insurance Institute for Highway Safety Highway Loss Data Institute, 2021). Sports- and recreation-related injuries remain an issue for the active teenager and young adult. Basketball and general exercise were reported as the most common activities that led to injury in those ages 15 to 24 years (Sheu et al., 2016).

Suicide (Self-harm)

Since 2016, suicide has been the second leading cause of death in teenagers (ages 14–18 years). A national study of high-schoolers identified that in 2019, approximately 1 in 5 (18.8%) considered attempting suicide, 1 in 6 made a suicide plan (15.7%), and 1 in 11 attempted suicide (8.9%)—this represents an increase between 2009 and 2019. The highest prevalence of suicidal ideation and behaviors was reported by females; White, non-Hispanic teens; those who had sexual contact with the same or both sexes; and those who identify as lesbian, gay, or bisexual. However, Black, non-Hispanic teens, both male and female, had the highest prevalence estimates for suicide attempts (Ivey-Stephenson et al., 2020). Comprehensive interventions, programs, and policies are needed to address suicide risk factors such as ACEs, stigma, access to lethal suicide means, media sensationalizing deaths, and a lack of individual/familial coping skills or community support. Recognition and effective intervention with evidence-based treatment (such as cognitive behavior therapy) requires formal and informal parental, school, and community training to increase awareness and provide opportunities for implementing suicide prevention strategies (Ivey-Stephenson et al., 2020).

Examples of Actual or Potential Health Problems and Needs

ADOLESCENCE

Actual or Potential Health Problem or Need	Possible Etiologic Factors	Potential Signs and Symptoms
Risky health behavior	• Insufficient resources (knowledge, finances, role models) • Insufficient social support • Social anxiety; difficulty forming peer relationships • Peer pressure	• Poor decision making • Engagement in unsafe behaviors • Smoking, vaping • Substance use, misuse, abuse
Disturbed Personal Identity	• Alteration in actual/perceived social role • Cultural incongruence • Sexual orientation or gender identity exploration or confirmation • Discrimination, prejudice, bias, disparities • Dysfunctional family processes • Low self-esteem	• Verbalizations regarding confusion, anger, frustration • Suicidal ideation or behaviors
Readiness for Positive Family Process	—	• Demonstrated engagement with family in social situations • Verbalized desire to seek formal therapy • Open conversations that focus on family roles and responsibilities

Substance Use, Misuse, and Abuse

Smoking and the use of illegal drugs pose serious health risks, and the use of alcohol is significantly related to risk-taking behavior for adolescents and young adults. According to the annual 2020 survey of 8th-, 10th-, and 12th-graders (Johnston et al., 2021; National Institute on Drug Abuse, 2021), most illicit drug use (including LSD, MDMA, cocaine, crack, heroin, oxycontin, amphetamines, and ketamine) has not changed since the last survey. OTC cough and cold medicines, most of which contain dextromethorphan, increased for all three grades. Although vaping *just flavoring* decreased, vaping *nicotine* and *marijuana* increased in 10th and 12th graders. Daily marijuana use, which is at or near the all-time high since 1991, may be impacted by social and legal changes occurring across the United States, as disapproval decreases and availability increases. Alcohol remains the most widely used substance by teenagers. The decline in alcohol use tracked from the 1980s through 2019 did not continue in 2020; there were significant increases in lifetime, annual 30-day, and daily alcohol use in all three groups. Young people tend to be moving away from narcotic misuse, which bodes well for the opioid crisis, but new substances and delivery devices, popularity driven by the internet and social media, and the rediscovery of older drugs all impact on the trends of substance use. Although general prevention strategies are helpful with younger children, drug-specific education and warnings tend to be more effective with this age group (Johnston et al., 2021; National Institute on Drug Abuse, 2021). Substance use disorder, including use of tobacco and alcohol, is further discussed in Chapter 28.

Pregnancy

Despite a 72% decline in the teen pregnancy rate in the United States since 1991, the U.S. teen pregnancy rate is substantially higher than in other western, industrialized countries (CDC, 2021d; Cox, 2020). The interplay among teen pregnancy, race and ethnicity, geographical location, community structures and support, and social determinants of health, particularly socioeconomic level, needs to be considered when interpreting teen pregnancy statistics. For example, when considering only age and socioeconomic status, White teens have a higher pregnancy rate than their Black counterparts, but there are no differences between the birth rates of Black and White teens (Dumas et al., 2020). Developing measures for funding, running, and promoting community-level interventions to mitigate risk need to consider socioeconomic factors (Cox, 2020; Dumas et al., 2020). Nurses should evaluate their own bias, consider their role in reducing stigma, support the unique needs of teen parents, and promote the teens' growth and development as parents and families (SmithBattle, 2020).

Nutritional Problems

Fad dieting and habitually eating fast foods are common among adolescents and young adults. Although eating disorders often surface during the teen years or young adulthood, they may also develop during childhood or later in life (National Institute of Mental Health, 2018). The most common eating disorders are anorexia nervosa (compulsive dieting to the point of self-starvation), bulimia nervosa (a destructive cycle of binge eating followed by self-induced vomiting in an effort to prevent weight gain), and binge eating disorder (excessive eating that is not followed by purging, excessive exercise, or fasting). The psychodynamics of these conditions are complex, but almost always involve a negative self-concept. Eating disorders may also be associated with anxiety or depression (National Institute of Mental Health, 2018).

Adolescents and young adults are consuming energy drinks with increasing frequency. These drinks have high levels of caffeine, which is not always clearly disclosed on the label, and are advertised to boost energy and improve mental and physical performance. Approximately 27% of students surveyed in the *Monitoring for the Future* 2010 to 2016 surveys (8th and 10th grades) reported consuming energy drinks or shots (Jackson & Leal, 2018). Because it is a stimulant, excessive caffeine levels can result in anxiety, rapid pulse, abnormal cardiac rhythms, and nervousness.

Sexually Transmitted Infections

Adolescents and young adults who engage in sexual intercourse without a condom are at a higher risk for contracting **sexually transmitted infections (STIs)** than adults. Although adolescents and young adults ages 15 to 24 years account for 50% of the 20 million new STIs in the United States, they represent only 25% of the sexually experienced population (Committee on Improving the Health, Safety, and Well-Being of Young Adults, 2015). Lack of knowledge, lack of psychosocial maturity, embarrassment, and a lack of planning ahead (e.g., not using condoms) are the most common reasons for this increased risk. Trichomonal and monilial infections, as well as HPV, are common.

Chlamydia, an infection of the genital tract, is the most common STI in the United States. Women younger than age 25 years and older women with key risk factors require screening every year (CDC, 2021f). Chlamydial infections occur in both biologic sexes, as do syphilis and herpes simplex type II (genital herpes). These STIs pose serious health threats.

Human immunodeficiency virus (HIV)/acquired immunodeficiency syndrome (AIDS) is the STI that poses the greatest single threat to people and society as a whole. Although HIV can be transmitted through means other than sexual contact, transmission is primarily through genital, oral, or anal sexual activities. HIV/AIDS is a major cause of death in the world, and its incidence is predicted to further increase still further. (See Chapter 43 for an in-depth discussion of STIs.)

Developmental and Situational Stressors

Adolescents and young adults deal with many stressors related to lifestyle, occupation, and relationships.

STRESSORS RELATED TO SEXUAL ORIENTATION

Peer pressure and fear of being different can be a source of stress for a young person who is questioning their gender identity or sexual orientation. Are they physically and emotionally attracted to a person of the same or opposite sex, or to both sexes? This attraction is an evolving process, but typically emerges between middle childhood and early adolescence. New research indicates that sexual orientation may be related to genetic, hormonal, developmental, social, or cultural influences, but irrespective of definitive evidence, there is agreement that a person has little or no choice regarding it. There is also consensus that sexual orientation cannot be changed by medication or therapy.

Terms commonly used to describe sexual orientation include *heterosexual* (attracted to members of the opposite sex), *gay* (attracted to members of the same sex; more commonly men who are attracted to men), *lesbian* (women who are attracted to women), and *bisexual* (attracted to both sexes). When a person's internal feelings of being male or female differ from their physical anatomy, the term *transgender* is used to describe that person's gender identity. The term *questioning* describes a person unsure of sexual orientation. The acronym LGBTQIA+ is commonly used in the United States to refer to all these alternatives collectively; however, there is a growing appreciation for the fact that sex, sexual assignment, gender identity, and sexual orientation occur on a spectrum and are not fixed for some people (see Chapter 43). For an excellent teaching and learning tool, check out the Genderbread Person at https://www.genderbread.org/resource/genderbread-person-v4-0.

People who identify as gay, lesbian, bisexual, and/or transgender may experience prejudice and discrimination that can have negative psychological outcomes. Some adolescents may be reluctant to reveal their sexual orientation or gender identity for fear of ridicule, rejection, or harassment from family and friends; others may receive unconditional support and love from both groups.

FAMILY STRESSORS

Family-centered stressors include both positive and negative factors, such as marriage, divorce, parenthood, and death of a parent. Stress may precipitate mental or physical health problems that are aggravated by ineffective coping mechanisms such as substance abuse, child abuse, spousal abuse, decreased nutrition and rest, and risk-taking behavior.

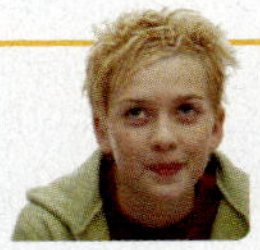

Consider **Darlene Schneider**, the 14-year-old pregnant adolescent described in the case file at the beginning of the chapter. Analysis of this patient's assessment reveals multiple developmental and situational stressors affecting Darlene that place her and her fetus at high risk for problems. Using this information, the nurse could develop a highly individualized care plan that focuses on these stressors (e.g., her lack of adequate supports, multiple sexual partners, poor nutritional habits), ultimately to the benefit of Darlene and her baby.

An increasing number of people are remaining single, either by choice or situation. Singlehood status has advantages and disadvantages. Being single gives people the freedom to come and go as they choose, to have more autonomy, to pursue or create their own career vision, and to spend money and time as they wish. On the other hand, external pressures to marry and the desire for love, to belong, and to raise a family may make young adults question the decision to remain single. Single-parent households are increasingly common, with individuals raising their children with or without the presence or support (financial or otherwise) of the other biologic parent. The stressors inherent in maintaining a household and raising children exist for these families, but their support systems are often different from those identified for the traditional nuclear family (two parents with one or more children). It is important to recognize that the definition of a *nuclear household*, one that contains a single-family nucleus (center), has evolved and specifically encompasses a married-couple family with or without children, a father with children, and a mother with children (United Nations Statistics Division, 2021).

Couples may encounter difficulties conceiving, delay childbearing until their careers are established, or choose not to have children. If they want to have children, infertility (defined as the inability to conceive after 1 year of coitus without contraception) may add even more stress. Women who have postponed having children may realize in their middle to late 30s that their so-called biologic clock is winding down; an increasing number of women in this age group are having their first child.

Divorce and separation are common in our society, with rates being highest among those marrying or cohabitating at a young age, having low income, and having low educational levels. It separates children from their families, has long-term emotional costs, and increases the number of single-parent families headed by women.

One-person, nuclear, composite/multi-person (friend or partner included), and extended households exist and thrive in the United States. Although for census and documentation purposes the term *family* refers to blood relatives (United Nations Statistics Division, 2021), informally, family has come to mean whomever the patient identifies as family. Recognizing and activating these resources and important people in their lives can make a difference in developing robust support systems for our patients.

Role of the Nurse in Promoting Health and Preventing Illness

A true assessment of adolescent development must include the profound changes in reproductive functioning. Beyond that consideration, perhaps one of the more significant nursing activities for people in this stage is facilitating healthy family relationships. Mutual respect, open communication, and accurate information exchange among family members pave the road for a healthy transition from adolescence to adulthood.

In this age group, acute illness is often more of an annoyance than a serious issue. If hospitalized, an adolescent's

Teaching Tips 23-5

ADOLESCENTS AND YOUNG ADULTS

Health Topic	Teaching Tip	Why Is This Important?
Safety	• Encourage drivers' education classes for adolescents, if available. • Discuss the relationship of alcohol and drug consumption to motor vehicle crashes. • Provide information about water safety, gun safety, and sports safety.	Most deaths in people between ages 15 and 24 years are the result of motor vehicle crashes, homicide, and suicide.
Nutrition	• Encourage a diet based on the food groups, with added calories during the adolescent growth spurt. • Refer for counseling for extremes in either underweight or overweight. • Discuss nutritional problems that may result from too much fast food and too many soft drinks. • A balance of food intake, exercise, and rest is important.	Nutritional needs increase to meet the accelerated physical growth and development during adolescence. Being underweight may result from an inadequate intake of calories, or in extreme cases from anorexia nervosa or bulimia. An intake of calories in excess of metabolic needs can lead to being overweight.
Sexual Development	• Secondary sex characteristics are fully developed. • Both males and females are physically capable of reproduction. • Discuss sexual behavior, biologic sex, and gender identification openly and honestly with adolescents.	The development of secondary sex characteristics that began in the school-aged child is completed during adolescence. Sexual behavior in adolescents and young adults may result in disease or pregnancy, as well as decreased self-esteem.
Growth and Development	• The adolescent is primarily influenced by the peer group. • Risk-taking behavior, especially in males, is common. • Maintaining open communication with teens is important. • Encourage increasing independence in the adolescent and young adult but continue to provide love and support. • Assist with clarifying values and goals for future occupation.	Peer groups may have positive or negative effects. The rapid physical and emotional changes of adolescence require revising self-concept and body image. These should stabilize by late adolescence. The young adult is usually living independently and has an occupation of choice.
Promoting Health and Preventing Illness	• Have immunizations and boosters as recommended. • Have regular physical, vision, and dental examinations. • Always have a physical examination before participating in sports activities. • Know your breasts and testicles and report any changes. • Learn to say "no" to pressures to have sexual activity. • Engage in safer-sex practices if sexually active. • Have an annual Pap test and pelvic examination if sexually active. • Know the dangers of STIs (from genital, oral, and anal sex) and have HIV testing especially if sex without a condom is practiced.	Immunizations and regular health-related examinations are essential to maintaining health. Chronic illnesses such as hypertension, cardiovascular disease, and diabetes mellitus may appear during adolescence and young adulthood. Sexual desires are high, and sexual activity is common. STIs are a major health problem, with more than two-thirds of those infected younger than 25. Untreated STIs may result in sterility in females and males or infection of an unborn fetus.

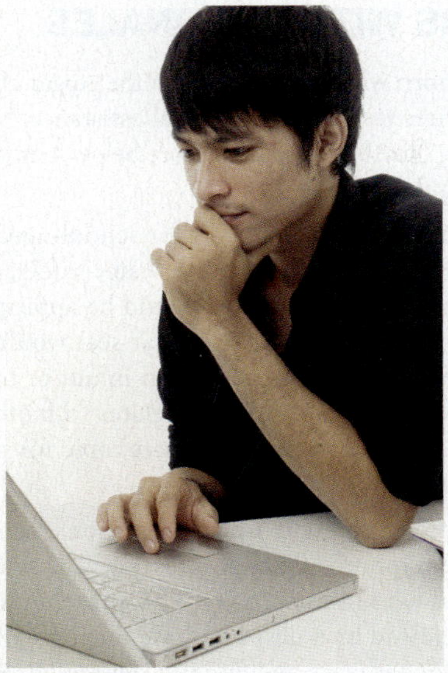

FIGURE 23-11. Adolescents with chronic illnesses can avoid feelings of isolation by using social networking sites to communicate with their peers.

and young adult's motivation to recover and to resume normal activities is strong. Because independence and self-sufficiency are important to adolescents and young adults, they will not easily accept the dependent sick role. Although chronic illnesses are less common, their occurrence can lead to delayed development, loss of independence, and permanent changes in personal and career goals. Prolonged hospitalization, long-term care, or home care increases the adolescent's feelings of isolation and may disrupt normal development. Educational and recreational activities should be provided, if at all possible (Fig. 23-11).

Unfolding Patient Stories: Christopher Parrish • Part 1

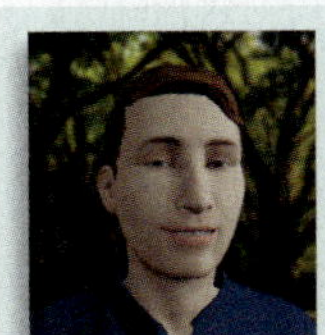

Christopher Parrish, age 18, is hospitalized for management of cystic fibrosis with weakness and weight loss. What areas of health promotion should the nurse discuss with Christopher? How can the nurse help an adolescent with a chronic illness avoid feelings of isolation? (Christopher Parrish's story continues in Chapter 32.)

Care for Christopher and other patients in a realistic virtual environment: ***vSim** for Nursing* (thepoint.lww.com/vSimFunds). Practice documenting these patients' care in DocuCare (thepoint.lww.com/DocuCareEHR).

Teaching activities to promote health for adolescents and young adults are listed in Teaching Tips 23-5.

DEVELOPING CLINICAL REASONING AND CLINICAL JUDGMENT

1. Based on the information presented in Chapters 22 and 23, describe nursing interventions to meet developmental needs for the following patients:
   - An infant hospitalized for treatment of a serious birth defect involving the heart and lungs
   - A toddler with a fracture of the left leg, treated in the emergency department and then sent home
   - A school-aged child, now in rehabilitation, with burns on both arms
   - A 20-year-old hospitalized for injuries resulting from an automobile accident after drinking alcohol
2. During your home visit to a 16-year-old girl with cancer, she says, "I don't believe in God." What would you reply? Why would you respond this way?
3. During a clinic visit, a 2-month-old infant appears listless and constantly cries. The mother tells you that he has colic, so she has been diluting his formula with water. What would you do now?

PRACTICING FOR NCLEX

1. The nurse assesses an Apgar score of 4 for a newborn. What action will the nurse take next?
   a. No intervention is necessary: this is a normal score.
   b. Provide respiratory assistance.
   c. Perform CPR.
   d. Wait 5 minutes and repeat the scoring process.
2. A school nurse is educating parents of school-aged children about safety issues at a parent–teacher meeting. What topics are appropriate for the nurse to include for this age group? Select all that apply.
   a. Childproofing the home
   b. Choosing a car seat
   c. Teaching pedestrian traffic safety
   d. Providing swimming lessons and water safety rules
   e. Discussing alcohol and drug consumption related to motor vehicle safety
   f. Teaching the child how to "stop, drop, and roll"
3. Nurses on a pediatric unit encourage parents of hospitalized infants and toddlers to remain with their children to help decrease what potential problem?
   a. Attachment
   b. Separation anxiety
   c. Risk for injury
   d. Failure to thrive
4. A nurse is teaching parents of toddlers how to spend quality time with their children. Which activity is developmentally appropriate for this age group?
   a. Playing video games
   b. Playing peek-a-boo
   c. Playing in a sand box
   d. Playing board games
5. A mother tells the nurse that she is worried about her 4-year-old daughter because she is "overly attached to her father and won't listen to anything I tell her to do." What information will the nurse convey to this parent?
   a. This is normal behavior for a preschooler.
   b. She and her family should see a counselor.
   c. Try to spend more time with her daughter.
   d. Her child should be tested for autism.

6. A school nurse is counseling parents of teenagers who are beginning high school. Which issues would be priority topics of discussion for this age group? Select all that apply.
   a. Influence of peer groups
   b. Bullying
   c. Water safety
   d. Eating disorders
   e. Risk-taking behavior
   f. Immunizations
7. A nurse working with adolescents in a group home discusses the developmental tasks appropriate for adolescents with the staff. What is an example of a primary developmental task of the adolescent?
   a. Working hard to succeed in school
   b. Achieving independence from parents
   c. Developing athletic activities and skills
   d. Accepting the decisions of parents
8. A school nurse at an elementary school is lobbying the school board to provide more fruits and vegetables on lunch menus and for snacks. Which rationale does the nurse give the board for this request?
   a. Children who are overweight tend to grow up and have chronic health problems.
   b. Children do not get sufficient vitamins, minerals, and proteins.
   c. The school exists in the center of a food desert.
   d. Children who are overweight are more prone to bullying.
9. A nurse is teaching new mothers about infant care and safety. What will the nurse include as a teaching point?
   a. Keep infants younger than 6 months out of direct sunlight.
   b. Use honey instead of sugar in homemade baby food.
   c. Place the baby on their stomach for sleeping.
   d. Keep crib rails down at all times.
10. The school nurse at a high school with a day care center identifies which of these individuals as at highest risk for abuse?
    a. 6-month-old baby who cries vigorously when their parent leaves
    b. Teen whose parents are divorcing
    c. Student with an STI displaying risky sexual behaviors
    d. Adolescent who sprained their ankle at soccer practice
11. The school nurse is speaking to the parent of a school-aged child who is returning to school after the death of the other parent. The nurse explains that which of these behaviors most likely indicates regression due to great stress on the child?
    a. Bedwetting when previously toilet trained
    b. Wanting to play video games
    c. Crying loudly when sad
    d. Being afraid of the dark

ANSWERS WITH RATIONALES

1. **b.** A newborn who scores 4 to 6 on the Apgar chart typically requires respiratory or special assistance. Normal Apgar scores are 7 to 10. Those who score below 4 are in need of life-saving measures.
2. **c, d, f.** Important safety topics for school-aged children include pedestrian traffic safety, water safety, and fire safety. Childproofing a home would be appropriate for parents of a toddler, choosing a car seat would be an appropriate topic for parents of an infant or toddler, and teaching drug and alcohol as it relates to motor vehicle safety would be a more appropriate topic for parents of adolescents.
3. **b.** Separation anxiety is a normal response when a young child (age 6 months through preschool) is separated from loved ones who offer security. This presents with initial crying followed by a despair phase during which the child no longer cries and appears depressed. Encouraging parents or guardians to remain with hospitalized children decreases this anxiety and promotes the child's trust in others.
4. **c.** Playing in a sand box with toys that emphasize gross motor skills and creativity is a developmentally appropriate activity for a toddler. Video games may be appropriate for school-aged children and adolescents but should be monitored. Playing peek-a-boo is developmentally appropriate for an infant, and playing board games usually begins with preschool and older children.
5. **a.** Preschoolers, according to Freud, are in the phallic stage, with the biologic focus primarily genital. The child has a sexual desire for the opposite-sex parent, but as means of defense strongly identifies with the same-sex parent. This is normal behavior for a preschooler; the family does not need counseling or autism testing. Spending more time with the child is always a good idea but is not the solution for normal behavior.
6. **a, b, d, e.** Appropriate topics of discussion for parents of adolescents include peer groups, bullying, eating disorders, and risk-taking behaviors. Discussing immunizations would be appropriate for parents of children from infants to school-age. Water safety should be taught in the preschool and school-age years.
7. **b.** Adolescence is a time to establish more mature relationships with both males and females of the same age.
8. **a.** Overweight school-aged children often become overweight adolescents and adults who are at risk for heart disease, high blood pressure, type 2 diabetes, stroke, cancer, asthma, and osteoarthritis. Primary prevention of obesity in children has far-reaching, long-term benefits. While it may be true that some children can have nutritional deficiencies, a school may be located in a food desert, and that overweight children are more prone to bullying, the overarching goal is primary prevention.
9. **a.** Infants younger than age 6 months should be kept out of direct sunlight and covered with protective clothing and hats. The nurse should also teach parents *not* to add honey or sugar to homemade baby food, to place the baby on the *back* for sleeping to prevent SIDS, and to keep the crib rails *up* at all times.

10. c. Psychological consequences of abuse or neglect can include behavioral manifestations including substance abuse, criminality, continuation of the abuse and neglect cycle, and sexual risk-taking. The other behaviors described are not specific for abuse.

11. a. Regression is manifested by behavior that is more characteristic of a younger age and can occur at any time in response to stressful circumstances. The most common regressive behaviors are excessive clinging to caregivers, loss of control over elimination, and the use of more infantile speech patterns.

Bibliography

American College of Obstetricians and Gynecologists. (2015, October/2021). *The Apgar score.* (Committee Opinion No. 644). Committee on Obstetric Practice, American Academy of Pediatrics—Committee on Fetus and Newborn. https://www.acog.org/clinical/clinical-guidance/committee-opinion/articles/2015/10/the-apgar-score

American College of Obstetricians and Gynecologists. (2018, October). *Optimizing support for breastfeeding as part of obstetric practice.* (Committee Opinion No. 756). https://www.acog.org/clinical/clinical-guidance/committee-opinion/articles/2018/10/optimizing-support-for-breastfeeding-as-part-of-obstetric-practice

American Psychiatric Association (APA). (2021, August). *Specific learning disorder.* https://www.psychiatry.org/patients-families/specific-learning-disorder/what-is-specific-learning-disorder

American SIDS Institute. (2022). *What is SIDS/SUID?* Retrieved March 9, 2022, from https://www.sids.org/what-is-sidssuid

Apgar, V. (1953). A proposal for a new method of evaluation of the newborn infant. *Current Researches in Anesthesia and Analgesia, 32*(4), 260–267. https://journals.lww.com/anesthesia-analgesia/pages/articleviewer.aspx?year=1953&issue=07000&article=00006&type=Citation

Centers for Disease Control and Prevention (CDC). (2015, April 15). *Division of nutrition, physical activity, and obesity—Growth chart training: Using the WHO growth charts.* https://www.cdc.gov/nccdphp/dnpao/growthcharts/who/recommendations/index.htm

Centers for Disease Control and Prevention (CDC). (2019, July 26). *Vaccines and preventable diseases: Meningococcal vaccine recommendations.* https://www.cdc.gov/vaccines/vpd/mening/hcp/recommendations.html

Centers for Disease Control and Prevention (CDC). (2020a, April 1). *Vaccine information statements (VISs): Tdap (tetanus, diphtheria, pertussis) VIS.* https://www.cdc.gov/vaccines/hcp/vis/vis-statements/tdap.html

Centers for Disease Control and Prevention (CDC). (2020b, July 15). *Substance use during pregnancy.* https://www.cdc.gov/reproductivehealth/maternalinfanthealth/substance-abuse/substance-abuse-during-pregnancy.htm?CDC_AA_refVal=https%3A%2F%2Fwww.cdc.gov%2Freproductivehealth%2Fmaternalinfanthealth%2Ftobaccousepregnancy%2Findex.htm

Centers for Disease Control and Prevention (CDC). (2020c, October 30). *Reproductive health: Premature birth.* https://www.cdc.gov/reproductivehealth/features/premature-birth/index.html

Centers for Disease Control and Prevention (CDC). (2021a, January 5). *Sudden unexpected infant death and sudden infant death syndrome: SUID and SDY case registry.* https://www.cdc.gov/sids/case-registry.htm

Centers for Disease Control and Prevention (CDC). (2021b, February 12). *Recommended children and adolescent immunization schedule for ages 18 years or younger, United States, 2021.* https://www.cdc.gov/vaccines/schedules/hcp/child-adolescent.html

Centers for Disease Control and Prevention (CDC). (2021c, March 15). *Violence prevention: Child abuse and neglect prevention.* https://www.cdc.gov/violenceprevention/childabuseandneglect/index.html?CDC_AA_refVal=https%3A%2F%2Fwww.cdc.gov%2Fviolenceprevention%2Fchildmaltreatment%2Findex.html

Centers for Disease Control and Prevention (CDC). (2021d, March 29). *Reproductive health: Teen pregnancy.* https://www.cdc.gov/teenpregnancy/index.htm

Centers for Disease Control and Prevention (CDC). (2021e, April 28). *Sudden unexpected infant death and sudden infant death syndrome: Data and statistics.* https://www.cdc.gov/sids/data.htm

Centers for Disease Control and Prevention (CDC). (2021f, July 22). *Chlamydia—CDC fact sheet (detailed).* https://www.cdc.gov/std/chlamydia/stdfact-chlamydia-detailed.htm

Chang, J. G., Cimino, F. M., & Gossa, W. (2020). ADHD in children: Common questions and answers. *American Family Physician, 102*(10), 592–602.

Child Welfare Information Gateway. (2019a, April). *Long-term consequences of child abuse and neglect.* U.S. Department of Health and Human Services, Children's Bureau. https://www.childwelfare.gov/pubPDFs/long_term_consequences.pdf

Child Welfare Information Gateway. (2019b, April). *What is child abuse and neglect? Recognizing the signs and symptoms.* U.S. Department of Health and Human Services, Children's Bureau. https://www.childwelfare.gov/pubPDFs/whatiscan.pdf

Committee on Improving the Health, Safety, and Well-Being of Young Adults; Board on Children, Youth, and Families; Institute of Medicine; National Research Council. (2015). *Investing in the health and well-being of young adults.* In R. J. Bonnie, C. Stroud, & H. Breiner (Eds.). National Academies Press (U.S.).

Cox, J. E. (2020). Understanding the differences in pregnancy and birth rates for Black and White teens. *The Journal of Adolescent Health, 67*(3), 313–314. https://doi.org/10.1016/j.jadohealth.2020.06.010

Dabbous, R. (2021). Hannah Arendt and Sigmund Freud on sexual identity in 2020. *Sexuality & Culture, 25*(3), 835–851. https://doi.org/10.1007/s12119-020-09796-4

De Kruijff, I., Veldhuis, M. S., Tromp, E., Vlieger, A. M., Benninga, M. A., & Lambregtse-van den Berg, M. P. (2021). Distress in fathers of babies with infant colic. *Acta Paediatrica, 110*(8), 2455–2461. https://doi.org/10.1111/apa.15873

Dumas, S. A., Chu, S., & Horswell, R. (2020). Analysis of pregnancy and birth rates among Black and White Medicaid-enrolled teens. *The Journal of Adolescent Health, 67*(3), 409–415. https://doi.org/10.1016/j.jadohealth.2020.04.026

Erikson, E. H. (1963). *Childhood and society* (2nd ed.). W. W. Norton.

Flanders, S., Ladame, F., Carlsberg, A., Heymanns, P., Naziri, D., & Panitz, D. (2016). On the subject of homosexuality: What Freud said. *The International Journal of Psychoanalysis, 97*(3), 933–950. https://doi.org/10.1111/1745-8315.12520

Fowler, J. W. (1981). *Stages of faith: The psychology of human development and the quest for meaning.* HarperCollins Publishers.

Franceschi, R., Rizzardi, C., Maines, E., Liguori, A., Soffiati, M., & Tornese, G. (2021). Failure to thrive in infant and toddlers: A practical flowchart-based approach in a hospital setting. *Italian Journal of Pediatrics, 47*(1), 62. https://doi.org/10.1186/s13052-021-01017-4

Freud, S. (1960). *The ego and the id: The standard edition of the complete psychological works of Sigmund Freud.* In J. Strachey (Ed.). W. W. Norton.

Fryar, C. D., Carroll, M. D., & Afful, J. (2021, January 29). *Prevalence of overweight, obesity, and severe obesity among children and adolescents aged 2–19 years: United States, 1963–1965 through 2017–2018.* NCHS Health E-Stats. https://www.cdc.gov/nchs/data/hestat/obesity-child-17-18/obesity-child.htm#Suggested%20citation

Gould, R. L. (1978). *Transformations: Growth and change in adult life.* Simon & Schuster.

Hagan, J. F., Jr, Balachova, T., Bertrand, J., Chasnoff, I., Dang, E., Fernandez-Baca, D., Kable, J., Kosofsky, B., Senturias, Y. N., Singh, N., Sloane, M., Weitzman, C., Zubler, J., Neurobehavioral Disorder Associated With Prenatal Alcohol Exposure Workgroup, & American Academy of Pediatrics (2016). Neurobehavioral disorder associated with prenatal alcohol exposure. *Pediatrics, 138*(4), e20151553. https://doi.org/10.1542/peds.2015-1553

Havighurst, R. J. (1972). *Developmental tasks and education* (3rd ed.). David McKay.

Hjern, A., Lindblom, K., Reuter, A., & Silfverdal, S. A. (2020). A systematic review of prevention and treatment of infantile colic. *Acta Paediatrica, 109*(9), 1733–1744. https://doi.org/10.1111/apa.15247

Hockenberry, M. J., Rodgers, C. C., & Wilson, D. (2022). *Wong's essentials of pediatric nursing* (11th ed.). Elsevier.

Homan, G. J. (2016). Failure to thrive: A practical guide. *American Family Physician, 94*(4), 295–299. https://www.aafp.org/afp/2016/0815/afp20160815p295.pdf

Insurance Institute for Highway Safety Highway Loss Data Institute. (2021, March). *Fatality facts 2019: Teenagers.* https://www.iihs.org/topics/fatality-statistics/detail/teenagers

Institute of Medicine (IOM) & National Research Council (NRC). (2015). *Investing in the health and well-being of young adults.* The National Academies Press. https://www.nap.edu/catalog/18869/investing-in-the-health-and-well-being-of-young-adults

Ivey-Stephenson, A. Z., Demissie, Z., Crosby, A. E., Stone, D. M., Gaylor, E., Wilkins, N., Lowry, R., & Brown, M. (2020). Suicidal ideation and behaviors among high school students—Youth Risk Behavior Survey, United States, 2019. *MMWR Supplements, 69*(1), 47–55. https://doi.org/10.15585/mmwr.su6901a6

Jackson, D. B., & Leal, W. E. (2018). Energy drink consumption and the perceived risk and disapproval of drugs: Monitoring the Future, 2010–2016. *Drug and Alcohol Dependence, 188*, 24–31. https://doi.org/10.1016/j.drugalcdep.2018.03.022

Jatana, K. R., Rhoades, K., Milkovich, S., & Jacobs, I. N. (2017). Basic mechanism of button battery ingestion injuries and novel mitigation strategies after diagnosis and removal. *Laryngoscope, 127*(6), 1276–1282. https://doi.org/10.1002/lary.26362

Johnston, L. D., Miech, R. A., O'Malley, P. M., Bachman, J. G., Schulenberg, J. E., & Patrick, M. E. (2021). *Monitoring the Future: National survey results on drug use 1975–2020: Overview, key findings on adolescent drug use.* Institute for Social Research, University of Michigan. http://www.monitoringthefuture.org//pubs/monographs/mtf-overview2020.pdf

Kable, J. A., & Mukherjee, R. A. S. (2017). Neurodevelopmental disorder associated with prenatal exposure to alcohol (ND-PAE): A proposed diagnostic method of capturing the neurocognitive phenotype of FASD. *European Journal of Medical Genetics, 60*(1), 49–54. https://doi.org/10.1016/j.ejmg.2016.09.013

Khalaf, R. T., Ruan, W., Orkin, S., Wilsey, M., Fishman, D. S., Mallon, D., Pan, Z., Hazleton, K. Z., Kramer, R. E., & Walker, T. (2020). Gastric injury secondary to button battery ingestions: A retrospective multicenter review. *Gastrointestinal Endoscopy, 92*(2), 276–283. https://doi.org/10.1016/j.gie.2020.04.037

Klaus, M. H., & Kennell, J. H. (1982). *Parent–infant bonding.* C. V. Mosby.

Levinson, D. J., Darrow, C. N., Klein, E. B., Levinson, M. H., & McKee, B. (1978). *The seasons of a man's life.* The Random House Publishing Group.

Mubarak, A., Benninga, M. A., Broekaert, I., Dolinsek, J., Homan, M., Mas, E., Miele, E., Pienar, C., Thapar, N., Thomson, M., Tzivinikos, C., & de Ridder, L. (2021). Diagnosis, management, and prevention of button battery ingestion in childhood: A European Society for Paediatric Gastroenterology Hepatology and Nutrition position paper. *Journal of Pediatric Gastroenterology and Nutrition*, *73*(1), 129–136. https://doi.org/10.1097/MPG.0000000000003048

National Institute on Drug Abuse. (2021, May 20). *Monitoring the future*. https://www.drugabuse.gov/drug-topics/trends-statistics/monitoring-future

National Institutes of Health (NIH): Eunice Kennedy Shriver National Institute of Child Health and Human Development. (2018, September 11). *About learning disabilities* https://www.nichd.nih.gov/health/topics/learning/conditioninfo

National Institute of Mental Health. (2018). *Eating disorders: About more than food*. https://www.nimh.nih.gov/health/publications/eating-disorders/

Norholt, H. (2020). Revisiting the roots of attachment: A review of the biological and psychological effects of maternal skin-to-skin contact and carrying of full-term infants. *Infant Behavior & Development*, *60*, 101441. https://doi.org/10.1016/j.infbeh.2020.101441

Oei, J. L. (2020). Alcohol use in pregnancy and its impact on the mother and child. *Addiction*, *115*(11), 2148–2163. https://doi.org/10.1111/add.15036

Piaget, J., & Inhelder, B. (1969). *The psychology of the child*. Basic Books.

Psychology Today. (2019, April 3). *Child abuse*. https://www.psychologytoday.com/conditions/child-abuse

Robert Wood Johnson Foundation. (2021, October 14). From crisis to opportunity: Reforming our nation's policies to help all children grow up healthy. https://media.stateofobesity.org/wp-content/uploads/2021/10/12132618/State-of-Childhood-Obesity-10-13-21-Final-WEB.pdf

Schölin, L., Mukherjee, R. A. S., Aiton, N., Blackburn, C., Brown, S., Flemming, K. M., Gard, P. R., Howlett, H., Plant, M., Price, A. D., Shields, J., Smith, L. A., Suttie, M., Zammitt, D. C., Cook, P. A., & UK FASD Research Collaboration. (2021). Fetal alcohol spectrum disorders: An overview of current evidence and activities in the UK. *Archives of Disease in Childhood*, *106*(7), 636–640. https://doi.org/10.1136/archdischild-2020-320435

Sheu, Y., Chen, L. H., & Hedegaard, H. (2016, November 18). Sports- and recreation-related injury episodes in the United States, 2011–2014. *National Health Statistics Reports*, (99), 1–12. https://www.cdc.gov/nchs/data/nhsr/nhsr099.pdf

SmithBattle, L. (2020). Walking on eggshells: An update on the stigmatizing of teen mothers. *The American Journal of Maternal Child Nursing*, *45*(6), 322–327. https://doi.org/10.1097/NMC.0000000000000655

Task Force on Sudden Infant Death Syndrome. (2016). SIDS and other sleep-related infant deaths: Updated 2016 recommendations for a safe infant sleeping environment. *Pediatrics*, *138*(5), e20162938. https://doi.org/10.1542/peds.2016-2938

Thomas, A., Chess, S., & Birch, H. G. (1968). *Temperament and behavior discussed in children*. New York University Press.

Topjian, A. A., Raymond, T. T., Atkins, D., Chan, M., Duff, J. P., Joyner, B. L. Jr, Lasa, J. J., Lavonas, E. J., Levy, A., Mahgoub, M., Meckler, G. D., Roberts, K. E., Sutton, R. M., Schexnayder, S. M., & Pediatric Basic and Advanced Life Support Collaborators. (2020). Part 4: Pediatric basic and advanced life support: 2020 American Heart Association guidelines for cardiopulmonary resuscitation and emergency cardiovascular care. *Circulation*, *142*(16_suppl_2), S469–S523. https://doi.org/10.1161/CIR.0000000000000901

United Nations Statistics Division. (2021). *Demographics and social statistics: Households and families*. https://unstats.un.org/unsd/demographic-social/sconcerns/family/index.cshtml

U.S. Food and Drug Administration (FDA). (2018, January 22). *FDA Drug Safety Communication: FDA requires labeling changes for prescription opioid cough and cold medicines to limit their use to adults 18 years and older*. https://www.fda.gov/drugs/drug-safety-and-availability/fda-drug-safety-communication-fda-requires-labeling-changes-prescription-opioid-cough-and-cold

Ward, Z. J., Bleich, S. N., Cradock, A. L., Barrett, J. L., Giles, C. M., Flax, C., Long, M. W., & Gortmaker, S. L. (2019). Projected U.S. state-level prevalence of adult obesity and severe obesity. *The New England Journal of Medicine*, *381*(25), 2440–2450. https://doi.org/10.1056/NEJMsa1909301

Wolke, D., Bilgin, A., & Samara, M. (2017). Systematic review and meta-analysis: Fussing and crying durations and prevalence of colic in infants. *Journal of Pediatrics*, *185*, 55–61.e4. https://doi.org/10.1016/j.jpeds.2017.02.020

Wolraich, M. L., Hagan, J. F., Jr, Allan, C., Chan, E., Davison, D., Earls, M., Evans, S. W., Flinn, S. K., Froehlich, T., Frost, J., Holbrook, J. R., Lehmann, C. U., Lessin, H. R., Okechukwu, K., Pierce, K. L., Winner, J. D., Zurhellen, W., & SUBCOMMITTEE ON CHILDREN AND ADOLESCENTS WITH ATTENTION-DEFICIT/HYPERACTIVE DISORDER (2019). Clinical practice guideline for the diagnosis, evaluation, and treatment of attention-deficit/hyperactivity disorder in children and adolescents. *Pediatrics*, *144*(4), e20192528. https://doi.org/10.1542/peds.2019–2528

Zeevenhooven, J., Koppen, I. J., & Benninga, M. A. (2017). The new Rome IV criteria for functional gastrointestinal disorders in infants and toddlers. *Pediatric Gastroenterology Hepatology & Nutrition*, *20*(1), 1–13. https://doi.org/10.5223/pghn.2017.20.1.1

24 Middle and Older Adulthood

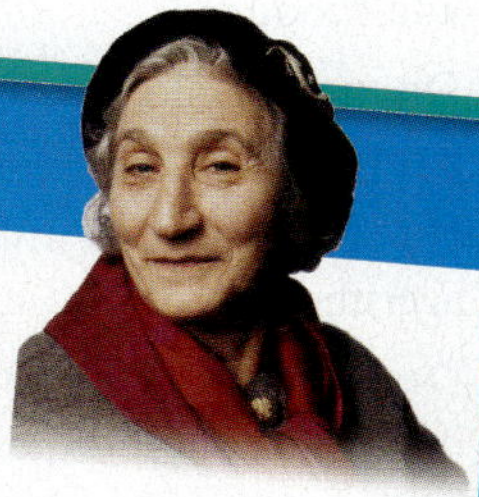

Ethel Peabody

Ethel, an 88-year-old single woman, is being discharged from the hospital. She shows signs of early dementia, and was treated for cardiac problems this hospitalization. She has no family and lives in a small, two-story house with her three cats. There is some concern about her safety at home. She depends on a neighbor for help and refuses to consider moving to a retirement community or extended-care facility.

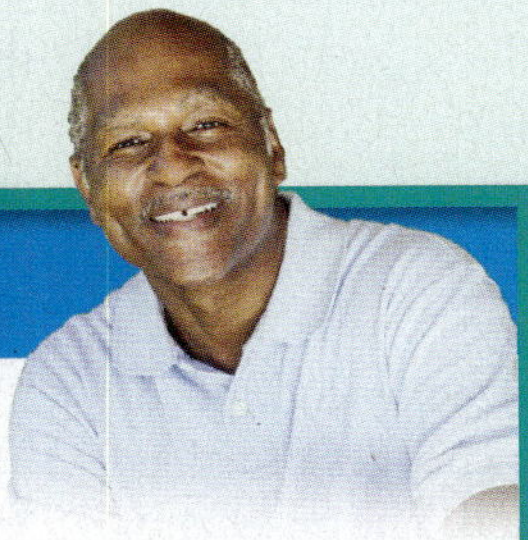

Larry Jenkins

Larry, a 67-year-old man with diabetes, states, "Everything's gone downhill since I retired 5 months ago." He reports being "bored out of my mind" and drinking more alcohol simply because "there's nothing else to do!"

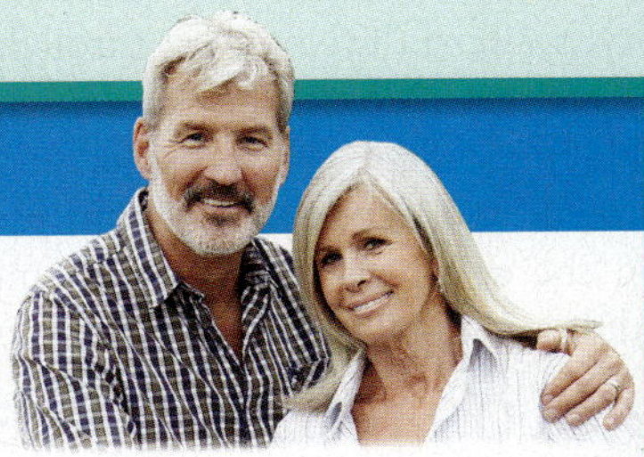

Rosemary Mason

Rosemary, a 49-year-old woman who comes to the clinic with her 54-year-old husband, confides that she wishes drugs that treat erectile dysfunction had never been discovered. "I was happier when we just cuddled at night. Now he wants to try all sorts of things, and I just don't have time or energy for this!"

Learning Outcomes

After completing the chapter, you will be able to accomplish the following:

1. Summarize the theories that describe how and why aging occurs.
2. Describe major physiologic, cognitive, psychosocial, moral, and spiritual developments and tasks of middle and older adulthood.
3. Describe common health problems in middle and older adulthood.
4. Discuss physiologic and functional changes that occur with aging.
5. Describe common myths and stereotypes that perpetuate ageism.
6. Describe nursing interventions to promote health for individuals in middle and older adulthood.
7. Identify the health care needs of older adults in terms of chronic illnesses, accidental injuries, and acute care needs.

Nursing Concepts

- Advocacy
- Cognition
- Development
- Family
- Identity
- Sexuality

Aging is a gradual process, characterized by continued development and maturation. The changes of aging begin as one enters middle adulthood. The onset and effects of those changes throughout the middle and older adult years are influenced by numerous biological, psychosocial, and environmental factors. The physiologic changes of aging, first experienced in middle adulthood, become more obvious in older adulthood. Continued cognitive and psychosocial development throughout adult life depends to a great extent on a person's sense of self-concept and prior ability to adapt. This chapter continues the discussion of growth and development from previous chapters, focusing on the aging years. For an example addressing the older adult, see the Reflective Practice box.

BIOLOGICAL THEORIES OF AGING

Although there are valid sociologic, psychological, and nursing theories of aging that will be embedded in our discussion of aging, this chapter will begin with the biological theories of aging. As a person ages, changes in cells, tissues, organs, and organ systems occur. Scientists do not fully understand why some people, even within the same family or environment, age much more rapidly than others. Although internal processes may influence aging, other factors, such as nutrition and the environment, also play a role. Numerous theories describe how and why aging occurs, but none is universally accepted. These nonstochastic (predetermined) and stochastic (by chance) biological theories of aging focus on a variety of factors, including genetic inheritance, cell metabolism and function, and the immune system (Eliopoulos, 2022; Miller, 2019).

Genetic Theory

The genetic theories of aging hold that lifespan depends to a great extent on genetic factors. In one theory, genes within the organism control *genetic or biological clocks*, which determine the occurrence and rate of metabolic processes, including cell division. This telomere–telomerase hypothesis is based on the understanding that a finite number of cell divisions are possible, so cellular death is essentially preprogrammed.

Neuroendocrine and Immunity Theories

Two other preprogrammed theories involve the neuroendocrine and immune systems. The neuroendocrine system contains the pituitary and hypothalamus that serve as control mechanisms for the entire body. As age advances, these control mechanisms fail, which leads to failure of the body's essential pacemaker, and death.

The immunity theory of aging focuses on the functions of the immune system. This system—composed primarily of the bone marrow, thymus, spleen, and lymph nodes—seeks out and destroys foreign agents (such as viruses, bacteria, and perhaps cells undergoing neoplastic changes). The immune response declines steadily after younger adulthood as the thymus loses size and function. Age-associated changes in the immune system, also known as *immunosenescence,* are thought to be responsible for the increase in infections such as pneumonia and septicemia, immune disorders, and cancer as adults age. There is also some evidence to support an increase in autoimmune disorders, with the body essentially attacking itself. Some authorities believe that nutrition plays an important role in maintaining the immune response; therefore, there is much interest in vitamin supplements (such as vitamin E) that are believed by some to improve immune function.

Stochastic Theories

Stochastic theories of aging are based on the idea that there is a randomness to cellular damage and errors that makes predicting aging and death impossible. One example is the *wear and tear theory* in which organisms wear out from increased metabolic functioning, and cells become exhausted from the constant energy depletion that occurs when the body continually adapts to stressors. The organism eventually wears out from use.

Cross-linkage, a chemical reaction that produces damage to the DNA and cell death, forms the basis for another theory. As a person ages, cross-links accumulate, leading to essential molecules in the cell binding together and

QSEN Reflective Practice: Cultivating QSEN Competencies

CHALLENGE TO ETHICAL AND LEGAL SKILLS

Mrs. Ethel Peabody is an 88-year-old single woman who is being discharged from the hospital. She shows signs of early dementia, and was treated for cardiac problems this hospitalization. She has no family and lives in a small, two-story house with her three cats. When the provider ordered her discharge, I had grave concerns about her ability to live safely on her own. When I asked if she had ever thought about moving to a long-term care facility or retirement community, she said, "I'd rather die than go to one of those places!" When I directly expressed that I was worried about her safety, she told me her cats would take care of her. When I repeated this conversation to the charge nurse, the charge nurse said, "There is nothing we can do if the patient isn't willing to explore other options."

Thinking Outside the Box: Possible Courses of Action

- Feel satisfied that I had reported my concerns to the charge nurse and let whatever happens happen.
- Explore hospital and other resources to determine realistic options for someone like Mrs. Peabody; consider the obligations of caregivers and the hospital.
- Find my instructor and seek their counsel.
- Seek out the unit's social worker, outline my concerns, and see if they have other recommendations.

Evaluating a Good Outcome: How Do I Define Success?

- Both Mrs. Peabody's safety and autonomy are protected.
- I feel at peace with the decision that was made for the patient and the role I played in this decision.
- My personal and professional integrity are intact.
- My legal responsibilities and those of the institution are met.

Personal Learning: Here's to the Future!

Sadly, I must confess that I was invited to accompany another patient for a diagnostic study off the unit, so I never followed through on my concerns. Mrs. Peabody was discharged to her home, and I never learned what happened to her. However, I was troubled by my inaction and discussed this situation with my instructor. As a result, I am now aware of more available options that I can use when faced with similar situations in the future. The number of older adults will continue to grow, presenting many similar challenges in the future. I want to make sure I'm prepared for my next "Mrs. Peabody." Meanwhile, I will be talking with our patient-relations person, the social worker, hospital risk manager, and our office on aging to increase my knowledge of support services for older adults.

QSEN SELF-REFLECTION ON QUALITY AND SAFETY COMPETENCIES DEVELOPING KNOWLEDGE, SKILLS, AND ATTITUDES FOR CONTINUOUS IMPROVEMENT

How do you think you would respond in a similar situation? Why? What does this tell you about yourself and about the adequacy of your skills for professional practice? Can you think of other ways to respond? What could the nursing student have done differently? What *knowledge, skills,* and *attitudes* do you need to develop to continuously improve quality and safety when caring for patients like Mrs. Peabody?

Patient-Centered Care: How might the student have interacted with the charge nurse, social worker, and other pertinent hospital personnel to promote a safe, structured home environment for Mrs. Peabody while respecting her preferences? What alternatives are available to allow this patient to remain in her home while ensuring her safety? If available options to assist Mrs. Peabody had been explored during her hospitalization, what nursing actions might be helpful as this information is shared with the patient?

Teamwork and Collaboration/Quality Improvement: What communication skills do you need to develop to facilitate your role as a patient advocate? What skills would be of particular importance when dealing with the charge nurse? What strategies might be appropriate to ensure that you function as a valued member of the health care team?

Safety/Evidence-Based Practice: How might the lack of any home care interventions affect the outcome for Mrs. Peabody? What safety measures could be enacted that would allow Mrs. Peabody the opportunity to request assistance when needed? What evidence in nursing literature provides guidance for decision making regarding patients living alone with impaired cognition?

Informatics: Can you identify essential information that must be documented in Mrs. Peabody's electronic record regarding her cardiac condition and treatment? Why is it important to document an assessment of the patient's current mental health status? Can you identify any other essential information that supports safe patient care and that should be included in the electronic record? Does the unit or hospital have a program where patients are called for follow-up? Will Mrs. Peabody follow up with her primary care provider? What documentation would be useful for these teams?

interfering with normal cell function. This manifests as a decrease in elasticity and flexibility.

The *free radical* theory is based on oxidative stress. Free radicals, formed during cellular metabolism, are molecules with unpaired, high-energy electrons that seek to combine with another molecule. This inappropriate electron pairing disrupts cell membranes and affects DNA and protein synthesis. Over time, irreversible damage results from the accumulated effects. Antioxidants are thought to protect against this type of free radical damage.

MIDDLE ADULTHOOD

The **middle adulthood** years are generally considered to be ages 40 to 65 years. This is a period of gradual, individualized changes in both physical and psychosocial dimensions. Because the average lifespan has increased, most people in this age range still consider themselves young compared with the older adult population. Visible signs of aging and a heightened awareness of the time left to live lead adults in middle adulthood to evaluate their achievement of goals, and influence their adaptation to older age.

Physiologic Development

In the early years of this period of life, physical functions are usually still effective. As time passes, gradual internal and external physiologic changes occur. These are not pathologic changes, but normal changes that result from aging. The person must modify self-image and self-concept to successfully adapt and accept these normal changes. Physical changes of the adult in middle adulthood are outlined in Box 24-1.

The hormonal changes that take place in midlife affect males and females differently. Females undergo menopause, a gradual decrease in ovarian function, with subsequent depletion of estrogen and progesterone. This change usually occurs between 40 and 55 years of age. With the cessation of ovulation, menstrual periods stop either gradually or abruptly, causing many females to experience hot flashes, mood swings, and fatigue. The loss of estrogen also increases the risk for osteoporosis and heart disease. The process can last for several years; afterward, the female can no longer become pregnant. Males do not experience physical symptoms from the decreased levels of hormones, called andropause. Androgen levels diminish slowly; males may have some loss of sexual potency, but are still capable of reproduction.

Box 24-1 Physical Changes in the Middle Adult Years

- Fatty tissue is redistributed; males tend to develop abdominal fat, females thicken through the middle.
- The skin is drier.
- Wrinkle lines appear on the face.
- Gray hair appears, and males may lose hair on the head.
- Cardiac output begins to decrease.
- Muscle mass, strength, and agility gradually decrease.
- There is a loss of calcium from bones, especially in perimenopausal females.
- Fatigue increases.
- Visual acuity diminishes, especially for near vision (presbyopia).
- Hearing acuity diminishes, especially for high-pitched sounds (presbycusis).
- Hormone production decreases, resulting in menopause or andropause.

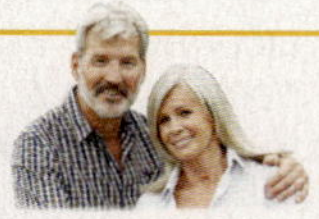

Remember **Rosemary Mason**, the 49-year-old woman described at the beginning of the chapter. The nurse could incorporate information about the differences in hormonal changes for males and females into a teaching plan to help Rosemary understand and adjust to the changes that are occurring.

Cognitive Development

Cognitive and intellectual abilities of middle-aged adults change little from young adulthood. There often is increased motivation to learn, especially if the knowledge gained can be applied immediately and has personal relevance. Problem-solving abilities remain consistent throughout adulthood, although response time may be slightly longer. This is not due to a decrease in ability, but may be related to having more memories to process or a desire to think a problem through before responding.

Psychosocial Development

The middle-aged adult years often are a time of increased personal freedom, economic stability, and deepening social relationships (Fig. 24-1). This is also a time of increased responsibility and an awareness of one's own mortality. The middle-aged adult realizes that their life may be half (or more) over and may feel many things are still undone. This realization can lead to a developmental crisis and situational stressors. Several theories regarding the developmental tasks of middle adulthood are described below.

Erikson's Theory

According to Erikson (1963), the middle-aged adult is in a period of generativity versus stagnation. The tasks are to establish and guide the next generation, accept middle-age changes, adjust to the needs of aging parents or other important people, and reevaluate goals and accomplishments. Adults who do not achieve these tasks tend to focus on themselves, becoming overly concerned with their own physical and emotional health needs.

Havighurst's Theory

The developmental tasks of the individual in middle adulthood described by Havighurst (1972) are learned behaviors arising from maturation, personal motives and values, and civic responsibility. To successfully master this developmental stage, the middle-aged adult must accept and adjust to physical changes, maintain a satisfactory occupation, assist children to become responsible adults, adjust to aging parents, and relate to their spouse or partner as a person.

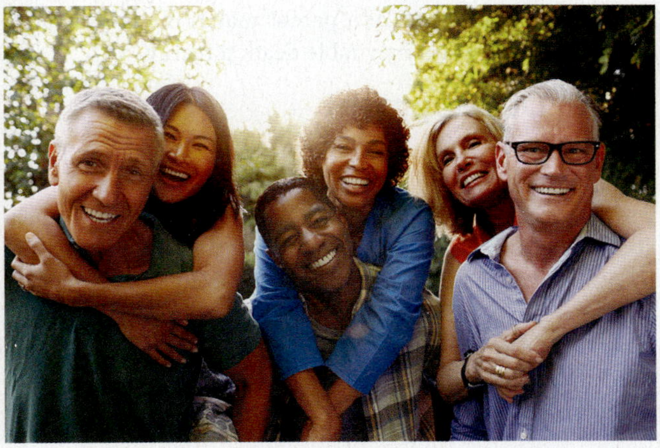

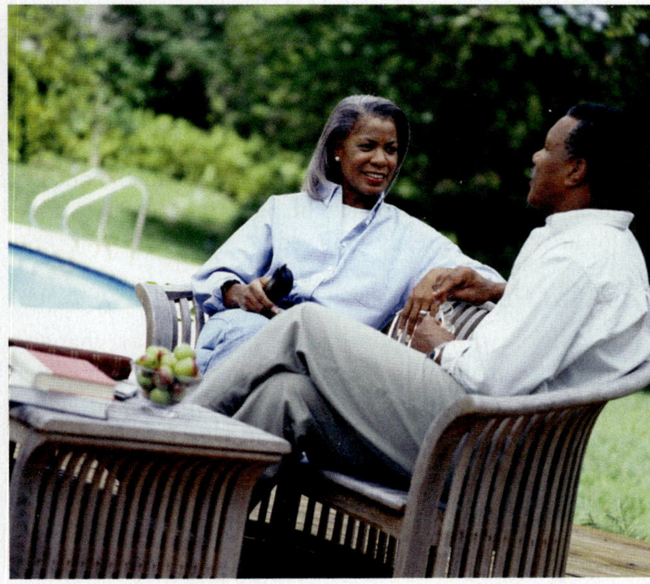

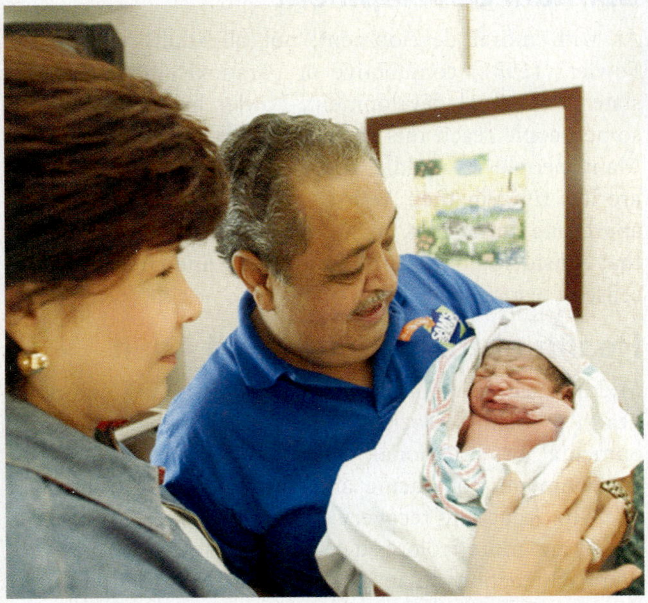

FIGURE 24-1. The middle adult years are generally characterized by expanded social relationships, renewed relationships with a spouse or partner, and expanded family roles. (*Source:* Top left: *Photo by Monkey Business Images/Shutterstock.*)

Levinson's Theory

Levinson (Levinson et al., 1978) theorized that the individual in middle adulthood may choose either to continue an established lifestyle or to reorganize their life in a period of midlife transition.

Gould's Theory

Gould (1978) viewed ages 35 to 43 years as a time when adults look inward. He considered ages 43 to 50 years as a time when adults accept their lifespan as having definite boundaries, and have a special interest in their spouse or partner, friends, and community. He viewed ages 50 to 60 years as the period when adults experience increased feelings of self-satisfaction, value the spouse or partner as a companion, and become more concerned with health.

Adjusting to the Changes of Middle Adulthood

Various changes can take place during the middle years. These include changes in employment, relationships with a spouse or partner, relationships with children who are becoming adults, and relationships with aging parents or other important people. Midlife transition may occur in people of all genders in their 40s. Although an individual may not feel that they are aging, the realization that others consider them "old" or "older" can be stressful.

Employment

Middle-aged adults may experience changes in employment. They may opt for a career change and return to school to obtain new knowledge and skills. These changes often result from a need for increased job satisfaction, satisfying a lifelong goal, or economic conditions. Some employees in this age group have lost their jobs because of company downsizing during the recent economic turmoil and have had to acquire new skills and additional education to find employment in other areas. Individuals who have been immersed in a career may decide to have children and either become stay-at-home parents or reduce their workload. Increasing numbers of middle-aged adults are self-employed, often working from home.

As the 50s approach, questions about retirement and economic security become more prevalent, with an increased interest in the benefits of financial and retirement plans. These concerns can be heightened by overall economic conditions. For example, many people who had planned on an early retirement may decide to continue their active employment status, whereas others who had planned to work longer are laid off and forced into an unplanned early retirement. The security of retirement investments and income is critical to ensure that people remain financially stable and that workers receive the pensions they are working toward or have already achieved.

Spousal Relationships

Relationships with a spouse or a partner may change. Although for many this is a time of greater security and stability with stronger emotional commitment and sharing, for some it is a time of disenchantment. Either partner may develop negative or critical feelings and attitudes as a result of changes in physical appearance, energy levels, or sexual needs and abilities. Dissatisfaction with not achieving career or family goals contributes to the stresses placed on the marriage. Extramarital affairs and divorce may result.

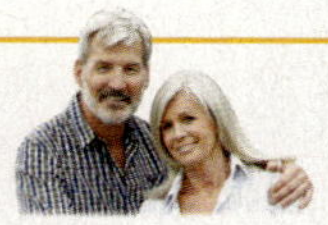

Recall **Rosemary Mason**, the 49-year-old woman, voicing displeasure with her husband's desire to "try all sorts of things" sexually. The nurse could use this information about spousal relationships to gather additional assessment data about the couple's relationship before her husband started medication to treat his erectile dysfunction. This would help develop an appropriate care plan that addresses Rosemary's current displeasure.

Loss of a spouse or a partner is more likely in middle adulthood. The loss is a major crisis and a threat to a person's self-concept, and may result in a major role change. Many changes may occur, including a reduced income, changes in lifestyle and social relationships, and the need for help to work through the loss and grief (see Chapter 44).

Relationships With Children and Aging Family Members

Middle-aged adults may be caught in a *generation sandwich*. Their children may be independent and married, with children of their own, or may be recent college graduates who have returned home to live. Difficulty finding employment coupled with the burden of student loans often necessitates the postponement of independent living. Providing ongoing support for adult children while simultaneously caring for aging family presents a unique set of financial, logistical, resource, and emotional stressors for middle-aged adults.

Although much has been written about the *empty-nest syndrome* that occurs when the last child leaves home, most middle-aged parents welcome the increased space, time, and independence they have when active parenting ceases. However, as their involvement with and responsibility for children decrease, middle-aged adults may be called upon to help care for aging parents and other family members. The physical aging or death of a parent makes the middle-aged adult's own aging and inevitable death a reality.

Moral Development

According to Kohlberg (1969), a middle-aged adult may either remain at the conventional level or move to the postconventional level of moral development. The person who has had sustained responsibility for the welfare of others and has consistently applied ethical principles developed in adolescence is more likely to move to the postconventional level. At this level, the adult believes that the rights of others take precedence, and takes steps to support those rights.

Spiritual Development

As with moral development, not all adults progress to Fowler's (1981) conjunctive or paradoxical–consolidative state of spiritual development. Fowler believed that only some people reach this stage, and only after age 30 years. Many people in middle adulthood who reach this stage are less rigid in their beliefs, recognize paradoxes in life, appreciate symbolism, engage in mutual perspective-taking that considers norms and implicit bias, and consider a new sense of justice.

Health of the Middle-Aged Adult

Middle-aged adults are subject to physical and emotional health problems associated with lifestyle behaviors, developmental or situational crises, family history, and the environment. Both acute and chronic illnesses are more likely to occur, and recovery takes longer. This is a result of slower and more prolonged responses to stressors, more pronounced reactions to an illness, and the possibility of more than one illness being present at a time.

The leading causes of death in the middle adult years (ages 45 to 64 years), according to 2019 statistics, are malignant neoplasms; cardiovascular/heart disease; unintentional injury, including poisoning, motor vehicle accidents, and falls; suicide; chronic lower respiratory disease; liver disease; diabetes mellitus; cerebrovascular causes; nephritis (kidney disease); and septicemia (infection; Centers for Disease Control and Prevention [CDC], 2021d). Other major health problems include rheumatoid arthritis, obesity, alcoholism, and depression.

The risk for these common health problems often depends on a combination of lifestyle factors and aging. As individuals get older, energy requirements decrease. Middle-aged adults tend to maintain previous eating patterns and caloric intake while being less physically active. This trend can result in obesity and atherosclerosis, with an increased risk for high blood pressure, coronary artery disease, renal failure, and diabetes. Additionally, smoking and alcohol consumption put the person at greater risk for cancer, chronic respiratory diseases, and liver disease.

Chronic illness in middle-aged adults has a major effect on self-concept and may precipitate changes in life structure. For example, after a serious heart attack, a person may face changes in family role, earning capacity, and social relationships. Such changes usually cause great stress.

Middle age does not automatically result in physical or emotional health problems. Many people remain healthy throughout their lives, but knowing preventive health care practices and their special needs at this age can help middle-aged adults have improved quality and quantity of life. In fact, many adults cultivate new eating and exercise habits when they personally experience the metabolic and functional changes associated with aging.

Role of the Nurse in Promoting Health and Preventing Illness

The nurse has a major role in promoting health and preventing illness in middle-aged adults by teaching, serving as a role model, and encouraging self-care responsibilities. See the accompanying display, Examples of Actual or Potential Health Problems and Needs: Middle Adulthood.

Health-related screenings, examinations, and immunizations for adults are outlined in Box 24-2 on page 636. Additionally, the following health promotion activities are recommended:

- Eat a diet low in fat and cholesterol, including fruits, vegetables, and fiber; use sugar, salt, and sodium in moderation.
- Make regular exercise a part of life.
- Drink alcohol in moderation, if at all.
- Do not smoke.

The middle-aged adult needs to know the dangers of substance use disorders and the potential sequelae. Alcohol consumption and binge drinking increased in adults in the United States during the COVID-19 pandemic due to heightened stress and boredom (Gorssman et al., 2020; Pollard et al., 2020; Weerakoon et al., 2021)—the long-term consequences of this are yet to be determined. Referrals to support groups and individual counseling may be necessary to strengthen a middle-aged adult's coping mechanisms and promote acceptance of personal and family changes. Having successfully met developmental tasks, the healthy middle-aged adult is ready to enjoy the rest of life. A sense of continuity and adaptability from the early 20s through the 50s is essential for a person to meet the developmental tasks of aging satisfactorily and to enjoy all remaining years.

OLDER ADULTHOOD

Society has arbitrarily labeled a person older than age 65 years as an **older adult**. To account for the diversity that exists among different age groups, the older adulthood is often further divided into the three age classifications: youngest-old (ages 65 to 74 years), middle-old (ages 75 to 84 years), and oldest-old (ages 85 years and older; Eliopoulos, 2022).

American society is aging—dramatically, rapidly, and largely well. With birthrates down and some baby boomers already reaching retirement age, we can estimate that 16.5% of the population is age 65 years or older (Unites States Census Bureau, 2021). In 2021, life expectancy projections for men who reach age 65 increased to age 83.2 and for women who reach age 65 to age 85.8 (CDC, 2021e). Health disparities become magnified in the older adult population. Race, ethnicity, immigration, sex and gender identification, physical and mental disabilities, and economic status all affect access to health care and health outcomes (He et al., 2016). Dwyer-Lindgren et al. (2017) analyzed data from 1980 to 2014 and identified three major sets of factors that explain

Examples of Actual or Potential Health Problems and Needs

MIDDLE ADULTHOOD

Actual or Potential Health Problem or Need	Possible Etiologic Factors	Potential Signs and Symptoms
Caregiver Fatigue	• Unrealistic expectations of themselves in the caregiver role • Competing role commitments—sandwich generation • Lack of caregiving experience • Insufficient coping strategies and resilience • Insufficient knowledge of individual, familial, or community resources	• Verbalizations of uncertainty, fatigue, and concern about the care of the person for whom they provide care • Physical manifestations such as yawning, GI upset, inattention, or excessive sleepiness • Decrease in professional productivity • Unwanted changes in physical, psychological, social, emotional, or spiritual self-care activities
Readiness for Positive Family Process	—	• Verbalizations related to family processing—establishing individuality and boundary-setting, while maintaining family connectedness • Adapting to an empty nest—recognition of positives and negatives • Engagement in activities that enhance family resilience • Establishment of adult relationships with children

Source: International Council of Nurses (ICN). (2019). *Nursing diagnosis and outcome statements.* https://www.icn.ch/sites/default/files/inline-files/ICNP2019-DC.pdf; Wolters Kluwer. (2022). Problem-based care plans. In *Lippincott Advisor.* Wolters Kluwer. https://advisor.lww.com/lna/home.do

Box 24-2 Guidelines for Health-Related Screenings, Examinations, and Immunizations for the Aging Adult

Physical Examination
- Every 3 years until age 40 years
- Every year after age 40 years

Breast Cancer Screening (for Average-Risk People With Female Anatomy)
- There is an emphasis on knowing your own breasts and reporting any changes.
- Mammography screening may be offered beginning at age 40 years but should be initiated every year beginning at age 45 years (American Cancer Society [ACS], 2021) or age 50 years (American College of Obstetricians and Gynecologists [ACOG], 2017/2021); those ages 55 years and older can switch to mammograms every 2 years (ACS, 2021); mammograms should continue through age 75 years (ACOG, 2017/2021).

Cervical Cancer Screening (Females, Beginning at Age 21 Years)
- Females should have a pelvic examination with Papanicolaou (Pap) exam every 3 years for ages 21 to 29 years, and every 5 years for ages 30 to 65 years.
- Females who have had a total hysterectomy (removal of the uterus and cervix) do not need cervical cancer screening, unless the surgery was for cervical precancer or cancer.
- Females over age 65 years with no abnormal Pap tests in the last 10 years should consult with their health care provider about continuing cervical cancer screening.

Prostate Exam (Males, Beginning Age 50 Years)
- The prostate-specific antigen (PSA) test should be discussed with the provider; recommend this conversation at age 45 years if the patient is African American or has a family history of prostate cancer.
- Digital rectal examination (DRE) should take place every year.
- Screening is individualized based on health care provider and the person's concerns.

Testicular Cancer Screening (Males)
- There is an emphasis on knowing the testicles and reporting any changes.
- Testicular clinical examination is part of the general physical exam.

Colorectal Cancer Testing (Beginning Age 45 Years)
- Fecal occult blood test should be done every year.
- Digital rectal examination (DRE) should be done every year.
- Flexible sigmoidoscopy should be done every 5 years, *or*
- Colonoscopy every 10 years, *or*
- Double contrast barium enema every 5 years, *or*
- CT colonography (virtual colonoscopy) every 5 years.
- For people **ages 76 through 85 years**, talk with your health care provider about whether continuing to get screened is right for you.
- People **older than age 85 years** should no longer get colorectal cancer screening.

Skin Cancer Exam
- Self-examination should be done every month.
- Clinical skin examination is part of the general physical exam.

Oral Cancer Exam
- Every year as part of medical or dental checkups

Bone Density Testing
- Menopausal and postmenopausal females younger than age 65 years with risk factors, or older than age 65 years
- Males aged 50 to 69 years with risk factors, or older than age 70 years
- Fracture after age 50 years
- Height loss

Vision Exam
- Eye examination, with a test for glaucoma, should be done every 1 to 2 years.

Immunizations (Healthy Adults)
- *Tdap or Td:* Administer one dose Tdap, then Td booster every 10 years.
- *MMR vaccine:* Administer one dose of MMR to adults who previously received ≤2 doses of mumps-containing vaccine and are identified by a public health authority to be at increased risk during a mumps outbreak.
- *Influenza:* Administer one dose every year.
- *Pneumococcal vaccine:* Administer one dose of PCV13 (13-valent pneumococcal conjugate vaccine) for adults ages 65 years and older if not previously received, followed by one dose of PPSV23 (23-valent pneumococcal polysaccharide vaccine) 1 year after dose of PCV13. For adults with certain medical conditions who received a dose of PPSV23 at ages 19 to 64 years, administer a second dose of PPSV23 at age 65 years, followed by a dose of PCV13 1 year later (if not previously received).
- *Zoster Vaccine Live (ZVL) or Recombinant Zoster Vaccine (RZV):* Administer two doses of RZV (Shingrix) 2 to 6 months apart to adults ages 50 years and older regardless of past episode of herpes zoster or receipt of ZVL (Zostavax). Administer two doses of RZV 2 to 6 months apart to adults who previously received ZVL at least 2 months after ZVL. For adults ages 60 years and older, administer either RZV or ZVL (RZV is preferred).

Source: Data from American Cancer Society (ACS). (2021). *Cancer screening guidelines by age.* https://www.cancer.org/healthy/find-cancer-early/screening-recommendations-by-age.html#All_ages; American Cancer Society (ACS). (2021). *American Cancer Society guideline for colorectal cancer screening for people at average risk.* https://www.cancer.org/cancer/colon-rectal-cancer/detection-diagnosis-staging/acs-recommendations.html; The American College of Obstetricians and Gynecologists (ACOG). (2017/2021). Breast cancer risk assessment in average-risk women. Practice Bulletin No. 179. *Obstetrics & Gynecology, 130,* e1–e16. https://www.acog.org/clinical/clinical-guidance/practice-bulletin/articles/2017/07/breast-cancer-risk-assessment-and-screening-in-average-risk-women; Centers for Disease Control and Prevention [CDC]. (2021c). *Recommended immunization schedules for adults by age.* https://www.cdc.gov/vaccines/schedules/hcp/adult.html; and National Osteoporosis Foundation. (2021). *Bone density exam/testing.* https://www.nof.org/patients/diagnosis-information/bone-density-examtesting

74% of the variation in life expectancy at the county level across the United States:

- *Socioeconomic and race/ethnicity factors:* 60% of variation explained by income, population below poverty level, graduation from high school/college, unemployment rate, and race/ethnicity
- *Behavioral and metabolic risk factors:* 74% of variation explained by hypertension, diabetes, obesity, smoking, and physical activity level
- *Health care factors:* 27% of variation explained by number of available health care providers in the area, quality of services, and insurance

Boing et al. (2020) found that more than three fourths of the total variation in life expectancy can be attributed to county of residence in the United States, and that race, education, and income were particularly relevant to explaining the variations in life expectancy. Between 2009 and 2019, the population of older adults (ages 65 and older) in the United States increased from 39.6 million to 54.1 million (16% of the population) and is projected to reach 94.7 million in 2060. Ethnic and racial minority older-adult populations have increased from 7.8 million (20% of older adults) to 12.9 million (24% of older adults), with 2040 projections at 27.7 million (34% of older adults). Although only 8.9% of older adults live below the poverty line, which is a dramatic change from 30% in 1966, economic disparities exist: 18% of Black older adults, 17.1% of Hispanic older adults, 9.3% of Asian older adults, and 6.8% of non-Hispanic White older adults live in poverty (Administration for Community Living, 2021). These numbers directly reflect the need to consider resource allocation as well as policies and programs to assist our aging population.

Unique Population

The older adult population is the most unique group in society today. They have lived the longest and have participated in and adapted to complex societal changes. Older adults have witnessed the development of society from a predominately rural agricultural culture, through industrialization, to a service-oriented, high-technology culture. Technology's influence in the past 50 years in household management, travel logistics, media access, and social connections has changed the way we live our lives. Information that once took weeks or months to be received now is available instantaneously. In fact, most older adults have had some exposure to personal computers and hand-held communication devices, and many are technologically savvy. Most older adults have lived through the trauma of world wars. Many had parents with strong ethnic ties to another country, and many were immigrants themselves. Older adults have lived through the repercussions of and rebuilding after the Great Depression of the 1930s and several recessions. Antiwar movements and experiences in the Vietnam war, Desert Storm, Desert Shield, and other conflicts impact their current views of war and terrorism. The civil rights movement of the 1960s and 1970s shaped their views of race, inequalities, and activism. Although their political affiliation varies, they represent the largest block of voters—52% of registered voters are ages 50 years and older and 24% are ages 65 years and older (Pew Research Center, 2020).

Further adaptations become necessary with advancing age because of physical or cognitive limitations, retirement, loss of a spouse or family members, or changing income. Older adults face numerous role changes related to their age or health status. Lost roles must be replaced with new roles and activities that are acceptable and satisfying to the person.

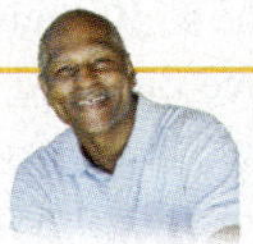

Recall **Larry Jenkins**, the 67-year-old lamenting that his life has been going "downhill" since he retired. The nurse could incorporate knowledge of role changes to develop an appropriate plan of care for the patient that fosters adjustment to his role changes.

Older people are living in a world that requires them to change and to adapt. Senior years are a time for people to reach their potential and to satisfy long-range goals that may have been delayed because of other responsibilities. It can also be a time for older adults to turn over to others certain tasks, such as career or community leadership. Because of recent economic challenges, some older adults have chosen to remain in the work force out of necessity, while others enjoy the socialization and intellectual stimulation that employment provides. Research has shown that most older adults do adjust and adapt to new roles, and most are satisfied with their lives and with what they have. Depending on the older adult's adaptability and supportive resources, older adulthood may be a time of happiness, peace, and understanding or of sorrow, conflict, and confusion.

Personal relationships evolve as people age. Increased mobility of families, multiple external influences, time drains on young families, and technologic advances can weaken intergenerational ties. Establishing new ways to communicate and engage among generations such as texting or social media can help fill this void.

Technology Alert

Adults learn best when the material being taught is relevant to their daily lives and is deemed important in the moment. Using technology to teach technology works to solidify learning and reinforce basic skills, so that more complex skills can be developed. Techboomers.com is a free educational website that serves older adults. Its purpose is to teach "older adults and other inexperienced Internet users . . . basic computer skills about websites that can help improve their quality of life" (Techboomers, 2018, "Who Are We"). Integrating these types of resources into health promotion activities can have a positive impact on the lives of older adults.

Ageism and Common Stereotypes

Sometimes, an older adult is the victim of ageism. **Ageism** is a form of prejudice, like racism or sexism, in which older adults are stereotyped and discriminated against. Fundamental to ageism is the view that older people are incapable and do not experience the same desires, needs, and concerns as younger adults. Although the process of aging is associated with some normal changes, not all people age at the same rate, and potential functional declines vary in type (e.g., cognitive or physical) and degree. Our industrial technologic world places a high priority on productivity, and some may think that older employees or retired people have outlived their usefulness. It is important to remember that older people are delaying retirement. In 2018, 24% of men and about 16% of women ages 65 years and older were in the labor force, and these numbers are expected to rise (Mather et al., 2019). Making assumptions simply based on a person's age is an example of implicit bias that can lead to discriminatory practices.

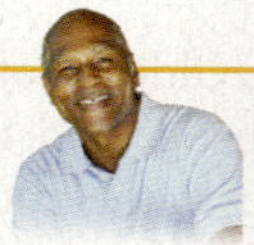

Think back to **Larry Jenkins**, the 67-year-old retiree. The nurse could incorporate knowledge of ageism as a basis for obtaining additional assessment data, examining possible factors contributing to the patient's feelings of boredom and uselessness.

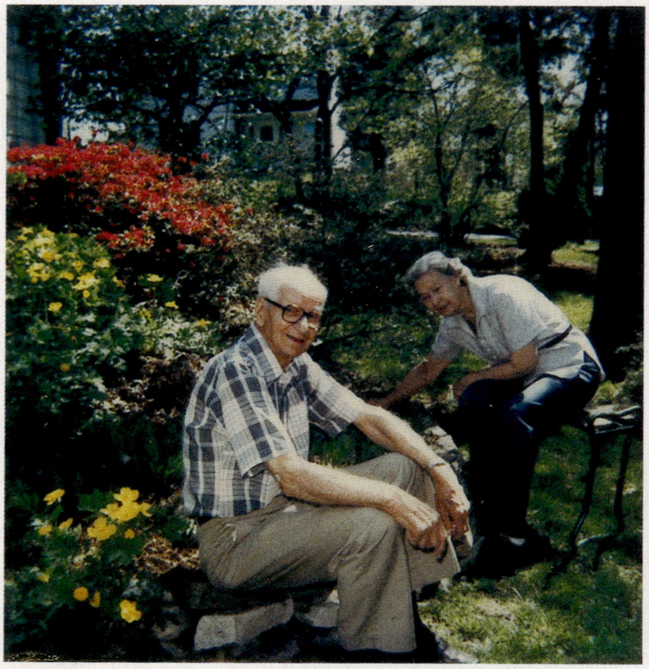

FIGURE 24-2. This couple, married 61 years, enjoys gardening together. They've found that they can continue most activities with only minor adjustments.

Older people may be incorrectly viewed as being rigid or narrow-minded, unable to learn, unreliable because of memory loss, too old to enjoy sexual pleasure, or childlike and dependent. Many people fear advancing age because of pervasive views that older people are living in poverty, lonely, in frail health, and headed for institutionalization in a long-term care facility. These descriptors are not true for most older adults (Fig. 24-2). Common myths about older adults are compared with the realities in Table 24-1.

Table 24-1 Myths and Realities About Older Adults

MYTH	REALITY
Old age begins at age 65 years.	Defining 65 years old as *old age* happened arbitrarily when age 65 years was set for Social Security payments in the 1930s, based on the labor market and the economy of that time.
Most older adults live in long-term care facilities.	Although the largest percentage of residents in long-term care facilities are older adults, many of whom have disabilities, only 1% of older adults ages 65–74 years, 2% of older adults ages 75–84 years, and 8% of adults older than age 85 years live in long-term care facilities (Administration for Community Living, 2021).
Most older adults are sick.	81% of older adults ages 65 to 74 years and 68% of older adults older than age 85 years rate their health *good*, *very good*, or *excellent* (Federal Interagency Forum on Aging-Related Statistics, 2020).
Old age means mental deterioration.	Although response time may be prolonged due to a longer processing time, neither intelligence nor personality normally change because of aging.
Older adults are not interested in sex.	Although sexual activity may be less frequent, the ability to perform and enjoy sexual activity lasts well into the 90s in healthy older adults.
Older adults do not care how they look.	Older adults want to be attractive to others.
Most older adults are isolated and lonely.	Loneliness results from death of loved ones or other losses, just as it does for people of all ages. Many older adults participate in social and community activities.
Bladder problems are a problem of aging.	Incontinence is not a part of aging; it generally has a root cause and requires medical attention.
Older adults do not deserve aggressive treatment for serious illnesses.	Older adults deserve aggressive treatment if they want it.
Older adults cannot learn new things.	Many older adults today are more educated than previous generations, and have had to adapt to technologic advances; they continue to use technology into old age.

Box 24-3 Normal Physiologic Changes of Older Adults

General Status

- Progressively decreasing efficiency of physiologic processes results in a fragile balance and hinders the body's ability to maintain homeostasis.
- Physical or emotional stressors cause the older adult to be more vulnerable because of decreased physiologic reserves.
- The older adult may continue to engage in all activities of middle age but intuitively adjusts to a modified pace and more frequent rest periods.

Integumentary System

- Wrinkling and sagging of skin occur with decreased skin elasticity; dryness and scaling are common.
- Balding becomes common in males, and females also experience thinning of hair; hair loses pigmentation.
- Skin pigmentation and moles are common, although the skin may become pale because of loss of melanocytes.
- Nails typically thicken, becoming brittle and yellowed.
- The blood vessels in the dermis become more fragile, causing increased bruising and purpura (hemorrhaging into the skin).

Musculoskeletal System

- Decreases in subcutaneous tissue and weight commonly are found in the oldest-old.
- Muscle mass and strength decrease.
- Bone demineralization occurs; bones become porous and brittle. Fracture is more common.
- Joints tend to stiffen and lose flexibility, and range of motion may decrease.
- Overall mobility commonly slows, and posture tends to stoop. Height may decrease 1 to 3 inches.

Neurologic System

- The central nervous system responds more slowly to multiple stimuli. Hence, the cognitive and behavioral response of the older adult may be delayed.
- Rate of reflex response decreases.
- Temperature regulation and pain/pressure perception become less efficient.
- There may be a loss of sensation in the extremities.
- The older adult may also experience difficulty with balance, coordination, fine movements, and spatial orientation, resulting in an increased risk for falls.
- Sleep at night typically shortens, and the older adult may awaken more easily. Catnaps become common.

Special Senses

- Diminished visual acuity (presbyopia) occurs, with increased sensitivity to glare, decreased ability to adjust to darkness, decreased accommodation, decreased depth perception, and decreased color discrimination. Cataracts may further obscure vision. As a result of these changes, the older adult may have difficulty reading small print, and daytime or night driving may be compromised.
- Diminished hearing acuity (presbycusis) occurs, particularly diminished pitch discrimination in the presence of environmental noises. Cerumen (wax) buildup is common. As a result of hearing problems or amplification issues with hearing aids, the older adult may withdraw from social events.
- The senses of taste and smell are decreased. Sweet and salty tastes diminish first. Sensitivity to odors may be reduced. Problems with nutrition may result.

Cardiopulmonary System

- Blood vessels become less elastic and often rigid and tortuous. Venous return becomes less efficient. Fatty plaque deposits continue to occur in the linings of the blood vessels. Lower-extremity edema and cooling may occur, particularly with decreased mobility. Peripheral pulses are not always palpable. Orthostatic hypotension can occur.
- The body is less able to increase heart rate and cardiac output with activity.
- Pulmonary elasticity and ciliary action decrease, so that clearing of the lungs becomes less efficient. Respiratory rate may increase, accompanied by diminished depth.

Gastrointestinal System

- Digestive juices continue to diminish, and nutrient absorption decreases.
- Malnutrition and anemia become more common.
- With reduced muscle tone and decreased peristalsis, constipation and indigestion are common complaints.
- Diminished saliva production leads to dry mouth problems.

Dentition

- Tooth decay and loss continue for most older adults.
- Eating habits may change, particularly if the older adult lacks teeth or has ill-fitting dentures.

Genitourinary System

- Blood flow to the kidneys decreases with diminished cardiac output.
- The number of functioning nephron units decreases by 50%; waste products may be filtered and excreted more slowly.
- Fluids and electrolytes remain within normal ranges, but the balance is fragile.
- Bladder capacity decreases by 50%. Voiding becomes more frequent; two or three times a night is usual (nocturia). A decrease in bladder and sphincter muscle control may result in stress incontinence or incomplete bladder emptying (overflow incontinence).
- About 75% of males over 65 years of age experience benign (not cancerous) hypertrophy of the prostate gland (BPH); surgery may be required if urinary retention occurs.
- The older female's genital tract atrophies and is associated with thinning and a decrease in vaginal secretions.

Physiologic Development

In older adults, all organ systems undergo some degree of decline in overall functioning, and the body becomes less efficient. Normal physiologic changes in structure and function of the body with aging are outlined in Box 24-3. Body functions that require integrated activity of several organ systems are affected the most. For example, aging of the cardiac muscles causes fluid retention in both peripheral tissues and the lungs, causing swelling of the legs and making breathing more difficult. The most commonly encountered chronic disorders are hypertension, arthritis, heart disease, cancer, diabetes, respiratory disorders (chronic obstructive pulmonary disease and asthma), and stroke (CDC, 2021e; Federal Interagency Forum on Aging-Related Statistics, 2020).

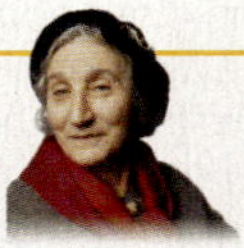

Recall **Ethel Peabody**, the 88-year-old woman with dementia and cardiac problems. Knowledge of physiologic changes associated with aging could help with developing an appropriate plan of care for this patient after discharge.

Most older adults regard themselves as healthy. In fact, 81% of older adults ages 65 to 74 years and 68% of older adults older than age 85 years rate their health *good*, *very good*, or *excellent* (Federal Interagency Forum on Aging-Related Statistics, 2020). There is growing evidence that aging is not synonymous with disability and loss of function. Like younger adults, older adults define their health in relation to how well they function. Functional health includes the ability to remain self-reliant, to compensate, and to maintain a sense of independence and control over self and environment.

There is a trend in health care today toward fostering increasing independence and self-care in older adults. Those who live alone are at greatest risk for loss of independence and increased need for assisted living or long-term care. Most older adults are never institutionalized, nor do they experience the effects of senility. Being healthy, however, does not necessarily mean living without disease. Most older adults have at least one chronic disorder and typically have at least two (Eliopoulos, 2022); their ability to adapt determines whether they are ill or healthy. Most older adults continue their activities from middle age and adapt intuitively to the gradual limitations of aging; it may take longer to complete an activity, or the activity may need to be modified. For example, an older adult with arthritis may need to use an electric can opener rather than a manual one, or a person with heart disease may need 3 hours to garden, resting several times, rather than the 1-hour gardening used to require.

Concept Mastery Alert

As people age, their ability to adapt, not the time it takes for them to adapt, is the key determinant for whether they will be ill or healthy.

Sarcopenia is the loss of muscle mass that frequently occurs in older adults as part of the natural aging process. The clinical definition of sarcopenia has been expanded to include a decrease in muscle mass that is assessed by handgrip strength, and a decrease in physical function that is assessed by gait speed (Eliopoulos, 2022). *Sarcopenic obesity* describes the muscle loss combined with obesity (an increase in body fat) as people age (Lee et al., 2016). This condition can result in loss of strength and function and a reduced quality of life that is significant for older adults. Since sarcopenia is mostly seen in inactive older adults, exercise that includes resistance training and adequate dietary protein are management strategies that can prevent or reverse this process.

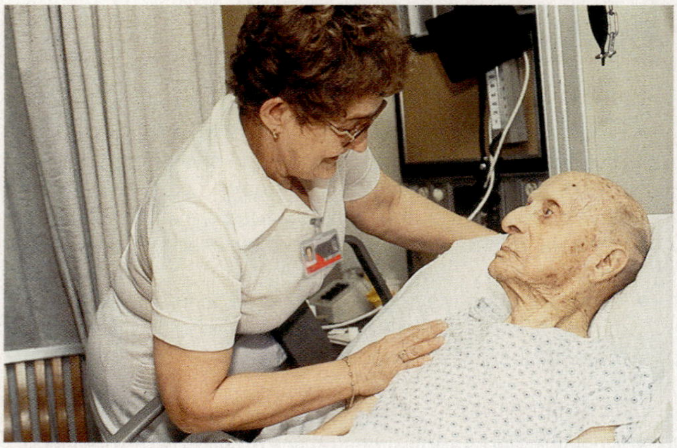

FIGURE 24-3. The hospitalized older adult requires nursing interventions to prevent complications. (*Source:* Used with permission from Shutterstock. *Photo by Kathy Sloane.*)

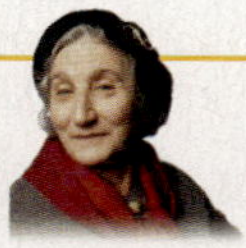

Remember **Ethel Peabody**, the woman described in the Reflective Practice box on page 631. The nurse can apply knowledge about functional health to determine the patient's needs for safety and independence while, at the same time, fostering a positive self-image.

The greatest threat to the health of older adults is loss of the physiologic reserve of the various organ systems. When illness occurs, increased physical and emotional stress places an older adult at risk for complex reactions. An older adult is more likely to develop complications and to recover more slowly (Fig. 24-3). For instance, an older adult with a hip fracture is at high risk for pneumonia and skin breakdown because of immobility, a decreased ability to mobilize pulmonary secretions, and thinner, more fragile skin.

Unfolding Patient Stories: Josephine Morrow • Part 1

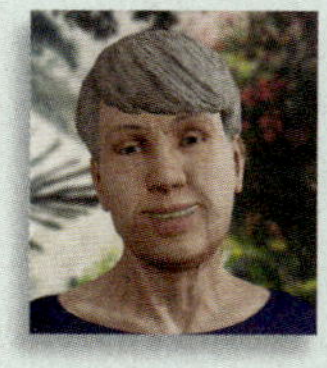

Josephine Morrow is 80 years old and developed a venous stasis ulcer on her lower extremity as a community-dwelling older adult. She recently moved to a skilled nursing home. What are normal physiologic changes the nurse should consider when caring for older adults? How can the nurse help Josephine adjust to long-term care and her loss of independence? (Josephine Morrow's story continues in Chapter 28.)

Care for Josephine and other patients in a realistic virtual environment: ***vSim** for Nursing* (thepoint.lww.com/vSimFunds). Practice documenting these patients' care in DocuCare (thepoint.lww.com/DocuCareEHR).

Cognitive Development

The term *cognition* indicates cerebral functioning, including a person's ability to perceive and understand their world.

Cognition does not change appreciably with aging. In fact, intelligence increases into the 60s, and learning continues throughout life. It is normal for an older adult to take longer to respond and react, particularly in new or unfamiliar surroundings. Knowing this, the nurse should slow the pace of care and allow older adults extra time to ask questions or complete activities. Mild short-term (recent) memory loss is common but can be remedied by an older adult using notes, schedules, and calendars. Long-term memory usually remains intact. Dementia, Alzheimer's disease (AD), depression, and delirium may occur and cause cognitive impairment. These conditions are discussed later in relation to the health of the older adult.

Psychosocial Development

Most theorists agree that a person's self-concept is relatively stable throughout adult life. An older adult who has a strong sense of self-identity and has successfully met challenges earlier in life will probably continue to do so. This person substitutes new roles for old roles and perhaps continues former roles in a new context. For example, business managers after retirement may continue to use their leadership talents in community or volunteer organizations. Older adults with a strong self-concept typically describe themselves as being healthier than others or "young for my years." Maslow, in his hierarchy of human needs, describes the level of self-actualization as the desire to become the most that one can be. A self-actualized person has realistic perceptions of self, is a problem solver, is usually spontaneous, needs time to focus on their individual potential, and views the world with a sense of appreciation. On the other hand, events that may accompany aging can threaten a person's self-concept. Depending on the person's outlook on life and past ability to cope, events such as retirement, loss of health or income, loss of ability to operate a motor vehicle, and isolation can be devastating. For example, a retired teacher whose sense of identity was closely tied to career may suddenly be in the position of having lost friends, income, and sense of accomplishment, and may consequently feel a loss of control and self-identity.

The loss of the privilege of driving has serious repercussions for older adults. Aging results in slower reaction times and changes in vision, such as increased sensitivity to the glare from approaching headlights as well as alterations in peripheral vision. Certain adjustments can prolong an older adult's ability to drive safely. These include driving only during daylight hours and avoiding travel at stressful times such as morning and evening rush hours. Keeping a safe distance from the car ahead and a watchful eye on unsafe weather conditions are also helpful.

When it becomes obvious for safety reasons that an older driver should stop driving altogether, it is best if family members address their concerns with the older adult in an honest, forthright manner. The U.S. Department of Transportation is an additional resource; state branches may request that an older driver be retested based on identification of a concern from a health care provider, a police or accident report, or written expressed concern from a family member. As the number of older drivers increases, so do the challenges to promote safe driving and find alternatives to driving (National Highway Traffic Safety Administration, n.d.).

Losing driving privileges is disheartening and can cause older adults to feel anxious and lonely, which may be viewed as another negative consequence of aging. This lack of independence may also result in less opportunity for activities or interactions with friends and family. The availability of alternative means of transportation should be explored. Some older adults take advantage of transportation services through their communities, or use ridesharing services such as Lyft or Uber.

Disengagement Theory

An early psychosocial theory, called the *disengagement theory*, maintained that older adults often withdraw from usual roles and become more introspective and self-focused. This withdrawal was theorized as intrinsic and inevitable, necessary for successful aging, and beneficial for both the person and for society.

Later studies showed that isolation is not desired or acceptable, and that as societal interactions decrease, healthy older adults increase their close relationships with family and friends. According to the *activity theory*, successful aging includes the ability to maintain high levels of activity and functioning. An older adult may substitute activities, but does not slow down or disengage from society. The *continuity theory* assumes that healthy aging is related to the older adult's ability to continue similar patterns of behavior from young and middle adulthood (Eliopoulos, 2022; Miller, 2019).

Erikson's Theory

Erikson (1963) identified ego integrity versus despair and disgust as the last stage of human development, which begins at about age 60 years. Older adults continue to look forward, but now also look back and begin to reflect on their lives. It is a time for realization of a *wholeness* perspective, with an inner search for meaning and order in the life cycle. Older adults search for emotional integration and acceptance of the past and present, as well as acceptance of physiologic decline without fear of death.

Older adults often like to tell stories of past events. This phenomenon, called **life review** or **reminiscence**, has been identified worldwide. Reminiscence is a way for older adults to relive and restructure life experiences, often in relation to their current situation, and with the added benefit of the perspective provided by life experience and wisdom. Although reminiscence therapy is often used in patients with mild to moderate dementia, reminiscence has value for older adults who do not have cognitive or memory impairments (Fig. 24-4 on page 642). Nurses use reminiscence therapy to encourage reflection and facilitate adaptation to present circumstances.

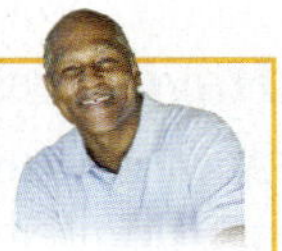

Think back to ***Larry Jenkins***, the 67-year-old man described at the beginning of the chapter. The nurse could use life review to foster Mr. Jenkins' ego integrity.

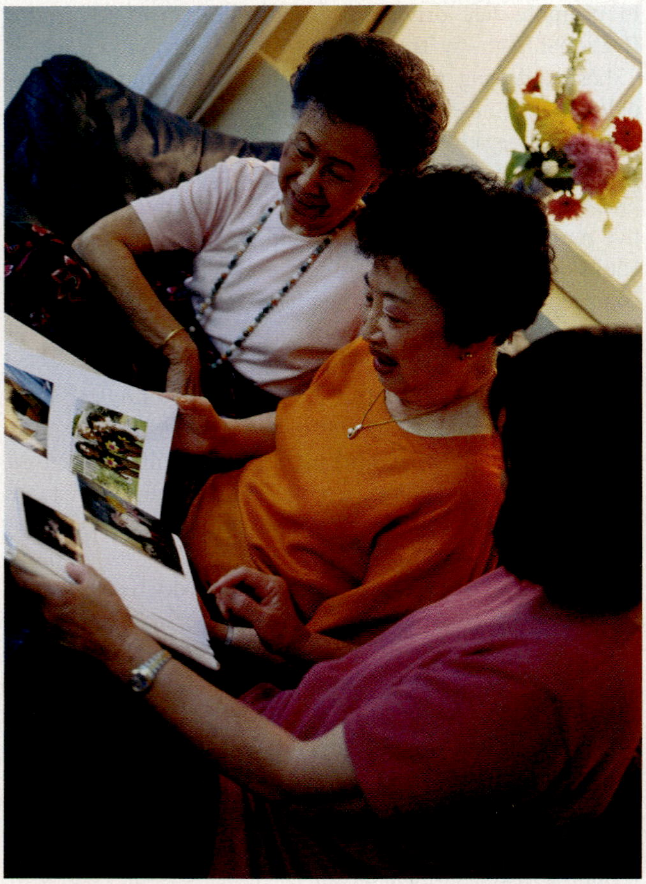

FIGURE 24-4. Reminiscing is a culturally universal phenomenon of aging. It is a way for the older adult to reassess life experiences and further develop a sense of accomplishment, fulfillment, and reward in life.

Ego integrity is facilitated when an older adult has successfully accomplished tasks that were identified earlier in life. Older adulthood can be a time for the person to look backward with pride and without regrets, and to look forward with optimism and enthusiasm. A person who regrets the past and sees current problems as insurmountable may despair. This person may view life as a series of unresolved problems and missed opportunities, and feel worthless or hopeless. A person in despair may want to do things over but fears the lack of time before death.

The tasks of midlife continue or may resurface. Older adults still strive to guide the coming generations and to leave something behind (generativity vs. stagnation). Their need for love and closeness continues (intimacy vs. isolation), as does a strong sense of who they are in relation to family and community (identity vs. role confusion). Because of physical and social changes associated with aging, older adults are repeatedly faced with the need to adapt and to repeat already completed tasks.

Havighurst's Theory

According to Havighurst (1972), the major tasks of old age are primarily concerned with the maintenance of social contacts and relationships. Successful aging depends on a person's ability to be flexible and adapt to new age-related roles. The person must find new and meaningful roles in old age while being reasonably comfortable with the social customs of the times.

Adjusting to the Changes of Older Adulthood

Older adults use their years of experience as a guide for adjusting to the changes that come with increasing age. These changes, based on Havighurst's tasks for later life, involve many areas of life, as described in the following sections.

Physical Strength and Health

Most older adults gradually modify their lifestyle to accommodate for declining strength and health. They rest more frequently, although continued activity and exercise are important for maintaining all physiologic functions. Diet modifications and prescribed medications may be necessary. Sleep disorders may develop, especially in women as they age (Sivertsen et al., 2021), and may contribute to daytime sleepiness, a slower response time, impaired memory, and behavior that may be mistaken for some form of cognitive impairment. Confusion and cognitive impairment in an older adult are not normal consequences of aging. An alteration in cognition or mental status that is new should be considered an acute problem and considered in relation to infection, polypharmacy, or other factors (Fitzgerald et al., 2017). An older adult is at high risk for accidents and falls and may need to curtail driving or use a cane or other aid to remain mobile.

Because of chronic illness, an older adult may need to adjust to living with some pain. Pain should not be assumed to be a normal consequence of aging, but it is often experienced by older adults and frequently is undertreated. Attitudes toward treating pain in this population may interfere with optimum pain relief. Providers and patients need to collaborate to differentiate mild chronic discomfort that may be related to the normal processes of aging, and acute or chronic pain that interferes with a functional lifestyle and requires intervention. Additional information about pain management for older adults can be found in Chapter 36. Delirium, sleep disturbances, cognitive changes, and diminished functional abilities may occur when pain is not managed adequately.

Because of the interplay between complex comorbidities, disease progression, and the expected changes with aging, loss of independence can occur. The loss of health is difficult to adjust to because it affects every aspect of life.

Retirement and Reduced Income

Retirement brings a change in a person's concept of time. Many older adults must learn to occupy their leisure time in ways that maintain their self-esteem while being personally satisfying. Satisfaction with retirement is closely tied to income and the relationships one has outside of work. While many older adults have adequate retirement income, for others, a lack of adequate income can affect their ability to meet their needs, such as for medical care and housing or social and creative interests.

Spouse or Partner Health

When a person's spouse or partner becomes ill, numerous and difficult adjustments must be made. An older adult may face new roles for the first time, such as cooking meals or handling family finances. These role changes come at a time when stress is already high. Providing physical care can be an overwhelming task if the caregiver is also frail or in poor health. Adaptations may be needed in living conditions and lifestyle, and one spouse may need to plan social and recreational events alone. Take a moment and reflect on the poem by Amy Haadad in the Poetry Nook.

The need for love and belonging does not diminish with age, and may become acute with the loss of the spouse or partner through illness or institutionalization. Humans are sexual beings, and sexual behavior does not necessarily stop in old age. Like younger adults, older adults need to experience intimacy physically by touching and sexual activity, and emotionally by sharing joys, sorrows, ideas, and values (Fig. 24-5).

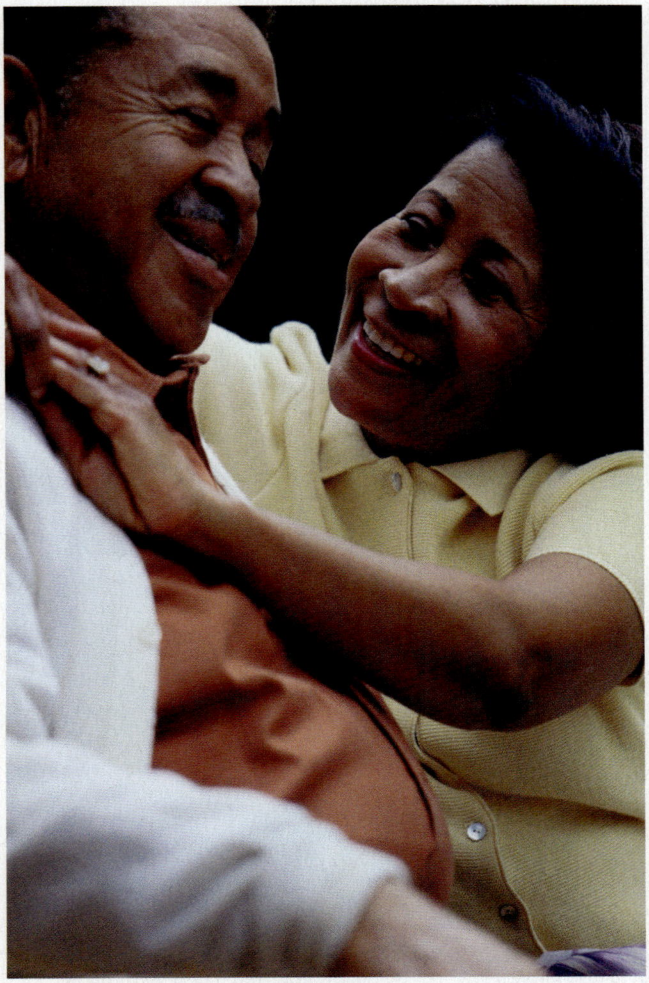

FIGURE 24-5. Stereotypical images of the older adult as narrow-minded, forgetful, sexless, and dependent are untrue of most older adults. This couple exhibits the vitality, sensuality, joy, and playfulness of a young couple.

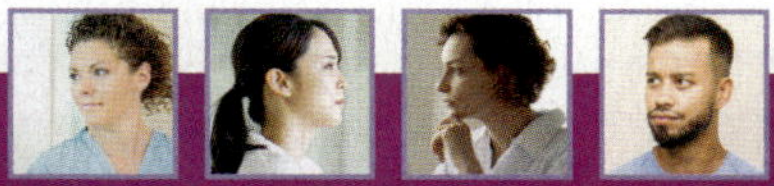

Poetry Nook

Landlines

Stubborn to the point of silence
she was determined to live on her own,
willing to let strangers into her home
to help her shower, see her naked.
These invasions into her privacy
were the price she paid to be free
to roam from room to room and be
alone at night. Nights were the worst
for me. I would clutch the ragged worry
each night, imagine her somewhere in
her house injured and helpless, lying
by the oxygen concentrator till dawn.
I put two phones in her bedroom.
I would reason she could crawl to one
for help. One next to her recliner where
she often slept, the other a red, rotary
phone hard-wired in the bathroom
with a ring like an air raid siren.
Her body failed her in diverse ways
but never her mind. No matter the number
of calls in a day, we always talked
at bedtime. When she didn't answer
right away I'd hang up, wait a bit
counting her slow steps in my head,
then try again. One night, I got no
answer. Too late for her to be out.
I pictured her motionless
on the kitchen floor, oxygen tubing
spaghettied around the legs of her walker,
a hazard we feared but lived with.
I dialed again, let it ring
forever. No answer. I drove, too fast,
to her house punched in the garage code,
flew inside, yelled, *Mom! Mom!*
The house was still except for the murmur
of the oxygen concentrator.
Night lights like luminaries marked
the way to the bedroom. She was not
on the floor or in her chair or bed.
I turned to the bathroom. There she was,
on the toilet, arms resting
on the metal safety rails, softly snoring,
her pink nylon underpants
around her ankles, the red phone planted
squarely between her bare feet.

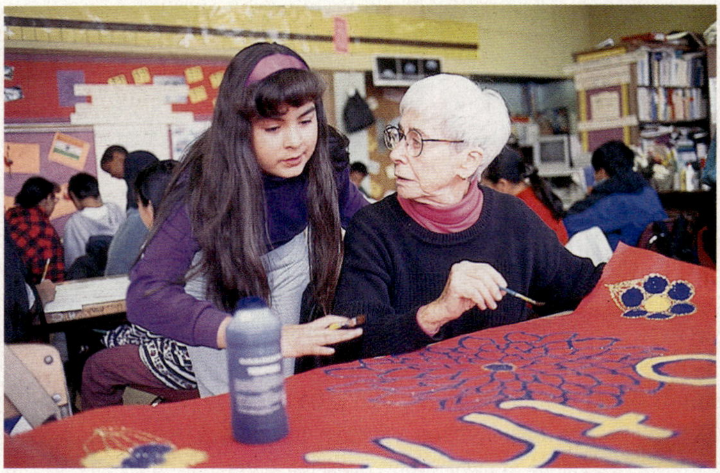

FIGURE 24-6. Social relationships and satisfying leisure activities remain important throughout life. This older adult volunteers in art class with sixth-grade students. (*Source:* Used with permission from Shutterstock. *Photo by Kathy Sloane.*)

Relating to Age Group

As the population ages, social organizations for older adults are becoming more numerous. For example, most communities have senior citizens' centers that offer meals, social and informational programs, and other activities for a nominal fee. Other organizations offer opportunities for travel, cultural events, and political involvement. Affiliation with people of the same age allows older adults to share common interests and concerns, and to find status among their peers. Some adults reside in retirement communities that provide a multitude of opportunities for social engagement. It should not be assumed, however, that older adults want to associate only with others their age; intergenerational friendships can be mutually beneficial and extremely rewarding (Fig. 24-6).

Concept Mastery Alert

Social isolation is different from ineffective coping. Social isolation is the feeling of being alone; ineffective coping refers to difficulty in adapting or responding to the changes associated with the situation. Ineffective coping can lead to social isolation.

Social Roles

Social roles change with the developmental tasks and adjustments of older adulthood, but the need to feel valued, useful, and productive continues. Older adults may develop new hobbies or increase their involvement in community, church, or family affairs (Fig. 24-7). They may do volunteer work or even begin a new career. If an older adult cannot adjust and form new relationships, social isolation can become a problem. **Social isolation** is a sense of being alone and lonely as a result of having fewer meaningful relationships. It may occur because of declining health or income, transportation problems, or ageism. Whatever the cause, prolonged social isolation has been associated with declining health and higher mortality rates. Unfortunately, the COVID-19 pandemic provided insight into the negative effects of social isolation on older adults caused by the social distancing and quarantining imposed by local/state/national mandates and health care policies intended to minimize transmission of the virus. The effects of social isolation on older adults included anxiety, depression, and despair. Older adults with dementia who were isolated suffered further cognitive decline (Chu et al., 2020). For older adults, reported sources of joy and comfort during the pandemic involved strengthened family relationships and friendships; the discovery of digital social contact; and a resurgence of hobbies fueled by re-engagement with self-care, exercise, faith, and nature (Whitehead & Torossian, 2021).

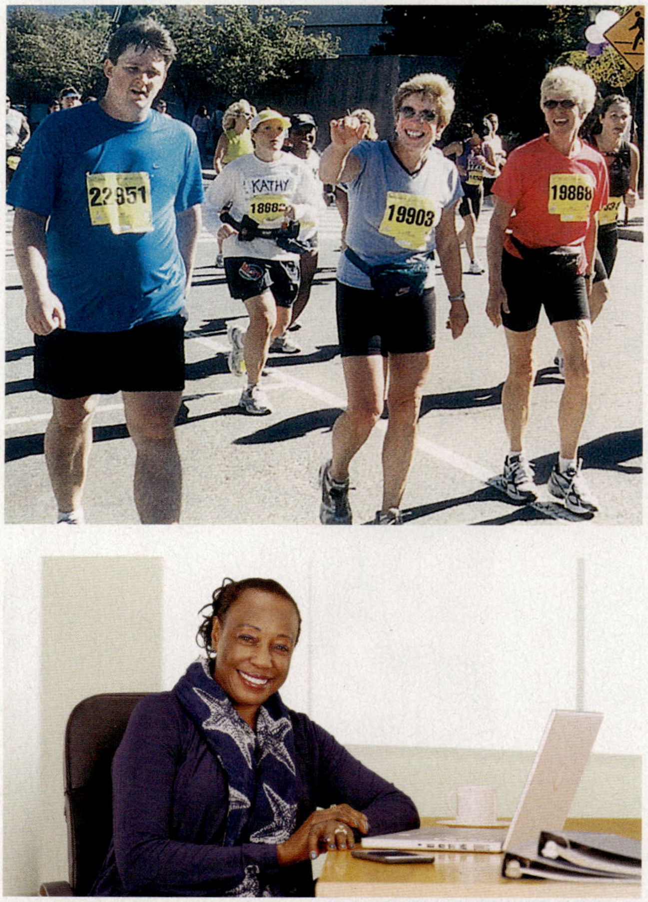

FIGURE 24-7. Older adults who exercise regularly improve their physical strength as well as overall stamina, mood, and mental health. Opportunities for engagement outside the home may involve the use of technology, which stimulates continued growth in the older adult, and may increase their feelings of personal control and engagement. (*Source: Bottom Photo by Rocketclips, Inc./Shutterstock.*)

Vulnerable Population Alert: Residents of Long-Term Care Facilities

If we learned anything during the COVID-19 pandemic, it is how vulnerable the residents in nursing homes are as well as their caregivers. About 5% of U.S. cases and nearly 40% of deaths attributed to COVID-19 have occurred in these long-term facilities, making them "ground zero" in the crisis. Sadly, the problems COVID-19 highlighted were hardly the beginning of what we know about deficient care in long-term care facilities. A stunning article in *The New York Times* (Silver-Greenberg & Gebeloff, 2021), described how nursing homes manipulate the rating systems about the quality of care provided by nursing homes and deceive the public. You may be choosing a five-star (top rating) nursing home for a loved one and have no idea about the fact that homes that received this rating masked serious problems, such as residents developing bed sores so severe that their bones were exposed. Others lost the ability to move.

Highlighting the challenges of staffing these homes, the *NYT* article describes a nursing home operating in 2017 with a skeleton crew. "Overwhelmed employees of the 120-bed facility would wake some residents as early as 3:30 AM to get them dressed for breakfast and they would put the residents back to bed to wait the hours until mealtime." In a lawsuit brought by a resident, charges included:

> More than a week passed before Ms. Johnson was first given a shower, her medical records show. Her surgical wound was not treated. No one came when she rang her call bell for help going to the toilet, so she sat for hours in her own urine and feces. At one point, . . . a passing maintenance man changed her diaper.

Silver-Greenberg, J., & Gebeloff, R. (March 14, 2021). To life ratings, nursing home shroud neglect. *The New York Times.*

Kolanowski, A., Cortes, T. A., Mueller, C., Bowers, B., Boltz, M., Bakerjian, D., Harrington, C., Popejoy, L., Vogelsmeier, A., Wallhagen, M., Fick, D., Batchelor, M., Harris, M., Palan-Lopez, R., Dellefield, M., Mayo, A., Woods, D. L., Horgas, A., Cacchione, P. Z., . . . Gerdner, L. (2021). A call to the CMS: Mandate adequate professional nurse staffing in nursing homes. *The American Journal of Nursing, 121*(3), 24–27. https://doi.org/10.1097/01.NAJ.0000737292.96068.18

Living Arrangements

Most older adults live in a community. In 2020, 61% of older adults living in a community lived with their spouse or partner, and 27% lived alone (20% of older men and 33% of older women). The number of older adults living alone increases with age. Relatively few older adults live in long-term care facilities (1% of older adults ages 65 to 74 years; 2% of older adults ages 75 to 84 years), but that number increases with age (8% for adults older than age 85 years), and as their needs increase (Administration for Community Living, 2021). When a person moves to a long-term care facility, the loss of home and possessions and the need to conform to the routines of institutional living can be traumatic for the person and family. Some people, however, choose to move for convenience, social relationships, or needed health care. Reflect on the Vulnerable Populations Alert that focuses on standards related to staffing and quality care in long-term care facilities.

Various types of housing options for older adults are outlined in Box 24-4 on page 646. The ability to function safely and independently at home depends a great deal on a person's functional health, transportation, income, and family. An older adult, for example, may need assistance with home repairs, housecleaning, or grocery shopping. Architectural barriers, such as steps, may need to be modified. Easy access to medical and recreational facilities and churches may become more important. Many older adults in poor health can continue living at home with some assistance from visiting nurses or with the aid of other services, such as home-delivered meals and senior transportation. Assisted-living housing is becoming more common, providing such requirements as meals, health care services, and cleaning services. Additional options for older adults include quality patient-centered programs with a focus on providing long-term care to older adults who want to remain in the community. Several examples are listed in Box 24-5 on page 647.

Retirement centers and senior citizens' housing have become common. For the family members of older adults who need health care, alternative methods of care have become available. Examples include respite care facilities, which allow the family a needed rest by temporarily housing and caring for an ailing older family member, and adult day services (ADS) centers, which provide a safe, stimulating environment during the day when family caregivers must work. Nurses should be knowledgeable about what health care and social services are available in the patient's community so that the patient and family can be referred (AARP, 2019).

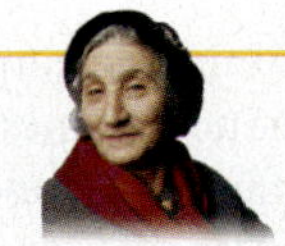

Remember **Ethel Peabody**, the 88-year-old woman with early dementia who lives alone. The nurse could work with social services to investigate possible community support resources available for the patient so that she can safely maintain her independence as much as possible.

Family and Role Reversal

An older adult's spouse or partner and other family members are natural support systems that help the person maintain functional health and independence to meet the developmental tasks of old age. Most older adults maintain close ties with their families; however, 38% of Medicare beneficiaries report feeling less socially connected to their families and friends (Administration for Community Living, 2021). Supportive assistance may include providing transportation, food, shelter, social interactions, and even complex medical and nursing treatments. Significant others, such as close friends and neighbors, may also take on tasks formerly assumed to be the responsibilities of the immediate family.

Not all families can assist an aged member satisfactorily because of geographic distance, low income, poor health, strained marital relationships, or infringement on career or lifestyle. Adult children may feel "sandwiched" between responsibilities for their own children and careers and the needs of older parents. It can be a guilt-ridden and emotionally

Box 24-4 Housing Options for Older Adults

Home modification: By making changes, older adults may be able to stay in their own homes. Examples of modifications are replacing doorknobs with handles, replacing faucet handles with levers, and installing grab bars in bathtubs. Older adults with disabilities may require additional modifications and support resources.

Accessory apartment: A separate apartment is constructed in part of an existing house, such as a basement, attic, or converted garage, or as a home addition. This allows older adults to live independently and privately while not being alone.

Assisted-living facility: These facilities generally provide housing, group meals, personal care, support services, and social activities in a social setting. Some health care may be provided. Costs vary from around $29,000 to $66,000 annually depending on location. Some states pay for personal care services for those with limited incomes.

Board and care homes, adult family homes, and adult group homes: Smaller in scale than assisted-living facilities, these services provide a room, meals, and help with daily activities. They may be licensed or unlicensed. Costs average $33,000 per year for a private room; Supplemental Security Income (SSI) will help pay for those with very limited incomes.

Continuing care retirement community (CCRC): This type of housing community offers several options and services, depending on the needs of the resident. Residents usually begin by living independently in apartments, and then move to an assisted-living facility on the same grounds. A skilled nursing center is also part of the community and available when needed. Sometimes called "aging-in-place" models, this type of housing tends to be expensive.

Elderly cottage housing opportunities (ECHO): ECHO homes are small portable cottages that are placed (most often) in the yard of an adult child's home. These units typically cost $28,000 or more, but do allow living independently while still close to support.

Home sharing: Two or more people may share an apartment or house. Each person usually has a private bedroom and shares the other living spaces. These homes may be sponsored by faith-based groups or community facilities.

Long-term care facilities: These facilities provide skilled nursing care or long-term care, including meals, personal care, and medical care. Bedrooms and bathrooms may be shared. Costs average $66,000 per year, but many are more expensive. Medicare provides only short-term coverage following a hospitalization. Medicaid provides coverage for low-income, low-asset people.

Naturally occurring retirement community (NORC): NORCs are neighborhoods or locations that happen to have a significant number of older adults in residence. Although they may occur naturally, their existence provides an opportunity to focus funding and other resources for older adults in the community.

Senior retirement communities, niche retirement communities, and villages: A grouping of rental apartments, condominiums, townhomes, or houses for residents who can take care of themselves and are mobile. Meals, grocery shopping, home repair, and housekeeping services may be offered (at additional cost). Social and recreational activities are usually offered.

Additional information about these housing options is provided by AARP at https://www.aarp.org/livable-communities/archives/info-2014/housing.html

draining time for all involved when an older adult's physical or emotional illness causes a reversal of roles. This situation can strain family resources.

Although moving in with adult children creates changes in roles and authority and can lead to stress on the adult child(ren), older adults often remain in the caretaking role. In 2019, approximately 1.1 million grandparents older than age 60 years lived in a home with one or more grandchildren and provided their basic needs. Of the 5.37 million people with intellectual and developmental disabilities who live with a family caregiver, 24% have adult caregivers ages 60 years and older (Administration for Community Living, 2021).

The nurse must view the whole family as the recipient of care and assess the family for capabilities and limitations for assisting the aged member. The nurse can help ease the strain by listening to the patient's and family's concerns and by validating the importance of family needs. The nurse assists the patient and family to find workable solutions and may refer the family to community support services.

Moral and Spiritual Development

Older adults, according to Kohlberg (1969), have completed their moral development. Most are at the conventional level, following society's rules in response to others' expectations. Spiritually, an older adult may remain at an earlier level, often at the individuative–reflective level. Many older adults, however, demonstrate conjunctive faith, where they integrate faith and truth to see the reality of their own beliefs, or universalizing faith, where they trust a greater power and believe in the future.

Another perspective on moral and spiritual development in older adults is the theory of **gerotranscendence**, which describes the transformation of a person's view of reality from a rational, social, individually focused, materialistic perspective to a more transcendent vision. This new vision is manifest by maturity, wisdom, spirituality, changes in perceptions of time and space (disappearance of distance), a decreased emphasis on superficial relationships, and, ultimately, life satisfaction (Tornstam, 1994). As a person ages, spirituality and transcendence are a resource and a source of strength when the person is faced with inevitable change and loss.

Health of the Older Adult

As the number of older adults increases, nurses will spend more time providing care for this population. Older adults can require care across all spheres of practice, including hospitals, long-term care facilities, emergency departments, outpatient surgeries, and homes. Nursing care for older adults should be based on two principles:

- Most older people are not impaired. They are functional members of the community who benefit from health-oriented interventions.
- Older people are more vulnerable to physical, emotional, and socioeconomic problems than people in other age

Box 24-5 Resources for Older Adults

AARP
https://www.aarp.org/caregiving/local/info-2019/national-resources-for-caregivers.html?cmp=RDRCT-9f9c190c-20210202
Identification of agencies, groups, and organizations focused on the care and support of older adults and their caregivers

Administration on Aging (AOA)
https://www.acl.gov/about-acl/administration-aging
Provides home- and community-based services to older adults through programs funded under the Older Americans Act

Aging and Disability Resource Center, National Association for Area Agencies on Aging (N4A)
https://www.n4a.org/adrcs
Helps older people and those with disabilities to live with dignity and choices in their homes and communities for as long as possible

Centers for Medicare and Medicaid Services (CMS)
http://www.cms.gov
U. S. Department of Health and Human Services (HHS) facility assigned to maintain health care security for its beneficiaries

Community Resource Finder
http://www.communityresourcefinder.org
The Alzheimer's Association Community Resource Finder searches a current list of licensed assisted-living residences, long-term care facilities, and other types of senior housing

Lotsa Helping Hands
http://www.lotsahelpinghands.com
Provides communication resources to support family caregivers, including help from volunteers and community

Meals on Wheels Association America
https://www.mealsonwheelsamerica.org
Provides lunch and dinner to older adults and people with disabilities

National Eldercare Locator
https://eldercare.acl.gov/Public/Index.aspx
Connects older adults and families by zip code, city, state, or county to eldercare resources in the community

National Institute on Aging
https://www.nia.nih.gov/
Includes health and wellness information for older adults

NORCs (Naturally Occurring Retirement Communities)
https://aging.ny.gov/naturally-occurring-retirement-community-norc
Formal organizations structured around a model of support services that are geographically based rather than service based

PACE (Program of All-Inclusive Care for the Elderly)
https://www.cms.gov/Medicare-Medicaid-Coordination/Medicare-and-Medicaid-Coordination/Medicare-Medicaid-Coordination-Office/PACE/PACE
Medicare/Medicaid-funded program for adults aged 55 years or older (specific criteria) to receive comprehensive interdisciplinary care to maintain living in the community

REACH (Racial and Ethnic Approaches to Community Health)
https://www.cdc.gov/nccdphp/dnpao/state-local-programs/reach/index.htm
Community-based, culturally appropriate programs focused on eliminating socially determined barriers to achieving health by supporting and funding community-based strategies, providing infrastructure, supporting national and international organizations, and increasing evidence-based strategies that address health disparities

U.S. Department of Health and Human Services (DHHS)
http://www.hhs.gov
Government facility charged with protecting health through the delivery of human services

groups. They may require special attention to health promotion and maintenance.

This section provides a broad introduction to the health care needs of the older adult in terms of chronic illness, accidental injuries, and acute illness.

Chronic Illness

The probability of a person becoming ill increases with age. Chronic health problems or disability also may result from acute illnesses or accidents such as pneumonia, fractures, motor vehicle accidents, and falls. The leading causes of death in adults ages 65 years and older are heart disease, cancer, chronic respiratory disease, stroke, AD, and diabetes (CDC, 2021d).

Although illness affects all dimensions of a person regardless of age, older adults have to contend with a variety of problems as they live with chronic illness. Aging is a normal process, and chronic illness is a pathologic process, but both often occur at the same time. Compensatory mechanisms that may have worked when older adults were younger are no longer sufficient because of the cumulative effects of chronic disease and the negative effects of aging on physiologic compensation. The interrelated changes of aging and the needs imposed by chronic illness increase the risk for problems in all areas of life, including—but not limited to—self-care, lifestyle, economics, social factors, and living arrangements. Chronic health conditions can negatively affect an older adult's functioning and quality of life, but many of these negative outcomes can be prevented or modified with behavioral interventions.

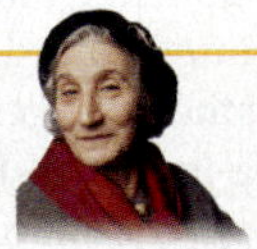

Think back to **Ethel Peabody**, the 88-year-old woman with early dementia and cardiac disease. The nurse could use knowledge about chronic illness as a basis for a teaching plan that addresses the patient's increased needs for safety.

IMPLICATIONS FOR HEALTH CARE

Consider the following:

- In 2020, 94% of community-dwelling older adults (ages 65 years and older) were covered by Medicare, which covers approximately half of acute health care costs. This is important because most older adults have at least one chronic illness, and many have multiple chronic diseases or conditions (Administration for Community Living, 2021).
- Hospitalization costs continue to rise, and the price of high-quality, long-term care may well be beyond the patient's or family's ability to pay.
- Special diets, special equipment, and medical supplies increase economic difficulties.
- In 1966, 29% of older adults (ages 65 years and older) lived below the poverty level. Although this percentage decreased to 10% in 2014 and 8.9% in 2020, meeting the expenses of health care is often difficult for older adults and their families. Women and those 75 years and older are more likely to live in poverty. Non-Hispanic White older adults are less likely than their Black, Asian, and Hispanic counterparts to live in poverty (Administration for Community Living, 2021; Federal Interagency Forum on Aging-Related Statistics, 2020).
- Medication costs related to chronic illness typically continue for the rest of a person's life, with multiple medications being the rule rather than the exception.
- **Polypharmacy**, the use of many medications at the same time, can pose many hazards for older adults. Complicated regimens need careful review to minimize risks and complications and maximize benefits. Polypharmacy, drug duplication, and unmonitored or unreported use of nonprescription medications can lead to negative outcomes. Pharmacists and other members of the interprofessional health care team need to educate and counsel older adults on these potential issues to minimize the risk for adverse effects, toxicities, and drug–drug interactions (Kinsey & Nykamp, 2017; see Research in Nursing: Bridging the Gap to Evidence-Based Practice).
- Nurses must be able to recognize adverse drug reactions in the older adult population instead of mistaking them for age-related changes. Refer to Chapter 30 for

Research in Nursing

BRIDGING THE GAP TO EVIDENCE-BASED PRACTICE

Interprofessional Collaborative Practice (IPCP) Models

Our population is aging. Older adults are projected to outnumber children younger than age 18 years by the year 2034 (U.S. Census Bureau, 2019). Although Interprofessional Collaborative Practice (IPCP) models, such as Programs of All-Inclusive Care for the Elderly (PACE) or the Doctors Assisting Seniors at Home (DASH) program, provide an effective means for supporting and keeping older adults in the community setting, they continue to be underutilized in the Unites States.

Related Research

Montano, A. R., Shellman, J., Malcolm, M., McDonald, D., Rees, C., Fortinsky, R., & Reagan, L. (2020). A mixed methods evaluation of GOT care!. *Geriatric Nursing*, *41*(6), 822–831. https://doi.org/10.1016/j.gerinurse.2020.04.016

Geriatric Outreach and Training with Care! (GOT Care!) began as a quality improvement project; this study used convergent parallel mixed methods (quantitative and qualitative) design to explore Emergency Department (ED) visit frequency and the related perceptions of stakeholders. GOT Care! required collaboration between geriatric nurse navigators (a new position within the community health system created for this program) and nursing, medicine, dentistry, pharmacy, physical therapy, public health, and social work students and faculty from a public university. After an interprofessional education (IPE) 2-day intensive for the students, geriatric nurse practitioner–led teams completed a geriatric-focused, comprehensive, in-home assessment on community-dwelling older adults. The interprofessional team then crafted a care plan that was shared with the older adult's primary care provider (PCP). The geriatric nurse navigator coordinated care. Weekly meetings over the course of the semester and a follow-up in-home visit by the interprofessional team focused on enacting community resources in an effort to decrease ED visits. Five cohorts (five semesters) of students and 51 community-dwelling older adults participated in GOT Care!. Although the ED visits did not decrease significantly at 6 or 12 months, a decrease was seen at 18 months. Combined with the qualitative data collected regarding perceptions of GOT Care!, this finding indicates that there may be significant long-term benefits of IPCP. Findings of the mixed methods study also indicate that GOT Care! may be more effective for high-risk (multiple comorbids, polypharmacy, diabetes, high-frequency ED visits baseline) community-dwelling older adults with specific demographics, which will help in future implementations of this and similar initiatives.

Relevance to Nursing Practice

The integration of IPE and IPCP teams in practice provides opportunities for growth and development for the professionals involved. One of the key themes identified in this study reinforces what is documented in the literature: "when the client benefits, the team benefits" (p. 828). Although the formation of IPCP teams requires intentionality and consideration of logistics, IPCP interventions can lead to improved outcomes for community-dwelling older adults, specifically surrounding ED visits and hospitalizations. Training students to capitalize on the strengths of their teammates facilitates the development of effective nurse-led IPCP teams in practice.

additional information regarding altered drug response in older adults.

- Family members must learn how to cope with the needs of the ill person. These needs include personal hygiene, medication administration, special diets, elimination, activities of daily living, and recognition of symptoms that necessitate medical attention.
- Family members must also adapt to psychological stressors such as changes in communication, changes in roles (e.g., an older parent becoming dependent on their adult children), and changes in their own lifestyles as they become the caregivers or share caregiving responsibilities.

QSEN POLYPHARMACY

Polypharmacy, the use of many medications at the same time, requires careful monitoring to minimize the risk for adverse effects, toxicities, and drug–drug interactions.

DIVERSITY AND CHRONIC ILLNESS

As the U.S. population ages dramatically and becomes more diverse, it is important to consider how cultural differences can affect future patterns of disease, disability, and health care use. Minority populations continue to grow. Projections indicate that by 2060, 23% of Americans will be ages 65 years and older. In 2018, 77% of older adults identified as non-Hispanic White; this percentage is projected to drop to 55% by 2060 (Mather et al., 2019).

The prevalence of certain diseases varies among racial and ethnic groups. Research continues to focus on the potential effects of genetics, genomics, and epigenetics (see Chapter 22), as well as the effects of early individual health behaviors and cultural practices, on the disease patterns of older adults in these various groups. The environment and constructs such as bias; social determinants of health; and **structural racism**, defined as "the combination of institutions, culture, history, ideology, and codified practices that generate and perpetuate inequity among racial and ethnic groups" (American Cancer Society [ACS], 2019, p. 2), play a huge role in the development of health care disparities (CDC, 2021f), which nurses are called to address (American Association of Colleges of Nursing [AACN], 2021). Health disparities that exist between nonminority populations and racial and ethnic minorities are particularly prevalent in the older population. Poverty, the presence of chronic illnesses, and difficulty accessing the health care system make older adults much more vulnerable to a diminished quality of life caused by disease. COVID-19 and the associated pandemic highlighted disparities in the social, economic, and secondary health issues that stemmed from the crisis. Social determinants of health played a role in the exposure, severity of illness, hospitalizations, and deaths associated with the virus (CDC, 2020b). This time was also punctuated by political and social upheaval in response to structural racism and the pronounced access and health disparities.

Profiles of various racial and ethnic groups, as classified by the U.S. government, indicate the following patterns of diseases:

- Heart disease is the leading cause of death for African American men and women. The prevalence of hypertension in Black adults ages 20 years and older in the United States is the highest in the world, with age-adjusted numbers reflecting 58.3% prevalence in non-Hispanic Black males and 57.6% prevalence in non-Hispanic Black females. Hypertension is associated with stroke, heart disease, and other vascular diseases (Virani et al., 2021). African Americans have the highest mortality rate and shortest survival of any minority for most major cancers. Black men have the highest incidence of cancer. Despite lower incidence rates than their non-Hispanic White female counterparts, non-Hispanic Black women have the highest death rates of all racial and ethnic groups for breast and uterine cancer; colorectal and prostate cancers are more common and faster growing (prostate) in Black men than in other racial or ethnic groups (ACS, 2019; CDC, 2013).
- The leading causes of illness and death for Hispanic or Latino Americans are heart disease and cancer. Although Hispanic Americans have lower death rates than non-Hispanic Whites in most areas, they have more deaths from diabetes and chronic liver disease, and a similar number of deaths from kidney disease. Hispanic American adults (ages 20 years and older) have 6.5% more obesity than non-Hispanic Black adults, 12.2% more obesity than non-Hispanic White adults, and 33.1% more obesity than Asian adults. Colorectal screening for adults ages 50 to 75 years shows wide variation based on race and ethnicity: White only 68.2%, Black/African American only 65.2%, Asian only 58.2%, American Indian/Alaska Native only 56%, Hispanic or Latino 57.9%, and Mexican (specifically) 52.5% (CDC, 2021c). It is important to note that Hispanic subgroups have different degrees of risk. For example, Hispanic adults who are of Mexican or Puerto Rican descent are twice as likely to die from diabetes as their White counterparts.
- Asian American individuals comprise many subgroups, with the six largest subgroups (Asian Indian, Chinese, Filipino, Japanese, Korean, and Vietnamese) often considered independently in analyses when reported. Overall, cancer is the leading cause of death for Asian Americans; however, heart disease is the leading cause of death among men of Asian Indian, Filipino, and Japanese descent. Stroke is the overall third leading cause of death (CDC, 2021b). AD mortality increased in Asian Americans, just as it had across all other racial and ethnic groups between 2003 and 2011 (Hastings et al., 2015).
- Heart disease, cancer, unintentional injuries, and diabetes are the leading causes of death in American Indian or Alaska Native people. Members of the 573 federally recognized tribes and their descendants have lingering heath disparities that result in a life expectancy 5.5 years less than all other races or ethnicities (Indian Health Service, 2019).
- Native Hawaiian or Other Pacific Islanders (from Guam, Samoa, or other islands) generally have higher reported

rates of smoking, alcohol consumption, and obesity compared with other ethnic or racial groups. This group shares the leading causes of death with the other groups (i.e., cancer, heart disease, unintentional injuries, stroke, and diabetes), but also has an increase in specific risks and diseases including hepatitis B, HIV/AIDS, and tuberculosis (Office of Minority Health, 2021).

Refer to Chapter 5 for additional discussion of cultural variations and influences on health care.

Accidental Injuries

The older adult is at increased risk for accidental injury because of changes in vision and hearing, loss of mass and strength of muscles, slower reflexes and reaction time, and decreased sensory ability.

Many older adults limit their activities because of their fear of falls that might result in serious health consequences. Falls are the most common cause of injuries and hospital admissions in older adults. More than 25% of older adults fall each year, but less than half tell their health care providers (CDC, 2020a). Fear of falling, personality traits of high neuroticism and low conscientiousness, and indicators of frailty have been shown to contribute to falls in older adults (Bromfield et al., 2017; Canada et al., 2020; Jehu et al., 2021; Makino et al., 2017). Falling once doubles the chance of the older adult falling again. One out of five falls causes serious injury, such as traumatic brain injury (TBI) or a fracture, and over 800,000 patients are hospitalized annually because of fall injuries. More than 95% of hip fractures are caused by falling, typically sideways. When adjusted for inflation, the direct medical costs related to falls average $50 billion annually (CDC, 2020a). Chapters 28 and 34 have additional information regarding the risk for falls and developmental considerations related to ambulation; see also the CDC's fall prevention information, available online at https://www.cdc.gov/homeandrecreationalsafety/falls/adultfalls.html.

In addition to the risk of falls, the combined effects of chronic illness and medications may make an older adult more prone to accidents. Older adults with reduced income may live in inadequate housing in neighborhoods with heavy traffic or high crime rates. They may be isolated from family members, and many live alone. Combined with the normal changes of aging and the effects of any illness, older people not only are at increased risk but also have a more difficult time regaining health after an injury. Refer to the PICOT in Practice display on preventing falls and to Chapter 28 for additional information related to risk for accidental injuries in older adults.

Dementia, Delirium, and Depression

Nurses and the health care team need to be attuned to abnormal processes that may occur in older adults. Often referred to as the "3Ds," dementia, delirium, and depression require specific assessment and management.

DEMENTIA

When a serious mental impairment occurs, the effect on the patient and family can be devastating. The term **dementia** refers to various organic disorders that progressively affect cognitive functioning. Dementia is chronic and usually develops gradually. Many people think of Alzheimer's disease (AD) when dementia is mentioned, but dementia may also occur more suddenly following a stroke or other vascular event. Referred to as *vascular dementia*, this form is often related to hypertension, and is the second most common type of dementia. Other dementias include Lewy body dementia and frontotemporal disorders. Differentiating the specific type of dementia affecting an older adult may be difficult, and many people have a form of *mixed dementia* consisting of two or more types (National Institute on Aging, 2021b).

Of the dementias that affect older adults, **Alzheimer's disease (AD)** is the most common degenerative neurologic illness and the most common cause of cognitive impairment. It is irreversible and progresses from deficits in memory and thinking skills to an eventual inability to perform basic self-care. The first indications of AD usually occur in a person's mid-60s, and nearly half of 85-year-old adults have the disease (National Institute on Aging, 2021b). There are 5.8 million people living with AD today, and this number is expected to more than double to 13.8 million by 2050 (Mather et al., 2019).

Although further research needs to be done to identify potential and actual causes and to find a cure for AD, we now know that the formation of amyloid plaques and tangles of tau proteins have an impact on the brain structure and function in older adults with AD. It is a progressively serious and ultimately fatal disorder. In mild or early AD, forgetfulness and impaired judgment may be evident. Over a period of several years, the person progresses to moderate or middle AD, and becomes progressively more confused, forgetting family and becoming disoriented in familiar surroundings. When the ability to perform simple activities of daily living is lost, and the older adult enters the severe or late stage of AD, the person requires constant supervision and care, often in a long-term care facility. There is no effective medical treatment for AD at this time. Reflect on the Vulnerable Populations Alert on persons with AD and their caregivers.

A common problem in patients with dementia is **sundowning syndrome**, in which an older adult habitually becomes confused, restless, and agitated after dark. Wandering may occur, and coping may be negatively affected by hallucinations, delusions, or paranoia. People with dementia are hospitalized more frequently than other older adults. The precipitating factor may be a medical-surgical problem, or the behavioral or psychiatric symptoms that occur with dementia. Often, a medical or nursing intervention can trigger a sequence of adverse events in a frail older adult. This downward spiral and decline is referred to as **cascade iatrogenesis**. Here is an example of cascade iatrogenesis: an episode of confusion and wandering at night may lead to a fall that results in a hip fracture. During the resulting hospitalization, the insertion of an indwelling catheter can precipitate a urinary tract infection that requires use of an antibiotic and possibly the development of antibiotic-resistant organisms. This is, unfortunately, not an uncommon scenario for nurses to encounter.

PICOT in Practice

ASKING CLINICAL QUESTIONS: PREVENTING FRAGILITY HIP FRACTURES

Scenario: You work as a nurse for an organization that offers preventive health care services for residents in a small, rural community. Recently, several 65-year-old and older residents living independently in the community have fallen in their homes. Many of the residents had to be hospitalized for broken hips following their falls. The falls were from low-energy trauma, such as falls from standing height, also known as fragility hip fractures.

As team leader for gerontology services, you want to help reduce the number of hip fractures in older adults in the community and increase bone health. You have read that consumption of dairy products can promote bone health. Other members of the team wonder if certain medications predispose older adults to falls and might be responsible for the risks and rates of falls in the community. You have offered to evaluate the evidence for effectiveness of both of these interventions.

- **Population:** Older adults living independently in the community
- **Intervention:** Dairy consumption
- **Comparison:** Prescribed medication
- **Outcome:** Hip fractures
- **Time:** 12 months

PICOT Question: Among older adults living independently in the community, does consumption of dairy products compared to prescribed medication result in decreased risk of hip fractures over 12 months?

Findings:

1. Hidayat, K., Du, X., Shi, B. M., & Qin, L. Q. (2020). Systematic review and meta-analysis of the association between dairy consumption and the risk of hip fracture: critical interpretation of the currently available evidence. *Osteoporos International, 31*(8), 1411–1425. https://doi.org/10.1007/s00198-020-05383-3

Nine articles were included in the meta-analysis with a total of 9,564 hip fracture events among 363,383 participants. The evidence from prospective cohort studies reassuringly suggests that the risk of hip fracture may not be elevated among people who consume milk, yogurt, and cheese, and that a greater consumption of milk or yogurt may even be associated with a lower risk of hip fracture depending on the factors that may differ across the population of interest.

2. Mortensen, S. J., Mohamadi, A., Wright, C. L., Chan, J. J., Weaver, M. J., von Keudell, A., & Nazarian, A. (2020). Medications as a risk factor for fragility hip fractures: A systematic review and meta-analysis. *Calcified Tissue International, 107*(1), 1–9. https://doi.org/10.1007/s00223-020-00688-1

Thirty-eight studies comprising 1,244,155 subjects and 188,966 cases of fragility hip fractures were included in this study. Hormone replacement therapy (HRT) with estrogen was associated with decreased risk of hip fracture. In contrast, the following medications were significantly associated with fragility hip fractures:

- Antidepressants
- Antiparkinsonian drugs
- Antipsychotic drugs
- Anxiolytic drugs
- Benzodiazepines
- Sedatives
- Systemic corticosteroids
- H2 Antagonists
- Proton-pump inhibitors
- Thyroid hormone

Strength of Evidence: Level I systematic reviews

Recommendation: You recommend that the team offer a bone health program that includes information about osteoporosis and fracture prevention. The program targets older adults taking medications associated with higher risk of hip fractures. In addition, the benefits of incorporating dairy products into a healthy, balanced diet are discussed as well as their unique package of valuable nutrients that are important for bone health.

Vulnerable Population Alert

The 2020 Alzheimer's Disease Facts and Figures

- Alzheimer's disease is the sixth leading cause of death in the United States.
- More than 5 million Americans are living with Alzheimer's disease.
- One in three older adults dies with Alzheimer's disease or another dementia.
- Fifty percent of primary care physicians believe the medical profession is not ready for the growing number of people with dementias.
- Sixteen million Americans provide unpaid care for people with dementias.
- These caregivers provided an estimated 18.6 billion hours valued at nearly $244 billion.
- Between 2000 and 2018, deaths from heart disease have decreased 7.8%, while deaths from Alzheimer's disease have increased 146% (https://www.alz.org/media/Documents/alzheimers-facts-and-figures-infographic.pdf).

Alzheimer's disease takes a devastating toll on caregivers. Compared with caregivers of people without dementia, twice as many caregivers of those with dementia indicate substantial emotional, financial, and physical difficulties. Do you make it a point to talk with the family caregivers of your patients with Alzheimer's disease or other dementias to ask how they are doing?

Caregiver Support Resources

Alzheimer's Association
https://alz.org/help-support/caregiving

Family Caregiver Alliance
https://www.caregiver.org/

For the patient with dementia, communication with family members and a systematic approach to assessment is required. Comprehensive and empathetic nursing care is important. Both the patient and family/caregivers need emotional support and teaching and may benefit from community resources that can ease the family's burden.

DELIRIUM

Sometimes delirium and depression in an older adult are mistaken for true dementia. **Delirium** is an acute syndrome of brain failure that can last from hours to weeks, has a specific cause, and resolves with treatment of the identified underlying cause. Symptoms of delirium include variable deficits in attention, awareness, and cognition that may have hyperactive, hypoactive, or mixed presentations (Thom et al., 2019). Delirium may not have one specific cause, and in older adults may be due to drug interactions, circulatory or metabolic problems, nutritional deficiencies, or a worsening illness that triggers inflammatory processes and disrupts neurotransmitters. During acute illness, older adults are particularly at risk for delirium because of their decreased cognitive reserve (Mattison, 2020; Wan & Chase, 2017).

Prevention is the first step in managing delirium. Incidences of delirium are more likely to occur with six key risk factors: cognitive impairment, sleep deprivation, immobility, visual or hearing impairment, and dehydration (Wan & Chase, 2017). Nurses should focus on these six issues as a starting point for preventive interventions. For example, providing frequent reorientation immediately after surgery serves to reorient and also comfort the patient. Ensuring glasses and hearing aids are at the bedside minimizes the isolation and confusion that may occur when the person awakens from anesthesia in an unfamiliar environment. Medications, such as antipsychotics, are used carefully in delirium because they can inadvertently exacerbate the problem.

When assessing behavioral changes, remember that an older adult with dementia may also develop delirium. This *delirium superimposed on dementia* can be difficult to differentiate. Family members and regular caregivers often serve as the best resources for the identification of a change in the trajectory of dementia in the patient. The focus in this instance is on treating the underlying cause of the delirium and returning the patient to their current (baseline) cognitive function. Key activities include interventions that are person centered, including assessing the patient's baseline cognitive function, integrating the patient's values and interests, enhancing the sensory abilities of the patient to communicate, encouraging the presence of family at the bedside, individualizing cognitive stimulation for that patient, and enhancing behavioral approaches to comfort and sleep (Bellelli et al., 2021; Yevchak et al., 2017).

Box 24-6 lists online resources for assessing for dementia and delirium.

Box 24-6 Online Tools for Assessment of Delirium and Dementia

Confusion Assessment Method (CAM)

https://help.agscocare.org/table-of-contents/delirium-instruments/H00101

Identifies delirium quickly. Long and short versions are available.

Delirium Observation Screening (DOS) Scale/ Delirium Observation Screening Scale (DOSS)

https://deliriumnetwork.org/wp-content/uploads/2018/05/DOSS.pdf

Consists of 13 items focused on routine observation of verbal and nonverbal behaviors.

Mini-Cog

https://mini-cog.com

Two-part test to determine if dementia or cognitive impairment is present (even in early stages). Takes 3 to 5 minutes to administer.

Mini-Mental Status Exam (MMSE)

http://www4.parinc.com/Products/Product.aspx?ProductID=MMSE

The original MMSE contains 30 questions and screens for cognitive impairment, estimates the severity of cognitive impairment, and documents changes over time with respect to decline or response to treatment.

MMSE Second Edition

http://www4.parinc.com/Products/Product.aspx?ProductID=MMSE-2

The second edition may be useful in populations with milder forms of cognitive impairment.

Neecham Confusion Scale

https://www.ncbi.nlm.nih.gov/pmc/articles/PMC1852304

Consists of nine items and is used to detect early stages of delirium; does not differentiate between dementia and delirium.

Simple Question for Easy Evaluation of Consciousness (SQEEC) and Single Question in Delirium (SQiD)

https://deliriumnetwork.org/wp-content/uploads/2019/05/SQUEEC.pdf

Two-question (SQiD has one question) screening that requires a narrative reflection.

DEPRESSION

Extreme or prolonged sadness in an older adult may be a warning sign of depression. Depression is not a normal part of aging. Death of a spouse or friends, coupled with changes in living environment or financial resources can precipitate feelings of grieving that, if unresolved, may result in depression. There is usually a distinct change of behavior accompanied by other specific signs and symptoms of depression, such as sleep disturbances, weight loss (sometimes gain), difficulty with concentration, irritability or anger, loss of interest in once pleasurable activities, vague pains, crying, fatigue, and suicidal thoughts or preoccupation with death (National Institute on Aging, 2021a).

Depression occurs in 6.3 million older adults worldwide secondary to ageism (World Health Organization, 2021a). Symptoms of depression are often inappropriately attributed to normal aging, drugs, the progression of chronic disease, or cognitive decline. The short form of the Geriatric Depression Scale (GDS), a 15-question screening tool (available online at https://consultgeri.org/try-this/general-assessment/issue-4.pdf), can be used effectively in older adults in any setting. When combined with a mental health assessment by a professional, it can facilitate a diagnosis of depression (Greenberg, 2012). Treatment of depression usually involves psychotherapy or counseling along with antidepressant medication. In an older adult, hopelessness rather than sadness is more often associated with suicidal intent. Depression in older adults varies in its presentation depending on a person's cultural background, stress level, and underlying medical conditions (National Institute on Aging, 2021a). Depression in older adults must be recognized by nurses and treated by the interprofessional team.

Elder Abuse

The increase in the number of older adults coupled with increasing lifespan has resulted in greater awareness about the problem of **elder abuse**, which is defined as, "an intentional act or failure to act by a caregiver or another person in a relationship involving an expectation of trust that causes or creates a risk of harm to an older adult" (Hall et al., 2016, p. 23). Elder abuse is experienced by 1 in 10 community-dwelling, older adults (ages 60 years and older) living in the United States (CDC, 2021a; U.S. Department of Justice, n.d.). An estimated 58% of perpetrators who commit nonfatal assaults against older adults (ages 60 years and older) have a personal relationship (family, friend, acquaintance) with the older adult. Based on the data collected, these cases may meet CDC criteria for elder abuse, which means elder abuse needs to be recognized as an underreported and widespread public health issue. Compared with women, men have higher rates of death by homicide (increased 7% 2010–2016) and experiencing nonfatal assaults (increased more than 75% 2002–2016), especially among men ages 60 to 69 years (CDC, 2021d; Logan et al., 2019). Environmental, social, financial, educational, and employment-based inequities amplify the risks of experiencing violence across the lifespan, particularly for racial and ethnic minorities. Addressing and reducing health disparities and structural inequities could decrease the violence perpetrated on older adults (Logan et al., 2019). The United States is not alone in managing this global public health priority. Estimates are that 15.7% of older adults (ages 60 years and older) worldwide have experienced some form of abuse (Yon et al., 2017). Worldwide, elder abuse rates have increased during the COVID-19 pandemic. Globally, elder abuse is experienced both in the community (1 in 6) and in long-term care facilities (World Health Organization, 2021b).

Elder abuse includes physical abuse, sexual abuse, psychological or emotional abuse, financial abuse or exploitation, and neglect (Hall et al., 2016).

- *Physical abuse* is the intentional use of physical force that results in acute or chronic illness, physical injury, pain that can range from physical discomfort to agony, functional impairment, distress in the form of mental or physical suffering, or death. Physical abuse includes the inappropriate use of medication, inappropriate use of physical restraints, and physical punishment.
- *Sexual abuse* involves forced or unwanted sexual interaction of any kind with an older adult, including touching and nontouching acts (such as photography, voyeurism, verbal or behavioral sexual harassment, or forced viewing of pornographic materials).
- *Emotional or psychological abuse* includes verbal or nonverbal behavior that results in the caregiver or trusted person inflicting anguish, mental pain, fear, or distress. This type of abuse can include humiliation and disrespect, threats (physical, psychological, or sexual), harassment, and isolation or coercive control.
- *Financial abuse* or *financial exploitation* involves the illegal, improper, or unauthorized use of the resources of an older adult by the caregiver or trusted person for the benefit of someone other than the older adult.
- *Neglect* involves failure by the caregiver or person in a trusted relationship to protect an elder from harm, or failure to meet the need for essential medical care, nutrition and hydration, activities of daily living (hygiene, clothing), or shelter that results in serious risk of compromised health or safety. This risk is considered relative to age, baseline health status, and cultural norms.

Unfortunately, only 1 out of every 23 cases of elder abuse is reported to the appropriate protective services (U.S. Department of Justice, n.d.).

Identification of elder abuse requires an alert health care provider. Indications of abuse are often misinterpreted as normal signs of aging. Careful observation of the relationship between the older adult and the caregiver may be the first evidence that the older adult is a victim of abuse. Pay attention to interactions involving voice tone, caring behaviors, and personal touch. Older adults who have been physically abused present with injuries that are incompatible with the older adult's or caregiver's version of how the injury occurred. Evidence of previously untreated injuries or suspicious cuts and bruises should alert health care providers to the possibility of physical abuse. If you suspect abuse, attempt to speak to the older adult in a private setting away from the caregiver; the suspected abuser should be interviewed only by professionals specifically trained in this type of interview. A victim may deny abuse or choose not to report it because of shame, fear of abandonment, worry about retaliation, or dementia. All assessment data should be objectively documented, including direct quotes from both parties. Most states require that health care professionals report any suspected cases of elder abuse to designated official facilities.

There is a lack of high-quality research studies in the literature, but clinical experience and documented best practice can guide multifaceted screening and intervention (Logan et al., 2019; Moore & Browne, 2016; U.S. Department of Justice, n.d.).

QSEN MULTIDISCIPLINARY TEAMS

The U.S. Department of Justice provides a guide designed to facilitate the development and growth of multidisciplinary teams (MDTs) dedicated to the review of elder abuse cases. This living document is designed to provide a structure for case review that any community can use (available online at https://www.justice.gov/elderjustice/mdt-toolkit).

The International Association of Forensic Nurses (2021) created a nursing curriculum (available at https://www.forensicnurses.org/page/AboutCurriculum) designed to provide nurses with foundational knowledge and skills in basic forensics focused on older adults. Box 24-7 lists various organizations that provide additional information and support about elder abuse.

Older Adults and the Health Care System

Our knowledge of aging has increased dramatically in the past 50 years. **Gerontology** is the scientific and behavioral study of all aspects of aging and its consequences. Normal changes that occur with aging result from complex interactions among genetics, biological systems, and physical and social environments. Disease complicates a person's ability to adapt and maintain **functional health** (the ability to carry out usual and desired daily activities). Mental or physical decline in older adults often may not be directly related to the aging process, but may result from the absence of supportive care and services that could prevent disease and help maintain the older adult's ability to function. The Fulmer SPICES tool (Fulmer, 2019) has proved effective in identifying common problems experienced in older adults that can lead to negative outcomes. It provides information on hospitalized older adults that may assist in preventing and detecting common complications. The acronym SPICES facilitates assessment and information gathering about the following:

- **S**—Sleep disorders
- **P**—Problems with eating or feeding
- **I**—Incontinence
- **C**—Confusion
- **E**—Evidence of falls
- **S**—Skin breakdown

This instrument can be used in many settings and alerts nurses to quickly identify interventions to individualize an older adult's care.

The increasing aging population has greatly strained a health care system that has traditionally focused on cures and acute disease processes. For an older adult with chronic disorders, the focus of care should include shared goals and promote functional health and independent living to the greatest extent possible. **Gerontologic nursing** combines the basic knowledge and skills of nursing with a specialized knowledge of aging in both illness and health. The terms *geriatrics* and *gerontology* are sometimes used interchangeably. *Geriatrics* is a branch of medicine that focuses on the study of health and disease later in life, while *gerontology* represents the multidisciplinary, scientific study of the effects of aging and age-related diseases on humans. Due in large part to the aging population nurses serve, there has been a shift to include coursework focused on older adults in undergraduate nursing curricula, and to provide postgraduate certifications in gerontology and nurse practitioner tracks focused on geriatrics. Given the increasing numbers of older adults, it is imperative for nurses to address the challenges of an aging population, be competent in geriatric care, integrate developmentally appropriate interventions, and be prepared to make a difference in outcomes for this unique population.

Box 24-7 Elder Abuse Resources

Law Enforcement Agencies

Phone: Dial 911

For use when an older adult is in immediate, life-threatening danger or when reporting suspected abuse is mandatory

National Center on Elder Abuse

Website: https://ncea.acl.gov

Phone: 1-855-500-3537

This site is a gateway to resources on elder abuse, neglect, and exploitation.

U.S. Administration on Aging, Eldercare Locator

Website: https://www.usa.gov/federal-agencies/eldercare-locator

Phone: 1-800-677-1116

Connects older adults and caregivers with sources of information on senior services

Role of the Nurse in Promoting Health and Preventing Illness

The nurse should teach the older adult patient and family/caregivers general health promotion activities. This is important because older people may consider themselves "too old" to worry about nutrition, exercise, health screenings, and immunizations. In addition to the recommended screenings, examinations, and immunizations outlined in Box 24-2 on page 636, the following should be emphasized:

- Eat a diet that includes all food groups; is low in fat, saturated fat, and cholesterol; balances calories with physical activity; has recommended amounts of fruits, vegetables, and grains; and uses sugar and salt in moderation.
- Make exercise a part of daily activities. This will decrease your risk of falls and may improve your core strength and focus.
- Discuss with your primary provider whether to include nutritional supplements as part of your daily routine. Although supplementation with vitamins, minerals, and herbs may be beneficial, a provider should guide your supplement plan so that side effects and toxicities are avoided (Eliopoulos, 2022).
- Drink alcohol in moderation.
- Do not smoke.

Box 24-8 Nursing Actions to Promote Health in Older Adults

Physiologic Function

- Maintain physiologic reserves. Maintain ongoing assessments for early detection of problems.
- Review perceptions of current health status, health problems, and prescribed or over-the-counter medications.
- Include nursing care that maintains physical status, such as skin care and planned rest and activity.

Cognitive Function

- Slow pace of activity and wait for responses.
- Be sure eyeglasses and hearing aids are used; ensure that lenses are clean and batteries are strong.

Psychosocial Needs

- Be aware that illness, hospitalization, or changes in living arrangements are major stressors.
- Assess and support sources of strength, including cultural and spiritual values and rituals.
- Encourage use of support systems: family (whomever they identify), friends, community resources, and pets.
- Set mutual goals and encourage the patient's role in making decisions about care.
- Encourage life review and reminiscence.
- Encourage self-care.
- Consider the patient's background, interests, capabilities, values, culture, and lifestyle when planning care.

Nutrition

- Assess for lost or damaged teeth; ensure that dentures fit properly. Provide foods appropriate to the patient's ability to chew.
- Assess height, weight, eating patterns, and food choices.
- Assess for malnutrition, especially in older adults impacted by cognitive, psychological, or social factors such as the 3Ds, isolation, limited income or access to nutritious food, and the need for assistance with food preparation or eating (Mangels, 2018).
- Assess swallowing ability.
- Consider using supplements under the direction of a provider.

Sleep and Rest

- Discourage excessive napping.
- Assess normal bedtime, time for rising, bedtime rituals, effects of pain, medications, anxiety, and depression.

Elimination

- Assess frequency of bladder elimination as well as problems with incontinence.
- Assess normal times for bowel movements while considering changes in activity, privacy, and medications.
- Ensure that the floor is not cluttered, the toilet is easily accessible, lighting is adequate, and privacy is provided.
- Suggest having safety bars installed in the bathroom.
- Review diet for necessary fluid and fiber content.

Activity and Exercise

- Assess ability to walk; ensure that assistive devices (such as a walker or cane) are available.
- Consider effects of illness, surgery, medications, and changes in diet and fluid intake on strength and motor function.
- Ensure an uncluttered environment with good lighting; suggest using a night light and removing rugs.
- Slow the pace of care, allowing extra time to carry out activities.

Sexuality

- Assist as necessary with hygiene, hair care, oral care, clean clothing and bedding, makeup, and shaving.
- Maintain a clean, odor-free environment.
- Demonstrate genuine caring: ask preferred name, listen carefully, and respect belongings.
- Discuss sex practices that involve a condom or other barrier device, if appropriate.
- Discuss water-soluble lubricants with females; refer males for evaluation if erectile dysfunction is a concern.

Meeting Developmental Tasks

- Promote continued development and maintenance of functional health by identifying unmet tasks, feelings of isolation, and physical or sensory limitations.
- Assist in finding creative solutions to developmental tasks.
- Collaborate with other health care providers to provide information and referral to community resources for the patient and family.

Concept Mastery Alert

Nurses working with older adults must understand that many changes that are seen are the result of normal interactions and processes of the body. This knowledge is broader than just having knowledge of illness and the older adult.

An older adult who requires surgery or medical treatment for chronic or acute illness has special, age-related needs regardless of the setting for care. Nursing care to meet age-related and developmental needs in any setting is outlined in Box 24-8. Although nursing care adapted to the needs of older adults is described throughout this text, general principles for care are included here. Nurses must recognize physiologic and psychosocial interrelationships and view older adults holistically. See the accompanying display, Examples of Actual or Potential Health Problems and Needs: Older Adult on page 656.

Illness can severely disrupt an older adult's ability to function independently. The ill patient is under increased physical and emotional stress, which increases the risk for complications because of the lack of physiologic reserves. When a patient is hospitalized or institutionalized, family and community interactions are severely inhibited. The acute care environment itself adds new stressors such as diagnostic tests, treatments, and surgery. In the face of new and unfamiliar routines and sensory stimulation, prior coping skills may not work, and an older adult may feel less able to understand and control the new environment. An older adult is more likely than a younger patient to suffer multisystem dysfunctions,

Examples of Actual or Potential Health Problems and Needs

OLDER ADULT

Actual or Potential Health Problem or Need	Possible Etiologic Factors	Potential Signs and Symptoms
Impaired Older Adult Development	• Inability to maintain or establish ties with friends, family, and acquaintances • Difficulty finding a place in life • Comorbidities affecting daily functional ability • Lack of control over finances, living situation, or other required resources	• Disturbed sleep pattern • Disengagement from activities and people • Frequent ED visits or hospitalizations • Focus on deficits and effects of aging • Difficulty making required role transitions

Injury Risk	• Inadequate intake or poor nutritional value of food
	• Community immunization level
	• Community resource deficit or lack of ability to access existing sources of support
	  • Unsafe or abusive living situation
	  • Social isolation secondary to transportation, social, financial, or community issues
		—

Readiness for Effective Spiritual Status	—	• Articulates contentment with status and life • Exhibits gerotranscendence • Has a sustained purpose in life • Adapts to expected and unexpected changes associated with aging and loss • Identifies sources of support, resources in the community, and mutually beneficial interactions with others

Source: International Council of Nurses (ICN). (2019). *Nursing diagnosis and outcome statements.* https://www.icn.ch/sites/default/files/inline-files/ICNP2019-DC.pdf; Wolters Kluwer. (2022). *Problem-based care plans.* In Lippincott Advisor. Wolters Kluwer. https://advisor.lww.com/lna/home.do

iatrogenic complications (caused by medications or treatments), delirium, increasing dependence with changes in their baseline, and accidents such as falls. Hospitalization of an older adult can also substantially accelerate cognitive decline.

The focus of nursing care is to assist older adults to function as independently as possible and to support their individual strengths. The nurse collaborates with the family and other members of the caregiving team to prevent complications of illness, to secure a safe and comfortable environment, and to promote the patient's return to health.

CARING FOR AN AGING POPULATION

Medical advances have enabled older adult and frail patients with serious and chronic illnesses and disabilities to survive much longer than they could in the past. American society faces the dilemma of how to care for this population. Already, millions of American families are struggling nobly to provide steady and demanding long-term care for their incapacitated loved ones, often with little respite or communal support, and usually for many years. It seems unlikely that increasing paid caregiving will be able to alleviate the growing strains on family caregivers. The pool of workers available for paid home health care is shrinking. Factors reducing the number of home health aides and nurses include the strenuousness of the work involved, inadequate financial compensation, difficult relationships with patients, language and cultural barriers, an aging nursing workforce, and the lack of health insurance and other benefits. Caring for older adults is complicated, but rewarding. The challenge for nurses is to incorporate the patient and family into the team and then work to identify, implement, and evaluate strategies to promote health and diminish or postpone frailty in this older population.

DEVELOPING CLINICAL REASONING AND CLINICAL JUDGMENT

1. Complete the following sentences, then analyze the reasons for your answers:
   a. When my parents can no longer care for themselves, I will ____________.
   b. If my parents were living in a long-term care facility, I would want the nurses to ____________.
   c. When I am old, I want my family to ____________.
2. Consider your own family. Can you identify developmental tasks for family members who are middle-aged adults and older adults? What factors in your family facilitate or impede meeting these tasks?

PRACTICING FOR NCLEX

1. A nurse caring for older adults in a provider's office researches aging theories to help determine why some people age more rapidly than others. Which statements describe the immunity theory of the aging process? Select all that apply.

a. Immunosenescence likely promotes the increase in infections in the older adult.
b. Free radicals have adverse effects on adjacent molecules.
c. Decreases in size and function of the thymus result in more infections.
d. Nutrition likely plays an important role in maintaining the immune response.
e. Lifespan depends to a great extent on genetic factors.
f. Organisms wear out from increased metabolic functioning.

2. A nursing student caring for older adults in a skilled nursing facility is completing an assignment identifying physical changes that are part of normal aging. What changes will the student include in this assignment? Select all that apply.
   a. Fatty tissue is redistributed.
   b. Skin is drier and wrinkles appear.
   c. Cardiac output increases.
   d. Muscle mass increases.
   e. Hormone production increases.
   f. Visual and hearing acuity diminishes.
3. A nurse researcher interviews adults to validate Erikson's theory that middle-aged adults who do not achieve their developmental tasks may be in the stage of stagnation. Which patient statement will the nurse correlate to this theory?
   a. "I am helping my parents move into an assisted-living facility."
   b. "I spend all of my time going to the doctor to be sure I am not sick."
   c. "I have enough money to help my son and his wife when they need it."
   d. "I earned this gray hair and I like it!"
4. A nurse providing health services for a community setting for people age 55 years and older considers health problems for these residents. Which of the following problems is most appropriate for many middle-aged adults?
   a. Adequate nutrition
   b. Mental health problems
   c. Abuse
   d. Caregiver role strain
5. The charge nurse in a long-term care facility discusses ageism with new nurse employees. Nurses are asked to intervene if they observe which of these examples demonstrating ageism?
   a. The AP encourages older adults to apply makeup or aftershave to promote positive self-image.
   b. The activity director explains to an older adult they could learn to use video conferencing to speak to their grandchildren.
   c. A nurse colleague states that older adult should not think about having a boyfriend or girlfriend after age 70 years.
   d. A nurse recognizes the patient who lost their partner of 45 years may be experiencing loneliness.
6. A nurse is caring for older adults in a senior adult day services (ADS) center. Which findings require follow up with the health care provider?
   a. Skin pigmentation caused by exposure to sun over the years
   b. Thin toenails with a bluish tint to the nail beds
   c. Using a walker while healing from a hip fracture related to brittle bones
   d. Bruising on forearms due to fragile blood vessels in the dermis
7. A nursing instructor teaching a gerontology class to nursing students discusses myths related to the aging of adults. Which statement will the students identify as a myth about older adults?
   a. Most older adults live in their own homes.
   b. Healthy older adults enjoy sexual activity.
   c. Aging results in mental deterioration.
   d. Older adults want to be attractive to others.
8. A nurse is helping to prepare a calendar for an older adult patient with cognitive impairment. Which type of cognitive impairment is non-reversible?
   a. Post-stroke speech issues
   b. Malnutrition
   c. Alzheimer's disease
   d. Loss of cardiac reserve
9. A nurse caring for an older adult living in a long-term care facility uses reminiscence to help the patient adapt to the changes of aging. The nurse uses which question to encourage reminiscence?
   a. "Tell me about how you celebrated Christmas when you were young."
   b. "Tell me how you plan to spend your time this weekend."
   c. "Did you enjoy the choral group that performed here yesterday?
   d. "Why don't you want to talk about your feelings?"
10. Following a fall that left an older adult temporarily bedridden, the nurse is using the SPICES assessment tool to evaluate for cascade iatrogenesis. Which are correct aspects of this tool? Select all that apply.
    a. S—Senility
    b. P—Problems with feeding
    c. I—Irritability
    d. C—Confusion
    e. E—Edema of the legs
    f. S—Skin breakdown
11. The nurse in a long-term care facility states in report that an older adult resident is quite frail. The oncoming caregiver prioritizes prevention of what problem?
    a. Confusion
    b. Falls
    c. Delirium
    d. Dementia
12. A patient is admitted to the acute care medical center with change in mental status, dehydration, and electrolyte

imbalances. Which of these reflects a reversible cause of the changes in mental status?
a. Alzheimer's disease
b. Delirium
c. Dementia
d. Delirium superimposed on dementia

ANSWERS WITH RATIONALES

1. **a, c, d.** The immunity theory of aging focuses on the functions of the immune system and states that the immune response declines steadily after younger adulthood as the thymus loses size and function, resulting in more infections. Vitamin supplements (such as vitamin E) may improve immune function. The cross-linkage theory proposed that a chemical reaction produces damage to the DNA and cell death. The free radical theory states that free radicals—molecules with separated high-energy electrons—formed during cellular metabolism can have adverse effects on adjacent molecules. The genetic theory of aging holds that lifespan depends to a great extent on genetic factors. According to the wear-and-tear theory, organisms wear out from increased metabolic functioning, and cells become exhausted from continual energy depletion from adapting to stressors.
2. **a, b, f.** Physical changes occurring with aging include these: fatty tissue is redistributed, the skin is drier and wrinkles appear, and visual and hearing acuity diminishes. Cardiac output decreases, muscle mass decreases (sarcopenia), and hormone production decreases, causing menopause or andropause.
3. **b.** According to Erikson (1963), the middle adult is in a period of generativity versus stagnation. The tasks are to establish and guide the next generation, accept middle-age changes, adjust to the needs of aging parents, and reevaluate goals and accomplishments. Middle adults who do not reach generativity tend to become overly concerned about their own physical and emotional health needs.
4. **d.** Many middle-aged adults help care for aging parents and have concerns about their own health and ability to continue to care for an older family member. Caregivers often face 24-hour care responsibilities for extended periods of time, which creates physical and emotional problems for the caregiver. Nutritional issues are more common in the childhood years and possibly in older adults. Mental health issues and abuse can occur in multiple age groups.
5. **c.** *Ageism* is a form of prejudice in which older adults are stereotyped by characteristics found in only some of their age group. The other statements are positive, building on the older adults' strengths and resilience.
6. **b.** Older adults' toenails may become thicker (not thinner), with a yellowish tint (not a bluish tint) to the nail beds; a blue tint may indicate hypoxemia. Exposure to sun over the years can cause older adults' skin to be pigmented. Bone demineralization occurs with aging, causing bones to become porous and brittle, making fractures more common. The blood vessels in the dermis become more fragile, causing an increase in bruising and purpura.
7. **c.** Although response time may be longer, intelligence does not normally decrease because of aging. Most older adults live in their own homes. Although sexual activity may be less frequent, the ability to perform and enjoy sexual activity lasts well into the 90s in healthy older adults. Older adults want to be attractive to others.
8. **c.** Alzheimer's disease causes progressive, irreversible cognitive impairment. It is the most common degenerative neurologic illness and the most common cause of cognitive impairment. With therapeutic intervention, speech therapy, proper diet, and pharmacologic intervention, the other problems can be managed and potentially improved.
9. **a.** Use of life review or reminiscence encourages reflection; the older adult can restructure life experiences and better adapt to life circumstances. Asking about a recent event, upcoming plans, or feelings would be unlikely to encourage reminiscence.
10. **b, d, f.** The SPICES acronym is used to identify common problems in older adults and stands for:
    S—Sleep disorders
    P—Problems with eating or feeding
    I—Incontinence
    C—Confusion
    E—Evidence of falls
    S—Skin breakdown
11. **b.** Fear of falling, indicators of frailty, and personality traits of high neuroticism and low conscientiousness contribute to falls in older adults. Falling once doubles the chance of the older adult falling again.
12. **b.** Delirium, an acute syndrome of brain failure, can last from hours to weeks, has a specific cause, and resolves with treatment of the identified underlying cause. Symptoms of delirium include deficits in attention, awareness, and cognition. Dementia refers to various organic disorders affecting cognitive function that are progressive and irreversible.

Bibliography

AARP. (2019, October 28). National agencies, groups and organizations for caregivers. https://www.aarp.org/caregiving/local/info-2019/national-resources-for-caregivers.html?cmp=RDRCT-9f9c190c-20210202
Administration for Community Living. (2021, May). *2020 profile of older Americans*. U.S. Department of Health and Human Services. https://acl.gov/sites/default/files/Aging%20and%20Disability%20in%20America/2020ProfileOlderAmericans.Final_.pdf
American Association of Colleges of Nursing (AACN). (2021, April 6). *The essentials: Core competencies for professional nursing education*. https://www.aacnnursing.org/Portals/42/AcademicNursing/pdf/Essentials-2021.pdf
American College of Obstetricians and Gynecologists (ACOG). (2017/2021). *Breast cancer risk assessment and screening in average-risk women*. Practice Bulletin No. 179. https://www.acog.org/clinical/clinical-guidance/practice-bulletin/articles/2017/07/breast-cancer-risk-assessment-and-screening-in-average-risk-women
American Cancer Society. (2019). *Cancer facts & figures for African Americans 2019–2021*. https://www.cancer.org/research/cancer-facts-statistics/cancer-facts-figures-for-african-americans.html
American Cancer Society (ACS). (2021). *American Cancer Socierty guideline for colorectal cancer screening for people at average risk*. https://www.cancer.org/cancer/colon-rectal-cancer/detection-diagnosis-staging/acs-recommendations.html
American Cancer Society (ACS). (2021). *Cancer screening guidelines by age*. https://www.cancer.org/healthy/find-cancer-early/screening-recommendations-by-age.html#All_ages
Bellelli, G., Brathwaite, J. S., & Mazzola, P. (2021). Delirium: A marker of vulnerability in older people. *Frontiers in Aging Neuroscience*, *13*, 626127. https://doi.org/10.3389/fnagi.2021.626127
Boing, A. F., Boing, A. C., Cordes, J., Kim, R., & Subramanian, S. V. (2020). Quantifying and explaining variation in life expectancy at census tract, county, and state levels in the United States. *Proceedings of the National Academy of Sciences of the United States of America*, *117*(30), 17688–17694. https://doi.org/10.1073/pnas.2003719117
Bromfield, S. G., Ngameni, C. A., Colantonio, L. D., Bowling, C. B., Shimbo, D., Reynolds, K., Safford, M. M., Banach, M., Toth, P. P., & Muntner, P. (2017). Blood pressure, antihypertensive polypharmacy, frailty, and risk for serious fall injuries among older treated adults with hypertension. *Hypertension*, *70*(2), 259–266. https://doi.org/10.1161/HYPERTENSIONAHA.116.09390
Canada, B., Stephan, Y., Sutin, A. R., & Terracciano, A. (2020). Personality and falls among older adults: Evidence from a longitudinal cohort. *The Journals of Gerontology. Series B, Psychological Sciences*

and Social Sciences, 75(9), 1905–1910. https://doi.org/10.1093/geronb/gbz040
Centers for Disease Control and Prevention (CDC). (2013). CDC health disparities and inequalities report—United States, 2013. *Morbidity and Mortality Weekly Report, 62*(3), 1–187. https://www.cdc.gov/minorityhealth/CHDIReport.html
Centers for Disease Control and Prevention (CDC). (2020a, July 9). *Cost of older adult falls.* https://www.cdc.gov/falls/data/fall-cost.html
Centers for Disease Control and Prevention (CDC). (2020b, December 10). *Introduction to COVID-19 racial and ethnic health disparities.* https://www.cdc.gov/coronavirus/2019-ncov/community/health-equity/racial-ethnic-disparities/index.html
Centers for Disease Control and Prevention (CDC). (2021a). *Elder abuse resources.* https://www.cdc.gov/violenceprevention/pdf/elder/preventingElderAbuseFactsheet.pdf
Centers for Disease Control and Prevention (CDC). (2021b, February 11). *Health of Asian or Pacific Islander population.* https://www.cdc.gov/nchs/fastats/asian-health.htm
Centers for Disease Control and Prevention (CDC). (2021c, February 12). *Health, United States, 2019—Data finder.* https://www.cdc.gov/nchs/hus/contents2019.htm?search=,Hispanic_or_Latino
Centers for Disease Control and Prevention (CDC). (2021d, March 2). *Injury prevention & control: Leading causes of death and injury.* https://www.cdc.gov/injury/wisqars/LeadingCauses.html
Centers for Disease Control and Prevention (CDC). (2021e, March 26). *National Center for Health Statistics: Older persons' health.* https://www.cdc.gov/nchs/fastats/older-american-health.htm
Centers for Disease Control and Prevention (CDC). (2021f, May 7). *Racism and health.* https://www.cdc.gov/healthequity/racism-disparities/index.html
Centers for Disease Control and Prevention (CDC). (2021g, July 8). *Recommended immunization schedules for adults ages 19 years or older, United States, 2021.* https://www.cdc.gov/vaccines/schedules/hcp/adult.html
Chu, C. H., Donato-Woodger, S., & Dainton, C. J. (2020). Competing crises: COVID-19 countermeasures and social isolation among older adults in long-term care. *Journal of Advanced Nursing, 76*(10), 2456–2459. https://doi.org/10.1111/jan.14467
Dwyer-Lindgren, L., Bertozzi-Villa, A., Stubbs, R. W., Morozoff, C., Mackenbach, J. P., van Lenthe, F. J., Mokdad, A. H., & Murray, C. J. L. (2017). Inequalities in life expectancy among US counties, 1980 to 2014: Temporal trends and key drivers. *JAMA Internal Medicine, 177*(7), 1003–1011. https://doi.org/10.1001/jamainternmed.2017.0918
Eliopoulos, C. (2022). *Gerontological nursing* (10th ed.). Wolters Kluwer.
Erikson, E. H. (1963). *Childhood and society* (2nd ed.). W. W. Norton & Company, Inc.
Federal Interagency Forum on Aging-Related Statistics. (2020). *Older Americans 2020: Key indicators of well-being.* U.S. Government Printing Office. https://www.agingstats.gov/docs/LatestReport/OA20_508_10142020.pdf
FitzGerald, J. M., O'Regan, N., Adamis, D., Timmons, S., Dunne, C. P., Trzepacz, P. T., & Meagher, D. J. (2017). Sleep-wake cycle disturbances in elderly acute general medical inpatients: Longitudinal relationship to delirium and dementia. *Alzheimer's & Dementia (Amst), 7*, 61–68. https://doi.org/10.1016/j.dadm.2016.12.013
Fowler, J. W. (1981). *Stages of faith: The psychology of human development and the quest for meaning.* HarperCollins Publishers.
Fulmer, T. (2019). Fulmer SPICES: An overall assessment tool for older adults. *Hartford Institute for Geriatric Nursing, New York University College of Nursing, 1*, 1–2. https://hign.org/sites/default/files/2020-06/Try_This_General_Assessment_1.pdf
Gould, R. L. (1978). *Transformations: Growth and change in adult life.* Simon & Schuster.
Greenberg, S. A. (2012). The geriatric depression scale (GDS). *Hartford Institute for Geriatric Nursing, New York University College of Nursing, 4*, 1–2. https://wwwoundcare.ca/Uploads/ContentDocuments/Geriatric%20Depression%20Scale.pdf
Grossman, E. R., Benjamin-Neelon, S. E., & Sonnenschein, S. (2020). Alcohol consumption during the COVID-19 pandemic: A cross-sectional survey of US Adults. *International Journal of Environmental Research and Public Health, 17*(24), 9189. https://doi.org/10.3390/ijerph17249189
Hall, J., Karch, D. L., Crosby, A. (2016). *Elder abuse surveillance: Uniform definitions and recommended core data elements, Version 1.0.* National Center for Injury Prevention and Control, Centers for Disease Control and Prevention. https://www.cdc.gov/violenceprevention/elderabuse/index.html
Hastings, K. G., Jose, P. O., Kapphahn, K. I., Frank, A. T., Goldstein, B. A., Thompson, C. A., Eggleston, K., Cullen, M. R., & Palaniappan, L. P. (2015). Leading causes of death among Asian American subgroups (2003-2011). *PLoS One, 10*(4), e0124341. https://doi.org/10.1371/journal.pone.0124341
Havighurst, R. J. (1972). *Developmental tasks and education* (3rd ed.). David McKay.
He, W., Goodkind, D., & Kowal, P. (2016, March 28). *An aging world: 2015.* U.S. Census Bureau (Report No. P95/16-1). U.S. Government Publishing Office.
Indian Health Service. (2019, October). *Disparities.* https://www.ihs.gov/newsroom/factsheets/disparities/
International Association of Forensic Nurses. (2021). *Nursing response to elder mistreatment curriculum.* https://www.forensicnurses.org/page/AboutCurriculum
Jehu, D. A., Davis, J. C., Falck, R. S., Bennett, K. J., Tai, D., Souza, M. F., Cavalcante, B. R., Zhao, M., & Liu-Ambrose, T. (2021). Risk factors for recurrent falls in older adults: A systematic review with meta-analysis. *Maturitas, 144*, 23–28. https://doi.org/10.1016/j.maturitas.2020.10.021
Kinsey, J. D., & Nykamp, D. (2017). Dangers of nonprescription medicines: Educating and counseling older adults. *Consultant Pharmacist, 32*(5), 269–280. https://doi.org/10.4140/TCP.n.2017.269
Kohlberg, L. (1969). Stage and sequence: The cognitive–developmental approach to socialization. In D. A. Gaslin (Ed.). *Handbook of socialization: Theory and research* (pp. 347–380). Rand McNally.
Lee, D. C., Shook, R. P., Drenowatz, C., & Blair, S. N. (2016). Physical activity and sarcopenic obesity: Definition, assessment, prevalence and mechanism. *Future science OA, 2*(3), FSO127. https://doi.org/10.4155/fsoa-2016-0028
Levinson, D. J., Darrow, C. N., Klein, E. B., Levinson, M. H., & McKee, B. (1978). *The seasons of a man's life.* The Random House Publishing Group.
Logan, J. E., Haileyesus, T., Ertl, A., Rostad, W. L., & Herbst, J. H. (2019). Nonfatal assaults and homicides among adults aged ≥60 years – United States, 2002-2016. *Morbidity and Mortality Weekly Report, 68*(13), 297–302. https://doi.org/10.15585/mmwr.mm6813a1
Mangels, A. R. (2018). Malnutrition in older adults. *The American Journal of Nursing, 118*(3), 34–41. https://doi.org/10.1097/01.NAJ.0000530915.26091.be
Makino, K., Makizako, H., Doi, T., Tsutsumimoto, K., Hotta, R., Nakakubo, S., Suzuki, T., & Shimada, H. (2017). Fear of falling and gait parameters in older adults with and without fall history. *Geriatrics & Gerontology International, 17*(12), 2455–2459. https://doi.org/10.1111/ggi.13102
Mather, M., Scommegna, P., & Kilduff, L. (2019, July 15). *Aging in the United States.* https://www.prb.org/resources/fact-sheet-aging-in-the-united-states/
Mattison, M. L. P. (2020). Delirium. *Annals of Internal Medicine, 173*(7), ITC49–ITC64. https://doi.org/10.7326/AITC202010060
Miller, C. A. (2019). *Nursing for wellness in older adults* (8th ed.). Wolters Kluwer.
Moore, C., & Browne, C. V. (2016). Emerging innovations, best practices, and evidence-based practices in elder abuse and neglect: A review of recent developments in the field. *Journal of Family Violence, 32*, 383–397.
National Highway Traffic Safety Administration. (n.d.). *Talking with older drivers about safe driving.* Retrieved August 13, 2021, from https://one.nhtsa.gov/Driving-Safety/Older-Drivers/Talking-with-Older-Drivers-about-Safe-Driving
National Institute on Aging. (2021a, July 6). *Alzheimer disease fact sheet.* https://www.nia.nih.gov/alzheimers/publication/alzheimers-disease-fact-sheet
National Institute on Aging. (2021b, July 7). *Depression and older adults.* https://www.nia.nih.gov/health/depression-and-older-adults
National Osteoporosis Foundation. (2021). *Bone density exam/testing.* https://www.nof.org/patients/diagnosis-information/bone-density-examtesting
Pew Research Center. (2020, June 2). *The changing composition of the electorate and partisan coalitions.* https://www.pewresearch.org/politics/2020/06/02/the-changing-composition-of-the-electorate-and-partisan-coalitions/
Pollard, M. S., Tucker, J. S., & Green, H. D., Jr. (2020). Changes in adult alcohol use and consequences during the COVID-19 pandemic in the US. *JAMA Network Open, 3*(9), e2022942. https://doi.org/10.1001/jamanetworkopen.2020.22942
Sivertsen, B., Pallesen, S., Friborg, O., Nilsen, K. B., Bakke, Ø. K., Goll, J. B., & Hopstock, L. A. (2021). Sleep patterns and insomnia in a large population-based study of middle-aged and older adults: The Tromsø study 2015–2016. *Journal of Sleep Research, 30*(1), e13095. https://doi.org/10.1111/jsr.13095
Techboomers. (2018). *Learn how to use popular websites.* https://techboomers.com
Thom, R. P., Levy-Carrick, N. C., Bui, M., & Silbersweig, D. (2019). Delirium. *The American Journal of Psychiatry, 176*(10), 785–793. https://doi.org/10.1176/appi.ajp.2018.18070893
Tornstam, L. (1994). Gerotranscendence: A theoretical and empirical exploration. In L. E. Thomas, & S. A. Eisenhandler (Eds.). *Aging and the religious dimension* (pp. 203–225). Greenwood Publishing Group.
U.S. Census Bureau. (2019, December 10). *2020 census will help policymakers prepare for the incoming wave of aging boomers.* https://www.census.gov/library/stories/2019/12/by-2030-all-baby-boomers-will-be-age-65-or-older.html
U. S. Census Bureau. (2021, July 1). *Quick facts: United States.* https://www.census.gov/quickfacts/US
U. S. Department of Health and Human Services: Office of Minority Health. (2021, April). *Profile: Native Hawaiians/Pacific Islanders.* https://minorityhealth.hhs.gov/omh/browse.aspx?lvl=3&lvlid=65
U.S. Department of Justice. (n.d.). *Elder justice initiative (EJI): About elder abuse.* Retrieved March 27, 2022, from https://www.justice.gov/elderjustice/about-elder-abuse
Virani, S. S., Alonso, A., Aparicio, H. J., Benjamin, E. J., Bittencourt, M. S., Callaway, C. W., Carson, A. P., Chamberlain, A. M., Cheng, S., Delling, F. N., Elkind, M. S. V., Evenson, K. R., Ferguson, J. F., Gupta, D. K., Khan, S. S., Kissela, B. M., Knutson, K. L., Lee, C. D., Lewis, T. T., … American Heart Association Council on Epidemiology and Prevention Statistics Committee and Stroke Statistics Subcommittee. (2021). Heart disease and stroke statistics-2021 update: A report from the American Heart Association. *Circulation, 143*(8), e254–e743. https://doi.org/10.1161/CIR.0000000000000950
Wan, M., & Chase, J. M. (2017). Delirium in older adults: Diagnosis, prevention, and treatment. *British Columbia Medical Journal, 59*(3), 165–170. https://bcmj.org/articles/delirium-older-adults-diagnosis-prevention-and-treatment
Weerakoon, S. M., Jetelina, K. K., & Knell, G. (2021). Longer time spent at home during COVID-19 pandemic is associated with binge drinking among US adults. *The American Journal of Drug and Alcohol Abuse, 47*(1), 98–106. https://doi.org/10.1080/00952990.2020.1832508
Whitehead, B. R., & Torossian, E. (2021). Older adults' experience of the COVID-19 pandemic: A mixed-methods analysis of stresses and joys. *The Gerontologist, 61*(1), 36–47. https://doi.org/10.1093/geront/gnaa126
World Health Organization. (2021a, March 18). *Ageism is a global challenge: UN.* https://www.who.int/news/item/18-03-2021-ageism-is-a-global-challenge-un
World Health Organization. (2021b, June 15). *Elder abuse.* https://www.who.int/news-room/fact-sheets/detail/elder-abuse
Yevchak, A., Fick, D. M., Kolanowski, A. M., McDowell, J., Monroe, T., LeViere, A., & Mion, L. (2017). Implementing nurse-facilitated person-centered care approaches for patients with delirium superimposed on dementia in the acute care setting. *Journal of Gerontological Nursing, 43*(12), 21–28. https://doi.org/10.3928/00989134-20170623-01
Yon, Y., Mikton, C. R., Gassoumis, Z. D., & Wilber, K. H. (2017). Elder abuse prevalence in community settings: A systematic review and meta-analysis. *The Lancet Global Health, 5*(2), e147–e156. https://doi.org/10.1016/S2214-109X(17)30006-2

UNIT V

Actions Basic to Nursing Care

Unit V focuses on the actions basic to practice—the nursing interventions planned, implemented, and evaluated to meet the health care needs of diverse patients across the lifespan, at any point along the health–illness continuum, and in all settings. Nursing interventions discussed in this unit include reducing and preventing transmission of pathogens, assessing vital signs, conducting a health history and physical assessment, maintaining safety, integrating complementary health approaches and integrative health concepts, administering medications, and providing perioperative care.

Chapter 25 explains medical and surgical aseptic techniques necessary to prevent and control the spread of microorganisms. Chapter 26 describes assessing vital signs, and Chapter 27 discusses conducting a health history and physical assessment. Nursing assessment is both an art and a science. The art of performing a skill is integrated into the science of nursing so that variations from normal are identified and evaluated, and necessary nursing interventions are implemented. The findings from assessments provide a database necessary to maintain or restore health and promote wellness.

Nurses are responsible for meeting basic human needs for physical safety and security. Chapter 28 discusses promoting environmental safety (including threats from bioterrorism), identifying risk factors for patients at any age, and implementing teaching and other nursing actions to prevent accidents. Chapter 29 discusses complementary health approaches and integrative health concepts, an ever-increasing component of health care.

Chapters 30 and 31 focus on collaborative and independent nursing interventions used to accurately and safely administer medications and provide perioperative care. In most instances, the advanced-practice professional prescribes the medications, and the surgeon performs the surgery. The nurse implements nursing interventions to promote patient safety and knowledge, and to facilitate optimal function or recovery in both hospital and community settings. Although facility procedures and protocols are often used in these situations, nursing interventions are individualized to the unique needs of each person requiring care.

"Our intent when we lay hands on the patient in bodily care is to comfort."

Lydia Hall (1906–1969), *an innovator in nursing practice, developed the theory that the direct nurse-to-patient relationship is itself therapeutic and that nursing care is the chief therapy for critically ill patients.*

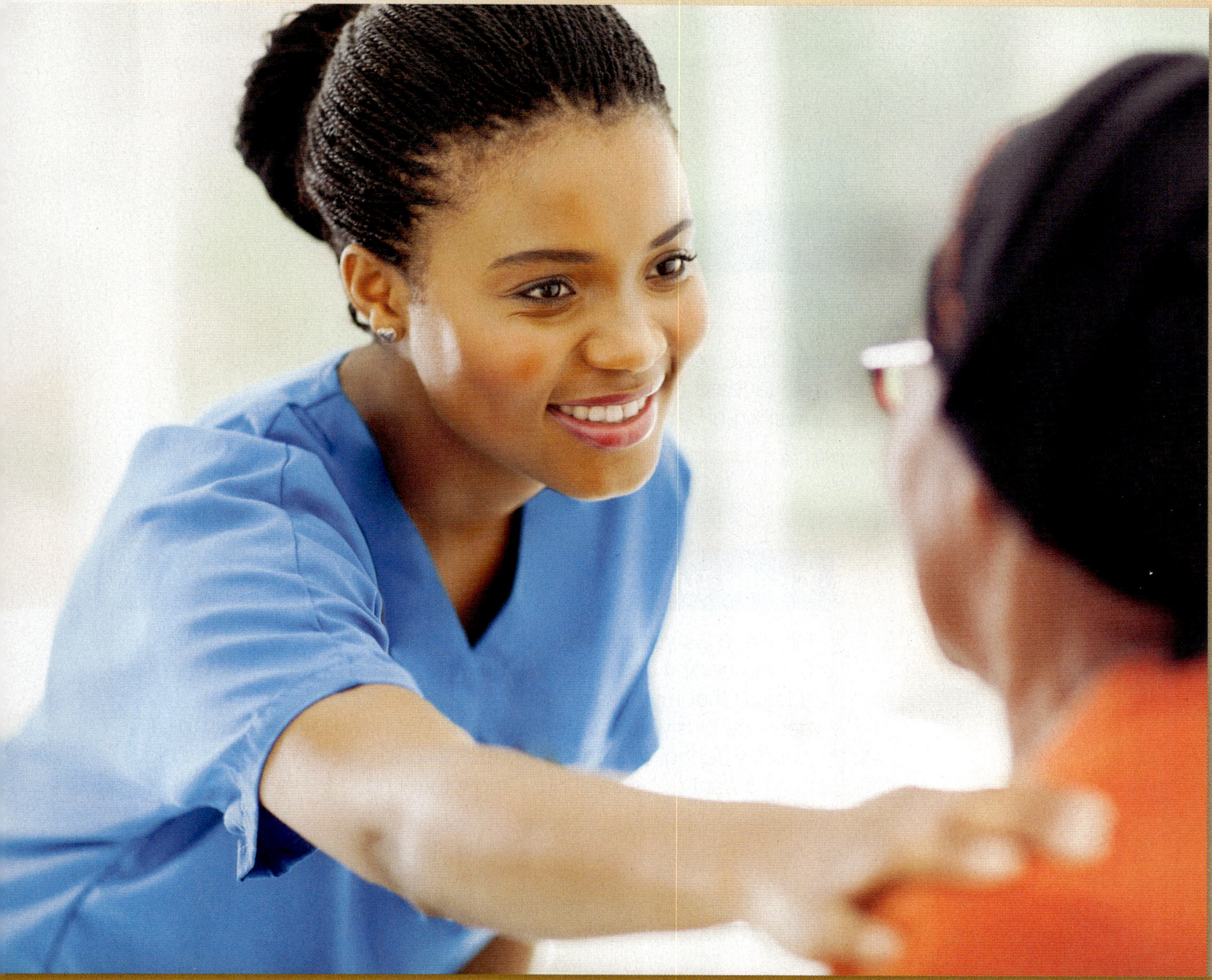

25 Asepsis and Infection Control

Jackson Ray Ivers

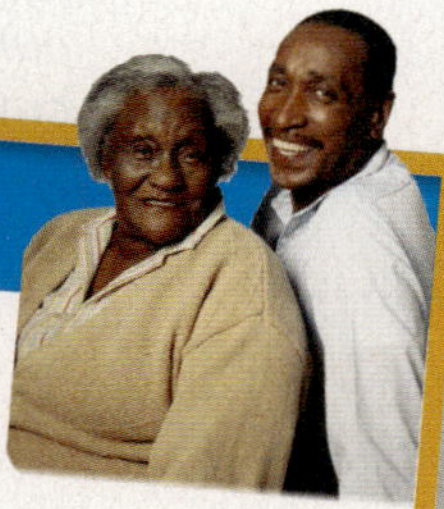

Jackson Ray comes to visit his mother, who has been hospitalized for a new-onset fever and cough after exposure to a friend with a highly communicable respiratory virus. He notices a sign on the door to check at the nurse's desk before entering. He asks, "What's going on? Why do I have to wash my hands and wear a mask?"

Esther Bailey

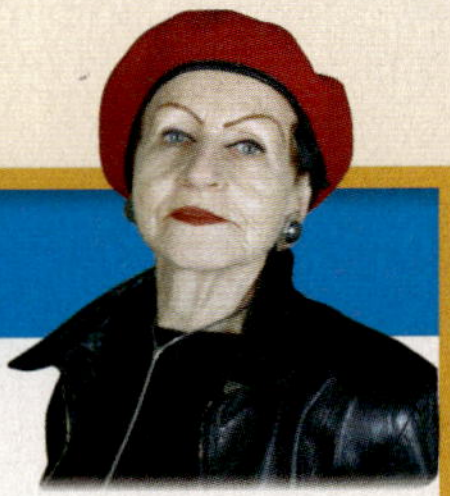

Esther, a 72-year-old patient has developed a postoperative wound infection after abdominal surgery. She also demonstrates new-onset, postoperative urinary retention and an inability to void. The standard of care in this situation requires insertion of an indwelling urinary catheter.

Giselle Turheis

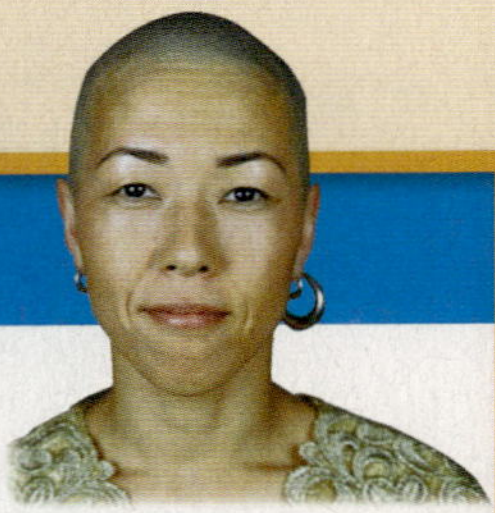

Giselle, a 38-year-old woman undergoing chemotherapy treatment for leukemia, states, "I know that my risk for infection is really high because of my poor immune status. But how do I respond to my Sunday school students, who are used to greeting me with a big hug? I want to be safe, but I know that I need these hugs too!"

Learning Outcomes

After completing the chapter, you will be able to accomplish the following:

1. Explain the infection cycle.
2. List the stages of an infection.
3. Identify patients at risk for developing an infection.
4. Describe nursing interventions used to break the chain of infection.
5. Identify situations in which hand hygiene is indicated.
6. Identify multidrug-resistant organisms that are prevalent in hospitalized patients and community settings.
7. List actual and potential problems and needs for a patient who has or is at risk for infection.
8. Describe strategies for implementing CDC guidelines for standard and transmission-based precautions when caring for patients.
9. Implement recommended techniques for medical and surgical asepsis.

Nursing Concepts

- Evidence-based practice
- Immunity
- Infection
- Inflammation
- Safety

A major concern for health care providers is the danger of spreading microorganisms from person to person and from place to place. Microorganisms are naturally present in almost all environments. Not all microorganisms are harmful—it depends on the type of organism, its location, the **host** (living being where an infectious, parasitic, or pathogenic agent resides and receives sustenance), and the circumstances. The Centers for Disease Prevention and Control (CDC, 2019g) defines **antimicrobials** as "drugs that treat infections by killing or slowing the growth of microbes causing infection.... bacterial infections are treated with drugs called antibiotics" (p. 7). Although *antimicrobial* and *antibiotic* are occasionally used interchangeably, antimicrobials technically include antifungals and drugs that treat parasites and viruses.

Government facilities at the international, national, state, and local levels, health care personnel, and laypeople recognize the need for an organized, systematic approach to the control of infections. For example, the CDC is the US government facility responsible for investigating, preventing, and controlling disease. Efforts by these facilities and people include mass immunization programs, laws concerning safe sewage disposal, regulations for the control of communicable diseases, and hospital infection–surveillance programs. Medical science continues to grapple with problems caused by increasingly virulent organisms that have become drug resistant, and problems related to patients who are vulnerable, including those who are immunologically compromised.

Prevention of infection is a major focus for nurses. The Quality and Safety Education for Nurses (QSEN Institute, 2020) initiative has identified safety as one of the leading issues in health care. The focus on safety includes effective infection control practices. As primary caregivers, nurses are involved in identifying, preventing, controlling, and teaching the patient about infection (see the accompanying Reflective Practice box on page 664). Applying infection prevention and control principles is the first critical step in breaking the cycle of infection.

INFECTION

Infection Cycle

An **infection** is a disease state that results from the presence of **pathogens** (disease-producing microorganisms) in or on the body. An infection occurs as a result of a cyclic process, consisting of six components, as shown in Figure 25-1 (on page 665). These components are:

- Infectious agent
- Reservoir
- Portal of exit
- Means of transmission
- Portals of entry
- Susceptible host

Infectious Agent

Some of the more prevalent agents that cause infection are bacteria, viruses, and fungi. **Bacteria**, the most significant and most commonly observed infection-causing agents in health care institutions, can be categorized in various ways. They are categorized by shape: spherical (cocci), rod shaped (bacilli), or corkscrew shaped (spirochetes). Bacteria can be categorized as either gram positive or gram negative based on their reaction to the Gram stain. For example, gram-positive bacteria have a thick cell wall that resists decolorization (loss of color) and are stained violet. However, gram-negative bacteria have chemically more complex cell walls and can be decolorized by alcohol. Thus, gram-negative bacteria do not stain. This information is crucial for providers when prescribing the most appropriate antibiotic therapy because antibiotics are classified as specifically effective against only gram-positive organisms or as broad spectrum and effective against several groups of microorganisms. Another distinguishing characteristic of (or way of categorizing) bacteria is their need for oxygen. Most bacteria require oxygen to live and grow and are, therefore, referred to as **aerobic**. Those that can live without oxygen are **anaerobic** bacteria.

A **virus** is the smallest of all microorganisms, visible only with an electron microscope. Viruses cause many infections, including the common cold, hepatitis A, B, and C (Centers for Disease Control and Prevention [CDC], 2020d), and human immunodeficiency virus (HIV). Antibiotics have no effect on viruses. However, there are some antiviral medications that decrease the severity and duration of viral

QSEN Reflective Practice: Cultivating QSEN Competencies

CHALLENGE TO ETHICAL AND LEGAL SKILLS

This is my last clinical rotation before graduation, and it has been a difficult year. My focus has been somewhat lacking for a while, and I haven't been as prepared as I should have been for my clinical and classroom experiences. My clinical instructor has been on my case for the last few weeks. I'm also realizing that in no time at all I will be out of school and providing patient care on my own. So, all of a sudden, I'm eager for as many clinical experiences as I can get. To make a long story short, I'm thrilled when offered the opportunity to catheterize Esther Bailey, a 72-year-old female patient on my unit. I quickly review the procedure and go to the patient's room, with the catheterization supplies in hand, feeling semi-confident. After introducing my clinical instructor and myself, and explaining what I'm about to do, I open the sterile package, prepare the sterile field, and cleanse the meatus. All of a sudden, as the patient asks a question and diverts my instructor's gaze, I realize (to my horror!) that I've contaminated the catheter. I've got a split second to decide what to do. I can tell my instructor what happened, obtain a new kit, and proceed anew, or pretend nothing happened and continue. After everything that has been drilled into us about the importance of sterility and the consequences of health care–associated infections (HAIs), I don't like that I'm even considering not admitting the mistake. But I'm also aware that it is time to leave the unit and the rest of the group is waiting for post-conference. Plus, after all, there are financial costs to obtaining another tray. But what if I do not admit the error and the instructor did see me contaminate the catheter? I run the risk of violating our university honor code!

Thinking Outside the Box: Possible Courses of Action

- Obviously the simplest solution: admit my error and accept the consequences.
- Request a new catheter and inform my instructor later that the patient moved just as I was preparing to enter the meatus (a bit of deception but this makes the error not MY fault).
- Alternatively, pretend that nothing happened and pray that no harm comes to the patient. (After all, how much bacteria do you need to contaminate a catheter? The patient is receiving antibiotic therapy postoperatively anyway.)
- Continue and not even be bothered by the contamination. (Life is one big risk for everyone, right? All that matters is that you take care of yourself first.)

Evaluating a Good Outcome: How Do I Define Success?

- Patient benefited from my actions or, at the very least, was not harmed.
- No one's integrity is compromised or sacrificed.
- No violations of the standards of practice or our nursing code of ethics (American Nurses Association [ANA], 2015) occurred.

Personal Learning: Here's to the Future!

At least I can say there was a happy ending to this story. I did stop, explain what happened, and waited while someone ran for a new catheterization tray. Amazingly, my instructor told me later that she valued my maturity, honesty, and ability to put the needs of the patient ahead of my own needs, stating that I "might just have what it takes after all!" I'm not sure how often I'll be called upon to put the needs of a patient ahead of my own needs, but hopefully I'll be ready to respond selflessly each time.

QSEN SELF-REFLECTION ON QUALITY AND SAFETY COMPETENCIES DEVELOPING KNOWLEDGE, SKILLS, AND ATTITUDES FOR CONTINUOUS IMPROVEMENT

How do you think you would respond in a similar situation? Why? Do you agree with the criteria that the nursing student used to evaluate a successful outcome? Why or why not? What *knowledge, skills,* and *attitudes* do you need to develop to continuously improve quality and safety when caring for patients like Mrs. Bailey?

Patient-Centered Care: What information regarding this procedure needs to be communicated to the patient? Does Mrs. Bailey understand why the urinary catheter is being inserted and the preferred target time for its removal?

Teamwork and Collaboration/Quality Improvement: What communication skills do you need to provide clear, comprehensive information to Mrs. Bailey? Did you explain to Mrs. Bailey why there was a pause in the procedure? Was your request for the additional supplies clearly and respectfully communicated to a team member? How was the charge/billing for the additional supplies handled?

Safety/Evidence-Based Practice: Is there anything you could have done to anticipate the unexpected? How do you think your response affected the situation? What evidence in nursing literature provides guidance for decision making regarding infection control?

Informatics: Can you identify the essential information that must be available in Mrs. Bailey's electronic record to support safe patient care? Is it important to electronically document daily the reasons why the urinary catheter is still in place?

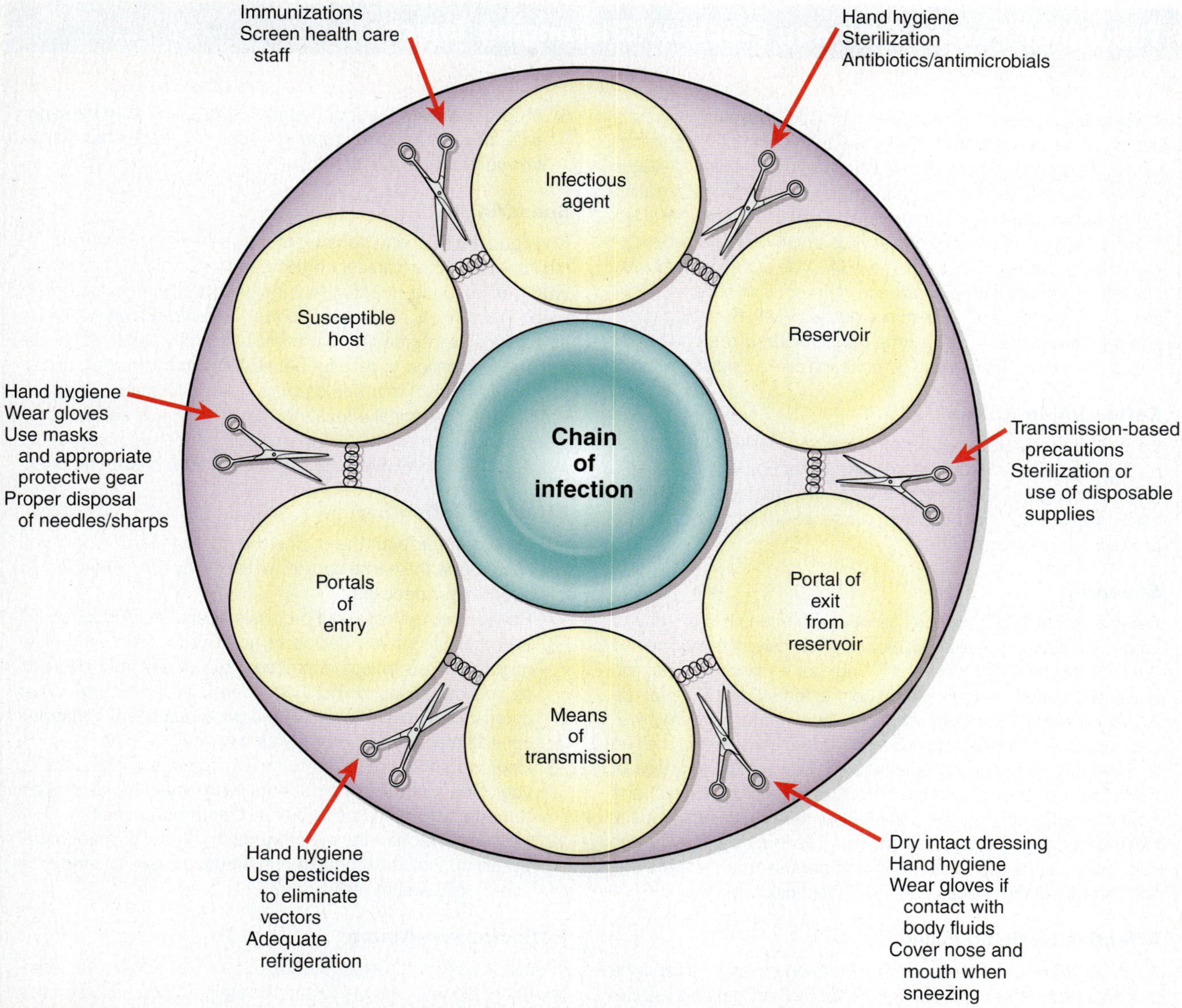

FIGURE 25-1. The infection cycle is demonstrated as a chain. The goal is to break the links of the chain to end the cycle. (*Source:* Adapted from Murphy, D. [1998]. Infectious microbes and disease: General principles. *Nursing Spectrum*, *7*[2], 12–14.)

infections such as influenza. The exact antiviral prescribed varies depending on the strain of influenza most prevalent in a given season and does not replace annual immunization (*flu shot*; CDC, 2019b). When given in the prodromal stage (infection/disease has begun, but the symptoms are just beginning and may be vague), antivirals can shorten the course of the illness with certain viruses such as herpes simplex virus type 1 (HSV-1; cold sores). With HIV specifically, antiretroviral therapy (ART) regimens are initiated as soon as possible after diagnosis because they effectively disturb the life cycle of the virus to block HIV replication and, ultimately, render the virus undetectable (Saag, 2019).

Fungi, plantlike organisms (molds and yeasts) that also can cause infection, are present in the air, soil, and water. Some examples of infections caused by fungi include athlete's foot, ringworm, and yeast infections. These infections are treated with antifungal medications; however, many infections due to fungi are resistant to treatment. **Parasites** are organisms that live on or in a host and rely on it for nourishment. Malaria is a serious disease that occurs when a parasite infects a certain type of mosquito that then feeds on humans.

Not all organisms to which a person is exposed cause disease. An organism's potential to produce disease in a person depends on a variety of factors, including:

- Number of organisms
- **Virulence** of the organism, or its ability to cause disease
- Competence of the person's immune system
- Length and intimacy (extent) of the contact between the person and the microorganism

IDENTIFICATION OF INFECTIOUS AGENTS

Identifying the type of infection and infectious agent is not always an easy process. Sometimes new diseases appear, and health care workers race to identify them so that treatment can begin. This is the process that occurred with AIDS and with severe acute respiratory syndrome (SARS). Other times, a disease that is **endemic** (occurs with predictability in one specific region or population) can appear in a different

Thoughtful Person-Centered Practice: Challenging Topics

Pandemic Considerations

Nursing is a profession. Among the hallmarks of professions are a certain degree of altruism and the quality of being self-regulating. When the coronavirus presented globally and in the United States in 2020, nurses were understandably on the frontlines of caring for the public. They cared for those who had contracted the virus, those at high risk of contracting the virus, and those who had exposure to persons with COVID-19. The ANA *Code of Ethics for Nurses* instructs nurses that our primary commitment is to patients, while at the same time telling us we have duties to self. Balancing these primary commitments during the pandemic became particularly stressful for many nurses and other health care professionals.

Reflection-in-Action

As you read, think about what the nurse needs to consider, both personally and professionally. What were the nurse's original thoughts? What factors were weighed in the decision making process? How did the nurse prioritize personal and professional responsibilities?

Scenario

Carol, a critical care nurse practitioner with three children, one of whom is a newborn, got a call to come back to work early. She had 3 weeks of maternity leave remaining, but a coworker was self-quarantining after feeling sick and getting tested, and the practice was short-staffed. Carol's husband was an emergency room physician already working extra shifts. If she went back to work, she had to think about how to stay safe (she knew about the shortage of personal protective equipment [PPE], N95 masks, gowns, etc.) and how to arrange care for her children. Her oldest was age 4 years. Her mother, age 65 years, was going to help, but this was now too risky given her mother's history of lung disease. Her mother's age and chronic condition put her in the highest-risk category.

Effective Noticing (Cues)

1. What did you notice about the situation initially? What information/observations are significant? What makes this situation different from a regular work assignment?

Effective Interpreting

2. How would you describe the obligations Carol has to "the patients who need her," her employer and team members, her family, herself, others?
3. If she cannot fulfill each of these obligations, how should she prioritize them? What basis/rationale would you use for prioritization?

Scenario

Remember that the ANA *Code of Ethics for Nurses* reminds us that "the nurse's primary commitment is to the patient," while at the same time states that "the nurse owes the same duties to self as to others, including the responsibility to promote health and safety, preserve wholeness of character and integrity, maintain competence, and continue personal and professional growth. In order to calculate her risk Carol needs to know more about the coronavirus and COVID-19. She also needs to know how to stay safe at work.

Effective Responding

4. Where is the best place to turn for guidelines? What resources should she tap?
5. If Carol believes that her hospital lacks the PPE to keep her safe, how should she respond? Does this lessen her obligation to work for this employer?

Scenario

Carol and her husband debated the pros and cons of her returning to work. After careful consideration, Carol, in partnership with her husband, made the anguished decision to return to work. "I know my patients need me." She would put whatever safeguards were needed to protect her family and loved ones, but she was called to care for her patients in this hugely uncertain time of need. In times of crisis, resource scarcity and the associated intentional allocation may become a serious consideration. The weight of a prolonged pandemic also affects individual and collective decision making and tolerance of risk.

Effective Reflecting

6. Do you agree with the choice the nurse made? Would you have made the same choice, why or why not? What would inform your decision?
7. How do you evaluate your professional and moral judgments?
8. Whether or not you decide to go back to work early, how might you use reflective practice to evaluate your decision so you can respond more confidently in the future? What criteria will you use to evaluate a good response? What personal characteristics inform your practice?
9. How would you respond to having to deny critical care to your oldest and sickest patients who would be least likely to benefit from scarce equipment and resources?
10. How do we handle exemptions to vaccine mandates? When do individual beliefs and practices take precedence over public health measures?

Reflection-on-Action

Then look back at the nurse's decisions and reflect on your learning—how did your knowledge and/or skills expand based on this scenario? What attitude, value, or belief shifts did you experience (if any) after reading this scenario? What would you do differently if you were in this situation? What more do you need to know to be able to manage this or a similar situation in the future?

Emmanuel, E. J., Persad, G., Upshur, R., Thome, B., Parker, M., Glickman, A., Zhang, C., Boyle, C., Smith, M., & Phillips, J. P. (2020). Fair allocation of scarce medical resources in the time of Covid-19. *The New England Journal of Medicine, 382*(21), 2049–2055.

Gostin, L. O., Friedman, E. A., & Wetter, S. A. (2020). Responding to COVID-19: How to navigate a public health emergency legally and ethically. *Hastings Center Report, 50*(2), 8–12.

Truog, R. D., Mitchell, C., & Daley, G. Q. (2020). The toughest triage—allocating ventilators in a pandemic. *The New England Journal of Medicine, 382*(21), 1973–1975.

For additional bioethics resources, we recommend this excellent, recent analysis of the ethical issues related to pandemics and have appended a short bibliography with hotlinks (https://www.thehastingscenter.org/responding-to-covid-19-how-to-navigate-a-public-health-emergency-legally-and-ethically/). Here is ethics guidance for health care institutions (https://www.thehastingscenter.org/ethicalframeworkcovid19/) and a resource hub on ethical issues in pandemics (https://www.thehastingscenter.org/publications-resources/ethics-resources-on-the-coronavirus/).

geographic location. For example, malaria that is endemic in Africa, particularly south of the Sahara and in parts of Oceania, is tracked to allow for ongoing assessment of the malaria situation around the world (CDC, 2020f). In cases like these, countries collaborate to learn about and implement diagnostic, control, and treatment options (World Health Organization [WHO], 2020b). **Pandemics**, like the one experienced with novel coronavirus (SARS-CoV-2) and the disease it causes (COVID-19) starting in 2019, are global outbreaks of a novel (new or not previously identified) virus that did not initially not have a known immunization or treatment (National Institute of Allergy and Infectious Disease, 2020). See the Challenging Topics feature.

COLONIZATION VERSUS INFECTION

Under normal conditions, some organisms may not produce disease. Microorganisms that commonly inhabit various body sites and are part of the body's natural defense system are referred to as normal flora. However, in certain situations, a typically harmless organism may generate an infection, especially in susceptible people. These bacteria are referred to as opportunists. For example, one type of *Escherichia coli* (*E. coli*) normally resides in the intestinal tract and causes no harm. However, if it migrates to the urinary tract, it can lead to urinary tract infection (UTI). Another example is the *Clostridioides difficile* organism (*C. diff*; formerly known as *Clostridium difficile*). If the *C. diff* organism resides in a person's body, but there are no clinical signs of an infection, this is referred to as *C. diff* **colonization**. An infection is present once the person exhibits specific manifestations of the disease. With both *E. coli* and *C. diff*, microscopic examinations reveal the presence of the bacteria. If a person's defense mechanisms are ineffective in responding to the bacterial invasion (colonization), infection will result.

Reservoir

The **reservoir** for growth and multiplication of microorganisms is the natural habitat of the organism. Possible reservoirs that support organisms pathogenic to humans include other people, animals, soil, food, water, milk, and inanimate objects.

OTHER PEOPLE

Some people who act as reservoirs for an infectious agent demonstrate signs and symptoms of the disease. Other people act as reservoirs for the infectious agent, but do not exhibit any manifestations of the disease. These people are considered carriers. Carriers, although asymptomatic, can transmit the disease. For example, a person who has tested positive for the HIV antibody/antigen may not exhibit any signs and symptoms of the disease at the time of testing. However, even the asymptomatic person may transmit the virus to others by activities such as condomless intimate sexual contact or sharing a contaminated needle and syringe. An infected pregnant woman may transmit the virus to her child during pregnancy, birth, or breastfeeding.

OTHER RESERVOIRS

Many other reservoirs exist and are encountered on a daily basis. The rabies virus is an example of a pathogen whose reservoir is various animals, notably dogs, squirrels, bats, and raccoons. A person contracts the rabies virus when bitten by an infected animal. The West Nile virus (WNV) is an example of an arbovirus (transmitted between arthropod [insect] vectors and a vertebrate host) whose reservoir is usually an infected mosquito or tick (McDonald et al., 2019). Mosquitoes feed on infected birds, become infected, and pass the infection on to people when feeding on their blood. The first local transmission of Zika virus infection was reported in December 2015 in the Caribbean. Zika is also transmitted by mosquitoes, which means that methods to prevent transmission of WNV (primarily prevention of mosquito bites) apply to Zika virus as well. Sexual and maternal–fetal transmission of Zika virus have been documented; poor pregnancy outcomes and microcephaly (a brain defect) can occur (CDC, 2020e), so preconception counseling is recommended (Polen et al., 2018).

Water can harbor *Giardia*, *E. coli* 0157-H7, and *Shigella*. Drinking or swimming in contaminated water can begin the infectious cycle in a person. Soil can act as a reservoir for the organisms that cause gas gangrene and tetanus. Food can also be a reservoir. Undercooked ground beef and fresh leafy vegetables have been identified as responsible for recent outbreaks of *E. coli* infections. The CDC recommends that all ground beef be cooked until well done and new laws keep fruits and vegetables safer when they are grown, picked, and washed. Milk can contain *Listeria* unless it is pasteurized. Reporting infectious disease outbreaks, including domestic foodborne illnesses with their associated recalls (e.g., lettuce and poultry) and current diseases international travelers may encounter, remains the responsibility of the CDC (2020i). Inanimate objects can also harbor organisms, such as the influenza virus, which may be spread if a person touches a contaminated article and then touches their nose or eyes. Nurses need to pay special attention to transferring organisms. For example, a nurse with artificial nails may harbor a large number and variety of microbes under the nails. Ineffective handwashing or improper glove use may also result in exposing an immunocompromised patient to the risk of infection.

Portal of Exit

The portal of exit is the point of escape for the organism from the reservoir. The organism cannot exert its influence unless it moves away from its original reservoir. Each type of microorganism has a typical primary exit route. In humans, common portals of exit include the respiratory, gastrointestinal (GI), and genitourinary (GU) tracts as well as breaks in the skin. Blood and tissue can also be portals of exit for pathogens.

Means of Transmission

An organism may be transmitted from its reservoir by various means or routes. Some organisms can be transmitted by more than one route. Organisms can enter the body by way of contact transmission, either directly or indirectly. **Direct contact** requires close proximity between the susceptible host and an infected person or a carrier, and includes activities such as touching, kissing, and sexual intercourse. Health care workers have the potential to directly transmit organisms to susceptible people through touching. **Indirect contact** involves personal contact with either: (1) a **vector**, a living creature that transmits an infectious agent to a human, usually an insect; or (2) an inanimate object, called a **fomite**, such as equipment or countertops (Brunette & Nemhauser, 2019). Keep in mind that nurses use stethoscopes many times of the course of day—stethoscopes, especially when unclean, have the potential to act as fomites of infection. In addition to providing education and addressing misconceptions and negative attitudes, best-practice recommendations, infection control policies and procedures, and functional systems need to be in place to support stethoscope hygiene practices (Breen & Hessels, 2017). Proper hand hygiene and glove use can interrupt the transmission of dangerous bacteria from nurses to patients. Ongoing work is being done to evaluate the effectiveness of antimicrobial surfaces, such as copper, in preventing and reducing health care–associated infections (HAIs; Muller et al., 2016; Zingg et al., 2019).

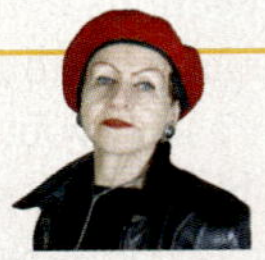

Recall **Esther Bailey**, the woman described at the beginning of the chapter in the Reflective Practice box on page 664, who was catheterized. In this situation, the catheter becomes contaminated. Indirect contact occurs if this contaminated catheter is inserted, predisposing her to an infection.

Microorganisms can also be spread through the airborne route when an infected host coughs, sneezes, or talks, or when the organism becomes attached to dust particles. Another means of transmission is through droplets. **Droplet transmission** is similar to **airborne transmission**. However, airborne particles are smaller than 5 μm (micrometer), and droplet particles are greater than 5 μm. This distinction matters when designing prevention strategies. For example, once there were data to support droplet transmission of the virus that causes COVID-19 (WHO, 2020d), frequent handwashing, disinfection of high-touch areas, social distancing (6 ft), and cloth masks for the general public became the cornerstones of transmission prevention (CDC, 2020g). These prevention recommendations continued even after vaccines became available because of the virus variants. Recommendations from WHO (2020) and other national and international guidelines specified that health care environments need to consider airborne transmission precautions with COVID-19, in addition to contact and droplet precautions (PPE required), with aerosol-generating procedures. Table 25-1 summarizes the means of transmission for several organisms, their reservoirs, and examples of diseases they transmit.

Portal of Entry

The portal of entry is the point at which organisms enter a new host. The organism must find a portal of entry to a host or it may die. The entry route into the new host is often the same as the exit route from the prior reservoir. The skin and urinary, respiratory, and GI tracts are common portals of entry.

Concept Mastery Alert

The skin and respiratory, gastrointestinal, and genitourinary tracts are common portals for organism entry and exit.

Table 25-1 Organisms Capable of Causing Disease

ORGANISM	RESERVOIR	MEANS OF TRANSMISSION	DISEASE TRANSMITTED
Borrelia burgdorferi	Ticks (sheep, cattle, deer, mice)	Contact (indirect, vectors)	Lyme disease
Escherichia coli (E. coli)	Feces Contaminated food or water	Contact (direct/indirect)	*E. coli* infection (Most common manifestation is diarrhea)
Hepatitis B virus (HBV)	Blood Feces Body fluids and excretions	Contact (direct; indirect possible, but unlikely)	Hepatitis B
Human immunodeficiency virus (HIV)	Blood Semen Vaginal secretions Breast milk	Contact (direct)	Acquired immunodeficiency syndrome (AIDS)
Mycobacterium tuberculosis (*M. tuberculosis* [TB])	Sputum (respiratory tract)	Contact (airborne)	Tuberculosis
Salmonella	Intestinal tracts of humans and other animals, including birds	Contact (direct/indirect)	Diarrheal illness
Staphylococcus aureus	Skin surface Mouth Nose Throat	Contact (direct/indirect)	• Minor skin infections: Carbuncle, boil, pimple, abscess • Respiratory infection • Endocarditis (infection of the heart valves) • Osteomyelitis (bone infection) • Bacteremia (bloodstream infections)

Susceptible Host

Microorganisms survive only in a source that provides shelter and nourishment (a host), and only if the microorganisms overcome any resistance mounted by the host's defenses. Susceptibility is the degree of resistance the potential host has to the pathogen. People who are hospitalized are often in a weakened state of health because of illness, and have less resistance. Thus, they are more susceptible to infection. Many factors influence a host's susceptibility; these are discussed later in the chapter.

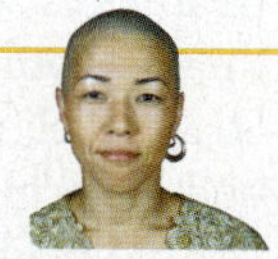

Remember **Giselle Turheis**, the woman with leukemia and a compromised immune status. Her susceptibility to infection is increased because of the lack of an adequate functioning immune system.

Stages of Infection

An understanding of the stages in the development of an infection is necessary to intervene and disrupt the infection cycle. An infection progresses through the following phases:

- Incubation period
- Prodromal stage
- Full (acute) stage of illness
- Convalescent period

The course and severity of the infection, as well as the patient's response, influence the type and extent of nursing care provided.

Incubation Period

The incubation period is the interval between the pathogen's invasion of the body and the appearance of symptoms of infection. During this stage, the organisms are growing and multiplying. The length of incubation may vary. For example, the common cold has an incubation period of 1 to 2 days, whereas tetanus has an incubation period ranging from 2 to 21 days.

Prodromal Stage

A person is most infectious during the prodromal stage. Early signs and symptoms of disease are present, but these are often vague and nonspecific, ranging from fatigue and malaise to a low-grade fever. This period lasts from several hours to several days. During this phase, the patient often is unaware of being contagious. As a result, precautions are not taken, and the infection spreads to other hosts.

Full Stage of Illness

The presence of infection-specific signs and symptoms indicates the full stage of illness. The type of infection determines the length of the illness and the severity of the manifestations. Symptoms that are limited or occur in only one body area are referred to as *localized* symptoms, whereas symptoms manifested throughout the entire body are referred to as *systemic* symptoms.

Convalescent Period

The convalescent period involves the recovery from the infection. Convalescence may vary according to the severity of the infection and the patient's general condition. The signs and symptoms disappear, and the person returns to a healthy state. Depending on the type of infection, there may be a temporary or permanent change in the patient's previous health state even after the convalescent period.

A person may continually pass through the four phases with the same infectious process, such as with HSV-1. Although there may have been only one infectious exposure, the infection may continue to cycle through the phases.

Infection Defense Mechanisms

Several defense mechanisms protect the body from invasion. The skin and mucous membranes are considered first-line defenses. One of the other first-line defenders is the body's normal flora, particularly the flora found in the GI tract. Flora help to keep potentially harmful bacteria from invading the body. If a pathogen makes it past these first-line defenses, the inflammatory response and immune response help the body combat infection.

Inflammatory Response

The inflammatory response is a protective mechanism. Inflammation helps the body neutralize, control, or eliminate the offending agent, and prepare the site for repair (Hinkle et al., 2022). In addition to infection, the inflammatory response also occurs in response to injury. It is either an acute or chronic process.

The hallmark signs of acute infection are redness, heat, swelling, pain, and loss of function, usually appearing at the site of the injury/invasion. The body's response occurs in two phases that are responsible for these hallmark signs: the vascular and cellular phases. In the vascular phase, small blood vessels constrict in the area, followed by vasodilatation of arterioles and venules that supply the area. This increase in blood flow results in redness and heat in the area. Histamine is released, leading to an increased permeability of vessels, which allows protein-rich fluid to pour into the area. At this point, swelling, pain, and loss of function can occur (Norris, 2019).

During the cellular stage, white blood cells (leukocytes) move quickly into the area. Neutrophils, the primary phagocytes, engulf the organism and consume cell debris and foreign material. Exudate, composed of fluid, cells, and inflammatory byproducts is released from the wound. The exudate may be clear (serous), contain red blood cells (sanguineous), or contain pus (purulent). The amount of exudate depends on the size and location of the wound. The damaged cells then are repaired by either regeneration (replacement with identical cells) or the formation of scar tissue (Norris, 2019). Refer to Chapters 33 and 43 for additional discussion of the inflammatory response.

Immune Response

Another protective mechanism is the immune response. The normal immune response involves the collective reaction of the immune system to an invading organism. The complex mechanisms that constitute the immune response occur as the body attempts to protect and defend itself. The foreign material is called an **antigen**, and the body commonly responds to the antigen by producing an **antibody**. This antigen–antibody reaction, also known as humoral immunity, is one component of the overall immune response. The other component that also helps the body defend against invaders is cell-mediated immunity. This type of immunity involves an increase in the number of lymphocytes (white blood cells) that destroy or react with cells the body recognizes as harmful (Norris, 2019). Although these complicated chemical and mechanical responses are not completely understood, it is known that they help to defend the body specifically against bacterial, viral, and fungal infections as well as malignant (cancerous) cells.

Factors Affecting the Risk for Infection

The susceptibility of the host depends on various factors:

- Integrity of skin and mucous membranes, which protect the body against microbial invasion
- pH levels of the GI and GU tracts, as well as the skin, which help to ward off microbial invasion
- Integrity and number of the body's white blood cells, which provide resistance to certain pathogens
- Age, sex, and heredity, which influence susceptibility—neonates and older adults appear to be more vulnerable to infection (see the accompanying box: Focus on the Older Adult)
- Immunity, natural or acquired, which acts to resist infection
- Level of fatigue, nutritional and general health status, the presence of preexisting illnesses, previous or current treatments, and certain medications, which play a part in the susceptibility of a potential host
- Stress level, which if increased may adversely affect the body's normal defense mechanisms
- Use of invasive or indwelling medical devices, which provides exposure to and entry for more potential sources of disease-producing organisms, particularly in a patient whose defenses are already weakened by disease

Health habits that promote wellness can reduce potential risk factors, thus decreasing the susceptibility of a host. Sensible nutrition, adequate rest and exercise, stress-reduction techniques, and good personal hygiene habits can help maintain optimum bodily function and immune response. Condomless anal or vaginal sex, sex between an

Focus on the Older Adult

AGE-RELATED CHANGES PREDISPOSING TO INFECTION

Infection Risk	Age-Related Changes	Nursing Strategies
Pulmonary infections	• Decreased cough reflex • Decreased elastic recoil of lungs • Decreased activity of cilia • Abnormal swallowing reflexes	• Place patient in sitting position to eat and drink. • Encourage patient to drink plenty of fluids, unless contraindicated. • Encourage patient to cough and deep breathe or use incentive spirometer. • Recommend pneumococcal vaccination (per guidelines) and influenza vaccination annually.
Urinary tract infections (UTI)	• Incomplete emptying of bladder • Decreased sphincter control • Bladder-outlet obstruction due to enlarged prostate gland • Pelvic floor relaxation due to estrogen depletion • Reduced renal blood flow	• Discuss with patient need to void at regular intervals. • Encourage patient to drink plenty of fluids, unless contraindicated. • Administer medications for enlarged prostate (benign prostate hypertrophy; BPH) and estrogen depletion as prescribed. • If patient wears absorbent product such as incontinence pad, instruct patient to change pad frequently and perform good perineal care. • Assess for UTIs (may be atypical clinical presentation in older adults). • Discuss the need for patient to void after sexual intercourse.
Skin infections	• Loss of elasticity • Increased dryness • Thinning of epidermis • Slowing of cell replacement • Decreased vascular supply	• Encourage patient to drink plenty of fluids, unless contraindicated. • Help patient to perform good hygiene practices daily. • Apply lotion to skin as needed. • Assess frequently for any breaks in skin integrity, rashes, or changes in skin.

Note: Atypical clinical manifestations of infection in an older adult include confusion, disorientation, lethargy, anorexia, delayed fever response, falls, incontinence, and failure to thrive.

Box 25-1 Laboratory Data Indicating an Infection

- Elevated white blood cell (leukocyte) count—normal value is 5,000 to 10,000/mm^3
- Increase in specific types of white blood cells—referred to as a differential or differential count (percentage of each cell type)

• Neutrophils	Normal = 60%–70%	Increased in acute infections that produce pus; increased risk for acute bacterial infection if decreased; may also be increased in response to stress
• Lymphocytes	Normal = 20%–40%	Increased in chronic bacterial and viral infections
• Monocytes	Normal = 2%–8%	Increased in severe infections: function as a scavenger or phagocyte
• Eosinophils	Normal = 1%–4%	May be increased in allergic reaction and parasitic infection
• Basophils	Normal = 0.5%–1%	Usually unaffected by infections

- Elevated erythrocyte sedimentation rate—red blood cells settle more rapidly to the bottom of a tube of whole blood when inflammation is present
- Presence of pathogen(s) in cultures of urine, blood, sputum, or other (wound) drainage

HIV-uninfected person and a person living with HIV with an unsuppressed viral load (Marcus & Snowden, 2020), and sharing intravenous (IV) needles are potentially dangerous, providing an opportunity for pathogens to enter a host and cause an infection.

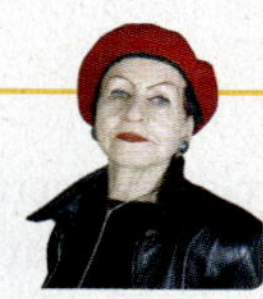

Think back to **Esther Bailey**, the woman being catheterized who also has developed a postoperative wound infection. Undergoing abdominal surgery disrupts the integrity of the skin and mucous membranes, thereby increasing her risk for a wound infection.

NURSING PROCESS FOR INFECTION PREVENTION AND CONTROL

It is imperative that health care providers safeguard the people entrusted to their care by controlling diseases and preventing the spread of infection. Vigilant preventive care can limit exposure to potentially harmful infectious organisms and reduce the occurrence of infection. Public health nurses and other professionals often initiate follow-up including **contact tracing**, which involves identifying people with an infectious disease and locating individuals and groups with whom they have come into direct contact to interrupt actual or potential transmission of the infectious disease (CDC, 2020j).

Assessing

The nurse plays a critical role in preventing and controlling infection. This role begins with early detection and surveillance techniques. The extent of nursing interventions depends on the susceptibility of the host, the virulence of the organism, and the patient's signs and symptoms.

Inquire about the patient's immunization status and previous or recurring infections. Observe nonverbal cues and gather information about the history of the current disease. Nursing assessments include observing for signs and symptoms of a local or systemic infection. A localized infection can result in redness, swelling, warmth in the involved area, pain or tenderness, and loss of function of the affected part. Manifestations of a systemic infection include fever, often accompanied by an increase in pulse and respiratory rate, lethargy, tenderness and enlargement of lymph nodes, and anorexia. Laboratory data can provide further insight into the presence of an infectious process. Any of the laboratory test results outlined in Box 25-1 may indicate the presence of an infection.

Compilation of these assessment data leads to the development of a unique nursing database that outlines potential nursing interventions for patients at risk for infection or those in whom an infection is already present.

Diagnosing

The potential for infection or the presence of an infection in a patient may lead to diagnosing actual or potential health problems or needs. These identified problems and needs guide the development and communication of a coordinated plan that often involves the interprofessional team. Examples of health problems and needs with related etiology and signs and symptoms can be found in the box titled Examples of Actual or Potential Health Problems or Needs: Asepsis and Infection Control on page 672.

Outcome Identification and Planning

The nurse develops appropriate patient outcomes after reviewing the assessment data, considering the cycle of events resulting in an infection, and incorporating the principles of infection control. Planning outcomes that prevent infection or disrupt the infection cycle presents an exciting challenge. Nursing interventions focused on controlling or preventing infection can positively impact patient outcomes. The following examples of expected patient outcomes are appropriate for preventing infection and using infection control techniques. The patient will:

- Demonstrate effective hand hygiene and good personal hygiene practices
- Identify the signs of an infection
- Maintain adequate nutritional and fluid intake
- Demonstrate proper disposal of soiled articles
- Use appropriate cleansing and disinfecting techniques

Examples of Actual or Potential Health Problems or Needs

ASEPSIS AND INFECTION CONTROL

Actual or Potential Health Problem or Need	Possible Etiologic Factors	Potential Signs and Symptoms
Dehydration	• Insufficient fluid intake • Insufficient knowledge about fluid needs • Fluid loss secondary to underlying infection	• Decrease in blood pressure, pulse pressure, and pulse volume • Dry mucous membranes • Increase in body temperature • Sudden weight loss • Weakness and other neurologic symptoms
Infection risk	• Alteration in skin integrity • Inadequate vaccination • Insufficient knowledge to avoid exposure to pathogens	—
Knowledge deficiency	• New and evolving standards of care and infection control practices	• Inability to articulate current infection control standards • Unwillingness to adhere to guidance regarding infection control

Source: Wolters Kluwer. (2020). Problem-based care plans. In *Lippincott advisor*. Wolters Kluwer. https://advisor.lww.com/lna/home.do

- Verbalize awareness of the necessity of proper immunizations
- Implement stress-reduction techniques
- Adhere to infection control precautions (isolation, equipment, visitors)
- Verbalize an understanding of health risks associated with a latex allergy

Implementing

The practice of **asepsis** includes all activities to prevent infection or break the chain of infection. The nurse uses aseptic techniques to halt the spread of microorganisms and minimize the threat of infection. There are two asepsis categories: medical asepsis and surgical asepsis. **Medical asepsis**, or clean technique, involves procedures and practices that reduce the number and transfer of pathogens. Medical asepsis procedures include performing hand hygiene and wearing gloves. **Surgical asepsis**, or sterile technique, includes practices used to render and keep objects and areas free from microorganisms. Surgical asepsis procedures include inserting an indwelling urinary catheter or inserting an IV catheter.

Using Medical Asepsis

Medical asepsis techniques are used continuously both within and outside health facilities, based on the assumption that pathogens are likely to be present. For example, shared drinking cups are considered unsanitary because a person harboring pathogens may transfer those pathogens to the cup. In a health care facility, if a specific pathogen is known to be present, special methods of medical asepsis are used to prevent further spread of the organism. Nearly every nursing activity includes practices of medical asepsis. Therefore, the nurse assumes responsibility for breaking the cycle of infection by providing safe patient care that protects the patient and the nurse from microorganisms that may cause disease. Box 25-2 highlights the basic practices of medical asepsis for nurses to routinely use when providing care to patients.

Limiting the dissemination of pathogens will decrease the transfer of pathogens from person to person. The most practical way to accomplish this is through the use of barriers that prevent transmission of the pathogens. Barriers are ways to decrease the spread of pathogens and include hand hygiene, personal protective equipment (PPE, discussed later), and other barrier techniques. Figure 25-2 shows how barriers break the infection cycle. Nurses must understand the various precautions or barrier techniques if they are to use them correctly and minimize infection risks to patients as well as to themselves (see Promoting Health 25-1 on page 674).

PERFORMING HAND HYGIENE

Hand hygiene is the most effective way to help prevent the spread of infectious agents. There is consensus that most health care–associated pathogens are transmitted via the contaminated hands of health care workers. According to an ongoing survey supported by the CDC, there were an estimated 1 in 31 hospitalized patients with an HAI, which has decreased since the original survey in 2011 (Magill et al., 2018). The CDC's initial guidelines for hand hygiene in health care settings remain largely unchanged (Healthcare Infection Control Practices Advisory Committee, 2017). The term *hand hygiene* applies to either handwashing with plain soap and water, the use of antiseptic handrubs including waterless alcohol-based products, or surgical hand antisepsis. Although there is agreement that hand hygiene is the most important procedure for preventing infections, hand hygiene is still not performed consistently in health care

Box 25-2 Practicing Basic Principles of Medical Asepsis in Patient Care

- Practice good hand hygiene.
- Carry soiled linens or other used articles/equipment so that they do not touch your clothing.
- Do not place soiled bed linen or any other items on the floor, which is grossly contaminated. It increases contamination of both surfaces.
- Avoid allowing patients to cough, sneeze, or breathe directly on others. Provide them with disposable tissues, and instruct them to cover their mouth and nose to prevent spread by airborne droplets.
- Move equipment away from you when brushing, dusting, or scrubbing articles. This helps prevent contaminated particles from settling on the hair, face, and clothing.
- Avoid raising dust. Use a specially treated cloth or a dampened cloth. Do not shake linens. Dust and lint particles constitute a vehicle by which organisms may be transported from one area to another.
- Clean the least soiled areas first and then the more soiled ones. This helps prevent having the cleaner areas soiled by the dirtier areas.
- Dispose of soiled or used items directly into appropriate containers. Wrap items that are moist from body discharge or drainage in waterproof containers, such as plastic bags, before discarding into the refuse holder so that handlers will not come in contact with them.
- Pour liquids that are to be discarded, such as bath water or mouth rinse, directly into the drain to avoid splattering in the sink and onto you.
- Sterilize equipment suspected of containing pathogens.
- Use practices of personal grooming that help prevent spreading microorganisms. Examples include shampooing the hair regularly, keeping hair short or pinned up to limit the possibility of carrying microorganisms on hair shafts, keeping fingernails short and free of broken cuticles and ragged nail edges, and avoiding wearing rings with grooves and stones that may harbor microorganisms.
- Follow guidelines conscientiously for standard and transmission-based precautions as prescribed by your facility.

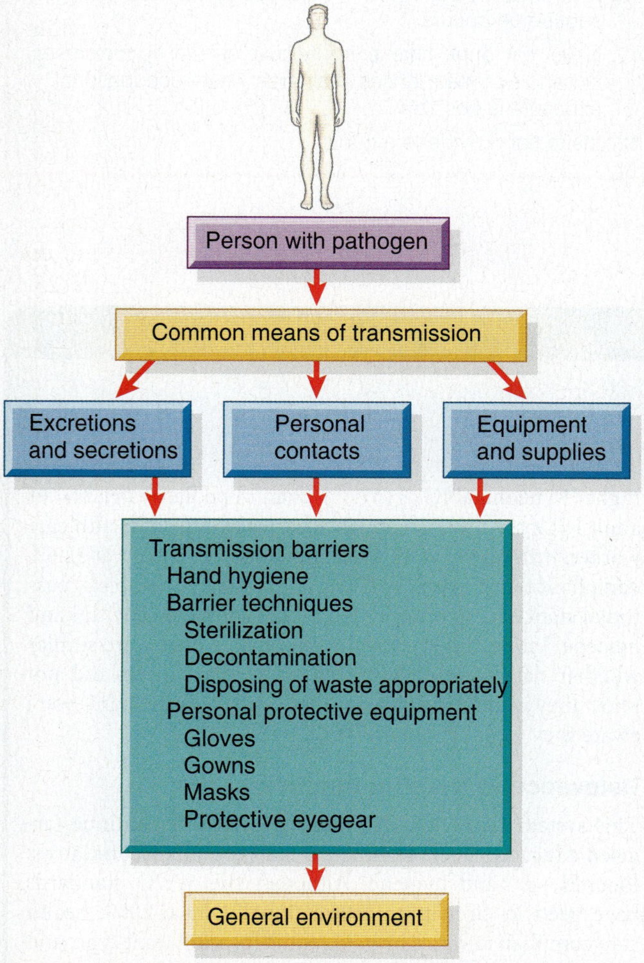

FIGURE 25-2. Transmission barriers help prevent the transporting of pathogens from the infected person to the general environment.

settings. A recent review of the literature found that the average baseline compliance rate for handwashing (based on the results from 16 studies performed primarily in the United States and Europe 2009–2014) was only 34.1%. The average compliance rate for handwashing increased to 56.98% after the implementation of various multimodal, multifaceted educational, and motivational interventions (Kingston et al., 2016). Other initiatives to support the evidence-based practice of handwashing highlight the benefits of positive role models (including leaders and managers), establishing a socially and culturally supportive clinical environment, the provision of ongoing education and training, and readily available supplies (Hammerschmidt & Manser, 2019; Kingston et al., 2017). Review the Research in Nursing box (on page 674) for another perspective on improving hand hygiene.

The WHO (2020c) defined *My 5 Moments for Hand Hygiene*. These include:

- Moment 1—Before touching a patient
- Moment 2—Before a clean or aseptic procedure
- Moment 3—After a body fluid exposure or risk of exposure
- Moment 4—After touching a patient
- Moment 5—After touching patient surroundings

The Joint Commission Center for Transforming Healthcare continues its campaign inviting all Joint Commission–accredited organizations to improve patient safety and lower the cost of health care. The Hand Hygiene Project takes advantage of their Targeted Solutions Tool (TST) that facilitates a "step-by-step process to accurately measure their organization's actual performance, identify their barriers to excellent performance, and direct them to proven solutions that are customized to address their particular barriers" (The Joint Commission Center for Transforming Healthcare, 2020, p. 1).

Promoting Health 25-1

INFECTION CONTROL PRECAUTIONS AND BARRIER TECHNIQUES

Use the assessment checklist to determine how well you are observing infection control or barrier precautions as you care for patients in a health care facility or in a community setting. Then develop a prescription for self-care by choosing appropriate behaviors from the list of suggestions.

Assessment Checklist

☐ almost always ☐ sometimes ☐ almost never

☐ ☐ ☐ 1. I perform hand hygiene before and after contact with a patient.

☐ ☐ ☐ 2. I choose the evidence-based option for hand hygiene depending on the situation (e.g., alcohol-based, pain soap and water, antimicrobial/antiseptic soap and water).

☐ ☐ ☐ 3. I wear PPE if contact with blood or body fluids is a possibility.

☐ ☐ ☐ 4. I cover my nose and mouth when coughing and sneezing and properly dispose of tissues.

☐ ☐ ☐ 5. I use additional protective equipment (gowns, masks, goggles, face shields) as appropriate.

☐ ☐ ☐ 6. I avoid recapping any used or contaminated needles.

☐ ☐ ☐ 7. I place needles or other sharp objects in a puncture-proof disposable container.

☐ ☐ ☐ 8. I dispose of used or contaminated objects and equipment in a leak-resistant plastic trash bag.

☐ ☐ ☐ 9. I am a role model for hand hygiene.

☐ ☐ ☐ 10. I collaborate with leadership to hold people accountable, identify access points for hand hygiene, and establish places to store items to accommodate hand hygiene.

Self-Care Behaviors

1. Read infection control standards published by OSHA and CDC.
2. Attend programs that provide updates on current CDC/OSHA policies and survey literature regularly to determine best practices.
3. Maintain strict personal hygiene habits.
4. Obtain immunizations when available.
5. Assess for any signs and symptoms of an infection.
6. Perform hand hygiene frequently.
7. Perform hand hygiene immediately after removing gloves.
8. Practice cough etiquette to prevent transmission of respiratory infections.
9. Protect myself with the barriers necessary to prevent exposure to blood, body fluids, or secretions.
10. Follow facility policy if any exposure to blood or body substance occurs.
11. Never eat, drink, smoke, apply cosmetics or lip moistener, or handle contact lenses in an area where occupational exposure is possible.
12. Make hand hygiene a habit.

Research in Nursing

BRIDGING THE GAP TO EVIDENCE-BASED PRACTICE

Hand Hygiene Compliance in the ICU: A Systematic Review

Despite the fact that hand hygiene is recognized as a key element in preventing the spread of infection, there are still significant issues with compliance in health care, even in ICUs where patients are already compromised. Hand hygiene noncompliance persists despite global efforts to impact change.

Related Research

Lambe, K. A., Lydon, S., Madden, C., Vellinga, A., Hehir, A., Walsh, M., & O'Connor, P. (2019). Hand hygiene compliance in the ICU: A systematic review. *Critical Care Medicine*, *47*(9), 1251–1257. https://doi.org/10.1097/CCM.0000000000003868

A systematic review considered 61 peer-reviewed studies focused on hand hygiene compliance, primarily in high-income countries (60.7%) and in adult intensive care units (ICUs; 85.2%). Overall, mean hand hygiene compliance internationally is 59.6%, which falls below the accepted standard that ranges from 80% to 90%. Of note is that compliance was higher in neonatal ICUs (67.0%) than in pediatric (41.2%) or adult ICUs (58.2%). Compliance varies by type of health care worker, with nurses at 43.4% compliance, physicians at 32.6% compliance, and other staff (e.g., respiratory therapists, custodial staff, and technicians) at 53.8% compliance with hand hygiene. Interestingly enough, compliance rates were similar whether data were collected covertly (participants did not know they were being observed) or overtly (participants were aware they were being observed).

Relevance to Nursing Practice

This systematic review highlights the need to continue targeted educational, environmental, and compliance initiatives focused on hand hygiene. Although the WHO standards have been in circulation internationally since 2009, health care compliance varies by geographic location, unit type, and composition of providers.

Table 25-2 Bacterial Flora on the Hands

TYPES OF BACTERIAL FLORA	CHARACTERISTICS	EFFECTIVE HAND HYGIENE MEASURES
Transient	• Occur on hands with activities of daily living • Relatively few in number on clean and exposed areas of the skin • Attached loosely on skin usually in grease, fats, and dirt • Found in greatest number under the fingernails • Can be pathogenic or nonpathogenic	Can be removed relatively easily by frequent and thorough handwashing
Resident	• Normally found in skin creases • Usually stable in number and type • Cling tenaciously to skin by adhesion and absorption	Considerable friction with a brush is required to remove them Less susceptible to antiseptics than transient bacteria

The targeted solutions tool and associated increase in hand hygiene has resulted in a 45% reduction in HAIs (up from 26% reduction) and saved up to 2.8 million dollars in direct medical costs (The Joint Commission Center for Transforming Healthcare, 2020).

The CDC Foundation forged an ongoing relationship with GOJO, the inventors of PURELL Instant Hand Sanitizer, to enhance hand hygiene educational outreach to patients, health care providers, and caregivers in various health care settings in the United States. The tools and educational materials are designed to improve hand hygiene practices and ultimately reduce the number of HAIs in the United States (CDC Foundation, 2016; GOJO Industries, 2020).

Bacteria

Two types of bacterial flora are normally found on the hands: transient bacteria and resident bacteria (Table 25-2). Transient bacteria, although usually easily removed by thorough handwashing, have the potential to adjust to the environment of the skin when they are present in large numbers over a long period of time, and become resident bacteria. If pathogenic organisms become resident bacteria on the skin, the hands then become carriers of that particular organism. Therefore, to help prevent transient bacteria from becoming resident bacteria, it is important to clean the hands promptly when they are visibly soiled, after each contact with contaminated materials, and after removing gloves. In addition, the seminal CDC guideline for hand hygiene in health care settings (2002) specifies that health care personnel involved in patient care should not wear artificial nails because they are more likely to be associated with higher bacterial counts. In fact, wearing artificial nails in the operating room (OR) is a citable offense during The Joint Commission accreditation process. Natural nails should be less than 1/4 inches long.

Cleansing Agents

Various hand hygiene products are available. Soaps and detergents, also referred to as nonantimicrobial agents, are considered adequate for routine mechanical cleansing of the hands and removal of most transient microorganisms. They work by lowering surface tension and acting as emulsifying agents. Bar, liquid, leaflet, and powdered soaps are all effective. Use of a particular product in a health care facility often depends on personnel or facility preference.

Using handwashing products that contain an antimicrobial or antibacterial ingredient is recommended in any setting where the risk for infection is high. When present in certain concentrations, these agents can kill bacteria or suppress their growth. Numerous studies that informed the landmark 2006 Institute for Healthcare Improvement (IHI, 2020b) guidance documented that alcohol-based handrubs, in most situations, more effectively reduce bacterial and viral counts on the hands of health care personnel than antimicrobial soap (IHI, 2020b). Alcohol-based handrubs have an alcohol concentration between 60% and 95% and are available as foam, gel, or lotions.

Techniques

If the health care worker's hands are not visibly soiled, alcohol-based handrubs are recommended because they save time, are more accessible and easy to use, and reduce bacterial count on the hands. The following are clinical situations when an alcohol-based handrub can be used to decontaminate hands (IHI, 2020b.)

- Before direct contact with patients
- After direct contact with patient's skin
- After contact with body fluids, mucous membranes, nonintact skin, and wound dressings, if hands are not visibly soiled
- After removing gloves
- Before inserting urinary catheters, peripheral vascular catheters, or invasive devices that do not require surgical placement
- Before donning sterile gloves prior to an invasive procedure (e.g., inserting a central venous access device)
- When moving from a contaminated body site to a clean body site during patient care
- After contact with objects (including equipment) located in the patient's environment

When used repeatedly, alcohol-based handrubs cause less dryness and skin irritation than soap products. Those who have sensitive or dry skin may benefit from use of an alcohol-based product that contains humectants, such as glycerine,

Guidelines for Nursing Care 25-1

HAND HYGIENE: USING AN ALCOHOL-BASED HANDRUB

- Apply product to the palm of one hand, using the amount of product recommended on the package (it will vary according to the manufacturer but usually is 3 mL and may require dispensing two pumps).
- Rub hands together, making sure to cover all surfaces of the hands, fingers, and in between the fingers. Also, clean the fingertips and the area beneath the fingernails.
- Continue rubbing until the hands are completely dry (at least 20 seconds).

or other emollients or moisturizers (Berardi et al., 2020; Gold & Avva, 2020). See Guidelines for Nursing Care 25-1 for directions on how to use an alcohol-based handrub.

Concept Mastery Alert

Alcohol-based handrubs are a quick way to remove germs when hands are not visibly soiled.

Alcohol-based hand sanitizers are effective against gram-positive and gram-negative bacteria including multidrug-resistant pathogens such as methicillin-resistant *Staphylococcus aureus* (MRSA) or vancomycin-resistant enterococci (VRE), HIV, influenza, HBV, and hepatitis C virus (HCV). They are also highly effective in halting the spread of seasonal flu, rhinovirus (the most common cause of colds), and many emerging viral pathogens such as Ebola virus disease (EVD), Zika virus, and severe acute respiratory syndrome coronavirus (SARS-CoV-2). The use of alcohol-based handrubs are less effective with *Cryptosporidium* (a waterborne parasite), norovirus (related to contaminated food), and *C. diff*, so soap and water are recommended. For example, *C. diff* is a gram-positive, anaerobic, spore-forming bacterium that is a common cause of diarrhea. It affects children, adults, and older adults. The morbidity and mortality associated with *C. diff* infections (CDIs) has motivated health care providers to improve prevention strategies. Alcohol does not kill *C. diff* bacterial spores; it only kills the vegetative form of the cell. One theory posits that when exposed to water, the endospore swells and the protective walls of the endospore burst (Yoo, 2018), but other theories posit the soap and rubbing associated with handwashing cause spore death. Either way, in the absence of definitive research, soap and water are the preferred hand hygiene method when these infections are suspected or diagnosed (Berardi et al., 2020; Gold & Avva, 2020). Glove use remains the cornerstone for preventing transmission, and contact precautions including a private/cohorted room and gown use are recommended until diarrhea stops. CDI is discussed later in this chapter.

If a health care worker's hands are visibly soiled or contaminated with blood or body fluids, washing the hands with antimicrobial soap and water is required. Handwashing is also required before eating and after using the restroom. Effective handwashing requires at least a 20-second scrub with plain soap or disinfectant and warm water. Hands that are visibly soiled need a longer scrub. Recommended handwashing techniques for medical asepsis are listed in Skill 25-1 on pages 692–694.

Hand antisepsis before assisting with a surgical procedure involves a lengthier scrub to reduce resident and transient flora on the forearms and hands. This procedure, known as a surgical hand scrub, incorporates surgical asepsis and is described in texts that deal with operating and delivery room procedures. Since 2002, CDC guidelines recommend using an antimicrobial soap or alcohol-based surgical hand scrub product for surgical hand antisepsis. Scrub time is also reduced significantly when alcohol-based scrub agents are used.

Preventing Health Care–Associated Infections

For various reasons and sometimes despite best efforts, certain patients in health care facilities develop **health care–associated infections (HAIs)**. The term HAI encompasses and has replaced the term nosocomial, which was used specifically to indicate something originating or taking place in a hospital. Infections that are community acquired and not associated with health care are differentiated from HAIs. An HAI develops as a result of medical care and may occur in many health care settings including hospitals, rehabilitation facilities, outpatient settings, and dialysis centers. The source of an HAI may be either exogenous or endogenous. An infection is referred to as **exogenous** when the causative organism is acquired from other people. An **endogenous** infection occurs when the causative organism comes from microbial life harbored in the person. An infection is referred to as **iatrogenic** when it results from a treatment or diagnostic procedure.

Prevention of HAIs is a major challenge for health care providers. Although this number has been on the decline since 2014, HAIs account for tens of thousands of deaths and billions of dollars in additional health care costs annually (Agency for Healthcare Research and Quality [AHRQ], 2019). The cost of the additional hospital care days necessary to treat an HAI is staggering, particularly in light of the efforts to control spiraling health care expenses. With its focus on patient safety, The Joint Commission mandated that death or serious injury caused by an infection-related event must be reported as a sentinel event (see Chapter 28 for a discussion of sentinel events; The Joint Commission, 2020). As of 2013, the Centers for Medicare and Medicaid Services (CMS) no longer reimburses hospitals for specific preventable *hospital-acquired conditions* (HACs). These HACs are high cost and/or high-volume occurrences that could be reasonably prevented with adherence to evidence-based guidelines; when they occur, HACs result in higher costs. Specific HAIs (catheter-associated UTIs, vascular catheter–associated infections, and various surgical site infections [SSIs]) are included in CMS's current 14 categories of HACs (CMS, 2020). As part of the Hospital-Acquired Condition Reduction Program (HACRP), CMS payments for 2019–2020 were reduced 1% for hospitals ranked in the 25% of worst-performing hospitals with respect to risk-adjusted HAC quality measures. Although this is an evolving process, there is potential that the critical impact that nurses have on decreasing the number of HAIs will be recognized and more easily verified.

Healthy People 2030 (2021) identifies opportunities for addressing existing infection control policies and practices in outpatient settings. These settings include ambulatory surgical centers, dialysis centers, traditional outpatient offices and clinics, and long-term care facilities. Expanding prevention efforts across the continuum of care is essential to the prevention of HAIs.

Based on the premise that most HAIs are preventable, in 2008 the U.S. Department of Health and Human Services (USDHHS; 2021), in conjunction with multiple other federal facilities, formed a Federal Steering Committee committed to coordinating strategies to reduce the transmission of HAIs. The most recent HAI action plan for 2015–2020 recently completed, with seven targets tracked. These include:

- Catheter-associated urinary tract infection (CAUTI)
- Surgical site infection (SSI)
- Central line–associated bloodstream infection (CLABSI)
- Invasive health care–associated and hospital-onset methicillin-resistant *Staphylococcus aureus* (MRSA) infections
- *Clostridioides difficile* (*C. diff*) infections (CDIs) and CDI hospitalizations

USING INVASIVE MEDICAL DEVICES

Most HAIs are caused by bacteria, such as *C. diff, E. coli, S. aureus, Streptococcus faecalis, Pseudomonas aeruginosa,* and *Klebsiella* species. Many HAIs can be traced to an invasive device, such as a urinary catheter or venous access catheter. For example, UTIs represent more than 9.5% of the infections reported by hospitals, and virtually all health care–associated UTIs are related to procedures and instrumentation involving the urinary tract. Approximately 12% to 16% of hospitalized adults have an indwelling urinary catheter placed; each patient has a 3% to 7% increased risk of acquiring a CAUTI each day the catheter remains in place (CDC, 2020b). Infection control measures include adherence to recommended best practices, or bundles. **Bundles** are typically three to five evidence-based practices that, when implemented together, improve patient outcomes (IHI, 2020a). The American Nurses Association (ANA, n.d.) initiative to prevent CAUTI outlines three areas of focus: (1) prevention of inappropriate short-term urinary catheter use, (2) timely removal of catheters that is nurse driven, and (3) catheter care during placement. Focused initiatives, like the one from the ANA, have resulted in changes in practice; however, surveillance, reporting, and prevention initiatives are still mandated and important. CLABSIs have a high mortality rate and are very costly. Central line insertion and maintenance guidelines, like those from the CDC and The Joint Commission (2013), clearly outline handwashing and aseptic technique when handling central lines. The 5-year target goal for CLABSI is a 50% reduction in the number of cases; recent figures show a 9% reduction between 2017 and 2018, with an 11% decrease reported in intensive care units (ICUs; CDC, 2019c).

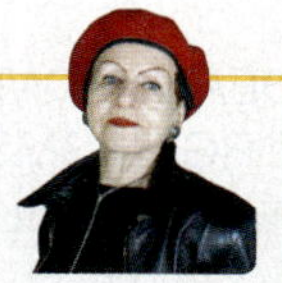

Consider **Esther Bailey**, the 72-year-old woman who has had abdominal surgery and developed a wound infection. The patient already has one infection. However, insertion of the catheter increases her risk for an additional infection, directly related to the use of the catheter.

The USDHHS Federal Steering Committee's (2020) target of 30% reduction in surgical site infections is on track, with a 17% decrease seen in targeted SSIs between 2008 and 2014 (CDC, 2016). Patients receiving mechanical ventilation are especially at risk for ventilator-associated pneumonia (VAP). This infection occurs when pathogens gain access to a patient's lungs via either an endotracheal or tracheostomy tube. VAP bundles provide an excellent example of how simultaneous implementation of seemingly simple interventions such as elevating the head of the bed to 30 to 45 degrees, providing regular oral care, and changing the ventilator circuit (tubing) only as needed, can be effective in preventing infection (Hinkle et al., 2022; Klompas, 2014). With all invasive devices, whether a venous access device, urinary catheter, or endotracheal tube, the interprofessional team collaborates to determine and document the necessity of a device, adheres to standards of care for insertion, and implements protocols (including bundles and guidelines) that address evidence-based infection prevention interventions.

REPORTING HEALTH CARE–ASSOCIATED INFECTIONS

Mandatory public reporting of HAI rates is required in the majority of states (CDC, 2019f). These reports contain specific data on CLABSI, CAUTI, SSI, MRSA, and *C. diff*, with additional information provided on antibiotic resistance and emerging infections. Check this link to see if your state is required by law to report HAI data: https://www.cdc.gov/HAI/state-based/required-to-report-hai-NHSN.html (see Additional Resources). Advocates of mandatory reporting believe that all facilities should report HAI rates. This public disclosure allows consumers to make more informed choices regarding their selection of a health care facility based on an institution's efforts to prevent HAIs. The expectation is that electronic medical records will serve as a surveillance system for tracking these events, thus streamlining the processes and providing an infrastructure for tracking. Keep in mind that several factors influence the speed with which initiatives like this one are embraced (AHRQ, 2014):

- Environmental factors: Who does this change benefit? Is the change mandatory?
- The nature of the innovation: Is it easy to understand? Is there strong evidence to support the change?
- Whether or not people can make the change: Can one person make a difference? Can we individualize the decision making?
- Organizational factors: Are there competing priorities, resource issues, and/or multiple decision makers?

DEALING WITH MULTIDRUG-RESISTANT ORGANISMS

A significant and disturbing trend continues to be the development of microorganisms, primarily bacteria (but also parasites, viruses, and fungi), resistant to one or more classes of antibiotics (or antimicrobials) that were originally effective to treat these infections (WHO, 2020a). The indiscriminate use of broad-spectrum antibiotics has allowed once-susceptible bacteria to develop defenses against antibiotics. While antibiotics kill bacteria that cause illness, they also affect good bacteria that protect the body from infection. As a result, the drug-resistant bacteria continue to grow and can even share their drug resistance with other bacteria, which further complicates treatment (CDC, 2019g). Resistant organisms MRSA, VRE, and carbapenem-resistant Enterobacteriaceae (CRE) have emerged. The CDC (2019g) lists four core actions to fight resistant strains:

- Preventing infections, thereby preventing the spread of resistance
- Tracking
- Improving antibiotic prescribing/stewardship
- Developing new drugs and diagnostic tests

Although this chapter will review some of the more urgent threats and most commonly known resistant infections, data and the associated prevention and treatment guidelines are always evolving. A good resource is the CDC's 2019 *Antibiotic Resistance Threats in the United States* that can be found at: https://www.cdc.gov/drugresistance/pdf/threats-report/2019-ar-threats-report-508.pdf; the 2013 version is also available on the site for comparison data.

Methicillin-Resistant *Staphylococcus aureus*

S. aureus bacteria are normally found in the nasal mucous membranes, on the skin, and in the respiratory and GI tracts. Approximately one third of the people in the United States are colonized with *S. aureus*, meaning that the organism is present (typically in the nose), but the person does not have symptoms and remains healthy and uninfected. They can, however, pass the organism on to others (CDC, 2019a). In the 1960s, a strain of *S. aureus* emerged that was resistant to the broad-spectrum antibiotic methicillin, which is the drug of choice used to treat these infections. The very powerful antibiotic, vancomycin, had to be used to treat the MRSA infections that, at that time, primarily occurred in health care settings. In the late 1990s, a type of MRSA appeared in the wider community. The prevalence of community-associated MRSA (CA-MRSA), a common cause of skin and soft tissue infections in the United States, has been increasing rapidly. Those most at risk are young children, older adults, and people in close physical proximity to others, including athletes, military personnel, inmates, and daycare attendees (CDC, 2019c; Gupta et al., 2015).

Treatment options for CA-MRSA begin with the use of good handwashing, PPE, and disinfection/sterilization of equipment by health care providers who come into contact with CA-MRSA. Guidelines currently recommend incision and drainage of abscesses in patients who are afebrile and healthy with mild, uncomplicated abscesses. Antimicrobial therapy may not be required. If incision and drainage are not effective and systemic or serious infection results, antimicrobial therapy may be necessary. Prior to antibiotic therapy, wound drainage should be sent for culture and sensitivity testing. Patient follow-up education includes encouraging frequent handwashing and maintenance of good personal hygiene, reviewing wound care techniques and the necessity of completion of prescribed treatment, and developing a prevention plan based on the identification of potential sources of infection (Gupta et al., 2015).

The health care–associated MRSA strain, on the other hand, has more serious implications. Patients who have surgery, have invasive devices, are immunocompromised, or who have longer hospital stays are at risk for developing an MRSA infection (Wang et al., 2015). MRSA can be responsible for bloodstream infections, wound infections, VAP, and multidrug resistance. IV vancomycin remains one of the first-line medications for the treatment of health care–associated MRSA (Cong et al., 2019; Pryor et al., 2020). In a health care setting, the main mode of transmission is through direct contact with the contaminated hands of health care personnel or indirect contact with equipment (CDC, 2019a). National data indicate that there was a 17% decrease in hospital-onset MRSA bloodstream infection rate each year between 2005 and 2013, but no significant changes occurred between 2013 and 2016. There were an estimated 323,700 cases in 2017, with 10,600 deaths (CDC, 2019g). Basic infection control practices remain the key to the prevention and control of MRSA.

Vancomycin Intermediate-Resistant *Staphylococcus aureus*, Vancomycin-Resistant *Staphylococcus aureus*, and Vancomycin-Resistant Enterococci

In the 1990s, following the increased use of vancomycin to treat MRSA, vancomycin intermediate-resistant *Staphylococcus aureus* (VISA) emerged in the United States, followed in 2002 by VRSA that was totally resistant to vancomycin (Pryor et al., 2020). Once bacteria develop drug resistance, they progress from being sensitive to an antibiotic, to an intermediate resistance, followed by complete resistance to the antibiotic. Since October 2010, all cases of VISA and VRSA have been successfully treated with other drugs approved by the U.S. Food and Drug Administration, and cases remain extremely rare. Patients most at risk of developing VISA and VRSA are those with a history of kidney disease or diabetes, a previous MRSA infection, presence of an invasive catheter, or recent exposure to vancomycin. Effective infection control measures are imperative to control the spread of VISA and VRSA; prudent use of vancomycin is an important preventive measure (Virginia Department of Health, 2018).

VRE are another serious pathogen in hospitals. Enterococci, a species of *Streptococcus* found in normal GI and GU tracts, can cause HAIs with a high mortality rate if the organism is vancomycin resistant. As the enterococci mutate and develop acquired and intrinsic resistance to mainstay drugs such as vancomycin, ampicillin, and gentamycin, providers continue to give targeted therapy (such as the synthetic antibiotic linezolid or daptomycin) in an effort to treat the infection and reduce complications (Levitus et al., 2020; see Table 25-1 on page 668). Risk factors for VRE are similar to other HAIs and include compromised immune systems, recent surgery, invasive devices, prolonged antibiotic use (especially vancomycin), and prolonged hospitalization.

VRE is spread via contact with the feces, urine, or blood of an infected or colonized person. In 2017, there were an estimated 54,500 cases of VRE in hospitalized patients, with 5,400 estimated deaths (CDC, 2019g). Health care providers must work to ensure prompt recognition, diagnosis, isolation, management, and infection control. Nursing assessment, intervention, and evaluation of high-risk patients and situations help to minimize infection and reduce the unnecessary suffering imposed on patients. To control the transmission of both MRSA and VRE, the CDC and a large volume of published evidence continue to support contact precautions along with meticulous hand hygiene, reducing the use of invasive devices, environmental cleaning, and decolonizing high-risk patients. Some institutions have removed contact precautions from this bundle and instead include standard precautions; they have noted no significant change in the incidence of MRSA or VRE (Pryor et al., 2020).

Carbapenem-Resistant Enterobacteriaceae

CRE are very difficult to treat and represent a public health threat. This disease was first reported in 2001 in the United States and is associated with a 40% to 50% mortality rate. *Klebsiella* species and *E. coli* are examples of Enterobacteriaceae normally found in the human intestine. Carbapenem antimicrobial drugs are broad-spectrum antimicrobials and the agents of choice for serious infections when an organism is resistant to other primary antibiotics. Resistance to carbapenems leaves few other treatment options. These organisms are readily passed from patient to patient, but rarely impact healthy people. People who have bladder or venous catheters in place, those who require ventilator assistance to breathe, patients with open surgical wounds, those taking antibiotics for a lengthy period of time, or people who have frequent hospitalizations (especially in an ICU) or long-term care facility stays are at risk for developing CRE. The plan of care requires laboratory testing to detect resistance to carbapenems; decisions on treatment of infections with CRE are based on these results. In 2017, there were an estimated 13,100 cases of CRE in hospitalized patients, with 1,100 deaths (CDC, 2019g). The CDC (2019g) recommends that the patient be placed on contact precautions. A focus on hand hygiene and education regarding prevention of CRE transmission are vital to prevent transmission of the deadly infection.

Acinetobacter Baumannii

Carbapenem-resistant *Acinetobacter baumannii* (CRAB) is a gram-negative bacterium found primarily in hospitals; those with immune issues, chronic lung disease, or diabetes may be more susceptible. It has spread through health care facilities, infecting 8,500 people that resulted in 700 deaths in 2017 (CDC, 2019g). CRAB has developed resistance to many antibiotic regimens, severely limiting treatment options and resulting in myriad clinical trials and observational studies to investigate alternative approaches to treat CRAB (Piperaki et al., 2019). When patients transition from one level of care to another, acute care, long-term care, and rehabilitation health care workers must maintain high-quality contact precautions to minimize the transfer of CRE (including CRAB) to another facility (Pryor et al., 2020). Because *A. baumannii* can also sustain itself in the environment, the patient's room and all mechanical equipment must be cleaned and disinfected to eliminate fomite transmission.

Clostridioides Difficile

Although not an antibiotic resistant infection, *C. diff* is caused by similar factors and is directly related to antibiotic use and resistance. National data indicate almost 223,900 people in the United States required hospitalization for *C. diff*, with at least 12,800 deaths attributed to *C. diff* (CDC, 2019g). While health care–associated (hospital and long-term care facilities) cases of CDIs are decreasing, community-associated cases of CDI are not. Although adults and children are both affected, CDI is seen largely in older adults. Both symptomatic and asymptomatic people serve as reservoirs for *C. diff*, as do any surfaces or objects contaminated with feces. This organism normally resides in the intestinal tract. When antibiotics (particularly broad-spectrum antibiotics) are prescribed or taken for a prolonged period of time, helpful bacteria are destroyed, and *C. diff* bacteria can grow out of control, creating a bacterial imbalance. Watery diarrhea, fever, and mild abdominal cramping are some of the more common signs and symptoms, but the severity of CDI depends on the specific strain (CDC, 2019e; Dubberke et al., 2014). Prevention is the key. General strategies to reduce the indirect transmission of CDI include (CDC, 2019e; Dubberke et al., 2014):

- Confirming CDI in patients with appropriate diagnostic testing protocols
- Avoiding the use of electronic equipment that is difficult to clean (electronic thermometers)
- Disinfecting dedicated patient care items and equipment (stethoscopes) between patients
- Using terminal cleaning protocols (including *C. diff* sporicidal agents) for patient-care areas and equipment with patient transfers and discharge

- Using full-barrier contact precautions (gown and gloves)
- Placing patients in private rooms; cohort patients with the same strain of CDI
- Performing meticulous hand hygiene (discussed earlier in this chapter on pages 672–675)
- Performing environmental contamination of rooms
- Educating health care providers (and patients/families as appropriate) on clinical presentation, transmission, and epidemiology of CDI
- Facilitating antibiotic stewardship (prescribing only when needed; minimizing high-risk antibiotic use)

QSEN *CLOSTRIDIOIDES DIFFICILE* (*C. DIFF*) INFECTION

Remember that CDI is not killed by alcohol-based handrubs, so soap and water are required.

In addition to recognition of CDI and prevention of transmission, keep in mind that best practice involves the measured use of antimicrobials—prescribing them at an appropriate dose and only when indicated. Antibody-based therapies may be used to manage patients with recurrent *C. diff* infections (CDC, 2019g).

STERILIZING AND DISINFECTING

Cleansing, disinfection, and sterilization help break the cycle of infection and prevent disease. Several processes are used to destroy microorganisms. **Disinfection** destroys all pathogenic organisms except spores; **sterilization** destroys all microorganisms, including spores/endospores (Yoo, 2018). Disinfection can be used when preparing the skin for a procedure or cleaning a piece of equipment that does not enter a sterile body part. Sterilization is usually performed on equipment that is entering a sterile portion of the body. Disinfection and sterilization of contaminated or infected objects and good hand hygiene diminish and often eliminate microorganisms as potential sources of infection.

Method Selection

Various factors influence the choice of sterilization and disinfection methods, including the following:

- Nature of organisms present: The CDC recommends that all supplies, linens, and equipment in a health care setting should be treated as if the patient were infectious. Some organisms are easily destroyed, whereas others can withstand certain common sterilization and disinfection methods.
- Number of organisms present: The more organisms present on an item, the longer it takes to destroy them.
- Type of equipment: Equipment with small lumens, crevices, or joints requires special care. Certain articles that may be damaged by various sterilization and disinfection methods require special handling.
- Intended use of equipment: The need for medical or surgical asepsis influences the preparation and cleaning of equipment. In the home, it may be safe to use equipment and supplies that are clean, but most health care facilities use sterilized articles for patient care.
- Available means for sterilization and disinfection: The choice of chemical or physical means of sterilization and disinfection depends on the nature and number of organisms, the type and intended use of the equipment, and the availability and practicality of the means. Table 25-3 lists the types of methods for sterilization and disinfection.
- Time: Time is a key factor when sterilizing or disinfecting articles. Failure to follow the recommended time periods is grossly negligent.

USING PERSONAL PROTECTIVE EQUIPMENT AND SUPPLIES

According to the 1992 Occupational Safety and Health Administration (OSHA) ruling, health care facilities must provide employees with the equipment and supplies necessary to minimize or prevent exposure to infectious material. This **personal protective equipment (PPE)** includes gloves, gowns, masks, and protective eye gear. Skill 25-2 on pages 695–700 illustrates the proper use of this equipment.

Gloves

Gloves are not a substitute for good hand hygiene. They are worn only once and discarded appropriately according to facility policy. Then hands are thoroughly decontaminated with meticulous hand hygiene. When nursing care activities do not involve the possibility of soiling the hands with body fluids, gloves are not necessary. Activities such as turning a patient, feeding a patient, taking vital signs, and changing IV fluid bags do not require the use of gloves as long as the potential contact with body fluids is not present. However, when there is a possibility of soiling the hands with body fluids, gloves must be worn.

Each patient interaction requires a clean pair of gloves. Some care activities for an individual patient may necessitate changing gloves more than once. Gloves should always be changed prior to moving from a contaminated task to a clean one. While wearing gloves, never leave the patient's room (unless transporting a contaminated item or moving a patient requiring transmission-based precautions), never write in the patient's chart, and never use the computer keyboard or telephone in the nurses' station. Also, health care workers should not touch their pagers, cell phones, or other facility-based communication devices without first performing good hand hygiene. Mobile phones, which are ubiquitous, fit easily into lab coat or scrub pockets where dirty hands can come into contact with the device. The dark, warm pockets are a breeding ground for thousands of microbes. Several studies confirm that touch screens and phones have microbe growth in 82% to 88% of the mobile phones tested. The good news is that hand hygiene is an effective means to stop the cycle of contamination (Cobb & Lazer, 2020).

Wearing gloves does not eliminate the need for proper hand hygiene. In reality, the warmth and moisture inside gloves create an ideal environment for bacteria to multiply, making it even more important to perform good hand hygiene before and after using gloves. Evidence-based practice

Table 25-3 Methods of Sterilization and Disinfection

METHOD	DISCUSSION	CAUTION
Physical		
Steam	Higher temperature caused by higher pressure destroys organisms (e.g., autoclaving)	Most plastic and rubber devices are damaged by autoclaving
Boiling water	Frequently used in the home—simple and inexpensive; boil item for at least 10 minutes	Spores and some viruses are not destroyed by boiling
Dry heat	Alternative sterilization method for home Used for metal items Heat oven to 350°F for 2 or more hours	Insufficient to destroy all microorganisms; not used in health care facilities
Radiation	Used for pharmaceuticals, foods, plastics, and other heat-sensitive items	Object must be directly exposed to ultraviolet radiation on all surfaces Poses risk to personnel
Chemical		
Ethylene oxide gas	Destroys microorganisms and spores/endospores by interfering with metabolic processes in cells Gas is released while items (oxygen and suction gauges, blood pressure equipment) are contained in autoclave	Precautions necessary because gas is toxic to humans
Chemical solutions	Generally used for instrument and equipment disinfection and for housekeeping disinfection Chlorines are useful for disinfecting water and for housekeeping purposes A solution of sodium hypochlorite (household bleach) in a 1:100 dilution effectively inactivates human immunodeficiency virus. Betadine and alcohol are also used as disinfectants	Method does not destroy all spores and may cause corrosion on metal surfaces

supports that gloving does not guarantee complete protection from infectious organisms. Gloves provide a barrier but are not impenetrable. It has been shown that many times glove-barrier failure goes undetected by the health care worker. Double gloving (putting on two gloves on one hand) is recommended if the health care worker is involved in a procedure during which exposure to blood or body fluids is expected, such as in an operating room (OR) setting where evidence indicates that glove perforations were reduced by 71% with double gloving (Association of periOperative Registered Nurses, 2020).

Sensitization to latex varies among health care workers based on their role and actual exposure to latex. Approximately 10% of health care workers and 1% to 2% of the general population are sensitized to traditional latex (Burkhart et al., 2015; Occupational Safety and Health Administration [OSHA], n.d.). Reactions to latex fall into three categories: (1) irritant contact dermatitis that results from contact with gloves where the hands become irritated and dry—this is not actually not an allergy; (2) allergic contact dermatitis (a type IV sensitivity), which is an actual reaction to the latex that results in localized pruritus (itching), erythema (redness or rash), and urticarial lesions 24 to 96 hours after the contact; and (3) a true latex allergy (a type I hypersensitivity) where there is an immediate systemic response that may result in anaphylaxis (Burkhart et al., 2015; National Institute for Occupational Safety and Health [NIOSH], 2012a). The cornstarch powder or talc used to make gloves easier to put on is a causative factor in latex allergy development, which is why there has been a move to powder-free gloves in the clinical setting. The powder binds with the latex protein and becomes airborne, thus contaminating the environment (Henry et al., 2020). Powder particles may be inhaled or absorbed into skin or mucous membranes or enter the bloodstream. It is important to remember that repeated exposures to latex have been shown to lead to a latex sensitivity. If a person continues to be exposed to latex after a sensitivity has developed, that person may demonstrate signs of a latex allergy. At present, there is no cure for a latex allergy.

The NIOSH (2012a) recommends that nonlatex gloves or powder-free, low-allergen latex gloves (if latex gloves are used) be available for use. Also, according to the OSHA Personal Protective Equipment Standard 1910.132 (2016), employers must provide alternative gloves if necessary. Because a completely *latex-free* environment is considered unattainable given the ubiquitous nature of latex, a *latex-safe* health care environment is essential for patients and health care providers with a latex allergy. All health care facilities are required to have a written policy that identifies how to deal with latex-sensitive employees and patients. Awareness of an allergy to latex is also important for safe home care. See Box 25-3 (on page 682) for information on latex allergy for health care personnel and patients.

Gowns

Gowns are usually worn to prevent soiling of the health care worker's clothing by the patient's blood and body fluids. They

Box 25-3 Latex Allergy Summary

Risk Factors

- Occupational exposure to latex (includes health care professionals)
- People with allergic tendencies
- People with food allergies, specifically banana, papaya, avocado, potatoes, kiwi fruit, chestnuts, and pineapples
- People with asthma, spina bifida, or a history of multiple surgical procedures or exposures to latex

Frequently Used Products that Contain Latex

- Gloves
- Blood pressure cuffs
- Electrode pads
- Stethoscopes
- IV tubing
- Urinary catheters
- Tourniquets
- Syringes
- Surgical masks
- Baby bottle nipples and pacifiers

Types of Reactions

- *Irritant contact dermatitis:* most common reaction usually restricted to hands that have come into contact with latex; symptoms include dry, irritated skin associated with pruritus
- *Allergic contact dermatitis or delayed hypersensitivity:* allergic contact dermatitis, displayed as dry, crusty bumps, erythema, pruritus, scaling vesicles, papular lesions at site of contact, including the palms; symptoms usually appear in 24 to 96 hours
- *Latex allergy or immediate hypersensitivity:* systemic reactions usually happen within minutes of exposure; displayed as rhinitis, conjunctivitis, angioedema, bronchospasm, shock, and/or systemic anaphylactic reactions; this is a life-threatening sensitivity that is rarely the first reaction to latex exposure

Diagnosis

- RAST (radioallergosorbent test): blood test for IgE antibodies to latex
- Skin prick: small amount of serum derived from latex placed on small prick in skin

Treatment

- Prevention: avoidance of latex-containing products
- Localized reaction: treat with oral diphenhydramine, cool compresses, and hydrocortisone 1% cream
- Systemic reaction: possibly treated with epinephrine subcutaneously, systemic steroids, antihistamines, with transport to the emergency department
  - Remove all latex-containing articles from the room
  - Place three-way stopcocks in IV lines for medication administration; place tape over any injection ports on IV tubing

Patient Teaching (If Diagnosed With Latex Allergy)

- Avoid all latex-containing products and avoid inhaling powder used in latex gloves
- Inform employer and other health professionals of latex allergy
- Wear medical alert bracelet
- Follow doctor's recommendations
- Inform health care provider/nurse of allergy prior to any injections/immunizations; a latex-free vial stopper should be used
- Ensure that health care provider is aware of allergy prior to any medical procedure or surgery

Source: Adapted from National Institute for Occupational Safety and Health (NIOSH). (2012a). *NIOSH Fast Facts–Home healthcare workers: How to prevent latex allergy.* DHHS (NIOSH) Publication No. 2012–119. http://www.cdc.gov/niosh/docs/2012-119/pdfs/2012-119.pdf

provide barrier protection and are donned immediately before entering the patient's room. Individual gown technique is recommended. This technique involves wearing a gown only one time and then discarding it appropriately according to facility policy. A waterproof or impervious gown is used if there is an increased likelihood of contact with a patient's blood or body fluids. If a gown becomes heavily soiled or moistened with blood or body fluids when caring for a patient, remove it, perform thorough hand hygiene, and put on a clean gown. There is no single special technique for applying a gown used as a barrier, but recommended practices for removing a soiled gown are described in Skill 25-2 on pages 695–700.

Masks

Surgical masks, which are FDA approved, and procedure/isolation masks help prevent biologic particles from being disseminated into the air by the wearer. Masks help prevent the wearer from coming into direct contact with known or suspected infected body fluids (such as blood) that may spray or splash. When worn properly, masks also protect the wearer from exposure to large particle pathogens (>5 μm in size) spread through close respiratory or mucous membrane contact with respiratory droplets. These droplets are generated by coughing, sneezing, or talking, and they typically travel less than 3 ft but may reach 6 ft in certain instances. (See Transmission-Based Precautions later in this chapter.) Particulate respirators are used to prevent the inhalation of either airborne droplet nuclei or small particle aerosols (≤5 μm in size), which can remain suspended in the air and travel longer distances (see Transmission-Based Precautions later in this chapter; Siegel et al., 2019).

Various mask practices are used. In some instances, all personnel and all the patient's visitors wear masks while in the patient's room. In other situations, the patient wears the mask when transported outside their room to either protect health care personnel and other patients from exposure to pathogens, or to protect the patient.

In the clinical setting, a mask is typically worn only once and not lowered around the neck and then brought back over the mouth and nose for reuse. How long one can wear a mask while caring for one patient is the subject of debate. Regardless of the time worn, a mask must be changed before it becomes damp from the wearer's exhalations. See Skill 25-2, pages 695–700 for the recommended practice for applying and removing a mask.

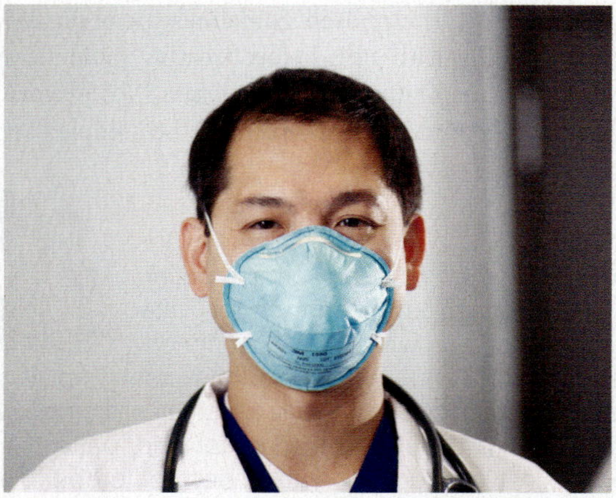

FIGURE 25-3. The N95 health care particulate respirator is NIOSH approved. It meets CDC guidelines for tuberculosis exposure control and is designed specifically for use in a health care setting. *(Source: Courtesy of 3M Health Care.)*

A particulate respirator filters inspired air; surgical masks filter only expired air. One of the most commonly used respirators is the N95 respirator, which is designed to filter airborne particles as small as 1 μm with 95% efficiency and fits comfortably against the face (Fig. 25-3). The elastic straps on these respirators provide more protection and a better fit than the ties on regular surgical masks, but fit-testing is required to ensure health care workers are using the appropriate mask size (CDC, 2020h; OSHA, 2011; Siegel et al., 2019). Once a fit test has been completed to determine the best respirator size, a seal check should be done every time the respirator is worn to ensure an adequate seal (Krah et al., 2018).

The serious increase in the number of multidrug-resistant tuberculosis cases prompted new guidelines to prevent the transmission of this disease. According to CDC guidelines, a NIOSH-certified N95 respirator or higher-level respirator must be worn when entering the airborne infection isolation (AII) room of a patient with known or suspected tuberculosis. These AII rooms are single-occupancy patient rooms designed for airborne transmission with environmental controls including negative pressure, an air flow rate of 6 to 12 air changes per hour, and direct venting of exhaust to the outside or the use of a high efficiency particulate air (HEPA) filter. Other infections or conditions that may be airborne such as EVD, influenza, coronavirus (MERS-CoV and SARS-CoV-2), and Zika viruses require standard, contact, droplet, and/or airborne precautions (CDC, 2019d; Siegel et al., 2019). We will address some of these specific cases later in this chapter.

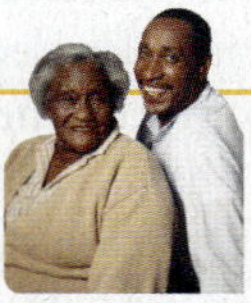

Think back to **Jackson Ray Ivers**, the son coming to visit his mother who is hospitalized with a new-onset fever and cough after exposure to a friend with a highly communicable respiratory virus. The nurse would incorporate knowledge of respiratory transmission and appropriate barriers to explain to Mr. Ivers why they need to wear a mask or a respirator while visiting.

Protective Eyewear

Protective eyewear, such as goggles or a face shield, must be available whenever there is a risk of contaminating the mucous membranes of the eyes. For example, suctioning a tracheostomy or assisting with an invasive procedure that may result in splattering of blood or other body fluids requires protection for the caregiver. Plain glasses are unacceptable because side shields are required.

HANDLING AND DISPOSING OF SUPPLIES

Used equipment may be disposed of after use or, if reusable, bagged according to facility policy, sent to a central cleaning area, and sterilized or disinfected. Double bagging may be required if the single bag is not secure or is soiled on the outside. A contaminated item must never be used for another patient.

Some linen bags are water soluble and dissolve in hot water, making it unnecessary for workers to handle the contaminated linen. The use of paper trays and plastic eating utensils does not prevent transmission of organisms and is no longer recommended. The combined hot water and detergent used in commercial dishwashers sufficiently decontaminates dishes, glasses, and utensils. All spills of body fluids or substances must be immediately cleaned with the appropriate chemical germicide or disinfectant.

When collecting a specimen, take care to prevent the outside of the container from becoming contaminated with any secretions or body fluids. Place all laboratory specimens in plastic bags and seal the bags to prevent leakage during transportation. A red bag marked *BIOHAZARD* is used to dispose of trash that contains liquid or semiliquid blood or other potentially infective material (OPIM), trash contaminated with blood or OPIM that would release these substances if compressed, and trash that is caked with dried blood or OPIM and is capable of releasing these materials during handling.

USING STANDARD AND TRANSMISSION-BASED PRECAUTIONS

In addition to barriers, specific precautions have been established to prevent the transmission of infection. Historically, health care workers employ **isolation**, a protective procedure that limits the spread of infectious diseases among hospitalized patients, hospital personnel, and visitors. Infection control programs, interprofessional teams, and other health care workers require a shared understanding of core principles to guide the development of and adherence to policies and procedures designed to create an environment dedicated to infection control and prevention.

Current Centers for Disease Control and Prevention Guidelines

The 2007 CDC guideline (Siegel et al., 2019) recognizes that health care delivery occurs in other settings beside acute care hospitals. This guideline, focused on preventing transmission of infectious agents in myriad health care settings, replaces the 1996 guideline and is updated periodically online as new information becomes available. This publication marks the transition from the narrow term *nosocomial infection* (hospital-acquired) to the broader term, *health care–associated infection* (associated with health care delivery in any setting). These guidelines reflect the emergence of new pathogens, methods to prevent transmission of multidrug-resistant organisms, and the CDC's concern regarding biologic terrorism. Nurses must understand the various precautions or barrier techniques if they are to use them correctly and minimize infection risks to patients as well as to themselves (see Promoting Health 25-1 on page 674).

The long-standing CDC guidelines (Siegel et al., 2019) continue to designate two tiers of precautions:

- **Standard precautions:** precautions used in the care of all hospitalized patients regardless of their diagnosis or possible infection status. These precautions apply to blood, all body fluids, secretions, excretions (except sweat), nonintact skin, and mucous membranes. New elements included in standard precautions are respiratory hygiene/cough etiquette, safe injection practices, and directions to use a mask when performing high-risk prolonged procedures involving spinal canal punctures. Elements of respiratory hygiene and cough etiquette include education of staff and patients, posted instructions for the population served, review of source control measures (e.g., using masks on patients who are coughing and appropriate use of tissues with sneezes), reinforcement of hand hygiene (especially with managing secretions), and spatial separation when possible.
- **Transmission-based precautions:** precautions used in addition to standard precautions for patients in hospitals with suspected infection with pathogens that can be transmitted by airborne, droplet, or contact routes. The 2007 CDC guidelines include a directive to don PPE when entering the room of a patient with transmission-based precautions, and to remove the PPE only when leaving the room. These categories recognize that a disease may have multiple routes of transmission.

The three types of transmission-based precautions (airborne, droplet, or contact) may be used alone or in combination, but always in addition to standard precautions. Box 25-4 summarizes the current CDC guidelines along with a listing of specific recommendations for both tiers of precautions. Hospitals are encouraged to tailor these recommendations as needed for implementation of their infection control strategy.

Although supported by the CDC and other infection control facilities, the efficacy of using contact precautions to prevent the spread of multidrug-resistant organisms, such as MRSA, continues to be considered. For example, there is little support in the literature for the routine use of contact precautions in MRSA, especially when it is endemic and colonization rates are high. Recommendations continue to support ongoing education of standard precautions and good handwashing (Pryor et al., 2020). As diseases, infections, or conditions emerge or their prevalence increases, guidelines need to evolve. For example, when EVD emerged as an impending issue in 2014, the CDC issued revised guidelines for health care workers caring for these patients. The revised guidelines focus on repeated hands-on training with PPE before treating patients, avoidance of skin or respiratory exposure when PPE is worn, and supervision by a trained monitor during the complex application and removal of PPE.

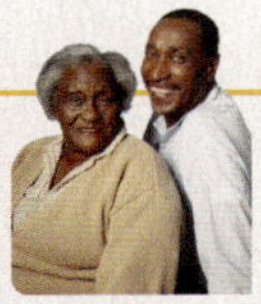

Recall ***Jackson Ray Ivers***, the son of a patient with a new-onset fever and cough after exposure to a friend with a highly communicable respiratory virus. Based on the nurse's knowledge of disease transmission, the nurse institutes droplet (with occasional airborne) precautions for the patient and instructs Mr. Ivers regarding the need for proper hand hygiene and the use of a mask or respirator.

In late 2019, SARS-CoV-2 and the disease it causes (COVID-19) created a pandemic unlike anything we have seen in the modern world. Since COVID-19 so greatly affected people worldwide, chances are good the section on masks was particularly interesting. Let's take a moment to talk about the underlying infection control principles that guided the experts during COVID-19. Since it is a novel virus, data and the associated specific recommendations were changing rapidly, but the underlying principles were fairly consistently applied. For example, when this first started and the mechanism for transmission was largely unknown, acute care facilities moved to requiring standard, contact, and airborne precautions (respirators and AII rooms) for patients with suspected or diagnosed COVID-19. Finite resources complicated the situation in health care, and there was a move to reuse, reallocate, and reconsider possible alternatives in the move to crisis planning. As experts surveyed the pandemic and had some evidence that COVID-19 was predominantly spread via contact and/or droplet routes, the move was made to consider droplet precautions (masks and face shields) in general health care interactions, as dictated by resources. Respirators were reserved for aerosol-generating procedures (e.g., during endotracheal intubation, a bronchoscopy, or suctioning), where the virus was thought to become airborne and be transmitted via fine/small particle aerosols over greater than 3 ft within a defined airspace. In these instances, the nose and mouth are protected by a particulate respirator, the eyes protected by goggles or a face shield, and the rest of the body protected with gloves and a gown (Siegel et al., 2019). The combination of the rapid spread, previous experience with SARS, an overwhelmed health care system, and core infection control principles, led experts to make some clear infection control recommendations for the general public that included: (1) handwashing, the foundation of all infection control practices, to decrease potential fomite and mucous membrane transfer (especially with untrained mask donning and doffing); (2) handmade cloth masks to prevent the spread of droplets, while protecting the supply of health care grade products for health care workers; (3) social distancing of 6 ft to reflect the estimated distance seen with SARS transmission; and (4) restrictions on large group, especially indoor, activities

Box 25-4 Summary of 2007 CDC Guidelines for Isolation Precautions in Health Care Settings

Standard Precautions (Tier 1)

- *Follow hand hygiene techniques.*
- *Wear clean nonsterile gloves* when touching blood, body fluids, excretions or secretions, contaminated items, mucous membranes, and nonintact skin. Change gloves between tasks on the same patient as necessary and remove gloves promptly after use.
- *Wear personal protective equipment* such as mask, eye protection, face shield, or fluid-repellent gown during procedures and care activities that are likely to generate splashes or sprays of blood or body fluids. Use gown to protect skin and prevent soiling of clothing.
- *Follow respiratory hygiene/cough etiquette.* Any patients, family members, and visitors with undiagnosed, transmissible respiratory infections require education to cover their mouth and nose with a tissue when coughing and promptly dispose of the tissue. During periods of increased occurrence of respiratory infections, offer a surgical mask to coughing patients and other symptomatic people upon entry to the health care facility or office. Encourage the coughing patient to maintain more than a 3-ft separation from other people in the health care facility or office.
- *Avoid recapping used needles.* Choose needles with safety devices that can be activated with one hand. If you must recap, never use two hands. Use a needle-recapping device or the one-handed scoop technique. Place needles, sharps, and scalpels in appropriate puncture-resistant containers after use.
- *Use safe injection practices* including single-dose vials when possible; use disposable needles and syringes for each injection, and prevent contamination of injection equipment and medication.
- *Wear face mask* if placing a catheter or injecting material into the spinal or epidural space.
- *Handle used patient care equipment that is soiled with blood or identified body fluids, secretions, and excretions carefully* to prevent transfer of microorganisms. Clean and reprocess items appropriately if used for another patient.
- *Use adequate environmental controls* to ensure that routine care, cleaning, and disinfection procedures are followed.
- *Review room assignments carefully.* Place patients who may contaminate the environment in private rooms (such as a patient who is incontinent).

Transmission-Based Precautions (Tier 2)

The following precautions are recommended in addition to standard precautions:

Airborne Precautions

Use these for patients who have infections that spread through the air such as tuberculosis, varicella (chicken pox), and rubeola (measles).

- Place patient in a private room that has monitored negative air pressure in relation to surrounding areas, 6 to 12 air changes per hour, and appropriate discharge of air outside, or monitored filtration if air is recirculated. Keep door closed and patient in room.
- Wear a respirator when entering room of patient with known or suspected tuberculosis. If patient has known or suspected rubeola (measles) or varicella (chicken pox), respiratory protection should be worn unless the person entering room is immune to these diseases.
- Transport patient out of room only when necessary and place a surgical mask on the patient if possible.
- Consult CDC guidelines for additional prevention strategies for tuberculosis.

Droplet Precautions

Use these for patients with an infection that is spread by large-particle droplets such as rubella, mumps, diphtheria, and the adenovirus infection in infants and young children.

- Use a private room, if available. Door may remain open.
- Wear PPE upon entry into the room for all interactions that may involve contact with the patient and potentially contaminated areas in the patient's environment.
- Transport patient out of room only when necessary and place a surgical mask on the patient if possible.
- Keep visitors 3 ft from the infected person.

Contact Precautions

Use these for patients who are infected or colonized by a multidrug-resistant organism (MDRO).

- Place the patient in a private room, if available.
- Wear PPE whenever you enter the room for all interactions that may involve contact with the patient and potentially contaminated areas in the patient's environment. Change gloves after having contact with infective material. Remove PPE before leaving the patient environment, and wash hands with an antimicrobial or waterless antiseptic agent.
- Limit movement of the patient out of the room.
- Avoid sharing patient-care equipment.

Source: Adapted from Siegel, J. D., Rhinehart, E., Jackson, M., Chiarello, L., & The Healthcare Infection Control Practices Advisory Committee. (2019, July). *2007 Guideline for isolation precautions: Preventing transmission of infectious agents in healthcare settings (Last update: July 2019).* https://www.cdc.gov/infectioncontrol/pdf/guidelines/isolation-guidelines-H.pdf

where transmission was more likely to occur via droplet or airborne mechanisms.

PREVENTING OCCUPATIONAL EXPOSURES

OSHA developed the Bloodborne Pathogens Standard in 1991 to protect health care workers from exposure or risk of exposure to pathogens such as HIV and HBV. This was revised in 2000 by the passage of The Needlestick Safety and Prevention Act that had more specifications for employers and more detail about how health care providers should participate in decisions and ensure safe practice regarding needlestick injuries and bloodborne exposures (Occupational Safety and Health Administration, 2012). The Needlestick Safety and Prevention Act requires health care providers to:

- Identify and provide safer medical devices that reduce or eliminate injuries from sharps
- Involve health care workers in the selection process of these safer devices

- Provide engineering controls for sharps disposal containers, self-sheathing needles, and other safety devices to reduce or eliminate sharps injuries
- Educate employees regarding how to safely use these devices
- Develop a sharps injury surveillance log

Although sharps injuries declined following the implementation of the revised standards in 2001, that decline has not continued (International Safety Center, 2020). Results from a national survey indicate that, based on data received from 170 hospitals in 2016 and 224 hospitals in 2017, the rate of injuries from sharps has risen every year for the last 3 years and now matches rates reported in 2001 to 2005. Close to 40% of these injuries occurred in surgery, and teaching hospitals had higher rates than nonteaching hospitals (Grimmond & Good, 2019). In an effort to highlight this ongoing issue, many nursing and health care organizations, including the ANA, developed a Consensus Statement and Call to Action that originally focused on: (1) improving sharps safety in the surgical setting, (2) understanding and reducing exposure risks in nonhospital settings, (3) involving front-line health care workers when choosing safety devices, (4) addressing gaps in safety devices and consider innovations, and (5) enhancing education and training. These consensus statements that began in 2010 continue to provide broad recommendations that target health care facilities, professional associations, organizations that set standards, manufacturers, regulatory agencies, and accrediting organizations. The group focuses on a system-level approach that is data-driven and proactive (International Safety Center, 2020).

Needlestick injuries are also a significant occupational hazard for health care workers visiting private homes (see Box 25-5). Keep in mind that although nurses may suffer the largest proportion of needlestick injuries (Grimmond & Good, 2019), it is not always the nurse or original person using the device who sustains the injury. Other clinicians, housekeeping, or laundry staff could also come in contact with these devices and sustain an injury.

The most serious risk associated with needlestick injuries or mucous membrane exposure is the possible risk of infection with pathogens such as HBV, HCV, and HIV. Health care facilities now purchase needles with built-in safety features and needleless, protected, or recessed IV systems. Although this equipment is more expensive, the higher costs may be budget neutral due to fewer needlestick injuries. Knowledge of safety devices and prevention of bloodborne pathogen exposures create a safer workplace environment and protect nurses from potentially life-threatening injuries.

REPORTING ACCIDENTAL EXPOSURES

Although system-level controls must work to minimize exposures and establish a safe work environment (International Safety Center, 2020; NIOSH, 2015), nurses also bear responsibility for their own safety. Any needlestick injury or accidental exposure to blood or body fluids must be reported immediately so that appropriate action can be taken. Underreporting of exposures is believed to be widespread. Reasons for not reporting exposures include belief that the injury is insignificant or that the actual risk is relatively small, reporting it requires too much time, concern about negative consequences if the injury is reported, and belief that these types of injuries are to be expected. It is imperative that nurses and other health care workers report these injuries promptly so that they receive any appropriate postexposure treatment and prophylaxis. A facility's plan for this type of exposure typically includes the following recommendations supported by the CDC and NIOSH (National Clinician Consultation Center, 2020):

- Immediate management of the exposure site—wash the exposed area immediately with warm water and soap, flush mucous membranes, or irrigate eyes
- Immediate, detailed report of the incident to the facility, with likely completion of an incident or injury report
- Baseline testing of the source person first, with permission, to determine HCV, HBV, and HIV status (rapid HIV testing preferred); baseline testing of the exposed person indicated with positive results from the source person; note if the exposed person is considered immune to HBV with documented positive titer and requires no further testing or follow-up
- Postexposure prophylaxis (PEP), if recommended; consideration of pregnancy and lactation

Box 25-5 Preventing Needlestick Injuries to Home Health Care Workers

Nurses working in private homes need to be aware of the factors that contribute to risks in these settings. They include:

- Avoid using needles whenever safe and effective alternatives are available.
- Use needles with safety devices; void recapping or bending needles that might be contaminated.
- Bring standard-labeled, leak-proof, puncture-resistant sharps containers to the patients' homes and promptly dispose of used needles and sharps in this container.
- Plan for safe handling and disposal of needles before use.
- Keep sharps container out of the reach of children, pets, and anyone not needing access to it.
- Ensure that sharps container is secure to prevent spilling before transporting it.
- Follow standard precautions, infection prevention, and general hygiene practices consistently.
- Participate in your employer's bloodborne pathogens training program.
- Help your employer elect and evaluate safety devices and equipment.
- Use devices with safety features provided by your employer.
- Report any needlestick or other sharps injury immediately to your employer.

Source: Adapted from National Institute for Occupational Safety and Health (NIOSH). (2012b). *NIOSH Fast Facts–Home healthcare workers: How to prevent needlestick and sharps injuries.* DHHS (NIOSH) Publication No. 2012–123. http://www.cdc.gov/niosh/docs/2012-123/pdfs/2012-123.pdf

- Follow-up testing as recommended—can be at 6 weeks, 3 months, and/or 12 months, depending on the exposure
- Counseling sessions regarding safe practices to protect self and others

PROVIDING CARE IN SPECIAL SITUATIONS

Occasionally, nurses need to use neutropenic precautions for a patient whose immune system is compromised (e.g., recovering from transplantation surgery or receiving chemotherapy). Those who are immunosuppressed more often than not become infected by organisms harbored in their own bodies, rather than by pathogens present in the environment or transmitted from other people. As with all hospitalized patients, standard precautions are required, but some additional measures are helpful when a patient's ability to withstand any bacterial invasion is compromised.

Recommendations in this situation include the following:

- Ensure that health care provider is healthy
- Restrict visits from friends and family members who have colds or contagious illnesses
- Avoid collection of standing water in the room (e.g., humidifiers) to prevent bacteria typically found in this water
- Avoid plants and flowers—soil is a source of bacteria and mold
- Follow hospital protocols regarding PPE for neutropenic precautions

The latest CDC (Siegel et al., 2019) guideline also addresses environmental controls that foster a *protective environment* to decrease the risk of infection in the most severely immunocompromised patients.

The increasing number of people who are ill or immunocompromised, coupled with increasingly virulent organisms, poses sterilization and disinfection concerns for home environments. Common measures that reduce the risk of infection at home include the following (OncoLink, 2020):

- Wash hands frequently—for the affected person and everyone who comes in contact with the affected person—especially before preparing food, before eating, and after using the restroom
- Maintain a clean home and frequently use household disinfectants and antibacterial wipes
- Avoid sharing personal items
- Perform regular, thorough oral care using a soft-bristled toothbrush
- Minimize the risk of injury—avoid sunburn, cuts, suppositories, tampons, and intercourse/penetration with sexual paraphernalia/oral sex
- Do not handle animal waste
- Avoid crowds, public pools, and adults or children who are sick or recently vaccinated
- Clean and disinfect kitchen surfaces, especially when preparing meat, chicken, and fish
- Cook food to the proper internal temperature; promptly refrigerate or freeze perishables, prepared foods, and leftovers
- Avoid raw meat and fish; wash all fresh fruits and vegetables; avoid soft cheese; use only pasteurized products; pay attention to sell-by dates

Controlling disease and preventing infections from spreading is a vital home care consideration for everyone.

Using Surgical Asepsis

Surgical asepsis techniques, used regularly in the operating room, labor and delivery areas, and certain diagnostic testing areas, are also used by the nurse at the patient's bedside. Procedures that involve the insertion of a urinary catheter, sterile dressing changes, or preparing an injectable medication are examples of surgical asepsis techniques. An object is considered sterile when all microorganisms, including pathogens and spores/endospores, have been destroyed. For example, the needle for an injection must be handled so that it is sterile when inserted into a patient. Sterile forceps or gloves are used to handle sterile dressings to protect against contamination. The basic principles of surgical asepsis are listed in Box 25-6 (on page 688).

When observing *medical asepsis* (clean technique), areas are considered contaminated if they bear or are suspected of bearing pathogens; whereas when following *surgical asepsis* (sterile technique), areas are considered contaminated if they are touched by any object that is not also sterile. One of the most important aspects of surgical and medical asepsis is that the effectiveness of both depends on faithful and conscientious practice by those performing them. It is far better to err on the side of safety when using surgical asepsis than to take the slightest chance of possible contamination. Being a patient advocate requires vigilant aseptic technique and a willingness to speak up if the patient's safety has been compromised by improper procedures.

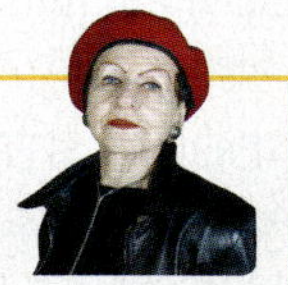

Think back to **Esther Bailey**, the woman described in the Reflective Practice box (on page 664). The nurse acted appropriately by speaking up about the possible contamination of the catheter. Had this catheter been used, the patient's safety would have been compromised.

Explaining the surgical asepsis procedure to patients facilitates their cooperation. Inform the patient about which objects and areas may not be touched and direct the patient to avoid sudden movements that might contaminate the equipment. This helps the patient assist in maintaining the sterility of the procedure.

OPENING A STERILE PACKAGE AND PREPARING A STERILE FIELD

Commercially prepared sterile items may be sealed in paper or packaged in plastic containers. Sterile packages may be opened on a flat surface or while held in the hands. Skill 25-3 on pages 701–705 illustrates how to open a sterile package and prepare a sterile field. A sterile item should be covered if

Box 25-6 Practicing Basic Principles of Surgical Asepsis

- Allow only a sterile object to touch another sterile object. Unsterile touching sterile means contamination has occurred.
- Open sterile packages so that the first edge of the wrapper is directed away from the worker to avoid the possibility of a sterile surface touching unsterile clothing. The outside of the sterile package is considered contaminated. Opening a sterile package is shown and described in Skill 25-3 on pages 701–705.
- Avoid spilling any solution on a cloth or paper used as a field for a sterile setup. The moisture penetrates through the sterile cloth or paper and carries organisms by capillary action to contaminate the field. A wet field is considered contaminated if the surface immediately below it is not sterile.
- Hold sterile objects above the level of the waist. This will ensure keeping the object within sight and preventing accidental contamination.
- Avoid talking, coughing, sneezing, or reaching over a sterile field or object. This helps to prevent contamination by droplets from the nose and the mouth or by particles dropping from the worker's arm.
- Never walk away from or turn your back on a sterile field. This prevents possible contamination while the field is out of the worker's view.
- Keep all items sterile that are brought into contact with broken skin or used to penetrate the skin to inject substances into the body or to enter normally sterile body cavities. These items include dressings used to cover surgical incisions, needles for injection, and tubes (catheters) used to drain urine from the bladder.
- Use dry, sterile forceps when necessary. Forceps soaked in disinfectant are not considered sterile.
- Consider the edge (outer 1 inch) of a sterile field to be contaminated.
- Consider an object contaminated if you have any doubt as to its sterility.

it is not used immediately. Reapply the cover by touching only the outside of the wrapper and reversing the opening order.

POURING STERILE SOLUTIONS

Care is necessary when pouring sterile liquids onto a sterile dressing or into a sterile basin. The outer surfaces of the bottle and cap are considered unsterile, whereas the inside areas and the solution are considered sterile. After a solution has been opened, the outer bottle should be labeled with date and time if it is to be reused. Most solutions are considered sterile for 24 hours after they are opened. When pouring from a bottle, grasp the bottle so that the label is in the palm of your hand. This action prevents any of the liquid from running over the label and making it illegible. Avoid splashing the liquid since this would contaminate the sterile field (see Skill 25-3, pages 701–705).

ADDING STERILE SUPPLIES TO A STERILE FIELD

After establishing a sterile field, it may be necessary to add items such as instruments or additional supplies to the sterile field. Item 6 in Skill 25-3 on pages 701–705 demonstrates this technique. Once a sterile field is established, objects on a field may be handled only by using sterile forceps or with hands wearing sterile gloves.

PUTTING ON STERILE GLOVES

Sterile gloves are donned in a way that allows only the inside of the gloves to come in contact with the hands. Skill 25-4 on pages 706–709 describes the proper technique for putting on sterile gloves.

After the gloves are on, only sterile items may be handled with the sterile-gloved hands. Careful removal of the gloves reduces any hand contact with contaminated materials. Good hand hygiene technique before and after putting on sterile gloves is imperative.

POSITIONING A STERILE DRAPE

The sterile drape, which ideally is waterproof, may be used to extend the sterile working area. Using sterile gloves allows the nurse to handle the entire drape surface. For protection when positioning, fold the upper edges of the drape over the sterile-gloved hands (Fig. 25-4). When sterile gloves are not worn, the nurse can touch only the outer 1 inch (2.5 cm) of the drape. Use caution when gently shaking the drape open so as not to touch one's clothing or an unsterile object. Hold the drape by the 1-inch upper edge and position the drape over the desired area. Do not reach over the drape because this would contaminate the sterile area.

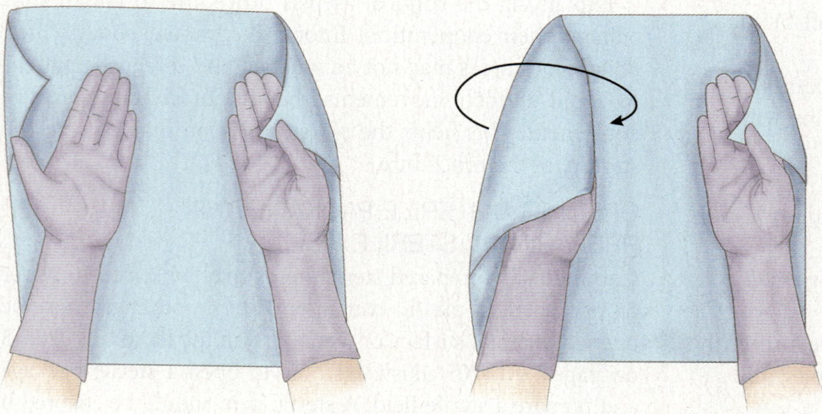

FIGURE 25-4. Techniques for cuffing a sterile drape over gloved hands.

Through the Eyes of a Student

She was the cutest little girl I have ever known. She was infected with HIV from birth. Her mother used illicit IV drugs and engaged in condomless vaginal sex with multiple partners. This little girl, who came into the world with an innocent, fresh, new face full of unconditional love, could not walk, could not talk, could not chew, and could not control her urine or bowel movements—but she could smile unlike any other child! In the beginning, I was so terrified of contracting HIV that I couldn't walk into her room without a mask, gown, gloves, protective eyewear, and basically a full protective body spacesuit. At the end of my time with her, I wanted to take her into my home and give her all the love, support, and care she needed. I am not saying that I didn't wear gloves when I changed her diapers or when I flushed her saline lock because I did … I was very careful. But I realized that she is a person, a person full of feelings, a person who needed me, and from whom I could learn. People with the HIV virus are just that—people. We need to learn to treat them as such.

I also learned not to fear the person who is diagnosed with HIV infection or AIDS. I know that I will remember to take the proper safety precautions with this person. But I also need to have a healthy respect for the virus and check any unconscious bias when I happen to think a particular patient is or isn't the "type of person" to have HIV. If I don't consistently use standard precautions, it is possible that one day I'll become infected through contact with someone who is "not the type." If that should ever happen, I hope everyone who cares for me will treat me as a real person and not be afraid.

—Karmi N. Soder, Georgetown University, Washington, DC

Meeting Needs of Patients Requiring Infection Control Precautions

The psychological implications of infection control precautions are usually great, whether the patient is strictly separated from others or needs only to observe relatively simple precautions (see the accompanying box, Through the Eyes of a Student).

The current CDC standard precautions treat all people in a similar manner and greatly minimize the psychological trauma of feeling unclean and undesirable, which often occurred with earlier measures. However, sensory deprivation and loss of self-esteem may occur with transmission-based precautions. For example, during the pandemic that began in 2019, when shelter in place orders were in effect, when high-risk populations were encouraged to remain home, when nursing homes were in lockdown, and when family was relegated to online socialization, older adults around the world experienced profound social isolation. Unfortunately, social isolation can lead to poor physical and mental health. Specific strategies to mitigate this loneliness and build social connections included public health positive messaging, mobilizing family and community-based resources, developing accessible technology-based interventions to engage older adults, and encouraging the health care team to consider social isolation and loneliness in their health care systems (Wu, 2020). For hospitalized patients in isolation at any time, friends and relatives may be forbidden to visit. Visitors as well as health care personnel may be inclined to spend less time with the patient because they are afraid that they will contract the disease or because of the inconvenience (and discomfort) of donning, wearing, then doffing the required PPE (e.g., gowns, masks, respirators, shoe covers, and face shields). This may lead to inconsistent recording of vital signs, irregular documentation, and less patient monitoring on the part of caregivers. Research has also verified that patients placed in isolation because of the presence of a communicable disease may suffer unintended consequences such as an increase in incidents of depression and/or anxiety, fewer and shorter visits from health care providers, and a decrease in satisfaction (Kullar et al., 2016). Nursing measures to help prevent the sensory deprivation and loss of self-esteem associated with isolation precautions are discussed in Chapters 42 and 45.

Health teaching about transmission-based precautions can ease the fears of patients and family members. Both must understand the pertinent epidemiologic facts and how to carry out the specific precautions. It is helpful to emphasize the following:

- Precautions are temporary
- A clear description of the precautions and protective equipment worn by the staff to protect the patient, the caregiver, and other patients
- Proper hand hygiene before and after visiting the patient is the most effective measure to prevent spread of the disease
- Continued explanations about procedures and continued updates on progress help to empower the patient

Nurses must document their health teaching about barrier precautions in the patient's care plan. A well-informed nurse who understands how to protect both self and patients, and a well-informed patient who is cooperating in one's own care, create the best infection-prevention team.

Raising Ethical Concerns About Infection Risks

Infection control and precautions minimize infection risks for patients as well as health care workers. However, the increasing numbers of people infected with HIV, HBV, and HCV have led to serious ethical concerns and controversy related to the risk for transmitting these diseases. The rights of the patient may conflict with the rights of the health care worker and the health care facility. Refer to the accompanying box, Nursing Advocacy in Action (on page 690), for an example of a situation in which the nurse must reconcile the patient's right to make choices versus the well-being of family members.

Nursing Advocacy in Action

Patient Scenario

Mrs. Samol is a 38-year-old patient in the medical ICU who is dying of AIDS-related complications. Since being diagnosed with AIDS, she has refused to inform her husband and family of her AIDS status. She even has an advance directive, which forbids the disclosure of her diagnosis when she can no longer advocate for herself. Her husband and mother cannot understand why the doctors and nurses cannot treat her "pneumonia"—the only diagnosis she gave them. The doctors and nurses caring for Mrs. Samol believe that her husband has the right to know his wife's diagnosis so that he can make decisions in his own best interest about being tested, having their children tested, etc.

Implications for Nursing Advocacy

What would you do if you were Mrs. Samol's nurse? Talk with your classmates and experienced nurses about the questions that follow.

- If you elect to advocate for the Samols, what practical steps can you take to ensure better health outcomes? Are there any legal guidelines for what you can and cannot do?
- What is reasonable to expect of a student nurse, a graduate nurse, and an experienced nurse in this situation?
- What advocacy skills are needed to effectively respond to this challenge?

Questions such as the following are being debated:

- Should all hospitalized patients be routinely tested for HCV infection?
- Should HBV testing be mandatory for all foreign-born residents of the United States?
- Should health care workers infected with HIV be permitted to perform exposure-prone invasive procedures?
- Should you address hand hygiene with another RN who you have observed never washes their hands after removing gloves?
- Should pregnant health care providers be expected to care for patients with infectious diseases?
- Since standard precautions are sufficient to protect health care workers from HIV, is there a need to include this information in SBAR report? Were it not for the family dynamics should this even be mentioned?

The CDC and various medical and nursing groups are seeking consensus on these issues, based on scientific information and valid statistical evidence. Although the CDC has issued guidelines related to these topics, not all states have adopted the guidelines. In addition, some states have revised them. All agree, however, that health care workers who conscientiously adhere to appropriate infection control precautions significantly reduce the risk for infection for patients and themselves.

Working With the Infection Preventionist

In the hospital, the nurse is responsible for the collection of statistics about infection and for educating patients and staff about effective infection control techniques. Many hospitals rely on this specialized practitioner, referred to as the infection preventionist, who has demonstrated expertise in specific competencies including (Billings et al., 2019):

- Epidemiology and surveillance
- Leading investigations and surveillance programs (using surveillance technology as appropriate)
- Preventing and controlling the transmission of infectious agents
- Managing and communicating plans and feedback, as well as performance improvement and patient safety initiatives
- Leading institutions through risk assessment and implementation stages
- Leading education, research, and performance improvement activities
- Overseeing employee/occupational health

Intensive investigative strategies create a positive environment that significantly reduces the incidence of HAIs in health care facilities. The infection preventionist knows the devastating effects of infection and is intent on promoting a safe environment while fostering a systematic approach to infection control.

In the home, the infection preventionist's duties include surveillance for facility-associated infections, education, consultation, epidemiologic investigation, quality-improvement activities, and policy and procedure development. OSHA regulations state that home care facilities must have an infection control program and that OSHA infection control standards and policies must be available to all staff for reference.

Teaching About Infection Control

Teaching about medical asepsis and infection control is a challenging nursing responsibility. Patients need to be aware of techniques that prevent the spread of infection and their rationale. COVID-19 provides a good exemplar of how misconceptions about mask requirements/recommendations belied the altruistic nature and adherence to the social contract exhibited by donning a mask in public—cloths masks did not necessarily protect the masked, they protected the community and individuals with whom the masked person came into contact. Use of the nursing process in infection control protects both the patient and the nurse.

Medical aseptic techniques are appropriate for most procedures in the home, except for self-injection technique and venous or dialysis catheter care, which require surgical asepsis. The patient frequently must make adjustments and improvise with the resources and supplies available for their use. In addition, the nurse emphasizes effective hand hygiene and other hygiene practices that interrupt the infection cycle. To satisfy OSHA requirements, many home care facilities have either a full-time or part-time infection preventionist. The Association for Professionals in Infection Control and Epidemiology (APIC, n.d.), an interprofessional organization dedicated to improving patient safety and health by reducing the risk of infection, has specific implementation guides that may be useful for educational initiatives: http://www.apic.org/Professional-Practice/Implementation-guides (see Additional Resources).

Teach patients to use basic principles of asepsis at home and in public facilities. These involve the activities of daily living (see Chapter 32 for a discussion of personal hygiene). Here are examples of medical asepsis practices recommended in the home:

- Wash hands before preparing food and before eating
- Prepare foods at temperatures high enough to ensure that they are safe to eat (e.g., preparation of fresh meat)
- Wash hands, cutting boards, and utensils with hot, soapy water before and after handling raw poultry and meat
- Keep foods refrigerated, especially those containing mayonnaise
- Wash raw fruits and vegetables before serving them
- Use pasteurized milk and fruit juices
- Wash hands after using the bathroom
- Use individual personal care items, such as washcloths, towels, and toothbrushes, rather than sharing

Note that neutropenic precautions and practices associated with medical asepsis are similar in many respects. The principles of medical asepsis are general and form a solid foundation for the more specific neutropenic precautions.

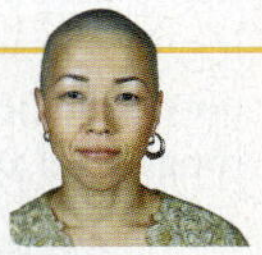

Think back to **Giselle Turheis**, the woman with leukemia and a compromised immune system. When teaching the patient about measures to prevent infection, the nurse would stress the use of proper practices in the home to reduce the patient's risk for infection.

Teach patients about ways to prevent infection in public facilities, such as the following:

- Wash hands after using any public bathroom
- Use paper towels or hot-air dryers in restrooms
- Use individually wrapped drinking straws
- Use tongs to lift food from common service trays in cafeterias, food stores, and salad bars

The community reinforces medical asepsis practices in various ways, including the following:

- Using sterilized combs and brushes in barber and beauty shops
- Performing examination of food handlers for evidence of disease
- Encouraging food handlers to receive the hepatitis A vaccination
- Enforcing frequent handwashing by food handlers

Evaluating

Nurses as primary caregivers can intervene in and positively affect a patient's outcome. By assessing the person at risk, identifying actual and potential health problems and needs, planning, and intervening to maintain a safe environment, the nurse can reduce a patient's potential for developing an infection.

Evaluation of the care plan determines whether the person's need for safety is being met effectively. Ongoing systematic evaluation is crucial for nurses who strive to maintain a secure environment for their patients as well as for themselves. If patient goals have been met and evaluative criteria have been satisfied, the patient will accomplish the following:

- Correctly use techniques of medical asepsis
- Identify health habits and lifestyle patterns that promote health
- State the signs and symptoms of an infection
- Identify unsafe situations in the home environment

REFLECTIVE PRACTICE LEADING TO PERSONAL LEARNING

Remember that the object of reflective practice is to look at an experience, understand it, and learn from it. As you begin to develop your expertise in evaluating the care plan, reflect on your experiences—successes and failures—in order to improve your practice. How can you do it better next time? What did you learn today that can help you tomorrow? Begin your reflection by paying close attention to the following:

- How consistently do you personally adhere to asepsis and infection control practices? How would you respond to constructive/critical feedback from a peer regarding your aseptic technique?
- What value do you attach to involving the patient in infection control practices? How do you individualize the care for patients when so many guidelines, policies, and procedures dictate your care?
- Did your experience with asepsis and infection control techniques change your perspective on the necessity of guidelines? What plan do you have to stay abreast of evolving recommendations at the facility, local, state, national, and global levels?
- How did you prioritize the data you collected? What patterns in the data did you identify? What knowledge from your learning, personal experience and intuition did you use to make decisions and develop your plan of care regarding infection control and prevention practices?

Keeping up with the latest evidence-based practice guidelines can be challenging. Multi-resistant organisms, evolving patterns of transmission, and the spread of disease and infection outside of endemic areas require diligence on the part of the health care professional. Balancing the needs of your individual patients with these responsibilities requires mindfulness and intentionality.

Perhaps the most important questions to reflect on are: Are your patients and their families/caregivers better for having had *you* share in the critical responsibility of partnering with them to ensure appropriate aseptic and infection control practices? Are your patients now receiving thoughtful, person-centered, prioritized, holistic, evidence-based treatment and care because of your efforts?

Skill 25-1 Performing Hand Hygiene Using Soap and Water (Handwashing)

DELEGATION CONSIDERATIONS

The application and use of hand hygiene using soap and water are appropriate for all health care providers.

EQUIPMENT

- Antimicrobial or nonantimicrobial soap (if in bar form, soap must be placed on a soap rack)
- Paper towels
- Moisturizing hand lotion or cream approved by health care facility (optional)

IMPLEMENTATION

ACTION	RATIONALE
1. Gather the necessary supplies. Stand in front of the sink. Do not allow your clothing to touch the sink during the washing procedure (Figure 1).	The sink is considered contaminated. Clothing may carry organisms from place to place.
2. Remove jewelry prior to patient contact, if possible, and secure in a safe place. A plain band may remain in place, based on facility policy.	Microorganisms may accumulate in settings of jewelry and underneath rings (CDC, 2019b), so it should not be worn during patient care. If jewelry was worn during care, it should be left on during handwashing.
3. Turn on water and adjust force (Figure 2). Regulate the temperature until the water is warm.	Water splashed from the contaminated sink will contaminate clothing. Warm water is more comfortable and is less likely to open pores and remove oils from the skin. Organisms can lodge in roughened and broken areas of chapped skin.

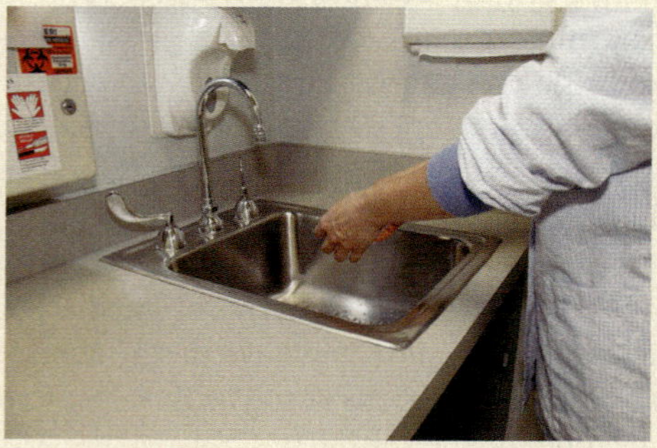

FIGURE 1. Standing in front of sink.

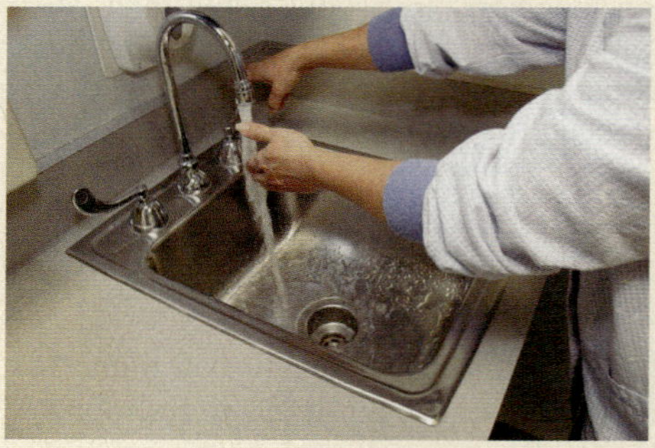

FIGURE 2. Turning on the water at the sink.

ACTION	RATIONALE
4. Wet the hands and wrist area. Keep hands lower than elbows to allow water to flow toward fingertips (Figure 3).	Water should flow from the cleaner area toward the more contaminated area. Hands are more contaminated than forearms.
5. Use about 1 teaspoon liquid soap from dispenser or rinse bar of soap and lather thoroughly, using a firm circular motion (Figure 4). Alternatively, use the amount of product recommended by the manufacturer. Cover all areas of hands with the soap product. If using bar soap, rinse soap bar again and return to soap rack without touching the rack.	Rinsing the soap before and after use removes the lather, which may contain microorganisms.

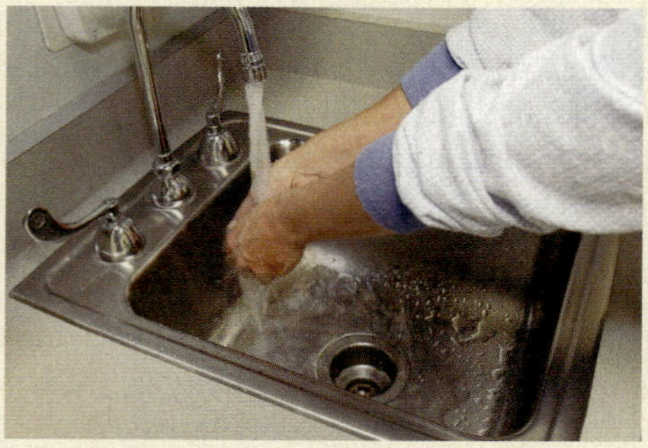

FIGURE 3. Wetting hands to the wrist.

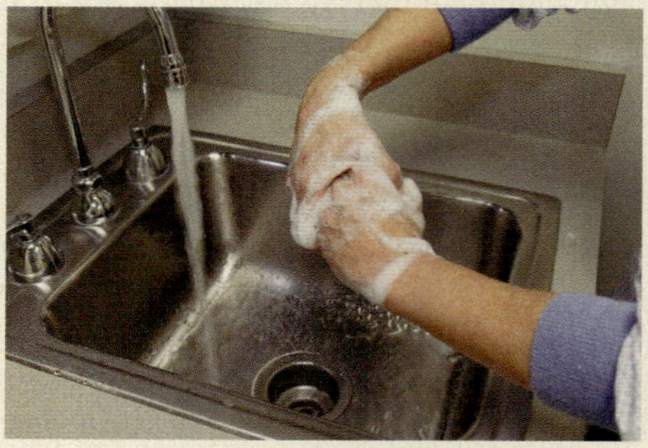

FIGURE 4. Lathering hands with soap and rubbing with firm circular motion.

ACTION

6. Continuing with firm rubbing and circular motions. Wash the palms and backs of the hands; each finger; the areas between the fingers (Figure 5); and the knuckles, wrists, and forearms. **Wash at least 1 inch above area of contamination.** If hands are not visibly soiled, wash to 1 inch above the wrists (Figure 6).

RATIONALE

Friction caused by firm rubbing and circular motions helps to loosen dirt and organisms that can lodge between the fingers, in skin crevices of knuckles, on the palms and backs of the hands, and on the wrists and forearms. Cleaning less contaminated areas (forearms and wrists) after hands are clean prevents spreading microorganisms from the hands to the forearms and wrists.

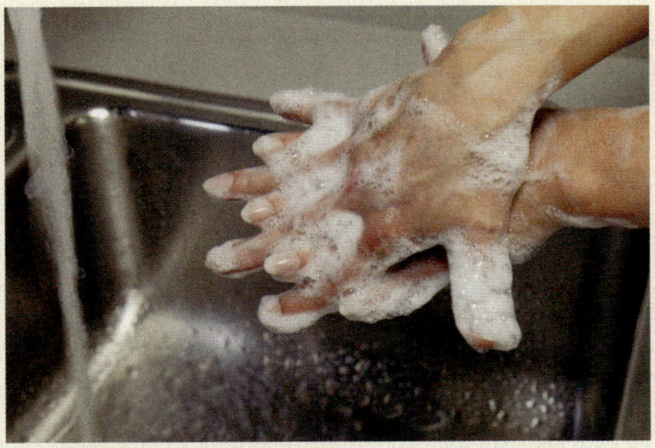

FIGURE 5. Washing areas between fingers.

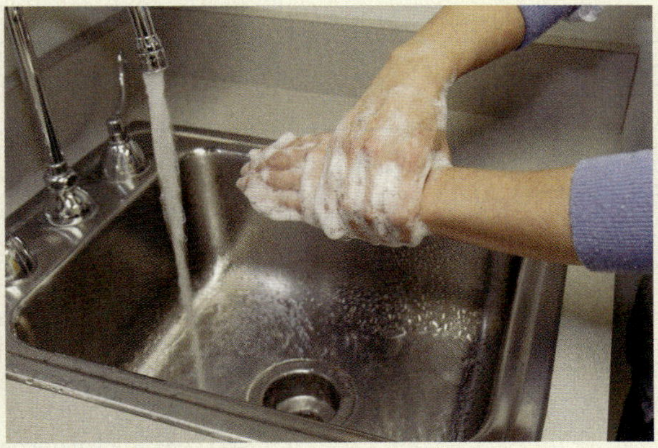

FIGURE 6. Washing to 1 inch above the wrist.

7. Continue this friction motion for at least 15 to 20 seconds.

Effective handwashing requires at least a 15- to 20-second scrub with plain soap or disinfectant and warm water (CDC, 2019b). Hands that are visibly soiled need a longer scrub.

8. Use fingernails of the opposite hand to clean under fingernails (Figure 7).

The area under nails has a high microorganism count, and organisms may remain under the nails, where they can grow and be spread to other people.

9. Rinse hands thoroughly under running water with water flowing toward fingertips (Figure 8).

Running water rinses microorganisms and dirt into the sink.

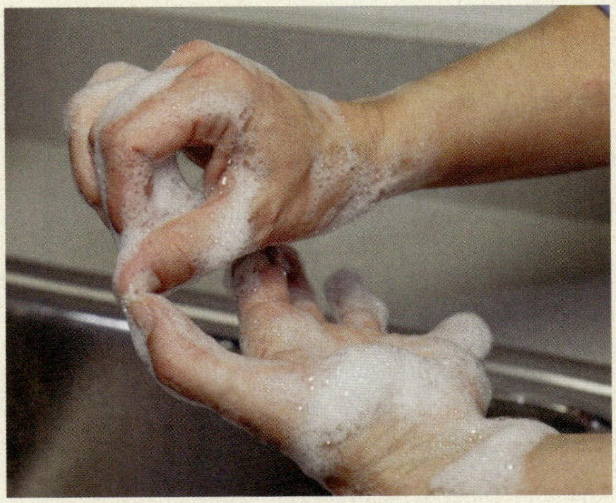

FIGURE 7. Using fingernails to clean under nails of opposite hand.

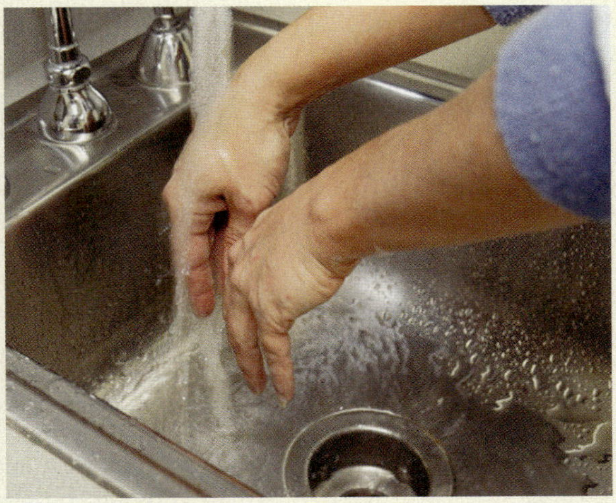

FIGURE 8. Rinsing hands under running water with water flowing toward fingertips.

10. Pat hands dry with a paper towel, beginning with the fingers and moving upward toward forearms, and discard it immediately. Use another clean towel to turn off the faucet. Discard towel immediately without touching other clean hand.

Patting the skin dry prevents chapping. Dry hands first because they are considered the cleanest and least contaminated area. Turning the faucet off with a clean paper towel protects the clean hands from contact with a soiled surface.

(continued on page 694)

Skill 25-1 Performing Hand Hygiene Using Soap and Water (Handwashing) *(continued)*

ACTION	RATIONALE
11. Use moisturizing hand lotion or cream, as approved by facility policy.	Moisturizing hand lotion or cream helps to increase skin hydration to keep the skin soft and prevents dermatitis. It is best applied after patient care is complete, from a small, personal container, according to facility policy. Avoid use of unapproved lotions or creams because they can cause deterioration of gloves or decrease the efficacy of som providers should educate patients, family Follow facility policy.

DOCUMENTATION

The performance of handwashing is not generally documented.

DEVELOPING CLINICAL REASONING AND CLINICAL JUDGMENT

SPECIAL CONSIDERATIONS

General Considerations

- The use of gloves does not eliminate the need for hand hygiene.
- The use of hand hygiene does not eliminate the need for gloves.
- Ensure hands are dry before gloves are donned to decrease risk of dermatitis (Halm & Sandau, 2018).
- Hand hygiene performance by patients is an important intervention to reduce acquisition and transmission of HAIs (Srigley et al., 2020; Wong et al., 2020).
- Hand hygiene performance by family and non-family visitors to health care facilities is an important intervention to reduce acquisition and transmission of HAIs (Kim & Lee, 2019; Lary et al., 2020).
- Health care providers should educate patients, family, and nonfamily visitors on the importance of hand hygiene. Informed patients, families, and visitors have the ability to be better engaged as members of the health care team and are better able to advocate for themselves (Kim & Lee, 2019; Lary et al., 2020).
- Health care consumers in all settings should be encouraged to "speak up for clean hands" and advocate for the use of hand hygiene by health care providers, family, and friends (CDC, 2016a; Gesser-Edelsburg et al., 2020).
- Germs can live under artificial fingernails before and after hand hygiene interventions. Health care providers should not wear artificial fingernails or extensions when having direct contact with patients at high risk (e.g., patients in intensive care units or operating rooms) (CDC, 2019b).
- Health care providers should keep natural nail tips less than ¼-inch long (CDC, 2019b)

Community-Based Care Considerations

- Proper hand hygiene, including the use of alcohol-based hand sanitizers, is useful to reduce the risk of spread of microorganisms among family members and friends (CDC, 2016a). Patients, family members, and caregivers should be encouraged to perform hand hygiene, preferably by washing their hands; washing with soap and water is the best way to remove germs in most situations (CDC, 2020b). If soap and water are not readily available, alcohol-based hand sanitizer should be used (CDC, 2020b). Instruct patients, family members, and caregivers to perform hand hygiene (CDC, 2016a):
  - before preparing or eating food
  - before touching eyes, nose, or mouth
  - before and after changing wound dressings or bandages
  - after using the restroom
  - after blowing their nose, coughing, or sneezing
  - after touching hospital or other health care–setting surfaces such as doorknobs, phones, tables, and bed rails

Skill 25-2 Using Personal Protective Equipment

DELEGATION CONSIDERATIONS

The application and use of PPE are appropriate for all health care providers.

EQUIPMENT

- Gloves
- Mask (surgical or particulate respirator)
- Impervious gown
- Goggles or face shield (protective eye wear; does not include eyeglasses)

Note: Equipment for PPE may vary depending on level of precautions required and facility policy.

IMPLEMENTATION

ACTION	RATIONALE
1. Check medical record and plan of care for type of precautions and review precautions in infection control manual.	Mode of transmission of organism determines type of precautions required.
2. Plan nursing activities before entering patient's room.	Organization facilitates performance of task and adherence to precautions.
3. Provide instruction about precautions and use of PPE to patient, family members, caregivers, and visitors.	Explanation encourages cooperation of patient, family, and caregivers and reduces apprehension about precaution procedures.
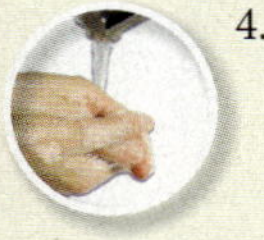 4. Perform hand hygiene.	Hand hygiene prevents the spread of microorganisms.
5. Put on gown, mask (surgical or particulate respirator), protective eyewear, and gloves based on the type of exposure anticipated and category of isolation precautions.	Use of PPE interrupts chain of infection and protects patient and nurse. Gown should protect all clothing and exposed skin on upper extremities. Gloves protect hands and wrists from microorganisms. Masks and particulate respirators protect wearer from direct contact with body fluids that may spray or splash; masks protect wearer from exposure to large-particle aerosols and particulate respirators protect wearer from inhalation of airborne droplet nuclei, and small-particle aerosols. Eyewear protects mucous membranes in the eye from splashes.
a. Put on the gown, with the opening in the back. Tie gown securely at neck and waist (Figure 1).	Gown should fully cover the torso from the neck to knees, arms to the end of wrists, and wrap around the back.
b. Put on the mask or respirator over your nose, mouth, and chin (Figure 2). Secure ties or elastic bands at the middle of the head and neck. Fit mask snug to face and below chin. Fit flexible band to nose bridge. If respirator is used, perform a fit check. Inhale: The respirator should collapse. Exhale: Air should not leak out.	Masks protect nurse or patient from droplet nuclei and large-particle aerosols. A mask must fit securely to provide protection.

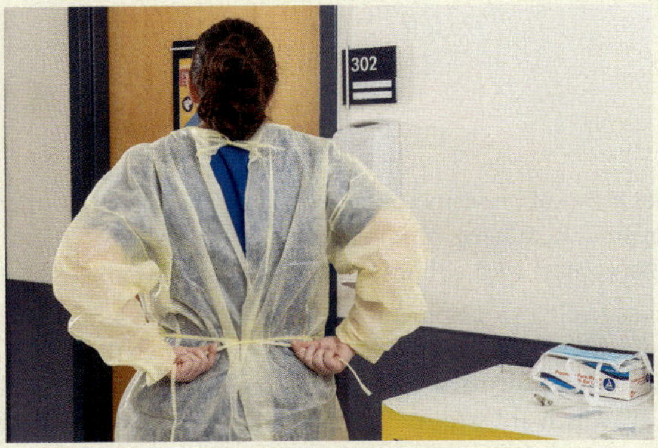

FIGURE 1. Tying gown at neck and waist.

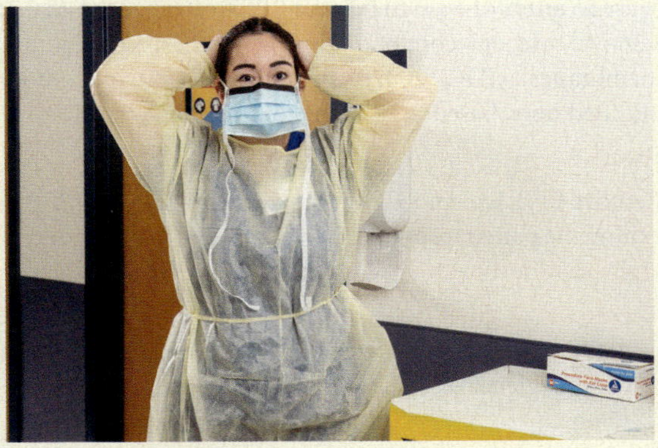

FIGURE 2. Applying mask over nose, mouth, and chin.

(continued on page 696)

Skill 25-2 Using Personal Protective Equipment *(continued)*

ACTION | **RATIONALE**

c. Put on goggles (Figure 3). Place over eyes and adjust to fit. Alternatively, a face shield could be used (Figure 4).

Eyewear protects mucous membranes in the eye from splashes; it must fit securely to provide protection.

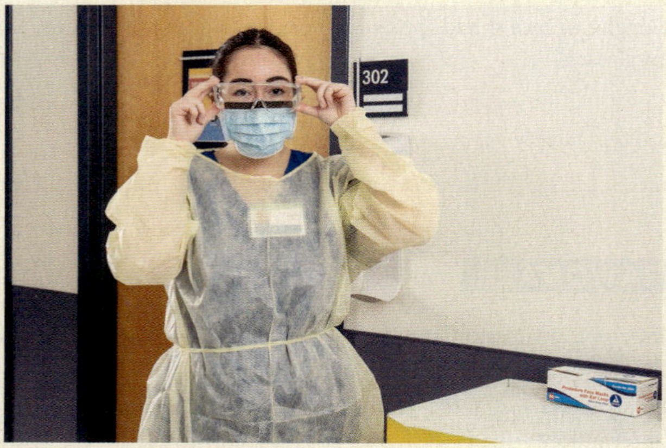

FIGURE 3. Putting on goggles.

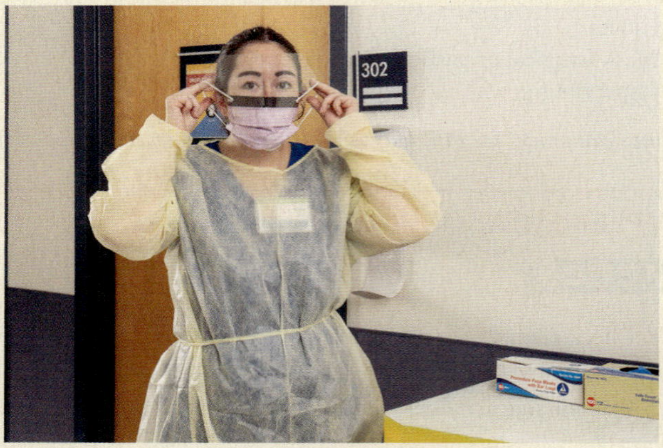

FIGURE 4. Putting on face shield.

d. Put on clean disposable gloves. Extend gloves to cover the wrist of the gown (Figure 5).

Gloves protect hands and wrists from microorganisms.

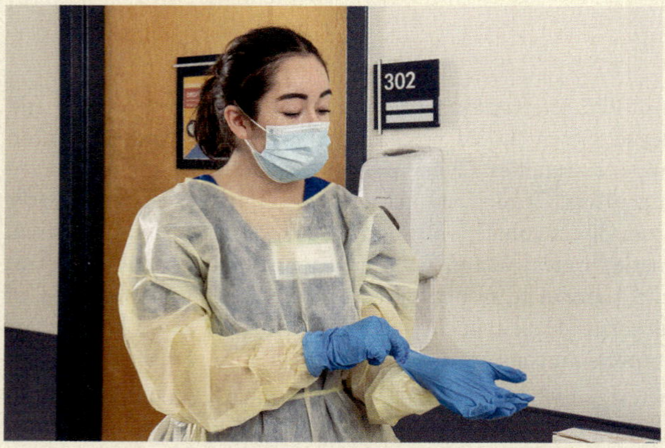

FIGURE 5. Putting on gloves, ensuring gloves cover gown cuffs.

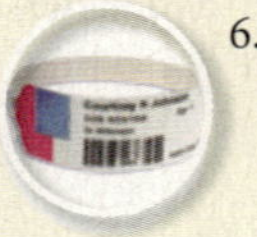

6. Identify the patient. Explain the procedure to the patient. Continue with patient care as appropriate.

Patient identification validates the correct patient and correct procedure. Discussion and explanation help allay anxiety and prepare the patient for what to expect.

Remove PPE

There are a variety of ways to remove PPE to achieve the goal of safe removal without contamination of clothes, skin, or mucous membranes (CDC, 2007; updated 2019). Two methods are outlined here, based on CDC recommendations.

Method A

7. Remove PPE: Except for respirator, if worn, remove PPE before exiting the patient room or in an anteroom. **Remove respirator after leaving the patient's room and closing the door**.

Proper removal prevents contact with and the spread of microorganisms. Removing respirator outside the patient's room prevents contact with airborne microorganisms.

a. **Outside of gloves are contaminated.** If hands are contaminated during gown or glove removal, immediately perform hand hygiene.

Outside front of equipment is considered contaminated. Hand hygiene prevents transmission of microorganisms.

The inside, outside back, and ties on head and back are considered clean, which are areas of PPE that are not likely to have been in contact with infectious organisms.

Skill 25-2 Using Personal Protective Equipment (continued)

ACTION

b. Grasp the palm area of one gloved hand with the opposite gloved hand and peel off first glove, turning the glove inside out as you pull it off (Figure 6). Hold the removed glove in the remaining gloved hand.

RATIONALE

Outside of gloves are contaminated. This process contains the contaminated areas.

ACTION

c. Slide fingers of ungloved hand under the remaining glove at the wrist, **taking care not to touch the outer surface of the glove** (Figure 7).

RATIONALE

Ungloved hand is clean and should not touch contaminated areas.

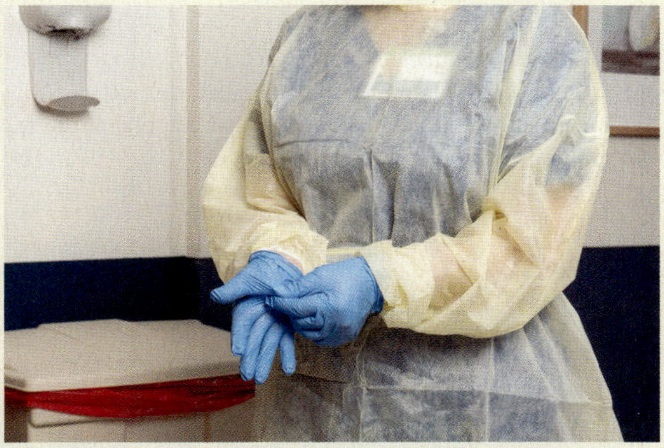

FIGURE 6. Grasping the palm area of one glove and peeling off.

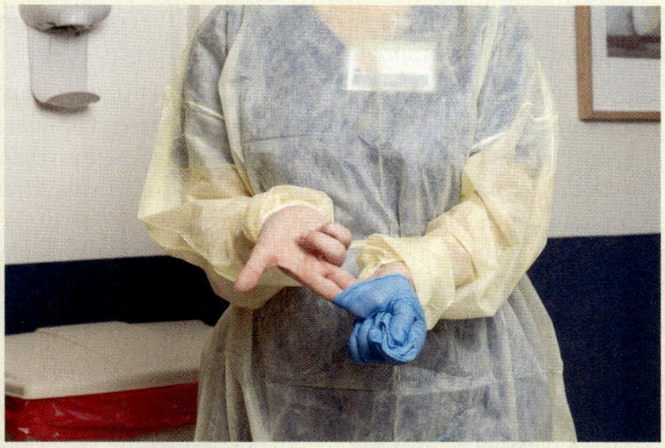

FIGURE 7. Sliding fingers of ungloved hand under the remaining glove at the wrist.

ACTION

d. Peel off the second glove over the first glove, containing the first glove inside the other (Figure 8). Discard in appropriate container.

RATIONALE

This process contains the outside, contaminated areas of gloves. Proper disposal prevents transmission of microorganisms.

ACTION

e. To remove the goggles or face shield: **Outside of goggles or face shield is contaminated—do not touch.** If hands are contaminated during goggle or face shield removal, immediately perform hand hygiene. Handle by the headband or earpieces and remove from the back (Figure 9). Lift away from the face. **Do not touch the front of goggles or face shield.** Place in designated receptacle for reprocessing or in an appropriate waste container.

RATIONALE

Outside of goggles or face shield is contaminated; do not touch. Hand hygiene prevents transmission of microorganisms.

Handling by headband or earpieces and lifting away from face prevents transmission of microorganisms. Proper disposal prevents transmission of microorganisms.

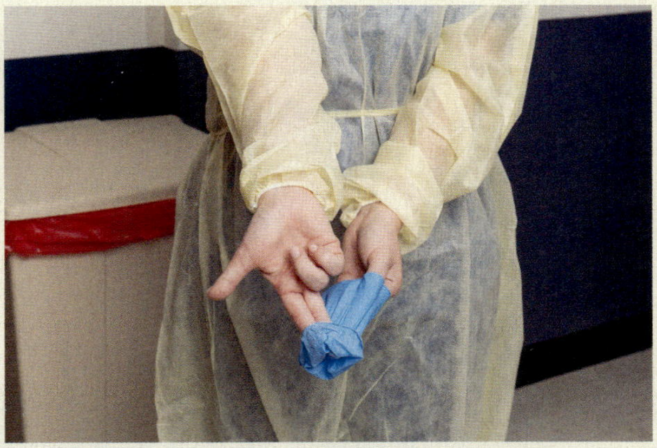

FIGURE 8. Peeling off the second glove, containing the first glove inside the other.

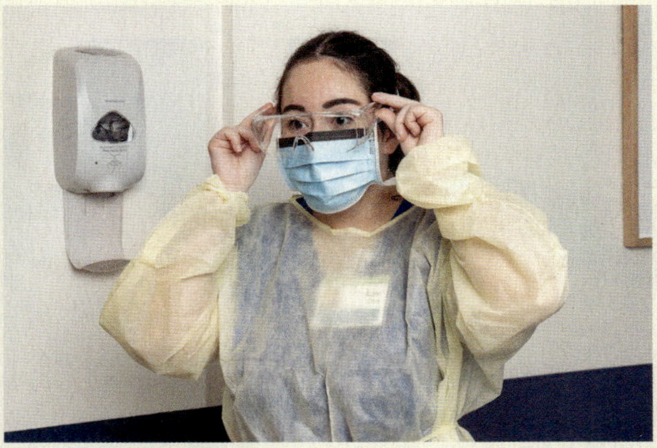

FIGURE 9. Removing goggles by grasping earpieces.

(continued on page 698)

Skill 25-2 Using Personal Protective Equipment *(continued)*

ACTION	RATIONALE
f. To remove gown: **Gown front and sleeves are contaminated.** If hands are contaminated during gown removal, immediately perform hand hygiene. Unfasten ties, if at the neck and back, taking care that sleeves of gown do not contact the body. Allow the gown to fall away from shoulders. **Touching only the inside of the gown**, pull away from the neck and shoulders (Figure 10). Keeping hands on the inner surface of the gown, pull gown from arms (Figure 11). Turn gown inside out. Fold or roll into a bundle (Figure 12) and discard in an appropriate waste container.	Gown front and sleeves are contaminated. Hand hygiene prevents transmission of microorganisms. Touching only the inside of the gown and pulling it away from the torso prevents transmission of microorganisms. This process contains the outside, contaminated areas of gown. Proper disposal prevents transmission of microorganisms.
g. To remove mask or respirator: **Front of mask/respirator is contaminated—do not touch.** If hands are contaminated during mask/respirator removal, immediately perform hand hygiene. Grasp the bottom ties or elastic of the mask/respirator, then top ties or elastic and remove. **Do not touch the front of mask or respirator** (Figure 13). Discard in an appropriate waste container. If using a reusable respirator, save for future use in the designated area.	Front of mask or respirator is contaminated; do not touch. Not touching the front of the mask and proper disposal of the mask prevent transmission of microorganisms.

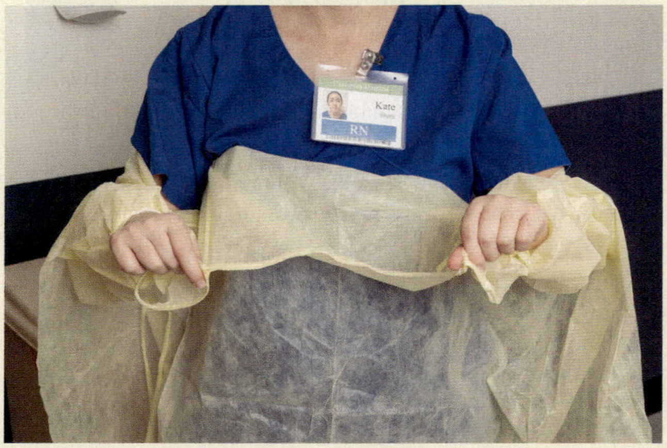

FIGURE 10. Touching only the inside of the gown, pull away from the neck and shoulders.

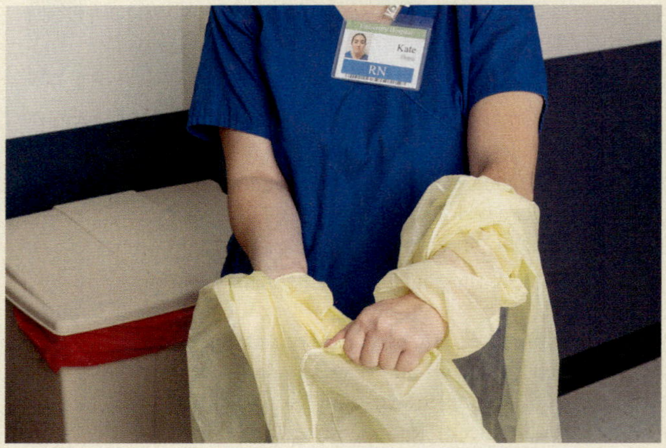

FIGURE 11. Keeping hands on the inner surface of the gown, pull gown from arms.

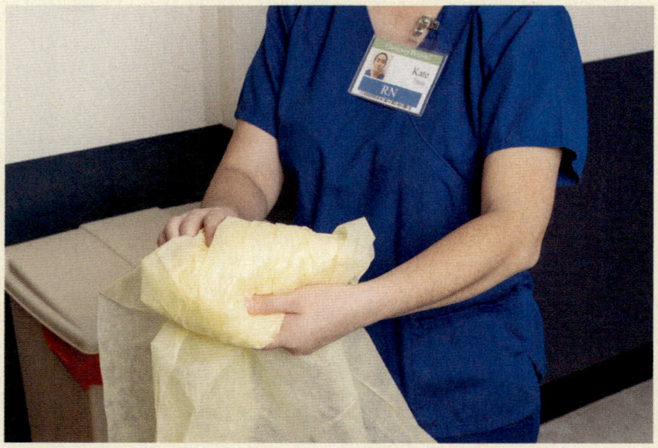

FIGURE 12. Turning gown inside out, rolling into a bundle.

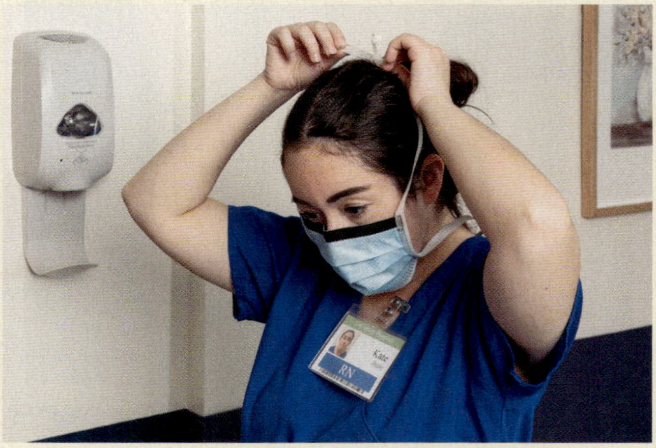

FIGURE 13. Removing mask or respirator, grasping the neck ties or elastic, taking care to avoid touching the front.

ACTION

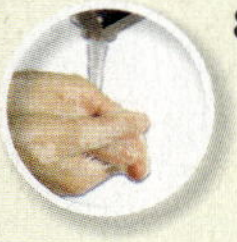

8. Perform hand hygiene immediately after removing all PPE.

RATIONALE

Hand hygiene prevents spread of microorganisms.

Remove PPE

There are a variety of ways to remove PPE to achieve the goal of safe removal without contamination of clothes, skin, or mucous membranes (CDC, 2007; update, 2019).

Method B

7. To remove gown and gloves: **Gown front and sleeves and the outside of gloves are contaminated.** If hands are contaminated during gown and glove removal, immediately perform hand hygiene. **Touching outside of gown only with gloved hands**, grasp the gown in the front and pull away from the body, breaking the ties in the back (Figure 14). While removing the gown, fold or roll the gown inside-out into a bundle (Figure 15). As gown is being removed, peel off gloves at the same time, **only touching the inside of the gloves and gown with bare hands** (Figure 16). Discard gown and gloves in an appropriate waste container.

Front of gown and sleeves, including waist strings, are contaminated. Hand hygiene prevents transmission of microorganisms.

Front of gown and outside of gloves are contaminated.

This process contains the outside, contaminated areas of gown.

Proper disposal prevents transmission of microorganisms.

Outside of goggles or face shield is contaminated; do not touch. Hand hygiene prevents transmission of microorganisms.

Handling by headband or earpieces and lifting away from face prevents transmission of microorganisms. Proper disposal prevents transmission of microorganisms.

Front of mask or respirator is contaminated; do not touch. Not touching the front of the mask and proper disposal of the mask prevent transmission of microorganisms.

Hand hygiene prevents spread of microorganisms.

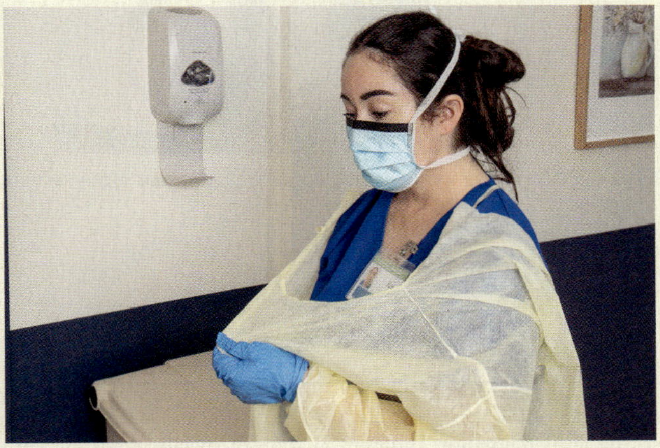

FIGURE 14. Grasping the outside of the front of gown and pulling away from the body.

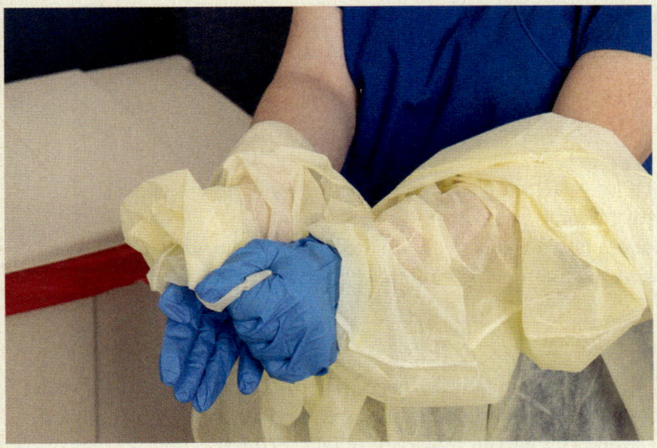

FIGURE 15. Rolling gown inside-out into a bundle.

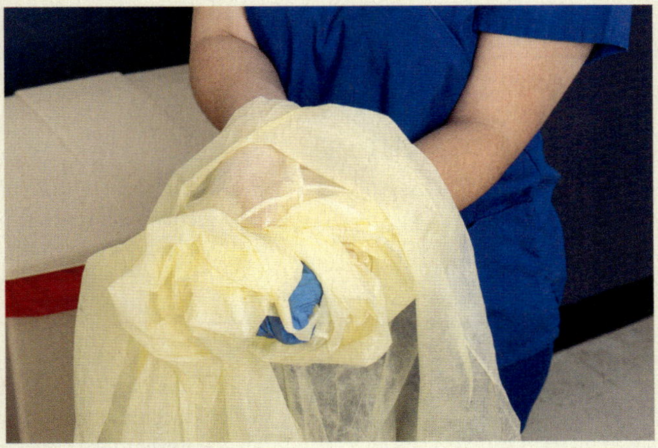

FIGURE 16. Peeling off gloves as gown is being removed, touching only the inside of the gloves and gown.

(continued on page 700)

Skill 25-2 Using Personal Protective Equipment *(continued)*

ACTION | **RATIONALE**

8. To remove the goggles or face shield: **Outside of goggles or face shield is contaminated—do not touch.** If hands are contaminated during goggle or face shield removal, immediately perform hand hygiene. Grasp the headband or earpieces and remove from the back (Figure 17). Lift away from the face. **Do not touch the front of goggles or face shield.** Place in designated receptacle for reprocessing or in an appropriate waste container.
9. To remove mask or respirator: **Front of mask/respirator is contaminated—do not touch.** If hands are contaminated during mask/respirator removal, immediately perform hand hygiene. Grasp the bottom ties or elastic of the mask/respirator, then top ties or elastic, lift away from face, and remove (Figure 18). **Do not touch the front of mask or respirator.** Discard in an appropriate waste container. If using a reusable respirator, save for future use in the designated area.

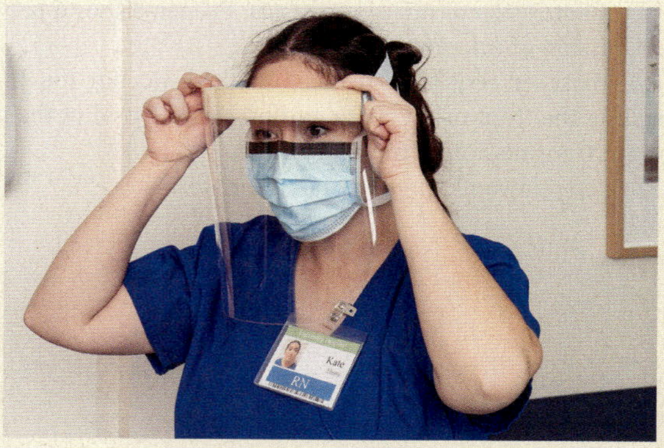

FIGURE 17. Removing the goggles or face shield, grasping the headband or earpieces.

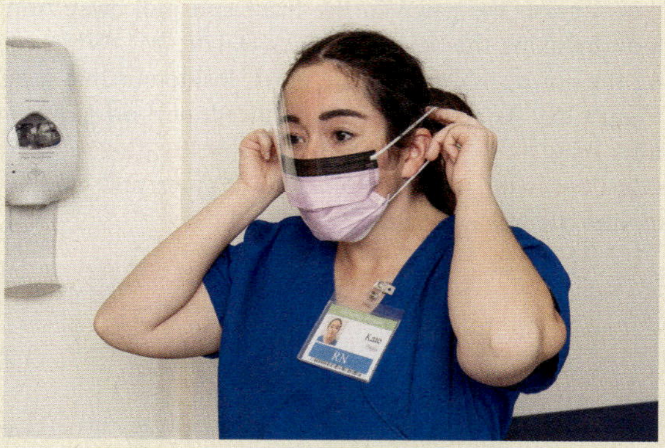

FIGURE 18. Removing the mask or respirator, grasping the bottom ties or elastic, and then the top ties or elastic.

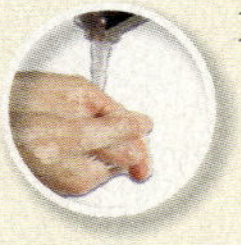

10. Perform hand hygiene immediately after removing all PPE.

DOCUMENTATION

It is not usually necessary to document the use of specific articles of PPE or each application of PPE. However, document the implementation and continuation of specific transmission-based precautions as part of the patient's care.

DEVELOPING CLINICAL REASONING AND CLINICAL JUDGMENT

UNEXPECTED SITUATIONS AND ASSOCIATED INTERVENTIONS

- *You did not realize the need for protective equipment at beginning of task:* Stop task and obtain appropriate protective wear.
- *You are accidentally exposed to blood and body fluids:* Stop task and immediately follow facility protocol for exposure, including reporting the exposure.

SPECIAL CONSIDERATIONS

Community-Based Care Considerations

- *Standard Precautions* are used for all patient care, based on risk assessment, and make use of common-sense practices and PPE to protect health care providers from infection and prevent the spread of infection from person to person (CDC, 2016b).
- Measures related to Respiratory Hygiene/Cough Etiquette should be implemented in community settings for any person with signs of illness including cough, congestion, rhinorrhea, or increased production of respiratory secretions (CDC, 2016b).

Skill 25-3 Preparing a Sterile Field and Adding Items to a Sterile Field

DELEGATION CONSIDERATIONS

Procedures requiring the use of a sterile field and other sterile items are not delegated to assistive personnel (AP). Depending on the state's nurse practice act and the organization's policies and procedures, these procedures may be delegated to licensed practical/vocational nurses (LPN/LVNs). The decision to delegate must be based on careful analysis of the patient's needs and circumstances, as well as the qualifications of the person to whom the task is being delegated. Refer to the Delegation Guidelines in Appendix A.

EQUIPMENT

- Sterile-wrapped drape
- Additional sterile supplies, such as dressings, containers, or solutions, as needed
- PPE, as indicated

IMPLEMENTATION

ACTION	RATIONALE
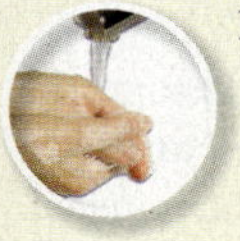 1. Perform hand hygiene and put on PPE, if indicated.	Hand hygiene and PPE prevent the spread of microorganisms. PPE is required based on transmission precautions.
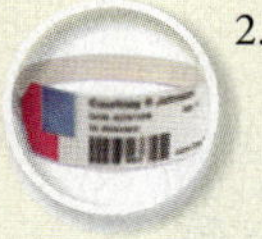 2. Identify the patient. Explain the procedure to the patient.	Patient identification validates the correct patient and correct procedure. Discussion and explanation help allay anxiety and prepare the patient for what to expect.
Preparing a Sterile Field	
3. Check that the packaged sterile drape is dry and unopened. Also note expiration date, making sure that the date is still valid.	Moisture contaminates a sterile package. Expiration date indicates period that package remains sterile.
4. Select a work area that is waist level or higher.	Work area is within sight. Bacteria tend to settle, so there is less contamination above the waist.
For a Prepackaged Sterile Drape	
a. Open the outer covering of the drape. Remove sterile drape, lifting it carefully by its corners. Hold away from body and above the waist and work surface.	Outer 1 inch (2.5 cm) of drape is considered contaminated. Any item touching this area is also considered contaminated.
b. Continue to hold only by the corners. Allow the drape to unfold, away from your body and any other surface (Figure 1).	Touching the outer side of the wrapper maintains the sterile field. Contact with any surface would contaminate the field.

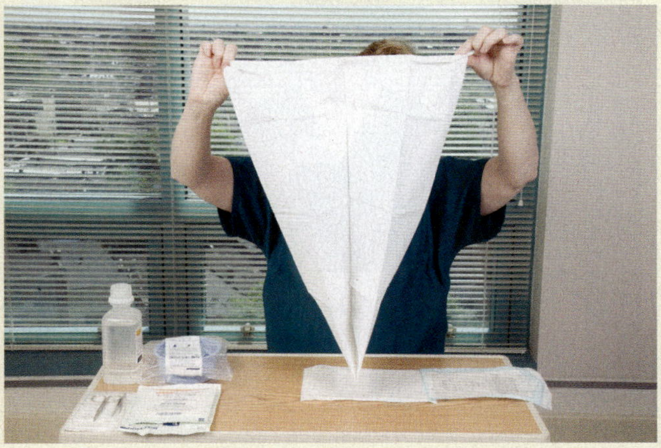

FIGURE 1. Holding drape by corners and allowing it to unfold away from body and surfaces.

(*continued on page 702*)

Skill 25-3 Preparing a Sterile Field and Adding Items to a Sterile Field *(continued)*

ACTION	RATIONALE
c. Position the drape on the work surface with the moisture-proof side down (Figure 2). This would be the shiny or blue side. Avoid touching any other surface or object with the drape. If any portion of the drape hangs off the work surface, that part of the drape is considered contaminated.	Moisture-proof side prevents contamination of the field if it becomes wet. The moisture penetrates the sterile cloth or paper and carries organisms by capillary action to contaminate the field. A wet field is considered contaminated if the surface immediately below it is not sterile.
For a Commercially Prepared Kit or Tray	
a. Open the outside cover of the package (Figure 3) and remove the kit or tray. Place in the center of the work surface, with the topmost flap positioned on the far side of the package. Discard outside cover.	This allows sufficient room for sterile field.
b. Reach around the package and grasp the outer surface of the end of the topmost flap, holding no more than 1 inch from the border of the flap. Pull open away from the body, keeping the arm outstretched and away from the inside of the wrapper (Figure 4). Allow the wrapper to lie flat on the work surface.	This maintains sterility of inside of wrapper, which is to become the sterile field. Outer surface of the wrapper is considered unsterile. Outer 1-inch border of the wrapper is considered contaminated.
c. Reach around the package and grasp the outer surface of the first side flap, holding no more than 1 inch from the border of the flap. Pull open to the side of the package, keeping the arm outstretched and away from the inside of the wrapper (Figure 5). Allow the wrapper to lie flat on the work surface.	This maintains sterility of inside of wrapper, which is to become the sterile field. Outer surface of the wrapper is considered unsterile. Outer 1-inch border of the wrapper is considered contaminated.

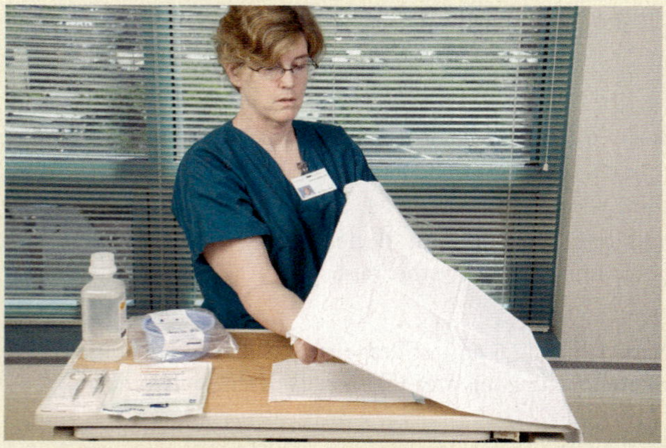

FIGURE 2. Positioning drape on work surface with the moisture-proof side down.

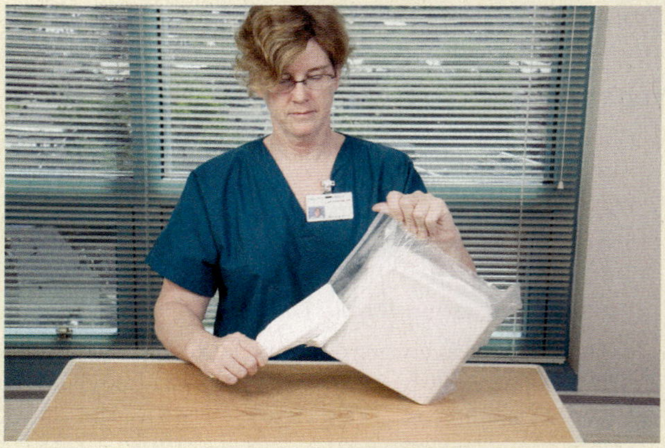

FIGURE 3. Opening outside cover of package.

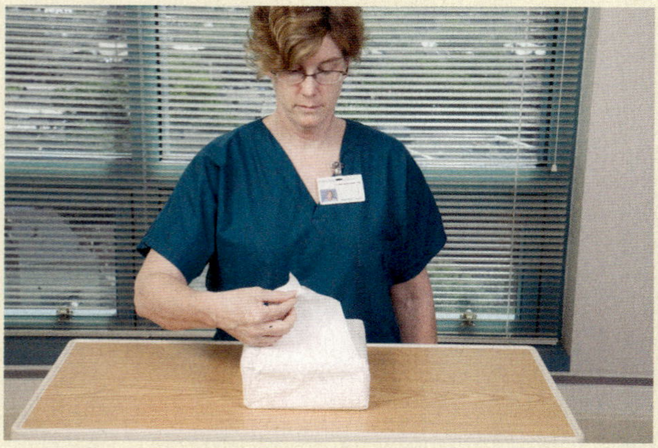

FIGURE 4. Pulling top flap open, away from body.

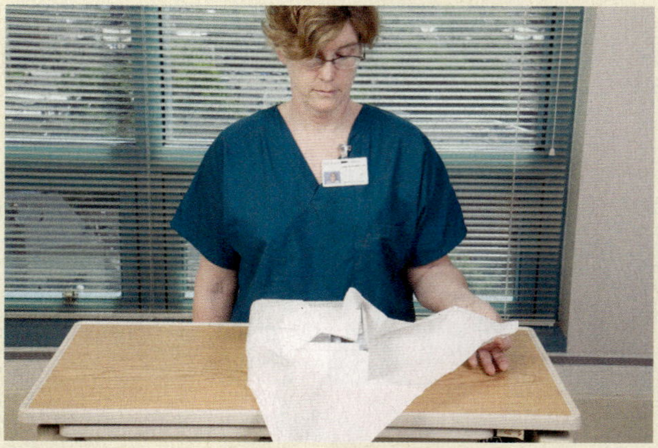

FIGURE 5. Pulling open the first side flap.

ACTION	RATIONALE
d. Reach around the package and grasp the outer surface of the remaining side flap, holding no more than 1 inch from the border of the flap. Pull open to the side of the package, keeping the arm outstretched and away from the inside of the wrapper (Figure 6). Allow the wrapper to lie flat on the work surface.	This maintains sterility of inside of wrapper, which is to become the sterile field. Outer surface of the wrapper is considered unsterile. Outer 1-inch border of the wrapper is considered contaminated.
e. Stand away from the package and work surface. Grasp the outer surface of the remaining flap closest to the body, holding not more than 1 inch from the border of the flap. Pull the flap back toward the body, keeping arm outstretched and away from the inside of the wrapper (Figure 7). Keep this hand in place. Use other hand to grasp the wrapper on the underside (the side that is down to the work surface). Position the wrapper so that when flat, edges are on the work surface, and do not hang down over sides of work surface (Figure 8). Allow the wrapper to lie flat on the work surface.	
f. The outer wrapper of the package has become a sterile field with the packaged supplies in the center (Figure 9). Do not touch or reach over the sterile field. Place additional sterile items on field as needed. Continue with the procedure as indicated.	Sterility of the field and contents are maintained.

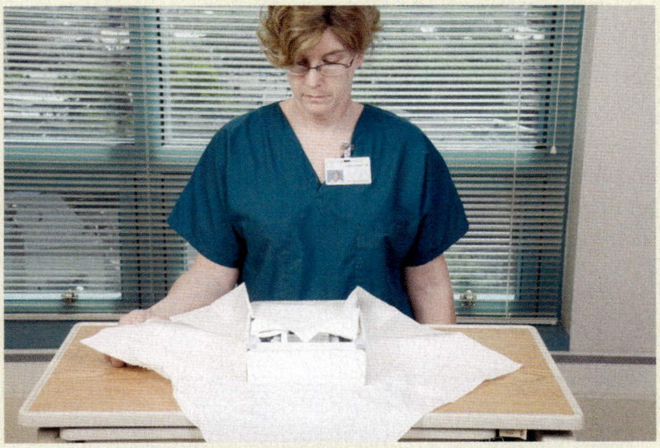

FIGURE 6. Pulling open the remaining side flap.

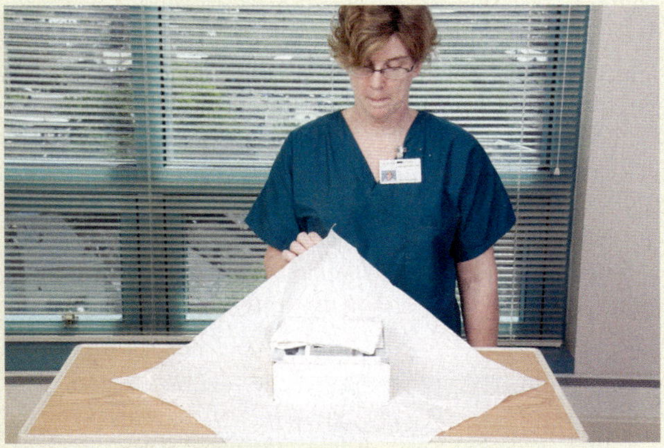

FIGURE 7. Pulling open flap closest to body.

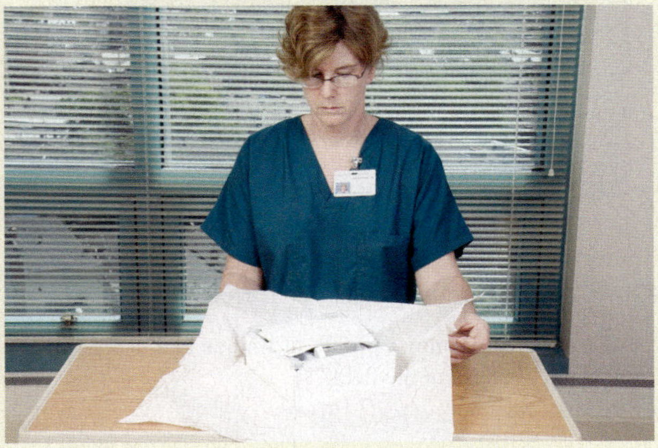

FIGURE 8. Positioning wrapper on work surface.

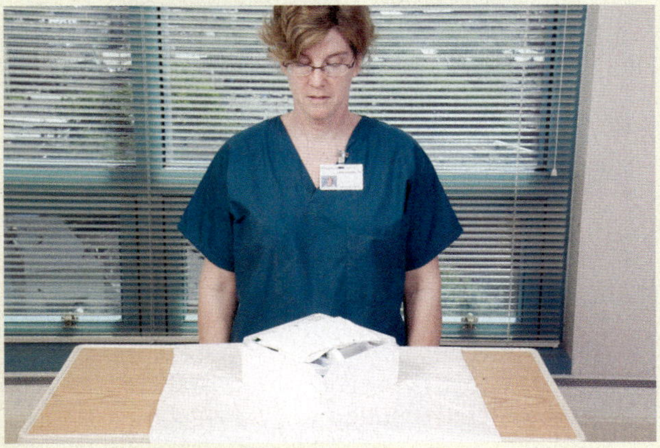

FIGURE 9. Outside wrapper of package is now sterile field.

(continued on page 704)

Skill 25-3 Preparing a Sterile Field and Adding Items to a Sterile Field *(continued)*

ACTION	RATIONALE
Adding Items to a Sterile Field	
5. Place additional sterile items on field as needed.	
To Add a Facility-Wrapped and Sterilized Item	
a. Hold facility-wrapped item in the dominant hand, with top flap opening away from the body. With other hand, reach around the package and unfold top flap and both sides.	Only sterile surface and item are exposed before dropping onto sterile field.
b. Keep a secure hold on the item through the wrapper with the dominant hand. Grasp the remaining flap of the wrapper closest to the body, taking care not to touch the inner surface of the wrapper or the item. Pull the flap back toward the wrist, so the wrapper covers the hand and wrist.	Only sterile surface and item are exposed before dropping onto sterile field.
c. Grasp all the corners of the wrapper together with the non-dominant hand and pull back toward wrist, covering hand and wrist. Hold in place.	Only sterile surface and item are exposed before dropping onto sterile field.
d. Hold the item 6 inches above the surface of the sterile field and drop onto the field. **Be careful to avoid touching the surface or other items or dropping any item onto the 1-inch border.**	This prevents contamination of the field and inadvertent dropping of the sterile item too close to the edge or off the field. Any items landing on the 1-inch border are considered contaminated.
To Add a Commercially Wrapped and Sterilized Item	
a. Depending on the type of package, hold package in one hand. Pull back top cover with other hand. Alternatively, carefully peel the edges apart using both hands (Figure 10).	Contents remain uncontaminated by hands.
b. After top cover or edges are partially separated, hold the item 6 inches above the surface of the sterile field. Continue opening the package and drop the item onto the field (Figure 11). **Be careful to avoid touching the surface or other items or dropping an item onto the 1-inch border.**	This prevents contamination of the field and inadvertent dropping of the sterile item too close to the edge or off the field. Any items landing on the 1-inch border are considered contaminated.

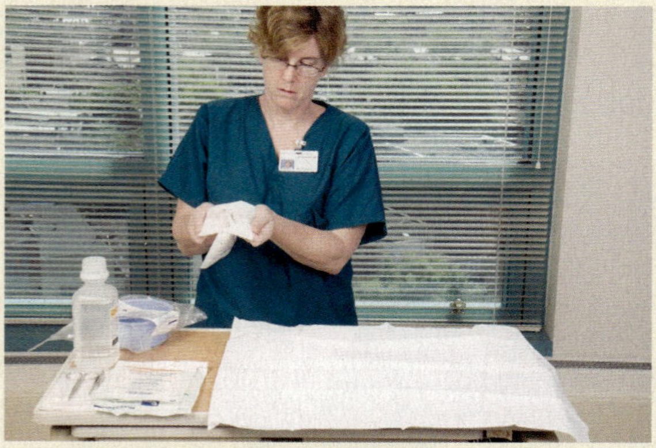

FIGURE 10. Carefully peeling edges apart.

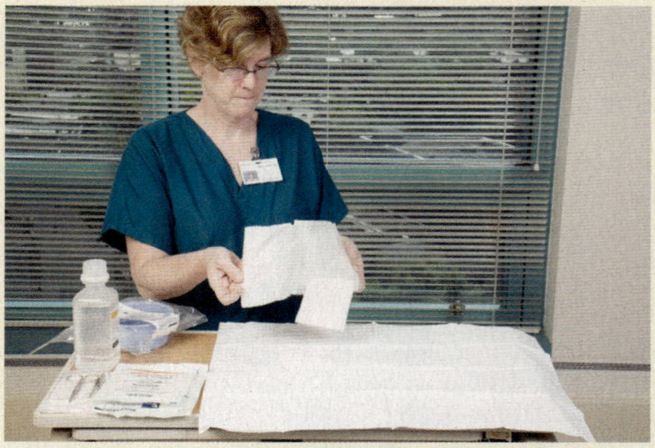

FIGURE 11. Dropping sterile item onto sterile field.

ACTION	RATIONALE
c. Discard wrapper.	A neat work area promotes proper technique and avoids inadvertent contamination of the field.
To Add a Sterile Solution	
a. Obtain appropriate solution and check expiration date.	Once opened, label any bottles with date and time. Solution may be kept for use for 24 hours once opened.

ACTION	RATIONALE
b. Open solution container according to directions and **place cap on table away from the field with edges up** (Figure 12).	Sterility of inside cap is maintained.
c. Hold bottle outside the edge of the sterile field with the label side facing the palm of your hand and prepare to pour from a height of 4 to 6 inches (10 to 15 cm). **Do not touch the tip of the bottle to the sterile container or field.**	Label remains dry, and solution may be poured without reaching across sterile field. Minimal splashing occurs from that height. Accidentally touching the tip of the bottle to a container or dressing contaminates them both.
d. Pour required amount of solution steadily into sterile container previously added to the sterile field and positioned at side of sterile field or onto dressings (Figure 13). **Avoid splashing any liquid.**	A steady stream minimizes the risk of splashing; moisture contaminates sterile field.

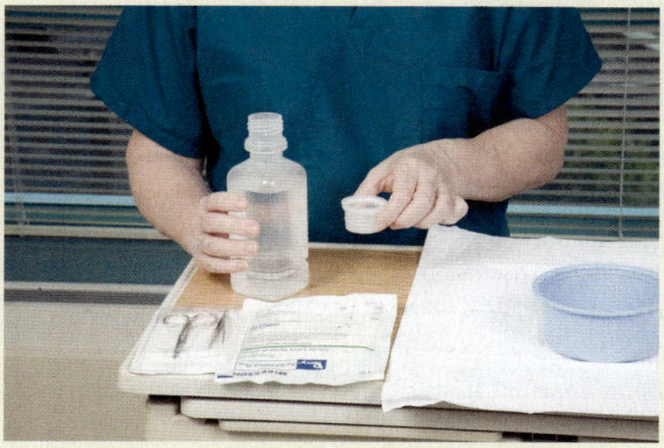

FIGURE 12. Opening bottle of sterile solution and placing cap on table with edges up.

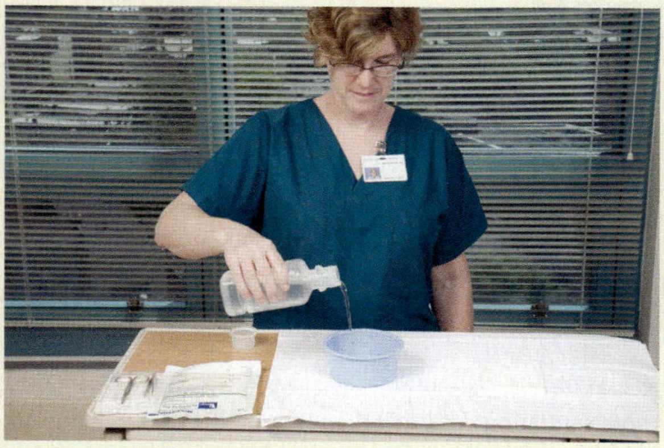

FIGURE 13. Pouring solution into sterile container.

ACTION	RATIONALE
6. Continue with procedure as indicated.	
7. When procedure is completed, remove PPE, if used. Perform hand hygiene.	Proper removal of PPE reduces the risk for infection transmission and contamination of other items. Hand hygiene prevents the spread of microorganisms.

DOCUMENTATION

It is not usually necessary to document the addition of sterile items to a sterile field. However, document the use of performing sterile technique for any procedure.

UNEXPECTED SITUATIONS AND ASSOCIATED INTERVENTIONS

- A part of the sterile field becomes contaminated: *When any portion of the sterile field becomes contaminated, discard the sterile field and any items on the field and start over.*
- You realize a supply is missing after setting up the sterile field: *Call for help. Do not leave the sterile field unattended. If you are unable to see the sterile field at all times, it is considered contaminated.*
- The patient touches the sterile field: *If the patient touches the sterile field, discard the supplies and prepare a new sterile field. If the patient is confused, have someone assist by holding the patient's hands and/or reinforcing what is happening.*

Skill 25-4 Putting on Sterile Gloves and Removing Soiled Gloves

DELEGATION CONSIDERATIONS

Procedures requiring the use of sterile gloves and other sterile items are not delegated to assistive personnel (AP). Depending on the state's nurse practice act and the organization's policies and procedures, these procedures may be delegated to licensed practical/vocational nurses (LPN/LVNs). The decision to delegate must be based on careful analysis of the patient's needs and circumstances, as well as the qualifications of the person to whom the task is being delegated. Refer to the Delegation Guidelines in Appendix A.

EQUIPMENT

- Sterile gloves of the appropriate size
- PPE, as indicated

IMPLEMENTATION

ACTION	RATIONALE
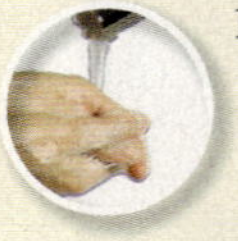 1. Perform hand hygiene and put on PPE, if indicated.	Hand hygiene and PPE prevent the spread of microorganisms. PPE is required based on transmission precautions.
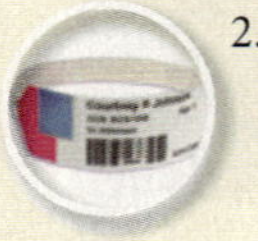 2. Identify the patient. Explain the procedure to the patient.	Patient identification validates the correct patient and correct procedure. Discussion and explanation help allay anxiety and prepare the patient for what to expect.
3. Check that the sterile glove package is dry and unopened. Also note expiration date, making sure that the date is still valid.	Moisture contaminates a sterile package. Expiration date indicates the period that the package remains sterile.
4. Place sterile glove package on clean, dry surface at or above your waist.	Moisture could contaminate the sterile gloves. Any sterile object held below the waist is considered contaminated.
5. Open the outside wrapper by carefully peeling the top layer back (Figure 1). Remove inner package, handling only the outside of it.	This maintains sterility of gloves in inner packet.
6. Place the inner package on the work surface with the side labeled "cuff end" closest to the body.	Allows for ease of glove application.
7. Carefully open the inner package. Fold open the top flap, then the bottom and sides (Figure 2). **Do not touch the inner surface of the package or the gloves.**	The inner surface of the package is considered sterile. The outer 1-inch border of the inner package is considered contaminated. The sterile gloves are exposed with the cuff end closest to the nurse.

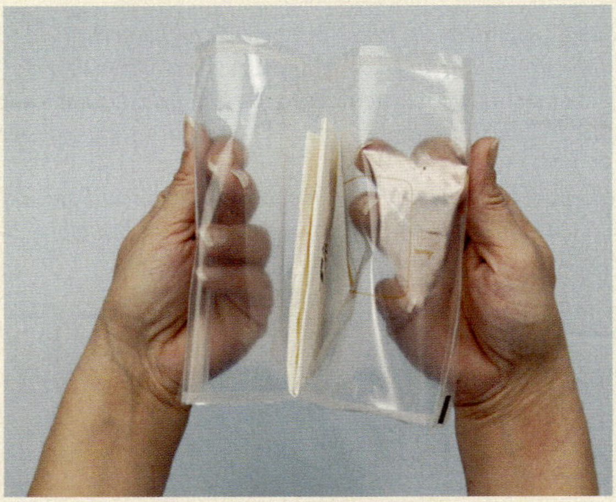

FIGURE 1. Pulling top layer of outside wrapper back.

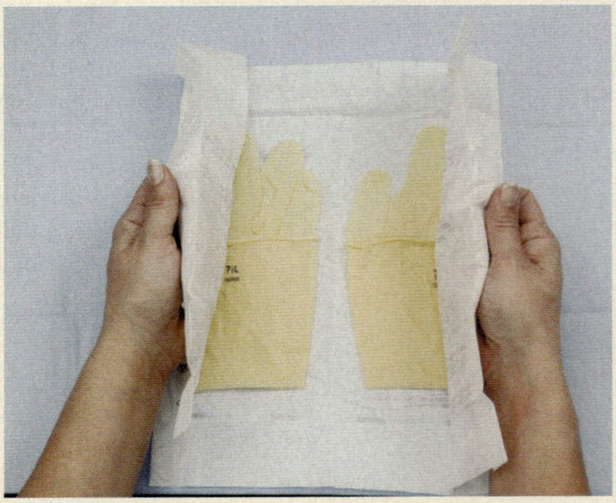

FIGURE 2. Folding back side flaps.

ACTION	RATIONALE
8. With the thumb and forefinger of the nondominant hand, grasp the folded cuff of the glove for the dominant hand, touching only the exposed inside of the glove (Figure 3).	Unsterile hand touches only inside of glove. Outside remains sterile.
9. Keeping the hands above the waistline, lift and hold the glove up and off the inner package with fingers down (Figure 4). **Do not let it touch any unsterile object.**	Glove is contaminated if it touches any unsterile objects.
10. Carefully insert dominant hand palm up into glove (Figure 5) and pull glove on. Leave the cuff folded until the opposite hand is gloved.	Attempting to turn upward with unsterile hand may result in contamination of sterile glove.
11. Hold the thumb of the gloved hand outward. Place the fingers of the gloved hand inside the cuff of the remaining glove (Figure 6). Lift it from the wrapper, taking care not to touch anything with the gloves or hands.	Thumb is less likely to become contaminated if held outward. Sterile surface touching sterile surface prevents contamination.

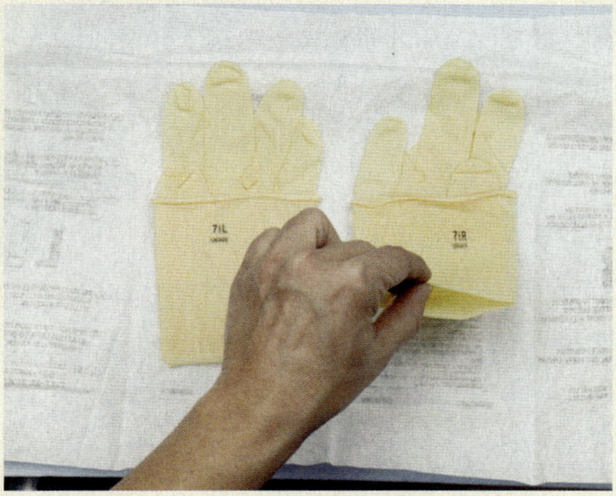

FIGURE 3. Grasping cuff of glove for dominant hand.

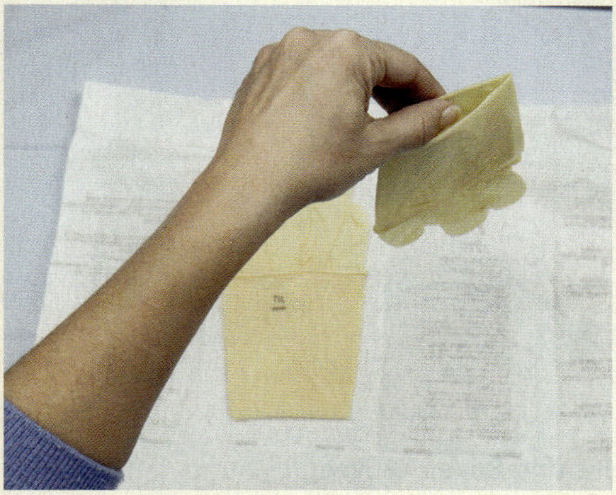

FIGURE 4. Lifting glove from package.

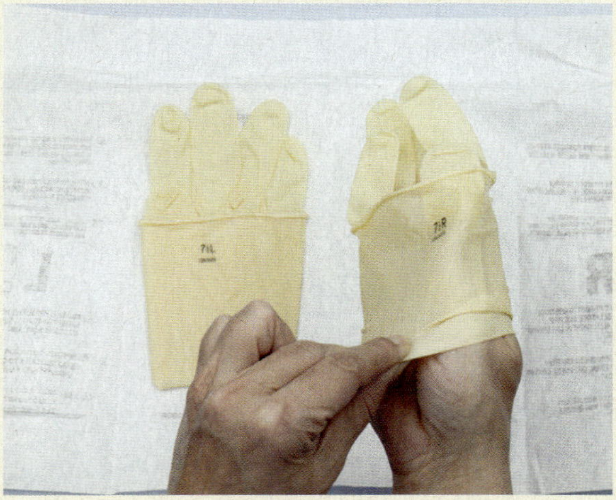

FIGURE 5. Inserting dominant hand into glove.

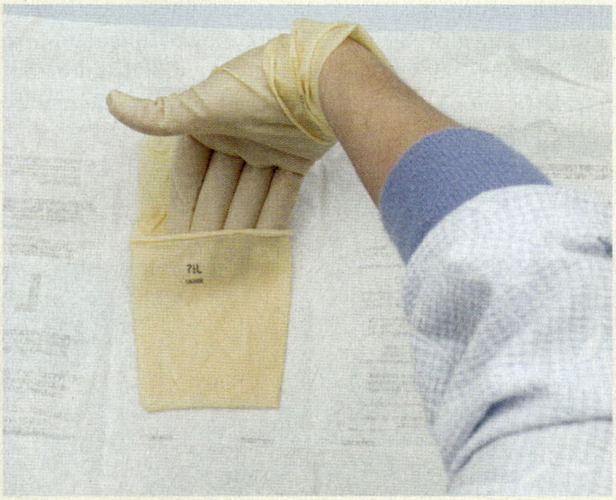

FIGURE 6. Sliding fingers under cuff of glove for nondominant hand.

(*continued on page 708*)

Skill 25-4 Putting on Sterile Gloves and Removing Soiled Gloves *(continued)*

ACTION	RATIONALE
12. Carefully insert nondominant hand into glove. Pull the glove on, taking care that the skin does not touch any of the outer surfaces of the gloves.	Sterile surface touching sterile surface prevents contamination.
13. Slide the fingers of one hand under the cuff of the other and fully extend the cuff down the arm, **touching only the sterile outside of the glove** (Figure 7). Repeat for the remaining hand.	Sterile surface touching sterile surface prevents contamination.
14. Adjust gloves on both hands, if necessary, **touching only sterile areas with other sterile areas** (Figure 8).	Sterile surface touching sterile surface prevents contamination.

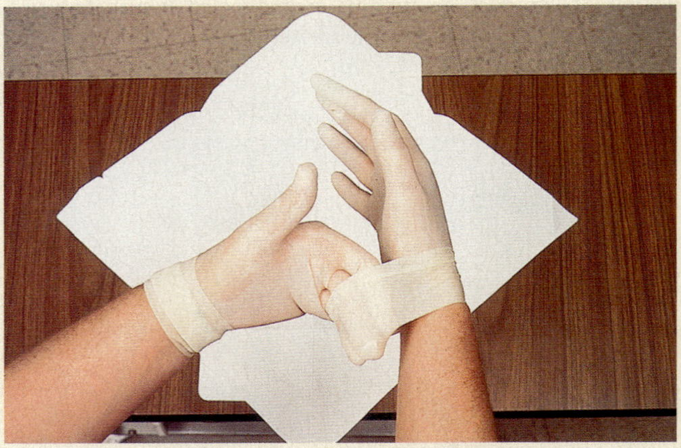

FIGURE 7. Sliding fingers of one hand under cuff of other hand and extending cuff down the arm.

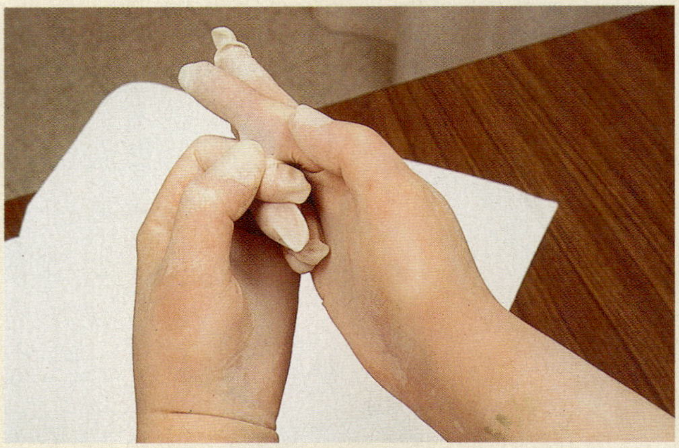

FIGURE 8. Adjusting gloves as necessary.

15. Continue with procedure as indicated.

Removing Soiled Gloves

16. **Outside of gloves is contaminated.** If hands are contaminated during gown or glove removal, immediately perform hand hygiene. Grasp the palm area of one gloved hand with the opposite gloved hand. Remove it by pulling it off, inverting it as it is pulled, keeping the contaminated area on the inside (Figure 9). Hold the removed glove in the remaining gloved hand.	Hand hygiene prevents the spread of microorganisms. Contaminated area does not come in contact with hands or wrists.

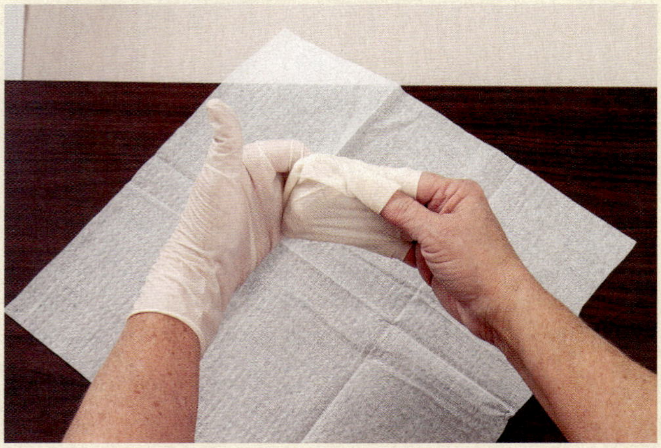

FIGURE 9. Inverting glove as it is removed.

ACTION

17. Slide fingers of ungloved hand between the remaining glove and the wrist (Figure 10). **Take care to avoid touching the outside surface of the glove.** Remove it by pulling second glove over the first glove, inverting it as it is pulled, keeping the contaminated area on the inside, and securing the first glove inside the second (Figure 11).

RATIONALE

Contaminated area does not come in contact with hands or wrists.

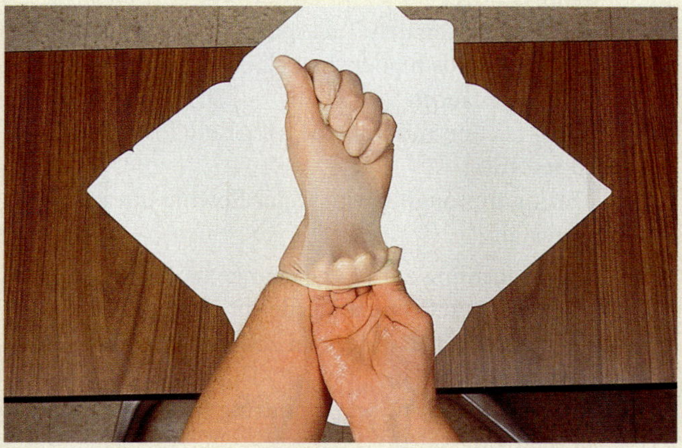

FIGURE 10. Sliding fingers of ungloved hand inside remaining glove.

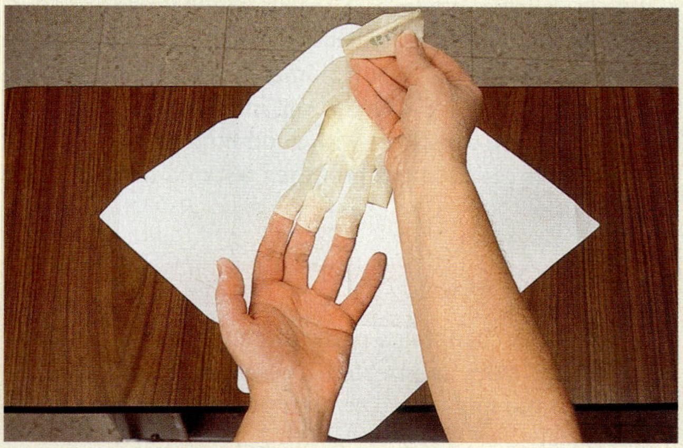

FIGURE 11. Inverting glove as it is removed, securing first glove inside it.

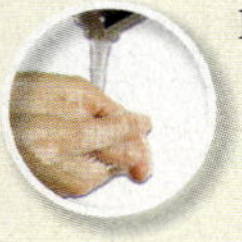

18. Discard gloves in appropriate container. Remove additional PPE, if used. Perform hand hygiene.

Proper removal and disposal of PPE reduces the risk for infection transmission and contamination of other items. Hand hygiene prevents the spread of microorganisms.

DOCUMENTATION

It is not usually necessary to document the application of sterile gloves and removal. However, document the use of sterile technique for any procedure performed using sterile technique.

DEVELOPING CLINICAL REASONING AND CLINICAL JUDGMENT

UNEXPECTED SITUATIONS AND ASSOCIATED INTERVENTIONS

- *Contamination occurs during application of the sterile gloves:* Discard gloves and open new package of sterile gloves.
- *A hole or tear is noticed in one of the gloves:* Discard gloves and open a new package of sterile gloves.
- *A hole or tear is noticed in one of the gloves during the procedure:* Stop procedure. Remove damaged gloves. Perform hand hygiene and put on new sterile gloves.
- *The patient touches the nurse's hand:* If the patient touches your hands and nothing else, you may remove the contaminated gloves and put on new sterile gloves. It may be a good idea to bring two pairs of sterile gloves into the room, depending on facility policy, so that you will not have to leave the procedure to get a new pair.
- If the patient touches the sterile field, discard the supplies and prepare a new sterile field. If the patient is confused, have someone assist you by holding the patient's hands or reinforcing what is happening.
- *Patient has a latex allergy:* Obtain latex-free sterile gloves.

DEVELOPING CLINICAL REASONING AND CLINICAL JUDGMENT

1. A nurse cannot help but notice that whenever a particular surgeon makes rounds, he ignores basic principles of asepsis. He moves from one patient to another, touching dressings without washing his hands between patients. He is also inconsistent in his practice of sterile technique. You have anecdotal information that leads you to suspect that there is a higher rate of postoperative infection among his patients. What do you do?
2. A friend who is a nursing student always wears gloves when doing anything for ill patients. You are more selective in your use of gloves. She tells you that you are a fool for "taking chances" because you never know what you may pick up and bring home. Is this a matter of personal preference? What about human touch? Is one position more consistent with good nursing? Are your instructors consistent in how they respond to these questions?

PRACTICING FOR NCLEX

1. A nurse is changing a patient's bed linens after drainage from an infected abdominal wound leaked. Which nursing action reflects proper use of medical asepsis?
   a. Carrying soiled bed linens close to the body to prevent spreading microorganisms into the air
   b. Placing soiled bed linens and hospital gowns on the floor when making the bed
   c. Moving the patient table away from the body when wiping it off
   d. Cleaning the most soiled items at the bedside first, followed by cleaner items
2. An outbreak of measles has occurred at the local elementary school. The parents of a child in the prodromal phase of the illness are told the child should stay home until well. What is important for the nurse to teach the parents about the prodromal phase?
   a. The organisms enter the body and multiply while the patient is asymptomatic.
   b. A person typically has vague, nonspecific symptoms and is highly contagious.
   c. The presence of infection-specific signs and symptoms develop, manifesting as local or systemic responses.
   d. The signs and symptoms of the illness disappear, and the person returns to their preillness state.
3. A nursing unit has multiple patients with MRSA infections requiring contact isolation. In which situations is it appropriate for the nurses to use an alcohol-based hand sanitizer to decontaminate their hands? Select all that apply.
   a. Before providing a bed bath
   b. Having visibly soiled hands after patient contact
   c. Removing gloves after patient care
   d. Inserting a urinary catheter
   e. Assisting with a surgical placement of a cardiac stent
   f. Removing old magazines from a patient's table
4. A nursing student is performing hand hygiene after providing care to a patient who is in isolation for *C. diff* related to antibiotic therapy. Which actions by the nursing student will the primary nurse need to correct? Select all that apply.
   a. Removing all jewelry including a platinum wedding band
   b. Decontaminating the hands with an alcohol-based hand sanitizer
   c. Using approximately 1 teaspoon of liquid soap
   d. Keeping hands higher than elbows when placing under the faucet
   e. Using friction motion when washing for at least 20 seconds
   f. Rinsing thoroughly with water flowing toward the fingertips
5. When performing a dressing change requiring surgical asepsis, a nurse opens sterile supplies and dons sterile gloves. What additional action by the nurse is appropriate?
   a. Avoiding splashing while pouring irrigant onto the sterile field
   b. Covering the nose and mouth with gloved hands if a sneeze is imminent
   c. Using forceps soaked in a disinfectant to place dressings on the sterile field
   d. Considering the outer 1 inch of the sterile field contaminated
6. The nurse on a medical-surgical unit is admitting a patient with a diagnosis of active tuberculosis. Which infection control precautions will the nurse put in place?
   a. Wearing sterile gloves for patients with visible body fluids
   b. Placing the patient on airborne precautions
   c. Wearing an N95 respirator mask when in the room
   d. Placing the patient in a single-occupancy room
   e. Ensuring the room provides positive pressure
   f. Restricting visitors for the duration of the patient's stay
7. Nursing students enrolled in a medical-surgical nursing course are learning about infection control measures. They have learned that nurses use droplet precautions for patients with which infections? Select all that apply.
   a. Rubella
   b. Herpes simplex
   c. Varicella
   d. Tuberculosis
   e. MRSA
   f. Adenovirus

8. A nurse and health care provider are preparing for insertion of a central venous catheter when the patient accidentally touches the sterile field. What action will the nurse take next?
   a. Ask another nurse to hold the patient's hand and continue setting up the field
   b. Remove any objects the patient touched and resume setting up the sterile field
   c. Have someone hold the patient's hand, discard the supplies, and prepare a new sterile field
   d. No action since the patient has touched their own sterile field
9. When performing sterile wound irrigation and dressing change for a postoperative patient, a new graduate nurse creates a sterile field. Which actions require correction by the preceptor? Select all that apply.
   a. Placing the bottle cap for the irrigating solution off the sterile field with the edges down
   b. Holding the bottle of irrigating solution inside the edge of the sterile field
   c. Applying the second sterile glove by lifting it from beneath the cuff with the thumb held away from the glove
   d. Pouring the irrigating solution into a sterile container from a height of 4 to 6 inches (10 to 15 cm)
   e. Opening packages of sterile gauze dressings, prior to applying sterile gloves
10. A nurse has finished providing care for a patient in contact isolation for a MRSA infection. Place the steps the nurse should follow to remove PPE in the correct order.
    a. Untie gown at the front waist
    b. Remove mask
    c. Remove gloves
    d. Remove gown
    e. Remove goggles
11. A nurse administering an injection to a patient who tested positive for HIV sustains a needlestick. What action should the nurse take first?
    a. Report the incident to the nurse manager and file an injury report
    b. Wash the exposed area with warm water and soap
    c. Consent to postexposure prophylaxis (PEP) at the appropriate time
    d. Set up counseling sessions regarding safe practice to protect self
12. During morning huddle, a nurse manager and some nurses are identifying patients on the unit who are at risk for hospital-acquired infections (HAIs). Which patients will the nurses identify? Select all that apply.
    a. Smoker, two packs of cigarettes daily
    b. White blood cell count of 2,000/mm^3
    c. Indwelling urinary catheter in place
    d. Vegetarian and slightly underweight
    e. Central venous catheter present
    f. Postoperative colostomy
13. A nurse is caring for a patient who is incontinent of stool and has developed a stage 3 pressure wound on the buttocks. What intervention will the nurse set as the priority of care?
    a. Increasing nutrition
    b. Promoting mobility
    c. Managing chronic pain
    d. Preventing infection
14. A home health nurse teaches a patient to a change the dressing for a chronic venous stasis ulcer using clean technique. Which principle of asepsis will the nurse consider when preparing the teaching plan?
    a. The nurse chooses clean or sterile technique based on personal preference.
    b. The use of clean technique is considered safe in the home setting.
    c. Surgical asepsis is the safest method to use in a home setting.
    d. The patient can use clean technique; their partner must wear sterile gloves.
15. When bathing a patient with *C. diff* infection, the nurse wears personal protective equipment (PPE). Which additional intervention promotes safe, effective care?
    a. Donning PPE after entering the patient room
    b. Bathing the perianal area last
    c. Personalizing care by substituting glasses for goggles
    d. Removing PPE after bathing the patient to talk with them in the room
16. A nurse is preparing to admit a patient with urinary sepsis related to vancomycin-resistant enterococci (VRE). While awaiting the patient's arrival, which of these actions will the nurse take?
    a. Prepare a negative-pressure room
    b. Ask the AP to get a supply of protective gowns
    c. Post a sign that visitors must wear a mask
    d. Obtain sterile gloves for personal care

ANSWERS WITH RATIONALES

1. **c.** According to the principles of medical asepsis, the nurse should move equipment and soiled items away from the body to prevent contaminated particles from settling on the hair, face, or uniform. The nurse should not put soiled items on the floor, as it is highly contaminated. The nurse should also clean the least soiled areas first, then move to the more soiled ones to prevent contamination.
2. **b.** During the prodromal stage, the person has vague signs and symptoms, such as fatigue and a low-grade fever. There are no obvious symptoms of infection during the incubation period, and symptoms are more specific and apparent during the full stage of illness, disappearing in the convalescent period.
3. **a, c, d, f.** An alcohol-based handrub is used in the following situations: before direct contact with patients; after direct contact with patient skin; after contact with body fluids *if hands are not visibly soiled;* after removing gloves; before

inserting urinary catheters, peripheral vascular catheters, or invasive devices *not requiring surgical placement;* before donning sterile gloves prior to an invasive procedure; when moving from a contaminated body site to a clean body site; and after contact with objects contaminated by the patient. It is essential to note that handrubs are not appropriate for use after caring for a patient with *C. diff* infection.

4. **b, d.** After caring for patients with *C. diff* infection, proper handwashing includes using soap and water, then rinsing thoroughly with water flowing toward fingertips. Proper hand hygiene permits a plain wedding band to be worn; other jewelry is removed. The nurse uses about 1 teaspoon (5 mL) of liquid soap, using friction motion for at least 20 seconds, washing to 1 inch above the wrists using friction.
5. **a, d.** Considering the outer inch of a sterile field as contaminated is a principle of surgical asepsis. Moisture, such as from splashes contaminates the sterile field, and sneezing would contaminate the sterile gloves. Forceps soaked in disinfectant are not considered sterile.
6. **b, c, d.** Airborne precautions are used for patients who have infections with small particles that spread through the air, for example, tuberculosis, varicella, and rubeola. An N95 respirator mask is worn and the patient placed in a private room, preferably with negative air pressure. Sterile gloves are used for procedures requiring surgical asepsis. Standard precautions are for all patient care when contact with blood or body fluids, nonintact skin, and mucous membranes are likely. Visitors must wear PPE, including a mask.
7. **a, f.** Rubella, diphtheria, and adenovirus infection are illnesses transmitted by large-droplet particles; droplet precautions and standard precautions are indicated. Airborne precautions refer to small, infectious particles spread through the air; for example, tuberculosis, varicella, and rubeola. Contact precautions are used for patients who are infected or colonized by a multidrug-resistant organism (MDRO), such as MRSA.
8. **c.** If a patient touches a sterile field, the nurse should discard all supplies and prepare a new sterile field. If the patient is restless or confused, the nurse obtains an assistant to hold the patient's hands and explain what is happening.
9. **a, b.** To add a sterile solution to a sterile field, the nurse opens the solution container according to directions and places the cap on the table away from the field with the edges up. The nurse then holds the bottle outside the edge of the sterile field with the label side facing the palm of the hand and pours from a height of 4 to 6 inches (10 to 15 cm) to prevent splashing.
10. **a, c, e, d, b.** If an impervious gown has been tied in front of the body at the waist, the nurse should untie the waist strings before removing gloves. Gloves are removed first because they are most likely to be contaminated, followed by the goggles, gown, and mask. Hands should be washed thoroughly after the equipment has been removed and before leaving the room.
11. **b.** When a needlestick injury occurs, the nurse should wash the affected area immediately with warm water and soap, report the incident to the nurse manager or appropriate person and complete an injury report, consent to and await the results of blood tests, consent to PEP, and attend counseling sessions regarding safe practice to protect self and others.
12. **b, c, e, f.** Leukopenia (low white blood cell count), indwelling urinary catheters, central venous catheters, and surgeries in which the wound is classified as dirty have been implicated in most HAIs. Cigarette smoking and a vegetarian diet have not been implicated as risk factors for HAIs.
13. **d.** The priority in this situation is to prevent infection through contamination of the wound by stool. The other actions may be taken as needed, after infection prevention is addressed.
14. **b.** Medical asepsis, or clean technique, involves procedures and practices that reduce the number and transfer of pathogens. This is usually recommended in the home setting, where the patient's environment is more controlled. Injections require surgical asepsis. The patient and partner share the same home; medical asepsis is appropriate.
15. **b.** When using PPE, the nurse should work from clean areas to soiled ones, don PPE before entering the patient room, always use goggles instead of personal glasses, and remove PPE in the doorway or anteroom just before exiting.
16. **b.** VRE is spread via contact with the feces, urine, or blood of an infected or colonized person. Contact precautions, meticulous hand hygiene, reducing the use of invasive devices, environmental cleaning, and decolonizing high-risk patients are indicated. Some institutions have discontinued using contact precautions and use standard precautions, with no significant change in the incidence of MRSA or VRE.

Bibliography

Agency for Healthcare Research and Quality (AHRQ). (2014). *Advances in the prevention and control of HAIs*. AHRQ Publication No. 14-0003. Prepared by IMPAQ International, LLC, Columbia, MD, under contract no. HHSA290200710071T. Agency for Healthcare Research and Quality. https://www.ahrq.gov/hai/patient-safety-resources/advances-in-hai/index.html

Agency for Healthcare Research and Quality (AHRQ). (2019, August). *AHRQ's healthcare-associated infections program*. https://www.ahrq.gov/hai/index.html

American Nurses Association (ANA). (n.d.). ANA CAUTI prevention tool. Retrieved July 3, 2020, from https://www.nursingworld.org/practice-policy/work-environment/health-safety/infection-prevention/ana-cauti-prevention-tool/

American Nurses Association (ANA). (2015). Code of ethics for nurses with interpretive statements. American Nurses Association. https://www.nursingworld.org/practice-policy/

Association for Professionals in Infection Control and Epidemiology, Inc. (APIC). (n.d.). APIC implementation guides. Retrieved July 7, 2020, from http://www.apic.org/Professional-Practice/Implementation-guides

Association of periOperative Registered Nurses. (2020). *Guidelines for perioperative practice*. AORN, Inc. MAN-020.

Berardi, A., Perinelli, D. R., Merchant, H. A., Bisharat, L., Basheti, I. A., Bonacucina, G., Cespi, M., & Palmieri, G. F. (2020). Hand sanitizers amid CoViD-19: A critical review of alcohol-based products on the market and formulation approaches to respond to increasing demand. *International Journal of Pharmaceutics, 584*, 119431. https://doi.org/10.1016/j.ijpharm.2020.119431

Billings, C., Bernard, H., Caffery, L., Dolan, S. A., Donaldson, J., Kalp, E., & Mueller, A. (2019). Advancing the profession: An updated future-oriented competency model for professional development in infection prevention and control. *American Journal of Infection Control, 47*(6), 602–614. https://doi.org/10.1016/j.ajic.2019.04.003

Breen, A., & Hessels, A. (2017). Stethoscopes: Friend or fomite? *Nursing Management, 48*(12), 9–11. https://doi.org/10.1097/01.NUMA.0000526917.85088.eb

Brunette, G. W. & Nemhauset, J. B. (Eds.). (2019). *CDC yellow book 2020: Health information for international travel*. Oxford University Press.

Burkhart, C., Schloemer, J., & Zirwas, M. (2015). Differentiation of latex allergy from irritant contact dermatitis. *Cutis, 96*(6), 369–371, 401. https://www.mdedge.com/dermatology/article/105157/contact-dermatitis/differentiation-latex-allergy-irritant-contact

CDC Foundation. (2016, January 21) CDC foundation and GOJO to enhance hand hygiene educational outreach in U.S. healthcare settings. https://www.cdcfoundation.org/pr/2016/cdc-foundation-and-gojo-enhance-hand-hygiene-educational-outreach-us-healthcare-settings

Centers for Disease Control and Prevention (CDC). (2002). Guideline for hand hygiene in health-care settings: Recommendations of the healthcare infection control practices advisory committee and the HICPAC/SHEA/APIC/IDSA hand hygiene task force. *Morbidity and Mortality Weekly Report, 51*(RR–16), 1–45. https://www.cdc.gov/mmwr/PDF/rr/rr5116.pdf

Centers for Disease Control and Prevention (CDC). (2007; updated 2019). *Guideline for isolation precautions: Preventing transmission of infectious agents in healthcare settings.* https://www.cdc.gov/infection-control/guidelines/isolation/index.html

Centers for Disease Control and Prevention (CDC). (2016). *National and state healthcare-associated infections progress report.* http://www.cdc.gov/HAI/pdfs/progress-report/hai-progress-report.pdf

Centers for Disease Control and Prevention (CDC). (2016a). *Hand hygiene in healthcare settings. Patients. Clean hands count for patients.* https://www.cdc.gov/handhygiene/patients/index.html

Centers for Disease Control and Prevention (CDC). (2016b). *Healthcare-associated infections. Outpatient settings. Guide to infection prevention in outpatient settings:Minimum expectations for safe care.* https://www.cdc.gov/hai/settings/outpatient/outpatientsettings.html

Centers for Disease Control and Prevention (CDC). (2019a, February 28). *Methicillin-resistant Staphylococcus aureus (MRSA): Healthcare settings.* https://www.cdc.gov/mrsa/healthcare/index.html

Centers for Disease Control and Prevention (CDC). (2019b, April 22). *Influenza (flu): What you should know about flu antiviral drugs?* https://www.cdc.gov/flu/treatment/whatyoushould.htm

Centers for Disease Control and Prevention (CDC). (2019c, June 26). *Methicillin-resistant Staphylococcus aureus (MRSA): General information.* https://www.cdc.gov/mrsa/community/index.html

Centers for Disease Control and Prevention (CDC). (2019d, August 2). *Interim infection prevention and control recommendations for hospitalized patients with Middle East respiratory syndrome coronavirus (MERS-CoV).* http://www.cdc.gov/coronavirus/mers/infection-prevention-control.html

Centers for Disease Control and Prevention (CDC). (2019e, August 7). *Healthcare-associated infections: Strategies to prevent Clostridioides difficile infection in acute care facilities.* https://www.cdc.gov/hai/prevent/cdi-prevention-strategies.html

Centers for Disease Control and Prevention (CDC). (2019f, November 30). *States with HAI reporting mandates.* https://www.cdc.gov/HAI/state-based/required-to-report-hai-NHSN.html

Centers for Disease Control and Prevention (CDC). (2019g, December). *Antibiotic resistance threats in the United States 2019.* U.S. Department of Health and Human Services, CDC. http://dx.doi.org/10.15620/cdc:82532

Centers for Disease Control and Prevention (CDC). (2020a, January). *Urinary tract infection (catheter-associated urinary tract infection [CAUTI] and non-catheter-associated urinary tract infection [UTI]) events.* https://www.cdc.gov/nhsn/pdfs/pscmanual/7psccauticurrent.pdf

Centers for Disease Control and Prevention (CDC). (2020d, April 22). *Viral hepatitis: What is viral hepatitis?* https://www.cdc.gov/hepatitis/abc/index.htm

Centers for Disease Control and Prevention (CDC). (2020e, April 23). *Zika and pregnancy: General Zika information.* https://www.cdc.gov/pregnancy/zika/general-information.html

Centers for Disease Control and Prevention (CDC). (2020f, April 24). *Parasites—Malaria.* https://www.cdc.gov/parasites/malaria/index.html

Centers for Disease Control and Prevention (CDC). (2020g, June 16). *Coronavirus disease 2019 (COVID-19): How COVID-19 spreads.* https://www.cdc.gov/coronavirus/2019-ncov/prevent-getting-sick/how-covid-spreads.html

Centers for Disease Control and Prevention (CDC). (2020h, June 19). *NIOSH-approved N95 particulate filtering facepiece respirators.* https://www.cdc.gov/niosh/npptl/topics/respirators/disp_part/n95list1.html

Centers for Disease Control and Prevention (CDC). (2020i, June 24). *CDC current outbreak list.* https://www.cdc.gov/outbreaks/

Centers for Disease Control and Prevention (CDC). (2020j, June 24). *Coronavirus disease 2019 (COVID-19): Frequently asked questions.* https://www.cdc.gov/coronavirus/2019-ncov/faq.html#Contact-Tracing

Centers for Medicare & Medicaid Services. (2020b, February 11). *Hospital-acquired conditions.* https://www.cms.gov/Medicare/Medicare-Fee-for-Service-Payment/HospitalAcqCond/Hospital-Acquired_Conditions

Centers for Medicare & Medicaid Services. (2020c, February 11). *Hospital-acquired condition reduction program (HACRP).* https://www.cms.gov/Medicare/Medicare-Fee-for-Service-Payment/AcuteInpatientPPS/HAC-Reduction-Program

Cobb, A., & Lazar, B. (2020). Mobile device usage contributes to nosocomial infections. *Radiologic Technology, 91*(3), 303–307.

Cong, Y., Yang, S., & Rao, X. (2019). Vancomycin resistant *Staphylococcus aureus* infections: A review of case updating and clinical features. *Journal of Advanced Research, 21*, 169–176. https://doi.org/10.1016/j.jare.2019.10.005

Dubberke, E. R., Carling, P., Carrico, R., & Donskey, C. J. (2014). Strategies to prevent Clostridium difficile infections in acute care hospitals: 2014 update. *Infection Control & Hospital Epidemiology, 35*(6), 628–645. https://doi.org/10.1017/S0899823X00193857

Gesser-Edelsburg, A., Cohen, R., Zemach, M., & Halavi, A. M. (2020). Discourse on hygiene between hospitalized patients and health care workers as an accepted norm: Making it legitimate to remind health care workers about hand hygiene. *American Journal of Infection Control, 48*(1), 61–67. https://doi.org/10.1016/j.ajic.2018.10.026

GOJO Industries, Inc. (2020, May 22). CDC offers strong safety recommendations—Including measures for hygiene and surface disinfection—As businesses welcome back employees and customers. https://www.gojo.com/en/Newsroom/Corporate-Statements/CDC-Offers-Measures-Hygiene-and-Surface-Disinfection-Businesses-Welcome-Back-Employees-and-Customers?sc_lang=en

Gold, N. A., & Avva, U. (2020, February 6). Alcohol sanitizer. In *StatPearls [Internet]*. StatPearls Publishing. https://www.ncbi.nlm.nih.gov/books/NBK513254/

Grimmond, T., & Good, L. (2019). EXPO-S.T.O.P. 2016 and 2017 blood exposure surveys: An alarming rise. *American Journal of Infection Control, 47*(12), 1465–1470. https://doi.org/10.1016/j.ajic.2019.07.004

Gupta, A. K., Lyons, D. C., & Rosen, T. (2015). New and emerging concepts in managing and preventing community-associated methicillin-resistant Staphylococcus aureus infections. *International Journal of Dermatology, 54*(11), 1226–1232. https://doi.org/10.1111/ijd.13010

Halm, M., & Sandau, K. (2018). Skin impact of alcohol-based hand rubs vs handwashing. *American Journal of Critical Care, 27*(4), 334–337. https://doi.org/10.4037/ajcc2018727

Hammerschmidt, J., & Manser, T. (2019). Nurses' knowledge, behaviour and compliance concerning hand hygiene in nursing homes: A cross-sectional mixed-methods study. *BMC Health Services Research, 19*(1), 547. https://doi.org/10.1186/s12913-019-4347-z

Healthcare Infection Control Practices Advisory Committee. (2017, March 15). *Core infection prevention and control practices for safe healthcare delivery in all settings—Recommendations of the Healthcare Infection Control Practices Advisory Committee.* Centers for Disease Control and Prevention. https://www.cdc.gov/hicpac/pdf/core-practices.pdf

Healthy People 2030. (2021). Healthcare-associated infections workgroup. https://health.gov/healthypeople/about/workgroups/healthcare-associated-infections-workgroup

Henry, N., Icot, R., & Jeffery, S. (2020). The benefits of latex-free gloves in the operating room environment. *British Journal of Nursing, 29*(10), 570–576. https://doi.org/10.12968/bjon.2020.29.10.570

Hinkle, J. L., Cheever, K. H., & Overbaugh, K. J. (2022). *Brunner & Suddarth's textbook of medical-surgical nursing* (15th ed.). Wolters Kluwer.

Institute for Healthcare Improvement (IHI). (2020a). *Bundles: Evidence-based care bundles.* http://www.ihi.org/Topics/Bundles/Pages/default.aspx

Institute for Healthcare Improvement (IHI). (2020b). *Tools—How-to guide: Improving hand hygiene.* http://www.ihi.org/resources/Pages/Tools/HowtoGuideImprovingHandHygiene.aspx

International Safety Center. (2020, December). *Moving the sharps safety agenda forward in the United States: 2020 consensus statement and call to action.* https://internationalsafetycenter.org/wp-content/uploads/2020/12/Moving_The_Sharps_Safety_In_Healthcare_Agenda_Forward_In_The_US.pdf

The Joint Commission Center for Transforming Healthcare. (2020). *Hand hygiene targeted solutions tool.* https://www.centerfortransforminghealthcare.org/what-we-offer/targeted-solutions-tool/hand-hygiene-tst/

The Joint Commission. (2013, November 20). *Preventing central line–associated bloodstream infections: Useful tools, an international perspective.* https://www.jointcommission.org/-/media/tjc/documents/resources/health-services-research/clabsi-toolkit/clabsi_toolkit_tool_2-5_review_of_joint_commission_and_jci_requirementspdf.pdf?db=web&hash=3C898CAD009F6029354C8DBF20BC0DAA

The Joint Commission. (2020). *Sentinel event policy and procedures.* https://www.jointcommission.org/resources/patient-safety-topics/sentinel-event/sentinel-event-policy-and-procedures/

Kim, D., & Lee, O. (2019). Effects of audio-visual stimulation on hand hygiene compliance among family and non-family visitors of pediatric wards: A quasi-experimental pre-post intervention study. *Journal of Pediatric Nursing, 46*, e92–e97. https://doi.org/10.1016/j.pedn.2019.03.017

Kingston, L. M., Slevin, B. L., O'Connell, N. H., & Dunne, C. P. (2017). Hand hygiene: Attitudes and practices of nurses, a comparison between 2007 and 2015. *American Journal of Infection Control, 45*(12), 1300–1307. https://doi.org/10.1016/j.ajic.2017.08.040

Kingston, L., O'Connell, N. H., & Dunne, C. P. (2016). Hand hygiene-related clinical trials reported since 2010: A systematic review. *Journal of Hospital Infection, 92*(4), 309–320. https://doi.org10.1016/j.jhin.2015.11.012

Klompas, M., Branson, R., Eichenwald, E. C., Greene, L. R., Howell, M. D., Lee, G., Magill, S. S., Maragakis, L. L., Priebe, G. P., Speck, K., Yokoe, D. S., & Berenholtz, S. M. (2014). Strategies to prevent ventilator-associated pneumonia in acute care hospitals: 2014 update. *Infection Control and Hospital Epidemiology, 35*(Suppl 2), S133–S154. https://doi.org/10.1017/s0899823x00193894

Krah, J., Shamblin, M., & Shaffer, R. (2018). Filtering out confusion: Frequently asked questions about respiratory protection, user seal check. U.S. Department of Health and Human Services, Centers for Disease Control and Prevention, National Institute for Occupational Safety and Health, DHHS (NIOSH) Publication 2018–130, https://doi.org/10.26616/NIOSHPUB2018130

Kullar, R., Vassallo, A., Turkel, S., Chopra, T., Kaye, K. S., & Dhar, S. (2016). Degowning the controversies of contact precautions for methicillin-resistant Staphylococcus aureus: A review. *American Journal of Infection Control, 44*(1), 97–103. https://doi.org/10.1016/j.ajic.2015.08.003

Lambe, K. A., Lydon, S., Madden, C., Vellinga, A., Hehir, A., Walsh, M., & O'Connor, P. (2019). Hand hygiene compliance in the ICU: A systematic review. *Critical Care Medicine, 47*(9), 1251–1257. https://doi.org/10.1097/CCM.0000000000003868

Lary, D., Calvert, A., Nerlich, B., Segal, J., Vaughan, N., Randle, J., & Hardie, K. R. (2020). Improving children's and their visitors' hand hygiene compliance. *Journal of Infection Prevention, 21*(2), 60–67. https://doi. org/10.1177/1757177419892065

Levitus, M., Rewane, A., & Perera, T. B. (2020, April 22). Vancomycin-resistant Enterococci (VRE). In *StatPearls [Internet]*. StatPearls Publishing. https://www.ncbi.nlm.nih.gov/books/NBK513233/

Magill, S. S., O'Leary, E., Janelle, S. J., Thompson, D. L., Dumyati, G., Nadle, J., Wilson, L. E., Kainer, M. A., Lynfield, R., Greissman, R., Ray, S. M., Beldavs, Z., Gross, C., Bamberg, W., Sievers, M., Concannon, C., Buhr, N., Warnke, L., Maloney, M., . . . for the Emerging Infections Program Hospital Prevalence Survey Team. (2018). Changes in prevalence of health care–associated infections in U.S. hospitals.

New England Journal of Medicine, *379*(18), 1732–1744. https://pubmed.ncbi.nlm.nih.gov/30380384/
Marcus, J. L., & Snowden, J. M. (2020). Words matter: Putting an end to "unsafe" and "risky" sex. *Sexually Transmitted Diseases*, *47*(1), 1–3. https://doi.org/10.1097/OLQ.0000000000001065
McDonald, E., Martin, S. W., Landry, K., Gould, C. V., Lehman, J., Fischer, M., & Lindsey, N. P. (2019). West Nile virus and other domestic nationally notifiable arboviral diseases—United States, 2018. *Morbidity and Mortality Weekly Report*, *68*(31), 673–678. https://www.cdc.gov/mmwr/volumes/68/wr/mm6831a1.htm
Muller, M. P., MacDougall, C., Lim, M.; Ontario Agency for Health Protection and Promotion, & Provincial Infectious Diseases Advisory Committee on Infection Prevention and Control. (2016). Antimicrobial surfaces to prevent healthcare-associated infections: a systematic review. *Journal of Hospital Infection*, *92*(1), 7–13. https://doi.org/10.1016/j.jhin.2015.09.008
National Clinician Consultation Center. (2020, April 22). *PEP quick guide for occupational exposures*. http://nccc.ucsf.edu/clinical-resources/pep-resources/pep-quick-guide-for-occupational-exposures/
National Institute for Occupational Safety and Health (NIOSH). (2012a). *NIOSH fast facts–Home healthcare workers: How to prevent latex allergies*. DHHS (NIOSH) Publication No. 2012–119. http://www.cdc.gov/niosh/docs/2012-119/pdfs/2012-119.pdf
National Institute for Occupational Safety and Health (NIOSH). (2012b). *NIOSH Fast Facts–Home healthcare workers: How to prevent needlestick and sharps injuries.* . DHHS (NIOSH) Publication No. 2012–123. http://www.cdc.gov/niosh/docs/2012-123/pdfs/2012-123.pdf
The National Institute for Occupational Safety and Health (NIOSH). (2015, January 13). *Hierarchy of controls*. https://www.cdc.gov/niosh/topics/hierarchy/default.html
National Institute of Allergy and Infectious Diseases. (2020, April 22). *NIAID strategic plan for COVID-19 research FY2020-2024*. https://www.niaid.nih.gov/sites/default/files/NIAID-COVID-19-Strategic-Plan-2020.pdf
Norris, T. L. (2019). *Porth's pathophysiology: Concepts of altered health states*. (10th ed.). Wolters Kluwer.
Occupational Safety and Health Administration (OSHA). (2011, June 8). *Regulations (Standards—29 CFR)—Personal protective equipment: Respiratory protection*. Standard No. 1910.134. https://www.osha.gov/laws-regs/regulations/standardnumber/1910
Occupational Safety and Health Administration (OSHA). (2012, April 3). *Regulations (Standards—29 CFR)—Toxic and hazardous substances: Bloodborne pathogens*. Standard No. 1910.1030. https://www.osha.gov/laws-regs/regulations/standardnumber/1910
Occupational Safety and Health Administration (OSHA). (2016, November 18). *Regulations (Standards—29 CFR)—Personal protective equipment: General requirements*. Standard No. 1910.132. https://www.osha.gov/laws-regs/regulations/standardnumber/1910
Occupational Safety and Health Administration (OSHA). (n.d.). *Safety and health topics: Latex allergy*. Retrieved July 6, 2020, from https://www.osha.gov/SLTC/latexallergy/index.html
OncoLink. (2020, February 12). *Low white blood cell count (neutropenia)*. https://www.oncolink.org/support/side-effects/low-blood-counts/neutropenia
Piperaki, E. T., Tzouvelekis, L. S., Miriagou, V., & Daikos, G. L. (2019). Carbapenem-resistant Acinetobacter baumannii: in pursuit of an effective treatment. *Clinical Microbiology and Infection*, *25*(8), 951–957. https://doi.org/10.1016/j.cmi.2019.03.014
Polen, K. D., Gilboa, S. M., Hills, S., Oduyebo, T., Kohl, K. S., Brooks, J. T., Adamski, A., Simeone, R. M., Walker, A. T., Kissin, D. M., Peterson, L. R., Honein, M. A., & Meany-Delman, D. (2018). Update: Interim guidance for preconception counseling and prevention of sexual transmission of Zika virus for men with possible Zika virus exposure—United States, August 2018. *Morbidity and Mortality Weekly Report*, *67*(31), 868–871. https://www.cdc.gov/mmwr/volumes/67/wr/mm6731e2.htm?s_cid=mm6731e2_w
Pryor, R., Viola-Luqa, C., Hess, O., & Bearman, G. (2020). Barrier Precautions in the Era of Multidrug Pathogens. *Current Treatment Options in Infectious Diseases*, 1–11. Advance online publication. https://doi.org/10.1007/s40506-020-00230-9
QSEN Institute. (2020). *Quality and safety education for nurses: QSEN competencies*. Retrieved June 24, 2020, from https://qsen.org/competencies/pre-licensure-ksas/
Saag M. S. (2019). HIV 101: fundamentals of antiretroviral therapy. *Topics in Antiviral Medicine*, *27*(3), 123–127. https://www.ncbi.nlm.nih.gov/pmc/articles/PMC6892619/
Siegel, J. D., Rhinehart, E., Jackson, M., Chiarello, L., & The Healthcare Infection Control Practices Advisory Committee. (2019, July). *2007 Guideline for isolation precautions: Preventing transmission of infectious agents in healthcare settings [Last update: July 2019]*. https://www.cdc.gov/infectioncontrol/pdf/guidelines/isolation-guidelines-H.pdf
Srigley, J. A., Cho, S. M., O'Neill, C., Bialachowski, A., Ali, R. A., Lee, C., & Mertz, D. (2020). Hand hygiene knowledge, attitudes, and practices among hospital inpatients: A descriptive study. *American Journal of Infection Control*, *48*(5), 507–510. https://doi. org/10.1016/j.ajic.2019.11.020
U.S. Department of Health & Human Services (USDHHS). (2021, August 24). *National HAI targets and metrics*. https://health.gov/our-work/health-care-quality/health-care-associated-infections/targets-metrics
Virginia Department of Health. (2018, September). *VISA/VRSA infections*. https://www.vdh.virginia.gov/epidemiology/epidemiology-fact-sheets/vancomycin-intermediate-staphylococcus-aureus-visa-and-vancomycin-resistant-staphylococcus-aureus-vrsa-infections/
Wang, S. H., Hines, L., van Balen, J., Mediavilla, J. R., Pan, X., Hoet, A. E., Kreiswirth, B. N., Pancholi, P., & Stevenson, K. B. (2015). Molecular and clinical characteristics of hospital and community onset methicillin-resistant Staphylococcus aureus strains associated with bloodstream infections. *Journal of Clinical Microbiology*, *53*(5), 1599–1608. https://doi.org/10.1128/JCM.03147-14
Wong, M. W. H., Xu, Y. Z., Bone, J., & Srigley, J. A. (2020). Impact of patient and visitor hand hygiene interventions at a pediatric hospital: A stepped wedge cluster randomized controlled trial. *American Journal of Infection Control*, *48*(5), 511–516. https://doi. org/10.1016/j.ajic.2019.09.026
World Health Organization (WHO). (2020a). *Antimicrobial resistance*. https://www.who.int/health-topics/antimicrobial-resistance
World Health Organization (WHO). (2020b). *Global Health Observatory (GHO) data: Malaria*. https://www.who.int/gho/malaria/en/
World Health Organization (WHO). (2020c). *Infection prevention and control: My 5 moments for hand hygiene*. https://www.who.int/infection-prevention/campaigns/clean-hands/5moments/en/
World Health Organization (WHO). (2020d, March 29). *Modes of transmission of virus causing COVID-19: Implications for IPC precaution recommendations*. https://www.who.int/news-room/commentaries/detail/modes-of-transmission-of-virus-causing-covid-19-implications-for-ipc-precaution-recommendations
Wu, B. (2020). Social isolation and loneliness among older adults in the context of COVID-19: A global challenge. *Global Health Research and Policy*, *5*, 27. https://doi.org/10.1186/s41256-020-00154-3
Yoo J. H. (2018). Review of disinfection and sterilization—Back to the basics. *Infection & Chemotherapy*, *50*(2), 101–109. https://doi.org/10.3947/ic.2018.50.2.101
Zingg, W., Park, B. J., Storr, J., Ahmad, R., Tarrant, C., Castro-Sanchez, E., Perencevich, E., Widmer, A., Krause, K. H., Kilpatrick, C., Tomczyk, S., Allegranzi, B., Cardo, D., Pittet, D., & 2017 Geneva IPC-Think Tank (2019). Technology for the prevention of antimicrobial resistance and healthcare-associated infections; 2017 Geneva IPC-Think Tank (Part 2). *Antimicrobial Resistance and Infection Control*, *8*, 83. https://doi.org/10.1186/s13756-019-0538-y

26 Vital Signs

Noah Shoolin

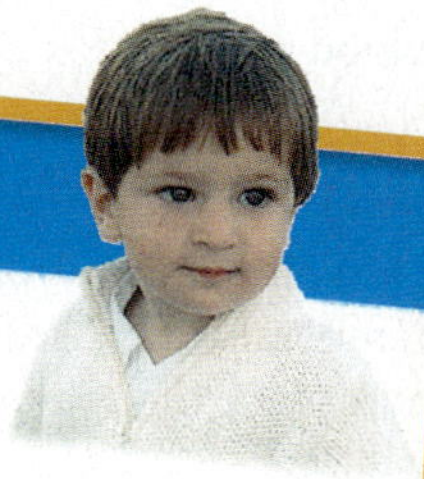

Noah is a 2-year-old who is brought to the emergency department by his mother. When the nurse attempts to obtain a tympanic temperature, the child begins to scream uncontrollably, crying and pushing the device away from his ear.

Tomas Esposito

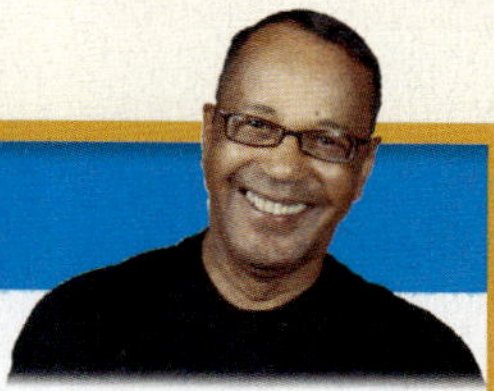

Tomas is a middle-aged man admitted to the hospital. He is placed in a private room with transmission-based infection control precautions, requiring staff to put on a gown and gloves when entering the room. A morning assessment, including vital signs, is needed.

Doretha Renfrow

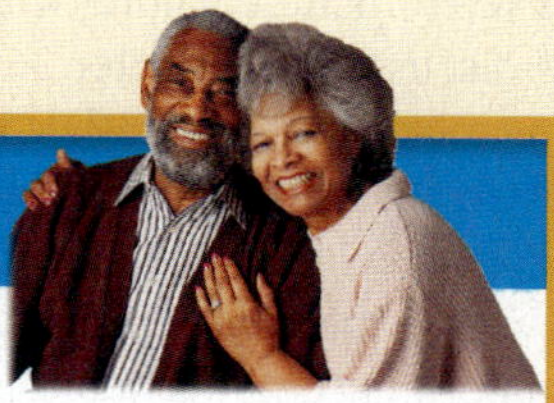

Doretha brings her 65-year-old husband, who is overweight and has high blood pressure, to the clinic for evaluation. Mrs. Renfrow states, "I really would like to learn how to take my husband's blood pressure so that I can keep track of his progress. Can you teach me how to do it?"

Learning Outcomes

After completing the chapter, you will be able to accomplish the following:

1. Explain the physiologic processes involved in homeostatic regulation of temperature, pulse, respirations, and blood pressure.
2. Compare and contrast factors that increase or decrease body temperature, pulse, respirations, and blood pressure.
3. Identify sites for assessing temperature, pulse, and blood pressure.
4. Assess temperature, pulse, respirations, and blood pressure accurately.
5. Demonstrate knowledge of the normal ranges for temperature, pulse, respirations, and blood pressure across the life span.
6. Provide information to patients about measuring temperature, pulse, and blood pressure at home.

Nursing Concepts

- Assessment
- Clinical Decision Making/Clinical Judgment
- Safety
- Thermoregulation
- Oxygenation
- Perfusion

Vital signs are indicators of physiologic functioning and reflect the health status of a person. Vital signs include a person's temperature, pulse, respiration, and blood pressure (abbreviated as T, P, R, BP). Pain assessment is often included along with measurement of vital signs and is discussed in Chapter 36. Pulse oximetry, the noninvasive measurement of arterial oxyhemoglobin saturation, is also often included with the measurement of vital signs and is discussed in Chapter 40.

Assessing vital signs as part of a nursing assessment is an important component of care in all health care settings. Nurses assess vital signs in a wide variety of instances, and compare findings with accepted normal values, the patient's usual patterns, with consideration to potential variations related to specific health conditions, illnesses and complications, medications, environmental factors, and therapies. Monitoring and analysis of the significance vital signs are important nursing responsibilities and are crucial to identifying changes in patient status (Dalton et al., 2018). Monitoring and evaluation of trends in intermittently measured vital signs is an important part of early identification of risk for a serious adverse event, contributing to timely intervention and improved patient outcomes (Brekke et al., 2019; Churpek et al., 2016).

Examples of appropriate times to measure vital signs include, but are not limited to, screenings at health fairs and clinics, in the home, upon admission to a health care setting, when medications are given that affect cardiac rate and rhythm, before and after invasive diagnostic and surgical procedures, and in emergency situations. Nurses obtain vital signs as often as a patient's condition requires such assessment, prioritizing, and adapting assessment of vital signs to address the patient's unique situation (Box 26-1). Frequency of assessment should be based on the patient's medical diagnosis, comorbidities, types of treatments and medications received, the patient's level of acuity and risk for complications, trends in the patient's vital signs, prescribed interventions, and facility policies (Burchill et al., 2015). Identification of a change in data related to assessment of vital signs is a crucial part of determining and recognizing deterioration in the status of a patient (Dalton et al., 2018). A patient's vital signs, along with oxygen saturation level (see Chapter 40), have been identified as the best indicators of cardiopulmonary arrest, unplanned intensive care unit (ICU) admission, and unexpected death (Malycha et al., 2019; Souza et al., 2019).

Box 26-1 When to Assess Vital Signs

- On admission to any health care facility or institution
- Based on facility or institutional policies and procedures
- Any time there is a change in the patient's condition
- Any time there is a loss of consciousness
- Before and after any surgical or invasive diagnostic procedure
- Before and after activity that may increase risk, such as ambulation after surgery
- Before administering medications that affect cardiovascular and respiratory function

In addition, institutional and facility policies provide guidance as to when and how frequently vital signs are assessed. For example, vital signs are assessed at 4-hour intervals, at a minimum, in hospitalized patients with elevated temperatures, with high or low blood pressures, with changes in pulse rate or rhythm, or with respiratory difficulty. In critical care settings, technologically advanced devices are used to continually monitor patients' vital signs. Regulations require monthly vital sign measurements in long-term care residents, but for residents classified as Medicare A (meaning they have been discharged from the hospital and now Medicare is paying for their stay to receive skilled nursing care) vital signs are taken daily. In the home and in some self-care and psychiatric units, assessments may be made only as frequently as the nurse judges necessary.

Although vital sign assessment may be delegated to other health care personnel when the condition of the patient is stable, it is the nurse's responsibility to ensure the accuracy of the data, interpret vital sign findings, and report abnormal findings. Principles of delegation should be followed. (Delegation is discussed in Chapters 10 and 18.) If a patient has abnormal or unusual physical signs or symptoms (e.g., chest pain or dizziness) or has unexpected changes in vital signs, the nurse should validate the findings and further assess the patient. See the accompanying Reflective Practice box for an example. The nurse should know the normal

QSEN Reflective Practice: Cultivating QSEN Competencies

CHALLENGE TO ETHICAL AND LEGAL SKILLS

At clinical 2 weeks ago, I had four patients for the first time, and I was very busy. One of my patients, Tomas Esposito, required transmission-based infection control precautions. So, every time I entered his room, I had to put on a gown and gloves. It was getting to be late in the morning and I still had not completed this patient's full assessment, including his vital signs. Upon entering the patient's room, I discovered that the separate stethoscope usually found in isolation rooms was not there. As a result, I had to remove my gown and gloves and go find the nurse to help me locate the stethoscope. Ultimately, the nurse had to get me a new isolation stethoscope set and put it together for me. Unfortunately, these stethoscopes are often poor in quality.

I went back to the patient's room and put on a new gown and gloves. By this time, Mr. Esposito was very irritable, and just wanted me to do the assessment quickly and leave him alone. I attempted to listen to measure his blood pressure, but I couldn't hear any sound after opening the valve on the blood pressure cuff. I played with the stethoscope for a few minutes and tried again, but I still couldn't hear anything. My patient kept telling me to leave him alone. Being a fourth-year nursing student and self-sufficient in doing the basic patient assessment, I felt stupid going to get the nurse or my instructor and telling her I couldn't obtain a blood pressure. I was really pressed for time and now was faced with a critical decision.

Thinking Outside the Box: Possible Courses of Action

- Remove my gown and gloves, get my instructor and the nurse and tell them that I was unable to hear any sounds to obtain a blood pressure measurement, and request their assistance.
- Leave the patient alone as he requested, saving precious time, pretending that I completed vital signs and his assessment, and charting the same findings as the previous shift's assessment.
- Explain to the nurse that the patient wasn't cooperating and ask her to do the blood pressure and assessment without my instructor knowing about it.
- Try to complete the vital signs and assessment using my own stethoscope and risk transmission of potentially infectious microorganisms to other patients on the unit.

Evaluating a Good Outcome: How Do I Define Success?

- Patient receives the highest quality of care.
- Professional integrity of all health care team members involved is maintained.
- All documented information is accurate.
- Professional, ethical, and legal principles are maintained.

Personal Learning: Here's to the Future!

Luckily, my conscience and my desire to always give the best care to my patients pushed me to the right decision. I took the time to remove my gown and gloves and went to find my instructor and the nurse. I told the nurse that I was having trouble hearing the patient's blood pressure. She was very understanding and came to the room with me and tried herself. Upon further investigation, we found that the problem was a broken stethoscope, not my incompetence to complete an assessment. After assessing the patient with a properly functioning stethoscope, I obtained his blood pressure, and also found expiratory wheezing and documented it. This finding provided a clue that I should probably keep a very close eye on this patient. Mr. Esposito ended up experiencing increasing difficulty breathing and his oxygen saturation levels began to drop. As a result, I realized just how important the initial assessment is when caring for a patient throughout the day. Hopefully, the lesson about how important it is to do the "right" thing for the patient will stick with me forever.

Catherine Barrell, Georgetown University

QSEN SELF-REFLECTION ON QUALITY AND SAFETY COMPETENCIES DEVELOPING KNOWLEDGE, SKILLS, AND ATTITUDES FOR CONTINUOUS IMPROVEMENT

How do you think you would respond in a similar situation? Why? Do you agree with the criteria that the nursing student used to evaluate a successful outcome? Why or why not? What *knowledge, skills, and attitudes* do you need to develop to continuously improve the quality and safety of care for patients like Mr. Esposito?

Patient-Centered Care: What information should be communicated to the patient about the care provided? How could you involve Mr. Esposito as a partner in coordinating his care to minimize frustration on the part of the patient and student? What might you have done to prevent the numerous trips in and out of the patient's room?

Teamwork and Collaboration/Quality Improvement: What communication skills do you need to improve to ensure that you function as a member of the patient-care team and to obtain assistance when needed? How should you follow up regarding the defective equipment?

Safety/Evidence-Based Practice: What might you have done to determine whether the stethoscope was functioning properly? How do you think your time management and organizational skills affect the situation? What evidence in nursing literature provides guidance for decision making regarding infection control?

Informatics: Can you identify the essential information that must be available in Mr. Esposito's electronic record to support safe patient care and coordination of care? Can you think of other ways to respond to or approach the situation?

Table 26-1 Age-Related Variations in Normal Vital Signs

AGE	TEMPERATURE °F °C	PULSE beats/min	RESPIRATIONS breaths/min	BLOOD PRESSURE mm Hg
Newborns	97.2–99.9 36.2–37.7	95–170	30–60	60–70/40
Infants	96–99.7 35.6–37.6	85–170	30–50	85/37
Toddler	96–99 35.6–37.2	70–150	20–40	88/42
Child	96–99 35.6–37.2	65–130	15–25	95/57
Adolescent	96.4–99.5 35.8–37.5	60–115	12–20	102/60
Adult	96.4–99.5 35.8–37.5	60–100	12–20	<120/80

Source: Adapted from Chiocca, E. M. (2019). *Advanced pediatric assessment* (3rd ed.). Springer Publishing Company; Hogan-Quigley, B., Palm, M. L., & Bickley, L. S. (2017). *Bates' nursing guide to physical examination and history taking* (2nd ed.). Wolters Kluwer; and Kyle, T., & Carman, S. (2021). *Essentials of pediatric nursing* (4th ed.). Wolters Kluwer.

variations in vital signs that occur at various ages as listed in Table 26-1 and understand potential variations related to specific health conditions and illnesses.

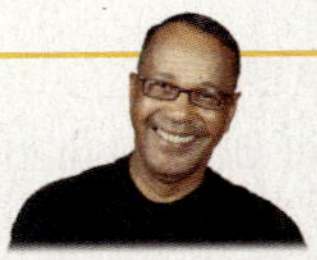

Recall **Tomas Esposito**, the patient requiring initial assessment described in the Reflective Practice display. The nurse's inability to auscultate heart and lung sounds would be an important finding that requires additional assessment. The nurse would need to evaluate these findings in conjunction with the patient's other vital signs and symptoms.

The skills of assessing each of the vital signs, with rationale for each action, and a discussion of normal and abnormal findings are presented in this chapter. See Chapter 27 for additional information about vital signs and health assessment.

TEMPERATURE

Body **temperature** is the difference between the amount of heat produced by the body and the amount of heat lost to the environment measured in degrees. Heat is generated by metabolic processes in the core tissues of the body, transferred to the skin surface by the circulating blood, and then dissipated to the environment. Core body temperature (intracranial, intrathoracic, and intraabdominal) is higher than surface body temperature. Normal body temperature, inclusive of the different routes that may be used for measurement, ranges from 96.7° to 100.5°F (35.9° to 38°C) (Jensen, 2019).

There are individual variations of these temperatures as well as variations related to age, biologic sex, physical activity, state of health, and environmental temperatures. Body temperature also varies during the day, with temperatures being lowest in the early morning and highest in the late afternoon (Boron & Boulpaep, 2016, as cited in Norris, 2019).

Physiology of Body Temperature

The core body temperature of a healthy person is maintained within a fairly constant range by the thermoregulatory set point of the thermoregulatory center in the hypothalamus. This center receives messages from cold and warm thermal receptors located throughout the body, compares that information with its temperature set point, and initiates responses to either produce or conserve body heat or to increase heat loss.

Heat Production

The primary source of heat in the body is metabolism, with heat produced as a by-product of metabolic activities that generate energy for cellular functions. Various mechanisms increase body metabolism, including hormones and exercise. When additional heat is required to maintain balance, epinephrine, and norepinephrine (sympathetic neurotransmitters) are released to rapidly alter metabolism so that energy production decreases and heat production increases. Thyroid hormone, produced by the thyroid gland, also increases metabolism and heat production, but over a much longer period. Shivering, a response that increases the production of heat, is initiated by the hypothalamus and results in muscle tremors, causing the production of heat. In addition, the contraction of pilomotor muscles of the skin, as occurs with shivering, causes piloerection, or "goose bumps," and reduces the surface area of skin available for heat loss. Physical exertion increases heat production through muscle movements.

Heat Loss

The skin is the primary site of heat loss. The circulating blood brings heat to the small connections between the arterioles and the venules, which lie directly below the skin's surface. These connections, called arteriovenous shunts, may remain

Table 26-2 Mechanisms of Heat Transfer

	RADIATION	CONVECTION	EVAPORATION	CONDUCTION
Definition	The diffusion or dissemination of heat by electromagnetic waves	The dissemination of heat by motion between areas of unequal density	The conversion of a liquid to a vapor	The transfer of heat to another object during direct contact
Example	The body gives off waves of heat from uncovered surfaces.	An oscillating fan blows currents of cool air across the surface of a warm body.	Body fluid in the form of perspiration and insensible loss is vaporized from the skin.	The body transfers heat to an ice pack, causing the ice to melt.

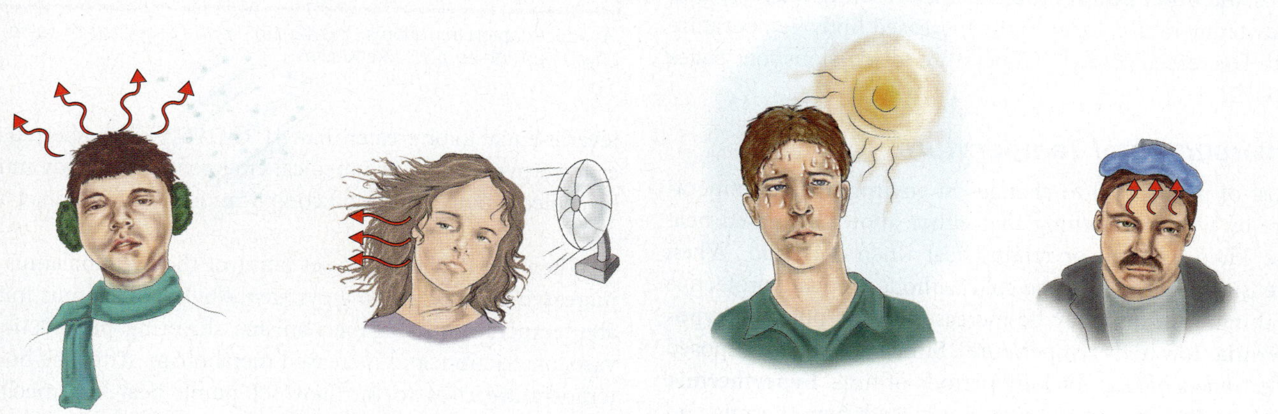

Radiation Convection Evaporation Conduction

open to allow heat to dissipate (e.g., during exercise in hot environmental temperatures) to the skin and then to the external environment, or they may close and retain heat in the body (e.g., when the body is exposed to cold environmental temperatures). The sympathetic nervous system controls the opening and closing of the shunts in response to changes in core body temperature and in environmental temperature (Norris, 2019). Heat is transferred to the external environment through the physical processes of radiation, convection, evaporation, and conduction. These processes are defined and illustrated in Table 26-2. Other heat losses occur through evaporation of sweat, through warming and humidifying of inspired air, and through elimination of urine and feces.

Factors Affecting Body Temperature

A variety of factors affect body temperature. These factors include time of day (circadian rhythms), age, biologic sex, physical activity, state of health, and environmental temperatures.

Circadian Rhythms

Many environmental and physiologic processes occur in repeated cycles of time. Some events in humans recur at 24-hour intervals, referred to as circadian (meaning nearly every 24 hours) rhythms. Predictable fluctuations in measurements of body temperature and blood pressure are examples of functions that have a circadian rhythm. For instance, body temperature can vary as much as 1.0°F (0.5°C) during the course of a day and is usually lower in the early morning than in the late afternoon and early evening (Jensen, 2019). This variation tends to be somewhat greater in infants and children. The peak elevation of a person's temperature occurs between 3 and 6 PM.

Age and Biologic Sex

Older adults lose some thermoregulatory control with aging; body temperatures in older adults may be lower than the average adult temperature (Touhy & Jett, 2018). Both the very old and the very young are more sensitive to changes in environmental temperature. Older adults are at risk for harm from extremes of temperature due to impaired thermoregulatory responses. The body temperature of infants and children changes more rapidly in response to both hot and cold air temperatures.

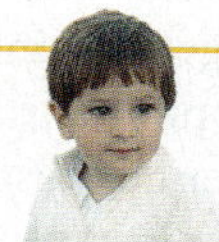

Consider **Noah Shoolin**, the 2-year-old brought to the emergency department by his mother. The nurse assessing the child's temperature would need to keep in mind the effect of environmental temperature changes on a child of this age. Efforts to prevent chilling and overheating would be incorporated into the child's care plan.

Women tend to experience more fluctuations in body temperature than do men, probably as the result of changes in hormones. The increase in progesterone secretion at ovulation increases body temperature as much as 0.5° to 1.0°F (0.3° to 0.5°C) (Jensen, 2019).

Physical Activity

Physical exertion increases body temperature. Increased metabolism resulting from muscle activity results in the production of heat. When evaluating temperature measurements, the nurse should consider whether the patient has participated in recent physical activity.

State of Health

Alterations in a person's health can contribute to variations in body temperature. The presence of certain disease conditions and other health problems may result in alterations in body temperature. Refer to the Increased Body Temperature and Decreased Body Temperature discussions on pages 720–721.

Environmental Temperature

Most of us respond to changes in environmental temperature by wearing clothing that either allows increased heat loss when it is hot or retains heat when it is cold. When one is exposed to extreme cold without adequate protective clothing, heat loss may be increased to the point of **hypothermia** (low body temperature). Similarly, if one is exposed to extremes of heat for long periods of time, **hyperthermia** (high body temperature) may result. Both hypothermia and hyperthermia may cause serious illness or death.

Normal Body Temperature

Body temperature varies among people, with a range of 0.3° to 0.6°C (0.5° to 1.0°F) from the average temperature considered to be within normal limits. However, wider variations from the average temperature may be normal for some people. A person with a normal body temperature is referred to as **afebrile** (without fever). Refer to Table 26-1 (on page 718) for the normal temperature ranges for various age groups.

Increased Body Temperature

Fever or **pyrexia** is an increase above normal in body temperature. A person with a fever is said to be **febrile**. Fever occurs in response to an upward displacement of the thermoregulatory set point in the hypothalamus, caused by pyrogens (substances that cause fever). Substances that can trigger this increase in temperature include bacteria, bacterial products, and whole microorganisms, such as viruses. Fever may also occur as a result of chemicals produced in the body in response to tissue injury, such as from myocardial infarction (MI), pulmonary emboli, cancer, trauma, and surgery. Although the purpose of fever is not fully understood, it signals increased immune function and inflammation, and is a valuable indicator of health status.

Most fevers, unless extremely high (above 40°C [104°F]), are not harmful (Norris, 2019). In fact, there are many beneficial effects of fever, including destruction of disease-causing microorganisms, increased susceptibility of disease-causing microorganisms to anti-infective agents, and enhanced response by the immune system (Norris). However, when fever is equal to or greater than 41°C (106°F), it is referred to as hyperpyrexia and is a medical emergency. The body must be cooled rapidly to prevent complications (Wasserman et al., 2021).

When the thermostatic set point of the hypothalamus is increased in response to a pyrogen, the hypothalamus initiates temperature-rising mechanisms: shivering, piloerection, vasoconstriction, and increased metabolism. After the body temperature rises to the new set point, heat-loss mechanisms (sweating, vasodilation, increased respirations) keep the body temperature from rising to dangerous levels. Most fevers are self-limiting, and the temperature returns to normal after the factors causing it are controlled. Box 26-2 lists terms used to describe types of fever.

Box 26-2 Terms and Definitions for Types of Fever

Intermittent: The body temperature returns to normal at least once every 24 hours.
Remittent: The body temperature does not return to normal and fluctuates a few degrees up or down.
Sustained or Continuous: The body temperature remains above normal with minimal variations.
Relapsing or Recurrent: The body temperature returns to normal for one or more days with one or more episodes of fever, each as long as several days.

Source: Adapted from Norris, T. L. (2019). *Porth's essentials of pathophysiology* (5th ed.). Wolters Kluwer.

The onset and significance of a fever from an illness differs according to age. The onset of a fever, which can be sudden or gradual, typically is more rapid in children than in adults. A mild elevation in temperature might indicate a serious infection in infants younger than 3 months of age who do not have well-developed temperature-control mechanisms. Older adults often have a lower baseline body temperature. Therefore, fever may be one of the later signs of illness with temperature elevations of only slightly above normal, even in a serious infection. It is important to assess baseline norm for body temperature when an older adult is well, in order to be able to identify unique manifestations of fever (Toughy & Jett, 2018).

Other types of increased body temperature are hyperthermia, neurogenic fever, and fever of unknown origin (FUO). Hyperthermia differs from fever in that the hypothalamic set point is not changed, but in situations of extreme heat exposure or excessive heat production (e.g., during strenuous exercise), the mechanisms that control body temperature are ineffective. Neurogenic fever is the result of damage to the hypothalamus from pathologies such as intracranial trauma, intracranial bleeding, or increased intracranial pressure. This type of fever does not respond to antipyretic medications (Norris, 2019). A fever of 38.3°C (101°F) or higher that lasts for 3 weeks or longer without an identified cause after a minimal diagnostic workup is identified as a FUO (Fusco et al., 2019; Mulders-Manders et al., 2015). Infections, such as tuberculosis or human immunodeficiency virus, malignancies, cirrhosis, and noninfectious inflammatory diseases are causes of FUO (Fusco et al., 2019; Norris, 2019).

Physical Effects of Fever

Patients with fever may experience loss of appetite; headache; hot, dry skin; flushed face; thirst; muscle aches; and fatigue. Respirations and pulse rate increase. Infants and children may experience febrile seizures as a result of a fever (Schellack, N., & Schellack, G., 2019). Older adults may experience periods of confusion and delirium related to an increased body temperature (Hinkle et al., 2022). Fever blisters may develop in some people as the fever activates the type I herpes simplex virus. Fluid, electrolyte, and acid–base imbalances are potentially dangerous complications of fever.

Treatment of Fever

Fever is an important part of a person's defense mechanisms against infection. Determining the cause of the fever and treating its underlying cause is an important part of patient care. Nursing care related to fever focuses on increasing patient comfort and preventing complications.

If the fever is the result of a bacterial or other type of microbial infection, the appropriate antibiotic or anti-infective may be prescribed. Antipyretic (fever-reducing) drugs, such as aspirin, ibuprofen, or acetaminophen, may be administered in certain circumstances, but routine antipyretic administration is usually avoided (Ludwig & McWhinnie, 2019). These drugs reset the elevated set point regulated by the hypothalamus. However, the National Reye's Syndrome Foundation, the U.S. Surgeon General, the U.S. Food and Drug Administration (FDA), the Centers for Disease Control and Prevention (CDC), the American Academy of Pediatrics (AAP), and the World Health Organization (WHO) recommend that aspirin and combination products containing aspirin not be taken by anyone younger than 19 years of age during fever-causing or flulike illnesses (American Academy of Pediatrics, 2021; National Reye's Syndrome Foundation, n.d.).

Modifications of the external environment may be implemented to increase heat transfer from the internal to the external environment, including the use of cool sponge baths, cool packs, and hypothermia (cooling) blankets. Guidelines for Nursing Care 26-1 (on page 722) outlines the procedure for using a hypothermia blanket. Oral fluids are increased to maintain cellular and intravascular status and prevent dehydration. Simple carbohydrates are included in the diet to prevent tissue breakdown from the hypermetabolic state.

QSEN PATIENT-CENTERED CARE

The health practices and beliefs of patients and/or family members/caregivers related to fever and other symptoms may be influenced by cultural beliefs and practices. Culturally and ethnically sensitive strategies must be considered when providing interventions and patient education related to fever.

Decreased Body Temperature

Hypothermia is a core body temperature below 35°C (95°F). Hypothermia occurs when the compensatory physiologic responses meant to produce and retain heat are overwhelmed by unprotected exposure to cold environments. This may be a result of accidental exposure or impaired perception of cold, which occurs particularly in older adults or the disabled. Chronic conditions—such as alcoholism, malnutrition, and hypothyroidism—increase the risk of hypothermia. Patients in the perioperative period and newborn infants are also at increased risk. Death may occur when body temperature falls below 35°C (95°F), but survival has been reported in isolated cases (such as in drowning in very cold water or burial in snow) when body temperatures have fallen in the range of severe hypothermia (26°C [78.8°F]) (Kuhnke et al., 2019). Survival is possible because rates of chemical reactions in the body are slowed, thereby decreasing the metabolic demands for oxygen.

Therapeutic hypothermia, the purposeful lowering of the core body temperature, has been used to improve outcomes after brain injury, during certain surgeries and after cardiac arrest (Morton & Fontaine, 2018; Norris, 2019). This decreased body temperature reduces metabolic rate and oxygen demand of the body to improve survival and neurologic outcomes (Alne, 2020).

Physical Effects of Hypothermia

Patients with hypothermia may experience poor coordination, slurred speech, poor judgment, amnesia, hallucinations, and stupor. Respirations decrease and the pulse becomes weak and irregular with lowering blood pressure.

Treatment of Hypothermia

Treatment of hypothermia includes rewarming the patient. Rewarming can be accomplished by covering with additional clothing and blankets, the use of heating blankets and pads, and radiant warmers. Warm fluids are administered either orally or through the intravenous route. Additional treatments include support of vital functions and the prevention and treatment of complications (Norris, 2019).

Assessing Temperature

To accurately assess body temperature, the nurse must know what equipment to use, which site to choose, and what method is appropriate. Although the measurement of temperature may be delegated to assistive personnel (AP), the nurse is responsible for assessing the findings, assessing the effect(s) of changes in body temperature, and implementing appropriate interventions. The nurse is also responsible for teaching the patient and caregiver(s) about methods of temperature measurement, normal values, and the need to communicate abnormal findings.

Equipment

Body temperature, measured in degrees, may be assessed with a variety of devices—electronic and digital thermometers, tympanic membrane thermometers, disposable single-use

Guidelines for Nursing Care 26-1

USING A HYPOTHERMIA BLANKET TO REGULATE BODY TEMPERATURE

A hypothermia blanket, or cooling pad, is a blanket-sized aquathermia pad that conducts a cooled solution, usually distilled water, through coils in a plastic blanket or pad. It operates much like an aquathermia pad (discussed in Chapter 33), except that the liquid is cooled instead of heated. Placing a patient on a hypothermia blanket or pad helps to lower body temperature. The nurse monitors the patient's body temperature and can reset the blanket setting accordingly. The blanket also can be preset to maintain a specific body temperature; the device continually monitors the patient's body temperature using a temperature probe (which is inserted rectally or in the esophagus or placed on the skin) and adjusts the temperature of the circulating liquid accordingly. When applying a hypothermia blanket, follow these steps:

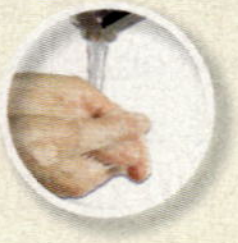

- Perform hand hygiene and put on PPE, if indicated.
- Review the prescribed intervention for the application of the hypothermia blanket. Obtain consent for the therapy per facility policy.
- Check that the water in the electronic unit is at the appropriate level. Check the temperature setting on the unit to ensure it is within the safe range.
- Apply lanolin or a mixture of lanolin and cold cream to the patient's skin where it will be in contact with the blanket.
- Turn on the blanket and make sure the cooling light is on. **Verify that the temperature limits are set within the desired safety range.**
- Place the hypothermia blanket on the bed and cover it with a sheet so that the patient's skin does not come in direct contact with the cold blanket. Position the blanket under the patient so that the top edge of the pad is aligned with the patient's neck.
- Put on gloves. Lubricate the rectal probe and insert it into the patient's rectum unless contraindicated. Or tuck the skin probe deep into the patient's axilla and tape it in place. For patients who are comatose or anesthetized, use an esophageal probe. Remove gloves and perform hand hygiene. Attach the probe to the control panel for the blanket.
- Wrap the patient's hands and feet in gauze if prescribed, or if the patient desires. For male patients, elevate the scrotum off the hypothermia blanket with towels.
- Recheck the thermometer and settings on the control panel.
- **Turn and position the patient regularly (every 30 minutes to 1 hour).** Keep linens free from condensation. Reapply cream, as needed. Observe the patient's skin for change in color, changes in lips and nail beds, edema, pain, and sensory impairment.
- **Monitor vital signs and perform a neurologic assessment, per facility policy, usually every 15 minutes, until the body temperature is stable.** In addition, monitor the patient's skin integrity, peripheral circulation, and fluid and electrolyte status, per facility policy.
- Observe for signs of shivering, including verbalized sensations, facial muscle twitching or twitching of extremities, or hyperventilation.
- Turn off the blanket according to facility policy, usually when the patient's body temperature reaches 1 degree above the desired temperature. **Continue to monitor the patient's temperature until it stabilizes.**

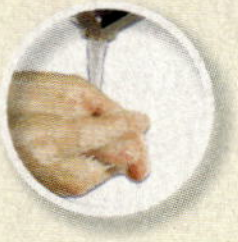

- Remove PPE, if used. Perform hand hygiene.

thermometers, temporal artery thermometers, noncontact infrared skin thermometers, and automated monitoring devices. Figure 26-1 illustrates several different types of thermometers. Each type of device has factors to consider when deciding the choice of appropriate thermometer when measuring a patient's temperature. The patient's health status may also influence the choice of device and measurement site, such as in situations requiring absolute accuracy in temperature measurement, including neonates or critically ill patients (Brosinski et al., 2018; Backer Mogensen et al., 2018; Fitzwater et al., 2019; Franconi, et al., 2018; Gates et al., 2018; Kiekkas et al., 2019). Refer to the discussions related to each type of thermometer (on pp. 723–724). No matter which type of thermometer is used, it is very important to follow the manufacturer's instructions to ensure an accurate measurement. Body temperature is documented in either Celsius or Fahrenheit degrees. Table 26-3 provides equivalent Celsius and Fahrenheit values as well as a method for conversion.

Glass thermometers with mercury-filled bulbs are not used in health care institutions to measure body temperature

Table 26-3 Equivalent Celsius and Fahrenheit Temperatures[a]

CELSIUS	FAHRENHEIT
35.0	95.0
36.0	96.8
36.5	97.6
37.0	98.6
37.5	99.5
38.0	100.4
38.5	101.3
39.0	102.2
40.0	104.0
41.0	105.8

[a]To convert Fahrenheit to Celsius, subtract 32 and multiply by 5/9. To convert Celsius to Fahrenheit, multiply by 9/5 and add 32.

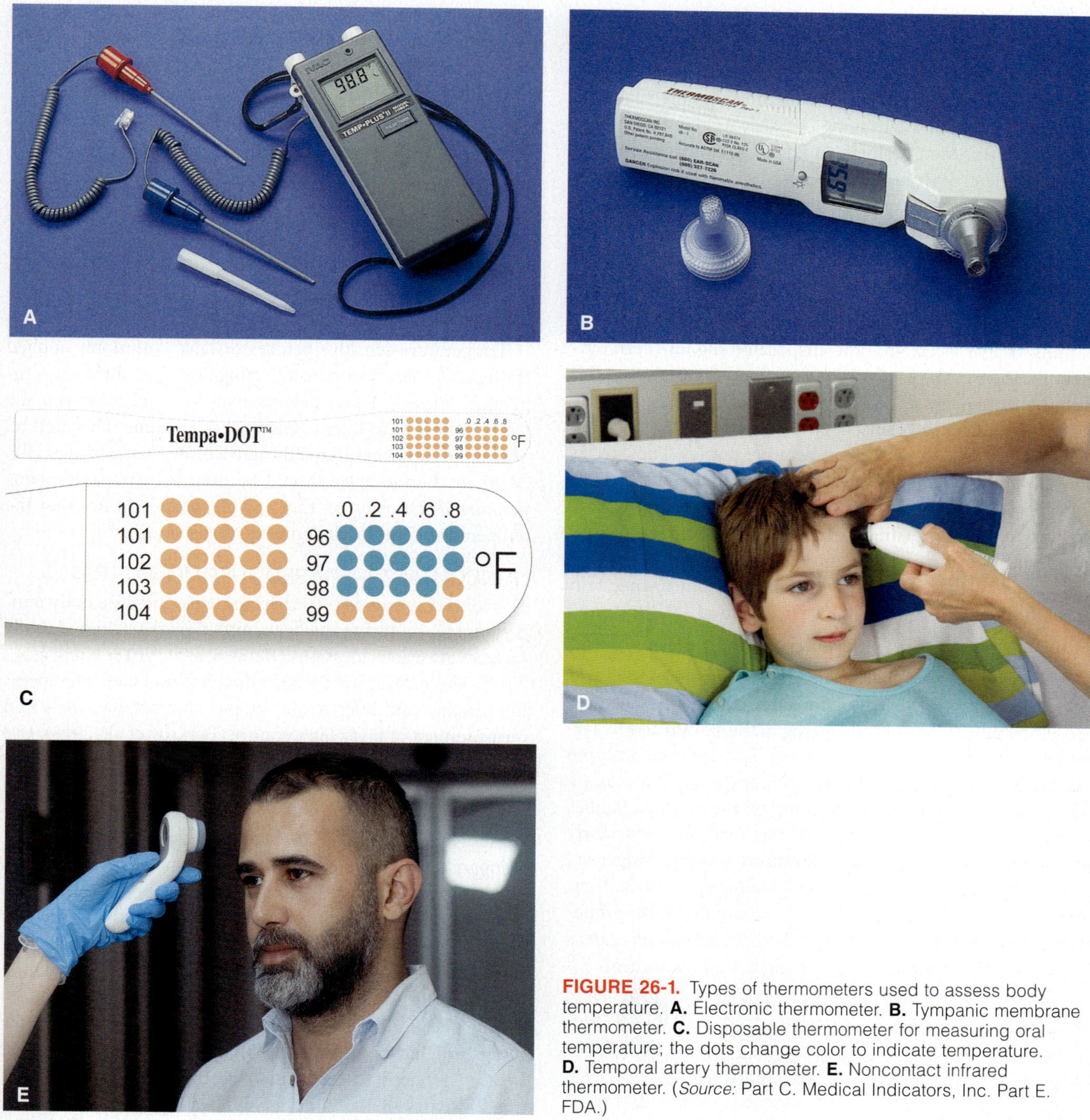

FIGURE 26-1. Types of thermometers used to assess body temperature. **A.** Electronic thermometer. **B.** Tympanic membrane thermometer. **C.** Disposable thermometer for measuring oral temperature; the dots change color to indicate temperature. **D.** Temporal artery thermometer. **E.** Noncontact infrared thermometer. (*Source:* Part C. Medical Indicators, Inc. Part E. FDA.)

due to federal safety recommendations (U.S. Environmental Protection Agency [EPA], n.d.). Some states and municipalities have laws or ordinances barring the sale and/or distribution of mercury fever thermometers (U.S. EPA). However, patients may still be using mercury thermometers at home. Nurses should encourage patients to use alternative devices, such as digital thermometers, to measure body temperature and include patient teaching as part of the plan of care. Bulb-type glass thermometers containing liquids other than mercury are available. This type of thermometer is prone to breakage and should never be used to take a temperature for a person who is unconscious or irrational, or for infants and young children.

Technology Alert

Neonates are at risk for hypothermia due to an immature temperature regulation mechanism. Hypothermia is one of the most important risk factors for morbidity and mortality in newborn infants (World Health Organization, n.d., as cited in Tanigasalam et al., 2019). The use of a novel hypothermia monitoring and alert bracelet device (BEMPU Bracelet) has been suggested as a screening tool to detect and alert for neonatal hypothermia. Use of the BEMPU can aid in identification of hypothermia and facilitate prompt management, preventing complications associated with hypothermia (Tanigasalme et al., 2019).

Equipment that is shared among patients is potentially contaminated and can contribute to the spread of disease-causing microorganisms (John et al., 2017). Nondisposable thermometers used to measure body temperature for more than one individual have been shown to be a possible source of transfer of microorganisms from equipment to room surfaces, other health care equipment, other health care providers, and patients (John et al., 2018). Effective strategies to reduce the risk for microbial transmission related to use of nondisposable thermometers are important considerations. Cleaning and disinfection of thermometers before and after use are critical interventions.

ELECTRONIC AND DIGITAL THERMOMETERS

Nondisposable electronic and disposable digital thermometers measure oral, rectal, or axillary body temperature over a period from a few seconds to 60 seconds, depending on the site and product used (Jensen, 2019). These battery-operated devices provide a numerical temperature display. The devices also have disposable probe covers to reduce the risk of transmission of microorganisms. Some models also provide memory recall of previous temperature measurements, a full 60-second pulse timer, and automatic conversion from the Fahrenheit to the Celsius scale. It is important to maintain calibration and charging of the device (Jensen, 2019).

TYMPANIC MEMBRANE THERMOMETERS

Tympanic membrane thermometers use infrared sensors to detect heat given off by the tympanic membrane, reflecting the temperature of the blood flowing in the carotid artery. The probe is covered with a probe cover and inserted into the ear canal tightly enough to seal the opening. The reading takes from 1 to 3 seconds, depending on the product. Studies conflict regarding the accuracy of this method, particularly in patients with temperature elevations (Backer Mogensen et al., 2018; Gates et al., 2018; Kurnat-Thoma et al., 2018; Ryan-Wenger et al., 2018). As such, it is important to use proper technique, maintain calibration, and adhere to manufacturer's guidelines for use and consider the method of assessment.

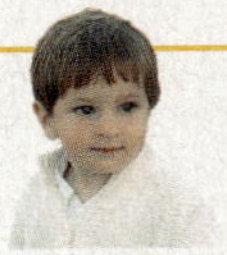

Remember **Noah Shoolin**, the toddler described at the beginning of the chapter? Although a tympanic thermometer yields a quick reading, the nurse would need to verify the accuracy of the reading, especially in light of the child's current upset state, possibly by asking the mother if she had taken the child's temperature before coming to the emergency department or by using an alternative method.

TEMPORAL ARTERY THERMOMETERS

Temporal artery thermometers measure body temperature by capturing the heat emitted by the skin over the temporal artery. These devices are battery operated and have a temperature display. Kurnat-Thoma et al. (2018) and Opersteny et al. (2017) found temporal artery measurements are an accurate method for noninvasive temperature assessment. However, operator technique and cleanliness of the thermometer lens can influence the reading (Furlong et al., 2015). Additional studies conflict regarding the accuracy of this method, particularly in patients with temperature elevations (Backer Mogensen et al., 2018; Brosinski et al., 2018; Fitzwater et al., 2019; Gates et al., 2018; Ryan-Wenger et al., 2018). As such, it is important to use proper technique and adhere to manufacturer's guidelines for use, and to consider the method of assessment (Brosinski et al., 2018; Fitzwater et al., 2019; Kiekkas et al., 2019).

DISPOSABLE SINGLE-USE THERMOMETERS

Disposable single-use thermometers are nonbreakable and register the temperature within seconds. Because they are used only once, they eliminate the danger of cross-infection and are sometimes used for patients requiring transmission-based precautions.

Temperature-sensitive patches or tape, commonly applied to the abdomen or forehead, change color at different temperature ranges. These devices may be used to screen the temperature of a toddler or young child at home. This method of temperature measurement is inaccurate (Robertson & Hill, 2019). A thermometer should be used to reassess the temperature if the color on the tape or patch indicates that the temperature is out of the normal average range.

NONCONTACT INFRARED THERMOMETERS

Noncontact infrared (IFR) thermometers measure body temperature by capturing the heat emitted by the skin over body surfaces at various locations (Berksoy et al., 2018; Wang et al., 2013). These devices are battery operated and have a temperature display, and offer a safe, simple, comfortable, and rapid measurement of body temperature (Berksoy et al., 2018). Use of a noncontact IFR thermometer does not require any body surface contact, no disposable probe covers are needed, and the risk of cross-infection is negligible (U.S. Food and Drug Administration [FDA], 2020a; Wang et al., 2013). However, comparisons of noncontact IFR thermometer measurements with tympanic, temporal artery and axillary body temperature measurement have resulted in inconsistent findings (Berksoy et al., 2018; Franconi et al., 2018). This method of temperature measurement has been suggested for use as screening for fever, not for ongoing monitoring of body temperature (Bayhan et al., 2014; Berksoy et al., 2018; Canadian Agency for Drugs and Technologies in Health, 2014). These devices must be used properly to get accurate readings and are not effective if used as the only means of detecting infection, such as screening to detect COVID-19 infections (U.S. FDA, 2020b). It is important to consider facility policy and procedures related to use; consider the method of assessment; and adhere to manufacturer's guidelines for use.

AUTOMATED MONITORING DEVICES

Automated monitoring devices are used in various health care settings to measure body temperature, pulse, respirations, and blood pressure simultaneously. These devices require less of the nurse's time, especially when these assessments need to be conducted frequently. Temperature sensors may be part of certain invasive devices used in critical care settings, such as pulmonary artery catheters, special rectal probes, and bladder catheters, allowing for continuous measurement of body temperature (Morton & Fontaine, 2018).

Technology Alert

Frequent monitoring of body temperature is an important aid in early detection of changes in the condition of critically ill patients (Schell-Chaple et al., 2018). Standard thermometry methods used in intensive care settings are invasive, may have barriers to use, may be contraindicated, or may not be available (Schell-Chaple et al.). The SpotOn system (3M Healthcare) uses a control unit, cable, and small disposable sensor applied to the lateral part of the patient's forehead to provide a continuous, noninvasive estimate core temperature and is an alternative to invasive temperature monitoring methods.

Sites and Methods of Assessing Body Temperature

The nurse is expected to choose an alternate, appropriate site, and the correct equipment for temperature measurement based on the patient's condition, facility policy, and prescribed interventions. Factors affecting site selection include the patient's age, state of consciousness, amount of pain, and other care or treatments (such as oxygen administration) being provided. Health facility policies and procedures may also provide guidance related to the site to be used for assessing patients' temperatures. If a temperature reading is obtained from a site other than the oral route, it is important to document the site of the measurement along with the result to ensure accurate comparison of data. If no site is listed with the documentation, it is generally assumed to be the oral route.

The sites most commonly used to assess body temperature are oral (sublingual), tympanic, temporal artery, rectal, and axillary. The probe is placed under the tongue (sublingual area) of a person's mouth to assess an oral temperature, in the anal canal to assess a rectal temperature, or in an axilla (armpit) to assess an axillary temperature. A probe is placed in the ear to assess a tympanic temperature. Temporal artery thermometers are swiped over the skin covering the temporal artery. For many clinical purposes, it is satisfactory to assess an oral, tympanic, temporal artery, axillary, or rectal temperature, provided proper technique is used, the site of the temperature is documented, and normal variations among the methods are considered. Comparing the recordings using two different sites is a method for double-checking the validity of an unusual measurement. The procedures for assessing body temperature at the oral, tympanic, temporal artery, axillary, and rectal sites, with rationale for each step, are outlined in Skill 26-1 (on pp. 747–754). The procedure for measuring temperature using a noncontact infrared thermometer is outlined in the Skill Variation included in Skill 26-1.

ASSESSING AN ORAL TEMPERATURE

When selecting the oral site, the patient must be able to close their mouth around the probe. Therefore, this site is not suitable for use with children younger than 6 years old, for some children with developmental delay, with patients who are unable to follow directions, with patients with changes in or inflammation of the oral mucosa, or for confused and comatose patients (Jensen, 2019; Mason et al., 2017; Opersteny et al., 2017). If a patient has had either hot or cold food or fluids or has been smoking or chewing gum, the general recommendation is to wait 15 to 30 minutes to allow the oral tissues to return to normal temperature. Mouth breathing can influence the results (Jensen, 2019). Oral temperatures should not be taken in people with diseases of the oral cavity, in those who have had surgery of the nose or mouth, or when there is a risk of seizures (Sund-Levander & Grodzinsky, 2013). In addition, oral temperatures should not be assessed in patients receiving oxygen by mask, because the time it takes to assess a reading is likely to result in a serious drop in the patient's blood oxygen level. Normal oral temperature readings range from 96.6° to 99.5°F (35.9° to 37.5°C) (Jensen, 2019; Weber & Kelley, 2018). The probe must remain in the sublingual pocket for the full period of measurement. Refer to Skill 26-1 (on pp. 747–754).

ASSESSING A TYMPANIC MEMBRANE TEMPERATURE

Infrared sensors in the thermometer sense heat from the body given off by the tympanic membrane. The thermometer does not touch the tympanic membrane. This site allows easy and safe measurement of temperature and is readily accessible. However, it should not be used for patients who have drainage from the ear, ear pain, ear infection, or scars on the tympanic membrane (Jensen, 2019). Temperature readings may be impacted by the presence of cerumen (earwax) (Oguz et al., 2018; Robertson & Hill, 2019). Normal tympanic temperature readings range from 98.2° to 100.9°F (36.8° to 38.3°C) (Jensen, 2019; Weber & Kelley, 2018). Refer to Skill 26-1 (on pp. 747–754).

Concept Mastery Alert

If a patient has drainage from the ear, ear pain, ear infection, or scarring on the tympanic membrane on one side, then the opposite ear may be used to measure the tympanic temperature.

ASSESSING A TEMPORAL ARTERY TEMPERATURE

Measurement on the right or left side of the forehead is equally effective. When taking a temporal artery temperature, assess for head coverings. Anything covering the area—such as a hat, hair, wigs, or bandages—would insulate the area, resulting in falsely high readings. If a patient is lying on the side, measure only the side of the head exposed to the environment. Do not measure temporal artery temperature over scar tissue, open lesions, or abrasions. Diaphoresis or sweat can impair the reading (Jensen, 2019). Move the thermometer across the forehead slowly and remain in contact with the skin to ensure accurate results. Temporal artery temperature readings are more accurate than axillary temperature measurement (Opersteny et al., 2017). Normal temporal artery temperature readings range from 98.7° to 100.5°F (36.3° to 38.1°C) (Jensen; Weber & Kelley, 2018). Refer to Skill 26-1 (on pp. 747–754).

ASSESSING AN AXILLARY TEMPERATURE

The axillary site may be used when both oral and rectal sites are contraindicated or when these sites are inaccessible but may provide readings that are less accurate than these sites (Jensen, 2019). As a result, axillary measurement should not be used where accurate temperature measurement is required. The axilla remains the most common place for temperature measurement in the neonate (Oguz et al., 2018). Axillary readings are affected by local blood flow, placement of the probe and closure of the axillary cavity, and the measurement time must be sufficient (Oguz et al., 2018; Sund-Levander & Grodzinsky, 2013). Place the probe in the center of the axilla; hold the patient's arm by the patient's side until the measurement is complete. Normal axillary temperature readings range from 95.6° to 98.5°F (35.4° to 36.9°C) (Jensen, 2019; Weber & Kelley, 2018). Refer to Skill 26-1 (on pp. 747–754).

ASSESSING A RECTAL TEMPERATURE

The rectal temperature is considered to be reflective of core body temperature and one of the most accurate routes (Jensen, 2019). The rectal route may be used when other routes are not practical or when an accurate measurement is required (Jensen, 2019). However, many patients are embarrassed at having their temperature taken rectally. The rectal site should not be used in newborns, children with diarrhea, and in patients who have undergone recent rectal, anal, vaginal, or prostate surgeries or have a disease of the rectum (Weber & Kelley, 2018). Because the insertion of the thermometer into the rectum can slow the heart rate by stimulating the vagus nerve, assessing a rectal temperature for patients with heart disease or after cardiac surgery may not be allowed in some institutions. In addition, assessing a rectal temperature is contraindicated in patients who are neutropenic (have low white blood cell counts, such as in leukemia) and in patients who have certain neurologic disorders (e.g., spinal cord injuries). Do not insert a rectal thermometer into a patient who has a low platelet count (thrombocytopenia). The rectum is very vascular, and a thermometer could cause rectal bleeding. Normal rectal temperature readings range from 97.4° to 100.5°F (36.3° to 38.1°C) (Jensen, 2019; Weber & Kelley, 2018). Refer to Skill 26-1 (on pp. 747–754).

ASSESSING TEMPERATURE WITH A NONCONTACT INFRARED THERMOMETER

Noncontact infrared (IFR) thermometers measure body temperature by capturing the heat emitted by the skin over body surfaces. This method of temperature measurement has been suggested for use as screening for fever, not for ongoing monitoring of body temperature (Bayhan et al., 2014; Berksoy et al., 2018; Canadian Agency for Drugs and Technologies in Health, 2014). Locations recommended for use for measurement include over the forehead (temporal artery), the neck (carotid artery), umbilicus, axilla, and nape of the neck (Berksoy et al., 2018; U.S. FDA, 2020a; Wang et al., 2013). Accuracy of measurement may be affected by the technique used during measurement, including positioning of the thermometer, as well as the presence of head covers and the environment (U.S. FDA, 2020a). Temperature measurement should be performed in a draft-free space, out of direct sun, and away from radiant heat sources (U.S. FDA, 2020a). The noncontact IFR thermometer should be placed in the testing environment or room for 10 to 30 minutes prior to use to allow the device to adjust to the environment (U.S. FDA, 2020a). Refer to the Skill Variation included in Skill 26-1 on page 747.

PULSE

The peripheral **pulse** is a throbbing sensation that can be palpated (felt) over a peripheral artery, such as the radial artery or the carotid artery. Peripheral pulses result from a wave of blood being pumped into the arterial circulation by the contraction of the left ventricle. As the heart contracts to eject blood into an already full aorta, smooth muscle in the arteries expands to compensate for the increase in pressure of the blood. This rhythmic distention of the arterial walls is the result of surges of blood as the heart beats. The distention of the arteries moves along the arterial system until it reaches the capillaries, where vessel walls lack elasticity and peripheral resistance to blood flow. The strength of the pulse reflects the amount of blood ejected with each beat of the heart (Jensen, 2019). The peripheral pulses may be felt wherever an artery passes over a solid structure, such as a bone or cartilage.

Characteristics of the peripheral pulse include rate, rhythm, strength (amplitude), and elasticity. These characteristics are indicators of the effectiveness of the heart as a pump, the volume of blood ejected with each heartbeat (stroke volume), and the adequacy of peripheral blood flow. The heart rate affects the amount of blood ejected by the heart with each beat and is determined by the frequency with which the ventricle contracts. The strength and rhythm affect how much blood is ejected and whether the beat is regular in rhythm. Further information about the control and mechanisms involved with blood flow and stroke volume is provided later in this chapter with the discussion of blood pressure and in Chapter 40.

An apical pulse may also be auscultated (listened to) over the apex of the heart as the heart beats. Heart sounds, which are produced by closure of the valves of the heart, are characterized as "lub-dub." The apical pulse is the result of closure of the mitral and tricuspid valves ("lub") and aortic and pulmonic valves ("dub"). The combination of the two sounds is counted as one beat.

Further information related to the characteristics of pulses is discussed later in this chapter.

Physiology of the Pulse

The pulse is regulated by the autonomic nervous system through the sinoatrial (SA) node (the pacemaker) of the heart. Parasympathetic stimulation of the SA node via the vagus nerve decreases the heart rate, and sympathetic stimulation of the SA node increases the heart rate and force of contraction. Additional information about the conduction system and function of the heart is discussed in Chapter 40. The pulse rate is the number of pulsations felt over a peripheral artery or heard over the apex of the heart in 1 minute. This rate normally corresponds to the same rate at which the heart is beating.

Table 26-4 Factors Affecting Pulse Rate

Age	Older adults may have a decreased pulse rate. Aging affects metabolic rate and can decrease the pulse rate.
Biologic sex	Women on average have slightly higher pulse rates than men.
Physical activity	Pulse rate increases with exercise to meet increased metabolic demands and ensure adequate oxygenation of tissues. Well-conditioned athletes may have a significantly decreased pulse rate. Regular cardiovascular exercise contributes to greater efficiency and strength of the heart muscle
Body Temperature	Elevated body temperature (fever/pyrexia) causes increased pulse rate due to increased metabolic demands and compensatory mechanisms to increase heat loss. With lowered body temperature (hypothermia), metabolism slows down with a corresponding decrease in pulse rate.
Stress	Increased levels of stress cause an increased pulse rate. Common sources of stress associated with increased pulse rate include pain, fear, and anxiety.
Medications	Many medications can cause alterations in pulse rate. Some medications increase a patient's pulse rate and others decrease a patient's pulse rate. Changes in pulse related to medication use can be an intended effect or an unintended adverse effect.
Presence of Disease and/or Health Conditions	Many acute and chronic health conditions affect a patient's pulse rate. Some diseases, such as chronic obstructive pulmonary disease and pneumonia, impair oxygenation and alter the pulse rate. Other health problems, such as sepsis, alter the pulse rate as a result of the body's response to infection. Peripheral vascular disease and heart failure affect the circulatory system and, as a result, affect the pulse.

Factors Affecting the Pulse

Many factors can affect both the heart rate and volume; however, compensatory mechanisms attempt to maintain a sufficient supply of blood to the cells at all times. For example, when the stroke volume decreases, such as when the blood volume is decreased because of hemorrhage, the heart rate increases to try to maintain the same cardiac output. Conversely, in a physically fit athlete whose heart pumps a maximum volume of blood per stroke, the heart rate may be at the low range or below the range of normal, yet the body cells remain adequately supplied. When assessing a patient's pulse, consider factors that could influence the pulse rate, including age, biologic sex, physical activity, fever, stress, medication use, and the presence of disease and/or health conditions. Table 26-4 identifies details related to each of these factors.

Normal Pulse Rate

The normal pulse rate for adolescents and adults ranges from 60 to 100 beats per minute (beats/min). The pulse rate increases and decreases in response to a variety of physiologic mechanisms. Pulse rate might also be altered by any of the factors discussed previously (Table 26-4). Normal pulse rates change across the life span, gradually diminishing from birth to adulthood (see Table 26-1 on page 718).

Increased Pulse Rate

As the heart rate increases, cardiac output usually also increases. However, **tachycardia**, a rapid heart rate, decreases cardiac filling time, which, in turn, decreases stroke volume and cardiac output, potentially leading to decreased tissue perfusion. An adult has tachycardia when the pulse rate is greater than 100 beats/min. Tachycardia is a normal response to exercise and emotion (Burns & Delgado, 2019). Tachycardia that persists at rest usually indicates some underlying problem (Burns & Delgado). Box 26-3 (on page 728) lists factors that may contribute to tachycardia.

Decreased Pulse Rate

Bradycardia is a pulse rate below 60 beats/min in an adult. A decrease in heart rate decreases cardiac output, potentially leading to a decrease in tissue perfusion. Bradycardia can be a normal finding in athletes and during sleep (Burns & Delgado, 2019). Bradycardia may not require treatment unless the patient is symptomatic (Burns & Delgado). Box 26-3 (on page 728) identifies factors that may contribute to bradycardia.

Pulse Strength (Amplitude)

The pulse strength (amplitude) refers to and describes the quality of the pulse in terms of its fullness; indicates the volume of blood flowing through the vessel; and reflects the strength of left ventricular contraction. Pulse strength is assessed by the feel of the blood flow through the vessel. The strength of each pulse beat is normally strong at all areas where an artery can be palpated (felt). There are several systems for grading the strength (amplitude) of arterial pulses. Nurses should be familiar with the system in use at their facility or institution. Table 26-5 (on page 728) presents one scale that is used to describe and document pulse strength (amplitude). In addition, the peripheral pulse may be described and documented as full and bounding when it is forceful or weak and thready when it is decreased in quality. Bounding pulses may occur with early stages of septic shock, exercise, fever, fluid volume excess, and anxiety (Jensen, 2019; Norris, 2019). Heart failure, hypovolemia, shock, hypernatremia (elevated plasma sodium level), and arrhythmias can cause decreased pulse strength (Jensen, 2019; Norris, 2019).

Box 26-3 Factors Contributing to Tachycardia and Bradycardia

Tachycardia	Bradycardia
• A decrease in blood pressure, such as occurs with blood loss, shock, trauma	• Coronary artery disease; myocardial infarction (MI; heart attack)
• An elevated body temperature	• Decreased body temperature
• Any condition resulting in poor oxygenation of blood, for example, chronic pulmonary disease or anemia	• Hypoxemia, obstructive sleep apnea
• Exercise	• Acute altered mental status, such as delirium
• Hyperthyroidism	• Hypothyroidism
• Pain	• Increased intracranial pressure and other central nervous system conditions, such as cerebral vascular accident ([CVA]; stroke)
• Strong emotions, such as fear, anger, anxiety, and surprise	• Response to vagal stimulation, such as ocular pressure or vomiting
• Some medications (e.g., atropine, epinephrine)	• Some medications (e.g., digitalis, antiarrhythmics)

Source: Adapted from Burns, S. M., & Delgado, S. A. (2019). *AACN essentials of critical care nursing* (4th ed.). McGraw-Hill Education; Norris, T. L. (2019). *Porth's essentials of pathophysiology* (5th ed.). Wolters Kluwer; Hinkle, J. L., Cheever, K. H., & Overbaugh, K. J. (2022). *Brunner & Suddarths's Textbook of medical-surgical nursing* (15th ed.). Wolters Kluwer; and Jensen, S. (2019). *Nursing health assessment. A best practice approach* (3rd ed.). Wolters Kluwer.

Pulse Rhythm

Pulse rhythm is the pattern of the beats and the intervals between them. Pulse rhythm is normally regular; the pulsations and the pauses between occur at evenly spaced intervals. An irregular pulse rhythm occurs when the beats and pauses between beats occur at unequal, varied intervals. An irregular pattern of heartbeats is called a **dysrhythmia**. Minor variations in regularity of the pulse may occur with respirations, with the rate increasing during inhalation and slowing during exhalation. This irregularity in rhythm occurs most commonly in children and young adults (Hinckle & Cheever, 2018; Jensen, 2019).

Pulse Elasticity

The normal artery feels smooth, straight, and resilient (springy); this finding is referred to as the elasticity of the artery or blood vessel (Jensen, 2019; Weber & Kelley, 2018). Arterial blood vessels become less elastic with increased age, resulting in a more rigid, less-resilient, and crooked arterial blood vessel (Eliopoulos, 2018; Jensen, 2019; Weber & Kelley, 2018).

Table 26-5 Pulse Strength (Amplitude)

GRADE	DESCRIPTION
0	Absent, unable to palpate
+1	Diminished, weaker than expected
+2	Normal; brisk, expected
+3	Bounding

Source: Adapted from Gerhard-Herman, M. D., Gornik, H. L., Barrett, C., Barshes, N. R., Corriere, M. A., Drachman, D. E., Fleisher, L. A., Gowkes, F. G. R., Hamburg, N. M., Kinlay, S., Lookstein, R., Misra, S., Mureebe, L., Olin, J. W., Patel, R. A. G., Regensteiner, J. G., Schanzer, A., Shishehbor, M. H., Stewart, K. J., … Wijeysundera, D. N. (2017). 2016 AHA/ACC Guideline on the management of patients with lower extremity peripheral artery disease: Executive Summary. *Vascular Medicine*, *22*(3), NPI–NP43. https://doi.org/10.1177/1358863X17701592.

Assessing the Pulse

The pulse may be assessed by palpating peripheral arteries, by auscultating the apical pulse with a stethoscope, or by using a portable Doppler ultrasound. It is important to know how to use a stethoscope and which site and method are appropriate for an individual patient at any particular moment.

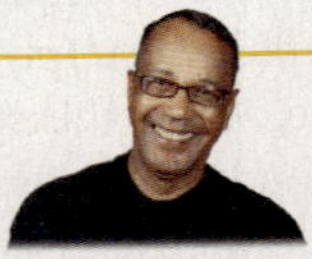

Remember **Tomas Esposito**, the middle-aged man requiring transmission-based infection-control measures and assessment? Although the nurse had difficulty auscultating his heart and lung sounds, the nurse would need to assess both his radial and apical pulse. It is possible that by palpating his radial pulse and then attempting to auscultate his apical pulse and not hearing anything, the nurse might have a clue leading her to suspect that the stethoscope was not functioning properly.

Equipment

Nurses most often use their fingers to assess the pulse by palpation, feeling the artery. However, various types of equipment may be used to assess a pulse. For example, the stethoscope is typically used to auscultate (listen to) the apical pulse. Doppler ultrasound may be used to assess pulses that are difficult to palpate. Electrocardiography is a graphic or digital recording of the electrical activity of the heart and may be used to assess the pulse rate and rhythm. Cardiac monitoring provides continuous observation of the patient's heart rate and rhythm. Additional basic information related to electrocardiography is discussed in Chapter 40 (p. 1599). Details of assessment with electrocardiography and cardiac monitoring are beyond the scope of this discussion. Refer to a medical-surgical or health assessment textbook for additional information regarding these interventions.

STETHOSCOPE

The stethoscope conducts sound from the patient's body to the listener and is used to auscultate (listen to) sounds not

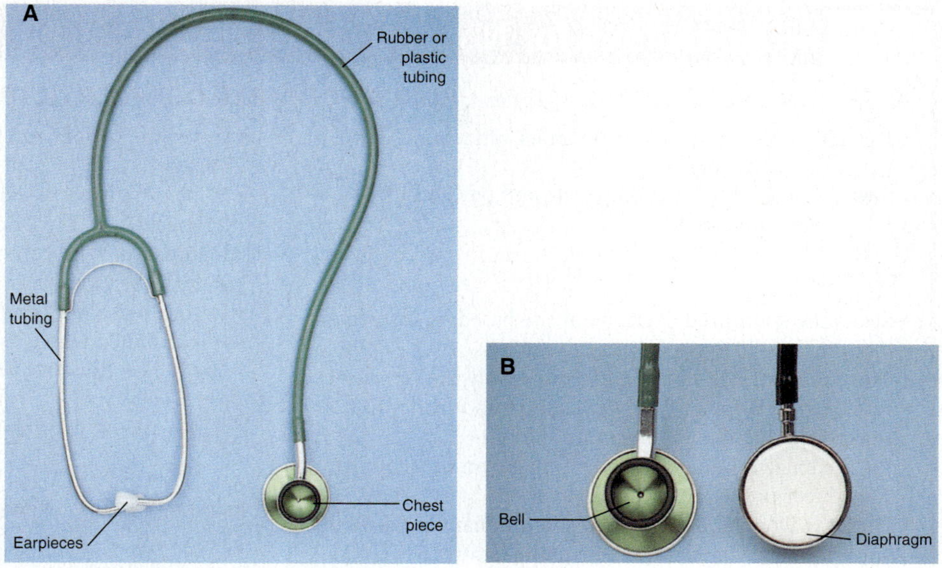

FIGURE 26-2. A stethoscope. **A.** Parts of a stethoscope. **B.** Parts of the chest piece; the bell and diaphragm. (*Source:* Used with permission from Weber, J. R., & Kelley, J. H. [2018]. *Health assessment in nursing* [6th ed.]. Wolters Kluwer, p. 43.)

audible to the unaided ear (Jensen 2019; Weber & Kelley, 2018). Environmental noise is also blocked to help more clearly discern the sounds (Jensen). The acoustical stethoscope, the most common type used, has an amplifying mechanism connected to earpieces by tubing. The stethoscope has a chest piece, which includes the *diaphragm* and *bell*, flexible tubing, earpieces, and ear tips. The diaphragm is a large, flat disk, and the bell has a hollowed, upright, curved appearance (Fig. 26-2). The diaphragm is more useful for hearing high-frequency sounds, such as respiratory sounds, because it screens out low-frequency sounds. The bell screens out high-frequency sounds and is more useful for hearing low-frequency sounds, such as those commonly made by the heart and the blood within the vessels.

The earpieces of the stethoscope should be selected to fit one's ear canals comfortably and snugly for the most effective auscultation. The ear pieces should be directed into the ear canal, toward the tympanic membrane, not against the ear itself. The ear tips should be large enough to fit snugly, but comfortably, to block out extraneous noises in the environment when the stethoscope is being used.

DOPPLER ULTRASOUND

A Doppler ultrasound device may be used to assess pulses that are difficult to palpate or auscultate. The device has an audio unit with an ultrasound transducer. Techniques for assessing pulses with a Doppler ultrasound device are outlined in Guidelines for Nursing Care 26-2 on page 730.

Sites and Methods of Assessing the Pulse

Nurses must know the correct site and method for assessing the pulse for individual patients. Although peripheral pulses are most frequently assessed as part of measurement of vital signs, an apical pulse or an apical–radial pulse should be assessed in certain situations, as described later.

ASSESSING PERIPHERAL ARTERIAL PULSES

Many peripheral artery sites might be used to assess the pulse by palpation. Figure 26-3 (on page 730) illustrates the most commonly used sites. Of these sites, the radial pulse site is assessed most often in children and adults. However, the radial pulse is difficult to palpate accurately in children younger than 2 years of age; the apical pulse should be auscultated for 1 minute for these patients (Jarvis & Eckhardt, 2020; Kyle & Carmen, 2021). Skill 26-2 (on pp. 755–757) describes the steps for assessing a peripheral pulse via palpation.

Circulation to the legs and feet may be assessed at the femoral, popliteal, posterior tibial, or dorsalis pedis sites. The carotid pulse site is used during emergency assessments, such as for patients who are in shock or have had a cardiac arrest. When taking a carotid pulse, lightly palpate only one side at a time to prevent any decrease in cerebrovascular circulation. The brachial pulse site is used most often for infants in these emergency situations.

ASSESSING THE APICAL PULSE

The apical pulse is obtained by listening with a stethoscope at the fifth intercostal space, left midclavicular line on the chest, and provides for assessment of a pulse rate and rhythm. In adults, the apical pulse is counted for 1 full minute. (Refer to the Guidelines for Nursing Care 26-3 on page 731.) Alternately, Jensen (2019) suggests it may be easier to assess the apical pulse on some patients at the second or third intercostal space, left sternal border (Erb's point). At this position on the chest, the heart is closer to the chest wall, so heart sounds may more easily be heard, and avoids exposing the breast in women (Jensen, 2019). The apical rate of an infant can also be easily palpated with the fingertips in addition to auscultation.

An apical pulse rate and rhythm should be assessed when a peripheral pulse is difficult to assess accurately because it is irregular, weak, or very rapid. An apical pulse is also assessed when giving medications that alter heart rate and rhythm. Apical pulse measurement is the preferred method of pulse assessment for children less than 2 years of age (Jarvis & Eckhardt, 2020; Kyle & Carmen, 2021).

Guidelines for Nursing Care 26-2

ASSESSING PERIPHERAL PULSE USING A PORTABLE DOPPLER ULTRASOUND DEVICE

- Determine the need to use a Doppler ultrasound device for pulse assessment.

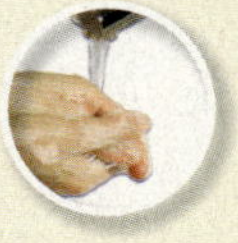

- Perform hand hygiene and put on PPE, if indicated.
- Select the appropriate peripheral site based on assessment data.
- Move the patient's clothing to expose only the site chosen.
- Remove the Doppler from the charger and turn it on. Make sure that the volume is set at low.
- Place a small amount of conducting gel on the Doppler transducer probe. Turn the Doppler on.
- Hold the Doppler base in your nondominant hand. With your dominant hand, touch the probe lightly to the skin with the probe tip in the gel. Adjust the volume, as needed. Hold the probe perpendicular to the skin. Slowly move the Doppler tip around until the pulse is heard (see figure).
- **Using a watch with a second hand, count the heartbeat for 1 minute. Note the rhythm of the pulse.**
- Remove the Doppler tip and turn the Doppler off. Wipe excess gel off the patient's skin with a tissue.
- Place a small × over the spot where the pulse is located with an indelible pen, depending on facility policy. Marking the site allows for easier future assessment. It can also make palpating the pulse easier since the exact location of the pulse is known.
- Cover the patient and help the patient to a position of comfort.
- Wipe off any gel remaining on the Doppler probe with a tissue. Clean the Doppler probe per facility policy or manufacturer's recommendations.
- Return the Doppler to the charge base.
- Record pulse rate, rhythm, and site, and the fact that it was obtained with a Doppler ultrasound device.

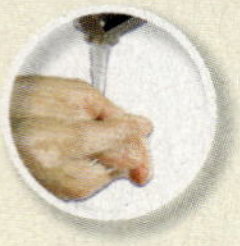

- Remove PPE, if used. Perform hand hygiene.

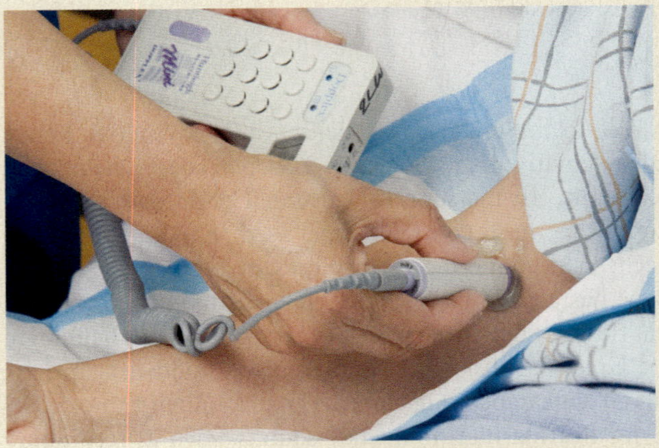

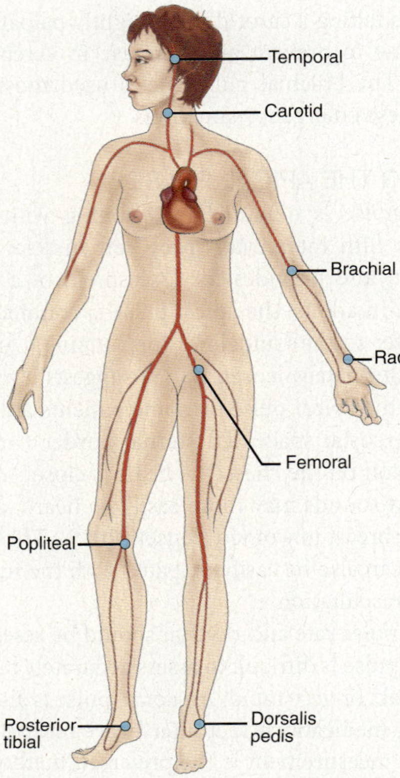

FIGURE 26-3. These arteries are located near the surface of the body. The pulse can be detected in any of these sites by light palpation.

ASSESSING THE APICAL–RADIAL PULSE

Counting of the pulse at the apex of the heart and at the radial artery simultaneously is used to assess the apical–radial pulse rate. Comparison of these two pulse rates provides an indirect evaluation of the ability of each heart contraction to eject enough blood into the peripheral circulation to create a pulse (Jensen, 2019). A difference between the apical and radial pulse rates is called the **pulse deficit** and indicates that all of the heartbeats are not reaching the peripheral arteries or are too weak to be palpated. This deficit suggests in insufficient cardiac force or volume, leading to decreased tissue perfusion. Guidelines for Nursing Care 26-4 outlines the technique for taking an apical–radial pulse.

RESPIRATIONS

Respiration involves ventilation, diffusion, and perfusion. Ventilation (or breathing) is movement of gases in and out of the lungs; inspiration (or inhalation) is the act of breathing in, and expiration (or exhalation) is the act of breathing out. Unlike heart rate, which is controlled by the autonomic nervous system, ventilation (breathing) has both autonomic and voluntary control. Diffusion is the exchange of oxygen and carbon dioxide between the alveoli of the lungs and the circulating blood. Perfusion is the exchange of oxygen and carbon dioxide between the circulating blood and tissue cells.

Guidelines for Nursing Care 26-3

ASSESSING THE APICAL PULSE

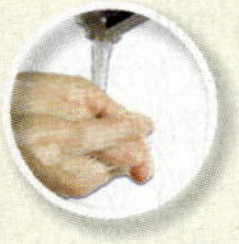

- Perform hand hygiene and put on PPE, if indicated.
- Use an alcohol swab to clean the diaphragm of the stethoscope. Use another swab to clean the earpieces, if necessary.
- Assist the patient to a sitting or reclining position and expose the chest area; move the patient's clothing to expose only the apical site.
- Hold the stethoscope diaphragm against the palm of your hand for a few seconds (to warm it).
- **Palpate the space between the fifth and sixth ribs (fifth intercostal space), and move to the left midclavicular line.** Place the diaphragm over the apex of the heart (see figure). Alternatively, auscultate an apical pulse in the second or third intercostal space left sternal border (Erb point) (Jensen, 2019).
- Listen for heart sounds ("lub-dub"). Each "lub-dub" counts as one beat.
- Using a watch with a second hand, count the heartbeat for 1 minute.
- Note the rhythm of the beats.
- Clean the diaphragm of the stethoscope with an alcohol swab.

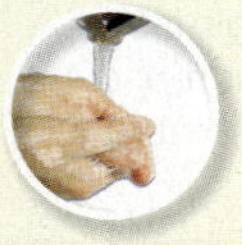

- Remove PPE, if used. Perform hand hygiene.

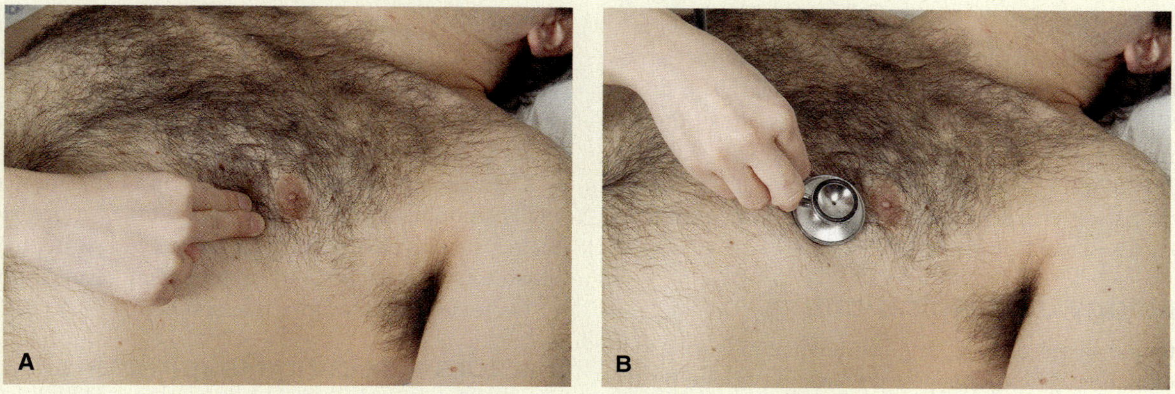

The apical pulse is usually found at (**A**) the fifth intercostal space just inside the midclavicular line and can be heard (**B**) over the apex of the heart.

Although nurses assess the manifestations of changes in all of these respiratory events, the component that is measured as a vital sign is ventilation, more commonly called **respirations**. Respiratory system assessment is described further in Chapter 27. Measuring respirations allows for baseline assessment of respiratory function, as well as providing insight into the status of the patient's homeostatic control (the body's internal environment) and presence of physiologic conditions, such as hypoxia (Rolfe, 2019). Respiratory rate abnormalities are important predictors of deteriorating

Guidelines for Nursing Care 26-4

TAKING AN APICAL–RADIAL PULSE

The following techniques are recommended to assess an apical–radial pulse rate:

- Two nurses are needed; one listens with a stethoscope over the apex of the heart for the heartbeat, and the other counts the rate at the radial artery.

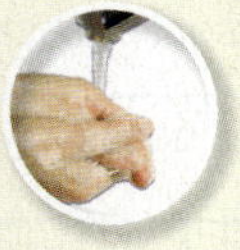

- Perform hand hygiene and put on PPE, if indicated.
- Expose the patient's chest wall so that the stethoscope can be placed directly on the skin of the chest wall.
- One watch with a sweep second hand is placed, so that both nurses can read it simultaneously.
- The nurses determine where they can best hear and feel the pulse and decide on a time to start counting, such as when the second hand on the watch is at a specified place (e.g., the number 12).
- Both nurses count for 1 full minute and record their counts. The difference between the apical and radial pulse rates is the pulse deficit.

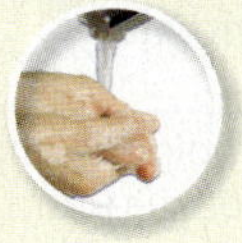

- Remove PPE, if used. Perform hand hygiene.

Box 26-4 Factors Affecting Respiratory Rate, Depth, and Movements

- **Age:** The respiratory rate decreases with age, ranging from a normal range of 30 to 60 breaths/min in a newborn to 12 to 20 breaths/min in an adult.
- **Exercise:** Exercise increases respiratory rate and depth.
- **Acid–base balance:** Alterations in acid–base balance (especially acidosis) commonly result in increased rate and depth of respirations (hyperventilation).
- **Brain lesions:** Lesions of the brain (such as hemorrhage or tumors) or brainstem can cause a change in both the depth and rate of respirations, most commonly manifested as Cheyne–Stokes respirations.
- **Increased altitude:** As an adaptation to higher altitudes, healthy people may exhibit Cheyne–Stokes respirations, especially when asleep. Higher altitudes also increase respiratory rate and depth prior to adaptation by increasing hemoglobin levels.
- **Respiratory diseases:** Any alterations in the normal respiratory structures may result in changes in respiratory rate, depth, and patterns, most often manifested as difficult breathing, using accessory muscles of respiration (such as the intercostal muscles), and increased rate. The depth may be shallower. Smoking can alter the pulmonary airways, resulting in an increase in respiratory rate at rest.
- **Anemia:** Anemia, a decrease in oxygen-carrying hemoglobin, may result in an increased rate of respirations.
- **Anxiety:** Anxiety can cause sighing type respirations (increased depth) and increased rate.
- **Medications:** Medications—such as narcotics, sedatives, and general anesthetics—slow respiratory rate and depth. Other drugs, including amphetamines and cocaine, may increase rate and depth.
- **Acute pain:** Acute pain increases respiratory rate but may decrease respiratory depth.

patient conditions and serious events, including cardiac arrest and intensive care admission (Malycha et al., 2019; Souza et al., 2019). Respiratory rate measurement is one of the few vital signs that is not easily measured by a monitor (Elliott & Baird, 2019). Accurate assessment and interpretation of respirations as part of vital sign measurement are important parts of clinical assessment (Rolfe, 2019).

Physiology of Respirations

The rate and depth of breathing can change in response to tissue demands. These changes are brought about by the inhibition or stimulation of the respiratory muscles by the respiratory centers in the brain. Activation of the respiratory centers occurs via impulses from chemoreceptors located in the aortic arch and carotid arteries, via stretch and irritant receptors in the lungs, and via receptors in muscles and joints. An increase in carbon dioxide is the most powerful respiratory stimulant, causing an increase in respiratory depth and rate. The cerebral cortex of the brain allows voluntary control of breathing, such as when singing or playing a musical instrument. See Chapter 40 for a further discussion of respiratory physiology.

The rate and depth of inhalation and exhalation are normally smooth, easy, and without conscious effort. However, factors such as environmental changes and pathophysiologic alterations in various body systems may result in increases or decreases in respiratory rate and depth.

Factors Affecting Respirations

Many different factors affect respiratory rate and depth. These factors include exercise; respiratory and cardiovascular disease; alterations in fluid, electrolyte, and acid–base balances; medications; trauma; infection; pain; and emotions. Box 26-4 outlines the factors that affect respiratory rate, depth, and movements. Table 26-6 describes and illustrates various respiratory patterns.

Table 26-6 Patterns of Respirations

	DESCRIPTION	PATTERN	ASSOCIATED FEATURES
Normal	12–20 breaths/min Regular	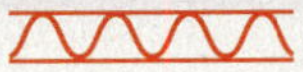	Normal pattern
Tachypnea	>24 breaths/min Shallow	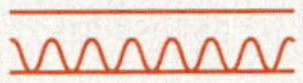	Fever, anxiety, exercise, respiratory disorders
Bradypnea	<10 breaths/min Regular	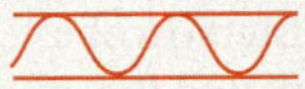	Depression of the respiratory center by medications, brain damage
Hyperventilation	Increased rate and depth	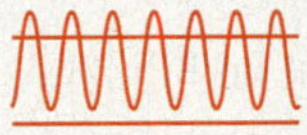	Extreme exercise, fear, diabetic ketoacidosis (Kussmaul's respirations)
Hypoventilation	Decreased rate and depth; irregular	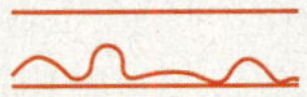	Overdose of narcotics or anesthetics
Cheyne–Stokes respirations	Alternating periods of deep, rapid breathing followed by periods of apnea; regular	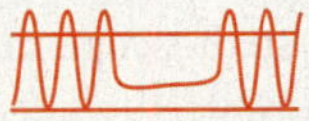	Drug overdose, heart failure, increased intracranial pressure, renal failure
Biot's respirations	Varying depth and rate of breathing, followed by periods of apnea; irregular	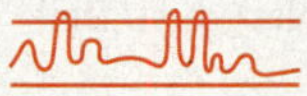	Meningitis, severe brain damage

Normal Respiratory Rate

Under normal conditions, healthy adults breathe about 12 to 20 times each minute; infants and young children breathe more rapidly (see Table 26-1 on page 718) (Hess et al., 2021). Normal, unlabored respiration is called **eupnea**. The relationship of one respiration to four heartbeats is fairly consistent in healthy people.

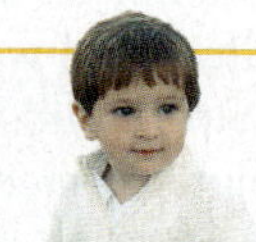

Think back to **Noah Shoolin**, the 2-year-old brought to the emergency department. The nurse would anticipate that the child's respiratory rate would be increased most likely as a result of his screaming and emotional upset.

Increased Respiratory Rate

Tachypnea, an increased respiratory rate of more than 24 breaths per minute (breaths/min), may occur in response to an increased metabolic rate, such as when a person has a fever. Cells require more oxygen at this time and produce more carbon dioxide that must be removed. Tachypnea may be present in patients who have hypoxia (decreased oxygen to body tissues) and who have pain in the thoracic area. An increase in both the rate and depth of respirations is **hyperventilation**. Hyperventilation may result from hypoxia, anxiety, exercise, or metabolic acidosis (Jensen, 2019). Respiratory diseases such as acute pneumonia may cause tachypnea or hyperventilation.

Decreased Respiratory Rate

Bradypnea, a decrease in respiratory rate, less than 10 breaths/min. Bradypnea may result from increased intracranial pressure, neurologic disease, or sedation (Jensen, 2019). Certain drugs, such as opioids (e.g., morphine, hydromorphone), can depress the respiratory rate, as well as respiratory depth. **Hypoventilation** refers to shallow, slow respiration and may be related to increased intracranial pressure or sedation (Jensen).

Respiratory Depth and Rhythm

The depth of respirations normally varies from shallow to deep. The depth of each respiration is about the same when resting or sleeping. Periodically, each person automatically inhales deeply (sighs), filling the lungs with more air than with the usual depth of respiration.

Respiratory rhythm is the pattern of the breaths and the intervals between them. Respiratory rhythm is normally regular; the breaths and the pauses between occur at evenly spaced intervals. An irregular respiratory rhythm occurs when the breaths and pauses between beats occur at unequal, varied intervals.

Abnormal breathing patterns with alterations in depth, rate, and rhythm include Cheyne–Stokes respirations, associated with cerebral vascular disease and severe traumatic brain injuries, and Biot's respirations, associated with severe brain stem injury and meningitis (Hess et al., 2021). Table 26-6 describes and illustrates these two abnormal breathing patterns.

There are additional terms used to describe the nature of respirations. **Apnea** refers to periods during which there is no breathing. Apnea can be caused by an obstructive defect or be mediated by the central nervous system (Hess et al., 2021). Without intervention, death will occur within a few minutes of onset of apnea (Hess et al.). **Dyspnea** is difficult or labored breathing (shortness of breath). Dyspnea may be the result of heavy exercise or exertion or from a health condition. Dyspnea can be perceived only be the person experiencing it and is characterized by an increased effort to breathe (Hess et al., 2021). A situation in which a patient can breathe more easily and most comfortably in an upright position, but experiences shortness of breath when lying flat, is known as **orthopnea**. While a person is sitting or standing, gravity lowers organs in the abdominal cavity away from the diaphragm. This gives the lungs more room for expansion within the chest, allowing the intake of more air with each breath. Orthopnea may be associated with pulmonary edema, heart disease, and various chronic respiratory diseases, such as chronic obstructive pulmonary disease (COPD) (Hess et al., 2021; Hinkle & Cheever, 2018).

Assessing Respirations

The nurse assesses respiratory rate (breaths per minute), depth (deep or shallow), and rhythm (regular or irregular) by inspection (observing and listening) or by listening with the stethoscope. Other methods of assessing respiratory effectiveness include using a pulse oximeter to determine oxygenation of blood and monitoring arterial blood gas results. A description of a pulse oximeter and a procedure for using it are found in Chapter 40. Arterial blood gas monitoring is discussed in Chapter 41. Skill 26-3 (on pp. 757–759) describes how to assess the respiratory rate. Further assessments of respirations are described in Chapters 27 and 40.

BLOOD PRESSURE

Blood pressure refers to the force of the moving blood against arterial walls. Maximum blood pressure is exerted on the walls of arteries when the left ventricle of the heart contracts and pushes blood through the aortic valve into the aorta at the beginning of systole. The pressure rises as the ventricle contracts (systole) and falls as the heart relaxes (diastole). This continuous contraction and relaxation of the left ventricle creates a pressure wave that is transmitted through the arterial system (Norris, 2019). The highest pressure, created during ventricular contraction, is the **systolic pressure**. When the heart rests between beats during ventricular diastole, the pressure drops. The lowest pressure present on arterial walls at this time is the **diastolic pressure**. The difference between the systolic and diastolic pressures is called the **pulse pressure**. Additional information about the function of the heart is discussed in Chapter 40.

Stroke volume and heart rate determine cardiac output (discussed in Chapter 40). Cardiac output and peripheral resistance determine both systolic and diastolic pressures. Peripheral resistance reflects the viscosity (thickness of the blood) and the changes in the radius of the arterioles.

Blood pressure is measured in millimeters of mercury (mm Hg) and is recorded as a fraction. The numerator is the systolic pressure; the denominator is the diastolic pressure. For example, if the blood pressure is 120/80 mm Hg, 120 represents the systolic pressure, and 80 represents the diastolic pressure. The pulse pressure, in this case, is 40 mm Hg.

Physiology of Blood Pressure

Arterial walls contain elastic tissue that allows them to stretch and distend (called compliance) as blood enters with each ventricular contraction. When the heart rests between each beat, the walls of the arteries return to their original position (recoil), although pressure in them does not drop to zero. The arterioles offer resistance to the pressure of the blood and keep the blood entering the capillaries in a continuous flow rather than in spurts. Therefore, the elasticity of the arterial walls, in addition to the resistance of the arterioles, helps to maintain normal blood pressure. With increased age, the walls of arterioles become less elastic, which interferes with their ability to stretch and dilate. This can subsequently limit adequate blood flow and contribute to rising pressure within the vascular system.

Although blood moves through the circulatory system from areas of higher pressure to areas of lower pressure, blood pressure is controlled by various short- and long-term mechanisms. These mechanisms regulate the blood pressure so that blood flow and blood pressure remain relatively constant.

Short-Term Regulation of Blood Pressure

The mechanisms for short-term blood pressure regulation (occurring over minutes or hours) are primarily neural (nerve) and humoral (pertaining to body fluids). These mechanisms correct temporary changes in pressure that occur during activities such as changing position or exercising and are also responsible for maintaining blood pressure during life-threatening situations. In addition, increased cardiac output (from a stronger contraction and increased stroke volume) results in an increased blood pressure while a weak contraction of the heart with decreased cardiac output causes a decrease in blood pressure.

The neural centers for blood pressure regulation are located in the brain in an area called the cardiovascular center. The cardiovascular center transmits parasympathetic impulses to the heart via the vagus nerve and sympathetic impulses to the heart and blood vessels via the spinal cord and peripheral sympathetic nerves. Stimulating the vagus nerve slows the heart rate; sympathetic stimulation increases the heart rate.

Pressure-sensitive receptors, called baroreceptors, are located in the heart and walls of arteries (such as the aortic arch and carotid). They are stimulated by changes in stretch of the blood vessel as blood pressure changes and send impulses to the cardiovascular center to initiate the appropriate changes in heart rate and vascular smooth muscle. For example, blood pressure normally decreases when rising from a lying to an upright position, resulting in decreased stretch of baroreceptors. In response, heart rate and peripheral vascular resistance increase to raise blood pressure. During life-threatening situations, such as a serious hemorrhage, the same mechanisms are activated.

Many different humoral mechanisms, along with hormones, also help regulate blood pressure. Epinephrine, a sympathetic neurotransmitter, is released by the adrenal gland to increase heart rate and contractility, thereby increasing cardiac output. The renin–angiotensin–aldosterone system, through angiotensinogen II, causes vasoconstriction in the arterioles. This leads to increased peripheral vascular resistance as a short-term mechanism, and also increases sodium and water retention by the kidneys to increase circulatory fluid volume, thus increasing blood pressure as a long-term mechanism (see discussion in the next section). Vasopressin (antidiuretic hormone [ADH]) is released from the posterior pituitary when stimulated by decreased blood volume and blood pressure, or by an increased osmolality of body fluids. It has a direct vasoconstricting effect on blood vessels, increasing peripheral resistance.

Long-Term Regulation of Blood Pressure

Certain long-term mechanisms are responsible for the ongoing regulation of blood pressure. These mechanisms regulate extracellular fluid volume through the kidneys. They function by regulating blood pressure for an individual person's equilibrium point. Arterial pressure rises when the body contains too much extracellular fluid. In response, increased amounts of sodium and fluid are excreted by the kidneys to return the blood pressure to the person's equilibrium point. When blood pressure decreases due to decreased extracellular fluid, the opposite effect occurs. Extracellular fluid volume regulates blood pressure directly by increasing cardiac output and renal blood flow and indirectly by autoregulation of blood flow, in which autoregulatory mechanisms redirect blood flow to various blood tissues.

Factors Affecting Blood Pressure

A single blood pressure measurement is not necessarily significant because of the many factors that influence blood pressure. Box 26-5 lists factors that commonly cause variations in blood pressure.

Normal Blood Pressure

Studies of healthy people indicate that blood pressure can be within a wide range and still be normal. Because of individual differences, it is important to know the normal blood pressure range of a particular person. A rise or fall of 20 to 30 mm Hg in a person's blood pressure is significant, even if it is within the generally accepted normal range. Although blood pressure varies constantly, sustained long-term changes are not considered normal. Normal blood pressure is defined as a systolic pressure <120 mm Hg and diastolic pressure <80 mm Hg (Whelton et al., 2018). Table 26-7 identifies the categories for blood pressure levels in adults.

Increased Blood Pressure

Many factors influence blood pressure; a single elevated blood pressure measurement is not necessarily significant. Patients may have elevated blood pressure levels as a result of various factors, including pain, anxiety, and acute health

Box 26-5 Factors Contributing to Blood Pressure Variations in Healthy People

- **Age:** The older adult has decreased elasticity of the arteries, which increases peripheral resistance and, therefore, increases blood pressure.
- **Circadian rhythm:** Normal fluctuations occur during the day. The blood pressure is usually lowest on arising in the morning. Blood pressure has been noted to rise as much as 5 to 10 mm Hg by late afternoon, and gradually falls again during sleep.
- **Biologic sex:** Women usually have lower blood pressure than men of the same age until menopause.
- **Food intake:** Blood pressure increases after eating food.
- **Exercise:** Systolic blood pressure rises during periods of exercise and strenuous activity.
- **Weight:** Blood pressure is usually higher in people who are obese than in those who are thin.
- **Emotional state:** Emotions, such as anger, fear, excitement, and pain, generally cause the blood pressure to rise, but the pressure falls to normal when the situation passes.
- **Body position:** Blood pressure tends to be lower in a prone or supine position than when sitting or standing.
- **Race:** Race is a factor in increased blood pressure (hypertension), which is more prevalent and more severe in African American men and women.
- **Drugs/Medications:** Oral contraceptives cause a mild increase in blood pressure in many women.

conditions (refer to Box 26-5). **Hypertension**, one of the most common health problems, is blood pressure that is above normal for a sustained period. A diagnosis of hypertension is made when the systolic pressure is 130 mm Hg or higher or the diastolic pressure is 80 mm Hg or higher, based on the average of two or more readings obtained on two or more occasions to estimate the patient's level of blood pressure (Whelton et al., 2018). The guidelines related to high blood pressure in adults were updated in 2017 to reflect a lower definition of high blood pressure to account for complications that can occur at lower pressure numbers, and to allow for earlier intervention (Whelton et al., 2018). These changes in the definition of hypertension will result in almost half of the U.S. adult population (46%) having high blood pressure, with the greatest impact expected among younger people (Whelton et al., 2018). The prevalence of hypertension is greater in African American and Hispanic adults than in White adults (Whelton et al., 2018). Elevated blood pressure also progressively increases with age (Whelton et al., 2018). Hypertension is a major risk factor for cardiovascular disease, cerebral vascular accident (CVA) (stroke), myocardial infarction (MI), heart failure (HF), peripheral vascular disease, and abdominal aortic aneurysm (Whelton et al., 2018). It is called a "silent killer" because there are often few symptoms beyond increased blood pressure (World Health Organization [WHO], 2019). Refer to Table 26-7 for blood pressure categories.

The basis for hypertension is thought to be dysfunction of the neurohormonal system. Over activation of both angiotensin and aldosterone result in an increase in blood pressure. Over time, this sustained increase results in a permanent remodeling and thickening of the blood vessels. As a result, there is increased peripheral resistance and a back-up of pressure to organs affected by the vascular system, such as the brain, heart, and kidneys. Disorders resulting from hypertension include those previously identified as well as thickening of the myocardium, enlargement of the ventricles, and kidney damage (chronic kidney disease or kidney failure).

There are many risk factors for the development of hypertension in adults. Significant risks are a family history of hypertension, race, aging, obstructive sleep apnea, and metabolic disorders such as metabolic syndrome, type 2 diabetes mellitus, obesity, and high cholesterol (Hinckle & Cheever, 2018). Lifestyle risk factors include a sedentary lifestyle; excessive alcohol consumption; and high dietary intake of salt, fats, and calories (Hinckle & Cheever, 2018).

Table 26-7 Categories for Blood Pressure Levels in Adults (Ages 18 and Older)

CATEGORY	BLOOD PRESSURE LEVEL (mm Hg)		
	Systolic		*Diastolic*
Normal	<120	*and*	<80
Elevated	120–129	*and*	<80
Hypertension Stage 1	130–139	*or*	80–89
Hypertension Stage 2	≥140	*or*	≥90
Hypertensive crisis	>180	*and/or*	>120

Source: Reprinted with permission. *Hypertension.* 2017; HYP.0000000000000066 ©2017 American Heart Association, Inc. Whelton, P. K., Carey, R. M., Aronow, W. S., Casey, D. E., Aronow, W. S., Casey, D. E., Collins, K. J., Himmelfarb, C. D., DePalma, S. M., Gidding, S., Jamerson, K. A., Jones, D. W., MacLaughlin, E. J., Muntner, P., Ovbiagele, B., Smith, Jr., S. C., Spencer, C. C., Stafford, R. S., Taler, S. J., … Wright, Jr., J. T. (2018). 2017 ACC/AHA/AAPA/ABC/ACPM/AGS/APhA/ASH/ASPC/NMA/PCNA Guideline for the prevention, detection, evaluation, and management of high blood pressure in adults: A Report of the American College of Cardiology/American Heart Association Task Force on Clinical Practice Guidelines. *Hypertension, 71*(6), e13–e115. https://doi.org/10.1161/HYP.0000000000000065

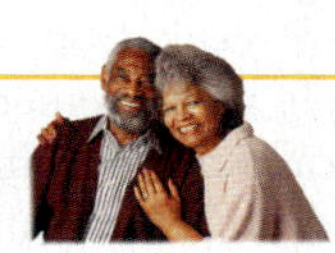

Remember **Mrs. Renfrow**, the wife of a man who is overweight and diagnosed with hypertension? The nurse would need to incorporate information about various risk factors for developing hypertension as well as information about risk related to hypertension in the teaching plan for Mrs. Renfrow and her husband.

Promoting Health Literacy

IN PATIENTS WITH HYPERTENSION

Patient Scenario

Harry Miller, 66 years old, went to his primary health care provider for his annual health assessment. He had gained 15 lb in the past year. When the office nurse took his blood pressure, it was 166/92 mm Hg. The nurse took Mr. Miller's blood pressure again and then repeated it later after his health assessment was completed. Although the reading varied by a few points, it remained consistently high. Mr. Miller was obviously surprised at having hypertension, because he said, "It has never been this high before. There must be something wrong with your machine." His health care provider tried to discuss the need for changes in his lifestyle as well as the need to take the medication prescribed for his blood pressure, but Mr. Miller said he had no questions and rushed out of the examining room.

Nursing Considerations: *Tips for Improving Health Literacy*

Provide Mr. Miller with printed literature about high blood pressure, including causes and risks. Explain that it is important to control his high blood pressure to prevent serious risks, such as heart attack and stroke. Urge Mr. Miller and his wife to talk to a dietitian about a nutritious diet that would help him lose weight; contains recommended servings of fiber, fruits, and vegetables; and contains less salt. Explain the action of the prescribed medication and the importance of taking the medication to reduce and control his blood pressure. Teach Mr. Miller and his wife about home blood pressure monitoring (HBPM). Encourage Mr. Miller to make an appointment to return to the office on a regular basis and to be prepared to ask his provider the following three questions:

- What is my main problem?
- What do I need to do?
- Why is it important for me to do this?

What additional measures can you take to help maintain health literacy in this patient and his wife? What other measures would be helpful for Mr. Miller if he did not speak English, could not read, or had other learning deficits?

Hypertension can be controlled by medications and lifestyle changes. Some of the categories of antihypertensive medications include diuretics (to decrease fluid volume), angiotensin-converting enzyme (ACE) inhibitors (to prevent vasoconstriction and aldosterone release by blocking the conversion of angiotensin I to angiotensin II), angiotensin II receptor blockers (ARB) (by selectively binding with the angiotensin II receptors in vascular smooth muscle and the adrenal cortex to block vasoconstriction and the release of aldosterone), vasodilators and calcium channel blockers (to relax smooth muscles of arterioles and decrease peripheral vascular resistance), and beta-adrenergic blockers (to block sympathetic stimulation and decrease cardiac output) (Karch, 2020). Lifestyle changes include weight loss for overweight or obese patients; a heart healthy diet (reduced sodium; low in saturated fat and total fat; increase in fruits, vegetables, and grains); limiting alcohol intake (no more than two alcohol drinks per day for men and no more than one for women); managing and coping with stress; and engaging in regular physical activity (Whelton et al., 2018). Nurses can influence the health of the public through screenings, education, and referrals. See Promoting Health Literacy in Patients with Hypertension for more information.

Screening for hypertension is recommended in children beginning at the age of 3 years. False elevations in pressures can result from anxiety or caffeine intake; checking multiple measurements over time is recommended (American Academy of Pediatrics, 2020). Hypertension is diagnosed if a child has auscultatory-confirmed blood pressure readings ≥95th percentile on 3 different visits (American Academy of Pediatrics, 2020). Lifestyle interventions, related to nutrition, sleep, and physical activity are initiated initially, with close monitoring. Refer to the Clinical Practice Guideline from the American Academy of Pediatrics (2020) for additional discussion related to and treatment of pediatric hypertension (Flynn et al., 2017).

Decreased Blood Pressure

Hypotension is below-normal blood pressure. Hypotension is blood pressure that is lower than 90/60 mm Hg (NHLBI, n.d.). The body uses the previously discussed mechanisms to maintain consistent blood pressure. Hypotension occurs primarily as a result of the inability of the body's control mechanisms to maintain or return blood pressure back to normal or the inability to do it quickly enough. Hypotension may also occur as a result of pathology (disease process), such as Parkinson disease (related problems with the autonomic nervous system contribute to low blood pressure) (NHLBI). Pathologic hypotension might result from vasodilation of the arterioles, failure of the heart to function as an effective pump, or loss of blood volume (such as with a hemorrhage). Hypotension can be a side effect of some medications, including antihypertensives, certain antidepressants, antianxiety medication, and analgesics. A consistently low blood pressure is normal in some adults, with no signs or symptoms. Hypotension is a concern if it causes signs or symptoms or is linked to a disease or health process. The nurse should immediately communicate assessments of hypotension and associated symptoms of dizziness, tachycardia, pallor, syncope, increased sweating, blurred vision, nausea, and confusion.

Orthostatic hypotension (postural hypotension) is a common form of low blood pressure (Cheshire, 2019). It results from an inadequate physiologic response to postural (positional) changes in blood pressure. *Classical orthostatic hypotension* is a sustained decrease in systolic blood pressure of ≥20 mm Hg or a decrease in diastolic blood pressure of ≥10 mm Hg *within* 3 minutes of standing or during a head-up tilt test to at least 60 degrees (Freeman et al., 2018). *Delayed orthostatic hypotension* (DOH) is a sustained reduction in blood pressure that occurs *after* 3 minutes of standing or upright tilt (Freeman et al.). *Initial orthostatic hypotension* is a transient reduction in systolic blood pressure of ≥40 mm Hg and/or a transient decrease in diastolic blood pressure of ≥20 mm Hg *within* 15 seconds of standing (Freeman et al., 2018). Orthostatic hypotension may be acute or chronic as well as symptomatic or asymptomatic.

Orthostatic hypotension occurs when a person rises to an erect position, either supine to sitting, supine to standing, or sitting to standing. It is caused by dehydration or blood loss; problems of the neurologic, cardiovascular, or endocrine systems; and/or use of certain classes of medications. Orthostatic hypotension may be associated with dizziness, confusion, lightheadedness, blurred vision, weakness, fatigue, nausea, tachycardia, palpitations, and headache, but the presence of symptoms is not necessary for the diagnosis (Freeman et al.). Symptoms occur with postural change, are exacerbated by standing, and relieved by sitting or lying flat (Freemen et al.). Aging is also a risk factor for developing orthostatic hypotension (Godbole & Aggarwal, 2018). Older adults who experience orthostatic hypotension are at increased risk for falls (McDonald et al., 2017). Orthostatic blood pressure measurements should be included in the clinical evaluation of all older adults (Lipsitz, 2017).

Several nonpharmacologic interventions may be used to control or prevent orthostatic hypotension. Educate patients about the need to arise and move about slowly, especially after a period of bed rest (Godbole & Aggarwal, 2018). When ambulating patients after surgery or prolonged bed rest, first raise the head of the bed, then assist the patient to a sitting position on the side of bed (often called "dangling") for a few minutes to assess for dizziness or faintness, and then assist to a standing position. If the patient becomes dizzy or feels faint, return the patient to bed and place in a supine position, which restores blood flow to the brain. Administer contributing medications at bedtime if possible, especially antihypertensives. Patients should ensure adequate hydration. Compression stockings and abdominal compression support garments may be implemented (Godbole & Aggarwal, 2018). There are also numerous medications that are used to treat orthostatic hypotension, with the goal to alleviate symptoms and avoid adverse effects, not necessarily restore normotension (Freeman et al., 2018). Guidelines for Nursing Care 26-5 describes one method to obtain blood pressure measurements to assess for orthostatic hypotension.

Assessing Blood Pressure

Measurement of blood pressure is an important part of vital sign measurement; identification of a patient's baseline status; and identification of changes in a patient's status. Accurate measurement of blood pressure (BP) is essential

Guidelines for Nursing Care 26-5

ASSESSING ORTHOSTATIC HYPOTENSION

Use the following guidelines to assess for orthostatic hypotension:

Assess for signs and symptoms of hypotension, such as dizziness, lightheadedness, pallor, diaphoresis, or syncope throughout the procedure. If the patient is attached to a cardiac monitor, assess for arrhythmias. Immediately return the patient to a supine position if symptoms appear during the procedure. Do not have the patient stand if symptoms of hypotension occur when the patient is sitting.

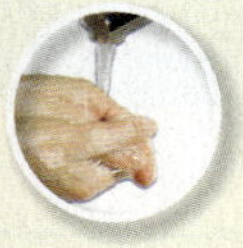

- Perform hand hygiene and put on PPE, if indicated.
- Lower the head of the bed. Place the bed in a low position.
- Ask the patient to lie in a supine position for 3 to 10 minutes. At the end of this time, take initial blood pressure and pulse measurements.
- Assist the patient to sit on the side of the bed with legs dangling. After 1 to 3 minutes, take the blood pressure and pulse measurements.
- Assist the patient to stand (unless contraindicated). Thirty seconds after standing, take blood pressure and pulse measurements, then a second set of measurements at 60 seconds (Godbole & Aggarwal, 2018). Wait 1 minute and take a third set of measurements, and a fourth set after one additional minute, for a total of 3 minutes (Godbole & Aggarwal).
- Record the measurements for each position. A decrease in systolic blood pressure of ≥20 mm Hg or a decrease in diastolic blood pressure of ≥10 mm Hg within 3 minutes of standing when compared with blood pressure from the sitting or supine position is significant for orthostatic hypotension (Godbole & Aggarwal). In patients with hypertension (supine systolic BP ≥160 mm Hg), a drop of systolic BP of at least 30 mm Hg is more appropriate (Godbole & Aggarwal).

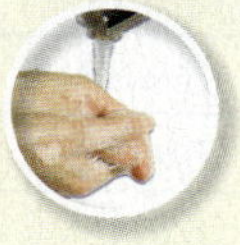

- Remove PPE, if used. Perform hand hygiene.

Source: Adapted from Freeman, R., Abuzinadah, A. R., Gibbons, C., Jones, P., Miglis, M. G., & Sinn, D. I. (2018). Orthostatic hypotension. JACC State-of-the-art review. *Journal of the American College of Cardiology*, *72*(11), 1294–1309. https://doi.org/10.1016/j.jacc.2018.05.079; Godbole, G. P., & Aggarwal, B. (2018). Review of management strategies for orthostatic hypotension in older people. *Journal of Pharmacy Practice and Research*, *48*(5), 483–491. https://doi.org/10.1002/jppr.1484; and Pickering, T. G., Hall, J. E., Appel, L. J., Falkner, B. E., Graves, J., Hill, M. N., Jones, D. W., Kurtz, T., Sheps, S. G., & Roccella, E. J. (2005). Recommendations for blood pressure measurement in humans and experimental animals. Part 1: Blood pressure measurement in humans: A statement for professionals from the subcommittee of professional and public education of the American Heart Association Council on High Blood Pressure Research. *Circulation*, *111*(5), 697–716. https://doi.org/10.1161/01.CIR.0000154900.76284.F6.

for the diagnosis and management of hypertension (Mutner et al., 2019). Blood pressure measurements should be obtained as two or more readings on two or more occasions and the measurements averaged to estimate the person's level of blood pressure (Whelton et al., 2018).

Blood pressure may be assessed with different types of devices and at several locations on the body. The nurse must know the appropriate equipment to use, including choosing the appropriate blood pressure cuff; how to accurately obtain the measurement; how to describe the sounds that are heard during the auscultatory method of measurement; and which site to choose in order to accurately assess blood pressure.

The auscultatory method has been the standard clinical method of measurement of blood pressure using a stethoscope and sphygmomanometer to detect the appearance and disappearance of the Korotkoff sounds, which represent systolic and diastolic blood pressure. Advances in technology have contributed to increased accuracy in automated, electronic oscillometric devices for measurement of BP; there is growing evidence supporting the use of these devices in clinical settings (Whelton et al., 2018). Many oscillometric devices have been validated that allow accurate BP measurement while reducing human errors associated with the auscultatory approach (Muntner et al., 2019; Myers et al., 2018). "Out-of-office" measurement of blood pressure can contribute to confirmation and improved management of hypertension (Muntner et al., 2019; Whelton et al., 2018). Ambulatory blood pressure monitoring (ABPM) and home blood pressure monitoring (HBPM) (self-monitoring) are two methods used to obtain blood pressure measurements outside the clinical practice areas. Systolic BP pressure can be estimated with a Doppler ultrasound device (described in the discussion of pulse measurement) or by palpation. Direct electronic measurement of BP is accomplished through direct arterial access and used primarily in intensive care areas.

Blood pressure measurement results are most commonly recorded with two numbers, written as a fraction. The first number in the fraction represents the systolic pressure—for example, if the blood pressure reading is 120/80 mm Hg, 120 is the systolic pressure. The second number in the fraction represents the diastolic pressure, in this case, a diastolic pressure of 80 mm Hg.

Blood Pressure Cuffs

The initial step in measuring blood pressure is determining the appropriate cuff size. Blood pressure cuffs are used in both the auscultatory and oscillometric methods of BP measurement. The cuff contains an airtight, flat, rubber bladder covered with cloth. Selecting a cuff of the proper size (ranging from neonate to adult thigh) is essential to obtain an accurate blood pressure reading. The correct cuff should have a bladder length that is 75% to 100% of the patient's arm circumference and a width that is 37% to 50% of the arm circumference, with a length-to-width ratio of 2:1 (Muntner et al., 2019).

The cuff should be pulled taut when placed on the bare limb, with comparable tightness at the top and bottom edges of the cuff. Check the tightness: one finger should fit easily at the top and bottom of the cuff; two fingers should fit but be very snug (Muntner et al., 2019).

Incorrect cuff size contributes to the most frequent error in measurement in nonacute care settings (Muntner et al., 2019). *If the cuff is too narrow*, the reading could be erroneously high because the pressure is not evenly transmitted to the artery. This occurs, for example, when an average-sized cuff is used on an obese person. Based on size and shape dimensions, an appropriately sized cuff as closely aligned to the AHA's guidelines as possible should be selected to ensure accurate readings in this patient population. A cone-shaped cuff may be necessary to accommodate the size and shape of the arm for these patients (Muntner et al., 2019). If a cuff cannot be fitted correctly, the wrist should be used (Muntner et al., 2019). Refer to the discussion Sites of Assessing the Blood Pressure later in this section. *If a cuff is too wide* (e.g., using an adult cuff on the arm of a child), the reading may be erroneously low because pressure is dispersed over a

Table 26-8 Recommended Blood Pressure Cuff Sizes

CUFF SIZE	CUFF BLADDER DIMENSIONS (cm)	ARM CIRCUMFERENCE[a] (cm)
Neonates, Infants, Children	Cuff bladder length should encircle 80–100% of arm Cuff bladder width-to-arm circumference ration of 0.45–0.55	
Small adult size	12 × 22	22–26
Adult size	16 × 30	27–34
Large adult size	16 × 36	35–44
Adult thigh size	16 × 42	45–52

[a]Select a blood pressure cuff that has a bladder length 75%–100% of the arm circumference and a width that is 37%–50% of the arm circumference.
Source: Adapted from Flynn, J. T., Kaelber, D. C., Baker-Smith, C. M., Blowey, D., Carroll, A. E., Daniels, S. R., de Ferranti, S. D., Dionne, J. M., Falkner, B., Flinn, S. K., Gidding, S. S., Goodwin, C., Leu, M. G., Powers, M. E., Rea, C., Samuels, J., Simasek, M., Thaker, V. V., Urbina, E. M., ... SUBCOMMITTEE ON SCREENING AND MANAGEMENT OF HIGH BLOOD PRESSURE IN CHILDREN. (2017). Clinical practice guideline for screening and management of high blood pressure in children and adolescents. *Pediatrics*, *140*(3), e2 0171904. https://doi.org/10.1542/peds.2017-1904; Muntner, P., Shimbo, D., Carey, R. M., Charleston, J. B., Gaillard, T., Misra, S., Myers, M. G., Ogedegbe, G., Schwartz, J. E., Townsend, R. R., Urbina, E. M., Viera, A. J., White, W. B., & Wright, J. T. Jr. (2019). Measurement of blood pressure in humans. A scientific statement from the American Heart Association. *Hypertension*, *73*(5), e35–e66. https://doi.org/10.1161/HYP.0000000000000087; and Pickering, T. G., Hall, J. E., Appel, L. J., Falkner, B. E., Graves, J., Hill, M.N., Jones, D. W., Kurtz, T., Sheps, S. G., & Roccella, E. J. (2005). Recommendations for blood pressure measurement in humans and experimental animals. Part 1: Blood pressure measurement in humans: A statement for professionals from the subcommittee of professional and public education of the American Heart Association Council on High Blood Pressure Research. *Circulation*, *111*(5), 697–716. https://doi.org/10.1161/01.CIR.0000154900.76284.F6

disproportionately large surface area. Recommendations by the AHA for the selection of an appropriately sized cuff are given in Table 26-8.

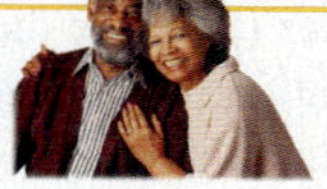

Think back to **Mrs. Renfrow**, the wife of a patient with hypertension who is overweight. The nurse would need to caution Mrs. Renfrow to make sure that the device she uses to measure her husband's blood pressure is sized adequately. Otherwise, the readings may be erroneous, possibly leading to inappropriate management based on inaccurate readings or a false sense of security that the hypertension is being controlled.

Depending on the product, cuffs may be disposable or reusable. They are closed around the limb with contact closures, such as nylon fabric that can be fastened to itself with Velcro. One or two tubes are attached to the bladder within the cuff, depending on the device used. Cuffs for the device used for the auscultatory method (sphygmomanometer) have two tubes; one is connected to a manometer and a second tube is attached to a bulb used to inflate the bladder in the cuff. Cuffs used with the oscillometric device have one tube connecting the cuff to the device. The cuff bladder is inflated enough to obstruct the flow of blood through the artery. A valve on the cuff bulb allows the cuff to be deflated while the pressure is being read during use of the auscultatory device.

Patient Preparation for Blood Pressure Measurement

Blood pressure measurement should take place in a quiet environment. The patient should not have consumed caffeine, exercised, or smoked for 30 minutes before the measurement (Muntner et al., 2019). The patient should not talk or move during the procedure. The patient may be supine or sitting; systolic BP may be as much as 10 mm Hg higher and diastolic BP as much as 5 mm Hg higher in the supine than the seated position (Tolonen et al., 2015, as cited in Muntner et al., 2019). In the supine position, the patient's arm should be supported with a pillow at heart level (Muntner et al., 2019). When sitting, the patient's arm should be supported on a table at heart level or held up by the health care provider (midpoint of the sternum). The patient's feet and back should be supported as well (Whelton et al., 2018). Adequate support and proper positioning prevent inaccurately high readings (Muntner et al., 2019). Lack of back support can lead to an increase in systolic readings of up to 15 mm Hg and diastolic reading up to 6 mm Hg (Pan et al., 2014, as cited in Muntner et al., 2019). Legs should not be crossed during BP measurement to avoid raising of the systolic BP by as much as 8 mm Hg and diastolic BP by as much as 5 mm Hg (Liu et al., 2016, as cited in Muntner et al., 2019).

Errors in Blood Pressure Measurement

Regardless of the method used to measure blood pressure, health care providers must ensure the use of validated and calibrated devices and use careful, accurate technique to avoid errors in BP measurement (Muntner et al., 2019; Pickering et al., 2005; Whelton et al., 2018). Retraining of health care professionals every 6 months to 1 year has been suggested to ensure accurate measurement (Muntner et al., 2019). Box 26-6 identifies potential sources of blood pressure measurement error.

Box 26-6 Sources of Error in Blood Pressure Measurement

- Use of noncalibrated, nonvalidated, nonmaintained device
- Use of a cuff of incorrect size
- Patient movement during measurement
- Patient talking during the measurement
- Incorrect placement and/or orientation of the cuff
- Incorrect positioning of the patient
- Use of inaccurate measurement technique
  - Incorrect positioning of the limb used for measurement
  - Inflation of cuff that is too rapid
  - Deflation of cuff that is too rapid (faster than 2 to 3 mm Hg per second)
- Environmental noise
- Failure to allow for a rest period prior to measurement
- Incorrect interpretation
- Reliance on blood pressures measured at a single occasion

Source: Adapted from Muntner, P., Shimbo, D., Carey, R. M., Charleston, J. B., Gaillard, T., Misra, S., Myers, M. G., Ogedegbe, G., Schwartz, J. E., Townsend, R. R., Urbina, E. M., Viera, A. J., White, W. B., & Wright, J. T. Jr. (2019). Measurement of blood pressure in humans. A scientific statement from the American Heart Association. *Hypertension, 73*(5), e35–e66. https://doi.org/10.1161/HYP.0000000000000087; Whelton, P. K., Carey, R. M., Aronow, W. S., Casey, D. E. Jr., Collins, K. J., Dennison Himmelfarb, C., DePalma, S. M., Gidding, S., Jamerson, K. A., Jones, D. W., MacLaughlin, E. J., Muntner, P., Ovbiagele, B., Smith, S. C. Jr., Spencer, C. C., Stafford, R. S., Taler, S. J., Thomas, R. J., Williams, K. A. Sr., ... Wright, J. T. Jr. (2018). 2017 ACC/AHA/AAPA/ABC/ACPM/AGS/APhA/ASH/ASPC/NMA/PCNA Guideline for the prevention, detection, evaluation, and management of high blood pressure in adults: A Report of the American College of Cardiology/American Heart Association Task Force on Clinical Practice Guidelines. *Hypertension, 71*(6), e13–e115. https://doi.org/10.1161/HYP.0000000000000065

Oscillometric Method of Measurement

Automated, electronic oscillometric blood pressure monitors determine blood pressure by analyzing the sounds of blood flow or measuring the amplitude of the oscillations (fluctuations) in blood flow upon deflation or inflation of the cuff (Fig. 26-4 on page 740). These devices can be set to take and record blood pressure readings at preset intervals. As previously discussed, there has been a shift away from manual auscultatory BP measurement to the use of oscillometric measurement method, supported by improved device technology, as well as the recommendation to obtain multiple BP readings to increase accuracy (Muntner et al., 2019). Oscillometric devices are commonly used to measure BP in a variety of settings, including clinics, ambulatory, home, and acute care (Muntner et al., 2019). Calibration of devices at regular intervals, based on manufacturer guidelines, is

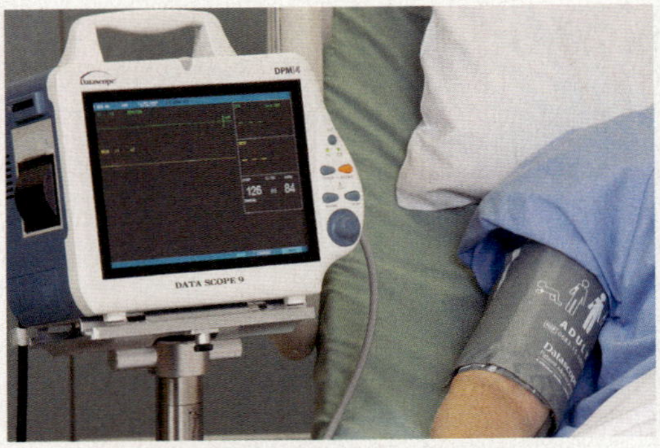

FIGURE 26-4. The electronic oscillometric blood pressure monitor reports systolic and diastolic blood pressure, as well as mean blood pressure. (*Source:* Used with permission from Shutterstock. *Photo by B. Proud.*)

recommended to ensure accuracy (Muntner et al., 2019). Health care providers must ensure use of validated and calibrated devices and use careful, accurate technique to avoid errors in BP measurement.

Many of these devices have additional integrated equipment, such as a thermometer and pulse oximetry, to perform multiple vital sign measurements.

Refer to Skill 26-4 on pp. 759–763 for a detailed description of the accurate use of the oscillometric method of BP measurement.

Auscultatory Method of Blood Pressure Measurement

The auscultatory method of measuring BP has been the traditional approach to measurement of systolic and diastolic blood pressure and remains an acceptable method for measuring blood pressure (Muntner et al., 2019). However, many of the sphygmomanometers available for use are susceptible to error and loss of calibration and require frequent calibration to ensure accuracy (Muntner et al., 2019). In addition, accuracy of BP readings relies on precise measurement technique (Muntner et al.). There are numerous potential sources of BP error and the use of inaccurate measurement technique is common (Kallioinen et al., 2017). As mentioned previously, this method is being replaced more and more by the use of oscillometric devices in clinical practice (Muntner et al., 2019).

A sphygmomanometer, along with a stethoscope, is used to assess blood pressure in the auscultatory method of BP measurement. The sphygmomanometer consists of a cuff (with an air compartment), a pump, and the manometer (pressure dial) (Fig. 26-5). The BP cuff is placed on the patient's limb and inflated, causing the underlying artery to be occluded and flow to stop; as the cuff is gradually deflated, blood flow is reestablished, accompanied by sounds that can be heard with a stethoscope placed at a pulse site corresponding with the underlying artery (Muntner et al., 2019). The nurse listens to a series of these sounds when assessing the blood pressure using the auscultatory method. These sounds are called **Korotkoff sounds**, described and illustrated in Table 26-9. These sounds are only heard when using a stethoscope to assess blood pressure. In some adults, each of these sounds is distinct, whereas in others only the beginning and ending sounds are heard. It is important to determine facility policy for recording blood pressure sounds and to be consistent in taking and documenting the readings.

The first sound heard through the stethoscope, which is the onset of Phase I, represents the systolic pressure. It is recorded as the first number in the fraction—for example, if the blood pressure reading is 120/80 mm Hg, 120 is the systolic pressure. The second number, which represents the diastolic pressure (in this case, 80), notes the level at which the sounds disappear completely, Phase V. Read measurements to the nearest even number (nearest 2 mm Hg) (Flynn et al., 2017; Whelton et al., 2018). In situations in which sounds were heard all the way down to zero—for example, in pregnant women and patients with arteriovenous fistulas—the blood pressure recording would include phase IV (e.g., 112/62/0) (Flynn et al., Muntner et al., Pickering et al., Whelton et al., 2018).

Refer to Skill 26-5 on pp. 763–768 for a detailed description of the accurate use of the auscultatory method of BP measurement.

Ambulatory Blood Pressure Monitoring

ABPM is a noninvasive, fully automated method of blood pressure measurement that allows for BP measurement to be recorded over an extended period of time, such as over 24 hours, while the patient is awake or asleep. The digital

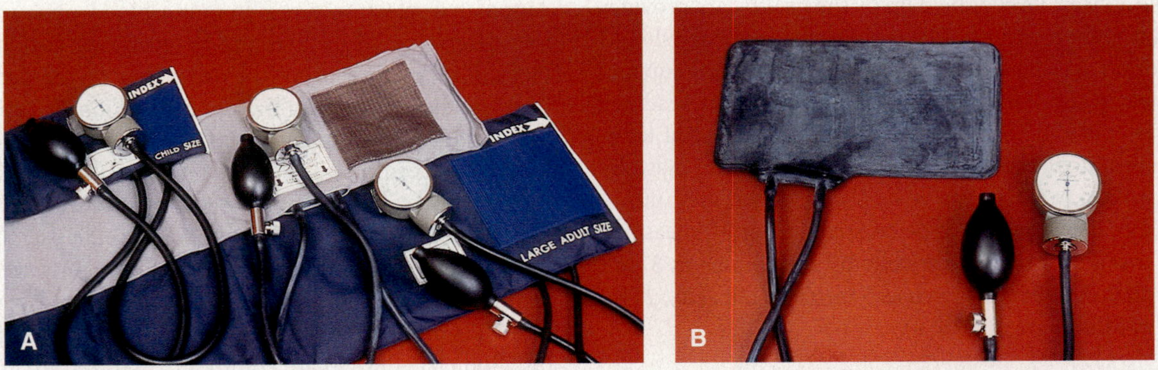

FIGURE 26-5. Sphygmomanometer. **A.** Three cuff sizes: a small cuff for a child or a small or frail adult, a normal-sized cuff, and a large adult cuff. A cuff sized for use on the thigh is also available. **B.** Parts of a sphygmomanometer. (*Source:* Part B used with permission from Weber, J. R., & Kelley, J. H. [2018]. *Health assessment in nursing* [6th ed.]. Wolters Kluwer, p. 135.)

Table 26-9 Korotkoff Sounds

PHASE	DESCRIPTION	ILLUSTRATION
Phase I	Characterized by the first appearance of faint but clear tapping sounds that gradually increase in intensity; the first tapping sound is the systolic pressure	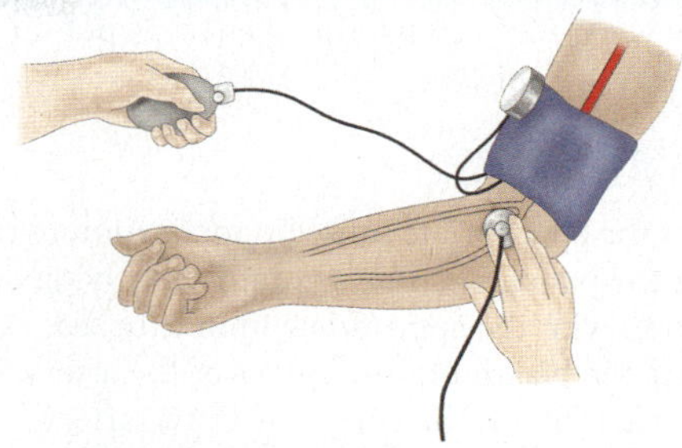 Blood flow interrupted by inflated cuff.
Phase II	Characterized by muffled or swishing sounds; these sounds may temporarily disappear, especially in hypertensive people; the disappearance of the sound during the latter part of phase I and during phase II is called the ***auscultatory gap*** and may cover a range of as much as 40 mm Hg; failing to recognize this gap may cause serious errors of underestimating systolic pressure or overestimating diastolic pressure	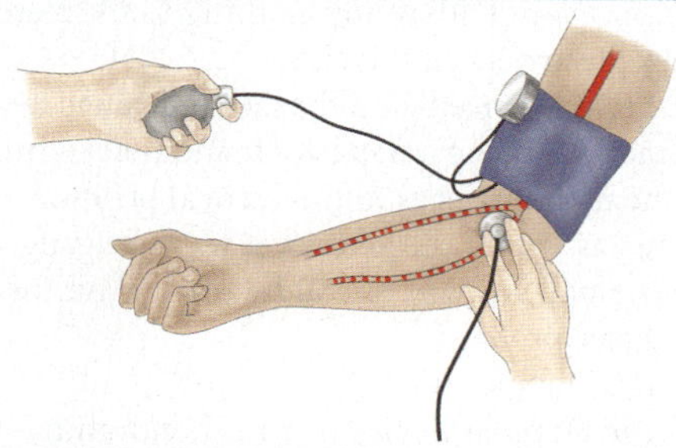 As the pressure in the cuff is released, blood starts flowing again and Korotkoff sounds are audible.
Phase III	Characterized by distinct, loud sounds as the blood flows relatively freely through an increasingly open artery	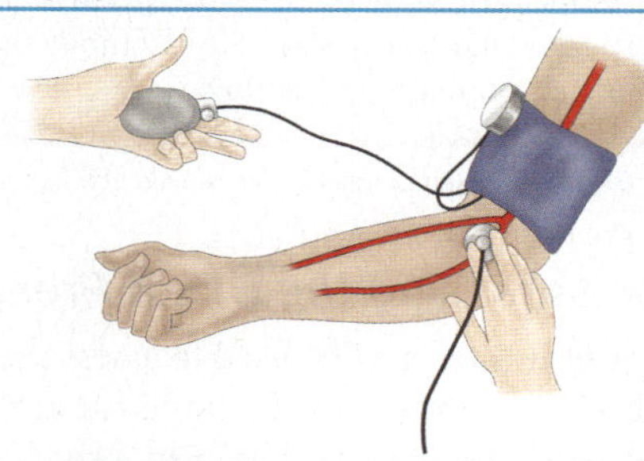 Cuff is completely deflated after Phase V, restoring complete blood flow.
Phase IV	Characterized by a distinct, abrupt, muffling sound with a soft, blowing quality	
Phase V	The last sound heard before loss of all sounds; the pressure at which the last sound is heard is the second diastolic pressure	

device consists of a cuff placed on the patient's arm, and the machine is small enough to be worn on a belt around the patient's waist. Readings are usually taken and recorded by the device every 20 to 30 minutes during the day and every hour at night (Cleveland Clinic, 2020). Patients must avoid bathing and swimming while wearing the device. ABPM may be used to supplement blood pressure readings obtained in nonacute care settings to detect abnormal fluctuations that may not be noted in single measurements. ABPM is useful in confirming a diagnosis of hypertension; identifying patterns in blood pressure measurements; and monitoring the effectiveness of antihypertensive drug therapy (Cleveland Clinic; Muntner et al., 2019). There is increased recognition of inconsistencies between office and out-of-office blood pressure readings, with office blood pressure readings often higher than ambulatory or home measurements (Muntner et al., 2019; Whelton et al., 2018). Studies have shown substantial differences in blood pressure when measured outside versus in the office or clinic setting (Muntner et al.). ABPM can be used to increase accuracy of BP readings and monitor blood pressure levels over time.

Doppler Ultrasound

An indirect blood pressure measurement may be obtained with a Doppler ultrasound device, which amplifies sounds. This device is especially useful if the sounds are indistinct or are inaudible with a regular stethoscope. This method only provides an estimate of systolic blood pressure. See Guidelines for Nursing Care 26-6 (on page 742) for this assessment technique.

Direct Electronic Measurement of Blood Pressure

It is possible to measure blood pressure directly through the insertion of a thin catheter into an artery, most commonly the radial or femoral artery (an arterial line [A-line]) (Burns & Delgado, 2019). The tip of the catheter senses the pressure and transmits this information to a machine that displays the systolic pressure and diastolic pressure in a waveform. This technique is used primarily in intensive care areas.

Guidelines for Nursing Care 26-6

ASSESSING BLOOD PRESSURE USING A DOPPLER ULTRASOUND

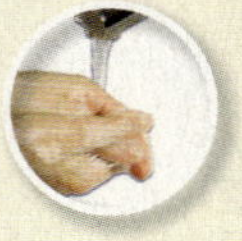

- Perform hand hygiene and put on PPE, if indicated.
- Select the appropriate limb for application of cuff.
- Have the patient assume a comfortable lying or sitting position with the appropriate limb exposed.
- Center the bladder of the cuff over the artery, lining the artery marker on the cuff up with the artery.
- Wrap the cuff around the limb smoothly and snugly, then fasten it. Do not allow any clothing to interfere with the proper placement of the cuff.
- Check that the needle on the aneroid gauge is within the zero mark. If using a mercury manometer, check to see that the manometer is in the vertical position and that the mercury is within the zero level with the gauge at eye level.
- Place a small amount of conducting gel on the Doppler transducer probe.
- Turn the Doppler on.
- Hold the Doppler device in your nondominant hand. Touch the probe lightly to the skin with the probe tip in the gel. Adjust the volume, as needed. Move the probe so it is perpendicular to the skin. Slowly move the Doppler tip around until you hear the pulse.
- Once the pulse is found using the Doppler, close the valve to the sphygmomanometer. Tighten the screw valve on the air pump.
- Inflate the cuff while continuing to use the Doppler on the artery. Note the point on the gauge where the pulse disappears.
- Pump the cuff another 20 to 30 mm Hg.
- Slowly open the valve on the manometer and deflate the cuff and note the reading for the systolic BP when the pulse returns.
- Repeat any suspicious reading, but wait at least 1 minute between readings to allow normal circulation to return in the limb. Deflate the cuff completely between attempts to check the blood pressure.
- Remove the Doppler tip and turn the Doppler off. Wipe excess gel off the patient's skin with tissue. Remove the cuff.
- Wipe off any gel remaining on the Doppler probe with a tissue. Clean the Doppler according to facility policy or manufacturer's recommendations.
- Return the Doppler to the charge base.

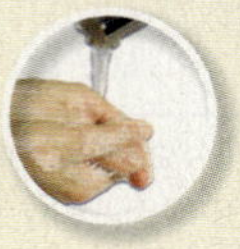

- Remove PPE, if used. Perform hand hygiene.

Source: Adapted from Jensen, S. (2019). *Nursing health assessment. A best practice approach* (3rd ed.). Wolters Kluwer.

Sites for Assessing the Blood Pressure

Although various sites may be used to assess the blood pressure, the brachial artery and the popliteal artery are most commonly used. Equipment has also been developed to measure blood pressure at the forearm; the radial site may be used with individuals who have very large upper arms or who are obese (Muntner et al., 2019). Some patients cannot have blood pressure measured in their upper arms because of obesity and/or various health conditions; blood pressure measurement may be obtained at their ankle (Sheppard et al., 2019). Refer to the accompanying Research in Nursing box addressing the relationship between arm and ankle blood pressure measurements.

ASSESSING BLOOD PRESSURE AT THE BRACHIAL ARTERY

The brachial artery is used most frequently for noninvasive blood pressure monitoring. It is recommended that blood pressure should be checked in each arm at an initial examination and that the arm with the higher blood pressure reading should be used for subsequent measurement (Williams et al., 2018, as cited in Muntner et al., 2019). It has been shown that most people have differences in blood pressure readings between arms. Persistent differences in measurements between arms may indicate coarctation of the aorta or upper extremity arterial obstruction (Muntner et al.). A brachial artery blood pressure assessment should not be taken on an arm with an intravenous line or with an arteriovenous fistula or shunt. Blood pressure assessment should also be avoided in the arm on the side of an axillary node dissection or mastectomy because the pressure may increase the risk of lymphedema developing in the affected arm.

The brachial artery must be palpated to identify its location; the BP cuff is placed on the arm with the center of the bladder length of the cuff in alignment with the brachial pulse. The lower end of the cuff should be 2 to 3 cm (Muntner et al.) above the antecubital fossa, allowing room for placement of the stethoscope.

Skill 26-4 (on pp. 759–763) describes how to assess the blood pressure using the auscultatory method at the brachial artery.

ASSESSING BLOOD PRESSURE AT THE RADIAL ARTERY

The radial artery is used to auscultate the Korotkoff sounds when assessing blood pressure in the forearm. The BP cuff is placed on the forearm and the stethoscope is placed over the radial artery at the wrist. Automated electronic oscillometric wrist monitors have been developed as well. However, evidence is conflicting on correlation of measurements from this site with upper arm measurements and the accuracy of measurements from this site (Arnold & McNaughton, 2018; Muntner et al., 2019). If this site is used, the wrist should be elevated and supported at the level of the heart (Muntner et al., 2019).

Research in Nursing

BRIDGING THE GAP TO EVIDENCE-BASED PRACTICE

Arm versus Leg/Ankle Blood Pressure Measurement

Assessment of vital signs is an important component of assessment in almost every health care setting. Blood pressure measurement is an essential element of this assessment. Standard practice includes obtaining this measurement in the upper arm, with the heart used as the reference for leveling. However, many treatments and health conditions limit the use of the arm for blood pressure measurements. The lower extremities may be considered as an alternative site. What is the relationship between blood pressure measurement in the arm and leg at the ankle? What are the implications of leg/ankle blood pressure measurement?

Sheppard, J. P., Albasri, A., Franssen, M., Fletcher, B., Pealing, L., Roberts, N., Obeid, A., Pucci, M., McManus, R. J., Martin, U., & British and Irish Hypertension Society. (2019). Defining the relationship between arm and leg blood pressure readings: A systematic review and meta-analysis. *Journal of Hypertension, 37*(4), 660–670. https://doi.org/10.1097/HJH.0000000000001958

The objective of this systematic review and meta-analysis was to define the relationship between arm and leg blood pressure to inform the interpretation of leg blood pressure readings in routine clinical practice, in instances when arm readings are not possible. Articles were included in the systematic review if the study measured and reported arm and leg blood pressure measured in the supine position and/or the difference between the two sites. A total of 44 articles were included in the review. Mean values for arm/leg blood pressure difference and confidence intervals or standard deviations were entered into a meta-analysis. Readings taken at the ankle in the supine position were 16 to 18 mm Hg higher than those taken in the arm. The researchers concluded ankle blood pressure measurements and arm blood pressure measurements are not interchangeable, and measurement location must be taken into consideration. Based on the study results, the researchers suggested that, when using ankle measurements rather than measurements taken in the arm, health care providers should consider adding 15 mm Hg to the systolic treatment threshold for hypertension, effectively making the threshold 155/90 mm Hg.

Relevance to Nursing Practice

Blood pressure measurement is a frequently used assessment. It may be necessary to obtain measurements from alternate locations, based on patient circumstances. Location of measurement and circumstances must be documented as well as taken into account when the patient's arms are not available and ankle measurements are considered.

Forearm measurements tend to be higher than the upper arm measurements (Halm, 2014).

This site has been suggested as an alternative for obtaining blood pressure readings for individuals who are obese, as it is often difficult to obtain the appropriately sized cuff for the upper arm, given arm circumference and conical-shaped upper arms common in obesity. The conical shape of the upper arm makes it difficult to fit the cuff to the arm, increasing the likelihood of inaccurate blood pressure measurement (Halm, 2014). Measurement in the forearm is a possible solution to this problem (Muntner et al., 2019; Palatini, 2018).

ASSESSING BLOOD PRESSURE AT THE POPLITEAL ARTERY

When the patient's brachial artery is inaccessible and/or the use of the upper arm is contraindicated, the nurse can assess the blood pressure using the popliteal artery in the leg. The systolic pressure is normally 10 to 40 mm Hg higher at this site than the arm, although the diastolic pressure is the same (Jensen, 2019). The technique for assessment is outlined in Guidelines for Nursing Care 26-7 on page 744.

PALPATING THE BLOOD PRESSURE

Assessing the blood pressure through palpation requires only the use of the sphygmomanometer. The cuff is inflated 30 mm Hg above the point at which the pulsation in the artery disappears. As the air in the cuff is released, the nurse feels for the return of the pulse. Usually, no diastolic pressure is recorded because the artery continues to pulsate as long as blood flows through it.

DIAGNOSING ACTUAL OR POTENTIAL HEALTH PROBLEMS AND NEEDS

The assessment of the patient may lead to the identification of one or more actual or potential health problems and needs related to alterations in vital signs. Following the formulation of the actual or potential health problems and needs, the nurse communicates findings to other nursing and health care professionals through the use of written and spoken word. The written actual or potential health problem or need becomes a permanent part of the patient's health record. Examples of health problems and needs with related etiology and signs and symptoms can be found in Examples of Actual or Potential Health Problems and Needs: Altered Vital Signs (on page 744).

TEACHING VITAL SIGNS FOR SELF-CARE AT HOME

Patients and/or their family members/caregivers often need to check their own temperature, pulse, and/or blood pressure at home. Guidelines for teaching self-assessment are presented in Teaching Tips 26-1 (on pages 745–746).

Guidelines for Nursing Care 26-7

ASSESSING BLOOD PRESSURE AT THE POPLITEAL ARTERY

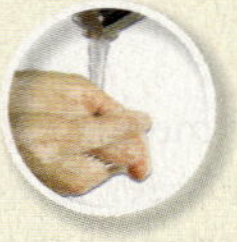

- Perform hand hygiene and put on PPE, if indicated.

- Place the patient in the prone position, if possible. If that position is not possible, place the patient in the supine position, with the knee slightly flexed.
- Use a cuff that is specifically made for this assessment, or one that is large enough to make an accurate assessment.
- Place the cuff around the lower third of the thigh, centered over and 2.5 cm (1 inch) above the popliteal artery, with the bladder over the posterior of the midthigh (see figure).
- Follow the same procedure for auscultation as for the brachial artery.

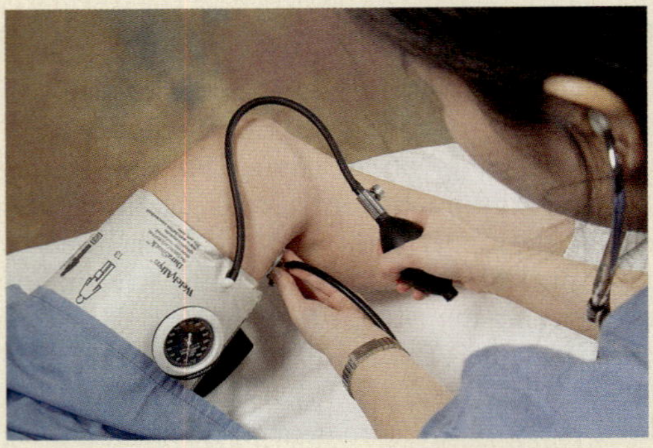

Thigh blood pressure. (*Source:* From Jensen, S. [2019]. *Nursing health assessment. A best practice approach* [3rd ed.]. Wolters Kluwer.)

HBPM refers to regular measurement of BP by an individual in the patient's home or usual environment (Muntner et al., 2019; Stergiou et al., 2018; Whelton et al., 2018). HBPM is being increasingly recommended. Research has shown that readings at home are reliable, are often lower than those taken in a health care provider setting, contribute to better adherence treatment, and provide multiple readings taken over prolonged periods, giving a better picture of the patient's status and response to treatment (Muntner et al., 2019; Stergiou et al., 2018; Whelton et al., 2018). Patient education related to HBPM includes the rationale for its use, as well as steps to obtain an accurate pressure reading. It is important to ensure that an appropriate device is used by the patient (Whelton et al., 2018). Measurements are averaged to identify the mean home BP level. Patients should record readings as directed by their healthcare provider according to the recommended monitoring schedule. Many devices automatically store and average readings, and results can be downloaded or accessed with telemonitoring, eliminating errors related to a lack of or inaccuracy in patient documentation. Suggested guidelines for HBPM include:

- Advising patients to buy validated oscillometric BP monitors that measure BP on the upper arm with an appropriate cuff size (Harvard Medical School, 2020; Stergiou et al., 2018).
- Explaining that home monitoring devices should be checked for accuracy every 1 to 2 years. Readings should be compared with auscultated measurement by a health care provider to ensure accuracy.
- Explaining that frequency of measurement is based on the individual patient's circumstances and intended outcomes.
- When HBPM is used for diagnosing hypertension, explaining that two readings are taken, at least 1 minute apart, while in a sitting position, in both the morning and at night, for a minimum of 3 days, with a preferred period of 7 days (Muntner et al., 2019; Stergiou et al., 2018).
- Instructing the patient to record measurements as directed to show to the health care provider.

Examples of Actual or Potential Health Problems and Needs

ALTERED VITAL SIGNS

Actual or Potential Health Problems and Needs	Possible Etiologic Factors	Potential Signs and Symptoms
Impaired Comfort	Dehydration Illness Infection	Flushed skin, tachycardia, tachypnea, increase in body temperature above normal range, body aches, headache
Altered Tissue Perfusion	Hypertension, smoking, diabetes mellitus	Absent or diminished pulses, blood pressure changes in extremities, capillary refill time >3 seconds, altered skin characteristics
Altered Breathing Pattern	Anxiety, hyperventilation, pain, neurologic impairment	Alterations in rate/rhythm/depth of breathing, dyspnea, pain, cough, use of accessory muscles to breathe, pulse oximetry <93%

Source: Wolters Kluwer. Problem-based care plans. (2020). *In Lippincott Advisor.* Wolters Kluwer. https://advisor.lww.com/lna/home.do

Teaching Tips 26-1

SELF-CARE: MEASURING TEMPERATURE, PULSE, AND BLOOD PRESSURE

Health Topic	Teaching Tips	Why Is This Important?
Measuring Temperature	• Body temperature varies during the day. It is lower in the morning and higher in the evening. It may vary somewhat based on the method used to take the temperature, the person's condition, and the time of day. • Measure temperature the same way every time. • Read the thermometer and write the numbers down on paper. • Clean the thermometer with soap and water, or alcohol. • When reporting temperature measurements to a health care provider, be sure to say which method was used.	If the temperature is very high or low, or if you have any concerns, contact your health care provider. Ensures accuracy and provides accurate information.
Using a Thermometer in the Mouth	• Wait 20 to 30 minutes after drinking or eating to measure oral temperature. • Turn the thermometer on. • Put the thermometer in the mouth and under the tongue in the back. Close the lips around the thermometer. Do not bite down with the teeth. • Listen for the signal or beep. • Remove the thermometer.	Consuming hot or cold foods can affect the reading.
Using a Tympanic Membrane Thermometer	• Turn the thermometer on. • Insert the ear probe snugly into the ear canal using gentle but firm pressure, angling toward the jaw. If the person is younger than 3 years, pull the ear lobe back and down. • Push the button to take the temperature and hold until reading is obtained. • Remove the thermometer.	Using equipment properly ensures accurate measurements.
Using a Temporal Artery Thermometer	• Turn the thermometer on. • Place it firmly against the center of the forehead. • Push the "on" button. Keep the button depressed while taking the temperature. • Slowly slide the thermometer straight across the forehead to the hairline. • Lift the thermometer from the forehead and touch it to the neck just behind the ear lobe. • Release the button.	
Using a Thermometer Under the Arm	• Turn the thermometer on. • Put the thermometer under the arm. • Fold the arm down and across the chest to hold it in place. • Listen for the signal or beep. • Remove the thermometer.	
Measuring the Pulse	• The pulse is often taken before taking certain medications, such as those to make the heartbeat slower or stronger. People who exercise and want to monitor the effect of the exercise on heart function may also take their pulse. • It is necessary to be able to see a watch or a clock with a second hand when taking the pulse. • Place one arm on a firm surface so that the palm is upward. Using the middle three fingers of the other hand, gently feel the outside of the arm just below the wrist with the fingertips. Do not press hard. When pulsations are felt, observe the second hand of the watch or clock and begin to count when the second hand reaches 12 (any number is fine, but it is often easier to remember to always begin counting when the second hand is on 12). Count each pulsation (beat) for 1 minute (when the second hand again reaches 12), and write the number down.	If the pulse is very fast, very slow, or irregular, or if you have any concerns, contact your health care provider.

(continued)

Teaching Tips 26-1 (continued)

SELF-CARE: MEASURING TEMPERATURE, PULSE, AND BLOOD PRESSURE

Health Topic	Teaching Tips	Why Is This Important?
Measuring Blood Pressure	• The blood pressure is often taken to determine how well medications are working to control high blood pressure. The blood pressure is usually checked once a week, or as instructed. Readings may be taken in the morning and evening. A record of blood pressure readings over time is more important than one reading. • Use a validated monitor with an automatic inflation cuff. • Avoid food, caffeine, tobacco, and alcohol for 30 minutes before taking a measurement. • Take your blood pressure before (not after) you eat. • Rest 3 to 5 minutes before taking your blood pressure. • Sit comfortably with your back supported and both feet on the floor (don't cross your legs). • Elevate your arm to heart level on a table or a desk. • Use the proper-sized cuff. It should fit smoothly and snugly around your bare upper arm. There should be enough room to slip a fingertip under the cuff. The bottom edge of the cuff should be 1 inch above the crease of the elbow. • Follow instructions that come with the home device.	Home blood pressure monitoring is the ideal method for monitoring the response to treatment for high blood pressure. If the blood pressure numbers increase or decrease by more than 10, or if you have any concerns, contact your health care provider. Ensures accuracy of readings.

REFLECTIVE PRACTICE LEADING TO PERSONAL LEARNING

Remember that the goal of reflective practice is to look at an experience, understand it, and learn from it. As you begin to develop expertise in assessing patients' vital signs, reflect on your experiences—successes and failures—in order to improve your practice. How can you do it better next time? What did you learn today that can help you tomorrow? Begin your reflection by paying close attention to the following while assessing vital signs and providing nursing care:

- Did your preparation and practice related to the measurement and assessment of vital signs result in your feeling confident in your ability to gather reliable, accurate data? Did your competence and confidence inspire the patient's and family/caregiver's trust?

  How did you prioritize the data you collected? What patterns in the data did you identify?

  What knowledge from your learning, personal experience and intuition did you use to make decisions and develop your plan of care?

- How confident are you that the data you communicated and recorded accurately communicates the health status of the patient? How successfully have you communicated this information to other members of the health care team?
- Were you aware of any cultural and/or ethnic beliefs or practices that may have influenced the health practices and beliefs of patients and/or family members/caregivers related to vital signs? Were you aware of any stereotypes or prejudices that might have negatively influenced the clinical encounter? If so, how did you address these?
- Was the patient/family/caregiver participation in the process at an optimal level? How might you have better engaged the patient and family/caregivers? Did the patient sense that you are respectful, caring, and competent to obtain accurate and relevant data?

Perhaps the most important questions to reflect on are: Are your patients and their families/caregivers better for having had *you* share in the critical responsibility of assessing their health status through assessment of vital signs? Are your patients now receiving thoughtful, person-centered, prioritized, holistic, evidence-based treatment and care because of your efforts?

Skill 26-1 Assessing Body Temperature

Skill Variation: *Assessing Body Temperature Using a Noncontact Infrared Thermometer*

DELEGATION CONSIDERATIONS

Measurement of body temperature may be delegated to assistive personnel (AP) as well as to licensed practical/vocational nurses (LPN/LVNs). The decision to delegate must be based on careful analysis of the patient's needs and circumstances as well as the qualifications of the person to whom the task is being delegated. Refer to the Delegation Guidelines in Appendix A.

EQUIPMENT

- Digital or electronic thermometer, appropriate for site to be used
- Disposable probe covers
- Water-soluble lubricant for rectal temperature measurement
- Nonsterile gloves, if appropriate
- Additional personal protective equipment (PPE), as indicated
- Toilet tissue, if needed
- Electronic record or pen and paper or flow sheet

IMPLEMENTATION

ACTION	RATIONALE
1. Check the prescribed interventions or plan of care for frequency of measurement and route. More frequent temperature measurement may be appropriate based on nursing judgment.	Assessment and measurement of vital signs at appropriate intervals provide important data about the patient's health status.
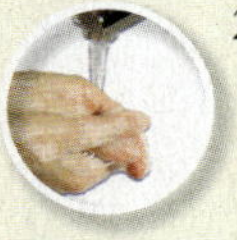 2. Perform hand hygiene and put on PPE, if indicated.	Hand hygiene and PPE prevent the spread of microorganisms. PPE is required based on transmission precautions.
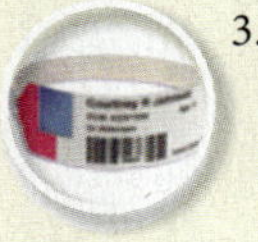 3. Identify the patient.	Identifying the patient ensures that the right patient receives the intervention and helps prevent errors.
4. Close the curtains around the bed and close the door to the room, if possible. Discuss the procedure with the patient and assess the patient's ability to assist with the procedure.	This ensures the patient's privacy. Explanation relieves anxiety and facilitates cooperation. Dialogue encourages patient participation and allows for individualized nursing care.
5. Assemble equipment on the overbed table within reach.	Organization facilitates performance of task.
6. Ensure that the electronic or digital thermometer is in working condition.	Improperly functioning thermometer may not give an accurate reading.
7. Put on gloves, if indicated.	Gloves prevent contact with blood and body fluids. Gloves are usually not required for an oral, axillary, or tympanic temperature measurement, unless contact with blood or body fluids is anticipated. Gloves should be worn for rectal temperature measurement.
8. Select the appropriate site based on assessment data.	This ensures safety and accuracy of measurement.
9. Follow the steps as outlined below for the appropriate type of thermometer.	
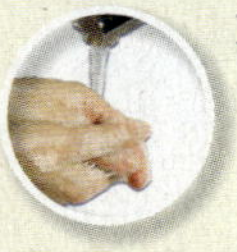 10. When measurement is completed, remove gloves, if worn. Remove additional PPE, if used. Perform hand hygiene.	Proper removal of PPE reduces the risk for infection transmission and contamination of other items. Hand hygiene prevents the spread of microorganisms.
Measuring an Oral Temperature	
11. Remove the electronic unit from the charging unit and remove the probe from within the recording unit.	Electronic unit must be taken into the patient's room to assess the patient's temperature. On some models, the machine is turned on when the probe is removed.

(continued on page 748)

Skill 26-1 Assessing Body Temperature *(continued)*

ACTION	RATIONALE
12. Cover thermometer probe with disposable probe cover, sliding it on until it snaps into place (Figure 1).	Using a cover prevents contamination of the thermometer probe.
13. **Place the probe beneath the patient's tongue in the posterior sublingual pocket (Figure 2). Ask the patient to close their lips around the probe.**	When the probe rests deep in the posterior sublingual pocket, it is in contact with blood vessels lying close to the surface.
14. Continue to hold the probe until you hear a beep (Figure 3). Note the temperature reading.	If left unsupported, the weight of the probe tends to pull it away from the correct location. The probe must remain in the sublingual pocket for the full period of measurement to ensure accurate measurement. The signal indicates that the measurement is completed. The electronic thermometer provides a digital display of the measured temperature.
15. Remove the probe from the patient's mouth. Dispose of the probe cover by holding the probe over an appropriate receptacle and pressing the probe-release button (Figure 4).	Disposing of the probe cover ensures that it will not be reused accidentally on another patient. Proper disposal prevents spread of microorganisms.
16. Return the thermometer probe to the storage place within the unit. Return the electronic unit to the charging unit, if appropriate.	The thermometer needs to be recharged for future use. If necessary, the thermometer should stay on the charger so that it is ready to use at all times.

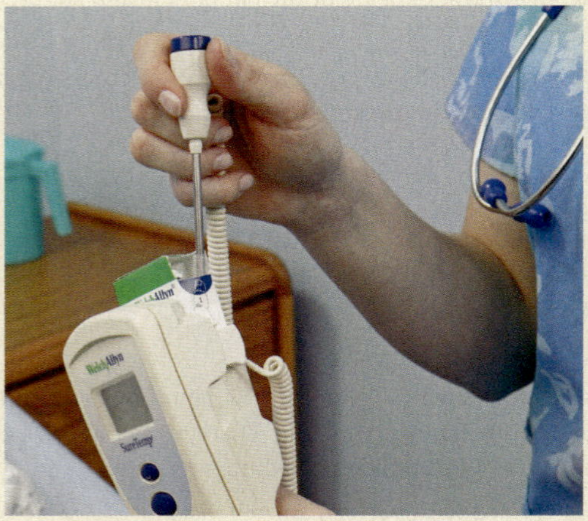

FIGURE 1. Putting probe cover on the thermometer.

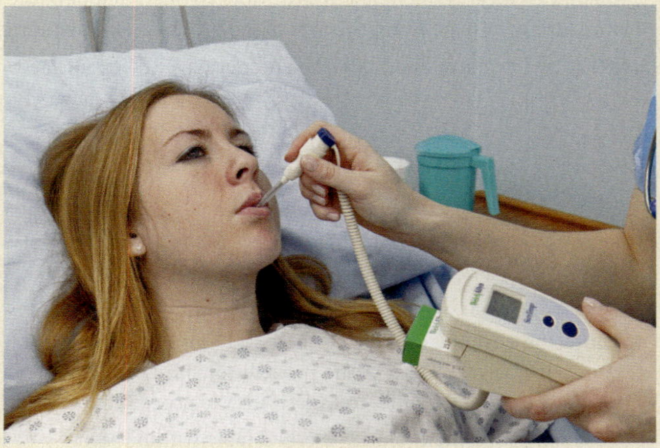

FIGURE 2. Placing thermometer under the tongue in the posterior sublingual pocket.

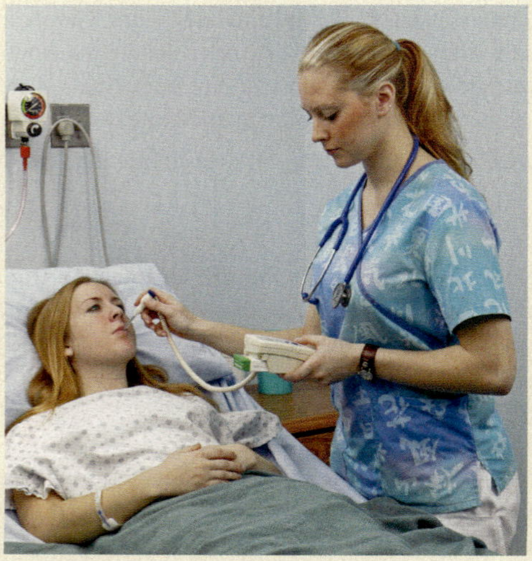

FIGURE 3. Holding probe in the patient's mouth.

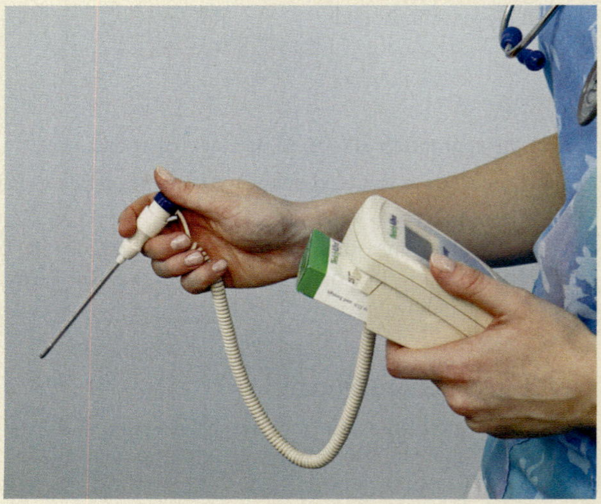

FIGURE 4. Pushing button to dispose of cover.

ACTION | **RATIONALE**

Measuring a Tympanic Membrane Temperature

17. If necessary, push the "ON" button and wait for the "ready" signal on the unit.

For proper function, the thermometer must be turned on and warmed up.

18. Attach the disposable cover onto the tympanic probe (Figure 5).

Use of a disposable cover deters the spread of microorganisms.

19. **Insert the probe snugly into the external ear using gentle but firm pressure, angling the thermometer toward the patient's jaw line. Pull the pinna up and back to straighten the ear canal in an adult (Figure 6).**

If the probe is not inserted correctly, the patient's temperature may be noted as lower than normal.

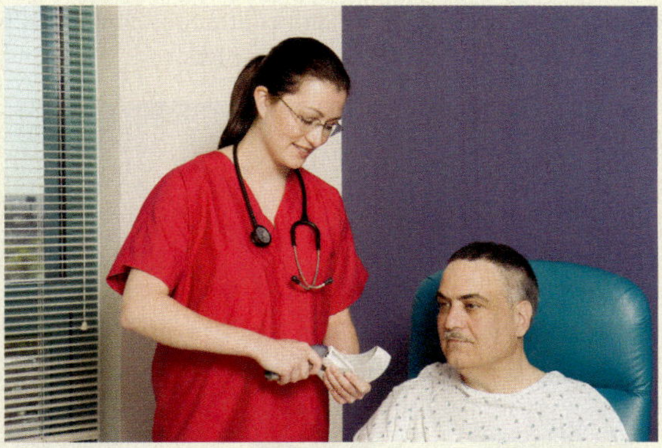

FIGURE 5. Attaching the disposable cover onto the tympanic probe.

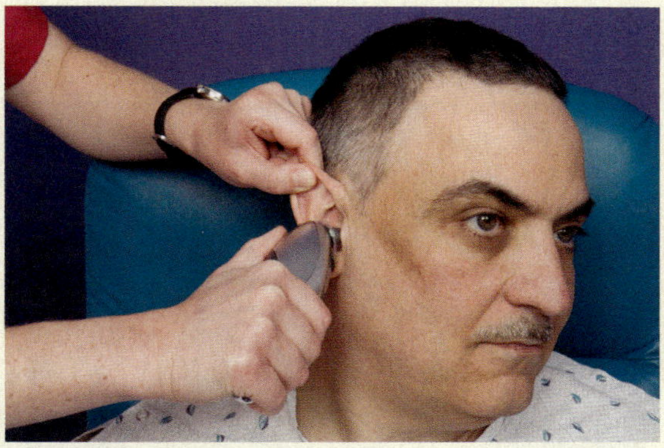

FIGURE 6. Thermometer in patient's ear canal with pinna pulled up and back.

20. Activate the unit by pushing the trigger button. The reading is immediate (usually within 2 seconds). Note the reading.

The digital thermometer must be activated to record the temperature.

21. Discard the probe cover in an appropriate receptacle by pushing the probe-release button or use the rim of cover to remove it from the probe (Figure 7). Replace the thermometer in its charger, if necessary.

Discarding the probe cover ensures that it will not be reused accidentally on another patient. Proper disposal prevents the spread of microorganisms. If necessary, the thermometer should stay on the charger so that it is ready to use at all times.

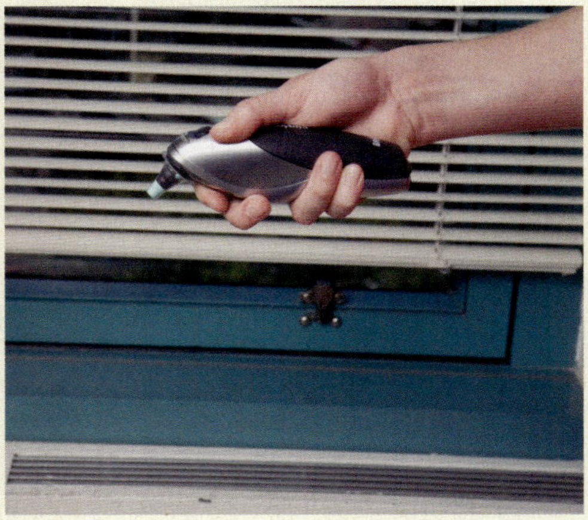

FIGURE 7. Disposing of probe cover.

Measuring Temporal Artery Temperature

If the temporal artery and behind the ear locations are not accessible, the femoral artery, lateral thoracic artery, and axillary sites may be used to assess body temperature using a temporal artery thermometer (Exergen, n.d.b).

22. Brush the patient's hair aside if it is covering the temporal artery area.

Anything covering the area—such as a hat, hair, wigs, or bandages—would insulate the area, resulting in falsely high readings. Measure only the side of the head exposed to the environment.

23. Apply a probe cover.

Using a cover prevents contamination of the thermometer probe.

(*continued on page 750*)

Skill 26-1 Assessing Body Temperature (continued)

ACTION	RATIONALE
24. Hold the thermometer like a remote-control device, with your thumb on the red "ON" button. Place the probe flush on the center of the forehead, with the body of the instrument sideways (not straight up and down) so that it is not in the patient's face (Figure 8).	Allows for easy use of the device and reading of the display. Holding the instrument straight up and down could be intimidating for the patient, particularly young patients and/or those with alterations in mental status.
25. Depress the "ON" button. Keep the button depressed throughout the measurement.	
26. **Slowly slide the probe straight across the forehead, midline, to the hairline, maintaining contact with the skin (Figure 9). Do not move the probe down the side of the face.**	Midline on the forehead, the temporal artery is less than 2 mm below the skin, whereas at the side of the face, the temporal artery is much deeper. Measuring there would result in falsely low readings. Slow movement and continuous contact with the skin are necessary to ensure accurate results.

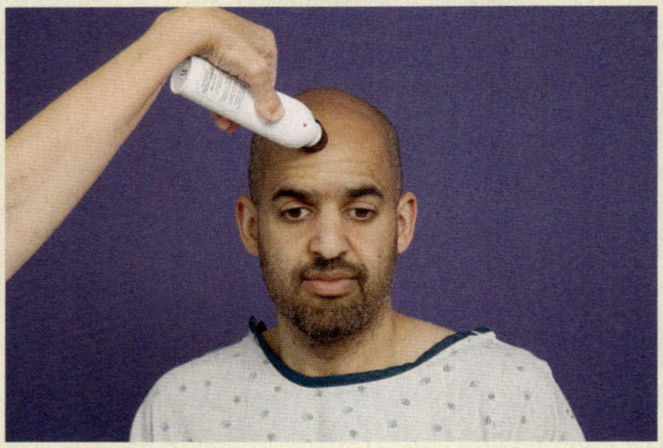

FIGURE 8. Placing the thermometer probe on the center of the forehead.

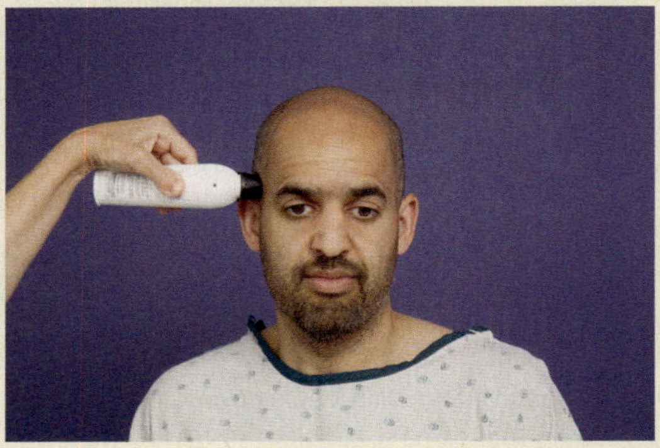

FIGURE 9. Sliding the probe across the forehead to the hairline.

ACTION	RATIONALE
27. If required, based on specific thermometer in use, brush hair aside if it is covering the ear, exposing the area of the neck under the ear lobe. Keeping the button depressed, lift the probe from the forehead and touch on the neck just behind the ear lobe, in the depression just below the mastoid (Figure 10).	Sweat causes evaporative cooling of the skin on the forehead, possibly leading to a falsely low reading. During diaphoresis, the area on the head behind the ear lobe exhibits high blood flow necessary for the arterial measurement; it is a double check for the thermometer (Exergen, n.d.a).

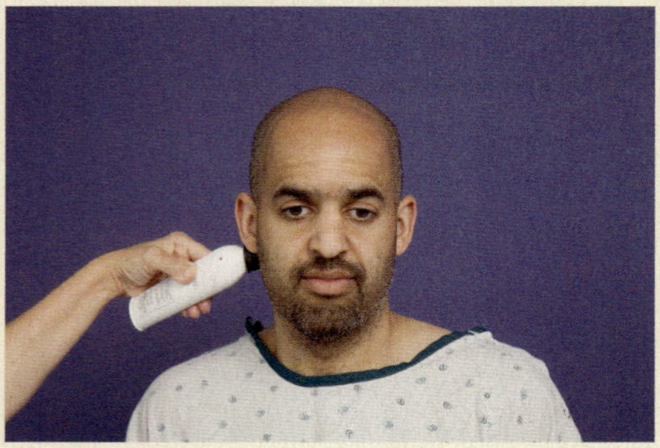

FIGURE 10. Touching the probe behind the ear.

ACTION	RATIONALE
28. Release the button and read the thermometer measurement.	
29. Hold the thermometer over a waste receptacle. Gently push the probe cover with your thumb against the proximal edge to dispose of the probe cover.	Discarding the probe cover ensures that it will not be reused accidentally on another patient.
30. The instrument will automatically turn off in 30 seconds, or press and release the power button.	Turns thermometer off.

Measuring Axillary Temperature

ACTION	RATIONALE
31. Remove the probe from the recording unit of the electronic thermometer. Place a disposable probe cover on by sliding it on and snapping it securely.	Using a cover prevents contamination of the thermometer probe.

ACTION | **RATIONALE**

32. Move the patient's clothing to expose only the axilla (Figure 11).

The axilla must be exposed for placement of the thermometer. Exposing only the axilla keeps the patient warm and maintains their dignity.

33. **Place the end of the probe in the center of the axilla (Figure 12). Have the patient bring the arm down and close to the body.** Hold the patient's arm by the patient's side until the measurement is complete.

The deepest area of the axilla provides the most accurate measurement; surrounding the bulb with skin surface provides a more reliable measurement.

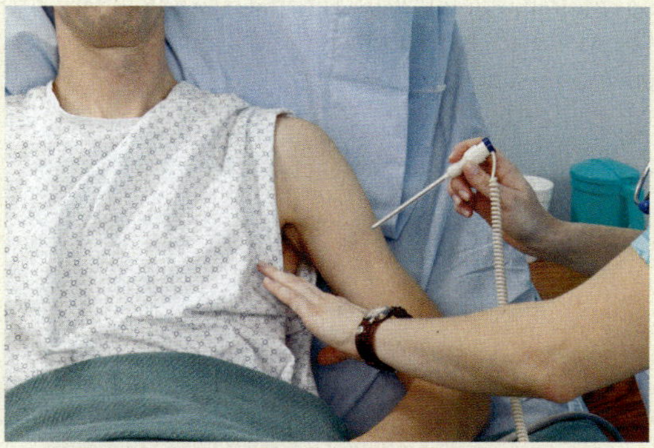

FIGURE 11. Exposing axilla to assess temperature.

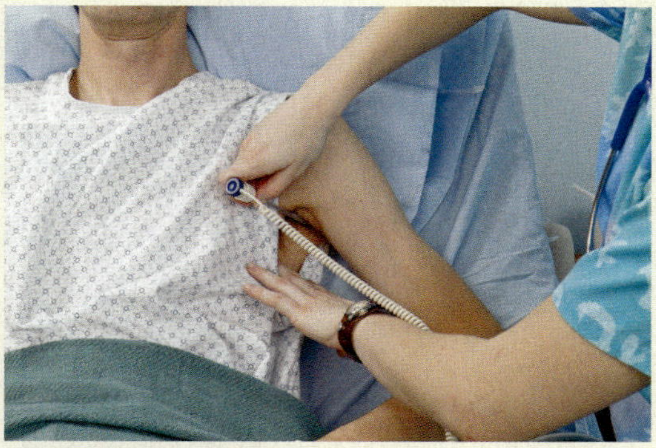

FIGURE 12. Placing thermometer in the center of the axilla.

34. Hold the probe in place until you hear a beep, and then carefully remove the probe. Note the temperature reading.

Axillary thermometers must be held in place to obtain an accurate temperature.

35. Cover the patient and help them to a position of comfort.

This ensures patient comfort.

36. Dispose of the probe cover by holding the probe over an appropriate waste receptacle and pushing the release button.

Discarding the probe cover ensures that it will not be reused accidentally on another patient.

37. Place the bed in the lowest position and elevate rails, as needed. Leave the patient clean and comfortable.

Low bed position and elevated side rails provide for patient safety.

38. Return the electronic thermometer to the charging unit.

The thermometer needs to be recharged for future use.

Measuring Rectal Temperature

39. Adjust the bed to a comfortable working height (VHACEOSH, 2016). Put on nonsterile gloves.

Having the bed at the proper height prevents back and muscle strain. Gloves prevent contact with contaminants and body fluids.

40. Assist the patient to a side-lying position. Pull back the covers sufficiently to expose only the buttocks. Position a young infant supine with legs flexed (Kyle & Carmen, 2021).

The side-lying position allows the nurse to see the buttocks. Exposing only the buttocks keeps the patient warm and maintains their dignity. Rectal temperatures are not normally taken in newborns, infants, and young children (Jensen, 2019; Silbert-Flagg & Pillitteri, 2018), but may be indicated. Refer to the Special Considerations section at the end of the skill.

41. Remove the rectal probe from within the recording unit of the electronic thermometer. Cover the probe with a disposable probe cover, sliding it on until it snaps in place (Figure 13).

Using a cover prevents contamination of the thermometer.

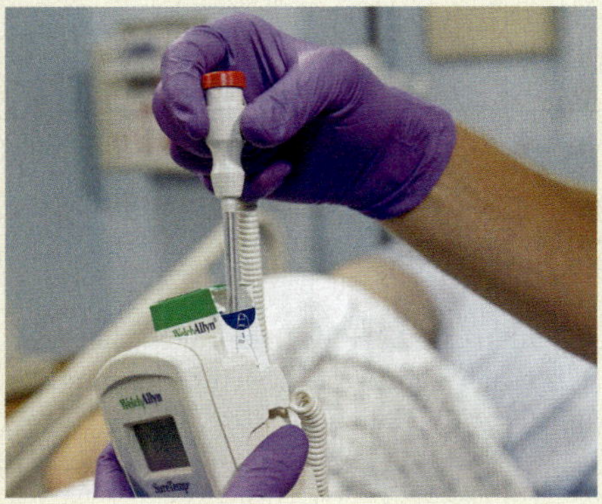

FIGURE 13. Removing appropriate probe and attaching disposable probe cover.

(continued on page 752)

Skill 26-1 Assessing Body Temperature *(continued)*

ACTION	RATIONALE
42. **Lubricate about 1 inch of the probe with a water-soluble lubricant (Figure 14).**	Lubrication reduces friction and facilitates insertion, minimizing the risk of irritation or injury to the rectal mucous membranes.
43. Reassure the patient. Separate the buttocks until the anal sphincter is clearly visible.	If not placed directly into the anal opening, the thermometer probe may injure adjacent tissue or cause discomfort.
44. **Insert the thermometer probe into the anus about 1.5 inches in an adult or no more than 1 inch in children (Figure 15)** (Kyle & Carmen, 2021).	Depth of insertion must be adjusted based on the patient's age. Rectal temperatures are not normally taken in newborns, infants, and young children (Jensen, 2019; Silbert-Flagg & Pillitteri, 2018), but may be indicated. Refer to the Special Considerations section at the end of the skill.

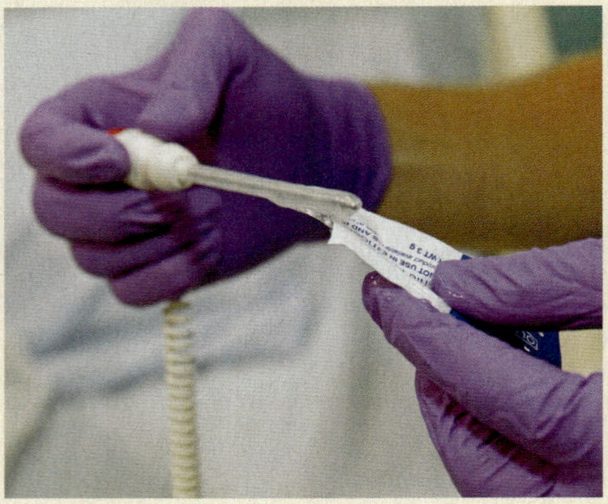

FIGURE 14. Lubricating thermometer tip.

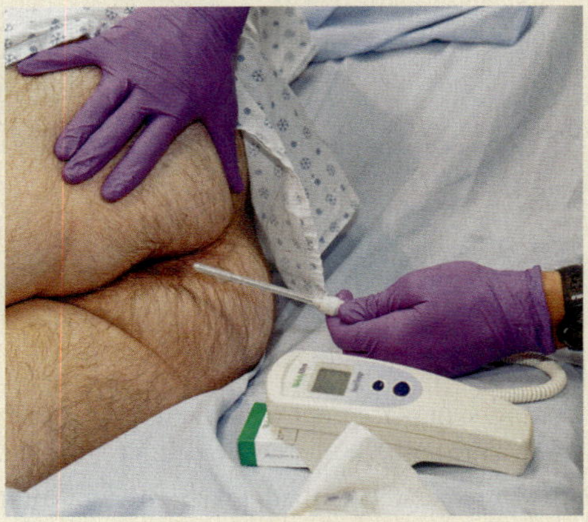

FIGURE 15. Inserting thermometer into the anus.

ACTION	RATIONALE
45. Hold the probe in place until you hear a beep, then carefully remove the probe. Note the temperature reading on the display.	If left unsupported, movement of the probe in the rectum could cause injury and/or discomfort. The signal indicates that the measurement is completed. The electronic thermometer provides a digital display of the measured temperature.
46. Dispose of the probe cover by holding the probe over an appropriate waste receptacle and pressing the release button.	Proper probe cover disposal reduces risk of microorganism transmission.
47. Using toilet tissue, wipe the anus of any feces or excess lubricant. Dispose of the toilet tissue. Remove gloves and discard them. Perform hand hygiene.	Wiping promotes cleanliness. Disposing of the toilet tissue avoids transmission of microorganisms.
48. Cover the patient and help them to a position of comfort.	This ensures patient comfort.
49. Place the bed in the lowest position; elevate rails as needed.	These actions provide for the patient's safety.
50. Perform hand hygiene.	Hand hygiene prevents the spread of microorganisms.
51. Return the thermometer to the charging unit.	The thermometer needs to be recharged for future use.

DOCUMENTATION

Guidelines

Record temperature in the electronic record or flow sheet. Communicate abnormal findings to the appropriate person. Identify the site of assessment used if other than oral.

Sample Documentation

Lippincott DocuCare **Practice documenting body temperature and other vital signs in *Lippincott DocuCare.***

10/20/25 Tympanic temperature assessed. Temperature 102.5°F. Patient states she has "a pounding" headache; denies chills, malaise. Physician notified. Received order to give 650 mg PO acetaminophen now. Incentive spirometer × 10 q 2 hours.

—M. Evans, RN

DEVELOPING CLINICAL REASONING AND CLINICAL JUDGMENT

UNEXPECTED SITUATIONS AND ASSOCIATED INTERVENTIONS

- *Temperature reading is higher or lower than expected based on your assessment:* Reassess temperature with a different thermometer. The thermometer may not be calibrated correctly. If using a tympanic thermometer, improper positioning of the probe can contribute to errors (Jensen, 2019).
- *During rectal temperature assessment, the patient reports feeling light-headed or passes out:* Remove the thermometer immediately. Quickly assess the patient's blood pressure and heart rate. Vagal stimulation during insertion of the probe may cause reduction in the patient's heart rate (Jensen, 2019). Notify the health care provider. Do not attempt to take another rectal temperature on this patient.

SPECIAL CONSIDERATIONS

General Considerations

- Glass thermometers with mercury-filled bulbs are not used in health care institutions to measure body temperature due to federal safety recommendations (U.S. Environmental Protection Agency [EPA], n.d.).
- If the patient smoked, chewed gum, or consumed hot or cold food or fluids recently, wait 15 minutes before taking an oral temperature to allow the oral tissues to return to baseline temperature (Mayo Clinic, 2020a).
- Nasal oxygen is not thought to affect oral temperature readings. Do not assess oral temperatures in patients receiving oxygen by mask. Removal of the mask for the time period required for assessment could result in a serious drop in the patient's blood oxygen level.
- When using a tympanic thermometer, make sure to insert the probe into the ear canal sufficiently tightly to seal the opening to ensure an accurate reading.
- A dirty probe lens and cone on the temporal artery thermometer can cause a falsely low reading. If the lens is not shiny in appearance, clean the lens with an alcohol swab or gauze moistened in alcohol (Exergen, n.d.b).
- If the temporal artery and behind the ear locations are not accessible, the femoral artery, lateral thoracic artery, and axilla sites may be used to assess body temperature using a temporal artery thermometer (Exergen, n.d.b).
- If the patient's axilla has been washed recently, wait 15 to 30 minutes before taking an axillary temperature to allow the skin to return to baseline temperature.

Infant and Child Considerations

- Pull the pinna back and down when measuring tympanic temperature on a child younger than 3 years of age. For children older than 3 years of age, there is no need to manipulate the pinna (Kyle & Carman, 2021).
- Small children have a limited attention span and difficulty keeping their lips closed long enough to obtain an accurate oral temperature reading. Based on an assessment of the child's ability to cooperate, it may be more appropriate to use the temporal or tympanic site.
- For children under 3 months (90 days) old, the axillary method is safest and is good for screening (Seattle Children's, 2022). If the axillary temperature is above 99 F, recheck with a rectal measurement. The rectal or temporal method should be used for children 3 months to 4 years old; the tympanic method can be used after 6 months of age (Seattle Children's, 2022). In children age 4 years or older, it is safe to measure temperature orally, in addition to tympanic and axillary methods (Seattle Children's, 2022).

(*continued on page 754*)

Skill 26-1 Assessing Body Temperature *(continued)*

Community-Based Care Considerations

- Teach patients who use electronic or digital thermometers to clean the probe after use to prevent transmission of microorganisms among family members/caregivers. Clean according to the manufacturer's directions.
- Patients may still be using glass mercury thermometers at home. Encourage patients to use alternative devices, such as digital thermometers.
- Teach patients using nonmercury glass thermometers to clean the thermometer after use in lukewarm soapy water and rinse in cool water. Store it in an appropriate place to prevent breakage and injury from the glass. Encourage patients to use alternative devices, such as digital thermometers.
- Teach patients that glass thermometers should never be used to take a temperature for a person who is unconscious or for infants and young children.
- Pacifier thermometers are not recommended for use (Mayo Clinic, 2020).

Skill Variation Assessing Body Temperature Using a Noncontact Infrared Thermometer

Noncontact infrared (IFR) thermometers measure body temperature by capturing the heat emitted by the skin over body surfaces at various locations. Comparisons of noncontact IFR thermometer measurements with tympanic, temporal artery, and axillary body temperature measurement have resulted in inconsistent findings related to accuracy of measurements (Aw, 2020; Berksoy et al., 2018; Franconi et al., 2018; Wang et al., 2013). As a result, this method of temperature measurement has been suggested for possible use as screening for fever, not for ongoing monitoring of body temperature (Aw, 2020; Bayhan et al., 2014; Berksoy et al., 2018; Canadian Agency for Drugs and Technologies in Health, 2014). Locations recommended for use for measurement include over the forehead (temporal artery), the neck (carotid artery), umbilicus, axilla, and nape of the neck (Berksoy et al., 2018; U.S. FDA, 2020a; Wang et al., 2013). **Proper use of the noncontact thermometer is essential to achieve as accurate measurement as possible and prevent inaccurate measurement** (U.S. FDA, 2020a).

1. Ensure the noncontact IFR thermometer has been exposed to the testing environment or room for 10 to 30 minutes prior to use to allow the thermometer to adjust to the environment.
2. Refer to Steps 1–8 in Skill 26-1.
3. Follow specific manufacturer instructions for use.
4. Use in a draft-free space that is out of direct sun and away from radiant heat sources (U.S. FDA, 2020a).
5. The patient's forehead should not be blocked or covered during measurement.
6. Clean and dry the patient's forehead.
7. Power the thermometer on.
8. Change mode setting, if necessary, based on thermometer features, to "Body."

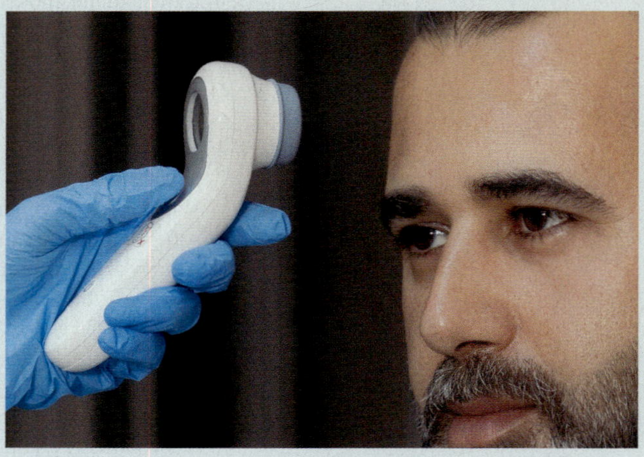

FIGURE A. Holding the device perpendicular from the patient's forehead. (*Source:* Used with permission from iStock. *Photo by ozgurdonmaz.*)

9. Hold the device perpendicular and 1 to 2 inches from the patient's forehead, or the distance recommended by the manufacturer (Figure A).
10. Press the "Scan" button. Measurement is almost instantaneous; note temperature measurement.
11. If a repeat measurement is necessary, follow the manufacturer's directions for the appropriate time interval between readings.

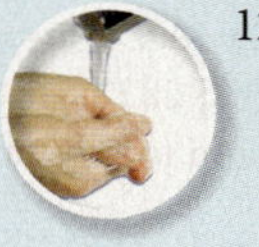

12. When measurement is completed, remove gloves, if worn. Remove additional PPE, if used. Perform hand hygiene.

Skill 26-2 Assessing a Peripheral Pulse by Palpation

DELEGATION CONSIDERATIONS

The measurement of the radial and brachial peripheral pulses may be delegated to assistive personnel (AP). The measurement of peripheral pulses may be delegated to licensed practical/vocational nurses (LPN/LVNs). The decision to delegate must be based on careful analysis of the patient's needs and circumstances as well as the qualifications of the person to whom the task is being delegated. Refer to the Delegation Guidelines in Appendix A.

EQUIPMENT

- Watch with second hand or digital readout
- Electronic record or pen and paper or flow sheet
- Nonsterile gloves, if appropriate; additional PPE, as indicated

IMPLEMENTATION

ACTION	RATIONALE
1. Check prescribed interventions or plan of care for frequency of pulse assessment. More frequent pulse measurement may be appropriate based on nursing judgment.	Assessment and measurement of vital signs at appropriate intervals provide important data about the patient's health status.
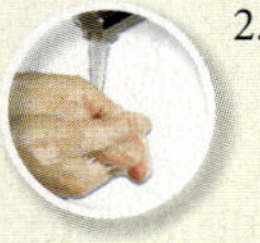 2. Perform hand hygiene and put on PPE, if indicated.	Hand hygiene and PPE prevent the spread of microorganisms. PPE is required based on transmission precautions.
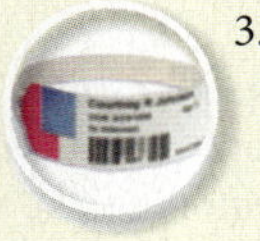 3. Identify the patient.	Identifying the patient ensures the right patient receives the intervention and helps prevent errors.
4. Close the curtains around the bed and close the door to the room, if possible. Discuss the procedure with the patient and assess the patient's ability to assist with the procedure.	This ensures the patient's privacy. Explanation relieves anxiety and facilitates cooperation.
5. Put on gloves, if indicated.	Gloves are not usually worn to obtain a pulse measurement unless contact with blood or body fluids is anticipated. Gloves prevent contact with blood and body fluids.
6. Select the appropriate peripheral site based on assessment data.	This ensures safety and accuracy of measurement.
7. Move the patient's clothing to expose only the site chosen.	The site must be exposed for pulse assessment. Exposing only the site keeps the patient warm and maintains their dignity.
8. Place your first, second, and third fingers over the artery (Figure 1). Place your fingers over the artery so that the ends of your fingers are flat against the patient's skin when palpating peripheral pulses. Do not press with the tip of the fingers only. **Lightly compress the artery so pulsations can be felt and counted.**	The sensitive fingertips can feel the pulsation of the artery.

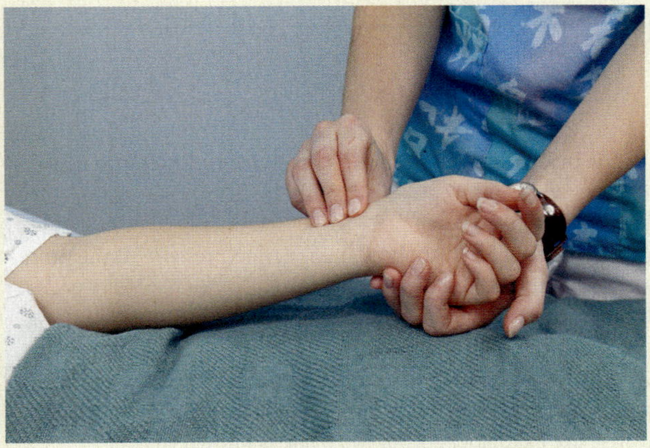

FIGURE 1. Placing fingers over the artery.

(*continued on page 756*)

Skill 26-2 Assessing a Peripheral Pulse by Palpation *(continued)*

ACTION	RATIONALE
9. Using a watch with a second hand, count the number of pulsations felt for 30 seconds (Figure 2). Multiply this number by 2 to calculate the rate for 1 minute. **If the rate, rhythm, or amplitude of the pulse is abnormal in any way, palpate and count the pulse for 1 minute.**	Ensures accuracy of measurement and assessment.

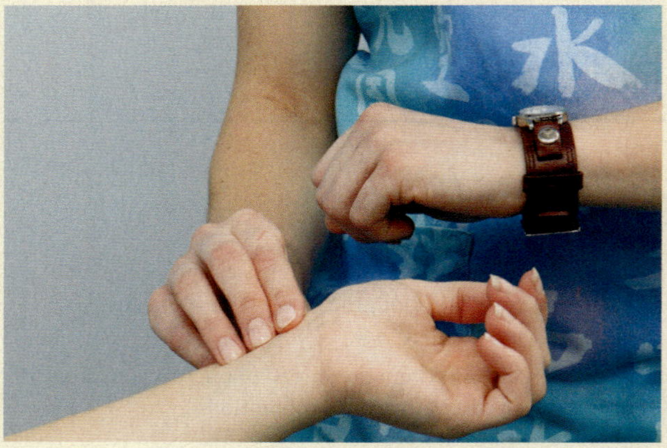

FIGURE 2. Counting the pulse.

ACTION	RATIONALE
10. Note the rhythm and amplitude of the pulse, as well as the elasticity of the blood vessel.	This provides additional assessment data regarding the patient's cardiovascular status.
11. When measurement is completed, remove gloves, if worn. Perform hand hygiene. Cover the patient and help them to a position of comfort.	Proper removal of gloves reduces the risk for infection transmission and contamination of other items. Hand hygiene prevents the spread of microorganisms. Covering and positioning the patient ensures patient comfort.
12. Remove additional PPE, if used. Perform hand hygiene.	Proper removal of PPE reduces the risk for infection transmission and contamination of other items. Hand hygiene prevents the spread of microorganisms.

DOCUMENTATION

Guidelines

Record pulse rate, strength, rhythm and elasticity in the electronic record or flow sheet. Identify site of assessment. Communicate abnormal findings to the primary care provider.

Sample Documentation

Lippincott DocuCare **Practice documenting pulse and other vital signs in *Lippincott DocuCare.***

2/6/125 1000 Pulses 84, regular, 2+, normal elasticity; equal bilaterally in radial, popliteal, and dorsalis pedis sites.

—M. Evans, RN

DEVELOPING CLINICAL REASONING AND CLINICAL JUDGMENT

UNEXPECTED SITUATIONS AND ASSOCIATED INTERVENTIONS

- *The pulse is irregular:* Monitor the pulse for a full minute. If the pulse is difficult to assess, validate pulse measurement by taking the apical pulse for 1 minute. If this is a change for the patient, notify the primary care provider.
- *The pulse is palpated easily, but then disappears:* Apply only moderate pressure to the pulse. Applying too much pressure may obliterate the pulse.
- *You cannot palpate a pulse:* Use a portable Doppler ultrasound to assess the pulse. If this is a change in assessment or if you cannot find the pulse using a Doppler ultrasound, notify the primary care provider. If you can find the pulse using a Doppler ultrasound, place a small X over the spot where the pulse is located, based on facility policy. This can make palpating the pulse easier because the exact location of the pulse is known.

SPECIAL CONSIDERATIONS

General Considerations

- The normal heart rate varies by age.
- The carotid pulse should be palpated only in the lower third of the neck to avoid stimulation of the carotid sinus (Jensen, 2019, p. 95). When palpating a carotid pulse, lightly press only one side of the neck at a time. Never attempt to palpate both carotid arteries at the same time. Bilateral palpation could result in reduced cerebral blood flow and cause the patient to lose consciousness (Jensen, 2019).
- If a peripheral pulse is difficult to assess accurately because it is irregular, feeble, or extremely rapid, assess the apical rate.

Infant and Child Considerations

- In children younger than 2 years of age, auscultate an apical pulse rate (refer to the Guidelines for Nursing Care 26-3 on page 731) (Jarvis & Eckhardt, 2020; Kyle & Carmen, 2021).
- In children older than age 2 years, use the radial site for pulse assessment and count for 1 minute (Jarvis & Eckhardt, 2020; Kyle & Carmen, 2021).
- Measure the apical rate if the child has a cardiac problem or congenital heart defect (see Guidelines for Nursing Care 26-3 on page 731).

Community-Based Care Considerations

- Teach the patient and family members/caregivers how to take the patient's pulse, if appropriate.
- Inform the patient and family/caregivers about digital pulse monitoring devices.
- Teach family members/caregivers how to locate and monitor peripheral pulse sites, if appropriate.

Skill 26-3 ▶ Assessing Respiration

DELEGATION CONSIDERATIONS

The measurement of respirations may be delegated to assistive personnel (AP) as well as to licensed practical/vocational nurses (LPN/LVNs). The decision to delegate must be based on careful analysis of the patient's needs and circumstances as well as the qualifications of the person to whom the task is being delegated. Refer to the Delegation Guidelines in Appendix A.

EQUIPMENT

- Watch with second hand or digital readout
- Electronic record or pen and paper or flow sheet
- PPE, as indicated

IMPLEMENTATION

ACTION	RATIONALE
1. **While your fingers are still in place for the pulse measurement, after counting the pulse rate, observe the patient's respirations (Figure 1).**	The patient may alter the rate of respirations if they are aware they are being counted (Hill et al., 2018).

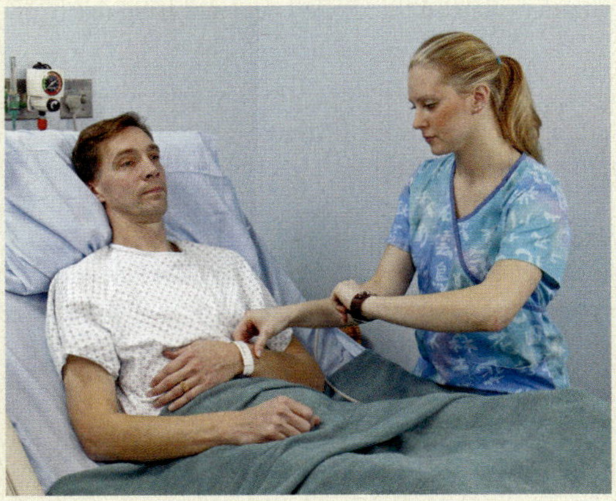

FIGURE 1. Assessing respirations.

(continued on page 758)

Skill 26-3 Assessing Respiration *(continued)*

ACTION	RATIONALE
2. Note the rise and fall of the patient's chest.	A complete cycle of an inspiration and an expiration composes one respiration.
3. Using a watch with a second hand, count the number of respirations for 30 seconds. Multiply this number by 2 to calculate the respiratory rate per minute. **Avoid counting for a 15-second interval.**	Sufficient time is necessary to observe the rate, depth, and other characteristics (Hill et al., 2018; Jarvis & Eckhardt, 2020). Use of a 15-second interval and multiplying by 4 can result in a respiratory count that is significantly incorrect (Hill et al., 2018; Jarvis & Eckhardt, 2020). Some literature suggests 60-second counts should be implemented whenever possible to ensure accuracy (Kallioinen et al., 2017).
4. **If respirations are abnormal in any way, count the respirations for at least 1 full minute** (Jarvis & Eckhardt, 2020).	Increased time allows the detection of unequal timing between respirations.
5. Note the depth and rhythm of the respirations.	This provides additional assessment data regarding the patient's respiratory status (Jarvis & Eckhardt, 2020).
6. When measurement is completed, remove gloves, if worn. Perform hand hygiene. Cover the patient and help them to a position of comfort.	Proper removal of gloves reduces the risk for infection transmission and contamination of other items. Hand hygiene prevents the spread of microorganisms. Covering and positioning the patient ensures patient comfort.
7. Remove additional PPE, if used. Perform hand hygiene.	Proper removal of PPE reduces the risk for infection transmission and contamination of other items. Hand hygiene deters the spread of microorganisms.

DOCUMENTATION

Guidelines

Document respiratory rate, depth, and rhythm on electronic record or flow sheet. Communicate any abnormal findings to the appropriate person.

Sample Documentation

Lippincott DocuCare Practice documenting respiration and other vital signs in *Lippincott DocuCare.*

10/23/25 0830 Patient breathing at a rate of 16 respirations per minute. Respirations regular and unlabored.

—M. Evans, RN

DEVELOPING CLINICAL REASONING AND CLINICAL JUDGMENT

UNEXPECTED SITUATIONS AND ASSOCIATED INTERVENTIONS

- *The patient is breathing with such shallow respirations that you cannot count the rate:* Sometimes it is easier to count respirations by auscultating the lung sounds. Auscultate lung sounds and count respirations for 30 seconds. Multiply by 2 to calculate the respiratory rate per minute. If the respiratory rate is irregular, count for a full minute. Notify the primary health care provider of the respiratory rate and the shallowness and irregularity of the respirations.

SPECIAL CONSIDERATIONS

- If respiratory rate or depth is irregular, count respirations for 1 minute.
- If respirations are very shallow and difficult to detect, observe the sternal notch, where respiration is more apparent.
- If respirations are difficult to detect, such as with patients who are obese or with children, place a hand on the upper chest or abdomen to feel the respiratory rate (Jarvis & Eckhardt, 2020). Alternatively, place a hand on the patient's shoulder to feel the respiratory rate (Jensen, 2019).

General Considerations

- If respiratory rate or depth is irregular, count respirations for 1 minute.
- If respirations are very shallow and difficult to detect, observe the sternal notch, where respiration is more apparent.
- If respirations are difficult to detect, such as with patients who are obese or with children, place a hand on the upper chest or abdomen to feel the respiratory rate (Jarvis & Eckhardt, 2020). Alternatively, place a hand on the patient's shoulder to feel the respiratory rate (Jensen, 2019).

Infant and Child Considerations

- For infants and children, count respirations for 1 full minute to ensure accuracy (Kyle & Carmen, 2021).
- Infants' respirations are primarily diaphragmatic; count abdominal movements to assess respiratory rate for infants (Jensen, 2019; Kyle & Carmen, 2021).
- Count thoracic movements to assess respiratory rate for infants and children older than 1 year of age (Kyle & Carmen, 2021).
- Assess respirations before taking the temperature so that the child is not crying, which would alter the respiratory status.
- Assess respirations in infants and children when the child is resting or sitting quietly, because respiratory rate often changes when infants or young children cry, feed, or become more active. The most accurate respiratory rate is obtained when the infant or child is at rest (Jensen, 2019; Kyle & Carmen, 2021).

Skill 26-4 Assessing Blood Pressure Using an Automated, Electronic Oscillometric Device

DELEGATION CONSIDERATIONS

The measurement of brachial artery blood pressure may be delegated to assistive personnel (AP) as well as to licensed practical/vocational nurses (LPN/LVNs). The decision to delegate must be based on careful analysis of the patient's needs and circumstances as well as the qualifications of the person to whom the task is being delegated. Refer to the Delegation Guidelines in Appendix A.

EQUIPMENT

- Blood pressure cuff of appropriate size
- Automated, electronic oscillometric blood pressure device
- Electronic record or pen and paper or flow sheet
- PPE, as indicated

IMPLEMENTATION

ACTION	RATIONALE
1. Check the prescribed interventions or plan of care for frequency of blood pressure measurement. More frequent measurement may be appropriate based on nursing judgment.	Provides for patient safety.
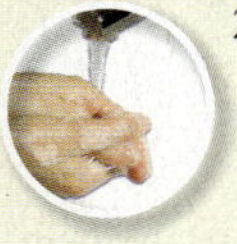 2. Perform hand hygiene and put on PPE, if indicated.	Hand hygiene and PPE prevent the spread of microorganisms. PPE is required based on transmission precautions.
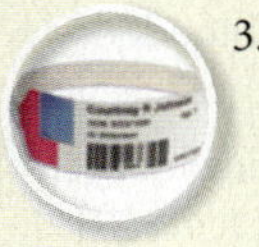 3. Identify the patient.	Identifying the patient ensures the right patient receives the intervention and helps prevent errors.

(continued on page 760)

Skill 26-4 Assessing Blood Pressure Using an Automated, Electronic Oscillometric Device *(continued)*

ACTION	RATIONALE
4. Close the curtains around the bed and close the door to the room, if possible. Discuss the procedure with the patient and assess patient's ability to assist with the procedure. Validate that the patient has relaxed for several minutes.	This ensures the patient's privacy. Explanation relieves anxiety and facilitates cooperation. Activity immediately before measurement can result in inaccurate results.
5. Put on gloves, if indicated.	Gloves prevent contact with blood and body fluids. Gloves are usually not required for measurement of blood pressure, unless contact with blood or body fluids is anticipated.
6. Select the appropriate arm (or alternate site) for measurement and blood pressure cuff (refer to Table 26-8 on page 738).	Decision on measurement site and cuff size is based on nurse's assessment of individual patient circumstances. Incorrect cuff size contributes to the most frequent error in measurement in nonacute care settings (Muntner et al., 2019).
7. Have the patient assume a comfortable lying or sitting position with the forearm supported at the level of the heart and the palm of the hand upward (Figure 1). If the measurement is taken in the supine position, support the arm with a pillow. In the sitting position, support the arm yourself or by using the bedside table. If the patient is sitting, have the patient sit back in the chair so that the chair supports their back. In addition, make sure the patient keeps the legs uncrossed.	The position of the arm can have a major influence when the blood pressure is measured; if the upper arm is below the level of the right atrium, the readings will be too high. If the arm is above the level of the heart, the readings will be too low (Muntner et al., 2019; Pickering et al., 2005). This position places the brachial artery on the inner aspect of the elbow so that the bell or diaphragm of the stethoscope can rest on it easily. Support for the patient's arm prevents isometric exercise that will affect the blood pressure level (Muntner et al., 2019). If the back is not supported, the diastolic pressure may be elevated falsely; if the legs are crossed, the systolic pressure may be elevated falsely (Muntner et al., 2019; Pickering et al., 2005).

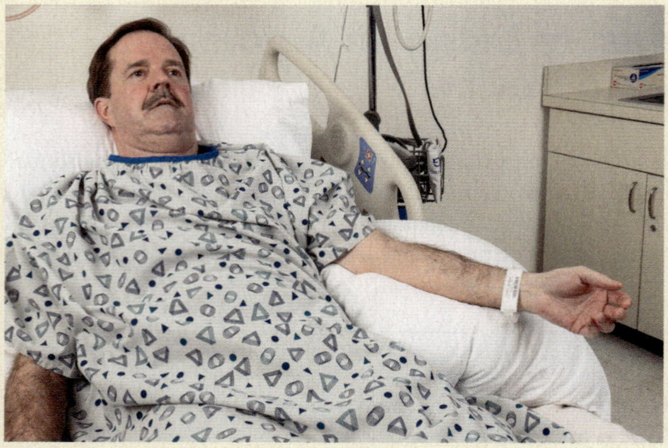

FIGURE 1. Proper positioning for blood pressure assessment using brachial artery.

ACTION	RATIONALE
8. Expose the brachial artery by removing garments or move a sleeve if it is not too tight, above the area where the cuff will be placed.	Clothing over the artery interferes with the ability to hear sounds and can cause inaccurate blood pressure readings. A tight sleeve would cause congestion of blood and possibly inaccurate readings (Muntner et al., 2019).
9. Palpate the location of the brachial artery. Center the bladder of the cuff over the brachial artery, about midway on the upper arm, so that the lower edge of the cuff is about 2.5 to 5 cm (1 to 2 inches) above the inner aspect of the elbow (Figure 2). **Line up the artery marking on the cuff with the patient's brachial artery.** The tubing should extend from the edge of the cuff nearer the patient's elbow (Figure 3).	Pressure in the cuff applied directly to the artery provides the most accurate readings. If the cuff gets in the way of the stethoscope, readings are likely to be inaccurate. A cuff placed upside down with the tubing toward the patient's head may give a false reading.
10. Wrap the cuff around the arm smoothly and snugly, and fasten it (Figure 4). Do not allow any clothing to interfere with the proper placement of the cuff.	A smooth cuff and snug wrapping produce equal pressure and help promote an accurate measurement. A cuff wrapped too loosely results in an inaccurate reading.
11. Turn on the machine. **If the machine has different settings for infants, children, and adults, select the appropriate setting.** Push the start button. Instruct the patient to hold the limb still and refrain from speaking.	Keeping the limb still and refraining from talking provide for accurate measurement of blood pressure levels (Muntner et al., 2019).

ACTION | **RATIONALE**

12. Wait until the machine beeps and the blood pressure reading appears. Note the reading (Figure 5).

Beep signals completion of reading.

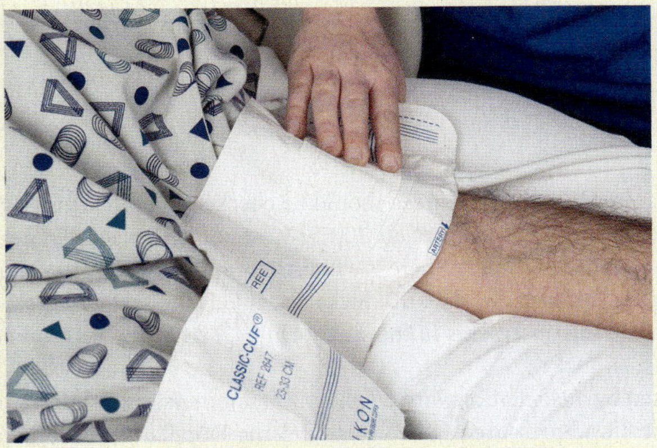

FIGURE 2. Centering the bladder of the cuff over the brachial artery.

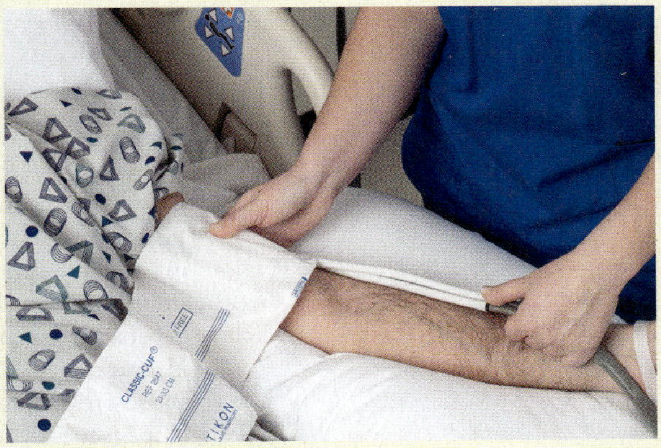

FIGURE 3. Cuff tubing extending from the edge of the cuff nearer the patient's elbow.

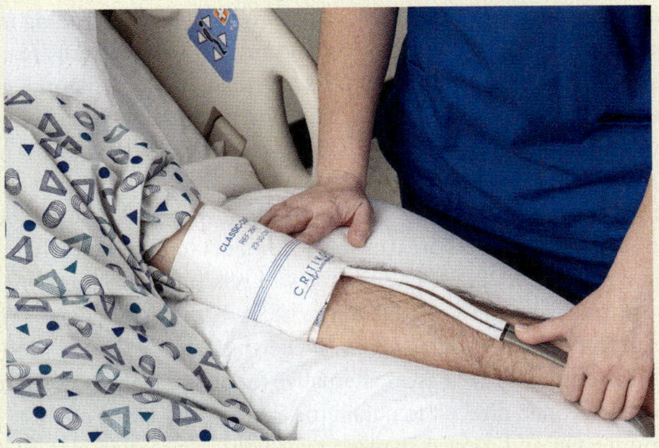

FIGURE 4. Wrapping the cuff around the arm smoothly and snugly.

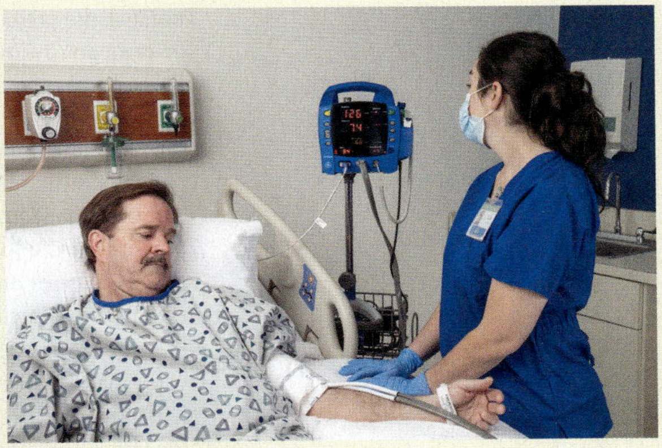

FIGURE 5. Noting the blood pressure reading.

13. Remove the cuff from the patient's limb and clean and store the equipment.

Cleaning of equipment prevents transmission of microorganisms and prepares equipment for future use.

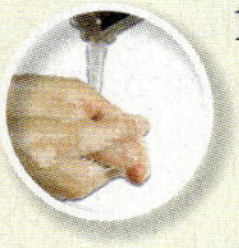

14. Remove gloves, if worn. Perform hand hygiene. Cover the patient and help them to a position of comfort.

Removing gloves properly reduces the risk for infection transmission and contamination of other items. Hand hygiene prevents the spread of microorganisms. Covering and positioning the patient ensures patient comfort.

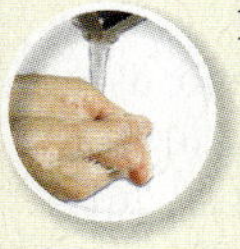

15. Remove additional PPE, if used. Perform hand hygiene.

Proper removal of PPE reduces the risk for infection transmission and contamination of other items. Hand hygiene deters the spread of microorganisms.

DOCUMENTATION GUIDELINES

Record the findings on the electronic record or flow sheet. Communicate abnormal findings to the primary health care provider. Identify arm used or site of assessment if other than brachial.

(continued on page 762)

Skill 26-4 Assessing Blood Pressure Using an Automated, Electronic Oscillometric Device *(continued)*

Sample Documentation

DocuCare Practice documenting blood pressure and other vital signs in *Lippincott DocuCare.*

10/18/25 0945 Blood pressure taken in right arm 180/88. Dr. Brown notified. Patient denies dizziness, headache. Captopril 25 mg PO twice a day prescribed. Blood pressure to be repeated 30 minutes after administering medication.

—*M. Evans, RN*

DEVELOPING CLINICAL REASONING AND CLINICAL JUDGMENT

SPECIAL CONSIDERATIONS

General Considerations

- It is recommended that blood pressure measurements should be checked in both arms at the first examination (Muntner et al., 2019; Pickering et al., 2005). Most people have differences in blood pressure readings between arms. When there is a consistent interarm difference, use the arm with the higher pressure (Muntner et al., 2019; Pickering et al., 2005).
- Separate repeated blood pressure measurements in the same arm by 1 to 2 minutes to avoid inaccurate results (Muntner et al., 2019).
- Blood pressure can be assessed by auscultation with a sphygmomanometer and stethoscope (see Skill 26-5); systolic blood pressure can be assessed using Doppler ultrasound (refer to the Guidelines for Nursing Care 26-6 on page 742).
- Incorrect cuff size contributes to the most frequent error in measurement in nonacute care settings (Muntner et al., 2019). *If the cuff is too narrow*, the reading could be erroneously high because the pressure is not evenly transmitted to the artery. *If a cuff is too wide,* the reading may be erroneously low because pressure is dispersed over a disproportionately large surface area.
- Diastolic blood pressure measured while the patient is supine is approximately 1 to 5 mm Hg higher than when measured while the patient is sitting; systolic blood pressure measured while the patient is supine is approximately 3 to 10 mm Hg higher than when measured while the patient is sitting (Muntner et al., 2019).
- Automated electronic oscillometric wrist monitors have been developed that measure blood pressure in the forearm using the radial artery. Forearm measurements tend to be higher than the upper arm measurements (Halm, 2014). The accuracy of readings with forearm monitors is affected by the position of the wrist relative to the heart. This can be avoided if the wrist is always at heart level when the reading is taken (Pickering et al., 2005).
- The wrist site for measurement has been suggested as an alternative for obtaining blood pressure readings in people who are obese. It is often difficult to obtain the appropriately sized cuff for the upper arm, given arm circumference and conical-shaped upper arms common in obesity. The conical shape of the upper arm makes it difficult to fit the cuff to the arm, increasing the likelihood of inaccurate blood pressure measurement (Halm, 2014). Thus, measurement in the forearm can be a possible solution to this problem (Muntner et al., 2019; Palatini, 2018).
- When the patient's brachial artery is inaccessible and/or the use of the upper arm is contraindicated, you can assess the blood pressure using the popliteal artery in the leg. The systolic blood pressure is at least 15 to 20 mm Hg higher at this site than the arm, although the diastolic pressure is the same (Muntner et al., 2019; Sheppard et al., 2019).

Infant and Child Considerations

- Use oscillometric devices that have been validated for use with children and adolescents (Muntner et al., 2019).
- In children, if elevated blood pressure is present when measure with an oscillometric device, auscultation should be performed to define blood pressure levels (Muntner et al., 2019).
- The use of wrist monitors is not recommended for pediatric patients (Muntner et al., 2019).
- Blood pressure should be taken in the right arm for children to align with normative data (Muntner et al., 2019).
- In infants and small children, the lower extremities are commonly used for blood pressure monitoring at the popliteal, dorsalis pedis, and posterior tibial sites. In children older than 1 year of age, the systolic pressure in the thigh tends to be 10 to 40 mm Hg higher than in the arm; the diastolic pressure remains the same (Kyle & Carman, 2021).
- Infants and children presenting with cardiac complaints may have blood pressures assessed in all four extremities. Large differences among blood pressure readings between the upper and lower extremities can indicate heart defects, such as coarctation of the aorta (Kyle & Carman, 2021).

Community-Based Care Considerations

- Patient and family/caregiver education related to home blood pressure monitoring (HBPM) should include information about hypertension, selection of equipment, appropriate procedures, and interpretation of results (Whelton et al., 2018).
- Automated blood pressure devices in public locations are generally inaccurate and inconsistent. In addition, the cuffs on these devices are inadequate for people with large arms (Pickering et al., 2005).
- Explain to the patient that it is important to use a cuff size appropriate for limb circumference. Inform the patient that cuff sizes range from a pediatric cuff to a large thigh cuff and that a poorly fitting cuff can result in an inaccurate measurement.
- Use of an automated validated digital monitoring device is suggested as best practice for HBPM (Whelton et al., 2018). Inform the patient about digital blood pressure monitoring equipment. Although more costly than manual cuffs, most provide an easy-to-read recording of systolic and diastolic measurements. Use of auscultatory devices is not recommended for HBPM because patients, family, and/or caregivers rarely master the technique required for accurate use of these devices (Whelton et al., 2018).
- Optimally, patients should measure and record blood pressure daily. Explain that two readings, at least 1 minute apart, should be taken in the morning before taking medications and in the evening (Muntner et al., 2019; Whelton et al., 2018). Measurement should occur following the guidelines detailed in Skill 26-4. Ideally, patients should measure weekly blood pressure readings beginning 2 weeks after a change in the treatment regimen and during the week before a follow-up visit (Whelton et al., 2018). The readings should be recorded to show to the health care provider. If possible, monitor with built-in memory should be brought to all health care visits.
- Explain that home monitoring devices should be checked for accuracy every 1 to 2 years. Readings should be compared with auscultated measurement by a health care provider to ensure accuracy.

Skill 26-5 Assessing Blood Pressure by Auscultation

DELEGATION CONSIDERATIONS

The measurement of brachial artery blood pressure may be delegated to assistive personnel (AP) as well as to licensed practical/vocational nurses (LPN/LVNs). The decision to delegate must be based on careful analysis of the patient's needs and circumstances as well as the qualifications of the person to whom the task is being delegated. Refer to the Delegation Guidelines in Appendix A.

EQUIPMENT

- Stethoscope
- Sphygmomanometer
- Blood pressure cuff of appropriate size
- Electronic record or pen and paper or flow sheet
- Alcohol swab
- PPE, as indicated

IMPLEMENTATION

ACTION	RATIONALE
1. Check the prescribed interventions or plan of care for frequency of blood pressure measurement. More frequent measurement may be appropriate based on nursing judgment.	Provides for patient safety.
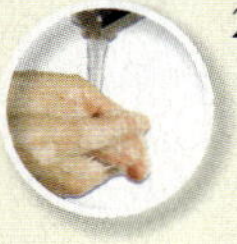 2. Perform hand hygiene and put on PPE, if indicated.	Hand hygiene and PPE prevent the spread of microorganisms. PPE is required based on transmission precautions.

(*continued on page 764*)

Skill 26-5 Assessing Blood Pressure by Auscultation *(continued)*

ACTION	RATIONALE
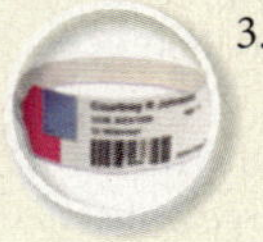 3. Identify the patient.	Identifying the patient ensures the right patient receives the intervention and helps prevent errors.
4. Close the curtains around the bed and close the door to the room, if possible. Discuss the procedure with the patient and assess patient's ability to assist with the procedure. Instruct the patient to hold the limb still and refrain from speaking during the measurement. Validate that the patient has relaxed for several minutes.	This ensures the patient's privacy. Explanation relieves anxiety and facilitates cooperation. Keeping the limb still and refraining from talking provide for accurate measurement of BP levels (Muntner et al., 2019). Activity immediately before measurement can result in inaccurate results.
5. Put on gloves, if indicated.	Gloves prevent contact with blood and body fluids. Gloves are usually not required for measurement of blood pressure, unless contact with blood or body fluids is anticipated.
6. Select the appropriate arm (or alternate site) for measurement and blood pressure cuff (refer to Table 26-8).	Decision on measurement site and cuff size is based on nurse's assessment of individual patient circumstances. Incorrect cuff size contributes to the most frequent error in measurement in nonacute care settings (Muntner et al., 2019).
7. Have the patient assume a comfortable lying or sitting position with the forearm supported at the level of the heart and the palm of the hand upward (Fig. 1). If the measurement is taken in the supine position, support the arm with a pillow. In the sitting position, support the arm yourself or by using the bedside table. If the patient is sitting, have the patient sit back in the chair so that the chair supports their back. In addition, make sure the patient keeps the legs uncrossed.	The position of the arm can have a major influence when the blood pressure is measured; if the upper arm is below the level of the right atrium, the readings will be too high. If the arm is above the level of the heart, the readings will be too low (Muntner et al., 2019; Pickering et al., 2005). This position places the brachial artery on the inner aspect of the elbow so that the bell or diaphragm of the stethoscope can rest on it easily. Support for the patient's arm prevents isometric exercise that will affect the BP level (Muntner et al., 2019). If the back is not supported, the diastolic pressure may be elevated falsely; if the legs are crossed, the systolic pressure may be elevated falsely (Muntner et al., 2019; Pickering et al., 2005).
8. Expose the brachial artery by removing garments or move a sleeve if it is not too tight, above the area where the cuff will be placed.	Clothing over the artery interferes with the ability to hear sounds and can cause inaccurate blood pressure readings. A tight sleeve would cause congestion of blood and possibly inaccurate readings (Muntner et al., 2019).
9. Palpate the location of the brachial artery. Center the bladder of the cuff over the brachial artery, about midway on the upper arm, so that the lower edge of the cuff is about 2.5 to 5 cm (1 to 2 inches) above the inner aspect of the elbow. **Line up the artery marking on the cuff with the patient's brachial artery.** The tubing should extend from the edge of the cuff nearer the patient's elbow (Fig. 2).	Pressure in the cuff applied directly to the artery provides the most accurate readings. If the cuff gets in the way of the stethoscope, readings are likely to be inaccurate. A cuff placed upside down with the tubing toward the patient's head may give a false reading.

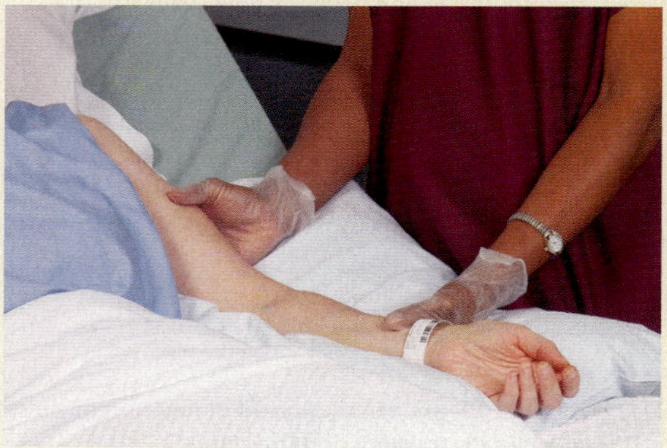

FIGURE 1. Positioning for blood pressure assessment using brachial artery. (*Source:* Used with permission from Shutterstock. *Photo by B. Proud.*)

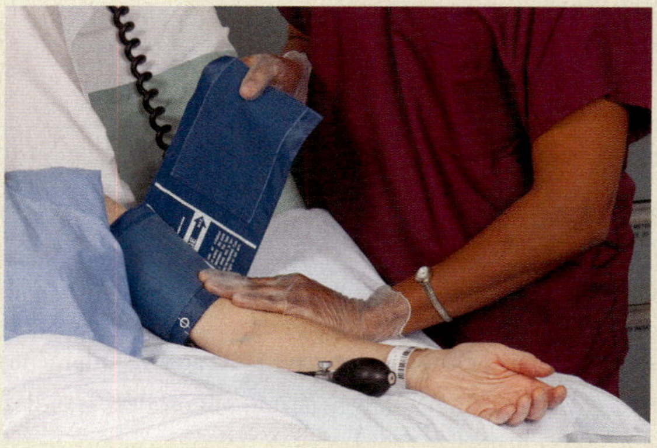

FIGURE 2. Placing the blood pressure cuff on the upper arm. (*Source:* Used with permission from Shutterstock. *Photo by B. Proud.*)

ACTION	RATIONALE
10. Wrap the cuff around the arm smoothly and snugly, and fasten it. Do not allow any clothing to interfere with the proper placement of the cuff.	A smooth cuff and snug wrapping produce equal pressure and help promote an accurate measurement. A cuff wrapped too loosely results in an inaccurate reading.
11. Check that the needle on the aneroid gauge is within the zero mark (Fig. 3).	If the needle is not in the zero area, the blood pressure reading may not be accurate.

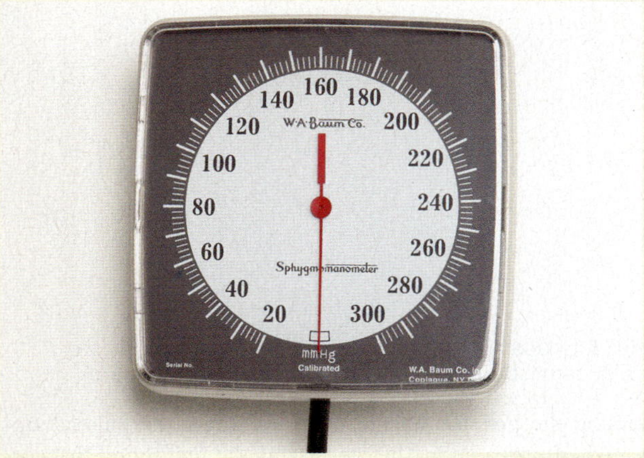

FIGURE 3. Ensuring gauge starts at zero. (*Source:* Used with permission from Shutterstock. *Photo by B. Proud.*)

Estimating Systolic Pressure

ACTION	RATIONALE
12. Palpate the pulse at the brachial or radial artery by pressing gently with the fingertips (Fig. 4).	To identify the first Korotkoff sound accurately, the cuff must be inflated 20 to 30 mm Hg above the point at which the pulse can no longer be felt (Muntner et al., 2019).

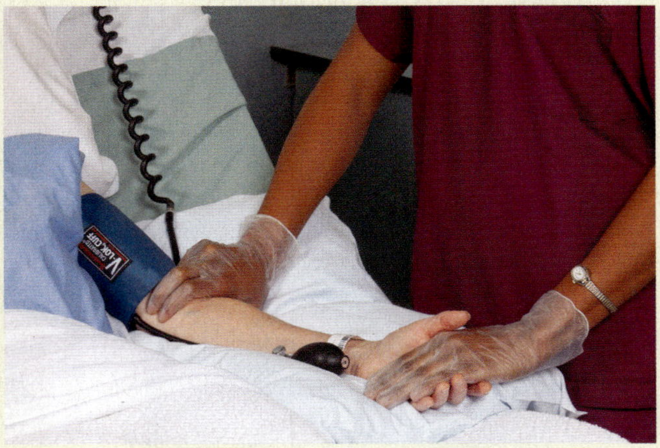

FIGURE 4. Palpating the brachial pulse. (*Source:* Used with permission from Shutterstock. *Photo by B. Proud.*)

ACTION	RATIONALE
13. Tighten the screw valve on the air pump.	The bladder within the cuff will not inflate with the valve open.
14. **Inflate the cuff while continuing to palpate the artery. Note the point on the gauge where the pulse disappears.**	The point where the pulse disappears provides an estimate of the systolic pressure. To identify the first Korotkoff sound accurately, the cuff must be inflated to a pressure above the point at which the pulse can no longer be felt.
15. Deflate the cuff and wait 1 minute.	Allowing a brief pause before continuing permits the blood to refill and circulate through the arm.

Obtaining Blood Pressure Measurement

ACTION	RATIONALE
16. Assume a position that is no more than 3 ft away from the gauge.	A distance of more than about 3 ft can interfere with accurate reading of the numbers on the gauge.
17. Place the stethoscope earpieces in your ears. Direct the earpieces forward into the canal and not against the ear itself.	Proper placement blocks extraneous noise and allows sound to travel more clearly.

(*continued on page 766*)

Skill 26-5 Assessing Blood Pressure by Auscultation *(continued)*

ACTION	RATIONALE
18. Place the bell or diaphragm of the stethoscope firmly but with as little pressure as possible over the brachial artery (Fig. 5). Do not allow the stethoscope to touch clothing or the cuff.	Having the bell or diaphragm directly over the artery allows more accurate readings. Heavy pressure on the brachial artery distorts the shape of the artery and the sound. Placing the bell or diaphragm away from clothing and the cuff prevents noise, which would distract from the sounds made by blood flowing through the artery.

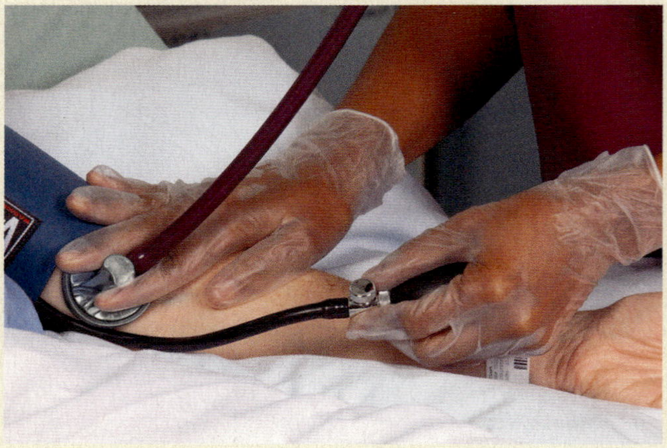

FIGURE 5. Placement of diaphragm of stethoscope. (*Source:* Used with permission from Shutterstock. *Photo by B. Proud.*)

ACTION	RATIONALE
19. Pump the pressure 20 to 30 mm Hg above the point at which the systolic pressure was palpated and estimated. Open the valve on the manometer and allow air to escape slowly (allowing the gauge to drop 2 mm Hg per second) (Muntner et al., 2019).	Increasing the pressure above the point where the pulse disappeared ensures a period before hearing the first sound that corresponds with the systolic pressure. It prevents misinterpreting phase II sounds as phase I sounds.
20. **Note the point on the gauge at which the first of at least two consecutive beats appears (Fig. 6). Read the pressure to the closest 2 mm Hg. Note this number as the systolic pressure.**	Systolic pressure is the point at which the blood in the artery is first able to force its way through the vessel at a similar pressure exerted by the air bladder in the cuff. The first sound is phase I of Korotkoff sounds.
21. Do not reinflate the cuff once the air is being released to recheck the systolic pressure reading.	Reinflating the cuff while obtaining the blood pressure is uncomfortable for the patient and can cause an inaccurate reading. Reinflating the cuff causes congestion of blood in the lower arm, which lessens the loudness of Korotkoff sounds.
22. **Note the point at which the sound completely disappears (Fig. 7). Read the pressure to the closest 2 mm Hg. Note this number as the diastolic pressure.**	The point at which the sound disappears corresponds to the beginning of phase V Korotkoff sounds and is generally considered the diastolic pressure reading (Muntner et al., 2019; Pickering et al., 2005).

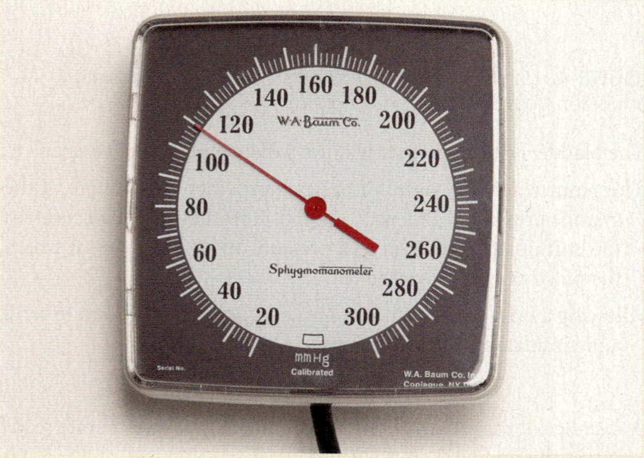

FIGURE 6. Noting the point on the gauge at which the first of at least two consecutive beats appears. (*Source:* Used with permission from Shutterstock. *Photo by B. Proud.*)

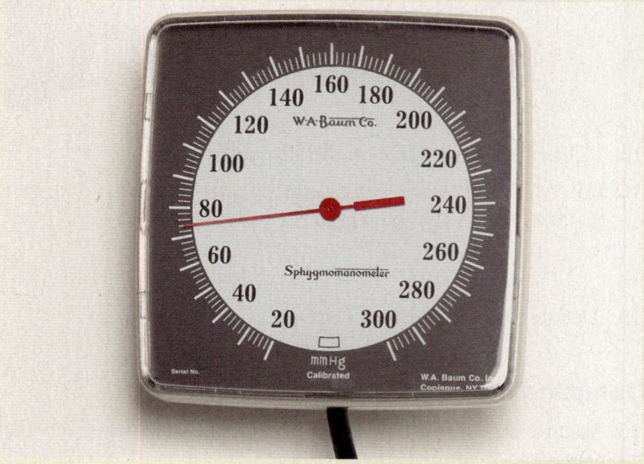

FIGURE 7. Noting the point at which the sound completely disappears. (*Source:* Used with permission from Shutterstock. *Photo by B. Proud.*)

ACTION	RATIONALE
23. Allow the remaining air to escape quickly. Repeat any suspicious reading, but wait at least 1 to 2 minutes. Deflate the cuff completely between attempts to check the blood pressure.	False readings are likely to occur if there is congestion of blood in the limb while obtaining repeated readings.
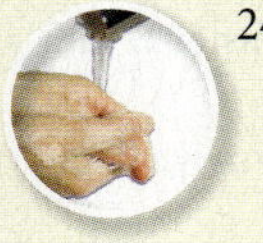 24. When measurement is completed, remove the cuff. Remove gloves, if worn. Perform hand hygiene. Cover the patient and help them to a position of comfort.	Removing gloves properly reduces the risk for infection transmission and contamination of other items. Hand hygiene prevents the spread of microorganisms. Covering and positioning the patient ensures patient comfort.
25. Clean the bell or diaphragm of the stethoscope with the alcohol wipe. Clean and store the sphygmomanometer, according to facility policy.	Appropriate cleaning deters the spread of microorganisms. Equipment should be left ready for use.
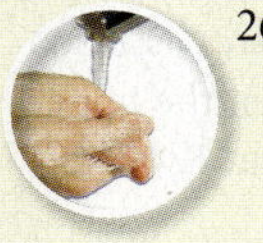 26. Remove additional PPE, if used. Perform hand hygiene.	Proper removal of PPE reduces the risk for infection transmission and contamination of other items. Hand hygiene deters the spread of microorganisms.

DOCUMENTATION GUIDELINES

Record the findings on the electronic record or flow sheet. Communicate abnormal findings to the primary health care provider. Identify arm used and site of assessment if other than brachial.

Sample Documentation

Lippincott DocuCare **Practice documenting blood pressure and other vital signs in *Lippincott DocuCare.***

10/18/25 0945 Blood pressure taken in right arm 180/88. Patient denies headache, dizziness. Dr. Brown notified. Captopril 25 mg PO twice per day prescribed. Blood pressure to be repeated 30 minutes after administering medication.

—*M. Evans, RN*

DEVELOPING CLINICAL REASONING AND CLINICAL JUDGMENT

SPECIAL CONSIDERATIONS

General Considerations

- It is recommended that blood pressure measurements be checked in both arms at the first examination (Muntner et al., 2019; Pickering et al., 2005). Most people have differences in blood pressure readings between arms. When there is a consistent interarm difference, use the arm with the higher pressure (Muntner et al., 2019; Pickering et al., 2005). Separate repeated blood pressure measurements in the same arm by 1 to 2 minutes to avoid inaccurate results (Muntner et al., 2019).
- Incorrect cuff size contributes to the most frequent error in measurement in nonacute care settings (Muntner et al., 2019). *If the cuff is too narrow,* the reading could be erroneously high because the pressure is not evenly transmitted to the artery. *If a cuff is too wide,* the reading may be erroneously low because pressure is dispersed over a disproportionately large surface area.
- Blood pressure can be assessed using an automatic electronic blood pressure monitor (see Skill 26-4); systolic blood pressure can be assessed using Doppler ultrasound.
- Diastolic blood pressure measured while the patient is supine is approximately 1 to 5 mm Hg higher than when measured while the patient is sitting; systolic blood pressure measured while the patient is supine is approximately 3 to 10 mm Hg higher than when measured while the patient is sitting (Muntner et al., 2019).
- The wrist site for measurement has been suggested as an alternative for obtaining blood pressure readings in people who are obese. It is often difficult to obtain the appropriately sized cuff for the upper arm, given arm circumference and conical-shaped upper arms common in obesity. The conical shape of the upper arm makes it difficult to fit the cuff to the arm, increasing the likelihood of inaccurate blood pressure measurement (Halm, 2014). Thus, measurement in the forearm can be a possible solution to this problem (Muntner et al., 2019; Palatini, 2018).

(*continued on page 768*)

Skill 26-5 Assessing Blood Pressure by Auscultation *(continued)*

- When the patient's brachial artery is inaccessible and/or the use of the upper arm is contraindicated, you can assess the blood pressure using the popliteal artery in the leg. The systolic blood pressure is at least 15 to 20 mm Hg higher at this site than the arm, although the diastolic pressure is the same (Muntner et al., 2019; Sheppard et al., 2019).

Infant and Child Considerations

- In children, if elevated blood pressure is present when measuring with an oscillometric device, auscultation should be performed to define blood pressure levels (Muntner et al., 2019).
- Blood pressure should be taken in the right arm for children to align with normative data (Muntner et al., 2019).
- In infants and small children, the lower extremities are commonly used for blood pressure monitoring at the popliteal, dorsalis pedis, and posterior tibial sites. In children older than 1 year of age, the systolic pressure in the thigh tends to be 10 to 40 mm Hg higher than in the arm; the diastolic pressure remains the same (Kyle & Carman, 2021).
- Infants and children presenting with cardiac complaints may have blood pressures assessed in all four extremities. Large differences among blood pressure readings between the upper and lower extremities can indicate heart defects, such as coarctation of the aorta (Kyle & Carman, 2021).

Community-Based Care Considerations

- Patient and family/caregiver education related to home blood pressure monitoring (HBPM) should include information about hypertension; selection of equipment; appropriate procedures; and interpretation of results (Whelton et al., 2018).
- Automated blood pressure devices in public locations are generally inaccurate and inconsistent. In addition, the cuffs on these devices are inadequate for people with large arms (Pickering et al., 2005).
- Use of an automated validated digital monitoring device is suggested as best practice (Whelton et al., 2018). Use of auscultatory devices is not recommended for HBPM because patients, family, and/or caregivers rarely master the technique required for accurate use of these devices (Whelton et al., 2018). Refer to information in Skill 26-4.

DEVELOPING CLINICAL REASONING AND CLINICAL JUDGMENT

1. Take your own pulse several times a day, such as when you first get up, before and after meals, and before and after exercise. Write down the rate, rhythm, and quality of the pulse. What changes did you see? What are the physiologic rationales for these changes?
2. Describe differences you might expect to find in the vital signs of the following individuals, and include the physiologic reasons for these differences:
   - A teenager who has his first football practice in 95°F (35°C) heat
   - An infant with a bacterial ear infection
   - A young woman arriving at the emergency department after an attempted assault
   - A middle-aged man who sustained serious trauma and bleeding in an automobile crash
   - A 92-year-old woman with a chronic respiratory disease

PRACTICING FOR NCLEX

1. A nurse receives information during shift report that a patient is afebrile. What action will the nurse take in response?
   a. Checking the MAR for prescribed antipyretic medication
   b. Reporting the finding to the primary care provider
   c. Taking the patient's temperature using a different method
   d. No action is necessary; this is a normal reading
2. A nurse is assessing the vital signs of a group of patients in the emergency department. Which patients require follow-up by the nurse? Select all that apply.
   a. Infant whose temperature is 100.5°F (38.1°C)
   b. Toddler whose blood pressure is 118/80
   c. School-age child whose temperature is 102.2°F (39°C)
   d. Adolescent whose pulse rate is 70 beats/min

e. Adult whose respiratory rate is 20 breaths/min
f. Older adult whose pulse rate is 42 beats/min

3. A nurse is caring for a newborn with hypothermia. What action does the nurse take to prevent heat loss from convection?
a. Wrapping the newborn in a blanket
b. Placing the newborn on a warmed surface
c. Reducing the temperature in the room
d. Increasing the temperature in the room

4. A charge nurse working on a medical-surgical unit stops the AP from taking rectal temperatures on patients with which problems? Select all that apply.
a. Hypothermia
b. Pneumonia
c. Bradycardia
d. Leukemia
e. Thrombocytopenia
f. Pancreatitis

5. While taking an adult patient's pulse, a nurse obtains a heart rate of 140 beats/min. What should the nurse do next?
a. Reassess the pulse in 1 hour
b. Measure the blood pressure
c. Document the information, noting tachycardia
d. Report the rate to the health care provider

6. During assessment of vital signs, a patient reports severe abdominal pain. Which pain-related changes in vital signs may be present? Select all that apply.
a. Pulse rate of 102
b. Body temperature 98.8°F
c. Blood pressure 154/86
d. Increased respiratory depth
e. Respiratory rate of 24
f. Body temperature 100.8°F

7. A nurse is caring for a group of patients on a cardiac unit. Which finding will prompt the nurse to assess the apical–radial pulse?
a. Bounding radial pulse
b. Immediately postoperative
c. Rapid, irregular pulse
d. Fluid volume deficit

8. A nurse is assessing the blood pressure of a patient with traumatic injuries using a Doppler device. Which information does the nurse expect to obtain?
a. Amplitude of the brachial pulse
b. Mean arterial blood pressure
c. Estimation of the systolic blood pressure
d. Apical–radial pulse rate

9. A nurse enters a room and finds a patient who is unable to catch their breath, has a respiratory rate of 28, and is using accessory muscles to breathe. What intervention will the nurse use to relieve dyspnea?
a. Remove pillows from under the head
b. Raise the head of the bed
c. Elevate the foot of the bed
d. Reassess the respiratory rate

10. A nurse has assessed an older adult for orthostatic hypotension as shown in the electronic health record (EHR). What action will the nurse take?
Exhibit: Electronic health record (EHR)
Graphic sheet
8:00 AM BP lying 124/76
BP sitting 118/74
BP standing 98/58
a. Encourage the patient to rise from a sitting position quickly to improve blood flow
b. Suggest that in the future the patient "dangle" for a few minutes before standing
c. Return the patient to bed and place them in Fowler position
d. Administer medication to increase blood pressure

11. A nurse is caring for a postoperative patient who experienced hypovolemic shock necessitating transfer to the ICU. The nurse manager reviews the medical record and suspects which situation contributed to the emergency?
Exhibit: Electronic health record (EHR)
Graphic sheet
2:00 PM T 99.2, P 88, RR 16, BP 106/54
2:15 PM T 99.6, P 94, RR 16, BP 100/52
2:30 PM T 99.4, P 110, RR 18, BP 96/50
2:45 PM T 99.2, P 120, RR 20, BP 84/48
a. Using an inappropriate format to document the vital signs
b. Failing to report tachycardia and hypotension to the provider
c. Not following the postoperative vital sign protocol
d. Failing to reflect a pain assessment in the documentation

12. A patient has a blood pressure reading of 130/90 mm Hg during a clinic visit. What recommendation for follow-up will the nurse make?
a. Follow-up measurements of blood pressure
b. Immediate treatment by a health care provider
c. No action, because the nurse considers this reading is due to anxiety
d. Change in dietary intake

13. A nurse participating in community blood pressure screening tells the patient their blood pressure is 120/80 mm Hg. When the patient asks what the numbers mean, what information does the nurse provide?
a. Rhythmic distention of the arterial walls from increased pressure due to surges of blood with ventricular contraction
b. Systolic pressure represents ventricular contraction causing high pressure on arterial walls; the bottom number or diastolic pressure reflects ventricular relaxation with a lower pressure on the arteries
c. Normal blood pressure
d. Difference between the pressure on arterial walls with ventricular contraction and relaxation

14. A nurse observes a nursing student is taking the blood pressure on a patient with a cuff that is too large for the patient's arm. What explanation does the nurse give to the student for why errors of measurement may result?
    a. "Using the wrong cuff will result in an incorrect reading."
    b. "This cuff will cause an elevation in diastolic blood pressure."
    c. "Using the wrong cuff will cause dangerous pressure on the arm."
    d. "An overly large cuff will cause an inaccurate low reading."
15. A nursing student is caring for a patient who has intravenous fluids infusing in the right arm. What action will the student take to correctly obtain the blood pressure?
    a. Take the blood pressure in the right arm
    b. Assess blood pressure using the left arm
    c. Use the smallest possible cuff
    d. Document an inability to take the blood pressure
16. The nurse must assess a patient's blood pressure using a thigh cuff, due to presence of a right antecubital IV and a left arm dialysis access. Which of these arteries will the nurse use for auscultation?
    a. Brachial
    b. Carotid
    c. Popliteal
    d. Radial

ANSWERS WITH RATIONALES

1. **d.** Afebrile means without fever, or a temperature is within the normal range. No additional actions are needed.
2. **a, d, e, f.** The normal temperature range for infants is 98.7° to 100.5°F (37.1° to 38.1°C). The normal pulse rate for an adolescent is 55 to 105. The normal respiratory rate for an adult is 12 to 20 breaths/min and the normal pulse for an older adult is 40 to 100 beats/min. The normal blood pressure for a toddler is 89/46, and the normal temperature for a child is 98.2° to 100°F (36.8° to 37.8°C; refer to Table 26-1).
3. **a.** Convection refers to heat disseminated by motion between areas of unequal density, for example, a fan blowing cool air over the body or an uncovered body. Placing the baby on a warmed surface would prevent heat loss via conduction. Reducing the temperature may decrease heat loss via perspiration (evaporation); increasing the temperature in the room may increase heat loss via evaporation.
4. **c, d, e.** The rectal site should not be used in newborns, children with diarrhea, and in patients who have undergone rectal or vaginal surgery. Inserting a rectal thermometer can stimulate the vagus nerve causing or worsening bradycardia; this route may be contraindicated in certain cardiac patients. The rectal route is also contraindicated in patients who have neutropenia (low white blood cell counts, such as in leukemia or those receiving chemotherapy), thrombocytopenia (low platelet counts), and certain neurologic disorders.
5. **d.** A pulse rate of 140 beats/min in an adult, tachycardia, is abnormally fast, and should be reported to the primary nurse or health care provider immediately. Tachycardia at rest often reflects an underlying issue and can lead to decreased tissue perfusion; additional assessments are needed.
6. **a, c, e.** The pulse, blood pressure, and respiratory rate often increase when a person is experiencing pain; respiratory depth decreases. Pain does not affect body temperature.
7. **c.** The nurse assesses the apical–radial pulse when dysrhythmia exists or is suspected, manifested by tachycardia or irregular pulse. The difference between the apical and radial pulse rates, called the pulse deficit, captures heart beats not reaching the peripheral arteries.
8. **b.** A Doppler provides an estimation of the systolic blood pressure when the pulse is inaudible. Diastolic pressure cannot be calculated because oscillations of the pulse will be audible during the entire BP assessment; recall the nurse can auscultate a pulse with the Doppler. The pulse amplitude obtained with palpation, the mean arterial pressure reflects the average blood pressure during a cardiac cycle, and the apical–radial pulse is assessed to detect a pulse deficit, often present with a dysrhythmia.
9. **b.** Elevating the head of the bed facilitates lung expansion by allowing the abdominal contents to descend, which facilitates lung expansion and oxygenation. Elevated respiratory may occur due to distress or hypoxemia; assessing the respiratory rate does not resolve the problem of dyspnea.
10. **b.** Allowing the patient to "dangle" on the edge of the bed prior to rising may prevent orthostatic hypotension, by allowing time to adjust to the upright position. Arising and moving about slowly, especially after a period of bed rest, might also prevent orthostatic hypotension. If a patient becomes dizzy or faint, the nurse should return the patient to bed and place them in a supine position, which restores blood flow to the brain. A β-blocker is given to decrease blood pressure for a patient with hypertension; the nurse will question this prescription when hypotension is present.
11. **b.** Pathologic hypotension, especially when associated with tachycardia, can result from vasodilation of the arterioles, failure of the heart to pump effectively, loss of blood (such as with a hemorrhage or shock), or poor oxygenation. The nurse reports such changes to the health care provider immediately and anticipates prescriptions to restore perfusion.
12. **a.** A single blood pressure reading that is mildly elevated is not significant, but the measurement should be monitored over time to determine if hypertension exists. The nurse will recommend a follow-up visit with the health care provider for a recheck.
13. **c.** The systolic pressure, 120 mm Hg, occurs when ventricular contraction causes the highest pressure on arterial walls. The diastolic pressure, 80 mm Hg, correlates with the lowest pressure on arterial walls as the heart rests between beats. The difference between systolic and diastolic pressures is called the pulse pressure. The rhythmic distention of the arterial walls as ventricular contraction pumps blood to the body creates the pulse.
14. **a.** A blood pressure cuff that is too large will cause a falsely low reading; a cuff that is too small will cause a falsely high reading. The wrong size cuff will not injure the patient, but pressure may be felt on the arm from a too tight cuff.
15. **b.** The blood pressure should be taken in the arm opposite of the arm with intravenous access or infusion.
16. **c.** When the patient's brachial artery is inaccessible and/or the use of the upper arm is contraindicated, blood pressure can be assessed using the popliteal artery of the leg. The blood pressure in that area, in both adults and children, is generally higher.

Bibliography

Allan, J., & Sheppard, K. (2018). Monitoring a pulse in adults. *British Journal of Nursing, 27*(1), 1237–1239.

Alne, T. (2020). Therapeutic hypothermia. Comparing surface vs intravascular cooling. *Dimensions of Critical Care Nursing, 39*(1), 12–22. https://doi.org/10.1097/DCC.0000000000000398

American Academy of Pediatrics (AAP). (2020). *AAP pediatric hypertension guidelines*. https://www.mdcalc.com/aap-pediatric-hypertension-guidelines

American Academy of Pediatrics (AAP). (2021, April 20). *Using over-the-counter medicines with your child*. https://www.healthychildren.org/English/safety-prevention/at-home/medication-safety/Pages/Using-Over-the-Counter-Medicines-With-Your-Child.aspx

American Heart Association. (2021). *Understanding blood pressure readings*. http://www.heart.org/HEARTORG/Conditions/HighBloodPressure/KnowYourNumbers/Understanding-Blood-Pressure-Readings_UCM_301764_Article.jsp#.WrZcg4jwaUl

Andrews, M., Boyle, J. S., & Collins, J. (2020). *Transcultural concepts in nursing care* (8th ed.). Wolters Kluwer.

Arnold, A., & McNaughton, A. (2018). Accuracy of non-invasive blood pressure measurements in obese patients. *British Journal of Nursing, 27*(1), 35–40. https://doi.org/10.12968/bjon.2018.27.1.35

Aw, J. (2020). The non-contact handheld cutaneous infra-red thermometer for fever screening during the COVID-19 global emergency. *Journal of Hospital Infection, 104*(4), 451. https://doi.org/10.1016/j.jhin.2020.02.010

Backer Mogensen, C., Wittenhoff, L., Fruerhøj, G., & Hansen, S. (2018). Forehead or ear temperature measurement cannot replace rectal measurements, except for screening purposes. *BMC Pediatrics, 18*(1), 15. https://doi.org/10.1186/s12887-018-0994-1

Bayhan, C., Özsürekçi, Y., Tekçam, N., Güloğlu, A., Ehliz, G., Ceyhan, M., & Kara, A. (2014). Comparison of infrared tympanic thermometer with non-contact infrared thermometer. *Journal of Pediatric Infectious Diseases, 8*, 52–55. https://doi.org/10.5152/ced.2014.1698

Berksoy, E. A., Bağ, Ö, Yazici, S., & Çelik, T. (2018). Use of noncontact infrared thermography to measure temperature in children in a triage room. *Medicine (Baltimore), 97*(5), e9737. http://doi.org/10.1097/MD.0000000000009737

Brekke, I. J., Puntervoll, L. H., Pedersen, P. B., Kellett, J., & Brabrand, M. (2019). The value of vital sign trends in predicting and monitoring clinical deterioration: A systematic review. *PLoS One, 14*(1), e0210875. https://doi.org/10.1371/journal.pone.0210875

Broskinski, C., Valdez, S., Riddell, A., & Riffenburgh, R. H. (2018). Comparison of temporal artery versus rectal temperature in emergency department patients who are unable to participate in oral temperature assessment. *Journal of Emergency Nursing, 44*(1), 57–63. http://doi.org/10.1016/j.jen.2017.04.015

Burchill, C., Anderson, B., & O'Connor, P. C. (2015). Exploration of nurse practices and attitudes related to postoperative vital signs. *Medsurg Nursing, 24*(4), 249–255.

Burns, S. M., & Delgado, S. A. (2019). *AACN essentials of critical care nursing* (4th ed.). McGraw-Hill Education.

Canadian Agency for Drugs and Technologies in Health. (2014, November 20). *Non-contact thermometers for detecting fever: A review of clinical effectiveness*. https://www.ncbi.nlm.nih.gov/books/NBK263237/pdf/Bookshelf_NBK263237.pdf

Centers for Disease Control and Prevention (CDC). (2020). *High blood pressure. Facts about hypertension*. https://www.cdc.gov/bloodpressure/facts.htm?CDC_AA_refVal=https%3A%2F%2Fwww.cdc.gov%2Fdhdsp%2Fdata_statistics%2Ffact_sheets%2Ffs_bloodpressure.htm

Cheng, R. Z., Bhalla, V., & Chang, T. I. (2019). Comparison of routine and automated office blood pressure measurement. *Blood Pressure Monitoring, 24*(4), 174–178. https://doi.org/10.1097/MBP.0000000000000392

Cheshire, W. P. (2019). Chemical pharmacotherapy for the treatment of orthostatic hypotension. *Expert Opinion on Pharmacotherapy, 20*(2), 187–199. https://doi.org/10.1080/14656566.2018.1543404

Churpek, M. M., Adhikari, R., & Edelson, D. P. (2016). The value of vital sign trends for detecting clinical deterioration on the wards. *Resuscitation, 102*, 1–5. https://doi.org/10.1016/j.resuscitation.2016.02.005

Cleveland Clinic. (2020, August 14). *24-hour ambulatory blood pressure monitoring*. https://my.clevelandclinic.org/health/diagnostics/16330-24-hour-ambulatory-blood-pressure-monitoring

Dalton, M., Harrison, J., Malin, A., & Leavey, C. (2018). Factors that influence nurses' assessment of patient acuity and response to acute deterioration. *British Journal of Nursing, 27*(4), 212–218. https://doi.org/10.12968/bjon.2018.27.4.212

Eliopoulos, C. (2018). *Gerontological nursing* (9th ed.). Wolters Kluwer.

Elliott, M., & Baird, J. (2019). Pulse oximetry and the enduring neglect of respiratory rate assessment: A commentary on patient surveillance. *British Journal of Nursing, 28*(19), 1256–1259. https://doi.org/10.12968/bjon.2019.28.19.1256

Exergen. (n.d.a). *Exergen temporal artery thermometry*. Retrieved July 17, 2021, from https://www.exergen.com/tathermometry/index.htm

Exergen. (n.d.b). *Temporal artery temperature measurement. Training handout for nursing staff.* Retrieved July 17, 2021, from https://www.exergen.com/wp-content/uploads/2018/05/TAT-5000-Training-Trifold.pdf

Fitzwater, J., Johnstone, C., Schuppers, M., Cordoza, M., & Norman, B. (2019). A comparison of oral, axillary, and temporal artery temperature measuring devices in adult acute care. *Medsurg Nursing, 28*(1), 35–41.

Flynn, J. T., Kaelber, D. C., Baker-Smith, C. M., Blowey, D., Carroll, A. E., Daniels, S. R., de Ferranti, S. D., Dionne, J. M., Falkner, B., Flinn, S. K., Gidding, S. S., Goodwin, C., Leu, M. G., Powers, M. E., Rea, C., Samuels, J., Simasek, M., Thaker, V. V., Urbina, E. M., ... SUBCOMMITTEE ON SCREENING AND MANAGEMENT OF HIGH BLOOD PRESSURE IN CHILDREN. (2017). Clinical practice guideline for screening and management of high blood pressure in children and adolescents. *Pediatrics, 140*(3), e20171904. https://doi.org/10.1542/peds.2017-1904

Franconi, I., La Cerra, C., Marucci, A. R., Petrucci, C., & Lancia, L. (2018). Digital axillary and non-contact infrared thermometers for children. *Clinical Nursing Research, 27*(2), 180–190. https://doi.org/10.1177/1054773816676538

Freeman, R., Abuzinadah, A. R., Gibbons, C., Jones, P., Miglis, M.G., & Sinn, D. I. (2018). Orthostatic hypotension. JACC State-of-the-art review. *Journal of the American College of Cardiology, 72*(11), 1294–1309. https://doi.org/10.1016/j.jacc.2018.05.079

Furlong, D., Carroll, D. L., Finn, C., Gay, D., Gryglik, C., & Donahue, V. (2015). Comparison of temporal to pulmonary artery temperature in febrile patients. *Dimensions of Critical Care Nursing, 34*(1), 47–52. https://doi.org/10.1097/DCC.0000000000000090

Fusco, F. M., Pisapia, R., Nardiello, S., Cicala, S. D., Gaeta, G. B., & Brancaccio, G. (2019). Fever of unknown origin (FUO): Which are the factors influencing the final diagnosis? A 2005–2015 systematic review. *BMC Infectious Diseases, 19*(1), 653. https://doi.org/10.1186/s12879-019-4285-8

Gates, D., Horner, V., Bradley, L., Fogle Sheperd, T., John, O., & Higgins, M. (2018). Temperature measurements. Comparison of different thermometer types for patients with cancer. *Clinical Journal of Oncology Nursing, 22*(6), 611–617. https://doi.org/10.1188/18.CJON.611-617

Gerhard-Herman, M. D., Gornik, H. L., Barrett, C., Barshes, N. R., Corriere, M. A., Drachman, D. E., Fleisher, L. A., Gowkes, F. G. R., Hamburg, N. M., Kinlay, S., Lookstein, R., Misra, S., Mureebe, L., Olin, J. W., Patel, R. A. G., Regensteiner, J. G., Schanzer, A., Shishehbor, M. H., Stewart, K. J., ... Wijeysundera, D. N. (2017). 2016 AHA/ACC Guideline on the management of patients with lower extremity peripheral artery disease: Executive Summary. *Vascular Medicine, 22*(3), NPI–NP43. https://doi.org/10.1177/1358863X17701592

Godbole, G. P., & Aggarwal, B. (2018). Review of management strategies for orthostatic hypotension in older people. *Journal of Pharmacy Practice and Research, 48*(5), 483–491. https://doi.org/10.1002/jppr.1484

Halm, M. A. (2014). Arm circumference, shape, and length: How interplaying variables affect blood pressure measurement in obese persons. *American Journal of Critical Care, 23*(2), 166–170. https://doi.org/10.4037/ajcc2014364

Harvard Medical School. (2020, June 1). *Reading the new blood pressure guidelines*. Harvard Health Publishing. https://www.health.harvard.edu/heart-health/reading-the-new-blood-pressure-guidelines

Hess, D. R., MacIntyre, N. R., Galvin, W. F., & Mishoe, S. C. (2021). *Respiratory care. Principles and practice* (4th ed.). Jones & Bartlett Learning.

Hill, A., Kelly, E., Horseill, M. S., & Watson, M. O. (2018). The effects of awareness and count duration on adult respiratory rate measurements: An experimental study. *Journal of Clinical Nursing, 27*(3-4), 546–554. https://doi.org/10.1111/jocn.13861

Hinkle, J. L., Cheever, K. H., & Overbaugh, K. J. (2022). *Brunner & Suddarths's Textbook of medical-surgical nursing* (15th ed.). Wolters Kluwer.

International Council of Nurses (ICN). (2019). *Nursing diagnosis and outcome statements*. https://www.icn.ch/sites/default/files/inline-files/ICNP2019-DC.pdf

Jarvis, C., & Echkardt, A. (2020). *Physical examination & health assessment* (8th ed.). Elsevier.

Jensen, S. (2019). *Nursing health assessment. A best practice approach* (3rd ed.). Wolters Kluwer.

John, A., Alhmidi, H., Cadnum, J. L., Jencson, A. L., & Donskey, C. J. (2017). Contaminated portable equipment is a potential vector for dissemination of pathogens in the Intensive Care Unit. *Infection Control Hospital Epidemiology, 38*(10), 1247–1249. https://doi.org/10.1017/ice.2017.160

John, A. R., Alhmidi, H., Cadnum, J. L., Jencson, A. L., Gestrich, S., & Donskey, C. J. (2018). Evaluation of the potential for electronic thermometers to contribute to spread of healthcare-associated pathogens. *American Journal of Infection Control, 46*(6), 708–710. https://doi.org/10.1016/j.ajic.2017.12.005

Kallioinen, N., Hill, A., Horswill, M S., Ward, H. E., & Watson, M. O. (2017). Sources of inaccuracy in the measurement of adult patients' resting blood pressure in clinical settings: A systematic review. *Journal of Hypertension, 35*(3), 421–441. https://doi.org/10.1097/HJH.0000000000001197

Karch, A. M. (2020). *Focus on nursing pharmacology* (8th ed.). Wolters Kluwer.

Kersey-Matusiak, G. (2019). *Delivering culturally competent nursing care. Working with diverse and vulnerable populations* (2nd ed.). Springer Publishing Company.

Kiekkas, P., Aretha, D., Almpani, E., & Stefanopoulos, N. (2019). Temporal artery thermometry in pediatric patients; systematic review and meta-analysis. *Journal of Pediatric Nursing, 46*, 89–99. https://doi.org/10.1016/j.pedn.2019.03.004

Kuhnke, M., Albrecht, R., Schefold, J. C., & Paal, P. (2019). Successful resuscitation from prolonged hypothermic cardiac arrest without extracorporeal life support: A case report. *Journal of Medical Case Reports, 13*(1), 354. https://doi.org/10.1186/s13256-019-2282-6

Kurnat-Thoma, E., Edwards, V., & Emery, K. (2018). Axillary, tympanic and temporal thermometry comparison in a community hospital pediatric unit. *Pediatric Nursing, 44*(5), 235–246.

Kyle, T., & Carman, S. (2021). *Essentials of pediatric nursing* (4th ed.). Wolters Kluwer.

Lipsitz, L. A. (2017). Orthostatic hypotension and falls. *Journal of the American Geriatrics Society, 65*(3), 470–471. https://doi.org/10.1111/jgs.14745

Ludwig, J., & McWhinnie, H. (2019). Antipyretic drugs in patients with fever and infection: Literature review. *British Journal of Nursing, 28*(10), 610–618. https://doi.org/10.12968/bjon.2019.28.10.610

Malycha, J., Bonnici, T., Clifton, D. A., Ludbrook, G., Young, J. D., & Watkinson, P. J. (2019). Patient centred variables with univariate associations with unplanned ICU admission: A systematic review. *BMC Medical Informatics and Decision Making, 19*(98). https://doi.org/10.1186/s12911-019-0820-1

Mason, T. M., Boubekri, A., Lalau, J., Patterson, A., Hartranft, S. R., & Sutton, S. K. (2017). Equivalence study of two temperature-measurement methods in febrile adult patients with cancer. *Oncology Nursing Forum, 44*(2), E82–E87. https://doi.org/10.1188/17.ONF.E82-E87

Mayo Clinic. (2020a, November 20). *Thermometer basics: Taking your child's temperature.* https://www.mayoclinic.org/healthy-lifestyle/infant-and-toddler-health/in-depth/thermometer/art-20047410

Mayo Clinic. (2020b, September 18). *Get the most out of home blood pressure monitoring.* https://www.mayoclinic.org/diseases-conditions/high-blood-pressure/in-depth/high-blood-pressure/art-20047889

McDonald, C., Pearce, M., Kerr, S. R., & Newton, J. (2017). A prospective study of the association between orthostatic hypotension and falls: Definition matters. *Age and Ageing, 46*(3), 439–445. https://doi.org/10.1093/ageing/afw227

Morton, P. G., & Fontaine, D. K. (2018). *Critical care nursing. A holistic approach* (11th ed.). Wolters Kluwer.

Mulders-Manders, C., Simon, A., & Bleeker-Rovers, C. (2015). Fever of unknown origin. *Clinical Medicine (Lond), 15*(3), 280–284. https://doi.org/10.7861/clinmedicine.15-3-280

Muntner, P., Shimbo, D., Carey, R. M., Charleston, J. B., Gaillard, T., Misra, S., Myers, M. G., Ogedegbe, G., Schwartz, J. E., Townsend, R. R., Urbina, E. M., Viera, A. J., White, W. B., & Wright, J. T. Jr. (2019). Measurement of blood pressure in humans. A scientific statement from the American Heart Association. *Hypertension, 73*(5), e35–e66. https://doi.org/10.1161/HYP.0000000000000087

Myers, M. G., Asmar, R., & Staessen, J. A. (2018). Office blood pressure measurement in the 21st century. *Journal of Clinical Hypertension (Greenwich), 20*(7), 1104–1107. https://doi.org/10.1111/jch.13276

National Heart, Lung, and Blood Institute (NHLBI). (n.d.). *Low blood pressure. Also known as hypotension.* Retrieved July 17, 2021, from http://www.nhlbi.nih.gov/health/health-topics/topics/hyp

National Reye's Syndrome Foundation. (n.d.). Reye's syndrome. What is the role of aspirin in triggering Reye's? Retrieved July 17, 2021, from https://www.reyessyndrome.org/blank-2

Norris, T. L. (2019). *Porth's essentials of pathophysiology* (5th ed.). Wolters Kluwer.

Oguz, F., Yildiz, I., Varkal, M. A., Hizli, Z., Toprak, S., Kaymakci, K., Saygili, S. K., Kilic, A., & Unuvar, E. (2018). Axillary and tympanic temperature measurement in children and normal values for ages. *Pediatric Emergency Care, 34*(3), 169–173. https://doi.org/10.1097/PEC.0000000000000693

Opersteny, E., Anderson, H., Bates, J., Davenport, K., Husby, J., Myking, K., & Oron, A. P. (2017). Precision, sensitivity and patient preference of non-invasive thermometers in a pediatric surgical acute care setting. *Journal of Pediatric Nursing, 35*, 36–41. http://doi.org/10.1016/j.pedn.2017.02.003

Palatini, P. (2018, August 15). Blood pressure measurement in the obese: Still a challenging problem. *E-Journal of Cardiology Practice, 16*(21). https://www.escardio.org/Journals/E-Journal-of-Cardiology-Practice/Volume-16/Blood-pressure-measurement-in-the-obese-still-a-challenging-problem

Pickering, T. G., Hall, J. E., Appel, L. J., Falkner, B. E., Graves, J., Hill, M.N., Jones, D. W., Kurtz, T., Sheps, S. G., & Roccella, E. J. (2005). Recommendations for blood pressure measurement in humans and experimental animals. Part 1: Blood pressure measurement in humans: A statement for professionals from the subcommittee of professional and public education of the American Heart Association Council on High Blood Pressure Research. *Circulation, 111*(5), 697–716. http://doi.org/10.1161/01.CIR.0000154900.76284.F6

Problem-based care plans. (2020). In *Lippincott Advisor.* Wolters Kluwer. https://advisor.lww.com/lna/home.do

Robertson, M., & Hill, B. (2019). Monitoring temperature. *British Journal of Nursing, 28*(6), 344–347. https://doi.org/10.12968/bjon.2019.28.6.344

Rolfe, S. (2019). The importance of respiratory rate monitoring. *British Journal of Nursing, 28*(8), 504–508. https://doi.org/10.12968/bjon.2019.28.8.504

Ryan-Wenger, N. A., Sims, M. A., Patton, R. A., & Williamson, J. (2018). Selection of the most accurate thermometer devices for clinical practice: Part 1: Meta-analysis of the accuracy of non-core thermometer devices compared to core body temperature. *Pediatric Nursing, 44*(3), 116–133.

Schellack, N., & Schellack, G. (2019). An overview of the management of fever and its possible complications in infants and toddlers. *Professional Nursing Today, 23*(1), 25–33.

Schell-Chaple, H. M., Liu, K. D., Matthay, M. A., & Puntillo, K. A. (2018). Rectal and bladder temperatures vs forehead core temperatures measured with SpotOn monitoring system. *American Journal of Critical Care, 27*(1), 43–50. https://doi.org/10.4037/ajcc2018865

Seattle Children's. (2022, April 6). Fever – How to take the temperature. https://www.seattlechildrens.org/conditions/a-z/fever-how-to-take-the-temperature/

Sheppard, J. P., Albasri, A., Franssen, M., Fletcher, B., Pealing, L., Roberts, N., Obeid, A., Pucci, M., McManus, R. J., Martin, U., & British and Irish Hypertension Society. (2019). Defining the relationship between arm and leg blood pressure readings: A systematic review and meta-analysis. *Journal of Hypertension, 37*(4), 660–670. https://doi.org/10.1097/HJH.0000000000001958

Silbert-Flagg, J., & Pillitteri, A. (2018). *Maternal and child health nursing* (8th ed.). Wolters Kluwer.

Souza, B. T., Lopes, M. C. B. T., Okuno, M. F. P., Batista, R. E. A., de Góis, A. F. T., & Campanharo, C. R. V. (2019). Identification of warning signs for prevention of in-hospital cardiorespiratory arrest. *Revista Latino-Americana de Enfermagem, 27*, e3072. DOI: 10.1590/1518-8345.2853.3072

Stergiou, G. S., Kario, K., Kollias, A., McManus, R. J., Ohkubo, T., Parati, G., & Imai, Y. (2018). Home blood pressure monitoring in the 21st century. *Journal of Clinical Hypertension (Greenwich), 20*(7), 1116–1121. https://doi.org/10.1111/jch.13284

Sund-Levander, M., & Grodzinsky, E. (2013). Assessment of body temperature measurement options. *British Journal of Nursing, 22*(15), 880, 882–888. https://doi.org/10.12968/bjon.2013.22.16.942

Tanigasalam, V., Vishnu Bhat, B., Adhisivam, B., Balachander, B., & Kumar, H. (2019). Hypothermia detection in low birth weight neonates using a novel bracelet device. *The Journal of Maternal-Fetal & Neonatal Medicine, 32*(16), 2653–2656. https://doi.org/10.1080/14767058.2018.1443072

Toughy, T. A., & Jett, K. (2018). *Ebersol and Hess' gerontological nursing & healthy aging* (5th ed.). Elsevier.

U.S. Environmental Protection Agency (EPA). (n.d.). *Mercury thermometers.* Retrieved July 17, 2021, from https://www.epa.gov/mercury/mercury-thermometers

U.S. Food and Drug Administration (FDA). (2020a, April 23). *Non-contact infrared thermometers.* https://www.fda.gov/medical-devices/general-hospital-devices-and-supplies/non-contact-infrared-thermometers

U.S. Food and Drug Administration (FDA). (2020b, June 19). *Non-contact temperature assessment devices during the COVID-19 pandemic.* https://www.fda.gov/medical-devices/coronavirus-covid-19-and-medical-devices/non-contact-temperature-assessment-devices-during-covid-19-pandemic

U. S. National Library of Medicine. (2020, February 25). *Low blood pressure.* MedlinePlus. https://medlineplus.gov/ency/article/007278.htm

VHA Center for Engineering & Occupational Safety and Health (CEOSH). (2016). *Safe patient handling and mobility guidebook.* http://www.tampavaref.org/safe-patient-handling/implementation-tools.htm

Wang, K., Gill, P., Wolstenholme, J., Heneghan, C., Thompson, M., Price, C. P., Van den Bruel, A., & Plüddemann, A. (2013). *Non-contact infrared thermometers.* National Institute for Health Research. https://www.community.healthcare.mic.nihr.ac.uk/reports-and-resources/horizon-scanning-reports/hs-report-0025

Wasserman, D. D., Creech, J. A., & Healy, M. (2021, October 20). *Cooling techniques for hyperthermia.* StatPearls. U. S. National Library of Medicine. https://www.ncbi.nlm.nih.gov/books/NBK459311/

Weber, J. R., & Kelley, J. H. (2018). *Health assessment in nursing* (6th ed.). Wolters Kluwer.

Whelton, P. K., Carey, R. M., Aronow, W. S., Casey, D. E. Jr, Collins, K. J., Himmelfarb, C. D., DePalma, S. M., Gidding, S., Jamerson, K. A., Jones, D. W., MacLaughlin, E. J., Muntner, P., Ovbiagele, B., Smith, S. C. Jr, Spencer, C. C., Stafford, R. S., Taler, S. J., Thomas, R. J., Williams, K. A. Sr, … Wright, J. T. Jr. (2018). 2017 ACC/AHA/AAPA/ABC/ACPM/AGS/APhA/ASH/ASPC/NMA/PCNA Guideline for the prevention, detection, evaluation, and management of high blood pressure in adults. *Hypertension, 71*(6), 1269–1324. https://doi.org/10.1161/HYP.0000000000000066

World Health Organization (WHO). (2019). Hypertension. https://www.who.int/news-room/fact-sheets/detail/hypertension

27 Health Assessment

Billy Collins

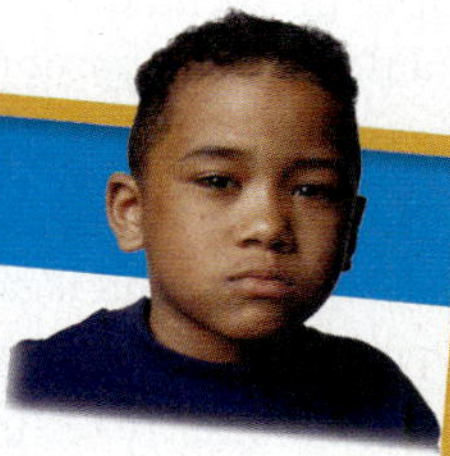

Billy, a 9-year-old boy with a history of allergies, including an allergy to insect stings, is spending a week at summer camp. He reports to the camp counselor that he was just stung by a bee.

Tammy Browning

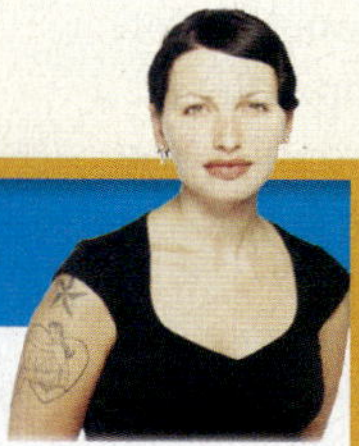

Tammy, who is expecting her first child, has arrived at the birthing center in labor. She and her partner, both in their late 20s, have a history of substance abuse, primarily alcohol and marijuana. A urine specimen is to be collected for routine evaluation and a drug screen. Tammy is unaware that drug testing will be done.

Ramona Lewis

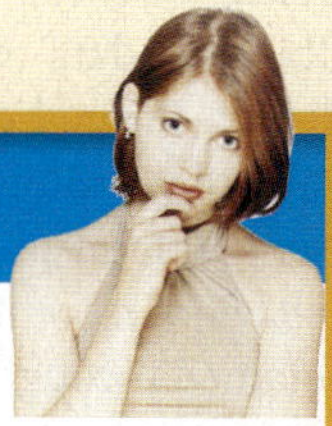

Ramona, a 22-year-old college student, was recently discharged from the inpatient unit with a diagnosis of anorexia nervosa. She is living with her partner, Karen, and her mother, in her mother's home. A home health nurse is visiting Ramona for follow-up services.

Lippincott DocuCare **Additional patient scenarios available in *Lippincott DocuCare*.**

Learning Outcomes

After completing the chapter, you will be able to accomplish the following:

1. Explain the components, purposes, and types of health assessments.
2. Prepare the patient and the environment for a health assessment.
3. Conduct a health history.
4. Use the techniques of inspection, palpation, and auscultation appropriately during a physical assessment.
5. Conduct a physical assessment in a systematic manner.
6. Document health assessment findings in a concise, descriptive, and legally appropriate manner.
7. Describe nursing responsibilities related to diagnostic and laboratory testing as part of health assessment.

Nursing Concepts

- Assessment
- Clinical Decision Making/Clinical Judgment
- Communication
- Therapeutic Communication

Conducting a health assessment involves collecting, validating, and analyzing subjective data and objective data to determine the patient's overall level of physical, psychological, sociocultural, developmental, functional, and spiritual health. Subjective data are based on patient experiences and perceptions, are known only by the patient (e.g., pain and nausea), and are reported by the patient (the patient's own words; sensations, symptoms, perceptions, desires, preferences, beliefs, ideas, values, and personal information). Objective data are measurable and are directly observed or elicited through general observation and physical examination (physical characteristics, body functions, and measurements [blood pressure, height, respiratory rate], appearance, behavior, laboratory results). Objective data may also be obtained through the patient's health record and observations reported by the patient's family, significant others, or care givers about the patient (Weber & Kelley, 2018).

Although most components of a health assessment are described in this chapter, some of the assessments included in a comprehensive or focused examination (such as an internal eye examination, a vaginal examination, or a rectal examination) are usually carried out by advanced practice professionals, health care providers with advanced education. Refer to a health assessment text for details of these advanced assessment skills.

HEALTH ASSESSMENT

Nursing health assessment involves gathering information about the health status of the patient. The nurse then evaluates and synthesizes the information (**data**). The nurse plans appropriate nursing interventions based on this data and evaluates patient care outcomes to deliver the best possible care for each patient. A health assessment includes a health history and a physical assessment. A **health history** is a collection of subjective information that provides information about the patient's health status. **Physical assessment** is a collection of objective data that provides information about changes in the patient's body systems.

A health assessment may be comprehensive, ongoing or partial (follow-up), focused, or emergency. The amount and type of information collected and frequency of assessment vary based on the patient's needs and health care setting and circumstances (Jensen, 2019). Nursing knowledge, expertise, judgment, and clinical experience guide decisions about which assessments are a priority for an individual patient and health care situation.

A **comprehensive health assessment** is broad and includes a complete health history and physical assessment. A comprehensive assessment is usually conducted when a patient first enters a health care setting, with information providing a baseline for comparing later assessments. An **ongoing or partial health assessment**, or **follow-up assessment**, is one that is conducted at regular intervals (e.g., at the beginning of each home health visit or each hospital shift) during care of the patient. This type of assessment concentrates on identified health problems to monitor positive or negative changes and evaluate the effectiveness of interventions. In addition, a brief reassessment of the patient's body systems and functional abilities is performed to detect any new problems (Weber & Kelley, 2018).

Clinical nurses must be organized and focused to complete meaningful health assessment, usually a partial health assessment, on all assigned patients within the first hour of the nursing shift (Haugh, 2015). This requires the nurse to assess each patient quickly and efficiently, incorporating assessments directed at basic bodily functions as well as assessment based on individual patient priorities. Nurses must use clinical judgment to adapt this assessment for each patient and based on the patient population served (Haugh, 2015). Any additional in-depth information about the patient can be obtained once the baseline status for each patient has been established. This prioritized initial assessment may also identify specific findings to follow-up on later. Box 27-1 (on page 776) provides an example of a brief, general assessment that can be used to gather pertinent data to be used provide a basis for prioritizing nursing care. Nurses should use clinical judgment to adapt this generic assessment to the individual circumstances of an individual patient and to monitor for changes that might require further intervention (Haugh, 2015).

A **focused health assessment** is conducted to assess a specific health issue. This type of assessment "usually involves one or two body systems and is smaller in scope than a comprehensive assessment, but more in depth on the specific issue or issues" (Jensen, 2019, p. 10). For example, if a woman is having abdominal pain, the nurse asks questions about urinary problems, bowel problems, allergies,

QSEN Reflective Practice: Cultivating QSEN Competencies

CHALLENGE TO ETHICAL AND LEGAL SKILLS

I have always been interested in labor and delivery, so I was very excited to have the opportunity to follow a nurse in labor and delivery and assist and witness the beginning of life. I had no idea that the whole process could be so complicated.

It was here that I met Tammy Browning, who was expecting her first child. She and her partner were in their late 20s or early 30s. She was in labor and had arrived at the birth center late last night. Before entering the room, the nurse gave me a brief rundown of what we were expected to do throughout the morning.

On entering the patient's room for the first time, I was shocked at what I saw. The room was dark and extremely cluttered with food, candy wrappers, and trash overflowing onto the floor. The patient's partner had been sleeping in the room and both of their belongings were all over the place. I could not believe it! When we left the room, the nurse told me that both the patient and her partner had a history of drug use, mainly alcohol and marijuana. We had to get a urine sample from her to do a dipstick test. The specimen was also going to be used for a drug screen, but the patient was not going to be told about this. I was shocked and confused by this action. I thought that we had to tell the patient everything we were going to do—right?

Thinking Outside the Box: Possible Courses of Action

- Go along with what the nurse decided to do, and when we get out of the patient's room, ask why she decided to take this course of action.
- Inform myself of the legality of taking this route of action.
- Inform my instructor and head nurse about the case, asking if this was a usual occurrence and requesting that they tell or educate me on what basis they were allowed to do this.

Evaluating a Good Outcome: How Do I Define Success?

- Safety of patient and neonate is ensured.
- Patient and baby benefit from the decided-on course of action.
- No breach of duty or harm is done.
- Patient receives proper care and treatment regardless of her past drug use and results of the drug tests.
- Respect for patient is maintained.

Personal Learning: Here's to the Future!

I really had no idea what to do. Because I did not feel legally competent to challenge the nurse and suggest a different course of action, I followed her and went along with her story. Afterward, I asked her if we were allowed to do this. Her answer was that she was doing it because the patient had a history of drug use and she suspected that she had been smoking marijuana up to the time she arrived. The test was not going to harm the baby or the mother; if anything, the test was going to be beneficial in providing the most adequate care for her and her baby. It was also going to assist in preparing for any complications that may arise during the delivery.

When she gave me this explanation, I figured that her reasons were valid and it was all right to do this since no one was going to get hurt and it would be beneficial. However, I was left with the thought that we were violating the patient's privacy. I also spoke with my clinical instructor about the situation. Through this experience, I realized that I need to educate myself more on the legal aspects of nursing. I had never paid much attention to the fact that I am exposed to many legal situations every day as a health care provider. Therefore, I must be prepared to confront them. I think that it is vital to be skilled as well as to be competent medically and legally. By having this knowledge, many difficult situations may be avoided and/or resolved. With this knowledge, I will also be a better advocate for my patients.

Stephanie Cuellar, Georgetown University

QSEN SELF-REFLECTION ON QUALITY AND SAFETY COMPETENCIES DEVELOPING KNOWLEDGE, SKILLS, AND ATTITUDES FOR CONTINUOUS IMPROVEMENT

How do you think you would respond in a similar situation? Why? What does this tell you about yourself and about the adequacy of your skills for professional practice? Do you agree with the criteria that the nursing student used to evaluate a successful outcome? Are there any other criteria that would be appropriate to use? Did the nursing student meet the criteria? Why or why not? What knowledge, skills, and attitudes do you need to develop to continuously improve the quality and safety of care for patients like Ms. Browning?

Patient-Centered Care: What do you think might have happened if the patient were told about the drug testing? Do you feel that the nurse's action of not telling the patient was based on appropriate ethical and legal principles? Why or why not? If so, what ethical and legal principles formed the basis for the action? If not, what ethical and legal principles were violated?

Teamwork and Collaboration/Quality Improvement: What communication skills do you need to improve to ensure that you function as a member of the patient care team? What skills do you need to implement effective strategies for communicating and resolving conflict? What skills do you need to assert your own position/perspective in discussions about patient care?

Safety/Evidence-Based Practice: What evidence in nursing literature provides guidance for decision making regarding care of this patient?

Informatics: Can you identify the essential information that must be available in Ms. Browning's electronic health record to support safe patient care and coordination of care? Can you identify the appropriate process to protect confidentiality of protected health information in the patient's health records? Can you think of other ways to respond to or approach the situation?

Box 27-1 Brief General Physical Assessment

Type of Assessment	Assessment Components
Safety	Bed position, call bell location, appropriate emergency equipment, assistive devices, fall risk/ hazards
Vital signs	Temperature, pulse, respirations, blood pressure, oxygen saturation, pain assessment
Mental status	Level of consciousness; orientation to person, place, and time; speech
Psychosocial	Behavior and affect
Head, eyes, ears, nose	Eyes, pupils, mouth, carotid arteries, swallowing, throat, neck facial color, moisture, lesions, wounds, glasses, hearing aid, ability to hear conversation, ability to see
Chest	Chest color, moisture, lesions, wounds, quality of respirations, heart sounds, lung sounds, cough, sputum
Abdomen	Abdomen color, moisture, lesions, wounds, bowel sounds, tenderness, distention, pain/discomfort, ability to eat, urine elimination pattern and urine characteristics, bowel elimination pattern, and stool characteristics
Upper and lower extremities	Skin, color, pulses, temperature, tenderness, edema, capillary refill, strength, sensation, range of motion, lesions, wounds
Activity	Movement and ambulation, ability to move in bed, ability to get out of bed, ability to walk and distance, gait
Therapeutic devices	Peripheral and central venous access devices, supplemental oxygen setting, pacemaker, cardiac monitor, urinary catheters, gastric tubes, chest tubes, dressings, braces, slings

Nurses should use clinical judgment to adapt this generic assessment to the individual circumstances of each patient and to monitor for changes that might require further intervention (Haugh, 2015).

Source: Adapted from Haugh, K. H. (2015). Head-to-toe: Organizing your baseline patient physical assessment. *Nursing, 45*(12), 58–61, Wolters Kluwer. Reprinted from Elsevier: Anderson, B., Nix, E., Norman, B., & McPike, H. D. (2014). An evidence based approach to undergraduate physical assessment practicum course development. *Nurse Education in Practice, 14*(3), 242–246; with permission from Elsevier.

and menstrual history during the health history and then assesses vital signs and abdominal structures during the physical assessment. Focused assessments may also be used to address the immediate and highest priority concerns for an individual patient.

An **emergency health assessment** is a type of rapid focused assessment conducted when addressing a life-threatening or unstable situation. Assessment of the airway, breathing, and circulation when encountering a patient with traumatic injury as a result of a motor vehicle accident is an example of an emergency assessment.

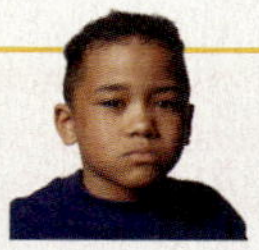

Consider **Billy Collins**, the 9-year-old who was stung by a bee. In this situation, the nurse would conduct an emergency assessment to determine the immediate effects of the bee sting, assessing for indications of an allergic reaction such as respiratory difficulty. Once this emergency assessment is completed and any immediate treatments initiated, the nurse would complete a health history to identify the boy's history of allergies and other relevant health issues.

Health assessment is an integral component of preventive health care. A preventive health assessment includes the patient's health history, risk for depression, functional ability, and level of safety; a physical examination; and patient education and counseling. Annual wellness visits include the patient's health history, blood pressure, height, weight, screening for cognitive impairment and potential risk factors related to depression, functional ability, and safety, as well as health education and preventive counseling. These services are part of the benefits offered for patients covered by Medicare, for example, as part of health promotion and disease prevention and detection (Centers for Medicare and Medicaid Services [CMS], 2018).

A nursing health assessment differs from other types of health assessments (e.g., one performed by a medical health care provider) in that it is a holistic collection of information about factors that affect or are affected by one's level of health. Nurses focus on how a person's health status is affecting activity levels and abilities to perform tasks, as well as how patients are coping with their health issues and any related loss of function or change in ability to function (Jensen, 2019). Accurate health assessment provides the foundation for therapeutic nursing care (Jensen, 2019). Health assessment is part of the foundation of the nursing process. The information from the nursing health assessment is used to formulate diagnoses or patient problems that require nursing care. Assessments are used to plan, implement, and evaluate teaching and care to promote an optimal level of health through interventions to prevent illness, restore health, and facilitate coping with disabilities or death. The information is also used to identify health problems that require interdisciplinary care or immediate referral to other health care providers.

This chapter provides information necessary to identify risks for or actual alterations in health, perform the skills of physical examination, and identify normal age-related variations in physical structures and functions. Health assessments are a part of nursing care for patients across the lifespan and may be conducted in any setting. Refer to the accompanying Reflective Practice box for an example. Additional information about assessment is found in Chapter 14.

Lifespan Considerations

A comprehensive assessment includes cognitive, psychosocial, and emotional development in addition to physical growth (Jensen, 2019). The nurse should identify growth and development patterns, expected variations and deviations from infancy through adolescence, adulthood, and into older age. Refer to Chapters 22, 23, and 24 for more information related to these assessments.

Cultural Considerations and Sensitivity

Each person is a unique individual. Culture influences a person's definition of health and illness (Jensen, 2019). Culture includes a person's racial or ethnic background and nonethnic culture, such as cultural identities based on socioeconomic status (e.g., culture of poverty), ability or disability (e.g., culture of the visually impaired), sexual orientation (e.g., LGBTQIA+ cultures), age (e.g., culture of the elderly), and occupational and professional cultures (e.g., culture of the military) (Jensen, 2019).

Nurses must consider patients within the context of family, culture, and community to meet the needs of an increasingly diverse population. Nurses and other health care professionals need to provide health care services in a sensitive, knowledgeable, and nonjudgmental manner with respect for people's health beliefs and practices, identifying patient specific needs based on the patient's current situation (Kersey-Matusiak, 2019). Nurses should be familiar with the general health beliefs and variances of various groups to improve the effectiveness of health care services and provide care within a cultural context. Nurses should know risk factors for alterations in health that are based on racial inheritance and ethnic backgrounds, as well as normal variations that occur within races. In addition, it is important to consider how cultural characteristics, such as religion and spirituality, may impact health. Cultural assessment is integrated into the overall assessment of the patient, family, and caregivers, incorporating questions aimed at gathering cultural data into the health assessment process (Andrews et al., 2020).

Concept Mastery Alert

All patients, regardless of their race or culture, have the same basic human needs. However, the nurse needs to keep in mind any cultural influences or factors affecting anatomy and physiology, health beliefs, and alterations in health.

Significant disparities exist for vulnerable populations, groups, and communities at a higher risk for poor health as a result of the barriers they experience to social, economic, political, and environmental resources. This also includes potential and actual limitations due to illness or disability (Joszt, 2018; National Collaborating Centre for Determinants of Health, 2020). For example, during the COVID-19 pandemic of 2020, groups of people were identified as vulnerable simply because of their specific risk of profound illness or even death with exposure to the virus. In 2020, these groups included people age 65 years and older; people of any age who have serious underlying medical conditions, such as chronic lung disease, diabetes, or liver disease, or who are obese or immunocompromised; and people with barriers to health care access, due to factors such as insurance status or immigration status (Berlinger et al., 2020; Centers for Disease Control and Prevention, 2020a). Cultural data, as part of health assessment, helps nurses identify patients who are most at risk and plan specific and individualized person-centered interventions that take mutually identified vulnerabilities into consideration. Vulnerable Population Alert 27-1 (on page 778) provides information and resources to support evidence-based practice related to an identified vulnerable population.

Chapter 5 provides information about cultural diversity, transcultural assessment, and the importance of providing culturally sensitive nursing care. Box 8-4 in Chapter 8 provides information about respectful ways to relate to patients from different cultures.

Patient Preparation

When conducting a nursing health assessment, it is important to consider and remain sensitive to the patient's physiologic needs (e.g., pain or decreased stamina because of age or illness) and psychological needs (e.g., anxiety about having the examination). Explain that the first part of the assessment will involve questions about the patient's health concerns, health habits, and lifestyle and that the information will only be shared with the patient's other health care providers. Inform the patient that after the health history is completed, body structures will be examined.

The patient may be anxious for various reasons. Reassure the patient by explaining that the assessments should not be painful. Explaining the assessment in general terms can help decrease the patient's embarrassment, fear of possible abnormal physical findings, or fear of "failing" a test. Be sure to then explain each assessment in greater detail as it is performed. Explain that drapes (covers) will be used during the examination, and only the area being assessed will be exposed. Answer the patient's questions directly and honestly.

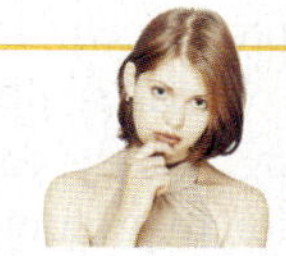

Think back to **Ramona Lewis**, the college student who was recently discharged after treatment for anorexia nervosa. The nurse would need to incorporate knowledge of the emotional and physical effects of eating disorders when communicating with Ms. Lewis. In addition, the patient's anxiety is likely to be high; thus, using empathy, taking the time to explain things slowly, and establishing a trusting nurse–patient relationship are important.

Vulnerable Population Alert 27-1: Lesbian, Gay, Bisexual, Transgender, Questioning/Queer, Intersex, Ally/Asexual (LGBTQIA) Individuals

LGBTQIA individuals encompass all races and ethnicities, religions, and social classes (Healthy People 2020, n.d.). The LGBTQIA community is a vulnerable populace that accounts for 4.5% of the U.S. population (Aisner et al., 2020; The Williams Institute, UCLA School of Law, 2019). Research suggests that LGBTQIA individuals encounter health disparities linked to social stigma, discrimination, and denial of their civil and human rights (Healthy People 2020, n.d.). Fear of discrimination causes many LGBTQIA people to avoid seeking care and when they do get treatment, they are often not treated with the respect or cultural consideration that all patients deserve (Human Rights Campaign, n.d.). LGBTQIA health requires focused attention from health care and health care professionals to address health disparities, including:

- Increased risk for psychiatric disorders, substance abuse, and suicide
- LGBT youth are more likely to be homeless
- Increased experiences of violence and victimization
- Discrimination in access to health insurance, employment, housing, marriage, adoption, and retirement benefits
- Increased experiences of discrimination and prejudice
- Inadequate training and education contributing to a shortage of health care providers who are knowledgeable and culturally competent in LGBT health

Source: Adapted from Aisner, J., Zappas, M., & Marks, A. (2020). Primary care for lesbian, gay, bisexual, transgender, and queer/questioning (LGBTQ) patients. *The Journal for Nurse Practitioners, 16*(4), 281–285; Healthy People 2020. (n.d.). *Lesbian, gay, bisexual, and transgender health.* Office of Disease Prevention and Health Promotion. https://www.healthypeople.gov/2020/topics-objectives/topic/lesbian-gay-bisexual-and-transgender-health; Human Rights Campaign. (n.d.). Explore: Health & aging. https://www.hrc.org/explore/topic/health-and-aging; and The Williams Institute, UCLA School of Law. (2019). *LGBT data & demographics.* https://williamsinstitute.law.ucla.edu/visualization/lgbt-stats/?topic=LGBT#density

Resources

Centers for Disease Control and Prevention (CDC).
Lesbian, gay, bisexual, and transgender health.
https://www.cdc.gov/lgbthealth/

Do Ask, Do Tell
https://doaskdotell.org/

GLMA: Health Professionals Advancing LGBT Equality
http://www.glma.org/

The GLMA Handbook on LGBT Health.
Schneider, J. S., Silenzio, V., and Erickson-Schroth, L. (Eds.). Praeger. http://glma.org/index.cfm?fuseaction=Page.viewPage&pageId=1177&parentID=534&nodeID=1

Human Rights Campaign
https://www.hrc.org/

National Coalition for Sexual Health
https://nationalcoalitionforsexualhealth.org/

Environmental Preparation

Privacy and respect for the patient are primary concerns when conducting a health assessment. In an outpatient setting, such as a clinic or primary care provider office, separate examination rooms provide a quiet, private space for assessment. Prepare the examination room before the health assessment is conducted by preparing the examination table, providing a gown and drape for the patient, and gathering instruments and special supplies needed for the assessment. In a hospital or community-based facility, the health assessment usually takes place in the patient's room. If the area is open to others, an enclosure with a curtain or screen is essential. The room should be warm enough to prevent chilling, and the area or room should be adequately lit, either by sunlight or overhead lighting.

When patients are seen in their home, an assessment may be performed in the patient's bedroom or another private area. Direct the patient to a private dressing area or to a comfortable area in the home and ask the patient to change into a gown, if possible.

For all settings, if necessary, assist the patient with undressing. Ask the patient to empty the bladder before the examination to promote patient comfort during the assessment and to facilitate assessment of the abdomen by the nurse.

Nurse's Role in Diagnostic and Laboratory Testing

Diagnostic procedures and laboratory tests provide crucial information about a patient's health; these results become a part of the total health assessment. Nurses assist before, during, and after some diagnostic tests, and complete other testing as prescribed. The nurse is also responsible for other activities associated with diagnostic tests, such as witnessing the patient's consent, scheduling the test, preparing the patient physically and emotionally for the test, providing care, and teaching the patient and/or caregivers about the prescribed procedures or tests.

Discussion of relevant diagnostic procedures and laboratory testing related to specific health issues can be found in each clinical chapter. Normal findings for many laboratory tests are found in Appendix C in online Student Resources for this text.

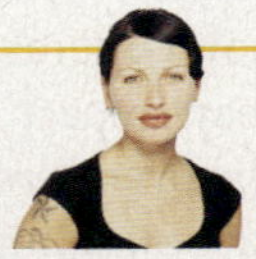

Consider **Tammy Browning**, the pregnant woman with a history of substance abuse. A urine specimen was to be obtained for routine testing. In addition, the specimen was to be used for drug testing without the patient's knowledge. Typically, a signed consent form is not necessary for urine specimens. However, the nurse would need to know the facility's policy and legal statutes of the area regarding consent for drug testing before obtaining the specimen.

HEALTH HISTORY

A health history is a collection of data that provides a detailed profile of the patient's health status. Nurses use therapeutic communication skills and interviewing techniques during the health history to establish an effective nurse–patient relationship and to gather data to identify actual and potential health problems as well as health-promotion activities and sources of strength. Effective interviewing skills are described in Chapters 8 and 14.

Information is collected during an interview with the patient, who is the primary source of data. The patient's family members and/or caregivers may also be an important source of data. They can sometimes offer insight that cannot be gained from patients who may be acutely ill, in pain, or cognitively impaired. Fawcett and Rhynas (2012) suggest, "Nurses need to balance the benefits of obtaining information from family members with the potentially conflicting motivations of patients and their families." The health records of the patient, if available, can also be used to collect additional information. Nurses should know and be sensitive to cultural differences that influence how both verbal and nonverbal communications are interpreted.

Components of the health history include biographical data, the reason the patient is seeking health care, present health or history of present health concern, past health history, family health history, functional health and a **review of systems** (a series of questions about all body systems that helps to reveal concerns or problems as part of the health history). The nurse should adapt questions to the individual patient, omitting questions that do not apply and adding questions that seem pertinent, based on the setting, situation, and ongoing information as the health assessment proceeds. Be sure to use language the patient can understand; avoid using medical terms and jargon. Refer to Focused Assessment Guide 27-1 (on page 780) for examples of appropriate questions related to these components. Examples of health history questions related to each body system (review of systems) are included in the discussion of each region of the physical examination later in the chapter.

Biographical Data

Depending on the health care setting, some biographical data may be collected by people other than the nurse. For example, someone in the admissions department or a receptionist in a medical office may obtain demographic data, including the patient's name, address, and billing and insurance information. Additional biographical information may include biologic sex, sexual orientation, gender identity, age and birth date, marital status, occupation, race, ethnic origin, religious preference, presence of an advance directive/living will, and the patient's primary health care provider. The source of the information is also recorded. Differences in language and culture may have an effect on the quality and safety of health care. Language has been identified as contributing to health disparities, as a significant barrier to access to health care, and a barrier to quality health care and appears to increase the risks to patient safety (Ali & Watson, 2018; Chung et al., 2020; Kersey-Matusiak, 2019; Ku & Jewers, 2013). Language barriers negatively impact the nurse's ability to effectively assess and meet patient care needs (Ali & Watson, 2018). It is important to note the patient's preferred language for discussing health care, as well as any sensory or communication needs. Hospitals are required to address unique patient needs, meet patient-centered communication standards, and comply with cultural competence requirements as outlined by The Joint Commission (2010; updated 2014). Box 8-4 in Chapter 8 provides information about respectful ways to relate to patients from different cultures, including communication techniques.

Reason for Seeking Health Care

The reason for requesting care is a statement in the patient's own words that describes the patient's reason for seeking care. This can help to focus the rest of the assessment. Ask an open-ended question, such as, "Tell me why you are here today." *Try to record whatever the person has to say in the person's exact words. Avoid paraphrasing or interpreting.* For example, if a patient comes into the clinic and tells you "I am having trouble sleeping. At night, I can't seem to stop my thoughts. All I do is worry," it is important to document the patient's own words. It would be incorrect to document the following: "Patient complains of insomnia and anxiety." Correct documentation may include the following: "Patient states, 'I am having trouble sleeping. At night, I can't seem to stop my thoughts. All I do is worry.'"

History of Present Health Concern

When taking the patient's history of present health concern, be sure to explore the symptoms thoroughly. Encourage the patient to describe and explain any symptoms. The description should include information regarding the onset of the problem, location, duration, intensity, quality/description, relieving/exacerbating factors, associated factors, past occurrences, any treatments, and how the problem has affected the patient. Refer to Focused Assessment Guide 27-1 (on page 780) for examples of appropriate questions related to this component.

Past Health History

A patient's past health history may provide insight into causes of current symptoms. It also alerts the nurse to certain risk factors. A past health history includes childhood and adult illnesses, chronic health problems and treatment, and previous surgeries or hospitalizations. This history should also include accidents or injuries, obstetric history, allergies, and the date of most recent immunizations. Vaccine recommendations are updated each year by the Centers for Disease Control and Prevention (CDC). Current guidelines for different age groups can be found on the CDC's website at www.cdc.gov (CDC, n.d.a). Ask the patient about health maintenance screenings, such as routine mammograms and colorectal tests, including dates and results, as well as the use of safety measures. Ask the patient about prescribed and over-the-counter medications, including vitamins, supplements, and any home or herbal remedies. Include the name, dose, route, frequency, and purpose for each medication. Refer to Focused Assessment Guide 27-1 (on page 780) for examples of appropriate questions related to this component.

Focused Assessment Guide 27-1

HEALTH HISTORY

Factors to Assess	Questions and Approaches
Present health history	"When did you first begin having this problem?" "Did it happen suddenly or slowly?" "Show me exactly where you are having this problem." "What other symptoms have you had with this problem?" "How have you treated this problem?"
Past health history	"Tell me about the childhood illnesses, such as measles or mumps, that you had." "What are you allergic to?" "Describe any accidents, injuries, and surgeries you have had." "What prescribed or over-the-counter medications do you use?" "Do you take any herbal or dietary supplements?" "What is the date of your most recent immunization for tetanus; pertussis; polio; measles; rubella; mumps; influenza; hepatitis A, B, and C; and pneumococcus?"
Family history	"How old are the members of your family?" "If any members of your family are not living, what caused their death?" "Is there any history of this health problem you have in other family members?" "Do any family members have long-term illnesses?"
Functional health	"Describe a typical day." "Do you have difficulty or require assistance with bathing or dressing?" "Do you have difficulty or require assistance with toileting or moving around?" "Do you have difficulty or require assistance with eating or preparing meals?" "Do you have difficulty or require assistance with shopping or administering your own medications?" "Tell me about your driving. Who provides transportation?" "Do you have difficulty or require assistance with housekeeping, finances, or laundry?" "Do you smoke or drink alcohol? If so, what kind, for how long, and how much?" "Do you use recreational drugs such as marijuana, tranquilizers, crack, cocaine, or methamphetamine? If so, how much do you use and how often? Have you been exposed to any environmental toxins, such as pesticides, herbicides, or occupational chemicals? "Describe the foods you eat during a typical day." "Tell me about your sleep patterns." "How much exercise do you get each day?" "Who in your family or community is available to help you with health problems if you need it?" "What religious affiliations do you have?" "Does your religious faith or spirituality play an important part in your life?" "Tell me about how you deal with stress." "Describe any changes that you have had in your mood or feelings." "Have you ever been treated for any problems with your mood or behavior?" "How do you feel about the future?" "Do you feel unsafe in your home?" "Tell me about your use of seat belts in cars." "Tell me about your family's use of sports helmets, padding, or other protective equipment." "Are you currently in a relationship? Are the aspects of sex satisfactory to you and your partner?"

QSEN EVIDENCE-BASED PRACTICE (EBP)

Health screening tests can identify health problems and diseases early when they are easier to treat. Individualized patient education is an important part of nursing care. Knowledge of current recommendations from reliable and expert sources is imperative when providing interventions and patient education related to health screening tests.

Family History

Information about a person's family history will provide insight into diseases and conditions for which an individual patient may be at increased risk. Certain disorders have genetic links. For example, a family history of cancer is a risk factor for cancer. Information regarding contact with family members with communicable diseases or environmental hazards can provide clues to the patient's current health or risk factors for health issues. For example, it would be important to note that a family member had recently recovered from pertussis (whooping cough), especially if the patient is presented with respiratory symptoms. This information can also identify important topics for health teaching and counseling. For example, if a child with asthma is living in a household with family members who smoke, the child is at great risk for exacerbations of the disease. Family counseling regarding asthma and smoking would be an important health care intervention. Refer to Focused Assessment Guide 27-1 for examples of appropriate questions related to this component.

Functional Health

Information about a patient's functional health helps to identify the effects of health or illness on a patient's self-care abilities and quality of life including the strengths of the patient and areas that need to improve (Jarvis & Eckhardt, 2020; Jensen, 2019). Psychosocial factors and lifestyle and health practices can contribute to and influence a patient's overall health and well-being. For example, smoking is related to many health problems. Discussion of one or more of these topics may cause strong personal reactions by a patient. It is very important to be nonjudgmental and explain why you need to know certain information (Hogan-Quigley et al., 2017). Consider assessing these factors at the end of the interview, because these issues may naturally arise during the review of systems and a trusting relationship has been established, making the discussion of personal issues easier (Jensen, 2019).

Social determinants of health, the conditions (social, economic, and physical) in the environments in which people live their lives, affect a wide range of health, functioning, and quality-of-life outcomes and risks (Healthy People 2030, n.d.). Ask about the patient's social support, interpersonal relationships, and resources for assistance. Ask about confidants, supporters, and people that are able to help the patient to cope with any health alteration, illness, or other change. Support provided by caregivers, family, friends, and social organizations can positively impact health promotion, improve coping with stress, enhance self-esteem, and support healthy lifestyle behaviors (Mayo Clinic, 2018a).

Ask about additional sociocultural factors that may impact a patient's health and use of health care, such as:

- Language barriers
- Literacy
- Limited access to food market and ability to obtain food
- Access to transportation
- Job opportunities
- Stable housing/safe environment

This information helps us to understand factors that may influence a patient's health and use of health care and shape more effective interventions (Healthy People, 2030, n.d.).

Ask about the patient's level of activity and exercise (Chapter 34), sleep and rest (Chapter 35), and nutrition (Chapter 37). Assess the patient's ability to perform **activities of daily living (ADLs)** or self-care activities. Eating, bathing, dressing, and toileting are examples of ADLs. Assess the patient's ability to perform **instrumental activities of daily living (IADLs)** or those activities needed for independent living. Housekeeping, meal preparation, management of finances, and transportation are examples of IADLs. Functional ability may be further assessed using a formal tool, such as the Katz Index of Independence in Activities of Daily Living, which is used with older adults. This tool can be found in Chapter 34. Refer to Focused Assessment Guide 27-1 for examples of appropriate questions related to these components.

Obtain information related to the patient's values, beliefs, and spiritual resources (Chapter 47); self-esteem and self-concept (Chapter 42); and coping and stress management (Chapter 43). Ask about personal habits, including use of alcohol, illicit drugs, and/or tobacco; exposure to environmental and occupational hazards; and intimate partner and family/caregiver (domestic) violence. Intimate partner violence (IPV) is physical violence, sexual violence, stalking, or psychological harm by a current or former partner or spouse, which can occur among heterosexual or same-sex couples and does not require sexual intimacy (Centers for Disease Control and Prevention [CDC], 2018). The Focused Assessment Guide 27-1 provides examples of appropriate questions related to these components. Refer to Chapter 28 for additional discussion of intimate partner violence and an example of an assessment screening tool.

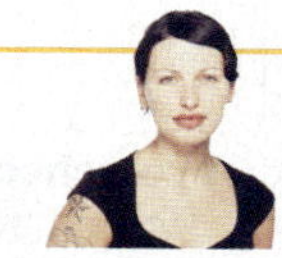

Remember **Tammy Browning**, the young woman who is expecting her first child. The nurse would include an assessment of current and past use of alcohol and drugs as part of Tammy's admission to the birthing unit. This assessment would include questions regarding the type and amount of drugs and alcohol she has used or is using as well as the frequency of use.

Obtain information about the patient's mental health. "Mental health is an integral part of a patient's well-being; thus, the assessment of mental health status is essential" (Jensen, 2019, p. 185). Regular screenings in primary care and other health care settings enable earlier identification of mental health and substance use disorders, leading to earlier treatment and care. There are many assessment tools available to assist with screening for mental health disorders. Specific tools are available to screen for depression or suicide, for example, and to be used with specific populations, such as adolescents or older adults. The Patient Health Questionnaire-9 (PHQ-9), the most common screening tool to identify depression, is one example of a mental health assessment tool (Box 27-2 on page 782). Refer to Focused Assessment Guide 27-1 for examples of appropriate questions related to this component.

Sexual health is an essential element of overall health and well-being (Altarum Institute, 2019). Use neutral and inclusive terms (e.g., partner) and a nonjudgmental manner to obtain information about the patient's sexual history, sexual activity, gender identity, and sexual orientation. This information will help identify the needs of individual patients and provide patient-centered, culturally considerate care (Altarum Institute, 2019; Cahill et al., 2020). Box 27-3 (on page 782) provides some suggested strategies and essential health questions for assessment of sexual health. Additional points related to assessment of sexual and reproductive health are included in the "Assessing Female Genitalia" and

Box 27-2 The Patient Health Questionnaire-9 (PHQ-9)

Over the last 2 weeks, how often have you been bothered by any of the following problems? (Use "✓" to indicate your answer)	Not At All	Several Days	More Than Half the Days	Nearly Every Day
1. Little interest or pleasure in doing things	0	1	2	3
2. Feeling down, depressed, or hopeless	0	1	2	3
3. Trouble falling or staying asleep, or sleeping too much	0	1	2	3
4. Feeling tired or having little energy	0	1	2	3
5. Poor appetite or overeating	0	1	2	3
6. Feeling bad about yourself—or that you are a failure or have let yourself or your family down	0	1	2	3
7. Trouble concentrating on things, such as reading the newspaper or watching television	0	1	2	3
8. Moving or speaking so slowly that other people could have noticed. Or the opposite—being so fidgety or restless that you have been moving around a lot more than usual.	0	1	2	3
9. Thoughts that you would be better off dead or of hurting yourself in some way	0	1	2	3
FOR OFFICE CODING 0 + ______ + ______ + ______ = Total Score: ______				

If you checked off any problems, how difficult have these problems made it for you to do your work, take care of things at home, or get along with other people?

Not difficult at all	Somewhat difficult	Very difficult	Extremely difficult
☐	☐	☐	☐

How to Score PHQ-9

Major Depressive Syndrome is suggested if:

- Of the 9 items, 5 or more are checked as at least "More than half the days"
- Either item #1 or #2 is positive, that is, at least "More than half the days"

Other Depressive Syndrome is suggested if:

- Of the 9 items, 2, 3, or 4 are checked as at least "More than half the days"
- Either item #1 or #2 is positive, that is, at least "More than half the days"

Source: From Patient Health Questionnaire (PHQ) Screeners. Developed by Dr. Robert L. Spitzer, Dr. Janet B. W. Williams, Dr. Kurt Kroenke, and colleagues, with an educational grant from Pfizer Inc. No permission required to reproduce, translate, display, or distribute. http://www.phqscreeners.com

Box 27-3 Strategies and Health Questions for Assessment of Sexual Health

In a matter-of-fact manner, inform the patient that sexual health is important to overall health and these questions are asked of everyone.

Ask the patient's partner, relative, or caregiver to step out of the room for the assessment.

Give the patient the opportunity to ask questions or voice concerns.

Assure the patient that all information is confidential.

Ask the following questions in a nonjudgmental manner, using neutral and inclusive terms:

- Have you been sexually active in the last year? If yes, what types of sex do you have? With men, women, or both? How many partners have you had?
- If no, have you ever been sexually active?
- How do you think of yourself? Lesbian, gay, straight, bisexual; something else (specify); don't know
- What is your current gender identity? Male, female, female-to-male/transgender male/trans man, male-to-female/transgender female/trans woman, nonbinary or nonconforming, genderqueer, additional category (specify), decline to answer
- What sex were you assigned at birth, as shown on your birth certificate? Male, female, decline to answer
- What are your pronouns? He/him, she/her, they/their, something else (specify)
- What do you do to protect yourself from STIs?
- Have you been vaccinated against HPV? Hepatitis A? Hepatitis B?
- What questions do you have about your body and/or sex?

Source: Adapted from Altarum Institute. (2019). Sexual health and your patients: A provider's guide. National Coalition for Sexual Health. https://nationalcoalitionforsexualhealth.org/tools/for-healthcare-providers; Cahill, S., Baker, K., & Makadon, H. (2020). Do ask, do tell: A toolkit for collecting sexual orientation and gender identify information in clinical settings. The Fenway Institute and the Center for American Progress. https://doaskdotell.org/

"Assessing Male Genitalia" later in this chapter. Refer also to Chapter 46 for additional information.

Review of Systems

The review of systems is a series of questions about all body systems that helps to reveal concerns or problems as part of the health history. Many times, these questions can be incorporated into the physical examination of each region, such as asking about bowel habits when listening to bowel sounds in the abdomen. In addition, many questions relate to one or more body systems, thus the information obtained may pertain to more than one area. For example, asking about recent changes in weight is part of the overall health state, but it also provides information about fluid balance, and may offer information about appetite and functional ability. Examples of health history questions related to each body system are included in the discussion of each region of the physical examination later in the chapter.

PHYSICAL ASSESSMENT

Physical assessment is the systematic collection of objective information. The physical assessment is usually conducted in a head-to-toe sequence or a system sequence but can be adapted to meet the needs of the patient. It is often necessary to modify the sequence, positions, and specific assessments based on the patient's age, energy level, and cognitive and physical state, as well as time constraints. Even when modified, it is important to conduct the physical assessment in an organized and knowledgeable manner. Conducting an accurate physical assessment takes time and practice. Note that not all assessments included in a comprehensive physical assessment are covered in this chapter. The information reviewed here addresses the assessments that may be used by beginning and general health care providers. Consult an assessment textbook for additional information related to more advanced assessment procedures.

Preparing for a Physical Examination

Prior to beginning a physical examination, think about how to make the patient comfortable and relaxed. Be sure to use appropriate verbal and nonverbal communication techniques. Refer to the discussion earlier in this chapter. Think about the appropriate and essential components of the examination for the individual patient and circumstances, as well as the sequence of the examination—what order will be used to assess the areas required by the examination. Refer to the discussion of focused assessments earlier in the chapter.

Adjust the lighting and the environment; good lighting and a quiet environment are important, but not always possible. Do the best you can to make the conditions as favorable as possible (Hogan-Quigley et al., 2017). Refer also to the discussion of environmental preparation earlier in the chapter. Gather and check the equipment needed for the examination. Assist the patient to the appropriate position to start the examination. Use proper hand hygiene techniques and standard precautions when performing physical examinations. Transmission-based precautions are implemented in addition as needed. Refer to Chapter 25 for information about hand hygiene, standard precautions, and transmission-based precautions.

Equipment

The equipment used in a physical assessment should be readily accessible, clean, and in proper working order. Equipment that will touch the patient should be warmed (by the examiner's hands or warm water) before use. Following are details about the equipment most likely used by beginning health care providers. However, beginning health care providers may observe or assist with more advanced assessments. Refer to Figure 27-1 for equipment that may be used by more advanced health care providers. Nurses will need a watch with a second hand in addition to the materials identifies below. Clean equipment after use with each patient, based on facility policies, to prevent transmission of microorganisms between patients or between

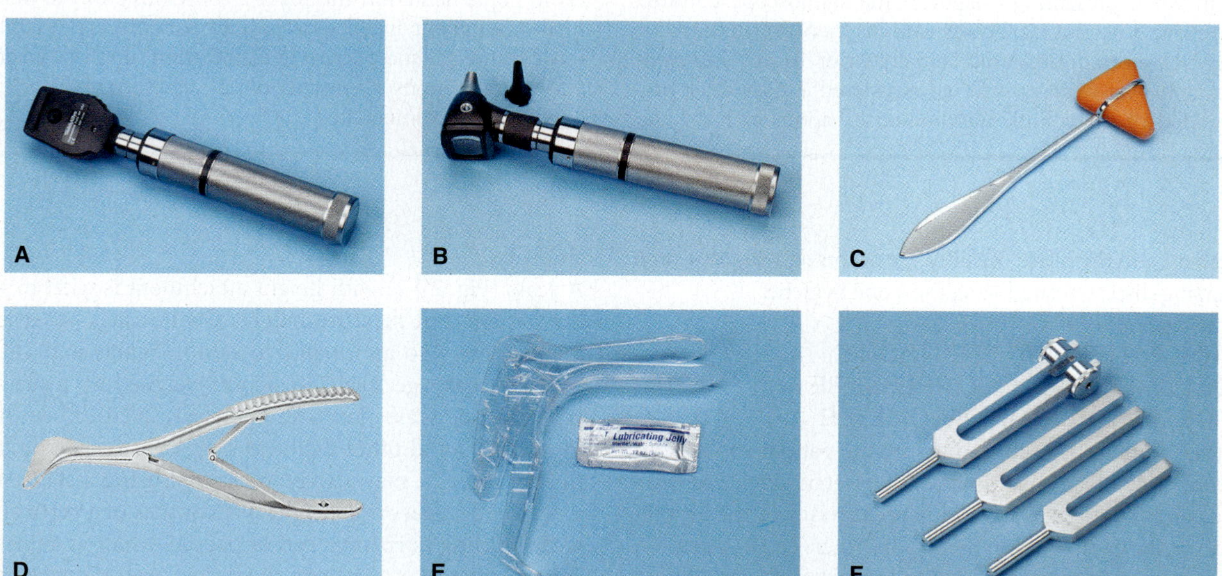

FIGURE 27-1. Equipment used in advanced assessment. **A.** Ophthalmoscope. **B.** Otoscope. **C.** Percussion hammer. **D.** Nasal speculum. **E.** Vaginal speculum and water-soluble lubricant. **F.** Tuning forks.

Research in Nursing

BRIDGING THE GAP TO EVIDENCE-BASED PRACTICE

Stethoscope Hygiene

Stethoscopes, like other patient care equipment, should be cleaned between patients and undergo routine disinfection to prevent the spread of microorganisms. This simple intervention is rarely done despite guideline recommendations (Holleck et al., 2020). What can be done to improve compliance by health care professionals?

Related Evidence

Holleck, J. L., Campbell, S., Alrawili, H., Frank, C., Merchant, N., Rodwin, B., Perez, M. F., Gupta, S., Federman, D. G., Chang, J. J., Vientos, W., & Dembry, L. (2020). Stethoscope hygiene: Using cultures and real-time feedback with bioluminescence-based adenosine triphosphate technology to change behavior. *American Journal of Infection Control*, 48(4), 380–385. https://doi.org/10.1016/j.ajic.2019.10.005

The purpose of this quality improvement project was to determine whether demonstrating what is growing on the stethoscopes of providers via culture or bioluminescence technology alters perceptions and improves compliance with stethoscope hygiene. In addition, the researchers sought to gain a better understanding of the beliefs and the barriers to stethoscope hygiene. Participants included medical students, house staff, and attending physicians on the medical wards at a Department of Veterans Affairs (VA) tertiary care teaching hospital. Beginning with the first week of their medicine inpatient rotations at the VA, providers were given the opportunity to culture their stethoscopes and swab for bioluminescence-based adenosine triphosphate testing before and after disinfection with alcohol pads, alcohol-based hand rub, or hydrogen peroxide disinfectant wipes. Beginning with the second week of their rotations, actual photographic images of stethoscope culture plates before and after disinfection were presented for visual impact at a morning report. Bioluminescence scores of stethoscopes before and after disinfection were provided in real-time and again when presenting images of the stethoscope cultures. Pre-surveys exploring beliefs and barriers to stethoscope hygiene were administered initially prior to any intervention and post-surveys were administered 2 days after presentation of the results. Baseline observations of hand and stethoscope hygiene rates were discreetly recorded at the start of rotations, after presenting the culture images and bioluminescence scores during the second week and during the fourth week of provider rotations. The bacteria isolated, colony-forming units (CFUs), and bioluminescence scores were tracked. This 4-week period was repeated for a total of three cycles. A total of 1,245 observed hand hygiene opportunities showed that compliance improved from 72.5% to 82.3% ($p < .001$). Observed patient–provider encounters (590) revealed no significant change in stethoscope hygiene rates of 10% initially and 5% afterward ($p = .08$), although self-reported rates trended from 56% to 67% postintervention ($p = .06$). Perceptions regarding stethoscope hygiene importance improved 8.5/10 to 9.3/10; $p = .04$. Disinfection with alcohol pads, alcohol-based hand rub, and hydrogen peroxide disinfectant wipes were equivalent in CFU reduction ($p = .21$). The top three barriers to stethoscope hygiene were forgetfulness, time constraints, and limited access to supplies. The authors concluded that showing providers what is growing on their stethoscopes improved "buy in" regarding stethoscope hygiene importance. Objective observations failed to show improvement in stethoscope hygiene rates, but hand hygiene performance improved. The authors noted a significant gap between what providers think they are doing and what they are actually doing.

Relevance to Nursing Practice

Disinfection of patient care equipment, such as stethoscopes, reduces bacteria on the equipment, including the potential to reduce and limit transmission of pathogens. Stethoscopes, like other patient care equipment, should be cleaned between patients and undergo routine disinfection. Nurses and other health care providers need to be aware of the potential barriers to implementation and make a conscious effort to implement equipment hygiene as part of patient care. Facilities must ensure adequate access to disinfection supplies and consider interventions to support use of disinfectants to reduce barriers to implementation.

the patient and the nurse. Refer to the accompanying Research in Nursing display related to stethoscope hygiene.

THERMOMETER AND ELECTRONIC OSCILLOMETRIC BLOOD PRESSURE DEVICE OR SPHYGMOMANOMETER

The thermometer is used to measure the patient's body temperature. Use of an electronic oscillometric device is used to measure blood pressure and is preferred over the auscultatory method of measurement (Muntner et al., 2019). A sphygmomanometer is required to complete an auscultatory measurement of blood pressure. Refer to Chapter 26 for a more detailed discussion of equipment to measure vital signs.

SCALE

A scale (Fig. 27-2) with height attachment is used to weigh the patient and measure height. Chair scales are available for patients who are unable to stand. Infants and children younger than age 2 or 3 years are weighed on a platform-type balance scale (Jarvis & Eckhardt, 2020). Beds for use in hospitals and other facilities may have a scale built into the bed. Height may also be measured using a stadiometer, a device for measuring height that consists of a vertical ruler with a sliding horizontal rod or paddle, which is adjusted to rest on the top of the head. It is often wall mounted but is used horizontally on a tabletop for infants and young children to measure length.

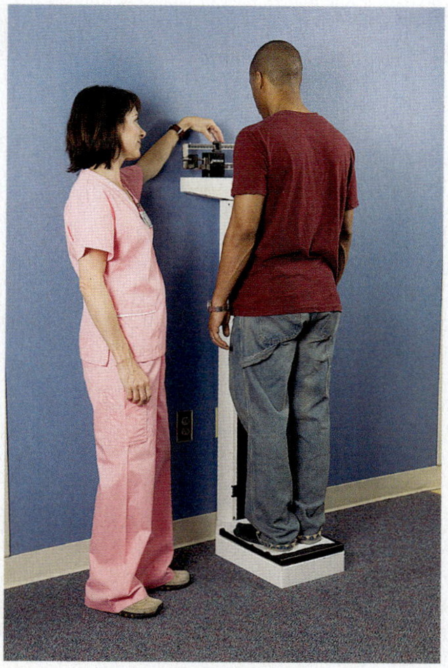

FIGURE 27-2. A scale with height attachment is used to weigh the patient and measure height. (*Source:* Jensen, S. [2019]. *Nursing health assessment: A best practice approach* [3rd ed.]. Wolters Kluwer Health.)

FLASHLIGHT OR PENLIGHT

A light source is used to assist in viewing inside the mouth and nose. It is also used to determine the reactions of the pupils of the eyes.

STETHOSCOPE

The stethoscope, illustrated and described in Chapter 26, is used to measure blood pressure. It is also used to auscultate (listen to) heart, lung, abdomen, and cardiovascular sounds (Fig. 27-3). When using the stethoscope, expose the body part to be auscultated and try to minimize environmental noises. Use the *bell* of the stethoscope to detect low-pitched sounds. Hold the bell lightly against the body part being auscultated. Use the *diaphragm* of the stethoscope to detect high-pitched sounds (such as normal heart sounds, breath sounds, and bowel sounds). Hold the diaphragm firmly against the body part being auscultated.

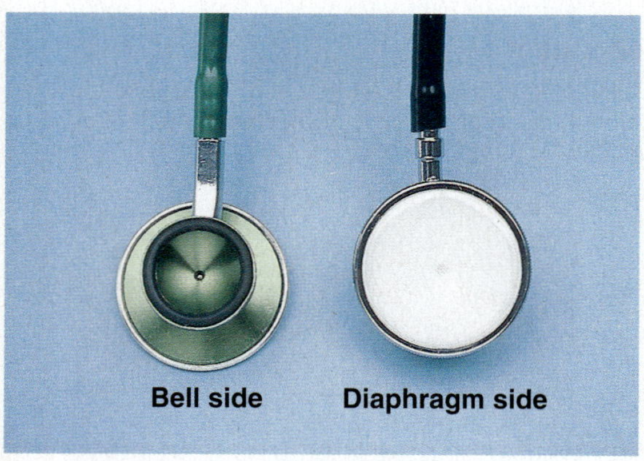

FIGURE 27-3. Stethoscope bell and diaphragm.

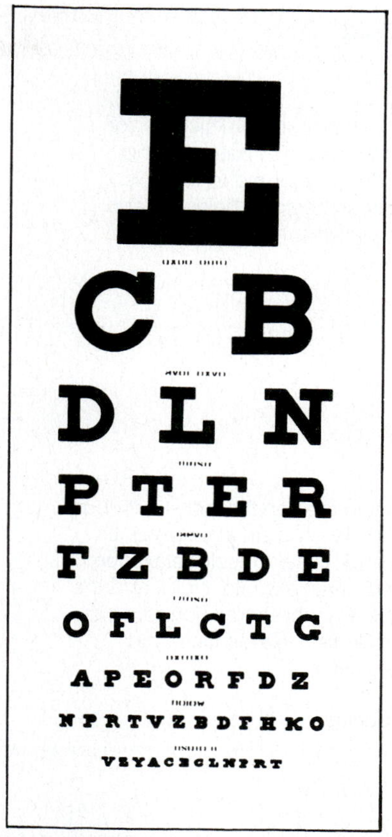

FIGURE 27-4. Snellen chart.

METRIC TAPE MEASURE AND RULER

A tape measure is used to measure waist circumference in adults. It is also used to measure head circumference in infants and children, as well as chest circumference in infants. A ruler is used to measure abnormal findings on the skin, such as wounds, incisions, or lesions.

EYE CHART

A Snellen eye chart (Fig. 27-4), or other vision assessment tool, is used to screen for distant vision. The Snellen chart consists of characters arranged in lines of different-sized type; the line of largest characters is at the top of the chart and the line of smallest characters is at the bottom. Scores ranging from 20/10 (the smallest line of characters) to 20/200 (the largest line of characters) indicate visual acuity.

A handheld vision screener, such as a Jaeger card, can be used to test near vision. The Jaeger card also consists of characters arranged in lines of different-sized type, like the Snellen chart. A distance equivalent based on the Snellen chart is shown on the side of the card.

Positioning and Draping

A variety of positions may be used during a physical assessment (see Box 27-4 on page 786). During positioning, it is important to consider the patient's age, culture, health status, mobility, physical condition, energy level, and privacy. Positioning patients who are weak or have physical limitations may require assistance. Position should be adjusted to accommodate patient limitations, such as arthritis, confusion,

Box 27-4 Positions Used During Physical Assessment

Standing

The patient stands erect. This position should not be used for patients who are weak, dizzy, or prone to fall. It is used to assess posture, balance, and gait (while walking upright).

Standing

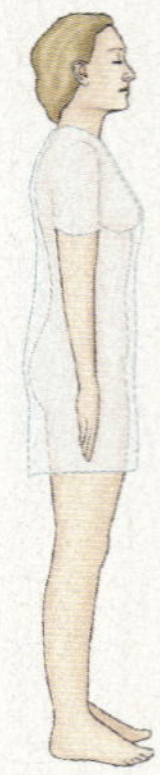

Sitting

The patient may sit in a chair or on the side of the bed or examining table, or remain in bed with the head elevated. It allows visualization of the upper body, facilitates full lung expansion, and is used to assess vital signs and the head, neck, anterior and posterior thorax, lungs, heart, breasts, and upper extremities.

Sitting

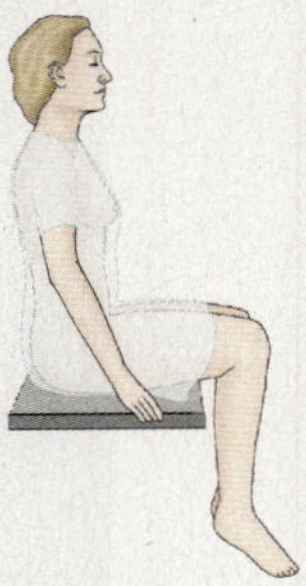

Supine

The patient lies flat on the back with legs extended and knees slightly flexed. It facilitates abdominal muscle relaxation and is used to assess vital signs and the head, neck, anterior thorax, lungs, heart, breasts, abdomen, extremities, and peripheral pulses.

Supine

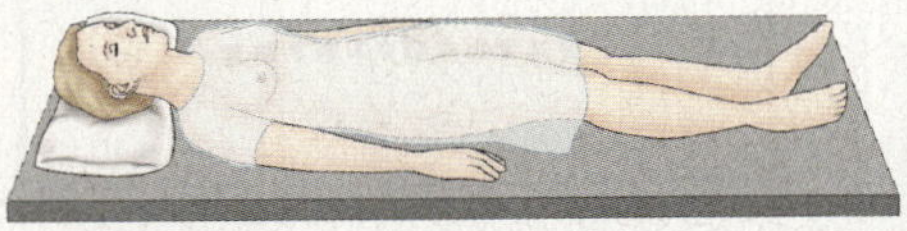

Dorsal Recumbent

The patient lies on the back with legs separated, knees flexed, and soles of the feet on the bed. It is used to assess the head, neck, anterior thorax, lungs, heart, breasts, extremities, and peripheral pulses. It should not be used for abdominal assessment because it causes contraction of the abdominal muscles.

Dorsal recumbent

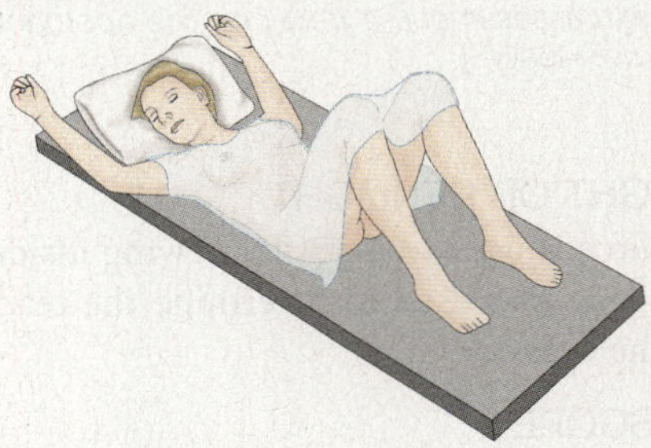

Sims Position

The patient lies on either side with the lower arm below the body and the upper arm flexed at the shoulder and elbow. Both knees are flexed, with the upper leg more acutely flexed. It is used to assess the rectum or vagina.

Sims position

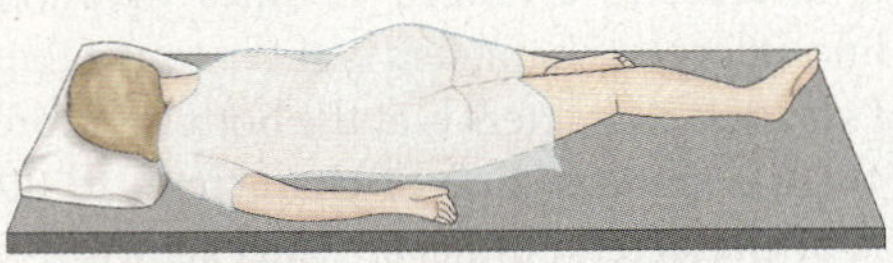

Prone

The patient lies flat on the abdomen with the head turned to one side. It is used to assess the hip joint and the posterior thorax.

Prone

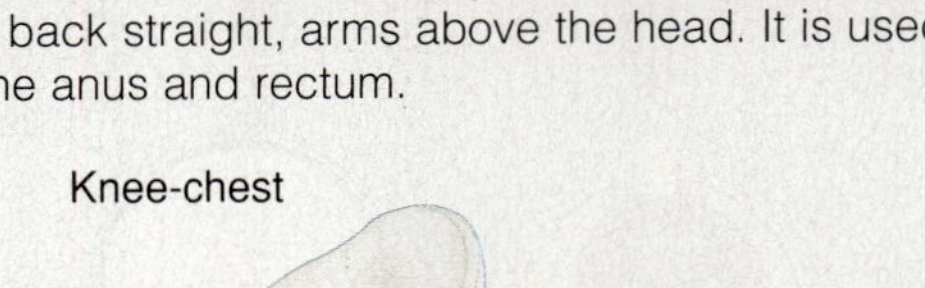

Lithotomy

The patient is in the dorsal recumbent position with the buttocks at the edge of the examining table and the heels in stirrups. It is used to assess female genitalia and rectum.

Lithotomy

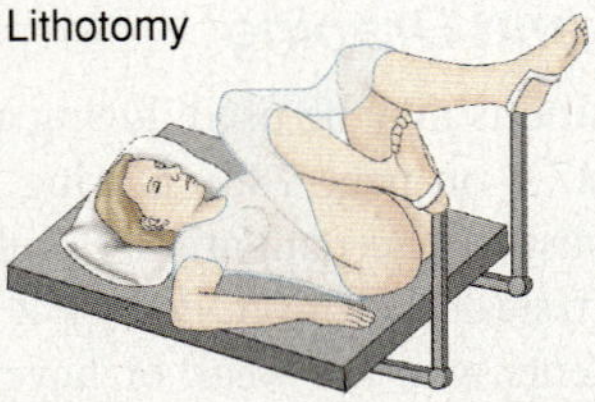

Knee–Chest

The patient kneels, with the body at a 90-degree angle to the hips, back straight, arms above the head. It is used to assess the anus and rectum.

Knee-chest

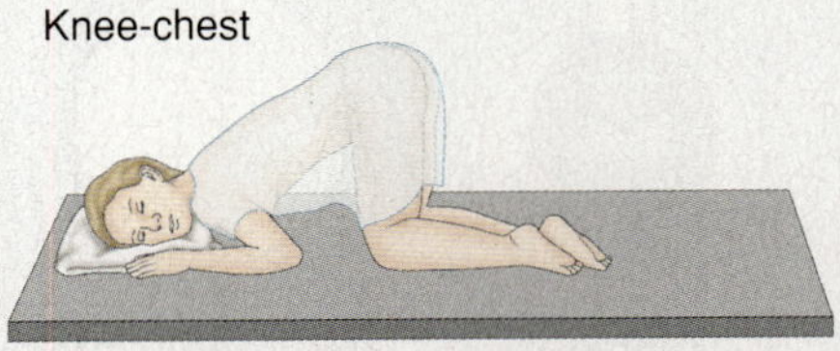

pain, or respiratory problems. Uncomfortable or embarrassing positions should not be maintained for long periods. The assessment should be organized so that several body systems can be assessed with the patient in one position, thus minimizing unneeded and possibly tiring movements.

Draping prevents unnecessary exposure, provides privacy, and keeps the patient warm during the physical assessment. Drapes may be paper, cloth, or bed linens. When conducting an assessment, expose only the body parts being assessed to maintain the patient's modesty and comfort.

Techniques of Physical Assessment

The four primary assessment techniques are inspection, palpation, percussion, and auscultation. These techniques are most often used in the sequence listed; variations are noted in the discussion of specific body areas later in the chapter. Bilateral body parts are always compared; for example, the assessment findings of one leg are compared with those of the other leg. Bilateral body parts are normally symmetric; that is, they have the same size and shape as well as the same characteristics, such as movement or pulses. Wait until the end of the examination to assess any areas that are likely to be painful or cause the patient extreme discomfort.

Inspection

Inspection is the process of performing deliberate, purposeful observations in a systematic manner. Closely observe visually but also use hearing and smell to gather data throughout the assessment. Assess details of the patient's appearance, behavior, and movement. Inspection begins with the initial patient contact and continues through the entire assessment. Adequate natural or artificial lighting is essential for distinguishing the color, texture, and moisture of body surfaces.

Inspect each area of the body for size, color, shape, position, movement, and symmetry, noting normal findings and any deviations from normal. Inspection is usually followed by palpation during the assessment of each body part.

Palpation

Palpation uses the sense of touch. The hands and fingers are sensitive tools that can assess skin temperature, turgor, texture, and moisture, as well as vibrations within the body (such as the heart) and shape or structures within the body (e.g., the bones). Specific parts of the hand are more effective at assessing different qualities (Fig. 27-5). The dorsum (back) surfaces of the hand and fingers are used for gross measure of temperature. The palmar (front) surfaces of the fingers and fingerpads are used to assess firmness, contour, shape, tenderness, and consistency. The fingerpads are best at fine discrimination. Use fingerpads to locate pulses, lymph nodes, and other small lumps, and to assess skin texture and edema. Vibration is palpated best with the ulnar, or outside, surface of the hand.

The nurse's hands should be warmed and the fingernails short. Prior to any assessment involving palpation, inform the patient about the areas to be palpated and ask for permission to use touch. When conducting palpation, any area of tenderness is palpated last. Light or deep palpation may be used, controlling the depth by the amount of pressure applied. For light palpation, apply pressure with the fingers together and lightly depressing the skin and underlying structures about 1 to 2 cm (0.5 inch to 0.75 inch) (Fig. 27-6). Light palpation is used to feel for pulses, tenderness, surface skin texture, temperature, moisture, and muscular resistance (Jarvis & Eckhardt, 2020; Jensen, 2019; Weber & Kelley, 2018). Deep palpation is used to assess organs, masses, structures that are covered by thick muscle and tenderness (Jensen, 2019; Weber & Kelley, 2018). Deep palpation should be used cautiously and only by experienced advanced health care providers. Refer to a health assessment text for details of this advanced physical assessment skill.

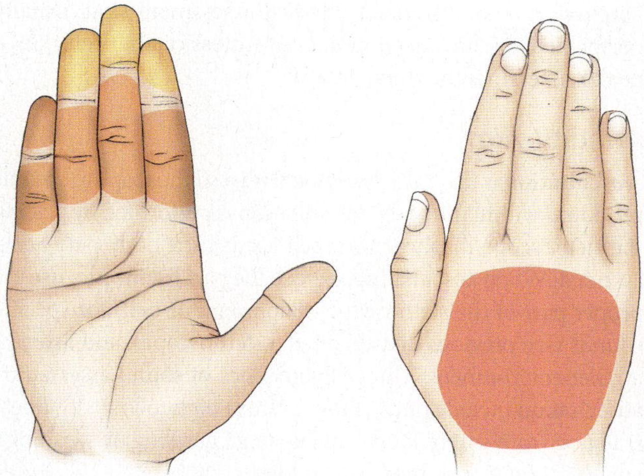

FIGURE 27-5. (**Left**) Palmar surfaces of the examiner's fingertips and fingerpads are used for discriminatory sensation such as firmness, tenderness, and shape. (**Right**) The dorsum, or back of the hand, is used to assess surface temperature. Fingers and fingerpads are used to assess firmness, contour, shape, tenderness, and consistency.

Percussion

Percussion is the act of striking one object against another to produce sound. The fingertips are used to tap the body over body tissues to produce vibrations and sound waves. The characteristics of the sounds produced are used to assess the location, shape, size, and density of tissues. Abnormal sounds suggest alteration of tissues or the presence of a mass.

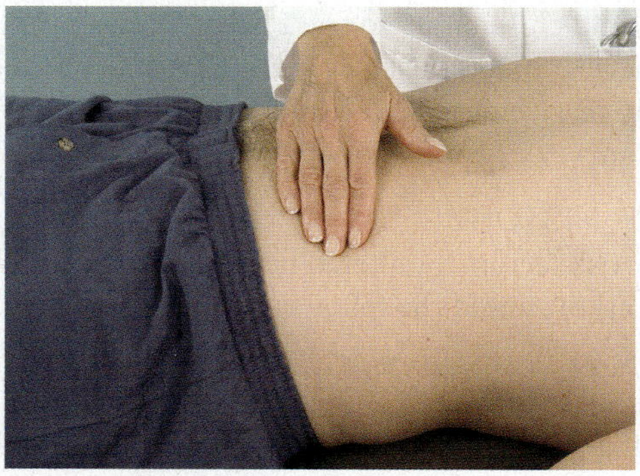

FIGURE 27-6. In light palpation, light pressure is applied by placing the fingers together and depressing the skin and underlying structures about 1 to 2 cm (0.5 inch to 0.75 inch). (*Source:* Used with permission from Shutterstock. *Photo by B. Proud.*)

Percussion is an advanced physical assessment skill, usually performed by advanced practice professionals. Refer to a health assessment text for details.

Auscultation

Auscultation is the act of listening with a stethoscope to sounds produced within the body. Auscultation is performed by placing the stethoscope diaphragm or bell against the body part being assessed. When auscultating, expose the part listened to, use the proper part of the stethoscope (diaphragm or bell) for specific sounds (see previous discussion of a stethoscope), and listen in a quiet environment. The characteristics of sound assessed by auscultation include pitch (ranging from high to low), loudness (ranging from soft to loud), quality (e.g., gurgling or swishing), and duration (short, medium, or long).

Conducting a Physical Assessment

There are various organizing structures for conducting a physical assessment. Health care providers often proceed in a head-to-toe, body system approach, including all or some of the assessments, based on the circumstances and needs for an individual patient. Think about the appropriate and essential components of the examination for the individual patient and circumstances, as well as the sequence of the examination. Refer to the discussion of focused assessments on page 780. Although each body system is discussed individually here, in reality, nurses usually combine several systems (e.g., while assessing the head and neck they also assess the cranial nerves, which are part of the neurologic system). As identified earlier in the discussion of the review of systems, questions about a body system are often incorporated into the physical examination of each region. Examples of health history questions related to each body system are included in the discussion of each region of the physical examination later in the chapter. The accompanying head-to-toe assessment video demonstrates one potential sequence as well as proper technique.

Performing a General Survey

The general survey contributes to an overall impression of the patient. It includes observing the patient's overall appearance and behavior, taking vital signs, measuring height, weight, and waist circumference, head circumference (infants and children up to age 2 years [American Academy of Pediatrics, 2020; Weber & Kelley, 2018]), and calculating the body mass index (BMI). Information obtained from the general survey provides clues to the patient's overall health.

HEALTH HISTORY

Identify risk factors for altered health during the health history by asking about the following:

- History of changes in weight
- History of pain or discomfort
- Sleeping patterns, difficulty sleeping

APPEARANCE AND BEHAVIOR

Observation of the patient's appearance and behavior provides information about various aspects of the patient's health. While collecting information during the health history, inspect the patient's body build, posture, and gait. Note proportion of height to weight, which provides insight into nutritional status. Observe whether the patient has an erect or slumped posture, and evaluate movements and gait pattern for coordination. Uncoordinated or spontaneous movements may suggest neurologic problems. Note signs of illness and/or distress, such as changes in posture, skin color, and respirations; nonverbal communication of pain; and a short attention span.

Observe hygiene and grooming (cleanliness, body odors) and note any deficits, which may indicate other problems. For example, patients with inappropriate dress (e.g., wrong for the season) or worn or dirty clothing may be experiencing feelings of depression or have inadequate financial resources. Assess cognitive processes (speech content and patterns; orientation to person, place, and time; appropriate verbal responses). As cognitive processes are controlled by the neurologic system, these are discussed later in the chapter.

Clues to mood and mental health are provided by speech, facial expressions, ability to relax, eye contact, and behavior. If depression, anxiety, or other mental health disorders are suspected, use appropriate screening tools and refer the patient to the appropriate health care professionals as necessary. The PHQ-9, a common screening tool to identify depression, was mentioned earlier in the chapter in the discussion of psychosocial and lifestyle factors (Box 27-2 on page 782). Box 27-5 presents the Geriatric Depression Scale, a useful tool in screening older adults for depression. This tool is completed by the patient and reviewed by the health care provider.

HEIGHT AND WEIGHT

The ratio of height to weight is an assessment of overall health and potential overnutrition or undernutrition. Measure height and weight using accurate scales and measuring devices. Ask the patient to remove shoes and heavy clothing if the measurements are taken before undressing (Guidelines for Nursing Care 27-1). If the patient cannot stand erect, obtain weight using a chair or bed scale. Refer to Skill 27-1 (on pp. 822–824) for instructions to obtain a patient's weight using a portable bed scale. Make sure to measure the height (length) of children age 2 years and younger in the recumbent position with the legs fully extended (Jarvis & Eckhardt, 2020). Weigh infants without any clothing, and weigh children in their underwear.

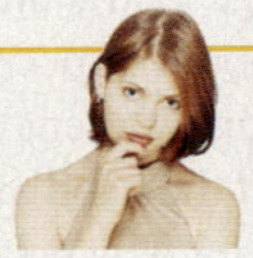

Remember **Ramona Lewis**, the young woman with anorexia nervosa. The nurse would use baseline data, including Ramona's height and weight, to monitor Ramona's health status.

HEAD CIRCUMFERENCE

Head circumference is measured at birth and each physical examination for infants and children up to age 2 years (American Academy of Pediatrics, 2020; Weber & Kelley, 2018). Circle the tape measure around the infant or child's head (not including the ears), beginning at the forehead just above the eyebrows, bringing the tape around the head just above the occipital prominence at the back of the head, using the

Box 27-5 Geriatric Depression Scale (GDS)

Instructions: Circle the answer that best describes how you felt over the past week.

1. Are you basically satisfied with your life?	yes	no
2. Have you dropped many of your activities and interests?	yes	no
3. Do you feel that your life is empty?	yes	no
4. Do you often get bored?	yes	no
5. Are you in good spirits most of the time?	yes	no
6. Are you afraid that something bad is going to happen to you?	yes	no
7. Do you feel happy most of the time?	yes	no
8. Do you often feel helpless?	yes	no
9. Do you prefer to stay at home, rather than going out and doing things?	yes	no
10. Do you feel that you have more problems with memory than most?	yes	no
11. Do you think it is wonderful to be alive now?	yes	no
12. Do you feel worthless the way you are now?	yes	no
13. Do you feel full of energy?	yes	no
14. Do you feel that your situation is hopeless?	yes	no
15. Do you think that most people are better off than you are?	yes	no

Total Score ________

Scoring Instructions: Score 1 point for "no" to questions 1, 5, 7, 11, and 13. Score 1 point for "yes" to other questions. A total score of 5 or more suggests possible depression and warrants further assessment.

Source: Republished with permission of Taylor and Francis Group LLC Books, from Sheikh, J. I., & Yesavage, J. A. (1986). Geriatric Depression Scale (GDS): Recent evidence and development of a shorter version. In T. L. Brink (Ed.), *Clinical gerontology: A guide to assessment and intervention* (pp. 165–173). Haworth Press; permission conveyed through Copyright Clearance Center, Inc.

widest span (Jarvis & Eckhardt, 2020; Kyle & Carmen, 2021). Measurements are used to show the pattern of head growth.

BODY MASS INDEX AND WAIST CIRCUMFERENCE

BMI (adults and children) and waist circumference (adults) are the preferred methods to establish ideal body weight (National Heart, Lung, and Blood Institute, n.d.a). **Body mass index (BMI)** is a ratio of weight to height. BMI is used as an initial assessment of nutritional status and is an indicator of obesity or malnutrition. BMI also provides an estimation of relative risk for some diseases, such as heart disease, high blood pressure, type 2 diabetes, gallstones, breathing

Guidelines for Nursing Care 27-1

OBTAINING HEIGHT AND WEIGHT WITH AN UPRIGHT BALANCE SCALE

Obtaining Height

- Ask the patient to remove shoes.
- Raise L-shaped sliding arm on the measuring device attached to the scale somewhat higher than the patient's approximate height.
- Ask the patient to step on the platform of the scale and stand erect with the back to the measuring device and the heels together.
- Lower the L-shaped sliding arm until it rests on top of the patient's head.
- Read the height in inches and record.
- Ask the patient to step down from the platform.

Obtaining Weight

- Balance the scale on "zero."
- Ask the patient to remove shoes (and coat, if appropriate) and step onto the platform.
- Move the sliding indicator to the left until the scale balances.
- Read the weight in pounds and record.
- Ask the patient to step down from the platform.
- Return the scale weight indicator to zero.
- Considerations: Daily weights should be obtained at the same time each day (usually early morning), with the patient wearing the same clothing, and using the same scale.

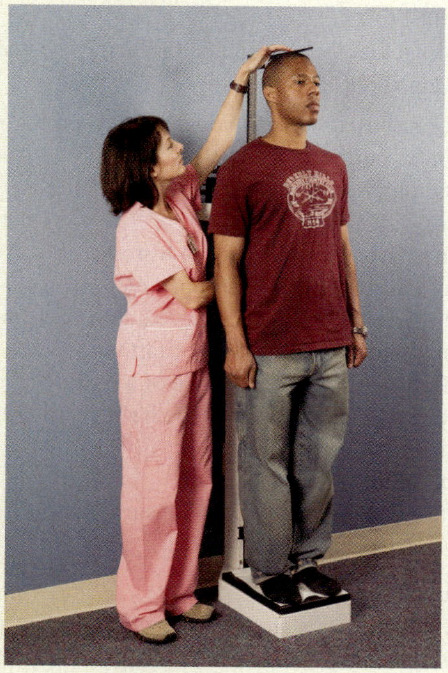

Source: Used with permission from Shutterstock. *Photo by B. Proud.*

problems, and certain cancers (National Heart, Lung, and Blood Institute, n.d.a). Calculate the BMI after obtaining the patient's height and weight. Refer to the discussion of BMI, including method for calculation, in Chapter 37.

Waist circumference is the measurement around a patient at the level of the umbilicus and is a good indicator of abdominal fat. The location of excess body fat is thought to be an important and reliable indicator of risk for diseases. Refer to the discussion of waist circumference in Chapter 37.

VITAL SIGNS

Vital signs are measured to establish a baseline for the database and to detect actual or potential health problems. Some facilities, particularly acute care facilities, may include measurement of oxygen saturation as part of the vital signs. Vital signs are discussed in detail in Chapter 26. Oxygen saturation is discussed in Chapter 40.

PAIN

Pain assessment is often considered the fifth vital sign. Assessment of pain is part of the initial assessment of a patient and continues throughout the nurse–patient relationship. Assessment of pain is discussed in Chapter 36.

Assessing the Integument

The integument is comprised of the skin, nails, hair, scalp and sweat and sebaceous glands. Assessing the integumentary structures provides information about the patient's overall health status, as well as clues to local or systemic health problems. It also provides data about self-care activities to maintain health, hygiene, and nutrition. Assessing for skin cancer is essential and provides the base for teaching skin cancer prevention. Refer to Box 27-6 for guidelines on assessing for melanoma. Additional information related to assessment of the integument is discussed in Chapter 33.

HEALTH HISTORY

Identify risk factors for altered health during the health history by asking about the following:

- History of rashes, lesions, change in color, or itching
- History of bruising or bleeding in the skin
- History of allergies to medications, plants, foods, or other substances
- Exposure to the sun and sunburn history
- History of bathing routines and products
- Presence of lesions (wounds, bruises, abrasions, or burns)
- Presence of body piercings and/or tattoos
- Change in the color, size, or shape of a mole
- Exposure to chemicals that may be harmful to the skin, hair, or nails
- Degree of mobility
- Types of food eaten and liquids consumed each day
- Cultural practices related to skin

PHYSICAL ASSESSMENT

The skin, hair, and nails are assessed by inspection and palpation. Assessment of the skin should begin with the general survey and continue throughout the physical examination. Protect the patient's privacy by exposing only the body part being examined. If the patient has lesions of the skin (including the scalp) or an infestation of the hair with lice, wear gloves during palpation.

The skin is a general indicator of the patient's health status and provides information that might indicate an underlying disease. Begin the assessment with an overall inspection of the skin's condition. Assess specific areas of the skin during assessment of other body systems (e.g., you may assess the skin on the abdomen while performing other abdominal assessments). Ensure adequate lighting, which is essential for accurate assessments. Inspect the skin for color, vascularity, and lesions (Fig. 27-7), and palpate for temperature, moisture, turgor, and texture.

Box 27-6 Assessing for Melanoma

Warning Signs: The ABCDEs of Melanoma

A: Asymmetry

If a line is drawn through a mole, the two halves will not match.

B: Border

The borders of an early melanoma tend to be uneven. The edges may be scalloped or notched.

C: Color

Having a variety of colors is another warning signal. A number of different shades of brown, tan, or black could appear. A melanoma may also become red, white, or blue.

D: Diameter

Melanomas usually are larger in diameter than the size of the eraser on your pencil (1/4 inch or 6 mm), but they may sometimes be smaller when first detected.

E: Evolving

Any change—in size, shape, color, elevation, or another trait, or any new symptom such as bleeding, itching, or crusting—points to danger.

Source: Skin Cancer Foundation. (2019). Melanoma overview. https://www.skincancer.org/skin-cancer-information/melanoma/ Copyright The Skin Cancer Foundation All Rights Reserved. For more information on skin cancer visit SkinCancer.org.

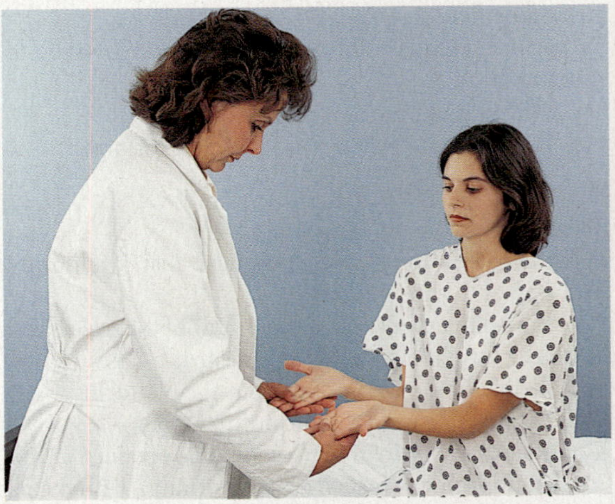

FIGURE 27-7. The skin is inspected for color, vascularity, and lesions. (*Source:* Used with permission from Shutterstock. *Photo by B. Proud.*)

Table 27-1 Skin Color Assessment

COLOR VARIATIONS	ASSESSMENT AREAS	POSSIBLE CAUSES
Redness (erythema, flushing)	Facial area, localized area of skin on the body	Blushing, alcohol intake, fever, injury trauma, infection
Bluish (cyanosis)	Exposed areas, particularly the ears, lips, inside of the mouth, hands and feet, and nail beds	Cold environment, cardiac or respiratory disease (decreased oxygenation)
Yellowish (jaundice)	Overall skin areas, mucous membranes, and sclera	Liver disease (increase in bilirubin levels)
Paleness (pallor)	Exposed areas, particularly the face and lips, conjunctivae, and mucous membranes Shock (decreased blood volume)	Anemia (decreased hemoglobin)
Vitiligo (whitish patchy areas on the skin)	Overall skin areas, lips, nail beds, and conjunctivae	Depigmentation (congenital or autoimmune conditions)
Tanned or brown	Sun-exposed areas	Overexposure (increased melanin production), pregnancy (brown spots)

Inspecting Skin Color

Skin color varies among races and among people, ranging from a pinkish white to various shades of brown. Skin areas that are normally exposed, such as the face and hands, may have a somewhat different color from areas that are usually covered by clothing, but otherwise skin color is relatively consistent. Some body areas of people with darker skin tones, such as the palms of the hands and the soles of the feet, normally have less pigmentation than other body areas.

Changes in skin color include erythema, cyanosis, jaundice, and pallor (Table 27-1). These color changes are often easier to assess in people with light skin tones. **Erythema**, redness of the skin, is caused by dilation of superficial blood vessels. It is associated with sunburn, inflammation, fever, trauma, and allergic reactions. When assessing for erythema in people with darker skin tones, it is important to assess skin temperature; areas of erythema will feel warm when compared with surrounding skin.

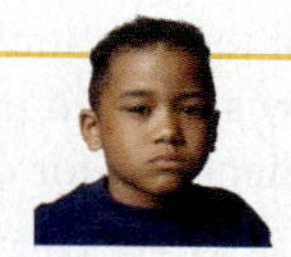

Think back to **Billy Collins**, the child who was stung by a bee. The nurse would use inspection skills to observe for erythema in the area of the sting.

Cyanosis is a bluish or grayish discoloration of the skin in response to inadequate oxygenation. Cyanosis is assessed as a blue tinge in patients with lighter skin and as dullness in patients with dark skin tones. **Jaundice** is a yellow color of the skin resulting from elevated amounts of bilirubin in the blood. It is associated with liver and gallbladder disease, some types of anemia, and excessive hemolysis (breakdown of red blood cells). It usually develops first in the sclera of the eyes and then in the skin and mucous membranes. It is more difficult to observe jaundice on the trunk of the body in patients with darker skin tones, but the sclera, oral mucous membranes, palms, and soles appear yellow to yellow-orange. **Pallor**, or paleness of the skin, often results from a decrease in the amount of circulating blood or hemoglobin, causing inadequate oxygenation of the body tissues. Depending on severity, pallor may be visible over the entire skin surface or only in the lips, nail beds, mucous membranes, and conjunctiva. Pallor in patients with dark skin tones is seen as an ashen gray or yellow tinge.

Inspecting Skin Vascularity and Lesions

Inspect the skin for vascularity, bleeding, or bruising; these signs might relate to a cardiovascular, hematologic, or liver dysfunction. **Ecchymosis** is a collection of blood in the subcutaneous tissues, causing purplish discoloration. **Petechiae** are small hemorrhagic spots caused by capillary bleeding. If they are present, assess their location, color, and size.

Lesions are areas of diseased or injured tissue such as bruises, scratches, cuts, burns, insect bites, and wounds (breaks in the continuity of the skin). Assess lesions and wounds for size, shape, depth, location, and presence of drainage or odor. Refer to a health assessment text for details of terms used to describe different types of lesions. Wounds are discussed in Chapter 33. Scars are healed wounds. Describe rashes (skin eruptions) in terms of their type, size, elevation, coloring, and presence of drainage or itching. Assess the location and condition of body piercings and/or tattoos. Document the exact body surface areas involved.

Palpating Skin Temperature, Texture, Moisture, and Turgor

The skin is normally warm and dry. An increase in skin temperature and moisture can indicate an elevated body temperature. The texture of the skin varies from smooth and soft to rough and dry. In the dehydrated patient, the texture is dry, loose, and wrinkled, and the mucous membranes are cracked and dry. An excessive amount of perspiration, such as when the entire skin is moist, is called **diaphoresis**.

Turgor is the fullness or elasticity of the skin. It is usually assessed on the sternum or under the clavicle by lifting a fold of skin with the thumb and first finger (Fig. 27-8 on page 792). Skin turgor is considered normal when the fold

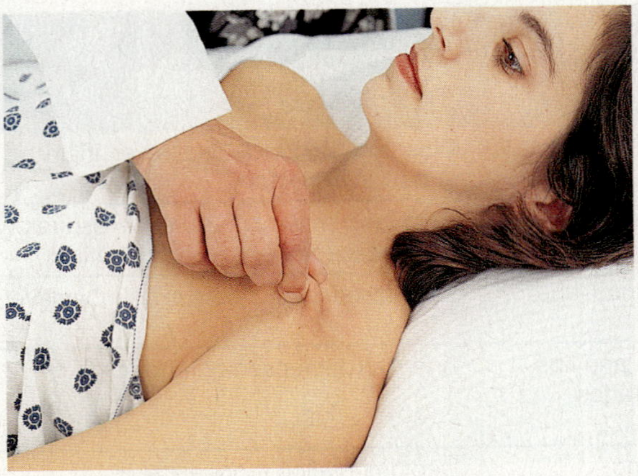

FIGURE 27-8. To assess skin turgor, a small fold of skin is picked up and then released to return to its normal shape. Difficulty in lifting a skin fold may indicate presence of edema. (*Source:* Used with permission from Shutterstock. *Photo by B. Proud.*)

returns to its usual shape when released. When the patient is dehydrated, the skin's elasticity is decreased, and the skin fold returns slowly. Decreased skin turgor may be a normal finding in older adults as a result of decreased elasticity and thinning of the dermis as a person ages.

Difficulty in lifting a skin fold may indicate **edema** (excess fluid in the tissues). Edema is characterized by swelling, with taut and shiny skin over the edematous area. If the area of edema is palpated with the fingers, an indentation (measured in millimeters for depth of the indentation) may remain after the pressure is released; if the indentation is very deep, it is called pitting edema. Edema may be graded; refer to Chapter 41 for a visual representation of a grading system (p. 1680). Edema may be the result of overhydration, heart failure, kidney failure, trauma, or peripheral vascular disease.

Inspecting the Nails

Inspect the nails for shape, angle, texture, and color. The nails should be somewhat convex and should follow the natural curve of the finger. The angle between the nail and its base should be about 160 degrees. The nails should be smooth, and the nail base, when palpated, should be firm and nontender. Abnormal findings include infection, painless separation of the nail plate from the nail, increased brittleness or thickness, and clubbing (bulging of the last part of the finger with curved, convex nails related to reduced oxygen in the blood).

Inspecting the Hair and Scalp

Hair may be found on all body surfaces except the palms of the hands, the soles of the feet, and parts of the genitalia. Assess the hair for color, texture, and distribution. The hair is normally resilient, evenly distributed, and neither excessively dry nor oily. Abnormal findings include unusual balding (alopecia) and excessive amounts of hair on the face and body (hirsutism). Hair loss may be normal or may be the result of chemotherapy, radiation therapy, infection, hormonal disorders, or inadequate nutrition. Decreased oxygenation of peripheral tissues, especially of the lower extremities, may cause loss of hair. Excessive hair growth may occur in people with hormonal disorders.

Separate the hair to inspect the scalp for color, dryness, scaliness, lumps, lesions, or lice. Nits, which are the white eggs of lice, can be differentiated from dandruff or lint because they are attached to the hair shaft. If lumps or masses are palpated, note their location, size, tenderness, and mobility.

NORMAL AGE-RELATED VARIATIONS: INFANT/CHILD

Common skin variations in newborns and children include:

- Jaundice and milia (whiteheads) in newborns
- Fine downy hair (lanugo) for the first 2 weeks of life
- Smooth, thin skin at birth
- Pubic hair development at the onset of puberty

NORMAL AGE-RELATED VARIATIONS: OLDER ADULT

Common skin variations in the older adult include:

- Wrinkles, dryness, scaling, decreased turgor
- Raised dark areas (senile keratosis)
- Flat, brown age spots (senile lentigines)
- Small, round red spots (cherry angioma)
- Fine, brittle gray or white hair
- Hair loss
- Coarse facial hair in women, decreased body hair in men and women
- Thick, yellow toenails

Assessing the Head and Neck

Assessment of the head and neck includes the skull, face, eyes, ears, nose and sinuses, mouth and pharynx, trachea, thyroid gland, and lymph nodes. During the health history, note any health problems such as headaches or dizziness. If the patient smokes, include a discussion about ways to stop smoking in the care plan. Physical examination of the structures of the head and neck provides data about the shape and structure of cranial bones, function of special senses (sight, hearing, taste, smell), nasal and oral structures, and any swelling or pain in the lymph nodes in the neck. Assessment of the size and consistency of the thyroid gland is performed by advanced practice professionals. Refer to a health assessment text for details.

HEALTH HISTORY

Identify risk factors for altered health during the health history by asking about the following:

- Changes in vision or hearing with aging
- History of use of corrective lenses or hearing aids
- History of allergies
- History of disturbances in vision or hearing
- History of chronic illnesses such as hypertension, diabetes mellitus, or thyroid disease
- Exposure to harmful substances or loud noises
- History of smoking (how long, how many packs/day), chewing tobacco, or cocaine use
- Presence of body piercings and/or tattoos
- History of eye or ear infections
- History of head trauma
- Oral and dental care practices

PHYSICAL ASSESSMENT

Inspecting and Palpating the Head and Face

Inspect and palpate the head for size and shape. The parts of the head and face should be in proportion to each other and symmetric. Although the shape of the normal skull varies considerably, generally the shape is gently curved with prominences at the frontal and parietal bones. Abnormal findings include lack of symmetry or unusual size or contour of the skull (either may be the result of trauma or diseases affecting the growth of bone) and tenderness. If the skull of a child or an adult appears disproportionately large or small, measure the circumference. Measuring head circumference is a normal part of infant assessment to the age of 2 years and should be conducted at each health-related visit.

Inspect the face for color, symmetry, and distribution of facial hair. Edema of the face, especially around the eye (periorbital edema), and involuntary facial movements (e.g., tics, tremors) are abnormal findings. If abnormalities are noted, document the location, amount, duration, and timing.

Inspecting the Eyes

Assess the structures and functions of the eyes using a penlight and an eye chart. Inspection is the primary assessment technique used. Assessment includes the external eye structures, visual acuity, extraocular movements, and peripheral vision. Advanced health care providers usually perform assessment of the internal eye structures with an ophthalmoscope, which is an advanced assessment skill. Refer to a health assessment text for details.

Inspecting External Eye Structures. Inspect the eyes, eyebrows, eyelids, eyelashes, lacrimal glands, pupils, and iris for position and alignment (Fig. 27-9). Asymmetry of position and alignment of the eyes may be caused by muscle weakness

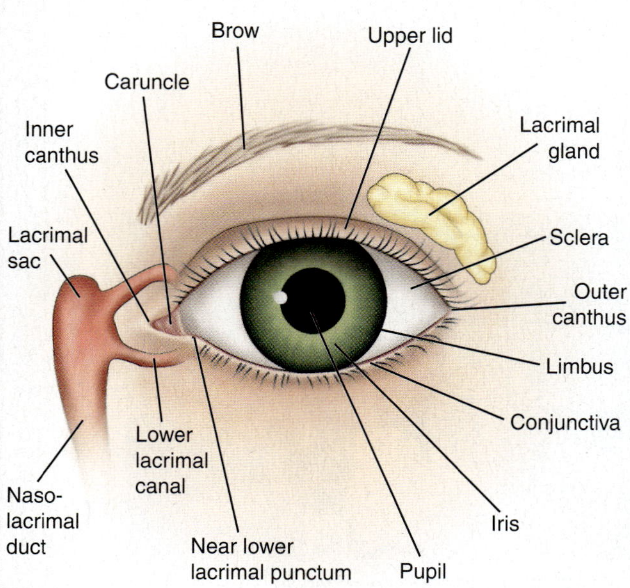

FIGURE 27-9. The eye and surrounding structures.

or a congenital abnormality. The eyebrows should be equally distributed; the eyelashes should curl outward.

Inspect the eyelids for color, edema, and equal coverage of the eyeball. Abnormal findings include drooping of the upper lids (ptosis), which may be attributable to damage to the oculomotor nerve, myasthenia gravis, or a congenital disorder; inward turning of the lower lid and lashes (entropion); outward turning of the lower lid and lashes (ectropion); and redness or drainage (from infection of the lid margins, conjunctivae, or hair follicles). Inspect and palpate the lacrimal glands for edema and pain.

The pupils are normally black, equal in size, round, and smooth. The pupils may be pale and cloudy if the patient has cataracts (loss of opacity of the lens). Injury to the eye, glaucoma, and certain medications may cause the pupil to dilate (mydriasis); certain drugs can cause constriction (miosis), and unequal pupils may result from central nervous system injury or illness.

Assess the pupils for reaction to light and accommodation and for convergence (Guidelines for Nursing Care 27-2 on page 794). Decreased or absent pupillary response indicates blindness or serious brain damage. Inability of the eyes to accommodate or converge is abnormal.

Assessing Visual Acuity, Extraocular Movements, and Peripheral Vision. Assess visual acuity with the Snellen chart. Have the patient stand 20 ft from the chart and ask the patient to read the smallest line of letters possible, first with both eyes and then with one eye at a time (with the opposite eye covered). Note whether the patient's vision is being tested with or without corrective lenses.

Visual acuity is measured by using the standardized numbers listed on the side of the chart. The numerator is 20, representing the distance in feet the patient was from the test. The denominator represents the smallest line read accurately by the patient. Visual acuity is recorded as a fraction and is written as 20 over the smallest line read by the patient with no more than two inaccurate readings (such as "20/30–2 with glasses"). Thus, the larger the denominator, the poorer the patient's vision (Jensen, 2019). Use a Snellen picture chart or Snellen E-chart to test vision in patients who are unable to read English and in young children. The E-chart uses the capital letter E in varying sizes pointing in different directions. The patient points their fingers in the direction the legs of the E are pointing.

Test near vision with a handheld vision screen with varying sizes of print. A Jaeger card can be used for this measurement. The patient holds the card 14 inches from the eyes. Ask the patient to read the smallest line of letters possible, with one eye at a time (with the opposite eye covered), and corrective lenses in place, if used. The results are recorded as a fraction and written as 14 over the smallest line read by the patient. A normal result is 14/14.

Test extraocular movements by assessing the cardinal fields of vision for coordination and alignment. Normally both eyes move together, are coordinated, and are parallel. Tests for peripheral vision (or visual fields) are used

Guidelines for Nursing Care 27-2

MEASURING PUPILLARY REACTION, SIZE, ACCOMMODATION, AND CONVERGENCE

Pupillary Reaction

- Darken the room.
- Ask the patient to look straight ahead.
- Bring the penlight from the side of the patient's face and briefly shine the light on the pupil (Figure A).

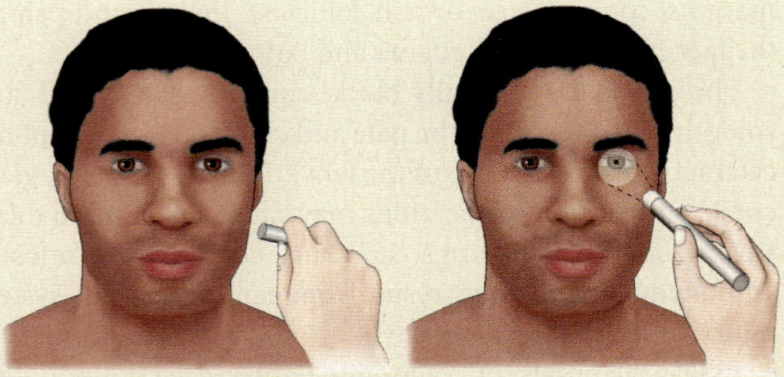

FIGURE A. Assessing pupillary reaction.

- Observe the pupil's reaction; it normally rapidly constricts (direct response). Also observe pupil size (Figure B).
- Repeat the procedure and observe the other eye; it too normally will constrict (consensual reflex).
- Repeat the procedure with the other eye.

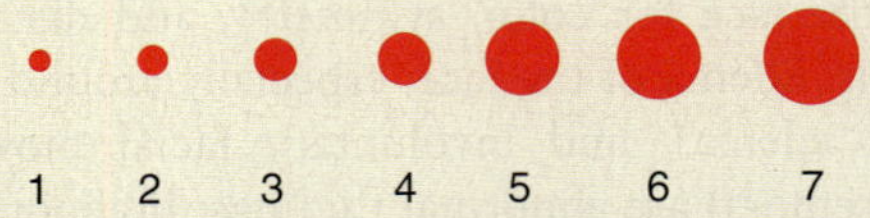

FIGURE B. Pupillary gauge measures pupils (dilation or constriction) in millimeters (mm).

Accommodation

- Hold the forefinger, a pencil, or other straight object about 10 to 15 cm (4 to 6 inches) from the bridge of the patient's nose.
- Ask the patient to first look at the object, then at a distant object, then back to the object being held. The pupil normally constricts when looking at a near object and dilates when looking at a distant object (Figure C).

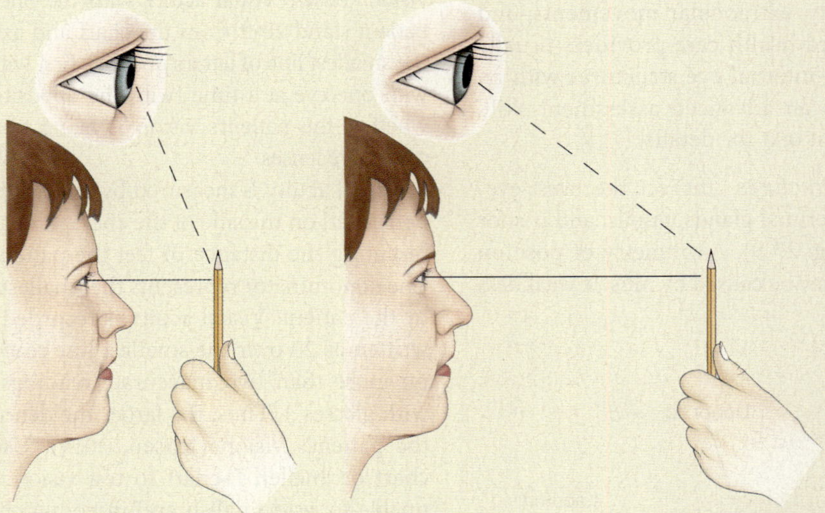

FIGURE C. Assessing accommodation.

Convergence

- Hold your finger about 6 to 8 inches from the bridge of the patient's nose.
- Move your finger toward the patient's nose to assess convergence (Figure D). The patient's eyes should normally converge (assume a cross-eyed appearance).

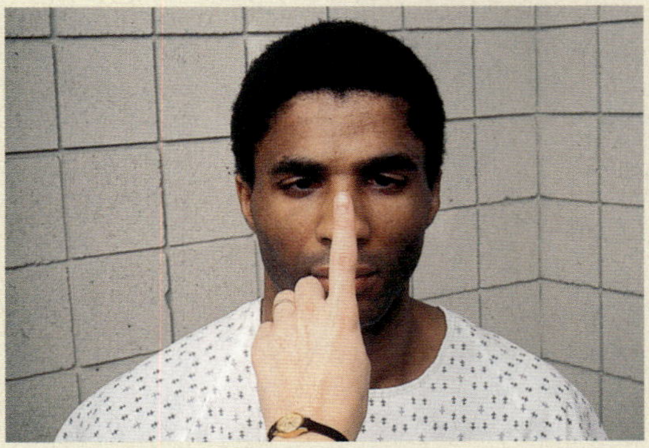

FIGURE D. Assessing convergence.

Guidelines for Nursing Care 27-3

ASSESSING EXTRAOCULAR MOVEMENTS AND PERIPHERAL VISION

Extraocular Movements

- Ask the patient to sit or stand about 2 ft away, facing you sitting or standing at eye level with the patient.
- Ask the patient to hold the head still and follow the movement of your forefinger or a penlight with the eyes.
- Keeping your finger or light about 1 foot from the patient's face, move it slowly through the cardinal positions: up and down, left and right, diagonally up and down to the left, diagonally up and down to the right (see figure).

Peripheral Vision

- Have the patient stand or sit about 2 ft away, facing you at eye level.
- Ask the patient to cover one eye with a hand or an index card.
- Ask the patient to look directly at your nose and fix the eyes on that spot.
- Cover your own eye opposite the patient's closed eye.
- Hold one arm outstretched to one side (right or left) equidistant from you and the patient, and move your fingers into the visual fields from various peripheral points.
- Ask the patient to tell you when the fingers are first seen (both you and the patient should see the fingers at the same time).
- Repeat the procedure for the other eye.

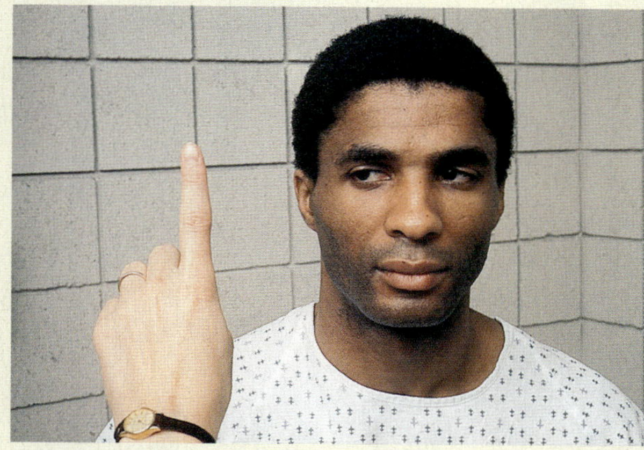

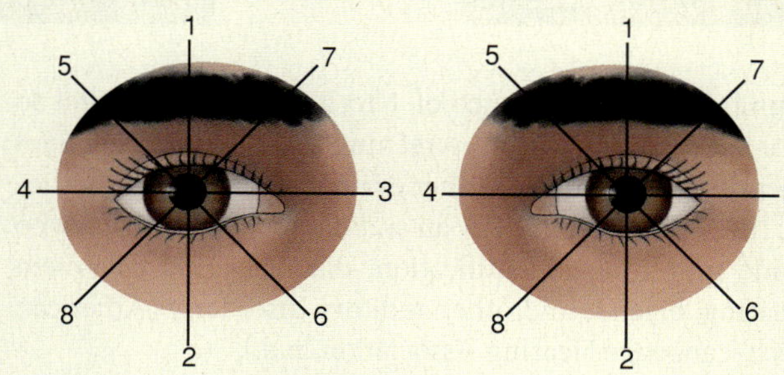

Testing extraocular movement of the eye.

to assess retinal function and optic nerve function. Full peripheral vision is normal. Guidelines for Nursing Care 27-3 describes how to assess extraocular movements and peripheral vision.

Inspecting and Palpating the Ears

Assess the external ear by inspection and palpation. Advanced health care providers usually perform assessment of the structures of the ear canal and tympanic membrane with an otoscope, which is an advanced assessment skill. Refer to a health assessment text for details.

Inspecting and Palpating the External Ear. Inspect the external ear (Fig. 27-10) for shape, size, and lesions. The external surfaces of the ear should be smooth, and the shape and size of the ears should be symmetric and proportional to the head. Abnormal findings include unequal height and size, uneven color, and lesions. Inspect the visible portion of the ear canal. Note the presence of cerumen (wax), edema, discharge, or foreign bodies. Gently palpate the external ear for pain, edema, or presence of lesions. Pain when manipulating the pinna is a symptom of an infection of the external ear.

Assessing Hearing and Sound Conduction. General hearing screening tests that are useful include self-report questionnaires and the whisper test. Self-report questionnaires can be administered in a verbal, written or computerized format and collect information related to patient reports of hearing ability and deficits, and associated impact on activities of daily living and quality of life. Screening of hearing using the whisper test is accomplished as follows: test hearing in one ear at a time by determining whether the patient can hear a whispered voice. Assess hearing acuity out of the patient's line of vision (to prevent lip reading), with the opposite ear covered. Determine whether the patient can hear a whispered sentence or group

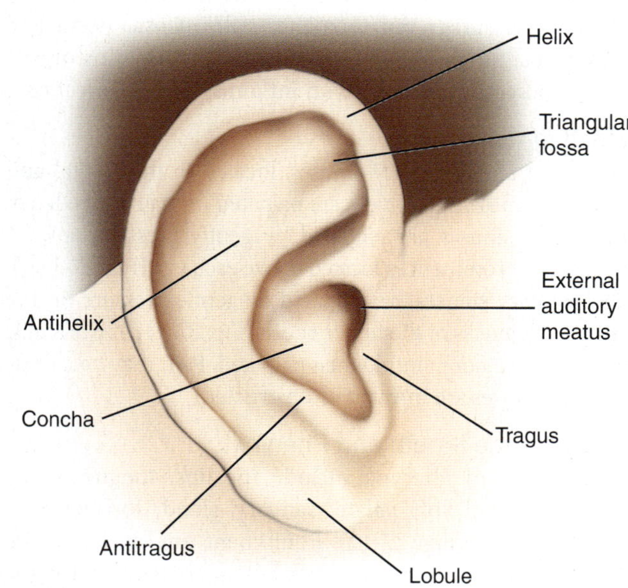

FIGURE 27-10. External structures of the ear.

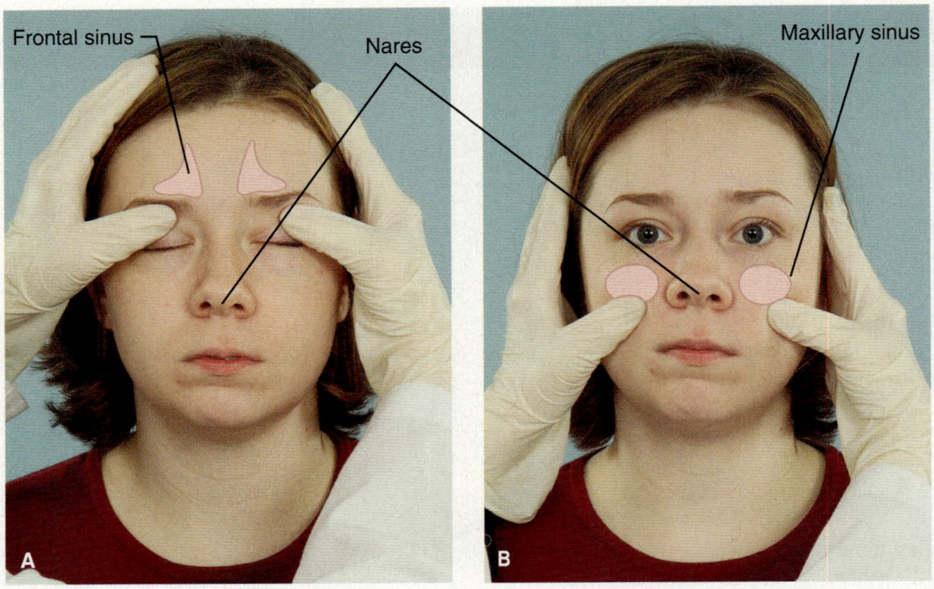

FIGURE 27-11. **A.** Nares and frontal sinuses. The frontal sinuses are palpated by gently pressing upward on the bony prominences above each eye. **B.** The maxillary sinuses are palpated by applying gentle pressure on the bony prominences of the upper cheek. (*Source:* Used with permission from Shutterstock. *Photos by B. Proud.*)

of numbers from a distance of 1 to 2 ft. Ask the patient to repeat what you said. Both screening tests can provide clues to identifying a need for further evaluation, such as an audiologic (hearing) evaluation by an audiologist (professional who provide prevention, identification, diagnosis and treatment of hearing, balance and other auditory disorders) (American Speech-Language Hearing Association, n.d.).

Inspecting the Nose

Assessment of the nose involves examining the external nose and the nares (Fig. 27-11A). Inspect the nose and inspect and palpate the sinuses with the patient sitting and their head slightly tilted back, if possible.

Assess the nose for patency by occluding one nostril at a time and asking the patient to inhale and exhale through the nose. Inspect each anterior nares by tipping the patient's head back slightly and shining a light into the nares. Examine the mucous membranes for color and the presence of lesions, exudate, or growths. Normally, the nasal mucosa is moist and darker red than the oral mucosa. Abnormal findings include swelling of the mucosa, and bleeding or discharge (indicating allergies with inflammation or infection).

Palpating the Sinuses

The frontal and maxillary sinuses, located in the frontal and maxillary bones, respectively, are palpated for pain and edema. The frontal sinuses are palpated by gently pressing upward on the bony prominences located above each eye (Fig. 27-11A). The maxillary sinuses are palpated by gentle pressure on the bony prominences of the upper cheek (Fig. 27-11B). Normally, the sinuses are not painful when palpated. Pain may be a finding if the sinuses are infected or obstructed.

Inspecting the Mouth and Pharynx

The mouth and pharynx include the lips, tongue, teeth, gums, hard and soft palate, salivary gland, tonsillar pillars, and tonsils (Fig. 27-12). Equipment used to assess the mouth, pharynx, and neck includes a penlight, a tongue blade, a 4 × 4-inch gauze sponge, and gloves.

Assess the mouth and pharynx by inspecting the lips, gums and teeth, tongue, under the tongue, and hard and soft palates. Have the patient sit with the head tilted backward, if possible, and the mouth opened wide. Use palpation if any abnormalities are noted during inspection. Wear gloves when assessing a patient's mouth and use 4 × 4-inch gauze to hold the tongue for palpation.

The lips should be pink, moist, and smooth. The tongue and mucous membranes are normally pink, moist, and free of swelling or lesions. If the patient wears dentures, ask the patient to remove them for inspection of the gums and roof of the mouth. The gums should be pink and smooth. With the patient's tongue relaxed on the floor of the mouth, examine the mucous membrane of the oropharynx while depressing the base of the tongue with a tongue depressor. The uvula is normally centered and freely movable. The tonsils, if present, are small, pink, and symmetric in size. The

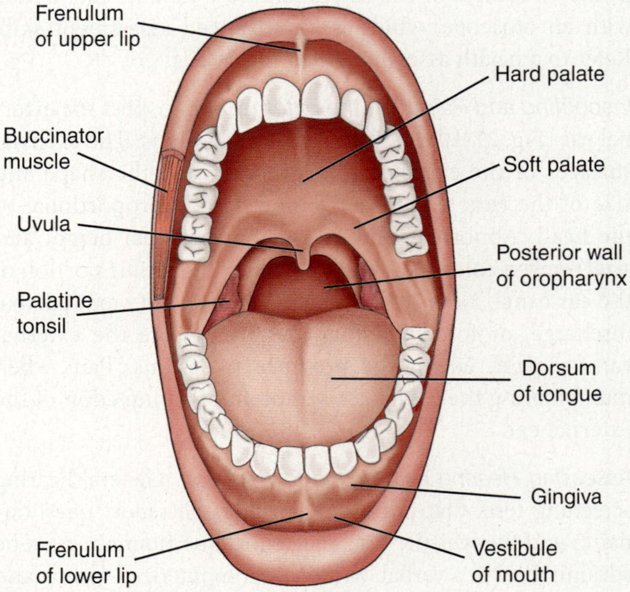

FIGURE 27-12. Structures of the mouth.

teeth should be regular and free of cavities or have dental restoration.

Abnormal findings include pallor, cyanosis, or redness and swelling of the mucous membranes; lesions of the mucosa and lips; swollen, red tonsils (indicating infection); swollen, red, and bleeding gums (from nutritional deficits, inflammation or infection, poorly fitted dentures, or poor oral hygiene); poorly aligned, missing, or carious teeth; a white coating on the tongue (from poor oral hygiene, irritation, or smoking); a fissured tongue (from dehydration); a bright-red tongue (seen in deficiencies of iron, vitamin B_{12}, or niacin); or a black, hairy tongue (from antibiotic use).

Inspecting and Palpating the Neck

Assessments of the neck include the trachea, lymph nodes, and thyroid gland (Fig. 27-13). Assess the neck with the patient sitting and the neck slightly hyperextended, if possible. Ask the patient to tilt the head backward, forward, and side to side to assess range of motion (ROM). The neck should be symmetric, with smooth and controlled ROM. Also assess the neck for venous distention. No neck vein distention (indicating heart problems) should be visible. Palpation of the thyroid is an advanced assessment skill, usually performed by advanced health care providers. Refer to a health assessment text for details.

Inspecting and Palpating the Trachea. Assess the position of the trachea in the neck. Inspect and palpate the trachea. The trachea should be midline and symmetrical.

Inspecting the Thyroid Gland. Assess the thyroid gland with the neck slightly hyperextended. Observe the lower portion of the neck overlying the thyroid gland. Assess for symmetry and visible masses. Ask the patient to swallow. Observe the area while the patient swallows. Offer a glass of water, if necessary, to make it easier for the patient to swallow.

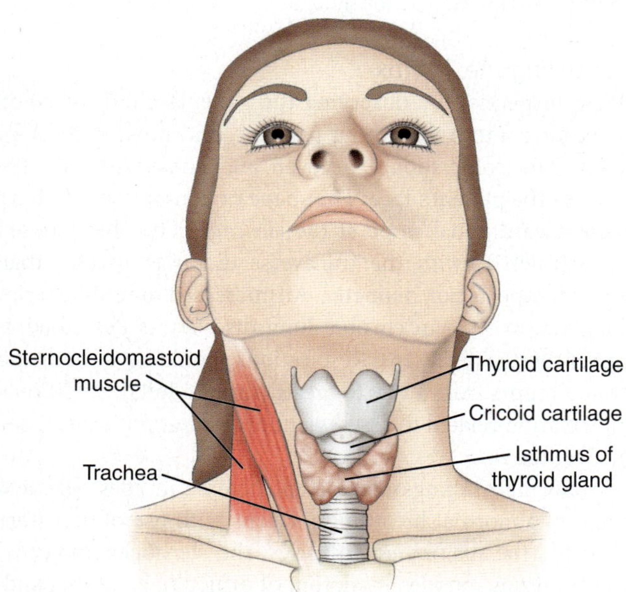

FIGURE 27-13. Structures of the neck.

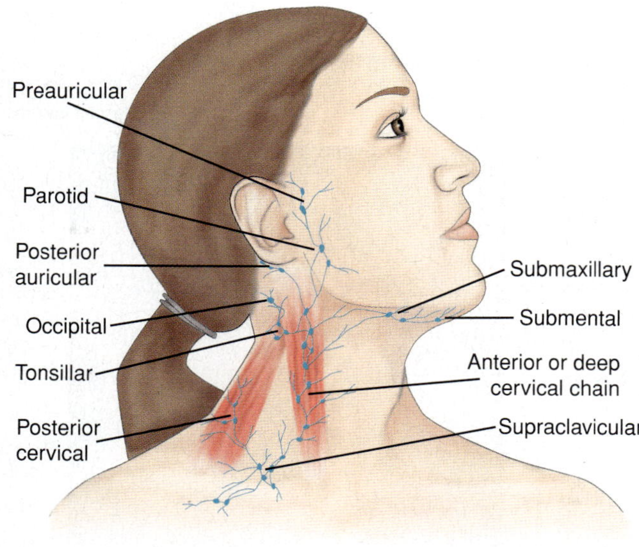

FIGURE 27-14. Location of the lymph nodes of the neck.

Abnormal findings include asymmetry, enlargement, lumps, and bulging. These findings may indicate the presence of enlargement of the thyroid (a goiter), inflammation of the thyroid (thyroiditis), or cancer of the thyroid.

Palpating the Lymph Nodes. Palpate the lymph nodes (Fig. 27-14) with the pads of the fingers for enlargement, tenderness, and mobility. The nodes are generally not palpable; if palpable, they should be small, mobile, smooth, and nontender. If lymph nodes are palpable, assess location, size, consistency, mobility, and tenderness. Enlarged lymph nodes (lymphadenopathy) may indicate infection, autoimmune disorders, or metastasis of cancer.

NORMAL AGE-RELATED VARIATIONS: INFANT/CHILD

Common head and neck variations in newborns and children include:

- Closing of posterior fontanel at age 8 weeks, soft anterior fontanel at about age 18 months
- Gazing at and following bright objects by age 1 month
- Focusing with both eyes by age 6 months
- Pupils at the inner folds (pseudostrabismus)
- Startle reflex in newborns

NORMAL AGE-RELATED VARIATIONS: OLDER ADULT

Common head and neck variations in the older adult include:

- Impaired near vision (presbyopia)
- Decreased color vision and peripheral vision
- Decreased adaptation to light and dark
- A white ring around the cornea (arcus senilis)
- Entropion (eyelid turns inward) and ectropion (eyelid turns outward)
- Hearing loss (presbycusis)
- Elongated ear lobes
- Decreased neck ROM
- Smaller, more easily palpated lymph glands

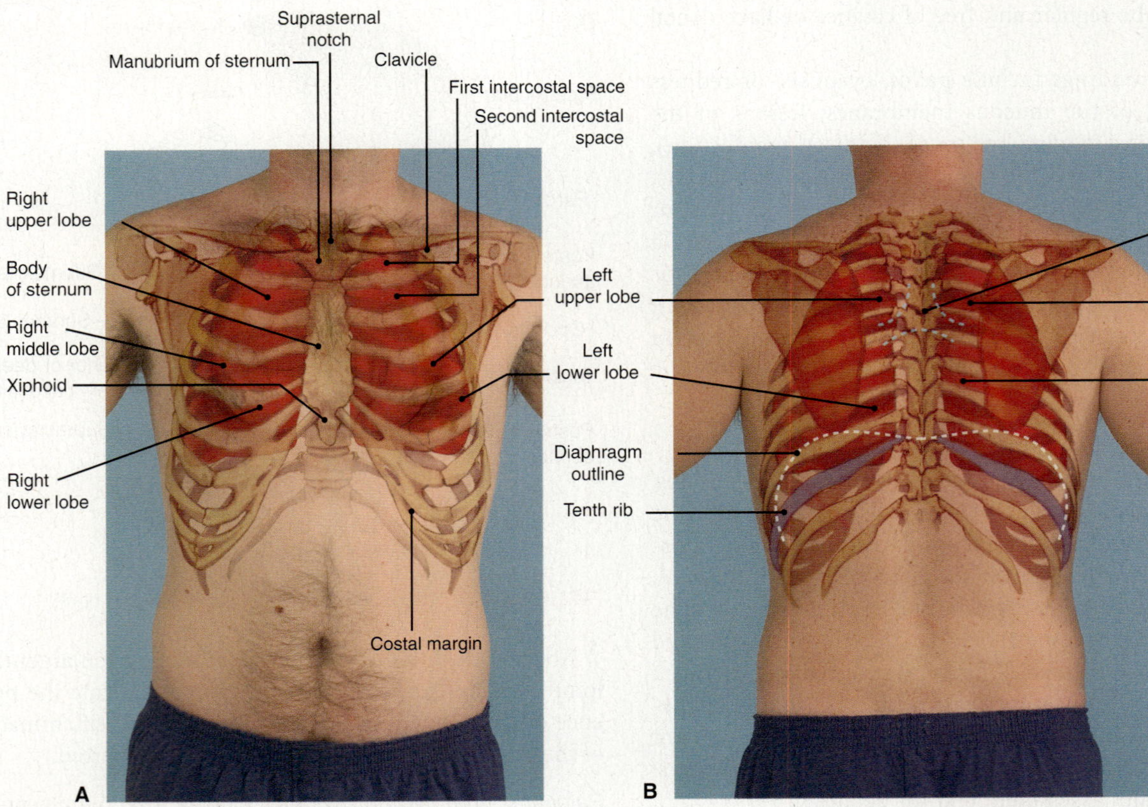

FIGURE 27-15. Thoracic landmarks. **A.** Anterior. **B.** Posterior.

Assessing the Thorax and Lungs

The thorax (Fig. 27-15) comprises the lungs, rib cage, cartilage, and intercostal muscles. Data from the health history may elicit a health problem, such as dyspnea or chest pain, as well as information about sleep patterns, cough, and sputum. A history of smoking indicates the need to include ways to stop smoking in the care plan. Environmental exposure to certain inhalants (such as secondhand smoke, paint, air pollution, or asbestos fibers) in the home or workplace may increase the risk of respiratory diseases and cancer. Physical examination provides data about the bony structures of the thorax, respiratory effort, chest expansion, and breath sounds. Additional information related to assessment of the thorax and lungs is discussed in Chapters 26 and 40.

HEALTH HISTORY

Identify risk factors for altered health during the health history by asking about the following:

- History of trauma to the ribs or lung surgery
- Number of pillows used when sleeping
- History of chest pain with deep breathing
- History of persistent cough with or without producing sputum
- History of allergies
- Environmental exposure to chemicals, asbestos, or smoke
- History of smoking (how long, how many packs/day)
- History of lung disease in family members or self
- History of frequent or chronic respiratory infections

PHYSICAL ASSESSMENT

Physical assessment of the thorax and lungs requires a stethoscope and a watch. Make sure that the environment is warm and adequately lit. The techniques for this assessment include inspection, palpation, percussion, and auscultation. The patient may be in a sitting position or in a supine position with the head raised about 30 degrees, if possible. Percussion of the thorax is an advanced assessment technique, usually performed by advanced health care providers. Refer to a health assessment text for details.

Inspecting the Thorax

Begin inspection by observing the patient's chest for color, shape or contour, breathing patterns, and muscle development. The color should be even and consistent with the color of the patient's face. The shape or contour should have a downward equal slope at the rib cage. The chest should be symmetric, with the transverse diameter greater than the anteroposterior diameter. An increased anteroposterior diameter, as seen in chronic lung diseases, is described as barrel chest (Fig. 27-16). Respirations should be smooth and even, ranging from 12 to 20 breaths/min (adults). Additional information related to assessment of respiration is discussed in Chapter 26.

Abnormal findings include an increase in chest size and contour, abnormal breathing patterns with use of accessory muscles (the major neck muscles, the sternocleidomastoid and trapezius muscles; symptom of difficulty breathing and/or respiratory disease, such as chronic obstructive pulmonary

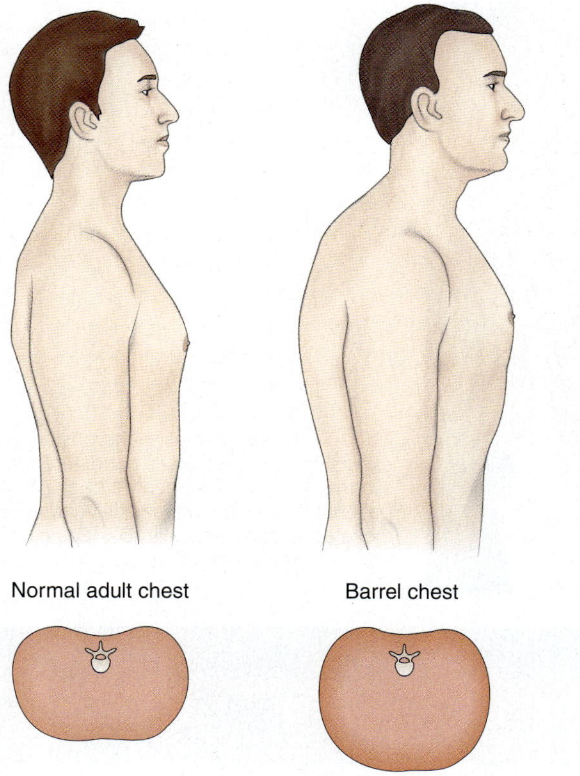

FIGURE 27-16. Profile and anteroposterior diameter of normal adult chest and barrel chest.

disease or asthma), unequal chest expansion (may occur in chest trauma or pneumonia), and abnormal respirations.

Palpating the Thorax

Palpation is used to detect areas of sensitivity, chest expansion during respirations, and vibrations (fremitus). Use the palmar surface of the hands to palpate the anterior and posterior thoracic landmarks (Fig. 27-17) in a sequential pattern for temperature, moisture, muscular development, and any tenderness or masses. The skin should be warm and dry, with symmetric muscular development, and no tenderness, masses, or vibrations. Abnormal findings may be cool or excessively dry or moist skin, muscle asymmetry, tenderness, masses, and vibrations.

Chest expansion is determined by placing the hands over the posterior chest wall, with the fingers at the level of T9 or T10 (Fig. 27-18A on page 800). Ask the patient to take a deep breath, and observe the movement of your thumbs. The thorax should expand symmetrically (Fig. 27-18B on page 800).

Auscultating Breath Sounds

Auscultation is used to detect airflow within the respiratory tract. Ask the patient to breathe slowly and deeply through the mouth. Place the warmed diaphragm of the stethoscope over the thoracic landmarks and auscultate breath sounds in the same sequential pattern as used for palpation (see Fig. 27-17). Normally, breath sounds result from the free movement of air into and out of all parts of the bronchial tree. Listen for the duration, pitch, and intensity of the sounds.

Normal breath sounds (Table 27-2 on page 800) vary over different parts of the lungs. **Bronchial breath sounds** heard over the larynx and trachea are high-pitched, harsh "blowing" sounds, with sound on expiration being longer than inspiration. **Bronchovesicular breath sounds** are heard over the mainstem bronchus and are moderate blowing sounds, with inspiration equal to expiration. **Vesicular breath sounds** are soft, low-pitched, whispering sounds, heard over most of the lung fields, with sound on inspiration being longer than expiration.

Adventitious breath sounds (extra, abnormal sounds) are not normally heard in the lungs and result from air moving through moisture, mucus, or narrowed airways. These abnormal sounds also result from sudden opening of collapsed alveoli. Refer to Table 27-3 (on page 801) for an explanation of these abnormal sounds. If any of these sounds are heard, listen for the loudness, pitch, duration, timing in the respiratory cycle (inspiration vs. expiration), location on

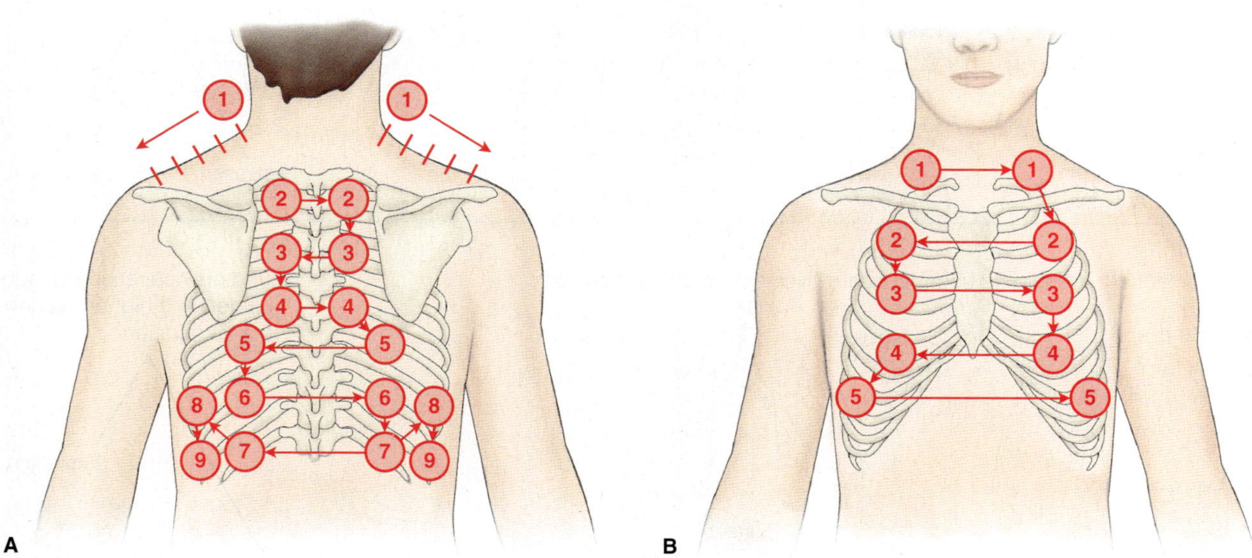

FIGURE 27-17. Posterior (**A**) and anterior (**B**) chest—landmarks and systematic sequence of assessment. The pattern is used for palpation, percussion, and auscultation of the chest.

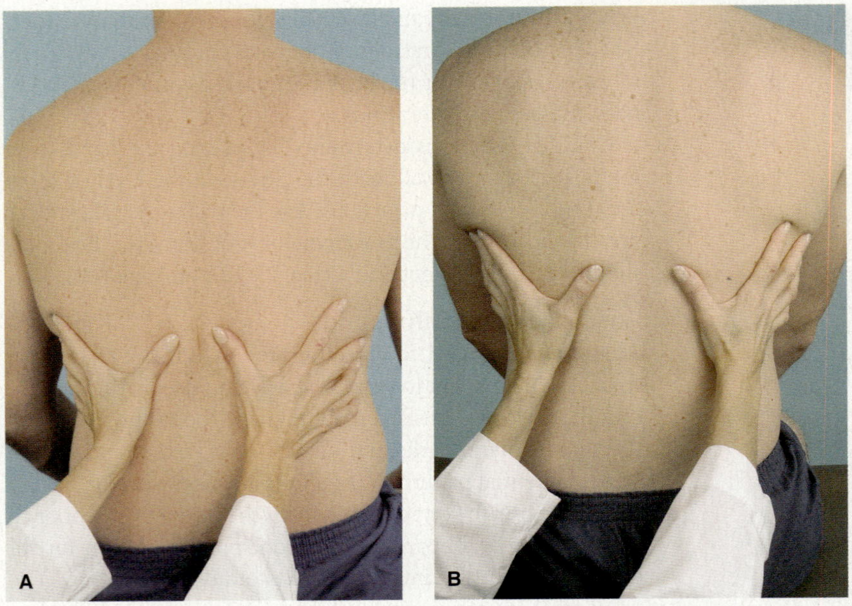

FIGURE 27-18. Palpating the posterior thorax excursion. The examiner's hands are placed symmetrically on the patient's back (**A**). As the patient inhales, the examiner's hands should move apart symmetrically (**B**). (*Source:* Used with permission from Shutterstock. *Photos by B. Proud.*)

Table 27-2 Normal Breath Sounds

TYPE, DESCRIPTION, AND LOCATION	RATIO OF INSPIRATION TO EXPIRATION
Bronchial or Tubular Blowing, hollow sounds; auscultated over the larynx and trachea 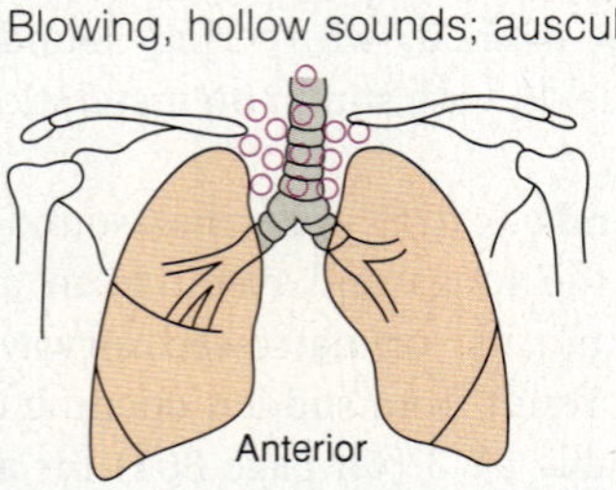	Sound on expiration is longer, lower, and higher pitched than inspiration 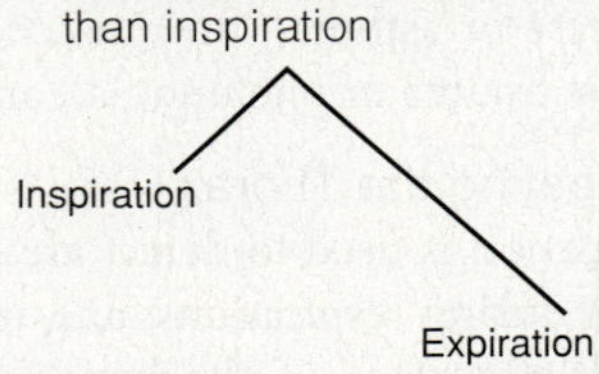
Bronchovesicular Medium-pitched, medium intensity, blowing sounds; auscultated over the first and second interspaces anteriorly and the scapula posteriorly 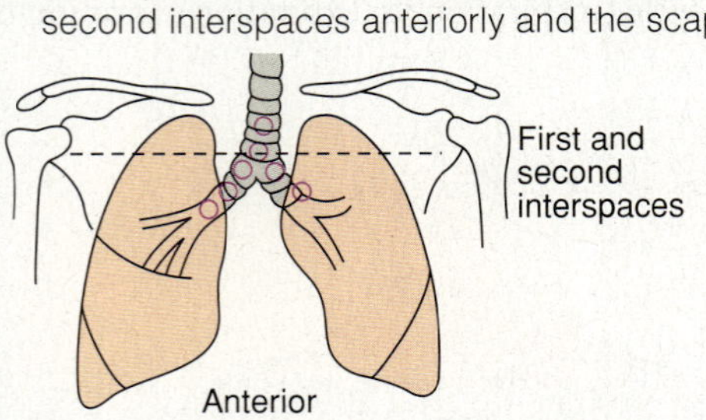 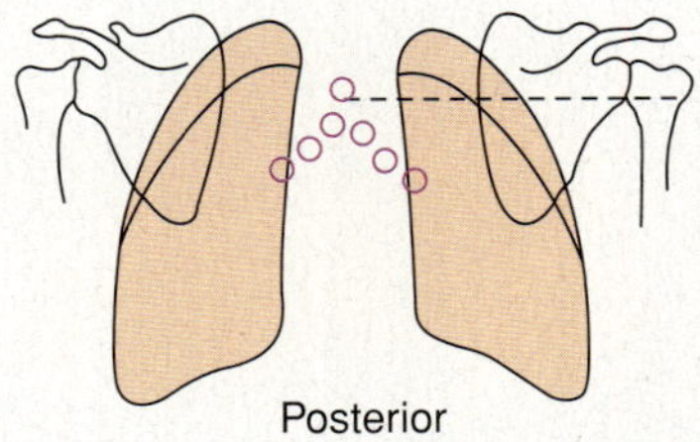	Inspiration and expiration sounds have similar pitch and duration 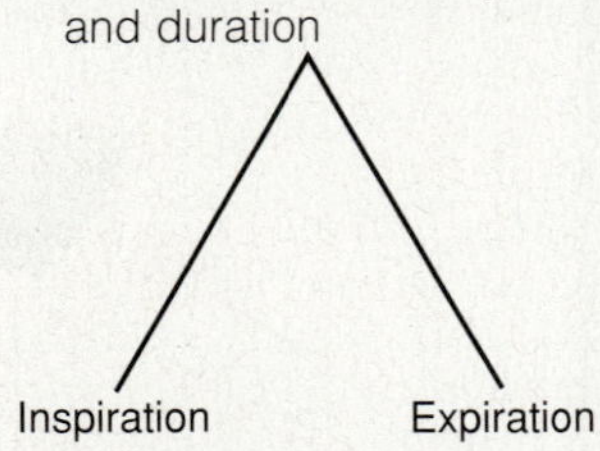
Vesicular Soft, low-pitched, whispering sounds; heard over most of the lung fields 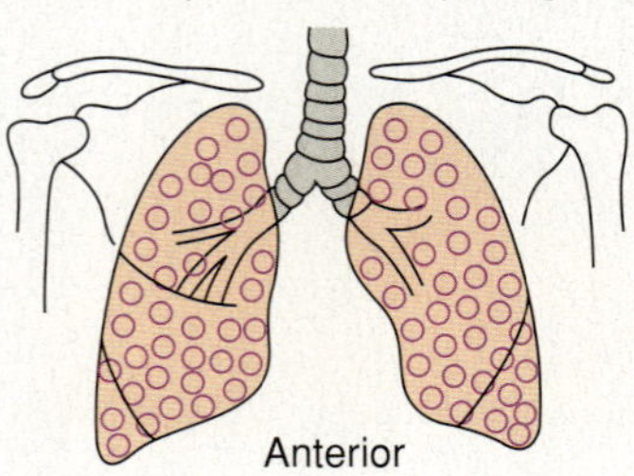 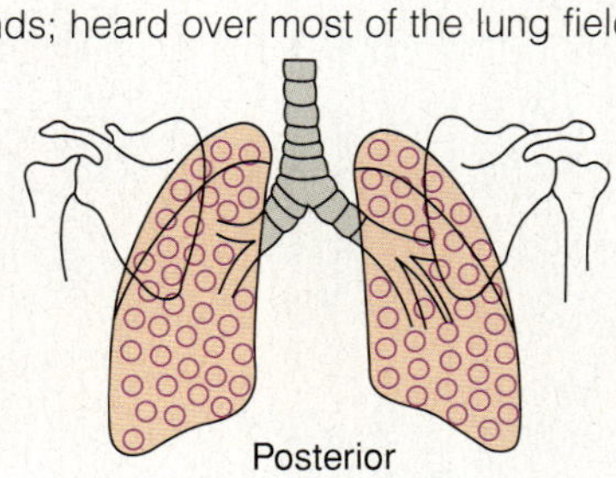	Sound on inspiration is longer, louder, and higher pitched than expiration 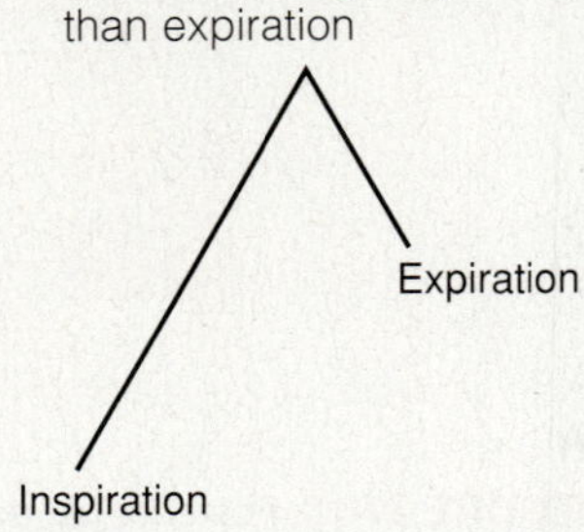

Table 27-3 Adventitious Breath Sounds

TYPE AND CHARACTERISTICS	ILLUSTRATION
Wheeze (Sibilant) Musical or squeaking High-pitched, continuous sounds Auscultated during inspiration and expiration Air passing through narrowed airways	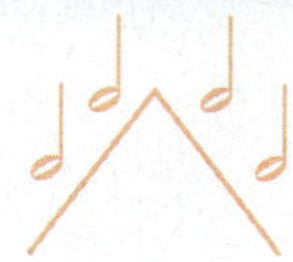
Rhonchi (Sonorous Wheeze) Sonorous or coarse; snoring quality Low-pitched, continuous sounds Auscultated during inspiration and expiration Coughing may clear the sound somewhat Air passing through or around secretions	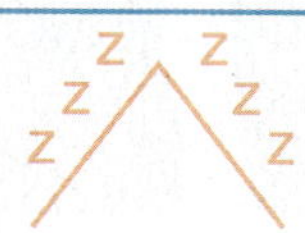
Crackles Bubbling, crackling, popping Low- to high-pitched, discontinuous sounds Auscultated during inspiration and expiration Opening of deflated small airways and alveoli; air passing through fluid in the airways	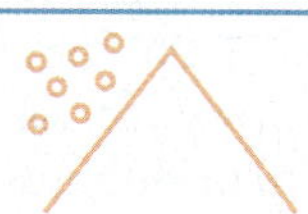
Stridor Harsh, loud, high-pitched Auscultated on inspiration Narrowing of upper airway (larynx or trachea); presence of foreign body in airway	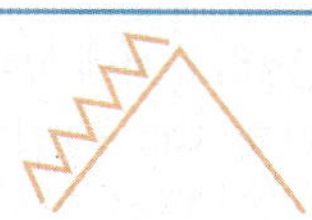
Friction Rub Rubbing or grating Loudest over lower lateral anterior surface Auscultated during inspiration and expiration Inflamed pleura rubbing against chest wall	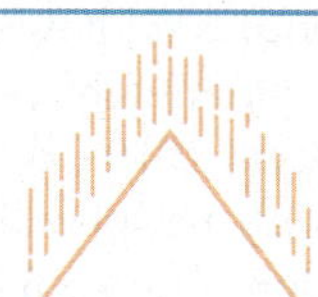

the chest wall, variations with breathing, and any change after a cough or deep breath (Jensen, 2019). If a productive cough occurs during assessment of the thorax and lungs, the sputum should be assessed for color, consistency, and amount.

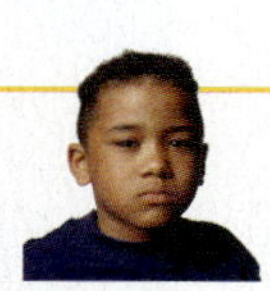

Think back to **Billy Collins**, the 9-year-old who was stung by a bee. Incorporating knowledge of the signs and symptoms of an allergic reaction, the nurse would inspect Billy's chest for accessory muscle use and auscultate his lungs, noting any evidence of wheezing, which is commonly observed with allergic reactions.

NORMAL AGE-RELATED VARIATIONS: INFANT/CHILD

Common thorax and lung variations in newborns and children include:

- Louder breath sounds on auscultation
- More rapid respiratory rate (until ages 8 to 10 years)
- Use of abdominal muscles during respiration (infants and young children up to school age)

NORMAL AGE-RELATED VARIATIONS: OLDER ADULT

Common thorax and lung variations in older adults include:

- Increased anteroposterior chest diameter
- Increase in the dorsal spinal curve (kyphosis)
- Decreased thoracic expansion
- Use of accessory muscles to exhale

Assessing the Cardiovascular and Peripheral Vascular Systems

Cardiovascular and peripheral vascular assessment includes assessment of the heart and the extremities. Questions in the health history can identify supporting subjective data such as leg pain, chest pain, or dyspnea on exertion. Data can also be used to identify ADLs and health behaviors that increase the risk of cardiovascular disease, including smoking, lack of exercise, and a diet high in calories, fats, and salt. If these risks are identified, the plan of care should include referral for additional diagnostic testing and teaching about health-promotion activities. The physical examination is used to identify signs and symptoms of heart disease and peripheral vascular disease (most often found in the lower extremities). Additional information related to assessment of the cardiovascular and peripheral vascular systems is discussed in Chapters 26 and 40.

HEALTH HISTORY

Identify risk factors for altered health during the health history by asking about the following:

- History of chest pain, palpitations, or dizziness
- Swelling in the ankles and feet
- Number of pillows used to sleep
- Type and amount of medications taken daily
- History of heart defect, rheumatic fever, or chest or heart surgery
- Personal or family history of hypertension (high blood pressure), myocardial infarction (heart attack), coronary artery disease, high blood cholesterol levels, or diabetes mellitus
- History of smoking (how long, how many packs/day)
- Type and amount of exercise
- Usual foods eaten each day
- Changes in color or temperature of the extremities
- History of pain in the legs when sleeping or pain that is worsened by walking
- History of blood clots or sores on the legs that do not heal

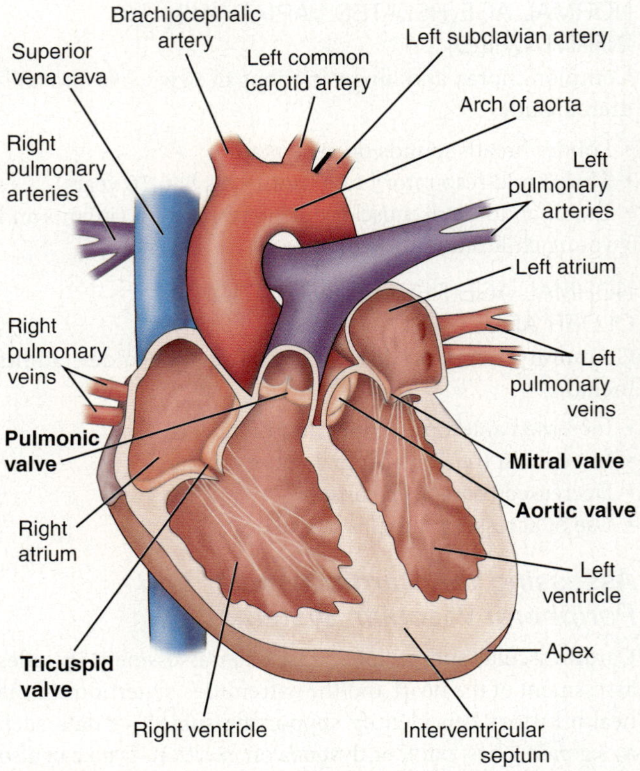

FIGURE 27-19. View of the interior of the heart showing the atrioventricular and semilunar valves responsible for heart sounds.

PHYSICAL ASSESSMENT

The techniques used for cardiovascular assessment are inspection, palpation, and auscultation. Necessary equipment includes a stethoscope with a bell and diaphragm, an electronic oscillometric device or sphygmomanometer to measure blood pressure, and a watch. The patient may be in a sitting position or in a supine position with the head raised about 30 degrees, if possible. Adequate lighting is essential for inspection of color and for pulsations. A quiet environment is necessary for accurate auscultation of heart sounds. Figure 27-19 provides a view of the heart, including the heart valves responsible for heart sounds.

Peripheral vascular assessment includes measuring the blood pressure and assessing the skin and perfusion of the extremities and the peripheral pulses. Assessments are made by inspection and palpation, with the patient sitting or supine. Use of an electronic oscillometric device to measure blood pressure is preferred over the auscultatory method of measurement (Muntner et al., 2019). Refer to Chapter 26 for a detailed discussion of measurement of blood pressure.

Peripheral vascular assessments may be combined with assessment of other body areas. Many health care providers assess the neuromuscular, musculoskeletal, and peripheral vascular systems as an integrated assessment. Refer to Skill 27-2 (on pp. 824–830) for an example of a systematic, integrated assessment of these systems.

Inspecting the Neck and Precordium

Observe the neck and **precordium** (the portion of the body over the heart and lower thorax, encompassing the

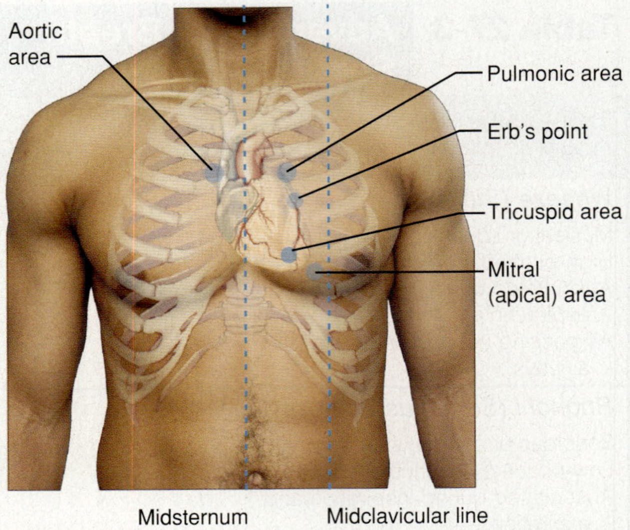

FIGURE 27-20. The precordium with the traditional cardiac landmarks and areas for auscultation.

aortic, pulmonic, tricuspid, and apical areas, and Erb's point) (Fig. 27-20) for visible pulsations. Pulsations usually are absent except for the apical impulse, located at about the fourth or fifth intercostal space at the left midclavicular line. Inspect the epigastric area at the tip of the sternum for pulsation of the abdominal aorta. Findings of neck vein distention (indicating heart disease) or visible pulsations in precordial areas other than the apical impulse (which may result from abnormalities of the ventricle) are considered abnormal.

Palpating the Neck and Precordium

Palpate the carotid artery medial to the sternomastoid muscle in the neck between the jaw and the clavicle, in the lower third of the neck (Fig. 27-21) (Jensen, 2019). Palpate the carotid arteries one at a time to avoid obstructing both arteries simultaneously, reducing blood flow to the brain and potentially causing dizziness or loss of consciousness (Jensen, 2019). Note the strength of the pulse and grade it as with peripheral pulses (refer to discussion later in this section on page 804). Normal findings include equal pulses bilaterally, with a strength of +2. Abnormal findings include

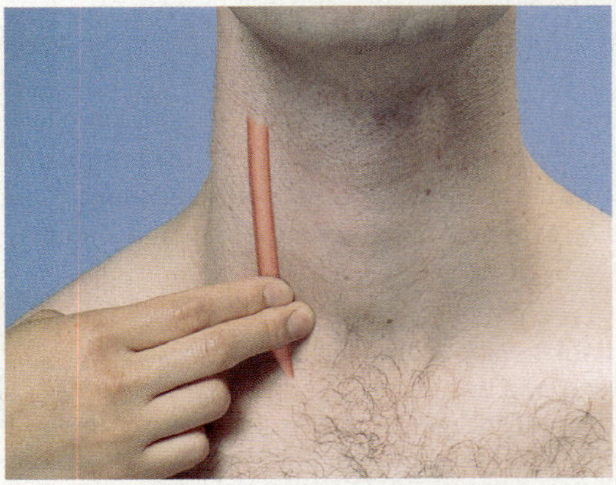

FIGURE 27-21. Palpate the carotid artery medial to the sternomastoid muscle in the neck between the jaw and the clavicle. (*Source:* Jensen, S. [2010]. *Nursing health assessment: A best practice approach* [1st ed.]. Wolters Kluwer Health.)

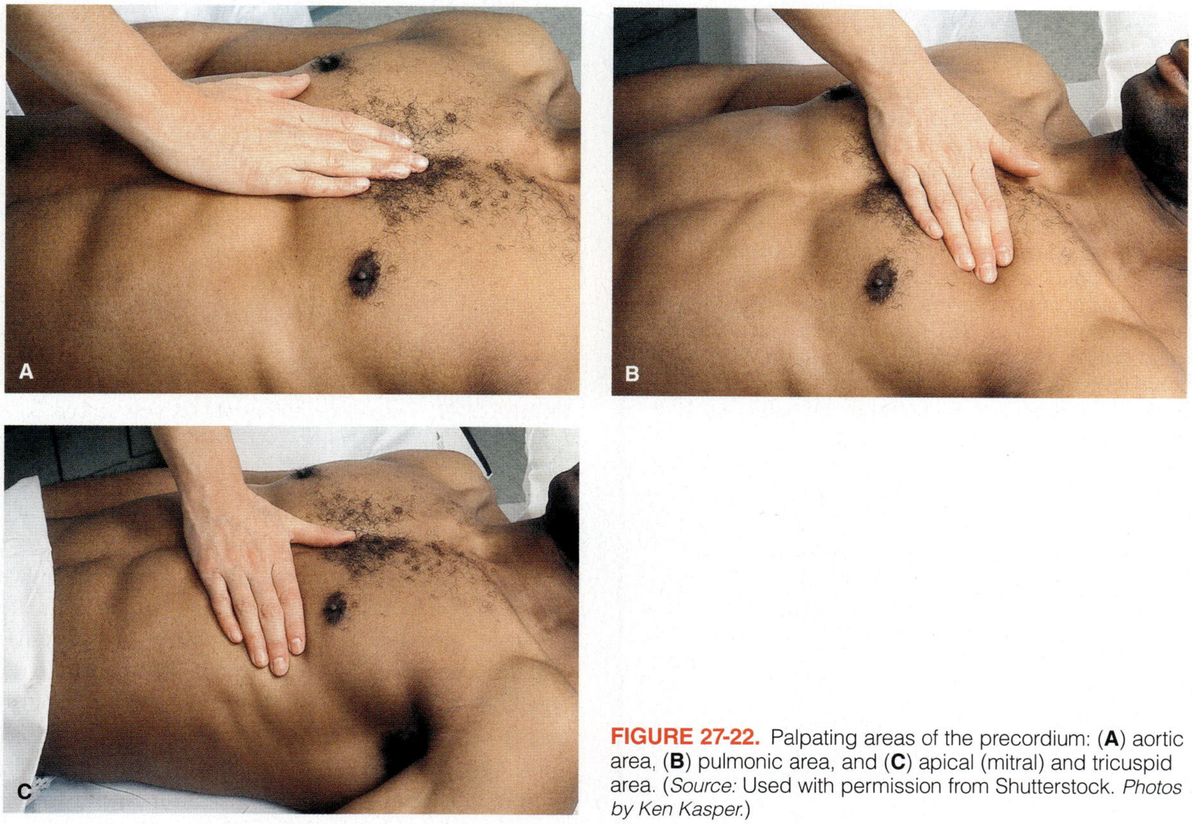

FIGURE 27-22. Palpating areas of the precordium: (**A**) aortic area, (**B**) pulmonic area, and (**C**) apical (mitral) and tricuspid area. (*Source:* Used with permission from Shutterstock. *Photos by Ken Kasper.*)

an absent pulse; a diminished (weak) or thready pulse (which may indicate decreased cardiac output); a forceful or bounding pulse (seen in hypertension and circulatory fluid overload); and an asymmetric pulse (related to impaired circulation). Additional information related to assessment of the pulses is discussed in Chapter 26.

Using the palmar surface of the hand with the four fingers held together, gently palpate the precordium for pulsations (Fig. 27-22). Palpate in a systematic manner, assessing specific cardiac landmarks—the aortic (A), pulmonic (B), tricuspid, and mitral areas (C), as well as Erb's point. Palpate the apical impulse in the mitral area. Note size, duration, force, and location in relationship to the midclavicular line. Normal findings include no pulsation palpable over the aortic and pulmonic areas, with a palpable apical impulse. Abnormal findings include precordial thrills, which are fine, palpable, rushing vibrations over the right or left second intercostal space, and lifts or heaves, which involve a rise along the border of the sternum with each heartbeat.

Auscultating the Carotid Arteries

Using the bell of the stethoscope, auscultate over the carotid arteries for bruits. Bruits are abnormal "swooshing or blowing" sounds heard over a blood vessel, caused by blood that is swirling in the vessel rather than normal smooth flow. A bruit may be heard in the presence of stenosis (narrowing) or occlusion of an artery. Bruits may also be caused by abnormal dilation of a vessel. Report and document changes in vascular sounds.

Auscultating Heart Sounds

Auscultation is used to determine the heart sounds caused by closure of the heart valves. Ask the patient to breathe normally. Use systematic auscultation, beginning at the aortic area, moving to the pulmonic area, then to Erb's point, then to the tricuspid area, and finally to the mitral area (see Fig. 27-20). Use the diaphragm of the stethoscope first to listen to high-pitched sounds. Then use the bell to listen to low-pitched sounds. Focus on the overall rate and rhythm of the heart and the normal heart sounds (Box 27-7 on page 804).

Abnormal findings include extra heart sounds at any of the cardiac landmarks and abnormal rate or rhythm. Extra heart sounds are often heard when the patient has anemia or heart disease. A wide variety of conditions may alter the normal heart rate or rhythm, including serious infections, diseases of the heart muscle or conducting system, dehydration or overhydration, endocrine disorders, respiratory disorders, and head trauma. Extra heart sounds may be S_3, S_4, or murmurs.

S_3, known as the third heart sound, follows S_2 and is often represented by a "lub-dub-dee" pattern ("dee" being S_3). This sound is best heard with the stethoscope bell at the mitral area, with the patient lying on the left side. S_3 is considered normal in children and young adults and abnormal in middle-aged and older adults. S_4 is the fourth heart sound, occurring right before S_1, and is often represented by a "dee-lub-dub" pattern ("dee" being S_4). S_4 is considered normal in older adults but abnormal in children and adults. Heart murmurs are extra heart sounds caused by some disruption

Box 27-7 Normal Heart Sounds

During auscultation, the first heart sound, called S_1, is heard as the "lub" of "lub-dub." This sound occurs when the mitral and tricuspid valves close and corresponds to the onset of ventricular contraction (see figure). The sound, low-pitched and dull, is heard best at the apical area. The second heart sound, S_2, occurs at the termination of systole and corresponds to the onset of ventricular diastole. The "dub" of "lub-dub" represents the closure of the aortic and pulmonic valves. The sound of S_2 is higher pitched and shorter than S_1. The two sounds occur within 1 second or less, depending on the heart rate.

Normal findings include S_1, that is louder at the tricuspid and apical areas, with S_2 louder at the aortic and pulmonic areas.

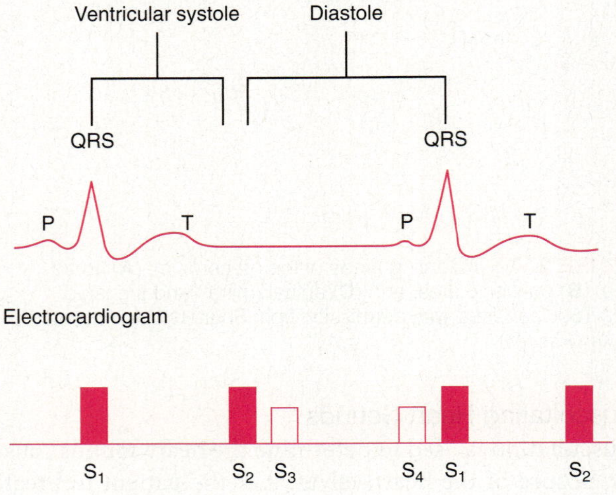

Heart sounds

Heart sounds in relation to the cardiac cycle and an electrocardiogram.

of blood flow through the heart. The characteristics of a murmur and grading depend on the adequacy of valve function, rate of blood flow, and size of the valve opening. In clinical practice, nurses are more concerned with recognizing changes in murmurs rather than in diagnosing and labeling them (Jensen, 2019, p. 467). Refer to a health assessment text for grading details and additional information related to assessment of heart sounds.

Inspecting the Extremities

Inspect the skin of the extremities for color, temperature, continuity, lesions (as described previously for assessment of the integument), venous patterns, and edema. Normally, venous patterns, varicosities, rashes, ulcers, or edema are absent on the lower extremities. However, if the patient has peripheral vascular disease (resulting in decreased blood flow and oxygenation of tissues), the skin of the lower extremities is typically pale and cool, shiny with brown discolorations, and hairless. The toenails are thickened. Phlebitis (inflammation of a vein) of the lower extremity is indicated by pain, redness, and swelling of the affected calf or thigh.

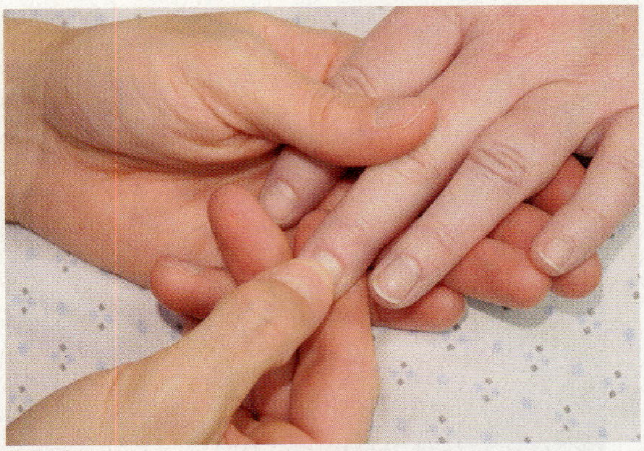

FIGURE 27-23. Assessing capillary refill. (*Source:* Jensen, S. [2019]. *Nursing health assessment: A best practice approach* [3rd ed.]. Wolters Kluwer Health.)

Palpating Peripheral Pulses and Capillary Refill

Use the pads of the index and middle fingers to palpate peripheral pulses for amplitude and symmetry. Palpate, carefully and one at a time, the carotid, brachial, radial, femoral, popliteal, dorsalis pedis, and posterior tibial pulses (see Fig. 26-3 on page 730). These pulses should be strong and equal bilaterally. The strength (amplitude) of the pulses, with a scale that may be used for documentation, is described in Table 26-5 on page 728. Assess capillary refill by using your thumb and forefinger to squeeze the patient's fingernail or toenail until it blanches (turns white). Release the pressure and observe the time it takes for normal color to return (Fig. 27-23). Normal capillary refill is <3 seconds (Jensen, 2019). Additional information related to assessment of pulses is discussed in Chapter 26.

Abnormal findings include an absent, weak, or thready pulse (which may indicate a decreased cardiac output), a forceful or bounding pulse (seen in hypertension and circulatory fluid overload), and an asymmetric pulse (related to impaired circulation). Prolonged capillary refill is associated with alterations in peripheral perfusion, edema, and cardiac output.

Other assessments to determine arterial blood flow include Allen's test and Buerger's test, which are usually performed by advanced practice professionals and are not discussed here. Refer to an assessment text for details.

Assessing Neurovascular Status

Assessment of neurovascular status is an important nursing intervention leading to early identification of neurovascular impairment and timely intervention (Agency for Clinical Innovation, 2018; Johnston-Walker & Hardcastle, 2011; Turney et al., 2013). Musculoskeletal trauma, crush injuries, orthopedic surgery, and external pressure from a cast or tight-fitting bandage can cause damage to blood vessels and nerves. This damage causes localized inflammation and tissue edema, which can lead to significantly diminished perfusion and severe ischemia, with resulting severe and permanent dysfunction of the affected area and/or loss of a limb. A neurovascular assessment includes assessing for changes in circulation, motor function, and sensation. Box 27-8 outlines the components of a neurovascular assessment.

Box 27-8 Components of a Neurovascular Assessment

- **Pain:** Extreme pain, especially on passive motion, is a significant sign of probable neurovascular impairment in an extremity. Subjective and objective assessments should be included. Opioid analgesia is unlikely to relieve the pain.
- **Pallor (perfusion):** Comparison between affected and unaffected limb is important. Assess color and temperature of the extremity. Pale skin, decreased tone, or white color may indicate poor arterial perfusion. Cyanosis may indicate venous stasis. Coolness or decreased temperature may indicate decreased arterial supply. Compare distal to proximal temperature variation in affected limb. Assess capillary refill.
- **Peripheral pulses:** Comparison between affected and unaffected limb is important. Assess the consistency of arterial blood flow (pulse presence, rate, quality) to and past the affected area. Assess capillary refill, especially in patients whose pulses cannot be palpated due to casts or bandages and in nonverbal patients.
- **Paresthesia (sensation):** May be first symptom of changes in sensory nerves to appear. Numbness, tingling, or "pins and needles" sensations may be reported. Evaluate the areas above and below the affected area.
- **Paralysis (movement):** The ability of the patient to move the extremity distal to the injury. Paralysis of an extremity may be the result of prolonged nerve compression or irreversible muscle damage.
- **Pressure:** Comparison between affected and unaffected limb is important. Swelling occurs as a physiologic response to injury. Affected area may become taut and firm to the touch, with surrounding skin appearing shiny. The feeling of tightness or pressure may be present.
- **Blood loss/ooze:** Assess blood loss on dressings, casting materials any surgical drains.

Source: Adapted from Hinkle, J. L., Cheever, K. H., & Overbaugh, K. J. (2022). *Brunner & Suddarth's Textbook of medical-surgical nursing* (15th ed.). Wolters Kluwer; Johnston-Walker, E., & Hardcastle, J. (2011). Neurovascular assessment in the critically ill patient. *Nursing in Critical Care*, *16*(4), 170–177 with permission from John Wiley and Sons.

NORMAL AGE-RELATED VARIATIONS: INFANT/CHILD

Common cardiovascular and peripheral vascular variations in newborns and children include:

- Visible cardiac pulsation if the chest wall is thin
- Sinus dysrhythmia (the rate increases with inspiration and decreases with expiration)
- Presence of S_3 (in about one third of all children)
- More rapid heart rate (until about age 8 or 10 years)

NORMAL AGE-RELATED VARIATIONS: OLDER ADULT

Common cardiovascular and peripheral vascular variations in older adults include:

- Difficult to palpate apical pulse
- Difficult to palpate distal arteries
- More prominent and tortuous blood vessels; varicosities common
- Increased systolic and diastolic blood pressure
- Widening pulse pressure (refer to Chapter 26)

Assessing the Breasts and Axillae

Although the assessments and disorders described here focus on the female breast, men also are at risk for breast disease. Figure 27-24 provides a lateral cross section of the breast, including the underlying structures. Each breast has a lymphatic network that drains into the underlying axilla (Fig. 27-26 on page 807). Physical assessment of the breasts and axilla is primarily conducted to identify any lumps in the breasts and/or enlargement or pain in axillary lymph nodes; if assessed, the patient should have further diagnostic tests.

Research does not show a clear benefit of regular physical breast exams, and as a result regular clinical breast exam and breast self-exam are not recommended (American Cancer Society, 2020; U.S. Preventive Services Task Force and the American Congress of Obstetricians and Gynecologists, as cited in Johns Hopkins Medicine, n.d.). Early detection tests, such as breast cancer screening, are based on an individual woman's risk for breast cancer and include risk assessment tools, mammograms, magnetic resonance imaging (MRI), ultrasound, and other tests. The American Cancer Society provides recommendations for early breast cancer detection. These recommendations can be accessed on the American Cancer Society's website at www.cancer.org. Women should be familiar with how their breasts normally look and feel as a result of everyday self-care and promptly report changes

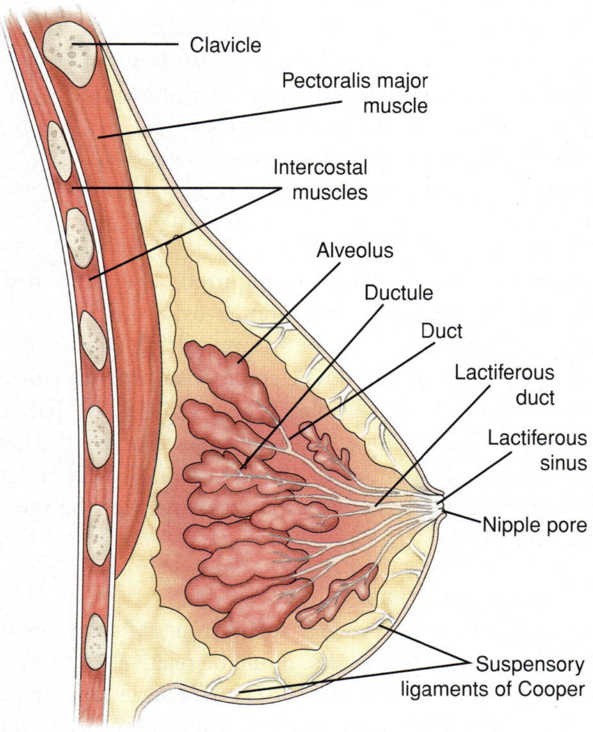

FIGURE 27-24. Lateral view of the female breast.

Box 27-9 Breast Self-Awareness

All women should be familiar with how their breasts normally look and feel. This helps in noticing any changes. Instruct patients to contact a health care provider for any changes in their breasts.

Changes to look for:

- Lumps
- Change in size or shape
- Skin irritation, such as redness, thickening, dimpling of skin
- Pain or redness of a nipple
- Nipple discharge other than breast milk
- Swelling

Source: Adapted from Johns Hopkins Medicine. (n.d.). *Health. Wellness and prevention. Breast self-awareness.* https://www.hopkinsmedicine.org/health/wellness-and-prevention/breast-self-awareness; American College of Obstetricians and Gynecologists. (2017). *Mammography and other screening tests for breast problems. Frequently asked questions: Gynecologic problems.* https://www.acog.org/patient-resources/faqs/gynecologic-problems/mammography-and-other-screening-tests-for-breast-problems.

to a health care provider (American Cancer Society, 2020). Review information related to breast self-awareness with the patient after completion of the physical exam. Box 27-9 outlines information related to breast self-awareness.

HEALTH HISTORY

Identify risk factors for altered health during the health history by asking about the following:

- History of pain in one or both breasts, including relationship to menstrual period
- History of lumps or swelling, redness, change in size, or dimpling in the breasts
- History of discharge from the breast
- Family history of ovarian or breast cancer
- History of breast disease, biopsy, or surgery
- Menstrual and pregnancy history, breastfeeding
- Use of hormones, oral contraceptives
- Knowledge related to breast self-awareness
- Most recent mammogram

PHYSICAL ASSESSMENT

If assessment of the breasts is required, assess the breasts and axilla in both men and women using inspection and palpation. The patient can be sitting or lying supine. When sitting, the patient should sit erect, with arms at sides or raised overhead, if possible. When supine, the patient's hand on the side being examined is placed under the head, if possible. Examination of the breast and axilla is often performed sequentially with the assessment of the thorax, lungs, and heart.

Inspecting the Breasts

Inspect the breasts for size, shape, symmetry, color, texture, and skin lesions. The breasts should be relatively symmetric, although variations are normal. The size varies among people. The shape of the breasts is round and smooth, and there should be no skin depressions (retraction) or puckering (dimpling). The color should be consistent with the rest of the skin, and the texture of the skin should be soft.

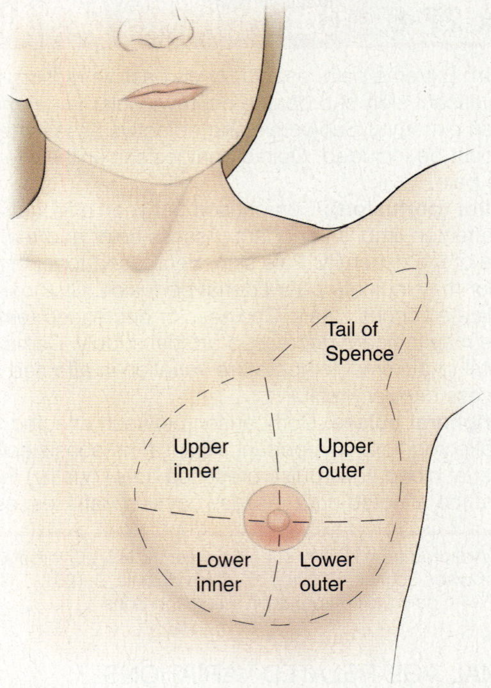

FIGURE 27-25. Location of assessment findings of the breast is identified by quadrant.

Inspect the areola and nipples for size and shape and the nipples for discharge, crusting, and inversion. The areolar and nipple areas should be equal in size, round or oval, with a smooth surface. Montgomery's tubercles (sebaceous glands on the areolae of the breasts) are a normal component of the areola. The nipples are normally everted. Discharge from the nipples is an abnormal finding except in pregnancy (leaking is normal during pregnancy and breastfeeding). Other abnormal findings include dimpling, lesions, and asymmetry.

Palpating the Breasts and Axillae

Palpate the breasts in each of the four quadrants (the upper outer quadrant, the lower outer quadrant, the upper inner quadrant, and the lower inner quadrant) to detect any abnormal lumps (Fig. 27-25). Guidelines for Nursing Care 27-4 provides instructions for palpation.

Palpate the nipple and areola, and gently compress the nipple between the thumb and forefinger to assess for discharge. The breast tissue should be smooth and firm, with a granular consistency. If a mass is detected, carefully assess its location, size, shape, consistency, and tenderness. The breasts are normally tender during the week before menstruation.

An increase in the nodularity and tenderness of the breasts may be associated with the menstrual period or may indicate fibrocystic disease. Discharge, lumps, lesions, dimpling, asymmetry, and palpable lymph nodes may be indicative of breast cancer.

Palpate the axillary areas for lymph nodes (Fig. 27-26), which normally are nonpalpable and nontender. If any

Guidelines for Nursing Care 27-4

PALPATING THE BREASTS

Palpate each quadrant of each breast in a systematic method, either the circular, wedge, or vertical strip technique. The patient should be supine with a small pillow or towel beneath her back, and the arm on the side of the breast to be examined, raised above her head.

Circular

- Start at the tail of Spence and move in increasingly smaller circles (Figure A).
- Use the pads of the first three fingers to gently compress the breast tissue against the chest wall.

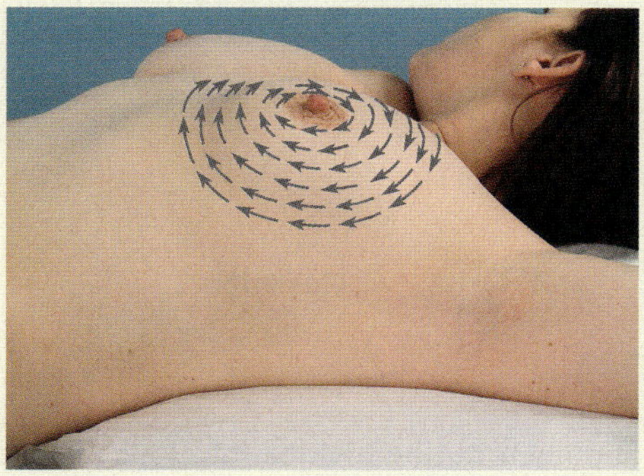

FIGURE A. Circular technique.

Wedge

- Work in a clockwise direction and palpate from the periphery toward the areola (Figure B).
- Use the pads of the first three fingers to gently compress the breast tissue against the chest wall.

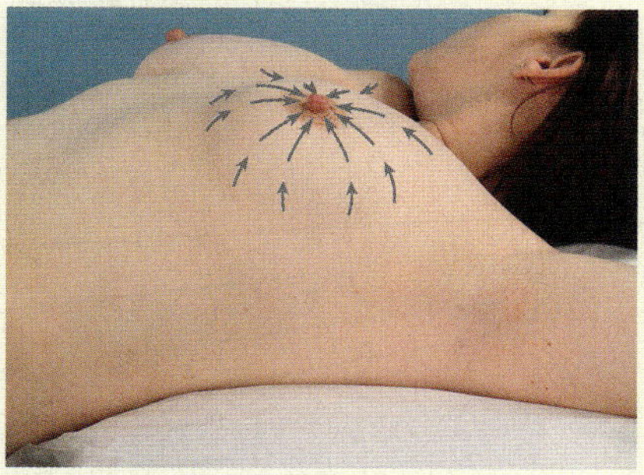

FIGURE B. Wedge technique.

Vertical Strip

- Start at the outer edge of the breast and palpate up and down the breast (Figure C).
- Use the pads of the first three fingers to gently compress the breast tissue against the chest wall.

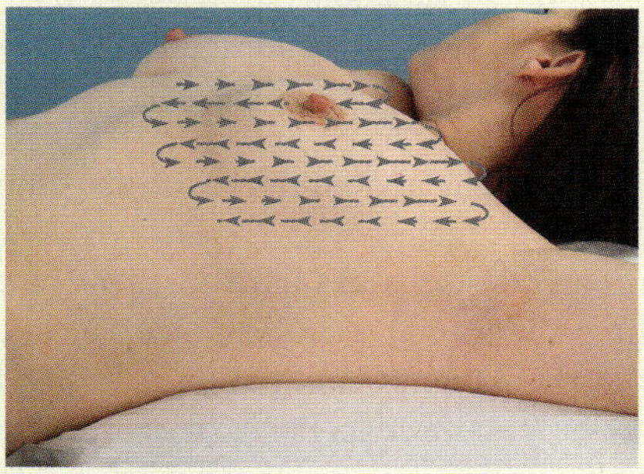

FIGURE C. Vertical strip technique.

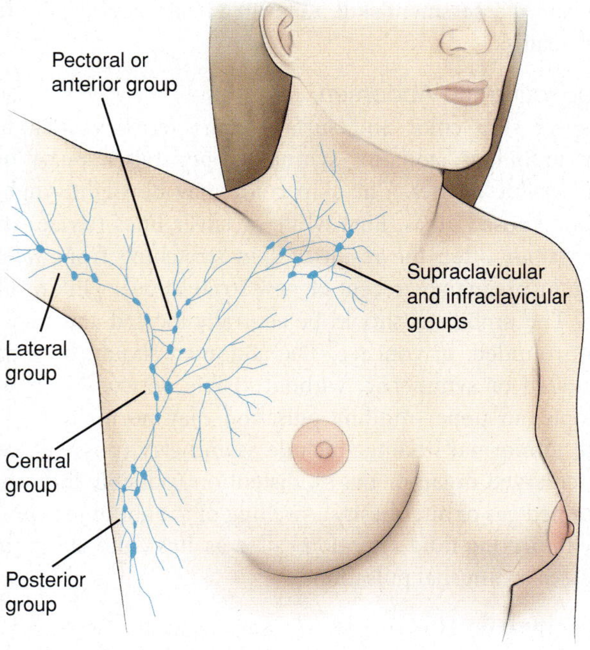

FIGURE 27-26. Location of the cervical, axillary, and mammary lymph nodes.

nodes are palpable, assess their location, size, shape, consistency, tenderness, and mobility. Palpable lymph nodes are an abnormal finding.

NORMAL AGE-RELATED VARIATIONS: INFANT/CHILD

Common breast and axillae variations in newborns and children include:

- Breast enlargement and a white discharge from the nipples (up to age 2 weeks)
- Female breast growth beginning at age 10 or 11 years
- Temporary enlargement of one or both breasts (gynecomastia) in pubescent boys

NORMAL AGE-RELATED VARIATIONS: OLDER ADULT

Common breast and axillae variations in older adults include granular, pendulous breasts in women.

Assessing the Abdomen

The abdominal cavity (Fig. 27-27 on page 808) contains the stomach, the small intestine, the large intestine, the liver, the gallbladder, the pancreas, the spleen, the kidneys, and

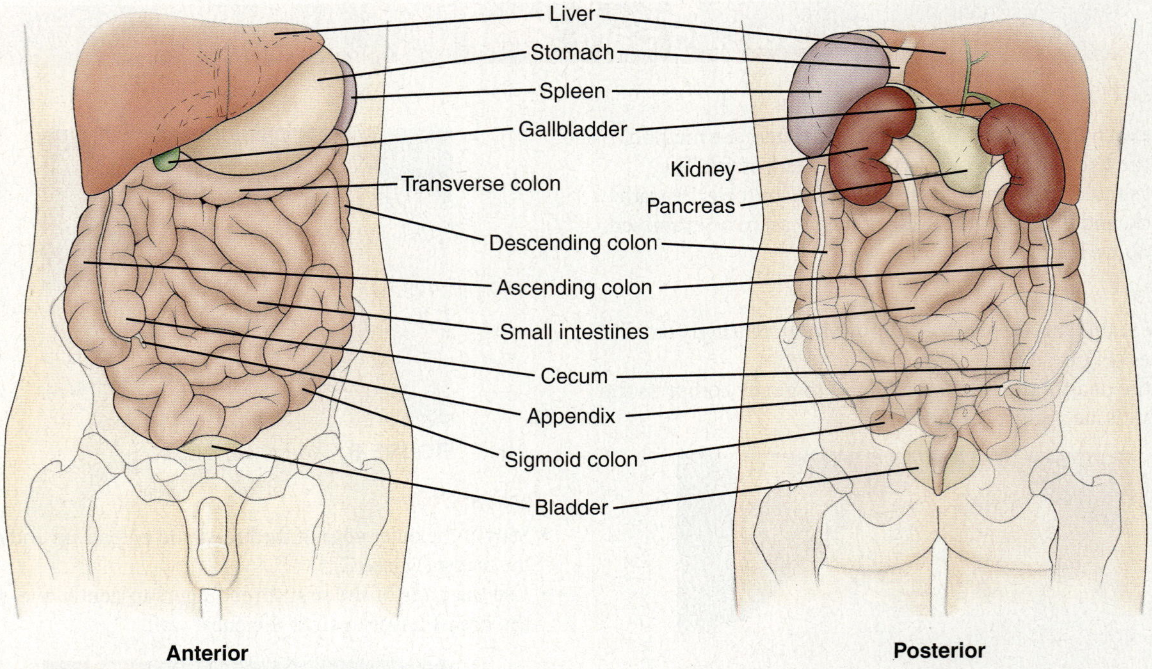

FIGURE 27-27. Organs of the abdominal cavity.

the urinary bladder. The abdominal cavity also contains the female reproductive organs.

Health history questions are used to identify subjective data, including abdominal pain and nausea, and to collect data about the patient's elimination patterns, fluid and nutritional intake, and lifestyle. Physical examination is conducted to further assess problems with pain and to identify abdominal masses. Abdominal assessments are also used to assess for the presence of bowel sounds (e.g., the return of bowel sounds after surgery) and retention of urine in the urinary bladder.

HEALTH HISTORY

Identify risk factors for altered health during the health history by asking about the following:

- History of abdominal pain
- History of indigestion, nausea or vomiting, constipation or diarrhea
- History of food allergies or lactose intolerance
- Appetite and usual food and fluid intake
- Usual bowel and bladder elimination patterns
- History of gastrointestinal disorders
- History of urinary tract disorders
- History of abdominal surgery or trauma
- Amount and type of alcohol ingestion
- For women, menstrual history

PHYSICAL ASSESSMENT

Ask the patient to empty the bladder. Place the patient in the supine position with the head slightly elevated and arms at the sides, if possible. Place small pillows under the head and knees for comfort. Make sure that the patient is warm and comfortable to help prevent contraction of the abdominal muscles, which makes palpation difficult.

The abdomen can be divided into four quadrants: right upper, right lower, left upper, and left lower (Fig. 27-28). The sequence of techniques used to assess the abdomen is inspection, auscultation, percussion, and palpation. *Percussion and palpation are done after auscultation because they stimulate bowel sounds.* Ask the patient to breathe slowly and deeply through the mouth during the examination to promote relaxation. Ask the patient to identify painful areas of the abdomen and explain that you will assess these at the end of the examination. Advanced health care providers usually perform percussion of the abdomen, which is an advanced assessment skill. Refer to a health assessment text for details.

Inspecting the Abdomen

Inspect skin color and surface characteristics, including the umbilicus, contour, symmetry, peristalsis, pulsations, and visible masses. The skin color may be slightly lighter than exposed areas. Fine white or silver lines (striae) may be visible, often the result of skin stretching from weight gain or pregnancy; recent or new striae appear pink or bluish. The umbilicus should be centrally located and may be flat, rounded, or concave. The abdomen should be evenly rounded or symmetric, without visible peristalsis. In thin people, an upper midline pulsation may normally be visible. Abnormal findings include asymmetry (possibly from an enlarged organ or mass), distention (possibly indicating retained gas or air; obesity), swelling of the abdomen (possibly indicating fluid retention called ascites), and abdominal masses or unusual pulsations.

Auscultating Bowel Sounds and Vascular Sounds

Auscultation is used to assess bowel sounds and vascular sounds. Warm the stethoscope. Traditionally, bowel sounds

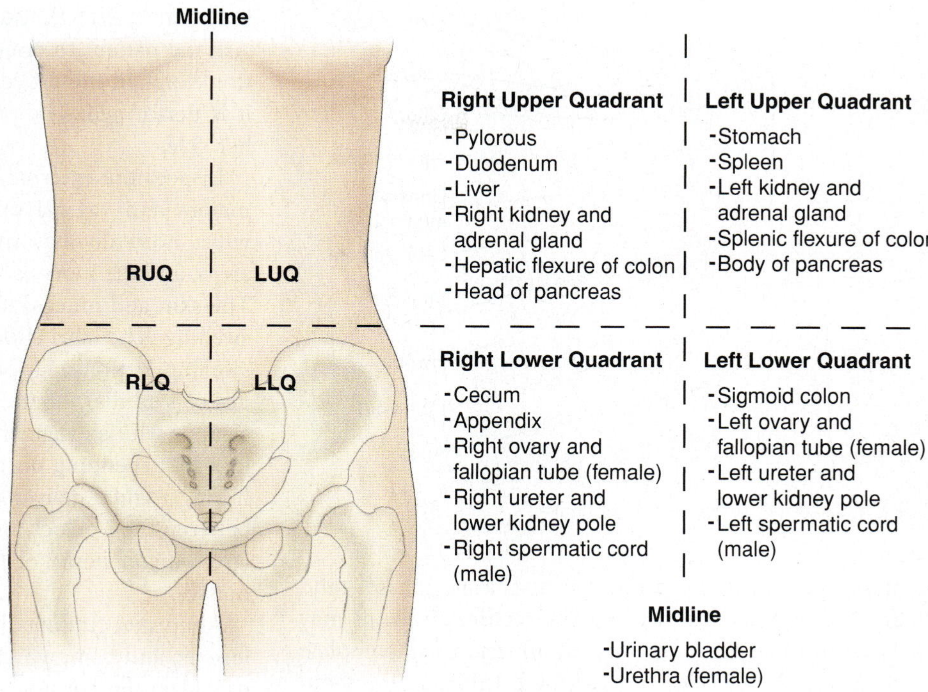

FIGURE 27-28. Diagram of abdominal quadrants and outline of underlying organs.

are assessed in all four quadrants of the abdomen. Using light pressure, place the flat diaphragm on the right lower quadrant of the abdomen, then move to right upper quadrant, left upper quadrant, and finally to the left lower quadrant. Listen carefully for bowel sounds (gurgles and clicks), and note their frequency and character (usually occur every 5 to 15 seconds). Before documenting bowel sounds as absent, the nurse must listen for 1 minute or longer in each abdominal quadrant (Jensen, 2019; Weber & Kelley, 2018). Some sources suggest bowel sounds radiate widely over the abdomen, and listening in all four quadrants is not necessary; assessment of presence and hypoactivity (decreased)/hyperactivity (increased) is sufficient (Jarvis & Eckhardt, 2020; McGee, 2018). Abnormal findings include increased bowel sounds (often heard with diarrhea or in early bowel obstruction), decreased bowel sounds (heard after abdominal surgery or late bowel obstruction), or absent bowel sounds (indicating peritonitis or paralytic ileus). Bowel sounds of high-pitched tinkling or rushes of high-pitched sounds indicate a partial bowel obstruction.

Using the bell of the stethoscope, auscultate over the abdominal aorta, femoral arteries, and iliac arteries for bruits. Bruits are abnormal "swooshing or blowing" sounds heard over a blood vessel, caused by blood that is swirling in the vessel, rather than normal smooth flow. A bruit may be heard in the presence of stenosis (narrowing) or occlusion of an artery. Bruits may also be caused by abnormal dilation of a vessel. Report and document changes in or absence of bowel and vascular sounds.

Palpating the Abdomen

Use light palpation to assess the abdomen; apply pressure with the fingers together and lightly depressing the skin and underlying structures about 1 to 2 cm (0.5 to 0.75 inch) (Jarvis & Eckhardt, 2020; Jensen, 2019; Weber & Kelley, 2018). Watch the patient's face for nonverbal signs of pain during palpation. Palpate each quadrant in a systematic manner, noting muscular resistance, tenderness, or masses. If the patient reports abdominal pain, palpate the area of pain last. The abdomen should normally be soft, relaxed, and free of tenderness. Abnormal findings include involuntary rigidity, spasm, masses, and pain (which may indicate trauma, peritonitis, infection, tumors, or enlarged or diseased abdominal organs).

NORMAL AGE-RELATED VARIATIONS: INFANT/CHILD

Common abdominal variations in newborns and children include:

- Umbilical cord in newborns; dries and falls off within the first few weeks of life
- A "potbelly" (younger than age 5 years)
- Visible peristaltic waves

NORMAL AGE-RELATED VARIATIONS: OLDER ADULT

Common abdominal variations in older adults include:

- Decreased bowel sounds
- Decreased abdominal tone
- Fat accumulation on the abdomen and hips

Assessing Female Genitalia

The external female genitalia consist of the mons pubis, labia majora and minora, clitoris, vestibular glands, vaginal vestibule, vaginal orifice, and urethral opening (Fig. 27-29 on page 810). Information collected during the health history is especially helpful in identifying risk factors for cancer and health-related behaviors that increased risk for sexually transmitted infections. During the physical assessment, the external genitalia may be examined. The female

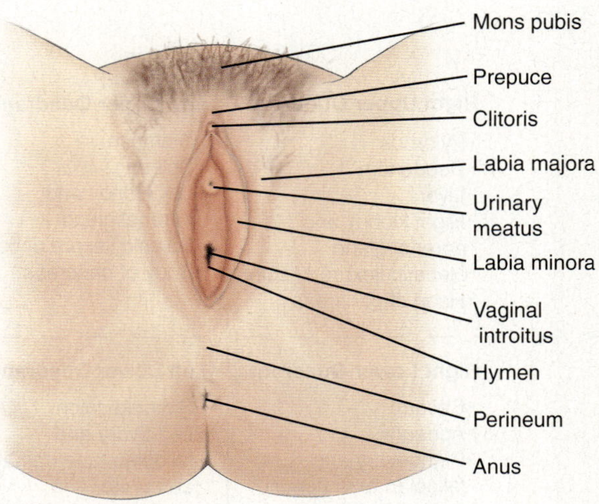

FIGURE 27-29. External female genitalia.

genitalia are assessed for lesions, discharge, masses, and enlargement of internal organs. The rectum and anus may be assessed during part of this examination if a complete health assessment is being performed. Information about rectal examination is provided later in this chapter. The internal pelvic examination is an advanced skill, usually performed by an advanced practice professional. Refer to a health assessment text for details of this advanced assessment skill.

HEALTH HISTORY

Identify risk factors for altered female health during the health history by asking about the following:

- Menstrual history (age of first and last period, length of flow, type of flow, pain)
- Sexual history (age at which sexual activity began, number and biologic sex of partners, practices)
- Pain with intercourse, difficulty achieving orgasm
- Number of pregnancies and live births
- History of sexually transmitted infection
- Use of contraceptives/protection from sexually transmitted infections (STIs)
- Frequency of pelvic examinations and Pap smears
- History of vaginal discharge, itching, or pain on urination
- Use of hormones and tobacco (how long, how much, how many packs/day)

PHYSICAL ASSESSMENT

Assess the genitalia by inspection and palpation. A description of an internal pelvic assessment of women is included in this chapter. This is an advanced assessment technique, but nurses often assist in performing vaginal examinations and need to be familiar with the procedure. In many instances, male health care providers will ask that a female be present in the room during the examination. Women from some cultures or who practice certain religions may agree to a physical examination of the genitalia only by a female nurse or female health care provider. Equipment required includes a good light source and disposable gloves.

Inspecting and Palpating the External Genitalia

Ask the patient to empty her bladder before the examination. Explain the procedure to her and help her to relax as it is performed. The patient should be supine or lying on her side.

Inspect the external genitalia for color, size of the labia majora and vaginal opening, lesions, and discharge. The vulva normally has more pigmentation than other skin areas, and the mucous membranes are dark pink and moist. The skin and mucosa should be smooth, without lesions or swelling. The labia should be symmetric without lesions or swelling. Lesions may be the result of infections (such as herpes or syphilis). There may normally be a small amount of clear or whitish vaginal discharge. The vaginal orifice varies in size, depending on the woman's age, sexual history, and having vaginal delivery. In children, loss of hymenal tissue between the 3 o'clock and 9 o'clock position indicates trauma (from digits, penis, or foreign objects). Palpate the labia for masses.

Abnormal findings include redness, swelling, discharge, lesions, and pain, which may indicate infection, an abscess, or cancer. For related assessments of the urinary tract and sexually transmitted infections, see Chapters 38 and 46.

Inspecting Internal Genitalia

Examination of the internal genitalia is an advanced assessment technique and usually performed by advanced health care providers. The examination is outlined here to provide the student with an understanding of the examination if asked to assist. The patient is placed in the lithotomy position on the examination table, with the legs in stirrups, and draped so that only the genitalia are exposed. Explain the procedure and help the patient to relax as it is performed. A speculum, consisting of two blades and an adjustment device, is lubricated and inserted into the vagina. This allows inspection of the cervix and other internal genitalia for abnormalities. Specimens for a Papanicolaou (Pap) test for cervical and vaginal cancer can be obtained, as well as specimens for gonorrhea and chlamydia cultures, and to test for human papillomavirus (HPV). The vaginal wall is inspected as the speculum is removed. With lubricated fingers, the advanced practice professional palpates the internal genitalia for location, size, mobility, tenderness, and masses. Refer to a health assessment text for additional details of this advanced assessment skill. The examination of the rectum is often included at this time. This examination is discussed later in the chapter.

NORMAL AGE-RELATED VARIATIONS: INFANT/CHILD

Common genitalia variations in newborns (resulting from exposure to maternal hormones in utero, normally seen in the first week after birth and subsiding by the second week after birth) and children include:

- Enlarged labia and clitoris
- Breast enlargement
- Vaginal discharge in girls, called pseudomenstruation

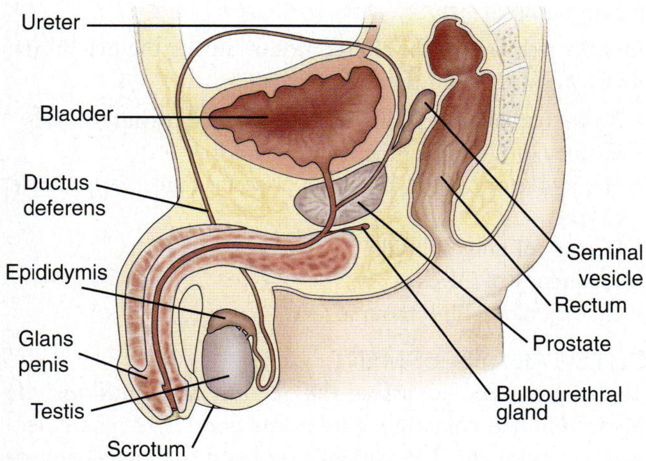

FIGURE 27-30. Organs of the male genital system.

- Pubic hair and breast development occur at puberty and follow a regular sequence of development
- Menstruation begins about 2.5 years after puberty begins
- Irregular menstrual cycle for first 2 years

NORMAL AGE-RELATED VARIATIONS: OLDER ADULT

Common genitalia variations in older women include:

- Decreased size of labia and clitoris
- Decreased amount of pubic hair
- Decreased vaginal secretions
- Pale, thin, and dry vaginal mucosa

Assessing Male Genitalia

The male genitalia (Fig. 27-30) include the penis, testicles, epididymis, scrotum, prostate gland, and seminal vesicles. In addition, the inguinal area may be examined as part of this assessment. Information from the health history is helpful in identifying self-care and lifestyle factors that increase the risk of illnesses, such as testicular cancer or sexually transmitted infections. The physical examination is focused on detecting abnormal findings so that early identification and treatment can be initiated. Review or teach the procedure for testicular self-examination after completion of the physical exam. Figure 27-31 reviews the procedure for testicular self-examination.

HEALTH HISTORY

Identify risk factors for altered male health during the health history by asking about the following:

- Frequency of digital rectal examinations (DREs)
- Frequency of testicular self-examination
- Use of contraceptives/protection from sexually transmitted infections (STIs)
- Occupational exposure to chemicals (tire and rubber manufacturing, farming, mechanics)
- Sexual history (age at which sexual activity began, number and biologic sex of partners, practices)
- History of sexually transmitted infection
- History of discharge from the penis

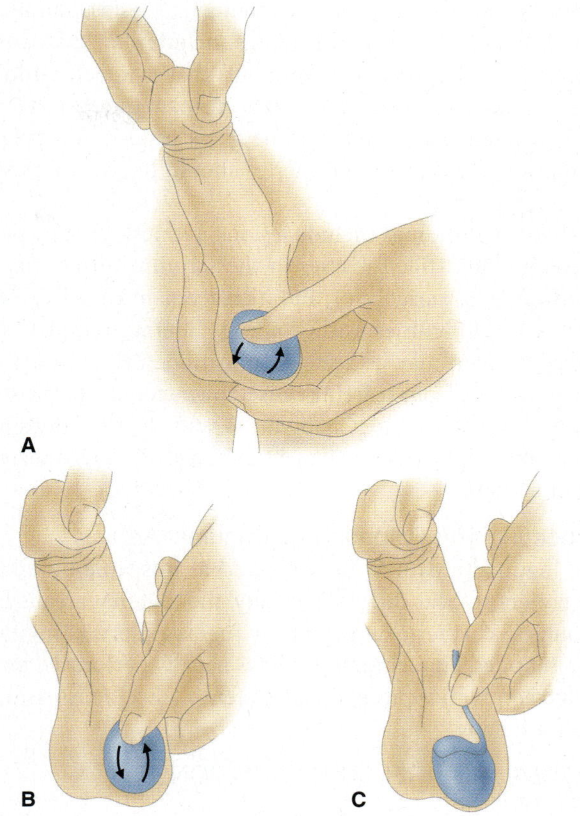

FIGURE 27-31. Testicular self-examination. A convenient time is after a warm bath or shower when the scrotum is relaxed. Both hands are used to palpate the testis; the normal testicle is smooth and uniform in consistency. **A.** With the index and middle finger under the testis and the thumb on tip, roll the testis gently in a horizontal plane between the thumb and fingers, feeling for any evidence of a small lump or abnormality. **B.** Follow the same procedure for palpation in a vertical plane. **C.** Locate the epididymis (small, coiled tube) on the top and back of the testicle that may feel like a small bump. Repeat the examination for the other testis; it is normal to find one testis larger than the other. Any changes should be reported to a health care provider. (*Source:* Adapted from American Cancer Society. [2018]. *Testicular cancer early detection, diagnosis and staging.* https://www.cancer.org/content/dam/CRC/PDF/Public/8845.00.pdf; Mayo Clinic. [2018]. *Testicular exam.* https://www.mayoclinic.org/tests-procedures/testicular-exam/about/pac-20385252.)

- Difficulty with urination (incontinence, hesitancy, frequency, voiding at night)
- History of erectile dysfunction, pain with intercourse

PHYSICAL ASSESSMENT

The patient may be standing or supine. Gloves are worn during this assessment.

Inspecting and Palpating the External Genitalia

The external genitalia are inspected for size, placement, contour, appearance of the skin, redness, edema, and discharge. If the patient is uncircumcised, retract the foreskin for inspection of the glans penis and return foreskin back over the glans penis after inspection. Assess the location of the urinary meatus. Inspect the scrotum for symmetry; it is not unusual for the left testicle to lie lower in the scrotal sac than the right testicle. Palpate the testes. The size, shape, and consistency of the scrotal contents (i.e., testes) should be similar bilaterally. Normal findings include skin that is free of lesions, and a foreskin (if present) that is intact, uniform in color, and easily retracted. The urinary meatus is normally located in the center of the glans penis and is free of discharge. The scrotum and testes should be free of masses and nontender.

Abnormal findings include lesions, redness, edema, pain, discharge, fluid-filled masses in the scrotum (symptoms of a hydrocele or varicocele), and displacement of the urinary meatus or difficulties with voiding. Edema, redness, discharge, or pain may indicate an infection. Voiding difficulties may result from scarring caused by infections or prostate enlargement. Refer to Chapters 38 and 46 for additional discussion of the male urinary tract and sexually transmitted infections.

Inspecting and Palpating the Inguinal Area

The inguinal area may be inspected at this time by asking the patient to bear down. Normally, the inguinal area is free of bulges. Further assessment for inguinal hernia, inguinal lymph nodes, and femoral hernia is usually performed by an advanced practice professional. Refer to a health assessment text for details.

NORMAL AGE-RELATED VARIATIONS: INFANT/CHILD

Common genitalia variations in newborns (resulting from exposure to maternal hormones in utero, normally seen in the first week after birth and subsiding by the second week after birth) and children include:

- Breast enlargement
- Development of pubic hair and enlargement of the scrotum, testes, and penis occurs at puberty and follows a regular sequence to adult configuration
- Spontaneous nocturnal emission of seminal fluid occurs at puberty

NORMAL AGE-RELATED VARIATIONS: OLDER ADULT

Common genitalia variations in older adults include:

- Decreased penis size
- Decreased pubic hair
- Decreased size and firmness of testes

Assessing the Rectum and Anus

Although the rectum and anus are not assessed in all patients, this assessment is a part of a total health assessment for both men and women. Assessments of the rectum and anus are usually performed by advanced practice professionals. Information from the health history provides information about normal patterns of bowel elimination and identifies risks for illness (such as colon cancer) and health behaviors (such as frequency of DREs to assess for cancer or engaging in anal intercourse). Physical examination provides information to support teaching about risk for colon cancer and the risks of sexually transmitted infections (including AIDS) associated with unprotected anal sex.

HEALTH HISTORY

Identify risk factors for altered health during the health history by asking about the following:

- Bowel patterns, including constipation, diarrhea, or pain
- History of blood or mucus in the stool
- Family history of polyps, colon or rectal cancer, or prostate cancer
- History of hemorrhoids
- Frequency of DREs
- History of anal intercourse

PHYSICAL ASSESSMENT

Techniques used to assess the rectum and anus include inspection and palpation. Gloves and good lighting are necessary equipment. The patient may be in the knee–chest or side-lying position.

Inspection is used to assess the anal area, which normally has increased pigmentation and some hair growth. Assess for lesions, ulcers, fissures, inflammation, and external hemorrhoids (dilated veins appearing as reddened protrusions). Ask the patient to bear down as though having a bowel movement. Assess for the appearance of internal hemorrhoids or fissures. Normally, there is no protrusion of tissue. Abnormal findings include relaxed sphincter tone; skin cracks, nodules, or hemorrhoids at the anal sphincter; and bleeding (which may indicate hemorrhoids or colorectal cancer). Advanced practice professionals usually perform palpation of the anal canal and sphincter and the prostate gland in men. Refer to a health assessment text for details.

NORMAL AGE-RELATED VARIATIONS: INFANT/CHILD

Normally physical examination of the rectum and anus is not performed in young children or adolescents.

NORMAL AGE-RELATED VARIATIONS: OLDER ADULT

Common variations in older adults include:

- Anus is darker in color
- Hemorrhoids

Assessing the Musculoskeletal System

The primary structures of the musculoskeletal system are the bones, muscles, cartilage, ligaments, tendons, and joints. Health history information is used to evaluate the patient's ability to carry out ADLs and to collect data about areas such as pain, stiffness, and ability to move. Physical examination provides information about posture, gait, bone size and structure, joint range of motion (ROM; the maximum degree of movement of which a joint is normal capable), and muscle strength. Normally, the joints are bilaterally equal in size, shape, and color; are free of swelling, pain, nodules, or crepitus (grating sounds on movement); and can move through full ROM. Abnormal findings include deformity, crepitus, and limited ROM (indicating injury, inflammation and/or arthritis of the affected joints or bones, and muscle pain and/or weakness caused by injury or disease). *Many health care providers assess the neuromuscular, musculoskeletal, and peripheral vascular systems as an integrated assessment.* Refer to Skill 27-2 (on pp. 824–830) for an example of a systematic, integrated assessment of these systems.

HEALTH HISTORY

Identify risk factors for altered health during the health history by asking about the following:

- History of trauma, arthritis, or neurologic disorder
- History of pain or swelling in the muscles and/or joints
- Frequency and type of usual exercise
- Dietary intake of calcium
- History of any surgery on muscles or joints
- History of smoking (how long, how many packs/day)
- History of alcohol intake

PHYSICAL ASSESSMENT

Assess the patient's ability to assume a variety of positions, including standing, sitting, and supine, if possible. *Assessments of the musculoskeletal system can be integrated into assessment of other body systems.*

Inspecting and Palpating the Muscles

Examine the muscles by inspection and palpation of muscle groups and by testing muscle tone and strength. Muscle groups are observed for bilateral symmetry and palpated for tenderness. Normally, they are symmetric and nontender. Evaluate muscle tone (the normal condition of a muscle at rest) by putting each joint and extremity through passive ROM. Assess muscle strength. Guidelines for Nursing Care 27-5 (on pages 814–815) describes testing muscle strength.

Abnormal findings include atrophy (a decrease in size), tremors (involuntary movements), and flaccidity (without tone) of muscles. Other abnormal findings are loss of strength and tone, decreased ROM, uncoordinated movements, swelling, and pain. Abnormal findings may indicate a musculoskeletal disease, trauma, or a neurologic disease.

Palpating the Bones

Palpate the bones for normal contour and prominence and for bilateral symmetry. Abnormal findings include pain, enlargement, asymmetry, and changes in contour. Abnormal findings may indicate trauma, degenerative joint disease, musculoskeletal disease, or a neurologic disease.

Inspecting and Palpating the Joints

Each joint is put through its full ROM to assess the degree of movement. Joint movements include flexion, extension, hyperextension, abduction, adduction, supination, and pronation. Normally, each joint has full ROM, is nontender, and moves smoothly. Palpate joints for the abnormal findings of pain, swelling, nodules, and crepitation (a grating sound heard or felt on movement).

Inspecting Spinal Curves

With the patient standing, inspect the spine from the back and from the side. The spine normally has concave curves at the cervical and lumbar spine and convex curves at the thoracic and sacrococcygeal spine. Kyphosis (an increased thoracic spinal curve) is more often seen in older adults. An exaggerated lumbar curve (lordosis) is often seen during pregnancy or in obesity. Scoliosis is a lateral curvature of the spine with increased convexity on the side that is curved. School nurses often first identify scoliosis during screenings, which are recommended twice for girls at ages 10 and 12, and once for boys at ages 13 to 14 years (Hresko et al., 2015). Findings indicating scoliosis are illustrated in Figure 27-32.

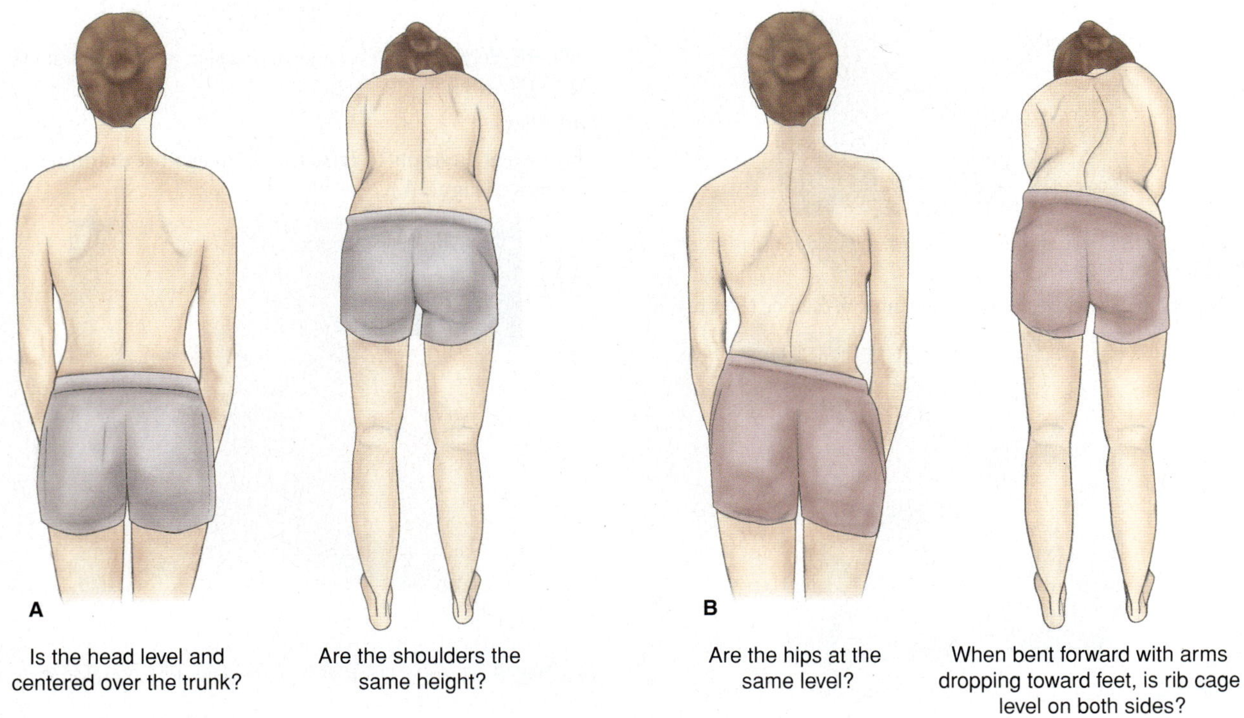

FIGURE 27-32. Screening for scoliosis. **A.** Normal position and spinal curves. **B.** Scoliosis indicators.

Guidelines for Nursing Care 27-5

ASSESSING MUSCLE STRENGTH

Assess muscle strength by asking the patient to move against resistance. Bilateral equal resistance should be present. Observe muscle contraction and determine muscle strength exerted. Muscle strength should be bilaterally equal, with a slight increase on the dominant side. Techniques for assessing the muscles include:

Shoulder Flexion

The patient flexes shoulder muscle against resistance of the examiner's hand (Figure A).

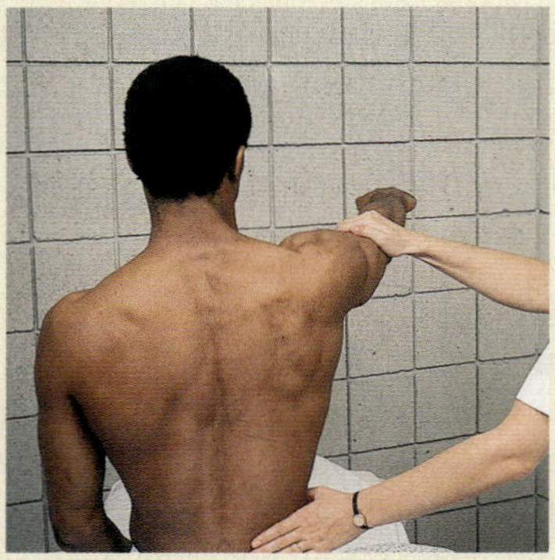

FIGURE A. *Source:* Used with permission from Shutterstock. *Photo by Ken Kasper.*

Elbow Extension and Flexion

- The patient first extends the elbow against resistance by the examiner (Figure B).

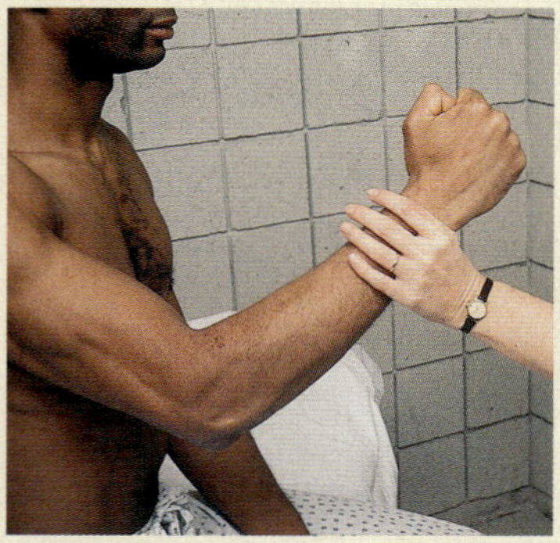

FIGURE B. *Source:* Used with permission from Shutterstock. *Photo by Ken Kasper.*

- Then the patient flexes the elbow against resistance (Figure C).

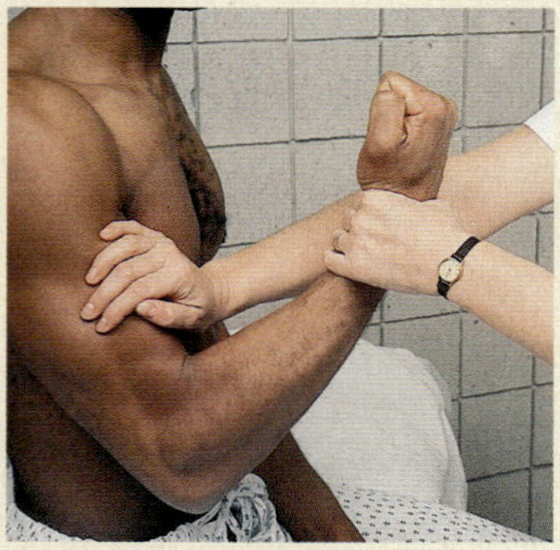

FIGURE C. *Source:* Used with permission from Shutterstock. *Photo by Ken Kasper.*

Wrist Extension

The patient makes a fist and resists examiner's attempts to pull down wrist (Figure D).

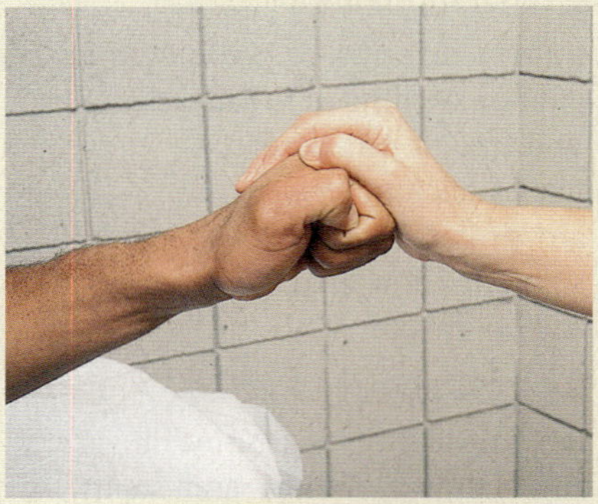

FIGURE D. *Source:* Used with permission from Shutterstock. *Photo by Ken Kasper.*

Grip

The patient squeezes the examiner's index and middle fingers (Figure E).

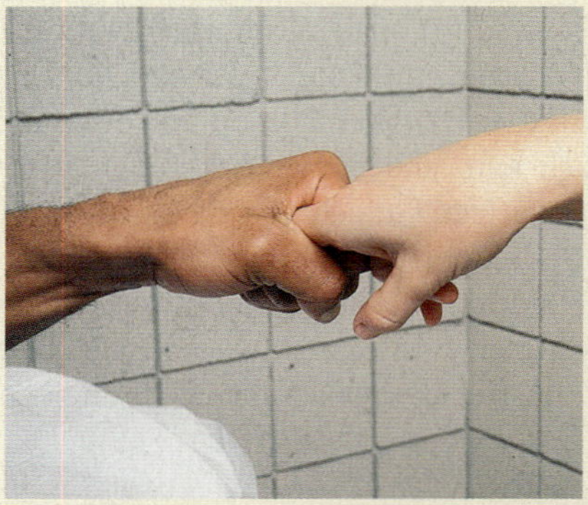

FIGURE E. *Source:* Used with permission from Shutterstock. *Photo by Ken Kasper.*

Hip Flexion

The patient attempts to raise the thigh against examiner's resistance (Figure F).

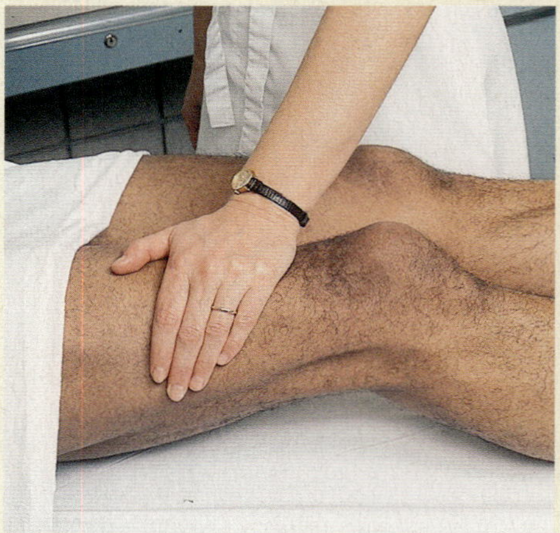

FIGURE F. *Source:* Used with permission from Shutterstock. *Photo by Ken Kasper.*

Guidelines for Nursing Care 27-5 (continued)

ASSESSING MUSCLE STRENGTH

Knee Flexion and Extension

- With the patient's knee bent and foot on the examining table, the patient attempts to keep foot down while the examiner attempts to straighten the patient's leg to test flexion (Figure G).

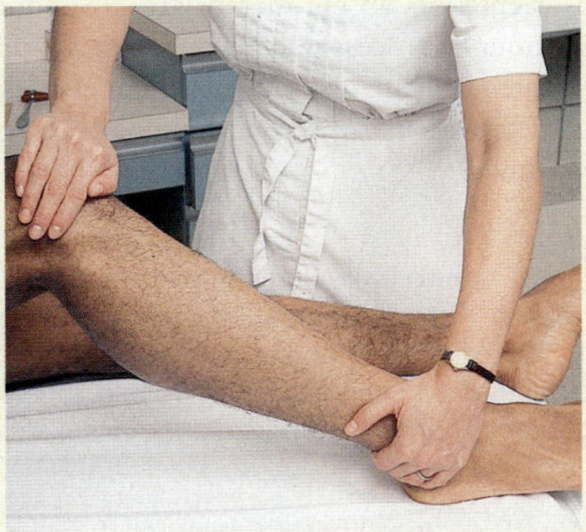

FIGURE G. *Source:* Used with permission from Shutterstock. *Photo by Ken Kasper.*

- To test extension, the examiner supports the patient's knee, and the patient attempts to straighten the leg against resistance at the ankle (Figure H).

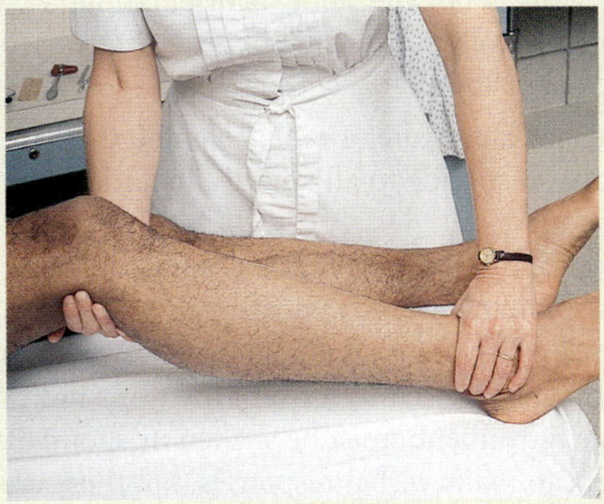

FIGURE H. *Source:* Used with permission from Shutterstock. *Photo by Ken Kasper.*

Ankle Plantar Flexion and Dorsiflexion

- The patient first pushes the balls of the feet against resistance of the examiner's hands (Figure I).

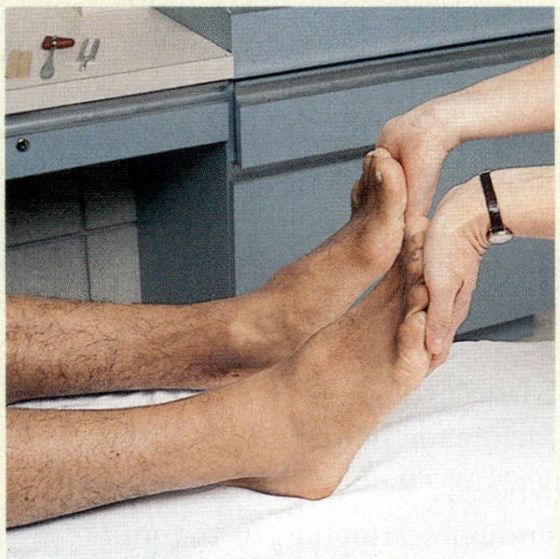

FIGURE I. *Source:* Used with permission from Shutterstock. *Photo by Ken Kasper.*

- Then, the patient attempts to pull against examiner's resistance (Figure J).

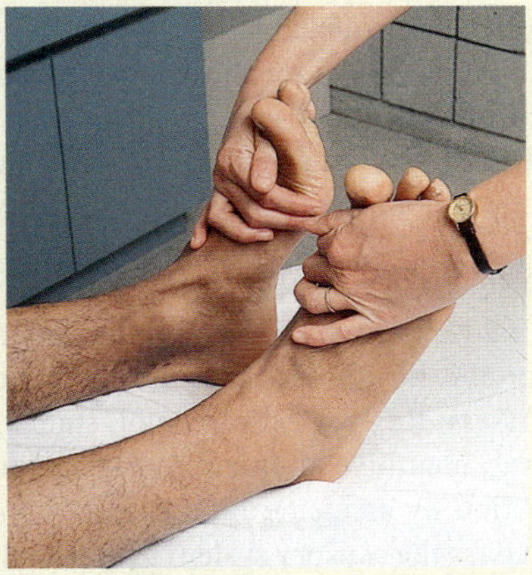

FIGURE J. *Source:* Used with permission from Shutterstock. *Photo by Ken Kasper.*

NORMAL AGE-RELATED VARIATIONS: INFANT/CHILD

Common musculoskeletal variations in newborns and children include:

- C-shaped curve of spine at birth; the anterior cervical curve develops at about ages 3 to 4 months, and the anterior lumbar curve develops between ages 12 and 18 months
- Lordosis (an exaggerated lumbar curve)
- Pronation of the feet in children between ages 12 and 30 months
- Genu varum (bowleg) for 1 year after learning to walk

NORMAL AGE-RELATED VARIATIONS: OLDER ADULT

Common musculoskeletal variations seen in older adults include:

- Loss of muscle mass and strength
- Decreased ROM
- Kyphosis
- Decreased height
- Osteoarthritic changes in joints

Assessing the Neurologic System

Neurologic assessment includes cerebral function, cranial nerve function, cerebellar function, motor and sensory function, and reflexes. The health history is useful in obtaining information about ADLs and other pertinent data, such as dizziness, loss of sensation, headaches, and ability to see, hear, taste, and detect sensations. Physical examination is conducted to identify mental status and level of consciousness, cranial nerve function, muscle strength and coordination, and reflexes. Normally, the patient is alert and responsive, has full sensory function, and all muscle groups are bilaterally strong. Abnormal findings are discussed with specific parts of the examination that follow. Many health care providers assess the neuromuscular, musculoskeletal, and peripheral vascular systems as an integrated assessment. Refer to Skill 27-2 (on pp. 824–830) for an example of a systematic, integrated assessment of these systems.

HEALTH HISTORY

Identify risk factors for altered health during the health history by asking about the following:

- History of numbness, tingling, or tremors
- History of seizures
- History of headaches or dizziness
- History of trauma to the head or spine
- History of high blood pressure or stroke
- Changes in the ability to hear, see, taste, or smell
- Loss of ability to control bladder and bowel
- History of smoking (how long, how many packs/day)
- History of chronic alcohol use
- History of diabetes mellitus or cardiovascular disease
- Use of prescription and over-the-counter medications

PHYSICAL ASSESSMENT

Evaluate cerebral function by observing the patient's behavior throughout the health history interview and physical assessment. Assess the patient's mental status, memory, emotional status, cognitive abilities, and behavior. Evaluate cerebellar function by assessing motor skills, coordination, and balance. Assess the sensory system by having the patient identify various sensory stimuli, and evaluate the reflexes by contraction of specific muscles.

Equipment for a neurologic assessment includes a visual acuity chart, a penlight, a sharp object (e.g., a large safety pin), cotton balls, a tongue depressor, and familiar objects, such as a key or coin. The patient should be sitting, if possible, and the environment should be quiet. Advanced practice professionals typically perform assessment of deep tendon reflexes to determine the functional ability of specific spinal segment levels. Refer to a health assessment text for details.

Assessing Mental Status

Mental status assessment includes level of consciousness, level of awareness, behavior and appearance, memory, and language. On initial contact, assess the patient's level of consciousness and begin to evaluate the patient's orientation to person, place, and time, as well as cognitive abilities and affect (whether the patient knows who they are, where they are, and the day or month or year). Observe the patient's appearance, general behavior, ability to speak clearly, and their ability to respond to questions.

Assess the patient's overall appearance. The patient should have a clean, neat appearance with erect posture; should be oriented to person, place, and time; should have memory recall (both short- and long-term memory); and should be able to demonstrate coherent and logical thought processes. Abnormal findings include poor hygiene, inappropriate dress, disorientation, absent memory recall, and incoherent or illogic thought processes. These abnormal findings may indicate a mental health disorder, developmental delay, brain disease, cerebrovascular disorder, alcohol or drug intoxication, or a tumor.

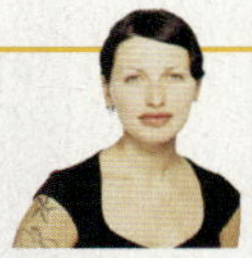

Think back to **Tammy Browning**, the pregnant woman with a history of substance abuse. The nurse would assess the patient's mental status for clues suggesting recent drug use, incorporating knowledge of abnormal findings into the assessment.

The following discussion of each of the mental status components includes sample questions or specific assessments to use during the assessment.

Assessing Level of Consciousness. Consciousness is the degree of wakefulness or the ability of a person to be aroused. This is not the same as orientation; a patient may be conscious but not oriented. Level of consciousness is described as follows:

- Awake and alert: fully awake; oriented to person, place, and time; responds to all stimuli, including verbal commands
- Lethargic: appears drowsy or asleep most of the time but makes spontaneous movements; can be aroused by gentle shaking and saying patient's name
- Stuporous: unconscious most of the time; has no spontaneous movement; must be shaken or shouted at to arouse; can make verbal responses, but these are less likely to be appropriate; responds to painful stimuli with purposeful movements
- Comatose: cannot be aroused, even with use of painful stimuli; may have some reflex activity (such as gag reflex); if no reflexes present, is in a deep coma

The Glasgow Coma Scale (GCS) (Table 27-4) is a standardized assessment tool that assesses level of consciousness. The GCS is used as a rapid evaluation of the status of acutely ill patients at risk of acute brain damage (Derbyshire & Hill, 2018). Some limitations to using the GCS include the inability to assess the verbal score after the patient has been intubated; a lack of assessment of respiration and brainstem reflexes; inability to assess a possible developing vegetative state; and inability to recognize pseudocoma.

The FOUR (Full Outline of UnResponsiveness) score coma scale (Table 27-5) is an assessment tool for adult

Table 27-4 Glasgow Coma Scale

The Glasgow Coma Scale (GCS) is a tool used to assess arousal and level of consciousness and coma (Morton & Fontaine, 2018). The GCS evaluates three key categories of behavior that most closely reflect activity in the higher centers of the brain: eye opening, verbalization, and movement (Morton & Fontaine, 2018; Waterhouse, 2005). Within each category each level of response is given a numerical value. The maximal score is 15 indicating a fully awake, alert, and oriented patient; an overall score of 8 or below is associated with coma (Hickey, 2020; Morton & Fontaine, 2018).

COMPONENT	SCORE	RESPONSE
Eye opening	4	Spontaneous eye opening
	3	Eyes open to speech
	2	Eyes open to pain
	1	No eye opening
Motor response	6	Obeys commands fully
	5	Localizes to noxious stimuli
	4	Withdraws from noxious stimuli
	3	Abnormal flexion (i.e., decorticate posturing; flexes elbows and wrists while extending lower legs to pain)
	2	Abnormal extensor response (i.e., decerebrate posturing; extends upper and lower extremities to pain)
	1	No motor response
Verbal response	5	Alert and oriented
	4	Confused yet coherent speech
	3	Inappropriate words and jumbled phrases consisting of words
	2	Incomprehensible sounds
	1	No verbal response

Source: Adapted from Hickey, J. V. (2020). *The clinical practice of neurological and neurosurgical nursing* (8th ed.). Wolters Kluwer; reprinted from *The Lancet*, Teasdale, G., & Jennett, B. Assessment of coma and impaired consciousness. A practical scale. *Lancet*, *2*(7872), 81–84, Copyright 1974, with permission from Elsevier.

Table 27-5 Full Outline of Un-Responsiveness (FOUR) Coma Scale

The FOUR coma scale combines the most important neurologic signs into an easy-to-use scale with four components. The maximum score in each of these components is 4. The components are not totaled or summed and can be used to detect decreasing consciousness, increasing intracranial pressure, and brain herniation, as well as predict patient outcome (Iyer et al., 2009; Mercy et al., 2013; Oh et al., 2019; Sadaka et al., 2012; Wijdicks et al., 2005; Zappa et al., 2020).

	0	1	2	3	4
Eye response	E0: Eyelids remain closed with pain	E1: Eyelids closed but open to pain	E2: Eyelids closed but open to loud voices	E3: Eyelids open but not tracking	E4: Eyelids open or opened, tracking or blinking to command
Motor response *Note: Ask patients to make a peace sign, a fist, and show thumbs up*	M0: No response to pain	M1: Extension response to pain	M2: Flexion response to pain	M3: Localizing to pain	M4: Thumbs up, fist, or peace sign
Brainstem reflexes	B0: Absent pupil, corneal, and cough reflex	B1: Pupil and corneal reflexes absent	B2: Pupil or corneal reflexes absent	B3: One pupil wide and fixed	B4: Pupil and corneal reflexes present
Respiration	R0: Breathes at ventilator rate or apnea	R1: Breathes above ventilatory rate	R2: Not intubated, irregular breathing	R3: Not intubated, Cheyne–Stokes breathing pattern	R4: Not intubated, regular breathing pattern

Source: Reprinted from Elsevier, Iyer, V. N., Mandrekar, J. N., Danielson, R. D., Zubkov, A. Y., Elmer, J. L., & Wijdicks, E. F. (2009). Validity of the FOUR score coma scale in the medical intensive care unit. *Mayo Clinic Proceedings*, *84*(8), 694–701, with permission from Elsevier; and Sadaka, F., Patel, D., & Lakshmanan, R. (2012). The FOUR score predicts outcome in patients after traumatic brain injury. *Neurocritical Care*, *16*(1), 95–101.

and pediatric patients with severe neurologic impairment (Hickey, 2020). It includes information not assessed by the GCS, including measurement of brainstem reflexes; determination of eye opening, blinking, and tracking; a broad spectrum of motor responses; and the presence of abnormal breath rhythms and a respiratory drive, providing a more comprehensive neurologic assessment (Jalali & Rezaei, 2014; Zappa et al., 2020). The FOUR score tool does not include an assessment of verbal response and may be more useful for assessing critically ill patients with depressed level of consciousness (Almojuela et al., 2019). Because the FOUR score, unlike the GCS, does not include an assessment of verbal response, it is more useful for assessing critically ill patients who have undergone intubation (Iyer et al., 2009; Sadaka et al., 2012).

Assessing Level of Awareness. Assess awareness by evaluating orientation to time, place, and person. The following questions may be used:

- *Time:* What is today's date? What day of the week is it? What season of the year is this? What was the last holiday?
- *Place:* Where are you now? What is the name of this city? What state are we in?
- *Person:* What is your name? How old are you? Who came to visit you this morning?

Although exceptions may occur, people who have impaired awareness first lose time orientation, followed by place orientation, and then person orientation. Remember that it is often difficult to know the exact date when one is ill, in pain, or in unfamiliar surroundings.

Assessing Memory. Assess memory by asking questions that require answers demonstrating immediate recall and recall for past events. To assess immediate memory, ask the patient to repeat a series of numbers forward or backward (e.g., 3, 6, 9). Start with three numbers and gradually increase the digits until the patient cannot respond correctly. Most adults can repeat a series of five to eight numbers forward and four to six digits backward. You might also ask, "What did you eat for breakfast this morning?" To assess past memory, ask, "When is your birthday?" or "When is your wedding anniversary?"

Assessing Language

The cerebral cortex controls the ability to express self through writing, words, or gestures and to understand the spoken and written word. Some simple methods of assessing language capabilities include asking the patient to name items in the room (e.g., bed, flowers, gown, pajamas), to follow simple commands (such as "Point to your head"), to read a short sentence aloud, or to match printed and spoken words with appropriate pictures. Injury to the cortex can cause aphasia, which is a disorder of language ability. Aphasia may be expressive (the person understands written and spoken words but cannot write or speak to communicate effectively) or receptive (the person cannot understand written or spoken words). These aphasias may also be combined.

Assessing Cranial Nerve Function

The function of the 12 cranial nerves is assessed primarily during the neurologic assessment, although parts of cranial nerve function are assessed with other body systems (e.g., capillary response during assessment of the face). Each nerve has a specific function and is evaluated individually. Table 27-6 outlines the cranial nerves, with their function and assessment methods.

Assessing Motor and Sensory Function

Motor ability is evaluated by assessing balance, gait, and coordination. Sensory function is assessed by testing sensory discrimination of pain, light touch, and vibrations.

Inspecting Balance and Gait. Evaluate balance and gait by having the patient walk across the room on the toes, on the heels, and heel to toe. Observe posture, balance, and arm and leg movements. The posture should be erect, with slight swaying in the standing position. Walking (gait) should be smooth and rhythmic, with arms swinging at the sides.

Assessing Motor Function and Coordination. Evaluate motor function and coordination by having the patient rapidly touch each finger with the thumb, rapidly pat the hand on the thigh, and tap the foot on the floor (or against your hand, if the patient is supine). Repeat the sequence on the opposite limb. Normally, the movements are coordinated. If the patient is unable to perform these movements, it may indicate disease of the upper motor neurons or cerebellum.

Assessing Sensory Perception. Test sensory perception by evaluating the patient's response to pain, light touch, and normal shapes. With the patient's eyes closed, randomly touch the skin on the upper and lower extremities and the trunk with a sharp object and a soft object. The assessment proceeds from distal (hands, arms, feet, or legs) to proximal (the trunk). The patient should be able to distinguish between sharp (painful) and soft or dull touch. Sensory perception may also be assessed by asking the patient to close the eyes and identify familiar objects (such as a coin or key) by touching them. Abnormal findings include inability to perceive pain or light touch, inability to identify the location of touch, and inability to identify familiar objects.

Neurovascular Assessment. Assessment of neurovascular status is an important nursing intervention leading to early identification of neurovascular impairment and timely intervention (Agency for Clinical Innovation, 2018; Johnston-Walker & Hardcastle, 2011; Turney et al., 2013). Refer to the discussion of neurovascular assessment earlier in the chapter. See Box 27-8 (on page 805) for an outline of the components of a neurovascular assessment.

Table 27-6 Summary of Cranial Nerves

NERVE (NUMBER)	TYPE	FUNCTIONS	METHODS FOR EXAMINING NERVE
Olfactory (I)	Sensory	Sense of smell	Test each nostril for smell reception with various agents and interpretation
Optic (II)	Sensory	Sense of vision	Test vision for acuity and visual fields
Oculomotor (III)	Motor	Pupil constriction	
	Raise eyelids	Test pupillary reaction to light and ability to open and close eyelids	
Trochlear (IV)	Motor/ proprioceptor	Downward, inward eye movement	Test for downward and inward movement of the eye
Trigeminal (V)	Motor	Jaw movements—chewing and mastication	Ask patient to open and clench jaws while you palpate the jaw muscles
	Sensory	Sensation on the face and neck	Test face and neck for pain sensations, light touch, and temperature
Abducens (VI)	Motor	Lateral movement of the eyes	Test ocular movement in all directions
Facial (VII)	Motor	Muscles of the face	Ask the patient to raise eyebrows, smile, show teeth, and puff out cheeks
	Sensory	Sense of taste on the anterior two thirds of the tongue	Test for the taste sensation with various agents
Acoustic (VIII)	Sensory	Sense of hearing	Test hearing ability
Glossopharyngeal (IV) and vagus (X)	Motor/sensory	Palate, pharynx, vocal cords, gag reflex, swallowing	Ask the patient to open mouth and say "ah," and/or yawn; observe upward movement of the soft palate and uvula; note ability to swallow; elicit gag response in an unconscious patient
			Ask the patient to speak; note that the voice sounds smooth and not strained or hoarse
Accessory (XI)	Motor/sensory	Movement of shoulder muscles	Ask the patient to shrug shoulders against your resistance
Hypoglossal (XII)	Motor	Movement of the tongue; strength of the tongue	Ask the patient to protrude tongue; ask patient to push tongue against cheek

Sources: Delgado, S.A. (2024). *AACN essentials of critical care nursing* (5th ed.). McGraw Hill; Hickey, J.V., & Strayer, A.L. (2020). *The clinical practice of neurological and neurosurgical nursing* (8th ed.). Wolters Kluwer; Hogan-Quigley, B., & Palm, M. L. (2022). *Bates' nursing guide to physical examination and history taking* (3rd ed.). Wolters Kluwer; Jarvis, C., & Eckhardt, A. (2024). *Physical examination & health assessment* (9th ed.). Elsevier.

NORMAL AGE-RELATED VARIATIONS: INFANT/CHILD

Common neurologic variations for newborns and children include:

- Positive Babinski sign (normal in children less than 24 months) (Jensen, 2019)
- Grasp reflex (present at birth)
- Motor control develops in head, neck, trunk, and extremities sequence

NORMAL AGE-RELATED VARIATIONS: OLDER ADULT

Common neurologic variations for older adults include:

- Slower thought processes and verbal responses
- Decreased sensory ability (hearing, sight, smell, taste, temperature, pain)
- Slower coordination and voluntary movements
- Decreased reflex responses
- Appearance of confusion in unfamiliar surroundings
- Slower gait, with a wider base and flexed hips and knees

DOCUMENTATION OF DATA

After completing the health history and physical assessment, organize all health assessment data to identify actual and potential health problems, identify diagnoses or patient problems, plan appropriate care, and evaluate the patient's responses to interventions. Document the data, with each system recorded individually. Box 27-10 (on page 820) illustrates an example of a health history and physical assessment documentation.

A pattern is often established that begins during the history and is confirmed during the physical assessment. For example, a health history of a woman diagnosed with multiple sclerosis (a neurologic disorder) might include data about fatigue and increased weakness and muscle spasms in the legs. Physical examination findings would include decreased muscle strength in the lower extremities. These data may be used to support the identification of a health problem of Activity Intolerance.

Box 27-10 Documenting a Health Assessment

Mrs. D. comes to a local community outpatient facility for intolerance of eating fatty foods. She says, "I just started having a lot of gas and was sick to my stomach after eating fried foods." The nurse makes the following assessments.

Health History

Mrs. D. is a 52-year-old woman who lives with her 54-year-old husband on a farm in a rural midwestern area. She graduated from high school and is employed as a secretary for a local

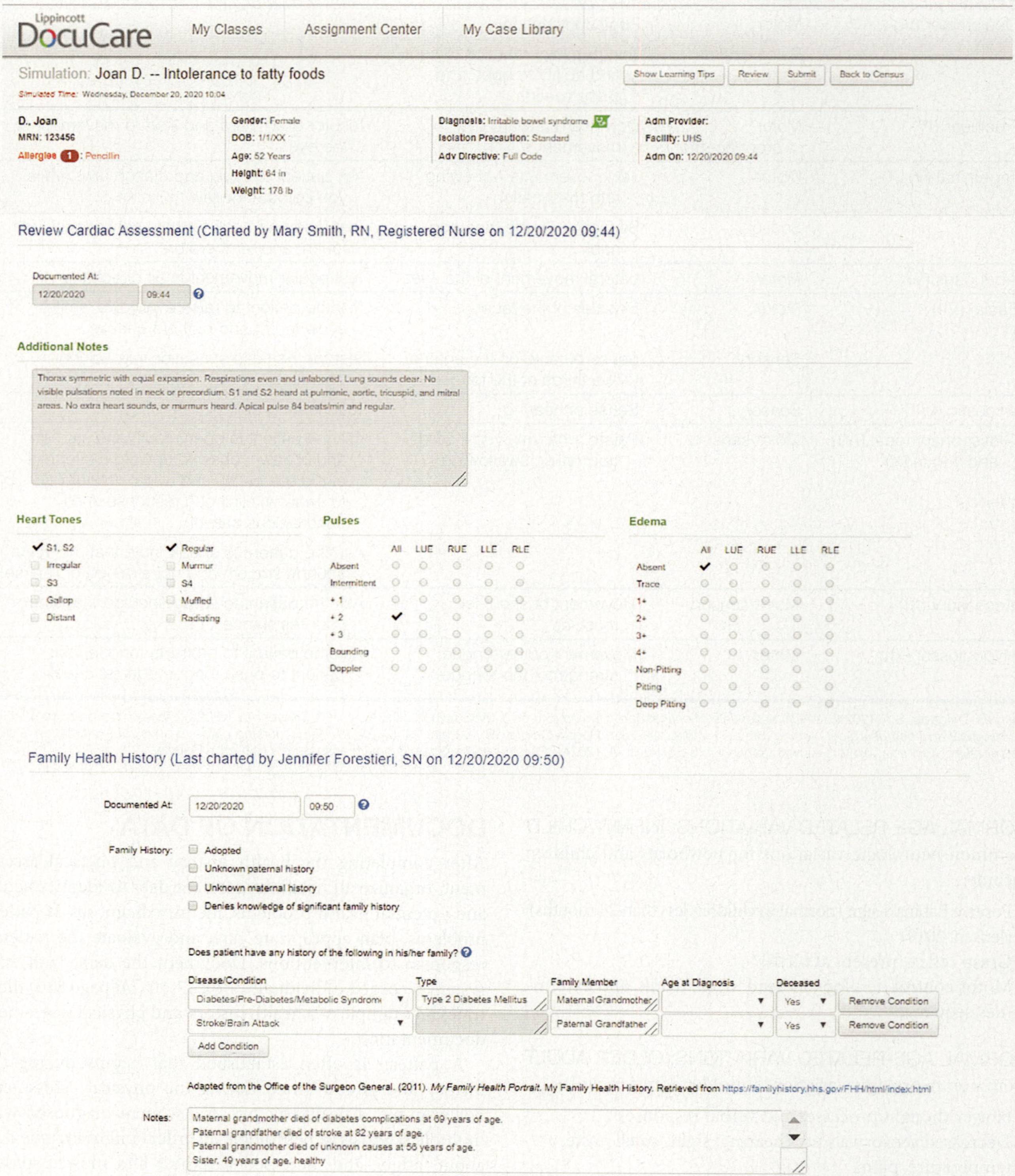

Lippincott DocuCare | My Classes | Assignment Center | My Case Library

Simulation: Joan D. -- Intolerance to fatty foods

Show Learning Tips | Review | Submit | Back to Census

Simulated Time: Wednesday, December 20, 2020 10:04

D., Joan
MRN: 123456
Allergies (1): Penicillin

Gender: Female
DOB: 1/1/XX
Age: 52 Years
Height: 64 in
Weight: 178 lb

Diagnosis: Irritable bowel syndrome
Isolation Precaution: Standard
Adv Directive: Full Code

Adm Provider:
Facility: UHS
Adm On: 12/20/2020 09:44

Review Cardiac Assessment (Charted by Mary Smith, RN, Registered Nurse on 12/20/2020 09:44)

Documented At: 12/20/2020 09:44

Additional Notes

Thorax symmetric with equal expansion. Respirations even and unlabored. Lung sounds clear. No visible pulsations noted in neck or precordium. S1 and S2 heard at pulmonic, aortic, tricuspid, and mitral areas. No extra heart sounds, or murmurs heard. Apical pulse 84 beats/min and regular.

Heart Tones

✔ S1, S2	✔ Regular
☐ Irregular	☐ Murmur
☐ S3	☐ S4
☐ Gallop	☐ Muffled
☐ Distant	☐ Radiating

Pulses

	All	LUE	RUE	LLE	RLE
Absent	○	○	○	○	○
Intermittent	○	○	○	○	○
+1	○	○	○	○	○
+2	✔	○	○	○	○
+3	○	○	○	○	○
Bounding	○	○	○	○	○
Doppler	○	○	○	○	○

Edema

	All	LUE	RUE	LLE	RLE
Absent	✔	○	○	○	○
Trace	○	○	○	○	○
1+	○	○	○	○	○
2+	○	○	○	○	○
3+	○	○	○	○	○
4+	○	○	○	○	○
Non-Pitting	○	○	○	○	○
Pitting	○	○	○	○	○
Deep Pitting	○	○	○	○	○

Family Health History (Last charted by Jennifer Forestieri, SN on 12/20/2020 09:50)

Documented At: 12/20/2020 09:50

Family History:
☐ Adopted
☐ Unknown paternal history
☐ Unknown maternal history
☐ Denies knowledge of significant family history

Does patient have any history of the following in his/her family?

Disease/Condition	Type	Family Member	Age at Diagnosis	Deceased	
Diabetes/Pre-Diabetes/Metabolic Syndrome	Type 2 Diabetes Mellitus	Maternal Grandmother		Yes	Remove Condition
Stroke/Brain Attack		Paternal Grandfather		Yes	Remove Condition

Add Condition

Adapted from the Office of the Surgeon General. (2011). *My Family Health Portrait.* My Family Health History. Retrieved from https://familyhistory.hhs.gov/FHH/html/index.html

Notes:
Maternal grandmother died of diabetes complications at 69 years of age.
Paternal grandfather died of stroke at 82 years of age.
Paternal grandmother died of unknown causes at 56 years of age.
Sister, 49 years of age, healthy

Box 27-10 Documenting a Health Assessment *(continued)*

insurance facility. Mrs. D. is well groomed, alert, and oriented. She occasionally takes over-the-counter medications for constipation and colds. She takes a prescription medication twice a day for "high blood pressure." She says she has about two mixed drinks a week and does not smoke. She has had five pregnancies, resulting in five living children.

Mrs. D. had her tonsils removed at age 5 years, had an appendectomy at age 22 years, and is allergic to penicillin (causes rash and difficulty breathing). She has had all her immunizations, but her last tetanus shot was 10 years ago. Her family history of illness is as follows:

Maternal grandfather died of heart problems at age 77 years.
Maternal grandmother died of diabetes complications at age 69 years.
Paternal grandfather died of stroke at age 82 years.
Paternal grandmother died of unknown causes at age 56 years.
Sister, age 49 years, healthy.
Brother died at age 22 years in a car accident.

Physical Assessment

Vital signs: T = 98.8°F (orally), P = 82 beats/min, R = 16 breaths/min, BP = 150/88 mm Hg

Height/weight: 5 ft, 4-inch tall, 178 lb

Integument: Skin warm and dry, normal turgor. Numerous freckles over face and arms. Old scar, RLQ (appendectomy). Nails convex and smooth. Hair dark brown, shiny, normal distribution.

Head and neck: Skull size and shape normal. Facial features symmetric. Can raise eyebrows, close eyes, smile, and puff out cheeks. External eye structures symmetric. Sclera white, conjunctiva pink. Wears glasses to correct near-sightedness. Vision with glasses 20/30-2 on Snellen chart. Pupils equal, round, and react to light bilaterally. Demonstrates accommodation, convergence, and peripheral vision. External ears symmetric. Canals smooth and pink without excess cerumen. Right nostril clear, left nostril occluded with mucus. Left maxillary sinus slightly tender on palpation. Teeth in good repair with six fillings. Oral mucous membranes pink. Tonsils absent. Trachea midline. No lymph nodes palpable.

Thorax/lungs/heart: Thorax symmetric with equal expansion. Respirations even and unlabored. Lung sounds clear. No visible pulsations noted in neck or precordium. S_1 and S_2 heard at pulmonic, aortic, tricuspid, and mitral areas. No extra heart sounds, or murmurs heard. Apical pulse 84 beats/min and regular.

Breasts and axilla: Skin pink. No dimpling or retraction noted. Areolae and nipples dark brown, no crusting or drainage. No masses palpated in breasts. Axillary lymph nodes are not palpable. To have mammogram at next visit.

Abdomen: Obese, rounded. Umbilicus midline. No pain on light palpation. Bowel sounds heard in all four quadrants. No bruits heard on auscultation.

Peripheral vascular: Pulses equal in both arms. Pulses equal in both legs. No edema present. Superficial varicose veins present on both lower extremities between ankle and knee. Toenails thick and yellow.

Genitalia: Will be assessed at next visit with pelvic and Papanicolaou smear.

Rectum and anus: Inspected only. Small external hemorrhoids noted.

Musculoskeletal: Stands erect. Normal spinal curves. No joint deformities, tenderness, or crepitation. Full active ROM in all joints. Muscle strength equal bilaterally, slightly stronger on the right (dominant side).

Neurologic: Alert and oriented to time, place, and person. Facial expressions appropriate. Speech clear and appropriate. Demonstrates long- and short-term memory. All cranial nerves tests were intact. Gait even.

REFLECTIVE PRACTICE LEADING TO PERSONAL LEARNING

Remember that the goal of reflective practice is to look at an experience, understand it, and learn from it. As you begin to develop expertise in performing health assessments, reflect on your experiences—successes and failures—in order to improve your practice. How can you do it better next time? What did you learn today that can help you tomorrow? Begin your reflection by paying close attention to the following while performing health assessment and providing nursing care:

- Did your preparation and practice related to performing health assessment result in your feeling confident in your ability to gather reliable, accurate data? Did your competence and confidence inspire the patient's, family's, and caregiver's trust?
- How did you prioritize the data you collected? What patterns in the data did you identify? What knowledge from your learning, personal experience, and intuition did you use to make decisions and develop your plan of care?
- How confident are you that the data you reported and recorded accurately communicates the health status, health problems, issues, risks, and strengths of the patient? How successfully have you communicated this information to other members of the health care team? How successfully have you communicated who this patient/family is to the interdisciplinary team?
- Were you aware of any cultural and/or ethnic beliefs or practices that may have influenced the health assessment? Were you aware of any stereotypes or prejudices that might have negatively influenced the clinical encounter? If so, how did you address these?
- Was the patient/family/caregiver participation in the process at an optimal level? How might you have better engaged the patient, family, and caregivers? As you concluded your assessment, did the patient/family/caregivers know your name, and know what to expect of you and your nursing care? Did the patient sense that you are respectful, caring, and competent to obtain accurate and relevant data?

Perhaps the most important questions to reflect on are: Are your patients and their families/caregivers better for having had *you* share in the critical responsibility of assessing their health status? Are your patients now receiving thoughtful, person-centered, prioritized, holistic, evidence-based treatment and care because of your efforts?

Skill 27-1 Using a Portable Bed Scale

DELEGATION CONSIDERATIONS

Measurement of body weight may be delegated to assistive personnel (AP) as well as to licensed practical/vocational nurses (LPN/LVNs). The decision to delegate must be based on careful analysis of the patient's needs and circumstances as well as the qualifications of the person to whom the task is being delegated. Refer to the Delegation Guidelines in Appendix A.

EQUIPMENT

- Bed scale with sling
- Cover for sling
- Sheet or bath blanket
- PPE, as indicated

IMPLEMENTATION

ACTION	RATIONALE
1. Check the prescribed interventions or plan of care for frequency of weight measurement. More frequent measurement of the patient's weight may be appropriate based on nursing judgment. Obtain the assistance of a second caregiver, based on the patient's mobility and ability to cooperate with the procedure.	This provides for patient safety and appropriate care.
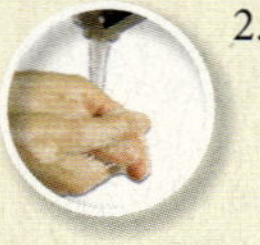 2. Perform hand hygiene and put on PPE, if indicated.	Hand hygiene and PPE prevent the spread of microorganisms. PPE is required based on transmission precautions.
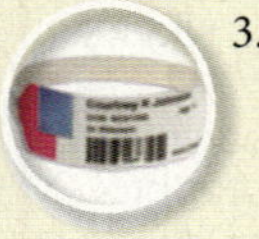 3. Identify the patient.	Identifying the patient ensures that the right patient receives the intervention and helps prevent errors.
4. Close the curtains around the bed and close the door to the room if possible. Discuss the procedure with the patient and assess the patient's ability to assist with the procedure.	This ensures the patient's privacy. Explanation relieves anxiety and facilitates cooperation.
5. Place a cover over the sling of the bed scale.	Using a cover deters the spread of microorganisms.
6. Attach the sling to the bed scale. Lay the sheet or bath blanket in the sling. Turn on the scale. **Balance the scale so that weight reads 0.0.**	Scale will add the sling, blanket, and cover into the weight unless it is zeroed with the sling, blanket, and cover.
7. Adjust the bed to a comfortable working position (VHA-CEOSH, 2016). Position one caregiver on each side of the bed, if two caregivers are present. Raise side rail on the opposite side of the bed from where the scale is located, if not already in place. Cover the patient with the sheet or bath blanket. Remove other covers and any pillows.	Having the bed at the proper height prevents back and muscle strain. Having one caregiver on each side of the bed provides for patient safety and appropriate care. Side rail assists patient with movement. Blanket maintains patient's dignity and provides warmth.
8. Turn the patient onto their side facing the side rail, keeping their body covered with the sheet or blanket. Remove the sling from the scale. Place the cover on the sling. Roll cover and sling lengthwise. Place rolled sling under the patient, making sure the patient is centered in the sling.	Rolling the patient onto their side facilitates placing the patient onto the sling. Blanket maintains patient's dignity and provides warmth.
9. Roll the patient back over the sling and onto the other side. Pull the sling through, as if placing sheet under patient, unrolling the sling as it is pulled through.	This facilitates placing the patient onto the sling.
10. Roll the scale over the bed so that the arms of the scale are directly over the patient. **Spread the base of the scale.** Lower the arms of the scale and place the arm hooks into the holes on the sling.	By spreading the base, you are giving the scale a wider base, thus preventing the scale from toppling over with the patient. Hooking sling to scale provides secure attachment to the scale and prevents injury.

ACTION | **RATIONALE**

11. Once the scale arms are hooked onto the sling, gradually elevate the sling so that the patient is lifted up off the bed (Figure 1). **Assess all tubes and drains, making sure that none have tension placed on them as the scale is lifted. Once the sling is no longer touching the bed, ensure that nothing else is hanging onto the sling (e.g., ventilator or IV tubing). If any tubing is connected to the patient, raise it up so that it is not adding any weight to the patient.**

The scale must be hanging free to obtain an accurate weight. Any tubing that is hanging off the scale will add weight to the patient.

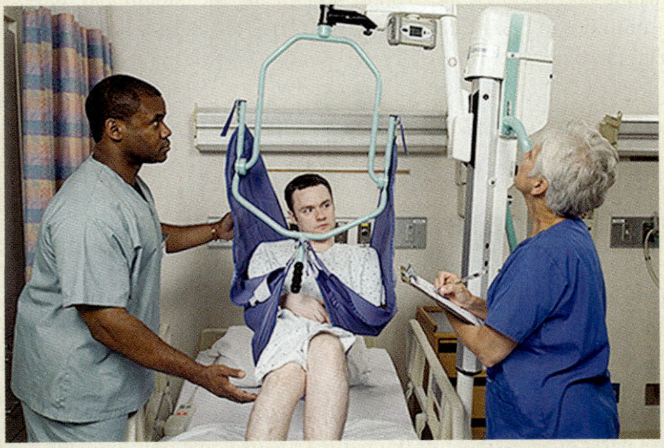

FIGURE 1. Using a bed scale.

12. Note the weight reading on the scale. Slowly and gently, lower the patient back onto the bed. Disconnect the scale arms from the sling. Close the base of the scale and pull it away from the bed.

Lowering the patient slowly does not alarm the patient. Closing the base of the scale facilitates moving the scale.

13. Raise the side rail. Turn the patient to the side rail. Roll the sling up against the patient's backside.

Raising the side rail is a safety measure.

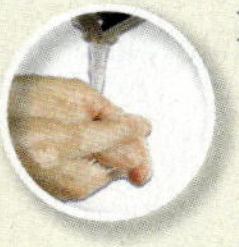

14. Raise the other side rail. Roll the patient back over the sling and up facing the other side rail. Remove the sling from the bed. Remove gloves, if used. Raise the remaining side rail. Perform hand hygiene.

The patient needs to be removed from the sling before it can be removed from the bed. Hand hygiene deters the spread of microorganisms.

15. Cover the patient and help them to a position of comfort. Place the bed in the lowest position.

Ensures patient comfort and safety.

16. Remove the disposable cover from the sling and discard in the appropriate receptacle.

Using a cover deters the spread of microorganisms.

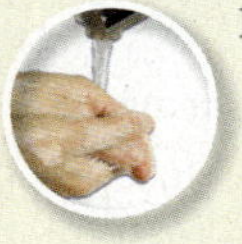

17. Remove additional PPE, if used. Clean equipment based on facility policy. Perform hand hygiene.

Proper removal of PPE reduces the risk for infection transmission and contamination of other items. Cleaning equipment prevents transmission of microorganisms. Hand hygiene deters the spread of microorganisms.

18. Replace the scale and sling in the appropriate spot. Plug the scale into the electrical outlet.

Scale should be ready for use at any time.

DOCUMENTATION

GUIDELINES

Document weight, unit of measurement, and scale used.

SAMPLE DOCUMENTATION

10/15/25 0230 Patient reports pain in legs 5/10. Premedicated with oxycodone 5 mg and acetaminophen 325 mg 2 tabs PO before obtaining weight per order. Patient weighed using bed scale, 75.2 kg.

—M. Evans, RN

(*continued on page 824*)

Skill 27-1 Using a Portable Bed Scale *(continued)*

DEVELOPING CLINICAL REASONING AND CLINICAL JUDGMENT

UNEXPECTED SITUATIONS AND ASSOCIATED INTERVENTIONS

- *As the patient is being lifted, the scale begins to tip over:* Stop lifting the patient. Slowly lower the patient back to the bed. Ensure that the base of the scale is spread wide enough before attempting to weigh the patient.
- *Weight differs from the previous day's weight by more than 1 kg:* Weigh the patient using the same scale at the same time each day. Check scale calibration. Make sure that the patient is wearing the same clothing. Make sure that no tubes or containers are hanging on the scale. If the patient is incontinent, make sure undergarments are clean and dry.
- *Patient becomes agitated as the sling is raised into the air:* Stop lifting the patient and reassure them. If the patient continues to be agitated, lower them back to the bed. Reevaluate necessity of obtaining weight at that exact time.

Skill 27-2 Assessing the Neurologic, Musculoskeletal, and Peripheral Vascular Systems

DELEGATION CONSIDERATIONS

The assessment of the patient's neurologic, musculoskeletal, and peripheral vascular systems should not be delegated to assistive personnel (AP). Some items may be noticed while providing care and noted by the AP. The nurse must then validate, analyze, document, communicate, and act on these findings, as appropriate. Depending on the state's nurse practice act and the organization's policies and procedures, the licensed practical/vocational nurses (LPN/LVNs) may perform some or all the parts of assessment of the patient's neurologic, musculoskeletal, and peripheral vascular systems. The decision to delegate must be based on careful analysis of the patient's needs and circumstances as well as the qualifications of the person to whom the task is being delegated. Refer to the Delegation Guidelines in Appendix A.

EQUIPMENT

- PPE, as indicated
- Bath blanket or other drape
- Tongue depressor
- Examination gown
- Gloves
- Containers of odorous materials (e.g., coffee or chocolate), as indicated
- Miscellaneous items (e.g., pin, cotton, paper clip)
- Cotton-tipped applicators

IMPLEMENTATION

ACTION	RATIONALE
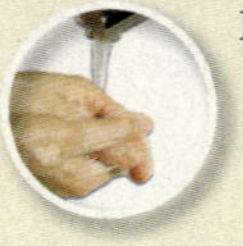 1. Perform hand hygiene and put on PPE, if indicated.	Hand hygiene and PPE prevent the spread of microorganisms. PPE is required based on transmission precautions.
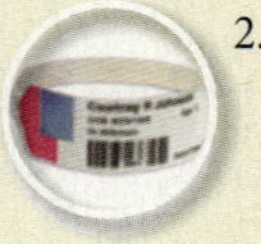 2. Identify the patient.	Identifying the patient ensures the right patient receives the intervention and helps prevent errors.
3. Close the curtains around the bed and close the door to the room, if possible. Explain the purpose of the neurologic, musculoskeletal, and peripheral vascular examinations and what you are going to do. Answer any questions.	This ensures the patient's privacy. Explanation relieves anxiety and facilitates cooperation.

ACTION	RATIONALE
4. Help the patient undress, if needed, and provide a patient gown. Assist the patient to a supine position, if possible. Use the bath blanket to cover any exposed area other than the one being assessed.	Having the patient wear a gown facilitates examination of the neurologic, musculoskeletal, and peripheral vascular systems. Use of a bath blanket provides for comfort and warmth.
5. Begin with a survey of the patient's overall hygiene and physical appearance.	This provides initial impressions of the patient. Hygiene and appearance can provide clues about the patient's mental state and comfort level.
6. Assess the patient's mental status.	
a. Evaluate level of consciousness.	This helps identify the patient's level of awareness.
b. Evaluate the patient's orientation to person, place, and time.	The patient should be awake and alert. Patients with altered level of consciousness may be lethargic, stuporous, or comatose.
c. Assess memory (immediate recall and past memory).	Memory problems may indicate neurologic impairment.
d. Evaluate the patient's ability to understand spoken and written word.	Evaluation of the patient's ability to understand spoken and written word helps assess for aphasia.
7. Test cranial nerve (CN) function, as indicated.	It is not necessary to assess every cranial nerve for every patient. Assessment should be individualized based on the patient's needs and health care setting and circumstances (Jensen, 2019).
a. Ask the patient to close the eyes, occlude one nostril, and then identify the smell of different substances, such as coffee, chocolate, or alcohol. Repeat with the other nostril.	This action tests the function of CN I (olfactory nerve).
b. Test visual acuity and pupillary constriction. Refer to previous discussion in the assessment of the head and neck.	This tests function of CN II and CN III (optic and oculomotor nerves).
c. Move the patient's eyes through the six cardinal positions of gaze. Refer to previous discussion in the assessment of the head and neck.	This testing evaluates the function of tests CN III, CN IV, and CN VI (oculomotor, trochlear, and abducens nerves).
d. Ask the patient to smile, frown, wrinkle the forehead, and puff out cheeks (Figure 1).	This maneuver evaluates the motor function of CN VII (facial nerve).

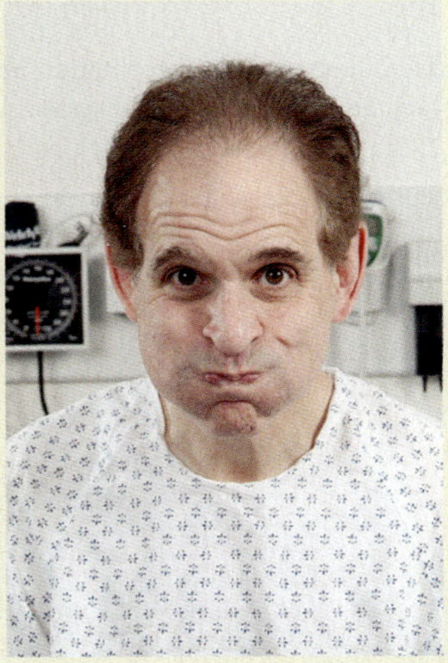

FIGURE 1. Puffing out cheeks.

ACTION	RATIONALE
e. Ask the patient to protrude tongue and push against the cheek with the tongue.	This evaluates function of CN XII (hypoglossal nerve).
f. Palpate the jaw muscles. Ask the patient to open and clench jaws. Stroke the patient's face with a cotton ball.	This evaluates function of CN V (trigeminal nerve).
g. Test hearing with the whispered voice test. Refer to previous discussion in the assessment of the head and neck.	This evaluates function of CN VIII (acoustic nerve).

(*continued on page 826*)

Skill 27-2 Assessing the Neurologic, Musculoskeletal, and Peripheral Vascular Systems *(continued)*

ACTION	RATIONALE
h. Put on gloves. Ask patient to open mouth. While observing soft palate, ask patient to say "ah"; observe upward movement of the soft palate. Test the gag reflex by touching the posterior pharynx with the tongue depressor. Explain to patient that this may be uncomfortable. Ask the patient to swallow. Remove gloves.	Gloves prevent contact with blood and body fluids. An intact gag reflex and swallowing indicate normal functioning of CNs IX and X (glossopharyngeal and vagus nerves).
i. Place your hands on the patient's shoulders (Figure 2) while they shrug against resistance. Then place your hand on the patient's left cheek, then the right cheek, and have the patient push against it.	These actions check CN XI (spinal accessory nerve) function and trapezius and sternocleidomastoid muscle strength.
8. Check the patient's ability to move their neck. Ask the patient to touch their chin to the chest and to each shoulder, then move each ear to the corresponding shoulder (Figure 3), and then tip the head back as far as possible.	These actions assess neck ROM, which is normally smooth and controlled.

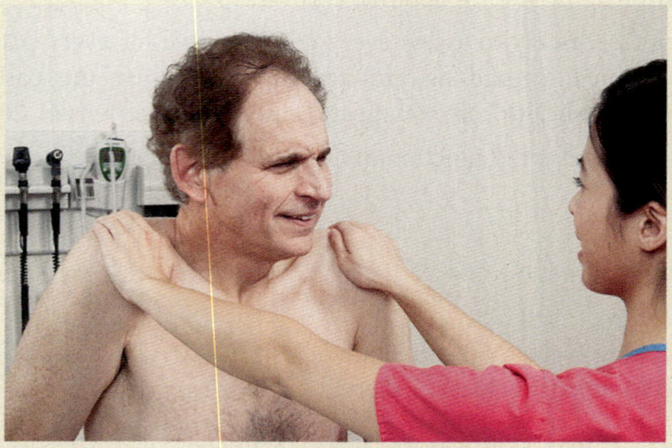

FIGURE 2. Assessing function of the spinal accessory nerve (CN XI) and muscular strength. (*Source:* From Weber, J. R., & Kelley, J. H. (2018). *Health assessment in nursing* [6th ed., p. 585]. Wolters Kluwer.)

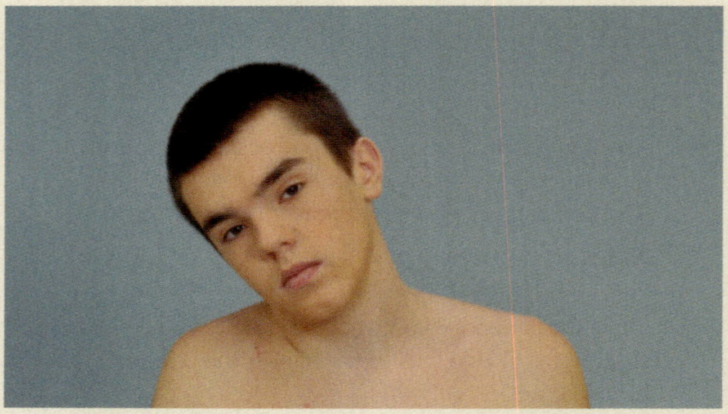

FIGURE 3. Moving each ear to the corresponding shoulder. (*Source:* From Jensen, S. [2019]. *Nursing health assessment* [3rd ed., p. 601]. Wolters Kluwer.)

ACTION	RATIONALE
9. Inspect the upper extremities. Observe for skin color, presence of lesions, rashes, and muscle mass. Palpate for skin temperature, texture, and presence of masses.	Examination of the upper extremities provides information about the circulatory, integumentary, and musculoskeletal systems.
10. Ask the patient to extend arms forward and then rapidly turn palms up and down.	This maneuver tests proprioception and cerebellar function.
11. Ask the patient to flex upper arm and to resist examiner's opposing force (Figure 4).	This technique assesses the muscle strength of the upper extremities.

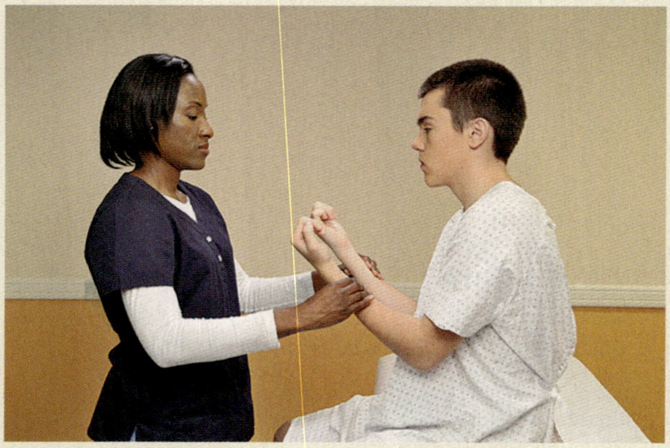

FIGURE 4. Assessing muscle strength of the upper extremities. (*Source:* From Jensen, S. [2019]. *Nursing health assessment* [3rd ed., p. 604]. Wolters Kluwer.)

ACTION | **RATIONALE**

12. Inspect and palpate the hands, fingers, wrists (Figure 5), and elbow joints.

Inspection and palpation provide information about abnormalities, tenderness, and ROM.

13. Ask the patient to bend and straighten the elbow, and flex and extend the wrists and hands.

This tests ROM of elbow joint and wrists.

14. Palpate the skin and the radial and brachial pulses. Assess the pulse rate, quality or amplitude, and rhythm. Test capillary refill.

Pulse palpation and capillary refill evaluate the peripheral vascular status of the upper extremities.

15. Cross your index and middle fingers. Have the patient squeeze your index and middle fingers (Figure 6).

This maneuver tests the muscle strength of the hands.

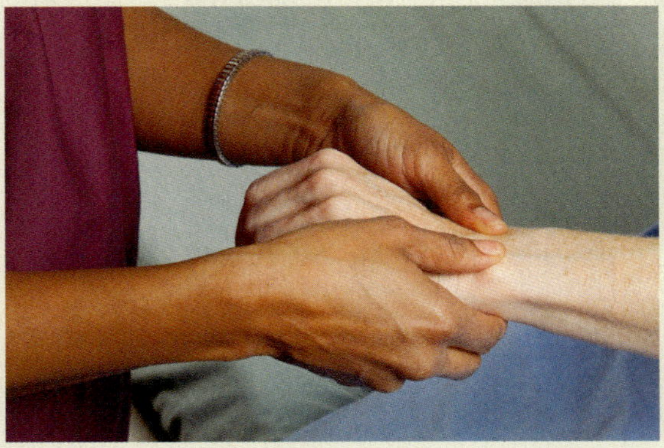

FIGURE 5. Palpating the wrist. (*Source:* Used with permission from Shutterstock. *Photo by B. Proud.*)

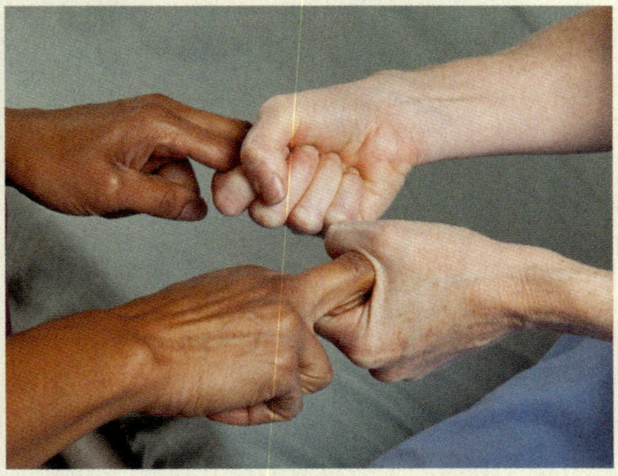

FIGURE 6. Testing grip. Patient squeezes nurse's crossed index and middle fingers. (*Source:* Used with permission from Shutterstock. *Photo by B. Proud.*)

16. Assist the patient to a supine position. Palpate (Figure 7A) and then use the bell of the stethoscope to auscultate the femoral pulses in the groin (Figure 7B), if not done during assessment of the abdomen. Note the strength of the pulse and grade it as with peripheral pulses.

This technique assesses flow of blood through the arteries. Auscultation can detect a bruit.

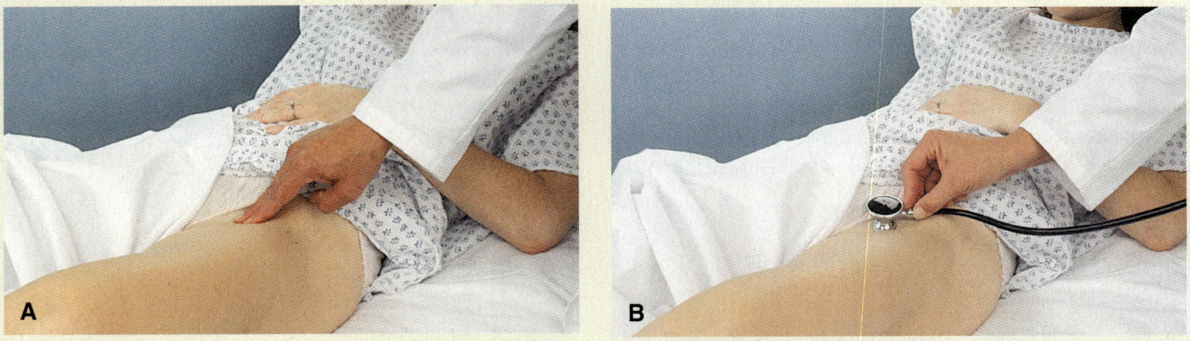

FIGURE 7. Palpating (**A**) and auscultating (**B**) the femoral pulses. (*Source:* Used with permission from Shutterstock. *Photos by B. Proud.*)

17. Examine the lower extremities. Inspect the legs and feet for color, lesions, varicosities, hair growth, nail growth, edema, and muscle mass.

Inspection provides information about peripheral vascular function.

(*continued on page 828*)

Skill 27-2 Assessing the Neurologic, Musculoskeletal, and Peripheral Vascular Systems *(continued)*

ACTION	RATIONALE
18. Assess for pitting edema in the lower extremities by pressing fingers into the skin at the pretibial area and dorsum of the foot (Figure 8A). If an indentation remains in the skin after the fingers have been lifted, pitting edema is present (Figure 8B).	This technique reveals information about excess interstitial fluid. Refer to an edema scale in assessing the amount of edema: 1+ about 2 mm deep to 4+ about 8 mm deep.

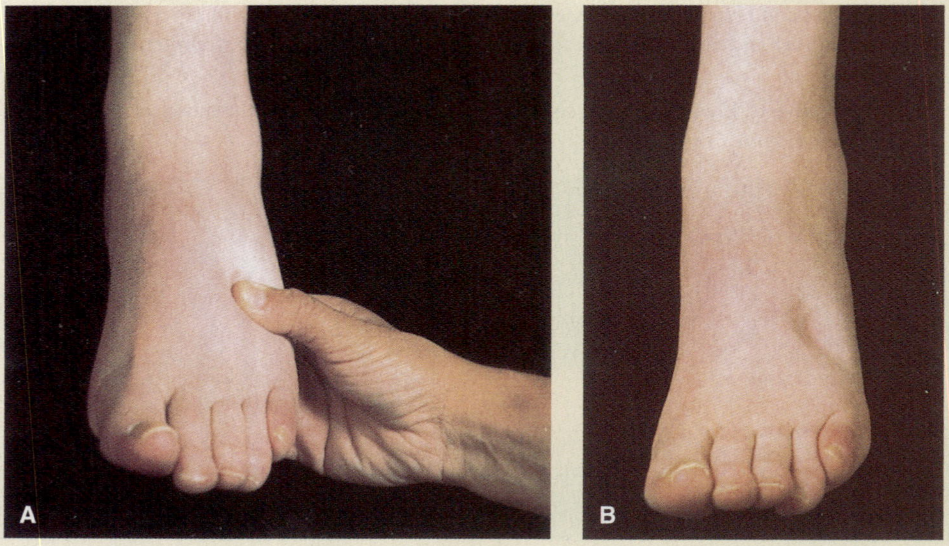

FIGURE 8. Assessing for pitting edema in lower extremities. (*Source:* From Hogan-Quigley, B., Palm, M. L., & Bickley, L. [2017]. *Bates' nursing guide to physical examination and history taking* [2nd ed., p. 453]. Wolters Kluwer.)

ACTION	RATIONALE
19. Palpate for pulses and skin temperature at the posterior tibial, dorsalis pedis, and popliteal areas. Assess the pulse rate, quality or amplitude, and rhythm. Test capillary refill.	Pulses, skin temperature, and capillary refill provide information about the patient's peripheral vascular status.
20. Ask the patient to move one leg laterally with the knee straight to test abduction of the hip. Keeping knee straight, move leg medially to test adduction of the hip. Repeat with other leg.	This maneuver assesses ROM and provides information about joint problems.
21. Ask the patient to raise the thigh against the resistance of your hand (Figure 9); next have the patient push outward against the resistance of your hand; then have the patient pull backward against the resistance of your hand. Repeat on the opposite side.	These measures assess motor strength of the upper and lower legs.

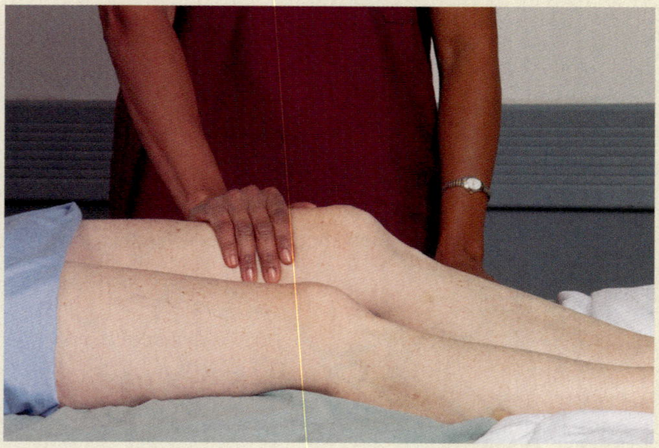

FIGURE 9. Testing motor strength of upper leg. Patient attempts to raise thigh against nurse's resistance. (*Source:* Used with permission from Shutterstock. *Photo by B. Proud.*)

ACTION	RATIONALE
22. Ask the patient to dorsiflex and then plantarflex both feet against opposing resistance (Figure 10).	These measure ankle flexion and dorsiflexion.

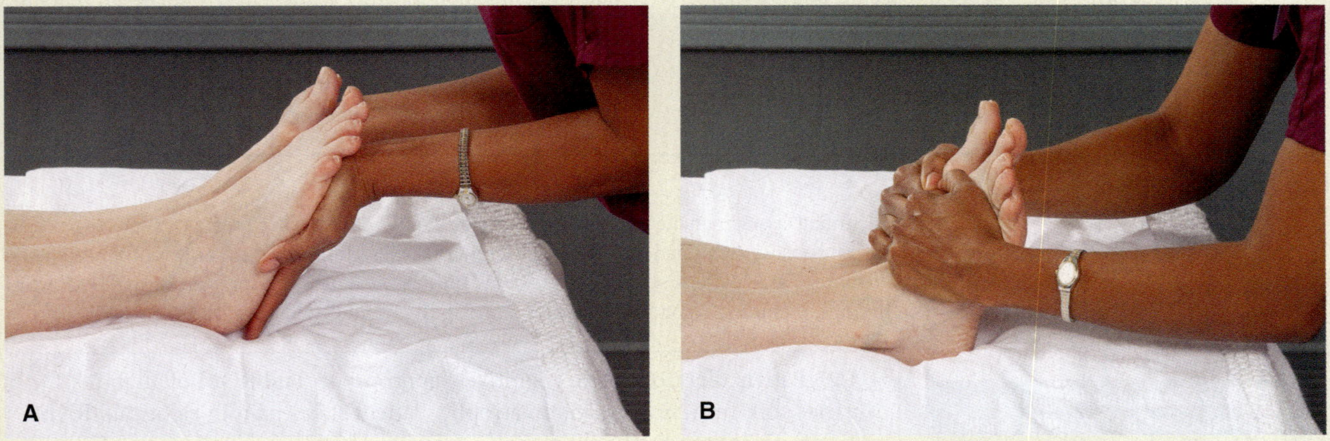

FIGURE 10. **A.** Testing ankle flexion and dorsiflexion. The patient first pushes the balls of the feet against resistance of the nurse's hands. **B.** Then attempts to pull against nurse's resistance. (*Source:* Used with permission from Shutterstock. *Photos by B. Proud.*)

ACTION	RATIONALE
23. As needed, assist the patient to a standing position. Observe the patient as they walk with a regular gait, on the toes, on the heels, and then heel to toe (Figure 11).	This procedure evaluates cerebellar and motor function.
24. Perform the Romberg's test; ask the patient to stand straight with feet together, both eyes closed with arms at side (Figure 12). Wait 20 seconds and observe for patient swaying and ability to maintain balance. Be alert to prevent a patient fall or injury related to losing balance during this assessment.	This test checks cerebellar functioning and evaluates balance, equilibrium, and coordination. Slight swaying is normal, but patient should be able to maintain balance.
25. Assist the patient to a comfortable position.	This ensures the patient's comfort.

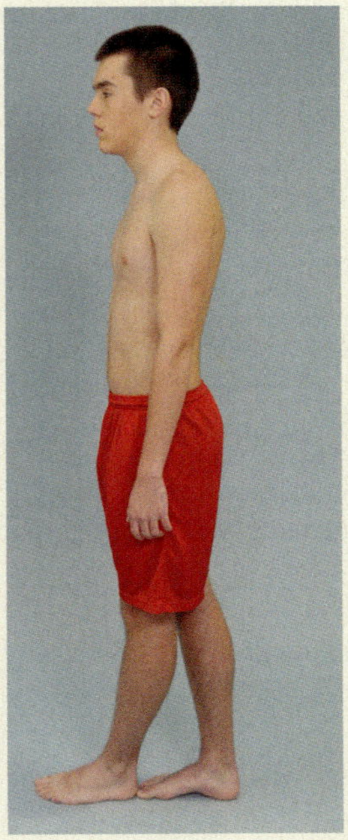

FIGURE 11. Testing heel to toe walking. (*Source:* From Jensen, S. [2019]. *Nursing health assessment* [3rd ed., p. 652]. Wolters Kluwer.)

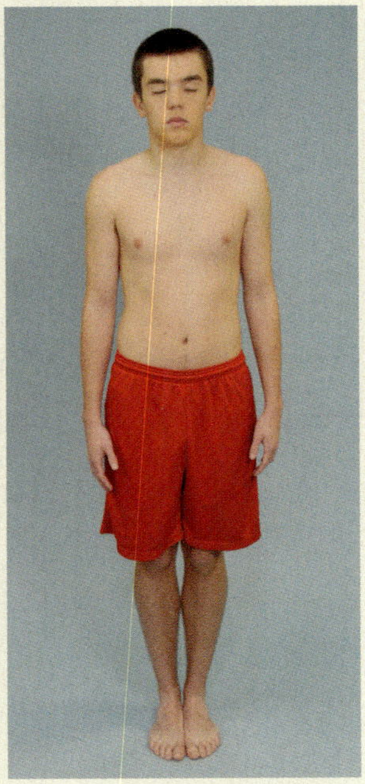

FIGURE 12. Positioning for the Romberg's test. (*Source:* From Jensen, S. [2019]. *Nursing health assessment* [3rd ed., p. 653]. Wolters Kluwer.)

(continued on page 830)

Skill 27-2 Assessing the Neurologic, Musculoskeletal, and Peripheral Vascular Systems *(continued)*

ACTION	RATIONALE
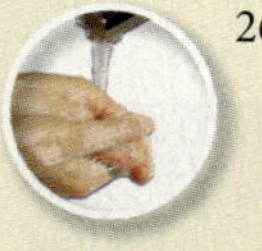 26. Remove PPE, if used. Perform hand hygiene. Continue with assessments of specific body systems, as appropriate, or indicated. Initiate appropriate referral to other health care providers for further evaluation, as indicated.	Proper removal of PPE reduces the risk for infection transmission and contamination of other items. Hand hygiene prevents the spread of microorganisms. Additional assessments should be completed, as indicated, to evaluate the patient's health status. Intervention by other health care providers may be indicated to evaluate and treat the patient's health status.

DOCUMENTATION

GUIDELINES

Document assessment techniques performed, along with specific findings. Note the cognitive responses of the patient, the tested cranial nerves, and sensation and motor responses. Document any patient statements of pain, muscle weakness, or joint abnormality. Record findings, including color, turgor, temperature, pulses, and capillary refill.

SAMPLE DOCUMENTATION

Lippincott DocuCare **Practice documenting assessment techniques and findings in *Lippincott DocuCare*.**

<u>4/4/25</u> Patient alert, oriented, cognitively appropriate. Full ROM of all joints. Muscles soft, firm, nontender, no atrophy. Patient states pain in right calf. Right calf skin paler tone and slightly cooler compared with left calf. Peripheral pulses 72, +2, regular rhythm, equal bilaterally; exception—right posterior tibial and dorsalis pedis pulses +1. Capillary refill right lower extremity sluggish, >3 seconds, +sensation in feet, equal bilaterally.

—S. Moses, RN

DEVELOPING CLINICAL REASONING AND CLINICAL JUDGMENT

SPECIAL CONSIDERATIONS

General Considerations

- Before performing the mental status examination, inform the patient that some of the questions may seem unusual, but that you are attempting to evaluate overall cognitive function.

Infant and Child Considerations

- In an infant, jerky and brief twitching of the extremities may be noted and considered a normal finding.
- The Babinski sign is a normal finding in children age 24 months and younger (Jensen, 2019).
- The infant's extremities move symmetrically through ROM but lack full extension.
- Motor control develops in head, neck, trunk, and extremities in sequence.
- Coordination of movement varies according to the developmental level of the young child.

Older Adult Considerations

- Be aware that short-term memory, such as recall of recent events, may diminish with age. Older adults may also experience slowed reaction time as well.
- In the older adult patient, expect to find decreased musculoskeletal function, such as loss of muscle strength.
- Slower gait, with a wider base and flexed hips and knees.
- Keep in mind that older adults may take longer to perform certain actions, such as completing activities for testing coordination.

DEVELOPING CLINICAL REASONING AND CLINICAL JUDGMENT

1. Describe how you would explain a cardiovascular assessment to the following patients:
   - A healthy 5-year-old
   - A college student who has never been ill
   - A 50-year-old man who has never had a physical assessment
   - An 85-year-old woman with heart problems
2. When you are conducting a health history, your patient gives you strange answers. Later, during the mental status assessment, she gives you the wrong answers for the date and place. She also cannot remember what medications she takes. How would you document this information? What would you do next?
3. When you make a home visit to conduct an initial health history and physical assessment, the patient refuses to let you do more than assess vital signs. What would you do?

PRACTICING FOR NCLEX

1. A nurse on a medical-surgical unit is caring for a group of patients. For which patient will the nurse perform a focused assessment?
   a. Newly admitted
   b. Recent application of a wrist cast
   c. Signs of acute respiratory distress
   d. Post-abdominal surgery without complications
2. A nurse admitting a patient to a long-term care facility performs a functional assessment. Which questions will the nurse include as part of the assessment? Select all that apply.
   a. "Are you able to dress yourself?"
   b. "Do you have a history of smoking?"
   c. "What is the problem for which you are seeking care?"
   d. "Do you prepare your own meals?"
   e. "Do you manage your own finances?"
   f. "Whom do you rely on for support?"
3. A nurse in the neurology clinic is assessing a patient's eyes for extraocular movements. Which correctly describes the procedure for this test?
   a. Ask the patient to sit about 3 ft away, facing the nurse.
   b. Have the patient follow a penlight held 1 ft from their face slowly through the cardinal positions.
   c. Move a penlight in concentric circular motion in front of the patient's eyes.
   d. Ask the patient to cover one eye with a hand or index card.
4. A nursing student is learning to perform physical assessments. When will the student use the technique of palpation? Select all that apply.
   a. Assessing temperature of a patient's feet
   b. Counting the apical pulse
   c. Assessing for skin turgor
   d. Evaluating lymph nodes
   e. Assessing for dullness over a tumor
   f. Finding a heart murmur
5. When inspecting the skin of a patient who has cirrhosis of the liver, the nurse notes the skin has a yellow tint. What term will the nurse use to document the skin assessment in the electronic health record?
   a. Jaundice
   b. Cyanosis
   c. Erythema
   d. Pallor
6. The nurse places a patient in the dorsal recumbent position during a physical assessment. Which nursing assessments can the nurse perform with the patient in this position? Select all that apply.
   a. Assessing the abdomen
   b. Taking peripheral pulses
   c. Performing a breast examination
   d. Auscultating the heart
   e. Assessing vital signs
   f. Assessing balance and gait
7. A school nurse assesses adolescents' visual acuity using a Snellen eye chart. Which explanation does the nurse provide to the student whose vision is 20/40 in both eyes?
   a. "They see better than 50% of people."
   b. "Double vision is present."
   c. "Vision is less than normal."
   d. "They have normal vision."
8. The nurse is caring for a patient experiencing bronchospasm due to an exacerbation of asthma. During auscultation, the nurse anticipates the presence of which breath sound?
   a. Sibilant
   b. Wheezes
   c. Rhonchi
   d. Crackles
9. A nurse in the emergency department is using the Glasgow coma scale to assess a patient who was struck in the head and upper body with a baseball bat. Based on the information in the neurologic assessment, what numerical value will the nurse assign?
   Electronic heath record (EHR)
   Neurologic assessment
   The patient opens his eyes to painful stimulus, does not speak, and withdraws to painful stimulus. Unable to assess orientation to person, time, and place.
   a. 3
   b. 7
   c. 11
   d. 15
10. A nurse is caring for a patient with exacerbation of COPD and pneumonia. When auscultating the lungs, coarse expiratory, low-pitched, and continuous sounds that clear with coughing are present. How will the nurse document this breath sound in the electronic health record?
    a. Rhonchi
    b. Bronchovesicular breath sounds
    c. Stridor
    d. Bronchial breath sounds

11. A nurse is assessing a patient's eyes for accommodation. Place the steps of this assessment in order they are performed.
    a. Document the results in the electronic health record.
    b. As the patient to look at a distant object, then back to the object held.
    c. Hold a straight object 0 to 15 cm (4 to 6 inches) from the bridge of the patient's nose.
    d. Observe for pupillary constriction when looking at the near object and for pupillary dilation when looking at the distant object held.
    e. Ask the patient to look at the object.
12. A nurse is performing a breast assessment using the circular technique for palpation, gently compressing the breast tissue against the chest wall. How does the nurse proceed with the examination?
    a. Begins at the tail of Spence and moves in increasing smaller circles
    b. Starts at the outer edge of the breast and palpates up and down the breast
    c. Works in a counterclockwise direction and palpates from the periphery toward the areola
    d. Proceeds from the inner edge of the breast and palpates up and down the breast
13. During physical assessment, a nurse inspects a patient's abdomen. What assessment technique does the nurse perform next?
    a. Percussion
    b. Palpation
    c. Auscultation
    d. Whichever provides patient comfort
14. A nurse and AP are caring for a patient who just returned from the operating room after a femoral–popliteal arterial bypass graft. The nurse is getting another admission. What activity can the nurse safely delegate to the AP?
    a. Determining if pedal pulses are present
    b. Evaluating the patient's pain
    c. Reinforcing the sterile dressing
    d. Ordering dressing supplies
15. A patient has come to the emergency department with symptoms of a stroke. During the assessment, the nurse asks the patient to raise their eyebrows, smile, and show their teeth to evaluate which cranial nerve?
    a. Olfactory
    b. Optic
    c. Facial
    d. Vagus

ANSWERS WITH RATIONALES

1. **b.** After application of a cast, the nurse performs a focused neurovascular assessment, to assess circulation, sensation, and motor ability. A newly admitted patient requires a comprehensive assessment. The nurse performs an emergency assessment on a patient who presents with signs of acute respiratory difficulty. A postoperative patient without complications will receive ongoing assessments at regular intervals to evaluate the effectiveness of care and to assess for new problems.
2. **a, d, e.** A functional health assessment including strengths and areas needing improvement focuses on the effects of health or illness on a patient's quality of life. Questions about the patient's ability to perform ADLs and IADLs such as dressing, grooming, preparing meals, and managing finances are included. A history of smoking is a lifestyle factor, and the chief complaint is the reason for seeking health care; both are assessed during the health history. Social networks and support psychosocial factors are also assessed during the health history.
3. **b.** The steps in testing for extraocular movement are: (1) Ask the patient to sit or stand about 2 ft away, facing the nurse, who is sitting or standing at eye level with the patient; (2) ask the patient to hold the head still and follow the movement of a forefinger or a penlight with the eyes; (3) keeping the finger or light about 1 foot from the patient's face, move it slowly through the cardinal positions of gaze—up and down, left and right, diagonally up and down to the left, diagonally up and down to the right.
4. **a, c, d.** During palpation, the nurse uses the sense of touch to compare bilateral pulses for symmetrical temperature, assess skin turgor, and check for enlarged lymph nodes. During percussion, the fingertips are used to tap the body over body tissues to produce vibrations and sound waves. The characteristics of the sounds provide information about the location, shape, size, and density of tissues, such as dullness over a mass or fluid accumulation. Auscultation refers to listening with a stethoscope to sounds produced in the body; counting the apical pulse or auscultating heart sounds/murmurs are examples.
5. **a.** Jaundice refers to a yellowish skin color caused by liver, gallbladder, or pancreatic exocrine diseases. Cyanosis is a bluish skin color caused by a cold environment or decreased oxygenation. Erythema is a reddish color caused by blushing, alcohol intake, fever, injury trauma, or infection. Pallor is a paleness caused by anemia or shock.
6. **b, c, d.** In the dorsal recumbent position, the patient lies on the back with legs separated, knees flexed, and soles of the feet on the bed. It is used to assess the head, neck, anterior thorax, lungs, heart, breasts, extremities, and peripheral pulses. It should not be used for abdominal assessment because it causes contraction of the abdominal muscles. Vital sign assessment should be done in the sitting position, and evaluating balance and gait is done with the patient in the standing position.
7. **c.** Normal vision is 20/20. The higher the denominator indicates increasingly worse vision; 20/40 vision indicates less than normal vision.
8. **d.** Wheezes are musical or squeaking high-pitched, continuous sounds heard as air passes through narrowed airways, such as with bronchospasm found in asthma or COPD. Rhonchi are low-pitched, continuous sounds with a snoring quality, which may clear with coughing; they occur when air passes through secretions. Crackles are discontinuous bubbling, cracking, or popping, low- to high-pitched sounds, that occur when air passes through fluid in the airways.
9. **b.** Eye opening to painful stimulus = 2 points, no speech = 1 point; and withdrawal to painful stimulus = 4 points, for a total score of 7. A score of 8 or less is associated with coma.

10. a. Rhonchi are abnormal low-pitched, continuous breath sounds auscultated during inspiration and occasionally expiration, indicating that air is passing through or around secretions. Bronchovesicular breath sounds are normal sounds heard on inspiration and expiration. Stridor is a harsh, loud, high-pitched sound auscultated on inspiration indicating narrowing of the upper airway or presence of a foreign body. Bronchial sounds are normal blowing, hollow sounds, auscultated over the larynx and trachea.

11. c, e, b, d, a. To test accommodation the nurse holds the forefinger, a pencil, or other straight object about 10 to 15 cm (4 to 6 inches) from the bridge of the patient's nose. The patient is asked to look at the object, then at a distant object, then back to the object being held. The pupil normally constricts when looking at a near object and dilates when looking at a distant object. The patient must be cooperative to complete this assessment.

12. a. During breast assessment, the nurse palpates each quadrant of the breasts in a systematic method using the pads of the first three fingers to gently compress the breast tissue against the chest wall. In the circular method, the nurse begins at the tail of Spence and move in increasingly smaller circles. In the wedge method, the nurse works in a clockwise direction and palpates from the periphery toward the areola. In the vertical strip method, the nurse begins at the outer edge of the breast, palpating up and down the breast.

13. c. When assessing the abdomen, the sequence for assessment is: inspection, auscultation, percussion, and palpation. Auscultation follows inspection to avoid stimulating bowel sounds during percussion.

14. d. The nurse can delegate noncomplex activities to the AP such as obtaining (dressing) supplies, bedmaking, bathing, I & O, toileting, and ambulation. The nurse must perform assessments, provide teaching, perform sterile procedures, and develop the care plan.

15. c. Motor function of the facial nerve (cranial nerve VII) is assessed by asking the patient to raise their eyebrow, smile, and show their teeth. The olfactory nerve (cranial nerve I) is tested by testing the sense of smell using various familiar substances. The nurse tests the optic nerve (cranial nerve II) for acuity and visual fields and the vagus nerve (cranial nerve X) by asking the patient to swallow and speak, noting hoarseness.

Bibliography

Agency for Clinical Innovation (ACI). ACI Musculoskeletal Network. (2018). Neurovascular assessment. New South Wales Government. https://aci.health.nsw.gov.au/__data/assets/pdf_file/0004/458185/ACI_0147-MSK-compartment-guide_V4.pdf

Aisner, A. J., Zappas, M., & Marks, A. (2020). Primary care for lesbian, gay, bisexual, transgender, and queer/questioning (LGBTQ) patients. *The Journal for Nurse Practitioners, 16*(4), 281–285. https://doi.org/10.1016/j.nurpra.2019.12.011

Ali, P. A., & Watson, R. (2018). Language barriers and their impact on provision of care to patients with limited English proficiency: Nurses' perspectives. *Journal of Clinical Nursing, 27*(5–6), e1152–e1160. https://doi.org/10.1111/jocn.14204

Almojuela, A., Hasen, M., & Zeiler, F. A. (2019). The Full Outline of UnResponsiveness (FOUR) Score and its use in outcome prediction: A scoping systematic review of the adult literature. *Neurocritical Care, 31*(1), 162–175. https://doi.org/10.1007/s12028-018-0630-9

Altarum Institute. (2019). Sexual health and your patients: A provider's guide. National Coalition for Sexual Health. https://nationalcoalitionforsexualhealth.org/tools/for-healthcare-providers

American Academy of Pediatrics. (2020). Recommendations for preventive pediatric health care. https://downloads.aap.org/AAP/PDF/periodicity_schedule.pdf

American Cancer Society. (2018). *Testicular cancer early detection, diagnosis and staging.* https://www.cancer.org/content/dam/CRC/PDF/Public/8845.00.pdf

American Cancer Society. (2020). *Breast cancer. American Cancer Society recommendations for early the detection of breast cancer.* https://www.cancer.org/cancer/breast-cancer/screening-tests-and-early-detection/american-cancer-society-recommendations-for-the-early-detection-of-breast-cancer.html

American College of Obstetricians and Gynecologists. (2017). *Mammography and other screening tests for breast problems. Frequently asked questions: Gynecologic problems.* https://www.acog.org/patient-resources/faqs/gynecologic-problems/mammography-and-other-screening-tests-for-breast-problems

American Speech-Language-Hearing Association (n.d.). *Adult hearing screening. Screening for disability (activities and participation). Self-assessment tools.* Retrieved July 17, 2021, from https://www.asha.org/practice-portal/professional-issues/adult-hearing-screening/

Anderson, B., Nix, E., Norman, B., & McPike, H. D. (2014). An evidence based approach to undergraduate physical assessment practicum course development. *Nurse Education in Practice, 14*(3), 242–246. https://doi.org/10.1016/j.nepr.2013.08.007

Andrews, M., Boyle, J. S., & Collins, J. (2020). *Transcultural concepts in nursing care* (8th ed.). Wolters Kluwer.

Berlinger, N., Wynia, M., Powell, T., Hester, M., Milliken, A., Fabi, R., Cohn, F., Guidry-Gries, L. K., Watson, J. C., Bruce, L., Chuang, E. J., Oei, G., Abbott, J., & Jenks, N. P. (2020, March 16). *Ethical framework for health care institutions & guidelines for institutional ethics services responding to the coronavirus pandemic. The Hastings Center.* https://www.thehastingscenter.org/ethicalframeworkcovid19/

Boyd, M. A. (2018). *Psychiatric nursing: Contemporary practice* (6th ed.). Wolters Kluwer.

Burns, S. M., & Delgado, S. A. (2019). *AACN Essentials of critical care nursing* (4th ed.). McGraw-Hill Education.

Cahill, S., Baker, K., & Makadon, H. (2020). *Do ask, do tell: A toolkit for collecting sexual orientation and gender identify information in clinical settings.* The Fenway Institute and the Center for American Progress. https://doaskdotell.org/

Centers for Disease Control and Prevention (CDC). (n.d.a). *Immunization schedules.* Retrieved June 19, 2020, from https://www.cdc.gov/vaccines/schedules/

Centers for Disease Control and Prevention (CDC). (n.d.b). *A guide to taking a sexual history.* [Brochure]. Retrieved June 19, 2020, from https://www.cdc.gov/std/treatment/sexualhistory.pdf

Centers for Disease Control and Prevention (CDC). (2018). *Violence prevention. Intimate partner violence.* https://www.cdc.gov/violenceprevention/intimatepartnerviolence/index.html

Centers for Disease Control and Prevention (CDC). (2020a). *Coronavirus disease 2019. People who are at higher risk.* https://www.cdc.gov/coronavirus/2019-ncov/need-extra-precautions/people-at-higher-risk.html

Centers for Disease Control and Prevention (CDC). (2020b). *HIV. Taking a sexual history.* https://www.cdc.gov/hiv/clinicians/transforming-health/health-care-providers/sexual-history.html

Centers for Medicare and Medicaid Services. (2018). *Initial preventive physical examination (IPPE).* https://www.cms.gov/Outreach-and-Education/Medicare-Learning-Network-MLN/MLNProducts/downloads/MPS_QRI_IPPE001a.pdf

Chung, S., Huang, Q., LaMori, J., Doshi, D., & Romanelli, R. J. (2020). Patient-reported experiences in discussing prescribed medications with a health care provider: Evidence for racial/ethnic disparities in a large health care delivery system. *Population Health Management, 23*(1), 78–84. https://doi.org/10.1089/pop.2018.0206

Dalton, M., Harrison, J., Malin, A., & Leavey, C. (2018). Factors that influence nurses' assessment of patient acuity and response to acute deterioration. *British Journal of Nursing, 27*(4), 212–218. https://doi.org/10.12968/bjon.2018.27.4.212

Derbyshire, J., & Hill, B. (2018). Performing neurological observations. *British Journal of Nursing, 27*(19), 1110–1114. https://doi.org/10.12968/bjon.2018.27.19.1110

Douglas, C., Windsor, C., & Lewis, P. (2015). Too much knowledge for a nurse? Use of physical assessment by final-semester nursing students. *Nursing & Health Sciences, 17*(4), 492–499. https://doi.org/10.1111/nhs.12223

Dudek, S. (2022). *Nutrition essentials for nursing practice* (9th ed.). Wolters Kluwer.

Eliopoulos, C. (2018). *Gerontological nursing* (9th ed.). Wolters Kluwer.

Fawcett, T., & Rhynas, S. (2012). Taking a patient history: The role of the nurse. *Nursing Standard, 26*(24), 41–46. https://doi.org/10.7748/ns2012.02.26.24.41.c8946

Greenshields, S. (2019). Neurological assessment in children and young people. *British Journal of Nursing, 28*(16), 1056–1059. https://doi.org/10.12968/bjon.2019.28.16.1056

Hall, A. (2018). Heart sounds: Auscultation for valvular heart disease. *British Journal of Cardiac Nursing, 13*(1), 12–18. https://doi.org/10.12968/bjca.2018.13.1.12

Haugh, K. H. (2015). Head-to-toe: Organizing your baseline patient physical assessment. *Nursing, 45*(12), 58–61.

Healthy People 2030. (n.d.a). *Social determinants of health.* Office of Disease Prevention and Health Promotion. Retrieved April 9, 2022, https://health.gov/healthypeople/priority-areas/social-determinants-health

Healthy People 2020. (n.d.). *Lesbian, gay, bisexual, and transgender health.* Office of Disease Prevention and Health Promotion. Retrieved June 9, 2020, from https://www.healthypeople.gov/2020/topics-objectives/topic/lesbian-gay-bisexual-and-transgender-health

Hess, D. R., MacIntyre, N. R., Galvin, W. F., & Mishoe, S. C. (2021). *Respiratory care: Principles and practice* (4th ed.). Jones & Bartlett Learning.

Hickey, J. V. (2020). *The clinical practice of neurological and neurosurgical nursing* (8th ed.). Wolters Kluwer.

Hinkle, J. L., Cheever, K. H., & Overbaugh, K. J. (2022). *Brunner & Suddarth's Textbook of medical-surgical nursing* (15th ed.). Wolters Kluwer.

Hogan-Quigley, B., Palm, M. L., & Bickley, L. (2017). *Bates' nursing guide to physical examination and history taking* (2nd ed.). Wolters Kluwer.

Holleck, J. L., Campbell, S., Alrawili, H., Frank, C., Merchant, N., Rodwin, B., Perez, M. F., Gupta, S., Federman, D. G., Chang, J. J., Vientos, W., & Dembry, L. (2020). Stethoscope hygiene: Using cultures and real-time feedback with bioluminescence-based adenosine triphosphate technology to change behavior. *American Journal of Infection Control, 48*(4), 380–385. https://doi.org/10.1016/j.ajic.2019.10.005

Hresko, M. T., Talwalkar, V. R., & Schwend, R. M. (2015). *Position statement-Screening for the early detection for idiopathic scoliosis in adolescents. SRS/POSNA/AAOS/AAP position statement.* Scoliosis Research Society. https://www.srs.org/about-srs/news-and-announcements/position-statement—screening-for-the-early-detection-for-idiopathic-scoliosis-in-adolescents

Human Rights Campaign. (n.d.). Explore: Health & aging. Retrieved June 9, 2020, from https://www.hrc.org/explore/topic/health-and-aging

Iyer, V. N., Mandrekar, J. N., Danielson, R. D., Zubkov, A. Y., Elmer, J. L., & Wijdicks, E. F. M. (2009). Validity of the FOUR score coma scale in the medical intensive care unit. *Mayo Clinic Proceedings, 84*(8), 694–701. https://doi.org/10.1016/S0025-6196(11)60519-3

Jalali, R., & Rezaei, M. (2014). A comparison of the Glasgow Coma Scale Score with Full Outline of Unresponsiveness Scale to predict patients' traumatic brain injury outcomes in intensive care units. *Critical Care Research and Practice. 2014*(2014), 289803. https://doi.org/10.1155/2014/289803

Jarvis, C., & Echkardt, A. (2020). *Physical examination & health assessment* (8th ed.). Elsevier.

Jensen, S. (2019). *Nursing health assessment: A best practice approach* (3rd ed.). Wolters Kluwer.

Johns Hopkins Medicine. (n.d.). *Health. Wellness and prevention. Breast self-awareness.* Retrieved July 28, 2020, from https://www.hopkinsmedicine.org/health/wellness-and-prevention/breast-self-awareness

Johnston-Walker, E., & Hardcastle, J. (2011). Neurovascular assessment in the critically ill patient. *Nursing in Critical Care, 16*(4), 170–177. https://doi.org/10.1111/j.1478-5153.2011.00431.x

The Joint Commission. (2011). *Advancing effective communication, cultural competence, and patient-and-family-centered care for the lesbian, gay, bisexual, and transgender (LGBT) community: A field guide.* https://www.jointcommission.org/-/media/enterprise/tjc/imported-resource-assets/documents/lgbtfieldguide_web_linked_verpdf.pdf?db=web&hash=1EC363A65C710BCD1D4E14ED120CB237

The Joint Commission. (2014). *Advancing effective communication, cultural competence, and patient- and family-centered care: A roadmap for hospitals.* http://www.jointcommission.org/roadmap_for_hospitals

The Joint Commission. (2015, May 28). *Quick safety 13: Overcoming the challenges of providing care to LEP patients.*https://www.jointcommission.org/en/resources/news-and-multimedia/newsletters/newsletters/quick-safety/quick-safety-issue-13-overcoming-the-challenges-of-providing-care-to-lep-patients/overcoming-the-challenges-of-providing-care-to-lep-patients/

Joszt, L. (2018, July 20). *5 vulnerable populations in healthcare.* Newsroom. American Journal of Managed Care. https://www.ajmc.com/newsroom/5-vulnerable-populations-in-healthcare

Keltner, N. L., & Steele, D. (2019). *Psychiatric nursing* (8th ed.). Elsevier.

Kersey-Matusiak, G. (2019). *Delivering culturally competent nursing care: Working with diverse and vulnerable populations* (2nd ed.). Springer Publishing Company.

Keveric, J., Jelinek, G. A., Knott, J., & Weiland, T. J. (2011). Validation of the Full Outline of Unresponsiveness (FOUR) Scale for conscious state in the emergency department: Comparison against the Glasgow Coma Scale. *Emergency Medicine Journal, 28*(6), 486–490. https://doi.org/10.1136/emj.2009.085845

Ku, L., & Jewers, M. (2013). *Health care for immigrant families: Current policies and issues.* Migration Policy Institute. https://www.migrationpolicy.org/research/health-care-immigrant-families-current-policies-and-issues

Kyle, T., & Carman, S. (2021). *Essentials of pediatric nursing* (4th ed.). Wolters Kluwer.

Lynn, P. (2023). *Taylor's clinical nursing skills: A nursing process approach* (6th ed.). Wolters Kluwer.

Mayo Clinic. (2018a). *Healthy lifestyle. Stress management.* https://www.mayoclinic.org/healthy-lifestyle/stress-management/in-depth/social-support/art-20044445

Mayo Clinic. (2018b). *Testicular exam.* https://www.mayoclinic.org/tests-procedures/testicular-exam/about/pac-20385252

McCormick, R., Robin, A. T., Gluch, J., & Lipman, T. H. (2019). Oral health assessment in acute care pediatric nursing. *Pediatric Nursing, 45*(6), 299–309.

McGee, S. R. (2018). *Evidence-based physical diagnosis* (4th ed.). *Chapter 51. Auscultation of the abdomen.* Elsevier.

Mercy, A. S., Thakur, R., Yaddanapudi, S., & Bhagat, H. (2013). Can FOUR Score replace GCS for assessing neurological status of critically ill patients-An Indian study. *Nursing and Midwifery Research Journal, 9*(2), 63–72. http://doi.org/10.33698/NRF0154

Mitchell, A., & Elbourne, S. (2020). Lower limb assessment. *British Journal of Nursing 29*(1), 18–21. https://doi.org/10.12968/bjon.2020.29.1.18

Moore, A., & Merrill, E. (2019). Evaluating older adult self-care capacity. *Nursing made incredibly easy! 17*(2), 34–41.

Morton, P. G., & Fontaine, D. K. (2018). *Critical care nursing: A holistic approach* (11th ed.). Wolters Kluwer.

Moscrop, A., Ziebland, S., Roberts, N., & Papanikitas, A. (2019). A systematic review of reasons for and against asking patients about their socioeconomic contexts. *International Journal for Equity in Health, 18*(1), 112. https://doi.org/10.1186/s12939-019-1014-2

Muntner, P., Shimbo, D., Carey, R. M., Charleston, J. B., Gaillard, T., Misra, S., Myers, M. G., Ogedegbe, G., Schwartz, J. E., Townsend, R. R., Urbina, E. M., Viera, A. J., White, W. B., & Wright, J. T. Jr. (2019). Measurement of blood pressure in humans: A scientific statement from the American Heart Association. *Hypertension, 73*(5), e35–e66. https://doi.org/10.1161/HYP.0000000000000087

National Cancer Institute. (2021, June 18). *Breast cancer prevention (PDQ®)—Health professional version.* https://www.cancer.gov/types/breast/hp/breast-prevention-pdq

National Collaboration Centre for Determinants of Health. (2020). Glossary. Vulnerable populations. http://nccdh.ca/glossary/entry/vulnerable-populations

National Heart, Lung, and Blood Institute (NHLBI). (n.d.a). *Aim for a health weight. Assessing your weight and health risk.* Retrieved July 17, 2021, from https://www.nhlbi.nih.gov/health/educational/lose_wt/risk.htm

National Heart, Lung, and Blood Institute (NHLBI). (n.d.b). Overweight and obesity. Retrieved July 17, 2021, from https://www.nhlbi.nih.gov/health-topics/overweight-and-obesity

Norris, T. L. (2019). *Porth's essentials of pathophysiology* (5th ed.). Wolters Kluwer.

Oh, H. S., Shin, S. Y., Kim, S. H., & Seo, W. S. (2019). Construct validity and reliability of the Full Outline of UnResponsiveness (FOUR) score in spontaneous subarachnoid haemorrhage caused by aneurysm rupture. *Journal of Clinical Nursing, 28*(21–22), 3776–3785. https://doi.org/10.1111/jocn.14877

Sadaka, F., Patel, D., & Lakshmanan, R. (2012). The FOUR score predicts outcome in patients after traumatic brain injury. *Neurocritical Care, 16*(1), 95–101. https://doi.org/10.1007/s12028-011-9617-5

Senger, B. A., & Smith, D. W. (2020). Augmenting a focused bedside history for prelicensure nursing students. *Journal of Nursing Education, 59*(3), 178. https://doi.org/10.3928/01484834-20200220-14

Silbert-Flagg, J., & Pillitteri, A. (2018). *Maternal and child health nursing* (8th ed.). Wolters Kluwer.

Skin Cancer Foundation. (2019). *Melanoma overview.* https://www.skincancer.org/skin-cancer-information/melanoma/

Squires, A. (2018). Strategies for overcoming language barriers in healthcare. *Nursing Management, 49*(4), 20–27. https://doi.org/10.1097/01.NUMA.0000531166.24481.15

Squires, A., & Youdelman, M. (2019). Section 1557 of the Affordable Care Act: Strengthening language access rights for patients with limited English proficiency. *Journal of Nursing Regulation, 10*(1), 65–67. https://doi.org/10.1016/S2155-8256(19)30085-7

Taylor, E. J. (2020). Initial spiritual screening and assessment: Five thing to remember. *Korean Journal of Hospice & Palliative Care, 23*(1), 1–4. https://doi.org/10.14475/kjhpc.2020.23.1.1

Teasdale, G., & Jennett, B. (1974). Assessment of coma and impaired consciousness. A practical scale. *Lancet, 2*(7872), 81–84. https://doi.org/10.1016/S0140-6736(74)91639-0

Toughy, T. A., & Jett, K. (2018). *Ebersol and Hess' gerontological nursing & healthy aging* (5th ed.). Elsevier.

Townsend, M., & Morgan, K. I. (2018). *Psychiatric mental health nursing: Concepts of care in evidence-based practice* (9th ed.). F.A. Davis Company.

Tuohy, D. (2019). Effective intercultural communication in nursing. *Nursing Standard, 34*(2), 45–50. https://doi.org/10.7748/ns.2019.e11244

Turney, J., Raley Noble, D., & Kim, S. C. (2013). Orthopaedic nurses' knowledge and interrater reliability of neurovascular assessments with 2-point discrimination test. *Orthopaedic Nursing, 32*(3), 167–172. https://doi.org/10.1097/NOR.0b013e3182920abb

VHA Center for Engineering & Occupational Safety and Health (CEOSH). (2016). *Safe patient handling and mobility guidebook.* http://www.tampavaref.org/safe-patient-handling.htm

Videbeck, S. L. (2020). *Psychiatric mental health nursing* (8th ed.). Wolters Kluwer.

Waterhouse, C. (2005). The Glasgow Coma Scale and other neurological observations. *Nursing Standard, 19*(33), 55–64; quiz 66–67. https://doi.org/10.7748/ns2005.04.19.33.56.c3857

Weber, J. R., & Kelley, J. H. (2018). *Health assessment in nursing* (6th ed.). Wolters Kluwer.

Wijdicks, E. F. M., Bamlet, W. R., Maramattom, B. V., Manno, E. M., & McClelland, R. L. (2005). Validation of a new coma scale: The FOUR Score. *Annals of Neurology, 58*(4), 585–593. https://doi.org/10.1002/ana.20611

The Williams Institute, UCLA School of Law. (2019). *LGBT data & demographics.* https://williamsinstitute.law.ucla.edu/visualization/lgbt-stats/?topic=LGBT#density

Winchester, S. B. (2019). Social Determinants of Health Assessment Tool: Implications for healthcare practice. *Social Work in Public Health, 34*(5), 395–408. https://doi.org/10.1080/19371918.2019.1614507

Yesavage, J. A. (1986). The use of self-rating depression scales in the elderly. In L. W. Poon (Ed.), *Handbook for clinical memory assessment of older adults.* American Psychological Association.

Zappa, S., Fagoni, N., Bertoni, M., Selleri, C., Venturini, M. A., Finazzi, P., Metelli, M., Rasulo, F., Piva, S., Latronico, N. (2020). Determination of imminent brain death using the Full Outline of Unresponsiveness Score and the Glasgow Coma Scale: A prospective, multicenter, pilot feasibility study. *Journal of Intensive Care medicine, 35*(2), 203–207. https://doi.org/10.1177/0885066617738714

28 Safety, Security, and Emergency Preparedness

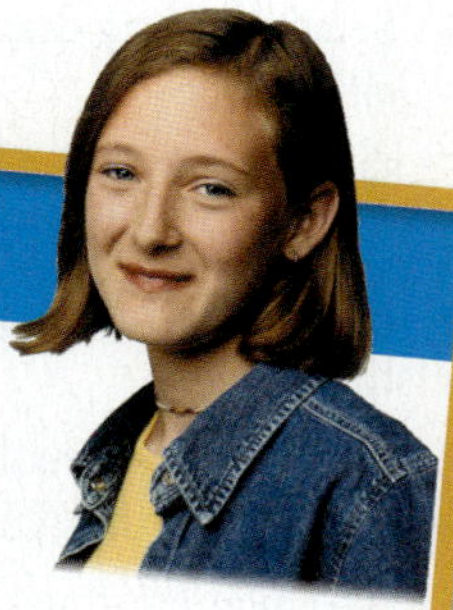

Kara Greenwood

Kara, a high school junior class representative and peer counselor, comes to the local community health center for a routine examination. During the interview, she says, "My guidance counselor has asked me and a few of my friends to develop a talk for our classmates on the dangers we face as adolescents. I know everybody is worried about terrorism, but I want to make sure that we talk about other safety issues, too."

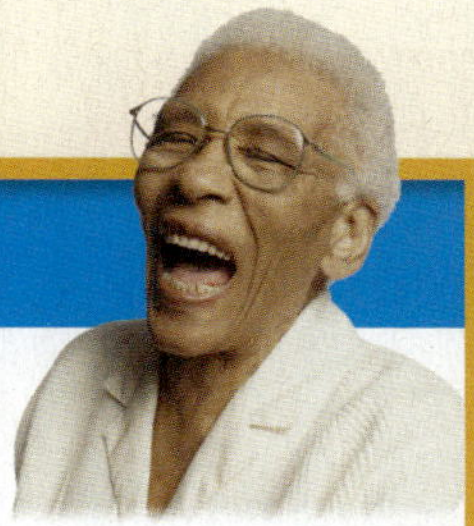

Bessie Washington

Bessie, a 77-year-old woman, was recently discharged to her home after suffering a cerebrovascular accident (stroke). She lives alone in a small, one-bedroom apartment and uses a walker to ambulate. She says, "I have so much stuff crammed into this small apartment! I almost fell this morning going from my bedroom to the kitchen."

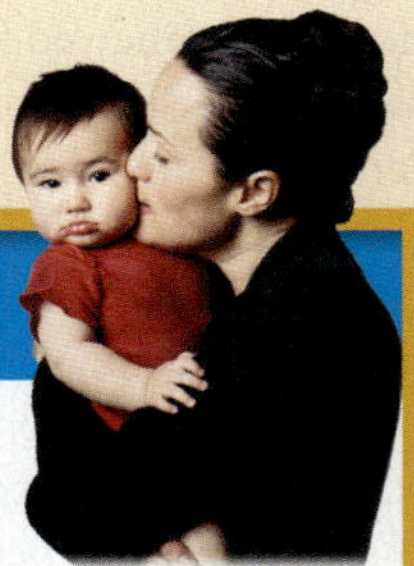

Juanita and Inez Flores

Juanita is a young mother of a 1-year-old girl, Inez. Today, they are at the clinic for a well-child visit. Juanita is sitting on a cot with her daughter, whose legs are dangling off the edge of the cot, about a foot above ground level. Juanita turns to get something out of her purse when Inez falls to the floor and begins to cry loudly.

Learning Outcomes

After completing the chapter, you will be able to accomplish the following:

1. Identify person-centered aspects of safety and security.
2. Identify patients at risk for injury.
3. Describe specific safety risk factors for each developmental stage.
4. Select nursing diagnoses for patients in unsafe situations.
5. Describe health-teaching interventions to promote safety for each developmental stage.
6. Describe strategies to decrease the risk for injury in the home.
7. Describe systems-based aspects of safety and security, specifically in relation to the health care setting.
8. Articulate population-based aspects of safety and security.
9. Explore resources for developing and evaluating an emergency management plan.
10. Evaluate the effectiveness of safety interventions.

Nursing Concepts

- Medical Emergencies
- Safety
- Communication
- Health Policy
- Violence

Safety and security are basic human needs. **Safety**—or freedom from danger, harm, or risk—is a paramount concern that underlies all nursing care. In addition, individual patient safety is a responsibility of all health care providers. The Institute of Medicine (IOM; renamed National Academy of Sciences, Engineering, and Medicines in 2015) report *To Err is Human*, introduced in 2000, recognized the need for a renewed focus on a culture of safety that promotes safe, effective, person-centered delivery of care. The IOM identified safety as an organizational priority and emphasized that medical errors are more frequently due to system problems rather than human error. Evidence-based research has identified tools and techniques designed to facilitate the elimination of errors and promote a safer health care environment (U.S. Department of Labor, OSHA, 2016). However, the impact each person has on the collective development of a culture of safety should not be minimized. Since nurses comprise the largest number of health care workers, their role is prominent and they have an unparalleled opportunity to influence the lives of their patients. The American Nurses Association (ANA) defines a **culture of safety** as an organizational environment where "core values and behaviors—resulting from a collective and sustained commitment by organizational leadership, manager and workers—emphasize safety over competing goals" (ANA, n.d.b, para 3). This idea of a culture of safety originated in the business world, but has been translated to health care and includes these key features: (1) acknowledgment of the high-risk nature of health care and the commitment to safe operations, (2) maintenance of a blame-free environment where reporting is protected and expected, (3) promotion of teamwork and collaboration to prevent and seek solutions to patient safety issues, and (4) a systems-based perspective where the organization commits resources to address actual/potential safety issues (U.S. Department of Health and Human Services, Agency for Healthcare Research and Quality, 2019a). Safety is a focus in all health care facilities as well as in the home, workplace, and community. Many safety and security concerns are universal for all age groups, but there are unique considerations for each developmental stage. We will focus on the nurse's role in individual-person-centered and system-based aspects of safety in the first two parts of this chapter.

In addition to consideration at the individual and health care systems levels, safety and security in the broader sense of our community will be explored in the third part of this chapter. Since the mass casualties that occurred in the terrorist attacks of September 11, 2001, as well as terrorist attacks around the world since then and the pandemic, the health care community has become increasingly aware of the need to be prepared should future incidents occur. Nurses are a vital part of any emergency response team and need knowledge about biologic, chemical, and radioactive agents as well as the skills and competencies required to respond safely and effectively.

The Institute for Healthcare Improvement (IHI, 2020) convened a steering committee comprising 27 national organizations to devise *A National Action Plan to Advance Patient Safety* and an associated assessment plan and implementation resource guide. The four foundational and interconnected areas identified for collaboration include: (1) culture, leadership and governance by leaders, governing bodies, and policymakers focused on safety; (2) patient and family engagement that includes partnering in all aspects of their care; (3) workforce safety and resilience using a systems perspective; and (4) establishing a network that supports continuous learning and information sharing. This call to action and associated competencies connect person-centered care, the systems perspective, and population health in an effort to advance patient safety.

This chapter provides practical information on the nurse's role in addressing safety and security from the person-centered, system, and population perspectives. Safety is one of the foundational principles of nursing care—watch for examples related to safety throughout this textbook and reflect on the clear application of principles related to safety in the situations presented in each chapter. Understanding the fundamental principles of safety and security provides the basis for the delivery of nursing care and should guide your thinking as a member of the profession. (See the accompanying Reflective Practice box.)

QSEN Reflective Practice: Cultivating QSEN Competencies

CHALLENGE TO ETHICAL AND LEGAL SKILLS

I first met Juanita Flores while working at a children's hospital two summers ago in a nurse externship program. Juanita was the mother of a 1-year-old girl, Inez, who had been diagnosed with failure to thrive and had been on the rehabilitation unit for some time. The child was very small and had a feeding program prescribed. One day while I was in the room, Juanita was sitting on the cot with her daughter, whose legs were dangling off the edge of the cot, about 1 foot above ground level. I was taking the child's vital signs. As the mother turned her back for a minute to grab something from her bag, I turned away to wash my hands in the sink. All of a sudden, I heard a thud and crying as Inez fell to the floor. Juanita tried to comfort her, picking her up and rocking and singing to her. Although I knew it was not completely my fault, I felt horrible about turning my back on the child for only a few seconds to wash my hands. Although Juanita and I were both in the room, the child had been left unsupervised. I was not watching Inez for only a few seconds . . . and she fell. I wanted to tell my preceptor right away and knew I *should* in case anything had happened to the child, but I was nervous and afraid that I would get into trouble.

Thinking Outside the Box: Possible Courses of Action

- Tell my preceptor immediately that the child had fallen, and risk being asked why I had turned my back on the child.
- Report later that morning that the child had fallen earlier, and not make a big deal of it.
- Not mention it at all.

Evaluating a Good Outcome: How Do I Define Success?

- Patient benefits from my actions, or at least is not harmed.
- My professional integrity is not compromised, nor is the personal integrity of the patient.
- A level of respect is maintained between the preceptor and student.
- Institutional policy for incident reporting is not violated.

Personal Learning: Here's to the Future!

Although I did tell my preceptor what had happened, I was not pleased by the way I handled the situation. Instead of reporting the incident right away, I waited until my preceptor was in the room with me, a half-hour or so later. I casually mentioned that the child had fallen earlier that morning but seemed to be fine. When my preceptor asked why I did not inform her earlier, I said that I couldn't find her and assumed that she was busy—plus, the child seemed fine and her mother was with her.

I was disappointed in how I dealt with this situation. Although I did not get formally reprimanded for the situation, an incident report was written documenting that the child had fallen. The health care provider also came to examine Inez to ensure that the child was indeed okay. My preceptor stressed the importance of reporting incidents as soon as they happen, rather than delaying or ignoring them. This time the child was uninjured, but I learned that in the future I will report any problem immediately. It is very important to follow the institution's policy for reporting incidents to ensure both your professional integrity and the well-being of the patient.

Anne Hrynko, Georgetown University

QSEN SELF-REFLECTION ON QUALITY AND SAFETY COMPETENCIES DEVELOPING KNOWLEDGE, SKILLS, AND ATTITUDES FOR CONTINUOUS IMPROVEMENT

How do you think you would respond in a similar situation? Why? What does this tell you about yourself and about the adequacy of your skills for professional practice? Is the nurse extern's fear justification for the action? Please explain. What ethical and legal principles, if any, were violated in this situation? What liability would the nurse extern be required to assume? Can you think of other ways to respond? What knowledge, skills, and attitudes do you need to develop to continuously improve quality and safety when caring for patients like Juanita and Inez Flores?

Patient-Centered Care: How might the nurse extern have interacted with the mother to promote the child's safety? What information should the nurse extern discuss with Juanita Flores concerning providing a safe environment for her child at various developmental stages? How could the nurse extern further involve the mother as a partner in maintaining safety through all hospital encounters?

Teamwork and Collaboration/Quality Improvement: What communication skills do you need to improve to ensure that you function as a member of the patient care team and minimize risk of harm to patients? How do you think this incident affected the relationship between the nurse extern and her preceptor?

Safety/Evidence-Based Practice: How might the delay in reporting the child's fall have affected the outcome of this situation? Should the extern initiate a discussion with her preceptor to review personal accountability and reporting procedures in a timely manner for any safety violations or incidents? What evidence in nursing literature provides guidance for decision making regarding ensuring a safe patient care environment? Given the focus on a culture of safety, should the health care team review what went wrong to allow this incident to occur, rather than who let it happen?

Informatics: Can you identify essential information that must be documented in the child's electronic health record regarding the fall she experienced? What other actions should be documented regarding the institution's response to the incident?

PERSON-CENTERED ASPECTS OF SAFETY AND SECURITY

Promoting safety and preventing injury are dual responsibilities of the nurse. Being aware of individual factors that affect a patient's safety, such as developmental level, lifestyle, mobility, sensory perception, knowledge level, communication ability, physical health state, and psychosocial state allows nurses to identify potential hazards and promote wellness. Injuries and deaths from motor vehicle accidents, falls, fire, suffocation, poisoning, and abuse/interpersonal violence occur with alarming regularity across the lifespan, but they tend to be associated with a specific age group/developmental level. Many of these injuries and deaths can be prevented with appropriate safety awareness and precautions. Patient safety is integral to the nursing plan of care. It is important to empower patients to make changes to their own environment, but depending on the situation, nurses may need to intervene in order to control or modify the patient's environment.

DEVELOPMENTAL CONSIDERATIONS

Each developmental level carries its own particular risks. Physical and cognitive changes reflect the sequential developmental stages of infancy through older adulthood. Health care needs and safety risks change as people progress from infancy to the older adult stage. For children, potential hazards multiply as their motor skills develop and their environment expands. Nurses promote safe sleeping practices for infants when they advise parents and caregivers to avoid stuffed animals and crib bumpers that increase the risk for suffocation. The risk of falling is noticeably higher for children. Toddlers are increasingly active and need appropriate safeguards to prevent falls in the home. Outdoor play and the associated injuries become an issue in the years between toddlerhood and adolescence. Adolescents face great dangers when they take illegal drugs, drink alcohol, take medications not prescribed for them, or engage in sex without a condom. These unsafe behaviors can result in alcohol-related motor vehicle accidents, pregnancy, and sexually transmitted diseases. Drug and/or alcohol use disorders are a concern for young and middle-aged adults employed in stressful work environments. Older adults experiencing altered balance or decline in cognitive abilities are increasingly vulnerable to falls and episodes of confusion. Nurses have first-hand experience with the specific hazards confronting each age group and situation. Education to promote awareness of potentially dangerous situations must begin as early as possible and continue throughout the lifespan.

Prompt recognition of a potential or actual threat to safety is crucial; the nursing assessment may play a vital role in identifying hazards in the environment. Teaching Tips 28-1 lists common types of safety risks according to developmental age, along with sample teaching tips to discuss with patients and families. Although some risks are universal and occur across the lifespan, developmental stages need to be considered when developing a safety teaching plan.

Neonate and Infant

FETAL CONSIDERATIONS

Safety considerations begin with an awareness of behaviors that may harm the developing fetus. Newborns of mothers who smoke have a lower birth weight. Excessive alcohol consumption and use of drugs may cause adverse effects that are readily apparent at birth. Reinforce a pregnant person's knowledge of the risks associated with excess alcohol consumption, smoking, drug use, and exposure to other dangers in the environment (Centers for Disease Control and Prevention [CDC], 2020d). It is also important to stress the importance of regular prenatal visits and the use of prenatal vitamins.

MOBILITY

The nurse has many opportunities to educate parents/caregivers about safety and accident prevention for infants. Young infants' lack of mobility limits opportunities for hazardous activity, but safeguards are vital to prevent accidents. Safe care includes never leaving the infant unattended, using crib rails, and monitoring the setting for objects that the infant could place in the mouth and swallow. As the child becomes more active, parents and caregivers must be alert to hazards that a curious, mobile child may encounter. All items within reach must be carefully inspected and, if dangerous, kept in a safe place, out of the child's reach. Because infants frequently climb or pull up on objects, hot liquids and sharp instruments must be placed out of their reach. Also, remind parents/caregivers that items that are small enough to fit through a standard toilet paper tube represent a potential choking hazard for young children.

CAR SEATS

All 50 states mandate the use of infant carriers and car seats when transporting a child in a motor vehicle. In 2018, the American Academy of Pediatrics (AAP) reaffirmed published guidelines recommending that infants and toddlers remain in a rear-facing safety seat until they reach the highest height or weight allowed by the car safety seat manufacturer. This position provides more support for the head, neck, and spine should a crash occur. Children should then progress to a forward-facing seat with a five-point harness until they reach the maximum height and weight limit for that seat. Children should use a belt-positioning booster seat until they are 4 ft, 9 inches tall and between 8 and 12 years old (80 to 100 lb). Due to the force of a deployed airbag, sitting in the front seat is not recommended until the child is 13 years old (Durbin et al., 2018). If no other arrangement is possible and an older child must ride in the front seat, move the vehicle seat as far back as possible away from the air bag and restrain the child properly based on the child's size. Most parents/caregivers do not secure the car seat tightly enough with the seat belt or latch system, or they fail to tighten the car seat's harness straps. These seemingly simple omissions can lead to tragic consequences.

Teaching Tips 28-1

PREVENTING ACCIDENTS AND PROMOTING SAFETY AT VARYING DEVELOPMENTAL STAGES

Developmental Stage/ Safety Risks	Teaching Tip	Why This Is Important
Fetus Abnormal growth and development	• Abstain from alcohol and caffeine while pregnant. • Stop smoking or reduce the number of cigarettes smoked per day. • Avoid all drugs, including OTC drugs, unless prescribed by a health care provider. • Avoid exposure to pesticides and certain environmental chemicals. • Avoid exposure to radiation.	Any factors, chemical or physical, can adversely affect the fertilized ovum, embryo, and developing fetus. A fetus is extremely vulnerable to environmental hazards.
Neonate (first 28 days of life) Infection Falls Accidental suffocation and strangulation in bed (ASSB)	• Wash hands frequently. • Never leave infant unsupervised on a raised surface without side rails. • Use appropriate infant car seat that is secured in the back seat facing the rear of the car. • Handle infant securely while supporting the head. • Place infant on back to sleep.	Physical care for the newborn includes maintaining a patent airway, protecting the baby from infection and injury, and providing optimal nutrition.
Infant Falls Injuries from toys Burns Suffocation or drowning Inhalation or ingestion of foreign bodies	• Supervise child closely to prevent injury. • Select toys appropriate for developmental level. • Use appropriate safety equipment in the home (e.g., locks for cabinets, gates, electrical outlet covers). • Never leave child alone in the bathtub. • Childproof the entire house.	Infants progress from rolling over to sitting, crawling, and pulling up to stand. They are very curious and will explore everything in their environment that they can.
Toddler Falls Cuts from sharp objects Burns Suffocation or drowning Inhalation or ingestion of foreign bodies/poisons	• Have poison control center phone number in readily accessible location. • Use appropriate car seat for toddler. • Supervise child closely to prevent injury. • Childproof house to ensure that poisonous products, drugs, guns, and small objects are out of toddler's reach. • Never leave child alone and unsupervised outside. • Keep all hot items on stove out of child's reach.	Toddlers accomplish a wide variety of developmental tasks and progress to walking and talking. They become more independent and continue to explore their environment.
Preschooler Falls Cuts Burns Drowning Inhalation or ingestion Guns and weapons	• Teach child to wear proper safety equipment when riding bicycles or scooters. • Ensure that playing areas are safe. • Begin to teach safety measures to child. • Do not leave child alone in the bathtub or near water. • Practice emergency evacuation measures. • Teach about fire safety.	Though more independent, preschoolers still have an immature understanding of dangerous behavior. They may strive to imitate adults and thus attempt dangerous behavior.
School-Age Child Burns Drowning Broken bones Concussions (TBI) Inhalation or ingestion Guns and weapons Substance use Bullying	• Teach accident prevention at school and home. • Teach child to wear safety equipment when playing sports and when riding a bicycle. • Reinforce teaching about symptoms that require immediate medical attention. • Continue immunizations as scheduled. • Provide drug, alcohol, and sex education. • Reinforce use of seat belts and pedestrian safety. • Support social relationships and watch for changes in the child that may indicate bullying or being bullied.	School-age children have developed more refined muscular coordination, but increasing involvement in sports and play activities increases their risk for injury. TBI can cause disruption in brain function and death. Cognitive maturity improves their ability to understand safety instructions.

(*continued*)

Teaching Tips 28-1 *(continued)*

PREVENTING ACCIDENTS AND PROMOTING SAFETY AT VARYING DEVELOPMENTAL STAGES

Developmental Stage/ Safety Risks	Teaching Tip	Why This Is Important
Adolescent Motor vehicle accidents Drowning Guns and weapons Inhalation and ingestion Bullying	• Teach responsibilities of new freedoms that accompany being a teenager. • Enroll teen in safety courses (driver education, water safety, emergency care measures). • Emphasize gun safety. • Get physical examination before participating in sports. • Make time to listen to and talk with your adolescent (helps with stress reduction). • Follow healthy lifestyle (nutrition, rest, etc.). • Teach about sexuality, intercourse, sexually transmitted diseases, and birth control. • Encourage child to report any sexual harassment or abuse of any kind. • Engage in open dialogue about events relative to social media, personal relationships, and school activities.	Adolescence is a critical period in growth and development. The adolescent needs increasing freedom and responsibility to prepare for adulthood. During this time, the mind has a great ability to acquire and use knowledge. The teen's peer group is a greater influence than families during this stage.
Adult Stress Domestic violence Motor vehicle accidents Industrial accidents Drug and alcohol use disorders	• Practice stress reduction techniques (e.g., meditation, exercise). • Enroll in a defensive driving course. • Evaluate the workplace for safety hazards and utilize safety equipment as prescribed. • Practice moderation when consuming alcohol. • Avoid use of illegal drugs. • Provide options and referrals to those experiencing intimate partner violence (IPV).	As people progress through the adult years, visible signs of aging become apparent. Lifestyle behaviors and situational or family crises can also impact an adult's overall health and cause stress. Preventive health practices help adults improve the quality and duration of life.
Older Adult Falls Motor vehicle accidents Elder abuse Sensorimotor changes Fires	• Identify safety hazards in the environment. • Modify the environment as necessary. • Attend defensive driving courses or courses designed for older drivers. • Encourage regular vision and hearing tests. • If prescribed, ensure that eyeglasses and hearing aids are available and functioning. • Wear appropriate footwear. • Have operational smoke detectors in place. • Objectively document and report any signs of neglect and abuse.	Accidental injuries occur more frequently in older adults because of decreased sensory abilities, slower reflexes and reaction times, changes in hearing and vision, and loss of strength and mobility. Collaboration between family and health care providers can ensure a safe, comfortable environment, and promote healthy aging.

Toddler and Preschooler

ENVIRONMENT

To prevent accidental injury and death in toddlers and preschoolers, parents/caregivers need to consider the environment. Play areas should allow for exploration, but still provide for safety. Children's overconfidence, curiosity, and impulsiveness make them more likely to dart into the street while chasing a ball, climb into a discarded refrigerator, or play with matches. Vigilant supervision by parents/caregivers should anticipate hazards in the environment, protect the child, and capitalize of teaching moments to model and instill good decision making in the child. Childproofing products are available that help parents/caregivers and children recognize dangerous items in the home and prevent injury. **Poison control centers (PCCs)** provide checklists for poison proofing a home and provide lists of toxic household items. Such lists are helpful when assessing and teaching the family about poisonous materials (see Box 28-1).

POISONING

Ingestion of poisons or medications is a major threat for preschoolers, due in part to the unprecedented amount of medication in the average home today. Concerted efforts by people, communities, state governments, and the federal government have reduced the number of accidental deaths by poisoning. The **PR**evention of **O**verdoses and **T**reatment **E**rrors in **C**hildren **T**askforce (PROTECT) Initiative is one collaborative among public health agencies, private companies, professional organizations, consumer/patient advocates, and

Box 28-1 Home Safety Checklist

Fire and Burn Safety

- ☐ Have a list of emergency phone numbers posted near the phone.
- ☐ Install smoke detectors in each room (or at a minimum, on each floor).
- ☐ Replace smoke detector batteries when you reset your clock.
- ☐ Have a fire extinguisher available on each floor and know how to use it.
- ☐ Practice a fire escape plan with your family.
- ☐ Teach all family members to stop, drop, and roll if clothing catches on fire.
- ☐ Keep matches and lighters out of children's reach.
- ☐ Keep lighted candles out of children's reach.
- ☐ Buy flame-resistant children's clothing, particularly sleepwear.
- ☐ Keep bedroom doors closed while sleeping (use monitor to listen for a child).
- ☐ Have ashtrays readily available if there is a smoker in the house.
- ☐ Enforce a strict "no smoking in bed" policy.
- ☐ After a party, check wastebaskets, ashtrays, furniture, and carpets for carelessly discarded cigarettes.
- ☐ Turn off a kerosene heater when no one is in the room and at bedtime.
- ☐ Operate your fireplace or wood-burning stove safely (flue open, fire screen covering the opening, annual chimney cleaning, proper disposal of ashes).
- ☐ Prevent trash or paint-saturated rags from accumulating in your garage.
- ☐ Store oily rags, gasoline, or other flammables away from heating sources or open flames, such as the pilot light of the water heater.
- ☐ Cook on back burners and turn pot handles toward the back of the stove.
- ☐ Keep hot dishes away from the edges of tables and counters.
- ☐ Set water heater at a safe temperature (below 120°F).
- ☐ Check bath water temperature with the back of your wrist before placing a child in bath.
- ☐ Use sunscreen and protective clothing to minimize exposure to the sun and prevent sunburn.

Electrical Safety

- ☐ Maintain electrical cords in good condition.
- ☐ Protect unused electric outlets with safety covers.
- ☐ Use the proper replacement for a blown fuse.
- ☐ Keep an electric space heater away from curtains and flammable material.
- ☐ Turn off appliances before going to bed or leaving the house.
- ☐ Hire a professional to do electrical repairs.
- ☐ Never overload wall outlets or extension cords.
- ☐ Unplug appliances that are not in use.
- ☐ Do not permit young children to use the microwave.

Preventing Poisoning

- ☐ Keep the phone number for the local poison control center next to the phone.
- ☐ Color-code medication bottles for those who are visually impaired.
- ☐ Syrup of ipecac is no longer recommended if poisoning should occur. Immediately contact the Poison Control Center (1-800-222-1222).
- ☐ Store all medicines in child-resistant containers in a locked medicine cabinet.
- ☐ Destroy old medicines (flush down the toilet or drop off at appropriate facilities).
- ☐ Keep all poisonous plants out of a child's reach.
- ☐ Avoid eating any fresh or prepared foods that look or smell spoiled.
- ☐ Store cleaning products, insecticides, and corrosives safely out of a child's reach.
- ☐ Avoid mixing caustic products with any other household product (dangerous chemical reactions may occur).
- ☐ Keep shampoos and cosmetics in a safe place.
- ☐ Use safety latches on cabinets.
- ☐ Store alcoholic beverages out of a child's reach.
- ☐ Check that paint or finish on furniture and toys is nontoxic.
- ☐ Install a carbon monoxide detector in your home.
- ☐ Have your furnace professionally inspected each year.
- ☐ Keep vents and chimneys clear of debris and have them checked seasonally.
- ☐ Don't operate cars, motorized equipment, or charcoal or gas grills in enclosed spaces.

Preventing Falls and Other Injuries

- ☐ Keep stairways clear and uncluttered.
- ☐ Maintain walkways, stairs, and railings in good repair.
- ☐ Keep stairs, hallways, outside walkways, and working areas well lit.
- ☐ Install safety gates at tops and bottoms of stairways.
- ☐ Paint the bottom step of the stairs a different color.
- ☐ Apply nonslip adhesive strips to the bottom surface of the tub or shower.
- ☐ Have a raised toilet seat with support arms available if necessary.
- ☐ Provide grab bars next to the toilet and in the tub or shower area.
- ☐ Use sturdy chairs that have armrests.
- ☐ Eliminate scatter rugs or secure them with adhesive strips on the underside.
- ☐ Use a handheld device, such as pincers, when reaching for inaccessible items.
- ☐ Buckle a child into an approved automobile safety seat even when making short trips.

Firearm Safety

- ☐ Keep guns and ammunition stored separately and locked up.
- ☐ Install trigger locks on all guns.
- ☐ Make certain that the key to the locked gun storage area is not available to a child.
- ☐ Discuss the risk for injury from guns and gun safety with your children.
- ☐ Instruct your child never to touch a gun or remain in a friend's house where a gun is accessible.

Preventing Asphyxiation or Choking

- ☐ Keep plastic bags out of a child's reach.
- ☐ Check that crib slats are no more than 2 3/8 inches apart.
- ☐ Ensure that the mattress fits the sides of the crib snugly.
- ☐ Remove soft pillows or thick blankets from your infant's crib.
- ☐ Never place an infant on a waterbed to sleep.
- ☐ Cut food into small pieces before giving it to a young child.
- ☐ Supervise young children when eating and drinking.
- ☐ Avoid giving peanuts, hard candy, or other small treats to a young child.
- ☐ Keep small objects, such as jewelry, buttons, and safety pins, out of a child's reach.
- ☐ Use toys appropriate for the child's age.
- ☐ Always watch a child who is in the tub.
- ☐ Cover wading pools and sandboxes when not in use.
- ☐ Check that nearby swimming pools are enclosed with a fence that your child cannot easily climb over.
- ☐ Keep pool rescue equipment nearby.
- ☐ Supervise your child closely when near water.
- ☐ Know how to perform cardiopulmonary resuscitation and the Heimlich maneuver.

other experts focused on developing strategies to keep children safe from unintentional medication overdoses. Their focus is on a three-pronged approach involving safer (child-resistant) packaging, safer use, and safer storage (CDC, 2020g). Although the number of children seen in the emergency department (ED) has steadily decreased since it peaked in 2010, each year, more than 47,500 children younger than age 6 years are treated for accidental poisoning from ingestion of medications (Safe Kids Worldwide, 2020). Dosing errors constitute fewer of the medication cases and involve giving the medication twice by mistake, giving the medication doses too close together, giving the incorrect dose, confusing the units of measurement, and using the dispensing cup incorrectly (Safe Kids Worldwide, 2020). Factors that put children most at risk for exposure to toxic substances include unsafe storage in the home, spending time in environments other than the home, lack of attention on the part of the caregiver, the rise in multigenerational families, and the presence of multiple pharmaceuticals, vitamins, and dietary supplements in the home (Safe Kids Worldwide, 2020).

Nursing interventions involve health education aimed at preventing accidental poisoning in the home. Every household must have the telephone number of the nearest PCC readily available. Emphasize that parents/caregivers should call the PCC immediately, before attempting any home remedy. Parents/caregivers may be instructed to bring the child immediately to an emergency facility for treatment. The focus of emergency treatment of poisoning is to stabilize vital body functions, prevent the absorption of the poison, and encourage excretion of the toxic substance.

Activated charcoal is considered the most effective agent for preventing absorption of the ingested toxin. It is not recommended for storage or use at home. Activated charcoal can be administered through a nasogastric tube in the ED for serious poisonings after the risks and benefits have been determined (Juurlink, 2016). Syrup of ipecac is no longer recommended because vomiting may be dangerous. A toxic substance may prove more hazardous coming up rather than when it was swallowed. Gastric lavage is no longer prescribed routinely for treatment of ingestion of a toxic substance because it may propel the poison into the small intestine, where absorption will occur. The amount of toxin removed by gastric lavage is relatively small.

ASPHYXIATION

Suffocation, or **asphyxiation**, may occur at any age, but the incidence is greater in children. In suffocation, air does not reach the lungs and breathing stops. Common causes of suffocation are drowning, choking on a foreign substance inhaled into the trachea, and gas or smoke poisoning. The leading cause of preventable-injury death in infants younger than one year is mechanical suffocation (82%), which is most frequently attributed to soft bedding (69%), bedding overlays (blankets, persons; 19%), and wedging (entrapped between a mattress and a wall; 12%; Lambert et al., 2019). A young child may be strangled accidentally by the shoulder harness of a seat belt or become trapped while playing in a discarded refrigerator and suffocate.

Drowning is a form of suffocation. For children ages 1 to 14 years, fatal drowning is the second-leading cause of unintentional, injury-related death, second only to motor vehicle crashes (CDC, 2021b). Drowning is second only to birth defects for cause of death in children ages 1 to 4 years (CDC, 2019c). Most drowning deaths in young children occur because of inadequate adult supervision of a child in or near a bathtub or pool, even a small wading pool. Older children are more likely to drown while swimming or boating. Other factors include missing or ineffective fences around water, not wearing life jackets, drinking alcohol, and using drugs and prescription medication (CDC, 2021b). Disparity persists with the rates of drowning deaths between some racial and ethnic groups. Black children ages 5 to 9 years drown at 2.6 times the rate of White children, and Black children ages 10 to 14 years drown at 3.6 times the rates of White children. This number jumps to 7.6 times the rate of White children when considering death in swimming pools (CDC, 2021b).

Educating the public about the causes of suffocation can save many lives. Assessing the knowledge level of people, especially parents, is vital. Nurses need to be alert to hazards that might cause a child to asphyxiate or choke (see Box 27-1 on page 778). Unconsciousness, respiratory failure, and cardiac arrest can occur as a result of suffocation. Emergency measures must start without delay, beginning with the removal of any obstruction and administration of cardiopulmonary resuscitation (CPR). When teaching parents, the nurse should emphasize careful supervision of children and should outline specific situations that place children at risk for suffocation. Health education is a valuable preventive force (see Box 28-1, on page 841, for specific interventions).

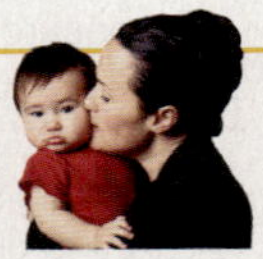

Recall **Juanita Flores**, the mother of the child who fell off a cot. As part of the plan of care, review safe infant care with Juanita and provide anticipatory guidance related to toddler safety in preparation for the child's discharge home.

CHILD ABUSE

Protecting a child also includes being alert to manifestations that indicate *child maltreatment or abuse* (Box 28-2). In the United States in 2018, child protective services (CPS) agencies received an estimated 4.3 million referrals involving 7.8 million children, with approximately 67.3% of those reports coming from professionals (educators, legal/law enforcement, social services). Based on these reports, 3.5 million children were screened in, which means they received an investigation or an alternative response from the CPS agency. In 2018, 28.7% of the estimated 678,000 victims of maltreatment were younger than 3 years old. An estimated 1,770 children died of abuse and neglect, with 70.6% of child fatalities younger than 3 years old, and those younger than age 1 year accounting for almost half (46.6%) of total child fatalities (U.S. Department of Health and Human Services,

Box 28-2 Manifestations of Child Maltreatment

The four common types of child abuse or maltreatment include:

Physical Abuse

Unexplained or repeated injuries resulting from physical force.

Manifestations include bruises, fractures (arms, legs, facial, ribs), burns, bite marks, head injuries, and any other indications of force.

Sexual Abuse

Engaging a child in sexual acts including fondling, rape, and exposing a child to other sexual activities.

Can be manifested by vaginal discharge, urinary tract infection, difficulty walking or sitting, sexually transmitted infections, and genital pain.

Emotional Abuse

Behaviors that harm a child's self-worth or emotional well-being.

Manifestations can include extremes in behavior, sleep problems, headaches or stomachaches, avoiding activities.

Neglect

Failure to meet a child's basic needs including housing, food, clothing, education, and access to medical care.

Source: Adapted from Fortson, B. L., Klevens, J., Merrick, M. T., Gilbert, L. K., & Alexander, S. P. (2016). Preventing child abuse and neglect: A technical package for policy, norm, and programmatic activities. National Center for Injury Prevention and Control, Centers for Disease Control and Prevention. https://www.cdc.gov/violenceprevention/pdf/CAN-Prevention-Technical-Package.pdf

Administration for Children and Families, Administration on Children, Youth and Families, Children's Bureau, 2020). Maltreatment includes physical (46.1%), sexual, or psychological abuse; includes sex trafficking; and may be a result of neglect, which is the most common form of maltreatment (72.8%). All 50 states have laws that require health care personnel to report suspected child abuse. To report abuse, contact The National Child Abuse Hotline at 1-800-422-4453 (1-800-4-A-Child).

School Age

ACCIDENTS

Although school-age children are increasingly independent, they still need help avoiding activities that are potentially dangerous. Accidents continue to be a leading cause of death. The nurse should counsel parents of school-age children about specific interventions for safety at home, at school, and in the neighborhood. All school-age children need to continue to be secured in safety seats, belt-positioning booster seats, or shoulder lap belts for their size. Use the Safety Belt Fit Test to determine when a child may safely use a seat belt without a booster (Box 28-3).

Each year, a significant number of children younger than 10 years are injured in *bicycle accidents.* Many of these

Box 28-3 Safety Belt Fit Test

Parents often ask, "When is it OK for a child to move from a booster seat to a seat belt?" If a child meets all of the following criteria, the child may sit in the back seat of a vehicle with a properly adjusted seat belt:

- Have the child sit in a back seat with their entire back and bottom against the vehicle's seat back. If the child's knees bend at the edge of the seat, go on with the test.
- Buckle the seat belt. If it stays low on the hips and is not resting on the soft part of the stomach, go on with the test.
- Check the shoulder belt. If it lays on the collarbone and shoulder, go on with the test.
- If the child is able to maintain the correct seating position with the shoulder belt on the shoulder and the lap belt low across the hips, then the child is ready to move from a booster seat to a seat belt.

If your child does not meet all four criteria, continue using a booster seat and retest again next month.

Source: Adapted from Safe Kids Worldwide. (2022). *Seat belt safety for big kids.* http://www.safekids.org/tip/seat-belt-safety-big-kids

injuries involve the head or face. The protective effect of bicycle helmets among children is well documented. Studies indicate that legislation and injury prevention strategies have had a positive impact on increasing helmet use and decreasing the number and severity of bicycle accidents that result in a head injury in this very vulnerable population. However, their use is far from universal. Because of their multiple experiences with children and parents, nurses—whether in the ED or a well-child setting—have many opportunities for health teaching related to bicycle safety and helmet use. Points to include in any teaching session include the following:

- Children should wear helmets at all times when riding a bicycle.
- Young children who are secured in a child seat as a passenger on a bicycle should also wear a properly sized helmet.
- The helmet should rest flat on the top of the child's head (approximately 1 inch above the eyebrows) and fit snugly.
- The chinstrap on the helmet should be adjusted so that it fits securely. If you can slide two fingers under the strap, the helmet is too loose.
- Any helmet that is involved or damaged in a crash should be discarded and replaced.
- Parents are effective role models for their children when they also wear helmets while riding a bicycle.

Playground activity promotes the development of social skills, reduces anxiety, encourages creativity and independence, increases confidence and resilience, and has physical benefits (Bergeron et al., 2019). Strategies to reduce the risk and severity of playground injury to children, especially traumatic brain injury (TBI) in children ages 5 to 9 years, include attentive adult supervision, employing methods to reduce high-risk behavior, designing age-appropriate playground equipment, and creating an environment that is well designed and maintained (Cheng et al., 2016). Although the majority (56%) of playground-related injuries treated in EDs are fractures, contusions, and abrasions (CDC, 2019d), sport- or recreation-related activities (fall or interpersonal contact, roller sports, equestrian and related activities, skiing/snowboarding, water sports) can also result in TBI. TBI usually results from a blow, bump, or jolt to the head that causes disruption in brain function. The direct blow to the head causes the brain to accelerate into the skull and then return and bounce off the opposite side of the skull. The brain can also rotate inside the skull, resulting in further damage. Every year in the United States, over 500,000 children present to the ED with TBI, with more than 60,000 children requiring hospitalization (Yue et al., 2016). A *concussion* is a milder form of TBI that is usually sports related (CDC, 2020e). Nurses in a variety of settings need to be alert for indications of concussion. The common manifestations can be subtle, but parents, teachers, and nurses need to be aware of the following descriptions of symptoms by category that may require a 911 call and immediate ED attention:

- Physical: headache, vomiting, problems with balance, fatigue, dazed or stunned appearance
- Cognitive: mentally foggy, difficulty concentrating and remembering, confusion, forgets recent activities
- Emotional: irritability, nervousness, very emotional behavior, any change in personality
- Sleep: drowsiness, difficulty falling asleep, sleeping more or less than usual

Technology Alert

In an effort to minimize the risk of concussion and other TBIs, the Centers for Disease Control and Prevention (CDC) created the HEADS UP program. HEADS UP provides tools resources for parents, health care providers, and leaders/coaches associated with schools, school sports, and community youth sports. Check out the CDC website at: https://www.cdc.gov/headsup/index.html for useful videos, informational PDFs, mobile apps, graphics, podcasts, and social media links.

Evaluation immediately following a concussion includes assessment of airway, breathing, and circulation (ABCs) and any indication of a cervical spine injury. The Sport Concussion Assessment Tool (5th edition; SCAT5) is one of the more widely used tools; it is available in adult and child versions (Child SCAT5 for ages 5 to 12) and designed to be used by medical professionals (Davis et al., 2017; Echemendia et al, 2017). Treatment for an uncomplicated concussion includes monitoring, avoidance of medications (alcohol, sleeping tablets, aspirin, anti-inflammatories, narcotics), and physical and cognitive rest until a licensed practitioner medically clears the athlete to return to activity. Cognitive rest entails avoidance of any computer-based activity, reading, watching television, and playing games of any kind.

CHILD ABDUCTION

The possibility of child abduction also needs to be addressed with parents and children for this age group. Abduction occurs for a number of reasons and is a tragedy that devastates parents, families, and communities. Strangers, family members, friends, or neighbors may kidnap children. Some children suffer sexual assault or are murdered by their captors. Adults who prey on children often take advantage of the innocent and trusting nature of children to persuade the child to accompany them. Children, even the very young, need basic instructions on how to recognize and respond to a potentially dangerous situation. Health teaching should also emphasize the need for parents to be alert and vigilant at all times regarding the whereabouts of their children.

Teach parents and caregivers about the AMBER Alert System, which can be activated when a child is missing and believed to be kidnapped. This critical response program uses the resources of law enforcement and the media to notify the public about an abduction. As of January 1, 2013, any Wireless Emergency Alerts–activated phone is automatically enrolled to receive alerts regarding the President, any imminent threat, and AMBER Alerts (U.S. Department of Justice, Office of Justice Programs, n.d.). The AMBER Alert is a powerful tool that helps enlist the public to help recover kidnapped children and return them to their families.

BULLYING

According to the American Psychological Association (2020), an estimated 40% to 80% of school-age children experience bullying at some point and 10% to 15% may be either chronic victims or bullies themselves. **Bullying** is generally defined as a form of direct or indirect aggression that includes hostile physical, verbal, psychological, and/or relational behaviors. It is intentional, repeated over time, and commonly occurs in the context of a relationship, which means there is usually a power differential involved. Children who are bullied are different or perceived to be different by their peers for any number of reasons including economic status, religious affiliation, weight, minority or immigrant status, learning or behavioral issue, sexuality or sexual orientation, exposure to trauma, lack of close relationships or familial issues, and child maltreatment (Hornor, 2018). Bullying results in immediate harm and/or negative social, mental health, and physical health consequences for the victimized child.

Cyberbullying contains similar elements and is often seen in conjunction with in-person bullying. Cyberbullying involves using information and communication technologies to bully (text messages, chat rooms, photos, social media), which means it can be perpetrated from anywhere at any time, is pervasive, has the capacity for an unlimited audience, has the perceived veil of anonymity, and often involves severe privacy violations (Waasdorp & Mehari, 2019). Because of the methods used, cyberbullying can be more difficult to detect and address; the perception of anonymity makes the perpetrators bolder and decreases their ability to see the results of their actions and develop empathy.

Children who are bullied are at risk for developing physical health consequences, somatic issues (headaches, stomach aches, irritable bowel syndrome), school absenteeism, depression, anxiety, low self-esteem, eating and sleep disorders, substance use, delinquent behavior, academic failure, and suicidal ideation. Perpetrators of bullying may have similar issues, but often display less empathy and more conduct issues than their peers. The consequences of bullying often extend through adolescence and young adulthood, into middle age and beyond (Hornor, 2018).

Adolescent

DRIVING

Much of the adolescent's time is spent away from home with their peer group. Adolescents are particularly at risk for motor vehicle accidents because they spend so much time in automobiles and are prone to distracted driving and driving under the influence of substances. The CDC (2019g) lists motor vehicle accidents as the number one cause of death for adolescents. Teens ages 16 to 19 years are three times more likely to be in a fatal crash than drivers older than age 20 years, with the death rate for males in that age group twice as high as that of females. Graduated driver licensing systems facilitate adult supervision and limit high-risk situations by mandating a learner stage, an intermediate stage (limits on number/type of passengers and curfews), and an unrestricted stage that varies by state (Insurance Institute for Highway Safety & Highway Loss Data Institute, 2020).

Distracted driving is a troubling trend for all age groups, but particularly for adolescents who comprise the largest percentage of distracted drivers. According to a report sponsored by the AAA Foundation for Traffic Safety (Carney et al., 2015), the most common forms of distraction for teens in the 6 seconds prior to a crash include: interacting with one or more passengers (15%), cell phone use (12%), looking at someone in the vehicle (10%), looking at something outside the window (9%), singing/dancing to music (8%), grooming (6%), and reaching for something (6%). According to a 2019 brief sponsored by the AAA Foundation for Traffic Safety (Arnold et al., 2019), distracted driving is underreported and on the rise. In their various roles, nurses have the potential to educate teenagers about this very dangerous risk to themselves and others by highlighting existing and emerging countermeasures. Education and/or behavioral countermeasures should focus on awareness campaigns, safe driving skills, the importance of wearing a seat belt, limited nighttime driving, obeying speed limits, never using a cell phone or texting while driving, and limiting the number of other teenagers in the car. Legislative countermeasures include handheld bans for all, texting bans for all, and complete cellphone bans for teens. Technology countermeasures that can be employed to assist teens include cellphone-blocking technology and driver monitor/feedback systems (Arnold et al., 2019).

SUBSTANCE USE, MISUSE, AND ABUSE

Alcohol use among teenagers is more common than use of tobacco or illicit drugs. Based on findings from a 2018 report (Substance Abuse and Mental Health Services Administration [SAMHSA], 2019), 9% of people ages 12 to 17 years currently use alcohol (2.2 million adolescents drank in the past month), 4.7% engage in binge alcohol drinking (five or more drinks on the same occasion at least once in the past month), and 0.5% drink heavily (five or more drinks more than 5 days in the past 30 days). By age 15 years, approximately 24.6% of teens have had at least one drink. People ages 12 to 20 years drink 4% of all alcohol consumed in the United States, with more than 90% of that alcohol consumed through binge drinking (National Institute on Alcohol Abuse and Alcoholism [NIAAA], 2021).

Nurses and parents should collaborate to reinforce safety behaviors in adolescents. Enforcement of zero tolerance laws regarding drinking age and driving while under the influence of alcohol, prevention programs in schools, and family efforts to influence whether their children consume alcohol are all significant factors aimed at preventing underage drinking. Successful approaches are comprehensive and consider social and environmental factors, genetics, personality, rate of maturation and development, and level of risk (NIAAA, 2021).

Illicit drug use increased among adolescents (ages 12 to 17 years) the past three reporting cycles: 2016 (15.8%), 2017 (16.3%), and 2018 (16.7%). An average of 4.2 million adolescents used illicit drugs in 2018 (SAMHSA, 2019). Teenagers abuse legally available drugs such as prescription medications (pain relievers, tranquilizers, stimulants, and sedatives) and over-the-counter (OTC) cough, cold, sleep, and diet medications. They also use illegal substances such as marijuana, cocaine, heroin, inhalants, and hallucinogens such as LSD. *Designer drugs*, synthetic/chemical derivatives of known illegal drugs, have seen a resurgence in the past 10 years. These total unregulated and typically legal designer drugs have a high potential for abuse and make their way onto the market under the guise of harmless names (Foundation for a Drug-Free World, 2020). The most popular synthetic and designer drugs include:

- MDMA: *Ecstasy, Molly, X, Hug Drug, Lover's Speed, Peace*; stimulant (euphoria) and mild hallucinogen/psychedelic (U.S. Department of Justice: Drug Enforcement Administration, 2020)
- Fentanyl analogues (acetyl fentanyl, carfentanil, valeryl fentanyl, fluoroisobutyryl fentanyl: *Apache, China Girl, China White, Dance Fever, Friend, Goodfellas, Jackpot, Murder 8, Tango & Cash*; synthetic opioid most commonly involved drug in overdose deaths) (National Forensic Laboratory Information System, 2021; National Institute on Drug Abuse, 2019a)
- 2C-B: psychedelic/psychostimulant (Papaseit et al., 2018); popular on the dark web
- NBOMe: *N-bomb, N-boom, Dots, 251-NBOMe*; hallucinogen (Zawilska et al., 2020)
- Desomorphine: *Krokodil, Crocodil, Crocodile, Russian Magic, Poor Man's Heroin, Zombie Drug*; highly addictive opioid derivative of codeine with narcotic and analgesic effects

that is more common internationally (U.S. Department of Justice: Drug Enforcement Administration, 2019)
- Bath salts: *Bliss, Blue Silk, Cloud Nine, Drone, Energy-1, Ivory Wave, Lunar Wave, Meow Meow, Ocean Burst, Pure Ivory, Purple Wave, Red Dove, Snow Leopard, Stardust, Vanilla Sky, White Dove, White Knight, White Lightning*; stimulant (U.S. Department of Justice: Drug Enforcement Administration, 2020)
- Synthetic cannabinoids (THC): *Spice, K2, Blaze, RedX Dawn, Paradise, Demon, Black Magic, Spike, Mr. Nice Guy, Ninja, Zohai, Dream, Genie, Sence, Smoke, Skunk, Serenity, Yucatan, Fire, Crazy Clown*; psychoactive (U.S. Department of Justice: Drug Enforcement Administration, 2020)

Warning signs of alcohol and drug abuse during adolescence include physical fatigue, personality change, poor judgment, sudden mood changes, withdrawal from the family, a variety of school-related issues (negative attitude, drop in grades, failure), and social problems. Parents need to focus on open communication with their teenagers, role model appropriate behavior, and seek help and guidance once a problem with alcohol or drug use is recognized.

Cigarette smoking in adolescents (ages 12 to 17 years) in 2002 was at 13%. This percentage has declined every year since then and is currently at an all-time low of 2.7% (SAMHSA, 2019). However, e-cigarette use, also called *vaping*, with flavored nicotine, nicotine, and marijuana continues to rise in this population (CDC, 2020c). In 2018, 27.1% of high school students and 7.2% of middle school students reported current tobacco use, most commonly via e-cigarettes. Federal law mandates a minimum age of 18 years to purchase tobacco products and bans billboard advertising within 1,000 ft of schools and playgrounds. However, campaigns for e-cigarettes and the flavoring that was banned in refillable devices but not disposable ones (U.S. Food and Drug Administration, 2020), tends to appeal to teens. Teenagers and younger children may be influenced to use tobacco products by the Internet, music, television, and movies, but parents can be the greatest influence. Conversations regarding the risks of smoking should begin as early as ages 5 to 6 years because many children start using tobacco products at age 11 years and may be addicted by age 14 years (American Cancer Society [ACS], 2019).

PIERCINGS AND TATTOOS

Body piercing has become increasingly popular with adolescents and young adults. Common sites for piercing include the ears, nose, eyebrows, lips, tongue, nipples, navel, and genitals. If not performed in a professional, clean environment, there is a risk for contracting hepatitis B or C, tetanus, or HIV. Even in a sterile environment, some common risks of piercing include chronic infection, skin allergies, abscess formation, inflammation, nerve damage, or prolonged bleeding (Gardner, 2019).

Although the U.S. Food and Drug Administration (FDA) has opted not to control piercings, it has provided some safety and regulatory guidance for *tattoos*, which have become increasingly popular (2019). Tattoos are permanent markings on skin surfaces viewed as a form of body art. Risks involved in tattooing include infection (similar to piercings), allergic reactions, granulomas (nodules), keloid formation (scarring), complications with MRIs, dissatisfaction, and problems associated with removal (FDA, 2019b). Although still regulated at the state (not federal) level, the FDA continues to collect data on pigments used in tattoo inks that are not approved for skin contact. Teens and their parents, who may be required to issue consent, need to be careful with both permanent and temporary tattoos. In particular, the FDA issued a warning statement about black and blue henna tattoos and other inks that also contain only hair dye. Meticulous post-piercing and tattoo care reduce the risk for developing an infection. Nurses need to be informed about the health risks in order to be effective and well-informed health educators.

FIREARMS

There are significant security issues related to adolescents and the use of guns. International studies indicate that when considering all high-income countries, 91% of firearm deaths of children ages 0 to 14 years occur in the United States. Nearly 1,300 children (ages 0 to 17 years) in the United States die from gunshot wounds, and 5,790 children are treated for gunshot wounds each year. Boys (82% to 84%), adolescents (ages 13 to 17 years), and minorities are more likely to be affected. In all cases, a handgun is the most common firearm used. Younger children are more likely to be involved in multivictim events or in family disputes and killed in a home (85%). Older children are more likely to die in the context of crime and violence (self-directed 38%, homicides 53%, or unintentional 6%) and have approximately the same likelihood of being killed in a home (39%) as on the streets (38%). Firearm-related deaths are the second-leading cause of injury-related death in children (ages 1 to 17 years), second only to motor vehicle accidents, and the third leading cause of death in children overall (Fowler et al., 2017). Adolescents need encouragement and education about ways to solve arguments without guns and violence, and guidance and direction for developing resources to cope with the stresses of daily living. Strategies to minimize firearm injuries should consider more global violence prevention strategies, poverty, social relationships, the environment, and other contextual factors related to social determinants of heath that contribute to a culture of violence.

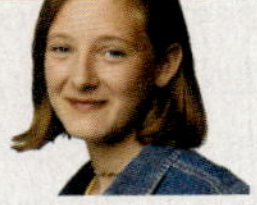

Think back to **Kara Greenwood**, the adolescent who is to present a discussion on adolescent dangers. Numerous issues face adolescents today; providing safety information is crucial to help adolescents make mature decisions about health hazards they are likely to encounter.

INTERNET AND SOCIAL MEDIA

The use of the Internet has grown, particularly among teenagers. This has prompted legitimate safety concerns by parents/caregivers. Certain people take advantage of the vulnerability of young children, teenagers, and adults with intellectual disabilities by stalking them online and exploiting them sexually and financially (Buijs et al., 2017). Meeting someone with whom the person has communicated online poses the greatest safety risk for children. Since online and offline safety risks are very similar, educational programs should focus on the integration of online dangers into long-standing efficacious programs that address things such as offline bullying, dating abuse, and sexual abuse/predators (Finkelhor et al., 2020). Safety guidelines for parents include addressing the following with their children:

- Remind adolescents that anything posted on the Internet is available to the public at large in perpetuity and can resurface at any time. Posts or tweets made today may impact on their ability to secure a job in the future.
- Keep identifying information private (e.g., full name, address, telephone number). Use a screen name that does not contain any identifying information.
- Investigate filtering software or methods of blocking out objectionable information.
- Ask for access to phone, social media accounts, and email, and maintain friend-status on your teen's Facebook, Instagram, Snapchat, and other online accounts.
- Ask teens to avoid public chat rooms and forums where they do not have a personal contact. Computer sex offenders often use chat rooms to contact potential victims.
- Never allow a child to arrange a meeting alone with someone the child has met online.
- Never respond to e-mails or messages that are suggestive, obscene, threatening, or inappropriate in any way. Be alert for downloaded files with suffixes that indicate images or pictures (e.g., .jpg, .gif, .bmp, .tif, or .pcx). If a parent/caregiver becomes aware of the transmission or viewing of child pornography while online, the adult should report this immediately to the local FBI office and the CyberTipline at the National Center for Missing and Exploited Children (1-800-843-5678).
- Emphasize that a good amount of what is said or written online may not be true. Teach tips for evaluating sites and promote online literacy.
- Monitor and set rules regarding the amount of time that adolescents spend on the computer or with their other devices (tablets, cell phones).
- Respect your teen's privacy as possible. Recognize that the Internet provides them the ability to socialize and connect with people—allow them space and provide them the tools they need to maintain their personal safety.

SEX TRAFFICKING

An amendment to the Justice for Victims of Trafficking Act of 2015 includes the need for identification, assessment, and reporting of suspected sex trafficking for anyone younger than age 24 years. Victims of sex trafficking may be younger than age 3 years (1%), but the percentages increase for older victims, with 71.9% of victims ages 14 to 17 years. The majority of the victims of sex trafficking are one of three races: White (41.6%), Black (23.5%), and Hispanic (19.3%), which is similar to the distribution for other maltreatment types. Although 16.1% of perpetrators are parents and 34.5% are known to be non-parents, more than half (54.3%) of the victims of sex trafficking have an unknown/missing relationship to their trafficker (U.S. Department of Health and Human Services, Administration for Children and Families, Administration on Children, Youth and Families, Children's Bureau, 2020). Although sex trafficking affects teens disproportionally, this is a public health issue that requires community engagement and monitoring, especially in communities where trafficking is more prevalent.

Adult

DRUG USE AND POISONING

Drug use trends among college-age adults (ages 19 to 22 years) has changed significantly over the past few years. Marijuana use is at an all-time 35-year high for college students and their non-college counterparts (43%), with daily/near daily use approximately twice as high among the non-college group. Nicotine vaping increased dramatically between 2017 and 2018, with numbers topping 15.5% for the college students and 12.5% for non-college students. Opioid misuse and binge drinking declined significantly in this age group. Adderall® misuse is higher among college students in general but varies in that college men and non-college women had higher rates than their counterparts (National Institute on Drug Abuse, 2019b).

In 2018, there were 67, 367 drug poisoning (overdose) deaths in the United States, which is a 4.1% drop from 2017. Causes were classified as unintentional (87.4%), suicides (7.2%), undetermined intent (5.2%) or homicides (less than 1%). Types of drugs involved included heroin, opioids (natural, synthetic, and semisynthetic), methadone, cocaine, psychostimulants with abuse potential, and combinations of these drugs. Increases in deaths attributed to drugs such a fentanyl or their analogs, cocaine, and psychostimulants were noted in 2018 (Hedegaard et al., 2020).

INTIMATE PARTNER VIOLENCE

Intimate partner violence (IPV) involves: physical violence (hitting kicking, or other physical force), sexual violence (forcing a sex act, sexual touching, or a nonphysical event without consent), stalking (a pattern of repeated, unwanted attention and contact) and/or psychological aggression (verbal and nonverbal communication intended to mentally or emotionally harm and/or exert control by a current or former intimate partner, such as a spouse, dating partner, or sexual partner). It is not uncommon for several types of IPV to occur in tandem (CDC, 2019e). For about 11 million women and 5 million men, IPV began in adolescence and is referred to as teen dating violence (TDV). In the United States, 36.4% of women experienced sexual violence, physical violence, and/or stalking by an intimate partner during their lifetime, with 25.1% of women reporting some

Vulnerable Population Alert

Intimate partner violence (IPV) most frequently occurs before age 25 years; many men and women first encounter IPV before age 18 years. This is a public health problem that requires a multifaceted approach to primary prevention and early intervention. The CDC has published technical packages that outline the *strategy*, the *approach*, and the *evidence* to prevent or reduce public health problems. Check out the violence prevention packages at https://www.cdc.gov/violenceprevention/pub/technical-packages.html.

residual IPV-related impact. More than one third (36.4%) of women experienced psychological aggression by an intimate partner during their lifetime. Men are also affected by IPV with 33.6% of men experiencing sexual violence, physical violence, and/or stalking; 34.2% experienced psychological aggression by an intimate partner during their lifetime (Smith et al., 2018).

The nurse is often the initial health care provider in contact with a victim of IPV or child abuse. Prompt recognition of the potential or actual threat to safety is crucial, and the nursing assessment may play a vital role in identifying a harmful environment. It is not always easy to confirm that a person has sustained injuries as a result of IPV. Many victims of IPV are reluctant to admit any abuse and may even deny that it has occurred. In fact, few victims of IPV ever seek help from the legal or health care systems (Breiding et al., 2015). Some studies have suggested that routine screening is effective, but most experts agree that asking simple, specific questions in a private setting (even the restroom, if the perpetrator is present) can also be helpful. Box 28-4 is an example of an assessment tool that the nurse can use to identify victims of IPV.

There are special clinical considerations for IPV in LGBTQ relationships. Although most aspects of IPV are similar to those identified in heterosexual and/or cisgender relationships, one aspect that is unique is the power inherent in *outing* a survivor's sexual or gender identity that may be used as a wedge to isolate the victim from family and other support system. Baseline discrimination based on sexual orientation or gender identity is compounded for those from racial/ethnic minority groups and those who are socioeconomically disadvantaged. Fears of the LGBTQ IPV survivor include fear of generating further negativity toward the LGBTQ community, fear of rejection from family members or friends who do not accept the underlying relationship, fear of the impact on their identity or future LGBTQ relationships, and fear of engaging with health care professionals or institutions who do not accept LGBTQ relationships (American Psychiatric Association, 2019). Assessment methods for identification of perpetrators and victims of IPV "should focus not on the sex, gender identity, or gender expression of the person but instead focus on a thorough assessment of empathy, agency, and entitlement" (American Psychiatric Association, 2019, p. 3). At least 49% of transgender and gender nonconforming people killed in 2019 were killed by someone known to the victim, or a friend, family member, or intimate partner. Young transgender women of color who live in the South are disproportionately affected (Human Rights Campaign Foundation, 2019). This provides an excellent example of **intersectionality**, where race, sex, gender, class, and other individual characteristics intersect and overlap with one another, often leading to an increased burden of discrimination on several fronts and other negative outcomes (Crenshaw, 1989). As with all cases of IPV, providers must work to understand the relationship as a whole and consider patterns that indicate a power differential, controlling behaviors, expressions of fear, decision-making dominance, and/or barriers to social engagement.

Nurses may assist in outlining the components of a safety plan (The National Domestic Violence Hotline, n.d.). IPV is a complex issue and simply leaving may not be an immediately viable option. Safety plans can include information on the following:

- Safety while living with an abusive partner: remove weapons, keep phone accessible, develop a signal to notify trusted friends and family, teach your children how to get help and how to get out safely, keep the car keys accessible and the car full of gas, minimize online footprint that can be used for location purposes, do not wear jewelry or scarves that could pose a threat to your safety, keep copies of important documents, create a *go-bag* with copies of important documents, medications, and other essentials.

Box 28-4 E-HITS Intimate Partner Violence Screening Instrument

Extended–Hurt, Insulted, Threaten, Scream

Over the last 12 months, how often did your partner:

1. Physically hurt you?
2. Insult your or talk down to you?
3. Threaten you with harm?
4. Scream or curse at you?
5. Force you to have sexual activities?

Each item is answered on a 5-point Likert scale:

- 1 = never
- 2 = rarely
- 3 = sometimes
- 4 = fairly often
- 5 = frequently

Score range: 5–25
Cutoff for IPV: ≥7

Source: Iverson, K. M., King, M. W., Gerber, M. R., Resick, P. A., Kimerling, R., Street, A. E., & Vogt, D. (2015). Accuracy of an intimate partner violence screening tool for female VHA patients: a replication and extension. *J Trauma Stress*, *28*(1), 79–82. https://doi.org/10.1002/jts.21985

- Safety planning with children: teach them how to call 911, teach them not to intervene, involve them in the plans for physical safety, teach them IPV is not their fault.
- Safety planning for pets: stock extra supplies, copy their medical records.
- Safety planning during pregnancy: recognize the heightened risk, utilize time with your provider to discuss IPV issues, take a female-only prenatal class.
- Emotional safety planning: seek out supportive people, identify and work toward goals, create a peaceful space in your environment for yourself, value yourself, remember you deserve to be kind to yourself.
- Leaving a relationship: keep evidence of abuse, plan with your children, use identified community resources, grab your go-bag, communicate your history and needs to new support systems, protect yourself and avoid the perpetrator after leaving, and consider your legal options.

Nurses must follow any policies or procedures outlined by their facility and document any interactions with victims of IPV. Many institutions have a trained victim advocate available. The nurse must keep in mind that regardless of the outcome, the victim of IPV has the right to self-determination without judgment—they often know what is best and their agency should be respected. Additional resources include the National Domestic Violence Hotline (1-800-799-SAFE), which will provide contact information regarding local domestic violence shelters and other resources, including those networks that are LGBTQ-focused.

Older Adult

FALLS

Although one of every four older people (age >65 years) falls each year, fewer than half of them tell their provider (CDC, 2017). Many falls at home go unreported because they do not cause injuries requiring medical attention. However, injuries from falls may also go unreported because older adults fear activity restrictions, loss of independence, or placement in a long-term care facility. The fear of falling can also cause anxiety and panic, which may make an older adult more vulnerable to a fall. One out of five falls causes a serious injury such as broken bones or a head injury. Interestingly, more than 95% of hip fractures are caused by falling, usually sideways from a ground-level fall. At least 300,000 older adults are hospitalized for hip fracture every year. This means that, when adjusted for inflation, the direct medical costs for fall injuries are $50 billion annually, with Medicare and Medicaid covering 75% of these costs (CDC, 2021a).

Assessment of the risk for falling includes the use of nursing history and physical examination. Ask about any previous falls—evidence shows that self-reported history of falls is a significant predictor of future falls and risk of fracture (Soh et al., 2020). Note any assistive devices that the patient uses (e.g., a cane or walker). Be alert to any history of drug or alcohol use disorder. Consider comorbidities such as obesity, osteoarthritis, diabetes, hypertension, chronic pain, depression, and any associated medications (Noohu et al., 2017). Characteristics of older adults most strongly associated with fall risk are depression, difficulty completing routine errands, and difficulty with ADLs (bathing or bathing); injuries from a fall are most strongly associated with depression, difficulty with ADLs, and single/unmarried status (Bergen et al., 2019). Family members and significant others are often valuable resources. Knowledge of family support systems and the home environment is crucial for the nurse to plan protective health measures. Since the mid-1980s, a fall is generally categorized as either an *accidental fall* (fall of otherwise low-risk adults; clutter or a spill cause a person to trip), an *anticipated physiologic fall* (a direct consequence of gait imbalances, effects of medication, or dementia), or an *unanticipated physiologic fall* (caused by unknown or unexpected medical issues such as a stroke or seizure; Morse et al., 1987). An initiative from the CDC, STEADI (Stopping Elderly Accidents, Deaths & Injuries; CDC, 2019b) provides an excellent algorithm for health care provider fall risk screening, assessment, and intervention (Table 28-1 on page 850 and Fig. 28-1 on page 850).

Major causes of falls in the home include slippery surfaces, poor lighting, clutter, and improperly fitting clothing or slippers. Common traffic pathways in the home, the bathroom, and access areas to and from the home are hazardous areas for older adults. Measures as simple as installing handrails in bathrooms and on stairs, ensuring good lighting, and discarding or repairing broken equipment around the home help prevent accidents (see Box 28-1, page 841). Assessments by the nurse can play a vital role in promoting safety in the home.

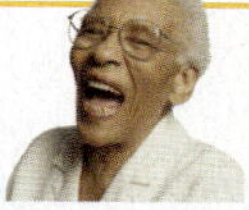

Consider **Bessie Washington**, the older woman who ambulates with a walker after suffering a stroke. A thorough home safety assessment by the home care nurse is essential when developing the patient's plan of care. This assessment would be valuable in identifying areas that promote patient safety and hazards that need to be addressed.

Evidence supports the positive role that calcium supplementation and vitamin D play in promoting skeletal health and reducing fall risk for this population (CDC, 2019b). Regular exercise has a positive effect on bone and muscle strength, balance, and flexibility of joints. Exercise, particularly regimens including stability-challenging exercises, has been proven to reduce the number of falls by 32% and the number of people who fall by 22% (Hamed et al., 2018).

MOTOR VEHICLE ACCIDENTS

Most accidents that involve older adults are preventable. Although older adults tend to wear safety belts, observe speed limits, drive fewer miles, and abstain from drinking while driving, due to age-related vulnerabilities, medical conditions, and prolonged recovery risks, seniors have the highest crash death rate after adolescents (AAA, 2022). Vision changes, slowed reaction time, alterations in judgment, and decreased range of motion affect the older driver. Some become overly cautious, whereas others are prone to careless behavior. Teach the following interventions to help older adults drive safely: maintain the automobile in optimal

Table 28-1 Fall Risk Factors

MODIFIABLE	
• Poor gait and balance • Strength issues • Visual impairment • Problems with feet and/or shoes • Comorbidities documented (depression, osteoporosis)	• Use of medications that increase falls risk • Orthostatic hypotension • Hazards in the home (and community) • Vitamin D deficiency
Start by addressing these modifiable issues that can be either intrinsic or extrinsic	
INTRINSIC (PERSON-BASED)	**EXTRINSIC (ENVIRONMENT-BASED)**
Advanced age	Lack of stair handrails
Previous falls	Poor stair design
Muscle weakness	Lack of bathroom grab bars
Gait and balance problems	Dim lighting or glare
Poor vision	Obstacles and tripping hazards
Postural hypotension	Slippery or uneven surfaces
Comorbidities and vitamin D deficiencies	Medications
Fear of falling	Improper use of assistive devices (canes, walkers)

Source: Adapted Centers for Disease Control and Prevention (CDC). (2019b). *Resource algorithm for fall risk screening, assessment, and intervention.* https://www.cdc.gov/steadi/pdf/STEADI-Algorithm-508.pdf

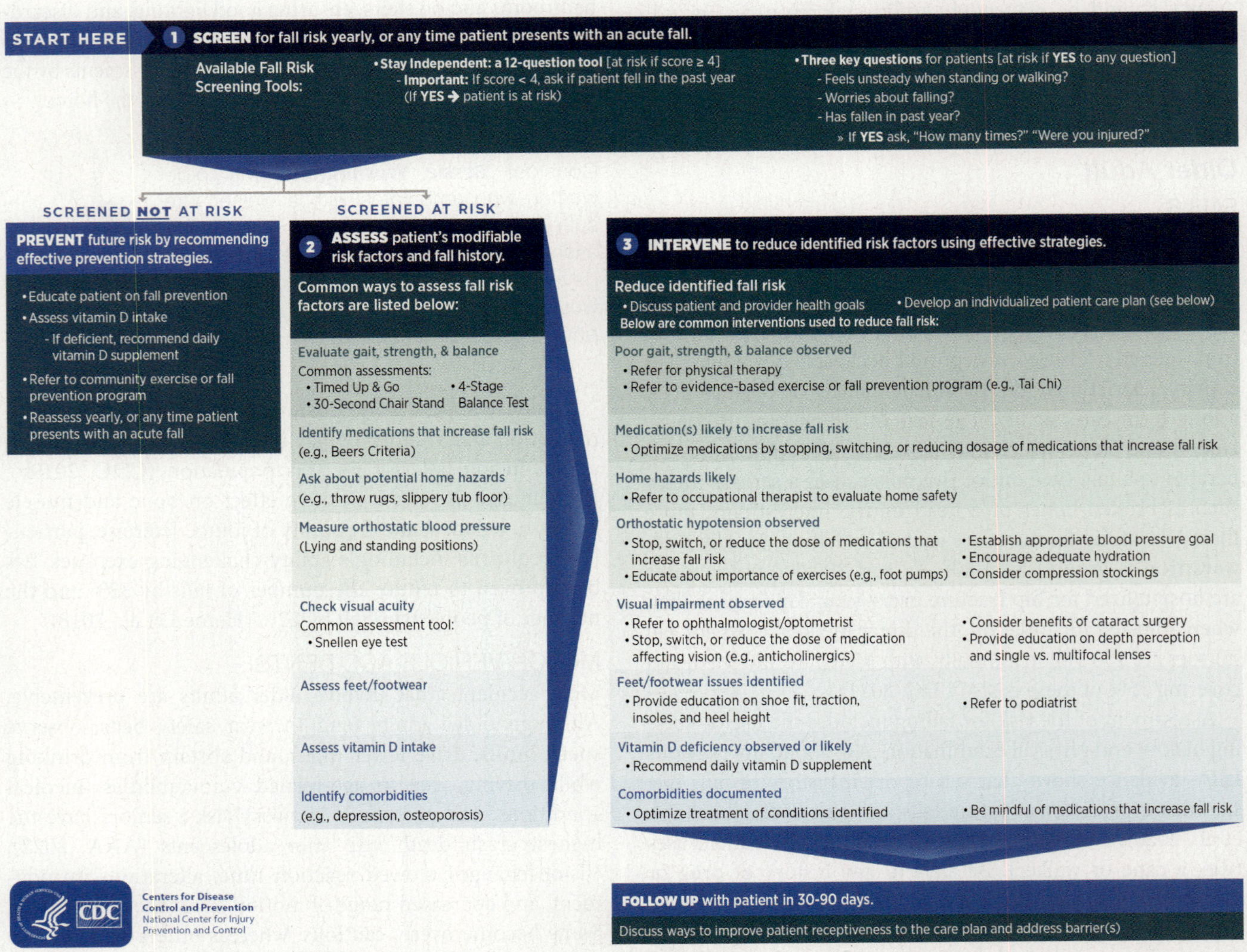

FIGURE 28-1. Algorithm for Fall Risk Assessment and Interventions. (*Source:* From the Centers for Disease Control and Prevention [CDC, 2019b] and Stopping Elderly Accidents, Deaths & Injuries [STEADI]. https://www.cdc.gov/steadi/pdf/STEADI-Algorithm-508.pdf)

Focus on the Older Adult

TEACHING TIPS TO PREVENT MEDICATION-RELATED POISONING

Age-Related Changes	Nursing Strategies
Confusion	• Do not hesitate to call the provider, nurse, or pharmacist with any questions. • Develop good communication with your provider, nurse, and pharmacist. • Use a medication calendar or diary to keep track of your dosing schedule. • Use a pill dispenser or pre-filled medication packs as a reminder tool.
Reduced vision	• Request large-print labels from your pharmacist.
Polypharmacy	• Report side effects from medications to your health care provider. • Do not share medications with others or take their pills. • When a drug is discontinued, discard any remaining medication appropriately. • Fill all your prescriptions at one pharmacy.
Effect of drugs in the aging body	• Keep the telephone numbers for your health care providers and the PCC in a readily accessible place. • Do not stop taking any prescription drug or change the dose without first consulting the provider or nurse. • Avoid doubling a dose if you forget a medication. Check with the health care provider or nurse first. • Avoid mixing alcohol with medicines without first checking with the pharmacist.

driving condition, schedule regular eye examinations, wear corrective lenses when necessary, drive less after dark, avoid driving in bad weather, avoid difficult roads during peak traffic times, and keep noise from the radio and other equipment to a minimum. Some states require additional testing for older adults before they can renew their driver's license.

FIRE

Fires also are a significant hazard for older adults, representing 40% of all fire deaths, with 2.7 times (age >65 years) and 3.8 times (age >85 years) greater risk of dying in a fire than the total population (U.S. Fire Administration, 2020). Factors such as confusion, forgetfulness, and diminished visual and olfactory senses place them at greater risk for burn injuries. Health teaching should include additional safety precautions if the older adult smokes in the home. Because it may be difficult to distinguish the intensity of temperatures, heating devices often used by older adults need to be carefully monitored and regulated. Smoke detectors indicate the presence of a fire that may not be recognized by an older adult with a diminished sense of smell.

POLYPHARMACY AND POISONING

Accidental overdosing on medications is also a safety risk, possibly related to poor eyesight or confusion. Special devices such as medication trays or electronic dispensing systems can be prefilled to help prevent older adults from taking additional doses (see Remote Medication Monitoring System in Chapter 30 on p. 940).

Nursing education efforts can also change behaviors that place older adults at risk for medication-related poisoning. Although poisonings happen more frequently in children, providers receive many calls from adults, particularly older adults, regarding accidental poisonings. Suggestions for preventing poisoning in older adults are included in the accompanying box, Focus on the Older Adult.

ELDER ABUSE

Elder abuse has no universally accepted definition, but legal, professional, and governmental definitions include elements of physical, sexual, and/or psychological abuse, neglect (including abandonment), and/or financial exploitation. The perpetrator is generally known and trusted by the vulnerable elder, the perpetrator's actions are intentional, and the end-result is a serious risk of harm to an older adult (U.S. Department of Health and Human Services, Administration for Community Living, n.d.; See Chapter 23 for a more complete description of the types of elder abuse.) Given the expanding number of people older than age 65 years, the incidence of maltreatment in this vulnerable population is expected to escalate. In most of the reported cases, a family member is the one who abused the older adult. Disability, dementia, and place of residence (private home or community setting) all impact the type, duration, and residual physical, psychological, financial, social, and other effects of elder abuse (U.S. Department of Health and Human Services, Administration for Community Living, n.d.). Nurses must be alert to any indications of elder abuse, document any injuries or behaviors that suggest elder abuse, and report suspected incidents to appropriate facilities in states where it is required. It is important to observe and objectively document voice tone, interactions, and personal touch between the older adult and a caregiver. If abuse is suspected, speak to the older adult in a private setting away from the caregiver, and work with the interprofessional team to coordinate expertise, resources, and interventions. Follow all guidelines and protocols regarding reporting and best practices (U.S. Department of Health and Human Services, Administration for Community Living, n.d.). When possible, addressing caregiver stress and caregiver substance abuse issues may help to prevent elder abuse.

Patient Environments

Certain work, social, and home environments inherently place people in more hazardous situations. Habits and routines fostered by the environment also directly impact safety risks. For example, following the law and wearing a seatbelt, if taught from a young age, becomes second nature. Do not forget to consider developmental issues discussed earlier in this chapter within the context of environment. For example, young and middle-aged adults need to be reminded about the effects of stress on their lifestyle and health. Coping with the demands of raising a family and succeeding in a career may lead to unsafe health habits and an often socially acceptable use of drugs or alcohol.

Work Environment

Occupation and work environment often affect a person's safety. People who work in certain occupations may experience exposure to health hazards, such as excessive noise, pollution, toxic chemicals or vapors, or infectious agents. For example, a worker who operates industrial machinery or works with chemicals has a greater risk for accidental injury. Exposure to excessive noise (e.g., a construction site, extremely loud music) may lead to hearing loss. Health care staff who suffer sleep deprivation due to extended work hours and variable shift assignments are more likely to commit errors and be a factor in adverse events (see further discussion in Chapter 34). Nurses working in the operating room are regularly exposed to surgical smoke, a byproduct of laser and electrocautery procedures. Surgical smoke contains chemicals that cause upper respiratory tract irritation and inflammation.

> **Self-Care Alert**
>
> Nurses working the operating room who are exposed to surgical smoke must complete competency validation, participate in ongoing education and training, and engage in the review of policies and procedures to promote the health and well-being of themselves and the entire surgical team.

Operating room personnel must be empowered to use smoke-evacuation practices (Association of periOperative Registered Nurses [AORN], 2020). Reproductive hazards may exist for females with long-term exposure to certain anesthetic agents. Certain drugs can also pose risks to health care professionals, but regulations and standards exist to protect health care personnel. For example, General Chapter <800> outlines a standard generated by the U.S. Pharmacopeial (USP) Convention (2019) that describes quality and practice standards for health care personnel, including nurses, who handle hazardous drugs. Nurses remain at increased risk for musculoskeletal (back) injuries, needlestick and sharp injuries, exposure to hazardous and toxic chemicals, radiation exposure, exposure to infectious diseases, stress that includes moral distress, and workplace violence. Workplace violence, consisting of both physical and psychological damage, has been identified as a major issue for health care providers (American Nurses Association, 2019). The Joint Commission has issued a sentinel event alert on workplace violence that specifically addresses the prevention of physical and verbal violence, and promotes reporting of violence in the health care setting (The Joint Commission, 2018).

Nurses need to adhere to standards, guidelines, recommendations, and policies to promote safety and minimize preventable injury.

Social Environment

Some people by nature are more inclined to take risks and jeopardize their safety. For example, some people do not use appropriate protective equipment, such as wearing a helmet when riding a motorcycle or bicycle. Such behaviors, whether voluntary (refusal) or involuntary (cannot afford) increase the risk for injury.

Stress may precipitate an unhealthy lifestyle that involves drug or alcohol abuse. For example, a high school student involved in multiple school activities and intent on maintaining excellent grades may turn to an addictive substance such as methamphetamine as a stimulant. This drug temporarily allows the student to remain alert for more hours each day and complete required class assignments but has significant negative consequences. See the PICOT in Practice box for more information.

Vulnerable populations also need support and attention, regardless of the circumstances that made them vulnerable. Social determinants of health include aspects of social and physical environments that involve key issues related to economic stability, neighborhood and built environment, social and community context, health and health care, and education (see Chapter 3, p. 56). A person's sense of security and well-being are directly tied to conditions in the environment where they reside. Addressing the health disparities and inequities in an environment, particularly those at the system or institutional level (e.g., racism or discrimination against LGBTQIA+ persons), requires a change in practice, policies, research, and community partnerships that will directly affect health outcomes, as well as public safety, social isolation, education, violence, and unequal access to resources (CDC, 2019h; U.S. Department of Health and Human Services, Office of Disease Prevention and Health Promotion, 2020a). Nurses have always been strong patient advocates regarding safety concerns for vulnerable populations. See Nursing Advocacy in Action for an example of a nurse supporting a vulnerable patient's safety and health.

Home Environment

Environmental safety hazards can result in poisoning and fires. Nursing assessment includes identifying people at risk and recognizing unsafe situations that involve both physical and interpersonal dangers (see discussions of abuse and IPV earlier in this chapter). Recognizing these factors helps the

PICOT in Practice

ASKING CLINICAL QUESTIONS

Scenario: You are a public health nurse working for the local Health Department. As part of a national smoking cessation initiative, you are planning a presentation on different options to help those who want to quit smoking. Previous presentations have concentrated on nicotine replacement therapies (NRTs) and/or counseling to assist those interested in smoking cessation. You wonder if electronic cigarettes (e-cigarettes) that typically contain nicotine, have any role in helping people stop smoking.

E-cigarettes have become popular, especially with younger smokers, and you wonder if you could leverage this popularity and use e-cigarettes (with nicotine) in place of other NRTs. You decide to research the topic further to see if the use of e-cigarettes (with nicotine) can help an individual quit smoking.

- **Population:** Smokers who wish to quit
- **Intervention:** Use of electronic cigarettes
- **Comparison:** Nicotine replacement therapy
- **Outcome:** Smoking cessation
- **Time:** 12 months

PICOT Question: In smokers who wish to quit, does the use of e-cigarettes (with nicotine) compared to NRTs help achieve smoking cessation in a 12-month period?

Findings:

1. Hartmann-Boyce, J., McRobbie, H., Lindson, N., Bullen, C., Begh, R., Theodoulou, A., Notley, C., Rigotti, N. A., Turner, T., Butler, A. R., & Hajek, P. (2020). Electronic cigarettes for smoking cessation. *Cochrane Database of Systematic Reviews.* Issue 10, Art. No.: CD004346. https://doi.org/10.1002/14651858.CD010216.pub4

Included 50 completed studies, representing 12,430 participants, of which 26 are randomized controlled trials (RCTs). Thirty-five of the 50 included studies were new to this review update. There was moderate-certainty evidence that e-cigarettes (with nicotine) increase quit rates compared to e-cigarettes without nicotine and compared to NRTs. Evidence comparing e-cigarettes (with nicotine) with usual care/no treatment also suggests a benefit, but it was less certain.

2. Grabovac, I., Oberndorfer, M., Fischer, J., Wiesinger, W., Haider, S., & Dorner, T. E. (2021). Effectiveness of electronic cigarettes in smoking cessation: A systematic review and meta-analysis. *Nicotine & Tobacco Research, 23*(4), 625–634. https://doi.org/org/10.1093/ntr/ntaa181

The search yielded 13,950 publications with 12 studies being identified as eligible for systematic review ($N = 8{,}362$) and 9 for random-effects meta-analyses (range: 30 to 6,006 participants). The results suggest that e-cigarettes (with nicotine) may be more effective in smoking cessation when compared to placebo electronic cigarettes or NRT. When compared to counseling alone, e-cigarettes (with nicotine) are more effective short term, but its effectiveness appears to diminish with later follow-ups.

Level of Evidence: Level I: systematic review

Recommendations: There is moderate-certain evidence that e-cigarettes (with nicotine) increase smoking cessation rates. Though there is some research to suggest that quit rates are short term, the combination of counseling and adjunct therapies might assist individuals long term. You include these findings in your presentation to the community along with additional information on counseling services as well as adjunct nicotine therapies to help reach smoking cessation.

nurse develop an individualized plan of care and nursing interventions for protecting the patient in the home.

All health care providers should recommend that a carbon monoxide (CO) detector be installed to alert family members to toxic levels of the gas. Gas or oil companies and the local health authority can help identify and remove sources of contamination. Many states and communities now require installation of CO detectors in residences. (See Box 28-1, page 841, for additional tips for preventing poisoning.)

Most exposures to toxic fumes occur in the home. Poisoning may result from improper mixing of household substances, prolonged use of strong cleaning products, or

Nursing Advocacy in Action

Patient Scenario

Ms. Jackson was admitted to the labor and delivery unit in active labor. She is in prison for killing her husband and is accompanied to the hospital by two armed guards. She is in shackles in the labor room "to prevent her escape." When you begin your shift, you find a woman in hysterics who has been in labor for 12 hours because of the position of the baby. You want to get her shackles off to try to make her more comfortable, but the guards aren't willing to help. They explain that it is policy to keep them on for felons like Ms. Jackson. You are horrified.

Implications for Nursing Advocacy

How will you respond if you are Ms. Jackson's nurse? Talk with your classmates and experienced nurses about the questions that follow:

- If you elect to advocate for Ms. Jackson and other women like her, what practical steps can you take to reflect your moral agency and work to develop policies and procedures that meet the requirements of law enforcement, but allow for compassionate, person-centered nursing care?
- What is reasonable to expect of a student nurse, a graduate nurse, and an experienced nurse in this situation?
- What advocacy skills are needed to effectively respond to this challenge?

malfunctioning household appliances (gas, oil, and kerosene heaters) that can release CO. CO is a poisonous gas that is also colorless, odorless, and tasteless, which makes it especially dangerous. Exposure can result in mild symptoms or progress to a life-threatening problem or long-term effects. CO toxicity can cause severe organ damage in a very short period of time. More than 150 people in the United States die each year from (non–fire-related) accidental CO poisoning (U.S. Consumer Product Safety Commission, n.d.).

Nurses need to review existing fire prevention strategies and escape plans in their home safety assessment. Ensuring homes have a working, high-quality smoke alarm that is tested regularly is the highest priority. Box 28-1 (on page 841) lists important fire safety issues as well as other safety issues that should be addressed when assessing for risk factors in the home. Fire, injury from fire, and fire-related deaths increased by 2% from 2008 to 2017 but are still less than a third the rate in the late 1970s. Based on data collected by the U.S. Fire Administration (2019), residential fires (29%) are second in prevalence only to outdoor fires (43%). It is important to note that 78% of all fire deaths occur in the home (U.S. Fire Administration). Cooking is the leading cause of residential building fires (52%). Heating caused 9% of residential fires. Residential fires that result in fatalities are most often related to careless actions (17%), followed by causes under investigation (14%), intentional actions (13%), and smoking (12%; U.S. Fire Administration). Most fatal home fires occur while people are sleeping, and most people who die in house fires die of smoke inhalation rather than burns. The widespread availability and use of home smoke alarms is considered the primary reason for the significant decline in fire-related injury and death. Low-cost smoke alarm options increase home-prevention accessibility for all people, including those for whom cost is a consideration. Work is being done to fine-tune smoke detectors to minimize nuisance alarms that sound with the detection of any smoke aerosol particles, even those created by routine cooking. This is important because these nuisance alarms result in people disconnecting the wires or removing the batteries from their smoke alarm, thereby rendering it useless (Warmack et al., 2015).

Accidents in the home frequently result from careless use of equipment or from malfunctioning or poorly maintained equipment. Many injuries and deaths from electric shock can be prevented. Overloaded electrical circuits, faulty appliances, frayed wires, careless use of electrical equipment, and handling of electrical devices and cords with wet hands or while wearing wet shoes can result in injury or death. (See Box 28-1, page 841, for specific guidelines to prevent electrical injury.)

Functional Ability

Mobility

Any limitation in mobility is potentially unsafe. An older adult with an unsteady gait is more prone to falling. Furthermore, if the patient is in an unfamiliar setting, such as a health care facility, the problem may be aggravated. Someone with paralysis or a spinal cord injury may require assistance with even simple movements. Supportive devices—such as canes, walkers, and wheelchairs—may facilitate movement, but they require careful patient instruction and preparation for safe use. Recent surgery or a prolonged illness can temporarily affect a patient's mobility and necessitate special precautions to prevent falls or injuries. Nurses must assess a patient's risk for injury with a view toward maintaining independence and fostering self-esteem while providing a safe and predictable environment.

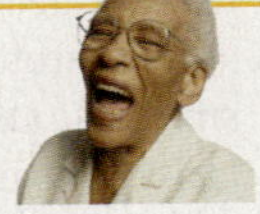

Think back to **Bessie Washington**, the 77-year-old woman who experienced a stroke, lives alone in a small apartment, and requires a walker to ambulate. To ensure that the patient remains safe, the nurse needs to assess the patient's home environment closely for hazards. This is especially important for Bessie based on her statement that she almost fell recently.

Sensory Perception

Alterations in sensory perception can have a devastating effect on safety. Any impairment in sight, hearing, smell, taste, or touch can reduce a person's sensitivity to the environment. Vision changes may cause a person to stumble, lose their balance, and fall. In 2014, a CDC analysis determined that the state-specific annual prevalence of falls among older adults (age >65 years) with severe vision impairment ranged from 30.8% to 59.1%. Prevalence of falls in older adults without severe vision impairment ranged from 20.4% to 32.4% (Crews et al., 2016). Declines in visual acuity, contrast sensitivity, depth perception, visual field, and visual motion perception related to the illusion of self-motion, postural control, and balance control all contribute to the risk of injury related to visual changes (Saftari & Kwon, 2018). A patient with a hearing deficit may not be able to hear safety alarms, automobile horns, or sirens and may not hear health care instructions. A patient with a reduced ability to distinguish odors may fail to detect leaking gas or smoke. A patient with a loss of taste may have unsafe eating habits or may eat tainted food. A patient whose tactile sense is impaired may not perceive temperature extremes that are a threat to safety.

Ability to Communicate

The ability to communicate is basic to many safety practices. The nurse must assess any factor that influences the patient's ability to receive and send messages. Fatigue, stress, medication, aphasia, and language barriers are examples of factors that can affect personal communication and prevent the patient from accurately perceiving events. For example, a medication side effect of drowsiness may interfere with a health teaching session between the nurse and the patient taking this medication. A valid assessment by the nurse not only identifies the patient's level of understanding, but also facilitates a positive communication experience.

Knowledge

An awareness of safety and security precautions is crucial for promoting and maintaining wellness throughout the lifespan. For example, patients need instructions to adhere to a medical regimen or to follow safety precautions when oxygen is in use. They require a certain amount of knowledge to manage new equipment and unfamiliar procedures. Nursing assessment includes identifying and recognizing potentially threatening circumstances caused by a lack of knowledge regarding safety and security precautions. Patient teaching about safety is crucial and must be individualized, take into account health literacy, and be leveled appropriately for patients and families.

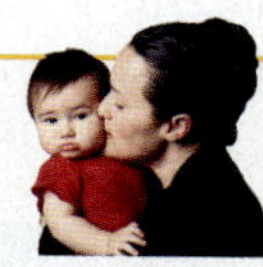

Recall **Juanita Flores**, the young mother of the 1-year-old who fell from a cot. The nurse's knowledge of potential threats to safety for infants, in conjunction with providing anticipatory guidance to the mother about safety issues for infants, would be essential to prevent future potential injury.

Health

Physical Health State

When a person is chronically ill or in a weakened state, the focus of health care includes preventing accidents as well as promoting wellness and restoring the person to a healthy state. For example, the nurse caring for a patient who is recovering from a stroke (cerebral vascular accident) identifies the patient's neuromuscular impairment, pays particular attention to health teaching concerning the person's ability to maintain a sense of balance, and carefully assists the patient with ambulation to prevent falls. Many patients who fall have a primary or secondary diagnosis of cardiovascular disease. Prevention of complications and return to the optimal level of functioning require attention to safety and become primary concerns in a rehabilitation program. The nurse strives to maximize the patient's potential by considering safety factors in all phases of the illness and recovery experience.

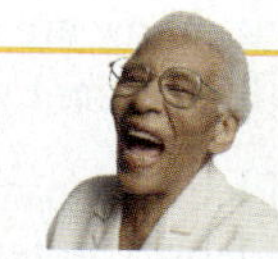

Consider **Bessie Washington**, the woman who is now at home after having a stroke. The nurse would incorporate knowledge of safety factors along with knowledge of Bessie's mobility limitations to develop a plan of care that maximizes her potential while maintaining her safety.

Psychosocial Health State

Stressful situations tend to narrow a person's attention span and make the person more prone to accidents. Stress may occur over a long period, but the effects tend to be more devastating in the person's later years, when there is typically less adaptive and coping capacity. Depression may result in confusion and disorientation, accompanied by reduced awareness or concern about environmental hazards. Social isolation or lack of social contact may lead to a reduced level of concentration, errors in judgment, and a diminished awareness of external stimuli.

Nursing Process

An assessment of the patient may lead to the identification of one or more diagnoses or patient problem related to actual or potential safety issues. Following the formulation of the diagnoses or patient problems, the nurse communicates findings to other nursing and health care professionals through the use of the written and spoken word. The written diagnosis or patient problem becomes a permanent part of the patient's health record. Examples of health problems and needs with related etiology and signs and symptoms can be found in the box titled Examples of Actual or Potential Health Problems and Needs: Safety and Security.

Many accidental injuries and deaths are preventable. Consider the various factors and the environment that affect the patient's safety, and formulate expected outcomes uniquely suited to each situation and circumstance. Nursing

Examples of Actual or Potential Health Problems and Needs

SAFETY AND SECURITY

Actual or Potential Health Problems and Needs	Possible Etiologic Factors	Potential Signs and Symptoms
Risk for Fall	• Absence of stairway gate or window guard (children) • Difficulty with gait • Inadequate supervision • Insufficient knowledge of modifiable factors • Unsafe home environment	—
Risk for Poisoning	• Access to dangerous product • Access to pharmaceutical agent • Insufficient knowledge of pharmacologic agents • Occupational setting without adequate safeguards • Insufficient vision	—

Source: International Council of Nurses (ICN). (2019). *Nursing diagnosis and outcome statements.* https://www.icn.ch/sites/default/files/inline-files/ICNP2019-DC.pdf

interventions focus on meeting these safety needs. Some expected outcomes for patients that promote safety and prevent injury are as follows.

The patient will:

- Identify unsafe situations in their environment
- Identify potential hazards in their environment
- Demonstrate safety measures to prevent falls and other accidents
- Establish safety priorities with family members or significant others
- Demonstrate familiarity with their environment
- Identify resources for safety information

Nursing interventions are designed for each developmental level as well as for specific hazards in the environment. Adults who are developmentally disabled or who are experiencing dementia or delirium may require the same safety measures typically considered for children. Injury control includes preventing injuries, providing acute care for injured patients, and rehabilitation services. The emphasis needs to be on injury prevention, which promotes the reduction of injuries through eliminating risky events, measuring the consequences of these events, and reducing the severity of injuries. Skill 28-1 on pages 871–872 demonstrates the proper method for performing a situational assessment. Interventions that include modification of the environment and education for at-risk people have proven effective.

Teaching is an important intervention for accident prevention and health promotion. Many teaching opportunities concerning safety measures arise while the nurse performs regular patient care, and many resources are available to supplement health teaching (Fig. 28-2). Also, remember that

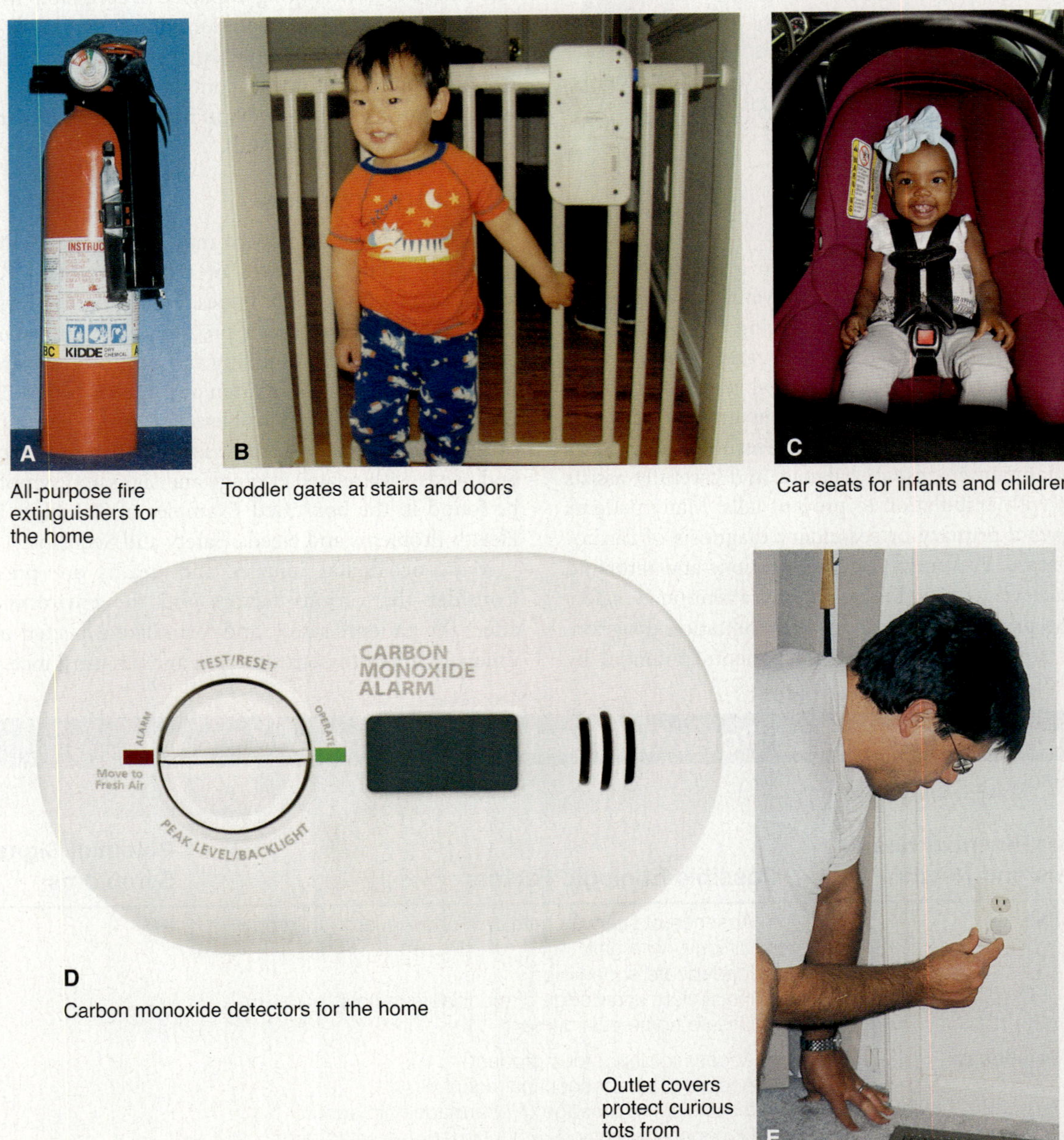

A All-purpose fire extinguishers for the home

B Toddler gates at stairs and doors

C Car seats for infants and children

D Carbon monoxide detectors for the home

E Outlet covers protect curious tots from electrical shock

FIGURE 28-2. The nurse's responsibilities in home safety are primarily that of education and counseling, including providing information about home safety devices and sources for additional information. (*Source:* C. Courtesy of K. Bartlett.)

nurses who role model good health behaviors are more effective teachers. Careful assessment, diagnosis, and planning prepare nurses to use these opportunities wisely. Assessment data and statistical information often provide helpful information for health care personnel who are developing a safety program for patients at risk. Safety education classes, in addition to situational health teaching, can be worthwhile for hospitalized patients and their family members. Studies have demonstrated that early assessment of vulnerable patients and preventive education programs can decrease the incidence of falls and promote safety.

Evaluation is the final step of the nursing process. Nurses must evaluate the effectiveness of their interventions to promote environmental safety, prevent injury, and promote emergency preparedness. If the expected patient outcomes have been met and evaluative criteria have been satisfied, the patient should be able to accomplish the following:

- Correctly identify real and potential unsafe environmental situations
- Implement safety measures in the environment
- Use available resources to obtain safety information
- Incorporate accident prevention practices into activities of daily living
- Remain free of injury

ASPECTS OF SAFETY AND SECURITY

All four spheres of practice-prevention and promotion of health and well-being, chronic disease care, regenerative (critical and trauma) care, and hospice and palliative care (American Association of Colleges of Nursing, 2021)-involve interactions with patients, families, and communities where safety and security must be considered. Health care encompasses interactions that occur in primary, secondary, and tertiary settings. This section will highlight these points of contact and specifically consider the acute care (hospital) setting as an exemplar.

Patient Safety

Admission to a heath care facility requires intentional consideration of person-centered risks and injury prevention strategies. The initial assessment performed by the nurse upon admission to a health care facility summarizes all of this information (refer to Nursing History in Chapter 15).

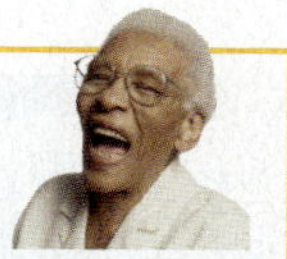

Recall **Bessie Washington**, the older adult woman described at the beginning of the chapter. Based on the assessment of the patient, the nurse would identify Bessie's risk for falls as high. It would be crucial to incorporate this information into her plan of care to ensure her safety.

Orienting the Person to Surroundings

A person who is familiar with one's surroundings is less likely to experience an accidental injury. As part of the hospital admission routine, orient the patient to the safety features and equipment in the room. An explanation and demonstration of the adjustable bed and side rails, call system, telephone, television, and bathroom help the patient adjust to the new environment. The patient identification bracelet and a discussion of facility routine further ensure safety and assist the patient to adapt to the unfamiliar setting. Disruption in routine, unfamiliar surroundings, competing priorities, and the physiologic and psychological effects of illness contribute to the stress experienced by all patients. Use this orientation as an opportunity to demonstrate the importance of orienting an older adult to new surroundings when the older adult moves in with a family member or moves to a new residential community.

Technology Alert

As part of the admission process, many electronic health records (EHRs) have embedded one or more questions regarding safety: *Do you feel safe in your home? Do you feel safe in your relationships? Do you feel like you may be in danger in your home?* The challenge for providers is to attribute meaning and context for these questions, and to ask them at an appropriate time (Hunt et al. 2017).

Preventing Falls in the Health Care Facility

Health care facilities have fall prevention programs that are enacted for the duration of the patient's stay and are designed to facilitate discussion regarding safety at home and in the community. National initiatives encourage health care providers to ask these three questions at every encounter with older adults:

1. Have you fallen in the past year?
2. Do you feel unsteady when standing or walking?
3. Do you worry about falling?

Figure 28-1 (on page 850) depicts the CDC's STEADI decision-making algorithm for determining and addressing fall risk. Nurses are responsible for identifying patients who are at high risk for falls, documenting pertinent assessments on the chart, and planning appropriate interventions to ensure their safety. A nurse whose behavior is reasonable, prudent, and similar to the behavior that would be expected of another nurse in similar circumstances is unlikely to be found liable if a patient falls, even if the fall results in an injury.

Concept Mastery Alert

Of the many ways to avoid falls in the acute care setting, the best outcome for a patient at risk for falling is that the patient will not experience a fall and remains free of injury.

The Joint Commission requires that hospitals implement fall prevention assessments and programs; they also require reporting, with a root cause analysis, of falls deemed a **sentinel event**, which is an unexpected occurrence involving death or serious physical or psychological injury, or

Box 28-5 Nursing Interventions to Prevent Falls in a Health Care Facility

- Complete a risk assessment.
- Indicate risk for falling on patient's door and chart.
- Keep bed in low position.
- Keep wheels on bed and wheelchair locked.
- Leave call bell within patient's reach.
- Instruct patient regarding use of call bell.
- Answer call bells promptly.
- Leave a night light on.
- Eliminate all physical hazards in the room (clutter, wet areas on the floor).
- Provide nonskid footwear.
- Leave water, tissues, bedpan/urinal within patient's reach.
- Move bedside commode out of sight to discourage attempts at independent transfer (as appropriate).
- Document and report any changes in patient's cognitive status to the health care team at the change of shift.
- Use alternative strategies when necessary instead of restraints.
- As a last resort, use the least restrictive restraint according to facility policy.
- If restraint is applied, assess patient at the required intervals.

the risk of death or injury (The Joint Commission, 2022c); see "Sentinel Events" on page 164 in Chapter 7, Legal Dimensions of Nursing Practice. The Centers for Medicare and Medicaid Services (CMS) has identified falls as a *never event* (medical error that should never occur) and includes falls and trauma on its list of Hospital Acquired Conditions (HAC) for which reimbursement will be limited, specifically for falls that result in fractures, dislocations, and/or intracranial injuries (U.S. Department of Health and Human Services, Agency for Healthcare Research and Quality, 2019b). Safety measures recommended to reduce the number of falls in acute and extended-care facilities are given in Box 28-5.

A simple evaluation tool can help identify hospitalized patients at risk for falling. According to accreditation standards, the Hendrich II Fall Risk Model™, which can be administered quickly, evaluates eight independent risk factors. This tool also includes the Get Up and Go Test that measures a person's ability to rise from a seated position. Performance on each physiologic factor merits a specific score and identifies those most at risk for falls. The Morse Fall Scale is another tool frequently used. Institutions can use the score on the Morse Fall Scale, derived from the answers to six questions, to identify patients at risk for falls. View the Hendrich II Fall Risk Model™ and the Morse Fall Scale in Student Resources online for this text.

In response to The Joint Commission's mandate that accredited health care organizations must reduce the risk of harm to patients resulting from falls, hospitals have implemented effective programs to safeguard their patients from falls. Examples of these improvement strategies include:

- *Preventing Falls Targeted Solutions Tool (TST)*: An online application from The Joint Commission for Transforming Healthcare (2022) that provides a systematic approach to reduce the rate of falls.
- *Falls Toolkit*: A comprehensive toolkit that contains elements such as a falls notebook (with instructions, policies, and training materials), post-fall huddle guides, hospital/staff/community assessment tools, podcasts, website links, and other tools (U.S. Department of Veterans Affairs, 2019).
- *Falls Prevention Training Program:* A program highlighting the importance of staff orientation and periodic, ongoing training; includes education for staff on the intrinsic and extrinsic risks of falling, environmental assessments, and falls prevention strategies (ECRI, 2018).
- *Root Cause Analysis (RCA):* A tool used to study health care–related (actual) *adverse events* and *close calls*. The RCA process is designed to find out what happened, why it happened, and how to prevent it from happening again. The RCA process supports the development of a culture of safety at an institution (United States Department of Veteran Affairs, 2018).

Polypharmacy has long been listed as a risk factor for falls—the changes in medication regimen while hospitalized further compound this issue. Research indicates that adverse effects related to the specific medication categories of antiepileptics and benzodiazepines are more predictive of falling. Some common safety devices used in health care facilities are shown in Figure 28-3.

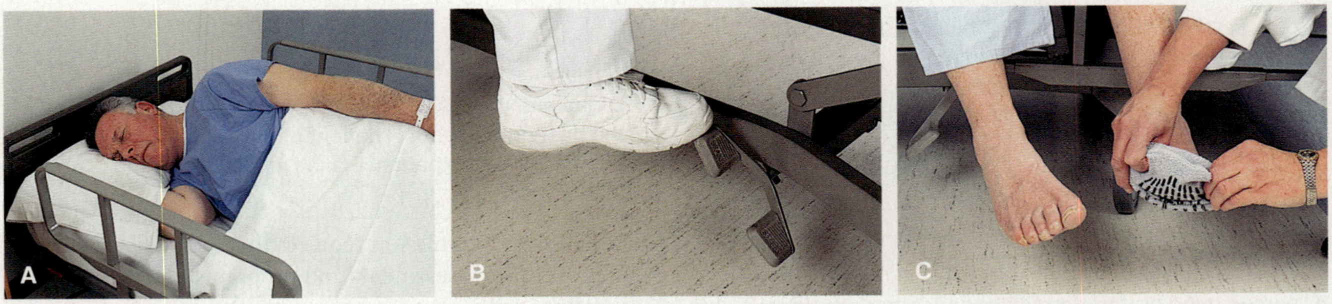

FIGURE 28-3. Some of the safety devices used in health care facilities and in the home to prevent falls. **A.** Side rails on bed raised at the patient's request; the patient must be able to raise and lower the side rail without help. **B.** Locking devices on wheeled equipment. **C.** Nonskid slippers. (*Source:* Used with permission from Shutterstock. *Photos by B. Proud*).

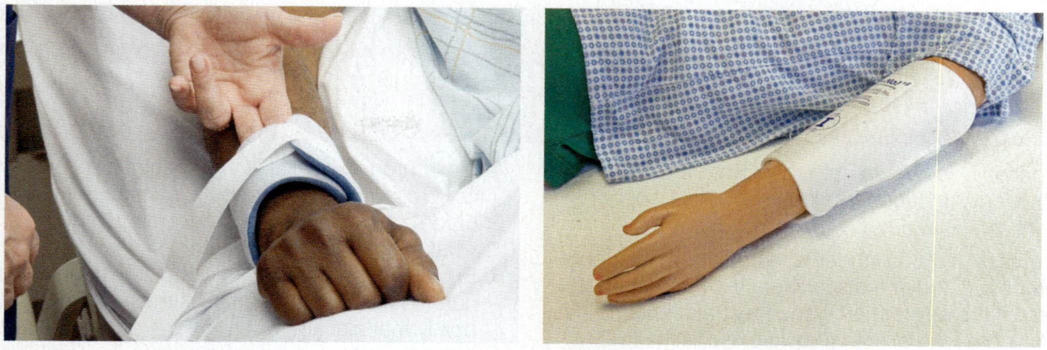

FIGURE 28-4. Restraints used for adults and children. The purpose of restraints is to help prevent the patient from being harmed. Restraints should not interfere with physiologic functioning by impairing circulation, limiting muscular activity to the point of immobilization, or interfering with respiration. Restraints that can be adjusted to the desired activity limitation are most likely to be accepted by the patient and family.

Unfolding Patient Stories: Josephine Morrow • Part 2

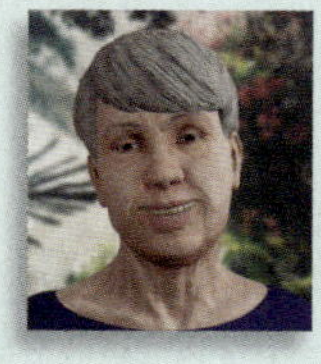

Recall from Chapter 24, **Josephine Morrow**, an 80-year-old with a venous stasis ulcer on her lower extremity who recently moved to a skilled nursing home. She has an unsteady gait and forgets to call for assistance when getting out of bed. How can the nurse promote patient safety and prevent falls? Why would the nurse refrain from using restraints for Josephine?

Care for Josephine and other patients in a realistic virtual environment: ***vSim** for Nursing* (thepoint.lww.com/vSimFunds). Practice documenting these patients' care in DocuCare (thepoint.lww.com/DocuCareEHR).

Using Restraints in Health Care Facilities

Restraints are physical devices or chemical means used to limit a patient's freedom and movement that cannot be easily removed (or eliminated) by the patient. Side rails, geriatric chairs with attached trays, and appliances tied at the wrist, ankle, or waist are types of physical restraints. Figure 28-4 shows examples of physical restraints that can be used for adults and children. Drugs that are used to control behavior and are not included in the person's normal medical regimen can be considered chemical restraints.

In the past, it was considered acceptable bedside care to restrain patients to protect them from harm, but the use of restraints for this purpose is potentially dangerous. Physical restraints can increase the possibility of serious injury due to a fall—they do not prevent falls. Negative outcomes of restraint use include skin breakdown and contractures, incontinence, depression, delirium, anxiety, aspiration and respiratory difficulties, and even death. Older adults with dementia are most at risk of being restrained, in general; in the ICU setting, younger adults are restrained at approximately the same rate as older adults. The use of restraints is declining as health care providers become more educated about the risks associated with their use.

Since 1987, the federal government and accrediting agencies have worked to reduce or eliminate the use of restraints. Initial guidelines formulated by the Health Care Financing Administration as part of the 1987 Omnibus Budget Reconciliation Act encouraged the limited use of restraints in long-term settings. The current standard for long-term care facilities is to provide safe care without the use of physical or chemical restraints. Federal and state mandates, as well as The Joint Commission, recommend that acute care facilities use restraints only as a last resort.

Federal guidelines reinforce that in all settings, the primary responsibility is to protect and promote patient's rights, and that restraints may only be used to protect the patient, staff, or others. They must be discontinued at the earliest possible time. Any health care facility that accepts Medicare and Medicaid reimbursement must abide by the federal guidelines for the use of restraints. In addition to labeling preventing falls and fall-related injuries a sentinel event (Sentinel Event Alert #55), The Joint Commission (2022c) identified preventing restraint death as a sentinel event (Sentinel Event Alert #8). These events signal the need for an immediate investigation and response. The American Nurses Association (2012) approved a revised position statement defining the nurse's role in reducing restraint use in health care. Their recommendations are included in Box 28-6 on page 860.

USING SIDE RAILS AS A RESTRAINT

In the past, side rails were used to provide support and aid equilibrium, but it is now recognized that they can pose serious risks for a confused or agitated patient. A 1995 FDA Safety Alert informed health care facilities of the hazards associated with side rail use. A person of small stature has a greater risk for entrapment or injury. Death from asphyxiation has occurred when patients have become wedged between the mattress and the bed frame or side rail. Although patient entrapment is uncommon, it can be fatal. Most of the victims of side rail fatalities are frail, of advanced age, or confused, and many exhibit uncontrolled body movement. Most incidents of entrapment occur in a long-term care setting.

A side rail is not considered a restraint if the patient requests that it be raised to aid in getting in or out of bed. Some patients may request that side rails be used at night

Box 28-6 American Nurses Association (ANA) Board of Directors Position Statement: Reduction of Patient Restraint and Seclusion in Health Care Settings

Recommendations: To ensure safe, quality care for all patients in the least restrictive environment, ANA supports nursing efforts to:

1. Educate nurses, nursing students, assistive personnel, other members of the interdisciplinary team, and family caregivers on the appropriate use of restraint and seclusion, and on the alternatives to these restrictive interventions;
2. Ensure sufficient nursing staff to monitor and individualize care with the goal of only using restraint when no other viable option is available;
3. Ensure policies and environment support services are in place to provide feasible alternatives to physical and chemical restraints;
4. Move progressively toward a restraint-free environment while providing a therapeutic sanctuary for all;
5. Enforce documentation requirements and education about what should be documented;
6. Explore the ethical implications of restraining patients with nursing students and discuss the need for institutional policy that clarifies when, where, and how patients are to be restrained and monitored while restrained;
7. Be aware of all implications of allowing the application of restraints in health care settings. The nurse administrator should make consultation available to nurses, including ethical consultation about decisions to restrain; and
8. Develop clear policies based on accepted national standards to guide decision making regarding restraints.

Source: American Nurses Association. (2012, March 12). *Reduction of patient restraint and seclusion in health care settings.* https://www.nursingworld.org/~4af287/globalassets/docs/ana/ethics/ps_reduction-of-patient-restraint-and-seclusion-in-health-care-settings.pdf

while they sleep so that they feel more secure (see Fig. 28-3A on page 858). Patients requesting side rails must be able to raise and lower the side rails themselves. Side rails that are raised with the *intent* to prevent the patient from voluntarily attempting or actually getting out of bed, would be considered a restraint; if the *intent* of raising the side rails is to prevent a patient from inadvertently falling out of bed, or if the patient lacks the physical ability to even attempt to get out of bed, side rails would not be considered a restraint (The Joint Commission, 2021). If a family member requests the use of side rails for a patient, it is the nurse's responsibility to review benefits and risks associated with their use and periodically evaluate the reason for their use. Side rails are not routinely recommended for all situations. It is the responsibility of health care facilities to evaluate existing bed systems for entrapment risks and investigate corrective actions that may be necessary to provide a safe environment for patients.

USING ALTERNATIVES TO RESTRAINTS

Careful nursing assessment is the key to identifying appropriate alternatives to restraint use and finding an individualized solution (Box 28-7). Nursing interventions may be

Box 28-7 Choosing Alternatives to Restraints

- Determine whether a behavior pattern exists.
- Assess for pain and treat appropriately.
- Rule out causes for agitation. Assess respiratory status, vital signs, blood glucose level, fluid and electrolyte issues, and medications. Use standardized screening tools to evaluate change in function.
- Involve the family and other people important to the individual in the patient's care.
- Ask family members or significant other to stay with the patient.
- Reduce stimulation, noise, and light.
- Distract and redirect, using a calming voice.
- Use simple, clear explanations and directions.
- Check environment for hazards.
- Use night light.
- Identify door of room (e.g., use of balloon, sign, patient's picture, ribbon).
- Use an electronic alarm system on a temporary basis (e.g., bed or position-sensitive alarms) to warn of unassisted activity.
- Allow restless patient to walk after ensuring that environment is safe.
- Use a large plant or piece of furniture as a barrier to limit wandering from designated area.
- Use low-height beds.
- Place floor mats on each side of the bed.
- Ensure the use of glasses and hearing aids, if necessary.
- Use pillows wedged against the side of the chair to keep patient positioned safely.
- Use full-length body pillows, a swimming pool noodle, or a rolled blanket to indicate the edge of the bed.
- Assist with toileting at frequent intervals.
- Arrange for a bedside commode.
- Make the environment as homelike as possible; provide familiar objects.
- Provide a warm beverage.
- Provide comfortable rocking chairs.
- Use therapeutic touch.
- Play music or video selections of the patient's choice.
- Offer diversional activities, such as games and books.
- Encourage daily exercise/provide exercise and activities or relaxation techniques.
- Consider relocation of the patient to a room closer to the nursing station.
- Conceal tubing necessary for care. Anchor tubing securely. Conceal tubing with gauze wrap; unwrap regularly to assess site for complications.
- Investigate possibility of discontinuing bothersome treatment devices (e.g., intravenous line, catheter, feeding tube).

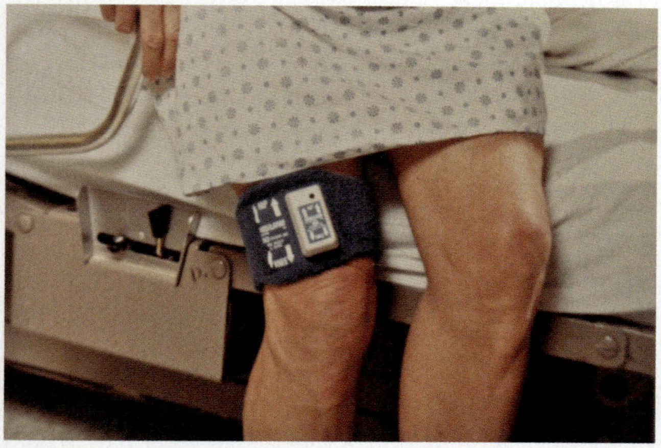

FIGURE 28-5. Ambularm device. (*Source:* Reprinted with permission of AlertCare, Inc.)

used to reduce confusion or agitation and provide a safe environment. Using a restraint on an older adult who tends to wander is unjustified because a variety of alternative options can be used to keep such patients safe. Figure 28-5 shows an example of a position-sensitive electronic device that is an alternative to using restraints. A variety of electronic alarms and monitors are available for chairs, beds, and doors.

USING RESTRAINTS AS A LAST RESORT

Despite all efforts, restraints may be the only solution in some situations. The least restrictive restraint should be the first option. Restraints must never be applied for the convenience of the staff. The patient's family must be consulted and involved in the plan of care before applying restraints in a long-term care setting. They must be informed of the facility's policy regarding applying and removing restraints and may be asked to sign a release form to protect the facility from liability. Facility policy, The Joint Commission, and state and federal guidelines require an order from a provider permitted to provide specific oversight of restraints, such as a physician or other licensed practitioner (U.S. Department of Health and Human Services, Centers for Medicare and Medicaid Services, 2019). The order should include the type of restraint, justification for the restraint, and criteria for removal. The order must never be written for PRN (as needed) use.

In an emergency, the physical restraint can be applied if an established protocol is followed, but an order from a provider must be obtained immediately or within a few minutes according to Joint Commission Standards. The order must state the intended duration of use. The patient must be monitored and assessed at least every hour or according to facility policy. An inpatient psychiatric patient in restraints requires continual observation, including specific assessments every 15 minutes. Initial documentation must reflect the date and time the restraint is applied, the type of restraint, alternatives that were attempted (including their results), and notification of the patient's family and health care provider. Ongoing documentation includes the frequency of assessment and release intervals, assessment findings, and other nursing interventions such as toileting. Constant reevaluation of the need for the restraint is vital. Chapter 7 discusses the legal issues involved when restraints are used. Student nurses, from their earliest clinical experiences, need help to identify and assess the cause of a patient's behavior and not just the behavior itself. Careful patient assessment is needed to develop creative alternative strategies. Skill 28-2 on pages 873–876 demonstrates the proper method for applying restraints should they be necessary.

Concept Mastery Alert

Restraints may be applied, per protocol, without a provider's order only if the situation is an emergency and the threat to safety is imminent. However, restraints should only be used as a last resort and an order must be obtained immediately afterward.

Facility Safety

In addition to individual patient safety, the safety of the facility itself and its employees must also be intentionally considered—establishing a safe and secure environment promotes the delivery of safe, quality care. Laws or regulations, such as those imposed by Occupational Safety and Health Administration (U.S. Department of Labor, OSHA, 2016), help promote modification of at-risk behavior of health care workers. Initiatives that consider smooth transitions of care (see Chapter 12, Interprofessional Collaborative Practice and Care Coordination Across Settings) promote safety as patients navigate the complex health care system. An agency's policies and procedures foster the development and maintenance of a safe, predictable work environment, and provide recourse for employees should actions potentially or actually affect the safety of patients, health care workers, or the communities they serve.

Fire Safety

Fire prevention and emergency response programs in health care facilities are sometimes viewed by staff as time-consuming or unnecessary exercises, but nurses must be prepared at all times to protect patients from injury. Hospitals are required by law to establish safety boards and to inspect the facility regularly for possible hazards. Equipment must be checked periodically, and escape routes must be kept open. Nurses, as part of their daily care procedures, must be aware of their facility's policies, review equipment and its proper functioning, and assess when and how often drills are performed.

Careless smoking, faulty electrical equipment, and combustion of anesthetic agents are the most common causes of hospital fires. Orientations in health care facilities emphasize fire prevention information and the facility's smoking policy. Nurses are responsible for patients' safety and need to be familiar with the facility's fire safety plan, exits, the location and operation of fire extinguishers, and any special instructions for reporting a fire.

Most hospital procedures emphasize the following priorities and recommend that staff members remember the acronym RACE as a guide:

- **R**escue anyone in immediate danger
- **A**ctivate the fire code system and notify the appropriate person
- **C**onfine the fire by closing doors and windows
- **E**vacuate patients and other people to a safe area

ABC (universal, dry chemical) fire extinguishers are the most common extinguishers used in health care facilities. In the home setting, cigarettes, grease, and electrical problems are most often responsible for fires. Educating parents about home fire safety includes having a plan of action similar to that used in health care settings. (See Box 28-1, on page 841, for priorities and practical suggestions for fire and burn safety.)

Alarm Management

The hospital is a very noisy place, but that is sometimes necessary. Overhead announcements that are fairly universal cue health care staff to a variety of events such as a medical emergency (Code Blue), child abduction (Code Pink), a bomb threat (Code Black), or even hazardous spill (Code Orange; The Joint Commission, n.d.). There are also almost ubiquitous alarms from any variety of monitoring systems throughout the hospital. Staff conversations and medical device alarms contribute to the cacophony of sounds that can be disconcerting to patients, at the very least, and perhaps even detrimental to their health and healing. Safety initiatives have focused on improving the hospital soundscape by training staff in noise reduction, enforcing noise reduction programs (such as the quiet time instituted on some units to allow for an afternoon respite for patients), rethinking and reworking alarms and considering their necessity in the clinical setting to decrease desensitization and alarm fatigue of staff, and researching the effects of noise on patient and staff (Oleksy & Schlesinger, 2019).

Preventing Equipment-Related Accidents

With the marked increase in the use of highly sophisticated electronic equipment in health care settings, all members of the health care team must learn to use the equipment properly and recognize signs of malfunctioning equipment. Suction devices with inadequate vacuum, and rate regulators or infusion pumps that deliver erratic amounts of solution, have resulted in equipment-related accidents. Failure to use protective belts or side rails on stretchers and to lock wheelchair wheels can result in patient injury.

Electrical equipment can present a safety hazard to both the patient and health care practitioner when safety measures are ignored. Most electrical equipment used in hospitals is equipped with three-prong plugs. The third prong, when inserted into a properly wired wall outlet, provides a ground for the piece of equipment. A ground is a connection from an electricity source to the earth through which electric current leakage can be harmlessly conducted.

Box 28-8 Decreasing Equipment-Related Accidents

- Use equipment only for the use for which it was intended.
- Do not operate equipment with which you are unfamiliar.
- Handle equipment with care to prevent damaging it.
- Use three-prong electric plugs whenever possible.
- Do not twist or bend electric cords. The wires inside the cord may break.
- Be alert to signs that indicate equipment is faulty such as breaks in electric cords, sparks, smoke, electric shocks, loose or missing parts, and unusual noises or odors. Report signs of trouble immediately.
- Make certain that electric cords are not in a position to be trapped as beds are raised or lowered. This can strip insulation covering the electric wires.
- Be alert for wet surfaces on areas where electric cords or connections are present.
- Make certain when charging defibrillator batteries that charging indicator light is on.
- Implement a process for reporting and addressing problems with equipment.

Box 28-8 lists guidelines to help reduce the number of equipment-related accidents. Hospitals and long-term care facilities are required by federal law and U.S. Food and Drug Administration (FDA, 2019) regulations to report to the FDA and the manufacturer of a device any suspected deaths or serious injuries related to use of the device.

Preventing Procedure-Related Accidents

The nurse must always be cautious and alert to prevent procedure-related accidents. Errors are possible when administering medications or intravenous solutions, transferring a patient, changing a dressing, or applying external heat to a patient's extremity. Therefore, nurses must follow correct procedures when administering care. Safeguards to prevent errors include making sure that the patient is identified correctly (Fig. 28-6), calling a time-out in the operating suite, and following protocols and policies designed to protect patients.

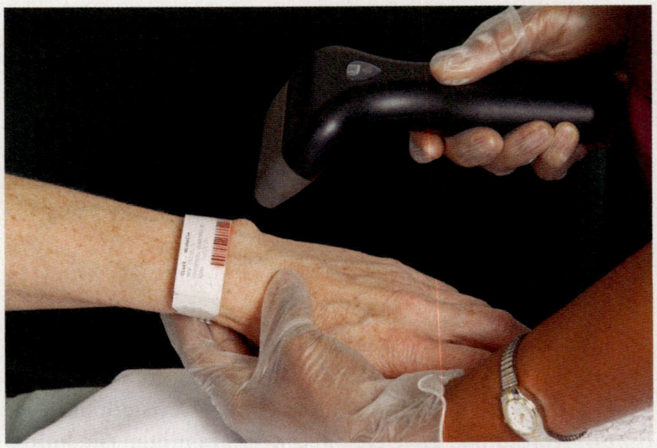

FIGURE 28-6. An essential nursing responsibility is checking the patient's identification bracelet before any procedure. Here, the nurse checks the patient's identification before administering medications.

In an effort to promote a culture of safety, The Joint Commission (2022b) publishes an annual list of National Patient Safety Goals. These are established based on sentinel events that have been reported and include the corrective actions recommended as a response to these sentinel events. Some goals are ongoing while others may get removed from the annual list once hospitals have incorporated the recommended practices to meet a particular safety goal into their standards of operation. The goals and related requirements are specific to each accreditation program (e.g., ambulatory care, assisted living, long-term care). Accreditation by The Joint Commission requires that a health care organization provide evidence that these goals have been addressed and requirements have been met. Effective alternatives may be acceptable, depending on the services provided by the particular health care organization. National Patient Safety Goals are available on The Joint Commission website at http://www.jointcommission.org/standards_information/npsgs.aspx (see Additional Resources).

Filing a Safety Event Report

An accident or incident that compromises safety in a health care facility requires the completion of a **safety event report**.

Recall ***Juanita Flores***, the young mother whose child fell off the cot. As a result of the fall, a safety event report was completed.

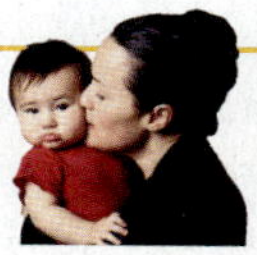

This is a confidential document, formerly referred to as an incident report, which objectively describes the circumstances of the accident or incident. The report also details the patient's response and the examination and treatment of the patient after the incident. The nurse completes the event report immediately after the incident and is responsible for recording the circumstances and the effect on the patient in the medical record. The safety event report is not a part of the medical record and should not be mentioned in the documentation. Because laws vary by state, nurses must know their own state law regarding safety event reports. All safety event reports are reviewed carefully to detect any potentially threatening situation or pattern. These reports are discussed in more detail in Chapter 7. When an incident results in a patient injury, the nurse has a responsibility to speak openly and honestly with the patient and family.

POPULATION-BASED ASPECTS OF SAFETY AND SECURITY

Ideally, the nurse, the patient, and the family should work together to eliminate or reduce accident risks in the home and health care setting. Engagement with partners in the community, provides nurses the opportunity to impact change at the local, state, national, and global levels. Nationally, community-based nurses and emergency nurses are establishing partnerships and venturing into the community to offer injury prevention activities to children and families. A good resource for nurses is the CDC's WISQARS (Web-based Injury Statistics Query and Reporting System) available at http://www.cdc.gov/injury/wisqars. This site is an interactive, online database that provides fatal and nonfatal injury, violent death, and cost of injury data from a variety of trusted sources. Population health is interprofessional in nature and involves engaging at the community level to connect practice to policy. These interprofessional partnerships include public health experts, educators, industry leaders, health care providers, and government representatives. Population health initiatives focus on collaborative efforts of systems, agencies, and organizations to work together on resource allocation and community-based initiatives designed to overcome barriers and improve the health outcomes for a population (CDC, 2019f).

Safety in Schools

A school nurse has many opportunities and a ready audience for health teaching about safety, including screening programs (e.g., vision and hearing), fire prevention sessions, drug and alcohol prevention programs, firearm safety, and classes on various accident prevention techniques. Managing minor accidents at school often provides an opportunity for additional preventive teaching. In this setting, the school nurse has the opportunity for formal or informal health teaching with children and parents/caregivers that should include parental encouragement to do the following:

- Monitor the child's use of the Internet
- Get involved in school activities and ask pertinent questions
- Volunteer for safety committees that include staff and parents
- Ensure that the school's emergency preparedness plan is current

For many children, school meal programs effectively reduce food insecurity, support healthy development, address obesity, and promote learning. Need-based programs are historically based on the individual applying for free or reduced-cost school meals, but there is a move toward entire schools participating in *community eligibility*, a program that allows schools to offer both breakfast and lunch to all students at no charge. Districts that participate in this collaborative effort recognize the academic, health, and administrative benefits; participation of eligible schools rose by 6.6% from 2018 to 2019 (FitzSimons et al., 2020). Formal programs like this have the added benefits of minimizing the stigma for children unable to pay for meals (even at reduced prices) and demonstrating a mechanism by which to provide food to children when school has scheduled or unexpected closures (Food Research & Action Center, 2020). The Healthy, Hunger-Free Kids Act of 2010 was signed into law in 2010, but rules set forth by the United States that went into effect for the 2020–2021 school year relaxed some of the nutrition standards (U.S. Department of Agriculture, Food and Nutrition Service, 2018;

U.S. Department of Agriculture, Food and Nutrition Service, 2020). It is important for nurses to appreciate their role in supporting or advocating changes to governmental rules, acts, and laws that determine nutrition and access standards for school breakfasts and lunches.

Schools are charged with creating a safe and supportive learning environment for students. Check out SchoolSafety.gov for action plans and resources on school safety topics including bullying and cyberbullying, threat assessment and reporting, security personnel, physical security and mental health, emergency planning with training and drills, school climate, and recovery.

Environmental Pollutants

Although much has been done to identify and control environmental pollutants, many U.S. residents still remain at risk for exposure to potentially unhealthy substances in the environment. In addition, certain environmental areas, such as dense urban areas, have proven to be more hazardous. Air pollution, in addition to its evidence-based link to climate change, has been shown to also increase the prevalence and severity of respiratory diseases, cardiovascular events, nervous system dysfunction, and diseases of the skin (Manisalidis et al., 2020; Vilcassim et al., 2019).

Community Violence

Living in an area where crime is prevalent can pose a threat to physical security and emotional well-being. Violence, acts of aggression, and terrorism are components of 21st-century life. Security measures such as locks, security systems, and exterior lighting can promote safety.

Home Health Nursing

It is imperative that nurses are aware of risks or hazards in certain settings that have the potential to result in violence and cause personal injury. Nurses include patient safety when assessing the home environment and neighborhood, and they consider access to and resources in the patient's community to develop a person-centered home health care plan. Nurses also need to consider their own safety. For example, in high-crime areas, a personal security escort may be provided to ensure a safe nurse visit (Irani et al., 2020). The Occupational Safety and Health Administration (U.S. Department of Labor, OSHA, 2016) identifies possible safety controls for home settings and specifies the use of a cell phone with GPS tracking, identification of exit routes and areas for patient de-escalation, assessment of outdoor and indoor lighting, use of a lock for supplies and equipment, and use of a well-maintained vehicle. Regulations also describe the responsibility of the employer to draft and enforce workplace violence policies, track workers, employ a system for documenting violent behavior of patients and families, provide a means for employees to receive backup assistance, and provide discretion to the employee to leave the situation if they feel threatened or unsafe (U.S. Department of Labor, OSHA, 2016). Use Promoting Health 28-1 as a tool for self-evaluation of safety behaviors in the community setting before using it with others.

Firearm Injuries

Preventing injuries caused by firearms has become a major concern for health care professionals. Intentional injuries caused by firearms are a leading cause of mortality in children. Some people believe that keeping a gun in the home provides protection for family and property. However, when a gun is available, it is more likely that the owner or a family member, rather than an intruder, will suffer a fatal injury. If not stored properly, guns can be extremely dangerous. Young children are curious and like to explore their surroundings—most children who die of unintentional firearm injury are shot by a peer in the same age range. When children encounter a loaded gun, even if instructed not to touch the weapon, the outcome is often tragic (Fowler et al., 2017).

Promoting Health 28-1

SAFETY IN THE COMMUNITY

Use the assessment checklist to determine how well you are meeting your needs for maintaining personal safety as you assist with health care delivery in the community.

Assessment Checklist

☐ almost always ☐ sometimes ☐ almost never

☐ ☐ ☐ 1. I wear a badge or clothing that identifies me as a health care worker.

☐ ☐ ☐ 2. I dress in an unobtrusive, professional manner with minimal jewelry.

☐ ☐ ☐ 3. I keep my car in good working order.

☐ ☐ ☐ 4. I am aware of neighborhoods where personal safety and security may be a problem.

☐ ☐ ☐ 5. I notify my patient of my planned visit and confirm directions to the home.

☐ ☐ ☐ 6. I communicate with my agency regarding the timing and location of my home visits.

☐ ☐ ☐ 7. I request pets be secured before my visit.

☐ ☐ ☐ 8. I assess the environment, noting lighting and establishing an exit strategy.

☐ ☐ ☐ 9. I ensure equipment, supplies, and personal items are secured and not visible in my vehicle.

☐ ☐ ☐ 10. I enter patients' homes only when invited in by a responsible adult.

Also, having a gun in the house increases the risk for domestic homicide threefold.

Recent multivictim/mass shootings, gang violence incidents, activities related to drug procurement, interpersonal disagreements, and activities associated with law enforcement are examples of potential risks for injuries and fatalities associated with firearms. An estimated 4% of children ages 0 to 17 years in the United States in 2014 were in a place where they could see or hear people being shot, bombs going off, or street riots (Fowler et al., 2017)—this number may have increased since the mass, global protests in 2020 in response to the death of George Floyd and the call for police reform. Gun ownership is a sensitive issue; therefore, nurses need to approach this topic in a nonjudgmental manner with the focus on injury prevention. Nurses function as prevention partners by educating the public on the epidemic of gun-related injuries and deaths and informing families about the risks of firearm injury while discussing appropriate safety measures (see Box 28-1 on page 841).

Nurses are in a unique position to raise awareness and to help reduce high-risk behavior that may lead to firearm injuries and deaths. In homes, schools, and other health care settings, nurses can provide information on how parents/caregivers can keep guns out of the hands of children. Parents/caregivers may be unaware of how common gunshot injuries are or the dangers that can occur when a gun is accessible to children and young adults. Healthy People 2020 identified objectives related to injury and violence prevention, several of which involve the use of firearms. This is important because it identifies violence as a public health issue that needs to be addressed at the community level (U.S. Department of Health and Human Services, Office of Disease Prevention and Health Promotion, 2020b).

Emergency Preparedness

Emergency preparedness has always been a concern for health care workers. Nurses, as members of emergency response teams, need to be aware of their role when an emergency or disaster occurs. Existing community resources are usually sufficient to respond to an emergency situation, such as a multiple vehicle collision, a fire in an apartment complex involving a significant number of burn injuries, an explosion, or plane crash. Since the September 11, 2001, terrorist attacks in New York, Washington, DC, and Pennsylvania, attention has been focused on national security and strategies for sustaining emergency preparedness levels. These events highlighted the need for communities to step up the level of their involvement in emergency preparedness for any disaster.

A **disaster** is broadly defined as a tragic event of great magnitude that requires the response of people outside the involved community. Disasters can be categorized as natural (e.g., massive flooding following a hurricane or an earthquake) or manmade (e.g., a toxic spill, war, or a terrorist event). In any disaster, the lives of the victims, their families, the affected community, and even the entire nation are affected in incalculable ways.

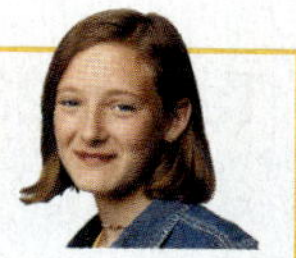

Think back to ***Kara Greenwood***, the adolescent described in the beginning of the chapter. Her statement revealed her peer group's awareness of terrorism. Kara would need to obtain additional information about terrorism from community sources when preparing the discussion.

Based on national and world events, the efforts of government facilities, nongovernmental facilities, the private sector, communities, and individuals are all vital components of health and emergency response systems when a disaster occurs. In addition, accreditation bodies such as The Joint Commission (2022a) have contributed to the considerable progress that hospitals have made in disaster preparedness (U.S. Department of Health and Human Services, Office of Disease Prevention and Health Promotion, 2022). Disaster training is now more rigorous and standardized, and it encompasses the entire community and its resources. These health care coalitions provide the foundation for improved response capacity.

The National Disaster Medical System (NDMS) coordinates health care practitioners who supplement local disaster responses in large-scale disasters. In collaboration with USDHHS, Homeland Security, Veterans Affairs, and the Defense Department, they supply funds, equipment, training, and medical and support personnel (U.S. Department of Health and Human Services, 2019). Nurses have a critical role in caring for victims of a disaster.

The CDC is also committed to responding rapidly to mass trauma events and chemical, biologic, radiologic, and nuclear agents. The CDC's Health Alert Network (HAN), available at http://emergency.cdc.gov/han, has improved the ability of state and local health facilities to detect and communicate varying health threats (CDC, 2020b). The CDC has also collaborated with pharmaceutical companies and other partners to create regional stockpiles of the drugs that would be needed to treat manmade outbreaks of disease, such as anthrax, plague, and other diseases. It is dangerous for the United States to not continue to develop the optimal emergency preparedness capabilities that it needs to protect its communities. As we have seen with previous disasters, older Americans are particularly vulnerable. The age-85-years-and-older population is the fastest-growing segment of older adults, and they are at high risk during a disaster. Deficits in strength and mobility, vision and hearing loss, multiple chronic illnesses, and possible dependence on life-saving equipment make it challenging to meet their many needs (CDC, 2019a).

Addressing Biologic Threats

Bioterrorism involves the deliberate spread of pathogenic organisms into a community to cause widespread illness, fear, and panic (CDC, 2018b). The organisms used in a mass attack may not be routine, and the clinical manifestations may be vague and nonspecific. Table 28-2 (on page 866) outlines some of the more common biologic agents, including symptoms and interventions. If an unusual number of

Table 28-2 Biologic Agents of Concern

AGENTS	CLINICAL MANIFESTATIONS	TREATMENT/PROTECTION
Anthrax (*Bacillus anthrax*)	Symptoms variable based on form of anthrax: • Cutaneous: Skin lesion with local edema that progresses, enlarges, ulcerates, and becomes necrotic • Gastrointestinal: Nausea, vomiting, fever, abdominal pain, hematemesis, severe diarrhea • Inhalational: Fever, fatigue, cough, dyspnea, pain; may progress to meningitis, septicemia, shock, and death	Standard precautions Decontamination possibly required for recent exposure Rapid administration of antimicrobial therapy Supportive therapy for shock, fluid volume deficit, and airway management Vaccine available; currently recommended only for high-risk populations
Botulism (*Clostridium botulinum*)	Possible release via airborne method, or contaminated food supplies Ocular symptoms such as blurred vision Skeletal muscle paralysis that progresses symmetrically and in a descending manner Muscle weakness that can result abruptly in respiratory failure	Standard precautions Passive immunization with botulinum antitoxin Supportive respiratory care
Brucellosis	Acute or insidious onset of fever and one or more of the following: night sweats, arthralgia, headache, fatigue, anorexia, myalgia, weight loss, arthritis/spondylitis, meningitis, or focal organ involvement (endocarditis, orchitis/epididymitis, hepatomegaly, splenomegaly)	PPE Supportive care Multidrug antimicrobial regimens
Plague or "black death" (*Yersinia pestis*)	Expected attack most likely airborne (inhalation of bacilli) with sudden appearance in ED of multiple patients with respiratory symptoms Symptoms similar to a severe respiratory infection Progresses rapidly to severe pneumonia, sepsis, and death	Standard precautions with droplet precautions until 48 hours after initiation of antibiotic therapy Antibiotic of choice: streptomycin (IM) or gentamicin sulfate (IM or IV); possible use of oral antibiotics (effective when mass numbers of people are ill) Fatality rate of 100% for those not receiving treatment within 24 hours of onset of symptoms
Smallpox (*Variola major*, viral agent)	Spread via direct contact or inhalation of respiratory droplets; most likely to be spread via aerosol route Flulike symptoms Characteristic rash that progresses to crusted scabs in 5 days, most prominent on face and extremities	Strict contact and airborne precautions for duration of illness—vaccination for those exposed No proven treatment Supportive care including possible antibiotics if secondary infections develop Use of antiviral agents under investigation Vaccine available; currently recommended only for high-risk populations
Tularemia (*Francisella tularensis*)	Transmission via contaminated water, food, and soil; most likely aerosolization of bacteria for use as a biologic weapon Fever Nonproductive or productive cough Possible progression to respiratory failure	Standard precautions Drug therapy such as streptomycin or gentamicin sulfate Fluid and respiratory support measures Vaccine under investigation
Viral hemorrhagic fevers (e.g., Lassa, Ebola, Marburg, yellow, and dengue fevers)	Possible spread via aerosol infection Fever Myalgias Conjunctival symptoms Mild hypotension Petechial hemorrhages Progresses to shock and hemorrhage	Standard, droplet, and contact precautions for the duration of illness; additional precautions, including use of negative-pressure room, N95, or higher respirator Use of personal protective equipment (PPE) (see Chapter 24) No proven treatment other than supportive care Avoidance of aspirin or other anticlotting drugs

Source: Adapted from Centers for Disease Control and Prevention (CDC). (2017, August 2). *Emergency preparedness and response: Bioterrorism.* https://emergency.cdc.gov/bioterrorism/

people suddenly experience similar signs and symptoms, health care personnel should consider whether they may have been exposed to a biologic agent.

Health care personnel must adhere to the Standard Precautions recommended by the CDC. For certain diseases, additional safeguards may be necessary. If a contagious disease is suspected, the patient should be isolated accordingly. Although not usually required with biologic agents, decontamination may be necessary if a patient's exposure status is uncertain. The patient may need to bathe or shower with soap and place their clothing in sealed plastic bags. The CDC routinely posts a list of nationally notifiable conditions that include infectious diseases, noninfective conditions, and outbreaks of immediate concern (CDC, 2020a).

Addressing Chemical Threats

The use of chemical agents as a terrorist weapon is a growing concern. A **chemical emergency** could be triggered by the deliberate or unintentional release of a chemical compound that has the potential for harming people's health (CDC, 2018a). The chemical would probably be dispersed in an enclosed space, such as a subway or a closed sports arena, to cause the maximum effect. Chemical agents act rapidly, and immediate decontamination is crucial before patients are transported to a hospital. Emergency preparedness requires the swift transfer of portable decontamination units, equipment, and trained personnel to the site of the chemical attack.

Several categories of chemicals can be used as weapons of mass destruction (CDC, 2018a):

- **Biotoxins**—poisons from plants or animals
- **Blister agents/vesicants**—chemicals that severely blister the eyes, respiratory tract, and skin on contact
- **Blood agents**—poisons that are absorbed into the blood
- **Caustics (acids)**—chemicals that burn or corrode the skin, eyes, and mucous membranes on contact
- **Choking/lung/pulmonary agents**—chemicals that cause severe irritation or swelling of the respiratory tract
- **Incapacitating agents**—drugs that affect the ability to think clearly or that cause an altered state of consciousness or even unconsciousness
- **Long-acting anticoagulants**—poisons that cause bleeding by preventing blood from clotting properly
- **Metals**—agents that consist of metallic poisons
- **Nerve agents**—highly poisonous chemicals that prevent the nervous system from working properly
- **Organic solvents**—agents that damage the tissues by dissolving fats and oils
- **Riot control agents/tear gas**—highly irritating agents normally used by law enforcement for crowd control or by individual people for protection
- **Toxic alcohols**—poisonous alcohols that can damage the heart, kidneys, and nervous system
- **Vomiting agents**—chemicals that cause nausea and vomiting

Addressing Radiation Threats

Nuclear terrorism involves intentional introduction of radioactive materials into the environment for the purpose of causing injury and death. Nuclear terrorism is the most immediate and extreme threat to our global security (U.S. Department of Homeland Security, 2019). The attack might involve use of a radiation dispersion device (*dirty bomb*), a planned assault at a nuclear power station or weapons facility, or dispersal of radioactive material into the food or water supply. Even a small amount of radioactive material can have devastating effects.

Radiation burns occur as a result of exposure to a radioactive source. The severity of injury depends on a variety of factors, including the duration of the exposure and the distance between the source and the person. A higher dose increases the likelihood of developing later effects such as bone marrow depression and cancer. Lymph tissue and bone marrow are the tissues most sensitive to radiation while the skin, kidneys, intestines, and gonads are the most radiation-sensitive organs (CDC, 2020f). Although the likelihood of a nuclear attack may be small, nurses need to be well informed, familiar with their facility's emergency response plan, and prepared to deal with a nuclear emergency.

Nurses serving on a radiologic emergency response team must protect themselves and wear the necessary equipment, including a radiation detection device. They will assess patients in a radiation emergency area (REA) designated by the hospital's emergency response plan. If patients have not been decontaminated at the scene of the attack, decontamination will occur at the medical facility.

Addressing Cyber Terror

Cyber terror involves the use of high technology to disable or delete critical infrastructure data or information. It is a serious threat to national security and very difficult to identify a perpetrator who resides in cyberspace. Cyberspace is particularly difficult to secure due to many factors including: (1) the ability of perpetrators to operate from anywhere in the world; (2) the linkages between cyberspace and physical systems, especially those involving critical infrastructure; and (3) and the difficulty of reducing vulnerabilities and minimizing consequences in complex cyber networks (U.S. Department of Homeland Security, 2020). The federal facilities responsible for investigating cyber terror must remain vigilant because it is difficult to predict such attacks. Authorities agree that strengthening the resilience and security of cyberspace has emerged as an important concern for national security (U.S. Department of Homeland Security, 2020). These criminals are constantly searching for vulnerabilities and looking for opportunities to launch an attack. Intruders can break into supposedly secure systems to alter files and steal confidential information. An attack on a hospital network could potentially compromise the ability of providers and nurses to care for patients and respond to health care emergencies, which could directly impact on patient safety.

Cybersecurity awareness needs to be part of the conversation with patients, families, communities, and community partners. A federally supported toolkit, updated annually, provides key messaging, engagement ideas, resources, and information on social media. The overarching theme for 2019 of "OWN IT. SECURE IT. PROTECT IT." (National Initiative for Cybersecurity Careers and Studies, n.d.) provides the framework for specific actions involving understanding, securing, and maintaining your digital profile. Internet use continues to grow in the United States and is currently at 95% or 310 million users as of January 2019. Globally there was a 75% growth between 2014 and 2019, and there are currently more than 4.39 billion global Internet users (Kemp, 2019). On average, individuals are online more than 6.5 hours every day, with some users accessing their devices hundreds of times each day. The three most popular sites are Google, YouTube, and Facebook, with Twitter losing ground and e-commerce (online shopping) steadily rising (Kemp, 2019). Gaming online and systems that support massively multiplayer online role-playing games (MMORPGs) are changing the way people socialize worldwide. The open access enjoyed by individuals comes with some responsibilities. Nurses can focus on the physical risks of increased screen time, the impact of social media on interpersonal relationships, the advantages and disadvantages of access and smart devices, the socioeconomic and generational barriers to access, the need to develop media literacy to vet sites and posts for accuracy and authenticity, and the ramifications of the globalization of communication on individual communities.

Preparing for Mass Trauma Terrorism

Terrorists have used bombs and other explosives in a variety of ways (e.g., roadside devices, on public transportation) to inflict mass trauma injuries and cause multiple fatalities. Proximity to the detonation determines the severity of injuries and mortality rates. Blast lung injury (BLI) has recently been recognized as a direct consequence of the blast wave from a high explosive detonation. Once the condition is diagnosed, the patient may require complex care and should be admitted to an intensive care unit. Key signs include a low blood pressure (hypotension), a slow heartbeat (bradycardia), and temporary pause in breathing (apnea). Few emergency health care providers in the United States have experience treating patients with explosion-related injuries.

Technology Alert

To address this lack of experience with explosion-related injuries, the CDC funded a grant for an online curriculum to address *Bombings: Injury Patterns and Care* that can be found at https://www.acep.org/imports/clinical-and-practice-management/resources/ems-and-disaster-preparedness/disaster-preparedness-grant-projects/bombings-injury-patterns-and-care/ (American College of Emergency Physicians, 2020). The CDC also released a mobile application specifically to provide immediate access to key information for providers. Download the app at https://apps.apple.com/au/app/cdc-blast-injury/id890434999?ign-mpt=uo%3D2.

Pandemic Preparation

The initial draft of this chapter for the 10th edition of the textbook was written while we were in the middle of the Coronavirus (COVID-19) pandemic and associated quarantine in the United States. I am choosing to *break the "fourth wall"* and tell you this because this is a unique situation that the average person did not expect, and it is taking a toll on people worldwide. Nurses talk about *tolerance of ambiguity*, *mindfulness*, and *resilience*—these words are part of our vernacular and things we intentionally build in response to the (ethical) stresses inherent in our work. What is striking is that because of the pandemic, the public experienced compassion fatigue and moral fatigue right along with health care providers. This pandemic has brought to light the importance of collaboration and coordination between: (1) individuals and their communities, the social contract of wearing masks; (2) individuals and their states, guidance that is geographically based; (3) states and public health experts, guidance based on data trends germane to the area; (4) states and national government, resource allocation and sharing; (5) government writ large and scientists, the CDC and the WHO are good examples; and (6) our nation and the global world—economic-, resource-, and science-based decision making. Response time, resource allocation (appropriate equipment and re-shuffling of health care providers), crisis plans (based on trends and available resources), economic impact (from unemployment to global trade), and public safety (especially of vulnerable populations) all affect decisions made by leaders and individuals. In 2019 and 2020, the intention of a united, measured response was complicated by the evolving science, the related ever-changing guidance, and inaccurate and confusing data reports. Crisis planning in moments of uncertainty is not ideal. It is far better to have a general plan in place with contingencies; funding for contact tracing and testing earmarked; resources stockpiled with production/trade agreements drafted; and a means for clear, cogent, concise dissemination of information to the public. Nurses need to lead the way in an evaluation of our collective response to the pandemic and work to shape the plan for the next global challenge.

Identifying Disaster Resources

Each health care facility should determine in advance how to deliver care should an emergency or disaster occur. This involves collaboration with internal committees and external facilities. Organizations that serve as resources for recommendations and updated information are listed in Table 28-3.

In any disaster, nurses will have multiple roles. In addition to clinical expertise, nurses may be responsible for triage, various treatments, counseling, and assistance with distribution of resources. There are many unresolved issues regarding the legal, ethical, and personal responsibilities of a nurse when a disaster occurs. There may be concerns about personal safety, legal implications, and the ethical decisions they may be

Research in Nursing

BRIDGING THE GAP TO EVIDENCE-BASED PRACTICE

Staying Abreast of the Science During a Pandemic

Evolving science, the availability of massive amounts of unvetted information through nontraditional dissemination mediums (e.g., social media), varied levels of health literacy, ineffective and misleading communication, and other factors have forced health care providers to educate and make decisions in a tense environment. The application of best evidence requires the ability to locate, appraise, synthesize, and articulate findings of scientific research. Nurses routinely stay abreast of new developments and integrate current guidelines and principles into their delivery of nursing care. A change in nursing practice is typically based on peer-reviewed research that informs facility-based guidelines, protocols, and policies. The sheer volume of information available to nurses in their personal and professional lives, and the speed with which this information is accessible, challenges nurses to identify reliable sources of information.

Related Research

Science brief: COVID-19 vaccines and vaccination. (2021). In National Center for Immunization and Respiratory Diseases (NCIRD), Division of Viral Diseases, *CDC COVID-19 Science Briefs*. Centers for Disease Control and Prevention (US). https://www.ncbi.nlm.nih.gov/books/NBK570435/

The CDC routinely disseminates a summary of recent changes to document the current state of vaccination and provide up-to-date recommendations. Although previous science briefs addressed the efficacy of vaccination in general, this report from September 15, 2021 reiterates the efficacy of vaccination against COVID-19 hospitalization and death caused by the biggest, current issue, the Delta variant of SARS-CoV-2. The brief integrates new data from studies published since the last update regarding the benefit of a third dose of vaccine in specific populations, mixed vaccine schedules, duration of protection from vaccination, and clinical transmissibility in fully vaccinated persons. To explain the scope of this work, the International Vaccine Access Center, Johns Hopkins Bloomberg School of Public Health and World Health Organization publish weekly summary tables that contribute to their ongoing systematic review of the results of students on COVID-19 vaccination effectiveness (https://view-hub.org/resources). Their October 14, 2021, systematic review table contained 105 studies regarding post-authorization COVID-19 vaccine effectiveness that met inclusion criteria. They also identified 133 studies that may be of interest but did not meet inclusion criteria. This is just one of the myriad resources that inform the CDC's science briefs and guidance documents for vaccination and for fully vaccinated people.

Relevance to Nursing Practice

It is important that nurses reflect on lesson learned during the pandemic and use that information to inform the collective response to future issues. Although staying abreast of developments is important for all health care providers, independently completing an ongoing systematic review and analysis of an evolving pandemic is unrealistic. Best practice involves leveraging expert synthesis and analysis to inform decision making and drive the creation of up-to-date guidance at the facility and national levels.

Table 28-3 Emergency Preparedness Resources

ORGANIZATION	ACTIVITIES
National Disaster Medical System (NDMS) http://www.phe.gov/Preparedness/responders/ndms/Pages/default.aspx	Has responsibility for managing and coordinating the federal medical response to major emergencies and federally declared disasters
Federal Emergency Management Agency (FEMA) http://www.fema.gov	Works to build and support the national emergency management system
Centers for Disease Control and Prevention (CDC) http://www.cdc.gov	Acts as the lead federal facility for disease prevention and control activities; provides backup support to state and local health departments
The Joint Commission http://www.jointcommission.org	Accredits facilities according to established safety and quality standards; revises the emergency management standards for health care facilities
American Red Cross http://www.redcross.org	Acts as the lead nongovernmental facility that provides safety information and disaster response
Department of Homeland Security http://www.dhs.gov/index.shtm	Protects the nation against further terrorist attacks and coordinates the response for future emergencies

called on to make in a disaster. The ANA is partnering with government facilities, employers, and individual nurses to resolve these issues and allow nurses to respond confidently with their usual compassionate attitude (American Nurses Association, n.d.c). Nurses came face-to-face with difficult decisions, challenging training, and the need to remain adaptable and flexible with evolving protocols and policies in the Ebola crisis and in the Coronavirus (COVID-19) pandemic. The ANA Enterprise created an online COVID-19 Resource Center that includes clinical information, legislative and regulatory advocacy information, licensure information, ethical considerations, other nurse-specific resources (American Nurses Association, n.d.a). These experiences provided nurses the opportunity to engage in the creation of plans and strategies for the proper management of future epidemics and mass disaster situations.

Disaster preparedness is imperative at all levels. In order to reduce confusion and lessen the impact of a disaster, people need to take responsibility, include the family in all discussions, and develop a personal disaster plan. The American Red Cross (2022) recommends a very straightforward plan of action for emergency preparedness: get a kit, make a plan, and be informed. Emergency food, supplies, and medications should be assembled; a communication routine should be established, and sources for reliable information should be monitored when disaster strikes. Multiple resources are available to assist in this preparation including one from the CDC (http://emergency.cdc.gov/preparedness).

Addressing Psychological Aspects of Disasters

Disasters affect the lives of victims, family members, and health care personnel in many ways. Fear and panic can be expected. Other potential emotions include anger, horror, as well as real and exaggerated concerns about possible future events. Nurses and other health care providers (as first responders), rescue and recovery workers, and staff at a medical facility, can help to minimize panic by addressing risks and providing careful explanations. Anxiety and moral fatigue can be addressed with reassurance and emotional support. The impact of a disaster on each person varies, and it can have lingering effects. Most disaster survivors experience normal stress reactions, but some may exhibit acute stress disorder or posttraumatic stress disorders that require treatment. Emergency preparedness education and planning must also address mental health issues.

REFLECTIVE PRACTICE LEADING TO PERSONAL LEARNING

Remember that the object of reflective practice is to look at an experience, understand it, and learn from it. As you begin to develop your expertise in evaluating the plan of care, reflect on your experiences—successes and failures—in order to improve your practice. How can you do it better next time? What did you learn today that can help you tomorrow? Begin your reflection by paying close attention to the following:

- How aware are you of the developmental considerations regarding safety? Are you able to articulate them and teach at the appropriate level?
- What value do you attach to involving the patient in safety and security? How do you individualize the care for patients when so many guidelines, policies, and procedures dictate your care?
- How can nurses impact change at the system and population levels? What is the role of the nurse in health care and population- or community-based initiatives? How do you see nurses' agency manifest in these situations?
- What plan do you have to stay abreast of evolving statistics on national issues? How do you plan to be aware of current global security issues and the associated recommendations at the facility, local, state, national, and global levels?

Keeping up with the latest evidence-based practice guidelines can be challenging. Global shifts and evolving statistics change the emphasis of our nursing care. Balancing the needs of your individual patient with these responsibilities requires mindfulness and intentionality.

Perhaps the most important questions to reflect on are: Are your patients and their families/caregivers better for having had *you* share in the critical responsibility of partnering with them to ensure appropriate safety and security practices? Are your patients now receiving thoughtful, person-centered, prioritized, holistic, evidence-based treatment and care because of your efforts?

Skill 28-1 Performing a Situational Assessment

DELEGATION CONSIDERATIONS

A situational assessment should not be delegated to assistive personnel (AP). However, the AP may notice some items while providing care. The nurse must then validate, analyze, document, communicate, and act on these findings, as appropriate. Depending on the state's nurse practice act and the organization's policies and procedures, the licensed practical/vocational nurses (LPN/LVNs) may perform some or all of the parts of a situational assessment. The decision to delegate must be based on careful analysis of the patient's needs and circumstances as well as the qualifications of the person to whom the task is being delegated. Refer to the Delegation Guidelines in Appendix A.

EQUIPMENT

- PPE, as indicated

IMPLEMENTATION

ACTION	RATIONALE
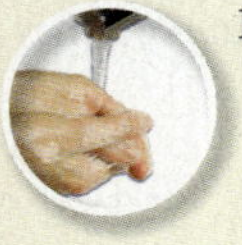 1. Perform hand hygiene and put on PPE, if indicated.	Hand hygiene and PPE prevent the spread of microorganisms. PPE is required based on transmission precautions.
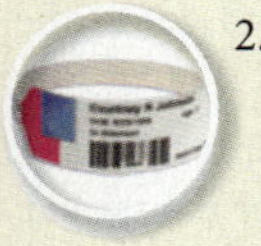 2. Identify the patient. Explain the purpose of the assessment to the patient.	Identifying the patient ensures the right patient receives the intervention and helps prevent errors. Explanation helps reduce anxiety and promotes engagement and understanding.
3. Assess for data that suggest a problem with the patient's airway, breathing, or circulation. If a problem is present, identify if it is urgent or nonurgent in nature. Refer to Chapter 27 for specific related assessments.	Problems with the patient's airway, breathing, or circulation may signal a situation requiring immediate action. It is important to determine the importance of information, focus on the most relevant and important data, act on that which is important and develop plans for interventions that can be justified in relation to their likelihood of success (Lasater, 2007).
4. Assess the patient's level of consciousness, orientation, and speech. Observe the patient's behavior and affect (Figure 1). If a problem is present, identify if it is urgent or nonurgent in nature. Refer to Chapter 27 for specific related assessments.	Problems with the patient's level of consciousness, orientation, speech, behavior, or affect may signal a situation requiring immediate action. It is important to determine the importance of information, focus on the most relevant and important data, act on that which is important and develop plans for interventions that can be justified in relation to their likelihood of success (Lasater, 2007).

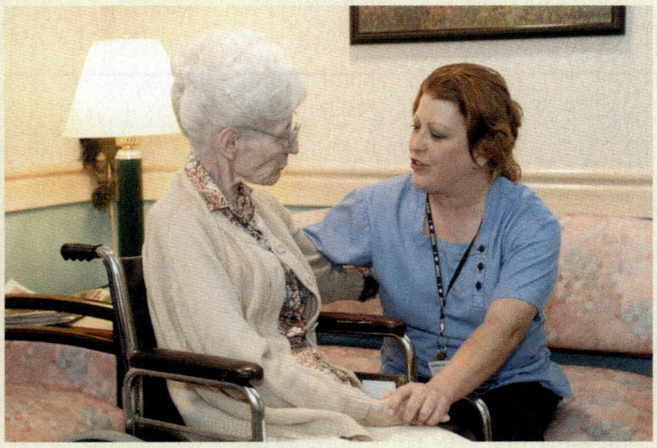

FIGURE 1. Observing the patient's behavior and affect. (*Source:* Used with permission from Shutterstock. *Photo by Rick Brady.*)

ACTION	RATIONALE
5. Assess the patency of an oxygen delivery device, if in use. Refer to Chapter 40 for specific related assessments.	Properly functioning equipment is required to maintain delivery of oxygen.
6. Assess other relevant *priority* body systems as appropriate, based on individual patient circumstances.	Nurses must use clinical judgment to adapt this assessment for each patient, based on the individual circumstances of an individual patient (Henley Haugh, 2015).
7. Survey the patient's environment. Assess the bed position and call bell location. The bed should be in the lowest position, and the call bell (based on specific patient care setting) should be within the patient's reach.	Environmental survey identifies problems that may harm the patient (Cohen, 2013).

(*continued on page 872*)

Skill 28-1 Performing a Situational Assessment *(continued)*

ACTION	RATIONALE
8. Assess for clutter and hazards. Remove excess equipment, supplies, furniture, and other objects from rooms and walkways. Pay particular attention to high traffic areas and the route to the bathroom.	All are possible hazards and could cause the patient to fall.
9. Note the presence and location of appropriate emergency equipment, based on individual patient situation.	Emergency equipment must be immediately available if needed.
10. Note the presence and location of appropriate assistive devices and mobility aids, based on individual patient situation. Ensure any devices are within the patient's reach.	Assistive devices should be available for patient use.
11. Assess for the presence of an intravenous (IV) access and/or infusion. Assess patency of the device and the insertion site. If an infusion is present, assess the solution and rate. Refer to Chapter 41 for specific related assessments.	Assessment allows for identification of problems and ensures administration of intravenous fluids as prescribed.
12. Assess for the presence of any tubes, such as gastric tubes, chest tubes, surgical drains, or urinary catheters. Assess patency of the device and insertion site. Refer to Chapters 33 and 37 to 40 for specific related assessments.	Assessment allows for identification of problems and ensures patency of devices.
13. Provide a bedside commode and/or urinal/bedpan, if appropriate. Ensure that it is near the bed at all times.	This prevents falls related to incontinence or trying to get to the bathroom.
14. Ensure that the bedside table, telephone, and other personal items are within the patient's reach at all times.	This prevents the patient from having to overreach for a device or items, and/or possibly attempt ambulation or transfer unassisted.
15. Consider what further assessments should be completed and additional interventions that may be indicated. Identify problems that need to be communicated and whom to contact.	Early detection of problems allows for corresponding interventions to prevent adverse occurrences, supporting improved patient outcomes (Large & Aldridge, 2018).
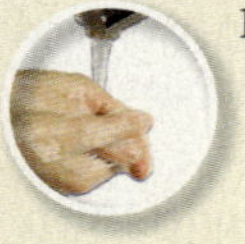 16. Remove PPE, if used. Perform hand hygiene.	Proper removal of PPE reduces the risk for infection transmission and contamination of other items. Hand hygiene prevents transmission of microorganisms.

DOCUMENTATION GUIDELINES

Document significant assessment findings as directed by facility policy and protocol. Include associated interventions and/or related communication.

DEVELOPING CLINICAL REASONING AND CLINICAL JUDGMENT

SPECIAL CONSIDERATIONS

Community-Based Care Considerations

- Examine the home for objects on the floor, the presence of wires or cords, objects on the steps, and loose or torn carpet. Encourage residents to keep walkways, floors, and stairs clear.
- Assess for adequate lighting, especially at the top and bottom of stairs and pathways from the bedroom to bathroom.
- Assess for the presence of working smoke detectors at a minimum on every floor of the home, ideally in every room. Provide education regarding safe use as appropriate.
- Assess for the presence of a carbon monoxide detector.
- Assess for the presence of firearms in the home. Provide education regarding safe storage as appropriate.
- Assess for the presence of space heaters. Provide education regarding safe use as appropriate.
- If there are children in the home, evaluate the method used to store medications, cleaning products, insecticides, and corrosives. Provide education regarding safe storage as appropriate and Poison Control Center contact information.

Skill 28-2 Applying an Extremity Restraint

DELEGATION CONSIDERATIONS

After assessment of the patient by the RN, the application of an extremity restraint may be delegated to assistive personnel (AP) as well as to licensed practical/vocational nurses (LPN/LVNs). The decision to delegate must be based on careful analysis of the patient's needs and circumstances as well as the qualifications of the person to whom the task is being delegated. Refer to the Delegation Guidelines in Appendix A.

EQUIPMENT

- Appropriate cloth restraint for the extremity that is to be immobilized
- Padding, if necessary, for bony prominences
- PPE, as indicated

IMPLEMENTATION

ACTION	RATIONALE
1. Determine the need for restraints. Assess the patient's physical condition, behavior, and mental status.	Restraints should be used only as a last resort when alternative measures have failed, and the patient is at increased risk for harming self or others.
2. Confirm facility policy for the application of restraints. **Secure an order from the physician or other licensed practitioner who is permitted to order restraint or seclusion in that health care facility, or validate that the order has been obtained within the required time frame (CMS, 2020).**	Policy protects the patient and the nurse and specifies guidelines for application as well as the type of restraint and duration. **Each order for restraint or seclusion used for the management of violent or self-destructive behavior that jeopardizes the immediate physical safety of the patient, a staff member, or others may only be renewed in accordance with the following limits for up to a total of 24 hours: (A) 4 hours for adults 18 years of age or older, (B) 2 hours for children and adolescents 9 to 17 years of age, or (C) 1 hour for children under 9 years of age. After 24 hours, before writing a new order for the use of restraint or seclusion for the management of violent or self-destructive behavior, a physician or other licensed practitioner who is permitted to order restraint or seclusion in that health care facility and responsible for the care of the patient must see and assess the patient** (CMS, 2006).
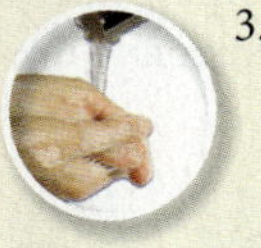 3. Perform hand hygiene and put on PPE, if indicated.	Hand hygiene and PPE prevent the spread of microorganisms. PPE is required based on transmission precautions.
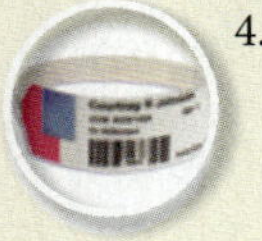 4. Identify the patient.	Identifying the patient ensures the right patient receives the intervention and helps prevent errors.
5. Explain the reason for restraint use to patient and family/caregivers. Clarify how care will be given and how needs will be met. Explain that restraint is a temporary measure.	Explanation to the patient and family/caregivers may lessen confusion and anger and provide reassurance. A clearly stated facility policy on the application of restraints should be available for the patient and family/caregivers to read. In a long-term care facility, the family/caregivers must give consent before a restraint is applied.
6. Include the patient's family and/or caregivers in the plan of care.	Promotes person-centered, individualized care and engagement, continuity of care and understanding.
7. Inspect the restraint before use. Do not use a restraint that is soiled or damaged (TIDI Products, 2018a).	Always inspect the device before each use, checking for broken stitches or parts, torn, cut or frayed material; or locks, buckles or hook-and-loop fasteners that do not hold securely. Do not use soiled or damaged restraints to prevent injury or death (TIDI Products, 2018a).

(continued on page 874)

Skill 28-2 Applying an Extremity Restraint *(continued)*

ACTION	RATIONALE
8. Apply restraint according to the manufacturer's directions:	Proper application reduces the risk for injury.
a. Choose the least restrictive type of device that allows the greatest possible degree of mobility.	This provides minimal restriction.
b. Pad bony prominences.	Padding helps prevent skin injury.
c. Wrap the restraint around the extremity with the soft part in contact with the skin (Figure 1). If a hand mitt is being used, pull over the hand with cushion to the palmar aspect of the hand (Figure 2).	Prevents excess pressure on the extremity.

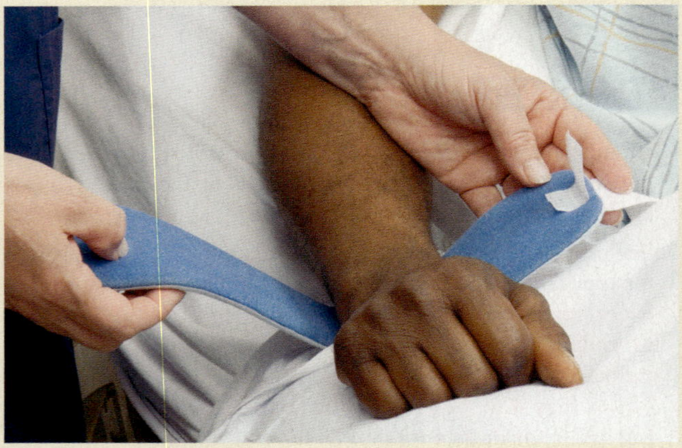

FIGURE 1. Wrapping the restraint around the extremity with the soft part in contact with the skin.

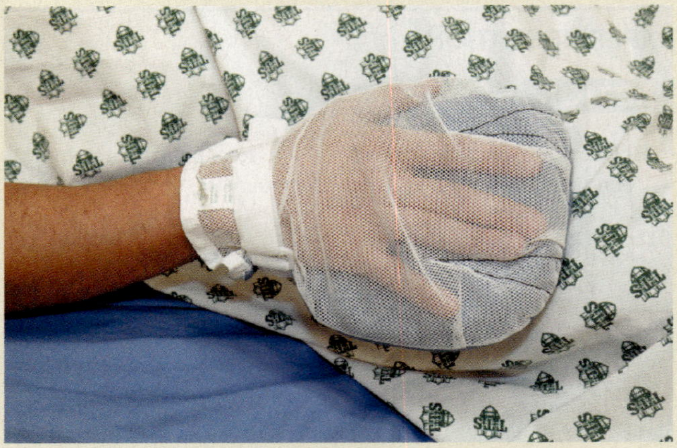

FIGURE 2. Using a hand mitt, with cushion to the palmar aspect of hand.

ACTION	RATIONALE
9. Secure in place with the hook-and-loop fastener straps or other mechanism, depending on specific restraint device (Figure 3). Depending on the characteristics of the specific restraint, close the quick-release buckle on the cuff.	Proper application secures the restraint and ensures that there is no interference with the patient's circulation and potential alteration in neurovascular status.
10. **Ensure that one to two fingers can be inserted between the restraint and patient's extremity (Figure 4).**	The restraint must be snug, but not compromise circulation (TIDI Products, 2018b). Proper application ensures that nothing interferes with the patient's circulation and potential alteration in the neurovascular status.

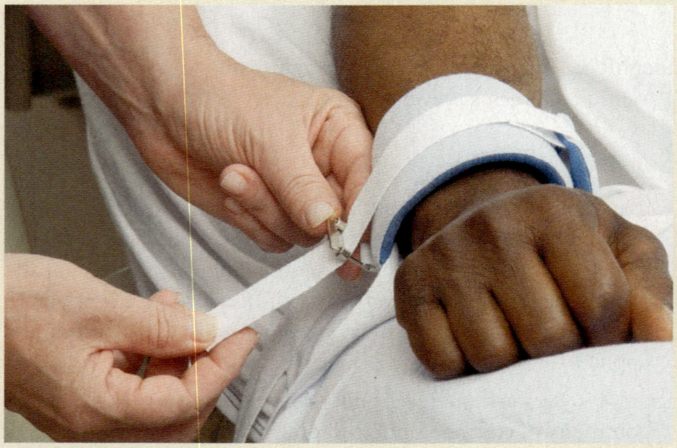

FIGURE 3. Securing restraint on extremity.

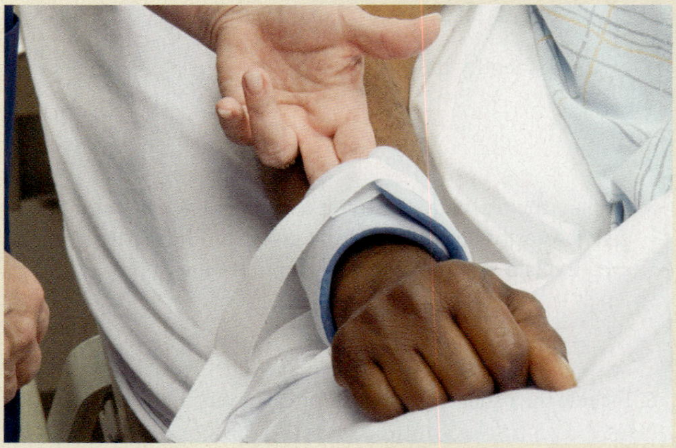

FIGURE 4. Ensuring that two fingers can be inserted between the restraint and the patient's extremity.

Skill 28-2 Applying an Extremity Restraint (continued)

ACTION	RATIONALE
11. Maintain restrained extremity in normal anatomic position. **Use a quick-release knot to tie the restraint to the bed frame that moves with the patient, not side rail, bed rail, mattress, or head/footboard (Figure 5).** The restraint may also be attached to a chair frame. The site should not be readily accessible to the patient.	Maintaining a normal position lessens the possibility of an injury. A quick-release knot ensures that the restraint will not tighten when pulled and can be removed quickly in an emergency. Securing the restraint to a side rail may injure the patient when the side rail is lowered. Tying the restraint out of the patient's reach promotes security.

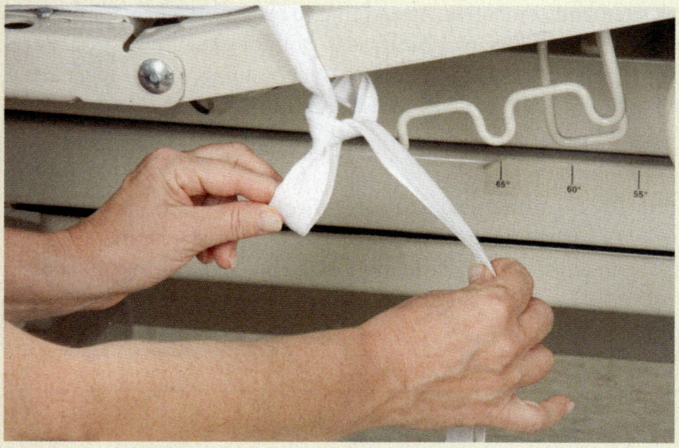

FIGURE 5. Securing restraint to bed frame.

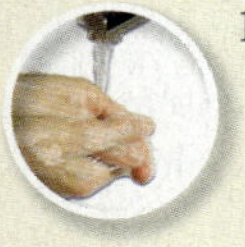

ACTION	RATIONALE
12. Remove PPE, if used. Perform hand hygiene.	Proper removal of PPE reduces the risk for infection transmission and contamination of other items. Hand hygiene prevents transmission of microorganisms.
13. **Assess the patient according to facility policy, or more often, based on the individual patient circumstances and nursing judgment.** Assessment should include the placement of the restraint, neurovascular assessment of the affected extremity, and skin integrity. In addition, assess for signs of sensory deprivation, such as increased sleeping, daydreaming, anxiety, panic, and hallucinations. Monitor the patient's vital signs.	The condition of the restrained patient must be continually assessed, monitored, and reevaluated (CMS, 2006). The frequency of monitoring should be made on an individual basis, which includes a rationale that reflects consideration of the individual patient's medical needs and health status (CMS, 2006). Improperly applied restraints may cause skin tears, abrasions, or bruises. Decreased circulation may result in paleness, coolness, decreased sensation, tingling, numbness, or pain in extremity. The use of restraints may decrease environmental stimulation and result in sensory deprivation. Monitoring vital signs provides information about the status of the patient.
14. **Remove restraint at least every 2 hours or according to facility policy, individual patient circumstances, and nursing judgment. Remove the restraint at least every 2 hours for children 9 to 17 years of age and at least every 1 hour for children under 9 years of age, or according to facility policy, individual patient circumstances, and nursing judgment.** Perform range-of-motion (ROM) exercises. Provide for hydration, nutritional, and elimination needs.	Removal allows you to assess the patient and reevaluate the need for a restraint. It also allows interventions for toileting, provision of nutrition and liquids, exercise, and change of position. Exercise increases circulation in the restrained extremity.
15. **Evaluate the patient for continued need of restraint.** Reapply restraint only if continued need is evident and order is still valid.	Continued need must be documented for reapplication.
16. Reassure the patient at regular intervals. Provide continued explanation of rationale for interventions, reorientation if necessary, and plan of care. **Keep the call bell within the patient's easy reach.**	Reassurance demonstrates caring and provides an opportunity for sensory stimulation as well as ongoing assessment and evaluation. The patient can use the call bell to summon assistance quickly.

(continued on page 876)

Skill 28-2 Applying an Extremity Restraint *(continued)*

DOCUMENTATION

Guidelines

Document alternative measures attempted before application of the restraint and that less restrictive interventions have been determined to be ineffective. Document patient assessment before application. Record patient and family/caregiver education and understanding regarding restraint use. Document family/caregiver consent, if necessary, according to facility policy. Document reason for restraining patient, date and time of application, type of restraint, times when removed, and frequency and result of nursing assessments.

Sample Documentation

7/10/25 0830 Patient disoriented and combative. Attempting to remove tracheostomy and indwelling urinary catheter; verified with primary physician both devices are necessary at this time. Patient continued to tug at catheter and pull on tracheostomy while supervised at bedside. Family unwilling to sit with patient. Wrist restraints applied bilaterally as prescribed.

—K. Urhahn, RN

7/10/25 1030 Patient continues to be disoriented and combative. Wrist restraints removed for 30 minutes during patient's bath; skin intact, hands warm, even skin tone, +radial pulses, +movement; passive and active range of motion completed. Wrist restraints reapplied.

—K. Urhahn, RN

DEVELOPING CLINICAL REASONING AND CLINICAL JUDGMENT

UNEXPECTED SITUATIONS AND ASSOCIATED INTERVENTIONS

- *Patient has an IV catheter in the right wrist and is trying to remove a drain from a wound:* The left wrist may have a cloth restraint applied. Due to the IV in the right wrist, alternative forms of restraints could be tried, such as a cloth mitt or an elbow restraint.
- *Patient cannot move left arm:* Do not apply the restraint to an extremity that is immobile. If the patient cannot move the extremity, there is no need to apply a restraint. Restraint may be applied to right arm after obtaining an order from the physician or other licensed practitioner who is permitted to order restraint or seclusion in that health care facility and is responsible for the care of the patient.

SPECIAL CONSIDERATIONS

General Considerations

- Do not position patient with wrist restraints flat in a supine position due to an increased risk for aspiration (Springer, 2015). If supine position is necessary, be aware that constant monitoring may be required to reduce risk for complications for those at risk of vomiting while restrained (TIDI Products, 2018a).
- Check restraint for correct size before applying. Extremity restraints are available in different sizes. If restraint is too large, patient may free the extremity. If restraint is too small, circulation may be affected.
- Avoid use on an extremity restraint on a limb with a dislocation or fracture (TIDI Products, 2018b).
- Do not use on an extremity with an IV or wound site that could be compromised by the device (TIDI Products, 2018b).
- Always inspect the device before each use, checking for broken stitches or parts, torn, cut or frayed material; or locks, buckles or hook-and-loop fasteners that do not hold securely. Do not use soiled or damaged restraints (TIDI Products, 2018a).

Community-Based Care Considerations

- In long-term care facilities, patients have the right to be free from physical or chemical restraint not required to treat the resident's medical symptoms. When the use of restraints is indicated, the facility must use the least restrictive alternative for the least amount of time and document ongoing re-evaluation of the need for restraints (2020b).

DEVELOPING CLINICAL REASONING AND CLINICAL JUDGMENT

1. You are the visiting nurse for a frail older adult who lives alone in her own home and prizes her independence. You assess her to be at high risk for falls because of her general weakness, the medication she takes, and a long history of indifference to safety counseling. What instruments can you use to determine her falls risk? What is the benefit of using a standardized instrument/tool for risk assessment? What nursing interventions are likely to be most effective in ensuring her safety?
2. You are the nurse lobbying for improvement in state and federal emergency preparedness. What do you see as your top three priorities? Which federal agencies would be the best partners? What state and community resources should be considered? Why is emergency preparedness so important?

PRACTICING FOR NCLEX

1. The nurse manager and nurses in an acute care hospital are participating in a safety huddle to identify patients at risk for falling. Which patients will the nurses determine require follow-up? Select all that apply.
   a. Age >50 years
   b. History of falling
   c. Taking antibiotics
   d. Presence of postural hypotension
   e. Nausea from chemotherapy
   f. Transferred from long-term care
2. A school nurse is teaching parents about home and fire safety. What information will be included in the teaching plan? Select all that apply.
   a. Sixty percent of U.S. fire deaths occur in the home.
   b. Most fatal fires occur when people are cooking.
   c. Most people who die in fires die of smoke inhalation.
   d. Fire-related injury and death have declined due to the availability and use of smoke alarms.
   e. Fires are more likely to occur in homes without electricity or gas.
   f. Fires are less likely to spread if bedroom doors are kept open when sleeping.
3. A community health nurse is providing education on child safety. Who does the nurse identify as at highest risk for choking and suffocation?
   a. A toddler playing with his older brother's wooden blocks
   b. A 4-year-old eating yogurt and strawberries for lunch
   c. An infant sleeping in the prone position
   d. A 3-year-old drinking a glass of juice
4. While discussing home safety with the nurse, a patient admits that they smoke a cigarette in bed before falling asleep at night. Which health problem is the priority for this patient?
   a. Impaired gas exchange: etiology, cigarette smoking
   b. Acute anxiety: etiology, inability to stop smoking
   c. Nonadherence: etiology, nonadherence to recommendation to stop smoking
   d. Knowledge deficiency: etiology, risk for burn and suffocation in a house fire
5. A nurse working in a pediatrician's office receives calls from parents whose children have ingested a toxic substance from under the sink. How will the nurse advise the parents?
   a. Administer activated charcoal in tablet form and take child to the ED.
   b. Administer syrup of ipecac and take child to the ED.
   c. Bring the child in to the primary care provider for gastric lavage.
   d. Call the PCC immediately before attempting any home remedy.
6. A nurse is teaching parents in a parenting class about the use of car seats and restraints for infants and children. What should be the focus of this education?
   a. Booster seats should be used for children until they are 4′9″ tall and weigh between 80 and 100 lb.
   b. Most U.S. states mandate the use of infant car seats and carriers when transporting a child in a motor vehicle.
   c. Infants and toddlers up to age 2 years (or the maximum height and weight for the seat) should be in a front-facing safety seat.
   d. Children age older than 6 years may be restrained using a car seat belt in the back seat.
7. A nurse in a long-term care facility is on an interprofessional safety committee focusing on protecting older adults from injury and trauma. Which action does the nurse suggest they prioritize?
   a. Ensuring proper function of fire alarms
   b. Preventing exposure to temperature extremes
   c. Screening for partner or elder abuse
   d. Maintaining clutter free rooms and hallways
8. An experienced nurse and new graduate nurse are caring for a confused older adult who gets out of bed and wanders. The preceptor intervenes when observing which action by the graduate nurse?
   a. Raising all four side rails to keep the patient in bed
   b. Performing documentation in the patient's room
   c. Suggesting obtaining a patient "sitter"
   d. Using a bed alarm to alert staff the patient leaving the bed
9. The hospital's fire alarm sounds, and an announcement is made that there is a fire in a patient room. What is the priority for nurses on the unit?
   a. Removing patients from the room or vicinity
   b. Attempting to put out the fire with water or appropriate extinguishers
   c. Closing all the doors on the unit to contain the fire
   d. Running to the closest unit and requesting help

10. A nurse is filing a safety event report for a confused patient who fell while getting out of bed. Which action is most appropriate during documentation?
   a. Including suggestions on how to prevent the incident from recurring
   b. Providing minimal information about the incident
   c. Discussing the details with the patient before documenting them
   d. Recording the circumstances and effect on the patient in the health record
11. Nursing students are invited to participate in the clinical agency's annual disaster drill, simulating the release of an airborne infectious agent and ensuing panic. Which assignment is most appropriate for the students?
   a. Cleansing and dressing wounds sustained during the panic
   b. Triaging patients with respiratory symptoms and traumatic injuries
   c. Providing information to families of missing loved ones
   d. Ensuring everyone entering and working has an N95 mask
12. A disoriented older resident likes to wander the halls of their long-term care facility but becomes agitated when they cannot find their room. Which action is most appropriate as an alternative to restraints?
   a. Placing them in a geriatric chair near the nurses' station
   b. Using the sheets to secure them snugly in the bed
   c. Keeping the bed in the high position
   d. Identifying their door with his photograph and a balloon
13. A nurse has exhausted every effort to keep a confused, postoperative patient safe and in bed. Following The Joint Commission guidelines for use of restraints, which nursing action reflects safe practice?
   a. Positioning the patient in the supine position prior to applying wrist restraints
   b. Ensuring that two fingers can be inserted between the restraint and patient's wrist
   c. Applying a cloth restraint to the left hand of the patient with an IV catheter in the right wrist
   d. Tying an elbow restraint to the raised side rail of the patient's bed
14. During the admission process, a nurse orients an older adult to their hospital room. What is the current safety priority?
   a. Explaining how to use the telephone
   b. Introducing the patient to their roommate
   c. Reviewing the hospital policy on visiting hours
   d. Demonstrating how to operate the call bell
15. A nurse works in a facility stating they support a culture of safety. What will the nurse expect to find operationalized in this culture? Select all that apply.
   a. Support for reporting errors and near misses without blame
   b. Nurses being the employees responsible for safety in the organization
   c. Commitment of resources to address actual/potential safety issues
   d. Emphasis placed on individuals, their departments, and resources
   e. Promotion of teamwork and collaboration throughout the organization
   f. Administrators' and managers' commitment to safe operations
16. A school nurse is teaching about adolescent safety with students entering high school. What will the nurse include in the discussion about the major causes of death in this group? Select all that apply.
   a. Choking
   b. Diving accidents
   c. Car accidents
   d. Suicide
   e. Intimate partner violence
   f. Cigarette smoking

ANSWERS WITH RATIONALES

1. **b, d, f.** Risk factors for falls include age >65 years, documented history of falls, postural hypotension which can cause dizziness, and unfamiliar environment. A medication regimen that includes diuretics creating urinary urgency and tranquilizers, sedatives, hypnotics, or analgesics causing altered mental status and impaired judgment are also risks. Chemotherapy or antibiotics are not included as factors leading to falls.
2. **c, d, e.** Eighty percent of fire deaths in the United States occur in the home. Most fatal home fires occur while people are sleeping, and most deaths result from smoke inhalation rather than burns. The widespread availability and use of home smoke alarms is considered the primary reason for the decline in fire-related injury and death. People with limited financial resources may use space or kerosene heaters, wood stoves, or a fireplace as the sole source of heat if utilities are turned off. Bedroom doors should be kept closed when sleeping and monitors used to listen for children.
3. **c.** Infants should be placed on their backs to sleep. A young child may place small or loose parts in the mouth. Anything that will fit through the average toilet paper roll is not safe for a toddler. A 3-year-old and a 4-year-old drinking juice and eating yogurt are developmentally appropriate.
4. **d.** Because the patient is not aware or denies that smoking in bed poses a danger for fire and toxic fumes, education about the risk for burns and suffocation is needed. The other three nursing diagnoses are correctly stated but are not a priority in this situation.
5. **d.** The nurse tells the parents to call the PCC immediately, before attempting a home remedy. Parents may be instructed to bring the child to an emergency facility for immediate treatment. Activated charcoal is not appropriate to use at home but under medical supervision, after the risks and benefits have been assessed. Syrup of ipecac is no longer recommended because vomiting may exacerbate the hazard as it vomited up. Gastric lavage is no longer prescribed routinely for the treatment of ingestion of a toxic substance because it may propel the poison into the small intestine, where absorption will occur. The amount of toxin removed by gastric lavage is relatively small.

6. a. Booster seats should be used for children until they are 4′9″ tall and weigh between 80 and 100 lb. All 50 U.S. states mandate the use of infant car seats and carriers when transporting a child in a motor vehicle. Infants and toddlers up to age 2 years (or up to the maximum height and weight for the seat) should be in a rear-facing safety seat. Many children older than age 6 years should still be in a booster seat.
7. **d.** Falls among older adults are the most common cause of hospital admissions for trauma, therefore rooms and hallways should be free of clutter. Elder abuse, fires, and temperature extremes are also significant hazards for older adults but are not the most common cause of trauma admissions. IPV occurs more frequently in adults as opposed to older adults.
8. a. The desire to prevent a patient from wandering is not sufficient reason for the use of side rails. People of small stature are more likely to be injured slipping through or between the side rails. A history of falls from a bed with raised side rails carries a significant risk for a serious incident. The nurse uses creative measures while promoting safety and respect for the patient's dignity.
9. a. The nurse uses the acronym RACE and rescues and/or removes the patient and those in nearby rooms as the safety priority. Sounding the alarm and extinguishing the fire are important after the patient is safe. Remaining on the unit allows you to assist patients and is more appropriate; assistance can be summoned by phone.
10. d. A safety event report objectively describes the circumstances of the accident or incident. The report also details the patient's response and the examination and treatment of the patient after the incident. The nurse completes the event report immediately after the incident and is responsible for recording the circumstances and the effect on the patient in the medical record. The safety event report is not a part of the medical record and should not be mentioned in the documentation. Because laws vary in different states, nurses must know their own state law regarding safety event reports.
11. **d.** Rapid assessment and triage are essential during a disaster. Delegating tasks appropriate to students are based on skill level and ability to complete skills independently. Ensuring masks are worn and the education for this, if needed, are within the educational and clinical skills of nursing students.
12. d. This allows the resident to be on the move and be more likely to find their room when they want to return. Many facilities use this kind of approach, rather than restrict patients' movements. Identifying the patient's door with their photo and a balloon may resolve the issue without restraints. Using the geriatric chair and sheets are forms of physical restraint. Leaving the bed in the high position is a safety risk and would likely result in a fall.
13. **b.** The nurse should be able to place two fingers between the restraint and a patient's wrist or ankle. Restraining the patient in a supine position increases the risk of aspiration. Due to the IV in the right wrist, alternative forms of restraints should be tried, such as a cloth mitt or an elbow restraint. Securing the restraint to a side rail may injure the patient when the side rail is lowered.
14. **d.** Teaching the patient to use the call bell is a safety priority; knowing how to use the phone, meeting the roommate, and knowledge of visiting hours will not necessarily prevent an accidental injury.
15. **a, c, e, f.** The key features of a culture of safety include: (1) acknowledging the high-risk nature of health care and the commitment to safe operations, (2) maintaining a blame-free environment where reporting is protected and expected, (3) promoting teamwork and collaboration to prevent and seek solutions to patient safety issues, and (4) valuing safety as a focus in all health care facilities, the home, workplace, and community.
16. **c, d.** Car accidents and suicide are common causes of death in adolescents. Choking is more typical in children younger than age 3 years. While diving accidents can occur in adolescents due to poor judgment, this is not as common. Intimate partner violence is more common in adults. Smoking, while ill advised, takes many years or decades to become a cause of death.

Bibliography

AAA. (2022). Senior driving: Facts and figures. Retrieved June 9, 2022, from https://seniordriving.aaa.com/resources-family-friends/conversations-about-driving/facts-research/

American Academy of Child and Adolescent Psychiatry. (2016, April). *Bullying*. (Report No. 80). American Academy of Child and Adolescent Psychiatry. https://www.aacap.org/AACAP/Families_and_Youth/Facts_for_Families/FFF-Guide/Bullying-080.aspx

American Association of College of Nursing. (2021, April 6). *The essentials: Core competencies for professional nursing education*. https://www.aacnnursing.org/AACN-Essentials

American Cancer Society (ACS). (2019, April 18). *Keeping your kids tobacco free: What parents need to know*. https://www.cancer.org/healthy/stay-away-from-tobacco/keeping-your-kids-tobacco-free.html

American College of Emergency Physicians. (2020). *Bombings: Injury patterns and care*. https://www.acep.org/imports/clinical-and-practice-management/resources/ems-and-disaster-preparedness/disaster-preparedness-grant-projects/bombings-injury-patterns-and-care/

American Nurses Association. (n.d.a). *COVID-19 resource center*. Retrieved June 10, 2020, from https://www.nursingworld.org/practice-policy/work-environment/health-safety/disaster-preparedness/coronavirus/

American Nurses Association. (n.d.b). *Culture of safety*. Retrieved May 26, 2020, from https://www.nursingworld.org/practice-policy/work-environment/health-safety/culture-of-safety/

American Nurses Association. (n.d.c). *Disaster preparedness*. Retrieved June 10, 2020, from https://www.nursingworld.org/practice-policy/work-environment/health-safety/disaster-preparedness

American Nurses Association. (2012, March 12). *Reduction of patient restraint and seclusion in health care settings*. https://www.nursingworld.org/~4af287/globalassets/docs/ana/ethics/ps_reduction-of-patient-restraint-and-seclusion-in-health-care-settings.pdf

American Nurses Association. (2019, June). *Workplace violence*. https://www.nursingworld.org/practice-policy/advocacy/state/workplace-violence2/

American Psychiatric Association (APA). (2019). *Treating LGBTQ patients who have experienced intimate partner violence*. Retrieved April 9, 2020, from https://www.psychiatry.org/File%20Library/Psychiatrists/Cultural-Competency/IPV-Guide/APA-Guide-to-IPV-Among-LGTBQ-Communities.pdf

American Red Cross. (2022). *How to prepare for emergencies*. Retrieved June 9, 2022, from https://www.redcross.org/get-help/how-to-prepare-for-emergencies.html

Arnold, L. S., Benson, A. J., Tefft, B. C., Barragan, D., Jin, L., Kolek, S., & Horrey, W. J. (2019, November). *Effectiveness of distracted driving countermeasures: A review of the literature* (Research Brief). AAA Foundation for Traffic Safety. https://aaafoundation.org/wp-content/uploads/2019/11/19-0553_AAAFTS-DD-Countermeasures-Brief_r3.pdf

Association of periOperative Registered Nurses (AORN). (2020). *Management of surgical smoke*. Retrieved June 9, 2022, from https://www.aorn.org/guidelines/clinical-resources/tool-kits/management-of-surgical-smoke-tool-kit

Bergen, G., Stevens, M. R., Kakara, R., & Burns, E. R. (2019). Understanding modifiable and unmodifiable older adult fall risk factors to create effective prevention strategies. *American Journal of American Lifestyle Medicine, 15*(6), 580–589. https://doi.org/10.1177%2F1559827619880529

Bergeron, N., Bergeron, C., Lapointe, L., Kriellaars, D., Aubertin, P., Tanenbaum, B., & Fleet, R. (2019). Don't take down the monkey bars: Rapid systematic review of playground-related injuries. *Canadian Family Physician Medecin De Famille Canadien, 65*(3), e121–e128. https://www.cfp.ca/content/65/3/e121.long

Breiding, M. J., Basile, K. C., Smith, S. G., Black, M. C., & Mahendra, R. R. (2015). *Intimate partner violence surveillance: Uniform definitions and recommended data elements, version 2.0*. National Center for Injury Prevention and Control, Centers for Disease Control and Prevention. http://www.cdc.gov/violenceprevention/pdf/intimatepartnerviolence.pdf

Buijs, P. C. M., Boot, E., Shugar, A., Fung, W. L. A., & Bassett, A. S. (2017). Internet safety issues for adolescents and adults with intellectual disabilities. *Journal of Applied Research in Intellectual Disabilities, 30*(2), 416–418. https://doi.org/10.1111/jar.12250

Carney, C., McGehee, D., Harland, K., Weiss, M., & Raby, M. (2015, March 25). *Using naturalistic driving data to assess the prevalence of environmental factors and driver behaviors in teen driver crashes*. AAA Foundation for Traffic Safety. http://newsroom.aaa.com/wp-content/uploads/2015/03/TeenCrashCausation_2015_FINALREPORT.pdf

Centers for Disease Control and Prevention (CDC). (2017, February 10). *Home and recreational safety: Important facts about falls.* https://www.cdc.gov/homeandrecreationalsafety/falls/adultfalls.html

Centers for Disease Control and Prevention (CDC). (2018a, January 18). *Emergency preparedness and response: Chemical emergencies overview.* http://emergency.cdc.gov/chemical/overview.asp

Centers for Disease Control and Prevention (CDC). (2018b, April 4). *Emergency preparedness and response: Bioterrorism.* https://emergency.cdc.gov/bioterrorism/

Centers for Disease Control and Prevention (CDC). (2019a, May 21). *Alzheimer's disease and healthy aging: Emergency preparedness for older adults.* https://www.cdc.gov/aging/publications/features/older-adult-emergency.html

Centers for Disease Control and Prevention (CDC). (2019b). *Resource algorithm for fall risk screening, assessment, and intervention.* https://www.cdc.gov/steadi/pdf/STEADI-Algorithm-508.pdf

Centers for Disease Control and Prevention (CDC). (2019c, February 6). *A national action plan for child injury prevention: Reducing drowning injuries in children.* https://www.cdc.gov/safechild/nap/index.html

Centers for Disease Control and Prevention (CDC). (2019d, February 6). *Playground safety.* https://www.cdc.gov/safechild/playground/index.html

Centers for Disease Control and Prevention (CDC). (2019e, February 26). *Preventing intimate partner violence.* https://www.cdc.gov/violenceprevention/intimatepartnerviolence/fastfact.html

Centers for Disease Control and Prevention (CDC). (2019f, July 23). *What is population health?* https://www.cdc.gov/pophealthtraining/whatis.html

Centers for Disease Control and Prevention (CDC). (2019g, October 30). *Motor vehicle safety – Teen drivers: Get the facts.* https://www.cdc.gov/motorvehiclesafety/teen_drivers/teendrivers_factsheet.html

Centers for Disease Control and Prevention (CDC). (2019h, December 19). *NCHHSTP social determinants of health.* https://www.cdc.gov/nchhstp/socialdeterminants/index.html

Centers for Disease Control and Prevention (CDC). (2020a). *National notifiable disease surveillance system (NNDSS): 2020 national notifiable conditions.* Retrieved June 9, 2022, from https://wwwn.cdc.gov/nndss/conditions/notifiable/2020/

Centers for Disease Control and Prevention (CDC). (2020b, January 22). *Emergency preparedness and response: Health alert network (HAN).* https://emergency.cdc.gov/han/

Centers for Disease Control and Prevention (CDC). (2020c, February 3). *Quick facts on the risks of e-cigarettes for kids, teens, and young adults.* https://www.cdc.gov/tobacco/basic_information/e-cigarettes/Quick-Facts-on-the-Risks-of-E-cigarettes-for-Kids-Teens-and-Young-Adults.html

Centers for Disease Control and Prevention (CDC). (2020d, February 26). *Pregnancy.* https://www.cdc.gov/pregnancy/during.html

Centers for Disease Control and Prevention (CDC). (2020e, March 16). *HEADS UP.* https://www.cdc.gov/headsup/index.html

Centers for Disease Control and Prevention (CDC). (2020f, April 16). *Radiation emergencies: Radiation and your health.* https://www.cdc.gov/nceh/radiation/emergencies/index.htm?CDC_AA_refVal=https%3A%2F%2Femergency.cdc.gov%2Fradiation%2Findex.asp

Centers for Disease Control and Prevention (CDC). (2020g, April 30). *PROTECT initiative: Advancing children's medication safety.* https://www.cdc.gov/MedicationSafety/protect/protect_Initiative.html

Centers for Disease Control and Prevention (CDC). (2021a, August 6). *Older adult fall prevention: Facts about falls.* https://www.cdc.gov/falls/facts.html

Centers for Disease Control and Prevention (CDC). (2021b, July 17). *Drowning facts.* https://www.cdc.gov/drowning/facts/index.html

Centers for Medicare & Medicaid Services (CMS). (2006, December 8). Department of Health and Human Services. Federal Register. Part IV. 42 CFR Part 482. *Medicare and Medicaid programs; Hospital conditions of participation: Patients' rights; Final rule.* https://www.cms.gov/Regulations-and-Guidance/Legislation/CFCsAndCoPs/downloads/finalpatientrightsrule.pdf

Centers for Medicare & Medicaid Services (CMS). (2020, December 21). Department of Health and Human Services. CMS manual system. Pub. 100-07. Appendix A. Survey protocol, regulations and interpretive guidelines for hospitals. §482.13 *Conditions of participation: Patients' rights.* https://www.cms.gov/Regulations-and-Guidance/Guidance/Manuals/downloads/som107ap_a_hospitals.pdf

Cheng, T. A., Bell, J. M., Haileyesus, T., Gilchrist, J., Sugerman, D. E., & Coronado, V. G. (2016). Nonfatal playground-related traumatic brain injuries among children, 2001–2013. *Pediatrics, 137*(6), e20152721. https://doi.org/10.1542/peds.2015-2721

Crenshaw, K. (1989). Demarginalizing the intersection of race and sex: A Black feminist critique of antidiscrimination doctrine, feminist theory and antiracist politics. *University of Chicago Legal Forum, Vol. 1989*, Article 8. https://chicagounbound.uchicago.edu/uclf/vol1989/iss1/8

Crews, J. E., Chou, C. F., Stevens, J. A., Saaddine, J. B. (2016). Falls among persons aged ≥65 years with and without severe vision impairment—United States, 2014. *Morbidity and Mortality Weekly Report, 65*(17), 433–437. http://dx.doi.org/10.15585/mmwr.mm6517a2external

Davis, G. A., Purcell, L., Schneider, K. J., Yeates, K. O., Gioia, G. A., Anderson, V., Ellenbogen, R. G., Echemendia, R. J., Makdissi, M., Sills, A., Iverson, G. L., Dvorak, J., McCrory, P., Meeuwisse, W., Patricios, J., Giza, C. C., & Kutcher, J. S. (2017). The Child Sport Concussion Assessment Tool 5th edition (Child SCAT5). *British Journal of Sports Medicine, 51*(11), 859–861. http://dx. doi. org/ bjsports- 2017- 097492childscat5

Durbin, D. R., Hoffman, B. D., & Aap Council on Injury, Violence, and Poison Prevention. (2018). Child passenger safety. *Pediatrics, 142*(5), e20182460. https://doi.org/10.1542/peds.2018-2460

Echemendia, R. J., Meeuwisse, W., McCrory, P., Davis, G. A., Putukian, M., Leddy, J., Makdissi, M., Sullivan, S. J., Broglio, S. P, Raftery, M., Schneider, K., Kissick, J., Mccrea, M., Dvorak, J., Sills, A., Aubry, M., Engebretsen, L., Lossemore, M., Fuller, G., … Herring, S. (2017). The Sport Concussion Assessment Tool 5th edition (SCAT5). *British Journal of Sports Medicine, 51*(11), 848–850. http://dx.doi.org/bjsports-2017-097506SCAT5

ECRI. (2018, September 26). *Healthcare risk, quality, & safety guidance: Falls prevention training program.* https://www.ecri.org/search-results/member-preview/hrc/pages/edutrain14

Finkelhor, D., Walsh, K., Jones, L., Mitchell, K., & Collier, A. (2020). Youth internet safety education: Aligning programs with the evidence base. *Trauma Violence Abuse, 22*(5), 1233–1247. http://dx.doi.org/10.1177/1524838020916257

FitzSimons, C., Maurice, A., & Osbourne, M. (2020, May 27). *Community eligibility: The key to hunger-free schools—School year 2019–2020.* Food Research & Action Center. https://frac.org/?s=The+key+to+hunger-free

Food Research & Action Center. (2020, March). Ensuring access to the child nutrition programs in the event of school closures. https://frac.org/wp-content/uploads/two-pager-child-nutritionfinalfinalMarch20-1-1.pdf

Fortson, B. L., Klevens, J., Merrick, M. T., Gilbert, L. K., & Alexander, S. P. (2016). *Preventing child abuse and neglect: A technical package for policy, norm, and programmatic activities.* National Center for Injury Prevention and Control, Centers for Disease Control and Prevention. https://www.cdc.gov/violenceprevention/pdf/CAN-Prevention-Technical-Package.pdf

Foundation for a Drug-Free World. (2020). *Synthetic drugs.* http://www.drugfreeworld.org/drugfacts/synthetic.html

Fowler, K. A., Dahlberg, L. L., Haileyesus, T., Gutierrez, C., & Bacon, S. (2017). Childhood firearm injuries in the United States. *Pediatrics, 140*(1), e20163486. https://doi.org/10.1542/peds.2016-3486

Gardner, S. S. (2019, February 12). *Teen body piercings: Risks, safety, and more.* https://teens.webmd.com/teen-girls-body-ear-piercing#3

Hamed, A., Bohm, S., Mersmann, F., & Arampatzis, A. (2018). Follow-up efficacy of physical exercise interventions on fall incidence and fall risk in healthy older adults: A systematic review and meta-analysis. *Sports Medicine Open, 4*(1), 56. https://doi.org/10.1186/s40798-018-0170-z

Healthy, Hunger-Free Kids Act of (2010). Public Law No. 111–296. https://www.congress.gov/bill/111th-congress/senate-bill/3307

Hedegaard, H., Miniño, A. M., & Warner, M. (2020, January). *Drug overdose deaths in the United States 1999–2018 (NCHS Data Brief No. 356).* U.S. Department of Health and Human Services, Centers for Disease Control and Prevention, National Center for Health Statistics. https://www.cdc.gov/nchs/data/databriefs/db356-h.pdf

Henley Haugh, K. (2015). Head-to-toe: Organizing your baseline patient physical assessment. *Nursing, 45*(12), 58–61.

Hornor, G. (2018). Bullying: What the PNP needs to know. *Journal of Pediatric Health Care, 32*(4), 399–408. https://doi.org/10.1016/j.pedhc.2018.02.001

Human Rights Campaign Foundation. (2019). *A national epidemic: Fatal anti-transgender violence in the United States in 2019.* https://assets2.hrc.org/files/assets/resources/Anti-TransViolenceReport2019.pdf?_ga=2.129631498.722345101.1591737857-999813957.1591737857

Hunt, L. M., Bell, H. S., Baker, A. M., & Howard, H. A. (2017). Electronic health records and the disappearing patient. *Medical Anthropology Quarterly, 31*(3), 403–421. https://doi.org/10.1111/maq.12375

Insurance Institute for Highway Safety, & Highway Loss Data Institute. (2020, May). *Graduated licensing laws by state.* https://www.iihs.org/topics/teenagers/graduated-licensing-laws-table?topicName=teenagers

Irani, E., Hirschman, K. B., Cacchione, P. Z., & Bowles, K. H. (2020). The role of social, economic, and physical environmental factors in care planning for home health care recipients. *Research in Gerontological Nursing, 13*(3), 130–137. http://dx.doi.org/10.3928/19404921-20191210-01

The Joint Commission. (n.d.). *Overhead emergency codes.* Retrieved June 7, 2020, from https://www.jointcommission.org/-/media/tjc/documents/resources/emergency-management/em-overhead-emergency-codes-posterpdf.pdf

The Joint Commission. (2021, November 22). *Restraint and seclusion—Enclosure beds, side rails and mitts.* https://www.jointcommission.org/en/standards/standard-faqs/critical-access-hospital/provision-of-care-treatment-and-services-pc/000001668/

The Joint Commission. (2018, April 17). *Sentinel event alert 59: Physical and verbal violence against health care workers.* https://www.jointcommission.org/-/media/tjc/documents/resources/patient-safety-topics/sentinel-event/sea_59_workplace_violence_4_13_18_final.pdf

The Joint Commission. (2022a). *Emergency management.* Retrieved June 9, 2022, from https://www.jointcommission.org/en/resources/patient-safety-topics/emergency-management/

The Joint Commission. (2020b). *National patient safety goals: 2022 national patient safety goals.* Retrieved June 9, 2022, from https://www.jointcommission.org/standards/national-patient-safety-goals/

The Joint Commission. (2022c). *Sentinel event alert newsletters.* Retrieved June 9, 2022 from https://www.jointcommission.org/resources/patient-safety-topics/sentinel-event/sentinel-event-alert-newsletters/

The Joint Commission Center for Transforming Healthcare. (2022). *Targeted solutions tool for preventing falls.* Retrieved June 9, 2022 from https://www.centerfortransforminghealthcare.org/what-we-offer/targeted-solutions-tool/preventing-falls-tst/

Juurlink, D. N. (2016). Activated charcoal for acute overdose: A reappraisal. *British Journal of Clinical Pharmacology, 81*(3), 482–487. https://doi.org/10.1111/bcp.12793

Kemp, S. (2019, January 31). *Digital 2019: Global digital overview.* https://datareportal.com/reports/digital-2019-global-digital-overview

Lambert, A. B. E., Parks, S. E., Cottengim, C., Faulkner, M., Hauck, F. R., & Shapiro-Mendoza, C. K. (2019). Sleep-related infant suffocation deaths attributable to soft bedding, overlay, and wedging. *Pediatrics, 143*(5), e20183408. https://doi.org/10.1542/peds.2018-3408

Large, C., & Aldridge, M. (2018). Non-technical skills required to recognise and escalate patient deterioration in acute hospital settings. *Nursing Management (Harrow), 25*(2), 24–30.

Lasater, K. (2007). Clinical judgment development: Using simulation to create an assessment rubric. *Journal of Nursing Education, 46*(11), 496–503.

Manisalidis, I., Stavropoulou, E., Stavropoulos, A., & Bezirtzoglou, E. (2020). Environmental and health impacts of air pollution: A review. *Frontiers in Public Health, 8*, 14. https://doi.org/10.3389/fpubh.2020.00014

Morse, J. M., Tylko, S. J., & Dixon, H. A. (1987). Characteristics of the fall-prone patient. *Gerontologist, 27*(4), 516–522. https://doi.org/10.1093/geront/27.4.516

The National Domestic Violence Hotline. (n.d.). *Path to safety: What is a safety plan?* Retrieved June 1, 2020, from http://www.thehotline.org/help/path-to-safety/#tab-id-8

National Forensic Laboratory Information System. (2021, September). *Snapshot: Newly reported substances*. https://www.nflis.deadiversion.usdoj.gov/nflisdata/docs/NFLIS_Snapshot_092021.pdf

National Initiative for Cybersecurity Careers and Studies. (n.d.). *National cybersecurity awareness month 2019*. Retrieved June 10, 2020, from https://niccs.us-cert.gov/national-cybersecurity-awareness-month-2019

National Institute for Healthcare Improvement. (2022, May). *National action plan to advance patient safety*. http://www.ihi.org/Engage/Initiatives/National-Steering-Committee-Patient-Safety/Pages/National-Action-Plan-to-Advance-Patient-Safety.aspx

National Institute on Alcohol Abuse and Alcoholism. (2021, May). *Underage drinking*. https://www.niaaa.nih.gov/sites/default/files/publications/NIAAA_Underage_Drinking_1.pdf

National Institute on Drug Abuse. (2019a, February). *Fentanyl*. https://www.drugabuse.gov/publications/drugfacts/fentanyl

National Institute on Drug Abuse. (2019b, September). *Drug and alcohol use in college-age adults in 2018*. https://www.drugabuse.gov/related-topics/trends-statistics/infographics/drug-alcohol-use-in-college-age-adults-in-2018

Noohu, M. M., Dey, A. B., Sharma, S., & Hussain, M. E. (2017). International Classification of Function, Disability and Health framework for fall risk stratification in community dwelling older adults. *Geriatric Care, 3*(6526), 1–7. https://doi.org/10.4081/gc.2017.6526

Oleksy, A. J., & Schlesinger, J. J. (2019). What's all that noise—Improving the hospital soundscape. *Journal of Clinical Monitoring and Computing, 33*(4), 557–562. https://doi.org/10.1007/s10877-018-0215-3

Papaseit, E., Farré, M., Pérez-Mañá, C., Torrens, M., Ventura, M., Pujadas, M., de la Torre, R., & González, D. (2018). Acute pharmacological effects of 2C-B in humans: An observational study. *Frontiers in Pharmacology, 9*, 206. https://doi.org/10.3389/fphar.2018.00206

Safe Kids Worldwide. (2020, March). *Keeping kids safe around medicine: Insights and implications*. https://www.safekids.org/sites/default/files/medicine_safety_study_2020-v14.pdf

Safe Kids Worldwide. (2022). *Seat belt safety for big kids*. Retrieved on June 9, 2022 from http://www.safekids.org/tip/seat-belt-safety-big-kids

Saftari, L. N., & Kwon, O. S. (2018). Ageing vision and falls: A review. *Journal of Physiological Anthropology, 37*(1), 11. https://doi.org/10.1186/s40101-018-0170-1

Smith, S. G., Zhang, X., Basile, K. C., Merrick, M. T., Wang, J., Kresnow, M., & Chen, J. (2018, November). *The National Intimate Partner and Sexual Violence Survey (NISVS): 2015 Data brief—Updated release*. National Center for Injury Prevention and Control, Centers for Disease Control and Prevention. https://www.cdc.gov/violenceprevention/pdf/2015data-brief508.pdf

Soh, S. E., Barker, A. L., Morello, R. T., & Ackerman, I. N. (2020) Applying the International Classification of Functioning, Disability and Health framework to determine the predictors of falls and fractures in people with osteoarthritis or at high risk of developing osteoarthritis: Data from the Osteoarthritis Initiative. *BMC Musculoskeletal Disorders, 21*(1), 138. https://doi.org/10.1186/s12891-020-3160-5

Springer, G. (2015). When and how to use restraints. *American Nurse Today, 10*(1), 26–27. https://www.myamericannurse.com/wp-content/uploads/2015/01/ant1-Restraints-1218.pdf

Substance Abuse and Mental Health Services Administration. (SAMHSA). (2019, August). *Key substance use and mental health indicators in the United States: Results from the 2018 National Survey on Drug Use and Health (HHS Publication No. PEP19-5068, NSDUH Series H-54)*. Center for Behavioral Health Statistics and Quality, Substance Abuse and Mental Health Services Administration. https://www.samhsa.gov/data/sites/default/files/cbhsq-reports/NSDUHNationalFindingsReport2018/NSDUHNationalFindingsReport2018.pdf

TIDI Products. (2018a). *Posey®. Safety information for the use of Posey® restraining products*. https://f.hubspotusercontent40.net/hubfs/8218994/IFU/Restraints%20and%20Restraint%20Alternatives/Posey-Soft-Limb-Holder-2530-2540-25281.pdf

TIDI Products. (2018b). *Posey® limb holders. Application instructions for wrist and ankle*. Retrieved on June 9, 2022, from https://f.hubspotusercontent40.net/hubfs/8218994/IFU/Restraints%20and%20Restraint%20Alternatives/Posey-Soft-Limb-Holder-2530-2540-25281.pdf

U.S. Consumer Product Safety Commission. (n.d.). *Carbon monoxide information center*. Retrieved June 6, 2020, from https://www.cpsc.gov/Safety-Education/Safety-Education-Centers/Carbon-Monoxide-Information-Center/Carbon-Monoxide-Questions-and-Answers-

U.S. Department of Agriculture, Food and Nutrition Service. (2018, December 12). Child nutrition programs: Flexibilities for milk, whole grains, and sodium requirements. 7 CFR Parts 210, 215, 220, and 226 [FNS–2017–0021] RIN 0584–AE53. *Federal Register, 83*(238), 63775–63794. https://www.govinfo.gov/content/pkg/FR-2018-12-12/pdf/2018-26762.pdf

U.S. Department of Agriculture, Food and Nutrition Service. (2020, January 23). Simplifying meal service and monitoring requirements in the National School Lunch and School Breakfast Programs. 7 CFR Parts 210, 215, 220, 226, and 235 [FNS–2019–0007] RIN 0584–AE67. *Federal Register, 85*(15), 4094–4134. https://www.govinfo.gov/content/pkg/FR-2020-01-23/pdf/2020-00926.pdf

U.S. Department of Health and Human Services (USDHHS). (2019, December 10). *Public health emergency: National disaster medical system*. http://www.phe.gov/Preparedness/responders/ndms/Pages/default.aspx

U.S. Department of Health and Human Services, Administration for Community Living. (n.d.). *National Center on Elder Abuse*. Retrieved June 4, 2020, from https://ncea.acl.gov/What-We-Do/Research/Statistics-and-Data.aspx

U.S. Department of Health and Human Services, Administration for Children and Families, Administration on Children, Youth and Families, Children's Bureau. (2020, January 15). *Child maltreatment 2018*. https://www.acf.hhs.gov/cb/resource/child-maltreatment-2018

U.S. Department of Health and Human Services, Agency for Healthcare Research and Quality. (2019a, September). *Culture of safety*. https://psnet.ahrq.gov/primer/culture-safety

U.S. Department of Health and Human Services, Agency for Healthcare Research and Quality. (2019b, September). *Patient safety primer: Never events*. https://psnet.ahrq.gov/primer/never-events

U.S. Department of Health and Human Services, Centers for Medicare and Medicaid Services. (2019, September 30). *Medicare and Medicaid programs; regulatory provisions to promote program efficiency, transparency, and burden reduction; fire safety requirements for certain dialysis facilities; hospital and critical access hospital (CAH) changes to promote innovation, flexibility, and improvement in patient care* [RIN 0938-AT23]. https://s3.amazonaws.com/public-inspection.federalregister.gov/2019-20736.pdf

U.S. Department of Health and Human Services, Office of Disease Prevention and Health Promotion. (2020a, June 5). *Healthy People 2020: Social determinants of health*. https://www.healthypeople.gov/2020/topics-objectives/topic/social-determinants-of-health

U.S. Department of Health and Human Services, Office of Disease Prevention and Health Promotion. (2020b, June 9). *Healthy People 2020: Injury and violence prevention*. https://www.healthypeople.gov/2020/topics-objectives/topic/injury-and-violence-prevention/objectives

U.S. Department of Health and Human Services, Office of Disease Prevention and Health Promotion. (2022, February 6). *Healthy People 2020: Preparedness*. https://www.healthypeople.gov/2020/topics-objectives/topic/preparedness/objectives

U.S. Department of Homeland Security. (2019, March 13). *Nuclear attack fact sheet*. https://www.dhs.gov/publication/nuclear-attack-fact-sheet

U.S. Department of Homeland Security. (2020, March 17). *Cybersecurity*. https://www.dhs.gov/topic/cybersecurity

U.S. Department of Justice, Office of Justice Programs. (n.d.). *AMBER alert – America's missing: Broadcast emergency response*. Retrieved May 30, 2020, from http://www.amberalert.gov

U.S. Department of Justice, Drug Enforcement Administration. (2019, December). *Desomorphine*. https://www.deadiversion.usdoj.gov/drug_chem_info/desomorphine.pdf

U.S. Department of Justice, Drug Enforcement Administration. (2020). *Drugs of abuse: A DEA resource guide/2020 edition*. Retrieved on June 9, 2022, from https://www.dea.gov/sites/default/files/2020-04/Drugs%20of%20Abuse%202020-Web%20Version-508%20compliant-4-24-20_0.pdf

U.S. Department of Labor, Occupational Safety and Health Administration (OSHA). (2016). *Guidelines for preventing workplace violence for healthcare and social service workers*. OSHA 3148-06R 2016. Retrieved June 9, 2022, from https://www.osha.gov/Publications/osha3148.pdf

U.S. Department of Veteran Affairs. (2018, November 29). *VA national center for patient safety: Root cause analysis*. https://www.patientsafety.va.gov/professionals/onthejob/rca.asp

U.S. Department of Veteran Affairs. (2019, July 18). *VA national center for patient safety: Falls toolkit*. https://www.patientsafety.va.gov/professionals/onthejob/falls.asp

U.S. Fire Administration. (2019, November). Fire in the United States 2008–2017. https://www.usfa.fema.gov/downloads/pdf/publications/fius20th.pdf

U.S. Fire Administration. (2020, March 9). Fire safety outreach materials for older adults. https://www.usfa.fema.gov/prevention/outreach/older_adults.html

U.S. Food and Drug Administration (FDA). (2019a, October 31). *Tattoos & permanent makeup: Fact sheet*. https://www.fda.gov/cosmetics/cosmetic-products/tattoos-permanent-makeup-fact-sheet

U.S. Food and Drug Administration (FDA). (2019b, July 8). *Medical device reporting (MDR): How to report medical device problems*. https://www.fda.gov/medical-devices/medical-device-safety/medical-device-reporting-mdr-how-report-medical-device-problems

U.S. Food and Drug Administration (FDA). (2020, January 2). *FDA finalizes enforcement policy on unauthorized flavored cartridge-based e-cigarettes that appeal to children, including fruit and mint*. https://www.fda.gov/news-events/press-announcements/fda-finalizes-enforcement-policy-unauthorized-flavored-cartridge-based-e-cigarettes-appeal-children

U.S. Pharmacopeial Convention. (2020, June 26). *USP <800>FAQs*. https://go.usp.org/General-Chapter-800-FAQ

Vilcassim, M. J. R., Thurston, G. D., Chen, L. C., Lim, C. C., Saunders, E., Yao, Y., & Gordon, T. (2019). Exposure to air pollution is associated with adverse cardiopulmonary health effects in international travellers. *Journal of Travel Medicine, 26*(5), taz032. https://doi.org/10.1093/jtm/taz032

Warmack, R. J., Wolf, D., & Frank, S. (2015, January). *Smart smoke alarm: Using linear discriminant analysis. Sponsored by the U.S. Fire Administration (USFA) and the U.S. Consumer Product Safety Commission (CPSC) and prepared under DOE Contract # DE-AC05-00OR22725 between Department of Energy Oak Ridge Office and UT-Battelle, LLC*. https://www.usfa.fema.gov/downloads/pdf/publications/smart_smoke_alarm_lda.pdf

Waasdorp, T. E., & Mehari, K. R. (2019). Cyberbullying: Building the research in context. *Journal of Adolescent Health, 65*(5), 575–576. https://doi.org/10.1016/j.jadohealth.2019.08.006

Yue, J. K., Winkler, E. A., Burke, J. F., Chan, A. K., Dhall, S. S., Berger, M. S., Manley, G. T., & Tarapore, P. E. (2016). Pediatric sports-related traumatic brain injury in United States trauma centers. *Neurosurgical Focus, 40*(4), E3. https://doi.org/10.3171/2016.1.FOCUS15612

Zawilska, J. B., Kacela, M., & Adamowicz P. (2020). NBOMes-highly potent and toxic alternatives of LSD. *Frontiers in Neuroscience, 14*, 78. https://doi.org/10.3389/fnins.2020.00078

29 Complementary and Integrative Health

Brian Legett

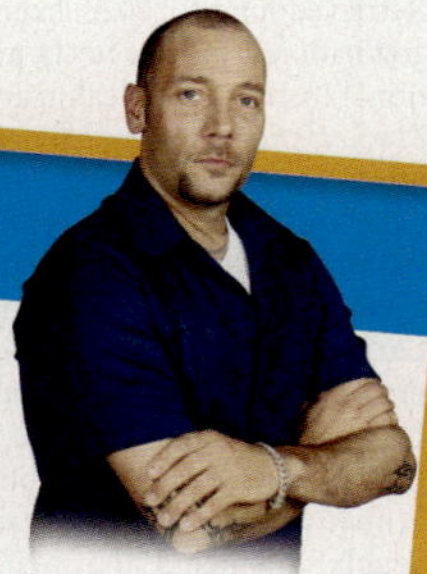

Brian, a 30-year-old man with a long history of back problems due to a work injury, comes to the clinic for evaluation. He states, "I've had so many kinds of treatment, and nothing seems to work. Maybe, I should see a chiropractor?"

Sylvia Puentes

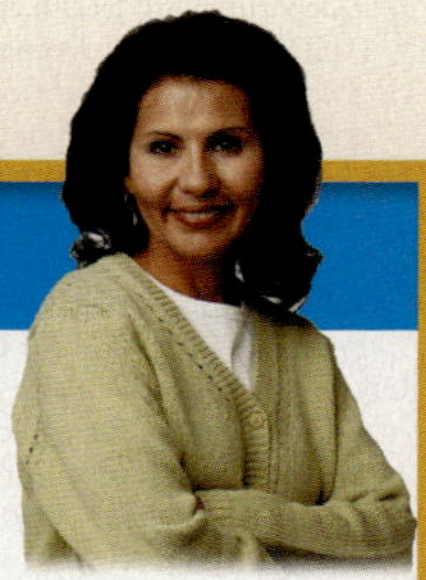

Sylvia, a middle-aged woman, is scheduled for abdominal surgery next week. She comes to the outpatient clinic for preoperative evaluation and laboratory testing and says, "I'm really anxious about the surgery, but I don't want to take any medicines. Is there anything I can do to help me relax?"

Lee Chen

Lee, a 65-year-old man dying of lung cancer, was brought to the United States from China by his two daughters, who believed that U.S. medicine would cure him. Mr. Chen did not respond to any of the therapies that were attempted, and the team wants to transition to palliative care. The daughters are unwilling to authorize removal of ventilatory support or sign a do-not-resuscitate order. They request an acupuncturist, but their health care provider refuses their request.

Learning Outcomes

After completing the chapter, you will be able to accomplish the following:

1. Differentiate complementary health approaches and integrative health from allopathic/conventional medicine.
2. Compare and contrast the beliefs about the origin of disease and ways to promote health of each of the three main categories of complementary health approaches.
3. Describe ways in which nurses can use knowledge of complementary health approaches and integrative health in providing patient care.
4. Identify the knowledge the public should possess about complementary health approaches and integrative health if they wish to be informed consumers.
5. Describe ways in which nurses can use selected complementary health approaches for self-care and health promotion.

Nursing Concepts

- Clinical Decision Making/Clinical Judgment
- Health
- Wellness
- Illness

Many people in the United States are using complementary health approaches (CHAs) and integrative health (IH) care to promote health and assist with healing from illness. The term **complementary health approaches (CHAs)** refers to health care interventions that are not typically part of conventional medical care that are used together with conventional medical interventions (NCCIH, 2020a). The term **integrative health (IH)** refers to the combination of complementary health and conventional health approaches in a coordinated way (NCCIH, 2020a). If a nonmainstream practice is used in place of conventional medical care, it is considered an alternative modality. However, most people who use health care approaches that are not typically part of conventional medical care also use conventional health care (NCCIH, 2020a) and therefore alternative care will not be discussed in this chapter. The term *complementary and alternative medicine* (CAM) is also still sometimes used; however, this terms does not accurately reflect the fact that CHAs and IH care are not "medicines" and people without medical degrees practice CHAs/IH. This chapter discusses basic CHA and IH concepts that a practicing nurse needs to understand to provide safe nursing care.

Nurses need to be knowledgeable about CHAs for several reasons. The World Health Organization's definition of health identifies, "Health is a complete physical, mental and social well-being and not merely the absence of disease or infirmity" (WHO, n.d., para 1). Health and illness are affected by all components of an individual, including their body, mind and spirit and efforts to promote health and treat illness benefit from an integration of conventional Western medicine with complementary and alternative therapies (Eliopoulos, 2018a). The use of integrative approaches to health and wellness has grown within care settings across the United States (NCCIH, 2020a, para 8). Consumers increasingly desire and are using care options beyond conventional medicine (Eliopoulos, 2018a) and patients, families, other health care providers, and health care institutions increasingly expect practicing nurses to be knowledgeable about CHA. Patients may use these types of therapies as outpatients and want to continue their use as inpatients. They or family members/caregivers may expect nurses to administer herbal preparations or nutritional supplements or ask advice regarding the use of these therapies. Also, it is not uncommon for people to retain health care practices brought from other countries although they reside in the United States. In these situations, nurses can assist patients by accommodating CHA/IH healing practices as much as possible. In addition, as evidence grows demonstrating the effectiveness of selected CHAs, many institutions now provide complementary therapies to inpatients as part of total patient care in an effort to provide IH care. Refer to the accompanying Reflective Practice display box on page 884.

Another reason nurses need to be knowledgeable about CHAs is that many nurses are expanding their clinical practice by incorporating CHAs. Many state boards of nursing recognize select complementary modalities as part of nursing practice and have provisions for the safe practice of these modalities by registered nurses.

Finally, although CHAs may seem totally safe, some therapies have led to harmful and, at times, potentially lethal outcomes. Nurses play an important role in educating the public about how these therapies can be used safely and effectively. This chapter will provide helpful resources for education.

QSEN PATIENT-CENTERED CARE

It is important for the nurse to recognize and consider personally held attitudes and beliefs regarding complementary and integrative health approaches and not allow personal values to interfere with the provision of individualized care that respects individual patient values, preferences, and expressed needs.

INTRODUCTION TO COMPLEMENTARY HEALTH APPROACHES

Although the use of most CHAs predates modern medicine, it was not until recently that nursing and medical schools began to teach about their use. The sharp divide between conventional Western medicine and CHAs has now softened, and successful practitioners know how to combine the two successfully.

QSEN Reflective Practice: Cultivating QSEN Competencies

CHALLENGE TO COGNITIVE SKILLS

This spring, while working on an oncology floor, I was caring for Lee Chen, a 65-year-old man dying of lung cancer. His two daughters, who were living in the United States, had brought him from China to the United States, believing that U.S. medicine would cure him. Unfortunately, Mr. Chen's cancer had not responded to any of the therapies that were attempted. All of his professional caregivers believed that the goal of treatment should now be preparation for a comfortable and dignified death using compassionate palliative care. His daughters, however, were unwilling to accept this goal and would not authorize removing him from ventilatory support or issuing a do-not-resuscitate order. Mr. Chen could no longer speak on his own behalf. One afternoon, one of his daughters informed Mr. Chen's health care provider that she was going to bring an acupuncturist in to work on her father. The health care provider told her in no uncertain terms that he would not allow "voodoo medicine" on his unit. I wasn't sure what to do because both daughters were growing more and more upset, and this answer seemed like the "last straw."

Thinking Outside the Box: Possible Courses of Action

- Accept the status quo and try to comfort the daughters.
- Support the health care provider's judgment and try to get the daughters to see things his way.
- Learn more about acupuncture and related benefits and harms (I have never seen it done and know very little about what to expect).
- Find out if the health care provider really had the authority to forbid acupuncture on this patient.
- Advocate for the patient and his family if there is a possibility that acupuncture will benefit him.

Evaluating a Good Outcome: How Do I Define Success?

- Patient receives culturally appropriate, thoughtful person-centered care consistent with the goals of compassionate palliative care.
- The patient is not harmed.
- Mr. Chen's daughters feel supported as they struggle with decisions and anticipatory grieving.
- All health care team members (including Mr. Chen's health care provider) learn about acupuncture and other CHAs, as well as about the hospital's policies regarding their use.
- The health care provider is confronted in a professional manner about the behavior, as it increased stress on the family caregivers.
- I grow in my knowledge of how to incorporate CHA into my care.

Personal Learning: Here's to the Future!

I was so upset by the daughters' distress that I decided to learn more about acupuncture. After searching the Internet and talking with a nurse who was receiving acupuncture treatments, I decided that acupuncture treatments were unlikely to harm the patient; in fact, the treatments just might help to increase his comfort level. At the very least, Mr. Chen's daughters would believe that we respected and supported their efforts to help their father. I was also hopeful that the professional caregiving team would learn more about culturally competent care. When I spoke with the nurse manager for the unit, she understood my goals, discussed the situation with Mr. Chen's health care provider, and secured his approval for having the acupuncturist visit. I learned that the acupuncturist had to be credentialed by our hospital. While Mr. Chen's cancer did not respond to the acupuncture treatment, he did seem more comfortable, and his daughters couldn't thank me enough. I talked with them about how impressive their devotion to their father was and also mentioned that they may need to give him one last gift, the gift of "letting go." Unfortunately, I never saw this family again because this was my last week on this unit.

Melinda Ventura, Georgetown University

QSEN SELF-REFLECTION ON QUALITY AND SAFETY COMPETENCIES
DEVELOPING KNOWLEDGE, SKILLS, AND ATTITUDES FOR CONTINUOUS IMPROVEMENT

How do you think you would respond in a similar situation? Why? What does this tell you about yourself and about the adequacy of your competencies for professional practice? Can you think of other ways to respond?

What *knowledge, skills,* and *attitudes* do you need to develop to continuously improve the quality and safety of care for patients like Mr. Chen?

Patient-Centered Care: How can you establish a successful partnership with family members discouraged by a patient's worsening condition who want to try CHAs? How did the nursing student promote respectful, person-centered, culturally competent care?

Teamwork and Collaboration/Quality Improvement: What factors do you think may have played a role in the health care provider's answer? Imagine if the nursing student (rather than the nurse manager) had approached the health care provider to allow the acupuncturist to visit. Do you think that the health care provider's answer would have been the same as it was when the manager conferred with him? Explain why or why not. What competencies do you need to develop to get the team to work well together? What needs to change to improve quality in this setting?

Safety/Evidence-Based Practice: What does the evidence point to as "best practice" in a situation like this? What safety needs does Mr. Chen have and how can you meet them?

Informatics: Can you identify the essential information that must be available in Mr. Chen's record to support safe patient care and coordination of care?

Can you think of other ways to respond to or approach the situation? What else might the nursing student have done to ensure a successful outcome?

Allopathic Medicine and Complementary Health Approaches

Allopathic medicine is a system in which medical doctors and other health care professionals, such as nurses, pharmacists, and therapists, treat symptoms and diseases using drugs, radiation, or surgery (NCI, n.d.a). Other terms for this type of approach are conventional medicine, biomedicine, mainstream medicine, orthodox medicine, and Western medicine (NCI, n.d.a). Allopathic medicine has been dominant for about 100 years in the United States and has spearheaded remarkable advances in biotechnology, surgical interventions, pharmaceutical approaches, and diagnostic tools. Allopathic medical care is particularly effective when aggressive treatment is needed in emergency or acute situations. However, allopathic medical care has not been totally effective in addressing the health of the whole person or in dealing with persistent symptoms related to chronic illness and patient quality of life (Helming et al., 2022). The CHA and allopathic systems differ fundamentally in several ways (Table 29-1). Until recently, the majority of decision making in CHAs has been based on observation, experience, and traditional healing manuscripts, in contrast to allopathic medicine, which has moved away from these methodologies to evidence-based practice. However, holistic nurses and other practitioners continue to advance the scientific knowledge base of evidence for holistic practice and for the effectiveness of holistic interventions (Helming et al., 2022).

Many CHAs are based on a theory and philosophy of holism upon which holistic nursing also is based. Many practitioners and consumers of health care choose to combine allopathic modalities and CHAs using an integrative approach. These concepts are discussed in the following sections.

Holism

Holism is a theory and philosophy that focuses on connections and interactions between parts of the whole; interrelationships of the physical, mental, emotional, sexual, cultural, social, spiritual, and energetic dimensions of the person (Helming et al., 2022). In contrast, the conventional scientific approach has focused on reductionism, reducing the human body to isolated parts rather than a unified whole, and in which treatment of health conditions focus on an individual organ or system rather than the whole being (Eliopoulos, 2018a). Using a holistic perspective, all living organisms, including humans, are continuously connecting and interacting with their environment. Further, parts of the organism, whether they are systems, subsystems, or cells, are also continuously interacting and changing. This continual interaction and change means that the body is not the sum of its parts (as in reductionism), but that it is a unified, dynamic whole.

Although someone might view holism as a recently developed belief system, holism in fact was the predominant belief throughout history until sometime before Descartes, a French philosopher who lived in the early part of the 17th century. Descartes and other influential thinkers asserted that the mind and body were separate from each other—mind–body dualism (Thibaut, 2018). That belief lasted until the early 20th century, when researchers began to prove that there was a connection between the mind and the body.

One of the 20th-century researchers, Selye (1976), developed the term *general adaptation syndrome* (GAS) to describe the general holistic pattern that emerges when people experience stress/illness. The GAS reflects a general response that occurs in various parts of the body. This theory holds that when someone is sick, that person is "sick all over," not just where symptoms manifest. Selye also demonstrated that adrenal exhaustion can be caused by emotional tension, such as suppressed rage or frustration. (For more on the GAS, see Chapter 43.)

A holistic philosophy underlies many CHA. People have a mind, body, emotions, and spirit that are connected and function as a unified whole. A change in any part of the

Table 29-1 Beliefs Underlying Complementary and Alternative Therapies and the Allopathic Therapies

COMPLEMENTARY AND INTEGRATIVE HEALTH APPROACHES	ALLOPATHIC THERAPIES
Mind, body, and spirit are integrated and together influence health and illness.	Illness occurs in either the mind or the body, which are separate entities.
Health is a balance of body systems: mental, social, and spiritual, as well as physical.	Health is the absence of disease.
Illness is a manifestation of imbalance or disharmony.	The main causes of illness are considered to be pathogens (bacteria or viruses) or biochemical imbalances.
Symptoms are a sign or reflection of a deeper instability within the person; restoring physical and mental harmony will alleviate the symptoms. Healing is a slow process that involves the whole person.	Curing seeks to destroy the invading organism or repair the affected part.
Emphasis is on health. Healing is done by the patient; care is individualized.	Emphasis is on disease and high technology. Drugs, surgery, and radiation are among the key tools for dealing with medical problems.

Through the Eyes of a Nurse

Healing is a lifelong journey into understanding the wholeness of human existence. Along this journey, our lives mesh with those of patients, families, and colleagues, where moments of new meaning and insight emerge in the midst of crisis. Healing occurs when we help patients, families, and ourselves embrace what is feared most. It occurs when we seek harmony and balance. Healing is learning how to open what has been closed, so that we can expand our inner potentials. It is the fullest expression of oneself that is demonstrated by the light and shadow and the male and female principles that reside in each of us. It is accessing what we have forgotten about connections, unity, and interdependence. With a new awareness of these interrelationships, healing becomes possible, and the experience of the nurse as an instrument of healing and as a nurse healer becomes actualized. A nurse healer is one who facilitates another person's growth toward wholeness (body–mind–spirit) or who assists another with recovery from illness or transition to peaceful death. Healing is not just curing symptoms. Rather, it is the exquisite blending of technology with caring, love, compassion, and creativity (p. xxiv).

—*Barbara Montgomery Dossey, Lynn Keegan*

Source: Dossey, B. M., & Keegan, L. (2016). *Holistic nursing: A handbook for practice* (7th ed.). Jones & Bartlett Learning. Used with permission.

organism will be reflected in other parts. When someone feels the emotion of sadness, that person may have a physical response of crying. In addition, when a person feels stressed and overwhelmed, the face and body language frequently reflect these conditions. However, there are also times when a person experiences physical symptoms, such as pain and fatigue, when there is no underlying pathophysiology in the body; rather, there may be psychosocial stressors which impact the body and a person's experience of daily life. Holism acknowledges that the body and mind interact as one; the healing of a person's symptoms in the body must also involve healing in the mind, and vice versa. "The goal is not to treat diseases but to serve the needs of the total person through the healing of the body, mind and spirit" (Eliopoulos, 2018b, p. 92).

Holistic nursing is nursing practice built on a holistic philosophy. Healing the whole person is its goal. Since holism is a philosophy and not a specific nursing role, holistic nurses can be found in all varieties of health care settings as well as in independent practice settings. In addition, holistic nurses frequently add CHAs to their practice. Most holistic nurses use CHAs for self-care, an essential component of holistic practice (AHNA, n.d.). The American Holistic Nurse Association (AHNA) promotes the education of nurses, other health care professionals, and the public in all aspects of holistic caring and healing (AHNA, n.d.).

Self-Care Alert

Nurses should practice self-care behaviors that promote wellness and resilience (American Association of Colleges of Nursing [AACN], 2021). Intentional use of holistic behaviors can be helpful in leading a healthful and less stressful life. What are you doing to support your well-being? Investigate various CHAs and consider how you might integrate CHAs into your plan for self-care.

Nurses are challenged to explore three questions in relation to uniting contemporary medical and surgical therapies with health rituals and complementary modalities (Helming et al., 2022, p. xxii):

1. What do we know about the meaning of healing?
2. What can we do each day to facilitate healing?
3. How can we be an instrument in the healing process?

Read through the accompanying Through the Eyes of a Nurse and reflect on your commitment to holistic, person-centered nursing and healing. Holistic nursing is recognized as a nursing specialty by the American Nurses Association (AHNA, n.d.). The AHNA also provides published standards for holistic nursing practice (AHNA & ANA, 2019). Registered nurses can become certified in basic and advanced holistic nursing through the American Holistic Nurses Credentialing Corporation (AHNCC, 2020).

Integrative Care

A person who uses integrative care uses some combination of allopathic medicine and CHAs (Table 29-2). There are several types of integrative care models used throughout the United States that can be housed in virtually all health care delivery structures. Optimally, these models include sensitive and knowledgeable health care providers who work with patients to design a plan of care that is responsive to the patient's and family's/caregiver's preferences and needs and combines the best of allopathic medicine and CHAs while avoiding harmful interactions (Helming et al., 2022).

Table 29-2 Integrative Care of the Common Cold[a]

COMPLEMENTARY AND INTEGRATIVE HEALTH APPROACHES	ALLOPATHIC APPROACHES
Acupuncture to appropriate areas to reduce sinus congestion	Decongestant over-the-counter medications
Rest and fluids	Rest and fluids

[a]In this example, adding herbs and/or acupuncture to a typical allopathic approach would represent integrative care.

Complementary Health Approaches and Nursing

CHAs consist of a large variety of therapies that are based on a set of beliefs different from those of allopathic medicine. Some of these modalities have developed fairly recently (e.g., guided imagery), while others have been used for thousands of years as components of ancient healing systems (e.g., Ayurveda or traditional Chinese medicine). Some therapies can be used effectively without assistance (e.g., nutritional approaches, deep breathing exercises), while others (e.g., naturopathy, acupuncture) are more effective when used with guidance from practitioners who have particular knowledge and expertise.

Many people use CHAs for stress management/reduction (NCCIH, 2020b). Techniques such as relaxation with focused breathing, meditation, imagery, biofeedback, and massage are used in all stages of health and illness to promote healing and/or manage symptoms. Because stress can contribute to illness, CHAs can sometimes be effective in reducing symptoms and enhancing quality of life. Nurses can assist patients—and themselves—with these therapies. Refer to the Research in Nursing display regarding the use of yoga and mindfulness in relation to stress in children and adolescents with asthma.

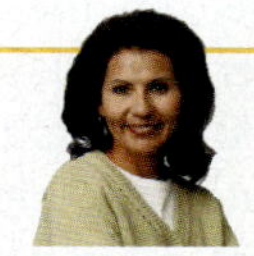

Recall **Sylvia Puentes**, the anxious patient scheduled for surgery. The nurse's knowledge of CHAs would be important in helping this patient to reduce her preoperative anxiety. The nurse could discuss various methods available, allowing the patient to select the one that seems best for her. Such actions help develop a trusting nurse–patient relationship and foster a sense of self-esteem in the patient by allowing her to participate in the plan of care and decision making.

Use of Complementary Health Approaches in the United States

The most comprehensive and reliable findings to date on Americans' use of CHAs are released by the National Center

Research in Nursing

BRIDGING THE GAP TO EVIDENCE-BASED PRACTICE

Yoga and Mindfulness

Stress is considered a significant trigger for physical and mental health issues, including asthma in children (Lack et al., 2020). Children with asthma experience impaired quality of life, symptoms of anxiety and impaired ability to participate in physical activity (Lack et al., 2020). Many therapies maybe helpful in reducing stress, resulting in enhanced health management and improved quality of life for these patients.

Related Research

Lack, S., Brown, R., & Kinser, P. A. (2020). An integrative review of yoga and mindfulness-based approaches for children and adolescents with asthma. *Journal of Pediatric Nursing, 52*, 76–81. https://doi.org/10.1016/j.pedn.2020.03.006

The purpose of this integrative review was to examine the use of yoga and mindfulness for children and adolescents with asthma. A comprehensive search of five databases was completed to identify studies addressing the physiologic and psychological health effects of yoga and mindfulness in children and adolescents (aged 19 years and younger) with asthma. Data bases searched included PubMed/MEDLINE, PsychINFO, Web of Science, EMBASE, and CINAHL, from the launch of the database through January 2020. Keywords included "yoga," mindfulness," and "asthma." The authors also searched the reference lists of articles (ancestry approach) to identify publications in addition to those identified as a result of the database searches. An initial review of titles and abstracts was followed by full-text review. Studies were included if the participants were ages 19 years and younger and if the study examined yoga and asthma, mindfulness and asthma, and yoga and mindfulness and asthma. Studies were excluded if the participants were adults or mixed data of children and adults; and if the articles were review articles, commentaries, editorials, abstracts, and poster sessions. A total of 11 articles met the criteria for review from the years 1991 to 2019.

A variety of study designs were used in the reviewed articles, including pilot, single-subject, and correlational studies. Four studies used a control group, and one was longitudinal. The studies were carried out in eight countries. Two of the studies assessed mindfulness in adolescents with asthma; nine studies evaluated yoga as intervention for children and adolescents with asthma. The majority of studies of a yoga-based intervention identified that the use of yoga by children and adolescents is associated with improved lung function, anxiety, and quality of life. The studies of a mindfulness intervention suggested that higher rates of trait mindfulness were associated with lower rates of wheezing and coughing and were related to decreased asthma-specific stress and improved asthma control and quality of life. The authors concluded that there are preliminary indications to support the use of yoga and mindfulness for enhancing the physical and psychological health of children and adolescents with asthma.

Relevance to Nursing Practice

The use of CHAs, such as yoga and mindfulness, offer the potential help decrease stress and anxiety resulting in positive effects on the physical and psychological health of patients. Nurses have an important role in helping patients to manage self-care and health problems and issues. Yoga and mindfulness are inexpensive and easy to implement approaches that offer the potential for symptom management and self-regulation of asthma triggers and other effects of stress and anxiety.

for Complementary and Integrative Health (NCCIH), part of the National Institutes of Health, and the National Center for Health Statistics (NCHS), part of the Centers for Disease Control and Prevention (CDC). The following findings are based on the 2017 edition of the NCHS National Health Interview Survey (NHIS), a study in which tens of thousands of Americans are interviewed about their health- and illness-related experiences. The report is available, along with a press release and graphics, at https://www.nccih.nih.gov/research/statistics/nhis/2017.

Prevalence of Complementary Health Approaches

The annual NHIS by the NCCIH includes a special section on CHAs every 5 years. The 2012 NHIS found that, in the United States, approximately 30% of adults (about 3 in 10) and approximately 12% of children (about 1 in 9) were using some form of CHAs in the 12 months before the survey (Clarke et al., 2015). In 2012, CHA use was more prevalent among women, adults ages 30 to 69 years, adults with higher levels of education, adults who were not poor, adults living in the West, former smokers, and adults who were hospitalized in the last year. Adults younger than age 65 years and those with private health insurance were more likely than those with public health insurance or uninsured adults to use CHAs. There also are cultural variations. In 2012, the use of CHAs in non-Hispanic Whites was 37.9%, in Hispanics was 22%, and non-Hispanic Blacks was 19.3% (Clarke et al., 2015). There was a decrease in use of CHAs by poor adults (those who have an annual income at the national poverty threshold) from 26.6% in 2007 to 20.6% in 2012 (Clarke et al., 2015).

Past NHIS research identified yoga, meditation, and seeing a chiropractor as some of the most commonly used CHAs (Clarke et al., 2015). The 2017 NHIS examined changes over time in the percentage of adults who used yoga, meditation, and chiropractors in the 12 months before the survey as well as variation by biologic sex, age, and race and Hispanic origin (Clarke et al., 2018). This survey data identified increases from 2012 to 2017 in the use of yoga, meditation, and chiropractors (Clarke et al., 2018). Yoga was the most commonly used CHA among adults ages 18 years and older, increasing from 9.5% (2012) to 14.3% (2017) (Clarke et al., 2018). Participants who identified as women were more likely to use yoga, meditation, and chiropractors during the survey period than participants who identified as men (Clarke et al., 2018). Non-Hispanic White adults were more likely to use yoga, meditation, and chiropractors compared with Hispanic and non-Hispanic Black adults (Clarke et al., 2018). Other commonly used CHAs are nonvitamin, nonmineral, and natural products (17.7%); deep breathing exercises (10.9%); yoga (9.5%); chiropractic or osteopathic manipulation (8.4%); meditation (8%); and massage (6.9%) (Clarke et al., 2015). Of all the natural products, fish oil and glucosamine, chondroitin, or a combination supplement were the products most commonly used by adults in 2012 (Clarke et al., 2015).

The NHIS is an annual survey conducted by the NCHS about health and health care use (Clarke et al., 2015; Jou & Johnson, 2016). One component of this survey is a CHA supplement, asking adults in the United States older than age 18 years about communication and disclosure with their primary care physician in relation to the use of CHAs. One third of the 7,493 participants indicated they use CHAs; however, 42.3% of these CHA users indicated that they do not discuss CHA use with their primary care physician (Clarke et al., 2015; Jou & Johnson, 2016). Participants reported most nondisclosure was related to physicians not asking about CHA use or to concerns about physician knowledge regarding CHAs (Clarke et al., 2015; Jou & Johnson, 2016). These findings highlight the need for nurses to ask about CHA use at every patient visit and to emphasize that it is important to discuss CHA use with their health care providers. Patients should be proactive and initiate conversation about their use of CHAs, providing information about any CHAs they are using or considering for use (NCCIH, 2020e).

Reasons for Using Complementary Health Approaches

People use CHAs for an array of conditions and reasons. In general, people who choose CHAs are seeking ways to improve their health and well-being or to relieve symptoms associated with chronic, even terminal, illnesses or the side effects of conventional treatments for them. Other reasons for choosing to use CHAs include having a holistic health philosophy or a transformational experience that changes one's worldview and wanting greater control over one's own health. For example, people may use CHAs for pain conditions such as back, neck, or joint pain. The type of CHA implemented appears to be related to the most common outcomes of their use. For example, studies suggest possible benefits of yoga for several aspects of wellness, with practitioners of yoga commonly reporting positive stress management; mental and emotional health; healthy activity habits; promotion of sleep; and positive effects on relief of back and neck pain (NCCIH, 2019a).

Use of Complementary Health Approaches With Children

In 2012, the CHAs most commonly used by U.S. children in the 12 months prior to the survey included nonvitamin, nonmineral, and natural products (4.9%); chiropractic or osteopathic manipulation (3.3%); yoga (3.1%); deep breathing (2.7%); and homeopathic treatment (1.8%) (Black et al., 2015). Back or neck pain, head or chest cold, other musculoskeletal conditions, anxiety or stress, and attention-deficit hyperactivity disorder were the most common reasons for use of a CHA reported in children (Black et al., 2015).

Similar to the NHIS survey results indicating an increase in use of yoga and meditation in adults older than age 18 years, data from the 2017 NHIS found that the use of yoga and meditation significantly increased among U. S. children ages 4 to 17 years (Black et al., 2018). The percentage of children using yoga in the 12 months prior to the survey increased from 3.1% (2012) to 8.4% (2017) (Black et al., 2018).

Box 29-1 Complementary Health Approaches: Be an Informed Consumer

- Take charge of your health by being an informed consumer.
- Talk with your health care providers when making any decisions about using complementary health approaches. Your health care providers can give you advice based on your medical needs.
- If you are thinking about using a CHA therapy, learn the facts. Is it safe? Does it work?
- Find out what scientific studies have been done. It is not a good idea to use a CHA therapy simply because you have seen it in an advertisement or on a website or because people have told you that it worked for them.
- Keep in mind that the number of websites offering health-related resources grows every day. Many sites provide valuable information, while others may have information that is unreliable or misleading. To evaluate the quality of a website, take a look at who runs the site, who pays for it, and the purpose of the site. Also, check out where the information comes from, how it is selected, and how current it is.
- Scientific research on many CHA therapies is relatively new, so information about safety and effectiveness may not be available for every therapy. However, many studies of CHA treatments are underway, and researchers are always learning more about CHA.
- You can find reliable information on CHA through the National Institutes of Health's National Center for Complementary and Integrative Health (NCCIH). The NCCIH website (http://nccih.nih.gov) provides a variety of useful information as well as links to other trustworthy sources.

Source: Adapted from NCCIH. (2015). Be an informed consumer. https://nccih.nih.gov/health/decisions; National Center for Complementary and Integrative Health (NCCIH). (2020, February). *Be an informed consumer.* https://www.nccih.nih.gov/health/be-an-informed-consumer

The use of meditation increased from 0.6% (2012) to 5.4% (2017) (Black et al., 2018).

Growth of the Complementary Health Approaches Industry

In 2012, 59 million Americans spent $30.2 billion out-of-pocket on CHAs (NCCIH, 2016e). The AACN identifies the need for nursing students to develop an understanding of holistic person-centered care that has healing the whole person as its goal (AACN, 2021). Approximately one half of medical schools in the United States offer at least one CAM course or clinical practice rotation (Cowen & Cyr, 2015). Insurers increasingly pay for selected CHAs for particular identified conditions (American Cancer Society, 2015). Scores of private organizations provide classes and workshops for consumers as well as education and practical experience for health care providers.

Many private and governmental organizations have been developed to address CHAs. The NCCIH funds research on CHAs and is a great first resource for professionals and the public seeking information about CHAs. Health care professionals and consumers can find valuable information about the safety and efficacy of CHAs on the NCCIH website at https://www.nccih.nih.gov/. Refer to Box 29-1 for additional advice to the public about being an informed consumer.

The U.S. Food and Drug Administration (FDA) regulates dietary supplements and provides guidance for consumers seeking health-related information about dietary supplements. The FDA (n.d.) offers consumers "5 Things to Consider Before Taking a Dietary Supplement," a guide to making informed decisions about using supplements (Fig. 29-1 on page 890). The guideline includes a warning that if "claims sound too good to be true, they probably are" and a reminder that the term "natural" does not always mean "safe" (U.S. FDA, n.d.). Even with these tips, fraudulent health products are not always easy to spot. The FDA recommends that people check with a physician or other health care provider when tempted to purchase or use an unproven product or one with questionable claims. Consumers can subscribe to the FDA Podcasts and News Feeds to access up-to-date information on fraudulent and/or tainted products as well as other drug, food, and health topics to help keep from being duped or hurt by these products (U.S. FDA, 2020).

COMPLEMENTARY HEALTH APPROACHES CATEGORIES

NCCIH (2020a) classifies the major CHAs into three categories: mind–body practices, natural products, and other CHAs. Each category contains several therapies. For example, meditation is a therapy included in the mind–body category. Box 29-2 describes each of these categories. Table 29-3 (on pages 891–892) lists examples of therapies from these categories that are used to address pain, describing what they help and how they work. Information

Box 29-2 Complementary Health Approach Categories

Mind–body practices use a variety of techniques designed to enhance the mind's ability to affect bodily function and symptoms. Examples include yoga, chiropractic and osteopathic manipulation, meditation, acupuncture, relaxation techniques (e.g., breathing exercises, guided imagery), tai chi, Pilates, energy medicine, and others.

Natural products include the use of botanicals (herbs), vitamins, minerals, fatty acids, amino acids, proteins, prebiotics and probiotics, whole diets, and functional foods.

Other CHAs do not fit into either of the two previous groups and include traditional healers, Ayurveda medicine, homeopathy, traditional Chinese medicine, naturopathy, and functional medicine.

Source: National Center for Complementary and Integrative Health (NCCIH). (2020a). https://www.nccih.nih.gov/health/complementary-alternative-or-integrative-health-whats-in-a-name

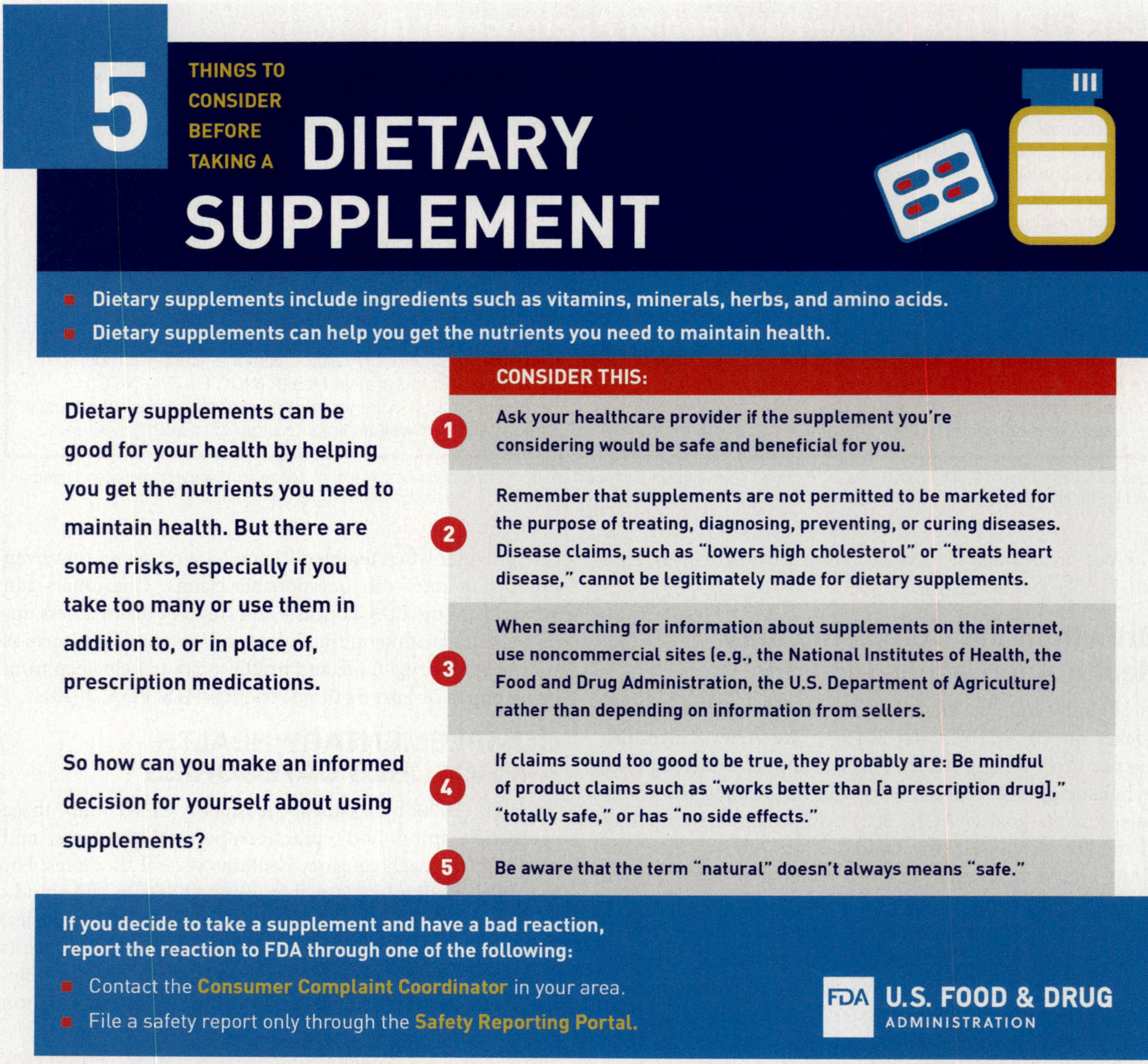

FIGURE 29-1. A guide to making informed decisions about the use of supplements. (*Source:* U.S. Food and Drug Administration (FDA). [n.d.]. *5 things to consider before taking a dietary supplement.* https://www.fda.gov/media/106435/download)

on some of the most widely used CHAs of interest to nurses is discussed in the following sections.

Mind–Body Practices

Many people recognize that there is a strong mind–body connection. Common everyday occurrences indicate that some connection does indeed exist. For example, students may experience insomnia related to anxiety the night before a major examination or suffer a migraine headache triggered by a fight with a spouse or good friend. Recent research has expanded our knowledge of how the mind and body communicate with each other. The scientific field of psychoneuroimmunology (PNI) addresses the effect of the mind on health and resistance to disease, investigating the connections among psychology, neuroendocrinology, and immunology (Helming et al., 2022). Chemicals such as cortisol have been found to be associated with stress and immunosuppression during anaphylaxis allergic reaction (Moraes et al., 2018). Neuropeptides are another chemical found to have properties that allow them to affect neurologic and physiologic tissue receptors. Many neuropeptide receptor sites lie along the gastrointestinal (GI) tract; this explains why people can experience a large variety of GI symptoms in response to emotional situations.

Knowing how this communication between the mind and body occurs assists in the understanding of the mind–body modalities, which may be useful for patients and others as well as self-care for nurses. Psychoneuroimmunology-based interventions can be used to control symptoms and improve a patient's quality of life (Moraes et al., 2018). Intentional

Table 29-3 Complementary and Integrative Health Approaches That Work on Pain

TYPE	WHAT THEY HELP	HOW THEY HELP	EXAMPLES
Mind–body practices that are movement-based: Physical exercises and practices	Musculoskeletal pain, joint pain, and lower-back pain	By strengthening muscles, supporting joints, improving alignment, and releasing endorphins	• *Physical therapy:* Specialized movements to strengthen weak areas of the body, often through resistance training • *Yoga:* An Indian practice of meditative stretching and posing • *Pilates:* A resistance regimen that strengthens core muscles • *Tai chi:* A slow, flowing Chinese practice that improves balance • *Feldenkrais:* A therapy that builds efficiency of movement
Natural products—nutritional and herbal remedies: Food choices and dietary supplements (ask your doctor before using supplements)	All chronic pain but especially abdominal discomfort, headaches, and inflammatory conditions, such as rheumatoid arthritis	By boosting the body's natural immunity, reducing pain-causing inflammation, soothing pain, and decreasing insomnia	• *Anti-inflammatory diet:* A Mediterranean eating pattern high in whole grains, fresh fruits, leafy vegetables, fish, and olive oil • *Omega-3 fatty acids:* Nutrients abundant in fish oil and flaxseed that reduce inflammation in the body • *Ginger:* A root that inhibits pain-causing molecules • *Turmeric:* A spice that reduces inflammation • *MSM:* Methylsulfonylmethane, a naturally occurring nutrient that helps build bone and cartilage
Other mind–body approaches: Using the powers of the mind to produce changes in the body	All types of chronic pain	By reducing stressful (and, hence, pain-inducing) emotions such as panic and fear and by refocusing attention on subjects other than pain	• *Meditation:* Focusing the mind on something specific (such as breathing or repeating a word or phrase) to quiet it • *Guided imagery:* Visualizing a particular outcome or scenario with the goal of mentally changing one's physical reality • *Biofeedback:* With a special machine, becoming alert to body processes, such as muscle tightening, to learn to control them • *Relaxation:* Releasing tension in the body through exercises such as controlled breathing
Energy healing: Manipulating the electrical energy—called *chi* in Chinese medicine—emitted by the body's nervous system	Pain that lingers after an injury heals, as well as pain complicated by trauma, anxiety, or depression	By relaxing the body and the mind, distracting the nervous system, producing natural painkillers, activating natural pleasure centers, and manipulating chi	• *Acupuncture:* The insertion of hair-thin needles into points along the body's meridians, or energetic pathways, to stimulate the flow of energy throughout the body; proven helpful for postsurgical pain and dental pain, among other types • *Acupressure:* Finger pressure applied to points along the meridians, to balance and increase the flow of energy • *Qi gong:* Very slow, gentle physical movements, similar to tai chi, that cleanse the body and circulate chi • *Reiki:* Moving a practitioner's hands over the energy fields of the patient's body to increase energy flow and restore balance

(*continued*)

Table 29-3 Complementary and Integrative Health Approaches That Work on Pain *(continued)*

TYPE	WHAT THEY HELP	HOW THEY HELP	EXAMPLES
Physical manipulation: Hands-on massage or movement of painful areas	Musculoskeletal pain, especially lower back and neck pain; pain from muscle underuse or overuse; and pain from adhesions or scars	By restoring mobility, improving circulation, decreasing blood pressure, and relieving stress	• *Massage:* The manipulation of tissue to relax clumps of knotted muscle fiber, increase circulation, and release patterns of chronic tension • *Chiropractic:* Physically moving vertebrae or other joints into proper alignment, to relieve stress • *Osteopathy:* Realigning vertebrae, ribs, and other joints, as with chiropractic; osteopaths have training equivalent to that of medical doctors
Lifestyle changes: Developing healthy habits at home and work	All types of chronic pain	By strengthening the immune system and enhancing well-being and by reframing one's relationship to (and, thus, experience of) chronic pain	• *Sleep hygiene:* Creating an optimal sleep environment to get deep, restorative rest; strategies include establishing a regular sleep–wake schedule and minimizing light and noise • *Positive work environment:* Having a comfortable workspace and control over one's activities to reduce stress and contribute to the sense of mastery over pain • *Healthy relationships:* Nurturing honest and supportive friendships and family ties to ease anxiety that exacerbates pain • *Exercise:* Regular activity to build strength and lower stress

Source: Research suggests these therapies can ease discomfort. For more information, visit the website of the National Center for Complementary and Integrative Health (www.nccih.nih.gov).

use of mind–body interventions to invoke the relaxation response has been suggested to help patients control stress, manage pain, fatigue, and anxiety, and improve sleep quality (Georga et al., 2019; Kiley et al., 2018; Labus et al., 2019).

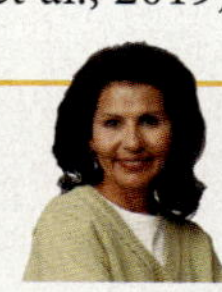

Think back to **Sylvia Puentes**, the anxious preoperative patient. The nurse would need to incorporate an understanding of the mind–body connection when discussing possible suggestions for anxiety relief.

Relaxation

Relaxation techniques promote parasympathetic nervous system activity, helping to reduce sympathetic activity and restore the balance of the two systems. The complex psychophysiologic processes that activate to deal with a real or perceived emergency, characterized by increased sympathetic nervous system activity, can contribute to symptoms such as increased blood pressure, cool hands and feet, tight muscles, increased heart rate, and increased anxiety. The ultimate goal is to increase the parasympathetic system influence in the mind–body and thus reduce the effect of stress and stress-related illness on the body.

Relaxation can be useful whether a patient is experiencing a single stressful event, such as surgery or chronic stress. Patient benefits include reduced anxiety, reduced muscle tension and pain, improved functioning of the immune system, enhanced sleep and rest, and an improved overall sense of well-being (NCCIH, 2021). Relaxation techniques include progressive muscle relaxation, guided imagery, deep breathing exercises, autogenic training, biofeedback, and self-hypnosis (NCCIH, 2021). Because these modalities are quite different, the type of relaxation modality chosen needs to be individually suited to the patient, based on their health status, personal preferences, and available time.

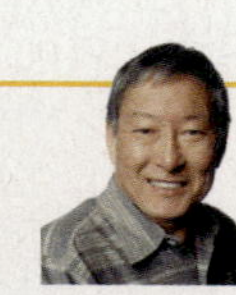

Recall **Mr. Chen**, the 65-year-old man dying of lung cancer. The nurse needs to include the patient's daughters when developing the plan of care. Therefore, when interacting with the patient's daughters, the nurse would also assess their stress level as they cope with their father's deteriorating condition. This assessment could provide valuable information about the cultural beliefs and values of each daughter, leading the nurse to suggest possible culturally appropriate methods for relaxation.

Nurses can assist patients and others to begin to achieve a relaxation response by focusing on their breathing. Patients can lengthen their breathing or focus on abdominal or diaphragmatic breathing. Benson (1975) found it helpful to use a mental device such as a repetitive phrase to remind the body to relax. Nurses can also practice relaxation as part of their self-care, enabling them to better deal with personal and work-related stress. Relaxation exercises can be done anywhere, at any time, and without cost.

Meditation

Meditation has been part of many spiritual and healing traditions for hundreds of years. Meditation refers to a group of techniques, such as mantra meditation, relaxation response, mindfulness meditation, and Zen Buddhist meditation. In meditation, a person learns to focus attention. Some forms of meditation instruct the practitioner to become mindful of thoughts, feelings, and sensations and to observe them in a nonjudgmental way. This practice is believed to result in a state of greater calmness and physical relaxation, as well as psychological balance (NCCIH, 2021). Practicing meditation can change how a person relates to the flow of emotions and thoughts.

Most types of meditation have four elements in common (NCCIH, 2016b):

- *A quiet location:* Meditation is usually practiced in a quiet place with as few distractions as possible. This can be particularly helpful for beginners.
- *A specific, comfortable posture:* Depending on the type being practiced, meditation can be done while sitting, lying down, standing, walking, or in other positions.
- *A focus of attention:* Focusing one's attention is usually a part of meditation. For example, the meditator may focus on a mantra (a specially chosen word or set of words), an object, or the sensations of the breath. Some forms of meditation involve paying attention to whatever is the dominant content of consciousness.
- *An open attitude:* Having an open attitude during meditation means letting distractions come and go naturally without judging them.

Patients seeking inpatient care might have a meditation practice they want to continue. Nurses should provide the time necessary for this to occur. Nurses could benefit from a meditation practice as well and could practice a brief meditation during breaks from patient care activities.

Guided Imagery

Guided imagery focuses on evoking pleasant images to replace negative or stressful feelings and to promote relaxation. Guided imagery involves using all five senses to imagine an event or body process unfolding according to a plan. When all senses are involved in the experience, the imaginary situation is more fully encoded in the body and more likely to take place. A relaxation technique is frequently used to prepare the mind and body before beginning an imagery session. Nurses can assist patients and others with imagery in several ways (Quinn, 2019):

- Many kinds of recorded imagery material with scripts are available so that people can use them independently. If some of these are available on the nursing unit, patients can determine what types of recorded material they would like to use or purchase. Patients can also be assisted to write a script and record it for their own use.
- Nurses can work with patients using a picture or photograph to visualize the desired outcome in a body part or in a situation. Patients can add to the visual cue and develop a total image.
- During a painful or stressful event, such as an intravenous line being started, the patient can "go to a favorite place" and imagine being there with all the pleasant experiences related to that space.

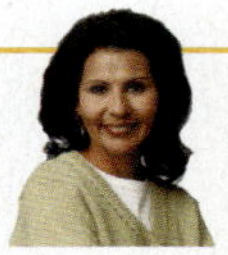

Think back to **Sylvia Puentes**, the anxious patient scheduled for surgery. Any of these types of imagery techniques would be appropriate suggestions for the patient. However, the nurse needs to assess the patient's preferences, beliefs, and ability to participate in these techniques to determine the best recommendation.

Yoga

Yoga is a mind and body practice with historical origins in ancient Indian philosophy. In the United States, yoga is practiced independently or paired with other health-promoting activities that assist people to achieve unity and wholeness. In general, in the United States, yoga involves the combination of physical movements, breathing practices, and relaxation practices/meditation (NCCIH, 2019a). Yoga promotes strength and flexibility, increases endurance and relaxation, reduces a person's response to stress, promotes healthy eating/activity habits, and promotes sleep (NCCIH, 2019a; Sivaramakrishnan et al., 2019). Yoga has been incorporated into comprehensive integrative pain management interventions (Pearson et al., 2020) and supportive interventions to address the negative side effects of cancer treatment (Johnson & Haag, 2019). Breathing exercises, posture awareness, spiritual practices, and mind–body centering can be added to the basic postures. Basic yoga postures are illustrated in Figure 29-2 on page 894. Common styles or traditions of yoga include (Yoga Alliance, n.d.):

- Iyengar, which focuses on proper alignment of the body and use of poses and breathing to address specific needs of the practitioner
- Kripalu or "gentle yoga," which focuses on relaxation and coming into balance
- Ashtanga, which focuses on synchronizing breathing with a fast-paced series of postures
- Bikram, which is done in a studio heated to 105°F and involves 26 set postures

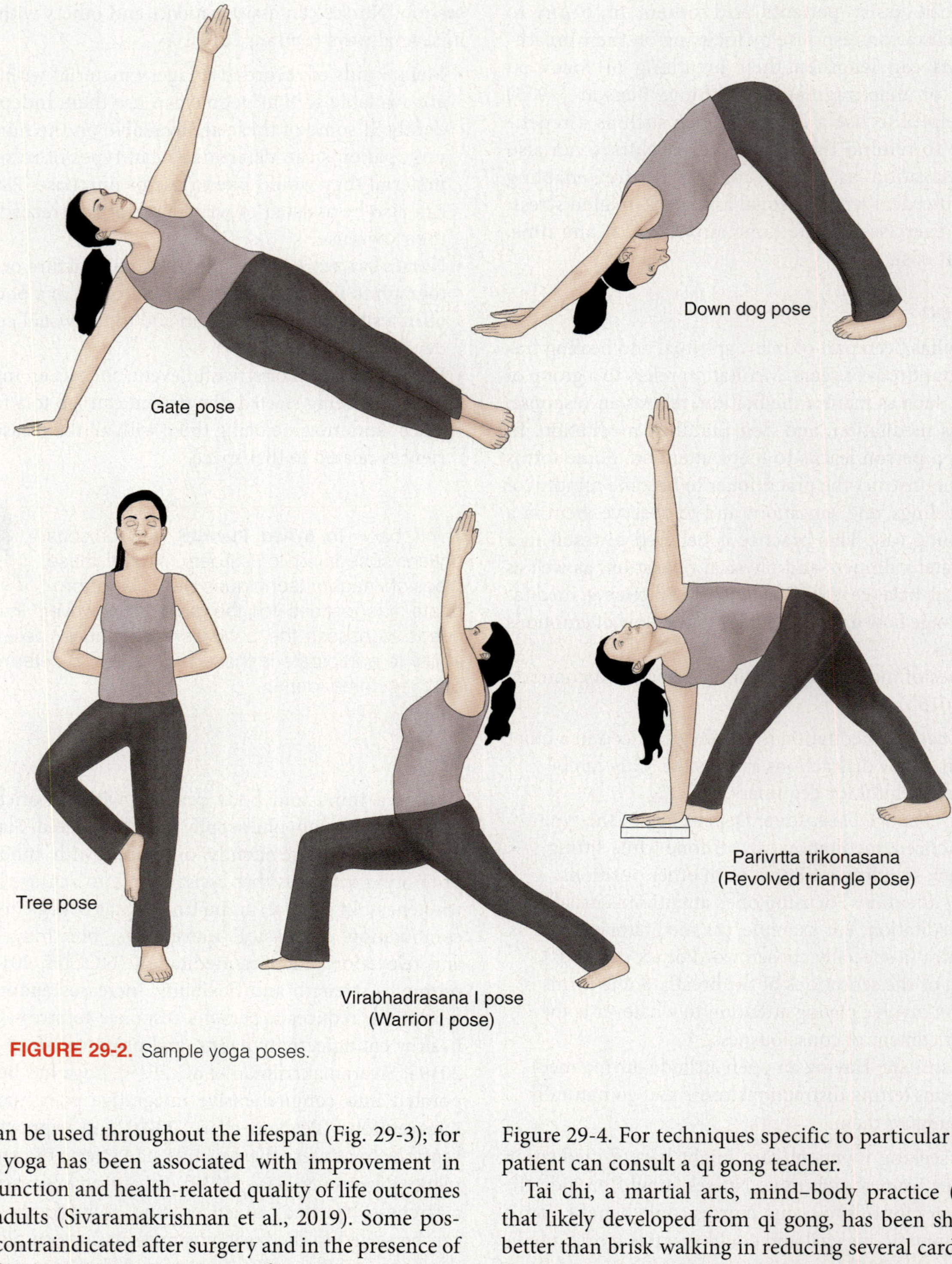

FIGURE 29-2. Sample yoga poses.

Yoga can be used throughout the lifespan (Fig. 29-3); for example, yoga has been associated with improvement in physical function and health-related quality of life outcomes in older adults (Sivaramakrishnan et al., 2019). Some postures are contraindicated after surgery and in the presence of disease. Consumers can stream yoga classes or attend yoga classes in-person. Encourage patients to find a type of yoga that is compatible with their physical condition and goals.

Qi Gong and Tai Chi

Qi gong is a system of postures, exercises (both gentle and dynamic), breathing techniques, and visualization. The majority of qi gong exercises or meditations enhance systemic health. They are designed to restore the healing system, the body's innate intelligence, so it knows how to correct and heal itself. Qi gong postures are illustrated in Figure 29-4. For techniques specific to particular diseases, a patient can consult a qi gong teacher.

Tai chi, a martial arts, mind–body practice (Fig. 29-5) that likely developed from qi gong, has been shown to be better than brisk walking in reducing several cardiovascular disease risk factors and improving psychosocial well-being (Chan et al., 2018). Both tai chi and qi gong (also known as qigong) have origins in China and involve physical movement, mental focus, deep breathing, and relaxation (NCCIH, 2016b). As with yoga, qi gong and tai chi can be learned through the use of streamed or face-to-face classes. Various tai chi and qi gong organizations offer training and certification programs, with differing criteria and levels of certification for instructors (NCCIH, 2016b). Encourage those interested to ask potential instructors about their background and knowledge.

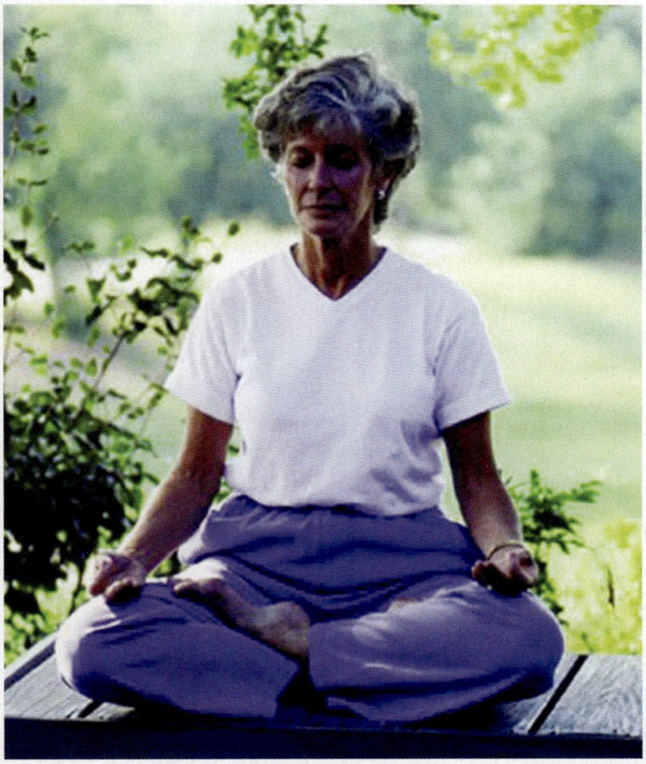

FIGURE 29-3. A woman practicing yoga.

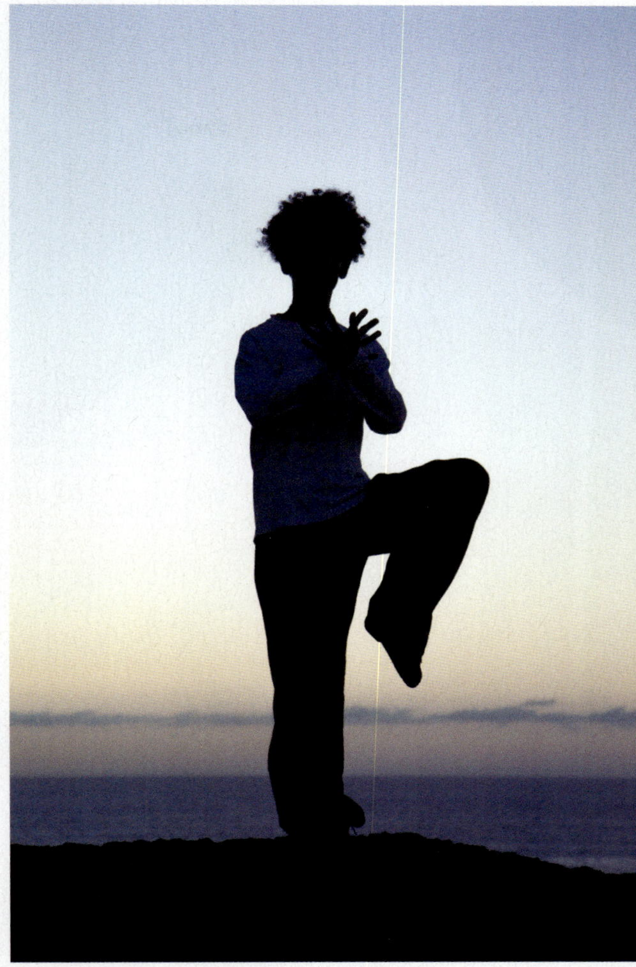

FIGURE 29-5. A woman practicing tai chi. (*Source: Photo by Tamara Kulikova/Shutterstock.*)

Acupuncture

Acupuncture addresses a person's qi. Traditionally, Qi (*chi* in Japanese) is believed to flow vertically in the body through an intricate structure of 12 primary meridians, energy circuits that nourish and support all cells and organs of the body (Fig. 29-6). Acupuncture consists of placing very thin, short, sterile needles at particular acupoints, believed to be centers of nerve and vascular tissue, along a meridian (Figs. 29-7 on page 896 and 29-8 on page 896). Acupuncture either increases or decreases the flow of qi along the meridian, restoring the balance of yin and yang. This change in the

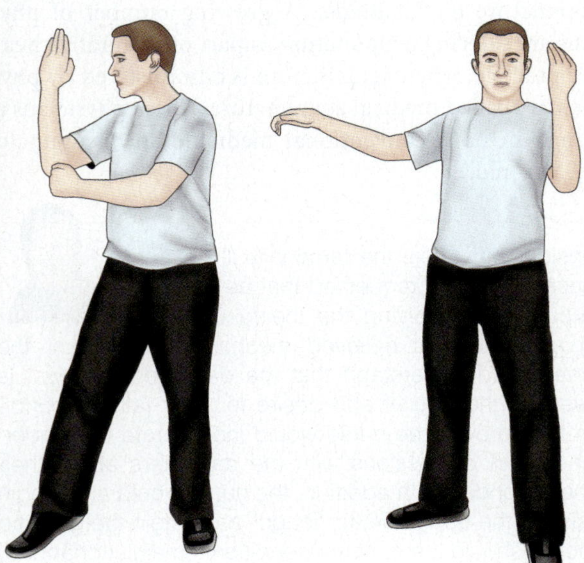

FIGURE 29-4. Qi gong postures.

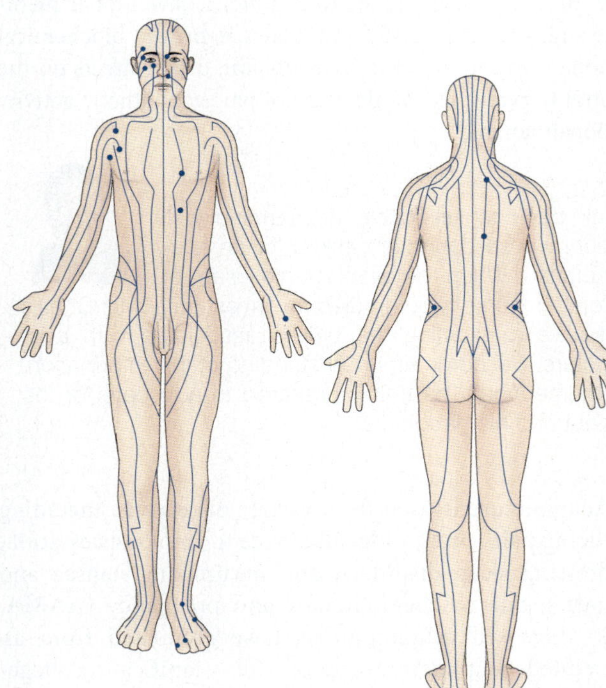

FIGURE 29-6. Acupuncture meridians.

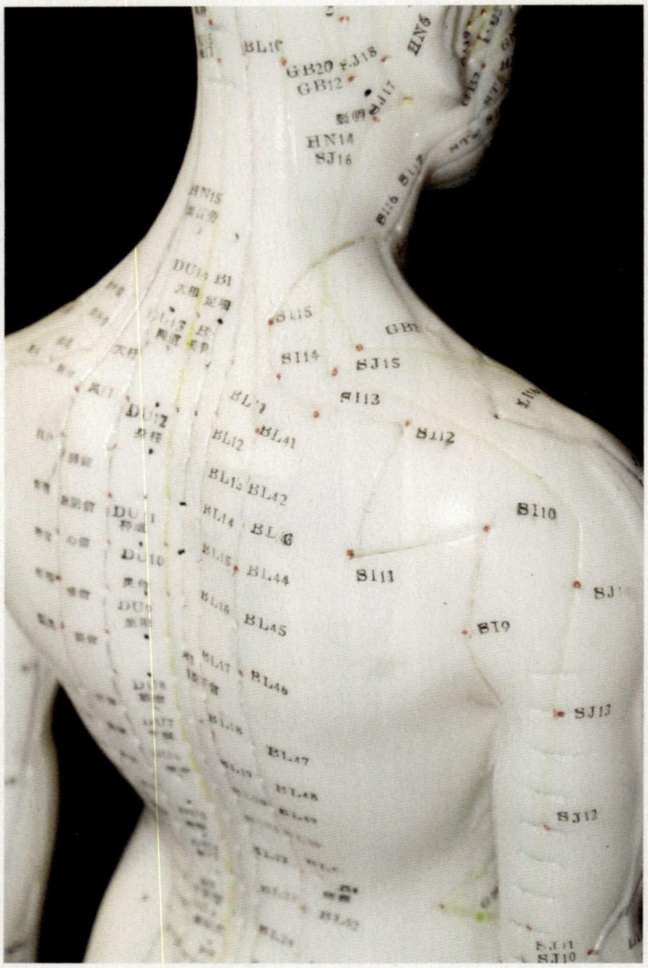

FIGURE 29-7. Model of acupuncture points on the body. (*Source: Photo by Cora Reed/Shutterstock.*)

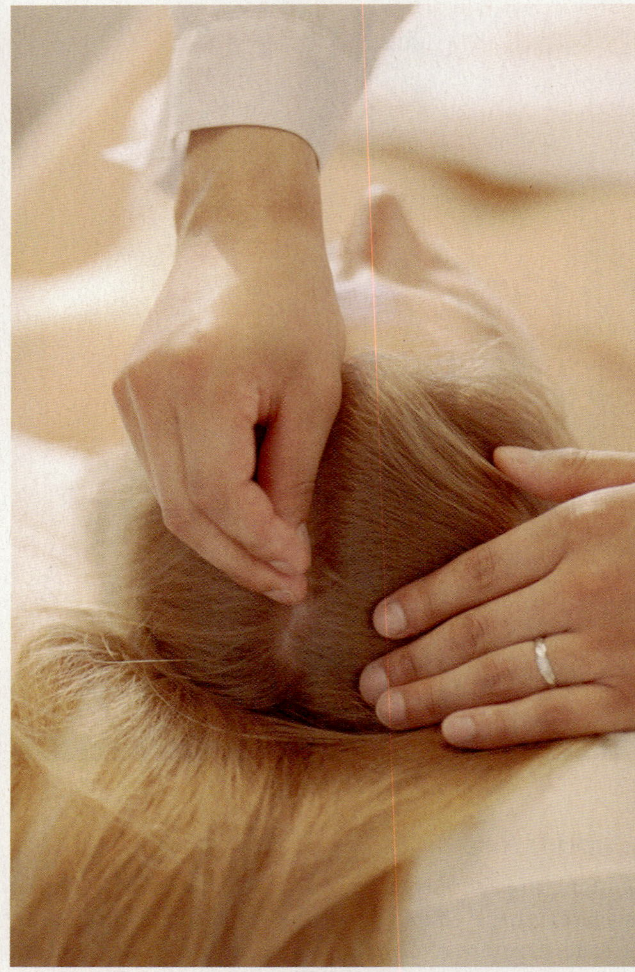

FIGURE 29-8. An acupuncture needle applied to a woman's scalp. (*Source: Photo by Cultura Motion/Shutterstock.*)

flow of energy contributes to healing. Conventional medicine suggests acupuncture stimulates improved biochemical actions involved in nerve transmission, direct effects on the central nervous and modulation of parasympathetic activity (Koppelman, n.d.).

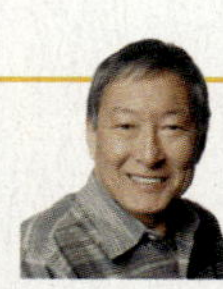

Think back to **Lee Chen**, the terminally ill patient whose daughters asked for an acupuncturist. When developing the plan of care, the nurse would need to investigate Mr. Chen's culture and examine the beliefs associated with acupuncture. Based on an understanding of this information, the nurse would be better prepared to advocate for the patient and his daughters.

Acupuncture is used for a variety of reasons, including reducing pain, promoting adherence to smoking cessation, addressing sleep disorders, and minimizing nausea and vomiting due to chemotherapy and pregnancy (AAMA, n.d.). Licensed acupuncturists have graduated from an accredited acupuncture school after significant college-level coursework. In addition, they have passed a licensure examination. However, education and training standards and requirements vary from state to state (NCCIH, 2016c). Acupuncture is generally provided in clinics or private offices, although it is possible for acupuncturists to provide acupuncture on inpatients. A growing number of physicians are offering acupuncture as part of integrative health care practice; when acupuncture is administered by physicians, it's called medical acupuncture. These physicians are trained in both conventional medicine and acupuncture (AAMA, n.d.).

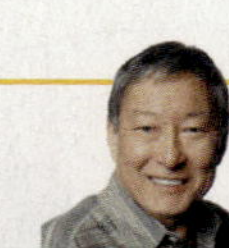

Consider **Mr. Chen**, the terminally ill patient whose daughters requested that he receive acupuncture. Applying the theory underlying acupuncture's believed mechanism of action, the nurse would understand that the daughters' request is based on their belief and desire for their father's condition to improve. The nurse would incorporate this understanding in discussions with the daughters about their father's condition. In addition, the nurse would also begin assisting the daughters to "let go" and begin the grieving process should the patient's condition remain unchanged, even after the acupuncture.

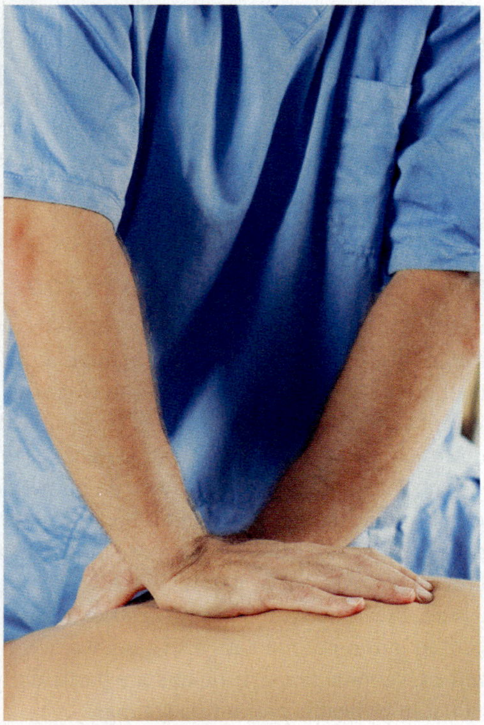

FIGURE 29-9. A chiropractic health care professional provides an adjustment. (*Source: Photo by Microgen/Shutterstock.*)

Chiropractic Health Care

Chiropractic health care is a profession that focuses on the relationship between the body's structure—mainly the spine—and its functioning (NCCIH, 2019c). Chiropractic practitioners primarily perform adjustments (manipulations) to the spine or other parts of the body with the goal of correcting alignment problems, alleviating pain, improving function, and supporting the body's natural ability to heal itself (Fig. 29-9). The NCCIH reports that most research on chiropractic health care has focused on spinal manipulation (NCCIH, 2019c). Spinal manipulation appears to benefit some people with low-back pain and may also be helpful for headaches, neck pain, upper- and lower-extremity joint conditions, and whiplash-associated disorders. Chiropractors may combine the use of spinal adjustments and other manual therapies with several other treatments and approaches, such as exercise and nutritional counseling (NCCIH, 2019c).

Doctors of chiropractic medicine (DC) are licensed and attend 4 years of chiropractic school after prerequisite undergraduate coursework and pass a national licensing exam. The types of services chiropractors are allowed to provide vary from state to state (NCCIH, 2019c). At this time, most chiropractic treatment is conducted on outpatients. A good understanding of chiropractic medicine will allow you to answer patients' questions and ask questions about a patient's current treatments. This knowledge also helps you to be able to refer patients asking questions about chiropractic medicine to reliable sources of information.

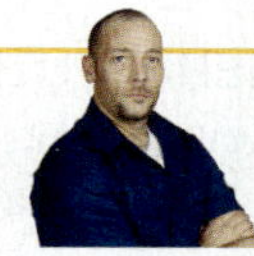

Recall **Brian Legett**, the patient with chronic back problems who has experienced little relief and is asking about seeing a chiropractor. When responding to Mr. Legett, the nurse would need to explain the underlying principles of chiropractic science. In addition, the nurse, in conjunction with other health care team members involved in the patient's plan of care, would need to review the patient's history thoroughly to identify (if possible) the underlying cause of his back problems and the various treatments attempted. This review would be important in determining if a referral to a chiropractor would be appropriate.

Aromatherapy

Aromatherapy is the use of essential oils of plants as a therapy to improve physical, emotional, and spiritual well-being (Fontaine, 2019). The fragrance of these oils is believed to ultimately affect the very sensitive amygdala of the limbic system in the brain, where emotional memories are stored and released (Johns Hopkins Medicine, n.d.). Laboratory and animal studies have shown that certain oils have antibacterial, antiviral, antifungal, calming, and energizing effects. Essential oils can be absorbed by the body through in halation and topical applications (Helming et al., 2022). Aromatherapy practices have been utilized in the management of pain, sleep disorders, anxiety, depression, nausea and vomiting, and increased general well-being (Dilek & Necmiye, 2020). Commonly used essential oils in a health care setting are ginger for nausea and lavender for insomnia (Fontaine, 2019). Essential oils vary in quality and potency depending on the manufacturing processes. If specific essential oils are approved for use in an inpatient setting, provide education on these oils. Some people are highly sensitive to strong fragrances, particularly concentrated essential oils. This might preclude their use in some patient settings.

Certification in Aromatherapy for health professionals is available. Standards for professional aromatherapy education are set by the National Association for Holistic Aromatherapy (n.d.b).

Energy-Healing Therapies

Energy-healing therapies include many diverse practices, with a fundamental underlying assumption that all life is sustained by universal life energy that moves freely within and without a person's being (Helming et al., 2022). Energy-healing therapy techniques are based on the belief that this primary life force can be influenced and thus contribute to physiologic healing. These techniques involve channeling healing energy through the hands of a practitioner into the patient's body to restore a normal energy balance and, therefore, health (Clarke et al., 2015). Energy-healing therapies are used in treating a wide variety of ailments and health problems and may often be used with other CHAs as well as conventional medical treatments (Clarke et al., 2015).

THERAPEUTIC TOUCH

Therapeutic touch (TT) is the process of energy exchange; practitioners focus on healing by use of their hands on or near the body with the intent to help or heal (Bagci & Cinar Yucel, 2020). The TT process consists of centering, assessing the energy field, and rebalancing the field using modulation, *unruffling*, and other techniques (Krieger, 1993).

TT uses four primary scientific premises (Krieger, 1993, pp. 12–13):

1. All the life sciences agree that, physically, a human being is an open energy system.
2. Anatomically, a human being is bilaterally symmetrical.
3. Illness is an imbalance in a person's energy field.
4. Human beings have natural abilities to transform and transcend their conditions of living.

TT has been used to manage pain and anxiety as well as other symptoms (Bagci & Yucel, 2020). Registered nurses can become credentialed in TT (TTIA, 2003).

HEALING TOUCH

Healing touch (HT) uses gentle intentional touch to assist in balancing physical, emotional, mental, and spiritual well-being (Healing Beyond Borders, 2020). The goal of HT is to restore wholeness through harmony and balance, enhancing the person's ability to self-heal (Hausladen Foley et al., 2016). Treatment involves the health care provider placing their hands either on or slightly above the body to assess for disturbances in the energy field, then working with the energy fields (auras) and energy centers (chakras) to clear and balance the energy (Healing Beyond Borders, n.d.). Certification in HT for people of various backgrounds is available through several Healing Touch organizations.

SOUND HEALING

Sound is an ancient form of healing. Examples include the central importance of drum and flutes for American Indians and Tibetan singing bowls. Sound, using the vibrational energy of tones, music, chants, song, and a variety of sound-producing instruments, is used to promote relaxation and healing (Fontaine, 2019). Music has been used to help patients relax, to increase sleep quality (Kavurmaci et al., 2020), decrease anxiety (Langer Bro et al., 2019) is increasingly used in hospice to comfort the dying. Music can be used to promote positive outcomes in several ways. Patients can listen to their favorite music prior to surgery or other stressful events, during imagery, and while relaxing. Music is frequently played in operating rooms with positive effects on the performance of the surgical team (Rastipisheh et al., 2019), and harp or piano music is played in patient lounges and lobbies. Music is also implemented to improve the quality of life for patients with communication impairment, such as later-stage dementia, and increase nonverbal communication (Clare et al., 2020).

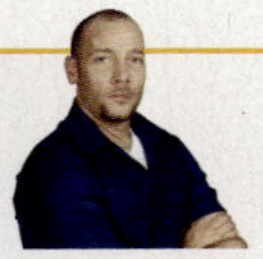

Think about **Brian Legett**, the man with chronic back pain described at the beginning of the chapter. Based on an assessment of the patient's likes and dislikes, the nurse might suggest music therapy as a means to help Brian relax and reduce his discomfort.

Manipulative and Body-Based Practices

This group of therapies includes therapeutic massage—an assortment of techniques that involve manipulation of soft tissues of the body through pressure and movement, as well as a variety of techniques such as Rolfing, shiatsu, Feldenkrais method, Alexander technique, myofascial release (MFR), and others. The goal is to break up tension held in body structures, promote communication between mind–body structures, promote detoxification, and generally improve body functioning. Some of these therapies can be painful while they work to oxygenate tissues, break up lymphatic congestion, release muscle tightness, and promote circulation. These therapies require specialized educational preparation and are particularly useful in rehabilitation or health-promotion settings.

Natural Products

Botanical agents (herbs) and nutritional supplements are chemical compounds that are ingested with the hope of achieving a therapeutic goal. They are becoming increasingly popular with consumers, who can buy many of these preparations over the counter (OTC) or from company distributors. Currently, dietary supplements (which include herbs and nutritional supplements) are considered foods, thus manufacturers need to follow FDA labeling requirements (FDA, 2019). Some product sample analyses have revealed inconsistencies in the amount of active ingredients. The National Institutes of Health Office of Dietary Supplements (ODS) works to strengthen knowledge and understanding of dietary supplements and provides dietary supplement fact sheets for both health professionals and consumers (ODS, n.d.a). These fact sheets and other up-to-date information regarding dietary supplements, including consumer protection updates from the FDA may be accessed from this site at https://ods.od.nih.gov/factsheets/list-all/ (ODS, n.d.b).

Botanicals (Herbal Products) and Nutritional Supplements

Some consumers and practitioners are attracted to herbs because they are "natural" plant products, which may be perceived as more compatible with the body than manufactured pharmaceutical agents. In fact, some pharmaceutical agents (e.g., digitalis) were first produced as natural products derived from plants and now are produced chemically. In many countries, herbal products are regulated and available through the primary health care system. In Germany, for example, the Federal Institute for Drugs and Medical Devices Commission E reviews scientific data and establishes prescriptive standards for herbs and plant products used for healing (NCI, n.d.b).

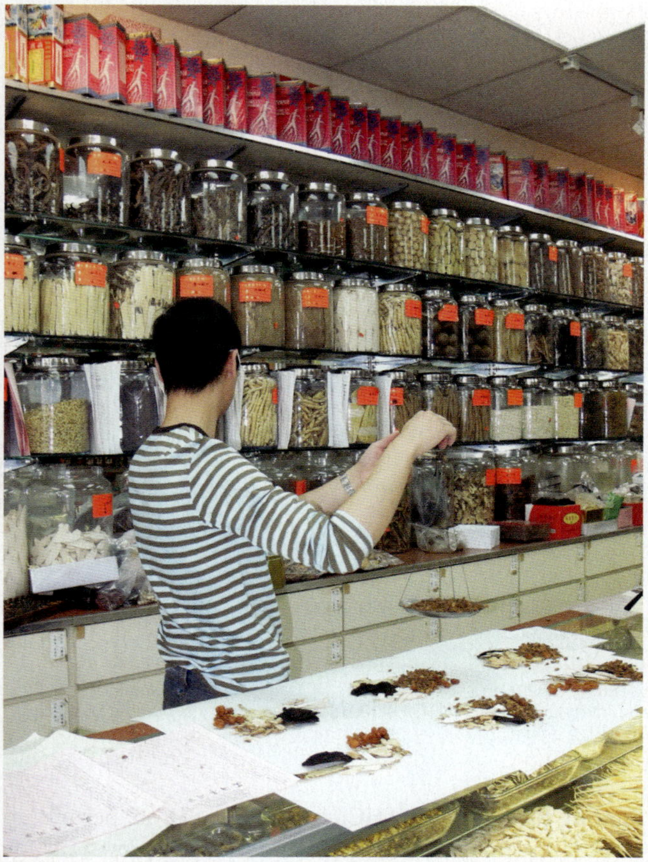

FIGURE 29-10. Herbs may be used as part of a treatment plan for patients who choose a whole medical system. (*Source:* Hood, L. [2018]. *Leddy & Pepper's professional nursing* [9th ed.]. Wolters Kluwer.)

In the United States, the FDA classifies herbs as a food and not a drug, falling under the category of dietary supplements (MFMER, 2017a). This is important because herbs are not regulated for quality and potency as drugs are, and herbal formulas can be sold without being studied to see if they are helpful or harmful (MFMER, 2017a).

Many whole medical systems use herbs as part of their treatment system for disease and reduction of symptoms (Fig. 29-10) (whole medical systems are discussed in the Other Complementary Health Approaches section). For example, echinacea and goldenseal (separately or in combination) may be used for infections, and ginkgo biloba is used to dilate blood vessels and reduce symptoms of memory loss and mental confusion (Fontaine, 2019).

Nutritional (dietary) supplements are chemical compounds that contain ingredients (vitamins, minerals, enzymes, amino acids, essential fatty acids) believed to promote health. These products have a wide range of safety and effectiveness.

Extensive specialized education is required before a nurse can be competent to advise patients on the use of herbs and supplements. However, as increasing numbers of patients are using herbs and supplements, nurses need to be aware of the various products available and provide education to patients to ensure safety with their use. For example, some herbs and/or supplements may interact with prescribed medications patients are taking. Ginkgo biloba, used by people to improve memory, affects platelet function and should not be used concurrently with other antiplatelet drugs and anticoagulants (MFMER, 2017b). The herb kava, used by patients for anxiety, has been linked to serious liver damage (Mayo Clinic, 2019). Women who are pregnant or nursing and children are particularly at risk and should be especially cautious about using herbal supplements either alone or in mixtures. Many supplements have not been well tested for safety in pregnant women, nursing mothers, or children (ODS, 2020). Herbals/health supplements should not be given to a child unless recommended by their health care provider (ODS, 2020). Teaching Tips 29-1 (on page 900) provides important patient education information related to herbs and supplements.

Medical Cannabis

Multiple products from the cannabis plant species have been promoted as "natural" products to alleviate numerous symptoms and increase wellness (Long, 2020; Trentham, 2019b). Patients are increasingly using prescribed medical marijuana and cannabidiol products that are available without a prescription to treat their conditions (Brown, 2020). However, despite marketing for the treatment of a variety of conditions, conclusive evidence regarding safety and efficacy of cannabis for therapeutic purpose is, for the most part, lacking (Dill & Kurkowski, 2020). Therapeutic uses for cannabis or cannabinoids include for antiemetic effects in chemotherapy-induced nausea and vomiting, chronic pain in adults, multiple sclerosis–related spasticity, and reduction of seizure frequency associated with severe epilepsy (National Academies of Sciences, Engineering, and Medicine, 2017; U.S. FDA, 2018b). Nurses need to have an understanding of the endocannabinoid system and understand cannabis pharmacology and the research associated with use of these products (Brown, 2020; NCSBN, 2018). Nurses must also remain aware of the current legal status of cannabis products and be able to answer patients' questions and provide patients accurate information related to their safety and effectiveness (Brown, 2020; NCSBN, 2018).

The marijuana components tetrahydrocannabinol (THC) and cannabidiol (CBD) are the most commonly known compounds of the marijuana (cannabis) plant. THC is the active psychoactive compound in marijuana and is what is tested for in a urine drug screen. The biologic effects of cannabinoids are mediated by cannabinoid (CBI) receptors, located throughout the body, and especially focused near the nervous system, and are part of the endocannabinoid system in the body (Benson, 2019; Long, 2020). The endocannabinoid system is an internal regulatory system that functions to maintain homeostasis and equilibrium (Benson, 20109; Long, 2020; Meletis, 2020; Theisen & Konieczny, 2019). The most common and well-studied CBI receptors include CB1 and CB2 (Theisen & Konieczny, 2019). CB1 receptors are predominantly found in the central and peripheral nervous systems as well as other organs of the body and, when activated, can help alleviate anxiety, stress, pain, and inflammation (Theisen & Konieczny, 2019). CB2 receptors are concentrated in the

Teaching Tips 29-1

USING HERBS AND SUPPLEMENTS

Teaching Tip	Why Is This Important?
Get information from knowledgeable and reliable sources.	Advertising media and many sources on the Internet frequently seek primarily to sell the product, not educate the consumer.
Buy products that are produced by reputable companies and include label logos that identify dietary supplements and herbals that have been tested for ingredient quality and contaminants.	Since this industry is not regulated, contamination and inconsistency in the amount of product sometimes occur.
Whenever possible, buy single products.	If the product contains several ingredients and you have a reaction or positive response, you won't know which ingredient was the causative agent.
Follow the label instructions and monitor for adverse effects.	Herbal remedies and supplements can be toxic in higher-than-recommended doses.
Become knowledgeable about the product and your reason for using it.	Consumers who initiate any type of self-care tend to make better decisions if they are well informed.

Source: Modified from Helming, M. A. B., Shields, D. A., Avino, K. M., & Rosa, W. E. (Eds.). (2022). *Dossey & Keegan's Holistic nursing. A handbook for practice* (8th ed.). Jones & Bartlett Learning; National Center for Complementary and Integrative Health (NCCIH). (2019). *Using dietary supplements wisely.* https://www.nccih.nih.gov/health/using-dietary-supplements-wisely#hed6

peripheral immune cells as well as in the central and peripheral nervous systems and the lungs and, when activated, can help alleviate inflammation (Theisen & Konieczny, 2019). In addition to CBI receptors, this system also consists of ligands and enzymes that regulate sleep, pain perception, memory, mood, and appetite. The receptors can be stimulated by endogenous cannabinoids as well as plant-derived and synthetic cannabinoids (Theisen & Konieczny, 2019). The ligands act as chemical messengers to stimulate cannabinoids to interact at the receptor sites, and the enzymes break down cannabinoids after they have completed their function (Theisen & Konieczny, 2019). Cannabinoids are chemical compounds that can influence the cannabinoid receptors and promote the release of neurotransmitters. Tetrahydrocannabinol (THC) and CBD are the most abundant cannabinoids (Theisen & Konieczny, 2019).

Marijuana is listed in the Schedule I of the federal Controlled Substances Act because of the psychoactive effects of THC and the potential for abuse. The U.S. Drug Enforcement Administration (DEA) considers all cannabinoids, including marijuana and CBD, a Schedule I drug and they remain illegal under federal law (Benson, 2019; Trentham, 2019a), with one exception. FDA-approved drugs that contain CBD derived from cannabis and no more than 0.1% THC have been placed in Schedule V (U.S. DEA, 2018). Hemp is regulated by the U.S. Department of Agriculture, and, if it is produced in a manner consistent with federal and state regulations and the THC content is negligibly low (not more than 0.3% THC), is considered legal (Agriculture Improvement Act of 2018, 2018). State laws regarding any of these substances vary and range from making it legal for prescribers to recommend CBD oils for certain conditions, limiting the allowable THC content in CBD oil, permitting clinical research, and making or not making provisions for legal sale or purchase of CBD (Bemben, 2019).

The FDA has approved a new drug class of medications called cannabinoids (Brown, 2020). FDA-approved cannabinoids include an oral CBD-based drug (Epidiolex), which has been shown to reduce the frequency of seizures when compared with a placebo and has been approved to treat severe forms of epilepsy (Brown, 2020; U.S. FDA, 2018b). Dronabinol is a synthetic cannabinoid approved to treat chemotherapy-induced nausea and vomiting and anorexia and weight loss secondary to AIDS (Bemben, 2019). Nabilone is another synthetic cannabinoid similar to THC and is approved for refractory chemotherapy-induced nausea and vomiting (Bemben, 2019). FDA regulations indicate that products that contain THC or CBD cannot be sold as dietary supplements (Gottlieb, 2018).

MARIJUANA

Marijuana plants contain high levels of THC and lower levels of CBD (Trentham, 2019b). THC is the most abundant cannabinoid in the cannabis plant. The FDA has not approved the plant marijuana for the treatment of health problems (Trentham, 2019b). Fifteen states, two territories, and the District of Columbia have legalized medical and recreational marijuana (ProCon, 2020b). Another 34 states and 2 more territories have legalized medical marijuana only to treat certain medical conditions (ProCon, 2020b).

Medical marijuana is available in several forms for consumption, dictated by state law. Available forms may include pills containing oil to be swallowed and digested; extracts that are inhaled or vaporized; liquids and tinctures for use under the tongue or as an oral spray; topical gels, creams, and ointments for localized effect; patches for transdermal absorption; and flowers/dry leaf to be consumed through vaporization. THC produces euphoric, psychoactive effects that influence mood, consciousness, and behavior. Side effects are dose dependent and may include hypotension, hallucinations, tachycardia, central nervous system depression, euphoria, dizziness, drowsiness, somnolence, confusion, new or worsening nausea and vomiting, and seizures and can lead to substance use disorder (Theisen & Konieczny, 2019).

The use of substances with THC to treat certain health problems or for recreational use could be legal based on State law but may still result in violation of the law (Trentham, 2019b). For example, persons employed in safety sensitive positions, such as nurses, in which use of marijuana may negatively impact the work performance and constitute a threat to health or safety, cannot test positive for marijuana or its constituents. A positive test may result in disciplinary action by an employer. Many state and professional regulations do not differentiate between consumption of marijuana for medical purposes while not working and use during work hours/employment (Trentham, 2019b).

CANNABIDIOL

CBD is the second most active ingredient and a natural component found in marijuana plants. CBD is one of many chemicals in the cannabis plant and is also a compound found in hemp (Trentham, 2019b). It is derived from the stalks, leaves, and buds of the hemp plant (Trentham, 2019b). CBD is a mood-altering substance (Theisen & Konieczny, 2019) but is considered a nonpsychoactive chemical (Long, 2020; Trentham, 2019b). It does not produce a "high" or euphoric effect (Brown, 2020). There is a lack of large-scale clinical trials showing the efficacy of CBD as well as evidence-based recommendations and in-depth understanding of risks and benefits (Hande, 2017; Whiting et al., 2015, as cited in Bonn-Miller et al., 2017). Seventeen states have laws specifically addressing CBD (Bemben, 2019; ProCon, 2020a).

There is growing consumer demand for CBD constituents of the cannabis plant due to purported medicinal benefits (Whiting et al., 2015, as cited in Bonn-Miller et al., 2017). CBD has been shown to improve mood by decreasing anxiety and depression and is effective for treating nausea and vomiting, seizures, and pain (Theisen & Konieczny, 2019). CBD is being studied as a treatment for other conditions, including chronic pain, Parkinson disease, schizophrenia, diabetes, multiple sclerosis, irritable bowel syndrome, movement disorders due to Tourette syndrome, posttraumatic stress disorder, and sleep disorders, but research supporting benefits remains limited (Bauer, 2018; Long, 2020; NCCIH, 2019h). Consumers report use of CBD for potential therapeutic effect, either alone or in combination with other therapies, in treating seizure disorders, psychotic symptoms, anxiety, depression, inflammation, cancer, cardiovascular diseases, neurodegeneration, symptoms of multiple sclerosis, sleep disorders, and chronic pain (Benson, 2019; Carroon & Phillips, 2018). Side effects are dose dependent, including dizziness, anxiety, diarrhea, jitteriness, decreased appetite, hepatocellular injury, dry mouth, fatigue, somnolence, sedation, nausea, vomiting, changes in appetite or mood, and suicidal ideation (Bemben, 2019; Theisen & Konieczny, 2019; Trentham, 2019b).

CBD is available in several forms. CBD capsules, pills, and gummies are available for oral consumption with absorption via the GI tract (Benson, 2019). Oral products allow for convenient dosing, with slow absorption (Brown, 2020). CBD is also suspended in oil or alcohol (tincture), which is placed under the tongue with a dropper and absorbed via capillaries. This results in quicker absorption and more rapid effects (Benson, 2019). CBD is also available as a vaporization liquid for inhalation using an e-cigarette, with quick absorption from the lungs into the bloodstream (Benson, 2019; Brown, 2020). This route of administration is associated with damage to the lungs (Brown, 2020). Topical CBD is available in creams and lotions. Administration via this route results in localized effects but has been associated with localized skin reactions (Brown, 2020).

There is a lack of precision in product labeling that may contribute to a false sense of safety (Trentham, 2019a). There are few studies to support CBD products obtained without a prescription to treat any medical conditions (Brown, 2020). The CBD products that are sold in the United States are not regulated by the FDA. Discrepancies between federal and state cannabis laws result in inadequate regulation and oversight leading to inaccurate labeling of some products. Most CBD products claim to have under 0.3% THC, classified as hemp, but a lack of regulation in the manufacturing process, consistent dosing, testing standards, and oversight may also contribute to unreliable THC levels (Bonn-Miller et al., 2017; Trentham, 2019b). A 2017 study by Bonn-Miller et al. examined 84 products from 31 companies available via online retail that included CBD content on the packaging. A blind analysis of cannabinoid content identified a wide range and inconsistent CBD concentrations: 26% contained less CBD than labeled; 21% contained THC; and 43% were underlabeled (CBD concentrations were higher than listed on the product). The authors concluded the findings highlight the need for additional monitoring of products sold on the Internet and for manufacturing and testing standards, as well as oversight of medicinal cannabis products (Bonn-Miller et al., 2017).

CBD Safety

Most patients tolerate CBD products (Brown, 2020). However, there is a lack of quality scientific studies on the use and effects of CBD, and the long-term effects of using CBD products are unknown at this time, as there have been no long-term studies to date (Brown, 2020). CBD use may cause increased activity of anticoagulants (Brown, 2020); increased serum concentrations of selective serotonin-reuptake inhibitors, antipsychotics, beta-blockers, opioids, tricyclic antidepressants, benzodiazepines, antihistamines, some statins, macrolides, and antiretrovirals (Fugh-Berman et al., n.d.); and increased liver enzymes (Fugh-Berman et al., n.d.). There is also some concern for unreliability of the purity of CBE products; concentrations of CBD oil vary widely from brand to brand and bottle to bottle within brands (Trentham). Companies use different CBD sources, extraction methods, and production techniques, and not all resulting products are equal (Trentham). Some state regulations allow for up to 5% THC in CBD oil (Trentham, 2019b). Patients and health care providers should be aware that consumption of CBD oil or products with CBD oil may result in a positive urine drug screen for THC; consumption of CBD with higher concentrations will result in a positive urine test for THC (Brown, 2020; Trentham, 2019b).

HEMP OIL

Hemp oil is derived from industrial hemp, a variety of cannabis plant species, which has a lower concentration of THC compared to marijuana (Trentham, 2019b). The amount of THC in hemp is to be less than 0.3%, in order to be sold legally (Andres, 2019; Trentham, 2019b). Hemp oil is low in saturated fat and high in antioxidants, vitamin E, and omega-3 and -6 fatty acids and may be used as an ingredient in cooking. Manufacturers of shampoos, soaps, and body lotions may include hemp oil as an ingredient. Patients and healthcare providers should be aware that consuming hemp foods can cause positive results in urine drug screening testing for THC (Trentham, 2019b).

PATIENT EDUCATION

As with any health-related issue, patient education related to the use of cannabis and CBD products is an important nursing intervention. Patients need to be aware that CBD products available online and OTC without prescription are not regulated and not proven to treat any medical condition (Brown, 2020). Patients should be encouraged to consider products with full disclosure regarding the ingredients of the product, to carefully examine product labels (Bensen, 2019; Epstein, 2020), and review the certificate of analysis (COA) for any OTC product (Theisen & Konieczny, 2019). Patients should look for products with certification from outside agencies, such as the National Science Foundation International (Benson, 2019). Discussions with patients should include information about cannabis, marijuana, and CBD safety, effectiveness, and potential side effects (Brown, 2020; Hande, 2017). It is also important to identify all medications (prescription and OTC) and supplements the patient is using to identify and discuss potential drug interactions (Brown, 2020). Patient education should also address the potential for positive urine drug screening and related consequences, as indicated (Brown, 2020).

Nurses frequently care for patients who use or who are considering use of therapeutic cannabis products and must have adequate knowledge about these products and clinical implications to better serve patients. Theisen and Konieczy (2019) suggest nurses can help patients make smart decisions by educating themselves. As more patients decide to explore cannabis as a CHA, nurses may be faced with making clinical judgments to balance promoting and safeguarding personal integrity and respecting the values and preferences of patients and others. Refer to the Thoughtful, Person-Centered Practice: Challenging Topics Medical Cannabis to work through one possible patient care scenario.

QSEN Thoughtful, Person-Centered Practice: Challenging Topics

Medical Cannabis

Many controversial issues make it challenging to know how to respond as a professional nurse in select scenarios. Often, the nurse's personal and/or professional values may conflict with options desired by patients, families, employers, and communities. Not infrequently, nurses have to make clinical judgments balancing promoting and safeguarding personal integrity and respecting the values and preferences of patients or others.

Read the scenario below and see if you can articulate what you believe, why you believe this, and how these beliefs are likely to inform the decisions you make and your behavior, especially when you are confronted with competing obligations. Based on Tanner's Clinical Judgment Model (2006), consider reflection-in-action and reflection-on-action (Nielson, Stragnell, & Jester, 2007):

Reflection-in-Action: As you read, consider what the nurse is thinking in the moment—What happened? How did the patient, family/caregiver, and or healthcare provider respond? What did the nurse do next?

Scenario

You are a camp nurse and administering the children's prescribed medications is one of your responsibilities. On Johnny's first day, he hands you a bottle hand-labeled as "Cod Liver Oil," which his mother wants administered by mouth, twice a day. You contact the mother and tell her you need a physician's order to administer anything, even over-the-counter or holistic medicine. She sends you back the child's physical with clearly photo-shopped instructions to give two droppers full. You call the physician who did the physical to clarify the order, and he confirms that he did not write it. When you inform the mother, she is irate that you violated her privacy by contacting the physician. Suspicious about the mother's behavior, you smell the bottle and suspect it is cannabis based.

Effective Noticing (Cues)

1. What did you notice about the situation initially? What information/observations are significant? What information deviates from what is expected/normal/usual?

Scenario

When you call the mother back, she admits that the "Cod Liver Oil" is really a full-spectrum cannabidiol (CBD) oil that she had been administering to her son twice daily for his attention-deficit/hyperactivity disorder (ADHD). You think that CBD is a schedule 1 controlled substance, but you are not sure; you know that different forms of cannabis have been legalized on both state and federal levels. You have kept your manager informed, and she seems more

Thoughtful, Person-Centered Practice: Challenging Topics (*continued*)

concerned about placating the mother than promoting Johnny's well-being—or yours! Do you administer the oil to Johnny? Is administering this drug within your scope of practice?

You want to talk with Johnny to learn what he knows about the "cod liver oil," but his mother tells you that she does not want him to know that he is taking CBD oil. She was adamant that Johnny be told it is a vitamin supplement.

You wonder if you have an obligation to report this mother to child protective services.

Effective Interpreting

1. How would you prioritize this data? What other assessment data, evidence and/or information would you need to consider the situation? How would you obtain this additional information?
2. What do you think about this situation? Consider personal and previous nursing experiences that you have had and formal knowledge (physiology, psychology, communication skills) that may be of assistance in providing care in this situation.
3. Once the nurse suspects that the "cod liver oil" is actually some form of cannabis, she is less certain of how to proceed because she has never been in a situation like this before. What sort of "fact finding" would you recommend and what resources can you tap? How could you best learn what you need to know about the oil; your scope of practice and legal obligations about administering a cannabis-based oil; your ethical obligations to protect the patient, especially if it turns out, as it did in this case, that your initial research showed that children with ADHD do well with stimulants but not with depressants, which the oil was?

Now, see if you can articulate what you believe, why you believe this, and how these beliefs are likely to inform the decisions you make and your behavior, especially when you confronted with competing obligations.

Effective Responding

4. How would you describe the obligations you have in this scenario to your patient and his mother, to yourself, and to your employer?
5. If you cannot fulfill each of these obligations, how will you prioritize them? What basis/rationale do you use for prioritization? Remember that the ANA *Code of Ethics for Nurses* reminds us that "the nurse's primary commitment is to the patient," while at the same time states that "the nurse owes the same duties to self as to others, including the responsibility to promote health and safety, preserve wholeness of character and integrity, maintain competence, and continue personal and professional growth.
6. What are a nurse's reporting obligations when a child or other vulnerable party is at risk? What resources will you consult to learn more about this? Is your duty to report the mother's behavior trumped by another consideration/obligation?

Effective Reflecting

7. Which statement below best captures your beliefs?
   a. Parents should be able to make decisions for their children and a nurse does not have the right to challenge these decisions.
   b. Parents do not have unlimited rights over their children. If I believe their decisions are likely to harm a child, I have an obligation to advocate for the well-being of the child.

How will your belief inform your response in this scenario?

8. Whether you decide to administer the oil as directed by the boy's mother and your employer or refuse, how might you use reflective practice to evaluate your decision so you can respond more confidently in similar situations in the future? What criteria will you use to evaluate a good response?
9. What personal attributes and competencies are most likely to lead to a good response?

Reflection-on-Action

Then look back at the nurse's decisions and reflect on your learning—how did your knowledge and/or skills expand based on this scenario? What attitude, value, or belief shifts did you experience (if any) after reading this scenario? What would you do differently if you were in this situation? What more do you need to know to be able to manage this or a similar situation in the future?

Nielson, A., Stragnell, S., & Jester, P. (2007). Guide for reflection using the Clinical Judgment Model. *Journal of Nursing Education, 46*(11), 513–516. https://doi.org/10.3928/01484834-20071101-06

Tanner, C. A. (2006). Thinking like a nurse: a research-based model of clinical judgment in nursing. *Journal of Nursing Education, 45*(6), 204–211. https://doi.org/10.3928/01484834-20060601-04

Nutritional Therapy

The eating habits of people in the United States are being scrutinized because of the alarming increase in obesity, particularly in children, and chronic illnesses in all age groups. A diet consisting of prepared and processed foods and large amounts of meat, dairy products, and sugar has been associated with various diet-related chronic diseases and unfortunately represents the dietary habits of many Americans (U.S. Department of Health and Human Services and U.S. Department of Agriculture, 2020). People with a variety of credentials have endorsed many eating plans that purport to address these health problems. The diversity of these approaches is understandably very confusing to the consumer. An examination of these popular diets is beyond the scope of this book. Holistic nutrition approaches health and healing from a whole-person, individualistic perspective, providing advice on how to improve diet, lifestyle, and attitude to promote optimal health (NANP, n.d.). This belief has been a cornerstone of holistic nutritional approaches for centuries in traditional Chinese medicine (TCM) and Ayurvedic systems (discussed in the next sections). Many of these approaches are endorsed by naturopathic practitioners (naturopathy is discussed on page 905).

Other Complementary Health Approaches

Whole medical systems (or alternative medical systems) are other CHAs and consist of a philosophy and theory about health and illness along with specific types of treatment. These systems have developed independently from allopathic medicine and are generally culturally based. Ayurveda, TCM, shamanism (which includes native traditions), homeopathy, and naturopathy are examples of whole medical systems.

Ayurveda

Ayurveda originated in the ancient civilization of India and is considered one of the world's oldest medical systems (NCCIH, 2019e). The aim of Ayurvedic medicine is to integrate and balance the body, mind, and spirit (Fontaine, 2019). Key concepts include universal interconnectedness among people, their health, and the universe; and the body's constitution and life forces (Helming et al., 2022). Ayurvedic practitioners prescribe individualized treatments that include herbs, metals, minerals, and other materials; diet and exercise; and lifestyle recommendations (NCCIH, 2019e). Ayurvedic products are regulated as dietary supplements in the United States, and some have the potential to be toxic due to the present of metals (NCCIH, 2019e).

Special considerations may be necessary for patients who want to continue their Ayurvedic program while hospitalized. For example, some people may have special dietary (e.g., vegetarian) needs, some may need time set aside for self-care such as meditation, and some may desire to continue taking an herbal supplement. All precautions related to herbal and pharmaceutical interactions should be followed when using Ayurvedic herbal preparations.

Traditional Chinese Medicine

Underlying the practice of **traditional Chinese medicine (TCM)** is a unique view of the world and the human body that is different from Western medicine concepts. This view is based on the ancient Chinese belief of a natural order in the universe and an interconnectedness between the body and the cosmos, with a search for balance and harmony; a perception of humans as a small part of the larger surrounding universe—interconnected with nature and subject to its forces. The human body is regarded as an organic entity in which the various organs, tissues, and other parts have distinct functions but are all interdependent. In this view, health and disease relate to balance of the functions, as well as a balance of yin and yang energy (two opposing, yet complementary forces that shape the world and all life) (Cancer Research UK, 2018).

The goal of TCM is health promotion and quality of life, with an emphasis on the patient, not the illness (Fontaine, 2019). TCM practitioners use various mind and body practices, such as acupuncture and tai chi, as well as herbal products to address health problems (NCCIH, 2019b).

Shamanism

Shamanism is the oldest of all healing therapies concerned with the nature of creation, the natural flow of life, and with showing respect to our fellow creatures and one another (Fontaine, 2019). Shamanism developed in widely separated areas of the world, including North, Central, and South America, Africa, Australia, Indonesia, Malaysia, Bali, Tibet, Korea, Siberia, and across Europe (Fontaine, 2019). In shamanism, illness and other forms of distress are thought to originate in the spirit world (Vadala, 2019). The shaman or medicine man/woman possesses the ability to access the spirit world, which is done on behalf of people or the community, and return to "ordinary reality" with information on the proper treatment (Society for Shamanic Practice, n.d.). Particular emphasis is on the classic shamanic journey, one of the most remarkable visionary methods used by humankind to explore the hidden universe otherwise known mainly through myth and dream. Treatment may consist of retrieving lost soul energy, restoring the person to the right relationship with the spirit world, and treating symptoms (Andrews et al., 2020). General healing techniques involve native plants and herbs, animals, rituals, ceremonies, and purification techniques. In the United States, shamanic healing is gaining in popularity as Americans turn back to the old cultures for help and guidance in finding a better balance with nature and with themselves (Fontaine, 2019).

Homeopathy

Homeopathy is a medical system that was developed in Germany more than 200 years ago (NCCIH, 2018). The allopathic approach to dealing with illness is frequently to suppress symptoms; for example, acetaminophen can be given to reduce a fever. In contrast, homeopaths believe that when symptoms are suppressed in this manner, the condition "goes deeper" into the body, making it ultimately more difficult to cure. Supporters of homeopathy point to two unconventional theories (NCCIH, 2018):

- "Like cures like": The notion that a disease can be cured by a substance that produces similar symptoms in healthy people.
- "Law of minimum dose": The notion that the *lower* the dose of the medication, the *greater* its effectiveness. Many homeopathic remedies are so diluted that no molecules of the original substance remain.

Homeopathic remedies are derived from substances that come from plants, minerals, or animals, and include things such as red onion, arnica (mountain herb), crushed whole bees, white arsenic, poison ivy, belladonna (deadly nightshade), and stinging nettle (NCCIH, 2018). Homeopathic remedies are often formulated as sugar pellets to be placed under the tongue; they may also be in other forms, such as ointments, gels, drops, creams, and tablets. Treatments are "individualized" or tailored to each person—it is not uncommon for different people with the same condition to receive different treatments (NCCIH, 2018). There is little evidence to support homeopathy as an effective treatment for any specific condition (NCCIH, 2018). Although people sometimes assume that all homeopathic remedies are highly

Focused Assessment Guide 29-1

HOLISTIC CARE

Factors to Assess	Questions and Approaches
Stress	What measures does the patient use to reduce stress? If the patient wants to continue a meditation, relaxation, or imagery practice while receiving care, explore ways in which that can be accomplished.
Music/sound preferences	What preferences does the patient have for music or environmental sounds (e.g., ocean waves, birds) either while meditating or relaxing? Music could be provided by the patient if preferred music is not available.
Diet	What dietary preferences does the patient have (e.g., vegetarian, no processed foods)? Communicate these preferences to nutritional services.
Environmental sensitivity	Is the patient sensitive to environmental odors or fragrances? If so, can an air purifier be brought to the room?
Use of herbs and supplements	Is the patient taking any herbs or supplements as directed by a CHA practitioner or purchased over the counter? If so, obtain the names of the herbs/supplements, dosages, and reasons for their use. If these substances are in the patient's possession, follow applicable institutional policies.
Use of CHA health care provider	Is the patient planning to use a primary CHA provider while receiving allopathic care? If so, convey appropriate information to the primary allopathic provider.

diluted and therefore unlikely to cause harm, some products labeled as homeopathic can contain substantial amounts of active ingredients, thus could cause side effects and drug interactions (NCCIH, 2018).

Naturopathy

Naturopathy has evolved from traditional practices and health care approaches popular in Europe during the 19th century (NCCIH, 2017). Naturopaths believe that health is a dynamic state of being that provides abundant energy for people to deal with life in our complex society. Naturopathic medicine holds that the body innately knows how to maintain health and heal itself (Fontaine, 2019). The naturopathic provider's role is to support and restore the body using techniques and medicines that are geared to strengthen the body's own healing ability (Fontaine, 2019). Naturopathic practitioners use many different treatment approaches, including dietary and lifestyle changes, stress reduction, herbs and other dietary supplements, manipulative therapies, practitioner-guided detoxification, psychotherapy, and counseling (NCCIH, 2017). In the United States, naturopathic medicine is practiced by naturopathic physicians, traditional naturopaths, and other health care providers who also offer naturopathic services (NCCIH, 2017, para 3).

NURSING IMPLICATIONS OF COMPLEMENTARY HEALTH APPROACHES

The development of CHAs continues to be a market-driven and, in some respects, a patient-driven phenomenon. Many patients/consumers are unsatisfied with allopathic treatments and are turning to CHAs for relief of symptoms and healing. Since health care currently operates on a business model, it is probable that more CHAs will become available to deal with real or perceived market needs. Third-party payers do not cover many of these therapies, which means that consumers must pay out of pocket for them. In addition, government and professional groups do not regulate most of the therapies. Because of this lack of regulation, there can be inconsistencies among the preparation and care provided by practitioners.

Nursing is expanding its knowledge base to include information that addresses CHAs. For example, pharmacology courses in schools of nursing frequently include information on herbs. Certifications in basic holistic nursing for nurses with a baccalaureate degree and in advanced holistic nursing for nurses with a master's degree are available through the AHNCC. It is expected that CHAs will become a larger part of practice for nurses. See the accompanying PICOT in Practice on page 906. There is a great opportunity for nurses to expand their practice to meet existing patient needs as well as to promote health. See the Focused Assessment Guide 29-1: Holistic Care for identification of areas in which a holistic nurse can approach patient care.

Patient education about CHA is essential. Patients and the public need to know about the safe and effective use of CHA. Numerous resources exist to educate health care professionals and the public. The NCCIH health topics page is always a good place to start. The NCCIH encourages patients to talk with health care providers about their use of CHAs (NCCIH, 2020c). Box 29-3 (on page 906) outlines tips nurses can use with patients from the NCCIH

PICOT in Practice

ASKING CLINICAL QUESTIONS: ACUPUNCTURE/ACUPRESSURE

Scenario: You are a nurse working with a large maxillofacial surgery group who attended a conference on integrative nursing. One presenter that stood out discussed the benefits of acupuncture/acupressure in managing gag reflex in patients undergoing dental procedures. Gagging is a common problem encountered during dental treatment, making therapeutic procedures distressing and often difficult or even impossible to perform. One of the surgeons asks if you learned something new at the conference and you discuss the results of the presentation.

The office currently only uses sedatives to facilitate sedation in patient undergoing procedures. You wonder if acupuncture/acupressure compared to sedatives has any benefit in the care of patients specifically pediatric patients undergoing procedures.

- **Population:** Patients receiving sedation for dental procedure
- **Intervention:** Use of acupuncture/acupressure
- **Comparison:** Use of sedatives
- **Outcome:** Decreased gag reflex
- **Time:** During dental procedures

PICOT Question: Does the use of acupuncture/acupressure by a nonanesthesiologist compared to administration of sedatives result in depression of gag reflex in children and adults undergoing dental treatment and improved experience?

Findings:

1. Ashley, P. F., Chaudhary, M., & Lourenço-Matharu, L. (2018). Sedation of children undergoing dental treatment. *Cochrane Database of Systematic Reviews, 12*(12), CD003877. https://doi.org/10.1002/14651858.CD003877.pub5.

Included 50 studies with a total of 3,704 children up to age 16 years. Thirty-four different sedatives were used, often with inhalational nitrous oxide as well. Dosages, mode of administration and time of administration varied widely. Studies were grouped into placebo-controlled, dosage and head-to-head comparisons. Meta-analysis of the available data for the primary outcome (behavior) was possible for studies investigating oral midazolam versus placebo only. There was moderate-certainty evidence that oral midazolam is an effective sedative agent for children undergoing dental treatment. There is a need for further well-designed and well-reported clinical trials to evaluate other potential sedation agents.

2. Eachempati, P., Kumbargere Nagraj, S., Kiran Kumar Krishanappa, S., George, R. P., Soe, H. H. K., & Karanth, L. (2019). Management of gag reflex for patients undergoing dental treatment. *Cochrane Database of Systematic Reviews, 2019*(11), CD011116. https://doi.org/doi: 10.1002/14651858.CD011116.pub3

The interventions used to manage gagging include antinausea medicines, sedatives, local and general anesthetics, herbal remedies, behavior therapy, and cognitive behavior therapy, acupressure, acupuncture, laser, and prosthetic devices. This systematic review included four trials with 328 people (263 adults and 65 children who were age 4 years or older). Of the trials reviewed, one compared acupuncture and acupressure (with thumb, device, and sea band) at P6 (point located three-finger breadths below the wrist on the inner forearm in between the two tendons) to sham acupuncture and acupressure with and without sedation. One trial compared acupuncture at P6 point to sham acupuncture. P6 is an important acupuncture point in the Jueyin Pericardium Meridian of Hand. These trials reported both completion of dental procedure and reduction in gagging as their outcomes.

Strength of Evidence: Level I: systematic review

Recommendations: Conscious sedation or moderate sedation is the ability of the patient to independently maintain an open mouth and respond sensibly to verbal commands. In addition, the patient will retain adequate function of protective reflexes such as the gag reflex. There is a fine line between a sedated patient to an anaesthetized patient. The ideal sedative agent would reduce anxiety and improve behavior. Oral midazolam probably improves behavior of children during dental treatment. Acupuncture at P6 point (a point located in the inside of the wrist) when compared to acupressure to reduce gagging when undergoing dental procedures is appropriate. The same intervention with sedation did not show a difference. You discuss these findings with the maxillofacial surgery group and suggest offering integrative therapies for patients undergoing dental procedures.

Box 29-3 Tips for Talking With Health Care Providers

Patients can stay in better control and effectively manage their health when they share their use of complementary health practices. This information also ensures health care providers are better able to help patients make wise health care decisions (NCCIH, 2020e).

Encourage patients to:

- List the complementary health practices used to provide a full picture of what they do to manage their health when completing a patient history form.
- Tell their health care provider about any complementary health approaches used at every health care visit. Include over the counter and prescription medicines, and dietary and herbal supplements.
- Ask questions about any new complementary health practice they may be considering for use.
- Be proactive. Don't wait for their health care provider to ask about any complementary health practice they are using—start the conversation.

Source: Adapted from National Center for Complementary and Integrative Health (NCCIH). (2020, October 8). *4 tips: Start talking with your health care providers about complementary health approaches.* https://www.nccih.nih.gov/health/tips/tips-start-talking-with-your-health-care-providers-about-complementary-health-approaches to help patients begin a conversation with their health care provider. The National Cancer Institute's Office of Cancer Complementary and Alternative Medicine (OCCAM, 2013) provides a valuable teaching resource entitled *Talking about Complementary and Alternative Medicine with Health Care Providers: A Workbook and Tips.* This resource is available for patients and professionals on their website at https://cam.cancer.gov/health_information/talking_about_cam.htm.

REFLECTIVE PRACTICE LEADING TO PERSONAL LEARNING

Remember that the goal of reflective practice is to look at an experience, understand it, and learn from it. As you begin to develop expertise in implementing measures related to complementary and integrative health practices, reflect on your experiences—successes and failures—in order to improve your practice. How can you do it better next time? What did you learn today that can help you tomorrow? Begin your reflection by paying close attention to the following while performing interventions related to CHAs and integrative health care and providing nursing care:

- Were you aware of any cultural and/or ethnic beliefs or practices that may have influenced the health practices and beliefs of patients and/or family members/caregivers related to CHA/IH? Were you aware of any stereotypes or prejudices that might have negatively influenced the clinical encounter? If so, how did you address these?
- Was the patient/family/caregiver participation in the process at an optimal level? How might you have better engaged the patient and family/caregivers? Did the patient sense that you are respectful, caring, and competent to obtain accurate and relevant data?
- What knowledge from your learning, personal experience, and intuition did you use to make decisions and develop your plan of care?
- Did your preparation and practice related to performing interventions related to CHA/IH result in your feeling confident in your ability to provide care? Did your competence and confidence inspire the patient's and family's/caregiver's trust?
- As you concluded your care, did the patient/family/caregivers know your name and know what to expect of you and your nursing? Did the patient sense that you are respectful, caring, and competent to provide care?

Perhaps the most important questions to reflect on are: Are your patients and their families/caregivers better for having had *you* share in the critical responsibility of partnering with them to address their CHA/IH needs? Are your patients now receiving thoughtful, person-centered, prioritized, holistic, evidence-based treatment and care because of your efforts?

DEVELOPING CLINICAL REASONING AND CLINICAL JUDGMENT

1. You are caring for a culturally diverse population. How would you appropriately assess for and implement CHA into your nursing care, simultaneously demonstrating respect for your patients' beliefs and preferences while honoring your commitment to evidence-based nursing/medicine?
2. The family of a woman dying of cancer approaches you with a brown paper bag of ground herbs and asks you to mix them with the patient's next tube feeding. They are very upset that she isn't healing and believe the herbs might help. How do you respond and what is the basis for your response? Talk with other students about what they would do and compare your responses.
3. A nurse who practices TT tells you that she finds it very helpful for all sorts of patients. When you press her for details, you learn that she even practices this technique on patients without their consent while they are sleeping. Are you troubled by this? Is patient consent needed for CHA in the same way it is needed for allopathic treatments?
4. A patient brings you a newspaper article discussing some potential alternative therapies. Part of the article states: "Thanks to a $374,000 taxpayer-funded grant, we now know that inhaling lemon and lavender scents doesn't do a lot for our ability to heal a wound. With $666,000 in federal research money, scientists examined whether distant prayer could heal AIDS. It could not. The National Center for Complementary and Integrative Health also helped pay scientists to study whether squirting brewed coffee into someone's intestines can help treat pancreatic cancer (a $406,000 grant) and whether massage makes people with advanced cancer feel better ($1.25 million). The coffee enemas did not help. The massage did." He asks you how he can know "what works?" How do you reply?

PRACTICING FOR NCLEX

1. A patient recovering from a myocardial infarction tells the nurse: "My life feels out of control since I had the heart attack. I'd like to try yoga, but I don't think I'm strong enough to hold poses for long." What response by the nurse is most appropriate?
   a. "Concentrate on relaxing and taking your blood pressure medicine regularly; don't worry about doing yoga."
   b. "Yoga can lower stress. Seek a slow-paced, gentle class when you are cleared for activity."
   c. "Ashtanga yoga is a gently paced yoga that can help with breathing and blood pressure."
   d. "Yoga is contraindicated for patients who have had a heart attack."

2. A nurse is providing education on CHAs to a group of patients in a rehabilitation facility. Which statement is appropriate for the nurse to include?
   a. "CHAs are safe interventions used to supplement traditional care."
   b. "Many patients use CHAs as outpatients but do not wish to continue as inpatients."
   c. "Many nurses incorporate CHAs; could we try a relaxation exercise together?"
   d. "Most CHAs are newer, and effectiveness has not been established.
3. A nurse mentor is teaching a new nurse about the underlying beliefs of CHAs versus allopathic therapies. Which statements by the new nurse indicate that teaching was effective? Select all that apply.
   a. "CHA proponents believe the mind, body, and spirit are integrated and together influence health and illness."
   b. "CHA proponents believe that health is a balance of body systems: mental, social, and spiritual as well as physical."
   c. "Allopathy proponents believe that the main cause of illness is an imbalance or disharmony in the body systems."
   d. "Curing, according to CHA proponents, seeks to destroy the invading organism or repair the affected part."
   e. "Allopathic proponents place emphasis on disease, and drugs, surgery, and radiation are key tools for curing."
   f. "According to CHA proponents, health is the absence of disease."
4. A nurse plans to include integrative care for a patient who has many functional limitations related to painful rheumatoid arthritis. Which nursing intervention best represents the use of integrative care?
   a. The nurse administers naproxen and uses guided imagery to promote relaxation and promote pain relief.
   b. The nurse prepares the patient's health care provider–approved herbal tea and uses meditation to relax the patient prior to bed.
   c. The nurse administers naproxen and performs prescribed range-of-motion exercises.
   d. The nurse arranges for acupuncture for the patient and designs a menu high in omega-3 fatty acids.
5. A nurse works in a practice with naturopathic health care providers. What nursing actions would this nurse perform? Select all that apply.
   a. Treating the symptoms of the disease
   b. Providing patient education
   c. Focusing on treating individual body systems
   d. Suggesting interventions to prevent illness
   e. Incorporating the healing power of nature
   f. Encouraging patients' responsibility for their own health
6. A nurse cares for patients in a chiropractic office. What patient education would the nurse perform? Select all that apply.
   a. Proper application of heat or ice
   b. Explaining the purpose of electrical stimulation
   c. Teaching relaxation techniques
   d. Educating about a prescription medication
   e. Teaching before an invasive procedure
   f. Using safety with dietary supplements
7. A nurse colleague with severe arthritis of the hip tells you they would like to incorporate use of medical marijuana into their pain relief regimen. What is most appropriate to share with your colleague?
   a. Marijuana is a controlled substance.
   b. Even where marijuana is legal, employees testing positive for THC may be disciplined.
   c. This is an effective tool for many people for pain management.
   d. The regulation of marijuana for recreation use is different than for employment.
8. A nurse is guiding a group of patients in a meditation practice. Which teaching point is most appropriate to help the patients achieve a state of calmness, physical relaxation, and psychological balance?
   a. Always lie down in a comfortable position during meditation.
   b. Focus on multiple problems that they feel demands attention.
   c. Allow distractions to come and go naturally without judging them.
   d. Suppress distracting or wandering thoughts to maintain focus.
9. A nurse working in an inpatient hospice facility incorporates aromatherapy into their practice. For which patient problem will ginger be most helpful?
   a. Insomnia
   b. Nausea
   c. Dementia
   d. Pain
10. A nurse manager working in a hospital setting is researching the use of energy healing as an integrative care practice. Which patient would most likely benefit from this type of CHA?
    a. One who is anxious about residual pain from cervical spinal surgery
    b. One who is experiencing abdominal discomfort
    c. One who is experiencing chronic pain from diabetes
    d. One who has frequent cluster headaches
11. A nurse in the pain management clinic is explaining complementary health approaches to a patient with severe back pain who is interested in holistic health. What approaches could the nurse include in the discussion? Select all that apply.
    a. Acupressure or acupuncture
    b. Qi gong or tai chi
    c. Minimally invasive surgery
    d. Gentle yoga
    e. Aromatherapy

12. A patient with chronic pain tells the nurse they are very tired and sleeping fitfully. What actions promoting sleep hygiene will the nurse suggest?
    a. Sleep with a night light on.
    b. Play soft, pleasing music.
    c. Perform a relaxation exercise.
    d. Establish a regular sleep–wake schedule.
    e. Minimize noise.

ANSWERS WITH RATIONALES

1. **b**. Kripalu, or "gentle yoga," focuses on relaxation and coming into balance. Ashtanga focuses on synchronizing breath with a fast-paced series of postures. The nurse should not discourage the use of yoga in patients who are healthy enough to participate. Yoga is not contraindicated in patients with controlled high blood pressure. Post-MI patients should resume activity with guidance from the health care provider.
2. **c**. Many nurses are expanding their clinical practice by incorporating CHAs. Although many CHAs seem safe, some therapies have led to harmful or lethal outcomes. Patients should seek guidance from the provider. Many patients use these types of therapies as outpatients and choose to continue them as inpatients. Most complementary and alternative therapies predate modern medicine; it was not until recently that nursing and medical schools began to teach about their use.
3. **a, b, e**. With CHAs, mind, body, and spirit are integrated and together influence health and illness; illness is a manifestation of imbalance or disharmony. Allopathic beliefs include: The main causes of illness are considered to be pathogens (bacteria or viruses) or biochemical imbalances, curing seeks to destroy the invading organism or repair the affected part, and emphasis is on disease and high technology. Drugs, surgery, and radiation are among the key tools for dealing with medical problems. According to allopathic beliefs, health is the absence of disease.
4. **a.** Patient participation in guided imagery (a CHA) with the administration of pain medications (allopathy) is an example of integrative care. Integrative care uses some combination of allopathic medicine and CHAs.
5. **b, d, e, f.** Naturopathic medicine is a system of medicine and a way of life. Emphasis is on patient responsibility, patient education, health maintenance, and disease prevention. Its principles include minimizing harmful side effects and avoiding suppression of symptoms, educating patients and encouraging them to take responsibility for their own health, treating the whole person, preventing illness, believing in the healing power of nature, and treating the cause of a disease or condition rather than its symptoms.
6. **a, b, c, f.** Chiropractors may combine the use of spinal adjustments and other manual therapies with several approaches including heat and ice, electrical stimulation, relaxation techniques, rehabilitative and general exercise, counseling about weight and diet, and using dietary supplements. Chiropractors do not prescribe medication or perform invasive procedures.
7. **b.** THC is the psychoactive substance found in marijuana. Marijuana used for health problems or recreational use may be legal based on state law. However, for persons employed in safety-sensitive positions, such as nursing, the presence of THC or its constituents may pose a threat to health and safety. A positive test for THC may result in disciplinary action by an employer.
8. **c.** Meditators are encouraged to let distractions come and go naturally without judging them. Assuming a comfortable posture lying down, sitting, standing, or walking is appropriate, as is focusing attention on a mantra, object, or breathing. The individual should not suppress distracting or wandering thoughts; instead, they should gently bring attention back to focus.
9. **b.** Commonly used essential oils in a health care setting are ginger or peppermint for nausea and lavender or chamomile for insomnia.
10. **a.** Energy healing is focused on pain that lingers after an injury heals as well as pain complicated by trauma, anxiety, or depression. Nutritional and herbal remedies treat all chronic pain, but especially abdominal discomfort, headaches, and inflammatory conditions, such as rheumatoid arthritis.
11. **a, b, d, e.** Holistic nursing is based on the philosophy of holism, which incorporates the mind, body, and emotions. Further, the interrelationships of the bio-psycho-social-spiritual dimensions of the person are greater than and not separate from their parts. Conventional scientific models focus on treatment of health conditions, individual organs, or organ systems rather than the whole dynamic being as part of their environment. Surgical procedures do not address body, mind, and emotions.
12. **b, c, d, e, f.** Creating an optimal sleep environment for deep, restorative rest includes establishing a regular sleep–wake schedule and minimizing light and noise. Music can promote relaxation and increase sleep quality, as can relaxation exercises.

Bibliography

Agriculture Improvement Act of 2018, 132 Stat. 4490, Public Law 115-334-, 115th Congress. (2018, December 20). https://uscode.house.gov/statutes/pl/115/334.pdf

American Academy of Medical Acupuncture (AAMA). (n.d.). *The benefits of medical acupuncture. Acupuncture: An overview*. Retrieved October 3, 2020, from https://www.medicalacupuncture.org/For-Patients/Acupuncture-in-the-News

American Association of Colleges of Nursing (AACN). (2021). *The essentials: Core competencies for professional nursing education*. https://www.aacnnursing.org/AACN-Essentials

American Cancer Society. (2015, March 31). *Will my insurance cover alternative and complementary therapies?* https://www.cancer.org/treatment/treatments-and-side-effects/complementary-and-alternative-medicine/complementary-and-alternative-methods-and-cancer/insurance-coverage-for-cam.html

American Holistic Nurses Association (AHNA). (n.d.). *Welcome to AHNA!* Retrieved September 30, 2020, from https://www.ahna.org/

American Holistic Nurses Association (AHNA) & American Nurses Association (ANA). (2019). *Holistic nursing. Scope and standards of practice* (3rd ed.). https://www.ahna.org/Shop/Publications

American Holistic Nurses Credentialing Corporation (AHNCC). (2020). *Certification overview*. https://www.ahncc.org/certification/

Andres, C. (2019). Important legislative and regulatory changes impacting the commercialization of cannabis, hemp, and CBD. *Alternative Therapies in Health and Medicine, 25*(S2), 36–38.

Andrews, M., Boyle, J. S., & Collins, J. (2020). *Transcultural concepts in nursing care* (8th ed.). Wolters Kluwer.

Bagci, H., & Cinar Yucel, S. (2020). A systematic review of the studies about Therapeutic Touch after the year of 2000. *International Journal of Caring Sciences, 13*(1), 231–241.

Bauer, B. A. (2018, December 20). *What are the benefits of CBD—and is it safe to use?* Mayo Clinic. Mayo Foundation for Medical Education and Research (MFMER). https://www.mayoclinic.org/healthy-lifestyle/consumer-health/expert-answers/is-cbd-safe-and-effective/faq-20446700

Bemben, N. M. (2019, May 21). *CBD oil and medical marijuana: Pharmacists need to know the high points*. https://www.wolterskluwer.com/en/expert-insights/

cbd-oil-and-medical-marijuana-pharmacists-need-to-know-the-high-points
Benson, H. (1975). *The relaxation response.* William Morrow & Co.
Benson, D. (2019). Should CBD be part of my patients' treatment? *Alternative Therapiesin Health and Medicine, 25*(1). 8–11.
Black, L. I., Barnes, P. M., Clarke, T. C, Stussman, G. J., & Nahin, R. L. (2018). *Use of yoga, medication, and chiropractors among U.S. children aged 4–17 years. NCHS Data Brief, no. 324.* National Center for Health Statistics. https://www.nccih.nih.gov/research/research-results/national-survey-reveals-increased-use-of-yoga-and-meditation-among-us-children.
Black, L. I., Clarke, T. C., Barnes, P. M., Stussman, B. J., & Nahin, R. L. (2015). *Use of complementary health approaches among children aged 4–17 years in the United States: National Health Interview Survey, 2007–2012. National Health Statistics Reports. No. 78.* National Center for Health Statistics.
Bonn-Miller, M. O., Loflin, M. J. E., Thomas, B. F., Marcu, J. P., Hyke, T., & Vandrey, R. (2017). Labeling accuracy of cannabidiol extracts sold online. *JAMA, 318*(17), 1708–1709. https://doi.org/10.1001/jama.2017.11909
Brown, N. (2020). Implications of cannabidiol on your practice. *The Journal for Nurse Practitioners, 16*(5), 400–401. https://doi.org/10.1016/j.nurpra.2019.11.007
Cancer Research UK. (2018, December 5). *Traditional Chinese medicine.* https://www.cancerresearchuk.org/about-cancer/cancer-in-general/treatment/complementary-alternative-therapies/individual-therapies/traditional-chinese-medicine
Chan, A. W. K., Chair, S. Y., Lee, D. T. F., Leung, D. Y. P., Sit, J. W. H., Cheng, H. Y., & Taylor-Piliae, R. E. (2018). Tai Chi exercise is more effective than brisk walking in reducing cardiovascular disease risk factors among adults with hypertension: A randomised controlled trial. *International Journal of Nursing Studies, 88,* 44–52. https://doi.org/10.1016/j.ijnurstu.2018.08.009
Clare, A., Camic, P. M., Crutch, S. J., West, J., Harding, E., & Brotherhood, E. (2020). Using music to develop a multisensory communicative environment for people with late-stage dementia. *The Gerontologist, 60*(6), 1115–1125.
Clarke, T. C., Barnes, P. M., Black, L. I., Stussman, B. J., & Nahin, R. L. (2018). *Use of yoga, meditation, and chiropractors among U. S. adults aged 18 and over. NCHS Data Brief, no. 325.* National Center for Health Statistics.
Clarke, T. C., Black, L. I., Stussman, B. J., Barnes, P. M., & Nahin, R. L. (2015, February 10). Trends in the use of complementary health approaches among adults: United States, 2002–2012. National Health Statistics Reports. No. 79. National Center for Health Statistics. http://www.cdc.gov/nchs/data/nhsr/nhsr079.pdf
Corroon, J., & Phillips, J. A. (2018). A cross-sectional study of cannabidiol users. *Cannabis and Cannabinoid Research, 3*(1), 152–161. https://doi.org/10.1089/can.2018.0006
Cowen, V. S., & Cyr, V. (2015). Complementary and alternative medicine in U. S. medical schools. *Advances in Medical Education and Practice, 6,* 113–117. https://doi.org/10.2147/AMEP.S69761
Dilek, B., & Necmiye, C. (2020). Usage of aromatherapy in symptom management in cancer patients: A systematic review. *International Journal of Caring Sciences, 13*(1), 537–546.
Dill, J. L., & Kurkowski, A. (2020). CBD: Considerations for use within the health system. *Hospital Pharmacy, 55*(1), 9–11. https://doi.org/10.1177/0018578719873870
Doğan, M. D. (2020). The effect of laughter therapy on anxiety. A meta-analysis. *Holistic Nursing Practice, 34*(1), 35–39. https://doi.org/10.1097/HNP.0000000000000363
Eliopoulos, C. (2018a). *Invitation to holistic health* (4th ed.). Jones & Bartlett Learning.
Eliopoulos, C. (2018b). *Gerontological nursing* (9th ed.). Wolters Kluwer.
Epstein, E. C. (2020). Is CBD appropriate for pediatric disorders? *Journal of Clinical Chiropractic Pediatrics, 19*(1), 1619–1620.
Fontaine, K. L. (2019). *Complementary & alternative therapies for nursing practice* (5th ed.). Pearson.
Fugh-Berman, A., Wood, S., Kogan, M., Abrams, D., Mathre, M. L., Robie, A., Raveendran, J., Onumah, K., Mehta, R. S., White, S., & Kasimu-Graham, J. (n.d.). *Medical cannabis. Adverse effects & drug reactions.* Government of the District of Columbia. Department of Health. https://doh.dc.gov/sites/default/files/dc/sites/doh/publication/attachments/Medical%20Cannabis%20Adverse%20Effects%20and%20Drug%20Interactions_0.pdf
Georga, G., Chrousos, G., Artemiadis, A., Panagiotis, P. P., Bakakos, P., & Darviri, C. (2019). The effect of stress management incorporating progressive muscle relaxation and biofeedback-assisted relaxation breathing on patients with asthma: A randomised controlled trial. *Advances in Integrative Medicine, 6*(2), 73–77. https://doi.org/10.1016/j.aimed.2018.09.001
Gottlieb, S. (2018, December 20). *FDA statement. Statement from FDA Commissioner Scott Gottlieb, M.D., on signing of the Agriculture Improvement Act and the agency's regulation of products containing cannabis and cannabis-derived compounds.* U.S. FDA. https://www.fda.gov/news-events/press-announcements/statement-fda-commissioner-scott-gottlieb-md-signing-agriculture-improvement-act-and-agencys
Hande, K. (2017). Pain management: Strategies for screening and monitoring patients receiving chronic opioid therapy. *Clinical Journal of Oncology Nursing, 21*(6), 669–672. https://doi.org/10.1188/17.CJON.669-672
Hausladen Foley, M. K., Anderson, J., Mallea, L., Morrison, K., & Downey, M. (2016). Effects of healing touch on postsurgical adult outpatients. *Journal of Holistic Nursing, 34*(3), 271–279. https://doi.org/10.1177/0898010115609486
Healing Beyond Borders. (n.d.). *What is healing touch?* Retrieved October 3, 2020, from https://www.healingbeyondborders.org/index.php/about/what-is-healing-touch
Healthwise. (2015, February 18). *Health library. Comfrey. Michigan Medicine.* University of Michigan. https://www.uofmhealth.org/health-library/d04502a1
Helming, M. A. B., Shields, D. A., Avino, K. M., & Rosa, W. E. (Eds.). (2022). *Dossey & Keegan's Holistic nursing. A handbook for practice* (8th ed.). Jones & Bartlett Learning.
Johns Hopkins Medicine. (n.d.). *Health. Aromatherapy: Do essential oils really work?* Retrieved March 26, 2022, https://www.hopkinsmedicine.org/health/wellness-and-prevention/aromatherapy-do-essential-oils-really-work#:~:text=When%20inhaled%2C%20the%20scent%20molecules,be%20absorbed%20by%20the%20skin.
Johnson, P., & Haag, C. (2019). The yoga mat, where East meets West: A pilot and feasibility study evaluating a structured yoga practice on common side effects of chemotherapy/biotherapy in cancer patients. *Journal of Oncology Navigation & Survivorship, 10*(9), 340–348.
Jou, J., & Johnson, P. J. (2016). Nondisclosure of complementary and alternative medicine use to primary care physicians: Findings from the 2012 National Health Interview Survey. *JAMA Internal Medicine, 176*(4), 545–546. https://doi.org/10.1001/jamainternmed.2015.8593
Kavurmaci, M., Dayapoğlu, N., & Tan, M. (2020). Effect of music therapy on sleep quality. *Alternative Therapies in Health & Medicine, 26*(4), 22–26.
Kiley, K. A., Sehgal, A. R., Neth, S., Dolata, J., Pike, E., Spilsbury, J. C., & Albert, J. M. (2018). The effectiveness of guided imagery in treating compassion fatigue and anxiety of mental health workers. *Social Work Research, 42*(1), 33–43. https://doi.org/10.1093/swr/svx026
Koppelman, M. H. (n.d.). *Acupuncture: An overview of scientific evidence.* Evidence Based Acupuncture. Retrieved October 3, 2020, from https://www.evidencebasedacupuncture.org/acupuncture-scientific-evidence/
Krieger, D. (1993). *Accepting your power to heal.* Bear & Company.
Labus, N., Wilson, C., & Arena, S. (2019). Mind-body therapies as a therapeutic intervention for pain management. *Home Healthcare Now, 37*(5), 293–294. https://doi.org/10.1097/NHH.0000000000000809
Lack, S., Brown, R., & Kinser, P. A. (2020). An integrative review of yoga and mindfulness-based approaches for children and adolescents with asthma. *Journal of Pediatric Nursing, 52,* 76–81. https://doi.org/10.1016/j.pedn.2020.03.006
Langer Bro, M., Johansen, C., Vuust, P., Enggaard, L., Himmelstrup, B., Mourits-Anderson, T., Brown, P., d'Amore, F., Wreford Anderson, E. A., Abildgaard, N., & Gram, J. (2019). Effects of live music during chemotherapy in lymphoma patients: A randomized, controlled, multi-center trial. *Supportive Care in Cancer, 27*(10), 3887–3896. https://doi.org/10.1007/s00520-019-04666-8
Lindquist, R., Tracy, M. F., & Snyder, M. (Eds.). (2018). *Complementary and alternative therapies in nursing* (8th ed.). Springer Publishing Company.
Long, T. (2020, August). CBD: Weeding through the controversy. *Nevada RNformation, 29*(3), 12–14. https://d3ms3kxrsap50t.cloudfront.net/uploads/publication/pdf/2090/Nevada_RN_8_20.pdf
Mayo Clinic News Network. (2019, October 17). *Home remedies: Anxiety and herbal remedies.* https://newsnetwork.mayoclinic.org/discussion/home-remedies-anxiety-and-herbal-remedies/
Mayo Foundation for Medical Education and Research (MFMER). (2017a, November 8). *Nutrition and healthy eating.* https://www.mayoclinic.org/healthy-lifestyle/nutrition-and-healthy-eating/in-depth/herbal-supplements/art-20046714#:~:text=Herbal%20supplements%20are%20regulated%20by,a%20category%20called%20dietary%20supplements
Mayo Foundation for Medical Education and Research (MFMER). (2017b, October 12). *Ginkgo.* https://www.mayoclinic.org/drugs-supplements-ginkgo/art-20362032
Meletis, C. (2020). CBD for pain: Is cannabidiol a natural alternative to opioid drugs? *Alternative Therapies in Health and Medicine, 26*(S1), 6–7.
Moraes, L. J., Miranda, M. B., Loures, L. F., Mainieri, A. G., & Mármora, C. H. C. (2018). A systematic review of psychoneuroimmunology-based interventions. *Psychology, Health & Medicine, 23*(6), 635–652. https://doi.org/10.1080/13548506.2017.1417607
National Academies of Sciences, Engineering, and Medicine. (2017). *The health effects of cannabis and cannabinoids: The current state of evidence and recommendations for research.* The National Academies Press. https://doi.org/10.17226/24625.
National Association for Holistic Aromatherapy (NAHA). (n.d.a). *About aromatherapy.* Retrieved March 26, 2022, https://naha.org/explore-aromatherapy/about-aromatherapy/
National Association for Holistic Aromatherapy (NAHA). (n.d.b). *Approved standards for professional aromatherapy education.* Retrieved October 3, 2020, from https://naha.org/education/standards/
National Association of Nutrition Professionals (NANP). (n.d.). *What is holistic nutrition?* Retrieved March 26, 2022, https://www.nanp.org/what-is-holistic-nutrition-
National Cancer Institute (NCI). (n.d.a). *NCI dictionaries. Allopathic medicine.* Retrieved September 29, 2020, from https://www.cancer.gov/publications/dictionaries/cancer-terms/def/allopathic-medicine
National Cancer Institute (NCI). (n.d.b). *German Commission E.* Retrieved November 6, 2021, from https://www.cancer.gov/publications/dictionaries/cancer-terms/def/german-commission-e
National Cancer Institute (NCI). Office of Cancer Complementary and Alternative Medicine. (2013, April 12). *Talking about complementary and alternative medicine with health care providers: A workbook and tips.* https://cam.cancer.gov/health_information/talking_about_cam.htm
National Center for Complementary and Integrative Health (NCCIH). (2016a). *Meditation: In depth.* https://www.nccih.nih.gov/health/meditation-in-depth
National Center for Complementary and Integrative Health (NCCIH). (2016b). *Tai chi and qi gong: In depth.* https://www.nccih.nih.gov/health/tai-chi-and-qi-gong-in-depth
National Center for Complementary and Integrative Health (NCCIH). (2016c, January). *Acupuncture: In depth.* https://www.nccih.nih.gov/health/acupuncture-in-depth

National Center for Complementary and Integrative Health (NCCIH). (2016d, May 17). *Tai chi and physical therapy were equally helpful for knee osteoarthritis.* https://www.nccih.nih.gov/research/research-results/study-shows-tai-chi-and-physical-therapy-were-equally-helpful-for-knee-osteoarthritis

National Center for Complementary and Integrative Health (NCCIH). (2016e, June 22). *Americans spend $30 billion a year out-of-pocket on complementary health approaches.* https://www.nccih.nih.gov/research/research-results/americans-spend-30-billion-a-year-outofpocket-on-complementary-health-approaches

National Center for Complementary and Integrative Health (NCCIH). (2017). *Naturopathy.* https://www.nccih.nih.gov/health/naturopathy

National Center for Complementary and Integrative Health (NCCIH). (2018, July). *Homeopathy.* https://www.nccih.nih.gov/health/homeopathy

National Center for Complementary and Integrative Health (NCCIH). (2019a, May). *Health information. Yoga: What you need to know.* https://www.nccih.nih.gov/health/yoga-what-you-need-to-know

National Center for Complementary and Integrative Health (NCCIH). (2019b, April). *Traditional Chinese medicine: What you need to know.* https://www.nccih.nih.gov/health/traditional-chinese-medicine-what-you-need-to-know

National Center for Complementary and Integrative Health (NCCIH). (2019c, April). *Chiropractic: In depth.* https://www.nccih.nih.gov/health/chiropractic-in-depth

National Center for Complementary and Integrative Health (NCCIH). (2019d, April). *Traditional Chinese medicine: What you need to know.* https://www.nccih.nih.gov/health/traditional-chinese-medicine-what-you-need-to-know

National Center for Complementary and Integrative Health (NCCIH). (2019e, January). *Ayurvedic medicine: In depth.* https://www.nccih.nih.gov/health/ayurvedic-medicine-in-depth

National Center for Complementary and Integrative Health (NCCIH). (2019f, May). *Yoga: What you need to know.* https://www.nccih.nih.gov/health/yoga-what-you-need-to-know

National Center for Complementary and Integrative Health (NCCIH). (2019g, January). *Using dietary supplements wisely.* https://www.nccih.nih.gov/health/using-dietary-supplements-wisely#hed6

National Center for Complementary and Integrative Health (NCCIH). (2019h, November). *Cannabis (marijuana) and cannabinoids: What you need to know.* https://www.nccih.nih.gov/health/cannabis-marijuana-and-cannabinoids-what-you-need-to-know

National Center for Complementary and Integrative Health (NCCIH). (2020a, September 29). *Health information. Complementary, alternative or integrative health: What's in a name?* https://nccih.nih.gov/health/integrative-health#cvsa

National Center for Complementary and Integrative Health (NCCIH). (2020b, January). *Health information. Stress.* https://www.nccih.nih.gov/health/stress

National Center for Complementary and Integrative Health (NCCIH). (2020c, February). *Be an informed consumer.* https://www.nccih.nih.gov/health/be-an-informed-consumer

National Center for Complementary and Integrative Health (NCCIH). (2020d, January). *Aromatherapy.* https://www.nccih.nih.gov/health/aromatherapy

National Center for Complementary and Integrative Health (NCCIH). (2020e, October 8). *4 tips: Start talking with your health care providers about complementary health approaches.* https://www.nccih.nih.gov/health/tips/tips-start-talking-with-your-health-care-providers-about-complementary-health-approaches

National Center for Complementary and Integrative Health (NCCIH). (2020f, October 8). *Health information.* https://www.nccih.nih.gov/

National Center for Complementary and Integrative Health (NCCIH). (2020g, October 8). *Terms related to complementary and integrative health.* https://www.nccih.nih.gov/health/providers/terms-related-to-complementary-and-integrative-health

National Center for Complementary and Integrative Health (NCCIH). (2021, June). *Relaxation techniques: What you need to know.* https://www.nccih.nih.gov/health/relaxation-techniques-what-you-need-to-know

National Council of State Boards of Nursing (NCSBN). (2018). The NCSBN National Nursing Guidelines for medical marijuana. *Journal of Nursing Regulation, 9*(2), S1–S60. https://ncsbn.org/The_NCSBN_National_Nursing_Guidelines_for_Medical_Marijuana_JNR_July_2018.pdf

Office of Dietary Supplements (ODS). National Institutes of Health. (n.d.a). *Strengthening knowledge and understanding of dietary supplements.* Retrieved November 6, 2021, from https://ods.od.nih.gov/

Office of Dietary Supplements (ODS). National Institutes of Health. (n.d.b). *Dietary supplement fact sheets.* Retrieved November 6, 2021, from https://ods.od.nih.gov/factsheets/list-all/

Office of Dietary Supplements (ODS). National Institutes of Health. (2020, September 3). *What you need to know. Dietary supplements.* https://ods.od.nih.gov/factsheets/WYNTK-Consumer/

Pearson, N., Prosko, S., Sullivan, M., & Taylor, M. J. (2020). *Yoga therapy and pain. How yoga therapy serves in comprehensive integrative pain management, and how it can do more. An IAYT white paper.* International Association of Yoga Therapists. https://cdn.ymaws.com/www.iayt.org/resource/resmgr/docs_whitepapers/iayt_pain_white_paper.pdf

ProCon. (2020a, April 14). *States with legal cannabidiol (CBD).* ProCon.org. https://medicalmarijuana.procon.org/states-with-legal-cannabidiol-cbd/

ProCon. (2020b, March 24). *Legal medical marijuana states and DC. Laws, fees, and possession limits.* ProCon.org. https://medicalmarijuana.procon.org/legal-medical-marijuana-states-and-dc/

Quinn, C. (2019). Guided imagery: An effective pain management tool for total joint replacement? *Nursing, 49*(10), 57–59. https://doi.org/10.1097/01.NURSE.0000580712.40392.cc

Rastipisheh, P., Choobineh, A., Razeghi, M., Kazemi, R., Ghaem, H., Taheri, S., & Maghsoudi, A. (2019). The effects of playing music during surgery on the performance of the surgical team: A systematic review. *Work, 64*(2), 407–412. https://doi.org/10.3233/WOR-192984

Selye, H. (1976). *The stress of life* (revised ed.). McGraw-Hill.

Sivaramakrishnan, D., Fitzsimons, C., Kelly, P., Ludwig, K., Mutrie, N., Saunders, D. H., & Baker, G. (2019). The effects of yoga compared to active and inactive controls on physical function and health related quality of life in older adults – Systematic review and meta-analysis of randomised controlled trials. *International Journal of Behavioral Nutrition and Physical Activity, 16*(1), 33. https://doi.org/10.1186/s12966-019-0789-2

Society for Shamanic Practice. (n.d.). *What is shamanism?* Retrieved October 7, 2020, from https://shamanicpractice.org/about/what-is-shamanism/

Stutley, M. (2003). *Shamanism. An introduction.* Taylor & Francis Group.

Theisen, E., & Konieczny, E. (2019). Medical cannabis: What nurses need to know. *American Nurse Today, 14*(11).

Therapeutic Touch International Association (TTIA). (n.d.). *Therapeutic Touch International Association.* Retrieved March 26, 2022, https://therapeutictouch.org/

Therapeutic Touch International Association (TTIA). (2003). *Position on credentialing.* https://therapeutictouch.org/policies/position-on-credentialing/#:~:text=Credentialing%20is%20an%20essential%20mechanism,practice%2C%20education%2C%20and%20research

Thibaut, F. (2018). The mind-body Cartesian dualism and psychiatry. *Dialogues in Clinical Neuroscience, 20*(1), 3.

Thornton, L. (2019). A brief history and overview of holistic nursing. *Integrative Medicine, 18*(4), 32–33.

Trentham, M. A. (2019a). CBD oil and your nursing license. *ABSN Update, 23*(5), 12–14.

Trentham, M. A. (2019b). Natural products- Are they safe for my license? *ABSN Update, 23*(2), 21–23.

U.S. Department of Health and Human Services and U.S. Department of Agriculture. (2020). *Dietary guidelines for Americans 2020–2025.* https://www.dietaryguidelines.gov/sites/default/files/2020-12/Dietary_Guidelines_for_Americans_2020-2025.pdf

U.S. Drug Enforcement Administration (DEA). (2018, September 28). *Schedules of controlled substances: Placement in Schedule V of certain FDA-approved drugs containing cannabidiol; Corresponding change to permit requirements.* https://www.federalregister.gov/documents/2018/09/28/2018-21121/schedules-of-controlled-substances-placement-in-schedule-v-of-certain-fda-approved-drugs-containing

U.S. Food and Drug Administration (FDA). (n.d.). *5 things to consider before taking a dietary supplement.* https://www.fda.gov/media/106435/download.

U.S. Food and Drug Administration (FDA). (2013, March 4). *6 tip-offs to rip-offs: Don't fall for health fraud scams.* https://www.fda.gov/consumers/consumer-updates/6-tip-offs-rip-offs-dont-fall-health-fraud-scams

U.S. Food and Drug Administration (FDA). (2018a, February 23). *Tips for dietary supplement users.* https://www.fda.gov/food/information-consumers-using-dietary-supplements/tips-dietary-supplement-users

U.S. Food and Drug Administration (FDA). (2018b, June 25). *FDA approves first drug comprised of an active ingredient derived from marijuana to treat rare, severe forms of epilepsy.* https://www.fda.gov/news-events/press-announcements/fda-approves-first-drug-comprised-active-ingredient-derived-marijuana-treat-rare-severe-forms

U.S. Food and Drug Administration (FDA). (2019, August 16). *Dietary supplements.* https://www.fda.gov/food/dietary-supplements

U.S. Food and Drug Administration (FDA). (2020, July 23). *Subscribe to podcasts and news feeds.* https://www.fda.gov/about-fda/contact-fda/subscribe-podcasts-and-news-feeds

Vadala, J. (2019, March 27). *Cross-culturally exploring the concept of shamanism.* Human Relations Area Files. https://hraf.yale.edu/cross-culturally-exploring-the-concept-of-shamanism/

World Health Organization (WHO). (n.d.). *About WHO. Who we are. Constitution.* Retrieved September 30, 2020, from https://www.who.int/about/who-we-are/constitution#:~:text=Health%20is%20a%20state%20of,belief%2C%20economic%20or%20social%20condition

Yoga Alliance. (n.d.). *Learn about yoga. Types of yoga.* https://www.yogaalliance.org/LearnAboutYoga/AboutYoga/Typesofyoga

30 Medications

Regina Sauder

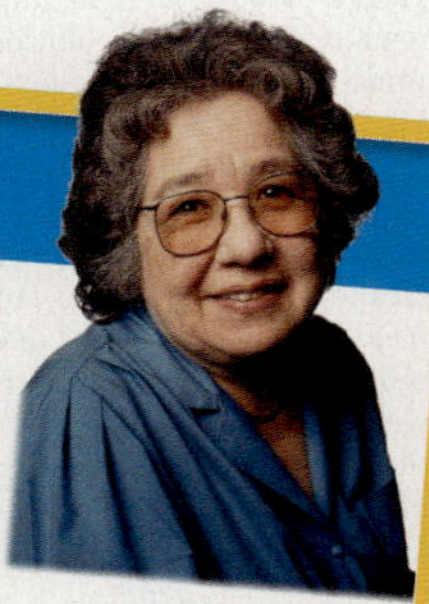

Regina, a 73-year-old woman with a history of lymphoma, has presented to the emergency department with pain, swelling, and erythema (redness) of her left calf. She has been diagnosed with a left leg deep vein thrombosis (DVT). She is receiving intravenous heparin and oral warfarin. When she is discharged, she will need to have weekly blood testing to ensure therapeutic levels of the warfarin.

Mildred Campbell

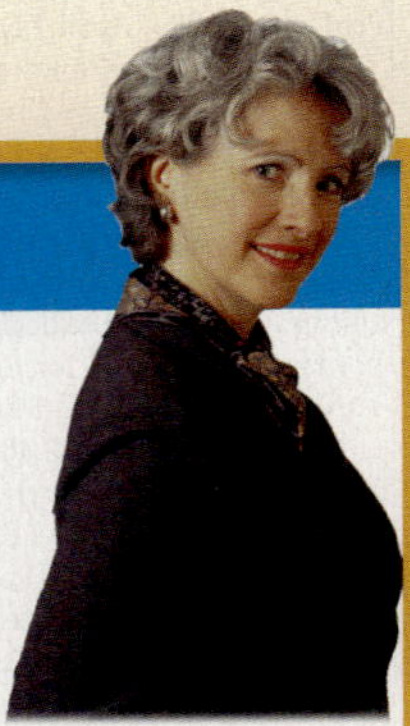

Mildred, a 65-year-old woman with a history of arthritis and hypertension (high blood pressure), comes to the clinic for evaluation of her painful joints. She states, "I just saw this new medicine advertised on television that is supposed to be really helpful in relieving joint pain. What do you think? Is it something I should try?"

François Baptiste

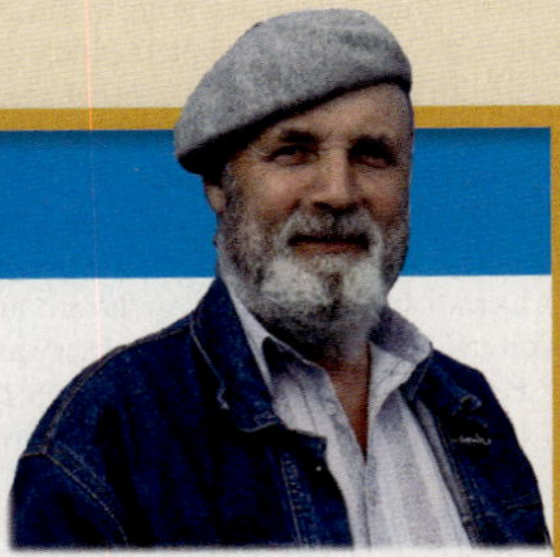

François is an older adult with a wound infection requiring intravenous antibiotic therapy. He is scheduled to receive his next dose at 1000. The medication delivered by the pharmacy is labeled with the correct drug and dose, but with a different patient's name.

Lippincott DocuCare **Additional patient scenarios available in *Lippincott DocuCare.***

Learning Outcomes

After completing the chapter, you will be able to accomplish the following:

1. Discuss drug legislation in the United States.
2. Describe basic principles of pharmacology, including drug nomenclature and types of drug preparations.
3. Develop an understanding of basic principles of pharmacology, including mechanisms of drug action, adverse drug reactions, and factors affecting drug action.
4. Discuss principles of medication administration, including an understanding of medication orders, dosage calculations, and medication safety measures.
5. Obtain patient information necessary to establish a medication history.
6. Describe principles used to prepare and administer medications safely by the oral, parenteral, topical, and inhalation routes.
7. Use a systematic process for medication administration such as the Nursing Process to safely administer medications.
8. Develop teaching plans to meet patient needs specific to medication administration.

Key Concepts

- Addiction
- Pharmacology
- Clinical Decision Making/Clinical Judgment
- Safety

A drug or medication is any substance that modifies body functions when taken into the body. The study of drugs and their effect on the body's functioning is called **pharmacology**. A pharmacist is a person licensed to prepare and dispense drugs. Physicians, dentists, psychiatrists, podiatrists, physician assistants, and advanced practice nurses have prescriptive authority. Prescriptive authority for advanced practice nurses (clinical nurse specialists, nurse practitioners, certified nurse anesthetists, nurse midwives) and physician assistants varies in the degree of independence and the medications that may be prescribed from state to state. Nurses must be familiar with the laws relative to prescriptive authority in their state of practice. The prescriber conveys medication plans to others by an order called a *prescription*. In a hospital or other health care facility, after the pharmacist prepares the medication, the nurse administers the medication to the patient. This chain provides a system of checks-and-balances for medication administration. If an error is made when the order is written, the pharmacist or nurse administering the medication has the opportunity to note the discrepancy. If an error occurs when the pharmacy dispenses the medication, the administering nurse has the opportunity to note this discrepancy. See the accompanying Reflective Practice box (on pages 914–915) for an example.

Medication administration is a core nursing function that involves skillful technique and consideration of safety principles that consider the patient's developmental state, individual characteristics, and health status. The nurse administering medications needs to have knowledge of drugs, including drug names, preparations, classifications, adverse effects, and physiologic factors that affect drug action. Information about specific drugs is available in pharmacology texts and drug reference books. Computer programs and electronic databases are available for up-to-date medication information. Nurses must have sufficient knowledge about the drugs being administered to safely care for their patients. The Joint Commission has made several recommendations regarding safe practice when administering medications. Up-to-date information about these recommendations can be found at https://www.jointcommission.org/standards/national-patient-safety-goals/.

The nursing process can be applied to medication administration. Assessment includes a comprehensive medication history, awareness of the patient's allergies, and patient assessment, as well as ongoing assessments of the patient's response during and after medication administration. Diagnoses are developed and problem identification stems from the assessment data. Patient-centered outcomes are evaluated after implementation of the plan of care and are tailored to the patient's needs.

PRINCIPLES OF PHARMACOLOGY

An overview of basic pharmacology includes drug nomenclature, types of drug preparations, drug classification, drug indication, mechanisms of drug action, adverse drug reactions, side effects, and factors affecting drug action, as well as drug blood level monitoring and pertinent U.S. drug legislation.

Drug Nomenclature

Drugs have several names, and are most commonly referred to by their generic and trade names. The **generic name**, which identifies the drug's active ingredient, is the name assigned by the manufacturer that first develops the drug. Often, the generic name is derived from the chemical name, which is a precise description of the drug's chemical composition that identifies the drug's atomic and molecular structure using exact chemical language and terminology. The generic name is not owned by any drug company and is universally accepted. The official name (also known as a *monograph*) is the name by which the drug is identified in publications such as the United States Pharmacopeia (USP) and National Formulary (NF; USP-NF, 2020). The official name is typically the generic name. The **trade name**, also referred to as the *brand name*, is selected by the pharmaceutical company that sells the drug and is protected by trademark. A drug can have several trade names when produced by different manufacturers.

QSEN Reflective Practice: Cultivating QSEN Competencies

CHALLENGE TO ETHICAL AND LEGAL SKILLS

During my clinical rotation for complex care a few weeks ago, I met François Baptiste, an older adult with a wound infection requiring intravenous antibiotic therapy. He was due for a certain IV antibiotic to be hung at 1000. When I checked his drawer at 0800 and 0900, the antibiotic was not there. However, the nurse I was working with told me not to call pharmacy about it yet since the pharmacy staff often comes and replaces the drawers in the medication carts before 1000 anyway. Sure enough, a pharmacy representative came up that hour and changed the medication drawers. At 1000, I went to look in my patient's drawer. What I found confused me a great deal! Yes, the bag of medication was in there. Yes, it was the right drug and the right dose. However, it was the wrong patient! The label on the bag in my patient's drawer had another patient's name on it. I looked up information on that other patient, and it turned out he was also a patient on the unit. This patient was also receiving the same drug, at the same dose, but at a different time. I wondered if I should hang this bag for my patient because he was due for it, even though it had someone else's name and medical record number on the label. It was, after all, the same drug and the same dose.

Thinking Outside the Box: Possible Courses of Action

- Change the patient's name on the label and hang the bag.
- Call pharmacy to ask about the mix-up. If the bag really did contain the same medication at the same dose, then change the patient's name on the label and hang it for my patient.
- Check the other patient's medication administration record (MAR) to confirm that he is, indeed, receiving the same drug at the same dose as my patient, and if so, use this bag for my patient (since it is in my patient's drawer and my patient is due for it).
- Ask my nurse and/or preceptor what to do. Is it okay, safe, and legal to use this bag if someone else's name is on the label? If they say yes, check with the nurse caring for the patient whose name is on the label to make sure they don't not need the medication right now.
- Send the bag back to pharmacy, requesting they send up a new one with an accurate label.
- Call pharmacy, ask them to send up a new bag with an accurate label, and tell them I am giving the other bag to the other patient's nurse.

Evaluating a Good Outcome: How Do I Define Success?

- The right patient receives the right drug, at the right dose, at the right time, via the right route, with the right documentation, understanding the right rationale.
- The patient feels comfortable and safe with the drug being administered to him.
- The needs of my patient and those of the patient whose name was on the bag are assessed and met. Both patients have the medication available to them when they are due to receive it.
- My education and my license are not put at risk by an avoidable medication error.
- My legal skills are sharpened by thinking and working through the situation.

Personal Learning: Here's to the Future!

Ultimately, I addressed the situation step-by-step to make sure all the bases were covered. First, I checked the other patient's drawer to see if he had a bag of this IV antibiotic. He did not, which led me to believe that either his bag was placed in my drawer by accident, or his bag had not been made yet. Then I checked my patient's MAR and that of the other patient. Indeed, both were scheduled to receive the same drug, at the same dose, via the same route. However, my patient was due for it at 1000, the other patient was due for it at 1400. Next, I brought the medication bag, the MARs, and my other paperwork to my clinical instructor and to the nurses caring for my patient and the other patient. They all agreed that the bag that was in my drawer was the right drug at the right dose, even though it had the wrong name on the label. However, it is not the nurse's responsibility or legal right to dispense medication. For this reason, the bag of medication needed to be returned to the pharmacy because it was labeled with the wrong name. The pharmacist must relabel the medication, thus preparing and dispensing a correctly labeled dose for each patient. I called the pharmacy, explained what I had found, and told them I would be returning the dose that had been delivered to my patient. I requested a correct dose for 1000 for my patient. The pharmacy delivered a new bag of medication, correctly labeled, in time for the patient's 1000 dose. After checking everything again, I administered the medication to my patient. My patient did not have an adverse reaction, the other patient got his medication when it was due, and no mistakes were made by any of the nurses. The only mistake that was made was by pharmacy—they put the wrong label on the bag and then put the bag in the drawer.

I learned that checking and double-checking medication labels is extremely important. After a while, we all have a tendency to get into the habit of glancing at things when we are in a hurry, especially when it involves labels we look at all the time, feeling confident that we would recognize a problem. This is not the first time I could have missed a change on the label—there have been several times when I did not think to check every single thing on a label. That's because after giving it so many times, I felt it had become routine. But every time I am tempted not to double-check a label, I am reminded of this situation. As a result, I triple-check things because those are the times when I may not be paying as close attention as I need to be. Because I do not have my license yet, I am still learning all the laws and regulations surrounding medication administration. However, as a student nurse, I am careful to avoid any mistakes that could place me in jeopardy legally for areas of which I *am* aware. In addition, I am always careful to

QSEN Reflective Practice: Cultivating QSEN Competencies *(continued)*

CHALLENGE TO ETHICAL AND LEGAL SKILLS

protect my education and my future as a nurse by not doing things about which I am uncertain. I always ask my preceptor or my nurse for help or advice when I need it. While my legal skills probably need some work, they are certainly not terrible, and my skills and I are moving in the right direction.

Tracey Sara Miller, Georgetown University

QSEN SELF-REFLECTION ON QUALITY AND SAFETY COMPETENCIES
DEVELOPING KNOWLEDGE, SKILLS, AND ATTITUDES FOR CONTINUOUS IMPROVEMENT

How do you think you would respond in a similar situation? Why? What does this tell you about yourself and about the adequacy of your skills for professional practice? Do you agree with the criteria to evaluate a successful outcome? Did the nursing student validate the rationale for the outcome? What *knowledge, skills, and attitudes* do you need to develop to continuously improve the quality and safety of care for patients like Mr. Baptiste?

Patient-Centered Care: Would it have been appropriate for the nursing student to change the name on the label? Why or why not? How did the nursing student's actions adhere to ethical and legal principles? Did the nursing student act as an advocate for Mr. Baptiste?

Teamwork and Collaboration/Quality Improvement: What communication skills do you need to improve to ensure that you communicate appropriately in situations like this? What communication skills do you need to improve to ensure that you could address this issue as a member of the patient-care team? How can you ensure that this event is used to prevent similar issues in the future to improve the quality of care?

Safety/Evidence-Based Practice: How can you communicate observations or concerns related to hazards and errors to patients, families, and the health care team? What is your role in preventing errors? What legal principles did the nursing student adhere to with the described actions? Suppose the nursing student had given the medication without double-checking all of the information. What legal principles might have been violated? What evidence in nursing literature provides guidance for decision making regarding care of this patient? What does this tell you about yourself and about the adequacy of your skills for professional practice?

Informatics: Can you identify the essential information that must be available in Mr. Baptiste's electronic health record (EHR) to support safe patient care and coordination of care? What information should be documented in the EHR regarding the student's assessment and interventions? Can you think of other ways to respond to or approach the situation?

Nurses should be familiar with both generic and trade names. For example, acetaminophen (generic name) has trade names such as Tylenol, Tempra, and Liquiprin. The generic name is universal and is not likely to change; however, the trade name will change depending on the specific company and manufacturer. Health care entities vary in their use of generic-only or both the generic and trade names. Electronic medication administration records (eMARs) typically default to the generic names, but may include both the generic and trade names. In conversations with interprofessional/intraprofessional teams and with patients, the trade name is often used because it is frequently easier than the generic name to articulate or spell. In drug literature and in clinical practice, trade names are capitalized and generic names are presented in lowercase unless they are in a list or used at the beginning of a sentence (Frandsen & Pennington, 2021; Karch, 2020). Developing a working knowledge of the generic and trade names of drugs is an important part of the nurse's responsibilities when transcribing orders and administering medication therapies.

Types of Drug Preparations

Drugs are available in many forms, or preparations. The form in which the drug is prepared may determine the route of administration. Drug preparations are available for enteral (oral), topical, and parenteral (injection, infusion, implantation) administration. Some drugs may be prepared in only one form to be administered by a certain route. Others may be supplied in several preparations, allowing them to be given through various routes. One type of preparation may be desirable in a given situation. For example, a liquid preparation of a medication would be indicated for a young child who cannot swallow solid preparations, such as tablets. A suppository may be indicated to deliver a medication for a patient who cannot take anything by mouth. Table 30-1 (on page 916) describes drug preparations commonly used by nurses.

Drug Classifications

Drug classifications, or drug classes, refer to groups of drugs that share similar characteristics. Drugs are classified in two primary ways: pharmaceutical class and therapeutic class. The pharmaceutical class refers to the mechanism of action (MOA), physiologic effect (PE), and chemical structure (CS) of the drug (U.S. Food and Drug Administration [FDA], 2018a). The therapeutic class refers to the clinical indication for the drug or therapeutic action (e.g., analgesic, antibiotic, or antihypertensive). General knowledge related to the class of drug can assist with understanding specific drugs in that same class.

Drug Indications

Pharmacotherapeutics is a subtopic of pharmacology that considers the "therapeutic uses and effects of drugs"

Table 30-1 Common Types of Drug Preparations

PREPARATION	DESCRIPTION
Capsule	Powder or gel form of an active drug enclosed in a gelatinous container; may also be called liquigel
Elixir	Medication in a clear liquid containing water, alcohol, sweeteners, and flavor
Enteric coated	A tablet or pill coated to prevent stomach irritation
Extended release (ER)	Preparation of a medication that allows for slow and continuous release over a predetermined period; may also be referred to as CR or CRT (controlled release), SR (sustained or slow release), SA (sustained action), LA (long acting), or TR (timed release)
Liniment	Medication mixed with alcohol, oil, or soap that is rubbed on the skin
Lotion	Drug particles in a solution for topical use
Lozenge	Small oval, round, or oblong preparation containing a drug in a flavored or sweetened base that dissolves in the mouth and releases the medication; also called *troche*
Ointment	Semisolid preparation containing a drug to be applied externally; also called an *unction*
Pill	Mixture of a powdered drug with a cohesive material; may be round or oval
Powder	Single or mixture of finely ground drugs
Solution	A drug dissolved in another substance (e.g., in an aqueous solution)
Suppository	An easily melted medication preparation in a firm base such as gelatin that is inserted into the body (rectum, vagina, urethra)
Suspension	Finely divided, undissolved particles in a liquid medium; should be shaken before use
Syrup	Medication combined in a water and sugar solution
Tablet	Small, solid dose of medication, compressed or molded; may be any color, size, or shape (e.g., caplets are elongated/oval in shape and are often coated); *enteric-coated tablets* are coated with a substance that is insoluble in gastric acids to reduce gastric irritation by the drug
Transdermal patch	Unit dose of medication applied directly to skin for diffusion through skin and absorption into the bloodstream

(Merriam-Webster, n.d.). It addresses *why* we administer a specific drug, which is more commonly known as the *clinical indication(s)*. Understanding the desired outcome of administering a drug is an important part of nursing responsibilities related to medication administration. Nurses are legally responsible for understanding the pharmacotherapeutics of all drugs they administer. This knowledge is required for the practicing nurse to assess the appropriateness of the medication, as well as provide appropriate and accurate patient education (Frandsen & Pennington, 2021; Karch, 2020).

Mechanisms of Drug Action

Pharmacokinetics

Pharmacokinetics is the effect the body has on a drug once the drug enters the body. It is the movement of drug molecules in the body in relation to the drug's absorption, distribution, metabolism, and excretion.

ABSORPTION

Absorption is the process by which a drug is transferred from its site of entry into the body to the bloodstream. Absorption of a drug is influenced by the following factors.

Route of Administration

The rate of absorption depends on the route of administration. Drugs given orally usually take the longest to be absorbed, with liquids that do not need to be dissolved having a faster absorption rate than capsules or tablets. Drugs injected intramuscularly or subcutaneously are usually absorbed more rapidly than oral medications. Drugs administered intravenously are placed directly into the bloodstream, thus technically are not absorbed and take effect quickly. Drugs administered through intact skin, unless formulated specifically for systemic absorption (transdermal patches), tend to have primarily local effects. However, drugs administered via a mucous membrane (oral mucosa, eye, nose, vagina, or rectum) are absorbed both locally and systemically, which means the drug acts right at the site of administration, but also passes directly into the bloodstream. The portion of a drug that reaches the systemic circulation and can act on the cells is called the drug's **bioavailability** (Frandsen & Pennington, 2021).

Lipid Solubility

Cell membranes have a fatty acid layer. A drug that is more lipid soluble can be absorbed more readily and pass more easily through the cell membrane.

pH

Acidic drugs are well absorbed in the stomach. Drugs that are alkalotic remain ionized or insoluble in an acidic environment. These drugs are not absorbed before reaching the small intestine. The concept of acid–base balance is further discussed in Chapter 42.

Blood Flow

Absorption is increased with increased blood flow. Patients with impaired circulatory function absorb drugs less rapidly than patients with normal circulatory function.

Local Conditions at the Site of Administration

The more extensive the absorbing surface, the greater the absorption of the drug and the more rapid the effect. For example, a patient with burns would have poor absorption from an intramuscular injection because of the damage to the blood supply typically present in muscle. Food, especially fatty food that slows gastric emptying, can slow the rate of absorption of some drugs; but food may enhance the rate of absorption of poorly soluble drugs. Since most of the absorption in the gastrointestinal tract takes place in the small intestine, the length of time a drug is present in the intestinal tract (diarrhea or vomiting) affects absorption and drug bioavailability. Drug absorption can be manipulated with sustained-release preparations or enteric-coated preparations, which are primarily absorbed in the small intestine (Le, 2019). Enteric-coated preparations are resistant to the digestive action of the stomach.

Drug Dosage

When determining a drug dosage, providers consider absorption, distribution, metabolism, and elimination. The amount of a drug administered directly impacts its bioavailability. For example, a loading dose, or a larger than normal dose, is usually given when a patient is in acute distress and the maximum therapeutic effect is desired as quickly as possible. Serum drug levels (which require a blood-draw and laboratory analysis) help determine dosage by reflecting absorption, bioavailability, and drug half-life, as well as metabolic and excretory rates. Serum drug levels ultimately indicate the onset, peak, and duration of action (Frandsen & Pennington, 2021). These laboratory values become especially important when the margin of error between a therapeutic level and toxic level is narrow. If drug toxicity occurs, it can be detected quickly and treated in the controlled hospital environment. A maintenance dose is a lower dosage that becomes the usual or daily dosage. Patients who receive digoxin or phenobarbital, for example, may receive loading doses when therapy is initiated and then transition to a maintenance dose. The goal of drug dosing is to give a dose that achieves the desired therapeutic effect of the drug (pharmacotherapeutics) without causing other undesirable or adverse reactions (discussed later in this chapter).

DISTRIBUTION

Distribution occurs after a drug has been injected or absorbed into the bloodstream—the drug molecules are transported throughout the body to where they take action. Metabolism and excretion occur after distribution. Distribution depends on: (1) the adequacy of blood circulation; (2) protein binding, which affects the drug's ability to leave the bloodstream or storage areas (such as muscle, fat, or other tissues) and enter the cells; and (3) the selectively permeable blood–brain barrier that protects the central nervous system (CNS) with its capillary wall, but can also limit the passage of drugs intended to act on the CNS (Frandsen & Pennington, 2021). In the case of pregnancy and lactation, some drugs readily cross the placenta and/or enter breast milk. These factors must be considered when planning and implementing drug therapies. Any concern about the safe use of a medication during pregnancy can be identified in a pharmacology text, through consultation with a pharmacist, or from trusted computer programs and electronic databases.

METABOLISM

Metabolism, or biotransformation, is the change of an active drug from its original form to an inactivated or new form (Frandsen & Pennington, 2021; Karch, 2020). The liver is the primary site for drug metabolism. Various processes and enzymes are involved in metabolism. Most drugs are inactivated by the liver and transformed to inactive substances for excretion (discussed in the next section). Physiologic changes associated with aging, the presence of liver disease, or other factors that impair the functioning of the liver decrease its ability to metabolize drugs. Other tissues, such as those of the gastrointestinal tract, lungs, and kidneys, also have a role in drug metabolism (Frandsen & Pennington, 2021; Karch, 2020).

Drugs given orally move from the intestinal lumen to the liver by way of the portal vein. Some drugs are extensively metabolized in the liver and do not make it to the systemic circulation. This reduction in bioavailability is referred to as the *first-pass effect* or presystemic metabolism (Frandsen & Pennington, 2021; Karch, 2020). Drugs with extensive or variable first-pass effects, such as nitroglycerin, are not given orally because most of the drug would be destroyed by the liver, with little or no drug left to work in the body. This is why nitroglycerin is only given via sublingual, transdermal, or intravenous routes (McCuistion et al., 2021). Some drugs are metabolized by the liver to an inactive form, reducing the amount of active drug left in the body. Other drugs may be metabolized to an active drug metabolite (another form), and may be more active than the original drug. Pharmacology texts provide more detailed explanations of the metabolism of drugs.

EXCRETION

After the drug is broken down to an inactive form, excretion of the drug occurs. **Excretion** is the process of removing a drug, or its metabolites (products of metabolism), from the body. The kidneys excrete most drugs through urine. The lungs are the primary route for the excretion of gaseous substances, such as inhalation anesthetics. Some drugs or their metabolites are excreted through bile—either directly through feces or returned to the liver and then eventually excreted by the kidney. The skin has minimal excretory function (Frandsen & Pennington, 2021). Some medications may be contraindicated, or dosages may need to be adjusted, if renal excretion is impaired. Changes associated with aging, disease, or the presence of other factors that impair the functioning of the kidneys can decrease their ability to excrete drugs. Manufacturers are required by law to include specific information regarding implications for specific populations, including geriatric or pregnant patients, on the package inserts of prescription drugs and biologic products (FDA, 2020). Of particular concern are details concerning the excretion of these drugs in older adults whose renal function has declined.

Pharmacodynamics

Drugs act at the cellular level to achieve the desired effects. The process by which drugs act on target cells, resulting in alterations in cellular reactions and functions, is called **pharmacodynamics**. Pharmacodynamics represents what a drug does to the body (Farinde, 2019). Drugs turn on, turn off, promote, or block responses that are part of the body's processes. One mechanism of drug action is a drug–receptor interaction, in which the drug interacts with one or more cellular structures to alter cell function. These specialized structures are called receptor sites. The drug fits the receptor just like a key fits a lock. Drugs may also combine with other molecules in the body to achieve their effect. For example, a drug may combine with an enzyme to achieve the desired effect, which is referred to as a drug–enzyme interaction. Other drugs achieve their effect by acting on the permeability of the cell membrane, or altering the cellular environment via neurohormones that regulate key physiologic processes (Frandsen & Pennington, 2021).

Adverse Drug Reactions

Although a therapeutic effect is the desired outcome in medication administration, sometimes secondary undesirable effects occur. Harmful effects that lead to injury are known as adverse effects, adverse drug events (ADEs), and **adverse drug reactions (ADRs**; Frandsen & Pennington, 2021; Karch, 2020; Marsh, 2018).

Some unintended, secondary effects are mild, predictable, and may be tolerated as part of the therapy. These are often referred to as *side effects*. For example, morphine, an opioid agonist, is used to treat moderate to severe and chronic pain. A known side effect of morphine is constipation. However, the benefit of pain relief usually outweighs the side effect of constipation, so that side effect is often accepted and managed with stool softeners and laxatives. On the other hand, adverse reactions can be severe and may require discontinuation of the drug, depending on whether the benefit of the drug outweighs the harm from the adverse effect. For example, should the morphine cause a sudden drop in blood pressure, this may be considered an ADR and require intervention and discontinuation of the morphine.

Another example of an ADR is the development of an iatrogenic disorder caused unintentionally by drug therapy. Neutropenia caused by chemotherapy is an example of an ADR. Other types of ADRs to be discussed include allergic effects, drug tolerance, toxic effects, idiosyncratic effects, and drug interactions.

It is important for nurses and other health care professionals to monitor for ADRs. Serious ADRs, considered *adverse events* or sentinel events (discussed in Chapter 28), must be documented according to facility policy and should be reported to a national database, such as MedWatch. MedWatch is a safety information and voluntary adverse events reporting program, sponsored by the U.S. Food and Drug Administration (FDA, 2020). This program provides nationwide tracking of all serious ADRs, along with up-to-date information about medication errors and potential or actual medical-product problems and errors. According to FDA (2019) criteria, a serious ADE is defined as an action that is life threatening, requires intervention to prevent death or permanent impairment, and/or leads to death, hospitalization, disability, or congenital anomaly. Reporting of serious adverse effects is necessary for corrective action to take place to protect patients. This information is used to revise drug labels, add warnings for health care providers, create patient medication guides, or withdraw a drug from the market (FDA, 2019). One example of how this information is used is the addition of a Boxed Warning (formerly known as Black Box Warnings). These boxed warnings are placed on the label of certain prescription drugs (such as specific antidepressant and cancer-treatment drugs), to indicate the risk for serious ADRs and provide safety information (Delong & Preuss, 2020; Frandsen & Pennington, 2021). Additional information regarding reporting adverse events is discussed at the end of the chapter, in the section on Preventing and Responding to Medication Errors.

Unfolding Patient Stories: Mona Hernandez • Part 2

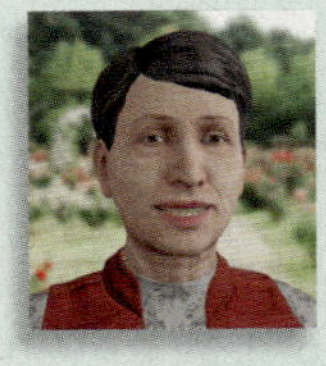

Remember **Mona Hernandez** from Chapter 18, the 72-year-old female admitted with pneumonia. She has a history of hypertension controlled with hydrochlorothiazide 25 mg daily, continues to smoke a half pack of cigarettes per day, and is 20 lb overweight. The provider has ordered moxifloxacin 400 mg IV as a secondary line infusion (piggyback) daily to treat the pneumonia. What factors affecting drug action and potential adverse effects should the nurse consider before administering the antibiotic to Mona?

Care for Mona and other patients in a realistic virtual environment: ***vSim** for Nursing* (thepoint.lww.com/vSimFunds). Practice documenting these patients' care in DocuCare (thepoint.lww.com/DocuCareEHR).

Allergic Effect

An **allergic effect** is an immune system response that occurs when the body interprets the administered drug as a foreign substance and forms antibodies against the drug. A drug allergy manifests differently depending on the drug, the allergy, and the patient. Clinical manifestations of allergic reactions range from mild to severe. The reaction can occur immediately after the patient receives the medication or be delayed for hours to days. Symptoms may become more severe each time the drug is introduced into the body.

Some of the signs and symptoms of a drug allergy are rash, urticaria, fever, diarrhea, nausea, and vomiting. The most serious allergic effect is called an **anaphylactic reaction** (anaphylaxis). **Anaphylaxis** is life threatening and results in respiratory distress, sudden severe bronchospasm, and cardiovascular collapse. This reaction is treated with vasopressors, bronchodilators, corticosteroids, oxygen therapy, intravenous fluids,.and antihistamines.

Drug Tolerance

Drug tolerance occurs when the body becomes accustomed to the effects of a particular drug over a period of time. Larger doses of the drug must be taken to produce the desired effect. For example, patients using morphine for an extended period of time become tolerant to the drug's therapeutic effects and eventually need higher and higher doses to control their pain.

Toxic Effect

Toxic effects (toxicities) are specific groups of symptoms related to drug therapy that carry risk for permanent damage or death (Frandsen & Pennington, 2021). The organ or system affected by the toxicity is used to name the toxicity, such as with nephrotoxicity, or damage to the kidney. Toxicities can occur from a cumulative effect. A cumulative effect occurs when the body cannot metabolize one dose of a drug before another dose is administered. A mismatch between absorption and excretion means that each new dose increases the total quantity in the body. Older adults are especially at risk for experiencing a cumulative effect. This is related to altered drug metabolism and elimination due to impaired hepatic metabolism and renal clearance related to normal changes in these systems associated with aging. Researchers are working to quantify this risk and develop risk prediction models to improve early detection and prevent progressive organ damage in this vulnerable population (Tecklenborg et al., 2020).

Idiosyncratic Effect

An **idiosyncratic effect** (sometimes called *paradoxical effect*) is any unusual or peculiar response to a drug that may manifest itself by overresponse, underresponse, or even the opposite of the expected response. Idiosyncratic effects are related to a patient's unique response to a drug and are thought to be the result of genetic enzyme deficiencies that lead to an abnormal mechanism of drug breakdown. This term may become obsolete as ADR reporting continues and the specific mechanisms of ADRs are discovered (Marsh, 2018). Older adults often have unpredictable or erratic responses to medications.

Drug Interactions

Drug interactions occur when one drug is affected in some way by another drug, a food, or another substance that is taken at the same time. There are times when known drug interactions may be advantageous. For example, one medication may be given to offset or counteract another medication's side effects. Some medications are given together when their actions are synergistic or when one drug potentiates (increases) the therapeutic effects of another drug. Other drug interactions are not beneficial, especially when the drug interaction decreases the therapeutic effect and/or increases the adverse effects. In a drug–drug interaction, the combined effect of two or more drugs acting simultaneously can produce several effects (Frandsen & Pennington, 2021):

- Additive effect—drugs with similar pharmacologic actions; results in an increase in the overall effect
- Synergistic effect—drugs with different sites or MOA; results in greater effects when taken together (one drug potentiates the other)
- Antagonistic effect—combined drugs alter the overall sum effect or negate each other; results in an effect less than that of each drug alone
- Interference—one drug interferes with the metabolism of another; leads to the buildup of a medication (that cannot be metabolized) and can result in toxicity or an ADR
- Displacement—one drug binds to protein-binding sites and forces another drug to be displaced; results in the released drug becoming pharmacologically active and can lead to an increase in the effect of the unbound drug

For example, ingesting alcohol and barbiturates together creates an unbeneficial **synergistic effect** with the potential for significantly increased CNS depression. It is important to be knowledgeable about and watch for drug interactions and the effects of drug therapy.

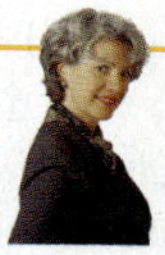

Think back to **Mildred Campbell**, the 65-year-old woman with arthritis and hypertension (high blood pressure) asking about a recently advertised medication for joint pain relief. The nurse should assess the patient's medication history to determine her current medication regimen and keep in mind that many older adults see more than one health care provider. The nurse must consider possible polypharmacy (taking of more than two medications at a time) and potential risks for drug interactions, even before discussing whether the advertised medication would be appropriate.

Dietary supplements, herbs, and other *natural* remedies are another potential problem area for drug interactions. Many patients do not consider dietary supplements, herbs, and natural remedies to be medications because they can purchase these items at a store selling nutritional products. However, many of these products have recognized pharmacologic effects, unexpected allergic reactions, and problematic drug–supplement interactions (Dudek, 2017; National Center for Complementary and Integrative Health [NCCIH], 2022). When asking patients if they are taking any medications, specifically ask if they are taking any herbal or natural supplements. Health care providers need to identify viable resources (Gregory et al., 2016) and be aware of the intended benefits, possible adverse effects, potential drug interactions, and perioperative implications related to these types of supplements. Further information related to dietary supplements, and natural and herbal products can be found at the FDA's website (https://www.fda.gov/food/dietary-supplements) and the NCCIH website (https://nccih.nih.gov).

Factors Affecting Drug Action

Certain variables can influence the action or effect of a medication. These variables include developmental considerations, patient's body weight, patient's biologic sex, genetic and cultural factors, psychological factors, pathology, environment, and timing of medication administration. In addition, social determinants of health play a role when considering availability of resources, access to education and health care, community resources, social support, health literacy, and access to emerging technologies.

Developmental Considerations

During pregnancy, many drugs are contraindicated because of their possible adverse effects on the fetus. Certain drugs, referred to as **teratogenic**, are known to have the potential to cause developmental defects in the embryo or fetus and are contraindicated. Examples of teratogenic drugs include cocaine, alcohol, neurologic medications (e.g., phenytoin and valproate), antimicrobials (e.g., tetracyclines and fluoroquinolones), anticoagulants (e.g., coumadin), antithyroid medications, and the hormonal medication, diethylstilbestrol (Arfman et al., 2020; Kobaly & Mandel, 2019; Tsamantioti & Hashmi, 2020). In 2015, the FDA (2020) replaced the drug classification categories (A, B, C, D, and X) with a new labeling system, the Pregnancy and Lactation Labeling Rule (PLLR), that addresses pregnancy, lactation, and females and males with reproductive potential. The timing (trimester, weeks) of administration during pregnancy, the dose of the medication, and a risk–benefit analysis inform decisions made by the pregnant person and their health care provider. Some drugs cross into breast milk, putting breastfed infants at risk for adverse effects from drugs in the breast feeding person's circulation. Small body size, reduced weight, and reduced body water also alter distribution, as do decreases in cardiac output and organ perfusion. Therefore, a child's medication dose is smaller than an adult's dose. Infants are especially sensitive to medications because of the immaturity of their organs and immaturity of the blood–brain barrier. Older people are sensitive to medications because their bodies have experienced physiologic changes associated with the aging process, including decreased gastric motility, muscle mass, acid production, and blood flow, which affect drug absorption. They may also be more susceptible to certain adverse effects. Liver function declines with advancing age, and changes occur in the hepatic enzymes involved in drug metabolism. Blood flow to the liver decreases secondary to a decrease in cardiac output. Drugs are excreted more slowly from the body as a result of changes in kidney function. Receptor sensitivity is altered in older people, and their sensitivity to certain drugs increases. The physiologic changes in older people that increase drug susceptibility are summarized in the accompanying display, Focus on the Older Adult.

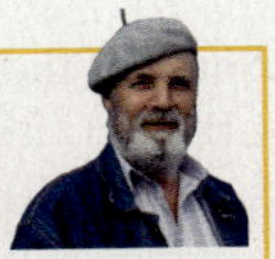

Recall **Mr. Baptiste**, the older adult receiving intravenous antibiotics for a wound infection. The nurse would need to consider age-related changes that might interfere with the drug action, and be especially alert for signs and symptoms of drug toxicity.

Weight

Expected responses to drugs are based largely on the reactions that occur when the drugs are given to healthy adults (ages 18 to 65 years, 150 lb [~68 kg]). It is important to know the usual dose for a medication before administering it. Body surface area (BSA) is the area of the external surface of the body, expressed in square meters (m^2). BSA is the initial factor considered when calculating the drug dose for infants, children, older adults, patients receiving oncologic medications, and patients with low body weight (Frandsen & Pennington, 2021; Karch, 2020). Drug doses for children are calculated by weight in kilograms or BSA.

Biologic Sex

The difference in the distribution of body fat and fluids in males and females is a minor factor affecting the action of some drugs. To date, most research on drugs and their actions and effects has been conducted on males. Future clinical drug trials are expected to include more females/women to document the effects of hormonal fluctuations, and determine the safety and efficacy of specific drugs during pregnancy (Fairlie et al., 2019).

Cultural and Genetic Factors

Religious restrictions and beliefs or cultural practices may affect the patient's acceptance of, response to, and adherence to certain drug therapies. Health care providers need an understanding of a patient's cultural values, beliefs, and practices to provide culturally competent care that reflects cultural humility (Giger & Haddad, 2020). For example, Christian Scientists place their faith in a system of spiritual healing; therefore, they do not take medicine. A Christian Scientist would not participate in a childhood vaccination program or seek pharmaceutical therapy to manage disease (The Christian Science Board of Directors, 2020). Herbal treatments that are popular in some cultures may interfere with or counteract the action of prescribed medication.

Ethnopharmacology is a relatively new field of study composed of several interrelated aspects. "Combining the approaches of medical anthropology, phytotherapy, and pharmaceutical science, this discipline examines medicinal plants in indigenous cultures, their bioactive compounds, and the sustainable development and production of nature-derived therapeutics" (Transcultural C.A.R.E. Associates, 2020, Ethno Pharmacology). Although standardized classification systems do not universally exist, discussions around ethnopharmacology and ethnomedicine involve cultural perceptions and values that impact medical systems, cross-cultural comparisons of terms and medicinal uses, and drug

Focus on the Older Adult

NURSING STRATEGIES TO ADDRESS AGE-RELATED CHANGES IN DRUG RESPONSE

Age-Related Changes	Implication or Response	Nursing Strategies
Decreased gastric motility and slowed gastric emptying; increased gastric pH	Stomach irritation; nausea and vomiting; gastric ulceration; altered absorption of drugs	• Assess for symptoms of gastrointestinal discomfort. • Assess stool for blood.
Decreased lean body mass; decreased total body water	Decreased distribution of water-soluble drugs and higher plasma concentrations, leading to increased possibility of drug toxicity	• Assess for signs of drug interactions or toxicity. • Monitor blood levels of drugs. • Monitor fluid balance—intake and output.
Increased adipose tissue	Accumulation of fat-soluble drugs; delay in elimination and accumulation of drug in the body, leading to prolonged action and increased possibility of toxicity	• Assess for signs of drug interactions or toxicity. • Monitor blood levels of drugs.
Decreased number of protein-binding sites	Higher drug plasma concentrations, leading to increased possibility of drug toxicity	• Assess for signs of drug interactions or toxicity. • Monitor blood levels of drugs. • Monitor laboratory values—albumin and prealbumin.
Decreased liver function; decreased enzyme production for drug metabolism; decreased hepatic perfusion	Decreased rate of drug metabolism; higher drug plasma concentrations, leading to prolonged action and increased possibility of drug toxicity	• Assess for signs of drug interactions or toxicity. • Monitor blood levels of drugs. • Monitor laboratory values—hepatic enzymes.
Decreased kidney function, renal mass, and blood flow	Decreased excretion of drugs, leading to possible increased serum levels/toxicity	• Assess for signs of drug interactions or toxicity. • Particularly monitor NSAID use, which may decrease renal blood flow and function. • Monitor blood levels of drugs. • Monitor laboratory values—creatinine clearance, blood urea nitrogen, serum creatinine.
Alterations in normal homeostatic responses; altered peripheral venous tone	Exacerbated response to cardiovascular drugs; more pronounced hypotensive effects from medications	• Assess for signs of drug interactions or toxicity. • Monitor blood levels of drugs. • Monitor vital signs. • Take orthostatic hypotension precautions.
Alterations in blood–brain barrier and sensitivity of receptor sites	Enhanced central nervous system penetration of fat-soluble drugs; increased possibility for alterations in mental status, dizziness, gait disturbances	• Assess for signs of drug interactions or toxicity. • Assess for dizziness and lightheadedness. • Take fall safety precautions.
Decreased central nervous system efficiency	Prolonged effect of drugs on the central nervous system; exacerbated response to analgesics and sedatives	• Assess for signs of drug interactions or toxicity • Assess for alterations in neurologic status • Monitor vital signs and pulse oximetry.
Decreased production of oral secretions; dry mouth	Difficulty swallowing oral medications	• Monitor ability to swallow medications, especially tablets and capsules. • Discuss changing medications to forms that can be crushed and/or liquid forms with prescribing practitioner.
Decreased lipid content in skin; decreased blood supply to the skin	Possible decrease in absorption of transdermal medications	• Monitor effectiveness of transdermal preparations.

Source: Adapted from Frandsen, G., & Pennington, S. S. (2021). *Abrams' clinical drug therapy: Rationales for nursing practice* (12th ed.). Wolters Kluwer; Hinkle, J. L., Cheever, K. H., & Overbaugh, K. J. (2022). *Brunner & Suddarth's textbook of medical-surgical nursing* (15th ed.). Wolters Kluwer; Miller, C. A. (2019). *Nursing for wellness in older adults* (8th ed.). Wolters Kluwer; and Norris, T. L. (2020). *Porth's essentials of pathophysiology* (5th ed.). Wolters Kluwer.

Box 30-1 Tips for Culturally Respectful Communication

- Encourage cultural sensitivity in health care workers in your particular setting. Acquire basic information about health beliefs and practices of various cultural groups in your health care setting. This provides a basis for assessing a patient's beliefs and practices. Recognize, however, that within all cultures and ethnic groups, there are members who do not hold all the values of the group.
- Consider biologic variations (e.g., color, body structure, pharmacogenetics) when performing a baseline assessment and administering medications.
- Be alert to atypical drug responses or unexpected adverse effects that may occur in certain racial or ethnic groups. This knowledge helps you direct assessment questions as appropriate.
- Ask specifically about the use of folk or home remedies prescribed by a nontraditional healer.
- Ask specific questions about possible adverse effects, rather than asking general questions or waiting for the patient to voice concerns. For example, do not ask, "Are you having any problems with your medicine?" Instead, ask, "Have you noticed any unusual, involuntary movements?"
- Practice cultural humility. Consider individual cultural health practices, values, and definitions of health and illness when teaching patients and families. Ask, "What do you think caused your health problem?" and "What treatment do you think will help?"
- Include culturally sensitive information in all basic health teaching. For example, consider the patient's perception of time and space when teaching.
- Consider the impact of their social organization and roles when presenting information. Involve the family and other members of the community as appropriate.
- Determine the patient's language preferences for spoken and written communication. Use trained medical interpreters as needed.
- Use printed or audiovisual information that is in the language spoken by your patients. Recognize that diversity exists within cultural groups. For example, the Hispanic population includes Mexicans, Cubans, Puerto Ricans, and other Latino groups.
- Help culturally diverse patients to value and understand the importance of communicating concerns and asking questions about prescribed medications. Patients and families need to know how to identify major adverse effects of the medications they are taking and the appropriate person(s) to contact if these effects are noted.

Source: Adapted from Giger, J. N., & Haddad, L. G. (2020). *Transcultural nursing: Assessment and intervention* (8th ed.). Elsevier Inc; Muñoz, C., & Hilgenberg, C. (2006). Ethnopharmacology: Understanding how ethnicity can affect drug response is essential to providing culturally competent care. *Holistic Nursing Practice, 20*(5), 227–234. https://doi.org/10.1097/00004650-200609000-00004; and Woods, D. L., Mentes, J. C., Cadogan, M., & Phillips, L. R. (2017). Aging, genetic variations, and ethnopharmacology: Building cultural competence through awareness of drug responses in ethnic minority elders. *Journal of Transcultural Nursing, 28*(1), 56–62. https://doi.org/10.1177/1043659615606202.

discovery (Bruhn & Rivier, 2019; Staub et al., 2015). The more recent use of the term *ethnopharmacology* (or *ethnic pharmacology*) involves the study of the effect of ethnicity on responses to prescribed medication, especially drug absorption, metabolism, distribution, and excretion. This is often associated with **pharmacogenetics** where differences in the responses of patients receiving the same medication may result from genetic differences, such as genetic variations in certain enzymes, that may cause differing drug responses. Ethnicity and race influence responses to certain medications. Certain ethnic groups and races have more of these variations than do others (Muñoz & Hilgenberg, 2006; Woods et al., 2017). Specifically, there may be important variations in the therapeutic dose and/or incidence of adverse effects. Some patients in certain groups obtain therapeutic responses at lower doses than those usually prescribed, while other patient groups require a larger dose to have the same therapeutic response. For example, angiotensin-converting enzyme (ACE) inhibitors have been found to more frequently cause an ACE inhibitor–induced cough in Asian American patients, and there is a higher risk of angioedema (severe swelling) with African American patients. ACE inhibitors are generally less effective with African American patients; thiazide-type diuretics and calcium channel blockers (CCBs) are more effective in controlling their hypertension (Whelton et al., 2018). Care must be taken, however, to avoid making sweeping generalizations and assumptions. Ethnicity and race influence responses to certain medications, but no two people are alike.

General and specific cultural knowledge allows the health care provider to ask the right questions when interacting with patients of varying backgrounds. Nurses who are aware of the specific needs and beliefs of culturally diverse patient populations are better able to communicate effectively and provide holistic, person-centered care that reflects cultural humility. Box 30-1 gives guidelines for effective, culturally respectful communication about medication.

Psychological Factors

The patient's expectations of the medication may affect the response to the medication. A **placebo** is a pharmacologically inactive substance. In clinical drug trials, one group of patients receives the active drug, whereas another group receives a placebo to study the drug's effects. Some patients appear to have the same response with the placebo as with the active drug–this is referred to as the *placebo effect* (McCuistion et al., 2021). Psychological factors such as attitudes and expectations of drug therapy also directly impact adherence to the medication plan, especially with long-term drug therapy (Frandsen & Pennington, 2021).

Pathology

The presence of disease can affect drug action. For example, the liver is the primary organ for drug breakdown, so pathologic conditions that involve the liver may slow metabolism and alter the dosage of the drug needed to reach a therapeutic level. Drugs taken orally may be impacted if a gastrointestinal disorder interferes with absorption. Cardiovascular disorders that affect blood flow potentially impact all pharmacokinetic processes. The kidneys excrete most drugs and their byproducts from the body. Pathologic conditions that involve the kidneys would change excretion and alter the dosage of the drug required to obtain a therapeutic level. Even the endocrine system, particularly thyroid disorders, has an effect on metabolism. These types of conditions also influence the presence of adverse effects, such as toxicities.

Environment

A patient's environment may influence that individual's response to medications. Sensory deprivation and overload may affect drug responses. The patient who receives pain medication or a sedative in an active, noisy environment may not be able to benefit fully from the medication's effects; those receiving pain medication in a quiet environment and using an additional relaxation method, such as guided imagery, may benefit from the pain medication for a longer period of time. The relative oxygen deprivation at high altitudes may increase sensitivity to some drugs.

In addition, nutritional state can also affect the body's reaction to certain drugs. When dietary factors are altered, drug therapy may produce different effects in the body than would normally occur. For example, many drugs normally bind to proteins in the plasma. Lowered protein levels in the body means less drug bound to plasma proteins, which impacts on biotransformation and excretion of the drug. This leads to a higher concentration of free (unbound) drug in the body. A higher drug concentration increases the drug's effect in the body and the risk for adverse effects (Frandsen & Pennington, 2021; Karch, 2020).

Timing of Administration

The presence of food in the stomach can delay the absorption of orally administered medications. Alternatively, some medications should be given with food to prevent gastric irritation; the nurse should consider this when establishing a patient's medication schedule. Other medications may have enhanced absorption if taken with certain foods. Circadian rhythms and cycles may also influence drug action.

Drug Dose and Serum Drug Levels

Serum (blood) drug levels were reviewed earlier in this chapter in relation to drug dosage (see Absorption). The goal is to maintain a therapeutic level of a drug in the body. In addition to using serum drug levels to initiate and monitor drug therapy, they are also used to assess peak and trough levels of certain drugs, particularly antibiotics that are known to be toxic to the kidney (nephrotoxic). After a drug has been absorbed, its serum level can be monitored by drawing a blood specimen and measuring the level of the drug in the serum. A drug's **therapeutic range** is the concentration of drug in the blood serum that produces the desired effect without causing toxicity. The **peak level**, or highest plasma concentration, of the drug should be measured when absorption is complete. The peak level may be affected by factors that affect drug absorption as well as the route of administration. The peak level is typically drawn 1 hour after a drug has been administered (depending on the route). The **trough level** is the point when the drug is at its lowest concentration, indicating the rate of elimination. The trough level is typically drawn 30 minutes before the next dose is scheduled to be administered. The dosage schedule, as well as the half-life of the drug, can affect the trough level. A drug's **half-life** is the amount of time it takes for 50% of the serum concentration of a drug to be eliminated from the body. When a drug is given at a consistent dose, it takes four or five half-lives to achieve a steady concentration and develop balance between tissue and serum concentrations. This is when maximal therapeutic effects occur (Frandsen & Pennington, 2021; Karch, 2020). Monitoring these levels ensures that therapeutic ranges are obtained without reaching toxic levels.

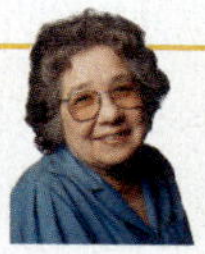

Consider **Regina Sauder**, the adult admitted to the hospital with a DVT. She is receiving intravenous heparin and oral warfarin, both of which are monitored using blood tests. Her dose of each drug is adjusted based on the laboratory results to ensure the appropriate therapeutic effect.

Drug Legislation

In 1906, the Pure Food and Drug Act designated the U.S. Pharmacopeia and National Formulary as the official drug resource in the United States (USP-NF, 2020), which set national standards for drug quality. This act also empowered the federal government to enforce these standards. This legislation was updated in 1938 by the Federal Food, Drug and Cosmetic Act, prohibiting adulterated or mislabeled drugs from being made available. The FDA enforces this law. Extensive testing of new drugs is required before they may be marketed for use. The Durham-Humphrey amendment to the Federal Food, Drug and Cosmetic Act enacted in 1952 distinguished prescription drugs from nonprescription (over-the-counter [OTC]) drugs and provided directions for dispensing prescription drugs.

The Kefauver-Harris Amendment of 1962 increased controls on drug safety, requiring tighter testing of drugs and written inclusion in the drug literature of adverse reactions and contraindications for approved drugs. The Comprehensive Drug Abuse Prevention and Control Act, also known as the Controlled Substances Act, was passed in 1970. This law regulates the distribution of narcotics and other drugs of abuse. Such drugs have been categorized according to their therapeutic usefulness and potential for misuse or abuse (U.S. Department of Justice, Drug Enforcement Administration, 2020). Government programs for the prevention and treatment of **substance use disorder** (a term that encompasses drug/substance abuse and substance dependence/addiction) were established. In 1983, the Drug Enforcement Administration (DEA), a part of the Department of Justice, was identified as the nation's sole legal drug enforcement facility (Karch, 2020). See the Thoughtful, Person-Centered Practice: Challenging Topics (on page 924) feature for a discussion of clinical judgment as it relates to the challenging topic of patients who are drug-seeking.

Thoughtful, Person-Centered Practice: Challenging Topics

Patients Who Are Drug-Seeking

Many controversial issues make it challenging to know how to respond as a professional nurse in select scenarios. Often, the nurse's personal and/or professional values may conflict with options desired by patients, families, employers, and communities. Not infrequently, nurses have to make clinical judgments, balancing promoting and safeguarding personal integrity and respecting the values and preferences of patient. The *Essentials* for entry-level professional nursing education, a document that guides curriculum development and outcomes, identifies a competency within Domain 9 (Professionalism) focused on demonstrating "awareness of personal and professional values and conscious and unconscious biases" (p. 57). The *Essentials* also addresses biases in Domain 10 (Personal, Professional, and Leadership Development) with respect to self-awareness and "developing capacity for leadership" (p. 59) and in Domain 6 (Interprofessional Partnerships) in relation to the "mutual respect and communication" (p. 47) required when working with other professions (AACN, 2021).

Read the scenario below and see if you can articulate what you believe, why you believe this, and how these beliefs are likely to inform the decisions you make and your behavior, especially when you are confronted with competing obligations. Based on Tanner's Clinical Judgment Model (2006), consider reflection-in-action and reflection-on-action (Nielson, Stragnell, & Jester, 2007):

Reflection-in-Action

As you read, consider what the new nurse is thinking in the moment—what happened? How did the patient, family, and health care provider respond? What did the nurse do next?

Scenario

As a new graduate nurse in residency in a busy Emergency Department (ED), I wouldn't be doing triage for some time, but the team assigned me to the triage nurse for the day to assess my progress and hone my assessment skills. With the support of the very experienced triage nurse, I had appropriately (and quickly) identified a *Code Stroke*, wrapped a laceration while comforting both the father and child, and expedited the admission of a patient undergoing cancer treatment who had spiked a fever. The flow of patients was steady, which kept us busy, but I noted occasional muffled crying coming from what I thought was a middle-age woman in the corner of the room. She had already been triaged by my preceptor, but I had stepped away during the interaction and didn't know the full story. Between patients, I asked the triage nurse, "What's going on with the woman who is crying? I can't see her face because she's got a blanket over her head, but I can hear her periodically crying. Should I check on her again…bring her back for re-assessment?" The triage nurse rolled their eyes in response. I followed-up with, "What am I missing?" The triage nurse explained, "She's reporting severe, unexplained pain in her back. Her assessment is totally unremarkable. She verbalized the need for IV Dilaudid because nothing else works. That's three red flags." In that moment, I realized that I still had a lot to learn regarding how to synthesize information obtained subjectively from the patient and objectively from the health care professional. The triage nurse encouraged me to go do a re-assessment and report back. I centered myself, considered my personal biases, thought about what I knew about drug-seeking behavior, and approached the patient in the now-empty waiting room.

Effective Noticing (Cues)

1. What did you notice about the situation initially? What information/observations are significant? What information deviates from what is expected/normal/usual?

Effective Interpreting

2. How would you prioritize this data? What other assessment data, evidence and/or information would you need to consider the situation? How would you obtain this additional information?
3. What do you think about this situation? Consider personal and previous nursing experiences that you have had and formal knowledge (physiology, psychology, communication skills) that may be of assistance in providing care in this situation.

Scenario

I chose to give the patient the benefit of the doubt and tried hard to ignore the seeds planted by the triage nurse—there was a good chance this patient was really in pain and needed medical intervention. As I approached the patient, I could hear her talking on the phone: she was laughing and very interactive with the person on the other end of the call. Since her head was under the blanket, and she did not respond to my verbal requests for attention, I briefly touched her arm to get her attention. She immediately uncovered her head, told the person on the phone she would call them back, and grabbed her lower back, wincing in pain. I appreciate that the experience of pain is individual and the experience is what the patient says it is, so I proceeded with my assessment. The patient reported new onset, sudden back pain and requested hydromorphone (Dilaudid) IV. I let her know that I was the nurse performing the triage assessment and could not prescribe any medications. I indicated that, based on our assessment, it was likely going to be an hour wait, but that we would get her back to a room as soon as possible. She began to moan loudly and stood up, verbalizing that she "didn't deserve to be treated this way." The patient approached another nurse walking through the waiting room, who briefly engaged with the patient and then gestured to me to meet him behind the nurse's station with the triage nurse. As the three of us came together, the nurse who was approached by the patient in the waiting room revealed that he knew this patient from the other EDs where he picked up shifts, and that the patient was flagged as drug-seeking and prescriber-shopping in the system. I listened but asked

Thoughtful, Person-Centered Practice: Challenging Topics *(continued)*

if I could go finish my interaction with the patient before making my final clinical judgment. As I entered the waiting room, I realized that the blanket was on the floor, and the patient was gone.

Reflection-in-Action

Now, consider the nurses' decisions and reflect on your learning. See if you can articulate what you believe, why you believe this, and how these beliefs are likely to inform the decisions you make and your behavior, especially when you're confronted with competing obligations.

Effective Responding

4. How would you describe the obligations you have in this scenario to your patient, to yourself, to your team, and to the community?
5. If you cannot fulfill each of these obligations how will you prioritize them? What basis/rationale do you use for prioritization? Remember that the ANA *Code of Ethics for Nurses* reminds us that "health is a universal right," which includes access to emergency care. Has this patient received adequate access through the triage process?
6. What policies, procedures, and guidelines could you use in this specific situation? What are the requirements regarding reporting and follow-up at the hospital, local, and national level?

Effective Reflecting

As you think about this case, is your assumption that the patient left to seek treatment elsewhere because she needed timely intervention for her indescribable pain that she did not think she would get in your ED or because she realized that she had been outed as drug-seeking? As nurses, we have to differentiate between making assumptions or viewing patients as stereotypes, and using our experience to inform our clinical judgment.

7. Do you think the triage nurse used their experience to inform their decision or was it based on a jaded response or assumption? Did the triage nurse provide adequate support/rationale for their decision?
8. Do you agree with the criteria the nurse used to evaluate their decision? How do you evaluate your clinical and moral judgments?
9. What resources can you access to better inform your decision?
10. What personal attributes and competencies are most likely to lead to a good response?

Reflection-on-Action

Then look back at the scenario and reflect on your learning—how might this have been different if you did not have the additional information from the third-party nurse who happened to walk through the waiting room? How did your knowledge and/or skills expand based on this scenario? What attitude, value, or belief shifts did you experience (if any) after reading this scenario? What would you do differently if you were in this situation? What more do you need to know to be able to manage this or a similar situation in the future?

Lasater, K. (2007). Clinical judgment development: Using simulation to create an assessment rubric. *Journal of Nursing Education, 46*(11), 496–503. https://case.edu/nursing/sites/case.edu.nursing/files/2018-06/Clinical-Judgement-Development.pdf.

Nielson, A., Stragnell, S., & Jester, P. (2007). Guide for reflection using the Clinical Judgment Model. *Journal of Nursing Education, 46*(11), 513–516.

Tanner, C. A. (2006). Thinking like a nurse: A research-based model of clinical judgment in nursing. *Journal of Nursing Education, 45*(6), 204–211.

More current drug-related legislation includes the Food and Drug Administration Modernization Act of 1997. This act provides for accelerated review and use of new drugs and approves drug testing in children before marketing. In addition, it necessitates the inclusion of clinical trial data for experimental drug use for serious or life-threatening health conditions and requires drug companies to provide information related to *off-label* drugs (drugs not approved by the FDA), including their uses and costs. The act requires that drug companies planning to discontinue drugs must inform health professionals and patients at least 6 months before stopping drug production (McCuistion et al., 2021).

In 2003, the Pediatric Research Equity Act was signed into legislation. This act authorizes the FDA to require testing by drug manufacturers of drugs and biologic products for their safety and effectiveness in children. Drug manufacturers must not assume that children are small adults (McCuistion et al., 2021). Also in 2003, Congress approved the Medicare Prescription Drug Improvement and Modernization Act (MMA). This legislation provides financial assistance to seniors to purchase needed prescription medications.

PRINCIPLES OF MEDICATION ADMINISTRATION

Medication Prescriptions and Orders

Prescription and *order* both refer to the means by which a provider communicates information regarding medications (and other procedures and therapies) to the health care team. When considering medication administration, both terms refer to a prescription written or entered into the EHR by a provider with prescriptive rights. In health care, the word *order* is typically used in the inpatient setting, with *prescription* primarily used in the outpatient and community settings. No medication may be given to a patient without a medication order from a licensed practitioner. Each health facility has a policy specifying the manner in which the practitioner writes an order. In some instances, prescriptions are written on a form designed specifically for a primary care provider's order. This becomes part of a patient's permanent record. Prescribers are able to make use of electronic prescribing systems, sending medication prescriptions electronically to outpatient pharmacies. Most health care facilities are beginning to use computer provider order-entry (CPOE) systems. CPOE systems allow the prescribing provider to enter medication orders in a standard format. CPOE systems guide the prescriber in complete, accurate, and appropriate prescribing. The computer sends the prescription directly to the pharmacy and enters the prescription into the patient's permanent record. This prevents any guessing when handwriting is illegible or drug names are similar (Frandsen & Pennington, 2021). Some of the information this system provides includes recommended dosing of medications, drug-specific information, current patient information, laboratory tests that monitor the action of the drug, and potential interactions that may occur with other medications or food. A CPOE system can make medication administration safer and reduce ADEs.

Safe practice dictates that a nurse follows only a written order or an order entered into a CPOE system because these types of orders are less likely to result in error or misinterpretation. Under certain circumstances, such as in an emergency, a verbal order from the prescribing provider may be given to a registered nurse or a pharmacist. In most settings, a student nurse is not permitted to accept a verbal order from a provider. The legal implications for dispensing and administering an agent without a written order vary, and nurses must be familiar with the exact facility policy whenever called on to administer therapeutic agents. The legal implications of verbal orders are discussed in Chapter 7.

Usual hospital policy dictates that when a patient is admitted, unless specific orders to the contrary are written, all drugs that may have been prescribed while the patient was at home are discontinued. To avoid the possibility of having the patient continue to take the home medications while receiving the same ones or others under new orders, all medications should be sent home with the family or removed from the patient's bedside. In some inpatient facilities, patients keep their medications at their bedside and learn, or continue, to administer them as they would at home. It is believed that this approach helps to promote patients' independence. This practice is also seen with drugs that are not available at a health care institution (such as oral contraceptives and certain antidiabetic agents). Careful labeling and adherence to institution-based policies and procedures must be ensured. Nurses continue to be involved with the medication self-administration process, verifying the medications are understood by the patient, are taken appropriately, and that the medications are documented in the patient's permanent record.

When a patient has had surgery, is transferred to another clinical service, is transferred to another health facility, or has any other transition in care, it is a general practice that all orders related to drugs are discontinued and new orders are written in the new setting. **Medication reconciliation** is a process used by the health care team where the current medication orders are compared to patient report, the patient's medical record, and prescriptions that may have been in place prior to the transition of care (Barnsteiner, 2008). Although most often a responsibility of the nurse, pharmacists and other members of the health care team play a valuable role in the medication reconciliation process (Choi & Kim, 2019; Fernandes et al., 2020). The Joint Commission (2020a) includes medication reconciliation as part of the 2020 National Patient Safety Goals. Goal 3 identifies the collection of a patient's current medication list, informing patients of the importance of maintaining an accurate medication list, and comparison of medications taken with the newly prescribed medications to prevent duplications, omissions, or interactions (The Joint Commission). Implementation of medication reconciliation, especially at times of transitions in care, remains best practice despite the relative lack of evidence that medication reconciliation directly reduces the rate of ADEs or directly affects other patient outcomes (Anderson et al., 2019; Redmond et al., 2018; Rose et al., 2017; Tamblyn et al., 2019). Ideally, medication reconciliation involves more than simply a review of the medication lists. Reconciliation should address: (1) ensuring agreement among the clinicians on the patient's health care team, (2) ensuring agreement between the patient and clinician(s), (3) deprescribing any unnecessary medications, (4) decreasing the complexity of medication regimens to decrease patient burden and increase adherence, (5) assessing the cost of medications and out-of-pocket expenses, and (6) communicating with all involved health care team members (Rose et al., 2017). Standardization of the processes inherent in medication reconciliation is needed to support adequate measurement and targeted quality improvement initiatives (Rose et al., 2017; Rungvivatjarus et al., 2020; Zimmerman et al., 2017).

Types of Orders

There are several types of orders that a prescriber may write. A *routine order* is carried out as specified until it is canceled by another order. Many practitioners whose practices are limited to a particular clinical area have a specified set of written orders for all their hospitalized patients. These are also referred to as *standing orders*. A practitioner may write a routine or standing order with specified limitations; that is, the prescriber specifies that a certain order is to be carried out for a stated number of days or times. After the stated period has passed, the order is discontinued automatically.

The prescriber may write a **PRN order** (*as needed*) for medication. The patient receives medication when it is requested or required, and when the specifics of the order (particularly clinical parameters and timing between doses) are met. PRN orders are commonly written for the treatment of symptoms. For example, medications used for pain relief, to relieve nausea, and for sleep aids are often written as a PRN or as-needed order.

Another type of order is the *one-time* order. With this type of order, the directive is carried out only once, at a time specified by the prescriber. Medication to be administered immediately before surgery is an example of a one-time order. A **stat order** is also a single order, but it is carried out immediately. A stat order for a bronchodilator or an antihistamine would be carried out immediately for a patient who is experiencing an anaphylactic drug reaction.

Parts of the Medication Order

The medication order consists of seven parts:

1. Patient's name and a secondary identifier (date of birth, medical record number)
2. Date and time the order is written
3. Name of drug to be administered
4. Dosage of the drug
5. Route by which the drug is to be administered
6. Frequency of administration of the drug
7. Signature of the prescribing provider

Medication orders require the drug, dose, rate, route, frequency, and, when appropriate, duration to be explicit and specific to the needs of the patient in order to achieve the desired outcome. Although not to be used for identifying a patient, inpatient orders also contain information regarding the patient's location, such as unit and room number (Bowen, 2016).

PATIENT'S NAME AND A SECONDARY IDENTIFIER (DATE OF BIRTH, MEDICAL RECORD NUMBER)

The patient's full name is used. The middle name or initial should be included to avoid confusion with other patients. In facilities using paper records, the patient's full name, secondary identification number, and the primary care provider's name are labeled on all sheets on the patient's chart, including the medical order sheet. Be extremely careful when administering medications when there is more than one patient on the unit with the same last name. Not only can the nurse give the wrong patient the wrong medication, but a provider may enter an order in the wrong patient's medical record. A secondary identifier is used when verifying the patient's identity. If using the date of birth as a second identifier, the day, month, and year should all be included.

DATE AND TIME THE ORDER IS WRITTEN

The date and time the order is written are provided. Because the nursing staff in inpatient facilities changes several times during each 24-hour period, the date and time help to prevent errors of oversight as different nurses take charge of the patient's care. When an order is to be followed for a specified number of days, the date and time are important so that the discontinuation date and time can be determined accurately. State law determines the length of time an order for a narcotic remains valid, so the starting date and time must be clearly documented. Hospitals are utilizing many computer applications in patient care. Examples of such technology include a computer-generated database, computer-generated medication administration orders, and computer-generated flow sheets, as well as EHRs. This technology is helping to improve patient safety, but it also requires that nurses monitor the computer system for patient updates, including new medication orders.

NAME OF DRUG TO BE ADMINISTERED

The name of the drug is stated in the order, either by the trade (brand) name and/or by the generic name. Certain brand names are well known, but the practice of using the generic name is considered safest and is required by many health care facilities.

A nurse unfamiliar with a drug can use several sources to obtain information. The USP-NF (2020) is the official source in the United States. Most other countries have similar references that describe official therapeutic agents. Most facilities also provide their own formulary, listing the drugs stocked by the facility. Health care facilities also provide access to online medication information sites. The *Physicians' Desk Reference* (PDR) is another source of information that is supplied by pharmaceutical companies. In addition, information about drugs can be obtained from the hospital pharmacist, the prescriber, and any of several texts written specifically for the nursing role in the management of drug therapy. Many of these nursing-specific texts are available as software and can be loaded onto handheld devices such as tablets and smartphones.

DOSAGE OF THE DRUG

The dosage of a drug can be stated in either the metric or the household system. These systems are described in the Dosage Calculations section. The metric system has been adopted internationally, is the most widely used, and is the safest measurement system for drug dosages. Self-administered drugs are commonly labeled in household measurements to facilitate administration for the patient. The household system of measurement may also be used in community settings, such as a person's home (McCuistion et al., 2021). It is important to be familiar with common equivalent measurements when using household equipment, such as teaspoons and tablespoons, because the home is usually not equipped with special measuring devices. If administration equipment is not available, instruct patients to use measuring spoons and *not* silverware, due to the variability of the amount silverware can hold. The most common equivalents are in Appendix B. However, to prevent errors, best practice requires providing patients with commercially available oral syringes, droppers (infants), and cups printed with easy-to-read volumes using only the metric scale (Institute for Safe Medication Practices, 2020).

Certain standard abbreviations are used to indicate drug amounts; it is important to know the common abbreviations before administering drugs. Refer to Box 20-3 in Chapter 20 for common abbreviations used in drug orders. Several abbreviations used in the past have been identified as having the potential to cause errors. The Joint Commission has identified an official *do not use* list of abbreviations. See Table 20-3 on page 528 for this list. The use of ambiguous medical abbreviations has been identified by the Institute for Safe Medication Practices (ISMP) and the FDA as one of the most common but preventable sources of medication errors (ISMP, 2017). Refer to the website for the ISMP at https://www.ismp.org/Tools/abbreviations for more information about their campaign to eliminate the use of error-prone abbreviations. In addition, the ISMP has identified a list of error-prone abbreviations, symbols, and dose designations that should never be used when communicating medical information (ISMP, 2017). See Table 20-2 for this list.

Table 30-2 Routes for Administering Drugs

TERMS USED TO DESCRIBE ROUTE	HOW DRUG IS ADMINISTERED
Oral route	Having patient swallow drug
Enteral route	Administering drug through an enteral tube
Sublingual administration	Placing drug under tongue
Buccal administration	Placing drug between cheek and gum
Parenteral route	Injecting drug into the body
Subcutaneous injection	Subcutaneous tissue
Intramuscular injection	Muscle tissue
Intradermal injection	Corium (under epidermis)
Intravenous injection	Vein
Intra-arterial injection	Artery
Intracardial injection	Heart tissue
Intraperitoneal injection	Peritoneal cavity
Intraspinal injection	Spinal canal
Intraosseous injection	Bone
Topical route	Applying drug onto skin or mucous membrane
Vaginal administration	Vagina
Rectal administration	Rectum
Inunction	Rubbing drug into skin
Instillation	Placing drug into direct contact with mucous membrane
Irrigation	Flushing mucous membrane with drug in solution
Skin application	Applying transdermal patch
Pulmonary route	Having patient inhale drug

ROUTE OF ADMINISTRATION

The route to be used when administering a medication is stated clearly because some drugs can be given in more than one way, and others may be used safely through only one route. The route also affects the absorption of drug. Table 30-2 describes common routes by which medications are administered. Refer to The Nursing Process for Administering Medications beginning on page 935 for guidelines on administering drugs by these routes.

FREQUENCY OF ADMINISTRATION

The time and frequency with which a drug is to be administered are usually stated in standard abbreviations in the medication order. Keep in mind that only approved abbreviations are used, and care is taken to not use old abbreviations that have been phased out due to error and safety concerns (see Table 20-3 on page 528). Common abbreviations used in writing prescriptions, including time and frequency, are listed in Box 20-3 on page 524.

The nursing service, facility policy, and pharmacy departments of inpatient facilities usually determine the hours at which routine drugs are given. To lessen the risk for error, many health care facilities use the 24-hour clock (or military time), which designates midnight as 0000 hours and runs until 2400 hours. For example, an every-4-hour drug administration may be at the times of 1200, 1600, 2000, 0000, 0400, and 0800. Another facility may use the hours 1300, 1700, 1900, 0100, 0500, and 0900. If an administration order states that the drug is to be given before or after meals, the time of administration depends on the hours at which meals are served. It is a nursing and pharmacy responsibility to check that times for medication administration correspond to safe practice for that drug.

If a drug is to be given only once or twice a day, the decision about which hours to use depends on the nature of the drug and the patient's plan of care, as well as the standard facility administration times. Whenever possible, consider the patient's choice of time.

Administer drugs punctually, as ordered. A nurse administering medications to several patients cannot reasonably give all of the medications to all of the patients exactly on the hour indicated. Facility policies vary, but a common one is that drugs should be administered within a half-hour before or after the indicated hour. Thus, a drug to be administered at 0900 can be administered any time between 0830 and 0930 using this policy. However, it is important to note that this policy does not apply to all drugs. A preoperative medication ordered to be given at 0730 should be administered at that hour because the time was planned in relation to the time that surgery is to begin. Preoperative medications may also be given when the nursing unit receives a call from the operating room to premedicate the surgical patient. This also holds true when patients are given drugs before certain diagnostic procedures and with stat orders.

SIGNATURE OF THE PRESCRIBING PROVIDER

Prescribers using a CPOE access the system using a unique username and password. The identifying information of the prescribing provider, such as name and title, is automatically recorded when the system is accessed, and a handwritten signature is not necessary. When it is necessary to handwrite a prescription, the signature, title, and identifiers (such as the DEA or National Provider Identifier [NPI] numbers) of the prescriber must accompany the order. Many facilities require prescribers to also include their printed name and address with the signature, to facilitate contacting the prescriber as needed.

This identifying information is important for legal reasons because the authority to prescribe drugs is defined by state laws. Also, if there is a question about the prescription, the identifying information indicates who should be contacted.

Checking the Medication Order

Facility policy specifies the manner in which the medication order is checked. Various systems are used; nurses should be familiar with the system used in the facility where they work and should use it as trained to minimize errors.

The patient's medication record, often called an MAR (medication administration record) is a complete list of all medications prescribed for the patient. Increasing numbers of health care facilities are computerizing patient records, including medication records (eMARs [electronic medication administration record]). The nurse is responsible for checking that the medication order was transcribed correctly by comparing it with the original order, depending on the type of system in use. The nurse is also responsible for double-checking the dosage and appropriateness of the medication.

Questioning the Medication Order

Nurses are legally responsible for the drugs they administer. Therefore, it is important to question any drug order suspected to be in error. The suspected error may be in any part of the order. A study of neonatal nurses in Australia identified several things that impact on nurses questioning an order, including the working environment (whether positive or negative), their perceived responsibility to do the right thing, and their knowledge about medications (Aydon et al., 2016). When preparing to administer a medication, ask yourself why the patient is receiving the medication—is there a rationale you can provide as to why this medication has been prescribed? Do the therapeutic and pharmacologic classes link with your patient's condition(s)? If not, then ask the provider or pharmacist, and/or use an appropriate resource to further investigate. Perhaps the provider inadvertently prescribed the wrong medication—the only way to be sure is to ask. Take the time to look up the medication, especially if it is one you do not use on a daily basis, and consider whether the dose, route, frequency, and prescribed use are within the range of what your resource lists. Once in practice, nurses tend to become familiar with medications used frequently with the patient populations they serve, but learning what is a *reasonable* dose takes time and experience. There are potential legal implications if a medication error occurs when, based on education and experience, the nurse should have noted and reported the error. Confusion over the placement of a decimal point can lead to a medication error. A zero should always precede a decimal point (e.g., 0.1 mg) for clarity. The use of a trailing zero (e.g., 1.0) is not considered good practice and has been included in The Joint Commission's *Do not use* list. See Table 20-3 on page 528 for additional abbreviations included in this list.

A drug to which the patient is allergic may be prescribed inadvertently. In health care facilities, the allergy is listed in the chart/EHR, specifically on the eMAR/MAR, and may also be linked to the computerized medication dispensing system. The patient may wear a wristband (often red) that indicates specific allergies, so be sure to check for this when you first identify the patient. Before administering a medication, best practice is to question the patient about ever having received the medication and ask whether the patient is aware of any reaction to the medication. The patient may describe past adverse reactions with the drug. If the nurse suspects an undocumented allergy, the nurse should not give the drug and notify the provider. An allergic reaction can be life threatening to the patient.

In addition, a drug may be prescribed that would potentially interact with another medication the patient is taking. It is important that nurses verify all medications that they are unfamiliar with before administration to avoid possible drug interactions. If a nurse has difficulty deciphering a prescription, guessing is gross carelessness; checking with the provider who wrote the prescription is the only safe procedure.

Nurses have the right to refuse to administer any medication that, based on their knowledge and experience, may be harmful to the patient. Although this situation seldom occurs, it is important to understand that the patient's safety is a primary objective in the administration of medications. Always notify the primary care provider of the refusal to administer any medication. Document any concerns regarding medication orders in the patient's medical record, and note having contacted the primary care provider, the response of the primary care provider, and any related interventions. A standardized interprofessional approach to medication administration coupled with an emphasis on patient safety creates an environment that supports the nurse questioning an order, which may directly impact on patient outcomes.

Medication Supply Systems

Medications are supplied in a number of ways. Many facilities make use of one or more systems in conjunction with each other, or variations of systems. Unit dose dispensing on a patient-specific basis is now the standard of practice for most hospitals. Pharmaceutical manufacturers provide all medications in health systems in unit dose packages that are labeled with readable medication information and computer scannable bar-coding that includes the medication's unique identifier, lot number, and expiration date (American Society of Health-System Pharmacists [ASHP], 2009). Computerized automated dispensing cabinets are a technology based on stock supply of unit dose medications. A large cabinet containing stock medications for the unit is used. The nurse accesses the system with a user name and password, pulling up a medication list for a specific patient or a list of available medications. In many systems, only medications entered for a specific patient are available for withdrawal at any one time. A computerized medication dispensing system is shown in Figure 30-1 on page 930. With an individual unit dose supply system, each patient is supplied with the medication needed for a period of time. The nurse is responsible for accurately obtaining the prescribed medications from the patient's supply. In the unit dose system, the pharmacist simplifies medication preparation by packaging and labeling each dosage for a 24-hour period.

Some nursing units use a medication cart for the administration of medications. The standard cart contains individual drawers into which the medications for each patient are placed. If computers are not standard in every patient room and an EHR is used, there may also be a computer attached

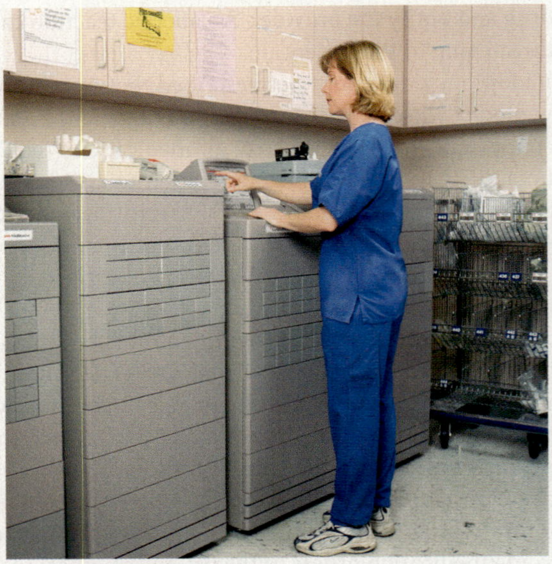

FIGURE 30-1. Computerized medication dispensing system.

to the cart that allows for ready access to the eMAR by the administering nurse. The nurse moves the cart from room to room when dispensing medications.

Bar-code medication administration (BCMA) involves a computerized bar-coded administration system, where each patient and each nurse is identified by a unique bar code. Each drug is also packaged with a bar code that includes its unique National Drug Code number to identify the form and dosage. The nurse scans their own ID, the patient's ID, and each package of medication to be administered. The system confirms the nurse's dispensing authority and the patient's ID, matching the patient with their medication profile. If any of the information is incorrect or does not match, an alert message will appear on the screen notifying the nurse of the discrepancy. The system also records the medication administration and stores the information (ASHP, 2009). The implementation of BCMA technology has the potential to reduce administration errors not related to timing, errors associated with transcription of orders, and total medication errors (Shah et al., 2016).

Technology Alert

Bar-Code Medication Administration (BCMA)

BCMA uses bar-code technology to provide a safeguard against human error. Although BCMA has contributed to a reduction in medication errors, work-arounds that deviate from institution policy and procedures need to be addressed. Identification of best-practice workflow needs to be compared to actual bedside observed workflow using processes such as root cause analysis (see Chapter 28). Clinical nurses must be engaged in the process of identification and removal of barriers to BCMA best practice and work to establish a culture of safety. Reinforcement and support by nurses' social networks in the clinical environment can positively affect nurses' compliance with appropriate use of BCMA (Yuan et al., 2020).

Dosage Calculations

Systems of Measurement

Nurses need to be proficient in the use of weights and measures as well as systems of measurement to calculate drug dosages and prepare medications for administration. Two systems of measurement are used in the United States for administering medications: the metric system and the household system. The apothecary system was used infrequently in the past and is no longer used for measurement of medications (McCuistion et al., 2021). The nurse may be called on to convert dosages from metric to household and household to metric. It is extremely important to be able to calculate commonly used equivalents, as listed in Appendix B. Practice the Medication Calculation Problems at the end of this chapter to develop your dose calculation skills.

METRIC SYSTEM

The metric system is the most widely accepted and convenient system of measurement. The basic units of measurement are the meter (linear), the liter (volume), and the gram (weight). The metric system is a decimal system, in which each unit can be divided into multiples of 10 (10, 100, 1,000). Calculations in the metric system often involve moving the decimal point to the right or left. In the preparation of medications, the following metric units are typically used:

Weight

- 1 kilogram = 1,000 grams
- 1 gram = 1,000 milligrams
- 1 milligram = 1,000 micrograms

Volume

- 1 liter = 1,000 milliliters or cubic centimeters

It may be necessary to convert drug dosages to a different unit in the metric system. To convert a larger unit into a smaller unit, move the decimal point to the right (the new number is larger than the original). To convert a smaller unit into a larger unit, move the decimal point to the left (the new number is smaller than the original). *Example 1:* 0.5 g equals how many milligrams? Move the decimal point three places to right; the answer is 500 mg. *Example 2:* 900 mg equals how many grams? Move the decimal point three places to the left; the answer is 0.9 g.

HOUSEHOLD SYSTEM

The household system is not widely used except in some community settings, such as a person's home. Teaspoon and tablespoon are commonly used household measures. The household system is not as accurate as the metric system because of the lack of standardization of spoons, cups, and glasses. The measurements are approximate, so the National Council for Prescription Drug Programs (NCPDP, n.d.) and other entities (American Academy of Pediatrics, 2015) advocate for the transition to the metric system in the United States for all dosing. Until this occurs, nurses need to reinforce that a teaspoon is considered to be equivalent to 5 mL. Three teaspoons equal one tablespoon. One ounce is considered to be equivalent to 30 mL. As discussed previously, teaspoon and tablespoon refer to measuring spoons, not silverware.

Methods for Computing Drug Dosages

Drugs are sometimes prepared and supplied in the amount ordered by the prescriber, and the nurse can see when checking the medication label that no calculation is necessary. At other times, drugs are not prepared and supplied in the exact quantities called for in the medication order, and the nurse must do a dosage calculation to determine what quantity of medication the patient is to receive.

FORMULA METHODS

Several formulas can be used to calculate drug dosages. One such formula consists of ratios to set up a proportion and can be used to calculate dosages for both solid and liquid preparations. A ratio shows the relation between numbers. A proportion contains two ratios. The nurse is usually seeking the quantity of on-hand medication that is equal to the desired dosage (the dosage ordered). The formula is as follows:

$$\frac{\text{dose on hand}}{\text{quantity on hand}} = \frac{\text{dose desired}}{x\,(\text{quantity desired})}$$

The dosage must be in the same unit of measurement. This applies to the quantity as well. Dosages are on the top line of the proportion, quantities on the bottom line. After the numbers are placed in the proportion, cross-multiply to find the desired quantity. The benefit of this method is that it is predictable and easy to recall: "I have 250 mg in 5 mL and I need 625 mg in I-don't-know-how-many mL." The proportion method of calculation works best with simple calculations.

Example: Amoxicillin, 625 mg PO, is ordered. It is supplied as a liquid preparation containing 250 mg in 5 mL. How much does the nurse administer?

$$\frac{250\text{ mg}}{5\text{ mL}} = \frac{625\text{ mg}}{x\text{ mL}}$$

Cross multiply:

$$250x = 3{,}125$$

Isolate x:

$$\frac{250x}{250} = \frac{3{,}125}{250}$$

$$x = 12.5\text{ mL}$$

Remember to *Drag-the-Tag* (the measurement associated with the x from the beginning formula)

Follow the standard rounding rules: For numbers >1, round to the 10th (tenth); for numbers <1, round to the 100th (hundredth).

Example: Digoxin 0.125 mg PO daily is prescribed. It is available as a liquid in a unit dose container labeled 500 mcg/10 mL. How many mL does the nurse administer? There are two systems of measurement in this problem and conversions cannot be built into this formula, so the conversion must take place before using the proportion method. The nurse knows that 1 mg is equal to 1,000 mcg; therefore, 0.125 mg equals 125 mcg.

$$\frac{500\text{ mcg}}{10\text{ mL}} = \frac{125\text{ mcg}}{x\text{ mL}}$$

Cross multiply:

$$500x = 1{,}250$$

Isolate x:

$$\frac{500x}{500} = \frac{1{,}250}{500}$$

$$x = 2.5\text{ mL}$$

Drag-the-Tag

Follow the standard rounding rules: For numbers >1, round to the 10th (tenth); for numbers <1, round to the 100th (hundredth).

Another formula that can be used to calculate drug dosages is as follows:

$$\frac{\text{dose desired}}{\text{dose on hand}} \times \text{quantity on hand} = \text{desired quantity}$$

Using this formula, the previous example would be solved as:

Don't forget to multiply by quantity on hand.

$$\frac{125\text{ mcg}}{500\text{ mcg}} \times 10\text{ mL} = x$$

$$\frac{125\ \cancel{\text{mcg}}}{500\ \cancel{\text{mcg}}} \times 10\text{ mL} = 2.5\text{ mL}$$

The mcg will cancel, leaving mL for labeling the answer.
Follow the standard rounding rules: For numbers >1, round to the 10th (tenth); for numbers <1, round to the 100th (hundredth).

This formula can be used for both liquid dosages and fractions of tablets. However, this formula can lead to errors if the carrier (10 mL in the example above) is not 1. The proportion (above) and dimensional analysis (below) methods are recommended.

DIMENSIONAL ANALYSIS

Another method that is used to compute medication dosages is dimensional analysis. Dimensional analysis, also known as factor-labeled method, is a systematic, straightforward approach to setting up and solving problems that require conversions. It is an excellent way to approach medication math because it can be used with both simple and complex medication calculations. A standard approach in chemistry, dimensional analysis is a way of thinking about problems that can be used when conversions are needed to move from an order to a dose. When using dimensional analysis, the first numerator must be what you are solving for, with the remaining part of the equation working to cancel out all unnecessary content.

For instance, in the amoxicillin example, you would set up the equation like this:

$$\text{mL} = \frac{5\ \text{mL}}{250\ \text{mg}} \times \frac{625\ \text{mg}}{1}$$

$$\text{mL} = \frac{5\ \text{mL}}{250\ \cancel{\text{mg}}} \times \frac{625\ \cancel{\text{mg}}}{1} = 12.5\ \text{mL}$$

Cancel out in multiplication.
Follow the standard rounding rules: For numbers >1, round to the 10th (tenth); for numbers <1, round to the 100th (hundredth).

Dimensional analysis can also include conversion factors in the same calculation. For instance, the nurse is to administer 50 mcg fentanyl. The pharmacy supplies the nurse with an ampule of fentanyl 0.1 mg/2 mL. How much should the nurse administer? To solve the problem, the mg needs to be converted to mcg. This can all be done in the same calculation with dimensional analysis.

Conversion from mcg to mg.

$$\text{mL} = \frac{2\ \text{mL}}{0.1\ \text{mg}} \times \frac{1\ \text{mg}}{1{,}000\ \text{mcg}} \times \frac{50\ \text{mcg}}{1}$$

$$\text{mL} = \frac{2\ \text{mL}}{0.1\ \cancel{\text{mg}}} \times \frac{1\ \cancel{\text{mg}}}{\underset{20}{\cancel{1{,}000}}\ \cancel{\text{mcg}}} \times \frac{\overset{1}{\cancel{50}}\ \cancel{\text{mcg}}}{1} = \frac{2\ \text{mL}}{2} = 1\ \text{mL}$$

Cancel out and reduce in multiplication.

Here is an example of what the starting formula would look like in the more traditional chemistry format:

2 mL	1 mg	50 mcg
0.1 mg	1,000 mcg	1

Pediatric Calculations

According to Kyle and Carman (2021), the most common method for calculating pediatric medication doses is based on body weight, due to the wide range of size differences from infants to toddlers to school-age children. The recommended dosage is usually expressed as the amount of drug to be given over a 24-hour period (mg/kg/day) or as a single dose (mg/kg/dose). When calculating pediatric drug dosages, check whether the prescribed amount is per dose or per 24-hour period. A medication overdose can occur if the nurse does not note that the calculation is per 24 hours and gives the total amount of medication in one dose. Weigh the child and, if necessary, convert the weight into kilograms by dividing the child's weight in pounds by 2.2 to compute the equivalent kilograms of weight. Then multiply the child's weight in kilograms by the prescribed dose to obtain the appropriate dose for the child. A drug reference book will identify the safe dose range for pediatric drug dosages based on weight.

Using Safety Measures While Preparing Drugs

The National Coordinating Council for Medication Error Reporting and Prevention (2020, para. 1) states,

> A medication error is any preventable event that may cause or lead to inappropriate medication use or patient harm while the medication is in the control of the health care professional, patient, or consumer. Such events may be related to professional practice, health care products, procedures, and systems, including prescribing, order communication, product labeling, packaging, and nomenclature, compounding, dispensing, distribution, administration, education, monitoring, and use.

Medication errors can occur with almost any type of drug. Errors are more common with certain classes of medications, such as analgesics, antibiotics, anticoagulants, chemotherapeutic agents, diabetic medications, and cardiovascular agents. This is thought to possibly be due to the pharmacologic properties of the drugs that result in more adverse effects, toxicities, and interactions. Medication errors are also common in drugs with narrow therapeutic levels and in drugs prescribed frequently (Frandsen & Pennington, 2021). Safety is of the utmost importance in preparing and administering medications. There are many interventions that can minimize the risk for medication errors. The following is a discussion of nursing interventions to reduce this risk.

Three Checks and the Rights of Medication Administration

Use of the three checks and the rights of medication administration when administering medications can assist with safe administration of medications. The use of the previously discussed technology, such as bar-code medication administration (BCMA) and medication dispensing systems, does not relieve the nurse of responsibility for ensuring safe medication administration. Check the label on the medication package or container three times during medication preparation and administration. The label should be read:

1. **When the nurse reaches for the unit dose package or container**
2. **After retrieval from the drawer and compared with the eMAR/MAR, or compared with the eMAR/MAR immediately before pouring from a multidose container**
3. **Just before giving the unit dose medication to the patient, or when returning the multidose container**

Figure 30-2 illustrates the comparison of a medication label with the eMAR (second label check) to ensure accuracy.

The rights of medication administration can help to ensure accuracy when administering medications. However, the ISMP (2007) reiterated a position taken in 1999 that, the rights of medication administration "are merely broadly stated goals or desired outcomes of safe medication practices that offer no procedural guidance on how to achieve these goals" (para. 1). The rights themselves do *not* ensure

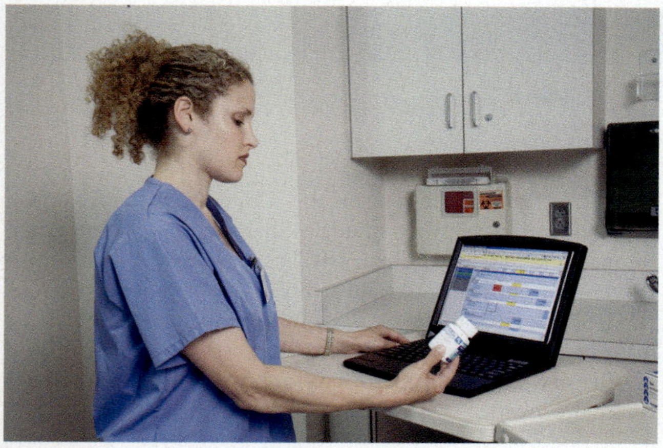

FIGURE 30-2. Comparing medication label with eMAR.

medication safety. The nurse assumes individual accountability for safe drug administration by collaborating with the patient and interprofessional team, and engaging in behavior that follows the standards of practice defined by the institution to achieve the goals of the rights (Frandsen & Pennington, 2021; Hanson & Haddad, 2020). Suggested rights of administration vary slightly between references, with anywhere from the classic 5 rights (listed first) through upward of 11 rights of medication administration common in the literature (Frandsen & Pennington, 2021; McCuistion et al., 2021; Smeulers et al., 2015). Nurses should integrate reliance on embedded, sometime rote, processes with intentional decision-making grounded in clinical judgment.

QSEN RIGHTS OF ADMINISTRATION

Keep in mind that nurses consider the rights of medication administration while adhering to standards of practice, policies, and procedures in order to promote safe medication administration.

Ensure that the (1) **right medication** is given to the (2) **right patient** in the (3) **right dosage** (in the right form) through the (4) **right route** at the (5) **right time** for the (6) **right reason** based on the (7) **right (appropriate) assessment data** using the (8) **right documentation** and monitoring for the (9) **right response** by the patient. Additional rights have been suggested to include (10) the **right to education**, ensuring that patients receive accurate and thorough information about the medication, and (11) the **right to refuse**, acknowledging that patients can and do refuse to take a medication. The first five rights are included in most references to the rights of medication administration and are the ones verified at each of the three checks. Validating the right reason requires the nurse to understand the rationale for administration and answer the questions, "Does it make sense?" and "Is it appropriate for this person?" The right documentation refers to accurate and timely documentation of administration. The right response refers to the evaluation by the nurse related to the effectiveness of the medication's intended purpose and monitoring the patient for the desired response. When a patient refuses to take a medication, the nurse should try to determine the reason for the refusal and take reasonable measures to convince the patient to take the medication, explaining the risk of refusal and reinforcing the reason for the medication. The patient's refusal and any education and/or explanation provided related to trying to facilitate administration must be documented. The primary care provider should be informed of the refusal, especially when the omission poses a specific threat to the patient (McCuistion et al., 2021).

In addition, it is important to acknowledge that nurses are not the only professionals responsible for the medication administration process. Medication administration is a process with many interconnected players, including clinical nurses, physicians, advanced practice professionals, pharmacists, and patients. All involved in the process share the responsibility for a safe medication system (Hanson & Haddad, 2020). Education and training should focus on interprofessional roles and responsibilities, communication techniques, and other initiatives that foster the teamwork required to promote patient safety in medication administration processes (Bartlett & Kinsey, 2020).

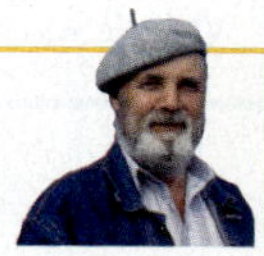

Think back to ***Mr. Baptiste***, the patient described in the beginning of the chapter and the Reflective Practice display. By adhering to the rights of medication administration, the nurse would be able to determine that the medication delivered by the pharmacy was labeled incorrectly.

Maintaining a Safe Environment

An environment that promotes safety and good working habits contributes to accuracy in the preparation of drugs for administration. Refer to the Research in Nursing display Practice Environments and Medication Errors on page 934. Nurses should be aware of the higher risk of making an error when their work flow is distracted or interrupted. Bravo, Cochran, and Barrett (2016) discuss physical working conditions that can influence the nurse's ability to perform safely, highlighting the need to decide whether to deflect, defer, or address distractions. An international study (Cottell et al., 2020) reported that participants identified the following as causes of medication incidents: (1) shortcoming in their individual knowledge, skills, and/or abilities; (2) patient and medication regimen complexities; (3) team factors related to communication, supervision, or support; (4) lack of clarity regarding policies, procedures, or protocols; and (5) the work environment including heavy workload, staffing mix, and availability of equipment. The hospital/unit structure, leadership, teamwork, communication, and required safety measures also impact on the environment, either positively or negatively affecting the probability of medication errors.

After beginning to prepare drugs for administration, do not leave them unattended. If it is imperative to leave for a short time, place the prepared drugs in a locked area, such as in the medication cart. The nurse who prepares the

Research in Nursing

BRIDGING THE GAP TO EVIDENCE-BASED PRACTICE

Practice Environments and Medication Errors

Medication preparation and administration is primarily a nursing responsibility in the acute care setting. How do nurses cope when an error is made and how do they use this experience to prevent future errors?

Related Research

Athanasakis, E. (2019). A meta-synthesis of how registered nurses make sense of their lived experiences of medication errors. *Journal of Clinical Nursing, 28*(17–18), 3077–3095. https://doi.org/10.1111/jocn.14917

This meta-synthesis presents an analysis of published, sound qualitative studies that met defined inclusion criteria and focused on an exploration of nurses' lived experience with medication errors. Themes identified through this synthesis included: (1) human fallibility related to personal stress, workload, and distractions; (2) the emotional impact (ranged from self-doubt to shame, fear, and powerlessness) that resulted in symptoms often associated with post-traumatic stress disorder; (3) constructive learning that addressed individual as well as organizational accountability; (4) impact on licensure (registration in the United Kingdom) and employment; (5) copying strategies that stemmed from reassurance and support from trusted colleagues; (6) consideration of the patient status and safety; (7) root cause analysis; and (8) identification of preventative measures moving forward. Medication errors are a multifaceted issue with both positive and negative implications for nurses and the facilities where they work.

Relevance to Nursing Practice

Although the classification of a medication error can vary (error of omission through wrong dose/route/patient) and the associated ramifications for patients range from minor to severe, the impact of a medication error often extends past the immediate patient outcome. Nurses harbor feelings regarding the incident and must intentionally reflect on the lessons learned and clinical judgment processes, while also allowing themselves the space to grow and the grace to continue in the profession.

medication also administers the drug and records the drug administration. When not working at the medication dispensing system or medication cart, keep it locked. This is a requirement of the certifying bodies of hospitals.

Handling Controlled Substances Safely

Medication dispensing systems should be locked; this includes securement of controlled substances. Depending on the system used, controlled substances may be kept in an internal locked drawer or container as an added safety measure, providing for a *double locked* system. Opioids or other controlled substances may be prescribed only by physicians; in some states, nurse practitioners and physician assistants who are registered with the Department of Justice, Bureau of Narcotics, and Dangerous Drugs may prescribe them as well. According to federal law, a record must be kept for each narcotic that is administered. Although methods of recording may differ, the following information usually is required:

- Name of the patient receiving the controlled substance
- Amount of the substance used
- Hour the controlled substance was given
- Name of the prescribing provider
- Name of the nurse who administered the substance

It is a common practice to check controlled substances daily at specified intervals. In hospitals, this check is usually performed at each shift change. The number of doses of all controlled substances stored in the dispensing system is counted and must match the number of doses accounted for in the administration records. Many facilities use various computerized systems for dispensing narcotics and other controlled substances. Tracking controlled substances is often supported by the computerized automated dispensing cabinets that store unit dose medications for the unit. The nurse has a secure identification code that provides access to the system, identifies the patient by name or identification number, and prompts verification of the expected count of each drug as it is removed. Because the nurse's secure identification code is equivalent to the nurse's signature, it should never be given out to other staff members. Manual counting is warranted if a nurse discovers the controlled substance count is incorrect. A controlled substance count that does not match the count expected by the administration records must be reported and rectified immediately. The law requires these special precautions to aid in the control of substance use disorder by patients and health care workers.

The nurse administering controlled substances has an important responsibility to see that the federal law is observed. If for any reason a controlled substance prepared for administration has to be discarded, a second nurse should act as a witness. This validation by two nurses is recorded based on the requirements of the medication system in use. Document with a witness any time a full dosage is not given and some of the controlled substance needs to be discarded. For instance, if 3 mg of an opioid has been prescribed and the opioid is available in a vial of 4 mg/4 mL, the remaining 1 mg (1 mL) should be disposed of (also known as *wasted*) while a witness is watching, and both registered nurses should record the transaction according to facility policy and medication system in use.

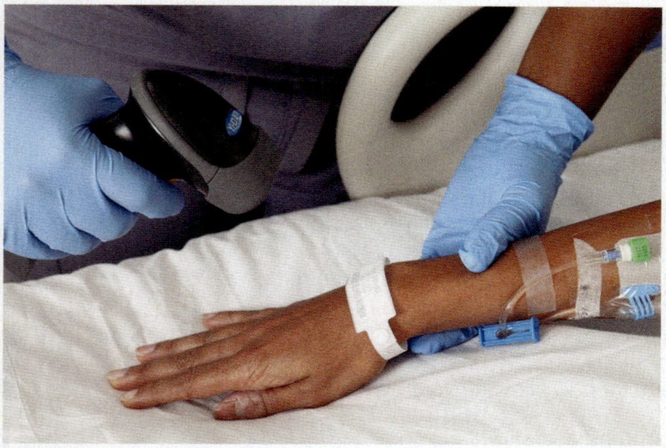

FIGURE 30-3. Scanning the name-band as part of checking patient's identity. In addition to scanning, the patient should also verbally confirm two identifiers such as name and birthday (when possible).

Identifying the Patient

Positive identification of the patient is essential to safe drug administration. Before administering the drug, check carefully to see that the right drug is being given to the right patient. The 2020 National Patient Safety Goals established by The Joint Commission (2020a) states that whenever administering patient medications, at least two patient identifiers should be used. The patient's room number or physical location may not be used to validate patient identification. Patients in inpatient health care facilities usually wear identification bracelets, sometimes referred to as a *name-band* or *arm band.* Identify the patient by checking the identification wristband, as shown in Figure 30-3. Before referring to the patient by name, ask the patient (when possible) to verbally state their name and birthdate to verify they are wearing the correct arm band. Then validate the patient's name (first identifier) and identification number, medical record number, and/or birth date (second identifier), comparing with the eMAR or MAR. Specific identifiers used depend on facility policy. If using a bar-code system, the nurse will also scan the patient's bracelet. Scanning, although an important safety step in the medication administration process, does *not* replace the need for verbal and visual confirmation of the patient's identity using two identifiers. The computer system will validate the patient's identification, but this does not replace the manual name-band and eMAR/MAR verification the nurse should perform. In some long-term care facilities, a current photograph of the resident, displayed above the resident's bed, can also be used for identification.

NURSING PROCESS FOR ADMINISTERING MEDICATIONS

Assessing

Assessment of the patient receiving medications begins during a nursing history. One component of this is the medication history, which informs the medication reconciliation process. During the interview, the nurse can adapt questions to meet the patient's needs and level of understanding. Avoid using medical jargon that the patient may not understand; use familiar terms as possible. For instance, the patient may refer to a diuretic as the "water pill" or to an anticoagulant as a "blood thinner." Areas to be included in the medication history are listed in the accompanying Focused Assessment Guide 30-1 on page 936.

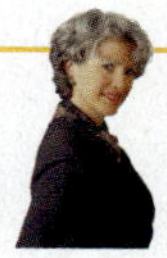

The nurse caring for **Mildred Campbell** would need to incorporate the information the patient shared regarding her interest in an advertised medication when assessing the patient. This information is extremely important to prevent possible drug interactions should the patient decide to use the medication advertised on television.

Additional information to be assessed includes the patient's health status, current and past illnesses, laboratory test results, known drug allergies, and religious beliefs and/or cultural practices. Assess the patient with regard to medications during the nursing history and continue the assessment during and after medication administration.

Diagnosing Actual or Potential Health Problems and Needs

Data that the nurse collect may lead to diagnosing one or more actual or potential health problems or needs related to medication administration. Following diagnosing actual or potential health problems or needs, the nurse communicates their findings to other nursing and health care professionals through the use of the written and spoken word. The written health problem becomes a permanent part of the patient's health record. The actual and potential problems are verbally communicated during hand-off and interprofessional team meetings as part of the SBAR report. Examples of patient problems and needs with related etiology and signs and symptoms can be found in the box titled Examples of Actual or Potential Health Problems and Needs: Medication Administration on page 937.

Outcome Identification and Planning

Nursing measures for patients receiving medication are directed toward the patient's achievement of the following goals:

- Expected therapeutic effects will be demonstrated within a specified time frame
- Expected change in symptoms: for example, the patient's pain will be relieved, or vital signs will return to baseline
- Maintenance of therapeutic blood levels of medication
- The patient will correctly identify key information regarding prescribed medications

Implementing

Remain with the patient and make sure that the medication is taken. If the patient receives several drugs, offer them separately so that if one is refused or dropped, positive

Focused Assessment Guide 30-1

MEDICATIONS

Factors to Assess	Questions and Approaches
Previous and current drug use	• What medications are you taking that the primary care provider prescribed for you? • What over-the-counter medications and natural or herbal supplements are you taking on a regular basis? • Do you use nonmedicinal drugs (e.g., alcohol, caffeine, home remedies)? • How often do you use them? • What is the reason for taking the medications? • What medications have you taken during the past year and for what reasons? • Is there anything else you have tried to alleviate your symptoms?
Medication schedule	• At what times do you take your medications? • Is there a special way any of your medications has to be prepared (e.g., crushing and mixing with applesauce)? • Do you have any special method for remembering to take your medications?
Response to medications	• Do you have any allergies to medications? • Have the medications had the expected effects? • Have you ever experienced any adverse or unexpected reactions to the medications? • Is there a family history of this type of reaction to medications?
Attitude toward drugs and use of drugs	• How do you feel about taking medications? • Do you have any emotional responses regarding your medications (e.g. anxiety, distrust, fear, body image disturbance, anger, etc.) that may interfere with your desire to take the medications? • Why do you take the medications?
Adherence to regimen	• Can you tell me your understanding of the reason for taking the medications? • Can you describe how you follow the medication schedule? • Are there any problems that prevent you from following the medication regimen? • Can you afford your medications? • Do you have a reliable means for obtaining your medications (e.g. online delivery, pharmacy pick-up, transportation)? • Do you have adequate knowledge of how to take or administer your medications? • Have you performed a return demonstration for any complex administration procedures?
Storage	• Where are your medications stored at home? • How long do you keep medications in the home? • Can you show me any medications you have on hand?

identification can be made, and the drug can be recorded or replaced. Open each medication package after providing any necessary teaching and confirming the patient will take the medication. Never leave medications at the bedside for the patient to take later. This is an unsafe practice because the patient may forget to take the medication, or someone else may take the medication. Record medication administration while or immediately after the patient takes the medication. Some facilities allow patients to self-administer certain drugs. Be familiar with facility policy on this matter.

Table 30-3 (on page 938) summarizes questions to ask and actions to take when administering drugs by any route to ensure the correct administration of medications, as well as examples of nursing interventions to promote safe medication administration and appropriate outcomes.

Administering Oral Medications

Drugs given orally are intended for absorption in the stomach and small intestine. The oral route is the most common route of administration. PO, the common shorthand for oral administration, is based on the Latin *per os*, which means "by mouth" (Frandsen & Pennington, 2021). It is usually the most convenient and comfortable route for the patient. Drugs administered orally have slower onset and a more prolonged, but less potent, effect than drugs administered via other routes. There are certain situations in which oral medications should not be administered, such as when the patient has difficulty swallowing, is unconscious, is to receive nothing by mouth (NPO), or is vomiting. Occasionally, a patient may unintentionally or intentionally hide a medication in the mouth. Ensure that the medication was actually swallowed before recording that it has been taken.

Oral medications are available in solid and liquid form. Solid preparations include tablets, capsules, and pills. Some tablets are scored (intentionally grooved by the manufacturer) for easy breaking if a partial quantity is needed. Unless a tablet is scored, do not break it by hand because doing so could result in an inaccurate dose. Enteric-coated tablets are

Examples of Actual or Potential Health Problems and Needs

MEDICATION ADMINISTRATION

Actual or Potential Health Problem or Need	Possible Etiologic Factors	Potential Signs and Symptoms
Knowledge Deficiency	• Introduction of new medication(s) • Varied drug interactions, side effects, adverse effects, and toxicities • Actual/potential person-centered implications related to class, action, administration, distribution, metabolism, or excretion of medication(s) • Complex directions regarding administration route and process	• Verbalizations of confusion • Anxiety regarding new medications • Inability to describe medication action, side effects, risk factors, or how to administer the medication
Risk for Alterations in Gastrointestinal Motility	• Eating habit change • Potential/actual drug interactions and absorption variations • Immobility • Stressors • Side effects associated with pharmaceutical agent and treatment regimen	—
Impaired Ability to Manage Medication Regime	• New medication regimen • Complex medication regimen • Lifestyle/role changes associated with medication regimen • Adherence issues involving social determinants of health such as access, affordability, and patient/caregiver engagement	• Inability to make choices of daily living that support medication regimen management • Failure to take medications as prescribed • Verbalization of difficulty in managing medication regimen • Manifestations of disease/disorder progression, lack of symptom management, and/or unintended signs and symptoms

Source: International Council of Nurses (ICN). (2019). *Nursing diagnosis and outcome statements.* https://www.icn.ch/sites/default/files/inline-files/ICNP2019-DC.pdf; Wolters Kluwer. (2022). Problem-based care plans. In *Lippincott Advisor.* Wolters Kluwer. https://advisor.lww.com/lna/home.do

covered with a hard surface that impedes absorption until the tablet has left the stomach; thus, the medication is released in the small intestine. Enteric-coated tablets are used when the active ingredient of the drug is irritating to the stomach mucosa. As a result, less gastrointestinal irritation occurs and the medication is protected from destruction by gastric acid. Enteric-coated tablets should not be chewed or crushed because crushing the medication destroys the protective coating. Other forms of oral medications that should not be chewed or crushed without checking with the prescriber include any of the extended-release forms, such as SR (sustained release), ER (extended release), CR or CRT (controlled release), SA (sustained action), or LA (long acting). Chewing and/or crushing these medications destroys their extended-release delivery mechanism and may result in potentially toxic peaks and low troughs.

Liquid preparations include elixirs, spirits, suspensions, and syrups. Some are water-based solutions, and others are alcohol-based solutions. If the patient has had a previous drug or alcohol addiction, it is important to carefully consider the administration of medications containing alcohol. Disposable, calibrated cups are available for the administration of liquid medications. For patients who find it difficult to take liquids from a cup, the medication can be placed in the mouth directly using a plastic, needleless, oral syringe. Place the syringe between the gum and cheek and give the liquid to the patient slowly—most adults can tolerate 5 mL at a time without issue. This technique, in addition to having the patient in an upright or side-lying position, helps prevent the patient from choking and aspirating the medication. Shake emulsions and suspensions well and administer them promptly to ensure an accurate dosage.

Liquids are available in multidose bottles and single-dose containers. If a label becomes difficult to read or accidentally comes off the container, return the container to the pharmacy. Never give a medication from a bottle without a label or with a label that cannot be read with accuracy. Because of the danger of error and contamination, do not return unused medications to their bottles. Exercise care in pouring to prevent unnecessary loss. Do not transfer medications from one pharmacy container to another. Many medication bottles now have an identification code number on them. If similar medications were mixed and a patient had a reaction, it would be difficult to identify which drug was responsible. Do not use a medication with an unexpected precipitate, or one that has changed color. Skill 30-1 on pages 970–976 describes the techniques for preparing and administering oral medications.

SPECIAL TECHNIQUES

Certain drugs that are given orally can discolor the teeth or damage the enamel. The administration technique for this medication is to mix it well with water or some

Table 30-3 Ensuring Correct Administration of Medications

"RIGHT" TO ENSURE	QUESTIONS TO ASK	ACTIONS TO TAKE
When Preparing to Give Medication		
Right drug	• Has the patient been given this medication before? • Given the patient's symptoms and diagnosis, does it make sense for the patient to have this medication?	• Determine if the patient has any known drug allergies or sensitivities. • Assess the patient's other medications to detect possible contraindications. • Make sure it is the right medication; packaging, labeling, and spelling of some drugs look alike—watch for visual cues on packing or in how the drug name is written. • Have another person double-check medications and mathematical calculations (per policy).
Right reason	• Do the patient's condition, symptoms, and health status warrant receiving this medication?	• Determine if the patient has the condition the medication is used for and if rationale for the administration can be verified.
Right dose, route, and preparation	• Is the correct dose being administered? • How is the medication administered? • Does administration require medication math to calculate the dose?	• Ensure that labeling is legible and clearly understood. • Follow institution medication protocols as written.
Immediately before Administering the Medication		
Right patient	• Is this the right patient to receive this medication?	• Verify the identity of the patient using at least two identifiers: name and date of birth (check wristband, ask patient to state name).
Right time	• Is this the correct time for the medication to be administered?	• Check when the medication was last administered. If the drug is new, document when it is first given. Consider the facility's routine administration schedule.
Right route	• Is it appropriate to administer the medication orally, intravenously, by injection, or other route?	• Check the original orders to verify the route of administration.
Right assessment data	• Is it appropriate to administer the medication, based on the specific data collected?	• Collect appropriate assessment data related to mechanism of action and/or therapeutic effect.
Right education	• Is the patient familiar with the medication? Does the patient understand the purpose, dosing, and administration information, as well as other information specific to medication?	• Assess patient's level of knowledge. Provide patient education as necessary. Consider the health literacy of the patient when teaching.
Right to refuse	• Has the patient verbally agreed to take the medication? Has the patient expressed any concern with the medication?	• Acknowledge the patient's right to self-determination. Provide education, then verify, document, and notify the provider about the refusal as needed.
After the Medication has been Administered		
Right documentation	• Has the correct documentation been completed according to facility policy?	• Complete documentation according to facility policy immediately after administering any medication. • Document and communicate to the appropriate health care provider any signs and symptoms indicative of any adverse effects.
Right response	• How is the patient responding to the medication?	• Monitor the patient to determine the efficacy of the drug, detect and prevent complication, and evaluate and document changes in health status. • When applicable, assess the patient's laboratory values to detect changes. • Provide patient education, when possible, so patient is alert to adverse effects and changes in how they feel.

Source: Modified from Frandsen, G., & Pennington, S. S. (2021). *Abrams' clinical drug therapy: Rationales for nursing practice* (12th ed.). Wolters Kluwer; McCuistion, L. E., Vuljoin-DiMaggio, K., Winton, M. B., & Yeager, J. J. (2018). *Pharmacology: A patient-centered nursing process approach* (9th ed.). Saunders, an imprint of Elsevier Inc.; and Smeulers, M., Verweij, L., Maaskant, J. M., de Boer, M., Krediet, C. T., Nieveen van Dijkum, E. J., & Vermeulen, H. (2015). Quality indicators for safe medication preparation and administration: A systematic review. *PLoS ONE*, *10*(4), e0122695. https://doi.org/10.1371/journal.pone.0122695.

other liquid, have the patient take the medication mixed with liquid through a drinking straw, then encourage the patient to drink water after administration. This practice reduces the strength of the drug that comes in contact with the teeth.

Some patients object to the taste of certain medications. The following techniques help disguise or mask an objectionable taste:

- Crush the medication (if appropriate for type of medication) and mix with food or a drink so that the patient can swallow it. Many times the food or drink will mask the flavor of the medication. However, as previously discussed, some drugs cannot be crushed (e.g., enteric-coated and sustained-release capsules). Check with the pharmacist or a pharmacology reference if you are uncertain about crushing a medication.
- Allow the patient to suck on a small piece of ice for a few minutes before taking the medication. The ice numbs the taste buds, and the objectionable taste is less discernible.
- Store oily medications in the refrigerator. Cold oil is less aromatic than oil at room temperature.
- Place the medication in a syringe, and place the syringe on the back portion of the tongue (near the cheek), being careful not to trigger the patient's gag reflex. This places the medication on the part of the tongue with few taste buds.
- Offer oral hygiene immediately after giving the medication.
- Give the medication with generous amounts of water or other liquids, if permitted, to dilute the taste.

Children

It can be challenging to administer medications to infants and children. Children younger than 5 years have difficulty swallowing tablets and capsules. Therefore, most medications are available in liquid form. Nursing responsibilities includes teaching and preparing caregivers to administer medications to a child at home. In addition to understanding the medication prescription and the reason for the medication, the caregiver should be able to demonstrate any special techniques involved in administering the prescribed drugs. Question caregivers about their experiences giving medications to their children, about access to proper dosing devices, and previous use of the devices. Demonstrate how to use the appropriate dosing device that will be used at home. Ensure that the caregivers give a correct return demonstration. Help caregivers plan for the times of the day to give the medication. In addition, provide written instructions that clearly state the dose and times of the day for administration. Helpful strategies for administering oral medications to children include the following:

- Use a dropper to give infants or very young children liquid medications while holding them in a sitting or semi-sitting position. Place the medication between the gum and cheek to prevent aspiration.
- Crush uncoated tablets or empty a soft capsule (if appropriate for form of medication) and mix the medication with a bite of soft foods—such as potatoes, pudding, ice cream, or cooked or hot cereal—for children who are likely to aspirate liquids. However, as previously discussed, some drugs cannot be crushed (e.g., enteric-coated and sustained-release capsules). Check with the pharmacist or a pharmacology reference if you are uncertain about crushing a medication.
- Take care when selecting the food to be mixed with the medication. The item should not be an essential part of the child's diet, such as formula or the child's favorite food. The child may refuse to eat a food associated with medications.
- If a medication has an objectionable taste, warn the child if they are old enough to understand. Failing to warn the child is likely to decrease the child's trust in the nurse. Do not lie to a child about medication administration.
- Offer the child a flavored ice pop or frozen fruit bar immediately before taking the medication. It numbs the tongue, making the taste of the medication less evident.
- Praise the child for a job well done after the child swallows the medication.

Older Adults

Techniques for administering medications to older people include the following:

- Allow extra time to administer medications to older adults because their reflexes may be slowed and they may require additional explanation of the treatment regimen.
- Older adults may have difficulty swallowing medications and may find it easier to take their medications when crushed or given in liquid form. Initiate swallowing by gently massaging the laryngeal prominence or the area just below the chin prominence. The pressure from the gentle massage creates the desire to swallow. A speech therapist may offer additional suggestions for patients who have difficulty swallowing, such as a chin-to-chest position to increase the strength of the swallow.
- Reevaluation of the drug dosage is necessary with the older adult, especially when considering potential interactions and toxicities. Weight and age should be used as criteria for determining the dosage.
- Assist the older adult to set up a schedule as a reminder to take medications as scheduled at home. Associate medication with activities (such as breakfast or a television show) and not a specific time.
- Monitor the patient carefully for adverse effects that may result from the drug regimen. Encourage the patient to have all prescriptions filled at one pharmacy to facilitate appropriate management of the patient's entire medication regimen.
- Teach patients the names of drugs, rather than distinguishing them by color. Manufacturers may vary the colors of generic drugs, and the visual changes associated with aging may make it more difficult to identify medications by their color.
- Empower patients to take control of their health by providing education and ongoing support focused on adherence to the medication regimen.

Technology Alert

Remote Medication Monitoring System

Telehealth is an emerging technology that allows for remote communication between a patient and the provider. Remote monitoring of vital signs, weight, and patient-reported symptoms frequently occurs with telehealth monitoring. Hale et al. (2016) describe a specific remote medication monitoring system piloted with older adults diagnosed with heart failure, a complex disease process that requires diligent ongoing medication and symptom management. The technology used includes (1) a device (outfitted with daily dispensing bins, sensors for each bin, and a camera) that alerts the patient with lights and sounds when medications are due; and (2) a monitoring center staffed by advisors who provide reminders to refill the system each week and follow-up calls to the patient and an appointed caregiver when medications are not taken. Although the results are mixed and more studies need to be done, this type of relatively low-cost technology shows promise in supporting patients with medication adherence.

ADMINISTERING MEDICATIONS THROUGH AN ENTERAL FEEDING TUBE

Patients with a gastrointestinal tube (nasogastric, nasointestinal, percutaneous endoscopic gastrostomy [PEG], or jejunostomy [J] tube) often receive medication through the tube. The insertion of the tube and care of the patient with an enteral feeding tube are described in Chapter 37. Current recommendations support the use of enteral feeding connections that comply with the International Organization for Standardization (ISO) 80369-1 or ISO 80369-3 standard (FDA, 2018b). These connectors, such as ENFit®, are designed to provide secure and unique (different from intravenous) adaptors and connections specifically designed for enteral feeding systems. Suggestions for preparing and administering medications through the tube have been fairly consistent for the past 10 to 15 years:

- Verify the current feeding tube's placement (distal location) and patency—note that tubes that terminate in the stomach can tolerate larger boluses than tubes that sit in the intestines (Reber et al., 2019).
- Verify the dosage form, drug, formulation, and any preparation steps with the prescription/order (Boullata et al., 2017).
- Use liquid medications if they are appropriate for enteral administration. In liquid medication not specifically formulated for enteral administration, sugars, preservatives, and agents that thicken the solution may cause gastrointestinal disturbances and impact on medication absorption (Bandy et al., 2019; Boullata et al., 2017; Zoeller et al., 2020). Dilute thick suspensions as needed, typically with equal parts medication and (purified) water (Boullata et al., 2017).
- Certain immediate-release solid dosage medications can be crushed and made into a slurry. Grind medication to a fine powder and mix it with 30 mL of (purified) water immediately before administration through the tube (Bandy et al., 2019; Boullata et al., 2017; Zoeller et al., 2020).
- Certain capsules may be opened, the powder emptied into (purified) water, and the medication administered through the tube. Check manufacturer recommendations and/or with a pharmacist to verify (Boullata et al., 2017).
- Attach a clean oral/enteral syringe (≥20 mL) for administering flushes and medication(s) (Boullata et al., 2017).
- Flush the tube with at least 15 mL (purified)water (at least 5 mL for children) before giving each medication and immediately after giving each medication (Boullata et al., 2017; Zoeller et al., 2020). Flushing helps to maintain tube patency.
- Give medications separately and flush with water between each drug (Boullata et al., 2017). The medications may not be physically or chemically compatible—mixing them can lead to tube obstruction or altered therapeutic actions (Boullata et al., 2017).
- Although the research is not conclusive, if a medication needs to be administered down a nasogastric tube connected to suction, keep it disconnected from the suction and clamped for 30 minutes after administration of the medication to allow absorption (Bandy et al., 2019).
- If the patient is receiving tube feedings, review information about the drugs to be administered. Absorption of some drugs is affected by tube-feeding formulas. Discontinue a continuous tube feeding and leave the tube clamped for the required period of time before and after the medication has been given, according to the reference and facility protocol.
- Document the total water and liquid medication volume on the intake and output record. Adjust the amount of water used if the patient's fluid intake is restricted. Always follow institution policy and procedure regarding administering medications through an enteral feeding tube (Boullata et al., 2017).
- Keep in mind the importance of interprofessional collaboration between the prescribing provider, the pharmacist, and the nurse to ensure safe enteral medication prescribing, preparation, and administration (Bandy et al., 2019; Boullata et al., 2017; Reber et al., 2019).

Concept Mastery Alert

When administering medications via an enteral tube, the same amount of purified water—at least 30 mL—is used to mix the medication and to flush the tube (15 mL before and 15 mL after medication administration).

ADMINISTERING SUBLINGUAL AND BUCCAL MEDICATIONS

Certain drugs, such as nitroglycerin, are administered sublingually. This means a tablet is placed under the patient's tongue. Another method is to administer the medication between the cheek and gum, known as buccal administration. These areas are rich in superficial blood vessels, which allow the drug to be absorbed relatively rapidly into the bloodstream for quick systemic effects. Sublingual and buccal medications should not be swallowed, but rather held in place so that complete absorption can occur. Before administering a sublingual or buccal drug, offer the patient a drink of water (if the patient is permitted to have fluids) or oral care (if the patient is NPO). This ensures that the tablet will dissolve appropriately. Certain opioids that were previously available for parenteral administration only can now also be administered in a lollipop or oral-transmucosal form.

Administering Parenteral Medications

The word **parenteral** means outside the intestines or alimentary canal. Several methods to administer a medication by the parenteral route involve injecting the medication into those body tissues outside of the intestines or alimentary canal and into the circulatory system. Table 30-2 on page 928 defines terms used to describe various types of parenteral injections. Advanced injection techniques consist of injecting medications into an artery, the peritoneum, heart tissues, the spinal canal, and bones. Intraosseous administration continues to be supported by the American Heart Association (2020) and certifications they support include this training. Techniques for injecting medications into all of these areas are discussed in advanced clinical texts. In most instances, physicians, advanced practitioners, or specially trained providers are responsible for these procedures.

EQUIPMENT

Needles and Syringes

Needles are available in various lengths and gauges, with different sizes of bevels. The needle length used depends on the route of administration. The gauge refers to the diameter of the needle. Needle gauges are numbered 18 through 30. As the diameter of the needle increases, the gauge number decreases. For example, an 18-gauge needle is larger in diameter than a 30-gauge needle. The bevel of the needle is its sloped edge, designed to make a narrow, slit-like opening that closes quickly.

Concept Mastery Alert

Opposites rule. The larger the gauge of a needle, the smaller the diameter.

Syringes are supplied in various sizes. Most syringes are plastic and disposable. Some syringes are supplied with the needle attached; others are not, in which case you should select an appropriate needle. Figure 30-4 shows the parts of a needle and the parts of a syringe.

Choose the equipment needed for an injection based on the following criteria:

- *Route of administration:* A longer needle is required for an intramuscular injection than for an intradermal or a subcutaneous injection. See the discussion related to each individual route for specific guidelines regarding needle length and gauge.

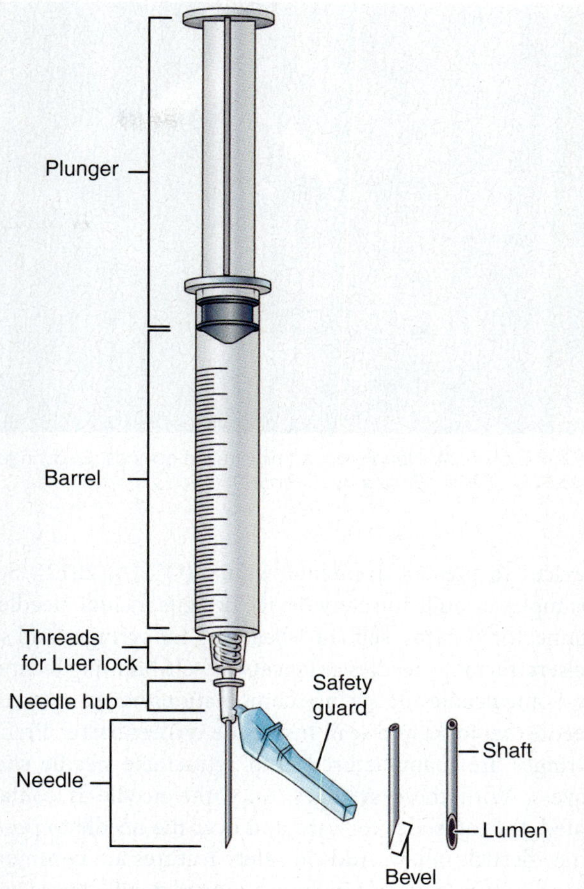

FIGURE 30-4. Parts of a needle and syringe.

- *Viscosity of the solution:* Some medications are more viscous (thick) than others and require a needle with a large lumen to inject the drug.
- *Quantity to be administered:* The larger the amount of medication to be injected, the larger the syringe needs to be. Smaller syringes should be used as needed for precise dosing because they provide smaller increments of measurement—never estimate a dose. For example, a 1-mL syringe provides increments of 0.01 mL, but a 5-mL syringe allows for precise measures only down to 0.2 mL.
- *Body size:* An obese person requires a longer needle to reach muscle tissue than does a thin person. A thin person or an older adult with decreased muscle mass requires a shorter needle.
- *Type of medication:* There are special syringes for certain uses. An example is the insulin syringe used only to inject insulin.

Once used on a patient, do not recap needles. After use, activate the safety device to cover the tip of the needle and place the needle with the syringe attached in an approved puncture-resistant container. Because most needlesticks are related to unsafe needle devices, and not unsafe or careless behavior by healthcare workers, health care facilities are required by the Occupational Safety and Health Administration (OSHA) Needlestick Safety and Prevention Act of 2001 to provide needles with built-in or add-on safety control

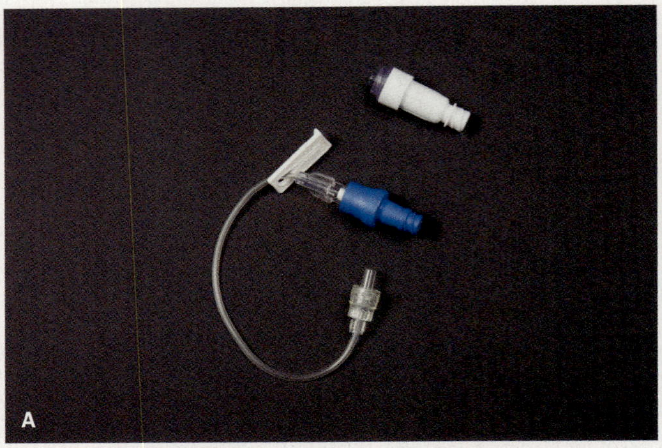

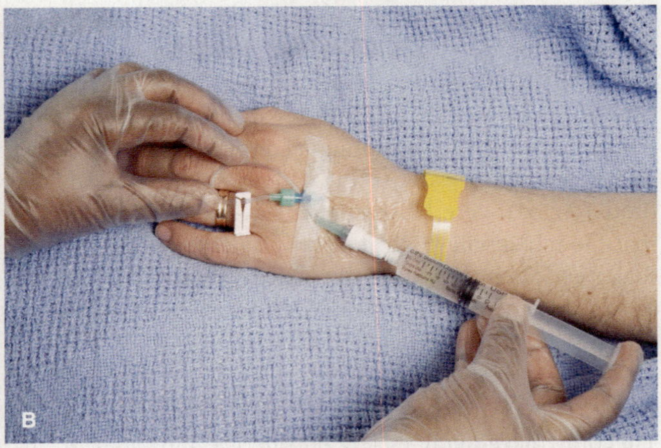

FIGURE 30-5. **A.** Needleless administration devices. **B.** Syringe attached to needleless administration device. (*Source:* Used with permission from Shutterstock. *Photos by B. Proud.)*

devices to prevent accidental injury (OSHA, 2012). Some examples of built-in safety device designs include needleless connector systems, self (re-)sheathing for syringes and scalpels, retractable needles or lancets, or self-blunting technology. Some needle and syringe combinations have a retractable needle that locks and seals inside the syringe barrel. Prefilled syringes are manufactured with retractable needle sheath covers. With these syringes, once the needle is contaminated, the top slides forward and over the needle to prevent a needlestick injury. Add-on safety features are common in the clinical setting and include a hinged needle guard safety feature. After the injection is given, push the needle guard into place using the one-handed technique recommended by manufacturers to prevent injury (OSHA, n.d.).

When administering parenteral injections, maintain surgical asepsis and use strict sterile technique to avoid introducing organisms into the body. The parts of the syringe and needle that must be kept sterile during the procedure of preparing and administering an injection include the inside of the barrel, the part of the plunger that enters the barrel, the tip of the barrel (threads for Luer lock), and the needle, except for the exterior of the needle hub. Never open and set down a syringe or needle. To maintain sterility, first open the syringe (being careful not to handle the tip of the barrel) and then open the needle (or needleless adapter) from the hub side, screwing the needle onto the syringe threads while the covered tip of the needle is still in the package. Surgical asepsis also applies to cleaning the skin for an injection. Cleanse the skin with alcohol in a circular motion, working from the center of the designated site outward. Follow manufacturer recommendations when preparing the site using other antimicrobials (e.g., back and forth motion with chlorhexidine products).

Needleless Systems

The risk for accidental needlesticks and exposure to bloodborne pathogens is reduced significantly with the use of needleless devices or protected needles. Chapter 25 describes the rationale for these systems of protection for health care workers. Needleless systems are available for intravenous use, including recessed and shielded intravenous needle connectors, as well as blunt cannulas that are inserted into special receptor sites on tubing or lock setups. Discard all needleless devices or blunt cannulas in special containers that are puncture-proof, leak-proof, and labeled clearly. Figure 30-5 shows an example of a needleless administration device.

PREPARING MEDICATIONS FOR ADMINISTRATION BY INJECTION

Drugs that are administered by injection are packaged in several ways. Those that deteriorate in solution are usually dispensed as powders and are reconstituted immediately before injection. Drugs that remain stable in solution are usually dispensed in ampules, bottles, prefilled cartridges, or vials in an aqueous or oily solution or suspension. Drugs may be dispensed in single-dose glass ampules, single-dose rubber-capped vials, multidose rubber-capped vials, and prefilled cartridges.

Removing Medication From an Ampule

An **ampule** is a glass flask that contains a single dose of medication for parenteral administration. Figure 30-6 shows an example of an ampule. There is no way to prevent airborne contamination of any unused portion of medication after the ampule is opened; if not all the medication is used, discard

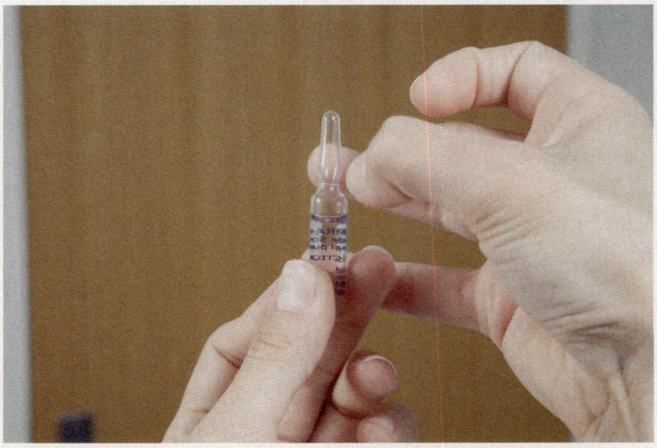

FIGURE 30-6. Ampule. (*Source:* Used with permission from Shutterstock. *Photo by B. Proud.*)

the remainder. Medication is removed from an ampule after its thin neck is broken. Take special care when breaking the ampule so that you do not get cut. If you cut yourself on the ampule, discard the ampule and medication. Because of the risk of small glass shards falling into the ampule, use a filter needle to remove the medication from the vial and then discard it appropriately. Invert the ampule or place it on a flat surface to draw the solution into the syringe. Care must be taken not to contaminate the needle by touching the rim of the ampule. Replace the filter needle with an unfiltered needle of appropriate size on the syringe before administering the medication. Skill 30-2 on pages 976–979 shows how to remove medication from an ampule.

Removing Medication from a Vial

A **vial** is a plastic or glass bottle with a self-sealing stopper through which the medication is removed (Fig. 30-7). For safety in transporting and storing, the vial is usually covered with a soft metal or plastic cap that can be removed easily. The self-sealing rubber stopper under the removed cap is the means of entrance into the vial.

Some drugs are dispensed in vials that contain several doses. This means that the nurse can remove several doses from the same container. To prevent microbial growth in the vial, each multidose vial is usually good for only 24 hours. Label the vial with the time and date when first used. To facilitate removal of medication from a multiuse vial, inject air into the vial; single-use vials often do not require instillation of air. The amount of air injected into the vial is the same amount as the desired quantity of solution. The Centers for Disease Control and Prevention (CDC, 2015) recommends that medications packaged as multiuse vials be assigned to a single patient whenever possible. In addition, it is recommended that the top of the vial be cleaned prior to each entry and that a new sterile needle and syringe is used with each entry. Skill 30-3 on pages 980–982 details how to remove medication from a vial.

Using a Prefilled Cartridge or Syringe

Prefilled cartridges provide a single dose of medication. Insert the cartridge into a reusable holder or injection device. Before giving the injection, check the dosage in the cartridge and clear the cartridge of excess air. Most prefilled cartridges are overfilled; therefore, eject any excess medication to give an exact dose and avoid a medication error. Tubex and Carpuject are two types of prefilled cartridges. Figure 30-8 shows examples of prefilled cartridges and injector devices. Integration of safety principles associated with these devices requires nurse and leadership engagement, adequate education, and policies and procedures to guide practice (Prentiss et al., 2016). Prefilled cartridges should not be used as vials in routine practice (Institute for Safe Medication Practices, 2018).

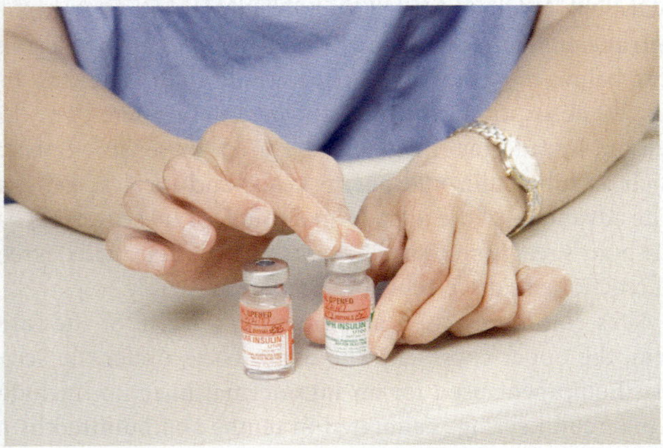

FIGURE 30-7. Vials. (*Source:* Used with permission from Shutterstock. *Photo by B. Proud.*)

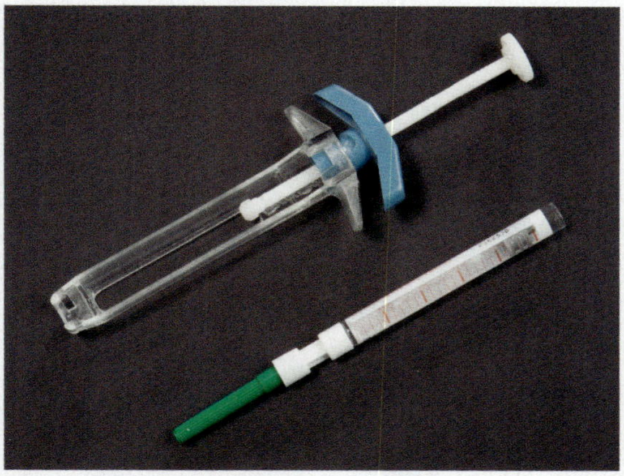

FIGURE 30-8. Prefilled cartridge and injector device. (*Source:* Used with permission from Shutterstock. *Photo by B. Proud.*)

Similar to prefilled cartridges are prefilled syringes. These are syringes that are already filled with a medication and usually have their own needle attached. Like prefilled cartridges, these syringes also come with excess air. In some cases, this air should *not* be expelled before administering the medication. Enoxaparin is an example of a syringe for which the air should not be expelled before administering (Sanofi-Aventis, 2020).

Mixing Medications in One Syringe

When considering mixing two medications in one syringe, first ensure that the two drugs are compatible. Certain medications, such as diazepam, are incompatible with other drugs in the same syringe. Other drugs have limited compatibility and should be administered within 15 minutes of preparation. Incompatible drugs may become cloudy or form a precipitate in the syringe. Discard these medications and re-prepare the drugs in separate syringes. Mixing more than two drugs in one syringe is not recommended. If it must be done, contact the pharmacist to determine the compatibility of the three drugs, as well as the compatibility of their pH values and the preservatives that may be present in each drug. A drug compatibility table should be available to nurses who are preparing medications.

Preparation of medications in one syringe depends on how the medication is supplied. When using a single-dose vial and a multidose vial, inject air into the multidose vial and draw the medication in the multidose vial into the syringe first. This prevents the contents of the multidose vial from being contaminated with the medication in the single-dose vial. The

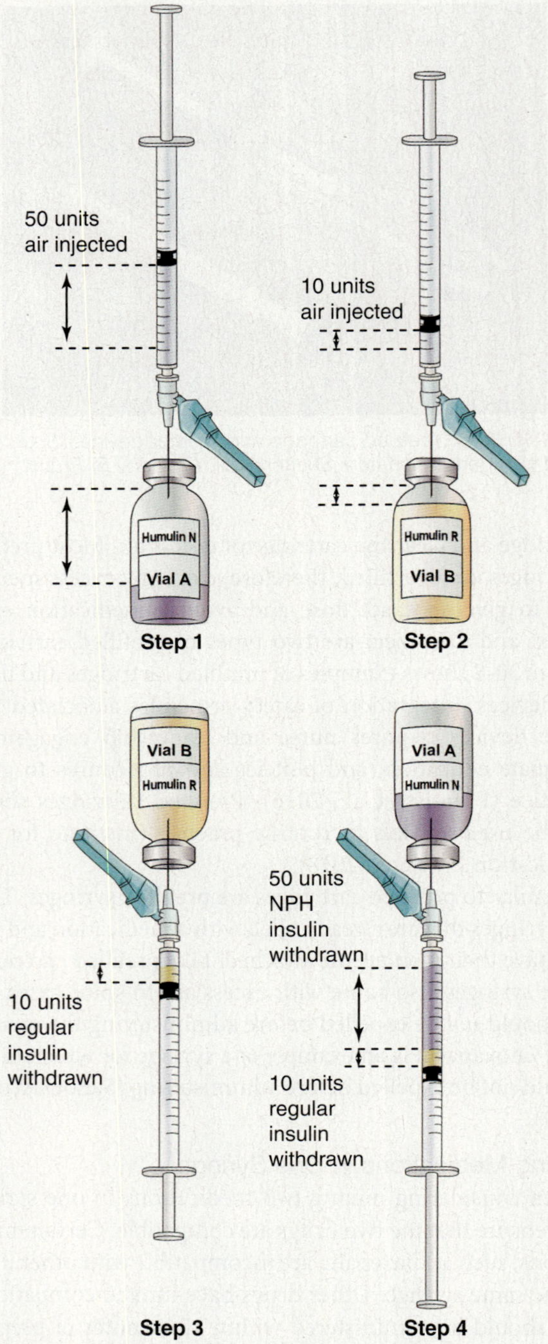

FIGURE 30-9. Mixing medications (insulin) in one syringe.

steps to follow when preparing medications from two multidose vials in one syringe are illustrated in Figure 30-9. When preparing medications from an ampule and a vial, prepare the medication in the vial first. Draw up the medication in the ampule after the medication in the vial.

Mixing Insulins in One Syringe

Insulin, a naturally occurring hormone produced by the pancreas, enables cells to use carbohydrates. Two of the issues relative to insulin in patients with diabetes mellitus include no insulin production or insufficient insulin production. Many types of insulin are available for use by patients with diabetes mellitus. Insulins vary in their onset and duration of action and are classified as rapid acting, short acting, intermediate acting, and long acting (Frandsen & Pennington, 2021). A patient may receive more than one type of insulin. A patient may be treated with a basal insulin, such as insulin glargine, insulin detemir, or NPH insulin to cover the body's basal metabolic needs. In addition, the patient will probably also be treated with a prandial (with a meal) or preprandial (before a meal) insulin, such as insulin lispro or insulin aspart, to prevent postprandial (after meal) hyperglycemia (high blood glucose). Glargine and detemir cannot be mixed with other insulins. Patients treated with other insulins may require the mixing of the two insulins in one syringe. Before administering any insulin, be aware of the onset time, peak, and duration of effects and ensure that proper food is available. Refer to a drug reference for a listing of the different types of insulin and action specific to each type.

Insulin is typically available in multidose vials, and dosages are calculated in units. The scale commonly used is U100, which is based on 100 units of insulin contained in 1 mL of solution. An insulin syringe is also calibrated in units. Insulin is also available in injection pens. Before administering insulin, check the dosage with the prescription. Skill 30-4 on pages 983–986 gives the steps for mixing two types of insulin in the same syringe. Insulin administration is discussed below in the Administering Medications Subcutaneously section.

Reconstituting Powdered Medications

Occasionally, a drug is supplied as a powder in a vial. A liquid, or diluent, must be added to the powder before it is administered as a solution. The technique of adding a diluent to a powdered drug is called *reconstitution*. Information needed for reconstitution, such as the specific solution to use for the diluent and dosage calculation, is usually found on the vial label or a package insert. Additional sources of information about reconstitution of medications are the pharmacist and electronic resources, such as a medication database.

Another form that powdered medications may come in is an Act-O-Vial (Pfizer). Act-O-Vials have the diluent and powder in the same vial but separated by a rubber stopper. When the nurse is ready to administer the medication, the rubber stopper is deployed, and the Act-O-Vial is agitated gently to mix the diluent and powder.

ADMINISTERING MEDICATIONS INTRADERMALLY

Intradermal injections are administered into the dermis, just below the epidermis. The intradermal route has the longest absorption time of all the parenteral routes. For this reason, intradermal injections are used for sensitivity tests, such as tuberculin and allergy tests, and local anesthesia. The advantage of the intradermal route for these tests is that the body's reaction to substances is easily visible, and degrees of reaction are discernible by comparative study.

Sites commonly used are the inner surface of the forearm, the upper chest, and the upper back, under the scapula. Equipment used for an intradermal injection includes a tuberculin syringe calibrated in tenths and hundredths of a milliliter. A ⅜″ to ½″, 26- or 27-gauge needle is typically available. The dosage given intradermally is small, usually less than 0.5 mL. The angle of administration for an intradermal injection is 5 to 15 degrees. Skill 30-5 on pages 987–991 demonstrates how to administer an intradermal injection.

ADMINISTERING MEDICATIONS SUBCUTANEOUSLY

Subcutaneous injections are administered into the adipose tissue layer just below the epidermis and dermis. This tissue has few blood vessels, thus drugs administered here have a slow, sustained rate of absorption into the capillaries. This route is used to administer drugs such as insulin and heparin.

Subcutaneous Injection Sites

Various sites may be used for subcutaneous injections, including the outer aspect of the upper arm, the abdomen (from below the costal margin to the iliac crests), the anterior aspects of the thigh, the upper back, and the upper ventral or dorsogluteal area (Fig. 30-10). In general, avoid sites that are bruised, tender, hard, swollen, inflamed, or scarred. Absorption rates differ among the various sites. Injections in the abdomen are absorbed most rapidly; ones in the arms are absorbed somewhat more slowly; those in the thighs, even more slowly; and those in the upper ventral or dorsogluteal areas have the slowest absorption (American Diabetes Association [ADA], 2022).

Equipment

It is important to choose the right equipment to ensure depositing the medication into the intended tissue layer and not the underlying muscle. Equipment used for a subcutaneous injection includes a syringe of appropriate volume for the amount of drug being administered. A 25- to 30-gauge, 3/8″ to 1″ needle can be used. The 25-gauge 5/8″ needles are most commonly used for adults. Needle length ranges exist because patients present with different amounts of subcutaneous tissue that varies based on age, body mass index, sex, and general build—choose the needle length that ensures the needle terminates in the subcutaneous tissue. Usually, no more than 1 mL of solution is given subcutaneously. Giving larger amounts adds to the patient's discomfort and may predispose to poor absorption. Some medications are packaged in prefilled cartridges with a needle attached. Enoxaparin, for example, is provided this way. Confirm that the provided needle is appropriate for the patient before use.

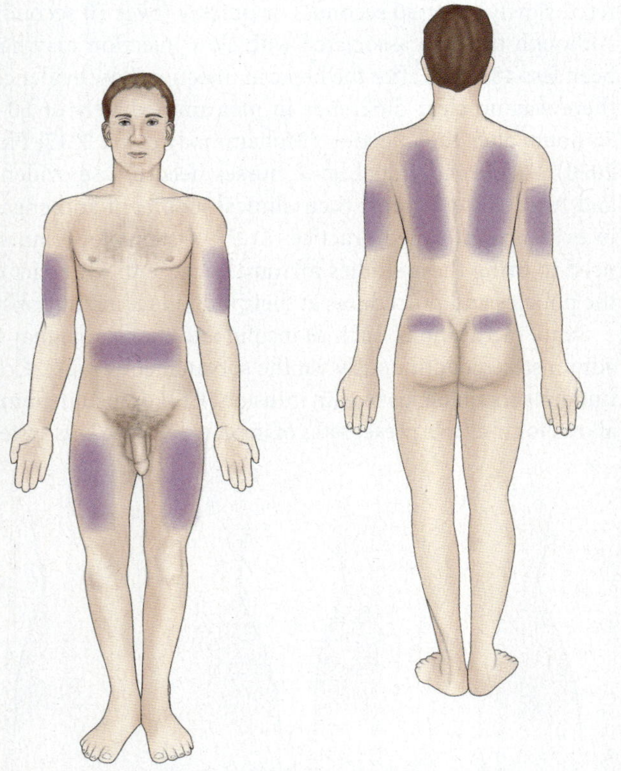

FIGURE 30-10. Sites on the body where subcutaneous injections can be given.

Procedure

Subcutaneous injections are administered at a 45- to 90-degree angle, with the 45-degree angle used only for small patients with a limited amount of subcutaneous tissue. Choose the angle of needle insertion based on the amount of subcutaneous tissue present and the length of the needle. In general, the shorter, 3/8″ needle should be inserted at a 90-degree angle (common on prefilled and insulin syringes), and the longer, 3/8″ needle may be inserted at a 45-degree angle. Recommendations differ regarding pinching or bunching of a skin fold for administration (Centers for Disease Control and Prevention, 2015/2020). Pinching is advised for thinner patients and when a longer needle is used to lift the adipose tissue away from underlying muscle and tissue. If pinching is used, once the needle is inserted, release the skin and stabilize the base of the needle to avoid injecting into compressed tissue.

If blood or clear fluid appears at the site after withdrawing the needle, apply gentle pressure. Massaging the site is not necessary and can damage underlying tissue as well as increase the absorption of the medication. Massaging after heparin administration can contribute to hematoma formation.

It is necessary to rotate sites or areas for injection if the patient is to receive frequent injections. This helps to prevent buildup of fibrous/adipose tissue and permits complete absorption of the medication. Because absorption rates vary from site to site, it is recommended that patients administering their own insulin use the same area of the body at the same time every day to ensure more consistent absorption and prevent tissue changes from repeated use of the same site (American Diabetic Association, 2022; Frandsen & Pennington, 2021; Karch, 2020). For instance, every morning the patient may use the abdomen for insulin injection, and every evening before dinner, the patient may inject the insulin into the arms or thighs. Keep in mind that the best absorption occurs in the abdomen. In each case, the injections should be given an inch away from the previous injection site. A small spot bandage or piece of tape can be used to mark the first injection site, with subsequent injections rotated in a circle around that site. After this area has been used, an adjacent site, an inch away, can be selected, using the same rotation format. A marked diagram incorporated into the patient's plan of care is also helpful for noting alternative sites. Do not rely on memory. The patient cannot always recall the site of

Box 30-2 Reducing Discomfort in Subcutaneous and Intramuscular Administrations

The following are recommended techniques for reducing discomfort when injecting medications subcutaneously or intramuscularly:

- Select a needle of the smallest gauge that is appropriate for the site and solution to be injected, and select the correct needle length.
- Be sure the needle is free of medication that may irritate superficial tissues as the needle is inserted. The recommended procedure is to use two needles—one to remove the medication from the vial or ampule and a second one to inject the medication. If medication is in a prefilled syringe with a nonremovable needle and has dripped back on the needle during preparation, gently tap the barrel to remove the excess solution.
- Use the Z-track technique for intramuscular injections to prevent leakage of medication into the needle track, thus minimizing discomfort.
- Inject the medication into relaxed muscles. There is more pressure and discomfort when the medication is injected into a contracted muscle.
- Do not inject areas that feel hard on palpation or tender to the patient.
- Insert the needle with a dart-like motion without hesitation, and remove it quickly at the same angle at which it was inserted. These techniques reduce discomfort and tissue irritation.
- Do not administer more solution in one injection than is recommended for the site. Injecting more solution creates excess pressure in the area and increases discomfort.
- Inject the solution slowly so that it may be dispersed more easily into the surrounding tissue (10 seconds per 1 mL).
- Apply gentle pressure after injection, unless this technique is contraindicated.
- Allow patients who are fearful of injections to talk about their fears. Answer patients' questions truthfully, and explain the nature and purpose of the injection. Taking the time to offer support often allays fears and decreases discomfort.
- Rotate sites when the patient is to receive repeated injections. Injections in the same site may cause undue discomfort, irritation, or abscesses in tissues.
- For children, provide age-appropriate support and involve their parent, guardian, or other support person when possible.

the previous injection; therefore, the site of administration must be recorded in the patient's record.

Skill 30-6 on pages 991–996 shows the procedure for administering medications subcutaneously. Techniques for reducing discomfort in subcutaneous administrations are listed in Box 30-2.

Drug-Specific Equipment and Techniques

Various drugs require very specific equipment and/or techniques. Insulin is prepared using an insulin syringe. Other drugs are never administered with an insulin syringe. Insulin syringes are available with 28- to 31-gauge, 5/16″ and ½″ length needles, and in 3/10-mL to 1-mL sizes. The shorter needles (5/16″) are the most common length used. Shorter needles cause less pain, and there is less risk for inadvertent injection into muscle tissue. Insulin pens are also available for insulin administration. Insulin injection pens are prefilled devices that combine the insulin container and syringe. Patients attach a needle for each administration, dial a dose of insulin, and depress a plunger to administer the dose. See Guidelines for Nursing Care 30-1: Using an Insulin Injection Pen.

Heparin is also administered subcutaneously. The abdomen is the most commonly used site. Avoid the area 2″ around the umbilicus and the belt line. Certain medications have specific manufacturer-recommended administration requirements. For example, low–molecular-weight heparin (enoxaparin) should be administered in the alternating "left and right anterolateral and left and right posterolateral abdominal wall[s]" (Sanofi-Aventis, 2020, section 2.5 Administration; Fig. 30-11). To administer the medication, pinch the tissue gently and insert the needle at a 90-degree angle. In addition, enoxaparin is packaged in a prefilled syringe with an air bubble. Do not expel the air bubble before administration. A Cochrane review considered data from four randomized control trials regarding the effects of speed of administration of heparin and low molecular weight heparin (enoxaparin) on pain, bruising, and hematoma formation. The evidence shows that there is essentially no difference in the patient experience whether the injection is administered slowly (over 30 seconds) or quickly (over 10 seconds). Although the pain associated with slow injection may have been less 48 hours after the heparin injection (low evidence), there was no clear difference in pain immediately or 60 to 72 hours after the injection (Mohammady et al., 2017; Pich, 2020). At the individual level, nurses need to use evidence and research to support their clinical judgment and engage in evidence-informed practice. At the systems level, nurses need to bring these studies forward because they impact on the policies and procedures at their individual institutions.

Some medications, such as insulin and morphine, may be administered continuously via the subcutaneous route. Continuous subcutaneous insulin infusion (CSII or insulin pump) allows for multiple preset rates of insulin delivery. This system

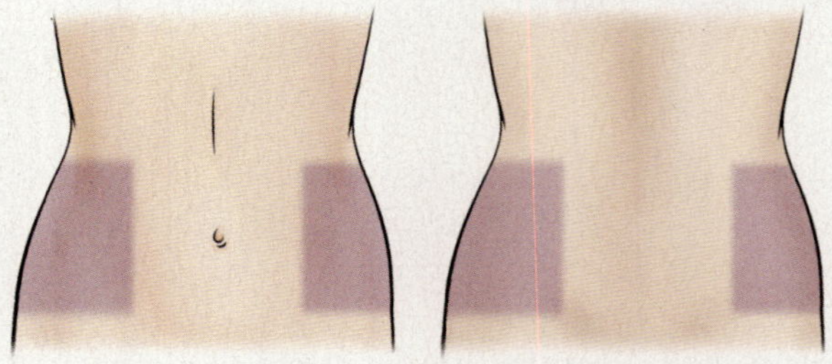

FIGURE 30-11. Sites for administration of enoxaparin.

Guidelines for Nursing Care 30-1

USING AN INSULIN INJECTION PEN

- Perform hand hygiene and put on PPE, as indicated.
- **Identify the patient. Compare the information with the eMAR/MAR. The patient should be identified using at least two methods** (The Joint Commission, 2020a).
- Explain procedure to the patient.
- Close the door to the room or pull the bedside curtain.
- **Complete necessary assessments before administering medications. Check the patient's allergy bracelet or ask the patient about allergies. Explain the purpose and action of the medication to the patient.**
- Scan the patient's bar code on the identification band, if required.
- **Based on facility policy, the third check of the label may occur at this point. If so, recheck the labels with the eMAR/MAR before administering the medications to the patient.**
- Select an appropriate administration site.
- Assist the patient to the appropriate position for the site chosen. Drape, as needed, to expose only area of site to be used.
- Identify the appropriate landmarks for the site chosen.
- Remove the pen cap.
- Insert an insulin cartridge into the pen, if necessary, following the manufacturer's directions.
- If administering an insulin suspension, gently roll the pen 10 times and invert the pen 10 times to mix the insulin.
- Scrub the self-sealing seal end of the pen cartridge holder with an antimicrobial swab.
- Remove the protective paper tab from the needle.
- Screw the needle onto the reservoir. (Patients at home should reserve the outer shield for later use.) Dial the dose selector to 2 units to prime the pen (perform an *air shot*) to get rid of air and make certain the pen is working properly.
- Hold the pen upright and tap to force any air bubbles to the top.
- Hold the pen upright and press the injection button or plunger firmly. Watch for a drop of insulin at the needle tip.
- Check the drug reservoir to make sure enough insulin is available for the dose.
- Check that the dose selector is at 0 (zero), then dial the units of insulin for the dose.
- Put on gloves.
- Clean the injection site. If the pen needle is longer than 5 mm, gently pinch the skin at the injection site to form a skin fold (Becton, Dickinson and Company [BD], 2020).
- Hold the pen in the palm of your hand, perpendicular to the forearm, with your thumb at the injection button end of the pen. Use your thumb for injection.
- Administer the subcutaneous injection. Press the injection button on the pen all the way in. Keep the button depressed and count to 10 before removing from the skin.
- The safety shield automatically covers the needle when the needle is removed from the skin. Remove the needle from the pen; a second safety shield automatically covers the back end of the needle when removed from the pen. Dispose of the needle in a sharps container.
- Alternatively, patients at home should replace the reserved outer shield on the needle before removing the needle from the pen. Other needle removal devices and procedures exist; patients should follow the instructions provided by their health care provider related to their specific insulin pen.
- Remove gloves and additional PPE, if used.
- Perform hand hygiene.
- Document administration on the eMAR/MAR, including the injection site.

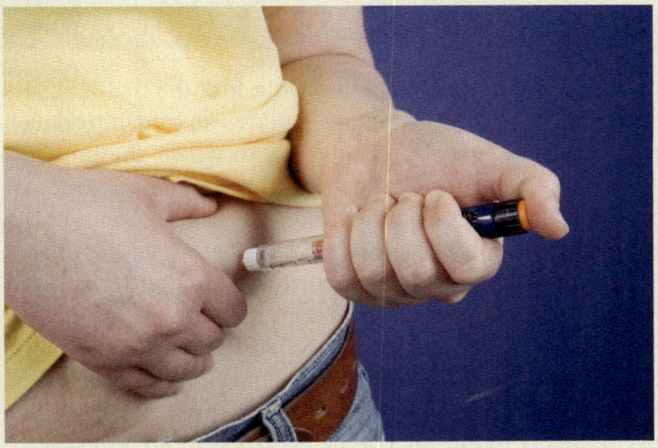

Patient using an insulin pen. (*Source:* Used with permission from Shutterstock. *Photo by B. Proud.*)

Source: Adapted from Becton, Dickinson and Company (BD). (2020/2016a). BD AutoShield Duo™ pen needle How to inject with a pen. https://www.bd.com/en-us/offerings/capabilities/diabetes-care/pen-needles/bd-autoshield-duo-pen-needlehttps://www.bd.com/us/diabetes/page.aspx?cat=7001&id=7259

uses a small computerized reservoir that delivers insulin via tubing through a small plastic cannula or needle inserted into the subcutaneous tissue. The pump is programmed to deliver a continuous dose of insulin (basal) and allows for the administration of on-demand (bolus) administration as needed for meals or an elevation in blood glucose. The settings may be adjusted as needed for things such as exercise and illness. This type of insulin administration more closely mirrors the body's normal function and promotes better blood glucose control, increases quality of life, and reduces potential microvascular and macrovascular complications of diabetes (Nimri et al., 2020). Sites are changed every 2 to 3 days according to the manufacturer's recommendations. Figure 30-12 (on page 948) shows a patient wearing an insulin pump. Another

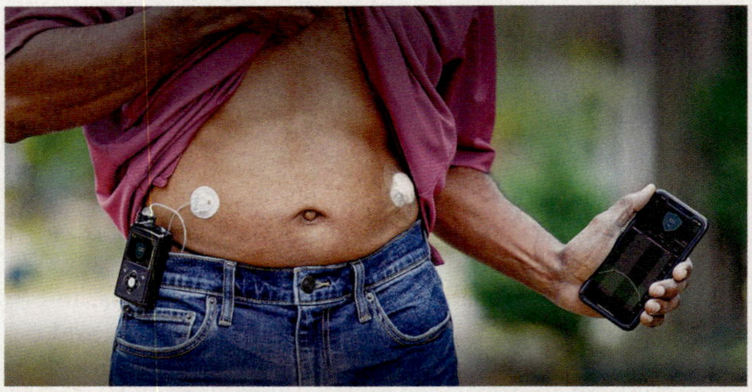

FIGURE 30-12. Patient wearing an insulin pump. (Courtesy of Medtronic.)

example of a medication given via continuous subcutaneous infusion is morphine. Subcutaneous morphine infusion can be used for palliative dyspnea and pain management. Advantages of continuous subcutaneous medication infusion include the sustained rate of absorption via the subcutaneous route and convenience for the patient.

Technology Alert

Insulin pump therapy can also be integrated with continuous blood glucose monitoring, which allows for responsive insulin administration, downloading of trends and information regarding glucose and insulin needs, and direct transmission of data to health care providers. Many insulin pumps are waterproof and interface with a smartphone.

ADMINISTERING MEDICATIONS INTRAMUSCULARLY

Intramuscular injections deliver medication through the skin and subcutaneous tissues into certain muscles. Muscles have larger and a greater number of blood vessels than subcutaneous tissue, allowing faster onset of action than with subcutaneous injections. Some medications administered intramuscularly are formulated to have a longer duration of effect. The deposit of medication creates a depot at the site of injection, designed to deliver slow, sustained release over hours, days, or weeks. This route is used to administer drugs such as antibiotics, hormones, and vaccines, such as the pneumococcal and hepatitis vaccines. The accompanying box, Through the Eyes of a Student, relates one student's experience administering an intramuscular injection.

Aspiration, or pulling back on the plunger to check if a blood vessel has been entered, is not necessary and has not proved to be a reliable indicator of needle placement. Despite a tradition of aspiration, if correct technique is used and recommended anatomic injection sites are used, the likelihood of injecting into a blood vessel is small and there is no scientific evidence to support aspiration (Centers for Disease Control and Prevention, 2019; Sisson, 2015). The World Health Organization (WHO, 2020) and CDC (2015/2020) do not include aspiration in their steps for intramuscular injection of vaccines. The wide-spread use of auto-disable (AD) syringes encouraged by WHO (2020) further reinforces no aspiration with IM vaccine administration, since most AD syringes are not designed to aspirate (Sepah et al., 2017). In

Through the Eyes of a Student

I entered my patient's room, knowing that she had had surgery less than 12 hours before my arrival, and introduced myself. I asked how she was feeling, to which she immediately responded, "I feel really sick. I think I'm going to throw up. I need something—now!" I told her that I would check the medication orders and be back as soon as possible. I walked quickly to the medication administration record, and there it was glaring at me in black and white on the eMAR: "Prochlorperazine, 10 mg IM q 6 hr PRN nausea or vomiting." My mind raced as I thought, "I have never given an IM injection. There has to be something else prescribed." I knew there wasn't. I found my clinical instructor and announced, "My patient needs an IM injection." Given the anxiety I was feeling, everything went surprisingly well as we prepared the medication. I went over the procedure one last time before entering the patient's room.

We approached the patient just in time for her to look at us in sheer terror and cry, "I hope that shot isn't for me; I hate them," which did nothing for my already shaking hands. I explained that she couldn't take a pill because she could not have anything by mouth because of the nature of her surgery and that this would help. She was agreeable after hearing the rationale. My instructor and I positioned the patient on her side so that I could give her the shot in the (preferred) ventrogluteal area. I marked the landmarks at least half a dozen times, wiped the area with alcohol, and asked her if she was ready for the injection. *Big mistake!* She swiftly replied, "No, but get it over with." I took a minute to reassure her (and silently, me) again.

A little voice in my head repeated the words my *technologies* professor had said a million times, "Darting action is the key to a successful injection." So, I aimed at the bull's-eye that appeared in front of my eyes. My hand, which seemed to be moving in slow motion, propelled downward at a 90-degree angle. Secretly, I prayed that I would not hit my own hand. I looked down and it was a bull's-eye, thank goodness, but the needle had not penetrated the muscle! The patient successfully tensed her muscle tight enough to intercept the needle midflight. At that moment, she relaxed, probably because she thought the worst was over, and I pushed the needle into place. I stabilized the syringe at the end of the barrel, and began injecting the prochlorperazine slowly, watching my hands shake. Then I withdrew the needle, activated the needle safety device, and gently applied pressure over the site. It was over and I wanted to scream, "I did it!" but I kept my composure to feign the experience I lacked. Giving my first IM injection was not as bad as I thought it would be!

—Alison L. Moriarty, Georgetown University, Washington, DC

addition, aspiration causes increased pain when performed over the standard 5 to 10 seconds (Sisson, 2015); aspiration, even when performed, is not always performed over the recommended time-frame (Sisson, 2015; Thomas et al., 2016). Some medication manufacturers indicate that aspiration may be recommended when administering certain medications, at certain dosages, at certain rates, but more research needs to be done on this topic in the adult setting (Sepah et al., 2017; Thomas et al., 2016). Consult facility policy and manufacturer recommendations to ensure safe administration.

Intramuscular Injection Sites

Various sites may be used for intramuscular injections. To avoid complications, it is important to be able to identify anatomic landmarks and site boundaries and to use an accurate, careful technique when administering intramuscular injections. If care is not taken, possible complications include abscesses; cellulitis; injury to blood vessels, bones, and nerves; lingering pain; tissue necrosis; and periostitis (inflammation of the membrane covering a bone). Avoid any site that is bruised, tender, hard, swollen, inflamed, or scarred. After using the appropriate landmarks, always palpate the muscle to ensure the location identified is appropriate for each individual patient.

Consider the age of the patient, medication type, and medication volume when selecting a site for intramuscular injection. See Table 30-4 for information related to intramuscular site selection. Rotate the sites used to administer intramuscular medications when therapy requires repeated injections. Whatever pattern of rotating sites is used, provide a description of it in the patient's plan of nursing care.

The *ventrogluteal site* (see Fig. 30-13A on page 950) involves the gluteus medius and gluteus minimus muscles in the hip area. This site offers a large muscle mass that is relatively free from major nerves and blood vessels, the site is associated with less pain (Şanlialp Zeyrek et al., 2019), the area is clean (fecal contamination is rare at this site), and the patient can be on the back, abdomen, or side for the injection. To relax the gluteal muscle, the patient may flex the knees while lying on the back, point the toes inward while lying in the prone position, and flex the upper leg in front of the lower leg in the side-lying position. Although any of these three positions may be used when injecting into the ventrogluteal site, most nurses prefer the side-lying position.

To locate the ventrogluteal site, place the palm of your hand over the greater trochanter, with your fingers facing the patient's head. The right hand is used for the patient's left hip, or the left hand for the right hip, to identify landmarks. Place the index finger on the anterosuperior iliac spine and extend the middle finger dorsally, palpating the iliac crest. A triangle is formed, and the injection is given in the center of the triangle.

The *vastus lateralis* (see Fig. 30-13B on page 950) involves the quadriceps femoris muscle and is located along the anterolateral aspect of the thigh. There are no large nerves or vessels in its proximity, and it does not cover a joint. To locate the site, divide the thigh into thirds horizontally and vertically and administer the injection in the outer middle third. This space provides a large number of injection sites. The vastus lateralis site is particularly desirable for infants and children, whose gluteal muscles are poorly developed. Caregivers and nurses can use the cuddle position (semi-recumbent on caregiver's lap), the bed position (lying on back), the upright position (lap-sitting), or the straddle position (infant facing the caregiver) to promote access to the preferred site, while keeping the infant still and comforted (WHO, 2020).

The *deltoid muscle* is located in the lateral aspect of the upper arm (see Fig. 30-13C on page 950). It is the recommended site for vaccines for adults and may be used for children between ages 3 and 18 years for vaccine administration (CDC, 2019). The deltoid muscle is not developed enough in infants and toddlers to absorb medication adequately.

Table 30-4 Intramuscular Site Selection

CRITERIA	RECOMMENDED SITE
Age of Patient	
Infants and toddlers	Vastus lateralis
Children	Vastus lateralis or deltoid
Adults	Ventrogluteal or deltoid
Medication Type	
Biologicals (infants and toddlers)	Vastus lateralis
Biologicals (children and adults)	Deltoid
Medications that are known to be irritating, viscous, or oily solutions	Ventrogluteal

Source: Adapted from Centers for Disease Control and Prevention (CDC). (2015/2020). *Epidemiology and prevention of vaccine-preventable diseases* (13th ed.). J. Hamborsky, A. Kroger, & S. Wolfe (Eds.). Public Health Foundation. http://www.cdc.gov/vaccines/pubs/pinkbook/index.html

Concept Mastery Alert

The deltoid is the recommended site for vaccines for adults. The ventrogluteal site is recommended for general IM injections in adults.

Damage to the radial nerve and artery is a risk with use of the deltoid site. Intramuscular injections into the deltoid muscle should be limited to 1 mL of solution, but up to 2 mL may be administered, depending on the size of the muscle. Locate the deltoid muscle by palpating the lower edge of the acromion process. The deltoid site is typically three fingerbreadths below the acromium process. Visualize a triangle formed at the midpoint in line with the axilla on the lateral aspect of the upper arm, with the base of the triangle at the acromion process.

The dorsogluteal site has been previously identified as a possible site to be used for intramuscular medication administration. However, this site has been associated with inadvertent injection into subcutaneous tissue because the area

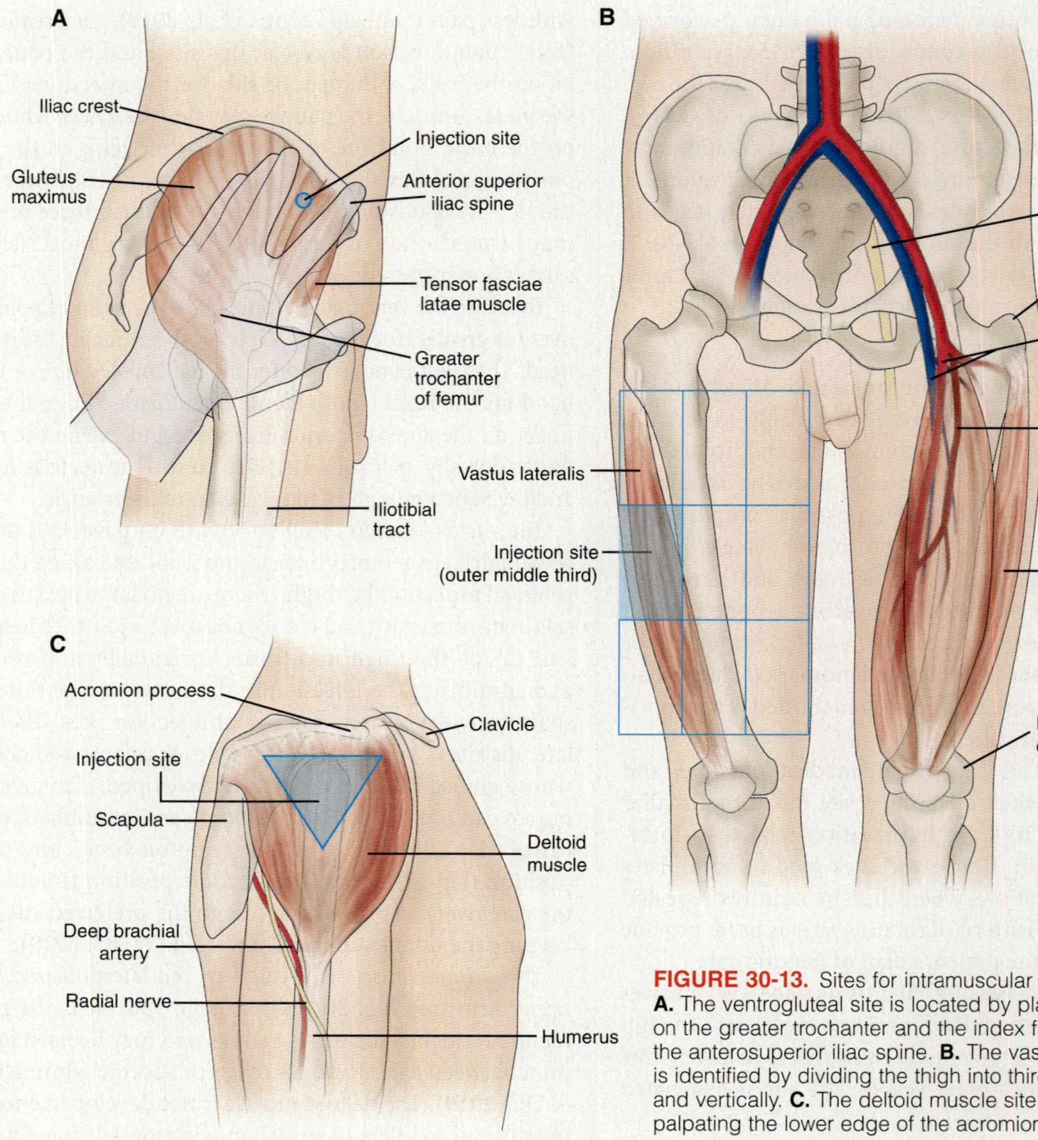

FIGURE 30-13. Sites for intramuscular injections. **A.** The ventrogluteal site is located by placing the palm on the greater trochanter and the index finger toward the anterosuperior iliac spine. **B.** The vastus lateralis site is identified by dividing the thigh into thirds, horizontally and vertically. **C.** The deltoid muscle site is located by palpating the lower edge of the acromion process.

is covered with subcutaneous tissue in many people. Injection into subcutaneous tissue alters drug absorption and can cause tissue irritation, pain, infection, neuropathy, bleeding, abscess formation, or necrosis (Ozen et al., 2019). It is also near the gluteal artery. More importantly, this site has been associated with significant injury, including pain and temporary or permanent paralysis, caused by damage to the sciatic nerve and other small nerves (Wu et al., 2020). Therefore, the dorsogluteal site is no longer recommended for use for intramuscular injections (Arslan & Özden, 2018; Frandsen & Pennington, 2021; Sisson, 2015; WHO, 2020). Discontinuing use of this site is linked to the elimination of aspiration during IM injections as routine practice (Sisson, 2015). It should be noted that despite the current recommendations to not use the dorsogluteal site (unless absolutely necessary; CDC, 2019), nurses continue to use this site in practice. Focused education and training on use of the ventrogluteal site increases the knowledge of nurses and may alleviate anxiety and change their opinions of outdated practice traditions (Arslan & Özden, 2018). More research needs to be done to generate definitive empirical evidence and universal, clear guidance on this topic (Brown et al., 2015; CDC, 2015/2020; Mraz et al., 2018). Follow the policies and procedures outlined by your health care facility.

Equipment

It is important to choose the right equipment for a particular intramuscular injection. Needle length should be based on the individual patient (see Table 30-5 for intramuscular needle length recommendations). Patients who are obese may require a longer needle (CDC, 2015/2020) and those who are emaciated may require a shorter needle. Appropriate gauge is determined by the medication being administered. In general, biologic agents and medications in aqueous solutions should be administered with a 20- to 25-gauge needle. Medications in oil-based solutions should be administered with an 18- to 25-gauge needle. Many medications come in prefilled syringe units. If a needle is provided on the prefilled unit, ensure that the needle on the unit is the appropriate length for the patient and situation.

Table 30-5 Intramuscular Injection Needle Length

SITE/AGE[a]	NEEDLE LENGTH
Vastus lateralis	5/8″ to 1″
Deltoid (children)	5/8″ to 1″
Deltoid (adults)	5/8″ to 1½″
Ventrogluteal (adults)	1″ to 1½″

[a]Biologic sex and weight are directly related to needle length choice; the size of the muscle, the adipose tissue thickness at the injection site, the volume of medication to be administered, and the injection technique also need to be considered. (Smart Sense Link: CDC PinkBook: http://www.cdc.gov/vaccines/pubs/pinkbook/vac-admin.html)

Source: Adapted from Centers for Disease Control and Prevention (CDC). (2015/2020). *Epidemiology and prevention of vaccine-preventable diseases* (13th ed.). J. Hamborsky, A. Kroger, & S. Wolfe (Eds.). Public Health Foundation. http://www.cdc.gov/vaccines/pubs/pinkbook/index.html

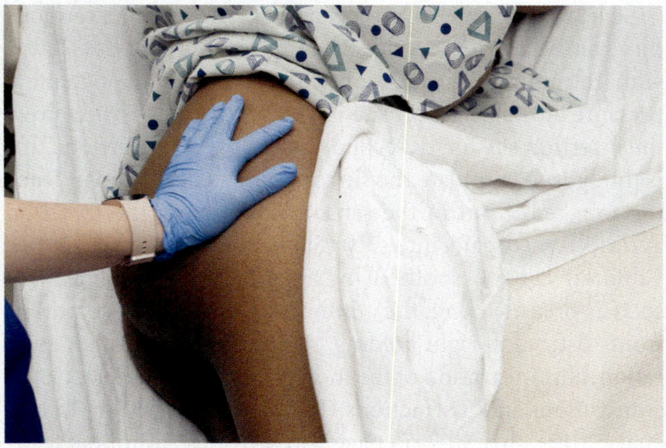

FIGURE 30-14. Spreading the skin taut at ventrogluteal site.

Procedure

The volume of medication that can be administered intramuscularly varies based on the intended site. In general, 1 to 5 mL is the accepted volume range. The less-developed muscles of children and older adults limit the intramuscular injection to 1 to 2 mL. Administer the intramuscular injection so that the needle is perpendicular to the patient's body. This should ensure that it is given using a 90-degree angle of injection (CDC, 2019).

Many of the drugs given intramuscularly can cause irritation to subcutaneous tissues when backflow into the tissues occurs along the injection track. Therefore, the **Z-track technique** is recommended for all intramuscular injections (particularly nonvaccine injections) to ensure that medication does not leak back along the needle track and into the subcutaneous tissue (Karch, 2020; Yilmaz et al., 2016). This technique reduces pain and discomfort (Şanlialp Zeyrek et al., 2019), particularly for patients receiving injections over an extended period. The Z-track method is also suggested for older adults who have decreased muscle mass. Some agents, such as iron, are best given via the Z-track method due to the irritation and discoloration associated with this agent (Karch, 2020).

In the Z-track technique, attach a clean needle to the syringe after the syringe is filled with the medication to prevent the injection of any residual medication on the needle into superficial tissues. Pull the skin down or to one side 1 to 2 cm (Yilmaz et al., 2016; Karch, 2020), spread the skin taut at the injection site, and hold in this position with the nondominant hand. Insert the needle and inject the medication slowly. After 10 seconds, withdraw the needle steadily and release the displaced tissue to allow it to return to its normal position. Massage of the site is *not* recommended because it may cause irritation by forcing the medication to leak back into the needle track. However, gentle pressure may be applied with a dry sponge. The procedure for administering an intramuscular injection using the Z-track technique is outlined in Skill 30-7 on pages 996–1002. An alternative method for intramuscular injection is to stretch the skin flat between two fingers and hold it taut for needle insertion. This technique for administering an intramuscular injection is illustrated in Figure 30-14. Figure 30-15 compares the angles for needle insertion for different forms of injections. The decision to simply stretch the skin taut or use the Z-track method is based on the individual patient and clinical judgment. Knowledge of landmarks and risks, along with an assessment of muscle size and consideration of the medication itself, are of paramount importance for the nurse.

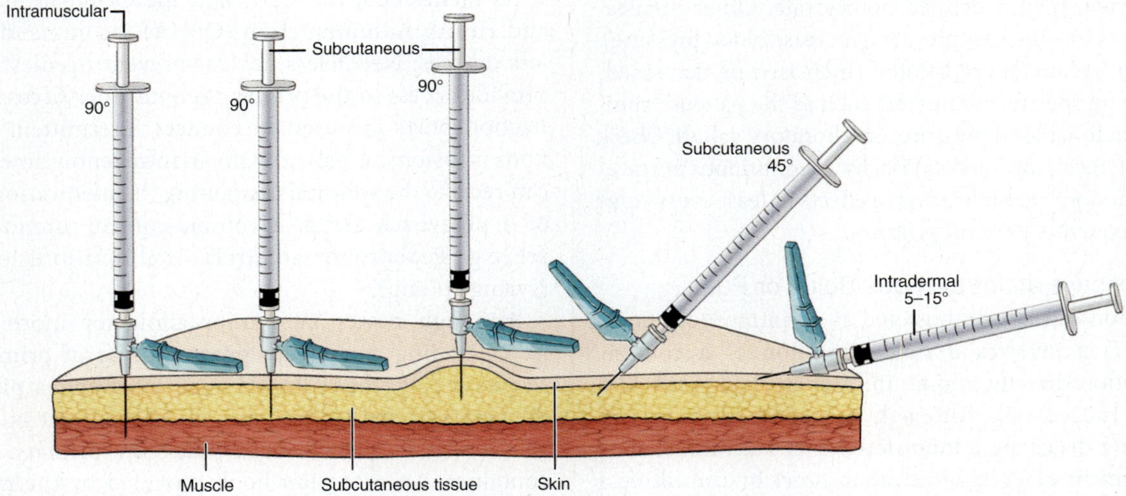

FIGURE 30-15. Comparison of insertion angles for intramuscular, subcutaneous, and intradermal injections.

Several techniques have been suggested as interventions that can be used to reduce discomfort and pain associated with intramuscular injections. The application of manual pressure at the insertion site is one suggestion. Firmly press the insertion site for 10 seconds before needle insertion. This is thought to stimulate the surrounding nerve endings, leading to a reduction in the sensory input from the injection and decreased pain intensity (Şanlialp Zeyrek et al., 2019). Children can be soothed by nonpharmacologic methods such as breastfeeding, the administration of sweet solutions, front-to-front upright holding, rapid injection without aspiration, administration of the most painful vaccine last, tactile stimulation, and distractions (Harrison et al., 2014; Taddio et al., 2010). Box 30-2 on page 946 provides additional techniques for reducing discomfort when injecting medications subcutaneously or intramuscularly.

ADMINISTERING MEDICATIONS INTRAVENOUSLY

Intravenous administration of medications delivers the drug directly into the bloodstream. Medications administered intravenously have an immediate effect. The **intravenous route** is the most dangerous route of administration because the drug is placed directly into the bloodstream, it cannot be recalled, and its actions cannot be slowed. Intravenous administration is the route used in most emergency situations when immediate onset of action is required. There also are many nonemergency clinical situations in which drugs are administered intravenously. Patient-controlled analgesia (PCA) allows the patient to control administration of an intravenous analgesic for pain management (refer to Chapter 35). There are several ways to administer medications intravenously. Observe aseptic technique when administering medications intravenously to prevent introduction of microorganisms.

Medications via Intravenous Solution

Medications may be added to the patient's infusion solution. In most facilities, the pharmacist adds the prescribed drug to a large volume of intravenous solution.

When medication is administered by infusion, the patient receives it at a defined rate (mL/hr) over a defined period of time. IV fluid, such as 0.9% or 0.45% Sodium Chloride, may run continuously at a defined hourly rate. Other medications, such as insulin, vasopressors (increase blood pressure), heparin, or sedatives, are titrated (increased or decreased) depending on specific parameters such as the patient's clinical presentation, blood pressure, or laboratory values. Check the patient receiving medication by a continuous intravenous infusion for possible adverse effects at least every hour or more frequently per unit protocol.

Medications via an Intravenous Bolus or Push

A medication can be administered as an intravenous bolus or push. This involves a single injection of a concentrated solution directly into an intravenous line (Skill 30-8 on pages 1002–1008). Although the administration rate varies, many drugs are administered over a 2-minute time frame. Confirm exact administration times by consulting a pharmacist or drug reference.

Medications via Intermittent Intravenous Infusion

Medications can be administered by intermittent intravenous infusion. The drug is mixed with a small amount of an intravenous solution, such as 50 to 100 mL of saline or dextrose, and administered over a short period at the prescribed interval (e.g., every 4 hours). The administration time is dictated by the dose and classification of the prescribed medication. For example, many antibiotics and electrolytes are administered over 30 to 90 minutes. The administration is most often performed using an intravenous infusion pump, which requires the nurse to program the infusion rate (mL/hr) and prescribed volume into the pump. *Smart (computerized) pumps* are being used by many facilities for intravenous infusions, including intermittent infusions. Smart pumps also require programming of infusion rates by the nurse, but also are able to identify dosing limits and practice guidelines to aid in safe administration (Institute for Safe Medication Practices, 2020). More information about intravenous infusions and smart pumps is provided in Chapter 41. Administration may be achieved by gravity infusion, which requires the nurse to calculate the infusion rate in drops per minute (gtt/min). The formula for this requires knowledge of the drop factor, which represents the number of drops per mL a specific IV tubing set delivers—this drop factor is determined by the manufacturer and printed on the IV tubing packaging.

The formula for calculating gtt/min =

$$\frac{\text{Drop Factor (gtt/mL)} \times \text{Volume to be Infused (mL)}}{\text{Time in Minutes (min)}}$$

An easy way to remember this formula is $\frac{D \times V}{M}$—no one relishes going to the DMV, but this acronym is familiar to anyone who has a driver's license in the United States. The calculated flow rate of a medication administered via gravity can be altered when the patient bends the extremity proximal to the intravenous insertion site, lifts the extremity, or has an infiltration at the insertion site. Best practice is to use an intravenous infusion pump whenever possible. Knowing how to calculate drops per minute is invaluable when equipment is scare or in an emergency situation.

As mentioned, the CDC and the Occupational Safety and Health Administration (OSHA) recommend needleless devices. Needleless devices prevent needlesticks and provide access to the primary venous line. Access or connection ports are used to connect intermittent intravenous infusions. A patient with an intravenous line in place can receive the solution containing the medication by way of a piggyback setup, a volume-control administration set (e.g., Pediatrol or Volutrol), or a mini-infusion pump (syringe pump).

Although newer IV pumps allow for more flexibility (including concurrent programming of primary and secondary/piggyback lines), some intravenous **piggyback delivery systems** still require the intermittent or additive solution to be placed higher than the primary solution container. An extension hook provided by the manufacturer provides for easy lowering of the main intravenous

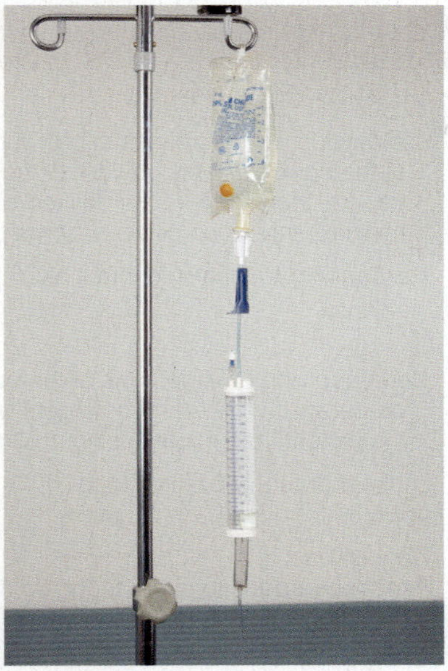

FIGURE 30-16. Volume-control administration set and IV solution for dilution of medication. (*Source:* Used with permission from Shutterstock. *Photo by B. Proud.*)

container. The port on the primary intravenous line has a back-check valve that automatically stops the flow of the primary solution, allowing the secondary or piggyback solution to flow when connected. Because manufacturers' designs vary, check the directions carefully for the systems used in the facility. Intravenous administration of medications using a gravity-based piggyback setup is explained in Skill 30-9 on pages 1008–1014.

Medications can also be placed in a volume-control administration set for intermittent intravenous infusion. The medication is diluted with a small amount of solution and administered through the patient's intravenous line (Fig. 30-16). This type of equipment may be used for infusing solutions into children, the critically ill, and older adults when the volume of fluid infused is a concern.

The mini-infusion pump (syringe pump) for intermittent infusion is battery operated and allows medication mixed in a syringe to be connected to the primary line (Fig. 30-17). The medication is delivered when the pump applies mechanical pressure to the syringe plunger.

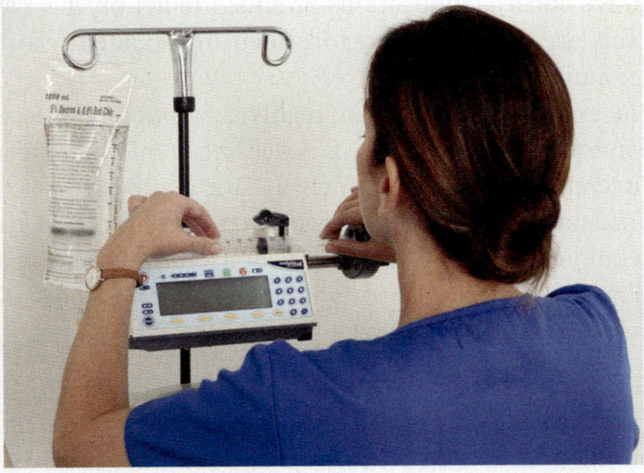

FIGURE 30-17. Inserting syringe into mini-infusion pump.

A medication or drug infusion lock, also known as an intermittent peripheral venous access device or *saline lock*, is used for patients who require intermittent intravenous medication, but not a continuous intravenous infusion. This device consists of a catheter connected to a short length of extension tubing capped with a sealed injection port. A peripheral venous access device is shown in Skill 30-10 on pages 1015–1020. After the catheter is in place in the patient's vein, anchor the catheter and tubing to the patient's arm so that the catheter remains in place until the patient no longer requires the medication intravenously.

An intermittent peripheral venous access device allows the patient more freedom than a continuous intravenous infusion. The patient is connected to the intravenous line when it is time to receive the medication and disconnected when the medication is completed. It is important to keep the device patent (working) by flushing with small amounts of saline pushed through the device on a routine basis. Do not start an intermittent infusion until intravenous placement is confirmed. Flush the peripheral venous access device before the infusion is begun and after the infusion is completed to clear the vein of any medication and to prevent clot formation in the catheter. The procedure for flushing this device with saline is discussed in Skill 30-10 on pages 1015–1020. A medication prescribed as an intravenous bolus or push (discussed on page 1012) may also be administered via a medication lock (refer to Skill 30-10). Assess the intravenous site for complications (see Chapter 41). If infiltration or phlebitis occurs, remove the device and insert a new catheter in a new site.

In addition to a peripheral intravenous line, intermittent intravenous medication may be administered through a central venous access device (CVAD). Many of these devices have particular specifications to be followed when using for administration of fluids or medication. It is important to be aware of the specifics for the device being used. Facilities have specific policies in place for reference. CVADs are discussed in more detail in Chapter 41.

Administering Topical Medications

Medications delivered via the topical route are applied to the skin or mucous membranes, including the eyes, ears, nose, rectum, vagina, and lungs. **Topical applications** are usually intended for direct action at a particular site, although some can have systemic effects and may be prescribed for that systemic effect. The action depends on the type of tissue and the nature of the agent.

If the site of application is readily accessible, such as the skin, an agent can easily be placed onto it. If it is a cavity, such as the nose, or is enclosed, such as the eye, a mechanical applicator may be needed to introduce the drug. Topical medications should not be shared. For medications administered routinely, patients in the hospital will have their own medications labeled with their names for individual use.

SKIN APPLICATIONS

The skin is a mechanical and chemical barrier that protects the underlying tissues. It is a sense organ, with receptors

Box 30-3 Typical Preparations Applied to the Skin

Preparation	Use	Nursing Considerations
Powder	Promote drying of the skin. Prevent friction on the skin.	Use caution when applying to prevent inhalation of the powder. Apply powder to the gauze square, then apply to the desired site to minimize inhalation of the airborne particles.
Ointment	Provide prolonged contact of a medication with the skin. Soften the skin.	Massage thoroughly into intact skin.
Creams and oils	Lubricate and soften skin. Prevent drying of skin.	When applying to large parts of the body, warm preparation in the hand or fingers to prevent the patient from experiencing chilling.
Lotions	Protect and soothe the skin.	Shake thoroughly before using. Apply with cotton balls or gauze.
Transdermal: reservoirs, microreservoirs, adhesives, matrices	These systems contain multiple layers, each with a specific job. An impermeable backing prevents drug diffusion from the exposed portion. The drug layer of the system contains drug, with a rate-controlling layer (or microneedles) to slow the release of the drug over time, ending with an adhesive layer to enhance the attachment of the system to the patient's skin (Rabiei et al., 2020).	Wear gloves. Handle by edges to avoid touching drug when handling system. Rotate application sites to avoid skin irritation.

that respond to touch, pain, pressure, and temperature. The skin helps in excretion, in regulating body temperature, and in storing essentials to the body such as water, salts, and glucose.

When a drug is incorporated in an agent such as an ointment and rubbed into the skin for absorption, the procedure is referred to as an inunction. On intact skin, drugs are absorbed into the lining of the sebaceous glands. Absorption is hindered because of the protective outer layer of the skin, which makes penetration difficult, and because of the fatty substances that protect the lining of the glands. Cleaning the skin thoroughly with soap or detergent and water before administration and then rubbing the medicated preparation into the skin can enhance absorption. Absorption can also be improved by using a drug mixed in an ointment or added to a liniment that will mix with the fat in the gland lining. When indicated, local heat applied to the application area can improve blood circulation and promote absorption. To prevent any absorption by the nurse's skin, wear gloves during the application of topical medications. Refer to Box 30-3 for information related to typical preparations applied to the skin.

The transdermal route is being used more frequently to deliver medication. This involves applying to the skin a disk or patch that contains medication intended for daily use or for longer intervals. Transdermal patches are commonly used to deliver hormones, narcotic analgesics, cardiac medications, and nicotine. These devices should not be massaged or moistened, have heat or cold applied, or be kept on during procedures such as an MRI or defibrillation. Transdermal patches that contain estrogen should not be applied to breast tissue due to the associated risks of breast cancer. Medication errors have occurred when patients applied multiple patches at once or failed to remove the overlay on the patch that exposes the skin to the medication. Opioid analgesic patches are associated with the most adverse drug effects and require careful monitoring for advancing sedation and respiratory depression (Jungquist et al., 2020; see Chapter 36 for more information on opioids). Clear patches have a cosmetic advantage but can be difficult to find on the patient's skin when they need to be removed or replaced. Despite a slow onset of action, transdermal drug patches maintain consistent serum drug levels. See Guidelines for Nursing Care 30-2: Applying Transdermal Patches.

EYE INSTILLATIONS AND IRRIGATIONS

The receptors for the sense of sight are located in the eye. The outer layer of the eyeball is called the sclera (the white of the eye). The cornea is the transparent part of the sclera in front of the eyeball. The sclera is fibrous and tough, but the cornea is injured easily by trauma. For this reason, applications to the eye seldom are placed directly onto the eyeball. Because direct application cannot be made onto the sensitive cornea, applications intended to act on the eye or the lids are placed onto, or instilled or irrigated into, the lower conjunctival sac.

The eye is a delicate organ, highly susceptible to infection and injury. Although the eye is never free of microorganisms, the secretions of the conjunctiva have a protective action against many pathogens. For maximum safety for the patient, the equipment, solutions, and ointments introduced into the conjunctival sac should be sterile. If this is not possible, follow the most careful guidelines for medical asepsis.

Eye Drops

Eye drops are instilled for their local effects, such as for pupil dilation or constriction when examining the eye, for treating an infection, or for controlling intraocular pressure

Guidelines for Nursing Care 30-2

APPLYING TRANSDERMAL PATCHES

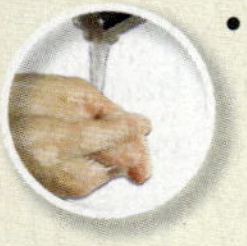

- Perform hand hygiene and put on PPE, as indicated.

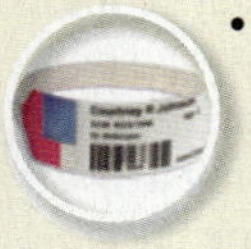

- **Identify the patient. Compare the information with the eMAR/MAR. The patient should be identified using at least two methods** (The Joint Commission, 2020a).
- **Complete necessary assessments before administering medications. Check the patient's allergy bracelet or ask the patient about allergies. Explain the purpose and action of the medication to the patient.**
- Scan the patient's bar code on the identification band, if required.
- **Based on facility policy, the third check of the label may occur at this point. If so, recheck the labels with the eMAR/MAR before administering the medications to the patient.**
- Put on gloves.
- Assess patient's skin where patch is to be placed, looking for any signs of irritation or breakdown. Site should be clean, dry, and free of hair. Rotate application sites.
- **Remove any old transdermal patches of the same medication from the patient's skin.** Fold patch in half with adhesive sides sticking together and discard according to facility policy.
- Gently wash the area where the old patch was.
- Remove the patch from its protective covering.
- Remove the covering on the patch without touching the medication surface. Apply the patch to the patient's skin. Smooth the edges down, and use the palm of your hand to press firmly for 30 seconds. Do not massage.
- Depending on facility policy, initial and write the date and time of administration on a piece of medical tape. Apply the tape to the patient's skin in close proximity to the patch. **Do not write directly on the medication patch.**
- Remove gloves and additional PPE, if used. Perform hand hygiene.
- Document the administration of medication immediately after administration including date, time, dose, route of administration, and site of administration on eMAR/MAR or record.
- Evaluate patient's response to medication within appropriate time frame for early detection of adverse effects.
- Check for dislodgement of the patch if the patient is active. Read information about the patch or consult with the prescriber or pharmacist to determine reapplication schedule and procedure.
- Assess for any skin irritation at application site. If necessary, remove the patch, wash the area carefully, and allow skin to air dry. Apply a new patch at a different site. Assess the potential for adverse reaction.
- Aluminum backing on a patch necessitates precautions if defibrillation is required. Burns and smoke may result. These patches should be removed before an MRI is performed to avoid burning of the skin.

in patients with glaucoma. The type and amount of solution depend on the purpose of the instillation. See Guidelines for Nursing Care 30-3: Instilling Eye Drops on page 956.

Ointments

Various types of medication in ointment form may be prescribed for the eye. These ointments are usually used for a local infection or irritation. Eye ointments are dispensed in a tube. A small amount of ointment is distributed along the exposed lower conjunctival sac after the eyelids and eyelashes have been cleansed. About ½ inch of ointment is squeezed from the tube along the exposed sac moving from the inner canthus to the outer canthus of the eye. After the application, the eyes should be closed. The warmth helps to liquefy the ointment. Instruct the patient to move the eye because this helps to spread the ointment under the lids and over the surface of the eyeball. Explain that the ointment may temporarily blur vision; encourage the patient not to rub the eye.

Eye Irrigation

Eye irrigation is performed to remove secretions or foreign bodies or to cleanse and soothe the eye. In an emergency, eye irrigation can be used to remove chemicals that may burn the eye. Copious amounts of tap water should be used to remove chemicals such as acid. The irrigation should continue for at least 15 minutes, and then professional help should be sought. Many emergency departments have eye flush stations to help with eye irrigations. Care should be taken so that the overflowing irrigation fluid does not contaminate the other eye.

Eye Medication Disks

An eye medication disk is flexible and resembles a small contact lens. These disks contain medication that is released gradually into the conjunctival sac. Once applied, the disk remains in place for as long as a week before being removed and discarded. When properly placed, the disk is completely covered by the lower eyelid, allowing the patient to wear contact lenses, swim, and sleep with the disk in place. Eye medication disks are usually applied at bedtime because they initially cause blurring of vision.

EAR INSTILLATIONS AND IRRIGATIONS

The ear contains the receptors for hearing and equilibrium. It consists of the external ear, the middle ear, and the inner ear. The external ear consists of the auricle or pinna and the exterior auditory canal. The auditory canal serves as a passageway for sound waves. Drugs or irrigations are instilled into the auditory canal for their local effect. They are used to soften wax, relieve pain, apply local anesthesia, destroy organisms, or destroy an insect lodged in the canal, which

Guidelines for Nursing Care 30-3

INSTILLING EYE DROPS

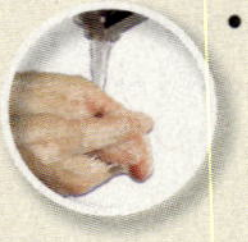

- Perform hand hygiene.

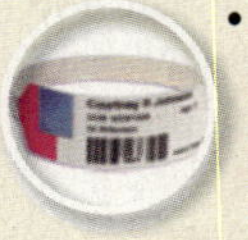

- **Identify the patient. Compare the information with the eMAR/MAR. The patient should be identified using at least two methods** (The Joint Commission, 2020a).
- **Complete necessary assessments before administering medications. Check the patient's allergy bracelet or ask the patient about allergies. Explain the purpose and action of the medication to the patient.**
- Scan the patient's bar code on the identification band, if required.
- **Based on facility policy, the third check of the label may occur at this point. If so, recheck the labels with the eMAR/MAR before administering the medications to the patient.**
- Put on gloves.
- Offer the patient paper tissues to remove solution and tears that may spill from the eye during the procedure.
- Clean the eyelids and eyelashes of any drainage with cotton balls or gauze squares moistened with water or normal saline solution, as needed. Debris can be carried into the eye when the conjunctival sac is exposed. Use each area of the cleaning surface once, moving from the inner toward the outer canthus to prevent carrying debris to the lacrimal ducts.
- Tilt the patient's head back slightly if sitting, or place the patient's head over a pillow if lying down. **Tilting the patient's head should be avoided if the patient has a condition that limits range of motion.** The head may be turned slightly to the affected side to prevent solution or tears from flowing toward the opposite eye.
- Remove the cap from the medication bottle, being careful not to touch the inner aspect of the cap or the tip of the bottle.
- Invert the monodrip plastic container that is commonly used to instill eye drops.
- Have the patient look up while focusing on something on the ceiling.
- Place the thumb or two fingers near the margin of the lower eyelid immediately below the eyelashes, and apply pressure downward over the bony prominence of the cheek. The lower conjunctival sac is exposed as the lower lid is pulled down.
- **Hold the dropper close to the eye but avoid touching the eyelids or lashes.** Rest the lateral side of your hand on the patient's forehead, just above the eyebrow, as needed for stability. Touching the eye, eyelids, or lashes can contaminate the medication in the bottle, startle the patient, causing blinking, or injure the eye.
- Squeeze the container and allow the prescribed number of drops to fall in the lower conjunctival sac. Do not allow medication to fall onto the cornea. This may injure the cornea or cause the patient to have an unpleasant sensation.
- Release the lower lid after the eye drops are instilled. Ask the patient to close the eyes gently.
- Apply gentle pressure with your gloved finger over the inner canthus to prevent the eye drops from flowing into the tear duct. This minimizes the risk of systemic effects from the medication.
- Replace the cover on the medication bottle.
- Instruct the patient not to rub the affected eye.
- Remove gloves and additional PPE, if used. Perform hand hygiene and assist the patient to a comfortable position.
- Document the administration of medication immediately after administration including date, time, dose, route of administration, and site of administration on the eMAR/MAR or record.
- Evaluate the patient's response to the medication within the appropriate time frame.

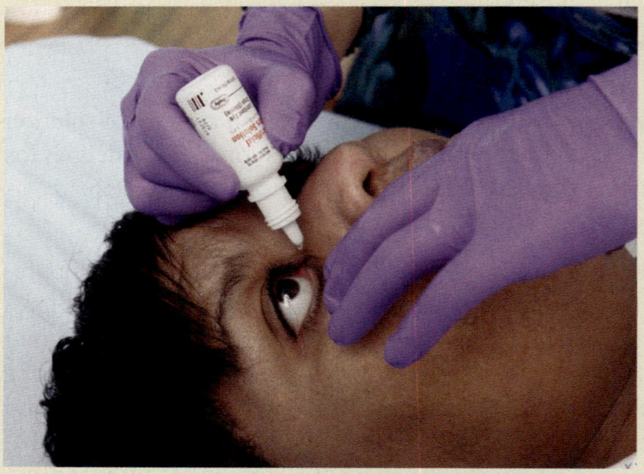

With the lower lid pulled down, the nurse prepares to administer the eye drops on the lower conjunctival sac.

can cause almost intolerable discomfort. If the ear canal has swollen to the point that medication cannot pass, a long piece of cotton material called a wick is inserted so that one end is near the middle ear and the other end is external to the ear. This cotton then acts as a wick to help medication get into the canal.

The tympanic membrane separates the external ear from the middle ear. Normally, it is intact and closes the entrance to the middle ear completely. If it is ruptured or has been opened by surgical intervention, the middle ear and the inner ear have a direct passage to the external ear. When this occurs, instillations and irrigations should be performed with the greatest of care to prevent forcing materials from the outer ear into the middle ear and the inner ear. Sterile technique is used to prevent infection.

Ear Drops

Follow the techniques listed in Guidelines for Nursing Care 30-4: Instilling Ear Drops when placing drops in the external auditory canal.

Guidelines for Nursing Care 30-4

INSTILLING EAR DROPS

- Perform hand hygiene and put on PPE, as indicated.
- **Identify the patient. Compare the information with the eMAR/MAR. The patient should be identified using at least two methods** (The Joint Commission, 2020a).
- **Complete necessary assessments before administering medications. Check the patient's allergy bracelet or ask the patient about allergies. Explain the purpose and action of the medication to the patient.**
- Scan the patient's bar code on the identification band, if required.
- **Based on facility policy, the third check of the label may occur at this point. If so, recheck the labels with the eMAR/MAR before administering the medications to the patient.**
- Put on gloves.
- Clean the external ear of drainage with cotton balls moistened with water or normal saline solution, as needed.
- Place the patient on the unaffected side in bed, or if ambulatory, have the patient sit with the head well tilted to the side so that the affected ear is pointed upward. This positioning prevents the drops from escaping from the ear.
- Remove the cap from the medication bottle, being careful not to touch the inner aspect of the cap or the tip of the container.
- Straighten the auditory canal by pulling the cartilaginous portion of the pinna up and back in an adult (Fig. A), straight back for a child older than 3 (Fig. B), and down and back in an infant or a child under age 3 years (Fig. C). Pulling on the pinna as described helps to straighten the canal properly for ear instillation.
- Invert and hold the dropper in the ear with its tip above the auditory canal.
- **Squeeze the bottle and allow drops to fall on the side of the canal. Avoid instilling in the middle of the canal, to avoid instilling directly onto the tympanic membrane.**
- Release the pinna after instilling the drops, and have the patient maintain the position to prevent the medication from escaping.
- Gently press on the tragus a few times to help move the medication from the canal toward the tympanic membrane.
- If ordered, loosely insert a cotton ball to prevent medication from leaking out.
- Replace the cap on the medication bottle.
- Instruct patient to remain lying down with the affected ear upward for 5 minutes. Wait 5 minutes before instilling drops in the second ear, if prescribed.
- Remove gloves and additional PPE, if used. Perform hand hygiene and assist the patient to a comfortable position.
- Document the administration of medication immediately after administration including date, time, dose, route of administration, and site of administration on the eMAR/MAR or record.

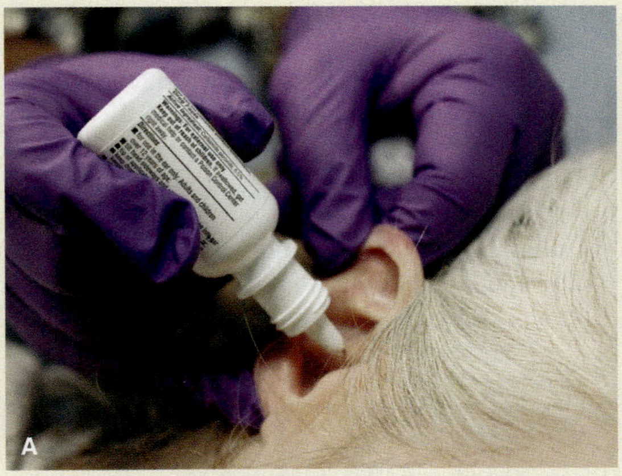

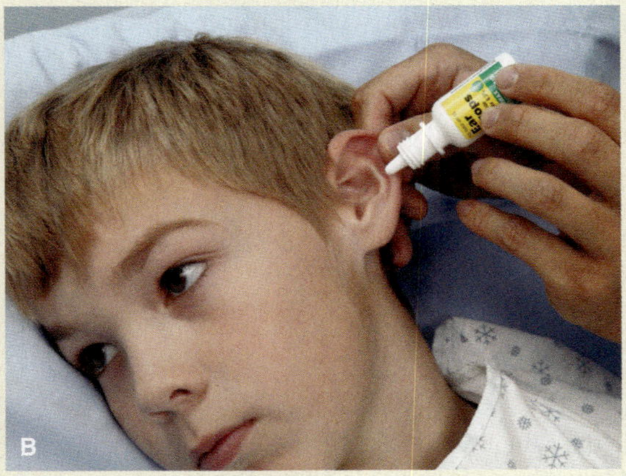

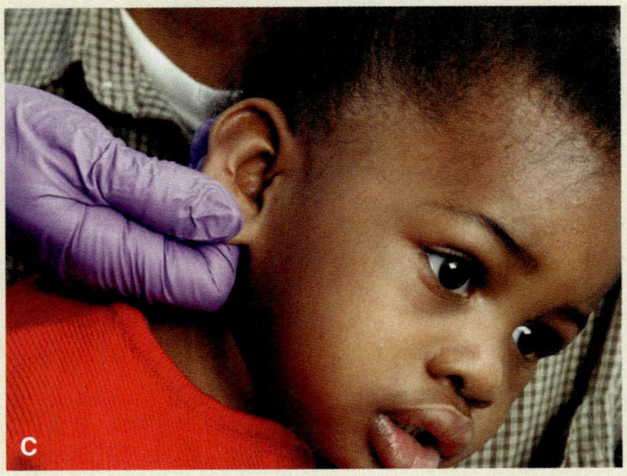

A. Adult patient positioned for ear drop instillation; nurse straightens the auditory canal by pulling the cartilaginous portion of the pinna up and back.
B. School-aged child positioned for ear drop instillation; nurse straightens the auditory canal by pulling the cartilaginous portion of the pinna straight back.
C. Child younger than age 3 years ready for ear drop instillation; the nurse straightens the auditory canal by pulling the cartilaginous portion of the pinna down and back. Child can be held by parent.

EAR IRRIGATIONS

Irrigations of the external auditory canal are ordinarily done for cleaning purposes or for applying heat to the area. Typically, normal saline solution is used, although an antiseptic solution may be indicated for local action. To prevent pain, the irrigation solution should be at least at room temperature. An irrigation syringe is used in most instances. An irrigating container with tubing and an ear tip may also be used, especially if the purpose of the irrigation is to apply heat to the area.

NASAL INSTILLATIONS

Besides serving as the olfactory organ, the nose functions as an airway to the lower respiratory tract and protects the tract by cleaning and warming the air taken in by inspiration. Cilia project on most of the surfaces of the nasal mucous membrane, which help remove particles of dirt and dust from the inspired air. The nose also serves as a resonator when speaking and singing.

Nasal instillations are used to treat allergies, sinus infections, and nasal congestion. Medications with a systemic effect, such as vasopressin or naloxone, may also be prepared as a nasal instillation. The nose is normally not a sterile cavity, but, because of its connection with the sinuses, it is important to observe medical asepsis carefully when using nasal instillations. See Guidelines for Nursing Care 30-5: Instilling Nose Spray.

Medications may also be applied to the nasal mucous membrane via nasal drops. The patient should blow the nose before instilling the drops. Have the patient sit up with head tilted well back and maintain this position for a few minutes after instillation. This position allows the solution to flow well back into the nares. Hold up the tip of the nose and place the dropper just inside the naris, about one third of an inch, without touching the naris. Instill the prescribed number of drops in one naris and then into the other. Avoid touching the nares with the dropper; inadvertent contact may cause the patient to sneeze and contaminate the dropper.

Guidelines for Nursing Care 30-5

INSTILLING NOSE SPRAY

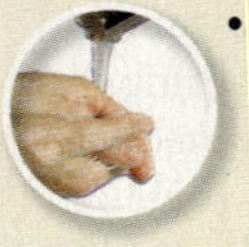

- Perform hand hygiene and put on PPE, as indicated.

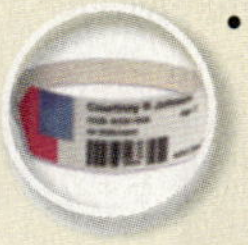

- **Identify the patient. Compare the information with the eMAR/MAR. The patient should be identified using at least two methods** (The Joint Commission, 2020a).
- **Complete necessary assessments before administering medications. Check the patient's allergy bracelet or ask the patient about allergies. Explain the purpose and action of the medication to the patient.**
- Scan the patient's bar code on the identification band, if required.
- **Based on facility policy, the third check of the label may occur at this point. If so, recheck the labels with the eMAR/MAR before administering the medications to the patient.**
- Put on gloves.
- Provide the patient with paper tissues and ask that the patient blow the nose before instilling the nose drops.
- Have the patient sit up with head tilted back. **Tilting the patient's head should be avoided if the patient has a condition that limits range of motion.**
- Instruct the patient that, depending on the medication, it may be necessary to inhale gently through the nose as the spray is being administered.
- Agitate the bottle gently, if required for specific medication. Insert the tip of the nose piece of the bottle into one nostril.
- Close the opposite nostril with a finger. Instruct the patient to breathe in gently through the nostril, if required. Compress or activate the bottle to release one spray at the same time the patient breathes in.
- Keep the medication container compressed and remove from the nostril. Release the container from the compressed state. Do not allow the container to return to its original position until it is removed from the patient's nose.
- Instruct the patient to hold their breath for a few seconds, and then breathe out slowly through the mouth. Repeat in the other nostril, as prescribed or indicated.
- Wipe the outside of the bottle nose piece with a clean, dry tissue or cloth and replace the cap. Instruct the patient to avoid blowing the nose for 5 to 10 minutes, depending on the medication.
- Remove gloves and additional PPE, if used. Perform hand hygiene and assist the patient to a comfortable position.
- Document the administration of medication immediately after administration including date, time, dose, route of administration, and site of administration on the eMAR/MAR or record.

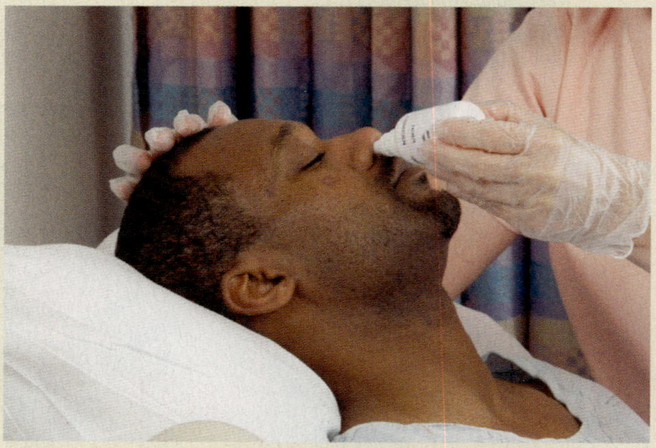

Inserting tip of bottle into nostril. (*Source:* Craven, R. F., Himle, C. J., & Henshaw, C. M. [2017]. *Fundamentals of Nursing: Human Health and Function* [8th ed]. Wolters Kluwer.)

Guidelines for Nursing Care 30-6

INSERTING VAGINAL CREAM OR SUPPOSITORY

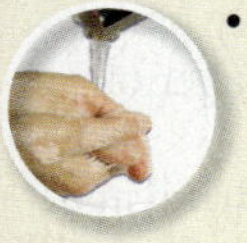

- Perform hand hygiene and put on PPE, if indicated.

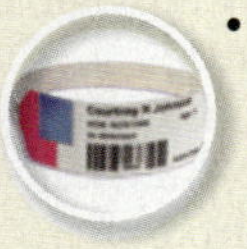

- **Identify the patient. Compare the information with the eMAR/MAR. The patient should be identified using at least two methods** (The Joint Commission, 2020a).
- **Complete necessary assessments before administering medications. Check the patient's allergy bracelet or ask the patient about allergies. Explain the purpose and action of the medication to the patient.**
- Scan the patient's bar code on the identification band, if required.
- **Based on facility policy, the third check of the label may occur at this point. If so, recheck the labels with the eMAR/MAR before administering the medications to the patient.**
- Ask the patient to void before inserting medication.
- Put on gloves.
- Position the patient so that they are lying on their back with knees flexed. Maintain privacy with draping. Provide adequate light to visualize vaginal opening.
- Perform perineal care. Spread labia with fingers and clean area at vaginal orifice. Wipe from front to back, using a different portion of the disposable cloth/washcloth with each stroke.
- Remove gloves and put on new gloves.
- Fill a vaginal applicator with the prescribed amount of cream, or have a suppository ready (Fig. A).
- Lubricate the applicator with lubricant, as necessary. The rounded end of a suppository may be lubricated with a water-soluble lubricant (Fig. B).
- For a vaginal cream, spread the labia and introduce the applicator gently in a rolling manner while directing it downward and backward to follow the normal contour of the vagina for its full length. Push the plunger to its full length, then gently remove the applicator with the plunger depressed. For a vaginal suppository, lubricate your gloved index finger on your dominant hand. Spread the labia and insert the rounded end of the suppository along the posterior wall of the canal to the length of your finger.
- **Ask the patient to remain in the supine position for a minimum of 5 to 10 minutes after insertion.**
- Offer the patient a perineal pad to collect drainage.
- Remove gloves and additional PPE, if used. Perform hand hygiene and assist the patient to a comfortable position.
- Document the administration of medication immediately after administration including date, time, dose, route of administration, and site of administration on the eMAR/MAR or record.

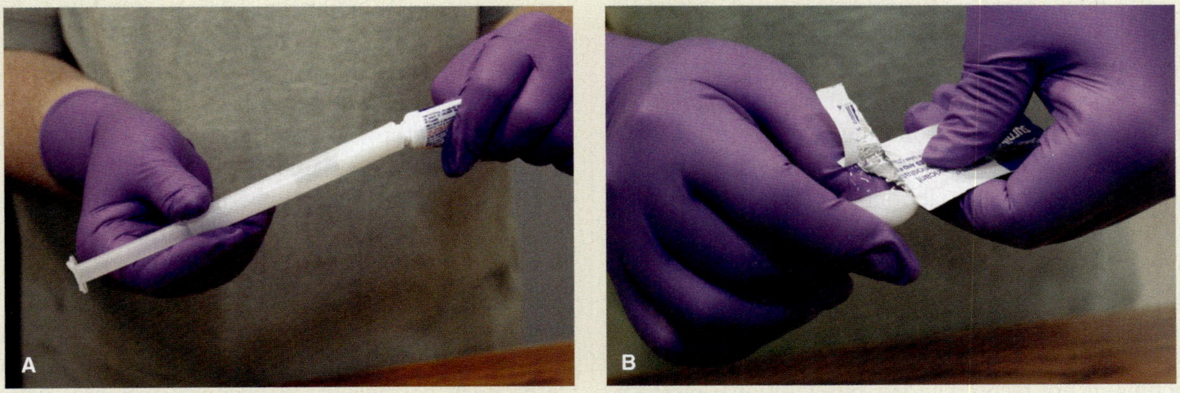

A. Filling vaginal applicator with cream. **B.** Lubricating vaginal suppository.

VAGINAL APPLICATIONS

A healthy vagina contains few pathogens, but many nonpathogenic organisms. The nonpathogens are important because they protect the vagina from the invasion of pathogens. The normal secretions in the vagina are acidic and further serve to protect the vagina from microbial invasion. Therefore, the normal mucous membrane is its own best protection.

Creams, foams, and tablets can be applied intravaginally using a narrow, tubular applicator with an attached plunger. Suppositories that melt when exposed to body heat are also administered by vaginal insertion. Refrigerate suppositories for storage. Evidence shows that perineal talc use and the instillation of non-prescription douches—incorrectly presumed to clean the vagina after menstruation, minimize the contraction of sexually transmitted infections (STIs), or prevent pregnancy—are contraindicated and may lead to vaginal and endometrial infections; pelvic inflammatory disease; pregnancy complications; and cervical, uterine, and endometrial cancers (Gondwe et al., 2020; Hamoonga et al., 2019; O'Brien et al., 2019).

Ask the patient to void before inserting the medication. Position the patient so that they are lying on their back with knees flexed. Maintain privacy with draping. Provide adequate light to visualize the vaginal opening. See Guidelines for Nursing Care 30-6: Inserting Vaginal Cream or Suppository.

Guidelines for Nursing Care 30-7

INSERTING A RECTAL SUPPOSITORY

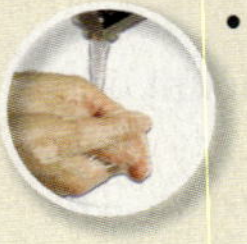

- Perform hand hygiene and put on PPE, if indicated.

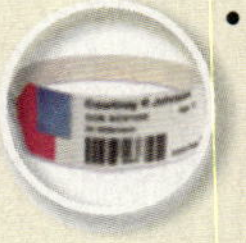

- **Identify the patient. Compare the information with the eMAR/MAR. The patient should be identified using at least two methods** (The Joint Commission, 2020a).
- **Complete necessary assessments before administering medications. Check the patient's allergy bracelet or ask the patient about allergies. Explain the purpose and action of the medication to the patient.**
- Scan the patient's bar code on the identification band, if required.
- **Based on facility policy, the third check of the label may occur at this point. If so, recheck the labels with the eMAR/MAR before administering the medications to the patient.**
- Put on gloves.
- Assist the patient to their left side in a Sims position. Drape accordingly to expose only the buttocks.
- Remove the suppository from its wrapper. Apply lubricant to the rounded end. Lubricate the index finger of your dominant hand.
- Separate the buttocks with your nondominant hand and instruct the patient to breathe slowly and deeply through the mouth while the suppository is being inserted.
- Using your index finger, insert the suppository, round end first, along the rectal wall. Insert about 3 to 4 inches.
- Use toilet tissue to clean any stool or lubricant from around the anus. Release the buttocks. Encourage the patient to remain on their side for at least 5 minutes and retain the suppository for the appropriate amount of time for the specific medication.

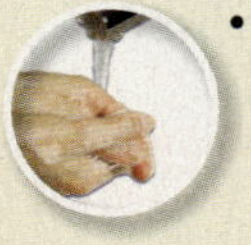

- Remove gloves and additional PPE, if used. Perform hand hygiene and assist the patient to a comfortable position.
- Document the administration of medication immediately after administration including date, time, dose, route of administration, and site of administration on the eMAR/MAR or record.

RECTAL INSTILLATIONS

Rectal suppositories and enemas are used primarily for their local action, such as laxatives and fecal softeners. Systemic effects are also achieved with rectal suppositories. Acetaminophen suppositories are used for an antipyretic effect, and many antiemetics are available in suppository form to relieve nausea and vomiting. Do not administer suppositories to patients who have had recent rectal or prostate surgery. Assess recent laboratory values, particularly the patient's white blood cell and platelet counts. Patients who have thrombocytopenia or are neutropenic should not receive rectal suppositories. Do not administer rectal suppositories to patients at risk for cardiac arrhythmias due to the risk of a vasovagal response. Rectal douching, like vaginal douching, is not recommended, but additional research is needed to better understand the risks, associations with STIs and HIV transmission, social and cultural practices, and sexual contexts of rectal douching, which is practiced by men who have sex with men (MSM) and transwomen (Dangerfield II et al., 2020; Reeders et al., 2020).

Use clean disposable gloves to prevent contamination with feces and microorganisms. Refer to Guidelines for Nursing Care 30-7: Inserting a Rectal Suppository. After the suppository is inserted, the patient should remain in that position for 5 minutes. If the suppository is for laxative purposes, it must remain in position for 35 to 45 minutes, or until the patient feels the urge to defecate.

Administering Medications by Inhalation

Drugs for **inhalation** are aerosolized, delivered in small particles, and breathed in by the patient. The lungs are supplied richly with blood and have a large surface area. These characteristics allow drugs to be absorbed easily from the lower respiratory tract. Inhalation may be used to administer several different classes of drugs with varying properties and indications. The smaller the particles of inhaled medication, the lower in the respiratory tract the medication tends to travel. A disadvantage of using this route is that the drug dosage is difficult to establish.

Drugs classified as bronchodilators are an example of a medication administered by inhalation. Bronchodilators act to decrease resistance to airflow by enlarging air passageways. Bronchodilators promote relaxation of musculature in the tracheobronchial tree. The relaxed passages produce less resistance to airflow and provide an opened respiratory passageway. Bronchodilators are further discussed in Chapter 40.

Drugs for inhalation may be administered at home, in the hospital, or in another facility by a nebulizer. Nebulizers facilitate administration of the medication by dispersing the liquid medication in compressed air (*medical air*) or high-flow oxygen. This method is valuable for patients who require inhalation of a drug several times a day when the hand atomizer is fatiguing. Infants and toddlers can also benefit from nebulized medications. With the use of an oxygen mask, children can receive medications with minimal interruption of their activities. Oxygen masks for the pediatric population come in a variety of sizes and also have cute animals on them to make the mask less intimidating for the child. The oxygen stream is also useful in the production of vapors when high humidity is needed continuously for long periods. Refer to the Guidelines for Nursing Care 30-8.

Guidelines for Nursing Care 30-8

USING AN INHALED MEDICATION DEVICE

- Assess the patient's ability to manage a metered-dose inhaler, dry powder inhaler, or small-volume nebulizer.
- Explain, demonstrate, and encourage the patient to manipulate the inhaler or nebulizer apparatus.
- Encourage the patient to wash hands thoroughly before using device.

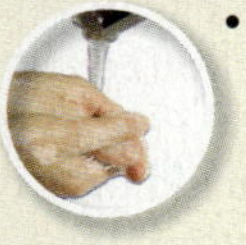

- Perform hand hygiene.

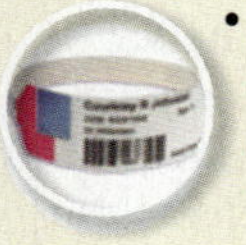

- **Identify the patient. Compare the information with the eMAR/MAR. The patient should be identified using at least two methods** (The Joint Commission, 2020a).
- **Complete necessary assessments before administering medications. Check the patient's allergy bracelet or ask the patient about allergies. Explain the purpose and action of the medication to the patient.**
- Scan the patient's bar code on the identification band, if required.
- **Based on facility policy, the third check of the label may occur at this point. If so, recheck the labels with the eMAR/MAR before administering the medications to the patient.**

Metered-Dose Inhaler (MDI)

- Shake the inhaler well.
- Remove the mouthpiece covers from the MDI and the spacer. Attach the MDI to the spacer by inserting it in the open end of the spacer, opposite the mouthpiece.
- Have the patient place the spacer's mouthpiece into their mouth, grasping securely with the teeth and sealing the lips tightly around the mouthpiece lips. Have the patient breathe normally through the spacer.
- If no spacer is used, patient takes a deep breath, exhales, holds the inhaler between the lips or 1 to 2 inches away from the mouth (based on guidance from the provider and manufacturer), inhales slowly and deeply while depressing the medication canister and continues to inhale for a full breath.
- Have the patient breathe normally through the spacer.

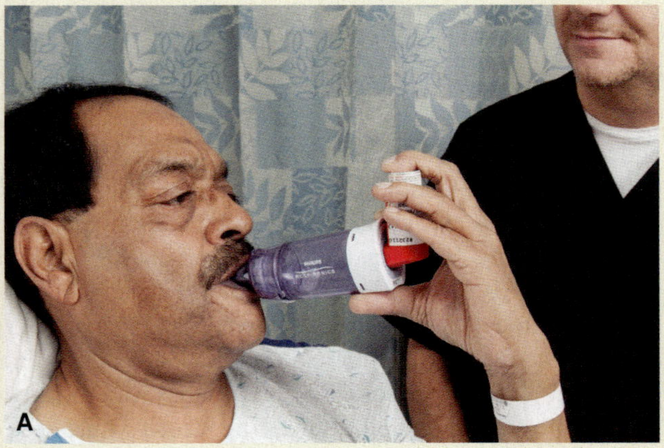

A. Patient using a metered-dose inhaler with a spacer.

- Instruct the patient to exhale completely, then depress the canister once, releasing one puff into the spacer, and inhale slowly and deeply through the mouth. **Instruct the patient to hold their breath for 5 to 10 seconds, or as long as possible, then to exhale slowly through pursed lips.**
- **Wait 1 to 5 minutes, as indicated by the medication, before administering the next puff, as prescribed.**
- After the prescribed number of puffs has been administered, have the patient remove the MDI from the spacer and replace the caps on both the MDI and spacer.
- Have the patient gargle and rinse with tap water after using an MDI, as indicated. Clean the MDI according to the manufacturer's directions.

Dry Powder Inhaler (DPI)

- Review the specific instructions the specific DPI to be administered.
- Remove the mouthpiece cover (if present) and load a dose if necessary. Alternatively, activate the inhaler, if necessary, according to the manufacturer's directions.
- Have the patient breathe out slowly and completely, without breathing into the DPI. **The patient should place teeth over, and seal lips around, the mouthpiece. It is important to not block the opening with the tongue or teeth.**
- **Have the patient breathe in strong, steady, and deeply through the mouth, for longer than 2 to 3 seconds.**
- Remove the inhaler from the mouth. Instruct the patient to hold their breath for 5 to 10 seconds, or as long as possible, and then to exhale slowly through pursed lips.
- Wait 1 to 5 minutes, as indicated by the medication, before administering the next puff. After the prescribed amount of puffs has been administered, have the patient replace the cap or storage container.
- Have the patient gargle and rinse with tap water after using a DPI, as indicated. Clean the DPI according to the manufacturer's directions.

Small-Volume Nebulizer

- Remove the nebulizer cup from the device and open it.
- Place premeasured unit dose medication in the bottom section of the cup or use a dropper to place concentrated dose of medication in the cup and add prescribed fluid to dilute if required.
- Screw the top portion of the nebulizer cup back in place and attach the cup to the nebulizer.
- Attach one end of tubing to the stem on the bottom of the nebulizer cuff and the other end to the air compressor or oxygen source.
- Turn on the air compressor or oxygen.
- Check that a fine medication mist is produced by opening the valve.
- Have the patient place the mouthpiece into mouth and grasp securely with teeth and lips.
- **Instruct the patient to inhale slowly and deeply through the mouth and hold each breath for a slight pause before exhaling. (A nose clip may be necessary if the patient is also breathing through the nose.)**

(*continued*)

Guidelines for Nursing Care 30-8 *(continued)*

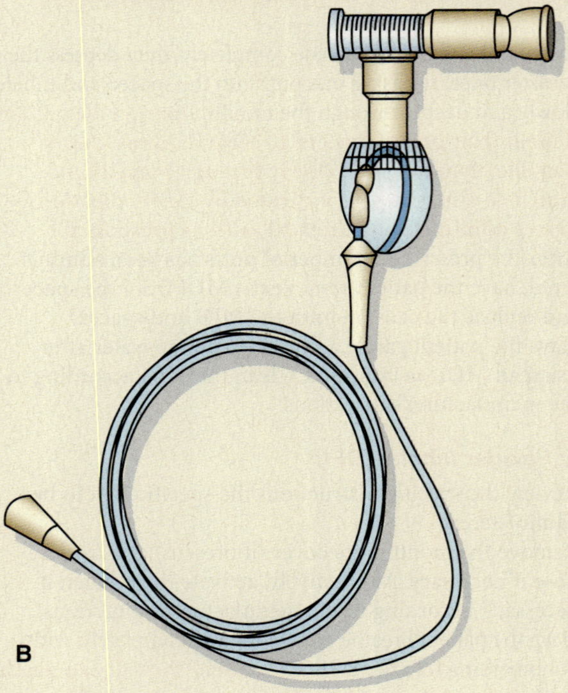

B. Small-volume nebulizer.

- Have patient continue this inhalation technique until all medication in the nebulizer cup has been aerosolized (usually about 15 minutes). When the medication in the nebulizer cup has been completely aerosolized, the cup will be empty.
- Have the patient remove the nebulizer from the mouth, and gargle and rinse with tap water, as indicated. Clean and store the nebulizer according to the manufacturer's directions and facility policies.

Home Considerations

- Patients should know how to tell when medication levels are getting low. The most reliable method is to look on the canister and see how many puffs the canister contains. Divide this number by the number of puffs used daily to ascertain how many days the MDI will last. For instance, if the MDI contains 200 puffs and the patient takes 6 puffs per day, the MDI should last for 33 days. Keep a diary or record of inhaler use and discard the inhaler on reaching the labeled number of doses. This method may be cumbersome and impractical for some patients, but it is a reliable way to determine how much medication remains in an MDI. Another accurate way to know when the canister is depleted is to use a dose counter, which counts down each time the canister is activated (Cleveland Clinic, 2020). **Floating the canister in water is not reliable and is contraindicated. Immersion in water can cause valve obstruction and threatens product integrity** (MedlinePlus, 2020).
- The plastic holder provided with the inhaler should be cleaned at least weekly. Remove the medication canister and clean with warm running water. Shake the holder and allow to air dry. Some medication canisters cannot be removed from the plastic holder. Wipe the mouthpiece with a cloth or dry cotton swab and/or refer to the manufacturer's directions for cleaning (Cleveland Clinic, 2020). Clean the spacer once a week by soaking in warm water with a mild detergent. Rinse well and shake off excess water. Allow to air dry (Cleveland Clinic, 2020). Do not store spacer in a plastic bag to prevent moisture retention and possible resulting microorganism growth.

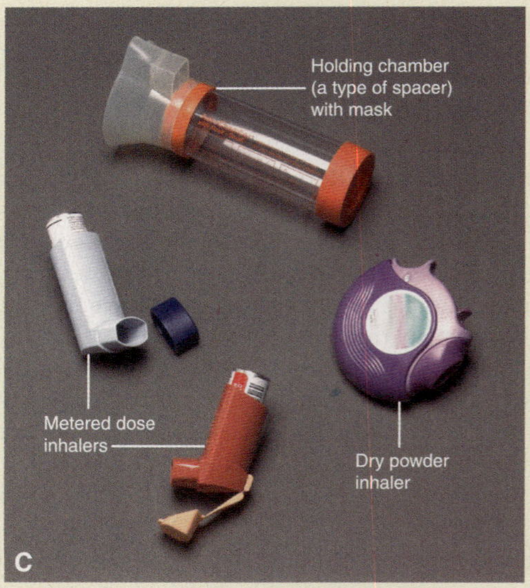

C. Examples of metered-dose inhalers, spacer, and dry powder inhaler.

What the public considers an inhaler is technically called a handheld, metered-dose inhaler (MDI). Unfortunately, the MDI is often used incorrectly (Price et al., 2017), and the correct dose of medication is not delivered. For better medication delivery, use a spacer whenever administering medication via an MDI, particularly with a child. Refer to Guidelines for Nursing Care 30-8: Using an Inhaled Medication Device.

Dry powder inhalers (DPIs) are another type of delivery method for inhaled medications. The medication is supplied in a powder form, either in a small capsule or disk inserted into the DPI, or in a compartment inside the DPI. DPIs are breath activated. A quick breath by the patient activates the flow of medication, eliminating the need to coordinate activating the inhaler (spraying the medicine) while inhaling the medicine at the same time. However, the drug output and size distribution of the aerosol from a DPI is more or less dependent on the flow rate through the device, thus the patient must be able to take a powerful, deep inspiration (Alismail et al., 2016; Price et al., 2017). Many types of DPIs are available, with distinctive operating instructions. Some have to be loaded with a dose of medication each time they are used and some hold a preloaded number of doses (referred to as a *diskus* in some cases). It is important to understand the particular instructions for the medication and particular delivery device being used. Refer to the Guidelines for Nursing Care 30-8.

Documenting Medication Administration

The medication administration record is a legal document. Recording each dose of medication as soon as possible after it is given provides a documented record that can be consulted if there are any questions about whether the patient received the medication. Do not record medications before they are given. If something changed and the medication was not actually given, the medication record would incorrectly show that the patient received the medication. Different forms are used for recording medications; an example of an eMAR is given in Figure 30-18.

The name of the medication, dosage, route of administration, time given, and name of the person administering the medication are noted in the record. Record the site used for an injection, the location of a topical or transdermal application, and the naris, eye, or ear used for those administrations. The identity of the nurse completing the documentation is recorded based on the unique user ID and password assigned to each nurse when an eMAR is used. Other specific patient information may be required. For instance, record the pulse rate when administering some cardiac drugs, or record a description of the effects on the patient's pain when administering analgesics.

OMITTED DRUGS

Drugs may be omitted intentionally or inadvertently. The omission and the reason for it are documented on the patient's record. The nurse should notify and collaborate with the prescribing provider regarding the planned or actual omission of drugs. Drugs may be omitted intentionally for the following reasons:

- The patient is to have a diagnostic test and is required to fast before the test. Oral drugs may be omitted, or their administration may be delayed, depending on the provider's orders.
- The problem for which the medication is intended no longer exists. For example, a laxative has been ordered for a patient. The patient has had a bowel movement and no longer needs the laxative. The laxative is then omitted.
- The medication does not meet prescribed administration guidelines or the clinical judgment of the nurse necessitates follow up with the prescribing provider. For example, it is standard practice to hold certain cardiac drugs if the heart rate or blood pressure fall below a certain level; these parameters may or may not be included with the order itself.
- The patient is suspected of having an allergy to the medication. Any suspected allergy should be reported to the primary care provider.

REFUSED DRUGS

If the patient refuses to take a drug that is considered essential to the therapeutic regimen, report this promptly. It is important to determine the reason for the refusal and to ensure the refusal is not related to a knowledge deficit. If the patient is not persuaded by reasonable efforts and adamantly refuses

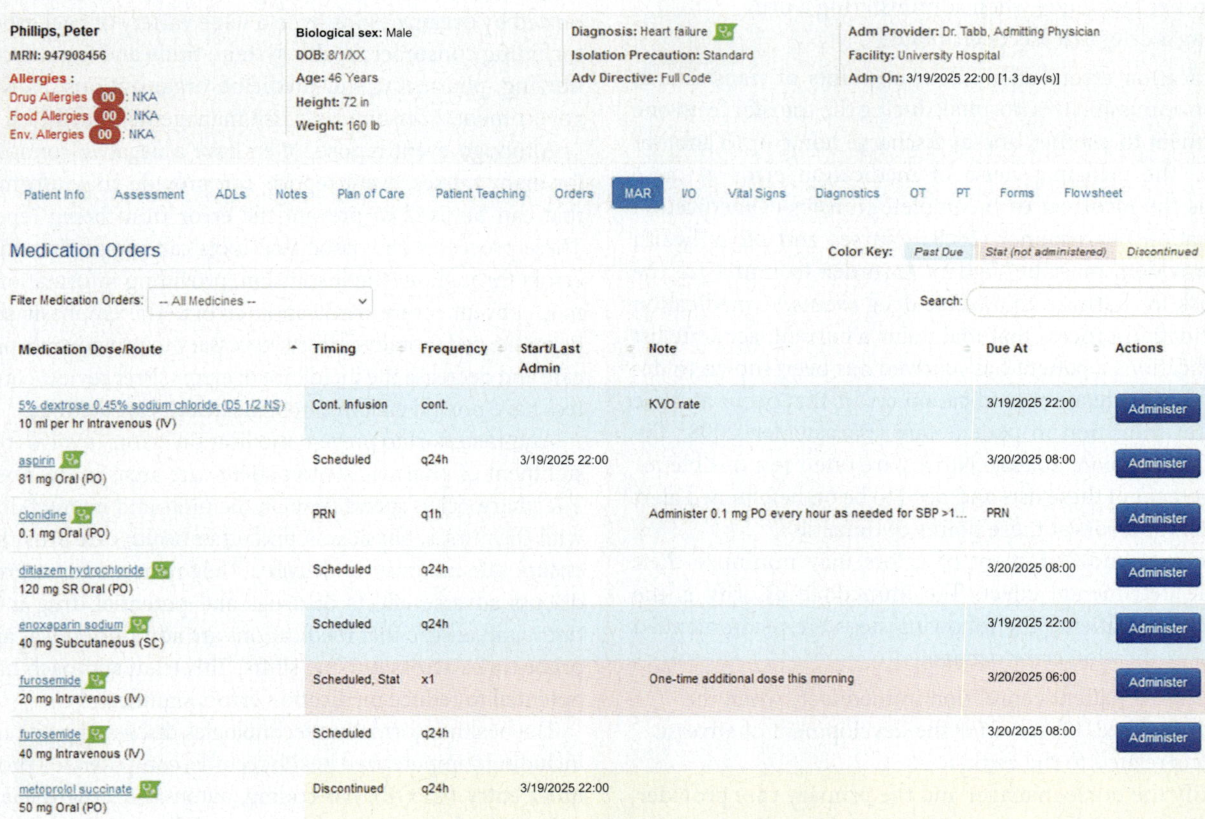

Phillips, Peter
MRN: 947908456
Allergies :
Drug Allergies 00 : NKA
Food Allergies 00 : NKA
Env. Allergies 00 : NKA

Biological sex: Male
DOB: 8/1/XX
Age: 46 Years
Height: 72 in
Weight: 160 lb

Diagnosis: Heart failure
Isolation Precaution: Standard
Adv Directive: Full Code

Adm Provider: Dr. Tabb, Admitting Physician
Facility: University Hospital
Adm On: 3/19/2025 22:00 [1.3 day(s)]

Patient Info | Assessment | ADLs | Notes | Plan of Care | Patient Teaching | Orders | MAR | I/O | Vital Signs | Diagnostics | OT | PT | Forms | Flowsheet

Medication Orders

Color Key: Past Due | Stat (not administered) | Discontinued

Filter Medication Orders: -- All Medicines --

Search:

Medication Dose/Route	Timing	Frequency	Start/Last Admin	Note	Due At	Actions
5% dextrose 0.45% sodium chloride (D5 1/2 NS) 10 ml per hr Intravenous (IV)	Cont. Infusion	cont.		KVO rate	3/19/2025 22:00	Administer
aspirin 81 mg Oral (PO)	Scheduled	q24h	3/19/2025 22:00		3/20/2025 08:00	Administer
clonidine 0.1 mg Oral (PO)	PRN	q1h		Administer 0.1 mg PO every hour as needed for SBP >1...	PRN	Administer
diltiazem hydrochloride 120 mg SR Oral (PO)	Scheduled	q24h			3/20/2025 08:00	Administer
enoxaparin sodium 40 mg Subcutaneous (SC)	Scheduled	q24h			3/19/2025 22:00	Administer
furosemide 20 mg Intravenous (IV)	Scheduled, Stat	x1		One-time additional dose this morning	3/20/2025 06:00	Administer
furosemide 40 mg Intravenous (IV)	Scheduled	q24h			3/20/2025 08:00	Administer
metoprolol succinate 50 mg Oral (PO)	Discontinued	q24h	3/19/2025 22:00			

FIGURE 30-18. Example from a web-based academic EHR simulation program.

to take a medication, it is unwise to continue urging the patient. Patients have the right to refuse therapy; recognize and respect that right. Describe the refusal to take prescribed drugs and the manner in which the situation was managed in the patient's record, then report the refusal to pharmacy and the prescribing provider according to facility policy.

Preventing and Responding to Medication Errors

Nurses should take every precaution to avoid errors when administering therapeutic agents. The safe nurse does not allow automatic habits of preparing medications or technology to replace constant thinking, purposeful action, and repeated checking for accuracy. It is important to make use of appropriate resources, including medication software, online medication databases, and consultation with a pharmacist (Choi & Kim, 2019; Fernandes et al., 2020).

Common types of medication errors include the following:

- Inappropriate prescribing of the drug (e.g., incorrect dose, quantity, or route; or inadequate instruction)
- Extra, omitted, or wrong doses
- Administration of a medication to a patient that was not ordered for that patient (see Focused Critical Thinking Guide 30-1)
- Administration of a drug by an incorrect route or at an incorrect rate
- Failure to give a medication within the prescribed time interval
- Incorrect preparation of a drug before administration
- Improper technique when administering a drug
- Giving a drug that has deteriorated

Medication errors often occur at points of transition in care: on admission to a hospital, during the transfer from one department to another, and at discharge home or to another facility. The principal cause of medication error at these times is the incorrect or incomplete transfer of medication information (Barnsteiner, 2008). Nurses and other health care providers must be vigilant in order to minimize the high risk for harm from adverse drug events. A medication reconciliation process that maintains a current, accurate list of medications a patient has received has been shown to decrease the incidence of medication errors that occur at these points of transition in patient care (Barnsteiner, 2008; The Joint Commission, 2020a). Nurses are often responsible for management of these lists and need to be on heightened alert to watch for errors at these points of transition.

Prompt acknowledgment of errors may minimize their possible detrimental effect. The immediate priority is the safety of the patient. The following steps are recommended when a medication error occurs:

1. Check the patient's condition immediately when the error is noted. Observe for the development of adverse effects related to the error.
2. Notify the nurse manager and the primary care provider to discuss possible courses of action, depending on the patient's condition.
3. Report the incident using whatever method is appropriate for your institution. These may include an incident report, a quality-assurance report, a risk assessment/root cause analysis report, or a variance report. These forms—generally called *special event*, *event*, or *unusual occurrence reports*—require an objective, complete account of the medication error. Include the steps taken after the error was recognized. For legal reasons, describe the error fully and accurately. Medication errors are a common allegation in nursing liability cases. Do not document in the patient's record the fact that an incident report was filed. Your institution is bound by state and national mandates to report certain incidents. Some of this reporting is voluntary and some is required. For example, reporting *near-miss* medication errors, where an error almost occurred, is voluntary in some instances, but *sentinel events*, where serious patient harm or death results from the error, require reporting (Wolf & Hughes, 2008; The Joint Commission, 2020b).

There are several voluntary external reporting programs that track medication errors. Nurses and other health care providers are encouraged to report medication errors to these organizations. Reporting errors to one of these programs assists in learning more about patient safety, enhancing patient safety standards, and implementing practices to reduce errors. MEDWATCH (www.fda.gov/Safety/MedWatch/default.htm) is administered by the FDA. The National Coordinating Council for Medication Error Reporting and Prevention (www.nccmerp.org) is a cooperative effort supported by organizations from a wide variety of backgrounds, including consumer, health system, trade and manufacturer, nursing, pharmacy, and medicine organizations, as well as government, licensing, and risk management facilities.

Although event reports often have a negative connotation for many nurses, event reports can provide vital information that can be used to prevent the error from being repeated. These processes and associated tools can provide tracking of errors throughout the institution, providing information that may prevent future medication errors. The emphasis should be on the collaborative efforts necessary to provide safe patient care and decrease the incidence of errors. Peer review committees have proved effective in some health care settings.

Another effort to prevent medication errors involves the assignment of pharmacists to patient care areas in the hospital. The pharmacists spend time on the units and interact directly with the nurses, physicians, and other health care providers to ensure safe medication delivery. They review patient profiles, discuss adverse effects of drugs and potential drug interactions, and ensure that medications are administered at appropriate times across nursing shifts. This team approach has the potential to reduce medication errors significantly.

The health information technologies discussed previously—including computerized health records, computerized provider order entry (CPOE), bar coding, automated drug-dispensing systems, and unit dosing—can potentially contribute to reducing medication errors. However, the person administering the

30-1 Focused Critical Thinking Guide

MEDICATIONS

You are caring for two residents in a long-term care facility. One of your residents is scheduled to receive a B_{12} injection, and because it will be your first intramuscular injection, it has you more than a little apprehensive. You are eagerly waiting for the moment when your instructor will be free to supervise your injection. Meanwhile, she has cleared you to administer the 1000 meds; you bring a multivitamin, a diuretic, and an antiinflammatory agent to one of your assigned residents. When you go to record the medications you administered, you suddenly realize that you gave them to the wrong resident. When you grab your peer and confide your error, she says, "Whatever you do, don't tell Miss McMullen (the clinical instructor). She gets spastic about med errors and has a reputation for gleefully failing students!" You remember that the resident who received the wrong medications has no known drug allergies and you think that she probably wouldn't suffer any adverse effects from the meds she received. What should you do?

1. Identify goal of thinking

Determine how you ought to respond to the realization that you administered medications to the wrong resident.

2. Assess adequacy of knowledge

Pertinent circumstances: A resident has received three medications that were not prescribed for her. *You are a nursing student in your first clinical rotation* and fear your clinical instructor's response should you inform her about your error. You are unsure of the harm that might result from the resident receiving the wrong medication.

Prerequisite knowledge: To decide how you should respond in this situation, you need to understand your professional obligations, which include your moral and legal accountability for having committed a medication error. You will need knowledge of the pharmacologic action of each of the medications you administered and their potential adverse effects on the resident who received them (possible interactions with other medications she is receiving, contraindications with related adverse effects, etc.). You recognize that there is no way for you to get the knowledge you need to make a morally and legally defensible response unless you admit your error to a responsible party.

Room for error/Time constraints: Because you do not know the effects of these medications, you are not in a position to judge how much room there is for error, nor are you able to make a prudent decision about how much time you have to act. The only defensible response is to seek help to clarify your position immediately because a resident's well-being is potentially at stake. No imagined personal costs would justify a delay in your admission of your error.

3. Address potential problems

The most serious obstacle to critical thinking in this situation would be an inability to think rationally about your obligation to report the error because of your fear of being censured by your clinical instructor. You will want to examine critically your friend's claim that your instructor will respond harshly because this may not, in fact, be the case. You will also want to test your peer's unstated assumption that your primary obligation in this sort of situation is to take care of yourself—even if this course of action results in harm to a patient. It would be helpful to think through the consequences of every health care professional behaving in this manner.

4. Consult helpful resources

Given that you are new to medication administration and are unable to assess the potential harm caused to the resident who received the wrong medications, you will find that your most helpful resource is your instructor, and you will need to enlist her assistance immediately. She will need to contact the resident's health care provider to determine whether there are any contraindications to this resident receiving the medications you administered or possible interactions with other medications. A pharmacist may also need to be consulted. You will want to be familiar with the institution's policy on medication errors and will need to know how to complete an incident report. If the long-term care facility has a risk manager, you may want to consult that person.

5. Critique judgment/decision

You have two options here: Admit your error and initiate appropriate follow-up or attempt to cover up your error and "hope for the best." Your decision will be made on the strength of your moral conviction that your primary obligation is to safeguard patient well-being, even if this involves some self-sacrifice. Once you recognize the potentially disastrous consequences of patients not being able to trust health care professionals to act in their best interests, you decide that there really is only one professionally acceptable response in this situation, and you inform your instructor. It turns out that the resident who received the wrong medications suffered no adverse reactions. You, on the other hand, spend an awful morning following up on your error and even have to delegate your B_{12} injection to another student while you are admitting your error to the resident, her attending, and the charge nurse, as well as completing the special event report. At the end of the day, your instructor compliments you for your honesty and sense of responsibility and cautions you not to repeat the mistake. You are grateful that your worst fears (*failing*) weren't confirmed and leave the unit having learned a powerful lesson about the costs of being accountable.

medication, the nurse, needs to remain vigilant in preventing errors.

Teaching about Medications

Teaching about medications is an ongoing process and should begin as soon as the patient is admitted to the health care facility. Developing a plan of care related to medications is an important part of nursing care. See the Nursing Care plan 30-1 for Regina Sauder on pages 968–969. In many cases, patients continue a prescribed medication regimen at home after discharge from the hospital. Education about prescribed medications influences the patient's adherence to the medication regimen at home. Teaching should be tailored to the patient's level of understanding and with an awareness of any cultural implications. Written instructions, based on an assessment of the patient's level of health literacy, can be used as a reference for the patient. Well-educated patients can act as a final safety net in the medication process when nurses encourage patient participation and use the patient's knowledge in the verification process through informal and formal processes (Garfield et al., 2016; Wang et al., 2019). Refer to Teaching Tips 30-1: Medications.

Explain the techniques of medication administration to the patient and caregivers. Before being discharged from a health care facility, the patient should practice the necessary techniques under the supervision of a nurse to acquire sufficient skill for safe administration. Many patients have learned to give themselves injections, as well as many other medications, when the teaching was planned well and the patient was able and willing to learn. A teach-back that includes a return demonstration provides valuable information regarding gaps in the patient's knowledge, skills, or attitudes.

Emphasize the importance of taking medications as prescribed and for as long as prescribed. A common error made by patients is simply omitting a drug, either through carelessness or because they believe that missing a dose is not important. Various aids are available to remind the patient to take medication on schedule. Medication containers that beep when a dose is due to be taken, scratch-off dots on a medication label, and an electronic cap that signals dosage time and records each time the cap is removed are available. Various smart phone applications (apps) and telehealth-related products are also making their way onto the market. Advise patients to keep their medications with them when they travel. If luggage is lost or misplaced, refilling the prescription may be difficult. Instruct the patient not to alter the dosage without consulting the primary care provider. Also, teach the patient not to discontinue medications when symptoms disappear. Drugs used to maintain health, such as those used to control high blood pressure, need to be continued as prescribed to avoid recurrence of symptoms. Medications such as antibiotics need to be taken as prescribed in their entirety to ensure maximal effect and minimize recurrence.

Teaching Tips 30-1

MEDICATIONS

Health Topic	Teaching Tip	Why Is This Important?
General information	• Medication name and dosage • Intended effects of medication • Expected side effects of medication	Patients should know the names and reasons for medications in case of medical emergencies. Patients should also know expected side effects of the medication so they do not stop taking the medication.
Taking the medication	• Medications should be taken at the same time every day. • Teach whether food, beverages, or other medications have any effect on the medication. • Teach what patient should do if a dose is missed. • Teach patient to take medications as prescribed for as long as prescribed. • Teach not to alter drug dosage without consulting health care provider.	If patients make taking medications a part of their daily routine, they are less likely to miss a dose. Some medications require food to prevent stomach irritation; absorption of other medications is impeded by food in the stomach. Patients are likely to miss a dose of medication and need to know what to do if this happens. Some medications have severe consequences if stopped abruptly; others need to be taken for a set period of time and at a recommended dosage to be effective.
Special instructions	• Teach what to do when adverse effects occur. • Keep medications with them when traveling. • Do not share medications with other people. • Store properly. • Keep a list of all medications, including OTC drugs, dietary supplements, herbs, and natural supplements.	Patients need to know whom to contact if any adverse effects occur. Luggage can be lost or misplaced. Teach patients that just because someone else has similar symptoms, it does not mean that the same medication should be taken. Medication should be kept out of the reach of children and pets. For labeling purposes, medications should be kept in the container in which they were dispensed. Some medications are sensitive to humidity and light; keep medications in a cool, dry place. Keep your health care providers up to date on your list of medications.

Nursing Advocacy in Action

Substance use disorder during pregnancy results in significant health problems for the pregnant person, fetus, and newborn. Recently, OxyContin has become a popular alternative to other street drugs such as heroin. In utero exposure to opiates is associated with neonatal abstinence syndrome in as many as 55% to 94% of exposed infants. The onset and severity of the infant's withdrawal from the drug varies with the type and duration of the drug taken by the pregnant person (Hudak et al., 2016).

Patient Scenario

Jasmine is a 24-year-old single mother who is experiencing homelessness. She has a history of injecting OxyContin (120 to 500 mg/day) intravenously for the past 2 years due to pain in her back. She has a history of barbiturate abuse during her last pregnancy. She has delivered two other infants prematurely at 32 weeks and 36 weeks. Both of these children are in foster care.

Implications for Nursing Advocacy

How will you respond if you are Jasmine's clinic nurse? Talk with your classmates and experienced nurses about the questions that follow.

- If you elect to advocate for Jasmine and her baby, what practical steps can you take to ensure better health outcomes?
- Who is your priority in this situation: Jasmine or the baby?
- How do we handle a situation where the needs of the individual may not be readily met by the resources available? Discuss potential/actual health disparities for Jasmine who is experiencing homelessness.
- What is reasonable to expect of a student nurse, a graduate nurse, and an experienced nurse in this situation?
- What advocacy skills are needed to effectively respond to this challenge?

Caution the patient not to share prescribed medications with other family members, friends, or neighbors. Inappropriate use of another person's drugs (diversion) can have serious consequences.

At the very least, a patient should be able to verbalize the following:

- How and when to administer the medication
- When to notify the health care provider
- Expected side effects and potential adverse effects

Nurses have a responsibility to teach about substance use disorder. Teaching may take place on an individual basis or on a family or community level. Substance use disorder is a major public health concern worldwide, especially among teenagers and young adults. Refer to the Nursing Advocacy in Action box. Continued public and individual education is indicated, and nurses are also expected to set high standards for their own behavior and use of drugs. Because substance use disorder is increasingly common in health care providers, nurses who suspect that a colleague is abusing drugs must observe, document, and intervene for the patients' safety.

Nurses working with patients to promote appropriate behaviors related to medication administration should examine their own behaviors as factors in the success of the plan. Nurses who role model good health behaviors are more effective teachers. Use the display, Promoting Health 30-1: Medications, for yourself before using it with others.

Promoting Health 30-1

MEDICATIONS

Use the assessment checklist to determine how well you are meeting your needs related to safe medication practices. Then develop a prescription for self-care by choosing appropriate behaviors from the list of suggestions.

Assessment Checklist

☐ almost always ☐ sometimes ☐ almost never

☐ ☐ ☐ 1. I store medications in a safe place (e.g., a cool, dry place, away from direct sunlight, out of the reach of children).

☐ ☐ ☐ 2. I discard medications that have passed their expiration date.

☐ ☐ ☐ 3. I wear a Medic-Alert tag or carry information that identifies a drug allergy or required medication.

☐ ☐ ☐ 4. I am cautious about combining prescribed medication with OTC drugs, herbal supplements, alcohol, or foods that can interact with the drug.

Self-Care Behaviors

1. Finish all prescriptions as ordered by your provider.
2. Avoid foods, alcohol, or over-the-counter drugs and herbal supplements that may interact with a prescribed drug.
3. Use available resources (textbooks, pharmacist, provider) to verify the potential for drug interactions or possible adverse effects of a medication.
4. Use a reminder system to maintain medication schedule.
5. Avoid sharing medications or taking someone else's prescribed pills.
6. Complete any laboratory tests necessary for maintenance or adjustment of a medication regimen.
7. Practice safe behaviors when storing medications.
8. Purchase drugs from the same pharmacy as an additional safeguard with multiple medication regimens.

Information to promote safe medication practices, such as information about prescription and over-the-counter medications, medication safety, medication administration, and alternative medications, is available online.

Evaluating

Assess the effectiveness of drugs in several ways. Clinical observation is the first method. Collect subjective data from the patient (e.g., “My pain has disappeared.”) and collect objective data (e.g., the patient’s vital signs) to evaluate effectiveness of the medication. It is also important to assess the patient for adverse drug effects.

Measurement of drug levels in body fluids provides data about the patient’s response to a particular medication. For many drugs—including digoxin, warfarin, anticonvulsants, and aminoglycoside antibiotics—monitoring blood levels is an important component of therapy (Frandsen & Pennington, 2021; McCuistion et al., 2021). Test the patient to determine whether the drug level in the blood is within the therapeutic range. Drug dosages may be adjusted based on the serum drug level. Monitoring systems can also assist the nurse in evaluating drug effectiveness. For the patient with an arrhythmia, for example, a cardiac monitor can show a change in heart rhythm.

REFLECTIVE PRACTICE LEADING TO PERSONAL LEARNING

Remember that the object of reflective practice is to look at an experience, understand it, and learn from it. As you begin to develop your expertise in evaluating the plan of care, reflect on your experiences—successes and failures—in order to improve your practice. How can you do it better next time? What did you learn today that can help you tomorrow? Begin your reflection by paying close attention to the following:

- How aware are you of the importance of the checks and rights in guiding your medication administration practices? Are you able to integrate your knowledge of medications into your patient teaching?
- What value do you attach to involving the patient in medication safety practices in the hospital, in the community, and in their homes? How do you individualize the care for patients when so many guidelines, policies, and procedures dictate your care?
- What plan do you have to stay abreast of evolving national guidelines and goals related to safe medication administration?

Keeping up with the latest evidence-based practice guidelines can be challenging. Global shifts and evolving statistics change the emphasis of our nursing care. Balancing the needs of your individual patient with these responsibilities requires mindfulness and intentionality.

Perhaps the most important questions to reflect on are: Are your patients and families/caregivers better for having had *you* share in the critical responsibility of partnering with them to ensure appropriate and safe medication administration practices? Are your patients now receiving thoughtful, person-centered, prioritized, holistic, evidence-based treatment and care because of your efforts?

Nursing Care Plan for *Regina Sauder* 30-1

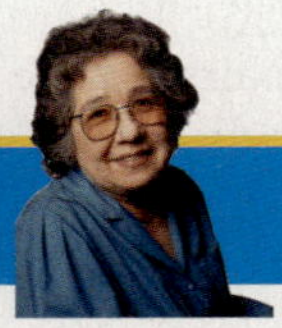

Regina Sauder, 73 years old, presented to the emergency department with pain, swelling, and erythema of her left calf. She has a history of lymphoma. Vascular studies of the lower extremities show a left leg deep vein thrombosis. She was admitted to the hospital and started on intravenous heparin. After 3 days of heparin therapy, she was started on warfarin, in addition to the heparin. Her warfarin dose is being adjusted based on her daily INR level. Daily assessment of her INR level will continue in the hospital until her level is therapeutic. Initially, weekly monitoring of the INR level will continue after discharge.

ASSESSMENT FINDINGS

- PTT is 60 seconds, within expected parameters for adequate hypercoagulation with heparin therapy.
- INR is 1.2, on the low end of expected parameter for adequate hypercoagulation with warfarin therapy.
- Patient’s left lower leg is without swelling, tenderness, and erythema.
- Patient states, “It feels so much better. I had so much pain, but not now. But, why am I taking two different medications? Am I going to have to go home with this tube in my arm?” Mrs. Sauder appears anxious, is fidgeting, and becomes tearful during the conversation with the nurse. She states, “I think this new pill sounds scary.” Her husband reports unease about his wife’s ability “to keep track of everything.”
- Patient and husband unable to verbalize knowledge regarding signs of bleeding, dosage, timing of administration, dietary guidelines, or need for scheduled follow-up blood work.
- Patient and her husband live in a two-story home, with the bathroom on the second floor.

Nursing Care Plan for *Regina Sauder* 30-1 *(continued)*

HEALTH PROBLEM Bleeding risk due to warfarin administration

EXPECTED OUTCOME By 3/20/24 the patient and her husband will:
- Identify signs and symptoms of bleeding

NURSING INTERVENTIONS	RATIONALE	EVALUATIVE STATEMENT
Provide instruction identifying signs and symptoms of bleeding.	Focuses teaching session on a single idea, allowing the patient to concentrate more completely on the material. Older adults and highly anxious patients may have reduced short-term memory and benefit from mastery of one concept at a time.	3/19/24 Outcome met. Mrs. Sauder and her husband are able to identify signs and symptoms of bleeding to report to their health care provider. *B. Huber, RN*
Give patient and husband written pamphlet from drug manufacturer.	Provide information using various media because different people take in information in different ways. Provides concrete reinforcement.	
Encourage questions.	Patients and family members often feel shy or embarrassed about asking questions. Gives permission to ask.	

EXPECTED OUTCOME By 3/20/24 the patient's husband will:
- Remove from their home potential hazards that could lead to falls and subsequent bleeding.

NURSING INTERVENTIONS	RATIONALE	EVALUATIVE STATEMENT
Review with patient and husband potential causes of falls at home.	Falls may cause internal bleeding.	3/18/24 Outcome met. Husband removed several loose rugs, repaired loose stairs, and improved the lighting at the stairs to the bathroom. *B. Clapp, RN*
Assist the patient and husband in evaluating their home environment to identify potential hazards.	Remove potential hazards to prevent falls and injury.	
Encourage the use of proper lighting, handrails on stairways, removal of small rugs, fastening loose carpet edges.	Remove potential hazards to prevent falls and injury.	

SAMPLE DOCUMENTATION

3/17/204 Nursing

Patient, husband, and nurse met to discuss potential effects of warfarin therapy and risk for injury. Discussion centered on importance of preventing injury while on warfarin at home. See care plan. Patient progress will be evaluated in 4 days, 3/21/24.

B. Clapp, RN

Skill 30-1 Administering Oral Medications

DELEGATION CONSIDERATIONS

The administration of oral medications is not delegated to assistive personnel (AP). The administration of specified oral medications to stable patients in some long-term care settings may be delegated to AP who have received appropriate training. Depending on the state's nurse practice act and the organization's policies and procedures, the administration of oral medications may be delegated to licensed practical/vocational nurses (LPN/LVNs). The decision to delegate must be based on careful analysis of the patient's needs and circumstances as well as the qualifications of the person to whom the task is being delegated. Refer to the Delegation Guidelines in Appendix A.

EQUIPMENT

- Medication in disposable cup or oral syringe
- Liquid (e.g., water, juice) with straw, if not contraindicated
- Electronic Medication Administration Record (eMAR) or Medication Administration Record (MAR)
- PPE, as indicated

IMPLEMENTATION

ACTION	RATIONALE
1. Gather equipment. Check each medication prescribed against the original in the health record, depending on facility policy and the medication order system in place. Clarify any inconsistencies. Check the patient's health record for allergies.	The prescription is the legal record of prescribed medication interventions. This comparison helps to identify errors that may have occurred when orders were transcribed. Computer provider order-entry (CPOE) systems allow prescribers to send electronic medication prescriptions directly to the pharmacy located in a health care facility and to outpatient pharmacies.
2. Know the actions, special nursing considerations, safe dose ranges, purpose of administration, and potential adverse effects of the medications to be administered. Consider the appropriateness of the medication for this patient.	This knowledge aids the nurse in evaluating the therapeutic effect of the medication in relation to the patient's health status and can also be used to educate the patient about the medication.
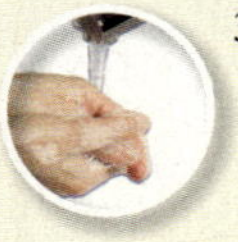 3. Perform hand hygiene.	Hand hygiene prevents the spread of microorganisms.
4. Move the medication supply system to the outside of the patient's room or prepare for administration at the medication supply system in the medication area. Alternatively, access the medication administration supply system at or inside the patient's room.	Organization facilitates error-free administration and saves time.
5. Unlock the medication supply system or drawer. Enter the passcode into the computer and scan employee identification, if required.	Locking the medication supply system or drawer safeguards each patient's medication supply. Facility accrediting organizations require medication supply systems to be locked when not in use. Entering the passcode and scanning ID allows only authorized users into the computer system and identifies the user for documentation by the computer.
6. **Prepare medications for one patient at a time.**	This prevents errors in medication administration.
7. Read the eMAR/MAR and read the label when selecting the proper medication from the medication supply system or patient's medication drawer.	This is the *first* check of the medication label.
8. Read the label and compare the medication label with the eMAR/MAR (Figure 1). Check expiration dates and perform calculations, if necessary. Scan the bar code on the package, if required.	This is the *second* check of the label. Verify calculations with another nurse to ensure safety, if necessary.

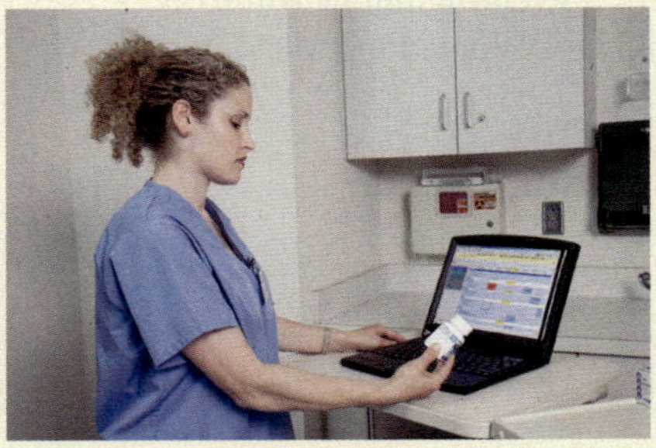

FIGURE 1. Comparing medication label with eMAR.

ACTION	RATIONALE
9. Prepare the required medications:	
a. *Unit dose packages:* **Do not open the wrapper until at the bedside.** Keep opioids and medications that require special nursing assessments separate from other medication packages.	Wrapper is kept intact because the label is needed for an additional safety check. Special assessments may be required before giving certain medications. These may include assessing vital signs and checking laboratory test results.
b. *Multidose containers:* When removing tablets or capsules from a multidose bottle, pour the necessary number into the bottle cap and then place the tablets or capsules in a medication cup. Break only scored tablets, if necessary, to obtain the proper dosage. Do not touch tablets or capsules with your hands.	Pouring medication into the cap allows for easy return of excess medication to the bottle. Pouring tablets or capsules into your hand is unsanitary.
c. *Liquid medication in multidose bottle:* When pouring liquid medications out of a multidose bottle, hold the bottle so the label is against the palm. Use the appropriate measuring device when pouring liquids and read the amount of medication at the bottom of the meniscus at eye level (Figure 2). Wipe the lip of the bottle with a paper towel.	Liquid that may drip onto the label makes the label difficult to read. Accuracy is possible when the appropriate measuring device is used and then read accurately.

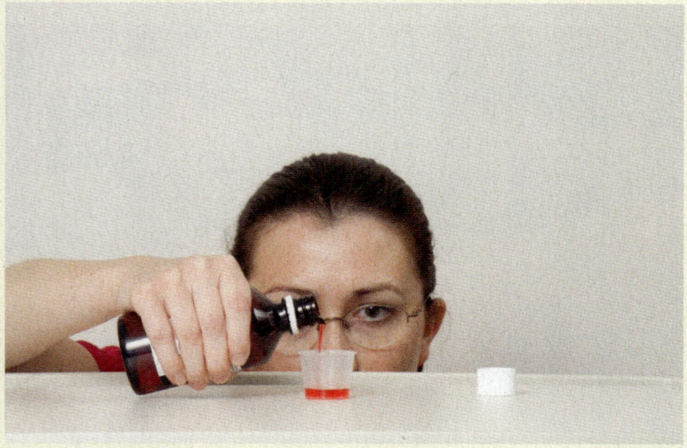

FIGURE 2. Measuring at eye level. (*Source:* Used with permission from Shutterstock. *Photo by B. Proud.*)

ACTION	RATIONALE
10. **Depending on facility policy, the third check of the label may occur at this point. If so, when all medications for one patient have been prepared, read the label and recheck the labels with the eMAR/MAR before taking the medications to the patient. However, many facilities require the third check to occur at the bedside, after identifying the patient.**	This *third* check ensures accuracy and helps to prevent errors. *Note:* Many facilities require the third check to occur at the bedside, after identifying the patient and before administration.
11. Replace any multidose containers in the patient's drawer or medication supply system. **Log out of and/or lock the medication supply system before leaving it.**	Locking the medication supply system or drawer safeguards the patient's medication supply. Facility accrediting organizations require medication supply systems to be locked when not in use.
12. Transport medications to the patient's bedside carefully and keep the medications in sight at all times.	Careful handling and close observation prevent accidental or deliberate disarrangement of medications.
13. **Ensure that the patient receives the medications at the correct time.**	Check facility policy, which may allow for administration within a period of 30 minutes before or 30 minutes after the designated time.
14. Perform hand hygiene and put on PPE, if indicated.	Hand hygiene and PPE prevent the spread of microorganisms. PPE is required based on transmission precautions.

(*continued on page 972*)

Skill 30-1 Administering Oral Medications *(continued)*

ACTION	RATIONALE
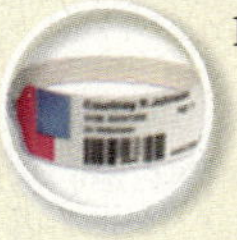 15. **Identify the patient. Compare the information with the eMAR/MAR. The patient should be identified using at least two of the following methods** (The Joint Commission, 2021):	Identifying the patient ensures the right patient receives the medications and helps prevent errors. The patient's room number or physical location is not used as an identifier (The Joint Commission, 2021). Replace the identification band if it is missing or inaccurate in any way.
a. Check the name on the patient's identification band (Figure 3).	
b. Check the identification number on the patient's identification band.	
c. Check the birth date on the patient's identification band.	
d. Ask the patient to state their name and birth date, based on facility policy.	This requires a response from the patient, but illness and strange surroundings often cause patients to be confused.
16. **Complete necessary assessments before administering medications. Check the patient's allergy bracelet, if present, or ask the patient about allergies. Explain the purpose and action of each medication to the patient.**	Assessment is a prerequisite to administration of medications.
17. Scan the patient's bar code on the identification band, if required (Figure 4) (The Joint Commission, 2021).	The bar code provides an additional check to ensure that the medication is given to the right patient.

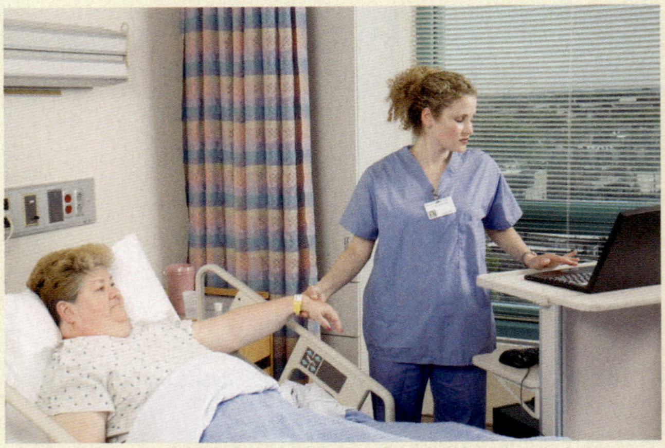

FIGURE 3. Comparing patient's name and identification number with eMAR.

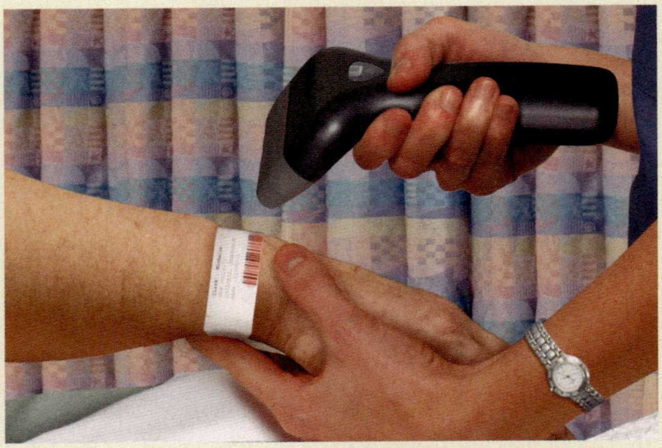

FIGURE 4. Scanning bar code on patient's identification bracelet. (*Photo by B. Proud.*)

ACTION	RATIONALE
18. **Based on facility policy, the third check of the medication label may occur at this point. If so, read the label and recheck the label with the eMAR/MAR before administering the medications to the patient.**	Many facilities require the *third* check to occur at the bedside, after identifying the patient and before administration. If facility policy directs the *third* check at this time, this *third* check ensures accuracy and helps prevent errors.
19. Assist the patient to an upright or lateral (side-lying) position.	Swallowing is facilitated by proper positioning. An upright or side-lying position protects the patient from aspiration.
20. Administer medications:	
a. Offer water or other permitted fluids with pills, capsules, tablets, and some liquid medications.	Liquids facilitate swallowing of solid drugs. Some liquid drugs are intended to adhere to the pharyngeal area, in which case liquid is not offered with the medication.
b. Ask whether the patient prefers to take the medications by hand or in a cup.	This encourages the patient's participation in taking the medications.

ACTION

RATIONALE

21. **Remain with the patient until each medication is swallowed. Never leave medication at the patient's bedside** (Figure 5).

Unless you have seen the patient swallow the drug, the drug cannot be recorded as administered. The patient's health record is a legal record. Medications can be left at the bedside only with a prescriber's order.

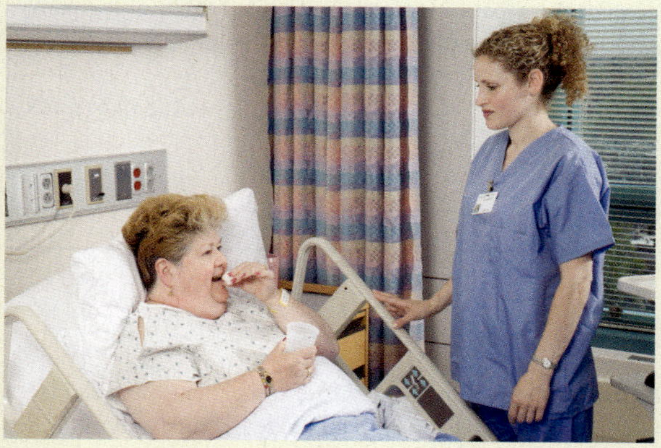

FIGURE 5. Remaining with patient until each medication is swallowed.

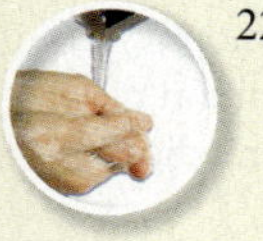

22. Assist the patient to a comfortable position. Remove PPE, if used. Perform hand hygiene.

Promotes patient comfort. Proper removal of PPE prevents transmission of microorganisms. Hand hygiene deters the spread of microorganisms.

23. Document the administration of the medication immediately after administration. See Documentation section below.

Timely documentation helps to ensure patient safety.

24. Evaluate the patient's response to the medication within the appropriate time frame.

The patient needs to be evaluated for therapeutic and adverse effects from the medication.

DOCUMENTATION

GUIDELINES

Record each medication immediately after it is administered on the eMAR/MAR or health record using the required format. Include the date and time of administration (Figure 6). If using a bar-code system, medication administration is automatically recorded when the bar code is scanned. PRN medications require documentation of the reason for administration. Prompt recording avoids the possibility of accidentally repeating the administration of the drug. If the drug was refused or omitted, record this in the appropriate area on the medication record and notify the health care team as appropriate. This verifies the reason medication was omitted and ensures that health care personnel providing care for the patient are aware of the occurrence. Recording administration of an opioid may require additional documentation on a controlled-substance record, stating drug count and other specific information. A record of fluid intake and output measurement is required.

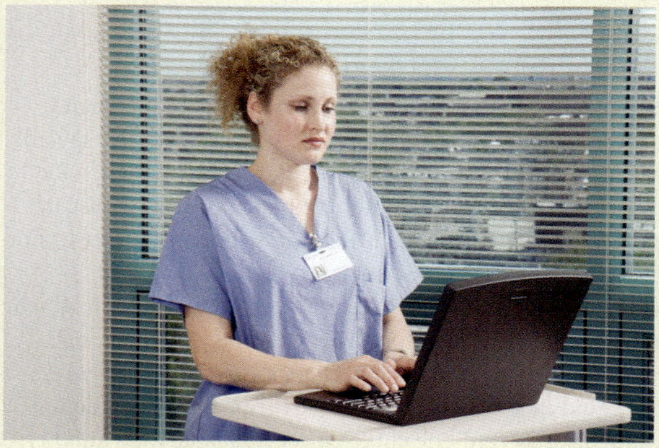

FIGURE 6. Recording each medication administered on eMAR.

(*continued on page 974*)

Skill 30-1 Administering Oral Medications (continued)

SAMPLE DOCUMENTATION

DocuCare Practice documenting medication administration in *Lippincott DocuCare.*

8/6/25 0835 Patient states he is having constant stabbing leg pains. Rates pain as an 8/10. Percocet 2 tabs administered.

—K. Sanders, RN

8/6/25 0905 Patient resting comfortably. Rates leg pain as a 1/10.

—K. Sanders, RN

8/6/25 1300 Patient states he does not want pain medication, despite return of leg pain. States, "It made me feel woozy last time." Feelings discussed with patient. Patient agrees to take Percocet 1 tab at this time.

—K. Sanders, RN

8/6/25 1320 Percocet, 1 tablet given PO.

—K. Sanders, RN

DEVELOPING CLINICAL REASONING AND CLINICAL JUDGMENT

UNEXPECTED SITUATIONS AND ASSOCIATED INTERVENTIONS

- *Patient states that it feels like medication is lodged in throat:* Offer the patient more fluids to drink. If allowed, offer the patient bread or crackers to help move the medication to the stomach.
- *It is unclear whether the patient swallowed the medication:* Check in the patient's mouth, under their tongue, and between their cheek and gum. Patients with altered cognition may not be aware that the medication was not swallowed. Also, patients may "cheek" medications to avoid taking the medication or to save it for later use.
- *Patient vomits immediately or shortly after receiving oral medication:* Assess vomit, looking for pills or fragments. Do not readminister the medication without notifying the health care team. If a whole pill is seen and can be identified, the prescriber may ask that the medication be administered again. If a pill is not seen or medications cannot be identified, do not readminister the medication in order to prevent the patient from receiving too large a dose.
- *Child refuses to take oral medications:* Some medications may be mixed in a small amount of food, such as pudding or ice cream. Do not add the medication to liquids because the medication may alter the taste of liquids; if the child then refuses to drink the rest of the liquid, you will not know how much of the medication was ingested. Use creativity when devising ways to administer medications to a child. See the section below, Infant and Child Considerations, for suggestions.
- *Capsule or tablet falls to the floor during administration:* Discard and obtain a new dose for administration. This prevents contamination and transmission of microorganisms.
- *Patient refuses medication:* Explore the reason for the patient's refusal. Review the rationale for use of the drug, explain the risk of refusal, and any other information that may be appropriate. If you are unable to administer the medication despite education and discussion, document the omission and any education and/or explanation provided related to attempts to facilitate administration according to facility policy. The health care team should be informed of the refusal, especially when the omission poses a specific threat to the patient (McCuistion et al., 2021).

SPECIAL CONSIDERATIONS

General Considerations

- Some liquid medication preparations, such as suspensions and emulsions, require agitation to ensure even distribution of medication in the solution. Be familiar with the specific requirements for medications you are administering.
- Place medications intended for sublingual absorption under the patient's tongue. Instruct the patient to allow the medication to dissolve completely. Reinforce the importance of not swallowing the medication tablet.
- Some oral medications are provided in powdered forms. Verify the correct liquid in which to dissolve the medication for administration. This information is usually included on the package. Verify any unclear instructions with a pharmacist or medication reference. If there is more than one possible liquid in which to dissolve the medication, include the patient in the decision process; patients may find one choice more palatable than another.

- Ongoing assessment is an important part of nursing care for both evaluation of patient response to administered medications and early detection of adverse drug reactions. If an adverse effect is suspected, withhold further medication doses and notify the health care team. Additional intervention is based on type of reaction and patient assessment.
- If the patient questions a medication order or states the medication is different from the usual dose, always recheck and clarify with the original prescription and/or prescriber.
- If the patient's level of consciousness is altered or their swallowing is impaired, check with the health care team to clarify the route of administration or alternative forms of medication. This may also be a solution for a pediatric or a confused patient who is refusing to take a medication.
- Patients with poor vision can request large-type labels on medication containers. A magnifying lens also may be helpful.
- Provide written medication information to reinforce discussion and education in the appropriate language, if the patient is literate. If the patient is unable to read, provide written information to family or caregiver, if appropriate. Written information should be at a 4th- to 6th-grade level, using short sentences and simple words, and incorporate pictures to increase ease of understanding (Patient Safety Network, 2019).
- If the patient has difficulty swallowing tablets, it may be appropriate to crush the medication to facilitate administration. Not all medications can be crushed or altered; long-acting and slow-release drugs are examples of medications that cannot be crushed. Check manufacturer's recommendations and/or with a pharmacist to verify (Anderson, 2019; Boullata, 2021; White & Bradnam, 2015).
- If the medication can be crushed, use a pill-crusher or mortar and pestle to grind the tablet into a powder. Crush each pill one at a time. Dissolve the powder with water or other recommended liquid in a liquid medication cup, keeping each medication separate from the others. Keep the package label with the medication cup for future comparison of information. Combine the crushed medication with a small amount of soft food, such as applesauce or pudding, to facilitate administration.
- Liquid medication not dispensed as unit dose should be administered in an oral syringe when available (ISMP, 2020) (Figure 7).

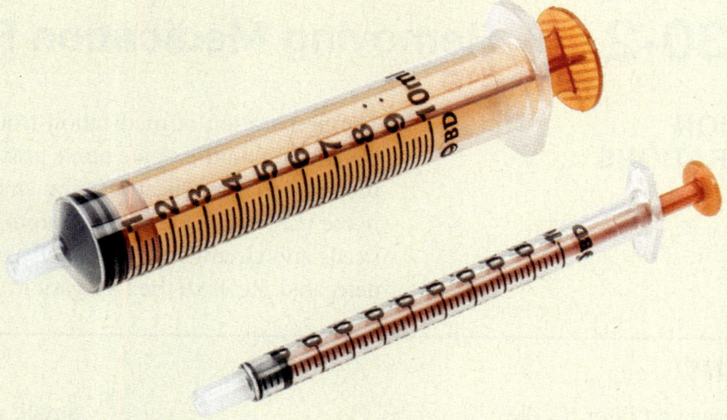

FIGURE 7. Monoject™ oral syringe. Note that specific syringes are designed for "ORAL USE ONLY." (Courtesy and © Becton, Dickinson and Company. Reprinted with permission.)

Infant and Child Considerations

- Special devices, such as oral syringes and calibrated nipples, are available in a pharmacy to ensure accurate dose calculations for young children and infants.
- Some creative ways to administer medications to children include the following: have a "tea party" with medicine cups; place a designated oral tip syringe or dropper in the space between the cheek and gum and slowly administer the medication (Kyle & Carman, 2021); save a special treat for after the medication administration (e.g., movie, playroom time, or a special food, if allowed).

(continued on page 976)

Skill 30-1 Administering Oral Medications *(continued)*

- If a medication has an objectionable taste, warn the child if they are old enough to understand. Failing to warn the child is likely to decrease the child's trust in the nurse. Do not lie to a child about medication administration.
- Caution caregivers to remove and dispose of plastic syringe caps present on the end of syringes before drug administration to reduce the risk of choking. Companies manufacture syringes labeled "oral use" without the caps on them and should be considered for use (ISMP, 2020).

Older Adult Considerations

- Older adults with arthritis may have difficulty opening childproof caps. On request, the pharmacist can substitute a cap that is easier to open. A rubber band twisted around the cap may provide a more secure grip for older adults.
- Consider large-print written medication information, when appropriate.
- Physiologic changes associated with the aging process, including decreased gastric motility, muscle mass, acid production, and blood flow, can affect the patient's response to the medication, including drug absorption and increased risk of adverse effects. Older adults are more likely to take multiple drugs. As a result, drug interactions in the older adult are a significant consideration that may affect mental status (Frandsen & Pennington, 2021).

Community-Based Care Considerations

- Encourage the patient to discard expired prescription medications based on label instructions or community guidelines.
- Discuss safe storage of medications when there are children and pets in the home environment.
- Discuss with parents the difference in over-the-counter medications made for infants and medications made for children. Many times, parents do not realize that there are different strengths to the actual medications, leading to under- or overdosing.
- Encourage patients to carry a card listing all medications they take, including dosage and frequency, in case of an emergency.
- Discuss the importance of using an appropriate measuring device for liquid medications. Caution patients not to use eating utensils for measuring medications; use a liquid medication cup, oral syringe, or measuring spoon to provide accurate dosing.

Skill 30-2 Removing Medication From an Ampule

DELEGATION CONSIDERATIONS

The preparation of medication from an ampule is not delegated to assistive personnel (AP). Depending on the state's nurse practice act and the organization's policies and procedures, the preparation of medication from an ampule may be delegated to a licensed practical/vocational nurse (LPN/LVN). The decision to delegate must be based on careful analysis of the patient's needs and circumstances as well as the qualifications of the person to whom the task is being delegated. Refer to the Delegation Guidelines in Appendix A.

EQUIPMENT

- Sterile syringe and filter needle
- New needle for replacing filter needle, if indicated
- Ampule of medication
- Antimicrobial swab
- Small, sterile gauze pad
- Gloves
- Electronic Medication Administration Record (eMAR) or Medication Administration Record (MAR)

IMPLEMENTATION

ACTION	RATIONALE
1. Gather equipment. Check each medication prescribed against the original in the health record, depending on facility policy and the medication order system in place. Clarify any inconsistencies. Check the patient's health record for allergies.	The prescription is the legal record of prescribed medication interventions. This comparison helps to identify errors that may have occurred when orders were transcribed. Computer provider order-entry (CPOE) systems allow prescribers to send electronic medication prescriptions directly to the pharmacy located in a health care facility and to outpatient pharmacies.

ACTION	RATIONALE
2. Know the actions, special nursing considerations, safe dose ranges, purpose of administration, and adverse effects of the medications to be administered. Consider the appropriateness of the medication for this patient.	This knowledge aids the nurse in evaluating the therapeutic effect of the medication in relation to the patient's health status and can also be used to educate the patient about the medication.
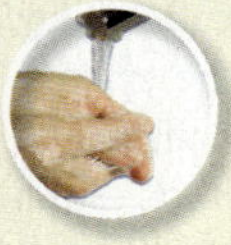 3. Perform hand hygiene.	Hand hygiene prevents the spread of microorganisms.
4. Move the medication supply system to the outside of the patient's room or prepare for administration at the medication supply system in the medication area. Alternatively, access the medication administration supply system at or inside the patient's room.	Organization facilitates error-free administration and saves time.
5. Unlock the medication supply system or drawer. Enter the passcode and scan employee identification, if required.	Locking the medication supply system or drawer safeguards each patient's medication supply. Facility accrediting organizations require medication supply systems to be locked when not in use. Entering the passcode and scanning ID allows only authorized users into the computer system and identifies the user for documentation by the computer.
6. **Prepare medications for one patient at a time.**	This prevents errors in medication administration.
7. Read the eMAR/MAR and read the label when selecting the proper medication from the medication supply system or the patient's medication drawer.	This is the *first* check of the label.
8. Read the label and compare the label with the eMAR/MAR. Check expiration dates and perform calculations, if necessary. Scan the bar code on the package, if required.	This is the *second* check of the label. Verify calculations with another nurse to ensure safety, if necessary.
9. Tap the stem of the ampule (Figure 1) or twist your wrist quickly (Figure 2) while holding the ampule vertically.	This facilitates movement of medication in the stem to the body of the ampule.
10. Put on gloves. Using the antimicrobial swab, scrub the neck of the ampule. Wrap a small sterile gauze pad around the neck of the ampule.	Gloves reduce risk of injury to hands from glass (Innovation Compounding, 2020). Scrubbing the neck is necessary to reduce the risk of contamination (Dolan et al., 2016; Innovation Compounding, 2020). Wrapping the neck of the ampule with gauze protects your fingers from the glass as the ampule is broken.
11. Breaking away from your body, use a snapping motion to break off the top of the ampule along the scored line at its neck (Figure 3). **Always break away from your body.**	This protects your face and fingers from any shattered glass fragments.

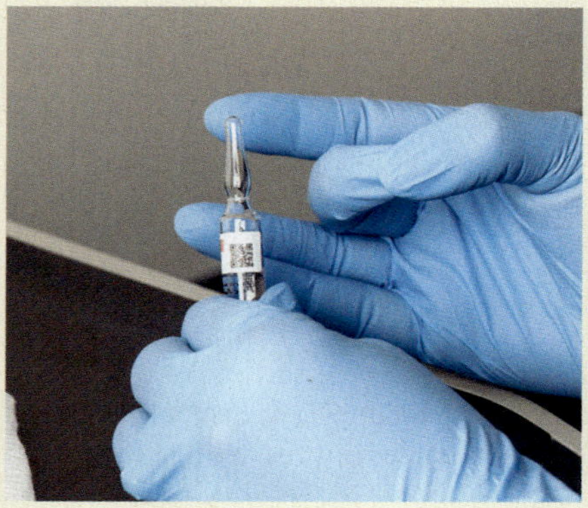

FIGURE 1. Tapping stem of the ampule.

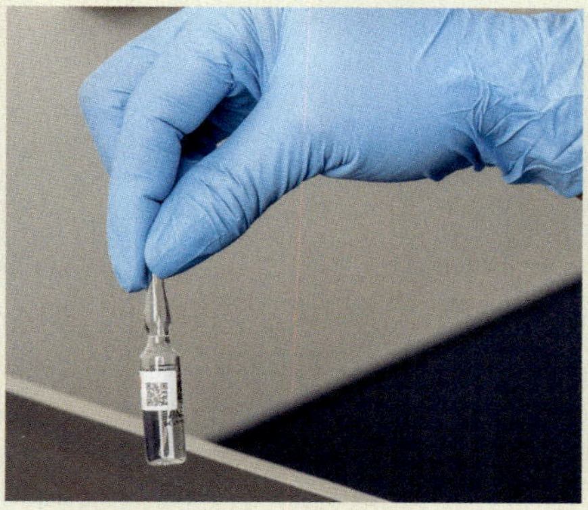

FIGURE 2. Twisting wrist quickly while holding ampule vertically.

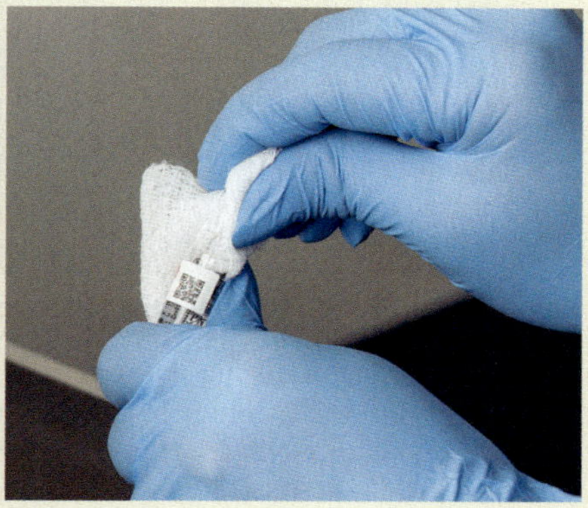

FIGURE 3. Using a snapping motion to break top of ampule.

(continued on page 978)

Skill 30-2 Removing Medication From an Ampule *(continued)*

ACTION

12. Attach the filter needle to the syringe. Remove the cap from the filter needle by pulling it straight off.

RATIONALE

Use of a filter needle prevents the accidental withdrawing of small glass particles with the medication (Innovation Compounding, 2020). Pulling the cap off in a straight manner prevents accidental needlestick.

ACTION

13. Withdraw the medication in the amount ordered plus a small amount more (approximately 30% more). **Do not inject air into the solution. While inserting the filter needle into the ampule, be careful not to touch the rim.** Use either of the following methods to withdraw the medication:

RATIONALE

By withdrawing an additional small amount of medication, any air bubbles in the syringe can be displaced once the syringe is removed while allowing ample medication to remain in the syringe. The contents of the ampule are not under pressure; therefore, air is unnecessary and will cause the contents to overflow. The rim of the ampule is considered contaminated.

ACTION

a. Insert the tip of the needle into the ampule, which is upright on a flat surface, and withdraw fluid into the syringe (Figure 4). **Touch the plunger only at the knob.**

RATIONALE

Handling the plunger only at the knob will keep the shaft of the plunger sterile.

ACTION

b. Insert the tip of the needle into the ampule and invert the ampule. Keep the needle centered and not touching the sides of the ampule. Withdraw fluid into the syringe (Figure 5). **Touch the plunger only at the knob.**

RATIONALE

Surface tension holds the fluids in the ampule when inverted. If the needle touches the sides or is removed and then reinserted into the ampule, surface tension is broken, and fluid runs out. Handling the plunger only at the knob will keep the shaft of the plunger sterile.

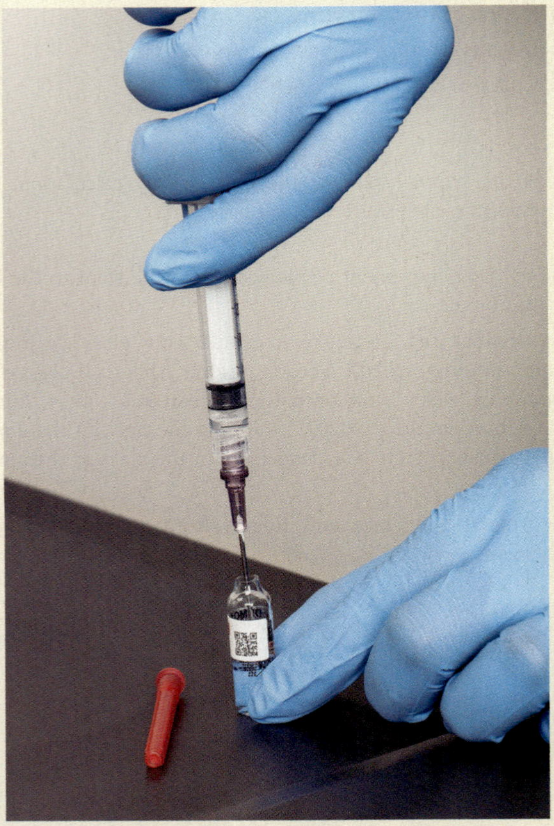

FIGURE 4. Withdrawing medication from upright ampule.

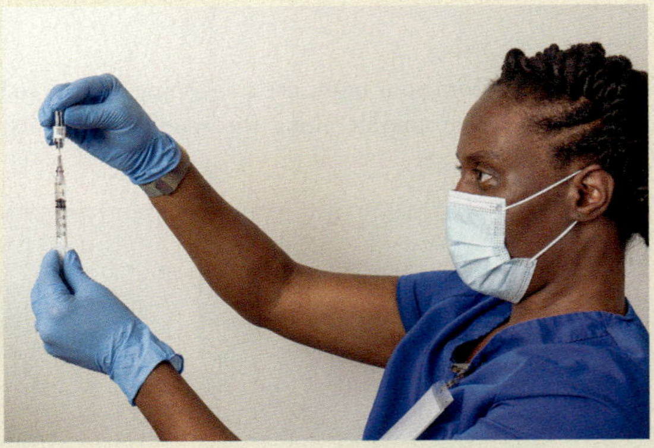

FIGURE 5. Withdrawing medication from inverted ampule.

ACTION

14. Wait until the needle has been withdrawn to tap the syringe and expel the air carefully by pushing on the plunger. **Check the amount of medication in the syringe with the medication dose and discard any surplus, according to facility policy.**

RATIONALE

Ejecting air into the solution increases pressure in the ampule and can force the medication to spill out over the ampule. Ampules may have overfill. Careful measurement ensures that the correct dose is withdrawn.

ACTION	RATIONALE
15. **Depending on facility policy, the third check of the label may occur at this point. If so, when all medications for one patient have been prepared, read the label and recheck the labels with the eMAR/MAR before taking the medications to the patient. However, many facilities require the third check to occur at the bedside, after identifying the patient.**	This *third* check ensures accuracy and helps to prevent errors. *Note:* Many facilities require the *third* check to occur at the bedside, after identifying the patient and before administration.
16. Label the syringe with the medication name, dose, and amount (The Joint Commission, 2021).	Unlabeled syringes are unidentifiable and may lead to a medication administration error (The Joint Commission, 2021).
17. **Engage the safety guard on the filter needle and remove the needle. Discard the filter needle in a suitable container. Attach the appropriate administration device to the syringe.**	The filter needle used to draw up medication should not be used to administer the medication. This will prevent any glass shards from entering the patient during administration.
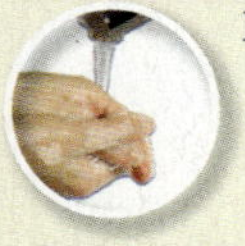 18. Discard the ampule in a suitable container. Remove gloves and perform hand hygiene.	Any medication that has not been removed from the ampule must be discarded because sterility of contents cannot be maintained in an opened ampule. Removing gloves and performing hand hygiene deters the spread of microorganisms
19. **Log out of and/or lock the medication supply system before leaving it.**	Locking the medication supply system safeguards the patient's medication supply. Facility accrediting organizations require medication supply systems to be locked when not in use.
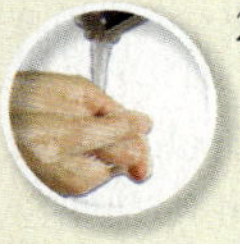 20. Perform hand hygiene.	Hand hygiene deters the spread of microorganisms.
21. Proceed with administration, based on prescribed route.	See appropriate skill for prescribed route.

DOCUMENTATION GUIDELINES

It is not necessary to record the removal of the medication from the ampule. Prompt recording of administration of the medication is required immediately after it is administered.

DEVELOPING CLINICAL REASONING AND CLINICAL JUDGMENT

UNEXPECTED SITUATIONS AND ASSOCIATED INTERVENTIONS

- *You cut yourself while trying to open the ampule:* Discard the ampule and medication in case contamination has occurred. Clean and bandage the wound and obtain a new ampule. Communicate the incident according to facility policy.
- *All of medication was not removed from the stem and insufficient medication remains in body of ampule for dose:* Discard the ampule and drawn medication. Obtain a new ampule and start over. Medication in the original ampule stem is considered contaminated once the neck of the ampule has been placed on a nonsterile surface.
- *You inject air into inverted ampule, spraying medication:* Wash your hands to remove any medication. If any medication has gotten into your eyes, perform eye irrigation. Obtain a new ampule for medication dose. Communicate the incident according to facility policy.
- *Plunger becomes contaminated before inserted into ampule:* Discard the needle and syringe and start over. If the plunger is contaminated after medication is drawn into the syringe, it is not necessary to discard and start over. The contaminated plunger will enter the barrel of the syringe when pushing the medication out, will not come in contact with the medication, and will not contaminate the medication.

SPECIAL CONSIDERATIONS

- When mixing medications in one syringe, preparation of medications in one syringe depends on how the medication is supplied. When preparing medications from an ampule and a vial, prepare the medication in the vial first. Draw up the medication in the ampule *after* the medication in the vial (see Skill 30-3).

Skill 30-3 Removing Medication From a Vial

DELEGATION CONSIDERATIONS

The preparation of medication from a vial is not delegated to assistive personnel (AP). Depending on the state's nurse practice act and the organization's policies and procedures, the preparation of medication from a vial may be delegated to licensed practical/vocational nurses (LPN/LVNs). The decision to delegate must be based on careful analysis of the patient's needs and circumstances as well as the qualifications of the person to whom the task is being delegated. Refer to the Delegation Guidelines in Appendix A.

EQUIPMENT

- Sterile syringe and needle or blunt cannula (size depends on medication being administered)
- Needleless access device (if available)
- Vial of medication
- Antimicrobial swab
- Second needle (optional)
- Filter needle (optional)
- Electronic Medication Administration Record (eMAR) or Medication Administration Record (MAR)

IMPLEMENTATION

ACTION	RATIONALE
1. Gather equipment. Check each medication prescribed against the original in the health record, depending on facility policy and the medication order system in place. Clarify any inconsistencies. Check the patient's health record for allergies.	The prescription is the legal record of prescribed medication interventions. This comparison helps to identify errors that may have occurred when orders were transcribed. Computer provider order-entry (CPOE) systems allow prescribers to send electronic medication prescriptions directly to the pharmacy located in a health care facility and to outpatient pharmacies.
2. Know the actions, special nursing considerations, safe dose ranges, purpose of administration, and adverse effects of the medications to be administered. Consider the appropriateness of the medication for this patient.	This knowledge aids the nurse in evaluating the therapeutic effect of the medication in relation to the patient's health status and can also be used to educate the patient about the medication.
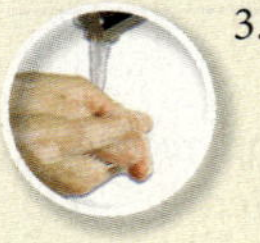 3. Perform hand hygiene.	Hand hygiene deters the spread of microorganisms.
4. Move the medication supply system to the outside of the patient's room or prepare for administration at the medication supply system in the medication area. Alternatively, access the medication administration supply system at or inside the patient's room.	Organization facilitates error-free administration and saves time.
5. Unlock the medication supply system or drawer. Enter the passcode and scan employee identification, if required.	Locking the medication supply system or drawer safeguards each patient's medication supply. Facility accrediting organizations require medication supply systems to be locked when not in use. Entering the passcode and scanning ID allows only authorized users into the system and identifies the user for documentation by the computer.
6. **Prepare medications for one patient at a time.**	This prevents errors in medication administration.
7. Read the eMAR/MAR and read the label when selecting the proper medication from the medication supply system or the patient's medication drawer.	This is the *first* check of the label.
8. Read the label and compare the label with the eMAR/MAR. Check expiration dates and perform calculations, if necessary. Scan the bar code on the package, if required.	This is the *second* check of the label. Verify calculations with another nurse to ensure safety, if necessary.
9. Remove the metal or plastic cap on the vial that protects the self-sealing stopper.	The cap needs to be removed to access the medication in the vial.
10. **Scrub the self-sealing stopper top with the antimicrobial swab and allow to dry.**	The antimicrobial swab removes surface microbial contamination. Allowing the antimicrobial solution to dry completely (5 to 20 seconds) ensures complete antimicrobial effectiveness (Gorski et al., 2021; Slater et al., 2018). Drying also prevents antimicrobial solution from entering the vial on the needle.

ACTION | **RATIONALE**

11. Remove the cap from the needle or blunt cannula by pulling it straight off. **If the vial in use is a multidose vial**, touch the plunger only at the knob and draw back an amount of air into the syringe that is equal to the specific dose of medication to be withdrawn. If the vial in use is a single-use vial, there is no need to draw air into the syringe.

Pulling the cap off in a straight manner prevents accidental needlestick injury. Handling the plunger only at the knob will keep the shaft of the plunger sterile. Because a vial is a sealed container, injection of an equal amount of air (before fluid is removed) is required to prevent the formation of a partial vacuum. If not enough air is injected, the negative pressure makes it difficult to withdraw the medication after repeated use.

12. Hold the vial on a flat surface. Pierce the self-sealing stopper in the center with the needle tip (Figure 1) or blunt cannula; alternatively, insert a needleless access device (Figure 2) into the stopper on the vial and connect the syringe. Inject the measured air into the space above the solution. **Do not inject air into the solution.** If the vial in use is a single-use vial, there is no need to inject air into the vial.

Air bubbled through the solution could result in withdrawal of an inaccurate amount of medication. Needleless access devices may be used to prevent needlestick injuries based on facility policy (Frandsen & Pennington, 2021).

13. Invert the vial. **Keep the tip of the needle or blunt cannula below the fluid level if in use (Figure 3).**

This prevents air from being aspirated into the syringe.

14. Hold the vial in one hand and use the other to withdraw the medication. **Touch the plunger only at the knob. Draw up the prescribed amount of medication while holding the syringe vertically and at eye level (Figure 4).**

Handling the plunger only at the knob will keep the shaft of the plunger sterile. Holding the syringe at eye level facilitates accurate reading, and the vertical position makes removal of air bubbles from the syringe easy.

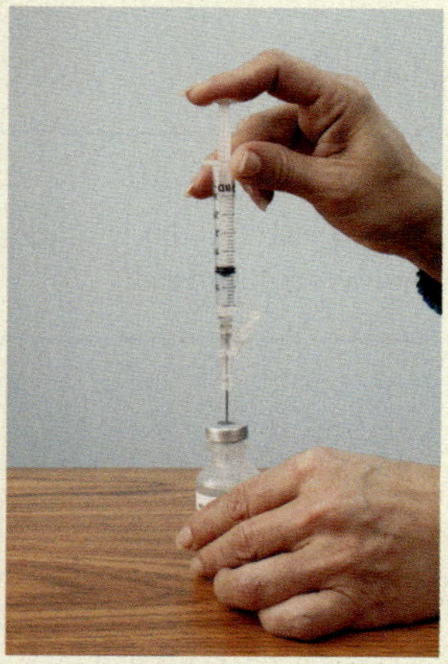

FIGURE 1. Injecting air with vial upright.

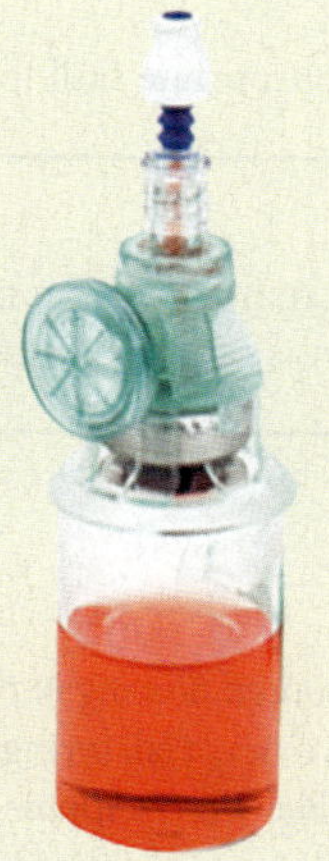

FIGURE 2. Example of a needleless system to access a medication vial.

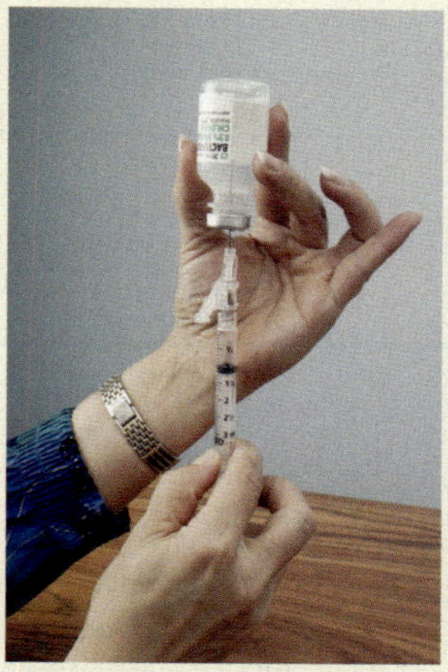

FIGURE 3. Positioning needle tip in solution.

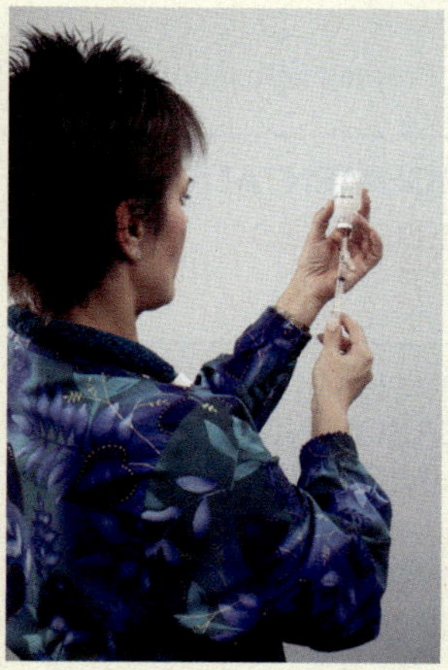

FIGURE 4. Withdrawing medication at eye level.

15. If any air bubbles accumulate in the syringe, tap the barrel of the syringe sharply and move the needle past the fluid into the air space to re-inject the air bubble into the vial. Return the needle tip to the solution and continue withdrawal of the medication.

Removal of air bubbles is necessary to ensure an accurate dose of medication.

16. After the correct dose is withdrawn, remove the needle or needleless access device from the vial; carefully replace the sterile cap over the needle if used. Alternatively, carefully attach a needle or syringe cap. Some facilities require changing the needle, if one was used to withdraw the medication, before administering the medication.

Capping prevents contamination and protects against accidental needlesticks. A one-handed recap method may be used as long as care is taken not to contaminate the needle during the process. Changing the needle may be necessary because passing the needle through the stopper on the vial may dull the needle. In addition, it ensures the tip of the needle is free from medication residue, significantly reducing pain intensity associated with the injection (Ağaç & Günes, 2010).

17. **Check the amount of medication in the syringe with the medication dose and discard any surplus.**

Careful measurement ensures that the correct dose is withdrawn.

(continued on page 982)

Skill 30-3 Removing Medication From a Vial *(continued)*

ACTION	RATIONALE
18. **Depending on facility policy, the third check of the label may occur at this point. If so, when all medications for one patient have been prepared, read the label and recheck the labels with the eMAR/MAR before taking the medications to the patient. However, many facilities require the third check to occur at the bedside, after identifying the patient.**	This *third* check ensures accuracy and helps to prevent errors. *Note:* Many facilities require the *third* check to occur at the bedside, after identifying the patient and before administration.
19. Label the syringe with the medication's name, dose, and amount (The Joint Commission, 2021).	Unlabeled syringes are unidentifiable and may lead to a medication administration error (The Joint Commission, 2021).
20. **If a multidose vial is being used, label the vial with the date and time opened and the beyond-use date (see Special Considerations), and store the vial containing the remaining medication according to facility policy.** Limit the use of multiple-dose vials and dedicate them to a single patient whenever possible (CDC, 2019).	Because the vial is sealed, the medication inside remains sterile and can be used for future injections. Labeling the opened vials with a date, time, and beyond-use date limits its use after a specific time period. Limiting use of multiple-dose vials and dedicating their use to a single patient when possible limits risk of contamination and transfer of microorganisms (CDC, 2019; Dolan et al., 2016).
21. **Log out of and/or lock the medication supply system before leaving it.**	Locking the medication supply system or drawer safeguards the patient's medication supply. Facility accrediting organizations require medication supply systems to be locked when not in use.
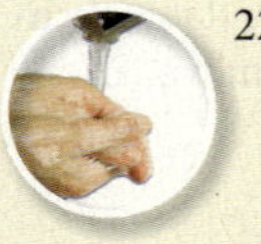 22. Perform hand hygiene.	Hand hygiene deters the spread of microorganisms.
23. Proceed with administration, based on prescribed route.	See appropriate skill for prescribed route.

DOCUMENTATION GUIDELINES

It is not necessary to record the removal of the medication from a vial. Prompt recording of administration of the medication is required immediately after it is administered.

DEVELOPING CLINICAL REASONING AND CLINICAL JUDGMENT

UNEXPECTED SITUATIONS AND ASSOCIATED INTERVENTIONS

- *A piece of self-sealing stopper is noticed floating in the medication in the syringe:* Discard the syringe, needle, and vial. Obtain a new vial, syringe, and needle and prepare the dose as ordered.
- *As the needle attached to the syringe filled with air is inserted into vial, the plunger is immediately pulled down:* If possible to withdraw medication, continue steps as explained above. If such a vacuum has formed that this is impossible, remove the syringe and inject more air into the vial.
- *Plunger is contaminated before injecting air into vial:* Discard the needle and syringe and start over.
- *Plunger is contaminated after medication is drawn into syringe*: It is not necessary to discard the needle and syringe and start over. The contaminated plunger will enter the barrel of the syringe when pushing the medication out, will not come in contact with the medication, and will not contaminate the medication.

SPECIAL CONSIDERATIONS

- When mixing medications in one syringe, preparation of medications in one syringe depends on how the medication is supplied. When using a single-dose vial and a multidose vial, inject air into the multidose vial and draw the medication from the multidose vial into the syringe first. This prevents the contents of the multidose vial from being contaminated with the medication in the single-dose vial. The steps to follow when preparing medications from two multidose vials in one syringe are outlined in Skill 30-4.
- Vials used to draw two or more medications into a single syringe must be discarded after use (Dolan et al., 2016).
- Do not administer medication from a single-dose vial to multiple patients (CDC, 2019).
- Limit the use of multiple-dose vials and dedicate them to a single patient whenever possible (CDC, 2019).
- Multiple-dose vials must be labeled with a beyond-use date when first opened, as indicated by facility policy (CDC, 2019).

Skill 30-4 Mixing Medications From Two Vials in One Syringe

DELEGATION CONSIDERATIONS

The preparation of medication from two vials is not delegated to assistive personnel (AP). Depending on the state's nurse practice act and the organization's policies and procedures, the preparation of medication from two vials may be delegated to licensed practical/vocational nurses (LPN/LVNs). The decision to delegate must be based on careful analysis of the patient's needs and circumstances as well as the qualifications of the person to whom the task is being delegated. Refer to the Delegation Guidelines in Appendix A.

EQUIPMENT

The preparation of two types of insulin in one syringe is used as the example in the following procedure.

- Two vials of medication (insulin in this example)
- Sterile syringe (insulin syringe in this example)
- Sterile needle (if not already packaged with syringe)
- Antimicrobial swabs
- Electronic Medication Administration Record (eMAR) or Medication Administration Record (MAR)

IMPLEMENTATION

ACTION	RATIONALE
1. Gather equipment. Check each medication prescribed against the original in the health record, depending on facility policy and the medication order system in place. Clarify any inconsistencies. Check the patient's health record for allergies.	The prescription is the legal record of prescribed medication interventions. This comparison helps to identify errors that may have occurred when orders were transcribed. Computer provider order-entry (CPOE) systems allow prescribers to send electronic medication prescriptions directly to the pharmacy located in a health care facility and to outpatient pharmacies.
2. Know the actions, special nursing considerations, safe dose ranges, purpose of administration, and adverse effects of the medications to be administered. Confirm the compatibility of the medications in one syringe. Consider the appropriateness of the medication for this patient.	This knowledge aids the nurse in evaluating the therapeutic effect of the medication in relation to the patient's health status and can also be used to educate the patient about the medication.
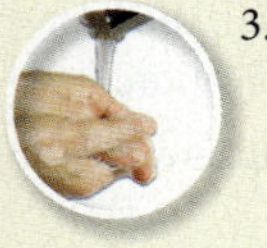 3. Perform hand hygiene.	Hand hygiene prevents the spread of microorganisms.
4. Move the medication supply system to the outside of the patient's room or prepare for administration at the medication supply system in the medication area. Alternatively, access the medication administration supply system at or inside the patient's room.	Organization facilitates error-free administration and saves time.
5. Unlock the medication supply system or drawer. Enter the passcode and scan employee identification, if required.	Locking the supply system or drawer safeguards each patient's medication supply. Facility accrediting organizations require medication supply systems to be locked when not in use. Entering the passcode and scanning ID allows only authorized users into the system and identifies the user for documentation by the computer.
6. **Prepare medications for one patient at a time.**	This prevents errors in medication administration.
7. Read the eMAR/MAR and read the label when selecting the proper medications from the medication supply system or the patient's medication drawer.	This is the *first* check of the label.
8. Read the label and compare the labels with the eMAR/MAR. Check expiration dates and perform dosage calculations, if necessary. Scan the bar code on the package, if required.	This is the *second* check of the labels. Verify calculations with another nurse to ensure safety, if necessary.
9. If necessary, remove the cap that protects the self-sealing stopper on each vial.	The cap protects the self-sealing top.

(*continued on page 984*)

Skill 30-4 Mixing Medications From Two Vials in One Syringe *(continued)*

ACTION / **RATIONALE**

10. **If the medication is a suspension (e.g., a modified insulin, such as NPH insulin), roll and agitate the vial to mix it well.**

There is controversy regarding how to mix insulin in suspension. Some sources advise rolling the vial; others advise shaking the vial. Consult facility policy or pharmacist. Regardless of the method used, it is essential that the suspension be mixed well to avoid administering an inconsistent dose.

11. **Scrub the self-sealing stopper top with the antimicrobial swab and allow it to dry.**

The antimicrobial swab removes surface microbial contamination. Allowing the antimicrobial solution to dry completely (5 to 20 seconds) ensures complete antimicrobial effectiveness (Gorski et al., 2021; Slater et al., 2018). Drying also prevents antimicrobial solution from entering the vial on the needle.

12. Remove the cap from the needle by pulling it straight off. Touch the plunger only at the knob. Draw back an amount of air into the syringe that is equal to the dose of modified insulin to be withdrawn.

Pulling the cap off in a straight manner prevents accidental needlestick. Handling the plunger only by the knob ensures sterility of the shaft of the plunger. Before fluid is removed, injection of an equal amount of air is required to prevent the formation of a partial vacuum, because a vial is a sealed container. If not enough air is injected, the negative pressure makes it difficult to withdraw the medication with repeated use.

13. Hold the modified vial on a flat surface. Pierce the self-sealing stopper in the center with the needle tip and inject the measured air into the space above the solution (Figure 1). Do not inject air into the solution. Withdraw the needle.

Unmodified insulin should never be contaminated with modified insulin. Placing air in the modified insulin first without allowing the needle to contact the insulin ensures that the second vial-entered (unmodified) insulin is not contaminated by the medication in the other vial. Air bubbled through the solution could result in withdrawal of an inaccurate amount of medication.

14. Draw back an amount of air into the syringe that is equal to the dose of unmodified insulin to be withdrawn.

A vial is a sealed container. Therefore, injection of an equal amount of air (before fluid is removed) is required to prevent the formation of a partial vacuum. If not enough air is injected, the negative pressure makes it difficult to withdraw the medication.

15. Hold the unmodified vial on a flat surface. Pierce the self-sealing stopper in the center with the needle tip and inject the measured air into the space above the solution (Figure 2). Do not inject air into the solution. Keep the needle in the vial.

Air bubbled through the solution could result in withdrawal of an inaccurate amount of medication.

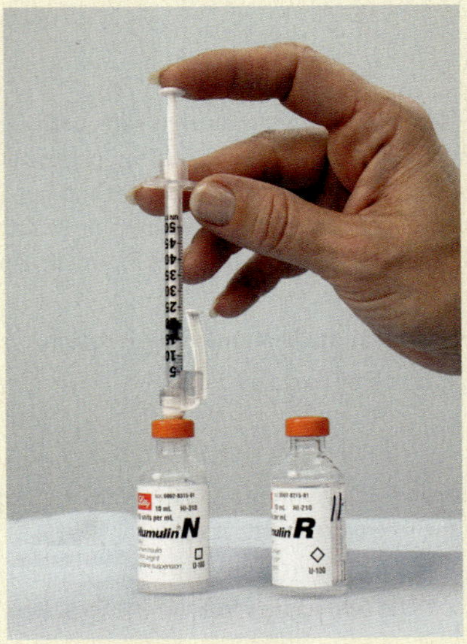

FIGURE 1. Injecting air into modified insulin preparation.

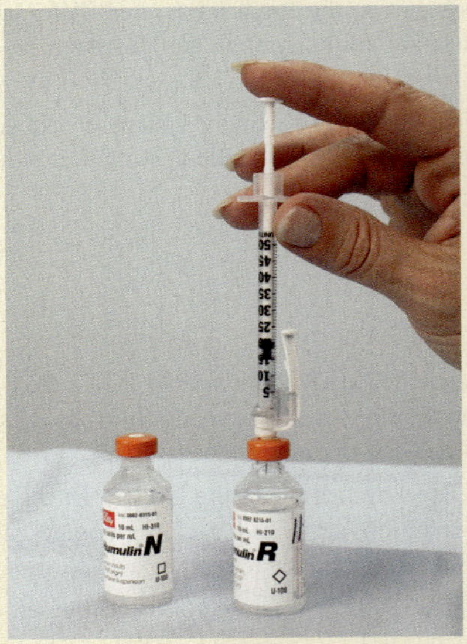

FIGURE 2. Injecting air into unmodified insulin vial.

ACTION

16. Invert the vial of unmodified insulin. Hold the vial in one hand and use the other to withdraw the medication. **Touch the plunger only at the knob. Draw up the prescribed amount of medication while holding the syringe at eye level and vertically** (Figure 3). Turn the vial over and then remove the needle from the vial.

RATIONALE

Holding the syringe at eye level facilitates accurate reading, and the vertical position allows easy removal of air bubbles from the syringe. First dose is prepared and is not contaminated by insulin that contains modifiers.

17. Check that there are no air bubbles in the syringe.

The presence of air in the syringe would result in an inaccurate dose of medication.

18. **Check the amount of medication in the syringe with the medication dose and discard any surplus.**

Careful measurement ensures that the correct dose is withdrawn.

19. **Recheck the vial label with the eMAR/MAR.**

This is the *third* check to ensure accuracy and to prevent errors. It must be checked now for the first medication in the syringe, as it is not possible to ensure accuracy once a second drug is in the syringe.

20. Calculate the endpoint on the syringe for the combined insulin amount by adding the number of units for each dose together.

This allows for accurate withdrawal of the second dose.

21. Insert the needle into the modified vial and invert it, **taking care not to push the plunger and inject medication from the syringe into the vial.** Invert the vial of modified insulin. Hold the vial in one hand and use the other to withdraw the medication. **Touch the plunger only at the knob. Draw up the prescribed amount of medication while holding the syringe at eye level and vertically (Figure 4). Take care to withdraw only the prescribed amount.** Turn the vial over and then remove the needle from the vial. Carefully recap the needle. Carefully replace the cap over the needle.

The previous addition of air eliminates the need to create positive pressure. Holding the syringe at eye level facilitates accurate reading. Capping the needle prevents contamination and protects the nurse against accidental needlesticks. A one-handed recap method may be used as long as care is taken to ensure that the needle remains sterile.

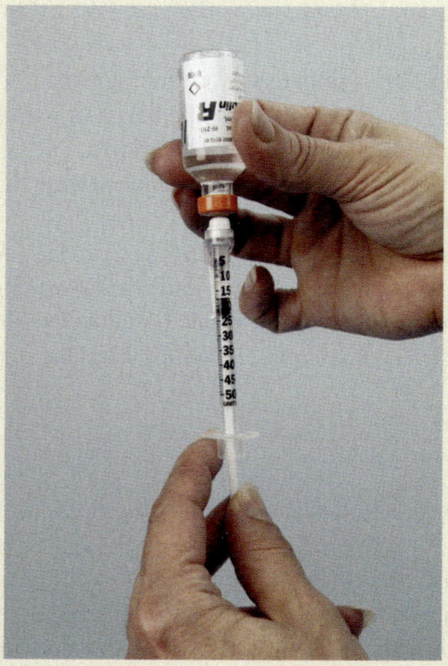

FIGURE 3. Withdrawing prescribed amount of unmodified insulin.

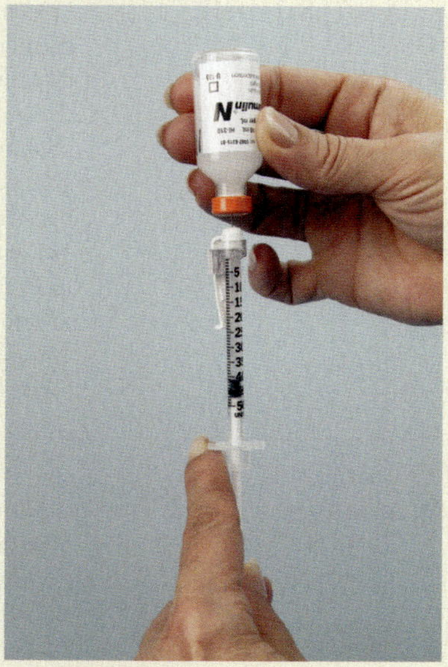

FIGURE 4. Withdrawing modified insulin.

22. **Check the amount of medication in the syringe with the medication dose.**

Careful measurement ensures that correct dose is withdrawn.

23. **Depending on facility policy, the third check of the label may occur at this point. If so, read the label and recheck the labels with the MAR before taking the medications to the patient. However, many facilities require the third check to occur at the bedside, after identifying the patient.**

This *third* check ensures accuracy and helps to prevent errors. *Note:* Many facilities require the *third* check to occur at the bedside, after identifying the patient and before administration.

(*continued on page 986*)

Skill 30-4 Mixing Medications From Two Vials in One Syringe *(continued)*

ACTION	RATIONALE
24. **Label the vials with the date and time opened and beyond-use date, and store the vials containing the remaining medication, according to facility policy.**	Because the vial is sealed, the medication inside remains sterile and can be used for future injections. Labeling the opened vials with a date and time limits its use after a specific time period. The CDC recommends that medications packaged as multiuse vials be assigned to a single patient whenever possible (CDC, 2019; Dolan et al., 2016).
25. Label the syringe with the medication's name, dose, and amount date (The Joint Commission, 2021).	Unlabeled syringes are unidentifiable and may lead to a medication administration error (The Joint Commission, 2021).
26. **Log out of and/or lock the medication supply system before leaving it.**	Locking the medication supply system or drawer safeguards the patient's medication supply. Facility accrediting organizations require medication supply systems to be locked when not in use.
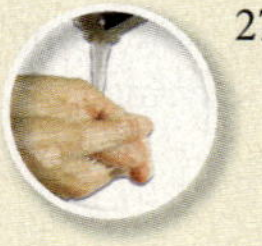 27. Perform hand hygiene.	Hand hygiene deters the spread of microorganisms.
28. Proceed with administration, based on prescribed route.	See appropriate skill for prescribed route.

DOCUMENTATION GUIDELINES

It is not necessary to record the removal of the medication from the vials. Prompt recording of administration of the medication is required immediately after it is administered.

DEVELOPING CLINICAL REASONING AND CLINICAL JUDGMENT

UNEXPECTED SITUATIONS AND ASSOCIATED INTERVENTIONS

- *You contaminate the plunger before injecting air into the insulin vial:* Discard the needle and syringe and start over.
- *The plunger is contaminated after medication is drawn into the syringe:* It is not necessary to discard and start over. The contaminated plunger will enter the barrel of the syringe when pushing the medication out and will not contaminate the medication.
- *You allow modified insulin to come in contact with the needle before entering the unmodified insulin vial:* Discard the needle and syringe and start over.
- *You notice that the combined amount is not the ordered amount (i.e., you have less or more units in combined syringe than ordered):* Discard the syringe and start over. There is no way to know for sure which dosage is wrong or which medication should be expelled.
- *You inject medication from the first vial (in syringe) into the second vial:* Discard the vial and syringe and start over.

SPECIAL CONSIDERATIONS

General Considerations

- A patient with diabetes who is visually impaired may find it helpful to use a magnifying apparatus that fits around the syringe.
- Before attempting to explain or demonstrate devices that help low-vision diabetic patients to prepare their medication, attempt to use the device yourself under similar circumstances. To detect any difficulties the patient may experience, practice using the aid with your eyes closed or in a poorly lit room.

Infant and Child Considerations

- School-age children are generally able to prepare and administer their own injections, such as insulin, with supervision (American Academy of Pediatrics, 2020). Parents/caregivers and the child should be involved in teaching.

Skill 30-5 Administering an Intradermal Injection

DELEGATION CONSIDERATIONS

The administration of an intradermal injection is not delegated to assistive personnel (AP). Depending on the state's nurse practice act and the organization's policies and procedures, the administration of an intradermal injection may be delegated to licensed practical/vocational nurses (LPN/LVNs). The decision to delegate must be based on careful analysis of the patient's needs and circumstances as well as the qualifications of the person to whom the task is being delegated. Refer to the Delegation Guidelines in Appendix A.

EQUIPMENT

- Prescribed medication
- Sterile syringe, usually a tuberculin syringe calibrated in tenths and hundredths, and a 3/8″ to ½″, 26- or 27-gauge needle
- Antimicrobial swab
- Disposable gloves
- Small gauze square
- Electronic Medication Administration Record (eMAR) or Medication Administration Record (MAR)
- PPE, as indicated
- Marking pen for indicating area for future assessment, if indicated

IMPLEMENTATION

ACTION	RATIONALE
1. Gather equipment. Check each medication prescribed against the original in the health record, depending on facility policy and the medication order system in place. Clarify any inconsistencies. Check the patient's health record for allergies.	The prescription is the legal record of prescribed medication interventions. This comparison helps to identify errors that may have occurred when orders were transcribed. Computer provider order-entry (CPOE) systems allow prescribers to send electronic medication prescriptions directly to the pharmacy located in a health care facility and to outpatient pharmacies.
2. Know the actions, special nursing considerations, safe dose ranges, purpose of administration, and adverse effects of the medications to be administered. Consider the appropriateness of the medication for this patient.	This knowledge aids the nurse in evaluating the therapeutic effect of the medication in relation to the patient's health status and can also be used to educate the patient about the medication.
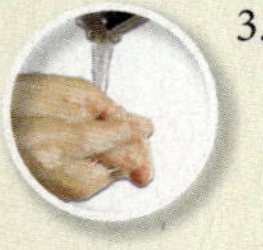 3. Perform hand hygiene.	Hand hygiene deters the spread of microorganisms.
4. Move the medication supply system to the outside of the patient's room or prepare for administration at the medication supply system in the medication area. Alternatively, access the medication administration supply system at or inside the patient's room.	Organization facilitates error-free administration and saves time.
5. Unlock the medication supply system or drawer. Enter the passcode and scan employee identification, if required.	Locking the medication supply system or drawer safeguards each patient's medication supply. Facility accrediting organizations require medication supply systems to be locked when not in use. Entering the passcode and scanning ID allows only authorized users into the system and identifies the user for documentation by the computer.
6. **Prepare medications for one patient at a time.**	This prevents errors in medication administration.
7. Read the eMAR/MAR and read the label when selecting the proper medication from the medication supply system or the patient's medication drawer.	This is the *first* check of the label.
8. Read the label and compare the label with the eMAR/MAR. Check expiration dates and perform calculations, if necessary. Scan the bar code on the package, if required.	This is the *second* check of the label. Verify calculations with another nurse to ensure safety.
9. If necessary, withdraw the medication from an ampule or vial as described in Skills 30-2 and 30-3.	

(*continued on page 988*)

Skill 30-5 Administering an Intradermal Injection *(continued)*

ACTION	RATIONALE
10. **Depending on facility policy, the third check of the label may occur at this point. If so, when all medications for one patient have been prepared, read the label and recheck the labels with the eMAR/MAR before taking the medications to the patient. However, many facilities require the third check to occur at the bedside, after identifying the patient.**	This *third* check ensures accuracy and helps to prevent errors. *Note:* Many facilities require the *third* check to occur at the bedside, after identifying the patient and before administration.
11. Label the syringe with the medication's name, dose, and amount (The Joint Commission, 2021).	Unlabeled syringes are unidentifiable and may lead to a medication administration error (The Joint Commission, 2021).
12. **Log-out of and/or lock the medication supply system before leaving it.**	Locking the medication supply system or drawer safeguards the patient's medication supply. Facility accrediting organizations require medication supply systems to be locked when not in use.
13. Transport medications to the patient's bedside carefully and keep the medications in sight at all times.	Careful handling and close observation prevent accidental or deliberate disarrangement of medications.
14. **Ensure that the patient receives the medications at the correct time.**	Check facility policy, which may allow for administration within a period of 30 minutes before or 30 minutes after the designated time.
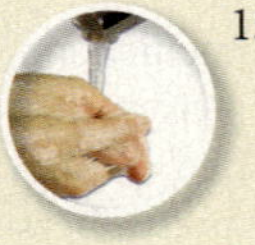 15. Perform hand hygiene and put on PPE, if indicated.	Hand hygiene and PPE prevent the spread of microorganisms. PPE is required based on transmission precautions.
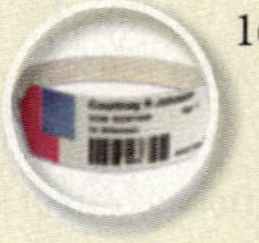 16. **Identify the patient. Compare the information with the eMAR/MAR. The patient should be identified using at least two of the following methods** (The Joint Commission, 2021):	Identifying the patient ensures the right patient receives the medications and helps prevent errors. The patient's room number or physical location is not used as an identifier (The Joint Commission, 2021). Replace the identification band if it is missing or inaccurate in any way.
a. Check the name on the patient's identification band.	This requires a response from the patient, but illness and strange surroundings often cause patients to be confused.
b. Check the identification number on the patient's identification band.	
c. Check the birth date on the patient's identification band.	
d. Ask the patient to state their name and birth date, based on facility policy.	
17. Close the door to the room or pull the bedside curtain.	This provides patient privacy.
18. **Complete necessary assessments before administering medications. Check the patient's allergy bracelet, if present, or ask the patient about allergies. Explain the purpose and action of the medication to the patient.**	Assessment is a prerequisite to administration of medications. Explanation provides rationale, increases knowledge, promotes patient engagement, and reduces anxiety.
19. Scan the patient's bar code on the identification band, if required (The Joint Commission, 2021).	This provides an additional check to ensure that the medication is given to the right patient.
20. **Based on facility policy, the third check of the label may occur at this point. If so, read the label and recheck the labels with the eMAR/MAR before administering the medications to the patient.**	Many facilities require the *third* check to occur at the bedside, after identifying the patient and before administration. If facility policy directs the *third* check at this time, this *third* check ensures accuracy and helps to prevent errors.
21. Put on gloves.	Gloves help prevent exposure to contaminants.
22. Select an appropriate administration site. Assist the patient to the appropriate position for the site chosen. Drape, as needed, to expose only site area to be used.	Using the appropriate site prevents injury and allows for accurate reading of the test site at the appropriate time. Draping provides privacy and warmth.
23. Cleanse the site with an antimicrobial swab while wiping with a firm, circular motion and moving outward from the injection site. Allow the skin to dry.	Pathogens on the skin can be forced into the tissues by the needle. Moving from the center outward prevents contamination of the site. Allowing the antimicrobial solution to dry completely (5 to 20 seconds) ensures complete antimicrobial effectiveness (Gorski et al., 2021; Slater et al., 2018), and prevents introducing alcohol into the tissue, which can be irritating and uncomfortable.

ACTION | **RATIONALE**

24. Remove the needle cap with the nondominant hand by pulling it straight off.
This technique lessens the risk of an accidental needlestick.

25. Use the nondominant hand to spread the skin taut over the injection site (Figure 1).
Taut skin provides an easy entrance into intradermal tissue.

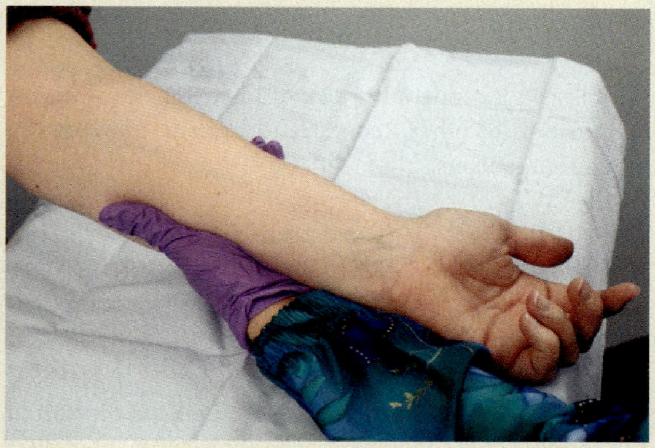

FIGURE 1. Spreading skin taut over injection site.

26. Hold the syringe in the dominant hand, between the thumb and forefinger with the bevel of the needle up.
Using the dominant hand allows for easy, appropriate handling of the syringe. Having the bevel up allows for smooth piercing of the skin and introduction of medication into the dermis.

27. Hold the syringe at a 5- to 15-degree angle from the site. Place the needle almost flat against the patient's skin (Figure 2), bevel side up, and insert the needle into the skin. Insert the needle only about ⅛ inch with entire bevel under the skin.
The dermis is entered when the needle is held as nearly parallel to the skin as possible and is inserted about ⅛ inch.

28. Once the needle is in place, steady the lower end of the syringe. Slide your dominant hand to the end of the plunger.
This prevents injury and inadvertent advancement or withdrawal of needle.

29. Slowly inject the agent while watching for a small wheal to appear (Figure 3).
The appearance of a wheal indicates the medication is in the dermis.

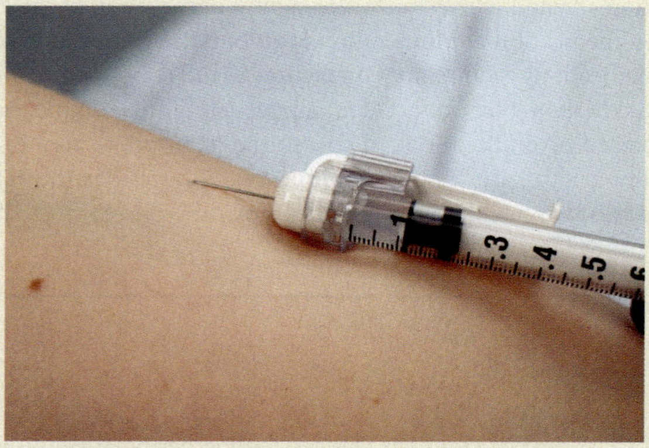

FIGURE 2. Inserting needle almost flat against the skin.

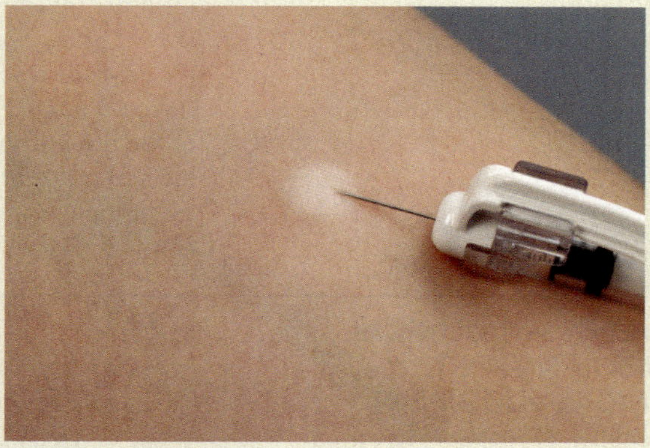

FIGURE 3. Observing for wheal while injecting medication.

30. Withdraw the needle quickly at the same angle that it was inserted. Do not recap the used needle. Engage the safety shield or needle guard.
Withdrawing the needle quickly and at the angle at which it entered the skin minimizes tissue damage and discomfort for the patient. Safety shield or needle guard prevents accidental needlestick injury.

31. **Do not massage the area after removing needle. Tell the patient not to rub or scratch the site. If necessary, gently blot the site with a dry gauze square. Do not apply pressure or rub the site.** Use the marking pen to mark the area for further assessment, if indicated.
Massaging or rubbing the area where an intradermal injection is given may spread the medication to underlying subcutaneous tissue.

(continued on page 990)

Skill 30-5 Administering an Intradermal Injection *(continued)*

ACTION	RATIONALE
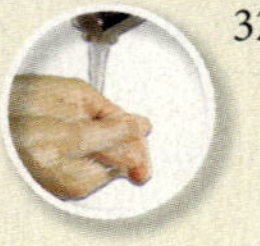 32. Remove gloves and perform hand hygiene. Assist the patient to a position of comfort.	Removing gloves and performing hand hygiene reduces risk for contamination of other items and the spread of microorganisms. Assisting the patient to a position of comfort promotes patient comfort.
33. Discard the needle and syringe in an appropriate container, such as a sharps receptacle.	Proper disposal of the needle prevents injury.
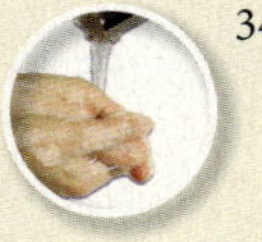 34. Remove additional PPE, if used. Perform hand hygiene.	Proper removal of PPE reduces the risk of infection transmission and contamination of other items. Hand hygiene prevents the spread of microorganisms.
35. Document the administration of the medication immediately after administration. See Documentation section below.	Timely documentation helps to ensure patient safety.
36. Evaluate the patient's response to the medication within the appropriate time frame.	The patient needs to be evaluated for therapeutic and adverse effects from the medication.
37. Observe the area for signs of a reaction at determined intervals after administration. Inform the patient of the need for inspection.	With many intradermal injections, you need to look for a localized reaction in the area of the injection at the appropriate interval(s) determined by the type of medication and purpose. Explanation provides rationale, increases knowledge, promotes patient engagement, and reduces anxiety.
38. If medication is intended for allergy skin testing, observe the patient for sensitivity to the injected allergen (Hoy & Ng, 2021).	Sensitivity to an allergen places the patient at risk for the development of anaphylaxis and may require the administration of epinephrine subcutaneously (Hoy & Ng, 2021). (Refer to Skill 30-6.)

DOCUMENTATION

GUIDELINES

Record each medication administered on the eMAR/MAR or health record using the required format, including date, time, and the site of administration, immediately after administration. Some facilities recommend circling the injection site with ink. Circling the injection site easily identifies the intradermal injection site and allows for future careful observation of the exact area. If using a bar-code system, medication administration is automatically recorded when the bar code is scanned. PRN medications require documentation of the reason for administration. Prompt recording avoids the possibility of accidentally repeating the administration of the drug. If the drug was refused or omitted, record this in the appropriate area on the medication record and notify the health care team as appropriate. This verifies the reason medication was omitted and ensures that health care personnel providing care for the patient are aware of the occurrence.

DEVELOPING CLINICAL REASONING AND CLINICAL JUDGMENT

UNEXPECTED SITUATIONS AND ASSOCIATED INTERVENTIONS

- *You do not note a wheal or blister at the injection site:* The medication has been inadvertently injected subcutaneously. Document according to facility policy and notify the health care team as appropriate. You may need to obtain an order to repeat the procedure.
- *Medication leaks out of the injection site before the needle is withdrawn:* The needle was inserted less than ⅛ inch. Document according to facility policy and notify the health care team as appropriate. You may need to obtain an order to repeat the procedure.
- *You stick yourself with the needle before injection:* Discard the needle and syringe appropriately. Follow facility policy regarding needlestick injury. Prepare a new syringe with medication and administer to the patient. Communicate and document the incident according to facility policy.
- *You stick yourself with the needle after injection:* Discard the needle and syringe appropriately. Follow facility policy regarding needlestick injury. Communicate and document the incident according to facility policy.

SPECIAL CONSIDERATIONS

- Fluzone® Intradermal is the only vaccine in the United States administered by the intradermal route and is available for patients ages 18 to 64 years (CDC, 2015; Prescriber's Digital Reference [PDR], 2021; Sanofi Pasteur, 2017). The site of administration for this vaccine is the deltoid region of the upper arm, and the needle is inserted perpendicular to the skin (PDR, 2021). **This vaccine should not be administered into the forearm or other site used to administer other intradermal medications.** The single-dose prefilled microinjection syringe administers a 0.1-mL dose (Sanofi Pasteur, 2017). **No other influenza vaccine formulations should be administered by the intradermal route.** Follow the manufacturer's directions for appropriate administration.
- Ongoing assessment is an important part of nursing care for both evaluation of patient response to administered medications and early detection of adverse reactions. If an adverse effect is suspected, withhold further medication doses and notify the health care team. Additional intervention is based on type of reaction and patient assessment.

Skill 30-6 Administering a Subcutaneous Injection

DELEGATION CONSIDERATIONS

The administration of a subcutaneous injection is not delegated to assistive personnel (AP). Depending on the state's nurse practice act and the organization's policies and procedures, the administration of a subcutaneous injection may be delegated to licensed practical/vocational nurses (LPN/LVNs). The decision to delegate must be based on careful analysis of the patient's needs and circumstances as well as the qualifications of the person to whom the task is being delegated. Refer to the Delegation Guidelines in Appendix A.

EQUIPMENT

- Prescribed medication
- Sterile syringe and needle. Needle size depends on the medication to be administered and patient body type (see previous discussion).
- Antimicrobial swab
- Nonlatex, disposable gloves
- Small gauze square
- Electronic Medication Administration Record (eMAR) or Medication Administration Record (MAR)
- PPE, as indicated

IMPLEMENTATION

ACTION	RATIONALE
1. Gather equipment. Check each medication prescribed against the original in the health record, depending on facility policy and the medication order system in place. Clarify any inconsistencies. Check the patient's health record for allergies.	The prescription is the legal record of prescribed medication interventions. This comparison helps to identify errors that may have occurred when orders were transcribed. Computer provider order-entry (CPOE) systems allow prescribers to send electronic medication prescriptions directly to the pharmacy located in a health care facility and to outpatient pharmacies.
2. Know the actions, special nursing considerations, safe dose ranges, purpose of administration, and adverse effects of the medications to be administered. Consider the appropriateness of the medication for this patient.	This knowledge aids the nurse in evaluating the therapeutic effect of the medication in relation to the patient's health status and can also be used to educate the patient about the medication.
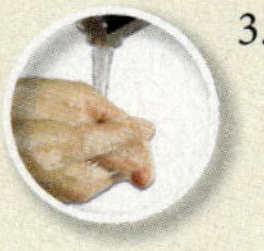 3. Perform hand hygiene.	Hand hygiene prevents the spread of microorganisms.
4. Move the medication supply system to the outside of the patient's room or prepare for administration at the medication supply system in the medication area. Alternatively, access the medication administration supply system at or inside the patient's room.	Organization facilitates error-free administration and saves time.

(continued on page 992)

Skill 30-6 Administering a Subcutaneous Injection *(continued)*

ACTION	RATIONALE
5. Unlock the medication supply system or drawer. Enter the passcode and scan employee identification, if required.	Locking the medication supply system or drawer safeguards each patient's medication supply. Facility accrediting organizations require medication supply systems to be locked when not in use. Entering the passcode and scanning ID allows only authorized users into the computer system and identifies the user for documentation by the computer.
6. **Prepare medications for one patient at a time.**	This prevents errors in medication administration.
7. Read the eMAR/MAR and read the label when selecting the proper medication from the medication supply system or the patient's medication drawer.	This is the *first* check of the label.
8. Read the label and compare the medication label with the eMAR/MAR. Check expiration dates and perform calculations, if necessary. Scan the bar code on the package, if required.	This is the *second* check of the label. Verify calculations with another nurse to ensure safety, if necessary.
9. If necessary, withdraw the medication from an ampule or vial as described in Skills 30-2 and 30-3.	
10. **Depending on facility policy, the third check of the label may occur at this point. If so, when all medications for one patient have been prepared, read the label and recheck the labels with the eMAR/MAR before taking the medications to the patient. However, many facilities require the third check to occur at the bedside, after identifying the patient.**	This *third* check ensures accuracy and helps to prevent errors. *Note:* Many facilities require the *third* check to occur at the bedside, after identifying the patient and before administration.
11. Label the syringe with the medication's name, dose, and amount (The Joint Commission, 2021).	Unlabeled syringes are unidentifiable and may lead to a medication administration error (The Joint Commission, 2021).
12. **Log out of and/or lock the medication supply system before leaving it.**	Locking the medication supply system or drawer safeguards the patient's medication supply. Facility accrediting organizations require medication supply systems to be locked when not in use.
13. Transport medications to the patient's bedside carefully and keep the medications in sight at all times.	Careful handling and close observation prevent accidental or deliberate disarrangement of medications.
14. **Ensure that the patient receives the medications at the correct time.**	Check facility policy, which may allow for administration within a period of 30 minutes before or 30 minutes after the designated time.
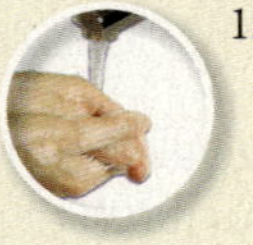 15. Perform hand hygiene and put on PPE, if indicated.	Hand hygiene and PPE prevent the spread of microorganisms. PPE is required based on transmission precautions.
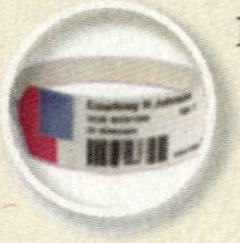 16. **Identify the patient. Compare the information with the eMAR/MAR. The patient should be identified using at least two of the following methods** (The Joint Commission, 2021):	Identifying the patient ensures the right patient receives the medications and helps prevent errors. The patient's room number or physical location is not used as an identifier (The Joint Commission, 2021). Replace the identification band if it is missing or inaccurate in any way.
a. Check the name on the patient's identification band.	
b. Check the identification number on the patient's identification band.	
c. Check the birth date on the patient's identification band.	
d. Ask the patient to state their name and birth date, based on facility policy.	This requires a response from the patient, but illness and strange surroundings often cause patients to be confused.
17. Close the door to the room or pull the bedside curtain.	This provides patient privacy.
18. **Complete necessary assessments before administering medications. Check the patient's allergy bracelet, if present, or ask the patient about allergies.** Explain the purpose and action of the medication to the patient.	Assessment is a prerequisite to administration of medications. Explanation provides rationale, increases knowledge, promotes patient engagement, and reduces anxiety.

ACTION

RATIONALE

19. Scan the patient's bar code on the identification band, if required (The Joint Commission, 2021) (Figure 1).

Scanning provides an additional check to ensure that the medication is given to the right patient.

20. **Based on facility policy, the third check of the label may occur at this point. If so, read the label and recheck the labels with the eMAR/MAR before administering the medications to the patient.**

Many facilities require the *third* check to occur at the bedside, after identifying the patient and before administration. If facility policy directs the *third* check at this time, this *third* check ensures accuracy and helps to prevent errors.

21. Put on gloves.

Gloves help prevent exposure to contaminants.

22. Select an appropriate administration site. Assist the patient to the appropriate position for the site chosen. Drape, as needed, to expose only site area to be used.

Using an appropriate site and positioning prevent injury. Draping helps maintain the patient's privacy.

23. Identify the appropriate landmarks for the site chosen.

Good visualization is necessary to establish the correct site location and to avoid complications (Taylor et al., 2023).

24. Cleanse the area around the injection site with an antimicrobial swab. Use a firm, circular motion while moving outward from the injection site (Figure 2). Allow the area to dry.

Pathogens on the skin can be forced into the tissues by the needle. Moving from the center outward prevents contamination of the site. Allowing the antimicrobial solution to dry completely (5 to 20 seconds) ensures complete antimicrobial effectiveness (Gorski et al., 2021; Slater et al., 2018), and prevents introducing alcohol into the tissue, which can be irritating and uncomfortable.

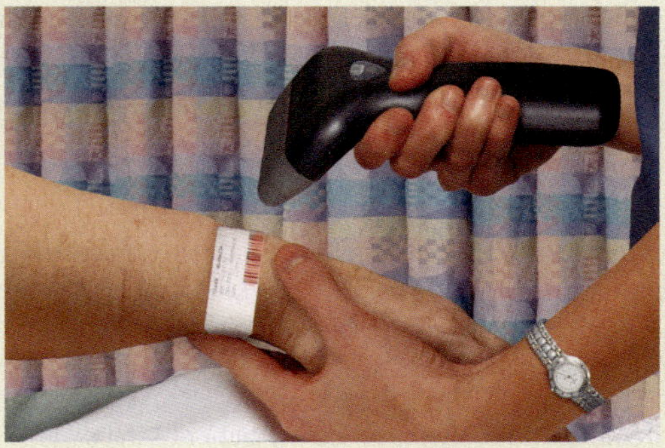

FIGURE 1. Scanning bar code on the patient's identification bracelet. (*Source:* Used with permission from Shutterstock. *Photo by B. Proud.*)

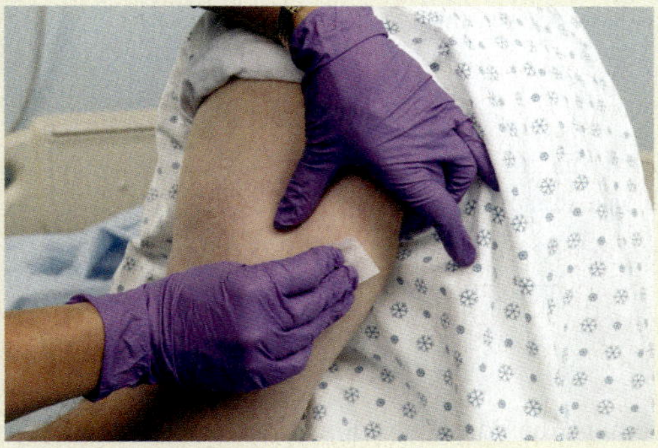

FIGURE 2. Cleaning injection site.

25. Remove the needle cap with the nondominant hand, pulling it straight off.

The cap protects the needle from contact with microorganisms. This technique lessens the risk of an accidental needlestick.

26. Hold the syringe in the dominant hand between the thumb and forefinger. Use the thumb, index finger and middle finger on the nondominant hand to pinch up the skin and underlying fatty tissue (Figure 3). Inject the needle quickly at a 45- or 90-degree angle, depending on the amount of underlying subcutaneous tissue (Figure 4).

Pinching up the skin and underlying fatty tissue lifts the adipose tissue away from underlying muscle and tissue (Wolicki & Miller, 2020; Shepard, 2018b). Inserting the needle quickly causes less pain to the patient. For a person with a limited amount of subcutaneous tissue, insert the needle at a 45-degree angle (Shepherd, 2018b).

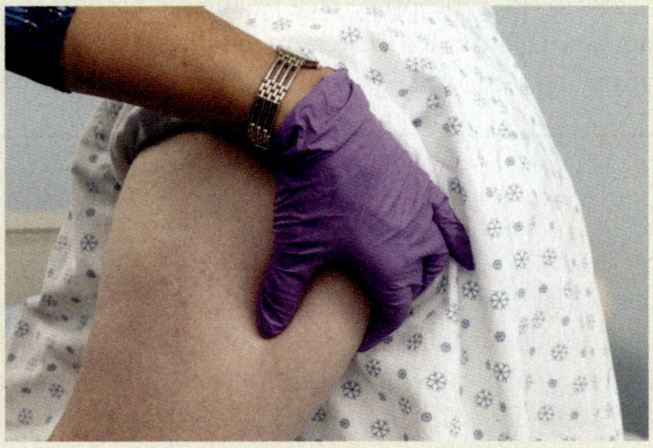

FIGURE 3. Pinching up the skin and underlying fatty tissue.

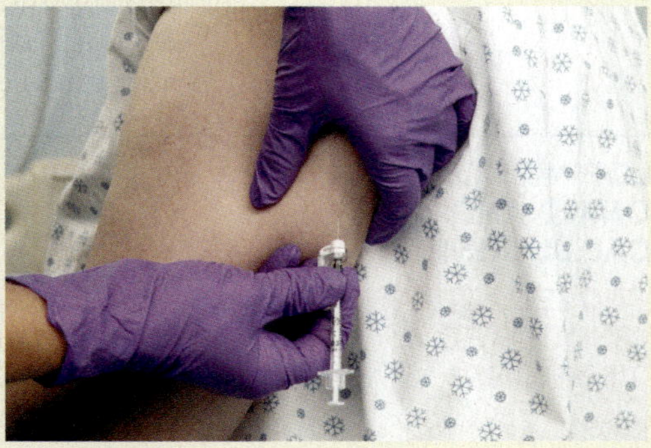

FIGURE 4. Inserting needle.

(*continued on page 994*)

Skill 30-6 Administering a Subcutaneous Injection *(continued)*

ACTION	RATIONALE
27. Move your nondominant hand to the lower end of the syringe and slide your dominant hand to the end of the plunger, taking care to avoid moving the syringe. Alternatively, move your middle finger into place on the syringe, holding the syringe with your thumb and middle finger, and move your index finger to the end of the plunger; taking care to avoid moving the syringe.	This allows for stabilization of the syringe and avoids movement. Moving the syringe could cause damage to the tissues and inadvertent administration into an incorrect area.
28. Inject the medication. Withdraw the needle quickly at the same angle at which it was inserted, while supporting the surrounding tissue with your nondominant hand.	Slow withdrawal of the needle pulls the tissues and causes discomfort. Applying counter traction around the injection site helps to prevent pulling on the tissue as the needle is withdrawn. Removing the needle at the same angle at which it was inserted minimizes tissue damage and discomfort for the patient.
29. Do not recap the used needle. Engage the safety shield or needle guard.	Safety shield or needle guard prevents accidental needlestick.
30. If blood or clear fluid appears at the site after withdrawing the needle, use a gauze square to apply gentle pressure to the site. **Do not massage the site.**	Massaging the site can damage underlying tissue and increase the absorption of the medication (Taylor et al., 2023). Massaging after heparin administration can contribute to hematoma formation.
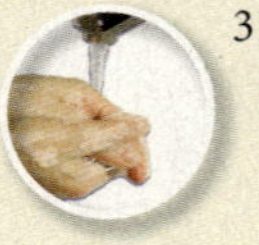 31. Remove gloves and perform hand hygiene. Assist the patient to a position of comfort.	Removing gloves and performing hand hygiene reduces the risk of contamination of other items and the spread of microorganisms. Assisting the patient to a position of comfort promotes patient comfort.
32. Discard the needle and syringe in an appropriate container, such as a sharps receptacle.	Proper disposal of the needle prevents injury.
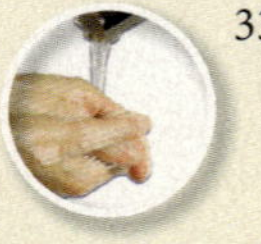 33. Remove additional PPE, if used. Perform hand hygiene.	Proper removal of PPE reduces the risk of infection transmission and contamination of other items. Hand hygiene prevents the spread of microorganisms.
34. Document the administration of the medication immediately after administration.	Timely documentation helps to ensure patient safety.
35. Evaluate the patient's response to the medication within the appropriate time frame for the particular medication.	The patient needs to be evaluated for therapeutic and adverse effects from the medication.

DOCUMENTATION GUIDELINES

Record each medication given on the eMAR/MAR or health record using the required format immediately after administration, including date, dose, time, and the site of administration. If using a bar-code system, medication administration is automatically recorded when the bar code is scanned. PRN medications require documentation of the reason for administration. Prompt recording avoids the possibility of accidentally repeating the administration of the drug. If the drug was refused or omitted, record this in the appropriate area on the medication record and notify the health care team as appropriate. This verifies the reason medication was omitted and ensures that health care personnel providing care for the patient are aware of the occurrence.

DEVELOPING CLINICAL REASONING AND CLINICAL JUDGMENT

UNEXPECTED SITUATIONS AND ASSOCIATED INTERVENTIONS

- *Patient refuses to let you administer medication in a different location:* Explain the rationale behind rotating injection sites. Discuss other available injection sites with the patient. If the patient will still not allow injection in another area, administer medication to patient, document the patient's refusal of rotation of the injection site and discussion, and notify the health care team.

- *You stick yourself with the needle before injection:* Discard the needle and syringe appropriately. Follow facility policy regarding needlestick injury. Prepare a new syringe with medication and administer to the patient. Communicate and document the incident according to facility policy.
- *You stick yourself with the needle after injection:* Discard the needle and syringe appropriately. Communicate and document the incident according to facility policy.
- *During injection, patient pulls away from the needle before the medication is delivered fully:* Remove and appropriately discard the needle. Attach a new needle to the syringe and administer the remaining medication at a different site. Document events and interventions according to facility policy.

SPECIAL CONSIDERATIONS

General Considerations

- Ongoing assessment is an important part of nursing care for both evaluation of patient response to administered medications and early detection of adverse drug reactions. If an adverse effect is suspected, withhold further medication doses and notify the health care team. Additional intervention is based on type of reaction and patient assessment.
- Injection speed does not seem to influence pain sensation associated with subcutaneous injection (Heise et al., 2014; Mohammady et al., 2017; Pich, 2020; Zijlstra et al., 2018).
- Because absorption rates vary from site to site, it is recommended that patients administering their own insulin use the same area of the body at the same time every day to ensure more consistent absorption and prevent tissue changes from repeated use of the same site (ADA, 2020; Frandsen & Pennington, 2021; Karch, 2020). For instance, every morning the patient may use the abdomen for insulin injection, and every evening before dinner, the patient may inject the insulin into the arms or thighs. Keep in mind that the best absorption occurs in the abdomen. In each case, the injections should be given an inch away from the previous injection site. A small spot bandage or piece of tape can be used to mark the first injection site, with subsequent injections rotated in a circle around that site. After this area has been used, an adjacent site, an inch away, can be selected, using the same rotation format. A marked diagram incorporated into the patient's plan of care is also helpful for noting alternative sites. Patients should be encouraged to not rely on memory. The patient cannot always recall the site of the previous injection, therefore, the site of administration should be recorded. When the patient is receiving care from a health care provider, the site of administration must be recorded in the patient's health record.
- Heparin is administered subcutaneously. The abdomen is the most commonly used administration site. Avoid the area 2 inches around the umbilicus and the belt line.
- Certain medications have specific manufacturer-recommended administration requirements. For example, enoxaparin (low–molecular-weight heparin) should be administered alternating between the left and right anterolateral and left and right posterolateral abdominal wall (Sanofi-Aventis, 2020) (Figure 5). To administer the medication, pinch the tissue gently to form a skin fold and insert the needle at a 90-degree angle (Sanofi-Aventis, 2020). Enoxaparin is packaged in a prefilled syringe with an air bubble. **Do not expel the air bubble before administration** (Sanofi-Aventis, 2020).

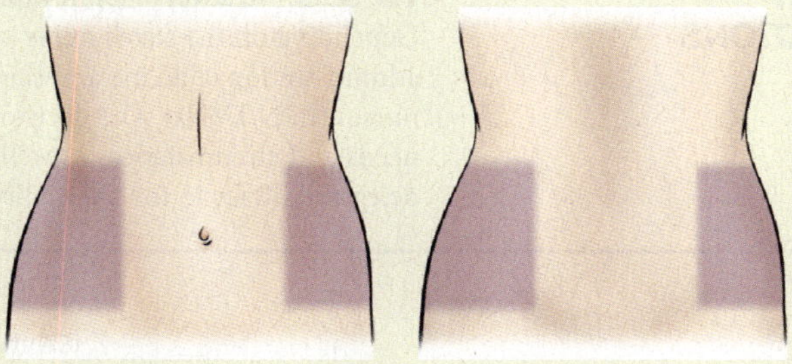

Anterior view   Posterior view

FIGURE 5. Sites for administration of enoxaparin.

(*continued on page 996*)

Skill 30-6 Administering a Subcutaneous Injection *(continued)*

Infant and Child Considerations

- Do not tell a child that an injection will not hurt. Describe the feel of the injection as a pinch or a sting. A child who believes you have been dishonest is less likely to cooperate with future procedures.

Older Adult Considerations

- Many older adults have less adipose tissue. Adjust the needle length and insertion angle accordingly. (Refer to discussion earlier in Skill.) You do not want to inadvertently give a subcutaneous medication intramuscularly.

Community-Based Care Considerations

- Reuse of syringes in the home setting is not recommended.
- The use of antimicrobial swabs to clean the injection site in home environments may be unnecessary; patients may use soap and water to clean the site if the area is visibly soiled (Sexson et al., 2016).
- Because absorption rates vary from site to site, it is recommended that patients administering their own insulin use the same area of the body at the same time every day to ensure more consistent absorption and prevent tissue changes from repeated use of the same site (ADA, 2020; Frandsen & Pennington, 2021). Refer to the information discussed in the "General Considerations" section of this Skill.
- Encourage patients to consult the policies of their local government regarding contaminated and sharps waste disposal.
- The U.S. Food & Drug Administration (FDA, 2021) recommends a two-step process for properly disposing of used needles and other sharps by patients, family members, and caregivers: (1) Needles and other sharps should be placed in a sharps disposal container immediately after they have been used to reduce the risk of needle sticks, cuts, and punctures from loose sharps. (2) Used sharps disposal containers should be disposed of according to community guidelines; guidelines and disposal programs vary depending on location. Patients should consult local trash removal services and the local health department to identify available disposal methods. Never use glass containers.
- Sharps disposal methods (depending on community location) include drop boxes or supervised collection sites, household hazardous waste collection sites, mail-back programs, and residential special waste pick-up services (FDA, 2021).
- If a patient, family member, or caregiver does not want to purchase a sharps container, an empty laundry detergent or bleach bottle may be used. It must be a strong plastic container with a screw-on lid, *not* an empty plastic water or soda bottle or other type of thin plastic container (SafeNeedleDisposal.org, 2021). Label the container as sharps and not for recycling. The screw-on top should be used to close the container for disposal, and containers should be sealed with strong tape (e.g., duct tape) (SafeNeedleDisposal.org, 2021).
- Sharps disposal containers should be kept out of reach of children and pets (FDA, 2021).
- The Safe Needle Disposal resource page provides information on needle disposal takeback programs and an interactive tool to locate state waste links (FDA, 2021; SafeNeedleDisposal.org, 2021).

Skill 30-7 Administering an Intramuscular Injection

DELEGATION CONSIDERATIONS

The administration of an intramuscular injection is not delegated to assistive personnel (AP). Depending on the state's nurse practice act and the organization's policies and procedures, the administration of an intramuscular injection may be delegated to licensed practical/vocational nurses (LPN/LVNs). The decision to delegate must be based on careful analysis of the patient's needs and circumstances as well as the qualifications of the person to whom the task is being delegated. Refer to the Delegation Guidelines in Appendix A.

EQUIPMENT

- Gloves
- Additional PPE, as indicated
- Prescribed medication
- Sterile syringe and needle of appropriate size and gauge
- Antimicrobial swab
- Small gauze square
- Electronic Medication Administration Record (eMAR) or Medication Administration Record (MAR)

IMPLEMENTATION

ACTION	RATIONALE
1. Gather equipment. Check each medication prescribed against the original in the health record, depending on facility policy and the medication order system in place. Clarify any inconsistencies. Check the patient's health record for allergies.	The prescription is the legal record of prescribed medication interventions. This comparison helps to identify errors that may have occurred when orders were transcribed. Computer provider order-entry (CPOE) systems allow prescribers to send electronic medication prescriptions directly to the pharmacy located in a health care facility and to outpatient pharmacies.
2. Know the actions, special nursing considerations, safe dose ranges, purpose of administration, and adverse effects of the medications to be administered. Consider the appropriateness of the medication for this patient.	This knowledge aids the nurse in evaluating the therapeutic effect of the medication in relation to the patient's health status and can also be used to educate the patient about the medication.
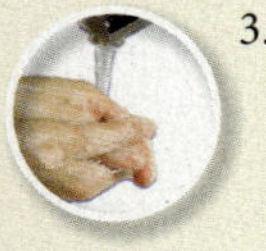 3. Perform hand hygiene.	Hand hygiene prevents the spread of microorganisms.
4. Move the medication supply system to the outside of the patient's room or prepare for administration at the medication supply system in the medication area. Alternatively, access the medication administration supply system at or inside the patient's room.	Organization facilitates error-free administration and saves time.
5. Unlock the medication supply system or drawer. Enter the passcode and scan employee identification, if required.	Locking the medication supply system or drawer safeguards each patient's medication supply. Facility accrediting organizations require medication supply systems to be locked when not in use. Entering the passcode and scanning ID allows only authorized users into the system and identifies the user for documentation by the computer.
6. **Prepare medications for one patient at a time.**	This prevents errors in medication administration.
7. Read the eMAR/MAR and read the label when selecting the proper medication from the medication supply system or the patient's medication drawer.	This is the *first* check of the label.
8. Read the label and compare the label with the eMAR/MAR. Check expiration dates and perform calculations, if necessary. Scan the bar code on the package, if required.	This is the *second* check of the label. Verify calculations with another nurse to ensure safety, if necessary.
9. If necessary, withdraw the medication from an ampule or vial as described in Skills 30-2 and 30-3.	
10. **Depending on facility policy, the third check of the label may occur at this point. If so, when all medications for one patient have been prepared, read the label and recheck the labels with the eMAR/MAR before taking the medications to the patient. However, many facilities require the third check to occur at the bedside, after identifying the patient.**	This *third* check ensures accuracy and helps to prevent errors. *Note:* Many facilities require the *third* check to occur at the bedside, after identifying the patient and before administration.
11. Label the syringe with the medication's name, dose, and amount (The Joint Commission, 2021).	Unlabeled syringes are unidentifiable and may lead to a medication administration error (The Joint Commission, 2021).
12. **Log out of and/or lock the medication supply system before leaving it.**	Locking the medication supply system or drawer safeguards the patient's medication supply. Facility accrediting organizations require medication supply systems to be locked when not in use.
13. Transport medications to the patient's bedside carefully and keep the medications in sight at all times.	Careful handling and close observation prevent accidental or deliberate disarrangement of medications.
14. **Ensure that the patient receives the medications at the correct time.**	Check facility policy, which may allow for administration within a period of 30 minutes before or 30 minutes after the designated time.

(continued on page 998)

Skill 30-7 Administering an Intramuscular Injection *(continued)*

ACTION	RATIONALE
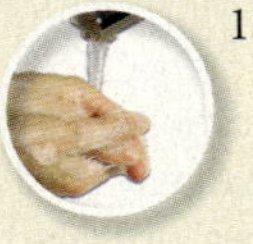 15. Perform hand hygiene and put on PPE, if indicated.	Hand hygiene and PPE prevent the spread of microorganisms. PPE is required based on transmission precautions.
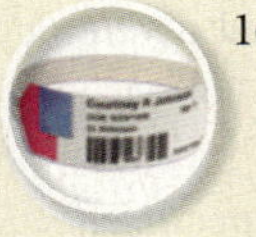 16. **Identify the patient. Compare the information with the eMAR/MAR. The patient should be identified using at least two of the following methods** (The Joint Commission, 2021):	Identifying the patient ensures the right patient receives the medications and helps prevent errors. The patient's room number or physical location is not used as an identifier (The Joint Commission, 2021). Replace the identification band if it is missing or inaccurate in any way.
a. Check the name on the patient's identification band.	This requires a response from the patient, but illness and strange surroundings often cause patients to be confused.
b. Check the identification number on the patient's identification band.	
c. Check the birth date on the patient's identification band.	
d. Ask the patient to state their name and birth date, based on facility policy.	
17. Close the door to the room or pull the bedside curtain.	This provides patient privacy.
18. **Complete necessary assessments before administering medications. Check the patient's allergy bracelet, if present, or ask the patient about allergies. Explain the purpose and action of the medication to the patient.**	Assessment is a prerequisite to administration of medications. Explanation provides rationale, increases knowledge, promotes patient engagement, and reduces anxiety.
19. Scan the bar code on the patient's identification band, if required (Figure 1) (The Joint Commission, 2021).	This provides an additional check to ensure that the medication is given to the right patient.
20. **Based on facility policy, the third check of the label may occur at this point. If so, read the label and recheck the labels with the eMAR/MAR before administering the medications to the patient.**	Many facilities require the *third* check to occur at the bedside, after identifying the patient and before administration. If facility policy directs the *third* check at this time, this *third* check ensures accuracy and helps to prevent errors.
21. Put on gloves.	Gloves help prevent exposure to contaminants.
22. Select an appropriate administration site. Assist the patient to the appropriate position for the site chosen. Drape, as needed, to expose only the site area being used.	Selecting the appropriate site and appropriate positioning prevent injury. Draping provides privacy and warmth.
23. **Identify the appropriate landmarks and site boundaries for the site chosen (Figure 2).**	Good visualization is necessary to establish the correct site location and to avoid complications (Taylor et al., 2023).

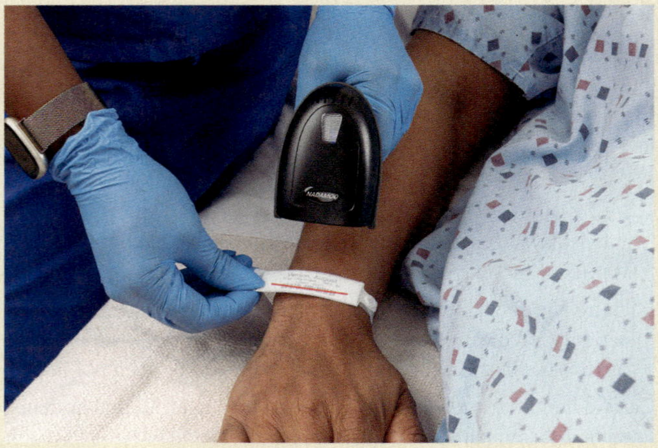

FIGURE 1. Scanning bar code on the patient's identification bracelet.

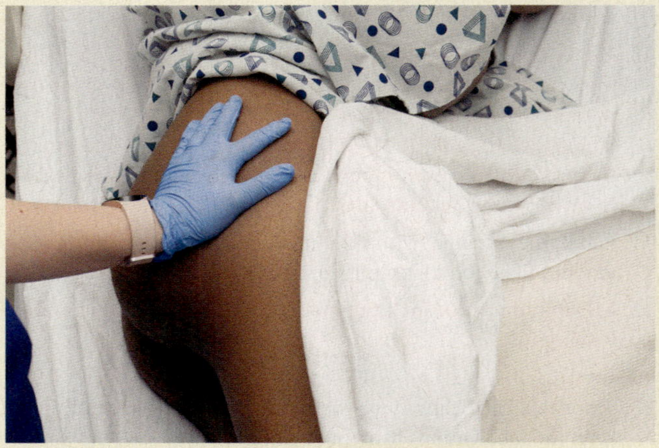

FIGURE 2. Identifying the appropriate landmarks.

ACTION	RATIONALE
24. Cleanse the site with an antimicrobial swab while wiping with a firm, circular motion and moving outward from the injection site. Consider leaving the alcohol pad on the skin with the tip of the pad pointing toward the center of the area you just prepared. Allow the skin to dry.	Pathogens on the skin can be forced into the tissues by the needle. Moving from the center outward prevents contamination of the site. Allowing the antimicrobial solution to dry completely (5 to 20 seconds) ensures complete antimicrobial effectiveness (Gorski et al., 2021; Slater et al., 2018), and prevents introducing alcohol into the tissue, which can be irritating and uncomfortable.
25. Remove the needle cap by pulling it straight off. Hold the syringe in your dominant hand between the thumb and forefinger.	This technique lessens the risk of an accidental needlestick and also prevents inadvertently unscrewing the needle from the barrel of the syringe.
26. Displace the skin in a Z-track manner. Pull or shift the skin and underlying tissue down or to one side 1 to 2 cm (Karch, 2020; Yilmaz et al., 2016) with your nondominant hand and hold the skin and tissue in this position (Figure 3). Alternatively, based on assessment of the particular circumstances for an individual patient, if the nurse decides not to use the Z-track technique, the skin should be stretched flat between two fingers and held taut for needle insertion.	Z-track technique is recommended for all intramuscular injections to ensure medication does not leak back along the needle track and into the subcutaneous tissue (Hopkins & Arias, 2013; Yilmaz et al., 2016). This technique reduces pain and discomfort, particularly for patients receiving injections over an extended period. The Z-track method is also suggested for older adults who have decreased muscle mass. Some agents, such as iron, are best given via the Z-track method due to the irritation and discoloration associated with this agent.
27. Quickly dart the needle into the tissue so that the needle is perpendicular to the patient's body, administering at an angle of 90 degrees (CDC, 2021) (Figure 4).	A quick injection is less painful. Inserting the needle at a 90-degree angle facilitates entry into muscle tissue.

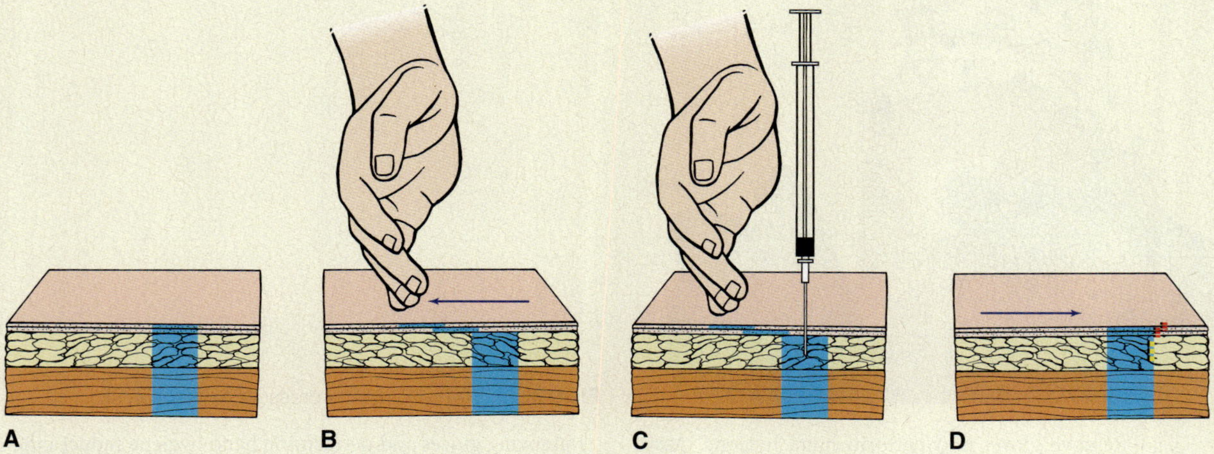

FIGURE 3. Z-track or zigzag technique is recommended for intramuscular injections. **A.** Normal skin and tissues. **B.** Pulling or shifting the skin and underlying tissue down or to one side. **C.** Needle is inserted at a 90-degree angle. **D.** Once needle is withdrawn, displaced tissue is allowed to return to its normal position, preventing solution from escaping from muscle tissue. Hand and finger positioning is adjusted for the specific administration site for accurate identification of landmarks and use of safe injection technique.

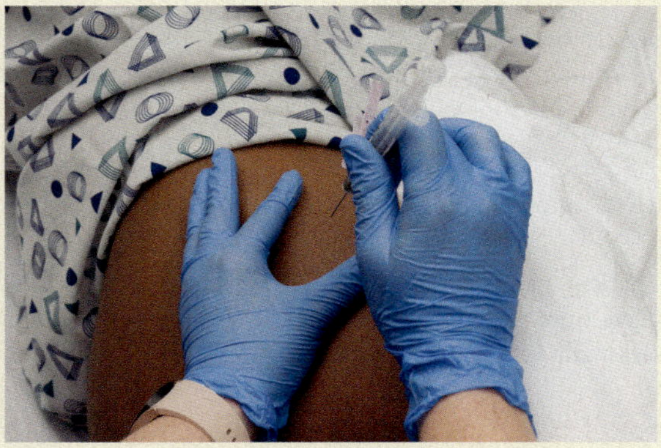

FIGURE 4. Darting needle into tissue.

(continued on page 1000)

Skill 30-7 Administering an Intramuscular Injection *(continued)*

ACTION / **RATIONALE**

28. As soon as the needle is in place, use the thumb and forefinger of your nondominant hand to hold the lower end of the syringe, taking care to maintain the displacement of the skin and tissue. Slide your dominant hand to the end of the plunger. Inject the solution slowly.

Moving the syringe could cause damage to the tissues and inadvertent administration into an incorrect area. Rapid injection of the solution creates pressure in the tissues, resulting in discomfort.

29. Once the medication has been instilled, wait 10 seconds before withdrawing the needle.

This allows medication to begin to diffuse into the surrounding muscle tissue (Gutierrez & Munakomi, 2021).

30. Withdraw the needle smoothly and steadily at the same angle at which it was inserted, supporting tissue around the injection site with your nondominant hand. **Remove the hand holding the displaced skin and tissue only after removal of the needle, allowing the displaced skin and tissue to return to its normal position.**

Slow withdrawal of the needle pulls the tissues and causes discomfort. Applying counter traction around the injection site helps to prevent pulling on the tissue as the needle is withdrawn. Removing the needle at the same angle at which it was inserted minimizes tissue damage and discomfort for the patient. Allowing displaced skin and tissue to move back into place while needle is still inserted causes damage to the tissues.

31. Do not recap the used needle. Engage the safety shield or needle guard.

A safety shield or needle guard prevents accidental needlestick.

32. Apply gentle pressure at the site with a dry gauze (Figure 5). **Do not massage the site.**

Light pressure causes less trauma and irritation to the tissues. Massaging can force medication into subcutaneous tissues and increase discomfort.

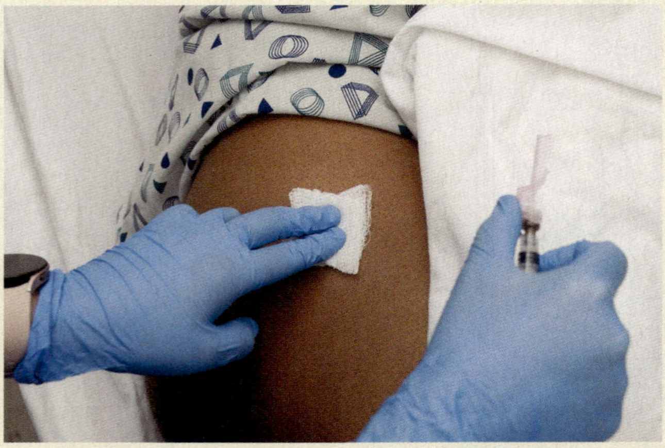

FIGURE 5. Applying gentle pressure at injection site.

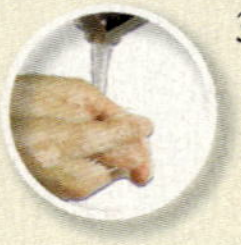

33. Remove gloves and perform hand hygiene. Assist the patient to a position of comfort.

Removing gloves and performing hand hygiene reduces the risk of contamination of other items and the spread of microorganisms. Assisting the patient to a position of comfort promotes patient comfort.

34. Discard the needle and syringe in the appropriate container, such as a sharps receptacle.

Proper disposal of the needle prevents injury.

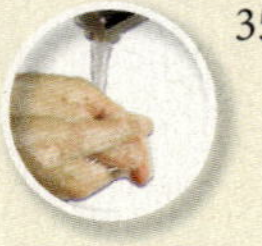

35. Remove gloves and additional PPE, if used. Perform hand hygiene.

Proper removal of PPE reduces the risk of infection transmission and contamination of other items. Hand hygiene prevents the spread of microorganisms.

36. Document the administration of the medication immediately after administration. See Documentation section below.

Timely documentation helps to ensure patient safety.

37. Evaluate the patient's response to the medication within the appropriate time frame. Assess site, if possible, within 2 to 4 hours after administration.

The patient needs to be evaluated for therapeutic and adverse effects from the medication. Visualization of the site allows for assessment of any untoward effects.

DOCUMENTATION GUIDELINES

Record each medication given on the eMAR/MAR or record using the required format, including date, time, and the site of administration, immediately after administration. If using a bar-code system, medication administration is automatically recorded when the bar code is scanned. PRN medications require documentation of the reason for administration. Prompt recording avoids the possibility of accidentally repeating the administration of the drug. If the drug was refused or omitted, record this in the appropriate area on the medication record and notify the health care team as appropriate. This verifies the reason medication was omitted and ensures that health care personnel providing care for the patient are aware of the occurrence.

DEVELOPING CLINICAL REASONING AND CLINICAL JUDGMENT

UNEXPECTED SITUATIONS AND ASSOCIATED INTERVENTIONS

- *You stick yourself with the needle before injection:* Discard the needle and syringe appropriately. Follow facility policy regarding needlestick injury. Prepare a new syringe with the medication and administer to the patient. Communicate and document the incident according to facility policy.
- *You stick yourself with the needle after injection:* Discard the needle and syringe appropriately. Follow facility policy regarding needlestick injury. Communicate and document the incident according to facility policy.
- *During injection, the patient pulls away from the needle before the medication is delivered fully:* Remove and appropriately discard the needle. Attach a new needle to the syringe and administer the remaining medication at a different site. Document events and interventions, according to facility policy.
- *While injecting the needle into the patient, you hit patient's bone:* Withdraw and discard the needle. Apply a new needle to the syringe and administer in an alternate site. Document the incident in the patient's health record. Notify the health care team. Communicate and document the incident according to facility policy.

SPECIAL CONSIDERATIONS

General Considerations

- Ongoing assessment is an important part of nursing care for both evaluation of patient response to administered medications and early detection of adverse drug reactions. If an adverse effect is suspected, withhold further medication doses and notify the health care team. Additional intervention is based on the type of reaction and patient assessment.
- The deltoid is the recommended site for vaccines for adults and may be used for children ages 3 to 18 years for vaccine administration (CDC, 2021).

Infant and Child Considerations

- The vastus lateralis is the preferred site for intramuscular injections in infants (age 12 months and younger) and young children (ages 1 to 2 years) (CDC, 2021). The deltoid can be used in children ages 1 to 2 years if the deltoid muscle mass is adequate (CDC, 2021).
- The deltoid is the preferred site for children ages 3 to 18 years (CDC, 2021).

Older Adult Considerations

- Muscle mass atrophies as a person ages. Take care to evaluate the patient's muscle mass and body composition. Use an appropriate needle length and gauge for patient's body composition. Choose an appropriate site based on the patient's body composition.

Community-Based Care Considerations

- The use of antimicrobial swabs to clean the injection site in home environments may be unnecessary; patients may use soap and water to clean the site if the area is visibly soiled (Sexson et al., 2016).
- Encourage patients to consult the policies of their local government regarding contaminated and sharps waste disposal.
- The U.S. Food & Drug Administration (FDA, 2021) recommends a two-step process for properly disposing of used needles and other sharps by patients, family members, and caregivers. (1) Needles and other sharps should be placed in a sharps disposal container immediately after they have been used to reduce the risk of needle sticks, cuts, and punctures from loose sharps. (2) Used sharps disposal containers should be disposed of according to community guidelines; guidelines and disposal programs vary depending on location.

(continued on page 1002)

Skill 30-7 Administering an Intramuscular Injection *(continued)*

Patients should consult local trash removal services and the local health department to identify available disposal methods. Never use glass containers.

- Sharps disposal methods (depending on community location) include drop boxes or supervised collection sites, household hazardous waste collection sites; mail-back programs, and residential special waste pick-up services (FDA, 2021).
- If a patient, family member, or caregiver does not want to purchase a sharps container, an empty laundry detergent or bleach bottle may be used; it must be a strong plastic container with a screw-on lid, *not* an empty plastic water or soda bottle or other type of thin plastic container (SafeNeedleDisposal.org, 2021). Label the container as sharps and not for recycling. The screw-on top should be used to close the container for disposal, and containers should be sealed with strong tape (e.g., duct tape) (SafeNeedleDisposal.org, 2021).
- Sharps disposal containers should be kept out of reach of children and pets (FDA, 2021).
- The Safe Needle Disposal resource page provides information on needle disposal takeback programs and an interactive tool to locate state waste links (FDA, 2021; SafeNeedleDisposal.org, 2021).

Skill 30-8 Administering Medications by Intravenous Bolus or Push Through an Intravenous Infusion

DELEGATION CONSIDERATIONS

The administration of medications by intravenous bolus is not delegated to assistive personnel (AP). Depending on the state's nurse practice act and the organization's policies and procedures, the administration of specified intravenous medications in some settings may be delegated to licensed practical/vocational nurses (LPN/LVNs) who have received appropriate training. The decision to delegate must be based on careful analysis of the patient's needs and circumstances as well as the qualifications of the person to whom the task is being delegated. Refer to the Delegation Guidelines in Appendix A.

EQUIPMENT

- Antimicrobial swab
- Watch or clock with second hand
- Gloves
- Additional PPE, as indicated
- Prescribed medication
- Two normal saline flushes prepared in a syringe (3 to 10 mL) according to facility policy
- Passive disinfection caps (based on facility policy)
- Syringe with a needleless device or 23- to 25-gauge, 1-inch needle (follow facility policy)
- Electronic Medication Administration Record (eMAR) or Medication Administration Record (MAR)

IMPLEMENTATION

ACTION	RATIONALE
1. Gather equipment. Check each medication prescribed against the original in the health record, depending on facility policy and the medication order system in place. Clarify any inconsistencies. Check the patient's health record for allergies. Check a drug resource to clarify whether the medication needs to be diluted before administration. Check the administration rate.	The prescription is the legal record of prescribed medication interventions. This comparison helps to identify errors that may have occurred when orders were transcribed. Computer provider order-entry (CPOE) systems allow prescribers to send electronic medication prescriptions directly to the pharmacy located in a health care facility and to outpatient pharmacies. Compatibility of medication and solution prevents complications. Delivers the correct dose of medication as prescribed.
2. Know the actions, special nursing considerations, safe dose ranges, purpose of administration, and adverse effects of the medications to be administered. Consider the appropriateness of the medication for this patient.	This knowledge aids the nurse in evaluating the therapeutic effect of the medication in relation to the patient's health status and can also be used to educate the patient about the medication.

ACTION	RATIONALE
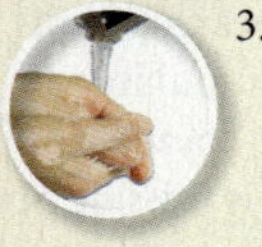 3. Perform hand hygiene.	Hand hygiene prevents the spread of microorganisms.
4. Move the medication supply system to the outside of the patient's room or prepare for administration at the medication supply system in the medication area. Alternatively, access the medication administration supply system at or inside the patient's room.	Organization facilitates error-free administration and saves time.
5. Unlock the medication supply system or drawer. Enter the passcode and scan employee identification, if required.	Locking the medication supply system or drawer safeguards each patient's medication supply. Facility accrediting organizations require medication supply systems to be locked when not in use. Entering the passcode and scanning ID allows only authorized users into the system and identifies the user for documentation by the computer.
6. **Prepare medications for one patient at a time.**	This prevents errors in medication administration.
7. Read the eMAR/MAR and select the proper medication from the medication supply system or the patient's medication drawer.	This is the *first* check of the label.
8. Compare the label with the eMAR/MAR. Check expiration dates and perform calculations, if necessary. Scan the bar code on the package, if required.	This is the *second* check of the label. Verify calculations with another nurse to ensure safety, if necessary.
9. If necessary, withdraw the medication from an ampule or vial as described in Skills 30-2 and 30-3.	
10. **Depending on facility policy, the third check of the label may occur at this point. If so, when all medications for one patient have been prepared, recheck the labels with the eMAR/MAR before taking the medications to the patient. However, many facilities require the third check to occur at the bedside, after identifying the patient.**	This *third* check ensures accuracy and helps to prevent errors. *Note:* Many facilities require the *third* check to occur at the bedside, after identifying the patient and before administration.
11. Label the syringe with the medication's name, dose, and amount (The Joint Commission, 2021).	Unlabeled syringes are unidentifiable and may lead to a medication administration error (The Joint Commission, 2021). Appropriately label all clinician-prepared syringes of IV push medications or solutions, unless the medication or solution is prepared at the patient's bedside and is immediately administered to the patient (ISMP, 2015, p. 12).
12. **Log out of and/or lock the medication supply system before leaving it.**	Locking the medication supply system or drawer safeguards the patient's medication supply. Facility accrediting organizations require medication supply systems to be locked when not in use.
13. Transport medications and equipment to the patient's bedside carefully and keep the medications in sight at all times.	Careful handling and close observation prevent accidental or deliberate disarrangement of medications. Having equipment available saves time and facilitates performance of the task.
14. **Ensure that the patient receives the medications at the correct time.**	Check facility policy, which may allow for administration within a period of 30 minutes before or 30 minutes after the designated time.
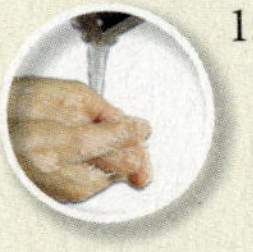 15. Perform hand hygiene and put on PPE, if indicated.	Hand hygiene and PPE prevent the spread of microorganisms. PPE is required based on transmission precautions.

(continued on page 1004)

Skill 30-8 Administering Medications by Intravenous Bolus or Push Through an Intravenous Infusion *(continued)*

ACTION	RATIONALE
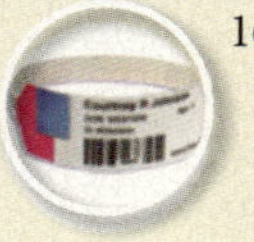 16. **Identify the patient. Compare the information with the eMAR/MAR. The patient should be identified using at least two of the following methods** (The Joint Commission, 2021):	Identifying the patient ensures the right patient receives the medications and helps prevent errors. The patient's room number or physical location is not used as an identifier (The Joint Commission, 2021). Replace the identification band if it is missing or inaccurate in any way.
a. Check the name on the patient's identification band.	This requires a response from the patient, but illness and strange surroundings often cause patients to be confused.
b. Check the identification number on the patient's identification band.	
c. Check the birth date on the patient's identification band.	
d. Ask the patient to state their name and birth date, based on facility policy.	
17. Close the door to the room or pull the bedside curtain.	This provides patient privacy.
18. **Complete necessary assessments before administering medications. Check the patient's allergy bracelet, if present, or ask the patient about allergies. Explain the purpose and action of the medication to the patient.**	Assessment is a prerequisite to administration of medications. Explanation provides rationale, increases knowledge, and reduces anxiety.
19. Scan the patient's bar code on the identification band, if required (The Joint Commission, 2021).	This provides an additional check to ensure that the medication is given to the right patient.
20. **Based on facility policy, the third check of the label may occur at this point. If so, recheck the label with the eMAR/MAR before administering the medications to the patient.**	Many facilities require the *third* check to occur at the bedside, after identifying the patient and before administration. If facility policy directs the *third* check at this time, this *third* check ensures accuracy and helps to prevent errors.
21. Assess the IV site for the presence of inflammation or infiltration or other signs of complications.	IV medication must be given directly into a vein for safe administration.
22. If the IV infusion is being administered via an infusion pump, pause the pump.	Pausing prevents infusion of fluid during bolus administration and activation of pump occlusion alarms.
23. Put on gloves.	Gloves prevent contact with blood and body fluids.
24. Select the injection port on the administration set that is closest to the patient. Close the clamp on the administration set immediately above the injection port (Figure 1). Do not disconnect the administration set from the venous access device hub (Gorski et al., 2021).	Using the port closest to the needle insertion site minimizes dilution of the medication. Closing the clamp immediately above the access port ensures the medication is administered to the patient and prevents the medication from backing up the tubing.

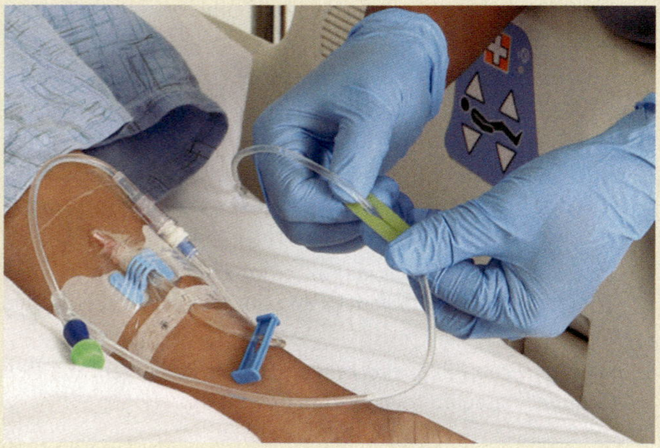

FIGURE 1. Closing the clamp on the administration set.

ACTION

25. Remove the passive disinfection cap from the needleless connector or end cap on the infusion set injection port (Figure 2). Alternatively, if a passive disinfection cap is not in place, use an antimicrobial swab to vigorously disinfect the connection surface and sides of the needleless connector or end cap on the injection port and allow it to dry.

RATIONALE

The passive disinfection caps contain an antiseptic-impregnated sponge that dispenses the antiseptic over the connector's top and threads, and provides continuous disinfection of the needleless connection versus intermittent disinfection when using antimicrobial wipes (Barton, 2019; Casey et al., 2018). Venous access device entry points, end caps, and needleless connectors must be vigorously scrubbed and disinfected prior to each access to reduce the risk for introduction of microorganisms and prevent venous access device–related infection (Flynn et al., 2019; Gorski et al., 2021). Friction is needed to physically remove microorganisms from the top, sides, and threads of the needleless connector or end cap. Allow the antiseptic to dry completely to ensure complete effectiveness (Gorski et al., 2021; Slater et al., 2018).

26. Uncap the saline flush syringe. Insert the saline flush syringe into the needleless connector or end cap on the injection port on the administration tubing (Figure 3).

Assessing patency of the venous access device is necessary to ensure IV administration of the medication.

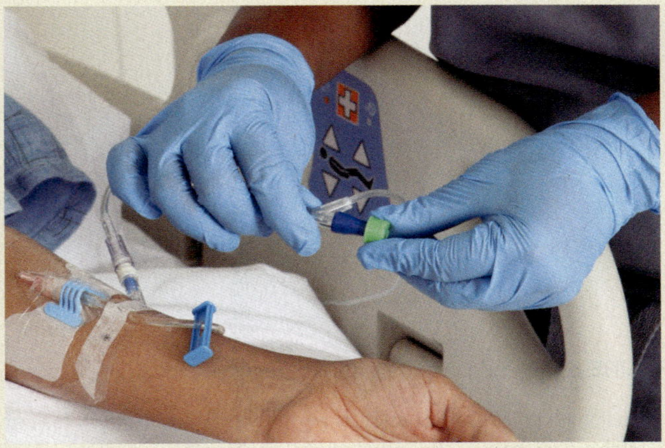

FIGURE 2. Removing the passive disinfection cap.

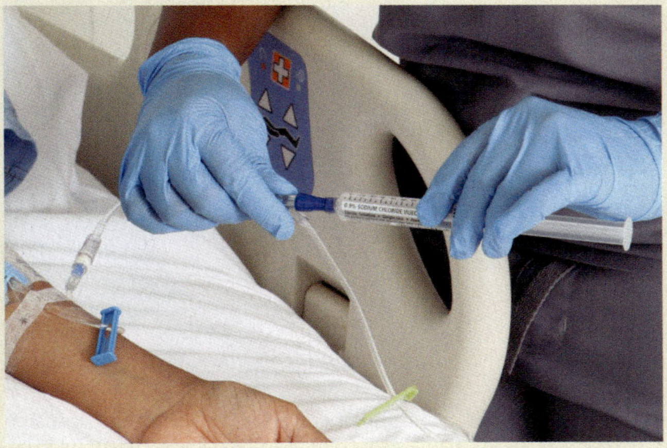

FIGURE 3. Inserting the saline flush syringe into the injection port.

27. Pull back on the syringe plunger to aspirate the catheter for positive blood return (Figure 4). If positive, instill the solution over 1 minute or according to facility policy. Remove the syringe.

Positive blood return confirms patency before administration of medications and solutions (Gorski et al., 2021). Flushing without incident ensures patency of the IV line and administration of the medication into the bloodstream.

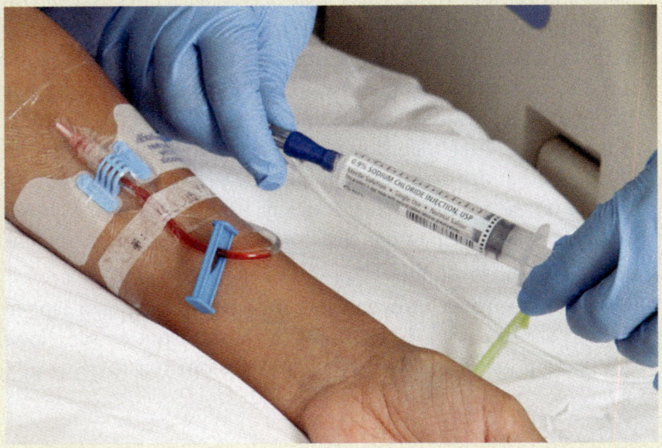

FIGURE 4. Pulling back on the plunger to aspirate for a blood return.

(continued on page 1006)

Skill 30-8 Administering Medications by Intravenous Bolus or Push Through an Intravenous Infusion *(continued)*

ACTION	RATIONALE
28. Use an antimicrobial swab to vigorously disinfect the connection surface and sides of the needleless connector or end cap on the injection port and allow it to dry.	Venous access device entry points, end caps, and needleless connectors must be vigorously scrubbed and disinfected prior to each access to reduce the risk for introduction of microorganisms and prevent venous access device–related infection (Flynn et al., 2019; Gorski et al., 2021). Friction is needed to physically remove microorganisms from the top, sides, and threads of the needleless connector or end cap. Allow the antiseptic to dry completely to ensure complete effectiveness (Gorski et al., 2021; Slater et al., 2018).
29. Uncap the medication syringe. Insert the medication syringe into the needleless connector or end cap on the injection port. Using a watch or clock with a second-hand to time the rate, **inject the medication at the recommended rate (Figure 5).**	This delivers the correct amount of medication at the proper interval.

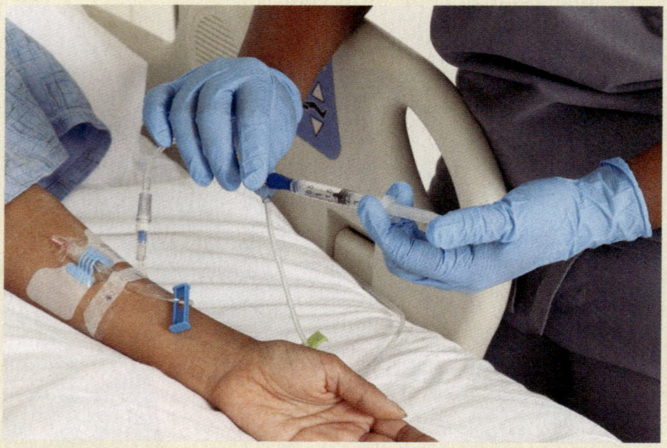

FIGURE 5. Injecting medication at the recommended rate.

ACTION	RATIONALE
30. While administering the medication, observe the infusion site and assess the patient for any adverse reaction. If signs of adverse reaction occur, stop the infusion immediately and notify the health care team.	Signs of adverse reaction, such as peripheral IV infiltration, rash or itching, or pain at the infusion site, necessitate stopping administration of the drug (Gorski et al, 2021).
31. Detach the medication syringe. Use a new antimicrobial swab to vigorously disinfect the connection surface and sides of the needleless connector or end cap on the injection port and allow it to dry. Uncap the second saline flush syringe. Insert the saline flush syringe into the needleless connector or end cap on the injection port. Instill the flush solution at the same rate as the administered medication (Gorski et al., 2021).	Venous access device entry points, end caps, and needleless connectors must be vigorously scrubbed and disinfected prior to each access to reduce the risk for introduction of microorganisms and prevent venous access device–related infection (Flynn et al., 2019; Gorski et al., 2021). Friction is needed to physically remove microorganisms from the top, sides, and threads of the needleless connector or end cap. Allow the antiseptic to dry completely to ensure complete effectiveness (Gorski et al., 2021; Slater et al., 2018). Flushing after medication administration ensures the entire drug dose has been cleared from the extension tubing on the venous access device or from the infusion system and prevents precipitation due to solution/medication incompatibility (Gorski et al., 2021).
32. Remove the flush syringe. Unclamp the administration set above the injection port.	Clamping prevents air from entering the extension set on a capped venous access device. Unclamping the administration set allows for resumption of the continuous IV infusion.

ACTION	RATIONALE
33. Using an antimicrobial swab, vigorously disinfect the connection surface and sides of the needleless connector or end cap on the injection port and allow it to dry. Attach a passive disinfection cap to the needleless connector or end cap on the extension tubing or the injection port on the administration set (Figure 6).	Venous access device entry points, end caps, and needleless connectors must be vigorously scrubbed and disinfected prior to each access to reduce the risk for introduction of microorganisms and prevent venous access device–related infection (Flynn et al., 2019; Gorski et al., 2021). Friction is needed to physically remove microorganisms from the top, sides, and threads of the needleless connector or end cap. Allow the antiseptic to dry completely to ensure complete effectiveness (Gorski et al., 2021; Slater et al., 2018). Passive disinfection caps contain an antiseptic-impregnated sponge that dispenses the antiseptic over the connector's top and threads and protect the hub from contamination by touch or airborne sources (Barton, 2019; Casey et al., 2018).

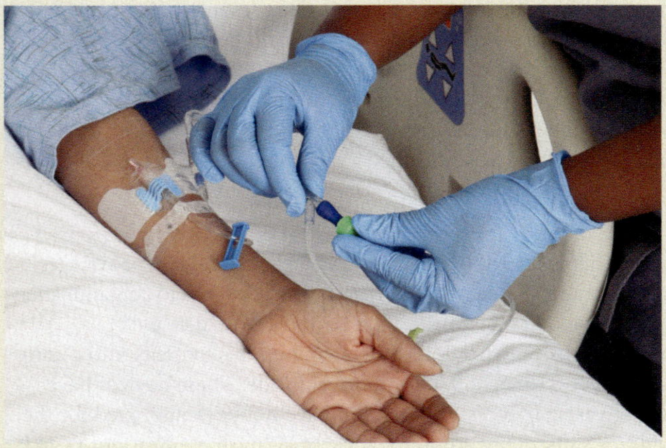

FIGURE 6. Attaching a passive disinfection cap.

ACTION	RATIONALE
34. Remove gloves and perform hand hygiene. Restart the infusion pump and check IV fluid infusion rate.	Removing gloves and performing hand hygiene prevents the spread of microorganisms. Restarting the infusion pump resumes the prescribed continuous infusion of fluid. Checking the IV fluid infusion rate assures accuracy in administration.
35. Discard the syringe in the appropriate receptacle.	Proper disposal prevents injury and spread of microorganisms.
36. Remove additional PPE, if used. Perform hand hygiene.	Proper removal of PPE reduces the risk of infection transmission and contamination of other items. Hand hygiene prevents the spread of microorganisms.
37. Document the administration of the medication immediately after administration. See Documentation section below.	Timely documentation helps to ensure patient safety.
38. Evaluate the patient's response to the medication within the appropriate time frame.	The patient needs to be evaluated for therapeutic and adverse effects from the medication.

DOCUMENTATION

GUIDELINES

Document the administration of the medication immediately after administration, including date, time, dose, route of administration, site of administration, and rate of administration on the eMAR/MAR or record using the required format. If using a bar-code system, medication administration is automatically recorded when the bar code is scanned. PRN medications require documentation of the reason for administration. Prompt recording avoids the possibility of accidentally repeating the administration of the drug. If the drug was refused or omitted, record this in the appropriate area on the medication record and notify the health care team as appropriate. This verifies the reason medication was omitted and ensures that health care personnel providing care for the patient are aware of the occurrence.

(*continued on page 1008*)

Skill 30-8 Administering Medications by Intravenous Bolus or Push Through an Intravenous Infusion *(continued)*

DEVELOPING CLINICAL REASONING AND CLINICAL JUDGMENT

UNEXPECTED SITUATIONS AND ASSOCIATED INTERVENTIONS

- *Upon assessing the IV site before administering medication, no blood return is visible upon aspiration:* If the IV appears patent, without signs of infiltration, and IV fluid infuses without difficulty, proceed with administration. Observe closely for signs and symptoms of infiltration during and after administration.
- *Upon assessing the patient's IV site before administering medication, you note that IV has infiltrated:* Stop the IV fluid and remove the IV from the patient's extremity. Restart the IV in a different location. Continue to monitor the new IV site as medication is administered.
- *While administering medication, you note a cloudy, white substance forming in the IV tubing:* Stop administering the medication. Clamp the IV at the site nearest to the patient. Change the administration tubing and restart the infusion. Check a drug resource or consult a pharmacist regarding compatibility of the medication and IV fluid before continuing with administration. Medication infusion may require a second IV site.
- *While you are administering the medication, the patient begins to complain of pain at the IV site:* Stop the medication. Assess the IV site for any signs of infiltration or phlebitis. Flush the IV with normal saline to check for patency. If the IV site appears within normal limits, resume medication administration at a slower rate.

SPECIAL CONSIDERATIONS

- Do not withdraw IV push medications from commercially available, cartridge-type syringes into another syringe for administration. Using the cartridge as a vial can lead to contamination and/or dosing errors, drug mix-ups, and other medication errors (ISMP, 2015, p. 11).
- Do not dilute or reconstitute IV push medications by drawing up the contents into a commercially available, prefilled flush syringe of 0.9% sodium chloride. These devices have been approved for flushing of vascular access devices, but have not been approved for the reconstitution, dilution, and/or subsequent administration of IV push medications (ISMP, 2015, p. 11).
- Appropriately label all clinician-prepared syringes of IV push medications or solutions, unless the medication or solution is prepared at the patient's bedside and is immediately administered to the patient (ISMP, 2015, p. 12).
- If the IV is a small gauge (22 to 24 gauge) placed in a small vein, a blood return may not occur even if the IV is intact. Also, the patient may report stinging and pain at the site while medication is being administered due to irritation of the vein. Slowing the rate of administration may relieve discomfort.
- Ongoing assessment is an important part of nursing care for both evaluation of patient response to administered medications and early detection of adverse drug reactions. If an adverse effect is suspected, withhold further medication doses and notify the health care team. Additional intervention is based on type of reaction and patient assessment.

Skill 30-9 Administering Medications by Intravenous Bolus or Push Through a Medication or Drug-Infusion Lock

DELEGATION CONSIDERATIONS

The administration of medications through an intermittent peripheral venous access device is not delegated to assistive personnel (AP). Depending on the state's nurse practice act and the organization's policies and procedures, the administration of specified IV medications in some settings may be delegated to licensed practical/vocational nurses (LPN/LVNs) who have received appropriate training. The decision to delegate must be based on careful analysis of the patient's needs and circumstances as well as the qualifications of the person to whom the task is being delegated. Refer to the Delegation Guidelines in Appendix A.

EQUIPMENT

- Prescribed medication
- Two normal saline flushes prepared in a syringe (3 to 10 mL) according to facility policy
- Antimicrobial swabs
- Passive disinfection caps (based on facility policy)
- Syringe with a needleless device or 23- to 25-gauge, 1-inch needle (follow facility policy)
- Watch or clock with a second hand
- Disposable gloves
- Electronic Medication Administration Record (eMAR) or Medication Administration Record (MAR)
- Additional PPE, as indicated

IMPLEMENTATION

ACTION	RATIONALE
1. Gather equipment. Check each medication prescribed against the original in the health record, depending on facility policy and the medication order system in place. Clarify any inconsistencies. Check the patient's health record for allergies. Check a drug resource to clarify whether medication needs to be diluted before bolus administration. Verify the recommended administration rate.	The prescription is the legal record of prescribed medication interventions. This comparison helps to identify errors that may have occurred when orders were transcribed. Computer provider order-entry (CPOE) systems allow prescribers to send electronic medication prescriptions directly to the pharmacy located in a health care facility and to outpatient pharmacies. Recommended administration rate delivers the correct dose of medication as prescribed.
2. Know the actions, special nursing considerations, safe dose ranges, purpose of administration, and adverse effects of the medications to be administered. Consider the appropriateness of the medication for this patient.	This knowledge aids the nurse in evaluating the therapeutic effect of the medication in relation to the patient's health status and can also be used to educate the patient about the medication.
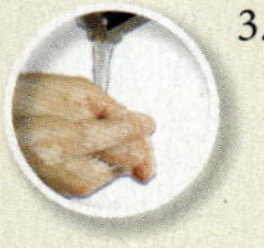 3. Perform hand hygiene.	Hand hygiene prevents the spread of microorganisms.
4. Move the medication supply system to the outside of the patient's room or prepare for administration at the medication supply system in the medication area. Alternatively, access the medication administration supply system at or inside the patient's room.	Organization facilitates error-free administration and saves time.
5. Unlock the medication supply system or drawer. Enter the passcode and scan employee identification, if required.	Locking the medication supply system or drawer safeguards each patient's medication supply. Facility accrediting organizations require medication supply systems to be locked when not in use. Entering the passcode and scanning ID allows only authorized users into the system and identifies the user for documentation by the computer.
6. **Prepare medications for one patient at a time.**	This prevents errors in medication administration.
7. Read the eMAR/MAR and select the proper medication from the medication supply system or the patient's medication drawer.	This is the *first* check of the label.
8. Compare the label with the eMAR/MAR. Check expiration dates and perform calculations, if necessary. Scan the bar code on the package, if required.	This is the *second* check of the label. Verify calculations with another nurse to ensure safety, if necessary.
9. If necessary, withdraw the medication from an ampule or vial as described in Skills 30-2 and 30-3.	Allows administration of medication.
10. **Depending on facility policy, the third check of the label may occur at this point. If so, when all medications for one patient have been prepared, recheck the labels with the eMAR/MAR before taking the medications to the patient. However, many facilities require the third check to occur at the bedside, after identifying the patient.**	This *third* check ensures accuracy and helps to prevent errors. *Note:* Many facilities require the *third* check to occur at the bedside, after identifying the patient and before administration.

(*continued on page 1010*)

Skill 30-9 Administering Medications by Intravenous Bolus or Push Through a Medication or Drug-Infusion Lock *(continued)*

ACTION	RATIONALE
11. Label the syringe with the medication's name, dose, and amount (The Joint Commission, 2021).	Unlabeled syringes are unidentifiable and may lead to a medication administration error (The Joint Commission, 2021).
12. **Log out of and/or lock the medication supply system before leaving it.**	Locking the medication supply system or drawer safeguards the patient's medication supply. Facility accrediting organizations require medication supply systems to be locked when not in use.
13. Transport medications and equipment to the patient's bedside carefully and keep the medications in sight at all times.	Careful handling and close observation prevent accidental or deliberate disarrangement of medications. Having equipment available saves time and facilitates performance of the task.
14. **Ensure that the patient receives the medications at the correct time.**	Check facility policy, which may allow for administration within a period of 30 minutes before or 30 minutes after the designated time.
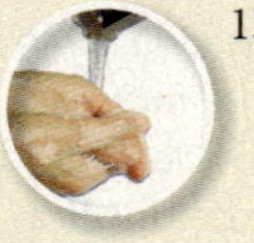 15. Perform hand hygiene and put on PPE, if indicated.	Hand hygiene and PPE prevent the spread of microorganisms. PPE is required based on transmission precautions.
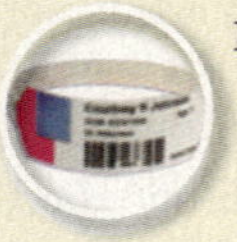 16. **Identify the patient. Compare the information with the eMAR/MAR. The patient should be identified using at least two of the following methods** (The Joint Commission, 2021):	Identifying the patient ensures the right patient receives the medications and helps prevent errors. The patient's room number or physical location is not used as an identifier (The Joint Commission, 2021). Replace the identification band if it is missing or inaccurate in any way.
a. Check the name on the patient's identification band.	This requires a response from the patient, but illness and strange surroundings often cause patients to be confused.
b. Check the identification number on the patient's identification band.	
c. Check the birth date on the patient's identification band.	
d. Ask the patient to state their name and birth date, based on facility policy.	
17. Close the door to the room or pull the bedside curtain.	This provides patient privacy.
18. **Complete necessary assessments before administering medications. Check the patient's allergy bracelet, if present, or ask the patient about allergies. Explain the purpose and action of the medication to the patient.**	Assessment is a prerequisite to administration of medications. Explanation provides rationale, increases knowledge, and reduces anxiety.
19. Scan the bar code on the patient's identification band, if required (The Joint Commission, 2021) (Figure 1).	Scanning provides an additional check to ensure that the medication is given to the right patient.

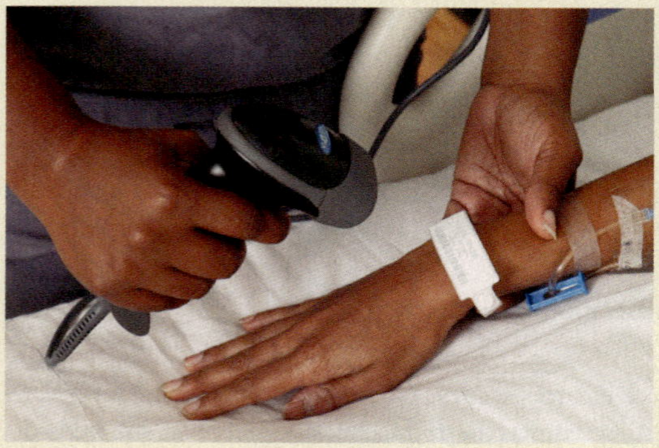

FIGURE 1. Scanning bar code on patient's identification bracelet.

ACTION	RATIONALE
20. **Based on facility policy, the third check of the label may occur at this point. If so, recheck the labels with the eMAR/MAR before administering the medications to the patient.**	Many facilities require the *third* check to occur at the bedside, after identifying the patient and before administration. If facility policy directs the *third* check at this time, this *third* check ensures accuracy and helps to prevent errors.

ACTION	RATIONALE
21. Assess the IV site for the presence of inflammation or infiltration.	IV medication must be given directly into a vein for safe administration.
22. Put on gloves.	Gloves protect the nurse's hands from contact with the patient's blood.
23. Remove the passive disinfection cap from the needleless connector or access port of the medication lock (Figure 2). Alternatively, if a passive disinfection cap is not in place, use an antimicrobial swab to vigorously disinfect the connection surface and sides of the needleless connector or end cap on the injection port and allow it to dry.	Passive disinfection caps contain an antiseptic-impregnated sponge that dispenses the antiseptic over the connector's top and threads and protects the hub from contamination by touch or airborne sources (Barton, 2019; Casey et al., 2018). Venous access device entry points, end caps, and needleless connectors must be vigorously scrubbed and disinfected prior to each access to reduce the risk for introduction of microorganisms and prevent venous access device–related infection (Flynn et al., 2019; Gorski et al., 2021). Friction is needed to physically remove microorganisms from the top, sides, and threads of the needleless connector or end cap. Allow the antiseptic to dry completely to ensure complete effectiveness (Gorski et al., 2021; Slater et al., 2018).
24. Uncap the saline flush syringe. Stabilize the port with your nondominant hand and insert the saline flush syringe into the needleless connector or end cap on the access port of the medication lock (Figure 3).	Assessing patency of the venous access device is necessary to ensure IV administration of the medication.
25. Release the clamp on the extension tubing of the medication lock (Figure 4). Pull back on the syringe plunger to aspirate the catheter for positive blood return (Figure 5). If positive, instill the solution over 1 minute or according to facility policy. Observe the insertion site while inserting the saline. Remove the syringe.	Positive blood return confirms patency before administration of medications and solutions (Gorski et al., 2021). Flushing without incident ensures patency of the IV line and administration of the medication into the bloodstream. Puffiness, pain, or swelling as the site is flushed could indicate infiltration of the catheter.

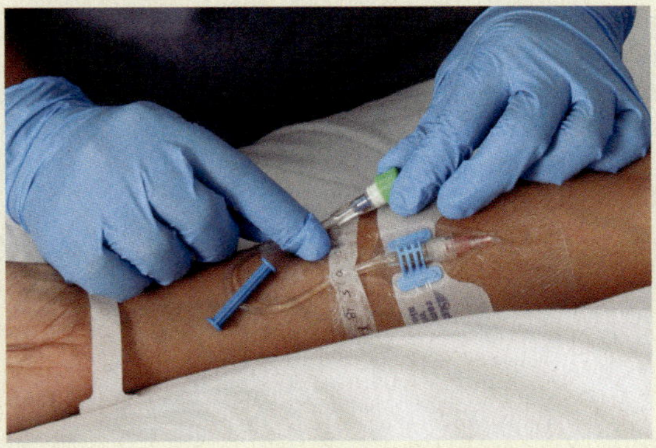

FIGURE 2. Removing the passive disinfection cap from the access port.

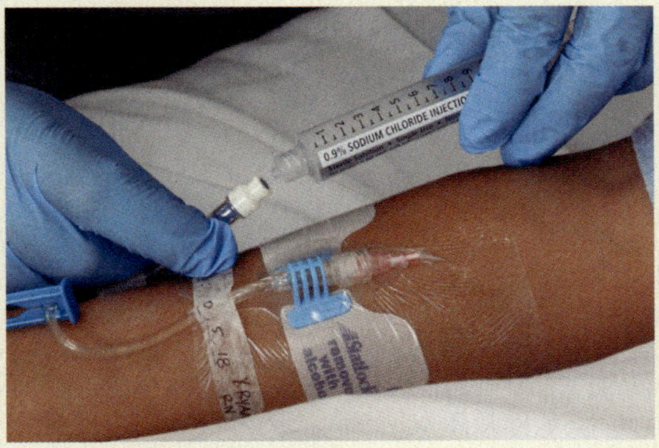

FIGURE 3. Inserting the saline flush syringe into the access port.

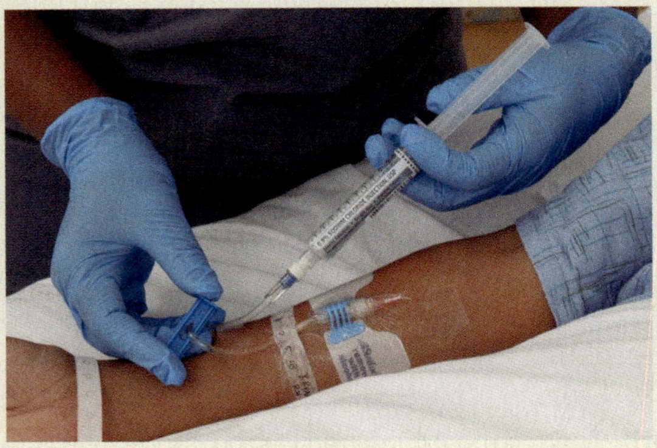

FIGURE 4. Releasing the clamp on the extension tubing.

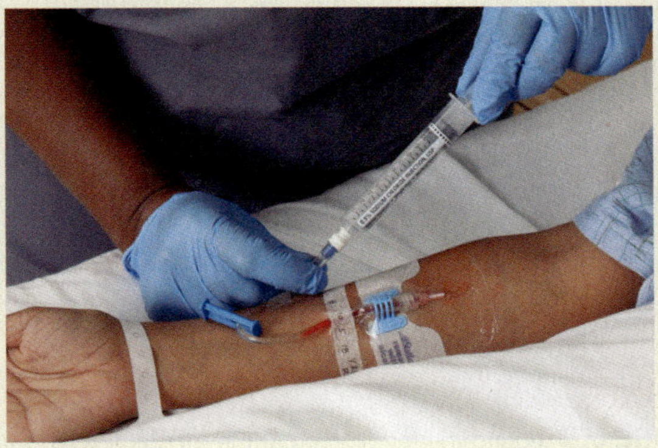

FIGURE 5. Pulling back on the plunger to aspirate for a blood return.

(continued on page 1012)

Skill 30-9 Administering Medications by Intravenous Bolus or Push Through a Medication or Drug-Infusion Lock *(continued)*

ACTION	RATIONALE
26. Use an antimicrobial swab to vigorously disinfect the connection surface and sides of the needleless connector or end cap on the injection port and allow it to dry.	Venous access device entry points, end caps, and needleless connectors must be vigorously scrubbed and disinfected prior to each access to reduce the risk for introduction of microorganisms and prevent venous access device–related infection (Flynn et al., 2019; Gorski et al., 2021). Friction is needed to physically remove microorganisms from the top, sides, and threads of the needleless connector or end cap. Allow the antiseptic to dry completely to ensure complete effectiveness (Gorski et al., 2021; Slater et al., 2018).
27. Uncap the medication syringe. Insert the medication syringe into the needleless connector or end cap on the access port of the medication lock. Using a watch or clock with a second-hand to time the rate, **inject the medication at the recommended rate (Figure 6). Do not force the injection if resistance is felt.**	This delivers the correct amount of medication at the proper interval. Easy installation of medication usually indicates that the lock is still patent and in the vein. If force is used against resistance, a clot may break away and cause a blockage elsewhere in the body.
28. While administering the medication, observe the infusion site and assess the patient for any adverse reaction. If signs of adverse reaction occur, stop the infusion immediately and notify the health care team.	Signs of adverse reaction, such as peripheral IV infiltration, rash or itching, or pain at the infusion site, necessitate stopping administration of the drug (Gorski et al., 2021).
29. Remove the medication syringe from the access port. Use a new antimicrobial swab to vigorously disinfect the connection surface and sides of the needleless connector or end cap on the injection port and allow it to dry. Stabilize the port with your nondominant hand. Uncap the second saline flush syringe. Insert the saline flush syringe into the needleless connector or end cap on the access port. Instill the flush solution at the same rate as the administered medication (Gorski et al., 2021).	Venous access device entry points, end caps, and needleless connectors must be vigorously scrubbed and disinfected prior to each access to reduce the risk for introduction of microorganisms and prevent venous access device–related infection (Flynn et al., 2019; Gorski et al., 2021). Friction is needed to physically remove microorganisms from the top, sides, and threads of the needleless connector or end cap. Allow the antiseptic to dry completely to ensure complete effectiveness (Gorski et al., 2021; Slater et al., 2018). Flushing after medication administration ensures the entire drug dose has been cleared from the extension tubing on the venous access device or from the infusion system and prevents precipitation due to solution/medication incompatibility (Gorski et al., 2021).
30. If the medication lock is capped with a positive pressure valve/device, remove the syringe, and then clamp the extension tubing (Figure 7). Alternatively, to gain positive pressure if positive pressure valve/device is not present, clamp the extension tubing as you are still flushing the last of the saline into the medication lock. Remove the syringe.	Positive pressure prevents blood from backing into the catheter and causing the medication lock to clot off.

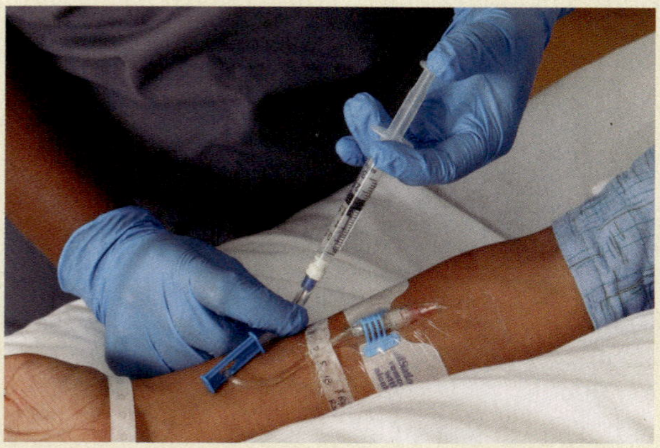

FIGURE 6. Injecting the medication at the recommended rate.

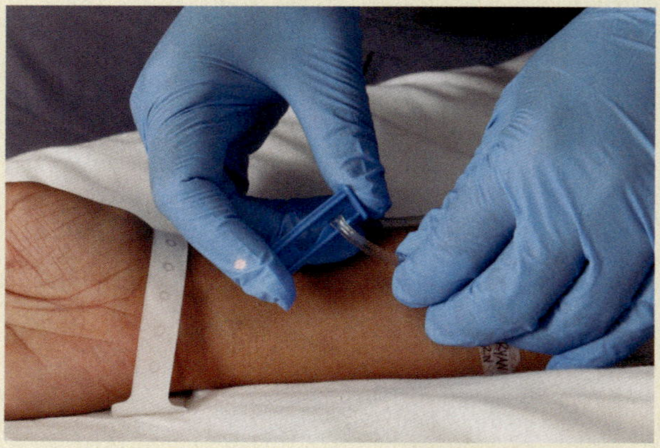

FIGURE 7. Clamping the extension tubing.

ACTION	RATIONALE
31. Using an antimicrobial swab, vigorously disinfect the connection surface and sides of the needleless connector or end cap on the injection port and allow it to dry. Attach a passive disinfection cap to the needleless connector or end cap on the access port of the medication lock (Figure 8).	Venous access device entry points, end caps, and needleless connectors must be vigorously scrubbed and disinfected prior to each access to reduce the risk for introduction of microorganisms and prevent venous access device–related infection (Flynn et al., 2019; Gorski et al., 2021). Friction is needed to physically remove microorganisms from the top, sides, and threads of the needleless connector or end cap. Allow the antiseptic to dry completely to ensure complete effectiveness (Gorski et al., 2021; Slater et al., 2018). Passive disinfection caps contain an antiseptic-impregnated sponge that dispenses the antiseptic over the connector's top and threads and protect the hub from contamination by touch or airborne sources (Barton, 2019; Casey et al., 2018).

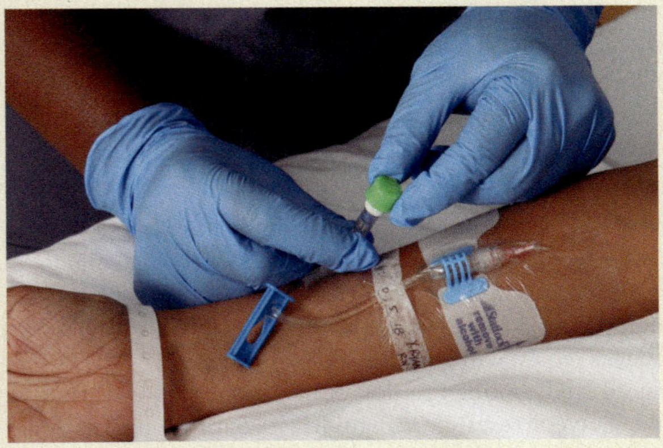

FIGURE 8. Attaching a passive disinfection cap to the access port.

32. Discard the syringe in the appropriate receptacle.	Proper disposal prevents injury and the spread of microorganisms.
33. Remove gloves and additional PPE, if used. Perform hand hygiene.	Proper removal of PPE reduces the risk of infection transmission and contamination of other items. Hand hygiene prevents the spread of microorganisms.
34. Document the administration of the medication immediately after administration. See Documentation section below.	Timely documentation helps to ensure patient safety.
35. Evaluate the patient's response to the medication within an appropriate time frame.	The patient needs to be evaluated for therapeutic and adverse effects from the medication.

DOCUMENTATION

GUIDELINES

Document the administration of the medication and saline flush, including date, time, dose, route of administration, site of administration, and rate of administration on the eMAR/MAR or record using the required format, immediately after administration. If using a bar-code system, medication administration is automatically recorded when the bar code is scanned. PRN medications require documentation of the reason for administration. Prompt recording avoids the possibility of accidentally repeating the administration of the drug. If the drug was refused or omitted, record this in the appropriate area on the medication record and notify the health care team as appropriate. This verifies the reason medication was omitted and ensures that the health care personnel providing care for the patient are aware of the occurrence.

(continued on page 1014)

Skill 30-9 Administering Medications by Intravenous Bolus or Push Through a Medication or Drug-Infusion Lock *(continued)*

DEVELOPING CLINICAL REASONING AND CLINICAL JUDGMENT

UNEXPECTED SITUATIONS AND ASSOCIATED INTERVENTIONS

- *Upon assessing the medication lock site before administering the medication, you note that the medication lock has infiltrated:* Remove the medication lock from the extremity. Restart the peripheral venous access in a different location. Continue to monitor the new site as the medication is administered.
- *While you are administering medication, the patient begins to complain of pain at the site:* Stop the medication. Assess the medication lock site for signs of infiltration and phlebitis. Flush the medication lock with normal saline again to recheck patency. If the IV site appears within normal limits, resume medication administration at a slower rate. If pain persists, stop, remove the medication lock, and restart in a different location.
- *As you are attempting to access the lock, the syringe tip touches the patient's arm:* Discard the syringe. Prepare a new dose for administration.
- *No blood return is noted upon aspiration:* If the medication lock appears patent, without signs of infiltration, and normal saline fluid infuses without difficulty, proceed with administration. Observe closely for signs and symptoms of infiltration during and after administration.

SPECIAL CONSIDERATIONS

General Considerations

- Vascular access devices should also be "locked" after completion of the flush solution at each use to decrease the risk of occlusion and catheter-related bloodstream infection (Gorski et al., 2021). According to the guidelines from the INS, vascular access devices are locked with normal saline solution (Gorski et al., 2021). If the device is not in use, periodic flushing according to facility policy is required to keep the catheter patent.
- Previously, recommendations suggested routine rotation of insertions sites at various intervals, usually 72 to 96 hours. Current research and guidelines support maintaining peripheral IV access devices until no longer clinically indicated or until a complication develops (Gorski et al., 2021; Weston, 2019). Nurses should use clinical assessment and judgment in deciding when to replace or discontinue a peripheral venous access device.
- The clinical need for the IV catheter should be assessed on a daily basis (Gorski et al., 2021). The device insertion site and dressing should be assessed every 4 hours at a minimum (Gorski et al., 2021; Weston, 2019).
- A peripheral venous access device that is no longer necessary should not be kept in place just in case it may be needed in a few days (Weston, 2019).
- Ongoing assessment is an important part of nursing care to evaluate patient response to administered medications and early detection of adverse reactions. If an adverse effect is suspected, withhold further medication doses and notify the health care team. Additional intervention is based on type of reaction and patient assessment.

Infant and Child Considerations

- The primary method for IV medication administration for infants and children is a mini-infusion (syringe) pump (Kyle & Carman, 2021). Refer to Skill 30-10.
- Administration of IV bolus or push medication is usually reserved for emergency situations and when therapeutic blood levels must be reached quickly to achieve the desired effect (Kyle & Carman, 2021).

Skill 30-10 Administering a Piggyback Intermittent Intravenous Infusion of Medication

DELEGATION CONSIDERATIONS

The administration of medications by intermittent IV infusion is not delegated to assistive personnel (AP). Depending on the state's nurse practice act and the organization's policies and procedures, the administration of specified IV medications in some settings may be delegated to licensed practical/vocational nurses (LPN/LVNs) who have received appropriate training. The decision to delegate must be based on careful analysis of the patient's needs and circumstances as well as the qualifications of the person to whom the task is being delegated. Refer to the Delegation Guidelines in Appendix A.

EQUIPMENT

- Medication prepared in labeled small-volume IV bag
- Short secondary infusion tubing
- Infusion pump
- Antimicrobial swab
- Needleless connector, if required, based on facility procedure
- Metal or plastic hook
- IV pole
- Watch or clock with a second hand (gravity infusion)
- Date label for tubing
- Electronic Medication Administration Record (eMAR) or Medication Administration Record (MAR)
- PPE, as indicated

IMPLEMENTATION

ACTION	RATIONALE
1. Gather equipment. Check each medication prescribed against the original in the health record, depending on facility policy and the medication order system in place. Clarify any inconsistencies. Check the patient's health record for allergies. Check the administration rate.	The prescription is the legal record of prescribed medication interventions. This comparison helps to identify errors that may have occurred when orders were transcribed. Computer provider order-entry (CPOE) systems allow prescribers to send electronic medication prescriptions directly to the pharmacy located in a health care facility and to outpatient pharmacies.
2. Know the actions, special nursing considerations, safe dose ranges, purpose of administration, and adverse effects of the medications to be administered. Consider the appropriateness of the medication for this patient. **Assess the compatibility of the ordered medication, diluent, and the infusing IV fluid.**	This knowledge aids the nurse in evaluating the therapeutic effect of the medication in relation to the patient's health status and can also be used to educate the patient about the medication. Compatibility of medication and solutions prevents complications.
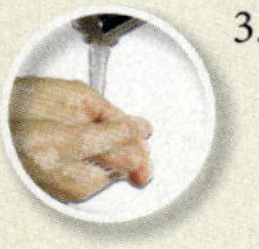 3. Perform hand hygiene.	Hand hygiene prevents the spread of microorganisms.
4. Move the medication supply system to the outside of the patient's room or prepare for administration at the medication supply system in the medication area. Alternatively, access the medication administration supply system at or inside the patient's room.	Organization facilitates error-free administration and saves time.
5. Unlock the medication supply system or drawer. Enter the passcode and scan employee identification, if required.	Locking the medication supply system or drawer safeguards each patient's medication supply. Facility accrediting organizations require medication supply systems to be locked when not in use. Entering the passcode and scanning ID allows only authorized users into the system and identifies the user for documentation by the computer.
6. **Prepare medications for one patient at a time.**	This prevents errors in medication administration.
7. Read the eMAR/MAR and read the label when selecting the proper medication from the medication supply system or the patient's medication drawer.	This is the *first* check of the label.
8. Read the label and compare the label with the eMAR/MAR. Check expiration dates. Confirm the prescribed or appropriate infusion rate. Calculate the drip rate if using a gravity system. Scan the bar code on the package, if required.	This is the *second* check of the label. Verify calculations with another nurse to ensure safety, if necessary. Infusing medication at an appropriate rate prevents injury.

(*continued on page 1016*)

Skill 30-10 Administering a Piggyback Intermittent Intravenous Infusion of Medication *(continued)*

ACTION	RATIONALE
9. **Depending on facility policy, the third check of the label may occur at this point. If so, when all medications for one patient have been prepared, read the label and recheck the labels with the eMAR/MAR before taking the medications to the patient. However, many facilities require the third check to occur at the bedside, after identifying the patient.**	This *third* check ensures accuracy and helps to prevent errors. *Note:* Many facilities require the *third* check to occur at the bedside, after identifying the patient and before administration.
10. **Log-out of and/or lock the medication supply system before leaving it.**	Locking the medication supply system or drawer safeguards the patient's medication supply. Facility accrediting organizations require medication supply systems to be locked when not in use.
11. Transport medications to the patient's bedside carefully and keep the medications in sight at all times.	Careful handling and close observation prevent accidental or deliberate disarrangement of medications.
12. **Ensure that the patient receives the medications at the correct time.**	Check facility policy, which may allow for administration within a period of 30 minutes before or 30 minutes after the designated time.
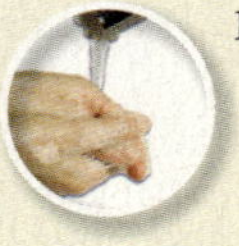 13. Perform hand hygiene and put on PPE, if indicated.	Hand hygiene and PPE prevent the spread of microorganisms. PPE is required based on transmission precautions.
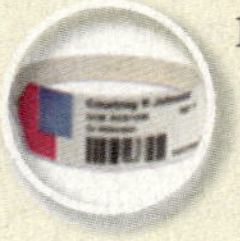 14. **Identify the patient. Compare the information with the eMAR/MAR. The patient should be identified using at least two of the following methods** (The Joint Commission, 2021):	Identifying the patient ensures the right patient receives the medications and helps prevent errors. The patient's room number or physical location is not used as an identifier (The Joint Commission, 2021). Replace the identification band if it is missing or inaccurate in any way.
a. Check the name on the patient's identification band.	This requires a response from the patient, but illness and strange surroundings often cause patients to be confused.
b. Check the identification number on the patient's identification band.	
c. Check the birth date on the patient's identification band.	
d. Ask the patient to state their name and birth date, based on facility policy.	
15. Close the door to the room or pull the bedside curtain.	This provides patient privacy.
16. **Complete necessary assessments before administering medications. Check the patient's allergy bracelet, if present, or ask the patient about allergies. Explain the purpose and action of the medication to the patient.**	Assessment is a prerequisite to administration of medications. Explanation provides rationale, increases knowledge, and reduces anxiety.
17. Scan the patient's bar code on the identification band, if required (The Joint Commission, 2021).	Scanning provides an additional check to ensure that the medication is given to the right patient.
18. **Based on facility policy, the third check of the label may occur at this point. If so, read the label and recheck the labels with the eMAR/MAR before administering the medications to the patient.**	Many facilities require the *third* check to occur at the bedside, after identifying the patient and before administration. If facility policy directs the *third* check at this time, this *third* check ensures accuracy and helps to prevent errors.
19. Assess the IV site for the presence of inflammation or infiltration or other signs of complications.	IV medication must be given directly into a vein for safe administration.
20. Close the clamp on the short secondary infusion tubing. Using aseptic technique, remove the cap on the tubing spike and the cap on the port of the medication container, taking care to avoid contaminating either end.	Closing the clamp prevents fluid from entering the system until the nurse is ready. Maintaining sterility of the tubing and the medication port prevents contamination.
21. Attach the infusion tubing to the medication container by inserting the tubing spike into the port with a firm push and twisting motion, taking care to avoid contaminating either end.	Maintaining sterility of the tubing and medication port prevents contamination.

ACTION	RATIONALE
22. Hang the piggyback container on the IV pole, positioning it higher than the primary IV if necessary, based on the type of IV infusion device in use and according to the manufacturer's recommendations. If necessary for the particular infusion pump in use, use the metal or plastic hook to lower the primary IV fluid container (Figure 1). If using gravity infusion, the primary IV fluid container must be lowered.	The position of the containers influences the flow of IV fluid into the primary setup.
23. If the secondary infusion tubing is being used for the first time, place a label on the administration tubing with the current date.	Most facilities allow the reuse of tubing, reducing the risk for contamination. The frequency of administration set tubing changes varies. The label identifies the date of the first use of the tubing. Intermittent administration sets disconnected after use should be replaced every 24 hours; repeated disconnection and reconnection increase the risk of contamination at the spike end, catheter hub, needleless connector, and the end of the administration set, potentially increasing the risk for catheter-related bloodstream infection (Gorski et al., 2021)
24. Squeeze the drip chamber on the administration tubing and release. Fill the chamber to the line or about half full. Open the clamp on the administration tubing and prime the tubing. Close the clamp. Place the needleless connector on the end of the tubing, using sterile technique, if required.	This removes air from tubing and preserves the sterility of the setup.
25. Remove the passive disinfection cap from the needleless connector or end cap on the infusion set injection port. Alternatively, if a passive disinfection cap is not in place, use an antimicrobial swab to vigorously disinfect the connection surfaces and sides of the access port or stopcock on the administration set above where the tubing enters the infusion pump or above the roller clamp on the primary IV infusion tubing (gravity infusion) (Figure 2).	Passive disinfection caps contain an antiseptic-impregnated sponge that dispenses the antiseptic over the connector's top and threads and protects the hub from contamination by touch or airborne sources (Barton, 2019; Casey et al., 2018). Venous access device entry points, end caps, and needleless connectors must be vigorously scrubbed and disinfected prior to each access to reduce the risk for introduction of microorganisms and prevent venous access device–related infection (Flynn et al., 2019; Gorski et al., 2021). Friction is needed to physically remove microorganisms from the top, sides, and threads of the needleless connector or end cap. Allow the antiseptic to dry completely to ensure complete effectiveness (Gorski et al., 2021; Slater et al., 2018).The backflow valve in the primary line secondary port stops flow of the primary infusion while the piggyback solution is infusing. Once completed, the backflow valve opens, and flow of the primary solution resumes.

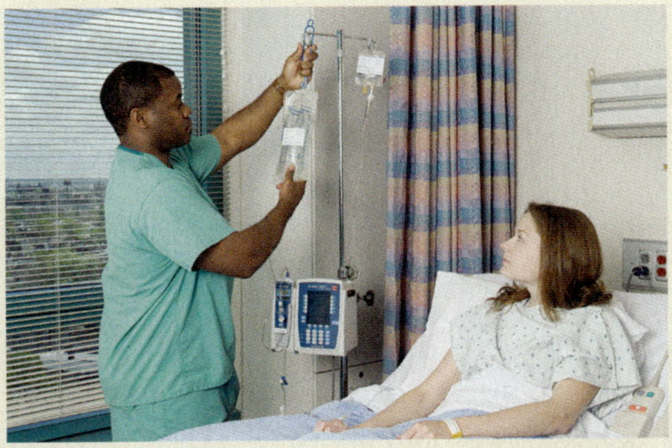

FIGURE 1. Lowering the primary IV fluid container to position the piggyback container higher than primary IV fluid container. (*Source:* Used with permission from Shutterstock. *Photo by B. Proud.*)

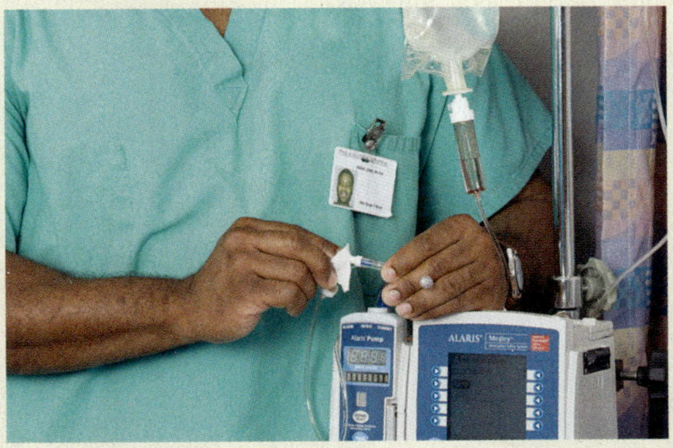

FIGURE 2. Vigorously scrubbing the access port. (*Source:* Used with permission from Shutterstock. *Photo by B. Proud.*)

(continued on page 1018)

Skill 30-10 Administering a Piggyback Intermittent Intravenous Infusion of Medication *(continued)*

ACTION

26. Connect the piggyback setup to the access port (Figure 3) or stopcock. If using, turn the stopcock to the open position.

RATIONALE

Needleless systems and a stopcock setup eliminate the need for a needle and are recommended by the CDC.

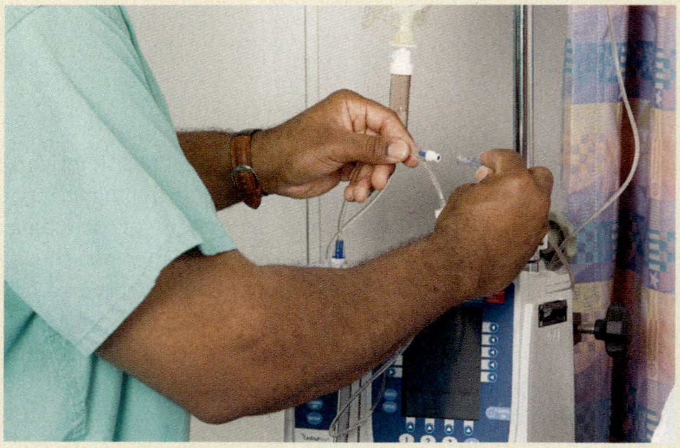

FIGURE 3. Connecting piggyback administration set to access port. (*Source:* Used with permission from Shutterstock. *Photo by B. Proud.*)

27. Alternatively, if the administration set is in place from a previous infusion, there is no need to disconnect the secondary tubing to connect the current dose of medication. The secondary tubing will be primed via "backfill" or "back prime" of the secondary tubing.

Most facilities allow the reuse of tubing, reducing the risk for contamination. "Back prime" is recommended as the method to use to prime a secondary administration set when there is compatibility with the primary fluid (Gorski et al., 2021). The frequency of administration set tubing changes varies.

28. Clamp the secondary infusion tubing and remove the previous, empty medication bag. Attach the current medication dose bag to the secondary infusion tubing, as outlined in Steps 20–22. Lower the medication bag below the main IV solution container and open the clamp on the secondary infusion tubing. This allows the primary IV solution to flow up the secondary tubing to the drip chamber, "back priming" or "backfilling" the tubing. Allow the solution to enter the drip chamber until the drip chamber is half full. Close the clamp on the secondary tubing and hang the medication container on the IV pole.

This "backfill" method keeps the infusion system intact, preventing both introduction of microorganisms and loss of medication when the tubing is primed. "Back prime" is recommended as the method to use to prime a secondary administration set when there is compatibility with the primary fluid (Gorski et al., 2021). Check facility policy regarding the use of "back prime."

29. Open the clamp on the secondary infusion tubing. Set the rate for the secondary infusion on the infusion pump and begin the infusion (Figure 4). If using gravity infusion, use the roller clamp on the primary infusion tubing to regulate the flow at the prescribed delivery rate (Figure 5). Monitor medication infusion at periodic intervals.

The backflow valve in the primary line secondary port stops the flow of the primary infusion while the piggyback solution is infusing. Once completed, the backflow valve opens, and flow of the primary solution resumes. It is important to verify the safe administration rate for each drug to prevent adverse effects.

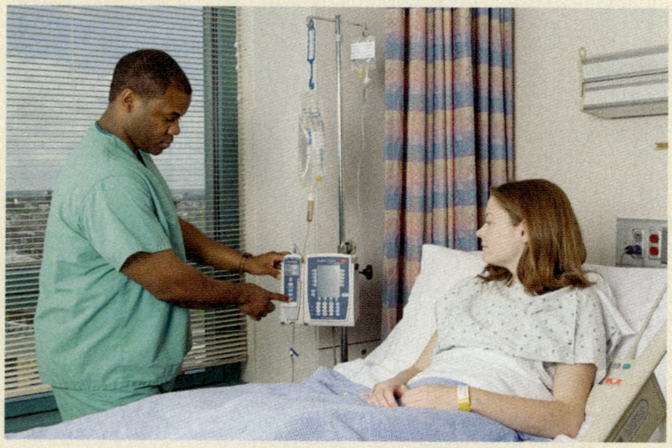

FIGURE 4. Setting rate for secondary infusion on infusion pump. (*Source:* Used with permission from Shutterstock. *Photo by B. Proud.*)

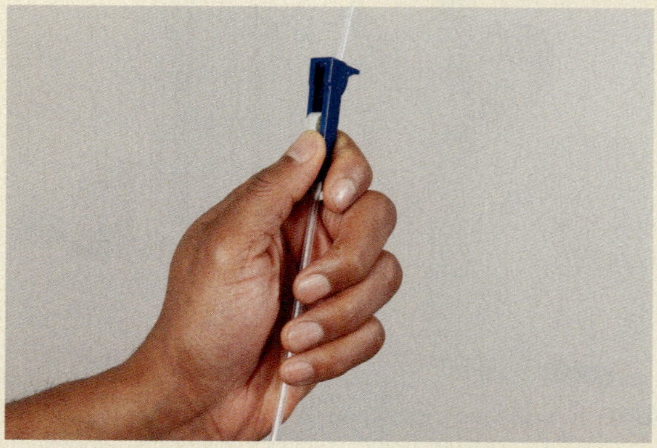

FIGURE 5. Using roller clamp on primary infusion tubing to regulate gravity flow. (*Source:* Used with permission from Shutterstock. *Photo by B. Proud.*)

ACTION	RATIONALE
30. Clamp the tubing on the piggyback set when the solution is infused and leave the setup in place.	Most facilities allow the reuse of tubing, reducing the risk for contamination. Leaving the secondary tubing and medication bag in place until the next dose keeps the infusion system intact, preventing both introduction of microorganisms and loss of medication when the tubing is primed. "Back prime" is recommended as the method to use to prime a secondary administration set when there is compatibility with the primary fluid (Gorski et al., 2021). Check facility policy regarding the use of "back prime." The frequency of administration set tubing changes varies.
31. Raise the primary IV fluid container to the original height, if lowered for the infusion. **Check the primary infusion rate on the infusion pump. If using gravity infusion, readjust the flow rate of the primary IV.**	Most infusion pumps automatically restart the primary infusion at the previous rate after the secondary infusion is completed. If using gravity infusion, piggyback medication administration may interrupt the normal flow rate of the primary IV. Rate readjustment may be necessary.
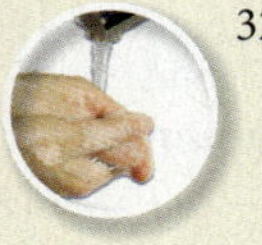 32. Remove PPE, if used. Perform hand hygiene.	Proper removal of PPE reduces the risk of infection transmission and contamination of other items. Hand hygiene prevents the spread of microorganisms.
33. Document the administration of the medication immediately after administration. See Documentation section below. Document the volume of fluid administered on the intake and output record, if necessary.	Timely documentation helps to ensure patient safety.
34. Evaluate the patient's response to the medication within an appropriate time frame.	The patient needs to be evaluated for therapeutic and adverse effects from the medication.

DOCUMENTATION

GUIDELINES

Document the administration of the medication immediately after administration, including date, time, dose, route of administration, site of administration, and rate of administration on the eMAR/MAR or record using the required format. If using a bar-code system, medication administration is automatically recorded when the bar code is scanned. PRN medications require documentation of the reason for administration. Prompt recording avoids the possibility of accidentally repeating the administration of the drug. If the drug was refused or omitted, record this in the appropriate area on the medication record and notify the health care team as appropriate. This verifies the reason medication was omitted and ensures that health care personnel providing care for the patient are aware of the occurrence. Document the volume of fluid administered on the intake and output record.

DEVELOPING CLINICAL REASONING AND CLINICAL JUDGMENT

UNEXPECTED SITUATIONS AND ASSOCIATED INTERVENTIONS

- *Upon assessing the IV site before administering medication, you note that the IV has infiltrated:* Stop the IV fluid and remove the IV from the extremity. Restart the IV in a different location. Continue to monitor the new IV site as the medication is administered.
- *While administering medication, you note a cloudy, white substance forming in the IV tubing:* Stop the IV from flowing and stop administering the medication to prevent precipitate from entering the patient's circulation. Clamp the IV at the site nearest to the patient. Replace tubing on primary and secondary infusions. Check a drug resource or consult a pharmacist regarding compatibility of the medication and IV fluid before continuing with administration. Medication infusion may require a second IV site or administration through an access port closer to the IV site and flushing of the tubing before and after administration.

(continued on page 1020)

Skill 30-10 Administering a Piggyback Intermittent Intravenous Infusion of Medication *(continued)*

- *While you are administering medication, the patient begins to complain of pain at the IV site:* Stop the medication. Assess the IV site for any signs of complications. Flush the IV with normal saline to check for patency. If the IV site appears within normal limits, resume medication administration at a slower rate.

SPECIAL CONSIDERATIONS

General Considerations

- Intermittent administration sets disconnected after use should be replaced every 24 hours; repeated disconnection and reconnection increases risk of contamination at the spike end, catheter hub, needleless connector, and the end of the administration set, potentially increasing the risk for catheter-related bloodstream infection (Gorski et al., 2021).
- Ongoing assessment is an important part of nursing care for both evaluation of patient response to administered medications and early detection of adverse reactions. If an adverse effect is suspected, withhold further medication doses and notify the patient's health care team. Additional intervention is based on type of reaction and patient assessment.

Infant and Child Considerations

- The primary method for IV medication administration for infants and children is a mini-infusion (syringe) pump (Kyle & Carman, 2021).
- Infants and small children with fluid restrictions may not tolerate the added IV fluid needed for administration with piggyback systems. For these children, consider using the mini-infusion pump.

DEVELOPING CLINICAL REASONING AND CLINICAL JUDGMENT

1. See the accompanying Nursing Care Plan for Regina Sauder for an example of the nursing process for medication administration.
2. You are scheduled to give an intramuscular injection in the ventrogluteal site and remember learning that it should be administered using the Z-track technique. When you mention this to the nurse in the hospital who has been taking care of your patient, she tells you there is no reason to use the Z-track technique. You remember your instructor telling you to use the Z-track technique. What should you do?
3. You are caring for two patients and have just completed giving medications to the first when you realize that you gave her the medications prescribed for your other patient. What should you do?

PRACTICING FOR NCLEX

1. A nurse administers a dose of an oral medication for hypertension to a patient who immediately vomits after swallowing the pill. What action will the nurse take first?
   a. Readminister the medication and notify the health care provider.
   b. Obtain the pill in a liquid form for administration.
   c. Assess the emesis, looking for the pill.
   d. Notify the primary care provider.
2. A nurse caring for a group of patients uses measures to reduce discomfort for the patients during injections. Which technique is recommended?
   a. Selecting a needle of the largest gauge that is appropriate for the site and solution to be injected
   b. Injecting the medication into contracted muscles to reduce pressure and discomfort at the site
   c. Using the Z-track technique for intramuscular injections to prevent leakage of medication into the needle track
   d. Applying vigorous pressure in a circular motion after the injection to distribute the medication to the intended site
3. A nurse is preparing medications for patients in the ICU. The nurse is aware that patient variables may affect the absorption of these medications. Which statements accurately describe these variables the nurse will use as a basis for practice? Select all that apply.
   a. Patients in certain ethnic groups obtain therapeutic responses at lower doses or higher doses than those usually prescribed.
   b. Some people experience the same response with a placebo as with the active drug used in studies.
   c. People with liver disease metabolize drugs more quickly than people with normal liver functioning.
   d. A patient who receives a pain medication in a noisy environment may not receive full benefit from the medication's effects.
   e. Oral medications should not be given with food as the food may delay the absorption of the medications.
   f. Circadian rhythms and cycles may influence drug action.

4. A nurse is administering a pain medication to a patient. In addition to checking the identification bracelet, which active identification strategy reflects best practice?
   a. Asking the patient their name and birthdate
   b. Reading the patient's name on the sign over the bed
   c. Asking the patient's roommate to verify the patient's name
   d. Asking, "Are you Mr. Brown?"

5. A nurse is administering a medication to a patient via an enteral feeding tube. Which are accurate guidelines related to this procedure? Select all that apply.
   a. Crushing the enteric-coated pill and mix it in a liquid
   b. Initially flushing the tube with 60 mL of very warm water
   c. Using the recommended policy to check tube placement in the stomach or intestine
   d. Giving each medication separately and flush with water between each drug
   e. Lowering the head of the bed to prevent reflux
   f. Adjusting the amount of water used if patient's fluid intake is restricted

6. A medication prescription reads: "Hydromorphone, 2 mg IV every 3 to 4 hours PRN pain." The prefilled cartridge is available with a label reading "Hydromorphone 2 mg/1 mL" and a statement that the cartridge contains 1.2 mL of hydromorphone. How should the nurse proceed?
   a. Give the entire contents of the cartridge sent by the pharmacy
   b. Call the pharmacy and request the proper dose
   c. Refuse to give the medication and document refusal in the EHR
   d. Discard 0.2 mL before administration; verify the waste with another nurse

7. A nurse prepares to administer insulin to a patient with diabetes. What is the correct procedure to carry out this prescription?
   MAR
   7:30 AM: 40 units of NPH insulin and 10 units of regular insulin daily subcutaneously.
   a. Inject air into the regular insulin vial and withdraw 10 units; then, using the same syringe, inject air into the NPH vial and withdraw 40 units of NPH insulin.
   b. Inject air into the NPH insulin vial, being careful not to allow the solution to touch the needle; next, inject air into the regular insulin vial and withdraw 10 units; followed by withdrawal of 40 units of NPH insulin.
   c. Inject air into the regular insulin vial, being careful not to allow the solution to touch the needle; next, inject air into the NPH insulin vial and withdraw 40 units; then, withdraw 10 units of regular insulin.
   d. Inject air into the NPH insulin vial and withdraw 40 units; then, using the same syringe, inject air into the regular insulin vial and withdraw 10 units of regular insulin.

8. A nurse is administering heparin subcutaneously to a patient. What technique is appropriate for this injection?
   a. Aspirating before giving and gently massage after the injection
   b. Avoiding aspirating; massaging the site for 1 minute
   c. Avoiding aspirating before and massaging after the injection
   d. Massaging the injection site; aspirating is unnecessary but will do no harm

9. A nurse discovers that a medication error occurred. What is the nurse's priority?
   a. Recording the error on the medication sheet
   b. Notifying the physician regarding course of action
   c. Assessing the patient for adverse effects of the error
   d. Completing an event report, explaining how the mistake was made

10. A nurse is teaching a patient how to use a meter-dosed inhaler to control asthma. What are appropriate guidelines for this procedure? Select all that apply.
    a. Shake the inhaler well and remove the mouthpiece covers from the MDI and spacer.
    b. Take shallow breaths when breathing through the spacer.
    c. Depress the canister releasing one puff into the spacer and inhale slowly and deeply.
    d. After inhaling, exhale quickly through pursed lips.
    e. Wait 1 to 5 minutes as prescribed before administering the next puff.
    f. Gargle and rinse with salt water after using the MDI.

11. A nurse in a rehabilitation facility is preparing to administer a skeletal muscle relaxant to a patient recovering from a motor vehicle accident. When the patient states, "I don't want that pill," what action will the nurse take next?
    a. Encourage the patient to take the pill to help reduce muscle spasm.
    b. Explain that the health care provider prescribes only necessary medications.
    c. Ask the patient to explain their concern about the medication.
    d. Question the patient about allergies and previous medication reactions.

12. A nurse is preparing to administer medications to a patient transferred from the intensive care unit just as lunch is served. Prior to administering medications to the patient, the nurse takes which action?
    a. Performing medication reconciliation
    b. morning care has been administered
    c. Ordering the patient a meal
    d. Taking a report from the nurse sending the patient

13. When administering an IVPB medication using gravity, what action is appropriate for the nurse take?
    a. Placing the primary IV bag below the level of the piggyback bag
    b. Disconnecting the tubing closest to the patient and flushing the intravenous access
    c. Ensuring the piggyback bag is below the main IV bag
    d. Closing the roller clamp to the secondary infusion
14. A nurse is administering enoxaparin subcutaneously using the manufacturer's prefilled syringe. Which action reflects correct practice?
    a. Administering the medication in the posterolateral abdomen
    b. Removing air bubble prior to injecting
    c. Gently rubbing the abdomen after injection to promote absorption
    d. Replacing the cap on the syringe before discarding it in the sharps container
15. A nurse is administering medications to an older adult with dysphagia. After crushing the pills, which action is most appropriate?
    a. Mixing the crushed medications with 120 mL of water before administering
    b. Mixing the medications into the patient's bowl of pudding
    c. Crushing each pill separately and administering each in a teaspoon of applesauce
    d. Asking the patient to chew the pills and providing juice after swallowing
16. A patient experiencing chest pain asks the nurse why a nitroglycerin tablet must be placed under their tongue instead of swallowed. Which answer by the nurse is appropriate?
    a. "We could put the tablet between the cheek and gum, instead."
    b. "The area is rich in superficial blood vessels, and helps with absorption."
    c. "Swallowing interferes with quick systemic effects."
    d. "This is an enteric-coated tablet, designed for absorption outside the stomach."
17. A nurse in the pediatric unit of an acute care hospital is awaiting a prescription for antibiotics for a toddler with a severe infection. Which information about the child is essential to document immediately?
    a. Beverage preference
    b. Whether a parent/guardian is present at the bedside
    c. Weight in kilograms
    d. Intake and output
18. A nurse in a pediatric practice teaches the mother of a toddler to administer antibiotic ear drops. What education by the nurse is correct?
    a. "It is best to pull the pinna of the affected ear up and back."
    b. "Place the child on their side of the affected ear and pull the pinna straight back."
    c. "When administering the ear drop, gently pull the pinna down and back."
    d. "Cleanse the ear canal with a cotton swab before administering."
19. A nurse is planning to administer digoxin to a patient. After reviewing the medical record, what action will the nurse take?

    Electronic Health Record

    Prescriptions
    - 11/22/2025 digoxin loading dose 0.25 mg IV twice today only
    - 11/23/2025 begin digoxin 0.125 mg orally daily

    Laboratory Studies
    - Digoxin level: 2.7 ng/mL (reference range 0.5–2 ng/mL)

    a. Administer the medication, recording the level in the MAR.
    b. Hold the medication and confer with the prescriber.
    c. Give the patient one half the dose.
    d. Evaluate the patient's kidney function studies.
20. A nurse notices that an older adult patient is malnourished, and blood tests reveal reduced plasma protein levels. For which of these pharmacodynamic effects will the nurse observe?
    a. Medication toxicities
    b. Failure to thrive
    c. Weight gain
    d. Mental confusion
21. A nurse on a medical-surgical unit is planning to administer an antibiotic to a patient with a kidney infection who is 10 weeks' pregnant. The drug reference states that the medication is teratogenic. Which action will the nurse take?
    a. Administer the medication, because the risk of illness is greater than the benefit of the medication.
    b. Hold the medication and collaborate with the health care provider to find an alternative.
    c. Ask the patient if they consent to receive the medication and document the response in the electronic health record.
    d. Collaborate with the pharmacist on dose reduction.
22. At 8 AM, a nurse receives a prescription for an analgesic to be administered every 4 hours PRN. The nurse plans to administer this medication at what times?
    a. 0800, 1200, 1600, 2000, 0000, 0400 hours
    b. Around the clock on even hours
    c. Six times daily
    d. Upon patient request, within prescribed time intervals

ANSWERS WITH RATIONALES

1. **c.** If a patient vomits immediately after swallowing an oral pill, the nurse should assess the emesis (vomit) for the pill or fragments of it. The nurse will collaborate with the health care provider to determine if another dose should be administered.

2. **c.** The nurse should use the Z-track technique for intramuscular injections to prevent medication from leaking into the needle track, minimizing discomfort. The nurse should select a needle of the smallest gauge that is appropriate for the site and solution to be injected, and select the correct needle length for the type of injection and patient size. The nurse should inject the medication into relaxed muscles since more pressure (causing discomfort) will be required to injected into contracted muscles. The nurse should apply gentle pressure after injection, unless this technique is contraindicated.
3. **a, b, d, f.** Nurses are responsible for applying pharmacologic knowledge during medication administration, including varied responses in patients from different ethnic groups (ethnopharmacology). The patient's expectations of the medication may affect the response to the medication; for example, when a placebo is given and a patient has a therapeutic effect. Environment may also influence the patient's response to medications; for example, sensory deprivation and overload may affect drug responses. Circadian rhythms and cycles may also influence drug action. The liver is the primary organ for drug breakdown, thus pathologic conditions that involve the liver may slow metabolism and alter the dosage of the drug needed to reach a therapeutic level. The presence of food in the stomach can delay the absorption of orally administered medications. Alternatively, some medications should be given with food to prevent gastric irritation, which the nurse should consider when establishing a patient's medication schedule. Other medications may have enhanced absorption if taken with certain foods.
4. **a.** The nurse should ask the patient to state their name and birthdate based on facility policy. A sign over the patient's bed may not be current or correct. The roommate is an unsafe source of information. The patient may not hear their name or may reply in the affirmative regardless of accuracy (e.g., a person with a hearing deficit).
5. **c, d, f.** The nurse should use the facility policy for checking tube placement prior to administering medications. The nurse should also give each medication separately and flush with water between each drug, adjusting the amount of water used if fluids are restricted. Enteric-coated medications should not be crushed, the tube should be flushed with 15 to 30 mL of water, and the head of the bed should be elevated to prevent reflux and aspiration.
6. **d.** Many prefilled medication cartridges are overfilled, requiring some medication to be discarded to prevent adverse effects. Always check correct dose compared to the volume in the syringe for accuracy. As this is a prefilled syringe, it is not necessary to call the pharmacy or refuse to give the medication. Wasting narcotics typically requires a second RN to witness the waste and verify the amount of narcotic discarded.
7. **b.** Regular or short-acting insulin (unmodified insulin) should never be contaminated with NPH or any insulin modified with added protein. Placing air in the NPH vial first without allowing the needle to contact the solution ensures that the regular insulin will not be contaminated.
8. **c.** When giving heparin subcutaneously, the nurse should not aspirate or massage, so as not to cause trauma or bleeding in the tissues.
9. **c.** The nurse's first responsibility is the patient—careful observation is necessary to assess for adverse effects of the medication error. The other nursing actions are pertinent but only after evaluating the patient's welfare.
10. **a, c, e.** The correct procedure for using a meter-dosed inhaler is: Shake the inhaler well and remove the mouthpiece cover; breathe normally through the spacer; depress the canister releasing one puff into the spacer and inhale slowly and deeply; after inhaling, hold breath for 5 to 10 seconds, or as long as possible, and then exhale slowly through pursed lips; wait 1 to 5 minutes as prescribed before administering the next puff; and gargle and rinse with tap water after using the MDI.
11. **c.** The nurse should first assess the patient's concern about the medication and provide education, if needed. If an allergy is the cause, the nurse should withhold the medication and notify the health care provider. Encouraging or manipulating a patient to take a pill undermines the patient's trust, especially if an adverse reaction occurs.
12. **a.** Medication reconciliation has been shown to decrease the incidence of medication errors that occur at points of transition in patient care. This process maintains a current, accurate list of medications a patient has received. Morning care can be delayed, if not yet given. Obtaining the patient's meal can be delegated to another person on the unit (e.g., AP). A report must be taken prior to accepting the patient for transfer.
13. **a.** Hang the piggyback container on the IV pole, positioning it higher than the primary IV bag. When infusing by gravity, the primary IV fluid container must be lowered. Closing the roller clamp to the secondary line will impede flow of the piggybacked medication.
14. **a.** Enoxaparin should be administered in the alternating "left and right anterolateral and left and right posterolateral abdominal wall[s]." Air, inserted by the manufacturer, should not be expelled prior to use. As this is a low–molecular-weight heparin, do not massage the area to prevent bruising. Recapping any syringe places the nurse at risk for needlestick injury and is not recommended.
15. **c.** Older adults may have difficulty swallowing medications and may find it easier to take their medications when crushed or given in liquid form. Combine the crushed medication with a small amount of soft food, such as applesauce or pudding; 120 mL or a bowl of pudding is a large amount; should the patient not finish all the food, an accurate assessment of medication taken cannot be assessed. Only medications designated as chewable can be used in this way.
16. **b.** Drugs with extensive or variable first-pass effects, such as nitroglycerin, are not given orally because most of the drug would be destroyed by the liver, with little or no drug left to work in the body. Sublingual medications should not be swallowed, but rather held in place so that complete absorption can occur. Before administering a sublingual or buccal drug, offer the patient water (if permitted) or oral care (if NPO). Placing a tablet between the cheek and gum is consistent with the buccal route of administration, not sublingual. Enteric-coated tablets are designed to dissolve after passing through the stomach.
17. **c.** Drug doses for children are calculated by weight in kilograms or BSA. The weight is needed for the provider to write the prescription.

18. **c.** For children ages 3 years and younger, the nurse teaches the parent or caregiver to pull the pinna down and back to straighten the auditory canal, then instill the medication. For adults, the pinna is pulled up and back; for school-age children, the pinna is pulled straight back. The nurse does not insert cotton swabs in the ear; rather, the nurse can wipe the external ear of drainage, if necessary.
19. **b.** The nurse is responsible for safe medication administration, including interpreting therapeutic serum drug levels. The nurse withholds the medication based on the toxic (high) drug level. Next, the nurse collaborates with the health care provider to determine if a dose adjustment is indicated. Prescribing is outside the nurse's scope of practice; determining a half dose is needed is a prescription. The patient's renal function will be evaluated periodically, but it is most important not to give a medication when the blood level demonstrates toxicity.
20. **a.** Lowered protein levels in the body means less drug bound to plasma proteins, which leads to a higher concentration of free (unbound) drug in the body. This higher drug concentration increases the risk for adverse effects.
21. **b.** Medications that are identified as teratogenic have the potential to cause developmental defects in the embryo or fetus and are contraindicated. The nurse must hold the medication and notify the health care provider of the pregnant person's pregnancy status. The patient is not the best person to determine the impact of this medication on the fetus; the medication is a teratogen, even with dose reduction.
22. **d.** When administering PRN medication, the patient receives medication when it is requested or required, and when the clinical parameters of the order, including timing between doses, are met. PRN orders are commonly written for the treatment of symptoms, in this instance, pain.

MEDICATION CALCULATION PROBLEMS

1. Metoprolol 25 mg PO is prescribed. Metoprolol is available as 50-mg tablets. How many tablets would the nurse administer?
2. Phenytoin 100 mg PO is prescribed to be given through a nasogastric tube. Phenytoin is available as 30 mg/5 mL. How much would the nurse administer?
3. Captopril 12.5 mg PO is prescribed. Captopril is available as 25-mg tablets. How many tablets would the nurse administer?
4. Potassium chloride, 20 mEq, is prescribed. Potassium chloride is available as 10 mEq per tablet. How many tablets would the nurse administer?
5. Digoxin 0.0625 mg PO is prescribed. Digoxin is available as 0.125-mg tablets. How many tablets would the nurse administer?
6. Propantheline bromide 15 mg is prescribed. Propantheline bromide is available as 7.5-mg tablets. How many tablets would the nurse administer?
7. Ciprofloxacin 500 mg PO is prescribed. Ciprofloxacin is available as 250-mg tablets. How many tablets would the nurse administer?
8. Heparin bolus of 65 units/kg IV × 1 now is prescribed. The patient weighs 220 lb. Heparin is available in 10,000 units/mL vials. How many mL would the nurse administer?
9. Theophylline elixir 100 mg PO is prescribed by way of a percutaneous endoscopic gastrostomy tube. Theophylline elixir is available as 80 mg/15 mL. How much would the nurse administer?
10. Clonidine 0.1 mg PO is prescribed. Clonidine is available as 0.2-mg tablets. How many tablets would the nurse administer?
11. Vitamin K 10 mg given IM is prescribed. Vitamin K is available as 5 mg/mL. How much would the nurse administer?
12. Morphine sulfate 10 mg IV is prescribed. Morphine is available as 4 mg/mL. How much would the nurse administer?
13. Midazolam 3 mg IM is prescribed. Midazolam is available as 5 mg/mL. How much would the nurse administer?
14. Ondansetron 0.15 mg/kg is prescribed. Ondansetron is available as 2 mg/mL. The patient weighs 30 kg. How much would the nurse administer?
15. Epoetin alfa 2,000 units SC is prescribed. Epoetin alfa is available in 4,000 units/mL. How much would the nurse administer?
16. Methylprednisolone 40 mg IV is prescribed every 8 hours. Methylprednisolone is available 125 mg/2 mL. How many mL would the nurse administer?
17. Octreotide acetate 50 mcg SC is prescribed. Octreotide is available as 100 mcg/mL. How much would the nurse administer?
18. Lisinopril 40 mg once a day is prescribed. Lisinopril is available as an oral solution 8 mg/mL. How much should the nurse administer via the enteral feeding tube?
19. Prochlorperazine 7.5 mg IM is prescribed. Prochlorperazine is available as 5 mg/mL. How much would the nurse administer?
20. Glycopyrrolate 0.4 mg IM is prescribed. Glycopyrrolate is available as 200 mcg/mL. How much would the nurse administer?
21. Gentamycin 80 mg in 100 mL IV is prescribed. The administration set delivers 10 gtt/mL. If the medication runs over 30 minutes, how many drops per minute (gtt/min) should the nurse administer?
22. The IV fluid 0.9% Sodium Chloride is prescribed to run continuously at 75 mL/hr. The administration set delivers 10 gtt/mL. How many drops per minute (gtt/min) should the nurse administer?

ANSWERS TO MEDICATION CALCULATION PROBLEMS

FORMULA METHOD ("Desire over have")	FORMULA METHOD (Proportions)	DIMENSIONAL ANALYSIS (Chemistry)
$\frac{\text{dose desired}}{\text{(quantity desired)}} \times \text{quantity on hand} = \text{desired quantity}$ ***Need to make sure to multiply by the quantity on hand, even if that quantity is one (1)*	$\frac{\text{dose on hand}}{\text{quantity on hand}} = \frac{\text{dose desired}}{x\ \text{(quantity desired)}}$ ***Need to make sure that dosages are in both numerators and quantities are in the denominators*	What you are solving for = dose desired × dose available ***This formula may also include conversions as needed. The goal is to rely on the mathematical principles associated with multiplying fractions.*
LEAST PREFERABLE…BUT ALIGNS WITH MENTAL MATH	PREFERRED FOR SIMPLE CALCULATIONS	RECOMMENDED FOR SIMPLE AND COMPLEX CALCULATIONS OR WHERE CONVERSIONS ARE REQUIRED
NUMBER 1		
$\frac{25\text{ mg}}{50\text{ mg}} \times 1\text{ tablet} = x$ $\frac{25\ \cancel{\text{mg}}}{50\ \cancel{\text{mg}}} \times 1\text{ tablet} = 0.5 \text{ or } \frac{1}{2}\text{ tablet}$	$\frac{50\text{ mg}}{1\text{ tablet}} = \frac{25\text{ mg}}{x\text{ (tablet)}}$ $50x = 25$ $\frac{50x}{50} = \frac{25}{50}$ $x = 0.5 \text{ or } \frac{1}{2}\text{ tablet}$	$\text{tablet} = \frac{1\text{ tablet}}{50\text{ mg}} \times \frac{25\text{ mg}}{1}$ $\text{tablet} = \frac{1\text{ tablet}}{\cancel{50}^{2}\ \cancel{\text{mg}}} \times \frac{\cancel{25}^{1}\ \cancel{\text{mg}}}{1} = 0.5 \text{ or } \frac{1}{2}\text{ tablet}$
NUMBER 2		
$\frac{100\text{ mg}}{30\text{ mg}} \times 5\text{ mL} = x$ $\frac{100\ \cancel{\text{mg}}}{30\ \cancel{\text{mg}}} \times 5\text{ mL} = 16.6\overline{6} = 16.7\text{ mL}$	$\frac{30\text{ mg}}{5\text{ mL}} = \frac{100\text{ mg}}{x\text{ (mL)}}$ $30x = 500$ $\frac{30x}{30} = \frac{500}{30}$ $x = 16.6\overline{6} = 16.7\text{ mL}$	$\text{mL} = \frac{5\text{ mL}}{30\text{ mg}} \times \frac{100\text{ mg}}{1}$ $\text{mL} = \frac{5\text{ mL}}{30\ \cancel{\text{mg}}} \times \frac{100\ \cancel{\text{mg}}}{1} = 16.6\overline{6} = 16.7\text{ mL}$
**Follow the standard rounding rules: For numbers > 1, round to the 10th (tenth); for numbers < 1, round to the 100th (hundredth).		
NUMBER 3		
$\frac{12.5\text{ mg}}{25\text{ mg}} \times 1\text{ tablet} = x$ $\frac{12.5\ \cancel{\text{mg}}}{25\ \cancel{\text{mg}}} \times 1\text{ tablet} = 0.5 \text{ or } \frac{1}{2}\text{ tablet}$	$\frac{25\text{ mg}}{1\text{ tablet}} = \frac{12.5\text{ mg}}{x\text{ (tablet)}}$ $25x = 12.5$ $\frac{25x}{25} = \frac{12.5}{25}$ $x = 0.5 \text{ or } \frac{1}{2}\text{ tablet}$	$\text{tablet} = \frac{1\text{ tablet}}{25\text{ mg}} \times \frac{12.5\text{ mg}}{1}$ $\text{tablet} = \frac{1\text{ tablet}}{\cancel{25}^{2}\ \cancel{\text{mg}}} \times \frac{\cancel{12.5}^{1}\ \cancel{\text{mg}}}{1} = 0.5 \text{ or } \frac{1}{2}\text{ tablet}$

(continued)

ANSWERS TO MEDICATION CALCULATION PROBLEMS *(continued)*

FORMULA METHOD ("Desire over have")	FORMULA METHOD (Proportions)	DIMENSIONAL ANALYSIS (Chemistry)
$\frac{\text{dose desired}}{\text{(quantity desired)}} \times \text{quantity on hand} = \text{desired quantity}$ ***Need to make sure to multiply by the quantity on hand, even if that quantity is one (1)*	$\frac{\text{dose on hand}}{\text{quantity on hand}} = \frac{\text{dose desired}}{x \text{ (quantity desired)}}$ ***Need to make sure that dosages are in both numerators and quantities are in the denominators*	What you are solving for = dose desired × dose available ***This formula may also include conversions as needed. The goal is to rely on the mathematical principles associated with multiplying fractions.*
NUMBER 4		
$\frac{20\text{ mEq}}{10\text{ mEq}} \times 1\text{ tablet} = x$ $\frac{20\text{ m}\cancel{\text{Eq}}}{10\text{ m}\cancel{\text{Eq}}} \times 1\text{ tablet} = 2\text{ tablets}$	$\frac{10\text{ mEq}}{1\text{ tablet}} = \frac{20\text{ mEq}}{x\text{ (tablet)}}$ $10x = 20$ $\frac{10x}{10} = \frac{20}{10}$ $x = 2$ tablets	$\text{tablet} = \frac{1\text{ tablet}}{10\text{ mEq}} \times \frac{20\text{ mEq}}{1}$ $\text{tablet} = \frac{1\text{ tablet}}{\cancel{10}_1\ \cancel{\text{mEq}}} \times \frac{\cancel{20}^2\ \cancel{\text{mEq}}}{1} = 2\text{ tablets}$
NUMBER 5		
$\frac{0.0625\text{ mg}}{0.125\text{ mg}} \times 1\text{ tablet} = x$ $\frac{0.0625\ \cancel{\text{mg}}}{0.125\ \cancel{\text{mg}}} \times 1\text{ tablet} = 0.5$ or ½ tablet	$\frac{0.125\text{ mg}}{1\text{ tablet}} = \frac{0.0625\text{ mg}}{x\text{ (tablet)}}$ $0.125x = 0.0625$ $\frac{0.125x}{0.125} = \frac{0.0625}{0.125}$ $x = 0.5$ or ½ tablet	$\text{tablet} = \frac{1\text{ tablet}}{0.125\text{ mg}} \times \frac{0.0625\text{ mg}}{1}$ $\text{tablet} = \frac{1\text{ tablet}}{0.125\ \cancel{\text{mg}}} \times \frac{0.0625\ \cancel{\text{mg}}}{1} = 0.5$ or ½ tablet
NUMBER 6		
$\frac{15\text{ mg}}{7.5\text{ mg}} \times 1\text{ tablet} = x$ $\frac{15\text{ mg}}{7.5\text{ mg}} \times 1\text{ tablet} = 2\text{ tablets}$	$\frac{7.5\text{ mg}}{1\text{ tablet}} = \frac{15\text{ mg}}{x\text{ (tablet)}}$ $7.5x = 15$ $\frac{7.5x}{7.5} = \frac{15}{7.5}$ $x = 2$ tablets	$\text{tablet} = \frac{1\text{ tablet}}{7.5\text{ mg}} \times \frac{15\text{ mg}}{1}$ $\text{tablet} = \frac{1\text{ tablet}}{\cancel{7.5}_1\ \cancel{\text{mg}}} \times \frac{\cancel{15}^2\ \cancel{\text{mg}}}{1} = 2\text{ tablets}$
NUMBER 7		
$\frac{500\text{ mg}}{250\text{ mg}} \times 1\text{ tablet} = x$ $\frac{500\ \cancel{\text{mg}}}{250\ \cancel{\text{mg}}} \times 1\text{ tablet} = 2\text{ tablets}$	$\frac{250\text{ mg}}{1\text{ tablet}} = \frac{500\text{ mg}}{x\text{ (tablet)}}$ $250x = 500$ $\frac{250x}{250} = \frac{500}{250}$ $x = 2$ tablets	$\text{tablet} = \frac{1\text{ tablet}}{250\text{ mg}} \times \frac{500\text{ mg}}{1}$ $\text{tablet} = \frac{1\text{ tablet}}{\cancel{250}_1\ \cancel{\text{mg}}} \times \frac{\cancel{500}^2\ \cancel{\text{mg}}}{1} = 2\text{ tablets}$

FORMULA METHOD ("Desire over have")	FORMULA METHOD (Proportions)	DIMENSIONAL ANALYSIS (Chemistry)
$\frac{\text{dose desired}}{\text{(quantity desired)}} \times$ quantity on hand = desired quantity ***Need to make sure to multiply by the quantity on hand, even if that quantity is one (1)*	$\frac{\text{dose on hand}}{\text{quantity on hand}} = \frac{\text{dose desired}}{x\text{ (quantity desired)}}$ ***Need to make sure that dosages are in both numerators and quantities are in the denominators*	What you are solving for = dose desired × dose available ***This formula may also include conversions as needed. The goal is to rely on the mathematical principles associated with multiplying fractions.*
NUMBER 8		
Step one – Convert: 220 lb ÷ 2.2 lb/kg $220\ \cancel{\text{lb}} \div 2.2\ \cancel{\text{lb}}\text{/kg} = 100\text{ kg}$ Step two – Determine Dose: $65\text{ units/}\cancel{\text{kg}} \times 100\ \cancel{\text{kg}} = 6{,}500\text{ units}$ Step three – Calculate: $\frac{6{,}500\text{ units}}{10{,}000\text{ units}} \times 1\text{ mL} = x$ $\frac{6{,}500\ \cancel{\text{units}}}{10{,}000\ \cancel{\text{units}}} \times 1\text{ mL} = 0.65\text{ mL}$	Step one – Convert: $\frac{2.2\text{ lb}}{1\text{ kg}} = \frac{220\text{ lb}}{x\text{ (kg)}}$ $2.2x = 220$ $\frac{2.2x}{2.2} = \frac{220}{2.2}$ $x = 100\text{ kg}$ Step two – Determine Dose: $\frac{1\text{ kg}}{65\text{ units}} = \frac{100\text{ kg}}{x\text{ units}}$ $x = 6{,}500\text{ units}$ Step three – Calculate: $\frac{10{,}000\text{ units}}{1\text{ mL}} = \frac{6{,}500\text{ units}}{x\text{ (mL)}}$ $10{,}000x = 6{,}500\text{ units}$ $\frac{10{,}000x}{10{,}000} = \frac{6{,}500}{1}$ $x = 0.65\text{ mL}$	$\text{mL} = \frac{1\text{ mL}}{10{,}000\text{ units}} \times \frac{65\text{ units/kg}}{1} \times \frac{220\text{ lb}}{1} \times \frac{1\text{ kg}}{2.2\text{ lb}}$ $\text{mL} = \frac{1\text{ mL}}{10{,}000\ \cancel{\text{units}}} \times \frac{65\ \cancel{\text{units}}/\cancel{\text{kg}}}{1} \times \frac{220\ \cancel{\text{lb}}}{1} \times \frac{1\ \cancel{\text{kg}}}{2.2\ \cancel{\text{lb}}}$ $= \frac{6{,}500}{10{,}000} = 0.65\text{ mL}$
**Follow the standard rounding rules: For numbers >1, round to the 10th (tenth); for numbers <1, round to the 100th (hundredth).		
NUMBER 9		
$\frac{100\text{ mg}}{80\text{ mg}} \times 15\text{ mL} = x$ $\frac{100\ \cancel{\text{mg}}}{80\ \cancel{\text{mg}}} \times 15 = 18.75 = 18.8\text{ mL}$	$\frac{80\text{ mg}}{15\text{ mL}} = \frac{100\text{ mg}}{x\text{ (mL)}}$ $80x = 1{,}500$ $\frac{80x}{80} = \frac{1{,}500}{80}$ $x = 18.7 = 18.8\text{ mL}$	$\text{mL} = \frac{15\text{ mL}}{80\text{ mg}} \times \frac{100\text{ mg}}{1}$ $\text{mL} = \frac{15\text{ mL}}{80\ \cancel{\text{mg}}} \times \frac{100\ \cancel{\text{mg}}}{1} = 18.75 = 18.8\text{ mL}$
**Follow the standard rounding rules: For numbers >1, round to the 10th (tenth); for numbers <1, round to the 100th (hundredth).		

(*continued*)

ANSWERS TO MEDICATION CALCULATION PROBLEMS *(continued)*

FORMULA METHOD ("Desire over have")	FORMULA METHOD (Proportions)	DIMENSIONAL ANALYSIS (Chemistry)
$\frac{\text{dose desired}}{\text{(quantity desired)}} \times \text{quantity on hand} = \text{desired quantity}$ ***Need to make sure to multiply by the quantity on hand, even if that quantity is one (1)*	$\frac{\text{dose on hand}}{\text{quantity on hand}} = \frac{\text{dose desired}}{x\ \text{(quantity desired)}}$ ***Need to make sure that dosages are in both numerators and quantities are in the denominators*	What you are solving for = dose desired × dose available ***This formula may also include conversions as needed. The goal is to rely on the mathematical principles associated with multiplying fractions.*
NUMBER 10		
$\frac{0.1\text{ mg}}{0.2\text{ mg}} \times 1\text{ tablet} = x$ $\frac{0.1\cancel{\text{ mg}}}{0.2\cancel{\text{ mg}}} \times 1\text{ tablet} = 0.5$ or ½ tablet	$\frac{0.2\text{ mg}}{1\text{ tablet}} = \frac{0.1\text{ mg}}{x\text{ (tablet)}}$ $0.2x = 0.1$ $\frac{0.2x}{0.2} = \frac{0.1}{0.2}$ $x = 0.5$ or ½ tablet	$\text{tablet} = \frac{1\text{ tablet}}{0.2\text{ mg}} \times \frac{0.1\text{ mg}}{1}$ $\text{tablet} = \frac{1\text{ tablet}}{0.2\cancel{\text{ mg}}} \times \frac{0.1\cancel{\text{ mg}}}{1} = 0.5$ or ½ tablet
NUMBER 11		
$\frac{10\text{ mg}}{5\text{ mg}} \times 1\text{ mL} = x$ $\frac{10\cancel{\text{ mg}}}{5\cancel{\text{ mg}}} \times 1\text{ mL} = 2\text{ mL}$	$\frac{5\text{ mg}}{1\text{ mL}} = \frac{10\text{ mg}}{x\text{ (mL)}}$ $5x = 10$ $\frac{5x}{5} = \frac{10}{5}$ $x = 2\text{ mL}$	$\text{mL} = \frac{1\text{ mL}}{5\text{ mg}} \times \frac{10\text{ mg}}{1}$ $\text{mL} = \frac{1\text{ mL}}{\cancel{5}_{1}\cancel{\text{ mg}}} \times \frac{\cancel{10}^{2}\cancel{\text{ mg}}}{1} = 2\text{ mL}$
NUMBER 12		
$\frac{10\text{ mg}}{4\text{ mg}} \times 1\text{ mL} = x$ $\frac{10\cancel{\text{ mg}}}{4\cancel{\text{ mg}}} \times 1\text{ mL} = 2.5\text{ mL}$	$\frac{4\text{ mg}}{1\text{ mL}} = \frac{10\text{ mg}}{x\text{ (mL)}}$ $4x = 10$ $\frac{4x}{4} = \frac{10}{4}$ $x = 2.5\text{ mL}$	$\text{mL} = \frac{1\text{ mL}}{4\text{ mg}} \times \frac{10\text{ mg}}{1}$ $\text{mL} = \frac{1\text{ mL}}{4\cancel{\text{ mg}}} \times \frac{10\cancel{\text{ mg}}}{1} = 2.5\text{ mL}$
**Follow the standard rounding rules: For numbers >1, round to the 10th (tenth); for numbers <1, round to the 100th (hundredth).		
NUMBER 13		
$\frac{3\text{ mg}}{5\text{ mg}} \times 1\text{ mL} = x$ $\frac{3\cancel{\text{ mg}}}{5\cancel{\text{ mg}}} \times 1\text{ mL} = 0.6\text{ mL}$	$\frac{5\text{ mg}}{1\text{ mL}} = \frac{3\text{ mg}}{x\text{ (mL)}}$ $5x = 3$ $\frac{5x}{5} = \frac{3}{5}$ $x = 0.6\text{ mL}$	$\text{mL} = \frac{1\text{ mL}}{5\text{ mg}} \times \frac{3\text{ mg}}{1}$ $\text{mL} = \frac{1\text{ mL}}{5\cancel{\text{ mg}}} \times \frac{3\cancel{\text{ mg}}}{1} = 0.6\text{ mL}$

FORMULA METHOD ("Desire over have")	FORMULA METHOD (Proportions)	DIMENSIONAL ANALYSIS (Chemistry)
$\frac{\text{dose desired}}{\text{(quantity desired)}} \times \text{quantity on hand} = \text{desired quantity}$ ***Need to make sure to multiply by the quantity on hand, even if that quantity is one (1)*	$\frac{\text{dose on hand}}{\text{quantity on hand}} = \frac{\text{dose desired}}{x\text{ (quantity desired)}}$ ***Need to make sure that dosages are in both numerators and quantities are in the denominators*	What you are solving for = dose desired × dose available ***This formula may also include conversions as needed. The goal is to rely on the mathematical principles associated with multiplying fractions.*
NUMBER 14		
Step one – Determine Dose: $0.15\text{ mg}/\cancel{\text{kg}} \times 30\cancel{\text{kg}} = 4.5\text{ mg}$ Step two – Calculate: $\frac{4.5\text{ mg}}{2\text{ mg}} \times 1\text{ mL} = x$ $\frac{4.5\cancel{\text{ mg}}}{2\cancel{\text{ mg}}} \times 1\text{ mL} = 2.25 = 2.3\text{ mL}$	Step one – Determine Dose: $\frac{1\text{ kg}}{0.15\text{ mg}} = \frac{30\text{ kg}}{x\text{ mg}}$ $x = 4.5\text{ mg}$ Step two – Calculate: $\frac{2\text{ mg}}{1\text{ mL}} = \frac{4.5\text{ mg}}{x\text{(mL)}}$ $2x = 4.5$ $\frac{2x}{2} = \frac{4.5}{2}$ $x = 2.25 = 2.3\text{ mL}$	$\text{mL} = \frac{1\text{ mL}}{2\text{ mg}} \times \frac{0.15\text{ mg/kg}}{1} \times \frac{30\text{ kg}}{1}$ $\text{mL} = \frac{1\text{ mL}}{2\cancel{\text{ mg}}} \times \frac{0.15\cancel{\text{ mg}}/\cancel{\text{kg}}}{1} \times \frac{30\cancel{\text{ kg}}}{1} = 2.25 = 2.3\text{ mL}$
**Follow the standard rounding rules: For numbers >1, round to the 10th (tenth); for numbers <1, round to the 100th (hundredth).		
NUMBER 15		
$\frac{2{,}000\text{ units}}{4{,}000\text{ units}} \times 1\text{ mL} = x$ $\frac{2{,}000\cancel{\text{ units}}}{4{,}000\cancel{\text{ units}}} \times 1\text{ mL} = 0.5\text{ or }\frac{1}{2}\text{ mL}$	$\frac{4{,}000\text{ units}}{1\text{ mL}} = \frac{2{,}000\text{ units}}{x\text{(mL)}}$ $4{,}000x = 2{,}000$ $\frac{4{,}000x}{4{,}000} = \frac{2{,}000}{4{,}000}$ $x = 0.5\text{ or }\frac{1}{2}\text{ mL}$	$\text{mL} = \frac{1\text{ mL}}{4{,}000\text{ units}} \times \frac{2{,}000\text{ units}}{1}$ $\text{mL} = \frac{1\text{ mL}}{\cancel{4{,}000}_{2}\cancel{\text{ units}}} \times \frac{\cancel{2{,}000}^{1}\cancel{\text{ units}}}{1} = 0.5\text{ or }\frac{1}{2}\text{ mL}$
NUMBER 16		
$\frac{40\text{ mg}}{125\text{ mg}} \times 2\text{ mL} = x$ $\frac{40\cancel{\text{ mg}}}{125\cancel{\text{ mg}}} \times 2\text{ mL} = 0.64\text{ mL}$	$\frac{125\text{ mg}}{2\text{ mL}} = \frac{40\text{ mg}}{x\text{(mL)}}$ $125x = 80$ $\frac{125x}{125} = \frac{80}{125}$ $x = 0.64\text{ mL}$	$\text{mL} = \frac{2\text{ mL}}{125\text{ mg}} \times \frac{40\text{ mg}}{1}$ $\text{mL} = \frac{2\text{ mL}}{125\cancel{\text{ mg}}} \times \frac{40\cancel{\text{ mg}}}{1} = 0.64\text{ mL}$
**Follow the standard rounding rules: For numbers >1, round to the 10th (tenth); for numbers <1, round to the 100th (hundredth). **For numbers >1, round to the 10th (tenth); for numbers <1, round to the 100th (hundredth).		

(*continued*)

ANSWERS TO MEDICATION CALCULATION PROBLEMS *(continued)*

FORMULA METHOD ("Desire over have")	FORMULA METHOD (Proportions)	DIMENSIONAL ANALYSIS (Chemistry)
$\frac{\text{dose desired}}{\text{(quantity desired)}} \times$ quantity on hand = desired quantity ***Need to make sure to multiply by the quantity on hand, even if that quantity is one (1)*	$\frac{\text{dose on hand}}{\text{quantity on hand}} = \frac{\text{dose desired}}{x\text{ (quantity desired)}}$ ***Need to make sure that dosages are in both numerators and quantities are in the denominators*	What you are solving for = dose desired × dose available ***This formula may also include conversions as needed. The goal is to rely on the mathematical principles associated with multiplying fractions.*
NUMBER 17		
$\frac{50\text{ mcg}}{100\text{ mcg}} \times 1\text{ mL} = x$ $\frac{50\text{ }\cancel{\text{mcg}}}{100\text{ }\cancel{\text{mcg}}} \times 1\text{ mL} = 0.5$ or ½ mL	$\frac{100\text{ mcg}}{1\text{ mL}} = \frac{50\text{ mcg}}{x\text{(mL)}}$ $100x = 50$ $\frac{100x}{100} = \frac{50}{100}$ $x = 0.5$ or ½ mL	$\text{mL} = \frac{1\text{ mL}}{100\text{ mcg}} \times \frac{50\text{ mcg}}{1}$ $\text{mL} = \frac{1\text{ mL}}{\cancel{100}_{2}\text{ mcg}} \times \frac{\cancel{50}^{1}\text{ }\cancel{\text{mcg}}}{1} = 0.5$ or ½ mL
NUMBER 18		
$\frac{40\text{ mg}}{8\text{ mg}} \times 1\text{ mL} = x$ $\frac{40\text{ }\cancel{\text{mg}}}{8\text{ }\cancel{\text{mg}}} \times 1\text{ mL} = 5\text{ mL}$	$\frac{8\text{ mg}}{1\text{ mL}} = \frac{40\text{ mg}}{x\text{(mL)}}$ $8x = 40$ $\frac{8x}{8} = \frac{40}{8}$ $x = 5\text{ mL}$	$\text{mL} = \frac{1\text{ mL}}{8\text{ mg}} \times \frac{40\text{ mg}}{1}$ $\text{mL} = \frac{1\text{ mL}}{\cancel{8}_{1}\text{ }\cancel{\text{mg}}} \times \frac{\cancel{40}^{5}\text{ }\cancel{\text{mg}}}{1} = 5\text{ mL}$
NUMBER 19		
$\frac{7.5\text{ mg}}{5\text{ mg}} \times 1\text{ mL} = x$ $\frac{7.5\text{ }\cancel{\text{mg}}}{5\text{ }\cancel{\text{mg}}} \times 1\text{ mL} = 1.5\text{ mL}$	$\frac{5\text{ mg}}{1\text{ mL}} = \frac{7.5\text{ mg}}{x\text{(mL)}}$ $5x = 7.5$ $\frac{5x}{5} = \frac{7.5}{5}$ $x = 1.5\text{ mL}$	$\text{mL} = \frac{1\text{ mL}}{5\text{ mg}} \times \frac{7.5\text{ mg}}{1}$ $\text{mL} = \frac{1\text{ mL}}{5\text{ }\cancel{\text{mg}}} \times \frac{7.5\text{ }\cancel{\text{mg}}}{1} = 1.5\text{ mL}$

**For numbers >1, round to the 10th (tenth); for numbers <1, round to the 100th (hundredth).

FORMULA METHOD ("Desire over have")	FORMULA METHOD (Proportions)	DIMENSIONAL ANALYSIS (Chemistry)
$\frac{\text{dose desired}}{\text{(quantity desired)}} \times$ quantity on hand = desired quantity ***Need to make sure to multiply by the quantity on hand, even if that quantity is one (1)*	$\frac{\text{dose on hand}}{\text{quantity on hand}} = \frac{\text{dose desired}}{x\text{ (quantity desired)}}$ ***Need to make sure that dosages are in both numerators and quantities are in the denominators*	What you are solving for = dose desired × dose available ***This formula may also include conversions as needed. The goal is to rely on the mathematical principles associated with multiplying fractions.*
NUMBER 20		
Step one – Convert: 200 mcg = 200 mcg (÷1,000) = 0.2 mg Step two – Calculate: $\frac{0.4\text{ mg}}{0.2\text{ mg}} \times 1\text{ mL} = x$ $\frac{0.4\text{ }\cancel{\text{mg}}}{0.2\text{ }\cancel{\text{mg}}} \times 1\text{ mL} = 2\text{ mL}$	Step one – Convert: $\frac{1{,}000\text{ mcg}}{1\text{ mg}} = \frac{200\text{ mcg}}{x\text{(mg)}}$ $1{,}000x = 200$ $\frac{1{,}000x}{1{,}000} = \frac{200}{1{,}000}$ $x = 0.2\text{ mg}$ Step two – Calculate: $\frac{0.2\text{ mg}}{1\text{ mL}} = \frac{0.4\text{ mg}}{x\text{(mL)}}$ $0.2x = 0.4$ $\frac{0.2x}{0.2} = \frac{0.4}{0.2}$ $x = 2\text{ mL}$	$\text{mL} = \frac{1\text{ mL}}{200\text{ mcg}} \times \frac{0.4\text{ mg}}{1} \times \frac{1{,}000\text{ mcg}}{1\text{ mg}}$ $\text{mL} = \frac{1\text{ mL}}{200\text{ }\cancel{\text{mcg}}} \times \frac{0.4\text{ }\cancel{\text{mg}}}{1} \times \frac{1{,}000\text{ }\cancel{\text{mcg}}}{1\text{ }\cancel{\text{mg}}} = 2\text{ mL}$
OR	OR	
Step one – Convert: 0.4 mg = 0.400 (×1,000) = 400 mcg Step two – Calculate: $\frac{400\text{ mcg}}{200\text{ mcg}} \times 1\text{ mL} = x$ $\frac{400\text{ }\cancel{\text{mcg}}}{200\text{ }\cancel{\text{mcg}}} \times 1\text{ mL} = 2\text{ mL}$	Step one – Convert: $\frac{1\text{ mg}}{1{,}000\text{ mcg}} = \frac{0.4\text{ mg}}{x\text{ mcg}}$ $x = 400\text{ mcg}$ Step two – Calculate: $\frac{200\text{ mcg}}{1\text{ mL}} = \frac{400\text{ mcg}}{x\text{(mL)}}$ $200x = 400$ $\frac{200x}{200} = \frac{400}{200}$ $x = 2\text{ mL}$	

(continued)

ANSWERS TO MEDICATION CALCULATION PROBLEMS *(continued)*

FORMULA METHOD ("Desire over have")	FORMULA METHOD (Proportions)	DIMENSIONAL ANALYSIS (Chemistry)
$\frac{\text{dose desired}}{\text{(quantity desired)}} \times \text{quantity on hand} = \text{desired quantity}$ ***Need to make sure to multiply by the quantity on hand, even if that quantity is one (1)*	$\frac{\text{dose on hand}}{\text{quantity on hand}} = \frac{\text{dose desired}}{x\ \text{(quantity desired)}}$ ***Need to make sure that dosages are in both numerators and quantities are in the denominators*	What you are solving for = dose desired × dose available ***This formula may also include conversions as needed. The goal is to rely on the mathematical principles associated with multiplying fractions.*
Number 21		
Drop Factor (gtt/mL) × Volume to be Infused (mL)	$\frac{10\ \text{gtt}/\cancel{\text{mL}} \times 100\ \cancel{\text{mL}}}{30\ \text{minutes}} = 33.33333 = 33\ \text{gtt/min}$	Time in Minutes (min)
**Keep in mind that we are counting actual drops in the drip chamber, so gtt/min must be rounded to the whole number—we cannot visualize a third of a drop!		
Number 22		
Drop Factor (gtt/mL) × Volume to be Infused (mL)	$\frac{10\ \text{gtt}/\cancel{\text{mL}} \times 75\ \cancel{\text{mL}}}{60\ \text{minutes}} = 12.5 = 13\ \text{gtt/min}$	Time in Minutes (min)
**Keep in mind that you must provide minutes…not hours. There are 60 minutes in an hour, so use 60 in the formula.		

Bibliography

Alismail, A., Song, C. A., Terry, M. H., Daher, N., Almutairi, W. A., & Lo, T. (2016). Diverse inhaler devices: A big challenge for health-care professionals. *Respiratory Care, 61*(5), 593–599. https://doi.org/10.4187/respcare.04293

American Academy of Pediatrics. (2015). Metric units and the preferred dosing of orally administered liquid medications. *Pediatrics 135*(4), 784–787. http://pediatrics.aappublications.org/content/pediatrics/135/4/784.full.pdf

American Association of Colleges of Nursing (AACN). (2021, April 6). *The essentials: Core competencies for professional nursing education*. https://www.aacnnursing.org/Portals/42/AcademicNursing/pdf/Essentials-2021.pdf

American Diabetes Association (ADA). (2022). *Insulin routines*. Retrieved April 29, 2022 from https://www.diabetes.org/healthy-living/medication-treatments/insulin-other-injectables/insulin-routines

American Heart Association. (2020). *2020 American Heart Association guidelines for CPR and ECC*. Retrieved February 10, 2022, from https://cpr.heart.org/en/resuscitation-science/cpr-and-ecc-guidelines

American Society of Health-System Pharmacists (ASHP). (2009). ASHP statement on bar-code-enabled medication administration technology. *American Journal of Health-System Pharmacy, 66*(6), 588–590. https://www.ashp.org/-/media/assets/policy-guidelines/docs/statements/bar-code-enabled-medication-administration-technology.ashx

Anderson, L. J., Schnipper, J. L., Nuckols, T. K., Shane, R., Le, M. M., Robbins, K., Pevnick, J. M., & Members of the PHARM-DC group. (2019). Effect of medication reconciliation interventions on outcomes: A systematic overview of systematic reviews. *American Journal of Health-System Pharmacy, 76*(24), 2028–2040. https://doi.org/10.1093/ajhp/zxz236

Arfman, I. J., Wammes-van der Heijden, E. A., Ter Horst, P. G. J., Lambrechts, D. A., Wegner, I., & Touw, D. J. (2020). Therapeutic drug monitoring of antiepileptic drugs in women with epilepsy before, during, and after pregnancy. *Clinical Pharmacokinetics, 59*(4), 427–445. https://doi.org/10.1007/s40262-019-00845-2

Arslan, G. G., & Özden, D. (2018). Creating a change in the use of ventrogluteal site for intramuscular injection. *Patient Preference & Adherence, 12*, 1749–1756. https://doi.org/10.2147/PPA.S168885

Athanasakis, E. (2019). A meta-synthesis of how registered nurses make sense of their lived experiences of medication errors. *Journal of Clinical Nursing, 28*(17-18), 3077–3095. https://doi.org/10.1111/jocn.14917

Aydon, L., Hauck, Y., Zimmer, M., & Murdoch, J. (2016). Factors influencing a nurse's decision to question medication administration in a neonatal clinical care unit. *Journal of Clinical Nursing, 25*(17–18), 2468–2477. https://doi.org/10.1111/jocn.13277

Bandy, K. S., Albrecht, S., Parag, B., & McClave, S. A. (2019). Practices involved in the enteral delivery of drugs. *Current Nutrition Reports, 8*(4), 356–362. https://doi.org/10.1007/s13668-019-00290-4

Barnsteiner, J. H. (2008, April). Medication reconciliation. In R. G. Hughes (Ed.). *Patient safety and quality: An evidence-based handbook for nurses (Chapter 38)*. Agency for Healthcare Research and Quality (US). http://www.ncbi.nlm.nih.gov/books/NBK2648

Bartlett, J. L., & Kinsey, J. D. (2020). Large-group, asynchronous, interprofessional simulation: Identifying roles and improving communication with student pharmacists and student nurses. *Currents in Pharmacy Teaching and Learning, 12*(6), 763–770. https://doi.org/10.1016/j.cptl.2020.01.023

Becton, Dickinson and Company (BD). (2020). *BD AutoShield Duo™ pen needle*. https://www.bd.com/en-us/offerings/capabilities/diabetes-care/pen-needles/bd-autoshield-duo-pen-needle

Boullata, J. I., Carrera, A. L., Harvey, L., Escuro, A. A., Hudson, L., Mays, A., McGinnis, C., Wessel, J. J., Bajpai, S., Beebe, M. L., Kinn, T. J., Klang, M. G., Lord, L., Martin, K., Pompeii-Wolfe, C., Sullivan, J., Wood, A., Malone, A., Guenter, P., & ASPEN Safe Practices for Enteral Nutrition Therapy Task Force, American Society for Parenteral and Enteral Nutrition. (2017). ASPEN safe practices for enteral nutrition therapy. *Journal of Parenteral and Enteral Nutrition, 41*(1), 15–103. https://doi.org/10.1177/0148607116673053

Bowen, J. F. (2016). Prescriptions and medication orders. In P. Agarwal (Ed.). *Pharmaceutical calculations* (pp. 17–29). Jones & Bartlett Learning, LLC, an Ascend Learning Company.

Bravo, K., Cochran, G., & Barrett, R. (2016). Nursing strategies to increase medication safety in inpatient settings. *Journal of Nursing Care Quality, 31*(4), 335–341. https://doi.org/10.1097/NCQ.0000000000000181

Brown, J., Gillespie, M., & Chard, S. (2015). The dorso-ventro debate: In search of empirical evidence. *British Journal of Nursing, 24*(22), 1132–1139. https://doi.org/10.12968/bjon.2015.24.22.1132

Bruhn, J. G., & Rivier, L. (2019). Ethnopharmacology—A journal, a definition and a society. *Journal of Ethnopharmacology, 242*, 112005. https://doi.org/10.1016/j.jep.2019.112005

Centers for Disease Control and Prevention (CDC). (2015/2020). *Epidemiology and prevention of vaccine-preventable diseases* (13th ed.). J. Hamborsky, A. Kroger, & S. Wolfe (Eds.). Public Health Foundation. http://www.cdc.gov/vaccines/pubs/pinkbook/index.html

Centers for Disease Control and Prevention (CDC). (2019, December 3). Injection safety: One & only campaign. https://www.cdc.gov/injectionsafety/one-and-only.html

Centers for Disease Control and Prevention (CDC). (2019, June 21). Vaccine recommendations and guidelines of the Advisory Committee on Immunization Practices (ACIP). https://www.cdc.gov/vaccines/hcp/acip-recs/general-recs/administration.html

Choi, Y. J., & Kim, H. (2019). Effect of pharmacy-led medication reconciliation in emergency departments: A systematic review and meta-analysis. *Journal of Clinical Pharmacy and Therapeutics, 44*(6), 932–945. https://doi.org/10.1111/jcpt.13019

The Christian Science Board of Directors. (2020). *What is Christian science?* http://christianscience.com/what-is-christian-science/beliefs-and-teachings/christian-science-brochure

Cleveland Clinic. (2020). Inhalers. http://my.clevelandclinic.org/health/articles/how-to-use-a-metered-dose-inhaler

Cottell, M., Wätterbjörk, I., & Hälleberg Nyman, M. (2020). Medication-related incidents at 19 hospitals: A retrospective register study using incident reports. *Nursing Open, 7*(5), 1526–1535. https://doi.org/10.1002/nop2.534

Dangerfield, D. T., II, Johnson, D., Hamlin-Palmer, S., Browne, D. C., Mayer, K. H., & Hickson, D. A. (2020). Prevalence and correlates of rectal douching and enema use among black sexual minority men and black transwomen in the Deep South. *Archives of Sexual Behavior, 49*(6), 1915–1922. https://doi.org/10.1007/s10508-019-01605-w

Delong C., & Preuss C. V. (2020, February 21). Black Box. *In StatPearls [Internet]*. StatPearls Publishing. https://www.ncbi.nlm.nih.gov/books/NBK538521/

Dudek, S. (2017). *Nutrition essentials for nursing practice* (8th ed.). Wolters Kluwer Health, Inc.

Fairlie, L., Waitt, C., Lockman, S., Moorhouse, M., Abrams, E. J., Clayden, P., Boffito, M., Khoo, S., Rees, H., Cournil, A., Venter, W. F., Serenata, C., & Chersich, M. (2019). Inclusion of pregnant women in antiretroviral drug research: what is needed to move forwards?. *Journal of the International AIDS Society, 22*(9), e25372. https://doi.org/10.1002/jia2.25372

Farinde, A. (2019, June). *Overview of pharmacodynamics*. In Merck manual: Professional version. https://www.merckmanuals.com/professional/clinical-pharmacology/pharmacodynamics/overview-of-pharmacodynamics?query=pharmacodynamics

Fernandes, B. D., Almeida, P. H. R. F., Foppa, A. A., Sousa, C. T., Ayres, L. R., & Chemello, C. (2020). Pharmacist-led medication reconciliation at patient discharge: A scoping review. *Research in Social & Administrative Pharmacy, 16*(5), 605–613. https://doi.org/10.1016/j.sapharm.2019.08.001

Frandsen, G., & Pennington, S. S. (2021). *Abrams' clinical drug therapy: Rationales for nursing practice* (12th ed.). Wolters Kluwer.

Garfield, S., Jheeta, S., Husson, F., Lloyd, J., Taylor, A., Boucher, C., Jacklin, A., Bischler, A., Norton, C., Hayles, R., & Franklin, B. D. (2016). The role of hospital inpatients in supporting medication safety: A qualitative study. *PLoS One, 11*(4), e0153721. https://doi.org/10.1371/journal.pone.0153721

Giger, J. N., & Haddad L. G. (2020). *Transcultural nursing: Assessment and intervention* (8th ed.). Elsevier Inc.

Gondwe, T., Ness, R., Totten, P. A., Astete, S., Tang, G., Gold, M. A., Martin, D., & Haggerty, C. L. (2020). Novel bacterial vaginosis-associated organisms mediate the relationship between vaginal douching and pelvic inflammatory disease. *Sexually Transmitted Infections, 96*(6), 439–444. https://doi.org/10.1136/sextrans-2019-054191

Gregory, P. J., Jalloh, M. A., Abe, A. M., Hu, J., & Hein, D. J. (2016). Characterization of complementary and alternative medicine-related consultations in an academic drug information service. *Journal of Pharmacy Practice, 29*(6), 539–542. https://doi.org/10.1177/0897190015579450

Hale, T. M., Jethwani, K., Kandola, M. S., Saldana, F., & Kvedar, J. C. (2016). A remote medication monitoring system for chronic heart failure patients to reduce readmissions: A two-arm randomized pilot study. *Journal of Medical Internet Research, 18*(4), e91. https://doi.org/10.2196/jmir.5256

Hamoonga, T. E., Olowski, P., & Musonda, P. (2019). Vaginal douching in Zambia: A risk or benefit to women in the fight against cervical cancer: A retrospective cohort study. *BMC Women's Health, 19*(1), 135. https://doi.org/10.1186/s12905-019-0834-y

Hanson, A., & Haddad, L. M. (2020, July 27). Nursing rights of medication administration. In StatPearls. StatPearls Publishing. https://www.ncbi.nlm.nih.gov/books/NBK560654/

Harrison, D., Sampson, M., Reszel, J., Abdulla, K., Barrowman, N., Cumber, J., Fuller, A., Li, C., Nicholls, S., & Pound, C. M. (2014). Too many crying babies: A systematic review of pain management practices during immunizations on YouTube. *BMC Pediatrics, 14*(1), 134. https://doi.org/10.1186/1471-2431-14-134

Hinkle, J. L., Cheever K. H., & Overbaugh, K. J. (2022). *Brunner & Suddarth's textbook of medical-surgical nursing* (15th ed.). Wolters Kluwer.

Hudak, M. L., Tan, R. C., & The Committee on Drugs, The Committee on Fetus and Newborn. (2016). Neonatal drug withdrawal. *Pediatrics, 129*(2): e540–e560. http://pediatrics.aappublications.org/content/129/2/e540. Reaffirmed May 2016 by the American Academy of Pediatrics. *Pediatrics, 137* (5). https://doi.org/10.1542/peds.2016-0592

Institute for Safe Medication Practices (ISMP). (2007). *The five rights: A destination without a map*. Retrieved http://www.ismp.org/newsletters/acutecare/articles/20070125.asp

Institute for Safe Medication Practices (ISMP). (2017, October). *List of error-prone abbreviations: ISMP's of error-prone abbreviations, symbols, and dose designations*. http://www.ismp.org/Tools/errorproneabbreviations.pdf

Institute for Safe Medication Practices (ISMP). (2018, December). Part II: Survey results suggest action is needed to improve safety with adult IV push medications. *NurseAdivseERR, 16*(12), 1–5. https://www.ismp.org/sites/default/files/attachments/2018-12/NurseAdviseERR201812.pdf

Institute for Safe Medication Practices (ISMP). (2020, February 21). *ISMP targeted medication safety best practices for hospitals*. https://www.ismp.org/sites/default/files/attachments/2020-02/2020-2021%20TMSBP-%20FINAL_1.pdf

International Council of Nurses (ICN). (2019). *Nursing diagnosis and outcome statements*. https://www.icn.ch/sites/default/files/inline-files/ICNP2019-DC.pdf

The Joint Commission. (2020a). *2020 National patient safety goals*. https://www.jointcommission.org/standards/national-patient-safety-goals/

The Joint Commission. (2020b). *Sentinel event policy and procedures*. https://www.jointcommission.org/sentinel_event_policy_and_procedures

Jungquist, C. R., Quinlan-Colwell, A., Vallerand, A., Carlisle, H. L., Cooney, M., Dempsey, S. J., Dunwoody, D., Maly, A., Meloche, K., Meyers, A., Sawyer, J., Singh, N., Sullivan, D., Watson, C., & Polomano, R. C. (2020). American Society for Pain Management Nursing Guidelines on Monitoring for Opioid-Induced Advancing Sedation and Respiratory Depression: Revisions. *Pain Management Nursing, 21*(1), 7–25. https://doi.org/10.1016/j.pmn.2019.06.007

Karch, A. M. (2020). *Focus on nursing pharmacology* (8th ed.). Wolters Kluwer.

Kobaly, K., & Mandel, S. J. (2019). Hyperthyroidism and pregnancy. *Endocrinology and Metabolism Clinics of North America, 48*(3), 533–545. https://doi.org/10.1016/j.ecl.2019.05.002

Kyle, T., & Carman, S. (2021). *ESSENTIALS of pediatric nursing* (4th ed.). Wolters Kluwer.

Lasater, K. (2007). Clinical judgment development: Using simulation to create an assessment rubric. *Journal of Nursing Education, 46*(11), 496–503. https://case.edu/nursing/sites/case.edu.nursing/files/2018-06/Clinical-Judgement-Development.pdf

Le, J. (2019, May). *Drug absorption*. In *Merck manual: Professional version*. http://www.merckmanuals.com/professional/clinical-pharmacology/pharmacokinetics/drug-absorption

Marsh, D. E. S. (2018, August). *Adverse drug reactions (adverse drug effects)*. In *Merck manual: Professional version*. https://www.merckmanuals.com/professional/clinical-pharmacology/adverse-drug-reactions/adverse-drug-reactions

McCuistion, L. E., DiMaggio, K. V., Winton, M. B., & Yeager, J. J. (2021). *Pharmacology: A patient-centered nursing process approach* (10th ed.). Elsevier Inc.

MedlinePlus. (2020, October 8). *How to use an inhaler – No spacer*. https://medlineplus.gov/ency/patientinstructions/000041.htm

Merriam-Webster. (n.d.). Pharmacotherapeutics. In *Merriam-Webster.com dictionary*. Retrieved August 2, 2020, from http://www.merriam-webster.com/medical/pharmacotherapeutics

Miller, C. A. (2019). *Nursing for wellness in older adults* (8th ed.). Wolters Kluwer.

Mohammady, M., Janani, L, & Akbari Sari, A. (2017). Slow versus fast subcutaneous heparin injections for prevention of bruising and site pain intensity. *Cochrane Database of Systematic Reviews, 10*(10), CD008077. https://doi.org/10.1002/14651858.CD008077.pub4

Mraz, M. A. I., Thomas, C., & Rajcan, L. (2018). Intramuscular injection CLIMAT pathway: A clinical practice guideline. *British Journal of Nursing, 27*(13), 752–756. https://doi.org/10.12968/bjon.2018.27.13.752

Muñoz, C., & Hilgenberg, C. (2006). Ethnopharmacology: Understanding how ethnicity can affect drug response is essential to providing culturally competent care. *Holistic Nursing Practice, 20*(5), 227–234. https://doi.org/10.1097/00004650-200609000-00004

National Center for Complementary and Integrative Health. (2022, April 23). *Herbs at a glance*. https://www.nccih.nih.gov/health/herbsataglance

National Coordinating Council for Medication Error Reporting and Prevention. (2020). *About medication errors*. http://www.nccmerp.org/about-medication-errors

National Council for Prescription Drug Programs (NCPDP). (n.d.). *Standardize the dosing designations on prescription container labels for oral liquid medications*. Retrieved August 23, 2020, from https://www.ncpdp.org/NCPDP/media/pdf/mL_WP_Resource_Document.pdf

Nielson, A., Stragnell, S., & Jester, P (2007). Guide for reflection using the Clinical Judgment Model. *Journal of Nursing Education, 46*(11), 513–516.

Nimri, R., Nir, J., & Phillip, M. (2020). Insulin pump therapy. *American Journal of Therapeutics, 27*(1), e30–e41. https://doi.org/10.1097/MJT.0000000000001097

Norris, T. L. (2020). *Porth's essentials of pathophysiology* (5th ed.). Wolters Kluwer.

O'Brien, K. M., D'Aloisio, A. A., Shi, M., Murphy, J. D., Sandler, D. P., & Weinberg, C. R. (2019). Perineal talc use, douching, and the risk of uterine cancer. *Epidemiology, 30*(6), 845–852. https://doi.org/10.1097/EDE.0000000000001078

Occupational Safety and Health Administration (OSHA). (n.d.). *Healthcare wide hazards: Needlestick/Sharps injuries*. Retrieved October 5, 2020, from https://www.osha.gov/SLTC/etools/hospital/hazards/sharps/sharps.html#safer

Occupational Safety and Health Administration (OSHA). (2012, April 3). Regulations (Standards—29 CFR)—Toxic and hazardous substances: Bloodborne pathogens. Standard No. 1910.1030. https://www.osha.gov/laws-regs/regulations/standardnumber/1910

Ozen, O., Gunaydin, M., Tosun, A., Coskun, Z. U., Aytekin, K., & Takir, S. (2019). Assessment rate of true dorsogluteal intramuscular drug injection using ultrasonography. *Pakistan Journal of Medical Sciences, 35*(4), 1132–1137. https://doi.org/10.12669/pjms.35.4.313

Pich, J. (2020). Slow versus fast subcutaneous heparin injections for prevention of bruising and site pain intensity: A Cochrane review summary. *International Journal of Nursing Studies, 103*, 103238. https://doi.org/10.1016/j.ijnurstu.2018.12.001

Prentiss, A. S., Cockerel, A., & Butler, E. (2016). Nurse perceptions and safety practices of the carpuject cartridge system. *Journal of Nursing Care Quality, 31*(4), 350–356. https://doi.org/10.1097/NCQ.0000000000000194

Price, D. B., Román-Rodríguez, M., McQueen, R. B., Bosnic-Anticevich, S., Carter, V., Gruffydd-Jones, K., Haughney, J., Henrichsen, S., Hutton, C., Infantino, A., Lavorini, F., Law, L. M., Lisspers, K., Papi, A., Ryan, D., Ställberg, B., van der Molen, T., & Chrystyn, H. (2017). Inhaler errors in the CRITIKAL Study: Type, frequency, and association with asthma outcomes. *The Journal of Allergy and Clinical Immunology. In Practice, 5*(4), 1071–1081.e9. https://doi.org/10.1016/j.jaip.2017.01.004

Problem-based care plans. (2020). In *Lippincott Advisor*. Wolters Kluwer. https://advisor.lww.com/lna/home.do

Rabiei, M., Kashanian, S., Samavati, S. S., Jamasb, S., & McInnes, S. (2020). Nanomaterial and advanced technologies in transdermal drug delivery. *Journal of Drug Targeting, 28*(4), 356–367. https://doi.org/10.1080/1061186X.2019.1693579

Reber, E., Messerli, M., Stanga, Z., & Mühlebach, S. (2019). Pharmaceutical aspects of artificial nutrition. *Journal of Clinical Medicine, 8*(11), 2017. https://doi.org/10.3390/jcm8112017

Redmond, P., Grimes, T. C., McDonnell, R., Boland, F., Hughes, C., & Fahey, T. (2018). Impact of medication reconciliation for improving transitions of care. *The Cochrane Database of Systematic Reviews, 8*(8), CD010791. https://doi.org/10.1002/14651858.CD010791.pub2

Reeders, D., Li, P., Yuan, T., Feng, A., Zhao, H., & Zou, H. (2020). Much a-douche about nothing? Rectal douching, HIV, and sexually transmitted infection risks among men who have sex with men. *Sexually Transmitted Diseases, 47*(10), 663–664. https://doi.org/10.1097/OLQ.0000000000001224

Rose, A. J., Fischer, S. H., & Paasche-Orlow, M. K. (2017). Beyond medication reconciliation: The correct medication list. *The Journal of the American Medical Association, 317*(20), 2057–2058. https://doi.org/10.1001/jama.2017.4628

Rungvivatjarus, T., Kuelbs, C. L., Miller, L., Perham, J., Sanderson, K., Billman, G., Rhee, K. E., & Fisher, E. S. (2020). Medication reconciliation improvement utilizing process redesign and clinical decision support. *Joint Commission Journal on Quality and Patient Safety, 46*(1), 27–36. https://doi.org/10.1016/j.jcjq.2019.09.001

Şanlialp Zeyrek, A., Takmak, Ş., Kurban, N. K., & Arslan, S. (2019). Systematic review and meta-analysis: Physical-procedural interventions used to reduce pain during intramuscular injections in adults. *Journal of Advanced Nursing, 75*(12), 3346–3361. https://doi.org/10.1111/jan.14183

Sanofi-Aventis. (2020, May). *Lovenox: Highlights of prescribing information*. http://products.sanofi.us/Lovenox/Lovenox.pdf

Sepah, Y., Samad, L., Altaf, A., Halim, M. S., Rajagopalan, N., & Javed Khan, A. (2017). Aspiration in injections: Should we continue or abandon the practice?. *F1000Research, 3*, 157. https://doi.org/10.12688/f1000research.1113.3

Shah, K., Lo, C., Babich, M., Tsao, N. W., & Bansback, N. J. (2016). Bar code medication administration technology: A systematic review of impact on patient safety when used with computerized prescriber order entry and automated dispensing devices. *The Canadian Journal of Hospital Pharmacy, 69*(5), 394–402. https://doi.org/10.4212/cjhp.v69i5.1594

Sisson, H. (2015). Aspirating during the intramuscular injection procedure: A systematic literature review. *Journal of Clinical Nursing, 24*(17–18), 2368–2375. https://doi.org/10.1111/jocn.12824

Smeulers, M., Verweij, L., Maaskant, J. M., de Boer, M., Krediet, C. T. P., Nieveen van Dijkum, E. J. M., & Vermeulen, H. (2015). Quality indicators for safe medication preparation and administration: A systematic review. *PLoS ONE, 10*(4), e0122695. https://doi.org/10.1371/journal.pone.0122695

Staub, P. O., Geck, M. S., Weckerle, C. S., Casu, L., & Leonti, M. (2015). Classifying diseases and remedies in ethnomedicine and ethnopharmacology. *Journal of Ethnopharmacology, 174*, 514–519. https://doi.org/10.1016/j.jep.2015.08.051

Taddio, A., Appleton, M., Bortolussi, R., Chambers, C., Dubey, V., Halperin, S., Hanrahan, A., Ipp, M., Lockett, D., MacDonald, N., Midmer, D., Mousmanis, P., Palda, V., Pielak, K., Riddell, R. P., Rieder, M., Scott, J., & Shah, V. (2010). Reducing the pain of childhood vaccination: an evidence-based clinical practice guideline (summary). *Canadian Medical Association Journal, 182*(18), 1989–1995. https://doi.org/10.1503/cmaj.092048

Tamblyn, R., Abrahamowicz, M., Buckeridge, D. L., Bustillo, M., Forster, A. J., Girard, N., Habib, B., Hanley, J., Huang, A., Kurteva, S., Lee, T. C., Meguerditchian, A. N., Moraga, T., Motulsky, A., Petrella, L., Weir, D. L., & Winslade, N. (2019). Effect of an electronic medication reconciliation intervention on adverse drug events: A cluster randomized trial. *JAMA Network Open, 2*(9), e1910756. https://doi.org/10.1001/jamanetworkopen.2019.10756

Tanner, C. A. (2006). Thinking like a nurse: a research-based model of clinical judgment in nursing. *Journal of Nursing Education, 45*(6), 204–211.

Tecklenborg, S., Byrne, C., Cahir, C., Brown, L., & Bennett, K. (2020). Interventions to reduce adverse drug event-related outcomes in older adults: A systematic review and meta-analysis. *Drugs & Aging, 37*(2), 91–98. https://doi.org/10.1007/s40266-019-00738-w

Thomas, C. M., Mraz, M., & Rajcan, L. (2016). Blood aspiration during IM injection. *Clinical Nursing Research, 25*(5), 549–559. https://doi.org/10.1177/1054773815575074

Transcultural C.A.R.E. Associates. (2020). *Ethnic & ethno pharmacology*. http://transculturalcare.net/ethnic-ethno-pharmacology

Tsamantioti, E. S., & Hashmi, M. F. (2020). Teratogenic medications. In *StatPearls*. StatPearls Publishing. https://www.ncbi.nlm.nih.gov/books/NBK553086/

U.S. Department of Justice, Drug Enforcement Administration. (2020). *Drugs of abuse: A DEA resource guide/2020 edition*. https://www.dea.gov/sites/default/files/2020-04/Drugs%20of%20Abuse%202020-Web%20Version-508%20compliant-4-24-20_0.pdf

U. S. Food and Drug Administration (FDA). (2018a, March 27). *Pharmacologic class*. https://www.fda.gov/industry/structured-product-labeling-resources/pharmacologic-class

U.S. Food and Drug Administration (FDA). (2018b, November 7). *Medical device connectors*. http://www.fda.gov/medical-devices/general-hospital-devices-and-supplies/medical-device-connectors

U.S. Food and Drug Administration (FDA). (2019, April 1). *Electronic code of federal regulations: Drugs for human use* § 312.32 (USFDA Title 21, Volume 5, Chapter 1, Subchapter D, Part 312, Subpart B, §312.32). U.S. Food and Drug Administration. https://www.accessdata.fda.gov/scripts/cdrh/cfdocs/cfcfr/cfrsearch.cfm?fr=312.32

U.S. Food and Drug Administration (FDA). (2020, August 1). *MedWatch: The FDA safety information and adverse event reporting program*. https://www.fda.gov/safety/medwatch-fda-safety-information-and-adverse-event-reporting-program

U.S. Food and Drug Administration (FDA). (2020, July 30). *Electronic code of federal regulations: Specific requirements on content and format of labeling for human prescription drug and biological products described in §201.56(b)(1)* (USFDA Title 21, Chapter 1, Subchapter C, Part 201, Subpart B, §201.57). U.S. Food and Drug Administration. http://www.ecfr.gov/cgi-bin/text-idx?SID=271c0d97a71e17e1bac24472e99138c2&mc=true&node=se21.4.201_157&rgn=div8

U.S. Food and Drug Administration (FDA). (2020, March 2). *Pregnancy and lactation labeling (drugs) final rule*. https://www.fda.gov/drugs/labeling-information-drug-products/pregnancy-and-lactation-labeling-drugs-final-rule

U.S. Pharmacopeial Convention. (2020). *USP–NF updates*. Retrieved August 2, 2020, from https://www.uspnf.com/

Wang, B. H., Zhang, J. J., Zhang, J., Zhu, Q., & Yan, Q. Y. (2019). The development and psychometric testing of Inpatients' Involvement in Medication Safety Scale (IIMSS). *Journal of Nursing Management*, *27*(8), 1648–1654. https://doi.org/10.1111/jonm.12852

Whelton, P. K., Carey, R. M., Aronow, W. S., Casey, D. E., Jr, Collins, K. J., Dennison Himmelfarb, C., DePalma, S. M., Gidding, S., Jamerson, K. A., Jones, D. W., MacLaughlin, E. J., Muntner, P., Ovbiagele, B., Smith, S. C., Jr, Spencer, C. C., Stafford, R. S., Taler, S. J., Thomas, R. J., Williams, K. A., Sr, … Wright, J. T., Jr. (2018). 2017 ACC/AHA/AAPA/ABC/ACPM/AGS/APhA/ASH/ASPC/NMA/PCNA Guideline for the prevention, detection, evaluation, and management of high blood pressure in adults: A report of the American College of Cardiology/American Heart Association Task Force on Clinical Practice Guidelines. *Journal of the American College of Cardiology*, *71*(19), e127–e248. https://doi.org/10.1016/j.jacc.2017.11.006

Wolf, Z. R., & Hughes, R. G. (2008). Medication reconciliation. In R. G. Hughes (Ed.). *Patient safety and quality: An evidence-based handbook for nurses (Chapter 35)*. Agency for Healthcare Research and Quality (US). http://www.ncbi.nlm.nih.gov/books/NBK2652

Woods, D. L., Mentes, J. C., Cadogan, M., & Phillips, L. R. (2017). Aging, genetic variations, and ethnopharmacology: Building cultural competence through awareness of drug responses in ethnic minority elders. *Journal of Transcultural Nursing*, *28*(1), 56–62. https://doi.org/10.1177/1043659615606202

World Health Organization (WHO). (2020). *Immunization in practice: A practical guide for health staff–Module 5: Managing and immunization session*. http://www.who.int/immunization/documents/training/en

Wu, J., Cai, Y., Cao, A., Bi, Y., Hu, X., & Yang, S. (2020). Recommendation of the best site based on the distribution pattern of extramuscular and intramusular nerves for gluteal muscle injection. *International Journal of Morphology*, *38*(4), 975–982. https://doi.org/10.4067/s0717-95022020000400975

Yilmaz, D., Khorshid, L., & Dedeoğlu, Y. (2016). The effect of the Z-track technique on pain and drug leakage in intramuscular injections. *Clinical Nurse Specialist*, *30*, E7–E12. https://doi.org/10.1097/NUR.0000000000000245

Yuan, C. T., Nembhard, I. M., & Kane, G. C. (2020). The influence of peer beliefs on nurses' use of new health information technology: A social network analysis. *Social Science & Medicine*, *255*, 113002. https://doi.org/10.1016/j.socscimed.2020.113002

Zimmerman, K. M., Salgado, T. M., & Dixon, D. L. (2017). Medication reconciliation vs medication review. *The Journal of the American Medical Association*, *318*(10), 965–966. https://doi.org/10.1001/jama.2017.10552

Zoeller, S., Bechtold, M. L., Burns, B., Cattell, T., Grenda, B., Haffke, L., Larimer, C., Powers, J., Reuning, F., Tweel, L., Guenter, P., & ASPEN Enteral Nutrition Task Force. (2020). Dispelling myths and unfounded practices about enteral nutrition. *Nutrition in Clinical Practice*, *35*(2), 196–204. https://doi.org/10.1002/ncp.10456

31 Perioperative Nursing

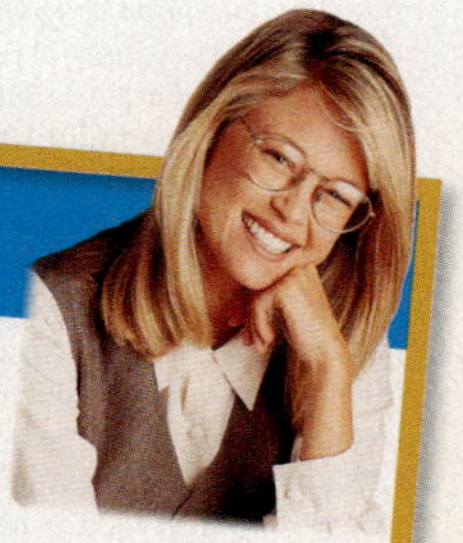

Molly Greenbaum

Molly, a 38-year-old female who is scheduled for a vaginal hysterectomy later in the day, arrives at the hospital at 0630. With tears in her eyes and wringing her hands, she states, "I really didn't sleep very much last night. I kept thinking about the surgery."

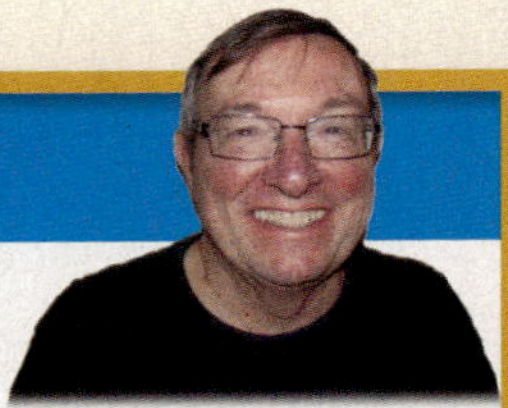

Marcus Benjamin

Marcus, a 73-year-old male, has just had a total hip replacement under general anesthesia and is transferred to the postanesthesia care unit (PACU). His vital signs are stable. He has an intravenous catheter in his right antecubital space, infusing at 125 mL/hr, and an indwelling urinary catheter in place, draining clear yellow urine. The dressing over the surgical site is clean and dry, without any drainage.

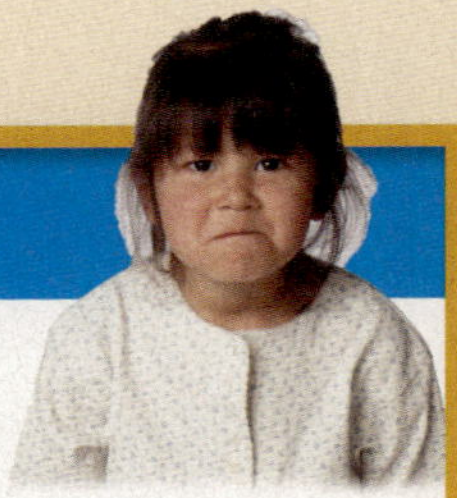

Gabrielle McAllister

Gabrielle McAllister is a 5-year-old female scheduled for a tonsillectomy and adenoidectomy at a hospital-based, same-day surgery unit. She was born with a congenital cardiac defect and has had six prior surgeries. She is small for her age and is allergic to latex but is an otherwise healthy kindergarten student.

Learning Outcomes

After completing the chapter, you will be able to accomplish the following:

1. Describe the surgical experience, including perioperative phases, classifications of surgery, types of anesthesia, informed consent and advance directives, and outpatient/same-day surgery.
2. Conduct a preoperative nursing history and physical assessment to identify patient strengths as well as factors that increase risks for surgical and postoperative complications.
3. Prepare a patient physically and psychologically for surgery.
4. Identify assessments and interventions specific to the prevention of complications in the immediate and early postoperative phases.
5. Use the nursing process to develop an individualized plan of care for the surgical patient during each phase of the perioperative period.

Nursing Concepts

- Management of care
- Evidence-based practice
- Teaching and learning/patient education
- Thermoregulation

The treatment of many illnesses and injuries includes some type of operative or other invasive procedure. In this chapter, we will refer to the myriad operative and other invasive procedures (Association of periOperative Registered Nurses [AORN], 2020) performed in the operating room or surgical suite, using the general term *surgery*. Surgery requires collaboration and the integration of role-specific knowledge and skills of multiple care providers to ensure patient safety and promote good outcomes. Surgery may be done for a variety of reasons: to cure or minimize disease; to diagnose the specific presence of a disease or condition; to reconstruct or eliminate a defect; to enhance form and function; to palliate, or offer comfort, when cure is not possible; to follow up or monitor an incurable disease process; or to offer a preventive option when disease is inevitable, such as an elective, prophylactic mastectomy for a person at high risk for breast cancer. Surgery may be planned or unplanned, elective/optional or necessary, major or minor, and may involve any body part or system. Surgery is a stressor that requires physical and psychosocial adaptations for both the patient and the family. The patient's recovery from a surgical procedure requires skillful and knowledgeable nursing care, whether the surgery is done on an outpatient basis or in the hospital. See the accompanying Reflective Practice box (on pages 1038–1039) for an example of nursing care for a patient who has undergone surgery.

Nursing care provided for the patient before, during, and after surgery is called **perioperative nursing**. All members of the interprofessional team use the term *perioperative* to describe the entire time surrounding an operative or other invasive procedure. The nursing process is used to guide assessments and interventions that promote the recovery of health, prevent further injury or illness, and facilitate coping with alterations in physical structure and function.

A conceptual model for perioperative nursing care is shown in Figure 31-1 (on page 1039). In this model, the patient is at the center of all care activities. Surrounding the patient are four domains. Three of these domains—safety, physiologic responses, and behavioral responses—are integral to patient care. The fourth domain, health system, represents the structural elements and other health system activities that must be present to support safe, effective, high-quality patient care (AORN, 2011).

With this model, each domain has desired outcomes. These outcomes are identified first in the model because perioperative nursing is preventive and outcome-focused in nature. This is in contrast to the usual progression of the nursing process, which begins with assessment. Thus, perioperative nurses base their plans of care on recognized desired outcomes. Perioperative nurses assess the patient for the relevance of the outcome, then identify actual or potential nursing problems and plan interventions. The Perioperative Nursing Data Set (PNDS) reflects AORN-designed, standardized nursing language that captures the perioperative patient experience from preadmission to discharge (AORN, 2020).

Technology Alert

Established in 2017, AORN Syntegrity® seamlessly integrates the language from the Perioperative Nursing Data Set (PNDS) and AORN's evidence-based Guidelines for Perioperative Practice with the Electronic Health Record (EHR) to help streamline the communication, scheduling, workflow, analytics, and documentation processes inherent in the perioperative phases (AORN, 2020).

One of the most significant roles of the perioperative nurse is that of collaborator—the nurse interfaces directly and indirectly with other nurses, surgeons, support personnel, anesthesia professionals, perioperative services executives, quality improvement personnel, and risk management experts. Evidence-based practice that considers patient and family preferences, clinical expertise of the health care provider, and the best evidence available informs decision making at all stages of the complex perioperative process. The ultimate, shared goal is to provide safe, quality care for the vulnerable perioperative patient (AORN, 2020).

The type of surgery scheduled influences the desired outcomes, health problem identification, assessments, and interventions carried out by the nurse. The perioperative

QSEN Reflective Practice: Cultivating QSEN Competencies

CHALLENGE TO ETHICAL AND LEGAL SKILLS

During a recent clinical experience on a level II ICU, I cared for Ron Johnson, a middle-aged male patient who had an extensive medical history that included gunshot wounds, bilateral leg amputations, paraplegia, and several surgeries. Because of this, he had lengthy hospital stays and was known by the staff as being a difficult and manipulative patient. During my encounter with him, he had just returned from the OR where they had performed a urinary diversion. He was ordered to be nothing by mouth (NPO) for 24 hours following surgery. However, he claimed that his surgeon had told him that he would be able to eat immediately after the surgery, and he was demanding that I give him food and fluids. "I want some food and I want it now!" I told the patient that I had to follow the orders in his chart and that it was unlikely that he would be able to have anything by mouth during my shift. He asked me to explain the reasons for being NPO after surgery, and I did my best under the time constraints by telling him that the bowel is affected by anesthesia, and it is not ready to handle the intake of food and fluids. In all honesty, I didn't know the major consequences of eating or drinking after surgery; however, I didn't admit this to him. He was obviously not satisfied with my explanation because when I returned from my lunch break, he was sitting in front of a lunch tray. He had talked a new nursing assistant into getting him the items. He made the decision to act against my instructions and the instructions of his surgeon, perhaps because I was not able to give him a clear, articulate explanation of his NPO status.

Thinking Outside the Box: Possible Courses of Action

- Tell the patient that I was unable to give him the best explanation of his NPO status, informing him that I would return in 5 to 10 minutes after consulting with a nurse, and deciding the best way to articulate to him the consequences of ignoring the order.
- Avoid giving him any explanation at all, assuming that because of his extensive surgical history, he knew the reasons why he must not eat or drink.
- Ask a nurse or the dietitian to explain the NPO order.
- Alert the surgeon that this patient was at risk for being nonadherent and ask her to come to see the patient as soon as possible.

Evaluating a Good Outcome: How Do I Define Success?

- The patient verbalizes an understanding of my explanation and the consequences of his actions.
- The patient complies with the health care provider's orders and with my instructions.
- The patient remains free of injuries/complications.
- I feel competent in my explanations and actions.
- I take responsibility for the impact of my (in)action with the patient and partner with him in decision making.

Personal Learning: Here's to the Future!

This patient taught me a great deal. He taught me that sometimes, rather than giving an inadequate explanation, it would be better to admit that you do not know or that your knowledge is not up to par in a particular area. I should have been honest with Mr. Johnson, admitting that I was unsure about why he wasn't allowed to eat or drink. It would have been more advantageous to consult with someone else before giving him a more thorough explanation. I also should have recognized that Mr. Johnson was exhibiting extreme frustration and depression, placing him at high risk for nonadherence. All he needed was someone to take extra time with him, offering compassion and support. Unfortunately, the patient did not comply with the order and thus was at risk for developing serious complications, such as a bowel obstruction. I alerted the surgeon of the patient's actions and, luckily, the surgeon was understanding. In the future, I will make a major effort to gather the appropriate information to give patients a thorough, understandable explanation when they ask for specific information.

Colleen Kilcullen, Georgetown University

QSEN SELF-REFLECTION ON QUALITY AND SAFETY COMPETENCIES DEVELOPING KNOWLEDGE, SKILLS, AND ATTITUDES FOR CONTINUOUS IMPROVEMENT

How would you respond in a similar situation? Why? What does this tell you about yourself and about the adequacy of your skills for professional practice? Can you think of other ways to approach this situation? What *knowledge, skills,* and *attitudes* do you need to develop in order to continuously improve quality and safety when caring for patients like Mr. Johnson?

Patient-Centered Care: What information about his postoperative instructions needs to be clearly communicated to Mr. Johnson? How might his past history have influenced the nursing student's actions? Explain. If you were this nursing student, would Mr. Johnson's past history have influenced you? Why or why not? How could you involve Mr. Johnson as a partner in coordinating his care, thus minimizing his frustration? How could you provide emotional support?

Teamwork and Collaboration/Quality Improvement: What communication skills do you need to provide clear, comprehensive information to Mr. Johnson? Would collaboration with your instructor or Mr. Johnson's nurse have resulted in another approach to communicating and explaining the health care provider's orders in a timely manner?

QSEN Reflective Practice: Cultivating QSEN Competencies *(continued)*

CHALLENGE TO ETHICAL AND LEGAL SKILLS

Safety/Evidence-Based Practice: Can you obtain any resources/articles from the nursing literature that provide information and guidance regarding risks associated with intake of food and fluids in the immediate postoperative period? Do you think your response to Mr. Johnson provided a safe environment for him?

Informatics: What information should be electronically documented regarding your interaction with Mr. Johnson? Is there a better way to describe this patient or is *noncompliant* appropriate? What about the word *nonadherence*? Do those words have different connotations? Can you identify the essential information that must be noted in his electronic record to support safe patient care?

nurse's goal is to promote and assist the patient and family to achieve a level of wellness equal to or greater than what they had prior to the surgical procedure (AORN, 2020).

THE SURGICAL EXPERIENCE

Regardless of the surgical or interventional procedure required or the setting in which it is performed, all patients progress through specific phases, all patients must provide informed consent for the surgery or procedure, and some surgeries and procedures require some type of anesthesia and monitoring support.

Perioperative Phases

The patient who is having surgery progresses through several distinct periods, called the **perioperative phases**. The three phases of perioperative patient care are:

- *Preoperative phase:* Begins when the patient and surgeon mutually decide that surgery is necessary and will take place; ends when the patient is transferred to the operating room (OR) or procedural bed.
- *Intraoperative phase:* Begins when the patient is transferred to the OR bed; ends with transfer to the

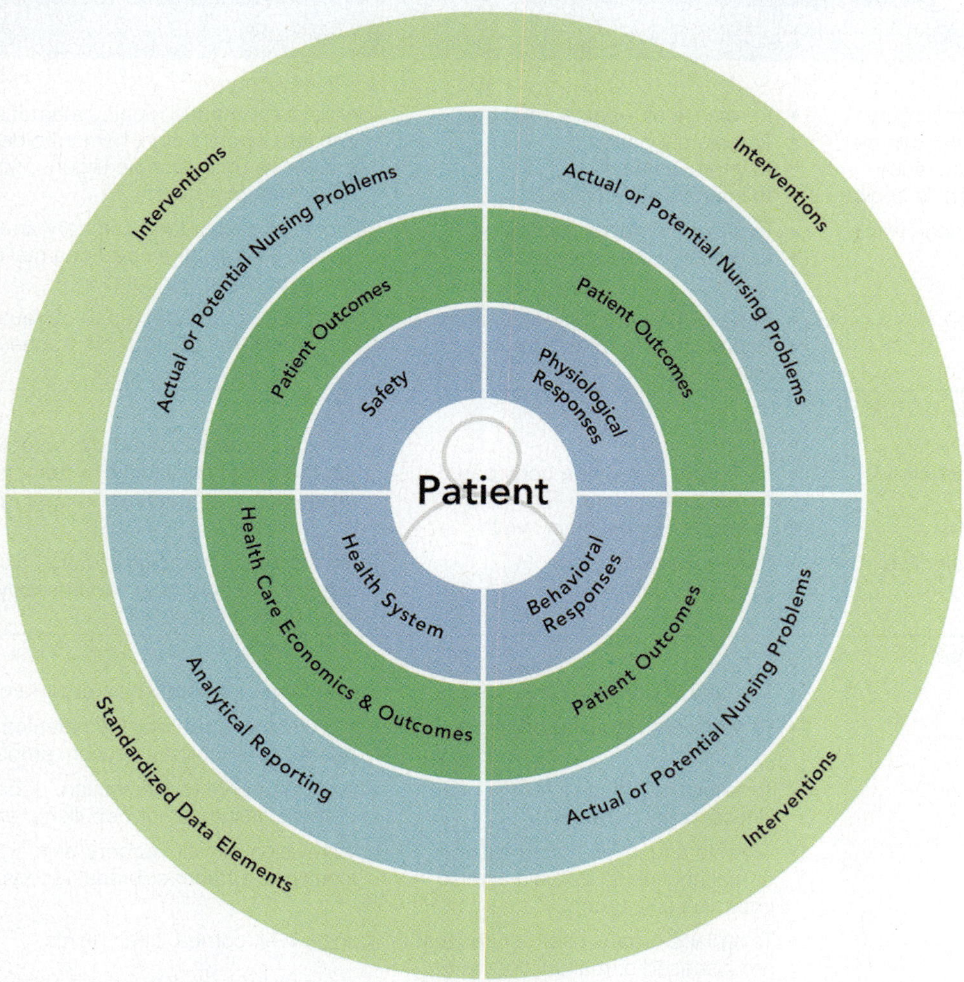

FIGURE 31-1. Perioperative Patient-Focused Model. (*Source:* Reprinted with permission from Guidelines for Perioperative Practice. Copyright © 2018, AORN, Inc, 2170 S. Parker Road, Suite 400, Denver, CO 80231. All rights reserved.)

postanesthesia care unit (PACU). The PACU is an area often adjacent to the surgical suite designed to provide care for patients recovering from anesthesia or moderate sedation/analgesia.

- *Postoperative phase:* Begins with admission to the PACU or other recovery area; ends with complete recovery from surgery and the last follow-up health care provider visit.

The postoperative phase can be further divided into phases that represent levels of care, not necessarily locations: (1) phase I, where close monitoring is required for management of airway, ventilation, hemodynamic monitoring, fluid and electrolyte balance, and pain control; (2) phase II, where the patient no longer requires acute care measures and is prepared for self-care, for family/caregiver care, or for care in an extended care environment (e.g., rehabilitation center); and (3) phase III (Extended Care) where the focus is on providing ongoing care for patients requiring extended observation or intervention after transfer or discharge from phase I or II (American Society of PeriAnesthesia Nurses [ASPAN], 2020).

With the increasing trend toward short-stay or same-day surgery, nursing interventions in each phase of perioperative nursing care may vary somewhat, but they remain basically the same. The nursing process is used during each phase to meet physical and psychosocial needs and to facilitate the patient's return to health. Each of these phases, with related patient needs and nursing activities, is described in detail in this chapter.

Surgical Procedure Classification

Surgical procedures usually are classified according to urgency, risk, and purpose. Table 31-1 lists each classification, with purposes and examples for each. No matter what the defined degree of risk, any surgical procedure imposes physical and psychological stress, and is seldom considered minor by the patient.

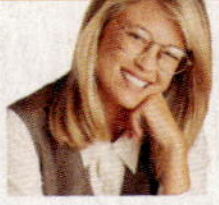

Recall **Molly Greenbaum**, the 38-year-old woman who is to undergo a vaginal hysterectomy. The nurse would incorporate knowledge about the various classifications of surgery to plan appropriate care before and after surgery.

Table 31-1 Classification of Surgical Procedures

CLASSIFICATION	PURPOSE	EXAMPLES
Based on Urgency		
Elective: Delay of surgery has no ill effects; can be scheduled in advance based on patient's choice	• To remove or repair a body part • To restore function • To improve health • To improve self-concept	Tonsillectomy, hernia repair, cataract extraction and lens implantation, hemorrhoidectomy, hip prosthesis (may also be urgent), scar revision, facelift, mammoplasty
Urgent: Usually done within 24–48 hours	• To remove or repair a body part • To preserve or restore health	Removal of gallbladder, coronary artery bypass graft (CABG), surgical removal of a malignant tumor, colon resection, amputation
Emergency: Done immediately	• To prevent further tissue damage • To preserve life (plus purposes listed above)	Control of hemorrhage; repair of trauma, perforated ulcer, intestinal obstruction; tracheostomy
Based on Degree of Risk		
Major: May be elective, urgent, or emergency	• To preserve life • To remove or repair a body part • To restore function • To improve or maintain health	Carotid endarterectomy, cholecystectomy, nephrectomy, colostomy, hysterectomy, radical mastectomy, amputation, trauma repair, CABG
Minor: Primarily elective	• To remove skin lesions • To correct deformities	Tooth extraction, removal of warts, skin biopsy, dilation and curettage, laparoscopy, cataract extraction, arthroscopy
Based on Purpose		
Diagnostic	• To make or confirm a diagnosis	Breast biopsy, laparoscopy, exploratory laparotomy
Ablative	• To remove a diseased body part	Appendectomy, subtotal thyroidectomy, partial gastrectomy, colon resection, amputation
Palliative	• To relieve or reduce intensity of an illness; is not curative	Colostomy, nerve root resection, debridement of necrotic tissue, tumor debulking, arthroscopy
Reconstructive	• To restore function to traumatized or malfunctioning tissue may also improve self-concept	Scar revision, plastic surgery, skin graft, internal fixation of a fracture, breast reconstruction
Transplantation	• To replace organs or structures that are diseased or malfunctioning	Kidney, liver, cornea, heart, joints
Constructive	• To restore function in congenital anomalies	Cleft palate repair, closure of atrial–septal defect

Surgery Based on Urgency

Surgery based on urgency is further categorized into broad categories that cross specialty areas:

- **Elective surgery** is a procedure that is preplanned and based on the patient's choice and availability of scheduling for the patient, surgeon, and facility. This is a nonurgent procedure that does not have to be done immediately.
- **Urgent surgery** must be done within a reasonably short time frame to preserve health but is not an emergency.
- **Emergency surgery** must be done immediately to preserve life, a body part, or function.

Surgery Based on Degree of Risk

Surgery is classified as minor or major based on the degree of risk for the patient. Minor surgery is almost always performed in settings such as a health care provider's office, an outpatient clinic, or a same-day/outpatient surgery setting (also referred to as ambulatory surgery). This classification means that the surgical procedure usually carries a low risk and results in few complications. In contrast, major surgery may require hospitalization and specialized care, has a higher degree of risk, involves major body organs or life-threatening situations, and has a greater risk for postoperative complications.

However, this major and minor nomenclature is not as descriptive of actual procedures today because of the remarkable evolution of surgical science and technology. Advances in the use of laser techniques and minimally invasive approaches, involving very small incisions, make major surgery less traumatic, which facilitates shortened hospital stays. New surgical approaches using minimally invasive techniques and robotic technology continue to evolve. Thus, many surgical procedures, even though they are classified as major, are now performed on an outpatient (same-day/ambulatory) basis or as a 23-hour hospital stay. Major procedures can be accomplished in short time frames. The patient can return home on the same day with nominal pain, allowing a quick return to normal daily activities.

Surgery Based on Purpose

Surgery may also be classified according to its purpose. Some terms used to classify surgical procedures based on purpose include *diagnostic, curative, preventive, ablative, palliative, reconstructive, transplantation,* and *constructive* (see Table 31-1).

Anesthesia

Anesthesia is a method and technique of making potentially uncomfortable interventions tolerable and safe. Anesthetic agents can be administered systemically (to the whole body) or regionally (to a specific region of the body) to block nerve conduction. General, or systemic, anesthesia is a balance of loss of consciousness, analgesia (pain relief), relaxation, and loss of reflexes (temporary paralysis). In contrast, regional anesthesia does not cause narcosis (sleepiness), but results in analgesia and reflex loss. Moderate sedation involves intravenous (IV) administration of sedatives and analgesics to produce analgesia and a degree of amnesia that can be promptly reversed, whereas topical or local anesthesia targets a specific tissue of the body. Anesthesiologists (medical doctors) or certified registered nurse anesthetists (CRNAs) administer anesthetic agents while monitoring the patient's physiologic response and maintaining homeostasis throughout the procedure and recovery. Nurse anesthesia is an advanced nursing specialty. Both physicians and nurses who administer anesthesia perform preoperative physical assessments, conduct preoperative teaching, administer anesthesia during the surgical procedure, and oversee the patient's postoperative recovery from the anesthetic. The pre-anesthetic evaluation (PAE) performed to assess medical readiness of a patient for surgery, may be performed in-person or remotely. The PAE routinely includes an evaluation of the patient's airway, a review of any laboratory or other diagnostic results, and a risk analysis. Early identification of an airway that may be difficult to manage allows for adequate preparation of equipment, the patient, and the interprofessional team (Apfelbaum et al., 2022). Advances in telehealth make the PAE using telehealth technology a reliable and resource-effective option that promotes patient satisfaction, especially for patients who reside in remote or rural areas (Schoen & Prater, 2019).

General (Systemic) Anesthesia

General anesthesia involves the administration of drugs by inhalation or the IV route to produce central nervous system depression. General anesthesia typically is a combination of both IV and inhalation anesthetics that allows for rapid induction, excretion, and reversal of effects. The desired actions of general anesthesia are loss of consciousness, amnesia (short-term loss of memory), analgesia (the brain does not respond to pain signals), relaxed skeletal muscles, and depressed reflexes. Choices of route and type of anesthesia are made primarily by the anesthesia provider after discussion with the patient. Many factors influence these choices, including the type and length of surgery and the physical and psychological status of the patient. For example, children, especially those who are uncooperative, may benefit from inhalation induction. Caregiver presence during induction varies and requires additional education and support of the caregiver (Nelson et al., 2018).

The three phases of general anesthesia are induction, maintenance, and emergence. Induction begins with administration of the anesthetic agent and continues until the patient is ready for the incision. Maintenance continues from this point until near the completion of the procedure. Emergence starts as the patient begins to awaken from the altered state induced by the anesthesia and usually ends when the patient is ready to leave the OR; the length of time depends on the depth and length of anesthesia. New anesthetic agents enable patients to emerge from anesthesia and *wake up* in a fraction of the time required in the past. When these agents are used, patients frequently bypass PACU stage 1 and move directly to PACU stage 2. This is referred to as *fast tracking*. This enables more surgical procedures to be safely done in health care providers' offices and in other ambulatory settings.

General anesthesia is advantageous because it can be used for patients of any age and for any surgical procedure, with the patient unaware of the physical trauma of the surgery. There are, however, major associated risks for circulatory and respiratory depression, postoperative nausea and vomiting (PONV), and alterations in thermoregulation. Postoperative bronchospasm is another risk, especially in patients with multiple comorbidities.

Children and young adults require greater attention as they emerge from general anesthesia because they may experience emergence agitation or emergency delirium. Evidence-based interventions to prevent or combat pediatric emergence agitation include monitoring with advanced technology, involving the family/caregiver(s) in the process, considering pharmacologic adjuncts, and using alternative methods of general anesthesia (Hoch, 2019).

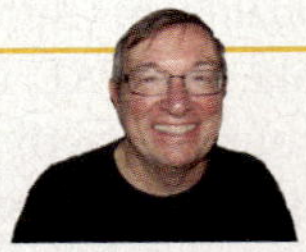

Remember **Marcus Benjamin**, the 73-year-old male who had a total hip replacement. When developing an appropriate care plan for this patient, the nurse would need to incorporate knowledge about the risks associated with general anesthesia along with knowledge of the physiologic changes associated with aging. Key to this care plan would be measures that prevent or minimize Mr. Benjamin's risk for complications.

Moderate Sedation/Analgesia

Moderate sedation/analgesia, also called *conscious* or *procedural sedation,* is used for short-term and minimally invasive procedures. The patient maintains cardiorespiratory function and can respond to verbal commands. The IV administration of sedatives and analgesics (or sedatives alone) produces a decrease in anxiety and discomfort/pain with some degree of amnesia (AORN, 2020). In moderate sedation/analgesia, the patient does not have large variations in vital signs and retains protective reflexes, spontaneous ventilation, and the ability to communicate, including the ability to purposefully respond to verbal and tactile stimulation (AORN, 2020). In addition to anesthesiologists and CRNAs, others who may administer moderate sedation/analgesia include: perioperative, endoscopy, interventional radiology, interventional cardiology, or other nurses with specialized training and competence in administering the medications and monitoring the patient's cardiac rate and rhythm, respiratory rate, oxygen saturation, level of consciousness, level of pain, blood pressure, and skin condition.

Regional Anesthesia

Regional anesthesia occurs when an anesthetic agent is injected near a nerve or nerve pathway in or around the operative site, inhibiting the transmission of sensory stimuli to central nervous system receptors. Pneumatic tourniquets may also be used to confine an intravenous anesthetic to a specific extremity, thus providing anesthesia only to that extremity (AORN, 2020). The patient receiving regional anesthesia remains awake but loses sensation in a specific area or region of the body. In some instances, reflexes may also be lost. Although regional anesthesia may be selected for numerous types of surgery and patients, it is especially useful in reducing postsurgical pain, bowel dysfunction, and length of hospital stay for older adult patients. It also reduces risks associated with general anesthesia for this population.

Regional anesthesia may be accomplished through nerve blocks, spinal anesthesia (subarachnoid block), epidural anesthesia, or intravenous (IV) anesthesia with pneumatic tourniqueting:

- *Nerve blocks* (peripheral) are accomplished by injecting a local anesthetic around a nerve trunk supplying the area of surgery such as the jaw, face, or extremities. Onset and duration of the block depend on the anesthetic drug, its concentration, the amount injected, and the addition of additional medications (such as epinephrine) that prolong the block.
- *Spinal anesthesia* is achieved by injecting a local anesthetic into the subarachnoid space through a lumbar puncture, causing sensory, motor, and autonomic blockage. This type of anesthesia is used for surgery of the lower abdomen, perineum, and legs. Adverse effects of spinal anesthesia may include hypotension, headache, and urine retention.
- *Epidural anesthesia* involves the injection of the anesthetic through the intervertebral spaces, usually in the lumbar region (although it may also be used in the thoracic or cervical regions). It is used for surgeries of the chest, abdomen, pelvis, and legs; epidurals are also commonly used in childbirth.
- *Intravenous anesthesia with pneumatic tourniqueting* primarily occurs with surgery or procedures involving an extremity. The equipment consists of a tourniquet cuff, tubing, and a pressure regulator. Risks include nerve injuries, skin integrity issues, pain, compartment syndrome, formation of a deep vein thrombosis, and systemic issues that may occur with deflation (AORN, 2020).

Local and Topical Anesthesia

Local anesthesia is the injection of an anesthetic agent such as bupivacaine, lidocaine, or tetracaine to a specific area of the body (AORN, 2020). It bathes the tissue around a targeted nerve or infiltrates the underlying tissue in the operative area. The surgeon administers local anesthesia for minor, short-term surgical, or diagnostic procedures such as tissue biopsy. Epinephrine may be mixed with the local anesthetic to minimize bleeding by causing local vasoconstriction. It also prolongs the length of analgesia by trapping the anesthetic in the tissue through slowed absorption that results from the vasoconstriction of the surrounding vessels (AORN, 2020). Local anesthesia may also be injected during general anesthetic procedures to prolong pain relief after the general anesthetic wears off.

Topical anesthesia is primarily applied to intact skin but may be used with mucous membranes and in some cases of wound care. Although its use as a topical anesthetic has declined since its introduction in the 1890s, cocaine in a 4% to 10% solution may be used topically in the mouth, larynx, or nasal cavities alone or in combination with other agents (Gwinnutt & Gwinnutt, 2017; Sikka et al., 2015). Other common topical anesthetics include lidocaine, tetracaine, and benzocaine. A lidocaine (2.5%)–prilocaine (2.5%) combination, frequently referred to as EMLA (eutectic mixture of local anesthetics), may be used on intact skin prior to injection, catheter placement, or laceration repair (Gwinnutt & Gwinnutt, 2017; Sikka et al., 2015). Topical anesthetics may be sprayed, spread, or applied with a compress of drug-saturated gauze or cotton-tipped applicators. Loss of feeling and sensation occur in the specific area where the topical anesthesia is applied.

Informed Consent and Advance Directives

Informed consent reflects a *process* of effective communication that results in the patient's voluntary agreement to undergo a particular procedure or treatment (such as surgery). In order to ensure the patient's understanding prior to giving consent, the health care provider performing the procedure should provide the following information in everyday language that considers the patient's health literacy level and is culturally sensitive (The Joint Commission, 2022):

- Description of the procedure or treatment (its name, site, and side if applicable), potential alternative therapies, and the option of nontreatment
- Underlying disease process and its natural course
- Name and qualifications of the health care provider performing the procedure or treatment—provide an emphasis on shared decision making between the patient and provider(s)
- Explanation of the risks (nature, magnitude, probability of the risks) and benefits
- Explanation that the patient has the right to refuse treatment and that consent can be withdrawn
- Explanation of expected (not guaranteed) outcome, recovery, and rehabilitation plan and course

Informed consent protects the patient, the health care providers, and the health care facility. The signed, dated, and timed form is a legal document as well as an ethical imperative. Regulatory bodies also consider the *quality* of informed consent as it relates to patient autonomy and other ethical and legal principles, and have implemented the use of a validated tool to assess the quality of informed consent documents (Centers for Medicare & Medicaid Services, 2020; Spatz et al., 2020). More detailed information about informed consent is included in Chapter 7.

Concept Mastery

Knowing the key elements of the informed consent *process* improves the *quality* of the informed consent as it relates to patient autonomy, the role of the nurse, and other ethical and legal considerations.

Advance directives, which are also legal documents, allow patients to specify instructions for health care treatment should they be unable to communicate these wishes postoperatively. This allows patients to discuss their wishes with family members in advance of the surgery. Suspension of a do-not-resuscitate (DNR) or allow-natural-death (AND) order, although not required for surgery, should be discussed as part of the informed consent process. Actions used in resuscitation (mechanical ventilation, vasoactive drips) are integral to the surgical process, and surgery itself poses specific risks where reversible cardiopulmonary arrest may occur (American Society of Anesthesiologists, 2018; Shapiro & Singer, 2019). It is important to discuss and document the exact wishes of the patient before surgery, especially related to resuscitation. See Chapter 44 for more information on advance care planning.

Outpatient/Same-Day Surgery

Surgical procedures performed in outpatient or same-day surgical settings are common. These include freestanding surgery centers, hospital-based surgery centers, interventional units, and health care providers' offices. Some freestanding surgery centers specialize in selected types of surgery, such as orthopedics, repair of cataracts, or hernia repair. Others perform a wide variety of surgical interventions, including major surgical procedures that formerly required a stay in a hospital.

Typically, patients are admitted to the ambulatory surgery center the morning of surgery. Allowing the patient to spend the night before surgery at home and to return home to recover reduces much of the stress associated with surgery and may also decrease the risk of infection. Patients who are older, chronically ill, or who do not have support systems or access to resources to provide the care needed after surgery may require additional teaching and referral for home care services. When possible, the nurse should arrange these types of referrals prior to the date of surgery.

NURSING PROCESS FOR PREOPERATIVE CARE

Patients who require surgical intervention and nursing care enter the health care setting due to a wide variety of situations, ranging from essentially healthy people who have planned elective procedures to emergency admissions for treatment of trauma or serious illness. Surgical patients may be of any age and at any point on the health–illness continuum. It is the nurse's responsibility to identify factors that affect the risk of a surgical procedure. This includes assessing

Box 31-1 Preoperative Information for Outpatient/Same-Day Surgery

Using simple language the patient can understand, instruct the patient (verbally and in writing) as follows:

- List medications routinely taken and ask the health care provider which should be taken or omitted the morning of surgery.
- Notify the surgeon's office if a cold or infection develops before surgery.
- List all allergies and be sure the OR staff is aware of them.
- Follow all instructions from your surgeon regarding bathing or showering with a special soap or solution.
- Remove nail polish and, depending on the surgical site, do not wear makeup, lotions, or deodorant on the day of the procedure.
- Leave all jewelry and valuables at home.
- Wear clothing that buttons in front; short-sleeved garments are better for surgery on the hands.
- Have a responsible adult available for transportation home after recovery from anesthesia.
- Inform the patient of limitations on eating or drinking before surgery, with a specific time to begin the limitations.
- Notify the patient about when and where to arrive for the procedure, as well as the estimated time when the procedure will be performed.

the physical and psychosocial needs of the patient and family, diagnosing actual or potential health problems or needs, and establishing a plan of care. Interventions are designed to meet the patient's physical and psychological needs and facilitate recovery as the patient progresses through the perioperative period.

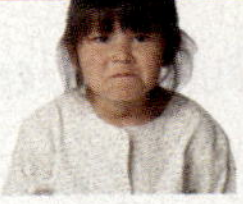

Consider **Gabrielle McAllister**, the 5-year-old child scheduled for tonsillectomy and adenoidectomy. As a child with a history of cardiac defects, prior surgeries, and latex allergy, she is at risk for anesthesia complications related to her congenital disability and allergic reaction if exposed to latex. The nurse would need to obtain a thorough history of her previous surgeries, what happens when she is exposed to latex, and how she responded after the surgeries to identify her risk for problems with the current surgical procedure and anesthesia.

Some outcomes that frame plans of care for surgical patients might include that patients:

- Receive respectful care that is developmentally and culturally appropriate
- Remain free from injury and adverse effects related to positioning, retained surgical items, or chemical, physical, or electrical hazards
- Experience no surgical site infection(s)
- Maintain fluid and electrolyte balance and skin integrity
- Maintain normal body temperature
- Collaborate in the management of their pain
- Demonstrate an understanding of the physiologic and psychological responses to their planned surgery
- Participate in their rehabilitation process following surgery

Assessing

The importance of preoperative assessment cannot be overemphasized. Surgery causes major trauma to the body, and preoperative assessments identify factors that may place the patient at greater risk for complications during and after surgery.

Assessment of the surgical patient includes:

- Obtaining a health history and performing a physical assessment to establish a baseline database
- Identifying risk factors and allergies that could cause surgical adverse events
- Identifying medications and treatments the patient is currently receiving
- Determining the teaching and psychosocial needs of the patient and caregivers
- Determining postsurgical support and referral needs for recovery

The assessment is often conducted several days before surgery as part of preoperative laboratory screening and teaching; this is referred to as preadmission testing. It may be conducted in the hospital, a surgical clinic, an office, in the patient's home, or by phone.

Preoperative nursing assessments and teaching are key care activities for patients who will be having outpatient or same-day surgery. Preoperative teaching can often be combined with preoperative screening tests, which are usually done up to 30 days before the scheduled surgery. Preoperative assessment and teaching for outpatient/same-day surgery includes providing important information and preoperative instructions to the patient and family (Box 31-1).

Unfolding Patient Stories: Edith Jacobson • Part 1

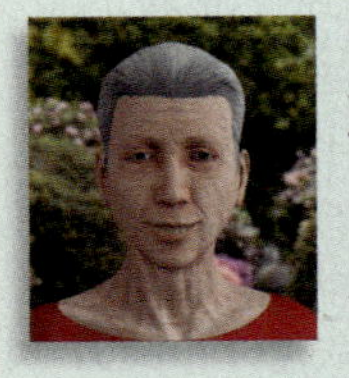

Edith Jacobson, an 85-year-old female, is scheduled for surgical repair of a left hip fracture under general anesthesia. What are the responsibilities of the nurse in the preoperative period to prepare the patient for surgery and minimize the risk of complications? What preoperative teaching should the nurse provide for Edith and her family?

(Edith Jacobson's story continues in Chapter 35.) Care for Edith and other patients in a realistic virtual environment: ***vSim** for Nursing* (thepoint.lww.com/vSimFunds). Practice documenting these patients' care in DocuCare (thepoint.lww.com/DocuCareEHR).

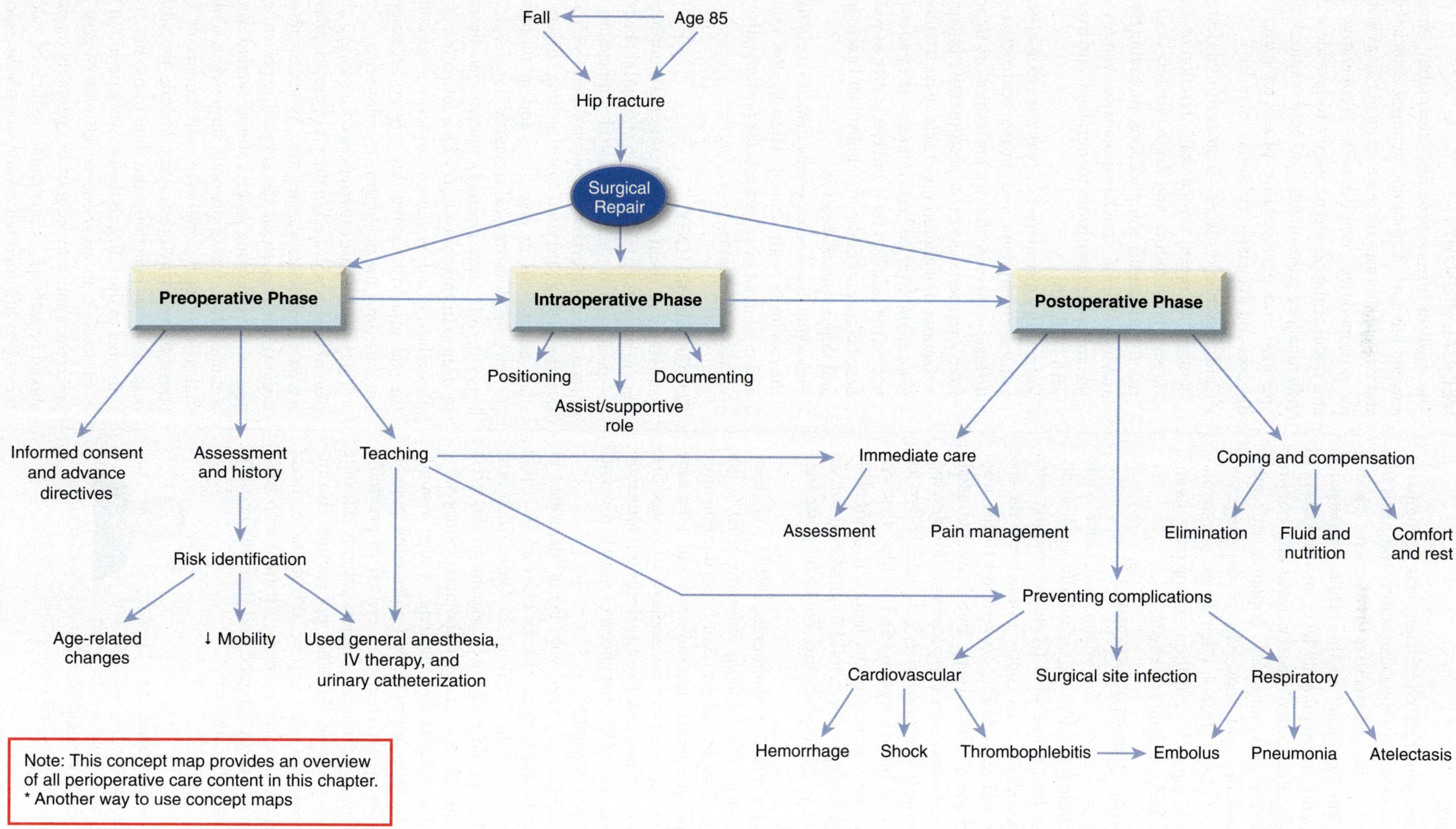

Concept map that provides an overview of the nursing foci for Edith Jacobson or any patient in the perioperative process. ↓, decreased; IV, intravenous/intravenous catheter.

Health History

The health history identifies risk factors and strengths in the patient's physical and psychosocial status, and helps the nurse individualize the preoperative assessment. Health history information significant to the surgical experience includes the patient's developmental level; medical history, including allergies; medication history, including nonprescription drugs; previous surgeries; implants; extremity limitations; perceptions and knowledge of the surgery to be done; nutrition; use of alcohol, illicit drugs, or nicotine; activities of daily living and occupation; coping patterns and support systems; and sociocultural needs.

DEVELOPMENTAL CONSIDERATIONS

Surgery poses a greater risk for infants and older adults than for older children and young or middle-aged adults. The infant has a lower total blood volume, making even a small loss of blood a serious concern because of the risk for dehydration and the inability to respond to the need for increased oxygen during surgery. Due to infants' small, soft, and pliable airways and their propensity for developing upper respiratory infections, they can quickly develop airway obstruction, bronchospasm, and stridor that can result in hypoxia and even respiratory failure. If an infant or young child exhibits signs of even mild respiratory infection on the day of surgery, the procedure might be postponed until a later date.

Infants also have difficulty maintaining stable body temperature during surgery because the shivering reflex is not well developed, making hypothermia or hyperthermia more likely. Their lower glomerular filtration rate and creatinine clearance can lead to a slower metabolism of drugs that require renal biotransformation. Because the liver is immature until after the first year of life, the effects of muscle relaxants and narcotics may be prolonged.

Physiologic changes associated with aging (described in Chapter 24) increase the surgical risk for older adults. These changes, summarized in the Focus on the Older Adult box, decrease the ability of older adults to respond to the stress of surgery, alter the effects of preoperative and postoperative medications and anesthesia, and prolong or alter wound-healing processes. With an increasing older adult population, assessing physiologic changes is crucial to providing safe, quality nursing care to older surgical patients. Chronic illnesses, more common in the older population, also increase surgical risk and may require alterations in usual perioperative procedures. For example, a patient with heart failure may be more easily fatigued and thus unable to be mobile immediately after surgery.

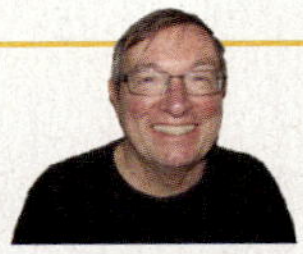

Consider **Marcus Benjamin**, the 73-year-old male who had a total hip replacement. Due to his age, the nurse would need to be alert to potential complications specifically associated with age-related changes, reduced mobility, and surgical equipment.

MEDICAL HISTORY

The medical history provides information about past and current illnesses. Pathologic changes associated with past and current illnesses increase surgical risk as well as the risk for postoperative complications. Preoperative assessments and documentation are necessary to provide a database for individualized assessments and interventions in the intraoperative and postoperative phases of care. Examples of diseases and associated risks may include:

- Cardiovascular diseases—such as thrombocytopenia, hemophilia, recent myocardial infarction or cardiac surgery, heart failure, and dysrhythmias—increase the risk for anesthesia complications, including hemorrhage and hypovolemic shock, hypotension, venous stasis, thrombophlebitis/thromboembolism, and overhydration with IV fluids.
- Respiratory disorders—such as pneumonia, bronchitis, asthma, emphysema, and chronic obstructive pulmonary diseases—increase the risk for respiratory depression from anesthesia as well as postoperative pneumonia, atelectasis, and alterations in acid–base balance.
- Kidney and liver diseases influence the patient's response to anesthesia, affect fluid and electrolyte as well as acid–base balance, alter the metabolism and excretion of drugs, and impair wound healing.
- Endocrine diseases, especially diabetes mellitus, increase the risk for hypoglycemia or acidosis, slow wound healing, and present an increased risk for postoperative cardiovascular complications.

SURGICAL HISTORY

Gathering data about previous surgeries is important for meeting the patient's physical and psychological needs throughout the perioperative period. Physical implications of previous surgeries are important to the intraoperative and postoperative phases (e.g., previous heart or lung surgery may necessitate adaptations in anesthesia and in positioning during surgery). Previous surgical complications—such as malignant hyperthermia, latex sensitivity, pneumonia, thrombophlebitis, or **deep vein thrombosis (DVT)**, a formation of a blood clot (thrombus) in a deep vein or surgical site infection—may put the patient at risk during this surgery, necessitating vigilant intraoperative and postoperative monitoring.

The patient's past experiences with surgery also affect the plan of care established in the preoperative phase, especially if a past experience was negative. When the interview elicits negative feelings about the surgical experience, pain management, or nursing interventions carried out to prevent complications during previous surgeries, teaching and mutual goal setting become even more important. For children, stressful events before surgery include the admission process, lab tests, injections, the time frame before and during transport to the OR, and the recovery period in the PACU.

In addition to experiences with past surgery, the patient's perceptions and knowledge of the upcoming surgical procedure should be assessed. The patient's questions or statements about the surgery are important for meeting psychological and family

Focus on the Older Adult

NURSING STRATEGIES TO ADDRESS AGE-RELATED CHANGES IN PERIOPERATIVE PATIENTS

Age-Related Changes	Nursing Strategies
Cardiovascular	
Decreased cardiac output, stroke volume, and cardiac reserve Decreased peripheral circulation Increased vascular rigidity	• Obtain and record baseline vital signs. • Assess peripheral pulses. • Teach leg exercises, turning, and explain the purpose of early ambulation after surgery. • Document baseline activity levels and tolerance of fatigue. • Monitor fluid administration rate. • Allow sufficient time for effects of medications to occur; administer the lowest dose possible of medications.
Respiratory	
• Reduced vital capacity • Diminished cough reflex • Decreased oxygenation of blood • Decreased chest expansion and strength of intercostal muscles and diaphragm	• Obtain and record baseline respiratory depth and rate. • Teach coughing and deep-breathing exercises. • Teach use of incentive spirometer. • Assess color of skin. • Explain use of pulse oximeter for monitoring postoperative oxygenation.
Central Nervous System	
Decreased reaction time and coordination Reduced short-term memory Sensory deficits Decreased thermoregulation ability	• Orient to surroundings. • Institute safety measures, such as keeping environment clear of clutter and using a night-light. • Allow additional time for teaching, *teach-back* activities, and questions and answers. • Use appropriate measures to conserve body heat.
Renal	
Decreased renal blood flow Reduced bladder capacity	• Monitor fluid and electrolyte status. • Maintain and record intake and output. • Provide ready access to toileting.
Gastrointestinal	
Increased gastric pH Prolonged gastric-emptying time Decreased hepatic blood flow and enzyme function	• Obtain baseline weight. • Monitor nutritional status (weight, laboratory data). • Observe for prolonged effects of medications.
Integumentary	
Decreased vascularity Decreased skin moisture and elasticity Decreased subcutaneous fat	• Assess skin status. • Monitor fluid status. • Pad and protect bony prominences. • Monitor skin for pressure areas. • Use minimal amounts of tape on dressings and intravenous sites. • Encourage active and passive range of motion, with repositioning as needed.

needs when preparing the patient for surgery, planning for patient and family teaching, and preparing for discharge.

MEDICATION HISTORY

The use of prescribed, over-the-counter, or herbal drugs can affect the patient's reaction to, and increase the risk from, the stress of surgery and the effects of the anesthetic agent. Some herbal products can increase bleeding while others may potentiate the actions of depressant anesthetic drugs. Medications in the following categories increase surgical risk:

- Anticoagulants (may precipitate hemorrhage)
- Diuretics (may cause electrolyte imbalances, with resulting respiratory depression from anesthesia)
- Tranquilizers (may increase the hypotensive effect of anesthetic agents)
- Adrenal steroids (abrupt withdrawal may cause cardiovascular collapse in long-term users)
- Antibiotics in the mycin group (when combined with certain muscle relaxants used during surgery, may cause respiratory paralysis)

Although some medications are discontinued before surgery, the nurse should know the purposes and actions of the patient's drugs as well as the health care provider's orders. Specific medications may be given the morning of surgery with sips of water (e.g., patients with heart or cardiovascular problems or diabetes mellitus).

NUTRITIONAL STATUS

Both malnutrition and obesity increase surgical risk. Surgery increases the body's need for nutrients necessary for normal tissue healing and resistance to infection. A patient who is malnourished is at greater risk for alterations in fluid and electrolyte balance, delay in wound healing, and wound infection. Patients who are obese are at increased risk for respiratory and cardiovascular compromise. The supine position, often used in surgery and other invasive procedures, negatively impacts on airway management, ventilation and oxygenation, pulmonary and cardiac blood flow, cardiac output, and work of the heart. Patients who are obese also have an increased incidence of gastroesophageal reflux disease (GERD), hiatal hernia, and abdominal pressure that puts them at risk for aspiration of stomach contents (AORN, 2020). Adipose tissue has a poor blood supply and, therefore, has less resistance to infection. As a result, postoperative complications of delayed wound healing, wound infection, and disruption in the integrity of the wound are more common.

USE OF ALCOHOL OR ILLICIT/PRESCRIPTION/OTHER DRUGS

Patients with a large habitual intake of alcohol require larger doses of anesthetic agents and postoperative analgesics, increasing the risk for drug-related complications. Although the exact mechanisms remain unclear, patients who use illicit drugs, opioids, or cannabis (tetrahydrocannabinol [THC]) are at risk for interactions with anesthetic agents and often require a multimodal approach for anesthesia (Maslonka et al., 2020). These are specific to the illicit drug used and should be noted on the medical record for safe anesthetic management. IV drug use may render veins hardened, inflamed, and unusable for anesthesia drug administration.

Patients who smoke or use electronic nicotine delivery systems (ENDS)/vaping products (ASPAN, 2020) are at higher risk for respiratory complications after surgery. All patients retain pulmonary secretions during anesthesia, but smokers, who already have increased mucous secretions and decreased ciliary action in the tracheobronchial tree, have more difficulty clearing the respiratory passages after surgery. In addition, the tracheobronchial mucosa is chronically irritated in people who smoke; anesthesia increases this irritation. Patients who smoke are at risk for hypoxia and postoperative pneumonia. Nicotine compromises wound healing by constricting blood vessels, impairing blood flow to healing tissues.

ACTIVITIES OF DAILY LIVING AND OCCUPATION

Exercise, rest, and sleep habits are important for preventing postoperative complications and facilitating recovery. A patient with a well-established exercise program has improved cardiovascular, respiratory, metabolic, and musculoskeletal function, which decreases the risks of surgery. Rest and sleep are essential to physical and emotional adaptation and recovery from the stress of surgery. Information from the health history allows the nurse to individualize interventions to promote rest and sleep.

Many surgical procedures require a delay in returning to a career/occupation/job or may affect how the patient earns a living. Knowledge of a patient's usual work and their concerns about returning to work helps the nurse plan necessary teaching and referrals.

COPING PATTERNS AND SUPPORT SYSTEMS

Assessing the patient's psychological, sociocultural, and spiritual dimensions is as important as the physical history and examination. Surgery is a major psychological stressor and affects coping patterns, support systems, and individual human needs. A surgical procedure, even a planned, minor procedure, can cause anxiety and fear. While obtaining the health history, the nurse uses cues from the patient's and family's verbal and nonverbal communication to identify fears and concerns, and to plan nursing interventions to provide the information and emotional support necessary for successful recovery from surgery.

Surgery is an unfamiliar experience over which a person has no control; the resulting anxiety and fear may be expressed in many ways such as anger, withdrawal, apathy, confrontation, or questioning. Patients often fear the unknown, pain or death, and changes in body image and self-concept. The patient typically has fears about the surgery itself—the anesthesia, the diagnosis, the future, financial and family responsibilities, response to pain, or possible disfigurement or disability. Common fears are that the anesthesia will not "put me to sleep," that death will occur during surgery, or that the patient will not be able to handle postoperative pain. Surgical procedures may leave the patient with permanent changes in body structure, function, or appearance. This may increase patients' fear of alterations in physical attractiveness, social relationships, lifestyle, and sexuality.

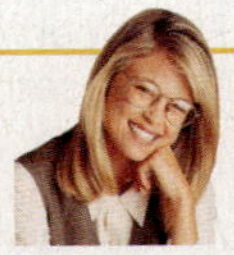

Remember **Molly Greenbaum**, the 38-year-old female who is fearful of surgery? Her statements about the inability to sleep, in conjunction with the tears in her eyes and wringing of hands, would be cues that she is experiencing stress. Exploring Molly's fears, past coping mechanisms, and support systems would be valuable in developing the patient's plan of care, both before and after surgery. Doing so would help promote a positive perioperative experience for her. In addition, the nurse would need to investigate what specific trepidation Molly may be experiencing related to a vaginal hysterectomy, such as changes in physical attractiveness, marital relationship, sexuality, and end of reproductive capability.

Therapeutic communication skills are essential for establishing the trusting nurse–patient relationship that is necessary to identify and resolve fear. Encourage the patient to identify and verbalize fears; often simply talking about fears helps to diminish their magnitude. At the same time, incorrect knowledge can be identified and corrected, strengths can be noted, and teaching can begin. The reduction of anxiety is of major importance in preoperative preparation; emotional

Research in Nursing

BRIDGING THE GAP TO EVIDENCE-BASED PRACTICE

Description of Missed Perioperative Nursing Care

A 2015 comprehensive review found that between 55% and 98% of nurses reported not completing at least one task during their assigned shift on their inpatient hospital unit. This identified missed care ranged from engaging in interprofessional care rounds to performing activities of daily living such as mouthcare or ambulation. Missed care could potentially also have detrimental effects on patient outcomes in the highly acute and well-defined perioperative period.

Related Research

Marsh, V., Kalisch, B., McLaughlin, M., & Nguyen, L. (2020). Nurses' perceptions of the extent and type of missed perioperative nursing care. *AORN Journal*, *112*(3), 237–247. https://doi.org/10.1002/aorn.13146

This study used a cross-sectional design with practicing operating room (OR) nurses who were members of their associated professional organization (AORN) to describe their reports of missed perioperative nursing care. The 1,693 participants completed the MISSCARE-OR Survey. This instrument was developed based on the Kalisch and Williams MISSCARE Survey from 2009; revised using published literature, a focus group, individual interviews; and validated through exploratory and confirmatory factor analyses. The five most frequently reported missed perioperative nursing care items were: (a) communication among the interprofessional team prior to transfer to the operating room (43.8%), (b) suspension of activities during the required surgical time out (39.9%), (c) use of isolation precautions for patients with infectious diseases (36.1%), (d) use of a standardized hand-off tool during transitions (33.7%), and (e) the reporting of abnormal laboratory values to the anesthesia provider (33.4%). It is noteworthy that OR nurses who reported adequate staffing reported fewer missed nursing care interventions than OR nurses who reported inadequate staffing.

Relevance to Nursing Practice

The emphasis of the World Health Organization (WHO), The Joint Commission, and AORN recommendations on checklists focused on *safety, closing,* and *legal considerations* may explain why fewer instances of missed care in these areas were reported. Perioperative nursing care items associated with communication were the most frequently reported missed. Education of the interprofessional team and future research needs to focus on strategies to improve communication and investigate the relationship between missed perioperative nursing care and patient surgical outcomes.

stress added to the physical stress of surgery increases the surgical risk. The nursing history should elicit the ways in which a patient provides self-support to reduce stress. These are discussed in Chapter 43 and range from listening to music to practicing active relaxation techniques. See the accompanying Research in Nursing box.

Coping with stress can be facilitated through the support systems identified in the assessment phase of preoperative nursing care. When appropriate and approved by the patient, family members or significant others should be part of the initial interview and should be included in discussions of fears and concerns. Encourage family members to provide support before and after surgery. When permitted, encourage parents/guardians to accompany their child to the preoperative waiting area and bring the parents/guardians to the recovery area when the child is awake.

Identifying the patient's spiritual beliefs aids in meeting individual spiritual needs. These needs can be met through acceptance, participation in prayer or other rituals, and/or referral to a spiritual leader. Faith in a higher being or source of personal strength may provide support and help to reduce fear in some people.

The need for other support systems can also be identified in the initial interview. For example, a patient having a colostomy, heart transplant, or mastectomy may have many questions answered and anxieties reduced by a preoperative visit from a person who has had the same operation and adapted successfully.

SOCIOCULTURAL NEEDS

A person's perceptions of and reactions to the surgical experience are influenced by several factors, including family health beliefs and practices, cultural/ethnic background, and social determinants of health. A patient who requires surgery, but lacks the requisite medical literacy and resources, may appear resistant to teaching and exhibit signs of nonadherence. Reactions to teaching, physical care, and pain are also influenced by a patient's background and experience. For example, a patient reared with the belief that it is inappropriate to acknowledge pain may demonstrate a stoic acceptance of pain and refuse needed medications postoperatively. Also keep in mind that a patient who had someone close to them die during the perioperative period may consciously or unconsciously associate the surgical experience with death.

Cultural and ethnic influences also affect the patient's responses to and perceptions of the surgical experience. The patient's cultural background may require that nursing interventions be individualized to meet needs in such areas as language, food preferences, family interactions and participation, personal space, and health beliefs and practices (see Chapter 5). For example, a patient from a culture that believes that bed rest is the most important treatment for illness or injury may have difficulty accepting the need for postoperative exercises and early ambulation. Language barriers require the use of formal interpreter services (not family members) that should be utilized at every phase of the perioperative period.

Focused Assessment Guide 31-1

PREOPERATIVE PHYSICAL ASSESSMENT

Factors to Assess	Questions and Approaches
General survey	• Note general state of health. • Note body posture and stature. • Take and record vital signs.
Integumentary system	• Inspect skin for color, characteristics, and location and appearance of any lesions. • Assess skin over bony prominences. • Determine skin turgor.
Respiratory system	• Observe chest excursion and diameter and shape of thorax. • Auscultate breath sounds. • Palpate for any pain or tenderness.
Cardiovascular system	• Inspect for jugular vein distention. • Auscultate apical rate, rhythm, and character. • Auscultate heart sounds. • Inspect for peripheral edema. • Palpate strength of peripheral pulses bilaterally.
Gastrointestinal system	• Inquire about time of last intake of fluid or food. • Inquire about time of last bowel movement. • Inspect abdominal contour. • Auscultate bowel sounds.
Neurologic system	• Note orientation, level of consciousness, awareness, and speech. • Assess reflexes. • Assess motor and sensory ability. • Assess visual and hearing ability.
Musculoskeletal system	• Inspect and note joint range of motion. • Palpate muscle strength. • Assess ability to ambulate.

Physical Assessment

Assessing the patient's current physical status provides data for interventions to decrease surgical risk and prevent potential postoperative complications. Depending on the situation, the physical assessment is conducted as described in Chapter 27. See also Focused Assessment Guide 31-1 for key areas to assess preoperatively.

Various presurgical screening tests provide objective data of normal body function. In cases of abnormalities, such tests provide data for medical interventions to improve the patient's physical status and thus decrease potential surgical complications. The nurse's role is to ensure that the tests are explained to the patient, appropriate specimens are collected, the results are documented in the patient's record before surgery, and abnormal findings are reported.

Usual presurgical screening tests include chest x-ray, electrocardiography (ECG/EKG), complete blood count (CBC), basic or complete metabolic panel (electrolytes, renal function), and urinalysis. Normal findings for laboratory tests are found in Appendix C. Significant abnormal findings include an elevated white blood cell count (presence of infection), decreased hematocrit and hemoglobin level (presence of bleeding, anemia), prolonged coagulation times (liver or medication-based), hyperkalemia or hypokalemia (increased risk for cardiac problems), and elevated blood urea nitrogen or urinalysis results (potential kidney issues). Additional cardiac clearance may be indicated for patients with a cardiac history or abnormal ECG/EKG results. Glucose testing is done as part of presurgical screening and often repeated the morning of surgery.

Diagnosing Actual or Potential Health Problems and Needs

Patient problems and needs identified in the preoperative period involve actual and potential problems and often focus on safety and mitigation of complications. These problems and needs are derived from the analysis of subjective and objective data obtained from the health history and physical examination as well as information from other health team members and screening tests. The actual and potential health problems and needs identified in the preoperative phase guide the entire perioperative plan of care. Although the plan is individualized, there are some risks and potential problems that exist for any patient undergoing an operative or other invasive procedure. The development and communication of a coordinated plan of care improves interprofessional collaboration and minimizes the risk of complications in the intraoperative and postoperative

Examples of Actual or Potential Health Problems and Needs

PREOPERATIVE PATIENT

Actual or Potential Health Problem or Need	Possible Etiologic Factors	Potential Signs and Symptoms
Knowledge Deficiency	• Lack of environmental and situational information regarding impending surgery • Surgical procedure—complexity, classification, preparation • Specific, universal perioperative outcomes	• Asking appropriate/inappropriate questions • Verbalizations of lack of understanding, complex information, processing of new information
Perioperative Injury Risk	• Alteration in cardiac and/or pulmonary function • Alteration in skin integrity—surgical positioning, immobility • Individualized risk factors—age, lifestyle (smoking, obesity), comorbidities • Stasis of body fluid • Expected and unexpected risks of anesthesia	

Source: Wolters Kluwer. (2022). *Problem-based care plans.* In *Lippincott Advisor.* Wolters Kluwer. https://advisor.lww.com/lna/home.do

phases. Examples of patient problems or needs with related etiology and signs and symptoms can be found in the box titled Examples of Actual or Potential Health Problems and Needs: Preoperative Patient.

Outcome Identification and Planning

Preoperative nursing care is affected by the length of the preoperative phase. There may not be enough time for comprehensive assessments and teaching for patients who enter the hospital through the emergency department needing immediate surgery and those who have outpatient/same-day surgery. In such cases, the nurse uses standardized preoperative plans and individualizes the plan for the particular patient and family. Outcomes are standard for all patients having surgery, but nursing interventions are designed to meet the priority needs of individual patients and situations.

Planning for the entire perioperative period is done in the preoperative phase and includes expected outcomes that are discussed and mutually agreed on by the nurse, the patient, and the family. Patient-specific outcomes may include that the patient:

- Verbalizes physical- and emotional-readiness for surgery
- Demonstrates coughing, turning, deep-breathing, and other postoperative exercises
- Verbalizes expectations of postoperative pain management
- Maintains fluid intake and nutritional balance to meet needs

Implementing

Preoperative nursing interventions provide the patient with the necessary psychological and physical preparation for surgery and the postoperative phase. This section discusses implementing the care plan to meet established patient goals. Skill 31-1 (on pages 1069–1074) outlines the actions and rationale for preoperative patient care.

Preoperative nursing care is specific and focused on addressing key aspects of care involving (Turunen et al., 2017):

- **Holistic preoperative screening:** complete medical, physical, social, psychological, and personal assessments
- **Coordination:** collaborate with the entire interprofessional team
- **Communication:** promote open, clear communication
- **Patient and family education:** provide specific pre- and postoperative instructions
- **Individual patient- and family-centered care:** promote empowerment and emotional support/comfort
- **Preoperative contact:** engage with the patient prior to surgery for screening and patient preparation, providing last-minute instruction as needed
- **Scheduling:** prioritize and communicate surgical scheduling plans

Preparing the Patient Psychologically Through Communicating

Surgery is almost always viewed as a life crisis and evokes anxiety and fear. Anxiety can be reduced and recovery facilitated by nursing actions that focus on therapeutic communication and patient and family teaching. Each patient is a unique person and responds to the surgical experience in a unique way. One note of caution: Avoid false reassurance. In an attempt to allay anxiety and fear, the nurse may be tempted to reassure patients that they will be fine. Such a response denies patients' emotional needs, shuts off therapeutic communications and trust, and may not be true.

The nurse uses therapeutic communication skills and techniques, as described in Chapter 8, to establish a supportive and trusting nurse–patient relationship and to facilitate psychological safety and security. Nursing interventions to meet the psychological needs of the surgical patient through communication are outlined in Box 31-2 on page 1052.

Box 31-2 Nursing Interventions to Meet Psychological Needs of Patients Having Surgery

- Practice intentional presence in which the focus is on being in the moment with the patient.
- Establish and maintain a therapeutic relationship, allowing the patient to verbalize fears and concerns.
- Use active listening skills to identify and validate verbal and nonverbal messages revealing anxiety and fear.
- Use touch, as appropriate, to demonstrate genuine empathy and caring.
- Be prepared to respond to common patient questions about surgery, including:
  - Will I lose control of body functions while I'm having surgery?
  - How long will I be in the operating room and PACU?
  - Where will my family be?
  - Will I have pain when I wake up?
  - Will the anesthetic make me sick?
  - Will I need a blood transfusion?
  - How long will it be before I can eat?
  - What kind of scar will I have?
  - When will I be able to be sexually active?
  - When can I go back to work?

Preparing the Patient Psychologically Through Teaching

Teaching about postoperative activities, a nursing responsibility, is implemented in the preoperative phase. Patients and families need to know about surgical events and sensations, how to manage pain, and how to perform the physical activities necessary to decrease the risk for postoperative complications and facilitate recovery. The teaching–learning process (see Chapter 9) is individualized to meet universal and individual patient needs. The success of preoperative teaching varies with the timing of the teaching, the patient and their support systems, the type of surgery, and group versus individual sessions. Preoperative teaching has proven beneficial in decreasing postoperative complications and length of stay, as well as positively influencing recovery. Patients who are well prepared with detailed preoperative instruction deal more effectively with their surgery and are better prepared to manage their pain and engage in appropriate self-care activities.

The timing of teaching is a significant consideration: Teaching too far in advance of surgery or when the patient is anxious is less effective. In today's health care system, patients often enter the hospital the day of surgery and teaching must be adapted to this schedule. Many institutions provide teaching sessions before admission to prepare the patient for surgery. Whether done before or after admission, a preoperative teaching checklist gives nurses organized, comprehensive guidelines for instruction. Box 31-3 provides a sample of preoperative teaching with associated surgical events.

TEACHING ABOUT SURGICAL EVENTS AND SENSATIONS

When surgery is scheduled, explain to patients and their families how long the surgery and postanesthesia care will last, as well as what will be done before, during, and after

Box 31-3 Sample Preoperative Teaching: Activities and Events for In-Hospital Surgery

Preoperative Phase

- Exercises and physical activities
  - Deep-breathing exercises
  - Coughing
  - Incentive spirometry
  - Turning
  - Leg exercises
  - Early mobility
- Pain management
  - Meaning of PRN orders for medications
  - Multimodal pain medication options
  - Timing for best effect of medications
  - Splinting incision
  - Nonpharmacologic pain management options
- Visit by anesthesiologist or CRNA
- Physical preparation
  - NPO
  - Medications the night before/day of surgery
  - Preoperative checklist (review items)
- Visitors and waiting room
- Transported to operating room

Intraoperative Phase

- Holding area
  - Skin preparation
  - Intravenous lines and fluids
- Medications
- Operating room
  - Operating room bed
  - Lights and common equipment (e.g., cardiac monitor, pulse oximeter, warming device)
  - Safety belt and other positing devices/equipment
  - Sensations
  - Health care team roles

Postoperative Phase

- Postanesthesia care unit
  - Frequent vital signs, assessments (e.g., orientation, movement of extremities, strength of grasp)
  - Dressings/drains/tubes/catheters
  - Intravenous lines
  - Pain medications/comfort measures
  - Family notification
  - Sensations
  - Airway/oxygen therapy/pulse oximetry
  - Health care team roles
- Transfer to unit
  - Frequent vital signs
  - Sensations
  - Pain medications/nonpharmacologic strategies
  - NPO, diet progression
  - Exercises
  - Early ambulation
- Visitation policies

surgery (e.g., procedures, medications, equipment). If the surgery is elective, an actual or computerized tour of the operating suite, or a video of the preoperative journey to the OR may be helpful in reducing anxiety and fear of the unknown. This is especially helpful for children. Provide an explanation of surgical events, including a description of the various members of the health care team; where and when to report for admission; instructions for preoperative skin preparation, fasting, and bowel prep, if prescribed; instructions for taking special medications; and the importance of bringing a responsible adult to drive the patient home. Explain to patients that they may not drive themselves home or take public transportation alone if they have had any anesthesia or sedatives.

Patients also benefit from knowing what sensory alterations they may experience during the perioperative period. Although the sensations differ depending on the type of surgery, teaching should include information about dry mouth and drowsiness from preoperative medications, a sore throat from the insertion of an endotracheal tube, a gradual return of feeling and movement after spinal anesthesia, and pain from the surgical incision. It is also important to make sure that patients are aware of the coolness of the environment, firmness of the OR bed, the sounds and sights of multiple care providers wearing surgical masks, and the bright overhead lights. Assure patients that they are the most important person in the room and will be well cared for and comforted. It is likely that the patient will receive antianxiety medication, which is also an amnesic. However, this medication should not prevent the nurse from clarifying information with patients and answering their questions.

TEACHING ABOUT PAIN MANAGEMENT

Pain is a normal part of the surgical experience and a major concern for the patient and family. Evidence-based guidelines for the management of acute surgical pain have been established by several professional organizations. The guidelines include references to: (1) individualized, developmentally appropriate patient teaching on pain management options, plans, and goals; (2) preoperative evaluation that guides postoperative pain management; (3) ongoing assessment of pain using validated assessment tools that include both subjective and objective components of assessment; (4) incorporation of multimodal anesthesia; and (5) individualized use of pharmacologic and nonpharmacologic methods of pain management (Chou et al., 2016). Continuing or unresolved pain can increase the patient's length of recovery and delay discharge. Treat unrelieved, severe postoperative pain as a serious complication of surgery, not as a normal expectation. The nurse is responsible for assessment, implementation, and evaluation of a pain management plan, and for teaching the patient preoperatively how to communicate and report pain (see Chapter 36) so that it is manageable. Keep in mind that the absence of pain (0 on a scale of 1–10) is unreasonable after surgery; the nurse works with the patient to establish a mutually agreed-upon postoperative pain goal. Introduce children and their families to an age-specific pain scale preoperatively.

Teach the patient and family that medications to relieve pain will be prescribed by the surgeon and administered by the nurse. The provider may prescribe pain medications to be given on a regular basis or on an as needed (PRN) basis. If medication is ordered PRN, there is a time restriction between doses (e.g., every 2 or 4 hours). Explain to patients that they need to ask for the medication before the pain becomes severe. If the medication does not control the pain or if the patient has unpleasant side effects (such as nausea and vomiting), a different medication can be prescribed. Current recommendations caution against routine opioid prescription postoperatively, focusing on oral opioid administration with acetaminophen and/or nonsteroidal anti-inflammatory drugs (NSAIDs) as needed, or the use of patient-controlled analgesia (PCA) when the parenteral route is necessary (Chou et al., 2016). The use of relaxation techniques (e.g., deep breathing, music, and guided imagery) enhances the effects of pain medications, as discussed in Chapter 29. Chapter 30 discusses spinal block.

Alternative methods of pain control that may be used after surgery include transcutaneous electrical nerve stimulation (TENS), pressure-controlled pain pumps filled with local anesthetics with soaker drains placed inside the incision, and PCA pumps. PCA infusion pumps allow patients to self-administer doses of pain-relieving medication within prescribed time and dose limits. Patients activate the delivery of the medication by pressing a button on a cord connected to the pump or a button directly on the pump. Teach the patient how to use these methods of pain control before surgery and monitor their effectiveness after surgery. A discussion of TENS and information about nursing interventions when using PCA are in Chapter 35.

TEACHING ABOUT PHYSICAL ACTIVITIES

The most common causes of postoperative complications are alterations in cardiovascular and respiratory function, including atelectasis, pneumonia, thrombophlebitis, DVT, and thromboembolism. Physical activities to reduce the risk for these complications include deep breathing, coughing, incentive spirometry, leg exercises, turning in bed, and early ambulation. These and other activities that will be required postoperatively are taught in the preoperative period. The patient should be able to state the purpose and demonstrate the activities before going to surgery. This section gives the rationale for the activities; postoperative complications are discussed later in the chapter.

Deep Breathing

During surgery, the cough reflex is suppressed, mucus accumulates in the tracheobronchial passageways, and the lungs do not ventilate fully. After surgery, respirations often are less effective as a result of the anesthesia, pain medications, and decreased voluntary respiratory effort because of incisional or other pain. Patients who have thoracic or high abdominal incisions are especially prone to shallow breathing because of incisional pain with deeper respirations.

Guidelines for Nursing Care 31-1

TEACHING DEEP-BREATHING TECHNIQUES

- Place the patient in semi-Fowler's position, with the neck and shoulders supported.
- Ask the patient to place the hands over the rib cage, so that the patient can feel the chest rise as the lungs expand.
- Ask the patient to:
  - Exhale gently and completely.
  - Inhale through the nose gently and completely.
  - Hold the breath for 3 to 5 seconds and mentally count "one, one thousand, two, one thousand," and so forth.
  - Exhale as completely as possible through the mouth with lips pursed (as if whistling).
  - Repeat three times.
- This exercise should be done every 1 to 2 hours while the patient is awake for the first 24 hours after surgery and as necessary thereafter, depending on risk factors and pulmonary status.

As a result, alveoli do not inflate or may collapse and secretions are retained, increasing the risk for atelectasis and respiratory infection. Deep-breathing exercises hyperventilate the alveoli and prevent them from collapsing again, improve lung expansion and volume, help to expel anesthetic gases and mucus, and facilitate oxygenation of tissues. See Guidelines for Nursing Care 31-1 for how to teach the patient deep-breathing techniques.

Coughing

Coughing helps remove retained mucus from the respiratory tract and usually is taught in conjunction with deep breathing—although it is recommended to write out the phrase, you may see nurses use the shorthand CDB (*cough and deep breathe*) in narrative notes. Coughing is especially important in patients with an increased risk for respiratory complications. Because coughing is often painful, teach the patient how to splint the incision (i.e., support the incision with a pillow or folded bath blanket) and to use the time after pain medication has been administered to their best advantage. See Guidelines for Nursing Care 31-2 on how to teach the patient how to cough effectively.

Incentive Spirometry

An incentive spirometer is often prescribed for patients having surgery. The proper technique for using it should be practiced preoperatively and reinforced by nurses and other members of the patient care team, including respiratory therapists. This device helps to increase lung volume, promote inflation of alveoli, and facilitate venous return. A gauge on the incentive spirometry device allows patients to measure their progress and provides immediate positive reinforcement for the breathing efforts. See Chapter 40 for more information.

Leg Exercises

During surgery, venous blood return from the legs slows. In addition, some surgical positions, such as having the legs elevated in the lithotomy position (see illustration in Box 27-2 on page 1052), decrease venous return. With circulatory stasis in the legs, thrombophlebitis, DVT, and the risk for emboli are potential complications. Leg exercises increase venous return through flexion and contraction of the quadriceps and gastrocnemius muscles. Leg exercises must be individualized to patient needs, physical condition, physician preference, and facility protocol. Figure 31-2 highlights how to teach the patient to perform leg exercises that engage the ankles and feet.

Turning in Bed

Turning in bed improves venous return, respiratory function, and intestinal peristalsis, while preventing the

Guidelines for Nursing Care 31-2

EFFECTIVE COUGHING

- Place the patient in a semi-Fowler's position, leaning forward.
- Provide a pillow or folded bath blanket to use in splinting the incision.
- Ask the patient to:
  - Inhale and exhale deeply and slowly through the nose three times.
  - Take a deep breath and hold it for 3 seconds.
  - "Hack" out for three short breaths.
  - With mouth open, take a quick breath.
  - Cough deeply once or twice.
  - Take another deep breath.
  - Repeat the exercise every 2 hours while awake.

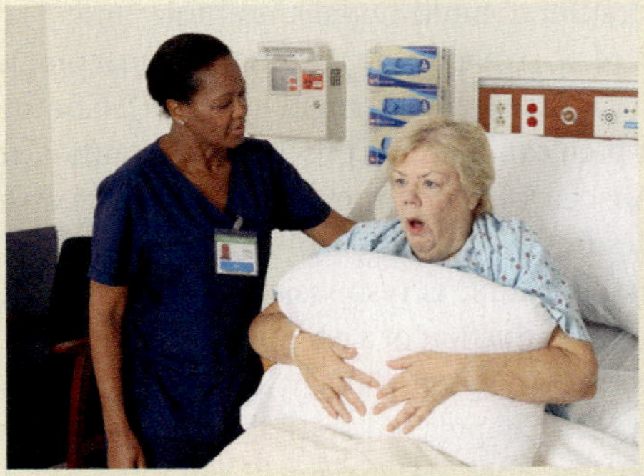

Encouraging the patient to "hack" out three short coughs after holding their breath.

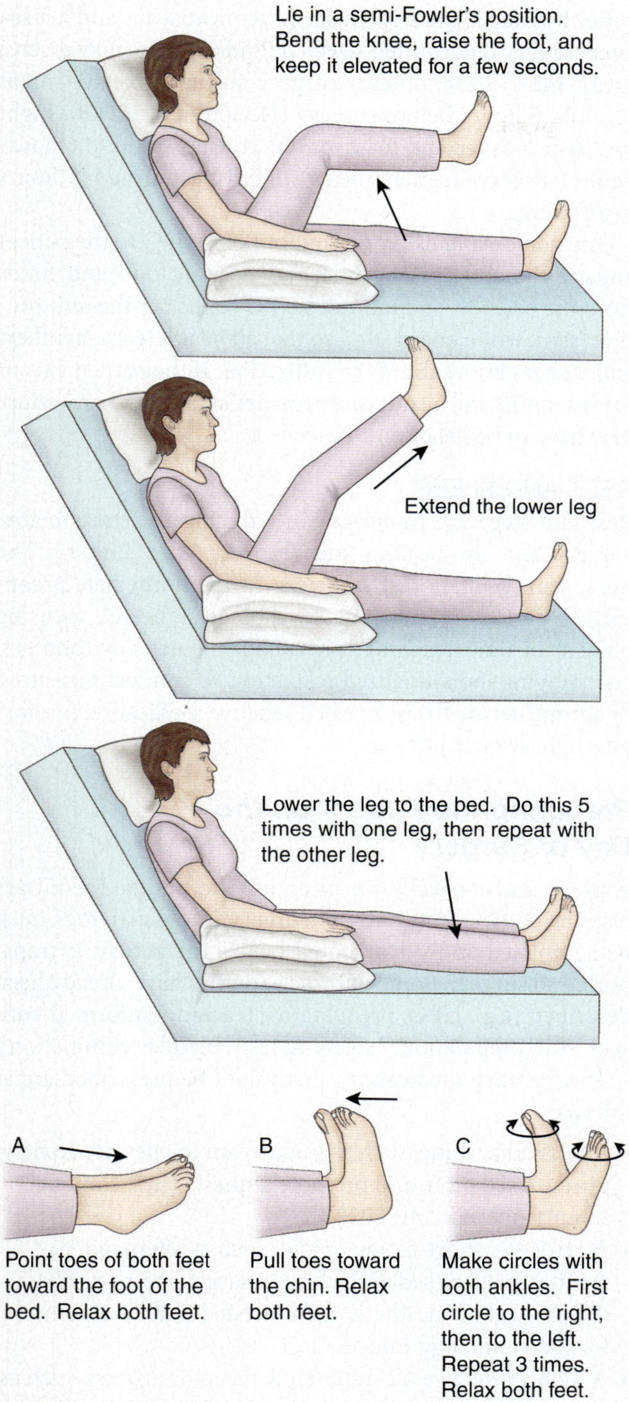

FIGURE 31-2. Leg exercises to increase venous return.

unrelieved skin pressure that would occur if the patient were to remain in only one position. Although turning in bed sounds like a simple procedure, incisional pain makes it difficult, underscoring the need for practicing it before surgery. To turn in bed, patients should raise one knee, reach across to grasp the side rail on the side toward which they are turning, and roll over while pushing with the bent leg and pulling on the side rail. A small pillow is useful for splinting the incision while turning. The patient should turn and change positions in bed every 2 hours when awake.

Early Ambulation

Although related to leg exercises and turning in bed, early ambulation has positive effects on the respiratory, cardiovascular, integumentary, musculoskeletal, gastrointestinal, and renal systems. Discussing the benefits during the preoperative period helps patients fully engage in this activity (as appropriate) postoperatively despite expected pain and discomfort.

Preparing the Patient Physically

The physical preparation of the patient for surgery varies, depending on the patient's physical status and special needs, type of surgery, and the health care provider's orders. Certain nursing interventions are appropriate for all surgical patients in the areas of hygiene and skin preparation, elimination, nutrition and fluids, and rest and sleep. The nurse is also responsible for the preparation and safety of the patient on the day of surgery.

HYGIENE AND SKIN PREPARATION

Intact skin is the body's first line of defense against microorganisms, and the surgical incision provides a potential entry for infection. Therefore, the skin is prepared to minimize skin contamination and decrease the risk for postoperative surgical site infection.

The skin is cleaned at the operative site with an antibacterial soap or solution to remove bacteria. The patient can do this while taking a bath or shower the day of or night before surgery. The specific choice of soap or antiseptic product depends on the patient, the procedure, and manufacturer recommendations (AORN, 2020; Cowperthwaite & Holm, 2015), but there is a renewed emphasis on protocols that include providing clear verbal and written instructions for patients, with electronic reminders sent as appropriate (Stanton, 2021). Although the evidence is mixed in the literature, many facilities have specific surgical bundles or protocols that include preoperative showers or baths using soap, followed by an antiseptic wash using some combination of FDA-approved iodine-, alcohol-, and/or chlorhexidine gluconate (CHG)-based products (AORN, 2020). Ideally, a tinted antiseptic that is visible on the skin should be used (Stanton, 2021). For example, the nurse may need to cleanse children and adult inpatients preoperatively with microfiber cloths impregnated with 2% CHG antimicrobial skin antiseptic. This skin antiseptic eliminates skin microorganisms and leaves an antimicrobial film on their skin. Shampooing the hair and cleaning the fingernails also help to reduce the number of organisms present on the body.

Leave hair at the surgical site in place if possible. Removal of hair at the surgical site depends on the amount of hair, the location of the incision, and the type of surgical procedure being performed. If ordered, this may be done on the unit or in the surgical suite immediately before the operation, usually in the surgical holding area. If hair must be removed, AORN (2020) recommends removing only the hair that will interfere with the surgical procedure using hair clippers as close to the time of surgery as possible. Document the condition of the skin, method of hair removal, and skin preparation site and agent. Instruct the patient not to shave the area of the surgical site prior to surgery unless so directed by the health care provider.

ELIMINATION

Emptying the bowel of feces is no longer a routine procedure before surgery. The nurse uses the preoperative assessment to determine the need for a prescription to facilitate bowel elimination. If the patient has not had a bowel movement for several days or has had preoperative barium diagnostic tests, an enema helps prevent postoperative constipation.

If the patient is scheduled for surgery of the lower gastrointestinal tract, a bowel prep and cleansing enema may be prescribed. Peristalsis does not return for 24 to 48 hours after the bowel is handled, so preoperative cleansing helps to decrease postoperative constipation. An empty bowel also prevents contamination of the surgical area during surgery.

Insertion of an indwelling urinary catheter may be prescribed before surgery, especially in patients having pelvic surgery, to prevent bladder distention or accidental injury. If an indwelling catheter is not in place, instruct the patient to void immediately before receiving preoperative medications to ensure an empty bladder during surgery.

NUTRITION AND FLUIDS

Patients need to be well-nourished and hydrated before surgery to counterbalance fluid, blood, and electrolyte loss during surgery; to facilitate anesthesia delivery; to counter the surgical stress response; and to promote tissue healing after surgery. The surgical stress response involves endocrine (hormonal), hematologic, metabolic, and immune changes that are triggered to compensate for intravascular volume depletion, cardiac output and oxygen consumption changes, and energy expenditures associated with the stress of surgery and the immune response (Gillis & Wischmeyer, 2019). Integration of a nutrition assessment, ideally performed by a registered dietician using a validated instrument, provides baseline information that informs preoperative and postoperative decisions regarding supplemental nutrition, fluids, or electrolytes (see Chapter 41). A patient who is undernourished or malnourished may require nutritional intervention to shore up their physiological reserve prior to surgery to increase their capacity to respond to surgical stress. This nutritional support should continue postoperatively (Gillis & Wischmayer, 2019). In emergencies, IV fluid and blood products are administered as needed to the patient prior to surgery.

Although maintaining an NPO status for at least 8 hours prior to surgery was formerly the standard, the American Society of Anesthesiologists (2017) revised the practice guidelines for preoperative fasting. Current practice guidelines allow patients to drink clear liquids up to 2 hours before surgery. If clear liquids are allowed by the health care provider, the patient should be taught that clear liquids include water, fruit juices without pulp, carbonated beverages, clear tea, and black coffee. These liquids do not include any alcohol. Patients, especially children, may be less anxious, better hydrated, and experience fewer headaches and nausea after surgery if permitted selected fluids. Infants may receive breast milk 4 hours before surgery and may receive infant formula 6 hours before surgery (Nelson et al., 2018). Light meals such as tea and toast may be consumed up to 6 hours before surgery; regular meals should be finished 8 hours before surgery.

The nurse explains the reason for being NPO to the patient and, at the appropriate time, removes all food and fluids from the bedside, and indicates NPO status per the unit routine (sign, white board, etc.) so that all health team members and visitors know about the restriction. If the patient eats or drinks, notify the health care provider at once; the procedure may have to be delayed or cancelled.

REST AND SLEEP

Rest and sleep are important in reducing the stress before surgery and for healing and recovery after surgery. The nurse can facilitate rest and sleep in the immediate preoperative period by meeting psychological needs, focusing on just-in-time teaching, providing a quiet environment, encouraging individualized relaxation or comfort measures, or administering the prescribed sedative medication for hospitalized surgical patients.

Preparing the Patient on the Day of Surgery

A preoperative checklist is often used to outline the nurse's responsibilities on the day of surgery; these activities must be completed and documented before the patient is transported to surgery. Some of these activities have already been described (e.g., NPO, preoperative teaching, informed consent, skin preparation, screening tests, bladder elimination).

Preoperative medications that might be prescribed are as follows:

- A benzodiazepine, such as midazolam to alleviate anxiety, produce sedation, and promote amnesia (U.S. National Library of Medicine, 2020)
- A synthetic short-acting opioid, such as alfentanil, to facilitate patient sedation and relaxation and to decrease the amount of anesthetic agent needed (National Center for Biotechnology Information, 2020)
- A highly selective α2-adrenergic receptor agonist, such as dexmedetomidine, to reduce anesthesia requirements and pain (Obara, 2018)

Guidelines for Nursing Care 31-3 provides further information about preoperative interventions the day of surgery for a hospitalized patient.

Evaluating

Evaluating the care plan for the preoperative phase is based on the expected outcomes. The plan is effective if the patient is physically and emotionally prepared for surgery, verbalizes expected events and sensations of the perioperative period, and demonstrates postoperative exercises and activities.

Guidelines for Nursing Care 31-3

PROVIDING PREOPERATIVE PATIENT CARE: HOSPITALIZED PATIENT (DAY OF SURGERY)

- Check that preoperative consent forms are signed and dated, witnessed, and correct. Verify advance directives are in the medical record (as applicable).
- Gather the needed equipment and supplies.
- Perform hand hygiene.
- **Check vital signs.** Notify the health care provider of any pertinent changes (i.e., rise or drop in blood pressure, elevated temperature, cough, symptoms of infection).
- Provide oral care. Assess for loose teeth. **Verify adherence to food and fluid restrictions before surgery.**
- Facilitate/verify bathing was completed the morning of or night before surgery. **Complete any skin antiseptic preparation per surgical protocol or bundle.**
- Instruct the patient to remove all personal clothing, including underwear, and put on a hospital gown.
- Ask patient to remove cosmetics, jewelry including body piercings, nail polish, and prostheses (e.g., contact lenses, false eyelashes, dentures). Some facilities allow a wedding band to be left in place, depending on the type of surgery, provided it is secured to the finger with tape.
- If possible, give valuables to a family member or place valuables in an appropriate area, such as the hospital safe.
- **Have the patient empty their bladder before surgery.**
- Attend to any special preoperative orders, such as starting an IV line.
- Complete the preoperative checklist and the record of the patient's preoperative preparation.
- **Administer preoperative medication as prescribed by the surgeon/anesthesia provider.**
- Raise the side rails of the bed; place the bed in the lowest position. Instruct the patient to remain in the bed or on the stretcher. If necessary, a safety belt may be used.
- Help move the patient from the bed to the transport stretcher if necessary. Reconfirm patient identification and ensure that all preoperative events and measures are documented.
- Tell the family of the patient where the patient will be taken after surgery and the location of the waiting area where the surgeon will come to explain the outcome of the surgery.
- After the patient leaves for the OR, prepare the room and make a postoperative bed for the patient. Anticipate any necessary equipment based on the type of surgery and the patient's history.

NURSING PROCESS FOR INTRAOPERATIVE CARE

The intraoperative phase of surgery begins with admission of the patient to the surgical area and lasts until the patient is transferred to the PACU or other recovery area. The perioperative nurse has critical responsibilities and roles in collaboratively meeting patient needs. The nursing process uses the preoperative data and plan as a basis for the intraoperative plan of care.

Assessing

The first room the patient enters when transferred to the surgical area is the preoperative holding area. Nurses in surgical scrub attire identify the surgical patient, assess the patient's emotional and physical status, and verify the information on the preoperative checklist, including assessment data, lab reports, and consents for surgery and blood transfusion. They may also carry out required immediate preoperative care, including performing skin preparation, starting IV fluids, placing intermittent pneumatic compression devices (IPCDs) to prevent DVT, determining pain level, reassuring patient and family, providing comfort, and giving preoperative medications. The nurse also assesses the patient's response to the procedures and explains the events of surgery. Review Figure 31-3 on page 1058, a surgical checklist from AORN that seamlessly incorporates the standards and requirements from Joint Commission and the World Health Organization (WHO; AORN, 2020).

When the OR is ready, the patient is transported to the OR. Once the patient transfers from the stretcher to the OR bed, the patient is identified again with the operative team using at least two identifiers (such as name, birth date). The patient is then anesthetized, positioned, prepped, and draped. The perioperative nurse assesses the patient and reviews preoperative data, paying particular attention to factors that increase surgical risk. To maintain patient safety, the nurse also assesses the patient during positioning, and monitors supplies used.

Diagnosing Actual or Potential Health Problems and Needs

Patient problems in the intraoperative period may occur as a result of the position of the patient, the effects of the anesthesia, equipment used, disruption of tissues during the operative or invasive procedure, and the incision. Examples of patient problems or needs with related etiology and signs and symptoms can be found in the box titled Examples of Actual or Potential Health Problems and Needs: Intraoperative Patient on page 1058.

Outcome Identification and Planning

The planning phase of the nursing process focuses on identifying interventions most effective for preventing complications, anticipating patient problems, and ensuring patient safety. Some expected outcomes are that the patient will:

- Remain free of neuromuscular injury
- Remain free from wrong-site, wrong-side, wrong-patient surgical procedure

COMPREHENSIVE SURGICAL CHECKLIST

Blue = World Health Organization (WHO) Green = The Joint Commission - Universal Protocol 2016 National Patient Safety Goals Teal = Joint Commission and WHO

PREPROCEDURE CHECK-IN	SIGN-IN	TIME-OUT	SIGN-OUT
In Preoperative Ready Area	Before Induction of Anesthesia	Before Skin Incision	Before the Patient Leaves the Operating Room
Patient or patient representative actively confirms with registered nurse (RN):	RN and anesthesia professional confirm:	Initiated by designated team member: All other activities to be suspended (except in case of life-threatening emergency)	RN confirms:
Identity ☐ Yes Procedure and procedure site ☐ Yes Consent(s) ☐ Yes Site marked ☐ Yes ☐ N/A by the person performing the procedure **RN confirms presence of:** History and physical ☐ Yes Preanesthesia assessment ☐ Yes Nursing assessment ☐ Yes Diagnostic and radiologic test results ☐ Yes ☐ N/A Blood products ☐ Yes ☐ N/A Any special equipment, devices, implants ☐ Yes ☐ N/A Include in Preprocedure check-in as per institutional custom: Beta blocker medication given ☐ Yes ☐ N/A Venous thromboembolism prophylaxis ordered ☐ Yes ☐ N/A Normothermia measures ☐ Yes ☐ N/A	Confirmation of the following: identity, procedure, procedure site, and consent(s) ☐ Yes Site marked ☐ Yes ☐ N/A by person performing the procedure Patient allergies ☐ Yes ☐ N/A Pulse oximeter on patient ☐ Yes Difficult airway or aspiration risk ☐ No ☐ Yes (preparation confirmed) Risk of blood loss (> 500 mL) ☐ Yes ☐ N/A # of units available ______ Anesthesia safety check completed ☐ Yes **Briefing:** All members of the team have discussed care plan and addressed concerns ☐ Yes	Introduction of team members ☐ Yes **All:** Confirmation of the following: identity, procedure, incision site, consent(s) ☐ Yes Site is marked and visible ☐ Yes ☐ N/A Fire Risk Assessment and Discussion ☐ Yes (prevention methods implemented) ☐ N/A Relevant images properly labeled and displayed ☐ Yes ☐ N/A Any equipment concerns ☐ Yes ☐ N/A **Anticipated Critical Events** **Surgeon:** States the following: ☐ Critical or nonroutine steps ☐ Case duration ☐ Anticipated blood loss **Anesthesia professional:** Antibiotic prophylaxis within 1 hour before incision ☐ Yes ☐ N/A Additional concerns ☐ Yes ☐ N/A **Scrub person and RN circulator:** Sterilization indicators confirmed ☐ Yes Additional concerns ☐ Yes ☐ N/A **RN:** Documented completion of time out ☐ Yes	Name of operative procedure: ______ Completion of sponge, sharp, and instrument counts ☐ Yes ☐ N/A Specimens identified and labeled ☐ Yes ☐ N/A Equipment problems to be addressed ☐ Yes ☐ N/A Discussion of Wound Classification ☐ Yes **To all team members:** What are the key concerns for recovery and management of this patient? ______ ______ ______ ______ **Debriefing with all team members:** Opportunity for discussion of – team performance – key events – any permanent changes in the performance card

The Joint Commission does not stipulate which team member initiates any section of the checklist except for site marking. The Joint Commission also does not stipulate where these activities occur. See the Universal Protocol for details on the Joint Commission requirements.

AORN SAFE SURGERY TOGETHER

FIGURE 31-3. Surgical checklist. (*Source:* Reprinted with permission from AORN.org. Copyright © 2019, AORN, Inc, 2170 S. Parker Road, Suite 400, Denver, CO 80231. All rights reserved.)

Examples of Actual or Potential Health Problems and Needs

INTRAOPERATIVE PATIENT

Actual or Potential Health Problem or Need	Possible Etiologic Factors	Potential Signs and Symptoms
Perioperative Injury Risk	• Unintended retained foreign objects • Tourniquet use • Surgical energy-generating devices—electrosurgical units, electrocauteries, ultrasonic instruments, and lasers	—
Perioperative Positioning Injury	• Length and type of surgical procedure • Patient-specific factors identified through screening—comorbidities, hypoperfusion, and oxygenation issues • Surgical positioning • Availability and correct use of positioning and pressure-reducing devices	• Stretching and compression injuries, pressure injuries, or shearing injuries • Tissue edema, ischemia, or neurologic impairment • Residual effects that result in a temporary or permanent functional restriction (or death)

Source: Association of periOperative Registered Nurses (AORN). (2020). *Guidelines for perioperative practice.* AORN, Inc. https://www.aorn.org/guidelines https://www.aorn.org/guidelines; International Council of Nurses (ICN). (2019). *Nursing diagnosis and outcome statements.* https://www.icn.ch/sites/default/files/inline-files/ICNP2019-DC.pdf; Wolters Kluwer. (2022). *Problem-based care plans.* In *Lippincott Advisor.* Wolters Kluwer. https://advisor.lww.com/lna/home.do

- Maintain fluid and electrolyte balance
- Maintain skin integrity (other than the incision)
- Have symmetric breathing patterns
- Be free of injury from burns, retained surgical items (inaccurate count of sharps, instruments, and soft goods such as surgical sponges used during the procedure), and medication errors
- Remain free from surgical site infection
- Maintain normothermia

Implementing

During surgery, nurses function as scrub nurses and perioperative registered nurse (RN) circulators, in an expanded role as registered nurse first assistants (RNFAs), or as advanced practice registered nurses (APRNs), including CRNAs.

The scrub nurse is a member of the sterile team who maintains sterile technique while draping and handling instruments and supplies. The perioperative RN circulator, assigned to a patient for the duration of the procedure, serves as a patient advocate. The RN circulator coordinates the plan of care, establishes collaborative relationships while supervising and evaluating the surgical team, facilitates transitions of care, and provides direction and intervention in emergency situations (AORN, 2019). The perioperative RN circulator is ultimately responsible for the nursing-specific patient outcomes of the operative or other invasive procedure (AORN, 2020) and facilitates the following: appropriate transfer and positioning of the patient; surgical site/skin antiseptic preparation; verifying and providing additional supplies or medications; anticipating needs of the surgical team to facilitate the procedure; maintaining environmental safety; and counting the number of instruments, sharp items such as needles, and soft goods such as sponges used during the surgery to prevent the accidental loss of an item in the surgical site. The RNFA actively assists the surgeon by providing exposure of the operative area, hemostasis (by using surgical clamps or other medical devices on bleeding tissue), and wound closure. The APRN coordinates care activities; collaborates with physicians and nurses in all phases of perioperative and postanesthesia care; and integrates case management, critical paths, and research into care of the surgical patient. A CRNA may be directly involved in administering anesthesia and anesthesia-related care. Additional educational preparation is required for the roles of the RNFA and the APRN.

Error Prevention

Despite current safeguards and processes, **never events** occur in the surgical setting. These never events are considered sentinel events by the Joint Commission, and the Centers for Medicare and Medicaid Services (CMS) does not reimburse hospitals for any expenses incurred as a result of a preventable patient injury. Public reporting of these errors improves the quality of care, and hospitals are under increased pressure to correct the problems that contribute to these events (Agency for Healthcare Research and Quality [AHRQ], 2019). Examples of these errors include leaving a foreign object in the patient's body, performing the wrong surgery, or operating on the incorrect body site (AHRQ, 2019). The Joint Commission (2020), an independent accrediting facility for health care organizations and facilities, has established the Universal Protocol to prevent wrong-site, wrong-procedure, and wrong-person surgery. The universal protocol has three components:

1. Preoperative patient identification verification process
2. Marking the operative site
3. Final verification just prior to beginning the procedure, referred to as the **time-out**

The time-out occurs immediately before starting the surgical procedure and is initiated by a designated member of the team. The surgeon, the anesthesia provider, the RN circulator, the OR technician, and any other active participants conduct the time-out assessment and ensure that there are no questions or concerns. During the time-out, all members of the surgical team must agree on the identity of the patient, the correct surgical site, and the procedure that will be performed. The completion of the time-out is documented appropriately. To further minimize patient risk in the dynamic perioperative setting and promote safe, quality care, AORN (2019) believes that a minimum of one perioperative RN circulator should be dedicated to each patient for the duration of that patient's intraoperative experience.

Positioning

Preoperative assessment findings guide the nurse in knowing extremity limitations and other functional needs to individualize patient care. The equipment in the room should be prepared prior to the procedure based on the planned procedure, the surgeon's preferences, and the status of the patient (AORN, 2020). The patient is placed in a specific operative position after anesthesia has produced loss of consciousness and reflexes. Using proper body mechanics and following the directions provided by the manufacturer for any equipment, the nurse works with the entire surgical team to coordinate any required movement and maintain body alignment. The risk for skin injury is avoided by lifting with a lateral-transfer device, rather than rolling or pulling the patient into the surgical position. Rolling or pulling can cause a shearing force, in which two or more tissue layers slide on each other, stretching subcutaneous blood vessels, obstructing blood flow, and contributing to pressure injuries (AORN, 2020). Although all of the operative positions are not described here, perioperative nurses need to know the position that will be used and significant nursing considerations for that position. Two examples are the Trendelenburg position and the lithotomy position. The Trendelenburg position requires lowering the upper torso and raising the feet. It is commonly used in minimally invasive surgery of the lower abdomen or pelvis. The displacement of the abdominal viscera toward the head decreases diaphragmatic movement and respiratory exchange; pooling blood increases intracranial and intraocular pressures; and hypotension can result with return to the supine position. When possible, patients should not be kept in this position for extended periods of time, and skin should be monitored for shearing. The lithotomy position is used for gynecologic, rectal, and urologic procedures. The placement of legs in stirrups causes pooling of blood in the legs, increasing the risk of DVT. Pressure can also damage the peroneal nerve, with resultant foot drop. Patients can experience lower back strain if they are not positioned slowly and carefully (AORN, 2020). Refer to Chapter 27 for additional information regarding body positions.

Draping

Drapes are used to create and maintain a sterile field around the operative site, preventing the passage of microorganisms, particulate matter, and fluids between sterile and nonsterile areas. The only area left exposed is the incision site. In some cases, plastic adhesive drapes may be used to form a complete seal over the skin. With these drapes, skin color is visible, and the incision is made through the impermeable adhesive drape.

Documenting

Throughout surgery, the perioperative nurse documents on the intraoperative record ongoing patient assessment, item counts (soft goods, sharps, instruments), monitoring data (e.g., vital signs, urine output, blood loss, pulse oximetry results, body temperature), positioning, medications, dressings and drains, specimens, equipment used (electrosurgery unit and settings, ultrasound, video, stirrups for positioning), and responses to care. This documentation includes planning and implementation of perioperative nursing activities and evaluation of the achievement of patient outcomes.

Transferring to the Postanesthesia Care Unit

After completion of the surgical procedure and emergence from anesthesia, the patient is moved carefully from the operating bed to a stretcher or bed. This is a critical time: sudden or rough handling can cause severe hypotension or potentially lethal cardiac or respiratory arrest. The patient is then transported to the PACU, and the OR nurse provides a hand-off report to the PACU nurse containing relevant preoperative and intraoperative assessments and interventions. The primary objective of the hand-off report from OR nurse to PACU nurse is to provide accurate information about the patient's care, procedure, tourniquet time, drains, medications used, presenting condition, and any important events that occurred during the procedure. It allows for communication, clarification and questions, and continuity of care.

Evaluating

Evaluation of the effectiveness of the care plan for the intraoperative phase is based on the expected outcomes. If met, the plan was effective.

POSTOPERATIVE NURSING CARE

The postoperative phase can be divided into two stages—immediate care (usually provided in the PACU in both in-hospital and outpatient/same-day surgery centers) and ongoing postoperative care (lasting from return to the unit through convalescence). Nursing assessments and interventions are consistent with those in the preoperative and intraoperative phases and are carried out to maintain function, promote recovery, and facilitate coping with alterations in structure or function. (See the accompanying Through the Eyes of a Student.) Assessments and nursing interventions are combined in discussing immediate postoperative care; the phases of the nursing process are used to describe ongoing postoperative care.

Immediate Postoperative Assessment and Care

Care in the PACU involves assessing the postoperative patient, with an emphasis on preventing complications from anesthesia and/or the surgery. Assessments are continuous, using preoperative and intraoperative data as the basis for comparison. The assessments made in the PACU include respiratory status (airway, pulse oximetry), cardiovascular

Through the Eyes of a Student

The first time I took care of a patient with "multiple tubes," I was horrified at the thought of actually touching the patient. I hadn't really been exposed to that many critically ill patients until my last semester as a student nurse. I remember being assigned a patient in the cardiothoracic intensive care unit. The patient was a "fresh heart"—a patient who just had a coronary artery bypass graft (CABG) that morning.

I remember walking into the room and thinking, "What do I do with all of these tubes?" and then with horror thinking, "What if one of them falls out?" Needless to say, I was overwhelmed and frightened, but at the same time excited at the challenge that faced me. I asked my preceptor what each tube was for, where it was hooked up, and whether it would fall out if I touched it. They answered all my questions with patience and understanding and asked me if I wanted to handle the tubes. I looked at them as if they were unhinged but went ahead and did it. Would you believe that nothing fell out! I must admit that the experience taught me a lot, but it also got me over the fear of tubes.

I now chuckle every time I see a nursing student's face with that same look of horror I had, and I try to answer every question with the same degree of patience and understanding that my preceptor had for me.

—Lynda L. Ullmer, RN, Gaithersburg, MD

status (blood pressure), temperature, central nervous system status (level of alertness, movement, shivering), fluid status, wound status, gastrointestinal status (nausea and vomiting), and general condition. These assessments initially are made every 10 to 15 minutes.

The average PACU stay is about 1 hour, but it will vary depending on the type of surgery, length of anesthesia, and patient response. Outpatient/same-day surgical patients return home after full recovery in the PACU or phase 2 recovery. The critical role functions of the PACU nurse include vigilant monitoring during emergence from anesthesia and the first hours after surgery, managing pain, maintaining fluid and electrolyte balance, stabilization of physiologic parameters (such as heart and respiratory rates), and preparation for the next level of care.

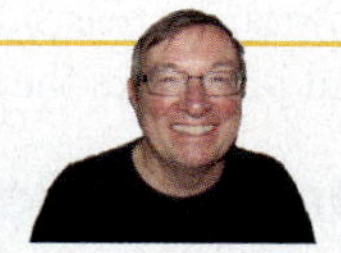

Mr. Benjamin, the older adult who has had a total hip replacement, will require frequent assessments during his stay in the PACU, specifically vital signs, cardiovascular status, respiratory status, IV therapy, wound status, and gastrointestinal status. If he had spinal anesthesia, neurologic assessments would be done every 15 minutes.

Respiratory Status

The nurse assesses respiratory function by monitoring respiratory rate, rhythm, and depth; auscultating breath sounds; noting the oxygen saturation level and PCO_2 levels; assessing skin color; and observing cardiovascular and mental status. During a surgical procedure with general anesthesia, an endotracheal tube may be inserted to administer the anesthetic gases and maintain patent air passages. This artificial airway is not removed until the laryngeal and pharyngeal reflexes return, allowing the patient to control the tongue, cough, and swallow. If newer short-acting anesthetic agents are used, the endotracheal tube is usually removed in the OR. The nurse assesses the patient's airway for patency, administers oxygen, and initiates pulse oximetry. Ineffective respiratory function is indicated by restlessness and anxiety; unequal chest expansion with use of accessory muscles; shallow, noisy respirations; cyanosis; and tachycardia.

Respiratory obstruction is the most common PACU emergency. It may occur as a result of secretion accumulation, obstruction by the tongue, laryngospasm (a sudden, violent contraction of the vocal cords and laryngeal closure), or laryngeal edema. Respiratory obstruction is diagnosed when there is ineffective respiratory function accompanied by wheezing or crowing sounds with respiratory effort. In the case of respiratory distress due to laryngospasm, call for help—early recognition and intervention is key. The recommended initial step involves maneuvers to open the airway: (1) firm pressure behind the angles of the jaw on both sides (Fink, 1956); or (2) firm upward pressure at the "laryngospasm notch bounded anteriorly by the condyle of the mandible, posteriorly by the mastoid process, and superiorly by the base of the skull" (Larson, 1998, p. 1293). Opening the airway is followed by the administration of oxygen, management of secretions, and, if respiratory distress is still unresolved, the administration of sedatives/paralytics and consideration of reintubation (Sibert et al., 2020). General nursing interventions, including positioning to promote drainage of secretions, administering humidified oxygen, encouraging the patient to take deep breaths, and suctioning, may be used to maintain a patent airway and tissue oxygenation.

Cardiovascular Status

Assess cardiovascular function by taking vital signs, monitoring electrocardiogram rate and rhythm, and observing skin color and condition. Compare blood pressure findings with baseline data from the preoperative period. Transient hypertension can occur as a result of anesthetic effects, respiratory insufficiency, the surgical procedure, or the excitement phase of recovery from anesthesia.

Hypotension may be the result of varied factors, including preoperative medications, anesthetic agents, position changes, blood loss, respiratory alterations, and peripheral blood pooling. Oxygen administration, deep breathing, leg exercises, verbal stimulation (to help expel anesthetic gases and facilitate increasing level of consciousness), and maintaining or increasing IV fluid administration rates can raise low blood pressure.

Patients are at risk for altered body temperature related to the surgical procedure, its length, anesthetic agents, a cool surgical environment, age, and use of cool irrigating or infusion fluids. Inadvertent **hypothermia** (temperature below 36°C [96.8°F]) can lead to complications of poor wound healing, hemodynamic stress, cardiac disturbances, coagulopathy, delayed emergence from anesthesia, and shivering with its associated discomfort (AORN, 2020). Routinely measure the patient's core body temperature using an invasive/noninvasive device, or estimate core body temperature with peripheral measurement (oral/axilla/rectum) using a thermometer or probe. Note that current guidelines do not recommend infrared methods, such as tympanic membrane measurement, for the perioperative patient (AORN, 2020). If the patient is hypothermic, warmed blankets placed on the patient's body and forced warm-air devices are used for rewarming.

Assess all pulses for bilateral equality, rhythm, rate, and character. Of special significance are assessments of abnormal function—an irregular rhythm, absence of pulses, or tachycardia. Carefully evaluate for tachycardia, an early symptom of shock. Other related assessments for shock are a decreasing blood pressure, cyanosis, a cool skin temperature, and a decrease in urine output. After surgery on an extremity, closely monitor pulse checks, neurologic checks, color, temperature, and sensation.

Central Nervous System Status

The return of central nervous system function is assessed through the patient's response to stimuli and orientation. Consciousness returns in reverse order, with the usual pattern being: (1) unconsciousness, (2) response to touch and sounds, (3) drowsiness, (4) awake but not oriented, then

(5) awake and oriented. Nurses in the PACU verbally reorient the patient by gently touching and calling the patient by name. If the patient had spinal anesthesia, neurologic checks are done every 15 minutes for the first hour. Differentiating alterations in level of consciousness that are expected during this phase from those that are unexpected or related to another underlying cause, such as delirium or hypoxia, requires experience and clinical judgment.

Fluid Status

Fluid imbalance may result from factors such as preoperative fluid restriction, fluid loss during surgery, wound drainage, or the surgical stress response (with retention of sodium and water). Imbalanced fluid volume (deficit or excess) is a risk for all surgical patients but is an especially important consideration in children and older adults. Monitor fluid status by assessing skin turgor, vital signs, urine output, wound drainage, and the OR's documentation of total intake and output. IV fluid administration assessments include the type of fluid or blood product infused, the rate, location of lines, condition of the IV insertion site, and the security and patency of the tubing.

Wound Status

The nurse in the PACU assesses the dressing over the incision for amount, consistency, and color of drainage, as well as for any tubes or drains and the amount and type of drainage by that route. Large amounts of bright-red drainage, combined with other abnormal physical status assessments (restlessness, pallor, cool moist skin, decreasing blood pressure, increasing pulse and respiratory rates), may indicate hemorrhage and hypovolemic shock. Report these symptoms immediately. Nurses in the PACU and throughout the postoperative period must turn patients to ensure that there is no drainage or blood pooling under the patient.

Concept Mastery Alert

If a large amount of fresh red drainage appears on a patient's dressing, the nurse should *not* remove the dressing and apply a new one. It is best to reinforce the dressing with additional bandages to reduce the possibility of hemorrhage resulting from dislodging clots that may be forming.

Pain Management

Pain is both a subjective and an objective experience. Pain management experts recommend the assessment of pain using a rating scale. The scale may be verbal (ranging from *no pain* to *worst possible pain*), numeric (with *10* on a scale of 0–10 being the worst possible pain), or a FACES rating scale, ranging from a smiley face indicating no pain to a face that has frowns and tears for worst possible pain (see Chapter 36). Initial pain management, using NSAIDs and opioids, occurs in the PACU. Opioids may be delivered by PCA, allowing the patient to control the analgesic administration. Nonpharmacologic methods to decrease pain and improve comfort include positioning, verbal reassurance, and touch. These should supplement, not substitute for, pharmacologic pain relief. Preoperative determination of mutually agreed upon, realistic pain goals and identification of methods that are personally effective for the patient assist in effective implementation in the PACU.

General Condition

Other assessments and interventions are made to ensure physical and emotional comfort and safety. Constant reorientation and reassurance that the surgery is completed provide psychological comfort. Careful assessments, proper positioning, and use of side rails maintain physical safety. The patient is discharged from the PACU when their physical status and level of consciousness are considered stable. The PACU nurse should notify visitors that the patient is being transferred back to the patient's room. Use of a standardized hand-over process, tool, or checklist decreases communication breakdowns, increases the quality of information communicated, and promotes the safe transition of care (AORN, 2020).

Ongoing Postoperative Care

Ongoing postoperative care is planned to facilitate recovery from surgery and coping with alterations. The plan includes promoting physical and psychological health, preventing complications, and teaching self-care for when the patient returns home. Skill 31-2 (on pages 1074–1080) outlines initial and ongoing postoperative patient care.

NURSING PROCESS FOR ONGOING POSTOPERATIVE CARE

Assessing

For hospitalized patients, the nurse on the unit assists PACU personnel in transferring the patient and performs an initial assessment using data from the preoperative and intraoperative phases. A postoperative checklist or flow sheet may be used. The initial assessment is often combined with the implementation of postoperative health care provider's orders. See Table 31-2 for focused assessments and interventions.

After conducting the assessment, document the time of arrival and all assessment data. Facility protocol is followed for assessment routines: Common time frames are every 15 minutes until stable, changing to every 1 to 2 hours for the first 24 hours, and every 4 hours thereafter. Although protocols are used as guidelines in the immediate postoperative period, the nurse is responsible for using their clinical judgment to adjust the frequency and priorities of assessment to meet the specific needs of each patient.

Diagnosing

The nurse uses assessment data, the plan of care established before and during an operative or other invasive procedure, and input from caregivers to identify actual and potential patient problems in the postoperative phase. Examples of patient problems or needs with related etiology and signs and symptoms can be found in the box titled Examples of Actual or Potential Health Problems and Needs: Postoperative Patient.

Table 31-2 Postoperative Assessments and Interventions Upon Return to the Unit

FACTORS TO ASSESS	ASSESSMENTS AND INTERVENTIONS
Vital signs and oxygen saturation	• Obtain temperature, blood pressure, pulse, respiratory rate, and oxygen saturation. • Note, report, and document deviations from preoperative and PACU data as well as symptoms of complications.
Color and temperature of skin	• Inspect skin for color (pallor, cyanosis), temperature, and moisture (diaphoresis).
Level of consciousness	• Verify type of anesthesia and any reversal agents administered. • Assess and reorient (as needed) to person, place, and time. • Assess reaction to stimuli and ability to move all four extremities.
Intravenous fluids	• Verify estimated blood loss in the OR. • Check infusion site(s). • Verify type and amount of solution, flow rate, security, and patency of tubing.
Surgical site	• Verify surgical procedure, location, approach, and any positioning requirements. • Assess dressing and dependent areas for drainage (color, amount, consistency). • Secure drains and tubes: be sure they are intact, patent, and properly connected to drainage systems.
Other tubes	• Assess indwelling urinary catheter, gastrointestinal suction, and other tubes for drainage, patency, and amount of output. • Ensure that dependent drainage bags are hanging properly and suction drainage is attached and functioning. • If oxygen is prescribed, ensure placement of prescribed application and flow rate.
Comfort	• Verify orders for pain medications including medication(s), dose, route, and frequency. • Assess pain (location, duration, intensity) and determine whether analgesics were given in the PACU. • Assess for nausea and vomiting. • Cover the patient with a blanket. • Reorient to the room as necessary. • Allow visitors to remain with the patient after the initial assessment is completed.
Position and safety	• Place the patient in an ordered position or, if the patient is not fully conscious, place in the side-lying position. • Elevate the side rails and place the bed in locked and low position. • Perform a focused or brief head-to-toe assessment to establish a baseline.

Examples of Actual or Potential Health Problems and Needs

POSTOPERATIVE PATIENT

Actual or Potential Health Problem or Need	Possible Etiologic Factors	Potential Signs and Symptoms
Acute Pain	• Surgical incision • Required surgical positioning • Required movement to prevent postoperative complications	• Change in physiologic parameters (pulse, respirations, blood pressure) • Self-report or evidence of pain characteristics using a standardized pain instrument • Instinctive, frequent repositioning or guarding • Reports of tissue, joint, neurologic discomfort • Hesitation or refusal to ambulate or engage in coughing and deep breathing exercises
Surgical Site Infection Risk	• Patient-specific factors—comorbidities, nutritional state, compensatory mechanisms, immune response • Contamination of sterile field during operative or invasive procedure • Environmental, personnel, or equipment failure	—

Source: Wolters Kluwer. (2022). *Problem-based care plans.* In *Lippincott Advisor.* Wolters Kluwer. https://advisor.lww.com/lna/home.do

Nursing Advocacy in Action

Patient Scenario

Alex is a 28-year-old male admitted to the surgical intensive care unit after undergoing a partial gastric bypass surgical procedure. He originally weighed 700 lb but lost 100 lb prior to being approved for the surgery. Patients undergoing bariatric surgery, like Alex, are usually admitted to the intensive care unit for airway management, and to ensure strict adherence to fluid intake restrictions needed to maintain the integrity of the suture line. You are assigned to care for Alex. The nurse giving the report says the following:

- "Alex is noncompliant with the fluid intake restrictions. He tries to sneak water. I don't know why we have to care for patients who are not willing to follow the medical treatment plan that they agreed to before surgery."
- "He should be repositioned hourly but since he's not motivated to participate with his ADLs, especially bathing and turning in bed, I wouldn't worry. Why should we risk hurting ourselves when he obviously doesn't care?"
- "His mother told the charge nurse yesterday that caregivers were making comments related to his size and were not providing the same quality of care as they gave to other patients."

Implications for Nursing Advocacy

How will you respond if you are Alex's nurse? Talk with your classmates and experienced nurses about the questions that follow.

- If you elect to advocate for Alex, what practical steps can you take to ensure better health outcomes?
- What is reasonable to expect of a student nurse, a graduate nurse, and an experienced nurse in this situation?
- What advocacy skills are needed to effectively respond to this challenge?

Outcome Identification and Planning

The plan of care in the postoperative phase begins in the preoperative phase, when nursing activities to reduce stress and teach postoperative activities are implemented. From admission, prepare the patient and family for uneventful recovery and self-care after discharge. Individualize specific expected outcomes based on risk factors, the surgical procedure, and the patient's unique needs. Examples of desired postoperative outcomes for a patient after major surgery are as follows:

The patient will:

- Carry out leg (including foot and ankle) exercises every 2 to 4 hours
- Perform effective coughing and deep breathing exercises every hour while awake
- Engage in early ambulation
- Verbalize decreasing levels of pain that meet pre-established pain goals
- Regain and maintain a balanced intake and output
- Regain normal bowel and bladder elimination
- Exhibit a healing surgical incision
- Remain free of infection—pulmonary, surgical site, or other
- Verbalize any concerns about appearance of wound
- Verbalize and demonstrate wound self-care

Implementing

Many nursing interventions in the postoperative phase have already been discussed in this chapter or are fully discussed in other chapters. Nursing care focuses on interventions that prevent complications, promote a return to health, and facilitate coping with alterations in function and/or body image.

A wide variety of factors increase the risk of postoperative complications, including age, health habits, physical condition, medical history, psychological status, and surgical intervention (e.g., anesthesia, positioning, wound). Ongoing postoperative assessments and interventions are implemented to decrease the risk for postoperative complications. If complications occur, perform focused physical assessments, provide care and emotional support to the patient and family, and carry out prescribed treatments. See Nursing Advocacy in Action for an example of a patient who may require an advocate.

Preventing Cardiovascular Complications

Nursing interventions to prevent or monitor for cardiovascular complications are listed in Box 31-4. Specific cardiovascular complications include hemorrhage, shock, thrombophlebitis and thromboembolism, and pulmonary embolus.

HEMORRHAGE

Hemorrhage is an excessive internal or external blood loss that may lead to hypovolemic shock. Nurses throughout the postoperative period must turn patients to ensure that there is no unseen blood pooling under the patient or flank ecchymosis, indicating internal bleeding. Hemorrhage and the resulting hypovolemic shock manifest as an increase in heart rate (earliest sign of shock) and associated hypotension; restlessness, anxiety, and apprehension; cold, clammy skin and cool, mottled extremities; deep, rapid respirations; and decreased urine output. The primary priorities for the patient experiencing a hemorrhage are to stop the bleeding and replace blood volume. Nursing interventions include applying a pressure dressing to the bleeding site, calling the medical intervention/rapid response team, notifying the surgeon immediately, and being prepared to have the patient return to the OR if bleeding cannot be stopped.

SHOCK

Shock is the body's reaction to inadequate organ perfusion. In shock, there is activation of compensatory mechanisms to address the resulting hypoperfusion, metabolic changes, and activation of the inflammatory response. The type of shock most commonly seen in postoperative patients is hypovolemic

Box 31-4 Nursing Interventions to Prevent or Monitor Postoperative Cardiovascular Complications

- Assess and document vital signs as ordered and as the patient's status dictates, using preoperative assessments as a baseline.
- Provide covers, forced warm air, or other warming device or techniques as necessary to prevent shivering and hypothermia.
- Maintain fluid balance.
- Maintain accurate intake and output.
- Monitor rate, type, and access site of IV fluids.
- Assess skin turgor and hydration of mucous membranes.
- Monitor amount, color, and consistency of wound drainage (dressings and drains or tubes).
- Implement leg exercises and turning in bed every 2 hours.
- Assist with ambulation—ambulation usually begins the evening of surgery and increases as tolerated; blood pressure and pulse and respiratory rates are used to monitor tolerance.
- Apply and follow protocols for graduated compression stockings or pneumatic compression devices, if prescribed.
- Administer anticoagulant medications, if prescribed.
- Measure bilateral calf and thigh circumference daily.
- Assess for leg swelling, tenderness, or palpable venous cord.
- Avoid positioning that impedes venous return (e.g., do not mechanically raise the knee portion of the bed or place pillows under the knees).

shock secondary to a profound loss of blood, plasma, and fluid, which decreases the circulating blood volume. Other forms of shock (cardiogenic, circulatory/distributive [septic, neurogenic, anaphylactic], obstructive) are possible depending on the surgery and patient. With all forms of shock, interventions focus on addressing the underlying cause and managing the patient's oxygenation–ventilation, fluid and nutritional balance, and blood pressure. Early recognition and treatment is the key to survival with shock.

Specific nursing interventions include calling for the medical intervention/rapid response team and notifying the surgeon immediately; establishing and maintaining the airway; placing the patient in a flat position with the legs elevated 30 to 45 degrees; administering oxygen; monitoring vital signs, hematocrit, and blood gas results; maintaining body warmth with covers; and administering medications. The nurse must also be prepared to assist with the insertion of IV lines and administer fluids, as well as packed red blood cells or other blood components.

Concept Mastery Alert

Monitoring urine output is an important nursing intervention because adequate urine output indicates adequate tissue perfusion.

THROMBOPHLEBITIS AND THROMBOEMBOLISM

Thrombophlebitis is an inflammation of a vein associated with thrombus (blood clot) formation. Thrombophlebitis is typically superficial and, in patients without an underlying condition, is often related to IV catheters. A thrombus that forms in a deep vein, particularly in the legs of postoperative patients, is called a deep vein thrombosis (DVT). The primary goal is DVT prevention. Postoperative nursing interventions include administering medications (e.g., low-molecular-weight heparin or low-dose unfractionated heparin); correctly applying graduated compression stockings, IPCDs (Box 31-5 on page 1066), or venous foot pumps; and increasing mobility (American Association of Critical Care Nurses, 2018). Manifestations of DVT are pain and cramping in the calf or thigh of the involved extremity, redness and swelling in the affected area, elevated temperature, and an increase in the diameter of the involved extremity. This increase in extremity circumference (typically the calf) is the most significant sign of a DVT and the provider should be notified. The priority for the patient with a known DVT is preventing a clot from breaking loose and becoming a **venous thromboembolism (VTE)** that propagates (travels) to the heart, brain, or lungs (called a *pulmonary embolism*; see Preventing Respiratory Complications for more details). It is important during every shift to assess the legs for swelling and tenderness; measure bilateral calf or thigh circumference; and determine if the patient experiences any unexplained anxiety, wheezing, chest pain, or dyspnea. Patients who receive anticoagulants or other medications to prevent or treat DVT/VTE also need to be monitoring for bleeding (AORN, 2020). Instruct the patient who has a known DVT to not massage the legs.

Preventing Respiratory Complications

Nursing interventions to prevent respiratory complications include monitoring vital signs; implementing deep breathing, coughing, and incentive spirometry; turning in bed every 2 hours; ambulating; maintaining hydration; avoiding positioning that decreases ventilation; and monitoring responses to narcotic analgesics. The postoperative pulmonary care program known as I COUGH has been adopted in several institutions since its inception in 2012 (Cassidy et al., 2013). The focus of this efficacious, yet simple program is to reduce respiratory complications. To mitigate the loss of initial gains and recommit the heath care team to this effective program, the current iteration focuses on implementing standardized pulmonary practices across all surgical services, ongoing education, and addressing the underlying cultural/environmental issues that may impede implementation at a health care facility (Cassidy et al., 2020). I COUGH stands for:

- **I**ncentive spirometry
- **C**oughing/deep breathing
- **O**ral care
- **U**nderstanding (patient and staff education)
- **G**etting out of bed at least three times daily
- **H**ead of bed (HOB) elevation

Box 31-5 Intermittent Pneumatic Compression Devices

Pneumatic compression devices are composed of an air pump, connecting tubes, and an extremity sleeve. The sleeve may cover the entire leg or may extend from the foot to the knee. A variety of types are available; the accompanying figure provides one example. The devices apply brief pressure to the legs to enhance blood flow and venous return, thereby decreasing the risk of DVT formation after surgery. The devices may apply either intermittent or sequential pressure. Intermittent pneumatic compression devices (IPCDs) fit over the entire leg, with inflation and deflation of the sleeve covering the leg alternating from one leg to the other by a preset timer. Sequential pneumatic compression devices are designed so that pressure moves up the leg in increments. They may inflate and deflate by alternating from one leg to the other, or they may do so for both legs at once.

Nursing Care

- Explain the purpose of the device to the patient.
- Apply the device according to the manufacturer's instructions, making sure that two fingers fit between the leg and the sleeve.
- Position the tubing so that the patient can move about without interrupting the airflow.
- Remove the sleeves at least once a day for skin care and assessment.
- Assess the extremities for peripheral pulses, edema, changes in sensation, and movement on a regular schedule.
- Ensure that all chambers are inflating in proper sequence once per shift.
- Craft a plan for safe removal and storage when exiting the bed; reinforce reapplication upon return to bed

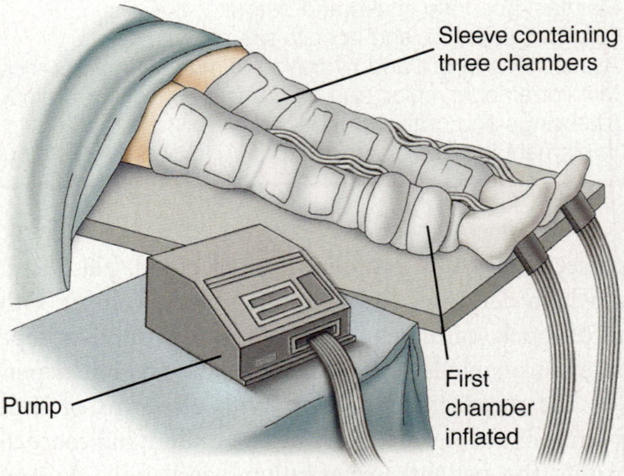

Intermittent or sequential pneumatic compression devices.

Specific respiratory complications include pulmonary embolus, atelectasis, and pneumonia.

PULMONARY EMBOLISM

A VTE is a blood clot or foreign substance that is dislodged and travels through the bloodstream until it lodges in a smaller vessel. In postoperative patients, the VTE is often part of a thrombus that breaks free from a vein wall. If the VTE lodges in the pulmonary vessels, it is called a **pulmonary embolism**. Manifestations of a pulmonary embolism include dyspnea, chest pain, cough, cyanosis, rapid respirations, tachycardia, and anxiety. This is a life-threatening condition and immediate treatment is necessary. The primary goals of care are to stabilize cardiovascular and respiratory function as well as prevent further emboli. Nursing interventions include notifying the health care provider immediately, calling the medical intervention/rapid response team, assessing vital signs frequently, administering oxygen for an oxygen saturation <90%, administering anticoagulants and other medications as prescribed (fluid and vasopressors if unstable), and preparing the patient for potential diagnostic and interventional procedures.

ATELECTASIS

Atelectasis is the incomplete expansion or collapse of alveoli with retained mucus that involves a portion of lung and results in poor gas exchange. Manifestations of atelectasis include decreased lung sounds over the affected area, dyspnea, cyanosis, crackles, restlessness, and apprehension. The primary goals of care are to ensure oxygenation of tissues, prevent further atelectasis, and expand involved lung tissues. Use of an incentive spirometer is particularly helpful in preventing atelectasis by promoting alveolar expansion. Nursing interventions include those used to prevent or monitor for respiratory complications, positioning the patient in semi-Fowler's position, administering oxygen, and administering analgesics for pain. For a sudden onset, notify the surgeon immediately and call the medical intervention/rapid response team.

PNEUMONIA

Pneumonia is an inflammation of the alveoli as the result of an infectious process or the presence of foreign material. Pneumonia may occur postoperatively as a result of aspiration, infection, depressed cough reflex, increased secretions from anesthesia, dehydration, and immobilization. Manifestations of pneumonia include fever, chills, a cough that produces rusty or purulent sputum, crackles and wheezes, dyspnea, and chest pain. The primary goals of care are to treat the underlying infection, maintain respiratory function, and prevent the spread of microorganisms. Nurses carefully monitor for sepsis which is where the infection causes a systemic inflammatory response and leads to organ dysfunction (Centers for Disease Control and Prevention [CDC], 2018). Although a slight elevation in temperature is expected after the trauma of surgery, an increase in temperature to ≥101°F or a decrease to ≤96.8°F with associated changes in white blood cell count, respiratory rate, heart rate, lactate, and/or blood glucose requires follow-up and monitoring for active infection (CDC, 2018). Nursing interventions include those used to prevent or monitor for respiratory complications, promoting full aeration of the lungs by positioning the patient in semi-Fowler's or Fowler's position, encouraging the use of incentive spirometry,

Box 31-6 Nursing Assessments and Interventions to Meet Postoperative Elimination Needs

Bowel Elimination

- Assess for the return of peristalsis by auscultating bowel sounds every 4 hours when the patient is awake.
- Assess abdominal distention, especially if bowel sounds are not audible or are high pitched (indicative of possible paralytic ileus, which is an absence of intestinal peristalsis).
- Assess ability to pass flatus and stool.
- Assist with movement in bed and ambulation to relieve gas pains, a common postoperative discomfort.
- Encourage food and fluid intake when ordered, especially fruit juices and high-fiber foods.
- Maintain privacy when patient is using the bedpan, commode, or bathroom.
- Administer suppositories, enemas, or medications, such as stool softeners, as prescribed.

Urinary Elimination

- Monitor patterns of intake and output.
- Assist in assuming normal position to void by using an upright position when on a bedpan and using a bedside commode or bathroom when able; assist the male patient to stand upright to void with a urinal.
- Assess for bladder distention by palpating above the symphysis pubis if the patient has not voided within 8 hours after surgery or if the patient has been voiding frequently in amounts of less than 50 mL; bladder scan PRN, notify the health care provider of abnormal assessment results.
- Maintain prescribed intravenous fluid infusion rates.
- Encourage oral fluid intake when prescribed.
- Provide privacy when the patient is using bedpan, bedside commode, urinal, or bathroom.
- Initiate urinary catheterization, if prescribed.

promoting ambulation, administering oxygen, administering medications (e.g., antibiotics, expectorants, analgesics), providing frequent oral hygiene, and ensuring rest and comfort. See the Surviving Sepsis Campaign (Society of Critical Care Medicine, n.d.) website at https://www.sccm.org/SurvivingSepsisCampaign/Home for more details on sepsis guidelines and bundles.

Preventing Surgical Site Complications

The nurse assesses and cares for the surgical site to promote healing and prevent complications such as infection, dehiscence (wound closure separation), and evisceration (protrusion of intra-abdominal organs). Wound care is discussed in Chapter 33. Nursing interventions to prevent surgical site complications are assessing vital signs (especially for fever); maintaining hydration; maintaining nutritional status; encouraging a diet high in protein, carbohydrates, calories, and vitamins; using proper hand hygiene; and following aseptic technique when changing dressings at the surgical site and exit sites for tubes and drains. Dispose of soiled gloves and dressings following standard precautions.

Promoting a Return to Health

Nurses provide interventions during postoperative recovery to promote physical and psychological functioning at as near a normal state as possible. The plan of care to achieve this objective includes activities to meet elimination, fluid and electrolyte balance, nutrition, rest and comfort, and pain management needs.

ELIMINATION NEEDS

Both urinary and bowel elimination are altered by anesthesia. Manipulation of organs during surgery, inactivity, pain medication, and altered fluid and food intake all impact baseline bowel and bladder routines during the perioperative period. Assessments and nursing interventions to promote the return of normal bowel and urinary elimination are outlined in Box 31-6.

FLUID AND NUTRITION NEEDS

Nursing assessments and interventions to meet fluid needs include monitoring trends and balance of intake and output, maintaining prescribed IV fluid infusion rates, encouraging fluid intake, and assessing skin turgor and mucous membranes for fluid volume deficit. Nutritional needs are met by monitoring weight, providing oral hygiene before meals and as needed, facilitating postoperative dietary progression, maintaining an environment conducive to appetite (clean, neat, free of odors), encouraging the patient to sit up in a chair for meals, and encouraging family presence during meals. Nurses employ clinical judgment regarding patient tolerance of fluids and food to advance the patient's diet—often from clear to full liquids, then from a soft to regular diet. Objective measures that inform decision-making postoperatively include presence of bowel sounds, flatus, diaphoresis, vomiting, diarrhea or constipation, abdominal distension, and review of an intake/output log. Subjective measures include the patient's reports of hunger, feelings of discomfort (nausea or pain), and interest in food. Refer to Chapter 37 for more insight into nutrition.

COMFORT AND REST NEEDS

Comfort is a priority after surgery. Factors that interfere with comfort include nausea, vomiting, thirst, hiccups, positioning in bed, room noise and temperature, and pain at the surgical site. Nursing interventions that promote rest and comfort by alleviating these problems are listed in Guidelines for Nursing Care 31-4 on page 1068. The nurse also promotes comfort by providing personal hygiene, keeping bed linens clean, maintaining a patient-preferred room temperature, providing quiet rest periods, and allowing family members to remain with the patient.

Helping the Patient Cope

Surgery may alter the patient's physical appearance as well as physiologic function, leading to the risk for or actual alterations in self-concept and body image. Changes in a person's

Guidelines for Nursing Care 31-4

PROMOTING POSTOPERATIVE REST AND COMFORT

Nausea and Vomiting

- Avoid giving large amounts of fluids or food at one time, especially after being NPO.
- Administer prescribed medications.
- Provide oral hygiene, as needed.
- Maintain a clean environment.
- Avoid use of a straw.
- Avoid strong-smelling food.
- Assess for possible allergy or intolerance to medications, such as antibiotics or analgesics.
- Maintain bowel elimination.

Thirst

- Offer sips of water or ice chips when NPO (if permitted).
- Maintain oral hygiene.

Hiccups

- Have the patient do the following:
  - Take several swallows of water while holding the breath (if not NPO).
  - Rebreathe into a paper bag.
  - Eat a teaspoon of granulated sugar.
- Provide medications as prescribed.

Surgical Pain

- Assess pain frequently; administer prescribed analgesics every 2 to 4 hours on a regular schedule during the first 24 to 36 hours after surgery.
- Reinforce preoperative teaching for pain management.
- Offer nonpharmacologic measures to supplement medications: massage, position changes, relaxation, guided imagery, meditation, music.

self-perception can influence all of the human dimensions and areas of human functioning, including self-esteem, relationships with others, sexual identity, spiritual beliefs, sociocultural values, and independent and fulfilling engagement in activities of daily living.

Many surgical patients have the same reaction to loss of a body part as to a death (see Chapter 44). The response and adaptation to the loss are influenced by multiple factors, including age, cultural values and beliefs, sociocultural background, significance of the body part, visibility of the body part, time to prepare for the change, and support people available. A surgical patient's grief is a normal and appropriate response. It is unique to the person experiencing it, and although there are stages and phases of grief, there is no timetable for it. The nurse must be aware of the patient's needs and provide interventions to meet those needs in coping with change. Nursing interventions to facilitate coping and adaptation are outlined in Box 31-7.

Providing Outpatient/Same-Day Surgery Postoperative Care

Evaluating the patient's postoperative status after outpatient/same-day surgery focuses on ensuring that the patient can be safely cared for at home. After surgery and recovery from the anesthetic, ask the patient to sit up and drink liquids. A patient who is no longer drowsy or dizzy, has stable vital signs, and has voided is allowed to go home accompanied by a responsible adult. The patient is not allowed to drive a car or go home alone on public transportation. The usual length of time from completion of surgery to discharge is 1 to 3 hours, provided that established criteria have been met. Give written and verbal instructions for home care to the patient and caregivers. Ask the patient and caregivers to *teach back* or provide a *return demonstration* to verify the patient's/caregiver's understanding. The patient and nurse both sign and date that these instructions were received, reviewed, and understood.

Evaluating

The nurse may evaluate the achievement of desired outcomes for postoperative recovery and rehabilitation in a number of ways. Because the final resolution of some desired outcomes may not be apparent or measurable at the time of discharge, many institutions use follow-up telephone calls or mailed surveys to patients. It may also be possible to collaborate with the health care provider's office to have a patient complete a survey on the first postoperative visit.

Box 31-7 Nursing Interventions to Facilitate Postoperative Coping and Adaptation

- Accept each patient as a unique person. Use appropriate pronouns and address the patient by their preferred name.
- Identify through verbal and nonverbal cues patients who are at risk for alteration in self-concept. The risk is increased if the patient has little support from others, a visible alteration, or an alteration that will seriously affect functional ability.
- Allow time for patients and families to verbalize their feelings about the alteration, and do not assume that all patients will have problems.
- Identify and support strengths and effective coping mechanisms.
- Encourage the patient and family to be part of goal setting and decision making throughout the surgical experience.
- Provide teaching and honest information to the patient and family about all aspects of care.
- Work collaboratively with other members of the health care team to provide referrals and resources as necessary to meet physical, psychological, and spiritual needs.

Whatever mechanism is selected, include the following important outcomes as part of evaluative criteria: absence of surgical site infection, patient satisfaction with pain management measures, return to former levels of mobility and activity, absence of postoperative nausea and vomiting (PONV) at discharge, and absence of other complications for which the patient was at risk.

REFLECTIVE PRACTICE LEADING TO PERSONAL LEARNING

Remember that the object of reflective practice is to look at an experience, understand it, and learn from it. As you begin to develop your expertise in evaluating the plan of care, reflect on your experiences—successes and failures—in order to improve your practice. How can you do it better next time? What did you learn today that can help you tomorrow? Begin your reflection by paying close attention to the following:

- How aware are you of the developmental considerations regarding the perioperative phases? Are you able to articulate the populations are greatest risk during surgery?
- What value do you attach to involving and empowering the patient throughout the perioperative process? How do you individualize the care for patients when so many guidelines, policies, and procedures dictate your care? What are the key elements of nursing care during the pre-, intra-, and postoperative phases?
- What plan do you have to stay abreast of evolving standards and surgical procedures? What are the core principles of perioperative nursing that will exist irrespective of evolving technologies?

Keeping up with the latest evidence-based practice guidelines can be challenging. Ensuring you are tuned into the appropriate professional organizations and governmental facilities can help you stay on the cutting edge. Balancing the needs of each patient with these responsibilities requires mindfulness and intentionality.

Perhaps the most important questions to reflect on are: Are your patients and families better for having had *you* share in the critical responsibility of partnering with them to ensure appropriate perioperative care? Are your patients now receiving thoughtful, person-centered, prioritized, holistic, evidence-based treatment and care because of your efforts?

Skill 31-1 Providing Preoperative Patient Care

DELEGATION CONSIDERATIONS

Preoperative assessment and teaching are not delegated to assistive personnel (AP). Depending on the state's nurse practice act and the organization's policies and procedures, preoperative teaching may be delegated to licensed practical/vocational nurses (LPN/LVNs) after an assessment of education needs by the registered nurse. The decision to delegate must be based on careful analysis of the patient's needs and circumstances as well as the qualifications of the person to whom the task is being delegated. Refer to the Delegation Guidelines in Appendix A.

EQUIPMENT (Varies, Depending on the Type of Surgery and Surgical Setting)

- Blood pressure cuff
- Electronic blood pressure monitor/sphygmomanometer
- Pulse oximeter
- IV infusion device
- Graduated compression stockings
- Pneumatic compression device
- Tubes, drains, vascular access tubing
- Incentive spirometer
- Small pillow
- PPE, as indicated

IMPLEMENTATION

ACTION	RATIONALE
1. Check the patient's health record for the type of surgery and review the prescribed interventions. Review the nursing database, history, and physical examination. Check that the baseline data are recorded; communicate any assessment abnormalities or areas of concern to the health care team.	These checks ensure that the care will be provided for the right patient and any specific teaching based on the type of surgery will be addressed. Also, this review helps to identify patients who are at increased surgical risk.
2. **Check that all diagnostic testing has been completed and results are available; identify and communicate abnormal results to the health care team.** Gather the necessary supplies.	This check may influence the type of surgery performed and anesthetic used, as well as the timing of surgery or the need for additional consultation. Preparation promotes efficient time management and an organized approach to the task.

(*continued on page 1070*)

Skill 31-1 Providing Preoperative Patient Care *(continued)*

ACTION	RATIONALE
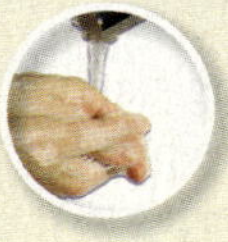 3. Perform hand hygiene and put on PPE, if indicated.	Hand hygiene and PPE prevent the spread of microorganisms. PPE is required based on transmission precautions.
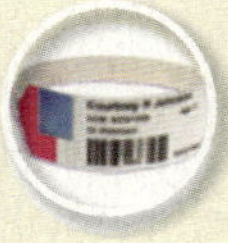 4. Identify the patient.	Identifying the patient ensures the right patient receives the intervention and helps prevent errors.
5. Close the curtains around the bed and close the door to the room, if possible. Explain what you are going to do and why you are going to do it to the patient and significant other. Place necessary supplies on the bedside stand, overbed table, or other surface within easy reach.	Closing the curtains and door ensures the patient's privacy. Explanation relieves anxiety and facilitates engagement. Bringing everything to the bedside conserves time and energy. Arranging items nearby is convenient, saves time, and avoids unnecessary stretching and twisting of muscles on the part of the nurse.
6. Explore the psychological needs of the patient and family/caregivers related to the surgery.	Meeting the psychological needs of the patient and family/caregivers before surgery can have a beneficial effect on the postoperative course.
a. Establish a therapeutic relationship, encouraging the patient to verbalize concerns or fears.	Use of therapeutic communication skills decreases anxiety (Croke, 2020a), promotes healing, enhances safety, and improves clinical outcomes.
b. Use active listening skills, answering questions and clarifying any misinformation.	
c. Use touch, as appropriate, to convey genuine empathy.	
d. Offer to contact spiritual counselor (e.g., priest, minister, rabbi) to meet spiritual needs.	Spiritual beliefs for some patients and family/caregivers can provide a source of support over the perioperative course.
7. **Identify learning needs of patient and family/caregivers.** Ensure that the informed consent of the patient for the surgery has been signed, timed, dated, and witnessed. Inquire if the patient has any questions regarding the surgical procedure (Figure 1). Check the patient's record to determine if an advance directive has been completed. If an advance directive has not been completed, discuss with the patient the possibility of completing it, as appropriate. If patient has had surgery before, ask about this experience.	Patient education enhances surgical recovery and allays anxiety by preparing the patient for postoperative convalescence, discharge plans, and self-care (Croke, 2020b). The surgeon is responsible for explaining the details of the surgical procedure and potential risks and complications. The nurse is responsible for clarifying what the surgeon has explained to the patient and contacting the surgeon if the patient does not understand or has further questions. An advance directive provides written communication of the patient's wishes to the health care team related to the patient's desire for extraordinary life-sustaining treatments if the patient's condition is deemed unsalvageable. Previous surgical experience may impact preoperative care positively or negatively, depending on the patient's experience.

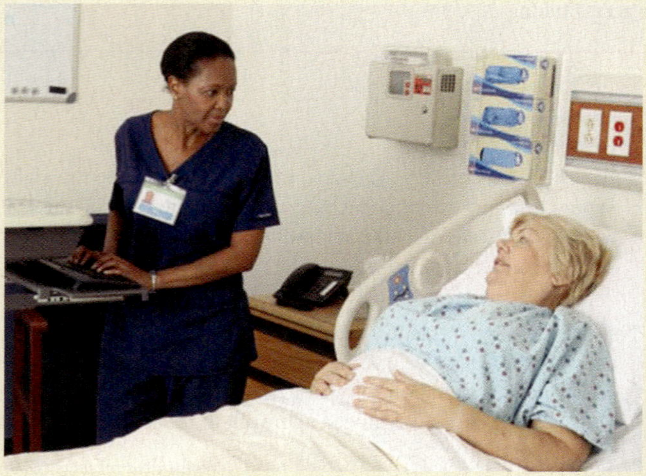

FIGURE 1. Identifying needs of patient and answering questions.

ACTION	RATIONALE
8. Teach deep-breathing exercises.	Deep-breathing exercises improve lung expansion and volume, help expel anesthetic gases and mucus from the airway, and facilitate the oxygenation of body tissues.
9. Teach coughing and splinting.	Coughing helps remove retained mucus from the respiratory tract. Splinting minimizes pain while coughing or moving.
10. Teach use of incentive spirometer, as prescribed or indicated.	Incentive spirometry improves lung expansion, helps expel anesthetic gases and mucus from the airway, and facilitates oxygenation of body tissues. Use of incentive spirometry may be based on patient risk factors and/or health care provider preference; evidence of effectiveness in prevention of postoperative pulmonary complications is controversial (Branson, 2013; Cassidy et al., 2020; Lumb, 2019; Strickland et al., 2013).
11. Teach leg exercises, as appropriate.	Physical activity reduces the risk of postoperative complications. Leg exercises assist in preventing muscle weakness, promote venous return, and decrease complications related to venous stasis. Leg exercises may be contraindicated for patients with certain conditions, such as lower extremity fractures.
12. Teach about early ambulation, as appropriate.	Physical activity reduces the risk of postoperative complications. Early ambulation has positive effects on the respiratory, cardiovascular, integumentary, musculoskeletal, gastrointestinal, and renal systems (Hinkle et al., 2022). Discussing the benefits during the preoperative period help patients fully engage in this activity (as appropriate) despite expected pain and discomfort postoperatively.
13. Assist the patient in putting on graduated compression stockings. Demonstrate how the pneumatic compression device operates.	Graduated compression stockings and pneumatic compression devices are used postoperatively for patients who are at risk for a deep vein thrombosis (DVT) and pulmonary embolism (AORN, 2018; Fan et al., 2020; Hinkle et al., 2022; Tubog, 2019).
14. Teach about turning in the bed.	Turning and repositioning of the patient is important to prevent postoperative complications and to minimize pain.
a. Instruct the patient to use a pillow or bath blanket to splint where the incision will be. Ask the patient to raise their left knee and reach across to grasp the right side rail of the bed. If the patient is turning to the left side, they will bend the right knee and grasp the left side rail.	
b. When turning the patient onto the right side, ask the patient to push with bent left leg and pull on the right side rail (Figure 2). Explain to the patient that you will place a pillow behind his/her back to provide support, and that the call bell will be placed within easy reach.	
c. Explain to the patient that position change is recommended every 2 hours.	

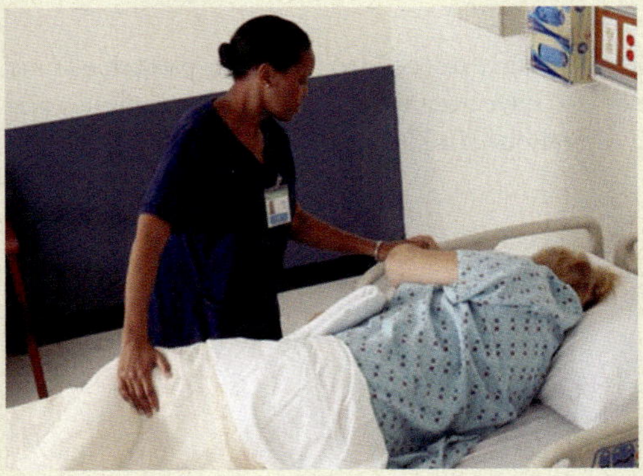

FIGURE 2. Helping the patient roll over to her right side while she pushes with left bent leg and pulls on the side rail.

(continued on page 1072)

Skill 31-1 Providing Preoperative Patient Care *(continued)*

ACTION	RATIONALE
15. Provide individualized, developmentally appropriate teaching about pain management options, plans and goals.	Individualized use of pharmacologic and nonpharmacologic methods of pain management is an important part of pain management guidelines related to surgery (Chou et al., 2016). Adequate pain control is important; continuing or unresolved pain can increase the patient's length of recovery and delay discharge.
a. Discuss past experiences with pain and interventions that the patient has used to reduce pain.	Past experiences with pain can impact the patient's ability to manage surgical pain. Pain is a subjective experience and the interventions effective in reducing pain vary from patient to patient.
b. Discuss the availability of analgesic medication post-operatively.	Depending on the prescribed interventions, the patient may need to request analgesic medication, as needed, or a patient-controlled analgesia (PCA) or epidural analgesia may be prescribed, for which the patient will need specific instruction on how to use.
c. Discuss the use of PCA, as appropriate.	Patient understanding of the use of PCA is crucial for effective, safe administration.
d. Explore the use of other alternative and nonpharmacologic methods to reduce pain, such as position change, massage, relaxation/diversion, guided imagery, and meditation.	These measures may reduce anxiety and may decrease the amount of pain medication that is needed. Analgesic therapy should involve a multimodal approach influenced by age, weight, and comorbidity.
16. Review equipment that may be used after surgery.	
a. Show the patient various equipment, such as IV infusion devices, electronic blood pressure cuff, tubes, urinary catheters, and surgical drains.	Knowledge can reduce anxiety about equipment and upcoming experiences. The patient may need an indwelling urinary catheter during and after surgery to keep the bladder empty and to monitor urinary output. Drains are frequently used to remove excess fluid around the surgical incision.
17. Provide skin preparation.	
a. **Ask the patient to bathe or shower with the antibacterial soap or solution. Remind the patient to clean the surgical site.** An antiseptic shower, bath, or cleansing with antimicrobial-impregnated wipes may be prescribed the evening before surgery and repeated the morning of surgery to begin the process of preparing the skin before surgery and to prevent infection (Mok et al., 2019; Parry, 2018). The skin is cleaned at the operative site with an antibacterial soap or solution to remove microorganisms. The patient can do this while taking a bath or shower. The specific choice of soap or antiseptic product depends on the patient, the procedure, and the manufacturer recommendations (AORN, 2020). This skin antiseptic eliminates skin microorganisms and leaves an antimicrobial film on their skin.	Evidence-based practice advises against hair removal at the surgical site due to increased potential for infection. If hair removal is necessary, it should be accomplished using hair clippers and be performed immediately before the surgery, in a patient care room outside the operating room, using disposable supplies and aseptic technique (AORN, 2020, as cited in Spruce, 2020a, p. 82). Follow facility policy regarding skin preparation of the surgical patient. In addition, immediately before the surgical procedure, the skin of the patient's operative site will be cleansed with a product that is compatible with the antiseptic used for showering.
18. Provide teaching about and follow dietary/fluid restrictions. **Explain to the patient that both food and fluid will be restricted before surgery to ensure that the stomach contains a minimal amount of gastric secretions. This restriction is important to reduce the risk of aspiration. Emphasize to the patient the importance of avoiding food and fluids during the prescribed time period, because failure to adhere may necessitate cancellation of the surgery.**	Ensure that fluid and dietary restrictions (NPO), as prescribed or as per facility protocol, have been followed. These restrictions assist in preventing aspiration (Hinkle et al., 2022).

ACTION	RATIONALE
19. Provide intestinal preparation, as appropriate. In certain situations, such as surgery of the lower gastrointestinal tract or pelvic surgery, the bowel will need to be prepared by administering enemas or laxatives.	A prescribed bowel prep and cleansing enema may be prescribed if the patient is scheduled for surgery of the lower gastrointestinal tract to evacuate the bowel and to reduce the intestinal bacteria to help prevent contamination of the surgical area during surgery. Peristalsis may not return for 24 to 48 hours after the bowel is handled, so preoperative cleansing also helps to decrease postoperative constipation.
a. As needed, explain the purpose of enemas or laxatives before surgery. If the patient will be administered an enema, clarify the steps as needed.	Enemas can be stressful, especially when repeated enemas are required to obtain a clear fluid return. Repeated enemas may cause fluid and electrolyte imbalance, orthostatic hypotension, and weakness.
20. **Check and verify administration of regularly scheduled medications.** Review with the patient routine medications, over-the-counter medications, and herbal supplements that are taken regularly. Check the prescribed interventions and review with the patient which medications they should take and those they should not take the day of surgery.	Many patients take medications for a variety of chronic medical conditions. Adjustments in taking these medications may be needed before surgery. Certain medications, such as aspirin, are stopped days before surgery due to their anticoagulant effect. Certain cardiac and respiratory drugs may be taken the day of surgery per prescribed intervention. If the patient has diabetes, oral hypoglycemic agent and/or insulin dosages may be reduced.
21. Provide information to the patient and family/caregivers regarding timing of surgical events and potential sensations that may be experienced. Explain to patients and their families how long the surgery and postanesthesia care will last, as well as what will be done before, during, and after surgery (e.g., procedures, medications, equipment). Explain to patients that they may not drive themselves home or take public transportation alone if they have had any anesthesia or sedation.	Patients and their families require this information to plan activities accordingly. Explanation and knowledge relieve anxiety and facilitates engagement.
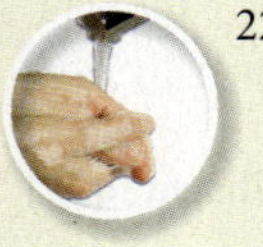 22. Remove PPE, if used. Perform hand hygiene.	Proper removal of PPE reduces the risk for infection transmission and contamination of other items. Hand hygiene prevents the spread of microorganisms.

DOCUMENTATION

Guidelines

Document that the patient's health records were reviewed, including the history, physical assessment, and any laboratory values and diagnostic studies. Record that the health care team was notified of any abnormal values. Document the components of perioperative teaching that were reviewed with the patient and family/caregivers, if present, such as use of the incentive spirometer, deep-breathing exercises, splinting, leg exercises, graduated compression stockings, and pneumatic compression devices. Record the patient's ability to demonstrate the skills and response to the teaching, and note if any follow-up instruction needs to be performed. Document other preoperative teaching, including pain management, intestinal preparation, medications, and preoperative skin preparation. Record any patient concerns about the surgery and whether the surgeon/health care team was contacted to provide any further explanations. Document the emotional support that was offered to the patient and if a spiritual counselor was notified per request of patient.

Sample Documentation

4/2/25 1030 Patient's health records were reviewed, and no abnormal results were identified. Perioperative teaching points reviewed with patient and his wife, including the rationale for each of these points. Patient demonstrated proper deep breathing, splinting while coughing, and leg exercises. Reviewed pain management, intestinal preparation, medications, and preoperative skin preparation. Patient stated that he was anxious about the surgery because this will be his first time to the OR. Emotional support and reassurance were provided.

—J. Grabes, RN

(continued on page 1074)

Skill 31-1 Providing Preoperative Patient Care *(continued)*

DEVELOPING CLINICAL REASONING AND CLINICAL JUDGMENT

UNEXPECTED SITUATIONS AND ASSOCIATED INTERVENTIONS

- *Patient's laboratory results are noted to be abnormal:* Notify health care team. Some abnormalities, such as an elevated international normalized ratio (INR) or abnormalities in the complete blood count (CBC), may postpone the surgery.
- *Patient says to you, "I'm not sure I really want this surgery":* Ask the patient to elaborate on their concerns. Discuss with the patient why they feel this way. Notify the health care team. Patients should not undergo surgery until any questions or doubts are resolved and they are sure that surgery is what they want.

SPECIAL CONSIDERATIONS

General Considerations

- Patients who are obese are at increased risk for respiratory and cardiovascular compromise as well as an increased incidence of gastroesophageal reflex disease, hiatal hernia, and abdominal pressure that puts them at increased risk for aspiration of stomach contents (AORN, 2020). In taking the history of these patients, be alert for other medical conditions, such as diabetes, cardiovascular disease, respiratory disease, kidney disease, and liver disease, which also increase the risk of surgical complications.
- Current recommendations caution against routine opioid prescription postoperatively, focusing on oral opioid administration with acetaminophen and/or nonsteroidal anti-inflammatory drugs (NSAIDs) as needed, or the use of patient-controlled analgesia (PCA) when the parenteral route is necessary (Chou et al., 2016).

Infant and Child Considerations

- Children have special needs related to their overall health, age, and size. Easing preoperative anxiety of the child is crucial and includes using simple and concrete terms when providing information (Aranha & Dsouza, 2019; Kyle & Carman, 2021).
- The nurse needs to be sensitive to the anxiety level of the parent and provide support, explanations, and patient teaching, as needed (Aranha & Dsouza, 2019; Kyle & Carman, 2021).
- Accurate weights are essential for correct medication dosages (Kyle & Carman, 2021).
- Developmentally appropriate pain assessment and management needs to be initiated to ensure adequate pain management (Kyle & Carman, 2021).

Older Adult Considerations

- Age-related changes and pre-existing chronic conditions can affect the postoperative course of the older adult patient (Eliopoulos, 2018).
- It is important to present preoperative teaching information slowly with reinforcement, because processing of information can be slower (Bastable, 2017).
- Management of postoperative pain in older adults may be complicated by a number of factors, including a higher risk of age- and disease-related changes in physiology and disease–drug and drug–drug interactions (Karch, 2020).

Skill 31-2 Providing Postoperative Care

DELEGATION CONSIDERATIONS

Postoperative measurement of vital signs may be delegated to assistive personnel (AP) as well as to licensed practical/vocational nurses (LPN/LVNs). Postoperative assessment and teaching are not delegated to AP. Depending on the state's nurse practice act and the organization's policies and procedures, postoperative teaching may be delegated to LPN/LVNs after an assessment of education needs by the registered nurse. The decision to delegate must be based on careful analysis of the patient's needs and circumstances as well as the qualifications of the person to whom the task is being delegated. Refer to the Delegation Guidelines in Appendix A.

EQUIPMENT (Varies, Depending on the Surgery)

- Electronic blood pressure monitor/sphygmomanometer
- Blood pressure cuff
- Electronic thermometer
- Pulse oximeter
- Stethoscope
- IV infusion device, IV solutions
- Graduated compression stockings (as prescribed/indicated)
- Pneumatic compression devices (as prescribed/indicated)
- Tubes, drains, vascular access tubing
- Incentive spirometer (as prescribed/indicated)
- PPE, as indicated
- Blankets and/or forced-air warming device, as needed

IMPLEMENTATION

ACTION	RATIONALE
Immediate Care	
1. When the patient returns from the PACU, participate in hand-off report from the PACU nurse and review the OR and PACU data. Gather the necessary supplies.	Obtaining a hand-off report ensures accurate communication and promotes continuity of care. Preparation promotes efficient time management and an organized approach to the task.
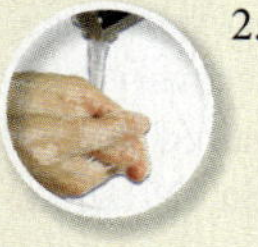 2. Perform hand hygiene and put on PPE, if indicated.	Hand hygiene and PPE prevent the spread of microorganisms. PPE is required based on transmission precautions.
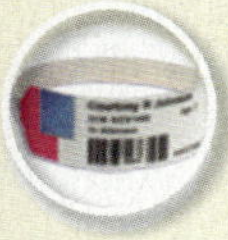 3. Identify the patient.	Identifying the patient ensures the right patient receives the intervention and helps prevent errors.
4. Close the curtains around the bed and close the door to the room, if possible. Explain what you are going to do and why you are going to do it to the patient or significant other. Place necessary supplies on the bedside stand, overbed table, or other surface within easy reach.	Closing the curtains and door ensures the patient's privacy. Explanation relieves anxiety and facilitates engagement. Bringing everything to the bedside conserves time and energy. Arranging items nearby is convenient, saves time, and avoids unnecessary stretching and twisting of muscles on the part of the nurse.
5. **Place the patient in safe position (semi- or high-Fowler's or side-lying). Note level of consciousness.**	A head of bed (HOB)-elevated position facilitates deep breathing; the side-lying position with neck slightly extended prevents aspiration and airway obstruction. Alternate positions may be appropriate based on the type of surgery.
6. **Obtain vital signs. Monitor and record vital signs frequently.** Prescribed assessment frequency may vary, but usual frequency includes taking vital signs every 15 minutes the first hour, every 30 minutes the next 2 hours, every hour for 4 hours, and finally every 4 hours. Refer to facility policy and adjust based on patient circumstances and nursing clinical judgment (AORN, 2019). Temperature measurement should be obtained using the same site and method of measurement (AORN, 2019). If continuous vital sign monitoring is used, apply monitor per manufacturer's directions.	Comparison with baseline preoperative vital signs may indicate impending shock, respiratory compromise, or hemorrhage. Although protocols are used as guidelines in the immediate postoperative period, the nurse is responsible for adjusting the frequency and priorities of assessment to the specific needs of each patient. Temperature measurement can vary significantly when temperatures are measured at different sites or by different methods; the same site and method of temperature measurement should be used throughout the perioperative phases when clinically feasible (AORN, 2019). Wireless continuous vital sign monitoring maybe used to aid in early detection of changes in the patient's condition (Downey et al., 2018; Verillo et al., 2019).

(continued on page 1076)

Skill 31-2 Providing Postoperative Care *(continued)*

ACTION	RATIONALE
7. Assess the patient's respiratory status. Measure the patient's oxygen saturation level (Figure 1). If oxygen is prescribed or warranted, ensure accurate delivery device and flow rate. Measure and monitor the patient's end-tidal carbon dioxide levels as prescribed or based on facility policy.	Comparison with baseline preoperative respiratory assessment may indicate impending respiratory complications. Pulse oximetry provides information about the patient's oxygenation status. Measurement of end-tidal carbon dioxide levels (capnography) provides information about the patient's ventilation status and may be used to monitor patients with known or suspected obstructive sleep apnea and those who receive sedation and opioids or other CNS depressants (Borczynski & Worobel-Luk, 2019; Burns & Delgado, 2019; Hess et al., 2021).
8. Assess the patient's cardiovascular status.	Comparison with baseline preoperative cardiovascular assessment may indicate impending cardiovascular complications.
9. Assess the patient's neurovascular status, based on the type of surgery performed.	Comparison with baseline preoperative neurovascular assessment may indicate impending neurovascular complications.
10. Provide for warmth, using heated or extra blankets, or forced-air warming device as necessary. Assess skin color and condition.	The OR is a cold environment. All perioperative patients are at risk for hypothermia (AORN, 2019). Hypothermia is uncomfortable, and it is associated with prolonged postoperative recovery, cardiac arrhythmias, impaired renal function, and impaired wound healing (Hinkle et al., 2022; Link, 2020; Nieh & Su, 2018; Xu et al., 2019).
11. Put on gloves. Assess the surgical site. Check dressings for color, odor, presence of drains, and amount of drainage (Figure 2). Mark the drainage on the dressing by circling the amount and include the time. Assess dependent areas, such as turning the patient to assess visually under the patient, for bleeding from the surgical site.	Hemorrhage and shock are life-threatening complications of surgery and early recognition is essential.

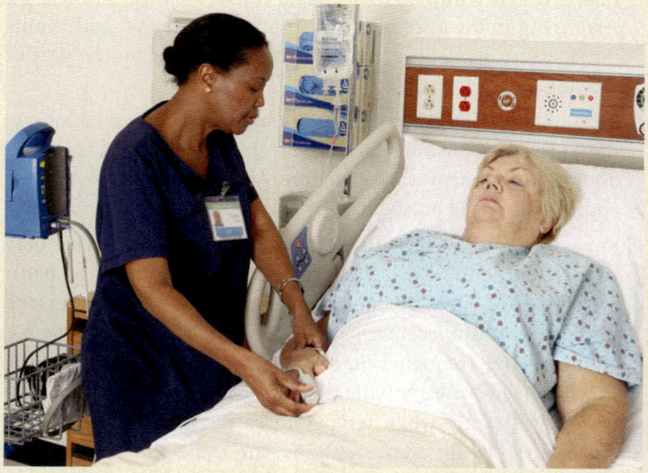

FIGURE 1. Obtaining postoperative oxygen saturation level.

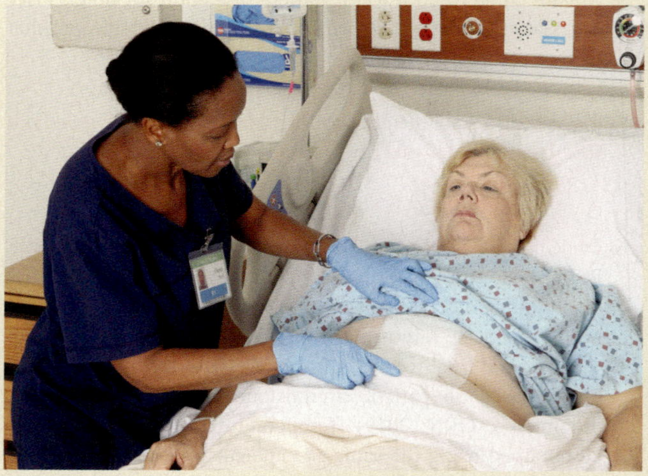

FIGURE 2. Checking dressings for color, odor, and amount of drainage.

ACTION	RATIONALE
12. Verify that all tubes and drains are patent, and the equipment is working; note the amount of drainage in collection device. If an indwelling urinary catheter is in place, note urinary output.	This ensures function of drainage devices.
13. Verify and maintain IV infusion at prescribed rate.	This replaces fluid loss and prevents dehydration and electrolyte imbalances.
14. Assess for pain. Check health record to verify if analgesic medication was administered in the PACU. Administer analgesics as indicated, prescribed, and appropriate. If the patient has been instructed in the use of PCA for pain management, review its use. Institute nonpharmacologic pain management interventions as appropriate and indicated.	Use a facility-approved pain scale (Chou et al., 2016). Observe for nonverbal behavior that may indicate pain, such as grimacing, crying, and restlessness. Analgesics and other nonpharmacologic pain strategies are used for relief of postoperative pain.

ACTION	RATIONALE
15. Assess for nausea and vomiting. Administer antiemetic medication as indicated, prescribed, and appropriate. Institute nonpharmacologic management interventions as appropriate and indicated.	General anesthesia can cause postoperative nausea and vomiting. Vomiting can lead to serious complications, including pulmonary aspiration, dehydration, and dysrhythmias secondary to electrolyte imbalances (Koyuncu et al., 2020). Aromatherapy has been suggested as a complementary intervention to decrease postoperative nausea and vomiting (Abril et al., 2019; Karaman et al., 2019; Spruce, 2020b).
16. Provide for a safe environment. Keep the bed in low position with the side rails up, based on facility policy. Have the call bell within patient's reach.	This adjustment to the bed prevents accidental injury. Easy access to the call bell permits the patient to call for nurse when necessary.
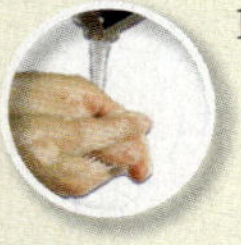 17. Remove PPE, if used. Perform hand hygiene.	Proper removal of PPE reduces the risk for infection transmission and contamination of other items. Hand hygiene prevents transmission of microorganisms.
Ongoing Care	
18. Promote optimal respiratory function.	The patient is at risk for respiratory complications postoperatively. Interventions can be implemented to prevent respiratory complications.
a. Assess respiratory rate, depth, quality, color, and capillary refill. Ask if the patient is experiencing any difficulty breathing.	The patient is at risk for pulmonary complications postoperatively. Postoperative analgesic medication can reduce the rate and quality of the respiratory effort. Interventions can be implemented to prevent cardiovascular complications.
b. Assist with coughing and deep-breathing exercises.	
c. Assist with incentive spirometry, as indicated/prescribed.	
d. Assist with early ambulation.	
e. Provide frequent position changes.	
f. Administer oxygen, as prescribed.	
g. Monitor pulse oximetry.	
19. Promote optimal cardiovascular function:	Patient is at risk for cardiovascular complications postoperatively. Interventions can be implemented to prevent cardiovascular complications.
a. Assess apical rate, rhythm, and quality and compare with peripheral pulses, color, and blood pressure. Ask if the patient has any chest pains or shortness of breath.	
b. Provide frequent position changes.	
c. Assist with early ambulation.	
d. Apply graduated compression stockings or pneumatic compression devices, if prescribed and not in place. If in place, assess for integrity.	
e. Provide leg and range-of-motion exercises if not contraindicated.	
20. Promote optimal neurologic function:	Anesthetic and pain management agents can alter neurologic function. Sedation scales are used to assess sedation levels and provide nurses with a useful tool to make decisions about the timing of medication interventions and when to intervene based on patients' sedation levels (Hall & Stanley, 2019).
a. Assess level of consciousness, movement, and sensation. Assess and monitor the patient's level of sedation using a sedation scale, particularly if opioids are used to treat postoperative pain (Hall & Stanley, 2019).	

(*continued on page 1078*)

Skill 31-2 Providing Postoperative Care *(continued)*

ACTION	RATIONALE
b. Determine the level of orientation to person, place, and time.	
c. Test motor ability by asking the patient to move each extremity.	Anesthesia alters motor and sensory function.
d. Evaluate sensation by asking the patient if they can feel your touch on an extremity.	
21. Promote optimal renal and urinary function and fluid and electrolyte status. Assess intake and output, evaluate for urinary retention and monitor serum electrolyte levels.	Anesthetic agents and surgical manipulation in the area may temporarily depress bladder tone and response causing urinary retention.
a. Promote voiding by offering bedpan/bedside commode, or assistance to bathroom at regular intervals, noting the frequency, amount, and if any burning or urgency symptoms.	Frequency, burning, or urgency may indicate possible urinary tract abnormality.
b. Monitor urinary catheter drainage if present.	Communicate with the health care team if the patient's urinary output is less than 30 mL/hr or 240 mL/8-hr period.
c. Measure intake and output.	Intake and output are good indicators of fluid balance.
22. Promote optimal gastrointestinal function and meet nutritional needs:	Anesthetic agents and opioids depress peristalsis and normal functioning of the gastrointestinal tract (Karch, 2020). Flatus indicates return of peristalsis.
a. Assess abdomen for distention and firmness. Ask if patient feels nauseated, any vomiting, and if passing flatus.	
b. Auscultate for bowel sounds.	Presence of bowel sounds indicates return of peristalsis.
c. Assist with diet progression; encourage fluid intake; monitor intake.	Patients may experience nausea after surgery and are encouraged to resume diet slowly, starting with clear liquids and advancing as tolerated.
d. Medicate for nausea and vomiting, as prescribed. Institute nonpharmacologic interventions as appropriate and indicated.	Antiemetics are frequently prescribed to alleviate postoperative nausea. Complementary interventions may be effective in decreasing nausea and vomiting.
23. Promote optimal wound healing.	Alterations in nutritional, circulatory, and metabolic status may predispose the patient to infection and delayed healing.
a. Assess condition of wound for presence of drains and any drainage.	
b. Use surgical asepsis for dressing changes and drain care.	Surgical asepsis reduces the risk of infection.
c. Inspect all skin surfaces for beginning signs of pressure injury and use pressure-relieving supports to minimize potential skin breakdown.	Lying on the OR table in the same position can predispose some patients to pressure injury formation, especially in patients who have undergone lengthy procedures.
24. Promote optimal comfort and relief from pain.	This shortens recovery period and facilitates return to normal function.
a. Assess for pain (location and intensity using pain scale).	Control of postoperative pain promotes patient comfort and recovery.
b. Provide for rest and comfort; provide extra blankets, as needed, for warmth.	Patients may experience chills in the postoperative period.
c. Administer analgesics, as needed, and/or initiate nonpharmacologic methods, as appropriate.	Multimodal analgesia, combining analgesic drugs from different classes, is recommended to reduce the risk of adverse drug effects (Polomano et al., 2017; Poulsen et al, 2019).
25. Promote optimal outcomes related to psychosocial needs:	This facilitates individualized care, anxiety reduction, and patient's return to normal health.
a. Provide emotional support to patient and family/caregivers, as needed.	
b. Explain procedures and offer explanations regarding postoperative recovery, as needed, to both patient and family members/caregivers.	

DOCUMENTATION

Guidelines

Document the time that the patient returns from PACU to the surgical unit. Record the patient's level of consciousness, vital signs, all assessments, and condition of dressing. If patient has oxygen in place, an IV, or any other equipment, record this information. Document pain assessment, interventions that were instituted to alleviate pain, and the patient's response to the interventions. Document any patient teaching that is reviewed with the patient, such as use of incentive spirometer.

Sample Documentation

4/10/25 1330 Patient returned to room at 1315, drowsy but easily aroused; answers to name. Patient's temperature 98.8°F, pulse 78, BP 122/84, O_2 sat 96% on O_2 2 L/min. Right lower abdominal dressing dry and intact. Rates pain at a "4" on a scale of 1 to 10, was medicated in PACU with 4-mg morphine sulfate IV at 1030. Incentive spirometry completed × 10 cycles, 750 mL each. Patient deep breathing and coughing without production and turned to right side with HOB elevated. See EHR for additional system assessments.

—J. Grabbs, RN

DEVELOPING CLINICAL REASONING AND CLINICAL JUDGMENT

UNEXPECTED SITUATIONS AND ASSOCIATED INTERVENTIONS

- *Vital signs are progressively increasing or decreasing from baseline:* Collaborate with the health care team. A continued decrease in blood pressure or an increase in heart rate could indicate internal bleeding or **hemorrhage**.
- *Dressing was clean before but now has large amount of fresh blood:* Do not remove dressing. Reinforce dressing with more bandages. Removing the bandage could dislodge any clot that is forming and lead to further blood loss. Consult with the health care team.
- *Patient reports pain that is not relieved by prescribed medication:* After fully assessing pain, consult with the health care team. Pain can be a clue to other problems, such as hemorrhage.
- *Patient is febrile within 12 hours of surgery:* Assist patient with coughing and deep breathing. If prescribed, encourage incentive spirometry. Continue to monitor vital signs and laboratory values such as complete blood count (CBC).
- *Adult patient has a urine output of less than 30 mL/hr:* Unless this is expected, consult with the health care team. Urine output is a good indicator of tissue perfusion. Patient may need more fluid or may need medication to increase blood pressure if blood pressure is low.

SPECIAL CONSIDERATIONS

General Considerations

- Be aware of baseline sensory deficits. Ensure appropriate aids are in place, such as glasses or hearing aids. Lack of appropriate aids may impact postoperative assessments, such as level of consciousness.
- For patients undergoing throat surgery, such as a tonsillectomy, evaluate swallowing pattern. A patient who has had throat surgery and swallows frequently may be bleeding from the incision site.
- Multimodal analgesia, which combines analgesic drugs from different classes and employs analgesic techniques that target different mechanisms of pain, is recommended in the treatment of acute postoperative pain. The synergistic effects maximize pain relief at lower analgesic doses, reducing the risk of adverse drug effects (Polomano et al., 2017, p. S12).
- Consider the need for a bariatric mattress or bariatric bed for a patient who is obese because this patient is at greater risk for alterations in skin integrity due to the poor vascular supply of adipose tissue and restrictions in movement (Hinkle et al., 2022).

(continued on page 1080)

Skill 31-2 Providing Postoperative Care *(continued)*

- Intermittent manual vital sign measurement as single data points may provide an incomplete picture of patients' postoperative physiologic status (Downey et al., 2018; Verrillo et al., 2019). Wearable sensor packs using wireless technology are being used in some settings for continuous measurement of vital signs. This monitoring provides trending of vital signs (such as heart rate, respiratory rate, noninvasive blood pressure, temperature, and pulse oximetry) and may help in early detection of patient deterioration and improve patient outcomes (Verrillo et al., 2019).
- Aromatherapy has been used successfully to decrease postoperative nausea and vomiting. Inhalers using essential oils, including peppermint, ginger, lavender, rose and spearmint oils, or a blend of these oils, have been shown to be effective (Abril et al, 2019; Karaman et al., 2019; Spruce, 2020b).
- Ensure that written postoperative instructions specific to the patient and follow-up appointments with the surgeon or other health care professionals are provided to each patient upon discharge from the hospital or outpatient center. Information, such as signs and symptoms to report to the health care team, as well as restrictions in activity and diet, are addressed. In addition, patients discharged the same day as their surgery are required to have a responsible person accompany them home, and a contact telephone number is to be provided in case of emergency. The patient should be alert and oriented, or mental status should be at the patient's baseline. The vital signs of the patient should be stable. Have the patient "teach back" important information/instructions in their own words.

Infant and Child Considerations

- Postoperative complications are often related to the respiratory system in this age group. After receiving general anesthesia, premature infants are at greater risk for apnea (Subramaniam, 2019).
- Infants and children are at great risk for temperature-related complications because their body temperature can change rapidly. It is essential to have warmed blankets and other warming equipment available to avoid this complication.

Older Adult Considerations

- Older adults may take longer to return to normothermia and their baseline level of orientation. Drugs and anesthetics may delay this return.
- Forced-air warming systems are suggested as the most effective means of rewarming older patients with postoperative hypothermia (Xu et al., 2019).

DEVELOPING CLINICAL REASONING AND CLINICAL JUDGMENT

1. Work through the Evolving Case Study 31-1 to help develop your clinical reasoning and clinical judgment skills.
2. You are providing the immediate preoperative care for a woman scheduled for surgery to remove a brain tumor. She tells you she does not want the surgery because she knows she is dying and just wants to go home to be with her husband and children. She also knows that her husband cannot accept the fact that she is dying and wants her to have the surgery. What do you do?
3. You are assigned to discharge a woman from your same-day surgery unit to her home. You strongly believe that she is not ready to go home, and there is no caregiver in her home. When you voice your concern to the surgeon, you are told that this is not your problem and that there is nothing anyone can do about the situation because her insurer will not approve hospitalization. How do you respond?

EVOLVING CASE STUDY 31-1

Scenario: Gabrielle McAllister, a 5-year-old admitted for removal of her tonsils and adenoids in same-day surgery, arrives at the outpatient surgery center with her mother. Gabrielle is clinging to her mother and quietly crying. Her mother says, "I don't think I can stand this again, but I know it has to be done."

QUESTION r/t CUES: As the initial point of contact for Gabrielle and her mother, what should the nurse say to begin the nurse–patient relationship?

A. "Mom, I know you are stressed, but you know the routine by now!"
B. "Hi, Gabrielle, my name is Emily, and I'm your nurse. Can you tell me something you like to do for fun with your family?"
C. "Gabrielle, this is my stethoscope. I'm going to listen to your heart and lungs."
D. "Hi, Gabrielle and Mom. I need you to calm down so we can get you ready for the big surgery."

Scenario: After some time and rapport formation, Gabrielle relaxes enough for the nurse to begin an assessment. The admitting nurse notes that Gabrielle is a 5-year-old female, who is small for her age. The child has a history of several previous surgeries for a congenital cardiac defect and a known latex allergy. Assessment parameters from a head-to-toe assessment are generally within normal limits. Gabrielle's lymph nodes in her neck are slightly swollen and her tonsils are visibly enlarged, but she denies difficulty breathing or swallowing at the moment. She reports a "little bit of a sore throat" and general throat/neck discomfort. Gabrielle has not had anything to eat or drink since she went to sleep last night.

QUESTION r/t ANALYZING CUES: Which information from this initial preoperative assessment is most important to convey to the professional administering the anesthesia and the intraoperative team?

A. Documented latex allergy
B. Gabrielle's emotional state
C. History of previous surgeries
D. System by system assessment data

Scenario: The nurse returns to the room and finds that Gabrielle is calm and cooperative, but still won't let go of her mother.

QUESTION r/t PRIORITIZING HYPOTHESIS: Based on the objective and subjective assessment of this patient, which priority problem should the nurse identify to guide the perioperative plan of care?

A. Bleeding risk
B. Activity intolerance
C. Acute anxiety
D. Thermal injury risk

Scenario: As they talk and the perioperative outcomes are identified, Gabrielle's mother starts talking about the transition of care to the operating room itself. Gabrielle climbs in her mom's lap and begins to yell, "No . . . No . . . you're not leaving me!"

QUESTION r/t GENERATING SOLUTIONS: Which solution is reasonable and safe for this transition of care?

A. Gabrielle's mom will be given time alone with Gabrielle in the preoperative room to provide comfort to Gabrielle
B. Gabrielle's mom will accompany Gabrielle to the surgical suite and remain with Gabrielle until the inhaled anesthesia takes effect
C. Gabrielle's mom will be at the preoperative bedside while the nurse initiates IV therapy and administers an IV sedative
D. Gabrielle's mom will administer an oral sedative to Gabrielle under the supervision of the nurse

Scenario: The nurse continues to build rapport with Gabrielle and her mother, and feels confident that they can review some key preoperative teaching that will be needed in the immediate postoperative phase.

QUESTION r/t TAKING ACTION: Which content and teaching modality best fit this particular situation?

A. Have Gabrielle use the incentive spirometer while providing direction and encouragement
B. Show Gabrielle the OR suite, taking time to point out the equipment and lights
C. Have Gabrielle perform a series of arm and neck stretches
D. Talk to Gabrielle and her mom about the likelihood of postoperative nausea and vomiting

Scenario: Gabrielle is taken to the OR suite. She is "nervous," but smiles when told by the CRNA that it's time to "get those tonsils out and eat lots of popsicles."

QUESTION r/t EVALUATING OUTCOMES: The nurse documents attainment of expected outcomes in the preoperative phase as part of the perioperative plan of care. Which outcomes were met for Gabrielle? Select all that apply.

A. Correct return demonstration of postoperative activities designed to prevent complications
B. Physical and emotional readiness for operative procedure; appropriate for age
C. Decreased risk for surgical site, catheter-based, and community-acquired infections
D. Caregiver articulation of when to call the provider for follow-up and/or intervention
E. Pulse oximetry >98% on room air

PRACTICING FOR NCLEX

1. A nurse in the PACU is preparing to receive a patient from surgery who sustained a ruptured spleen in a motor vehicle accident. Which of these system assessments will take priority?
   - Electronic Health Record: Operative Note
   - Splenectomy secondary to trauma
   - Estimated blood loss 900 mL

   a. Neurologic system, ambulatory function
   b. Cardiovascular system, vital signs
   c. GI system, bowel function
   d. Integumentary, skin breakdown

2. A nurse is preparing a patient for a cesarean birth using spinal anesthesia. Which effects of anesthesia will the nurse teach the patient to expect? Select all that apply.
   a. Loss of consciousness
   b. Inability to speak
   c. Reduction or loss of deep tendon reflexes
   d. Loss of sensation below the injection
   e. Inability to move the lower extremities
   f. Prolonged pain relief after other anesthesia wears off

3. A nurse has been asked to witness a patient signature on an informed consent form for surgery. What communication from the surgeon does the nurse expect the patient to receive before signing the form? Select all that apply.
   a. Option of nontreatment
   b. Underlying disease process and its natural course
   c. Notice that once the form is signed, the patient cannot withdraw the consent
   d. Explanation of the guaranteed outcome of the procedure or treatment
   e. Name and qualifications of the provider of the procedure or treatment
   f. Explanation of the risks and benefits of the procedure or treatment

4. An older adult who is scheduled for a hip replacement is taking several medications on a regular basis. Which group of medications does the nurse identify as a surgical risk for this patient?
   a. Anticoagulants
   b. Antacids
   c. Laxatives
   d. Sedatives

5. A nurse is caring for a patient who is obese and has had abdominal surgery. The nurse prioritizes a plan to prevent what postoperative complication?
   a. Anesthetic interactions
   b. Impaired wound healing
   c. Weight gain
   d. Flatulence

6. When caring for a patient who returned from the operating room 8 hours ago, which finding requires follow-up assessment by the nurse?
   a. Patient reports discomfort at surgical site, scale of 5/10
   b. Patient voids small amounts every 20–30 minutes
   c. Patient is sleepy and awakens only to touch
   d. Patient reports thirst and dry mouth

7. A nurse is providing teaching for a patient scheduled to have same-day surgery. Which teaching method would be most effective in preoperative teaching for ambulatory surgery?
   a. Lecture
   b. Discussion
   c. Audiovisuals
   d. Written instructions

8. An adult patient awaiting surgery says to the nurse, "I am so frightened—what if I don't wake up?" What is the nurse's best response?
   a. "Are you worried about the anesthesia?"
   b. "Tell me what concerns you most."
   c. "Your surgeon is great; she operated on my aunt!"
   d. "Many people are anxious before surgery."

9. During preoperative teaching about pain management, the patient asks the nurse to explain how a PCA pump works. What will the nurse teach the patient about PCA?
   a. "It allows the patient to be completely free of pain during the postoperative period."
   b. "It allows the patient to take unlimited amounts of medication as needed."
   c. "It allows the patient to choose the type of medication given postoperatively."
   d. "It permits the patient to self-administer limited doses of pain medication."

10. A nurse is planning caring for a patient who had thoracic surgery. Which nursing interventions are most appropriate for patients undergoing this type of surgery?
    a. Observing for incisional wound healing
    b. Monitoring vital signs, especially pulse and blood pressure
    c. Instructing the patient on the proper use of the incentive spirometer
    d. Applying antiembolism stockings

11. While assessing a patient in the PACU following abdominal surgery, a nurse promptly contacts the surgeon for which of these findings? Select all that apply.

    <u>Electronic Health Record</u>

    Vital signs
    - 1200: T 97.4, P-89, RR 12, BP/102/70
    - 1215: T 97.4, P-92, RR 12, BP/100/68
    - 1230: T 97.2, P-112, RR 12, BP/98/60

Intake Output/Hemovac
- 1200: 200 mL 0.9% saline infused 30 mL sanguineous material
- 1215: IV NSS 25 mL 45 mL serosanguineous material
- 1230: IV NSS 25 mL 250 mL bright red blood

a. Tachycardia
b. IV with normal saline solution
c. Wound drainage
d. Patient restless
e. Patient reports incisional pain 8/10

12. A nurse is caring for a postoperative patient who has been on bedrest for 5 days. What interventions will the nurse use to prevent deep vein thrombosis (DVT)? Select all that apply.
a. Administering analgesics
b. Documenting daily calf circumference
c. Assessing vital signs every 4 hours
d. Encouraging ambulation
e. Applying intermittent pneumatic compression devices (IPCDs)
f. Providing education on pain management

13. A scrub nurse is assisting a surgeon with a kidney transplant. What are the patient responsibilities of the scrub nurse? Select all that apply.
a. Maintaining sterile technique
b. Draping and handling instruments and supplies
c. Identifying and assessing the patient on admission
d. Integrating case management
e. Preparing the skin at the surgical site
f. Providing exposure of the operative area

14. A nurse on a surgical unit is aware that older adults develop reduced vital capacity as a result of normal physiologic changes. Based on these changes, which nursing intervention takes priority?
a. Taking and recording vital signs every shift
b. Turning, coughing, and deep breathing every 4 hours
c. Encouraging increased intake of oral fluids
d. Assessing bowel sounds daily

15. A nurse teaches a patient the rationale for performing leg exercises after surgery. How does the nurse best explain the purpose of the exercises to the patient?
a. Improves respiratory function
b. Maintains functional abilities
c. Provides diversional activities
d. Increases venous return

16. A nurse is preparing a patient for same-day surgery. Which of these patient-related findings must the nurse report immediately?
a. Asking how long after the surgery they can leave the hospital
b. Received an oral anticoagulant last night
c. Surgeon has not yet filled out the consent form
d. Blood pressure is 142/86

ANSWERS WITH RATIONALES

1. **b.** The priority assessment focuses on the ruptured organ, blood loss, and monitoring for early signs of shock. Tachycardia, the first sign of shock, and decreasing blood pressure must be immediately reported to the health care provider. The neurologic system may be affected due to anesthesia, but ambulatory function is not the immediate priority. The nurse anticipates reduced or absent bowel sounds after surgery, but risk for blood loss is the priority. The nurse plans to promote wound healing and repositions the patient to prevent skin breakdown; however, hemorrhage and early detection of shock is the priority at this time.

2. **d, e.** A localized loss of sensation, loss of motor function, and possible loss of reflexes occur with a regional anesthetic. Loss of consciousness, including speech and relaxation of skeletal muscles, occurs with general anesthesia. Prolonged pain relief after other anesthesia wears off and infiltration of the underlying tissues in an operative area occur with topical anesthesia.

3. **a, b, e, f.** The information communicated while obtaining informed consent includes the description of the procedure or treatment; potential alternative therapies; the option of nontreatment; the underlying disease process and its natural course; the name and qualifications of the health care provider performing the procedure or treatment; explanation of the risks and benefits; explanation that the patient has the right to refuse treatment; explanation that consent can be withdrawn; and explanation of expected (not guaranteed) outcome, recovery, and rehabilitation plan and course.

4. **a.** Anticoagulant medications increase the risk for hemorrhage intra- and postoperatively.

5. **b.** Adipose (fatty) tissue has poor blood supply, which places the obese patient at risk for delayed wound healing, wound infection, and disruption in the integrity of the wound. Medication interactions are not the primary concern and are managed by the nurse anesthetist or anesthesiologist. Postoperative bleeding and flatulence (gas) after anesthesia are concerns for all patients, not just those with obesity.

6. **b.** This patient is displaying typical signs of urinary retention, voiding small frequent amounts. Discomfort is expected and can be managed with prescribed analgesics. Anesthesia or opioid analgesia promotes sedation from which this patient awakens to touch. Dry mouth and thirst can result from NPO status and possible anticholinergic medication intended to dry respiratory secretions during surgery.

7. **d.** Written instructions are most effective in providing information for same-day surgery.

8. **b.** An open-ended question that allows the patient to express concerns, fears, and feelings is therapeutic and most appropriate. The other options suggest "yes/no" answers or suggest issues that may not be present. This type of communication does not allow the patient to clarify their thoughts.

9. **d.** The nurse educates the patient that the PCA pump allows patients to self-administer doses of pain-relieving medication within health care provider–prescribed times and dose limits. It is not realistic to promise absence of pain or unlimited access to medication nor allow the patient to select the pain medication prescribed.
10. **a.** A thoracic incision, near or overlying the lungs, makes it difficult or painful for patients to take deep breaths and cough. The nurse uses analgesics, repositioning, coughing and deep breathing, and an incentive spirometer to promote respiratory expansion and airway clearance to decrease the risk for respiratory complications.
11. **a, c, d.** Increased wound drainage, restlessness, increasing pulse, and decreasing blood pressure are symptoms of blood loss/hemorrhage and must be promptly identified to prevent shock. Diminished bowel sounds are expected after surgery and anesthesia. Incisional pain is anticipated; the nurse uses prescriptions for analgesia to help resolve pain. Due to NPO status and blood loss from surgery, IV fluids are administered.
12. **d.** To prevent DVT, the nurse plans to apply an IPCD and antiembolism stockings. Assessments such as vital signs and calf circumference will detect but not prevent DVT. Maintaining bedrest continues to promote risk, and early ambulation helps prevent DVT.
13. **a, b.** The scrub nurse is a member of the sterile team who maintains sterile technique while draping and handling instruments and supplies. Two duties of the circulating nurse are to identify and assess the patient on admission to the OR and prepare the skin at the surgical site. The perioperative registered nurse actively assists the surgeon by providing exposure of the operative area. The advanced practice registered nurse coordinates care activities, collaborates with physicians and nurses in all phases of perioperative and postanesthesia care, and integrates case management, critical paths, and research into care of the surgical patient.
14. **b.** Reduced vital capacity in older adults decreases respiratory expansion, increasing the risk for pneumonia and atelectasis. Encouraging the patient to turn, cough, and deep breathe every 4 hours helps to prevent complications.
15. **d.** Leg exercises promote venous return and decrease complications related to venous stasis causing DVT and help prevent muscle weakness. These exercises also decrease risk for thrombophlebitis and emboli.
16. **b.** Patients receiving anticoagulants are at risk for bleeding or hemorrhage during invasive and surgical procedures. Wanting to know an anticipated discharge date is expected, the surgeon can fill out the consent form prior to sedation, and a slight increase in blood pressure is possible related to anxiety before surgery.

Bibliography

Abril, K., Diaz, S., Yasui, T., Collins, K., & Elsabrout, K. (2019). Inhaled peppermint aromatherapy for treatment of postoperative nausea and vomiting: A complement to traditional pharmacologic treatments. *MEDSURG Nursing, 28*(6), 375–380.

Agency for Healthcare Research and Quality (AHRQ). (2019, September). *Never events*. https://psnet.ahrq.gov/primers/primer/3/never-events

American Association of Critical Care Nurses. (2018). AACN practice alert: Preventing venous thromboembolism in adults. *Critical Care Nurse, 38*(3), 88. https://aacnjournals.org/ccnonline/article-abstract/38/3/88/20820/Preventing-Venous-Thromboembolism-in-Adults?redirectedFrom=fulltext

American Society of Anesthesiologists. (2017). Practice guidelines for preoperative fasting and the use of pharmacologic agents to reduce the risk of pulmonary aspiration: Application to healthy patients undergoing elective procedures: An updated report by the American Society of Anesthesiologists Task Force on preoperative fasting and the use of pharmacologic agents to reduce the risk of pulmonary aspiration. *Anesthesiology, 126*(3), 376–393. https://doi.org/10.1097/ALN.0000000000001452

American Society of Anesthesiologists. (2018, October 17). Ethical guidelines for the anesthesia care of patients with do-not-resuscitate (DNR) orders or other directives that limit treatment. https://www.asahq.org/~/media/sites/asahq/files/public/resources/standards-guidelines/ethical-guidelines-for-the-anesthesia-care-of-patients.pdf

American Society of PeriAnesthesia Nurses (ASPAN). (2020). *2021–2022 Perianesthesia nursing standards, practice recommendations and interpretive statements*. American Society of PeriAnesthesia Nurses.

Apfelbaum, J. L., Hagberg, C. A., Connis, R. T., Abdelmalak, B. B., Agarkar, M., Dutton, R. P., Fiadjoe, J. E., Greif, R., Klock, P. A., Mercier, D., Myatra, S. N., O'Sullivan, E. P., Rosenblatt, W. H., Sorbello, M., & Tung, A. (2022). 2022 American Society of Anesthesiologists practice guidelines for management of the difficult airway. *Anesthesiology, 136*(1), 31–81. https://doi.org/10.1097/ALN.0000000000004002

Aranha, P. R., & Dsouza, S. N. (2019). Preoperative information needs of parents: A descriptive survey. *Journal of Research in Nursing, 24*(5), 305–314. DOI: 10.1177/1744987118821708

Association of periOperative Registered Nurses (AORN). (2011). *Perioperative nursing data set: The perioperative nursing vocabulary* (3rd ed.). AORN, Inc.

Association of periOperative Registered Nurses (AORN). (2018). Guideline summary: Prevention of venous thromboembolism. *AORN Journal, 107*(6), 750–754. http://doi.org/10.1002/aorn.12147

Association of periOperative Registered Nurses (AORN). (2019). AORN position statement on perioperative registered nurse circulator dedicated to every patient undergoing an operative or other invasive procedure. *AORN Journal, 110*(1), 82–85. https://doi.org/10.1002/aorn.12741

Association of periOperative Registered Nurses (AORN). (2020). *Guidelines for perioperative practice*. AORN, Inc. https://www.aorn.org/guidelines

Bastable, S. B. (2017). *Essentials of patient education* (2nd ed.). Jones & Bartlett Learning.

Borczynski, E., & Worobel-Luk, P. (2019). Capnography monitoring of patients with obstructive sleep apnea in the post-anesthesia care unit: A best practice implementation project. *JBI Database of Systematic Reviews and Implementation Projects, 17*(7), 1532–1547. https://doi.org/10.11124/JBISRIR-2017-003939

Branson, R. D. (2013). The scientific basis for postoperative respiratory care. *Respiratory Care, 58*(11), 1974–1984. https://doi.org/10.4187/respcare.02832

Burns, S. M., & Delgado, S. A. (2019). *AACN essentials of critical care nursing* (4th ed.). McGraw Hill Education.

Cassidy, M. R., Rosenkranz, P., McCabe, K., Rosen, J. E., & McAneny, D. (2013). I COUGH: Reducing postoperative pulmonary complications with a multidisciplinary patient care program. *JAMA Surgery, 148*(8), 740–745. https://doi.org/10.1001/jamasurg.2013.358

Cassidy, M. R., Rosenkranz, P., Macht, R. D., Talutis, S., & McAneny, D. (2020). The I COUGH multidisciplinary perioperative pulmonary care program: One decade of experience. *Joint Commission Journal on Quality and Patient Safety, 46*(5), 241–249. https://doi.org/10.1016/j.jcjq.2020.01.005

Centers for Disease Control and Prevention (CDC). (2018, May). *Hospital toolkit for adult sepsis surveillance*. https://www.cdc.gov/sepsis/pdfs/Sepsis-Surveillance-Toolkit-Aug-2018_508.pdf

Centers for Medicare & Medicaid Services. (2020, June 22). *Measure of informed consent quality prior to elective, hospital-performed procedures*. https://cmit.cms.gov/CMIT_public/ViewMeasure?MeasureId=5612#tab1

Chou, R., Gordon, D. B., de Leon-Casasola, O. A., Rosenberg, J. M., Bickler, S., Brennan, T., Carter, T., Cassidy, C. L., Chittenden, E. H., Degenhardt, E., Griffith, S., Manworren, R., McCarberg, B., Montgomery, R., Murphy, J., Perkal, M. F., Suresh, S., Sluka, K., Strassels, S., … Wu, CL. (2016). Management of postoperative pain: A clinical practice guideline from the American pain society, the American society of regional anesthesia and pain medicine, and the American society of anesthesiologists' committee on regional anesthesia, executive committee, and administrative council. *The Journal of Pain, 17*(2), 131–157. https://doi.org/10.1016/j.jpain.2015.12.008

Cowperthwaite, L., & Holm, R. L. (2015). Perioperative patient skin antisepsis. *AORN Journal, 101*(1), 71–80. https://doi.org/10.1016/j.aorn.2014.11.009

Croke, L. (2020a). Open communication and empathy during perioperative stage can ease patient anxiety. *AORN Journal, 111*(2), P5. http://dx.doi.org/10.1002/aorn.12968

Croke, L. (2020b). Nonpharmacologic strategies to help reduce preoperative patient anxiety. *AORN Journal, 111*(2), P8–P10. http://dx.doi.org/10.1002/aorn.12970

Downey, C., Randell, R., Brown, J., & Jayne, D. G. (2018). Continuous versus intermittent vital signs monitoring using a wearable, wireless patch in patients admitted to surgical wards: Pilot cluster randomized controlled trial. *Journal of Medical Internet Research, 20*(12), e10802. http://dx.doi.org/10.2196/10802:10.2196/10802

Eliopoulos, C. (2018). *Gerontological nursing* (9th ed.). Wolters Kluwer.

Fan, C., Jia, L., Fang, F., Zhang, Y., Faramand, A., Chong, W., & Hai, Y. (2020). Adjunctive intermittent pneumatic compression in hospitalized patients receiving pharmacologic prophylaxis for venous thromboprophylaxis: A systematic review and meta-analysis. *Journal of Nursing Scholarship, 52*(4), 397–405. http://dx.doi.org/10.1111/jnu.12566

Fink, B. R. (1956). The etiology and treatment of laryngeal spasm. *Anesthesiology, 17*(4), 569–577. https://doi.org/10.1097/00000542-195607000-00007

Gillis, C., & Wischmeyer, P. E. (2019). Pre-operative nutrition and the elective surgical patient: Why, how and what? *Anaesthesia, 74*(Suppl 1), 27–35. https://doi.org/10.1111/anae.14506

Gwinnutt, M., & Gwinnutt, C. L. (2017). *Clinical anaesthesia: Lecture notes* (5th ed.). John Wiley & Sons, Ltd.

Hess, D. R., MacIntyre, N. R., Galvin, W. F., & Mishoe, S. C. (2021). *Respiratory care: Principles and practice* (4th ed.). Jones & Bartlett Learning.

Hinkle, J. L., Cheever, K. H. & Overbaugh, K. J. (2022). *Brunner & Suddarth's Textbook of medical-surgical nursing* (15th ed.). Wolters Kluwer.

Hoch, K. (2019). Current evidence-based practice for pediatric emergence agitation. *American Association of Nurse Anesthetists (AANA) Journal, 87*(6), 495–499. https://www.aana.com/docs/default-source/aana-journal-web-documents-1/aana-journal-course-update-for-nurse-anesthetists-current-evidence-based-practice-for-pediatric-emergence-agitation.pdf?sfvrsn=48030e04_6

The Joint Commission. (2022, April). Informed consent: More than getting a signature. *Quick Safety, 21*. https://www.jointcommission.org/resources/news-and-multimedia/newsletters/newsletters/quick-safety/quick-safety–issue-21-informed–consent-more-than-getting-a-signature/informed-consent-more-than-getting-a-signature/

The Joint Commission. (2020). Universal protocol. https://www.jointcommission.org/standards_information/up.aspx

Karaman, S., Karaman, T., Tapar, H., Dogru, S., & Suren, M. (2019). A randomized placebo-controlled study of aromatherapy for the treatment of postoperative nausea and vomiting. *Complementary Therapies in Medicine, 42*, 417–421. https://doi.org/10.1016/j.ctim.2018.12.019

Karch, A. M. (2020). *Focus on nursing pharmacology* (8th ed.). Wolters Kluwer.

Koyuncu, O., Urfali, S., Hakimoğlu, S., & Taşdoğan, A. M. (2020). Strategies to prevent postoperative nausea and vomiting. *Turkish Journal of Oncology, 35*(3), 349–355. https://doi.org/10.5505/tjo.2020.2270

Kyle, T., & Carman, S. (2021). *Essentials of pediatric nursing* (4th ed.). Wolters Kluwer.

Larson, P. C. Jr. (1998). Laryngospasm—The best treatment. *Anesthesiology, 89*(5), 1293–1294. https://doi.org/10.1097/00000542-199811000-00056

Link, T. (2020). Guidelines in practice: Hypothermia prevention. *AORN Journal, 111*(6), 654–663. https://doi.org/10.1002/aorn.13038

Lumb, A. B. (2019). Pre-operative respiratory optimisation: An expert review. *Anaesthesia, 74*(Suppl 1), 43–48. https://doi.org/10.1111/anae.14508

Maslonka, M. A., Schertz, A. R., Markowski, L. M., & Miller, P. J. (2020). Sedation challenges in patients with E-cigarette, or vaping, product use-associated lung injury (EVALI). *BMJ Case Reports, 13*(9), e233866. https://doi.org/10.1136/bcr-2019-233866

Mok, W. Q., Ullal, M. J., Su, S., Yiap, P. L., Yu, L. H., Lim, S. M. M., Ker, S. Y. J., & Wang, J. (2019). An integrative care bundle to prevent surgical site infections among surgical hip patients: A retrospective cohort study. *American Journal of Infection Control, 47*(5), 540–544. https://doi.org/10.1016/j.ajic.2018.10.011

National Center for Biotechnology Information. (2020). *PubChem compound summary for CID 51263, Alfentanil*. https://pubchem.ncbi.nlm.nih.gov/compound/Alfentanil

Nelson, K., Nicholls, C., & Muckler, V. C. (2018). Pediatric review and perioperative considerations. *Journal of Perianesthesia Nursing, 33*(3), 265–274. https://doi.org/10.1016/j.jopan.2016.03.011

Nieh, H. C., & Su, S. F. (2018). Force-air warming for rewarming and comfort following laparoscopy: A randomized controlled trial. *Clinical Nursing Research, 27*(5), 540–559. https://doi.org/10.1177/1054773817708082journals.sagepub.com/home/cnr

Obara, S. (2018). Dexmedetomidine as an adjuvant during general anesthesia. *Journal of Anesthesia, 32*(3), 313–315. https://doi.org/10.1007/s00540-018-2509-5

Parry, A. (2018). Preventing infection in surgical patients. *British Journal of Nursing, 27*(21), 1218–1220.

Polomano, R. C., Fillman, M., Giordano, N. A., Vallerand, A. H., Wiltse Nicely, K. L., & Jungquist, C. R. (2017). Multimodal analgesia for acute postoperative and trauma-related pain. *American Journal of Nursing, 117*(3 Suppl 1), S12–S26. https://doi.org/10.1097/01.NAJ.0000513527.71934.73

Poulsen, M. J., Coto, J., & Cooney, M. F. (2019). Music as a postoperative pain management intervention. *Journal of PeriAnesthesia Nursing, 34*(3), 662–666. https://doi.org/10.1016/j.jopan.2019.01.003

Schoen, D. C., & Prater, K. (2019). Role of telehealth in pre-anesthetic evaluations. *AANA Journal, 87*(1), 43–49. https://nurseanesthesiology.aana.com/wp-content/uploads/2020/03/Schoen-R.pdf

Shapiro, M. E., & Singer, E. A. (2019). Perioperative advance directives: Do Not Resuscitate in the operating room. *The Surgical Clinics of North America, 99*(5), 859–865. https://doi.org/10.1016/j.suc.2019.06.006

Sibert, K. S., Long, J. L., & Haddy, S. M. (2020). Extubation and the risks of coughing and laryngospasm in the era of Coronavirus Disease-19 (COVID-19). *Cureus, 12*(5), e8196. https://doi.org/10.7759/cureus.8196

Sikka, P. K., Beaman, S. T., & Street, J. A. (Eds.) (2015). *Basic clinical anesthesia*. Springer-Verlag.

Society of Critical Care Medicine. (n.d.). *Surviving sepsis campaign*. Retrieved December 30, 2020, from https://www.sccm.org/SurvivingSepsisCampaign/Home

Spatz, E. S., Suter, L. G., George, E., Perez, M., Curry, L., Desai, V., Bao, H., Geary, L. L., Herrin, J., Lin, Z., Bernheim, S. M., & Krumholz, H. M. (2020). An instrument for assessing the quality of informed consent documents for elective procedures: Development and testing. *BMJ Open, 10*(5), e033297. https://doi.org/10.1136/bmjopen-2019-033297

Spruce, L. (2020b). Using a complementary intervention to decrease postoperative nausea and vomiting. *AORN Journal, 112*(4), 417–418. http://doi.org/10.1002/aorn.13193

Stanton, C. (2021). Guideline for preoperative patient skin antisepsis. *AORN Journal, 113*(4), P5–P7. https://doi.org/10.1002/aorn.13380

Strickland, S. L., Rubin, B. K., Drescher, G. S., Haas, C. F., O'Malley, C. A., Volsko, T. A., Branson, R. D., Hess, D. R., & American Association for Respiratory Care, Irving, Texas. (2013). AARC clinical practice guideline: Effectiveness of nonpharmacologic airway clearance therapies in hospitalized patients. *Respiratory Care, 58*(12), 2187–2193. https://doi.org/10.4187/respcare.02925

Subramaniam, R. (2019). Anaesthetic concerns in preterm and term neonates. *Indian Journal of Anaesthesia, 63*(9), 771–779. https://doi.org/10.4103/ija.IJA_591_19

Tubog, T. D. (2019). Combined intermittent pneumatic leg compression and pharmacological prophylaxis for prevention of venous thromboembolism. *Orthopaedic Nursing, 38*(4), 270–272. https://doi.org/10.1097/NOR.0000000000000574

Turunen, E., Miettinen, M., Setälä, L., & Vehviläinen-Julkunen, K. (2017). An integrative review of a preoperative nursing care structure. *Journal of Clinical Nursing, 26*(7–8):915–930. https://doi.org/10.1111/jocn.13448

U.S. National Library of Medicine. (2020, November 30). *Midazolam injection*. https://medlineplus.gov/druginfo/meds/a609014.html

Verrillo, S. C., Cvach, M., Hudson, K. W., & Winters, B. D. (2019). Using continuous vital sign monitoring to detect early deterioration in adult postoperative inpatients. *Journal of Nursing Care Quality, 34*(2), 107–113. https://doi.org/10.1097/NCQ.0000000000000350

Wolters Kluwer. (2022). Problem-based care plans. In *Lippincott Advisor*. Wolters Kluwer.

Xu, H., Xu, G., Ren, C, Liu, L., & Wei, L. (2019). Effect of forced-air warming system in prevention of postoperative hypothermia in elderly patients. A prospective controlled trial. *Medicine, 98*(22), 1–6. http://dx.doi.org/10.1097/MD.0000000000015895

UNIT VI

Promoting Healthy Physiologic Responses

The art and science of caring are blended when nurses implement actions to meet basic human needs and to promote healthy physiologic responses. The chapters in Unit VI focus on information and guidelines essential to nursing practice in a wide variety of clinical and community settings that involve both healthy and ill patients of all ages. Included are nursing interventions to basic physiologic needs: hygiene, skin integrity, activity and rest, nutrition, elimination, oxygenation, and fluid–electrolyte balance and to promote comfort and pain management.

Each basic physiologic need is discussed first with a review of concepts pertinent to the specific area of human function and response, then with an examination of factors that affect need satisfaction. The steps of the nursing process are used to provide guidelines and information necessary for making accurate assessments establishing outcomes; and planning, implementing, and evaluating specific nursing interventions to meet needs and promote wellness.

The chapters in Unit VI enable the beginning nurse to integrate the knowledge and skills necessary to promote healthy physiologic responses in patients in any practice setting. Nursing process skills are further refined to ensure that care is holistic, comprehensive, and person centered.

" . . . what nursing has to do is to put the patient in the best condition for nature to act upon him."

Florence Nightingale (1820–1910), *a philosopher, theorist, statistician, humanitarian, and inspirational leader who founded modern nursing through a systematic method of training well-qualified nurses. She also initiated important reforms in military sanitation and hospital construction that greatly improved patient survival.*

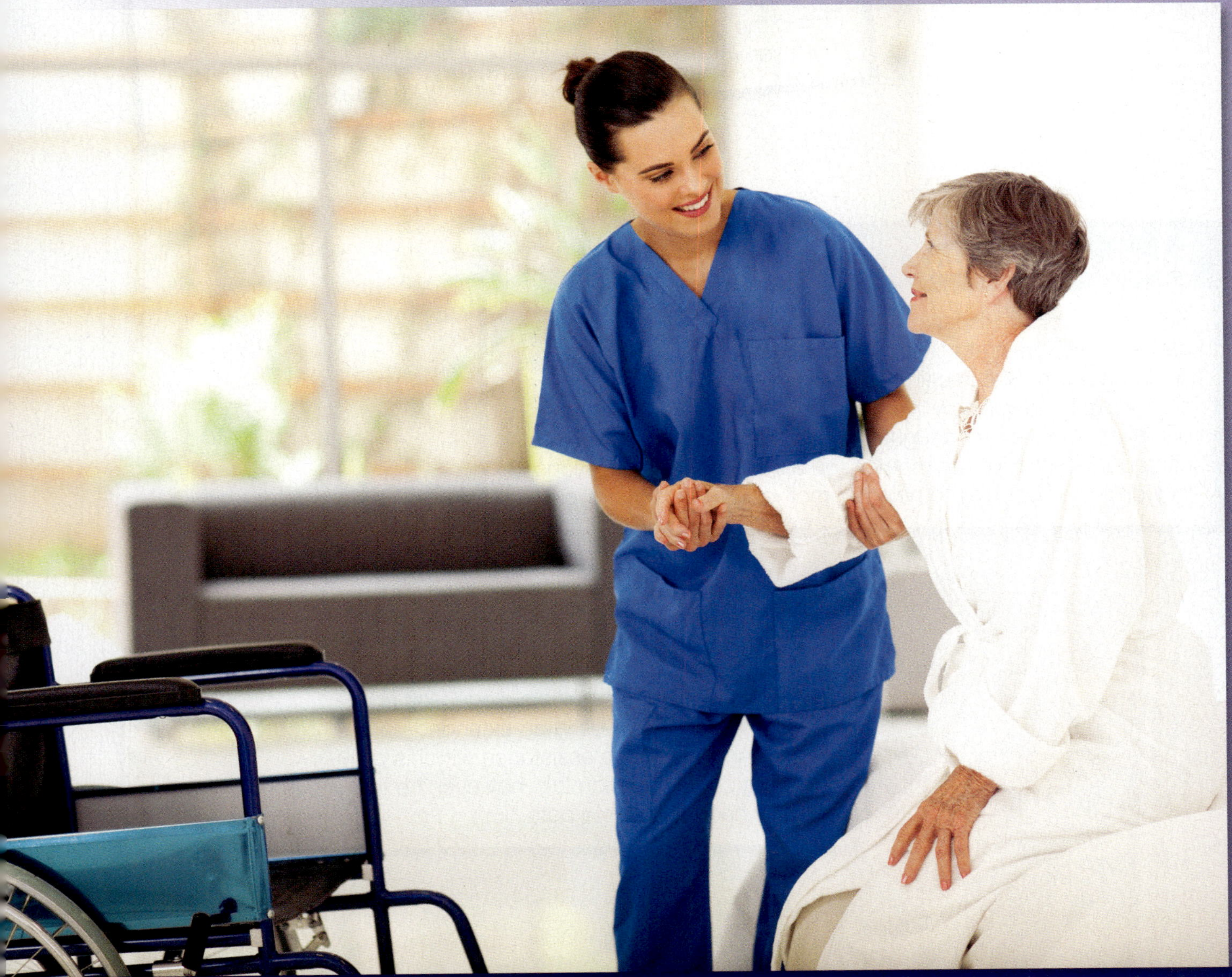

32 Hygiene

Kylie Simpson

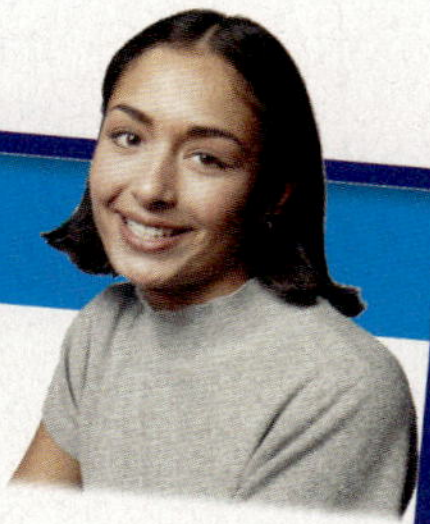

Kylie, age 20, is a student at a state university. After having vaginal itching and burning for 2 weeks, she visits the campus health clinic. She is diagnosed with a vaginal infection. She asks the nurse at the campus health clinic, "Is there something wrong with me? This is the second vaginal infection I have had in 7 months. Isn't there something I can do to keep this from happening again?"

Sonya Delamordo

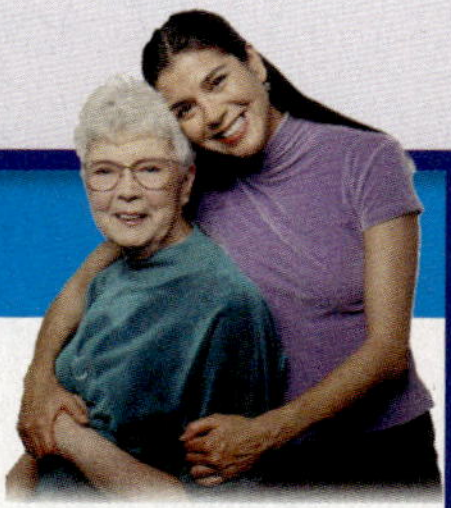

Sonya is an older Hispanic woman who has had a stroke (brain attack) resulting in right-sided paralysis. She is being discharged from the hospital and will now live with her daughter, who will be her primary caregiver. Her daughter is eager to learn everything she can about caring for her mother and asks numerous questions, including the best way to help her mother with personal hygiene.

Andrew Craig

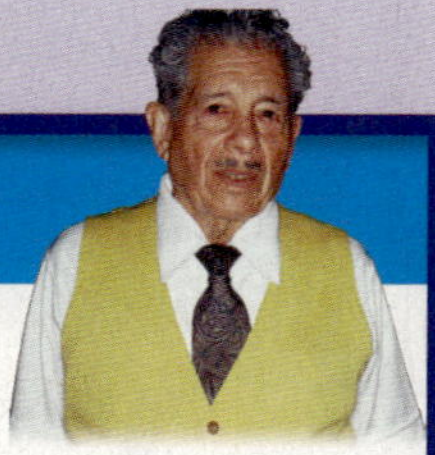

Andrew, age 68, has multiple diagnoses and limited mobility. He lives in an extended-care facility. Andrew needs assistance with his daily morning care. This morning, however, he tells the nurse, "I've already had a complete bath."

Learning Outcomes

After completing the chapter, you will be able to accomplish the following:

1. Identify factors affecting personal hygiene.
2. Assess the adequacy of hygiene practices and self-care behaviors using appropriate interview and physical assessment skills.
3. Assess the condition of the patient's skin, oral cavity, hair, and nails using appropriate interview and physical assessment skills.
4. Formulate diagnoses/patient problems related to hygiene amenable to nursing intervention.
5. Demonstrate techniques for assisting patients with hygiene measures, including those used when administering various types of baths and those used in cleaning each part of the body.
6. Describe agents commonly used on the skin and scalp, including any precautions related to their use.
7. Plan, implement, and evaluate nursing care related to diagnoses/patient problems involving alterations in and related to hygiene.

Nursing Concepts

- Assessment
- Clinical decision making/clinical judgment
- Safety
- Tissue integrity

Measures for maintaining a minimal level of personal cleanliness and grooming, called **personal hygiene**, promote physical and psychological well-being. Hygiene practices include bathing and care of the skin and specific body areas, including the oral cavity, eyes, ears, nose, hair, nails, feet, and perineal and vaginal areas. Personal hygiene practices vary widely among people. It is important that personal care be carried out conveniently and frequently enough to promote good hygiene and wellness. Acute and chronic illness, hospitalization, and institutionalization may make it necessary to modify hygiene practices. In these situations, the nurse helps the patient to continue sound hygiene practices and can teach the patient and family members/caregivers, when necessary, regarding hygiene. Nurses assisting patients with basic hygiene must respect individual patient preferences, providing only the care that patients cannot, or should not, provide for themselves. Nurses should value each patient as a person and take into consideration the patient's physical and psychological state of being. Social determinants of health, such as religion and culture, educational perspectives, and financial issues, and their impact on hygiene are important considerations when planning and assisting patients in meeting their hygiene needs (see the accompanying Reflective Practice box on pages 1090) (Moore & Merrill, 2019; Ramos-Morcillo et al., 2019).

This chapter discusses multiple factors that affect personal hygiene and nursing measures that promote personal hygiene. A practical guide for assessing the adequacy of personal hygiene is presented. The data collected when assisting with hygiene may lead to the identification of multiple diagnoses/patient problems and/or collaborative problems. Examples of such diagnoses/problems are provided in the chapter. In addition, patient outcomes are presented, as are specific nursing strategies used when performing care of the skin, mouth, eyes, ears, nose, hair, nails, feet, perineal areas, and vaginal areas. Nursing considerations related to maintaining an appropriate patient environment are discussed as well. The concluding plan of care related to feminine hygiene illustrates how the nurse uses knowledge of personal hygiene practices and the integumentary system, along with specific nursing interventions, to address diagnoses/patient problems and to promote the patient's general sense of well-being.

HYGIENE PRACTICES

Hygienic practices include caring for the skin, hair, nails, eyes, ears, nose, mouth, feet, and perineal area. There are strong links between good hygiene practices and a person's health. Inadequate hygiene practices can contribute to alterations in a person's health.

The skin, or integument, is the largest organ of the body and has multiple functions. The integumentary system is made up of the skin, the subcutaneous layer directly under the skin, and the appendages of the skin, including the hair and nails. Chapter 33 provides a description of the anatomy and physiology of the integumentary system and factors that affect skin integrity. Adequate skin hygiene, including foot care, contributes to maintaining skin condition and integrity, an important first line of defense, preventing the entry of pathogens, minimizing absorption of harmful substances, and preventing excessive water loss (Lichterfeld et al., 2015; Voegeli, 2019; Wounds UK, 2018).

Hair is an accessory structure of the skin. Good general health is essential for attractive hair and skin, and cleanliness is a positive influence. Illness affects the hair, especially when endocrine abnormalities, increased body temperature, poor nutrition, or anxiety and worry are present. Changes in the color or condition of the hair shaft are related to changes in hormonal activity or to changes in the blood supply to hair follicles.

The nails are an accessory structure of the skin composed of epithelial tissue. Healthy nail beds are pink, convex, and evenly curved. With certain pathologic conditions, and to some extent with aging, the nails become ridged and areas become concave. Hygienic care includes keeping the nails of fingers and feet trimmed and clean.

QSEN Reflective Practice: Cultivating QSEN Competencies

CHALLENGE TO INTERPERSONAL SKILLS

It was our first day of clinical, sophomore year, and we were instructed to provide complete personal care with our patients. My patient, Andrew Craig, was a 68-year-old man with multiple diagnoses and limited mobility. As I entered the room, he told me he had just had a bed bath a few hours earlier. I wasn't sure what to do, so I asked the tech if my patient had already had a complete bed bath. The tech pulled me into the patient's room and proceeded to scream at the patient, telling him not to lie to me and threatening to make him sit in the chair all day. This patient did not have a hip and had antibiotic beads in the area, so it was very painful for him to sit in a chair because the beads dug into his side. The tech then told me to do the bed bath and left the room. I was left in a very awkward position because the patient was mad at me and I was astounded by how the tech had treated this patient. I was extremely upset as a result of this confrontation.

The day was emotionally very difficult for me, and when I arrived home, I became even more upset. The manner in which the tech treated the patient, even though the patient may have been manipulative, was completely out of line.

Thinking Outside the Box: Possible Courses of Action

- Make the best of a bad situation, but do nothing to change the status quo: "Hey, I'm only a student, right?"
- Confront the tech and tell her about my outrage.
- Report the tech to her supervisor.
- Consult with my instructor about how a professional nurse should respond in a situation like this.
- Be prepared to "go to the top" if initial attempts to reform a bad system don't meet with success.

Evaluating a Good Outcome: How Do I Define Success?

- The patient's basic hygiene needs are met.
- The patient's humanity and integrity are respected.
- Health care professionals and technicians are held accountable for incompetent, unethical, and illegal behavior (the tech, nursing leadership, and administration in this long-term care facility).
- I learn how to be a successful patient advocate.

Personal Learning: Here's to the Future!

I proceeded to talk to my clinical instructor and the coordinator of the class about the incident. The coordinator contacted the long-term care facility and I had to give a formal statement about the incident. The nurse manager who took my statement was not very receptive and was actually very patronizing.

This entire experience helped me to recognize the type of nurse I want to be. First and foremost, I always want to ensure that I provide high-quality patient care. At the time of my unfortunate experience, I did not respond immediately to the tech's inappropriate comments. But now that I have gained more experience and become more confident, I would definitely respond immediately if a similar situation ever arose again. I realize that I can't let fear stand in my way when the quality of patient care is suffering. I would encourage any nurse who sees a colleague or anyone treating a patient without the utmost respect and care to speak up and contact appropriate personnel to discuss the situation.

In addition to this tech's inappropriate behavior, the overall conditions of this long-term care facility were appalling. I learned a lot this semester about the shortage of nurses (1 RN for 40 patients) and, consequently, how patient care is being jeopardized. During the unfortunate episode to which I was exposed, I was astonished and outraged, but I didn't take any steps to change the conditions except reporting this one incident. At the end of the semester, we reported the conditions to the class coordinator. Now I realize that as a person, I could have done more to change the conditions in the long-term care facility. In retrospect, I should have taken a leadership role and notified the outside licensing organization about these conditions (the long-term care facility ended up losing its accreditation that summer). All nurses are responsible for ensuring the quality of care given to patients, and we must contact whomever necessary to ensure changes are made.

This experience was very difficult for me, but in the end, I think it opened my eyes to the importance of nurses acting as advocates and leaders.

Catherine Barrell, Georgetown University

QSEN SELF-REFLECTION ON QUALITY AND SAFETY COMPETENCIES DEVELOPING KNOWLEDGE, SKILLS, AND ATTITUDES FOR CONTINUOUS IMPROVEMENT

How do you think you would respond in a similar situation? Why? What does this tell you about yourself and about the adequacy of your skills for professional practice? What *knowledge, skills,* and *attitudes* do you need to develop to continuously improve the quality and safety of care for patients like Mr. Craig?

Patient-Centered Care: What factors may have played a role in the tech's actions toward the patient and nursing student? What interventions should the nursing student implement to provide care based on respect for the patient's preferences, values, and needs? How did the nursing student's actions adhere to ethical and legal principles? Did the nursing student act as an advocate for Mr. Craig?

Teamwork and Collaboration/Quality Improvement: How could the nursing staff and other care providers collaborate to provide respectful care for Mr. Craig? What communication skills do you need to improve to ensure you function effectively as a member of the patient care team and to obtain assistance when needed?

QSEN Reflective Practice: Cultivating QSEN Competencies *(continued)*

CHALLENGE TO INTERPERSONAL SKILLS

Safety/Evidence-Based Practice: Is it within the nursing student's scope of practice to individually contact a higher authority such as a licensing facility about the situation? What evidence in nursing literature provides guidance for decision making regarding providing culturally competent health care?

Informatics: Can you identify the essential information that should be documented in Mr. Craig's electronic record to support safe patient care and coordination of care? Is there other documentation that should be part of the student's response to this incident? Can you think of other ways to respond to or approach the situation?

A person's general health influences the health of that person's mouth and teeth, and proper care of the mouth and teeth contribute to overall health. Maintaining good oral hygiene and dental care has several benefits. There is esthetic value in having a clean and healthy mouth. Having one's own teeth in good condition contributes to an intact body image. In addition, the beginning of the digestive process and tasting pleasure are enhanced when the mouth and teeth are in good condition. Oral health is directly related to systemic health, and poor oral health is associated with diabetes, cardiovascular disease, and metabolic syndrome (American Dental Association, 2019b). Oral health is an important concern in relation to overall health and quality of life.

The perineal area is dark, warm, and often moist, providing conditions that favor bacterial growth. The patient who cannot clean the perineal area needs the nurse's assistance for this important part of personal hygiene. Neglecting perineal cleaning for the patient who cannot provide self-care often results in physical and psychological discomfort for the patient, skin breakdown, and offensive odors.

FACTORS AFFECTING PERSONAL HYGIENE

Hygiene activities and practices can support health and prevent disease. However, hygiene practices vary widely among groups and people. It is important to respect differences in patient hygiene practices and provide care and information in a nonjudgmental manner. Social determinants of health may influence personal hygiene behaviors.

Culture

It is important to identify cultural variations that could affect a patient's personal hygiene preferences, such as typical bathing habits, and behaviors, such as use of various hygiene-related products (Andrews et al., 2020). For example, people from some cultures place a high value on personal cleanliness and feel unclean unless they shower or bathe at least once daily. Many consider bathing incomplete without the use of products to reduce or mask normal body odors. Other people often find a weekly bath sufficient and may feel no need to mask normal body odors. Culture may also influence whether bathing is a private or communal activity.

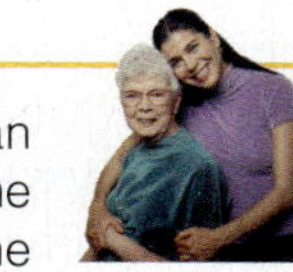

Consider **Sonya Delamordo**, the woman being discharged to her daughter's home after experiencing a stroke. Although the daughter is very eager to take care of her mother, the nurse explores the patient's culture to determine how the patient might feel about being cared for by her daughter. Often, hygiene is a personal matter. The nurse needs to discuss hygiene care with the patient and her daughter to ensure person-centered care.

Socioeconomic Status

A person's socioeconomic status and financial resources often define the hygiene options available to that person. A lack of funds to obtain toiletries or clean clothing may contribute to an inability to maintain personal hygiene needs. For example, someone renting a room in a boarding house may have limited or no access to a tub or shower and may have limited finances to buy soap, shampoo, shaving cream, and deodorant. People who are homeless, who often carry all their belongings in a car or shopping cart, may welcome the warm running water and soap available in roadside or public restrooms.

Spiritual Practices

Spiritual practices, including religious beliefs, may dictate ceremonial washings and purifications, sometimes as a prelude to prayer or eating. For example, in the Orthodox Jewish tradition, ritual baths are required for women after childbirth and menstruation. In some religions, contact with a deceased person or a deceased animal may make a person "unclean." Other religions dictate that no modern facilities be installed in homes. This would prohibit some people from having running water and toilets in their homes. As a result, they may bathe infrequently.

Developmental Level

Children learn hygiene practices while growing up. Family practices often dictate hygiene habits, such as morning or evening baths; the frequency of shampooing, tooth brushing, and clothing changes; feelings about nudity; and so on. As adolescents become more concerned about their personal appearance, they may adopt new hygiene measures, such as taking showers more frequently and wearing deodorant.

Bathing frequency commonly decreases as a person ages, possibly due to limitations in mobility and the natural tendency toward drier skin with age. Older adults may experience an increase in skin conditions or problems, increasing the need for education related to hygiene and skin care (Lichterfeld-Kottner et al., 2020; Moore & Merrill, 2019).

Health State

Disease, surgery, or injury may reduce a person's ability to perform hygiene measures or motivation to follow usual hygiene habits. Weakness, dizziness, and fear of falling may prevent a person from entering a tub or shower or from bending to wash the lower extremities. Illness may also create a demand for new or modified hygiene measures. For example, meticulous foot care becomes a priority for patients with peripheral vascular complications that often accompany diabetes mellitus. The presence of pain with an acute condition or chronic pain can affect a person's ability to perform and/or tolerate personal hygiene measures.

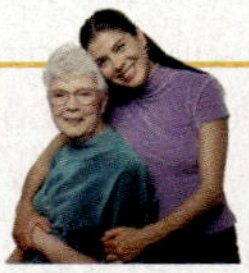

Remember ***Sonya Delamordo***, who has right-sided paralysis as a result of a stroke. She will have to adapt to caring for herself, dealing with the mobility limitations of her right side, especially if she is right handed. Both she and her daughter will have to learn how to adapt personal hygiene practices based on Sonya's abilities.

Personal Preferences

People have different preferences with regard to hygiene practices such as taking a shower versus a tub bath, using bar soap versus liquid soap, and washing to wake oneself or to relax before sleep. A person's self-concept and sexuality also influence personal hygiene practices. For example, in an effort to promote a positive self-image, older adults may use skin care products advertised to prevent wrinkles and diminish signs of aging. Women who are sexually active may use a variety of hygiene products following intercourse to promote cleanliness.

NURSING PROCESS FOR PERSONAL HYGIENE AND SKIN CARE

Assessing

The comprehensive nursing assessment uses interview and assessment skills to elicit data about the patient's hygiene status. When alterations in a patient's physical or mental health result in impaired ability to maintain acceptable personal hygiene, additional specific assessment skills are needed to determine the patient's limitations.

Nursing History

Bathing practices and cleansing habits and rituals vary widely. A clear threat to health must exist before a nurse decides that a person's hygiene practices are inadequate. The nurse assessing the adequacy of a patient's hygiene practices determines whether the patient has the knowledge, attitude, skills, and resources to care for the skin and mucous membranes. Use neutral and inclusive terms (e.g., partner) and a nonjudgmental manner to obtain information about the patient's gender identity, biologic sex, and sexual orientation. This information will help identify the needs of individual patients and provide thoughtful, person-centered care (Altarum Institute, 2019; Cahill et al., 2020). Focused Assessment Guide 32-1 provides additional suggested strategies, questions and approaches for an assessment of information related to hygiene practices. When documenting the nursing history, be specific, clearly describing the patient's typical hygiene practices and any issues or problems.

SKIN

Question the patient about any past or current skin problems and changes in their skin (e.g., rashes, lumps, itching, dryness, lesions) as well as recent surgeries, wounds, tattoos, or piercings. When skin problems are present, ask the patient the following:

- How long have you had this problem?
- Does it bother you?
- How does it bother you?
- Does it itch?
- Have you found anything that helps relieve these symptoms?

Additional information related to assessment of the skin is discussed in Chapter 27 and Chapter 33.

ORAL CAVITY

Identify the patient's normal oral hygiene practices and the variables influencing these practices. Note the history of any oral problems and related treatments.

Identify any variables known to cause oral problems, such as deficient self-care abilities, poor nutrition or excessive intake of refined sugars, family history of periodontal disease, or ingestion of chemotherapeutic agents that produce oral lesions. Patients at increased risk for oral problems include those who are seriously ill, comatose, dehydrated, confused, depressed, or paralyzed. Patients with mental health problems are also at risk for alterations in oral health (Griffiths et al., 2020; Kisely, 2016). Patients who are mouth breathers, those who can have no oral intake of nutrition or fluids, those with nasogastric tubes or oral airways in place, and those who have had oral surgery are also at increased risk.

Additional information related to assessment of the oral cavity is discussed in Chapter 27.

EYES, EARS, AND NOSE

Ask the patient to identify any special eye, ear, or nose care that the patient performs. Also, address any specific care measures related to the use and care of visual aids or prosthetics (glasses, contact lenses, artificial eye) and hearing aids. Inquire about any history of eye, ear, and nose problems, and related treatments.

Additional information related to assessment of the eyes, ears, and nose is discussed in Chapter 27.

Focused Assessment Guide 32-1

HYGIENE PRACTICES

Factors to Assess	Questions and Approaches
Daily and weekly bathing habits	Tell me about your daily and weekly bathing habits. Are there special bathing or hygiene products you routinely use or can't use? How can the nursing staff best help you to meet your hygiene needs?
Factors interfering with hygiene practices (sensory, cognitive, endurance, mobility, or motivation)	What recently or in the past has interfered with your hygiene practices? Does anything interfere with your ability to be as clean as you would like?
Pain	Do you have pain? Describe characteristics, onset, location, duration, associated symptoms, and intensity. Does the pain interfere with your ability to perform personal hygiene tasks? Does caring for yourself cause pain or discomfort?
Exposure history	Do you sunbathe? How much sun or tanning booth exposure do you get? Do you use sunscreen? Does your job or daily activities/hobbies expose you to chemicals, such as bleach, petroleum, paint, insecticides, or cleaning products?
History of skin or mucous membrane problems (nature, onset of problem and frequency, causes, severity, symptoms, interventions attempted, results)	Have you noticed any changes in your skin or mucous membranes? Describe any skin problems with rashes, lumps, itching, dryness, lesions, ecchymosis, or masses. What have you used to relieve these symptoms?
Special hygiene practices	
• Mouth	How do you clean your teeth and gums? How often do you have a dental examination? Do you have any dental appliances? Are there any tender areas or lesions in your mouth?
• Eyes, ears, and nose	Do you wear glasses or contact lenses to improve your vision? Do you wear a hearing aid? Have you noticed any changes in your eyes, ears, or nose? Have you experienced any discharge or bleeding from or swelling of your eyes, ears, or nose?
• Hair	Have you noticed any changes in your hair? Have you noticed any unusual dryness of the scalp or changes in hair texture and amount?
• Feet and nails	Have you noticed any changes in your feet or nails? Is the appearance of the nails normal? How do you normally care for and clean your nails? Is the skin intact on the feet? Have you noticed any swelling of one or both feet? Do you wear any special shoes?
• Perineum	Have you noticed any changes in your perineum? Have you noticed any unusual discharge, swelling, itching, or inflammation? Are you able to complete your own perineal care? Do you follow any special hygiene practices during menstruation? What type of feminine hygiene products (e.g., pads, tampons, douches) do you use?
• Piercings/Tattoos	Do you have any body piercings on your face, neck, arms, legs, torso, navel, or genitals? Have you experienced any problems related to the procedure? Do you have any tattoos? Are the tattoos healed? How do you care for your piercing(s) and/or tattoo(s)?

HAIR

Identify the patient's usual hair and scalp care practices, including styling preferences. Note any history of hair or scalp problems; possible causes of changes in the distribution, texture, or amount of hair; and related treatments. Be alert for any factors that are known to cause hair or scalp problems or that require special care such as deficient self-care abilities, immobility, malnutrition, and treatments known to result in hair loss (e.g., certain chemotherapeutic agents).

Additional information related to assessment of the hair is discussed in Chapter 27.

NAILS AND FEET

Gather information about the patient's normal nail and foot care practices. Include the type of footwear worn and any history of nail or foot problems and their treatments. Foot problems, particularly common in people with diabetes mellitus and peripheral vascular disease, often require hospitalization. A proactive educational approach can prevent many of the serious complications (e.g., ulcers, lower extremity amputations) associated with foot problems.

Identify any variables known to cause nail and foot problems, such as deficient self-care abilities, vascular disease, arthritis, diabetes mellitus, history of biting nails or trimming them improperly, frequent or prolonged exposure to chemicals or water, trauma, ill-fitting shoes, or obesity.

Additional information related to assessment of the nails and feet is discussed in Chapter 27.

Concept Mastery Alert

Diabetes mellitus can result in peripheral vascular disease; patients who have peripheral vascular disease may require hospitalization related to problems associated with the feet.

PERINEAL AND VAGINAL AREAS

Note any history of perineal or vaginal problems and related treatments. Identify any variables known to cause perineal or vaginal problems or to create a need for special care, such as urinary or fecal incontinence, an indwelling Foley catheter, childbirth, douching, rectal or genital surgery, and diseases such as urinary tract infection, diabetes mellitus, and certain sexually transmitted infections (STIs; e.g., herpes).

Additional information related to assessment of the perineal area is discussed in Chapter 27.

Physical Assessment

An assessment of pertinent body systems can provide data about the patient's hygiene status and the patient's ability to maintain personal hygiene.

MUSCULOSKELETAL SYSTEM

Impairment of the musculoskeletal system can interfere with a patient's ability to perform tasks related to personal hygiene. Many conditions produce muscle weakness, decreased range of motion, impaired balance, fatigue, and/or lack of coordination. The skills used to assess the musculoskeletal system are described in detail in Chapters 27 and 34.

SKIN

The inspection and palpation skills used to assess the integumentary system are described in detail in Chapters 27 and 33. Assisting patients with basic hygiene measures provides an excellent opportunity for examining a patient's skin. Many people are unaware that they have skin lesions, such as precancerous moles, that if untreated could prove fatal. Early detection and treatment of skin problems are important nursing functions.

When examining the skin, pay careful attention to cleanliness, color, texture, temperature, turgor, moisture, sensation, vascularity, and any lesions. Follow these general guidelines for assessing the skin:

- Incorporate assessment of the skin during the assessment of other body systems.
- Use a good source of light, preferably daylight.
- Compare bilateral parts for symmetry.
- Use standard terminology to communicate and record findings.
- Allow data obtained in the nursing history to direct the skin assessment.
- Identify any variables known to cause skin problems, such as deficient self-care abilities, immobility, malnutrition, decreased hydration, decreased sensation, sun exposure, vascular problems (altered tissue perfusion or venous return), or the presence of irritants (body secretions or excretions on the skin, other chemicals, mechanical devices).

Because lifestyle factors, changes in health state, illness, and certain diagnostic and therapeutic measures may adversely affect the skin, be alert for patients who may be at high risk for skin problems, and perform the appropriate skin assessment. Assessment may reveal dry skin, acne, or skin rashes. Recommended treatments for these skin problems are discussed in the Promoting Skin Health section on page 1102.

When documenting a physical assessment of the skin, describe exactly what is observed or palpated, including appearance, texture, size, location or distribution, and characteristics of any findings.

ORAL CAVITY

A physical assessment of the oral cavity involves inspection of the oral cavity and surrounding structures with attention to any unusual odors. When performing the physical assessment of the oral cavity, examine the following:

- *Lips:* color, moisture, lumps, ulcers, lesions, and edema
- *Buccal mucosa:* color, moisture, lesions, nodules, and bleeding
- *Color of the gums and surface of the gums:* lesions, bleeding, and edema
- *Teeth:* any loose, missing, or carious (decayed) teeth. Note the presence and condition of dentures or other orthodontic devices
- *Tongue:* color, symmetry, movement, texture, and lesions
- *Hard and soft palates:* intactness, color, patches, lesions, and petechiae (pinpoint round, red, purple, or brown spots that result from bleeding)
- *Oropharynx:* movement of the uvula and condition of tonsils, if present

Note unusual mouth odors and assess the adequacy of mastication and swallowing. An oral assessment tool can assist with assessment of the status of the oral cavity, as well as help to determine the frequency and procedure for oral care (Chick & Wynne, 2020). Identifying the problem and its cause and initiating appropriate treatment are imperative. This may require consultation with a dentist or health care provider. Refer to Chapter 27 for further description of nursing assessment of the oral cavity.

Dental Caries

The decay of teeth with the formation of cavities is called **caries**. Caries result from failure to remove **plaque**, an invisible, destructive, bacterial film that builds up on everyone's teeth and eventually leads to the destruction of tooth enamel. A successful plaque-fighting program includes limiting sweet snacks such as soft drinks, candy, gum, jams, and jellies between meals; thorough cleansing of the teeth; and regular dental checkups. The use of antiplaque fluoride toothpastes, mouth rinses, and flossing also help prevent dental caries.

Periodontal Disease

Periodontal diseases are the result of infections and inflammation of the gums and bone that surround and support the teeth (CDC, 2013). Periodontal disease and tooth decay are the two biggest threats to dental health (CDC, 2013). **Gingivitis** is an inflammation of the gingiva, the tissue that surrounds the teeth. **Periodontitis**, or periodontal disease, is a marked inflammation of the gums that also involves degeneration of the dental periosteum (tissues) and bone. Symptoms include bleeding gums; swollen, red, painful gum tissues; receding gum lines with the formation of pockets between the teeth and gums; pus that appears when gums are pressed; and loose teeth. If unchecked, plaque builds up and, along with dead bacteria, forms hard deposits called **tartar** at the gum lines. The tartar attacks the fibers that fasten teeth to the gums and eventually attacks bone tissue. The teeth then loosen and fall out. **Halitosis**, a strong mouth odor or a persistent bad taste in the mouth, may be the first indication of periodontal disease. Regular treatment by a dentist is imperative.

Other Oral Problems

Other oral problems that may be observed when inspecting the oral cavity include the following:

- **Stomatitis**, an inflammation of the oral mucosa, has numerous causes, such as bacteria, virus, mechanical trauma, irritants, nutritional deficiencies, and systemic infection. Symptoms may include heat, pain, increased flow of saliva, and halitosis.
- **Glossitis**, an inflammation of the tongue, can be caused by deficiencies of vitamin B_{12}, folic acid, and iron.
- **Cheilosis**, an ulceration and dry scaling of the lips with fissures at the angles of the mouth, can have multiple causes, including infections of the oral cavity (e.g., strep bacteria), a lack of iron or B vitamin deficiencies (especially riboflavin), and skin irritation (e.g., eczema).
- Dry oral mucosa may simply be related to dehydration or may be caused by mouth breathing, an alteration in salivary functioning, or certain medications (e.g., anticholinergic drugs).
- Oral malignancies, appearing as lumps or ulcers, must be distinguished from benign mouth problems because early detection may lead to cure; later detection can lead to radical surgery or death. Teach patients to see their dentist immediately if they notice white or red patches, persistent sores, swelling, bleeding, numbness, or pain in the mouth.

EYES, EARS, AND NOSE

During the eye examination, note the position, alignment, and general appearance of the eye. Check that eyelashes are distributed equally and curl outward. Note the presence of lesions, nodules, redness, swelling, crusting, flaking, excessive tearing, or discharge of eyelids. Check the color of the conjunctivae.

When examining the ear, note its position, alignment, and general appearance. Pay particular attention to a buildup of **cerumen** (wax) in the canal, dryness, crusting, or the presence of any discharge or foreign body. Older adults can have a buildup of cerumen that can cause impaired hearing. This is a result of harder, drier cerumen and decreased motility of the cilia in the ear canal.

While examining the nose, note its position and general appearance, patency of the nostrils, and presence of tenderness, dryness, edema, bleeding, discharge, or secretions.

Refer to Chapter 27 for additional information related to nursing assessment of the eyes, ears, and nose.

HAIR

Assess the condition of the hair. Inspect it for texture, cleanliness, and oiliness. Inspect the scalp for any scaling, lesions, inflammation, or infection. Note any abnormalities such as dandruff, hair loss, or infestations. Patients of African American descent may have very dry scalps and dry, fragile hair (Andrews et al., 2020). Patients of Asian descent may have straight hair that does not necessarily require special care (Andrews et al., 2020). When in doubt, ask the patient, a family member, or significant other about the specific manner in which hair care is performed. Refer to Chapter 27 for additional information related to nursing assessment of hair.

Dandruff

Dandruff is a condition characterized by itching and flaking of the scalp and may be complicated by the embarrassment it causes. Persistent, severe cases usually require medical attention, but daily brushing and shampooing with a medicated shampoo may be all that is needed to keep the scalp free of dandruff.

Hair Loss

Hair growth and hair loss are ongoing, daily processes. Hair loss becomes a potential problem only when it exceeds hair growth. Absence or loss of hair is called **alopecia**. Alopecia on the head is also referred to as baldness. Alopecia can be a partial or complete, local or generalized, loss of hair. Patchy hair loss can result from infections of the scalp. Hair loss from plaiting, excessive backcombing and teasing, or the use of hair rollers is usually temporary; hair returns when the tension on the hair shaft is halted.

Excessive generalized hair loss may occur with infection, nutritional deficiencies, hormonal disorders, childbirth, general anesthesia, drug toxicity, chemotherapy, thyroid disease, liver disease, hepatic and renal failure, and radiation. Alopecia can also occur as part of the aging process. Alopecia related to aging is more common in men than in women. There is no known cure for baldness. Although some medications are currently in use and others are being developed, their long-term efficacy is unknown. For example, minoxidil, a cardiovascular and antihypertensive drug, has reversed balding to some degree when applied to the scalp. Hairpieces, sometimes worn by people who are bald, require the same care as normal hair but less frequent washing.

Hair transplantation is a surgical procedure for baldness. Hair is taken from donor sites, usually from the back or sides of the scalp, and transplanted to areas with no hair. The procedure is long and expensive but reportedly has decided benefits for people who find baldness psychologically unpleasant. Complications include serious scalp infections.

Pediculosis

Infestation with lice is called **pediculosis**. There are three common types of lice: *Pediculus humanus capitis,* which infests the hair and scalp; *Pediculus humanus corporis,* which infests the body; and *Phthirus pubis,* which infests the shorter hairs on the body, usually the pubic and axillary hair. Lice lay eggs, called nits, on the hair shafts. Nits are white or light gray and look like dandruff but cannot be brushed or shaken off the hair. Frequent scratching and scratch marks on the body and the scalp suggest the presence of pediculosis. Pediculosis can be spread directly by contact with the hair of infested people. It is less common for transmission to occur indirectly through contact with clothing, bed linen, brushes, and combs of infested people. Treatment for pediculosis is discussed in the Providing Hair Care discussion on page 1111.

NAILS AND FEET

Examine nails for intactness and cleanliness. Assess capillary refill and the contour of the nail bed. Observe the nail base for redness, swelling, bleeding, discharge, and tenderness. Patients with dark skin tones may have freckles or pigmented streaks in their nails and nails may be thicker (Jarvis & Eckhardt, 2020). Examine the feet for cleanliness and intactness of skin, and note any swelling, inflammation, lesions, tenderness, or orthopedic problems. Carefully examine the skin between the toes. Refer to Chapter 27 for additional information related to nursing assessment of the nails and feet.

PERINEAL AND VAGINAL AREAS

Examine the male genitalia for color, lesions, swelling, inflammation, excoriation, tenderness, and discharge (amount, color, odor, source). Examine the female genitalia for color, lesions, masses, swelling, inflammation, excoriation, tenderness, and discharge (amount, color, odor, source). Inspect the anal area for cracks, nodules, distended veins, masses, or polyps. Note any perineal odors. Refer to Chapter 27 for additional information related to nursing assessment of the perineum.

Diagnosing Actual or Potential Health Problems and Needs

An assessment of a patient's hygiene practices and the skin, mucous membranes, and other body areas may lead to the identification of one or more diagnoses or patient problems related to hygiene. Following the formulation of the diagnoses or patient problems, the nurse communicates findings to other nursing and health care professionals through the use of the written and spoken word. The written diagnosis or patient problem becomes a permanent part of the patient's health record. Examples of health problems and needs with related etiology and signs and symptoms can be found in the box titled Examples of Actual or Potential Health Problems and Needs: Hygiene.

Examples of Actual or Potential Health Problems and Needs

HYGIENE

Actual or Potential Health Problems and Needs	Possible Etiologic Factors	Potential Signs and Symptoms
Bathing/hygiene ADL deficit	Sensory, cognitive, endurance, mobility, or motivation deficits; low value attached to regular bathing, brushing, flossing, and dental examinations; pain	"I don't need a bath. I'm not dirty." Five days postoperative from left thoracotomy. Transient confusion, generalized postoperative weakness. Unable to ambulate more than a few steps with assistance of two caregivers.
Impaired socialization	Negative body image	"I hate the way I look. Everyone stares at me. I don't even feel like going to school." Sixteen-year-old boy has come to the pediatrician's office for a physical for his driver's license permit. He has severe acne involving his face, neck, and back.
Risk for Impaired Oral Mucous Membrane Integrity	Inadequate oral hygiene, immunosuppression, inadequate nutrition, dehydration	—

Source: International Council of Nurses (ICN). (2019). *Nursing diagnosis and outcome statements.* https://www.icn.ch/sites/default/files/inline-files/ICNP2019-DC.pdf; Wolters Kluwer. (2020). *Problem-based care plans.* In Lippincott Advisor. Wolters Kluwer. https://advisor.lww.com/lna/home.do

Outcome Identification and Planning

The plan of care identifies nursing measures to assist the patient to develop or maintain hygiene practices that contribute to a sense of well-being. The following are examples of appropriate outcomes. The patient will:

- verbalize feeling comfortable and clean.
- participate fully in necessary hygiene measures according to cognitive, sensory, mobility, and endurance abilities.
- maintain intact skin and mucous membranes.
- demonstrate correct skin care measures (when indicated) such as oral care; care of eyes, ears, and nose; nail and foot care; and perineal and vaginal care.
- verbalize importance of good teeth-brushing habits, fluoride use, and regular dental examinations.
- demonstrate proper use and care of visual or auditory aids.
- participate in hair and scalp care as able.

Implementing

When performing general hygiene measures, respect the patient's personal preferences and encourage as much self-care as the patient can perform. Nurses should implement interventions to meet the patient's need for privacy, and promote physiologic and psychological wellness.

QSEN PATIENT-CENTERED CARE

Cultural, ethnic, family, and social backgrounds contribute to a patient's values regarding personal hygiene measures. Individualized care respects and encourages individual expression of patient values, preferences, and needs.

The following sections discuss hygiene measures, including providing scheduled care; assisting with bathing and skin care; massaging; providing routine hygiene care; providing environmental care, including making the bed; and teaching patients about skin care. Refer to the accompanying Focus on the Older Adult display for interventions related to hygiene for this age group.

Nurses who role model good health behaviors are more effective teachers. Use the Promoting Health 32-1 (on page 1098) display for yourself before using it with others.

Providing Scheduled Hygiene Care

When patients require nursing assistance with personal hygiene, provide this care at regular intervals. In most hospitals and long-term care settings, early morning care, morning care, afternoon care, hour of sleep care, and care as needed are provided. These are individualized according to the patient's personal and cultural preferences. Personal care

Focus on the Older Adult

NURSING STRATEGIES TO ADDRESS AGE-RELATED CHANGES IN HYGIENE

Age-Related Changes	Nursing Strategies
Impaired Oral Mucous Membrane	
• Loss of elasticity, atrophy of epithelial cells, diminished blood supply to connective tissue • Decreased salivation • Use of medications for chronic conditions that may cause dry mouth	• Floss and brush teeth with fluoride toothpaste twice a day; rinse after meals. • Brush dentures twice a day and rinse with cool water; remove and rinse dentures and rinse mouth after meals. • Avoid mouthwashes with alcohol content. • Inspect mouth daily for lesions and inflammation. • Use lubricant on lips. • Suck on sugar-free candies, chew sugarless gum, use salivary substitutes. • Continue with dental exams at the dentist every 6 months.
Impaired Physical Mobility	
• Decreased range of motion • Presence of chronic conditions that compromise functional ability • Decreased muscle strength and agility	• Use adaptive devices for hygiene such as toothbrush with a large or extended handle, long-handled body sponge, shower chair, and grab bars. • Provide for safety in the bathroom: use nonslip mats, grab bars.
Risk for Impaired Skin Integrity	
• Diminished secretion of natural oils and perspiration • Loss of elasticity • Thinning of epidermis, loss of elastin and subcutaneous fat	• Use safe water temperatures to bathe; warm water, not hot. • Avoid soap; use pH-balanced skin cleansers. • Shower instead of tub bath. • Use skin moisturizers and emollients at least daily. • Bath regularly, but less often (not every day).

Source: Adapted from Eliopoulos, C. (2018). *Gerontological nursing* (9th ed.). Wolters Kluwer; Lichterfeld-Lottner, A., El Genedy, M., Lahmann, N., Blume-Peytavi, U., Büscher, A., & Kottner, J. (2020). Maintaining skin integrity in the aged: A systematic review. *International Journal of Nursing Studies, 103*, 103509. https://doi.org/10.1016/j.ijnurstu.2019.103509; National Institute on Aging. (2020, March 13). *Taking care of your teeth and mouth.* https://www.nia.nih.gov/health/taking-care-your-teeth-and-mouth; National Institute on Aging. (n.d.). *Fall-proofing your home.* https://www.nia.nih.gov/health/fall-proofing-your-home; and Toughy, T. A., & Jett, K. (2018). *Ebersol and Hess' gerontological nursing & healthy aging* (5th ed.). Elsevier.

Promoting Health 32-1

HYGIENE

Use the assessment checklist to determine how well you are meeting your needs related to hygiene. Then develop a prescription for self-care by choosing appropriate behaviors from the list of suggestions.

Assessment Checklist

☐ almost always ☐ sometimes ☐ almost never

☐ ☐ ☐ 1. I keep my hair clean and neatly styled.

☐ ☐ ☐ 2. My skin is clean.

☐ ☐ ☐ 3. The condition of my mouth indicates satisfactory oral hygiene.

☐ ☐ ☐ 4. My nails are neatly manicured.

☐ ☐ ☐ 5. My body is free of unpleasant odors.

Self-Care Behaviors

1. Ensure that diet and exercise are appropriate, since this contributes to healthy skin.
2. Brush and floss teeth regularly and visit the dentist every 6 months.
3. Keep hair clean, combed, and brushed regularly.
4. Use certain hair care products (e.g., hair dyes) cautiously, since they may damage the hair.
5. Clean under nails and maintain nails at an appropriate length. Clip all nails straight across and shape or smooth with an emery board or file, if necessary.
6. Bathe and cleanse skin regularly. Apply lotion or cream to dry skin, as necessary. Cleanse the axilla and perineal area thoroughly and apply deodorant or antiperspirant as needed.
7. Appreciate the relationship between hygiene and overall well-being.

Information to promote healthy hygiene practices is available online.

assistance in the home and other community-based settings centers on patient preferences and routines. Personal care measures may be delegated to assistive personnel (AP). The nurse is responsible for ensuring that hygiene measures are performed satisfactorily and validates, analyzes, documents, communicates, and acts on any items noticed during care and communicated by AP.

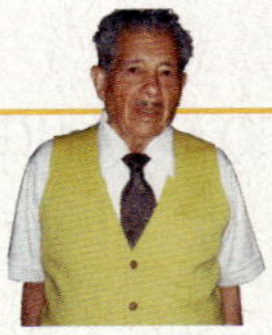

Remember **Andrew Craig**, the older man in the extended-care facility who reported that he had already had a complete bath. The nurse would need to investigate this to determine if he had indeed received care. If he had not, then the nurse would need to seek additional information to explain his statement; perhaps the patient was too tired or did not like having to be helped with his care. This information contributes to providing person-centered care.

EARLY MORNING CARE

Shortly after the patient awakens, assist with toileting if necessary and then provide comfort measures to refresh the patient and prepare them for breakfast (or diagnostic tests, procedures, or therapies). Nursing measures include washing the face and hands and providing mouth care.

MORNING CARE (AM CARE)

In many care environments, it is usual to complete morning care after breakfast. However, patient preferences and scheduled activities should be considered. For example, in rehabilitation settings, patients participate in physical and occupational therapy sessions for a majority of the daytime hours and patient bathing and other personal hygiene measures will be addressed in the evening.

Depending on the patient's self-care abilities, offer assistance with toileting, oral care, bathing, back massage, special skin care measures (e.g., pressure injury), hair care (includes shaving if indicated), cosmetics, dressing, and positioning for comfort. Facility policies are followed for refreshing or changing bed linens, and the patient's bedside area is tidied. In the home and other community-based settings, patient and/or family preferences and routines should be considered. When morning care is completed, the patient should feel refreshed and should be in a comfortable and safe environment.

Morning care is often categorized as self-care, partial care, or complete care. Patients identified as self-care are capable of managing their personal hygiene independently once oriented to the bathroom. However, offer a back massage and spend time assessing the patient's day-to-day needs. Patients identified as partial care often receive morning hygiene care at the bedside or seated near the sink in the bathroom. They usually require assistance with body areas that are difficult to reach. Patients identified as complete care require nursing assistance with all aspects of personal hygiene. A complete bed bath is done, or the patient may be taken to the shower.

AFTERNOON CARE (PM CARE)

Hospitalized patients frequently receive visitors in the afternoon or evening or use this time to rest when not scheduled for tests or therapies. Ensure the patient's comfort after lunch and offer assistance to nonambulatory patients with toileting, handwashing, and oral care. Bathing and other personal care activities may take place at this time, depending on individual patient circumstances.

HOUR OF SLEEP CARE (HS CARE)

In the evening, at the end of the day, again offer assistance with toileting, washing of the face and hands, and oral care. It may be appropriate to offer a back massage or other method of relaxation to help the patient to be calm and fall asleep. Change any soiled bed linens or clothing, and position the patient comfortably. Ensure that the call light and any other objects the patient desires (e.g., urinal, radio, water glass) are within easy reach.

AS NEEDED CARE (PRN CARE)

In addition to scheduled care, offer individual hygiene measures as needed. Some patients require oral care every 2 hours. Patients who are diaphoretic (sweating profusely) may need their clothing and bed linens changed several times a shift. At other times, a nurse may decide to forego hygiene measures because the patient's need for undisturbed rest may be a higher priority.

Assisting With Bathing and Skin Care

Bathing serves a variety of purposes, including:

- Cleansing the skin
- Acting as a skin conditioner
- Helping a person to relax
- Promoting circulation by stimulating the skin's peripheral nerve endings and underlying tissues
- Serving as a musculoskeletal exercise through activity involved with bathing, thereby improving joint mobility and muscle tonus
- Stimulating the rate and depth of respirations
- Promoting comfort through muscle relaxation and skin stimulation
- Providing sensory input
- Helping to improve self-image
- Providing an excellent opportunity to strengthen the nurse–patient relationship, to thoroughly assess the patient's integumentary system, to observe the patient's physiologic and emotional status closely, to teach the patient as indicated, and to demonstrate care and interest in the patient's general welfare

The simple act of bathing a patient is a vital and caring intervention. Although APs are increasingly performing hygiene measures, the nurse is responsible for ensuring that hygiene measures are performed satisfactorily. Refer to Chapters 10 and 17 for discussions of the nurse's accountability when care is delegated. Nurses whose primary focus is the patient, however, can use the time spent on assisting with bathing to establish a rapport with the patient and to further assess the patient's integumentary system. Bathing is performed in a matter-of-fact and dignified manner. Refer to the accompanying Through the Eyes of a Student.

SHOWER AND TUB BATHS

A shower may be the preferred method of bathing for patients who are ambulatory and able to tolerate the activity. Tub baths may be an option, particularly in long-term care or other community-based settings, depending on facility policy as well as in a patient's home environment. Tub, or immersion, bathing may be used for purposes other than

Through the Eyes of a Student

I entered the room with a feeling of dread. How could I possibly bathe the sick, older adult, helpless woman lying in this hospital bed? I had never bathed anyone older than age 2 years, other than myself, of course. How would I be able to move her limp, seemingly lifeless old body? What would an 85-year-old body look like? I could not imagine. I've read all the manuals that describe this procedure, I know what to do; so why am I so nervous? I must be worried that I will hurt her in some way. Maybe she has not been cared for properly before and her hygiene is poor. Well, I might as well get this over with because I'll be doing it the rest of my life. I've got to learn sometime.

I've mustered up enough courage to enter my patient's room. Michelle, her primary nurse, offers to help me because the patient is so difficult to move. Boy, am I relieved! Right before Michelle and I are about to begin, my patient, Mrs. Ash, asks for her teeth. I assume this must mean her dentures and reassure her that I have not seen them but will be happy to look for them as soon as we have completed her bath. Michelle and I each take a side and begin to bathe her. It's truly amazing how those range-of-motion exercises come to mind so easily. I had thought they were long forgotten with the rest of the past semester. Wouldn't my instructors love to hear me now! Suddenly Mrs. Ash yells, "I need the bedpan!" "Oh no!" I thought, as I rushed to the bathroom with soapy gloved hands trying frantically to locate her bedpan before there could be an accident. Michelle, who remained calm during my frenzy, simply stated, "Don't worry, she has an indwelling catheter. She says that every time I bathe her." I knew she had a catheter, how did I forget? Somewhat humbled, I returned to the procedure. I really wanted to put some lotion on her skin because it was so dry. When we were ready to do her back, we prepared to lift her. I pulled her toward me, and Michelle was to continue the bath. We were not prepared for what we saw underneath. Firmly cushioned in Mrs. Ash's lower left buttock were none other than her dentures! On removing them, Michelle and I had to smile at the periodontal grin implanted on Mrs. Ash's bottom. Michelle then asked her how her teeth had gotten to the location where we found them. All she seemed to know was that she needed those teeth back in her mouth NOW! She snatched the dentures from Michelle's hand and attempted to insert them. Michelle and I in unison blurted out, "No, Mrs. Ash, please wait until we clean your teeth before you put them back in your mouth!" Mrs. Ash, somewhat confused, begrudgingly handed over her teeth to be cleaned. Michelle had the honors while I finished the last touches of good hygiene for Mrs. Ash.

What a difference cleanliness can make, not only for the patient, but also for me, the student nurse. I felt better knowing that Mrs. Ash was clean and that this procedure was behind me. And to think that I was apprehensive! This was definitely an interesting learning experience.

—Marilyn Johnson, Holy Family College, Philadelphia

Box 32-1 Meeting the Bathing Needs of Patients With Dementia

- Shift the focus of the interaction from the "task of bathing" to the needs and abilities of the patient. Focus on comfort, safety, autonomy, and self-esteem, in addition to cleanliness.
- Individualize patient care. Consult the patient, the patient's record, family members, and other caregivers to determine patient preferences.
- Consider what can be learned from the behaviors associated with dementia about the needs and preferences of the patient. A patient's behavior may be an expression of unmet needs; unwillingness to participate may be a response to uncomfortable water temperatures or levels of sound or light in the room.
- Ensure privacy and warmth.
- Consider the use of music to soothe anxiety and agitation.
- Consider other methods for bathing. Showers and tub baths are not the only options in bathing. Towel baths, washing under clothes, and bathing "body sections" one day at a time are other possible options.
- Maintain a relaxed demeanor. Use calming language. Use one-step commands. Try to determine phrases and terms the patient understands in relation to bathing and make use of them. Offer frequent reassurance.
- Encourage independence. Use hand-over-hand or a guided hand technique to cue the patient regarding the purpose of the interaction and allow the patient to perform some of the activities independently.
- Explore the need for routine analgesia before bathing. Move limbs carefully and be aware of signs of discomfort during bathing.
- Wash the face and hair at the end of the bath or at a separate time. Water dripping in the face and having a wet head are often the most upsetting parts of the bathing process for people with dementia.

Source: Adapted from Gallagher, M., Hall, G. R., & Butcher, H. K. (2014). Bathing persons with Alzheimer's disease and related dementias. *Journal of Gerontological Nursing, 40*(2), 14–20; Konno, R., Kang, H. S., & Makimoto, K. (2014). A best-evidence review of intervention studies for minimizing resistance-to-care behaviours for older adults with dementia in nursing homes. *Journal of Advanced Nursing, 70*(10), 2167–2180; and Toughy, T. A., & Jett, K. (2018). *Ebersol and Hess' gerontological nursing & healthy aging* (5th ed.). Elsevier.

personal hygiene. Tub bathing can provide positive physical and mental effects, including mental and physical relaxation, decreased stress, and relief of menstrual cramps and labor contractions (Benfield et al., 2018; Goto et al., 2018). For the most part, even though many patients can bathe on their own, the following responsibilities apply:

- Check to see that the bathroom is available, clean, and safe. Showers should have mats or nonskid strips to prevent patients from slipping and falling.
- Ensure that necessary articles—such as skin cleanser, washcloth, towel, and gown—are available for the patient.
- Provide a place for a weak or physically disabled patient to sit in a shower. Most health facilities have a stool or chair that can be used in the shower, and handheld showerheads may facilitate the process. A commode chair with the pan removed serves effectively as a shower chair and may offer the patient more support than a stool or chair.
- Assist the patient to the shower or bathroom, as indicated. Patients who are beginning ambulation often need assistance to help prevent falling or fainting.
- Check to see that the water temperature is safe and comfortable—no more than 120°F. Use a thermometer to test the water coming out of the bath water tap (International Association of Fire Fighters [IAFF], n.d.).
- Ensure privacy for patients who can safely shower or bathe independently. See that a call device is handy, and make sure the patient knows what the button is for so the patient can obtain help if necessary.
- Help the patient get in and out of the bathtub, as indicated. Have the patient grasp the handrails at the side of the tub, or place a chair at the side of the tub. The patient sits on the chair and eases to the edge of the tub. After putting both feet into the tub, it is then relatively easy for the patient to reach the opposite side and ease down into the tub. The patient may kneel first in the tub and then sit in it; this process can be reversed when leaving the tub. Use a hydraulic lift, when available, to lower and lift patients who are unable to maneuver safely or completely bear their weight. Some community-based settings or homes have walk-in tubs available.
- Keep the bathroom door unlocked. Health personnel should be able to enter with ease if the patient needs help. A sign hung on the door ensures privacy. Never leave children or confused patients alone in the bathroom.
- Help to wash and dry areas of the body that the patient cannot reach, such as the back.
- Make any necessary adaptations to achieve person-centered bathing (Dementia Care Central, 2019; Gozalo et al., 2014; Scales et al., 2018; Whitehead & Golding-Day, 2019; Wolf & Czekanski, 2015). For example, if the patient is confused and becomes agitated as a result of overstimulation when bathing, reduce the stimuli. Turn down the lights and play soft music and/or warm the room before taking the patient into it (Konno et al., 2014). Another alternative is to consider bed bath variations to decrease agitation (Dementia Care Central, 2019). Box 32-1 outlines possible measures to implement to meet the bathing needs of patients with dementia.

Figure 32-1 illustrates several features that add to the safety of a patient taking a shower. Ensure proper cleaning of shower or tub between patient uses to comply with infection control measures, according to facility policy.

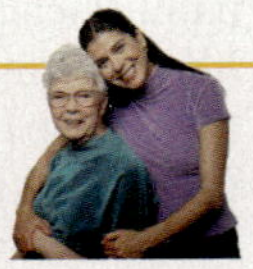

Recall **Sonya Delamordo**, the older woman who is going to live at her daughter's home after a stroke. The nurse should incorporate the responsibilities listed here into the teaching plan for Mrs. Delamordo's daughter to ensure the patient's safety with hygiene interventions.

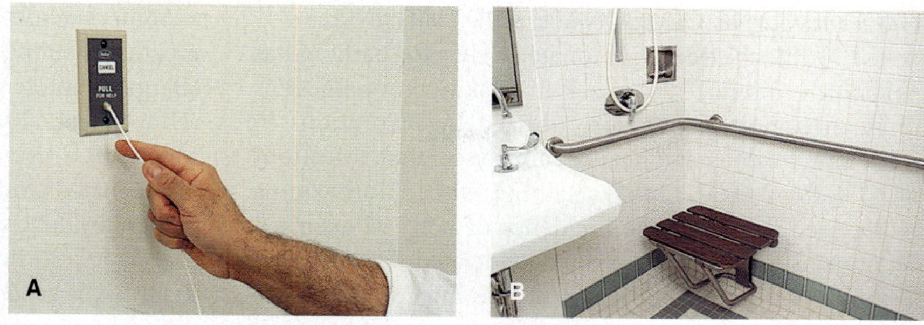

FIGURE 32-1. Examples of features that add to the safety of a patient taking a shower or bath. **A.** Call bell equipped with a pull cord. **B.** Shower equipped with a safety seat and hand rail. (*Source:* Used with permission from Shutterstock. *Photos by B. Proud.*)

BED BATHS

Some patients must remain in bed as a part of their therapeutic regimen but can still bathe themselves. Other patients are not on bed rest but require total or partial assistance with bathing in bed due to physical or mental deficits, such as fatigue or limited range of motion. Implement the following nursing measures to help patients take a bath in bed:

- Provide the patient with articles for bathing. If using a basin of water for bathing, ensure the water is a comfortable and safe temperature. Place these items conveniently for the patient on a bedside stand or overbed table.
- Provide privacy for the patient. Make sure the call device is within reach.
- Place cosmetics and other skin care products in a convenient place for the patient. Provide a mirror, a good light, and hot water for patients who wish to shave with a razor.
- Assist patients who cannot bathe themselves completely. For example, some patients can wash only the upper parts of the body. Nursing personnel then complete the remainder of the bath.

When bathing a patient, the wipe or washcloth removes some of the outermost skin layer. This sloughed skin may be evident on the wipe or washcloth and in the bathwater and will vary in color depending on the ethnic group of the patient (Andrews et al., 2020). This is important to note, as this does not mean that the patient was dirty—the normal sloughing of the skin is more evident in darkly pigmented people compared with patients with lighter pigmentation (Andrews et al., 2020).

Bathing procedures for patients who require total nursing assistance vary among health facilities. Skill 32-1 on pages 1121 offers one example as a guide. It assumes that the patient can be raised or lowered in bed and that, although the patient may have limited movement, the nurse can manage the patient alone.

DISPOSABLE BATH

The use of disposable bath products is an alternative to the traditional use of soap and water. Disposable bath products are prepackaged in single-use units, heated before use, do not require rinsing, and are equally effective at reducing skin bacteria (Matsumoto et al., 2019; Nøddeskou et al., 2015; Veje et al., 2020). There are several variations of this bath. One self-contained bathing system is a package containing 8 to 10 pre-moistened, disposable washcloths (Fig. 32-2). The unopened package is warmed in the microwave or stored in a warmer until use. Each part of the patient's body is cleansed with a fresh cloth. No rinsing is required. The skin is allowed to air dry (for about 30 seconds) so that the emollient ingredient of the cleaner remains on the skin. Other versions contain disposable wash gloves (Schoonhoven et al., 2015).

Feedback about use of disposable bathing products has been overwhelmingly positive. Nursing staff value the time savings when compared with a traditional bed bath and find it effective and easy to perform (Nøddeskou et al., 2015). These products also eliminate the cross-infection risk posed by soap, water, bath basins, and washcloths (Sturgeon et al., 2019). Most patients have commented favorably on the disposable bath and consider it a convenient alternative and preferred in certain circumstances (Nøddeskou et al., 2015; Veje et al., 2019). Patients with mild to moderate skin impairments demonstrated an improved skin condition with consistent use of the disposable bath (Matsumoto et al., 2019).

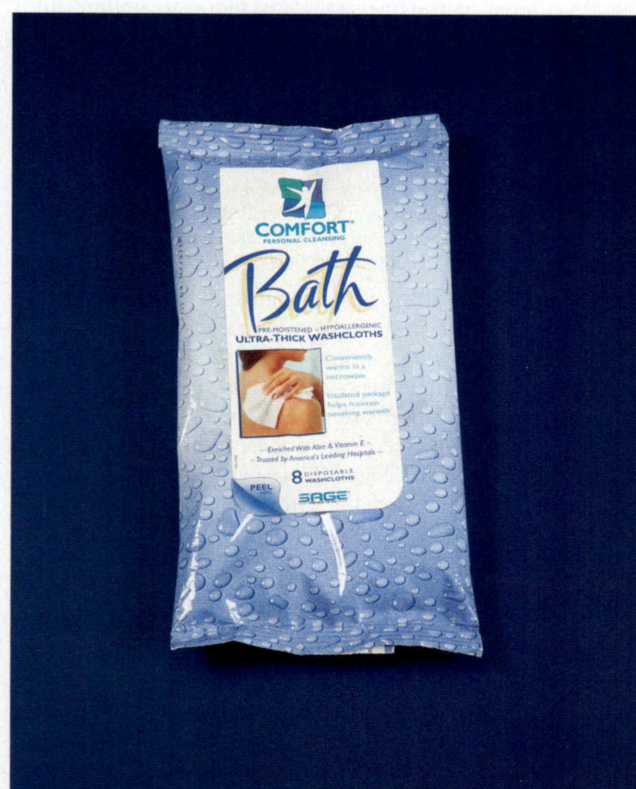

FIGURE 32-2. Commercial self-contained disposable bathing system.

CHLORHEXIDINE GLUCONATE AND BATHING

The use of chlorhexidine gluconate (CHG) for bathing has been shown to reduce colonization of skin with pathogens and is an important measure utilized by institutions in an attempt to decrease health care–associated infections (HAIs) (Hines et al., 2015). Bathing with chlorhexidine may be used to reduce the incidence of hospital-acquired infections, such as central line–associated bloodstream infections (CLABSIs) and surgical site infections, and to decrease rates of transmission and infection of resistant microorganisms, as well as to reduce the acquisition of or decolonization with multidrug-resistant organisms (Cassir et al., 2015; Martinez et al., 2020; Musuuza et al., 2019; Reynolds et al., 2019; Shah et al., 2016; Urias et al., 2018). Daily bathing with chlorhexidine has also been shown to decrease the incidence of the risk of ventilator-associated pneumonia (Chen et al., 2015).

Some facilities' policies include the use of CHG for all inpatient bathing, except for patients with a history of CHG allergy or intolerance or those younger than age 2 months (Hines et al., 2015). Chlorhexidine can be added to bath water, but is also available, and easier to use, in prepackaged impregnated cloths. CHG-impregnated cloths may result in higher residual skin concentrations after application compared to CHG liquid and water bathing (Rhee et al., 2018). Refer to the accompanying Research in Nursing box.

PROMOTING SKIN HEALTH

An easy and effective way to promote the barrier function of the skin and keep the skin healthy is the daily use of soap substitutes, topical moisturizers and emollients, and barrier products (Andriessen, 2013; Haesler et al., 2018; Lichterfeld et al., 2015; Voegeli, 2019). Soap cleans the skin, but at the same time it removes dirt from the surface, it affects the

Research in Nursing

BRIDGING THE GAP TO EVIDENCE-BASED PRACTICE

Bathing and Health Care–Associated Infections

Prevention of HAIs is a major challenge for health care providers. Health care facilities constantly strive to implement evidence-based practices to reduce the risk of HAIs for patients and promote patient health. Bathing using chlorhexidine gluconate (CHG) decreases preventable hospital-acquired central line–associated bloodstream infections (CLABSIs) (Reynolds et al., 2019). What interventions can improve implementation and increase consistency in use of bathing with CHG?

Related Research

Reynolds, S. S., Sova, C., McNalty, B., Lambert, S., & Granger, B. (2019). Implementation strategies to improve evidence-based bathing practices in a neuro ICU. *Journal of Nursing Care Quality, 34*(2), 133–138. https://doi.org/10.1097/NCQ.0000000000000347

The purpose of this observational study was to determine whether using tailored, multifaceted strategies would improve nurses' knowledge/perceptions of CHG bathing, improve compliance with implementation and documentation of daily CHG bathing, and decrease CLABSI rates in a large neuro ICU. Participants included the nurses and nursing assistants employed on the neurology ICU ($n = 85$) during implementation. Researchers used the Grol and Wensing Model of Implementation to guide the study. Potential barriers and facilitators to implementation of CHG bathing were identified through informal discussion with nursing staff. A knowledge deficit related to the appropriate procedure for bathing was identified as well as a lack of motivation and perceived importance of CHG bathing. Commitment to implementation of evidence-based practices to improve patient care was identified as a strong facilitator to change. Based on this information, staff participated in educational sessions related to the importance and use of CHG bathing, provided by the neuroscience clinical nurse specialist. Printed educational materials related to the use and importance of daily CHG bathing, which included pictures of directions for use of CHG cloths, were disseminated to the unit staff. Two nurse hospital–acquired infection "champions" acted as resources and role models for CHG bathing for the unit staff. Daily CHG bathing was audited for compliance beginning 2 months prior to and weekly for 6 months after implementation of the education; audit information and feedback were provided weekly to staff via email. Nurses' knowledge/perceptions of CHG bathing were measured via a survey prior to and after implementation of the strategies. Protocol compliance was measured using weekly audits of the documentation of use in the electronic health record. Data regarding the hospital's incidence of CLABSIs was provided by the hospital's infection prevention team, reported on a monthly basis, measured by the number of CLABSIs per 1,000 central line days.

Following implementation of the strategies, CLABSI infection rates decreased ($p = .031$). Statistically significant improvements were seen in bathing documentation (compliance) ($p = .013$), nurses' knowledge ($p = .001$), and perceived importance of CHG bathing ($p = .002$). The researchers concluded that use of tailored, multifaceted strategies can be used to improve knowledge of and compliance with the use of daily CHG bathing and reduce hospital-acquired infections such as CLABSIs.

Relevance to Nursing Practice

These results can be useful to other facilities in decreasing the risk of hospital-acquired infections such as CLABSIs. Nurses and nursing staff are the primary providers of bathing activities in many health care settings and should consider the implementation of tailored interventions to improve knowledge/perceptions and compliance with daily CHG bathing to improve patient health and decrease health care costs.

lipids that are present on the skin and the skin pH. This contributes to drier skin, damaging the barrier function of the skin. The use of mild cleansers with pH close to skin pH is recommended (Lichterfeld et al., 2015; Woods, 2019). The substitution of a nonsoap emollient cleaning agent is an easy way to prevent drying and damage to the skin. The rinseless products mentioned in the description of a disposable bath are examples of nonsoap emollient cleaning agents.

Topical emollient agents—also known as moisturizers—can be applied to the skin as a lotion, cream, gel, or ointment. They act to seal water into the skin and replace lipids in the skin, effectively hydrating the skin and recreating its waterproof barrier. Apply topical moisturizers after bathing. Ideally, they should be applied twice a day but may need more frequent application, depending on the skin condition and the product used.

Skin barrier products include creams, ointments, and films. These products are used to protect vulnerable skin and to protect skin at risk for damage caused by excessive exposure to water and irritants, such as urine and feces. They are also used to prevent skin breakdown around stomas and wounds with excessive exudate. Application of one of these products forms a thin layer on the surface of the skin to repel potential irritants. Apply these products by following the manufacturer's recommendations and facility policy. Box 32-2 outlines general skin care principles. Table 32-1 summarizes recommended treatments for dry skin, acne, and skin rashes.

Box 32-2 General Skin Care Principles

- Assess the patient's skin at least daily and after every episode of incontinence.
- Cleanse the skin when indicated, such as when soiled, using a no-rinse, pH-balanced skin cleanser.
- Avoid using soap and hot water; avoid excessive friction and scrubbing.
- Minimize skin exposure to moisture (incontinence, wound leakage); use a skin barrier product as necessary.
- Use skin emollients after bathing and as needed.

Table 32-1 Skin Care Problems

SKIN PROBLEM	DEFINITION	TREATMENT
Dry skin	The skin loses moisture and may crack and peel, or become irritated and inflamed. Symptoms include scaling, flaking, itching, and cracks in the skin.	• Keep baths or showers short, and/or bathe less frequently. • Use warm, not hot water to bathe. • Use as little soap as possible. Try mild cleansers or soaps. • Dry skin thoroughly and gently. • Use moisturizers at least daily. • Drink plenty of water throughout the day. Use a humidifier if the air is dry.
Acne	A skin condition that is characterized by clogged pores (blackheads, whiteheads, pimples), caused by dead skin cells and sebum (oil) sticking together in the pore. Sometimes bacteria that live on the skin also get inside the clogged pore. Inside the pore, the bacteria have a perfect environment for multiplying very quickly. With a large amount of bacteria inside, the pore becomes inflamed (red and swollen). If the inflammation goes deep into the skin, an acne cyst or nodule appears. Acne can appear on the face, back, chest, neck, shoulders, upper arms, and buttocks.	• Avoid squeezing or picking infected areas because this can spread the infection and cause scarring. • Gently wash the face twice a day and after sweating with a gentle nonabrasive cleanser using your fingertips and lukewarm (not hot) water. • Use oil-free, water-based moisturizers and makeup. Look for products that are "noncomedogenic" or "nonacnegenic." Use cosmetics sparingly to avoid further blockage of the sebaceous ducts. • Keep hair off the face and shampoo regularly. If hair is oily, shampoo daily. • Some acne treatments (both over-the-counter and prescription) can increase the skin's sensitivity to sunlight and ultraviolet light. Avoid sun/tanning booth exposure; use sunscreen. • Patients with a lot of acne, cysts, or nodules should consult a dermatologist. • Patients who feel shy or embarrassed as a result of acne; acne leaves scars or darkens skin; or for whom products used do not work should consult a dermatologist.
Skin rashes	Eruptions or inflammations of the skin that may be found anywhere on the body. May be precipitated by skin contact with an allergen, overexposure to the sun, and/or systemic causes, like a reaction to a medication.	• Wash area thoroughly with a mild cleansing agent and rinse well. • Use a moisturizing lotion on a dry rash to prevent itching and promote healing. • Use a drying agent on a wet rash. • Try tepid baths to help relieve inflammation and itching. • Use antiseptic sprays or lotions to help lessen itching, promote healing, and prevent skin breakdown. • Avoid exposure to causative agent, if known. • See a health care provider if symptoms do not respond to treatment or become worse.

PATIENTS WITH BARIATRIC NEEDS

Bariatrics is the science of providing health care for those who have extreme obesity, taking both a patient's weight and the distribution of this weight throughout the body into consideration (Muir & Archer-Heese, 2009). The number of patients who are overweight or obese with bariatric care needs remains a significant problem (Earlam & Woods, 2020; Williamson, 2020). Patients with bariatric care needs are at increased risk for skin integrity issues, including increased risk for alterations in skin integrity and therefore require focused nursing care to prevent skin issues (Earlam & Woods, 2020; Williamson, 2020). Assess the skin of bariatric inpatients twice a day, lifting and separating folds of skin to assess the area, utilizing extra help as necessary (Black & Hotaling, 2015). Nonsoap cleansers should be used and the skin should be dried to prevent retained moisture (Black & Hotaling, 2015; Williamson, 2020). Regular application of barrier creams or sprays can help protect skin from maceration in skin folds, the groin area, perineum and buttock cleft (Williamson, 2020). Currently, there is a lack of evidence related to bathing and hygiene needs or best practice recommendations related to skin hygiene for obese patients (Black & Hotaling, 2015; Cowdell & Radley, 2014; Williamson, 2020). Nurses and patients must work collaboratively to identify the best possible interventions to meet individual personal hygiene needs and preserve skin integrity (Cowdell & Radley, 2014; Dial et al., 2018).

PERINEAL CARE

Perineal cleaning should be performed in a matter-of-fact and dignified manner. Guidelines for Nursing Care 32-1 provides appropriate techniques related to general perineal care. In some cases, a sitz bath may be used to clean and soothe the perineal and anal areas. The procedure associated with administering a sitz bath is discussed in Chapter 33.

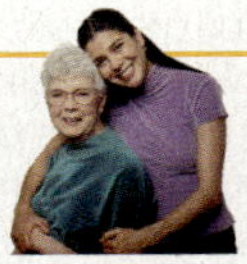

Remember **Sonya Delamordo**, who is going to live in her daughter's home after a stroke. The patient may be embarrassed to have her daughter help with perineal care. The nurse would encourage the patient to do as much as she is able, using her left hand. By doing so, the patient maintains some control over the situation, thereby promoting her self-esteem and fostering personal hygiene and independence.

If the patient has an indwelling catheter and the facility recommends daily care for the catheter, this is usually done after perineal care. Care of an indwelling catheter is discussed in Chapter 38.

Incontinent patients require special attention to perineal care. Patients with urinary or fecal incontinence are at risk for incontinence-associated dermatitis (perineal dermatitis), one type of moisture-associated skin damage (MASD) (Voegeli, 2019). This damage is related to excessive moisture, changes in the pH of the skin, overgrowth of bacteria and infection of the skin, and erosion of perineal skin from friction on moist skin. Early recognition of patients at risk for MASD is critical, along with good skin hygiene (Wounds UK, 2018). Skin care for these patients should include measures to reduce overhydration (excess exposure to moisture), contact with ammonia and bacteria, and friction. Remove soil and irritants from the skin during routine hygiene, and clean the area when the skin becomes exposed to irritants (Voegeli, 2019). Avoid using soap and excessive force for cleaning (Wounds UK, 2018). The use of perineal skin cleansers, moisturizers, and barriers is recommended for skin care for the incontinent patient (Voegeli, 2019). These products help promote healing and prevent further skin damage. Incontinence and nursing care of the patient with incontinence are discussed further in Chapters 33, 38, and 39.

Concept Mastery Alert

For the patient who is incontinent, it is important to keep the perineal area clean and dry. Use nonsoap cleansers and protect the area with moisture barriers.

MASSAGE

Massage has many benefits, including general relaxation and increased circulation. Massage can help alleviate pain (De Luca et al., 2020; Westman & Blaisdell, 2016). Massage of the back, hands, and/or feet may follow the patient's bath or may be provided as part of interventions to promote sleep or increase patient comfort and well-being (De Luca et al., 2020; Momeni et al., 2020; Sharma & Kumari, 2019). Some nurses forego the use of massage due to time constraints; however, in addition to the benefits stated previously, the use of massage provides an opportunity for the nurse to communicate and connect with the patient through touch.

Be aware of the patient's medical diagnosis and health issues when considering the use of massage. For example, a backrub is contraindicated if the patient has had back surgery or has fractured ribs. Refer to Skill 36-1 in Chapter 36 for details regarding giving a back massage.

Providing Vaginal Care

Vaginal mucous secretions are odor free until they combine with air and perspiration. Thus, for vaginal care, using plain soap and water is the most effective means to control odor. Douching is washing or cleaning out the inside of the vagina with water or other fluids (Office of Women's Health, 2019). In normal, healthy women, douching is believed to be unnecessary and is not recommended because it tends to remove normal bacterial flora from the vagina and alter the normal acidic environment. Douching can cause an overgrowth of harmful bacteria and lead to a yeast infection or bacterial vaginosis. If a woman already has a vaginal infection, douching can push the bacteria causing the infection up into the uterus, fallopian tubes and/or ovaries, leading to pelvic inflammatory disease (Office of Women's Health, 2019). Douching has also been linked to problems during pregnancy, STIs, and pelvic inflammatory disease. Douching is not recommended as a routine hygiene measure (Office of Women's Health, 2019).

Guidelines for Nursing Care 32-1

PROVIDING PERINEAL CARE

Perineal care may be carried out while the patient remains in bed. When performing perineal care, follow these guidelines:

- Assemble supplies, and provide for privacy.
- Explain the procedure to the patient, perform hand hygiene, and put on disposable gloves.
- Wash and rinse the groin area (both male and female patients). Use a small amount of a mild nonsoap cleaning agent and water, or disposable cleaning cloths.
- For a female patient, spread the labia and move the washcloth from the pubic area toward the anal area to prevent carrying organisms from the anal area back over the genital area (Figure A). Always proceed from the least contaminated area to the most contaminated area. Use a clean portion of the washcloth for each stroke. Rinse the washed areas well with plain water.

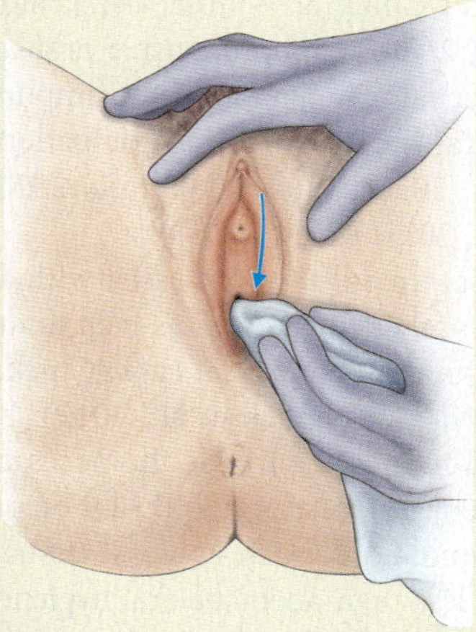

FIGURE A. Spreading the labia and moving the washcloth from the pubic area toward the anal area.

- For a male patient, clean the tip of the penis first, moving the washcloth in a circular motion from the meatus outward (Figure B). Wash the shaft of the penis using downward strokes toward the pubic area (Figure C). Always proceed from the least contaminated area to the most contaminated area. Rinse the washed areas well with plain water. In an *uncircumcised male patient* (teenage or older), retract the foreskin (prepuce) while washing the penis. Pull the uncircumcised male patient's foreskin back into place over the glans penis to prevent constriction of the penis, which may result in edema and tissue injury (MedlinePlus, 2020b). It is not recommended to retract the foreskin for cleaning during infancy and childhood, as injury and scarring could occur (MedlinePlus, 2020b). Wash and rinse the male patient's scrotum. Handle the scrotum, which houses the testicles, with care because the area is sensitive.

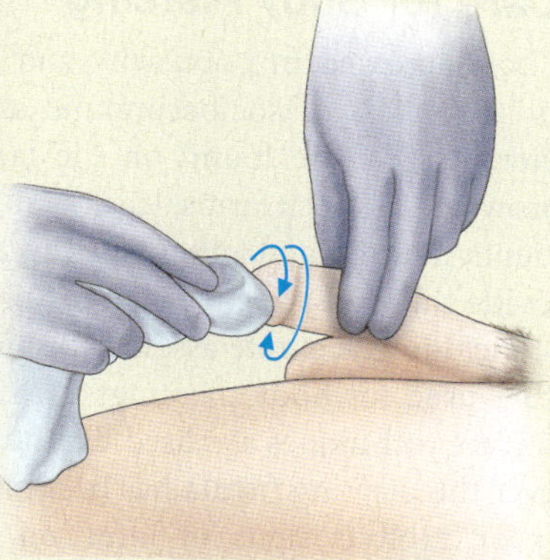

FIGURE B. Cleaning the tip of the penis, moving the washcloth in a circular motion from the meatus outward.

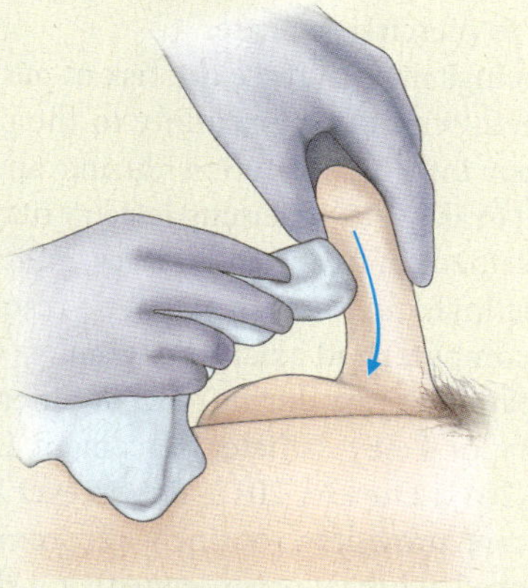

FIGURE C. Washing the shaft of the penis using downward strokes toward the pubic area.

- Dry the cleaned areas and apply an emollient as indicated. Avoid the use of powder. Powder may become a medium for the growth of bacteria.
- Turn the patient on their side and continue with cleansing the anal area. Continue in the direction of least contaminated to most contaminated area. In the female, cleanse from the vagina toward the anus. In both female and male patients, change the part of the washcloth being used with each stroke until the area is clean. Rinse and dry the area.

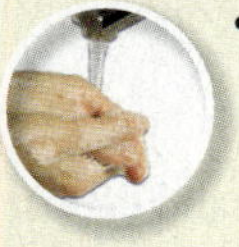

- Remove gloves and perform hand hygiene. Continue with additional care as necessary.

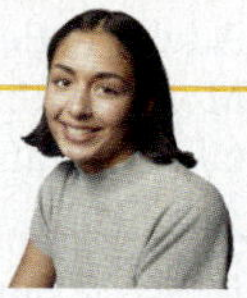

Consider **Kylie**, the university student who is concerned about recurring vaginal infections. The nurse at the campus health clinic should include teaching about feminine hygiene self-care behaviors in her care for Kylie.

Deodorants to control odor around the vaginal orifice are unnecessary. No therapeutic benefit from their use has been proven to date. Use of these special deodorants is not a substitute for keeping the area clean; female patients often require teaching on this subject. If patients insist on using them, explain they are intended for external use only. They should not be placed on sanitary napkins or tampons, should not be used on broken skin areas. Use is not recommended because of reported irritation and rashes, and urethral irritation (Mayo Foundation for Medical Education and Research, 2020a; Sparks, 2018).

Providing Care for Body Piercing

Body piercing has increased in popularity and acceptance in recent years, regardless of socioeconomic and cultural background. Piercings can be found on the face (tongue, lips, nose, eyebrows), ears, neck, arms, legs, torso, navel, and genitals of patients. Nurses and other health care providers need to provide safe and effective care for patients with body piercings, including accurate assessment and site care. Basic wound care used for body piercings is usually called "aftercare." Aftercare techniques are used for the new piercing and whenever the piercing fistula has become disrupted through injury or exhibits signs of infection or inflammation (Association of Professional Piercers, 2020; Mayo Foundation for Medical Education and Research, 2020b). Guidelines for Nursing Care 32-2 provides appropriate techniques related to piercing site care.

Tongue piercings may increase the risk of periodontal destruction in teeth with close proximity to the piercing, and should be taken into consideration during an oral assessment (Schmidt et al., 2019). Piercing jewelry may cause difficulty with placement of treatment devices, and can interfere with diagnostic imaging, such as magnetic resonance imaging (MRI) or computerized axial tomography (CT scan), or contribute to patient injury during MRI or other procedures, such as surgery or Foley catheter placement (Davis, 2014; DeBoer et al., 2011; Durkin, 2012; Rademeyer et al., 2020). Some health care providers routinely recommend that all jewelry is removed, whereas others state that it should not be removed unless necessary (D'Alesandro, 2014; Davis, 2014; Rademeyer et al., 2020). Various devices, such as plastic jewelry, are available to be used to keep the piercing tract open when removal is required (Van Hoover et al., 2017). The use of an intravenous catheter to maintain piercing patency has also been suggested (Rademeyer et al., 2020). Nurses should consult facility policies related to removal of body piercing jewelry.

Assisting With Oral Hygiene

The mouth requires care, particularly during illness, but sometimes care must be modified to meet a patient's needs. Adequate oral hygiene care is imperative to promote the patient's sense of well-being and comfort, and prevent deterioration of the oral cavity (Kisely, 2016; Riley, 2018). Poor oral hygiene contributes to the colonization of the oropharyngeal secretions by respiratory pathogens. Diligent oral hygiene care can improve oral health and limit the growth of pathogens in the oropharyngeal secretions, decreasing the incidence of aspiration pneumonia, community-acquired pneumonia, nonventilator health care–associated pneumonia (NV-HAP), and ventilator-associated pneumonia (VAP) (AACN, 2017; Chick & Wynne, 2020; Jenson et al., 2018; Quinn et al., 2020). Comprehensive oral care that includes thorough mechanical cleaning is an important part of care to achieve oral health outcomes for patients in all settings (Barbe et al., 2020; Chick & Wynne, 2020; Chicote, 2019; Gibney et al., 2019; Kisey, 2016).

An oral assessment tool can assist with assessment of the status of the oral cavity, as well as help to determine the frequency and procedure for oral care (Chick & Wynne, 2020; Chicote, 2019; McCormick et al., 2019). If the patient can assist with mouth care, provide the necessary materials and help the patient as necessary (Skill 32-2 on pages 1126–1131).

Physical limitations, such as those associated with aging, often lead to less-than-adequate oral hygiene (Thomas, 2019). The dexterity required for adequate brushing and flossing may decrease with age or illness. Older adults may be dependent on caregivers for oral hygiene. Patients with cognitive impairment, such as dementia, and mental illness are also at risk for inadequate oral hygiene (Brennan & Strauss, 2014; Jablonski et al., 2018; Kadia et al., 2014; Lee et al., 2013; Red & O'Neal, 2020). If

Guidelines for Nursing Care 32-2

PROVIDING BODY PIERCING CARE

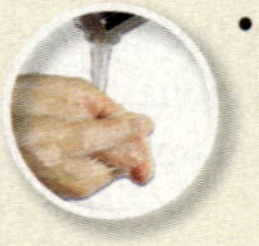

- Perform hand hygiene before providing care. Explain what you are going to do. Put on gloves.
- Clean the jewelry and the piercing site of all crust and debris. Clean the site with mild soap and warm water or normal saline solution. Use a cotton swab to gently remove any crusting. Rinse well. Remove gloves. Perform hand hygiene.
- Advise patients to avoid the use of alcohol, hydrogen peroxide, and ointments at the site.
- Advise patients to avoid immersion in unclean water such as baths, pools, hot tubs, or lakes during healing.
- Oral piercing aftercare includes rinsing with an antibacterial, alcohol-free mouthwash for 30 to 60 seconds after meals and at bedtime. The patient should brush the teeth with a new, soft-bristled toothbrush.
- Advise patients to avoid oral tobacco use.
- Most piercings take 6 to 8 weeks to heal, but some may take several months or a year to heal.

Source: Adapted from American Academy of Family Physicians. (2019, July 19). *Body piercing.* https://familydoctor.org/body-piercing/?adfree=true; McBride, D. L. (2018). Clinical guidance to tattooing and piercing among youth. *Journal of Pediatric Nursing, 39,* 83–84. https://doi.org/10.1016/j.pedn.2017.11.012; and Rademeyer, C., Farley, C. L., & Van Hoover, C. (2020). Health implications and counseling considerations for individuals with piercings and tattoos. *Nursing for Women's Health, 24*(3), 210–227. https://doi.org/10.1016/j.nwh.2020.03.006

Box 32-3 Meeting the Oral Hygiene Needs of Patients With Cognitive Impairments

- Choose a time of day when the patient is most calm and accepting of care.
- Enlist the aid of a family member or significant other.
- Break the task into small steps and provide short, simple instructions.
- Provide distraction, such as playing favorite music, while providing care.
- Allow the patient to participate. The nurse can put a hand over the patient's hand to guide the activity.
- Start the activity, showing the patient what to do, then let the patient take over.
- Withdraw and try again later if the patient strongly refuses care.
- Document effective and ineffective interventions to provide appropriate information for staff to give consistent, thoughtful, person-centered care.

Source: Adapted from Alzheimer's Association. (2020). *Dental care.* https://www.alz.org/help-support/caregiving/daily-care/dental-care; Eliopoulos, C. (2018). *Gerontological nursing* (9th ed.). Wolters Kluwer; and Konno, R., Kang, H. S., & Makimoto, K. (2014). A best-evidence review of intervention studies for minimizing resistance-to-care behaviours for older adults with dementia in nursing homes. *Journal of Advanced Nursing, 70*(10), 2167–2180.

the patient is unable to perform oral hygiene, make certain that the mouth receives care as often as necessary to keep it clean and moist, as often as every 1 or 2 hours if necessary. This is especially important for patients who cannot drink or are not permitted fluids by mouth. Refer to Box 32-3 for suggestions to meet the oral hygiene needs for patients with cognitive impairments. Skill 32-3 on pages 1131 identifies techniques for administering oral hygiene to dependent patients. Moisten the mouth with water, if allowed, and lubricate the lips frequently to keep the membranes well moistened.

The use of chlorhexidine gluconate (CHG) as part of oral hygiene has been integrated into oral hygiene regiments and is available as an oral rinse, oral spray, and dental gel (AACN, 2017; de Camargo et al., 2019). The use of CHG as part of protocols for systematic oral care for critically ill patients has been shown to reduce risk of ventilator-associated pneumonia (VAP) (AACN, 2017; Chen et al., 2015).

Patient education about oral hygiene is an important aspect of promoting good oral hygiene. Consider providing information about oral hygiene techniques and the importance of regular (twice yearly) dental visits to treat and prevent oral health problems. Emphasize that regular checkups aid in catching problems early and make any problems more manageable (Cleveland Clinic, 2019; MFMER, 2018). Refer to the PICOT in Practice box (on page 1108) for additional discussion related to oral hygiene and children.

TOOTHBRUSHING AND FLOSSING

Brush and floss teeth twice a day and rinse the mouth after meals. A soft-bristled toothbrush should be small enough to reach all teeth. Clean and dry all brushes between uses. Bacteria do most damage directly after eating, so make sure the patient brushes the teeth immediately after eating or drinking. In addition, clean the tongue with the toothbrush or a tongue scraper (MFMER, 2019a). Use a toothbrush even when the patient has no or few teeth. It is the only effective way to remove plaque (a thin film of bacteria that forms on teeth) and debris.

Automatic toothbrushes, electric or battery operated, are simple to use and can be used to removing debris and plaque and clean the teeth effectively. Use of an electric toothbrush provides superior oral hygiene care when oral hygiene is provided by a caregiver (Vannah & Sammarco, 2019). These devices are very useful for patients with arthritis or other conditions that make it difficult to brush effectively (MFMER, 2019a).

The toothbrush cannot reach areas between the teeth where food lodges and plaque can build up, so flossing at least once a day is recommended (American Dental Association [ADA], n.d.b). Flossing removes the debris that the toothbrush cannot and helps to break up colonies of bacteria. Other interdental cleaners may be used as well, such as cone-shaped brushes, and are particularly useful for patients who have a hard time handling dental floss or are unable to perform their own oral care (ADA, n.d.b). Pressurized water spray units (water flossing) are available to assist with oral hygiene to remove plaque and reduce gingivitis (ADA, n.d.d). Water flossing devices can be a useful option for patients who have trouble flossing by hand (ADA, n.d.d). However, if too much water pressure is used, particles of debris may be forced into tissue pockets, leading to gum damage. Therefore, patients should discuss use of these devices with a dentist.

Toothpastes and powders (dentifrices) aid the brushing process and usually have a pleasant taste that encourages brushing, especially by children. Most dentifrices are safe to use, but those containing harsh abrasives may scratch the enamel of the teeth and thus are not recommended. Salt and sodium bicarbonate are far less expensive than proprietary products on the market and just as effective for short-term use. However, these products lack fluoride and should not be used exclusively. Dentifrices containing stannous fluoride and antitartar agents, as well as antiplaque rinses, decrease dental caries and are recommended for use (ADA, 2019; ADA, n.d.e).

Unfolding Patient Stories: Christopher Parrish • Part 2

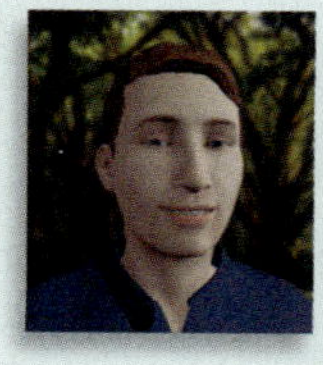

Recall from Chapter 23, **Christopher Parrish**, age 18, who has cystic fibrosis and frequent respiratory infections. He recently started college and is living in the dormitory. What questions can the nurse ask to identify his current hygiene practices and preferences? How would the nurse assess the adequacy of Christopher's personal hygiene behaviors? What education can the nurse provide to promote good hygiene and reduce his risk for infection?

Care for Christopher and other patients in a realistic virtual environment: ***vSim** for Nursing* (thepoint.lww.com/vSimFunds). Practice documenting these patients' care in DocuCare (thepoint.lww.com/DocuCareEHR).

PICOT in Practice

ORAL HEALTH AND SCHOOL DENTAL PROGRAM

Scenario: You are a school nurse discussing the importance of oral health with a group of parents and children at an after-school event. One area you have stressed is the importance of oral hygiene to reduce infection, plaque accumulation, and the risk of gum disease. Oral hygiene includes brushing to clean the surfaces of the teeth, flossing to clean the surfaces between the teeth, and regular dental checkups. Some parents share concerns that their children have developed cavities at their last dental visit. You notice there are inconsistencies in the regular intervals between dental checkups reported by the parents.

You consider if a school dental screening program for oral health would benefit parents and children living in the community.

- **Population:** Children at risk for gum disease
- **Intervention:** School dental screening programs
- **Comparison:** Regular interval dental checkups
- **Outcome:** Improved oral health status
- **Time:** 12 months

PICOT Question: Do school dental screening programs compared to regular interval dental checkups improve oral health status in children living in the community over 12 months?

Findings:

1. Arora, A., Khattri, S., Ismail, N. M., Kumbargere Nagraj, S., Eachempati, P. (2019). School dental screening programmes for oral health. *Cochrane Database of Systematic Reviews*. Issue 8. *Art. No.:* CD012595. https://doi.org/10.1002/14651858.CD012595.pub3

This included seven trials with 20,192 children ages 4 to 15 years and follow-up for 3 to 8 months. A very low certainty of evidence was found, which was insufficient to draw conclusions about whether there is a role for traditional school dental screening in improving dental care. Furthermore, when compared to traditional screening, there was no evidence of a difference in regular dental care (very low–certainty evidence).

2. Fee, P. A., Riley, P., Worthington, H. V., Clarkson, J. E., Boyers, D., Beirne, P. V. (2020). Recall intervals for oral health in primary care patients. *Cochrane Database of Systematic Reviews*. Issue 10. *Art. No.:* CD004346. https://doi.org/10.1002/14651858.CD004346.pub5

This included two studies with data from 1,736 participants. One study was conducted in a public dental service clinic in Norway and involved participants younger than age 20 years who were regular attenders at dental appointments. The other study was conducted in U.K. general dental practices and involved adults who attended regularly. It compared the effects of 6-month, 24-month, and risk-based recall intervals and measured outcomes at 4 years. For adults attending dental checkups in primary care settings, there is little to no difference between risk-based and 6-month checkups in the number of tooth surfaces with any caries, gingival bleeding, and oral health–related quality of life over a 4-year period (high-certainty evidence). The available evidence on recall intervals between dental checkups for children and adolescents was uncertain.

Strength of Evidence: Level I: systematic review

Recommendation: There is insufficient evidence to draw conclusions about whether there is a role for traditional school dental screening in improving dental care in children. Adults who see their dentist for a checkup every 6 months or at personalized intervals based on their dentist's assessment of their risk of dental disease does not affect tooth decay, gum disease, or quality of life. If parental dental care and preventative practices are any indication of childhood practices, children who see their dentist for a checkup every 6 months or at personalized intervals does not affect tooth decay, gum disease, or quality of life. High-quality studies that measure the impact of screening on oral health and are carried out over longer periods of time are needed.

MOUTHWASHES

Therapeutic mouth rinses that reduce bacteria can help reduce plaque, gingivitis, tartar (hardened plaque) and also freshen breath. Anticavity rinses with fluoride help protect tooth enamel to help prevent or control tooth decay (ADA, 2019). Swabs and mouthwash with alcohol should be avoided (Woon, 2020).

Halitosis is often a sign of something more serious than a strong smell that lingers after some foods (ADA, n.d.f). Halitosis may be the result of dental issues (cavities, gum disease); mouth, nose, and throat infections; dry mouth; or other chronic conditions (ADA, n.d.f). If the cause of halitosis is poor oral hygiene, a daily dental cleaning routine should reduce the odor.

Sometimes, halitosis may be systemic in nature. For example, the odor of onions and garlic on the breath comes from the lungs, where the oils are being removed from the bloodstream and eliminated with respiration. A mouthwash cannot remove halitosis when odors are being eliminated by respiration. If bad breath persists, a patient should consult with a dentist (ADA, n.d.f).

DENTURE CARE

Failing to wear dentures for a long period allows the gum line to change, thus affecting the fit of the dentures. It is not recommended, however, that dentures be worn continuously (24 hr/day) in order to reduce or minimize irritation of the oral tissues (American College of Prosthodontists, n.d.).

Patients with dentures are more likely to keep them in the mouth if they are kept clean. If the patient cannot care for them, the nurse must ensure that the dentures are clean. Use care when handling a patient's dentures because they represent a considerable financial investment, and replacement for damage or loss is expensive. Remove and rinse dentures and mouth after meals.

Dentures should be cleaned daily to reduce plaque and potentially harmful microorganisms (ADA, n.d.c). Daily cleaning includes brushing with a nonabrasive denture cleanser

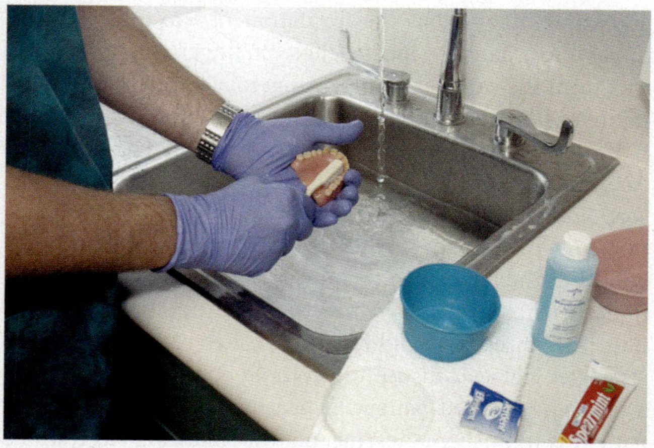

FIGURE 32-3. Cleaning dentures.

or mild dishwashing liquid with a denture brush (American College of Prosthodontists, n.d.).

When cleaning dentures for a patient, put on gloves and hold them over a basin of water or a sink lined with a washcloth or soft towel (Fig. 32-3) so that if they slip from your grasp, they will not fall onto a hard surface and break. If necessary, grasp the dentures with a 4″ × 4″ piece of gauze to help prevent them from slipping out of your gloved hands. Use cool or lukewarm water to cleanse them. Hot water may warp the plastic material of which most dentures are made. Use a denture brush and denture cleanser. Do not use toothpaste as it can be too harsh for denture surfaces (American College of Prosthodontists, n.d.). Rinse dentures thoroughly after soaking and brushing, prior to reinsertion into the mouth. Give the patient the opportunity to brush the gums and tongue and rinse the mouth before the dentures are replaced to stimulate circulation and help remove plaque (ADA, n.d.c). Assist the patient with care as necessary.

Store dentures in water when not in the patient's mouth (American College of Prosthodontists, n.d.). Leaving dentures to dry can cause warping. If the patient has been instructed to remove dentures while sleeping, a disposable denture cup is convenient and easy to use. A denture-cleaning tablet can be added to the water overnight (Woon, 2020). Advise the patient not to wrap dentures in toilet tissue or disposable wipes because these are likely to be thrown away.

Providing Eye Care

Normally, the eyes are kept clean with lacrimal secretions. During illness, the eyes may produce more secretions than normal and may appear glass-like. Use the following techniques when secretions adhere to the eyelashes and become dry and crusty or when discharge is present:

- Wear gloves during the cleaning procedure.
- Use water or normal saline and a clean washcloth or compress to clean the eyes. Never use soap to clean the eyes because soap is irritating to eye tissues.
- Dampen a cleaning cloth with the solution of choice and wipe once while moving from the inner canthus to the outer canthus of the eye. This technique minimizes the risk for forcing debris into the area drained by the nasolacrimal duct. Turn the cleaning cloth and use a different section for each stroke.
- Continue this technique, using a different section of the cleaning cloth for each stroke, until the eye is clean.
- If the eyelashes are matted with secretions or debris that cannot be removed by wiping, apply a warm, wet compress to the closed eye for 3 to 5 minutes to loosen the secretions so that they may be removed in a painless manner.

CARE OF THE UNCONSCIOUS PATIENT'S EYES

Patients with diminished or absent blink (corneal) reflexes and patients whose eyelids remain open require frequent eye care, at least every 4 hours. If the eye is not kept moist, corneal ulceration may result from excessive drying of the eye (Morton & Fontaine, 2018). Nursing measures include using saline or artificial tears or lubricant eye ointment based on the prescribed interventions or facility protocol, to lubricate the eye and a protective eye covering to keep the eye closed (Morton & Fontaine, 2018).

EYEGLASS CARE

Eyeglasses are essential for many people and represent a considerable financial investment. Take special precautions to prevent them from being broken or lost. Encourage patients who need glasses to wear them to avoid eyestrain.

Many eyeglasses have plastic lenses, which are considerably lighter in weight than glass lenses but correct vision just as well. Plastic lenses scratch easily. Whenever setting down glasses, make sure they are placed with the lenses up.

Clean eyeglasses over a towel, so that if they slip they will not become scratched or broken. Use warm water and soap or a special cleansing preparation. Hot water may warp plastic lenses and frames. Rinse the glasses well after cleaning them with soap and water; dry them with a clean, soft nonlint cloth (Cleveland Clinic, 2015). Paper products that are made of wood pulp increase the risk of scratching the lenses, so do not use a dry paper tissue to clean eyeglasses. Do not use silicone tissues to clean plastic lenses.

CONTACT LENS CARE

A contact lens is a small disc worn directly on the eyeball. It stays in place by surface tension of the eye's tears. Contact lenses are either rigid (hard) or soft. Rigid gas permeable (RGP) lenses are more inflexible than soft lenses. Soft lenses are made of a plastic material that absorbs water to become soft and pliable. They are brittle when dehydrated and absorb water when placed in a solution, usually normal saline, or when in contact with tears. Soft lenses may be used for daily wear or extended wear. Disposable soft lenses are also available.

People who wear contact lenses need to take special precautions to keep the lenses free of microorganisms that may lead to eye infections and to avoid injuring or scratching the surface of the eye. Patients should always perform hand hygiene before touching eye surfaces and lenses. Caution lens wearers about eye irritation in the presence of noxious vapors or smoke. Remind lens wearers that lenses should not come into contact with cosmetics, soaps, or hair sprays because eye irritation may result. Patients should use only commercially prepared, sterile contact lens solutions and discard the solution in the contact lens case each time the lenses are disinfected and stored (MFMER, 2019b). Patients should never rinse with tap water or saliva (Cleveland Clinic, 2020; MFMER, 2019b). Urge the patient to immediately report any adverse reaction related to contact lens use.

The cornea, which consists of dense connective tissue, does not have its own blood supply. It is nourished primarily by oxygen from the atmosphere and from tears. In a patient who wears contact lenses, the cornea requires more than its normal supply of oxygen because its metabolic rate increases. To allow the cornea to receive a maximal supply of oxygen, contact lenses should be worn and removed according to the type and manufacturer's recommendations. Excessive tearing, pain, and redness signal the need to remove lenses. Lenses should be cleaned and stored as prescribed. Different types of lenses require special care and certain types of cleaning/storage products. Sleeping without removing any contact lens is not recommended as the incidence of serious eye infections is greatly increased (Cleveland Clinic, 2020).

If a patient wears contact lenses but cannot remove them, the nurse may be responsible for removing them. This may occur, for example, when the nurse is caring for an unconscious patient. Whenever an unconscious patient is admitted without any family present, always assess to determine whether the patient wears contact lenses. If an eye injury is present, do not try to remove lenses because of the danger of causing an additional injury.

Providing Ear Care

Other than cleaning the outer ears, little intervention is needed for routine hygiene of the ear. After the ears are washed, dry them carefully with a soft towel so that water and cerumen (wax) are removed by capillary action. Forcing the towel into the ear for drying or using a cotton-tipped applicator may aid in the formation of wax plugs. Using bobby pins, hairpins, paper clips, or fingernails to remove wax from the ear is extremely dangerous because these may injure or puncture the eardrum.

If the patient uses a hearing aid, check the batteries routinely and clean the earpieces or ear mold daily with mild soap and water or according to the manufacturer's instructions. A whistling sound that is audible when the hearing aid is held in the hand with the power on and the volume high indicates that the battery is functioning properly. Figure 32-4 illustrates three types of hearing aids. Refer to Chapter 8 for strategies nurses can use to promote communication with a hearing-impaired patient. If hearing loss is mild and the patient is not using a hearing aid, the following suggestions may help to improve hearing and should be included in any patient teaching:

- Avoid noisy places for conversation.
- Choose well-lit places where it is easier to look at the speaker's face, lips, and hands for cues to the conversation.
- Cup your hand behind your ear.
- Ask people to face you when they are speaking to you.
- Ask people to repeat what they said, if it was not clear to you, and to speak slowly.
- Consider buying amplifying devices so that you can hear your television and radio without turning up the sound.

Providing Nose Care

The best way to clean the nose is to blow it gently. Both nostrils should be open while doing this. Closing one nostril adds to the danger of forcing debris into the eustachian tubes. Irrigations are usually contraindicated because of the danger of forcing material into the sinuses.

If the external nares are crusted, applying a warm, moist compress helps to soften and remove the crusts. Disposable paper tissues are recommended for nasal secretions. A cotton-tipped applicator may be used to clean the opening of the nares, but with great care to avoid injury. Never introduce the applicator into the nares.

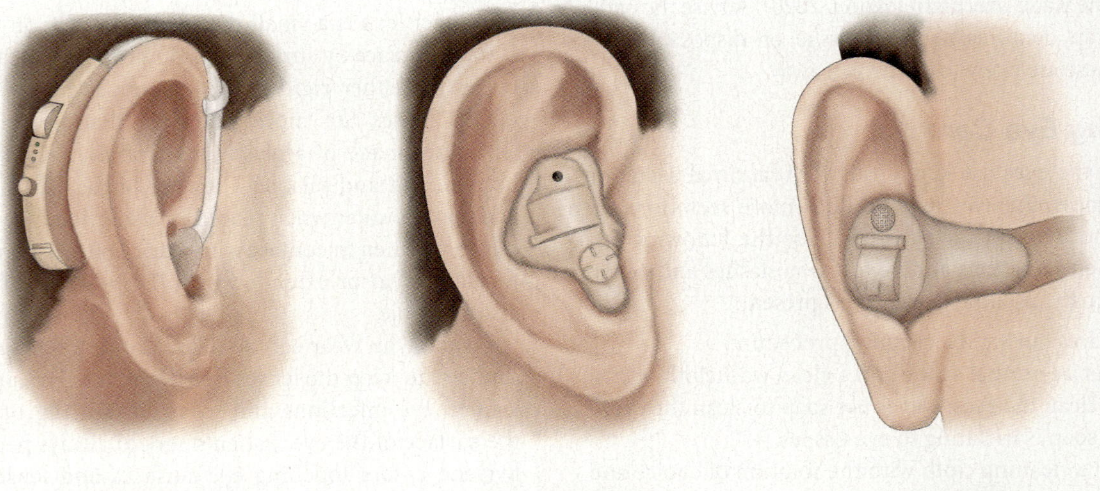

Behind the ear — In the ear — In the ear

FIGURE 32-4. Several types of hearing aids.

Providing Hair Care

Demonstrate cultural consideration by grooming the patient's hair in the manner and the style preferred by the patient. Hair that becomes entangled is difficult to comb. Combing tiny sections of hair at a time may be necessary if a patient's hair has not been combed for even 1 day. One way to protect long hair from matting and tangling is to ask the patient for permission to braid it. Parting the hair in the middle on the back of the head and making two braids, one on either side, prevents the discomfort of lying on one heavy braid on the back of the head. When braiding a patient's hair, ensure that the hair is not pulled too tightly.

Tightly curled (kinky) hair is normally dry and curly and becomes matted and tangled easily. Use a comb with wide-spaced teeth and work the hair through from the neckline upward toward the forehead. Some people have their hair straightened, but even after this process, it may be difficult to untangle the hair when the person is confined to bed. Some patients with this type of hair style their hair in small braids. The braids are not undone for shampooing and may need to have a lubricant or oil applied daily to prevent hair strands from breaking.

Occasionally, a patient's hair is almost hopelessly matted, and cutting the hair may be necessary. Usually the patient signs a written consent before a patient's hair is cut. Also, as appropriate, discuss with a member of the patient's immediate family the necessity of cutting the hair.

SHAMPOOING THE HAIR

The hair, which is exposed to the same dirt and oil as the skin, requires washing as often as necessary to keep it clean. Wash the comb and brush each time the hair is washed and as frequently as necessary between shampoos. Some health care facilities may have beauticians and barbers to assist with hair care, including shampooing, but this does not relieve the nurse of the responsibility.

Before shampooing the hair, brush or have the patient brush and comb the hair well to stimulate the scalp and undo tangled hair. The patient may then shampoo the hair while showering, if able. In some settings, shampooing a patient's hair is a prescribed intervention.

Shampoo caps are available and are being used with increasing frequency (Fig. 32-5). These commercially prepared, disposable caps contain a rinseless shampoo product.

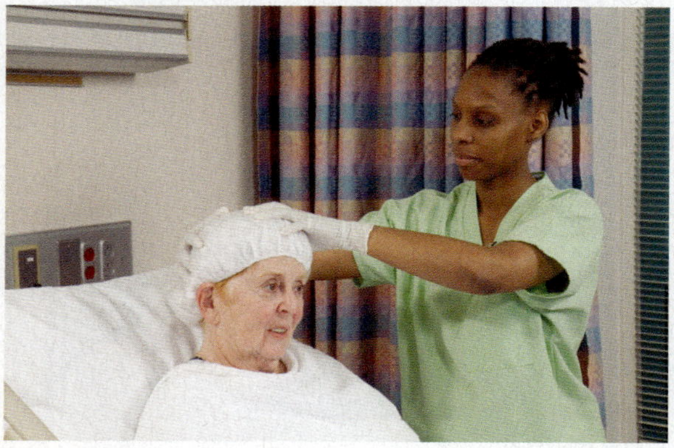

FIGURE 32-5. Using a shampoo cap to clean a patient's hair.

Warm the cap in the microwave or store it in a warmer until use. Place the cap on the patient's head and massage the hair and scalp through the cap, to lather the shampoo. After shampooing for the manufacturer's suggested length of time, remove and discard the cap.

If regular shampooing is inappropriate or is contraindicated by the patient's condition, other products for use at the bedside are available. These products do not require rinsing and are available as foams, concentrates, and dry powders. Apply the foam or concentrate cleaner and lather the product or distribute through hair according to the instructions on the label.

After shampooing or application of a foam or concentrate hair-cleaning product, towel-dry the patient's hair. Comb and style the hair according to the patient's preference. It may be appropriate to keep the head covered with a towel until the hair dries, to help minimize chilling of the patient. Guidelines for Nursing Care 32-3 on page 1112 provides one technique to shampoo hair for patients on bed rest at home or in a facility.

SHAVING

Grooming of body hair other than hair on the head can be an important part of a patient's self-esteem and well-being. Patients with beards or mustaches may require nursing assistance to keep the beard and mustache clean. Never trim or shave a patient's beard or mustache without the patient's consent. Female patients may require assistance with shaving underarm and leg hair, depending on the patient's personal preference and abilities. Standard razors with a blade tend to give a closer shave than do electric razors, but many patients find electric razors more convenient and practical. Electric shavers are usually recommended when the patient is receiving anticoagulant therapy or has a bleeding disorder (Hartford HealthCare, 2019) and are especially convenient for ill and bedridden patients. Shaving after a warm bath or shower softens the hair, making the process easier (Hartford HealthCare, 2019). The technique for shaving patients with a standard razor who cannot shave themselves is described in Guidelines for Nursing Care 32-4 (on page 1112).

TREATING PEDICULOSIS

Several commercial preparations, called pediculicides, are available for the treatment of pediculosis. These drugs destroy the lice and their eggs or nits. Two treatments may be necessary before all the nits are destroyed. The procedures and the medications used for the treatment of pediculosis vary among health facilities. The partners of patients with pubic infestation from within the previous month should be informed that they are at risk for infestation and should be treated (CDC, 2019a).

When educating the patient, stress the importance of carefully following the instructions and finishing the treatment, as indicated. Failure to comply with product instructions and/or finishing the treatment has produced lice that are resistant to pediculicides on the market. Drugs used to treat lice can be dangerous if they are misused or overused (CDC, 2019a). Additional interventions and patient education topics related to head lice are highlighted in Teaching Tips 32-1 on page 1113.

Guidelines for Nursing Care 32-3

SHAMPOOING A PATIENT'S HAIR IN BED

Follow these guidelines for shampooing the hair of patients on bedrest.

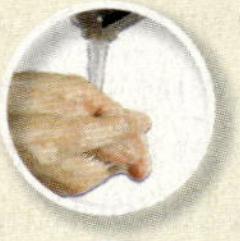

- Perform hand hygiene.

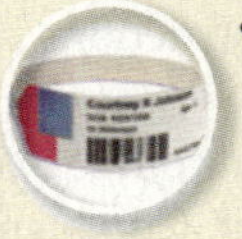

- Identify the patient. Explain procedure to the patient.
- Prepare several pitchers with comfortably warm (no more than 120°F) water for washing and rinsing, shampoo, one or two towels for drying, and a receptacle to receive wash and rinse water.
- Place a protective pad and a plastic hair-washing tray if one is available (see Figure) under the head. (Alternatively, a large trash bag can also be used under the patient's head and extended over the side of the bed to catch the water.)
- Place the patient in a position over the pad so that water drainage is directed into the receptacle.
- Wet the hair, apply shampoo, and massage the scalp well while washing the hair.
- Rinse the hair and reapply shampoo for a second washing, if indicated.
- Rinse the hair thoroughly.
- Apply conditioner if requested or if the scalp appears dry.
- Towel-dry the patient's hair. Apply additional hair product, such as leave-in conditioner, oil or pomade, based on patient preferences. Comb and style the hair according to the patient's preference.
- Keep the head covered with a towel until the hair dries, to help minimize chilling the patient.

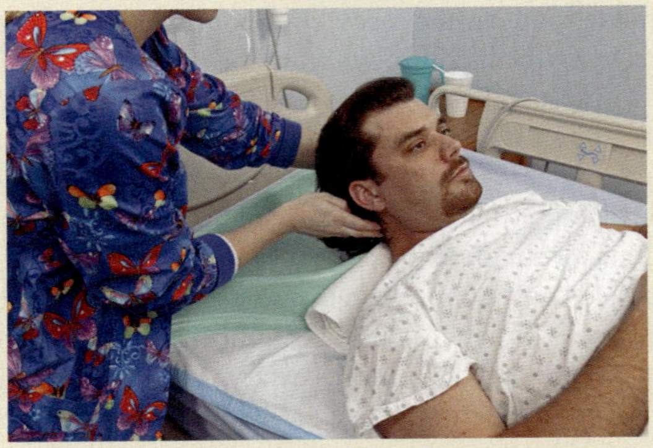

Providing Fingernail Care

The following are recommended techniques for the care of fingernails:

- Trim the nails straight across, then round the tips in a gentle curve. Do not trim so far down on the sides that the skin and cuticle are injured.
- Remove hangnails, which are broken pieces of cuticle, by carefully clipping them off. Do not pull or rip off hangnails (MFMER, 2019c).
- Gently push cuticles back off the nail when soft and pliable after washing in warm water, using a blunt instrument or a terry cloth.

Guidelines for Nursing Care 32-4

SHAVING WITH A STANDARD RAZOR

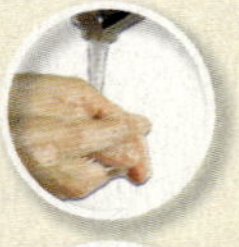

- Perform hand hygiene.

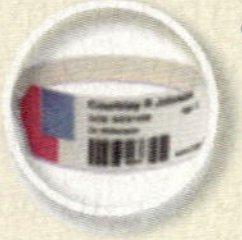

- Identify the patient. Explain procedure to the patient.
- Cover patient's chest with a towel or waterproof pad. Fill bath basin with comfortably warm (no more than 120°F) water.
- Press a warm washcloth on the patient's skin to soften the hair.
- Dispense shaving gel/cream into palm of hand. Rub hands together, then apply to area to be shaved in a layer approximately 0.5 inch thick.
- With one hand, hold the skin steady at the area to be shaved. Using a smooth stroke, begin shaving. *If shaving the face,* shave with the direction of hair growth in downward, short strokes (see Figure). *If shaving a leg,* shave against the hair in upward, short strokes.
- Remove residual shaving cream with a wet washcloth.
- If patient requests, apply aftershave or lotion to area shaved.
- Remove and discard gloves and perform hand hygiene.

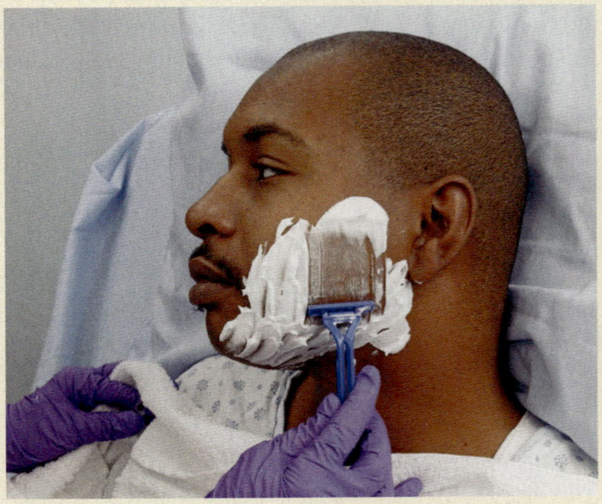

Shaving the face.

Teaching Tips 32-1

DEALING WITH HEAD LICE

Health Topic	Teaching Tip	Why Is This Important?
Who is at risk for getting head lice?	Preschool- and elementary-aged children and families/household members/caregivers are most often affected. Infection can occur after contact with someone who has lice.	Lice can infect any person, regardless of hygiene practices or social status.
How do you become infected with head lice?	Spread by direct contact with the hair of an infested person. Head-to-head contact provides greatest risk of transmission. Uncommonly spread by sharing clothing (hats, scarves, coats, sports uniforms) or belongings (hair ribbons, barrettes, combs, brushes, towels, stuffed animals). Uncommonly spread by lying on a bed, couch, pillow, or carpet that has recently been in contact with an infested person.	Avoid head-to-head (hair-to-hair) contact during play and other activities. Do not share clothing such as hats, scarves, coats, sports uniforms, hair ribbons, or barrettes. Do not share combs, brushes, or towels. Do not lie on beds, couches, pillows, carpets, or stuffed animals that have recently been in contact with an infested person.
What are the signs and symptoms of head lice infestation?	Tickling feeling on scalp; itching; sores on the head caused by scratching. Irritability and difficulty sleeping (head lice are most active in the dark). Lice may be seen especially behind the ears and near the neckline at the back of the neck.	The faster the lice are noticed, the easier they are to eradicate.
How is head lice infestation treated?	Apply a pediculicide[a] according to the manufacturer's directions. Hats, scarves, pillowcases, bedding, clothing, and towels worn or used by the infested person in the 2-day period just before treatment is started can be machine washed and dried using the hot water and hot air cycles (lice and eggs are killed by 5 minutes of exposure to temperatures greater than 128.3°F) Items that cannot be laundered may be dry-cleaned or sealed in a plastic bag for 2 weeks. Soak combs and brushes in hot water (at least 130°F) for 5 to 10 minutes. Vacuum the floor and furniture, particularly where the infested person sat or lay.	All head lice must be killed or removed or a reinfestation may occur. Retreatment of head lice usually is recommended because no approved pediculicide completely kills all lice eggs.

[a]Women who are pregnant or breastfeeding should not use pediculicides without consulting with their health care provider. Consult a health care provider before using pediculicides on a person who has allergies, asthma, or other medical conditions.

Source: Information obtained from Centers for Disease Control and Prevention (CDC). (2019, September 11). *Parasites—Lice*. https://www.cdc.gov/parasites/lice/

- Apply an emollient or moisturizer to the nails and cuticles to help prevent hangnails.
- Clean under the nails with a blunt instrument, being careful not to injure the area where the nail is attached to the underlying tissue.

Splitting and peeling of the nails can be caused by repeated or prolonged contact with water. Teach the patient to avoid contact with soap and water as much as possible, and to wear cotton-lined rubber gloves when washing dishes, cleaning, or using harsh chemicals. Encourage the frequent use of a good hand cream, and avoid using polish remover with acetone, which tends to dry the nails (MFMER, 2019c).

Providing Foot Care

Proper foot care is important at any age. It becomes even more so with aging and when conditions such as circulatory disturbances or diabetes mellitus are present. Keep toenails at a moderate length and cut toenails straight across the toes (MFMER, 2019d). Encourage patients with diabetes and peripheral vascular disease to schedule annual foot checks with their healthcare provider or podiatrist and to see an advanced practice provider or podiatrist for treatment related to bunions, corns, or calluses (American College of Foot and Ankle Surgeons, n.d.; Beuscher, 2019; MFMER, 2017). Guidelines for Nursing Care 32-5 on page 1114 highlights appropriate techniques related to foot care.

Providing Environmental Care

A patient's environment can improve or detract from the person's sense of well-being. A patient's environment can consist of a room in a facility, such as a hospital, one or more rooms in the patient's home or apartment, or something

Guidelines for Nursing Care 32-5

PROVIDING FOOT CARE

- Bathe the feet daily in a mild soap and lukewarm water solution. Avoid soaking the feet. Be sure to clean the interdigital area.
- Rinse the feet to remove soap residue that can dry and irritate the skin.
- Dry feet thoroughly, including the area between the toes.
- Apply a moisturizer to feet if they are dry. Patients with diabetes and peripheral artery disease should apply moisturizer on the tops and bottoms of the feet to keep the skin soft, but not between the toes. These patients should sprinkle talcum powder or cornstarch between the toes to keep the skin dry (MFMER, 2017).
- Consider using an antifungal foot powder if necessary to prevent fungal infections, such as athlete's foot.
- Patients with diabetes should file the nails; avoid using scissors or nail clippers, which may slip and injure tissues. Nondiabetic patients should avoid digging into or cutting the toenails at the lateral corners when trimming the nails.
- Do not cut off corns or calluses. Avoid commercial removers because they may contain ingredients that can lead to development of infection and ulcers. Consult a podiatrist, a health care provider who treats foot disorders, when corns or calluses are present.
- Explain the dangers of going barefoot. Skin on the feet may be injured, or athlete's foot may be acquired in public showers.
- Advise patients to wear appropriate footwear. Break in new shoes gradually. Improperly fitting shoes can lead to corns, calluses, bunions, and blisters. The soles should be flexible and nonslippery and the heel heights should be safe and offer appropriate support. Shoes with rough ridges, wrinkles, or tears in the linings should be discarded or repaired.
- Advise patients to wear cotton socks, which provide warmth and absorb perspiration.
- Teach patients to avoid wearing knee-high stockings, and to not sit with the knees crossed because this can obstruct the circulation to the lower extremities and feet.
- Prop the feet up above the level of the hips a few minutes several times a day if the feet swell.
- Avoid using heating pads and hot-water bottles because of the danger of blistering and burning the feet.
- Report any signs of foot problems to your primary care provider. This is especially important for patients with diabetes.

in-between. Regardless of the setting, ensure that the area is clean and clutter-free, safe, and pleasant. Patients may be in an individual "single" room or a multiple-bed room. Single rooms provide for patient privacy and dignity, and ensure confidentiality (Roos et al., 2020). Single rooms are also often part of infection control measures. However, patients in single rooms may feel isolated and experience loneliness (Roos et al., 2020). Multiple-bed rooms offer the opportunity for socialization, communication, and support, but may be associated with a loss of privacy, increased noise, and less control over the environment (Hasan Tehrani et al., 2018; Roos et al., 2020). Nurses must take these factors into consideration and implement actions to support patient-centered care in all room environments.

The patient's environment in a hospital or other facility consists of the bedside unit and the furnishings and equipment in the space around the bed. Basic furniture includes the bed, overbed table, bedside stand, and chairs. Standard equipment in the health care environment includes the call light, oxygen, suction, and electrical outlets; light fixtures; bath basin; emesis basin; bedpan or urinal; water pitcher and glass; and bed linens. One nursing responsibility is ensuring that necessary equipment and items are in their proper place and functioning properly. Patients usually store personal items in the bedside stand. Always request permission from alert patients or family members before opening the stand to obtain the bath basin, lotion, or other items. When assisting with hygiene, respecting the patient's right to privacy and ownership of personal goods decreases the patient's sense of powerlessness.

Good ventilation in patient rooms is imperative to limit pathogens and unpleasant odors associated with body secretions and excretions; for example, urine, stool, vomitus, draining wounds, or body odors. Decrease odors by emptying bedpans, urinals, and emesis basins promptly. When the waste receptacle in the patient's room is used to dispose of soiled dressings or anything with a strong odor, be sure to remove the trash before leaving the room. Dispose of the trash according to facility policy. Room deodorizers may need to be used.

Patient preferences for room temperature often vary widely. Whenever possible, respect the patient's preference when determining the room temperature. In general, the room temperature should be between 68°F and 74°F (20°C and 23°C).

Many patients find it difficult to sleep in a health care facility. Patients are often disturbed frequently for assessment or treatment purposes. Care should be taken to reduce harsh lighting and noises whenever possible, although adequate lighting is necessary for all nursing procedures. Whenever possible, avoid carrying on conversations immediately outside the patient's room. Many patients find this stressful because the noise disturbs them and because they believe whatever is being said involves them.

Before leaving the bedside, get into the habit of saying to the patient, "Is there anything else I can do to make you more comfortable?" Checking with the patient communicates genuine caring and can correct for any oversights.

BED SAFETY AND COMFORT

Many people who are ill and hospitalized or receiving care in other health care environments, or are being cared for at home may spend a large portion of the day in bed, so the bed is an important part of the patient's environment. Nursing responsibilities include ensuring a safe and comfortable bed.

The typical hospital bed has a motorized frame in three sections, which allows the height of the bed to be raised or lowered and the head and foot to be adjusted. Know how to operate the bed and be ready to explain it to the patient. Bed positions are described in Chapter 34. The height of the entire bed is usually adjustable as well, allowing the height to be adjusted to a comfortable level for the patient to move in and out of the bed (Morse et al., 2015). The bed elevation can also be adjusted to a comfortable level for caregivers to provide patient care. If the bed is elevated for any reason, for patient safety it is very important to place the bed in the lowest position after care is completed.

Bed size is an important consideration. Bed space must be sufficient to provide for patient comfort. Bed space must also be sufficient to allow for patient repositioning and participation in an almost unlimited number of care activities, such as wound inspection, dressing changes, cleaning or bathing, and linen changes. Research by Wiggermann et al. (2017) suggests BMI is a good predictor of the space required to turn from supine to lateral and provides guidance for choice of bed size for patients. Nurses should consider placing patients that are unable to laterally reposition themselves on a wider bed when the patient's BMI is greater than 35 kg/m^2 (Wiggerman et al., 2017). Patients with a BMI greater than 45 kg/m^2 should be placed on wider beds regardless of mobility (Wiggerman et al., 2017).

Newer bed designs include features to address patient satisfaction, patient safety, and caregiver efficiency (Wiggerman et al., 2019). For example, beds are available with frame designs that adjust for width and length of the patient and minimize patient migration (Ghersi et al., 2018; Wiggerman et al., 2019); lighted side rail handgrips to aid in visualization of bed rails when getting in and out of bed (Wiggerman et al., 2019); bed exit alarms and alarms that rearm when the patient returns to bed (Ghersi et al., 2018; Wiggerman et al., 2019); attachment points for the patient call bell to prevent it from falling out of reach (Wiggerman et al., 2019); and built-in USB ports so patients can charge personal electronic devices (Wiggerman et al., 2019).

Hospital beds can also be ordered for use in the home or other community-based care environments. Because certain positions may be harmful to some patients, instruct the patient and family/caregivers about advisable bed positions and the use of the bed controls. Side rails are used to provide assistance with moving in bed and movement in and out of bed (FDA, 2017a; Morse et al., 2015). Access to bed controls and is often on or in the side rails. See Chapter 28 for additional discussion about the use of side rails. Use side rails when indicated and according to facility policy. Also, lock the wheels or casters on the hospital bed whenever the bed is stationary to prevent the bed from moving when the patient is moving from the bed to an upright position or being transferred (FDA, 2017a). The headboard of most hospital beds is removable to allow close patient contact in an emergency situation.

Nurses are responsible for ensuring the safety and comfort of the patient at the bedside. To promote bed safety while maintaining patient comfort, ensure the following before leaving the patient's bedside:

- The bed is in its lowest position (FDA, 2017a). Low beds should be raised to the appropriate height for each patient to allow safe transition in and out of bed (Hester, 2015; Morse et al., 2015).
- The bed position is safe for the patient.
- The bed controls are functioning (bed is electrically safe).
- The call light is functioning and always within reach.
- Side rail(s) is/are raised if indicated or requested by the patient.
- The wheels or casters are locked (FDA, 2017a).

The hospital mattress is firm and generally covered with a water-repellent material that can be easily wiped with a bactericidal solution between patients. A variety of therapeutic beds and mattresses are available to reduce or relieve the effects of pressure on the skin (Fig. 32-6). These are discussed in more detail in Chapter 33. Other special beds are available for use in the care of patients with specific health issues, such as spinal injuries. Bariatric patient beds are extra-wide and designed to be used for patients who are very obese.

Facility policies usually dictate the availability and use of bed linens. Bed linens include mattress covers, sheets, incontinence pads, pillowcases, blankets, and bath blankets. Changing the bed linen is often not the nurse's responsibility and may be delegated. The nurse is responsible for coordinating with assistive personnel to ensure patient comfort. To promote bed comfort, ensure the following before leaving a patient:

- Linens are clean and free of crumbs and wrinkles.
- The patient feels comfortably warm.

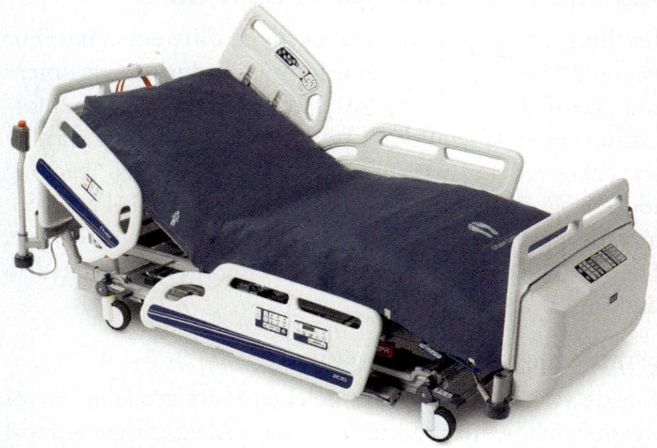

FIGURE 32-6. This special bed is an air-flotation, low–air-loss support surface to aid in prevention and support treatment of pressure injury; support treatment of severe or extensive burns, skin flaps and grafts; and as part of pain management, with a lateral turn and hold to assist in repositioning the patient. (*Source:* Image of Citadel® Patient Care System used with permission of Arjo Inc.)

Through the Eyes of a Student

One of my first patients was a man in his late 60s who had suffered a stroke. I was assigned to care for him, and his care included a bed bath and complete linen change—with him in the bed. I was determined to complete this task totally on my own, without asking anyone for help. This was my first mistake.

The patient yelled out a lot and had very rough mannerisms. I kept thinking to myself, "I must treat him with gentle care and not show any fear." Inside I was shaking furiously.

I managed to complete his bath and then began to change the sheets. I helped the patient to turn to one side, tucking the dirty linens close to him. I applied the fitted sheets to the upper portion of the bed . . . so far, so good. Immediately going to the foot of the bed, I applied the bottom portion. The top portion popped off—I ran to the top of the bed, reapplied the top portion—the bottom portion popped off—I reapplied it. . . . I must have spent 15 minutes running back and forth trying to get both ends to stay on. By this time, sweat was pouring off my face.

When I finally cried "Uncle," I discovered that certain fitted sheets just didn't fit all the mattresses. The usual routine in this case is to walk to the linen closet and get another fitted sheet. That probably takes about 15 seconds!

—Linda A. Keough; Delaware County Community College, Media, Pennsylvania

- Pressure areas are protected from rough sheets and water-repellent materials. This is especially important for patients with an increased risk for impaired skin integrity.

MAKING A BED

A comfortable bed and appropriate bedding contribute to a patient's sense of well-being. Bed linens are changed after the bath if the patient is bathed in the bed. Otherwise, many facilities change linens only when soiled. One method to change bed linen while the patient is out of the bed is described in Skill 32-4 on page 1134. A method to change bed linen with the patient in the bed is described in Skill 32-5 on page 1137.

Although there are variations in the procedure for making an occupied bed, these minor differences have no real effect on the patient's comfort. In some instances, creativity and flexibility are necessary when changing linens because of the patient's condition, orthopedic appliances on the bed, or treatments that may be in progress. Refer to Through the Eyes of a Student.

Teaching Patients About Skin Care

Teaching about skin care can occur at different times. For example, teaching can be done informally during assessment and personal care procedures. Here, the nurse shares information about general skin care measures, including ways to prevent or reduce a patient's risk for skin problems. Teaching addressing a specific topic, such as dry skin, diabetic foot care, or acne, may be addressed as part of the plan of care. The following section describes common topics related to skin care and skin problems.

SOAPS AND SKIN CLEANSERS

A wide variety of soaps and detergents are available. Soaps are often made from vegetable and animal fats, whereas most detergents are made from petroleum derivatives. For the most part, expensive cleansing agents are no more effective than their less expensive counterparts. Patients who experience dry skin or other alterations in skin health may benefit from using nonsoap skin cleansers. Refer to the discussion of these agents earlier in this chapter in the Promoting Skin Health section on page 1102.

DEODORANTS AND ANTIPERSPIRANTS

Perspiration is essentially odorless, although it contains some waste products, such as uric acid and ammonia. The odor of perspiration results when bacteria, normally present on everyone's skin, act on the skin's normal secretions.

Inform patients that keeping the body and clothing clean is the best way to prevent body odors. Recommend the use of deodorants and antiperspirants after the skin is clean. Deodorants eliminate odor by altering the pH of the skin to be more acidic, making it less attractive to bacteria (MFMER, 2019e). Antiperspirants contain aluminum-based compounds that temporarily block sweat pores, reducing the amount of perspiration that reaches the skin (MFMER, 2019e). Advise patients to use antiperspirants and deodorants with care and according to directions to prevent skin irritation. Keep in mind that these products are contraindicated in some situations; for example, before mammography and during the postoperative period for a patient who has a surgical wound under the arm, such as with a mastectomy.

COSMETICS

Cosmetics may be used to enhance the appearance of clean and healthy skin. Cosmetics may be used judiciously to help disguise blemishes, improve skin coloring, and make wrinkles appear less obvious. Some cultural and religious groups, however, may discourage their use.

Periodically, cosmetics containing harmful ingredients have appeared on the market. Be alert to such agents and help consumers avoid their use. The U.S. Department of Health and Human Services Food and Drug Administration (FDA) enforces federal laws on the purity of foods, drugs, and cosmetics and on the advertising claims of their manufacturers. The FDA is a good source of information regarding cosmetic safety. For example, the FDA maintains a list of color additives approved for use in cosmetics; encourage patients to check the ingredients of cosmetics, including color additives (FDA, 2017b).

Remind patients that cosmetics often become contaminated with bacteria and fungi. Teach patients not to share cosmetics and advise them to discard cosmetics after they are 2 to 4 months old, especially those applied near the eyes (FDA, 2016a). Encourage patients to keep makeup applicators and brushes immaculately clean.

SUNSCREEN

Spending time in the sun increases the risk of skin cancer and early skin aging (FDA, 2019b). Sun damage to the body is caused by invisible ultraviolet (UV) radiation. Patients of all skin tones are potentially at risk for sunburn and other harmful effects of exposure to UV radiation (FDA, 2019b). Everyone should take precautions to protect skin from sun damage. However, people who need to be especially careful in the sun are those who have pale skin; blond, red, or light brown hair; those who have been treated for skin cancer; or those who have a family member who's had skin cancer (FDA, 2019b). Others who need to be especially aware of sun-care precautions are patients who are prescribed certain medications that increase sun sensitivity, such as furosemide, glyburide, and quinolone antibiotics (e.g., ciprofloxacin). To reduce risk of sunburn and skin damage related to sun exposure, encourage patients to use sun protection measures. Refer to Box 32-4 for a list of suggested sun protection measures.

Box 32-4 Sun Protection Measures

Patients of all skin tones are potentially susceptible to sunburn and other harmful effects of exposure to UV radiation from the sun. Everyone should take precautions to protect skin from sun damage. To reduce risk of sunburn and skin damage related to sun exposure, encourage patients to use the following sun protection measures:

- Use broad-spectrum sunscreens with sun protection factor (SPF) values of 15 or higher regularly and as directed. Apply 15 minutes before you go outside for maximum benefit.
- Reapply sunscreen, even if labeled "water resistant," at least every 2 hours. Apply sunscreen more often if sweating, swimming, or jumping in and out of the water. Refer to individual product directions.
- Limit time in the sun, especially between the hours of 10 AM and 2 PM, when the sun's rays are most intense.
- Wear clothing to cover skin exposed to the sun; for example, long-sleeved shirts, pants, sunglasses, and broad-brimmed hats.
- Protect eyes with sunglasses. Choose sunglasses labeled with a UVA/UVB rating of 100%.
- Avoid using sunscreen for infants less than 6 months old. Keep infants under 6 months old out of the sun and in the shade. Dress infants in clothing that covers their sensitive skin, as well as a wide-brimmed hat.

Source: Adapted from U.S. Food and Drug Administration (FDA). (2019, August 29). *Sunscreen: How to help protect your skin from the sun.* https://www.fda.gov/drugs/understanding-over-counter-medicines/sunscreen-how-help-protect-your-skin-sun; U.S. Food and Drug Administration (FDA). (2019, February 21). *Tips to stay safe in the sun: From sunscreen to sunglasses.* https://www.fda.gov/consumers/consumer-updates/tips-stay-safe-sun-sunscreen-sunglasses; and U.S. Food and Drug Administration (FDA). (2016, July 6). *Should you put sunscreen on infants? Not usually.* https://www.fda.gov/consumers/consumer-updates/should-you-put-sunscreen-infants-not-usually

TICKS

Ticks are a significant problem because they can transmit serious diseases such as Lyme disease, Rocky Mountain spotted fever, and Colorado tick fever. Ticks attach themselves to a human host as the person brushes past leaves, brush, and tall grasses. Once on a person, ticks move to a warm and moist location, like the hairline, armpit, or groin, where they burrow into the host's skin and feed off the host's blood. Transmission of tick-borne diseases can be decreased if the tick is removed within 24 hours of becoming attached. To remove a tick, grasp it with clean fine-tipped tweezers close to the skin. Pull upward with steady, even pressure; do not twist or jerk the tick (CDC, 2019b). If mouth-parts break off and remain in the skin, remove the mouth-parts with the tweezer (CDC, 2019b). Once the tick is removed, cleanse the bite area and your hands with rubbing alcohol or soap and water (CDC, 2019b). Dispose of a live tick by putting it in alcohol, placing it in a sealed bag, wrapping tightly in tape, or flushing down the toilet (CDC, 2019b). A person should seek medical attention if a rash or fever develops within several weeks of removing a tick.

Information related to the prevention of tick bites is an important focus of patient education. Encourage patients to wear long sleeves, long pants, and long socks to help prevent ticks from coming in contact with the skin. Patients should apply insect repellent on clothing (permethrin) and exposed skin (product with at least 20% DEET) (National Institutes of Health [NIH], 2014). Clothing and skin should be checked frequently for ticks, which look like small black or brown spots. Encourage patients to bathe or shower as soon as possible after activities in an area where ticks are common and wash and/or dry clothes in a dryer on high heat (NIH).

Evaluating

Performing or assisting with the performance of hygiene measures provides a means of at least daily contact with the patient to determine whether the patient is achieving outcomes related to hygiene and skin care. Indicators that can be used to determine outcome achievement include the following:

- Level of patient's participation in hygiene program
- Elimination of, reduction in, or compensation for factors interfering with the patient's independent execution of hygiene measures; for example, weakness, decreased motivation, and lack of knowledge
- Changes related to specific skin problems; for example, healing of skin lesions, elimination or reduction in causative factors, and independent patient management of the prescribed treatment program

Ongoing evaluation helps adjust the plan of care. Refer to the accompanying Nursing Care Plan 32-1 (on pages 1118–1120) for Kylie Simpson and Female University Students for examples of the nursing process related to hygiene.

REFLECTIVE PRACTICE LEADING TO PERSONAL LEARNING

Remember that the goal of reflective practice is to look at an experience, understand it, and learn from it. As you begin to develop expertise in implementing hygiene measures, reflect on your experiences—successes and failures—in order to improve your practice. How can you do it better next time? What did you learn today that can help you tomorrow? Begin your reflection by paying close attention to the following while performing hygiene measures and providing nursing care:

- Did your commitment to engage your patients and families and to collaborate with your fellow students, instructor, and other members of the health care team as you implemented the plan of care result in successful partnerships?
- Did your preparation and practice related to performing interventions related to hygiene result in your feeling confident in your ability to provide care? Did your competence and confidence inspire the patient's and family's trust?
- How did you prioritize the data you collected? What patterns in the data did you identify? What knowledge from your learning, personal experience, and intuition did you use to make decisions and develop your plan of care?
- How confident are you that the data you reported and recorded accurately communicates the health status, health problems, issues, risks, and strengths of the patient? How successfully have you communicated this information to other members of the health care team?
- Were you aware of any cultural and/or ethnic beliefs or practices that may have influenced the patient's personal hygiene practices? Were you aware of any stereotypes or prejudices that might have negatively influenced the clinical encounter? If so, how did you address these issues?
- Did you need to modify the plan of care as a result of ongoing assessments? Did you think of better interventions to produce the expected outcomes?
- As you concluded your patient interactions, did the patient/family know your name, and know what to expect of you and your nursing care? Did the patient sense that you are respectful, caring, and competent to provide care?

Perhaps the most important questions to reflect on are: Are your patients and their families/caregivers better for having had *you* share in the critical responsibility of partnering with them to address their hygiene needs? Are your patients now receiving thoughtful, person-centered, prioritized, holistic, evidence-based treatment and care because of your efforts?

Nursing Care Plan for Kylie Simpson and University Students 32-1

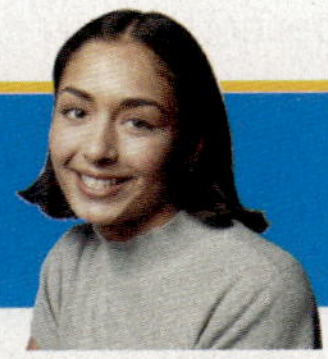

Glenda Davis is a nurse practitioner who works in a campus health clinic at a state university. Kylie Simpson met with Glenda Davis at the clinic. Kylie had been having vaginal itching and burning for 2 weeks. She was diagnosed with a vaginal infection. She asks Glenda, "This is terrible. It's the second infection in 7 months. Is there something wrong with me? Isn't there something I can do to keep this from happening again?"

Frequently, students ask Glenda questions about personal hygiene. Realizing that each student who presents with a question probably represents many other students with similar unvoiced questions, Glenda talks with Kylie, including patient teaching regarding personal hygiene and sexual health in their discussion. Glenda decides to develop an insert entitled *Self-Care: Personal Hygiene/Sexual Health* for the campus newspaper. The information she plans to include and the population she will address in her checklist are based on the following assessment data:

- Diverse population of various ages, cultures, religions, gender identities, sexual orientation, and family and lifestyle backgrounds.
- Knowledge about personal hygiene/sexual health varies widely from almost no knowledge to students who are well read or members of health professions.
- Students who present with questions are mostly concerned about the risk of acquiring a sexually transmitted infection (STI) or the dangers of certain products (e.g., tampons and toxic shock syndrome), or have questions related to intercourse and contraception.
- Numerous students report to the clinic with vaginal infections and urinary tract infections.
- Interest is high; ability to comprehend written materials is high.

Nursing Care Plan for Kylie Simpson and University Students 32-1 (continued)

HEALTH PROBLEM/NEED

Knowledge Deficiency: Personal hygiene/sexual health

Etiology: Information misinterpretation, lack of exposure, and unfamiliarity with information resources

Signs/Symptoms: Students presenting to the campus clinic with questions about personal hygiene/sexual health; high incidence of vaginal and urinary tract infections; negative attitudes about body frequently expressed

EXPECTED OUTCOME

Students will:

- express positive body image, valuing their uniqueness.

NURSING INTERVENTIONS	RATIONALE	EVALUATIVE STATEMENT
With each student who presents at the clinic for help with a gynecologic/sexual health concern or problem, take the time to assess their knowledge of the body and acceptance of their body and comfort with it.	The sexual health movement has encouraged feelings of ownership of their bodies, to appreciate their uniqueness, and to increase their awareness of their physical bodies and the feelings associated with them. Students may still feel that the genital area and cyclic phenomena such as the menstrual cycle and the sexual response cycle are "dirty"; and symptoms in this area may evoke fear, guilt, anxiety, and shame.	*Six-month evaluation:* 6/30/25 Outcome partially met: Students are beginning to discuss personal and sexual health concerns more freely, yet great hesitance persists. *G. Davis, RN*
Revision: Continue to help students to know, understand, and accept their bodies and to talk about their bodies. Make this a priority of the nursing staff at the clinic.		
Counsel appropriately.	It is important for nurses to provide students with information about their bodies.	

EXPECTED OUTCOME

Students will:

- correctly describe hygiene self-care behaviors they are willing to incorporate into their daily lifestyles.

NURSING INTERVENTIONS	RATIONALE	EVALUATIVE STATEMENT
Assess with each patient their knowledge of hygiene practices (correct any misconceptions) and motivation to use them consistently.	Many women have never been instructed about hygiene, and harmful practices may be "picked up" from the media and other sources (e.g., the use of frequent douching and deodorants to eliminate normal body odors).	6/30/25 Outcome met. Following publication of the *Self-Care: Feminine Hygiene* feature and one-on-one counseling using this printed handout, patients are knowledgeable about preventive hygiene measures. *G. Davis, RN*
Address specific concerns related to menstruation, intercourse, sexual health, other maturational events.	Maturational events, such as menstruation, becoming sexually active, and pregnancy, may result in a need for new or modified hygiene practices.	

(continued on page 1120)

Nursing Care Plan for Kylie Simpson and University Students 32-1 (continued)

NURSING INTERVENTIONS	RATIONALE	EVALUATIVE STATEMENT
Teach the importance of using preventive hygiene measures to reduce the likelihood of acquiring a urinary tract or vaginal infection. Distribute the *Self-Care: Personal Hygiene/Sexual Health* handout and discuss this with the patient.	It is better to prevent a genitourinary infection than to treat it.	

EXPECTED OUTCOME

Campus health clinic records will:

- demonstrate a reduction in both new and recurrent genitourinary infections.

NURSING INTERVENTIONS	RATIONALE	EVALUATIVE STATEMENT
Educate students regarding preventive hygiene measures (refer to the *Self-Care* handout).	It is better to prevent a genitourinary infection than to treat it.	6/30/25 Outcome met. Six months after publication and use of the *Self-Care: Personal Hygiene/Sexual Health* handout, the incidence of genitourinary infections is reduced 10%. Will continue to keep education in this regard a priority. *G. Davis, RN*
Educate students to distinguish normal from abnormal findings (vaginal discharge, pain, bleeding, problems with urination) and to seek help when appropriate. Nursing measures include teaching preventive measures, instructing in recognition of symptoms, and assisting with self-care activities to prevent and treat infections, including the securing of assistance when indicated.	Early treatment of genitourinary infections reduces the likelihood of residual problems.	
Document new and recurrent genitourinary infections; identify predisposing factors.	Documentation facilitates ongoing management of a recurring problem.	

SAMPLE DOCUMENTATION

6/15/25

Nursing student visited clinic and expressed need for information about feminine hygiene practices in general as well as those specific hygiene measures for use after intercourse. Also related concern about contracting an STI from partners. Reported that she became sexually active this year and has sexual intercourse once or twice weekly. Stated that "many of my friends use douches" and questioned whether any particular douche products are recommended. Discussed the *Self-Care: Feminine Hygiene* handout and reviewed various health care practices. Clarified for student her misconception regarding the advisability of douching. Also counseled her about her right to talk with a sexual partner about STIs and previous contacts with infected people. Advised that she refrain from contact or use a condom when she has intercourse. Student reported feeling more "in charge" of body and better able to care for it. Discussed all topics on care plan and encouraged her to revisit clinic in 6 months for further clarification and evaluation.

G. Davis, RN

Skill 32-1 Providing a Bed Bath

DELEGATION CONSIDERATIONS

The implementation of a bed bath may be delegated to assistive personnel (AP) as well as to licensed practical/vocational nurses (LPN/LVNs). The decision to delegate must be based on careful analysis of the patient's needs and circumstances as well as the qualifications of the person to whom the task is being delegated. Refer to the Delegation Guidelines in Appendix A.

EQUIPMENT

- Washbasin and warm water
- Personal hygiene supplies (deodorant, lotion, and others)
- Skin-cleaning agent
- Emollient and skin barrier, as indicated
- Towels (2)
- Washcloths (2)
- Bath blanket
- Gown, pajamas, or appropriate clothing
- Bedpan or urinal
- Laundry bag
- Nonsterile gloves; other PPE, as indicated

IMPLEMENTATION

ACTION	RATIONALE
1. Review the patient's health record for any limitations in physical activity.	Identifying limitations prevents patient discomfort and injury.
2. Perform hand hygiene and put on gloves and/or other PPE, if indicated.	Hand hygiene and PPE prevent the spread of microorganisms. PPE is required based on transmission precautions.
3. Identify the patient. Discuss the procedure with the patient and assess the patient's ability to assist in the bathing process, as well as personal hygiene preferences.	Identifying the patient ensures the right patient receives the intervention and helps prevent errors. Discussion promotes reassurance and provides knowledge about the procedure. Dialogue encourages patient participation and allows for individualized nursing care.
4. Assemble equipment on the overbed table or other surface within reach.	Organization facilitates performance of the task.
5. Close the curtains around the bed and close the door to the room, if possible. Adjust the room temperature, if necessary.	This ensures the patient's privacy and lessens the risk for loss of body heat during the bath.
6. Adjust the bed to a comfortable working height (VHA Center for Engineering & Occupational Safety and Health [VHACEOSH], 2016).	Having the bed at the proper height prevents back and muscle strain.
7. Remove sequential compression devices and graduated compression (antiembolism) stockings from lower extremities according to facility protocol.	Most manufacturers and facilities recommend removal of these devices before the bath to allow for assessment.
8. Put on gloves. Offer the patient a bedpan or urinal.	Gloves are necessary for potential contact with blood or body fluids. Voiding or defecating before the bath lessens the likelihood that the bath will be interrupted, because warm bath water may stimulate the urge to void.
9. Remove gloves and perform hand hygiene.	Hand hygiene deters the spread of microorganisms.
10. Put on a clean pair of gloves. Lower the side rail nearest to you and assist the patient to the side of bed where you will work. Have the patient lie on their back.	Gloves prevent transmission of microorganisms. Having the patient positioned near the nurse and lowering the side rail prevent unnecessary stretching and twisting of muscles on the part of the nurse.
11. Loosen top covers and remove all except the top sheet. Place a bath blanket over the patient and then remove the top sheet while the patient holds the bath blanket in place. If linen is to be reused, fold it over a chair. Place soiled linen in laundry bag. Take care to prevent linen from coming in contact with your clothing.	This ensures that the patient is not exposed unnecessarily, and warmth is maintained. If a bath blanket is unavailable, the top sheet may be used in its place.

(continued on page 1122)

Skill 32-1 Providing a Bed Bath *(continued)*

ACTION	RATIONALE
12. Remove the patient's gown or clothing and keep the bath blanket in place. If the patient has an IV line and is not wearing a gown with snap sleeves, remove gown from the other arm first. Pause the infusion pump and remove the tubing from the pump. Lower the IV container and pass the gown over the tubing and the container. **Rehang the IV container and insert the tubing into the infusion pump. Check the rate on the infusion pump and restart.**	This provides uncluttered access during the bath and maintains warmth of the patient. IV fluids must be maintained at the prescribed rate.
13. **Raise side rails and lower the bed.** Fill basin with a sufficient amount of comfortably warm water (no more than 120°F [49° C]). Add the skin cleanser, if appropriate, according to the manufacturer's directions. Change, as necessary, throughout the bath.	Side rails and lower bed height maintain patient safety. Adjusting the water temperature to no more than 120°F (49° C) decreases risk of burns and drying of the skin (International Association of Fire Fighters [IAFF], n.d.). Warm water is comfortable and relaxing for the patient. It also stimulates circulation and provides for more effective cleansing.
14. Raise the bed to a comfortable working height and lower the side rail nearest to you when you return to the bedside to begin the bath. Put on gloves, if indicated. Lay a towel across the patient's chest and on top of bath blanket.	Having the bed at the proper height prevents back and muscle strain. Gloves are necessary if there is potential contact with blood or body fluids. The towel prevents chilling and keeps the bath blanket dry.
15. With no cleanser on the washcloth, wipe one eye from the inner part of the eye, near the nose, to the outer part (Figure 1). Rinse or turn the cloth before washing the other eye.	Cleanser may be irritating to the eyes. Moving from the inner to the outer aspect of the eye prevents carrying debris toward the nasolacrimal duct. Rinsing or turning the washcloth prevents spreading organisms from one eye to the other.
16. Bathe the patient's face, neck, and ears. Apply appropriate emollient.	Use of emollients is recommended to restore and maintain skin integrity (Haesler et al., 2018; Lichterfeld et al., 2015; Voegeli, 2019).
17. Expose the patient's far arm and place towel lengthwise under it. Using firm strokes, wash hand, arm, and axilla, lifting the arm as necessary to access axillary region (Figure 2). Rinse, if necessary, and dry. Apply appropriate emollient. Cover the area with the bath blanket.	The towel helps to keep the bed dry. Washing the far side first eliminates contaminating a clean area once it is washed. Gentle friction stimulates circulation and muscles and helps remove dirt, oil, and organisms. Long, firm strokes are relaxing and more comfortable than short, uneven strokes. Rinsing is necessary when using some cleansing products. Use of emollients is recommended to restore and maintain skin integrity (Haesler et al., 2018; Lichterfeld et al., 2015; Voegeli, 2019). Re-covering the body maintains warmth.

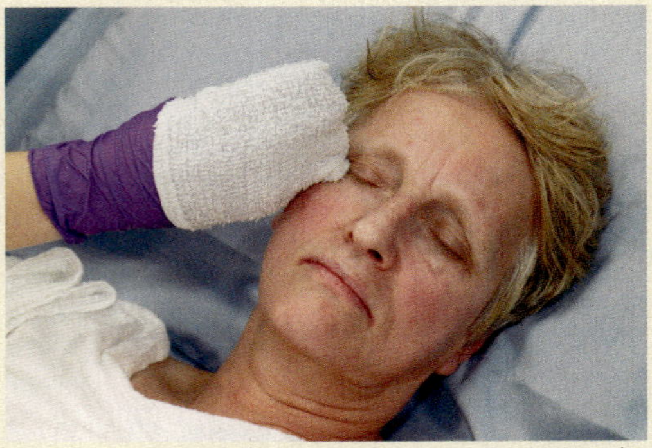

FIGURE 1. Washing from the inner corner of the eye outward.

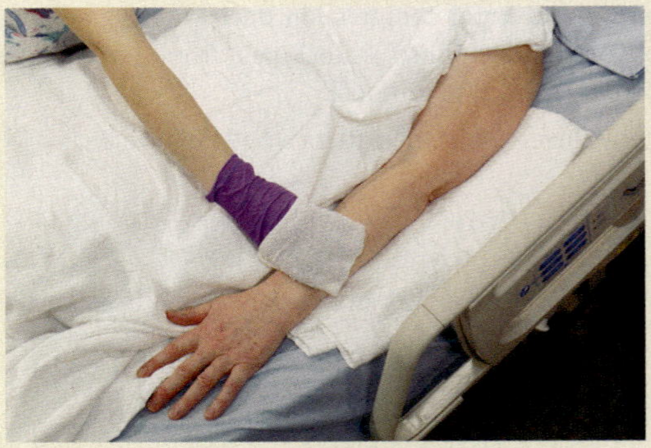

FIGURE 2. Exposing the far arm and washing it.

ACTION	RATIONALE
18. Repeat Step 17 for the arm nearest you. Another option might be to bathe one side of the patient first and then move to the other side of the bed to complete the bath.	
19. Spread a towel across the patient's chest. Lower the bath blanket to the patient's umbilical area. Wash, rinse, if necessary, and dry chest. Keep chest covered with towel between the wash and rinse. Pay special attention to the folds of skin under the breasts. Apply appropriate emollient.	Exposing, washing, rinsing, and drying one part of the body at a time avoids unnecessary exposure and chilling. Areas of skin folds may be sources of odor and skin breakdown if not cleaned and dried properly. Use of emollients is recommended to restore and maintain skin integrity (Haesler et al., 2018; Lichterfeld et al., 2015; Voegeli, 2019).

ACTION

RATIONALE

20. Lower the bath blanket to the perineal area. Place a towel over the patient's chest.

Keeping the bath blanket and towel in place avoids exposure and chilling.

21. Wash, rinse, if necessary, and dry abdomen (Figure 3). Carefully inspect and clean umbilical area and any abdominal folds or creases. Apply appropriate emollient.

Skin-fold areas may be sources of odor and skin breakdown if not cleaned and dried properly. Use of emollients is recommended to restore and maintain skin integrity (Haesler et al., 2018; Lichterfeld et al., 2015; Voegeli, 2019).

22. Return bath blanket to original position and expose far leg. Place towel under far leg. Using firm strokes, wash, rinse, if necessary, and dry leg from ankle to knee and knee to groin (Figure 4). Apply appropriate emollient.

The towel protects linens and prevents the patient from feeling uncomfortable from a damp or wet bed. Washing from ankle to groin with firm strokes promotes venous return. Use of emollients is recommended to restore and maintain skin integrity (Haesler et al., 2018; Lichterfeld et al., 2015; Voegeli, 2019).

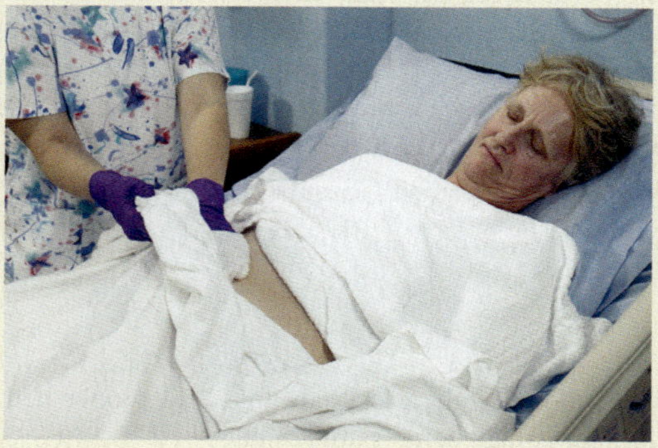

FIGURE 3. Washing the abdomen, with perineal and chest areas covered.

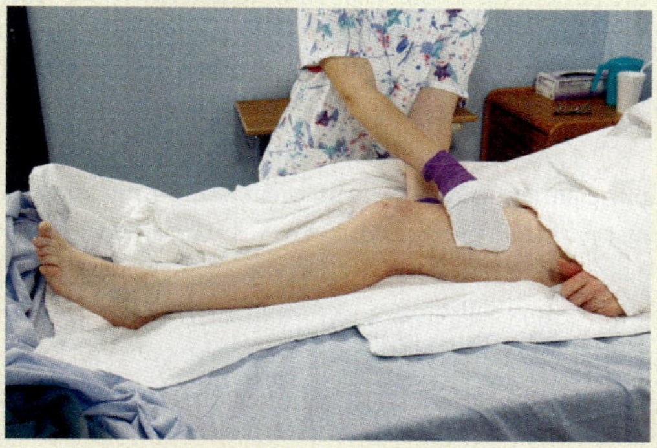

FIGURE 4. Washing and drying far leg, keeping the other leg covered.

23. Wash, rinse if necessary, and dry the foot. Pay particular attention to the areas between toes. Apply appropriate emollient.

Drying of the feet is important to prevent irritation, possible skin breakdown, and infections (Beuscher, 2019). Use of emollients is recommended to restore and maintain skin integrity (Haesler et al., 2018; Lichterfeld et al., 2015; Voegeli, 2019).

24. Repeat Steps 22 and 23 for the other leg and foot.

25. Make sure the patient is covered with the bath blanket. Change water and washcloth at this point or earlier, if necessary.

The bath blanket maintains warmth and privacy. Clean, warm water prevents chilling and maintains patient comfort.

26. Assist the patient to a prone or side-lying position. Put on gloves, if not applied earlier. Position bath blanket and towel to expose only the back and buttocks.

Positioning the towel and bath blanket protects the patient's privacy and provides warmth. Gloves prevent contact with body fluids.

27. Wash, rinse, if necessary, and dry back and buttocks area (Figure 5). **Pay particular attention to cleansing between gluteal folds and observe for any redness or skin breakdown in the sacral area.**

Fecal material near the anus may be a source of microorganisms. Prolonged pressure on the sacral area or other bony prominences may compromise circulation and lead to development of decubitus ulcer.

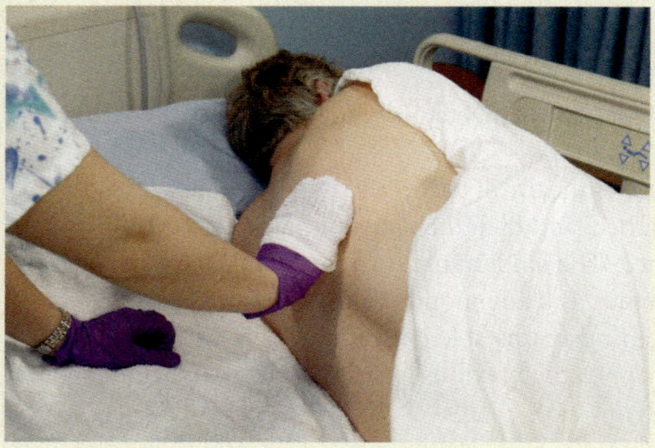

FIGURE 5. Washing the back.

(continued on page 1124)

Skill 32-1 Providing a Bed Bath *(continued)*

ACTION	RATIONALE
28. If not contraindicated, give the patient a backrub. Alternatively, back massage may be given after perineal care. Apply appropriate emollient and/or skin barrier product.	A backrub improves circulation to the tissues and is an aid to relaxation. A backrub may be contraindicated in patients with cardiovascular disease or musculoskeletal injuries. Use of emollients is recommended to restore and maintain skin integrity (Haesler et al., 2018; Lichterfeld et al., 2015; Voegeli, 2019). Skin barriers protect the skin from damage caused by excessive exposure to water and irritants, such as urine and feces (Williamson, 2020; Voegeli, 2019).
29. Remove gloves. Raise the side rail. Refill basin with clean water. Discard washcloth and towel. Put on clean gloves.	The washcloth, towel, and water are contaminated after washing the patient's gluteal area. Changing to clean supplies decreases the spread of organisms from the anal area to the genitals.
30. Set the patient up so they can complete perineal self-care. If the patient is unable to complete self-care, lower the side rail and complete perineal care. Apply skin barrier, as indicated. Raise the side rail, remove gloves, and perform hand hygiene.	Providing perineal self-care may decrease embarrassment for the patient. Effective perineal care reduces odor and decreases the risk for infection through contamination. Skin barriers protect the skin from damage caused by excessive exposure to water and irritants, such as urine and feces.
31. Help the patient put on a clean gown or clothing and assist with the use of other personal toiletries, such as deodorant or cosmetics. If the gown does not have snap sleeves and the patient has an IV, follow the steps in Action 12 to replace the gown.	This provides for the patient's warmth and comfort.
32. Protect pillow with towel, and groom the patient's hair.	
33. **When finished, make sure the patient is comfortable, with the side rails up and the bed in the lowest position.**	Proper positioning with raised side rails and proper bed height provides for patient comfort and safety.
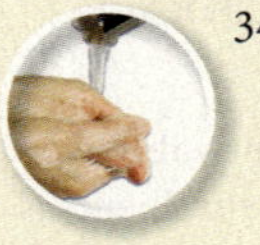 34. Change bed linens, as described in Skills 32-4 and 32-5. Dispose of soiled linens according to facility policy. Clean bath basin according to facility policy before returning to storage at bedside. Remove gloves and any other PPE, if used. Perform hand hygiene.	Proper disposal of linens and cleaning of bath basin reduce the risk for transmission of microorganisms. Proper removal of PPE reduces the risk for infection transmission and contamination of other items. Hand hygiene prevents the spread of microorganisms.

DOCUMENTATION

Guidelines

Record any significant observations and communication. Document the condition of the patient's skin. Record the procedure, amount of assistance given, and patient participation. Document the application of skin care products, such as a skin barrier.

Sample Documentation

> 07/06/2025 2130 Bath provided with complete assistance; reddened area (3 cm × 3 cm) noted on patient's sacral area; skin-care team consultation made.
>
> *—C. Stone, RN*

DEVELOPING CLINICAL REASONING AND CLINICAL JUDGMENT

UNEXPECTED SITUATIONS AND ASSOCIATED INTERVENTIONS

- *Patient becomes chilled during the bath:* If the room temperature is adjustable, increase it. Another bath blanket may be needed.
- *Patient becomes unstable during the bath:* Critically ill patients may need to be bathed in stages. For instance, the right arm is bathed, and then the patient is allowed to rest for a short period before the left arm is bathed. The amount of rest time needed depends on how unstable the patient is and which parameter is being monitored. For example, the nurse may watch the blood pressure while bathing an unstable patient and stop when it begins to decrease. Once the blood pressure returns to the previous level, the nurse can begin to bathe the patient again.

SPECIAL CONSIDERATIONS

General Considerations

- To remove the gown without snap sleeves from a patient with an IV line, take the gown off the uninvolved arm first, then pause the infusion pump and remove the tubing from the pump. Lower the IV container and pass the gown over the tubing and the container. **Rehang the IV container and insert the tubing into the infusion pump. Check the rate on the infusion pump and restart.** To replace the gown, follow the same steps, placing the clean gown on the unaffected arm first. **Never disconnect IV tubing to change a gown, because this causes a break in a sterile system and could introduce microorganisms.**
- Patients with bariatric care needs are at increased risk for skin integrity issues, including increased risk for alterations in skin integrity (Earlam & Woods, 2020; Williamson, 2020). Assess the skin of bariatric inpatients twice a day, lifting and separating the folds of skin to assess the area, utilizing extra help as necessary (Black & Hotaling, 2015). Nonsoap cleansers should be used, and the skin should be dried to prevent retained moisture (Black & Hotaling, 2015; Williamson, 2020).
- When bathing a patient, the wipe or washcloth removes some of the outermost skin layer. This sloughed skin may be evident on the wipe or washcloth and in the bathwater and will vary in color depending on the ethnic group of the patient (Andrews et al., 2020). This is important to note, as this does not mean that the patient was dirty—the normal sloughing of the skin is more evident in darkly pigmented people compared with patients with lighter pigmentation (Andrews et al., 2020).
- Lying flat in bed during the bed bath may be contraindicated for certain patients. The position may have to be modified to accommodate their needs.
- Incontinent patients require special attention to perineal care. Patients with urinary or fecal incontinence are at risk for incontinence-associated dermatitis (perineal dermatitis), one type of moisture-associated skin damage (MASD) (Voegeli, 2019). Remove soil and irritants from the skin during routine hygiene as well as cleansing when the skin becomes exposed to irritants (Voegeli, 2019). Avoid using soap and excessive force for cleaning (Wounds UK, 2018). Use perineal skin cleansers, moisturizers, and moisture barriers for skin care for these patients to promote healing and prevent further skin damage (Voegeli, 2019).
- If the patient has an indwelling catheter, use mild soap and water or a perineal cleanser to clean the perineal area; rinse the area well. Do not clean the periurethral area with antiseptics to prevent CAUTI while the catheter is in place (Gould et al., 2019). Routine hygiene (cleansing of the meatal surface during daily bathing or showering) is appropriate (Gould et al., 2019). Inspect the meatus for drainage and note the characteristics of the urine. Do not use powders and lotions after cleaning.
- The use of chlorhexidine gluconate (CHG) for bathing has been shown to reduce colonization of skin with pathogens and is an important measure utilized by institutions in an attempt to decrease health care–associated infections (HAIs), such as central line–associated bloodstream infections and surgical site infections (Hines et al., 2015; Martinez et al., 2020; Musuuza et al., 2019; Urias et al., 2018). Some facilities' policies include the use of CHG for all inpatient bathing, expect for patients with a history of CHG allergy or intolerance or those age less than 2 months (Hines et al., 2015). Chlorhexidine can be added to bath water but is also available in prepackaged impregnated cloths.
- If applying lotion, warm the lotion in your hands before applying it to the patient to prevent chilling.
- Soaking the patient's hands in a basin of water is an additional comfort measure for the patient. It facilitates thorough washing of the hands and between the fingers and aids in removing debris from under the nails. If appropriate and as indicated, place a folded towel on the bed next to the patient's hand and put the basin of water on it. Wash, rinse if necessary, and dry hand. Apply appropriate emollient. Use of emollients is recommended to restore and maintain skin integrity (Haesler et al., 2018; Lichterfeld et al., 2015; Voegeli, 2019).
- Basic wound care used for body piercings is usually called "aftercare." Aftercare techniques are used for the new piercing and whenever the piercing fistula has become disrupted through injury or exhibits signs of infection or inflammation (Association of Professional Piercers, 2020; Mayo Foundation for Medical Education and Research, 2020b). Clean the site with mild soap and warm water or normal saline solution (American Academy of Family Physicians, 2019). Use a cotton swab to gently remove any crusting. Rinse well.

(*continued on page 1126*)

Skill 32-1 Providing a Bed Bath *(continued)*

Infant and Child Considerations

- When bathing an infant or young child, have supplies within easy reach, and support or hold the child securely at all times to ensure safety.
- Never leave the child alone.
- Consider bathing a newborn using a reverse-order procedure, from "trunk to head," wetting the infant's head last to reduce the amount of time the infant's head is wet. The method supports a more rapid recovery of body temperature and decreased heat loss from evaporation during bathing (So et al., 2014).
- Delaying the newborn bath for 24 hours has been associated with multiple benefits, including increased likelihood of exclusive breastfeeding at discharge and decreased incidence of hypothermia and hypoglycemia in healthy newborns (Warren et al., 2020).

Older Adult Considerations

- Check the temperature of the water carefully before bathing an older adult, because sensitivity to temperature may be impaired in older adults.
- An older continent patient may not require a full bed bath with soap and water every day. If dry skin is a problem, water and skin lotion or bath oil may be used on alternate days.

Community-Based Care Considerations

- Use plastic trash bags or a plastic shower-curtain liner to protect the mattress when bathing or shampooing a patient in bed. Disposable washcloths may also be an option to consider. A large plastic container or baby bathtub can effectively serve as a shampoo basin.
- If linens are soiled with blood or body fluids, instruct family members/caregivers to wear gloves when handling them. The linens should be rinsed first in cold water and then washed separately from other household wash, using hot water, laundry detergent, and bleach.
- Teach a family member or caregivers how to perform comfort measures, such as a backrub.
- If patients are home with an indwelling catheter, instruct them or their caregivers to wash the urinary meatus and perineal area with mild soap and water.

Skill 32-2 Assisting the Patient With Oral Care

DELEGATION CONSIDERATIONS

The implementation of oral care may be delegated to assistive personnel (AP) as well as to licensed practical/vocational nurses (LPN/LVNs). The decision to delegate must be based on careful analysis of the patient's needs and circumstances as well as the qualifications of the person to whom the task is being delegated. Refer to the Delegation Guidelines in Appendix A.

EQUIPMENT

- Toothbrush
- Toothpaste
- Emesis basin
- Glass with cool water
- Disposable gloves
- Additional PPE, as indicated
- Towel
- Mouth rinse
- Washcloth or paper towel
- Lip lubricant (optional)
- Dental floss or other interdental cleaner
- Oral assessment tool, as indicated (Figure 1)

IMPLEMENTATION

ACTION	RATIONALE
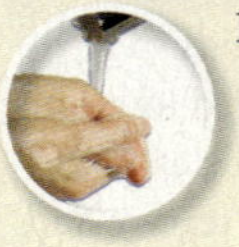 1. Perform hand hygiene and put on gloves if assisting with oral care, and/or other PPE, if indicated.	Hand hygiene and PPE prevent the spread of microorganisms. PPE is required based on transmission precautions.
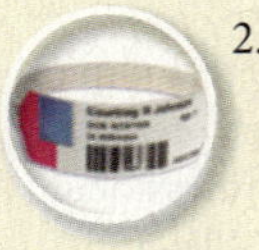 2. Identify the patient. Explain the procedure to the patient.	Identifying the patient ensures the right patient receives the intervention and helps prevent errors. Explanation facilitates engagement in care.
3. Assemble equipment on the overbed table or other surface within the patient's reach.	Organization facilitates performance of the task.

Oral Health Assessment Tool (OHAT) - Modified
Mouth Care Without a Battle©

Person Assessed:________________________ Assessed by:________________________ Date: ______________

For each category, circle the one best description. Then, in the column marked score, write the points for the assessment. Add the points in the bottom row. Problems ***underlined and in bold*** *are indications for immediate referral to a dentist, as they may represent a serious condition. For nursing home residents, problems in* ***bold*** *may require documentation on the MDS 3.0 and may trigger the Dental Care CAA, regardless of the total score.*

Category	0 = Healthy	1 = Minor Problems	2 = Major Problems	Score*
Lips	Smooth, pink, moist	Dry, chapped, or red at corners	**New or growing lump, ulcer, or lesion; white, red, and/or ulcerated patch; bleeding and/or ulcer at corners**	
Gums, palate, and insides of cheeks	Pink, moist, smooth, no bleeding	Dry, shiny, rough, red, and/or swollen area; **one small ulcer, lesion, and/or sore spot under dentures**	<u>**Swollen, tender area around a tooth or tooth root (suspected abscess);**</u> **swollen and/or bleeding ulcer; white, red and/or ulcerated patch; small pimple-like area with pus; widespread redness under dentures**	
Natural teeth	No decay or broken or worn down teeth	1-3 decayed or broken and/or very worn down teeth	<u>**One or more very loose teeth;**</u> **4 or more decayed or broken or very worn down teeth; fewer than 4 teeth**	
Dentures	No broken areas; teeth, dentures are regularly worn, and dentures are labeled with name	**1 broken area or tooth; denture loose, but adhesive not needed; denture uncleanable; denture not labeled with name;** dentures only worn for 1-2 hrs daily	**More than 1 broken area or tooth; denture so loose adhesive needed;** denture missing or not worn	
Quality of tooth hygiene	Clean and no food particles or tartar in mouth or on dentures	Food particles, tartar, and/or plaque in 1-2 areas of the mouth or on small area of dentures; bad breath (halitosis)	Food particles, tartar, and/or plaque in most areas of the mouth or on most of dentures; severe bad breath (halitosis)	
Tooth pain	No behavioral, verbal, or physical signs of dental pain	**Nonspecific verbal and/or behavioral signs of pain such as pulling at face, chewing lips, or not eating; unexplained aggression**	**Physical signs of pain (swelling of cheek or gum, broken teeth, ulcers); verbal and/or behavioral signs of pain specific to the mouth**	
Saliva / dry mouth	Moist tissues, watery and free flowing saliva	Dry, sticky tissues, little saliva present; person complains of dry mouth	Tissues parched and red; very little/no saliva present; saliva is thick	
Tongue	Normal, moist, roughness, pink	Patchy, fissured, red, coated	Patch that is red and/or white, ulcerated, and/or swollen	
			Total Score	

FIGURE 1. Oral Health Assessment Tool (OHAT). (Mouth Care Without a Battle, UNC Cecil G. Sheps Center for Health Services Research. Used by Permission.) *(continued)*

(*continued on page 1128*)

Skill 32-2 Assisting the Patient With Oral Care *(continued)*

Oral Health Assessment Tool (OHAT)

Patient: ______________________ **Scores at admission and regular reviews (date):** ______________

Completed by: ______________________

Category	0 = healthy	1 = changes*	2 = unhealthy*	Dates					
Lips	Smooth, pink, moist	Dry, chapped, or red at corners*	Swelling or lump, white/red/ulcerated patch: bleeding/ulcerated at corners						
Tongue	Normal, moist roughness, pink	Patchy, fissured, red, coated	Patch that is red &/or white, ulcerated, swollen						
Gums and tissues	Pink, moist, smooth, no bleeding	Dry, shiny, rough, red, swollen, one ulcer/sore spot under dentures	Swollen, bleeding, ulcers/white/red patches, generalized redness under dentures						
Saliva	Moist tissues, watery and free flowing saliva	Dry, sticky tissues, little saliva present, resident thinks they have dry mouth	Tissues parched and red, very little/no saliva present, saliva is thick, resident thinks they have a dry mouth						
Natural teeth Yes/No	No decayed or broken teeth/roots	1–3 decayed or broken teeth/roots or very worn down teeth	4+ decayed or broken teeth/roots, or very worn down teeth, or less than 4 teeth						
Dentures Yes/No	No broken areas or teeth, dentures regularly worn and labeled with name of resident	1 broken area/tooth or dentures only worn for 1-2 hours daily, or dentures not labeled with name, or loose	More than 1 broken area/tooth, denture missing or not worn, loose and needs denture adhesive or not labeled with name						
Oral cleanliness	Clean and no food particles or tartar in mouth or dentures	Food particles/tartar/plaque in 1–2 areas of the mouth or on small area of dentures or **halitosis** (bad breath)	Food particles/tartar/plaque in most areas of the mouth or on most of dentures or severe halitosis (bad breath)						
Dental pain	No behavioral, verbal, or physical signs of dental pain	Verbal &/or behavioral signs of pain such as pulling at face, chewing lips, not eating, aggression	Physical pain signs (swelling of cheek or gum, broken teeth, ulcers), as well as verbal &/or behavioral signs (pulling at face, not eating, aggression)						

Total Score: ______ ___/16 ___/16 ___/16 ___/16 ___/16 ___/16

_____ Arrange for resident to have a dental examination by a dentist

_____ Resident and/or family/guardian refused dental treatment

_____ Complete Oral Hygiene Care Plan and start oral hygiene care interventions for resident

_____ Review this resident's oral health again on: ____________

*If 1 or 2 scored for any category, please arrange for a dentist to examine the resident
Modified from Kayser-Jones et al., (1995) by Chalmers (2000b); Chalmers, King et al., (2005); Chalmers et al., (2004)

FIGURE 1. *(continued)*

ACTION	RATIONALE
4. Close the room door or curtains. Place the bed at an appropriate and comfortable working height (VHACEOSH, 2016).	Closing the door or curtains provides privacy. Proper bed height helps reduce back strain while performing the procedure.
5. Lower the side rail and assist the patient to a sitting position, if permitted, or turn the patient onto their side. Place a towel across the patient's chest.	The sitting or side-lying position prevents aspiration of fluids into the lungs. The towel protects the patient from dampness.
6. Encourage the patient to brush their own teeth according to the following guidelines. Assist, if necessary.	
a. Moisten the toothbrush and apply toothpaste to bristles.	Water softens the bristles.
b. Place the brush at a 45-degree angle to gum line (Figure 2) and brush from gum line to crown of each tooth (Figure 3). Brush outer and inner surfaces. Brush back and forth across the biting surface of each tooth.	Facilitates removal of **plaque** and **tartar**. The 45-degree angle of brushing permits cleansing of all tooth surface areas.
c. Brush the tongue gently with toothbrush or tongue scraper (MFMER, 2019a) (Figure 4).	This removes coating on the tongue. Gentle motion does not stimulate the gag reflex.
d. Have the patient rinse vigorously with water and spit into emesis basin (Figure 5). Repeat until clear. Suction may be used as an alternative for removal of fluid and secretions from the mouth.	The vigorous swishing motion helps to remove debris. Suction is appropriate if the patient is unable to expectorate well.

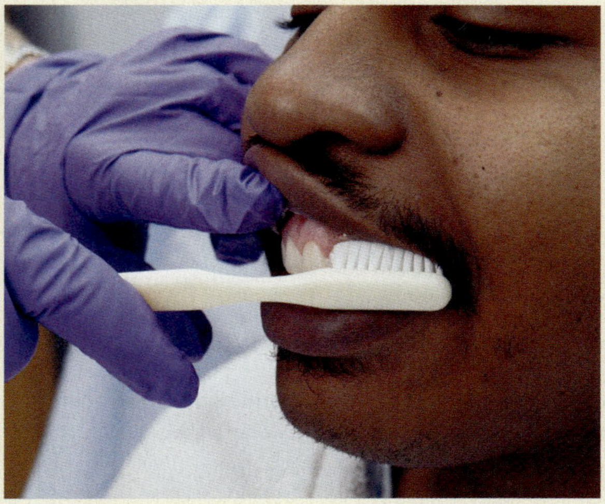

FIGURE 2. Placing brush at a 45-degree angle to gum line.

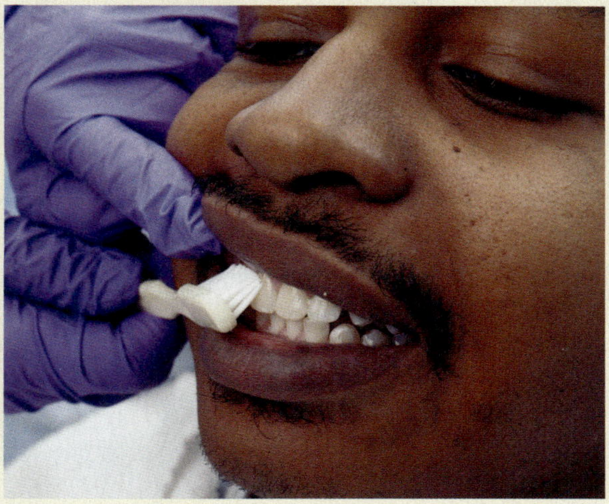

FIGURE 3. Brushing from gum line to the crown of each tooth.

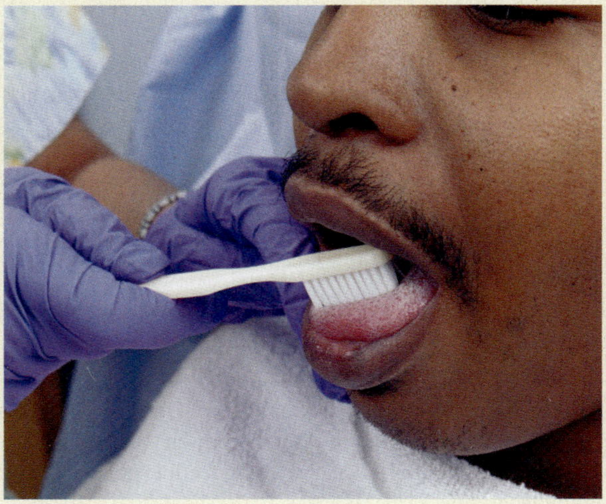

FIGURE 4. Brushing tongue.

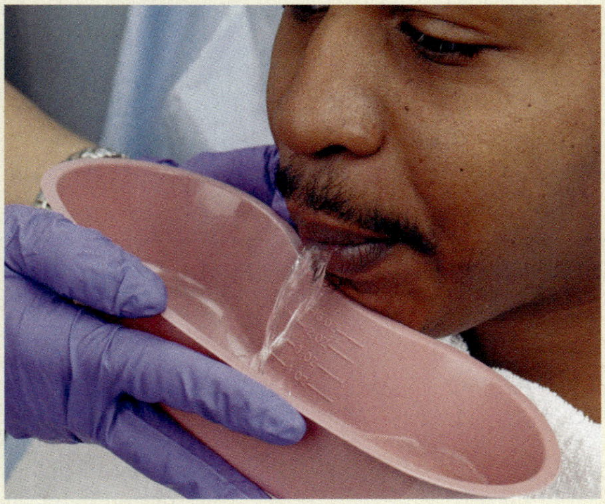

FIGURE 5. Holding emesis basin for patient to rinse and spit.

(*continued on page 1130*)

Skill 32-2 Assisting the Patient With Oral Care *(continued)*

ACTION	RATIONALE
7. Assist the patient to floss their teeth, if appropriate:	Flossing aids in removal of food and plaque and promotes healthy gum tissue (American Dental Association [ADA], n.d.b).
a. Remove approximately 18 inches of dental floss from container or use a plastic floss holder. Wrap most of the floss around one of the middle fingers. Wind the remaining floss around the same finger of the opposite hand, keeping about 1 to 1.5 inches of floss taut between the fingers.	The floss must be held taut to get between the teeth.
b. Insert floss gently between teeth, moving it back and forth downward to the gums.	Trauma to the gums can occur if floss is forced between teeth.
c. Move the floss up and down, first on one side of a tooth and then on the side of the other tooth, until the surfaces are clean (Figure 6). Repeat in the spaces between all teeth and the backside of the last teeth.	This ensures that the sides of both teeth are cleaned.
d. Instruct the patient to rinse mouth well with water after flossing.	Vigorous rinsing helps to remove food particles and plaque that have been loosened by flossing.

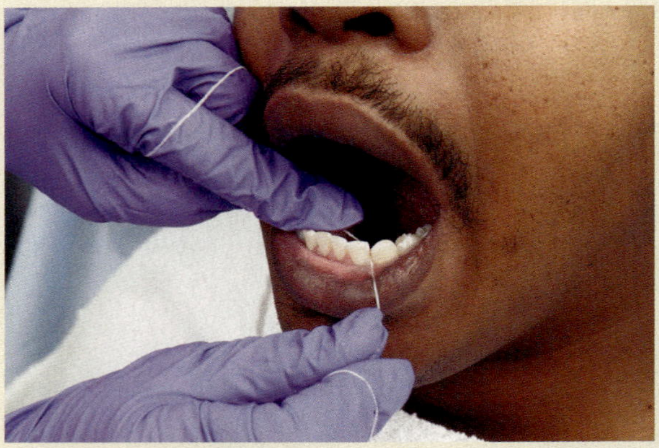

FIGURE 6. Flossing teeth.

ACTION	RATIONALE
8. Offer a mouth rinse if the patient prefers or if use has been recommended.	Use of a mouth rinse can reduce bacteria and can help reduce plaque, gingivitis, tartar (hardened plaque) and also freshen breath. Anticavity rinses with fluoride help protect tooth enamel to help prevent or control tooth decay (ADA, 2019).
9. Offer lip balm or petroleum jelly.	Lip balm lubricates lips and prevents drying.
10. Remove equipment. Remove gloves and discard. Perform hand hygiene. Raise the side rail and lower the bed. Assist the patient to a position of comfort.	Removing gloves properly reduces the risk for infection transmission and contamination of other items. These actions promote patient comfort and safety.
11. Remove any other PPE, if used. Perform hand hygiene.	Proper removal of PPE reduces the risk for infection transmission and contamination of other items. Hand hygiene prevents the spread of microorganisms.

DOCUMENTATION

Guidelines

Record oral assessment, significant observations, and unusual findings, such as bleeding or inflammation. Document any teaching done. Document procedure and patient response.

Sample Documentation

<u>10/2025</u> 0930 Patient performed oral care with minimal assistance. Oral cavity mucosa pink and moist. No evidence of bleeding or ulceration. Lips slightly dry; lip moisturizer applied. Reinforcement provided related to importance of flossing teeth every day. Patient demonstrates appropriate flossing technique.

—L. Schneider, RN

DEVELOPING CLINICAL REASONING AND CLINICAL JUDGMENT

UNEXPECTED SITUATIONS AND ASSOCIATED INTERVENTIONS

- *While cleaning the teeth, you notice a large amount of bleeding from the gum line:* Stop brushing. Allow the patient to gently rinse mouth with water and spit into emesis basin. Before brushing again, check the patient's most recent platelet level. Consider the use of a softer toothbrush to provide oral hygiene.
- *Patient has braces on their teeth:* Braces collect food particles. Brush extra thoroughly. Reinforce the importance of using an appropriate interdental cleaner.

SPECIAL CONSIDERATIONS

General Considerations

- Use a soft-bristled toothbrush with a small head even when the patient has no or few teeth. It is the only effective way to remove plaque and debris from the teeth, gums, and tongue.
- Automatic toothbrushes, electric or battery operated, are simple to use and can be used to removing debris and plaque and clean the teeth effectively. Use of an electric toothbrush provides superior oral hygiene care when oral hygiene is provided by a caregiver (Vannah & Sammarco, 2019).
- The use of chlorhexidine gluconate (CHG) as part of oral hygiene has been integrated into oral hygiene regimens and is available as an oral rinse, oral spray, and dental gel (AACN, 2017; de Camargo et al., 2019). The use of CHG as part of protocols for systematic oral care for critically ill patients has been shown to reduce risk of ventilator-associated pneumonia (VAP) (AACN, 2017; Chen et al., 2015).

Infant and Child Considerations

- Begin brushing children's teeth as soon as they begin to come into the mouth and begin flossing when the child has two teeth that touch (ADA, n.d.a).
- Clean an infant's gums by wiping with a clean, damp cloth (ADA, n.d.a).
- Young children should be supervised by an adult until they are between ages 7 and 10 years (Kyle & Carman, 2021); remind them not to swallow the toothpaste (ADA, n.d.a).
- Use smaller amounts of fluoride toothpaste on the toothbrush for children: a smear (size of a grain of rice) for children younger than age 3 years and a pea-sized amount for children ages 3 to 6 years (ADA, n.d.a).

Older Adults

- Physical limitations that may be associated with aging may interfere with the older adult's ability to perform adequate oral hygiene (Thomas, 2019). Pressurized water spray units (water flossing) are available to assist with oral hygiene to and can be a useful option for older adults and other patients who have trouble flossing by hand (ADA, n.d.d).

Skill 32-3 Providing Oral Care for the Dependent Patient

DELEGATION CONSIDERATIONS

The implementation of oral care for a dependent patient may be delegated to assistive personnel (AP) after assessment by the registered nurse as well as to licensed practical/vocational nurses (LPN/LVNs). The decision to delegate must be based on careful analysis of the patient's needs and circumstances as well as the qualifications of the person to whom the task is being delegated. Refer to the Delegation Guidelines in Appendix A.

EQUIPMENT

- Suction toothbrush (see Figure 4) or soft toothbrush
- Suction swab
- Suction catheter with suction apparatus
- Toothpaste or other oral cleanser
- Emesis basin
- Glass with cool water
- Disposable gloves
- Additional PPE, as indicated
- Towel
- Mouth rinse (optional)
- Dental floss in holder or other interdental cleaner
- Mouth-prop or second toothbrush (Figure 1)
- Denture-cleaning equipment (if necessary)
- Denture cup
- Denture cleaner
- 4 × 4 gauze
- Washcloth or paper towel
- Lip lubricant (optional)
- Oral health assessment tool (see Figure 1 in Skill 32-2)
- Additional care giver, as indicated

(*continued on page 1132*)

Skill 32-3 Providing Oral Care for the Dependent Patient *(continued)*

IMPLEMENTATION

ACTION	RATIONALE
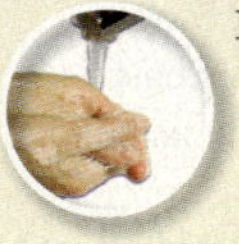 1. Perform hand hygiene and put on PPE, if indicated.	Hand hygiene and PPE prevent the spread of microorganisms. PPE is required based on transmission precautions.
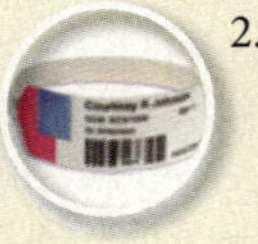 2. Identify the patient. Explain the procedure to the patient.	Identifying the patient ensures the right patient receives the intervention and helps prevent errors. Explanation facilitates engagement in care.
3. Assemble equipment on the overbed table or other surface within reach.	Organization facilitates performance of the task.
4. Close the room door or curtains. Place the bed at an appropriate and comfortable working height (VHACEOSH, 2016). Lower one side rail and position the patient on the side, with head tilted forward. Place towel across the patient's chest and emesis basin in position under chin. Depending on equipment in use, connect the suction toothbrush/swab or suction catheter to suction tubing and turn on suction. Put on gloves.	Closing the door or curtains provides privacy. Proper bed height helps reduce back strain while performing the procedure. The side-lying position with head forward prevents aspiration of fluid into lungs. Towel and emesis basin protect the patient from dampness. Suction provides means to remove oral hygiene products and saliva from oral cavity. Gloves prevent the spread of microorganisms.
5. Gently open the patient's mouth by applying pressure to the lower jaw at the front of the mouth. Do not use fingers to hold the patient's mouth open. Use another toothbrush or mouth prop (Figure 1) to keep the mouth open. Remove dentures, if present.	Patients with altered cognition may inadvertently bite fingers inserted into the mouth. Removal of dentures allows for cleaning of dentures and oral cavity.

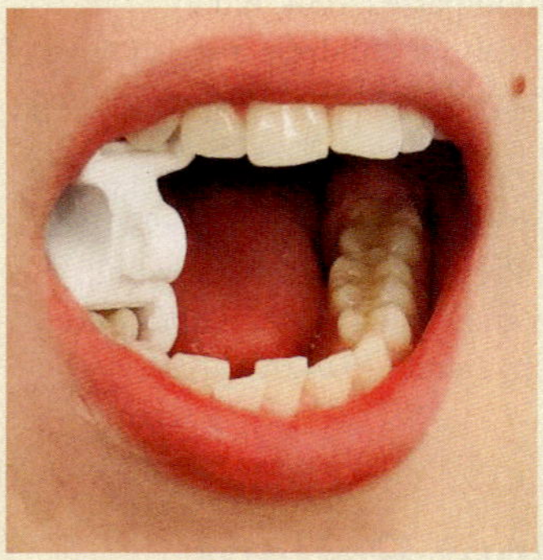

FIGURE 1. Example of a mouth prop. (*Source:* Used with permission from Neo-Health Services, Inc. © 2011 OrofacialMyology.com. All rights reserved.)

ACTION	RATIONALE
6. If using a regular toothbrush and suction catheter, one care giver provides oral cleaning and the other removes secretions with the suction catheter.	This allows for efficient care to reduce the risk of aspiration.
7. Brush the teeth and gums carefully with toothbrush and paste or other oral cleanser (Figure 2). Lightly brush the tongue.	The toothbrush provides friction necessary to clean areas where plaque and tartar accumulate.

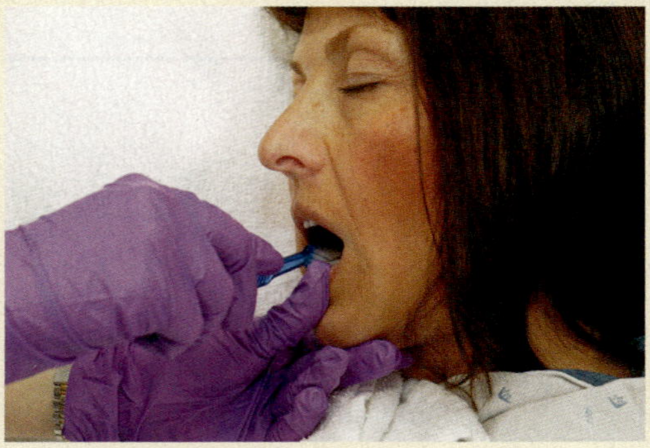

FIGURE 2. Carefully brushing patient's teeth.

ACTION

8. Moisten toothbrush with water to rinse the oral cavity. **Position the patient's head to allow for return of water. If using regular toothbrush, use suction catheter to remove the water and cleanser from oral cavity (Figure 3).**

RATIONALE

Rinsing helps clean debris from the mouth. Suction toothbrush removes fluids and cleansers.

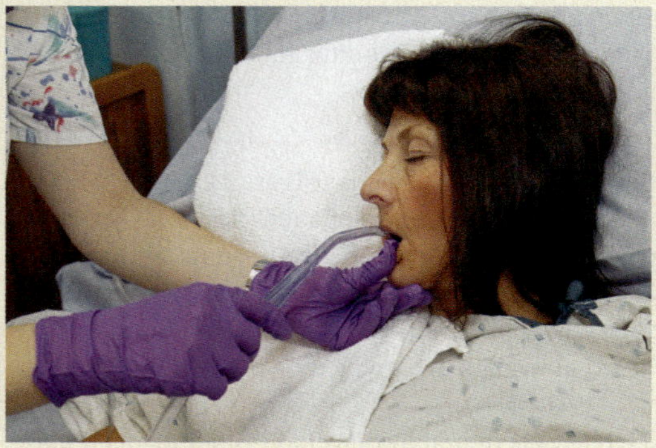

FIGURE 3. Using suction to remove excess fluid.

9. Brush the tongue gently with toothbrush or tongue scraper (MFMER, 2019a).

This removes coating on the tongue. Gentle motion does not stimulate the gag reflex.

10. Using the suction swab, apply a therapeutic antiseptic mouth rinse as indicated. Apply oral moisturizer as indicated.

Therapeutic and antiseptic mouth rinses reduce bacteria and reduce plaque, gingivitis, tartar, and reduce the incidence of health care–associated pneumonia (AACN, 2017; ADA, 2019; Chick & Wynne, 2020). Oral moisturizers provide moisture to the mucosa.

11. Clean the dentures before replacing.

Cleaning maintains dentures and oral hygiene. Plaque can accumulate on dentures and promote oropharyngeal colonization of pathogens.

12. Apply lubricant to the patient's lips.

This prevents drying and cracking of lips.

13. Remove equipment and return the patient to a position of comfort. Remove gloves. Perform hand hygiene. Raise the side rail and lower the bed.

Promotes patient comfort and safety. Removing gloves properly reduces the risk for infection transmission and contamination of other items. Hand hygiene prevents the spread of microorganisms.

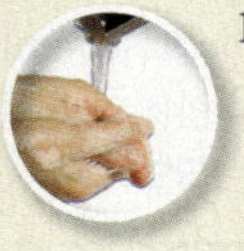

14. Remove additional PPE, if used. Perform hand hygiene.

Proper removal of PPE reduces the risk for infection transmission and contamination of other items. Hand hygiene prevents the spread of microorganisms.

DOCUMENTATION

Guidelines

Record oral assessment, significant observations, and unusual findings, such as bleeding or inflammation. Document any teaching done. Document care provided and patient response.

Sample Documentation

<u>7/10/25</u> 0945 Oral care performed. Oral cavity mucosa pink and moist. Small amount of bleeding noted from gums after using soft-bristled toothbrush. Resolved spontaneously when brushing completed. No evidence of ulceration. Lips slightly dry; lip moisturizer applied.

—*C. Stone, RN*

(*continued on page 1134*)

Skill 32-3 Providing Oral Care for the Dependent Patient *(continued)*

DEVELOPING CLINICAL REASONING AND CLINICAL JUDGMENT

UNEXPECTED SITUATIONS AND ASSOCIATED INTERVENTIONS

- *Patient begins to bite the toothbrush:* Do not jerk the toothbrush out. Wait for the patient to relax mouth before removing the toothbrush and continuing with care. Use distraction, gentle touch, or massage to divert the patient.
- *Mouth is extremely dry with crusts that remain after oral care provided:* Increase frequency of oral hygiene. Apply mouth moisturizer to oral mucosa. Monitor fluid intake and output to ensure adequate intake of fluid.

SPECIAL CONSIDERATIONS

- Suction toothbrushes may be used with patients with dysphagia (Figure 4).
- Use a soft bristled toothbrush with a small head even when the patient has no or few teeth. It is the only effective way to remove plaque and debris from the teeth, gums, and tongue.
- Automatic toothbrushes, electric or battery operated, are simple to use and can be used to removing debris and plaque and clean the teeth effectively. Use of an electric toothbrush provides superior oral hygiene care when oral hygiene is provided by a caregiver (Vannah & Sammarco, 2019).
- The use of chlorhexidine gluconate (CHG) as part of oral hygiene has been integrated into oral hygiene regimens and is available as an oral rinse, oral spray, and dental gel (AACN, 2017; de Camargo et al., 2019). The use of CHG as part of protocols for systematic oral care for critically ill patients has been shown to reduce risk of ventilator-associated pneumonia (VAP) (AACN, 2017; Chen et al., 2015).

FIGURE 4. Example of a suction toothbrush. (*Source:* Permission granted by Sage Products LLC.)

Skill 32-4 Making an Unoccupied Bed

DELEGATION CONSIDERATIONS

The making of an unoccupied bed may be delegated to assistive personnel (AP) as well as to licensed practical/vocational nurses (LPN/LVNs). The decision to delegate must be based on careful analysis of the patient's needs and circumstances as well as the qualifications of the person to whom the task is being delegated. Refer to the Delegation Guidelines in Appendix A.

EQUIPMENT

- One large flat sheet
- One fitted sheet
- Lifting/repositioning sheet or friction-reducing sheet (optional)
- Blankets
- Bedspread
- Pillowcases
- Linen hamper or bag
- Bedside chair
- Waterproof protective pad (optional)
- Disposable gloves
- Additional PPE, as indicated

IMPLEMENTATION

ACTION	RATIONALE
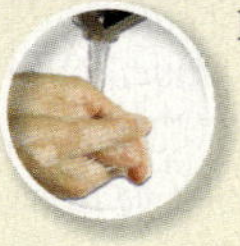 1. Perform hand hygiene. Put on PPE, as indicated.	Hand hygiene and PPE prevent the spread of microorganisms. PPE is required based on transmission precautions.
2. Explain to the patient what you are going to do and the reason for doing it, if the patient is present in the room.	Explanation facilitates engagement in care.

ACTION	RATIONALE
3. Assemble necessary equipment on the bedside stand, overbed table, or other surface within reach.	Arranging items nearby is convenient, saves time, and avoids unnecessary stretching and twisting of muscles on the part of the nurse.
4. Adjust the bed to a comfortable working height (VHACEOSH, 2016). Drop the side rails.	Having the bed at the proper height prevents back and muscle strain. Having the side rails down reduces strain on the nurse while working.
5. Disconnect the call bell or any tubes from bed linens.	Disconnecting devices prevents damage to the devices.
6. Put on gloves. Loosen all linen as you move around the bed, from the head of the bed on the far side to the head of the bed on the near side.	Gloves prevent the spread of microorganisms. Loosening the linen helps prevent tugging and tearing on linen. Loosening the linen and moving around the bed systematically reduce strain caused by reaching across the bed.
7. Fold reusable linens, such as sheets, blankets, or spread, in place on the bed in fourths and hang them over a clean chair.	Folding saves time and energy when reusable linen is replaced on the bed. Folding linens while they are on the bed reduces strain on the nurse's arms. Some facilities change linens only when soiled.
8. Snugly roll all the soiled linen inside the bottom sheet. Hold linen away from your body and place directly into the laundry hamper (Figure 1). **Do not place on floor or furniture. Do not hold soiled linens against your clothing.**	Rolling soiled linens snugly and placing them directly into the hamper helps prevent the spread of microorganisms. The floor is heavily contaminated; soiled linen will further contaminate furniture. Soiled linen contaminates the nurse's clothing, and this may spread organisms to another patient.
9. If possible, shift the mattress up to the head of the bed. If the mattress is soiled, clean and dry according to facility policy before applying new sheets.	This allows more foot room for the patient.
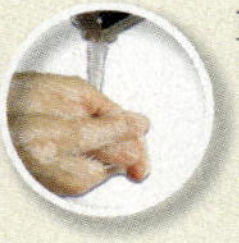 10. Remove your gloves, unless indicated for transmission-based precautions. Perform hand hygiene. Place the bottom sheet on the mattress and secure the bottom sheet over the corners at the head and foot of the mattress.	Gloves are not necessary to handle clean linen. Hand hygiene prevents the spread of microorganisms. Secures bottom sheet on one side of the bed.
11. Push the sheet open to the center of the mattress, pulling the sheet taut from the secured corners (Figure 2).	Making the bed on one side and then completing the bedmaking on the other side saves time. Pulling the sheet taut keeps it in place on the mattress. Having bottom linens free of wrinkles reduces patient discomfort.

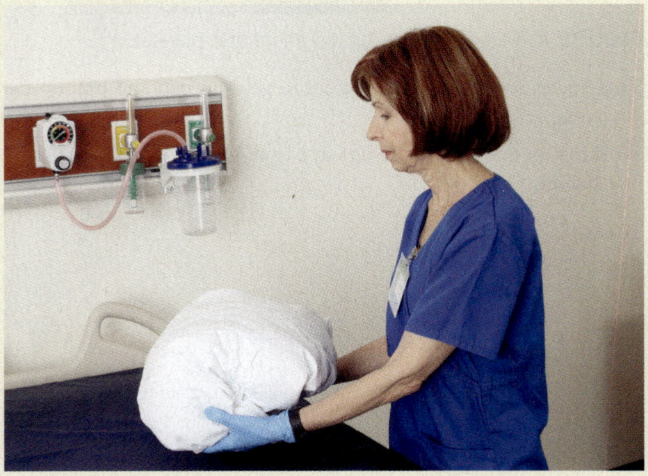

FIGURE 1. Bundling soiled linens in bottom sheet and holding them away from clothing.

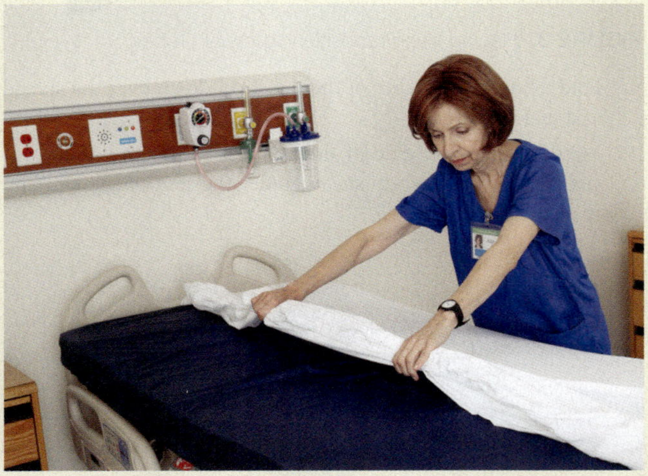

FIGURE 2. Pushing the bottom sheet open to the center of the mattress.

(continued on page 1136)

Skill 32-4 Making an Unoccupied Bed *(continued)*

ACTION	RATIONALE
12. If using, place the lifting/repositioning or friction-reducing sheet with its center fold in the center of the bed and positioned so it will be located under the patient's midsection; open it and fanfold to the center of the mattress (Figure 3). If a protective pad is used, place it over the lifting/repositioning or friction-reducing sheet in the proper area and open to the center fold. Not all facilities use lifting/repositioning sheets routinely. The nurse may decide to use one or a friction-reducing sheet based on patient circumstances. In some institutions, the protective pad doubles as a lifting/repositioning sheet. Tuck the lifting/repositioning or friction-reducing sheet securely under the mattress.	If the patient soils the bed, lifting/repositioning or friction-reducing sheet and pad can be changed without changing the bottom and top linens. Having all bottom linens in place before tucking them under the mattress avoids unnecessary moving about the bed. A lifting/repositioning or friction-reducing sheet can aid moving the patient in bed.
13. Move to the other side of the bed to secure bottom linens. Pull the bottom sheet tightly and secure over the corners at the head and foot of the mattress. Pull the lifting/repositioning or friction-reducing sheet tightly and tuck it securely under the mattress.	This removes wrinkles from the bottom linens, which can cause patient discomfort and promote skin breakdown.
14. Place the top sheet on the bed with its center fold in the center of the bed and with the hem even with the head of the mattress. Unfold the top sheet. Follow same procedure with top blanket or spread, placing the upper edge about 6 inches below the top of the sheet.	Opening linens by shaking them spreads organisms into the air. Holding linens overhead to open causes strain on the nurse's arms.
15. Tuck the top sheet and blanket under the foot of the bed on the near side. Miter the corners (Figure 4).	This saves time and energy and keeps the top linen in place.

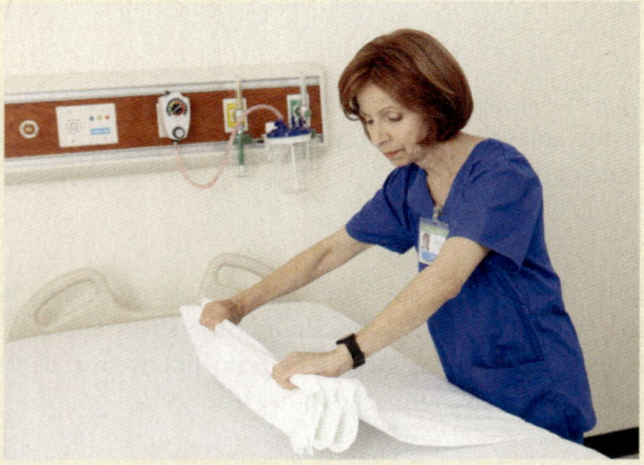

FIGURE 3. Placing lifting/repositioning sheet on bed.

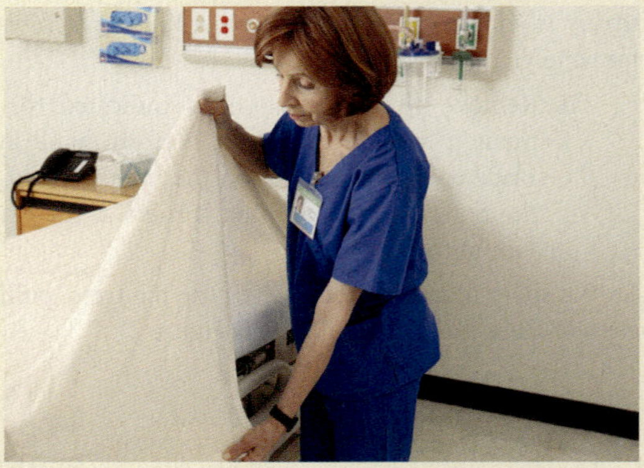

FIGURE 4. Mitering corner of top sheet and blanket.

ACTION	RATIONALE
16. Fold the upper 6 inches of the top sheet down over the spread and make a cuff.	This makes it easier for the patient to get into bed and pull up the covers.
17. Move to the other side of the bed and follow the same procedure for securing top sheets under the foot of the bed and making a cuff (Figure 5).	Working on one side of the bed at a time saves energy and is more efficient.

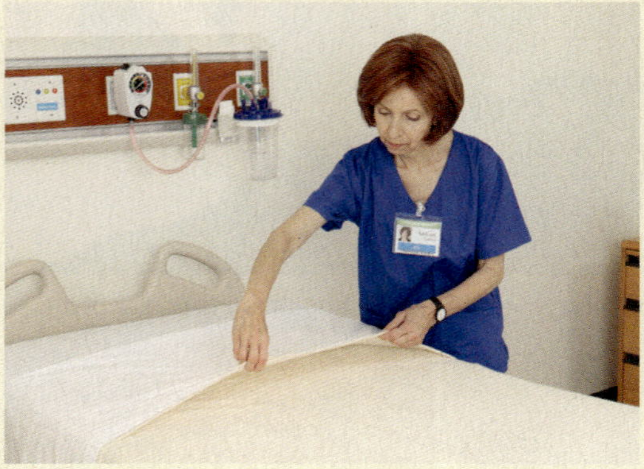

FIGURE 5. Cuffing top linens.

ACTION	RATIONALE
18. Place the pillows on the bed. Open each pillowcase in the same manner as you opened other linens. Gather the pillowcase over one hand toward the closed end. Grasp the pillow with the hand inside the pillowcase. Keep a firm hold on the top of the pillow and pull the cover onto the pillow. Place the pillow at the head of the bed.	Opening linens by shaking causes organisms to be carried on air currents. Covering the pillow while it rests on the bed reduces strain on the nurse's arms and back.
19. Fan-fold or pie-fold the top linens.	Having linens opened makes it more convenient for the patient to get into bed.
20. Secure the signal device on the bed, according to facility policy.	The patient will be able to call for assistance as necessary. Promotes patient comfort and safety.
21. Raise the side rail and lower the bed.	This promotes patient comfort and safety.
22. Dispose of soiled linen according to facility policy.	This deters the spread of microorganisms.
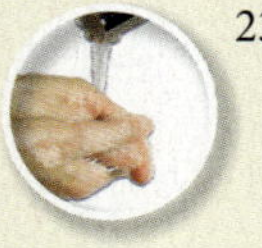 23. Remove any other PPE, if used. Perform hand hygiene.	Proper removal of PPE reduces the risk for infection transmission and contamination of other items. Hand hygiene prevents the spread of microorganisms.

DOCUMENTATION

Changing of bed linens does not require documentation. The use of a specialty bed or bed equipment should be documented.

DEVELOPING CLINICAL REASONING AND CLINICAL JUDGMENT

UNEXPECTED SITUATIONS AND ASSOCIATED INTERVENTIONS

- *Lifting/repositioning sheet is not available:* A flat sheet can be folded in half to substitute for a lifting/repositioning sheet, but extra care must be taken to avoid wrinkles in the bed.
- *Patient is frequently incontinent of stool or urine:* More than one protective pad can be placed under the patient to protect the bed, but take care to ensure that the patient is not lying on wrinkles from linens.

SPECIAL CONSIDERATIONS

- Many different types of specialty beds are available for use as part of treatment and prevention of many health issues, such as treatment of pressure injuries. Refer to the manufacturer's recommendations and instructions on use of specialty linens and products with these types of equipment.

Skill 32-5 Making an Occupied Bed

DELEGATION CONSIDERATIONS

The making of an occupied bed may be delegated to assistive personnel (AP) as well as to licensed practical/vocational nurses (LPN/LVNs). The decision to delegate must be based on careful analysis of the patient's needs and circumstances as well as the qualifications of the person to whom the task is being delegated. Refer to the Delegation Guidelines in Appendix A.

EQUIPMENT

- One large flat sheet
- One fitted sheet
- Lifting/repositioning sheet (optional) or friction-reducing sheet
- Blankets
- Bedspread
- Pillowcases
- Linen hamper or bag
- Bedside chair
- Protective pad (optional)
- Disposable gloves
- Additional PPE, as indicated

(*continued on page 1138*)

Skill 32-5 Making an Occupied Bed *(continued)*

IMPLEMENTATION

ACTION	RATIONALE
1. Check the health care record for limitations on the patient's physical activity.	This facilitates patient engagement in care, determines level of activity, and promotes patient safety.
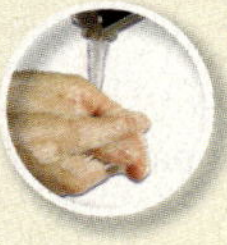 2. Perform hand hygiene. Put on PPE, as indicated.	Hand hygiene and PPE prevent the spread of microorganisms. PPE is required based on transmission precautions.
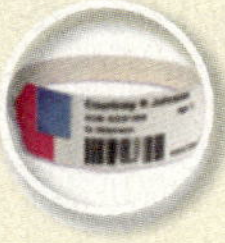 3. Identify the patient. Explain what you are going to do.	Patient identification validates the correct patient and correct procedure. Discussion and explanation allay anxiety and prepare the patient for what to expect.
4. Assemble equipment on the overbed table or other surface within reach.	Organization facilitates performance of the task.
5. Close the curtains around the bed and close the door to the room, if possible.	This ensures the patient's privacy.
6. Adjust the bed to a comfortable working height (VHACEOSH, 2016).	Having the bed at the proper height prevents back and muscle strain.
7. Lower the side rail nearest you, leaving the opposite side rail up. Place the bed in a flat position unless contraindicated.	Having the mattress flat makes it easier to prepare a wrinkle-free bed.
8. Put on gloves. Check bed linens for the patient's personal items. **Disconnect the call bell or any tubes/drains from bed linens.**	Gloves prevent the spread of microorganisms. It is costly and inconvenient when personal items are lost. Disconnecting tubes from linens prevents discomfort and accidental dislodging of the tubes.
9. Place a bath blanket over the patient. Have the patient hold on to the bath blanket while you reach under it and remove the top linen (Figure 1). Leave the top sheet in place if a bath blanket is not used and loosen from bottom of bed. Fold linen that is to be reused over the back of a chair. Discard soiled linen in a laundry bag or hamper. **Do not place on floor or furniture. Do not hold soiled linens against your clothing.**	The blanket provides warmth and privacy. Placing linens directly into the hamper helps prevent the spread of microorganisms. The floor is heavily contaminated; soiled linen will further contaminate furniture. Soiled linen contaminates the nurse's clothing, and this may spread organisms to another patient.

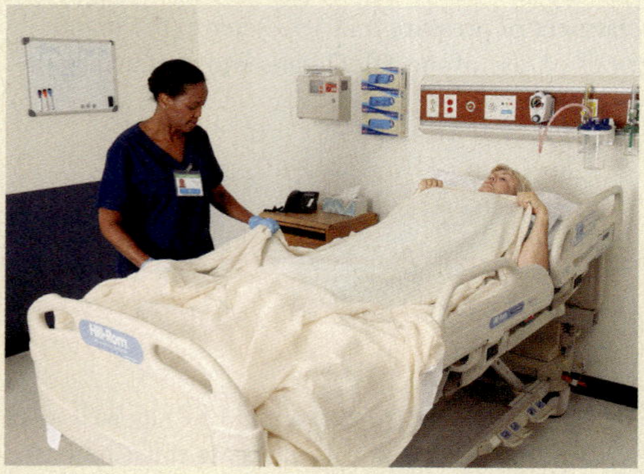

FIGURE 1. Removing top linens from under bath blanket.

ACTION	RATIONALE
10. If possible, and another person is available to assist, grasp the mattress securely and shift it up to head of bed.	This allows more foot room for the patient.
11. Assist the patient to turn toward the opposite side of the bed, and reposition the pillow under the patient's head. If the patient is partially able or unable to assist, friction-reducing devices, lifting/repositioning sheets, lateral transfer devices, and a full-body sling are potential equipment to consider, based on screening and assessment. Consider available bed features (turning, pressure release, rotation) to assist with the action (VA Mobile Health, n.d.).	This allows the bed to be made on the vacant side. Use of safe patient handling and mobility devices is best practice to prevent patient and health care provider injury (VA Mobile Health, n.d.; VHACEOSH, 2016).

ACTION	RATIONALE
12. Loosen all bottom linens from the head, foot, and side of the bed.	This facilitates removal of linens.
13. Fan-fold or roll soiled linens as close to the patient as possible (Figure 2).	This makes it easier to remove linens when the patient turns to the other side.
14. Use clean linen and make the near side of the bed. Place the bottom sheet in the center of the bed. Open the sheet and pull the bottom sheet over the corners at the head and foot of the mattress (Figure 3). Push the sheet toward the center of the bed, pulling it taut and positioning it under the old linens (Figure 4).	Opening linens on the bed reduces strain on the nurse's arms and diminishes the spread of microorganisms. Centering the sheet ensures sufficient coverage for both sides of the mattress. Positioning under the old linens makes it easier to remove linens.
15. If using, place the lifting/repositioning or friction-reducing sheet with its center fold in the center of the bed and positioned so it will be located under the patient's midsection. Open the lifting/repositioning or friction-reducing sheet and fan-fold it to the center of the mattress. Tuck it securely under the mattress (Figure 5). If a protective pad is used, place it over the lifting/repositioning or friction-reducing sheet in the proper area and open to the center fold. Not all facilities use lifting/repositioning sheets routinely. The nurse may decide to use one.	If the patient soils the bed, lifting/repositioning or friction-reducing sheet and pad can be changed without the bottom and top linens on the bed. A lifting/repositioning or friction-reducing sheet can aid in moving the patient in bed.

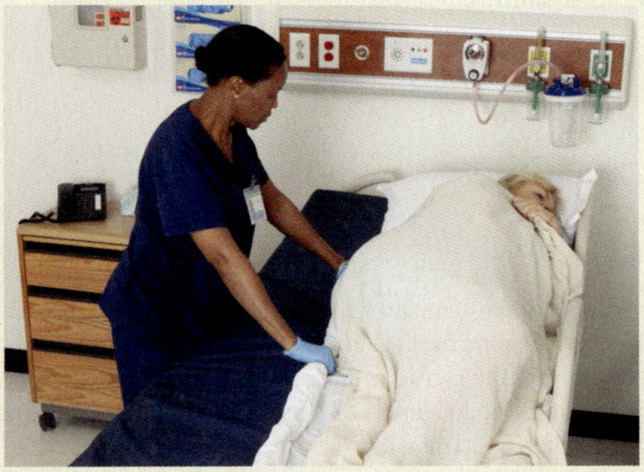

FIGURE 2. Moving soiled linen as close to patient as possible.

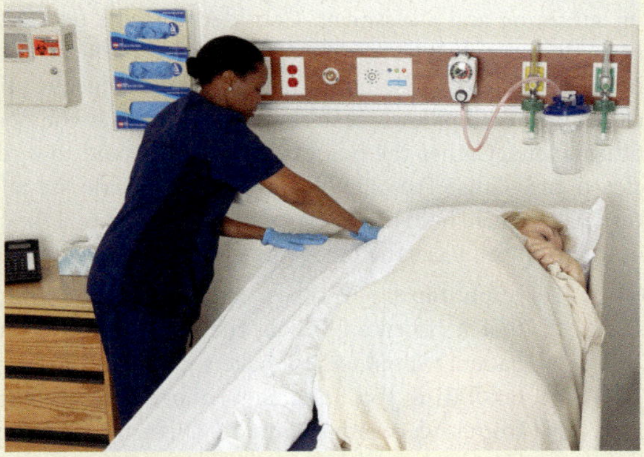

FIGURE 3. Pulling the bottom sheet over the corners at the head and foot of the mattress.

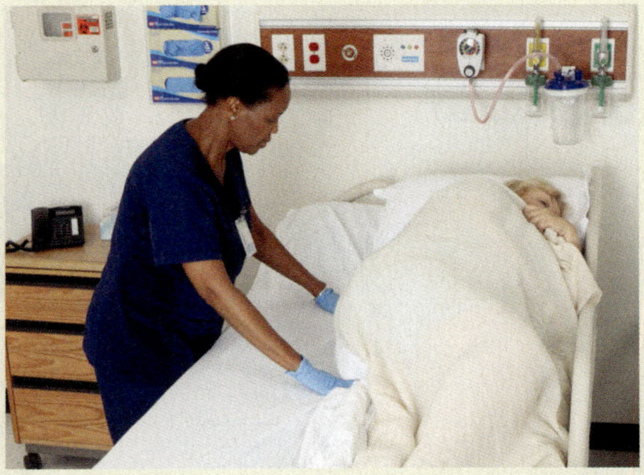

FIGURE 4. Pushing the bottom sheet toward the center of the bed, positioning it under old linens.

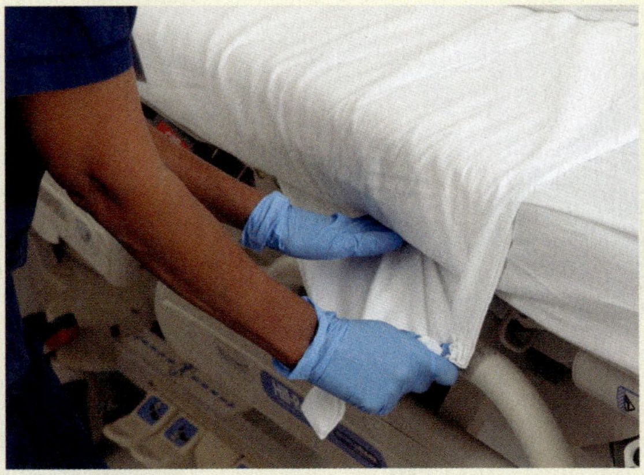

FIGURE 5. Tucking lifting/repositioning or friction-reducing sheet tightly.

(continued on page 1140)

Skill 32-5 Making an Occupied Bed *(continued)*

ACTION	RATIONALE
16. Raise the side rail. Assist the patient to roll over the folded linen in the middle of the bed toward you. If the patient is partially able or unable to assist, friction-reducing devices, lifting/repositioning sheets, lateral transfer devices, and a full-body sling are potential equipment to consider, based on screening and assessment. Consider available bed features (turning, pressure release, rotation) to assist with the action (VA Mobile Health, n.d.). Reposition pillow and bath blanket or top sheet. Move to other side of the bed and lower the side rail.	This ensures patient safety. The movement allows the bed to be made on the other side. Use of safe patient handling and mobility devices is best practice to prevent patient and health care provider injury (VA Mobile Health, n.d.; VHACEOSH, 2016). The bath blanket provides warmth and privacy.
17. Loosen and remove all bottom linen (Figure 6). Discard soiled linen in laundry bag or hamper. **Do not place on floor or furniture. Do not hold soiled linens against your clothing.**	Placing linens directly into the hamper helps prevent the spread of microorganisms. The floor is heavily contaminated; soiled linen will further contaminate the furniture. Soiled linen contaminates the nurse's clothing, and this may spread organisms to another patient.
18. Ease clean linen from under the patient. Pull the bottom sheet taut and secure at the corners at the head and foot of the mattress. Pull the lifting/repositioning or friction-reducing sheet tight and smooth. Tuck it securely under the mattress.	This removes wrinkles and creases in the linens, which are uncomfortable to lie on.
19. Assist the patient to turn back to the center of bed. If the patient is partially able or unable to assist, friction-reducing devices, lifting/repositioning sheets, lateral transfer devices, and a full-body sling are potential equipment to consider, based on screening and assessment. Consider available bed features (turning, pressure release, rotation) to assist with the action (VA Mobile Health, n.d.). Remove the pillow and change the pillowcase. Open each pillowcase in the same manner as you opened other linens. Gather the pillowcase over one hand toward the closed end. Grasp the pillow with the hand inside the pillowcase. Keep a firm hold on the top of the pillow and pull the cover onto the pillow. Place the pillow under the patient's head.	Use of safe patient handling and mobility devices is best practice to prevent patient and health care provider injury (VA Mobile Health, n.d.; VHACEOSH, 2016). Opening linens by shaking causes organisms to be carried on air currents.
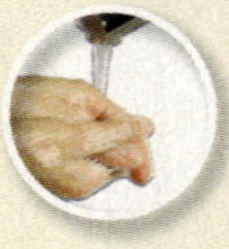 20. Apply top linen, sheet, and blanket, if desired, so that it is centered. Fold the top linens over at the patient's shoulders to make a cuff. Have the patient hold on to top linen and remove the bath blanket from underneath (Figure 7). Discard soiled linen in laundry bag or hamper. **Do not place on floor or furniture. Do not hold soiled linens against your clothing.** Remove gloves. Perform hand hygiene.	This allows bottom hems to be tucked securely under the mattress and provides for privacy. Placing linens directly into the hamper helps prevent the spread of microorganisms. The floor is heavily contaminated; soiled linen will further contaminate the furniture. Soiled linen contaminates the nurse's clothing, and this may spread organisms to another patient. Removing gloves properly reduces the risk for infection transmission and contamination of other items. Hand hygiene prevents the spread of microorganisms.

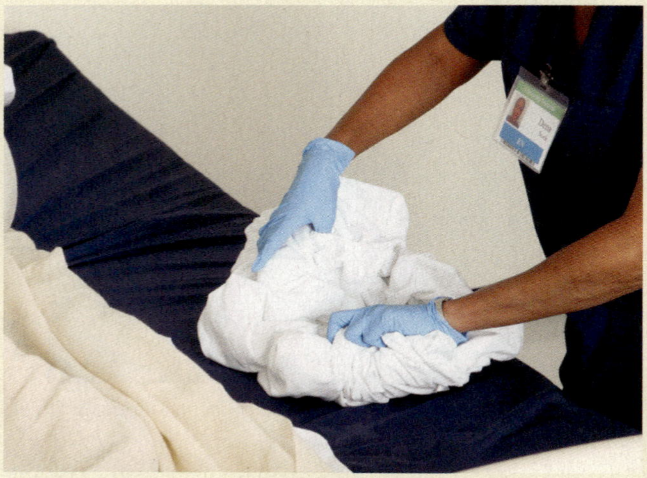

FIGURE 6. Removing soiled bottom linens from other side of bed.

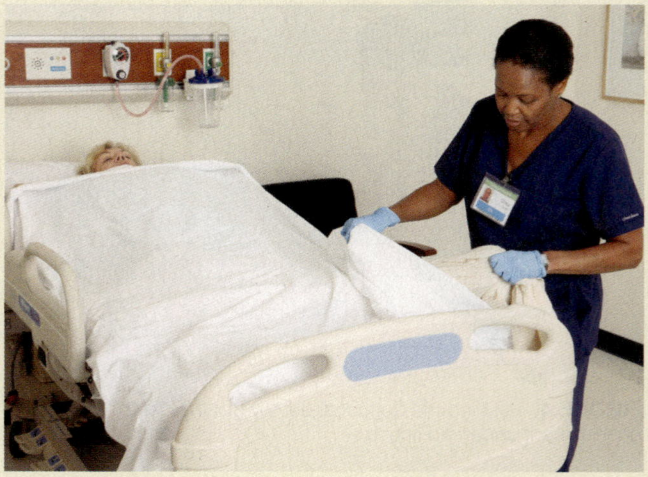

FIGURE 7. Removing bath blanket from under top linens.

ACTION	RATIONALE
21. Secure top linens under foot of mattress and miter corners. Loosen top linens over the patient's feet by grasping them in the area of the feet and pulling gently toward the foot of bed.	This provides for a neat appearance. Loosening linens over the patient's feet gives more room for movement.
22. Return the patient to a position of comfort. Raise the side rail and lower the bed. Reattach call bell.	This promotes patient comfort and safety.
23. Dispose of soiled linens according to facility policy.	This deters the spread of microorganisms.
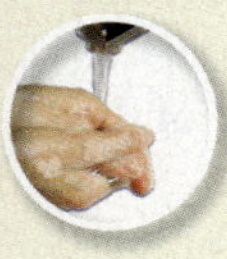 24. Remove any other PPE, if used. Perform hand hygiene.	Proper removal of PPE reduces the risk for infection transmission and contamination of other items. Hand hygiene prevents the spread of microorganisms.

DOCUMENTATION

Changing of bed linens does not require documentation. The use of a specialty bed or bed equipment should be documented. Document any significant observations and communication.

DEVELOPING CLINICAL REASONING AND CLINICAL JUDGMENT

UNEXPECTED SITUATIONS AND ASSOCIATED INTERVENTIONS

- *Dirty linens are grossly contaminated with urinary or fecal drainage:* Obtain an extra towel or protective pad. Place the pad under and over the soiled linens so that new linens will not be in contact with soiled linens. Clean and dry the mattress according to facility policy before applying new sheets.

SPECIAL CONSIDERATIONS

Older Adult Considerations

- Using a soft bath blanket or a flannelette blanket as a bottom sheet may solve the problem of "coldness" for older adult patients with vascular problems or arthritis.

DEVELOPING CLINICAL REASONING AND CLINICAL JUDGMENT

1. Work through the Nursing Care Plan for Kylie Simpson and University Students on pages 1118–1120 to help develop your clinical reasoning and clinical judgment skills.
2. Practice the art of back massage with a willing partner until you feel comfortable and confident including this nursing measure in your routine care. Discuss with other students the therapeutic benefits of massage, and identify nursing situations for which it may be the primary therapy.
3. Interview people of different ages and cultural backgrounds about their hygiene practices. Ask specific questions about the type of nursing assistance they would require if hospitalized and unable to meet their hygiene needs independently. Are there special products or equipment they would need? To what extent are nurses obliged to respect the hygiene preferences of patients?

PRACTICING FOR NCLEX

1. A nurse is scheduling hygiene for patients on the unit. What is the priority the nurse uses to guide planning for patient's personal hygiene?
   a. When the patient had their most recent bath
   b. The patient's usual hygiene practices and preferences
   c. Where the bathing fits in the nurse's schedule
   d. The time that is convenient for the AP
2. A nurse caring for patients in a critical care unit knows that providing good oral hygiene is an essential to good patient outcomes, especially for those receiving mechanical ventilation. What are positive outcomes expected from this care? Select all that apply.
   a. Promoting the patient's sense of well-being
   b. Preventing deterioration of the oral cavity
   c. Contributing to decreased incidence of aspiration pneumonia
   d. Eliminating the need for flossing
   e. Decreasing oropharyngeal secretions
   f. Compensating for an inadequate diet

3. A nurse assisting a patient with a bed bath observes the older adult has dry skin, which the patient states is "itchy." Which intervention is appropriate?
   a. Bathe the patient more frequently.
   b. Use an emollient on the dry skin.
   c. Explain that this is expected as people age.
   d. Limit the patient's fluid intake.
4. A charge nurse in a skilled nursing facility is working to reduce patients' foot and nail problems. The charge nurse reminds the nurses and APs to closely observe which of these patients at higher risk? Select all that apply.
   a. Patient taking antibiotics for chronic bronchitis
   b. Patient with type 2 diabetes
   c. Patient who has obesity
   d. Patient who frequently bites their nails
   e. Patient with prostate cancer
   f. Patient who frequently washes their hands
5. When assessing the skin, nurses use techniques to provide complete data and correct documentation. Which actions are appropriate during the skin assessment? Select all that apply.
   a. Comparing bilateral parts for symmetry
   b. Proceeding in a toe-to-head, systematic manner
   c. Using standard terminology to communicate and document findings
   d. Avoiding using data from the nursing history to direct the assessment
   e. Documenting only skin abnormalities on the health record
   f. When risk factors are identified, following up with a related skin assessment
6. A nurse is caring for an adolescent with severe acne. Which recommendations would be most appropriate to include in the teaching plan for this patient? Select all that apply.
   a. Wash the skin twice a day with a mild cleanser and warm water.
   b. Use cosmetics liberally to cover blackheads.
   c. Apply emollients on the area.
   d. Squeeze blackheads as they appear.
   e. Keep hair off the face and wash hair daily.
   f. Avoid tanning booth exposure and use sunscreen.
7. A nurse is performing oral care on a patient who has advanced dementia. The nurse notes that the mouth is extremely dry with crusts remaining after the oral care. What action will the nurse take next?
   a. Recommend a consultation with an oral surgeon.
   b. Communicate the condition to the health care team.
   c. Gently scrape the oral cavity with a tongue depressor.
   d. Increase the frequency of the oral hygiene and apply mouth moisturizer to oral mucosa.
8. A nursing student asks an experienced nurse why they provide massage for their patients. Which of these would be reflected in the nurse's response?
   a. To help with pain management
   b. To provide comfort
   c. To communicate to patients through touch
   d. To energize patients, especially those with dementia
   e. To facilitate healing after back or spinal surgery
   f. To help increase circulation
9. A nurse is caring for a patient with an eye infection with a moderate amount of discharge. What is the most appropriate technique for the nurse to use when cleansing this patient's eyes?
   a. Using diluted hydrogen peroxide on a clean washcloth to wipe the eyes
   b. Wiping the eye from the outer canthus toward the inner canthus
   c. Positioning the patient on the opposite side of the eye to be cleansed
   d. Cleansing the eye using a different section of the cloth for each stroke until clean
10. A nurse in a long-term care facility observes the AP providing foot care for patients. Which actions by the AP require the nurse to intervene? Select all that apply.
    a. Bathing the feet thoroughly in a mild soap and tepid water solution
    b. Soaking the resident's feet in warm water and bath oil
    c. Drying the feet and area between the toes thoroughly
    d. Applying an alcohol rub for odor and dryness to the feet
    e. Applying an antifungal foot powder
    f. Cutting the toenails at the lateral corners when trimming the nail
11. A nurse in a memory care unit is assisting a patient with dementia with bathing. Which nursing action will enhance patient comfort and prevent anxiety?
    a. Shifting the focus of the interaction to the "process of bathing"
    b. Washing the face and hair at the beginning of the bath
    c. Using music to soothe anxiety and agitation
    d. Avoiding towel baths or forms of bathing with which the patient is unfamiliar
12. A nurse is teaching a nursing student how to perform perineal care for patients. What actions are appropriate when performing this procedure? Select all that apply.
    a. For male and female patients, wash the groin area with a small amount of soap and water and rinse.
    b. For a female patient, spread the labia and move the washcloth from the anal area toward the pubic area.
    c. For male and female patients, always proceed from the most contaminated area to the least contaminated area.
    d. For male and female patients, use a clean portion of the washcloth for each stroke.
    e. For a male patient, clean the tip of the penis first, moving the washcloth in a circular motion from the meatus outward.
    f. In an uncircumcised male patient, avoid retracting the foreskin (prepuce) while washing the penis.

13. A home care nurse is assisting an older adult with an unsteady gait with a tub bath. Which action is recommended in this procedure?
    a. Adding bath oil to the water to prevent dry skin
    b. Allowing the patient to lock the door to guarantee privacy
    c. Assisting the patient in and out of the tub to prevent falling
    d. Keeping the water temperature very warm because older adults chill easily
14. A nurse is about to bathe a female patient who has an IV in the forearm. The patient's gown, which does not have snaps on the sleeves, needs to be removed prior to bathing. How will the nurse proceed?
    a. Quickly disconnecting the IV tubing closest to the patient and thread it through the gown sleeve
    b. Cutting the gown with scissors to allow arm movement
    c. Threading the bag and tubing through the gown sleeve, keeping the line intact
    d. Temporarily disconnecting the tubing from the IV container, threading it through the gown
15. A nurse is caring for a 25-year-old patient who is unresponsive following a head injury. The patient has several piercings in the ears and nose that appear crusted and slightly inflamed. What is the most appropriate action to care for this patient's piercings?
    a. Avoiding removing or washing the piercings until the patient is responsive
    b. Rinsing the sites with warm water and remove crusts with a cotton swab
    c. Washing the sites with alcohol and apply an antibiotic ointment
    d. Removing the jewelry and allow the sites to heal over
16. An RN in a long-term care facility supervises APs as they provide hygiene to older adults. What action by the AP will the nurse correct?
    a. When providing perineal care, washing the area from front to back
    b. Insisting the older adult must take a bath or shower each day
    c. Telling the patient to avoid soaking feet, helps the patient dry between the toes
    d. Covering areas not being bathed with a bath blanket

ANSWERS WITH RATIONALES

1. **b.** The patient's preferences, practices, and rituals should always be taken into consideration, unless there is a clear threat to health. The patient and nurse should work together to come to a mutually agreeable time and method to accomplish the patient's personal hygiene. The availability of staff to assist may be important, but the patient's preferences are a higher priority.
2. **a, b, c.** Adequate oral hygiene is essential for promoting the patient's sense of well-being and preventing deterioration of the oral cavity. Diligent oral hygiene and use of chlorhexidine gluconate (CHG) in critical care areas, can limit the growth of pathogens in oropharyngeal secretions, decreasing the incidence of ventilator-associated pneumonia, aspiration pneumonia, and other systemic diseases. Oral care does not eliminate the need for flossing, decrease oropharyngeal secretions, or compensate for poor nutrition.
3. **b.** An emollient soothes dry skin, whereas frequent bathing increases dryness. Telling the patient this is normal with aging and does not help resolve the issue. Limiting fluid intake can promote dehydration and exacerbate dry skin.
4. **b, c, d, f.** Variables known to cause nail and foot problems include deficient self-care abilities, vascular disease, arthritis, diabetes mellitus, history of biting nails or trimming them improperly, frequent or prolonged exposure to chemicals or water, trauma, ill-fitting shoes, and obesity. Antibiotic use and prostate cancer do not predispose to foot or nail problems.
5. **a, b, c, f.** During skin assessment, the nurse should compare bilateral parts for symmetry, use standard terminology to communicate and document findings, and perform the appropriate skin assessment when risk factors are identified. The nurse should proceed in a head-to-toe systematic manner, using cues/data from the nursing history to direct the assessment. When documenting a physical assessment of the skin, the nurse should describe exactly what is observed or palpated, including appearance, texture, size, location or distribution, and characteristics of any findings.
6. **a, e, f.** Washing the skin removes oil and debris, hair should be kept off the face and washed daily to keep oil from the hair off the face. Exposure to UV light should be avoided, especially when using acne treatments. Liberal use of cosmetics and emollients can clog the pores, worsening acne. Squeezing blackheads is discouraged because it may lead to infection.
7. **d.** If initial oral care results in continued dryness of the oral cavity with crusting, the nurse should increase frequency of oral hygiene, apply mouth moisturizer to oral mucosa, and monitor fluid intake and output to ensure adequate intake of fluid. It is not necessary to report this condition prior to providing the interventions mentioned above; however, mouth care and re-evaluation of the oral cavity is documented. The crusts should not be scraped with a tongue depressor.
8. **a, b, c, f.** The benefits of massage include general relaxation and increased circulation, pain relief, sleep promotion, and increased patient comfort and well-being. Massage also provides an opportunity for the nurse to communicate and connect with the patient through touch. Back massage is contraindicated if the patient has had back surgery or has fractured ribs.
9. **d.** The nurse applies gloves for the cleaning procedure, uses water or normal saline, and a clean washcloth or gauze to cleanse the eyes. After dampening a cleaning cloth with the solution of choice, the nurse wipes once while moving from the inner canthus to the outer canthus of the eye to reduce forcing debris into the area drained by the nasolacrimal duct. The nurse should turn the cleansing cloth and use a different section for each stroke until the eye is clean.
10. **b, d, f.** The nurse corrects the AP for soaking the feet or using alcohol and reminds them to use moisturizer if the feet are dry. Digging into or cutting the toenails at the lateral corners when trimming the nails requires correction; toenails should

be trimmed straight across. Guidelines for foot care include bathing the feet thoroughly in a mild soap and tepid water solution; drying feet thoroughly, including the area between the toes; and applying an antifungal foot powder when requested.

11. **c.** The nurse use music to soothe anxiety and agitation. The nurse should also shift the focus of the interaction from the "task of bathing" to the needs and abilities of the patient, and focus on comfort, safety, autonomy, and self-esteem, in addition to cleanliness. Wash the face and hair at the end of the bath or at a separate time. Water dripping in the face and having a wet head are often the most upsetting parts of the bathing process for people with dementia. The nurse should also consider methods for bathing aside from showers and tub baths. Towel baths, washing under clothes, and bathing "body sections" one day at a time, as well as dry shampoo or "shower cap" shampoos, are additional options.

12. **a, d, e.** Wash and rinse the groin area (both male and female patients) with a small amount of soap and water, and rinse. For male and female patients, always proceed from the least contaminated area to the most contaminated area and use a clean portion of the washcloth for each stroke. For a male patient, clean the tip of the penis first, moving the washcloth in a circular motion from the meatus outward. For a female patient, spread the labia and move the washcloth from the pubic area toward the anal area. In an uncircumcised male patient (teenage or older), retract the foreskin (prepuce) while washing the penis and return it to its original position when finished.

13. **c.** Safe nursing practice requires that the nurse assists a patient with an unsteady gait in and out of the tub. Adding bath oil to the bath water poses a safety risk because it makes the patient and tub slippery. Although privacy is important, if the patient locks the door, the nurse cannot help if there is an emergency. The water should be comfortably warm at 43° to 46°C. Older adults have an increased susceptibility to burns due to diminished sensitivity.

14. **c.** Threading the bag and tubing through the gown sleeve maintains a closed system and prevents contamination. No matter how quickly performed, any disconnection of IV tubing results in a breach of the sterile system, creating risk for infection. Cutting a gown is not an alternative except in an emergency.

15. **b.** When providing care for piercings, the nurse performs hand hygiene, applies gloves, then cleanses the site of all crusts and debris by rinsing the site with warm water and removing the crusts with a cotton swab. The nurse should then apply a dab of liquid-medicated cleanser, per policy, to the area, turn the jewelry back and forth to work the cleanser around the opening, rinse well, remove gloves, and perform hand hygiene. The nurse should not use alcohol, peroxide, or ointments at the site and should avoid removing piercings unless it is absolutely necessary (e.g., when an MRI is ordered.)

16. **b.** Older adults tend to develop dry skin; bathing frequency will change accordingly. Soaking adults' feet is not recommended. It is appropriate to keep a patient warm with bath blankets and provide perineal care washing from front to back.

Bibliography

Altarum Institute. (2019). *Sexual health and your patients: A provider's guide.* National Coalition for Sexual Health. https://nationalcoalitionforsexualhealth.org/tools/for-healthcare-providers

Alzheimer's Association. (2020). *Dental care.* https://www.alz.org/help-support/caregiving/daily-care/dental-care

American Academy of Dermatology (AAD). (n.d.). *Acne: Tips for managing.* Retrieved August 15, 2020, from https://www.aad.org/public/diseases/acne/skin-care/tips

American Academy of Family Physicians. (2019, July 19). *Body piercing.* https://familydoctor.org/body-piercing/?adfree=true

American Association of Critical-Care Nurses (AACN). (2017). *Practice alert: Oral care for acutely and critically ill patients. Critical Care Nurse, 37*(3), e19–e21.

American Association of Critical-Care Nurses (AACN). (2018). *Practice alert. Preventing venous thromboembolism in adults. Critical Care Nurse, 38*(3), 88. http://ccn.aacnjournals.org/content/36/5/e20.full.pdf.

American College of Foot and Ankle Surgeons. (n.d.). *Peripheral artery disease (PAD).* Retrieved August 25, 2020, from https://www.foothealthfacts.org/conditions/peripheral-arterial-disease-(p-a-d-)

American College of Prosthodontists. (n.d.). *Denture FAQs. Can I sleep in my dentures?* Retrieved July 31, 2020, from https://www.gotoapro.org/dentures-faq/#346

American Dental Association (ADA). (n.d.a). *Removable partial dentures.* Retrieved July 31, 2020, from https://www.mouthhealthy.org/en/az-topics/d/dentures-partial

American Dental Association (ADA). (n.d.b). *Flossing.* Retrieved August 15, 2020, from https://www.mouthhealthy.org/en/az-topics/f/flossing

American Dental Association (ADA). (n.d.c). *Dentures.* Retrieved August 15, 2020, from https://www.mouthhealthy.org/en/az-topics/d/dentures

American Dental Association (ADA). (n.d.d). *Water flossing.* Retrieved July 31, 2020, from https://www.mouthhealthy.org/en/az-topics/w/water-flossers

American Dental Association (ADA). (n.d.e). *Brushing your teeth.* Retrieved July 31, 2020, from https://www.mouthhealthy.org/en/az-topics/b/brushing-your-teeth

American Dental Association (ADA). (n.d.f). *Halitosis.* Retrieved July 31, 2020, from https://www.mouthhealthy.org/en/az-topics/h/halitosis

American Dental Association (ADA). (2019, August 29). *Oral health topics. Mouthrinse (Mouthwash).* https://www.ada.org/resources/research/science-and-research-institute/oral-health-topics/mouthrinse-mouthwash

American Dental Association (ADA). (2021a, December 23). *Oral-systemic health.* https://www.ada.org/resources/research/science-and-research-institute/oral-health-topics/oral-systemic-health

American Dental Association (ADA). (2021b, September 14). *Denture care and maintenance.* https://www.ada.org/resources/research/science-and-research-institute/oral-health-topics/dentures

Andrews, M., Boyle, J. S., & Collins, J. (2020). *Transcultural concepts in nursing care* (8th ed.). Wolters Kluwer.

Andriessen, A. (2013). Prevention, recognition and treatment of dry skin conditions. *British Journal of Nursing, 22*(1), 26–30.

Association of Professional Piercers. (2020). *Aftercare.* https://www.safepiercing.org/aftercare/

Barbe, A. G., Küpeli, L. S., Hamacher, S., & Noack, M. J. (2020). Impact of regular professional toothbrushing on oral health, related quality of life, and nutritional and cognitive status in nursing home residents. *International Journal of Dental Hygiene, 18*(3), 238–250. https://doi.org/10.1111/idh.12439

Bausch + Lomb. (2020). *Inserting and removing soft contact lenses.* https://www.bausch.com/reference/inserting-and-removing-contact-lenses#:~:text=Removing%20contact%20lenses%201%20Wash%2C%20rinse%2C%20and%20dry,the%20other%20lens%20by%20following%20the%20same%20procedure

Benfield, R., Heitkemper, M. M., & Newton, E. R. (2018). Culture, bathing and hydrotherapy in labor: An exploratory descriptive pilot study. *Midwifery, 64*, 110–114. https://doi.org/10.1016/j.midw.2018.06.005

Beuscher, T. L. (2019). Guidelines for diabetic foot care: A template for the care of all feet. *Journal of Wound Ostomy Continence Nursing, 46*(3), 241–245. https://doi.org/10.1097/WON.0000000000000532

Black, J., & Hotaling, T. (2015). Ten top tips: Bariatric skin care. *Wounds International, 6*(3), 17–21.

Brennan, L. J., & Strauss, J. (2014). Cognitive impairment in older adults and oral health considerations: Treatment and management. *Dental Clinics of North America, 58*(4), 815–828. https://doi.org/10.1016/j.cden.2014.07.001

Cadavona, J. J. P., Rimtepathip, P. P., & Jacob, S. E. (2018). Moisturization. *Journal of the Dermatology Nurses' Association, 10*(3), 158–160. https://doi.org/10.1097/JDN.0000000000000401

Cahill, S., Baker, K., & Makadon, H. (2020). *Do ask, do tell: A toolkit for collecting sexual orientation and gender identify information in clinical settings.* The Fenway Institute and the Center for American Progress. https://doaskdotell.org/

Cassir, N., Thomas, G., Hraiech, S., Brunet, J., Fournier, P. E., La Scola, B., & Papazian, L. (2015). Chlorhexidine daily bathing: Impact on health care-associated infections caused by gram-negative bacteria. *American Journal of Infection Control, 43*(6), 640–643. https://doi.org/10.1016/j.ajic.2015.02.010

Caya, T., Knobloch, M. J., Musuuza, J., Wilhelmson, E., & Safdar, N. (2019). Patient perceptions of chlorhexidine bathing: A pilot study using the health belief model. *American Journal of Infection Control, 47*(1), 18–22. https://doi.org/10.1016/j.ajic.2018.07.010

Centers for Disease Control and Prevention (CDC). (2013). *Oral health. Periodontal disease*. https://www.cdc.gov/oralhealth/conditions/periodontal-disease.html

Centers for Disease Control and Prevention (CDC). (2019a, September 11). *Parasites—Lice*. https://www.cdc.gov/parasites/lice/

Centers for Disease Control and Prevention (CDC). (2019b, September 6). *Ticks. Tick removal*. https://www.cdc.gov/ticks/removing_a_tick.html

Chen, W., Cao, Q, Li, S., Li, H., & Zhang, W. (2015). Impact of daily bathing with chlorhexidine gluconate on ventilator associated pneumonia in intensive care units: A meta-analysis. *Journal of Thoracic Disease, 7*(4), 746–753. https://doi.org/10.3978/j.issn.2072-1439.2015.04.21

Chick, A., & Wynne, A. (2020). Introducing an oral care assessment tool with advanced cleaning products into a high-risk clinical setting. *British Journal of Nursing, 29*(5), 290–296.

Chicote, A. (2019). Care aide abilities in oral care delivery and seniors' oral health outcomes. *Canadian Journal of Dental Hygiene, 53*(3), 178–181.

Cleveland Clinic. (2015, March 15). *Eyeglasses*. https://my.clevelandclinic.org/health/articles/8593-eyeglasses

Cleveland Clinic. (2017, December 8). *Ingrown toenails*. https://my.clevelandclinic.org/health/diseases/17664-ingrown-toenails

Cleveland Clinic. (2019, August 29). *Dental check-up*. https://my.clevelandclinic.org/health/treatments/11187-dental-check-up

Cleveland Clinic. (2020, June 16). *6 Do's and don'ts for contact lens wearers*. https://health.clevelandclinic.org/dos-and-donts-for-contact-lens-wearers/

Cowdell, F., & Radley, K. (2014). What do we know about skin-hygiene care for patients with bariatric needs? Implications for nursing practice. *Journal of Advanced Nursing, 70*(3), 543–552. https://doi.org/10.1111/jan.12208

Croney, S. (2018). Choosing an emollient. *British Journal of Nursing, 27*(11), 597–598.

D'Alesandro, M. A. (2014). Skin deep: Body piercings and dermal implants. *OR Nurse, 8*(6), 48. https://doi.org/10.1097/01.ORN.0000455910.23949.7d

Davis, C. (2014). Caring for … patients with tattoos and body piercings. *Nursing Made Incredibly Easy, 12*(6), 48–51. https://doi.org/10.1097/01.NME.0000454748.95582.1e

de Camargo, L., da Silva, S. N., & Chambrone, L. (2019). Efficacy of toothbrushing procedures performed in intensive care units in reducing the risk of ventilator-associated pneumonia: A systematic review. *Journal of Periodontal Research, 54*(6), 601–611. https://doi.org/10.1111/jre.12668

De Luca, E., Galizio, M., Resta, Daniela, & Papaleo, L. (2020). Integrating massage within oncology nursing care: An Italian pilot study. *International Journal of Caring Sciences, 13*(1), 194–206. https://internationaljournalofcaringsciences.org/docs/23_deluca_original_13_1.pdf

DeBoer, S., Seaver, M., Vidra, D., Robinson, B., & Klepacki, J. (2011). Breasts, bellies, below, and beyond: Body piercing jewelry and the transfer technique—when in doubt, don't necessarily take it out! *Journal of Emergency Nursing, 37*(6), 541–553. https://doi.org/10.1016/j.jen.2011.03.001

Dementia Care Central. (2019, September 23). How to safely and effectively assist an individual with dementia with bathing. https://www.dementiacarecentral.com/caregiverinfo/handsoncare/bathtime/

Dial, M., Holmes, J., McGownd, R., & Wendler, M. C. (2018). "I do the best I can:" Personal care preferences of patients of size. *Applied Nursing Research, 39*, 259–264. https://doi.org/10.1016/j.apnr.2017.11.028

Durkin, S. E. (2012). Tattoos, body piercing, and health-care concerns. *Journal of Radiology Nursing, 31*(1), 20–25. https://doi.org/10.1016/j.jradnu.2011.09.001

Earlam, A. S., & Woods, L. (2020). Obesity: Skin issues and skinfold management. *American Nurse Journal, 15*(6), 42–45.

Eliopoulos, C. (2018). *Gerontological nursing* (9th ed.). Wolters Kluwer.

Emery, K. P., & Guido-Sanz, F. (2019). Oral care practices in non-mechanically ventilated intensive care unit patients: An integrative review. *Journal of Clinical Nursing, 28*(13-14), 2462–2471. https://doi.org/10.1111/jocn.14829

Felton, D., Cooper, L., Duqum, I., Minsley, G., Guckes, A., Guckes, A., Meredith, P., Solie, C., Avery, D., Chandler, N. D.; American College of Prosthodontists, Academy of General Dentistry, American Dental Association Council on Scientific Affairs, American Dental Hygienists' Association, National Association of Dental Laboratories, & GlaxoSmithKline Consumer Healthcare. (2011). Evidence-based guidelines for the care and maintenance of complete dentures: A publication of the American College of Prosthodontists. *Journal of the American Dental Association, 142*(Suppl 1), 1S–20S.

Fisher, P., & Himan, C. (2020). Moisture-associated skin damage: A skin issue more prevalent than pressure ulcers. *Wounds UK, 16*(1), 58–63.

Gallagher, M., Hall, G. R., & Butcher, H. K. (2014). Bathing persons with Alzheimer's disease and related dementias. *Journal of Gerontological Nursing, 40*(2), 14–20. https://doi.org/10.3928/00989134-20131220-01

Ghersi, I., Mariño, M., & Miralles, M. T. (2018). Smart medical beds in patient-care environments of the twenty-first century: A state-of-art survey. *BMC Medical Informatics and Decision Making, 18*(1), 63. https://doi.org/10.1186/s12911-018-0643-5

Gibney, J. M., Wright, F. A., D'Souza, M., & Naganathan, V. (2019). Improving the oral health of older people in hospital. *Australasian Journal on Ageing, 38*(1), 33–38. https://doi.org/10.1111/ajag.12588

Goto, Y., Hayasaka, S., Kurihara, S., & Nakamura, Y. (2018). Physical and mental effects of bathing: A randomized intervention study. *Evidence-Based Complementary and Alternative Medicine*, 9521086. https://doi.org/10.1155/2018/9521086

Gould, C. V., Umscheid, C. A., Agarwal, R. K., Kuntz, G., & Pegues, D. A. and the Healthcare Infection Control Practices Advisory Committee (HICPAC). (2019 [update]). *Guideline for prevention of catheter-associated urinary tract infections 2009*. Centers for Disease Control and Prevention. https://www.cdc.gov/infectioncontrol/pdf/guidelines/cauti-guidelines-H.pdf

Gozalo, P., Prakash, S., Qato, D. M., Sloane, P. D., & Mor, V. (2014). Effect of the bathing without a battle training Intervention on bathing-associated physical and verbal outcomes in nursing home residents with dementia: A randomized crossover diffusion study. *Journal of the American Geriatrics Society, 62*(5), 797–804. https://doi.org/10.1111/jgs.12777

Greene, L. R. (2020). Non-ventilator health care-associated pneumonia (NV-HAP): Putting it all together. *American Journal of Infection Control, 48*(5S), A36–A38. https://doi.org/10.1016/j.ajic.2020.03.003

Griffiths, J., Jones, V., Leeman, I., Lewis, D., Patel, K., Wilson, K., & Blankenstein, R. (2020). Oral health care for people with mental health problems. Guidelines and recommendations. *British Society for Disability and Oral Health*. http://www.bsdh.org/documents/mental.pdf

Habibzadeh, H., Wosoi Dalavan, O., Alilu, L., Wardle, J., Khalkhali, H., & Nozad, A. (2020). Effects of foot massage on severity of fatigue and quality of life in hemodialysis patients: A randomized controlled trial. *International Journal of Community basede nursing & midwifery, 8*(2), 92–102. https://doi.org/10.30476/IJCBNM.2020.81662.0

Haesler, E., Frescos, N., & Rayner, R. (2018). The fundamental goal of wound prevention: Recent best evidence. *Wound Practice and Research, 26*(1), 14–22.

Hartford HealthCare. (2019, December 9). *Caregiving: Shaving an adult*. Hartford Hospital. https://hartfordhospital.org/health-wellness/health-resources/health-library/detail?id=abq1752

Hasan Tehrani, T., Bagher Maddah, S. S., Fallahi-Khoshknab, M., Ebadi, A., Mohammadi Shahboulaghi, F., & Gillespie, M. (2018). Respecting the privacy of hospitalized patients: An integrative review. *Nursing Ethics*, 969733018759832. https://doi.org/10.1177/0969733018759832

Hester, A. L. (2015). Preventing injuries from patient falls. *American Nurse Today, 10*(7), 36–37.

Hillery, S. (2019). Caring for patients with urinary incontinence-associated dermatitis. *British Journal of Nursing, 28*(9), S26–S28.

Hines, A. G., Nuss, S., Rupp, M. E., Lyden, E., Tyner, K., & Hewlett, A. (2015). Chlorhexidine bathing of hospitalized patients: Beliefs and practices of nurses and patient care technicians, and potential barriers to compliance. *Infection Control & Hospital Epidemiology, 36*(8), 993–994. https://doi.org/10.1017/ice.2015.92

Hinkle, J. L., Cheever, K. H., & Overbaugh, K. J. (2022). *Brunner & Suddarth's Textbook of medical-surgical nursing* (15th ed.). Wolters Kluwer.

International Association of Fire Fighters (IAFF). (n.d.). *The epidemic of liquid and steam burns*. National Scald Prevention Campaign. Retrieved July 29, 2020, from http://flashsplash.org/

Jablonski, R. A., Kolanowski, A. M., Azuero, A., Winstead, V., Jones-Townsend, C., & Geisinger, M. L. (2018). Randomised clinical trial: Efficacy of strategies to provide oral hygiene activities to nursing home residents with dementia who resist mouth care. *Gerontology, 35*(4), 365–375. https://doi.org/10.1111/ger.12357

Jarvis, C., & Echkardt, A. (2020). *Physical examination & health assessment* (8th ed.). Elsevier.

Jensen, S. (2019). *Nursing health assessment: A best practice approach* (3rd ed.). Wolters Kluwer.

Jenson, H., Maddux, S., & Waldo, M. (2018). Improving oral care in hospitalized non-ventilated patients: Standardizing products and protocol. *MEDSURG Nursing, 27*(1), 38–45.

Johns Hopkins All Children's Hospital. (n.d.). *Shaving*. Johns Hopkins Medicine. https://www.hopkinsallchildrens.org/Patients-Families/Health-Library/HealthDocNew/Shaving

Johnson, J., Suwantarat, N., Colantuoni, E., Ross, T. L., Aucott, S. W., Carroll, K. C., & Milstone, A. M. (2019). The impact of chlorhexidine gluconate bathing on skin bacterial burden of neonates admitted to the neonatal intensive care unit. *Journal of Perinatology, 39*(1), 63–71. https://doi.org/10.1038/s41372-018-0231-7

Jusino-Leon, G. N., Matheson, L., & Forsythe, L. (2019). Chlorhexidine gluconate baths: Supporting daily use to reduce central line-associated bloodstream infections affecting immunocompromised patients. *Clinical Journal of Oncology Nursing, 23*(2), E32–E38. https://doi.org/10.1188/19.CJON.E32-E38

Kadia, S., Bawa, R., Shah, H., Lippmann, S., & Narang, P. (2014). Poor oral hygiene in the mentally ill: Be aware of the problem, and intervene. *Current Psychiatry, 13*(7), 47–48.

Karch, A. M. (2020). *Focus on nursing pharmacology* (8th ed.). Wolters Kluwer.

Kemp, G., Hallbourg, M., Altounji, D., & Secola, R. (2019). Back to basics: CLABSI reduction through implementation of an oral care and hygiene bundle. *Journal of Pediatric Oncology Nursing, 36*(5), 321–326. https://doi.org/10.1177/1043454219849583

Kennedy, K. J., Price, K., Rando, T. L., Boylan, J., & Dyer, A. R. (2018). Ensuring healthy skin as part of wound prevention: An integrative review of health professionals' actions. *Journal of Wound Care, 27*(11), 707–715.

Kisely, S. (2016). No mental health without oral health. *The Canadian Journal of Psychiatry, 61*(5), 277–282. https://doi.org/10.1177/0706743716632523

Konno, R., Kang, H. S., & Makimoto, K. (2014). A best-evidence review of intervention studies for minimizing resistance-to-care behaviours for older adults with dementia in nursing homes. *Journal of Advanced Nursing, 70*(10), 2167–2180. https://doi.org/10.1111/jan.12432

Kyle, T., & Carman, S. (2021). *Essentials of pediatric nursing* (4th ed.). Wolters Kluwer.

Lee, B., Vangipuram, R., Peterson, E., & Tyring, S. K. (2018). Complications associated with intimate body piercings. *Dermatology Online Journal, 24*(7), https://escholarship.org/uc/item/5gp333zr

Lee, K. H., Wu, B., & Plassman, B. L. (2013). Cognitive function and oral health-related quality of life in older adults. *Journal of the American Geriatrics Society, 61*(9), 1602–1607. https://doi.org/10.1111/jgs.12402

Lichterfeld, A., Hauss, A., Surber, C., Peters, T., Blume-Peytavi, U., & Lottner, J., (2015). Evidence-based skin care: A systematic literature review and the development of a basic skin care algorithm. *Journal of Wound, Ostomy, and Continence Nursing, 42*(5), 501–524. https://doi.org/10.1097/WON.0000000000000162

Lichterfeld-Kottner, A., El Genedy, M., Lahmann, N., Blume-Peytavi, U., Büscher, A., & Kottner, J. (2020). Maintaining skin integrity in the aged: A systematic review. *International Journal of Nursing Studies, 103*, 103509. https://doi.org/10.1016/j.ijnurstu.2019.103509

Lim, Y. S. L., & Carville, K. (2019). Prevention and management of incontinence-associated dermatitis in the pediatric population: An integrative review. *Journal of Wound, Ostomy, Continence Nursing, 46*(1), 30–37. https://doi.org/10.1097/WON.0000000000000490

Lumbers, M. (2018). Moisture-associated skin damage: Cause, risk and management. *British Journal of Nursing, 27*(Suppl 12), S6–S14.

Magnani, C., Mastroianni, C., Giannarelli D., Stefanelli, M. C., Di Cienzo, V., Valerioti, T., & Casale, G. (2019). Oral hygiene care in patients with advanced disease: An essential measure to improve oral cavity conditions and symptom management. *American Journal of Hospice & Palliative Medicine, 36*(9), 815–819. https://doi.org/10.1177/1049909119829411

Martinez, T., Baugnon, T., Vergnaud, E., Duracher, C., Perie, A. C., Bustarret, O., Jugie, M., Rubinsztajn, R., Frange, P., Meyer, P., Orliaguet, G., & Blanot, S. (2020). Central-line-associated bloodstream infections in a surgical paediatric intensive care unit: Risk factors and prevention with chlorhexidine bathing. *Journal of Paediatrics and Child Health, 56*(6), 936–942. https://doi.org/10.1111/jpc.14780

Matsumoto, C., Nanke, K., Furumura, S., Arimatsu, M., Fukuyama, M., & Maeda, H. (2019). Effects of disposable bath and towel bath on the transition of resident skin bacteria, water content of the stratum corneum, and relaxation. *American Journal of Infection Control, 47*(7), 811–815. https://doi.org/10.1016/j.ajic.2018.12.008

Mayo Foundation for Medical Education and Research (MFMER). (2017, August 8). *Amputation and diabetes: How to protect your feet*. https://www.mayoclinic.org/diseases-conditions/diabetes/in-depth/amputation-and-diabetes/art-20048262

Mayo Foundation for Medical Education and Research (MFMER). (2018, February 1). *Dental exam for children*. https://www.mayoclinic.org/tests-procedures/dental-exam-for-children/about/pac-20393745

Mayo Foundation for Medical Education and Research (MFMER). (2019a, June 6). *Adult health. Oral health: Brush up on dental care basics*. https://www.mayoclinic.org/healthy-lifestyle/adult-health/in-depth/dental/art-20045536

Mayo Foundation for Medical Education and Research (MFMER). (2019b, March 27). *Contact lenses: What to know before you buy*. https://www.mayoclinic.org/healthy-lifestyle/adult-health/in-depth/contact-lenses/art-20046293

Mayo Foundation for Medical Education and Research (MFMER). (2019c, October 16). *Fingernails: Do's and don'ts for healthy nails*. https://www.mayoclinic.org/healthy-lifestyle/adult-health/in-depth/nails/art-20044954

Mayo Foundation for Medical Education and Research (MFMER). (2019d, December 10). *Ingrown toenails*. https://www.mayoclinic.org/diseases-conditions/ingrown-toenails/symptoms-causes/syc-20355903

Mayo Foundation for Medical Education and Research (MFMER). (2019e, September 24). *Sweating and body odor*. https://www.mayoclinic.org/diseases-conditions/sweating-and-body-odor/diagnosis-treatment/drc-20353898

Mayo Foundation for Medical Education and Research (MFMER). (2020a, July 18). *Piercings: How to prevent complications*. https://www.mayoclinic.org/healthy-lifestyle/adult-health/in-depth/piercings/art-20047317

Mayo Foundation for Medical Education and Research (MFMER). (2020b, March 31). *Ingrown hair*. https://www.mayoclinic.org/diseases-conditions/ingrown-hair/symptoms-causes/syc-20373893

Mayo Foundation for Medical Education and Research (MFMER). (2022, January 18). *Vagina: What's typical, what's not*. https://www.mayoclinic.org/healthy-lifestyle/womens-health/in-depth/vagina/art-20046562

McBride, D. L. (2018). Clinical guidance to tattooing and piercing among youth. *Journal of Pediatric Nursing, 39*, 83–84. https://doi.org/10.1016/j.pedn.2017.11.012

McCormick, R., Robin, A. T., Gluch, J., & Lipman, T. H. (2019). Oral health assessment in acute care pediatric nursing. *Pediatric Nursing, 45*(6), 299–309.

MedlinePlus. (2020a, July 8). *Rashes*. National Library of Medicine. https://medlineplus.gov/rashes.html

MedlinePlus. (2020b, July 2). *Penis care (uncircumcised)*. National Library of Medicine. https://medlineplus.gov/ency/article/001917.htm

Mitchell, A., & Hill, B. (2020). Moisture-associated skin damage: An overview of its diagnosis and management. *Community Wound Care, 25*(3), S12–S18.

Momeni, M., Arab, M., Dehghan, M., & Ahmadinejad, M. (2020). The effect of foot massage on pain of the intensive care patients: A parallel randomized single-blind controlled trial. *Evidence-Based Complementary and Alternative Medicine*. https://doi.org/10.1155/2020/3450853

Moncrieff, G., Van Onselen, J., & Young, T. (2015). The role of emollients in maintaining skin integrity. *Wounds UK, 11*(1), 68–74.

Moore, A., & Merrill, E. (2019, March/April). Evaluating older adult self-care capacity. *Nursing Made Incredibly Easy, 17*(2), 34–41. https://doi.org/10.1097/01.NME.0000553089.93831.33

Morse, J. M., Gervais, P., Pooler, C., Merryweather, A., Doig, A. K., & Bloswick, D. (2015). The safety of hospital beds: Ingress, egress, and in-bed mobility. *Global Qualitative Nursing Research, 2*, 1–20. https://doi.org/10.1177/2333393615575321

Morton, P. G., & Fontaine, D. K. (2018). *Critical care nursing. A holistic approach* (11th ed.). Wolters Kluwer.

Muir, M., & Archer-Heese, G. (2009). Essentials of a bariatric patient handling program. *The Online Journal of Issues in Nursing, 14*(1), Manuscript 5. https://doi.org/10.3912/OJIN.Vol14No1Man05

Musuuza, J. S., Guru, P. K., O'Horo, J. C., Bongiorno, C. M., Korobkin, M. A., Gangnon, R. E., & Safdar, N. (2019). The impact of chlorhexidine bathing on hospital-acquired bloodstream infections: A systematic review and meta-analysis. *BMC Infectious Diseases, 19*(1), 416. https://doi.org/10.1186/s12879-019-4002-7

National Institute on Aging. (n.d.). *Fall-proofing your home*. https://www.nia.nih.gov/health/fall-proofing-your-home

National Institute on Aging. (2020, March 13). *Taking care of your teeth and mouth*. https://www.nia.nih.gov/health/taking-care-your-teeth-and-mouth

National Institutes of Health (NIH). (2014). *Tick talk. Block tick bites and Lyme disease*. https://newsinhealth.nih.gov/2014/05/tick-talk

National Institutes of Health (NIH). (2015, October). *Keep your mouth healthy. Oral care for older adults*. NIH News in Health. https://newsinhealth.nih.gov/2015/10/keep-your-mouth-healthy

Nøddeskou, L. H., Hemmingsen, L. E., & Hørdam, B. (2015). Elderly patients' and nurses' assessment of traditional bed bath compared to prepacked single units—randomised controlled trial. *Scandinavian Journal of Caring Sciences, 29*(2), 347–352. https://doi.org/10.1111/scs.12170

Office of Women's Health. (2019, April 1). *Douching*. U.S. Department of Health and Human Services. https://www.womenshealth.gov/a-z-topics/douching

Parnham, A., Copson, D., & Loban, T. (2020). Moisture-associated skin damage: Causes and an overview of assessment, classification and management. *British Journal of Nursing, 29*(12), S30–S37.

Quinn, B., Giuliano, K. K., & Baker, D. (2020). Non-ventilator health care-associated pneumonia (NV-HAP): Best practices for prevention of NV-HAP. *American Journal of Infection Control, 48*(5S), A23–A27. https://doi.org/10.1016/j.ajic.2020.03.006

Rademeyer, C., Farley, C. L., & Van Hoover, C. (2020). Health implications and counseling considerations for individuals with piercings and tattoos. *Nursing for Women's Health, 24*(3), 210–227. https://doi.org/10.1016/j.nwh.2020.03.006

Ramos-Morcillo, A. J., Moreno-Martínez, F. J., Hernández Susarte, A. M., Hueso-Montoro, C., & Ruzafa-Martínez, M. (2019). Social determinants of health, the family, and children's personal hygiene: A comparative study. *International Journal of Environmental Research and Public Health, 16*(23), 4713.

Red, A., & O'Neal, P. V. (2020). Implementation of an evidence-based oral care protocol to improve the delivery of mouth care in nursing home residents. *Journal of Gerontological Nursing, 46*(5), 33–39. https://doi.org/10.3928/00989134-20200316-01

Reynolds, S. S., Sova, C., McNalty, B., Lambert, S., & Granger, B. (2019). Implementation strategies to improve evidence-based bathing practices in a neuro ICU. *Journal of Nursing Care Quality, 34*(2), 133–138. https://doi.org/10.1097/NCQ.0000000000000347

Rhee, Y., Palmer, L. J., Okamoto, K., Gemunden, S., Hammouda, K., Kemble, S. K., Lin, M. Y., Lolans, K., Fogg, L., Guanaga, D., Yokoe, D. S., Weinstein, R. A., Frendl, G., Hayden, M. K., & Centers for Disease Control and Prevention Epicenter Program. (2018). Differential effects of chlorhexidine skin cleansing methods on residual chlorhexidine skin concentrations and bacterial recovery. *Infection Control & Hospital Epidemiology, 39*(4), 405–411. https://doi.org/10.1017/ice.2017.312

Riley, E. (2018). The importance of oral health in palliative care patients. *Journal of Community Nursing, 32*(3), 57–61.

Roos, A. K. Ø, Skaug, E. A., Grønkahl, V. A., & Helgesenk, A. K. (2020). Trading company for privacy: A study of patients' experiences. *Nursing Ethics, 27*(4), 1089–1102. https://doi.org/10.1177/0969733019874497

Scales, K., Zimmerman, S., & Miller, S. J. (2018). Evidence-based nonpharmacological practices to address behavioral and psychological symptoms of dementia. *The Gerontologist, 58*(Suppl_1), S88–S102. https://doi.org/10.1093/geront/gnx167

Schmidt, J. C., Calderaro, S., Weiger, R., & Walter, C. (2019). On the association between oral piercings and periodontal conditions–A case series. *International Journal of Dental Hygiene, 17*(4), 318–326. https://doi.org/10.1111/idh.12403

Schoonhoven, L., van Gaal, B. G. I, Teerenstra, S., Adang, E., van der Vleuten, C., & van Achterberg, T. (2015). Cost-consequence analysis of "washing without water" for nursing home residents: A cluster randomized trial. *International Journal of Nursing Studies, 52*(1), 112–120. https://doi.org/10.1016/j.ijnurstu.2014.08.001

Schreiber, M. L. (2019). Tattoos and piercings: Considerations for nursing practice. *MEDSURG Nursing, 28*(2), 130–134.

Shah, H. N., Schwartz, J. L., Luna, G., & Cullen, D. L. (2016). Bathing with 2% chlorhexidine gluconate: Evidence and costs associated with central line-associated bloodstream infections. *Critical Care Nursing Quarterly, 39*(1), 42–50. https://doi.org/10.1097/CNQ.0000000000000096

Sharma, K., & Kumari, R. (2019). Study to assess the effectiveness of foot and hand massage on reducing pain among post-natal mothers who had undergone Caesarean section. *International Journal of Nursing Education, 11*(1), 79–84. https://doi.org/10.5958/0974-9357.2019.00017.5

Silbert-Flagg, J., & Pillitteri, A. (2018). *Maternal and child health nursing* (8th ed.). Wolters Kluwer.

So, H. S., You, M. A., Mun, J. Y., et al. (2014). Effect of trunk to head bathing on physiological responses in newborns. *Journal of Obstetric, Gynecological, & Neonatal Nursing, 43*(6), 742–751. https://doi.org/10.1111/1552-6909.12496

Sparks, D. (2018, October 4). *Women's wellness: Drink water to fight those urinary tract infections*. Mayo Clinic. https://newsnetwork.mayoclinic.org/discussion/womens-wellness-drink-water-to-fight-those-utis/

Sturgeon, L. P., Garrett-Wright, D., Lartey, G., Jones, M. S., Bormann, L., & House, S. (2019). A descriptive study of bathing practices in acute care facilities in the United States. *American Journal of Infection Control, 47*(1), 23–26. https://doi.org/10.1016/j.ajic.2018.07.007

Thomas, C. (2019). Dental care in older adults. *British Journal of Community Nursing, 24*(5), 233–235.

Toughy, T. A., & Jett, K. (2018). *Ebersol and Hess' gerontological nursing & healthy aging* (5th ed.). Elsevier.

U.S. Food and Drug Administration (FDA). (2016a, March 22). *Use eye cosmetics safely*. https://www.fda.gov/consumers/consumer-updates/use-eye-cosmetics-safely

U.S. Food and Drug Administration (FDA). (2016b, July 6). *Should you put sunscreen on infants? Not usually*. https://www.fda.gov/consumers/consumer-updates/should-you-put-sunscreen-infants-not-usually

U.S. Food and Drug Administration (FDA). (2017a, December 11). *A guide to bed safety bed rails in hospitals, nursing homes and home health care: The facts*. https://www.fda.gov/medical-devices/hospital-beds/guide-bed-safety-bed-rails-hospitals-nursing-homes-and-home-health-care-facts

U.S. Food and Drug Administration (FDA). (2017b, November 5). *Color additives permitted for use in cosmetics*. https://www.fda.gov/cosmetics/cosmetic-ingredient-names/color-additives-permitted-use-cosmetics

U.S. Food and Drug Administration (FDA). (2018a, August 30). *Bed rail safety*. https://www.fda.gov/medical-devices/consumer-products/bed-rail-safety?source=govdelivery&utm_medium=email&utm_source=govdelivery

U.S. Food and Drug Administration (FDA). (2018b, August 23). *Hospital beds*. https://www.fda.gov/medical-devices/general-hospital-devices-and-supplies/hospital-beds

U.S. Food and Drug Administration (FDA). (2019a, August 29). *Sunscreen: How to help protect your skin from the sun*. https://www.fda.gov/drugs/understanding-over-counter-medicines/sunscreen-how-help-protect-your-skin-sun

U.S. Food and Drug Administration (FDA). (2019b, February 21). *Tips to stay safe in the sun: From sunscreen to sunglasses*. https://www.fda.gov/consumers/consumer-updates/tips-stay-safe-sun-sunscreen-sunglasses

Urias, D. S., Varghese, M., Simunich, T., Morrissey, S., & Dumire, R. (2018). Preoperative decolonization to reduce infections in urgent lower extremity repairs. *European Journal of Truama and Emergency Surgery, 44*(5), 787–793. https://doi.org/10.1007/s00068-017-0896-1

VA Mobile Health. (n.d.). *Safe patient handling*. (Version 1.3.3). [Mobile app]. U. S. Department of Veteran Affairs. https://mobile.va.gov/app/safe-patienthandling

Van Hoover, C., Rademayer, C. A., & Farley, C. L. (2017). Body piercing: Motivations and implications for health. *Journal of Midwifery and Women's Health, 62*(5), 521–530. https://doi.org/10.1111/jmwh.12630

Vannah, C. E., & Sammarco, V. R. (2019). Electric brushes improve outcomes in caregiver-assisted oral hygiene. *Nursing, 49*(8), 56–60. https://doi.org/10.1097/01.NURSE.0000569764.96290.70

Veje, P. L., Chen, M., Jensen, C. S., Sørenen, J., & Primdahl, J. (2019). Bed bath with soap and water or disposable wet wipes: Patients' experiences and preferences. *Journal of Clinical Nursing, 28*(11-12), 2235–2244. https://doi.org/10.1111/jocn.14825

Veje, P. L., Chen, M., Jensen, C. S., Sørenen, J., & Primdahl, J. (2020). Effectiveness of two bed bath methods in removing microorganisms from hospitalized patients: A prospective randomized crossover study. *American Journal of Infection Control, 48*(6), 638–643. https://doi.org/10.1016/j.ajic.2019.10.011

VHA Center for Engineering & Occupational Safety and Health (CEOSH). (2016). *Safe patient handling and mobility guidebook*. http://www.tnpatientsafety.com/pubfiles/Initiatives/workplace-violence/sphm-pdf.pdf

Voegeli, D. (2019). Prevention and management of moisture-associated skin damage. *Nursing Standard, 34*(2), 77–82. https://doi.org/10.7748/ns.2019.e11314

VonStein, M., Buchko, B. L., Millen, C., Lampo, D., Bell, T., & Woods, A. B. (2019). Effect of a scheduled nurse intervention on thirst and dry mouth in intensive care patients. *American Journal of Critical Care, 28*(1), 41–46. https://doi.org/10.4037/ajcc2019400

Warren, S., Midodzi, W. K., Newhook, L. A. A., Murphy, P., & Twells, L. (2020). Effects of delayed newborn bathing on breastfeeding, hypothermia, and hypoglycemia. *Journal of Obstetric, Gynecologic & Neonatal Nursing, 49*(2), 181–189. https://doi.org/10.1016/j.jogn.2019.12.004

Weber, J. R., & Kelley, J. H. (2018). *Health assessment in nursing* (6th ed.). Wolters Kluwer.

Westman, K. F., & Blaisdell, C. (2016). Many benefits, little risk: The use of massage in nursing practice. *The American Journal of Nursing, 116*(1), 34–39. Doi: 10.10 HYPERLINK "https://doi.org/10.1097/01.naj.0000476164.97929.f2"97/01.NAJ.0000476164.97929.f2

Whitehead, P. J., & Golding-Day, M. R. (2019). The lived experience of bathing adaptations in the homes of older adults and their carers (BATH-OUT): A qualitative interview study. *Health and Social Care in the Community, 27*(6), 1534–1543. https://doi.org/10.1111/hsc.12824

Wiggerman, N., Rempel, K., Zerhusen, R. M., Pelo, T., & Mann, N. (2019). Human-centered design process for a hospital bed: Promoting patient safety and ease of use. *Ergonomics in Design, 27*(2), 4–12. https://doi.org/10.1177/1064804618805570

Wiggerman, N., Smith, K., & Kumpar, D. (2017). What bed size does a patient need? The relationship between body mass index and space required to turn in bed. *Nursing Research, 66*(6), 483–489. https://doi.org/10.1097/NNR.0000000000000242

Williamson, K. (2020). Nursing people with bariatric care needs: More questions than answers. *Wounds UK, 16*(1), 64–71. https://www.wounds-uk.com/journals/issue/608/article-details/nursing-people-with-bariatric-care-needs-more-questions-than-answers

Wolf, Z. R., & Czekanski, K. E. (2015). Bathing disability and bathing persons with dementia. *Medsurg Nursing, 24*(1), 9–14, 22.

Woods, M. (2019). Care of skin that is oedematous or at risk of oedema. *British Journal of Nursing, 28*(11), 674–676.

Woon, C. (2020). Improving oral care for hospitalised patients: Choosing appropriate products. *British Journal of Nursing, 29*(9), 520–525.

Wounds UK. (2018). *Best practice statement. Maintaining skin integrity*. https://www.wounds-uk.com/resources/details/maintaining-skin-integrity

33 Skin Integrity and Wound Care

Mary Biesicker

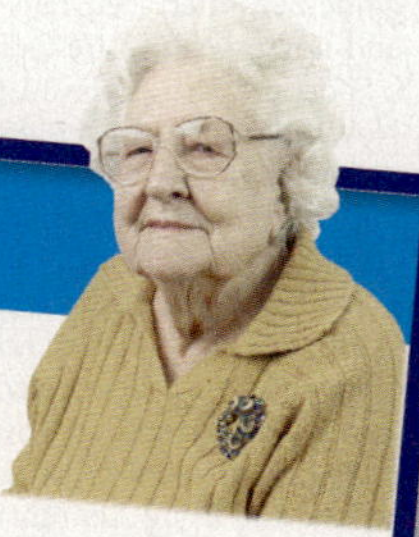

Mary, who is 84 years old, has been cared for at home by her daughter since being hospitalized last year for a cerebrovascular accident (stroke). She has been unable to take care of herself, finds it increasingly more difficult to get out of bed, and is having more frequent episodes of incontinence. According to her daughter, Mary has developed a "blister" on her back. Mary is being assessed by the home health care nurse at the request of her daughter, who is finding it difficult to care for her mother alone.

Lucius Everly

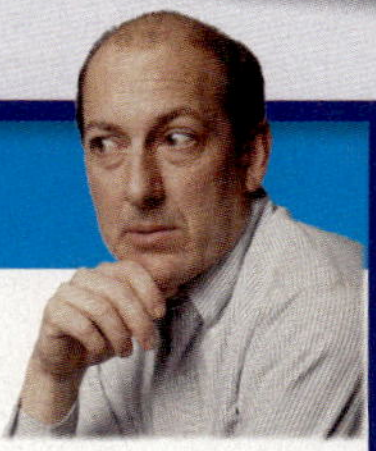

Lucius, a 52-year-old who has a history of diabetes and circulatory problems, underwent abdominal surgery several days ago and is in the critical care unit. He is slouched down in bed, his abdominal dressing is moist, and only part of the tape securing the dressing is adhering to the skin. His level of consciousness is decreased, and he responds only to moderate touch and pain. Further assessment reveals the beginning of a pressure injury on his heel.

Sam Bentz

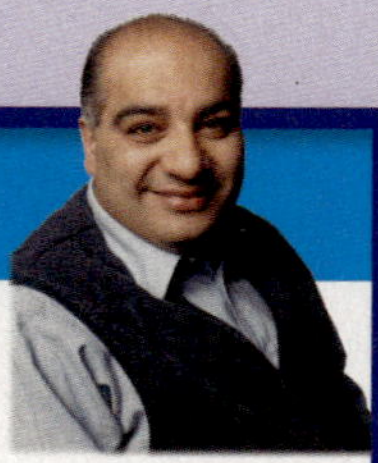

Sam, a 56-year-old, has been admitted to the hospital for aggressive treatment of a bone infection that has not responded to usual treatment methods. Sam is 5 ft 4 inches tall and weighs more than 300 lb. They tell you, "Last time I was here, my skin got really irritated and I developed several skin wounds."

Lippincott DocuCare **Additional patient scenarios available in *Lippincott DocuCare*.**

Learning Outcomes

After completing the chapter, you will be able to accomplish the following:

1. Discuss the processes involved in wound healing.
2. Identify factors that affect wound healing.
3. Identify patients at risk for pressure injury development.
4. Describe the method of staging of pressure injuries.
5. Accurately assess and document the condition of wounds.
6. Provide nursing interventions to prevent pressure injuries.
7. Implement appropriate dressing changes for different kinds of wounds.
8. Provide information to patients and caregivers for self-care of wounds at home.
9. Apply hot and cold therapy effectively and safely.

Nursing Concepts

- Cellular Regulation
- Evidence-Based Practice
- Infection
- Inflammation
- Tissue integrity

The skin is the body's first line of defense, protecting the underlying structures from invasion by organisms. Maintaining an intact skin surface is important because a break or disruption in this integrity is potentially dangerous and possibly life threatening. The nurse plays a major role in maintaining the patient's skin integrity, identifying risk factors that predispose a patient to a break in integrity, intervening to prevent or reduce a patient's risk for impaired skin integrity, and providing specific wound care when breaks in integrity arise. Additional information related to general skin care is discussed in Chapter 32.

Development and maintenance of the knowledge and skills necessary to implement evidence-based wound care is an essential component of nursing care. Using the nursing process, an individualized care plan is developed to assess the patient and the wound; identify and prevent complications; implement and evaluate skills essential to wound care; and provide physical and emotional support to facilitate healing, adaptation, and self-care. Wound care may be required in any health care setting and complex wound care at home is on the rise.

This chapter provides information about disruptions in skin and tissue integrity, including wounds and pressure injuries. Because applications of heat and cold are used to treat altered skin integrity, a discussion of those treatment modalities is also included. Refer to the Reflective Practice display for an illustration of nursing care issues related to skin integrity.

ANATOMY AND PHYSIOLOGY OF THE INTEGUMENTARY SYSTEM

Knowledge of the basic anatomy and physiology of the integumentary system and understanding the role of this system in the body provides a foundation for assessment. This knowledge also informs the analysis of data and provides rationale for planning and implementing interventions that promote and restore optimal skin integrity.

Structures of the Skin

The skin, or integument, is the largest organ of the body and has multiple functions. The skin covers the entire body and is continuous with mucous membranes at normal body orifices. It is essential for maintaining life.

The integumentary system is made up of the skin, the subcutaneous layer directly under the skin, and the appendages of the skin, including glands in the skin, hair, and nails. The integumentary system also includes the blood vessels, nerves, and sensory organs of the skin.

The skin has three layers: the epidermis, the dermis, and the subcutaneous tissue layer (Jensen, 2019; Norris, 2019). A cross-section of normal skin is illustrated in Figure 33-1 on page 1151.

The top layer, or outermost portion, is the **epidermis**. The epidermis is composed of layers of stratified epithelial cells. These cells fuse to form a protective, waterproof layer of keratin material. Epithelial cells have no blood vessels of their own and depend on underlying tissues for nourishment and waste removal. When well nourished, epithelium regenerates relatively easily and quickly.

The second layer of skin, the **dermis**, consists of a framework of elastic connective tissue comprised primarily of collagen. Nerves, hair follicles, glands, immune cells, and blood vessels are located in this layer (Norris, 2019). Each hair consists of the shaft, which projects through the dermis beyond the surface of the skin, and the hair follicle, which lies in the dermis.

The dermis rests on the **subcutaneous tissue**, the bottom layer that anchors the skin layers to the underlying tissues of the body. The subcutaneous tissue consists of adipose tissue, made up of lobules of fat cells, and connective tissue. This layer stores fat for energy, serves as a heat insulator for the body, and provides a cushioning effect for protection. This fatty tissue layer contains blood and lymph vessels, nerves, and fat cells.

Functions of the Skin and Mucous Membranes

The skin has multiple functions: protection, temperature regulation, psychosocial, sensation, vitamin D production, immunologic, absorption, and elimination. See Table 33-1 (on page 1152) for details of each of these functions.

Mucous membranes line body cavities that open to the outside of the body, joining with the skin. They can also be found in the digestive tract, the respiratory passages, and the urinary and reproductive tracts. Epithelium covers the

QSEN Reflective Practice: Cultivating QSEN Competencies

CHALLENGE TO ETHICAL AND LEGAL SKILLS

I had a tough clinical 2 weeks ago while caring for Lucius Everly, a critical care postop patient with a history of diabetes and circulation problems. The nurse I was working with had floated to the unit on this day, but I didn't know that at the time. Mr. Everly appeared to be neglected by other caregivers; because he was not communicating and had a decreased level of consciousness, he could not express his needs. In my opinion, he needed bathing, wound care, repositioning in bed, and some additional attention I was unable to provide independently. Although the nurse did their best to educate me on the history and status of the patient, the nurse spoke about Mr. Everly over the bed as if he wasn't even there. In my opinion, the nurse did not respect his inability to communicate. I became frustrated because she did not seem to share my sense of concern for him. The nurse was noncommittal when I asked specifically about foot care and what I could do to promote circulation in his feet. My frustration increased when I realized that he was developing a pressure ulcer on his heel.

Thinking Outside the Box: Possible Courses of Action

- Tell my clinical instructor of my frustrations earlier in the day so my patient's care could have been addressed earlier and my frustrations wouldn't have compounded.
- Go to the nurse and tell them that I wasn't comfortable with the care they were providing, insisting that more needed to be done for this patient.
- Ask the charge nurse to assess the quality of care that my patient was receiving compared to what he needed.

Evaluating a Good Outcome: How Do I Define Success?

- Patient receives a higher quality of care designed to maintain his dignity.
- The nurse responds positively to the constructive feedback, making changes to the care that is being provided to the patient.
- By addressing the problem earlier in the process, my frustrations do not interfere with my care of the patient or my development of working relationships with the health care team.
- The patient is not discriminated against and neglected based on his inability to communicate and his decreased level of consciousness.
- On a professional developmental level, I explore my agency and role in patient advocacy while I have the support of and guidance from my clinical faculty; I learn to effectively navigate a complex, interprofessional situation.

Personal Learning: Here's to the Future!

Happy and sad outcome. Although this patient was not verbally communicating, I held his hand, talked to him, and felt that he was able to recognize my caring presence. After interprofessional rounds that morning, I verbalized my frustration about the status of my patient to my clinical instructor and I asked if she would come meet him and help me provide the necessary care. Unlike my nurse, my clinical instructor involved Mr. Everly in his care, providing verbal and tactile support and comfort as we worked to make him as comfortable as possible. She provided me tips and tricks as she walked Mr. Everly and me through the interventions. My instructor demonstrated how to provide personal care focused on protecting and maintaining the dignity of the patient. In addition, my instructor called in the charge nurse to point out the lack of care this patient had been receiving, wanting to ensure that his future level of care improved. My instructor and the charge nurse, in a professional, nondegrading way, expressed to the assigned nurse that this patient needed a higher quality of care due to his critical condition. Having my instructor agree with my concerns for this patient and address the nurse and charge nurse made me feel much better about the care my patient would then receive. I later told my teacher that I was frustrated because I felt all the nurse was concerned about was "giving all the medications and signing off on the right pages," when in fact talking to this patient, holding his hand, and making him more comfortable were definitely as important. Two days later the patient died. I was sad but so honored to have been able to care for him and hold his hand in his last days.

Although I think I should have gone to my clinical instructor immediately to explain the problem I was having, telling her was the right decision. My instructor took my concerns seriously and first helped me care for the patient, then went straight to the charge nurse to ensure proper skin and wound care for the patient. Finally, she was able to address the nurse without insulting her to make sure we were all on the same page about the care this patient needed, but had not been receiving. By speaking up, I was able to leave my clinical assignment feeling positive about my actions and advocating for this patient. I still felt frustrated with how he had been cared for and realized that all too often as care providers, we get too involved in the routine of charting, distributing medications, and so on, and can forget how important some simple measures are such as offering a gentle touch, positioning, providing hygiene and wound care, and just spending time with the patient. I take comfort in knowing that I contributed, in a very small way, to Mr. Everly's dying with dignity.

Carrie Staines, Georgetown University

QSEN Reflective Practice: Cultivating QSEN Competencies *(continued)*

CHALLENGE TO ETHICAL AND LEGAL SKILLS

QSEN SELF-REFLECTION ON QUALITY AND SAFETY COMPETENCIES DEVELOPING KNOWLEDGE, SKILLS, AND ATTITUDES FOR CONTINUOUS IMPROVEMENT

How do you think you would respond in a similar situation? Why? What does this tell you about yourself and about the adequacy of your skills for professional practice? What factors might have affected the assigned nurse's response to the patient? Would the student have been affected by any of these same factors? Do you agree with the criteria to evaluate a successful outcome? Did the nursing student validate the rationale for the outcome? What *knowledge, skills,* and *attitudes* do you need to develop to continuously improve the quality and safety of care for patients like Mr. Everly?

Patient-Centered Care: What evidence from the scenario would lead you to suspect that the patient is at risk for impaired skin integrity? What preventive measures might be appropriate? What measures might be appropriate to ensure therapeutic person-centered care?

Teamwork and Collaboration/Quality Improvement: What communication skills do you need to improve to ensure that you communicate care provided and needed at each transition in care? What communication skills do you need to improve to ensure that you function as a member of the patient-care team? Can you think of other ways to respond? How can you frame advocating for the patient in a way that builds team relationships and promotes teamwork?

Safety/Evidence-Based Practice: What skills do you need to improve to ensure that patients in your care receive the best nursing care possible? What evidence in nursing literature provides guidance for decision making regarding care of this patient? What does this tell you about yourself and about the adequacy of your skills for professional practice? What, if any, ethical and legal principles were demonstrated by the nursing student's actions?

Informatics: Can you identify the essential information that must be available in Mr. Everly's electronic health record to support safe patient care and coordination of care? What information should be documented in the electronic health record regarding the student's assessment and interventions?

mucous membrane surfaces and contains cells that secrete mucus. Mucous membranes have receptors that offer the body protection. For example, an irritating substance in the upper respiratory tract causes a person to sneeze, and food caught in the larynx or trachea causes a person to cough. Sneezing and coughing are protective mechanisms that help rid the body of foreign materials. Mucous membranes are insensitive to temperature, except in the mouth and rectum, but are sensitive to pressure. Mucous membranes also function to absorb substances from their surface. For example, digested food is absorbed through the mucous membrane in the small intestine.

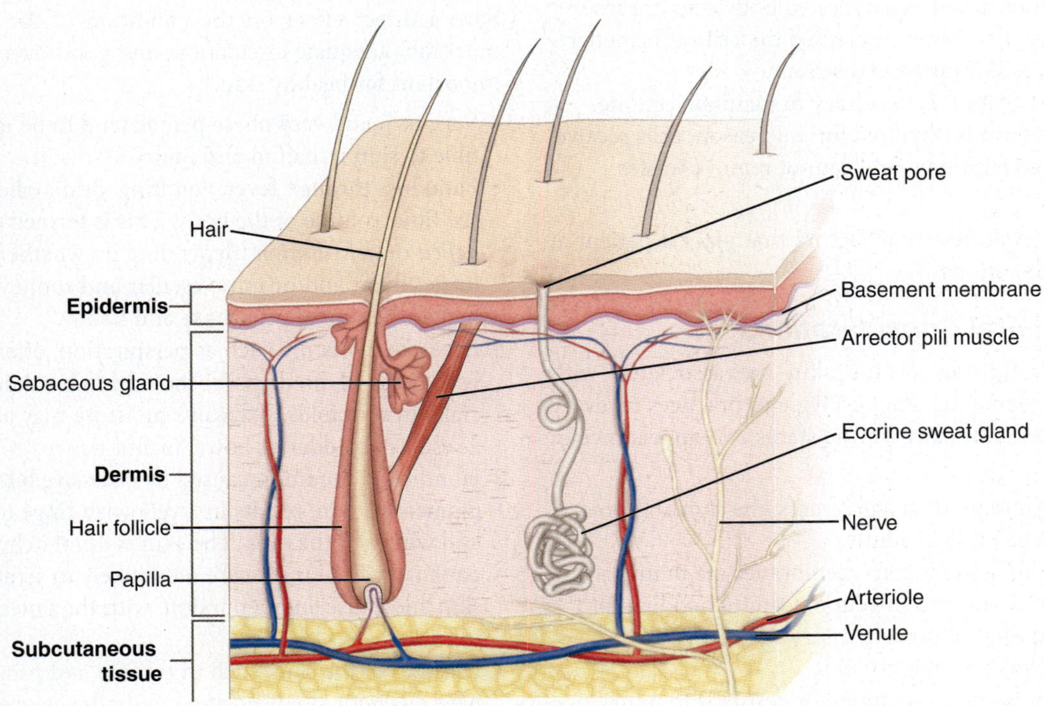

FIGURE 33-1. A cross section of normal skin.

Table 33-1 Functions of the Skin

FUNCTION	MECHANISMS
Protection	• Acts as a barrier to water, microorganisms, and damaging ultraviolet rays of the sun • Protects against infection • Protects against injury to underlying tissues and organs • Prevents loss of moisture from the surface and underlying structures
Temperature Regulation	• Draws heat from the skin as perspiration occurs and evaporates • Dissipates heat as blood vessels in the skin dilate • Compensates for cold conditions with the constriction of blood vessels in the skin to diminish heat loss • Compensates for cold through the contraction of pilomotor muscles that cause the hair to stand on end, forming a layer of air on the body for insulation (*gooseflesh* or *goose bumps*)
Psychosocial	• Contributes to the external appearance and is a major contributor to self-esteem • Plays an important role in identification and communication
Sensation	• Provides the sense of touch, pain, pressure, and temperature through millions of nerve endings • Allows the body to adjust to the environment through sensory impulses, in conjunction with the brain and spinal cord
Vitamin D Production	• Activated by ultraviolet rays from the sun to produce vitamin D
Immunologic	• Triggers immunologic responses when broken
Absorption	• Absorbs substances, such as medications, for local and systemic effects
Elimination	• Excretes small amounts of water, electrolytes, and nitrogenous wastes in sweat

Factors Affecting Skin Integrity

Basic principles related to integrity of the skin and mucous membranes include the following:

- Unbroken and healthy skin and mucous membranes serve as the first lines of defense against harmful agents.
- Resistance to injury of the skin and mucous membranes varies among people. Factors influencing resistance include the person's age, the amount of underlying tissues, and comorbidities.
- Adequately nourished and hydrated body cells are resistant to injury. The better nourished the cell is, the better able it is to resist injury and disease.
- Adequate circulation is necessary to maintain cell life. When circulation is impaired for any reason, cells receive inadequate nourishment and cannot remove wastes efficiently.

Table 33-2 identifies some factors that place a patient at risk for skin alterations.

Developmental Considerations

Specific characteristics of the skin are associated with different developmental stages. Hygiene practices at every age have a direct influence on the status and appearance of the skin.

- In children younger than age 2 years, the skin is thinner and weaker than it is in adults.
- An infant's skin and mucous membranes are injured easily and are subject to infection. Careful handling of infants is required to prevent injury to and infection of the skin and mucous membranes.
- A child's skin becomes increasingly resistant to injury and infection.
- The structure of the skin changes as a person ages. In older adults, the maturation of epidermal cells is delayed, leading to thin, easily damaged skin. Circulation and collagen formation are impaired, leading to decreased elasticity and increased risk for tissue damage from pressure. Changes that occur in the skin with aging are discussed in the Focus on the Older Adult feature (on page 1154).

State of Health

The state of a person's health and therapeutic treatments have a direct effect on the condition of the skin. Proper nutrition, adequate circulation, and good overall health are important for healthy skin.

- Very thin and very obese people tend to be more susceptible to skin irritation and injury.
- Fluid loss through fever, vomiting, or diarrhea reduces the fluid volume of the body. This is termed *fluid volume deficit* or *dehydration* (depending on whether there are intracellular and/or intravascular and sodium losses) and makes the skin appear loose and flabby.
- Excessive moisture such as perspiration, often associated with being ill, predisposes the skin to breakdown, especially in skin folds. Excessive moisture may also occur as a result of bladder or bowel incontinence.
- Jaundice, a condition caused by excessive bile in lightly pigmented skin, results in a yellowish tinge to the skin and whites of the eyes. The skin is often itchy and dry; patients with jaundice are more likely to scratch their skin and cause an open lesion, with the potential for infection.
- Diseases of the skin, such as eczema and psoriasis, may have a genetic predisposition and often cause lesions that require special care.

Table 33-2 Factors Placing a Person at Risk for Skin Alterations

FACTOR	NURSING IMPLICATIONS
Age	See text discussion regarding developmental issues related to skin and the Focus on the Older Adult feature on page 1154.
Lifestyle Variables	
Occupation or other activity that gives a person prolonged exposure to the sun	• Places person at high risk for developing skin cancer, which has an excellent prognosis if detected and treated in its early stages, but which may be fatal if treatment is delayed. • Assessment needs to include careful examination of a sore that does not heal, or a change in size or color of a wart or mole.
Body piercing	• Potential interference with airway management. Potential risk for bacterial and viral infections, scarring, nerve damage, tissue trauma, and deformity. • Assess patient's knowledge of symptoms of infection at the site and when to seek medical care. • Assess piercing site(s) for redness, swelling, discharge, or excessive pain at the site.
Changes in Health State	
Dehydration or malnutrition	• If fluid, protein, and vitamin C intake is deficient, skin loses elasticity and becomes prone to breakdown. • Nursing care is directed toward preventing skin breakdown: frequent changes of patient's position with skin assessment at each change, special mattresses and protection of bony prominences, use of lotions, and attention to fluid and nutritional status.
Reduced sensation (paralysis, local nerve damage, circulatory insufficiency)	• Patient's inability to sense temperature extremes, pressure, friction, and other such factors can easily result in injury. • Nursing care incorporates special attention to safety.
Illness	
Diabetes mellitus Impaired immune system	• Numerous factors combine to cause skin problems in patients with diabetes: cuts and sores that do not heal, lesions on the lower extremities that ulcerate and become necrotic, and recurrent bacterial and fungal infections. • The patient with diabetes must be taught special hygiene measures to prevent trauma to the skin and learn to assess the skin carefully to detect any alteration. • Patients with diagnoses that involve an alteration of the immune system (HIV, diabetes, autoimmune disorders) are predisposed to the development of skin breakdown and infections. • Treatments for underlying conditions may also affect the immune response essential for skin protection and wound healing (immunosuppressants, radiation).
Diagnostic Measures	
Gastrointestinal (GI) series	• The GI cleansing preparations administered to patients having GI studies done may result in diarrhea, which irritates the sensitive skin in the perianal area—especially if the patient had bouts of diarrhea before the studies; anticipating the problem, noting redness and inflammation, and beginning warm baths and ointments are welcome nursing measures that patients may be too embarrassed to seek.
Therapeutic Measures	
Bed rest	• Bed rest predisposes patients to skin breakdown; the harsh detergents used on hospital laundry compound this problem. • Pressure points need to be examined frequently and protected.
Casts	• Casts easily irritate the skin; careful assessment, covering the rough edges of the cast, and skin care are indicated.
Aquathermia unit	• Wet heat has therapeutic benefit but, if applied to the skin for too long, may macerate the skin; follow protocol in length of application, examine skin carefully between treatments, and allow to dry.
Medications	• Medications may cause allergic skin reactions, such as rashes. • When evaluating the patient's response to a new drug, examine the skin for redness and itching.
Radiation therapy	• Radiation therapy exposes normal skin cells as well as cancer cells in treatment field to effects of radiation, with the potential for erythema and dry/wet desquamation (loss of skin integrity).

Focus on the Older Adult

NURSING STRATEGIES TO ADDRESS AGE-RELATED CHANGES IN SKIN

Age-Related Changes	Nursing Strategies
Subcutaneous and dermal tissues become thin: • Skin is more easily injured. • Skin has less capacity to insulate. • Skin wrinkles more easily. • Sensation of pressure and pain is reduced.	• Do not apply tape to skin unless necessary. • Check skin frequently to observe for any signs of a pressure injury. • Pad bony prominences if necessary. • Assess pressure tolerance by checking pressure points for redness after 30 minutes.
Activity of the sebaceous and sweat glands decreases: • Skin becomes dryer. • Pruritus (itching) may occur.	• Clean perineal area daily but do not bathe full body on a daily basis. • Apply lotions and moisturizers as needed. • Encourage adequate hydration. • Eliminate the use of harsh soaps.
Cell renewal is shorter: • Healing time is delayed.	• Perform careful skin assessments, looking for signs of skin breakdown.
Melanocytes (cells that make the pigment that colors hair and skin) decline in number: • Hair becomes gray-white. • Skin may be unevenly pigmented.	• Assist patient with skin checks, observing for any signs of melanoma or other skin abnormalities.
Collagen fiber is less organized: • Skin loses elasticity.	• Check skin frequently for tears, irritation, or breakdown.

WOUNDS AND PRESSURE INJURIES

A **wound** is a break or disruption in the normal integrity of the skin and tissues. That disruption may range from a small cut on a finger to a third-degree burn covering almost all of the body. Wounds may result from mechanical forces (such as surgical incisions) or physical injury (such as a burn). Examples of types of wounds and their causes are highlighted in Table 33-3.

Wound Classification

The etiology, or cause, of a wound is considered when developing the plan of care for a patient. In general, most wounds can be classified as either surgical (intentional, controlled, sterile), traumatic (may require additional intervention such as fluid administration or a tetanus shot), neuropathic or vascular (related to an underlying neurologic and/or circulatory issue), or pressure related (Baranoski & Ayello, 2020). The underlying cause must be addressed. For example, in a patient with a diabetic foot ulcer, healing and prevention of future ulcers is predicated on the treatment of the underlying diabetes and associated neuropathies and circulatory issues. Wounds may also be defined as open or closed and acute or chronic, based on whether the wound follows the normal, timely healing process or not. Pressure injuries may be further classified as: (1) partial thickness where all or a portion of the dermis is intact; (2) full thickness where the entire dermis, sweat glands, and hair follicles are severed, which can expose bone, tendon, or muscle; (3) unstageable, a full-thickness loss where the true depth cannot be determined, or (4) deep pressure-induced tissue damage (European Pressure Ulcer Advisory Panel [EPUAP], National Pressure Injury Advisory Panel [NPIAP], & Pan Pacific Pressure Injury Alliance [PPPIA], 2019a/2019b).

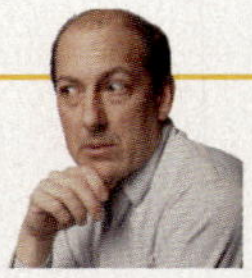

Think back to **Lucius Everly**, the patient who had abdominal surgery and is in the critical care unit. His postoperative treatments would necessitate the placement of one or more intravenous lines, which cause an intentional, controlled break in the skin. His abdominal incision would be considered a surgical wound. The nurse would incorporate an understanding of the principles of surgical asepsis when caring for these wound sites to prevent infection.

Open and Closed Wounds

An open wound occurs from intentional or unintentional trauma. The skin surface is broken, providing a portal of entry for microorganisms. Bleeding, tissue damage, an increased risk for infection, and delayed healing may accompany open wounds. Examples include incisions and abrasions.

A closed wound results from a blow, force, or strain caused by trauma such as a fall, an assault, or a motor vehicle crash. The skin surface is not broken, but soft tissue is damaged, and internal injury and hemorrhage may occur. Examples include ecchymosis and hematomas.

Acute and Chronic Wounds

Acute wounds, such as surgical incisions, usually heal within days to weeks. The wound edges are well approximated (edges meet to close skin surface), and the risk of infection is low.

Table 33-3 Types of Wounds

TYPE	CAUSE
Incision	Cutting or sharp instrument; wound edges well approximated and aligned; surrounding tissue undamaged; bleeds freely and least likely to become infected
Contusion	Blunt instrument, overlying skin remains intact, with injury to underlying soft tissue; possible resultant bruising and/or hematoma
Abrasion	Friction; rubbing or scraping epidermal layers of skin; top layer of skin scraped away; dirt and germs often embedded and can become infected
Laceration	Tearing of skin and tissue with blunt or irregular instrument; tissue not aligned, often with loose flaps of skin and tissue; frequently contaminated with dirt or other material ground into the wound and likely to become infected
Puncture	Blunt or sharp instrument puncturing the skin; intentional (such as venipuncture) or accidental; consider penetrating object when considering infection probability
Penetrating	Foreign object entering the skin or mucous membrane and lodging in underlying tissue; fragments possibly scattering throughout tissues
Avulsion	Tearing a structure from normal anatomic position; possible damage to blood vessels, nerves, and other structures
Chemical	Toxic agents such as drugs, acids, alcohols, metals, and substances released from cellular necrosis
Thermal	High or low temperatures; cellular necrosis as a possible result
Irradiation	Ultraviolet light or radiation exposure; can cause wet or dry desquamation
Pressure ulcers	Compromised circulation secondary to pressure or pressure combined with friction; classified by *Stages 1–4*, *Unstageable*, and *Deep Tissue* injury
Venous ulcers	Injury and poor venous return, resulting from underlying conditions, such as incompetent valves or obstruction; frequently have significant drainage; compression essential (after arterial flow verified)
Arterial ulcers	Injury and underlying ischemia, resulting from a lack of blood flow to the lower extremities secondary to conditions such as atherosclerosis or thrombosis; many have black eschar; increasing blood flow essential for treatment
Diabetic ulcers	Injury and underlying diabetic neuropathy, peripheral arterial disease, diabetic foot structure; located below the ankle

Source: Adapted from Corum, L. (2019). Ulcer and wound care: Getting to the depth of the issue. *National Center of Continuing Education.* https://nursece.com/pdfs/720_V2_Wound_Care.pdf; Baranoski, S., & Ayello, E. A. (2020). *Wound care essentials: Practice principles* (5th ed.). Wolters Kluwer; Norris, T. L. (2019). *Porth's pathophysiology: Concepts of altered health states* (10th ed.). Wolters Kluwer; and Hinkle, J. L., & Cheever, K. H. (2018). *Brunner & Suddarth's textbook of medical-surgical nursing* (14th ed., p. 2167 [Chart 72-4]). Wolters Kluwer Health.

Acute wounds usually progress through the healing process without interruption. Chronic wounds, in contrast, do not progress through the normal sequence of repair. The healing process is impeded. The wound edges are often not approximated, the risk of infection is increased, and the normal healing time is delayed (>30 days). Chronic wounds remain in the inflammatory phase of healing (discussed in the next section). Chronic wounds include any wound that does not heal along the expected continuum, such as wounds related to diabetes, arterial or venous insufficiency, and pressure injuries. Patients with chronic wounds report a diminished quality of life, chronic pain, and restricted mobility (sometimes related to the loss of a limb) and may even die because of their wound (Baranoski & Ayello, 2020; Hajhosseini et al., 2020).

Wound Healing

Wound healing is a process of tissue response to injury. Injured tissues are repaired by physiologic mechanisms that regenerate functioning cells and replace connective tissue cells with scar tissue. The healing process fills the gap caused by tissue destruction, restoring the structural integrity of the damaged tissue through the orderly release of growth factors and chemical mediators (Norris, 2019). These substances help to increase the blood supply to the damaged area, wall off and remove cellular and foreign debris, and initiate cellular development.

Normally, the healing process occurs without assistance. However, interventions can help to support the process. For example, tissue healing is promoted by keeping the injured area free of debris through proper cleaning. Positioning the wounded area to promote circulation to that part helps to promote tissue healing. These interventions are based on the principles of wound healing outlined in Box 33-1 on page 1156.

Wound repair occurs by primary intention, secondary intention, or tertiary intention. Wounds healed by primary intention are well approximated (skin edges tightly together). Intentional wounds with minimal tissue loss, such as those made by a surgical incision with sutured approximated edges, usually heal by primary intention. Wounds healed by secondary intention have edges that are not well approximated. Large, open wounds, such as from burns or major trauma, which require more tissue replacement and are often contaminated, commonly heal

Box 33-1 Principles of Wound Healing

- Intact skin is the first line of defense against microorganisms. A break in the integrity of the skin increases the risk for infection. Careful hand hygiene before caring for a wound is probably the single most effective method for preventing wound infections.
- The body responds systemically to trauma in any of its parts. For example, a surgical incision can cause a variety of systemic reactions, including increased body temperature, increased heart and respiratory rates, anorexia or nausea and vomiting, musculoskeletal tension, and hormonal changes.
- An adequate blood supply is essential for the body's normal response to any injury. The blood transports increased numbers of leukocytes, erythrocytes, and platelets to the site of injury. Antibodies are carried by the plasma. Increased circulation to the injured part removes toxins and debris and provides nutrients and oxygen. Areas of the body with a good blood supply, such as the head and the neck, heal faster than areas in which the blood supply is not as great, such as the distal part of an extremity.
- Normal healing is promoted when the wound is free of foreign material, such as excessive exudate, dead or damaged tissue cells, pathogenic organisms, or embedded fragments of bone, metal, glass, or other substances. In some situations, a collection of pus or foreign body is walled off and healing occurs around it to form an abscess.
- The ability to handle altered skin integrity depends on the extent of the damage and the person's general state of health. The capacity to deal adequately with a wound is limited when a healthy person sustains a massive injury, when the patient has a chronic illness or a depressed immune system, or when the patient is very young or very old.
- The body's response to a wound is more effective if proper nutrition has been maintained.
  - Undernourished patients are at greater risk for developing a wound infection because they have difficulty mounting their cell-mediated defense system associated with T-lymphocyte activity, and some leukocytic functions are diminished in the presence of protein deficiency.
  - Although the role of fatty acids in wound healing is not well understood, certain quantities of glucose are necessary to meet the energy requirements for wound healing.
  - Various vitamins, minerals, and trace elements are also needed for efficient wound healing. Vitamin A is necessary for collagen synthesis and epithelialization. Vitamin B complex serves as a cofactor of enzyme reactions needed for wound healing. Vitamin C is needed for collagen synthesis, capillary formation, and resistance to infection. Vitamin K is needed for the synthesis of prothrombin. Zinc, copper, and iron assist in collagen synthesis. Manganese serves as an enzyme activator.

by secondary intention. If a wound that is healing by primary intention becomes infected, it will heal by secondary intention. Wounds that heal by secondary intention take longer to heal and form more scar tissue (Norris, 2019). Connective tissue healing and repair follow the same phases in healing. However, differences occur in the length of time required for each phase and in the extent of new tissue formed. Wounds healed by tertiary intention, or delayed primary closure, are those wounds left open for several days to allow edema or infection to resolve or fluid to drain, and then are closed.

Phases of Wound Healing

The wound healing process can be divided into three or four phases, depending on the reference. In this chapter, four phases will be discussed: hemostasis, inflammation, proliferation, and maturation. These four phases systematically lead to repair of the injury (Baranoski & Ayello, 2020). If three stages are identified, hemostasis is included as part of the inflammatory stage (Norris, 2019).

HEMOSTASIS

Hemostasis occurs immediately after the initial injury primarily to stop the bleeding and activate the white blood cells to fight any invading bacteria. Involved blood vessels constrict and blood clotting begins through platelet activation and clustering. This coagulation results in the formation of a fibrin clot. The temporary clot forms, then the body releases substances that dissolve the clot (fibrinolysis) and stimulate other cells to migrate to the injury to participate in the other phases of healing (Baranoski & Ayello, 2020; Corum, 2019; Norris, 2019).

INFLAMMATORY PHASE

The inflammatory phase follows hemostasis and lasts about 2 to 3 days. White blood cells (WBCs), predominantly leukocytes and macrophages, move to the wound. Leukocytes arrive first to ingest bacteria and cellular debris. About 24 hours after the injury, macrophages (a larger phagocytic cell) enter the wound area and remain for an extended period. Macrophages are essential to the healing process. They not only ingest debris, but also release growth factors that are necessary for the growth of epithelial cells and new blood vessels. These growth factors also attract fibroblasts that help to fill in the wound, which is necessary for the next stage of healing. After a brief period of constriction during homeostasis, the blood vessels dilate and capillary permeability increases, allowing plasma and blood components to leak out into the area that is injured, forming a liquid called **exudate**. The accumulation of exudate and the increased perfusion result in acute inflammation, which is characterized by pain, heat, redness, and swelling at the site of the injury. Cytokines promote the repair process by increasing the inflammatory response. During the inflammatory phase, the patient has a generalized body response, including a mildly elevated temperature, leukocytosis (increased number of WBCs in the blood), and general malaise (Baranoski & Ayello, 2020; Corum, 2019; Norris, 2019).

PROLIFERATION/REPAIR PHASE

The proliferation phase, also known as the repair, fibroblastic, regenerative, or connective tissue phase, encompasses the processes that result in actual healing. The proliferation phase lasts for several weeks. New tissue is built to fill the wound space, primarily through the action of fibroblasts.

Fibroblasts are connective tissue cells that synthesize and secrete collagen and produce specialized growth factors responsible for inducing blood vessel formation as well as increasing the number and movement of endothelial cells. Capillaries grow across the wound, bringing oxygen and nutrients required for continued healing. Fibroblasts form fibrin that stretches through the clot. A thin layer of epithelial cells forms across the wound, and blood flow across the wound is reinstituted. The new tissue, called **granulation tissue**, forms the foundation for scar tissue development. It is highly vascular, red, and bleeds easily. In wounds that heal by first intention, epidermal cells seal the wound within 24 to 48 hours, thus the granulation tissue is not visible.

Collagen synthesis and accumulation continue, peaking in 5 to 7 days. Depending on the size of the wound, collagen deposit continues for several weeks or even years. By the end of the second week following the injury, most WBCs have left the wound area, and the wound is lighter in color. The systemic symptoms now typically disappear. During this phase, adequate nutrition, and oxygenation, as well as prevention of strain on the suture line, are important patient care considerations.

Wounds that heal by secondary intention eventually follow the same process but take longer to heal and form more scar tissue. Granulation tissue fills the wound and is then covered by skin cells that grow over the granulation tissue. Connective tissue healing and repair follow the same phases in healing. However, differences occur in the length of time required for each phase and in the extent of granulation tissue formed (Baranoski & Ayello, 2020; Corum, 2019; Norris, 2019).

MATURATION/REMODELING PHASE

The final stage of healing, maturation (or remodeling) begins about 3 weeks after the injury, possibly continuing for months or years. Collagen that was haphazardly deposited in the wound is remodeled, making the healed wound stronger and more like adjacent tissue. New collagen continues to be deposited, which compresses the blood vessels in the healing wound, so that the **scar** (avascular collagen tissue that does not sweat, grow hair, or tan in sunlight) eventually becomes a flat, thin line. Scar tissue is less elastic than uninjured tissue. The strength of the scar tissue remains less (70% to 80%) than that of normal tissue, even many years following injury, and it is never fully restored. Wounds that heal by secondary intention take longer to remodel and form a scar smaller than the original wound. If the scar is over a joint or other body structure, it may limit movement and cause disability (Baranoski & Ayello, 2020; Corum, 2019; Norris, 2019).

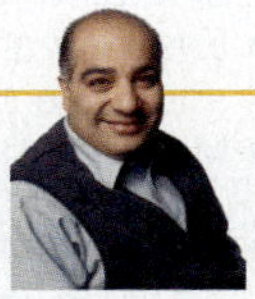

Recall ***Sam Bentz***, the 56-year-old admitted for treatment of a bone infection. The nurse would apply the knowledge about the phases of wound healing when reviewing this patient's past history, especially with respect to the wounds that developed during his last hospital admission. In addition, this knowledge would help form the basis for the patient's care plan should another wound occur during this hospitalization.

Factors Affecting Wound Healing

A variety of factors affect wound healing. Local factors, those occurring directly in the wound, include pressure, **desiccation** (dehydration), **maceration** (overhydration), trauma, edema, infection, excessive bleeding, **necrosis** (death of tissue), and the presence of **biofilm** (a thick grouping of microorganisms). Systemic factors, those occurring throughout the body, include age, circulation to and oxygenation of tissues, nutritional status, wound etiology, general health status and disease state, immunosuppression, proinflammatory conditions and extent of systemic inflammation, medication use and other therapies, and adherence to treatment plan (Baranoski & Ayello, 2020; Beyene et al., 2020; Norris, 2019).

LOCAL FACTORS

Factors occurring local to the wound itself can prolong wound healing. These factors are discussed in the following sections.

Pressure

Pressure disrupts the blood supply to the wound area. Persistent or excessive pressure interferes with blood flow to the tissue and delays healing.

Desiccation

Desiccation is the process of drying up. Cells dehydrate and die in a dry environment. This cell death causes a crust to form over the wound site and delays healing. Wounds that are kept moist (not wet) and hydrated experience enhanced epidermal cell migration, which supports **epithelialization** (epithelial cells form a new surface layer) and neovascularization (formation of new blood vessels; Hess, 2019).

Maceration

Maceration, tissue erosion, results from prolonged exposure to moisture. Overhydration of cells related to urinary and fecal incontinence can also lead to maceration and impaired skin integrity. This damage is related to moisture, changes in the pH of the skin, overgrowth of bacteria and infection of the skin, and erosion of skin from friction on moist skin. Moisture-associated skin damage (MASD) may be caused by drainage from the wound itself and can result in maceration of the areas surrounding the wound (Baranoski & Ayello, 2020).

Trauma

Repeated trauma to a wound area results in delayed healing or the inability to heal.

Edema

Edema at a wound site interferes with the blood supply to the area, resulting in an inadequate supply of oxygen and nutrients to the tissue.

Infection

Bacteria in a wound increase stress on the body, requiring increased energy to deal with the invaders. Infection requires large amounts of energy be spent by the immune system to fight the microorganisms, leaving little or no reserves to attend to the job of repair and healing. In addition, toxins produced by bacteria and released when bacteria die interfere with wound healing and cause cell death.

Excessive Bleeding

Excessive bleeding results in large clots. Large clots increase the amount of space that must be filled during healing and interferes with oxygen diffusion to the tissue. In addition, accumulated blood or drainage of any type is an excellent place for growth of bacteria and promotes infection (Baranoski & Ayello, 2020).

Necrosis

Dead tissue present in the wound delays healing. Dead tissue appears as slough—moist, yellow, stringy tissue—and **eschar** appears as dry, black, leathery tissue. Healing of the wound will not take place with necrotic tissue in the wound. Mechanical or chemical removal of the dead tissue must occur for healing to begin (Baranoski & Ayello, 2020; Hess, 2019).

Biofilm

Wound biofilms are the result of wound bacteria growing in clumps, embedded in a thick, self-made, protective, slimy barrier of sugars and proteins. This barrier contributes to decreased effectiveness of antibiotics against the bacteria (antibiotic resistance) and decreases the effectiveness of the normal immune response by the patient (Baranoski & Ayello, 2020). The bacteria also produce a protective matrix that attaches the biofilm to the wound surface. Biofilms impair wound healing and contribute to chronic wound inflammation and wound infection (Baranoski & Ayello, 2020; EPUAP, NPIAP, & PPPIA, 2019a/2019b; Hess, 2019).

SYSTEMIC FACTORS

Factors not related to the wound itself also can prolong wound healing. These factors are discussed in the following sections.

Age

The major skin layers arise from different embryologic origins, resulting in poor adherence between the epidermis and the dermis. This loose binding between the layers causes the layers to separate easily during an inflammatory process, placing infants and small children at risk for impaired skin integrity. Epidermal stripping, the unintentional removal of the epidermis with tape removal, is one type of such injury. Care should be taken to minimize tension, traction, and wrinkles on the skin when using tape on these young patients.

Children and healthy adults, however, heal more rapidly than do older adults, in whom physiologic changes caused by aging result in diminished fibroblastic activity and circulation. Older adults are more likely to have one or more chronic illnesses, with pathologic changes that impede the healing process. See the accompanying Focus on the Older Adult display for other age-related factors affecting wound healing.

Circulation and Oxygenation

Adequate blood flow to deliver nutrients and oxygen and to remove local toxins, bacteria, and other debris is essential for wound healing. Certain physical conditions, because of their effect on circulation and oxygenation, can affect wound healing. Circulation may be impaired in older adults and in people with peripheral vascular disorders, cardiovascular disorders, hypertension, or diabetes mellitus. Oxygenation of tissues is decreased in people with anemia or chronic respiratory disorders and in those who smoke.

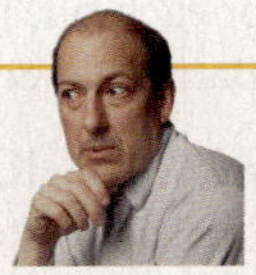

Recall ***Lucius Everly***, the patient described in the Reflective Practice display. The nurse's ability to integrate knowledge of the effects of diabetes on circulation would be important in planning measures to ensure adequate circulation to his extremities as a means to prevent skin breakdown.

Focus on the Older Adult

NURSING STRATEGIES TO ADDRESS AGE-RELATED CHANGES IN WOUND HEALING

Age-Related Changes	Nursing Interventions
Skin loses turgor and is more fragile.	• Maintain hydration with intravenous fluids as prescribed. • Maintain record of intake and output. • Use caution when removing tape.
Decreased secretion of enzymes and absorption of nutrients and minerals may increase risk for delayed wound healing.	• Maintain intake of adequate kilocalories with oral, enteral, or parenteral feedings. • Ensure that diet is high in protein, vitamin A, vitamin C, and trace elements (zinc and copper). • Monitor lab results such as serum albumin, total protein.
Risk of infection increases from: • Slower inflammatory response. • Reduced antibody production and endocrine system function. • Increased incidence of chronic illnesses, such as diabetes mellitus and cardiovascular disease, that compromise circulation and tissue oxygenation.	• Maintain careful hand hygiene and surgical asepsis with dressing changes and care of tubes or drains. • Take and record vital signs, noting and reporting increased temperature. • Monitor wound for manifestations of infection. • Administer medications as prescribed. • Administer supplemental oxygen as prescribed.

Large amounts of subcutaneous and tissue fat (which has fewer blood vessels) results in hypoperfusion and hypovascularity. This impaired oxygenation and perfusion leads to an alteration in cellular repair processes and the response of immune cells. People with obesity more frequently have tension on their wound edges that can result in wound dehiscence. Skin folds harbor bacteria and provide a moist environment well suited for the spread of fungal and bacterial infections. Skin-on-skin friction causes ulceration and is more common in people with obesity (Avishai et al., 2017).

Nutritional Status

Wound healing requires adequate proteins, carbohydrates, fats, vitamins, and minerals. Calories and protein are necessary to rebuild cells and tissues. Vitamins A and C are essential for epithelialization and collagen synthesis. Zinc plays a role in proliferation of cells. Fluids are necessary for optimal function of cells. All phases of the wound healing process are slowed or inadequate in the patient with poor nutritional status and fluid imbalance.

Some patients with obesity suffer from protein malnutrition, which interferes with healing. Patients who are undernourished may lack the nutritional stores to promote wound healing. Nutrition is further discussed in Chapter 37.

Wound Etiology (Cause)

Knowing the etiology (cause) of a wound directly impacts on assessment and treatment of the wound (Baranoski & Ayello, 2020). It may also indicate the general health status of the patient and the associated likelihood of future wounds. For example, a wound that stems from a decrease in arterial blood flow to the extremities, a systemic issue, may recur; however, a wound from a spider bite may be a one-time event.

The COVID-19 pandemic brought about two distinct etiologies: (1) unavoidable pressure injury, and (2) injury to baseline healthy heath care providers due to personal protective equipment (PPE). For patients, the hypercoagulable state inherent in COVID-19 resulted in skin changes that often appeared to be deep tissue pressure injury but were not. There was also an increase in the rate of deterioration and inability to prevent pressure injury in this critically ill population. This was compounded by multiorgan dysfunction, nutritional challenges, hemodynamic instability, proning and other position requirements, and the prolonged recovery period for some patients. Resource limitations and the shift to crisis care contributed to the inability of the interprofessional team to adhere to protocols and provide adequate classification of these microvascular-based injuries. Careful consideration needs to be given to resources and pressure injury prevention protocols during crisis situations (NPAIP, n.d.).

Nurses and other members of the interprofessional team also experienced unexpected skin injury during the COVID-19 pandemic. Although the benefits of wearing PPE far outweighed the risks, incorrectly worn PPE resulted in facial injury to health care professionals. Early in the pandemic, the NPIAP (2021) evidence-based recommendations included:

> (1) Prepare the skin before and after wearing PPE with skin sealants, barrier creams and moisturizers; (2) Frequent PPE offloading to relieve pressure and shear applied to the skin; (3) treat visible skin injuries immediately caused by PPE to minimize future infection; (4) non-porous dressings may provide additional skin protection, but lack current evidence; (5) health systems sound take care to educate frontline healthcare staff about placement and personal hygiene related to handling PPE (p. 5).

Nursing Self-Care Alert

Although the benefits of wearing a mask far outweighed the potential risks, nurses (and other members of the interprofessional health care team) had to take extra measures during the pandemic to protect their skin from breakdown due to prolonged use of masks and other necessary PPE.

Although these recommendations are evidence based, they need to be considered in the context of this crisis and include clinical judgment. Reflection on the pandemic is likely to result in additional practical, evidence-based recommendations, and drive the need for additional research on preventing PPE-related injuries (NPIAP, 2021).

Medications and Other Therapies

Patients who are taking corticosteroids or require postoperative radiation therapy are at high risk for delayed healing and wound complications. Corticosteroids decrease the inflammatory process, which may delay healing. Radiation depresses bone marrow function, resulting in decreased leukocytes and an increased risk of infection. The presence of a chronic illness (such as cardiovascular disease or diabetes mellitus) or impaired immune function can impair wound healing. Chemotherapeutic agents impair or stop proliferation of all rapidly growing cells, including cells involved in wound healing. Prolonged antibiotic therapy increases a patient's risk for secondary infection and superinfection.

Immunosuppression or Proinflammatory Conditions

Suppression of the immune system as a result of disease (e.g., HIV, lupus), medication (e.g., chemotherapy), or age (e.g., changes associated with advancing age) can delay wound healing. Proinflammatory conditions (e.g., vasculitis or rheumatoid arthritis) result in the release of proinflammatory cytokines, which prolong the inflammatory process (Baranoski & Ayello, 2020).

Adherence to Treatment Plan

Wound treatment plans will be discussed later in this chapter. Nonadherence to the treatment plan can negatively impact wound healing (Baranoski & Ayello, 2020). Fayne et al. (2020) explore the concept of *social genomics*, which considers the impact of social factors and processes on genome activity, as it relates to wound healing. Critical elements related to social determinants of heath and stress potentially directly (epigenetics, gene expression) or indirectly affect wound healing and, ultimately, impact on an individual's quality of life. The direct and indirect costs of wound care affect a patient's ability to adhere to a prescribed plan of care.

Wound Complications

Wound complications include infection, hemorrhage, dehiscence, evisceration, and fistula. These complications increase the risk for generalized illness and death, lengthen the patient's need for health care interventions, and add to health care costs.

INFECTION

Wound infection results when the patient's immune system fails to control the growth of microorganisms. Microorganisms can invade a wound at the time of trauma, during surgery, or at any time after the initial wound occurs. A contaminated wound is more likely to become infected than one that is not contaminated. In addition, the risk of infection is increased in a surgical wound created during a procedure involving the intestines because the risk for contamination with fecal material is high. Wound infections also occur as a result of hospital-acquired infections (HAIs). Symptoms of wound infection usually become apparent within 2 to 7 days after the injury or surgery; often, the patient is at home. Symptoms of infection include purulent drainage; increased drainage, pain, redness, and swelling in and around the wound; increased body temperature; and increased WBC count. Additional signs and symptoms include delayed healing and discoloration of granulation tissue in the wound (Baranoski & Ayello, 2020). In patients with infection in a chronic wound, pain and delayed healing may be the only symptoms (Baranoski & Ayello, 2020). Wound infections impair healing. Wound infections can lead to other complications, including development of chronic wounds, osteomyelitis (bone infection) and sepsis (presence of pathogenic organisms in the blood or tissues). See Box 33-2 for two helpful mnemonics to help you assess whether a patient has a wound infection (STONEES) or if the wound has undergone critical colonization (NERDS).

Box 33-2 Assessment of Degree of Wound Infection

Assessment of ≥3 signs/symptoms from the following list indicates superficial critical colonization:

NERDS

Nonhealing wound
Exudative wound
Red and bleeding wound
Debris in the wound
Smell from the wound

Assessment of ≥3 signs/symptoms from the following list indicates infection:

STONEES

Size is bigger
Temperature increased
OS—exposed bone
New areas of breakdown
Exudate
Erythema, **E**dema
Smell

HEMORRHAGE

Hemorrhage may occur from a slipped suture; a dislodged clot at the wound site; infection; or the erosion of a blood vessel by a foreign body, such as a drain. Check the dressing and the wound under the dressing, as possible, frequently the first 48 hours after the injury. Surgical sites and other wounds should be routinely checked at least every 8 hours and with position changes. If excessive bleeding does occur, additional pressure dressings or packing may be necessary, fluid replacement will be considered, and surgical intervention may be required. Internal hemorrhage causes the formation of a **hematoma**, a localized mass of usually clotted blood (Stedman, n.d.). If the bleeding leads to a large accumulation of blood, it can put pressure on surrounding blood vessels and cause tissue ischemia (deficiency of blood to an area). See Chapter 31 for more information about hemorrhage.

DEHISCENCE AND EVISCERATION

Dehiscence and evisceration (Fig. 33-2) are the most serious postoperative wound complications. **Dehiscence** is the partial or total separation of wound layers as a result of excessive stress on wounds that are not healed. **Evisceration** is the most serious complication of dehiscence. It occurs primarily with abdominal incisions (Baranoski & Ayello, 2020; Hinkle et al., 2022). In evisceration, the abdominal wound completely separates, with protrusion of viscera (internal organs) through the incisional area. Patients at greater risk for these complications include those who are obese or malnourished, smoke tobacco, use anticoagulants, have infected wounds, or experience excessive coughing, vomiting, or straining (Hinkle et al., 2022). An increase in the flow of (serosanguineous) fluid from the wound between postoperative days 4 and 5 may be a sign

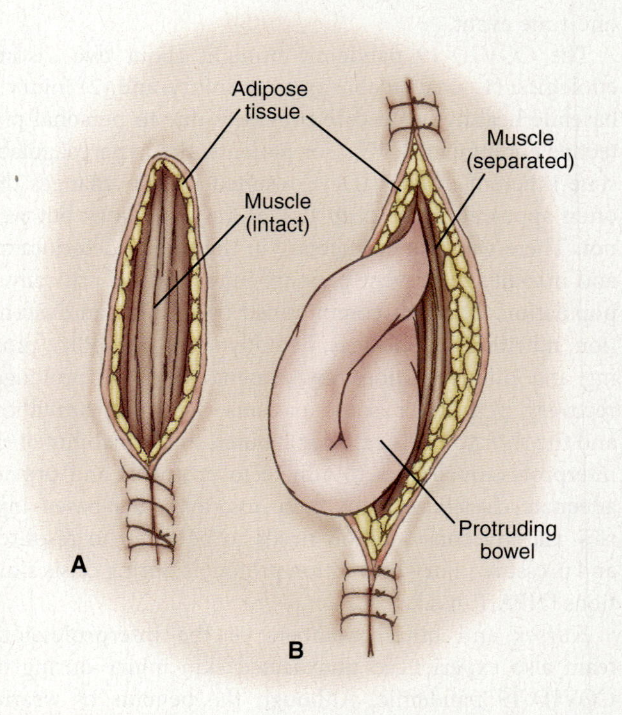

FIGURE 33-2. Wound complications. **A.** Dehiscence. **B.** Evisceration.

of an impending dehiscence. The patient may say that "something has suddenly given way." If dehiscence occurs, cover the wound area with sterile towels moistened with sterile 0.9% sodium chloride solution and notify the health care provider. Once dehiscence occurs, the wound is managed like any open wound. Dehiscence with evisceration of an abdominal incision is a medical emergency. Place the patient in the low Fowler's position and cover the exposed abdominal contents, as discussed previously, being sure to keep the exposed viscera moist. Do not leave the patient alone, and be sure to provide reassurance and intravenous pain medications as appropriate. Notify the primary care provider immediately. This situation is an emergency that requires prompt surgical repair, so the patient should be kept NPO (Baranoski & Ayello, 2020; Hinkle et al., 2022). Dehiscence results in a scary situation for a patient and those close to them. Consider the poem from Dr. Haddad and reflect on the patient experience.

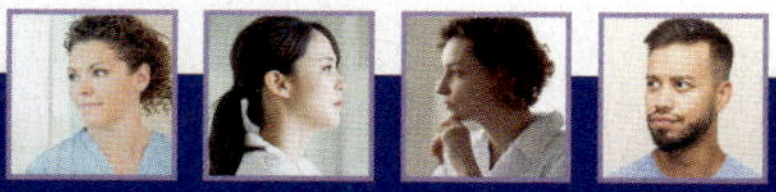

Poetry Nook

Dehiscence

You have come unstitched.

Holes appear on your threadbare abdomen.
Tunnels develop and connect bowel, liver, pancreas.
Enzymes ooze out and digest your skin,
no matter how hard we try to stem the flow.
A jerry-rigged system to
hold together our mistakes.
The stench is overwhelming, ever present
reminding everyone, but especially you,
that you have come undone.

Since the truth is too horrible to grasp,
since I can offer you nothing else,
I clean you up.
I wash your face,
brush your teeth,
comb your hair,
turn you on your side,
push soiled linens away,
roll clean sheets under you,
remove layers and layers of damp dressings,
and replace them with new dressings and tape.

I give you the certainty and calmness of my motions,
the competence and comfort of my touch
as I smooth the top sheet over my work.
Done.

For a few pristine moments, we allow ourselves
to be caught in the illusion of your wholeness.

FISTULA FORMATION

A **fistula** is an abnormal passage from an internal organ or vessel to the outside of the body, or from one internal organ or vessel to another. Fistulas may be created purposefully; for example, an arteriovenous (AV) fistula is created surgically to provide circulatory access for kidney dialysis. However, fistula formation is often the result of infection that has developed into an **abscess**, which is a collection of infected fluid that has not drained. Accumulated fluid applies pressure to surrounding tissues, leading to the formation of the unnatural passage between two visceral organs or an organ and the skin (Baranoski & Ayello, 2020). Figure 33-3 illustrates a rectovaginal fistula, which is an abnormal connection between the rectum and vagina. The presence of a fistula increases the risk for delayed healing, additional infection, fluid and electrolyte imbalances, and skin breakdown.

Pressure Injury

A **pressure injury** is defined as localized damage to the skin and underlying tissue that usually occurs over a bony prominence or is related to the use of a (medical or other) device (Edsberg et al., 2016). The National Pressure Injury Advisory Panel (Edsberg et al., 2016) recently updated their staging definitions, and the term **pressure ulcer** was replaced by ***pressure injury*** to better-represent the early stages of pressure injury where there is not an actual ulcer or break in the skin. A pressure injury may be acute or chronic. Most pressure injuries develop when soft tissue is compressed between a bony prominence and an external surface for a prolonged period of time, or when soft tissue undergoes pressure in combination with shear stress and/or friction (NPIAP, 2016a; EPUAP, NPIAP, & PPPIA, 2019b). The terms *decubitus ulcer, pressure sore,* and *bedsore* are also used to refer to this type of wound.

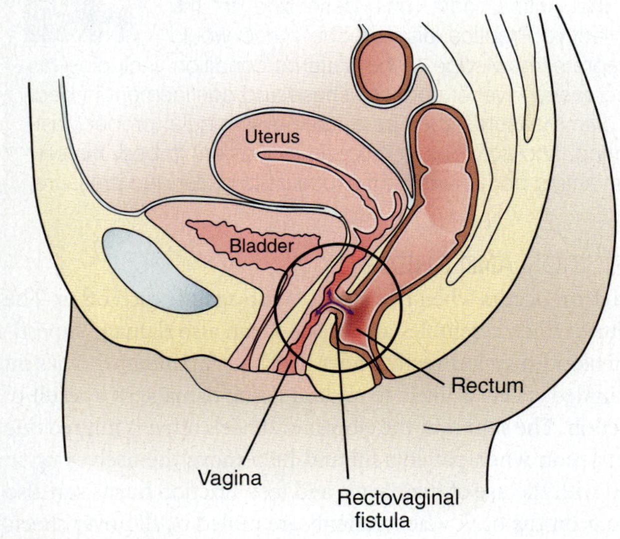

FIGURE 33-3. Fistula.

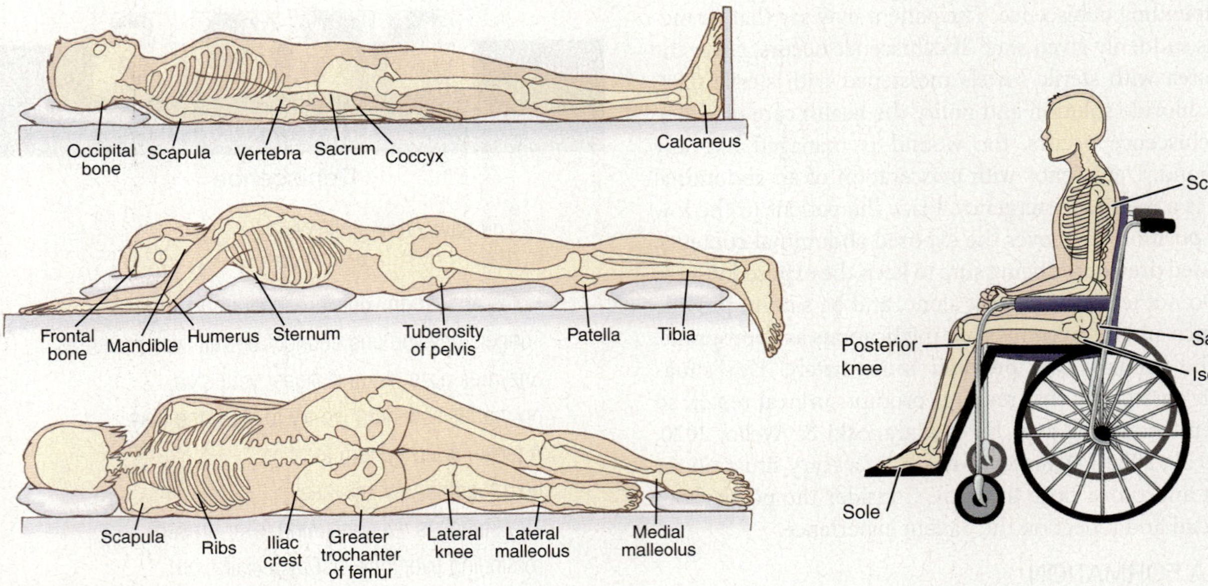

FIGURE 33-4. Common sites for development of pressure injuries.

Concept Mastery Alert

Pressure injury **is the current term that refers to what was previously known as a *pressure ulcer*.**

Pressure injuries are costly in terms of patient discomfort, disfigurement, decreased quality of life, and health care expenditures (Baranoski & Ayello, 2020; EPUAP, NPIAP, & PPPIA, 2019b). Most pressure injuries occur in older adults as a result of a combination of factors, including aging skin, chronic illnesses, immobility, malnutrition, fecal and urinary incontinence, and altered level of consciousness. Other significant at-risk populations include people with spinal cord injuries, traumatic brain injuries, or neuromuscular disorders where sensory perception may be altered. When pressure injuries occur, aggressive intervention and treatment can spare the patient unnecessary pain and discomfort, prevent further tissue deterioration, hasten wound healing, and save millions of health care dollars. It is important to keep in mind that "some pressure injuries are unavoidable despite provision of evidence-based care by the health care team" (NPIAP, 2017, p. 3).

Factors in Pressure Injury Development

Pathologic changes at a pressure injury site result from blood vessel collapse caused by pressure, usually from body weight. Necrosis eventually occurs, leading to the characteristic ulcer. Three mechanisms contribute to pressure injury development: (1) external pressure that compresses blood vessels, (2) friction and shearing forces that tear and injure blood vessels and abrade the top layer of skin, and (3) microclimate of the skin related to temperature and moisture on the skin (Corum, 2019).

EXTERNAL PRESSURE

Pressure injuries usually occur over bony prominences where body weight is distributed over a small area without much subcutaneous tissue to cushion damage to the skin. Common sites for pressure injuries are illustrated in Figure 33-4. Of the susceptible areas, most pressure injuries occur over the sacrum and coccyx, followed by the trochanter (hip) and the calcaneus (heel).

The major predisposing factor for a pressure injury is external pressure applied over an area, which results in occluded blood capillaries and poor circulation to tissues. Insufficient circulation deprives tissue of oxygen and nutrients, which leads to **ischemia** (deficiency of blood in a particular area), hypoxia (inadequate amount of oxygen available to cells), edema, inflammation, and, ultimately, necrosis and ulcer formation. A pressure injury may occur in as little as 1 to 2 hours if the patient has not moved or been repositioned to allow circulation to flow to dependent areas. Patients with casts, orthopedic devices, or support stockings require routine assessment of areas where inadequate circulation may be a contributing factor to the development of a pressure injury.

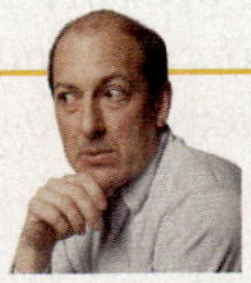

Consider ***Mr. Everly***, the postoperative patient in the critical care unit described in the Reflective Practice display. The nurse would integrate knowledge of the patient's condition, including his decreased level of consciousness and confinement in bed, to plan measures such as a turning schedule, proper positioning, and activities to promote movement in bed, thereby preventing body parts from exposure to prolonged pressure.

FRICTION AND SHEAR

Friction occurs when two surfaces rub against each other. The injury, which resembles an abrasion, can also damage superficial blood vessels directly under the skin. A patient who lies on wrinkled sheets is likely to sustain tissue damage as a result of friction. The skin over the elbows and heels often is injured due to friction when patients lift and help move themselves up in bed with the use of their arms and feet. Friction burns can also occur on the back when patients are pulled or slid over sheets while being moved up in bed or transferred onto a stretcher.

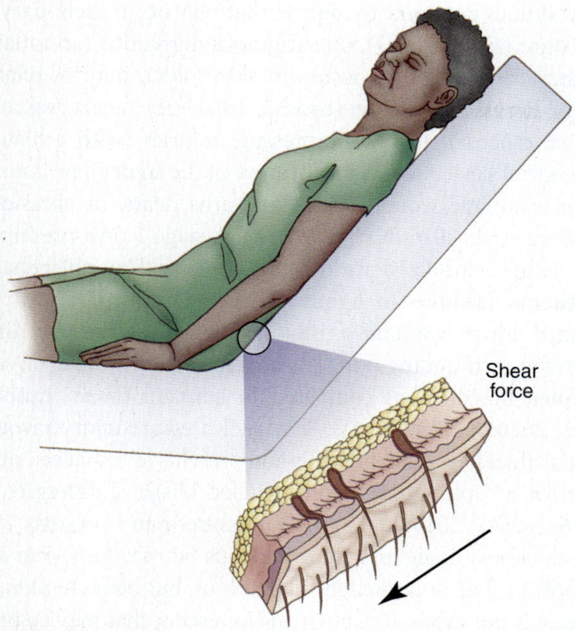

FIGURE 33-5. Shearing forces can occur when a patient is moved carelessly or slides down in bed.

Shear results when one layer of tissue slides over another layer. Shear separates the skin from underlying tissues. Shear includes shear stress, the force, and shear strain, the "distortion or deformation of tissue" (NPIAP, 2019, p. 5) secondary to shear stress. The small blood vessels and capillaries in the area are stretched and possibly tear, resulting in decreased circulation to the tissue cells under the skin. Figure 33-5 illustrates how shearing forces occur. Patients who are pulled, rather than lifted, when being moved up in bed, or from bed to chair or stretcher are at risk for injury from shearing forces. A patient who is partially sitting up in bed is susceptible to shearing force when the skin sticks to the sheet and underlying tissues move downward with the body toward the foot of the bed. This may also occur in a patient who sits in a chair but slides down.

MICROCLIMATE

Microclimate refers to the temperature and moisture (humidity) of the skin that comes into contact with a support surface, such as a bed or device (NPIAP, 2019). Skin that is moist does not have the same tolerance for pressure and shearing forces as skin that is dry (Corum, 2019). When skin is damp (from incontinence, perspiration, or drainage/exudate), it requires less friction to blister and abrade, which can lead to a pressure injury. Moisture from urinary and/or fecal incontinence has been linked to an increased likelihood of sacral pressure injury (Alvarez et al., 2016). There are four types of moisture-associated skin damage (MASD) identified in the literature: (1) incontinence-associated dermatitis (IAD) that results from chronic exposure to urine and/or stool, (2) perspiration-based (intertriginous) dermatitis (ITD), (3) periwound MASD due to exudate, and (4) peristomal MASD that occurs with ostomy output (McNichol et al., 2018).

Risks for Pressure Injury Development

In addition to pressure, friction, and shear, a combination of causes contributes to pressure injury development. These include immobility, nutrition, hydration, mental status, and age; these factors are addressed here. Additional risk factors are outlined in Box 33-3.

Box 33-3 Risk Factors for Pressure Injury Development

Mobility and activity limitations are required conditions for pressure injury development. In the absence of mobility issues, the risk factors listed here should not result in the formation of a pressure injury. Note that the development of a pressure injury may be unavoidable, even with preventative measures, in situations such as multiple organ dysfunction syndrome (MODS) where hemodynamic instability, inadequate nutrition/hydration, and immobility occur (Alvarez et al., 2016). Inadequate nutrition and dehydration, skin moisture, altered mental status, and advanced age are factors in the development of pressure injuries. In addition, patients compromised by the following conditions are at risk for pressure injury development:

- Poor skin hygiene
- Diabetes mellitus
- Diminished sensory perception (pain awareness)
- Fractures
- History of corticosteroid therapy
- General poor health
- Immobility secondary to paralysis or injury/illness
- Immunosuppression
- Incontinence—urinary or fecal
- Increased body temperature
- Microvascular dysfunction
- Multiple organ dysfunction syndrome (MODS)
- Previous pressure injuries
- Poor nutrition and hydration
- Sedation or coma
- Significant obesity or thinness
- Smoking
- Surgery
- Terminal illness/end-of-life/dying process

Source: Adapted from Alvarez, O. M., Brindle, C. T., Langemo, D., Kennedy-Evans, K. L., Krasner, D. L., Brennan, M. R., & Levine, J. M. (2016). The VCU pressure ulcer summit: The search for a clearer understanding and more precise clinical definition of the unavoidable pressure injury. *Journal of Wound, Ostomy and Continence Nursing, 43*(5), 455–463; Corum, L. (2019). Ulcer and wound care: Getting to the depth of the issue. *National Center of Continuing Education.* https://nursece.com/pdfs/720_V2_Wound_Care.pdf; and European Pressure Ulcer Advisory Panel (EPUAP), National Pressure Injury Advisory Panel (NPIAP), & Pan Pacific Pressure Injury Alliance (PPPIA). (2019b). *Prevention and treatment of pressure ulcers/injuries: Clinical practice guideline—The international guideline* (3rd ed.) E. Haesler (Ed.). Cambridge Media.

IMMOBILITY

Patients who spend long periods of time in bed or seated without shifting their body weight properly are at great risk for developing a pressure injury. People who are ambulatory usually do not develop this type of injury because no part of the body experiences prolonged pressure. In addition, when asleep, healthy people tend to move about in bed freely. Patients who are unconscious and paralyzed, those with cognitive impairments, those experiencing depression, or those with other physical limitations such as a fracture, are subject to pressure injuries if they are allowed to remain in any one position for an extended period. Additional factors that cause immobility and may result in this serious problem include surgery and the use of tranquilizers or sedatives.

NUTRITION AND HYDRATION

Protein–calorie malnutrition predisposes a person to pressure injury formation because poorly nourished cells are damaged easily. Protein deficiency leading to a negative nitrogen balance, electrolyte imbalances, and insufficient caloric intake also predisposes the skin to injury. Other deficiencies can increase risk. For example, vitamin C deficiency causes capillaries to become fragile, with resultant poor circulation to the area. The condition of the teeth or fit of dentures may also exacerbate the problem of inadequate dietary intake. Dehydration as well as edema can interfere with circulation and subsequent cell nourishment.

MENTAL STATUS

The more alert a person is, the more likely the person is to protect skin integrity by relieving pressure periodically and maintaining adequate skin hygiene. Apathy, confusion, or a comatose state can diminish these self-care abilities and increase the likelihood of skin breakdown.

AGE

Older adults are at a greater risk for pressure injury because the aging skin is more susceptible to injury. Chronic and debilitating diseases, more common in this age group, may adversely affect circulation and oxygenation of dermal structures. Other problems, such as malnutrition and immobility, compound the risk of pressure injury development in older adults.

Pressure Injury Staging

Although not a pressure injury, blanching (becoming pale and white) of the skin area under pressure may be an early warning sign of potential injury development. When pressure is relieved, blanching, which represents ischemia, is rapidly followed by hyperemia, a reddening in lightly pigmented skin. The body literally floods the area with blood to nourish and remove wastes from the cells. The area appears red and feels warm, but blanches when slight pressure is applied. After a patient who has been lying supine for 2 hours is repositioned onto the side, any reddened area due to reactive hyperemia should fade within 60 to 90 minutes. In patients with darkly pigmented skin, it may be best to assess for hyperemia by touch; the skin feels warm. Any potential change in color or temperature should be considered in relation to the surrounding tissue. Skin texture (taut, shiny, hardened) provides additional information for patients whose skin does not show blanching.

If the pressure is not removed when this ischemia occurs, circulation is further impaired, and a pressure injury develops. Appropriate intervention depends on early recognition of the stage of development of the pressure injury. Pressure injuries are commonly classified according to six stages (four numbered and two unnumbered): stage 1, stage 2, stage 3, stage 4, unstageable, and deep tissue pressure injury (DTPI; Edsberg et al., 2016; NPIAP, 2016a).

When assessing pressure injuries, it is important to note that this staging system should be used for pressure injuries only; it does not apply to injuries that may occur secondary to moisture (such as IAD), intertriginous dermatitis (an inflammatory condition that occurs in skin folds), injuries related to medical adhesive, neuropathic (diabetic) ulcers, vascular ulcers, mucosal membrane pressure injuries (with a history of medical device use at the location of the injury), or injuries from traumatic wounds (such as burns, tears, or abrasions; Edsberg et al., 2016; NPIAP, 2016a). A stage 1 pressure injury is a defined, localized area of intact skin with nonblanchable **erythema** (redness in lightly pigmented skin). Darkly pigmented skin may not have visible blanching; its color may differ from the surrounding skin. The area may be painful, firm, soft, warmer, or cooler as compared to adjacent tissue (Edsberg et al., 2016; NPIAP, 2016a). A stage 2 pressure injury involves partial-thickness loss of dermis and presents as a shallow, open ulcer or a ruptured/intact serum-filled blister (Edsberg et al., 2016; NPIAP, 2016a). A stage 3 pressure injury presents with full-thickness tissue loss. Subcutaneous fat may be visible and epibole (rolled wound edges) may occur, but bone, tendon, or muscle is not exposed. Slough and/or eschar that may be present do not obscure the depth of tissue loss. Ulcers at this stage may include undermining and tunneling (Edsberg et al., 2016; NPUAP, 2016a). Stage 4 injuries involve full-thickness tissue loss with exposed or palpable bone, cartilage, ligament, tendon, fascia, or muscle. Slough or eschar may be present on some part of the wound bed; epibole, undermining, and/or tunneling often occur (Edsberg et al., 2016; NPIAP, 2016a).

Concept Mastery Alert

The updated pressure injury staging system includes Arabic, not Roman numerals; the descriptions of the four stages (and two unstageable definitions) were formed based on a consensus of experts in 2016.

When the clinician is unable to visualize the extent of tissue damage due to slough or eschar, pressure injuries are classified as unstageable. Slough is yellow, tan, gray, green, or brown dead tissue; eschar is tan, brown, or black hardened dead tissue (necrosis) in the wound bed (EPUAP, NPIAP, & PPPIA, 2019b). Eschar and/or slough must be removed before the stage (3 or 4) can be determined. However, stable (dry, adherent, intact, without erythema or fluctuance) eschar on the heels or ischemic limb should not be removed or softened (NPIAP, 2016a).

Suspected deep-tissue injury presents as a persistent, nonblanchable purple or maroon discoloration of intact or nonintact skin, or separation of the epidermis that reveals a dark wound bed or blood-filled blister (NPIAP, 2016ab). The process that results in deep tissue injury begins about 48 hours before any visible deep red, purple, or maroon skin is evident, making it difficult to be sure of the cause of injury (NPIAP, 2021). It may initially present as a painful, firm, mushy, boggy, warmer, or cooler area as compared to adjacent tissue (EPUAP, NPIAP, & PPPIA, 2019b). This type of injury typically results from intense and/or prolonged pressure and shearing where the bone and muscle interface (NPIAP, 2016a).

Detailed descriptions of these stages and a visual representation are presented in Box 33-4.

Box 33-4 Pressure Injury Stages

Pressure Injury

A pressure injury is localized damage to the skin and underlying soft tissue usually over a bony prominence or related to a medical or other device. The injury can present as intact skin or an open ulcer and may be painful. The injury occurs as a result of intense and/or prolonged pressure or pressure in combination with shear. The tolerance of soft tissue for pressure and shear may also be affected by microclimate, nutrition, perfusion, comorbidities, and condition of the soft tissue.

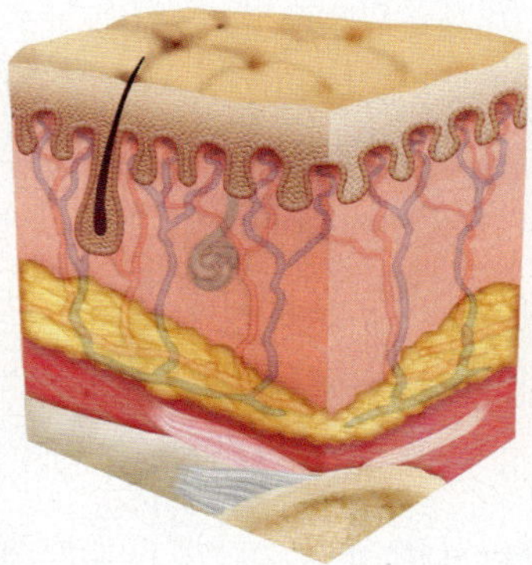

Healthy skin, lightly pigmented.[a]

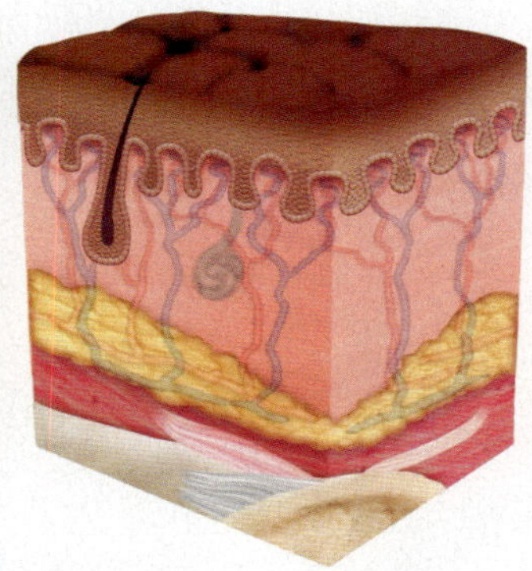

Healthy skin, darkly pigmented.[a]

Stage 1 Pressure Injury: Nonblanchable Erythema of Intact Skin

Intact skin with a localized area of nonblanchable erythema, which may appear differently in darkly pigmented skin. Presence of blanchable erythema or changes in sensation, temperature, or firmness may precede visual changes. Color changes do not include purple or maroon discoloration; these may indicate deep tissue pressure injury.

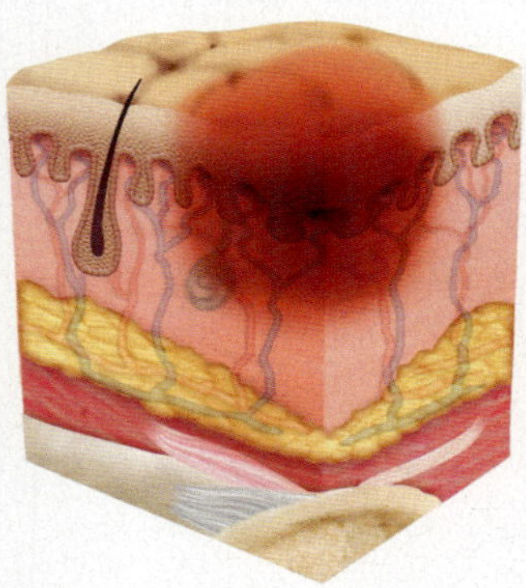

Stage 1 pressure injury, lightly pigmented.[a]

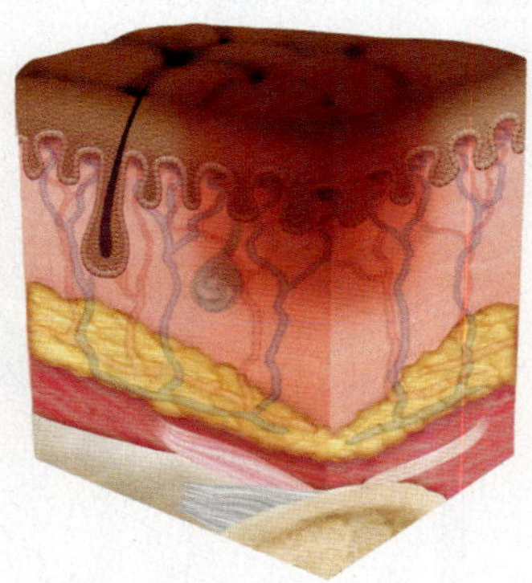

Stage 1 pressure injury, darkly pigmented.[a]

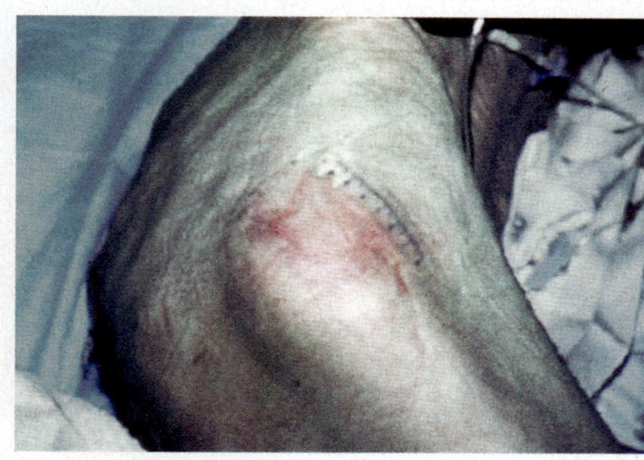

Stage 2 Pressure Injury: Partial-Thickness Skin Loss With Exposed Dermis

Partial-thickness loss of skin with exposed dermis. The wound bed is viable, pink or red, moist, and may also present as an intact or ruptured serum-filled blister. Adipose (fat) is not visible and deeper tissues are not visible. Granulation tissue, slough, and eschar are not present. These injuries commonly result from adverse microclimate and shear in the skin over the pelvis and shear in the heel. This stage should not be used to describe moisture-associated skin damage (MASD) including incontinence-associated dermatitis (IAD), intertriginous dermatitis (ITD), medical adhesive–related skin injury (MARSI), or traumatic wounds (skin tears, burns, abrasions).

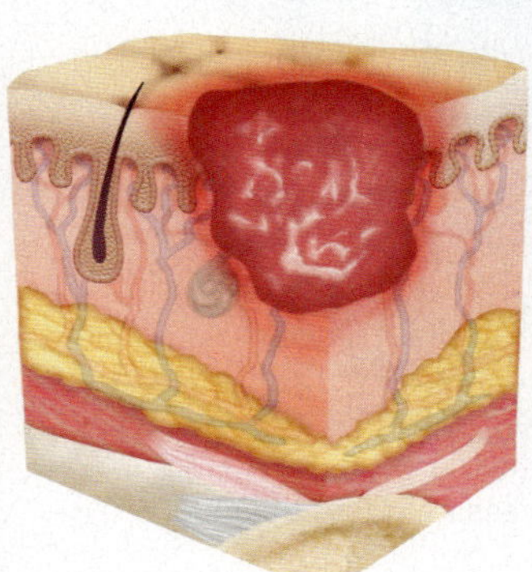

Stage 2 pressure injury.[a]

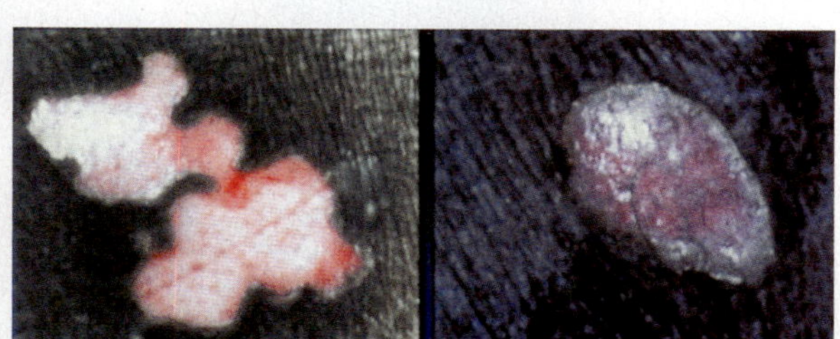

(continued)

Box 33-4 Pressure Injury Stages (*continued*)

Stage 3 Pressure Injury: Full-Thickness Skin Loss

Full-thickness loss of skin, in which adipose (fat) is visible in the ulcer and granulation tissue and epibole (rolled wound edges) are often present. Slough and/or eschar may be visible. The depth of tissue damage varies by anatomical location; areas of significant adiposity can develop deep wounds. Undermining and tunneling may occur. Fascia, muscle, tendon, ligament, cartilage, and/or bone are not exposed. If slough or eschar obscures the extent of tissue loss, this is an Unstageable Pressure Injury.

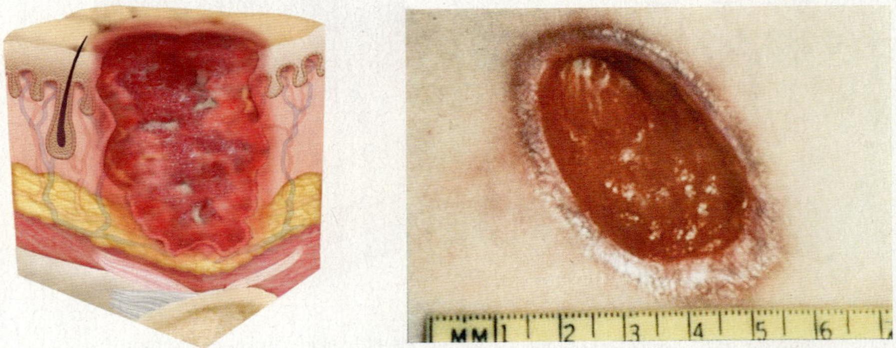

Stage 3 pressure injury.[a]

Stage 4 Pressure Injury: Full-Thickness Skin and Tissue Loss

Full-thickness skin and tissue loss with exposed or directly palpable fascia, muscle, tendon, ligament, cartilage or bone in the ulcer. Slough and/or eschar may be visible. Epibole (rolled edges), undermining, and/or tunneling often occur. Depth varies by anatomical location. If slough or eschar obscures the extent of tissue loss, this is an Unstageable Pressure Injury.

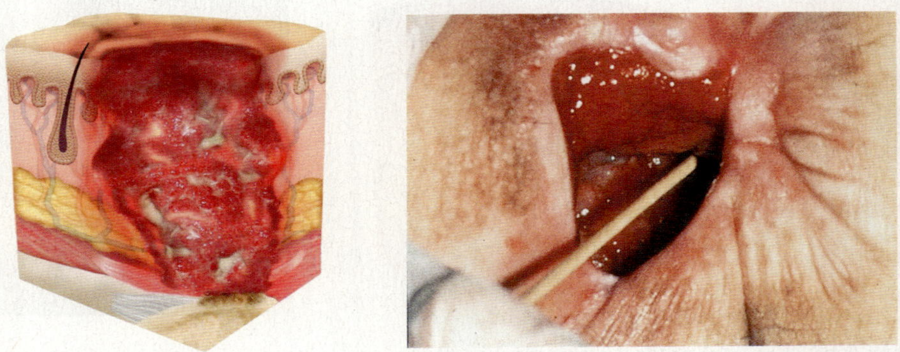

Stage 4 pressure injury.[a]

Unstageable Pressure Injury: Obscured Full-Thickness Skin and Tissue Loss

Full-thickness skin and tissue loss in which the extent of tissue damage within the ulcer cannot be confirmed because it is obscured by slough or eschar. If slough or eschar is removed, a stage 3 or stage 4 pressure injury will be revealed. Stable eschar (i.e., dry, adherent, intact without erythema or fluctuance) on the heel or ischemic limb should not be softened or removed.

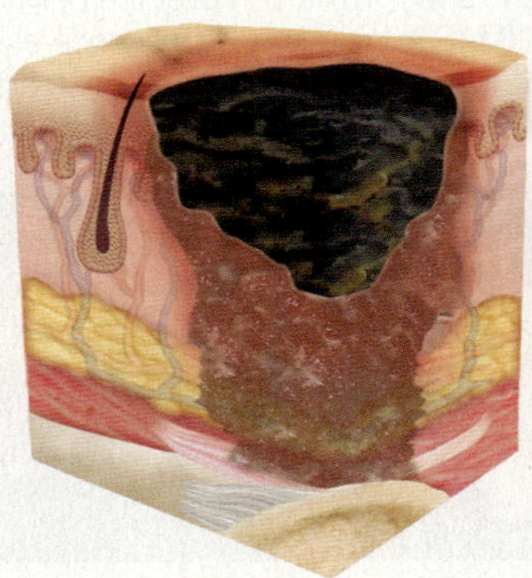

Unstageable pressure injury, dark eschar.[a]

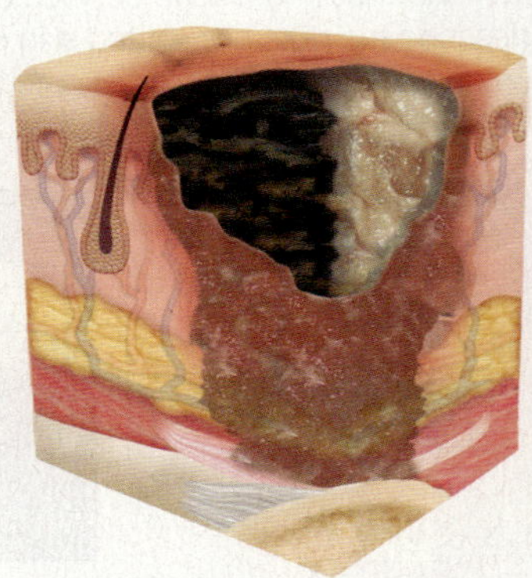

Unstageable pressure injury, slough and eschar.[a]

Box 33-4 Pressure Injury Stages (*continued*)

Deep Tissue Pressure Injury: Persistent Nonblanchable Deep Red, Maroon, or Purple Discoloration

Intact or nonintact skin with localized area of persistent nonblanchable deep red, maroon, or purple discoloration or epidermal separation revealing a dark wound bed or blood-filled blister. The process leading to deep tissue pressure injury (DTPI) begins 48 hours prior to any color changes. Pain and temperature change often precede skin color changes. Discoloration may appear differently in darkly pigmented skin. This injury results from intense and/or prolonged pressure and shear forces at the bone–muscle interface. The wound may evolve rapidly to reveal the actual extent of tissue injury, or may resolve without tissue loss. If necrotic tissue, subcutaneous tissue, granulation tissue, fascia, muscle, or other underlying structures are visible, this indicates a full-thickness pressure injury (unstageable, stage 3, or stage 4). Do not use DTPI to describe vascular, traumatic, neuropathic, or dermatologic conditions.

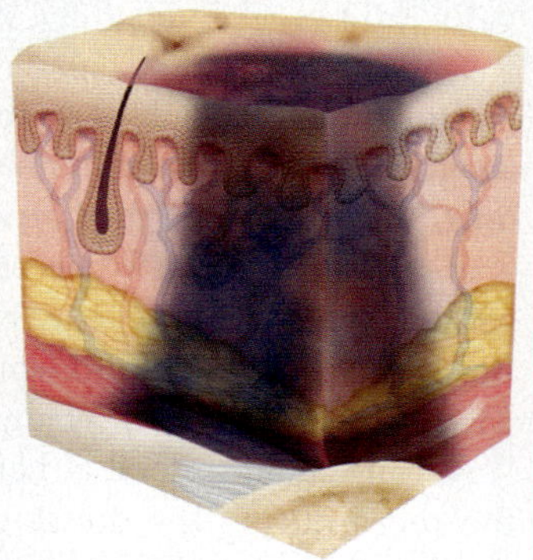

Deep tissue pressure injury.[a]

From National Pressure Injury Advisory Panel (NPUAP) (2016c). *Pressure injury illustrations.* Retrieved http://www.npuap.org/resources/educational-and-clinical-resources/pressure-injury-staging-illustrations/. Used with permission of the National Pressure. Ulcer Advisory Panel & date.)

Sources: Reprinted with permission from National Pressure Injury Advisory Panel (NPUAP). (2016a). *NPIAP Pressure injury stages.* Retrieved from https://npiap.com/page/PressureInjuryStages; National Pressure Injury Advisory Panel (NPIAP). (2021, January 8). *Evolution of deep tissue pressure injury.* https://npiap.com/news/546664/Evolution-of-Deep-Tissue-Pressure-Injury.htm. Used with permission from the National Pressure Injury Advisory Panel (NPIAP). Copyright 2021 NPIAP

Psychological Effects of Wounds and Pressure Injuries

Because the skin is a sensory organ and plays a major role in communication with others and self-image, wounds and pressure injuries require emotional as well as physical adaptation. Although stress and adaptation vary greatly among people, actual and potential emotional stressors are common in all patients with wounds. These stressors impact the quality of life of the patient and caregivers and include pain, anxiety, fear, activities of daily living, and changes in body image.

Pain

Pain is part of almost any trauma, from a small cut on the finger, to a chronic arterial ulcer or large incision made during abdominal surgery. Although pain can be considered a physical complication, it also has a large psychological component. Pain from wounds is often increased by activities such as ambulating, coughing, moving in bed, and dressing changes. The actual pain might be worsened by the patient's apprehension about such activities. Nursing interventions to reduce pain can greatly reduce emotional stress. See Chapter 36 for a more in-depth discussion of pain.

Anxiety and Fear

Anxiety and fear are common responses to a wound. Patients are apprehensive about the possibility of the wound opening, how much privacy will be lost as the wound is being cared for, and how they and others will react to the appearance and smell of the wound. When caring for patients with wounds, demonstrating acceptance and empathy, encouraging the expression of feelings, answering questions accurately and honestly, and avoiding excessive exposure of body parts when providing wound care are essential.

Activities of Daily Living

The presence of an acute or chronic wound or pressure injury can impact the ability of an individual to perform activities of daily living. Physical, financial, and medical restrictions can result in limitations on a person's ability to perform daily activities. The inability to perform any activity related to self-care (such as feeding oneself, bathing, dressing, grooming), work, homemaking, or leisure activities can negatively impact the person's quality of life.

Changes in Body Image

Body image reflects a person's view of oneself as a whole entity. When the skin and tissues are traumatized, that image is changed, requiring the person to adapt and reformulate their concept of self. Wounds and scars that are visible to others, especially on the face, can result in feelings of conspicuousness, ugliness, and diminished self-worth. Large scars, such as from removal of a breast or from creation of a colostomy opening, can seriously affect the person's sexuality, social relationships, and self-concept. Referral to support groups or counselors may be necessary to facilitate coping and acceptance of changes in body structure or function. See the Focused Critical Thinking Guide 33-1 on page 1168. In addition, Chapter 42 contains more information about self-concept.

NURSING PROCESS FOR WOUNDS AND PRESSURE INJURIES

Assessing

The patient's health history is an essential component for assessing the patient's integumentary status and identification of risk factors for problems with the skin. This information can be obtained from either the patient or a person identified

33-1 Focused Critical Thinking Guide

WOUND CARE: PROMOTING ACCEPTANCE OF CHANGES IN BODY IMAGE

During both clinical days in 1 week, you have been assigned to care for a middle-aged woman who has had a breast removed because of cancer. The patient, Mrs. Nola, is an attractive, usually cheerful woman who is eager to get better and return home. However, on both days, she turned her head away and would not look at the incision when her dressing was changed. She tells you that she "just can't stand to look at herself." Her husband has left the room during the dressing changes after telling you that "it makes me sick to see what happened to my wife." Mrs. Nola is to be discharged to her home the next day and needs to learn how to provide self-care for her wound. What do you do?

1. Identify goal of thinking

Determine the most effective way of ensuring wound care while also assisting Mrs. Nola in accepting her altered self-image.

2. Assess adequacy of knowledge

Pertinent circumstances: The diagnosis of cancer was made only 2 weeks before the surgical removal of the breast. The patient is to be discharged to her home the next day. The wound from her mastectomy has not completely healed and will require dressing changes for another 3 or 4 days. Mrs. Nola has had a disfiguring surgery and is coping with not only a change in body image, but also the diagnosis of cancer. She has never been seriously ill or had surgery. She has a strong, loving relationship with her husband, but he is unable to deal with the physical disfigurement at this time.

Prerequisite knowledge: Before you decide what to do in this situation, you need to know how Mrs. Nola is coping with her diagnosis of cancer. If she is still in denial about the disease, it is likely that she is also denying the surgical procedure and the changes in her body. You will need to review responses to the diagnosis of cancer as well as the stages of grief and loss. You will have to learn what her sources of support are and how she can best access and use them. You will need to assess how best to help her achieve wound care in the face of her continued refusal even to look at the wound.

Room for error: If she is forced to look at the wound or made to feel inadequate because of her inability to do so, she may feel threatened and may become angry in response to the perceived threat and retreat even further.

Time constraints: Some decision about wound care must be made before her discharge the next day.

3. Address potential problems

There are several potential obstacles to critical thinking in this situation. As a student, you want to exhibit safe, knowledgeable care, and the importance of teaching for home care has been an emphasis in this course. You have a sense of what the loss of a breast must mean, but know you cannot truly understand her lived experience. Having had a family member die of cancer, you find yourself wanting to do everything for Mrs. Nola. As a novice in nursing, you find it difficult to handle these emotional components of patient care and find yourself wanting to focus objectively on the task at hand and scold both the patient and her husband for being so silly about something as simple as a dressing change.

4. Consult helpful resources

You must first appreciate the loss and grief Mrs. Nola is experiencing, and you must then relate that to her response to self-care of the wound. Your best source of information about her coping methods and sources of personal strength is Mrs. Nola herself. You also discuss the most effective way of providing wound care at home with your instructor and the case manager for Mrs. Nola.

5. Critique judgment/decision

After talking to Mrs. Nola, your instructor, and the case manager, you mutually agree that Mrs. Nola cannot be hurried into acceptance of her medical diagnosis or her body changes. The case manager consults with Mrs. Nola's provider, who writes a prescription for a home health care nurse to visit for the next 4 days and complete the dressing change. After talking with Mrs. Nola, you identify that she is still very much in denial. You discuss with her the possibility of having a visitor from "Reach to Recovery," a support group for women with breast cancer who have had a mastectomy. Mrs. Nola tells you that she thinks she would like to talk to someone with the same diagnosis, and you call a referral for her. When you tell Mrs. Nola that a home health care nurse will be visiting her for the first few days at home to change her dressing and ensure Mrs. Nola can appropriately change the dressing herself, tears fill her eyes. She says, "I am so scared—I just don't know what to do." You realize that insisting that Mrs. Nola do her own dressing (in this moment) would have been extremely stressful for her. Focusing solely on the task would have been perceived as dismissive and could have negatively impacted on the trusting relationship you were trying to form with the patient. When you share the situation in postconference, your clinical group supports your clinical judgment.

Focused Assessment Guide 33-1

SKIN INTEGRITY

Factors to Assess	Questions and Approaches
Appearance of skin	• Do you have any skin areas that are discolored from your baseline coloration? Any gray (ashy) patches on your arms, elbows, lower legs, knees, or heels? • Have you noticed any texture changes in your skin? Bumps? Rough patches? Cracked thin lines? • Do some areas of skin on your body feel warmer or colder than others? • Describe the moisture in your skin: is it damp, dry, oily? • Have you noticed that your skin seems to be thinner? Where? • Have you noticed any swelling in your feet, ankles, or fingers? • Tell me about how you take care of your skin. For example, do you take a tub bath or shower? How often? Do you regularly use oils or lotions?
Recent changes in skin	• Do you have any sores on your body? If so, how many, and where are they? Have they changed in size? Do you have any drainage from them? • Have you noticed that the skin over your hips or backbone gets red/discolored if you sit or lie in one position for a long time? Any associated temperature changes in the skin? Does this disappear in a short time when you are up? • Have you gotten a piercing or tattoo recently? • Any recent surgical incisions or existing scars?
Activity/mobility	• Do you need assistance to walk or move? If so, how much? • Are you confined to your bed or a chair? • Can you independently change your position when you want to?
Nutrition	• Have you gained or lost weight recently? • Describe your usual meals each day. • How many glasses or cups of liquid do you drink each day? • Do you take any food supplements or vitamins? • Do you prepare your own meals? • Do you wear dentures? How do they fit? • Do you have any difficulty chewing or swallowing? • Has a doctor ever told you that you are anemic?
Pain	• If you have a sore, is it painful? • Do you take anything for pain? If so, what do you take, and how often? Does it help?
Elimination	• Have you noticed any problems (frequency, color, consistency, odor) with your bowels or urination? If so, describe. • Have you ever used pads or special pants because you can't control your urine or stools?

by the patient. The nursing examination combined with laboratory findings can provide information to identify a patient's strengths, as well as the nature of any problems, their course, related signs and symptoms, onset, frequency, and their effects on activities of daily living. The nurse decides, based on these findings, what problems can be treated independently by nursing. Other problems are referred to other members of the interprofessional team for decisions on treatment.

Nursing History

When obtaining the nursing history, include questions about the appearance of the skin and patient activities that may contribute to the development of a pressure injury. Often a combination of factors places the patient at greatest risk for a pressure injury.

Question the patient and family about recent changes in the appearance or condition of the skin and any skin care regimens. Also, assess activity status, nutritional state, elimination patterns, and cognitive state.

Evaluate the patient's general condition and laboratory test results. Be alert for signs and symptoms of infection, which may cause generalized malaise, increased pain, anorexia, and an elevated body temperature and pulse rate. Laboratory data indicating an infection include an elevated WBC count and, if a wound culture has been done, identification of a causative organism.

The accompanying Focused Assessment Guide 33-1 provides additional suggestions for gathering a nursing history.

Skin Assessment

Skin assessment should be an integral part of every patient's care. Physical assessment of the skin is included as part of the initial database collection. Skin assessment provides needed information for developing an appropriate plan of care. The inspection and palpation skills used to assess the integumentary system are described in detail in Chapter 27. Be sure to inspect the skin systematically in a head-to-toe fashion, including bony prominences, on admission and then at regular intervals for all at-risk patients. Reassessment is recommended (NPIAP, 2020), as follows:

- *Acute care setting:* On admission, then reassess every shift and with any change in condition
- *Long-term care setting:* On admission, then reassess weekly for 4 weeks, then quarterly and whenever the resident's condition changes
- *Home health care:* On admission, then reassess at every visit

Early detection and treatment of skin problems are important nursing functions. It is important to provide patients with a proactive strategy for skin care. Many conditions and wounds, particularly pressure injuries, can be prevented or minimized with early intervention. Interventions to promote skin health are discussed in Chapter 32.

Wound Assessment

Wound assessment involves inspection (sight and smell) and palpation for appearance, drainage, odor, and pain. Wound assessment determines the status of the wound, identifies barriers to the healing process, and identifies signs of complications. Accurate assessment provides essential baseline data and information to judge the effectiveness of treatment and wound healing progression. Skin integrity and wound assessment are performed at regular intervals, based on the nature of the wound and facility policy.

APPEARANCE OF THE WOUND

Note the location of the wound. Location is described in relation to the nearest anatomic landmark, such as bony prominences. Document the size of the wound. Measurements

Guidelines for Nursing Care 33-1

MEASURING WOUNDS AND PRESSURE INJURIES

Size of the Wound

- Draw the shape and describe it.
- Using agency protocol, measure the head-to-toe length, side-to-side width, and depth—use the greatest measurement for length, width, and depth.

Depth of the Wound

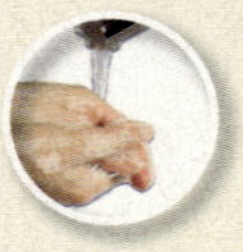

- Perform hand hygiene. Put on gloves.
- Moisten a sterile, flexible, cotton-tipped applicator with saline and insert it gently into the wound at a 90-degree angle with the tip down (Figure A).
- Mark the point on the swab that is even with the surrounding skin surface or grasp the applicator with the thumb and forefinger at the point corresponding to the wound's margin (Figure B).
- Remove the swab and measure the depth with a ruler (Figure C).

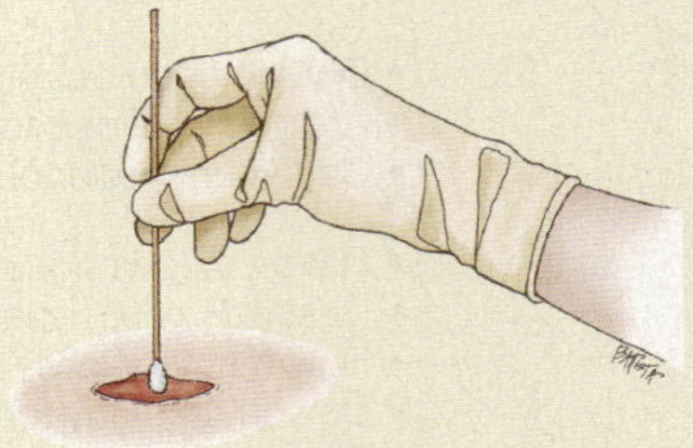

FIGURE A

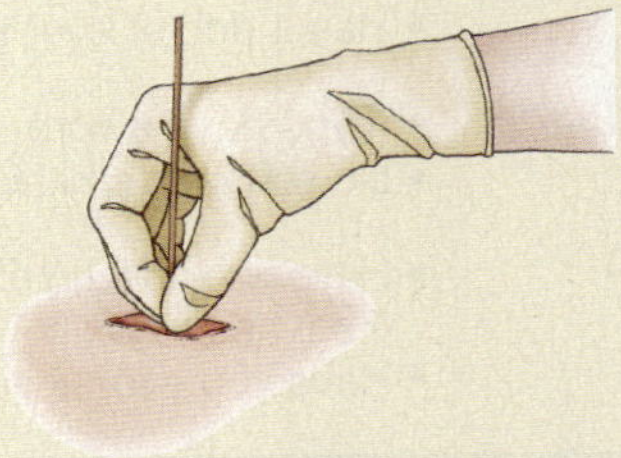

FIGURE B

Wound Tunneling

- Use standard precautions; use appropriate transmission-based precautions when indicated.

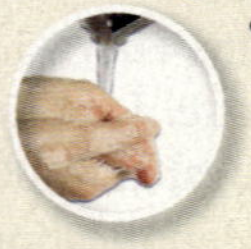

- Perform hand hygiene. Put on gloves.
- Determine direction: Moisten a sterile, flexible, cotton-tipped applicator with saline and gently insert a sterile applicator into the site where tunneling occurs. View the direction of the applicator as if it were the hand of a clock (Figure D). The direction of the patient's head represents 12 o'clock. Moving in a clockwise direction, document the deepest sites where the wound tunnels.
- Determine the depth: While the applicator is inserted into the tunneling, mark the point on the swab that is even with the wound's edge or grasp the applicator with the thumb and forefinger at the point corresponding to the wound's margin. Remove the swab and measure the depth with a ruler (see Figure C).
- Document both the direction and depth of tunneling.

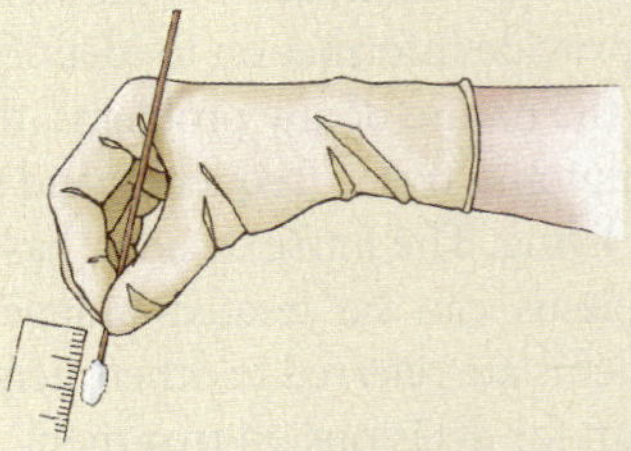

FIGURE C

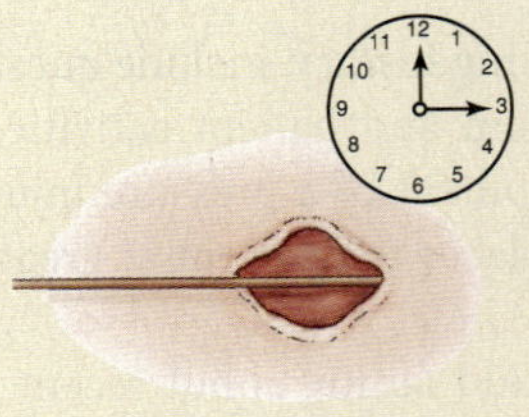

FIGURE D

Source: Adapted from Baranoski, S., & Ayello, E. A. (2020). *Wound care essentials: Practice principles* (5th ed.). Wolters Kluwer.

Box 33-5 RYB Wound Classification

A color classification system termed RYB (red-yellow-black) can be used for wound assessment and to help direct treatment for open wounds, or healing by secondary intention (Hess, 2019; Krasner, 1995; Stotts, 1990). This classification, with related interventions, is based on the assessment of wound color. However, many wounds have red, yellow, and black components and are categorized as mixed wounds (see Figure). When all colors are present, the wound is treated first for the most serious color: black, followed by yellow, and finally red.

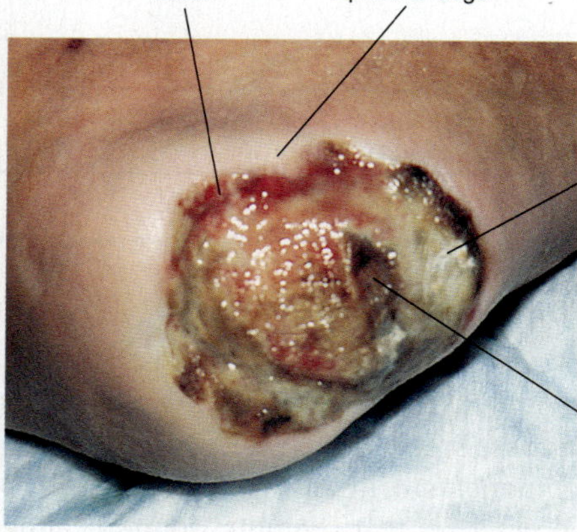

R = Red = Protect

Red wounds are in the proliferative stage of healing and reflect the color of normal granulation tissue. Wounds in this stage need protection with nursing interventions that include gentle cleansing, use of moist dressings, and changing of the dressing only when necessary, and/or based on product manufacturer's recommendations.

Y = Yellow = Cleanse

Yellow in the wound may indicate the presence of exudate (drainage) or slough and requires wound cleaning. These wounds are characterized by oozing from the tissue covering the wound, often accompanied by purulent drainage. Drainage can be whitish yellow, creamy yellow, yellowish green, or beige. To cleanse these wounds, nursing interventions include the use of wound cleansers and irrigating the wound.

B = Black = Debride

Black in the wound may indicate the presence of an eschar (necrotic tissue), which is usually black but may also be brown, gray, or tan. The eschar requires debridement (removal) before the wound can heal. These wounds are often cared for by advanced practice nurses who are educated in the care of more complex wounds. After debridement, the wound is treated as a yellow wound and then, as healing progresses, a red wound.

are taken in millimeters or centimeters, measuring length, width, and depth. Refer to Guidelines for Nursing Care 33-1 for details on measuring a wound.

Assess wounds for the approximation of the wound edges (edges meet) and signs of dehiscence or evisceration. Assess the color of the wound and surrounding area. Note the presence of drains, tubes, staples, and sutures. The edges of a healthy healing surgical wound appear clean and well approximated, with a crust along the wound edges. Initially, the edges are reddened and slightly swollen. After approximately 1 week, the skin is closer to normal in appearance, with wound edges healing together. The skin surrounding the wound may at first be bruised, but this too returns to normal as blood is reabsorbed.

When infection is present, the wound is swollen and deep red. It feels hot on palpation, and drainage is increased and possibly purulent. If dehiscence is impending or present, the wound edges are separated. If the wound edges have separated and the wound is open, describe the type of tissue in the wound: granulation, slough, or eschar (see Box 33-5).

Assess for the presence of odor, but only after the wound has been cleaned. The presence of odor can be indicative of certain types of bacteria.

DRAINAGE

The inflammatory response results in the formation of exudate which then drains from the wound. The exudate may contain fluid/serum, cellular debris, bacteria, and leukocytes (Baranoski & Ayello, 2020). This exudate is called wound drainage and is described as serous, sanguineous, serosanguineous, or, if infected, purulent.

- **Serous drainage** is composed primarily of the clear, serous portion of the blood and from serous membranes. Serous drainage is clear and watery.
- **Sanguineous drainage** consists of large numbers of red blood cells and looks like blood. Bright-red sanguineous drainage is indicative of fresh bleeding, whereas darker drainage indicates older bleeding.
- **Serosanguineous drainage** is a mixture of serum and red blood cells. It is light pink to blood tinged.
- **Purulent drainage** is made up of white blood cells, liquefied dead tissue debris, and both dead and live bacteria. Purulent drainage is thick, often has a musty or foul odor, and varies in color (such as dark yellow or green), depending on the causative organism.

Drains may be inserted in or near a wound to promote drainage, reducing the risk of abscess formation and promoting wound healing. Various types of drains are described in Table 33-4 on page 1172 and discussed later in this chapter.

Assess the amount, color, odor, and consistency of wound drainage. The amount and color depend on the wound location and size. Generally speaking, a small amount of exudate covers less than one third of the dressing, a moderate amount covers one third to two thirds of the dressing, and a large amount covers more than two thirds of the dressing (Baranoski & Ayello, 2020). Typically, larger wounds have more drainage than smaller wounds. Assess wound drainage on the wound, on the dressings, in drainage bottles or reservoirs, or—depending on the location of the wound and the amount of drainage—under the patient.

Table 33-4 Common Types of Drains

TYPE: OPEN	PURPOSE	EXAMPLE
Gauze, iodoform gauze, NuGauze—gauze dressings packed loosely so the wound is allowed to drain	Allow healing from base of wound	Infected wounds, after removal of hemorrhoids
Penrose: open drainage system consisting of a soft rubber tube that provides a sinus tract	Drains blood and fluid	After incision and drainage of abscess, in abdominal surgery
TYPE: CLOSED	**PURPOSE**	**EXAMPLE**
Blake: silicon tube with four chambers—similar to a JP externally	Drains blood and fluid	Used in cardiac surgery in place of a chest tube or JP drain
Chest tube: mediastinal placement (different from a chest tube used in the pleural space)	Drains blood	After cardiac surgery
Hemovac: portable negative pressure suction device	Drains blood and fluid	After abdominal, orthopedic surgery
Jackson-Pratt (JP): bulb suction device	Drains blood and fluid	After breast surgery or mastectomy, abdominal surgery
T-tube: T-shaped tube placed in the common bile duct	Collects bile	After gallbladder surgery

SUTURES AND STAPLES

Skin sutures are used to hold tissue and skin together. Sutures may be silk, synthetic material, or fine wire, and are classified as absorbable or nonabsorbable. Nonabsorbable sutures are removed when enough tensile strength has developed to hold the wound edges together during healing. The time frame varies depending on the patient's age, nutritional status, and wound location. Frequently, after skin sutures are removed, small wound-closure strips of adhesive are applied across the wound to give additional support as it continues to heal. New developments in sutures include drug-eluting (slow release) sutures, stem cell seeded sutures, antimicrobial sutures, and even elastic and electronic sutures (Dennis et al., 2016). Figure 33-6 shows an example of an incision with sutures. Retention sutures are used to provide extra support for patients with obesity and for wounds with an increased risk for dehiscence. The use of staples to close the skin may reduce the time required in the operating room, but there is some indication that the use of sutures may slightly reduce pain postoperatively, adverse events, and readmission rates. More research needs to be done on this topic (Cochetti et al., 2020).

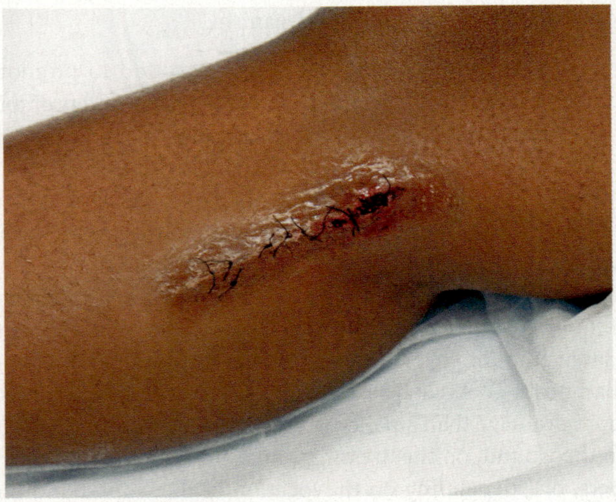

FIGURE 33-6. Incision with sutures.

Chronic Wound Assessment

Chronic wounds are often related to vascular or circulatory issues, with the lower extremities being the most frequently affected. Wound assessment of chronic wounds must address the unique components of these wounds and incorporate evidence-based practices that promote wound healing. The ABCESS acronym that was originally developed for students in podiatric medicine, provides an assessment framework that can be applied to chronic wounds of the lower extremity (McGuire et al., 2020):

- A: **A**ll of the patient—history, physical, and overview of patient status
- B: Wound **b**ed management—**b**ioload, **b**iofilm, **b**iomarkers, and **b**iopsy
- C: **C**irculation—arterial, venous, and lymphatic
- E: **E**dema, **e**xudate, and **e**rythema management—including dressing and compression
- S: **S**kin protection and treatment
- S: **S**ocial, **s**ocietal, and **s**piritual factors

Pressure Injury Assessment

It is a nursing priority to perform a comprehensive assessment in all settings. Nurses need to identify patients at risk for pressure injuries due to predisposing factors and recognize when there is evidence of actual pressure injuries.

RISK ASSESSMENT

Although no one risk assessment tool is universally recommended, these tools are part of an assessment that must be structured, comprehensive, and based on clinical judgment (EPUAP, NPIAP, & PPPIA, 2019b). A risk assessment form should be simple to use, reliable, cost effective, and supported by institutional policy (as applicable). Several scales are available to assess risk:

- Braden Scale: mental status, continence, mobility, activity, and nutrition (Braden & Maklebust, 2005; Fig. 33-7)

Braden Scale for Predicting Pressure Sore Risk

Sensory Perception: Ability to respond meaningfully to pressure-related discomfort — SCORE

1. **Completely Limited:** Unresponsive (does not moan, flinch, or grasp) to painful stimuli, due to diminished level of consciousness or sedation, OR limited ability to feel pain over most of body surface.
2. **Very Limited:** Responds only to painful stimuli. Cannot communicate discomfort except by moaning or restlessness, OR has a sensory impairment which limits the ability to feel pain or discomfort over half of body.
3. **Slightly Limited:** Responds to verbal commands but cannot always communicate discomfort or need to be turned, OR has some sensory impairment which limits ability to feel pain or discomfort in 1 or 2 extremities.
4. **No Impairment:** Responds to verbal commands. Has no sensory deficit which would limit ability to feel or voice pain or discomfort.

Moisture: Degree to which skin is exposed to moisture — SCORE

1. **Constantly Moist:** Skin is kept moist almost constantly by perspiration, urine, etc. Dampness is detected every time patient is moved or turned.
2. **Very Moist:** Skin is often but not always moist. Linen must be changed at least once a shift.
3. **Occasionally Moist:** Skin is occasionally moist, requiring an extra linen change approximately once a day.
4. **Rarely Moist:** Skin is usually dry: linen requires changing only at routine intervals.

Activity: Degree of physical activity — SCORE

1. **Bedfast:** Confined to bed.
2. **Chairfast:** Ability to walk severely limited or non-existent. Cannot bear own weight and/or must be assisted into chair or wheelchair.
3. **Walks Occasionally:** Walks occasionally during the day, but for very short distances, with or without assistance. Spends majority of each shift in bed or chair.
4. **Walks Frequently:** Walks outside the room at least twice and inside room at least once every 2 hours during waking hours.

Mobility: Ability to change and control body position — SCORE

1. **Completely immobile:** Does not make even slight changes in body or extremity position without assistance.
2. **Very Limited:** Makes occasional slight changes in body or extremity position but unable to make frequent or significant changes independently.
3. **Slightly Limited:** Makes frequent though slight changes in body or extremity position independently.
4. **No Limitation:** Makes major and frequent changes in position without assistance.

Nutrition: Usual food intake pattern — SCORE

1. **Very Poor:** Never eats a complete meal. Rarely eats more than 1/3 of food offered. Eats 2 servings or less of protein (meat or dairy products) per day. Takes fluids poorly. Does not take a liquid dietary supplement, OR is NPO and/or maintained on clear liquids or IV for more than five days.
2. **Probably Inadequate:** Rarely eats a complete meal and generally eats only about half of any food offered. Protein intake includes only 3 servings of meat or dairy products per day. Occasionally will take a dietary supplement, OR receives less than optimum amount of liquid diet or tube feeding.
3. **Adequate:** Eats over half of most meals. Eats a total of 4 servings of protein (meat, dairy products) each day. Occasionally will refuse a meal, but will usually take a supplement if offered, OR is on a tube feeding or TPN regimen, which probably meets most of nutritional needs.
4. **Excellent:** Eats most of every meal. Never refuses a meal. Usually eats a total of 4 or more servings of meat and dairy products. Occasionally eats between meals. Does not require supplementation.

Friction and Shear — SCORE

1. **Problem:** Requires moderate to maximum assistance in moving. Complete lifting without sliding against sheets is impossible. Frequently slides down in bed or chair, requiring frequent repositioning with maximum assistance. Spasticity, contractures, or agitation leads to almost constant friction.
2. **Potential Problem:** Moves feebly or requires minimum assistance. During a move skin probably slides to some extent against sheets, chair, restraints, or other devices. Maintains relatively good position in chair or bed most of the time but occasionally slides down.
3. **No Apparent Problem:** Moves in bed and in chair independently and has sufficient muscle strength to lift up completely during move. Maintains good position in bed or chair at all times.

3 or 4 = Moderate to Low Impairment
Total Points Possible: 23
Risk Predicting Score: 16 or Less

Risk Level
19-23 Not at risk
15-18 low risk
13-14 moderate risk
10-12 high risk
≤ 9 very high risk

NPO: Nothing by Mouth
IV: Intravenously
TPN: Total parenteral nutrition

Total Score:

FIGURE 33-7. Braden scale for predicting pressure ulcer risk. (*Source:* Copyright, Barbara Braden and Nancy Bergstrom, 1988. Reprinted with permission. All rights reserved.)

- Norton Scale: physical and mental conditions, activity, mobility, and incontinence (Norton, McLaren, & Exton-Smith, 1962/1975)
- Waterlow Scale: age and gender [sex], build and weight, continence, skin type, mobility, nutrition, and special population-specific risks (Waterlow, 1985)
- Jackson/Cubbin Pressure Area Risk Calculator: age, weight and tissue viability, medical history, general skin condition, mental status, mobility, hemodynamic status, respiratory status including oxygen requirements, incontinence, and hygiene—used primarily in the intensive care unit (Jackson, 1999); see the Research in Nursing box on page 1174

Research in Nursing

BRIDGING THE GAP TO EVIDENCE-BASED PRACTICE

Reducing the Incidence of Hospital-Acquired Pressure Injuries

Pressure injuries are costly in terms of patient discomfort, disfigurement, decreased quality of life, fatalities, and health care expenditures. Nurses play an important role in the prevention of pressure injuries. Pressure injury prevention for patients in the critical care environment poses unique challenges.

Related Research

Higgins, J., Casey, S., Taylor, E., Wilson, R., & Halcomb, P. (2020). Comparing the Braden and Jackson/Cubbin Pressure Injury Risk Scales in trauma-surgery ICU patients. *Critical Care Nurse, 40*(6), 52–61. https://doi.org/10.4037/ccn2020874

The purpose of this retrospective review of 366 medical records and associated analysis was to compare the predictive properties of the Braden and Jackson/Cubbin scales in critically ill patients from a trauma-surgical intensive care unit (ICU). Adult patients who were admitted to a trauma-surgical ICU, had an ICU stay of at least 72 hours, and did not have a preexisting pressure injury were included in the study. Irrespective of defined risk for pressure injury, all patients in the ICUs received interventions associated with a standard pressure injury prevention bundle. Although the Braden scale is widely used and provides efficacious predictive information, the critically ill patient demonstrates a higher propensity for oxygenation and perfusion issues, which are captured in the Jackson/Cubbin scale.

Those in the study who developed a pressure injury were older ($p = .05$), more often required vasopressors (to maintain blood pressure; $p < .001$) and mechanical ventilation (to support ventilation and oxygenation; $p < .001$), experienced incontinence ($p < .001$), and required assistance or were fully dependent for hygiene ($p < .001$). In general, the Braden scale was found to overpredict pressure injury risk, which impacts on resources and interventions, and can result in desensitization of the clinical staff. For this particular population, the Jackson/Cubbin scale outperformed the Braden scale in negative and positive predictive value, sensitivity, and specificity.

Relevance to Nursing Practice

The limitations of this study include the retrospective nature of data collection, the data collection time frame of 72 to 96 hours, the sampling strategy, and the use of one site for data collection. Although more research needs to be done to determine the best scale for determining pressure injury risk in specific populations, the clinical team associated with these trauma-surgical ICUs recommends the use of the Jackson/Cubbin scale to predict pressure injury risk.

With these tools, a numeric score is assigned to each assessment area. The degree of risk is based on the patient's total score. Using the Braden scale, a score of 19 to 23 indicates no risk; 15 to 18, mild risk; 13 to 14, moderate risk; 10 to 12, high risk; and 9 or lower, very high risk (Braden & Maklebust, 2005). Patients may have additional risk factors and/or other health problems not measured by the chosen assessment scale. Therefore, good nursing judgment may reveal the need for a higher intensity of preventive intervention than what may be identified by the scale alone (Baranoski & Ayello, 2020; Braden, 2012; Jackson, 1999).

Once a patient's risk has been identified, facilities use different approaches. Appropriate interventions are initiated based on the patient's identified risk. Many health care facilities use a pressure injury assessment form embedded in the electronic medical record that allows for trending. Documenting assessments is essential to maintaining a streamlined plan and ensuring continuity of care. All caregivers in the home or health care facility need to be aware of specific assessments, including assessment of mobility, nutritional status, and moisture and incontinence.

MOBILITY

Assessing a patient's mobility includes evaluating the patient's ability to move, turn, and reposition the body. A patient who is confined to bed or a chair or has limited range of motion is at increased risk for a pressure injury. This assessment of activity status is done upon admission to the health care facility or during the initial home care interview. The use of any assistive devices to maintain mobility and activity is noted. Additional suggestions for gathering information about mobility are described in Chapter 34.

NUTRITIONAL STATUS

The importance of sound nutrition in the prevention and treatment of a pressure injury is well established. Older adults, in particular, need adequate nutrition for optimal health and wound healing. Nutritional assessment is described in Chapter 37. Hydration and weight are important to consider, especially when unintended weight loss reaches 5% in 30 days or 10% over 180 days (Baranoski & Ayello, 2020). The following laboratory criteria that focus on diabetes and inflammatory markers (American Diabetes Association, 2022; Evans et al., 2022) indicate that a patient is nutritionally at risk for development of a pressure injury:

- Albumin level <3.2 mg/dL (normal, 3.4 to 5.4 g/dL)
- Prealbumin <15 mg/dL (normal 15 to 36 mg/dL)
- Total lymphocyte count <1,000/mm^3 (normal, 1,000 to 4,800/mm^3)
- Hemoglobin A1c >6.5% (normal <5.7%)
- Glucose >126 mg/dL (fasting normal <100 mg/dL)

MOISTURE AND INCONTINENCE

Many studies have documented that moisture makes the skin more susceptible to injury. Whether the moisture is from perspiration, wound drainage, urine, or stool, the skin is compromised. Moisture can create an environment in which microorganisms can multiply and the skin is more likely to blister, suffer abrasions, and become macerated. Chapters 38 and 39 have additional assessment information related to incontinence.

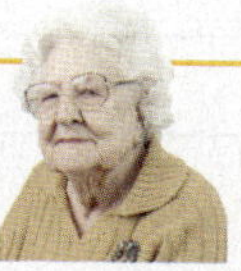

Remember **Mary Biesicker**, the woman who has been cared for at home by her daughter since being hospitalized last year for a cerebrovascular accident (stroke). Based on her daughter's report of Mary's increase in incontinence episodes and decreased level of functional independence, it is very likely that Mary developed a pressure injury. Keep Mary in mind as we move to explore prevention and treatment options for pressure injuries.

APPEARANCE OF EXISTING PRESSURE INJURY

Skin assessment for a pressure injury specifically includes inspection of the following (Baranoski & Ayello, 2020; NPIAP, 2020):

- Location of any lesion or ulcer
- Identification of the stage (see Box 33-4 on pages 1165–1167)
- Size of the ulcer: length, width, depth (see Guidelines for Nursing Care 33-1 on page 1170); presence of undermining, a hollow between the skin surface and the wound bed, resulting from death of the underlying tissue
- Color and type of wound tissue
- Presence of any abnormal pathways in the wound, such as a **sinus tract** (a cavity or channel underneath the wound that has the potential for infection) or *tunneling* (a passageway or opening that may be visible at skin level, but with most of the tunnel under the surface of the skin). See Guidelines for Nursing Care 33-1 on page 1170.
- Visible necrotic tissue; necrotic tissue that is in the process of separating from viable portions of the body is referred to as *slough*
- Presence of an exudate or drainage (amount and type)
- Presence of odor
- Presence or absence of granulation tissue
- Visible evidence of epithelialization
- Periwound skin condition

The Pressure Ulcer Scale for Healing (PUSH Tool) was developed by the National Pressure Ulcer Advisory Panel (NPUAP, 2016b) as a quick, reliable tool to monitor the change in pressure injury status over time (Fig. 33-8 on page 1176). Graphing the PUSH Tool scores over time for each pressure injury allows health care providers to track whether the injury/ulcer is healing, remains unchanged, or is deteriorating (NPUAP, 2016b).

The RYB Wound Classification (red-yellow-black; see Box 33-5 on page 1171) can also be used to aid in assessment and description of the pressure injury appearance.

Pain Assessment

Nurses have long recognized that patients with alterations in skin integrity—including surgical wounds, traumatic wounds, and pressure ulcers—experience pain. Focus assessment on whether dressing changes, positioning in bed or in a chair, or movement elicits any expressions of pain. Perform a pain assessment at each dressing change; measure and document the level of pain before, during, and after a procedure. Even if pain is never verbalized or expressed, always assume that pain is a definite possibility, and focus on comfort needs (EPUAP, NPIAP, & PPPIA, 2019b). Ask the patient about pain from the wound and determine if the pain is a one-time episode of pain, occurs with dressing changes, or is constant (Baranoski & Ayello, 2020). If the patient experiences increased or constant pain from the wound, perform further assessments. Increasing pain, especially when accompanied by an increased or purulent flow of drainage, may indicate delayed healing or an infection (EPUAP, NPIAP, & PPPIA, 2019b). Surgical incisional pain is usually most severe for the first 2 to 3 days and then progressively diminishes. Detailed assessment of pain is discussed in Chapter 36.

Diagnosing

Data that the nurse collect may lead to diagnosing actual or potential health problems or needs related to skin integrity and wound care. These identified problems and needs guide the development and communication of a coordinated plan that often involves the interprofessional team. Examples of patient problems and needs with related etiology and signs and symptoms can be found in the box titled Examples of Actual or Potential Health Problems and Needs: Patient with a Wound or Pressure Injury on page 1177.

Outcome Identification and Planning

When nurses care for patients who have or are at risk for altered skin and tissue integrity, nursing interventions are planned for returning the patient to health by facilitating wound healing, reducing the risk for complications, and promoting psychosocial adaptation. The following are examples of appropriate outcomes. The patient will:

- Maintain or restore skin integrity
- Demonstrate self-care measures to prevent pressure injury development
- Demonstrate self-care measures to promote wound healing
- Demonstrate evidence of wound healing
- Demonstrate increase in body weight and muscle size, if appropriate
- Remain free of infection at the site of the wound or pressure injury
- Remain free of signs and symptoms of infection
- Experience no new areas of skin breakdown
- Verbalize that the pain management regimen relieves pain to an acceptable level
- Demonstrate appropriate wound care measures before discharge
- Verbalize understanding of signs and symptoms to report and necessary follow-up care

NATIONAL PRESSURE ULCER ADVISORY PANEL

Pressure Ulcer Scale for Healing (PUSH)
PUSH Tool 3.0

Patient Name____________________ Patient ID# ____________

Ulcer Location ____________________ Date ____________

Directions:

Observe and measure the pressure ulcer. Categorize the ulcer with respect to surface area, exudate, and type of wound tissue. Record a sub-score for each of these ulcer characteristics. Add the sub-scores to obtain the total score. A comparison of total scores measured over time provides an indication of the improvement or deterioration in pressure ulcer healing.

LENGTH X WIDTH (in cm^2)	**0** 0	**1** < 0.3	**2** 0.3 – 0.6	**3** 0.7 – 1.0	**4** 1.1 – 2.0	**5** 2.1 – 3.0	**Sub-score**
		6 3.1 – 4.0	**7** 4.1 – 8.0	**8** 8.1 – 12.0	**9** 12.1 – 24.0	**10** > 24.0	
EXUDATE AMOUNT	**0** None	**1** Light	**2** Moderate	**3** Heavy			**Sub-score**
TISSUE TYPE	**0** Closed	**1** Epithelial Tissue	**2** Granulation Tissue	**3** Slough	**4** Necrotic Tissue		**Sub-score**
							TOTAL SCORE

Length x Width: Measure the greatest length (head to toe) and the greatest width (side to side) using a centimeter ruler. Multiply these two measurements (length x width) to obtain an estimate of surface area in square centimeters (cm^2). Caveat: Do not guess! Always use a centimeter ruler and always use the same method each time the ulcer is measured.

Exudate Amount: Estimate the amount of exudate (drainage) present after removal of the dressing and before applying any topical agent to the ulcer. Estimate the exudate (drainage) as none, light, moderate, or heavy.

Tissue Type: This refers to the types of tissue that are present in the wound (ulcer) bed. Score as a "4" if there is any necrotic tissue present. Score as a "3" if there is any amount of slough present and necrotic tissue is absent. Score as a "2" if the wound is clean and contains granulation tissue. A superficial wound that is reepithelializing is scored as a "1". When the wound is closed, score as a "0".

4 – Necrotic Tissue (Eschar): black, brown, or tan tissue that adheres firmly to the wound bed or ulcer edges and may be either firmer or softer than surrounding skin.

3 – Slough: yellow or white tissue that adheres to the ulcer bed in strings or thick clumps, or is mucinous.

2 – Granulation Tissue: pink or beefy red tissue with a shiny, moist, granular appearance.

1 – Epithelial Tissue: for superficial ulcers, new pink or shiny tissue (skin) that grows in from the edges or as islands on the ulcer surface.

0 – Closed/Resurfaced: the wound is completely covered with epithelium (new skin).

www.npuap.org
11F

PUSH Tool Version 3.0: 9/15/98

FIGURE 33-8. Pressure Ulcer Scale for Healing (PUSH) PUSH Tool 3.0 National Pressure Injury Advisory Panel (NPIAP). (2016b). *PUSH tool.* https://npiap.com/page/PUSHTool

Examples of Actual or Potential Health Problems and Needs

PATIENT WITH A WOUND OR PRESSURE INJURY

Actual or Potential Health Problem or Need	Possible Etiologic Factors	Potential Signs and Symptoms
Altered Skin Integrity	• External factors: pressure on bony prominences; surgical incision; use of mobility or assistive devices; exposure to heat/cold, radiation therapy, or other agents • Patient-based: age, weight, nutritional and hydration status, medical history, general skin condition, mental status, mobility, incontinence, and hygiene	• Acute pain • Unintentional Injury: Open wound, bleeding, hematoma/bruising, pressure injury/ulcer, shearing, burn • Intentional injury: surgical wound closed with staples, sutures, or another agent; open wound following surgical or chemical debridement
Pressure Injury Risk	• Pressure on bony prominences • Use of mobility-based or other equipment • Moisture and temperature variations on the skin • Debilitated or compromised state of the patient: mental or physical impairments, chronic or acute illness	—

Source: Wolters Kluwer. (2022). Problem-based care plans. In *Lippincott Advisor*. Wolters Kluwer. https://advisor.lww.com/lna/home.do

Implementing

Provide preventive measures for patients at risk for pressure injury. Teach patients about their health conditions and provide information and support to improve patients' health literacy. Refer to the accompanying Promoting Health Literacy display.

When caring for the patient with a wound or pressure injury, nursing interventions focus on preventing infection, promoting wound healing, preventing further injury or alteration in skin integrity, promoting physical and emotional comfort, and facilitating coping. It is often appropriate and necessary to consult with the wound care specialist, often a wound certified nurse specialist, to plan and coordinate the most effective care for the patient.

Preventing Pressure Injuries

Tissue load management refers to therapeutic means to manage pressure, friction, and shear on tissues (Baranoski & Ayello, 2020). Interventions to prevent injury to the skin and promote optimal health are outlined in Guidelines for Nursing Care 33-2 on page 1178. Additional interventions related to personal hygiene and maintaining skin health are discussed

Promoting Health Literacy

IN PATIENTS WITH BREAST CANCER

Patient Scenario

Tashana Douglas, 42, has been diagnosed with breast cancer. She had a modified mastectomy 3 weeks ago and has returned to the clinic to discuss the rest of her treatment. She is going to have several weeks of outpatient radiation therapy. She states, "I feel pretty good, and the surgeon said my cancer is gone. Why do I need more treatment? My neighbor told me her sister had radiation and had terrible side effects." Ms. Douglas appears anxious as she relates that the neighbor's sister was extremely tired and had a "terrible rash or burn with her treatment. It took a long time to get better and really hurt." She states, "I don't know if I want to risk having that happen to me!" Ms. Douglas verbalizes concern that she will "give the radiation to others in her home and make them sick." She asks, "Do you think I should have this radiation stuff?"

Nursing Considerations: *Tips for Improving Health Literacy*

Review with Ms. Douglas the appropriate interventions she should be using to ensure that her surgical site heals, including skin care. Provide Ms. Douglas with easy-to-read information about radiation therapy and potential side effects, as well as interventions she can implement to prevent and/or minimize the side effects of radiation therapy, particularly side effects related to skin integrity. Identify valid and reliable internet-based resources and discuss the importance of vetting the sites and information. Encourage her to ask her primary care provider, as well as the radiologist, as many questions as needed to understand her condition and the planned radiation treatment. Encourage Ms. Douglas to ask her primary care provider the following three questions:

- What is my main problem?
- What do I need to do?
- Why is it important for me to do this?

What additional measures can you take to help increase health literacy in this patient? What other measures would be helpful if Ms. Douglas does not speak English, cannot read, or has other learning deficits? How does her ability to *use* information, rather than just *understand* it, affect her autonomy, judgment, and decision making?

Guidelines for Nursing Care 33-2

PREVENTING PRESSURE INJURIES

- Assess the skin of patients at risk on a daily basis. Pay particular attention to bony prominences.
- Cleanse the skin routinely and whenever any soiling occurs. Use a mild cleansing agent, minimal friction, and avoid hot water.
- Maintain higher humidity in the environment and use skin moisturizers for dry skin.
- Avoid massage over bony prominences.
- Protect the skin from moisture associated with episodes of incontinence or exposure to wound drainage.
- Minimize skin injury from friction and shearing forces by using proper positioning, turning, and transferring techniques. Employ the use of appropriate equipment. Use lubricants, protective films, dressings, and padding to diminish the effects of friction on the skin.
- Use appropriate support surfaces (tissue load management surfaces).
- Investigate reasons for inadequate dietary intake of protein and calories. Administer nutritional supplements or more aggressive nutritional intervention as needed.
- Continue efforts to improve mobility and activity. If this is unrealistic, attempt to maintain current level of activity, mobility, and range of motion.
- Document measures used to prevent pressure injuries and the results of these interventions.

in Chapter 32. Implement interventions related to tissue load management as part of the nursing plan of care for patients at risk for developing pressure injuries or who have an existing pressure injury. This includes interventions that can be implemented while the patient is in bed and sitting in chairs or wheelchairs (see Skill 33-1, pages 1199–1201).

To protect patients at risk from the adverse effects of pressure, implement turning and positioning schedules, as well as the use of appropriate support surfaces (tissue load management surfaces). Follow facility protocols regarding repositioning, which may indicate turning bed-bound patients every two hours and repositioning chair-bound patients every hour. Teach patients to make subtle position changes frequently, including pressure-relieving maneuvers (such as lifts) as appropriate (EPUAP, NPIAP, & PPPIA, 2019b). Older adult patients tend to have less tissue tolerance, necessitating more frequent repositioning if redness on bony prominences is noted. The oblique position, an alternative to the side-lying position, results in significantly less pressure on the trochanter area. Do not position the head of the bed above 30 degrees unless medically contraindicated, and alternate right side, back, left side, and prone positions (when tolerated) using appropriate equipment to minimize friction and shearing (EPUAP, NPIAP, & PPPIA, 2019b). The best approach to turning and repositioning is to evaluate and reevaluate each patient to best determine an appropriate turning schedule (Baranoski & Ayello, 2020). See the accompanying Research in Nursing box on page 1174, which highlights the importance of the nurse's role in the prevention of pressure injuries.

Positioning devices such as pillows, foam wedges, or pressure-reducing boots can prove helpful to keep body weight off bony prominences. For example, unless contraindicated, a standard pillow placed under the length of the calves raises the heels off the bed and alleviates pressure. Never use ring cushions, or *donuts*, because they increase venous pressure. Minimize the effects of shearing force by limiting the amount of time the head of the bed is elevated, when possible.

Support surfaces are an important part of managing pressure, friction, and shear on tissues (Baranoski & Ayello, 2020). A support surface is a "specialized device for pressure redistribution designed for management of tissue loads, microclimate, and/or other therapeutic functions" (NPIAP, 2019, p. 5). Support surfaces are available in sizes and shapes to be used on beds, chairs, examination tables, and operating room tables. Support surfaces are pressure-reducing or pressure-relieving devices. The most common support surfaces are seating devices (air, fluid foam, or gel cushions); air-, gel-, or water-filled mattress overlays; static flotation mattresses; alternating air mattresses; low–air-loss beds; and air-fluidized beds. It is important to individualize the type of support surface based on the patient's needs. Some support surfaces allow for an extended length of time between position changes. Because none of these devices totally relieves pressure, continues to perform position changes at regular intervals.

The use of appropriate devices to ensure safe patient handling and movement is an important part of tissue load management. Use friction-reducing sheets and lifting devices with patients who cannot assist during transfers and position changes. These interventions and devices are discussed at length in Chapter 34.

Wound Care/Wound Management

The goal of wound care is to promote tissue repair and regeneration so that skin integrity is restored. Wounds can be treated by leaving them open to air; no **dressing** (protective covering placed over a wound) is applied. Wounds left open to air heal more slowly because wound drying produces a dried eschar or scab. If the scab is removed accidentally before healing is complete, reinjury occurs, and the new delicate cells are exposed. Wounds left open are exposed to more environmental factors and potential injury.

Closed wound care uses dressings to keep the wound moist, promoting healing. A moist environment is best for wound healing. When a dressing is placed over a wound, the wound fluid keeps the surface of the wound moist. As a result, epidermal cells migrate more rapidly, maximizing healing. In addition, covered wounds can help patients cope with alterations in body image.

In general, an ideal dressing should maintain a moist environment, be absorbent, provide thermal insulation, act as a bacterial barrier, reduce or eliminate pain at the wound site, and allow for pain-free removal (Baranoski & Ayello, 2020; Hess, 2019). Choosing a dressing or device for wound management needs to take into consideration wound- and skin-related factors, patient-related factors, and dressing-related factors (Hess, 2019). Many different types of dressings are available, but all have essentially the same purposes:

- Provide physical, psychological, and aesthetic comfort
- Prevent, eliminate, or control infection
- Absorb drainage (exudate)
- Maintain moisture balance of the wound
- Protect the wound from further injury
- Protect the skin surrounding the wound
- Debride (remove damaged/necrotic tissue), if appropriate
- Stimulate and/or optimize the healing response
- Consider ease of use and cost effectiveness

There is no standard frequency for how often dressings should be changed. It depends on the amount of drainage, the primary provider's preference, the nature of the wound, and the particular wound care product being used. It is customary for the surgeon or other advanced practice provider to perform the first dressing change on a surgical wound, usually within 24 to 48 hours after surgery.

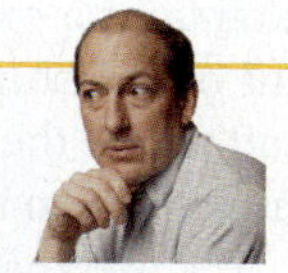

Consider the care needed by **Lucius Everly**, the patient in the critical care unit. Although he has multiple needs, performing incisional wound care cannot be overlooked; otherwise, his risk of infection may increase.

Wound contamination occurs through a moist medium. Microorganisms can move from the external surface through the dressing to the wound if a dressing remains in place until it is saturated. Microorganisms can also move from the wound to the outer surface of a saturated dressing. For these reasons, always replace dressings with fresh dressings or reinforce the dressing with additional dressings before drainage causes saturation.

Dressing changes provide an excellent opportunity for teaching, which is especially important when the patient will be changing dressings at home. Encourage the patient to help as much as possible, if appropriate.

The sight of the wound may disturb a patient. Listen carefully to what the patient is saying and observe nonverbal communication as well. In some instances, the patient may not want to look at the wound, particularly with a wound that involves a change in normal body functions or appearance, such as a wound resulting from the removal of a breast, the amputation of an extremity, or the placement of a tube in a draining wound. With patience and emotional support, patients can learn to cope with and adapt to their wound.

TYPES OF WOUND DRESSINGS

The items needed for a dressing change may be gathered individually or may be packaged in a sterile dressing tray, depending on the health care setting. Wound care in the home may depend on the supplies provided by the patient or family.

The number and type of dressings used depend on the location and size of the wound, type and depth of wound, the presence of infection, the need for **debridement** (removal of devitalized tissue and foreign material), and the amount and type of drainage. There are many dressing types and manufacturers (Hess, 2019)—the nurse needs to collaborate with the health care provider to ensure the correct dressing type is chosen, ongoing assessment occurs, and updates to the treatment plan (dressing choice) are made as the wound evolves.

There are three basic types of primary dressings: those that maintain moisture, those that absorb moisture, and those that add moisture (Baranoski & Ayello, 2020). Dry gauze dressings can be used to cover wounds, commonly closed surgical wounds. These dressings come in various sizes (2×2 inch, 4×4 inch, 4×8 inch) and are commercially packaged as single units or in packs. Gauze dressings often consist of three layers. The first layer of dressing material applied directly to a draining wound is often nonabsorbent but hydrophilic (i.e., capable of carrying moisture). This type of material allows drainage from the wound to move into overlying absorbent layers of dressing, helping to prevent maceration and reinfection. Moreover, this type of dressing is less likely to stick to the wound, making dressing changes more comfortable for the patient.

Material to absorb and collect drainage is then placed over the first layer of nonabsorbent material. This material acts as a wick, pulling drainage out by capillary action. Absorbent cotton has far greater capillarity than untreated cotton. Therefore, cotton-lined gauze sponges soak up more liquid than do unlined sponges. The number of gauze sponges used in the dressing depends on the amount of drainage. The wound may also be packed with gauze or another material. Loosely packed gauze, the threads of which act as numerous wicks, enhances capillarity, and directs drainage upward and away from the wound. Fluffed and loosely packed dressings are more absorbent than tightly packed dressings. The top of the dressing may be further protected by surgical or abdominal pads (ABDs), which are thick, absorbent pads that help to absorb profuse drainage (Fig. 33-9).

Nonadherent gauzes include sterile petrolatum gauze and Telfa gauze. Telfa's shiny outer surface is applied to the

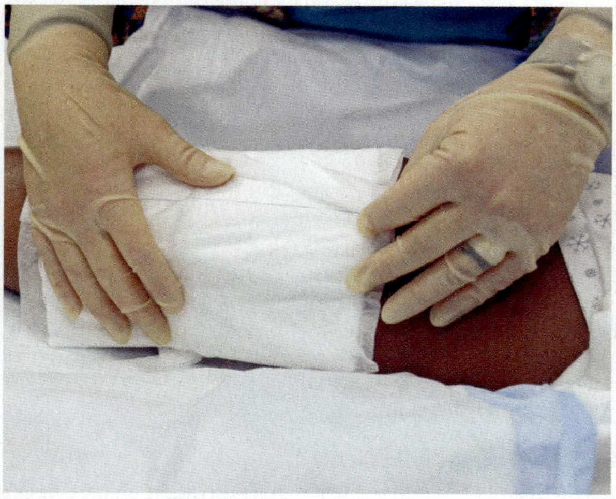

FIGURE 33-9. Surgical pad applied as last layer of wound dressing.

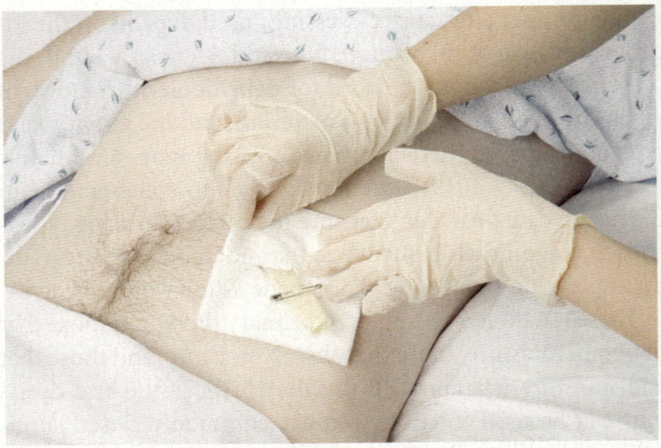

FIGURE 33-10. Precut dressing placed around surgical drain.

wound. These dressings allow drainage to pass through and be absorbed by the outer absorbent layer but prevent outer dressings from adhering to the wound and causing further injury when removed. These dressings are often used on incisions closed with sutures or staples.

Special gauze dressings (e.g., Sof-Wick) are precut halfway to fit around drains or tubes (Fig. 33-10). Larger dressings (8 × 10 bandages, abdominal pads [ABDs], Surgi-Pads) are placed over the smaller gauze dressings and absorb drainage and protect the wound from contamination or injury.

Transparent films (e.g., OPSITE) are semipermeable membrane dressings that are adhesive and waterproof. These dressings are occlusive, decreasing the possibility of contamination, while allowing visualization of the wound. This type of dressing is often used over peripheral intravenous sites, central venous access device insertion sites, and noninfected healing wounds (Fig. 33-11).

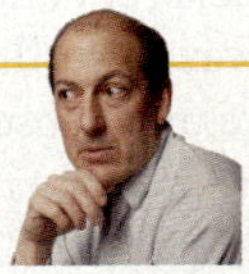

Think back to **Lucius Everly**, the patient in the critical care unit. The nurse most likely would use a transparent dressing on his venous access sites, thereby allowing frequent assessment of the sites.

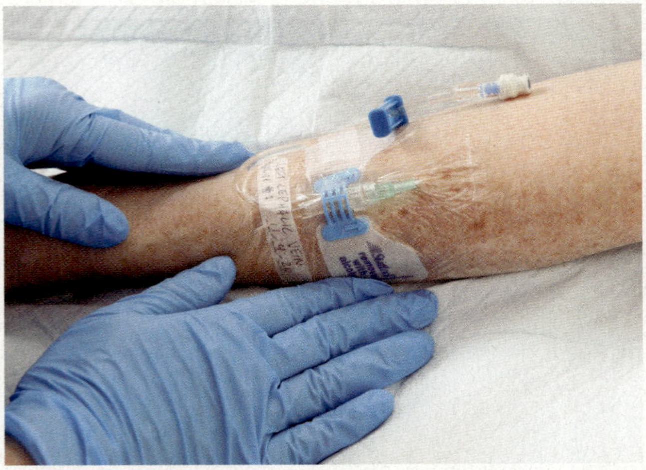

FIGURE 33-11. Transparent film dressing placed on intravenous access site.

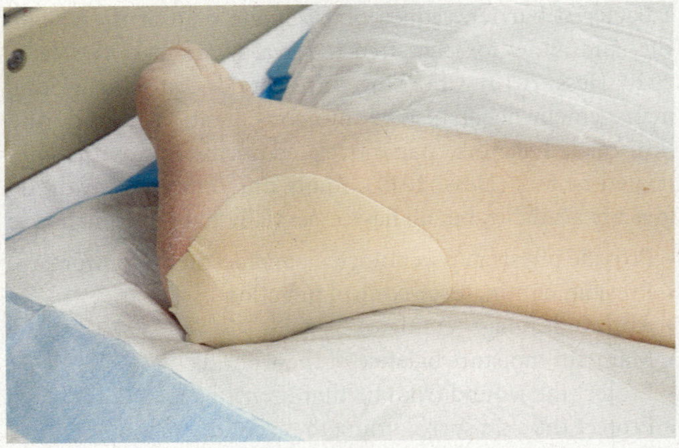

FIGURE 33-12. Hydrocolloid dressing in place on wound.

When caring for open wounds and pressure injuries, it is necessary to keep the wound tissue moist and the surrounding skin dry. Therefore, use dressings that continuously keep the wound moist, placing the moist dressing only on the wound surface and keeping the intact, healthy skin surrounding the ulcer dry because it is susceptible to damage. Select a dressing that absorbs exudate, if present, but still maintains a moist environment for healing. Use a skin sealant or moisture-barrier ointment on the surrounding skin and secure the dressing with the least amount of tape or other material to secure that is necessary.

The presence of foreign matter and/or devitalized, injured, infected tissue in a wound may indicate the need for debridement to promote wound healing (Baranoski & Ayello, 2020). Debridement can be accomplished through several different methods. Autolytic debridement uses occlusive dressings, such as hydrocolloids (Fig. 33-12) or transparent films, and uses the body's own enzymes and defense mechanisms to loosen and liquefy necrotic tissue. Enzymatic debridement involves the application of commercially prepared enzymes to speed up the body's autolytic process. Mechanical debridement uses external physical force to dislodge and remove debris and necrotic tissue. This could be achieved by wound irrigation with pulsed pressure lavage (washing), whirlpool therapy, ultrasound or laser treatment, or with surgical debridement. In the past, wet-to-dry gauze dressings have been used to debride wounds, but this is no longer considered good practice. This type of dressing damages healthy wound bed tissue and can be painful (Baranoski & Ayello, 2020). Concern exists that complete drying of the gauze disrupts angiogenesis. However, despite concerns by wound care experts, these dressings are still prescribed by health care providers for wound debridement. When possible, use a product designed to promote moisture balance; do not use dry gauze in an open wound.

There are many other wound care products/dressings available, each with distinctive actions, as well as indications, contraindications, advantages, and disadvantages. It is very important for the nurse to be aware of the products available in a particular facility and be familiar with the indications for, and correct use of, each type of dressing and wound care product. A wound with heavy exudate will need a more absorptive dressing, and a dry wound will require rehydration with a dressing that keeps the wound moist. Table 33-5 (on pages 1182–1183) outlines the purposes and uses for several wound dressing/product categories. Advances in wound care now include *smart* dressings, which have embedded sensors, microprocessors, and communication devices (O'Callaghan et al., 2020)—watch for continued advances in commercially available wound dressings.

Technology Alert

Smart dressings are changing the way we care for wounds by providing information through sensors, microprocessors, and communication devices.

CHANGING THE DRESSING

Prepare the patient for the dressing change before starting the procedure by explaining what will be done. If wound care is uncomfortable, administer a prescribed analgesic 30 to 45 minutes before changing the dressing. Also, plan to change the dressing midway between meals so that the patient's appetite and mealtimes are not disturbed.

Provide privacy by properly screening the patient; close the room door and curtain. Help the patient into a position that is comfortable but convenient for changing the dressing. Expose only the area necessary to perform the wound care while maintaining proper draping.

Using appropriate aseptic techniques when changing the dressing is crucial. The Aseptic Non Touch Technique (ANTT®, 2019) provides an international set of principles and specific framework designed to standardize safe aseptic practice and decrease the risk of infection. One component of the ANTT® framework addresses the essential nontouch technique. In the nontouch technique, the practitioner touches a site or equipment only as absolutely necessary, even when wearing sterile gloves. For example, when placing a dressing, the nurse will not touch the side of the dressing that will be in direct contact with the wound. Integrating core principles, such as the nontouch technique, into both routine nursing practice and agency guidelines, policies, and protocols is essential (ANTT®, 2019; Sonoiki et al., 2020). Be especially vigilant in performing hand hygiene thoroughly before and after changing dressings. Remember and adhere to standard precautions and transmission-based precautions, when necessary. Among the most common causes of hospital-acquired infections is carelessness in practicing asepsis during dressing changes. Surgical wounds that have dehisced require the use of sterile technique. Pressure injuries are nonsterile wounds, so there is no need to use sterile dressings on these wounds (Baranoski & Ayello, 2020; EPUAP, NPIAP, & PPPIA, 2019b). Nonsterile gloves can be used to perform clean wound care.

Concept Mastery Alert

A helpful way to remember which technique to use for wound care is this: Surgery occurs under sterile conditions, so open surgical wounds = sterile technique; pressure injuries = clean technique.

Removing a Dressing

Remove any dressing currently in place:

- Use standard precautions; use appropriate transmission-based precautions when indicated.
- Perform hand hygiene and put on clean (nonsterile) gloves.
- Remove tape and dressings in the direction of hair growth to minimize trauma to the skin. Using two hands and a low angle parallel to the skin, remove adhesives slowly while supporting the skin where it is attached to the tape/adhesive (Yates et al., 2017). Use a push–pull method; lift a corner of the dressing away from the skin, then gently push the skin away from the dressing/adhesive. Continue moving fingers of the opposite hand to support the skin as the product is removed (McNichol et al., 2013).
- Carefully lift the adhesive barrier from the surrounding skin to prevent medical adhesive–related skin injury (MARSI). Remove the sides/edges first, then the center. If there is resistance, use an adhesive remover (per manufacturer recommendations) for easy, rapid, and painless removal without the associated problems of skin stripping (McNichol et al., 2013; Yates et al., 2017).
- Slowly remove the dressing, noting the amount, type, color, and odor of the drainage.
- Discard the dressing according to facility policy.
- Remove gloves and perform hand hygiene.

Cleaning the Wound

Perform wound cleaning to remove microorganisms and debris with as little chemical and mechanical force as possible and protect healthy granulation tissue. Normal saline solution (0.9% sodium chloride) or cleansing solutions with antimicrobials are recommended, particularly when cleaning pressure injury wounds. There are also commercially prepared cleansing sprays, typically antiseptics or surfactants, available for use in wounds with debris, confirmed infection, or high levels of bacterial colonization (Baranoski & Ayello, 2020; EPUAP, NPIAP, & PPPIA, 2019b).

Wounds are cleaned initially and before applying any new dressing. Guidelines for Nursing Care 33-3 on page 1184 outlines the techniques for cleaning a wound with approximated edges, such as a surgical incision, and for cleaning a wound with edges that are not approximated to remove cellular debris and drainage. Wound irrigation is a directed flow of solution over tissues. Sterile equipment and solutions are required for irrigating an open wound, even in the presence of an existing infection. Sterile 0.9% sodium chloride or sterile water, a commercially prepared wound cleanser, an antiseptic, or an antibiotic solution may be used, depending on the condition of the wound and the primary health care provider's prescription. A sterile, large-volume syringe is used to direct the flow of the solution. After irrigation, open wounds may be packed and dressed with appropriate materials to absorb additional drainage and allow healing by secondary intention to take place (see Table 33-5 on pages 1182–1183). Nonsterile solutions are generally used to clean the skin surface if the wound edges are approximated.

(text continues on page 1184)

Table 33-5 Examples of Wound Dressings/Products

TYPE	PURPOSES	USE
Transparent films, such as: 3M™ Tegaderm™ BIOCLUSIVE™ Plus Transparent Film Dressing DermaView OPSITE™	• Allow exchange of oxygen between wound and environment • Are self-adhesive • Protect against contamination; waterproof • Prevent loss of wound fluid • Maintain a moist wound environment • Facilitate autolytic debridement • No absorption of drainage • Allow visualization of wound	• Wounds that are small; partial thickness • May remain in place for 4–7 days, resulting in less interference with healing • Stage 1 pressure injuries • Wounds with minimal drainage • Cover dressings for gels, foams, and gauze • Secure intravenous catheters, nasal cannulas, chest tube dressing, central venous access devices
Hydrocolloid dressings, such as: Comfeel® Plus Sacral Dressing DermaFilm Thin DuoDERM® CGF Dressing Hydrocolloid Dressing 3M™ Restore™ Hydrocolloid Dressing	• Are occlusive or semiocclusive, limiting exchange of oxygen between wound and environment • Inner layer is self-adherent, gel forming, and composed of colloid particles • Outer layer seals and protects the wound from contamination • Minimal to moderate absorption of drainage • Maintain a moist wound environment • Thermal insulation • Provide cushioning • Facilitate autolytic debridement • May remain in place for 3–7 days, depending on exudate	• Partial- and full-thickness wounds • Stage 2 and stage 3 pressure injuries • Prevention at high-risk friction areas • Wounds with light to moderate drainage • Wounds with necrosis or slough • First- and second-degree burns • Not for use with wounds that are infected
Hydrogels, such as: AquaDerm DermaGauze Elasto-Gel™ Island Hydrogel INTRASITE Gel Hydrogel Wound Dressing	• Polymer gels comprised of an 80–99% water base • Available in many sizes and forms (gels, sheets, gauze, strips) • Maintain a moist wound environment • Minimal absorption of drainage • Facilitate autolytic debridement • Thermal insulation • Do not adhere to wound • Less effective barrier than occlusive dressings • Reduce pain • Most require a secondary dressing to secure • May remain in place for 24–72 hours, depending on the gel form	• Partial- and full-thickness wounds • Stages 2–4 pressure injuries • Necrotic wounds • First- and second-degree burns • Dry wounds • Wounds with minimal exudate • Infected wounds • Radiation tissue damage
Alginates, such as: AQUACEL® EXTRA Wound Dressing Eclypse® Super Absorbent Dressing KALTOSTAT® Wound Dressing Melgisorb® Plus Alginate Dressing	• Contain alginic acid from brown seaweed; covered in calcium–sodium salts • Absorb exudate • Maintain a moist wound environment • Facilitate autolytic debridement • Require secondary dressing to secure	• Partial- and full-thickness wounds • May remain in place for 1–3 days • Stage 3 and stage 4 pressure injuries • Infected and noninfected wounds • Wounds with moderate to heavy exudate • Tunneling wounds; undermining • Moist red and yellow wounds • Not for use with wounds with minimal drainage or dry eschar
Foams, such as: 3M™ Tegaderm™ Foam Adhesive Dressing Advazorb® Heel Hydrophilic Foam Dressings Mepilex® Absorbent Foam Dressing Optifoam Gentle POLYDERM Plus Barrier Foam Dressing PolyMem® Dressing	• Foam covered by hydrophilic polyurethane or gel • Maintain a moist wound environment • Do not adhere to wound • Insulate wound • Highly absorbent • May require a secondary dressing to secure	• Partial- and full-thickness wounds • May remain in place 3–5 days (7 days for foams with silver), depending on exudate • Stages 2–4 pressure injuries • Surgical wounds • Absorb light to heavy amounts of drainage • Use around tubes and drains • Not for use with wounds with dry eschar

Table 33-5 Examples of Wound Dressings/Products *(continued)*

TYPE	PURPOSES	USE
Antimicrobials, such as: AQUACEL™ Ag Surgical Wound Dressing Mepilex® Ag Antimicrobial Foam Dressing Optifoam Ag+ Post-Op PolyMem® Silver™ Dressing	• Antimicrobial or antibacterial action (reduce and/or prevent infection) • Do not adhere to wound • Can be highly absorbent • May require a secondary dressing to secure • Antimicrobial action may last 7 days	• Partial- and full-thickness wounds • Stages 2–4 pressure injuries • Burns • Primary dressing over skin graft(s) and donor sites • Draining, exuding, and nonhealing wounds of any kind (pressure injury, venous/arterial, diabetic, surgical) • Acute and chronic wounds
Collagens, such as: DermaCOL PROMOGRAN™ Matrix Wound Dressing Stimulen™	• Protein (collagen derived from bovine, porcine, or avian sources) stimulates cellular migration and fosters new tissue development • Highly absorbent • Maintain a moist wound environment • Do not adhere to wound • Compatible with topical agents • Conform well to the wound surface • Require secondary dressing to secure • May remain in place 3–5 days (7 days for foams with silver), depending on exudate	• Partial- or full-thickness wounds • Stage 3 pressure injuries • Infected and noninfected wounds • Primary dressing over skin graft(s) and donor sites • Tunneling wounds • Moist red and yellow wounds
Contact layers, such as: ADAPTIC TOUCH™ Non-Adhering Silicone Dressing Profore WCL Silflex® Silicone Contact Layer	• Placed in contact with base of wound, protecting base from trauma during dressing change • Allow exudate to pass to a secondary dressing • Not intended to be changed with every dressing change • May be used with topical medication, wound filler, or gauze dressings	• Partial- and full-thickness wounds • Require secondary dressing to secure • Shallow, dehydrated wounds • Wounds with eschar • Wounds with viscous exudate
Composites, such as: 3M™ Tegaderm™ Absorbant Clear Acrylic Dressing Covaderm Plus Stratasorb	• Combine two or more physically distinct products in a single dressing with several functions • Allow exchange of oxygen between wound and environment • May facilitate autolytic debridement • Provide physical bacterial barrier and absorptive layer • Semiadherent or nonadherent	• Partial- and full-thickness wounds • Primary or secondary dressing • Stages 1–4 pressure injures • Wounds with minimal to heavy exudate • Necrotic tissue • Mixed (granulation and necrotic tissue) wounds • Infected wounds
Cellular and tissue-based products (CPTs) AlloSkin™ Grafix CORE®	• Nonviable or viable human or animal cells, tissue-based from humans and animals	• Partial- and full-thickness wounds • Venous and diabetic ulcers • Burns • Chronic wounds
Negative pressure wound therapy (NPWT), such as: Avelle™ Negative Pressure Wound Therapy System V.A.C.® Therapy	• Noninvasive device that applies pressure to the wound bed through a unit attached to a dressing/sponge (various foam densities) • Highly absorbent • Decreases bacterial colonization • Stimulates increased blood supply and granulation	• Partial- and full-thickness wounds • May remain in place 2–3 days, depending on manufacturer recommendations • Stage 3 and stage 4 pressure injuries • Draining, exuding, and nonhealing wounds of any kind (pressure injury, venous/arterial, diabetic, surgical, dehisced)

Source: Adapted from Baranoski, S., & Ayello, E. A. (2020). *Wound care essentials: Practice principles* (5th ed.). Wolters Kluwer; Hess, C. (2019). *Product guide to skin & wound care* (8th ed.). Wolters Kluwer; Hurd, T., Rossington, A., Trueman, P., & Smith, J. (2017). A retrospective comparison of the performance of two negative pressure wound therapy systems in the management of wounds of mixed etiology. *Advances in Wound Care*, *6*(1), 33–37. https://doi.org/10.1089/wound.2015.0679; and Norman, G., Goh, E. L., Dumville, J. C., Shi, C., Liu, Z., Chiverton, L., Stankiewicz, M., & Reid, A. (2020). Negative pressure wound therapy for surgical wounds healing by primary closure. *The Cochrane Database of Systematic Reviews*, *6*(6), CD009261. https://doi.org/10.1002/14651858.CD009261.pub6

Guidelines for Nursing Care 33-3

CLEANING WOUNDS

Cleaning Wounds With Approximated Edges

- Use standard precautions; use appropriate transmission-based precautions when indicated.
- Moisten a sterile gauze pad or swab with the prescribed cleansing agent.
- Use a new swab or gauze for each downward stroke.
- Clean from top to bottom.
- Work outward from the incision in lines parallel to it (Figure A).
- Wipe from the clean area toward the less clean area.

Cleaning Wounds With Edges That Are Not Approximated

- Use standard precautions; use appropriate transmission-based precautions when indicated.
- Moisten a sterile gauze pad or swab with the prescribed cleansing agent and squeeze out excess solution.
- Use a new swab or gauze for each circle.
- Clean the wound in full or half circles, beginning in the center and working toward the outside (Figure B).
- Clean to at least 1 inch beyond the end of the new dressing.
- If a dressing is not being applied, clean to at least 2 inches beyond the wound margins.

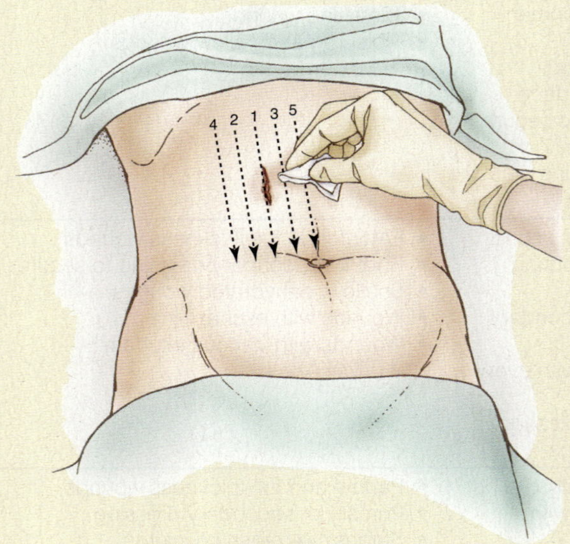

FIGURE A

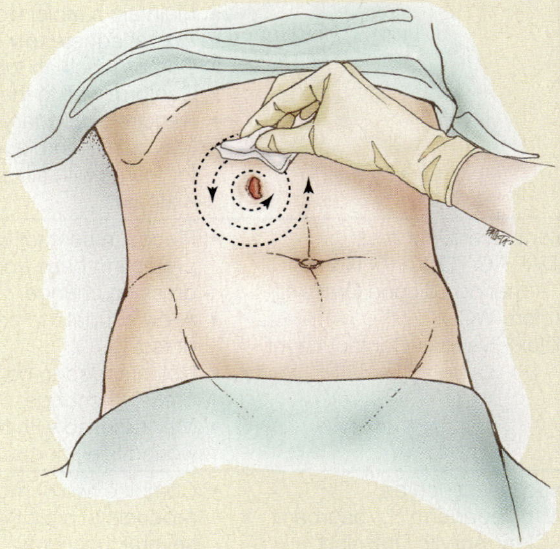
FIGURE B

Source: Hess, C. (2013). *Clinical guide to skin & wound care* (7th ed.). Wolters Kluwer.

Applying a New Dressing

Ensure that the area is clean and dry. Apply a skin protectant or barrier to the healthy skin around the wound. This is particularly important if there is drainage from the wound. The skin protectant prevents skin irritation and excoriation from tape, adhesives, and wound drainage (McNichol et al., 2013).

The nurse should be familiar with and follow the manufacturer's guidelines for the specific dressing in use (Hess, 2019). General guidelines for applying a new dressing include:

- Check the wound care order or nursing care plan.

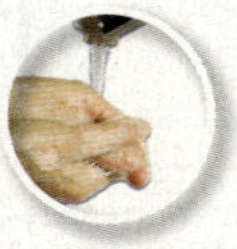

- Perform hand hygiene.
- Use standard precautions; use appropriate transmission-based precautions when indicated.

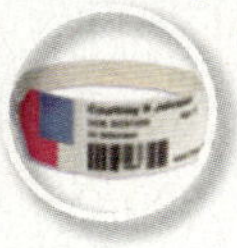

- Check the patient's identification.
- Explain what you are going to do to the patient.
- Provide privacy by closing the door to the room and pulling the bedside curtain.
- Put on gloves.
- Cleanse the wound, and periwound skin, as prescribed.
- Apply a skin barrier, such as Skin Prep, to the areas of skin where the dressing adhesive or tape will be placed and to areas around the wound where drainage may come in contact with skin.
- Apply any topical medications, foams, gels, and/or gauze to the wound as prescribed; ensure products stay confined to the wound and do not impact on intact surrounding tissue/skin.
- Gently place the dressing at the wound center and extend it at least 1 in beyond the wound in each direction. Alternatively, follow the manufacturer's directions for application.
- Remove gloves when the dressing is in place, before handling tape, if used.
- Do not apply tape under tension to prevent blisters and skin shearing.
- Perform hand hygiene.

Table 33-6 Popular Types of Tape

TYPE	PURPOSE
Micropore Paper Tape (hypoallergenic)	Paper tape Gentle, yet secure adhesion Good for sensitive skin Sticks to skin, other tape, and dressings Breathable and easy to tear
Transpore Polyethylene Tape (hypoallergenic)	Transparent plastic tape Adheres even when wet Often used to secure tubes and drains Breathable and perforated for easy tearing
Durable Cloth Tape	Silk-like cloth tape Flexible and comfortable Adheres well to skin Conforms to bony prominences Breathable and tears in any direction
Coban or Other Self Adherent Wrap	Sticks to itself—no adhesive, pins, or clips Breathable and lightweight Can be used for compression

Skill 33-2 on pages 1203–1208 describes cleaning a wound and applying a saline-moistened dressing. Skill 33-3 on pages 1208–1212 presents the technique for irrigating a wound.

Securing Wound Dressings

Many dressings are self-adhesive; therefore, no further material is needed to secure the dressing in place over the wound. However, other wound dressings require additional materials to hold the dressings in place, including tape, bandages and binders, and Montgomery straps.

Tape can be used to secure dressings in place. Tape comes in a wide variety of sizes and types, ranging in width from 1 to 4 inches (1-inch-wide tape is the most commonly used). Take care to protect the skin surrounding the wound from injury-related irritation or shearing or tearing of the skin during tape removal. Table 33-6 summarizes the types and purposes of different tapes.

Bandages and *binders* are used to secure dressings, apply pressure, and support the wound. **Bandages** are strips of cloth, gauze (e.g., roller gauze, Kerlix, Kling), or elasticized material (e.g., ACE bandages) used to wrap a body part. They come packaged in rolls and vary in width from 1 to 6 inches. Binders are designed for a specific body part and include slings, abdominal binders, chest binders, and T-binders. They may be made of cloth (flannel, muslin) or of an elasticized material that fastens together with Velcro. Guidelines for Nursing Care 33-4 highlights important principles for applying bandages and binders.

A *roller bandage* is a continuous strip of material wound on itself to form a cylinder or roll. Plain gauze, elastic webbing, and stretchable roller bandages are made in various widths and lengths. Begin applying the bandage to the distal part of the area. The free end is held in place with one hand while the other hand passes the roll around the body part. After the bandage is anchored, the roll is passed or rolled around the body part, taking care to exert equal tension in all turns and rolling toward the heart, to avoid causing venous stasis and resulting edema. Apply the bandage using a circular turn, spiral turn, or figure-of-eight turn (Fig. 33-13 on page 1186). For each technique, keep tension equal by unwinding the bandage gradually and only with as much length as is required. Evenly overlap one half to two thirds the width of the bandage with each turn, except for the circular turn. A circular turn is used primarily to anchor a bandage. In a circular turn, wrap the bandage around the body part, completely overlapping the previous bandage turn. Once the circular turn anchors the bandage, application continues, ascending in a spiral manner using a spiral turn. Each turn overlaps the preceding one by one half or two thirds the width of the bandage. The spiral turn is useful for the wrist, fingers, and trunk. The figure-of-eight turn consists of making oblique overlapping turns that ascend and descend alternatively. It is effective for use around joints, such as the knee, elbow, ankle, and wrist. When removing a roller bandage, cut the bandage with bandage scissors to prevent excessive manipulation of the part. Cut on the side opposite the injury or the wound, from one end to the other, so that the bandage can be folded open for its entire length. If the bandage is to be reused, it may be unwound by keeping the loose ends together and passing it as a ball from one hand to the other while unwinding it.

When applying a *recurrent bandage,* make a few circular turns to anchor the bandage, and place the initial end of the bandage at the center of the body part being bandaged, well back from the tip to be covered. Pass the bandage back and

Guidelines for Nursing Care 33-4

APPLYING BANDAGES AND BINDERS

- Clean the area to be covered and dry it thoroughly before applying a bandage or binder, because prolonged heat and moisture on the skin may cause skin breakdown.
- Bandage the body part in the normal functioning position to prevent deformities and discomfort.
- Apply the bandage or binder with sufficient pressure to provide the amount of immobilization or support desired, to remain in place, and to secure a dressing when present. Do not apply pressure to such a degree that circulation to the involved body part is impeded.
- Maintain equal tension with all bandage turns; avoid unnecessary and uneven overlapping of turns.
- After application, assess circulation and comfort at regular intervals.

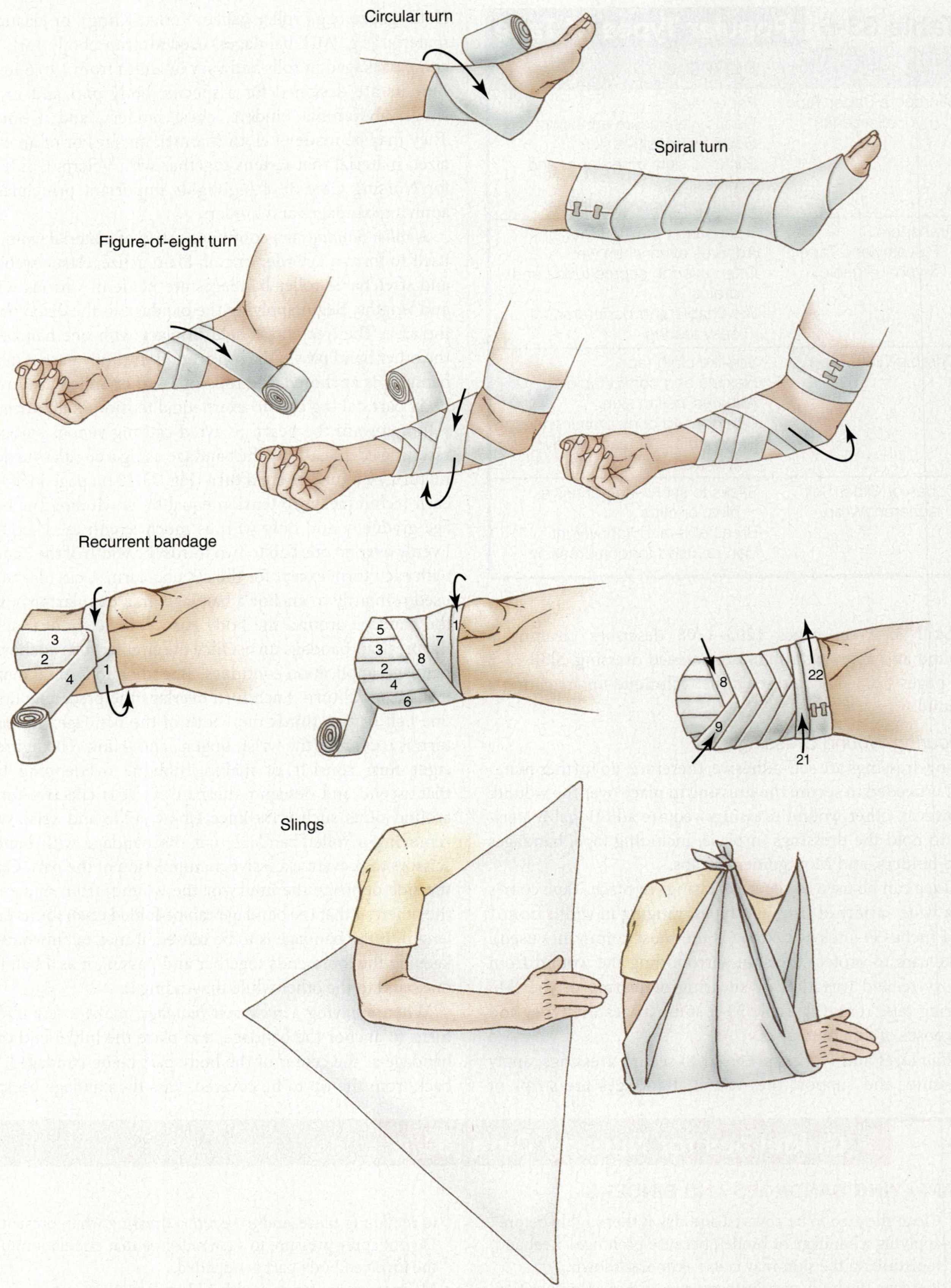

FIGURE 33-13. Techniques for applying various bandages.

forth over the tip, first on the one side and then on the other side of the centerpiece of the bandage. Figure 33-13 shows how to apply a recurrent bandage to a residual limb, using the figure-of-eight turn to finish the bandage. Recurrent bandages are used for fingers, for the head, and for a residual limb.

Of the many different kinds of *binders,* those used most commonly include straight binders, T-binders, and slings. A straight binder is a straight piece of material, usually about 15 to 20 cm (6 to 8 inches) wide and long enough to more than circle the torso. It is used for the chest and the abdomen. Straight binders may be pinned or, more commonly, fastened with Velcro.

A T-binder might be used to secure dressings on the rectum and perineum and in the groin. Although not used often in the hospital, these are sometimes used in the home care setting. The single T-binder is used for female patients, the double T-binder for male patients. Pass the belt around the waist and secure it, then pass the tails between the legs and fasten them to the belt.

A sling is used to support an arm. Most health care facilities use commercial strap slings or sleeve slings. In the home, a large piece of cloth folded into a triangle can be used as a sling (see Fig. 33-13).

Montgomery straps use ties attached to an adhesive backing to hold dressings in place. Newer devices and advances in skin care adhesives have led to a decreased use of Montgomery straps, but the concept is important to review. Protect the patient's skin with a skin barrier, such as Skin Prep, or a hydrocolloid dressing, prior to applying the Montgomery straps. Apply the adhesive backing to the skin adjacent to the wound, with the ties extending over the wound area. When the dressing is changed, untie the strips and turn them back to allow for wound care. After applying the new dressing, tie the straps over the dressing to hold it in place. Montgomery straps can be useful in preventing skin irritation and damage due to constant retaping with dressing changes. Change Montgomery straps only when they become moist or soiled.

Caring for Patients With Wound Drains

A variety of drains, catheters, or tubes may be inserted into or near a wound when it is anticipated that a collection of fluid in a closed area would delay healing. After a surgical procedure, the surgeon places one end of the tube or drain in or near the area to be drained and passes the other end through the skin, either directly through the incision or through a separate opening called a stab wound. Wound drains are either open systems that drain into dressings or closed systems that drain into a suction device. Drains and tubes may or may not be sutured in place.

OPEN DRAINAGE SYSTEMS

A Penrose drain is soft and flexible. This drain does not have a collection device. It empties into absorptive dressing material. It promotes drainage passively, with the drainage moving from the area of greater pressure, in the wound or surgical site, to the area of less pressure, the dressing. It is not sutured in place. A sterile, large safety pin or small tab is often attached to the outer portion to prevent the drain from slipping back into the incised area (Fig. 33-14). Care is necessary to ensure that these drains are not dislodged during dressing changes. Sometimes the health care provider orders a Penrose drain that is to be shortened each day. To do so, grasp the end of the drain with sterile forceps, pull it out a short distance while using a twisting motion, and cut off the end of the drain with sterile scissors. Place a new sterile pin or small tab at the base of the drain, as close to the skin as possible.

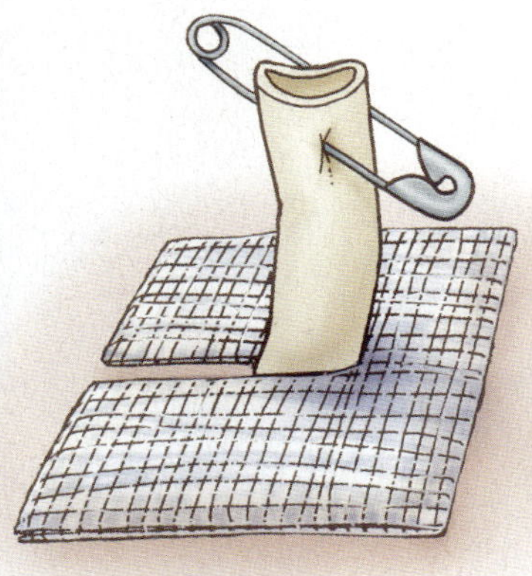

FIGURE 33-14. Penrose drain.

CLOSED DRAINAGE SYSTEMS

Closed drainage systems consist of a drainage tube that may be connected to an electrical suction device or have a portable built-in reservoir to maintain constant low suction. Examples include Jackson-Pratt drainage tubes (Fig. 33-15 on page 1188), Hemovacs (Fig. 33-16 on page 1188), and Blake drains, which have four drainage channels within the silicon tube. These tubes are usually sutured to the skin. The closed drainage system prevents microorganisms from entering the wound from saturated dressings. Closed drainage systems also allow accurate measurement of drainage. Be sure to know which type of drain or tube was inserted during surgery to ensure accurate assessments and interventions. These systems must be emptied, and the suction reestablished according to the directions for each device. This usually involves compressing the container while the port is open, then closing the port after the device is compressed. Skills 33-4 on pages 1212–1217 and 33-5 on pages 1217–1220 outline the procedures for caring for Jackson-Pratt and Hemovac drains. Wear gloves when emptying the drainage and do not touch the open port to avoid contaminating the port. If the device ever fully expands, meaning no suction is being applied, empty the device and reengage the suction. Although a surgical or percutaneous drain will likely always produce some output, drains are removed at different times, depending on the intention, location, and procedure. In general, drains are removed by the nurse or provider when the output color lightens (sanguineous, serosanguinous, then serous) or the amount of output decreases.

Collecting a Wound Culture

If assessment of the wound indicates a possible infection, it is important to culture the wound. Culturing the wound allows

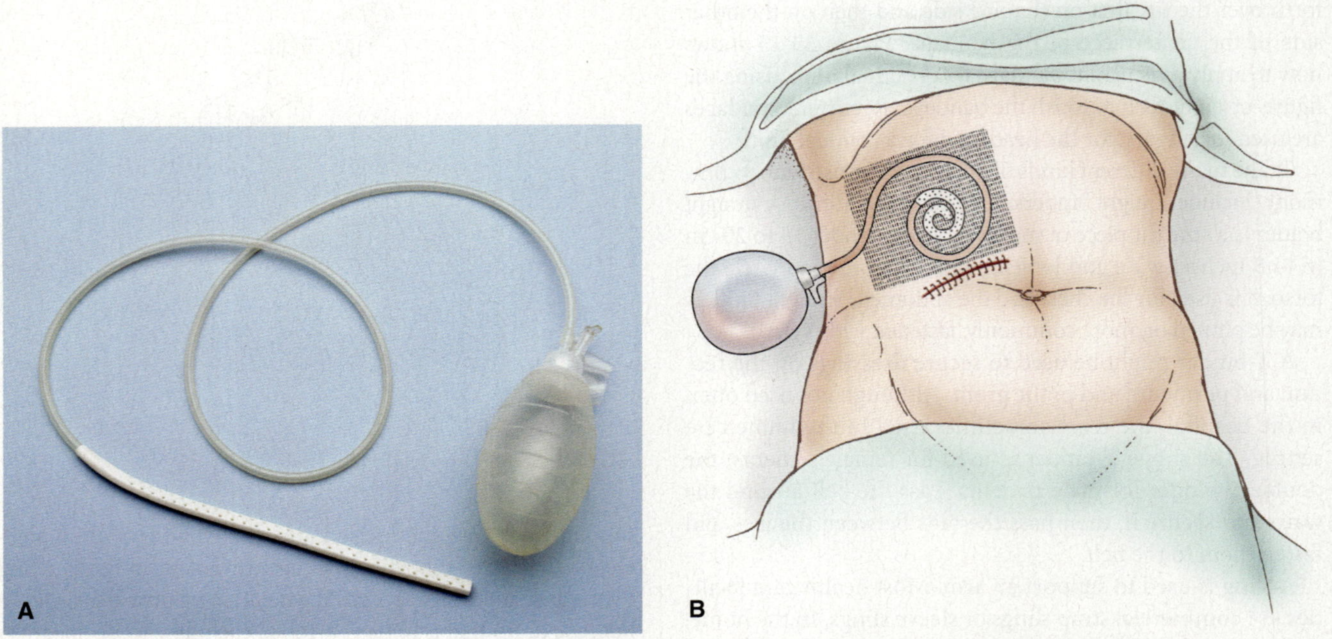

FIGURE 33-15. (A) Jackson-Pratt drain; (B) Jackson-Pratt drain inserted, with bulb compressed, which provides suction.

identification of the infecting organism(s) and appropriate interventions. Skill 33-6 on pages 1220–1224 reviews the process for obtaining a wound culture.

Using Additional Techniques to Promote Wound Healing

FIBRIN SEALANTS

Fibrin sealants are comprised of two substances found naturally in the human body: fibrinogen (a protein) and thrombin (an enzyme that acts on the fibrinogen to create a fibrin clot). Sealants are available in sponges, patches, and bandages; the glue is a liquid form that is applied using a gun or aerosol spray, which must be used per the manufacturer recommendations to prevent the introduction of an air or gas embolism (Edwards et al., 2016). The sealant is applied to tissues during an operative procedure to stop bleeding and glue together epidermal surfaces. This allows for wound closure with minimal drainage or scarring. The fibrin sealants have been shown to decrease the risk of hematoma (blood), decrease seroma (serous fluid) formation, and decrease the need for blood transfusion in some surgeries, but more research needs to be done on this topic (Daud et al., 2020; Edwards et al., 2016; Sircana et al., 2020). The glue is eventually metabolized and absorbed by the body. Dressings are not needed over these wounds because the skin is closed completely.

NEGATIVE PRESSURE WOUND THERAPY

Negative pressure wound therapy (NPWT) promotes wound healing and wound closure through the application of uniform negative pressure on the wound bed, reduction in bacteria in the wound, and the removal of excess wound fluid, while providing a moist wound healing environment. In clinical practice, this device is commonly referred to as a *wound V.A.C.* (vacuum-assisted closure) after one of the first devices approved by the U.S. Food and Drug Administration in 1995 (Hurd et al., 2017). The negative pressure results in mechanical tension on the wound tissues, stimulating cell proliferation, blood flow to wounds, and the growth of new blood vessels. There is some evidence that NPWT results in fewer surgical site infections for people experiencing primary wound closure, but until further evidence is published, the efficacy of NPWT with this type of

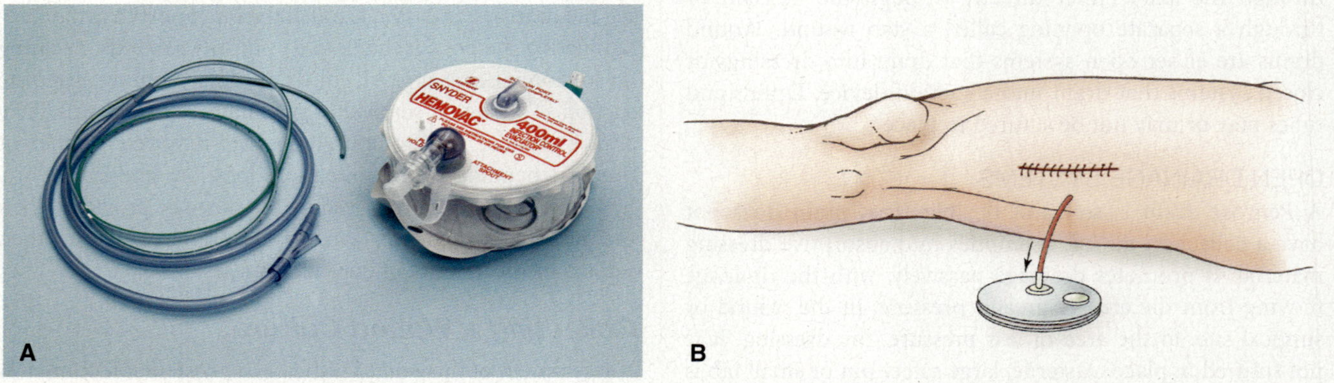

FIGURE 33-16. (A) Hemovac drain; (B) Hemovac drain inserted, with device compressed, which provides suction.

wound remains uncertain (Norman et al., 2020). The device typically requires a foam interface (in the wound) covered by a thin, transparent or hydrocolloid dressing that is connected to a plastic tube attached to a suction mechanism (Baranoski & Ayello, 2020). It is used to treat a variety of acute or chronic wounds, wounds with heavy drainage, wounds failing to heal, or wounds healing slowly. Examples of such wounds include stage 3 or stage 4 pressure injuries (EPUAP, NPIAP, & PPPIA, 2019b); arterial, venous, and diabetic ulcers; dehisced surgical wounds; infected wounds; skin graft sites; and full-thickness burns. NPWT is not considered for use in the presence of active bleeding; wounds with exposed blood vessels, organs, or nerves; malignancy in wound tissue; presence of dry/necrotic tissue; wounds with exposed vessels, nerves, tendons and ligaments; allergy to any component; or with fistulas of unknown origin (Baranoski & Ayello, 2020; Hurd et al., 2017). Assess candidates for preexisting bleeding disorders or the use of anticoagulants and other medications or supplements that prolong bleeding times (Baranoski & Ayello, 2020). Skill 33-7 on pages 1224–1229 outlines the procedure for applying NPWT.

GROWTH FACTORS

Growth factors are naturally occurring proteins. Recombinant platelet-derived growth factor (PDGF) is the only exogenous (introduced from outside the body) growth factor that has shown to be effective in wounds with delayed healing (EPUAP, NPIAP, & PPPIA, 2019b). PDGF activates the immune cells and fibroblasts and promotes the formation of the extracellular matrix (Baranoski & Ayello, 2020; Han & Ceilley, 2017).

HYPERBARIC OXYGEN THERAPY

Hyperbaric oxygen therapy (HBOT) is an advanced wound care technology used to facilitate repair of chronic wounds that occur secondary to diabetes, arterial or venous vascular issue, or pressure injury. These wounds are typically characterized by a lack of oxygen (hypoxia), impaired ability to generate new blood vessels (angiogenesis), and prolonged inflammation (Hajhosseini et al., 2020). HBOT involves placing patients in a hyperbaric, pressurized chamber, where they breathe 100% oxygen, which greatly increases the amount of oxygen dissolved in the plasma. The tissues are exposed to the high-concentration oxygen environment, which promotes cell proliferation and healing, increases wound metabolism, promotes an increased response to growth factors, stimulates angiogenesis, and has antibacterial and antioxidant effects that improve immune function (Baranoski & Ayello, 2020; Han & Ceilley, 2017). Based on a mix of evidence in the literature, the cost of this therapy, potential knowledge deficits related to inconsistent implementation, and a lack of high-quality studies (Hajhosseini et al., 2020), the use of HBOT as an adjunctive therapy is considered on a case-by-case basis.

HEAT AND COLD THERAPY

The application of heat or cold is sometimes used as part of the treatment of wounds. The application of heat accelerates the inflammatory response to promote healing. The local application of cold constricts peripheral blood vessels, reduces muscle spasms, and promotes comfort. The use of these therapies is discussed later in the chapter.

OTHER TREATMENT OPTIONS

When other treatment options have failed, surgery may be considered. Surgical procedures may include debridement, direct closure of the wound, skin grafting, various skin flap procedures, or limb amputation. The decision is based on the patient's condition and the severity of the wound or pressure injury. After surgery, vigilantly protect the surgical site from pressure and contamination.

Several other treatment modalities are being investigated. They include electrical stimulation, light therapy, ultrasonic energy, pulsed lavage, and miscellaneous topical agents (such as topical oxygen therapy) and systemic drugs (Baranoski & Ayello, 2020; EPUAP, NPIAP, & PPPIA, 2019b).

Removing Sutures or Staples

Sutures are removed when the wound has developed enough tensile strength to hold the wound edges together during healing. This stage varies from patient to patient, depending on age, nutritional status, and wound location. Silk sutures typically are removed within 6 to 8 days to prevent suture marks, even though collagen formation and remodeling take a total of at least 21 days. This means the scar may still stretch and widen after the silk sutures have been removed. Special subcutaneous techniques have been developed to minimize this problem.

Sutures are removed with a suture removal set; staples are removed with a special staple remover. The steps in removing sutures and staples are summarized in the accompanying Guidelines for Nursing Care 33-5 on page 1190. After the removal of skin sutures, small adhesive wound-closure strips that look something like tape are sometimes applied across the healing wound to help hold it together and give additional support as it continues to heal (Fig. 33-17). Unless otherwise directed, these adhesive strips are not removed during wound care.

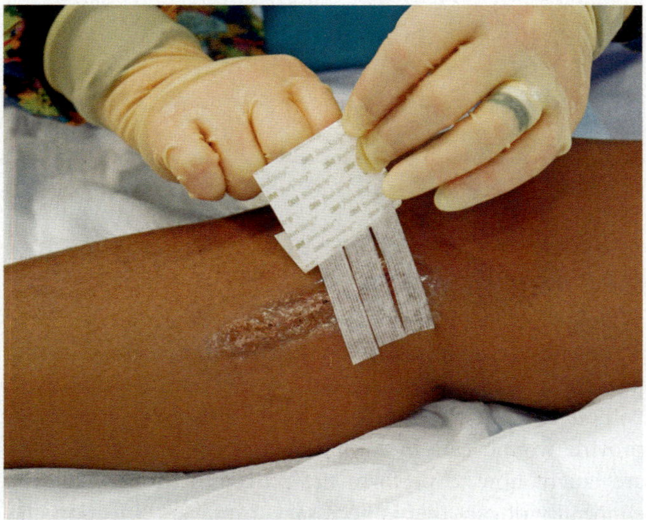

FIGURE 33-17. Applying Steri-Strips on an incision.

Guidelines for Nursing Care 33-5

REMOVING STAPLES AND SUTURES

The removal of staples or sutures may be done by the physician, an advanced practice professional, or by the nurse with a prescription/order. Always follow facility protocol; keep in mind these general guidelines:

- Use sterile technique, following recommended CDC guidelines for care of wounds.

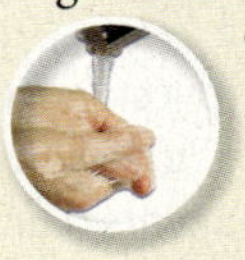

- Perform hand hygiene before and after the procedure.
- Explain the procedure to the patient. Describe the sensation that will be experienced as a pulling or pinching.
- Use proper technique to remove and dispose of old dressings.
- Clean the incision from the center of the wound outward, per facility policy and procedure for type of agent.
- Remove every other suture or staple to be sure wound edges are healed; if they are, remove remaining sutures or staples as ordered.
- Remove or reapply dressing, depending on health care provider preference and facility policy.
- Butterfly closure (Steri-Strip) application may be ordered for the healed wound after removal of staples or sutures to give additional support to the wound as it continues to heal. Follow facility protocol and primary care provider preference for placement of these tapes.

Specifics for Suture Removal

1. Use a sterile suture removal kit.
2. Using the sterile forceps, grasp the knot of the first suture and gently lift the knot.
3. Using the sterile scissors, cut one side of the suture below the knot close to the skin (Figure A).
4. Grasp the knot with the forceps and pull the cut suture through the skin (be sure to pull through the healed wound only the portion of the suture that has been inside the tissue).

Specifics for Staple Removal

1. As directed on the package, gently position the sterile staple remover under the staple to be removed.
2. Firmly close the staple remover to straighten the staple ends; do not lift upward while disengaging staple ends (Figure B).
3. Carefully lift upward with the closed staple remover to remove the staple from the incision line. It may be necessary to remove one end of the staple and then the other if it does not easily lift out.

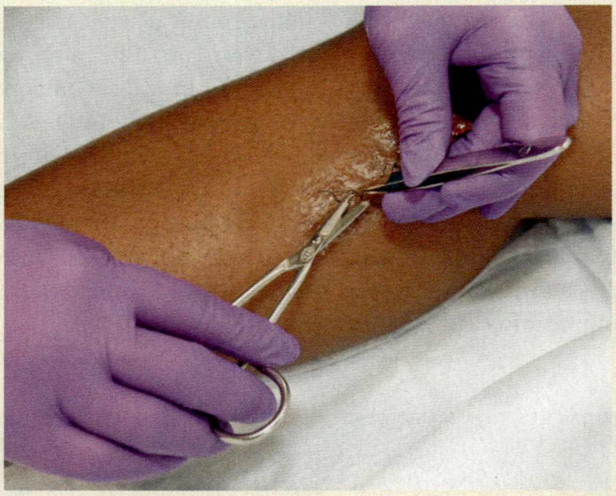

FIGURE A. Removing sutures.

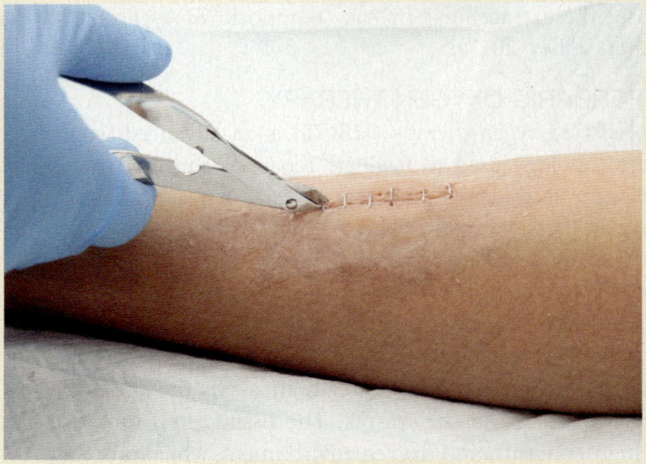

FIGURE B. Firmly closing the staple remover, bending the staple in the middle, and pulling the edges out of the skin.

Teaching Wound Care at Home

GENERAL GUIDELINES

With the increase in ambulatory surgery and earlier discharge of patients from inpatient settings to home care, teaching patients and their families about wound care is important. Although a nurse may be needed to change dressings and provide wound care in complex situations, caregivers often are taught how to perform the procedure. To provide the continuity of care that is necessary to prevent infection and promote healing, be sure to include teaching about wound care as part of discharge planning and in interactions with home care patients and caregivers. A summary of teaching content is outlined in Teaching Tips 33-1: Wound Care and Healing.

PRESSURE INJURY PREVENTION AND CARE

Teaching patients and caregivers how to prevent pressure injury requires a comprehensive, organized educational effort. Initially, the health care provider presents basic information that explains the terminology, identifies risk factors, explains where and how pressure injuries develop,

Teaching Tips 33-1

WOUND CARE AND HEALING

Health Topic	Teaching Tip	Why Is This Important?
Supplies	• Methods for obtaining dressing supplies such as purchasing from pharmacies, drug stores, discount stores, and medical supply stores • Considerations of costs and ease of use • Investigation about reimbursement by insurance or other source of health care financing	Patients need to be able to obtain appropriate supplies to perform prescribed care. Wound care will not be completed if supplies cannot be obtained for financial or other reasons, the wound care is complex, or the patient does not understand the wound care instructions.
Infection prevention	• Signs and symptoms of infection to be immediately reported to the health care provider • Need to watch for increased body temperature, flulike symptoms, red or separated wound edges, increased pain in the wound, and/or increased drainage that is thick and has a foul odor • Hand hygiene before putting on and after removing disposable gloves • Proper methods for disposal of old dressing, such as wrapping old dressing the used glove or in several layers of newspaper before putting it in a plastic bag for disposal in a trash container	Early detection of possible complications promotes early intervention and prevention of further complications. Preventative measures reduce transmission of microorganisms.
Wound healing	• Importance of eating well-balanced meals that are high in protein and vitamins • Need to drink six to eight glasses of fluids each day • Rest periods during the day • Modifications in activities of daily living and exercise until healing is complete and the health care provider recommends a return to regular activity	Promoting wound healing is essential.

and describes various prevention strategies and options. Illustrated instructions written at the level of the learner are a valuable resource. The protocols listed in the Guidelines for Nursing Care boxes serve as a model for development of a teaching plan that incorporates basic principles and targets people at risk. As new information becomes available, education for prevention of pressure injury requires updating.

Involve the patient and caregivers in the plan of care and provide them with a good understanding about causative factors for the pressure injury. Instruct them in proper hand hygiene techniques and how to identify the signs and symptoms of infection. Provide the patient and caregivers with simple, easy-to-read instructions. Encourage frequent consultation with the primary health care provider about the progress of wound healing and products used. In addition, ensure that the patient, family, or caregivers understand the need for adequate nutrition to aid in wound healing. Assess the patient's nutritional status and suggest consultation with a dietitian for dietary deficiencies, if necessary.

If dressing changes or wound care is painful, teach the patient to use pain medication as prescribed 30 to 45 minutes before the procedure. Reinforce the importance of hand hygiene before and after the dressing change.

Documenting Wound Care

Documentation related to wound care is an important nursing responsibility. Clear and accurate documentation is essential for communicating wound status and tracking the progression of healing. Precise documentation contributes to continuity of care, accurate evaluation of care, and appropriate changes in wound care, if necessary. Photographs of a wound contribute to accurate assessment documentation and measurement of changes over time. Figure 33-18 on page 1192 shows an example of an electronic documentation tool. Comprehensive wound documentation includes the following elements (Baranoski & Ayello, 2020):

- Any change in clinical status or wound healing
- Characteristics of the wound (see Fig. 33-18 on page 1192)
- Wound care and dressing(s)
- Nutritional status
- Support surfaces in use (bed and chair) and repositioning schedule
- Regular, scheduled reassessment of the wound
- Routine daily skin assessment and care using a standardized instrument
- Any other required forms for reimbursement

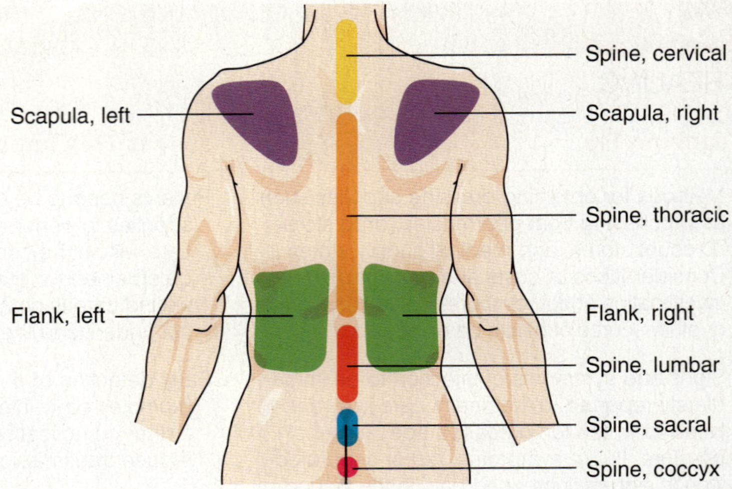

Region: Back

Specific location: Spine, sacral

Type: Pressure injury, stage 2

Length: 2

Width: 2

Depth: .5

Description: Open stage 2 pressure injury 2 cm x 2 cm x .5 cm, with partial-thickness skin loss and exposed dermis; dark red edges, pink interior, and small amount of serosanguineous drainage.

Peri-wound area: Stage 1 pressure injury surrounding ulcer: 5 cm x 6 cm area of non-blanchable erythema; reddened, but intact.

Dressing and wound care: Irrigated wound and with normal saline and applied hydrocolloid dressing per prescription to sacrum.

Focused notes: Patient reported pain 1/10 during assessment and dressing change; tolerated procedure without incident. Plan to ensure dressing remains intact and change every 3–7 days as needed.

FIGURE 33-18. Electronic wound and skin assessment/documentation example from a web-based academic EHR simulation.

Evaluating

Evaluation of wound and pressure injury care involves reassessment at regular intervals to monitor response to the treatment, determine the effectiveness of the treatment, and allow for necessary changes in the plan of care. When evaluating the effectiveness of a plan of care designed to prevent the development of pressure injuries or to treat pressure injuries or other wounds already present, the nurse uses each nurse–patient interaction to determine if the patient has met the individualized expected outcomes. Nursing care is considered effective if the patient, family member, or caregiver expresses satisfaction with prevention and treatment measures and can accomplish the following:

- Participate effectively in preventive and treatment regimens
- Prevent development of any additional areas of skin breakdown
- Demonstrate progressive healing of pressure injury or other wound
- Improve overall physical condition (including nutritional state and mobility status)
- Remain free of infection at any pressure injury or other wound site
- Communicate the need for additional support (environmental, physical, psychosocial)

Evaluation is a continuous process that involves ongoing assessment and revised plans and implementations. Color photographs are an excellent method of objectively evaluating the progression of wound healing, allowing visual comparison of the wound at the initial assessment and throughout the treatment and recovery stages.

HEAT AND COLD THERAPY

Heat and cold are applied to a specific part or all of a patient's body to bring about a local or systemic change in body temperature for various therapeutic purposes. Physiologic responses to heat and cold are modified by the method and duration of application, the degree of heat and cold applied, the patient's age and physical condition, and the amount of body surface covered by the application. Nurses use heat and cold as nursing interventions in both hospital- and community-based settings.

Body temperature is regulated by cells in the hypothalamus in response to signals from thermal (heat and cold) receptors located close to the skin's surface. Stimulation of these receptors sends sensory messages to the anterior hypothalamus to initiate mechanisms to dissipate heat (through vasodilation and sweating) or to preserve warmth through vasoconstriction and piloerection (*goose bumps*).

Pain receptors, also located near the skin's surface, are also affected by heat and cold as painful stimuli, with excessive heat perceived as burning and excessive cold experienced as numbness followed by pain.

Effects of Applying Heat

The application of local heat dilates peripheral blood vessels, increases tissue metabolism, reduces blood viscosity, increases capillary permeability, reduces muscle tension, and helps relieve pain. Vasodilation increases local blood flow. In turn, the supply of oxygen and nutrients to the area is increased, and venous congestion is decreased. As local blood flow increases, the viscosity of blood is reduced. Increased capillary permeability improves the delivery of leukocytes and nutrients, while also facilitating the removal of wastes and prolonging clotting time. These actions, combined with increased tissue metabolism, accelerate the inflammatory response to promote healing.

Heat reduces muscle tension to promote relaxation and helps to relieve muscle spasms and joint stiffness. Heat also helps relieve pain by stimulating specific nerve fibers, closing the gate that allows the transmission of pain stimuli to centers in the brain. Because of these local physiologic effects, heat in various forms is used to treat infections, surgical wounds, inflamed tissue, arthritis, joint and muscle pain, dysmenorrhea, and chronic pain.

The systemic effects of extensive, prolonged heat include increased cardiac output, sweating, increased pulse rate, and decreased blood pressure. This response occurs when heat is applied to a large body area, increasing the blood flow to that area while decreasing it to another part of the body, in effect, causing hypovolemic shock.

Effects of Applying Cold

The local application of cold constricts peripheral blood vessels, reduces muscle spasms, and promotes comfort. Cold reduces blood flow to tissues and decreases the local release of pain-producing substances such as histamine, serotonin, and bradykinin. This action in turn reduces the formation of edema and inflammation. Decreased metabolic needs and capillary permeability, combined with increased coagulation of blood at the wound site, facilitate the control of bleeding and reduce edema formation.

Cold also reduces muscle spasm, alters tissue sensitivity (producing numbness), and promotes comfort by slowing the transmission of pain stimuli. Cold, for these effects, is used after direct trauma, for dental pain, for muscle spasms, after sprains, and to treat some chronic pain syndromes.

Exposure to prolonged or extensive environmental cold produces systemic effects of increased blood pressure, shivering, and goose bumps. Although shivering is a normal body response to cold, prolonged exposure to cold temperatures may cause tissue injury.

Physiologic Considerations

The rebound phenomenon is important to the therapeutic value of heat and cold and to the safety of patients receiving such therapy. Heat produces maximum vasodilation in 20 to 30 minutes; if heat is continued beyond that time, tissue congestion and vasoconstriction occur (for unknown reasons). With cold, maximum vasoconstriction occurs when the skin reaches 60°F (15°C); then vasodilation begins.

The ability of the body to adapt to heat and cold is an important consideration when applying heat or cold and when teaching patients and caregivers about heat and cold therapy. Initially, heat and cold skin receptors are stimulated strongly by sudden changes in temperature. For the first few seconds after being stimulated, the response decreases rapidly. It then decreases more slowly for the next 30 minutes, as the receptors adapt to the temperature. A hot application, even if the temperature remains constant, does not feel as warm after adaptation has taken place. Be sure to inform patients that increasing the temperature or lengthening the time of application can seriously damage tissues.

NURSING PROCESS FOR HEAT AND COLD THERAPY

Assessing

Before initiating heat or cold therapy, assess the patient's physical and mental status, the condition of the body area to be treated with heat or cold, and the condition of the equipment to be used. Carefully evaluate factors influencing the patient's ability to tolerate heat and cold applications. These factors are the basis for the following considerations:

- How long will the heat or cold be applied? Prolonged exposure increases tolerance, and rebound effects are undesirable.
- What body part is involved? Some body areas, such as the neck, perineum, and inner aspects of the wrist and forearm, are more sensitive to thermal changes.
- Is the skin intact? Open tissue or abraded skin is more sensitive to thermal changes.
- How large is the area? Applications of heat or cold to large areas of the body cause systemic responses and lower tolerance of temperature change.
- What is the patient's age? Infants, children, and older adults do not tolerate temperature changes as well as adults.
- What is the patient's physical condition? Patients with certain alterations in health, such as those with cardiovascular or peripheral vascular diseases, might have reduced response to or tolerance of thermal changes.

Assessing Overall Status

Assessing the patient's overall status includes obtaining a health history and completing a physical examination. A history of cardiovascular or peripheral vascular impairment, sensory impairment, and alterations in mental status, such as confusion or decreased level of consciousness, indicates the need for caution when using heat or cold because of the danger of tissue damage. Assessments include response to stimuli (sharp and dull), color and appearance of body tissues, circulation (pulses, blanching sign, temperature, color), level of consciousness, and orientation.

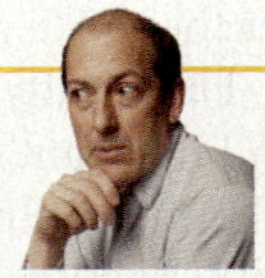

Consider **Mr. Everly**, the postoperative patient in the critical care unit. Imagine that the provider had prescribed heat or cold applications for this patient. The nurse would need to obtain a thorough assessment of his physical status when planning this care. His history of diabetes and circulation problems, coupled with his decreased level of consciousness, would place him at high risk for injury and tissue damage. In addition, the nurse would need to assess him frequently during the application of heat or cold to ensure his safety.

Do not apply heat to an open wound immediately after the trauma; during hemorrhage; over noninflammatory edema; to an acutely inflamed area, a localized malignant tumor, the testes, or the abdomen of a pregnant woman; or over metallic implants. Conversely, do not use cold for open wounds or for patients with impaired peripheral circulation or adverse reactions to cold.

Assessing the Area of Application

Perform baseline assessments to ensure safety and to evaluate the outcomes of therapy. The risk for damage to tissues is increased if the area is traumatized or has altered integrity. Assess for open lesions, blisters, wounds, edema, bleeding, or drainage. Also look for evidence of altered circulation such as changes in color, temperature, pulses, and sensation. As with any assessment, compare body parts bilaterally for changes. Tissues with decreased or absent pulses, those that appear pale or cyanotic, and those that feel cold to the touch indicate a decrease in circulation. Subsequently, the risk for injury from heat and cold applications increases.

When the heat or cold is applied, make ongoing assessments to ensure patient safety and comfort. When heat is applied, assess the patient for undesired responses, including localized redness, blistering, and pain (symptoms of burning), along with possible systemic responses, such as hypotension and changes in consciousness. When cold is applied, assess for localized responses, including pallor, cyanosis, numbness, and pain.

Assessing the Condition of Equipment

The nurse is responsible for checking the equipment used and for maintaining patient safety. Included in this responsibility is checking the condition of cords, plugs, and heating or cooling elements. In addition, inspect the equipment for fluid leaks. Also, check to ensure that the equipment distributes and maintains the constant temperature. Do not use faulty equipment; if faulty equipment is found, it should be returned for repair.

Diagnosing

The patient's need for and response to the heat or cold suggest possible nursing problems or needs, including the following:

- Acute or Chronic pain
- Altered tissue perfusion
- Thermal injury risk

Outcome Identification and Planning

Heat and cold are used for a variety of therapeutic purposes. When applications of heat or cold are part of a plan of care, the following outcomes are appropriate; specific outcomes should be chosen based on the purpose of the application. The patient will:

- Verbalize increased comfort
- Demonstrate evidence of wound healing, decreased muscle spasms, decreased edema, and increased comfort
- Verbalize and demonstrate safe hot or cold application

Implementing

Heat and cold applications may be moist or dry, using many forms and methods. The prescription for the heat and cold application should include the type of application, the body area to be treated, the frequency recommended, and length of time for the applications.

Explain to the patient the purpose and steps of the application and the sensations that will be experienced. In the hospital, provide a timer or clock and have the call bell within reach. In the home, teach the patient or caregiver to check the equipment each time to ensure that it is in good working order, avoid lying or leaning on the equipment, cover the heating device with a protective cloth, apply heat only for the prescribed time period, and report any changes in sensation or discomfort to the health care provider.

Applying Heat

Heat is applied by both dry and moist methods. Hot water bags, electric heating pads, aquathermia pads, or chemical heat packs provide local dry heat by conduction. Hot compresses or packs, sitz baths, or soaks provide moist heat by conduction.

DRY HEAT

Hot Water Bags

Hot water bags are a method of dry heat application. Although relatively easy and inexpensive to use, they have disadvantages. They may leak, and often the weight of the bag or bottle on the patient's body part can be uncomfortable. Moreover, there is a danger of burns from improper use.

Electric Heating Pads

An electric heating pad can be used to apply dry heat locally. It is easy to apply, is relatively safe to use, and provides constant and even heat. Improper use can, however, result in injury. When applying a heating pad, follow manufacturer-specific and these general recommendations:

- Avoid using pins to secure a heating pad. There is a danger of electric shock if a pin touches a wire.

- Place a covering over the pad, preferably one that is moisture proof. Also, prevent wet and moist conditions around the pad. Short-circuiting the heating element may cause an electric shock. Do not cover the heating pad with anything that might be heavy; heat may accumulate and burn the patient when it cannot dissipate normally from the pad.
- Place a heating pad anteriorly or laterally to, not under, the body part. If the heating pad is between the patient and the mattress, heat dissipation may be inadequate, leading to burning of the patient or the bed linens.
- Use a heating pad with a selector switch that cannot be turned up beyond a safe temperature. After the patient's receptors adapt to the initial application of heat, the patient may attempt to inappropriately increase the heat. Many people have been burned by turning up the heat in an electric pad because they thought the pad was too cool.
- Assess the skin at regular intervals for the effects of excessive exposure to heat such as increased skin redness, changes in sensation, or discomfort.
- Check facility protocol for the use of heating pads; a release form may need to be signed.

Aquathermia Pads

Aquathermia (Aqua-K) pads are commonly used in health care facilities and homes for various health problems, including back pain, muscle spasms, thrombophlebitis, and mild inflammation. These devices are safer to use than a heating pad, but they too must be checked carefully. Guidelines for using an aquathermia pad are given in Skill 33-8 on pages 1230–1232.

Hot Packs

Commercial hot packs provide a specified amount of dry heat for a specific period. Instructions on the package describe how to activate the pack, either by striking it on a firm surface, or by squeezing or kneading it. Follow the same precautions as for other types of dry heat applications.

MOIST HEAT

Warm Moist Compresses

Warm moist compresses are used to promote circulation and healing, and to reduce edema. Because moist heat evaporates and cools rapidly, change these compresses frequently and cover them with a heating agent (hot water bottle, heating pad, Aqua-K pad).

Sitz Baths

Sitz baths are a method of applying tepid or warm water to the pelvic, perineal, or rectal areas by sitting in a tub, special chair, or basin filled with sufficient water to reach the umbilicus. Special basins that fit onto the toilet seat are available. They are designed so that the patient's buttocks fit into a rather deep seat that is filled with water of the desired temperature; the legs and feet remain out of the water. The basins are disposable and economical for home or health care facility use. A regular bathtub is not as satisfactory for a sitz bath because the heat causes generalized vasodilation, altering the effect desired. Techniques for administering a sitz bath are given in Guidelines for Nursing Care 33-6 on page 1196.

Warm Soaks

The immersion of a body area into warm water or a medicated solution is called a soak. The purposes of soaks vary: to increase blood supply to a locally infected area; to aid in cleaning large, sloughing wounds, such as burns; to improve circulation; and to apply medication to a locally infected area. A soak has the added advantage of making manipulation of a painful area much easier because the body part is buoyed by the weight of water it displaces. Hydrotherapy, such as pulsatile lavage with suction, may be used to promote wound cleaning and debridement in pressure injuries (EPUAP, NPIAP, & PPPIA, 2019b). If a warm soak is prescribed, follow these general guidelines:

- If a soak is prescribed for a large wound (e.g., an entire arm or lower leg or even an area of the torso), expect to adapt sterile technique. For example, sterilize the container into which the body area is placed before use if possible; if not, clean the container scrupulously. Tap water may be used for soaks because it is accepted as being free from pathogens.
- Unless the temperature of the soak is prescribed otherwise, set the temperature of the water within a range of 105° to 109°F (40.5° to 43°C), which is considered to be physiologically effective and comfortable for the patient.
- Position the container holding the fluid so that the part to be immersed is comfortable and the patient is in good body alignment.
- During the treatment, which usually takes 15 to 20 minutes per soak, maintain the temperature of the soak as constant as possible. This may be done by discarding some of the fluid every 5 minutes and replacing it or by adding solutions at a higher temperature while agitating the water. When replacing or adding fluids, have the patient remove the extremity from the soak.

Applying Cold

Cold is applied by both dry and moist methods. Dry cold is provided with ice bags, cold packs, or a hypothermia blanket (or pad). Cold compresses are a method of applying moist cold.

DRY COLD

Ice Bags

An ice bag, like its counterpart the hot water bottle or bag, is a relatively easy and inexpensive method for applying cold to an area. It has essentially the same disadvantages as the hot water bag. Placing ice bags in the axilla, neck, and groin regions effectively lower the patient's core temperature quickly and are used when therapeutic hypothermia (32°C to 36°C) is indicated. When using an ice bag, follow these recommendations:

- Fill the bag with small pieces of ice to about two thirds full. This makes the bag lightweight. Using ice chips, rather than cubes, makes it easier to mold the bag to the body part.

Guidelines for Nursing Care 33-6

ASSISTING WITH A SITZ BATH

- Test the water in a sitz bath (Figure) with a thermometer before the patient enters the water.
- If the purpose of the sitz bath is to apply heat, use water at a temperature of 34° to 37°C (93° to 99°F) for 15 minutes to produce relaxation of the parts involved after a short initial period of contraction. Do not use warm water if considerable congestion is already present.

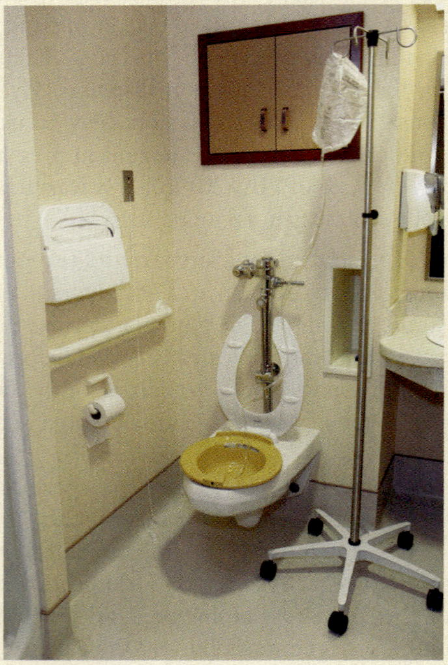

Sitz bath

- If the purpose of the sitz bath is to produce relaxation or to promote healing in a wound by cleansing it of discharge and debris, use water at a temperature of 34° to 37°C (93° to 99°F). Check facility protocols for the correct temperature.
- Assist the patient into the tub or onto the sitz bath and position properly. The patient should be able to sit in the basin or tub with the feet flat on the floor without any pressure on the sacrum or thighs.
- Wrap a blanket around the shoulders to protect from chilling and exposure.
- Monitor the patient closely for signs of weakness and fatigue, and discontinue the bath if faintness, pallor, a rapid pulse rate, or nausea is noted.
- Test the water in the tub several times and keep it at the desired temperature. Additional hot water may be added by pouring it slowly from a pitcher or by opening the hot water faucet slightly. Agitate the water by stirring it as the hot water is added to prevent burning the patient.
- Do not leave the patient alone if there are any questions about safety.
- Help the patient out of the tub when the bath is completed. A sitz bath should take 15 to 20 minutes. Help the patient dry and cover them adequately.

- Remove air from the ice bag in the same manner as removing air from a hot water bag.
- After securing the cap, test the ice bag for leaks and wipe off excess moisture.
- Place a cover on the ice bag to provide comfort and to absorb moisture that may accumulate on the outside of the bag.
- Apply an ice bag for 15 to 20 minutes, then remove it for about an hour before reapplying it. This technique prevents the effects of prolonged exposure to cold (Fig. 33-19).
- In the home setting, a bag of frozen vegetables (such as peas) makes a good substitute for an ice bag.

Cold Packs

Commercially prepared ice packs are available in many health care facilities and may be purchased for home use. These bags are sealed containers filled with a chemical or a nontoxic substance. Depending on the type, the bags are frozen in the freezer or (if not frozen) are squeezed to activate the chemical that produces the cold. These packs are advantageous because the frozen solution remains pliable and can be easily molded to fit the body part. They are covered with a ribbed cotton sleeve so that the bag can be slipped onto an extremity, or the bag can simply be placed on a body part,

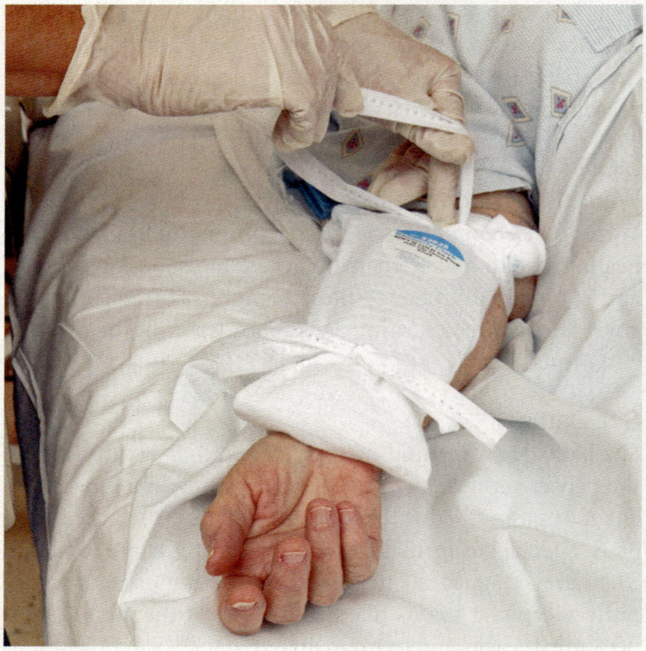

FIGURE 33-19. Cloth-wrapped ice bag. (*Source:* Reprinted with permission from Craven, R. F., Hirnle, C. J., & Henshaw, C. M. [2017]. *Fundamentals of nursing: Human health and function* [8th ed.]. Wolters Kluwer Health.)

such as the head. Assess the skin beneath the pack periodically for symptoms of numbness and pain.

MOIST COLD

Moist, cold local applications are called cold compresses. They might be used for an injured eye, a headache, a tooth extraction, and sometimes for hemorrhoids. The texture and thickness of the material used depend on the area to which it is applied. For example, eye compresses could be prepared from surgical gauze compresses, which have a small amount of cotton filling. A washcloth makes an excellent compress for the head or face.

Immerse the material used for the application in a clean basin that contains pieces of ice and a small amount of water. Wring the compress thoroughly before applying it to avoid dripping. Dripping is uncomfortable for the patient and may result in wetting the patient's clothing or bed linens. Change the compress frequently, continuing the application for 20 minutes. Repeat the application every 2 to 3 hours as ordered. Ice bags or commercial devices are available for keeping the compresses cold, helping to decrease the frequency with which they must be changed.

Evaluating

The expected outcomes for applying heat and cold are used to evaluate the effectiveness of the planned interventions. Although the specific outcomes depend on the purpose of the application, nursing care is considered effective if the patient is able to:

- Verbalize increased comfort
- Verbalize increased ability to rest and sleep
- Demonstrate evidence of wound healing
- Demonstrate a decrease in symptoms of muscle spasms, inflammation, and edema
- Verbalize and demonstrate safe hot and cold applications

Ongoing evaluation of skin integrity is needed to determine needs and the effectiveness of any interventions, including heat and cold therapy. (See the accompanying concept map for Lucius Everly and the Evolving Case Study for Sam Bentz, on pages 1233–1234.)

REFLECTIVE PRACTICE LEADING TO PERSONAL LEARNING

Remember that the object of reflective practice is to look at an experience, understand it, and learn from it. As you begin to develop your expertise in evaluating the plan of care, reflect on your experiences—successes and failures—in order to improve your practice. How can you do it better next time? What did you learn today that can help you tomorrow? Begin your reflection by paying close attention to the following:

- How aware are you of current initiatives to prevent the development of pressure injuries? What are some standard practices across the health care continuum designed to promote skin integrity in your at-risk patients?
- What value do you attach to involving and empowering the patient throughout the wound care process? How do you individualize the care for patients when so many guidelines, policies, and procedures dictate your care? How will you identify the resources, equipment, and supplies necessary to provide safe, quality wound care for your patient?
- What plan do you have to stay abreast of evolving standards and wound care procedures? What are the core principles of preventative skin care that will exist irrespective of evolving technologies?

Keeping up with the latest evidence-based practice guidelines can be challenging. Ensuring you are tuned into the appropriate professional organizations and governmental facilities can help you stay on the cutting edge. Balancing the needs of each patient with these responsibilities requires mindfulness and intentionality.

Perhaps the most important questions to reflect on are: Are your patients and their families/caregivers better for having had *you* share in the critical responsibility of partnering with them to ensure appropriate skin and wound care? Are your patients now receiving thoughtful, person-centered, prioritized, holistic, evidence-based treatment and care because of your efforts?

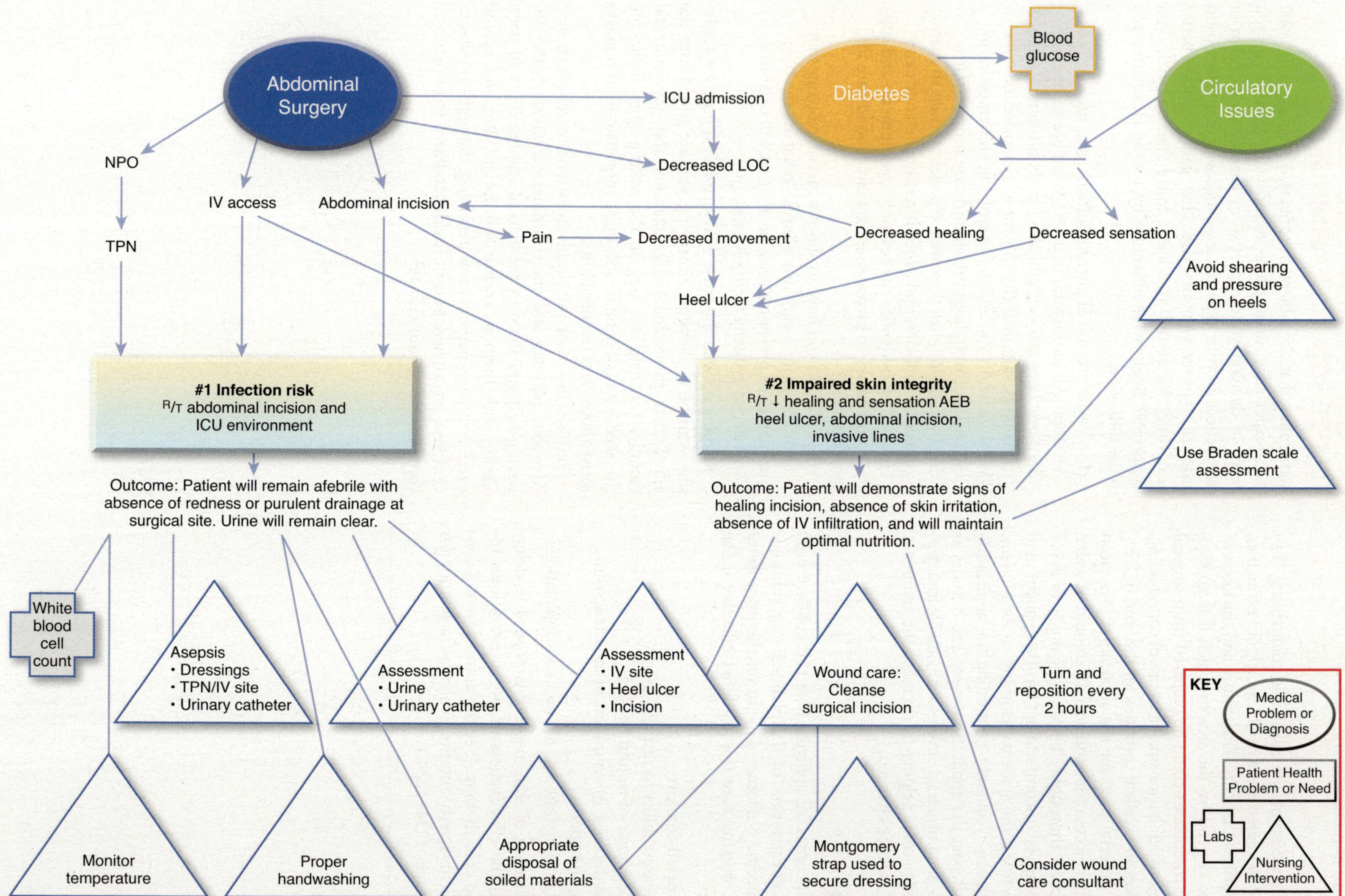

Evaluation
- **Diagnosis #1** Lucius is afebrile, urine is clear, no drainage noted from heel ulcer, serosanguineous drainage from incision. Continue interventions.
- **Diagnosis #2** Lucius has dressing changes done per protocol. Pink granulation tissue noted at surgical incision, no skin irritation. IV sites intact, TPN infusing. Continue interventions.

Concept map displaying the nursing process for Lucius Everly. Ø, no; Θ, negative; Δ, change; √, check; c̄, with; AEB, as evidenced by; DVT, deep vein thrombosis; hr, hours; INR, international normalized ratio; IV, intravenous/intravenous catheter; ROM, range of motion; Pt., patient; PT, physical therapy; PTT, partial thromboplastin time; q, each/every (from L., *quaque*); R/T, related to; US, ultrasound; w/d, withdraws; ×, times

Skill 33-1 Preventing Pressure Injury

DELEGATION CONSIDERATIONS

The assessment of a patient's skin is not delegated to assistive personnel (AP). Depending on the state's nurse practice act and the organization's policies and procedures, licensed practical/vocational nurses (LPN/LVNs) may perform some or all of the parts of assessment of the patient's skin. The use of interventions related to prevention of pressure injuries may be delegated to AP as well as to LPN/LVNs. The decision to delegate must be based on careful analysis of the patient's needs and circumstances as well as the qualifications of the person to whom the task is being delegated. Refer to the Delegation Guidelines in Appendix A.

EQUIPMENT

- Pressure injury assessment form and/or risk assessment tool
- Functional assessment tool, as indicated
- Support surfaces, such as integrated bed systems, specialized and/or low-pressure mattresses and overlays, seating surfaces and cushions, heel elevation devices, and foam positioning wedges, as indicated
- Safe patient handling and movement devices, as indicated
- Protective dressings, such as polyurethane foam dressing, as indicated
- Low-friction patient care textiles, such as bed linens and patient gowns
- Personal hygiene and skin barrier products, as indicated
- PPE, as indicated

IMPLEMENTATION

ACTION	RATIONALE
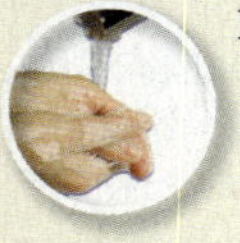 1. Perform hand hygiene and put on PPE, if indicated.	Hand hygiene and PPE prevent the spread of microorganisms. PPE is required based on transmission precautions.
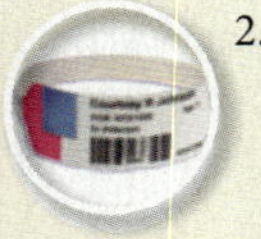 2. Identify the patient.	Identifying the patient ensures the right patient receives the intervention and helps prevent errors.
3. Discuss pressure injury prevention with the patient and/or patient family/caregivers. Explain what pressure injury is, the causes of pressure injuries, and the importance of a pressure injury prevention plan (McNichol et al., 2022).	These measures promote a collaborative relationship in which the patient is treated with respect. Explanation encourages patient understanding and reduces apprehension. Patient and caregiver education support engagement in care and assist patients to implement behaviors to meet goals for care (Joint Commission, 2018; Mitchell, 2018).
4. Assess the patient's skin at least daily, paying special attention to the skin over bony prominences and the skin in contact and under medical devices (Camacho-Del Rio, 2018; McNichol et al., 2022; EPUAP, NPIAP, & PPPIA, 2019a). Briefly assess the patient's skin at the pressure points during repositioning of the patient (EPUAP, NPIAP, & PPPIA, 2019a). Refer to Chapter 27 for additional skin assessment information.	Skin assessment provides information related to the patient's current status and detects impending or actual alterations in skin integrity (McNichol et al., 2022). Skin assessment provides information needed to develop an appropriate care plan. For patients at risk for pressure injury, the skin should be inspected as soon as possible upon admission to a health care service, as part of every pressure injury risk assessment, and additionally based on the individual's degree of pressure injury risk (EPUAP, NPIAP, & PPPIA, 2019a). Assessment of pressure points allows for identification of alterations in status and evaluation of the effectiveness of repositioning regimen; presence of persistent erythema may indicate the need to increase frequency of repositioning; pressure points onto which the patient will be repositioned should appear fully recovered from previous loading (EPUAP, NPIAP, & PPPIA, 2019a).
5. Assess the patient's risk for pressure injury upon entry to a health care setting and on a regularly scheduled basis or when there is a significant change in the patient's condition, incorporating appropriate assessment tools and scales, based on facility policy (WOCN, 2016).	Risk for pressure injury development should be determined on admission, as often as required based on the patient's acuity and as a result of any change in the patient's status (EPUAP, NPIAP, & PPPIA, 2019a). Identification of people at risk for developing pressure injury is a critical component of prevention (Baranoski & Ayello, 2020).

(continued on page 1200)

Skill 33-1 Preventing Pressure Injury *(continued)*

ACTION	RATIONALE
6. Utilize appropriate support surfaces to redistribute tissue loads, both while in bed and when seated, based on individual patient assessment and needs, facility policy, and availability (Baranoski & Ayello, 2020; Haesler, 2018). Appropriate support surfaces may include, but are not limited to, integrated bed systems, specialized and/or low-pressure mattresses and overlays, seating surfaces and cushions, heel elevation devices, and foam positioning wedges. Note: Pressure redistribution devices should serve as adjuncts and not replacements for repositioning of patients (WOCN, 2016). **Do not use foam rings, foam cut-outs or donut-type devices.** The Wound, Ostomy and Continence Nurses Society (WOCN, 2016) has developed a content-validated algorithm for support surface selection. Refer to the General Considerations below.	Support surfaces help prevent pressure injury by redistributing pressure and manage tissue loads; sequentially altering the parts of the body that bear load (to reduce the duration of loading on individual anatomical sites); managing the microclimate (moisture and temperature control); and friction and shear control (Baranoski & Ayello, 2020; Kalowes, 2018). Support surfaces also provide for proper body alignment and comfort (Baranoski & Ayello, 2020). Foam rings, foam cut-outs or donut-type devices concentrate pressure on the surrounding tissue and should be avoided (WOCN, 2016).
7. Routinely reposition the patient: determine frequency with consideration to the patient's level of activity, physical, cognitive, and psychological condition; ability to independently reposition; the type of support surface in use; general health condition; patient comfort and pain (EPUAP, NPIAP, & PPPIA, 2019a; McNichol et al., 2022).	Repositioning reduces or relieves pressure and limits the amount of time tissues are exposed to pressure and contributes to the patient's functional abilities (EPUAP, NPIAP, & PPPIA, 2019a; McNichol et al., 2022; WOCN, 2016).
8. Implement early mobilization to increase the patient's activity and mobility as tolerated. Develop a schedule for progressive sitting and ambulation as rapidly as tolerated by the individual patient. Collaborate with the physical and occupational therapists to develop an individualized intervention plan. Refer to Chapter 34 for additional discussion related to early mobilization and ambulation of patients.	Mobilization and ambulation relieve pressure, contributes to the patient's functional abilities, and may reduce risk for deterioration related to prolonged immobility (EPUAP, NPIAP, & PPPIA, 2019). Early mobility plays an important role in the patient's physical and psychological well-being (Arnold et al., 2018). Physical and occupational therapists are important resources for maximizing patient mobility (Baranoski & Ayello, 2020).
9. Use a 20- to 30-degree side-lying position or flat in bed (if not contraindicated) when positioning patients at risk for pressure injury in side-lying positions (EPUAP, NPIAP, & PPPIA, 2019; WOCN, 2016).	Avoid lying positions that increase pressure, such as the 90-degree position (EPUAP, NPIAP, & PPPIA, 2019a).
10. Maintain the head-of-bed elevation at or below 30 degrees, or at the lowest degree of elevation appropriate for the patient's medical condition.	Head-of-bed elevation at or below 30 degrees prevents shear-related injury (WOCN, 2016).
11. Consider the use of a prophylactic (preventative) dressing, such as a polyurethane foam dressing, on bony prominences, such as heels, hips, and the sacrum (Kalowes, 2018). Assess skin under a prophylactic dressing at least daily; replace prophylactic dressings that are damaged, loosened, displaced, excessively moist, or if the dressing or skin under the dressing becomes soiled and according to the manufacturer's directions (EPUAP, NPIAP, & PPPIA, 2019a).	Prophylactic dressings reduce friction, pressure and shear, protect fragile skin, and influence microclimate (Cornish, 2017; Kalowes, 2018; Lovegrove et al., 2020; EPUAP, NPIAP, & PPPIA, 2019a; WOCN, 2016).
12. Consider the use of low-friction patient care textiles, such as bed linens and patient gowns. Refer to Chapter 34 for additional information related to safe patient handling and the use of patient handling and mobility devices.	Low-friction textiles reduce shear, minimize skin irritation and dry quickly (EPUAP, NPIAP, & PPPIA, 2019a; WOCN, 2016).
13. Utilize safe patient handling interventions when moving a patient. Collaborate with the physical and occupational therapists to develop an individualized intervention plan. Refer to Chapter 34 for additional information related to safe patient handling and the use of patient handling and mobility devices.	Proper lifting, positioning, and repositioning techniques are critical to prevent injury from shearing forces (McNichol et al., 2022). Physical and occupational therapists are important resources for maximizing patient mobility (Baranoski & Ayello, 2020).

ACTION	RATIONALE
14. Provide appropriate skin and personal hygiene (Kalowes, 2018; Mitchell, 2018; Yilmazer et al., 2019). Utilize interventions to protect the skin from excessive exposure to moisture from wound exudate, perspiration, mucous, saliva, fistula or stoma effluent, and urinary and fecal incontinence. Refer to Chapters 32, 38, and 39 for additional information related to these interventions.	Exposure to excessive moisture contributes to skin damage and pressure injury development due to decreased tissue tolerance and increases susceptibility to friction, pressure, and shear (Baranoski & Ayello, 2020; Gray & Guiliano, 2018; Voegili, 2019; WOCN, 2016).
15. Provide appropriate interventions to support the patient's nutritional status and ensure adequate nutritional and fluid intake (Kalowes, 2018). Interventions may include strategies to enhance oral intake, high-calorie/high-protein nutritional supplements, fortified foods, and/or enteral or parenteral nutritional support (Baranoski & Ayello, 2020; Munoz et al., 2020). Collaborate with the registered dietician and dietary staff to develop an individualized nutrition intervention plan (Kawoles, 2018; EPUAP, NPIAP, & Pan Pacific Pressure Injury Alliance, 2019a).	Adequate calories, protein, fluids, vitamins, and minerals are required for health and tissue maintenance (Kalowes, 2018; McNichol et al., 2022). Nutritional management is an important aspect of a comprehensive care plan for pressure injury prevention (Bergstrom et al., 2018; EPUAP, NPIAP, & PPPIA, 2019; Lovegrove et al., 2020; Munoz et al., 2020; WOCN, 2016).
16. Implement interventions to prevent pressure injury related to the use of medical devices, based on the individual patient's situation.	Interventions are necessary to prevent pressure injury related to the use of medical devices (Camacho-Del Rio, 2018; Joint Commission, 2018; EPUAP, NPIAP, & PPPIA, 2019a; WOCN, 2016).
a. Ensure correct for patient size and application of devices in use.	Correct size and accurate application minimize pressure and shear.
b. Use prophylactic dressings under the device, as appropriate to the individual patient and clinical use (EPUAP, NPIAP, & PPPIA, 2019a).	Appropriate use of prophylactic dressing manages moisture and provides cushioning to reduce pressure (EPUAP, NPIAP, & PPPIA, 2019a).
c. Inspect the skin under the devices and observe for edema under the devices more than twice daily or more often, as indicated.	Presence of edema increases risk for alterations in skin integrity (EPUAP, NPIAP, & PPPIA, 2019a).
d. Remove device as soon as medically feasible. Routinely reposition or rotate any medical device daily when possible.	Removal prevents pressure injury. Repositioning or rotating redistributes pressure and decreases shear (EPUAP, NPIAP, & PPPIA, 2019a).
e. Keep the skin clean and dry under medical devices.	Moisture underneath medical device increases risk of alterations in skin integrity (Camacho-Del Rio, 2018).
17. Provide education to the patient and caregiver(s) about the prevention plan and ways to minimize the risk of pressure injury.	These measures promote a collaborative relationship in which the patient is treated with respect. Explanation encourages patient understanding and engagement and reduces apprehension. Patient and caregiver education assist patients to implement behaviors to meet goals for care (EPUAP, NPIAP, & PPPIA, 2019a; McNichol et al., 2022; WOCN, 2016).
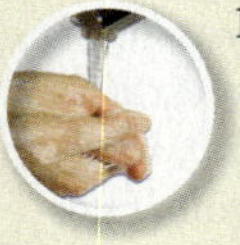 18. Remove gloves and additional PPE, if used. Perform hand hygiene.	Removing gloves and PPE properly reduces the risk for infection transmission and contamination of other items. Hand hygiene prevents the transmission of microorganisms.
19. Evaluate the patient's response to interventions. Reassess and alter care plan as indicated by facility policies and procedures, as appropriate.	Evaluation allows for individualization of care plan and promotes optimal patient comfort.

(continued on page 1202)

Skill 33-1 Preventing Pressure Injury *(continued)*

DOCUMENTATION GUIDELINES

Document risk and skin assessments, as well as other appropriate assessments, based on individual patient circumstances. Document interventions provided and patient responses. Record alternative treatments to consider, if appropriate. Document reassessment after interventions, at an appropriate interval, based on specific interventions used. Documentation related to pressure injury prevention is often completed on checklists or other tools on the patient's health record. Include any pertinent patient and family/caregiver education provided.

DEVELOPING CLINICAL REASONING AND CLINICAL JUDGMENT

UNEXPECTED SITUATIONS AND ASSOCIATED INTERVENTIONS

- *Patient develops a pressure injury:* Reassess the patient's condition. Perform assessment to differentiate pressure injuries from wounds and/or injuries due to other causes (WOCN, 2016). Consult with the patient's health care team regarding the injury and collaborate on a revised plan of care. Review and revise the current care plan to reflect the change in the patient's status and ensure implementation of appropriate nursing interventions. Implement appropriate wound care as prescribed and indicated in facility policy. Continue vigilant preventive interventions to avoid further pressure injury.

SPECIAL CONSIDERATIONS

General Considerations

- Preventive interventions related to pressure injury prevention should be based on nursing clinical judgment, the use of a reliable risk assessment tool, and assessment of individual patient extrinsic and intrinsic risk factors (EPUAP, NPIAP, & PPPIA, 2019a; WOCN, 2016). Interdisciplinary collaboration and communication are essential to pressure injury prevention in high-risk patient populations (Bergstrom et al., 2018).
- Extended use of prone positioning should be avoided unless required for management of the patient's medical condition; special consideration must be given to offloading of pressure points on the face, breast region, knees, toes, penis, clavicles, iliac crest and symphysis pubis, as well as the potential for uneven distribution of pressure and positioning of medical devices (EPUAP, NPIAP, & PPPIA, 2019a).
- Nurses must participate in continued pressure injury prevention and treatment education to ensure provision of evidence-based nursing care, achieve desired outcomes, and provide patients the best possible care (EPUAP, NPIAP, & PPPIA, 2019a).
- WOCN (2016) has developed a content-validated algorithm for support surface selection. This evidence- and consensus-based algorithm for support surface selection had a Content Validity Index (CVI) of 0.95 with an overall mean score of 3.72, indicating strong content validity and steps that are appropriate to the purpose of the algorithm (McNichol et al., 2015). Visit the WOCN website at https://www.wocn.org/learning-center/clinical-tools/ to access evidence for practice describing the Support Surface Algorithm, including the algorithm (McNichol et al., 2015); the interactive Support Surface Algorithm tool; and additional Support Surface Algorithm resources (WOCN, n.d.).

Infant and Child Considerations

- An age-appropriate risk assessment for pediatric, adolescent, and neonate populations considers risk factors of specific concern, including activity and mobility levels, skin texture and maturity, perfusion and oxygenation measures, presence of an external device, sensory perception, humidity, nutrition, friction and sheer, severity of illness, and duration of hospitalization (EPUAP, NPIAP, & PPPIA, 2019a; Ferreira et al., 2018).

Community-Based Care Considerations

- Pressure injury prevention in home settings can be challenging and may be compromised by access to resources and devices. Assessment of the patient and individual risk factors, as well as implementation of pressure injury prevention interventions in the home are critical in meeting patients' needs (Ellis, 2017; McGraw, 2018).
- Education of the patient, family, and caregivers is critical to ensure successful implementation of the pressure injury prevention care plan (Payne, 2016).

Skill 33-2 Cleaning a Wound and Applying a Dressing (General Guidelines)

DELEGATION CONSIDERATIONS

Wound care and procedures requiring the use of a sterile field and other sterile items are not delegated to assistive personnel (AP). Depending on the state's nurse practice act and the organization's policies and procedures, these procedures may be delegated to licensed practical/vocational nurses (LPN/LVNs). The decision to delegate must be based on careful analysis of the patient's needs and circumstances as well as the qualifications of the person to whom the task is being delegated. Refer to the Delegation Guidelines in Appendix A.

EQUIPMENT

- Sterile gloves, as indicated
- Gloves
- Additional PPE, as indicated
- Primary and secondary dressings (if indicated) as prescribed
- Sterile dressing set or suture set (for the sterile scissors and forceps)
- Sterile cleaning solution as prescribed (commonly 0.9% normal saline solution, or a commercially prepared wound cleanser)
- Skin protectant/barrier wipes
- Sterile basin (may be optional)
- Sterile drape (may be optional)
- Plastic bag or other appropriate waste container for soiled dressings
- Waterproof pad and bath blanket
- Bath blanket or other linens for draping patient
- Additional dressings and supplies needed or required based on the wound dressing/care prescribed for the patient

IMPLEMENTATION

ACTION	RATIONALE
1. Review the patient's health record for prescribed wound care or the care plan related to wound care. Gather necessary supplies.	Reviewing the health record and care plan validates the correct patient and correct procedure. Preparation promotes efficient time management and an organized approach to the task.
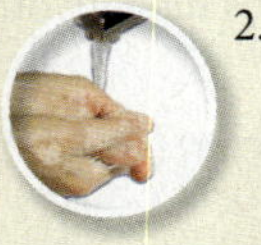 2. Perform hand hygiene and put on PPE, if indicated.	Hand hygiene and PPE prevent the spread of microorganisms. PPE is required based on transmission precautions.
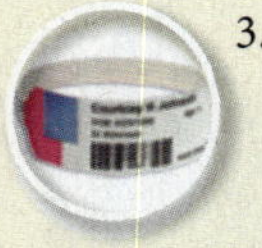 3. Identify the patient.	Identifying the patient ensures the right patient receives the intervention and helps prevent errors.
4. Assemble equipment on the overbed table or other surface within reach.	Organization facilitates performance of the task.
5. Close the curtains around the bed and close the door to the room, if possible. Explain to the patient what you are going to do and why you are going to do it.	This ensures the patient's privacy. Explanation relieves anxiety and facilitates engagement.
6. Assess the patient for the possible need for nonpharmacologic pain-reducing interventions or analgesic medication before wound care dressing change. Administer appropriate prescribed analgesic. Allow enough time for the analgesic to achieve its effectiveness.	Pain is a subjective experience influenced by past experience. Wound care and dressing changes may cause pain for some patients.
7. Place a waste receptacle or bag at a convenient location for use during the procedure.	Having a waste container handy means the soiled dressing may be discarded easily, without the spread of microorganisms.
8. Adjust the bed to a comfortable working height (VHA Center for Engineering & Occupational Safety and Health [CEOSH], 2016).	Having the bed at the proper height prevents back and muscle strain.
9. Assist the patient to a comfortable position that provides easy access to the wound area. Use the bath blanket to cover any exposed area other than the wound. Place a waterproof pad under the wound site.	Patient positioning and the use of a bath blanket provide for comfort and warmth. Waterproof pad protects underlying surfaces.

(continued on page 1204)

Skill 33-2 Cleaning a Wound and Applying a Dressing (General Guidelines) *(continued)*

ACTION

10. Check the position of drains, tubes, or other adjuncts before removing the dressing. Put on gloves and loosen the tape or adhesive edge on the old dressings by removing in the direction of hair growth and the use of a push–pull method (Fumarola et al., 2020) (Figure 1). Push–pull method: lift a corner of the dressing away from the skin, and then gently push the skin down and away from the dressing/adhesive (Fumarola et al., 2020). Continue moving fingers of the opposite hand to support the skin as the product is removed (Fumarola et al., 2020). Once all adhesive is loosened from the skin, carefully lift dressing from the surrounding skin to prevent medical adhesive–related skin injury (MARSI). Remove the sides/edges first, then the center. If the patient is at increased risk for MARSI, requires repeated application or removal of adhesive devices, or there is resistance, use an adhesive remover (Barton, 2020; Fumarola et al., 2020; Kelly-O'Flynn et al., 2020).

RATIONALE

Checking ensures that a drain is not removed accidentally if one is present. Gloves protect the nurse from contaminated dressings and prevent the spread of microorganisms. Removal of the tape in the direction of hair growth minimizes trauma to the skin (Fumarola et al., 2020). Pushing the skin down and away from the adhesive reduces the risk for medical adhesive–related skin injury (MARSI) (Fumarola et al., 2020). The use of adhesive remover allows for the easy, rapid, and painless removal without the associated problems of skin stripping and helps reduce patient discomfort (Barton, 2020; Fumarola et al., 2020; Kelly-O'Flynn et al., 2020).

11. Carefully remove the soiled dressings. If any part of the dressing sticks to the underlying skin, use small amounts of sterile saline to help loosen and remove it.

Cautious removal of the dressing is more comfortable for the patient and ensures that any drain present is not removed. Sterile saline moistens the dressing for easier removal and minimizes damage and pain.

12. After removing the dressing, note the presence, amount, type, color, and odor of any drainage on the dressings (Figure 2). Place soiled dressings in the appropriate waste receptacle. Remove your gloves and perform hand hygiene.

The presence of drainage should be documented. Proper disposal of soiled dressings and used gloves prevents the spread of microorganisms. Hand hygiene prevents the transmission of microorganisms.

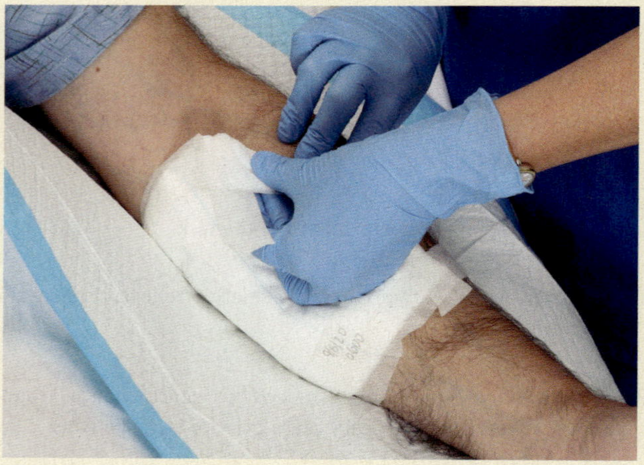

FIGURE 1. Loosening dressing tape or adhesive edge.

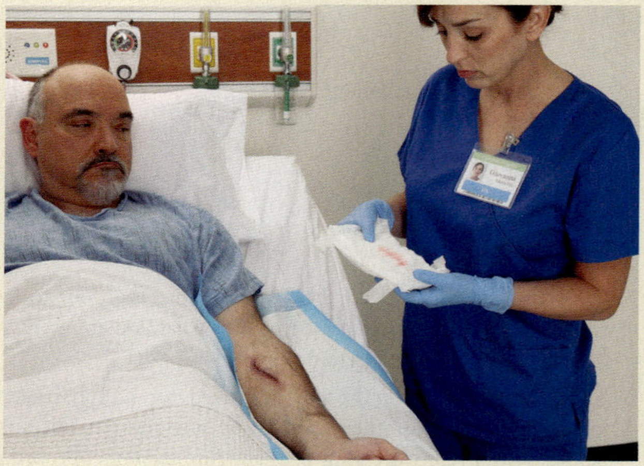

FIGURE 2. Noting characteristics of drainage on dressing that has been removed.

13. Inspect the wound site for size, appearance, and drainage. Assess if any pain is present. Check the status of sutures, adhesive closure strips, staples, and drains or tubes, if present. Note any problems to include in your documentation.

Wound healing or the presence of irritation or infection should be documented.

14. **Using sterile technique, prepare a sterile work area and open the needed supplies.**

Supplies are within easy reach and sterility is maintained.

15. Open the sterile cleaning solution. Moisten gauze for cleaning the peri-wound skin. Depending on the amount of cleaning needed, the solution might be poured directly over gauze sponges over a container for small cleaning jobs, or into a basin for more complex or larger cleaning.

Sterility of dressings and solution is maintained.

ACTION	RATIONALE
16. Put on sterile gloves. Alternatively, clean gloves (clean technique) may be used when cleaning a chronic wound or pressure injury.	The use of sterile gloves maintains surgical asepsis and sterile technique and reduces the risk for spreading microorganisms. Aseptic technique should be used to change dressings for surgical wounds and in the acute clinical setting, to reduce the risk of transfer of pathogens, likely to be present in an acute care setting, to the wound (Brown, 2018). Clean technique is appropriate for cleaning chronic wounds, wounds in the home, or pressure injuries (Baranoski & Ayello, 2020; EPUAP, NPIAP, & PPPIA, 2019a).
17. Clean the wound. Pour the cleaning solution over the wound from top to bottom. Alternatively, spray the wound from top to bottom with a commercially prepared wound cleanser. Wound irrigation is often used to clean open wounds and may also be used for other types of wounds. Refer to Skill 33-3.	Cleaning from top to bottom and center to outside ensures that cleaning occurs from the least to most contaminated area and a previously cleaned area is not contaminated again. Using a single gauze for each wipe ensures that the previously cleaned area is not contaminated again.
18. Clean the skin surrounding the wound. Clean from top to bottom and/or from the center to the outside, beginning at the wound edges (Figure 3). Use new gauze for each wipe, placing the used gauze in the waste receptacle.	Cleaning from top to bottom and center to outside ensures that cleaning occurs from the least to most contaminated area and a previously cleaned area is not contaminated again. Using a single gauze for each wipe ensures that the previously cleaned area is not contaminated again.
19. Once the wound and surrounding skin are cleaned, dry the surrounding skin area using a gauze sponge in the same manner.	Excess moisture on healthy skin increases risk for moisture-associated skin damage and interferes with proper adhesion of securement of dressings.
20. If a drain is in use at the wound location, clean around the drain. Refer to Skills 33-4 and 33-5.	Cleaning the insertion site helps prevent infection.
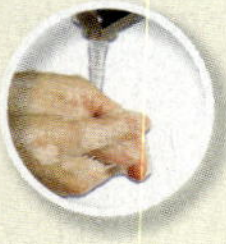 21. Remove gloves and place in the waste receptacle. Perform hand hygiene.	Proper disposal of used gloves and hand hygiene prevent the spread of microorganisms.
22. Put on sterile gloves. Alternatively, clean gloves (clean technique) may be used when cleaning a chronic wound or pressure injury. Apply a skin protectant or barrier to the healthy skin around the wound where the dressing adhesive or tape will be placed and where wound drainage may come in contact with the skin (Figure 4).	The use of sterile gloves maintains surgical asepsis and sterile technique and reduces the risk for spreading microorganisms. Clean technique is appropriate for cleaning chronic wounds, wounds in the home, or pressure injuries (Baranoski & Ayello, 2020; EPUAP, NPIAP, & PPPIA, 2019a). Skin barrier/protectant prevents skin irritation and excoriation from tape, adhesives, and wound drainage (Fumarola et al., 2020; Kelly-O'Flynn et al., 2020).

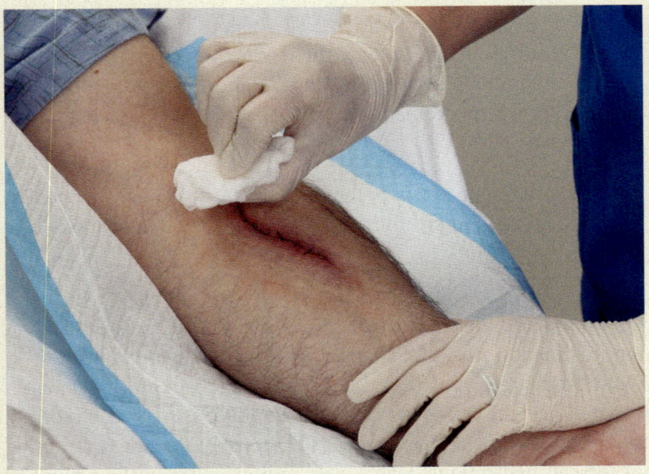

FIGURE 3. Cleaning the wound.

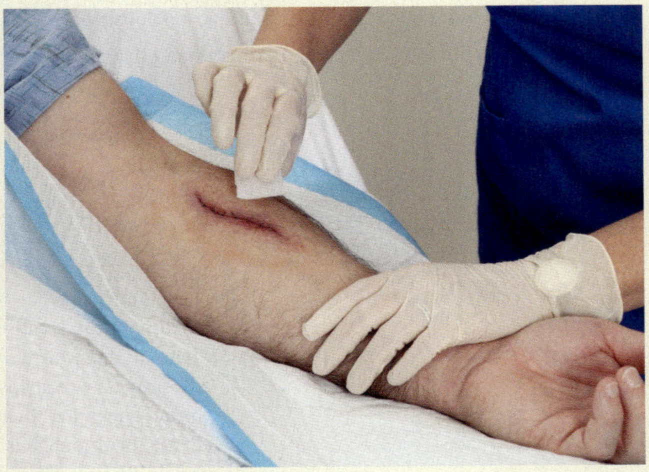

FIGURE 4. Applying skin protectant to skin surrounding wound.

(continued on page 1206)

Skill 33-2 Cleaning a Wound and Applying a Dressing (General Guidelines) *(continued)*

ACTION / **RATIONALE**

23. Apply any topical medications, foams, gels, and/or dressing product to the wound as prescribed; ensure products stay confined to the wound and do not impact on intact surrounding tissue/skin (Figure 5).

The growth of microorganisms may be inhibited and the healing process improved with the use of prescribed medications, foams, gels, and/or other wound care product.

24. Gently place the prescribed cover dressing at the wound center and extend it at least 1 inch beyond the wound in all directions. Alternatively, follow the manufacturer's directions for application (Figure 6).

Extending the dressing at least 1 inch past the wound edges ensures the dressing covers and protects the wound.

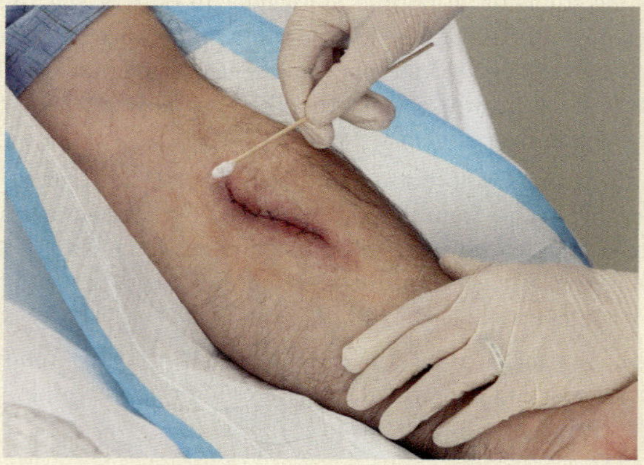

FIGURE 5. Applying prescribed wound care product.

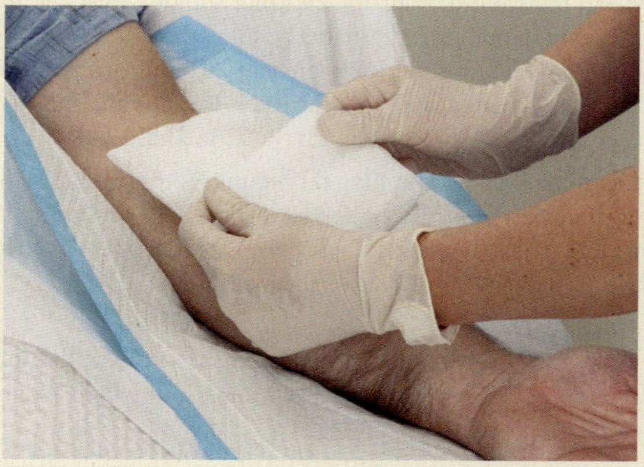

FIGURE 6. Applying cover dressing to site.

25. As necessary, apply a secondary dressing, based on products in use, prescribed interventions, and facility policy. Note: May not be necessary or appropriate, based on the cover dressing used in Step 23. Some dressings act as both primary and secondary dressings (Baranoski & Ayello, 2020).

Secondary dressings cover the primary dressing or secure the dressing (Baranoski & Ayello, 2020).

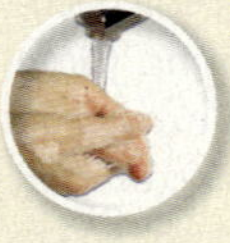

26. Apply additional materials, such as roller gauze, to secure the dressings as needed. Alternatively, many commercial wound products are self-adhesive and do not require additional tape. Remove gloves and perform hand hygiene.

Additional securing products keep the dressing in place. Proper disposal of gloves and hand hygiene prevent the spread of microorganisms.

27. Label the dressing with date and time. Remove all remaining equipment; place the patient in a comfortable position, with side rails up as indicated and bed in the lowest position.

Recording date and time provides communication and demonstrates adherence to care plan. Proper patient and bed positioning promotes safety and comfort.

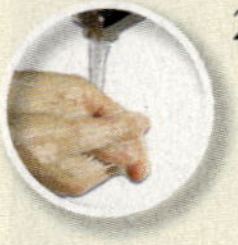

28. Remove PPE, if used. Perform hand hygiene.

Proper removal of PPE reduces the risk for infection transmission and contamination of other items. Hand hygiene prevents the spread of microorganisms.

29. Check all wound dressings at least every shift. More frequent checks may be needed if the wound is more complex.

Checking dressings ensures the assessment of changes in patient condition and timely intervention to prevent complications.

DOCUMENTATION

Guidelines

Document the location of the wound and that the dressing was removed. Record your assessment of the wound: size; approximation of wound edges; presence of sutures, staples, or adhesive closure strips if wound edges are approximated; record size and wound assessment if wound edges are not approximated; and the condition of the surrounding skin. Note if redness, edema, or drainage is observed and document characteristics if present. Document cleansing of wound and application of topical medications, foams, gels, and/or gauze to the wound as prescribed. Record the type of dressing that was reapplied. Note pertinent patient and family/caregiver education and any patient reaction to the procedure, including patient's pain level and effectiveness of nonpharmacologic interventions or analgesia if administered.

Sample Documentation

DocuCare Practice documenting wound care in *Lippincott DocuCare*.

9/8/25 0600 Dressing removed from left lateral calf incision. Scant purulent secretions noted on dressing. Incision edges approximately 1 mm apart, red, with ecchymosis and edema present. Small amount of purulent drainage from wound noted. Area cleansed with normal saline; antibiotic ointment applied as prescribed. Surrounding tissue red and ecchymotic. Redressed with nonadhering dressing and wrapped with stretch gauze. Patient reports adequate pain control after preprocedure analgesic; states pain is dull ache, 1/10 on pain scale.

—*N. Joiner, RN*

DEVELOPING CLINICAL REASONING AND CLINICAL JUDGMENT

UNEXPECTED SITUATIONS AND ASSOCIATED INTERVENTIONS

- *The previous wound assessment states that the incision was clean and dry, and the wound edges were approximated, with the staples and surgical drain intact. The surrounding tissue was without inflammation, edema, or erythema. After the dressing is removed, the nurse notes the incision edges are not approximated at the distal end, multiple staples are evident in the old dressing, the surrounding skin tissue is red and swollen, and purulent drainage is on the dressing and leaking from the wound:* Assess the patient for any other signs and symptoms, such as pain, malaise, fever, and paresthesias. Place a dry sterile dressing over the wound site. Report the findings to the health care team and document the event in the patient's record. Be prepared to obtain a wound culture and implement any changes in wound care as prescribed.
- *When removing a patient's dressing, the assessment reveals deterioration or significant improvement in the wound:* Notify the health care team or wound care specialist, as a different treatment modality and/or dressing product may be necessary.

SPECIAL CONSIDERATIONS

General Considerations

- Instruct the patient, if appropriate, and other members of the health care team to observe for excessive drainage that may overwhelm the dressing. They should also report when dressings become soiled or loosened from the skin.
- There are many dressing types and manufacturers—the nurse needs to collaborate with the health care team to ensure the correct dressing type is chosen, ongoing assessment occurs, and updates to the treatment plan (dressing choice) are made as the wound evolves. The choice of wound dressing will change during the healing period, based on a minimum of once-a-week wound assessment (more often with notable changes) (Baranoski & Ayello, 2020). The type of wound and status/characteristics of the wound influence the choice of the wound dressing, and several different types of products may be needed as the wound progresses through the stages of healing (Baranoski & Ayello, 2020, p. 191).
- Products designed to assist with dressing removal can reduce pain, avoid damaging the periwound skin and resulting skin stripping and MARSI and result in time savings (Fumarola et al., 2020; Kelly-O'Flynn et al., 2020; Reevell et al., 2016).
- When using adherent dressings, such as a hydrocolloid dressing, cut the dressing to size, allowing at least a 1-inch margin of healthy skin around the wound to be covered with the dressing (Baranoski & Ayello, 2020). Apply the dressing to the wound without stretching the dressing.
- Optimum and timely wound healing are supported by adequate nutrition and hydration (Dudek, 2018; Stuart, 2020). Collaborate with the registered dietician and dietary staff to develop an individualized nutrition intervention plan for the patient.

Infant and Child Considerations

- The skin of neonates is more fragile as a result of incomplete epidermal-to-dermal cohesion; use skin barrier products and adhesive removers, paper tape, or nonadherent dressings to prevent tearing of the skin (Baranoski et al., 2016; Fumarola et al., 2020; Kelly-O'Flynn et al., 2020).

(continued on page 1208)

Skill 33-2 Cleaning a Wound and Applying a Dressing (General Guidelines) *(continued)*

Older Adult Considerations

- The skin of older adults is less elastic and more fragile as a result of age-related changes; use skin barrier products and adhesive removers, paper tape, nonadherent dressings, or roller gauze (on extremities) to prevent tearing of the skin (Baranoski et al., 2016; Fumarola et al., 2020; Kelly-O'Flynn et al., 2020).

Community-Based Care Considerations

- Patients may shower to clean the wound before dressing changes in the community; patients should avoid using perfumed soaps, body wash, or antiseptics or soaps and instead use pH neutral shower and bath skin cleansers/emollients (Brown, 2018; Milne, 2019).
- Saline solution can be prepared at home by combining 1 teaspoon of noniodized salt with 1 quart of distilled water and stirring until the salt is completely dissolved (Baranoski & Ayello, 2020). This solution can be kept in a tightly covered glass or plastic container for up to 1 week at room temperature (Baranoski & Ayello, 2020).

Skill 33-3 Performing Irrigation of a Wound

DELEGATION CONSIDERATIONS

Irrigation of a wound and procedures requiring the use of a sterile field and other sterile items are not delegated to assistive personnel (AP). Depending on the state's nurse practice act and the organization's policies and procedures, these procedures may be delegated to licensed practical/vocational nurses (LPN/LVNs). The decision to delegate must be based on careful analysis of the patient's needs and circumstances as well as the qualifications of the person to whom the task is being delegated. Refer to the Delegation Guidelines in Appendix A.

EQUIPMENT

- An 18- to 19-gauge needle/angiocath and 30- to 35-mL syringe or a commercial cleanser packaged in a pressurized container (Baranoski & Ayello, 2020, p. 152; McLain & Moore, 2021; WOCN, 2016)
- Sterile irrigation solution as prescribed, warmed to body temperature, commonly 0.9% normal saline solution or other solution as prescribed
- Alternatively, irrigation solution may be packaged in individual, single-use syringe
- Plastic bag or other waste container to dispose of soiled dressings
- Sterile gloves
- Sterile drape (may be optional)
- Clean, disposable gloves
- Moisture-proof gown; mask, and eye protection or face shield
- Waterproof pad and bath blanket
- Bath blanket or other linens for draping patient
- Additional PPE, as indicated
- Additional dressings and supplies needed or required based on the wound dressing/care prescribed for the patient

IMPLEMENTATION

ACTION	RATIONALE
1. Review the patient's health record for prescribed wound care or the plan of care related to wound care. Gather necessary supplies.	Reviewing the health record and care plan validates the correct patient and correct procedure. Preparation promotes efficient time management and an organized approach to the task.
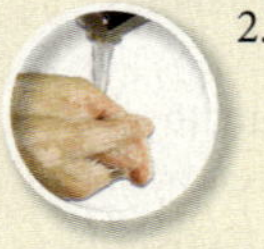 2. Perform hand hygiene and put on PPE, if indicated.	Hand hygiene and PPE prevent the spread of microorganisms. PPE is required based on transmission precautions.
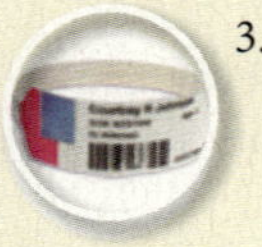 3. Identify the patient.	Identifying the patient ensures the right patient receives the intervention and helps prevent errors.
4. Assemble equipment on the overbed table or other surface within reach.	Organization facilitates performance of the task.
5. Close the curtains around the bed and close the door to the room if possible. Explain what you are going to do and why you are going to do it to the patient.	This ensures the patient's privacy. Explanation relieves anxiety and facilitates engagement.

ACTION	RATIONALE
6. Assess the patient for possible need for nonpharmacologic pain-reducing interventions or analgesic medication before wound care and/or dressing change. Administer appropriate prescribed analgesic. Allow enough time for the analgesic to achieve its effectiveness before beginning the procedure.	Pain is a subjective experience influenced by past experience. Wound care and dressing changes may cause pain for some patients.
7. Place a waste receptacle or bag at a convenient location for use during the procedure.	Having a waste container handy means the soiled dressing may be discarded easily, without the spread of microorganisms.
8. Adjust the bed to a comfortable working height (VHACEOSH, 2016).	Having the bed at the proper height prevents back and muscle strain.
9. Assist the patient to a comfortable position that provides easy access to the wound area. Position the patient so the irrigation solution will flow from the clean end of the wound toward the dirtier end or top to bottom. Use the bath blanket to cover any exposed area other than the wound. Place a waterproof pad under the wound site.	Patient positioning and the use of a bath blanket provide for comfort and warmth. Gravity directs the flow of liquid from the least contaminated to the most contaminated area. Waterproof pad protects underlying surfaces.
10. Put on a gown, mask, and eye protection or face shield.	Using PPE, such as gowns, masks, and eye protection, is part of *Standard Precautions.* A gown protects clothes from contamination should splashing occur. Appropriate personal protective equipment, including a mask and eye protection or face shield is essential when irrigating a wound with any degree of pressure (WOCN, 2016).
11. Check the position of drains, tubes, or other adjuncts before removing the dressing. Put on clean, disposable gloves and loosen the tape on the old dressings by removing in the direction of hair growth and the use of a push–pull method (see Figure 1, Skill 33-2) (Fumarola et al., 2020). Push–pull method: lift a corner of the dressing away from the skin, then gently push the skin away from the dressing/adhesive (Fumarola et al., 2020). Continue moving fingers of the opposite hand to support the skin as the product is removed (Fumarola et al., 2020). Once all adhesive is loosened from the skin, carefully lift dressing from the surrounding skin to prevent medical adhesive-related skin injury (MARSI). Remove the sides/edges first, then the center. If the patient is at increased risk for MARSI, requires repeated application or removal of adhesive devices, or there is resistance, use an adhesive remover (Barton, 2020; Fumarola et al., 2020; Kelly-O'Flynn et al., 2020).	Checking ensures that a drain is not removed accidentally if one is present. Gloves protect the nurse from contaminated dressings and prevent the spread of microorganisms. Removal of the tape in the direction of hair growth minimizes trauma to the skin (Fumarola et al., 2020). The use of adhesive remover allows for the easy, rapid, and painless removal without the associated problems of skin stripping and helps reduce patient discomfort (Barton, 2020; Fumarola et al., 2020; Kelly-O'Flynn et al., 2020).
12. Carefully remove the soiled dressings. If any part of the dressing sticks to the underlying skin, use small amounts of sterile saline to help loosen and remove it.	Cautious removal of the dressing is more comfortable for the patient and ensures that any drain present is not removed. Sterile saline moistens the dressing for easier removal and minimizes damage and pain.
13. After removing the dressing, note the presence, amount, type, color, and odor of any drainage on the dressings. Place soiled dressings in the appropriate waste receptacle.	The presence of drainage should be documented. Proper disposal of soiled dressings and used gloves prevents the spread of microorganisms.
14. Assess the wound for appearance, stage, presence of eschar, granulation tissue, epithelialization, undermining, tunneling, necrosis, sinus tract, and drainage. Assess the appearance of the surrounding tissue. Measure the wound.	This information provides evidence about the wound healing process and/or the presence of infection.
15. Remove your gloves and put them in the receptacle. Perform hand hygiene.	Discarding gloves prevents the spread of microorganisms. Hand hygiene prevents the spread of microorganisms.

(continued on page 1210)

Skill 33-3 Performing Irrigation of a Wound *(continued)*

ACTION	RATIONALE
16. Set up a sterile field, if indicated, and wound cleaning and irrigation supplies. Pour warmed sterile irrigating solution into the sterile container (based on supplies in use). Moisten gauze for cleaning the periwound skin. Put on the sterile gloves. Alternatively, clean gloves (clean technique) may be used when cleaning a chronic wound or pressure injury.	Using warmed solution prevents chilling the patient and may minimize patient discomfort. Aseptic technique should be used to change dressings for surgical wounds and in the acute clinical setting, to reduce the risk of transfer of pathogens, likely to be present in an acute care setting, to the wound (Brown, 2018). Clean technique is appropriate for cleaning chronic wounds, wounds in the home, or pressure injuries (Baranoski & Ayello, 2020; EPUAP, NPIAP, & PPPIA, 2019a).
17. Position the sterile basin below the wound to collect the irrigation fluid.	Patient and bed linens are protected from contaminated fluid.
18. Fill the irrigation syringe with solution (Figure 1). Alternatively, irrigation solution may be packaged in individual, single-use syringe; remove cap on syringe. Using your nondominant hand, gently apply pressure to the basin against the skin below the wound to form a seal with the skin (Figure 2).	The solution will collect in the basin and prevent the irrigant from running down the skin. Patient and bed linens are protected from contaminated fluid.

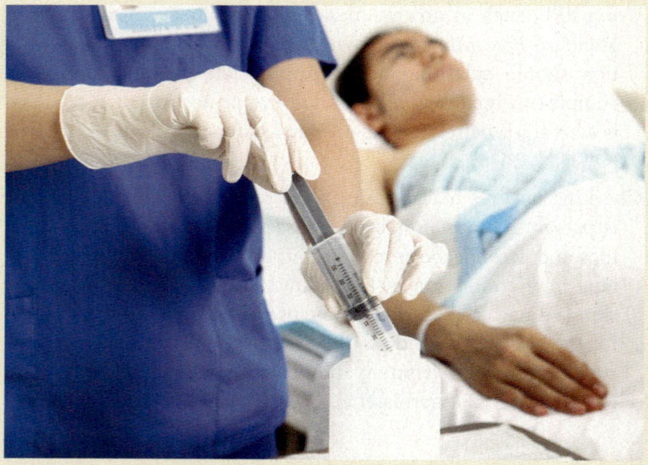

FIGURE 1. Drawing up sterile solution from sterile container into irrigation syringe.

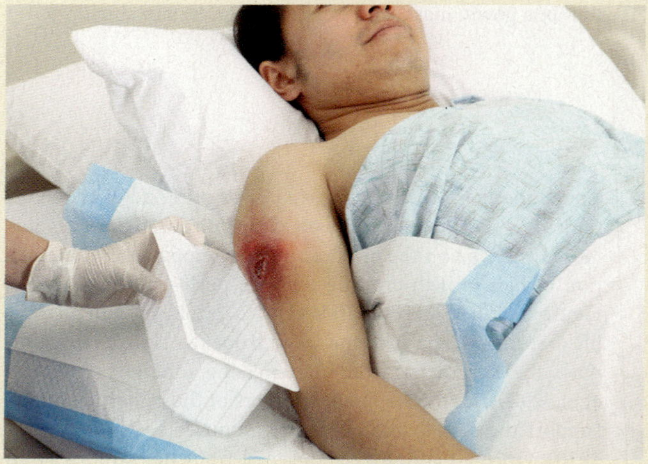

FIGURE 2. Applying pressure to basin to form seal.

ACTION	RATIONALE
19. Using either a pulsatile or continuous flow pattern, direct a stream of solution into the wound from top to bottom (Figure 3). Flush all wound areas.	The wound irrigating fluid stream can be delivered in either a pulsatile or continuous flow pattern (Baranoski & Ayello, 2020). Directing flow from top to bottom ensures that a previously cleaned area is not contaminated again.

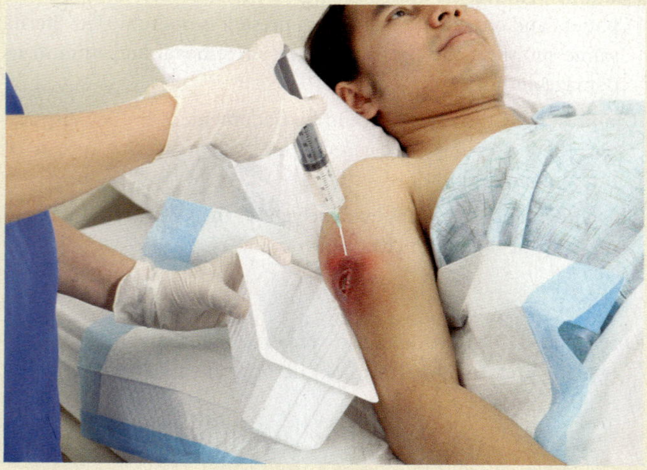

FIGURE 3. Irrigating wound with a stream of solution. Solution drains into collection container.

ACTION	RATIONALE
20. Watch for the solution to flow smoothly and evenly. When the solution from the wound flows out clear, discontinue irrigation.	Irrigation removes exudate and debris.
21. Once the wound is cleaned, clean the skin surrounding the wound and then dry the skin surrounding the wound (Figure 4). (Refer to Steps 18 and 19, Skill 33-2.)	Excess moisture on healthy skin increases risk for moisture-associated skin damage and interferes with proper adhesion of securement of dressings.
22. If a drain is in use at the wound location, clean around the drain. Refer to Skills 33-4 and 33-5.	Cleaning the insertion site helps prevent infection.
23. Remove gloves and perform hand hygiene.	Proper disposal of used gloves and hand hygiene prevent the spread of microorganisms.
24. Redress the wound, applying any topical medications, foams, gels, and/or gauze to the wound (Figure 5) and based on type of dressing prescribed or in use. (Refer to Skill 33-2 for general guidelines.)	Provides appropriate wound care to support plan of care.

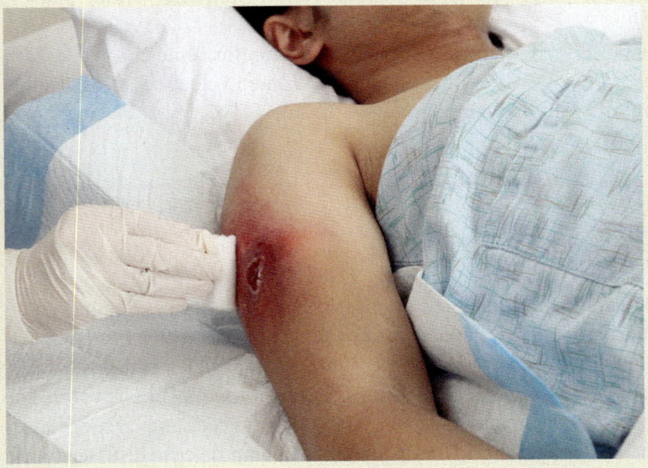

FIGURE 4. Drying around wound, not in wound, with gauze pad.

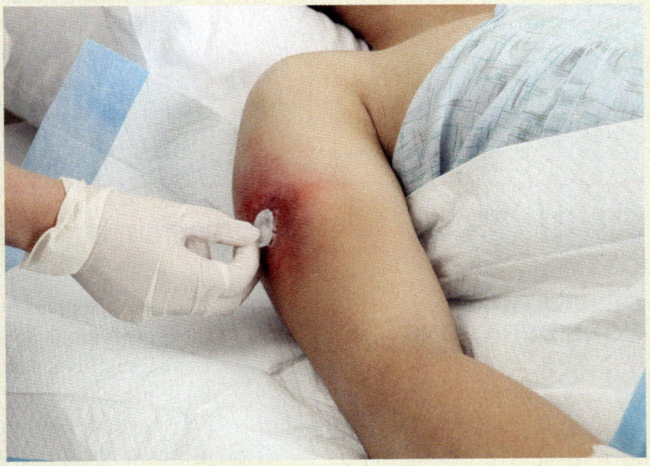

FIGURE 5. Applying wound contact material.

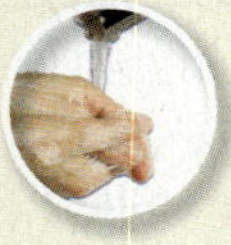

ACTION	RATIONALE
25. Remove PPE, if used. Perform hand hygiene.	Proper removal of PPE reduces the risk for infection transmission and contamination of other items. Hand hygiene prevents the spread of microorganisms.
26. Check all wound dressings at least every shift. More frequent checks may be needed if the wound is more complex.	Checking dressings ensures the assessment of changes in patient condition and timely intervention to prevent complications.

DOCUMENTATION

Guidelines

Document the location of the wound and that the dressing was removed. Record your assessment of the wound, including evidence of granulation tissue, presence of necrotic tissue, stage (if pressure injury), and characteristics of drainage. Include the appearance of the surrounding skin. Document the irrigation of the wound and solution used. Record the type of dressing that was applied. Note pertinent patient and family/caregiver education and any patient reaction to this procedure, including patient's pain level and effectiveness of nonpharmacologic interventions or analgesia if administered.

Sample Documentation

3/5/25 1700 Dressing removed from left outer heel area. Minimal serosanguineous drainage noted on dressings. Wound 4 cm × 5 cm × 2 cm, pink, with granulation tissue evident. Surrounding skin tone consistent with patient's skin, no edema or redness noted. Irrigated with normal saline and hydrogel dressing applied.

—J. Lark, RN

(continued on page 1212)

Skill 33-3 Performing Irrigation of a Wound *(continued)*

DEVELOPING CLINICAL REASONING AND CLINICAL JUDGMENT

UNEXPECTED SITUATIONS AND ASSOCIATED INTERVENTIONS

- *Patient experiences pain when the wound irrigation is begun:* Stop the procedure and administer an analgesic, as prescribed. Obtain new sterile supplies and begin the procedure after an appropriate amount of time has elapsed to allow the analgesic to begin working. Note the patient's pain on the plan of care so that pain medication can be given before future wound treatments.
- *During the wound irrigation, the nurse notes bleeding from the wound. This has not been documented as happening with previous irrigations:* Stop the procedure. Assess the patient for other symptoms. Obtain vital signs. Report the findings to the health care team and document the event in the patient's record.

SPECIAL CONSIDERATIONS

- Optimum and timely wound healing are supported by adequate nutrition and hydration (Dudek, 2018; EPUAP, NPIAP, & PPPIA, 2019a; Stuart, 2020). Collaborate with the registered dietician and dietary staff to develop an individualized nutrition intervention plan for the patient.
- A whirlpool bath may be prescribed as an alternative to irrigation for some chronic wounds (Baranoski & Ayello, 2020). The wound should not come in close contact with the water jets in the whirlpool to avoid tissue injury.

Skill 33-4 Caring for a Jackson-Pratt Drain

DELEGATION CONSIDERATIONS

Care for a JP drain insertion site is not delegated to assistive personnel (AP). Depending on the organization's policies and procedures, the drain may be emptied and reconstituted by AP. Depending on the state's nurse practice act and the organization's policies and procedures, these procedures may be delegated to licensed practical/vocational nurses (LPN/LVNs). The decision to delegate must be based on careful analysis of the patient's needs and circumstances as well as the qualifications of the person to whom the task is being delegated. Refer to the Delegation Guidelines in Appendix A.

EQUIPMENT

- Graduated container for measuring drainage
- Clean, disposable gloves
- Additional PPE, as indicated
- Cleansing solution, usually sterile normal saline
- Sterile gauze pads
- Skin protectant/barrier wipes
- Sterile drain sponges
- Sterile gloves
- Sterile cotton-tipped applicators, if appropriate
- Sterile container to hold cleaning solution
- Plastic bag or other appropriate waste container for soiled dressings
- Waterproof pad and bath blanket
- Additional dressings and supplies needed or as required for prescribed wound care

IMPLEMENTATION

ACTION	RATIONALE
1. Review the patient's health record for prescribed wound care or the plan of care related to wound/drain care. Gather necessary supplies.	Reviewing the health record and care plan validates the correct patient and correct procedure. Preparation promotes efficient time management and organized approach to the task.
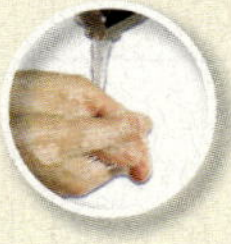 2. Perform hand hygiene and put on PPE, if indicated.	Hand hygiene and PPE prevent the spread of microorganisms. PPE is required based on transmission precautions.
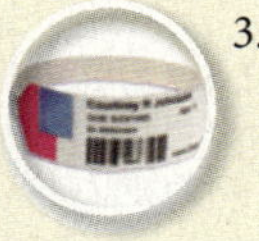 3. Identify the patient.	Identifying the patient ensures the right patient receives the intervention and helps prevent errors.

ACTION	RATIONALE
4. Assemble equipment on the overbed table or other surface within reach.	Organization facilitates performance of the task.
5. Close the curtains around the bed and close the door to the room, if possible. Explain what you are going to do and why you are going to do it to the patient.	This ensures the patient's privacy. Explanation relieves anxiety and facilitates engagement.
6. Assess the patient for possible need for nonpharmacologic pain-reducing interventions or analgesic medication before wound care dressing change. Administer appropriate prescribed analgesic. Allow enough time for the analgesic to achieve its effectiveness before beginning the procedure.	Pain is a subjective experience influenced by past experience. Wound care and dressing changes may cause pain for some patients.
7. Place a waste receptacle at a convenient location for use during the procedure.	Having a waste container handy means that the soiled dressing may be discarded easily, without the spread of microorganisms.
8. Adjust the bed to a comfortable working height (VHACEOSH, 2016).	Having the bed at the proper height prevents back and muscle strain.
9. Assist the patient to a comfortable position that provides easy access to the drain and/or wound area. Use a bath blanket to cover any exposed area other than the drain. Place a waterproof pad under the drain site.	Patient positioning and the use of a bath blanket provide for comfort and warmth. Waterproof pad protects underlying surfaces.
Emptying Drainage	
10. Put on gloves; put on mask or face shield, as indicated.	Gloves prevent the spread of microorganisms; mask reduces the risk of transmission should splashing occur.
11. Using sterile technique, open a gauze pad, making a sterile field with the outer wrapper.	Using sterile technique deters the spread of microorganisms.
12. Place the graduated collection container under the drain outlet. Without contaminating the outlet valve, pull off the cap. The chamber will expand completely as it draws in air. **Empty the chamber's contents completely into the container (Figure 1). Use the gauze pad to wipe the outlet. With one hand, fully compress the chamber along the long axis, side to side** (Mamuyac et al., 2019), **and replace the cap with your other hand (Figure 2).**	Emptying the drainage allows for accurate measurement. Cleaning the outlet reduces the risk of contamination and helps prevent the spread of microorganisms. Compressing the chamber along the long axis, side to side, reestablishes the suction. And generates higher negative pressure compared to the bottom-up methods (Mamuyac et al., 2019).

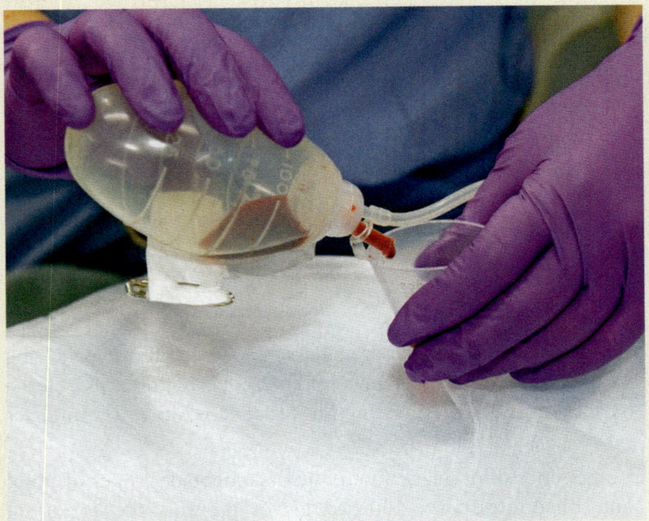

FIGURE 1. Emptying contents of Jackson-Pratt drain into collection container.

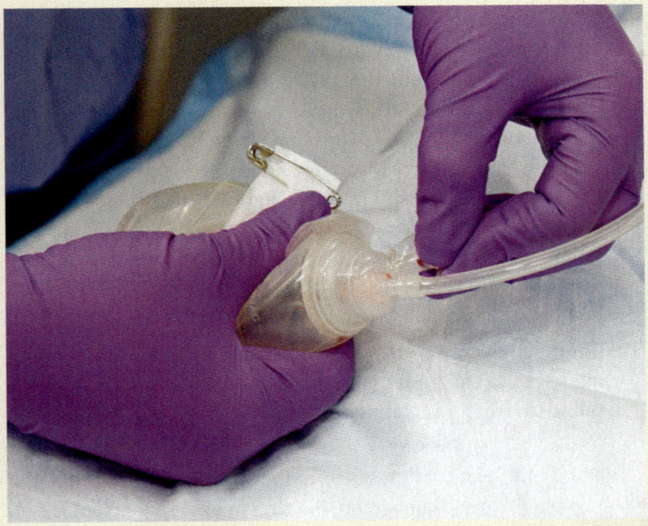

FIGURE 2. Compressing Jackson-Pratt drain and replacing cap.

(continued on page 1214)

Skill 33-4 Caring for a Jackson-Pratt Drain *(continued)*

ACTION	RATIONALE
13. Check the patency of the equipment. Bulb should remain compressed (Figure 3). **Check that the tubing is free from twists and kinks.**	Compressed chamber establishes suction. Patent, untwisted, or unkinked tubing promotes appropriate wound drainage.

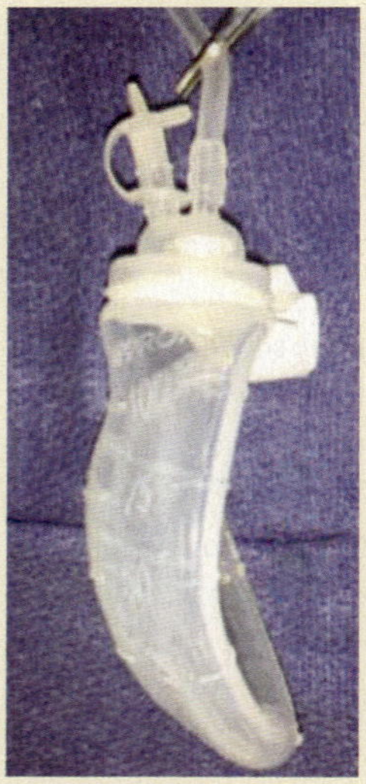

FIGURE 3. Compressed drain bulb.

ACTION	RATIONALE
14. Carefully measure and record the character, color, and amount of the drainage. Discard the drainage according to facility policy.	Documentation promotes continuity of care and communication. Appropriate disposal of biohazard material reduces the risk for microorganism transmission.
15. Remove gloves. Perform hand hygiene.	Removal of gloves and hand hygiene prevents the transmission of microorganisms.

Cleaning the Drain Site

ACTION	RATIONALE
16. Put on gloves. Check the position of the drain or drains before removing the dressing. Loosen the tape on the old dressings by removing in the direction of hair growth and the use of a push–pull method (Fumarola et al., 2020). Push–pull method: lift a corner of the dressing away from the skin, and then gently push the skin down and away from the dressing/adhesive (Fumarola et al., 2020). Continue moving fingers of the opposite hand to support the skin as the product is removed (Fumarola et al., 2020). Once all adhesive is loosened from the skin, carefully lift dressing from the surrounding skin to prevent medical adhesive–related skin injury (MARSI). Remove the sides/edges first, then the center. If the patient is at increased risk for MARSI, requires repeated application or removal of adhesive devices, or there is resistance, use an adhesive remover (Barton, 2020; Fumarola et al., 2020; Kelly-O'Flynn et al., 2020).	Gloves protect the nurse from contaminated dressings and prevent the spread of microorganisms. Dressing protects the site. Checking ensures that a drain is not removed accidentally. Removal of the tape in the direction of hair growth minimizes trauma to the skin (Fumarola et al., 2020). Pushing the skin down and away from the adhesive reduces the risk for medical adhesive–related skin injury (MARSI) (Fumarola et al., 2020). The use of adhesive remover allows for the easy, rapid, and painless removal without the associated problems of skin stripping and helps reduce patient discomfort (Barton, 2020; Fumarola et al., 2020; Kelly-O'Flynn et al., 2020).
17. Carefully remove the soiled dressings. If any part of the dressing sticks to the underlying skin, use small amounts of sterile saline to help loosen and remove it.	Cautious removal of the dressing is more comfortable for the patient and ensures that any drain present is not removed. Sterile saline moistens the dressing for easier removal and minimizes damage and pain.
18. Note the presence, amount, type, color, and odor of any drainage on the dressings. Place soiled dressings in the appropriate waste receptacle. Remove your gloves and perform hand hygiene.	The presence of drainage should be documented. Proper disposal of soiled dressings and used gloves prevents the spread of microorganisms. Hand hygiene prevents the transmission of microorganisms.

ACTION	RATIONALE
19. Inspect the drain site for appearance and drainage. Assess if any pain is present. Check the status of sutures, adhesive closure strips, and staples, if present. Note any problems to include in your documentation.	The wound healing process and/or the presence of irritation or infection must be documented.
20. Remove gloves and perform hand hygiene.	Removal of gloves and performance of hand hygiene prevent transmission of microorganisms.
21. **Using sterile technique, prepare a sterile work area and open the needed supplies.** Refer to facility policy and prescribed interventions regarding use of a sterile approach to site care.	Supplies are within easy reach and sterility is maintained. A sterile dressing is usually maintained for 24 to 48 hours; the use of a dressing after this time depends on the site assessment and amount of drainage (Orth, 2018). The site may be treated as an additional surgical wound, but often these sites are left open to air 24 hours after surgery. Refer to facility policy and prescribed interventions regarding need for sterile approach to site care and use of dressing.
22. Open the sterile cleaning solution. Pour it into the basin. Add the gauze sponges.	Sterility of dressings and solution is maintained.
23. Put on sterile gloves. Alternatively, clean gloves (clean technique) may be used based on facility policy and care setting.	The use of sterile gloves maintains surgical asepsis and sterile technique and reduces the risk of microorganism transmission. Clean technique is appropriate for cleaning chronic wounds, wounds in the home, or pressure injuries (Baranoski & Ayello, 2020; EPUAP, NPIAP, & PPPIA, 2019a).
24. Cleanse the drain site with the cleaning solution. Use the forceps and the moistened gauze or cotton-tipped applicators. **Start at the drain insertion site, moving in a circular motion toward the periphery. Use each gauze sponge or applicator only once.** Discard and use new gauze/applicator if additional cleansing is needed.	Cleaning is done from the least to most contaminated area so that a previously cleaned area is not contaminated again.
25. Dry with new sterile gauze in the same manner. Apply skin protectant/barrier to the skin around the drain; extend out to include the area of skin that will be taped.	Drying prevents skin irritation. Skin barrier/protectant prevents skin irritation and excoriation from tape, adhesives, and wound drainage (Fumarola et al., 2020; Kelly-O'Flynn et al., 2020).
26. Place a pre-split drain sponge under the drain. Apply gauze pads or other cover dressing, such as a transparent dressing, as indicated by facility policy, over the drain. Secure the dressings with tape, as needed. Remove and discard gloves. Perform hand hygiene.	The gauze absorbs drainage and prevents the drainage from accumulating on the patient's skin. Transparent dressing, tape or other securing products keep the dressing in place. Proper disposal of gloves prevents the spread of microorganisms. Hand hygiene prevents the transmission of microorganisms.
27. Secure the drain tubing to the patient's skin using a tape or a commercial securement/stabilization device, allowing slack in the tubing to avoid excessive tension. **Be careful not to kink the tubing and ensure the collection bag remains below the drain site.** Label the dressing with date and time.	Securing the tubing prevents accidental dislodgement or movement and avoids excessive tension on tube. Kinked tubing could block drainage. Maintaining the drain collection bag remains below the drain site facilitates proper drainage. Recording date and time provides communication and demonstrates adherence to plan of care.
28. Alternatively, if the drain site is open to air, observe the sutures that secure the drain to the skin. Look for signs of pulling, tearing, swelling, or infection of the surrounding skin. Gently clean the sutures with the gauze pad moistened with normal saline. Dry with a new gauze pad. Apply skin protectant/barrier to the surrounding skin. Remove and discard gloves. Perform hand hygiene.	Early detection of problems leads to prompt intervention and prevents complications. Gentle cleaning and drying prevent the growth of microorganisms. Skin barrier/protectant prevents skin irritation and excoriation from tape, adhesives, and wound drainage (Fumarola et al., 2020; Kelly-O'Flynn et al., 2020). Proper removal of gloves prevents the spread of microorganisms. Hand hygiene prevents the transmission of microorganisms.

(continued on page 1216)

Skill 33-4 Caring for a Jackson-Pratt Drain *(continued)*

ACTION | **RATIONALE**

29. Remove all remaining equipment; place the patient in a comfortable position, with side rails up as indicated and bed in the lowest position.

Proper patient and bed positioning promotes safety and comfort.

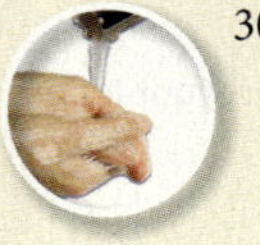

30. Remove additional PPE, if used. Perform hand hygiene.

Proper removal of PPE reduces the risk for infection transmission and contamination of other items. Hand hygiene prevents the spread of microorganisms.

31. Check drain status at least every 4 hours. Empty and reengage suction (compress device) when device is approximately 25% to 50% full (Mamuyac et al., 2019). Check all wound dressings at least every shift. More frequent checks may be needed if the wound is more complex, or dressings become saturated quickly.

Checking drain ensures proper functioning and early detection of problems. Emptying and compression ensure appropriate suction. Adequate suction pressure declines as bulb volume increases; bulb emptying should occur when the bulb is approximately 25% to 50% full for optimal accuracy and maintenance of adequate suction (Mamuyac et al., 2019; Yue et al., 2015). Checking dressings ensures the assessment of changes in patient condition and timely intervention to prevent complications.

DOCUMENTATION

Guidelines

Document the location of the drain, the assessment of the drain site, and patency of the drain. Note if sutures are intact. Document the presence and characteristics of drainage on the old dressing upon removal. Include the appearance of the surrounding skin. Document cleansing the drain site. Record any skin care and the dressing applied. Note that the drain was emptied and recompressed. Note pertinent patient and family/caregiver education and any patient reaction to this procedure, including patient's pain level and effectiveness of nonpharmacologic interventions or analgesia, if administered. Document the amount and characteristics of drainage obtained on the appropriate intake and output record.

Sample Documentation

2/7/25 2400 Right chest incision and drain open to air. Wound edges approximated, slight ecchymosis, no edema, redness, or drainage. Steri-Strips intact. JP drain patent and secured with suture. Exit site without edema, drainage, or redness; drain site cleaned with normal saline, and skin barrier applied. Drain emptied and recompressed. 40-mL sanguineous drainage recorded.

—C. White, RN

DEVELOPING CLINICAL REASONING AND CLINICAL JUDGMENT

UNEXPECTED SITUATIONS AND ASSOCIATED INTERVENTIONS

- *Patient has a JP drain in the right lower quadrant following abdominal surgery. The record indicates it has been draining serosanguineous fluid, 40 to 50 mL every shift. While performing your initial assessment, you note that the dressing around the drain site is saturated with serosanguineous secretions and there is minimal drainage in the collection chamber:* Inspect the tubing for kinks or obstruction. Assess the patient for changes in condition. Remove the dressing and assess the site. Often, if the tubing becomes blocked with a blood clot or drainage particles, the wound drainage will leak around the exit site of the drain. Cleanse the area and redress the site. Notify the health care team of the findings and document the event in the patient's record.
- *Patient calls you to the room and says, "I found this in the bed when I went to get up." He has his JP drain in his hand. It is completely removed from the patient:* Assess the patient for any new and abnormal signs or symptoms and assess the surgical site and drain site. Apply a sterile dressing the drain site. Notify the health care team of the findings and document the event in the patient's record.

SPECIAL CONSIDERATIONS

- A sterile dressing is usually maintained for 24 to 48 hours; the use of a dressing after this time depends on the site assessment and amount of drainage (Orth, 2018). The site may be treated as an additional surgical wound, but often these sites are left open to air 24 hours after surgery. Refer to facility policy and prescribed interventions regarding need for sterile approach to site care and use of dressing.
- Often patients have more than one JP drain. Number or letter the drains for easy identification. Record the drainage from each drain separately, identified by the number or letter, on the intake and output record.
- When the patient with a drain is ready to ambulate, empty and compress the drain before activity. Secure the drain to the patient's gown below the wound, making sure there is no tension on the drainage tubing. This removes excess drainage, maintains maximum suction, and avoids strain on the drain's suture line.
- Appropriate nutritional support is critical in achieving successful wound healing and may be overlooked (Quain & Khardori, 2015). Collaborate with the registered dietician and dietary staff to develop an individualized nutrition intervention plan for the patient (Baranoski & Ayello, 2020).

Community-Based Care Considerations

- Drain site care in the community setting is a clean, not sterile, procedure. Patients will use soap and water to clean the skin around the drain site (Memorial Sloan Kettering Cancer Center, 2019).

Skill 33-5 Caring for a Hemovac Drain

DELEGATION CONSIDERATIONS

Care for a Hemovac drain insertion site is not delegated to assistive personnel (AP). Depending on the organization's policies and procedures, the drain may be emptied and reconstituted by AP. Depending on the state's nurse practice act and the organization's policies and procedures, these procedures may be delegated to licensed practical/vocational nurses (LPN/LVNs). The decision to delegate must be based on careful analysis of the patient's needs and circumstances as well as the qualifications of the person to whom the task is being delegated. Refer to the Delegation Guidelines in Appendix A.

EQUIPMENT

- Graduated container for measuring drainage
- Clean, disposable gloves
- Additional PPE, as indicated
- Cleansing solution, usually sterile normal saline
- Sterile gauze pads
- Skin protectant/barrier wipes
- Sterile gloves
- Sterile cotton-tipped applicators, if appropriate
- Sterile container to hold cleaning solution
- Plastic bag or other appropriate waste container for soiled dressings
- Waterproof pad and bath blanket
- Additional dressings and supplies needed or as required for prescribed wound care

IMPLEMENTATION

ACTION	RATIONALE
1. Review the patient's health record for prescribed wound care or the plan of care related to wound/drain care. Gather necessary supplies.	Reviewing the health record and care plan validates the correct patient and correct procedure. Preparation promotes efficient time management and an organized approach to the task.
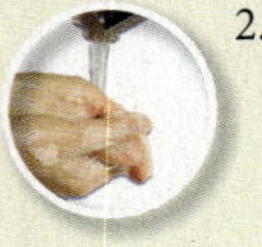 2. Perform hand hygiene and put on PPE, if indicated.	Hand hygiene and PPE prevent the spread of microorganisms. PPE is required based on transmission precautions.
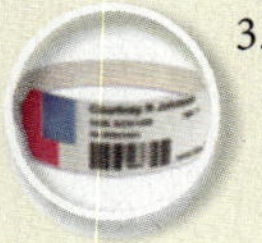 3. Identify the patient.	Identifying the patient ensures the right patient receives the intervention and helps prevent errors.

(continued on page 1218)

Skill 33-5 Caring for a Hemovac Drain *(continued)*

ACTION	RATIONALE
4. Assemble equipment on the overbed table or other surface within reach.	Organization facilitates performance of the task.
5. Close the curtains around the bed and close the door to the room, if possible. Explain what you are going to do and why you are going to do it to the patient.	This ensures the patient's privacy. Explanation relieves anxiety and facilitates engagement.
6. Assess the patient for possible need for nonpharmacologic pain-reducing interventions or analgesic medication before wound care dressing change. Administer appropriate prescribed analgesic. Allow enough time for analgesic to achieve its effectiveness before beginning the procedure.	Pain is a subjective experience influenced by past experience. Wound care and dressing changes may cause pain for some patients.
7. Place a waste receptacle at a convenient location for use during the procedure.	Having a waste container handy means that the soiled dressing may be discarded easily, without the spread of microorganisms.
8. Adjust the bed to a comfortable working height (VHACEOSH, 2016).	Having the bed at the proper height prevents back and muscle strain.
9. Assist the patient to a comfortable position that provides easy access to the drain and/or wound area. Use a bath blanket to cover any exposed area other than the drain. Place a waterproof pad under the drain site.	Patient positioning and the use of a bath blanket provide for comfort and warmth. Waterproof pad protects underlying surfaces.

Emptying Drainage

ACTION	RATIONALE
10. Put on gloves; put on mask or face shield, as indicated.	Gloves prevent the spread of microorganisms; mask reduces the risk of transmission should splashing occur.
11. Using sterile technique, open a gauze pad, making a sterile field with the outer wrapper.	Using sterile technique deters the spread of microorganisms.
12. Place the graduated collection container under the drain outlet. **Without contaminating the outlet, pull off the cap.** The chamber will expand completely as it draws in air. **Empty the chamber's contents completely into the container (Figure 1). Use the gauze pad to wipe the outlet. Place the container or a clean, flat surface. Fully compress the chamber by pushing down on the top until it meets the bottom and is flat** (Wechter, 2020b). **Keep the device tightly compressed while you apply the cap (Figure 2).**	Emptying the drainage allows for accurate measurement. Cleaning the outlet reduces the risk of contamination and helps prevent the spread of microorganisms. Compressing the chamber reestablishes the suction.

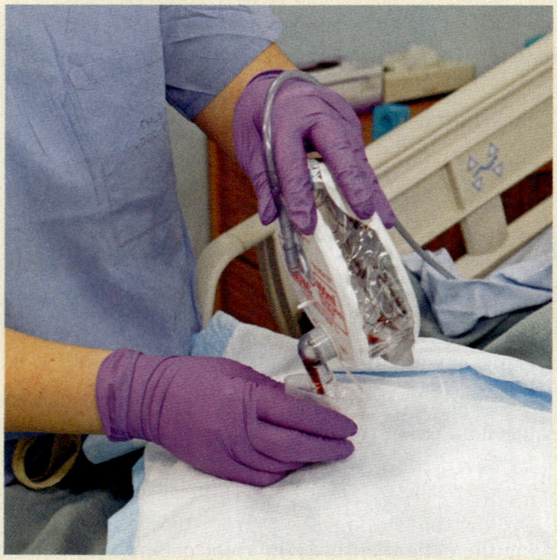

FIGURE 1. Emptying Hemovac drain into collection container.

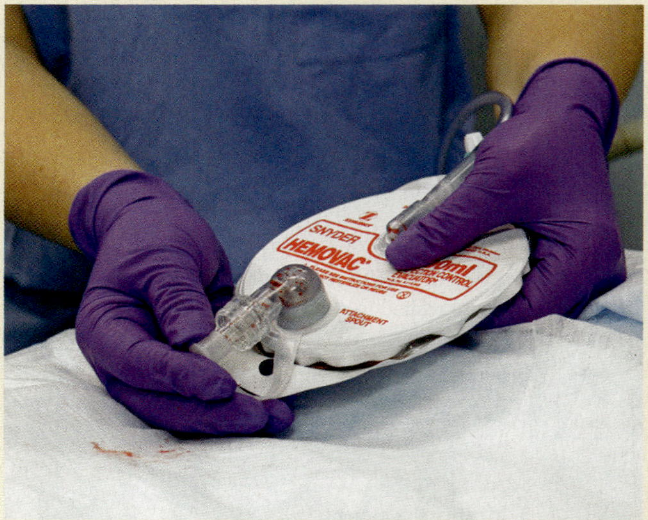

FIGURE 2. Compressing Hemovac and securing cap.

ACTION	RATIONALE
13. The device should remain compressed. Check the patency of the equipment. **Make sure the tubing is free from twists and kinks.**	Compressed device establishes suction. Patent, untwisted, or unkinked tubing promotes appropriate drainage from the wound.
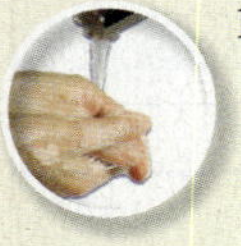 14. Carefully measure and record the character, color, and amount of the drainage. Discard the drainage according to facility policy. Remove gloves. Perform hand hygiene.	Documentation promotes continuity of care and communication. Appropriate disposal of biohazard material reduces the risk for microorganism transmission. Proper disposal of gloves deters transmission of microorganisms. Hand hygiene prevents the transmission of microorganisms.
Cleaning the Drain Site	
15. Put on gloves. If the drain site has a dressing, remove the dressing, assess and clean the site, and replace the dressing as outlined in Skill 33-4, Steps 16–26.	Dressing protects the site. Cleaning and drying sutures deters the growth of microorganisms.
16. Secure the drain tubing to the patient's skin using a tape or a commercial securement/stabilization device, allowing slack in the tubing to avoid excessive tension. **Be careful not to kink the tubing and ensure the collection bag remains below the drain site.** Label the dressing with date and time.	Securing the tubing prevents accidental dislodgement or movement and avoids excessive tension on tube. Kinked tubing could block drainage. Maintaining the drain collection bag remains below the drain site facilitates proper drainage. Recording date and time provides communication and demonstrates adherence to plan of care.
17. Alternatively, if the drain site is open to air, observe the sutures that secure the drain to the skin. Look for signs of pulling, tearing, swelling, or infection of the surrounding skin. Gently clean the sutures with the gauze pad moistened with normal saline. Dry with a new gauze pad. Apply skin protectant/barrier to the surrounding skin.	Early detection of problems leads to prompt intervention and prevents complications. Gentle cleaning and drying prevent the growth of microorganisms. Skin barrier/protectant prevents skin irritation and excoriation from tape, adhesives, and wound drainage (Fumarola et al., 2020; Kelly-O'Flynn et al., 2020).
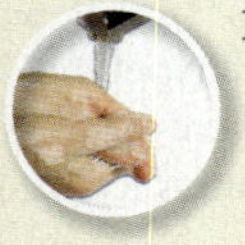 18. Remove and discard gloves. Perform hand hygiene.	Proper removal of gloves prevents the spread of microorganisms. Hand hygiene prevents the transmission of microorganisms.
19. Remove all remaining equipment; place the patient in a comfortable position, with side rails up as indicated and bed in the lowest position.	Proper patient and bed positioning promotes safety and comfort.
20. Remove additional PPE, if used. Perform hand hygiene.	Proper removal of PPE reduces the risk for infection transmission and contamination of other items. Hand hygiene prevents the spread of microorganisms.
21. Check drain status at least every 4 hours. Empty and reengage suction (compress device) every 2 to 4 hours (Bauldoff et al., 2020) and when it is half full of drainage or air. Check all wound dressings at least every shift. More frequent checks may be needed if the wound is more complex, or dressings become saturated quickly.	Checking the drain ensures proper functioning and early detection of problems. Emptying and compression ensure appropriate suction. Checking dressings ensures the assessment of changes in patient condition and timely intervention to prevent complications.

DOCUMENTATION

Guidelines

Document the location of the drain, the assessment of the drain site, and patency of the drain. Note if sutures are intact. Document the presence and characteristics of drainage on the old dressing upon removal. Include the appearance of the surrounding skin. Document cleansing of the drain site. Record any skin care and any dressing applied. Note that the drain was emptied and recompressed. Note pertinent patient and family/caregiver education and any patient reaction to this procedure, including patient's pain level and effectiveness of nonpharmacologic interventions or analgesia, if administered. Document the amount and characteristics of drainage obtained on the appropriate intake and output record.

(continued on page 1220)

Skill 33-5 Caring for a Hemovac Drain *(continued)*

Sample Documentation

> 1/18/25 1000 Hemovac drain in place at lateral aspect of left knee. Gauze dressing removed; no drainage noted on dressing. Suture intact; exit site slightly pink, without redness, edema, or drainage. Surrounding skin without edema, ecchymosis, or redness. Exit site and suture cleansed with normal saline and redressed with dry gauze dressing. Hemovac emptied of 90-mL sanguineous secretions and recompressed.
>
> *—A. Smith, RN*

DEVELOPING CLINICAL REASONING AND CLINICAL JUDGMENT

UNEXPECTED SITUATIONS AND ASSOCIATED INTERVENTIONS

- *Patient has a Hemovac drain placed in the left knee following surgery. The record indicates it has been draining serosanguineous secretions, 40 to 50 mL every shift. While performing your initial assessment, you note that the collection chamber is completely expanded. The nurse empties the device and compresses to resume suction. A short time later, the nurse observes that the chamber is completely expanded again:* Inspect the tubing for kinks or obstruction. Inspect the device, looking for breaks in the integrity of the chamber. Make sure the cap is in place and closed. Assess the patient for changes in condition. Remove the dressing and assess the site. Make sure the drainage tubing has not advanced out of the wound, exposing any of the perforations in the tubing. If you are not successful in maintaining the suction, notify the health care team of the findings and interventions and document the event in the patient's record.

SPECIAL CONSIDERATIONS

- A sterile dressing is usually maintained for 24 to 48 hours; the use of a dressing after this time depends on the site assessment and amount of drainage (Orth, 2018). The site may be treated as an additional surgical wound, but often these sites are left open to air 24 hours after surgery. Refer to facility policy and prescribed interventions regarding need for sterile approach to site care and use of dressing.
- When the patient with a drain is ready to ambulate, empty and compress the drain before activity. Secure the drain to the patient's gown below the wound, making sure there is no tension on the drainage tubing. This removes excess drainage, maintains maximum suction, and avoids strain on the drain's suture line.
- Appropriate nutritional support is critical in achieving successful wound healing and may be overlooked (Quain & Khardori, 2015). Collaborate with the registered dietician and dietary staff to develop an individualized nutrition intervention plan for the patient (Baranoski & Ayello, 2020).

Community-Based Care Considerations

- Drain site care in the community setting is a clean, not sterile, procedure. Patients will use soap and water to clean the skin around the drain site (Memorial Sloan Kettering Cancer Center, 2019).

Skill 33-6 Collecting a Wound Culture

DELEGATION CONSIDERATIONS

The collection of a wound culture is not delegated to assistive personnel (AP). Depending on the state's nurse practice act and the organization's policies and procedures, the collection of a wound culture may be delegated to licensed practical/vocational nurses (LPN/LVNs). The decision to delegate must be based on careful analysis of the patient's needs and circumstances as well as the qualifications of the person to whom the task is being delegated. Refer to the Delegation Guidelines in Appendix A.

EQUIPMENT

- A sterile culture kit (aerobic and/or anaerobic) with swab, or a culture tube with individual sterile swabs
- Sterile gloves
- Clean, disposable gloves
- Additional PPE, as indicated
- Plastic bag or appropriate waste receptacle
- Patient label for the sample tube
- Biohazard specimen bag
- Bath blanket (if necessary to drape the patient)
- Supplies to clean the wound with saline without preservatives (Baranoski & Ayello, 2020) and reapply the prescribed dressing after obtaining the culture. (Refer to Skills 33-2 and 33-3.)

IMPLEMENTATION

ACTION	RATIONALE
1. Review the patient's health record for prescribed intervention for obtaining a wound culture. Gather necessary supplies. If possible, obtain the wound culture prior to the start of antimicrobial therapy.	Reviewing the health record and care plan validates the correct patient and correct procedure. Preparation promotes efficient time management and an organized approach to the task. Antimicrobial therapy interferes with microorganism growth, so it is important to obtain the wound culture prior to the start of antimicrobial therapy, if possible (Huddleston Cross, 2014; Fischbach & Fischbach, 2018). If obtained after the initiation of antimicrobial therapy, provide information about the name of the antimicrobial, dose, and the date the therapy was initiated to the lab to aid in accurate interpretation of the culture findings (Baranoski & Ayello, 2020).
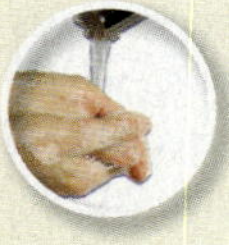 2. Perform hand hygiene and put on PPE, if indicated.	Hand hygiene and PPE prevent the spread of microorganisms. PPE is required based on transmission precautions.
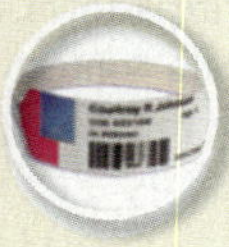 3. Identify the patient.	Identifying the patient ensures the right patient receives the intervention and helps prevent errors.
4. Assemble equipment on the overbed table or other surface within reach.	Organization facilitates performance of the task.
5. Close the curtains around the bed and close the door to the room, if possible. Explain to the patient what you are going to do and why you are going to do it.	This ensures the patient's privacy. Explanation relieves anxiety and facilitates engagement.
6. Assess the patient for possible need for nonpharmacologic pain-reducing interventions or analgesic medication before obtaining the wound culture. Administer appropriate prescribed analgesic. Allow enough time for the analgesic to achieve its effectiveness before beginning the procedure.	Pain is a subjective experience influenced by past experience. Wound care and dressing changes may cause pain for some patients.
7. Place an appropriate waste receptacle within easy reach for use during the procedure.	Having the waste container handy means that soiled materials may be discarded easily, without the spread of microorganisms.
8. Adjust the bed to a comfortable working height (VHACEOSH, 2016).	Having the bed at the proper height prevents back and muscle strain.
9. Assist the patient to a comfortable position that provides easy access to the wound. If necessary, drape the patient with the bath blanket to expose only the wound area. Place a waterproof pad under the wound site. Check the culture label against the patient's identification bracelet (Figure 1).	Patient positioning and the use of a bath blanket provide for comfort and warmth. Checking the culture label with the patient's identification ensures the correct patient and the correct procedure.

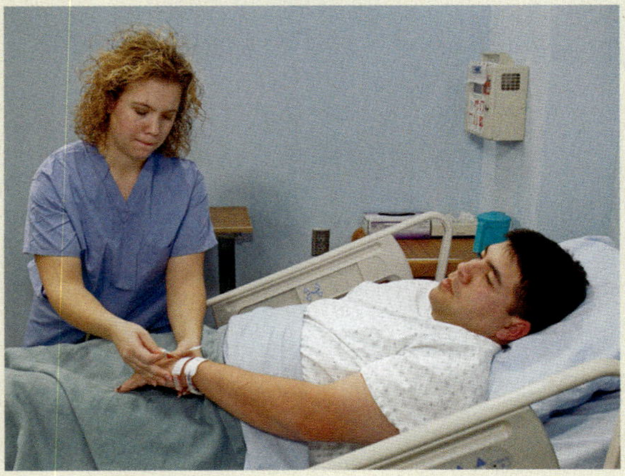

FIGURE 1. Checking culture label with the patient's identification band.

(*continued on page 1222*)

Skill 33-6 Collecting a Wound Culture *(continued)*

ACTION	RATIONALE
10. If there is a dressing in place on the wound, put on clean gloves and carefully remove the dressing. Refer to Skill 33-2. Note the presence, amount, type, color, and odor of any drainage on the dressings. Place soiled dressings in the appropriate waste receptacle.	Gloves protect the nurse from handling contaminated dressings. The dressing must be removed to allow access to the wound.
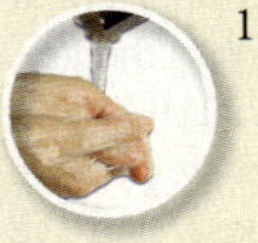 11. Remove gloves and perform hand hygiene.	Hand hygiene prevents the transmission of microorganisms.
12. Put on gloves. Assess and clean the wound, **using saline that has no preservative** (Baranoski & Ayello, 2020), as outlined in Skills 33-2 and 33-3.	Gloves prevent contact with blood and/or body fluids. This information provides evidence about the wound healing process and/or the presence of infection. Cleaning the wound removes wound exudate, topical therapies, and wound debris, which could introduce extraneous organisms into the collected specimen, resulting in inaccurate results (Baranoski & Ayello, 2020).
13. Dry the skin surrounding the wound with gauze. Put on clean gloves.	Excess moisture can contribute to skin irritation and breakdown. The use of a culture swab does not require immediate contact with the skin or wound, so clean gloves are appropriate to protect the nurse from contact with blood and/or body fluids.
14. Twist the cap to loosen the swab on the Culturette tube or open the separate swab(s) and remove the cap from the culture tube. **Keep the swab and inside of the culture tube(s) sterile (Figure 2).**	Supplies are ready to use and within easy reach, and aseptic technique is maintained.
15. If contact with the wound is necessary to separate wound margins to permit insertion of the swab deep into the wound, put a sterile glove on one hand to manipulate the wound margins. Clean gloves may be appropriate for contact with pressure injuries and chronic wounds.	If contact with the wound is necessary to collect the specimen, a sterile glove is necessary to prevent contamination of the wound. Clean technique may be appropriate for cleaning chronic wounds or pressure injuries (Baranoski & Ayello, 2020; EPUAP, NPIAP, & PPPIA, 2019a).
16. **Identify a 1-cm area of the wound that is free from necrotic tissue.** Carefully insert the swab into this area of clean viable tissue. **Press the swab to apply sufficient pressure to express fluid from the wound tissue and rotate the swab for 5 seconds** (Baranoski & Ayello, 2020). **Avoid touching the swab to intact skin at the wound edges (Figure 3).**	Cotton tip absorbs wound drainage. This technique (Levine technique) is considered to provide more accurate results and best practice for swab cultures (Baranoski & Ayello, 2020; WOCN, 2016). Contact with skin could introduce extraneous organisms into the collected specimen, resulting in inaccurate results.

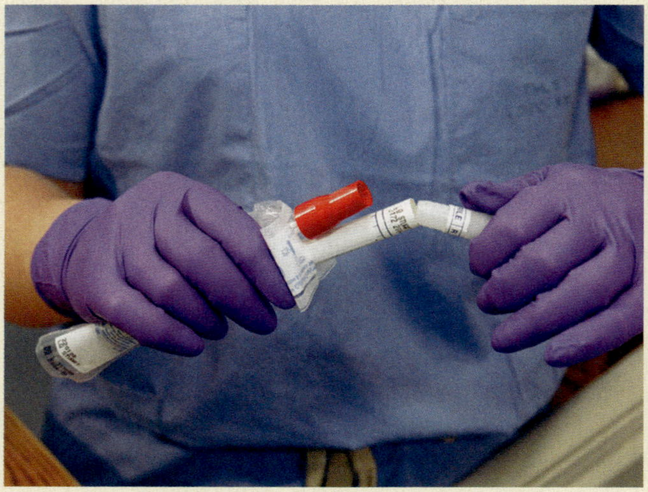

FIGURE 2. Removing cap from culture tube.

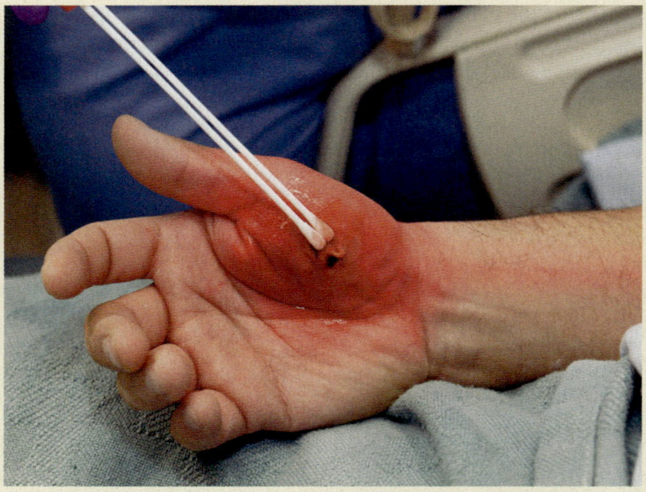

FIGURE 3. Rotating swab several times over wound surface.

ACTION

17. Place the swab back in the culture tube (Figure 4). **Do not touch the outside of the tube with the swab.** Secure the cap. Some swab containers have an ampule of medium at the bottom of the tube. It might be necessary to crush this ampule to activate. Follow the manufacturer's instructions for use.

Rationale: The outside of the container is protected from contamination with microorganisms, and the sample is not contaminated with organisms not in the wound. Surrounding the swab with culture medium is necessary for accurate culture results.

18. Use another swab if collecting a specimen from another area of the wound or site and repeat the procedure.

Rationale: Using another swab at a different site prevents cross-contamination of the wound.

19. Remove gloves and discard them accordingly. Perform hand hygiene.

Rationale: Removing gloves properly reduces the risk for infection transmission and contamination of other items. Hand hygiene prevents the transmission of microorganisms.

20. Put on gloves. Place a dressing on the wound, as appropriate, based on prescribed interventions and/or the plan of care. Refer to Skill 33-2. Remove gloves. Perform hand hygiene.

Rationale: Wound dressings protect, absorb drainage, provide a moist environment, and promote wound healing. Removing gloves and performing hand hygiene reduce the risk for transmission of microorganisms and contamination of other items.

21. After securing the dressing, label dressing with date and time. Remove all remaining equipment; place the patient in a comfortable position, with side rails up as indicated and bed in the lowest position.

Rationale: Recording date and time provides communication and demonstrates adherence to care plan. Proper patient and bed positioning promotes safety and comfort.

22. Label the specimen according to your institution's guidelines. Information included in addition to the patient's identification may include wound site, time the specimen was collected, any antimicrobials the patient is receiving, and the identity of the person who obtained the specimen (Baranoski & Ayello, 2020). Send or transport specimen to the laboratory in a biohazard bag immediately or within the optimal time from for transport as indicated by facility policy and guidelines (Figure 5).

Rationale: Proper labeling ensures proper identification of the specimen. Specimens must be sent to the laboratory immediately or within the optimal time from for transport as indicated by facility policy and guidelines to ensure accurate results (Baranoski & Ayello, 2020; Fischbach & Fischbach, 2018; WOCN, 2016).

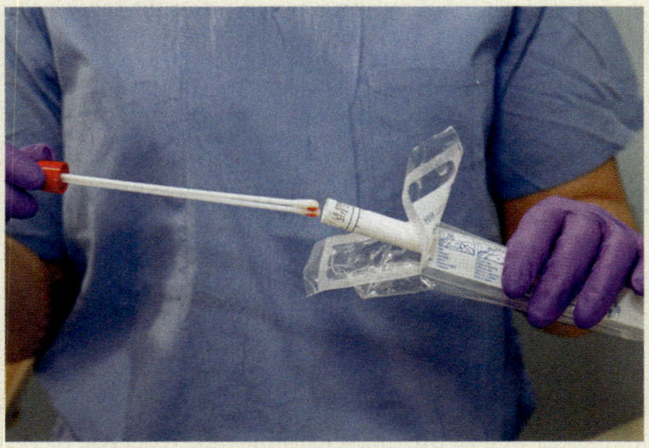

FIGURE 4. Placing swab in culture tube.

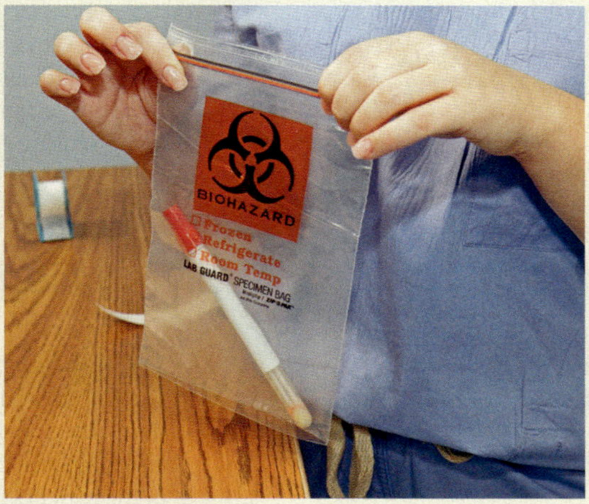

FIGURE 5. Labeled culture container in biohazard bag.

23. Remove PPE, if used. Perform hand hygiene.

Rationale: Proper removal of PPE reduces the risk for infection transmission and contamination of other items. Hand hygiene prevents the spread of microorganisms.

DOCUMENTATION

Guidelines

Document the location of the wound, the assessment of the wound, including the type of tissue present, presence of necrotic tissue, stage (if appropriate), and characteristics of drainage. Include the appearance of the surrounding skin. Document cleansing of the wound and the obtained culture. Record any skin care and/or dressing applied. Note pertinent patient and family/caregiver education and any patient reaction to this procedure, including patient's pain level and effectiveness of nonpharmacologic interventions or analgesia, if administered.

(continued on page 1224)

Skill 33-6 Collecting a Wound Culture *(continued)*

Sample Documentation

> 6/22/25 2100 Wound noted on patient's hand: 2 cm × 3 cm × 1 cm, red, tender, with purulent drainage present. Edges macerated, without erythema and tenderness. Wound cleaned with normal saline, culture obtained. Skin protectant/barrier applied to surrounding area, wound redressed with alginate, cover dressing, and roller gauze. Hand elevated. Culture labeled and sent to lab.
>
> *—J. Wentz, RN*

DEVELOPING CLINICAL REASONING AND CLINICAL JUDGMENT

UNEXPECTED SITUATIONS AND ASSOCIATED INTERVENTIONS

- *The nurse has inserted the culture swab into the patient's wound to obtain the specimen and realizes that the wound was not cleaned:* Discard this swab. Obtain the additional supplies needed to clean the wound according to facility policy and a new culture swab. Cleaning the wound removes wound exudate, topical therapies, and wound debris, which could introduce extraneous organisms into the collected specimen, resulting in inaccurate results (Baranoski & Ayello, 2020). Clean the wound using a using saline that has no preservative (Baranoski & Ayello, 2020) and then proceed to obtain the culture specimen.
- *As the nurse prepares to insert the culture swab into the wound, the nurse inadvertently touches the swab to the patient's bedclothes or other surface:* Discard this swab, obtain a new culture swab, and collect the specimen.

GENERAL CONSIDERATIONS

- Tissue biopsy is considered the "gold standard" of wound cultures; however, it and the aspiration technique are invasive and are performed by physicians and advanced practice professionals (Baranoski & Ayello, 2020; WOCN, 2016). Swab specimens are more commonly used because they are most easily collected, readily available, and may be collected by nurses in general practice (Baranoski & Ayello, 2020).
- Final culture results may take 24 to 72 hours depending on the method used and organism suspected; antimicrobial therapy based on the pathogens most commonly involved in a particular type of wound may be started immediately and changed if indicated when culture and sensitivity results are available (WOCN, 2016).

Skill 33-7 Applying Negative-Pressure Wound Therapy

DELEGATION CONSIDERATIONS

The application of negative pressure wound therapy is not delegated to assistive personnel (AP). Depending on the state's nurse practice act and the organization's policies and procedures, the application of negative pressure wound therapy may be delegated to licensed practical/vocational nurses (LPN/LVNs). The decision to delegate must be based on careful analysis of the patient's needs and circumstances as well as the qualifications of the person to whom the task is being delegated. Refer to the Delegation Guidelines in Appendix A.

EQUIPMENT

- Negative pressure unit
- Evacuation/collection canister (depending on specific system in use)
- Wound contact material, as indicated by wound care plan and device/materials in use
- Transparent adhesive drape
- Connection pad/tubing port
- Drainage tubing
- Skin protectant/barrier wipes
- Sterile gauze sponge
- An 18- to 19-gauge needle/angiocath and 30- to 35-mL syringe or a commercial cleanser packaged in a pressurized container (Baranoski & Ayello, 2020, p. 152; McLain & Moore, 2021; WOCN, 2016)
- Sterile irrigation solution as prescribed, warmed to body temperature, commonly 0.9% normal saline solution or other solution as prescribed
- Waste receptacle to dispose of contaminated materials
- Sterile gloves (two pairs)
- Sterile scissors
- Clean, disposable gloves
- Gown, mask, eye protection
- Additional PPE, as indicated
- Sterile scissors
- Waterproof pad and bath blanket

IMPLEMENTATION

ACTION	RATIONALE
1. Review the patient's health record for prescribed application of NPWT therapy, including the prescribed pressure setting for the device. Gather necessary supplies.	Reviewing the health record validates the correct patient and correct procedure. Preparation promotes efficient time management and an organized approach to the task.
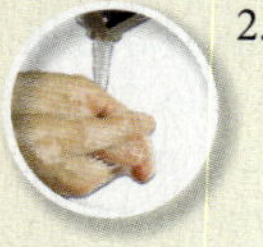 2. Perform hand hygiene and put on PPE, if indicated.	Hand hygiene and PPE prevent the spread of microorganisms. PPE is required based on transmission precautions.
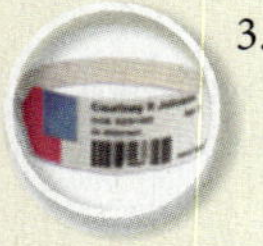 3. Identify the patient.	Identifying the patient ensures the right patient receives the intervention and helps prevent errors.
4. Assemble equipment on the overbed table or other surface within reach.	Organization facilitates performance of task.
5. Close the curtains around the bed and close the door to the room, if possible. Explain what you are going to do and why you are going to do it to the patient.	This ensures the patient's privacy. Explanation relieves anxiety and facilitates engagement.
6. Assess the patient for possible need for nonpharmacologic pain-reducing interventions or analgesic medication before wound care dressing change. Administer appropriate prescribed analgesic. Allow enough time for the analgesic to achieve its effectiveness before beginning the procedure.	Pain is a subjective experience influenced by past experience. Wound care and dressing changes may cause pain for some patients.
7. Adjust the bed to a comfortable working height (VHACEOSH, 2016).	Having the bed at the proper height prevents back and muscle strain.
8. Assist the patient to a comfortable position that provides easy access to the wound area. Position the patient so the cleaning/irrigation solution will flow from the clean end of the wound toward the dirty end. Expose the area and drape the patient with a bath blanket, if needed. Put a waterproof pad under the wound area.	Patient positioning and draping provide for comfort and warmth. Gravity directs the flow of liquid from the least contaminated to the most contaminated area. Waterproof pad protects the patient and the bed linens.
9. Have the disposal bag or waste receptacle within easy reach for use during the procedure.	Having a waste container handy allows for easy disposal of the soiled dressings and supplies, without the spread of microorganisms.
10. Using sterile technique, prepare a sterile field and add all the sterile supplies needed for the procedure to the field. Pour warmed, sterile irrigating solution into the sterile container, as indicated.	Proper preparation ensures that supplies are within easy reach and sterility is maintained. Warmed solution may result in less discomfort.
11. Put on a gown, mask, and eye protection.	The use of PPE is part of *Standard Precautions.* A gown protects your clothes from contamination if splashing should occur. Goggles protect mucous membranes of your eyes from contact with irrigant fluid.
12. If NPWT is currently in use, turn off the negative pressure unit. Consider turning off suction 5 to 10 minutes before dressing change to reduce pressure (Banasiewicz et al., 2019). Put on gloves. Loosen the tape on the old dressings by removing in the direction of hair growth and the use of a push–pull method (Fumarola et al., 2020). Push–pull method: lift a corner of the dressing away from the skin, and then gently push the skin down and away from the dressing/adhesive (Fumarola et al., 2020). Continue moving fingers of the opposite hand to support the skin as the product is removed (Fumarola et al., 2020). Once all adhesive is loosened from the skin, carefully lift dressing from the surrounding skin to prevent medical adhesive–related skin injury (MARSI). Remove the sides/edges first, then the center. If the patient is at increased risk for MARSI, requires repeated application or removal of adhesive devices, or there is resistance, use an adhesive remover (Banasiewicz et al., 2019; Barton, 2020; Fumarola et al., 2020; Kelly-O'Flynn et al., 2020).	Reduction in pressure reduces risk of pain associated with dressing removal (Banasiewicz et al., 2019). Gloves protect the nurse from contaminated dressings and prevent the spread of microorganisms. Removal of the tape in the direction of hair growth minimizes trauma to the skin (Fumarola et al., 2020). Pushing the skin down and away from the adhesive reduces the risk for medical adhesive–related skin injury (MARSI) (Fumarola et al., 2020). The use of adhesive remover allows for the easy, rapid, and painless removal without the associated problems of skin stripping and helps reduce patient discomfort (Banasiewicz et al., 2019; Barton, 2020; Fumarola et al., 2020; Kelly-O'Flynn et al., 2020).

(*continued on page 1226*)

Skill 33-7 Applying Negative-Pressure Wound Therapy *(continued)*

ACTION	RATIONALE
13. Carefully remove the soiled dressings. If any part of the dressing sticks to the underlying skin, use small amounts of sterile saline to help loosen and remove it.	Cautious removal of the dressing is more comfortable for the patient and ensures that any drain present is not removed. Sterile saline moistens the dressing for easier removal and minimizes damage and pain.
14. Note the presence, amount, type, color, and odor of any drainage on the dressings. **Note the number of pieces of wound contact material removed from the wound. Compare with the documented number from the previous dressing change.**	The presence and characteristics of drainage should be documented. All dressing materials must be removed from the wound bed during NPWT dressing changes (Baranoski & Ayello, 2020). Counting the number of pieces of wound contact material assures the removal of all foam that was placed during the previous dressing change (Schreiber, 2016).
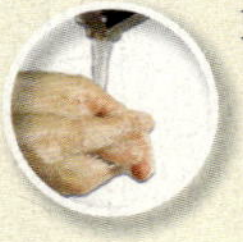 15. Discard the dressings in the receptacle. Remove your gloves and put them in the receptacle. Perform hand hygiene.	Proper disposal of dressings and used gloves prevents the spread of microorganisms. Hand hygiene prevents the transmission of microorganisms.
16. Put on sterile gloves. Using sterile technique, clean or irrigate the wound, based on wound care plan and prescribed wound care. Alternatively, clean gloves (clean technique) may be used when cleaning a chronic wound or pressure injury.	Aseptic technique maintains sterility of items to come in contact with wound. Cleaning and/or irrigation remove exudate and debris. Clean technique is appropriate for cleaning chronic wounds, wounds in the home, or pressure injuries (Baranoski & Ayello, 2020; EPUAP, NPIAP, & PPPIA, 2019a).
17. Clean the area around the wound with normal saline or prescribed skin cleanser. Dry the surrounding skin with a sterile gauze sponge.	Cleaning of skin removes debris and aids in adherence of dressing materials. Moisture provides a medium for the growth of microorganisms.
18. Assess the wound for appearance, stage, presence of eschar, granulation tissue, epithelialization, undermining, tunneling, necrosis, sinus tract, and drainage. Assess the appearance of the surrounding tissue. Measure the wound.	This information provides evidence about the wound healing process and/or the presence of infection.
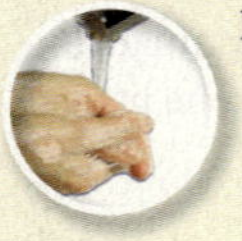 19. Remove gloves and perform hand hygiene.	Hand hygiene prevents the transmission of microorganisms.
20. Put on sterile gloves. **Wipe intact skin around the wound with a skin protectant/barrier wipe and allow it to dry.** Alternatively, clean gloves (clean technique) may be used when cleaning a chronic wound or pressure injury.	Aseptic technique maintains sterility of items to come in contact with wound. Skin barrier/protectant prevents skin irritation and excoriation from tape, adhesives, and wound drainage (Fumarola et al., 2020; Kelly-O'Flynn et al., 2020). Clean technique is appropriate for cleaning chronic wounds, wounds in the home, or pressure injuries (Baranoski & Ayello, 2020; EPUAP, NPIAP, & PPPIA, 2019a).
21. If the use of a wound contact layer (impregnated porous gauze or silicone adhesive contact layer) is indicated, use sterile scissors to cut the wound contact layer to fit the wound bed. Apply wound contact layer to the wound bed.	Impregnated porous gauze or silicone adhesive contact layer may be indicated, depending on wound filler material in use, to prevent adherence of wound filler to wound be to protect the wound bed (McNichol et al., 2022).
22. Fit the wound contact material to the shape of the wound. • If using foam wound contact material, use sterile scissors to cut the foam to the shape and measurement of the wound. **Do not cut foam over the wound.** More than one piece of foam may be necessary if the first piece is cut too small. Carefully place the foam in the wound (Figure 1). **Ensure foam-to-foam contact if more than one piece is required.** • **Note the number of pieces of wound filler placed in the wound.** • **Do not under- or overfill.**	Wound contact material should fill the wound, but not cover intact surrounding skin. Foam fragments may fall into the wound if cutting is performed over the wound. Foam-to-foam contact allows for even distribution of negative pressure. Recording the number of pieces of wound contact material aids in assuring the removal of all dressing material with next dressing change (Schreiber, 2016). Appropriate filling of wound is necessary to ensure safe and effective application of NPWT (Apelqvist et al., 2017; Schreiber, 2016).

ACTION

23. Trim and place the transparent adhesive drape or hydrocolloid to cover the wound contact material and an additional 3- to 5-cm border of intact periwound tissue (Figure 2). **Avoid stretching the transparent adhesive drape tight over the wound.**

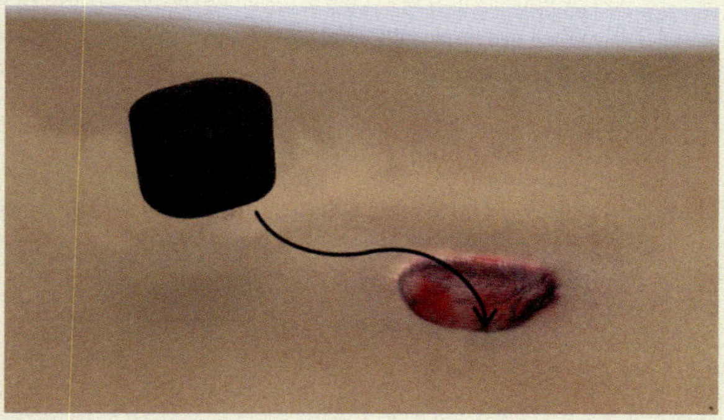

FIGURE 1. Cutting wound contact material (foam) to shape and measurement of wound. (*Source:* Used with permission. Courtesy of KCI, an Acelity Company.)

RATIONALE

The occlusive air-permeable adhesive drape or hydrocolloid provides a seal, allowing the application of the negative pressure. Tight stretching of transparent adhesive drape during application may cause periwound damage (Schreiber, 2016).

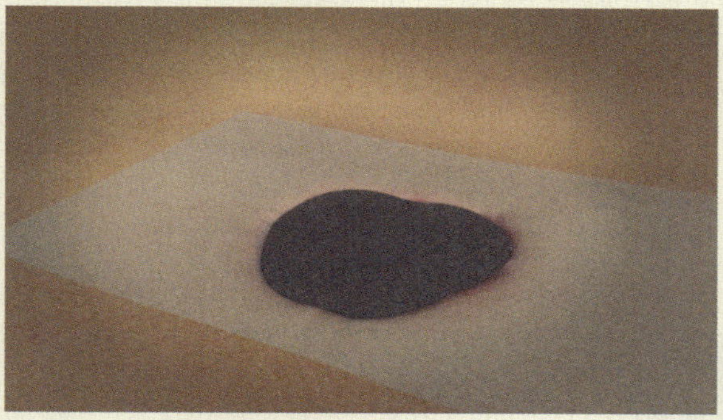

FIGURE 2. Placing transparent adhesive drape to cover the wound. (*Source:* Used with permission. Courtesy of KCI, an Acelity Company.)

24. Apply the connector pad/tubing port, if necessary, depending on the device and dressing materials in use. Choose an appropriate site to apply the connector pad/tubing port. Pinch the transparent adhesive drape and cut a hole through it (Figure 3). Apply the connector pad/tubing port and connective tubing over the hole (Figure 4). Position tubing away from the periwound area and anchor (Schreiber, 2016). Some devices, such as sNPWT, have integrated tubing, tubing port/connector pad and dressing, which do not require separate connection to the dressing.

Position the connector pad/tubing port and tubing to avoid placement over pressure areas, bony prominences, or skin creases to avoid excess pressure on the underlying skin and tissues (Schreiber, 2016). A hole in the drape and application of connector pad/tubing port and connective tubing are necessary for the application of negative pressure and removal of fluid and/or exudate. Securing the tubing prevents accidental excessive tension on the dressing (Schreiber, 2016).

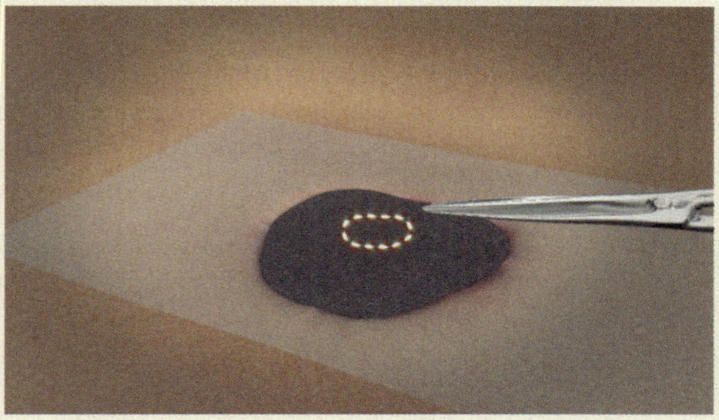

FIGURE 3. Cutting a hole in the drape.

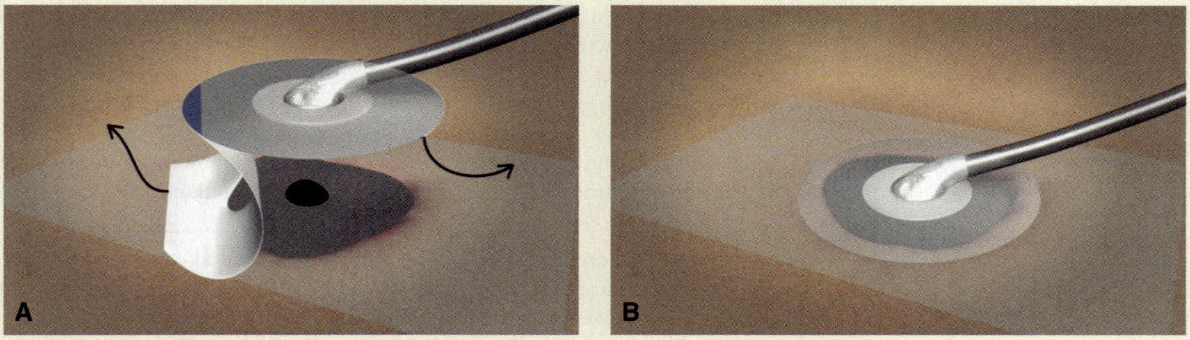

FIGURE 4. Applying the connecting pad over the hole.

(*continued on page 1228*)

Skill 33-7 Applying Negative-Pressure Wound Therapy *(continued)*

ACTION	RATIONALE
25. Attach the drainage cannister, depending on the device in use. Remove the drainage collection canister from the package and insert into the negative pressure unit until it locks into place. Attach the connective tubing to the canister and check that the clamps on the tubing are open, if present.	The tubing and canister provide means for the collection of drainage. Clamps must be open for the device to work properly.
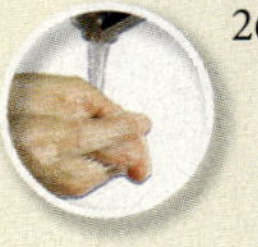 26. Remove gloves and discard. Perform hand hygiene. Turn on the power to the negative pressure unit. Select the prescribed therapy settings (suction and cycle type) and start the device.	Removal of gloves, proper disposal, and hand hygiene prevent transmission of microorganisms.
27. **Assess the dressing to ensure seal integrity. The dressing should be collapsed, shrinking to the wound contact material and skin (Figure 5). Observe drainage in tubing.**	Shrinkage confirms a good seal, allowing for accurate application of pressure and treatment. Observation of drainage in device tubing ensures proper flow (Schreiber, 2016).

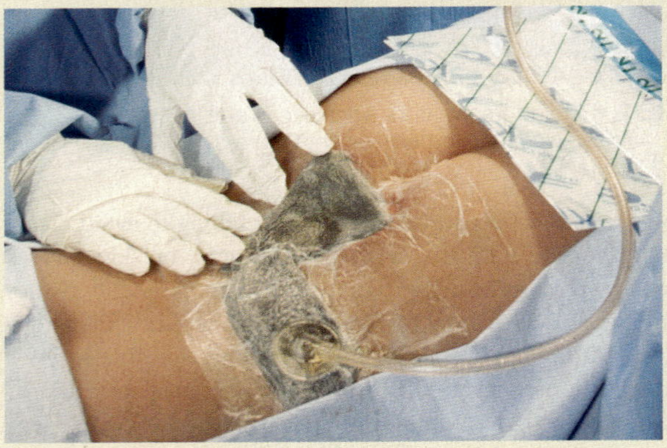

FIGURE 5. Dressing is collapsed, shrinking to wound contact material and skin. (*Source:* Used with permission. Courtesy of KCI, an Acelity Company.)

ACTION	RATIONALE
28. Label dressing with date and time. Remove all remaining equipment; place the patient in a comfortable position, with side rails up as indicated and bed in the lowest position.	Recording the date and time provides communication and demonstrates adherence to the care plan. Proper patient and bed positioning promotes safety and comfort.
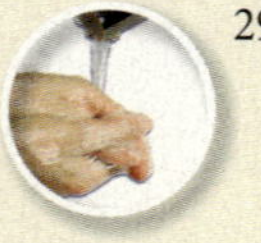 29. Remove PPE, if used. Perform hand hygiene.	Proper removal of PPE reduces the risk for infection transmission and contamination of other items. Hand hygiene prevents the spread of microorganisms.
30. Check all wound dressings at least every shift. More frequent checks may be needed if the wound is more. Check negative pressure settings at least every shift. Assess the patient's tolerance of and response to the therapy at least every shift.	Checking dressings, the device, and patient response ensures the assessment of changes in patient condition and timely intervention to prevent complications.

DOCUMENTATION

Guidelines

Record your assessment of the wound, including evidence of granulation tissue, stage (if appropriate), and characteristics of drainage. Include the appearance of the surrounding skin. Document the cleansing or irrigation of the wound and solution used. Document the application of the NPWT, noting the pressure setting, patency, and seal of the dressing. Describe the color and characteristics of the drainage in the collection chamber. Record pertinent patient and family/caregiver education and any patient reaction to this procedure, including the presence of pain and effectiveness or ineffectiveness of pain interventions.

Sample Documentation

4/5/25 0800 NPWT dressing intact with good seal maintained, system patent, pressure setting 80 mm Hg. Purulent, sanguineous drainage noted in collection chamber and tubing. Surrounding tissue without edema, redness, ecchymosis, or signs of irritation. Patient verbalizes an understanding of use of the device and movement limitations related to the system.

—B. Clark, RN

DEVELOPING CLINICAL REASONING AND CLINICAL JUDGMENT

UNEXPECTED SITUATIONS AND ASSOCIATED INTERVENTIONS

- *While assessing the patient, the nurse notes that the seal between the transparent adhesive drape and the wound contact material and skin is not tight:* Check the dressing seals, tubing connections, and canister insertion, and ensure the clamps are open. If a leak in the transparent drape is identified, the appropriate pressure is not being applied to the wound. Apply additional transparent dressing to reseal. If this application does not correct the break, change the dressing.
- *Patient reports acute pain while NPWT is operating:* Assess the patient for other symptoms, obtain vital signs, assess the wound, and assess the vacuum device for proper functioning. Report your findings to the health care team and document the event in the patient's health record. Administer analgesics, as prescribed. Continue or change the wound therapy, as prescribed. Some patients may be unable to tolerate NPWT and may require a change in the type of wound contact material used, addition of a wound contact layer, intermittent therapy cycling, a reduction in suction pressure, or discontinuation of the therapy (Apelqvist et al., 2017; Milne, 2015; Schreiber, 2016).

SPECIAL CONSIDERATIONS

- The wound should be debrided of as much necrotic tissue as possible before using NPWT; it is best to have the wound bed free of necrotic tissue (Baranoski & Ayello, 2020).
- Time dressing changes to allow for wound assessment by other members of the health care team.
- Dressings may need to be changed more often than 48 to 72 hours for wounds with heavy exudate (Baranoski & Ayello, 2020; EPUAP, NPIAP, & PPPIA, 2019a).
- Measure and record the amount of drainage each shift as part of the intake and output record.
- Check the fluid level in the canister periodically. Depending on the particular device in use, replace the canister whenever full or nearly full.
- The battery pack for sNPWT devices may contain a magnet; these devices should be kept at least 4 inches away from other medical devices to avoid disruption of nearby medical devices (Smith & Nephew, Inc., 2018; Watret et al., 2020).
- Be alert for audible and visual alarms on the vacuum device to alert you to problems, such as tipping of the device greater than 45 degrees, a full collection canister, an air leak in the dressing, or dislodgement of the canister.
- NPWT should operate for 24 hours a day. It should not be shut off for more than 2 hours in a 24-hour period. Remove the dressing any time therapy cannot be reestablished within the 2-hour time period (McNichol et al., 2022). When suction is lost, there is no mechanism for exudate control and allowing the dressing to remain in place without suction significantly increases the risk of wound infection (McNichol et al., 2022, p. 226). When NPWT is restarted, clean/irrigate the wound as prescribed or per facility policy and apply a new NPWT dressing.
- When maceration of the surrounding skin beneath the occlusive dressing occurs, this may be treated by placing a barrier/wafer dressing beneath the transparent dressing to protect the skin. Verify with facility policy, as needed.
- Approaches to NPWT continue to change, including the size of the vacuum pumps, types of wound contact materials and length of time recommended for the use of NPWT (Benbow, 2016).
- Appropriate nutritional support is critical in achieving successful wound healing and may be overlooked (Quain & Khardori, 2015). Collaborate with the registered dietician and dietary staff to develop an individualized nutrition intervention plan for the patient (Baranoski & Ayello, 2020).

Community-Based Care Considerations

- NPWT can be used in outpatient and home and other community settings (Edwards et al., 2018; EPUAP, NPIAP, & PPPIA, 2019a).
- Patients and caregivers must be educated about NPWT: how NPWT works, the risks and benefits of NPWT, device operation, signs of and actions for possible complications, response to alarms and emergencies, and when to seek and who to contact for assistance (Benbow, 2016; Schreiber, 2016).

Skill 33-8 Applying an External Heating Pad

DELEGATION CONSIDERATIONS

The application of an external heating pad may be delegated to assistive personnel (AP) as well as to licensed practical/vocational nurses (LPN/LVNs). The decision to delegate must be based on careful analysis of the patient's needs and circumstances as well as the qualifications of the person to whom the task is being delegated. Refer to the Delegation Guidelines in Appendix A.

EQUIPMENT

- Aquathermia heating pad with electronic unit
- Distilled water
- Cover for the pad, if not part of pad
- Gauze bandage or tape to secure the pad
- Bath blanket
- PPE, as indicated

IMPLEMENTATION

ACTION	RATIONALE
1. Review the patient's health record for prescribed intervention for the application of heat therapy, including frequency, type of therapy, body area to be treated, and length of time for the application. Gather necessary supplies.	Reviewing the health record and care plan validates the correct patient and correct procedure. Preparation promotes efficient time management and an organized approach to the task.
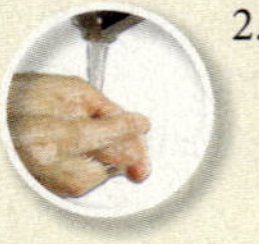 2. Perform hand hygiene and put on PPE, if indicated.	Hand hygiene and PPE prevent the spread of microorganisms. PPE is required based on transmission precautions.
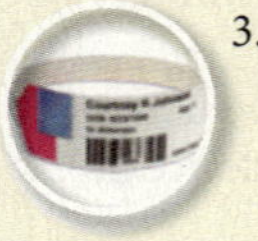 3. Identify the patient.	Identifying the patient ensures the right patient receives the intervention and helps prevent errors.
4. Assemble equipment on the overbed table or other surface within reach.	Organization facilitates performance of task.
5. Close the curtains around the bed and close the door to the room if possible. Explain what you are going to do and why you are going to do it to the patient.	This ensures the patient's privacy. Explanation relieves anxiety and facilitates engagement.
6. Adjust the bed to a comfortable working height (VHACEOSH, 2016).	Having the bed at the proper height prevents back and muscle strain.
7. Assist the patient to a comfortable position that provides easy access to the area where the heat will be applied; use a bath blanket to cover any other exposed area.	Patient positioning and the use of a bath blanket provide for comfort and warmth.
8. Assess the condition of the skin where the heat is to be applied.	Assessment supplies baseline data for posttreatment comparison and identifies conditions that may contraindicate the application.
9. Check that the water in the electronic unit (Figure 1) is at the appropriate level. Fill the unit two thirds full or to the fill mark, with distilled water, if necessary. Check the temperature setting on the unit to ensure it is within the safe range.	Sufficient water in the unit is necessary to ensure proper function of the unit. Tap water leaves mineral deposits in the unit. Checking the temperature setting helps to prevent skin or tissue damage.

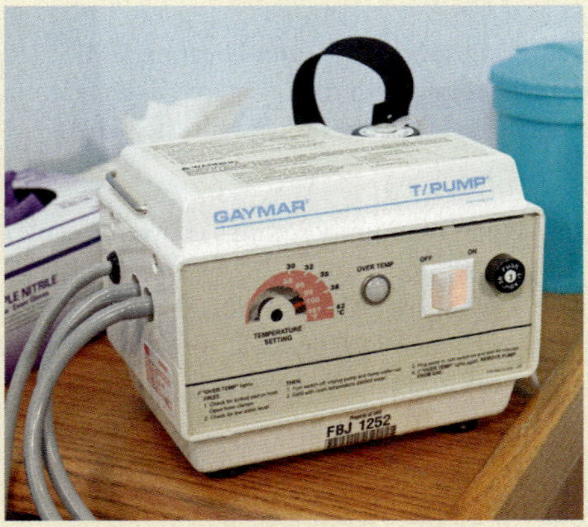

FIGURE 1. External heating pad electronic unit.

ACTION	RATIONALE
10. Attach pad tubing to the electronic unit tubing (Figure 2).	Allows flow of warmed water through the heating pad.
11. Plug in the unit and warm the pad before use. Apply the aquathermia pad to the prescribed area (Figure 3). Secure with roller gauze or tape.	Plugging in the pad readies it for use. Heat travels by conduction from one object to another. Gauze bandage or tape holds the pad in position; **do not use pins, as they may puncture and damage the pad.**

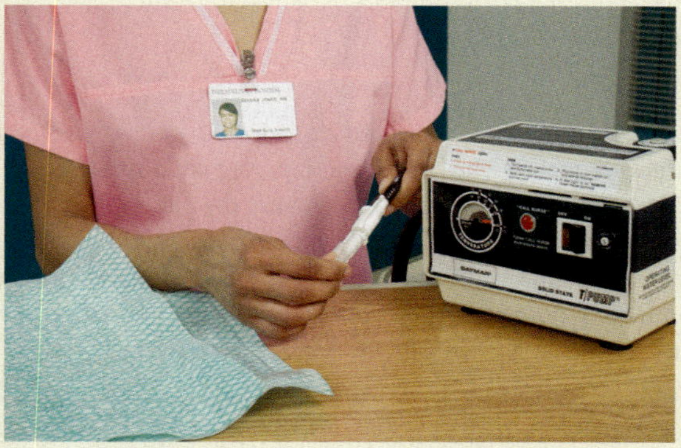

FIGURE 2. Attaching pad tubing to electronic unit tubing.

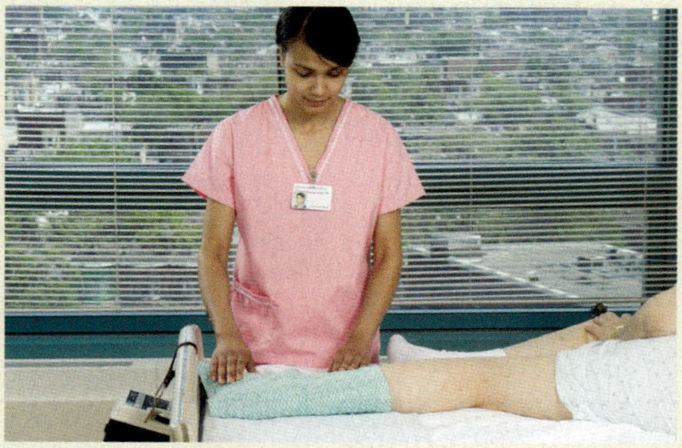

FIGURE 3. Applying heating pad to the prescribed area.

ACTION	RATIONALE
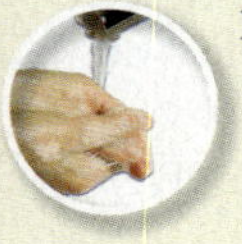 12. Remove PPE, if used, and perform hand hygiene.	Proper removal of PPE reduces the risk for infection transmission and contamination of other items. Hand hygiene prevents the spread of microorganisms.
13. **Monitor the condition of the skin and the patient's response to the heat at frequent intervals, according to facility policy. Do not exceed the prescribed length of time for the application of heat.**	Maximum **vasodilation** and therapeutic effects from the application of heat occur within 20 to 30 minutes. Using heat for more than this amount of time results in tissue congestion and **vasoconstriction**, known as the rebound phenomenon. Prolonged heat application may also result in an increased risk of burns and tissue damage. Assessment of the patient's skin is necessary for early detection of adverse effects, thereby allowing prompt intervention to avoid complications.
14. After the prescribed time for the treatment (up to 20 to 30 minutes) (Cleveland Clinic, 2020; Klein, 2019) remove the aquathermia pad. **Do not exceed the prescribed amount of time.** Reassess the patient and area of application, noting the effect and presence of any adverse effects.	Using heat for more than this amount of time results in tissue congestion and vasoconstriction, known as the rebound phenomenon. Prolonged heat application may also result in an increased risk of burns and tissue damage. Assessment provides input as to the effectiveness of the treatment.
15. Remove all remaining equipment; place the patient in a comfortable position, with side rails up as indicated and bed in the lowest position.	Proper patient and bed positioning promotes safety and comfort.
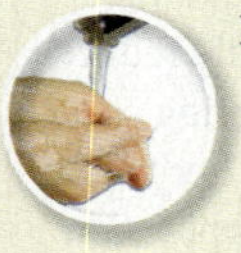 16. Remove additional PPE, if used. Perform hand hygiene.	Proper removal of PPE reduces the risk for infection transmission and contamination of other items. Hand hygiene prevents the spread of microorganisms.

DOCUMENTATION

Guidelines

Document the rationale for application of heat therapy. If the patient is receiving heat therapy for pain, document the assessment of pain pre- and postintervention. Specify the type of heat therapy and location where it is applied as well as the length of time applied. Record the condition of the skin, noting any redness or irritation before the heat application and after the application. Document the patient's reaction to the heat therapy. Record any appropriate patient or family/caregiver education.

(*continued on page 1232*)

Skill 33-8 Applying an External Heating Pad *(continued)*

Sample Documentation

9/13/25 2300 Patient states he has lower back pain, rating it 5 of 10, constant and aching. Aquathermia pad applied to patient's lower back for 30 minutes; patient now rating pain as 2 of 10 and intermittent. Skin without signs of redness or irritation before and after application.

—M. Martinez, RN

DEVELOPING CLINICAL REASONING AND CLINICAL JUDGMENT

UNEXPECTED SITUATIONS AND ASSOCIATED INTERVENTIONS

- *When performing a periodic assessment of the site during the application of heat, the nurse notes excessive swelling and redness at the site and the patient reports pain that was not present prior to the application of heat:* Remove the heat source. Assess the patient for other symptoms and obtain vital signs. Report your findings to the health care team and document the assessment and related interventions in the patient's record. Complete a variance or occurrence report, based on facility policy and procedures, to document the occurrence of an event that is out of the ordinary that has the potential to result in harm.

SPECIAL CONSIDERATIONS

General Considerations

- Direct heat treatment may be contraindicated for patients at risk for bleeding, patients with a sprained limb in the acute stage, or patients with a condition associated with acute inflammation (Klein, 2019). Use cautiously with children and older adults. Patients with diabetes, stroke, spinal cord injury, and peripheral neuropathy are at risk for thermal injury, as are patients with very thin or damaged skin. Be extremely careful when applying to heat-sensitive areas, such as scar tissue and stomas.
- Instruct the patient not to lean or lie directly on the heating device, as this reduces air space and increases the risk of burns.
- Check the water level in the aquathermia unit periodically. Evaporation may occur. If the unit runs dry, it could become damaged. Refill with distilled water periodically.

Older Adult Considerations

- Older adults are more at risk for skin and tissue damage because of their thin skin, loss of heat sensation, decreased subcutaneous tissue, and changes in the body's ability to regulate temperature (Eliopoulos, 2018; Touhy & Jett, 2018). Check these patients more frequently during therapy.

Community-Based Care Considerations

- A hot water bag or commercially prepared hot pack may be used in the home to apply heat. If using a hot water bag, fill with hot tap water to warm the bag, then empty it to detect any leaks. Check the temperature of the water with a thermometer or test on your inner wrist, adjusting the temperature as prescribed. Water used for heat applications needs to be at the appropriate temperature to avoid skin damage: set the temperature of the water within a range of 105° to 109°F (40.5° to 43°C), which is considered to be physiologically effective and comfortable for the patient. **Water temperature should not exceed 120°F (49°C)** (International Association of Fire Fighters, n.d.). Fill the bag one-half to two thirds full. Partial filling keeps the bag lightweight and flexible so that it can be molded to the treatment area. Squeeze the bag until the water reaches the neck; this expels air, which would make the bag inflexible and would reduce heat conduction. Fasten the top and cover the bag with an absorbent cloth. The covering protects the skin from direct contact with the bag. If using a commercially prepared hot pack, follow the manufacturer's directions and carefully assess skin before and after heat application.
- Electric heating pads may be used in the home to apply heat. Avoid the use of pins to prevent electric shocks. Use a dry covering over the pad to protect skin. Place a heating pad anteriorly or laterally to, not under, the body part. If the heating pad is between the patient and the mattress, heat dissipation may be inadequate, leading to burning of the patient or the bed linens. Caution the patient to use a heating pad with a selector switch that cannot be turned up beyond a safe temperature. The patient's receptors adapt to the initial application of heat, the patient may attempt to inappropriately increase the heat because the pad does not seem sufficiently warm, with the potential for burns.

DEVELOPING CLINICAL REASONING AND CLINICAL JUDGMENT

1. Work through the Evolving Case Study 33-1 to help develop your clinical reasoning and clinical judgment skills.
2. Review the Concept Map for Lucius Everly. Pay special attention to the interventions that address more than one actual or potential problem.
3. How would you individualize your teaching about needed supplies, wound care, and resources for the following patients?
   - A man who is currently unhomed admitted to the hospital for gangrene of the big toe; the toe has been amputated
   - A teenage gang member treated in the emergency department for a superficial (but long) knife wound
   - An infant who has had abdominal surgery and is now having diarrhea
   - A frail, 80-year-old man who needs daily dressing changes on a draining wound and lives with his wife who happens to be blind
4. Describe the nursing interventions you would include in a care plan to prevent pressure injuries in the following patients:
   - A middle-aged person, 70 lb over normal body weight, who has a fractured femur and is recovering at home (they live alone)
   - A 90-year-old man with cognitive impairment who is confined to bed
   - A 17-year-old girl who is paralyzed from the waist down after a diving accident and is wheelchair dependent

EVOLVING CASE STUDY 33-1

Scenario: Sam Bentz, a 56-year-old admitted to the hospital for management of nonhealing wounds and an infection mentions, "Last time I was here, my skin got really irritated and I developed several skin wounds."

QUESTION r/t CUES: Based on the patient's reason for admission, what initial question is the most important for the nurse to ask?

A. "Can you tell me about your wounds and what prompted you to come to the hospital?"
B. "Can you tell me why you were here for your last admission?"
C. "Is this admission due to your lack of follow-through after your last discharge?"
D. "Can you define irritated for me? Was this your interpretation or your provider's?"

Scenario: You note that Sam is 5 ft 4 in tall and weighs more than 300 lb with a BMI of >51.5, which means Sam falls into the obese category for adults of that same height. When you ask Sam to describe the wounds, including their size, location, and anything else they remember, Sam changes the subject and asks when dinner will be delivered.

QUESTION r/t ANALYZING CUES: What can the nurse determine from Sam's response?

A. Sam would benefit from a psychiatric consult to explore their issues.
B. Sam is dodging and is likely to be nonadherent with the treatment plan.
C. Sam is hesitant to talk about their wounds and may benefit from additional support.
D. Sam has a knowledge deficit and needs detailed information about their plan of care.

Scenario: The nurse sits down next to Sam, reframes, and asks the question again. Sam apologizes for reacting and admits that they felt "judged and fat-shamed" their last admission. Sam relaxes and begins describing their nonhealing wounds. Seizing the opportunity, the nurse performs an assessment and finds Sam's legs to be edematous, red, and macerated; weeping serous fluid; rough; and painful to the touch. There are also three large, round, deep, yellow, necrotic nonhealing wounds on the left lower leg near the ankle. When the nurse turns Sam to the side, the nurse notes a large, foul-smelling sacral wound that is covered with what appears to be an old duoderm dressing.

QUESTION r/t PRIORITIZING HYPOTHESIS: Based on the objective and subjective assessment of this patient, which priority problem should the nurse identify to guide the plan of care?

A. Altered skin integrity based on the nonhealing, chronic wounds
B. Bathing/hygiene ADL deficit based on the rash in the skin folds
C. Chronic low self-esteem based on their expression of feelings
D. Grief based on the likely role changes that occur with chronic issues

Scenario: The nurse reviews Sam's laboratory and diagnostic results and checks the medication administration record. The nurse sees that Sam has been prescribed a potent antibiotic to treat the diagnosed infection that has moved to the bone (osteomyelitis) and a topical antifungal to manage the severe dermatitis and skin breakdown in the abdominal skin folds.

(*continued on page 1234*)

EVOLVING CASE STUDY 33-1 *(continued)*

QUESTION r/t GENERATING SOLUTIONS: The nurse has 10 minutes before having to leave the room and administer blood to another patient. Which intervention is the priority for Sam?

A. Sitting quietly with Sam
B. Contacting Sam's partner and providing an update
C. Consulting wound care for a thorough assessment
D. Hanging the prescribed antibiotic

Scenario: Once the plan of care has been enacted to treat the immediate infection and existing wounds, the nurse moves to consider prevention.

QUESTION r/t TAKING ACTION: What interventions are most likely to be effective in engaging Sam in their treatment and prevention plan? Select all that apply.

A. Having Sam perform a return demonstration on active range of motion and repositioning
B. Facilitating the interaction with the wound care specialist and reinforcing any teaching points
C. Involving Sam's partner (with Sam's permission) in the dressing changes to increase their confidence before discharge
D. Providing a pressure-relief support surface for the bed and chair that Sam agrees to use
E. Instructing Sam on how to use the call bell and television remote in the room

Scenario: After 3 days of antibiotics, Sam is slated for discharge with ongoing home health care visits.

QUESTION r/t EVALUATING OUTCOMES: How will the nurse and Sam know that the treatment plan has been effective? Select all that apply.

A. The current wounds become smaller and show signs of healing.
B. Sam only occasionally has a fever and other signs of infection.
C. Sam is satisfied with the plan and expresses understanding and adherence.
D. Sam's partner can identify the early signs and symptoms of infection.
E. Sam can walk a mile without getting short of breath.

PRACTICING FOR NCLEX

1. Thirty-six hours after having surgery, a patient has a slightly elevated body temperature and generalized malaise as well as pain with redness at the surgical site. Which action is most appropriate?
   MAR
   - Acetaminophen 650 mg every 6 hours prn fever
   - Cefazolin (antibiotic) 1 g 1 hour preoperatively
   - Cefazolin 1 g, every 6 hours 3 times, postoperatively

   a. Documenting the findings and continuing to monitor the patient
   b. Administering antipyretics and contacting the provider for an antibiotic prescription
   c. Increasing the frequency of assessment to every hour and notifying the patient's primary care provider
   d. Obtaining a wound culture and increasing the frequency of wound care

2. A nurse on a surgical unit has assessed and documented a patient's wound and drainage. Which statements most accurately describe the characteristic of the wound drainage?
   Graphic Record
   - T 99.9 P100 RR 20 BP 138/88
   - Nursing note: Patient postoperative day 2. Dry sterile dressing changed on abdominal incision. Incision edges are well approximated with a slight ½-cm opening at inferior edge; incisional edges reddened. Hemovac draining sanguineous material, 60 mL for the shift. Patient reports moderate pain, relieved by oxycodone X1.

   a. Sanguineous drainage is composed of the clear portion of the blood and serous membranes.
   b. Sanguineous drainage is composed of a large number of red blood cells and looks like blood.
   c. Sanguineous drainage is composed of white blood cells, dead tissue, and bacteria.
   d. Sanguineous drainage is thin, cloudy, and watery and may have a musty or foul odor.

3. A postoperative patient who has a large abdominal incision suddenly calls out for help, shouting, "Something is falling out of my incision!" The nurse notes the wound is gaping open with tissue bulging outward. Place the nursing interventions in the order they should be performed, arranged from first to last.
   a. Notify the health care provider of the situation.
   b. Cover exposed tissue with sterile towels moistened with sterile 0.9% sodium chloride solution.
   c. Place the patient in the low Fowler position.
   d. Document the findings and outcome of interventions.
   e. Maintain NPO status for return to the OR for repair.

4. A patient was in an automobile accident and received a wound across the nose and cheek. After surgery to repair the wound, the patient says, "I am so ugly now." Based on this statement, psychosocial problem will the nurse plan to address?
   a. Pain
   b. Wound healing
   c. Body image
   d. Change in cognition

5. A patient is admitted with a nonhealing surgical wound. Which nursing interventions will the nurse use to promote wound healing? Select all that apply.
   a. Applying sterile dressing supplies
   b. Discussing zinc supplementation with the health care provider
   c. Maintaining bedrest
   d. Performing careful hand hygiene
   e. Teaching the patient to increase protein in the diet
   f. Suggesting the patient consume vitamin C–containing foods.
6. A nurse on a surgical unit is working with a nursing student and discussing various phases of wound healing for postoperative patients. Which statements accurately describe these stages? Select all that apply.
   a. Hemostasis occurs immediately after the initial injury.
   b. A liquid called exudate is formed during the proliferation phase.
   c. White blood cells move to the wound in the inflammatory phase.
   d. Granulation tissue forms in the inflammatory phase.
   e. During the inflammatory phase, the patient has generalized body response.
   f. A scar forms during the proliferation phase.
7. The nurse preceptor is supervising a new graduate nurse as they assess a patient with a pressure injury. The graduate nurse documents the presence of biofilm in the wound. The preceptor recognizes the graduate nurse understands this concept when the graduate makes which of these statements? Select all that apply.
   a. Enhanced healing occurs due to the presence of sugars and proteins.
   b. Delayed healing develops due to dead tissue present in the wound.
   c. Antibiotics against the bacteria become less effective.
   d. Skin loses its integrity due to overhydration of the cells of the wound.
   e. Delayed healing due to cells dehydrating and dying occurs.
   f. Decreased effectiveness of the patient's normal immune process results.
8. The nurse is cleaning an open abdominal wound that has edges that are not approximated. What are accurate steps in this procedure? Select all that apply.
   a. Use standard precautions or transmission-based precautions when indicated.
   b. Moisten a sterile gauze pad or swab with the prescribed cleansing agent and squeeze out excess solution.
   c. Clean the wound in full or half circles beginning on the outside and working toward the center.
   d. Work outward from the incision in lines that are parallel to it from the dirty area to the clean area.
   e. Clean to at least 1 inch beyond the end of the new dressing if one is being applied.
   f. Clean to at least 3 inches beyond the wound if a new dressing is not being applied.
9. A nurse is developing a care plan for an older adult patient who is recovering from a hip arthroplasty (hip replacement). Which assessment findings indicate a high risk for this patient to develop area(s) of pressure injury? Select all that apply.
   a. The patient takes time to think about responses to questions.
   b. The patient is an older adult with a poor appetite.
   c. The patient reports inability to control their urine.
   d. The patient's albumin level is <3.2 mg/dL (normal, 3.4 to 5.4 g/dL).
   e. Lab findings include BUN 12 (older adult, normal 8 to 23 mg/dL) and creatinine 0.9 (adult female, normal 0.61 to 1 mg/dL).
   f. The patient reports increased pain in right hip when repositioning in bed or chair.
10. A nurse is explaining to a patient the anticipated effect of the application of cold to an injured area. What response indicates that the patient understands the explanation?
    a. "There will be more discomfort in the area where the cold is applied."
    b. "I should expect more drainage from the incision after the ice has been in place."
    c. "Redness and swelling should decrease after cold treatment."
    d. "My incision may bleed more when the ice is first applied."
11. A nurse is providing education to a patient and their family regarding the use of negative pressure wound therapy (NPWT). The nurse documents that the teaching has been effective when the patient and family make which statement?
    a. "This therapy is used to collect excess blood loss and prevent formation of a scab."
    b. "The suction created will prevent infection and promote wound healing with less scar tissue."
    c. "Suction stimulates blood flow to the wound, removes excess fluid, and promotes a moist environment for healing."
    d. "This treatment irrigates the wound, suctions the irrigation fluid from the wound, and keeps it free from debris wound exudate."
12. After an initial skin assessment, the nurse documents the presence pressure area that is reddened and has a 1-cm blister. How will the nurse document the wound stage?
    a. Stage 1 dark maroon wound, skin intact
    b. Stage 2 with 1-cm blister noted
    c. Stage 3 wound base with red granulation tissue
    d. Stage 4 blanchable reddened area, 2 cm
13. A nurse notes a pressure wound base is red. Using the RYB system for documentation, what intervention is indicated?
    a. Irrigating the wound and applying an absorbent dressing
    b. Gently cleansing the wound and applying a moist dressing
    c. Discussing consultation for surgical debridement with the provider
    d. Performing frequent dressing changes to keep the wound and dressing dry

14. A nurse is developing education for nurses and UAPs related to prevention of pressure injuries for residents in a long-term care facility. Which action to prevent pressure injury will the nurses delegate to the UAP?
    a. Maintaining the head of the bed elevated consistently
    b. Massaging over bony prominences
    c. Repositioning bedbound patients every 4 hours
    d. Using a mild cleansing agent when cleansing the skin
15. A nurse caring for a patient with a stage 3 pressure wound with tunneling. How will the nurse best assess the tunneled area?
    a. Moisten a sterile, flexible applicator with saline and insert it gently into the wound at a 90-degree angle with the tip down.
    b. Photograph the wound per policy and describe the estimated depth in centimeters.
    c. Gently insert a sterile applicator into the wound and move it in a clockwise direction.
    d. Insert a calibrated probe gently into the wound and mark the point that is even with the surrounding skin surface.
16. Determine the patient's risk for pressure injury using the Braden scale found in Figure 33-7, based on information in the electronic health record (EHR).
    EHR 1430 Admission Assessment
    S: Patient admitted from nursing home for sepsis, confusion, ambulatory dysfunction.
    B: 87-year-old patient, with history of heart failure and hypertension; comes to ED with shortness of breath and yellow sputum.
    A: Lungs with crackles, pale, short of breath on exertion, pulse oximetry 88%, skin fragile.
    Bedrest maintained. States has not eaten nor drank fluids for last 36 hours; incontinent of small amount of urine × 2. Responding to painful stimuli, not participating in turning or care.
    R: Need orders for oxygen, sputum culture, activity level. Consider IV fluids. J. Smith RN.
    a. No risk
    b. Moderate risk
    c. High risk
    d. Very high risk
17. The nurse is caring for a patient 1 day postoperative abdominal surgery. The nurse identifies the patient is at risk for wound dehiscence. What patient risk factor is consistent with development of this problem?
    a. Cigar smoker
    b. Wound drainage 120 mL over 24 hours
    c. Height, 5′ 6″ and weight 240 lb
    d. WBC count 9,500 c/mm^3

ANSWERS WITH RATIONALES

1. **a.** The assessment findings are normal for this stage of healing following surgery. The patient is in the inflammatory phase of the healing process, which involves a response by the immune system. This acute inflammation is characterized by pain, heat, redness, and swelling at the site of the injury (surgery, in this case). The patient also has a generalized body response, including a mildly elevated temperature, leukocytosis, and generalized malaise.
2. **b.** Sanguineous drainage consists of large numbers of red blood cells and looks like blood. Bright-red sanguineous drainage is indicative of fresh bleeding, whereas darker drainage indicates older bleeding. Serous drainage, generally watery, is composed primarily of the clear, serous portion of the blood and serous membranes. Purulent drainage is made up of white blood cells, liquefied dead tissue debris, and both dead and live bacteria. It is thick, often has a musty or foul odor, and varies in color (such as dark yellow or green), depending on the causative organism.
3. **c, b, a. e. d.** The correct order of nursing interventions for this postoperative emergency is to place the patient in the low Fowler position (to prevent further damage or protrusion from increased intraabdominal pressure), cover exposed tissue with sterile towels moistened with sterile 0.9% sodium chloride solution (to protect the viscera), and notify the health care provider of the situation (to address the issue, likely with surgery). The patient is kept NPO, as prompt surgical repair will be needed. After the patient has received attention, the nurse documents all assessments and interventions in a timely manner.
4. **c.** Wounds cause emotional as well as physical stress.
5. **a, b, d, e, f.** Careful hand washing (medical asepsis) is the most important. The nurse will use sterile dressings and supplies and promote intake of vitamins, zinc, and protein. Depending on the site of the wound and condition of the patient, bedrest may be indicated.
6. **a, c, e.** Hemostasis occurs immediately after the initial injury, and exudate occurs in this phase as plasma and blood components leak out into the injured area. White blood cells, predominantly leukocytes and macrophages, move to the wound in the inflammatory phase to ingest bacteria and cellular debris. During the inflammatory phase, the patient has a generalized body response, including a mildly elevated temperature, leukocytosis (increased number of white blood cells in the blood), and generalized malaise. New tissue, called granulation tissue, forms the foundation for scar tissue development in the proliferation phase. New collagen continues to be deposited in the maturation phase, which forms a scar.
7. **c, f.** Wound biofilms are the result of wound bacteria growing in clumps, embedded in a thick, self-made, protective, slimy barrier of sugars and proteins. This barrier contributes to decreased effectiveness of antibiotics against the bacteria (antibiotic resistance) and decreases the effectiveness of the normal immune response by the patient (Baranoski & Ayello, 2020). Necrosis (dead tissue) in the wound delays healing. Maceration or overhydration of cells related to urinary and fecal incontinence can lead to impaired skin integrity. Desiccation is the process of drying up, in which cells dehydrate and die in a dry environment.
8. **a, b, e.** The correct procedure for cleaning an open wound with edges that are not approximated is: (1) use standard precautions and appropriate transmission-based precautions when indicated, (2) moisten sterile gauze pad or swab with prescribed cleansing agent and squeeze out excess solution, (3) use a new swab or gauze for each circle, (4) clean the wound in full or half circles beginning in the center and working toward the outside, (5) clean to at least 1 inch beyond the end of the new dressing, and (6) clean to at least 2 inches beyond the wound margins if a dressing is not being applied.

9. **b, c, d, f.** Pressure, friction, and shear, as well as other factors, usually combine to contribute to pressure injury development. The skin of older adults is more susceptible to injury; incontinence contributes to prolonged moisture on the skin, as well as negative effects related to urine in contact with skin; hip surgery involves decreased mobility during the postoperative period, as well as pain with movement, contributing to immobility; and increased pain in the hip may contribute to increased immobility. A low albumin level signals a risk for poor wound healing related to malnutrition. Apathy, confusion, and/or altered mental status are risk factors for pressure injury development; however, taking time to formulate responses is consistent with normal aging. This patient's BUN and creatinine are within normal range; however, dehydration (indicated by an elevated BUN and creatinine) is a risk for pressure injury development.
10. **c.** The local application of cold constricts peripheral blood vessels, reduces muscle spasms, and promotes comfort. Cold reduces blood flow to tissues, decreases the local release of pain-producing substances, decreases metabolic needs, and capillary permeability. The resulting effects include decreased edema, coagulation of blood at the wound site, promotion of comfort, decreased drainage from wound, and decreased bleeding.
11. **c.** Negative pressure wound therapy (NPWT) promotes wound healing and wound closure through the application of uniform negative pressure on the wound bed, reduction in bacteria in the wound, and the removal of excess wound fluid, while providing a moist wound healing environment. The negative pressure results in mechanical tension on the wound tissues, stimulating cell proliferation, blood flow to wounds, and the growth of new blood vessels. It is used to treat a variety of acute or chronic wounds, wounds with heavy drainage, wounds failing to heal, or healing slowly.
12. **b.** A stage 2 pressure injury involves partial-thickness loss of dermis and presents as a shallow open ulcer with a red–pink wound bed, without slough. It may also present as an intact or open/ruptured serum-filled blister. Dark maroon or purple wounds with intact skin represent deep tissue injury. Red granulation tissue is present in stage 3 or 4 pressure injuries that are healing. A blanchable, red area is a stage 1 pressure injury.
13. **b.** Red wounds are in the proliferative stage of healing and reflect the color of normal granulation tissue. Wounds in this stage need protection with nursing interventions that include gentle cleansing, use of moist dressings, and dressing changes only when necessary (or based on product manufacturer's recommendations). To cleanse yellow wounds, nursing interventions include the use of wound cleansers and irrigation. The eschar found in black wounds requires debridement (removal) before the wound can heal.
14. **d.** To prevent pressure injuries, the nurse teaches the UAP to cleanse the skin routinely and whenever soiling occurs by using a mild cleansing agent with minimal friction, and avoiding hot water. The nurse educates the UAP to minimize the effects of shearing force by limiting the amount of time the head of the bed is elevated, when possible. Bony prominences should not be massaged, and bed-bound patients should be repositioned every 2 hours.
15. **a.** To measure the depth of a wound, the nurse should perform hand hygiene and apply gloves; moisten a sterile, flexible applicator with saline and insert it gently into the wound at a 90-degree angle with the tip down; mark the point on the swab that is even with the surrounding skin surface, or grasp the applicator with the thumb and forefinger at the point corresponding to the wound's margin; and remove the swab and measure the depth with a ruler.
16. **d.** The patient is at very high risk for pressure injury. This patient responds only to painful stimulate (1); is occasionally moist (3); is bedridden (1); has not eaten (1), and requires maximum assistance for moving (1) for a total of 7 points. The Braden scale scoring is: a score of 19 to 23 indicates no risk; 15 to 18, mild risk; 13 to 14, moderate risk; 10 to 12, high risk; and 9 or lower, very high risk (Braden & Maklebust, 2005). In addition, nurses use clinical judgment to incorporate risk factors and/or other health problems into preventative interventions.
17. **a.** Wound dehiscence is the partial or total separation of wound layers as a result of excessive stress on unhealed wounds. Patients at greater risk include obese or malnourished individuals; tobacco smokers; and those taking anticoagulants, who have infected wounds, or who experience excessive coughing, vomiting, or straining (Hinkle & Cheever, 2018). An increase in the flow of (serosanguineous) fluid from the wound between postoperative days 4 and 5 may be a sign of an impending dehiscence. The patient may say that "something has suddenly given way."

Bibliography

Alvarez, O. M., Brindle, C. T., Langemo, D., Kennedy-Evans, K. L., Krasner, D. L., & Levine, J. M. (2016). The VCU pressure ulcer summit: The search for a clearer understanding and more precise clinical definition of the unavoidable pressure injury. *Journal of Wound, Ostomy and Continence Nursing, 43*(5), 455–463. https://doi.org/10.1097/WON.0000000000000255

American Diabetes Association (ADA). (2022). *Diabetes overview: Diagnosis.* Retrieved February 16, 2022, from https://www.diabetes.org/diabetes/a1c/diagnosis

Apelqvist, J., Willy, C., Fagerdah, A. M., Fraccalvieri, M., Malmsjö, M., Piaggesi, A., Probst, A., Vowden, P., & European Wound Management Association (EWMA). (2017). EWMA document: Negative pressure wound therapy. Overview, challenges and perspectives. *Journal of Wound Care, 26*(Suppl 3), S1–S154. https://doi.org/10.12968/jowc.2017.26.Sup3.S1

Arnold, M., Needham, D. M., & Nydahl, P. (2018). International round table discussion: Early Mobility. *International Journal of Safe Patient Handling & Mobility (SPHM), 8*(1), 57–64.

Aseptic Non Touch Technique (ANTT®). (2019). What is Aseptic Non Touch Technique (ANTT®)? http://antt.org/ANTT_Site/what_is_ANTT.html

Avishai, E., Yeghiazaryan, K., & Golubnitschaja, O. (2017). Impaired wound healing: Facts and hypotheses for multi-professional considerations in predictive, preventive and personalised medicine. *The EPMA journal, 8*(1), 23–33. https://doi.org/10.1007/s13167-017-0081-y

Baranoski, S., & Ayello, E. A. (2020). *Wound care essentials: Practice principles* (5th ed.). Wolters Kluwer.

Barton, A. (2020). Medical adhesive-related skin injuries associated with vascular access: Minimising risk with Appeel Sterile. *British Journal of Nursing, 29*(8), S20–S27. http://doi.org/10.12968/bjon.2020.29.8.S20

Benbow, M. (2016). Understanding safe practice in the use of negative pressure wound therapy in the community. *British Journal of Community Nursing, 21*(Suppl 12), S32–S34. https://doi.org/10.12968/bjcn.2016.21.Sup12.S32

Bergstrom, A., O'Harra, P., & Foster, W. M. (2018). Collaborative interdisciplinary teams and pressure injury prevention: High-acuity patient skin care requires consistent communication between perioperative and critical-care staff. *American Nurse Today, Supplement Pressure Injuries*, 27–28.

Beyene, R. T., Derryberry, S. L., Jr, & Barbul, A. (2020). The effect of comorbidities on wound healing. *The Surgical Clinics of North America, 100*(4), 695–705. https://doi.org/10.1016/j.suc.2020.05.002

Braden, B. J. (2012). The Braden Scale for predicting pressure sore risk: Reflections after 25 years. *Advances in Skin & Wound Care, 25*(2), 61. https://doi.org/10.1097/01.ASW.0000411403.11392.10

Braden, B., & Maklebust, J. (2005). Preventing pressure ulcers with the Braden scale. *American Journal of Nursing, 105*(6), 70–72. https://doi.org/10.1097/00000446-200506000-00031

Brown, A. (2018). Dispelling some myths and misconceptions in wound care. *Journal of Community Nursing, 32*(6), 24–32.

Camacho-Del Rio, G. (2018). Evidence-based practice: Medical device-related pressure injury prevention. *American Nurse Today, 13*(10), 50–52.

Cochetti, G., Abraha, I., Randolph, J., Montedori, A., Boni, A., Arezzo, A., Mazza, E., Rossi De Vermandois, J. A., Cirocchi, R., & Mearini, E. (2020). Surgical wound closure by staples or sutures? Systematic review. *Medicine, 99*(25), e20573. https://doi.org/10.1097/MD.0000000000020573

Cornish, L. (2017). The use of prophylactic dressings in the prevention of pressure ulcers: A literature review. *British Journal of Community Nursing, 22*(Suppl 6), S26–S32. https://doi.org/10.12968/bjcn.2017.22.Sup6.S26

Corum, L. (2019). Ulcer and wound care: Getting to the depth of the issue. *National Center of Continuing Education.* https://nursece.com/pdfs/720_V2_Wound_Care.pdf

Daud, A., Kaur, B., McClure, G. R., Belley-Cote, E. P., Harlock, J., Crowther, M., & Whitlock, R. P. (2020). Fibrin and thrombin sealants in vascular and cardiac surgery: A systematic review and meta-analysis. *European Journal of Vascular and Endovascular Surgery, 60*(3), 469–478. https://doi.org/10.1016/j.ejvs.2020.05.016

Dennis, C., Sethu, S., Nayak, S., Mohan, L., Morsi, Y. Y., & Manivasagam, G. (2016). Suture materials—Current and emerging trends. *Journal of Biomedical Materials Research. Part A, 104*(6), 1544–1559. https://doi.org/10.1002/jbm.a.35683

Dudek, S. (2018). *Nutrition essentials for nursing practice* (8th ed.). Wolters Kluwer.

Edsberg, L. E., Black, J. M., Goldberg, M., McNichol, L., Moore, L., & Sieggreen, M. (2016). Revised national pressure ulcer advisory panel pressure injury staging system: Revised pressure injury staging system. *Journal of Wound Ostomy Continence Nurses Society, 43*(6), 585–597. https://doi.org/10.1097/won.0000000000000281

Edwards, S. J., Crawford, F., van Velthoven, M. H., Berardi, A., Osei-Assibey, G., Bacelar, M., Salih, F., & Wakefield, V. (2016). The use of fibrin sealant during non-emergency surgery: A systematic review of evidence of benefits and harms. *Health Technology Assessment, 20*(94), 1–224. https://doi.org/10.3310/hta20940

Edwards, D., Bourke, N., Murdoch, J., & Verma, S. (2018). Using portable, single-use, canister-free, negative-pressure wound therapy for plastic surgery wounds. *Wounds UK, 14*(3), 56–62.

Eliopoulos, C. (2018). *Gerontological nursing* (9th ed.). Wolters Kluwer Health.

Ellis, M. (2017). Pressure ulcer prevention in care home settings. *Nursing Older People, 29*(3), 29–35.

European Pressure Ulcer Advisory Panel (EPUAP), National Pressure Injury Advisory Panel (NPIAP), & Pan Pacific Pressure Injury Alliance (PPPIA) (2019a, March 10). *Prevention and treatment of pressure ulcers/injuries: Quick reference guide* (3rd ed.). http://www.internationalguideline.com/static/pdfs/Quick_Reference_Guide-10Mar2019.pdf

European Pressure Ulcer Advisory Panel (EPUAP), National Pressure Injury Advisory Panel (NPIAP), & Pan Pacific Pressure Injury Alliance (PPPIA). (2019b). *Prevention and treatment of pressure ulcers/injuries: Clinical practice guideline—The international guideline.* (3rd ed.) E. Haesler (Ed.). Cambridge Media.

Evans, D. C., Corkins, M. R., Malone, A., Miller, S., Mogensen, K. M., Guenter, P., Jensen, G. L., & ASPEN Malnutrition Committee (2021). The use of visceral proteins as nutrition markers: An ASPEN position paper. *Nutrition in Clinical Practice, 36*(1), 22–28. https://doi.org/10.1002/ncp.10588

Fayne, R. A., Borda, L. J., Egger, A. N., & Tomic-Canic, M. (2020). The potential impact of social genomics on wound healing. *Advances in Wound Care, 9*(6), 325–331. https://doi.org/10.1089/wound.2019.1095

Ferreira, M., de Souza Gurgel, S., Lima, F., Cardoso, M., da Silva, V. (2018). Instruments for the care of pressure injury in pediatrics and hebiatrics: An integrative review of the literature. *Revista Latino-Americana de Enfermagem, 26*, e3034. https://doi.org/10.1590/1518-8345.2289.3034

Fischbach, F. T., & Fischbach, M. A. (2018). *A manual of laboratory and diagnostic tests* (10th ed.). Wolters Kluwer.

Fumarola, S., Allaway, R., Callaghan, R., Collier, M., Downie, F., Geraghty, J., Kiernan, S., & Spratt, F. (2020). Overlooked and underestimated: Medical adhesive-related skin injuries. Best practice consensus document on prevention. *Journal of Wound Care, 29*(Suppl 3c), S1–S24. https://doi.org/10.12968/jowc.2020.29.Sup3c.S1

Hajhosseini, B., Kuehlmann, B. A., Bonham, C. A., Kamperman, K. J., & Gurtner, G. C. (2020). Hyperbaric oxygen therapy: Descriptive review of the technology and current application in chronic wounds. *Plastic and Reconstructive Surgery. Global Open, 8*(9), e3136. https://doi.org/10.1097/GOX.0000000000003136

Han, G., & Ceilley, R. (2017). Chronic wound healing: A review of current management and treatments. *Advances in Therapy, 34*(3), 599–610. https://doi.org/10.1007/s12325-017-0478-y

Hess, C. (2013). *Clinical guide to skin & wound care* (7th ed.). Wolters Kluwer.

Hess, C. (2019). *Product guide to skin & wound care* (8th ed.). Wolters Kluwer.

Higgins, J., Casey, S., Taylor, E., Wilson, R., & Halcomb, P. (2020). Comparing the Braden and Jackson/Cubbin Pressure Injury Risk Scales in trauma-surgery ICU patients. *Critical Care Nurse, 40*(6), 52–61. https://doi.org/10.4037/ccn2020874

Hinkle, J. L., Cheever, K. H., & Overbaugh, K. J. (2022). *Brunner & Suddarth's textbook of medical-surgical nursing* (15th ed.). Wolters Kluwer.

Huddleston Cross, H. (2014). Obtaining a wound swab culture specimen. *Nursing, 44*(7), 68–69.

Hurd, T., Rossington, A., Trueman, P., & Smith, J. (2017). A retrospective comparison of the performance of two negative pressure wound therapy systems in the management of wounds of mixed etiology. *Advances in Wound Care, 6*(1), 33–37. https://doi.org/10.1089/wound.2015.0679

International Association of Fire Fighters. (n.d.). *The epidemic of liquid and steam burns.* National Scald Prevention Campaign. Retrieved August 22, 2020, http://flashsplash.org/

Jackson C. (1999). The revised Jackson/Cubbin Pressure Area Risk Calculator. *Intensive & Critical Care Nursing, 15*(3), 169–175. https://doi.org/10.1016/s0964-3397(99)80048-2

Jensen, S. (2019). *Nursing health assessment: A best practice approach* (3rd ed.). Wolters Kluwer.

The Joint Commission. (2018, July 23). *Quick safety 43: Managing medical device-related pressure injuries.* https://www.jointcommission.org/resources/news-and-multimedia/newsletters/newsletters/quick-safety/quick-safety-43-managing-medical-devicerelated-pressure-injuries/

Kalowes, P. (2018). Preventing pressure injuries in critically ill patients. *American Nurse Today,* Supplement Pressure Injuries, 14–40.

Kelly-O'Flynn, S., Mohamud, L., & Copson, D. (2020). Medical adhesive-related skin injury. *British Journal of Nursing, 29*(6), S20–S26. https://doi.org/10.12968/bjon.2020.29.6.S20

Klein, M. J. (2019, September 3). *Superficial heat and cold.* Medscape. https://emedicine.medscape.com/article/1833084-overview

Krasner, D. (1995). Wound care: How to use the red-yellow-black system. *American Journal of Nursing, 5*(95), 44–47.

Lovegrove, J., Fulbrook, P., & Miles, S. (2020). International consensus on pressure injury preventative interventions by risk level for critically ill patients: A modified Delphi study. *International Wound Journal, 17*(5), 1112–1127. https://doi.org/10.1111/iwj.13461

Mamuyac, E. M., Pappa, A. K., Thorp, B. D., Ebert, C. S. Jr, Senior, B. A., Zanation, A. M., Lin, F. C., & Kimple, A. J. (2019). How much blood could a JP suck if a JP could suck blood? *The Laryngoscope, 129*(8), 1806–1809. https://doi.org/10.1002/lary.27710

McGraw, C. A. (2018). Nurses' perceptions of the root causes of community-acquired pressure ulcers: Application of the model for examining safety and quality concerns in home health care. *Journal of Clinical Nursing, 28*(3–4), 575–588. https://doi.org/10.1111/jocn.14652

McGuire, J., Love, E., Vlahovic, T. C., Khan, K., Labbad, Z. G., Robinson, L., Magodia, S., Aljumail, A., Adler, L., & Stewart, J. (2020). The ABCESS system for chronic wound management: A new acronym for lower extremity wound management. *Wounds, 32*(suppl 11), S1–S25. https://online.fliphtml5.com/zxoes/aykr/#p=3

McLain, N. E. M., Moore, Z. E. H., & Avsar, P. (2021). Wound cleansing for treating venous leg ulcers. *Cochrane Database of Systematic Reviews, 3*(3), CD011675. https://doi.org/10.1002/14651858.CD011675

McNichol, L. L., Ayello, E. A., Phearman, L. A., Pezzella, P. A., & Culver, E. A. (2018). Incontinence-associated dermatitis: State of the science and knowledge translation. *Advances in Skin & Wound Care, 31*(11), 502–513. https://doi.org/10.1097/01.ASW.0000546234.12260.61

McNichol, L., Lund, C., Rosen, T., & Gray, M. (2013). Medical adhesives and patient safety: State of the science: Consensus statements for the assessment, prevention, and treatment of adhesive-related skin injuries. *Journal of Wound, Ostomy, and Continence Nursing, 40*(4), 365–380. https://doi.org/10.1097/WON.0b013e3182995516

McNichol, L. L., Ratliff, C. R., & Yates, S. S. (Eds). (2022). *Wound, Ostomy, and Continence Nurses Society™ (WOCN®). Core curriculum. Wound management* (2nd ed.). Wolters Kluwer.

McNichol, L., Watts, C., Mackey, D., Beitz, J. M., & Gray, M. (2015). Identifying the right surface for the right patient at the right time: Generation and content validation of an Algorithm for Support Surface selection. *Journal of Wound, Ostomy, and Continence Nursing, 42*(1), 19–37. https://doi.org/10.1097/WON.0000000000000103

Memorial Sloan Kettering Cancer Center. (2019, October 8). *Caring for your Penrose drain.* https://www.mskcc.org/cancer-care/patient-education/caring-your-penrose-drain

Milne, J. (2019). The importance of skin cleansing in wound care. *British Journal of Nursing, 28*(12), S20–S22. https://doi.org/10.12968/bjon.2019.28.12.S20

Mitchell, A. (2018). Adult pressure area care: Preventing pressure ulcers. *British Journal of Nursing, 27*(18), 1050–1052. https://doi.org/10.12968/bjon.2018.27.18.1050

Munoz, N., Posthauer, M. E., Cereda, E., Schols, J. M. G. A., & Haesler, E. (2020). The role of nutrition for pressure injury prevention and healing: the 2019 International Clinical Practice Guideline recommendations. *Advances in Skin & Wound Care, 33*(3), 123–136. https://doi.org/10.1097/01.ASW.0000653144.90739.ad

National Pressure Injury Advisory Panel (NPIAP). (2016a). *NPIAP Pressure injury stages.* https://npiap.com/page/PressureInjuryStages

National Pressure Injury Advisory Panel (NPIAP). (2016b). *PUSH tool.* https://npiap.com/page/PUSHTool

National Pressure Injury Advisory Panel (NPIAP). (2017). *NPUAP position statement on staging—2017 clarifications.* https://cdn.ymaws.com/npiap.com/resource/resmgr/npuap-position-statement-on-.pdf

National Pressure Injury Advisory Panel (NPIAP). (2019, November 19). *Support Surface Standards Initiative (S3I): Terms and definitions related to support surfaces.* https://cdn.ymaws.com/npiap.com/resource/resmgr/s3i/10-23_Terms_and_Defs_2019_We.pdf

National Pressure Injury Advisory Panel (NPIAP). (2020). *Pressure injury prevention points.* https://cdn.ymaws.com/npiap.com/resource/resmgr/online_store/1a._pressure-injury-preventi.pdf

National Pressure Injury Advisory Panel (NPIAP). (2021, January 8). *Evolution of deep tissue pressure injury.* https://npiap.com/news/546664/Evolution-of-Deep-Tissue-Pressure-Injury.htm

National Pressure Injury Advisory Panel (NPIAP). (n.d.). Unavoidable pressure injury during COVID-19 pandemic: A position paper from the National Pressure Injury Advisory Panel. Retrieved February 28, 2021, from https://cdn.ymaws.com/npiap.com/resource/resmgr/white_papers/Unavoidable_in_COVID_Pandemi.pdf

National Pressure Ulcer Advisory Panel (NPUAP) (2016b). *Pressure Ulcer Scale for Healing (PUSH). PUSH tool.* https://npiap.com/page/PUSHTool

Norman, G., Goh, E. L., Dumville, J. C., Shi, C., Liu, Z., Chiverton, L., Stankiewicz, M., & Reid, A. (2020). Negative pressure wound therapy for surgical wounds healing by primary closure. *The Cochrane Database of Systematic Reviews, 6*(6), CD009261. https://doi.org/10.1002/14651858.CD009261.pub6

Norris, T. L. (2019). *Porth's pathophysiology: Concepts of altered health states* (10th ed.). Wolters Kluwer.

Norton, D., McLaren, R., Exton-Smith, A. N. (1962/1975). *An investigation of geriatric nursing problems in hospital.* Churchill Livingstone.

O'Callaghan, S., Galvin, P., O'Mahony, C., Moore, Z., & Derwin, R. (2020). 'Smart' wound dressings for advanced wound care: A review. *Journal of Wound Care, 29*(7), 394–406. https://doi.org/10.12968/jowc.2020.29.7.394

Orth, K. (2018). Preventing surgical site infections related to abdominal drains in the intensive care unit. *Critical Care Nurse, 38*(4), 20–26. https://doi.org/10.4037/ccn2018254

Padula, W. V., Cuddigan, J., Ruotsi, L., Black, J. M., Brienza, D., Capasso, V., Cox, J., Delmore, B., Holden-Mount, S., Munoz, N., Nie, A. M., Pittman, J., Sonenblum, S., Tescher, A., & National Pressure Injury Advisory Panel (NPIAP). (2021). Best-practices for preventing skin injury beneath personal protective equipment during the COVID-19 pandemic: A position paper from the National Pressure Injury Advisory Panel (NPIAP). *Journal of Clinical Nursing.* https://doi.org/10.1111/jocn.15682

Payne, D. (2016). Strategies to support prevention, identification and management of pressure ulcers in the community. *British Journal of Community Nursing, 21*(Suppl 6), S10–S18. https://doi.org/10.12968/bjcn.2016.21.Sup6.S10

Problem-based care plans. (2022). In *Lippincott Advisor.* Wolters Kluwer. https://advisor.lww.com/lna/home.do

Quain, A. M., & Khardori, N. M. (2015). Nutrition in wound care management: A comprehensive overview. *Wounds, 27*(12), 327–335.

Reevell, G., Anders, T., & Morgan, T. (2016). Improving patients' experience of dressing removal in practice. *Journal of Community Nursing, 30*(5), 44–49.

Schreiber, M. L. (2016). Negative pressure wound therapy. *Med Surg Nursing, 25*(6), 425–428.

Sircana, G., Cauteruccio, M., Oliva, M. S., Piccirillo, N., Pesare, E., Minutillo, F., & Ziranu, A. (2020). Fibrin sealant reduces need for transfusions after hip hemiarthroplasty for femoral neck fractures. *Injury, 51*(Suppl 3), S23–S27. https://doi.org/10.1016/j.injury.2020.05.026

Sonoiki, T., Young, J., & Alexis, O. (2020). Challenges faced by nurses in complying with aseptic non-touch technique principles during wound care: A review. *British Journal of Nursing, 29*(5), S28–S35. https://doi.org/10.12968/bjon.2020.29.5.S28

Stedman T. L. (n. d.). *Stedman's online health and nursing dictionary.* Retrieved February 28, 2021, from thepoint.lww.com

Stotts, N. (1990). Seeing red, yellow and black: The three-color concept of wound care. *Nursing, 20*(2), 59–61.

Stuart, E. (2020). Nutrition and wound care: What community nurses should know. *Journal of Community Nursing, 34*(6), 58–62.

VHA Center for Engineering & Occupational Safety and Health (CEOSH). (2016). *Safe patient handling and mobility guidebook.* Author. http://www.tampavaref.org/safe-patient-handling.htm

Waterlow, J. (1985). Pressure sores: A risk assessment card. *Nursing Times, 81*(48), 49–55.

Woo, K. Y., & Sibbald, R. G. (2009). A cross-sectional validation study of using NERDS and STONEES to assess bacterial burden. *Wound Management & Prevention, 55*(8), 40–48. https://www.o-wm.com/content/a-cross-sectional-validation-study-using-nerds-and-stonees-assess-bacterial-burden

Wound, Ostomy and Continence Nurses Society (WOCN), Wound Guidelines Task Force. (2016). WOCH 2016 guideline for prevention and management of pressure injuries (ulcers). *Journal of Wound Ostomy & Continence Nursing, 44*(3), 241–246.

Wound, Ostomy and Continence Nurses Society (WOCN). (n.d.). *Clinical tools. Support Surface Algorithm.* Retrieved January 23, 2021, from https://www.wocn.org/learning-center/clinical-tools/

Yates, S., McNichol, L., Heinecke, S. B., & Gray, M. (2017). Embracing the concept, defining the practice, and changing the outcome: Setting the standard for medical adhesive-related skin injury interventions in WOC nursing practice. *Journal of Wound, Ostomy, and Continence Nursing, 44*(1), 13–17. https://doi.org/10.1097/WON.0000000000000290

34 Activity

Quan Hong Nguyen

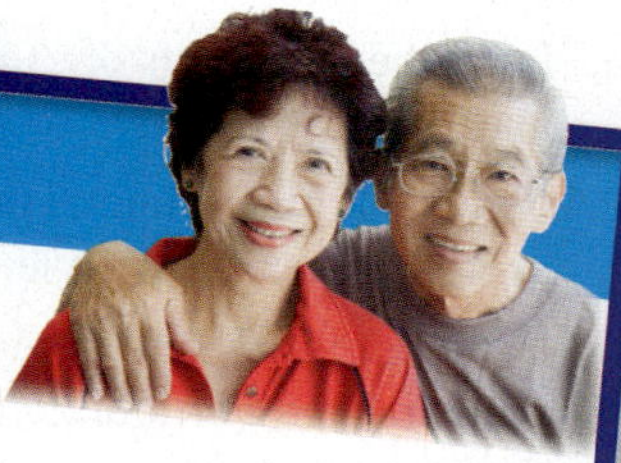

Mr. Nguyen is a 75-year-old man who had an ischemic stroke (cerebrovascular accident or brain attack) secondary to thrombosis (formation of a blood clot). His neurologic deficits have remained unchanged for the 2 days he has been in the hospital. He is alert but has hemiplegia (weakness) on his left side. His wife states, "It will be quite a bit of work for me to care for Quan at home. My bones and joints hurt all the time. He needs a lot of help turning, moving, and getting out of bed. How will I manage?"

Kelsi Lester

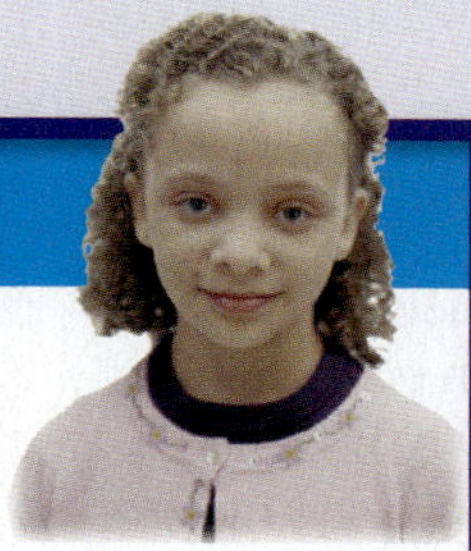

Kelsi is a 10-year-old girl in the pediatric unit as a result of a skiing accident. Unconscious at the present time, she may or may not regain consciousness. Kelsi is on bedrest. She requires frequent positioning to maintain correct body alignment as well as passive range-of-motion exercises to maintain her range of motion.

Maggie Wyatt

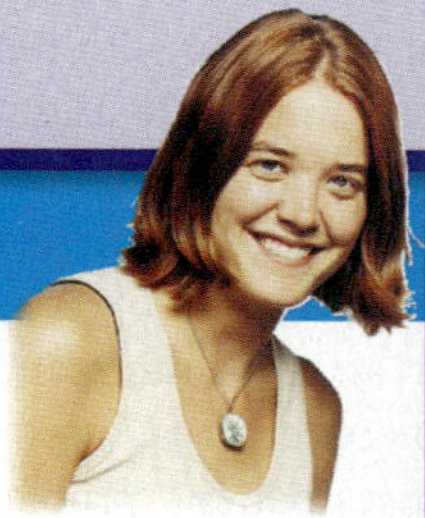

Maggie, a woman in her 30s, was hospitalized because the external fixation device used to treat her fractured right tibia caused an infection in her leg. Following therapy for the infection, the patient is being discharged and requires transfer from the wheelchair to her mother's car.

Learning Outcomes

After completing the chapter, you will be able to accomplish the following:

1. Describe the role of the skeletal, muscular, and nervous systems in the physiology of movement.
2. Identify variables that influence body alignment and mobility.
3. Differentiate isotonic, isometric, and isokinetic exercises.
4. Describe the effects of exercise and immobility on major body systems.
5. Assess body alignment, mobility, and activity tolerance, using appropriate interview and assessment skills.
6. Diagnose actual and potential health problems and needs related to mobility that may be addressed through nursing intervention.
7. Utilize principles of ergonomics when appropriate.
8. Use safe patient handling and mobility techniques and equipment when positioning, moving, lifting, and ambulating patients.
9. Develop exercise programs.
10. Plan, implement, and evaluate nursing care related to select diagnoses/patient problems involving alterations in and related to mobility.

Nursing Concepts

- Assessment
- Clinical decision making/clinical judgment
- Functional ability
- Health promotion
- Mobility

This chapter describes the physiology of movement and factors affecting body alignment and mobility. The effects of immobility on body systems are discussed along with related nursing interventions. A guide for assessing body alignment and mobility states is included, with pertinent interview questions and physical assessment techniques. Analysis of patient mobility data may lead to the identification of issues related to impaired physical mobility or activity intolerance or the effects of mobility problems on other areas of human functioning. Examples of diagnoses/patient problems are included, expected outcomes are identified, and specific nursing strategies are presented. Assessment criteria, screening for patient handling decisions, and proper use of patient handling equipment are discussed. A section on exercise differentiates the types of exercise, explores the role of exercise in disease prevention and health promotion, notes risks related to exercise, and assists in the design of individualized exercise programs. The concluding Concept Map and Nursing Care Plan illustrate how the nurse uses knowledge of mobility and safe patient handling techniques along with specific nursing interventions to promote fitness and address mobility problems. The accompanying Reflective Practice box highlights important considerations to keep in mind when caring for patients with alterations in mobility and activity deficits.

PHYSIOLOGY OF MOVEMENT AND ALIGNMENT

Purposeful, coordinated movement of the body and maintenance of alignment require the integrated functioning of the musculoskeletal and nervous systems. The following sections review concepts related to movement and alignment.

Skeletal System

The framework of bones, the joints between them, and cartilage that protects our organs and allows us to move is called the skeletal system. Functions of this system include:

- Supporting the soft tissues of the body (maintains body form and posture)
- Protecting crucial components of the body (brain, lung, heart, spinal cord)
- Furnishing surfaces for the attachments of muscles, tendons, and ligaments, which, in turn, pull on the individual bones and produce movement
- Providing storage areas for minerals (such as calcium) and fat
- Producing blood cells (hematopoiesis)

The 206 bones in the human body are classified by their shape. Long bones, found in the upper and lower extremities (e.g., humerus and femur), contribute to height and length. Short bones, located in the wrist and ankle, contribute to movement. Flat bones are relatively thin (e.g., ribs and several of the skull bones) and contribute to shape (structural contour). Irregular bones are all those bones not included in the preceding classifications (e.g., bones of the spinal column and jaw).

Bones are too rigid to bend without damage. Therefore, all movements that change the positions of the bony parts of the body occur at joints. The terms *articulation* and *joint* refer to the area where a bone meets another bone. Joints are classified according to the amount of movement they permit and on the basis of the material between the adjoining bones. Types of joints are outlined in Table 34-1 (on page 1242). Diarthroses or synovial joints, joints in which there is a potential space containing lubricating synovial fluid between the articulating bones, are freely moving joints. Freely movable joints are discussed here in relation to the topic of activity.

Several types of freely movable joints are found in the body. These include:

- *Ball-and-socket joint:* The rounded head of one bone fits into a cuplike cavity in the other; flexion–extension, abduction–adduction, and rotation can occur (e.g., shoulder and hip joints).

QSEN Reflective Practice: Cultivating QSEN Competencies

CHALLENGE TO TECHNICAL SKILLS

Last year during my medical-surgical clinical experience, I was taking care of Maggie Wyatt, a female patient in her 30s, with an external fixation device on her right leg. The patient had broken her tibia and had undergone three surgeries to try to correct the fracture. Maggie's current admission was for the treatment of an infection caused by the external device in place to treat the fracture. I was assigned to care for her on the day that she was being discharged. Throughout the day, I formed a close bond with her, and the nurse asked me to bring Maggie to her car when she was ready to leave. I was a little apprehensive about being able to help her into the car with the external fixator in place because she could not bend her leg at all. I had a couple of choices—I could take her down to the car myself and hope that there wouldn't be any problem helping her get into the car, or I could tell the nurse I didn't feel comfortable bringing the patient to the car because I didn't have any experience transferring patients with a device such as this one. However, I really wanted to bring this patient down and see her through the final stage of discharge.

Thinking Outside the Box: Possible Courses of Action

- Take the patient down to the car by myself and do the best I can to help transfer her to the car.
- Explain to the nurse that I don't feel that I have the skills to bring this patient down on my own and ask her to do it.
- Explain to the nurse that I would really like to bring the patient down to the car but that I do not feel that I have the experience to do it on my own; ask her to assist me.
- Ask the nurse about what the best way to transfer the patient to the car is before taking the patient to the car.

Evaluating a Good Outcome: How Do I Define Success?

- Patient receives the highest quality of care and has the least amount of pain possible during the transfer.
- I learn from the experience and gain skills and knowledge for the future.
- Patient is at least not harmed and is possibly benefitted by my action.

Personal Learning: Here's to the Future!

Unfortunately, in this case I did not make the right decision. I convinced myself that it could not be that difficult to transfer this very cooperative patient to her car with her mother's assistance. However, I definitely should have asked for assistance and screened the patient to identify appropriate safe patient handling and mobility equipment to use. The car was extremely small, and it was hard to get her to sit across the back seat while keeping her leg completely straight. The patient was experiencing a fair amount of pain from the device. So, every time we tried to get her into the car, she experienced more pain. Fortunately, a physical therapist came outside to help another patient and then also helped us. I realized that not only did I not have the skills to transfer her myself, but also that this was really a two-person job and required use of a transfer aid. The physical therapist showed me the best way to transfer this patient, and I learned a great deal from the experience. I was lucky that my patient was very understanding and accommodating in this situation. I gained some experience with transferring patients, but most importantly, I realized how important it is to trust your instincts and ask for help when you think you may need it—it's always better to be overprepared than underprepared.

Catherine Barrell, Georgetown University

QSEN SELF-REFLECTION ON QUALITY AND SAFETY COMPETENCIES DEVELOPING KNOWLEDGE, SKILLS, AND ATTITUDES FOR CONTINUOUS IMPROVEMENT

How do you think you would respond in a similar situation? Why? What does this tell you about yourself and about the adequacy of your skills for professional practice? Do you agree with the criteria that the nursing student used to evaluate a successful outcome? Are there any other criteria that would be appropriate to use? Did the nursing student meet the criteria? Why or why not? What *knowledge, skills,* and *attitudes* do you need to develop to continuously improve the quality and safety of care for patients like Ms. Wyatt?

Patient-Centered Care: What factors do you think might have influenced the nursing student's actions? Suppose that the patient was using crutches or a walker instead of having the fixation device in place. How might the nursing student's actions be different?

Teamwork and Collaboration/Quality Improvement: Imagine that the physical therapist did not arrive on the scene. What would have been the nursing student's next best action? What communication skills do you need to improve to ensure that you function as a member of the patient care team?

Safety/Evidence-Based Practice: What resources could the student have accessed to ensure the safe transfer of the patient? What evidence in nursing literature provides guidance for decision making regarding care of this patient? Can you think of other ways to respond to or approach the situation?

Table 34-1 Joints

TYPE	MOVEMENT	MATERIAL BETWEEN THE BONES	EXAMPLES
Fibrous 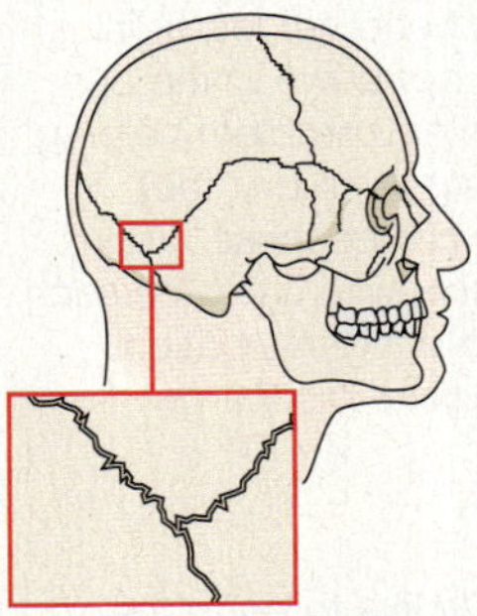	Immovable (synarthrosis)	No joint cavity; fibrous connective tissue between bones	Sutures between bones of skull
Cartilaginous 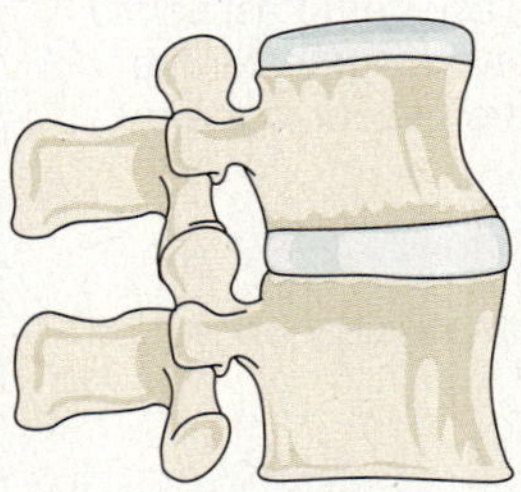	Slightly movable (amphiarthrosis)	No joint cavity; cartilage between bones	Pubic symphysis; joints between bodies of vertebrae
Synovial 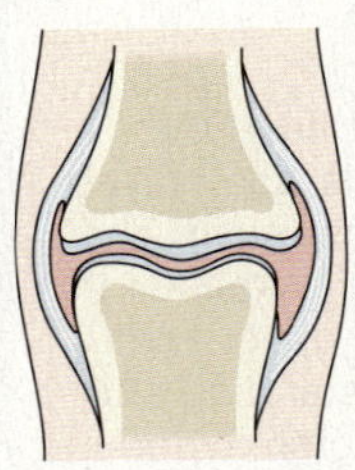	Freely movable (diarthrosis)	Joint cavity containing synovial fluid	Gliding, hinge, pivot, condyloid, saddle, ball-and-socket joints

Source: Reprinted with permission from Cohen, B. J., & Hull, K. L. (2019). *Memmler's structure and function of the human body* (12th ed.). Jones and Bartlett Learning.

- *Condyloid joint:* The oval head of one bone fits into a shallow cavity of another bone; flexion–extension and abduction–adduction can occur (e.g., wrist joint and joints connecting fingers to palm).
- *Gliding joint:* Flat surfaces of the bone slide over one another; flexion–extension and abduction–adduction can occur (e.g., carpal bones of wrist and tarsal bones of feet).
- *Hinge joint:* A spool-like (rounded) surface of one bone fits into a concave surface of another bone; only flexion–extension can occur (e.g., elbow, knee, ankle joints).
- *Pivot joint:* A ring-like structure that turns on a pivot; movement is limited to rotation (e.g., joints between the atlas and axis of the neck and between the proximal ends of the radius and the ulna at the wrist).
- *Saddle joint:* Bone surfaces are convex on one side and concave on the other; movements include flexion–extension, adduction–abduction, circumduction, and opposition (e.g., joint between the trapezium and metacarpal of the thumb).

Movements possible at diarthrodial joints include abduction, adduction, flexion, extension, and rotation. Special movements of the forearm, ankle, and clavicle include supination, pronation, inversion, and eversion. The thumb is the only joint that can perform opposition. These movements are defined in Table 34-2.

The strength and flexibility of the skeletal system also depend on ligaments, tendons, and cartilage. Ligaments are tough, fibrous bands of connective tissue that bind joints together and connect bones and cartilage. Tendons are strong, flexible, inelastic fibrous bands and flattened sheets of connective tissue that attach muscle to bone. Cartilage is hard, nonvascular connective tissue found in the joints as well as in the nose, ear, thorax, trachea, and larynx. Cartilage in joints functions as a shock absorber and provides a smooth surface that reduces friction between the moving parts of the joint. Fat may also provide padding at joints.

Muscular System

The muscular system is composed of three types of muscles: (1) skeletal, (2) cardiac, and (3) smooth or visceral muscles. Muscle tissue produces movement by contraction of its cells.

Table 34-2 Terms Commonly Used to Describe Body Positions and Movements

TERM	DEFINITION AND EXAMPLE
Abduction	Lateral movement of a body part away from the midline of the body. *Example:* A person's arm is abducted when it is moved away from the body.
Adduction	Lateral movement of a body part toward the midline of the body. *Example:* A person's arm is adducted when it is moved from an outstretched position to a position alongside the body.
Circumduction	Turning in a circular motion; combines abduction, adduction, extension, and flexion. *Example:* Circling the arm at the shoulder, as in bowling or a serve in tennis.
Flexion	The state of being bent. *Example:* A person's cervical spine is flexed when the head is bent forward, chin to chest.
Extension	The state of being in a straight line. *Example:* A person's cervical spine is extended when the head is held straight on the spinal column.
Hyperextension	The state of exaggerated extension. It often results in an angle greater than 180 degrees. *Example:* A person's cervical spine is hyperextended when looking overhead, toward the ceiling.
Dorsiflexion	Backward bending of the hand or foot. *Example:* A person's foot is in dorsiflexion when the toes are brought up as though to point them at the knee.
Plantar flexion	Flexion of the foot. *Example:* A person's foot is in plantar flexion in the footdrop position.
Rotation	Turning on an axis; the turning of a body part on the axis provided by its joint. *Example:* A thumb is rotated when it is moved to make a circle.
Internal rotation	A body part turning on its axis toward the midline of the body. *Example:* A leg is rotated internally when it turns inward at the hip and the toes point toward the midline of the body.
External rotation	A body part turning on its axis away from the midline of the body. *Example:* A leg is rotated externally when it turns outward at the hip and the toes point away from the midline of the body.
Special Movements	
Pronation	The assumption of the prone position. *Example:* A person is in the prone position when lying on the abdomen; a person's palm is prone when the forearm is turned so that the palm faces downward.
Supination	The assumption of the supine position. *Example:* A person is in the supine position when lying on the back; a person's palm is supine when the forearm is turned so that the palm faces upward.
Inversion	Movement of the sole of the foot inward (occurs at the ankle)
Eversion	Movement of the sole of the foot outward (occurs at the ankle)
Opposition	Rotation of the thumb around its long access (movement of the thumb across the palm to touch each fingertip of the same hand).

Skeletal muscle works with tendons and bones to move the body. Cardiac muscle forms the bulk of the heart and produces the contractions that create the heartbeat. Smooth muscle forms the walls of the hollow organs (such as the stomach and intestines) and is in the walls of blood vessels and other hollow tubes (such as ureters) that connect internal organs. Skeletal muscle is discussed here in relation to the topic of activity.

The skeletal muscle system includes the skeletal muscle tissue and connective tissue that comprise individual muscle organs, such as the biceps. Bones and joints provide form to the body and serve as the levers and fulcrums that make body movement possible. Movement results from a skeletal muscle contracting and exerting force on a tendon, which, in turn, pulls on a bone. Muscles have two differing points of attachment: (1) the attachment of a muscle to the more stationary bone is called the point of origin, and (2) the attachment to the more movable bone is the point of insertion. Between these two points is the fleshy "belly" of the muscle. The excitability, contractility, extensibility, and elasticity of muscles enable them to perform four important functions for the body through contraction:

- *Motion:* Skeletal muscle contractions pull on tendons and move the bones, creating movements as simple as extending the arm to as highly coordinated as swimming or skiing.
- *Maintenance of posture:* Skeletal muscle contractions hold the body in stationary positions.
- *Support:* Skeletal muscles support soft tissues in the abdominal wall and floor of the pelvic cavity.
- *Heat production:* Skeletal muscle contractions produce heat and help maintain body temperature.

Figure 34-1 (on page 1244) illustrates the relationship of skeletal muscles to bones and the use of bones as levers and of joints as fulcrums to produce body movement.

Nervous System

The skeletal and muscular systems cannot produce purposeful movement without a functioning nervous system.

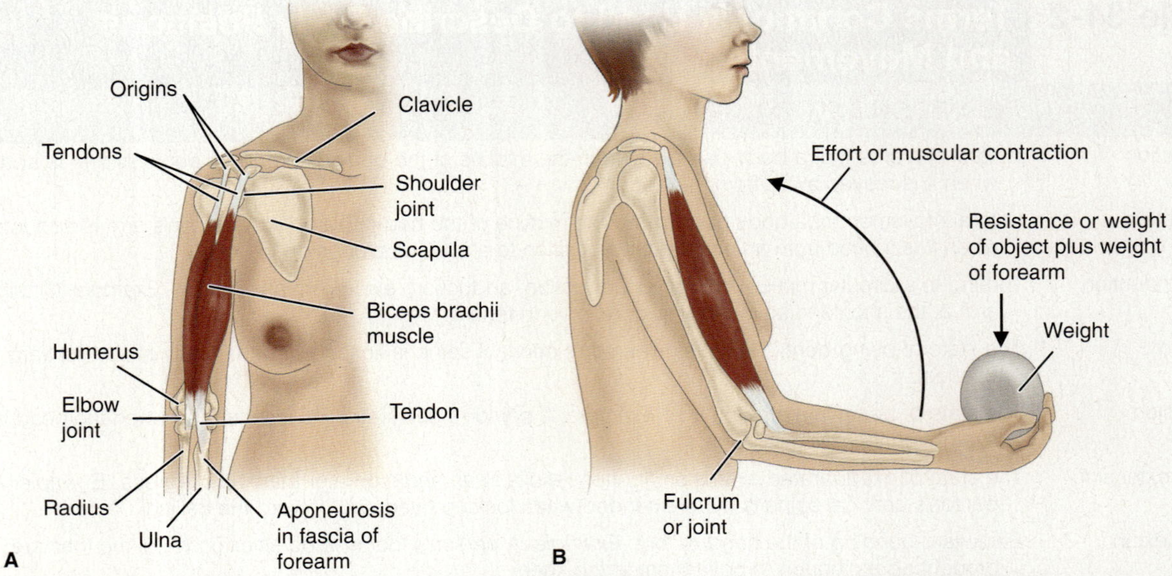

FIGURE 34-1. Relationship of skeletal muscles to bones. **A.** Skeletal muscles produce movements by pulling on bones. **B.** Bones serve as levers, and joints act as fulcrums for the levers. The lever and fulcrum principle is illustrated by the movement of the forearm lifting a weight.

Nerve impulses stimulate muscles to contract. More specifically:

- Nerve cells called neurons conduct impulses from one part of the body to another.
- The afferent neurons convey information from receptors in the periphery of the body to the central nervous system (CNS; e.g., light pressure on nose).
- This information is processed by the CNS, leading to a response (e.g., "There is a fly on my nose. I want to brush it off.").
- The efferent neurons convey the response from the CNS to skeletal muscles by way of the somatic nervous system (e.g., muscles in the arm, wrist, and hand contract, and the fingers brush the fly from the nose).

Normal Movement and Alignment

The following concepts are an important part of normal movement and musculoskeletal functioning and contribute to a person's overall well-being.

Body Alignment or Posture

Good posture, or proper body alignment, is the alignment of body parts that permits optimal musculoskeletal balance and operation and promotes healthy physiologic functioning. A person in correct alignment is experiencing no undue strain on the joints, muscles, tendons, or ligaments while balance is maintained.

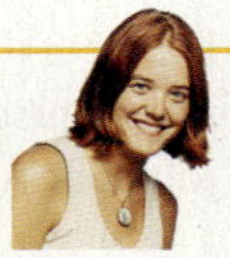

Consider ***Maggie Wyatt***, the woman being discharged with an external fixation device in place. Although the device is heavy and awkward and requires her to keep her right leg extended, body alignment is crucial for Maggie to prevent undue strain on other parts of her body.

The criteria for correct alignment in the standing, sitting, and reclining positions are described in the Assessing section on page 1257.

Balance

A body in correct alignment is balanced. An object is balanced when its center of gravity is close to its base of support, the line of gravity goes through the base of support, and the object has a wide base of support. The center of gravity of an object is the point at which its mass is centered. When the human is standing, the center of gravity is located in the center of the pelvis about midway between the umbilicus and the symphysis pubis. The line of gravity is a vertical line that passes through the center of gravity. The base of support is the foundation that provides for an object's stability. The wider the base of support and the lower the center of gravity, the greater the stability of the object will be. Figure 34-2 illustrates the effect of the base of support and gravity on body balance.

Body balance increases when people spread the feet farther apart and flex the hips and knees. This broadens the base of support and lowers the center of gravity. These two simple maneuvers are important interventions that can decrease the musculoskeletal strain that occurs with excessive stretching or overexertion of a muscle or muscle–tendon unit. Musculoskeletal strain most commonly affects the lower back and cervical spine region. Trauma to the musculoskeletal system is discussed on page 1249.

Coordinated Body Movement

Coordinated body movement is the ability of muscles to work together for purposeful movement. Using major and stronger muscle groups, rather than weaker ones, and taking advantage of the body's natural levers and fulcrums facilitates the actions of lifting, carrying, pushing, pulling, and

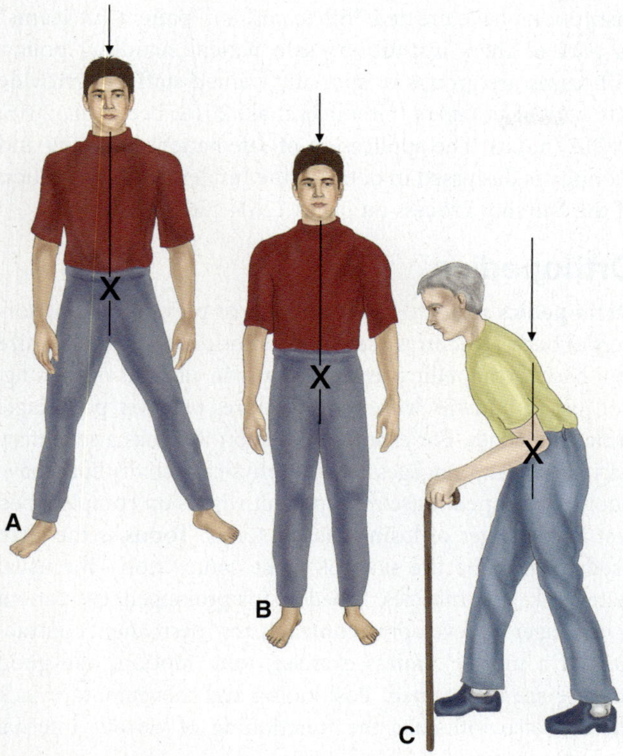

FIGURE 34-2. The effect of the base of support and gravity on balance is shown. **A.** The line of gravity passes through the wide base of support. This person is the most stable of the three. **B.** The line of gravity also passes through the base of support, although the base is narrower. This person is less stable than the person in **A**. **C.** The line of gravity does not pass through the base of support. This person is unstable.

moving objects. Major muscle groups include the flexors, extensors, and abductors of the thighs; flexors and extensors of the knees; and flexors and extensors of the upper and lower arms. For example, use of the arm bones as levers and the elbows as fulcrums facilitates lifting a weight against resistance, the force of gravity—the lever and fulcrum principle (see Fig. 34-1).

Postural Reflexes

Postural reflexes are the group of reflexes (automatic movements) that maintain body position and equilibrium, whether at rest or during movement. Integrated functioning of the musculoskeletal and nervous systems is essential for body alignment and balance. Postural tonus, the sustained contraction of select skeletal muscles that keeps the human body in an upright position against the force of gravity, depends on the functioning of several postural reflexes:

- The sensory organs in the inner ear provide a sense of position, orientation, and movement. Body movement (e.g., changes in head position) stimulates the sensory organs, which then transmit these impulses to the cerebellum.
- Joint movements stimulating special nerve endings in muscles, tendons, and fascia inform the brain of the location of a limb or body part.
- Visual impressions contribute to posture by alerting the person to spatial relationships with the environment (nearness of ceilings, walls, furniture, condition of floor, etc.).
- When extensor muscles are stretched beyond a certain point (e.g., when knees buckle under), their stimulation causes a reflex contraction that aids a person to reestablish erect posture (e.g., straighten the knee).

Safe Patient Handling and Mobility

Ergonomics is the practice of designing equipment and work tasks to conform to the capability of the worker and provides a means for adjusting the work environment and work practices to prevent injuries (OSHA, n.d.b). The use of proper body positions and avoidance of awkward postures provide protection from the stress of movement and activity (OSHA, n.d.b). Ergonomics includes proper body movement in daily activities, the prevention and correction of problems associated with posture, and the enhancement of coordination and endurance. It is important to use the principles of ergonomics during activity and during rest periods to prevent injury and to prevent sore muscles and joints. Many activities in which the nurse engages to move objects, from as simple an activity as moving a chair, repositioning the medication cart, or reaching to silence a monitor alarm, require understanding and using these principles. Nurses who consciously develop good habits when moving objects can demonstrate to others proper ways of using the musculoskeletal system. The application of ergonomics is discussed in the Implementing section of the Nursing Process on pages 1260–1262.

Ergonomics applied to activities associated with direct patient care is known as **safe patient handling and mobility (SPHM).** It is very important to incorporate safe patient handling and mobility interventions into nursing practice and patient care. Frequently, it is necessary to move patients who are weak or unable to move on their own. However, manual lifting, transferring, and repositioning of patients are high-risk activities for nurses and patients. Even routine repetitive care activities, such as changing bed linens and bathing patients, have the potential to cause back injury.

Self-Care Alert

Nurses are at high risk for musculoskeletal injuries from moving patients. Implement patient handling and mobility equipment as a best practice. Be familiar with the safe patient handling equipment available in your facility; understanding how to choose and use appropriate devices is a priority for self-care and safe patient care.

Injuries and musculoskeletal disorders are often caused by manually lifting patients, and nurses are at high risk every day (American Nurses Association [ANA], n.d.a). Patient handling injuries represent more than 20% of injuries to nurses (Hodgson et al., 2013). Nurses report musculoskeletal pain caused or exacerbated by their work and chronic back pain (Fragala et al., 2016). Of nurses in the United States, as many as 20% leave direct patient care positions because of risks associated with the work (OSHA, n.d.a). Many nurses say they have had episodes of occupation-related back problems and accept back pain as a routine consequence of the job—but this need not be. Variables that can lead to patient handling injuries include the following:

- Uncoordinated lifts
- High exertion (force required to life, move or handle patient) while in an awkward posture
- Assuming awkward and static postures
- Manual lifting and transferring of patients without assistive devices
- Lifting when fatigued
- Repetitive movements such as lifting, transferring, and repositioning patients
- Standing for long periods of time
- Transferring patients from beds to stretchers and chairs, wheelchairs, or operating tables; repositioning patients in bed
- Repetitive tasks
- Transferring/repositioning patients who have cognitive impairments, who are dependent/obese/overweight, or patients who are unable or unwilling to actively participate and promote their own movement (Fragala et al., 2016).

A more effective approach to safe patient transfers includes patient assessment criteria; screening and algorithms for patient handling and mobility decisions; specialized patient handling equipment used properly and operated using proper ergonomics; and the use of lift teams. The proper use of assistive devices to lift, move, reposition, and transport patients is key to SPHM (Fragala et al., 2016). In addition, the use of assistive patient handling equipment contributes to patient comfort and protects patient dignity, while increasing safety.

Research supports the consistent use of standardized protocols and assistive devices as an effective approach to decrease the risk of injury for health care workers (Nelson, 2015; Nelson et al., 2009). The National Institute for Occupational Safety and Health (NIOSH) (2013), Joint Commission and the Occupational Safety & Health Administration (OSHA) recommend a no-lift policy in conjunction with technology, assistive devices, education, and a culture of safety for all health care facilities (Fragala et al., 2016; OSHA and Joint Commission Resources Alliance, 2017). Implementing safe patient handling and mobility programs improves the quality of patient care and reduces the risk of harm for patients and health care workers (Nelson, 2015; OSHA and Joint Commission Resources Alliance, 2017).

Preventive measures should focus on careful assessment of the patient care environment so that patients can be moved safely and effectively. The use of a back-belt does not prevent back injury. In some institutions, specially trained staff members who function as "back injury resource nurses" are responsible for assisting nurses to assess patients. Other institutions have created "lift teams" or "patient lift teams" as part of their institution's safe patient handling policy. Lift teams are groups of specially trained staff that provide safe patient transfers (Graulich et al., 2018; Lee et al., 2015; OSHA, n.d.b). The application of safe patient handling and mobility is discussed in detail in the Implementation section of the Nursing Process on pages 1261–1262.

Orthopedics

Orthopedics refers to the correction or prevention of disorders of body structures used in locomotion. Nurses recognize that basic orthopedic principles apply in all areas of nursing, not just to patients with bone fractures or other pathologic skeletal changes. For example, a person who has a sedentary occupation and engages in little physical activity may have poorly developed muscles. A patient who is on complete bed rest is in danger of losing muscle tonus. **Tonus** is the term used to describe the state of slight contraction—the usual state of skeletal muscles. If bed rest is prolonged, the patient is in danger of developing **contractures** (permanent contraction of a muscle) unless exercise, joint motion, and good posture are maintained. Positioning and movement, or lack thereof, also influence the functioning of various internal body processes.

FACTORS AFFECTING MOVEMENT AND ALIGNMENT

Numerous factors, including growth and development, physical health, mental health, lifestyle variables, attitude and values, fatigue and stress, and external factors such as weather influence a person's posture, movement, and daily activity level.

Developmental Considerations

A person's age and degree of neuromuscular development markedly influence body proportions, posture, body mass, movements, and reflexes. To promote neuromuscular development in patients of all ages and to facilitate each patient's use of the body to perform self-care activities, nurses need to be familiar with developmental variations in body proportions and neuromuscular development. These variations are presented in Table 34-3 along with related nursing assessment priorities and nursing interventions.

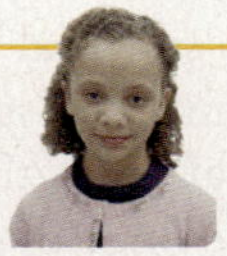

Recall ***Kelsi Lester***, the 10-year-old girl in a coma. Typically, children of this age are highly active and mobile. However, Kelsi is immobile and confined to bed due to her accident. The nurse would obtain a history of Kelsi's activity level before the accident to determine her neuromuscular development. The nurse would then use this information to develop an age-appropriate plan of care to maximize Kelsi's level of function.

Physical Health

Problems in the musculoskeletal or nervous systems can have a negative influence on body alignment and movement.

Table 34-3 Activity Variations Based on Developmental Level: Assessment Priorities and Nursing Interventions

DEVELOPMENTAL LEVEL	ASSESSMENT PRIORITIES	NURSING INTERVENTIONS
Infant		
• Periods of activity and alertness alternate with quiet periods and sleep. • At 3 months: May raise chest and head when prone. • By 5 months: Head control usually achieved.	Assess the following key developmental milestones at these ages: **3–6 months** • Ability to sit • Head control **6–9 months** • Sits steadily • Rolls over • Creeps on all fours • Pulls to a standing position • Has improved hand–eye coordination **9–12 months** • Progresses toward unassisted walking • Is able to pick up small objects	• Encourage parents to examine their baby. • Respond to concerns that parents have about minor variations in newborn's appearance or behavior. • Emphasize that individual variation in activity patterns and neuromuscular development should be expected. • Account for any prematurity when discussing normal developmental progression of preterm infants.
Toddler		
• Gross and fine motor development continues rapidly. • By 15 months: Most can walk unassisted. • At 18 months: Most can run. • At 2 years: Most can jump. • At 3 years: Most can stack blocks, work simple puzzles, and dress themselves.	• Assess progress in walking, running, and jumping. • Assess small-muscle coordination (e.g., ability to dress themselves, wash hands, brush teeth). • Distinguish slow developers who fall within normal range from those with developmental lags.	• Help parents to learn and accept their child's uniqueness. • Teach parents the importance of providing a safe environment. • Enthusiastically reinforce and praise toddler's mastery of new skills. • Set limits so that toddler does not overextend self in drive for mastery of skills.
Child		
• Greater gross and fine motor control. • By age 4: Negotiate stairs, walk backward, and hop on one foot. • By age 5: Skip, jump rope, and jump off heights of several steps. • Able to manipulate writing materials.	• Use developmental charts to assess gross and fine motor development. • Determine activity level and types of play that involve physical exertion.	• Teach parents that attitudes about the body and exercise are developed during this period. • Counsel as appropriate. • Assess safety issues and reinforce safety teaching at each stage.
Adolescent		
• Size increases: There is a growth spurt. • Secondary sex characteristics appear. • If physically fit: Can be a time of boundless energy and great athletic performance. • If inactive: May begin a lifelong pattern of unhealthy behavior.	• Determine activity level and type of regular exercise. • Evaluate safety of recreational choices. • Screen for scoliosis (lateral curvature of the spine). • Examine muscle mass, tone, and strength and joint mobility.	• Encourage physical activity, regular exercise, and limitation of sedentary hobbies. • Lifestyle counseling regarding the importance of exercise and fitness is critical. • Encourage to exercise regularly if necessary. • Caution about gauging physical limits and not "pushing too hard."
Adult		
• Stands and sits erect and is capable of balanced and coordinated purposeful movement. • During pregnancy: center of gravity shifts because of developing fetus. • Activity levels vary greatly.	• Assess balance between activity and rest in person's lifestyle. • Note any lifestyle factors or illnesses that interfere with mobility or ability to carry out activities of daily living.	• Fitness counseling is important. • Clarify misconceptions about exercise. • Design and monitor safe exercise programs. • Those with mobility alterations may require special care.
Older Adult		
• Increased convexity in the thoracic spine (kyphosis) from disk shrinkage and decreased height • Loss of muscle tone • Subcutaneous fat loss • Arthritic joint changes may be present	• Assess general ease of movement and gait. • Assess alignment. • Check joints and their function. • Assess muscle mass, tone, and strength.	• Teach and counsel about: • Importance of regular exercise • Need for high protein, calcium, and vitamin D–enriched diet • Pacing activities • Using assistive devices safely when needed • Safety-proof home to reduce falls

Similarly, illness or trauma involving other body systems may interfere with movement because of either the underlying pathology or the treatment regimen. Nurses must be sensitive to how both acute and chronic health problems affect a patient's general appearance (posture, body proportions, and movements), their ability to move purposefully to perform **activities of daily living (ADLs)** and **instrumental activities of daily living (IADLs)** or self-care activities, and maintain their quality of life (functional health) (Jarvis & Eckhardt, 2020; Jensen, 2019). Eating, bathing, dressing, and toileting are examples of ADLs. Housekeeping, meal preparation, management of finances, and transportation are examples of IADLs. When assessing a patient's response to a mobility deficit, work to:

- Encourage attempts at behaviors that promote self-care activities despite limitations (e.g., offer supportive suggestions to patients who attempt to feed themselves despite having hemiparesis).
- Reinforce behaviors that promote healthy functioning (e.g., congratulate a patient who manages transfers well despite left-sided weakness or paralysis).
- Correct behaviors that compound the mobility deficit over time (e.g., teach adaptive strategies that can be shared with other patients and families to a patient with arthritis who severely restricts movement because of joint stiffness and tenderness; or teach energy conservation measures to patients with emphysema who have greatly decreased activity tolerance).

Additional information related to activities of daily living, as well as functional health, is discussed in the Physical Assessment discussion later in this chapter and in Chapter 27.

Muscular, Skeletal, or Nervous System Problems

Problems with the musculoskeletal or nervous systems may involve one or more of the following health issues.

CONGENITAL OR ACQUIRED POSTURAL ABNORMALITIES

Postural abnormalities that affect appearance and mobility may be congenital in origin or acquired. Examples of patients experiencing one of these abnormalities include a newborn with developmental hip dysplasia, torticollis (lateral deviation of the neck) or a clubfoot; a teenager with lordosis (exaggerated anterior convex curvature of the spine) or scoliosis (lateral curvature of the spine); and an older adult with kyphosis (increased convexity in the curvature of the thoracic spine). Nursing responsibilities may include the following:

- Early detection of and referral for these problems
- Exploration and selection of patient education, counseling, and support as treatment options
- Careful attention to positioning, transfers, and exercise
- Education of the patient and family/caregivers regarding safe self-care activities

PROBLEMS WITH BONE FORMATION OR MUSCLE DEVELOPMENT

Problems with bone formation may include any of the following:

- Congenital problems, such as achondroplasia, in which premature bone ossification (bone tissue formation) leads to dwarfism or osteogenesis imperfecta, which is characterized by excessively brittle bones and multiple fractures both at birth and later in life
- Nutrition-related problems, such as vitamin D deficiency, which results in deformities of the growing skeleton (rickets)
- Disease-related problems, such as Paget's disease, in which excessive bone destruction and abnormal regeneration result in skeletal pain, deformities, and pathologic fractures
- Age-related problems, such as osteoporosis, in which bone destruction exceeds bone formation and in which the resultant thin, porous bones fracture easily

Problems with muscle development may be genetic in origin, a disease-related problem, or an age-related problem. The muscular dystrophies are a group of genetically transmitted disorders that share a common progressive degeneration and weakness of skeletal muscles. They vary in terms of the muscle groups involved and their clinical course. Myasthenia gravis is a weakness of the skeletal muscles caused by an abnormality at the neuromuscular junction that prevents muscle fibers from contracting. Myotonic muscular dystrophy involves prolonged muscle spasms or stiffening after use. Duchenne muscular dystrophy involves a muscle decrease in size, as well as weakening of muscles over time.

Nursing responsibilities for patients with problems of bone formation and muscle development and functioning include the following:

- Careful collaboration with the health care team to determine the motor capacities of the person
- Patient and family/caregiver education aimed at developing optimal mobility
- The ability to position, transfer, and exercise the patient safely, with attention to patient comfort

PROBLEMS AFFECTING JOINT MOBILITY

Inflammation, degeneration, and trauma can all interfere with joint mobility. The term *arthritis* describes more than 100 different diseases that affect areas in or around joints. Arthritis is characterized by inflammation, pain, damage to joint, stiffness and/or decreased range of motion (Arthritis Foundation, n.d.b; Centers for Disease Control and Prevention [CDC], 2020a). The most common type is osteoarthritis, also termed *degenerative joint disease.* Osteoarthritis is a noninflammatory, progressive disorder of movable joints, particularly weight-bearing joints, characterized by the deterioration of articular cartilage and pain with motion (Arthritis Foundation, n.d.a). Once the articular cartilage is damaged, bony deposits (bone spurs) may form in the joints, causing more pain with movement of the joint.

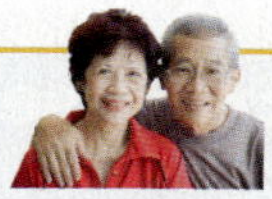

Remember **Mrs. Nguyen**, the older woman concerned about caring for her husband at home. The nurse would need to consider the impact of possible age-related issues as contributing to Mrs. Nguyen's current problems with bone and joint pain. Due to her older adult status, the likelihood of osteoporosis and degenerative joint disease is high. Therefore, teaching to minimize stress on the joints when assisting with her husband's care would be important in preventing possible bone and joint injuries and reducing pain.

Trauma to a joint may result in a sprain or a dislocation. A sprain occurs with the wrenching or twisting of a joint, resulting in a partial tear or rupture to its attachments. A dislocation is characterized by the displacement of a bone from a joint with tearing of ligaments, tendons, and capsules. Any condition restricting joint mobility has potentially crippling effects.

Nurses caring for patients with joint problems work collaboratively with physicians, other advanced practice professionals, physical therapists, and other health care professionals to maintain joint mobility. Patient education is directed to the patient's mastery of an exercise and care program, which fosters tissue repair and maximal independence in ADLs.

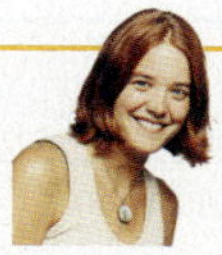

Think back to **Maggie Wyatt**, the woman being discharged after treatment for a fractured tibia. The nurse would need to work closely with other members of Maggie's health care team to ensure that joint mobility is maintained, even with the device in place. The discharge teaching plan would include measures to maintain function of the right leg while the external fixation device immobilizes the fractured area.

TRAUMA TO THE MUSCULOSKELETAL SYSTEM

Injury to the musculoskeletal system can result in fractures and soft tissue injuries. A fracture, a break in the continuity of a bone or cartilage, may result from a traumatic injury or some underlying disease process. Healing requires realignment of the bone fragment, immobilization, and restoration of the bone's function. Soft tissue injuries include sprains, strains, and dislocations (sprains and dislocations are discussed in the previous section, Problems Affecting Joint Mobility). A strain, the least serious of these injuries, is a stretching of a muscle. Nurses need to be knowledgeable in first aid measures for musculoskeletal trauma as well as in acute and rehabilitative care.

PROBLEMS AFFECTING THE CENTRAL NERVOUS SYSTEM

A problem in any of the parts of the brain or spinal cord involved with skeletal muscle control can affect mobility. The cerebral motor cortex assumes the major role of controlling precise, discrete movements. A cerebrovascular accident (stroke) or head trauma may damage the motor cortex and produce temporary or permanent voluntary motor impairment. Basal ganglia integrate semivoluntary movements such as walking, swimming, and laughing. In Parkinson's disease, there is progressive degeneration of the basal ganglia of the cerebrum, thus affecting walking and coordination. Unnecessary skeletal movements result in tremors and muscle rigidity, which interfere with voluntary movement. The cerebellum assists the motor cortex and basal ganglia by making body movements smooth and coordinated. In multiple sclerosis, the myelin sheaths of neurons in the central nervous system (CNS) deteriorate to hardened scars or plaques. Plaque formation in the cerebellum may produce lack of coordination, tremors, and/or weakness.

The pyramidal pathways of the nervous system convey voluntary motor impulses from the brain through the spinal cord by way of two major pathways: (1) the pyramidal pathway and (2) the extrapyramidal pathway. With trauma to the spinal cord, transection (severing) of these motor pathways results in complete bilateral loss of voluntary movement below the level of the trauma.

Nurses caring for patients with injury to the CNS need to be knowledgeable about the pathology and clinical course of these diseases to provide appropriate patient education and counseling. Education and counseling are directed at addressing how the disease may progress and how it may affect the patient's functioning.

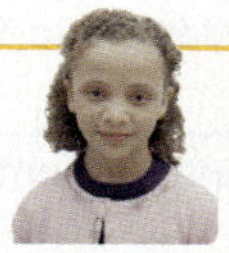

Recall **Kelsi Lester**, the 10-year-old in a coma after a skiing accident. Although Kelsi is unconscious, the nurse must communicate with her, making sure to explain everything that is happening to her and all that is being done. In addition, the nurse would need to communicate with Kelsi's family to ensure that they understand what is happening. For example, the nurse needs to explain the reasons for frequent turning, position changes, and exercises while Kelsi is unconscious.

Problems Involving Other Body Systems

The pathology of numerous other acute and chronic illnesses may also affect mobility. Chronic obstructive pulmonary disease and conditions such as ascites (accumulation of fluid in the peritoneal cavity) may alter posture. Any illnesses that interfere with oxygenation at the cellular level decrease the amount of oxygen available to the muscles for work and thus decrease activity tolerance. These illnesses include anemia, angina, cardiac arrhythmias, heart failure, and chronic obstructive pulmonary disease. Diseases characterized by a larger breakdown of protein than that which is manufactured, such as anorexia nervosa and certain cancers, lead to a negative nitrogen balance that results in muscle wasting and decreased physical energy for movement and work. Symptoms accompanying many illnesses, such as fatigue, muscle aches, and pain, may also lead to immobility. Bed rest is an important component of treatment for many diseases or trauma states, such as some surgeries and fractures. Although rest is essential for the healing process,

Table 34-4 Comparison of Effects of Exercise and Immobility on Body Systems

BODY SYSTEM	EFFECTS OF EXERCISE	EFFECTS OF IMMOBILITY
Cardiovascular System	↑ Efficiency of heart ↓ Resting heart rate and blood pressure ↑ Blood flow and oxygenation of all body parts	↑ Cardiac workload ↑ Risk for orthostatic hypotension ↑ Risk for venous thrombosis
Respiratory System	↑ Depth of respiration ↑ Respiratory rate ↑ Gas exchange at alveolar level ↑ Rate of carbon dioxide excretion	↓ Depth of respiration ↓ Rate of respiration Pooling of secretions Impaired gas exchange
Gastrointestinal System	↑ Appetite ↑ Intestinal tone	Disturbance in appetite Altered protein metabolism Altered digestion and utilization of nutrients ↓ Peristalsis
Urinary System	↑ Blood flow to kidneys ↑ Efficiency in maintaining fluid and acid–base balance ↑ Efficiency in excreting body wastes	↑ Urinary stasis ↑ Risk for renal calculi ↓ Bladder muscle tone
Musculoskeletal System	↑ Muscle efficiency ↑ Coordination ↑ Efficiency of nerve impulse transmission	↓ Muscle size, tone, and strength ↓ Joint mobility, flexibility Bone demineralization ↓ Endurance, stability ↑ Risk for contracture formation
Metabolic System	↑ Efficiency of metabolic system ↑ Efficiency of body temperature regulation	↑ Risk for electrolyte imbalance Altered exchange of nutrients and gases
Integument	Improved tone, color, and turgor, resulting from improved circulation	↑ Risk for skin breakdown and formation of pressure injuries
Psychological Well-Being	Energy, vitality, general well-being Improved sleep Improved appearance Improved self-concept Positive health behaviors	↑ Sense of powerlessness ↓ Self-concept ↓ Social interaction ↓ Sensory stimulation Altered sleep–wake pattern ↑Risk for depression Risk for learned helplessness

immobility associated with bed rest may cause its own problems. Table 34-4 outlines a comparison of the effects of immobility and exercise on body systems. Nurses need to be vigilant in determining the effects of any injury or illness on mobility and in providing care to facilitate optimal mobility as early as possible.

Mental Health

A person's mental health influences body appearance and movement as much as the person's physical health. Body processes tend to slow down with depression, and there is a lack of visible energy and enthusiasm. Body posture also may be affected. For example, the person with depression often sits with head bowed and shoulders slumped, and may lack the energy to eat or even to use the toilet. Even facial movement may be decreased to the point at which the person's face registers no emotion (termed a flat affect). Conversely, people who are not depressed are more likely to have erect posture, animated facial features, and energy for routine activities.

Lifestyle

Whether a person chooses an active or sedentary lifestyle is dependent on many variables, including occupation, leisure activity preferences, and cultural influences. Many occupations are sedentary (e.g., computer technician). Therefore, people in sedentary occupations wishing to exercise regularly need to plan ahead for these leisure activities by preparing to exercise before or after work hours or during a lunch break. People may also participate in leisure activities that are sedentary in nature such as reading, debating, crafts, and watching television. In addition, a person's diet and smoking history are other lifestyle variables that influence mobility.

Culture may also play a role, encouraging or discouraging exercise. Identifying culturally acceptable physical activities is an important step in planning a program of physical activity. Physical activities that are congruent with overall lifestyle and cultural context and planned in the context of a patient-centered approach will be easier to incorporate into daily living (Andrews et al., 2020; Lee & Im, 2010). The nurse should include the patient and family members/caregivers to determine preferred activities to devise a plan for increasing activity level.

Attitude and Values

In some families, such as those who hike, swim, or play ball together, children learn early to value regular exercise. As these children mature, they often continue to value exercise and find new ways to incorporate regular exercise into their daily routine. On the other hand, children may be raised in families who are sedentary and in which watching sports is the closest anyone comes to exercise. Attitudes and values learned early may be internalized for a lifetime. Individual values also influence the exercise options people make. People who place a high value on physical attractiveness may be highly committed to regular exercise because it helps produce the body they want. Another person may exercise because of the desire for physical strength, relating strength with power. However, someone more disposed to intellectual pursuits may perceive body development as simply wasting time that could be better used to develop the mind. Sometimes, people view exercise as too much of a chore, and thus avoid it. It is important to offer suggestions for how to incorporate exercise into the person's daily routine, making exercise less of a chore.

Fatigue and Stress

Chronic stress may deplete body energy to the point that fatigue makes even the thought of exercise overwhelming. Ironically, regular exercise is energizing and can better equip a person to deal with daily stresses. Excessive exercise, however, may stress the body and lead to injury as well as to fatigue.

External Factors

Many external factors can influence activity and mobility. Among these, weather probably exerts the greatest influence over outside exercise. A brisk, clear day is invigorating and invites increased activity. However, high humidity, very hot and very cold temperatures, rain, and snow discourage outdoor exercise. Nurses need to consider appropriate forms of exercise and social determinants when developing exercise recommendations to patients (Physiopedia, n.d.). Sufficient financial resources for gym memberships, access to exercise equipment, safe outdoor parks and sports areas, the availability of malls for early morning walkers, support people, and occupational or insurance rewards for exercise can all encourage regular exercise. Discouraging factors include lack of free time, insufficient financial resources for equipment purchase or gym membership, air pollution, unsafe neighborhoods, and lack of support and reinforcement. For example, walking is a commonly prescribed exercise. However, walking may pose a threat to the person who only has access to walk in unsafe environments, such as high-crime areas.

EXERCISE

Active exertion of muscles involving the contraction and relaxation of muscle groups is termed exercise. Each of the many different types of exercise can produce different physiologic and psychological benefits.

Types of Exercise

Exercise can be divided into two major types. One is based on the type of *muscle contraction* occurring during the exercise. The second is based on the type of *body movement* occurring and the health benefits achieved.

Muscle Contraction

Exercise may be categorized according to the type of muscle contraction involved as being isotonic, isometric, or isokinetic (Fig. 34-3 on page 1252).

Isotonic exercise involves muscle shortening and active movement. Examples include carrying out ADLs, independently performing range-of-motion exercises, and swimming, walking, jogging, and bicycling. Potential benefits include increased muscle mass, tone, and strength; improved joint mobility; increased cardiac and respiratory function; increased circulation; and increased osteoblastic or bone-building activity. These benefits do not occur when the nurse or family member/caregiver performs passive exercises for a patient because the patient's muscles do not exert effort. Therefore, although still beneficial, the overall potential benefits are reduced.

Isometric exercise involves muscle contraction without shortening (i.e., there is no movement or only a minimum shortening of muscle fibers). Examples include contractions of the quadriceps and gluteal muscles, such as what occurs when holding a yoga pose. Potential benefits are increased muscle mass, tone, and strength; increased circulation to the exercised body part; and increased osteoblastic activity. Nurses should encourage both isotonic and isometric exercises for hospitalized patients with limited mobility.

Isokinetic exercise involves muscle contractions with resistance. The resistance is provided at a constant rate by an external device, which has a capacity for variable resistance. Examples include rehabilitative exercises for knee and elbow injuries and lifting weights. Using the device, the person takes the muscles and joint through a complete **range of motion** (the maximum degree of movement of which a joint is normally capable) without stopping, meeting resistance at every point. A continuous passive motion (CPM) device used postoperatively after joint surgery (e.g., total knee replacement) performs these same type exercises passively for the patient.

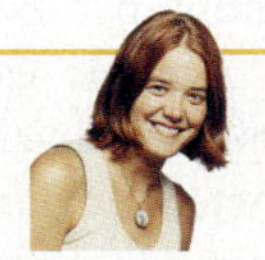

Consider **Maggie Wyatt**, the woman being discharged with an external fixation device in place. A specific exercise routine that includes isotonic and isometric exercises would most likely be prescribed for Maggie. Later in the course of Maggie's treatment, after her fracture has healed, isokinetic exercises may be included to strengthen her right leg.

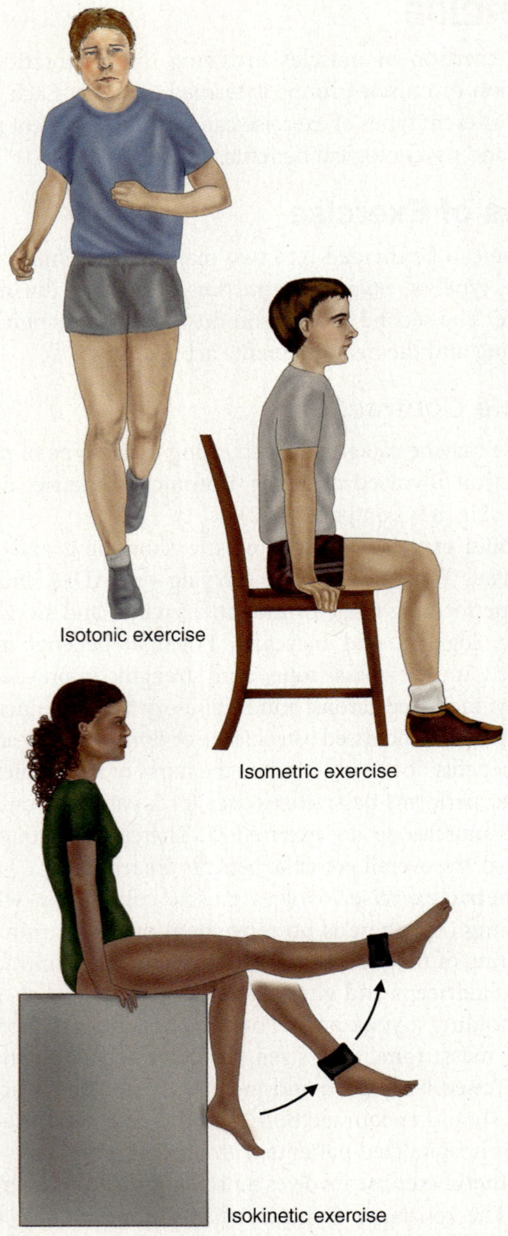

FIGURE 34-3. Three types of exercise. *Isotonic exercise* involves muscle shortening and active movement. *Isometric exercise* involves muscle contraction without shortening. *Isokinetic exercise* involves muscle contraction with resistance.

Body Movement

Exercise activities may also be categorized according to the type of body movement involved and the health benefits they produce. Types of exercise involving body movement include aerobic exercises, stretching exercises, strength and endurance exercises, and movement and ADLs.

Aerobic exercise refers to sustained (often rhythmic) muscle movements that increase blood flow, heart rate, and metabolic demand for oxygen over time, promoting cardiovascular conditioning. Examples of aerobic activities include swimming, walking, jogging, cross-country skiing, aerobic dancing, bicycling, jumping rope, and racquetball. Aerobic exercise may be further distinguished as having high or low impact. The number of injuries, such as shin splints, related to high-impact aerobic workouts led to the development of low-impact workouts that place less stress on the musculoskeletal system. Low-impact aerobic exercises include those activities in which at least one foot is on the ground at all times, like walking, rowing, or riding a stationary bicycle. High-impact exercises include activities that are more apt to jar the spine, like running, jumping, or kick-boxing.

Stretching exercise involves movements that allow muscles and joints to be stretched gently through their full range of motion, increasing flexibility. Specific warm-up and cool-down exercises, Hatha yoga, and some forms of dance are examples. Benefits include increased range-of-joint movements, improved circulation and posture, and relaxation.

Strength and endurance exercises are components of a variety of muscle-building programs. Weight training, calisthenics, and specific isometric exercises can build both strength and endurance, increasing the power of the musculoskeletal system, and generally improving the whole body. They may or may not have aerobic benefit.

Movement and ADLs include housecleaning, running after playful toddlers, climbing stairs instead of riding in elevators, and so on. Household activities can also contribute to an active lifestyle.

Effects of Exercise on Major Body Systems

The human body was designed for motion, and regular exercise is necessary for its healthy functioning. The effects of regular exercise on major body systems are explored in the following sections and outlined in Table 34-4. People differ in the benefits they receive from exercise based on the patient's age and overall health status. People who choose inactive lifestyles or who are forced into inactivity by illness or injury are at high risk for serious health problems (see Effects of Immobility on the Body section starting on page 1253).

Cardiovascular System

To meet the demand for oxygen created by the rhythmic contraction and relaxation of skeletal muscle groups, the supply of oxygenated blood to skeletal muscle needs to be increased. The cardiovascular system meets this challenge by increasing the heart rate, increasing the contractile strength of the myocardium, and increasing stroke volume (volume of blood ejected), thus increasing cardiac output. Arterial (systolic) blood pressure is increased, and blood is shunted from the nonexercising tissues to the heart and muscles. Exercise also improves venous return because the contracting muscles compress superficial veins and push blood back to the heart against gravity. Over time, regular exercise results in cardiovascular conditioning and produces the following benefits:

- Increased efficiency of the heart
- Decreased heart rate and blood pressure
- Increased blood flow to all body parts
- Improved venous return
- Increased circulating fibrinolysin (substance that breaks up small clots)

Respiratory System

The respiratory and cardiovascular systems work together to make increased oxygen available to the muscles. During exercise, the depth of respiration, respiratory rate, gas exchange at the alveolar level, and rate of carbon dioxide excretion are increased. Over time, regular exercise leads to improved pulmonary functioning. Improvements in pulmonary function include:

- Improved alveolar ventilation
- Decreased work of breathing
- Improved diaphragmatic excursion

Musculoskeletal System

The rhythmic contraction and relaxation of muscle groups during exercise result in increased muscle mass, tone, strength, and increased joint mobility. The more a person exercises, the more strength the person has to exercise or work in the future. Regular exercise produces the following benefits:

- Increased muscle efficiency (strength) and flexibility
- Increased coordination
- Reduced bone loss
- Increased efficiency of nerve impulse transmission

Regular exercise is also believed to slow the effects of aging. For example, exercise has been shown to help prevent osteoporosis (the process of bone demineralization) associated with aging (Fletcher et al., 2018).

Metabolic Processes

The metabolic rate increases during exercise so that sufficient glucose and fatty acids can be converted to provide the energy needed for increased muscle function. During strenuous exercise, the metabolic rate can increase to up to 20 times the person's normal rate. Increased body heat and waste products are also produced. With regular exercise, the efficiency of metabolism and body temperature regulation is increased. Other benefits of exercise on the metabolic processes include:

- Increased triglyceride breakdown
- Increased gastric motility
- Increased production of body heat

Gastrointestinal System

During exercise, blood is shunted away from the stomach and intestines to the exercising muscles. With regular exercise:

- Appetite is increased.
- Intestinal tone is increased, which improves digestion and elimination.
- Weight may be controlled.

Urinary System

Regular exercise increases blood circulation, including improved blood flow to the kidneys. This allows the kidneys to maintain the body's fluid balance and acid–base balance more efficiently and to excrete body wastes.

Skin

Increased circulation resulting from regular exercise nourishes the skin. Thus, regular exercise aids in promoting the overall general health of the skin.

Psychosocial Outlook

Some of the most important benefits of regular exercise are psychological. These benefits include:

- Increased energy, vitality, and general well-being
- Improved sleep
- Improved appearance (body image)
- Improved self-concept
- Increased positive health behavior

Risks Related to Exercise

A common reason many people give for not exercising is fear of experiencing personal harm. Personal harm can include cardiovascular events, muscle injuries, or falling. The nurse must be responsive to these fears with realistic knowledge of the risks associated with exercise and specific prevention strategies.

Precipitation of a Cardiac Event

Although the risk of exercise precipitating a major cardiac event in a healthy person is minimal, the risk is much higher for people with known or suspected cardiovascular (cardiac, peripheral vascular, or cerebrovascular disease), metabolic (type 1 and type 2 diabetes mellitus), or renal disease. Thus, the American College of Sports Medicine recommends physically inactive patients with known cardiovascular, metabolic, or renal disease and/or those with signs or symptoms suggestive of these diseases should seek medical clearance before starting an exercise program, regardless of the intensity of the exercise (Riebe et al., 2015).

Orthopedic Discomfort and Disability

Orthopedic problems caused by irritation of bones, tendons, ligaments, and sometimes muscles are the most common injuries associated with exercise. This irritation may result from added weight-bearing stress or from collision with the ground, an object, or another person.

Other Health Problems

Other types of health problems may be associated with different types of exercise, depending to a large extent on external factors (temperature on a given day, humidity, pollution index, safety of the neighborhood) as well as internal factors (age, history of previous injury, overuse, obesity, health history). Examples of other health problems related to exercise include heat exhaustion or heat stroke, exercise-induced asthma, and chest pain related to overexertion.

Effects of Immobility on the Body

Lack of exercise, inactivity, or immobility related to illness or injury place a person at high risk for serious health problems (Eanes, 2018). Immobility can affect the major body systems and has been linked to a predisposition to many chronic health problems (Johns Hopkins Medicine, n.d.). The effects of immobility on major body systems are explored in the following sections and outlined in Table 34-4 on page 1250. Like the benefits a person receives from exercise, complications resulting from immobility differ in their occurrence and severity based on the patient's age and overall health status.

Cardiovascular System

The primary and serious effects of immobility on the cardiovascular system include increased cardiac workload, orthostatic hypotension, and venous stasis, with resulting venous thrombosis. Immobility results in an increased workload for the heart. With immobility, the skeletal muscles that normally compress valves in the leg veins and help to pump the blood back to the right side of the heart do not adequately contract. There is less resistance offered by the blood vessels and blood pools in the veins, thus increasing the venous blood pressure and changing the distribution of blood in the immobile person. As a result, the heart rate, cardiac output, and stroke volume increase.

Immobility predisposes the patient to thrombi formation because of venous stasis, especially in the legs, where normal muscular activity helps move blood toward the central circulatory system. During periods of immobility, calcium leaves the bones and enters the blood, where it influences blood coagulation, leading to an increased risk of thrombus formation.

A person who is immobile is more susceptible to developing orthostatic hypotension. The normal neurovascular adjustments that occur to maintain systemic blood pressure with position changes are not used during periods of inactivity and become inoperative. A drop in blood pressure may occur as a result of a lack of vasoconstriction when changing from a supine to an upright position. The person tends to feel weak and faint when this condition occurs. See Chapter 26 for additional discussion of orthostatic hypotension.

Respiratory System

The effects of immobility on the respiratory system are related to decreased ventilatory effort and increased respiratory secretions. Immobility causes a decrease in the depth and rate of respirations, in part because of a reduced need for oxygen by body cells. When areas of lung tissue are not used over time, atelectasis (incomplete expansion or collapse of lung tissue) may occur. Immobility results in a poor exchange of carbon dioxide and oxygen, upsets their balance in the body, and eventually causes an acid–base imbalance.

When a person is immobile, the movement of secretions in the respiratory tract is decreased, causing secretions to pool and leading to respiratory congestion. These conditions predispose the person to respiratory tract infections. Hypostatic pneumonia is a type of pneumonia that results from inactivity and immobility. The situation worsens when the person is dehydrated or using pharmacologic agents that increase the tenacity of secretions, depresses the coughing mechanism and/or depresses respirations.

Decreased movement in the thoracic cage during respirations also occurs with immobility. This decrease may be due to loss of tonus in muscles involved with respirations, pressure on the chest wall because of the patient's position in bed, or depression of the respiratory system by various pharmaceutical agents.

Musculoskeletal System

Effects of immobility on the musculoskeletal system are rapidly seen in patients confined to bed. People attempting to walk after several days of bed rest are often surprised to find how weak their legs have become. Immobility (musculoskeletal disuse) leads to decreased muscle size (**atrophy**), tone, and strength; decreased joint mobility and flexibility; bone demineralization; and limited endurance, resulting in problems with ADLs.

Immobility is often the cause of contractures and ankylosis, a consolidation and immobilization of a joint. Contractures result from atrophy of muscles and from a decrease in the muscle's strength, coordination, and endurance, resulting in an inability to function. A joint can be permanently fixed when ankylosed.

The process of bone demineralization (osteoporosis) is also increased in immobile patients. Normally, the stress and strain of weight-bearing activity stimulate bone formation and balance it with the natural destruction of bone. With immobility, however, bone formation slows while breakdown increases, resulting in a net loss of bone calcium, phosphorus, and bone matrix. This condition, disuse osteoporosis, is characterized by bones that may be either spongy or brittle. Bone demineralization may result in pathologic fractures related to the bone's brittleness, bone deformities related to the bone's sponginess, arthropathy (joint disease) related to calcium depletion in the joints, or renal calculi (stones) related to the excessive excretion of calcium through the kidneys and urinary tract.

Metabolic Processes

Because the resting body requires less energy, the cellular demand for oxygen is decreased, leading to a decreased metabolic rate. In many immobilized patients, however, factors such as fever, trauma, chronic illness, or poor nutrition can actually increase the body's metabolic demands and increase catabolism (the breakdown of the body's protein stores to provide energy to meet the body's energy requirements). If unchecked, this process results in muscle wasting and a negative nitrogen balance. Anorexia, or decreased appetite, often accompanies and compounds this problem. Negative nitrogen balance and poor nutrition thus worsen the muscle atrophy and weakness already resulting from immobility. Numerous fluid and electrolyte imbalances, alterations in the exchange of nutrients and gases at the cellular level, and gastrointestinal (GI) problems can all result from metabolic disturbances.

Gastrointestinal System

Immobility leads to disturbances in appetite, decreased food intake, altered protein metabolism, and poor digestion and utilization of food. If people increase food intake while decreasing energy expenditure, weight gain will result. Normal muscular activity in the GI tract also slows down in an immobile person, which often results in constipation, poor defecation reflexes, and an inability to expel feces and gas adequately.

Urinary System

In a nonerect patient, the kidneys and ureters are level, and urine remains in the renal pelvis for a longer period of time before gravity causes it to move into the ureters and bladder. Urinary stasis favors the growth of bacteria that, when present in sufficient quantities, may cause urinary tract infections. Poor perineal hygiene, incontinence, decreased fluid intake, or an indwelling urinary catheter can increase the risk for urinary tract infection in an immobile patient.

Immobility also predisposes the patient to renal calculi, or kidney stones, which are a consequence of high levels of urinary calcium; urinary retention and incontinence resulting from decreased bladder muscle tone; the formation of alkaline urine, which facilitates growth of urinary bacteria; and decreased urine volume.

Skin

In patients who are immobile, especially those who are older or debilitated, the impaired circulation that accompanies immobility may result in serious skin breakdown. Prolonged pressure over bony prominences produces areas of breakdown, leading to pressure injuries. Pressure injuries are described in detail in Chapter 33.

Psychosocial Outlook

When a person can no longer move the body purposefully and needs to depend on someone else for assistance with simple self-care activities, the person's sense of self is often threatened. Skeletal deformities can influence body image, an inability to meet role expectations can decrease self-concept, and a prolonged period of lying dependent in bed can lead to feelings of worthlessness and diminished self-esteem.

Immobility can produce exaggerated emotional responses to the stresses of everyday living. Patients can become apathetic, possibly because of decreased sensory stimulation, and develop altered thought processes. Lack of mobility can also diminish a person's opportunities to interact socially and deprive that person of normal support systems. Coping difficulties are common for both immobilized patients and their families. Furthermore, the amount of time immobilized patients spend resting often disrupts their usual sleep–wake patterns and may interfere with both the quantity and quality of their sleep.

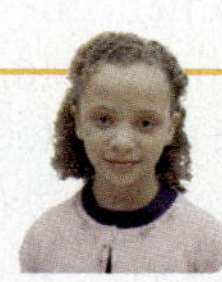

Remember **Kelsi Lester**, the 10-year-old girl who is unconscious. Due to her current state, Kelsi is at high risk for developing any or all of the possible complications associated with immobility, including thrombi, pneumonia, constipation, urinary tract infection, and skin breakdown. Although she is unconscious, the effects of immobility ultimately can affect her psychosocial outlook. The nurse would integrate knowledge of the effects of immobility when developing Kelsi's plan of care that would include close frequent assessment, early detection, and prompt intervention to prevent any possible complications.

NURSING PROCESS FOR ACTIVITY

Assessing

The comprehensive nursing assessment uses both interview and physical assessment skills to obtain data about the patient's mobility and activity status. When alterations in a patient's physical or mental health state result in impaired mobility, additional specific assessment skills are needed to determine the patient's physical limitations.

Nursing History

During the nursing history, interview patients regarding their daily activity level, endurance, exercise and fitness goals, mobility problems, physical or mental health alterations that affect mobility, and external factors affecting mobility. Questioning patients about their fitness goals is important to provide an indication of the patient's view of health. This interviewing strategy communicates to patients that you expect them to be exercising and is itself a powerful teaching tool.

Social determinants of health are conditions in the patients environments that may affect the patient's functioning and quality of life (Healthy People 2030, n.d.). Ask about sociocultural factors that may impact a patient's mobility and their ability to participate in activities, such as:

- Access to physical activity opportunities
- Safe neighborhoods and environments
- Income
- Services that provide practical support for participation in physical activities, such as child-care, advice and encouragement

This information helps us to understand factors that may influence a patient's health and use of health care and shape more effective interventions (Healthy People, 2030, n.d.).

The accompanying Focused Assessment Guide 34-1 (on page 1256) illustrates elements common to obtaining a mobility status history. When a problem exists, assess the nature of the problem, its onset and frequency, known causes, severity and symptoms, effects on everyday functioning, the interventions attempted by the patient, and the results.

Physical Assessment

Physical assessment of mobility status includes an assessment of general ease of movement and gait; alignment, joint structure, and function; muscle mass, tone, and strength; and endurance. Table 34-5 (on page 1257) provides normal findings and significant alterations related to these assessments. During this assessment, direct attention to both structure and function. The patient's ability to stand, walk, sit up, and grasp are important because these enable the patient to wash, dress, and feed oneself and perform other basic ADLs.

Focused Assessment Guide 34-1

MOBILITY AND EXERCISE

Factors to Assess	Questions and Approaches
Daily activity level	Describe the activities you normally carry out during a routine day and types of physical exercise that are part of your daily lifestyle. • Activities of daily living • Type, frequency, duration of physical exercise • Past history of activity and exercise; recent changes
Endurance	Describe how much and what type of activity makes you tired. • History of dizziness, dyspnea, frequent pauses in activity to rest, pounding heart, or marked increase in respiratory rate after moderate activity
Exercise/fitness goals	What exercise or fitness goals are you currently working on? • Attitudes about exercise and physical fitness • Knowledge of the benefits of exercise • Motivation to exercise
Mobility problems	Do you experience any problems with movement or with more vigorous activity or exercise? If yes, please describe these problems. • Nature of the problem (including symptoms) • Onset of disturbance and frequency • Known causes • Effect of problem on everyday functioning • Interventions attempted and results
Physical or mental health alterations	Are there any physical or mental health problems that may be affecting your mobility? • Decrease of strength or endurance (e.g., myocardial infarction, congestive heart failure, chronic obstructive pulmonary disease, cancer, gastrointestinal disorders) • Neuromuscular impairment (multiple sclerosis, Parkinson's disease, spinal injuries) • Musculoskeletal impairment (arthritis, fractures, muscular dystrophy) • Perceptual or cognitive impairment (cerebrovascular accident, brain tumor or trauma, vision disorders, dementia) • Pain or discomfort (burns, rheumatoid arthritis, chronic pain syndrome, postoperative pain) • Depression or severe anxiety (neurosis, schizophrenia)
External factors affecting mobility	Is there anything else you can think of that limits your ability to get around or participate in activities? • Environmental factors (stairs, lack of railings or other assistive devices, poor lighting, unsafe neighborhood) • Financial resources

Older adults make up an increasingly larger part of the general population. Functional decline and subsequent difficulties related to completion of ADLs and instrumental activities of daily living (IADLs) in older adults can have significant consequences (Yoo et al., 2020). Changes in mobility status contribute to this functional decline (Gray-Miceli, 2017; Tasheva et al., 2020). Moderate amounts of aerobic physical activity can reduce the risk of functional decline by as much as 30%, allowing older adults to continue with ADLs (American Geriatrics Society, 2016). Assessment of an older adult's ability to participate in physical activities and exercise and to care for themselves is an important part of a mobility assessment. This assessment can provide clues to changes in health and prevent, or prevent further, functional decline. See the accompanying Focus on the Older Adult (on page 1258) for an example of a tool (Katz Index of Independence in Activities of Daily Living) to use to measure the older adult's capacity to care for oneself and assist nurses to detect subtle changes in health and prevent functional decline. Additional information related to functional health is discussed in Chapter 27.

GENERAL EASE OF MOVEMENT AND GAIT

Begin the physical assessment of an ambulatory patient the moment the patient walks into the room. Voluntarily controlled, fluid, and coordinated body movements are key to the integrated functioning of the skeletal, muscular, and nervous systems. Note whether the patient's body movements are quick and sure or slow and deliberate. These observations communicate both a sense of the person's emotional status and self-care abilities. Common involuntary movements that may be observed include tremors (continuous quivering of whole muscles or major portions of a muscle) and tics (irregularly occurring spasmodic movements such as winking, grimacing, or shoulder shrugging).

Note the gait (manner of walking) of the patient who is ambulatory. The patient's movements while walking should be coordinated and the posture well balanced. The arms should

Table 34-5 Overview of Physical Assessment of Mobility Status

COMPONENT	NORMAL FINDING	SIGNIFICANT ALTERATIONS
General ease of movement	Body movements are: • Voluntarily controlled (purposeful) • Fluid • Coordinated	Involuntary movements: • Tremors • Tics • Chorea • Athetosis • Dystonia • Fasciculations • Myoclonus • Oral–facial dyskinesias
Gait and posture	Head erect, vertebrae are straight. Knees and feet point forward. Arms at side with elbows flexed. Arms swing freely in alternation with leg swings. While one leg is in the stance phase, the other is in the swing phase.	Abnormalities of gait and posture: • Spastic hemiparesis • Scissors gait • Steppage gait • Sensory ataxia • Cerebellar ataxia • Parkinsonian gait • Gait of old age • Use of assistive devices for ambulation
Alignment	Independent maintenance of correct alignment: • In the standing and sitting position, a straight line can be drawn from the ear through the shoulder and hip. • In bed, the head, shoulders, and hips are aligned.	Abnormal spinal curvatures Inability to maintain correct alignment independently
Joint structure and function	Absence of joint deformities Full range of motion	Limitation in the normal range of motion Increased joint mobility Swelling or tenderness in or around the joint Heat or redness Crepitation Deformities Muscle atrophy, nodules, skin changes Asymmetry of involvement
Muscle mass, tone, and strength	Adequate muscle mass, tone, and strength to accomplish movement and work	Atrophy, hypertrophy Hypotonicity (flaccidity), spasticity Paresis or paralysis
Endurance	Ability to turn in bed, maintain correct alignment when sitting and standing, ambulate, and perform self-care activities	Physiologic or psychological inability to tolerate an increase in activity: • Significantly increased pulse, respiration, blood pressure after rest • Shortness of breath, dyspnea • Weakness • Pallor • Confusion • Vertigo • Pain

swing freely in a rhythm alternating with the legs. Figure 34-4 (on page 1258) illustrates stance and swing, the two phases of the normal gait. The heel of the right foot strikes the ground (stance), while the toe of the left foot pushes off and leaves the ground, moving the leg from behind to in front of the body (swing). While one leg is in the stance phase, the other is in the swing phase. Detection of gait abnormalities is important because gait abnormalities may place the person at risk for injury and may indicate a neuromuscular disorder or intoxication.

Note whether the patient uses any assistive devices such as a wheelchair, brace, cane, walker, or crutches to aid in ambulation. Also, determine whether the assistive device is meeting the patient's needs, if it is required for mobility, and if it is being used safely.

ALIGNMENT

Correct body alignment permits optimal musculoskeletal balance and operation and promotes optimal physiologic functioning. Deviations in body alignment may result from chronic poor posture, trauma, muscle damage, or nerve dysfunction. Pain, fatigue, and a person's mental and emotional status may also influence alignment.

Observe alignment when a patient is standing, sitting, or lying (Fig. 34-5 on page 1258). Note whether the patient is able to maintain correct alignment independently.

Focus on the Older Adult

KATZ INDEX OF INDEPENDENCE IN ACTIVITIES OF DAILY LIVING

ACTIVITIES POINTS (1 OR 0)	**INDEPENDENCE:** (1 POINT)	**DEPENDENCE:** (0 POINTS)
	NO supervision, direction, or personal assistance	WITH supervision, direction, personal assistance, or total care
BATHING POINTS:____	(1 POINT) Bathes self completely or needs help in bathing only a single part of the body such as the back, genital area, or disabled extremity.	(0 POINTS) Needs help with bathing more than one part of the body or getting in or out of the tub or shower. Requires total bathing.
DRESSING POINTS:____	(1 POINT) Gets clothes from closets and drawers and puts on clothes and outer garments, complete with fasteners. May have help tying shoes.	(0 POINTS) Needs help with dressing self or needs to be completely dressed.
TOILETING POINTS:____	(1 POINT) Goes to toilet, gets on and off, arranges clothes, cleans genital area without help.	(0 POINTS) Needs help transferring to the toilet or cleaning self or uses bedpan or commode.
TRANSFERRING POINTS:____	(1 POINT) Moves in and out of bed or chair unassisted. Mechanical transferring aides are acceptable.	(0 POINTS) Needs help in moving from bed to chair or requires a complete transfer.
CONTINENCE POINTS:____	(1 POINT) Exercises complete self-control over urination and defecation.	(0 POINTS) Is partially or totally incontinent of bowel or bladder.
FEEDING	(1 POINT) Gets food from plate into mouth without help. Preparation of food may be done by another person.	(0 POINTS) Needs partial or total help with feeding or requires parenteral feeding.

TOTAL POINTS = ______ 6 = High (*patient independent*) 0 = Low (*patient very dependent*)

Source: Adapted from Katz, S., Down, T. D., Cash, H. R., & Grotz, R. C. (1970). Progress in the development of the index of ADL. *The Gerontologist, 10*(1), 20–30.

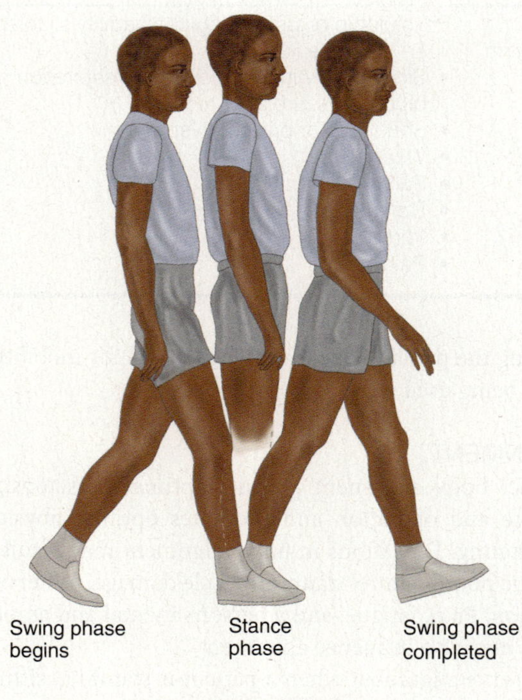

FIGURE 34-4. The stance and swing phases of normal gait.

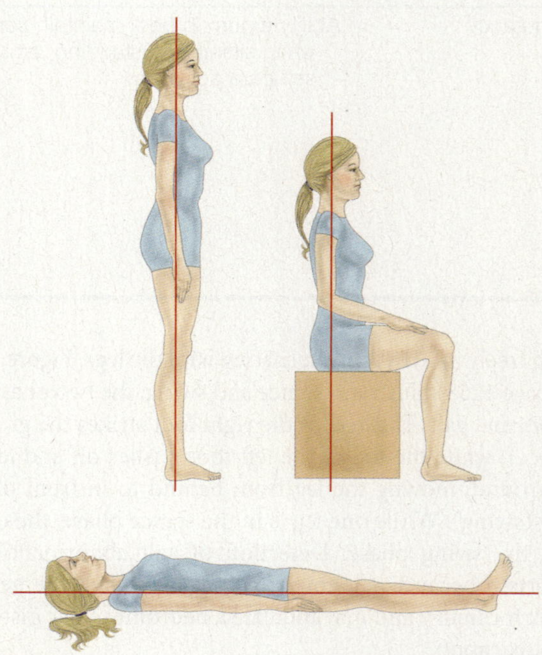

FIGURE 34-5. Adequate alignment (posture). In the sitting and standing positions, a straight line can be drawn from the ear through the shoulder and hip. In bed, the head, shoulders, and hips are aligned.

A patient's body is in correct body alignment in the standing position when:

- The head is held erect and in the midline.
- The face is in the forward position, in the same direction as the feet.
- The chest is held upward and forward.
- The spinal column is upright, and the curves of the spine are within normal limits.
- The abdominal muscles are held upward, with the abdomen comfortably tucked in and the buttocks downward.
- The arms hang comfortably at the sides.
- The knees are extended in a slightly flexed position—not bent or hyperextended in the knee-locked position.
- The feet are at right angles to the lower legs.
- The line of gravity goes through the midline, from the middle of the forehead to a midpoint between the feet; laterally the line of gravity runs vertically from the middle of the skull to the posterior of the foot.
- The base of support is on the soles of the feet, and weight is distributed through the soles and heels.

Correct body alignment when sitting is similar to correct alignment when standing except that the hips are flexed, the knees are flexed and not crossed, and the base of support is on the buttocks and upper thighs. The weight is distributed evenly on the buttocks and thighs. The thighs are parallel and the popliteal area should be free of the edge of the chair to prevent circulatory stasis and possible nerve injury. The patient's forearms are supported either on the armrests, lap, or on a flat surface in front of the chair.

JOINT STRUCTURE AND FUNCTION

Use inspection and palpation to examine joints, their range of motion, and the surrounding tissue. Range of motion is the maximum degree of movement of which a joint is normally capable. When assessing joint mobility, note the following:

- Size, shape, color, and symmetry of joints: note any masses, deformities, or muscle atrophy
- Range of motion of each joint
- Any limitation in the normal range of motion or any unusual increase in the mobility of a joint (instability); range of motion varies among people and decreases with aging
- Muscle strength when performing range-of-motion exercises against resistance
- Any swelling, heat, tenderness, pain, nodules, or crepitation (palpable or audible crunching or grating sensation produced by motion of the joint)
- Comparison of findings in one joint with those of the opposite joint

MUSCLE MASS, TONE, AND STRENGTH

Adequate skeletal muscle mass, tone, and strength are prerequisites to appropriate body movement and work performance. Mass refers to muscle size. Assess muscle mass throughout the body and compare one muscle group to another using tape measurements. Hypertrophy refers to increased muscle mass resulting from exercise or training. Atrophy describes muscle mass that is decreased through disuse or neurologic impairment. Patients experiencing muscle wasting as a result of a chronic disease process such as cancer may report visible changes in muscle mass.

The slight residual tension that remains in a resting normal muscle with an intact nerve supply is termed muscle tone. Assess muscle tone by flexing and extending the elbow or knee and noting the degree of resistance to these movements. Decreased tone, also known as hypotonicity or **flaccidity**, results from disuse or neurologic impairments and is described as a weakness of the involved area. **Spasticity** or hypertonicity, increased tone that interferes with movement, is also caused by neurologic impairments and is often described as a stiffness, tightness, or pulling of the muscle.

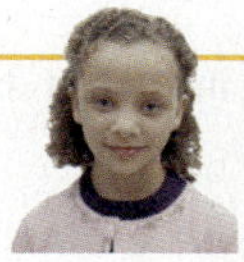

The nurse would need to assess closely the muscle tone of **Kelsi Lester**, the 10-year-old girl who is unconscious. The nurse would be alert for evidence of flaccidity, which could result from lack of use or possibly impairment of her nervous system due to the accident.

Muscle strength varies greatly from one person to another and even within the same person and is affected by muscle use. Test muscle strength by asking the patient to move actively against resistance. For example, instruct the patient to push the examiner's palms apart or to push the foot against the examiner's palm. When comparing muscle groups, remember that a person's dominant side tends to be stronger.

Impaired muscle strength or weakness is termed **paresis**. The absence of strength secondary to nervous impairment is called **paralysis**. Hemiparesis refers to weakness of one half of the body, and hemiplegia is paralysis of one half of the body. Paraplegia is paralysis of the legs, and quadriplegia is paralysis of the arms and legs.

Assess whether the patient's muscle strength is adequate for the performance of tasks the patient deems necessary. For example, a patient whose primary means of ambulation is a wheelchair requires upper body strength.

ENDURANCE

When assessing endurance, evaluate the patient's ability to turn in bed, maintain correct alignment when sitting or standing, ambulate, and perform self-care activities. When a physical or psychological factor is believed to be affecting endurance, evaluate the following:

- Vital signs while the patient is at rest
- Ability to perform the activity (e.g., ambulation)
- Patient's response during and after the activity
- Vital signs immediately after the activity
- Vital signs after the patient has rested for 3 minutes

Significant findings indicating that a person's exercise tolerance has been reached include noticeably increased pulse, respirations, and blood pressure; shortness of breath, dyspnea; weakness; pallor; confusion; and vertigo (sensation of spinning).

Examples of Actual or Potential Health Problems and Needs

MOBILITY/ACTIVITY

Actual or Potential Health Problems and Needs	Possible Etiologic Factors	Potential Signs and Symptoms
Activity intolerance	Any condition that interferes with the transport of oxygenated blood to tissue (e.g., cardiac problems such as congestive heart failure and arrhythmias; respiratory problems, especially chronic obstructive pulmonary disease; circulatory problems; diabetes mellitus) Immobility Generalized weakness Physical deconditioning	Altered response to activity: Exertional dyspnea, shortness of breath, excessive increase in respiratory rate Weak pulse, excessive increase in pulse rate, change in rhythm Blood pressure that fails to increase with activity or that decreases Weakness, pallor, confusion, vertigo Reports of fatigue or pain with activity
Impaired Ability to Transfer	Musculoskeletal impairment (fracture, arthritis) Neuromuscular impairment (muscular dystrophy, multiple sclerosis) Decreased strength and endurance Pain or discomfort Decreased muscle control, mass, or strength Joint stiffness Obesity	Physical inability to move purposefully or a reluctance to move Limited range of motion Limited ability to perform fine or gross motor skills Slowed, jerky, or uncoordinated movements Postural instability
Risk for Activity Intolerance	Imbalance between oxygen supply/demand Immobility Physical deconditioning Sedentary lifestyle	—

Diagnosing Actual or Potential Health Problems and Needs

An assessment of a patient's mobility and activity status may lead to the identification of one or more diagnoses or patient problems related to mobility, activity, and/or immobility. Following the formulation of the diagnoses or patient problems, the nurse communicates findings to other nursing and health care professionals through the use of the written and spoken word. The written diagnosis or patient problem becomes a permanent part of the patient's health record. Examples of diagnoses/patient problems with related etiology and signs and symptoms can be found in the box titled Examples of Actual or Potential Health Problems and Needs: Mobility/Activity.

Outcome Identification and Planning

If the patient is not experiencing any mobility or activity problems, expected patient outcomes are directed toward the promotion of physical fitness. For example, the patient will:

- Identify personal benefits of regular exercise
- List support systems that will reinforce exercise efforts
- Follow a program of regular physical exercise that improves cardiovascular function, endurance, flexibility, and strength

Patients at risk for specific mobility or activity problems may require different expected outcomes. For example, the patient will:

- Demonstrate correct body alignment
- Demonstrate full range of joint motion
- Demonstrate adequate muscle mass, tone, and strength to perform ADLs and/or IADLs

Patients who are immobile require outcomes directed toward preventing complications related to inactivity and its effects on the body systems. For example, the patient will:

- Be free from alterations in skin integrity
- Show signs of adequate circulation
- Maintain muscle mass, tone and strength

Individualize outcomes for more specific problems (e.g., for the patient learning to walk with crutches or needing to master transfer techniques with only upper body mobility).

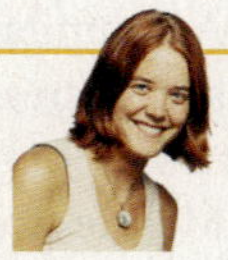

Consider ***Maggie Wyatt***, the woman being discharged after treatment for a fracture. An appropriate outcome for Ms. Wyatt would be that she demonstrates ability to transfer herself from the bed to the chair and then to the car, with the assistance of a support person.

Implementing

The use of ergonomics and safe patient handling and mobility strategies are discussed in the following sections. Nursing strategies designed to promote correct body alignment, mobility, and fitness are described, as well as interventions to prevent complications from immobility. Techniques for the use of graduated compression stockings and pneumatic compression devices, as well as performing range-of-motion exercises, are discussed.

It is important to remember that the National Institute for Occupational Safety and Health (NIOSH) (2013), Joint Commission, and the Occupational Safety & Health Administration (OSHA) recommend a no-lift policy in conjunction with technology, assistive devices, education, and a culture of safety for all health care facilities (Fragala et al., 2016; OSHA and Joint Commission Resources Alliance, 2017). Implementing safe patient handling and mobility programs improves the quality of patient care and reduces the risk of harm for patients and health care workers (Nelson, 2015; OSHA and Joint Commission Resources Alliance, 2017). Incorporating safe patient handling and mobility strategies, techniques for turning and moving a patient in bed, moving a patient from bed to stretcher and from bed to chair, and logrolling a patient are discussed. Also included are sections on preparing and helping patients to ambulate after bed rest and nursing strategies to promote exercise.

Application of Ergonomics to Prevent Injury

Providing patient care places demands on the nurse's musculoskeletal system. Musculoskeletal disorders plague the nursing profession, resulting in a significant burden on the health care sector and health care workers (Davis & Kotowski, 2015; OSHA, n.d.b). Ergonomics includes proper body movement in daily activities, the prevention and correction of problems associated with posture, and the enhancement of coordination and endurance.

Techniques to prevent back stress include:

- Develop a habit of erect posture (correct alignment). Slouching can strain neck and back muscles. When sitting, use the chair back to support the whole spine, keeping shoulders back but relaxed. Balance the head over the shoulders, avoid leaning forward, and hold in the stomach muscles.
- Use the longest and the strongest muscles of the arms and the legs to help provide the power needed in strenuous activities. The muscles of the back are less strong and more easily injured when used improperly.
- Use the internal girdle and a long midriff to stabilize the pelvis and to protect the abdominal viscera when stooping, reaching, lifting, or pulling. The internal girdle is made by contracting the gluteal muscles in the buttocks downward and the abdominal muscles upward. It is helped further by making a long midriff by stretching the muscles in the waist. Figure 34-6 illustrates correct and incorrect use of the internal girdle.
- Work as closely as possible to an object that is to be lifted or moved. This brings the body's center of gravity close to that of the object being moved, permitting most of the burden to be borne by the leg and arm muscles, rather than the back. Figure 34-7 illustrates a proper and an improper way to pick up an object.
- Face the direction of your movement. Avoid twisting your body.

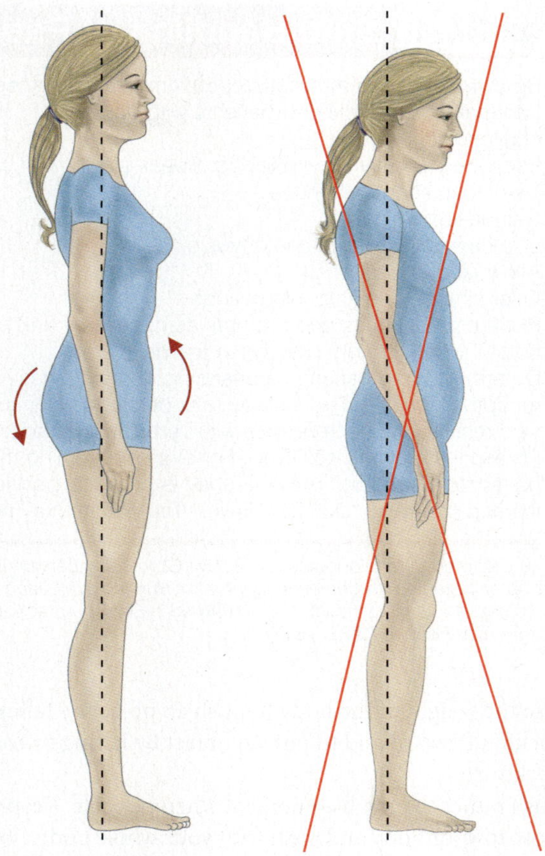

FIGURE 34-6. (*Left*) Correct. Internal girdle "on." Abdominal muscles contracted, giving a feeling of upward pull, and gluteal muscles contracted, giving a downward pull. (*Right*) Incorrect. Slouch position, showing abdominal muscles relaxed and body out of good alignment.

- Use the weight of the body as a force for pulling or pushing, by rocking on the feet or leaning forward or backward. This reduces the amount of strain placed on the arms and the back.
- Slide, roll, push, or pull an object, rather than lift it, to reduce the energy needed to lift the weight against the pull of gravity.

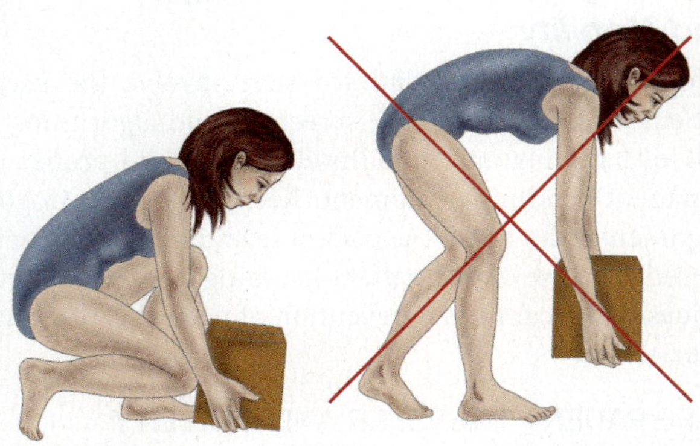

FIGURE 34-7. (*Left*) Correct. A good position for lifting is illustrated. This person is using the long and strong muscles of the arms and legs and holding the object so that the line of gravity falls within the base of support. (*Right*) Incorrect. This is an incorrect position for lifting because pull is exerted on the back muscles and leaning causes the line of gravity to fall outside the base.

Box 34-1 Safe Handling of Patients With Dementia

- Be aware that communication problems and weakness can make the handling of patients with dementia challenging.
- Face the patient when speaking. Speak slowly.
- Use clear, short sentences.
- Call patient by name.
- Use calm, reassuring tone of voice.
- Allow time for response.
- Offer simple, one-step instructions.
- Repeat verbal cues and prompts as necessary; this is helpful when thought processes are delayed.
- Determine if the patient experiencing dementia has receptive aphasia. This inability to understand what is being said results in noncompliance with verbal instructions.
- Phrase instructions positively. For example, remind the patient to "Stand up" until the chair is correctly positioned, instead of saying "Don't sit down." The patient may not register the "Don't" and will try to sit too early. Positive instructions are more likely to result in successful maneuvers.
- Ask one question at a time, allow the patient to answer, and repeat the question if necessary.
- Allow the patient to focus on the task; avoid correcting the process of the action unless it would be dangerous to the patient not to do so.
- Identify the patient's established patterns of behavior, customs, traits, and everyday habits and try to incorporate these habits into desired activities. For instance, a patient with dementia may resist or become frightened when a morning shower is attempted if the patient was accustomed to evening baths. Another patient may have difficulty getting out of bed in the morning for the simple reason that he is being asked to get out on what he considers the wrong side of the bed.

Source: Adapted from Eliopoulos, C. (2018). *Gerontological nursing* (9th ed.). Wolters Kluwer; Jootun, D., & Pryde, A. (2013). Moving and handling of patients with dementia. *Journal of Nursing Education and Practice, 3*(2), 126–131; Toughy, T. A., & Jett, K. (2018). *Ebersol and Hess' gerontological nursing & healthy aging* (5th ed.). Elsevier; and Varnam, W. (2011). How to mobilize patients with dementia to a standing position. *Nursing Older People, 23*(8), 31–36.

- Use the weight of the body to push an object by falling or rocking forward and to pull an object by falling or rocking backward.
- Push rather than pull equipment when possible. Keep arms close to your body and push with your whole body, not just your arms.
- Begin activities by broadening your base of support. Spread the feet to shoulder width.
- Make sure that the surface is dry and smooth when moving an object to decrease the effects of friction. Rough, wet, or soiled surfaces can contribute to increased friction, increasing the amount of effort required to move an object.
- Flex the knees, put on the internal girdle, and come down close to an object that is to be lifted.
- Break up heavy loads into smaller loads. Take breaks from lifting or moving to relax and recover.

Ensuring Safe Patient Handling and Mobility

Safe patient handling and transfers involve the use of patient assessment criteria, screening and algorithms for patient handling and mobility decisions, and proper use of patient handling equipment. Keep the patient in good alignment and protect the patient from injury while being moved. The use of safe patient handling devices and techniques is critical in the prevention of patient care–related injuries.

SAFE PATIENT TRANSFER AND MOBILITY

User training, device wear and tear, suitability of equipment, and correct operation of equipment are important factors related to prevention of patient injury and safe patient handling and mobility (Elnitsky et al., 2014; Monaghan, 2020a; Monaghan, 2019).

Follow these recommended guidelines when moving and lifting patients:

- Assess the patient. Know the patient's medical diagnosis and health issues, capabilities, and any movement not allowed. Apply braces or any device the patient wears before helping from bed.
- Assess the patient's ability to assist with the planned movement. Encourage patients to assist in their own transfers. Encouraging patients to perform tasks that are within their capabilities promotes independence. It is important to eliminate or reduce unnecessary tasks to reduce the risk of injury and increase the patient's self-esteem and mobility levels.
- Assess the patient's ability to understand instructions and cooperate with the staff to achieve the movement. Patient engagement during handling and mobility is an important factor in preventing adverse events (Elnitsky et al., 2014; Gallahger et al., 2019). Box 34-1 outlines general guidelines to consider related to mobility and safe handling of people with dementia.
- Ensure that enough staff are available and present to safely move the patient. See the Reflective Practice box at the beginning of the chapter (on page 1241).
- Assess the area for clutter, accessibility to the patient, and availability of devices. Remove any obstacles that may make moving and lifting inconvenient.
- Use a screening or assessment tool to aid in patient assessment and decision making regarding safe patient handling and mobility (Arnold, 2019; VA Mobile Health, n.d.). Use of a standardized tool supports consistency and appropriate use of SPHM equipment to assist patients with the appropriate level of mobility (Arnold, 2019; Boynton et al., 2020). Figures 34-8 and 34-9 (on page 1264) provide examples of screening/assessment tools.

Assessment Criteria and Care Plan for Safe Patient Handling and Movement

I. Patient's Level of Assistance:

_____ Independent—Patient performs task safely, with or without staff assistance, with or without assistive devices.

_____ Partial Assist—Patient requires no more help than standby, cueing, or coaxing, or caregiver is required to lift no more than 35 lb of a patient's weight.

_____ Dependent—Patient requires nurse to lift more than 35 lb of the patient's weight, or patient is unpredictable in the amount of assistance offered. In this case assistive devices should be used.

An assessment should be made prior to each task if the patient has varying level of ability to assist due to medical reasons, fatigue, medications, etc. When in doubt, assume the patient cannot assist with the transfer/repositioning.

II. Weight-Bearing Capability

_____ Full

_____ Partial

_____ None

III. Bilateral Upper-Extremity Strength

_____ Yes

_____ No

IV. Patient's level of cooperation and comprehension:

_____ Cooperative—may need prompting; able to follow simple commands.

_____ Unpredictable or varies (patient whose behavior changes frequently should be considered as unpredictable), not cooperative, or unable to follow simple commands.

V. Weight: _________ Height: _________

Body Mass Index (BMI) [needed if patient's weight is over 300 lb][1]:__________

If BMI exceeds 50, institute Bariatric Algorithms

The presence of the following conditions are likely to affect the transfer/repositioning process and should be considered when identifying equipment and technique needed to move the patient.

VI. Check applicable conditions likely to affect transfer/repositioning techniques.

_____ Hip/Knee/Shoulder Replacements	_____ Respiratory/Cardiac Compromise	_____ Fractures
_____ History of Falls	_____ Wounds Affecting Transfer/Positioning	_____ Splints/Traction
_____ Paralysis/Paresis	_____ Amputation	_____ Severe Osteoporosis
_____ Unstable Spine	_____ Urinary/Fecal Stoma	_____ Severe Pain/Discomfort
_____ Severe Edema	_____ Contractures/Spasms	_____ Postural Hypotension
_____ Very Fragile Skin	_____ Tubes (IV, Chest, etc.)	

Comments: ____

____

____

VII. Appropriate Lift/Transfer Devices Needed:

Vertical Lift: ____

____

Horizontal Lift: ____

____

Other Patient Handling Devices Needed: ____

____

Sling Type: Seated_____ Seated (Amputee)_____ Standing_____ Supine_____ Ambulation _____ Limb Support _____

Sling Size: ____________

Signature: ______________________________ **Date:** ____________

____

[1]If patient's weight is over 300 lb, the BMI is needed. For Online BMI table and calculator see: http://www.nhlbi.nih.gov/guidelines/obesity/bmi_tbl.htm.

FIGURE 34-8. Sample assessment tool for safe patient handling and movement. (*Source:* VHA Center for Engineering & Occupational Safety and Health [CEOSH]. [2016]. *Safe patient handling and mobility guidebook.* http://www.tnpatientsafety.com/pubfiles/Initiatives/workplace-violence/sphm-pdf.pdf)

- Decide which equipment to use. Protocols and algorithms are available to aid decision making to prevent injury to staff and patients. Figures 34-9 (on page 1264) and 34-10 (on page 1265) provide direction for selection of SPHM equipment/devices based on screening/assessment data.
- Plan carefully what you will do before moving or lifting a patient. Assess the mobility of attached equipment. You may injure the patient or yourself if you have not planned well. Communicate the plan with staff and the patient to ensure coordinated movement.

Test/Assessment Level	Description of Test	Pass Response	PASS =
Assessment Level 1 Assessment of: ▪ sitting balance ▪ upper extremity and core strength ▪ ability to sit upright without getting tachycardic, diaphoretic and/or light-headed; i.e., sitting tolerance	**Sit and Shake:** From semi-reclined position or at EOB, ask patient to sit upright for up to 1 minute (if there is any concern regarding orthostatic hypotension or postural intolerance); then reach across midline and shake hands with caregiver – repeat with other hand. (Patient's feet may either be flat on floor or dangling.) **Safe Mode:** Use sling and lift to assist to side of bed (e.g., sternal precautions, abdominal incision) or bed in chair position, then complete "Sit and Shake."	**Sit:** Able to follow commands and sit unsupported (i.e., unsupported by sling or bed surface) for up to 1 minute. **Shake:** Able to maintain seated balance while challenged by reaching across midline of trunk with one or both hands and shaking caregiver's hand.	**Pass** Assessment Level 1 "Sit and Shake" = **Proceed to Assessment Level 2, "Stretch"** **Fail = Mobility Level 1 Patient** *As appropriate, follow Critical Care Early/Progressive Mobility Program protocol to advance through BMAT Assessment Levels.*
Assessment Level 2 Assessment of: ▪ leg strength in preparation for weight bearing ▪ control and strength of leg muscles, including quadriceps and lower leg muscles ▪ foot drop	**Stretch:** While sitting upright unsupported, extend one leg and straighten knee (knee remains below hip level) and point toes/pump ankle between dorsiflexion/plantar flexion x 3 repetitions. (Patient's feet may either be flat on floor or dangling.) **Safe Mode:** Continue to use sling and lift (mobile or overhead/ceiling), bed in Fowler's or chair position to complete "Stretch."	**Stretch:** Able to extend leg and straighten knee = engage quadriceps; then able to pump ankle for 3 repetitions = AROM/move ankle between dorsiflexion/plantar flexion = engage calf muscles/skeletal muscle pump and assist with venous return/fluid shifts.	**Pass** Assessment Level 2 "Stretch" = **Proceed to Assessment Level 3, "Stand"** **Fail = Mobility Level 2 Patient**
Assessment Level 3 Assessment of: ▪ ability to shift forward, raise buttocks and rise smoothly; balance and strength to rise ▪ standing tolerance for up to 1 minute, which allows for fluid shifts and other compensatory changes to occur ▪ static standing balance	**Stand:** With feet flat on floor about shoulder width apart, shift forward, raise buttocks/rise and stand upright for up to 1 minute (if there is any concern regarding orthostatic hypotension, postural intolerance or syncope). **Safe Mode:** Use sit-to-stand lift and vest/sling, or ambulation vest/pants and lift. *Always default to using Safe Mode if concerned regarding orthostatic hypotension/syncopal event or other compensatory changes.*	**Stand:** Able to rise, maintain balance and upright standing position for up to 1 minute. *The majority of patients who exhibit orthostatic hypotension do so within the first minute of standing, which is the rationale for 1 minute.* Use walker, cane, crutches or prosthetic leg(s) as appropriate to assist.	**Pass** Assessment Level 3 "Stand" = **Proceed to Assessment Level 4, "Step"** **Fail = Mobility Level 3 Patient**
Assessment Level 4 Assessment of: ▪ pre-ambulation weight shift abilities ▪ further assessment of leg strength ▪ dynamic standing balance, which further allows for fluid shifts and other compensatory changes to occur ▪ cognitive ability to follow directions	**Step:** 1) March- or step-in-place taking small steps (not high-marching steps) x 3 repetitions; if able to pass then 2) Step forward with one foot, weight-bear/shift weight onto foot and return foot to starting position; repeat with other foot. **Safe Mode:** Use ambulation vest/pants and lift; consider use of bed in chair position and egress from end-of-bed. *Always default to using Safe Mode if concerned regarding orthostatic hypotension/syncopal event, other compensatory changes or falls.*	**Step:** Able to perform both marching-in-place and forward step and return with one foot and then the other. Use walker, cane, crutches or prosthetic leg(s) as appropriate.	**Pass Assessment Level 4 "Step" = Progress through Discharge Planning** Continue to complete BMAT per protocol; address medical issues and stability; use multidisciplinary approach: work on discharge goals for best destination/placement; consider functional status, ongoing equipment needs and ADL's **Fail = Remain a Mobility Level 4 Patient**

Patient's BMAT Mobility Level	Assessment Level					
	1. Sit & Shake*	2. Stretch*	3. Stand*	4. Step*	**Test Options in SAFE MODE** *(See Figure A, page one for Description of Basic Test)*	**Patient Care and Strengthening in SAFE MODE** SPHM Equipment to Consider for patient care/strengthening NOTE: Consult with PT/OT per facility protocol
Mobility Level 1 = Fails/unable to "Sit and Shake" ***As appropriate, follow Critical Care Early/ Progressive Mobility Program protocol.***	**FAIL**	NA	NA	NA	1) Perform with patient sitting upright in bed 2) Using lift and sling help patient sit at Edge of Bed (EOB) *As appropriate, follow Critical Care Early/Progressive Mobility Program protocol to advance through BMAT Assessment Levels.*	**Goals:** Avoid complications of immobility, engage and strengthen postural muscles and progress to Level 2. 1)Edge of Bed (EOB) dangling with sling and lift: work on sitting balance and reaching across midline; perform calf pump exercises 2)Bed in Fowler's or chair position: sitting supported or unsupported to cross midline and shake hands; also perform calf pump exercises 3)Lift and repo sheet: for boosting and turning 4)Lift and multistraps: for turning and limb holding 5)Lift and sling: for bed to chair/commode transfer 6)Friction Reducing Device (FRD): for PROM/AROM exercises
Mobility Level 2 = Passes "Sit and Shake;" Fails/unable to "Stretch"	PASS	**FAIL**	NA	NA	1) Perform with patient sitting upright in chair position 2) While at EOB dangling and secured by sling and lift	**Goals:** Avoid complications of immobility, engage and strengthen postural and lower extremity muscles, assist with fluid shifts and progress to Level 3. 1) FRD: partial squats and leg AROM exercises – bed flat or tilt position 2) Lift and repo sheet: boosting and turning 3) Lift and multistraps: limb holding or turning 4) Lift and sling: bed to chair/toilet transfer 5) In bed: perform additional calf pump exercises
Mobility Level 3 = Passes" Sit and Shake," and "Stretch;" Fails/unable to "Stand"	PASS	PASS	**FAIL**	NA	1)Using sit-to-stand lift with vest: evaluate patient's tolerance for standing upright and weight bearing; monitor patient's BP and HR; maintain balance for up to 1 minute. 2)Using standing/ambulation vest or pants and floor-based or ceiling lift: starting with patient's feet flat on floor, instruct patient to rise and stand; monitor patient's BP, HR, standing balance and tolerance for up to 1 minute. As appropriate, after testing in Safe Mode, use walker, cane, crutches, prosthetic leg(s) to evaluate standing tolerance and to progress to "Step."	**Goals:** Strengthen muscles in upright position, assist fluid shifts, avoid falls and progress to Level 4. 1)Sit-to-stand lift with vest/sling: stand for 1-2 minutes; shift weight from one foot/leg to the other, 2 – 3 deep breaths 2)Squats using FRD with bed in tilt position 3)Lift and multistraps: limb holding 4)Powered or non-powered sit-to-stand lift for bed to chair/toilet transfers (e.g., quick night-time transfer to and from toilet) 5)If using aid (walker, cane, crutches, prosthetic), after standing with sit-to-stand lift, work on standing with aid.
Mobility Level 4 = Passes "Sit and Shake," "Stretch" and "Stand;" Fails/unable to "Step"	PASS	PASS	PASS	**FAIL**	1) If a sit-to-stand lift with vest was used and patient passed "Stand:" evaluate first portion of "Step," march-in-place, while patient is still secure in vest attached to sit-to-stand lift. 2) Using ambulation vest or pants attached to lift: evaluate "Step" by instructing patient to march-in-place. If able to perform march-in-place, instruct patient to advance step with one foot and return foot to starting position. If able to pass, repeat with other foot. Use walker, cane, crutches or prosthetic leg(s) as appropriate.	**Goals:** Improve standing tolerance and endurance with stepping and weight-shifts, balance and ambulation; avoid falls; consider mobility, functional status, and discharge goals. 1)Lift and ambulation vest/pants for standing, stepping-in-place, weight-shifting/balance activities, and walking 2)Set distance goals to improve endurance and confidence with lift and without lift after passing "Step." 3)If using aid (walker, cane, crutches, prosthetic) to pass "Step," assure that aid is always easily accessible and used for transfers in-room and during hallway ambulation.
Progress through Discharge Planning = Passes all 4 Assessments Review Discharge Goals; Post-acute Discharge Planning	PASS	PASS	PASS	**PASS**	▪ Continue to complete BMAT per protocol; with any change in status adjust Mobility Level and goals as needed. ▪ While improving/maintaining mobility, continue to address medical issues and stability as needed; evaluate other medical conditions/treatment plan prior to physician release. ▪ Mobility goals may include: independence with bed mobility and transfers; improve balance, standing tolerance, endurance with walking; independence with aid(s) - walker, cane, crutches, prosthetic(s).	**Multidisciplinary approach:** ▪ Compare pre-admit status, including ability to perform ADLs, to discharge status; i.e., previous level of function (PLOF) compared to post-acute functional status; review rehabilitation goals – have they been met? ▪ Review discharge goals and guide discharge recommendations; appropriate post-acute discharge destination and equipment needs.

NOTE: *Always default to the safest testing/lifting/transfer method (e.g., total lift and sling) if there is any doubt in the patient's ability to perform the task.*

FIGURE 34-9. Bedside Mobility Assessment Tool (BMAT 2.0). Sample mobility assessment tool and associated SPHM equipment to consider. (Bedside Mobility Assessment Tool (BMAT 2.0) is a trademark of Hill-Rom Services, Inc.)

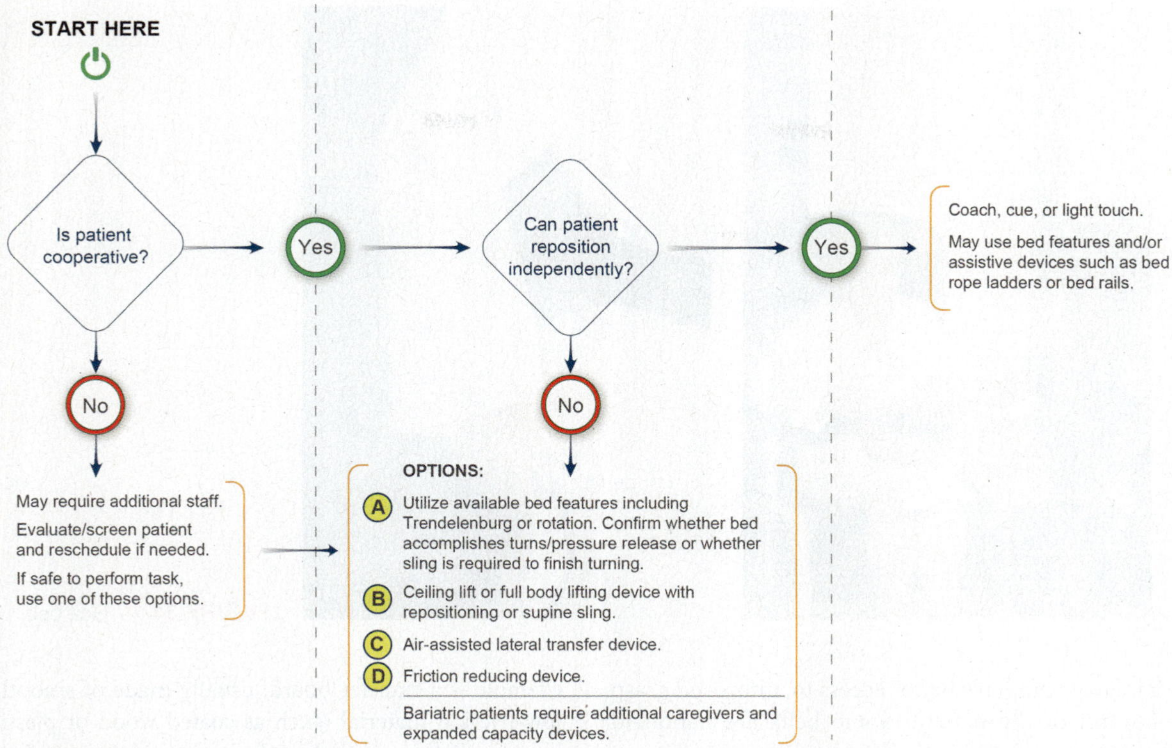

FIGURE 34-10. Example of an algorithm (assessment tool) to aid in decision making regarding safe patient handling and mobility to reposition a patient in bed. (*Source:* VA Mobile Health. [n.d.]. *Safe patient handling.* [Version 1.3.3]. Algorithm 3. [Mobile app]. U. S. Department of Veteran Affairs. https://mobile.va.gov/app/safe-patient-handling)

- Explain to the patient what you plan to do. Then use what abilities the patient has to assist you. This technique often decreases the effort required and the possibility of injury to you.
- If the patient is in pain, administer the prescribed analgesic sufficiently in advance of the transfer to allow the patient to participate in the move more comfortably.
- Elevate the bed as necessary so that you are working at a height that is comfortable and safe for you.
- Lock the wheels of the bed, wheelchair, or stretcher so that they do not slide while you are moving the patient.
- Be sure the patient is in good body alignment while being moved and lifted to protect the patient from strain and muscle injury.
- Support the patient's body properly. Avoid grabbing and holding an extremity by its muscles.
- Avoid friction on the patient's skin during moving.
- Use friction-reducing devices whenever possible, especially during lateral transfers.
- Move your body and the patient in a smooth, rhythmic motion. Jerky movements tend to put extra strain on muscles and joints and are uncomfortable for the patient.
- Use SPHM equipment/devices when moving patients. Be sure that you understand how the device operates and that the patient is properly secured and informed of what will occur. If you are not comfortable with the operation of the equipment, obtain assistance from a caregiver who is.
- Ensure that the equipment used meets weight requirements. Bariatric patients (BMI >50) require bariatric transfer aids and equipment. Bariatric transfer aids and equipment are designed to be used with people who are obese.

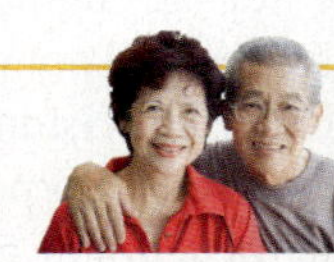

Consider **Mrs. Nguyen**, the woman caring for her husband at home. The nurse would evaluate the need for assistive devices and secure the identified items for patient care. The nurse would incorporate safe patient handling and moving guidelines when role modeling the proper techniques for moving and lifting Mr. Nguyen. In addition, the nurse would use these guidelines to develop a teaching plan for Mrs. Nguyen to ensure safety for all involved when moving and lifting Mr. Nguyen. After teaching Mrs. Nguyen, the nurse would observe her performing the technique to ensure understanding.

SPHM EQUIPMENT AND DEVICES

Many devices and equipment are available to aid in transferring, repositioning, lifting, and/or moving patients. It is important to use the right equipment and appropriate device based on patient assessment and desired movement and to use the equipment in the proper manner (Fragala et al., 2016). Several types and examples of SPHM equipment and devices are outlined here.

Gait Belts

A gait belt is a device used for transferring patients and assisting with ambulation (Fig. 34-11 on page 1266). The belt, which often has handles, is placed around the patient's waist and secured by Velcro fasteners or a buckle or clip. The handles can be placed in a variety of configurations so

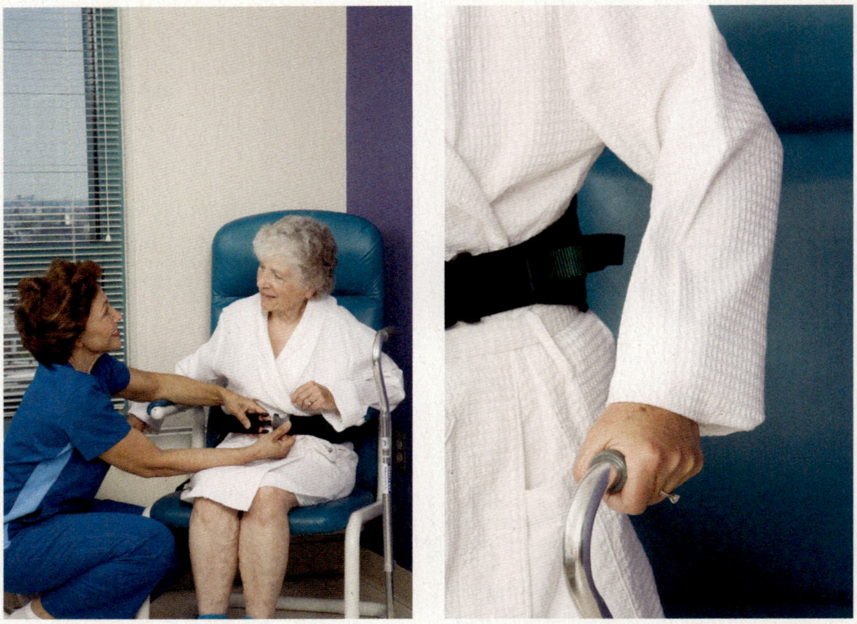

FIGURE 34-11. Gait belt.

that the caregiver can have better access to, improved grasp of, and control of the patient. Some belts are handheld slings that go around the patient, providing a firm grasp for the caregiver and facilitating the transfer. The gait belt is used to steady the patient, not to pull the patient up or as a lifting device stabilization during pivoting. Gait belts also allow the nurse to assist in ambulating patients who have leg strength, can cooperate, and require minimal assistance. Do not use gait belts on patients with abdominal or thoracic incisions or chest trauma. Gait belts should also not be used with patients exhibiting behavioral aggression, as the belt might be used as a weapon and for patients at risk for suicide, as the belt might be used for self-harm (Wintersgill, 2019).

Standing Assist and Repositioning Aids

Some patients need minimal assistance to stand up. With an appropriate support to grasp, they can lift themselves. Many types of non-powered standing assist and repositioning devices can provide leverage and help a patient to stand (VHACEOSH, 2016). These devices can be freestanding or attached to the bed or wheelchair. Other aids have a pull bar to assist the patient to stand, and then a seat unfolds under the patient. After the patient sits on the seat, the device can be wheeled to the toilet, chair, shower, or bed.

Lateral-Assist Devices

Lateral-assist devices reduce patient–surface friction during side-to-side transfers. Roller boards, slide boards, transfer boards, inflatable mattresses, and friction-reducing lateral-assist devices are examples of these devices, which make transfers safer and more comfortable for the patient. For example, an inflatable lateral-assist device is a flexible mattress that is placed under the patient. An attached, portable air supply then inflates the mattress, which provides a layer of air under the patient. This air cushion allows nursing staff to perform the move with much less effort. Another example is a transfer board, usually made of smooth, rigid, low-friction material (such as coated wood or plastic). The board, which is placed under the patient, provides a slick surface for the patient during transfers, reducing friction and the force required to move the patient. A third type of lateral sliding aid is made of a special fabric that reduces friction. Some devices have long handles that reduce reaching by staff to improve safety and make the transfer easier (Fig. 34-12).

Friction-Reducing Sheets

Friction-reducing sheets can be used under patients to prevent skin shearing when moving patients in bed and when assisting with lateral transfers. Their use reduces friction and the force required to move patients. However, use of these sheets may require excessive force and overexertion by the caregiver and increase the risk of musculoskeletal injuries for health care personnel (Battiste-McKinney & Halvorson, 2018; VHACEOSH, 2016). This possibility needs to be considered when planning patient handling and mobility interventions (VHACEOSH, 2016).

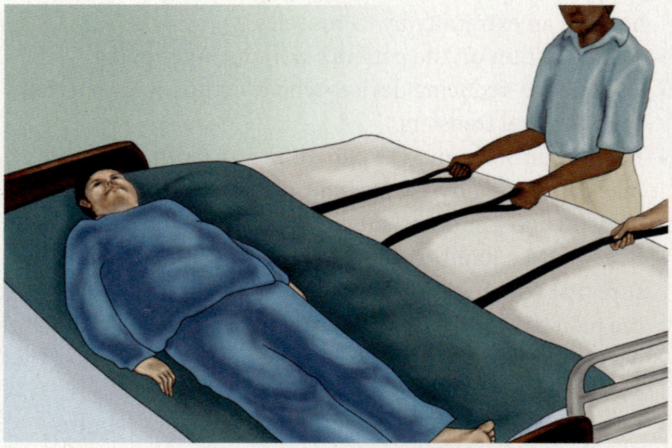

FIGURE 34-12. Lateral-assist device with long handles to reduce reaching by staff.

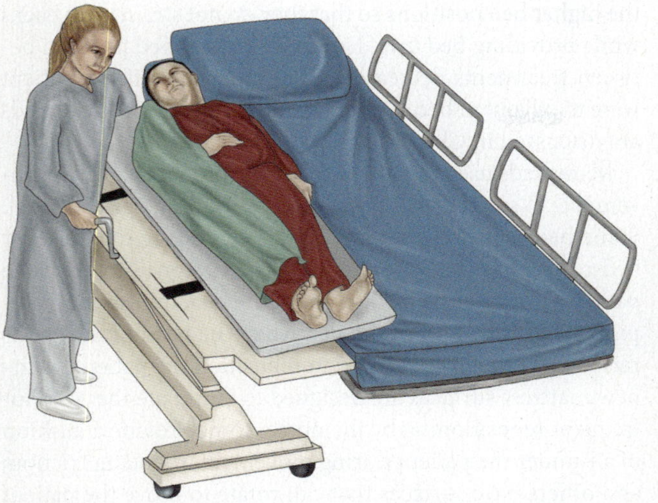

FIGURE 34-13. Mechanical lateral-assist device.

Mechanical Lateral-Assist Devices

Mechanical lateral-assist devices include specialized stretchers and eliminate the need to slide the patient manually. Some devices are motorized, whereas others use a hand crank. A portion of the device moves from the stretcher to the bed, sliding under the patient, bridging the bed and stretcher (Fig. 34-13). The device is then returned to the stretcher, effectively moving the patient without any pulling by staff members.

Transfer Chairs

Chairs that can convert into stretchers are available. These are useful with patients who have no weight-bearing capacity, cannot follow directions, and/or cannot cooperate. The back of the chair bends back, and the leg supports elevate to form a stretcher configuration, eliminating the need for lifting the patient. Some of these chairs have built-in mechanical aids to perform the patient transfer, as detailed previously.

Powered Stand-Assist and Repositioning Lifts

These devices can be used with patients who have some weight-bearing ability, can follow directions, and are cooperative. A simple sling is placed around the patient's back and under the arms. Some devices come with breathable slings that can remain under the patient, reducing the risk for the nurse in turning the patient to position the sling. Standing/ambulation vests may be used instead of a sling (Boynton et al., 2020); a vest may provide additional stability and security in the upper body area, distributing pressure over a larger area, often with extra padding at potential pressure areas and/or leg straps (Enos, 2019). Once in the sling or vest, the patient rests the feet on the device's footrest and places the hands on the handle. The device mechanically assists the patient to stand, without any assistance from the nurse (Fig. 34-14). Once the patient is standing, the device can be wheeled to a chair, the toilet, or bed. Some devices have removable footrests and can be used as a walker. Some have scales incorporated into the device that can be used to weigh the patient. Limb slings and turning bands can be used in conjunction with some lifts to support a body part, such as a limb during dressing changes, and to turn or reposition a patient in bed (Enos, 2019). The duration of time spent in slings should be limited to reduce risk for pressure injury, especially for vulnerable populations (Peterson et al., 2015).

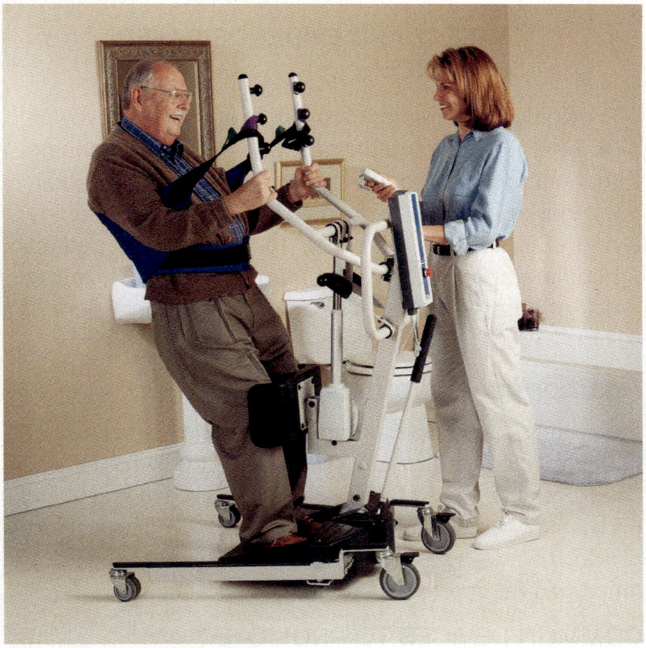

FIGURE 34-14. Stand-assist aid.

Powered Full-Body Lifts

These devices are used with patients who cannot bear any weight to move them out of bed, into and out of a chair, and to a commode or a stretcher. A full-body sling is placed under the patient's body, including head and torso, then the sling is attached to the lift (Fig. 34-15). As mentioned previously, some of these slings are made to stay under the patient to decrease strain on the staff during placement. The device slowly lifts the patient. Some devices can be lowered to the floor to pick up a patient who has fallen. These devices are available on portable bases and ceiling-mounted tracks. The duration of time spent in slings should be limited to reduce risk for pressure injury, especially for vulnerable populations (Peterson et al., 2015).

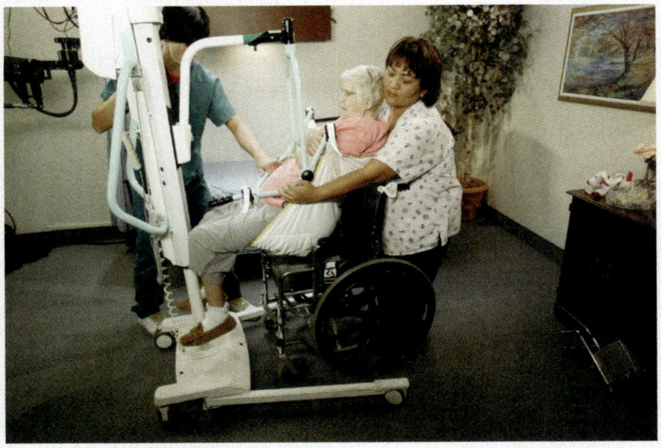

FIGURE 34-15. Powered full-body lift.

QSEN SAFETY AND EVIDENCE-BASED PRACTICE

Providing safe patient care involves the effective use of best-practice guidelines and safety-enhancing technologies related to patient handling and mobility. Nurses have a responsibility to use technology and standardized practices to ensure safe patient handling and mobility, and as a result, minimize the risk of harm to patients and health care providers.

Positioning Patients in Bed

Positioning that maintains correct body alignment and facilitates physiologic functioning contributes to the patient's psychological and physical well-being. The force of gravity pulls parts of the body out of alignment unless adequate support is provided. Various positions are, therefore, protective in nature only when the appropriate positions are maintained.

COMMON DEVICES TO PROMOTE CORRECT ALIGNMENT

Many devices can help maintain proper body alignment and muscle tonus while the patient is in bed and can alleviate discomfort or pressure on various parts of the body.

Foam Wedges and Pillows

Foam wedges and pillows are used primarily to provide support or to elevate a body part. Wedges and pillows of different sizes are useful for different parts. Pillows intended for the head are usually full-sized or large-sized pillows. Small wedges and pillows are ideal for support or elevation of the extremities, shoulders, or incisional wounds. Specially designed wedges and heavy pillows are useful to elevate the upper part of the body when an adjustable bed is unavailable, such as at home. When placing the support, assess for proper alignment. For example, excess cervical flexion would not be comfortable or useful in maintaining adequate respiratory patterns.

Mattresses

A mattress must be firm but have sufficient "give" to permit proper body alignment, as well as to be comfortable and supportive. A patient who must remain in a bed with a nonsupportive mattress may report backache and other discomforts.

Special mattresses, pads, and types of beds used to help prevent pressure injuries are discussed in Chapter 33.

Adjustable Beds

The nurse can elevate the head and/or foot of an adjustable bed to the desired degree. This positioning is discussed later in the chapter. Adjustable beds also allow the bed to be raised so that the mattress is flexed at the level of the knees. Flexion of the knees when the head of the bed is elevated 30 degrees helps to prevent shearing at the sacrum (Baranoski & Ayello, 2020).

It is also possible to alter the height of the bed, raising or lowering the bed to change the distance from the bed to the floor. Position the bed at the height that will let the patient stand with the least amount of effort. Health care workers use the higher bed positions so that they do not strain their backs while providing bed care. However, a lower bed position between treatments decreases the risk of injury if the patient were to fall out of bed. General guidelines for safe use of beds are discussed in Chapter 32.

Many beds used in patient care environments have improvements to support transfer and repositioning of the patient. Some beds easily convert to a chair, bypassing the need for bed-to-chair transfers. Other beds are designed to align the patient's hip with the pivot point in the bed, minimizing slippage toward the foot of the bed when the head of the bed is raised and reducing the need to reposition the patient. Many new mattress surfaces are designed to eliminate the need for frequent repositioning by the nurse; some provide a cushion of air under the patient during movement, reducing friction; and others have surfaces that can rotate to move the patient as needed for care. Some beds incorporate technology to reduce migration by the patient down in the bed as a result of head-of-bed elevation and the effects of gravity and resulting tissue shearing (Lustig et al., 2020). Additional discussion about patient care beds is provided in Chapter 32.

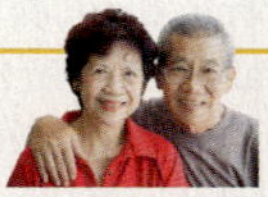

Consider ***Mrs. Nguyen***, the older woman caring for her husband after his stroke. If necessary and not already in the home, an adjustable bed or pressure-relieving mattress pads or coverings could be recommended to help her provide care to her husband. This would be beneficial to both Mrs. Nguyen and her husband.

Trapeze Bar

A trapeze bar (Fig. 34-16) is a handgrip suspended from a frame near the head of the bed. A patient can grasp the bar with one or both hands and raise one's trunk from the bed. The trapeze makes moving and turning considerably easier for many patients and facilitates transfers into and out of bed. It can also be used when a patient needs to perform exercises that strengthen some muscles of the upper extremities (e.g., biceps).

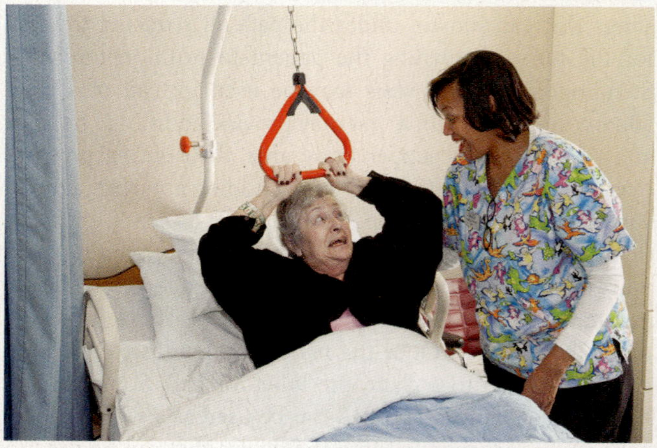

FIGURE 34-16. A trapeze device makes it possible for the patient to lift part of the body from the bed, facilitating turning and moving up in bed.

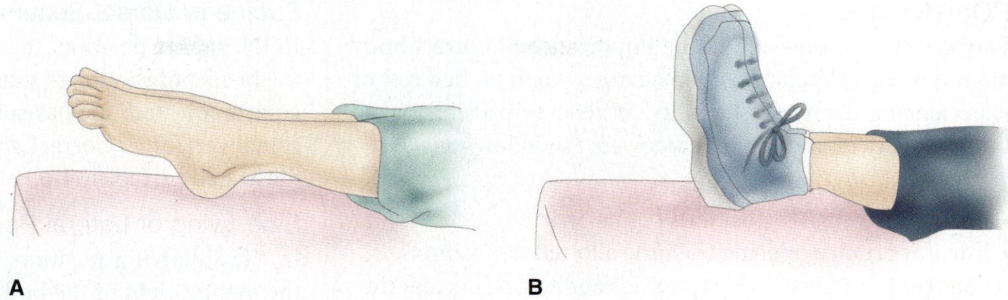

FIGURE 34-17. A. Plantar flexion occurs when the foot is not supported. B. When high-top sneakers support the feet, the dorsiflexion position is maintained.

Additional Equipment

The toes drop downward and the feet are in plantar flexion when the feet are unsupported in the dorsiflexion position. Because of the pull of gravity, this position of the feet occurs naturally when the body is at rest. If maintained for extended periods, plantar flexion can cause an alteration in the length of muscles, and the patient may develop a complication called **footdrop**. In this position, the foot is unable to maintain itself in the perpendicular position, heel–toe gait is impossible, and the patient experiences extreme difficulty in walking. The use of a foot support, such as a foot board, foot boot, splints, or high-top sneakers (Morton, 2018), helps avoid this complication. Figure 34-17 demonstrates a foot in plantar flexion versus the dorsiflexion position maintained by wearing a high-top canvas sneaker.

If top bedding must be kept off the patient's lower extremities, a device called a cradle is used. A cradle is usually a frame that supports the bed linens away from the patient to relieve pressure and to prevent anything from touching the legs and feet (Hinkle et al., 2022), while providing privacy and warmth. There are a number of sizes and shapes of cradles. If used, securely fasten the cradle to the bed so that it does not slide or fall on the patient.

Trochanter rolls are used to support the hips and legs to prevent external rotation of the hips (Hinkle et al., 2022). Figure 34-18 illustrates and describes how to use trochanter rolls. Properly placed pillows can also be used to help prevent this external rotation, but they tend to slip out of place and require frequent adjustment to be effective.

If a patient is paralyzed or unconscious, hand–wrist splints or hand rolls may be necessary to provide a means for keeping the thumb in the correct position, that is, slightly adducted and in apposition to the fingers. A hand roll can be created by folding a washcloth and rolling it. Once placed against the palm of the hand, it can effectively keep the hand in a functional position (Fig. 34-19). A commercial plastic or aluminum splint also may be used to hold the thumb in place regardless of the hand position. Encourage patients who are not moving their fingers to do finger exercises, with special attention to having the thumb touch the tip of each finger.

Side rails can assist the patient in rolling from one side to the other or to sitting up without calling for assistance. Using the side rails can help the patient retain or regain muscle efficiency. When using side rails, be sure to explain their use to patients and their families and follow the protocol of the health care facility. If a patient requests that side rails be raised for additional security, the patient must have the ability to raise and lower the side rails independently. Safe use of side rails is discussed in Chapters 28 and 32.

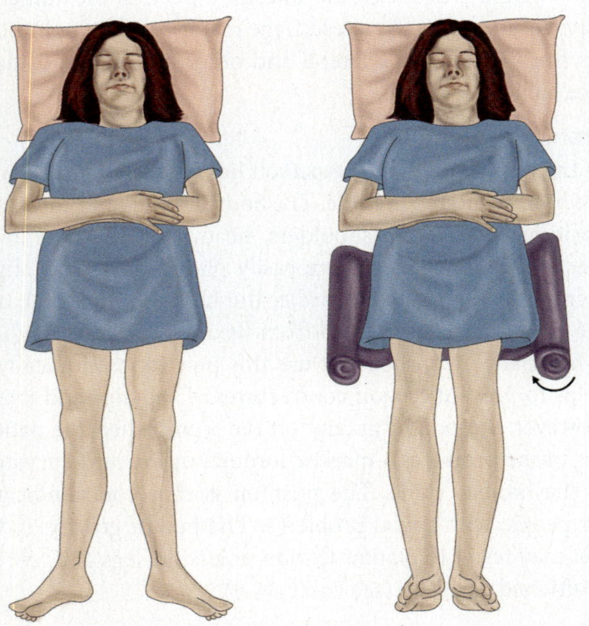

FIGURE 34-18. Trochanter rolls prevent external rotation of the hips of a bedridden patient. The patient is placed on a folded sheet so that the top edge is at the hips and the lower edge is about one third of the way down the thighs. Towels or bath blankets are rolled under each side until the roll is snugly against the patient's hips and thighs. The support cannot unroll, and the weight of the patient keeps it secure.

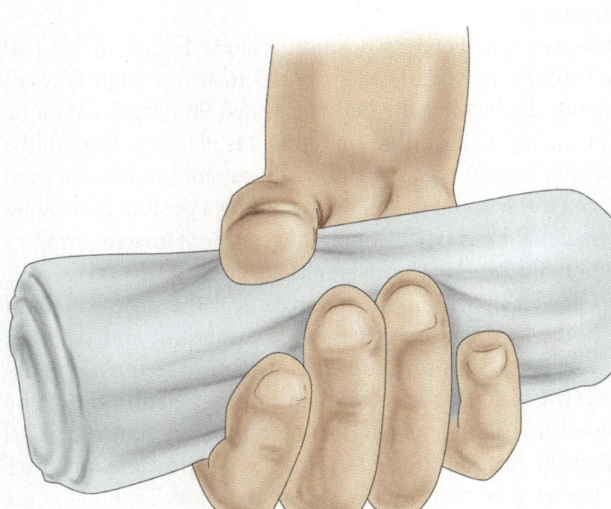

FIGURE 34-19. A hand roll helps maintain functional position.

POSITIONING

Patients may be unaware of the importance of correct body alignment and regular position changes when on bed rest or experiencing decreased mobility. Whenever possible, teach both the patient and family/caregivers the following:

- Correct positioning techniques
- The need to change positions regularly
- The importance of using the time allotted to position changes to exercise the extremities and to assess pressure areas

Regular repositioning redistributes the body's weight and provides pressure relief (Baranoski & Ayello, 2020; McNichol et al., 2021). Repositioning occurs when patients are moved into another position to relieve pressure off a particular part of the body or to redistribute the pressure on a body part (McNichol et al., 2021). Numerous studies have examined turning schedules; the traditional every-2-hour turn schedule may not be the most appropriate approach for every patient (Baranoski & Ayello, 2020). Individual patient characteristics and the use of support surfaces impact the effects of pressure redistribution. Research suggests the frequency of repositioning/turning should be evaluated and reevaluated and tailored to the specific needs of the individual patient based on the patient's unique responses to the care provided (Baranoski & Ayello, 2020; McNichol et al., 2021). When the patient is unable to change position independently, use a repositioning schedule, to assist with and document the rotation of positions. Chapter 33 provides additional discussion of pressure-relieving interventions and nursing care to prevent pressure injuries. Table 34-6 describes common body positions and measures to prevent potential complications associated with each position.

Fowler's Position

The semi-sitting position, or Fowler's position, calls for the head of the bed to be elevated 45 to 60 degrees. This position is often used to promote cardiac and respiratory functioning because abdominal organs drop in this position, providing maximal space in the thoracic cavity. This is also the position of choice for eating, conversation, and urinary and intestinal elimination.

Variations of Fowler's position include high-Fowler's and low-Fowler's, or semi-Fowler's position. In the high-Fowler's position, the head of the bed is elevated 90 degrees. When a bedside table with a pillow on top of it is placed in front of the patient in high-Fowler's position, the patient can lean forward and rest the arms on the pillow, assuming a posture that allows for maximal lung expansion. In low-Fowler's or semi-Fowler's position, the head of the bed is elevated only 30 degrees.

In Fowler's position, the buttocks bear the main weight of the body. In this position, the heels, sacrum, and scapulae are at risk for skin breakdown and require frequent assessment. The semi-Fowler's (semi-reclining) position should be avoided in patients at risk for alterations in skin integrity; raising the head of the bed even a few centimeters increases the shearing force over the sacral area. See Table 34-6 for information about correct positioning and nursing actions to prevent complications associated with this position.

Supine or Dorsal Recumbent Position

In the supine position, the patient lies flat on the back with the head and shoulders slightly elevated with a pillow unless contraindicated, such as spinal anesthesia or surgery on the spinal vertebrae. Correct alignment in the supine position is illustrated in Table 34-6.

Side-Lying or Lateral Position

In the side-lying position, the patient lies on the side and the main weight of the body is borne by the lateral aspect of the lower scapula and the lateral aspect of the lower ilium. Because many people routinely fall asleep in the side-lying position, this is a comfortable alternative to the supine position for the patient on bed rest. Although it relieves pressure on the scapulae, sacrum, and heels and allows the legs and feet to be comfortably flexed, support pillows are needed for correct positioning (see Table 34-6).

The oblique position or 30-degree side-lying position is a variation of the side-lying position. This position is recommended as an alternative to the side-lying position because it places significantly less pressure on the trochanter and sacrococcygeal areas (Baranoski & Ayello, 2020; McNichol et al., 2021). The patient turns toward the side with the hip of the top leg flexed at a 30-degree angle (instead of the 90 degrees side-lying position) and the knee flexed at 35 degrees. The calf of the upper leg is positioned slightly behind the body's midline. Pillows support the patient's back and calf of the top leg (Fig. 34-20 on page 1272).

Another variation of the lateral position is Sims' position. In this position, the patient again lies on the side, but the lower arm is behind the patient and the upper arm is flexed at both the shoulder and the elbow. In this position, the main body weight is borne by the anterior aspects of the humerus, clavicle, and ilium. As a result, the major pressure points differ from those in the lateral and other bed-lying positions (see Table 34-6).

Prone Position

In the prone position, the person lies on the abdomen with the head turned to the side. The body is straight in the prone position because the shoulders, head, and neck are in an erect position; the arms are easily placed in correct alignment with the shoulder girdle; the hips are extended; and the knees can be prevented from flexing or hyperextending. When patients on bed rest use this position periodically, it helps to prevent flexion contractures of the hips and knees. However, the pull of gravity on the trunk when the patient lies prone produces a marked lordosis or forward curvature of the lumbar spine. The position is thus contraindicated for people with spinal problems. The pull of gravity on the feet may result in plantar flexion unless the legs and feet are positioned carefully (see Table 34-6).

Using Graduated Compression Stockings and Pneumatic Compression Devices

Venous stasis, thrombophlebitis, and the development of venous thrombosis are potential complications of immobility (described in Chapter 31). Graduated compression stockings

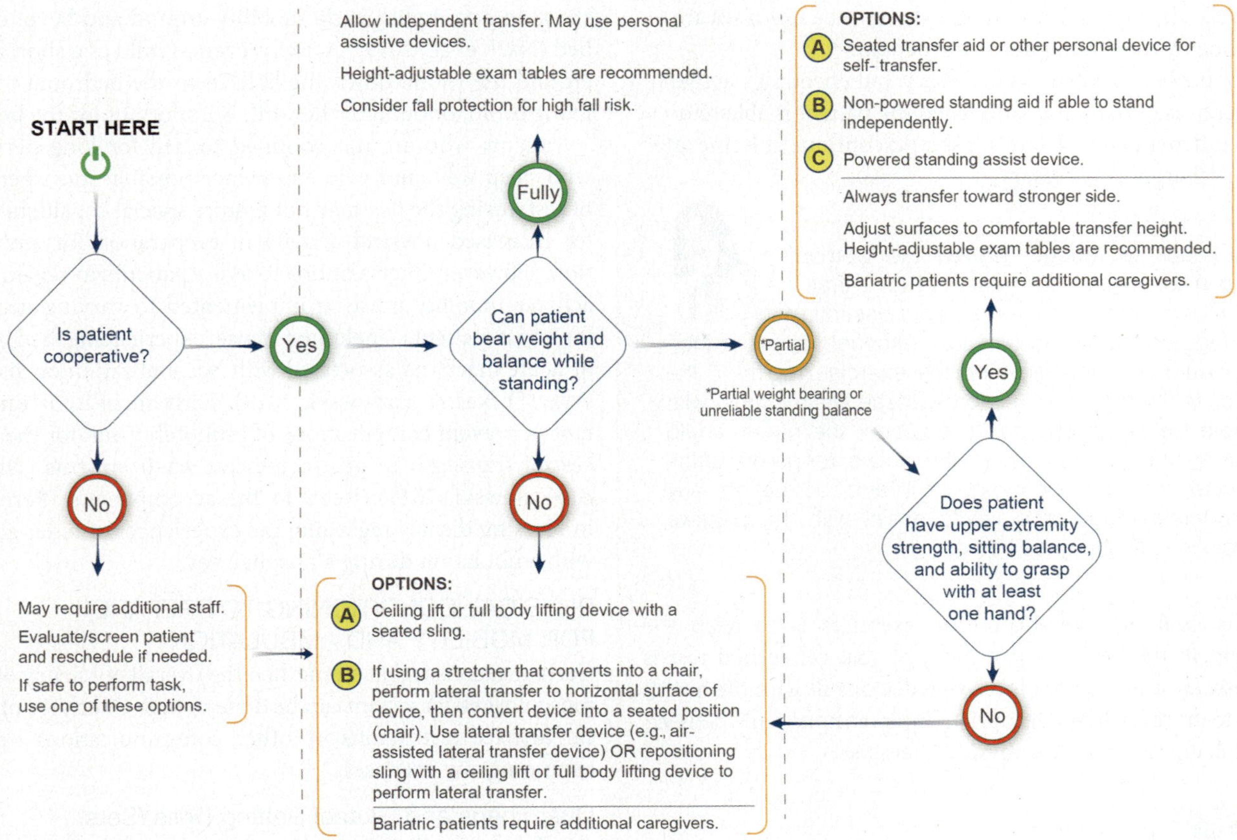

FIGURE 34-22. Example of an algorithm to aid in decision making regarding safe patient handling and mobility to transfer a patient from bed to a chair. (VA Mobile Health. [n.d.]. *Safe patient handling.* [Version 1.3.3]. Algorithm 1. [Mobile app]. U.S. Department of Veteran Affairs. https://mobile.va.gov/app/safe-patient-handling)

range of motion (isotonic exercise). In active-assistive exercise, the nurse may provide minimal support and assistance if the patient cannot do the exercise independently. In **passive exercise**, the patient is unable to move independently, and the nurse moves the joint through its range of motion. Both active and passive exercises improve joint mobility and increase circulation to the affected part, but only active exercise increases muscle mass, tone, and strength and improves cardiac and respiratory functioning. Thus, exercises should be as active as the patient's physical condition permits. It is also helpful to teach isometric exercises to patients to increase muscle mass, tone, and strength.

Include directives in the plan of care for range-of-motion exercises, specifying what, how, and when, so that all who care for the patient observe the same routine. In some care environments, nurses may work closely with physical therapists in designing and implementing exercise programs. Refer to Table 34-2 (on page 1243) for an explanation of terms related to movement. The following are basic guidelines to follow when helping to put the patient's joints through range of motion:

- Teach the patient what exercise is being undertaken, why, and how it will be done. A show-and-tell technique is often helpful.
- Avoid overexertion and continuing exercises to the point that the patient develops fatigue. The exercises are not meant to exhaust or tax the patient. It may be necessary to delay certain exercises until the patient's condition allows.
- Avoid neck hyperextension and attempts to achieve full range of motion in all joints with older adults. These movements may prove painful. Encourage adequate range of motion in those joints necessary to perform ADLs.
- Start gradually and work slowly. All movements should be smooth and rhythmic. Irregular and jerky movements are uncomfortable for patients.
- Move each joint until there is resistance but not pain. Report uncomfortable reactions and stop exercises until further instructions are obtained.
- Return the joint to a neutral position, that is, its normal position of alignment, when finishing each exercise.
- Keep friction at a minimum when moving extremities to avoid injuring the skin.
- Use range-of-motion exercises twice a day, and do the exercises regularly to build up muscle and joint capabilities. Perform each exercise two to five times. It is possible to perform many of the exercises when the patient is being bathed as part of that procedure. Encourage routine tasks such as eating, dressing, self-bathing, and writing to help to put certain joints through range of motion.
- Expect the patient's respiratory and heart rate to increase during exercise. These rates should return to usual resting

levels within 3 minutes. If they do not, the exercises are probably too strenuous for the patient.

- Use passive exercises as necessary, but encourage active exercises of the same kind when the patient is able to do so independently. Exercises should continue at home after a discharge, as necessary.

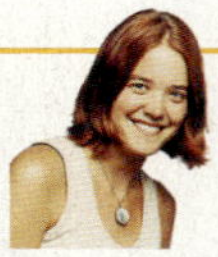

Think back to **Maggie Wyatt**, the woman being discharged after treatment for a fracture. Range-of-motion exercises are essential for Maggie to maintain function. Although physical therapy would probably develop the exercise regimen, the nurse would need to reinforce these instructions with Maggie before discharge. In addition, the nurse would observe Maggie performing the active range-of-motion exercises, giving encouragement and correcting any misunderstandings, and would assist with the passive exercises until she goes home.

The goal of range-of-motion exercises is to keep the patient in the best possible physical state when bed rest is necessary or movement is restricted. Consult with the health care team regarding appropriate interventions and the need for collaboration with a physical therapist.

Concept Mastery Alert

Caution is necessary when performing range-of-motion exercises with patients who are unresponsive because these patients are unable to report pain.

Patient Mobility

Fortunately, for most patients, prolonged periods of bed rest are no longer considered necessary during most illnesses. Routine activity and mobilization of patients is an important activity and is appropriate for most patient populations (Arnold et al., 2018; Liu et al., 2018; Nack et al., 2019; Tasheva et al., 2020). Early, routine mobilization of critically ill patients is safe and reduces hospital length of stay, shortens the duration of mechanical ventilation, shortens the length of stay, and improves muscle strength and functional independence (Campbell et al., 2015; Dammeyer et al., 2013; Dirkes & Kozlowski, 2019). Specialized equipment contributes to early mobilization and allows it to occur safely and comfortably for staff and patients (Arnold et al., 2018; Dirkes & Kozlowski, 2019). A wide variety of walking devices are available, such as wheeled walkers, knee walkers, platform walkers; platform walkers serve as a holder for medical equipment and also provide support for the patient while ambulating (Henecke et al., 2015; Nack et al., 2019).

Early mobility moves along a continuum, beginning when the patient may not be capable of active participation through activities in bed, such as scheduled turning or the bed-in-chair position. Upright-tilt beds progressively tilt from supine to full standing; edge-of-bed sitting helps the patient move toward physical independence (Nack et al., 2019). Ceiling and floor lifts may be paired with transfer or walking slings to accomplish early mobility around and beyond the bed (Nack et al., 2019). Activity, even as mild as a short walk around the room, down the hall, from the bedroom to the living room, or out into the yard, is important for the body.

Patients who are not confined to bed for long periods, who sleep well, and who experience possibly short periods of rest during the day may not require special considerations for increased physical activity in preparation for ambulation. However, interventions to assist patients to regain and achieve mobility must be implemented to varying degrees for most patients, including those experiencing bed reset or acute inactivity associated with hospitalization or disease state (Dirkes & Kozlowski, 2019). Early mobility is important to prevent complications of immobility and for the successful transition to post-acute care environments (Dirkes & Kozlowski, 2019). Refer to the accompanying Research in Nursing display regarding the experiences of older adults with ambulation during a hospital stay.

PHYSICAL CONDITIONING TO PREPARE FOR MOBILITY AND AMBULATION

Certain exercises that strengthen the overall efficiency of the musculoskeletal system can be done in bed. Check for physical activity restrictions or other contraindications before beginning any exercises.

Quadriceps and Gluteal Setting Drills (Sets)

Quadriceps drills are isometric exercises—exercises in which muscle tension occurs without a significant change in the length of the muscle. One of the most important muscle groups used in walking is the quadriceps femoris. This muscle group helps extend the leg and flex the thigh. To help reduce weakness and make first attempts at walking easier, encourage bedridden patients to contract this muscle group frequently. Following are techniques for quadriceps drills:

- Have the patient contract or tighten the muscles on the front of the thighs. The patient has the feeling of pushing the knees downward into the mattress and pulling the feet upward.
- Have the patient hold the position just described while counting slowly to four and then relax the muscles for an equal count. Emphasize that relaxation is important to prevent muscle fatigue.
- Caution the patient not to hold the breath during these exercises to avoid straining the heart.
- Teach the patient to do quadriceps drills two or three times each hour, four to six times a day, or as prescribed.
- Instruct the patient to stop the exercise short of muscle fatigue.

The muscles in the buttocks can be exercised in the same way by pinching the buttocks together and then relaxing them. This is called gluteal setting. Tightening and holding the abdominal muscles for 6 seconds and then relaxing them also strengthen this muscle group to facilitate walking.

Pushups

The muscles of the arms and shoulders may also need strengthening before the patient is ready to be out of bed.

Research in Nursing

BRIDGING THE GAP TO EVIDENCE-BASED PRACTICE

Older Adults Experiences With Ambulation During Hospitalization

Routine activity and mobilization of patients is an important activity and is appropriate for most patient populations. Early, routine mobilization of patients reduces hospital length of stay and improves muscle strength and functional independence. Older adults often lose their ability to independently ambulate during hospitalization (King et al., 2021), increasing the risk for complications associated with immobility. Best practice dictates that nurses encourage ambulation as part of the plan of care. What are the experiences of older adults with ambulation during hospital admission?

Related Research

King, B., Bodden, J., Steege, L., & Brown, C. J. (2021). Older adults experiences with ambulation during a hospital stay: A qualitative study. *Geriatric Nursing, 42*(1), 225–232. https://doi.org/10.1016/j.gerinurse.2020.08.005

The purpose of this qualitative study was to understand older adults' perceptions of and experiences with ambulation during a hospital admission. Community-swelling older adults ($n = 11$) who had a hospital admission within the past year were recruited to participate in five focus group meetings, each lasting 90 minutes. Two researchers conducted all focus groups, with one researcher conducting all interviews and one recording observations of the participants. The focus group meetings were audio recorded and transcribed verbatim. Observations of group interactions, pauses in the conversation, and non-verbal communications were recorded. Data analysis was conducted by two researchers using open coding, creating subcategories and categories. Weekly analysis meetings were used to compare and discuss consistency in coding, with joint reanalysis of disagreement in codes to reach consensus. Constant comparative analysis was used to compare data obtained from different participants. Data analysis resulted in a vivid understanding and description of the participants' experiences with walking during hospitalization. Member checking was used to verify accuracy of the data analysis. Participants described high complexity in deciding whether or not they could ambulate; six categories were identified, including *uncertainty*, *restriction messaging*, *non-welcoming space*, *caring for nurse and self*, *feeling isolated*, and *presenting self*. Numerous barriers influenced participants' decisions, including the physical environment, threats to personal dignity, a sense of isolation, and the desire to no burden the nursing staff with requests to ambulate. The researchers concluded that holder adults perceive hospitals as an unwelcoming space for physical movement and identify specific danger zones that exist within hospitals that preclude them from walking. The researchers suggested that this information provides critical insight into the need for interventions to improve older adult patient ambulation.

Implications for Nurses

The results of this study suggest that nurses need to consider possible barriers to ambulation by older adults in the hospital in order to implement appropriate interventions to address these barriers, support ambulation, and prevent complications of immobility. Nurses have a responsibility to improve older adult patient ambulation in the most efficient, effective, and safe manner possible.

Exercises should improve the strength needed to hold onto or get into a chair and to move about with greater ease. They are part of the preparation for patients who must learn to walk on crutches.

A trapeze attached to the bed of a patient who has limited use of the lower part of the body helps the patient to move about in bed and strengthens muscles in the upper part of the body. However, this does not strengthen the triceps, which is the muscle group necessary for crutch walking or for moving from a bed to a chair. More suitable exercises are pushups, which are done as follows:

- While sitting up in bed without support, the patient can do pushup exercises to strengthen the triceps. Instruct the patient to lift the hips off the bed by pushing down with the hands on the mattress. If the mattress is too soft, a block of books can be placed on the bed under the patient's hands.
- Pushups may also be done with the patient lying in bed on the abdomen. Instruct the patient to place the hands near the outstretched body at about shoulder level, with palms down on the mattress and elbows bent sharply. Then have the patient straighten the elbows to lift the head and shoulders off the bed.
- Pushups may also be done when the patient sits in an armchair or wheelchair. The patient places the hands on the arms of the chair and then raises the body out of the seat.
- Pushups should be done three or four times a day, increasing the number as upper body strength improves.

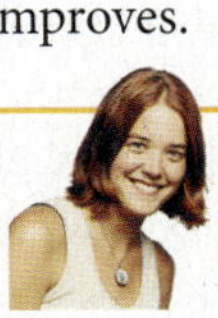

Remember **Maggie Wyatt**, the woman with a fracture being discharged? Due to bed rest, her physical conditioning may be less than what it was before the fracture. Therefore, exercises—such as quadriceps and gluteal setting exercises and pushups in bed—could help to improve Maggie's conditioning, allowing her to participate more fully in her care. These exercises will prepare Maggie for transferring from the bed to the chair or from the chair to the car.

Dangling

Dangling refers to the position in which the person sits on the edge of the bed with legs and feet over the side of the bed.

This exercise can help prepare patients for being out of bed. One method is carried out as follows:

- Place the patient in the sitting position in bed for a few minutes. This will accustom the patient to this position and help prevent feelings of faintness.
- Place the bed at a height that will allow the patient to reach the floor with their feet or the height to reach a footstool, on which the patient can rest their feet while dangling.
- Encourage the patient to make use of a stand-assist device, either freestanding or attached to the side of the bed to move toward the side of the bed and to a side-lying position, facing the side of the bed on which the patient will sit.
- Encourage the patient to make use of the stand-assist device to pivot a quarter of a turn and swing their legs over the side of the bed. Support the shoulders and legs if needed.
- Alternatively, use a sling and ceiling lift or floor lift to move the patient to a sitting position.
- Rest the patient's feet on the floor or on the footstool. This gives a sense of security and lessens the likelihood that the patient will slide off the bed.
- Have the patient move the feet using an up-and-down, marching motion. This promotes circulation in the legs.
- Assess for lightheadedness or other signs of orthostatic hypotension (dizziness, nausea, tachycardia, or pallor).
- Remain with the patient and be ready to place the patient back to a lying position if feeling faint, to prevent falling out of bed.

Daily Activities for Purposeful Exercise

Many activities can be carried out in ways that encourage patients to move and gain the benefit of exercise, improving physical conditioning. When patients understand the purpose, they often adopt other exercises for themselves. For example, position the over the bed table so that the patient must use shoulder and arm muscles to reach it, instead of placing it so that little effort is required to take things from it. Place the signal cord (call light) so that the patient must move either the arm or shoulder to reach it, as long as it is definitely within reach. Encourage patients to sit up and reach for the overbed table, to pull it close, and then to push it back in place. In addition, encourage patients to try to carry out self-care activities, including washing their back independently or putting on socks while still in bed.

In a hospital setting, ADLs may be one of the few independent activities that a patient can perform. Allowing patients to do as much as they can independently is vital. Be sure to offer encouragement and praise. Collaborate with the occupational therapist when necessary to determine types of adaptive equipment that would help the patient achieve maximal functional independence. Box 34-2 provides examples of adaptive equipment. Providing the necessary adaptive tools, coupled with encouraging independence, will create the optimal outcome.

Box 34-2 Adaptive Equipment to Assist With Activities of Daily Living

- Long-handled bath sponges
- Reachers
- Long-handled shoehorns and sock aids
- Elastic shoelaces
- Utensils that are enlarged, specially angulated, or have special grips
- Velcro devices
- Universal cuffs (to hold silverware, comb, toothbrush, and the like, in palm)
- Feeding devices such as plates or bowls with suction-cup bottoms and/or lips to help with scooping food
- Splints and positioning equipment
- Shower chairs
- Transfer benches
- Environmental adaptations (grab bars, ramps)

PROVIDING ASSISTANCE WITH WALKING

Physical inactivity associated with health conditions and health care can have many unfavorable consequences. Early mobility plays an important role in the patient's physical and psychological well-being (Arnold et al., 2018). Nurses caring for patients who have experienced physical deconditioning will often work in collaboration with physical medicine and rehabilitation health care providers. Before getting the patient out of bed, do the following:

- Use a screening or assessment tool to assess the patient's ability to walk and the need for SPHM devices and assistance to guide decision making (VA Mobile Health, n.d.; VHACDOSH, 2016). Suggested decision-making tools and suggested associated SPHM equipment are outlined in Figures 34-9 (on page 1264) and 34-22 (on page 1275).
- Consider use of a gait belt for any patient who is not independent to promote safety (Wintersgill, 2019). A gait belt is used to steady the patient, not as a lifting device (Wintersgill, 2019).
- Explain to the patient exactly what is to be done: transfer technique from bed to erect position, projected distance to be ambulated, assistance available, and the correct manner of using it. Instruct the patient to alert the nurse immediately if feeling dizzy or weak.
- Ensure that the patient has a clear path for ambulation.
- Provide skid-proof footwear.

Assist the patient to an erect position for ambulation, pausing after the patient is seated at the edge of the bed and again after the patient first stands to ensure that the patient feels steady. Use SPHM devices as necessary, to prevent injury to the nurse and patient. Reinforce the need to stand erect and to hold the head high to achieve the full benefits of walking. Patients who are fearful of walking often tend to look at their feet. Remind the patient to take deep breaths to aerate the lungs while walking. Because patients who are walking for the first time after prolonged bed rest often feel faint or weak, plan ambulation for a short distance, gradually increasing the distance as tolerated.

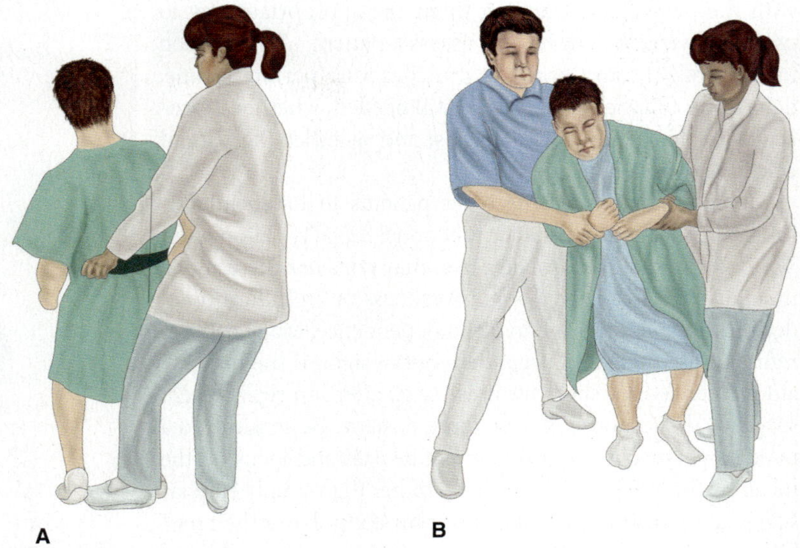

FIGURE 34-23. A. One nurse guiding a patient to the floor. B. Two nurses lowering a patient to the floor.

Should a patient faint or begin to fall while walking, stand with feet apart to create a wide base of support and rock the pelvis out on the side facing the patient. Use the gait belt and guide the patient slowly to the floor, supporting them on your thigh and your large quadriceps muscle, and protecting the patient's head (Wintersgill, 2019) (Fig. 34-23A). When two nurses are assisting a patient who starts to fall or faint, they both should use one hand to grasp the gait belt to support the patient and grasp the patient's hand or wrist with their other hand. After they have steadied the patient, they can slowly lower the patient to a chair or the floor (Fig. 34-23B).

One-Nurse Assist

Patients who require minimal nursing assistance may walk well with the nurse walking alongside. Provide support by standing at the patient's side and placing both hands at the patient's waist. Supporting the patient at the waist helps the patient to maintain an erect posture and prevents unintentionally pulling the patient to one side. Use of a gait belt snugly secured around the patient's waist also provides this type of support. Grasp the belt securely in the back, and walk behind and slightly to the side of the patient (Fig. 34-24).

Frequently, it is necessary to assist the patient with intravenous (IV) therapy equipment to walk. Secure a portable IV pole that moves easily. The patient walks with the assistance of the nurse and the portable IV pole. Ensure that all the equipment is secure before walking and be alert for any tension or sudden action that might dislodge or interfere with the infusion. Also, consider reviewing this technique with family members/caregivers who are assisting with ambulation and are unfamiliar with how to steady the patient, maneuver equipment, and navigate through crowded or narrow areas.

When a patient has weakness on one side, stand on the weaker or affected side and stabilize the patient by grasping the gait belt. Support the patient's weak arm by using one hand to support the patient's forearm and hand.

Two-Nurse Assist

A two-nurse assist is the safer method to use when there is uncertainty about the patient's ability to walk. Use of a gait belt snugly secured around the patient's waist provides assistance support the patient (Wintersgill, 2019). Each nurse should grasp the belt securely with the hand nearest the patient at the handle on each side of the patient. Support the patient's near arm by holding the patient's lower arm or hand. Walk slightly behind and to the side of the patient.

MOBILITY AIDS FOR WALKING

Various devices can assist a patient with walking. Some early mobilization devices were discussed earlier in the chapter. Other common devices to enhance the patient's balance and ability to bear weight include walkers, canes, braces, and crutches. Typically, a patient is fitted for one of these devices and instructed in its use in the department of physical medicine or physical therapy. In this instance, the nurse's concern is chiefly to reinforce the teaching the patient has received and to ensure that the patient continues to use the device properly to assist in safe ambulation. In some health care settings, however, nurses may be responsible for fitting patients

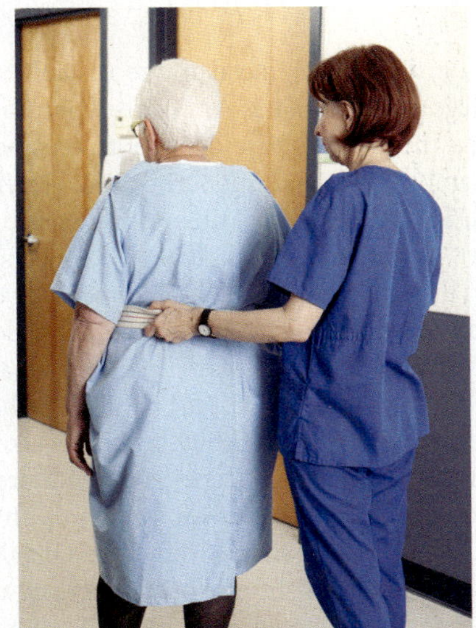

FIGURE 34-24. Assistance with ambulation. The nurse stands on the patient's weaker side and grasps the gait belt.

with the device and teaching them the appropriate way to use the device. Whenever you assess a patient who has been using a walker, cane, brace, or crutches for a period of time, determine whether the device is still needed, whether it continues to meet the patient's needs, and whether the patient continues to use it properly.

Mobility aids can enable older patients to independently fulfill their needs and enhance functional capacity (Eliopoulos, 2018). Some older adults, however, may consider the use of a mobility aid a visible symbol of weakness or an indication of decline in capabilities and loss of independence. Many patients refuse to use them and keep them out of sight. If the mobility aid is intended for short-term use (e.g., after hip replacement surgery), the response may be more positive. Be sensitive to a patient's perspective regarding these devices and focus on the meaning the aid has for the patient, rather than simply emphasizing how to use it. Allow patients some control over their mobility decisions while still ensuring a safe environment. General guidelines for helping patients who need the assistance of a walker, cane, brace, or crutches include the following:

- Whenever possible, instruct the patient and family members/caregivers in the correct use of the device before it is needed (e.g., before surgery). If family members/caregivers are knowledgeable, they can reinforce the teaching as needed.
- When ready to begin walking with the new device, make sure the patient is wearing rubber-soled, well-fitting shoes and that there is a clear path for ambulation (clean, flat, dry, well lit). Use a gait belt, especially if the patient is at high risk for falls.
- Before moving, make sure the patient is steady on the feet when standing; instruct the patient to stand erect, looking straight ahead. The nurse should walk behind and slightly to one side of the patient (in cases of hemiparesis or hemiparalysis, walk on the patient's affected side). Should the patient lose balance, be prepared to grasp the patient's shoulder and the gait belt to steady the patient.

Walker

A walker is a lightweight metal frame (usually aluminum) with four legs (see Fig. 34-25A). Walkers improve balance by increasing the patient's base of support, enhancing stability during ambulation, and supporting the patient's weight (Eliopoulos, 2018). The walker can provide a sense of security and support. There are several types of walkers, specified according to the arm strength and balance needs of the patient. Most walkers have four legs with rubber tips. Some walkers have wheels on the front legs. These walkers are best for patients with a gait that is too fast for a walker without wheels and for patients who have difficulty lifting a walker. Because lifting repeatedly is not required, energy expenditure and stress to the back and upper extremities is lower than with a standard walker. Walkers also are available with wheels on all four legs. Patients who require a larger base of support and do not rely on the walker to bear weight can use these. If full-body weight is applied to this type of walker, it could roll away, resulting in a fall. Wheeled walkers are best for patients who need minimal weight bearing from the walker. Walkers often prove to be difficult to maneuver through doorways and congested areas. They should not be used on stairs or an escalator (American Academy of Orthopedic Surgeons (AAOS), 2015).

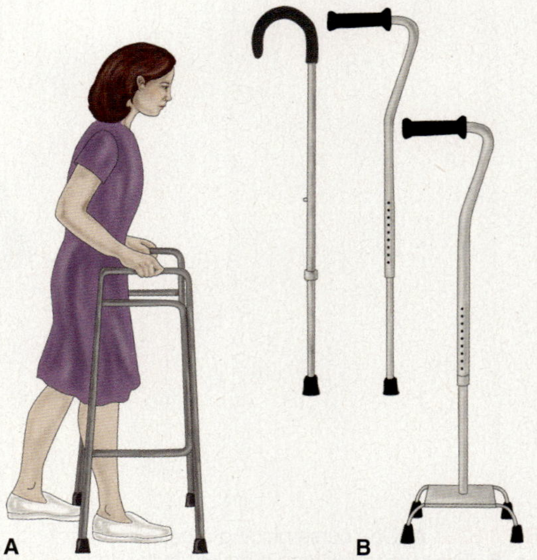

FIGURE 34-25. **A.** A walker is a lightweight metal frame with a broad, four-point base of support. **B.** Three types of canes: single-ended canes with half-circle handle; single-ended canes with straight handles; three- or four-prong canes are recommended for patients with poor balance.

When the patient stands between the back legs of the walker with arms relaxed at the side, the top of the walker should line up with the crease on the inside of the patient's wrist. When the patient's hands are placed on the grips, elbows should be slightly bent, flexed about 15 degrees (MFMER, 2019d). The walker's rubber tips should be intact to prevent slipping. In general, patients lift the walker without wheels ahead of themselves and step into it.

Instruct a patient using a walker to do the following:

- Wear nonskid shoes or slippers.
- When rising from a seated position, use the chair arms for support. Once standing, place one hand at a time on the walker and move forward into it.
- Begin by gripping the top of the walker at the grips, then lift and position or push the walker forward, about one step ahead, keeping the back upright—do not hunch over the walker (MFMER, 2019d). Place one leg inside the walker, keeping the walker in place. Do not step all the way to the front (AAOS, 2015). Push straight down on the grips of the walker and then step forward with the remaining leg into the walker, keeping the walker still. Repeat the process by moving the walker forward again.
- If the patient has an injured or weaker leg, the injured/weaker leg should be moved into the walker first, followed by the stronger or unaffected leg (American Academy of Orthopedic Surgeons, 2015; MFMER, 2019d).
- Caution the patient to avoid pushing the walker out too far in front and leaning over it. Patients should always step into the walker, rather than walking behind it, staying upright as they move (MFMER, 2019d).
- Never attempt to use a walker on stairs or an escalator.

Canes

Canes widen a person's base of support, providing improved balance (AAOS, 2015; Eliopoulos, 2018). Canes should not be used for bearing weight (Eliopoulos, 2018). Canes come in several variations (see Fig. 34-25B): single-ended canes with half-circle handles (recommended for patients requiring minimal support and those who will be using stairs frequently), single-ended canes with straight handles (recommended for patients with hand weakness because the handgrip is easier to hold but not recommended for patients with poor balance), or canes with three (tripod) or four prongs (quad cane) or legs to provide a wide base of support (recommended for patients with poor balance).

Many canes are adjustable. The cane should fit so that when the patient stands with the cane's tip 4 inches (10 cm) to the side of the foot, the cane extends from the floor to the crease in the patient's wrist. The elbow should be bent slightly, flexed 15 degrees when holding the cane (AAOS, 2015; MFMER, 2019e). Rubber tips on the cane prevent slipping and accidents. Inspect these regularly to ensure that they are intact. Teach patients to stand erect when walking with a cane and not to lean out over the cane.

When walking with a cane, instruct patients to hold the cane in the hand opposite the side that needs support (AAOS, 2015; MFMER, 2019e). If the cane is used for stability, the patient may hold it in either hand. Ambulation proceeds in the following fashion:

1. The patient stands with weight evenly distributed between the feet and the cane.
2. The cane is held on the patient's stronger side and is advanced one small stride ahead (AAOS, 2015).
3. Supporting weight on the stronger leg and the cane, the patient advances the weaker foot forward, parallel with the cane.
4. Supporting weight on the weaker leg and the cane, the patient brings the stronger leg forward to finish the step (AAOS, 2015).

Teach patients to position their canes within easy reach when they sit down so that they can rise easily.

Braces

Braces that support weakened leg muscles are available in many variations. Nursing responsibilities include knowing when the brace is to be worn and the correct technique for applying the brace, monitoring to ensure correct use of the brace by the patient, and observing for any untoward problems the brace might cause (e.g., skin irritation). Muscle changes such as those occurring with growth and development or brought about by illness (atrophy) may require the brace to be refitted to maintain its effectiveness.

Crutches

Sometimes it is necessary for patients to use crutches for a time to avoid putting any weight on one leg or foot. The two types of crutches most commonly used are axillary crutches and forearm crutches (Fig. 34-26).

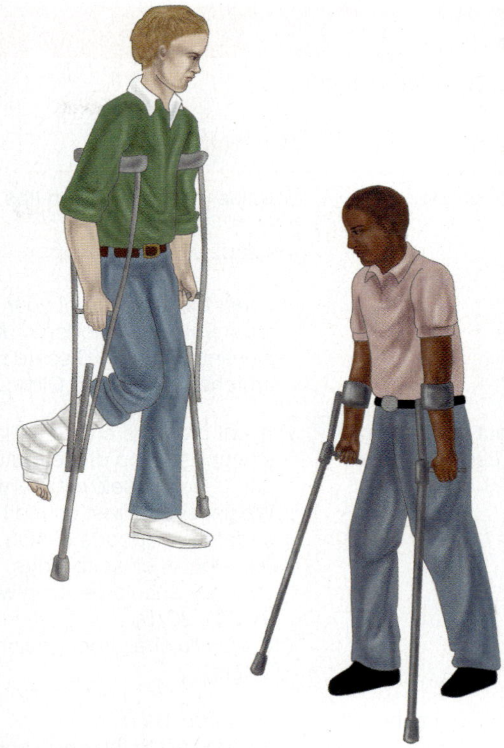

FIGURE 34-26. Axillary (*left*) and forearm (*right*) crutches.

Forearm crutches have a supportive frame extends beyond the handgrip for the lower arm to help guide the crutch. Axillary crutches require significant upper body and arm strength to use. Fitting of and the procedure for crutch walking is usually the responsibility of a physical therapist, but it is important for the nurse to be knowledgeable about the patient's progress and the gait being taught. Be prepared to guide the patient at home or in the hospital after the initial teaching is completed (Fig. 34-27). When using axillary crutches, remind the patient that the

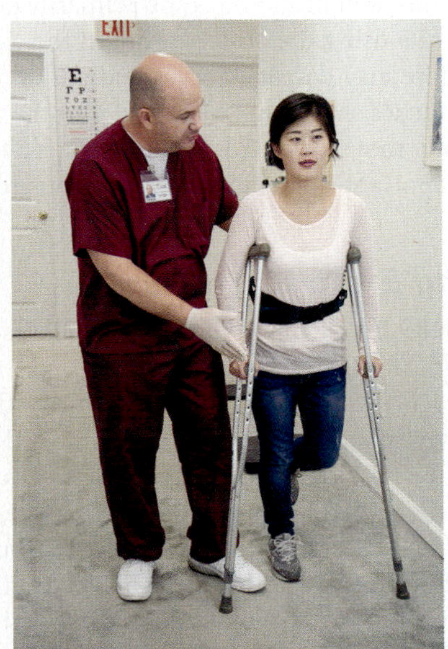

FIGURE 34-27. Assisting patient to stand erect facing forward in a tripod position.

Teaching Tips 34-1

CRUTCH WALKING

Health Topic	Teaching Tip	Why Is This Important?
Safety measures	Routinely inspect crutch tips.	Rubber crutch tips increase surface tension and help prevent slipping.
	Replace worn crutch tips.	Water decreases surface friction and increases the risk of slipping.
	Inspect the structure of your crutches routinely for cracks in a wooden crutch or bends in an aluminum crutch. Discard and replace damaged crutches (Cleveland Clinic, 2019).	Bends or cracks in crutches alter body alignment and decrease the ability to support weight, posing a safety hazard.
Correct positioning for use of crutches	Prevent pressure on the axillae. When standing up straight, the top of the crutches should be about 1 to 2 inches below the armpits (AAOS, 2015). Weight should rest on the hands, not on the underarm supports (AAOS, 2015).	Pressure placed on the axillae can cause damage to nerves and circulation.
	Keep elbows close to sides. The handgrips of the crutches should be even with the top of the hips (AAOS, 2015).	This helps stabilize the crutches to prevent the patient from falling.
	Prevent crutches from getting closer than 12 inches to feet.	This prevents the patient from tripping over the crutches.
Functioning at home	*To rise from a chair:* Slide forward to the edge of the chair. Extend the injured leg to prevent any weight bearing. Place crutches on unaffected side, lean forward, and push off using the crutches. *To climb stairs:* Advance unaffected leg past crutches, then place weight on unaffected leg. Advance affected leg and then crutches to the step. Continue with this order until top of stairs is reached. *To descend stairs:* Move crutches and affected leg first, followed by the unaffected leg.	Patient needs to learn that everyday occurrences may be challenging and, if not done correctly, may end up with injury to affected leg.

support of body weight should come primarily on the hands and arms while using the crutches, not in the axillary areas where pressure may damage nerves and cut off circulation. Also, the crutches should not be forced into the axillae each time the body moves forward. Teaching Tips 34-1 summarizes the important content to reinforce regarding crutch walking.

Promoting Exercise

PREVENTING ILLNESS AND PROMOTING WELLNESS THROUGH EXERCISE

The *Healthy People 2030* guidelines identify that regular physical activity can improve the health and quality of life of people of all ages and helps prevent certain chronic diseases such as hypertension, type 2 diabetes, and cardiovascular disease (USDHHS, n.d.). Vigorous physical activity is not always needed to achieve positive results. Studies have shown that moderate physical activity can be beneficial when incorporated into daily routines (MEFR, 2019c). Current recommendations encourage children and adolescents to be active through moderate-to-vigorous physical activity for 60 minutes or more a day and adults to minimally engage in activity that requires moderate effort, such as brisk walking for 2.5 to 5 hours or more a week (USDHHS, 2018).

An ongoing program of regular physical activity provides substantial health benefits and is essential for healthy aging (USDHHS, 2018). Physical activity guidelines for older adults who are fit and have no chronic conditions are the same as for all adults. Older adults should be as physically active as their abilities and conditions allow. Older adults should include exercises that maintain or improve balance (USDHHS, 2018). See the accompanying Focus on the Older Adult display for nursing strategies to promote exercise and activity in response to age-related changes.

Nurses who role model healthy behaviors are more effective teachers. Use Promoting Health 34-1 to assess yourself before using it with others. This display reflects on self-care behaviors vital for maintaining a healthy level of activity. Promoting exercise and emphasizing wellness behaviors are challenging opportunities for nurses. It is important to be committed to assisting and supporting

Focus on the Older Adult

NURSING STRATEGIES TO PROMOTE EXERCISE AND ACTIVITY FOR AGE-RELATED CHANGES

Age-Related Changes	Nursing Strategies
Activity Intolerance • Decreased respiratory vital capacity • Decreased transport of oxygenated blood to tissue (as in chronic obstructive pulmonary disease or decreased cardiac output)	• Encourage patient to gradually increase physical activity and to listen to cues from one's own body. • Teach effective breathing techniques. • Instruct patient to avoid sudden position changes that may cause dizziness. • Instruct patient to avoid extreme temperatures if exercising. • Provide for sufficient hydration. • Encourage patient to avoid exercise if weak or ill. • Instruct patient to stop exercising if chest pain occurs, and consult with the health care team before resuming activity. • Instruct patient to respect fatigue. Do not push to the point of exhaustion.
Impaired Physical Mobility • Decreased range of motion • Decreased stability of gait	• Encourage patient to warm up before beginning exercises and to cool down after exercising. • Encourage patient to modify exercises versus forcing joints beyond the natural range of motion. • Discuss safety precautions that patient may take when exercising, such as walking in a gym or mall versus on an uneven sidewalk, and walking with a partner. • Recommend that patient wear proper footwear when exercising.

patients to make lifestyle changes that improve the patients' health and well-being.

EXERCISE PROGRAMS

The benefits of exercise for each of the major body systems are so significant that developing individualized exercise programs for patients is an important nursing intervention, often in collaboration with the physical therapist and/or other health care providers. Such a program should incorporate ADLs and planned exercise sessions. Depending on the patient's physical condition, exercise is designed to promote optimal fitness.

Promoting Health 34-1

ACTIVITY

Use the assessment checklist to determine how well you are meeting your needs related to oxygenation. Then develop a prescription for self-care by choosing appropriate behaviors from the list of suggestions.

Assessment Checklist

☐ almost always ☐ sometimes ☐ almost never

☐ ☐ ☐ 1. My lifestyle demonstrates that I place a high value on exercise as a component of wellness (e.g., I use stairs instead of elevators).

☐ ☐ ☐ 2. I exercise for 30 to 45 minutes three or four times per week.

☐ ☐ ☐ 3. I have sufficient energy for each day's tasks.

☐ ☐ ☐ 4. I maintain my target weight/BMI.

Self-Care Behaviors

1. Decide to make the most of everyday opportunities for exercise: Use stairs instead of elevators, walk instead of ride, park the car farther from your destination than usual and walk the distance briskly, and so forth.
2. Choose exercise activities you enjoy and plan three or four 30- to 45-minute exercise sessions weekly.
3. Obtain medical clearance for exercise if you fall in a high-risk group. Learn and observe the appropriate exercise safeguards (e.g., wear running shoes with the proper support).
4. Alternate types of exercise to avoid boredom.
5. Use part of your lunchtime for brisk walking or other exercise.
6. Invite a friend to exercise with you so you have the added support of a buddy or join a spa, health club, or exercise group.
7. Consistently use principles of ergonomics in both leisure and work activities.
8. Build up exercise sessions gradually to avoid overexertion and injury to muscles.
9. Evaluate your lifestyle to see what prevents you from exercising regularly and address these factors (low value attached to health or exercise, low motivation, lack of time, lack of rest, or faulty nutrition).

Information to promote cardiovascular health and oxygenation is available online.

Box 34-3 Successful Exercise Programs

Characteristics to Promote Success

- The program is individually designed (considers the person's fitness goals, interests, skills, exercise opportunities, and exercise capacity).
- The program specifies warm-up and cool-down activities and a variety of major exercise activities—variety is preferable to a single-exercise activity.
- The program specifies frequency, intensity, and duration of exercise.
- The program is convenient to perform, compatible with the person's lifestyle, and fun!
- The person in such a program should understand the program and feel confident that exercise will result in definite health benefits.

Prevention Strategies to Avoid Risks

People beginning exercise programs should be familiar with the following guidelines:

- Physically inactive people with known cardiovascular, metabolic, or renal disease and/or those with signs or symptoms suggestive of these diseases should seek medical clearance before starting an exercise program, regardless of the intensity of the exercise (Riebe et al., 2015).
- Begin a new exercise program slowly and allow your body's support structure time to accommodate to the new stress.
- Know your body and respect its limitations. Never force a joint beyond its natural range of motion.
- Increase physical activity gradually over time to meet key guidelines or health goals.
- Follow the safety guidelines for specific exercises; for example, joggers are advised to run on soft surfaces as opposed to cement or asphalt, to wear well-constructed shoes with thick soles and arch supports, and to run in a safe environment with a low pollution index.
- People who develop new symptoms when increasing their levels of activity should consult a health care provider (USDHHS, 2018).

The person's commitment to a program of regular exercise depends on the following:

- Knowledge of the benefits of exercise and the problems related to immobility
- Appreciation of the fact that in society, sedentary lifestyles are common and most people must consciously choose to exercise
- Belief that each person is responsible for one's own health and that exercise is essential to one's well-being

Foster a commitment to regular exercise by teaching and counseling patients about exercise. To do this, be knowledgeable about the types and benefits of exercise as well as the risks associated with exercise.

When working with a patient to develop an individualized exercise prescription, use the following guidelines:

- Explore the patient's fitness goals, interests, skills, exercise opportunities, and exercise capacity.
- Assist the patient in obtaining medical clearance for exercise.
- Explore feasible exercise activities with the patient, considering the health benefits sought, the time involved, cost, any need for special equipment, precautions, and risks.
- Develop an exercise program that specifies warm-up and cool-down activities (walking, stretching) and three or four major exercise activities from which the patient can choose.
- Specify the frequency, duration, and intensity of the exercise activity. The recommended minimal frequency for activity that requires moderate effort, such as brisk walking, is two-and-a-half hours or more a week (USDHHS, 2018).
- Encourage the patient to complement the exercise program with everyday activities that require exercise.
- Try to identify with the patient any potential threats to the exercise program's successful implementation. Plan support strategies.
- Use ongoing evaluation to determine whether the exercise prescription is meeting the patient's needs and whether the patient is adhering to the prescription.
- Encourage the patient to have an exercise partner; they will encourage each other as well as keep each other company during the exercise.

Box 34-3 identifies characteristics of a successful exercise program and prevention strategies to avoid the risks associated with exercise.

Evaluating

When evaluating the effectiveness of a plan of care designed to help patients enhance, maintain, or regain mobility and fitness goals, use each nurse–patient interaction to evaluate the patient in the following respects:

- General ease of movement and gait
- Body alignment
- Joint structure and function
- Muscle mass, tone, and strength
- Endurance

An excellent time to assess these essential ingredients of well-being is when the patient is performing simple everyday tasks such as walking, undertaking hygiene measures, dressing, and eating. Because illness and enforced inactivity can affect these tasks negatively, ongoing evaluation is necessary if serious problems are to be avoided. For examples of the nursing process for activity, see the accompanying concept map for Kelsi Lester and Nursing Care Plan 34-1 (on pages 1286–1289) for Quan Hong Nguyen.

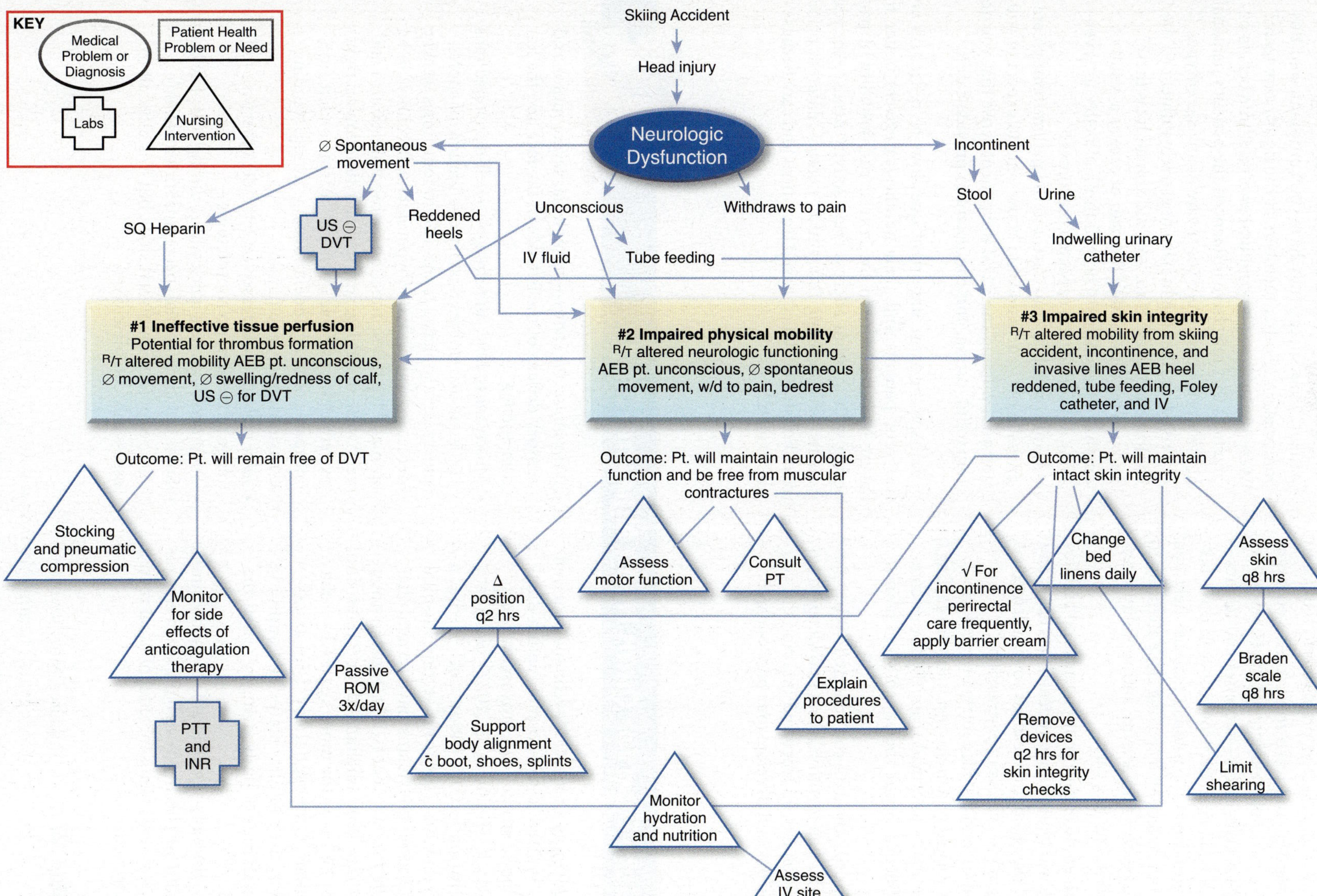

Evaluation

- **Diagnosis #1** Kelsi has no occurrences of DVT. Antiembolism stockings, sequential pneumatic compression devices, and activity have been maintained.
- **Diagnosis #2** Kelsi is being turned every 2 hours. Positioning devices are being used. No contractures or foot drop is noted. Parents are assisting in turning and ROM exercises.
- **Diagnosis #3** Kelsi's heels are no longer reddened. She shows no signs of skin breakdown.

Concept map that displays the use of the nursing process in designing a plan of care for Kelsi Lester. Ø, no; Θ, negative; Δ, change; √ check; c̄, with; AEB, as evidenced by; DVT, deep vein thrombosis; hrs, hours; INR, international normalized ratio; IV, intravenous/intravenous catheter; ROM, range of motion; Pt., patient; PT, physical therapy; PTT, partial thromboplastin time; q, each/every (from L., *quaque*); S/S, signs and symptoms; US, ultrasound; w/d, withdraws; ×, times.

REFLECTIVE PRACTICE LEADING TO PERSONAL LEARNING

Remember that the goal of reflective practice is to look at an experience, understand it, and learn from it. As you begin to develop expertise in implementing measures related to activity, reflect on your experiences—successes and failures—in order to improve your practice. How can you do it better next time? What did you learn today that can help you tomorrow? Begin your reflection by paying close attention to the following while performing activity and mobility interventions and providing nursing care:

- Did your commitment to engage your patients and families and to collaborate with your fellow students, instructor, and other members of the health care team as you implemented the plan of care result in successful partnerships?
- Did your preparation and practice related to performing interventions related to activity result in your feeling confident in your ability to provide care? Did your competence and confidence inspire the patient's and family/caregiver's trust?
- How did you prioritize the data you collected? What patterns in the data did you identify? What knowledge from your learning, personal experience and intuition did you use to make decisions and develop your plan of care?
- How confident are you that the data you communicated and recorded accurately communicates the health status, health problems, issues, risks, and strengths of the patient? How successfully have you communicated this information to other members of the health care team?
- Were you aware of any cultural and/or ethnic beliefs or practices that may have influenced the patient's personal activity practices? Were you aware of any stereotypes or prejudices that might have negatively influenced the clinical encounter? If so, how did you address these?
- Did you need to modify the plan of care as a result of ongoing assessments? Did you think of better interventions to produce the expected outcomes?
- As you concluded your care, did the patient/family/caregivers know your name and know what to expect of you and your nursing care? Did the patient sense that you are respectful, caring, and competent to provide care?

Perhaps the most important questions to reflect on are: Are your patients and their families/caregivers better for having had *you* share in the critical responsibility of partnering with them to address their activity needs? Are your patients now receiving thoughtful, person-centered, prioritized, holistic, evidence-based treatment and care because of your efforts?

Nursing Care Plan for *Quan Hong Nguyen* 34-1

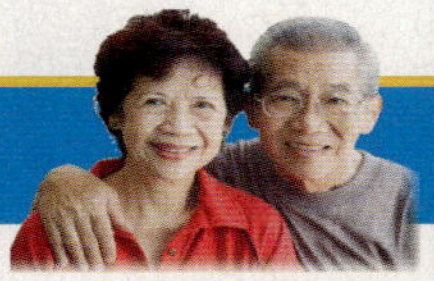

Quan Hong Nguyen is an alert, 75-year-old married man who was admitted to the hospital with a diagnosis of an ischemic stroke (cerebrovascular accident or brain attack; Hinkle et al., 2022) secondary to thrombosis (formation of a blood clot). He has a history of hypertension. This is his second hospital day, and the attending physicians have termed the stroke a *completed stroke;* that is, Mr. Nguyen's neurologic deficits have been unchanged for 2 days, and he is believed to be ready for more aggressive rehabilitative treatment. On hospital day 2, an assessment of Mr. Nguyen's mobility status and ability to participate in activities of daily living revealed the following data:

- *Mental status*—basically alert and able to follow simple commands; expresses his needs verbally when encouraged, but speech is slow; seems forgetful of usual routine for basic self-care activities
- *Neuromuscular status*—hemiplegia; severe motor and sensory deficits of the left side of the face and the left arm and leg
- *Muscle mass, tone, and strength*—well-developed muscles in all extremities; history of a lifetime of sports, most recently played tennis two to four times weekly; decreased muscle tone (hypotonicity, flaccidity) in left arm and leg motor function is absent in left arm and very weak in left leg; strong motor function on right extremities; incapable of weight bearing on left side; incapable of independent turning, sitting, standing, transferring, or ambulation
- *Joint mobility*—decreased on left side; otherwise full range of motion; no contractures
- *Endurance*—fatigues quickly (e.g., during complete bath)
- Some deficit in spatial–perceptual orientation (e.g., ignores objects on his left side), but it is difficult to assess this completely yet

HEALTH PROBLEM/ NEED

Impaired Mobility in Bed

Etiology: left hemiplegia and weakness

Signs/Symptoms: motor function absent in left arm and weak in left leg, decreased joint mobility in left extremities, fatigue.

Nursing Care Plan for *Quan Hong Nguyen* 34-1 *(continued)*

EXPECTED OUTCOME 1/25/25 Whenever observed, the patient will:

- Be in correct body alignment with (1) each joint on the left side higher than the joint proximal to it and (2) supportive devices in place (bed board, footboard, trochanter roll, hand–wrist splint, shoulder sling, pillows).

NURSING INTERVENTIONS	RATIONALE	EVALUATIVE STATEMENT
At each position change (as dictated by every-2-hour turn schedule posted at the bedside), ensure the patient is in correct alignment. Follow facility positioning guidelines for the supine, side-lying (lies on unaffected side), and prone positions.	Correct positioning prevents contractures, relieves pressures, and maintains alignment. Positioning each joint higher than the preceding one prevents edema and its resulting fibrosis. Placing the patient in the prone position for 30 minutes two or three times daily helps prevent knee and hip flexion contractures.	1/27/25 Outcome being met. Every-2-hour positioning schedule being followed with patient in correct body alignment to prevent contractures. *S. Beecher, RN*
Use the following supportive devices: firm mattress, footboard, trochanter roll, shoulder sling when the patient is in the upright position, volar resting splint, and pillows.	Support devices aid in maintaining the patient in correct positioning. Firm mattress provides skeletal support. Footboard during flaccid period prevents footdrop, heel cord shortening, and plantar flexion. Trochanter roll prevents external rotation of the hip when the patient is in the dorsal position. Shoulder sling during the flaccid period prevents shoulder subluxation and shoulder–hand syndrome. Volar resting splint supports the wrist and hand in a functional position. A pillow in the axilla of the left side prevents adduction of the affected side.	
Teach both the patient and family the importance of correct positioning.	Teaching promotes self-care and lays the foundation for successful rehabilitation.	
Allow the family to participate in helping the patient to get comfortable in the different positions.	Involving the family in the patient's care facilitates the coping process.	

EXPECTED OUTCOME By hospital day 7, 1/30/25, the patient will:

- Perform quadriceps, gluteal, and abdominal settings five times daily.

(continued on page 1288)

Nursing Care Plan for Quan Hong Nguyen 34-1 *(continued)*

NURSING INTERVENTIONS	RATIONALE	EVALUATIVE STATEMENT
Teach the patient and family how to tighten the quadriceps, gluteal, and abdominal muscles and hold them for 6 seconds (slow count to 4) before relaxing. A 2-minute rest should be allowed between contractions, and the patient should be cautioned not to hold his breath during these exercises. The exercises should be stopped short of muscle fatigue.	These exercises will maintain muscle mass, tone, and strength (while the patient is on bed rest); and prevent atrophy. They also increase circulation to the exercised body parts. Holding the breath places a strain on the heart.	1/30/25 Outcome partially met. Patient has demonstrated exercises correctly; however, he needs to be reminded to perform them. Family is effective in this regard. *Revision:* Compliment family on excellent job they are doing and reinforce importance of exercise to maximize rehabilitative potential. *S. Beecher, RN*

EXPECTED OUTCOME

By hospital day 7, 1/30/25, the patient will:

- Participate in the every-2-hour positioning schedule by assisting with turning to the degree he is able.

NURSING INTERVENTIONS	RATIONALE	EVALUATIVE STATEMENT
Teach the patient how he can help to reposition himself by grabbing onto the side rail with his right hand and also by placing his unaffected leg under the left one to move himself.	The more the patient can do independently, the more in control he will feel. These activities will pave the way to increasing independence in self-care activities.	1/27/25 Outcome met. Patient consistently assists in repositioning. *S. Beecher, RN*

HEALTH PROBLEM/NEED

ADL deficit

Etiology: decreased alertness and left-sided motor and sensory deficits

Signs/Symptoms: inability to use left arm (is right-handed), inability to ambulate, forgetfulness, fatigue.

EXPECTED OUTCOME

By hospital day 7, 1/30/25, the patient will:

- Demonstrate beginning ability to resume self-care activities despite motor and sensory deficits of left side; use right arm to (1) assist in morning hygiene; and (2) feed himself (finger foods, beverages).

NURSING INTERVENTIONS	RATIONALE	EVALUATIVE STATEMENT
Continue to assess extent of the patient's motor and sensory deficits and ability to perform self-care activities.	This facilitates recognition of any recovery of function and allows setting of appropriate goals.	1/29/25 Outcome met. For the past 2 days, patient has washed his left arm, abdomen, and legs; combed his hair; fed himself; and performed range-of-motion exercises. *S. Beecher, RN*
Set realistic short-term goals for each session with patient and reward progress: "This morning we'll see how much of your bath you are able to manage yourself!" "It must feel good to be able to do this for yourself again."	Adding *realistic* new tasks for each day gives the patient a goal to work toward; a pattern of *noticed* success encourages continued efforts.	

Nursing Care Plan for *Quan Hong Nguyen* 34-1 *(continued)*

NURSING INTERVENTIONS	RATIONALE	EVALUATIVE STATEMENT
Approach the patient from his unaffected side, and place call bell, bedside table, phone, and so on, on this side.	This helps the patient to compensate for alterations in sensory perception.	
Teach patient how to transfer all self-care activities to the unaffected side and how to use one-handed techniques and adaptive equipment.	There is never only one way to do anything.	
Encourage the patient to brush his teeth, comb his hair, bathe and feed himself, and to assist in toileting. Explain to the family why it is critical to allow him to do these things himself, even if movements are tiring, clumsy, and initially frustrating.	This improves the patient's sense of control of his own activities of daily living and improves morale.	

EXPECTED OUTCOME

On discharge to rehabilitation center, the patient will:

- Show signs of physical and mental readiness to acquire increasing independence in self-care.

NURSING INTERVENTIONS	RATIONALE	EVALUATIVE STATEMENT
Implement previously stated nursing actions.	These actions help the patient toward regaining control of his daily living and improve morale.	1/31/25 Outcome met. Patient's muscle strength and joint mobility maintained during hospitalization. Patient is now participating in self-care activities and is eager to learn skills to become more independent. *S. Beecher, RN*

SAMPLE DOCUMENTATION

1/25/25 1500, Nursing

- Dr. Steel examined the patient at 1300 and noted he is now "ready for more aggressive rehabilitative treatment." This was explained to the patient and his wife and son. The patient smiled and seemed to understand that he is out of immediate danger. Initial instructions given to the patient on how he can assist with position changes and actively exercise his left arm and leg. Correctly demonstrated these maneuvers with verbal cueing. Motor function still absent in left arm and weak in left leg. Care plan revised to incorporate new exercise goals.

S. Beecher, RN

Skill 34-1 Assisting a Patient With Repositioning in Bed

DELEGATION CONSIDERATIONS

Assisting a patient to turn in bed may be delegated to assistive personnel (AP) as well as to licensed practical/vocational nurses (LPN/LVNs). The decision to delegate must be based on careful analysis of the patient's needs and circumstances as well as the qualifications of the person to whom the task is being delegated. Refer to the Delegation Guidelines in Appendix A.

EQUIPMENT

- Friction-reducing sheet or lifting/repositioning sheet or other device (based on assessment)
- Lateral transfer device or full-body sling lift and cover sheet (based on assessment)
- Bed surface that inflates to aid in turning
- Pillows or other supports to help the patient maintain the desired position after turning and to maintain correct body alignment for the patient
- Additional caregivers and/or safe handling equipment to assist, based on assessment
- Nonsterile gloves, if indicated; other PPE as indicated

IMPLEMENTATION

ACTION	RATIONALE
1. Review the health record for prescribed interventions and plan of care for patient activity. Identify any movement limitations, conditions that may influence the patient's ability to move or be positioned, and the ability of the patient to assist with turning. **Consult a patient handling algorithm or other decision-making tool to plan an appropriate approach to moving the patient.**	Checking the health care record validates the correct patient and correct procedure. Identification of limitations and ability along with use of an algorithm helps to prevent injury and aids in determining the best plan for patient movement.
2. Gather any positioning aids or supports, if necessary.	Having aids readily available promotes efficient time management.
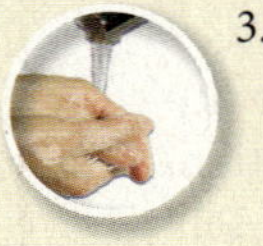 3. Perform hand hygiene. Put on PPE, as indicated.	Hand hygiene and PPE prevent the spread of microorganisms. PPE is required based on transmission precautions.
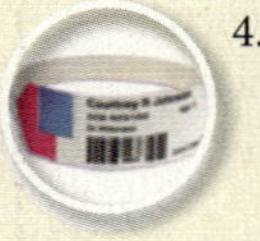 4. Identify the patient. Explain the procedure to the patient.	Patient identification validates the correct patient and correct procedure. Discussion and explanation help allay anxiety and prepare the patient for what to expect.
5. Close the curtains around the bed and close the door to the room, if possible. Position at least one nurse on either side of the bed. Place pillows, wedges, or any other support to be used for positioning within easy reach. Place the bed at an appropriate and comfortable working height (VHACEOSH, 2016). Lower both side rails.	Closing the door or curtains provides for privacy. Proper bed height helps reduce back strain while performing the procedure. Proper positioning and lowering of the side rails facilitate moving the patient and minimizes strain on the nurses.
6. If not already in place, position a friction-reducing sheet or lifting/repositioning sheet or other transfer device under the patient, based on assessment.	Friction-reducing/lifting/repositioning sheets and other transfer devices aid in preventing shearing and in reducing friction and the force required to move the patient.
7. Remove all pillows from under the patient's head, back, or legs. If moving the patient up in the bed, leave one pillow at the head of the bed, leaning upright against the headboard.	Removing pillows from under the patient facilitates movement; placing a pillow at the head of the bed prevents accidental head injury against the top of the bed.
8. Based on the screening and assessment information, position at least one nurse or other health care provider on either side of the bed, and lower both side rails.	Proper positioning and lowering the side rails facilitate moving the patient and minimize strain on the care providers.
9. If the patient is fully able to assist in repositioning, allow the patient to complete the move independently, with supervision.	Safe supervision allows for intervention by care giver if necessary and reduces the risk for injury.

ACTION	RATIONALE
10. If the patient is partially able or unable to assist, make use of friction-reducing devices, lifting/repositioning sheets (Figure 1), lateral transfer devices, full-body sling lift and/or engage the turning or rotation to assist with the action (VA Mobile Health, n.d.).	Use of SPHM equipment is necessary to reduce risk of injury to patient and care providers (Fragala et al., 2016; OSHA and Joint Commission Resources Alliance, 2017; VA Mobile Health, n.d.).

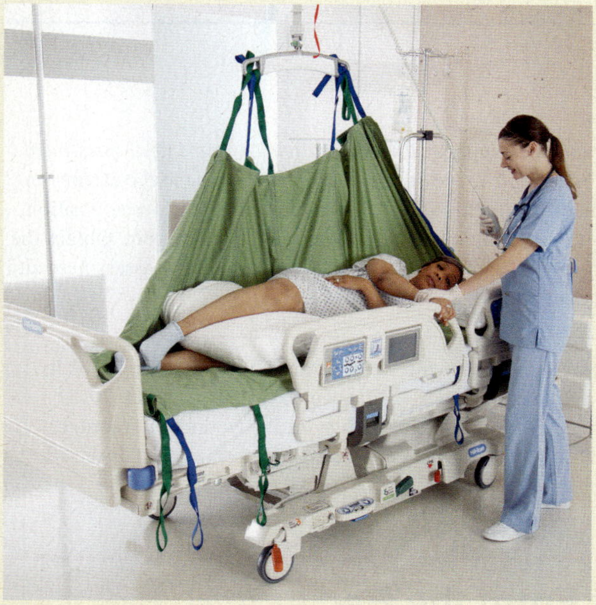

FIGURE 1. Example of a repositioning sheet for use with a lift.

ACTION	RATIONALE
11. If turning, activate the bed-turn mechanism to inflate the side of the bed behind the patient's back.	Activating the turn mechanism inflates the side of the bed for approximately 10 seconds, aiding in propelling the patient to turn, and reducing the work required by the nurse. This helps avoid injury to the nurse or other care provider.
12. Alternatively, follow manufacturer's directions to utilize the ceiling lift or full-body lifting device with the repositioning or supine sling or air-assisted transfer device.	Use of SPHM equipment is necessary to reduce risk of injury to patient and care providers (Fragala et al., 2016; OSHA and Joint Commission Resources Alliance, 2017; VA Mobile Health, n.d.).
13. Once the patient has been repositioned, make the patient comfortable and position in proper alignment, using pillows or other supports behind the patient's back (pull the shoulder blade forward and out from under the patient), under the leg and arm, as needed. Readjust the pillow under the patient's head. Elevate the head of the bed as needed for comfort.	Positioning in proper alignment with supports ensures that the patient will be able to maintain the desired position and will be comfortable. Positioning the shoulder blade removes pressure from the bony prominence.
14. Place the bed in the lowest position, with the side rails up, as indicated. Make sure the call bell and other necessary items are within easy reach.	Adjusting the bed height ensures patient safety. Having the call bell and essential items readily available helps promote safety.
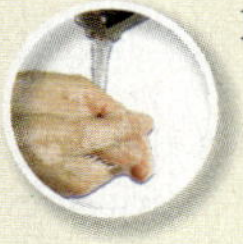 15. Clean transfer aids, per facility policy, if not indicated for single-patient use. Remove gloves and other PPE, if used. Perform hand hygiene.	Proper cleaning of equipment between patient use prevents the spread of microorganisms. Proper removal of PPE reduces the risk for infection transmission and contamination of other items. Hand hygiene prevents the spread of microorganisms.

DOCUMENTATION

Guidelines

Many facilities provide areas on the bedside flow sheet to document repositioning. Be sure to document the time the patient's position was changed, use of supports, and any pertinent observations, including skin assessment. Document the patient's tolerance of the position change. Document completed assessment algorithm for patient handling and movement decision and SPHM aids used to facilitate movement.

(continued on page 1292)

Skill 34-1 Assisting a Patient With Repositioning in Bed (continued)

Sample Documentation

11/10/25 1130 Patient repositioned from right side to left side; alignment maintained with wedge support behind back and pillow between legs. Skin on pressure points on right side without signs of irritation, edema, or redness. Patient reported no pain with movement. Bed-turn mechanism and friction-reducing sheet used to facilitate transfer; sheet left in place under patient. Patient partially able to assist with turn by pulling on bed rail.

—B. Clapp, RN

DEVELOPING CLINICAL REASONING AND CLINICAL JUDGMENT

UNEXPECTED SITUATIONS AND ASSOCIATED INTERVENTIONS

- *You are attempting to move a patient up in the bed when you realize your initial assessment was inaccurate and the patient is not able to participate with repositioning to the extent you thought:* Cover the patient, make sure all rails are up, lower the bed to the lowest position, and take a moment to reassess the situation using SPHM decision-making tool. Obtain the necessary equipment and number of personnel as indicated. Document the assessment and necessary equipment in the plan of care for continuity of care.

SPECIAL CONSIDERATIONS

- Institute Bariatric Algorithms for any patient who weighs more than 300 lb, or is 100 lb over ideal weight, or who has a body mass index (BMI) over 40 (VHA CEOSH, 2015).
- When moving a patient with a leg or foot problem, such as a cast, wound, or **fracture**, one caregiver should be assigned to monitor movement of that extremity to reduce risk of further injury.

Skill 34-2 Transferring a Patient From the Bed to a Stretcher

DELEGATION CONSIDERATIONS

The transfer of a patient from bed to stretcher may be delegated to assistive personnel (AP) as well as to licensed practical/vocational nurses (LPN/LVNs). The decision to delegate must be based on careful analysis of the patient's needs and circumstances as well as the qualifications of the person to whom the task is being delegated. Refer to the Delegation Guidelines in Appendix A.

EQUIPMENT

- Transport stretcher
- Ceiling lift or full-body lift
- Lateral-assist device, such as a transfer board, roller board, or air or mechanical lateral-assist device and cover sheet
- Bath blanket
- Regular blanket
- At least two assistants, depending on assessment and data
- Nonsterile gloves and/or other PPE, as indicated

IMPLEMENTATION

ACTION	RATIONALE
1. Identify any movement limitations, conditions that may influence the patient's ability to move or be positioned, and the ability of the patient to assist with the transfer. **Consult a patient handling algorithm, if available, to plan an appropriate approach to moving the patient.** Assess for tubes, IV lines, incisions, or equipment that may alter the positioning procedure. Gather transfer aids or supports as necessary.	Reviewing the health record and plan of care validates the correct patient and correct procedure. Checking for interfering equipment helps reduce the risk for injury. Identification of limitations and ability along with use of an algorithm helps to prevent injury and aids in determining the best plan for patient movement. Having aids readily available promotes efficient time management.

ACTION | **RATIONALE**

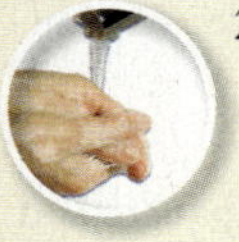

2. Perform hand hygiene and put on PPE, if indicated.

Hand hygiene and PPE prevent the spread of microorganisms. PPE is required based on transmission precautions.

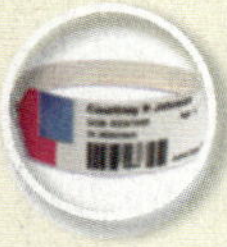

3. Identify the patient. Explain the procedure to the patient.

Patient identification validates the correct patient and correct procedure. Discussion and explanation help allay anxiety and prepare the patient for what to expect.

4. Close the curtains around the bed and close the door to the room, if possible. Adjust the head of the bed to a flat position or as low as the patient can tolerate. Raise the bed to a height that is even with the transport stretcher (VHACEOSH, 2016). Lower the side rails, if in place.

Closing the door or curtains provides for privacy. Proper bed height and lowering side rails make transfer easier and decrease the risk for injury.

5. Place the bath blanket over the patient and remove the top covers from underneath. Remove all pillows from under the patient's head, back, or legs.

Bath blanket provides privacy and warmth. Removing pillows from under the patient facilitates movement.

6. If not already in place, position a friction-reducing sheet or lifting/repositioning sheet or other transfer device under the patient, based on assessment.

Friction-reducing/lifting/repositioning sheets and other transfer devices aid in preventing shearing and in reducing friction and the force required to move the patient.

7. Follow manufacturer's directions to utilize the ceiling lift or full-body lifting device with the repositioning or supine sling or air-assisted transfer device (Figure 1).

Use of SPHM equipment is necessary to reduce risk of injury to patient and care providers (Fragala et al., 2016; OSHA and Joint Commission Resources Alliance, 2017; VA Mobile Health, n.d.).

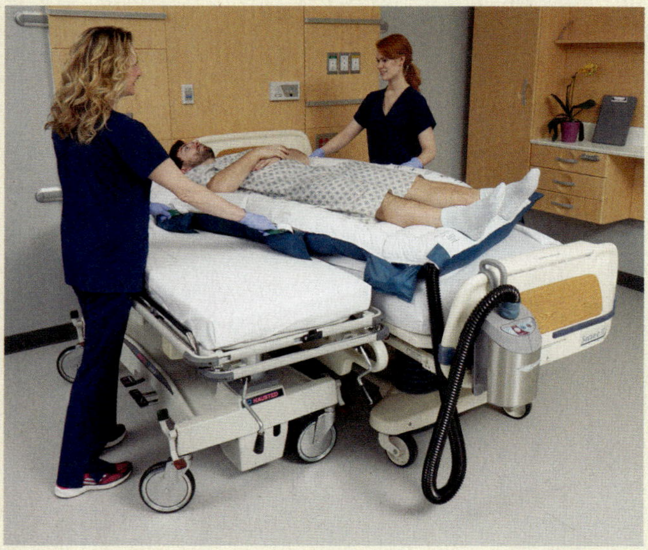

FIGURE 1. Example of an air-assisted transfer device.

8. Position the stretcher next (and parallel) to the bed. **Lock the wheels on the stretcher and the bed.**

Positioning equipment makes the transfer easier and decreases the risk for injury. Locking the wheels keeps the bed and stretcher from moving.

9. At a minimum, one caregiver should be positioned on the stretcher side of the bed, and another should stand on the side of the bed without the stretcher. Depending on the transfer device, other care givers should be positioned accordingly.

Team coordination provides for patient safety during transfer.

(continued on page 1294)

Skill 34-2 Transferring a Patient From the Bed to a Stretcher *(continued)*

ACTION	RATIONALE
10. Use the friction-reducing sheet to roll the patient away from the stretcher (Figure 2). Place the transfer device under the patient (Figure 3).	The transfer board or other lateral-assist device reduces friction, easing the workload to move patient.
11. **At a signal given by one of the caregivers and based on the manufacturer's directions for use of the device, move the patient from the bed to the stretcher (Figure 4).**	Working in unison distributes the work of moving the patient and facilitates the transfer.
12. Once the patient is transferred to the stretcher (Figure 5), remove the SPHM device or leave in place for future use, based on device type and facility policy. Provide a pillow and other supports as indicated. Secure the patient and raise the side rails. To ensure the patient's comfort, cover the patient with blanket and remove the bath blanket from underneath.	Positioning in proper alignment with supports ensures that the patient will be able to maintain the desired position and will be comfortable. Side rails promote safety. Blanket promotes comfort and warmth.

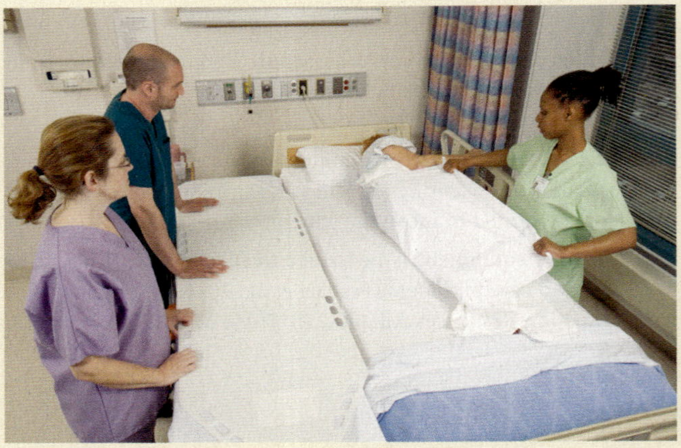

FIGURE 2. Using sheet to roll patient away from stretcher.

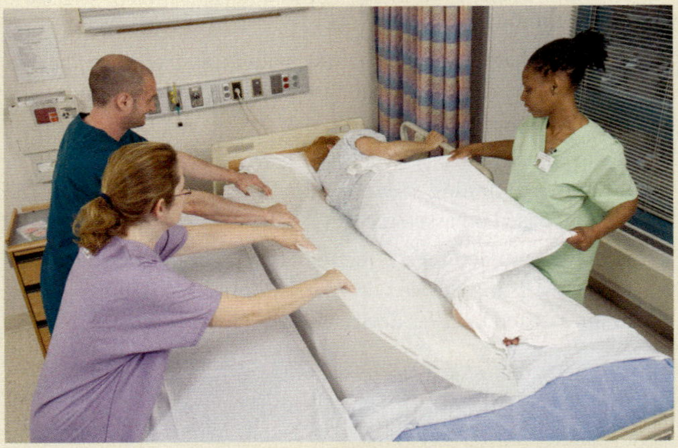

FIGURE 3. Positioning transfer device under patient.

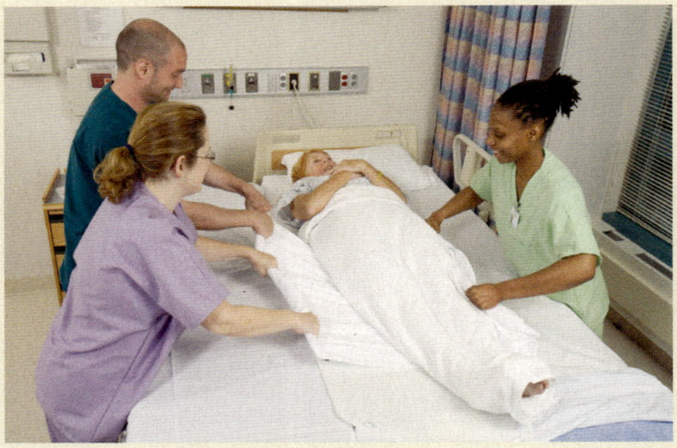

FIGURE 4. Transferring patient onto stretcher.

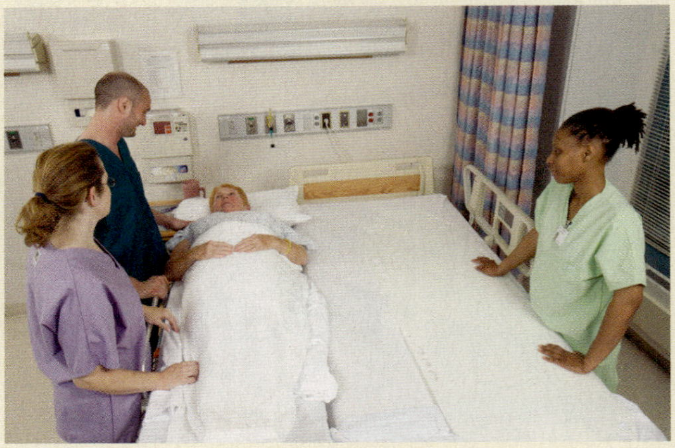

FIGURE 5. Patient on stretcher.

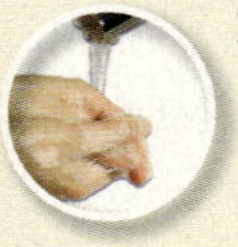

13. Clean transfer aids, per facility policy, if not indicated for single-patient use. Remove gloves and any other PPE, if used. Perform hand hygiene.	Proper cleaning of equipment between patient use prevents the spread of microorganisms. Proper removal of PPE reduces the risk for infection transmission and contamination of other items. Hand hygiene prevents the spread of microorganisms.

DOCUMENTATION

Guidelines

Document the time and method of transport, and patient's destination, according to facility policy. Document the completed assessment algorithm for patient handling and movement decision and the use of transfer aids and number of staff required for transfer.

Sample Documentation

5/12/25 1005 Patient transferred to stretcher via air-assisted lateral transfer device. Three caregivers required. Transported to radiology for chest x-ray. —*M. Joliet, RN*

DEVELOPING CLINICAL REASONING AND CLINICAL JUDGMENT

UNEXPECTED SITUATIONS AND ASSOCIATED INTERVENTIONS

- *Your patient needs to be transported to another department by stretcher. The patient is very heavy and somewhat confused, so you are concerned about his ability to cooperate with the transfer:* Consult a Bariatric Algorithm. Confirm that the patient handling equipment and stretcher meet weight, width, and height requirements of the patient (VHA CEOSH, 2015). Obtain the assistance of additional caregivers; bariatric patients and use of expanded capacity equipment requires more caregivers (VHA CEOSH, 2015). Use bariatric equipment and devices to move the patient (VHA CEOSH, 2015).

SPECIAL CONSIDERATIONS

- If the patient is unconscious or weakened, additional caregivers are needed to support the extremities and the head to reduce risk of further injury.
- Some mechanical lateral-transfer aids are motorized, and others use a hand crank. If a mechanical lateral-assist device is used, follow the manufacturer's directions for safe movement of the patient. Be familiar with weight restrictions for individual pieces of equipment.
- Keep in mind that the transfer of patients is often delegated to AP. Before moving patients, all personnel need to complete instructions about this skill and must be able to provide return demonstrations of transfer skills. When a patient is being transferred, communicate clearly any mobility restrictions or special care needs.
- Bariatric patients require additional caregivers and expanded capacity devices (VA Mobile Health, n.d; VHACEOSH, 2016). Institute Bariatric Algorithms for any patient who weighs more than 300 lb, or is 100 lb over ideal weight, or who has a BMI over 40 (VHA CEOSH, 2015).

DEVELOPING CLINICAL REASONING AND CLINICAL JUDGMENT

1. Work through the Concept Map for Kelsi Lester on page 1285 and the Nursing Care Plan for Quan Hong Ngyuen on pages 1286–1289 to help develop your clinical reasoning and clinical judgment skills.
2. Simulate a mobility impairment for yourself (i.e., you have to use crutches or a walker, cane, or wheelchair) and attempt to perform your usual daily activities, ideally including visiting a public place, such as a school or mall. How did you feel about the restriction of your movement? How can nurses best assist patients who are coping with these restrictions? How did the public respond to your impairment, and what effects might such responses have on people with mobility impairments? Are public spaces adequately adapted to meet the needs of those with mobility impairments? What measures are needed to address any deficiencies? Did you identify any safety needs?
3. Suppose a friend is confined to bed for several months after a motorcycle accident that resulted in severe orthopedic and internal injuries. What nursing measures would you recommend to avoid the hazards of immobility?

PRACTICING FOR NCLEX

1. A nurse is developing an exercise program for a patient who has COPD. Which instructions would the nurse include in a teaching plan for this patient? Select all that apply.
   a. Teach the patient to avoid sudden position changes that may cause dizziness.
   b. Recommend that the patient restrict fluid intake until after exercise.
   c. Instruct the patient to push a little further beyond fatigue each session.
   d. Tell the patient to avoid exercising in very cold or very hot temperatures.
   e. Encourage the patient to modify exercise if weak or ill.
   f. Recommend that the patient consume a high-carb, low-protein diet.

2. A nurse is providing active-assistive range-of-motion exercises for a patient who is recovering from a stroke. During the session, the patient reports that they are "too tired to go on." What actions are appropriate at this time? Select all that apply.
   a. Stop performing the exercises.
   b. Decrease the number of repetitions performed.
   c. Reevaluate the plan of care.
   d. Move to the patient's other side to perform exercises.
   e. Encourage the patient to finish the exercises and then rest.
   f. Assess the patient for additional symptoms of intolerance.
3. A nurse assists a patient with ambulation for the first time following a knee replacement. Shortly after beginning to walk, the patient tells the nurse that they are dizzy and feel like they might fall. Place these nursing actions in the order in which the nurse should perform them to protect the patient:
   a. Grasp the gait belt.
   b. Stay with the patient and call for help.
   c. Place feet wide apart with one foot in front.
   d. Gently slide the patient down to the floor, protecting their head.
   e. Pull the weight of the patient backward against your body.
   f. Rock your pelvis out on the side of the patient.
4. A nurse caring for patients in a pediatric office assesses children's achievement of developmental milestones. Which patient finding requires follow-up with the pediatrician?
   a. 4-month-old infant who is unable to roll over
   b. 6-month-old infant who is unable to hold head up
   c. 11-month-old infant who cannot walk unassisted
   d. 18-month-old toddler who cannot jump
5. A nurse is caring for a patient with lower extremity paralysis. Which action will the nurse take to prevent external rotation of the hip and foot?
   a. Use a trochanter roll.
   b. Apply SCDs.
   c. Obtain a prescription for antiembolism stockings.
   d. Have the patient maintain low-Fowler's position.
   c. Have the patient cross their arms on their chest and place a pillow between their knees.
   d. Place a cervical collar on the patient's neck and gently roll them to the other side of the bed.
6. A nursing student asks the primary nurse why an immobile patient developed two urinary tract infections (UTIs) in the 6 months. How does the nurse best explain this patient's risk for UTI?
   a. Improved renal blood supply to the kidneys
   b. Urinary stasis
   c. Decreased urinary calcium
   d. Acidic urine formation
7. A nurse on a medical-surgical unit notes a patient with pneumonia and is experiencing dyspnea. What action will the nurse take to improve the dyspnea?
   a. Encourage the patient to ambulate.
   b. Suggest the patient use music or television as distraction.
   c. Place the patient in Fowler's position.
   d. Tell the patient to take several deep breaths, then hold their breath for 5 seconds.
8. A nurse is assisting a postoperative patient with conditioning exercises to prepare for ambulation. Which instructions from the nurse are appropriate for this patient? Select all that apply.
   a. Do full-body pushups in bed six to eight times daily.
   b. Breathe in and out smoothly during quadricep-setting exercises.
   c. Place the bed in the lowest position or use a footstool for dangling.
   d. Dangle on the side of the bed for 30 to 60 minutes.
   e. Allow the nurse to bathe you completely to prevent fatigue.
   f. Perform quadriceps two to three times per hour, four to six times a day.
9. A nurse is caring for a patient who is on bedrest following a spinal injury. Which action is appropriate to prevent foot drop?
   a. Maintain the supine position with supination on the feet.
   b. Ask the family to bring in high-top sneakers to maintain foot dorsiflexion.
   c. Encourage hyperextension of the feet with adaptive devices or splints.
   d. Use pillows to keep the feet in the abducted position.
10. A nurse is instructing a patient recovering from a stroke on proper use of a cane. What information will the nurse include in the teaching plan?
    a. Support weight on the stronger leg and cane and advance weaker foot forward.
    b. Hold the cane in the same hand of the leg with the most severe deficit.
    c. Stand with as much weight distributed on the cane as possible.
    d. Avoid using the cane to rise from a sitting position, as this is unsafe.
11. A patient has a fractured left leg, which has been casted. Following teaching from the physical therapist for using crutches, the nurse reinforces which teaching point with the patient?
    a. Lean on the crutches using the axillae to bear body weight.
    b. Keep elbows close to the sides of the body.
    c. When rising, extend the uninjured leg to prevent weight bearing.
    d. To climb stairs, place weight on affected leg first.

12. A nurse working in a long-term care facility uses proper principles of ergonomics when moving and transferring patients to avoid back injury. Which action should be the focus of these preventive measures?
    a. Carefully assessing the patient care environment
    b. Using two nurses to lift a patient who cannot assist
    c. Wearing a back belt to perform routine duties
    d. Properly documenting the patient lift
13. A nurse is assisting a patient who is 2 days postoperative from a cesarean section dangle in preparation for sitting in a chair. After assisting the patient to stand up, the patient's knees buckle and she tells the nurse she feels faint. What is the appropriate nursing action?
    a. Supporting the patient as she stands, waiting a few moments, then continuing the move to the chair
    b. Calling for assistance and continuing the move with the assistance of another nurse
    c. Lowering the patient back to the side of the bed and pivoting her back into bed
    d. Having the patient sit down on the bed and dangle her feet before moving
14. A patient who injured the spine in a motorcycle accident is receiving rehabilitation services in a short-term rehabilitation center. The nurse caring for the patient tells the AP not to place the patient in which position?
    a. Side-lying
    b. Fowler's
    c. Sims'
    d. Prone
15. A nurse is using the Katz Index of Independence in Activities of Daily Living (ADLs) to assess the mobility of a hospitalized patient. During the patient interview, the nurse documents the following patient data: "Patient bathes self completely but needs help with dressing. Patient toilets independently and is continent. Patient needs help moving from bed to chair. Patient follows directions and can feed self." Based on this data, which score would the patient receive on the Katz index?
    a. 2
    b. 4
    c. 5
    d. 6
16. Two nurses are repositioning a patient and pulling the patient up in bed. Which of these steps is most appropriate to prevent injury to the nurses?
    a. Telling the patient to cross their arms and legs
    b. Pulling the patient from underneath the axilla toward the top of the bed
    b. Avoiding using a draw sheet to lift or reposition the patient
    c. Ensuring the bed is at the level of the nurses' hips
    d. Facing the head of the bed and rocking in synchrony
17. A nurse is getting a patient with right hemiparesis out of bed to the chair. What will the nurse say to the patient?
    a. "Stand on the weaker leg and pivot toward the chair."
    b. "I will call the lift team to carry you to the chair."
    c. "The chair is by your non-affected leg for smoother movement."
    d. "Avoid putting your hospital socks on, as that will restrict your feet moving."

ANSWERS WITH RATIONALES

1. **a, d.** Teaching points for exercising for a patient with COPD include avoiding sudden position changes that may cause dizziness and avoiding extreme temperatures. The nurse should also instruct the patient to remain adequately hydrated, respect fatigue as a sign of activity intolerance and not push to the point of exhaustion, and avoid exercise if weak or ill. Older adults should consume a high-protein, high-calcium, and vitamin D–enriched diet.
2. **a, c, f.** When a patient reports fatigue during range-of-motion exercises, the nurse should stop the activity, reevaluate the plan of care, and assess the patient for further symptoms indicating the activity is not tolerated. The exercises can be rescheduled for times of the day when the patient is feeling more rested, or spaced out at different times of the day.
3. **c, f, a, e, d, b.** When a patient is being moved or ambulated and starts to fall, the nurse places their feet wide apart with one foot in front, rocks their pelvis out toward the side of the patient, grasps the gait belt, supports the patient by pulling the patient's weight backward against their body, gently slides the patient down their body toward the floor while protecting the patient's head, and remains with the patient while calling for help.
4. **b.** By 5 months, head control is usually achieved. An infant usually rolls over by 6 to 9 months. By 15 months, most toddlers can walk unassisted. By 2 years, most toddlers can jump.
5. **a.** The trochanter roll is used to support the hips and legs to prevent external rotation. SCDs and antiembolism stockings are used to prevent DVT. Fowler's position allows for foot rotation and increases sacral pressure.
6. **b.** In a nonerect patient, the kidneys and ureters are level, limiting or delaying urinary drainage from the kidney pelvis to ureter and bladder. The resulting urinary stasis favors the growth of bacteria that can promote urinary tract infections. Regular exercise, not immobility, improves blood flow to the kidneys. Immobility predisposes the patient to bone demineralization, resulting in increased urinary calcium levels and alkaline urine, contributing to renal calculi and urinary tract infection, respectively.
7. **c.** High-Fowler's position promotes maximal lung expansion and is the position of choice during episodes of dyspnea. Encouraging ambulation during distress will increase dyspnea. Distracting the patient is not addressing the underlying cause of dyspnea, which is activity. Holding the breath increases demands on the heart.
8. **b, c, f.** Breathing in and out smoothly during quadricep-setting exercises maximizes lung inflation. The patient should perform quadricep-setting exercises two to three times per hour, four to six times a day, or as ordered. The patient should never hold their breath during exercise drills because this places a strain on the heart. Pushups are usually done three or four times a day and involve only the upper body. Dangling for a few minutes is done to adjust to the upright position; dangling for 30 to 60 minutes is impractical for the nurse to supervise and may prove unsafe. The nurse should

place the bed in the lowest position or use a footstool for dangling. The nurse should also encourage the patient to be as independent as possible to prepare for return to normal ambulation and ADLs.

9. **b.** To prevent foot drop, the nurse should support the feet in dorsiflexion using a footboard and/or high-top sneakers for further support. Supination involves lying patients on their back or facing a body part upward, and hyperextension is a state of exaggerated extension. Abduction involves lateral movement of a body part away from the midline of the body. These positions do not prevent foot drop.

10. **a.** The proper procedure for using a cane is to (1) stand with weight distributed evenly between the feet and cane; (2) support weight on the stronger leg and the cane and advance the weaker foot forward, parallel with the cane; (3) support weight on the weaker leg and cane and advance the stronger leg forward ahead of the cane; (4) move the weaker leg forward until even with the stronger leg and advance the cane again as in step 2. The patient should keep the cane within easy reach and use it for support to rise safely from a sitting position.

11. **b.** The patient should keep the elbows at the sides, prevent pressure on the axillae to avoid damage to nerves and circulation, extend the injured leg when rising to prevent weight bearing, and advance the unaffected leg first when climbing stairs.

12. **a.** Preventive measures should focus on careful assessment of the patient care environment so that patients can be moved safely and effectively. Using lifting teams and assistive patient handling equipment rather than two nurses to lift increases safety. The use of a back belt does not prevent back injury. The methods used for safe patient handling and mobility should be documented but are not the primary focus of interventions related to injury prevention.

13. **c.** If a patient becomes faint and their knees buckle when moving from bed to a chair or ambulating, the nurse should stop the activity, as the patient has demonstrated a clear risk for falling. The nurse should lower the patient back to the side of the bed, pivot her back into bed, cover her, and raise the side rails. Assess the patient's vital signs and for the presence of other symptoms. When vital signs are stable, another attempt can be made with the assistance of another staff. Instruct the patient to remain in the sitting position on the side of the bed for several minutes to allow the circulatory system to adjust to a change in position and prevent hypotension related to a sudden change from the supine position.

14. **d.** While placing the patient in the prone position for 30 minutes two or three times daily helps prevent knee and hip flexion contractures, it is contraindicated in patients who have spinal problems. The pull of gravity on the trunk when the patient lies prone produces a marked lordosis or forward curvature of the lumbar spine.

15. **b.** The total score for this patient is 4. On the Katz Index of Independence in ADLs, one point is awarded for independence in each of the following activities: bathing, dressing, toileting, transferring, continence, and feeding.

16. **d.** The nurses should face the direction the patient will move and rock in synchrony prior to moving the patient in that direction. A lifting or repositioning sheet or device is used to decrease friction and facilitate movement. While the patient can cross their arms, they can also be instructed to press their feet into the mattress to assist movement. The bed should be at the level of the nurses' elbows.

17. **c.** When transferring a patient, the chair is placed on the unaffected or stronger side, rather than the weaker or affected side. Lifting and carrying a patient unless absolutely necessary poses an unnecessary risk for injury to patient and staff. Patients should wear proper shoes, sturdy slippers, or hospital-issued socks with grips to prevent sliding and/or falling.

Bibliography

Adamczyk, M. A. (2018). Reducing intensive care unit staff musculoskeletal injuries with implementation of a safe patient handling and mobility program. *Critical Care Nursing Quarterly, 41*(3), 264–271.

Almutary, H., & Tayyib, N. (2020). Factors associated with exercise self-efficacy among people with chronic diseases. *Applied Nursing Research, 54*, 151275. https://doi.org/10.1016/j.apnr.2020.151275

American Academy of Orthopaedic Surgeons (AAOS). (2015, February). *How to use crutches, canes, and walkers.* https://orthoinfo.aaos.org/en/recovery/how-to-use-crutches-canes-and-walkers/

American Association of Critical-Care Nurses (AACN). (2016, October 1). *Practice alert. Preventing venous thromboembolism in adults.* https://www.aacn.org/clinical-resources/practice-alerts/venous-thromboembolism-prevention

American Geriatric Society. Health in Aging Foundation. (2016, November). *Physical activity.* https://www.healthinaging.org/a-z-topic/physical-activity/basic-facts

American Geriatric Society. Health in Aging Foundation. (2019a, June). *Choosing the right cane or walker.* https://www.healthinaging.org/tools-and-tips/choosing-right-cane-or-walker

American Nurses Association (ANA). (2015). *Safe patient handling and mobility. Understanding the benefits of a comprehensive SPHM program.* [Brochure]. https://www.nursingworld.org/~498de8/globalassets/practiceandpolicy/work-environment/health–safety/ana-sphmcover__finalapproved.pdf

American Nurses Association (ANA). (n.d.a). *Handle with care.* Retrieved December 17, 2021, from https://www.nursingworld.org/practice-policy/work-environment/health-safety/handle-with-care/

Andrews, M., Boyle, J. S., & Collins, J. (2020). *Transcultural concepts in nursing care* (8th ed.). Wolters Kluwer.

Anton, P., & Richard, C. (2018). A nurse-led mobility program on an acute rehabilitation unit. *Critical Care Nursing Quarterly, 41*(3), 282–288. https://doi.org/10.1097/CNQ.0000000000000207

Army Public Health Center. (2018, August 2). *Ergonomics. Safe patient handling.* https://phc.amedd.army.mil/topics/workplacehealth/ergo/Pages/Safe-Patient-Handling.aspx

Arnold, M. (2019). Functional assessments for safe patient mobilization across the continuum of care. *International Journal of Safe Patient Handling & Mobility (SPHM), 9*(3), 111–121.

Arnold, M., Needham, D. M., & Nydahl, P. (2018). International round table discussion: Early Mobility. *International Journal of Safe Patient Handling & Mobility (SPHM), 8*(1), 57–64.

Arthritis Foundation. (n.d.a). *Osteoarthritis.* https://www.arthritis.org/diseases/osteoarthritis

Arthritis Foundation. (n.d.b). *What is arthritis.* https://www.arthritis.org/health-wellness/about-arthritis/understanding-arthritis/what-is-arthritis

Bacharach, D. W., Miller, K., & von Duvillard, S. P. (2016). Saving your back: How do horizontal patient transfer devices stack up? *Nursing, 46*(1), 59–64.

Baptiste-McKinney, A., & Halvorson, B. (2018). The use of friction-reducing devices in a safe patient handling & mobility program. *International Journal of Safe Patient Handling & Mobility (SPHM), 8*(3), 132–141.

Baranoski, S., & Ayello, E. A. (2020). *Wound care essentials. Practice principles* (5th ed.). Wolters Kluwer.

Bartnik, L. M., & Rice, M. S. (2013). Comparison of caregiver forces required for sliding a patient up in bed using an array of slide sheets. *Workplace Health & Safety, 61*(9), 393–400.

Borrell, L. N. (2014). The effects of smoking and physical inactivity on advancing mortality in U.S. adults. *Annals of Epidemiology, 24*(6), 484–487.

Boyd, M. A. (2018). *Psychiatric nursing. Contemporary practice* (6th ed.). Wolters Kluwer.

Boynton, T., Kumpar, D., & VanGilder, C. (2020). The bedside mobility assessment tool 2.0. *American Nurse Journal, 15*(7), 18–22.

Burns, S. M., & Delgado, S. A. (2019). *AACN Essentials of critical care nursing* (4th ed.). McGraw-Hill Education.

Campbell, M. R., Fisher, J., Anderson, L., & Kreppel, W. (2015). Implementation of early exercise and progressive mobility: Steps to success. *Critical Care Nurse, 35*(1), 82–88.

Campo, M., Shiyko, M. P., Margulis, H., & Darragh, A. R. (2013). Effect of a safe patient handling program on rehabilitation outcomes. *Archives of Physical Medicine and Rehabilitation, 94*(1), 17–22.

Centers for Disease Control and Prevention (CDC). (2015a, May 15). *Healthy weight. Physical activity for a healthy weight.* https://www.cdc.gov/healthyweight/physical_activity/

Centers for Disease Control and Prevention (CDC). (2020a, May 13). *Arthritis.* https://www.cdc.gov/arthritis/

Clark, M., Phillips, L., & Knibbe, H. J. J. (2015). Lifting and transfer devices: A bridge between safe patient handling and pressure ulcer prevention. *American*

Journal of Safe Patient Handling and Movement, 5(4), 154–160.
Cleveland Clinic. (2019). *How to use crutches*. https://my.clevelandclinic.org/health/articles/15543-how-to-use-crutches
Dammeyer, J., Dickinson, S., Packard, D., & Ricklemann, C. (2013). Building a protocol to guide mobility in the ICU. *Critical Care Nursing Quarterly, 36*(1), 37–49.
Darragh, A. R., Shiyko, M., Margulis, H., Campo, M. (2014). Effects of a safe patient handling and mobility program on patient self-care outcomes. *The American Journal of Occupational Therapy, 68*(5), 589–596.
Davis, K. G., & Kotowski, S. E. (2015). Prevalence of musculoskeletal disorders for nurses in hospitals, long-term care facilities, and home health care: A comprehensive review. *Human Factors, 57*(5), 754–792.
de Castro, A. B. (2004). Handle With Care®: The American Nurses Association's campaign to address work-related musculoskeletal disorders. *Online Journal of Issues in Nursing, 9*(3), 3.
Dickinson, S., Taylor, S., & Anton, P. (2018). Integrating a standardized mobility program and safe patient handling. *Critical Care Nursing Quarterly, 41*(3), 240–252. https://doi.org/10.1097/CNQ.0000000000000202
Dirkes, S. M., & Kozlowski, C. (2019). Early mobility in the intensive care unit: Evidence, barriers, and future directions. *Critical Care Nurse, 39*(3), 33–42. https://doi.org/10.4037/ccn2019654
Drolet, A., DeJuillio, P., Harkless, S., Henricks, S., Kamin, E., Leddy, E. A., Lloyd, J. M., Waters, C., & Williams, S. (2013). Move to improve: The feasibility of using an early mobility protocol to increase ambulation in the intensive and intermediate care settings. *Physical Therapy, 93*(2), 197–207.
Dudek, S. (2022). *Nutrition essentials for nursing practice* (9th ed.). Wolters Kluwer.
Duff, J., Walker, K., Omari, A., & Stratton, C. (2013). Prevention of venous thromboembolism in hospitalized patients: Analysis of reduced cost and improved clinical outcomes. *Journal of Vascular Nursing, 31*(1), 9–14.
Eanes, L. (2018). Too much sitting: A newly recognized health risk. *American Journal of Nursing, 118*(9), 26–34.
Ecklund, M. M., & Bloss, J. W. (2015). Progressive mobility as a team effort in transitional care. *Critical Care Nurse, 35*(3), 62–68.
Eliopoulos, C. (2018). *Gerontological nursing* (9th ed.). Wolters Kluwer.
Elnitsky, C. A., Lind, J. D., Rugs, D., & Powell-Cope, G. (2014). Implications for patient safety in the use of safe patient handling equipment: A national survey. *International Journal of Nursing Studies, 51*(12), 1624–1633.
Enos, L. (2018). The role of ceiling lifts in a safe patient handling and mobility program. *International Journal of Safe Patient Handling and Movement, 8*(1), 25–45.
Enos, L. (2019). A comprehensive review of patient slings. *International Journal of Safe Patient Handling and Movement, 9*(1), 15–36.
Fletcher, G. F., Landolfo, C., Niebauer, J., Ozemek, C., Arena, R., & Lavie, C. J. (2018). Promoting physical activity and exercise. *Journal of the American College of Cardiology, 72*(23), 1622–1639. https://doi.org/10.1016/j.jacc.2018.10.025
Fragala, G., Boynton, T., Conti, M. T., Cyr, L., Enos, L., Kelly, D., McGann, N., Mullen, K., Salsbury, S., & Vollman, K. (2016). Patient-handling injuries: Risk factors and risk-reduction strategies. *American Nurse Today, 11*(5), 40–44.
Francis, R. (2020). What's new in SPHM. ANA's revised safe patient handling and mobility standards are coming soon. *American Nurse Journal, 15*(5), 66–70.
Francis, R., & Dawson, J. M. (2016). Special report: Preventing patient-handling injuries in nurses. *American Nurse Today, 11*(5), 37–38.
Gallagher, A., Dube, J., & Wawzyniecki, P. (2019). International round table discussion: Engaging patients and family in safe patient handling and early mobility decision-making. *International Journal of Safe Patient Handling & Movement (SPHM), 9*(1), 42–46.
Gillespie, T. (2018). Moving the bariatric patient. *Critical Care Nursing Quarterly, 41*(3), 297–301. https://doi.org/10.1097/CNQ.0000000000000209
Graulich, B., Labreche, M., Nydahl, P., & Strøm, T. (2018). Is there a need for lift or mobility teams within the ICU and beyond? *International Journal of Safe Patient Handling & Mobility, 8*(4), 182–186.
Gray-Miceli, D. (2017). Impaired mobility and functional decline in older adults: Evidence to facilitate a practice change. *Nursing Clinics of North America, 52*(3), 469–487. https://doi.org/10.1016/j.cnur.2017.05.002.
Harwood, K. J. (2015). Blazing a new trail: Advocacy for safe patient handling and mobility. *American Journal of Safe Patient Handling and Movement, 5*(1), 21–26.
Henecke, L., Hessler, K. L., & LaLonde, T. (2015). Inpatient ambulation. Use of an ambulation platform apparatus. *The Journal of Nursing Administration, 45*(6), 339–344.
Hess, D. R., MacIntyre, N. R., Galvin, W. F., & Mishoe, S. C. (2021). *Respiratory care. Principles and practice* (4th ed.). Jones & Bartlett Learning.
Hinkle, J. L., & Cheever, K. H., & Overbaugh, K. J. (2022). *runner & Suddarth's Textbook of medical-surgical nursing* (15th ed.). Wolters Kluwer.
Hodgson, M. J., Matz, M. W., & Nelson, A. (2013). Patient handling in the Veterans Health Administration: Facilitating change in the health care industry. *Journal of Occupational & Environmental Medicine, 55*(10), 1230–1237.
Hoogerduijn, J. G., Grobbee, D. E., & Schuurmans, M. J. (2014). Prevention of functional decline in older hospitalized patients: Nurses should play a key role in safe and adequate care. *International Journal of Nursing Practice, 20*(1), 106–113.
Huffman, G. M., Crumrine, J., Thompson, B., Mobley, V., Roth, K., & Roberts, C. (2014). On SHiPs and safety: A journey of safe patient handling in pediatrics. *Journal of Pediatric Nursing, 29*(6), 641–650.
Hurtado, D. A., Heinonen, G. A., Dumet, L. M., & Greenspan, S. A. (2018). Early career nurses with fewer patient handling supportive peers are likely to quit. *International Nursing Review, 65*(4), 596–600.
Jarvis, C., & Echkardt, A. (2020). *Physical examination & health assessment* (8th ed.). Elsevier.
Jensen, S. (2019). *Nursing health assessment. A best practice approach* (3rd ed.). Wolters Kluwer.
Johns Hopkins Medicine. (n.d.). *Risks of physical inactivity*. Retrieved August 31, 2020, from https://www.hopkinsmedicine.org/health/conditions-and-diseases/risks-of-physical-inactivity
Jootun, D., & Pryde, A. (2013). Moving and handling of patients with dementia. *Journal of Nursing Education and Practice, 3*(2), 126–131.
Kayser, S. A., Wiggermann, N. E., & Kumpar, D. (2020). Factors associated with safe patient handling practice in acute care and its relationship with patient mobilization: A cross-sectional study. *International Journal of Nursing Studies, 104*, 103508. https://doi.org/10.1016/j.ijnurstu.2019.103508
King, B., Bodden, J., Steege, L., & Brown, C. J. (2021). Older adults experiences with ambulation during a hospital stay: A qualitative study. *Geriatric Nursing, 42*(1), 225–232.. https://doi.org/10.1016/j.gerinurse.2020.08.005
Kotowski, S., & Davis, K. (2019). Factors impacting the patient migration in hospital beds: Pathway to reduce patient handling injuries. *International Journal of Safe Patient Handling & Mobility, 9*(3), 102–110.
Kresevic, D. M. (2015). Reducing functional decline in hospitalized older adults. *American Nurse Today, 10*(5), 8–10.
Kyle, T., & Carman, S. (2021). *Essentials of pediatric nursing* (4th ed.). Wolters Kluwer.
Larson, R. E., Murtagh, E. M., & Rice, M. S. (2018). Forces involved when sliding a patient up in bed. *Work, 59*(3), 439–448. https://doi.org/10.3233/WOR-182688
Latha, S., Wilson, K., Davis, K., & Kotowski, S. (2019. Reality of safe patient handling policies and programs across the United States. *International Journal of Safe Patient Handling & Mobility, 9*(2), 69–76.
Lee, S. J., Lee, J. H., & Gershon, R. R. M. (2015). Musculoskeletal symptoms in nurses in the early implementation phase of California's Safe Patient Handling legislation. *Research in Nursing & Health, 38*(3), 183–193.
Lee, S., & Im, E. (2010). Ethnic differences in exercise and leisure time physical activity among midlife women. *Journal of Advanced Nursing, 66*(4), 814–827.
Link, T. (2018). Guideline implementation: Safe patient handling and movement. *AORN Journal, 108*(6), 664–671. http://doi.org/10.1002/aorn.12423
Liu, B., Moore, J. E., Almaawiy, U., Chan, W. H., Khan, S., Ewusie, J., Hamid, J. S., & Straus, S. E. (2018). Outcomes of Mobilisation of Vulnerable Alders in Ontario (MOVE ON): A multisite interrupted time series evaluation of an implementation intervention to increase patient mobilisation. *Age and Ageing, 47*(1), 112–119. http://doi.org/10.1093/ageing/afx128
Lustig, M., Wiggermann, N., & Gefen, A. (2020). How patient migration in bed affects the sacral soft tissue loading and thereby the risk for a hospital-acquired pressure injury. *International Wound Journal, 17*(3), 631–640. http://doi.org/10.1111/iwj.13316
Mayeda-Letourneau, J. (2014). Safe patient handling and movement: A literature review. *Rehabilitation Nursing, 39*(3), 123–129.
Mayo Foundation for Medical Education and Research (MFMER). (2019a, May 22). *Back pain at work: Preventing pain and injury*. https://www.mayoclinic.org/healthy-lifestyle/adult-health/in-depth/back-pain/art-20044526
Mayo Foundation for Medical Education and Research (MFMER). (2019b, January 16). *Exercise: When to check with your doctor first*. https://www.mayoclinic.org/healthy-lifestyle/fitness/in-depth/exercise/art-20047414
Mayo Foundation for Medical Education and Resarech (MFMER). (2019c). *Exercise: 7 benefits of regular physical activity*. https://www.mayoclinic.org/healthy-lifestyle/fitness/in-depth/exercise/art-20048389
Mayo Foundation for Medical Education and Resarech (MFMER). (2019d, August 21). *Healthy lifestyle. Walker tips*. https://www.mayoclinic.org/healthy-lifestyle/healthy-aging/multimedia/walker/sls-20076469
Mayo Foundation for Medical Education and Resarech (MFMER). (2019e, August 21). *Healthy lifestyle. Cane tips*. https://www.mayoclinic.org/healthy-lifestyle/healthy-aging/multimedia/canes/sls-20077060
McMahon, A., Plambech, L., & Rush, A. (2019). International round table discussion: Are bariatric patients the new normal? *International Journal of Safe Patient Handling & Mobility (SPHM), 9*(2), 90–94.
McNichol, L. L., Ratliff, C, & Yates, S (Eds.). (2021). *Wound, Ostomy and Continence Nurses Society Core Curriculum: Wound management* (2nd ed.). Wolters Kluwer.
Mechan, P. (2014). Challenging the myth that it takes too long to use safe patient handling and mobility technology: A task time investigation. *American Journal of Safe Patient Handling and Movement, 4*(2), 46–51.
Mincer, A. (2007). Assistive devices for the adult patient with orthopaedic dysfunction. Why physical therapists choose what they do. *Orthopaedic Nursing, 26*(4), 226–233.
Monaghan, H. M. (2018). The role of mobile floor-based lifts in a safe patient handling and mobility program. *International Journal of Safe Patient Handling & Mobility (SPHM), 8*(2), 91–99.
Monaghan, H. M. (2019). Making safe patient handling and mobility training effective. Part 1. What to teach, where and when to teach it and how to teach it. *International Journal of Safe Patient Handling & Mobility, 9*(4), 143–148.
Monaghan, H. M. (2020a). Making safe patient handling and mobility training effective. Part 2. Assessing the competent practice. *International Journal of Safe Patient Handling & Mobility, 10*(1), 37–41.
Monaghan, H. M. (2020b). The challenge of change: Why are staff resistant to using safe patient handling equipment? *International Journal of Safe Patient Handling & Mobility, 10*(1), 7–12.
Morton, P. G., & Fontaine, D. K. (2018). *Critical care nursing. A holistic approach* (11th ed.). Wolters Kluwer.
Muir, M., & Archer-Heese, G. (2009). Essentials of a bariatric patient handling program. *The Online Journal of Issues in Nursing, 14*(1), Manuscript 5. http://doi.org/10.3912/OJIN.Vol14No1Man05
Muñoz-Figueroa, G. P., & Ojo, O. (2015). Venous thromboembolism: Use of graduated compression stockings. *British Journal of Nursing, 24*(13), 680–685.

Nack, B., Combs, J., & Herron-Foster, B. J. (2019). An interdisciplinary approach: Answering the how, when, and where of early mobility technology. *International Journal of Safe Patient Handling & Mobility (SPHM), 9*(2), 57–67.

National Institute for Occupational Safety and Health (NIOSH). (2013, August 2). *Safe patient handling and movement (SPHM)*. Centers for Disease Control and Prevention. https://www.cdc.gov/niosh/topics/safepatient/default.html

National Institutue for Health and Care Excellence (NICE) (UK). (2019). *Venous thromboembolism in over 16s: Reducing the risk of hospital-acquired deep vein thrombosis or pulmonary embolism. NICE Guideline*. https://www.nice.org.uk/guidance/ng89

National Osteoporosis Foundation. (n.d.). *What is osteoporosis and what causes it?* Retrieved August 10, 2020, from https://www.nof.org/patients/what-is-osteoporosis/

Nelson, A., Motacki, K., & Menzel, N. (2009). *The illustrated guide to safe patient handling and movement*. Springer Publishing Company. http://www.mtpinnacle.com/pdfs/Guide-to-Safe-Patient-Handling.pdf

Nelson, K. (2015). Safe patient handling and health care reform: An opportunity to link patient and worker safety. *American Journal of Safe Patient Handling & Movement, 5*(1), 9–12.

Noble, N. L., & Sweeney, N. L. (2018). Barriers to the use of assistive devices in patient handling. *Workplace Health & Safety, 66*(1), 41–48. http://doi.org/10.1177/2165079917697216

Nolen, J., Liu, H., Liu, H., McGee, M., & Grando, V. (2010). Comparison of gait characteristics with a single-tip cane, tripod cane, and quad cane. *Physical & Occupational Therapy in Geriatrics, 28*(4), 387–395.

Norris, T. L. (2019). *Porth's essentials of pathophysiology* (5th ed.). Wolters Kluwer.

Occupational Safety & Health Administration (OSHA) and Joint Commission Resource Alliance. (2017, August). *OSHA & worker safety. Handling with care. Practicing safe patient handling*. Environment of Care News. https://www.jcrinc.com/-/media/jcr/jcr-documents/about-jcr/osha-alliance/pages_from_ecn_20_2017_08-2.pdf?db=web&hash=E471E08D9AC494C0D2C740FD4103DACD

Occupational Safety & Health Administration (OSHA). U.S. Department of Labor. (2009). *Guidelines for Nursing Homes. Ergonomics for the prevention of musculoskeletal disorders*. https://www.osha.gov/sites/default/files/publications/final_nh_guidelines.pdf

Occupational Safety & Health Administration (OSHA). U.S. Department of Labor. (n.d.a). *Healthcare. Safe patient handling*. Retrieved August 10, 2020, from https://www.osha.gov/SLTC/healthcarefacilities/safepatienthandling.html

Occupational Safety & Health Administration (OSHA). U.S. Department of Labor. (n.d.b). *Safety and health topics. Ergonomics*. Retrieved April 29, 2022, https://www.osha.gov/ergonomics/control-hazards

Occupational Safety & Health Administration (OSHA). U.S. Department of Labor. (n.d.c). *Safe patient handling equipment*. Retrieved August 10, 2020, from https://www.osha.gov/dsg/hospitals/patient_handling_equipment.html

Owens, T., & Taplye, C. (2018). Pediatric mobility. The development of standard assessments and interventions for pediatric patients for safe patient handling and mobility. *Critical Care Nursing Quarterly, 41*(3), 314–322. http://doi.org/10.1097/CNQ.0000000000000210

Parchem, K., Peck, A., & Tales, K. (2018). A multidisciplinary approach to equipment use in pediatric patient mobilization. *Critical Care Nursing Quarterly, 41*(3), 330–339. http://doi.org/10.1097/CNQ.0000000000000211

Perry, S. E., Hockenberry, M. J., Lowdermilk, D. L., & Wilson, D. (2014). *Maternal child nursing care* (5th ed.). Elsevier Mosby.

Peterson, M. J., Kahn, J. A., Kerrigan, M. V., Gutmann, J. M., & Harrow, J. J. (2015). Pressure ulcer risk of patient handling sling use. *Journal of Rehabilitation Research & Development, 52*(3), 291–300.

Physiopedia. (n.d.). *Social determinants of physical activity*. https://www.physio-pedia.com/Social_Determinants_of_Physical_Inactivity

Purnell, L. D. (2013). *Transcultural health care. A culturally competent approach* (4th ed.). F. A. Davis Company.

Riebe, D., Franklin, B. A., Thompson, P. D., Ewing Garber, C., Whitfield, G. P., Magal, M., & Pescatello, L. S. (2015). Updating ACSMs recommendations for exercise preparticipation health screening. *Medicine & Science in Sports & Exercise, 47*(8), 2473–2479. http://doi.org/10.1249/MSS.0000000000000664

Ross, A., Touchton-Leonard, K., Perez, A., Wehrlen, L., Kazmi, N., & Gibbons, S. (2019). Factors that influence health-promoting self-care in registered nurses. *Advances in Nursing Science, 42*(4), 358–373. http://doi.org/10.1097/ANS.0000000000000274

Sachdeva, A., Dalton, M., & Lees, T. (2018). Graduated compression stockings for prevention of deep vein thrombosis. *Cochrane Database of Systematic Reviews, 11*(11), CD0011484. http://doi.org/10.1002/14651858.CD001484.pub4

Sadowski, C., & Jones, A. (2014). Ambulatory assistive devices. How to appropriately measure and use canes, crutches and walkers. *Pharmacy Practice, 1*(10), 24–31.

Schweickert, W. D., Pohlman, M. C., Pohlman, A. S., Nigos, C., Pawlik, A. J., Esbrook, C. L., Spears, L., Miller, M., Franczyk, M., Deprizio, D., Schmidt, G. A., Bowman, A., Barr, R., McCallister, K. E., Hall, J. B., & Kress, J. P. (2009). Early physical and occupational therapy in mechanically ventilated, critically ill patients: A randomized controlled trial. *Lancet, 373*(9678), 1874–1882.

Silbert-Flagg, J., & Pillitteri, A. (2018). *Maternal and child health nursing* (8th ed.). Wolters Kluwer.

Smith, S. R., Gibbs, R. L., Rosen, B. S., & Lee, J. T. (2015). The critical lift zone: Recognizing the need for safe patient handling equipment across the broader spectrum of patient weights. *American Journal of Safe Patient Handling and Movement, 5*(3), 108–116.

Spruce, L. (2020). Safe patient handling and movement. *AORN Journal, 112*(1), 63–71. http://doi.org/10.1002/aorn.13094

Stevens, L., Rees, S., Lamb, K., & Dalsing, D. (2013). Creating a culture of safety for safe patient handling. *Orthopaedic Nursing, 32*(3), 155–164.

Sturman-Floyd, M. (2013a). Moving and handling: Assessment of the resident. *Nursing & Residential Care, 15*(3), 150–156.

Sturman-Floyd, M. (2013b). Moving and handling: Supporting bariatric residents. *Nursing & Residential Care, 15*(6), 432–437.

Sturman-Floyd, M. (2013c). Moving and handling: support for residents with dementia. *Nursing & Residential Care, 15*(5), 276–280.

Swenson, S. L. (2020, May 6). 7 tips nurses should know about safe patient handling. *American Nurse, 15*(5). https://www.myamericannurse.com/7-tips-nurses-should-know-about-safe-patient-handling/

Tasheva, P., Vollenweider, P., Kraege, V., Roulet, G., Lamy, O., Marques-Vidal, P., & Méan, M. (2020). Association between physical activity levels in the hospital setting and hospital-acquired functional decline in elderly patients. *JAMA Network Open, 3*(1), e1920185. http://doi.org/10.1001/jamanetworkopen.2019.20185

Thompson, P. D., Arena, R. Riebe, D., & Pescatello, L. S.; American College of Sports Medicine (2013). ACSM's new preparticipation health screening recommendations from ACSM's Guidelines for Exercise Testing and Prescription. *Current Sports Medicine Reports, 12*(4), 215–217.

Timmerman, R. (2007). A mobility protocol for critically ill adults. *Dimensions of Critical Care Nursing, 26*(5), 175–179.

Toughy, T. A., & Jett, K. (2018). *Ebersol and Hess' gerontological nursing & healthy aging* (5th ed.). Elsevier.

U. S. Department of Veteran Affairs. (2016). *Public health. Safe patient handling and mobility (SPHM)*. https://www.publichealth.va.gov/employeehealth/patient-handling/index.asp

U.S. Department of Health and Human Services (USDHHS). Office of Disease Prevention and Health Promotion. (n.d.). *Healthy People 2030. Physical activity*. Retrieved December 17, 2021, from https://health.gov/healthypeople/objectives-and-data/browse-objectives/physical-activity

U.S. Department of Health and Human Services (USDHHS). Office of Disease Prevention and Health Promotion. (2018). *Physical activity guidelines for Americans* (2nd ed.). https://health.gov/sites/default/files/2019-09/Physical_Activity_Guidelines_2nd_edition.pdf

VA Mobile Health. (n.d.). *Safe patient handling*. (Version 1.3.3). [Mobile app]. U. S. Department of Veteran Affairs. https://mobile.va.gov/app/safe-patient-handling

VHA Center for Engineering & Occupational Safety and Health (CEOSH). (2016). *Safe patient handling and mobility guidebook*. http://www.tnpatientsafety.com/pubfiles/Initiatives/workplace-violence/sphm-pdf.pdf

VHA Center for Engineering & Occupational Safety and Health (CEOSH). (2015). *Bariatric safe patient handling and mobility guidebook: A resource guide for care of persons of size*. https://www.asphp.org/wp-content/uploads/2011/05/Baraiatrice-SPHM-guidebook-care-of-Person-of-Size.pdf

Waters, T. R., Nelson, A., Hughes, N., & Menzel, N. (2009). *Safe patient handling training for schools of nursing. Curricular materials*. http://www.cdc.gov/niosh/docs/2009-127/pdfs/2009-127.pdf

Weber, J. R., & Kelley, J. H. (2018). *Health assessment in nursing* (6th ed.). Wolters Kluwer.

Weiner, C., Alperovitch-Najenson, D., Ribak, J., & Kalichman, L. (2015). Prevention of nurses' work-related musculoskeletal disorders resulting from repositioning patients in bed. Comprehensive narrative review. *Workplace Health & Safety, 63*(5), 226–232.

Williams, J. W. Jr. (2016). Effectiveness of intermittent pneumatic compression devices for venous thromboembolism prophylaxis in high-risk surgical patients: A systematic review. *Journal of Arthroplasty, 31*(2), 524–532.

Wilson, K., Devito, D., Evanovich Zavotsky, K., Rusay, M., Allen, M., & Huang, S. (2018). Keep it moving and remember to P.A.C. (pharmacology, ambulation, and compression) for venous thromboembolism prevention. *Orthopaedic Nursing, 37*(6), 339–345. http://doi.org/10.1097/NOR.0000000000000497

Wintersgill, W. (2019). Gait belts 101: A tool for patient and nurse safety. *American Nurse Today, 14*(5), 31–34.

Wyatt, S., Meacci, K., & Arnold, M. (2020). Integrating safe patient handling and early mobility. *Journal of Nursing Care Quality, 35*(2), 130–134. http://doi.org/10.1097/NCQ.0000000000000425

Yeung, Y. L. (2015). Increase access to healthcare services with safe patient handling and mobility equipment. *American Journal of Safe Patient Handling and Movement, 5*(4), 140–147.

Yoder, A., Coley, K., Harrison, D., & Wright, K. (2014). Outcomes of a safe patient handling program implementation. *American Journal of Safe Patient Handling and Movement, 4*(4), 111–117.

Yoo, H. W., Kim, M. G., Oh, D. N., Hwang, J. H., & Lee, K. S. (2020). Factors associated with functional decline in older adults after discharge from an acute-care hospital. *Asian Nursing Research, 13*(3), 192–199. https://doi.org/10.1016/j.anr.2019.05.001

Zisberg, A., Shadmi, E., Gur-Yaish, N., Tonkikh, O., & Sinoff, G. (2015). Hospital-associated functional decline: The role of hospitalization processes beyond individual risk factors. *Journal of the American Geriatrics Society, 63*, 55–62.

35 Rest and Sleep

Jeanette and Abby Clark

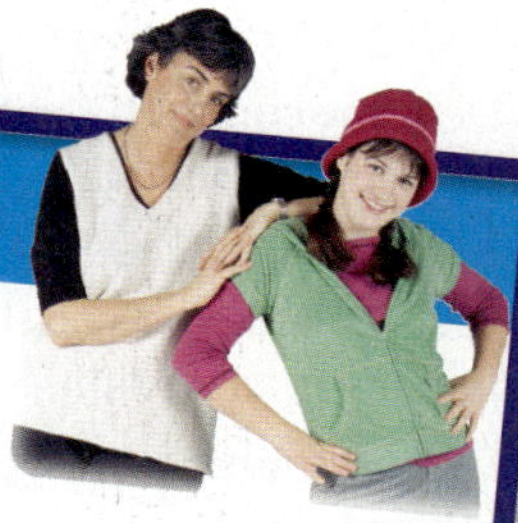

Jeanette accompanies her 15-year-old daughter, Abby, to the clinic. While the daughter is having some routine laboratory testing done in another department, Mrs. Clark says, "She always seems to be tired. When she was small, I could never get her to sleep. Now all she wants to do is sleep. It's all I can do to get her up for school each morning."

Charlie Bitner

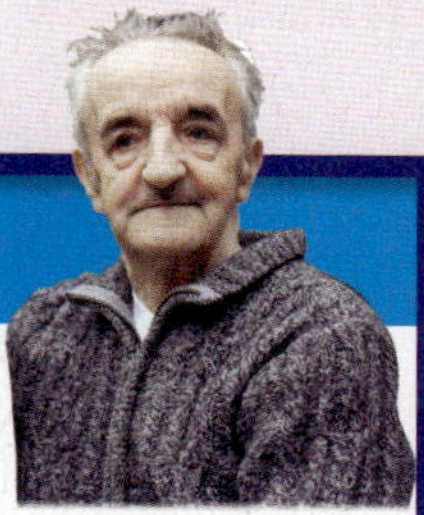

Charlie is an 86-year-old man who has recently been admitted to a long-term care facility. He tells his daughter that "even though I go to bed around 9 pm, I don't fall asleep until after midnight and then I'm up twice to go to the bathroom and have a lot of trouble falling back to sleep." His daughter has mentioned to the nurse that her father spends a lot of time napping during the day.

Omeara Family

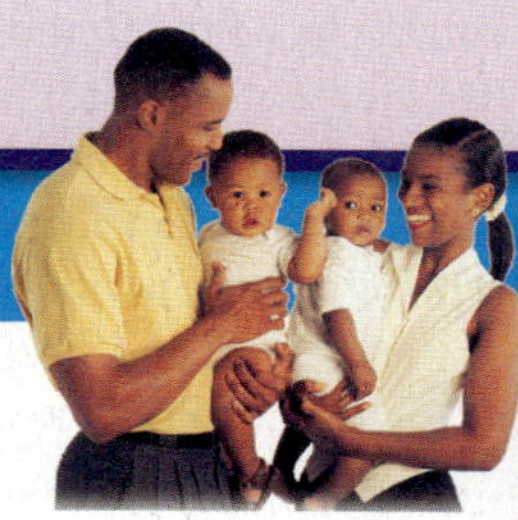

Lydia Omeara, age 30, asks the nurse at the well-baby clinic whether she should let her infant twins sleep in bed with her and her husband. "They have their own beds, of course, but at night, when they get up, they like to be in bed with us. Plus, I still breastfeed my babies, so having them nearby would really make it easier for me."

Learning Outcomes

After completing the chapter, you will be able to accomplish the following:

1. Describe the functions of rest and sleep.
2. Describe the physiology of sleep.
3. Identify variables that influence rest and sleep.
4. Describe nursing implications related to age-related differences in the sleep cycle.
5. Perform a comprehensive sleep assessment.
6. Describe common sleep disorders and associated assessment criteria.
7. Diagnose actual and potential health problems and needs related to sleep that may be addressed through nursing intervention.
8. Describe nursing strategies and interventions to promote rest and sleep.
9. Plan, implement, and evaluate nursing care related to alterations in rest and sleep.

Nursing Concepts

- Assessment
- Clinical decision making/clinical judgment
- Health promotion

Rest and sleep are vital for life and health—a person's body needs both sleep and rest, and rest is a vital component of restorative sleep (Helvig et al., 2016; National Sleep Foundation [NSF], n.d.a). However, various factors may affect a person's ability to obtain adequate sleep and/or find time for essential periods of rest. Deficiencies in rest and/or sleep can have a negative impact on a person's mental, physiologic, and emotional health (Helvig et al., 2016; Medic et al., 2017; NIH, 2019). Rest and sleep are often used synonymously; however, a person can sleep and not feel rested and can rest without sleeping (Helvig et al., 2016).

This chapter provides the nurse with knowledge of the functions of rest and sleep, as well as the physiology of sleep and factors affecting rest and sleep. Suggestions for performing a sleep assessment are included. Sample interview questions for a general sleep history are presented, along with information on sleep diaries and pertinent physical assessment data. The importance of analyzing these data is explained, and examples of potential health problems and needs related to rest and sleep are provided. Expected patient outcomes and specific nursing strategies for promoting rest and sleep are described. The concluding nursing care plan illustrates how the nurse's knowledge of rest and sleep, combined with skilled nursing interventions and caring, can resolve rest and sleep problems.

REST AND SLEEP

Rest is a basic need in health and illness (Helvig et al., 2016). **Rest** is a concept that is used in many disciplines; in this chapter, rest refers to a condition in which the body is in a decreased state of activity, with the consequent feeling of being refreshed.

Many factors affect a person's ability to rest. Adults juggling the demands of their job and family responsibilities often find little opportunity for rest and relaxation during the course of a day. Children involved in numerous extracurricular activities, as well as trying to excel academically, also do not have the opportunity to rest and relax during the day. Even when rest is possible, one's environment is not always conducive to physical and mental relaxation. Suggestions for preparing a restful environment and promoting relaxation are discussed later in the chapter.

Sleep is a state of rest accompanied by altered consciousness and relative inactivity. Sleep is part of what is called the sleep–wake cycle. Wakefulness is a time of mental activity and energy expenditure (Norris, 2019). Sleep is a period of inactivity and restoration of mental and physical function (Norris, 2019). It is a complex rhythmic state involving a progression of repeated cycles, each representing different phases of body and brain activity, and is crucial for physical, mental, and emotional well-being (Buysse, 2014). Although sensitivity to external stimuli is diminished during sleep as a result of diminished consciousness, this sensitivity can be reversed, as a person can be aroused by sensory or other stimuli (Norris, 2019).

The term *sleep health* has been proposed to express sleep as a positive, measurable attribute (Buysse, 2014, p. 12). Sleep health refers to a multidimensional pattern of multiple sleep characteristics, including sleep duration, continuity, timing, alertness, and satisfaction, that promotes physical and mental well-being (Hale et al., 2020).

Many people can fall asleep easily and remain asleep until the desired waking time. Conversely, others rarely fall asleep without a struggle; then when they do, sleep is fragmented. Insufficient sleep can seriously affect a person's physical and psychological health (see Physical and Psychological Effects of Insufficient Sleep). Consequently, nurses need to be vigilant in promoting good sleep health and detecting and addressing sleep disturbances. See the accompanying Reflective Practice display.

PHYSIOLOGY OF SLEEP

Two systems in the brainstem, the reticular activating system (RAS) and the bulbar synchronizing region, are believed to work together to control the cyclic nature of sleep. The RAS extends upward through the medulla, the pons, the midbrain, and into the hypothalamus; the bulbar synchronizing region is also located in the pons and medulla. It facilitates reflex and voluntary movements as well as cortical activities related to a state of alertness. The RAS comprises many nerve cells and fibers. The fibers have connections that relay impulses into the cerebral cortex and spinal cord.

QSEN Reflective Practice: Cultivating QSEN Competencies

CHALLENGE TO ETHICAL AND LEGAL SKILLS

I was working in our well-baby clinic today when a mother, Lydia Omeara, asked my advice about letting her infant twins sleep in bed with her and her husband: "They have their own beds, of course, but at night, when they get up, they seem to like to be in bed with us. Plus, I still breastfeed my babies, so having them nearby would really make it easier for me." She mentioned reading an article recently about this, noting that while this custom is usual in other countries, it had been discouraged until recently in the United States. According to the article, she said that it seems that more and more U.S. parents are doing this now. She asked for my advice, and I had no idea how to respond. Clearly, anything that resulted in better rest for the parents—who are up many times each night if the babies aren't sleeping well—would seem to be a good idea. However, I vaguely remembered learning that small children are at increased risk for sudden infant death syndrome (SIDS) in an adult bed. I needed to find the best way to respond to Mrs. Omeara.

Thinking Outside the Box: Possible Courses of Action

- Make up an answer: "Yes, it's OK" or "No way! What are you, crazy?"
- Refer her to a nurse with more experience.
- Tell her that I honestly don't know the answer, but I will find out more about this and then get back to her.

Evaluating a Good Outcome: How Do I Define Success?

- A decision is made about where the children sleep that protects them and promotes rest, health, and well-being for each member of the family.
- I learn more about the evidence for best practice to inform the best recommendation.
- I am faithful to my professional obligations to be knowledgeable about matters like this.

Personal Learning: Here's to the Future!

Since I don't have children myself and couldn't ever remember spending the night in my parents' bed or having a conversation with them about this, I certainly couldn't draw on personal experience in responding to this mother. In addition, we had never studied anything about this topic. I did remember a recent article in *Newsweek* magazine raising the issue, but I didn't remember this article proposing a scientifically-based recommendation. As a result, I did some research on this issue and learned that there are definitive recommendations for a safe infant sleeping environment from the American Academy of Pediatrics; these guidelines indicate that infants should sleep in the parent's room, close to the bed, but on a separate surface designed for infants, not in the parent's bed. I did my best to summarize the guideline and then I shared the guidelines with Mrs. Omeara so that she and her husband could make an informed decision.

This little experience has taught me a lot about the power of my profession to influence—literally—how people are born, live, and die. I want to have enough knowledge to help people make the best possible life choices, never leading them astray by virtue of my ignorance!

Amy Norris, Georgetown University

QSEN SELF-REFLECTION ON QUALITY AND SAFETY COMPETENCIES DEVELOPING KNOWLEDGE, SKILLS, AND ATTITUDES FOR CONTINUOUS IMPROVEMENT

How do you think you would respond in a similar situation? Why? What does this tell you about yourself and about the adequacy of your skills for professional practice? Do you agree with the criteria that the nursing student used to evaluate a successful outcome? Why or why not? What *knowledge, skills,* and *attitudes* do you need to develop to continuously improve quality and safety when caring for patients and their family like Lydia Omeara?

Patient-Centered Care: What information would be necessary for the nursing student to obtain from the patient to provide an overall picture of the family situation? How can you provide clear, reliable, and unbiased information to Ms. Omeara in a timely manner? What is the best way to communicate emotional support to Ms. Omeara as she struggles with making the right decision for her and her family?

Teamwork and Collaboration/Quality Improvement: What communication skills do you need to continue to function as a resource and advocate for your patient? Could collaboration with other nurses in the well-baby clinic result in a sleep history tool that you could use to assess Ms. Omeara's sleep needs and pattern?

Safety/Evidence-Based Practice: Can you identify any additional evidence in nursing literature that provides information related to the risk of SIDS when infants share a bed with their parents or other behaviors that increase risk? How do you think your response contributed to a safe environment for Ms. Omeara and her twins?

Informatics: What information should be electronically documented regarding your assessment of Ms. Omeara's sleep needs? Can you identify essential information that was provided in order for Ms. Omeara and her husband to make an informed decision?

During sleep, the RAS experiences few stimuli from the cerebral cortex and the periphery of the body. Wakefulness occurs when this system is activated with stimuli from the cerebral cortex and from periphery sensory organs and cells. For example, an alarm clock awakens us from sleep to a state of consciousness, in which we realize that we must prepare for the day. Sensations such as pain, pressure, and noise produce wakefulness by means of peripheral organs and cells.

The hypothalamus has control centers for several involuntary activities of the body, one of which concerns sleeping and waking. Injury to the hypothalamus may cause a person to sleep for abnormally long periods.

Various neurotransmitters are involved with the sleeping process. Norepinephrine and acetylcholine—in addition to dopamine, serotonin, and histamine—are involved with excitation. Gamma-aminobutyric acid (GABA) appears to be necessary for inhibition. However, research has yet to prove exactly how many of the biochemical changes and hormones function in sleep. **Melatonin**, a hormone, is thought to regulate the sleep–wake cycle and possibly circadian rhythms (see following discussion of circadian rhythms) (NSF, 2020a). It is also known that sleep and wake states are also characterized by distinct hormonal patterns that exert potential significant influences on metabolism and glucose homeostasis (Norris, 2019).

Circadian Rhythms

Rhythmic biologic clocks are known to exist in plants, animals, and humans. Influenced by both internal and external factors, they regulate certain biologic and behavioral functions in humans. Some cycles are monthly, such as a person's menstrual cycle. **Circadian rhythms** are predictable fluctuations in processes that occur in repeated cycles of time, completing a full cycle every 24 hours (Norris, 2019). Fluctuations in a person's heart rate, blood pressure, body temperature, hormone secretions, metabolism, and performance and mood display circadian rhythms.

Sleep is one of the body's most complex biologic rhythms. Circadian synchronization exists when a person's sleep–wake patterns follow the inner biologic clock located in the hypothalamus. When physiologic and psychological rhythms are high or most active, the person is awake; when these rhythms are low, the person is asleep. Light and dark are powerful regulators of the sleep–wake circadian rhythm; when there is interference with the normal cycle, circadian disruption (chrono disruption) occurs. For example, nurses who work the night shift may routinely sleep from 2 PM to 8 PM, and peak physiologic activity may occur between 2200 and 0600 during work. Problems of desynchronization occur when sleep–wake patterns are frequently altered, and the person attempts to sleep during high-activity rhythms or to work when the body is physiologically prepared to rest. A person's individual biologic clock also responds to numerous influences such as occupational demands and social pressures.

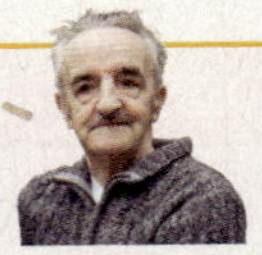

Think back to **Charlie Bitner**, the older man living in a long-term care facility. The nurse would need to assess Mr. Bitner, gathering data about his circadian rhythm. This knowledge would be important in developing an individualized plan of care for the patient to promote adequate sleep.

Stages of Sleep

Research reveals that there are two major stages of sleep: non–rapid eye movement (NREM) sleep and rapid eye movement (REM) sleep. These stages have been studied and analyzed with the help of the electroencephalograph (EEG), which receives and records electrical currents from the brain; the electrooculogram (EOG), which records eye movements; and the electromyograph (EMG), which records muscle tone. This combination of diagnostic recordings is referred to as a sleep study or polysomnogram. It is a noninvasive, pain-free study usually conducted over one or two nights in a sleep study facility. Once a health care provider interprets the results, treatments may be recommended for any conditions detected (NSF, 2020c).

Non–Rapid Eye Movement Sleep

Non–rapid eye movement (NREM) sleep, which comprises about 75% to 80% of total sleep time, consists of four stages. Stages I and II, consuming about 5% and 50% of a person's sleep time, respectively, are light-sleep states. During these stages, the person can be aroused with relative ease. Stages III and IV, each representing about 10% of total sleep time, are deep-sleep states, termed delta sleep or slow-wave sleep. The arousal threshold (intensity of stimulus required to awaken) is usually greatest in stage IV NREM. Throughout the stages of NREM sleep, the parasympathetic nervous system dominates, and decreases in pulse, respiratory rate, blood pressure, metabolic rate, and body temperature are observed. Characteristics of the four stages of NREM sleep are summarized in Box 35-1.

Rapid Eye Movement Sleep

It is more difficult to arouse a person during **rapid eye movement (REM) sleep** than during NREM sleep. In normal adults, the REM state consumes 20% to 25% of a person's nightly sleep time. People who are awakened during the REM state almost always report that they have been dreaming. They can usually vividly recall their dreams even if they were absurd or have no sensible meaning for them. Everyone dreams.

During REM sleep, the pulse, respiratory rate, blood pressure, metabolic rate, and body temperature increase, whereas general skeletal muscle tone and deep tendon reflexes are depressed. REM sleep is believed to be essential to mental and emotional equilibrium and to play a role in learning, memory, and adaptation.

A person who is deprived of REM sleep for several nights generally will spend more time in REM sleep on successive nights. This phenomenon, termed REM rebound, allows the total amount of REM sleep to remain fairly constant over time. See Box 35-1 for characteristics of REM sleep.

Box 35-1 Characteristics of NREM and REM Sleep

NREM Sleep

Stage I

- The person is in a transitional stage between wakefulness and sleep.
- The person is in a relaxed state but still somewhat aware of the surroundings.
- Involuntary muscle jerking may occur and waken the person.
- The stage normally lasts only minutes.
- The person can be aroused easily.
- This stage constitutes only about 5% of total sleep.

Stage II

- The person falls into a stage of sleep.
- The person can be aroused with relative ease.
- This stage constitutes 50% to 55% of sleep.

Stage III

- The depth of sleep increases, and arousal becomes increasingly difficult.
- This stage composes about 10% of sleep.

Stage IV

- The person reaches the greatest depth of sleep, which is called *delta sleep*.
- Arousal from sleep is difficult.
- Physiologic changes in the body include the following:
  - Slow brain waves are recorded on an EEG.
  - Pulse and respiratory rates decrease.
  - Blood pressure decreases.
  - Muscles are relaxed.
  - Metabolism slows and the body temperature is low.
  - This constitutes about 10% of sleep.

REM Sleep

- Eyes dart back and forth quickly.
- Small muscle twitching, such as on the face
- Large muscle immobility, resembling paralysis
- Respirations irregular; sometimes interspersed with apnea
- Rapid or irregular pulse
- Blood pressure increases or fluctuates
- Increase in gastric secretions
- Metabolism increases; body temperature increases
- Encephalogram tracings active
- REM sleep enters from stage II of NREM sleep and re-enters NREM sleep at stage II: arousal from sleep difficult
- Constitutes about 20% to 25% of sleep

Sleep Cycle

Normally during a **sleep cycle**, a person passes consecutively through the four stages of NREM sleep. This pattern is then reversed, and the person returns from stage IV to stage III to stage II. Instead of re-entering stage I and awakening, the person enters into the REM stage of sleep, after which the person re-enters NREM sleep at stage II and returns to stages III and IV. A person awakened from sleep at any time will return to sleep by starting at stage I of NREM sleep. Figure 35-1 illustrates the normal sleep pattern of young adults.

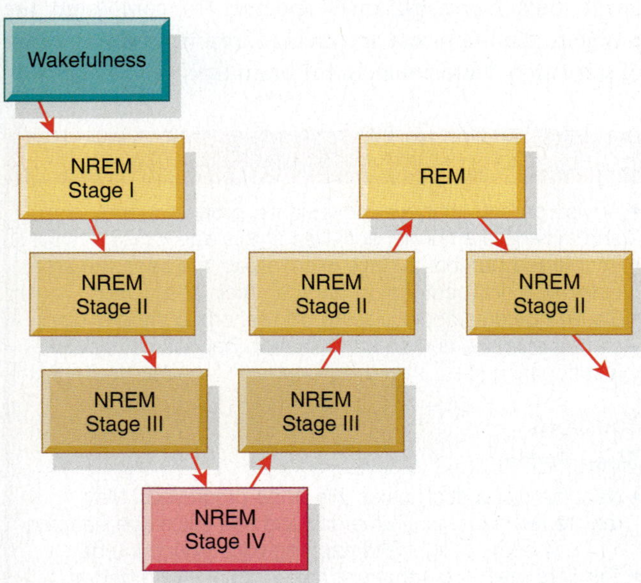

FIGURE 35-1. A single normal sleep cycle in a young adult. In the normal nocturnal pattern, the shaded cycle is repeated four or five times. Periods of REM sleep generally increase in duration; periods of deep sleep (stage IV) progressively decrease as morning approaches.

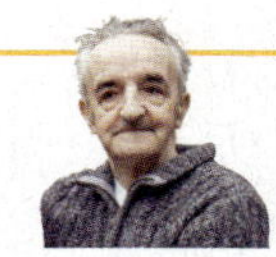

Consider **Charlie Bitner**, the long-term care resident described at the beginning of the chapter. When evaluating Mr. Bitner's sleep cycle, the nurse would need to keep in mind that each time Mr. Bitner awakes, his sleep cycle is starting all over again. Subsequently, he is experiencing light sleep, characteristic of sleep stages I and II.

Most people go through four or five cycles of sleep each night. On average, each cycle lasts about 90 to 110 minutes (Norris, 2019). The cycles tend to become longer as morning approaches. Ordinarily, more deep sleep occurs in the delta stage (NREM stages III and IV) in the first half of the night, especially if one is tired or has lost sleep. Variations in the sleep cycle occur according to age, as Figure 35-2 illustrates on page 1306.

REST AND SLEEP REQUIREMENTS AND PATTERNS

For no known reason, an average of 8 hours of sleep per night has been the accepted standard for adults, despite variations in individual requirements (see Box 35-2 on pages 1306–1307). No rigid formula exists for the regular intervals and duration of sleep. It is important, however, that each person follow a pattern of rest that maintains one's own well-being.

Despite individual variations, some generalities can be stated. On average, infants require 12 to 16 hours each day (including naps); toddlers, 11 to 14 hours (including naps); and preschoolers 10 to 13 hours (including naps) a day. School-aged children, ages 6 to 12 years, require from 9 to 12 hours of sleep, and teenagers 8 to 10 hours a day (American Academy of Sleep Medicine, 2016b; CDC, 2017).

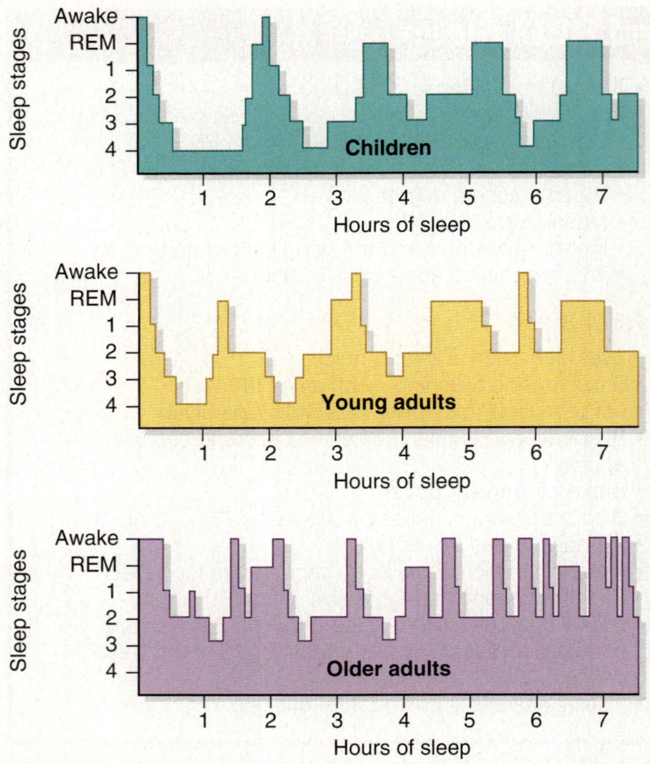

FIGURE 35-2. A comparison of developmental differences in NREM and REM cycles during nocturnal sleep for children, young adults, and older adults.

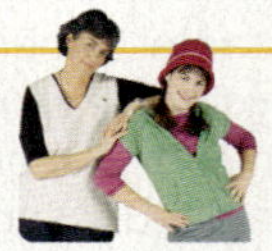

Recall ***Jeanette Clark***, the mother of an adolescent girl who seems to want to sleep all the time. When discussing this issue with Mrs. Clark, the nurse would need to integrate information about the adolescent's developmental stage—that is, that adolescence is a period of tremendous growth, which requires an increased amount of sleep.

The recommended amount of sleep for adults is 7 or more hours (CDC, 2017). Those who are able to relax and rest easily, even while awake, often find that less sleep is needed, whereas others may find that more sleep is required to overcome fatigue. Fatigue can be considered a normal, protective body mechanism and nature's warning that sleep is necessary. Chronic fatigue, however, is abnormal and is often a symptom of illness.

Sleep patterns of older adults vary, but the optimal recommendation for this age group is 7 to 8 or 9 hours (CDC, 2017). They may sleep less, however, because of insomnia and medical conditions that interrupt their sleep, and the quality of their sleep changes.

Patterns of sleep periodicity appear to be learned. For example, most people learn to sleep at night and to be awake and work during the day. However, many night workers learn to sleep equally well during the day.

PHYSICAL AND PSYCHOLOGICAL EFFECTS OF INSUFFICIENT SLEEP

Many people have sleep disturbances that go undetected for years, progressively undermining their energy and destroying their sense of self. One third of U.S. adults report that they usually get insufficient sleep (CDC, 2020). Insufficient sleep in children may affect normal growth and development and could be a contributing factor in performance deficits and behavioral problems. Furthermore, short sleep duration in childhood is associated with an increased risk of obesity during childhood or later in life (CDC, 2018a). The NSF (n.d.b) has also identified a link between insufficient sleep and obesity in adults and children; adults and children who slept less than the recommended hours per night were more likely to be overweight. This sleep–weight link is possibly related to two hormones: leptin and ghrelin (NSF, 2022a). Leptin signals the brain to stop eating, whereas ghrelin promotes continued eating. Research suggests that sleep deprivation lowers leptin levels and elevates ghrelin levels, thus increasing one's appetite. To compound the problem, the brain may interpret a drop in leptin as a sign of starvation. Unfortunately, the brain then signals the body

Box 35-2 Developmental Patterns of Sleep

Newborns and Infants

Sleep Pattern

- *Newborn:* Sleeps an average of 16 hr/24 hr; averages about 4 hours at a time.
- Each infant's sleep pattern is unique. On average, infants sleep 12 to 16 hours at night, with several naps during the day.
- Usually by age 8 to 16 weeks, an infant sleeps through the night.
- REM sleep constitutes much of the sleep cycle of a young infant.

Nursing Implications

- Teach parents to position infant on the back. This is the only safe sleeping position for infants younger than age 1 year. Sleeping in the prone position increases the risk for sudden infant death syndrome (SIDS).
- Advise parents that eye movements, groaning, grimacing, and moving are normal activities at this age.
- Encourage parents to have infant sleep in a separate area in the parents' bedroom rather than their bed.
- Caution parents about placing pillows, crib bumpers, quilts, stuffed animals, and so on in the crib because this poses a suffocation risk.

Toddlers

Sleep Pattern

- Need for sleep declines as this stage progresses. May require two naps during the day and end this stage sleeping 11 to 14 hours a night and napping once during the day.
- Toddlers may begin to resist naps and going to bed at night.
- They may move from crib to youth bed or regular bed at around age 2 years.

Box 35-2 Developmental Patterns of Sleep *(continued)*

Nursing Implications

- Establish a regular bedtime routine (e.g., reading a story, singing a lullaby, saying prayers).
- Advise parents of the value of a routine sleeping pattern with minimal variation.
- Encourage attention to safety once child moves from crib to bed. If child attempts to wander out of room, a folding gate may be necessary across the door of the room.

Preschoolers

Sleep Pattern

- Children in this stage generally sleep 10 to 13 hours at night.
- The REM sleep pattern is similar to that of an adult.
- Daytime napping decreases during this period, and by the age of 5 years, most children no longer nap.
- This age group may continue to resist going to bed at night.

Nursing Implications

- Encourage parents to continue bedtime routines.
- Advise parents that waking from nightmares or night terrors (awakening screaming about 20 minutes after falling asleep) are common during this stage. Waking the child and comforting the child generally helps. Sometimes use of a night light is soothing.

School-Aged Children

Sleep Pattern

- Younger school-aged children may require 9 to 12 hours nightly, whereas older children in this stage may average 9 to 11 hours.
- Sleep needs usually increase when physical growth peaks.

Nursing Implications

- Discuss the fact that the stress of beginning school may interrupt normal sleep patterns.
- Advise that a relaxed bedtime routine is most helpful at this stage.
- Inform parents about child's awareness of the concept of death possibly occurring at this stage. Encourage parental presence and support to help alleviate some of the child's concerns.

Teenagers

Sleep Pattern

- Sleep needs of teenagers vary widely, but the average requirement is 8 to 10 hours. The growth spurt that normally occurs at this stage may necessitate the need for more sleep; however, the stresses of school, activities, and part-time employment may cause adolescents to have a restless sleep. Adolescents tend to go to bed later than younger children and adults, but early morning start times for high school frequently require an early awakening time. This can result in an average of only 7 to 7.5 hours of sleep a night.
- Many adolescents do not get enough sleep.

Nursing Implications

- Advise parents that their adolescents' complaints of fatigue or inability to do well in school may be related to not enough sleep. *Excessive daytime sleepiness (EDS)* may also make the teenager more vulnerable to accidents and behavioral problems.

Young Adults

Sleep Pattern

- The amount of sleep required is 7 to 9 hours.
- Sleep is affected by many factors: physical health, type of occupation, exercise. Lifestyle demands may interfere with sleep patterns.
- REM sleep averages about 20% of sleep.

Nursing Implications

- Reinforce that developing good sleep habits has a positive effect on health, particularly as a person ages.
- If loss of sleep is a problem, explore lifestyle demands and stress as possible causes.
- Suggest use of relaxation techniques and stress-reduction exercises rather than resorting to medication to induce sleep. Sleep medications decrease REM sleep, may be habit forming, and frequently lose their effectiveness over time.

Middle-Aged Adults

Sleep Pattern

- Total sleep time decreases during these years, with a decrease in stage IV sleep.
- The percentage of time spent awake in bed begins to increase.
- People become more aware of sleep disturbances during this period.

Nursing Implications

- Encourage adults to investigate consistent sleep difficulties to exclude pathology or anxiety and depression as causes.
- Encourage adults to avoid use of sleep-inducing medication on a regular basis.

Older Adults

Sleep Pattern

- An average of 7 to 8 hours of sleep is usually adequate for this age group.
- Sleep is less sound, and stage IV sleep is absent or considerably decreased. Periods of REM sleep shorten.
- Older adults frequently have great difficulty falling asleep and have more complaints of problems sleeping.
- Decline in physical health, psychological factors, effects of drug therapy (e.g., nocturia), or environmental factors may be implicated as causes of inability to sleep.

Nursing Implications

- A comprehensive nursing assessment and individualized interventions may be effective in the long-term care of this age group.
- Emphasize concern for a safe environment because it is not uncommon for older adults to be temporarily confused and disoriented when they first awake.
- Use pharmacologic sleep aids with extreme caution because of declining physiologic function and concerns about polypharmacy.
- Encourage older adults to discuss sleep concerns with their health care provider.

to eat more while it simultaneously lowers the body's metabolic rate. When this happens, people are more likely to gain weight, even if food intake is decreased (Miller et al., 2015).

People who suffer sleep difficulties caused by working night shifts or constantly changing work shifts may experience adverse effects, including anxiety, personal conflicts, loneliness, depression, gastrointestinal (GI) symptoms, increase in type 2 diabetes, hypertension, and higher rates of cardiovascular disease including strokes, and substance abuse (Nena et al., 2018; National Institute for Occupational Safety and Health [NIOSH], n.d.). A person who has experienced shortened sleep by just a few hours a night can have a reaction time similar to someone intoxicated with alcohol (NSF, 2022b).

Sleep loss that results in fatigue and decreased competence increases the risk of a sleep-related motor vehicle accident. The NSF (n.d.c) reports that 55% of Americans admitted driving while feeling drowsy during the past year and drowsy driving is implicated in at least 100,000 motor vehicle accidents a year. A large study of critical care nurses reported that 43% of the nurses stated that they fell asleep while stopped at a traffic light and 20% had a traffic accident or a near miss directly associated with their fatigue (Johnson, 2011).

In addition, studies of physicians' and nurses' work habits have concluded that shift work sleep disorders (SWSDs) from extended work schedules are a causative factor in a substantial number of adverse medical events and errors (Weaver et al., 2018; Witkoski Stimpfel, 2020). Fatigue and sleepiness can compromise patient safety and increase the risk for adverse events such as medication errors. Sleep deprivation and the resulting consequences of decreased alertness and ability to perform tasks competently are well documented. The Office of Disease Prevention and Health Promotion (ODPHP) (2020) recognizes that improved attention to sleep health promotes a safer environment for health care workers and their patients. Objectives related to sleep health identified in *Healthy People 2030* include increasing the proportion of adults who get sufficient sleep; increasing the proportion of high school students who get sufficient sleep; increasing the proportion of people with sleep apnea symptoms who get evaluated by a health care provider; reducing the rate of motor vehicle crashes due to drowsy driving; increasing the proportion of children who get sufficient sleep; and increase the proportion of infants who are put to sleep on their backs (ODPHP, 2020). The Joint Commission (2018) acknowledges the impact of fatigue on health care workers and urges greater attention to the issue, suggesting actions for health care facilities to reduce fatigue-related risks. These include:

- Assess work schedules and staffing to address extended work shifts and hours.
- Review hand-off processes and procedures to ensure safe transfer of information.
- Request staff input in designing work schedules to minimize staff fatigue.
- Develop and implement a fatigue management plan.
- Educate staff about sleep hygiene and the effects of fatigue on patient safety.
- Address staff concerns about fatigue.
- Encourage teamwork to support staff who work extended shifts.
- Keep the effects of fatigue in mind when reviewing adverse events.

FACTORS AFFECTING REST AND SLEEP

A variety of factors influence both the quality and quantity of sleep. These factors help inform the assessment process as well as identification of appropriate interventions related to enhancing rest and sleep.

Developmental Considerations

Variations in sleep patterns are related to age. Box 35-2 highlights these variations and associated nursing implications. Routine assessment of sleepiness or short sleep patterns in children is a first step in identifying the existence of a sleep problem and factors interfering with a child's sleep. With a growing body of evidence linking inadequate sleep with obesity and other health concerns in children, health care practitioners must ask about patterns of sleep and sleep habits in children and discuss these issues with parents.

Many people ages 65 years and older report difficulty falling asleep, early awakening or waking frequently during the night, napping, or not feeling rested after a night's sleep (Hedges & Gotelli, 2020). Older adults often need more time to fall asleep and are less able to cope with changes in their usual sleep patterns compared to younger people. Many older adults nap during the day, which often results in sleeping fewer hours at night. Chronic illnesses in older adults may also affect their sleep patterns. For instance, many older men have enlargement of the prostate gland, which may cause them to awaken throughout the night to use the bathroom.

Motivation

A desire to be wakeful and alert helps overcome sleepiness and sleep. For example, a tired person may be wakeful and alert when at a party or when attending an interesting play or concert. The opposite is also true: When there is minimal motivation to be awake, sleep generally follows. For example, a student who is bored and disinterested in a lecture or class may doze during the lecture.

Culture

A person's cultural beliefs and practices can influence rest and sleep. Although developmental stages are similar, children's bedtime rituals, sleeping position and place, and pattern of sleep may vary based on culture. Methods to enhance or foster sleep may also be culturally influenced. A cultural orientation toward privacy and quiet makes sleep difficult in a busy special care unit. Sensitivity to a patient's culture must be included in the plan of care for preparing the patient for an evening's sleep.

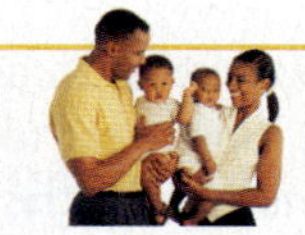

Think back to **Mrs. Omeara**, the mother of infant twins. She is wondering whether she should let her twins sleep in her and her husband's bed. The nurse should investigate the family's cultural background to determine any influences it may have on the patient's question. The nurse would then use this information to develop an individualized, culturally considerate plan of care for dealing with this question

Lifestyle and Habits

Various lifestyle factors can affect a person's ability to sleep well. People working a shift other than the day shift must reorganize their priorities, or sleep difficulties may occur. Based on the circadian cycle, the body prepares for sleep at night by decreasing the body temperature and releasing melatonin (a natural chemical produced at night that decreases wakefulness and promotes sleep). Working the night shift disrupts this natural process and can result in loss of sleep and other adverse effects (see Physical and Psychological Effects of Insufficient Sleep). Developing a sleep pattern is especially difficult if the work shift changes periodically. Nurses and others who work long hours and varying shifts have difficulty finding time to exercise, which can promote weight gain. The NIOSH (2020) offers information to educate nurses and their managers about the health and safety risks associated with shift work and long work hours and a training program to increase knowledge about personal behaviors and workplace systems to reduce associated risks.

The duration and quality of sleep can be affected by watching some types of television shows, participating in stimulating outside activities, and taking part in activity or exercise within 3 hours of the person's normal bedtime. A person's ability to relax from work-related pressures and to put aside home stresses are also important factors in the ability to fall asleep. Nurses who role model good health behaviors are more effective teachers. Use the Promoting Health 35-1 display for yourself before using it with others.

Physical Activity and Exercise

Activity and exercise increase fatigue and, in many instances, promote relaxation that is followed by sleep. It appears that physical activity increases both REM and NREM sleep. Moderate exercise is a healthy way to promote sleep, but exercise that occurs within a 3-hour interval before normal bedtime can hinder sleep. The fatigue that results from normal work activities or exercise is believed to contribute to a restful sleep, whereas excessive exercise or exhaustion can decrease the quality of sleep.

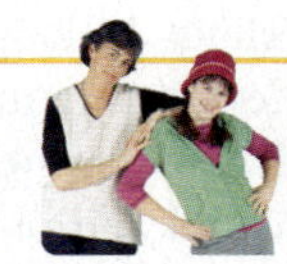

Remember **Jeanette Clark**, the mother of the adolescent girl who seems to be sleeping all the time. As part of the health promotion teaching plan, the nurse would need to explain to Mrs. Clark about the significant changes occurring during adolescence. In addition to this stage being a period of rapid growth, it is also a time of increased activity—physically, emotionally, and socially. All of these may be affecting her daughter's sleep patterns.

Dietary Habits

There is some evidence supporting a sleep moderating effect of the dietary amino acid L-tryptophan in promoting sleep (Binks et al., 2020). A small protein-containing snack (a source of tryptophan) before bedtime has been recommended for patients with insomnia. However, as nutritionists have studied the effects of various foods on mood, new information has emerged. Carbohydrates make tryptophan more available to the brain. This explains why

Promoting Health 35-1

REST AND SLEEP

Use the assessment checklist to determine how well you are meeting needs for rest and sleep. Then develop a prescription for self-care by choosing appropriate behaviors from the list of suggestions.

Assessment Checklist

☐ almost always ☐ sometimes ☐ almost never

☐ ☐ ☐ 1. I feel rested and refreshed when I get up in the morning.

☐ ☐ ☐ 2. I have energy to carry out normal activities of daily living.

☐ ☐ ☐ 3. I understand the normal changes in sleep and rest requirements and patterns that occur with aging.

☐ ☐ ☐ 4. I set aside time for quiet recreation and restful activities each day.

Self-Care Behaviors

1. Follow a regular routine for bedtime and morning awakening.
2. Accept individual differences in need for sleep.
3. Use relaxation exercises to relax before bedtime, especially if feeling stressed.
4. Avoid caffeine, smoking, and alcohol before bedtime.
5. Adjust bedcoverings, room temperature, and lighting to your preferences.
6. Eat a small protein and carbohydrate snack before going to bed.
7. Be aware of the potential dangers of sleeping pills.
8. Use some part of each day for quiet, enjoyable activities such as crafts, hobbies, reading, watching television, listening to music, and visiting with friends.
9. Incorporate periods of regular exercise into each week.

meals heavy in carbohydrate content tend to cause drowsiness. Combining foods that are high in tryptophan with healthy, complex carbohydrates improves sleep. Therefore, a small protein- and carbohydrate-containing snack such as peanut butter on toast or cheese and crackers about an hour before bed may be more effective (Binks et al., 2020; Sleep Foundation, 2020a).

Alcoholic beverages, when used in moderation, appear to induce sleep in some people. However, large quantities have been found to limit REM and delta sleep. Initially, alcohol consumption may help to induce sleep, but once the alcohol is cleared from the body, sleep is fragmented and disrupted often (Sleep Foundation, 2020b). Alcohol also interferes with entering deeper stages of sleep, which may result in feelings of fatigue upon wakening despite having spent an adequate amount of time in bed (Sleep Foundation, 2020a). Most recommendations to promote effective sleep state that alcohol and products containing alcohol should be avoided in the evening to promote better sleep habits.

Caffeine is a central nervous system stimulant. For many people, beverages containing caffeine interfere with the ability to fall asleep. Caffeine is thought to interfere with the action of adenosine, which is a compound found in every cell in the body. It binds to adenosine receptors in the brain, thus preventing the adenosine from entering nerve cells and causing drowsiness. Caffeine consumption should be avoided too close to bedtime as its effect may persist for several hours (Sleep Foundation, 2020b). Examples of beverages containing caffeine include coffee, tea, energy drinks, and most cola drinks. Chocolate also contains caffeine.

Smoking

Exposure to tobacco smoke is associated with poorer sleep quality (Zandy et al., 2020). Nicotine has a stimulating effect; smokers usually have a more difficult time falling asleep. They are more easily aroused once asleep and may describe themselves as light sleepers. Avoiding nicotine in any substance close to bedtime is suggested as part of good sleep hygiene practices (Sleep Foundation, 2020d). People usually report improved sleep patterns after discontinuing nicotine use.

Total withdrawal from smoking may be associated with temporary sleep disturbances. Patients who stop smoking often have more daytime sleepiness and report significantly more restlessness at night. Whether this is a short-term effect or is related to nicotine's effect on the central nervous system is uncertain.

Environmental Factors

Most people sleep best in their usual home environments. Sleeping in a strange or new environment tends to influence both REM and NREM sleep. People accustomed to sleeping in a noisy environment, such as a busy large city, actually have a hard time falling asleep in an area that is extremely quiet. By turning on soothing music or a fan or other background noise, the person may actually be able to rest in the new environment (Sleep Foundation, 2020c). Likewise, if a patient is accustomed to sleeping in a quiet environment, a room next to a high-traffic area, such as the nurse's desk, may not be the best place for this patient to rest.

Psychological Stress

Psychological stress, such as from illness and various life situations, tends to disturb sleep. In general, psychological stress affects sleep in two ways: (1) the person experiencing stress may find it difficult to obtain the amount of sleep needed; and (2) REM sleep decreases in amount, which tends to add to anxiety and stress.

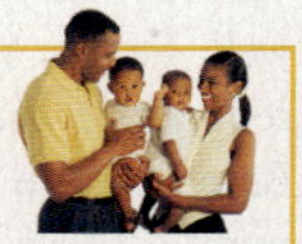

Consider **Mrs. Omeara**, the mother described in the beginning of the chapter and in the Reflective Practice display. The nurse would need to gather additional information about Mrs. Omeara's current situation to determine if any stressors might be affecting her ability to obtain adequate rest and sleep. Areas to address may include her typical daily activities, amount of time spent caring for each child, employment, and amount of assistance and support from others. In addition, the nurse would need to investigate the reasons underlying Mrs. Omeara's question about the babies sleeping in the parents' bed.

Illness

Illness, a physiologic as well as a psychological stressor, influences sleep. Certain illnesses are more closely related to sleep disturbances than others. For example:

- Gastric secretions increase during REM sleep. Many people with gastroesophageal reflux disease (GERD) awaken at night with heartburn or pain (NSF, 2020b). They find that using antacids to neutralize stomach acidity often relieves discomfort and promotes sleep.
- Certain epilepsy seizures are associated with certain stages of sleep; sleep deprivation is also associated with activation of seizures in some patients with epilepsy (Lanigar & Bandyopadhyay, 2017).
- Liver failure is associated with insomnia, excessive daytime sleepiness, and a reversal in day–night sleeping habits (disturbance of circadian rhythmicity) (Bruyneel & Sersté, 2018).
- Hypothyroidism is associated with sleep disturbances as a result of trouble tolerating cold at night and joint or muscle pain that disrupts sleep (Sleep Foundation, 2020c). Hyperthyroidism may result in difficulty sleeping due to arousals from nervousness or irritability, night sweats, or frequent urges to urinate (Sleep Foundation, 2020c). Thyroid disease may also be associated with restless legs syndrome (RLS) (see discussion on p. 1315), which may lead to significant sleep disruption (Sleep Foundation, 2020c).
- End-stage renal disease (ESRD) disrupts nocturnal sleep and leads to excessive daytime sleepiness. Patients with ESRD who receive dialysis also have a higher incidence of RLS (discussed later in the chapter) (Maung et al., 2016).

Medications

Health care practitioners must also take into account the effect that drugs used to treat health care problems may have on sleep. Drugs that can affect sleep include benzodiazepines, amphetamines, and antidepressants. Diuretics, antiparkinsonian drugs, some antidepressants and antihypertensives, steroids, decongestants, caffeine, and asthma medications are seen as additional common causes of sleep problems.

Chronotherapeutics is a growing field of study that involves the strategic use of time in the treatment of disease and administration of medications (Zaki et al., 2019). Researchers have determined that certain treatments for disease are more effective when circadian rhythms are taken into account. For example, an unequal dosing schedule including a greater intake of bronchopulmonary drugs and bronchodilators in the evening may be more effective in preventing asthma attacks that commonly occur at night during sleep (Zaki et al., 2019). The timing of antihypertensive medication administration may need to be adjusted to provide peak protection during early-morning hours, when heart attacks are more common (Hermida et al., 2019). Cancer chemotherapy appears to be less toxic when administered at certain times of the day (Mohammadi, 2016). Paying attention to biologic rhythms may influence drug tolerance and medication effectiveness, and reduce adverse effects, including those related to rest and sleep.

COMMON SLEEP DISORDERS

A nurse who interviews a patient to obtain a sleep history needs to understand common sleep disturbances to recognize significant data. The most recent classification of sleep disorders categorized by the International Classification of Sleep Disorders (ICSD) includes six major categories of disorders (American Academy of Sleep Medicine, 2014):

- Insomnia
- Sleep-related breathing disorders
- Central disorders of hypersomnolence
- Circadian rhythm sleep–wake disorders
- Parasomnias
- Sleep-related movement disorders

The more common sleep disorders are insomnia, sleep-related breathing disorders, circadian rhythm sleep–wake disorders, and parasomnias. A brief description of these disturbances follows, with the major focus on specific symptoms associated with the sleep disorder, as well as a brief discussion of possible treatments.

Insomnia

Insomnia is the most common sleep disorder (Hedges & Gotelli, 2020). **Insomnia** is characterized by difficulty falling asleep, intermittent sleep, or difficulty maintaining sleep, despite adequate opportunity and circumstances to sleep (American Academy of Sleep Medicine, 2014; Wilson et al., 2019). People experiencing insomnia report excessive daytime sleepiness (Wilson et al., 2019). As many as 30% to 35% of adults in the United States complain of insomnia (American Academy of Sleep Medicine, 2015). Older adults, women, people under stress, and people with certain health and mental health problems, such as depression are more likely to experience insomnia (American Academy of Sleep Medicine, 2015). Many cases of insomnia are related to disruptions in circadian rhythms. This sleep disorder can also occur during periods of stress; in situations involving some change in the normal environment such as shift work; as a result of pain, discomfort, or limited mobility; and as a result of the side effects of medications. Common medications that may result in insomnia include those taken for hypertension and cardiovascular disease, cold and allergies, attention-deficit hyperactivity disorder (ADHA), and depression (American Academy of Sleep Medicine, 2015).

Daytime consequences of insomnia include reports of feeling tired, lethargic, and irritable during the day. Difficulty concentrating is also a common manifestation. Older adults who experience insomnia while in an acute care setting may manifest delirium as a symptom of sleep deprivation (Hedges & Gotelli, 2020). It is a challenge for health care providers to understand the effects of age-related changes on sleep and be alert for the potential complications associated with insomnia in this growing population.

Insomnia may be a short-term or chronic in nature. Chronic insomnia is frequently listed as the motivating factor for a visit to a sleep disorder clinic. A growing number of health conditions have been associated with chronic insomnia. They include obesity; type 2 diabetes; psychiatric disorders such as depression; and cardiovascular disorders such as heart failure, stroke, hypertension, and myocardial infarction (heart attack) (CDC, 2018a; CDC, 2018b; Javaheri & Redline, 2017).

Nonpharmacologic approaches may be attempted initially to resolve the insomnia. Refer to the Teaching About Rest and Sleep discussion on page 1326. The misuse of alcohol or caffeine can have an adverse effect on sleep; stopping these behaviors may reduce or eliminate the insomnia. Cognitive behavioral therapy (CBT) is a safe, effective means of managing chronic insomnia and may include cognitive therapy, relaxation training, stimulus control therapy, or sleep restriction therapy (American Academy of Sleep Medicine, 2019; Brem, 2015; Chung et al., 2018). CBT is recommended as a first-line treatment of insomnia (Wilson et al., 2019). CBT involves meeting with a therapist and working through maladaptive sleep beliefs. It may also include biofeedback, additional relaxation techniques, and sleep hygiene measures (see Teaching About Rest and Sleep on page 1326). When used in conjunction with these other complementary therapies, CBT can be very successful (Brem, 2015). If, however, nonpharmacologic measures prove ineffective, pharmacologic treatment may be necessary. Refer to the Using Medications to Promote Sleep discussion on page 1325.

Sleep-Related Breathing Disorders

There are several sleep-related breathing disorders. The discussion here will focus on the more common OSAs. **Obstructive sleep apnea (OSA)** is a potentially serious sleep disorder in which the throat muscles intermittently relax and block the airway during sleep, causing breathing to repeatedly stop and start (Mayo Foundation for Medical Education and Research [MFMER], 2020b). OSA is further delineated as OSA (adult) and OSA (pediatric).

Adult OSA is characterized by five or more predominantly obstructive respiratory events (the absence of breathing [apnea] or diminished breathing efforts [hypopnea] or respiratory effort-related arousals) during sleep, accompanied by excessive daytime sleepiness, fatigue, insomnia, loud snoring, observed apnea, and/or gasping for air during sleep (MFMER, 2020b). Adults suffering from OSA may also present with associated health disorders (hypertension, coronary artery disease, atrial fibrillation, congestive heart failure, stroke, diabetes, cognitive dysfunction, or mood disorder) (American Academy of Sleep Medicine, 2014). OSA (adult) may be diagnosed based on a frequency of obstructive respiratory events that occur at a rate of >15 events per hour, even in the absence of associated symptoms or health disorders alone (American Academy of Sleep Medicine, 2014).

OSA (adult) is a common disorder, caused by recurrent collapse of the upper airway during sleep (Fig. 35-3). Breathing may cease for 10 to 20 seconds and possibly as long as 2 minutes. During long periods of apnea, the oxygen level in the blood drops, the pulse usually becomes irregular, and the blood pressure often increases. This decrease in ventilation and associated physiologic response activates the fight-or-flight response of the sympathetic nervous system and the sleeper startles and awakens (Simmons & Pruitt, 2012). This pattern may repeat 5 to 30 times or more each hour (MFMER, 2020b).

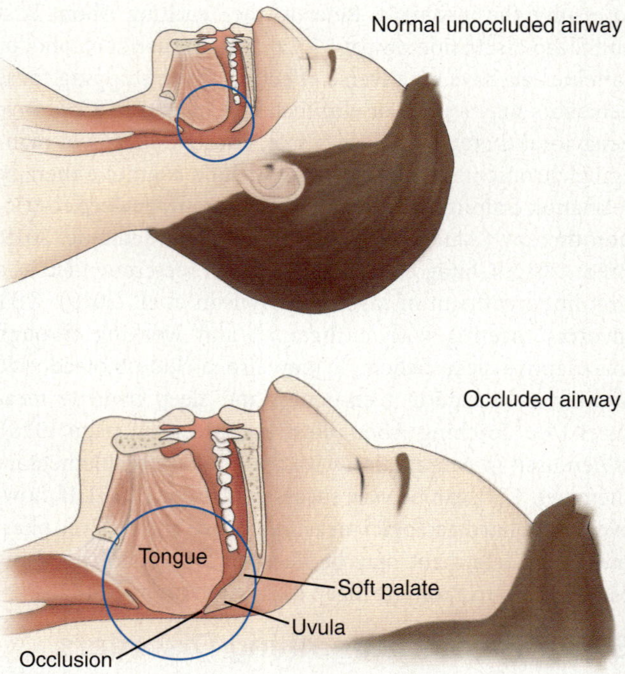

FIGURE 35-3. Obstructive sleep apnea occurs when the airway is occluded due to recurrent collapse of the upper airway. Normally, the airway remains open during sleep (see insets).

The incidence of OSA (adult) increases with age, obesity, large neck size, male, and family history and is associated with cardiovascular risk factors, cardiovascular disease, depression, increased risk of motor vehicle accidents, and increased mortality (American Academy of Sleep Medicine, 2016a; MFMER, 2020b; Norris, 2019).

Clinical information and nocturnal polysomnography can confirm the diagnosis of sleep apnea. This overnight sleep study also includes a video recording of sleep awakenings and movements. Cardiopulmonary monitoring of the arterial oxygen saturation and an electrocardiogram (ECG) to detect any cardiac arrhythmias can also assist in the diagnosis of OSA.

Adults with OSA may become irritable during the day, fall asleep during monotonous activities, have difficulty concentrating, and exhibit slower reaction times. Alcohol, tobacco, and sleeping pills increase the breathing disruption that occurs in sleep apnea and therefore should be avoided.

The definitive treatment of moderate or severe OSA involves use of a continuous positive airway pressure machine (CPAP). CPAP is noninvasive and consists of a mask connected to an air pump that is worn during sleep. This device delivers positive air pressure that holds the airway open. It can significantly improve the manifestations of OSA, but adherence and inconsistent use of the CPAP device is an issue for many patients. Patients may discontinue use of CPAP because of a sensation of claustrophobia, discomfort exhaling against air inflow, or dryness and skin irritation. Some patients who are unable to tolerate use of CPAP may be able to use a bilevel positive airway pressure (BPAP) machine (Hess et al., 2021; MFMER, 2020b). BPAP adjusts the air pressure delivered, providing more pressure when the patient inhales and less when the patient exhales. The decreased expiratory pressure may make exhalation more comfortable than with CPAP (Hess et al., 2021).

Mild OSA can be managed with a custom-made oral appliance (OA) that is used to enlarge the oropharynx by either advancing the mandible or keeping the tongue in a forward position (Hess et al., 2021). These hard, plastic devices are fitted by a dentist or orthodontist based on a mold of the patient's mouth. If a person is unable to tolerate CPAP, an OA is an alternative treatment, but OA are not considered first-line therapy for severe sleep apnea (Hess et al., 2021). OA may also be used with CPAP.

If medical treatment methods fail, several surgical procedures may be suggested to manage sleep apnea. Surgery is not without risks and poses significant postoperative issues for the patient. People who opt for these procedures need continued support and comprehensive teaching, including coping strategies, for the immediate postoperative period.

Pediatric OSA is a sleep disorder in which a child's breathing is partially or completely blocked repeatedly during sleep due to a narrowing or blockage of the upper airway during sleep. OSA (pediatric) is defined by the presence of one of these findings: snoring, labored/obstructed breathing, **enuresis** (urinating during sleep), or daytime consequences (hyperactivity or other neurobehavioral problems, sleepiness, fatigue) (American Academy of Sleep Medicine, 2014). Unlike adults, children with OSA are more likely to have behavioral problems than daytime sleepiness (MFMER, 2020a). A common underlying cause in children is enlargement of the adenoids and tonsils (MFMER, 2020a; Nierengarten, 2018). Obesity/overweight is also a risk factor in children as well as increased risk in children with neuromuscular disease, craniofacial dysmorphology, and certain genetic syndromes (Nierengarten, 2018).

Children and adolescents with symptoms of OSA, including snoring, should have a physical examination, polysomnography, overnight oximetry, and an electrocardiogram to confirm diagnosis (MFMER, 2020a; Marcus et al., 2012). Severe complications affecting a child's growth, cognitive development and behavior can occur if this disorder is untreated or ignored (MFMER, 2020a). Options for treatment in children include weight loss if obesity is present, adenotonsillectomy (removal of tonsils and adenoids), CPAP, BPAP, oral appliances, or intranasal corticosteroids (Marcus et al., 2012; MFMER, 2020a).

Central Disorders of Hypersomnolence

These disorders are characterized by excessive daytime sleepiness (hypersomnolence) that is not attributable to another sleep disorder, specifically those that result in disturbed sleep (e.g., sleep-related breathing disorders) or abnormalities of circadian rhythm (American Academy of Sleep Medicine, 2014).

Idiopathic **hypersomnia** is characterized by constant or recurrent episodes of extreme sleepiness, particularly during the day. A person may sleep for 10 or more hours at night and take naps during the day and still feel sleepy (NSF, n.d.). When they awake, they are often disoriented, irritated, restless, and have slower speech and thinking processes. Some people may have a genetic predisposition to hypersomnia. It appears most often in adolescents and young adults. Although not usually life threatening, hypersomnia can have some serious consequences, such as motor vehicle accidents that occur because of drowsiness or falling asleep while driving. These attacks may occur indefinitely (NSF, n.d.).

Treatment of hypersomnia is symptomatic in nature. Stimulant drugs may prove effective, or in some cases, antidepressants may be prescribed. Attention to diet (avoidance of alcohol and caffeine) and behavioral changes (avoidance of night work and social activities later in the evening) may offer some relief from such episodes. Additional interventions may include encouraging naps whenever possible and maintenance of a regular sleep schedule (NSF, n.d.).

Narcolepsy is a chronic neurologic disorder characterized by excessive daytime sleepiness and frequent overwhelming urges to sleep or inadvertent daytime lapses into sleep. Some people with narcolepsy also experience cataplexy, the sudden, involuntary loss of skeletal muscle tone lasting from seconds to 1 or 2 minutes (Norris, 2019). Additional symptoms include the presence of hallucinations or sleep paralysis (National Institute of Neurological Disorders and Stroke [NINDS], 2019b). A person with narcolepsy can literally fall asleep standing up, while driving a car, in the middle of a conversation, or while swimming. People with narcolepsy tend to fall asleep quickly, find it difficult to wake up, sleep fewer hours than others, and sleep restlessly. Symptoms usually appear in susceptible people during adolescence or early adulthood and are usually lifelong; symptoms may improve with treatment but never completely resolve (National Heart Lung and Blood Institute [NHLBI], n.d.a.; NINDS, 2019b).

Narcolepsy is caused by the brain's inability to regulate sleep–wake cycles and may have a genetic component (NINDS, 2019b; Norris, 2019). Many people with narcolepsy have been shown to have an unusually high rate of a specific human leukocyte antigen subtype and low hypocretin level has also been shown to be a possible contributor (NHLBI, n.d.a; Norris, 2019). Hypocretin is a neurotransmitter in the brain that causes alertness and wakefulness. It is unknown at this time what causes this low hypocretin level (American Academy of Sleep Medicine, 2014). Undiagnosed, a person with narcolepsy is potentially dangerous to self and others. In some countries, a person with a diagnosis of narcolepsy is not permitted to drive a motor vehicle. A sleep study is important to confirm the diagnosis of narcolepsy. At present, there is no cure. However, medications that restore alertness allow near-normal functioning for most patients.

A central nervous system stimulant (e.g., modafinil) that causes wakefulness may be used to control narcolepsy. Additional medications such as methylphenidate (a stimulant) and tricyclics and SSRI (antidepressants) have proved effective in treating narcoleptic symptoms (NINDS, 2019b). People using such drugs should take them faithfully because with discontinuation of use, the uncontrollable desire to sleep returns. In addition to medications, behavioral therapies should be implemented to help to control the symptoms of narcolepsy (NINDS, 2019b).

Circadian Rhythm Sleep–Wake Disorders

Circadian rhythm sleep–wake disorders are characterized by a chronic or recurrent pattern of sleep–wake rhythm disruption primarily caused by an alteration in the internal circadian timing system or misalignment between the internal circadian rhythm and the sleep–wake schedule desired or required; a sleep–wake disturbance (e.g., insomnia or excessive sleepiness); and associated distress or impairment, lasting for a period of at least 3 months (except for jet lag disorder) (American Academy of Sleep Medicine, 2014; Wilson et al., 2019). There are several disorders within this group of sleep disorders, with the most common being shift-work disorder and jet-lag disorder.

Shift-work disorder results from working on a schedule outside the traditional daytime workday (9:00 AM to 5:00 PM) that goes against the body's natural circadian rhythm (Cleveland Clinic, 2017a; Pacheco, 2020a). A constant or recurrent pattern of sleep interruption caused by difficulty adjusting to the different sleep and wake schedule results in excessive sleepiness during work and insomnia when trying to sleep between shifts (Wilson et al., 2019). Other symptoms may include ongoing tiredness, general feeling of discomfort or uneasiness, mood disorder, GI problems, and decreased sex drive (Cleveland Clinic, 2017a). Many industries and other occupations and professions rely on shift work, including nursing. The work schedule of shift workers may prevent attainment of sufficient sleep (Pacheco, 2020a). Shift workers are more likely to sleep fewer than 6 hours on workdays and experience drowsy driving at least once a month (Pacheco, 2020a). Not all shift workers experience sleep issues, but approximately 10% to 40% of shift workers experience symptoms of the disorder, including excessive sleepiness or insomnia (Cleveland Clinic, 2017a). In addition, shift work has been linked to problems with physical and mental health, performance, accidents, work-related errors, increased irritability or mood problems, and safety (Cleveland Clinic, 2017a; Nena et al., 2018; Pacheco, 2020a; Weaver et al., 2018).

Jet-lag disorder results from a conflict between the pattern of sleep and wakefulness between the internal biologic clock and that of a new time zone (Cleveland Clinic, 2020). This temporary disorder occurs as a result of travel across two or more time zones, producing difficulty adjusting and functioning optimally in the new time zone. Symptoms of jet lag include general tiredness, difficulty staying alert, an unwell feeling or discomfort, mood disturbance, and a change in appetite and other GI function (Cleveland Clinic, 2020; MFMER, 2020c).

Treatment for circadian rhythm sleep–wake disorders varies based on the type of disorder and the degree to which it affects a person, and usually includes a combination of interventions. Behavior therapy includes maintaining regular sleep–wake times, avoiding naps, keeping to a regular exercise routine, and avoiding caffeine, nicotine, and stimulating activities within several hours of bedtime (Cleveland Clinic, 2020). Light therapy helps ease the transition to a new schedule or time zone. It involves exposing the patient's eyes to an artificial bright light that simulates sunlight for a specific and regular amount of time during the time the person should be awake; exposure to sunlight can also be used to regulate the sleep–wake cycle (Cleveland Clinic, 2020; MFMER, 2020c; Wilson et al., 2019). Chronotherapy requires a commitment on the part of the patient to act over a period of weeks to progressively advance or delay the time of sleep for 1 to 2 hours per day. Over time, this results in a shift of the sleep–wake cycle (Cleveland Clinic, 2020). Medications such as melatonin (Wilson et al., 2019), modafinil (stimulant) or caffeine may also be used to adjust and maintain the sleep–wake cycle (Cleveland Clinic, 2020; MFMER, 2020c).

Parasomnias

Parasomnias are episodes or behaviors that occur during arousals from REM sleep or partial arousals from NREM sleep that disturb the patient or others (Cleveland Clinic, 2017b; Wilson et al., 2019). Parasomnias occur in both children and adults but are more common in children (DePietro, n.d.). Although parasomnias are commonly outgrown before adulthood, safety and prevention of injury are paramount concerns. These sleep disorders can occur rarely or on a regular basis. Examples of parasomnias include:

- ***Somnambulism*** or *sleepwalking* may range from sitting up in bed to walking around the room or the house to walking outside the house. The automatic behavior can also include behaviors which are very familiar to the patient, such as dressing, washing, or arranging objects in the house (Wilson et al., 2019). The sleepwalker is unaware of his environment and is unresponsive to other people.
- *REM Sleep Behavior Disorder (RBD)* is characterized by dramatic "acting out" and/or violent dreams during REM sleep (Cleveland Clinic, 2017b). While experiencing the dream episode, the sleeper can moan and thrash around in the bed, possibly causing harm to a bed partner or themselves (Wilson et al., 2019).
- *Sleep terrors/night terrors* are more common in children and occur during the deepest stages of sleep. Typical behavior involves waking up screaming, signs of intense fear, sitting up in bed accompanied by increased heart rate or breathing, sweating, and being unresponsive to comforting (Cleveland Clinic, 2017b; Wilson et al., 2019). They may appear to be awake and reasonable but are unable to communicate when they awaken from a sleep terror.
- *Nightmare disorder* involves frightening dreams that are vivid and disturbing. They occur more frequently in children and represent a normal developmental process.
- *Sleep enuresis* is urinating during sleep or bedwetting. Primary bedwetting occurs when a child at least 5 years old has never regularly stayed dry during sleep for 6 straight months (Pacheco, 2020b). It is more common in males. Secondary bedwetting occurs when a child or adult had earlier stayed dry for at least 6 straight months and then began bedwetting at least twice a week for a period of at least 3 months (American Academy of Sleep Medicine, n.d.). Secondary bedwetting can occur at any age and may be related to other health issues, such as a urinary tract problem, chronic constipation, OSA, social or psychological stress, or inability to concentrate urine, as in sickle cell disease or some forms of diabetes (American Academy of Sleep Medicine, n.d.). Children with secondary bedwetting have often recently faced a strong social or mental stress, such as parental divorce, physical or sexual abuse, or neglect (American Academy of Sleep Medicine, n.d.).
- *Sleep paralysis* is a brief state of involuntary immobility occurring on waking from a night's sleep or a nap, and may be accompanied by dreams (which may be of a frightening kind) (Wilson et al., 2019).
- *Sleep-related eating disorder* occurs when a person eats and drinks while sleeping but has no recollection of eating in the morning. It can occur during sleepwalking, and those affected can gain weight and experience injury

either from cooking in their sleep or eating potentially dangerous raw food or inedible or toxic substances, such as coffee grounds, cleaning solutions or cigarette butts (Cleveland Clinic, 2021). They may not be easily awakened or redirected during an episode and may exhibit signs of sleep disruption during waking hours.

There is little good evidence for treatment of parasomnias (Wilson et al., 2019). Parasomnias may be treated by improving sleep habits, including maintaining a regular sleep schedule; good sleep hygiene, and obtaining an adequate amount of sleep. Medication may be used to control symptoms based on the frequency and severity of the events (Wilson et al., 2019). It is important to safeguard against harm to the patient; locking of window and doors and sleeping on the ground floor may be considered. Interventions to increase the safety of a bed partner and children in the home should be considered as well (Wilson et al., 2019).

Sleep-Related Movement Disorders

There are several sleep-related movement disorders, which are characterized by physical movements during sleep. These movements may be irresistible or involuntary, occur during sleep or periods of rest and frequently result in insomnia and daytime fatigue (Kaiser Permanente, n.d.a). Some of the disorders in this group include sleep-related leg cramps and bruxism (grinding or clenching of the teeth), and restless legs syndrome (Kaiser Permanente, n.d.a).

Restless legs syndrome (RLS), also known as Willis–Ekbom disease (WED), is a common sleep-related neurologic disorder that affects approximately 7% to 10% of the people in the United States, including children and adults (NSF, 2020d; Restless Legs Syndrome Foundation, 2020). Abnormalities in the neurotransmitter dopamine have been associated with RLS (CDC, 2020). RLS involves involuntary movement of the legs when the body is at rest (NSF, 2020d). Patients with RLS cannot lie still and report unpleasant creeping, crawling, itching, aching, burning, throbbing, pulling, or tingling sensations and pain and discomfort in the legs (NSF, 2020d; RLS Foundation, 2020. Occasionally, RLS can occur in the arms, face, or torso. Patients describe an irresistible urge to move the legs when these sensations occur, usually during the evening and night, which may lead to kicking and/or the need to move around or pace, resulting in loss of sleep (CDC, 2020). Symptoms usually affect both sides of the body but can alternate between the left and right leg or occasionally occur only on one side of the body (NSF, 2020d). Women are at greater risk of having RLS, although both men and women can develop the condition, and it can begin at any age; research indicates that there is a genetic component to the disorder (NSF, 2020d). Additional risk factors include the use of antinausea medications and antidepressants, iron deficiency, renal disease, nerve damage, pregnancy, and rheumatoid arthritis or osteoarthritis. The use of alcohol, nicotine, and caffeine may also increase the risk for RLS (NSF, 2020d). This disorder has no specific diagnostic test and no known cure.

Nonpharmacologic measures to prevent or alleviate this discomfort include massaging the legs, walking, doing knee bends, and moving or gently stretching the legs. Research continues into additional treatment options, but the following may prove effective (Klingelhoefer et al., 2016):

- Avoiding high intake of caffeine and alcohol before bedtime
- Promoting good sleep habits (quiet, comfortable, cool sleeping environment; keeping regular bed and wake hours)
- Walking and stretching, massaging the affected limbs
- Using relaxation techniques; biofeedback and yoga may also relieve symptoms (see the accompanying Promoting Health Literacy display on page 1316).

Several medications may be used if symptoms are clinically significant with associated impairment of nighttime sleep, daytime alertness, and quality of life (Klingelhoefer et al., 2016). Medication to help correct the underlying dopamine abnormality combined with medication to promote sleep continuity may be prescribed (CDC, 2020). In general, the dosage is kept as low as possible and is administered as a single dose in the evening; medications recommended to treat RLS include ropinirole, pramipexole dihydrochloride, gabapentin enacarbil, and rotigotine transdermal system (Klingelhoefer et al., 2016). The Restless Legs Syndrome Foundation (http://www.rls.org) is a support group available for the millions of people with this disorder who experience chronic sleep loss.

Sleep Deprivation

Sleep deprivation describes the cumulative effect of a person not having sufficient sleep, a decrease in the amount, consistency, or quality of sleep. It may result from decreased REM sleep or NREM sleep. There are many causes, including the presence of a sleep disorder, such as insomnia, sleep apnea, or RLS, inadequate sleep behaviors, and insufficient total sleep time (Refer to the discussions related to common sleep disorders in this chapter). Manifestations of sleep deprivation progress from irritability and impaired mental abilities to a total disintegration of personality. Sleep deprivation may result in daytime fatigue and decreased alertness; impaired learning, focusing, memory, and reactions; trouble controlling emotions and behavior; difficulty interpreting other people's emotions and reactions; and feelings of worry, frustration, and anxiety (NHLBI, n.d.b). Children who are sleep deficient may have different reactions of deprivation, with resulting over activity, behavior issues, and difficulty paying attention as well as mood swings, anger, impulsivity, or lack of motivation (NHLBI, n.d.b). Sleep deficiency is associated with increased risk of injury, such as automobile accidents and fatalities, aviation accidents, and accidental falls and related fractures (NHLBI, n.d.b).

Partial sleep deprivation may result in loss of concentration, inattention, and impaired information processing, and poses serious safety risks. Excessive daytime sleepiness, a form of partial sleep deprivation, impairs performance at

Promoting Health Literacy

IN PATIENTS WITH RESTLESS LEGS SYNDROME

Patient Scenario

Mary Weymouth is a 40-year-old person who has an appointment to see her primary health care provider because of a "strange sensation in her legs that is keeping her awake at night." When asked by the nurse to further describe her symptoms, Mary explains that she has this feeling that "something is crawling up her lower leg." She keeps moving her leg from side to side until she finally just gets out of bed and walks around for a while. She states that movement seems to "make it better" but this does not work all the time. Sometimes, she also gets "pretty severe cramping pain" that can last several hours. Mary relates that this has been happening 2 or 3 nights a week for at least 1 month and she finds that she is "very sleepy" the following day. At times when she is at work, she said that she finds herself starting to "nod off" and is afraid that someone might notice, and she could lose her job. She's tried drinking a few glasses of wine at night to relax her and has also occasionally taken "some Tylenol PM" to see if that will help her sleep through the night. Nothing seems to help. After the health care provider examined Mary, he asked if anyone in her family had similar symptoms. Mary remembered that her mother used to tell her that she sometimes had "nervous legs" at night. The health care provider reviews her history and tells Mary that her symptoms indicate that she has restless legs syndrome (RLS). At this time, he prefers not to prescribe medication for her but wants her to try some nonpharmacologic measures to see if they ease her symptoms. As Mary is making another appointment, she tells the nurse that "she doesn't know how much longer she can manage without a good night's sleep most nights. I may just have to give Tylenol PM another try."

Nursing Considerations: *Tips for Improving Health Literacy*

Provide Mary with some specific information about measures that may ease her symptoms of RLS and allow her to get a restful sleep. Recommend that she avoid alcohol, caffeine, and any OTC sleeping medications because they contain antihistamines that may aggravate the symptoms of RLS. Encourage her to participate in and incorporate into her daily life regular, moderate physical activity to promote better sleep at night. Explain to Mary that there is no specific diagnostic test for RLS, but if her symptoms are not relieved by these other measures, there is medication that the health care provider might prescribe. Also, give her information about the online resource that is specifically for patients with RLS. When Mary returns for her follow-up appointment, she needs to be prepared to ask her health care provider the following questions:

- What is my main problem? Can anything else be associated with RLS?
- What else do I need to do?
- Why is it important for me to do this?
- What can you do if you prescribe a medication, but it does not help with my symptoms?

What additional measures can you take to help increase health literacy in this patient? What other measures would be helpful if Mary did not speak English, could not read, or had other learning deficits?

times when people need to be alert. The strange environment of the hospital, physical discomfort and pain, the effects of medications, and the need for 24-hour nursing care may also contribute to sleep deprivation in hospitalized patients (Delaney et al., 2018; Grimm, 2020).

As mentioned earlier in this chapter, recent research has indicated the possibility of a causal relationship between sleep deprivation and obesity, altered healing, depression, diabetes, and cardiovascular conditions. However, sleep deprivation clearly produces changes in physical and mental functioning, supporting the belief that sleep is essential for well-being. Whether it occurs as a result of a disorder or is due to voluntary sleep curtailment, sleep deprivation has wide-ranging negative consequences for human health and well-being (American Sleep Association [ASA], n.d.a). See also the earlier section, Physical and Psychological Effects of Insufficient Sleep.

The primary treatment of sleep deprivation is to increase total sleep time (ASA, n.d.a). Interventions are directed at the cause of deprivation for the individual patient and should also address improving sleep habits. Daytime naps may be beneficial but should be limited to earlier in the afternoon and, for adults, be no longer than 20 minutes to avoid troubles falling asleep at night (NHLBI, n.d.b). Napping in preschool-age children is normal and promotes healthy growth and development (NHLBI, n.d.b). Refer to the discussion of interventions to promote rest and sleep in the following sections.

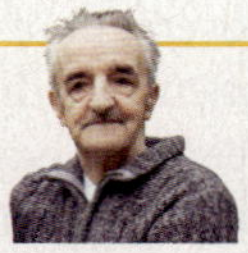

Recall **Charlie Bitner**, the long-term care facility resident complaining of sleep problems. From the patient's statements, the nurse would identify that Mr. Bitner is at risk for developing sleep deprivation. Therefore, the nurse would work with Mr. Bitner to establish measures that would promote effective sleep patterns.

Unfolding Patient Stories: Edith Jacobson • Part 2

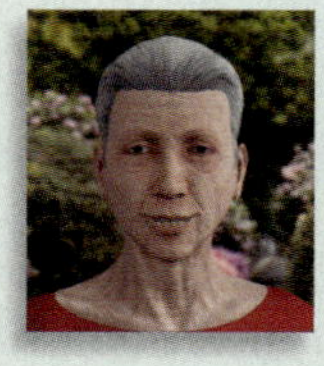

Recollect **Edith Jacobson** from Chapter 31, who is 85 and hospitalized for surgical repair of a left hip fracture. Are risk factors present for her to develop disordered sleep patterns or a lack of adequate sleep? How can insufficient sleep affect her physical and psychological health? What nursing interventions can promote adequate rest and sleep while Edith is hospitalized?

Care for Edith and other patients in a realistic virtual environment: ***vSim** for Nursing* (thepoint.lww.com/vSimFunds). Practice documenting these patients' care in DocuCare (thepoint.lww.com/DocuCareEHR).

NURSING PROCESS FOR REST AND SLEEP

Assessing

Sleep status can have a significant impact on health and a patient's ability to cope with illness. Nursing assessment of a patient's sleep and rest habits and status includes pertinent patient history and physical assessment. Sleep studies may be prescribed by an advanced practice professional and completed as part of the data collection process.

Rest and Sleep Nursing History

Health care providers in all settings should incorporate questions about sleep into routine health assessment. Interview questions help identify the patient's sleep–wakefulness patterns, the effect of these patterns on everyday functioning, the presence of factors that may be affecting the patient's sleep, the patient's use of sleep aids, and the presence of sleep disturbances and contributing factors. If the patient's sleep is adequate and poses no problems, the sleep history may be brief. At a minimum, ask the following questions of a patient (Weber & Kelley, 2018:

- Do you feel you are getting enough sleep?
- Do you feel rested when you awaken?
- How much sleep do you get each night?
- What do you do to help you fall asleep?
- Do you find it difficult to stay awake during the day?

When the patient's response to any of the interview questions indicates a potential problem, open-ended questions may be used to gather more data (Focused Assessment Guide 35-1).

Assess the patient's usual times for retiring and waking, bedtime rituals, and preferences regarding sleep environment

Focused Assessment Guide 35-1

REST AND SLEEP

Factors to Assess	Questions and Approaches
Usual sleep–wakefulness pattern: Recent changes	Do you set an alarm and hit "snooze" before getting up?
	How many hours of sleep do you usually get in a day?
Usual sleeping and waking times	Do you wake up earlier in the morning than you would like and find it difficult to fall back asleep?
	Have there been any recent changes in your usual sleep–wake patterns? If yes, describe them and tell me if they are causing any problems for you.
	Do you usually go to bed and wake up about the same time each day?
Number of hours of undisturbed sleep	How have you been sleeping?
	Do you have any difficulty falling asleep?
	Do you wake up frequently during the night?
	Do you dream at night?
	Are your dreams frightening?
Quality of sleep	How much sleep do you think you need to feel rested?
Number and duration of naps	Do you take naps throughout the day?
Effect of sleep pattern on everyday functioning	In what way does the sleep you get each day affect your everyday living?
	Has this sleep disturbance caused any change in your sex life?
Energy level (ability to perform activities of daily living)	Do you feel rested and ready to start the day when you wake up?
	Are there times during the day or certain activities when you feel especially tired?
	What happens when you don't get enough sleep?
	Are you having difficulty concentrating?
Sleep aids	What do you do to relax before you get ready for bed?
Means of relaxing before bedtime	Describe what you usually do to help yourself fall asleep.
Bedtime rituals	Tell me how you like your room (lights, noises, ventilation, position of door, temperature) and bed (mattress, pillows, blankets) when you are sleeping.
Sleep environment	Do you take any medications to help you sleep?
Pharmacologic aids	Are you taking any medicine at all?
Sleep disturbances and contributing factors	Tell me about your sleep problem.
	How often does it occur?
Nature of the sleep disturbance	Are you doing anything differently now that might be causing the problem?
Onset of disturbance	Do you wake up gasping for air?
Causes (physical, psychosocial, medicine related)	Do you snore?
	Do you recall changing your position frequently during the night?
Severity	What have you been doing to deal with the problem?
Symptoms	How effective were these measures?
Interventions attempted and results	

Nursing Advocacy in Action

Patient Scenario

Maria was born premature. After surgery on her bowel, she was placed on the transplantation list for a new liver and small bowel and started on total parenteral nutrition. She is now 9 months old but has spent the last 4 weeks in the hospital with fungemia, a fungus infection spread throughout the bloodstream. Her single mother, Ms. Gomez, practically lives at the hospital and in recent days has annoyed the nurses with her complaints about the nursing care. Her English is limited, but she is able to express her annoyance at the many times Maria is awakened during the night for treatment and care. "Why can't the nurses do several things at once so Maria can at least get a few hours of uninterrupted sleep?!" Recently the nurses complained to the medical director, and he informed Ms. Gomez that if she doesn't stop interfering with Maria's care, the doctors will take Maria off the transplantation list. The nurse giving you the report repeats this story and tells you "not to take any complaints or grief from the mom." When you meet Ms. Gomez and listen to her story, you admire her love for Maria and willingness to advocate for her. You also sense the mother's frustration with the system. She asks you tearfully, "They can't take Maria off the list, can they? I am only trying to be a good mother." Ms. Gomez appears to have no family or other support network.

Implications for Nursing Advocacy

How would you respond if you were the nurse assigned Maria as a patient? Talk with your classmates and experienced nurses about the questions that follow.

- Is it fair to say that Ms. Gomez is being threatened for trying to advocate for her baby? If you elect to advocate for Maria and her mother, what practical steps can you take to remedy this situation?
- What is it reasonable to expect of a student nurse, graduate nurse, and an experienced nurse in this situation?
- What advocacy skills are needed to effectively respond to this challenge?

so that these can be incorporated into the plan of care, if possible. Patients in hospitals or other care facilities often receive fragmented sleep. Their sleep may be disrupted by routine care measures, noise in the environment, and lighting (see the accompanying Nursing Advocacy in Action display). Paying attention to small matters can make the difference between a patient's having a good night of sleep or no sleep.

When a sleep disturbance is noted, ask about the following when obtaining the history:

- The nature of the problem
- The cause of the problem
- The related signs and symptoms
- When the problem began and how often it occurs
- How the problem affects everyday living
- The severity of the problem and whether it can be treated independently by nurses or needs to be referred to another health care professional
- How the patient is coping with the problem and the success of any treatments attempted

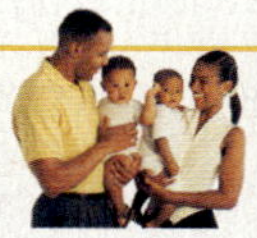

Think back to **Lydia Omeara**, the mother of twin infants who was asking about allowing the infants to sleep in their parents' bed. The nurse would need to obtain a sleep history from Mrs. Omeara to ascertain both her and her husband's sleep patterns. This information would be helpful in assisting Mrs. Omeara and her husband in making a decision about allowing the children to sleep in their parents' bed.

Assistance from the patient's bed partner may be needed to aid in data collection and provide more accurate information regarding the patient's sleep patterns. The patient's record may also contain pertinent information (e.g., a history of illnesses that influence sleep).

Sleep Diary

A sleep diary or log provides more specific data on the patient's sleep–wakefulness patterns over a period of time. It is completed over a period of time and provides information and insight about these patterns, possibly indicating activities and behaviors that affect the quality and quantity of sleep. In general, the diary is kept for 1 or 2 weeks and typically includes the total number of hours of sleep per day, the number of undisturbed hours of sleep, number of awakenings, and other details (Ibáñez et al., 2018). There are many versions of sleep diaries, and the information to be documented may include:

- Time patient retires
- Time patient tries to fall asleep
- Approximate time patient falls asleep
- Time of any awakenings during the night and when sleep was resumed
- Time of awakening in the morning
- Presence of any stressors the patient believes are affecting their sleep
- A record of any food, drink, or medication the patient believes has positively or negatively influenced their sleep (include time of ingestion)
- Record of physical activities—type, duration, and time
- Record of mental activities—type, duration, and time
- Record of activities performed 2 to 3 hours before bedtime, bedtime rituals, changes in sleep environment
- Presence of any worries or anxieties the patient believes are affecting their sleep

Sleep diaries are also available as mobile apps (Ibáñez et al., 2018) and offer the advantage of reducing the time needed for data entry and scoring (Tonetti et al., 2016).

It is helpful if the patient has a bed partner who can assist with the diary. The patient needs to understand that the diary is simply a diagnostic tool. If keeping the diary causes too much stress for the patient and further interferes with the ability to sleep restfully, it should be discontinued. A sample diary is available from the National Sleep Foundation.

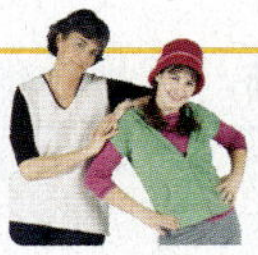

Remember **Jeanette Clark**, the mother of the adolescent girl who seems to be sleeping all the time. Having Mrs. Clark's daughter complete a sleep diary might be helpful in obtaining a better picture of what is happening and helping rule out other causes for the daughter's increased fatigue and sleeping. These underlying causes could be wide ranging, including such conditions as depression, physical illness, or increased activity or schoolwork.

Sleep Screening Tools

There are additional questionnaire screening tools that can be used to assess sleep disturbances and the quality of sleep. Some examples include:

- Epworth Sleepiness Scale
- Pittsburgh Sleep Quality Index (PSQI)
- STOP-Bang Questionnaire (OSA)
- Stanford Sleepiness Scale

Physical Assessment

The findings in the physical assessment may either confirm that the patient is getting sufficient rest to provide energy for the day's activities or validate the existence of a sleep disturbance that is decreasing the quantity or quality of sleep. Key findings include energy level (presence of physical weakness, fatigue, lethargy, or decreased energy), facial characteristics (narrowing or glazing of eyes, swelling of eyelids, decreased animation), or behavioral characteristics (yawning, rubbing eyes, slow speech, slumped posture). Physical data suggestive of potential sleep problems (e.g., obesity, enlarged neck, deviated nasal septum) may also be noted.

If the nurse or a bed partner can observe the patient sleeping, other sleep characteristics to assess include restlessness, sleep postures, and sleep activities such as snoring or leg jerking (RLS). Snoring is caused by an obstruction to airflow through the nose and mouth. Other than disturbing others in the same bedroom, snoring is not ordinarily a sleeping disorder. However, loud snoring or snoring accompanied by apnea can present a problem. When snoring changes from the characteristic sawing-wood sound to a more irregular silence followed by a snort, this indicates obstructive apnea. As mentioned earlier in the discussion of obstructive sleep apnea (OSA), snoring in children needs to be evaluated as a possible indication of OSA.

Additional Methods to Assess Sleep

There are several medical examinations and testing that can be done at a sleep clinic to assess sleep, sleep breathing, and sleep brain patterns to aid in evaluating sleep disturbances (Weber & Kelley, 2018).

The most used device to self-assess sleep is the smartphone (Ibáñez et al., 2018). Smartphones contain a microphone, camera, and an accelerometer (detects motion and determine tilt of the phone), and these features can be used to monitor sleep. As a result, many mobile apps have been developed and made available to assess sleep and support sleep self-management. Expert reviews have been completed and report high performance and reliability of these apps, but there is a lack of scientific validation studies to support clinical value and use (Choi et al., 2018; Ibáñez et al., 2018).

Diagnosing Actual or Potential Health Problems and Needs

An assessment of a patient's rest and sleep status may lead to the identification of one or more actual or potential health problems and needs related to rest and sleep. Following the formulation of the actual or potential health problems and needs, the nurse communicates findings to other nursing and health care professionals through the use of written and spoken word. The written actual or potential health problem or need becomes a permanent part of the patient's health record. Examples of health problems and needs with related etiology and signs and symptoms can be found in the Examples of Actual or Potential Health Problems and Needs: Rest and Sleep on page 1320.

Outcome Identification and Planning

Rest and sleep are essential components of well-being. Planning for patient care, especially in a health care facility, involves planning and collaborating with the patient to identify suitable goals in relation to rest and sleep. Nursing measures are directed toward the achievement of the following patient outcomes. The patient will:

- Maintain a sleep–wake pattern that provides sufficient energy for the day's tasks
- Demonstrate self-care behaviors that provide a healthy balance between rest and activity
- Identify stress-relieving rituals that enable the patient to fall asleep more easily
- Demonstrate decreased signs of sleep deprivation
- Verbalize feeling less fatigued and more in control of life activities

Implementing

In most cases, sleep problems are not the primary reason for a patient's interaction with the health care system. A key to detecting a patient's sleep problems is the use of appropriate communication skills while displaying a nonjudgmental, caring attitude. Patients who believe the nurse is generally concerned about their well-being are not reluctant to discuss their sleep concerns or problems. In order to correct a sleep problem, the patient needs to believe that the nurse cares and will provide help to promote rest and sleep. Interventions that promote good sleep and sleep hygiene

Examples of Actual or Potential Health Problems and Needs

REST AND SLEEP

Actual or Potential Health Problems and Needs	Possible Etiologic Factors	Potential Signs and Symptoms
Impaired sleep	Worries about family and lack of destressing rituals	• "At least 4 or 5 nights a week, I lay in bed awake for 3 or 4 hours before I finally fall asleep. Sometimes it is 2:00 or 3:00 in the morning, and I'm still awake worrying about the kids. I've tried getting up and reading or paying my bills, but even that doesn't make me sleepy." • Reports problem falling asleep for past 6 months; is widowed and very concerned about two teenage sons. Never sleeps until both sons are home. States she does nothing special to relax. Feels her worries are "her business"—no support person with whom she shares these. • Reports lack of energy and fatigue, difficulty completing activities of daily living.
Risk for impaired sleep	Noise of hospital environment and need for periodic treatments Frequent naps Post-surgical pain	—
Sleep deprivation	Frequent rotations of work shifts and overtime Inadequate sleep hygiene	• New graduate nurse, 24 years old, who has been working on a busy medical floor for 6 months; rotates 11–7 and 7–3 shifts; recently a problem with staffing has necessitated frequent rotations and often volunteers (two or three times a week) for overtime. • "I don't know what is wrong with me. I'm so tired anymore and don't feel at all like myself. All I want to do when I'm off is to sleep—but often I can't fall asleep when I lay down and often fall asleep when I should be awake. I can't concentrate. Please help!"

Source: International Council of Nurses (ICN). (2019). *Nursing diagnosis and outcome statements.* https://www.icn.ch/sites/default/files/inline-files/ICNP2019-DC.pdf; *Problem-based care plans.* (2020). In *Lippincott Advisor.* Wolters Kluwer. https://advisor.lww.com/lna/home.do

are important in maintaining health. **Sleep hygiene** is a set of behaviors or habits that may influence sleep quality (ASA, n.d.; Jansson-Fröjmark et al., 2019). Sleep hygiene involves the use of behaviors to facilitate sleep and avoidance of behaviors that interfere with sleep (Sleep Foundation, 2020d). Nursing care involves collaborating with the patient to identify suitable measures related to sleep hygiene and to promote rest and sleep.

QSEN EVIDENCE-BASED PRACTICE

It is important for the nurse to be able to identify evidence reports and guidelines related to appropriate and effective interventions to promote rest and sleep to support patients' health and well-being.

Preparing a Restful Environment

A comfortable bed (mattress and pillow) helps promote rest and sleep. The bottom linen should be tight and clean. The upper linen, while secure, should allow freedom of movement and should not exert pressure, especially over the legs and feet. Good body alignment is conducive to relaxation. For patients who must assume unusual positions because of their illness, ingenuity and skill are necessary to minimize muscle strain and discomfort. For example, patients who must sleep with their head and torso elevated to aid breathing should be well supported in a manner that relieves muscle strain.

A quiet and darkened room with privacy and a comfortable temperature promotes relaxation (ASA, n.d.b; NHLBI, n.d.b). Light-blocking curtains and/or an eye mask may be helpful in preventing light from interrupting sleep (Sleep Foundation, 2020d). In a strange environment, unfamiliar noises may be sources of distraction. Although some of these sounds are difficult to control, make every effort to reduce disturbances and to promote relaxation and sleep. Ear plugs or a fan or other background noise may be helpful in blocking disturbing noises (ASA, n.d.b; Sleep Foundation, 2020d; Sleep Foundation, 2020c). Many health care facilities have made attempts to transform their patient care areas into quieter settings that facilitate rest and sleep. Refer to the discussion related to minimizing sleep disturbances in health care settings on p. 1322.

Focus on the Older Adult

AGE-RELATED CHANGES AND NURSING STRATEGIES FOR REST AND SLEEP

Age-Related Changes	Nursing Strategies
Initiation of Sleep	
• Decreased physical activities	• Encourage patient to engage in some type of physical activity, such as walking or water aerobics.
• Tired and fatigued throughout day	• Discourage napping throughout day.
• Depression	• Arrange for assessment for depression and treatment.
• Polypharmacy	• Review medications that patient is taking and assess for any side effects of sleep pattern disturbances.
Maintaining Sleep	
• Nocturia	• Decrease fluids during the evening.
• Sleep-related movement disturbances (e.g., RLS)	• Take diuretics in the morning or early evening.
	• Discuss problems with health care provider.

The temperature of the room, the amount of ventilation, and the amount of bed covering are matters of individual choice. Meet the patient's wishes when at all possible. Many older adults cannot sleep if they feel cold. Thermal blankets or comforters, insulated bed socks, cotton flannel sheets, leg warmers, long underwear, and a cap help patients stay warm and promote comfort and sleep. Refer to Focus on the Older Adult for additional suggestions.

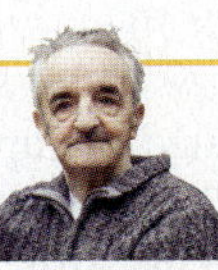

Recall **Charlie Bitner**, the older man living in a long-term care facility. The nurse would work with Mr. Bitner to ensure that his sleeping area is as comfortable and restful as possible. Making sure that he is warm enough, dimming the lights, closing the door (as appropriate), and minimizing disturbances outside his room would be key.

Promoting Bedtime Rituals

A comfortable pre-bedtime routine can promote good sleep (ASA, n.d.b). Many people have bedtime rituals to help them relax and promote sleep. Reading, listening to soft music, light stretching, relaxation exercises, talking to a family member, meditation or quite time, and praying are common before-sleep activities that can help put a person at ease and make it easier to fall asleep (ASA, n.d.b; Sleep Foundation, 2020d). Children may take a favorite doll, stuffed toy, or blanket to bed; listen to a bedtime story; kiss everyone good night; and say prayers before bed (Fig. 35-4). Readiness for sleep follows a personal hygiene routine for many people, such as brushing teeth, washing hands and face, voiding, or taking a warm bath or shower. Snacks are acceptable and are important elements in the bedtime rituals of many children and adults. Refer to the discussion below and to the previous discussion of dietary habits on page 1309.

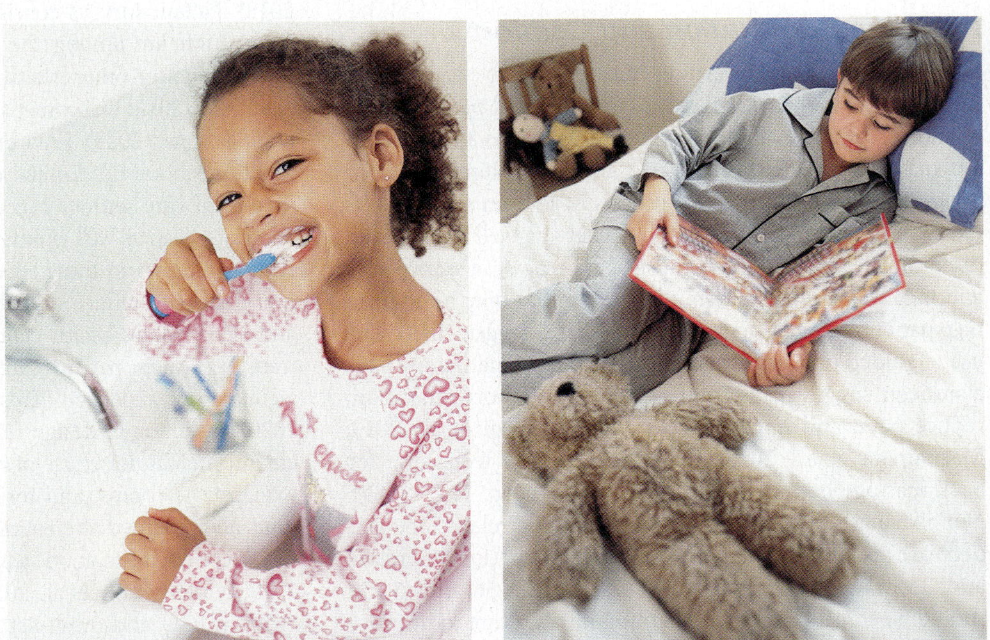

FIGURE 35-4. A bedtime routine helps promote sleep in children.

To promote relaxation and sleep, be alert to the patient's bedtime rituals and observe them as much as possible. Include these rituals in the patient's plan of care so that all health personnel can observe them.

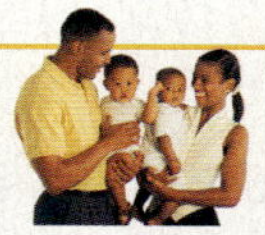

Teaching **Mrs. Omeara** about the importance of bedtime rituals for her twin infants may promote the children's sleep. In addition, the nurse would need to reinforce the need for Mrs. Omeara's bedtime rituals to ensure that the sleep she obtains is restful.

Offering Appropriate Bedtime Snacks and Beverages

A light snack is acceptable (NHLBI, n.d.b; Sleep Foundation, 2020d); going to bed hungry may interfere with sleep. As discussed earlier in the chapter, combining foods that are high in tryptophan with healthy, complex carbohydrates improves sleep (Binks et al., 2020; Sleep Foundation, 2020b). As a result, there appears to be justification for offering a snack that contains a protein and a carbohydrate before bedtime, if this is allowed in the patient's treatment regimen. Large, heavy or spicy meals within a few hours of bedtime may produce a bad night's sleep and should be avoided (NHLBI, n.d.b; Sleep Foundation, 2020d).

Recommend that the patient take fluids during the day but avoid excessive fluid intake before bedtime to prevent the need to use the bathroom during the night. Alcoholic beverages later in the evening should be avoided because they may interrupt the normal sleep cycle and interfere with deep sleep (Sleep Foundation, 2020b). For most patients, consumption of beverages containing caffeine should be reduced or avoided for at least 4 to 5 hours before bedtime; effects of caffeine can last as long as 8 hours (ASA, n.d.b; NHLBI, n.d.b; Sleep Foundation, 2020d).

Refer also to the previous discussion of dietary habits on page 1309.

Promoting Relaxation and Comfort

We can relax without sleeping but sleep rarely occurs until we are relaxed. Stress, anxiety, discomfort, and pain occur in relation to or as result of many health problems and interfere with a person's ability to relax, rest, and sleep. Numerous nonpharmacologic nursing interventions have been shown to be effective in alleviating stress and anxiety as well as pain and discomfort. A backrub, soft music, gentle noise, a warm bath, and face washing are nursing measures that may be used to help patients relax (Macnamara et al., 2018; Yeager, 2019). The use of guided imagery, visual imagery and aromatherapy have also been suggested as interventions to support relaxation, reduce pain, and improve sleep (Cheraghbeigi et al., 2019; Macnamara et al., 2018; Yeager, 2019). The technique for back massage is described in Skill 36-1 (on pp. 1377–1380). Nonpharmacologic interventions to aid in relaxation, and decrease discomfort and pain, including distraction and relaxation techniques, are described in Chapters 29, 36, and 43 and should be considered when planning nursing care to improve patient well-being and sleep.

Respecting Normal Sleep–Wake Patterns

A consistent sleep schedule, including sleep–wake regularity, is beneficial in achieving good sleep (ASA, n.d.b; Chung et al., 2018; Sleep Foundation, 2020d). Make every effort to allow patients to experience their normal period of sleep. In many instances, insisting that all patients retire and awaken at specific times is not necessary. For example, is there a good reason to wake a patient at 0700 if the patient ordinarily sleeps until 0800? The patient's normal napping habits should also be followed when possible. Sleep during morning naps consists primarily of light NREM and possibly REM sleep. Napping later in the evening when a person's sleep drive increases is comprised of more deep sleep, which may disrupt the person's ability to fall asleep at night (Pacheco, 2020c). With this knowledge, help patients plan napping periods that best fit their needs and interfere the least amount with nighttime sleeping. Additional information about napping is provided in the previous discussion related to sleep deprivation on page 1315.

Minimizing Sleep and Rest Disturbances in Health Care Settings

Factors associated with sleep disturbance in health care environments include light; noise made by health care staff, health care equipment/machines, and other patients; and care interactions (Delaney et al., 2018; Grimm, 2020; Hedges et al., 2019; Trossman, 2018). Studies have demonstrated that excessive noise on patient care units interferes with sleep and that these noise-related disruptions can increase patient anxiety, length of stay, and blood pressure; decrease oxygen saturation; increase pain and discomfort; diminish immune responses; and delay wound healing as well as having other negative effects (Crawford et al., 2018; Delaney, 2016; Reuter-Rice et al., 2020; Trossman, 2018; Wallis et al., 2019). Behavioral manifestations such as disorientation, restlessness, and irritability are also possible consequences, particularly in older adults (Hedges & Gotelli, 2020; Trossman, 2018). Patient surveys consistently report that noise and sleep deprivation are among the top concerns during admittance to a hospital or other health care facilities (Adatia et al., 2014; Anderson, 2012; Dobson et al., 2019; Fillary et al., 2015; Oleksy & Schlesinger, 2019). Environmental factors impacting a good night's sleep are not limited to acute care settings; residents in long-term care settings can encounter challenges in obtaining adequate sleep as well (Ellmers et al., 2013; Steiner et al., 2020). Although some of these sounds are difficult to control, make every effort to reduce disturbances and to promote relaxation and sleep. Many health care facilities have made attempts to transform their patient care areas into quieter settings that facilitate rest and sleep (Trossman, 2018; Winterbottom et al., 2020). Attention to design features with a focus on eliminating environmental noise, use of noise monitors, providing patients with private rooms, and formal quiet times (quiet hours) on units all are aimed at creating a more supportive environment that is conducive to good sleep (Hedges et al., 2019; Tabas et al., 2019; Winterbottom et al., 2020).

In an ICU and other settings, sleep is even further challenged by the level of light in the patient care areas as well

35-1 Focused Critical Thinking Guide

SLEEP

You have just arrived on the unit and checked your clinical assignment. You have two patients today and about 30 minutes before preconference. Your routine is to review their charts for pertinent information, go and introduce yourself to them, and take their morning vital signs before preconference. With 10 minutes to spare, you visit your second patient and find that he is sound asleep. Remembering that he had a fractured hip repaired 2 days ago and that the night nurse had stated in his note that the patient was restless and awake until 0400, you are reluctant to awaken him. On the other hand, at your midterm conference your instructor commented that you need to improve your organizational skills. If you don't have your vital signs recorded until after preconference, then breakfast arrives, doctors make rounds, and you're that much further behind in your morning care and documentation. When you look at the last set of vitals documented in the patient's EHR from midnight, you note the vital signs were within normal limits. You're attempting to reconcile several things—the importance of these morning vital signs, the patient's need for sleep, and your need to accomplish your tasks on time and receive a good evaluation. What should you do?

1. Identify goal of thinking

Determine whether it is more important to awaken your patient for morning vital signs or let him sleep at least until after your preconference.

2. Assess adequacy of knowledge

Pertinent circumstances: Your patient had major surgery 2 days ago, did not have a restful night, but is sleeping peacefully now. You realize that his vital signs can be an important indicator of a complication. You also need to accomplish your tasks in a timely and organized manner.

Prerequisite knowledge: To make your decision, you need knowledge about his postoperative condition and assessment data that indicate he is recovering or developing a complication. You are aware that sleep is vital to promote tissue repair, physical recovery, and mental well-being. You also need to review the tasks that you need to accomplish this morning and decide how and if priorities could be shifted.

Room for error/time constraints: Will a delay in taking vital signs cause injury to this patient? You are not planning to omit this task but just questioning whether to postpone it and allow the patient to have some additional sleep.

3. Address potential problems

Waking your patient for vital signs may be disturbing for him and interfere with his need for rest. A decision to postpone morning vital signs might also cause several problems. If the patient has developed a complication, such as an infection, his elevated temperature may go undetected for at least another hour. By the time you come out of preconference, the patient may be eating his breakfast, which further delays recording of vital signs. You perceive that you are already falling behind on your schedule and are really intent on completing your responsibilities on time today.

4. Consult helpful resources

Before you make your decision, you should check the patient's health record and note whether the previous set of vital signs were within normal limits. The primary nurse and your instructor may also help you sort through your priorities in this situation.

5. Critique judgment/decision

You have two choices here. If you wake your patient and take his vital signs, you are disturbing him when he is sleeping soundly, risking the fact that he may be angry with you, but you are on schedule for the day's activities. By postponing his vital signs at least until after postconference, you provide additional rest for the patient but know that you are already behind schedule and worry that your instructor will view you as disorganized. After reviewing your options and checking his EHR again, you decide to allow him to sleep and plan to take them as soon as possible after your preconference. During preconference, when your instructor reviews your priorities for the day, she comments positively that you have individualized care based on your particular patient's needs at the moment. In your mind, you determine that the vital signs are your next priority and will take minimal time, and you should still be able to complete care and documentation in a competent manner and on time.

as continuous exposure to light (Grimm, 2020; Trossman, 2018). Nighttime light can range from a level similar to that at twilight and peak at a level brighter than lighting in some television studios (Dave et al., 2015).

The scheduled nursing care can also be a source of disturbances to a patient's ability to achieve rest and sleep (Lampron & Copeland, 2019). Many patients report being awakened to take sleeping pills and are roused in the early morning to prepare for breakfast long before it is served. Consider these common complaints when developing the patient's plan of care; whenever possible, schedule nursing care to avoid unnecessary disturbances and to promote rest and sleep. Provide care during periods when the patient is normally awake. When this is not feasible, avoid awakening the patient during REM sleep, when the rapid eye movements can be observed. Because a patient's need for sleep is important, examine priorities for nursing care with the goal of decreasing staff interruptions (Dobson et al., 2019; Graham et al., 2021). For example, consider whether checking a vital sign or carrying out a particular nursing measure is more important than the patient's sleep (refer to the Focused Critical Thinking Guide 35-1).

Technology Alert

A sleep headband that actively cancels exterior sounds has been developed for use with patients to decrease environmental noise and promote sleep. The headband monitors a patient's vital signs and wirelessly transmits results to a central nursing station. The device consists of thin headband with two earpieces, a small plastic case that contains a wireless transmitter, pulse oximetry and thermometer sensors, and an auxiliary jack to enable optional playing of music (Vincensi et al., 2016).

Nursing interventions to manage factors associated with sleep disturbances in the health care environment to facilitate rest and sleep for patients should be based on individual patient needs and preferences and include:

- Maintaining a brighter room environment during daylight hours and reducing patients' light exposure during the night (Grimm, 2020; Trossman, 2018; Winterbottom et al., 2020).
- Decreasing the volume on alarms, telephones, and limiting staff conversations (Goeren et al., 2018; Grimm, 2020; Oleksy & Schlesinger, 2019
- Closing doors to patient rooms (Antonio, 2020).
- Bundling of care, scheduling and grouping care activities together so as not to awaken or disturb patients multiple times for interventions that can safely be postponed for a short time (Dobson et al., 2019; Graham et al., 2021; Grimm, 2020; Trossman, 2018).
- Medicating for pain as indicated and prescribed (Dobson et al., 2019).
- Keeping the room cool and providing sheets and blankets to the patient's comfort level (Dave et al., 2015; Dobson et al., 2019).
- Scheduling a quiet time, a period of rest overnight, in which patients are not awakened unless their condition or care specifically requires it (Graham et al., 2021; Lampron & Copeland, 2019).
- Providing ear plugs and/or eye masks, if requested and as appropriate (Antonio, 2020; Tabas et al., 2019). See the accompanying Research in Nursing display.

Additional interventions to minimize noise levels have been implemented at some health care facilities. These initiatives include innovative use of communication technology to target noise reduction, and campaigns titled "Shhh" (Silent Hospitals Help Healing), "Hush" (Help Us Support Healing), and institution of "Quiet Time" (Goeren et al., 2018; Hedges et al., 2019). It is difficult to guarantee rest and a good night's

Research in Nursing

BRIDGING THE GAP TO EVIDENCE-BASED PRACTICE

Earplugs and Eye Masks and Quality of Sleep in the Cardiac Care Unit

Sleep is essential for the well-being of a person. Many physiologic, psychological, and environmental factors contribute to sleep disruption for patients in health care settings, and particularly for patients in intensive care units (ICUs).

Related Research

Tabas, E. E., Khodadadi, F., Sarani, H., Saeedinezhad, F., & Jahantigh, M. (2019). Effect of eye masks, earplugs, and quiet time protocol on sleep quality of patients admitted to the cardiac care unit: A clinical trial study. *Medical Surgical Nursing Journal*, 8(3), e98762. https://doi.org/10.5812/msnj.98762

This quasi-experimental study aimed to compare the impact of applying eye masks and earplugs and the implementation of a quiet time (QT) protocol on the sleep quality of patients in the cardiac care unit of a hospital. Patients who met the eligibility criteria (n = 135) were assigned to three groups (n = 45 each) based on admission to the CCU. Participants were sequentially assigned first to the control group (usual care), the eye mask and earplugs group, and then the QT protocol group. The subjects were studied over 3 days after admission. The morning after the first night, the participants' sleep quality was measured using the Verran and Snyder-Halpern Sleep Scale (VSH). The VSH assesses the mental response of hospitalized adults to sleep and perceptions of the previous night's sleep, with questions divided into two domains: sleep effectiveness and sleep disturbance. On the second and third nights, the eye mask and earplugs and QT protocol were implemented for each group, respectively. The morning after the second and third nights, the participants' sleep quality was measured again. Results indicated the control group had scores indicating poor sleep quality, and the earplug and eye mask group had scores indicating decreased sleep disturbance and increased sleep efficacy. The mean score of sleep disturbance after the intervention was significantly different between the control and the two intervention groups ($p = .001$). The mean score of sleep efficacy was higher in the eye mask and earplugs group than the control group ($p = .002$). Patients' sleep quality improved after applying earplugs and using eye masks. Implementation of the QT protocol was effective in reducing sleep disturbance. The researchers concluded earplugs and eye mask are appropriate nonpharmacologic interventions to promote quality of sleep among CCU patients and nurses should use these tools to help reduce environmental factors which disturb patients' sleep.

Relevance to Nursing Practice

It is difficult to always completely control environmental factors in health care settings that may interfere with a patient's ability to sleep. Sleep is an important consideration in supporting patients' well-being and health. Nurses should consider strategies to incorporate into patient care to promote quality sleep. Earplugs and eye masks could be used as a sleep intervention for patients when appropriate.

sleep during admission to a health care facility but recognizing and listening to patients' concerns are critical to delivery of thoughtful person-centered care.

Using Medications to Promote Sleep

Medications may be prescribed as part of the plan of care to address disturbances in sleep. A thorough health history, drug history, and sleep history, as well as assessment of stress and coping patterns and any underlying medical conditions, are required prior to the use of medications to induce or maintain sleep. The underlying cause for the sleep disturbance must be determined; nonpharmacologic interventions should be tried first or in combination with pharmacologic therapy (Adams et al., 2019; Singh, 2016). Refer also to the discussion in the previous sections, as well as the Insomnia and Teaching About Rest and Sleep sections on pages 1326 and 1327.

When sleep disturbances cannot be managed by other means, medications may be prescribed (pharmacotherapy) to be used in combination with other therapies and interventions (Neubauer et al., 2018). Medications approved for use to induce sleep and maintain sleep include benzodiazepine-receptor agonists, a melatonin-receptor agonist, a selective histamine-receptor antagonist, and an orexin/hypocretin receptor antagonist (Neubauer et al., 2018; Reynolds & Adams, 2019). There are some other non–insomnia-indicated medications that are sometimes prescribed "off label" for sleep enhancement and include antidepressants, anxiolytics, antipsychotics, and antihypertensives; however, these medications have not been evaluated for efficacy or safety in subjects with insomnia (Neubauer et al., 2018). The characteristics of the most commonly prescribed sleep aids are highlighted in Box 35-3. Use of medication to treat sleep disturbances in older adults should be limited if possible; when prescribed, medication use and adverse effects should be reviewed frequently (Reynolds & Adams, 2019). It is important for the nurse and patient to know and understand the action and potential adverse effects of any prescribed medication to ensure responsible administration.

Sleep medications are often prescribed on an as needed (PRN) basis. Administer these medications only when indicated and always with the full knowledge of their limitations. Provide thorough patient education about these medications. In addition, help patients develop other self-care strategies, including developing healthy sleep and lifestyle behaviors. Use alternative nonpharmacologic measures to promote sleep when appropriate. Over-the-counter (OTC) sleep medications most often contain antihistamines and should only be used on a short-term basis because of the potential for adverse effects and their lack of effectiveness over a lengthy time period (Neubauer et al., 2018).

Some patients use complementary health approaches (CHAs) that include melatonin or hypnotic herbs. Evidence suggests melatonin can be of assistance in addressing select circadian rhythm sleep–wake disorders, for which insomnia may be a primary symptom. However, evidence is conflicting in regard to the use of melatonin at bedtime for the treatment of insomnia (Neubauer et al., 2018; Reynolds & Adams, 2019). Hypnotic herbal therapies include valerian and Pacific valerian (Fontaine, 2019). Nervines are another type of herb that have a mild effect on sleep and include passionflower, lemon balm, skullcap, and gotu kola (Yarnell, 2015). Complementary therapies are also used in combination, such as melatonin, passionflower, and lemon balm, and have been shown to be effective in treating mild-to-moderate insomnia (Lemoine et al., 2019). Herbs and other complementary health approaches may offer ways to improve sleep; it is important to include questions about use of these agents as part of a nursing assessment related to sleep, as some patients may not consider OTC herbs or other CHAs to be medication.

Box 35-3 Commonly Prescribed Pharmacologic Sleep Aids

Pharmacodynamic Category	Generic Name Example Medication	Indications	Potential Side Effects
Benzodiazepine receptor agonists, nonbenzodiazepines	zaleplon, eszopiclone, and zolpidem tartrate	Patients experiencing difficulty with sleep onset and maintenance, difficulty returning to sleep after awakening during the night	Somnolence, cognitive impairment, dizziness, fatigue, anterograde amnesia, parasomnias, confused behaviors Rebound insomnia may occur with abrupt discontinuation or intermittent use
Selective melatonin receptor agonist	ramelteon	Facilitates the onset of sleep but is not intended for sleep maintenance	
Orexin receptor antagonists	suvorexant	Insomnia characterized by difficulty with sleep onset and/or sleep maintenance	
Selective histamine receptor antagonist	doxepin	Patients experiencing difficulty with sleep maintenance	

Source: Neubauer, D. N., Pandi-Perumal, S. R., Spence, D. W., Buttoo, K., & Monti, J. M. (2018). Pharmacotherapy of insomnia. *Journal of Central Nervous System Disease*, *10*, 1–7. https://doi.org/10.1177/1179573518770672; Reynolds, A. C., & Adams, R. J. (2019). Treatment of sleep disturbance in older adults. *Pharmacy Practice and Research*, *49*, 296–304. https://doi.org/10.1002/jppr.1565

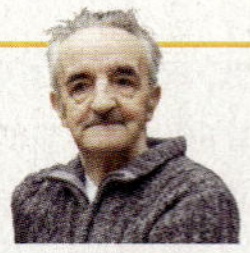

Remember ***Charlie Bitner***, the older man living in the long-term care facility. Nonpharmacologic measures would be helpful to promote sleep. Having Mr. Bitner consume a warm beverage before bedtime, listen to soft music, or receive a backrub may promote relaxation, thereby eliminating the need for and/or enhancing the effectiveness of the prescribed sleep medication.

Teaching About Rest and Sleep

A well-informed person is better able to cope with distressing situations. Teach patients and their families about the nature of rest and sleep and their importance to well-being, as the lack of sufficient and/or quality sleep affects not just the brain, but also the entire body (see Physical and Psychological Effects of Insufficient Sleep).

Also teach patients about normal variations in sleep patterns and common measures to promote relaxation and sleep (Teaching Tips 35-1). Review the patient's lifestyle and environment to identify possible changes to enhance sleep hygiene. Sleep hygiene suggestions include the following:

- Restricting the intake of caffeine, nicotine, and alcohol, especially later in the day
- Avoiding mental and physical activities after 5 PM that are stimulating
- Avoiding daytime naps
- Eating a light carbohydrate/protein snack before bedtime
- Avoiding high fluid intake in the evening so as to minimize trips to the bathroom during the night
- Sleeping in a cool, dark room
- Eliminating use of a bedroom clock
- Taking a warm bath before bedtime
- Trying to keep the sleep environment as quiet and stress-free as possible

Stimulus-control therapy is a CBT and works to reassociate the bed with sleepiness instead of awakening. Stimulus control therapy involves using the bedroom for sex and sleep only (Chawla et al., 2018). People with insomnia who have problems initiating sleep should go to bed only when sleepy and stay in the bedroom for only 15 to 20 minutes. If after this time they cannot fall asleep, they should leave the room, do something relaxing until sleepy, and return only when they feel sleepy. Getting up at the same time every day, no matter what time the person fell asleep, and refraining from napping during the day are recommended (Chawla et al., 2018).

Sleep restriction is another CBT and is designed to eliminate prolonged middle of the night awakenings. Sleep restriction initially restricts the time spent in bed, with subsequent steps gradually increasing the time spent in bed, limiting the time in bed to actual sleep time (Stanford Health Care, n.d.). It is thought that excessive time in bed may result in fragmented sleep, which may exacerbate the insomnia. A sleep diary helps to determine sleep patterns (Kaiser Permanente, n.d.b). The focus of sleep restriction is to avoid naps and early bedtimes and actually change the way a person sleeps. The initial time in bed is usually the average nightly total sleep time over the past week, with the minimum time not less than 5 to 5.5 hours (Kaiser Permanente, n.d.b; Stanford Health Care, n.d.). For example, if the average sleep time for a person is 6 hours, the person should be in bed for only 6 hours; after a week or so, there will be a marked decrease in time spent awake in the middle of the night. Then, the time spent in bed is gradually increased by 15 to 30 minutes if wakefulness in the middle of the night remains minimal. Increases may occur at weekly intervals, as long as 85% of the time spent in bed is spent sleeping (Stanford Health Care, n.d.). The procedure continues until no further extension is necessary because the person is sleeping better at night and feeling good during the day (Kaiser Permanente, n.d.b).

Teaching Tips 35-1

REST AND SLEEP

Health Topic	Teaching Tip	Why Is This Important?
Activity	• Find an activity that can be done daily and involves physical exertion, such as walking. • Do not participate in any physical activities right before bedtime.	• Sleep is easier to obtain if some physical activity has been completed. • Many people find it hard to rest and sleep right after a physical activity.
Nutrition	• Avoid food, beverages, or over-the-counter (OTC) medications that contain caffeine in the evening. • Eat a light dinner. • Eat a light protein and carbohydrate-containing snack at bedtime if hungry.	• Caffeine is a stimulant and may prolong the time it takes to fall asleep. • Eating a large meal before bedtime may produce heartburn, delaying sleep. • A small protein-containing snack (a source of tryptophan) combined with a carbohydrate (makes tryptophan more available to the brain) before bedtime has been recommended to improve sleep.
Sleep patterns	• Keep to usual waking time every day, even if previous night's bedtime was later than usual or sleep was restless. • Get out of bed if unable to fall asleep within 30 minutes and go into another room.	• Keeping the same pattern helps the body's circadian rhythms. • By using the bedroom for only sleep and sexual activity, the mind begins to associate this room with sleep.

Relaxation therapy involves any type of relaxation, such as progressive muscle relaxation, imagery training, or meditation. Not all relaxation methods are beneficial for all patients. Relaxation therapy and biofeedback are discussed in detail in Chapter 43.

Discuss the plan of care with the patient to make sure that the patient deems it acceptable. If a sleep disorder becomes a problem and common nursing measures are inadequate, the nurse may need to refer the patient to an advanced health care provider with the expertise to help the patient address their sleep concerns.

Evaluating

Evaluate the effectiveness of the plan of care to promote rest and sleep by determining whether the patient has met the individualized expected outcomes specified in the plan. See Nursing Care Plan 35-1 for Mr. Bitner.

Nursing care is considered effective if the patient is able to:

- Verbalize feeling rested or having had a restful night's sleep
- Identify factors that interfere with or disrupt the normal sleep pattern
- Use techniques that promote sleep and provide a restful environment
- Concentrate and function effectively during waking hours
- Eliminate behaviors related to sleep deprivation

REFLECTIVE PRACTICE LEADING TO PERSONAL LEARNING

Remember that the goal of reflective practice is to look at an experience, understand it, and learn from it. As you begin to develop use of and expertise in providing care to support patients' rest and sleep, reflect on your experiences—successes and failures—in order to improve your practice. How can you do it better next time? What did you learn today that can help you tomorrow? Begin your reflection by paying close attention to the following while performing interventions related to rest and sleep and providing nursing:

- How confident are you that the data you reported and recorded accurately communicates the status of the patient? How successfully have you communicated who this patient and family/caregivers are to the interdisciplinary team?
- Were you aware of any cultural and/or ethnic beliefs or practices that may have influenced the patient's rest and sleep practices? Were you aware of any stereotypes or prejudices that might have negatively influenced encounter? If so, how did you address these?
- How did you prioritize the data you collected? What patterns in the data did you identify? What knowledge from your learning, personal experience, and intuition did you use to make decisions and develop your plan of care?
- Did you need to modify the plan of care related to promoting rest and sleep as a result of ongoing assessments? Did you think of better interventions to produce the expected outcomes?
- As you concluded your care, did the patient/family/caregivers know your name, and know what to expect of you and nursing? Did the patient sense that you are respectful, caring, and competent to provide care?

Perhaps the most important questions to reflect on are: Are your patients and their families better for having had *you* share in the critical responsibility of being a part of their health care team? Are your patients now receiving thoughtful, person-centered, prioritized, holistic, evidence-based treatment and care because of your efforts?

Nursing Care Plan for *Mr. Bitner* 35-1

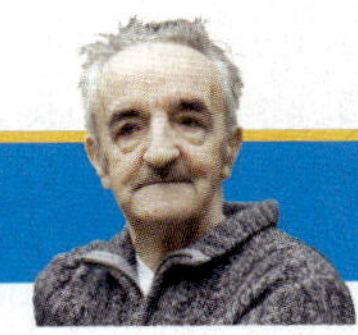

Mr. Bitner is an alert, widowed, 86-year-old man who was admitted to a long-term care facility 2 months ago. He is ambulatory and performs most of his own care. His admitting medical diagnoses include diabetes mellitus and hypertension. He adds to this list "a touch of arthritis." His daughter complains to the charge nurse that her father seems to be spending more and more time during the day napping and that he says he does not sleep well at night. A comprehensive sleep assessment of Mr. Bitner after his daughter's expression of concern reveals the following data:

- *Sleep–wakefulness pattern:* Patient goes to bed between 2000 and 2100 and gets out of bed between 0700 and 0800 because the staff are getting his roommate out of bed at this time. Patient states he never falls asleep before midnight because he always watched the late news at home. He usually wakes twice during the night to void and often cannot go back to sleep. During the day, patient is frequently observed dozing in his chair. If not discouraged, he returns to his room midmorning and afternoon for a 1-hour nap.
- *Effect of sleep pattern on everyday living:* Patient states: "I'm always tired. I don't seem to have much energy anymore." Patient has not socialized yet with other residents and, without strong encouragement, does not participate in group activities. From his point of view, the patient states that life holds little reason for him to be awake. "I worked for the railroad for almost 50 years and I never overslept once."
- *Sleep aids:* Patient denies ever using medication to fall asleep. States he often relaxed at home in the evening

(*continued on page 1328*)

Nursing Care Plan for *Mr. Bitner* 35-1 *(continued)*

with a couple of beers. Patient likes a dim light on during the night so that he can find the bathroom easily and likes his bedroom door ajar. He sleeps with two blankets and is often still cold.

- *Sleep disturbances and contributing factors:* Patient states: "Ever since my wife died, I'm just not getting enough sleep, and since I came here it's worse. I don't know why I don't fall asleep when I go to bed or why I wake up so much. It sure makes the nights long." Patient has no regular periods of exercise and drinks black coffee with every meal as well as one or two diet colas in the evening.

ACTUAL OR POTENTIAL HEALTH PROBLEMS AND NEED

Impaired sleep

Etiology: new sleep environment and schedule, evening caffeine intake, and insufficient meaningful daytime activity

Signs/Symptoms: difficulty falling asleep and remaining asleep

EXPECTED OUTCOME

By the next monthly assessment, 1/20/25, the patient will:

- Identify a routine hour of sleep and maintain retiring to bed at that time

NURSING INTERVENTIONS	RATIONALE	EVALUATIVE STATEMENT
Assess advisability of re-establishing Mr. Bitner's usual retiring pattern of going to bed after the 11 PM news. Assess how patient spends the time from the evening meal to 2300—explore relaxing alternatives with him. Investigate possibility that Mr. Bitner and his roommate might become social partners.	Strengthens the natural rhythm of his sleep–wake cycle. Elimination of evening naps will facilitate his falling asleep more easily.	1/18/25 Outcome met. Patient does not go to bed until after the news and has been observed talking with his roommate. *Recommendation:* Continue to develop evening activities with him—he finds that the time after supper "drags." *M. LeBon, RN*

EXPECTED OUTCOME

By the next monthly assessment, 1/20/25, the patient will:

- Report that he falls asleep within 1 hour of getting into bed

NURSING INTERVENTIONS	RATIONALE	EVALUATIVE STATEMENT
Continue to assess how long it takes patient to fall asleep after getting into bed.	In older adults, stage I time is increased.	1/18/25 Outcome partially met. Three or four nights a week, he falls asleep within 30 minutes of going to bed. States he really misses comfort of his wife. *Revision:* Investigate patient's sense of loss and need for touch. May be a good candidate for pet therapy program. *M. LeBon, RN*
Explore with patient means to relax before falling asleep—deep breathing, imagery, prayer.	Activities that calm and relax the person prepare the body for sleep.	
Teach the importance of using the bed only as a place to sleep. Advise patient when he cannot sleep to get out of bed and to go to another room, such as the common room, where he can perform some monotonous activity (watching television, listening to radio).	This maintains the bed as a powerful stimulus for sleep and helps to prevent "conditioned" insomnia ("Well, here I am in bed now and I know sleep won't come").	

Nursing Care Plan for Mr. Bitner 35-1 (continued)

EXPECTED OUTCOME

By the next monthly assessment, 1/20/25, the patient will:
- Decrease nighttime awakenings to one, after which he returns to a sound sleep

NURSING INTERVENTIONS	RATIONALE	EVALUATIVE STATEMENT
Assess and manipulate factors that contribute to nighttime awakenings: • Need to void (time of day diuretic is taken, amounts of fluid intake in the evening) • Roommate's wakefulness, snoring, or need for care • Uncomfortableness in strange environment • Comfort (e.g., temperature)	Individualizing the patient's bedtime environment and meeting comfort needs (warmth, soft light, and so forth) promote sleep onset and maintenance.	1/18/25 Outcome partially met. Nighttime awakenings vary from none to three nightly. See previous revision. *M. LeBon, RN*
Teach patient how, on awakening, to concentrate on breathing until he falls back to sleep.	This uses the power of relaxation and positive thinking to facilitate return to sleep.	

EXPECTED OUTCOME

By the next monthly assessment, 1/20/25, the patient will:
- Identify a preferred physical activity and participate on a routine basis

NURSING INTERVENTIONS	RATIONALE	EVALUATIVE STATEMENT
Assess whether patient understands the relation between daily exercise and his ability to sleep.	Regular exercise throughout the day is known to increase physical fatigue and to promote sleep. Exercise or stimulating activities immediately before retiring interfere with sleep's onset.	1/20/25 Outcome met. Patient has become an enthusiastic participant in exercise sessions—attends daily. *M. LeBon, RN*
Determine how his exercise needs can best be met (i.e., through a group program or an individualized program of walking or other program).	Exercise program must be individualized based on physical state and interests of patient.	
Use positive verbal reinforcement to communicate to patient that someone cares that he is using positive means to remedy his sleep disturbance and increase his well-being.	Activity provides the opportunity for socialization and improvement of a self-image. Positive reinforcement promotes continued participation.	
Encourage patient's daughter to go for walks with him when she visits and to question him about his exercise program.	Communications and interaction with family members helps the older adult to maintain self-esteem and to feel valuable and loved.	

EXPECTED OUTCOME

By the next monthly assessment, 1/20/25, the patient will:
- Verbalize an understanding of appropriate foods to avoid to enhance sleep. Substitute caffeine-free beverages for coffee and cola at supper and evening snack

(continued on page 1330)

Nursing Care Plan for Mr. Bitner 35-1 (continued)

NURSING INTERVENTIONS	RATIONALE	EVALUATIVE STATEMENT
Assess patient's willingness to substitute caffeine-free beverages for coffee and cola.	Caffeine is a stimulant that can cause difficulty sleeping.	1/20/25 Outcome met. Patient verbalizes an understanding of the importance of caffeine-free beverages at dinner and before bedtime. Patient now drinks decaffeinated coffee with meals and milk in the evening. Dislikes caffeine-free sodas. *M. LeBon, RN*
Consult with dietary department and his daughter about options. Experiment with options until his preferences are determined.	Caffeine-free versions of beverages are often available and can be used based on patient acceptance.	
Gradually reduce his caffeine intake, especially from evening meal onward. Offer a protein and carbohydrate evening snack.	The combination of a protein and carbohydrate snack appears to promote sleep.	

SAMPLE DOCUMENTATION

12/20/25 Nursing

Family conference to discuss Mr. Bitner's sleep disturbance—initiated by daughter's concern. Present were Mr. Bitner and his daughter (A. Jelner), K. Behner (social worker), W. Quing (activity director), and M. LeBon (primary nurse). Primary nurse presented findings from comprehensive sleep assessment: Actual Health Problem: Impaired sleep as a result of Mr. Bitner's new sleep environment and schedule, evening caffeine intake, and insufficient meaningful daytime activity.

Discussion centered on strategies to help Mr. Bitner develop interests in the center, including possibilities for increased physical exercise, decrease his evening caffeine intake (daughter to bring noncaffeinated sodas), and re-establish usual retiring and waking times. See plan of care. Patient's progress will be evaluated at next monthly assessment, 1/20/25.

M. LeBon, RN

DEVELOPING CLINICAL REASONING AND CLINICAL JUDGMENT

1. Interview three adults of varying ages (young, middle, older) about their sleep and rest patterns, using the Focused Assessment Guide in this chapter. Explore the special problems experienced by each of the adults, the efficacy of the self-help measures they use to cope, and helpful nursing interventions.
2. Interview three practicing nurses who are recent graduates. Using the Focused Assessment Guide in the text, ask them: if they are getting adequate rest, what factors are compromising their rest (e.g., working double or rotating shifts), how any lack of rest is affecting their practice, and what self-help measures they have used or would be appropriate. Discuss with your classmates the issue of practicing nurses with sleep alterations, the factors that place nurses at risk for sleep alterations, and what students can learn or actions to take to lower their risk.

PRACTICING FOR NCLEX

1. A nurse on a postpartum unit is teaching new parents about newborn safety and sleep patterns. Which comment from a parent indicates further teaching is required?
   a. "I can expect my newborn to sleep an average of 16 to 24 hours a day."
   b. "Eye movements or groans during my baby's sleep is an emergency."
   c. "It is essential that I place my infant on their back to sleep."
   d. "I will not place pillows or blankets in the crib to prevent suffocation."

2. A nurse observes involuntary muscle jerking in a sleeping patient. What action will the nurse take next?
   a. No action is necessary; this is normal in stage 1 sleep.
   b. Report the neurologic deficit to the health care provider.
   c. Lower the temperature in the patient's room.
   d. Awaken the patient, as this is an indication of night terrors.
3. A nurse working the night shift is watching the monitors on a telemetry unit and observes a slight increase in a patient's vital signs during sleep. Which of these points will the nurse correlate to changes in vital signs? Select all that apply.
   a. They are aware of his surroundings at this point.
   b. They are in delta sleep at this time.
   c. It would be most difficult to awaken them at this time.
   d. This is most likely an NREM stage.
   e. This stage constitutes around 20% to 25% of total sleep.
   f. The muscles are relaxed in this stage.
4. A nurse working in a sleep lab observes the developmental factors that may affect sleep. Which statements accurately describe these variations? Select all that apply.
   a. REM sleep constitutes much of the sleep cycle of a preschool child.
   b. By age 8 years, most children no longer take naps.
   c. Sleep needs usually decrease when physical growth peaks.
   d. Many adolescents do not get enough sleep.
   e. Total sleep decreases in adults with a decrease in stage IV sleep.
   f. Sleep is less sound in older adults, and stage IV sleep may be absent.
5. A nurse is providing education in a senior center on sleep and sleep hygiene in older adults. What teaching point will the nurse include?
   a. Drinking a cup of regular tea at night induces sleep.
   b. Using alcohol moderately promotes a deep sleep.
   c. Eating a bedtime snack high in tryptophan and carbohydrates improves sleep.
   d. Exercising right before bedtime can hinder sleep.
6. As part of interprofessional rounds, a nurse in a skilled facility assesses for sleep deficits. Patients with which health problems would the team identify as higher risk for sleep disturbances? Select all that apply.
   a. Uncontrolled hypothyroidism
   b. Anxiety
   c. GERD
   d. HIV
   e. Arthritis
   f. Urinary tract infection
7. A nurse is providing discharge teaching for patients regarding their medications. For which patients would the nurse recommend actions to promote sleep? Select all that apply.
   a. Patient taking iron supplements for anemia
   b. Patient with Parkinson's disease who is taking dopamine
   c. Older adult taking diuretics for congestive heart failure
   d. Child taking antibiotics for an ear infection
   e. Patient taking antidepressants
   f. Patient taking low-dose aspirin prophylactically
8. A nurse in a pediatric unit notes a school-aged child snores and appears to have labored breathing during sleep. Which assessment question could the nurse ask the patient or parents?
   a. "Do you have trouble sleeping?"
   b. "Have you missed a lot of school due to not feeling well?"
   c. "Have you been wetting the bed lately?"
   d. "Do you have a history of high blood pressure?"
9. At an annual health and wellness visit, the parent of an adolescent reports a teacher's concerns that their child is sleepy at school during class time. Which information will the nurse share with the parent and child? Select all that apply.
   a. Adolescents typically need 8 to 10 hours of sleep each night.
   b. Demands on the adolescent's time causes them to sleep longer hours.
   c. Insufficient sleep can lead to daytime sleepiness.
   d. Adolescents require reduced sleep in the teen years.
   e. The adolescent could benefit from a sleep study for insomnia.
10. A nurse recommends that a patient with a sleep disorder keep a sleep diary. Which data will the nurse ask the patient to document? Select all that apply.
    a. Daily mental activities
    b. Daily physical activities
    c. Morning and evening body temperature
    d. Daily measurement of fluid intake and output
    e. Presence of anxiety or worries affecting sleep
    f. Morning and evening blood pressure readings
11. A nurse in a rehabilitation facility develops a plan to help promote patients' sleep. What interventions will the nurse include in the plan? Select all that apply
    a. Maintain a consistent bedtime and time to awaken.
    b. Drink two or three glasses of water at bedtime.
    c. Have a large snack at bedtime.
    d. Take a sedative-hypnotic every night at bedtime.
12. A nurse is caring for an older adult who is having trouble falling asleep at night. What nursing interventions are appropriate for this patient? Select all that apply.
    a. Assess the patient for depression.
    b. Discourage napping during the day.
    c. Decrease fluids during the evening.
    d. Administer diuretics in the morning.
    e. Encourage the patient to engage in some type of physical activity.
    f. Assess medication for side effects of sleep pattern disturbances.

13. A nursing student is caring for an older adult with arthritis who states she did not sleep well and was "up all night to use the bathroom." To help promote sleep, the student plans to discuss re-timing which medication with the primary nurse?
   a. Furosemide (diuretic) 10:00 AM, 10:00 PM
   b. Melatonin 9:00 PM
   c. Acetaminophen 10:00 AM, 10:00 PM
   d. Artificial tears every 8 hours, 8:00 AM, 2:00 PM, 8:00 PM
14. A nurse caring for patients on a surgical unit should implement which recommendation to promote sleep? Select all that apply
   a. Keep the room light dimmed during the day.
   b. Maintain a cool temperature in the room for sleep.
   c. Keep the door of the room open for fresh air.
   d. Offer a hypnotic to patients on a regular basis.
   e. Offer pain medication prior to sleep, as needed.
   f. Provide earplugs if the patient agrees.
15. A nurse caring for patients in a long-term care facility is implementing interventions to help promote sleep in older adults. Which is the best action for these patients?
   a. Increase physical activities during the day.
   b. Encourage short periods of napping during the day.
   c. Increase fluids during the evening.
   d. Dispense diuretics during the afternoon hours.
16. A patient experiencing menopause tells the nurse at the medical clinic that she would like to try a CAH hormonal sleep aid like her friend uses. What information can the nurse give the patient?
   a. Melatonin, an over-the-counter hormonal sleep aid, has varied effectiveness.
   b. Lavender is a hormonal scented sleep aid.
   c. Lorazepam, a naturally occurring benzodiazepine, is recommended for sleep.
   d. Valerian is a natural hormonal sleep aid.
17. After reporting an adult patient's loud snoring and changes in vital signs occurring overnight the patient's health care provider, a nocturnal polysomnography study is prescribed. What teaching will the nurse provide about this test?
   a. This is a blood test, taken in the evening to evaluate leptin and ghrelin.
   b. The patient is monitored overnight to evaluate for sleep apnea.
   c. A patient is evaluated for leg jerking and awakenings during the night.
   d. Adults, rather than children, can be diagnosed with this test.

ANSWERS WITH RATIONALES

1. **b.** Eye movements, groaning, grimacing, and moving are normal activities at this age; no emergency exists. Newborns sleep an average of 16 to 24 hours a day. Infants should be placed on their backs for the first year to prevent SIDS. Parents should be cautioned about placing pillows, crib bumpers, quilts, stuffed animals, and other items in the crib as they pose a suffocation risk.
2. **a.** Involuntary muscle jerking occurs in stage I NREM sleep and is a normal finding. No further actions are needed for this patient.
3. **c, e.** This scenario describes REM sleep. During REM sleep, it is difficult to arouse a person, and the vital signs increase. REM sleep constitutes about 20% to 25% of sleep. In stage I NREM sleep, the person is somewhat aware of surroundings. In stage IV NREM sleep (delta sleep), the muscles are relaxed, whereas small muscle twitching may occur in REM sleep.
4. **d, e, f.** Many adolescents do not get enough sleep due to the demands of school, activities, and part-time employment. Total sleep time decreases during adult years, with a decrease in stage IV sleep. Sleep is less sound in older adults, and stage IV sleep is absent or considerably decreased. REM sleep constitutes much of the sleep cycle of a young infant, and by the age of 5 years, most children no longer nap. Sleep needs usually increase when physical growth peaks.
5. **c.** The nurse would teach that having a small bedtime snack high in tryptophan and carbohydrates improves sleep. Regular tea contains caffeine and increases alertness. Large quantities of alcohol limit REM and delta sleep. Physical activity within a 3-hour interval before normal bedtime can hinder sleep.
6. **a, b, c.** A patient who has uncontrolled hypothyroidism tends to have a decreased amount of NREM sleep, especially stages II and IV. Worries and anxiety can interfere with sleep, as can pain. A patient who has GERD may awaken at night with heartburn pain. Being HIV positive, taking corticosteroids, and having a urinary tract infection does not usually change sleep patterns.
7. **b, c, e.** Drugs that decrease REM sleep include barbiturates, amphetamines, and antidepressants. Diuretics, antiparkinsonian drugs, some antidepressants and antihypertensives, steroids, decongestants, caffeine, and asthma medications are seen as additional common causes of sleep problems.
8. **c.** OSA (pediatric) is defined by the presence of snoring, labored/obstructed breathing, enuresis, or daytime consequences (hyperactivity or other neurobehavioral problems, sleepiness, fatigue). Adults, children, and adolescents with symptoms of OSA, including snoring, should have polysomnography to confirm the diagnosis. Although OSA may cause insomnia, this is not the primary diagnosis in this case. Narcolepsy is a condition characterized by excessive daytime sleepiness and frequent overwhelming urges to sleep or inadvertent daytime lapses into sleep. Hypertension is a consequence of OSA in adults.
9. **a, c.** Adolescents require 8 to 10 hours of sleep nightly; however, demands on their time cut into the needed sleep. Insufficient sleep can lead to daytime sleepiness.
10. **a, b, e.** A sleep diary includes mental and physical activities performed during the day and the presence of any anxiety or worries the patient may be experiencing that affect sleep. A record of fluid intake and output, body temperature, and blood pressure is typically kept in the graphic record.
11. **a.** Keeping a consistent bedtime and awakening schedule, even when up late, helps promote sleep. Drinking two or three glasses of water at bedtime will probably cause the patient to awaken during the night to void. A large snack may be uncomfortable right before bedtime; instead, a small

protein and carbohydrate snack is recommended. Taking a sedative–hypnotic every night disturbs REM and NREM sleep, and sedatives also lose their effectiveness quickly.

12. **a, b, d, e, f.** For patients who are having trouble initiating sleep, the nurse should arrange for assessment for depression and treatment, discourage napping, promote activity, and assess medications for sleep disturbance side effects. Limiting fluids and administering diuretics in the morning are appropriate interventions.

13. **a.** It is best to administer diuretics in the morning or early evening to prevent nocturia. Melatonin promotes sleep and rest. Acetaminophen can relieve arthritis pain and help promote rest. Artificial tears, used for dry eyes, will not affect sleep.

14. **b, e, f.** The nurse should keep the room cool and provide earplugs and eye masks if desired. The nurse should maintain a bright room environment during daylight hours and dim lights in the evening, keeping the door of the room closed to keep out extraneous noise. Sleep aid medications should only be offered as prescribed with the knowledge that they can become habit forming.

15. **a.** In order to promote sleep in the older adult, the nurse should encourage daily physical activity such as walking or water aerobics. The nurse discourages napping during the day, decreases fluids at night, and dispenses diuretics in the morning (or early evening when necessary).

16. **a.** Melatonin, used as a complementary or alternate to traditional pharmacologic agents, is a hormone thought to regulate the sleep–wake cycle. Valerian is an herb; lavender is a plant used for aromatherapy and relaxation. Benzodiazepines are pharmacologic medications used to decrease anxiety and promote sleep and relaxation.

17. **b.** Polysomnography is an overnight sleep study to determine if an individual has sleep apnea and treatment. Leptin and ghrelin are hormones that regulate nutritional intake. Leptin signals the brain to stop eating, whereas ghrelin promotes continued eating. Research suggests that sleep deprivation lowers leptin levels and elevates ghrelin levels, increasing appetite; however, this does not help diagnose sleep apnea. Jerking legs in the early stage of sleep is expected. Both adults and children can benefit from diagnosis of sleep apnea with this test.

Bibliography

Adams, M., Holland, N., & Urban, C. (2019). *Pharmacology for nurses. A pathophysiologic approach* (6th ed.). Pearson.

Adatia, S., Law, S., & Haggerty, J. (2014). Room for improvement: Noise on a maternity ward. *BMC Health Services Research, 14*(1), 604.

American Academy of Pediatrics. (2016). SIDS and other sleep-related infant deaths: Updated 2016 recommendations for a safe infant sleeping environment. *Pediatrics, 138*(5), 1–12. https://doi.org/10.1542/peds.2016-2938

American Academy of Sleep Medicine. (n.d.). *Bedwetting—Overview & facts.* http://sleepeducation.org/sleep-disorders-by-category/parasomnias/bedwetting/overview-facts

American Academy of Sleep Medicine. (2014). *International classification of sleep disorders* (3rd ed.). (ICSD-3). https://learn.aasm.org/Public/Catalog/Details.aspx?id=%2FgqQVDMQIT%2FEDy86PWgqgQ%3D%3D&returnurl=%2fUsers%2fUserOnlineCourse.aspx%3fLearningActivityID%3d%252fgqQVDMQIT%252fEDy86PWgqgQ%253d%253d

American Academy of Sleep Medicine. (2015, March 4). *Sleep education. Insomnia.* http://sleepeducation.org/essentials-in-sleep/insomnia/overview-facts

American Academy of Sleep Medicine. (2016a, June 22). *Sleep education. Sleep apnea.* http://sleepeducation.org/essentials-in-sleep/sleep-apnea

American Academy of Sleep Medicine. (2016b, July 14). *Healthy sleep duration.* https://aasm.org/new-infographics-help-you-share-aasm-sleep-duration-recommendations/

American Academy of Sleep Medicine. (2019, May 6). *Insomnia. Treatment.* http://sleepeducation.org/essentials-in-sleep/insomnia/treatment

American Sleep Association (ASA). (n.d.a). *Sleep deprivation: Symptoms, causes, treatments.* https://www.sleepassociation.org/sleep-disorders/sleep-deprivation/

American Sleep Association (ASA). (n.d.b). *Children and sleep disorders.* https://www.sleepassociation.org/children-and-sleep/children-sleep-disorders/?highlight=enuresis

American Sleep Association (ASA). (n.d.c). *Sleep hygiene tips.* https://www.sleepassociation.org/about-sleep/sleep-hygiene-tips/

Anderson, P. (2012). Hospital noise, especially alarms, most disruptive to sleep. *Medscape Nurses..* http://www.medscape.com/viewarticle/767459

Andrews, M., Boyle, J. S., & Collins, J. (2020). *Transcultural concepts in nursing care* (8th ed.). Wolters Kluwer

Antonio, C. K. (2020). Improving quiet at night on a telemetry unit: Introducing a holistic sleep menu intervention. *American Journal of Nursing, 120*(10), 58–64. https://doi.org/10.1097/01.NAJ.0000718660.44502.86

Aparício, C., & Panin, F. (2020). Interventions to improve inpatients' sleep quality in intensive care units and acute wards: A literature review. *British Journal of Nursing, 29*(13), 770–776. https://doi.org/10.12968/bjon.2020.29.13.770

Binks, H., Vincent, G. E., Gupta, C., Irwin, C., & Khalesi, S. (2020). Effects of diet on sleep: A narrative review. *Nutrients, 12*(4), 936. https://doi.org/10.3390/nu12040936

Bombard, J. M., Kortsmit, K., Cottengim, C., & Johnston, E. O. (2018). Update from the CDC. Infant safe sleep practices in the United States. *American Journal of Nursing, 118*(12), 20–21. https://doi.org/10.1097/01.NAJ.0000549685.59006.ad

Boyd, M. A. (2018). *Psychiatric nursing. Contemporary practice* (6th ed.). Wolters Kluwer.

Brashears, K. A., & Erdlitz, K. (2020). Screening and support for infant safe sleep: A quality improvement project. *Journal of Pediatric Health Care, 34*(6), 591–600. https://doi.org/10.1016/j.pedhc.2020.07.002

Brem, S. (2015). Insomnia: Using CBT in primary care. *Clinical Advisor, 18*(2), 42–46.

Bruyneel, M., & Sersté, T. (2018). Sleep disturbances in patients with liver cirrhosis: Prevalence, impact, and management challenges. *Nature and Science of Sleep, 10*, 369–375. https://doi.org/10.2147/NSS.S186665

Buysse, D. J. (2014). Sleep health: Can we define it? Does it matter? *Sleep, 37*(1), 9–17.

Centers for Disease Control and Prevention (CDC). (2017, March 2). *How much sleep do I need?* https://www.cdc.gov/sleep/about_sleep/how_much_sleep.html

Centers for Disease Control and Prevention (CDC). (2018a, August 8). *Sleep and chronic disease.* https://www.cdc.gov/sleep/about_sleep/chronic_disease.html

Centers for Disease Control and Prevention (CDC). (2018b, December 3). *How does sleep affect your heart health?* https://www.cdc.gov/features/sleep-heart-health/index.html

Centers for Disease Control and Prevention (CDC). (2020, April 15). *Sleep and sleep disorders.* https://www.cdc.gov/sleep/index.html

Chawla, J., Park, Y., & Passaro, E. A. (2018, September 11). *What is stimulus-control therapy for insomnia? Medscape.* https://www.medscape.com/answers/1187829-70569/what-is-stimulus-control-therapy-for-insomnia

Cheraghbeigi, N., Modarresi, M., Rezaei, M., & Khatony, A. (2019). Comparing the effects of massage and aromatherapy massage with lavender oil on sleep quality of cardiac patients: A randomized controlled trial. *Complementary Therapies in Clinical Practice, 35*, 253–258. https://doi.org/10.1016/j.ctcp.2019.03.005

Choi, Y. K., Demiris, G., Lin, S. Y., Iribarren, S. J., Landis, C. A., Thompson, H. J., McCurry, S. M., Heitkemper, M. M., & Ward, T. M. (2018). Smartphone applications to support sleep self-management: Review and evaluation. *Journal of Clinical Sleep Medicine, 14*(10), 1783–1790. https://doi.org/10.5664/jcsm.7396

Chung, K. F., Lee, C. T., Yeung, W. F., Chan, M. S., Chung, E. W., & Lin, W. L. (2018). Sleep hygiene education as a treatment of insomnia: A systematic review and meta-analysis. *Family Practice, 35*(4), 365–375. https://doi.org/10.1093/fampra/cmx122

Cleveland Clinic. (2017a, April 22). *Shift work sleep disorder.* https://my.clevelandclinic.org/health/diseases/12146-shift-work-sleep-disorder

Cleveland Clinic. (2017b, April 22). *Parasomnias & disruptive sleep disorders.* https://my.clevelandclinic.org/health/diseases/12133-parasomnias–disruptive-sleep-disorders

Cleveland Clinic. (2020, April 1). *Circadian rhythm sleep disorders.* Ps://my.clevelandclinic.org/health/diseases/12115-circadian-rhythm-disorders

Cleveland Clinic. (2021, September 16). *Sleep-related eating disorders.* https://my.clevelandclinic.org/health/diseases/21730-sleep-related-eating-disorders

Crawford, K. J., Barnes, L. A., Peters, T. M., Falk, J., & Gehlbach, B. K. (2018). Identifying determinants of noise in a medical intensive care unit. *Journal of Occupational and Environmental Hygiene, 15*(12), 810–817. https://doi.org/10.1080/15459624.2018.1515491

Dave, K., Qureshi, A., & Gopichandran, L. (2015). Effects of earplugs and eye masks on perceived quality of sleep during night among patients in intensive care units. *Asian Journal of Nursing Education and Research, 5*(3), 319–322. https://doi.org/10.5958/2349-2996.2015.00065.8

Delaney, L. J. (2016). The role of sleep in patient recovery. *Australian Nursing & Midwifery Journal, 23*(7), 26–29.

Delaney, L. J., Currie, M. J., Huang, H. C. C., Lopez, V., & Van Haren, F. (2018). "They can rest at home": An observational study of patients' quality of sleep in an Australian hospital. *BMC Health Services Research, 18*(1), 524. https://doi.org/10.1186/s12913-018-3201-z

DePietro, M. A. (n.d.). *Children & sleep disorders.* American Sleep Association. Retrieved February12, 2021, from https://www.sleepassociation.org/children-and-sleep/children-sleep-disorders/?highlight=parasomnias

Dobson, L., Stutzman, S. E., Hicks. A. D., & Olson, D. M. (2019). Sleep hygiene in patients with chronic respiratory disease. *Nursing, 49*(2), 64–69. https://doi.org/10.1097/01.NURSE.0000549722.07316.42

Eliopoulos, C. (2018). *Gerontological nursing* (9th ed.). Wolters Kluwer Health.

Ellmers, T., Arber, S., Luff, R., Eyers, I., & Young, E. (2013). Factors affecting residents' sleep in care homes. *Nursing Older People, 25*(8), 29–32. https://doi.org/10.7748/nop2013.10.25.8.29.e466

Fillary, J., Chaplin, H., Jones, G., Thompson, A., Holme, A., & Wilson, P. (2015). Noise at night in hospital general wards: A mapping of the literature. *British Journal of Nursing, 24*(10), 536–540. https://doi.org/10.12968/bjon.2015.24.10.536

Fischbach, F. T., Fischbach, M. A., & Stout, K. (2022). *Fischbach's A manual of laboratory and diagnostic tests* (11th ed.). Wolters Kluwer.

Fontaine, K. L. (2019). *Complementary & alternative therapies for nursing practice* (5th ed.). Pearson.

Freeman, G. (2015). Nurse fatigue a 'huge' threat to patient safety. *Healthcare Risk Management, 37*(3), 25–28.

Frey, E., Hamp, N., & Orlov, N. (2020). Modelling safe infant sleep in the hospital. *Journal of Pediatric Nursing, 50*, 20–24. https://doi.org/10.1016/j.pedn.2019.10.002

Fry, A. (2020, October 23). *Sleep studies.* Sleep Foundation. https://health.gov/healthypeople/objectives-and-data/browse-objectives/sleep

Goeren, D., John, S., Meskill, K., Iacono, L., Wahl, S., & Scanlon, K. (2018). Quiet Time: A noise reduction initiative in a neurosurgical intensive care unit. *Critical Care Nurse, 38*(4), 38–45. https://doi.org/10.4037/ccn2018219

Graham, K., Ogbuji, G., Williams, Z., Crain, M., Rolin, B., Juala, J., Larbi, I., Bernard, N., Oster, C. A., Baird, M., & Gullatte, M. M. (2021). Challenges of implementing the Choosing Wisely Guideline to promote sleep and rest at night for hospitalized patients. *Journal of Nursing Care Quality, 36*(1), 50–56. https://doi.org/10.1097/NCQ.0000000000000494

Grimm, J. (2020). Sleep deprivation in the intensive care patient. *Critical Care Nurse, 40*(2), e16–e24. https://doi.org/10.4037/ccn2020939

Hale, L., Troxel, W., & Buysse, D. J. (2020). Sleep health: An opportunity for public health to address health equity. *Annual Review of Public Health, 41*, 81–99. https://doi.org/10.1146/annurev-publhealth040119-094412

Hedges, C., & Gotelli, J. (2020). Managing insomnia in older adults. *Nursing, 50*(9), 24–32. https://doi.org/10.1097/01.NURSE.0000694744.12428.d9

Hedges, C., Hunt, C., & Ball, P. (2019). Quiet Time improves the patient experience. *Journal of Nursing Care Quality, 34*(3), 197–202. https://doi.org/10.1097/NCQ.0000000000000363

Helvig, A., Wade, S., & Hunger-Eades, L. (2016). Rest and the associated benefits in restorative sleep: A concept analysis. *Journal of Advanced Nursing, 72*(1), 62–72. https://doi.org/10.1111/jan.12807

Hermida, R. C., Crespo, J. J., Domínguez-Sardiña, M., Otero, A., Moyá, A., Ríos, M. T., Sineiro, E., Castiñeira, M. C., Callejas, P. A., Pousa, L., Salgado, J. L., Durán, C., Sánchez, J. J., Fernández, J. R., Mojón, A., Ayala, D. E., & Hygia Project Investigators. (2019). Bedtime hypertension treatment improves cardiovascular risk reduction: The Hygia Chronotherapy Trial. *European Heart Journal, 41*(16), 1600. https://doi.org/10.1093/eurheartj/ehaa339

Hess, D. R., MacIntyre, N. R., Galvin, W. F., & Mishoe, S. C. (2021). *Respiratory care. Principles and practice* (4th ed.). Jones & Bartlett Learning.

Hinkle, J. L., Cheever, K. H. & Overbaugh, K. J. (2022). *Brunner & Suddarth's Textbook of medical-surgical nursing* (15th ed.). Wolters Kluwer.

Ibáñez, V., Silva, J., & Cauli, O. (2018). A survey on sleep assessment methods. *PeerJ, 6*, e4849. https://doi.org/10.7717/peerj.4849

International Council of Nurses (ICN). (2019). *Nursing diagnosis and outcome statements.* https://www.icn.ch/sites/default/files/inline-files/ICNP2019-DC.pdf

James, L., James, S. M., Wilson, M., Brown, N., Dotson, E. J., Edwards, C. D., & Butterfield, P. (2020). Sleep health and predicted cognitive effectiveness of nurses working 12-hour shifts: An observational study. *International Journal of Nursing Studies, 112*, 103667. https://doi.org/10.1016/j.ijnurstu.2020.103667

Jansson-Fröjmark, M., Evander, J., & Alfonsson, S. (2019). Are sleep hygiene practices related to the incidence, persistence and remission on insomnia? Findings from a prospective community study. *Journal of Behavioral Medicine, 42*(1), 128–138. https://doi.org/10.1007/s10865-018-9949-0

Jarvis, C., & Echkardt, A. (2020). *Physical examination & health assessment* (8th ed.). Elsevier.

Javaheri, S., & Redline, S. (2017). Insomnia and risk of cardiovascular disease. *Chest, 152*(2), 435–444. https://doi.org/10.1016/j.chest.2017.01.026

Jensen, S. (2019). *Nursing health assessment. A best practice approach* (3rd ed.). Wolters Kluwer.

Johnson, K. (2011). Sleep deprivation in medical caregivers has deadly results. *Medscape Nurses.* http://www.medscape.com/viewarticle/745022?src=mp&spon=24

The Joint Commission. (2018). *Sentinel Event Alert Issue 48: Health care worker fatigue and patient safety.* https://www.jointcommission.org/resources/patient-safety-topics/sentinel-event/sentinel-event-alert-newsletters/sentinel-event-alert-issue-48-health-care-worker-fatigue-and-patient-safety/

Kaiser Permanente. (n.d.a). *Sleep-related movement disorders.* Retrieved December 6, 2020, from https://thrive.kaiserpermanente.org/care-near-you/northern-california/eastbay/departments/sleep-clinic/common-sleep-problems/sleep-related-movement-disorders/

Kaiser Permanente. (n.d.b). *Sleep restriction therapy.* Retrieved December 8, 2020, https://thrive.kaiserpermanente.org/care-near-you/northern-california/sanjose/wp-content/uploads/sites/7/2015/10/sleep-restriction-rev2_tcm28-557887.pdf

Karch, A. M. (2020). *Focus on nursing pharmacology* (8th ed.). Wolters Kluwer.

Klingelhoefer, L., Bhattacharya, K., & Reichmann, H. (2016). Restless legs syndrome. *Clinical Medicine (Lond), 16*(4), 379–382. https://doi.org/10.7861/clinmedicine.16-4-379

Kyle, T., & Carman, S. (2021). *Essentials of pediatric nursing* (4th ed.). Wolters Kluwer.

Lampron, S., & Copeland, D. (2019). Using a sleep protocol to limit sleep interruptions on a medical-surgical unit. *Journal of Nursing Administration, 49*(7-8), 350–353. https://doi.org/10.1097/NNA.0000000000000766

Lanigar, S., & Bandyopadhyay, S. (2017). Sleep and epilepsy: A complex interplay. *Missouri Medicine, 114*(6), 453–457.

Lemoine, P., Bablon, J. C., & Da Silva, C. (2019). A combination of melatonin, vitamin B6 and medicinal plants in the treatment of mild-to-moderate insomnia: A prospective pilot study. *Complementary Therapies in Medicine, 45*, 104–108. https://doi.org/10.1016/j.ctim.2019.05.024

Macnamara, C. L., Cfejic, E., Parker, G. B., Lloyd, A. R., Lee, G., Beilharz, J. E., & Vollmer-Conna, U. (2018). Personalised relaxation practice to improve sleep and functioning in patients with chronic fatigue syndrome and depression: Study protocol for a randomised controlled trial. *Trials, 19*(1), 371. https://doi.org/10.1186/s13063-018-2763-8

Marcus, C. L., Brooks, L. J., Draper, K. A., Gozal, D., Halbower, A. C., Jones, J., Schechter, M. S., Sheldon, S. H., Spruyt, K., Ward, S. D., Lehmann, C., Shiffman, R. N., & American Academy of Pediatrics. (2012). Diagnosis and management of childhood obstructive sleep apnea syndrome. *Pediatrics, 130*(3), 576–584. https://doi.org/10.1542/peds.2012-1671

Maung, S. C., El Sara, A., Chapman, C., Cohen, D., & Cukor, D. (2016). Sleep disorders and chronic kidney disease. *World Journal of Nephrology, 5*(3), 224–232. https://doi.org/10.5527/wjn.v5.i3.224

Mayo Foundation for Medical Education and Research (MFMER). (2020a, October 3). *Pediatric obstructive sleep apnea.* https://www.mayoclinic.org/diseases-conditions/pediatric-sleep-apnea/symptoms-causes/syc-20376196

Mayo Foundation for Medical Education and Research (MFMER). (2020b, July 28). Sleep *apnea.* https://www.mayoclinic.org/diseases-conditions/sleep-apnea/symptoms-causes/syc-20377631

Mayo Foundation for Medical Education and Research (MFMER). (2020c, October 2). *Jet lag disorder.* https://www.mayoclinic.org/diseases-conditions/jet-lag/symptoms-causes/syc-20374027

Medic, G., Wille, M., & Hemels, M. E. H. (2017). Short- and long-term health consequences of sleep disruption. *Nature and Science of Sleep, 9*, 151–161. https://doi.org/10.2147/NSS.S134864

Miller, A. L., Lumeng, J. C., & LeBourgeois, M. K. (2015). Sleep patterns and obesity in childhood. *Current Opinion in Endocrinology Diabetes and Obesity, 22*(1), 41–47. https://doi.org10.1097/MED.0000000000000125

Mohammadi, D. (2016, February 19). Chronotherapy: Treating cancer at the right time. *The Pharmaceutical Journal.* The Royal Pharmaceutical Society. https://pharmaceutical-journal.com/article/feature/cancer-chronotherapy-timing-drug-administration-to-optimise-efficacy-and-reduce-toxicity

Morton, P. G., & Fontaine, D. K. (2018). *Critical care nursing. A holistic approach* (11th ed.). Wolters Kluwer.

National Heart Lung and Blood Institute (NHLBI). (n.d.a). *Narcolepsy.* https://www.nhlbi.nih.gov/health-topics/narcolepsy

National Heart Lung and Blood Institute (NHLBI). (n.d.b). *Sleep deprivation and deficiency.* https://www.nhlbi.nih.gov/health-topics/sleep-deprivation-and-deficiency

National Institute of Health (NIH). (2019, April 29). *About sleep.* Eunice Kennedy Shriver National Institute of Child Health and Human Development. https://www.nichd.nih.gov/health/topics/sleep/conditioninfo

National Institute of Neurological Disorders and Stroke (NINDS). (2019a, August 13). *Brain Basics: Understanding sleep.* https://www.ninds.nih.gov/Disorders/Patient-Caregiver-Education/Understanding-Sleep

National Institute of Neurological Disorders and Stroke (NINDS). (2019b, March 27). *Narcolepsy information page.* https://www.ninds.nih.gov/Disorders/All-Disorders/Narcolepsy-Information-Page

National Institute for Occupational Safety and Health (NIOSH). (n.d.). *Diseases and shift work.* https://www.cdc.gov/niosh/work-hour-training-for-nurses/longhours/mod3/15.html

National Institute for Occupational Safety and Health (NIOSH). (2020, April). *NIOSH training for nurses on shift work and long work hours.* CDC Course Numbers WB4217 and WB4218. DHHS (NIOSH) Publication Number 2015–115. https://www.cdc.gov/niosh/docs/2015-115/default.html

National Sleep Foundation (NSF). (n.d.). *Hypersomnia.* https://www.sleepfoundation.org/hypersomnia

National Sleep Foundation (NSF). (2020a, November 20). *How your circadian rhythm helps you sleep.* https://www.thensf.org/how-your-circadian-rhythm-helps-you-sleep/

National Sleep Foundation (NSF). (2020b, December 1). *Do I have insomnia?* https://www.thensf.org/do-i-have-insomnia/

National Sleep Foundation (NSF). (2020c, October 23). *Sleep studies.* https://www.sleepfoundation.org/sleep-studies

National Sleep Foundation (NSF). (2020d, December 3). *Do I have Restless Legs Syndrome?* https://www.thensf.org/do-i-have-restless-legs-syndrome/

National Sleep Foundation (NSF). (2021, March 16). *Resting vs. sleeping.* https://www.sleep.org/how-sleep-works/resting-vs-sleeping/

National Sleep Foundation (NSF). (2022a, April 15). *Weight loss and sleep.* https://www.sleepfoundation.org/physical-health/weight-loss-and-sleep

National Sleep Foundation (NSF). (2022b, April 18). *Drowsy driving.* https://www.sleepfoundation.org/drowsy-driving

Nena, E., Katsaouni, M., Steiropoulos, P., Theodorou, E., Constantinidis, T. C., & Tripsianis, G. (2018). Effect of shift work on sleep, health, and quality of life of health-care workers. *Indian Journal of Occupational and Environmental Medicine, 22*(1), 29–34. https://doi.org/10.4103/ijoem.IJOEM_4_18

Neubauer, D. N., Pandi-Perumal, S. R., Spence, D. W., Buttoo, K., & Monti, J. M. (2018). Pharmacotherapy of insomnia. *Journal of Central Nervous System Disease, 10*, 1–7. https://doi.org/10.1177/1179573518770672

Newberry, J. A. (2019). Creating a safe sleep environment for the infant: What the pediatric nurse needs to know. *Journal of Pediatric Nursing, 44*, 119–122. https://doi.org/10.1016/j.pedn.2018.12.001

Newsom, R. (2020, October 23). *Aging and sleep.* SleepFoundation.org. https://www.sleepfoundation.org/aging-and-sleep

Nierengarten, M B. (2018). Use guidelines to diagnose pediatric sleep apnea. *Contemporary Pediatrics, 35*(12). https://www.contemporarypediatrics.com/view/use-guidelines-diagnose-pediatric-sleep-apnea

Norris, T. L. (2019). *Porth's essentials of pathophysiology* (5th ed.). Wolters Kluwer.

Office of Disease Prevention and Health Promotion (ODPHP). (2020, October 8). *Healthy People 2030. Sleep.* https://health.gov/healthypeople/objectives-and-data/browse-objectives/sleep

Oleksy, A. J., & Schlesinger, J. J. (2019). What's all that noise – Improving the hospital soundscape. *Journal of Clinical Monitoring and Computing, 33*(4), 557–562. https://doi.org/10.1007/s10877-018-0215-3

Pacheco, D. (2020a, October 16). *What is shift work?* Sleep Foundation. Ps://www.sleepfoundation.org/shift-work-disorder/what-shift-work

Pacheco, D. (2020b, October 2). *Parasomnias.* Sleep Foundation. https://www.sleepfoundation.org/parasomnias

Pacheco, D. (2020c, October 9). *Does napping during the day affect your sleep at night?* https://www.sleepfoundation.org/articles/debunking-sleep-myths-does-napping-during-day-affect-your-sleep-night

Pacheco, D. (2020d, September 24). *Children and sleep.* https://www.sleepfoundation.org/children-and-sleep

Restless Legs Syndrome Foundation. (2020). *Understanding RLS.* https://www.rls.org/understanding-rls

Reuter-Rice, K., McMurray, M. G., Christoferson, E., Yeager, H., & Wiggins, B. (2020). Sleep in the intensive care unit: Biological, environmental, and pharmacologic implications for nurses. *Critical Care Nursing Clinics of North America, 32*(2), 191–201. https://doi.org/10.1016/j.cnc.2020.02.002

Reynolds, A. C., & Adams, R. J. (2019). Treatment of sleep disturbance in older adults. *Pharmacy Practice and Research, 49*, 296–304. https://doi.org/10.1002/jppr.1565

Simmons, S., & Pruitt, B. (2012). Sounding the alarm for patients with obstructive sleep apnea. *Nursing, 42*(4), 34–41; quiz 41–42. https://doi.org/10.1097/01.NURSE.0000412921.89889.ba

Singh, A. N. (2016). Recent advances in pharmacotherapy of insomnia. *International Medical Journal, 23*(6), 602–604.

Sleep Foundation. (2020a). *The best foods to help you sleep.* https://www.sleepfoundation.org/articles/food-and-drink-promote-good-nights-sleep

Sleep Foundation. (2020a). *Alcohol and sleep.* https://www.sleepfoundation.org/articles/alcohol-and-sleep

Sleep Foundation. (2020b). *The best foods to help you sleep.* https://www.sleepfoundation.org/articles/food-and-drink-promote-good-nights-sleep

Sleep Foundation. (2020c). *Effects of noise during sleep.* https://www.sleepfoundation.org/bedroom-environment/how-does-noise-affect-sleep

Sleep Foundation. (2020d). *Sleep hygiene.* https://www.sleepfoundation.org/articles/sleep-hygiene

Sleep Foundation. (2020e). *Thyroid issues and sleep.* https://www.sleepfoundation.org/physical-health/thyroid-issues-and-sleep

Stanford Health Care. (n.d.). *Sleep restriction and CBT. Cognitive Behavioral Therapy for insomnia (CBTI): Sleep restriction.* Retrieved December 8, 2020, from https://stanfordhealthcare.org/medical-treatments/c/cognitive-behavioral-therapy-insomnia/procedures/sleep-restriction.html

Steiner, V., Ames, A., Milz, S. A., & Dubin, S. (2020). Nursing home staff's perceptions of noise compared to measured noise levels: A Descriptive Study. *Journal of Gerontological Nursing, 46*(9), 37–45. https://doi.org/10.3928/00989134-20200706-03

Suni, E. (2020). *How much sleep do we really need?* https://www.sleepfoundation.org/articles/how-much-sleep-do-we-really-need

Tabas, E. E., Khodadadi, F., Sarani, H., Saeedinezhad, F., & Jahantigh, M. (2019). Effect of eye masks, earplugs, and quiet time protocol on sleep quality of patients admitted to the cardiac care unit: A clinical trial study. *Medical Surgical Nursing Journal, 8*(3), e98762. https://doi.org/10.5812/msnj.98762

Tonetti, L., Mingozzi, R., & Natale, V. (2016). Comparison between paper and electronic sleep diary. *Biological Rhythm Research, 47*(5), 743–753. https://doi.org/10.1080/09291016.2016.1191689

Trossman, S. (2018). Quiet please. Nurses offer strategies to promote patients' rest and sleep. *American Nurse Today, 13*(11), 46–48.

Vincensi, B., Pearch, K., Redding, J., Brandonisio, S., Tzou, S., & Meiusi, E. (2016). Sleep in the hospitalized patient: Nurse and patient perceptions. *Medsurg Nursing, 25*(5), 351–356.

Wallis, R., Harris, E., Lee, H., Davies, W., & Astin, F. (2019). Environmental noise levels in hospital settings: A rapid review of measurement techniques and implementation in hospital settings. *Noise & Health, 21*(102), 200–216. https://DOI: 10.4103/nah.NAH_19_18

Weaver, M. D., Vetter, C., Rajaratnam, S. M. W., O'Brien, C. S., Qadri, S., Benca, R. M., Rogers, A. E., Leary, E. B., Walsh, J. K., Czeisler, C. A., & Barger, L. K. (2018). Sleep disorders, depression, and anxiety are associated with adverse safety outcomes in healthcare workers: A prospective cohort study. *Journal of Sleep Research, 27*(6), e12722. https://doi.org/10.1111/jsr.12722

Weber, J. R., & Kelley, J. H. (2018). *Health assessment in nursing* (6th ed.). Wolters Kluwer.

Wilson, S., Anderson, K., Baldwin, D., Dijk, D. J., Espie, A., Espie, C., Gringras, P., Krystal, A., Nutt, D., Selsick, H., & Sharpley, A. (2019). British Association for Psychopharmacology consensus statement on evidence-based treatment of insomnia, parasomnias and circadian rhythm disorders: An update. *Journal of Psychopharmacology, 33*(8), 923–947. https://doi.org/10.1177/0269881119855343

Winterbottom, F. A., LeBlanc-Lucas, K., & Boylan, A. (2020). Nurses' influence on patient wellbeing. Noise reduction and Sunshine Therapy. *Critical Care Nursing Clinics of North America, 32*(2), 327–334. https://doi.org/10.1016/j.cnc.2020.02.012

Witkoski Stimpfel, A. (2020). Shift work and sleep disruption: Implications for nurses' health. *American Nurse, 15*(11), 23–25.

Wolters Kluwer. (2020). Problem-based care plans. In *Lippincott Advisor*. Wolters Kluwer.

Yarnell, E. (2015). Herbal medicine for insomnia. *Alternative and Complementary Therapies, 21*(4), 173–179. https://doi.org/10.1089/act.2015.29011.eya

Yeager, J. (2019). Relaxation interventions for antepartum mothers on hospitalized bedrest. *The American Journal of Occupational Therapy, 73*(1), 7301205110p1-7301205110p7. https://doi.org/10.5014/ajot.2019.025692

Zaki, N. F. W., Yousif, M., BaHammam, A. S., Spence, D. W., Bharti, V. K., Subramenian, P., & Pandi-Perumal, S. R. (2019). Chronotherapeutics: Recognizing the importance of timing factors in the treatment of disease and sleep disorders. *Clinical Neuropharmacology, 42*(3), 80–87. https://doi.org/10.1097/WNF.0000000000000341

Zandy, M., Chang, V., Rao, D. P., & Do, M. T. (2020). Tobacco smoke exposure and sleep: Estimating the association of urinary cotinine with sleep quality. *Health Promotion and Chronic Disease Prevention in Canada, 40*(3), 70–80. https://doi.org/10.24095/hpcdp.40.3.02

36 Comfort and Pain Management

Carla Potter

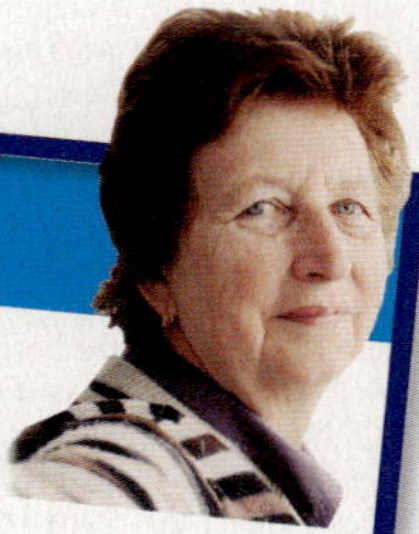

Carla is a 72-year-old adult who has a history of type 2 diabetes and associated diabetic neuropathy. She reports pain in her lower extremities that is at times sharp but, is generally dull. She also reports that she has relatively new periods of numbness and tingling. Carla is becoming increasingly worried that this constant pain is going to take over her life. She reports that an increase in stress and anxiety seems to be making the pain even worse.

Sheree Lincoln

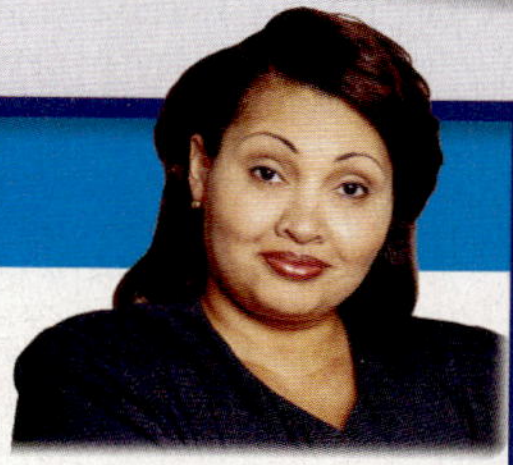

Sheree, a 42-year-old woman who has just undergone abdominal surgery, returns to the medical-surgical unit. Patient-controlled analgesia (PCA) is prescribed. Approximately 2 hours after returning from surgery, the patient reports unresolved pain. Assessment reveals that she has not been using the PCA device.

Xavier Malton

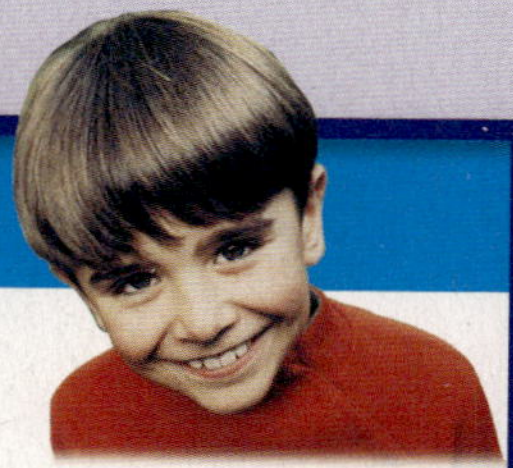

Xavier, a 5-year-old boy diagnosed with ulcerative colitis, is in the bathroom with his mother. He suddenly grabs his belly while on the toilet and starts to scream, "Something hurts really bad!" His mother pulls the emergency call bell. He is doubled over in pain and can't get off the toilet. After being assisted back to his bed and receiving the relatively small dose of pain medication prescribed by the provider, Xavier continues to scream for half an hour while curled up in a fetal position on his bed. "The pain is so bad; it will never go away!"

Learning Outcomes

After completing the chapter, you will be able to accomplish the following:

1. Describe specific elements in the pain experience.
2. Compare and contrast acute (nociceptive) and chronic (neuropathic, nociplastic) pain.
3. Identify factors that may affect a person's pain experience.
4. Obtain a complete pain assessment using appropriate interviewing and physical assessment skills.
5. Explain the relationship between pain and other areas of human functioning.
6. Use a holistic approach to pain management that considers a multimodal approach to the pharmacologic management of pain and includes nonpharmacologic methods.
7. Collaborate with the interprofessional team to develop, implement, and evaluate effective, individualized, evidence-based pain management regimens.
8. Use teaching and counseling skills to empower patients to direct their own pain management programs.

Nursing Concepts

- Cellular Regulation
- Evidence-Based Practice
- Infection
- Inflammation
- Tissue Integrity

Current reports indicate that 20.4% of adults in the United States experience chronic pain. High-impact chronic pain, chronic pain that frequently limits work, social, self-care, and recreational activities, impacts 7.4% of adults in the United States (Dahlhamer et al., 2018; Zelaya et al., 2020). Urbanization affected reports of chronic pain, with adults in rural areas experiencing the greatest percentage of chronic pain (28.1%) and high-impact chronic pain (10.9%). Older age, race, Hispanic origin, and biological sex also influence the percentage of adults who report chronic pain (Zelaya et al., 2020). When both direct (medical expenses) and indirect (missed days of work) costs are considered, the total financial impact of the use and misuse of alcohol, nicotine, and illicit (illegal) drugs, plus the misuse of prescribed drugs is more than $700 billion annually (National Institute on Drug Abuse, 2020). Additional costs of unrelenting, inadequately treated pain include physiologic, psychological, and social effects such as social isolation, disability and lost work productivity or advancement, change in the distribution of household chores, lower level of marital satisfaction, decrease in quality of life, limitations in performing complex activities, and feelings of fear, anxiety, depression, self-judgment, pain invalidation, stigmatization, and demoralization (Dahlhamer et al., 2018; Nicola et al., 2021; Suso-Ribera et al., 2020). Physiologic effects of pain include hyperglycemia, increased cardiac workload, immune system dysfunction, altered coagulation, gastrointestinal (GI) ileus, urinary retention, decreased lung volume, and fatigue (Hinkle et al., 2022; Karch, 2020).

Scientists and clinicians have united in their efforts to ensure that pain management is a high priority in our health care system. New advances in understanding and treating pain have focused on the possibility of safely managing most human pain. Hospital policies are required to include a comprehensive pain assessment that is consistent with the patient's scope of care, treatment, services, age, condition, and ability to understand. Hospitals must also reassess and respond to pain based on their established reassessment criteria. Hospitals can refer the patient for treatment of pain or employ pharmacologic and nonpharmacologic approaches that are patient-specific, consider the provider's clinical judgment, include a risk–benefit analysis, and comply with processes required for monitoring and education (The Joint Commission, 2021). Effective January 1, 2018, standards for hospitals from The Joint Commission (2017) specifically require hospitals to:

- **Identify pain assessment and pain management, including safe opioid prescribing, as an organizational priority:** involves a leader/leadership team; provides nonpharmacologic pain treatment modalities; provides staff and licensed independent practitioners educational resources, programs, and consultation services; identifies opioid treatment programs; facilitates practitioner and pharmacist access to the Prescription Drug Monitoring databases; and acquires equipment needed to monitor patients who are at high risk for adverse outcomes associated with opioid treatment
- **Actively involve the organized medical staff in leadership roles in organization performance improvement activities to improve quality of care, treatment, and services and patient safety:** medical staff participates in the establishment of protocols and quality metrics; and reviews performance improvement data
- **Assess and manage the patient's pain and minimize the risks associated with treatment:** employs accurate screening and assessment tools that are readily available and used appropriately; screens patients for pain during emergency department encounters and upon admission; treats the patient's pain or refers them for treatment; develops pain treatment plans based on evidence-based practices and patient involvement that considers the patient's condition, past medical history, treatment options, pain management goals; involves the patient in pain management treatment planning through the development of realistic expectations and goals, evaluation process, and education on pain management; monitors patients identified as high risk for adverse outcomes related to opioid treatment; reassesses and responds to the patient's pain through evaluation and documentation

QSEN Reflective Practice: Cultivating QSEN Competencies

CHALLENGE TO ETHICAL AND LEGAL SKILLS

While in my pediatrics rotation a local hospital, I was caring for Xavier Malton, a 5-year-old boy diagnosed with ulcerative colitis (UC), a form of inflammatory bowel disease (IBD). Suddenly, at the end of this relatively quiet shift, the emergency call bell alarm sounded. I realized that the call was coming from Xavier's bathroom. As I ran the 10 ft to his room, thoughts of him bleeding internally or perforating his bowel ran through my head. I got there at the same time his nurse did, only to discover that his mother had pulled the alarm because her son had suddenly grabbed his belly while on the toilet and had started screaming that something was "hurting really, really bad." He was so doubled over in pain that he could not even get off the toilet. Having Crohn disease myself (another form of IBD), I knew that the pain this boy was experiencing was excruciating and not imagined.

With help from Xavier's mother, his nurse and I got Xavier back into bed. We reviewed his chart only to learn Xavier did not have a PRN prescription for pain medication. We called the provider, who was hesitant to prescribe any pain medication. Pain is not unusual with UC, so the provider encouraged us to implement alternative methods of pain management such as distraction. We clearly presented Xavier's case and, based on our repeated recommendation, the provider agreed to prescribe pain medication, but only a very small dose. We immediately administered the pain medication, got Xavier as comfortable in bed as possible, and planned to routinely reassess his pain.

Although we had hoped the pain medication would relieve or at least alleviate some of his pain, Xavier continued to scream, curled up in a fetal position on his bed. I had to briefly leave the room, and even from across the hallway, I could hear him screaming that the pain was "so bad" and that it would "never go away."

Thinking Outside the Box: Possible Courses of Action

- I could give up and try not to care since this system clearly is not committed to meeting comfort needs, but this means abandoning my patient(s).
- I could be persistent about advocating for this patient until his pain is relieved, continuing to contact and work with key members of the interprofessional team to achieve pain relief for my patient.
- I could consult with a colleague who I respect regarding the best way to accomplish the goal of pain relief, since I don't want to alienate caregivers with whom I will need to continue to work.

Evaluating a Good Outcome: How Do I Define Success?

- Patient's pain is relieved and patient reports feeling comfortable.
- Colleagues are newly committed to the responsibility of everyone to adequately manage pain.
- My working relationships with other professional caregivers are not compromised by my advocacy for this patient.
- My personal and professional integrity remains intact.

Personal Learning: Here's to the Future!

Forty-five minutes after our shift had ended, Xavier's nurse and I were still following the provider around, basically demanding that she reassess the patient and prescribe additional pain medication for him. Finally, she performed a reassessment and prescribed a narcotic for pain management. Unfortunately, the narcotic she ordered was in short supply in the hospital. We spent the next 15 minutes tracking some down. Although it took more time than we had hoped, we did give Xavier additional pain medication, which, ultimately, did relieve his pain and allow him to fall asleep. However, we left the hospital almost an hour and a half after our shift had ended, time that was lost to Xavier and time for which we would not receive compensation.

Transforming the culture of health care is a daunting task. Demanding an unacceptable situation be remedied requires an absolute belief in the rights of the patient. The situation was indeed unacceptable—no child should be left to suffer. Interprofessional collaboration is challenging when members of the team have differing viewpoints. The nurse should be able to confidently and competently provide assessment data and a recommendation for the plan of care. This promotes safe, high-quality patient care and allows for the entire team to advocate for the patient. Any RN facing a situation that has the potential to transform the culture of health care for the better has the responsibility to take advantage of that situation, no matter what the perceived or actual professional risk. I would recommend that any RN in a similar situation take the same steps that Xavier's nurse and I did. Do not be afraid to challenge others who you think are wrong. Be confident in your opinions. Refuse to back down. Remember that you may be the only one who can ensure that your patient's needs are met. Always advocate for high-quality care; never settle for less.

Tracey Sara Miller, Georgetown University

QSEN Reflective Practice: Cultivating QSEN Competencies *(continued)*

CHALLENGE TO ETHICAL AND LEGAL SKILLS

QSEN SELF-REFLECTION ON QUALITY AND SAFETY COMPETENCIES DEVELOPING KNOWLEDGE, SKILLS, AND ATTITUDES FOR CONTINUOUS IMPROVEMENT

How do you think you would respond to or approach this situation? Why? What does this tell you about yourself and about the adequacy of your skills for professional practice? Do you agree with the criteria that the nursing student used to evaluate a successful outcome? Why or why not? What *knowledge, skills,* and *attitudes* do you need to develop to continuously improve quality and safety when caring for patients like Xavier?

Patient-Centered Care: What assurances should be given to Xavier and his mother about pain relief and control? What is the best way to communicate emotional support and a commitment to providing pain relief to Xavier and his mother? How could you involve Xavier's mother as a partner in coordinating Xavier's pain management?

Teamwork and Collaboration/Quality Improvement: What communication skills do you need to continue to function as an advocate for your patients? What strategies might be appropriate to ensure that you function as a valued member of the health care team? Can you think of other ways to communicate with team members regarding individual patients' responses to pain?

Safety/Evidence-Based Practice: Is there anything more you could have done to facilitate timely pain relief for Xavier? When are nonpharmacologic methods of pain relief most appropriate and effective? How do you think your response affected the situation? What evidence in nursing literature provides guidance for decision making regarding responses to pain and misconceptions about the pain experience?

Informatics: What information should be electronically documented regarding your assessment of the presence and severity of Xavier's pain? Can you identify other essential information that must be available in Xavier's electronic record to support safe patient care from the entire health care team?

of response to pain, progress toward pain management goals, side effects, and risk factors for adverse events; and educates patients and families on discharge plans related to pain management including plan, side effects, impact on activities of daily living, and safe storage, use, and disposal of opioids

- **Collect data to monitor its performance:** includes types of interventions and effectiveness
- **Compile and analyze data:** identifies areas that need change to increase safety and quality for patients; and monitors the use of opioids for safe use

A person in pain often experiences the pain as an all-consuming reality and wants only one intervention—pain relief. If pain relief were as simple as rubbing a back or administering a prescribed analgesic, the nurse's task would be easy. However, no two people experience pain exactly the same way. Differences in individual pain perception and response to pain, as well as the multiple and diverse causes of pain, require the nurse to use highly specialized knowledge and abilities to promote comfort and to relieve pain. The most essential of these are the nurse's knowledge and understanding that the patient's pain is real, the willingness to become involved in the patient's pain experience, and competence in developing effective pain management regimens. (See the accompanying Reflective Practice box for an example.)

Although pain is often all-consuming for patients, it can be missed or misjudged easily because it is intangible. As a result, it is often easier to overlook or minimize a patient's poorly communicated pain than it is to ignore a dressing that needs to be changed, the need for assistance with walking, or the routine administration of a prescribed medication. Nurses must draw upon empathy and sensitivity when caring for patients experiencing pain. In addition, when addressing pain, nurses should ensure they are implementing active interventions that extend beyond the assessment of pain, and include interventions focused on treating and managing pain. Carefully consider your interventions when developing a care plan focused on pain: *You must do more than assess to impact change*, especially with pain.

This chapter discusses the pain experience and factors that influence it. A detailed guide to assessing pain is presented, along with numerous examples of actual and potential problems, and specific nursing strategies for promoting comfort and assisting patients to achieve pain management goals. The Evolving Case at the end of the chapter illustrates the application of clinical judgment to promote pain management and patient comfort.

EXPERIENCE OF PAIN

Pain is an elusive and complex phenomenon. Despite its universality, its exact nature remains a mystery. It is one of the human body's defense mechanisms that indicate the person is experiencing a problem. Margo McCaffery offers the classic definition of pain that is probably of greatest benefit to nurses and their patients, "Pain is whatever the experiencing person says it is, existing whenever the experiencing person says it does" (1968, p. 95). This definition rests on the belief that the only one who can be a real authority on whether, and how, a person is experiencing pain is that person. Health care providers must respect the patient's description of the pain because it is a personal experience. The International Association for the Study of Pain (IASP) recently updated their 1979 definition of pain as "An unpleasant sensory and emotional experience associated with, or resembling that associated with, actual or potential tissue damage" (Raja et al., 2020, p. 1976). They expound on this definition with the following notes (p. 1978):

- Pain is always a personal experience that is influenced to varying degrees by biological, psychological, and social factors.
- Pain and nociception are different phenomena. Pain cannot be inferred solely from activity in sensory neurons.
- Through their life experiences, individuals learn the concept of pain.
- A person's report of an experience as pain should be respected.
- Although pain usually serves an adaptive role, it may have adverse effects on function and social and psychological well-being.
- Verbal description is only one of several behaviors to express pain; inability to communicate does not negate the possibility that a human or a nonhuman animal experiences pain.

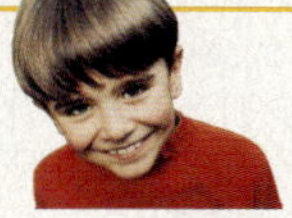

Consider **Xavier Malton**, the 5-year-old boy with ulcerative colitis who suddenly develops acute pain. The nurse appreciates that Xavier is indeed experiencing pain because of his screaming that something hurts. Furthermore, his pain is validated by his body posture and inability to get off the toilet.

Gate Control Theory of Pain

Many theories have attempted to explain the mechanism of pain. However, the **gate control theory**, originally proposed by Melzack and Wall in 1965, provides the most practical model regarding the concept of pain. It describes the transmission of painful stimuli and recognizes a connection between pain and the projection of pain information to the brain (Norris, 2020). The theory states that small nerve fibers conduct excitatory pain stimuli toward the brain, exaggerating the effect of the arriving impulses through a positive feedback mechanism. Large nerve fibers appear to inhibit the transmission of pain impulses from the spinal cord to the brain through a negative feedback system (Melzack & Wall). There is a transmission mechanism that is believed by some to be located in substantia gelatinosa cells in the dorsal horn of the spinal cord. This serves as the gate. Only a limited amount of sensory information can be processed by the nervous system at any given moment. When too much information is sent through, certain cells in the spinal column interrupt the signal as if closing a gate (Pasero & McCaffery, 2011). One concrete example of this is when a person rubs the site of an injury that has just occurred. This stimulation of the large fibers, which are largely inactive when the small-fiber activity is increased, can decrease the level of pain experienced by the person (Melzack & Wall). Figure 36-1 illustrates the gate control theory of pain.

Other factors thought to have an impact on the opening and closing of this gate are past experiences, the cultural and social environment, personal expectations, beliefs about pain, the emphasis placed on pain, and emotions. For example, a positive mood, distraction, or relaxation can work to close the gate; fear and anxiety have been shown to open the gate, thus increasing the pain experienced. Understanding gate theory can positively impact on a patient's development of skills that help in their self-management of chronic pain (LeFort et al., 2021). Although not everyone accepts the gate control theory, it appears to explain why mechanical and electrical interventions, or heat and pressure may provide effective pain relief. Nursing measures, such as massage or a warm compress to a painful lower back area, stimulate large nerve fibers to close the gate, thus blocking pain impulses from that area. Teaching self-management techniques that activate closing the gate may also minimize the experience of pain for patients (LeFort et al., 2021).

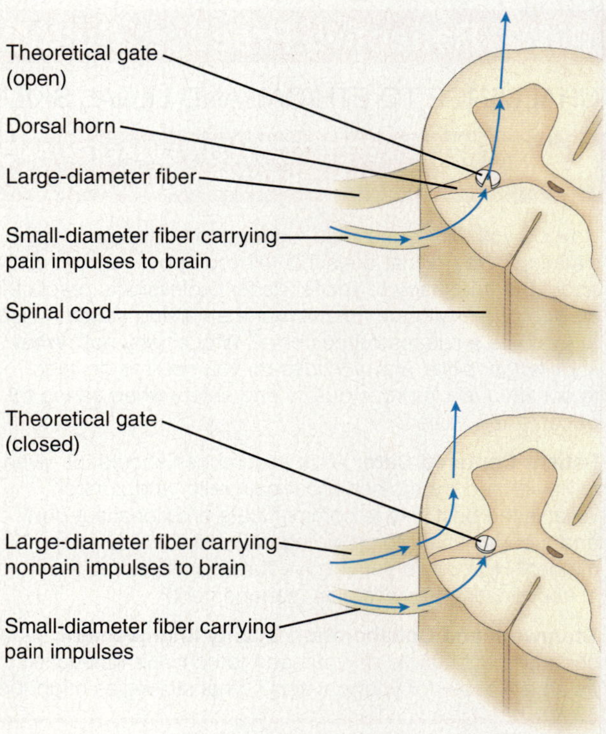

FIGURE 36-1. An illustration of the gate control theory of pain.

Theoretical models that explore pain also consider pain receptors, patterns of activity, the brain's role in managing inputs, and neurohormonal control of pain. There is no universally accepted explanation for the physiologic experience of pain. The mechanisms and pathways of pain are complex and continue to be explored (Norris, 2020).

Pain Process

The four specific physiologic processes involved in nociception (the ability to feel painful stimuli) include transduction, transmission, perception, and modulation of pain (Pasero & McCaffery, 2011). Nociceptive pain is initiated by nociceptors that are activated by injury to the peripheral tissue and is representative of the normal pain process (Norris, 2020).

Transduction

The activation of pain receptors is referred to as **transduction**. It involves conversion of painful stimuli into electrical impulses that travel from the periphery to the spinal cord at the dorsal horn. The **nociceptors**, or peripheral receptors, respond selectively to mechanical, thermal, and chemical stimuli that are noxious (Norris, 2020). In addition, when the threshold of perception for pain has been reached and when there is injured tissue, it is believed that the injured tissue releases chemicals that excite or activate nerve endings. For example, a damaged cell releases histamine, which excites nerve endings. Lactic acid accumulates in tissues injured by lack of blood supply and is believed to excite nerve endings, causing pain, or to lower the threshold of nerve endings to other stimuli (e.g., heat or pressure). The prolonged effect of pain stimuli acting on the central nervous system (CNS) can lead to sensitization, meaning that the threshold for activation of pain is lowered. At that point, even harmless stimuli can trigger pain; pain signals are faster and feel more intense.

Other substances are also released that stimulate nociceptors or pain receptors. These include bradykinin, prostaglandins, and substance P:

- Bradykinin, a powerful vasodilator that increases capillary permeability and constricts smooth muscle, plays an important role in the chemistry of pain at the site of an injury even before the pain message gets to the brain. It also triggers the release of histamine and, in combination with histamine, produces the redness, swelling, and pain typically observed when inflammation is present.
- Prostaglandins are important hormone-like substances that send additional pain stimuli to the CNS.
- Substance P, a neuropeptide, sensitizes receptors on nerves to feel pain and also increases the rate at which nerves fire.

Prostaglandins, substance P, and serotonin (a hormone that can act to stimulate smooth muscles, inhibit gastric secretion, and produce vasoconstriction) are **neurotransmitters**, substances that either excite or inhibit target nerve cells.

Receptors in the skin and superficial organs are incapable of responding selectively. However, mechanical, thermal, chemical, and electrical agents may stimulate them. Friction from bed linens and pressure from a cast are mechanical stimulants. Sunburn and cold water on a tooth with caries are thermal stimulants. An acid burn is the result of a chemical stimulant. The jolt of a static charge is an electrical stimulant (Norris, 2020; Pasero & McCaffery, 2011).

Transmission of Pain Stimuli

Pain sensations from the site of an injury or inflammation are conducted along pathways to the spinal cord and then on to higher centers. These pathways are clearly defined in certain areas but are still somewhat unclear in other areas. The overall process is known as **transmission**. No specific pain organs or cells exist in the body. Rather, an interlacing network of undifferentiated free nerve endings receives painful stimuli. Free nerve-ending pain receptors include the afferent (those fibers carrying impulses from the pain receptors toward the brain) fast-conducting A-delta–fibers and the slow-conducting C-fibers. The larger A-delta–fibers transmit acute, well-localized pain that is typically elicited by mechanical or thermal stimuli. The smaller C-fibers convey diffuse, longer-lasting pain that is triggered by chemical stimuli or persistent mechanical or thermal stimuli (Norris, 2020). It is estimated that there are several million of these nerve endings in the body, often embedded in the layers of the skin and in some internal tissues, such as the joint surfaces. In the deeper tissues of the body, the pain receptors are diffusely but unevenly spread (Pasero & McCaffery, 2011).

A protective pain reflex is responsible for withdrawal of an endangered tissue from a damaging stimulus. Sensory impulses travel over A-fibers through the dorsal root ganglion to the dorsal horn of the spinal cord. At this point, the sensory nerve impulse synapses with a motor neuron, and the impulse is carried along efferent nerve pathways back to the site of the painful stimulus in a reflex arc. This results in an immediate muscle contraction intended to withdraw/remove the injured body part from the source of the pain. As a concrete example, think about the reaction that occurs when a hot stove is touched. Figure 36-2 (on page 1342) illustrates the transmission of the pain sensation, the initiation of the protective reflex response, and conscious awareness of the location, intensity, and quality of the pain after the impulse reaches the cortex (Pasero & McCaffery, 2011).

Perception of Pain

The **perception** of pain involves the sensory process that occurs when a stimulus for pain is present. It includes the person's interpretation of the pain. The **pain threshold** is the "minimum intensity of a stimulus that is perceived as painful" (IASP, 2021). Adaptation may affect this perception of pain. For example, when a person's hand is immersed in warm water, a sensation of pain eventually occurs as the water is heated. However, the person can tolerate a higher temperature as water is gradually heated to the pain level than if the hand had been plunged into hot water without any preparation. Other factors that may impact perception, interpretation, and response to pain will be discussed later in this chapter.

Modulation of Pain

The process by which the sensation of pain is inhibited or modified is referred to as **modulation**. The sensation of pain appears to be regulated or modified by substances called neuromodulators. These **neuromodulators** are endogenous opioid compounds, meaning they are naturally present, morphine-like chemical regulators in the spinal cord and brain. They appear to have analgesic activity and alter the perception of pain. These endogenous opioid compounds are believed to produce their analgesic effects by binding to specific opioid receptor sites throughout the CNS, blocking the release or production of pain-transmitting substances. Both pain and stress appear capable of activating the endogenous opiate system.

Endorphins and enkephalins are opioid neuromodulators. **Endorphins** are produced at neural synapses at various points along the CNS pathway. They are powerful pain-blocking chemicals that have prolonged analgesic effects and produce euphoria. It is suggested that endorphins may be released when certain measures are used to relieve pain, such as skin stimulation and relaxation techniques, and

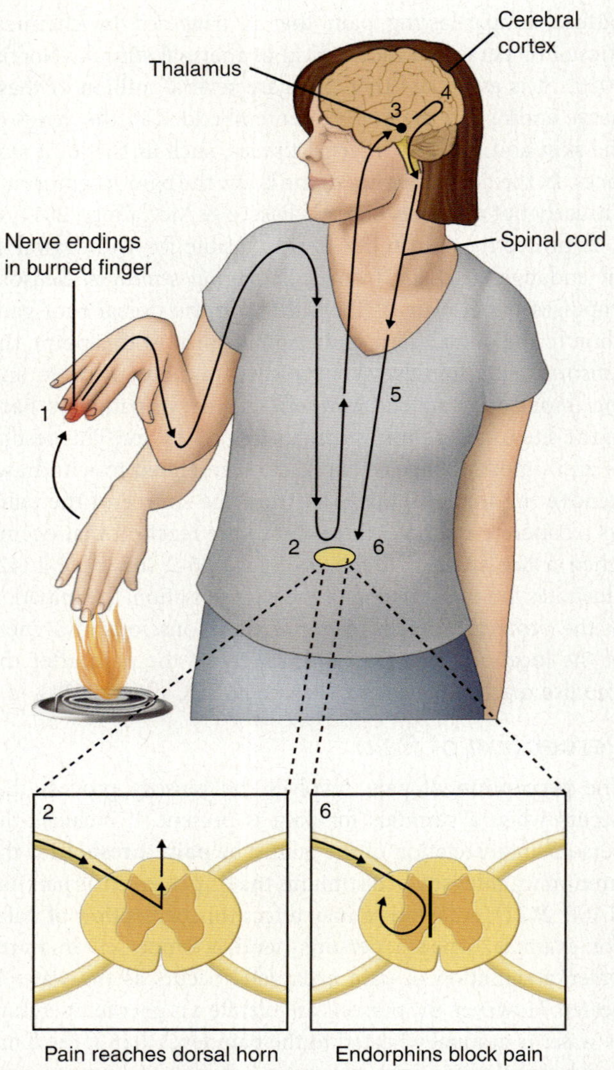

FIGURE 36-2. Pain sensation and relief. (*1*) Pain's path begins as a message and is received by nerve endings in a burned finger. (*2*) The pain signal from the burned finger travels as an electrochemical impulse along the length of the nerve to the dorsal horn on the spinal cord, a region that runs the length of the spine and receives signals from all over the body. (*3*) The message is relayed to the thalamus, a sensory center in the brain where sensations such as heat, cold, pain, and touch first become conscious. (*4*) It then travels on to the cortex, where the intensity and location of pain are perceived. (*5*) Pain relief begins as a signal from the brain and descends by way of the spinal cord. (*6*) In the dorsal horn, chemicals such as endorphins are released to diminish the pain message from the injured finger.

when certain pain-relieving drugs are used. The endorphin, dynorphin, has the most potent analgesic effect. However, many questions remain about endorphins.

Enkephalins, which are widespread throughout the brain and dorsal horn of the spinal cord, are considered less potent than endorphins. **Enkephalins** are thought to reduce pain sensation by inhibiting the release of substance P from the terminals of afferent neurons (Norris, 2020; Pasero & McCaffery, 2011).

Types of Pain

Pain may be classified according to its duration, its localization/location, or its etiology.

Duration of Pain

Perhaps the most common distinction involves the duration of pain. **Acute pain** is generally rapid in onset and varies in intensity from mild to severe. It is protective in nature. In other words, acute pain warns the person of tissue damage or organic disease and triggers autonomic responses such as increased heart rate, the fight-or-flight response, and increased blood pressure (Jungquist et al., 2017; Norris, 2020). After its underlying cause is resolved, acute pain disappears. It should end once healing occurs. Causes of acute pain include a pricked finger, sore throat, or surgery.

Chronic pain is maladaptive pain that persists or is recurrent for more than 3 months. When classified as chronic *primary* pain, the chronic pain itself is considered the disease—this includes diagnoses such as fibromyalgia or back pain. Chronic pain is classified as *secondary* when the chronic pain results from cancer, surgery or trauma, an issue in the nervous system (neuropathic), headache or orofacial issues, visceral (organ) conditions, or musculoskeletal diseases (Treede et al., 2019). Chronic pain presentation varies greatly and can include pain that is continuous, pain that is episodic with periods of **remission** (disease is present, but the person does not experience pain) and **exacerbation** (the symptoms reappear), or pain that is recurring and contains elements of both chronic and acute pain (Norris, 2020; Treede et al., 2019).

Patients have difficulty describing chronic pain because it may be poorly localized. The patient presentation will vary from person to person, which makes completing an accurate, objective assessment challenging for health care professionals. In addition, the misconceptions and personal biases of caregivers can adversely affect the management of patients with chronic pain. Chronic pain takes a toll on the person experiencing pain and may result in depression, anger, frustration, sleep and appetite disturbances, and dependency. Chronic secondary pain that is associated with a disease process, such as cancer, is more likely to be viewed as valid, while chronic primary pain that is not well defined may be misinterpreted or dismissed by health care providers. Health care providers who have experienced chronic pain or struggled through the experience with a loved one may have a special awareness of its debilitating, destructive nature. Improved classification and diagnostic coding (related to reimbursement) of chronic pain lends credibility to the consideration of chronic pain a stand-alone health condition, which positively impacts on the ability of patients to receive effective pain management (Treede et al., 2019).

Nurses need an awareness of their own personal feelings toward pain (especially chronic pain) and the factors that affect pain if they are to assess and manage their patient's pain creatively and effectively. See Promoting Health 36-1 for a checklist of behaviors to foster one's self-awareness of comfort needs and pain.

Localization/Location of Pain

Pain can also be categorized according to whether it is generalized or localized (IASP, 2021). **Cutaneous pain** (superficial pain) usually involves the skin or subcutaneous tissue. A

Promoting Health 36-1

COMFORT

Use the assessment checklist to determine how well you are meeting comfort needs. Then, develop a prescription for self-care by choosing appropriate behaviors from the list of suggestions.

Assessment Checklist

☐ almost always ☐ sometimes ☐ almost never

☐ ☐ ☐ 1. Obtain a medical evaluation when acute or chronic pain is present.

☐ ☐ ☐ 2. Respect pain as the body's means of signaling that all is not well.

☐ ☐ ☐ 3. Control stress in the environment.

☐ ☐ ☐ 4. Avoid excessive fatigue.

☐ ☐ ☐ 5. Implement stress reduction or diversionary behaviors when pain is present.

☐ ☐ ☐ 6. Maintain awareness of personal preconceived notions that affect my perception of pain in others.

Self-Care Behaviors

1. I seek medical attention when pain persists.
2. I am aware of my usual behavioral responses to pain.
3. I use stress reduction techniques regularly.
4. I sleep well at night.
5. I have a positive outlook about my present situation.
6. I am aware of how to use distraction strategies to deal with pain.
7. I have a self-care management regimen I use if pain requires intervention.

paper cut that produces sharp pain with a burning sensation is an example of cutaneous pain. Deep **somatic pain** is diffuse or scattered and originates in tendons, ligaments, bones, blood vessels, and nerves. Strong pressure on a bone or damage to tissue that occurs with a sprain causes deep somatic pain. **Visceral pain**, or splanchnic pain, is poorly localized and originates in body organs in the thorax, cranium, and abdomen. Visceral pain is one of the most common types of pain produced by disease, and occurs as organs stretch abnormally and become distended, ischemic, or inflamed (Norris, 2020). A reflex contraction or spasm of the abdominal wall, called guarding, may occur as a protective mechanism to prevent additional trauma to underlying structures. A person automatically tenses the abdomen when an acute abdominal pain condition is present. This prevents underlying tissues and organs from being palpated or touched.

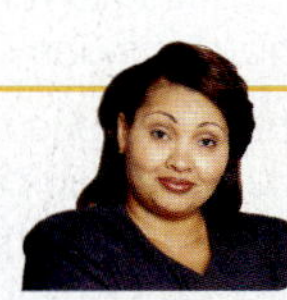

Think back to ***Sheree Lincoln***, the woman who has had abdominal surgery. Sheree was most likely experiencing visceral pain prior to surgery when her internal organs were undergoing injury, and the pain was vague and poorly localized. However, the postoperative pain she is experiencing now is more likely somatic pain because, although it may still be deep pain, it is now localized to the injury and incision site.

Pain can originate in one part of the body but be perceived in an area distant from its point of origin. This is known as **referred pain**. For example, pain associated with a myocardial infarction (heart attack) frequently refers to the neck, shoulder, chest, or arms (often the left arm). Referred pain is transmitted and perceived at a site different from the originating location but is referred to a place innervated by the same spinal segment. Figure 36-3 (on page 1344) illustrates areas to which pain from various organs is usually referred.

Etiology

Pain also is classified by its cause, which can be highly varied. Cancer-related pain and pain associated with end of life or palliation is generally considered separate from the following general pain classifications, and guidelines for treatment are specific to those types of pain. **Nociceptive pain** is initiated by nociceptors that are activated by actual or threatened damage to nonneural tissue and is representative of the normal pain process (IASP, 2021; Norris, 2020). **Nociceptors** are the peripheral somatosensory nerve fibers that transduce and encode noxious stimuli (IASP, 2021). Nociceptive pain is different from **neuropathic pain**, which is pain caused by a lesion or disease of the peripheral or central somatosensory nervous system (IASP, 2021; Norris, 2020; Raja et al., 2020). The exact cause of neuropathic pain is unknown, but it can originate either peripherally (e.g., phantom leg pain) or centrally (e.g., pain from spinal cord injury). Neuropathic pain can be of short duration but frequently is chronic. It is often described as burning, electric, tingling, or stabbing. Allodynia is an unexpected pain response that occurs after the introduction of a stimulus that is not normally known to provoke pain. Other characteristics of this pain include hyperalgesia, in which there is an increased pain response to a normally painful stimulus, and hyperesthesia, in which there is an increase in the level of sensitivity to a stimulus (IASP, 2021). Numerous pain syndromes have been identified that produce neuropathic pain. Several common examples are included in Table 36-1 (on page 1344).

In addition to nociceptive and neuropathic pain, patients may experience a combination of those two types of pain (mixed) or may have pain that is real but has no clear evidence

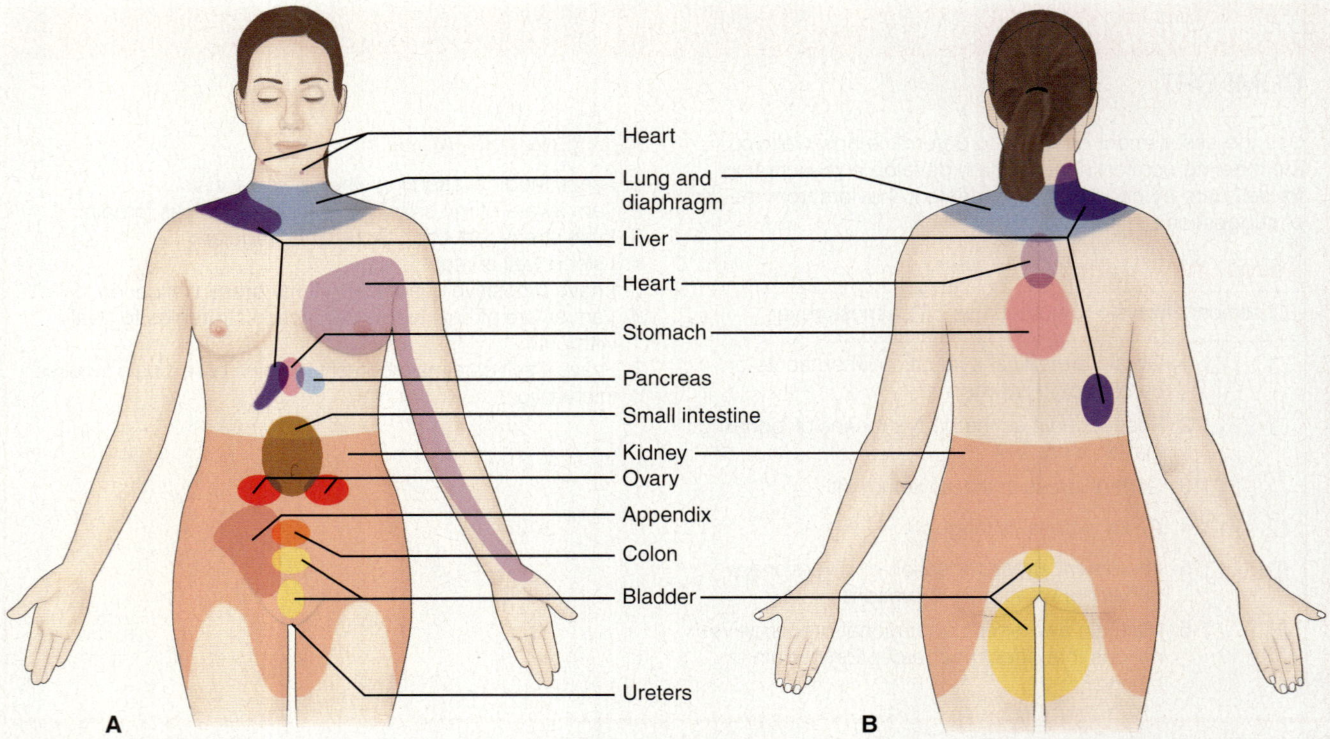

FIGURE 36-3. These drawings representing the anterior **(A)** and posterior **(B)** views of the body illustrate areas to which various organs refer pain.

of actual or threatened tissue damage. Pain that is not classified as nociceptive or neuropathic in nature is referred to as **nociplastic pain** and is addressed in the classification of chronic primary pain (Raja et al., 2020). Appropriate treatment of these syndromes is often delayed as a result of misdiagnosis, and they can prove difficult to treat. Nursing can play an important role in their early detection.

When pain is resistant to therapy and persists despite a variety of interventions, it is referred to as **intractable**. Nurses and other health care providers need to determine the appropriate pain treatment for each case of intractable pain so that a person can regain a healthy quality of life.

The pain that often occurs with an amputated leg where receptors and nerves are clearly absent, is a real experience

Table 36-1 Common Pain Syndromes Producing Neuropathic Pain

PAIN SYNDROME	DESCRIPTION
Complex regional pain syndrome (causalgia)	This pain occurs in the area of a partially injured peripheral nerve (the most common lesions are of the brachial plexus or median or sciatic nerve). The pain is described as burning, severe, diffuse, and persistent and is elicited by minimal movement or touch of the affected area. It increases with repeated stimulation and continues even after stimulation ceases.
Postherpetic neuralgia	This pain syndrome follows an acute central nervous system infection, such as herpes zoster (shingles). The herpes syndrome is characterized by a vesicular eruption and neuralgic pain, which is usually unilateral and encircles the body in band-like clusters. The severity of the pain may be mild to severe. Intractable pain may persist for months to years.
Phantom limb pain	This pain may occur in any person who has had a body part amputated either surgically or traumatically. Pain varies and may be a severe, burning, fiery sensation; crushing; cramping; a sense that the limb is edematous; or a sensation that the limb is being twisted and distorted. It may be triggered by the sensation of touching the residual limb, the occurrence of another illness, fatigue, atmospheric changes, and emotional stress.
Trigeminal neuralgia	This manifests as sudden, violent, lightning-like stabs of intense pain in one or more divisions of the trigeminal nerve, the fifth cranial nerve. Pain is usually experienced in the mouth, gums, lips, nose, cheek, chin, and surface of the head and may be triggered by everyday activities such as talking, eating, shaving, or brushing one's teeth.
Diabetic neuropathy	This is a common complication of long-term diabetes. Metabolic and vascular changes result in damage to peripheral and autonomic nerves. Sensory loss can result when peripheral nerves are involved and eventually lead to injury progressing to infection and gangrene. Symptoms include sensations of numbness, prickling, or tingling (paresthesias).

Box 36-1 Common Responses to Pain

Behavioral (Voluntary) Responses

Moving away from painful stimuli
Grimacing, moaning, and crying
Restlessness
Protecting the painful area and refusing to move

Physiologic (Involuntary) Responses

Typical Sympathetic Responses When Pain Is Moderate and Superficial

Increased blood pressure[a]
Increased pulse and respiratory rates[a]
Pupil dilation
Muscle tension and rigidity
Pallor (peripheral vasoconstriction)
Increased adrenaline output
Increased blood glucose

Typical Parasympathetic Responses When Pain Is Severe and Deep

Nausea and vomiting
Fainting or unconsciousness
Decreased blood pressure
Decreased pulse rate
Prostration
Rapid and irregular breathing

Affective (Psychological) Responses

Exaggerated weeping and restlessness
Withdrawal
Stoicism
Anxiety
Depression
Fear
Anger
Anorexia
Fatigue
Hopelessness
Insomnia and other sleep disturbances
Powerlessness

[a]An increase in vital signs may occur briefly in acute pain but may not occur when chronic pain is present.

for the patient. This type of pain is called **phantom pain** or phantom limb pain and does not have an identifiable physiologic or pathologic cause. One theory suggests that sensory misrepresentations from the missing limb may remain in the brain, thereby causing phantom pain.

Responses to Pain

Three types of responses to pain are physiologic, behavioral, and affective. Examples of these responses are listed in Box 36-1. The severity of pain and its duration affect responses to pain. Increases in vital signs may occur briefly in acute pain and may be absent in chronic pain states (Pasero & McCaffery, 2011).

Concept Mastery Alert

Physiologic responses are involuntary body responses; behavioral responses reflect body movements; affective responses reflect mood and emotions.

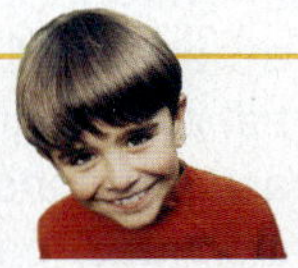

Recall **Xavier Malton**, the child with ulcerative colitis experiencing an acute episode of pain. The nurse is initially able to assess that Xavier is in pain by his screams. In addition, the nurse interprets his behavioral and affective responses, such as his body posture, inability to get off the toilet, and later his fetal position in bed. Moreover, the nurse would validate these findings with physiologic responses such as skin color, muscle tension, and possibly vital signs.

Mild pain experienced briefly may produce little or no behavioral response; intense pain experienced briefly usually results in reflex action to escape the cause. The patient is often able to accept pain that continues for a relatively short time, such as for a few days or a week, without it being all-consuming. The patient expects relief and believes the cause is self-limiting, but may experience some level of anxiety. On the other hand, chronic pain tends to consume the entire person. It demands total attention so that the patient has limited resources to take care of other matters of daily living. It is physically and emotionally exhausting and is associated with ongoing irritability, isolation, fatigue, fear, anger, feelings for helplessness, stress/anxiety, and depression (LeFort et al., 2021). Lack of an obvious response to pain does not mean the patient is without pain. Careful assessment is especially important to understand what the patient is experiencing.

FACTORS AFFECTING THE PAIN EXPERIENCE

Pain is a highly personal experience. Many factors influence the comfort status of a person at any given moment. When a person experiences pain, almost anything can influence how the painful stimulus is transmitted to the brain, how it is perceived, and the actual response. A biopsychosocial (BPS) model introduced in the late 1970s by Engel (1977) extended the existing biomedical model to consider the dynamic interaction between: (1) biological factors associated with the condition, including developmental and genetic components; (2) social influences of relationships, as well as cultural, situational, and adaptive factors; and (3) psychological influences of personality, coping skills, mental

Table 36-2 Additional Terms Used to Describe Pain

TERM	DESCRIPTION
Quality	
Sharp	Pain is stabbing in nature and intense.
Dull	Pain is not as intense or acute as sharp pain, possibly more annoying than painful. It is usually more diffuse than sharp pain.
Diffuse	Pain covers a large area. Usually, the patient is unable to point to a specific area without moving the hand over a large surface, such as the entire abdomen.
Shifting	Pain moves from one area to another, such as from the lower abdomen to the area over the stomach.
Other terms used to describe the quality of pain include sore, stinging, pinching, cramping, gnawing, cutting, throbbing, shooting, and vise-like pressure.	
Severity	
Severe or excruciating Moderate Slight or mild	These terms depend on the patient's interpretation of pain. Behavioral and physiologic signs help assess the severity of pain. On a scale of 0–10, slight pain could be described as being between 1 and 3; moderate pain, between 4 and 7; and severe pain, between 8 and 10.
Periodicity	
Continuous	Pain does not stop.
Intermittent	Pain stops and starts again.
Brief or transient	Pain is intermittent and passes quickly.

health, and past experiences. The BPS model was originally designed for psychiatry as a way to reframe research, teaching, and health care (Engel). Despite criticism, the model has been used, adapted, and extended to drive assessment and management of pain and suffering in many populations (Bolton & Gillett, 2019; Matteliano et al., 2014; Miaskowski et al., 2020; Murphy et al., 2020; Pickering et al., 2018).

A person learns what causes unpleasantness and what to interpret as pain. Each person's interpretation is influenced by background, such as how they have experienced and dealt with pain in the past, and what culture has taught the person about pain. Through past experiences, each person also learns to differentiate among the various types of pain and to associate pain with certain descriptive words. Table 36-2 lists common definitions for additional terms used by patients to describe pain.

Cultural and Ethnicity Variables

Cultural norms, or social norms, dictate much of our daily behavior, attitudes, and values. Therefore, it is natural that culture influences the person's response to pain. Ethnicity is a broad term that has many facets. Ethnicity generally refers to the social, religious, political, cultural, and/or psychological characteristics of a group of people that are maintained generation to generation. These characteristics provide a sense of identity and are rooted in ancestry, nationality, language, and a shared set of beliefs and values; sociocultural and environmental factors that are influenced by geographic location also need to be considered (Kim et al., 2020). Despite the understanding that the terms *ethnicity* and *race* do not capture all the complex factors that impact on the health or pain experience of people, they provide a means for: (1) beginning to describe the diversity present in the United States, (2) collecting complete data that can be shared across systems, and (3) developing a comprehensive picture of health care quality (Agency for Healthcare Research and Quality [AHRQ], 2018).

Nurses must appreciate that a patient's response to pain is based on a host of experiences and factors, and therefore requires an individualized plan of care. For example, one patient may present with a calm, objective, matter-of-fact approach to pain, while another patient may present with loud vocalizations, an emphasis on their unique experience, physical movements, and demands for relief. Both patients are experiencing pain. It is particularly important to avoid stereotyping responses to pain because the nurse frequently encounters patients who are either in pain or anticipating that it will develop. A form of pain expression that is frowned on in one culture may be desirable in another cultural group. For example, enduring pain stoically is a sign of strength among some groups (Cancio, 2020; Purnell, 2013). Be knowledgeable about cultural variations and develop an understanding of cultural influences on pain tolerance, expressions of pain, and alternative practices used to manage pain. Health care providers demonstrate respect and cultural humility if they acknowledge the potential effects of culture and ethnicity on the pain experience. Intentionally involve your patient in the pain assessment by asking questions and taking care to not make assumptions or generalizations based on ethnicity or race. It is important to note that the mixed ethnic heritage that is common in many patients today makes it more difficult to anticipate individual responses to pain based on their ethnicity. Asking direct questions regarding pain experiences, expectations, and management will serve you well when dealing with patients from any background.

QSEN PATIENT-CENTERED CARE

Intentionally involve your patient in the pain assessment, taking time to appreciate the potential effects of culture and ethnicity, without making assumptions or generalizations about the patient's individual pain experience.

By 2044, it is projected that more than half of all Americans will belong to a minority group, with the non-Hispanic White population comprising only 44% of the population of the United States (Colby & Ortman, 2015). This more diverse population will include people from many different ethnicities, who may express themselves in many different languages. This poses potential challenges for pain assessment and management. When the patient's language differs from that of the nurse, the nurse runs the risk of misinterpreting the patient's level of pain. For example, there are nuanced differences between the term *pain*, which usually describes the most severe discomfort, and *ache*, typically used to describe a dull, less severe type of discomfort. Communication is the cornerstone of a nurse's subjective assessment and associated teaching. Perceived and actual barriers to verbal and written communication should be considered and directly addressed with appropriate tools and resources including information sheets in different languages and the use of medical interpreters. It is important to remember that the greater the language differences or barriers, the poorer a patient's pain is controlled (Purnell, 2013).

Even though culture and ethnicity affect a patient's behavioral response to pain, consistent pain assessment is possible. Pain assessment tools have been translated into multiple languages and some assessments have empirical support for their "use across race/ethnicity and sex" (Rogers et al., 2020, p. 818). Pain rating scales are discussed later in this chapter.

Social determinants of health greatly impact on pain management outcomes. Recent research has confirmed that those who reside in low-income settings (Newman et al., 2018) and minority populations are less likely to receive the recommended treatments for pain in health care settings (Beletsky et al., 2021; Kim et al., 2020). Although pain is undertreated in the general population, minority patients often experience pain for a lengthy period of time before seeking treatment for it. There tends to be a disconnect between patients' beliefs, values, health behaviors, and individual preferences and what is available to them in the conventional/dominant health care system. Geographic location (whether a remote rural or densely populated urban setting) where physical barriers limit travel or where resources are lacking can also negatively impact on pain assessment and treatment. Language barriers, culturally inappropriate pain assessment tools, and prejudice and misconceptions may contribute to unsatisfactory pain outcomes. There is agreement that health care providers need to be aware of these inequities and make a concerted effort to confront these disparities (Beletsky et al., 2021; Newman et al., 2018; Purnell, 2013). Initiatives to address health care access and treatment disparities begin at the local and community level. Additional information on cultural influences on pain is presented in Chapter 5.

QSEN ENSURING HEALTH EQUITY

Initiatives to address treatment disparities and advance health equity begin at the local or community level, where assessments and interventions have a direct impact on the health-related social, policy, and economic needs of these vulnerable populations (National Academies of Sciences, Engineering, & Medicine, 2017).

Family, Biological Sex, Gender, and Age Variables

Other culturally related variables are family, biological sex, gender, and age. A person's response to pain or symptoms may be affected or influenced by the response of family members. Spouses also may reinforce pain behavior in their partners. Children growing up in different families may learn to *be brave* and ignore pain, or to use the pain experience to secure attention and service from caregivers. Family size and birth order do not appear to be significant in distinguishing those who suffer from chronic pain.

Similarly, children may learn that there are gender differences in pain expression. It may be acceptable for a little girl to run home crying with a scraped knee, but a little boy may be told that he should be brave and not cry. Adult men and women may hold on to gender expectations regarding pain communication and incorrectly interpret the presence or absence of pain expressions in others. Women are more comfortable communicating the discomfort associated with pain, but this ability to verbalize may cause some to view the pain as emotionally or psychologically based. Data suggest that there may be a biologic component to pain responses as well. The American Society of Anesthesiologists (2016) performed a review of the literature to describe the chronic pain experienced by females and discuss options to manage this pain. The triggers, experience of pain, recommended anesthesia, and other coping strategies may vary by biological sex and require more exploration.

In addition, different age groups have different beliefs and norms regarding pain sensation and response. At one time, the infant's inability to communicate pain led health care practitioners to the erroneous assumption that pain sensation was diminished or absent. More recently, it has been demonstrated that infants and small children are sensitive to and experience pain. Conditions normally painful in young adults (e.g., myocardial infarction) may result in minimal pain reports from older adults. An older adult not reporting pain may indicate that the person fears the treatment for the pain, the pain is dulled based on processes inherent in normal aging or chronic disease progression, or the older adult simply refuses to give in to the pain. For many older adults, pain has become accepted as a daily occurrence and is regarded as part of the normal aging process. Because of this false assumption, health care providers have often ignored or undertreated pain in older adults. These variables, which influence pain sensation, perception, and response, make pain assessment a complex task for the nurse.

Religious Beliefs and Spirituality

Religious beliefs can be a powerful influence on the person's experience of pain. In some religions, people view pain and suffering as a *lack of goodness* in themselves. Thus, pain and suffering are viewed as a means of purification or of making up for individual and community sin. This meaning helps the person to cope with pain, thus becoming a source of strength. Patients with this belief may refuse analgesics and other pain relief measures, feeling that this lessens their suffering. On the other hand, illness and pain may also be viewed as punishment from a vengeful God. People may find their faith shaken and question the existence of a loving God. Persistent pain, disability, and suffering can enhance spiritual awareness or may lead to anger and frustration. Spirituality includes a search for meaning in life and underpins many of the treatments identified as effective for managing addiction, such as the 12-step program identified by Alcoholics Anonymous. Recognizing these religious or spiritual manifestations as part of the biopsychosocial model provides patients and nurses space to recognize vulnerabilities and address intrinsic and extrinsic factors of pain and addiction (Matteliano et al., 2014). Patients may find it helpful to confer with a spiritual adviser about their pain experience.

Environment and Support People

A person's environment and the presence or absence of caring support people may also influence the experience of pain. Many people find that the strangeness of the health care environment, especially the lights, noise, lack of sleep, and constant activity of a critical care unit, compounds the experience of pain. The sense of powerlessness that accompanies admission to a health care facility may decrease the person's ability to cope with pain.

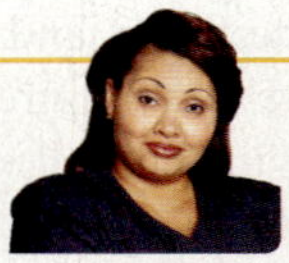

Recall ***Sheree Lincoln***, the postoperative patient in pain described at the beginning of the chapter. In addition to the pain related to surgery, the nurse would need to assess the effect of the environment on Sheree's pain. For example, she may be frightened by equipment being used postoperatively. In addition, she may feel alone and powerless due to her current condition. Assessment also would need to include information about past experiences with pain, support people available, and teaching she received preoperatively.

Depersonalization or separation from a favorite pillow, pet, or source of music may further decrease the person's sense of comfort. For some, the presence of a loved family member or friend is essential to their sense of well-being. Others prefer to be alone when in pain and may become agitated in the presence of a family member.

Some patients may use their pain to acquire secondary gains, such as special attention and services from their families. If unchecked, this tendency may lead to resentment and anger in family members and their eventual avoidance of the patient. Intervening and attempting an honest discussion of this problem is important.

Anxiety and Other Stressors

Anxiety, which is almost always present when pain is anticipated or being experienced, tends to increase the perceived intensity of pain. The threat of the unknown is ordinarily more devastating and anxiety-producing than a threat for which one has been prepared. Many studies have focused on the relationship between anxiety and pain (Rogers et al., 2020), or depression and pain. In chronic or persistent pain specifically, depressive symptoms are interrelated and often provide the impetus for seeking treatment (Kim et al., 2020; Newman et al., 2018).

Although a cause-and-effect relationship has not clearly been verified, pain may be aggravated with anxiety, muscular tension, and fatigue. The rested and relaxed person can often cope with more discomfort than someone who is suffering from a lack of sleep.

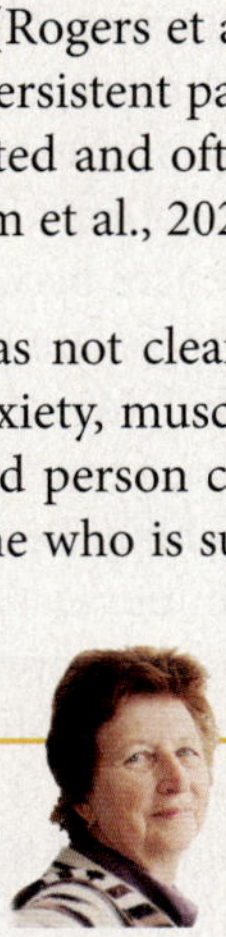

Think back to ***Carla Potter***, the woman experiencing complications from her diabetes. She also reports feeling stressed, fearful, and anxious over her constant pain and likely progression of her disease. In order to individualize her care plan, the nurse needs to gather additional data and investigate the possibility of specific measures that may effectively empower Carla Potter to reduce some of the anxiety and fear she reports.

A person who is greatly fatigued and who has no competing demands requiring their attention may experience pain more acutely. For example, many people have discovered that the pain of a foot ache or an ingrown toenail that was only mildly annoying during the day's work becomes unbearable at night when there is nothing else to distract the mind from the pain.

Past Pain Experience

A person's experience of pain in the past and the qualities of that experience profoundly affect new pain experiences:

- Some patients have never known severe pain and have no fear of pain, not realizing how intense the sensation can be.
- Some patients have experienced severe acute or chronic pain in the past but received immediate and adequate pain relief. These patients are generally unafraid of pain and initiate appropriate requests for assistance.
- Some patients have known severe pain in the past and were unable to secure relief. Even the suggestion of new pain can lead to acute feelings of fear, despair, and hopelessness.
- A person whose past pain experience led to correction of unhealthy behavior and produced a greater sense of health and well-being, may respect and value pain and consider the meaning and significance of new pain carefully.
- In general, people who have experienced more pain than usual in their lifetimes tend to anticipate more pain and exhibit increased sensitivity to pain.
- Some pain memories are virtually unforgettable. New contact with conditions similar to those that caused the earlier pain can provoke a violent response.

NURSING PROCESS FOR COMFORT AND PAIN MANAGEMENT

Assessing

Because the pain experience is unique to each person, the nurse who wants to help the patient achieve comfort and pain control needs sophisticated pain assessment skills. Assessing all factors that affect the pain experience—psychological, sociocultural, spiritual, and physiologic—is essential. Pain is complex and difficult to interpret and requires a reliable assessment tool.

Routine Pain Assessment

In an effort to improve patients' quality of life and make pain management a priority, the American Pain Society (1995) encouraged caregivers to include assessment for pain as the fifth vital sign. Routine measurement of vital signs accompanied by a pain assessment was thought to raise awareness of the existence of pain, place additional emphasis on optimizing pain relief, and move patients more quickly toward comfort and recovery. However, this framing led to the problematic interpretation that pain needed to be assessed *every* time vital signs were taken on *every* patient. This phrasing was removed from the Joint Commission Accreditation Standards in 2004 (Baker, 2017). Current emphasis is on pain assessment and management of acute and chronic pain that is individualized and includes recognition, management, and referral of patients with addiction (Baker, 2017). Effective pain management should be implemented and evaluated by the interprofessional team and the patient, not measured solely with patient satisfaction surveys or a numeric score on a pain scale. Realistic pain management goals need to be set with each patient.

Common Misconceptions

Many patient misconceptions interfere with the patient's ability to communicate pain. Some of these instances can lead to undertreatment of pain. It is important to assess for the following common patient beliefs related to pain and communicating it:

- The doctor has prescribed pain-relieving medication for me, which I will be given routinely.
- If I ask for something for my pain, I will immediately become addicted to the medication.
- Sometimes it is better to put up with the pain than to deal with the side effects of the pain medication.
- I should somehow be able to control my pain. It is immature to talk about pain.
- It is better to wait until the pain gets really bad before asking for help. If I take the medication now for moderate pain, it won't relieve severe pain later on.
- I don't want to bother anyone—I know how busy everyone is.
- It's natural for me to have excruciating pain after surgery. After a few days, I should notice it lessening.

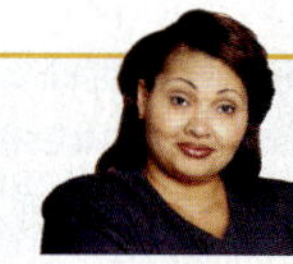

Recall **Sheree Lincoln**, the woman who has undergone abdominal surgery. It would be important for the nurse to investigate Sheree's understanding of her postoperative pain and what her expectations are. Doing so would provide clues for the nurse indicating possible patient misconceptions about pain and pain relief, thereby providing a basis for teaching and correcting these misconceptions.

Components of a Pain Assessment

The nurse will generally assess the following characteristics of pain:

- Patient's initial verbalization and description of the pain
- Onset of the pain: etiology or mechanism of injury (if known)
- Duration of the pain
- Location of the pain: localized, generalized, radiation
- Quality and character of the pain
- Intensity: severity of the pain
- Aggravating or causal factors: what triggers or makes it worse
- Alleviating/relieving factors: what makes it better
- Other contributing or related factors: anxiety, fear, depression, insomnia
- Effect on function: activities of daily living, recreation, work, quality of life
- Pain management goal

When assessing a person's pain, Pasero and McCaffery (2011) discuss these basic methods that are still relevant today:

1. Obtain the patient's self-report of pain.
2. Identify pathologic conditions or procedures that may be causing pain; consider physiologic measures (increased blood pressure and pulse). However, most research verifies that reliance on vital signs to indicate the presence of pain should be minimized. The absence of an increase in vital signs does not mean that pain is not present.
3. Consider patient behaviors that may indicate pain such as nonverbal behaviors (restlessness, grimacing, crying, clenching fists, protecting the painful area).
4. Take into account the report of a family member, another person close to the patient, or a caregiver who is familiar with the patient.
5. Attempt an analgesic trial and monitor the results.

Focused Assessment Guide 36-1 (on pages 1350–1351) suggests questions and approaches helpful in assessing pain factors.

Concept Mastery Alert

Assessment of pain requires information from a variety of sources. However, patients are the experts on their pain, and their ratings and descriptions of the pain are very important.

Focused Assessment Guide 36-1

THE PAIN EXPERIENCE

Factors to Assess	Questions and Approaches
Characteristics of the pain	
Location	*Where is your pain? Is it external or internal?* Asking the patient with acute pain to point to the painful area with one finger may help to localize the pain. Patients with chronic pain may have difficulty trying to localize their pain.
Severity	Ask the patient to indicate the degree (amount) of pain currently experienced on the following scale: 0 1 2 3 4 5 6 7 8 9 10 0 = No pain; 2 = Mild pain; 4 = Moderate pain; 7 = Severe pain; 10 = Pain as bad as it can be Note that it is important to give patients *zero/no pain* as an option. It is also helpful to ask how much pain the patient has (on the same scale) when the pain is at its least and at its worst: Least ___________ Worst ___________
Quality	*What words would you use to describe your pain?*
Duration	*How long have you been experiencing pain? How long does a pain episode last? How often does a pain episode occur?*
Aggravating or causal factors	*How does the pain develop and progress? Has the pain changed since it first began? If so, how? What makes the pain occur or increase in intensity?* If pattern can be identified, interventions early in a pain sequence will often be far more effective than those used after the pain is well established.
Alleviating factors	*What makes the pain go away or lessen? What methods of relief have you tried in the past? How long were they used? How effective were they?* Pharmacologic and nonpharmacologic methods of relief currently in effect for hospitalized patients should be apparent from the chart. It is important to verify the use of current prescriptions and their effectiveness with the patient. Outpatients may need to be asked to record a medication profile, a thorough and accurate account of all medications they are taking.
Contributing or related factors	*Are there any other factors that seem to relate consistently to your pain? Any other symptoms that occur just before, during, or after your pain?*
Physiologic responses	
Vital signs (blood pressure, pulse, respirations) Skin color Perspiration Pupil size Nausea	Signs of sympathetic stimulation may occur with acute pain but need not be present to verify the presence of pain. Signs of parasympathetic stimulation (decreased blood pressure and pulse, rapid and irregular respirations, pupil constriction, nausea and vomiting, and warm, dry skin) may occur, especially in prolonged, severe, visceral, or deep pain.
Muscle tension	Observe. Is the patient aware of any tight, tense muscles?
Anxiety	Are signs of anxiety evident? May include decreased attention span or ability to follow directions, frequent asking of questions, shifting of topics of conversation, avoidance of discussion of feelings, acting out, or somatization (physical symptoms arise from emotional or psychological distress).
Behavioral responses	
Posture, gross motor activities	Does patient rub or support a particular area? Make frequent position changes? Walk, pace, kneel, or assume a rolled-up position? Does patient rest a particular body part? Protect an area from stimulation? Lie quietly? In acute pain, postural and gross motor activities are often altered; in chronic pain, the only signs of change may be postures characteristic of withdrawal.

Focused Assessment Guide 36-1 (continued)

SKIN INTEGRITY

Factors to Assess	Questions and Approaches
Facial features	Does the patient have a pinched look? Are there facial grimaces? Knotted brow? Overall taut, anxious appearance? A look of fatigue is more characteristic of chronic pain.
Verbal expressions	Does the patient sigh, moan, scream, cry, or repetitively use the same words?
Affective responses	
Anxiety	*Do you feel anxious? Are you afraid? If so, how bad are these feelings?*
Depression	*Do you feel depressed, down, or low? If so, how bad are these feelings? Are your feelings about yourself mostly good or bad? Do you have feelings of failure? Do you see yourself or your illness as a burden to those you care about?*
Interactions with others	How does the patient act when in pain in the presence of others? How does the patient respond to others when not in pain? How do significant others and caregivers respond to the patient when the patient is in pain? When the patient is not in pain?
Degree to which pain interferes with patient's life (use past performance as baseline)	*Does the pain interfere with sleep? If so, to what extent? Is fatigue a major factor in the pain experience? Is the conduct of intimate or peer relationships affected by the pain? Is work function affected? Participation in recreational–diversional activities?* An activity diary is often helpful—sometimes crucial. One to several weeks of hourly activity recorded by the patient may be necessary. Levels of pain, intake of food, and sleep–rest periods are noted along with activities performed. Separate diaries for inpatient and outpatient episodes may be necessary because hospitalization markedly affects the nature and type of activities performed.
Perception of pain and meaning to patient	*Are you worried about your illness? Do you see any connection between your pain and the nature or course of illness? If so, how do you see them as related? Do you find any meaning in your pain? If so, is this beneficial or detrimental to you? Are you struggling to find some meaning for your pain?*
Adaptive mechanisms used to cope with pain	*What do you usually do to relieve stress? How well do these things work? What techniques do you use at home to help cope with the pain? How well have they worked? Do you use these in the hospital? If not, why not?*
Outcomes	*What would you like to be doing right now, this week, this month, if the pain were better controlled? How much would the pain have to decrease (on the 0–10 scale) for you to begin to accomplish these goals? What is your pain goal (on the 0–10 scale)?* Keep in mind that NO pain may not be an option for some patients. Helping them to identify a realistic goal promotes effective pain management.

Various forms used to help guide the assessment of pain have been described in the nursing literature. The primary purposes of using a guide to assess pain are to: (1) eliminate guesswork and biases when dealing with the patient's pain; (2) appreciate what the person is experiencing; (3) analyze findings that will help prepare an appropriate nursing response to the patient's pain; and (4) facilitate improved outcomes, such as fewer complications, shorter hospital stays, and improved quality of life.

For continued assessment of pain and evaluation of pain control measures, a pain scale allows the patient to rate pain experienced on a continual basis. A numerical pain scale that is currently the national standard is displayed in the Focused Assessment Guide 36-1. This scale is best for use with verbally communicative patients.

Do not overlook pain in patients who have difficulty with communication. Their pain requires adequate treatment. Examples of pain rating scales that can be used with patients who are nonverbal or have difficulty communicating verbally include the Behavioral Pain Scale (BPS) for use with critically ill patients who are intubated, and the Face Legs Activity Cry and Consolability (FLACC) pain scale for use with infants and young children (from ages 2 months to 7 years) and in children with cognitive impairment. Information about these pain-rating scales is included in Table 36-3 (on page 1352). The range of available scales and instruments allows the nurse or other interprofessional team member to choose a tool that is developmentally appropriate for each individual. Whichever tool is used, it is best to use the same tool to rate a patient's pain throughout a hospital stay.

A comprehensive pain assessment must also include discussion of the patient's expectations for pain relief. The patient and health care team need to set a realistic goal or a number on the pain scale that is acceptable and facilitates recovery. For example, it may not be possible to have a pain rating of zero after a surgical procedure when the movement

Table 36-3 Pain Assessment Scales

RESOURCE	WEBSITE	INDICATIONS
0–10 Numeric Rating Scale	https://www.sralab.org/rehabilitation-measures/numeric-pain-rating-scale	Adults and children (>9 years old) in all patient care settings who are able to use numbers to rate the intensity of their pain
Adult Nonverbal Pain Scale (NVPS)	https://com-jax-emergency-pami.sites.medinfo.ufl.edu/files/2015/02/Adult-nonverbal-pain-scale-University-of-Rochester-Medical-Center.pdf	Adults who are sedated and nonresponsive
Behavioral Pain Scale (BPS)	https://www.mdcalc.com/behavioral-pain-scale-bps-pain-assessment-intubated-patients	Useful with intubated, critically ill patients; measurement of bodily indicators of pain; and tolerance of intubation
Checklist of Nonverbal Indicators	http://prc.coh.org/PainNOA/CNPI_Tool.pdf	Adults who are unable to validate the presence of or quantify the severity of pain using either the Numeric Rating Scale or Wong–Baker FACES pain rating scale
COMFORT Behavior Scale	https://www.researchgate.net/publication/270804540_The_Comfort_Behavior_Scale	Infants, children, adults who are unable to use the numeric rating scale or Wong–Baker FACES pain rating scale
CRIES Instrument	http://prc.coh.org/pdf/CRIES.pdf	Neonates (ages 0–6 months)
Critical-Care Pain Observation Tool (CPOT)	https://kpnursing.org/professionaldevelopment/CPOTHandout.pdf	Adults who are sedated and nonresponsive
Faces Pain Scale—Revised (FPS-R)	http://www.iasp-pain.org/Education/Content.aspx?ItemNumber=1519	Children (4–16) in parallel with numerical self-rating scales (0–10); patients choose the depiction of a facial expression that best corresponds with their pain
FLACC Behavioral Scale	http://marshfieldclinic.libguides.com/ld.php?content_id=46985203	Infants and children (ages 2 months to 7 years) who are unable to validate the presence of or quantify the severity of pain
Iowa Pain Thermometer (IPT) & Revised Iowa Pain Thermometer (IPT-R)	http://www.painmanagementnursing.org/article/S1524-9042(14)00151-9/pdf	Older adults with cognitive impairment
Oucher Pain Scale	https://www.researchgate.net/figure/OUCHER-scale-Adapted-from-OUCHER-18-Explain-to-the-child-to-score-that-the-intensity-of_fig1_320001571	Young children who can point to a face to indicate their level of pain
Pain Assessment in Advanced Dementia Scale (PAINAD)	http://dementiapathways.ie/_filecache/04a/ddd/98-painad.pdf	Patients whose dementia is so advanced that they cannot verbally communicate
Wong–Baker FACES Pain Rating Scale	http://www.wongbakerfaces.org	Adults and children (>3 years old) in all patient care settings

required to prevent complications naturally causes some pain or discomfort. Having this conversation and setting a realistic, mutually agreed upon goal facilitates the patient's recognition and report of pain that is unacceptable. Setting pain management goals also provides the nurse the opportunity to establish rapport, discuss individualized pain management interventions, and evaluate the plan with the patient and caregivers.

Assessment of Special Populations

Pain rating scales attempt to confirm and, if possible, quantify the presence of pain in a variety of populations and situations. Alternative approaches to pain assessment for special populations ensure that unacceptable levels of pain are addressed and treated. For example, a nurse caring for a patient in an intensive care unit would use a valid and reliable pain assessment tool that considers the unresponsive and/or noncommunicative status of the patient. Recommended tools for critically ill patients unable to self-report pain include the Behavioral Pain Scale (BPS) and Critical-Care Pain Observation Tool (CPOT; see Table 36-3). Pain is common in critically ill patients when they are at rest, during routine care related to activities of daily living, and with the performance of specific procedures. Untreated severe pain

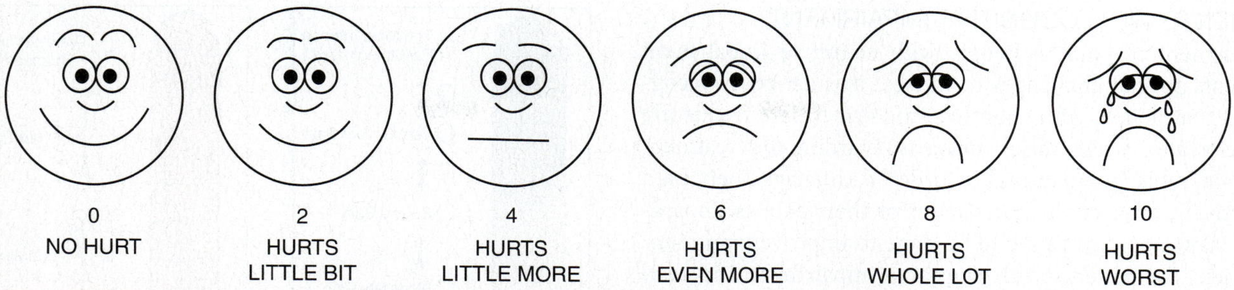

FIGURE 36-4. Wong–Baker FACES pain rating scale. Instructions: Explain to the person that each face is for a person who feels happy because he has no pain (hurt) or sad because he has some or a lot of pain. *Face 0* doesn't hurt at all. *Face 2* hurts just a little bit. *Face 4* hurts a little more. *Face 6* hurts even more. *Face 8* hurts a whole lot. *Face 10* hurts as much as you can imagine, although you don't have to be crying to have this worst pain. Ask the person to choose the face that best describes how much pain they have. Rating scale is recommended for people ages 3 years and older. (*Source:* ©1983 Wong-Baker FACES Foundation. www.WongBakerFACES.org. Used with permission.)

negatively affects critically ill patients; consistent, routine assessment and intervention should guide pain management. Pain should be treated in patients in the intensive care unit before a sedative agent is considered (Devlin et al., 2018).

CHILDREN

In recent years, health care personnel have become much more concerned about addressing pain and pain relief in infants and children. At one time, it was believed that young children lacked the neurologic development to sense pain the way adults do. Thus, pain relief was not a priority when children were hospitalized. Young children frequently received no treatment for pain for medical or surgical procedures during their entire hospital stay. Yet, infants, particularly premature infants, are as sensitive to painful stimuli as older children and adults.

Chronic pain in children represents a significant public health problem nationally and globally; there is the potential for significant impact on the child's social, emotional, and physical development and functional abilities. Family members and caregivers are also deeply affected. Chronic pain management in children requires an individualized, **multimodal approach** (using two or more different methods or medications to manage pain) that is collaborative, represents best practice, and is integrated (World Health Organization [WHO], 2021).

Current methods of assessing and measuring children's pain frequently involve use of more than one technique for assessment. A pain history provides information about the language the child uses to indicate pain, how and to whom this pain is usually reported, and indications of previous pain experiences and coping strategies. Self-report by the child is usually the most reliable account of pain. Communication with parents, guardians, or other people important to the patient is also vital for accurate pediatric pain assessment and management. In addition, the following observations may provide an indication of the presence and severity of pain in a child:

- Irritability and restlessness
- Crying, screaming, or other verbal expression of pain
- Grimacing, grinding of teeth, or clenching fists
- Touching or grabbing of painful body part
- Kicking, thrashing, or attempting to move away from a painful stimulus

Numerous scales and tools can be used to assess a child's pain. One commonly used pain assessment scale, the Wong–Baker FACES Pain Rating Scale (Fig. 36-4), asks children to compare their pain to a series of faces ranging from a broad smile to a tearful grimace. The Oucher Pain Scale, developed by Beyer et al. (1992) for use in young patients, combines a 0-to-100 scale with six photographic images of children in pain. This scale is helpful for use with older children. Adaptations of the Oucher pain scale are also available for various ethnic groups.

The CRIES Pain Scale is a tool intended for use with neonates and infants from ages 0 to 6 months. The COMFORT Scale, used to assess pain and distress in critically ill pediatric patients, relies on six behavioral and two physiologic factors that determine the level of analgesia needed to adequately relieve pain in these children. The FLACC Scale (F—Faces, L—Legs, A—Activity, C—Cry, C—Consolability), designed for infants and children from ages 2 months to 7 years who are unable to validate the presence or severity of pain, rates each of the five categories on a 0-to-2 scale. In addition, children may be asked to record their pain experiences in a daily diary. Detecting and accurately assessing pediatric pain have resulted in new and innovative approaches toward pain control in children.

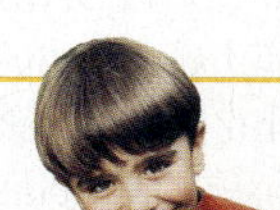

Think back to **Xavier Malton**, the 5-year-old with acute pain. Incorporating the use of an age-appropriate pain assessment tool would be crucial in assessing Xavier's pain. Because Xavier is 5 years old, he may have difficulty describing his pain and its severity. For example, according to Xavier, "Something was hurting very much." Using the FACES Scale or the Oucher Scale would help the nurse to quantify the severity of Xavier's pain, providing objective evidence from which to intervene appropriately. The tool also would be extremely useful in determining the effectiveness of pain relief interventions, providing objective evidence denoting any changes in the pain's severity. This evaluation would serve as a basis for continuing pain management.

PATIENTS WITH COGNITIVE IMPAIRMENT

Assessment of pain in people with cognitive impairment presents special challenges to nurses. It is generally recognized that people with cognitive impairment are frequently undertreated, which raises concerns regarding the treatment of vulnerable populations. In order to manage their pain effectively, an accurate assessment of their pain is imperative. Work must continue to be done to improve pain management for patients with cognitive impairment and residents of long-term care facilities (Fain et al., 2017). Nurses must also consider the potential negative impact of pain on cognitive function, specifically the impact of high levels of chronic pain on the development of memory impairment in older adults (van der Leeuw et al., 2018).

To manage pain effectively, nurses must rely on their own careful assessments, their empathic qualities, and the expectation that a patient with cognitive impairment will experience pain if a verbal patient usually reports this event as painful. Some common behaviors that can be assessed for indicators of pain in this population include (Pasero & McCaffery, 2011):

- Facial expressions
- Verbalizations and vocalizations
- Body movements
- Changes in interpersonal interactions
- Changes in activity patterns or routines
- Changes in mental status, such as agitation and aggression

The combination of a history of pain, observations of a patient's pain by families and caregivers, and the presence of medical diagnoses associated with pain also facilitates pain assessment in this population. Moreover, special efforts are needed to identify accurate methods for assessing pain in this population. The Pain Assessment in Advanced Dementia (PAINAD) Scale has been developed to assess pain in this population. It relies on observation of five specific items: breathing, vocalization, facial expression, body language, and consolability (Warden et al., 2003). Refer to Table 36-3 for additional information regarding the PAINAD scale.

OLDER ADULTS

Assessing pain in the older adult population can be challenging. Adults older than age 65 years experience pain more frequently than do younger adults. Up to 50% of older adults who live in the community and at least half of those who live in long-term care facilities report pain on a daily basis (Galicia-Castillo & Weiner, 2021). Pain negatively impacts the emotional well-being, functional ability, sleep, coping, and resources of older adults. Physiologic changes in older adults affect their sensation of pain and the pharmacokinetics and pharmacodynamics considerations of pain medications. Polypharmacy, especially with comorbidities, cognitive function, and misconceptions regarding pain and older adults influence decisions regarding multimodal pain management regimens (Rajan & Behrends, 2019). Although pain is not a normal part of aging, it is one of the most common health conditions in older adults and is associated with significant disability, primarily related to changes in mobility (Schwan et al., 2019).

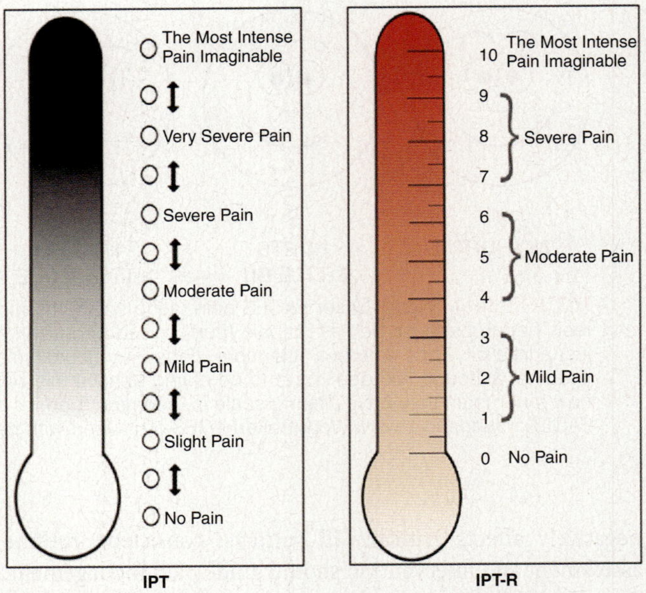

FIGURE 36-5. Iowa pain thermometer (IPT) and IPT-R (revised). (*Source:* Reprinted from Ware, L. J., Herr, K. A., Booker, S. S., Dotson, K., Key, J., Poindexter, N., Pyles, G., Siler, B., & Packard, A. [2015]. Psychometric evaluation of the Revised Iowa Pain Thermometer [IPT-R] in a sample of diverse cognitively intact and impaired older adults: A pilot study. *Pain Management Nursing, 16*[4], 475–482. http://dx.doi.org/10.1016/j.pmn.2014.09.004, Copyright [2015], with permission from Elsevier.)

Assessment of pain in the older adult can be problematic. Vision or hearing impairments may influence the assessment format. Multiple-drug regimens that are common in older people can also affect reliable reporting of pain. Many older adults view pain as a forecast of serious illness or death and thus are reluctant to admit its occurrence or report it. Boredom, loneliness, and depression may affect an older adult's perception and report of pain.

Experts agree that pain is best assessed using a comprehensive pain assessment that includes using a standardized tool, determining the impact of chronic pain on functional status (mood, mobility, ADLs, sleep, weight changes, and cognitive status), identifying attitudes and beliefs, including family members and caregivers in the data-gathering phase, identifying resources, and reviewing comorbidities and medications (Rajan & Behrends, 2019; Schwan et al., 2019). Although the Numeric Rating Scale is the most commonly used standardized tool, the Wong–Baker FACES Pain Rating Scale (see Fig. 36-4) or Faces Pain Scale–Revised (FPS-R) may also be effective for this age group. Some research has indicated that older adults prefer a vertical pain scale such as the Iowa Pain Thermometer (IPT) or Revised Iowa Pain Thermometer (IPT-R) shown in Figure 36-5, rather than the horizontal numeric pain scales (Herr et al., 2007; Ware et al., 2015). Special attention and consideration of an older adult's pain can positively affect the nurse's ability to assess pain accurately.

Diagnosing Actual or Potential Health Problems and Needs

Pain is such a complex phenomenon that its analysis often requires interprofessional collaboration. Although nursing has much to offer people experiencing both acute and chronic pain, the data collected by the nurse during the comprehensive pain assessment benefit the patient most when shared with physicians and other members of the health care team.

Attempting to intervene before an accurate assessment has been completed may mask the underlying cause of the patient's pain. False assumptions may result in progression of symptoms and the disease process. For example, the nurse who notes a pattern of headaches in a patient and relates this to the patient's description of recent stress (divorce, relocation, new job), may erroneously determine that the headaches are merely stress-related and implement a plan of relaxation exercises. A more careful analysis of patient data, however, may indicate that the headaches are of vascular origin or migraine in nature, and warrant further medical intervention. The headaches may also be symptomatic of intracranial disease such as a brain tumor, in which case delay in diagnosis could decrease the possibility of treatment and cure.

When diagnosing an actual or potential health problem or need related to acute or chronic pain, the coordinated care plan should identify the following:

- Type of pain
- Etiologic factors, to the extent that they are known and understood
- Patient's behavioral, physiologic, and affective responses
- Other factors affecting pain stimulus, transmission, perception, and response

Pain or Chronic Pain as the Problem

Problems related to pain require a nuanced approach. The importance of identifying these problems and including them as priorities in the care plan cannot be overstated. See the accompanying box, Examples of Actual or Potential Health Problems or Needs: Patients Experiencing Pain or Discomfort.

Pain or Chronic Pain as the Etiology

Because the experience of pain affects so many other aspects of human functioning, pain may be the etiology of numerous other problem statements (Wolters Kluwer, 2020), including but not limited to:

- Ineffective airway clearance related to unwillingness to ambulate secondary to postoperative incisional pain
- Acute anxiety related to pain anticipation and inadequate pain management in the past
- Constipation related to chronic use of narcotic analgesics
- Altered health maintenance related to loss of will to live secondary to prolonged chronic pain
- Grief related to belief that present pain means imminent death
- Injury risk related to decreased pain sensation
- Fatigue related to lack of relief from chronic pain
- Fear related to possible significance of pain
- Sleep deprivation from inability to fall asleep related to pain worsening at night

Examples of Actual or Potential Health Problems and Needs

PATIENT EXPERIENCING PAIN

Actual or Potential Health Problem or Need	Possible Etiologic Factors	Potential Signs and Symptoms
Acute Pain	• Nociceptive pain: Postoperative recovery, sports or other injury, sickle cell crisis	• Patient's report and description of pain using a standardized instrument, scale, or methodology • Nonverbal expressions of pain: grimacing, wincing, guarding or bracing, rubbing • Physiologic changes in heart rate, respirations, and blood pressure
Chronic Pain	• Unresolved acute injury, neuropathic pain (involving the nervous system), or nociplastic pain (fibromyalgia, low back pain, headache)	• Patient's report and description of pain using a standardized instrument, scale, or methodology • Clinical course of pain • Functional changes: mood, mobility, ADLs, sleep, weight changes, and cognitive status • Associated symptoms: depression, anxiety, social isolation
Difficulty Coping With Pain	• Inadequate pharmacologic and nonpharmacologic therapy based on evidence-based practice • Fear of medication/drug dependence • Mental state, fatigue, social stigma, • Lack of support from family, caregiver(s), partner, friends, or interprofessional team	• Verbal expressions of coping difficulty, stress, or pressure • Refusal of or apprehension with engagement with pharmacologic and nonpharmacologic interventions • Other sequelae: lack of problem-solving skills, change in life situation, or physiologic decline

Source: International Council of Nurses (ICN). (2019). *Nursing diagnosis and outcome statements.* https://www.icn.ch/sites/default/files/inline-files/ICNP2019-DC.pdf; Wolters Kluwer. (2022). Problem-based care plans. In *Lippincott Advisor.* Wolters Kluwer. https://advisor.lww.com/lna/home.do

- Psychosocial/spiritual needs related to belief that God is unfairly causing this pain as some sort of undeserved punishment
- Self-harm risk related to loss of will to live with unrelieved chronic pain

Outcome Identification and Planning

After the identification of a pain problem is made, developing and implementing a plan of care that demonstrates nursing's commitment to assist the patient in developing effective pain management strategies is crucial.

Nursing measures are directed toward the achievement of the following patient outcomes for people whose pain is acute in nature (i.e., it is expected that with healing the pain will subside and eventually disappear). The patient will:

- Describe a gradual reduction of pain, using a scale ranging from 0 (no pain) to 10 (pain as bad as it can be), clearly identifying numeric pain goals
- Demonstrate competent execution of successful pain management program (specify)

When pain or chronic pain is the etiology in a diagnosis or problem statement, outcomes will be specific to the underlying causes(s) and any functional changes associated with the pain.

For patients whose pain is chronic, an expected outcome may be contacting a center with expertise in pain management to explore options and develop a plan of care. Numerous practitioners and outpatient centers are available to support patients with chronic pain and to improve their pain management through a multimodal approach. Hospice care (also mentioned in Chapters 11 and 44) addresses the physical, spiritual, social, and economic needs of terminally ill patients and their families or caregivers in either the home or a hospice center. Pain relief is a priority in this setting. The provider, nurse, and other members of the health care team collaborate to develop the optimal pain management plan for each patient with chronic pain.

Implementing

After the care plan is developed, the nurse implements the nursing strategies that are most likely to assist the patient in achieving pain relief outcomes, whether at home or in a health care facility. Nursing interventions described in this chapter include establishing a trusting nurse–patient relationship, manipulating factors that affect the pain experience, initiating nonpharmacologic pain relief measures, managing pharmacologic interventions, reviewing additional pain control measures, ensuring ethical and legal responsibility to relieve pain, and teaching the patient about pain.

Establishing a Trusting Nurse–Patient Relationship

Most patients with pain feel better, suffer less, and experience less anxiety when they believe that a competent nurse cares about their experience of pain and is available for help and support. Without the confidence developed in a good nurse–patient relationship, fear and apprehension can make the patient feel like nothing seems to work. A good working relationship can increase the efficacy of basic nursing interventions. Measures that help strengthen the nurse–patient relationship and promote pain relief include discussing pain with the patient, setting pain goals together, listening to the patient about their preferred method of pain relief, and being intentionally present with the patient in pain. Being with them physically, psychologically, and spiritually, while focusing on their vulnerability and individual feelings, is one way we can provide holistic care that acknowledges their pain experience and improves their well-being. A provider's empathy, coupled with a patient's optimism, can positively impact on the chronic pain experience and associated outcomes (Cánovas et al., 2018). These measures promote a collaborative relationship in which the patient's pain is treated with respect (see the accompanying box, Through the Eyes of a Patient).

Manipulating Factors Affecting the Pain Experience

There are many ways to manage pain (Chou et al., 2021; Chou et al, 2022). In addition to a holistic approach that includes pharmacologic and nonpharmacologic measures,

Through the Eyes of a Patient

I've always thought of myself as a "take charge" kind of person. It's important for me in my business to be calm and always in control of my emotions. The *big C* changed everything for me. A recent hospitalization made me take time to think about what's happening to me.

Even in the hospital, I had a steady stream of visitors—some friends and some business associates. Even the mayor stopped by to see me. For all of them, I was my usual self—smiling, joking, and acting as if everything was normal. I made sure I took my pain medicine before they came. I kept all my fears about cancer and dying hidden behind my smiling face. I never broke down—not even in front of my wife. Men aren't supposed to cry, you know.

One nurse's simple gesture changed all that. One evening after all my visitors, my wife, and my son had left, she must have sensed something. She came over, stood next to me, put her arm around my shoulders and quietly said, "You know, Bob, it's all right to cry." It was like the dam opened up. I looked at her, my face cracked, and suddenly I couldn't stop sobbing. She must have known that I needed to talk about what was happening to me. I needed to say those words out loud to someone—"I'm afraid the pain will get too bad. I'm afraid of dying. I can't let my family see me this way!" She just let me cry, kept holding my hands, and just by being there and listening, helped me at that moment in ways that you will never know.

simple nursing interventions can positively alter patients' pain experience and speed their recovery.

REMOVING OR ALTERING THE CAUSE OF PAIN

Removing or altering the cause of the pain is ideal and sometimes possible. Possible measures that promote comfort and help in pain relief include removing or loosening a tight binder, if permissible; assisting the patient in emptying a full bladder; taking steps to relieve constipation and flatus; changing body positions and ensuring correct body alignment; and changing soiled linens and dressings that may be irritating the skin. Providing a needed snack or drink may help the patient feel more comfortable.

Certain medications are useful for removing or altering the intensity of painful stimuli. For example, drugs that decrease smooth-muscle spasms in the GI tract and those that decrease contractions of skeletal muscles reduce discomfort.

ALTERING FACTORS AFFECTING PAIN TOLERANCE

Pain tolerance level is the maximum intensity of a stimulus that produces pain a person is willing to accept in a given situation (IASP, 2021). By performing an accurate pain assessment and establishing a trusting relationship, the nurse is better-able to identify factors that contribute to the patient's pain experience. Alleviate the identified contributing factors whenever possible. For example, patients who have never had their pain acknowledged or who have repeatedly been told that their pain is all *in their head* may experience a greater ability to deal with their pain when someone finally takes the pain seriously. Nursing measures include communicating to the patient that their individual response to pain is acceptable and providing education to the patient's family and caregivers. A discussion of goals and expectations regarding pain also increases the amount of control the person feels and can impact their ability to tolerate a certain level of pain at a given moment in time.

Fatigue tends to increase pain, so promoting rest is helpful. The patient in pain usually feels more comfortable when the environment is quiet and restful. Although sensory restrictions—such as eliminating unnecessary noise and bright lights—are usually indicated, it is rarely helpful to leave the patient alone in an environment with little sensory input. The patient is then more likely to focus on themself and the discomfort.

Lack of knowledge, finding no meaning in the pain, being pessimistic about its relief, and fear may also interfere with the patient's ability to deal with pain. Common fears include a loss of control and embarrassment by being unable to deal with the pain maturely. Another fear may be a fear of taking pain relief medication. Patients, especially older adults, may view the need for medication as a sign of weakness, may fear addiction, or may be concerned about the medication losing its effectiveness, which could impact on future pain management needs.

Initiating Complementary Health Approaches and Integrative Health Care

Although analgesics are usually the primary treatment measure for pain, a growing trend is seen involving integration of complementary health approaches (CHA) and integrative health care (IH) concepts. These nonpharmacologic interventions are varied—they can be practiced in all health care settings as part of a holistic pain management strategy. Refer to Chapter 29 for additional discussion of complementary and alternative relief measures.

USING DISTRACTION

Focused attention on pain may increase the perception of pain, whereas preoccupation with other things has been observed to decrease the experience of pain. Distraction requires the patient to focus attention on something other than the pain. It is not entirely clear whether distraction raises the threshold of pain or increases pain tolerance. Many patients whose pain is relieved by distraction report being able to place pain in the periphery of awareness. This is compatible with the theory that if the reticular formation in the brainstem receives sufficient sensory input, it can ignore or block out select sensations such as pain. The Lamaze method of childbirth is one common example involving the use of distraction.

Distraction alone may relieve mild pain. However, it is most effective when used before pain begins or soon thereafter. It has also been proven effective when used with analgesics for treatment of a brief episode of severe pain (e.g., pain that accompanies a diagnostic procedure). Distraction may also be used successfully with children.

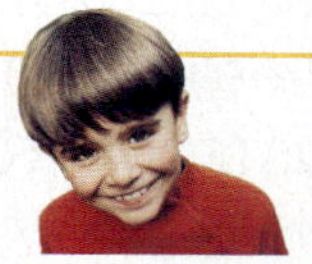

Recall **Xavier Malton**, the child with ulcerative colitis who was in severe pain. The nurse could incorporate the use of nonpharmacologic measures for pain relief, such as distraction, to enhance the effectiveness of analgesics.

Techniques that distract attention include the following:

- Visual distractions: counting objects, reading, or watching TV
- Auditory distractions: listening to music
- Tactile kinesthetic distractions: holding or stroking a loved person, pet, or toy; rocking; slow rhythmic breathing
- Interactive video games
- Project distractions: playing a challenging game, performing meaningful play or work

EMPLOYING HUMOR

Humor can be an effective distraction, can help a person cope with pain, and may even have a positive effect on the immune system. It has been proven beneficial in relieving acute painful procedural pain in children. Many pain, cancer, and ambulatory care centers encourage patients to view humorous videos before a painful, tedious procedure (IOM, 2011). Laughter may indeed be the best medicine. The potential physiologic and psychological benefits of laughter are highlighted in Box 36-2 (on page 1358).

Remember to use humor only with patients who are responsive to its use and wish to use it. Humor should not be used with patients in moderate to severe pain, nor should it be a replacement for pharmacologic analgesia. In addition, humor must be patient specific. The nurse will need to

Box 36-2 Therapeutic Effects of Laughter

Laughter causes the following physiologic and psychological effects:

- Increases the pain threshold
- Reduces arterial wall stiffness and improves endothelial function
- Reduces the risk of myocardial infarction (MI); reduces recurrence after MI in diabetes
- Improves lung function in patients with chronic obstructive pulmonary disease (COPD)
- Improves glycemic control; impacts on obesity
- Improves the success rate of in vitro fertilization
- Associated with satisfaction and an increased quality of life

Source: Adapted from Femer, R. E., & Aronson, J. K. (2013). Laughter and MIRTH (methodical investigation of risibility, therapeutic and harmful): Narrative synthesis. *The BMJ*, *347*, f7274. https://doi.org/10.1136/bmj.f7274; Noureldein, M. H., & Eid, A. A. (2018). Homeostatic effect of laughter on diabetic cardiovascular complications: The myth turned to fact. *Diabetes Research and Clinical Practice*, *135*, 111–119. https://doi.org/10.1016/j.diabres.2017.11.014

determine what makes a patient laugh, how the patient has used humor or play in the past, and how it helped. Let the patient select the humorous materials, and when possible, incorporate strategies that include the patient's family and friends.

LISTENING TO MUSIC

Listening to music can relax, soothe, decrease pain, and provide distraction. Music affects various neurotransmitters (such as epinephrine and norepinephrine), hormones (particularly cortisol), components of the immune system (especially with the cytokine interleukin-6), the autonomic nervous system (sympathetic and parasympathetic components), and psychological responses (Howland, 2016). Recent studies have confirmed that perioperative music therapy resulted in a decrease in postoperative pain, anxiety, and use of analgesics, with an increase in patient satisfaction (Hole et al., 2015; Kühlmann et al., 2018; Schneider, 2018). When used with patients experiencing self-reported chronic pain, there was also a decrease in depressive symptoms and other comorbidities associated with untreated pain (Garza-Villarreal et al., 2017). Acute pain guidelines recommend music and relaxation as interventions that, in combination with opioids, help to relieve moderate postoperative pain. Music therapy is a readily accessible therapy that is not associated with significant adverse effects. It should be considered a viable, potential treatment for many patients, including those in pain. Specific best practice recommendations include: (1) using music before, during, and after surgical procedures; (2) identifying calming music (60 to 80 BPM); (3) playing music continuously during the procedure or surgical intervention; and (4) playing music for 15 to 30 minutes at least twice a day during the pre- and postoperative periods (Poulsen & Coto, 2018).

USING IMAGERY

Patients who use imagery (an example of mind–body interaction) to decrease pain sensation imagine something that involves one or all of the senses, concentrate on that image, and gradually become less aware of the pain. Imagery may be as simple as a child thinking of happy things (a beloved pet, lollipops, Christmas morning, Grandma's lap) or as involved as an adult recreating a favorite place and then experiencing the healing presence or touch of a loved person, or the healing energies of nature in that setting. The imagery technique has also been used to create an image in which the cause of the pain is visualized and then overcome or counteracted by some more powerful image.

Imagery has been found to be more effective for patients with chronic pain than for patients with acute, severe pain. General techniques for successfully guiding a patient to use imagery include the following:

- Help the patient to identify the problem or goal.
- Suggest that the patient begin the imagery with several minutes of focused breathing, relaxation, or meditation.
- Help the patient to develop images of the problem, as well as personal internal resources (e.g., coping strategies) and external healing therapies (e.g., medications, treatments).
- Encourage images of the desired state of well-being at the end of the session.

If the patient becomes restless or upset, the imagery experience is terminated and attempted later when the patient seems better disposed. Guided imagery is also discussed in Chapter 43. Technology provides the opportunity to augment imagery or guided imagery techniques using virtual reality (VR), a computer-generated environment that may involve a screen or head-mounted display (HMD). Although more research needs to be done to determine the effectiveness of VR in varied situations with different populations, there is the potential for incorporating this specific modality into the holistic approach to acute and chronic pain management (Chuan et al., 2021).

MINDFULNESS PRACTICE

Mindfulness practice requires intentional presence in a nonjudgmental, accepting way using techniques such as centering, relaxation, meditation, and breath work. Mindfulness-Based Stress Reduction (MBSR), an evidence-based practice, was formalized by Dr. Kabat-Zinn (1982) in the late 1970s as a strategy to manage chronic pain. Since then, mindfulness practices have evolved to include health care professionals, patients, and the general public in myriad situations, including those related to chronic illnesses, the opioid crisis, and the stress of COVID-19. MBSR is often compared to or considered in relation to cognitive behavioral therapy (CBT), a psychotherapeutic treatment focused on challenging unhelpful thought or behavioral patterns through education; cognitive restructuring of thoughts and beliefs; problem resolution; relaxation; and, ultimately, a behavioral change that involves engagement in meaningful activities (Hawk et al., 2020; Pardos-Gascón et al., 2021). Although the results are mixed, with some studies showing a reduction in depression, disability, and chronic pain after an MBSR intervention (Marske et al., 2020) and others highlighting little support for the efficacy in managing acute or chronic pain

Research in Nursing

BRIDGING THE GAP TO EVIDENCE-BASED PRACTICE

Examination of the Effects of Implementing a Nurse-Led Pain Program for Patients With Nonmalignant Chronic Pain

Pain regimens require interprofessional collaboration to support implementation of a multimodal approach to pain management. Although nurses require prescriptions or orders for medication administration, there are a number of educational and nonpharmacologic interventions that are nurse-driven and support a holistic approach to pain management.

Related Research

Morales-Fernández, Á., Jimenez-Martín, J. M., Morales-Asencio, J. M., Vergara-Romero, M., Mora-Bandera, A. M., Aranda-Gallardo, M., & Canca-Sanchez, J. C. (2021). Impact of a nurse-led intervention on quality of life in patients with chronic non-malignant pain: An open randomized controlled trial. *Journal of Advanced Nursing, 77*(1), 255–265. https://doi.org/10.1111/jan.14608

This IRB-approved study used an experimental design, with the 279 participants randomly assigned to the usual care ($n = 105$) or intervention group ($n = 174$). The intervention consisted of an introductory one-on-one session, followed by six 90-minute weekly group sessions in which the 8 to 12 participants engaged in therapeutic dialogue and educational sessions with an advanced practice registered nurse (APRN) who specializes in chronic pain. The education deliverables were rooted in the principles of cognitive behavioral therapy (CBT) and focused on myriad topics including self-esteem, perceptions of pain, communication strategies, and relaxation techniques. The APRNs who ran the intervention all received a 2-month training course at a local university that collaborated on the study. Results were measured, using valid and reliable instruments, at baseline, then again at 3, 6, and 9 months after enrolling in the study. The nurse-led program led to improvements in several aspects of the patients' health-related quality of life and a (likely-related) decrease in the patient's self-reported levels of pain, anxiety, and depression. Patients reported satisfaction with the intervention, and the results were sustained over time.

Relevance to Nursing Practice

This article out of Spain reinforces that holistic pain management is not a U.S.-centric principle. Quality of life, pain level and description, and associated anxiety and depression are universal considerations because of their impact on patient well-being and satisfaction. Nurses make a difference in the patient chronic pain experience by providing patients the tools and confidence needed to take control and drive their own pain management program.

(Pei et al., 2021; Shires et al., 2020), mindfulness and related interventions have made their way into mainstream wellness discussions and are likely to continue to be used.

Relaxation practices are similar to mindfulness practices in that both decrease stress, tension, anxiety, depression, and pain. Both practices require intentionality and focus, augment the multimodal pain management plan, and can be used in tandem with each other. However, they differ in intention—mindfulness practices focus on acceptance in the moment, and relaxation practices are focused on strategies to change internal processes (Luberto et al., 2020). See Research in Nursing box. Relaxation techniques are also discussed in Chapters 29 and 43.

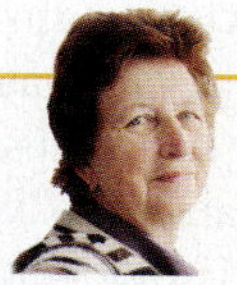

Consider **Carla Potter**, the older adult experiencing new-onset persistent pain in her lower extremities. Mindfulness practices may help her cope with the anxiety she is experiencing with this new pain. The first step is to assess her familiarity with mindfulness techniques and discuss which of these measures suit her current lifestyle and can be incorporated into her daily routine.

USING CUTANEOUS STIMULATION

The success of cutaneous stimulation (techniques that stimulate the skin's surface) in relieving pain is often explained using the gate control theory. The gate control theory of pain involves cutaneous nerve fibers, which are large-diameter fibers carrying impulses to the CNS. When the skin is stimulated, pain is believed to be controlled by closing the gating mechanism in the spinal cord. This decreases the number of pain impulses that reach the brain for perception. These techniques can be used in all health care settings to supplement a pain control regimen. Some forms of cutaneous stimulation include the following:

- Massage (with or without analgesic ointments or liniments containing menthol); see Skill 36-1 (on pp. 1377–1380)
- Application of heat or cold, or both intermittently (see detailed discussion in Chapter 33)
- Acupressure or trigger point release
- Transcutaneous electrical nerve stimulation (TENS) or electrical muscle stimulation (EMS, ESTIM, E-Stim)

Acupressure, a modern-day Western descendant of acupuncture, involves the use of the fingertips to apply gentle but firm pressure to usual acupuncture sites. This technique of holding and releasing various pressure points is rooted in traditional Chinese medicine (TCM) and focused on energy or *chi*. The calming effect of acupressure is most likely related to the body's release of endorphins and enkephalins. Members of the interprofessional team, particularly physical therapists, focus on trigger point release primarily to address referred pain. Trigger point release does not occur at the

PICOT in Practice

ASKING CLINICAL QUESTIONS: ACUPUNCTURE/ACUPRESSURE

Scenario: You are a nurse working with a large maxillofacial surgery group who attended a conference on integrative nursing. One presenter that stood out discussed the benefits of acupuncture/acupressure in managing the gag reflex in patients undergoing dental procedures. Gagging is a common problem encountered during dental treatment, making therapeutic procedures distressing and often difficult or even impossible to perform. One of the surgeons asks if you learned something new at the conference and you discuss the results of the presentation.

The office currently only uses sedatives to facilitate sedation in patient undergoing procedures. You wonder if acupuncture/acupressure compared to sedatives has any benefit in the care of patients "specifically pediatric patients" undergoing procedures.

- **Population:** Children receiving sedation
- **Intervention:** Use of acupuncture/acupressure
- **Comparison:** Use of sedatives
- **Outcome:** Decreased gag reflex
- **Time:** During dental procedures

PICOT Question: Does the use of acupuncture/acupressure by a nonanesthesiologist compared to administration of sedatives result in depression of gag reflex in children undergoing dental treatment and improved experience?

Findings:

1. Ashley, P. F., Chaudhary, M., Lourenço-Matharu, L. (2018). Sedation of children undergoing dental treatment. *Cochrane Database of Systematic Reviews*, (12), CD003877. https://doi.org/10.1002/14651858.CD003877.pub5

Included 50 studies with a total of 3,704 children up to age 16 years. Thirty-four different sedatives were used, often with inhalational nitrous oxide. There is moderate-certainty evidence that oral midazolam is an effective sedative agent for children undergoing dental treatment. There is a need for further well-designed and well-reported clinical trials to evaluate other potential sedation agents.

2. Eachempati, P., Kumbargere Nagraj, S., Kiran Kumar Krishanappa, S., George, R. P., Soe, H. H. K., Karanth, L. (2019). Management of gag reflex for patients undergoing dental treatment. *Cochrane Database of Systematic Reviews*, (11), CD011116. https://doi.org/10.1002/14651858.CD011116.pub3

The interventions used to manage gagging include antinausea medicines, sedatives, local and general anesthetics, herbal remedies, behavior therapy and cognitive behavior therapy, acupressure, acupuncture, laser, and prosthetic devices. This systematic review included four trials with 328 people (263 adults and 65 children who were ages 4 years and older). Of the trials reviewed, one compared acupuncture and acupressure (with thumb, device, and sea band) at P6 (point located three finger breadths below the wrist on the inner forearm in between the two tendons) to sham acupuncture and acupressure with and without sedation. One trial compared acupuncture at the P6 point to sham acupuncture. These trials reported both completion of dental procedure and reduction in gagging as their outcomes.

Level of Evidence I: systematic review.

Recommendations: Conscious sedation or moderate sedation is the ability of the patient to independently maintain an open mouth and respond sensibly to verbal commands. In addition, the patient will retain adequate function of protective reflexes such as the gag reflex. There is a fine line between a sedated patient and an anesthetized patient. The ideal sedative agent would reduce anxiety and improve behavior. Oral midazolam probably improves the behavior of children during dental treatment. Acupuncture at the P6 point when compared to acupressure to reduce gagging when undergoing dental procedures is appropriate. The same intervention with sedation did not show a difference.

same points as acupressure. Because patients, with training, can perform acupressure and trigger point release on themselves, it gives them a feeling of control in their care. See the accompanying PICOT in Practice box.

TENS is a noninvasive alternative technique that involves electrical stimulation of large-diameter fibers to inhibit transmission of painful impulses carried over small-diameter fibers. The TENS unit consists of a battery-powered portable unit, lead wires, and cutaneous electrode pads that are applied to the painful area (Fig. 36-6). The use of TENS requires a health care provider's prescription. TENS therapy has reportedly been effective in reducing postoperative pain and improving mobility after surgery. It is used for temporary relief of acute pain and for symptomatic chronic pain. Positive results have also been noted when it is used as an adjunct to physical therapy and for patients with low back pain. The TENS unit may be applied intermittently throughout the day or worn for extended periods of time, depending on the provider's order.

Although similar to a TENS unit, EMS tends to cause greater muscle contraction than a TENS unit. EMS is often used in conjunction with strength training to improve muscle strength and decrease pain in patients and athletes. It is associated with rehabilitation of neurologic or musculoskeletal issues and may be specifically referred to as functional (FES) or neuromuscular electrical stimulation (NMES; Johnston et al., 2021; Novak et al., 2020).

Use of cutaneous stimulation is limited because the pain must be localized. Otherwise, it is most likely too diffuse to be effective. In addition, most people cannot tolerate stimulation of the painful area; however, they may be helped by stimulation of the surrounding or contralateral area.

USING ACUPUNCTURE AND DRY NEEDLING

Traditional Chinese medicine (TCM) originated in ancient China and has evolved over the years. Chinese herbal medicine, acupuncture, and tai chi have integrated into Western

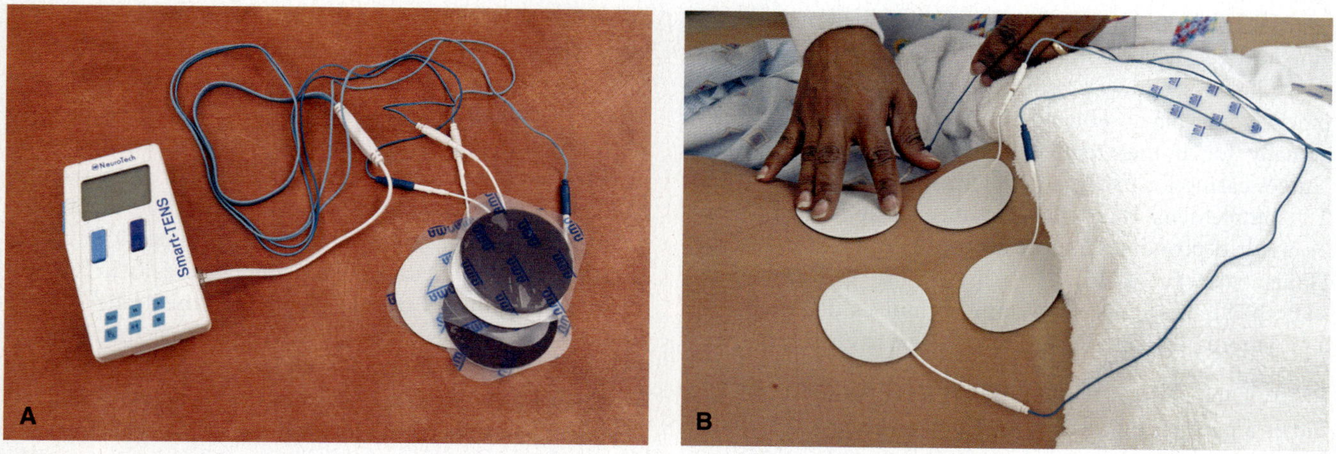

FIGURE 36-6. **A.** TENS unit. **B.** Applying TENS electrodes.

CHA (National Center for Complementary and Integrative Health [NCCIH], 2019). Acupuncture is a technique that uses thin needles of various lengths inserted through the skin at specific locations to produce insensitivity to pain by affecting meridians, *chi*, and energy flow. It has gained acceptance in the Western world as a CHA to help control discomfort from disorders such as headaches, low back pain, neck pain, osteoarthritis or knee pain, and cancer (NCCIH, 2019). The relief of pain by acupuncture is generally explained on the basis of the gate control theory; however, more research is needed on the efficacy of acupuncture. Licensed acupuncturists, usually chiropractors or those who hold a Doctor of Science in Oriental Medicine (DSOM)/Oriental Medical Doctorate (OMD), most often administer acupuncture. This therapy is considered safe when a licensed, experienced practitioner who uses sterile acupuncture needles performs it. Repeated treatments are often needed.

Trigger point dry needling (TDN) is a technique used by trained practitioners, including physical and occupational therapists. Although it uses sterile, filiform (solid, not hollow) needles such as acupuncture, TDN is based on Western medicine and began in the 1950s. The needles are inserted into key trigger points identified through a medical examination, the patient's report of pain and symptoms, and the practitioner's knowledge of anatomy. Dry needling involves penetration of the skin, followed by stimulation of myofascial trigger points, muscles, and connective tissues. This therapy focuses on the management of neuromusculoskeletal pain and impairments in movement (range of motion, strength, spasticity) that impact on the functional ability of the patient (Bynum et al., 2021; Institute of Advanced Musculoskeletal Treatments [IAMT], 2021; Sánchez-Infante et al., 2021).

USING HYPNOSIS

Hypnosis, a technique that produces a subconscious state accomplished by suggestions made by a hypnotist, has been used successfully in many instances to control pain. The person's state of consciousness is altered by suggestions so that pain is not perceived as it normally would be. According to many hypnotists, it also alters the physical signs of pain. Many people can be taught autohypnosis, that is, self-induced hypnosis, for the control of pain. It is generally believed that a successful response to hypnosis is related to the person's openness to suggestion, belief that hypnosis will work, and emotional readiness.

EMPLOYING BIOFEEDBACK

Biofeedback is a technique that uses a machine to monitor physiologic responses through electrode sensors on the patient's skin. The feedback signal or unit transforms the autonomic and neuromuscular physiologic data into visual, acoustic, and verbal feedback for the patient (Wagner et al., 2021). Upon seeing pain-related responses, such as increased muscle tension or elevated blood pressure, the patient is taught to regulate this physiologic response and control pain by practicing techniques such as deep-breathing exercises, progressive relaxation exercises, or visual imagery. Biofeedback decreases the person's pain by reducing the anxiety associated with lack of control over bodily functions, directing the person's attention away from the pain to the person's inner state and the feedback signal, and addressing the underlying, physiologic cause of the pain. Eventually, the person learns to recognize the sensations and employ measures to reduce pain without the use of the biofeedback machinery. The goal is to improve quality of life and increase physiologic function. Although biofeedback is safe and has not been shown to have adverse effects, limitations of this additive method include cost factors and limited availability of specialists (Wagner et al., 2021).

PROVIDING HEALING/THERAPEUTIC TOUCH

Healing Touch (HT) is an energy therapy that may be valuable as an adjunct to Western medicine. Some studies have indicated that it has been effective in reducing pain and anxiety in hospitalized patients and is recognized as an alternative therapy in end-of-life care for both adults and children (Weaver, 2017). It requires no equipment, uses light touch, and is appropriate for every level of care. Acceptance has been an obstacle for HT therapy, primarily because there is little evidence to support its use.

Although the terms are often used interchangeably, Therapeutic Touch (TT) historically is focused more on the universal field and directing life energy to patients. Patients who have received TT state that it helps with feelings of comfort, calmness, and well-being. It is derived from the ancient practice of laying on of hands, but nurses skilled in TT never actually touch their patients when using this technique. Nurses caring for patients with terminal diseases relate that TT complements their efforts to alleviate suffering and can be used to promote comfort during the final stages of life (Tabatabaee et al., 2016).

Both HT and TT were developed by nurses, do not require a provider's prescription, and can be used in any setting.

PROVIDING ANIMAL-ASSISTED INTERVENTION

Either a patient's own pet or an animal with an experienced handler can be used as complementary therapy to help relieve pain and provide a degree of comfort to people in various health care settings. Pet Partners (n.d.) is an organization that has been involved in therapy animal programs since 1977. These visits are either casual (*animal-assisted activities*—AAA) or more focused with a stated goal and documented results (*animal-assisted intervention*—AAI). Animals that visit patients include dogs, rabbits, guinea pigs, birds, cats, and even llamas. AAI has been used to relieve pain in children in acute care settings. Although evidence supports the use of AAI, acute and long-term care settings may have rules that preclude admitting animals. The introduction of pet-robot interventions (PRI), led to reductions in depression, anxiety, and loneliness in older adults with dementia. This innovation may represent a viable way to replicate the effects of AAI while eliminating barriers (Park et al., 2020).

Managing Pharmacologic Relief Measures

Pharmacologic pain management is a complex process that requires adequate assessment, consideration of guidelines and regulations, knowledge of medications, sufficient tracking and follow-up, patient teaching, and an interprofessional, multimodal approach. To make informed decisions and individualize care, nurses need updated information and ongoing education about drug therapy, the cornerstone of many pain-treatment regimens.

ADMINISTERING ANALGESICS

An **analgesic** is a pharmaceutical agent that relieves pain. Analgesics function to reduce the person's perception of pain and to alter the person's responses to discomfort. There are three general classes of drugs used for pain relief:

- **Opioid** analgesics (all controlled substances, e.g., morphine, codeine, oxycodone, meperidine, hydromorphone, methadone)
- Nonopioid analgesics (acetaminophen and nonsteroidal antiinflammatory drugs [NSAIDs])
- **Adjuvant** analgesics (anticonvulsants, antidepressants, multipurpose drugs)

The nurse administering analgesics needs to combine a healthy respect for the drug being administered with a thorough knowledge of its mechanism of action, side effects, and administration guidelines. This combination of knowledge of and respect for the drug should result in analgesics being used wisely to produce their desired effect.

Knowledge of common analgesics enables the nurse to tailor the patient's regimen and communicate professionally with prescribing health care providers about a patient who is being undermedicated, needs a different drug, or requires a different route of administration. Nurses should not independently decide to refrain from using an analgesic or reduce a prescribed dose because of a patient's unrealistic fear of a medication's potency or side effects. Pain medication choice and dosing requires a collaborative approach that includes the patient, nurse, pharmacist, and prescriber.

Repeated studies have confirmed improvement in pain assessment and documentation, but not in pain relief. Health care providers are questioning prescribing practices for opioids and admit a lack of confidence regarding how to prescribe opioids safely, how to detect abuse or emerging addiction, and how to broach these topics with their patients (Centers for Disease Control and Prevention [CDC], 2021b; Volkow & McLellan, 2016). This can lead to pain that is not appropriately managed. Nurses, who typically spend the most time with the patient and are trained in pain assessment and management, often compound this problem by further reducing an insufficient analgesic dose or by not administering the medication at all. Nurse variables include the low priority given to pain management, arbitrary pain assessments, erroneous judgments about a patient's pain and need for analgesia, and fear of being the person who administers the drug that causes respiratory depression or another serious side effect. Health care providers work to achieve optimum pain relief for all people (Karch, 2020). The inability of many patients to discuss their pain and to request pain assistance perpetuates this problem. However, consideration needs to be given as to whether reported pain is acute or chronic in nature. Nurses must employ best practices that consider evidence-based guidelines, position statements from associations, and consensus reports from expert panels to prevent the transition of acute pain to chronic pain (Jungquist et al., 2017). The interprofessional team must maintain responsibility for balancing reasonable, adequate pain relief with the actual and potential risks of pain medication prescription and use. Clear guidelines regarding the management of chronic pain exist and should guide practice (CDC, 2021b; National Institute on Drug Abuse, 2020).

Opioid Analgesics

Opioids, formerly called narcotic analgesics, are generally considered the major class of analgesics used in the management of moderate to severe nociceptive, neuropathic, and cancer-related pain. Although the term *opiates* refers to natural opioids such as heroin or morphine, and *opioids* refers to all natural, synthetic, and semisynthetic opioids, we use the broader term opioids in our discussion (CDC, 2021a). In sufficient dosage, opioids are considered effective in relieving pain that is peripheral/nociceptive in nature, such as acute pain due to injury, pain associated with rheumatoid arthritis, or cancer pain (National Institute on Drug

Abuse, 2020). Opioids produce analgesia by attaching to opioid receptors in the brain, similar to how a key fits a lock. Ongoing research on opioid analgesics also indicates that opioid receptors are present on cells of the immune system and may suppress immune function (Brejchova et al., 2021). Opioid receptor sites are further classified as mu-receptors that primarily block pain but are also involved in respiratory changes, euphoric feelings, pupil and GI changes, and physical dependence; delta-receptors that are thought to be involved with peripheral terminals; and kappa-receptors that block some pain but are also associated with pupil changes, dysphoria (profound unease that result in restlessness, anxiety, and depression), and sedation (Brejchova et al., 2021; Karch, 2020). The difference in opioid effects is related to their interaction with these three opioid types of receptors. Opioids that produce analgesia (agonists) can compete for binding sites on the receptors with opioids that do not produce analgesia (antagonists). An opioid agonist such as morphine binds to the mu-receptor site and produces analgesia (Norris, 2020). An opioid antagonist such as naloxone also competes for binding on the mu site, but it blocks the analgesic effect of morphine as well as its side effects. Most of the opioid analgesics commonly used in a clinical setting bind primarily to mu-receptor sites. Patients differ in their sensitivity to morphine because of genetic variability of the mu-receptor site.

There are many opioid analgesics that range from weak (codeine or tramadol) to strong (morphine, oxycodone, or hydromorphone). Health care providers individualize the choice of medication based on the disease process, level/type of pain, and other assessment factors. Current recommendations advise using evidence-based practice pain management that is multimodal and incorporates opioid-sparing therapies (Jungquist et al., 2020). Morphine, the prototype opioid, is often the opioid of choice because providers are familiar with it, it is readily available in multiple forms, and it is relatively inexpensive. Fentanyl, a synthetic opioid that is 50 to 100 times stronger than morphine, is available in a variety of forms that range from rapid-acting to long-acting (PDQ® Supportive and Palliative Care Editorial Board, 2021). Methadone is most commonly used to treat cancer pain (PDQ® Supportive and Palliative Care Editorial Board, 2021) and to manage detoxification in people with opioid dependence/addiction. If patients have continued uncontrolled pain, unmanageable side/adverse effects, a change in status that requires a change in route of administration, or develop toxicity, an opioid rotation (switch to another medication) may be initiated (PDQ® Supportive and Palliative Care Editorial Board, 2021).

QSEN DRUG SAFETY

Methadone is a mu-receptor agonist and an *N*-methyl-D-aspartate (NMDA) receptor antagonist that must be used cautiously because it has a rapid onset of action and a long half-life.

Nurses who are involved in the administration of opioids to manage acute and chronic pain must become familiar with equianalgesic opioid dosing, which involves using opioid conversion calculations that consider the dose, route, and potency of a medication. For example, although a patient may receive 4 mg of morphine IV, 4 mg of fentanyl IV would be lethal. This skill requires clinical judgment and is essential to determine safe and therapeutic dosage ranges of specific opioids (Curtis et al., 2021).

The most common side effects associated with opioid use are sedation, nausea, and constipation. Most side effects disappear with prolonged use, but if constipation persists, it usually responds to treatment with increased fluids and fiber and use of a mild laxative or stool softener. An opioid-naive person who has not developed tolerance may experience all of the side effects. This contrasts with an opioid-tolerant person who has taken opioids long enough and at sufficient levels to develop tolerance to the analgesic effect of the opioid and most of the side effects, except constipation.

Respiratory depression is a commonly feared adverse effect of opioid use. Opioid-induced respiratory depression can result in an increased length of stay and cost expenditures, readmission, and even death, especially with concurrent use of other respiratory depressant drugs such as alcohol or benzodiazepines (Khanna et al., 2020; National Institute on Drug Abuse, 2018). Current recommendations include integrating a comprehensive assessment of patient-specific, treatment-related, and environment-related risk factors before initiating opioid therapy, and for the duration of clinical care. Specific recommendations include electronic monitoring for patients deemed high-risk (Jungquist et al., 2020). A new predictive tool (PRODIGY), developed through international collaboration at 16 different sites with 1,266 patients, used continuous oximetry and capnography data to identify age ≥60 years (greatest risk for those ≥80 years old), male sex, opioid naivety, sleep disorders (such as sleep apnea), and chronic heart failure as predictive for an opioid-induced respiratory depression episode (Khanna et al., 2020). Another tool, the Pasero Opioid-Induced Sedation Scale, requires only nursing assessment and can be used to assess respiratory depression in adult and pediatric populations (Pasero & McCaffery, 2011; Hall & Stanley, 2019):

- S = sleep, easy to arouse: no action necessary
- 1 = awake and alert; no action necessary
- 2 = occasionally drowsy but easy to arouse; requires no action
- 3 = frequently drowsy and drifts off to sleep during conversation; decrease the opioid dose
- 4 = somnolent with minimal or no response to stimuli; discontinue the opioid and consider use of naloxone

If respiratory depression is suspected and the opioid dose is withheld, the patient may be physically stimulated by shaking or using a loud sound, along with reminders every few minutes to breathe deeply. If this is ineffective, naloxone, an opioid antagonist that reverses the respiratory-depressant effect of an opioid, can be used. Naloxone is administered intravenously in the hospital setting. Within 1 to 2 minutes, the patient usually opens their eyes and is able to respond to the nurse. When the patient is alert again and the respiratory rate is back to baseline, the opioid may be resumed. However, the half-life (time required for the concentration to decrease by half; duration of action) of naloxone is very short, so resedation may occur, and subsequent doses of naloxone may be required (every 5 minutes). Keep in mind that the naloxone works by blocking the action of the opioid, so if naloxone is required and/or the opioid cannot be resumed in a reasonable amount of time, the nurse must ensure another method of pain relief is administered.

There is a difference between opioid use short term (<3 weeks) for acute pain and long-term (>3 months) management of chronic pain with opioids. Patient education often needs to include a review of these key terms in order to allay fears and collaboratively develop a plan for pain management. Physical dependence and tolerance are frequently confused with addiction. **Physical dependence** is a phenomenon in which the body physiologically becomes accustomed to opioid therapy and suffers withdrawal symptoms if the opioid is suddenly removed, or the dose is rapidly decreased. **Tolerance** occurs when the body becomes accustomed to the opioid and needs a larger dose (up to 10 times the original dose) for pain relief. Tolerance can be avoided by administering smaller doses of a drug or using a multimodal approach. Physical dependence and tolerance are different from addiction primarily because physical dependence and tolerance are expected responses; addiction is not a typical or predictable result of opioid use (Karch, 2020; PDQ® Supportive and Palliative Care Editorial Board, 2021; Volkow & McLellan, 2016). **Addiction** is a "chronic, relapsing brain disease characterized by compulsive drug seeking and use despite adverse consequences" (National Institute on Drug Abuse, 2020, p. 4). If people are not misusing the prescribed drug(s), addiction occurs over time and in a small percentage of patients exposed to opioids, even if they have preexisting vulnerabilities such as long-term opioid use, a history of depression, or an existing substance use disorder. Key indicators of addiction include a profound craving for the drug, erosion of the inhibitory mechanisms that control efforts to refrain from drug use, and compulsive drug taking. The hallmark of addiction is this impairment to exert self-control. Addiction is associated with long-term opioid use, but surveillance with short-term use is also beneficial. Primary clinical efforts to prevent drug use, misuse, and addiction include performing an assessment of risk factors and protective factors before prescribing opioids, regular monitoring, referral to addiction treatment as needed, and prescription of amounts that minimize the risk of diversion (National Institute of Drug Abuse, 2020; Volkow & McLellan, 2016).

Opioid use disorder (OUD) and the opioid crisis have been at the center of public discourse for more than 15 years. Although prevention of OUD remains the primary goal, emergent intervention for opioid overdose and long-term pharmacologic treatment of OUD may be required. The U.S. Food and Drug Administration (FDA) has approved three forms of naloxone for community use: injectable, auto-injector, and nasal spray. Naloxone kits and the associated training are currently available to trained first responders and laypeople in the community either through prescriptions or state-based standing orders (FDA, 2019). The FDA (2021) actively seeks to increase the availability of naloxone by encouraging drug manufacturers to pursue approval for over-the-counter naloxone products, requiring manufacturers to include recommendations regarding naloxone with opioid-prescribing information, and extending the shelf life of naloxone from 24 to 36 months. Methadone, an opioid agonist; buprenorphine, a partial opioid agonist; and naltrexone, an opioid antagonist, are approved to support recovery from OUD and heroin use. Another common agent used to treat OUD, Suboxone®, contains both naloxone and buprenorphine. These medications all reduce opioid use and OUD-related symptoms, but they also increase adherence to a treatment plan, reduce the risk of HIV and HCV transmission, reduce legal issues and incarceration, and lead to a greater likelihood of maintaining employment (National Institute on Drug Abuse, 2018). See the Vulnerable Populations Alert on patients with an OUD.

National guidelines include a checklist for prescribing opioids for chronic pain. This guideline stems from the need to ensure safe, effective pain management for chronic pain while reducing the risk of OUD, overdose, and potential death (CDC, 2021b; Dowell et al., 2016). The checklist for prescribing opioids for chronic pain (that does not involve cancer-related, palliative, or end-of-life care) includes these three main patient-centered foci (CDC, 2021b):

- Determining when opioids should be started and continued to manage chronic pain; this includes using nonopioid and nonpharmacologic methods in conjunction with opioids, setting realistic treatment goals, and discussing the risk and benefits with patients
- Selecting the appropriate opioid (immediate-release, extended-release, long-acting), dose, duration of treatment, follow-up plan, and discontinuation parameters
- Assessing risk and mitigating harms of opioid use; this includes a review of the Prescription Drug Monitoring Program (PDMP) database, urine drug testing, co-prescribing benzodiazepines, and treating OUD as needed

The American Society of Pain Management Nurses and the American Pain Society (Drew et al., 2018) released a consensus statement on the nurse's role in interpreting and implementing as needed/PRN or titrated pain medications. The role of nurses in this process includes:

- Basing decisions on a complete pain assessment including (at least) pain intensity, temporal characteristics, and patient's previous response to this or other analgesics
- Using valid and reliable tools that are consistent and individualized to the patient
- Considering the pharmacokinetics of the opioid
- Avoiding administration issues such as giving partial doses more frequently or making a patient wait the full time interval after a partial dose; waiting until the peak effect of the first partial dose is reached before giving a subsequent dose

Vulnerable Population Alert

COVID-19 gave the world time to reflect on social injustice and racial disparities. There is a clarion call for a reckoning rising from bioethicists, legal experts, drug experts, sociologists, psychologists, researchers from many disciplines, physicians, and allied health professionals to end the war on drugs and begin to establish a system of racial justice. In addition to legalizing cannabis, which is well underway in many states, this group is in "favor of the ultimate legalization and careful regulation of MDMA (ecstasy), psychedelic drugs such as LSD and psilocybin, heroin, and other opioids, methamphetamine, and powder and crack cocaine—that is, all drugs used for nonmedical purposes that are currently deemed illicit" (Earp et al., 2021). But this group is not alone in their endeavors. MDMA, which is known to increase dopamine, norepinephrine, and serotonin, is being used in conjunction with manualized therapy (MDMA-assisted therapy) in a phase 3 clinical trial to address posttraumatic stress disorder (PTSD) with significantly positive results (Mitchell et al., 2021). This trial, part of the Multidisciplinary Association for Psychedelic Studies (MAPS) founded by Doblin in 1986, is moving MDMA toward U.S. Food and Drug Administration approval (Carpenter, 2020). Dr. Nate L. Hart, a professor of psychology of Columbia University, wrote a new book, *Drug Use for Grown-Ups: Chasing Liberty in the Land of Fear* that details his 5-year regular use of heroin for recreational purposes and combats the notion that drugs are inherently bad. Although the book provides much more nuance, it mentions that opioid overdoses are the product of mixing agents, not the opioids themselves, and that addiction does not happen with every person who ingests drugs, even drugs previously deemed highly addictive. The larger issue posited by Hart (Schwartz, 2021) and Earp et al. (2021) is that the war against drugs disproportionately affects poor and Black people. Criminal convictions trace back to slavery and Jim Crow–era tenets and are better handled by health care programs and social support, not the criminal justice system.

For your consideration:

- How does this framing change your attitudes toward what are currently consider illegal/illicit drugs?
- How does this affect your interactions with patients with opioid or substance abuse disorder?
- What are your perspectives regarding advocacy as a nurse regarding the U.S. criminal justice system? What can you use from our Code of Ethics to guide you?
- Pretend your patient presents you with these studies they read about on Twitter. How do you incorporate or counter this information?

Carpenter, D. E. (2020, May 12). Psychedelic pioneer Rick Doblin on FDA trials Of MDMA: Most important reality check Of MAPS' 34-year history. *Forbes*. https://www.forbes.com/sites/davidcarpenter/2020/05/12/psychedelic-pioneer-rick-doblin-on-fda-trials-of-mdma-most-important-reality-check-of-maps-34-year-history/?sh=46b7007230ad

Earp, B. D., Lewis, J., Hart, C. L., & with Bioethicists and Allied Professionals for Drug Policy Reform. (2021). Racial justice requires ending the war on drugs. *The American Journal of Bioethics, 21*(4), 4–19. https://doi.org/10.1080/15265161.2020.1861364

Mitchell, J. M., Bogenschutz, M., Lilienstein, A., Harrison, C., Kleiman, S., Parker-Guilbert, K., Ot'alora, G. M., Garas, W., Paleos, C., Gorman, I., Nicholas, C., Mithoefer, M., Carlin, S., Poulter, B., Mithoefer, A., Quevedo, S., Wells, G., Klaire, S. S., van der Kolk, B., … Doblin, R. (2021). MDMA-assisted therapy for severe PTSD: A randomized, double-blind, placebo-controlled phase 3 study. *Nature Medicine, 27*(6), 1025–1033. https://doi.org/10.1038/s41591-021-01336-3

Schwartz, C. (2021, January 12). When getting high is a hobby, not a habit. *The New York Times*. https://www.nytimes.com/2021/01/12/books/review/drug-use-for-grown-ups-carl-l-hart.html

- Teaching the patient the name of the drug, the dose administered, the monitoring process, and potential side effects to report
- Evaluating the patient's response to dose and dosing interval
- Ensuring complete documentation and communication during transitions of care
- Assisting with the development of policies that ensure patient comfort and safety

Prescribers should provide a fixed time interval (every 3 hours) but may provide a dosage range for a PRN opioid (e.g., 20 to 30 mg). Prescribing dosages based solely on a 0 to 10 numeric value reported by the patient does not consider other factors that the nurse considers when determining the appropriate dose for an individual patient. A registered nurse who is competent in pain assessment and medication administration can manage the pain management regimen using a correctly written prescription/order set (Drew et al., 2018).

Nonopioid Analgesics

Nonopioid analgesics, such as acetaminophen and NSAIDs, are usually the drugs of choice for both acute and persistent moderate chronic pain. The simplest dosage schedules and least invasive pain management modalities should be used first. Many times, these drugs alone can provide adequate pain relief. Many of these medications are OTC products, whereas some are available by prescription only. Some can cause gastric side effects, but these symptoms may be preventable if the drug is taken with food or antacids.

Acetaminophen has long been viewed as one of the safest and best-tolerated analgesics. It has proven to be an effective drug for acute pain treatment and is the most commonly used analgesic for children in the United States (Karch, 2020). It has a low incidence of adverse effects, but the risk of hepatotoxicity must be considered when acetaminophen is used for a lengthy period or at larger than the recommended dose (maximum of 4 grams/day). If pain is not controlled using the recommended dose of acetaminophen, NSAIDs or an opioid analgesic may be required to achieve pain relief.

NSAIDs have an antiinflammatory effect. Individual responses to NSAIDs vary, but these agents are contraindicated in patients with bleeding disorders (their action may interfere with platelet function), probable infections (NSAIDs can mask the signs of an infection), and in pregnancy at 20 weeks or later (potential fetal renal dysfunction; FDA, 2020b). The FDA (2020b) requires that NSAID labels contain information about the potential for GI bleeding and skin reactions associated with all NSAIDs, and a warning that all NSAIDs, except for aspirin, increase the risk of myocardial infarction (heart attack) or stroke. The combination of nonopioid analgesics and opioids provides more analgesia than either drug taken alone. Multimodal analgesic therapy is a relatively recent approach to pain management (Fig. 36-7). It combines two or more classes of analgesics that target different sites in the peripheral and central nervous systems to maximize pain relief with fewer adverse effects. The most common multimodal approach is a combination of nonopioid, opioid, and adjuvant analgesics (PDQ® Supportive and Palliative Care Editorial Board, 2021). The patient and caregivers will require an explanation regarding why multiple medications have been prescribed and how they work to relieve pain. Although often considered in relation to chronic pain, multimodal analgesia is also a valid approach to the management of acute pain. The pain associated with the postoperative period and trauma are positively impacted by the synergistic effect of multimodal analgesia, which maximizes pain relief at lower doses, thus reducing the risk of adverse effects of specific drugs (Polomano et al., 2017).

The COX-2 inhibitors, a class of NSAIDs, have a lower risk of GI bleeding but are thought to significantly increase cardiovascular risks. Celecoxib is available in the United States and used for treatment of osteoarthritis and rheumatoid arthritis (FDA, 2020b).

Adjuvant Analgesics

Adjuvant drugs are typically used for other purposes but are also integral to an optional pain management program. They may also reduce side effects from prescribed opioids or lessen anxiety about the pain experience. Adjuvant analgesics include antidepressants (venlafaxine, duloxetine, and tricyclics), anticonvulsants/gabapentinoids (gabapentin and pregabalin), alpha-2-agonists (clonidine and dexmedetomidine), local anesthetics (lidocaine), corticosteroids (dexamethasone, methylprednisolone, and prednisone), bisphosphonates (specifically for bone metastases), and NMDA agonists (ketamine and magnesium). They may be used to treat acute pain resulting from surgery, burns, or trauma; neuropathic pain syndromes such as diabetic neuropathy and postherpetic neuralgia; nociplastic pain such as fibromyalgia; and cancer-related pain (PDQ® Supportive and Palliative Care Editorial Board, 2021; Schwenk & Mariano, 2019).

APPLYING GENERAL PRINCIPLES FOR ANALGESIC ADMINISTRATION

When using medications for pain relief, the nurse must first assess the patient's pain and understand the patient's goals for pain relief. In the home as well as in acute care settings, nurses provide quality nursing care when they empower patients to take charge of their own pain relief measures. The following guidelines are recommended for effective, individualized pain management in any setting:

- Choose a pain scale or instrument that most accurately assists with assessment of pain.
- Try various pain control measures.
- Use pain control measures before pain increases in severity.
- Ask the patient what has been effective for pain relief in the past.
- Select and modify pain control measures based on the patient's response.
- Encourage the patient to try the pain treatment several times before labeling it ineffective.
- Be open minded about alternative, nonpharmacologic pain relief strategies.
- Be persistent.
- Be a safe practitioner.

Accurate documentation is imperative to determine effectiveness of the current regimen or the need to change pain control measures if relief is not obtained. Pain diaries or flow sheets provide a method for people to document their particular pain experience, list medication or alternative therapies that were used to treat the pain, and record the effectiveness of the interventions used. Attempts to recall particular aspects of a painful experience are not always accurate. Pain diaries can be used in a variety of settings and help improve the overall management of pain. Since more patients with acute and chronic pain are cared for in their home environment, effective patient and caregiver teaching is the cornerstone of pain relief therapy.

Ongoing Assessment

Just as the pain experience of each patient is unique, so too is the response of each patient to a prescribed analgesic. The nurse needs to continuously evaluate whether a medication is producing the desired analgesic effect; identify changes in the patient's condition (correction or worsening of pathology, increased drug tolerance) that necessitate changes in the analgesic agent, dose, or route of administration; and identify the development of side effects of the analgesic that may warrant its discontinuance. Assessment must include consideration of all agents integrated into the multimodal analgesia plan as well as any nonpharmacologic interventions. As long as the patient's pain exists, ongoing assessment and documentation of pain control is imperative. Fundamental to this assessment is the knowledge of the basic action, doses, and routes of administration; side effects; and administration guidelines of the analgesic(s) being administered.

Timing is an important consideration when administering analgesics. To time analgesics appropriately, know the average duration of action for the drug and time administration so that the peak analgesic effect occurs when the pain is expected to be most intense. For example, an analgesic would be offered before ambulating a patient postoperatively.

A PRN (as needed) drug regimen has not been proven effective for people experiencing acute pain. In the early postoperative period, when pain is expected, this protocol may result in an intense pain experience for the patient. Later, however, in the postoperative course, a PRN schedule may be acceptable to relieve occasional pain episodes. Continuous intravenous infusion has proved effective for the relief of acute postoperative pain. PCA and epidural analgesia are discussed later in the chapter.

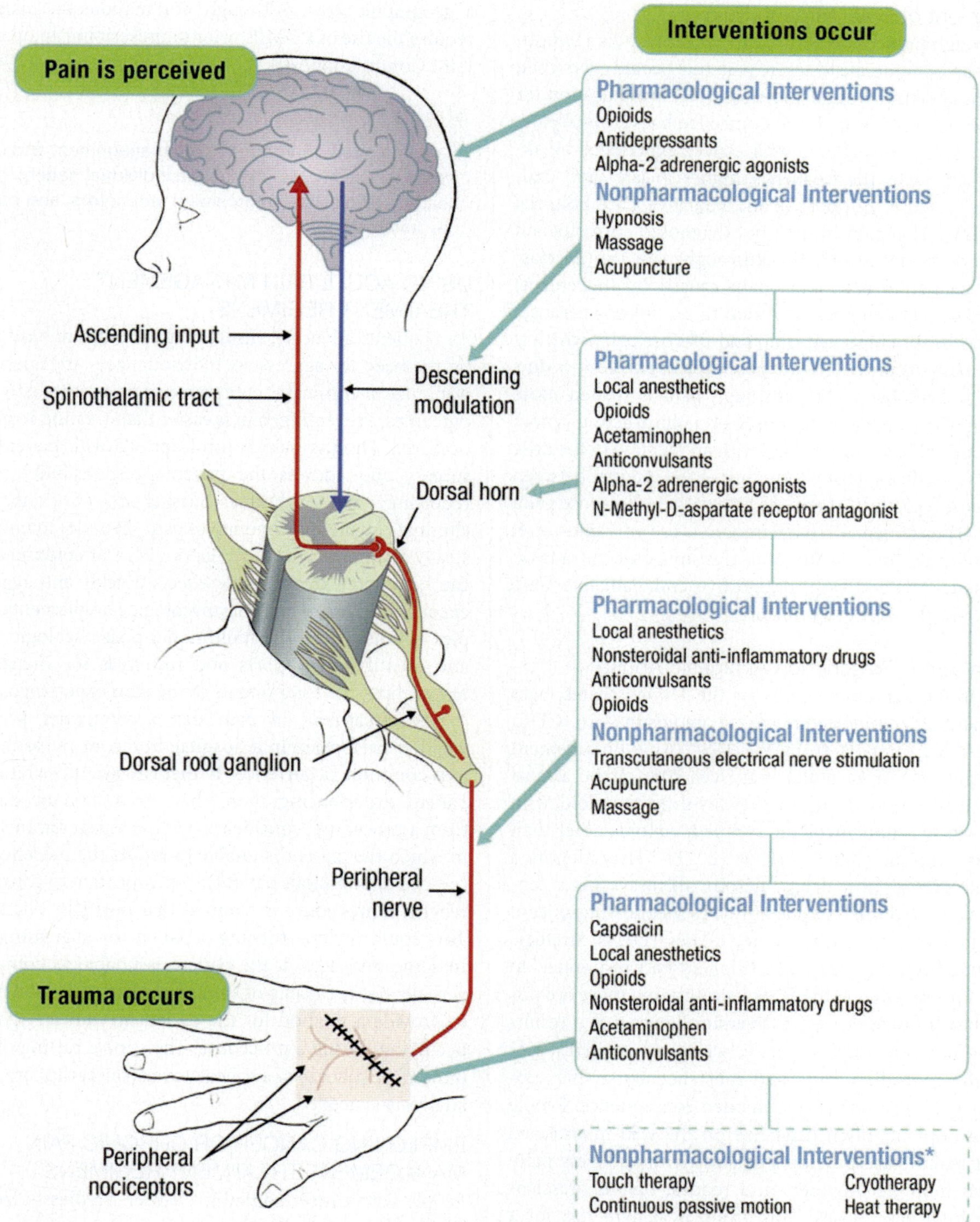

FIGURE 36-7. Multimodal pain management. (*Source:* Reprinted from Manworren, R. C. B. [2015]. Multimodal pain management and the future of a personalized medicine approach to pain. *AORN Journal*, *101*[3], 307–318.)

Nonpharmacologic and nonopioid pharmacologic therapies are the preferred choices for chronic pain that is not related to active cancer, palliative care, or end-of-life care. If progression to opioids becomes necessary, the lowest effective dose of an immediate-release opioid should be initiated first. Ongoing assessment and careful monitoring should guide the prescription of opioids for the management of chronic pain (CDC, 2021b; Dowell et al., 2016). Long-acting, controlled-release oral morphine or oxycodone or use of a fentanyl patch may be used in pain associated with cancer. Patients need instruction to apply the patch according to the time interval prescribed, avoid the application of heat in areas where the patch is in place, and dispose of used patches appropriately. Used and unneeded patches should be disposed of by folding together the adhesive side of the patch and flushing the patch down the toilet.

Management of Breakthrough Pain

Breakthrough pain, or breakthrough cancer pain, is a temporary flare-up of moderate to severe pain that occurs even when the patient is taking around-the-clock (ATC) medication for persistent pain and has had well-controlled background pain. As many as 75% of patients with cancer experience breakthrough pain, with the frequency higher in late- and end-stage cancer (PDQ® Supportive and Palliative Care Editorial Board, 2021). This pain is often not diagnosed correctly and is frequently undertreated. Breakthrough pain can be classified as incidental pain (e.g., pain caused by movement) or idiopathic (spontaneous pain due to an unknown cause) and should be differentiated from end-of-dose pain, which is when the pain occurs before the next dose of analgesic is due. Incident and idiopathic breakthrough pain is treated more effectively with supplemental doses of a short-acting opioid taken on a PRN basis, rather than with an increase in the dose of the ATC medication or shortening of the interval between doses, which typically is more effective with end-of-dose pain. Effective management of BTcP requires use of rapid-onset opioids administered via the oral, transmucosal, intranasal, or sublingual route (PDQ® Supportive and Palliative Care Editorial Board, 2021; FDA, 2020a).

Concern about Prescription Analgesic Abuse

More than 11.5 million people in the United States, ages 12 years and older, reported misusing opioids in 2016 (CDC, 2021b). A 2021 report from the U.S. Drug Enforcement Administration (DEA) noted that over 70% of the almost 71,000 drug overdose deaths in 2019 involved an opioid, with 72.9% of those deaths involving synthetic opioids other than methadone, typically fentanyl (CDC, 2021c). They identified controlled prescription drugs, heroin, illicit/synthetic fentanyl, cocaine, and methamphetamine as the most significant drug-related threats to the United States (DEA's Strategic Intelligence Section, 2021). Practitioners had responded to the need for improved pain relief by prescribing more opioids for patients. In some cases, the **diversion** (any act that results in a drug not reaching the person who was originally prescribed the controlled drug) and substance abuse that subsequently occurred was an unintended consequence. People who abuse opioids often capitalize on the well-intentioned desire of health care providers to sufficiently address pain. They visit multiple providers and request opioid prescriptions for high daily doses. This group is at high risk for a drug overdose, and some may even distribute drugs to others who are using them without a prescription (diversion). National guidelines and recommendations guide providers in the prescribing and dispensing of these high-risk medications. However, a multifaceted approach that involves collaboration between public health officials, law enforcement, educators, and community advocates is required to address this issue (DEA's Strategic Intelligence Section, 2021). One initiative is the creation of the Prescription Drug Monitoring Program (PDMP) database that allows prescribers to access prescription and dispensing data on prescription drugs for individual patients from multiple institutions within a geographic area. Although not mandatory, many states require the use of PDMPs prior to prescribing an opioid (The Joint Commission, 2017).

> **Concept Mastery Alert**
>
> A multifaceted approach to pain management and opioid abuse issues should involve the individual patient, public health officials, law enforcement, educators, and community advocates.

USING ACUTE PAIN MANAGEMENT TREATMENT REGIMENS

As a patient's advocate, ensure that a strong emphasis is placed on the need for aggressive, individualized strategies that can minimize or eliminate acute pain and promote positive patient outcomes. Preventing pain is easier than treating it once it has occurred. Discuss pain control options with patients before surgery and address the patient's responsibility regarding reporting pain. Additional nursing interventions that can eliminate acute postoperative pain include maintaining a steady serum level of the analgesic (PCA or epidural analgesia can help here), treating side effects quickly and aggressively, encouraging use of nonpharmacologic complementary therapies as adjuncts to the multimodal pharmacologic regimen, and identifying supports and resources for managing the biopsychosocial components of the pain experience.

Undertreatment of pain that accompanies procedures, whether performed in a hospital, home, or outpatient clinic, is a common occurrence. If there is any possibility of the patient experiencing more than mild pain or discomfort from a procedure, consider providing analgesia. In situations in which the patient is unable to report the presence of pain (e.g., an unconscious patient), it is important to consider pain relief if a procedure is planned that normally elicits a pain. This could include turning a patient or a dressing change. In some instances, if the patient is unable to communicate verbally but is capable of some response, it may be necessary to provide a method for the patient to indicate that pain is occurring during a procedure. The simple raising of a finger or hand or squeeze of a squeak toy can alert the caregiver that analgesia is needed.

EMPLOYING CANCER OR CHRONIC PAIN MANAGEMENT TREATMENT REGIMENS

People with cancer sometimes suffer needlessly from pain. The major principles that guide treatment for cancer or chronic pain include:

- Giving medications orally, if possible, for ease and convenience of administration
- Administering medication ATC rather than on a PRN basis
- Adjusting the dose to achieve maximum benefits with minimal side effects
- Allowing patients as much control as possible over their medication regimen

In an effort to alleviate unnecessary pain and suffering, the World Health Organization (WHO, 2019) supports a three-step analgesic ladder that outlines the appropriate

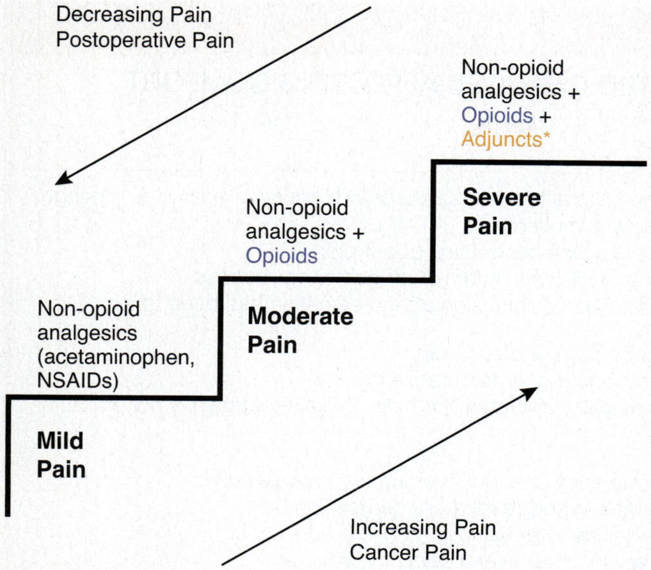

FIGURE 36-8. Various opioid (narcotic) and nonopioid medications may be combined with other medications. This adaptation of the WHO analgesic ladder for relieving cancer pain superimposes management of acute pain (indicated by arrows) on the original WHO stair-step model, which provides a visual representation of the basic differences between acute and chronic pain management. (*Source:* From Gai, N., Naser, B., Hanley, J., Peliowski, A., Hayes, J., & Aoyama, K. [2020]. A practical guide to acute pain management in children. *Journal of Anesthesia, 34*[3], 421–433. https://doi.org/10.1007/s00540-020-02767-x.)

progression of drugs and dosages that should be used to manage cancer-related pain effectively. Emphasis is on individualizing treatment and using the analgesic ladder to provide attentive, aggressive pain relief. The effectiveness of the WHO analgesic ladder is widely acknowledged; this regimen provides relief to 70% to 90% of patients with cancer pain. Movement through the analgesic ladder may not always progress through all steps in an orderly manner, depending on the intensity of the patient's pain. Some clinicians have suggested that the WHO three-step analgesic ladder may require some adjustment based on the clinical experience that has occurred in the 20 years since the ladder was proposed. A revised version (Fig. 36-8) superimposes management of acute pain (indicated by arrows) on the original WHO stair-step model, which provides a good visual representation of the basic differences between acute and chronic cancer pain management (Gai et al., 2020). The 10% to 30% of patients with severe pain who do not obtain satisfactory pain relief using this guideline may require alternative routes of drug administration, nerve blocks, or other invasive procedures to relieve their pain. The WHO ladder approach to pain management has also proved effective in treatment of patients with phantom limb pain and end-stage renal disease (Pasero & McCaffery, 2011).

PROVIDING PAIN TREATMENT IN SPECIAL POPULATIONS

Children and older adults need accurate assessment and treatment of pain. Their behavioral indicators of pain are unique, which necessitates special approaches to determine the presence and level of pain as well as individualized techniques to relieve the pain.

Children

Effective pain management in children requires careful assessment; good communication among patient, family, and caregivers; and a thorough understanding of the actions and side effects of drugs used to relieve pain. The child is still the best source of information about the pain; various assessment tools mentioned previously help to measure the intensity of the pain.

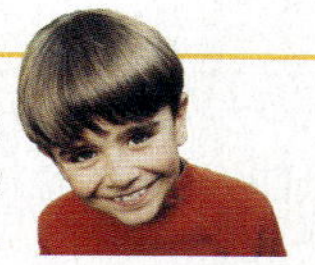

Think back to **Xavier Malton**, the child with ulcerative colitis in acute pain. The nurse needs to assess Xavier continually for effectiveness of the prescribed analgesic and request changes in any orders if the analgesic is not effective. Considering Xavier's current state, suggesting that the health care provider change the analgesic administration from PRN dosing to around-the-clock dosing may be appropriate for a short period of time.

In postoperative situations, children need analgesics ATC or by continuous infusion. Opioids are the drug of choice for moderate to severe pain, but intentional dispensing, identified disposal procedures, and proactive prescriptions for naloxone are essential, especially with adolescents who are particularly vulnerable to diversion and OUD (Yaster et al., 2020; WHO, 2021). Pain management for cancer pain or chronic pain in children follows the guidance outlined in the WHO analgesic ladder and requires a biopsychosocial, interprofessional, multimodal approach (WHO, 2021). Withholding opioid drugs from children with cancer because of fear of addiction is unjustified because current knowledge does not indicate that they are vulnerable to this problem.

Children also require pain management to minimize or alleviate the pain and distress associated with some procedures. The misconception persists that children experience pain differently. It is important to understand that if a procedure is painful for an adult, it is also painful for a child. Adequate education before the procedure and using drug and nondrug therapies to complement each other can take the pain and fear out of the experience. This is especially important for children with a chronic disease who must undergo multiple procedures as part of the treatment regimen.

Older Adults

Research on pain management in older adults has focused on pain associated with chronic illness and acute postoperative pain. Up to 50% of older adults who live in the community report that pain impacts on their normal daily function, and at least half of older adults who reside in a long-term care facility report having pain on a daily basis (Galicia-Castillo & Weiner, 2021). Pain management in this population needs to involve strategies used for all adults, including biopsychosocial considerations, multimodal pharmacologic interventions, and nonpharmacologic strategies but must also consider polypharmacy, pharmacokinetics, and pharmacodynamics. Physical therapy, exercise, and rehabilitation often provide strength, stability, and stamina training that

Focus on the Older Adult

NURSING STRATEGIES TO ADDRESS AGE-RELATED CHANGES AFFECTING COMFORT

Age-Related Changes	Nursing Strategies
Communication Difficulties	• Observe carefully for any behavioral manifestations or indications of pain (e.g., change in activity level or grimacing with movement). • Use open-ended questions to solicit information about pain. • Include family or caregiver to assist with information-gathering process. • Monitor for any behavior changes or confusion after medication has been taken.
Denial of Pain	• Clarify terms used to describe pain or discomfort. • Emphasize importance of reporting pain to caregivers. • Express concern about pain and a willingness to help. Explain that pain is not a normal consequence of aging.
Altered Physiologic Response to Analgesics	• Be aware of dosage and frequency to avoid oversedation and toxicity. • Monitor carefully for oversedation and respiratory depression. • Explain side effects of analgesics to patient. • Use memory aid if necessary to avoid overdosing. • Discourage self-medication of OTC medications. • Caution about use of alcohol with analgesics. • Caution about driving or operating machinery when taking analgesics.

can mitigate pain and improve function (Pickering et al., 2018; Schwan et al., 2019). Recommendations for analgesic administration for older adults include the following (Ali et al., 2018; Galicia-Castillo & Weiner, 2021):

- Use acetaminophen for older adults with mild to moderate pain.
- Use NSAIDs (oral or topical) when other treatments have failed; use for the shortest period of time possible.
- Progress to opioids for severe pain when other treatments have been unsuccessful and the pain is impacting on quality of life and functional issues; consider risk versus benefits.
- Consider adjuvants that address depression and neuropathic pain.
- Consider the use of legal cannabis and cannabinoids while considering the potential dysphoric effects.

Opioid drugs can be used safely for older adult patients as long as appropriate precautions are taken, pain is conscientiously assessed, and potential side effects are monitored. A general rule when administering pain medications to older adults is *start low and go slow*. Adjust dosage and dosing intervals for the older adult based on therapeutic response to the drug and the presence of adverse effects. The accompanying Focus on the Older Adult box describes additional strategies pertinent to this age group.

ADMINISTERING ANALGESICS BY OTHER METHODS

In addition to the variety of drugs used to treat pain, multiple options exist for drug delivery systems. PCA, epidural analgesia, and other advanced interventions have improved pain management and the quality of life for many people.

Patient-Controlled Analgesia

PCA provides effective individualized analgesia and comfort (Fig. 36-9). This method of analgesia therapy may be used to manage acute and chronic pain in a health care facility or the home. It is used less frequently with cancer pain, for which oral medication is the preferred route. This device is most commonly used to deliver analgesics intravenously, subcutaneously, or via the epidural route. The most frequently prescribed drugs for PCA administration are morphine, fentanyl, and hydromorphone.

The PCA system consists of a computerized, portable infusion pump containing a chamber for a syringe that is prefilled with the prescribed opioid analgesic. Both The Joint Commission and the Institute for Safe Medication Practices (ISMP) recommend standard doses and concentrations prepared in prefilled syringes. Initially, a loading dose is administered to raise blood levels to a therapeutic level and control the pain. Although a PCA pump can be set to deliver at a set rate (automatic dose or basal rate), these pumps are more typically used to deliver a dose when initiated by the patient, especially

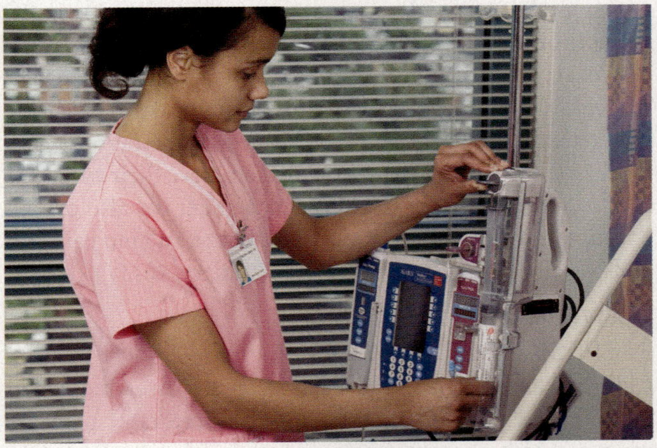

FIGURE 36-9. A patient-controlled analgesia unit allows the patient to regulate the intravenous infusion of small amounts of analgesic as needed.

in patients who are opioid-naïve (Gai et al., 2020; Polomano et al., 2017). When the sensation of pain reoccurs, the patient pushes a button that activates the PCA device to deliver a small preset bolus dose of the analgesic. A dose interval that is programmed into the PCA unit (usually 6 to 8 minutes) prevents reactivation of the pump and administration of another dose during that period of time. The pump mechanism can also be programmed to deliver only a specified amount of analgesic within a given time interval (the lock-out interval). These safeguards limit the possibility of possible overmedication. In addition, the preprogrammed intervals provide time for the patient to evaluate the effect of the previous dose. PCA pumps also have a locked safety system that prohibits any tampering with the device (Karch, 2020; Pasero & McCaffery, 2011). The goal with hospitalized patients who are using a PCA for acute pain management is to transition to an oral regimen prior to discharge. Adults and children weaning off a PCA to an oral opioid regimen may benefit from a hybrid PCA-oral administration model (Gai et al., 2020).

The proper selection of patients for PCA is vital for a positive experience. Suitable candidates for this type of delivery system include people who are alert and capable of controlling the unit. The Joint Commission and ISMP both identify people who are not recommended for this type of pain relief. These include confused older adults, infants and very young children, cognitively impaired patients, patients with conditions for which oversedation poses a significant health risk (e.g., asthma and sleep apnea), and patients who are taking other medications that potentiate opioids. PCA has proven safe for use in children as young as 4 years of age who do not have developmental delays (Pasero & McCaffery, 2011).

PCA has many advantages:

- Consistent analgesic blood level is maintained rather than the inconsistent analgesia obtained with periodic injections, which prevents in sharp rises and falls of serum opioid levels.
- The analgesic is delivered intravenously or epidurally so that absorption is faster and more predictable than with the intramuscular route.
- The patient is in charge of the pain management program.
- The patient is able to ambulate earlier, which causes fewer pulmonary complications.
- The patient is more satisfied and has improved pain relief.

PCA by proxy, which means that someone other than the patient activates the pump, continues to be a controversial issue. Unauthorized family members or caregivers (instead of the patient) who administer PCA by pushing the dosage button can cause serious analgesic overdoses resulting in oversedation, respiratory depression, and death. Some clinicians argue that in a pediatric or critical care setting (Benjenk et al., 2020), nurse-controlled analgesia or caregiver-controlled analgesia is appropriate. For this to be safe, rigid facility protocols need to be in place. The Joint Commission issued a sentinel event alert on PCA and does not recommend PCA by proxy; the ISMP (2016) recently reiterated a similar position based on their original recommendations from 1996. Institutions must verify that they have protocols in place to protect against unauthorized PCA delivery. It is also recommended that clear warning labels stating, "WARNING: BUTTON TO BE PRESSED ONLY BY THE PATIENT" be attached to PCA pumps (ISMP). Refer to Chapter 28 for a discussion of sentinel event alerts. The Joint Commission and ISMP also advise that health care providers need to carefully monitor patients for respiratory depression using pulse oximetry and capnography (measurement of carbon dioxide concentrations) as appropriate. The carbon dioxide level in a patient's expirations can be measured by a sensor contained in a mask or nasal cannula that the patient is wearing. This provides a more reliable measure of impending respiratory depression.

Setting up the PCA system and ensuring that it is functioning properly are nursing responsibilities. Improper programming of the pump is the most common human error associated with this therapy. Both The Joint Commission and the ISMP recommend that a second nurse checks the patient ID, drug dose and concentration, PCA pump settings, the infusion tubing, and site prior to the initiation of PCA. The ISMP (2020) identified targeted medication safety best practices that include ensuring appropriate antidotes, reversal agents, and rescue agents are readily available, and verifying that associated protocols and directions for use/administration permit emergency administration of these agents.

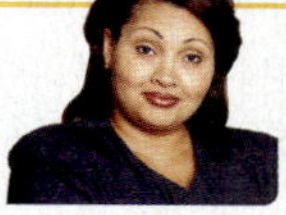

Recall **Sheree Lincoln**, the postoperative patient who is to use the PCA system for pain control. Two hours after surgery, the patient reports pain but has not used the PCA system. The nurse would need to determine the underlying reasons for not using the device. This assessment would include investigation of Sheree's knowledge base and what, if any, teaching she received preoperatively. For example, Sheree may have received teaching on how to use PCA but may not have understood when or why to use it. Possibly she may want to avoid use of any medication. The nurse would use this opportunity to reinforce instructions for using PCA, and also for other nonpharmacologic measures for pain relief such as distraction, relaxation, massage, or imagery.

There are now several manufacturers of oral PCA devices that allow hospitalized patients to self-administer oral doses of opioid analgesics. These systems utilize a wireless device that grants single-patient access to a prescribed medication. Use of these devices results in a significant reduction in administration time and significantly lower reported pain scores (Collins et al., 2020; Pizzi et al., 2020; Wirz et al., 2021).

Opioid analgesia via a continuous subcutaneous infusion is a safe, effective alternative when IV access is not available and oral analgesia is no longer possible. Candidates for subcutaneous infusion are often patients requiring hospice and palliative care. Equipment consists of a small-gauge needle inserted subcutaneously, an infusion pump, and an administration set that is clearly labeled *subcutaneous infusion*. This setup delivers the opioid in a small amount of fluid (typically

2 to 3 mL/hr). Nurses can initiate subcutaneous infusion therapy once competence has been validated. Assessment includes monitoring of vital signs, pain level, and the insertion site for leakage, bleeding, or other complications (Gorski et al., 2021).

Epidural Analgesia and Peripheral Nerve Blocks

Epidural analgesia can be used to provide pain relief during the immediate postoperative phase (particularly after thoracic, abdominal, orthopedic, and vascular surgery) and for chronic pain situations. Epidural pain management is also being used for children with terminal cancer and for children undergoing hip, abdominal, spinal, or lower extremity surgery (Gai et al., 2020). Absolute contraindications include an allergic response to analgesics being used, coagulation disorders, anticoagulants, and localized infection or sepsis; relative contraindications include hypotension or compromised cardiovascular system, increased intracranial pressure, spinal abnormalities, and certain neurologic conditions. The patient must agree to the analgesia and the intraprofessional team must be competent in the administration and management of epidural analgesia (Galligan, 2020). The anesthesiologist usually inserts the catheter in the midlumbar region into the epidural space between the walls of the vertebral canal and the dura mater or outermost connective tissue membrane surrounding the spinal cord. For temporary therapy, the catheter exits directly over the spine, and the tubing is positioned over the patient's shoulder, with the end of the catheter taped to the person's chest. For long-term therapy, the catheter is usually tunneled subcutaneously and exits on the side of the body or on the abdomen (Fig. 36-10).

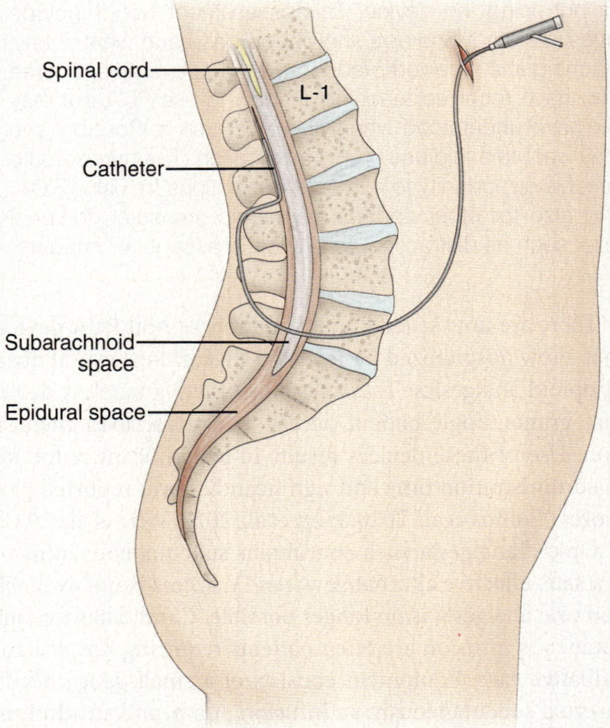

FIGURE 36-10. Placement of an epidural catheter for long-term use.

Typically, the opioid is combined with a local anesthetic (bupivacaine, levobupivicain, or ropivacaine). This combination improves pain management, and pain relief is achieved with smaller doses and less severe side effects (Galligan, 2020). The epidural analgesia can be administered as a bolus dose (either one time or intermittent) via a continuous infusion pump or by means of a patient-controlled epidural analgesia (PCEA) pump (Polomano et al., 2017; Wong & Lim, 2018). Because the epidural space contains blood vessels, nerves, and fat, lipid-soluble fentanyl is readily dissolved and has a rapid onset of action (5 minutes) but a short duration of action (approximately 2 hours). Hydromorphone has a 15- to 30-minute onset and a duration of action of up to 12 hours. Morphine has a slower onset of action (20 minutes) but may exert its analgesic effect for as long as 24 hours because it remains longer in the cerebrospinal fluid (CSF) and spinal tissue (Burchum & Rosenthal, 2019). Epidural catheters used for the management of acute pain are typically removed within 5 days of surgery, when oral medication can be substituted for relief of pain (Gai et al., 2020; Galligan, 2020).

Nursing responsibilities vary among institutions but must include careful monitoring and documentation of vital signs, laboratory values, pain intensity, motor and sensory block/function, the insert site and dressing, the delivery system, urinary output, and side effects related to surgery and opioid use (Gai et al., 2020; Galligan, 2020). See Guidelines for Nursing Care 36-1.

Peripheral nerve blocks produce a temporary loss of sensation and motor and autonomic function in a localized area. The local anesthetics work by chemically blocking the nerve pathways involved in pain sensation and response and are sometimes called *nerve blocks*. Many people have experienced nerve blocks during dental work, when having a wound sutured, during delivery of a newborn, or for some minor surgical procedures. Nursing measures include noting any allergic responses the patient has had in the past to anesthetic agents, alerting the patient to the pain associated with the initial injection of the anesthetic or numbing agent, offering emotional support to the patient during the procedure, observing for any untoward effects, and protecting the patient from injury until sensory and motor functions return.

Topical Anesthesia

Anesthetic agents may be applied topically to the skin or mucous membranes. Two topical anesthetic creams (EMLA, which contains 2.5% lidocaine and 2.5% prilocaine, and LMX-4, formerly ELA-Max, a 4% lidocaine cream) provide safe, effective analgesia for children before painful procedures such as phlebotomy, lumbar puncture, or bone marrow aspiration. EMLA cream is prescribed by the health care provider and must be covered by an occlusive dressing for at least 1 hour before the procedure to provide local pain relief. After the time period, the cream is removed. LMX-4 is an OTC preparation that takes effect in 30 minutes or less (Hsu et al., 2020).

Guidelines for Nursing Care 36-1

CARING FOR PATIENTS RECEIVING EPIDURAL OPIOIDS

Nursing Action	*Rationale*
Verify the health care provider's prescription for analgesia, drug preparation, and rate of infusion with another RN.	Verification provides for safe administration of the correct dose at the correct rate.
Keep an ampule of 0.4 mg of naloxone available on the unit.	Naloxone reverses the respiratory depressant effect of opioids.
Use epidural tubing. Label solution, tubing, and pump apparatus "For Epidural Infusion Only."	Labeling prevents inadvertent administration of other intravenous medications through this setup.
Assess and record sedation level (using a sedation scale) and respiratory status, including pulse oximetry continually for the first 20 minutes, at least q1h for the first 12 hours, every 2 hours up to 24 hours followed by q4h intervals until the epidural infusion is discontinued (or according to facility policy). Notify provider for the following: sedation rating of 3, ↓ in depth and respiratory rate below 8 breaths/min.	Opioids can depress respiratory center in the medulla. Change in level of consciousness is usually the first sign of altered respiratory function.
Keep head of bed elevated 30 degrees unless this is contraindicated.	Elevation of the patient's head minimizes upward migration of opioid in the spinal cord, thus decreasing risk for respiratory depression.
Record level of pain and effectiveness of pain relief.	Referencing helps in determining need for subsequent *breakthrough* pain medication.
Monitor urinary output and assess for bladder distention.	Opioids can cause urinary retention.
Assess movement and motor strength of lower extremities q4h.	Catheter may migrate into the intrathecal space and allow opioids to block transmission of nerve impulses completely through the spinal cord to the brain.
Monitor for side effects (pruritus, nausea, vomiting).	Opioids may spread into the trigeminal nerve, causing itching or resulting in nausea and vomiting due to slowed gastrointestinal function or stimulation of a chemoreceptor trigger zone in the brain. Medications are available to treat these side effects.
Assess for signs of infection, hematoma, or abscess at the insertion site.	Inflammation or local infection may develop at the catheter insertion site. Strict aseptic technique and sterile dressing and tubing changes according to facility policy can prevent infection. Monitor the site for bleeding.
Do not administer any other narcotics or adjuvant drugs without approval of clinician responsible for epidural management.	Additional medication may potentiate the action of the opioid, increasing the risk for respiratory depression.

Technology Alert

One system, ON-Q Pain Relief System, involves administration of local anesthetic medication directly at the affected surgical site. The benefit of this temporary system is earlier mobility and effective pain relief, with fewer side effects because of decreased opioid use postoperatively (Cinar et al., 2021; Porter et al., 2021).

Teaching the Patient and Family/Caregivers About Pain

Often, a well-informed person can cope better with the distress of pain and tends to experience less anxiety about pain. See the Promoting Health Literacy box (on page 1374) for suggestions regarding communicating with your health care provider to facilitate effective pain management.

Teaching about pain should include family members or caregivers so that they understand the concept of pain and are able to help the person in pain. The patient and anyone the patient identifies need information about the nature and causes of pain, explanation about a pain scale that can be used easily, practice with this assessment tool, and assistance to set goals for comfort and either optimal function or recovery. Encourage caregivers to be creative and specifically attuned to children's varied responses to pain. Play may be used effectively to discover a child's experience of pain

Promoting Health Literacy

IN PATIENTS WITH PAIN

Patient Scenario

Jennifer Tyler, 44, has had several visits to her primary provider about her pain. She told the office nurse that she "doesn't know how much more of this I can take." Her history reveals that she has had an "aching pain, literally all over my body" for the last 3 months. Jennifer states, "It's taking over my life now. Everything I do hurts, and to make matters worse, I don't sleep well at night, and I can't even think straight." Specific symptoms she reported include fatigue, occasional muscle spasms and pain in her legs, aching in her right shoulder, constant lower back pain, headaches that are occurring on a more frequent basis, and general anxiety about her health. Jennifer reports that initially she tried "Advil® off and on" with some mild relief and even admits taking some "old muscle relaxants" that her husband had from a back injury. Despite the antidepressants and sleeping pills that were prescribed for her, she has not been able to get much in the way of pain relief. After their initial examination, her provider has ordered a variety of laboratory studies to try and determine exactly what is causing Ms. Tyler's pain. At this visit, they told Ms. Tyler that they suspect fibromyalgia may be the cause of her pain and other symptoms. They prescribe pregabalin (Lyrica®) and want to see her again in 3 weeks to see how this medication is working for her. As she is making the next appointment, Jennifer tells the nurse, "I sure hope this new medicine works. I'm running out of hope here. What kind of a life is this?"

Nursing Considerations: *Tips for Improving Health Literacy*

Provide Ms. Tyler with printed literature about fibromyalgia. Explain that this disease is difficult to diagnose and that pregabalin (Lyrica®) was the first drug approved by the FDA to treat fibromyalgia. Tell Ms. Tyler that the provider may adjust her dose depending on how she tolerates the medicine and what kind of results she is getting from the drug. Caution her that dizziness and blurred vision may occur as side effects. Tell her if she has any signs of an allergic reaction, she should immediately stop taking the medication and report this to the health care provider. Inform her that she should avoid alcohol consumption while taking pregabalin and not drive if she experiences any dizziness or blurred vision. Explain to her that the provider may prescribe physical or occupational therapy for rehabilitation as she begins to rebuild her strength and stamina. Provide Ms. Tyler online resources, links, or apps to track her symptoms, locate a support group, and review other resources to increase the likelihood that Ms. Tyler is accessing appropriate, verified information on the internet. Encourage Ms. Tyler when she returns for her next visit to be prepared to ask her health care provider the following questions:

- What is my main problem?
- What do I need to do?
- Why is it important for me to do this?
- What can you do if this new medication is not working?
- What else can you or I do to treat my pain?

What additional measures can you take to help maintain health literacy in this patient? What other measures would be helpful if Ms. Tyler did not speak English, could not read, did not have access to electronic resources, or had a learning disability?

and to teach the child how to cope with pain. Children are usually receptive to using dolls to act out pain experiences. Teaching Tips 36-1 includes specific suggestions related to safety concerns about pain control in the home setting. In addition, provide the patient and caregivers with information about available resources, including reputable online sources for pain control and treatment, and encourage them to use them.

Teaching Tips 36-1

COMFORT

Health Topic	Teaching Tip	Why Is This Important?
Safety	Do not drive vehicle or operate heavy machinery after taking opioids or other medications that cause drowsiness.	Reflexes may be slowed and cognitive thinking decreased due to opioids and other medications.
	Avoid alcohol and other CNS depressants while taking pain medication.	Alcohol may interact with the pain medication and further depress the CNS, leading to respiratory failure.
	Do not smoke without someone else present while taking pain medication.	The patient may become tired due to the medication, fall asleep while smoking, and start a house fire.
	Get assistance with walking and other ADLs as needed	Some pain medications can cause drowsiness, dizziness, and blurred vision.
	Keep a record or pain diary of level of pain, medication taken, and effect of medication.	Provides more accurate documentation of pain experience, allows for appropriate prescribing, and prevents overdoses.
Diet	Do not take pain medication on an empty stomach.	Many patients become nauseated if pain medication is taken on an empty stomach.
Miscellaneous	Do not breastfeed without checking with your health care provider while taking pain medication.	Many pain medications can be found in breast milk and may harm the baby.

Ensuring the Ethical and Legal Responsibility to Relieve Pain

Quality pain management results when patients have access to safe, effective, evidenced-based, multimodal pain relief measures. Health care providers, in addition to monitoring, delivering, and documenting administration of analgesics, have a responsibility to inform patients that effective pain management is vital to their treatment. Patients also have the right to expect that their statements of pain will be heeded. Institutions must assign and educate clinicians to address these issues in a timely, knowledgeable manner. The rights of patients with pain recognize the multidimensional aspects of the pain experience and a person's right to have pain management strategies implemented in conjunction with the health care team. Keep in mind that our treatment of pain is evolving, especially our use of opioids and management of OUD. See Box 36-3 for information on the HEAL initiative. The interprofessional team provides ongoing clinical consultation, support, and education, while engaging the patient in discussions regarding pain management goals, interventions, and reasonable outcomes.

Legal Alert

Patients have the right to be treated with dignity and to be involved in developing their pain management plan of care.

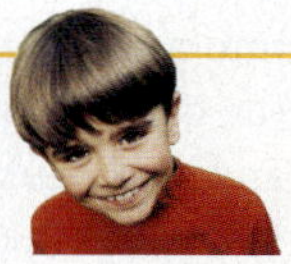

Consider **Xavier Malton**, the child with acute pain. The nurses in the scenario advocated for Xavier, reinforcing his rights to have pain controlled as soon as possible.

Pain assessment and management is complex and prevention, mitigating, and treatment strategies are ever-evolving. To meet the specific needs of patients and the populations nurses serve, health care facilities have committed to a focus on best practices and improved patient outcomes by supporting the use of clinical experts. The Pain Resource Nurse (PRN) has an expressed interest in pain management, is an effective interprofessional/intraprofessional communicator, and acts as a coach or mentor for colleagues. The PRN role, which has been around since the 1990s, requires specific training and is often filled by a staff nurse involved with direct patient care. Goals of these PRN programs include: (1) demonstrating pain management as an institutional priority; (2) increasing staff knowledge of pain and serving as a peer resource; (3) driving evidence-based pain management education that is reflected in protocols, policies, and procedures; (4) translating best practices into daily clinical practice, supported by sustainable program improvement processes; and (5) delivering safe, quality patient care (Allen et al., 2018; Crawford et al., 2016).

Box 36-3 National Institutes of Health (NIH) Helping to End Addiction Long-Term (HEAL) Initiative℠

The NIH HEAL Initiative℠ is an aggressive, transagency effort to fund and support projects nationwide to address the opioid epidemic. It focuses on:

1. Enhancing pain management strategies rooted in preclinical, clinical, and translational research—designed to foster better understanding, treatment, and management of pain
2. Improving treatments for opioid use disorder (OUD) and addiction through research that will help prevent OUD and provide evidence-based, holistic, treatment of OUD (and overdose) that can be replicated in myriad settings

Source: U.S. Department of Health and Human Services-National Institutes of Health. *NIH HEAL Initiative℠*. Retrieved February 18, 2022, from https://heal.nih.gov/

Understanding the Placebo Controversy

The term placebo comes from the Latin word meaning "I shall please." A **placebo** is any sham medication or procedure that is designed and known to not be of any therapeutic clinical value. The person receiving the placebo treatment, unaware of the placebo's properties, may find it to be effective for the relief of pain because of the perception that it will provide comfort and because of belief in the person administering it. This is referred to as the *placebo effect*. Many of the nonpharmacologic and multimodal pharmacologic strategies described in this chapter relied upon a sham intervention or placebo to test their efficacy. Various researchers have reported that a positive placebo effect may be related to a physiologic response (release of endorphins) or the patient's cultural expectations, attitudes, health beliefs, or anticipation of a positive response. Use of a placebo also has the potential to cause a harmful or undesirable response referred to as a *nocebo*. This negative outcome may involve mild discomforts such as nausea and pruritus or life-threatening complications.

The use of placebos outside of IRB-approved clinical trials, raises serious ethical questions. Is lying to a patient ever justifiable? A nurse who administers a hidden placebo must be willing to risk the possible consequence of the patient becoming aware of the duplicity and then refusing to trust the nurse or any other health care professional again. Patients who feel themselves to be in pain are vulnerable. If such patients discover a seeming plot to trick them into feeling better, it is unlikely that those patients will respect or appreciate the intentions of the physicians and nurses involved. The long-term negative effects of this practice far outweigh any of its benefits. Multiple facilities and professional organizations directly oppose placebo use outside of clinical trials, including the Oncology Nursing Society, the American Nurses Association, the American Society of Pain Management Nurses, and the American Pain Society (Arnstein et al., 2011). The nurse has firm legal and ethical grounds for refusing to administer a placebo to a patient who is not aware that receiving a placebo is possible.

Evaluating

As soon as a pain problem is identified and a treatment plan developed and implemented, evaluation becomes ongoing. Evaluation is directed toward the changing nature of the pain experience, the treatment modalities (pain management program), and the patient's and family's or caregiver's response(s) to the care plan, all of which overlap.

Experience of Evolving Pain

The pain the patient is experiencing may change in many ways, thus the nurse must be careful not to make a judgment about this too quickly. For example, if the pain lessens in intensity or disappears, it may mean that the underlying cause of the pain is diminished or absent and that treatment should be stopped, or it may mean that the pain management program is effective and should be continued. When pain intensity increases, it may simply indicate the need for more aggressive therapy, or it may be a warning that the underlying pathology has changed or worsened, and that new medical intervention is required. Often, a new problem amenable to treatment is masked by old or underlying pain, and its detection may be delayed to the point that treatment is useless.

Management Regimens

The use of both multimodal pharmacologic and nonpharmacologic therapies must be continually evaluated to determine whether they are the best possible means the patient could use to obtain pain relief, and whether they are effective with only minimal risk to the patient. Too often, a patient stays with the first analgesic prescribed without questioning whether it is the most effective drug for the particular pain, whether the dosage and timing guidelines are correct for the patient, and whether the analgesic is producing annoying or even harmful side effects that another drug would not produce. Patient and public safety are the priority when establishing and maintaining a pain management regimen.

Similarly, one patient may take to progressive relaxation exercises and find them helpful, whereas another patient may obtain similar benefits from a daily walking program. Nursing time spent evaluating the effectiveness of each pain relief therapy is well spent and results in a pain management program that is truly individualized for the patient.

Patient and Family Response

Ultimately, the plan of care is unsuccessful unless the patient and family (as defined by the patient) are satisfied with the results. But keep in mind that the elimination of pain is not always a reasonable goal. The interprofessional health care team needs to work directly with the patient and family to set and then evaluate reasonable, individualized goals for pain management. A successful plan of care results in the achievement of specified patient outcomes valued by the patient.

REFLECTIVE PRACTICE LEADING TO PERSONAL LEARNING

Remember that the object of reflective practice is to look at an experience, understand it, and learn from it. As you begin to develop your expertise in evaluating the care plan, reflect on your experiences—successes and failures—in order to improve your practice. How can you do it better next time? What did you learn today that can help you tomorrow? Begin your reflection by paying close attention to the following:

- How consistently do you personally incorporate pain assessment into your daily care? How have you worked to develop skills related to this assessment? How do you integrate your objective assessment with the subjective pain report from the patient?
- What value do you attach to involving the patient in establishing a pain management regimen? Which multimodal pharmacologic and nonpharmacologic interventions do you feel comfortable explaining and integrating into a recommended regimen? How do you individualize the care for patients when so many guidelines, policies, and procedures dictate your care?
- How does the public health issue of opioid abuse impact on your practice? How do you engage in pain management interventions while ensuring safety for your patient and the public?

Keeping up with the latest evidence-based practice guidelines can be challenging. Complex, multimodal pharmacologic regimens, a measured emphasis on nonpharmacologic interventions, the nature of pain as an individual experience, and national concerns and guidelines all impact on the nurse's ability to assist the patient in pain management. Balancing the needs of your individual patient with these responsibilities requires mindfulness and intentionality.

Perhaps the most important questions to reflect on are: Are your patients and their families/caregivers better for having had *you* share in the critical responsibility of partnering with them to ensure appropriate pain management practices? Are your patients now receiving thoughtful, person-centered, prioritized, holistic, evidence-based treatment and care because of your efforts?

Skill 36-1 Giving a Back Massage

DELEGATION CONSIDERATIONS

Providing a back massage may be delegated to assistive personnel (AP) as well as to licensed practical/vocational nurses (LPN/LVNs). The decision to delegate must be based on careful analysis of the patient's needs and circumstances as well as the qualifications of the person to whom the task is being delegated. Refer to the Delegation Guidelines in Appendix A.

EQUIPMENT

- Pain assessment tool and pain scale
- Lotion or oil, to which the patient has no allergy or aversion (Westman & Blaisdell, 2016)
- Bath blanket
- Towel
- Nonsterile gloves, if indicated
- Additional PPE, as indicated

IMPLEMENTATION

ACTION	RATIONALE
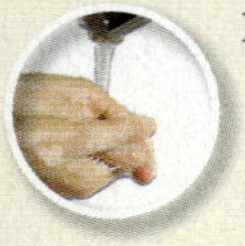 1. Perform hand hygiene and put on PPE, if indicated.	Hand hygiene and PPE prevent the spread of microorganisms. PPE is required based on transmission precautions.
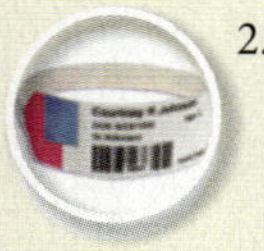 2. Identify the patient.	Identifying the patient ensures the right patient receives the intervention and helps prevent errors.
3. Offer a back massage to the patient and explain the procedure.	Explanation encourages patient understanding and engagement and reduces apprehension.
4. Put on gloves, if indicated.	Gloves are not usually necessary. Gloves prevent contact with blood and body fluid.
5. Close the room door and/or the curtain around the bed. Turn down the lights, if possible, and adjust the room temperature for patient comfort (Westman & Blaisdell, 2016).	Closing the door or curtain provides privacy, promotes relaxation, and reduces noise and stimuli that may aggravate pain and reduce comfort (Aparício & Panin, 2020; Goeren et al., 2018). Lowering the lights, reducing noise, and adjusting the temperature of the room create a calming environment (Westman & Blaisdell, 2016).
6. Assess the patient's pain using an appropriate assessment tool and measurement scale. Ask the patient if they have any aversion to touch (Westman & Blaisdell, 2016).	Accurate assessment is necessary to guide treatment and pain relief interventions and to evaluate the effectiveness of pain control measures. Patients with posttraumatic stress disorder or previous negative experience with massage may not want to receive massage (Westman & Blaisdell, 2016).
7. Raise the bed to a comfortable working position (VHA Center for Engineering & Occupational Safety and Health [CEOSH], 2016), and lower the side rail.	Having the bed at the proper height prevents back and muscle strain.
8. Assist the patient to a comfortable position, preferably the prone or side-lying position. Remove the covers and move the patient's gown just enough to expose the patient's back from the shoulders to sacral area. Drape the patient, as needed, with the bath blanket.	This position exposes an adequate area for massage. Draping the patient provides privacy and warmth.
9. Warm the lubricant or lotion in the palm of your hand, or place the container in small basin of warm water. During the massage, observe the patient's skin for reddened areas or injury. **Avoid areas of injury, such as wounds, burns, and pressure ulcers and areas with rashes, tubes, and IV access/lines** (Westman & Blaisdell, 2016). See Chapter 33 for detailed information regarding skin assessment.	Cold lotion causes chilling and discomfort. Massage of these areas could result in further injury and is contraindicated (Westman & Blaisdell, 2016).

(continued on page 1378)

Skill 36-1 Giving a Back Massage *(continued)*

ACTION	RATIONALE
10. Using light, gliding strokes (*effleurage*), apply lotion to patient's shoulders, back, and sacral area (Figure 1).	Effleurage relaxes the patient and lessens tension.
11. Place your hands beside each other at the base of the patient's spine and stroke upward to the shoulders and back downward to the buttocks in slow, continuous strokes (Figure 2). Continue for several minutes.	Continuous contact is soothing and stimulates circulation and muscle relaxation.
12. Massage the patient's shoulders, entire back, areas over iliac crests, and sacrum with circular, stroking motions, keeping hands in contact with the patient's skin. Continue for several minutes, applying additional lotion, as necessary.	A firm stroke with continuous contact promotes relaxation.
13. Knead the patient's back by gently alternating grasping and compression motions (*pétrissage*) (Figure 3).	Kneading increases blood circulation.
14. Complete the massage with additional long, stroking movements that eventually become lighter in pressure (Figure 4).	Long, stroking motions are soothing and promote relaxation; continued stroking with gradual lightening of pressure helps extend the feeling of relaxation.

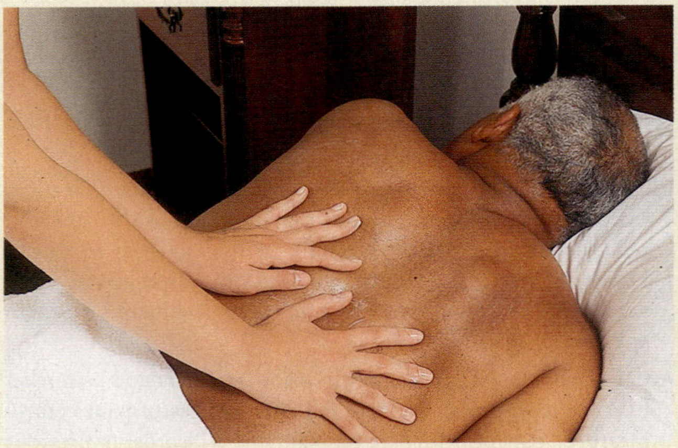

FIGURE 1. Using light, gliding strokes to apply lotion.

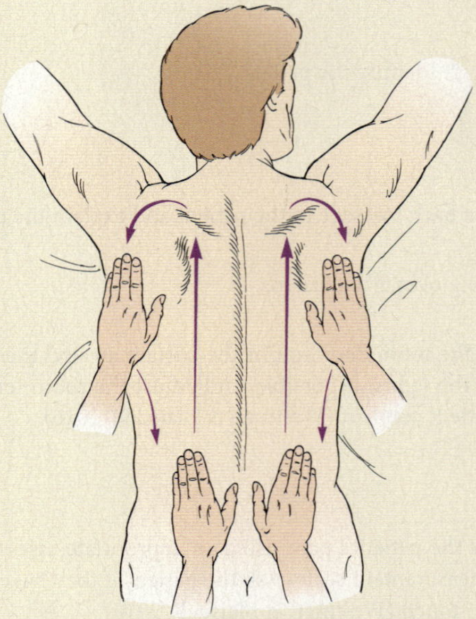

FIGURE 2. Stroking upward to shoulders and back downward to the buttocks.

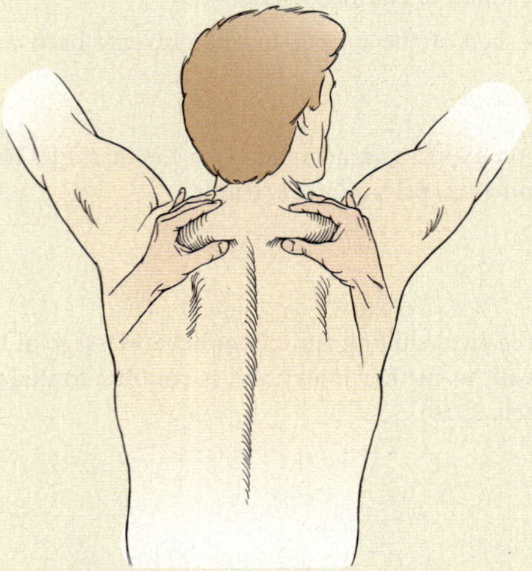

FIGURE 3. Kneading the patient's back.

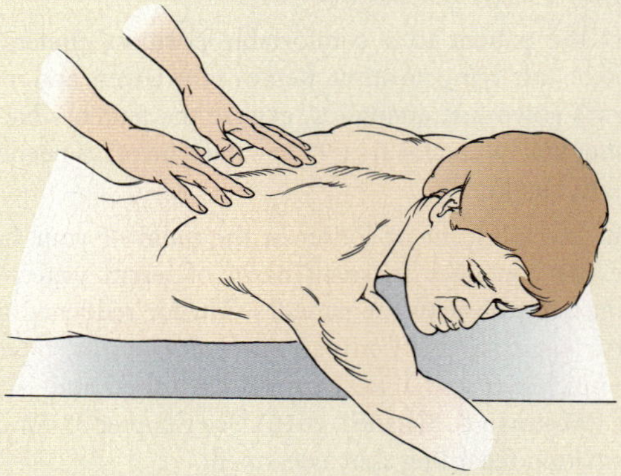

FIGURE 4. Using long strokes with lessening pressure.

ACTION	RATIONALE
15. If excess lotion remains, use the towel to pat the patient dry.	Drying provides comfort and reduces the feeling of moisture on the back.
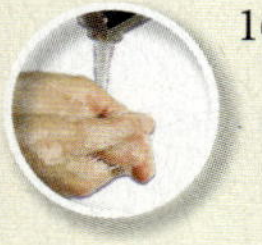 16. Remove gloves, if worn, and perform hand hygiene. Reposition patient's gown and covers. Raise side rail and lower bed. Assist patient to a position of comfort.	Removal of gloves and hand hygiene prevent transmission of microorganisms. Repositioning bedclothes, linens, and the patient helps to promote patient comfort and safety.
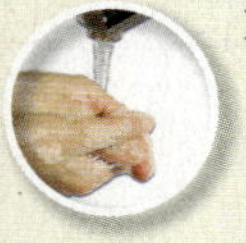 17. Remove additional PPE, if used. Perform hand hygiene.	Proper removal of PPE reduces the risk for infection transmission and contamination of other items. Hand hygiene prevents transmission of microorganisms.
18. Evaluate the patient's response to this intervention. Reassess level of discomfort or pain using original assessment tools. Reassess and alter care plan, as appropriate.	Reassessment allows for individualization of the patient's plan of care and promotes optimal patient comfort.

DOCUMENTATION

Guidelines

Document pain assessment and other significant assessments. Document massage use, length of time of massage, and patient response.

Sample Documentation

12/6/25 2330 Patient reports inability to sleep and increased pain at surgical site, rated 3/10. Medicated with acetaminophen 650 mg, as prescribed. Back massage administered ×10 minutes. Skin intact without redness. Patient reports increased comfort and relaxation; "I feel like I can sleep now."

—B. Black, RN

12/6/25 2400 Patient reports pain level 0/10.

—B. Black, RN

DEVELOPING CLINICAL REASONING AND CLINICAL JUDGMENT

UNEXPECTED SITUATIONS AND ASSOCIATED INTERVENTIONS

- *Patient cannot lie prone, so you are giving them a back massage while they are lying on their side. However, as you begin to massage the back, the patient cannot maintain the side-lying position:* If possible, have the patient hold on to the side rail on the side to which they are facing. If this is not possible or the patient cannot assist, use pillows and bath blankets to prevent the patient from rolling. If necessary, enlist the help of another person to maintain the patient's position. If possible, experiment with other positions based on the patient's condition and comfort, such as leaning forward against a pillow on the bedside table while sitting in a chair.
- *While massaging the patient's back, you notice a 5-cm reddened area on the patient's sacrum:* Note this observation in the patient's health record and communicate it to the health care team. Do not massage the area. When the back massage is completed, position the patient off the sacral area, using supports to maintain the patient's position, and institute a turning schedule.

SPECIAL CONSIDERATIONS

General Considerations

- Before giving a back massage, assess the patient's body structure and skin condition, and tailor the duration and intensity of the massage accordingly. If you are giving a back massage at bedtime, have the patient ready for bed beforehand so the massage can help them fall asleep.
- Massage only the hands, feet, or scalp of patients with sepsis, fever over 100°F, sickle cell or HIV crisis, thrombocytopenia, or meningitis (Westman & Blaisdell, 2016).
- Check in frequently with the patient during the massage, asking how the massage feels and adjust the pressure and technique based on the patient's preferences (Westman & Blaisdell, 2016).

(continued on page 1380)

Skill 36-1 Giving a Back Massage *(continued)*

Infant and Child Considerations

- Hold infants and small children in a comfortable, well-supported position, such as against the chest or across the lap.
- Oil or lotion should be odorless and edible in case the infant or child gets some in their mouth (MFMER, 2020).

Older Adult Considerations

- Be gentle with massage. The skin on older adults is often fragile and dry.
- Reduce pressure, provide short massage sessions, and consider alternative positions, such as supine or seated positions for massage with older adults (Durand, 2020).

DEVELOPING CLINICAL REASONING AND CLINICAL JUDGMENT

1. Work through the Evolving Case Study 36-1 to help develop your clinical reasoning and clinical judgment skills.
2. Interview a nurse who specializes in pain management. Ask the nurse to describe the various physiologic, psychological, and social responses to pain that the nurse has observed in patients with acute and chronic pain. Question the nurse about the different nursing interventions most likely to be effective for patients experiencing either acute or chronic pain. Inquire about specific pain management information and guidelines that the nurse usually includes in discharge planning and teaching.
3. Consider what you personally believe about pain: what it is, what causes it, what is most likely to relieve it. Determine how pain is currently being managed within the tradition of Western medicine and what role nursing plays in keeping patients pain-free. Visit nontraditional health centers where practitioners use a variety of noninvasive pain relief modalities, such as acupressure, mindfulness techniques, imagery, and dry needling. In what ways, if any, has this new learning experience modified your beliefs about pain? Will it change your ability to design effective pain management regimens for your patients?

EVOLVING CASE STUDY 36-1

Scenario: Carla is a 72-year-old woman who has a history of type 2 diabetes and associated diabetic neuropathy. Her wife is present at Carla's outpatient visit with the nurse practitioner, and Carla asks that she be included in all conversations. Carla is a retired schoolteacher with two grown daughters. She and her wife have been looking forward to traveling, but they are afraid that the complications from Carla's diabetes may impact on these plans. Carla has been followed by an endocrinologist for the past 8 years. The endocrinologist has documented that despite an A1c close to the goal range, Carla has complications from her diabetes, one of which is the direct cause of the persistent pain in Carla's legs.

QUESTION r/t CUES: Based on the patient's history, what initial question is the most important for the nurse to ask?

A. "Can you tell me about your pain?"
B. "So, what's new with you and your wife?"
C. "Have you been following the diet plan we outlined for you?"
D. "Tell me about your daily routine: what do you do on a daily basis?"

Scenario: Carla tells you that she has increased generalized discomfort—fatigue, anxiety, irritability—that she attributes to the stress of this new-onset, persistent pain. Carla tells you the pain is in both legs and began as occasional, sharp pain, but has evolved into a constant ache. Carla appears tense and her brow furrows as she reaches down to touch her legs.

QUESTION r/t ANALYZING CUES: Based on this opening description of pain, what other information would be helpful in determining the plan of care? Select all that apply.

A. Assessment of the quality of care provided by the endocrinologist
B. Carla's wife's objective view of the patient's pain progression
C. Identification of anything that seems to trigger the pain
D. Interventions that have been tried—what worked and what did not work
E. Other symptoms that may be related or associated with the pain experience

EVOLVING CASE STUDY 36-1 *(continued)*

Scenario: Carla shakes her head and tells you she is just trying to make it through the day; she is unable to describe any appropriate pain, stress, or anxiety management techniques. She admits she has occasionally taken some of her wife's "old tranquilizers" to ease her through a bad day, but she prefers not to take pain medication. Carla adheres to the general diet and medication regimen mandated by her type 2 diabetes but admits that the stress of these complications is impacting on her desire and ability to maintain control over her blood glucose.

QUESTION r/t PRIORITIZING HYPOTHESIS: Based on the objective and subjective assessment of this patient, where should the nurse focus the initial efforts of the interprofessional team?

A. Collaborating with the endocrinologist to manage the patient's blood glucose and A1c
B. Consulting psychiatry to set up a medication regimen to treat the patient's anxiety and depression
C. Working with the provider, the patient, and the patient's wife to address functional pain goals
D. Providing detailed information on the microvascular and macrovascular complications of type 2 diabetes

Scenario: The nurse works with Carla and her wife to determine the mutually agreed upon pain goal is 1/10 at rest and 3/10 with activity. Carla's functional goal is to have the stability and stamina to plan a walking tour of a new city without the pain impacting on her enjoyment of the trip.

QUESTION r/t GENERATING SOLUTIONS: Based on this information, the provider decides to add pharmacologic strategies to the plan of care. Which interventions are the ***priority*** for Carla? Select all that apply.

A. Provide information about a multimodal pain regimen
B. Focus on the side effects of high-dose immediate-release opioids
C. Discuss the significant risk for addiction with Carla and her wife
D. Teach adjuvant medications such as gabapentin for treatment of neuropathic pain
E. Integrate elements from the biopsychosocial model when designing interventions

Scenario: Carla's wife has been listening intently but has not yet said anything. You ask Carla's wife if she has any questions and she says, "I appreciate that, at this point, medications are probably necessary, but I was hoping for some other ideas about what we could do to help Carla."

QUESTION r/t TAKING ACTION: What other intervention(s) can be implemented for Carla?

A. Nothing quite yet—we need to see how the medications work before implementing other interventions.
B. The nurse could collaborate with Carla's wife to substitute the medications for placebos to see if the idea of medication helps the pain.
C. Carla could take any number of over-the-counter (OTC) and herbal supplements to augment the medications.
D. The nurse could ask Carla if she is willing to incorporate imagery, mindfulness, or other nonpharmacologic interventions.

Scenario: Carla is back in the office for an outpatient visit with the provider. As soon as you see Carla, she pulls out her phone to show you pictures of Helen, Georgia where she and her wife just vacationed.

QUESTION r/t EVALUATING OUTCOMES: How will the nurse and Carla know that the treatment plan has been effective?

A. Carla is completely pain free but is taking large doses of OTC acetaminophen.
B. Carla reports some pain but states she was able to engage in the full walking tour with occasional rest periods.
C. Carla admits that she is not taking the medication because she has just learned to live with the pain.
D. Carla tried a few nonpharmacologic recommendations but has opted to simply double the prescribed dose.

PRACTICING FOR NCLEX

1. During postconference, nursing students are exploring definitions of pain and its nature. Which statements should be included in this discussion? Select all that apply.
   a. "It is whatever the health care provider treating the pain says it is."
   b. "Pain exists whenever the person experiencing it says it is present."
   c. "It is an emotional and sensory reaction to tissue damage."
   d. "Pain is a simple, universal, and easy-to-describe phenomenon."
   e. "When a cause cannot be identified, pain is psychological in nature."
   f. "It is classified by duration, location, source, transmission, and etiology."

2. A nurse in a rehabilitation facility is evaluating patients with chronic pain to develop an interprofessional plan of care. Which patients would the nurse identify who could benefit from a multimodal approach to pain management? Select all that apply.
   a. Patient receiving chemotherapy for bladder cancer
   b. Adolescent who had an appendectomy
   c. Patient who is experiencing a ruptured aneurysm
   d. Patient with fibromyalgia requesting pain medication
   e. Patient having back pain related to an accident that occurred last year
   f. Patient experiencing pain from second-degree burns
3. A patient reports diffuse abdominal pain that is difficult to localize. The nurse documents this as which type of pain?
   a. Cutaneous
   b. Visceral
   c. Superficial
   d. Somatic
4. Which question by the nurse will be most helpful in determining whether a patient who is experiencing a myocardial infarction has referred pain?
   a. "Did your chest pain last 2 minutes or less?
   b. "Was the pain on the surface of your chest?"
   c. "Is this pain in your residual limb shooting or burning?"
   d. "Are you having any arm or shoulder pain?"
5. A nurse is caring for patients who are nonverbal. What are examples of behavioral responses to pain? Select all that apply.
   a. Cradling a wrist that was injured in a car accident
   b. Moaning and crying from abdominal pain
   c. Increasing pulse following a myocardial infarction
   d. Striking out at a nurse who attempts to provide a bath
   e. Acting depressed and withdrawn while experiencing chronic cancer pain
   f. Pulling away from a nurse trying to give an injection
6. A nurse is caring for patients in a hospital setting. Which patient would the nurse place at risk for pain related to the mechanical activation of pain receptors?
   a. Older adult on bedrest following cervical spine surgery
   b. Patient with a severe sunburn being treated for dehydration
   c. Industrial worker who has burns caused by a caustic acid
   d. Patient experiencing cardiac disturbances from an electrical shock
7. A nurse plans to promote a patient's natural pain mediators by using a whirlpool following intensive physical therapy to the legs. What is a potent pain-blocking neuromodulator, released through relaxation techniques?
   a. Prostaglandins
   b. Substance P
   c. Endorphins
   d. Serotonin
8. A postoperative patient asks the nurse about pain management following surgery. What teaching will the nurse provide?
   a. "Avoid asking for pain medication often, as it can be addictive."
   b. "It is better to wait until the pain is severe before asking for pain medication."
   c. "It's natural to have pain after surgery; it will lessen in intensity in a few days."
   d. "You will be more comfortable if you take the medication at regular intervals."
9. The nurse applies the gate control theory of pain to provide pain relief to a patient with chronic lower back pain. What nursing intervention will help relieve pain by "closing the gate"?
   a. Encouraging regular use of analgesics
   b. Applying moist heat to the area at intervals
   c. Reviewing the pain experience with the patient
   d. Ambulating the patient after administering medication
10. The nurse is assessing the pain of a neonate who is admitted to the NICU with a heart defect. Which pain assessment scale would be the best tool to use with this patient?
    a. CRIES
    b. COMFORT
    c. FLACC
    d. FACES
11. When the nurse assists a patient recovering from abdominal surgery to walk, the nurse observes that the patient grimaces, moves stiffly, and becomes pale. The nurse received in shift report that the patient has consistently refused pain medication. To help promote comfort, which additional data will the nurse gather? Select all that apply.
    a. Patient's understanding of or fear of taking prescribed analgesics
    b. Assessment of any current pain
    c. Presence of anxiety or additional stressors
    d. Assessment of the surgical incision for infection
    e. What the patient has eaten to this point
    f. Whether the patient is using the incentive spirometer
12. When developing the care plan for a patient with chronic pain, the nurse plans interventions based on the knowledge that chronic pain not related to cancer or palliative/end-of-life care is most effectively relieved through which method?
    a. Providing the highest effective dose of an opioid on a PRN (as needed) basis
    b. Using nonopioid drugs conservatively
    c. Applying multimodal nonpharmacologic and nonopioid pharmacologic therapies
    d. Administering a continuous intravenous infusion on a regular basis

13. When assessing pain in a child, the nurse needs to be aware of what considerations?
    a. Immature neurologic development results in reduced pain sensation
    b. Inadequate or inconsistent relief of pain is widespread
    c. Reliable assessment tools are currently unavailable
    d. Narcotic analgesic use should be avoided
14. A pregnant woman has received an epidural analgesic prior to delivery. Assessment for which outcome to the medication will the nurse prioritize?
    a. Pruritus
    b. Urinary retention
    c. Vomiting
    d. Respiratory depression
15. A nurse is assessing a patient receiving a continuous opioid infusion. For which outcome of treatment would the nurse immediately notify the primary care provider?
    a. A respiratory rate of 11/min with normal depth
    b. A sedation level of 4
    c. Mild forgetfulness
    d. Reported constipation
16. A patient is receiving a multimodal medication regimen as part of the treatment plan for neuropathic phantom limb pain. When the patient reports a bloody bowel movement, which medication prescription requires notification of the provider?
    a. Acetaminophen
    b. Nonsteroidal antiinflammatory
    c. Opioid medication
    d. Antianxiety medication
17. A nurse on an adult surgical floor enters a patient room and observes a family member pressing the button to administer a dose of PCA via the infusion pump. What response by the nurse is most appropriate?
    a. "That dose will sure be helpful after their type of surgery."
    b. "Having only the patient use the pump prevents respiratory complications."
    c. "If the patient asked you to press the button, then it's OK."
    d. "Since the pump has built in safeguards, you can help with pain management."
18. Students in a leadership class are discussing how social determinants of health affect pain management. Which statement is correct and should be included in the discussion?
    a. "Outcomes of pain management are generally satisfactory regardless of income."
    b. "Minority patients often receive excess medication."
    c. "Patients from minority groups often wait a long time before seeking treatment for pain."
    d. "Social determinants of health are unrelated to pain management."

ANSWERS WITH RATIONALES

1. **b, c, f.** Nurses must respect patients' reports of pain and consider the patient an expert on their pain experience. An accepted definition of pain is that pain is whatever the patient says it is, existing whenever the person says it does, even if the cause is not clearly established." Pain is a complex, unpleasant sensory and emotional experience associated with actual or potential tissue damage. Pain may be classified according to its duration, its location or source, its mode of transmission, or its etiology.
2. **a, d, e.** Chronic pain is pain that may be limited, intermittent, or persistent but that lasts beyond the normal healing period. Examples are cancer pain, fibromyalgia pain, and back pain. Acute pain is generally rapid in onset and varies in intensity from mild to severe, as occurs with an emergency appendectomy, a ruptured aneurysm, and pain from burns.
3. **b.** Visceral pain, which is poorly localized and can originate in body organs in the abdomen. Cutaneous pain (superficial pain) usually involves the skin or subcutaneous tissue. A paper cut that produces sharp pain with a burning sensation is an example of cutaneous pain. Deep somatic pain is diffuse or scattered and originates in tendons, ligaments, bones, blood vessels, and nerves. Strong pressure on a bone or damage to tissue that occurs with a sprain causes deep somatic pain.
4. **d.** Referred pain is perceived in an area distant from its point of origin, whereas transient pain is brief and passes quickly. One example is the pain of MI (heart attack) that can be felt in the shoulder or chest, among other areas. Superficial pain originates in the skin or subcutaneous tissue. Phantom pain may occur in a person who has had a body part amputated, either surgically or traumatically.
5. **a, b, f.** Physiologic responses are involuntary body responses; behavioral responses reflect body movements; affective responses reflect mood and emotions. Protecting or guarding a painful area, moaning and crying, and moving away from painful stimuli are behavioral responses. Examples of a physiologic or involuntary response would be increased blood pressure or dilation of the pupils. Affective responses, such as anger, withdrawal, and depression, are psychological in nature.
6. **a.** Receptors in the skin and superficial organs may be stimulated by mechanical, thermal, chemical, and electrical agents. Friction from bed linens causing pressure sores is a mechanical stimulant. Sunburn is a thermal stimulant. An acid burn is the result of a chemical stimulant. An electrical shock is an electrical stimulant.
7. **c.** Endorphins are produced at neural synapses at various points along the CNS pathway. They are powerful pain-blocking chemicals that have prolonged analgesic effects and produce euphoria. It is thought that endorphins are released through pain relief measures, such as relaxation techniques. Prostaglandins, substance P, and serotonin (a hormone that can act to stimulate smooth muscles, inhibit gastric secretion, and produce vasoconstriction) are neurotransmitters or substances that either excite or inhibit target nerve cells.
8. **d.** While many analgesics are ordered on a PRN (as needed) basis, patients should be taught that it is more difficult to relieve pain that prevent it. The patient should not wait until pain is severe or unbearable to request pain medication. Few people become addicted to the medications if used for a short

period of time. Pain following surgery can be controlled and should not be considered a natural part of the experience that will lessen in time.

9. **b.** The gate control theory states that a limited amount of sensory information can be processed by the nervous system at any given moment. When too much information is sent through, certain cells in the spinal column interrupt the signal as if closing a gate, interfering with pain perception. Nursing measures such as applying warmth to the lower back stimulate the large nerve fibers to close the gate and block the pain. The other choices do not involve attempts to stimulate large nerve fibers that interfere with pain transmission as explained by the gate control theory.

10. **a.** The CRIES Pain Scale is a tool intended for use with neonates and infants from 0 to 6 months. The COMFORT Scale, used to assess pain and distress in critically ill pediatric patients, relies on six behavioral and two physiologic factors that determine the level of analgesia needed to adequately relieve pain in these children. The FLACC Scale (F—Faces, L—Legs, A—Activity, C—Cry, C—Consolability) was designed for infants and children from age 2 months to 7 years who are unable to validate the presence or severity of pain. The FACES Scale is used for children who can compare their pain to the faces depicted on the scale.

11. **a, b, c, d.** While it seems the patient's immediate problem is unrelieved pain because the patient refuses to take pain medication, through further assessment, the nurse can plan to address fears of medication, teach about use of the pump, determine if anxiety is interfering with pain, or an infection is causing increased pain. While decreased oral intake may be a response to pain, the patient's dietary intake will not uncover the underlying reason for refusing medications. Use of the incentive spirometer is not included in pain assessment; rather, it is an intervention to prevent atelectasis.

12. **c.** Nonpharmacologic and nonopioid pharmacologic therapies (multimodal) are the preferred choices for chronic pain that is unrelated to active cancer, palliative care, or end-of-life care. If progression to opioids becomes necessary, the lowest effective dose of an immediate-release opioid should be initiated first. Ongoing assessment and careful monitoring should guide the prescription of opioids for the management of chronic pain (Dowell et al., 2016). A PRN (as needed) drug regimen has not been proven effective for people experiencing chronic or acute pain. When caring for a patient with acute pain, such as postoperative pain, medication should be offered or requested before pain becomes severe or unbearable. Once pain is adequately treated, such as later in the postoperative course, a PRN schedule may be effective.

13. **b.** Health care personnel are placing awareness of pain relief in children as a priority. The evidence supports the fact that children do indeed feel pain, and reliable assessment tools are available specifically for use with children. Opioid analgesics may be safely used with children as long as they are carefully monitored.

14. **d.** An opioid drug given by way of an epidural catheter or a displaced catheter may result in the occurrence of respiratory depression. Pruritus, urinary retention, and vomiting may occur but are not life threatening.

15. **b.** Sedation levels predict respiratory depression. The sedation scale uses: S = sleep, easy to arouse: no action necessary; 1 = awake and alert; no action necessary; 2 = occasionally drowsy but easy to arouse; requires no action; 3 = frequently drowsy and drifts off to sleep during conversation; decrease the opioid dose; and 4 = somnolent with minimal or no response to stimuli; discontinue the opioid and consider use of naloxone. A respiratory level of 11 with normal depth of breathing is usually not a cause for alarm. Mild forgetfulness or confusion may result from opioids; additional observation is necessary. Constipation is not life threatening; it should be reported to the health care provider but is not the priority.

16. **b.** The NSAIDs are contraindicated in patients with bleeding disorders (their action may interfere with platelet function). The nurse will hold the medication and collaborate with the provider to adjust the patient's prescriptions.

17. **b.** Unauthorized family members or caregivers (instead of the patient) who administer PCA by pushing the dosage button can cause serious analgesic overdoses resulting in oversedation, respiratory depression, and death. This is known as PCA by proxy. Institutions should have protocols in place to protect against unauthorized PCA delivery and clear warning labels attached to PCA pumps stating, "WARNING: BUTTON TO BE PRESSED ONLY BY THE PATIENT" (ISMP).

18. **c.** Social determinants of health greatly impact on pain management outcomes. Patients residing in low-income settings and minority populations are less likely to receive the recommended treatments for pain in health care settings. Minority patients often experience pain for a lengthy period of time before seeking treatment for it. Language barriers, culturally inappropriate pain assessment tools, and prejudice and misconceptions may contribute to unsatisfactory pain outcomes. Initiatives to address health care access and treatment disparities begin at the local and community level.

Bibliography

Agency for Healthcare Research and Quality (AHRQ). (2018, April). *Race, ethnicity, and language data: Standardization for health care quality improvement. 1. Introduction*. Agency for Healthcare Research and Quality. https://www.ahrq.gov/research/findings/final-reports/iomracereport/reldata1.html

Chou, R., Fu, R., Dana, T., Pappas, M., Hart, E., & Mauer, K. M. (2021, September). *Interventional treatments for acute and chronic pain: Systematic review*. Comparative Effectiveness Review No. 247. (Prepared by the Pacific Northwest Evidence-based Practice Center under Contract No. 75Q80120D00006.) AHRQ Publication No. 21-EHC030. Agency for Healthcare Research and Quality. https://effectivehealthcare.ahrq.gov/products/interventional-treatments-pain/research

Ali, A., Arif, A. W., Bhan, C., Kumar, D., Malik, M. B., Sayyed, Z., Akhtar, K. H., & Ahmad, M. Q. (2018). Managing chronic pain in the elderly: An overview of the recent therapeutic advancements. *Cureus, 10*(9), e3293. https://doi.org/10.7759/cureus.3293

Allen, E., Williams, A., Jennings, D., Stomski, N., Goucke, R., Toye, C., Slatyer, S., Clarke, T., & McCullough, K. (2018). Revisiting the pain resource nurse role in sustaining evidence-based practice changes for pain assessment and management. *Worldviews on Evidence-based Nursing, 15*(5), 368–376. https://doi.org/10.1111/wvn.12318

American Pain Society Quality of Care Committee. (1995). Quality improvement guidelines for the treatment of acute pain and cancer pain. *JAMA, 274*(23), 1874–1880. https://doi.org/10.1001/jama.1995.03530230060032

American Society of Anesthesiologists. (2016, February 24). Women's pain update. https://www.asahq.org/about-asa/newsroom/news-releases/2016/02/second-annual-asa-women-pain-update

Arnstein, P., Broglio, K., Wuhrman, E., & Kean, M. B. (2011). Position statement: Use of placebos in pain management. *Pain Management Nursing, 12*(4), 225–229. https://doi.org/10.1016/j.pmn.2010.10.033

Baker, D. W. (2017, May 5). The Joint Commission's pain standards: Origins and evolution. The Joint Commission. https://www.jointcommission.org/-/media/tjc/documents/resources/pain-management/pain_std_history_web_version_05122017pdf.pdf?db=web&hash=E7D12A5C3BE9DF031F3D8FE0D8509580

Beletsky, Burton, B. N., Finneran IV, J. J., Alexander, B. S., Macias, A., & Gabriel, R. A. (2021). Association of race and ethnicity in the receipt of regional anesthesia following mastectomy. *Regional Anesthesia and Pain Medicine*, *46*(2), 118–123. https://doi.org/10.1136/rapm-2020-101818

Benjenk, I., Messing, J., Lenihan, M. J., Hernandez, M., Amdur, R., Sirajuddin, S., Davison, D., Schroeder, M. E., & Sarani, B. (2020). Authorized agent-controlled analgesia for pain management in critically ill adult patients. *Critical Care Nurse*, *40*(3), 31–36. https://doi.org/10.4037/ccn2020323

Beyer, J., Denyes, M. J., & Villarruel, A. M. (1992). The creation, validation, and continuing development of the Oucher: A measure of pain intensity in children. *Journal of Pediatric Nursing*, *7*(5), 335–346.

Bolton, D., & Gillett, G. (2019) *The Biopsychosocial Model of health and disease: New philosophical and scientific developments*. Palgrave Pivot. https://doi.org/10.1007/978-3-030-11899-0_1

Brejchova, J., Holan, V., & Svoboda, P. (2021). Expression of opioid receptors in cells of the immune system. *International Journal of Molecular Sciences*, *22*(1), 315. https://doi.org/10.3390/ijms22010315

Burchum, J., & Rosenthal, L. (2019). *Lehne's pharmacology for nursing care* (10th ed.). Elsevier.

Bynum, R., Garcia, O., Herbst, E., Kossa, M., Liou, K., Cowan, A., & Hilton, C. (2021). Effects of dry needling on spasticity and range of motion: A systematic review. *The American Journal of Occupational Therapy*, *75*(1), 7501205030p1–7501205030p13. https://doi.org/10.5014/ajot.2021.041798

Cancio, R. (2020). Experiences with machismo and pain: Latino veterans. *American Journal of Men's Health*, *14*(6), 1557988320976304. https://doi.org/10.1177/1557988320976304

Cánovas, L., Carrascosa, A. J., García, M., Fernández, M., Calvo, A., Monsalve, V., Soriano, J. F., & Empathy Study Group. (2018). Impact of empathy in the patient-doctor relationship on chronic pain relief and quality of life: A prospective study in Spanish pain clinics. *Pain Medicine, 19*(7), 1304–1314. https://doi.org/10.1093/pm/pnx160

Carpenter, D. E. (2020, May 12). Psychedelic pioneer Rick Doblin on FDA trials of MDMA: Most important reality check Of MAPS' 34-year history. *Forbes*. https://www.forbes.com/sites/davidcarpenter/2020/05/12/psychedelic-pioneer-rick-doblin-on-fda-trials-of-mdma-most-important-reality-check-of-maps-34-year-history/?sh=46b7007230ad

Centers for Disease Control and Prevention (CDC). (2021a, January 26). *Opioids: Commonly used terms*. https://www.cdc.gov/opioids/basics/terms.html

Centers for Disease Control and Prevention (CDC). (2021b, February 17). *About CDC's opioid prescribing guideline*. https://www.cdc.gov/drugoverdose/prescribing/guideline.html

Centers for Disease Control and Prevention (CDC). (2021c, March 3). *Drug overdose deaths*. https://www.cdc.gov/drugoverdose/data/statedeaths.html

Chou, R., Wagner, J., Ahmed, A.Y., Blazina, I., Brodt, E., Buckley, D. I., Cheney, T. P., Choo, E., Dana, T., Gordon, D., Khandelwal, S., Kantner, S., McDonagh, M. S., Sedgley, C., & Skelly, A. C. (2022, March 25). *Treatments for acute pain: A systematic review*. Comparative Effectiveness Review No. 240. Prepared by the Pacific Northwest Evidence-based Practice Center under Contract No. 290-2015-00009-I. AHRQ Publication No. 20(21)-EHC006. Agency for Healthcare Research and Quality. https://effectivehealthcare.ahrq.gov/products/treatments-acute-pain/research

Chuan, A., Zhou, J. J., Hou, R. M., Stevens, C. J., & Bogdanovych, A. (2021). Virtual reality for acute and chronic pain management in adult patients: A narrative review. *Anaesthesia*, *76*(5), 695–704. https://doi.org/10.1111/anae.15202

Cinar, H. U., Celik, H. K., & Celik, B. (2021). The efficacy of the ON-Q elastomeric pump system in post-thoracotomy acute pain control. *Nigerian Journal of Clinical Practice*, *24*(5), 651–659. https://doi.org/10.4103/njcp.njcp_203_20

Colby, S. L., & Ortman, J. M. (2015, March). Projections of the size and composition of the U.S. population: 2014 to 2060. Current Population Reports, P25-1143. U.S. Census Bureau. https://www.census.gov/content/dam/Census/library/publications/2015/demo/p25-1143.pdf

Collins, L., Cata, D. M., & Conley, N. S. (2020). A comparison study-Oral patient-controlled analgesia versus traditional delivery of pain medication following orthopaedic procedures. *Orthopedic Nursing*, *39*(5), 324–332. https://doi.org/10.1097/NOR.0000000000000697

Crawford, C. L., Boller, J., Jadalla, A., & Cuenca, E. (2016). An integrative review of pain resource nurse programs. *Critical Care Nursing Quarterly*, *39*(1), 64–82. https://doi.org/10.1097/CNQ.0000000000000101

Curtis, M., McPherson, M. L., Swagger, S. M., & Matzo, M. (2021). Monitoring equianalgesic opioid dosing. *The American Journal of Nursing*, *121*(3), 60–63. https://doi.org/10.1097/01.NAJ.0000737312.95932.4d

Dahlhamer, J., Lucas, J., Zelaya, C., Nahin, R., Mackey, S., DeBar, L., Kerns, R., Von Korff, M., Porter, L., & Helmick, C. (2018). Prevalence of chronic pain and high-impact chronic pain among adults — United States, 2016. *Morbidity and Mortality Weekly Report (MMWR)*, *67*(36), 1001–1006. http://dx.doi.org/10.15585/mmwr.mm6736a2

DEA's Strategic Intelligence Section. (2021, March 2). 2020 Drug enforcement administration: NDTA national drug threat assessment. [DEA-DCT-DIR-008-21]. https://www.dea.gov/sites/default/files/2021-02/DIR-008-21%202020%20National%20Drug%20Threat%20Assessment_WEB.pdf

Devlin, J. W., Skrobik, Y., Gélinas, C., Needham, D. M., Slooter, A., Pandharipande, P. P., Watson, P. L., Weinhouse, G. L., Nunnally, M. E., Rochwerg, B., Balas, M. C., van den Boogaard, M., Bosma, K. J., Brummel, N. E., Chanques, G., Denehy, L., Drouot, X., Fraser, G. L., Harris, J. E., ... Alhazzani, W. (2018). Clinical practice guidelines for the prevention and management of pain, agitation/sedation, delirium, immobility, and sleep disruption in adult patients in the ICU. *Critical Care Medicine*, *46*(9), e825–e873. https://doi.org/10.1097/CCM.0000000000003299

Domenichiello, A. F., & Ramsden, C. E. (2019). The silent epidemic of chronic pain in older adults. *Progress in Neuro-psychopharmacology & Biological Psychiatry*, *93*, 284–290. https://doi.org/10.1016/j.pnpbp.2019.04.006

Dowell, D., Haegerich, T. M., & Chou, R. (2016). CDC guideline for prescribing opioids for chronic pain — United States, 2016. *Morbidity and Mortality Weekly Report*, *65*(1), 1–49. https://doi.org/10.15585/mmwr.rr6501e1

Drew, D. J., Gordon, D. B., Morgan, B., & Manworren, R. (2018). "As-needed" range orders for opioid analgesics in the management of pain: A consensus statement of the American Society for Pain Management Nursing and the American Pain Society. *Pain Management Nursing*, *19*(3), 207–210. https://doi.org/10.1016/j.pmn.2018.03.003

Durand, M. (2020, August 1). *Massage therapy for seniors*. American Massage Therapy Association. https://www.amtamassage.org/publications/massage-therapy-journal/massage-for-elderly/

Earp, B. D., Lewis, J., Hart, C. L., & with Bioethicists and Allied Professionals for Drug Policy Reform, (2021). Racial justice requires ending the war on drugs. *The American Journal of Bioethics*, *21*(4), 4–19. https://doi.org/10.1080/15265161.2020.1861364

Engel, G. L. (1977). The need for a new medical model: A challenge for biomedicine. *Science*, *196*(4286), 129–136. https://doi.org/10.1126/science.847460

Fain, K. M., Alexander, G. C., Dore, D. D., Segal, J. B., Zullo, A. R., & Castillo-Salgado, C. (2017). Frequency and predictors of analgesic prescribing in U.S. nursing home residents with persistent pain. *Journal of the American Geriatrics Society*, *65*(2), 286–293. https://doi.org/10.1111/jgs.14512

Femer, R. E., & Aronson, J. K. (2013). Laughter and MIRTH (methodical investigation of risibility, therapeutic and harmful): Narrative synthesis. *The BMJ*, *347*, f7274. https://doi.org/10.1136/bmj.f7274

Gai, N., Naser, B., Hanley, J., Peliowski, A., Hayes, J., & Aoyama, K. (2020). A practical guide to acute pain management in children. *Journal of Anesthesia*, *34*(3), 421–433. https://doi.org/10.1007/s00540-020-02767-x

Galacia-Castillo, M. C., & Weiner, D. K. (2021, March 21). Treatment of chronic non-cancer pain in older adults. *UpToDate*. https://www.uptodate.com/contents/treatment-of-chronic-non-cancer-pain-in-older-adults

Galligan, M. (2020). Care and management of patients receiving epidural analgesia. *Nursing Standard*, *35*(12), 77–82. https://doi.org/10.7748/ns.2020.e11573

Garza-Villarreal, E. A., Pando, V., Vuust, P., & Parsons, C. (2017). Music-induced analgesia in chronic pain conditions: A systematic review and meta-analysis. *Pain Physician*, *20*(7), 597–610.

Goeren, D., John, S., Meskill, K., Iacono, L., Wahl, S., & Scanlon, K. (2018). Quiet Time: A noise reduction initiative in a neurosurgical intensive care unit. *Critical Care Nursing*, *38*(4), 38–45. https://doi.org/10.4037/ccn2018219

Gorski, L., Hadaway, L., Hagle, M. E., Broadhurst, D., Clare, S., Kleidon, T., Meyer, B. M., Nickel, B., Rowley, S. Sharpe, E., & Alexander, M. (2021). *Infusion therapy standards of practice* (8th ed.). Infusion Nurses Society.

Hall, K. R., & Stanley, A. Y. (2019). Literature review: Assessment of opioid-related sedation and the Pasero Opioid Sedation Scale. *Journal of Perianesthesia*, *34*(1), 132–142. https://doi.org/10.1016/j.jopan.2017.12.009

Hawk, C., Whalen, W., Farabaugh, R. J., Daniels, C. J., Minkalis, A. L., Taylor, D. N., Anderson, D., Anderson, K., Crivelli, L. S., Cark, M., Barlow, E., Paris, D., Sarnat, R., & Weeks, J. (2020). Best practices for chiropractic management of patients with chronic musculoskeletal pain: A clinical practice guideline. *Journal of Alternative and Complementary Medicine*, *26*(10), 884–901. https://doi.org/10.1089/acm.2020.0181

Herr, K., Spratt, K., Garand, L., & Li, L. (2007). Evaluation of the Iowa Pain Thermometer and other selected pain intensity scales in younger and older adult cohorts using controlled clinical pain: A preliminary study. *Pain Medicine*, *8*(7), 585–600. https://doi.org/10.1111/j.1526-4637.2007.00316.x

Hinkle, J. L., Cheever, K. H., & Overbaugh, K. J. (2022). *Brunner & Suddarth's textbook of medical-surgical nursing* (15th ed.). Wolters Kluwer Health.

Hole, J., Hirsch, M., Ball, E., & Meads, C. (2015). Music as an aid for postoperative recovery in adults: A systematic review and meta-analysis. *Lancet*, *386*(10004), 1659–1671. https://doi.org/10.1016/S0140-6736(15)60169-6

Howland, R. H. (2016). Hey Mr. Tambourine Man, play a drug for me: Music as medication. *Journal of Psychosocial Nursing and Mental Health Services*, *54*(12), 23–27. https://doi.org/10.3928/02793695-20161208-05

Hsu, D. C., Stack, A. M., & Wiley, J. F. (2020). Clinical use of topical anesthetics in children. *UpToDate*. http://www.uptodate.com/contents/topical-anesthetics-in-children

Institute of Advanced Musculoskeletal Treatments (IAMT). (2021). *Curriculum*. https://www.iamt.org/curriculum

Institute of Medicine (IOM). (2011). *Relieving pain in America: A blueprint for transforming prevention, care, education, and research*. The National Academies Press. https://www.nap.edu/catalog/13172/relieving-pain-in-america-a-blueprint-for-transforming-prevention-care

Institute of Safe Medication Practices (ISMP). (2016, September 22). Worth repeating ... Recent PCA by proxy event suggests reassessment of practices that may have fallen by the wayside. https://www.ismp.org/resources/worth-repeating-recent-pca-proxy-event-suggests-reassessment-practices-may-have-fallen

Institute of Safe Medication Practices (ISMP). (2020, February 21). Targeted medication safety best practices for hospitals. https://www.ismp.org/guidelines/best-practices-hospitals

International Association for the Study of Pain. (2021). *Terminology*. Retrieved May 11, 2022, from https://www.iasp-pain.org/resources/terminology/?ItemNumber=1698

Johnston, T. E., Keller, S., Denzer-Weiler, C., & Brown, L. (2021). A clinical practice guideline for the use of ankle-foot orthoses and functional electrical stimulation post-stroke. *Journal of Neurologic Physical Therapy*, *45*(2), 112–196. https://doi.org/10.1097/NPT.0000000000000347

The Joint Commission. (2017, August 29). R3 report issue 11: Pain assessment and management standards for hospitals. https://www.jointcommission.org/assets/1/18/R3_Report_Issue_11_Pain_Assessment_8_25_17_FINAL.pdf

The Joint Commission. (2021, January 4). Pain assessment and management – Understanding the requirements. https://www.jointcommission.org/standards/standard-faqs/hospital-and-hospital-clinics/provision-of-care-treatment-and-services-pc/000002161/

Jungquist, C. R., Quinlan-Colwell, A., Vallerand, A., Carlisle, H. L., Cooney, M., Dempsey, S. J., Dunwoody, D., Maly, A., Meloche, K., Meyers, A., Sawyer, J., Singh, N., Sullivan, D., Watson, C., & Polomano, R. C. (2020). American Society for Pain Management Nursing guidelines on monitoring for opioid-induced advancing sedation and respiratory depression: Revisions. *Pain Management Nursing*, *21*(1), 7–25. https://doi.org/10.1016/j.pmn.2019.06.007

Jungquist, C. R., Vallerand, A. H., Sicoutris, C., Kwon, K. N., & Polomano, R. C. (2017). Assessing and managing acute pain: A call to action. *American Journal of Nursing*, *117*(3), S4–S11. https://doi.org/10.1097/01.NAJ.0000513526.33816.0e

Kabat-Zinn, J. (1982). An outpatient program in behavioral medicine for chronic pain patients based on the practice of mindfulness meditation: Theoretical considerations and preliminary results. *General Hospital Psychiatry*, *4*(1), 33–47. https://doi.org/10.1016/0163-8343(82)90026-3

Karch, A. M. (2020). *Focus on nursing pharmacology* (8th ed.). Wolters Kluwer.

Khanna, Bergese, S. D., Jungquist, C. R., Morimatsu, H., Uezono, S., Lee, S., Ti, L. K., Urman, R. D., McIntyre, R., Tornero, C., Dahan, A., Saager, L., Weingarten, T. N., Wittmann, M., Auckley, D., Brazzi, L., Le Guen, M., Soto, R., Schramm, F., . . . Overdyk, F. J. (2020). Prediction of opioid-induced respiratory depression on inpatient wards using continuous capnography and oximetry: An international prospective, observational trial. *Anesthesia and Analgesia*, *131*(4), 1012–1024. https://doi.org/10.1213/ANE.0000000000004788

Kim, H. J., Chang, S. J., Park, H., Choi, S. W., Juon, H. S., Lee, K. E., & Ryu, H. (2020). Intra-ethnic differences in chronic pain and the associated factors: An exploratory, comparative design. *Journal of Nursing Scholarship*, *52*(4), 389–396. https://doi.org/10.1111/jnu.12564

Kühlmann, A., de Rooij, A., Kroese, L. F., van Dijk, M., Hunink, M., & Jeekel, J. (2018). Meta-analysis evaluating music interventions for anxiety and pain in surgery. *The British Journal of Surgery*, *105*(7), 773–783. https://doi.org/10.1002/bjs.10853

LeFort, S., Lorig, K., Laurent, D., González, V., Sobel, D., Minor, M., Keefe, F., & Gecht-Silver, M. (2021). *Living a healthy life with chronic pain* (2nd ed.). Bull Publishing Company.

Luberto, C. M., Hall, D. L., Park, E. R., Haramati, A., & Cotton, S. (2020). A perspective on the similarities and differences between mindfulness and relaxation. *Global Advances in Health and Medicine*, *9*, 2164956120905597. https://doi.org/10.1177/2164956120905597

Marske, C., Shah, S., Chavira, A., Hedberg, C., Fullmer, R., Clark, C. J., Pipitone, O., & Kaiser, P. (2020). Mindfulness-based stress reduction in the management of chronic pain and its comorbid depression. *The Journal of the American Osteopathic Association*, *120*(9), 575–581. https://doi.org/10.7556/jaoa.2020.096

Matteliano, D., St Marie, B. J., Oliver, J., & Coggins, C. (2014). Adherence monitoring with chronic opioid therapy for persistent pain: A biopsychosocial-spiritual approach to mitigate risk. *Pain Management Nursing*, *15*(1), 391–405. https://doi.org/10.1016/j.pmn.2012.08.008

Mayo Foundation for Medical Education and Research (MFMER). (2020, April 8). *Infant massage: Understand this soothing therapy*. https://www.mayoclinic.org/healthy-lifestyle/infant-and-toddler-health/in-depth/infant-massage/art-20047151

Miaskowski, C., Blyth, F., Nicosia, F., Haan, M., Keefe, F., Smith, A., & Ritchie, C. (2020). A biopsychosocial model of chronic pain for older adults. *Pain Medicine*, *21*(9), 1793–1805. https://doi.org/10.1093/pm/pnz329

Mitchell, J. M., Bogenschutz, M., Lilienstein, A., Harrison, C., Kleiman, S., Parker-Guilbert, K., Ot'alora, G. M., Garas, W., Paleos, C., Gorman, I., Nicholas, C., Mithoefer, M., Carlin, S., Poulter, B., Mithoefer, A., Quevedo, S., Wells, G., Klaire, S. S., van der Kolk, B., … Doblin, R. (2021). MDMA-assisted therapy for severe PTSD: A randomized, double-blind, placebo-controlled phase 3 study. *Nature Medicine*, *27*(6), 1025–1033. https://doi.org/10.1038/s41591-021-01336-3

Morales-Fernández, Á., Jimenez-Martín, J. M., Morales-Asencio, J. M., Vergara-Romero, M., Mora-Bandera, A. M., Aranda-Gallardo, M., & Canca-Sanchez, J. C. (2021). Impact of a nurse-led intervention on quality of life in patients with chronic non-malignant pain: An open randomized controlled trial. *Journal of Advanced Nursing*, *77*(1), 255–265. https://doi.org/10.1111/jan.14608

Murphy, L. K., Rights, J. D., Ricciuto, A., Church, P. C., & Ahola Kohut, S. (2020). Biopsychosocial correlates of presence and intensity of pain in adolescents with inflammatory bowel disease. *Frontiers in Pediatrics*, *8*, 559. https://doi.org/10.3389/fped.2020.00559

National Academies of Sciences, Engineering, & Medicine. (2017). *Communities in action: Pathways to health equity*. The National Academies Press. http://nationalacademies.org/hmd/Reports/2017/communities-in-action-pathways-to-health-equity.aspx

National Center for Complementary and Integrative Health (NCCIH). (2019, April). Traditional Chinese medicine: What you need to know. https://www.nccih.nih.gov/health/traditional-chinese-medicine-what-you-need-to-know

National Institute on Drug Abuse. (2018, June). *Medications to treat opioid use disorder research report*. https://www.drugabuse.gov/download/21349/medications-to-treat-opioid-use-disorder-research-report.pdf?v=99088f7584dac93ddcfa98648065bfbe

National Institute on Drug Abuse. (2020, June). *Drugs, brains, and behavior: The science of addiction: The science of addiction*. NIH Pub No. 20-DA-5605. https://www.drugabuse.gov/sites/default/files/soa.pdf

Newman, A. K., Kapoor, S., & Thorn, B. E. (2018). Health care utilization for chronic pain in low-income settings. *Pain Medicine*, *19*(12), 2387–2397. https://doi.org/10.1093/pm/pny119

Nicola, M., Correia, H., Ditchburn, G., & Drummond, P. (2021). Invalidation of chronic pain: A thematic analysis of pain narratives. *Disability and Rehabilitation*, *43*(6), 861–869. https://doi.org/10.1080/09638288.2019.1636888

Norris, T. L. (2020). *Porth's essentials of pathophysiology* (5th ed.). Wolters Kluwer.

Noureldein, M. H., & Eid, A. A. (2018). Homeostatic effect of laughter on diabetic cardiovascular complications: The myth turned to fact. *Diabetes Research and Clinical Practice*, *135*, 111–119. https://doi.org/10.1016/j.diabres.2017.11.014

Novak, S., Guerron, G., Zou, Z., Cheung, G., & Berteau, J. P. (2020). New guidelines for electrical stimulation parameters in adult patients with knee osteoarthritis based on a systematic review of the current literature. *American Journal of Physical Medicine & Rehabilitation*, *99*(8), 682–688. https://doi.org/10.1097/PHM.0000000000001409

Pardos-Gascón, E. M., Narambuena, L., Leal-Costa, C., & van-der Hofstadt-Román, C. J. (2021). Differential efficacy between cognitive-behavioral therapy and mindfulness-based therapies for chronic pain: Systematic review. *International Journal of Clinical and Health Psychology*, *21*(1), 100197. https://doi.org/10.1016/j.ijchp.2020.08.001

Park, S., Bak, A., Kim, S., Nam, Y., Kim, H. S., Yoo, D. H., & Moon, M. (2020). Animal-assisted and pet-robot interventions for ameliorating behavioral and psychological symptoms of dementia: A systematic review and meta-analysis. *Biomedicines*, *8*(6), 150. https://doi.org/10.3390/biomedicines8060150

Pasero, C., & McCaffery, M. (2011). *Pain assessment and pharmacological management*. Mosby, Inc., Elsevier Inc.

PDQ® Supportive and Palliative Care Editorial Board. (2021, May 6). *Cancer pain (PDQ®)-Health professional version*. National Cancer Institute. https://www.cancer.gov/about-cancer/treatment/side-effects/pain/pain-hp-pdq#section/_58

Pei, J. H., Ma, T., Nan, R. L., Chen, H. X., Zhang, Y. B., Gou, L., & Dou, X. M. (2021). Mindfulness-based cognitive therapy for treating chronic pain a systematic review and meta-analysis. *Psychology, Health & Medicine*, *26*(3), 333–346. https://doi.org/10.1080/13548506.2020.1849746

Pet Partners. (n.d.). AAI for professionals. Retrieved May 20, 2021, from https://petpartners.org/learn/aat-professionals

Pickering, G., Zwakhalen, S., & Kaasalainen, S. (2018). *Pain management in older adults: A nursing perspective*. Springer.

Pizzi, L. J., Bates, M., Chelly, J. E., & Goodrich, C. J. (2020). A prospective randomized trial of an oral patient-controlled analgesia device versus usual care following total hip arthroplasty. *Orthopedic Nursing*, *39*(1), 37–46. https://doi.org/10.1097/NOR.0000000000000624

Polomano, R. C., Fillman, M., Giordano, N. A., Vallerand, A. H., Nicely, K. L., & Jungquist, C. R. (2017). Multimodal analgesia for acute postoperative and trauma-related pain. *American Journal of Nursing*, *117*(3), S12–S26. https://doi.org/10.1097/01.NAJ.0000513527.71934.73

Porter, A. C., Behrendt, N. J., Zaretsky, M. V., Liechty, K. W., Wood, C., Chow, F., & Galan, H. L. (2021). Continuous local bupivacaine wound infusion reduces oral opioid use for acute postoperative pain control following myelomeningocele repair. *American Journal of Obstetrics & Gynecology MFM*, *3*(2), 100296. https://doi.org/10.1016/j.ajogmf.2020.100296

Poulsen, M. J., & Coto, J. (2018). Nursing music protocol and postoperative pain. *Pain Management Nursing*, *19*(2), 172–176. https://doi.org/10.1016/j.pmn.2017.09.003

Purnell, L. (2013). *Transcultural health care: A culturally competent approach* (4th ed.). F. A. Davis.

Raja, S. N., Carr, D. B., Cohen, M., Finnerup, N. B., Flor, H., Gibson, S., Keefe, F. J., Mogil, J. S., Ringkamp, M., Sluka, K. A., Song, X. J., Stevens, B., Sullivan, M. D., Tutelman, P. R., Ushida, T., & Vader, K. (2020). The revised International Association for the Study of Pain definition of pain: Concepts, challenges, and compromises. *Pain*, *161*(9), 1976–1982. https://doi.org/10.1097/j.pain.0000000000001939

Rajan, J., & Behrends, M. (2019). Acute pain in older adults: Recommendations for assessment and treatment. *Anesthesiology Clinics*, *37*(3), 507–520. https://doi.org/10.1016/j.anclin.2019.04.009

Rogers, A. H., Gallagher, M. W., Garey, L., Ditre, J. W., Williams, M. W., & Zvolensky, M. J. (2020). Pain Anxiety Symptoms Scale-20: An empirical evaluation of measurement invariance across race/ethnicity, sex, and pain. *Psychological Assessment*, *32*(9), 818–828. https://doi.org/10.1037/pas0000884

Sánchez-Infante, J., Navarro-Santana, M. J., Bravo-Sánchez, A., Jiménez-Diaz, F., & Abián-Vicén, J. (2021). Is dry needling applied by physical therapists effective for pain in musculoskeletal conditions? A systematic review and meta-analysis. *Physical Therapy*, *101*(3), pzab070. https://doi.org/10.1093/ptj/pzab070

Schneider, M. A. (2018). The effect of listening to music on postoperative pain in adult orthopedic patients. *Journal of Holistic Nursing*, *36*(1), 23–32. https://doi.org/10.1177/0898010116677383

Schwan, J., Sclafani, J., & Tawfik, V. L. (2019). Chronic pain management in the elderly. *Anesthesiology Clinics*, *37*(3), 547–560. https://doi.org/10.1016/j.anclin.2019.04.012

Schwartz, C. (2021, January 12). When getting high is a hobby, not a habit. *The New York Times*. https://www.nytimes.com/2021/01/12/books/review/drug-use-for-grown-ups-carl-l-hart.html

Schwenk, E. S., & Mariano, E. R. (2019, October 25). Multimodal analgesia: The foundation of a successful perioperative experience. Anesthesiology News. https://www.anesthesiologynews.com/Review-Articles/Article/10-19/Multimodal-Analgesia-The-Foundation-of-a-Successful-Perioperative-Experience/56171?sub=657C4D13807ED3293D92B4AB63250B0D773C3BAFAC62F568FD1918F7529EFB5

Shires, A., Sharpe, L., Davies, J. N., & Newton-John, T. (2020). The efficacy of mindfulness-based interventions in acute pain: A systematic review and meta-analysis. *Pain*, *161*(8), 1698–1707. https://doi.org/10.1097/j.pain.0000000000001877

Substance Abuse and Mental Health Services Administration (SAMHSA). (2018, June). SAMHSA Opioid overdose prevention TOOLKIT: Opioid use disorder facts. HHS Publication No. (SMA) 18-4742PT1. https://store.samhsa.gov/sites/default/files/d7/priv/opioid-use-disorder-facts.pdf

Suso-Ribera, C., Yakobov, E., Carriere, J. S., & García-Palacios, A. (2020). The impact of chronic pain on patients and spouses: Consequences on occupational status, distribution of household chores and care-giving burden. *European Journal of Pain*, *24*(9), 1730–1740. https://doi.org/10.1002/ejp.1616

Tabatabaee, A., Tafreshi, M. Z., Rassouli, M., Aledavood, S. A., AlaviMajd, H., & Farahmand, S. K. (2016). Effect of therapeutic touch in patients with cancer: A literature review. *Medical Archives*, *70*(2), 142–147. https://doi.org/10.5455

Treede, R. D., Rief, W., Barke, A., Aziz, Q., Bennett, M. I., Benoliel, R., Cohen, M., Evers, S., Finnerup, N. B., First, M. B., Giamberardino, M. A., Kaasa, S., Korwisi, B., Kosek, E., Lavand'homme, P., Nicholas, M., Perrot, S., Scholz, J., Schug, S., … Wang, S. J. (2019). Chronic pain as a symptom or a disease: The IASP Classification of chronic pain for the International Classification of Diseases (ICD-11). *Pain*, *160*(1), 19–27. https://doi.org/10.1097/j.pain.0000000000001384

U.S. Department of Health and Human Services-National Institutes of Health. *NIH HEAL Initiative*SM. Retrieved May 26, 2021, from https://heal.nih.gov/

U.S. Food and Drug Administration (FDA). (2019, September 20). Statement on continued efforts to increase availability of all forms of naloxone to help reduce opioid overdose deaths. https://www.fda.gov/news-events/press-announcements/statement-continued-efforts-increase-availability-all-forms-naloxone-help-reduce-opioid-overdose

U.S. Food and Drug Administration (FDA). (2020a, December 29). *Transmucosal immediate-release fentanyl (TIRF) medicines*. https://www.fda.gov/drugs/information-drug-class/transmucosal-immediate-release-fentanyl-tirf-medicines

U.S. Food and Drug Administration (FDA). (2020b, December 31). *Nonsteroidal anti-inflammatory drugs (NSAIDs)*. https://www.fda.gov/drugs/postmarket-drug-safety-information-patients-and-providers/nonsteroidal-anti-inflammatory-drugs-nsaids

U.S. Food and Drug Administration (FDA). (2021, May 11). FDA approves higher dosage of naloxone nasal spray to treat opioid overdose. https://www.fda.gov/news-events/press-announcements/fda-approves-higher-dosage-naloxone-nasal-spray-treat-opioid-overdose

van der Leeuw, G., Ayers, E., Leveille, S. G., Blankenstein, A. H., van der Horst, H. E., & Verghese, J. (2018). The effect of pain on major cognitive impairment in older adults. *The Journal of Pain*, *19*(12), 1435–1444. https://doi.org/10.1016/j.jpain.2018.06.009

VHA Center for Engineering & Occupational Safety and Health (CEOSH). (2016). *Safe patient handling and mobility guidebook*. http://www.tnpatientsafety.com/pubfiles/Initiatives/workplace-violence/sphm-pdf.pdf

Volkow, N. D., & McLellan, A. T. (2016). Opioid abuse in chronic pain – Misconceptions and mitigation strategies. *The New England Journal of Medicine*, *374*(13), 1253–1263. https://www.nejm.org/doi/full/10.1056/nejmra1507771

Wagner, B., Steiner, M., Huber, D., & Crevenna, R. (2021). The effect of biofeedback interventions on pain, overall symptoms, quality of life and physiological parameters in patients with pelvic pain: A systematic review. *Wiener Klinische Wochenschrift*, *134*(Supp 1), 11–48. https://doi.org/10.1007/s00508-021-01827-w

Warden, V., Hurley, A. C., & Volicer, L. (2003). Development and psychometric evaluation of the Pain Assessment in Advanced Dementia (PAINAD) scale. *Journal of American Medical Directors Association*, *4*(1), 9–15. https://doi.org/10.1097/01.JAM.0000043422.31640.F7

Ware, L. J., Herr, K. A., Booker, S. S., Dotson, K., Key, J., Poindexter, N., Pyles, G., Siler, B., & Packard, A. (2015). Psychometric evaluation of the Revised Iowa Pain Thermometer (IPT-R) in a sample of diverse cognitively intact and impaired older adults: A pilot study. *Pain Management Nursing*, *16*(4), 475–482. https://doi.org/10.1016/j.pmn.2014.09.004

Weaver, M. (2017). Healing touch: Positively sharing energy in a pediatric hospital. *Journal of Pain and Symptom Management*, *54*(2), 259–261. https://doi.org/10.1016/j.jpainsymman.2016.12.340

Westman, K. F., & Blaisdell, C. (2016). Many benefits, little risk: The use of massage in nursing practice. *The American Journal of Nursing*, *116*(1), 34–39; quiz 40-41. https://doi.org/10.1097/01.NAJ.0000476164.97929.f2

Wirz, Seidensticker, S., & Shtrichman, R. (2021). Patient-controlled analgesia (PCA): Intravenous administration (IV-PCA) versus oral administration (Oral-PCA) by using a novel device (PCoA® Acute) for hospitalized patients with acute postoperative pain—A comparative retrospective study. *Pain Research & Management*, *2021*, 1–11. https://doi.org/10.1155/2021/2542010

Wolters Kluwer. (2020). Problem-based care plans. In *Lippincott Advisor*. Retrieved March 28, 2021, from https://advisor.lww.com/lna/home.do

Wong, J., & Lim, S. S. T. (2018). Epidural analgesia in a paediatric teaching hospital: Trends, developments, and a brief review of literature. *Proceedings of Singapore Healthcare*, *27*(1), 49–54. https://doi.org/10.1177/2010105817733997

World Health Organization (WHO). (2019, January). *WHO guidelines for the pharmacological and radiotherapeutic management of cancer pain in adults and adolescents*. https://www.who.int/publications/i/item/9789241550390

World Health Organization (WHO). (2021). *Guidelines on the management of chronic pain in children: Executive summary*. World Health Organization. https://www.who.int/publications/i/item/9789240021556

Yaster, M., McNaull, P. P., & Davis, P. J. (2020). The opioid epidemic in pediatrics: A 2020 update. *Current Opinion in Anaesthesiology*, *33*(3), 327–334. https://doi.org/10.1097/ACO.0000000000000865

Zelaya, C. E., Dahlhamer, J. M., Lucas, J. W., Connor, E. M. (2020, November 4). *Chronic pain and high-impact chronic pain among U.S. adults, 2019*. National Center for Health Statistics. https://www.cdc.gov/nchs/products/databriefs/db390.htm

37 Nutrition

Susan Oakland

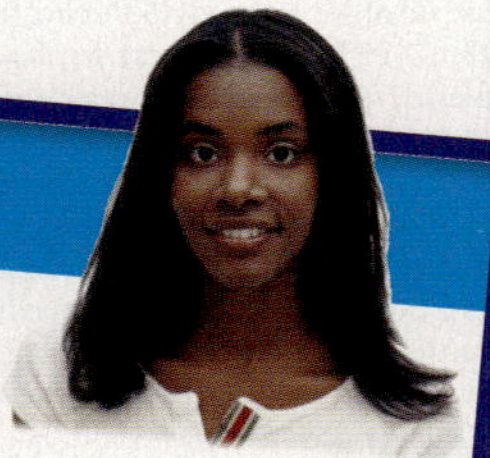

Susan Oakland, a 21-year-old student, is pregnant with her first child. Susan is in the ninth week of her pregnancy. She is experiencing persistent nausea, vomiting, and fatigue. She has had difficulty eating, with a resulting weight loss of 3 lb since her first prenatal visit at 5 weeks' gestation.

William Johnston

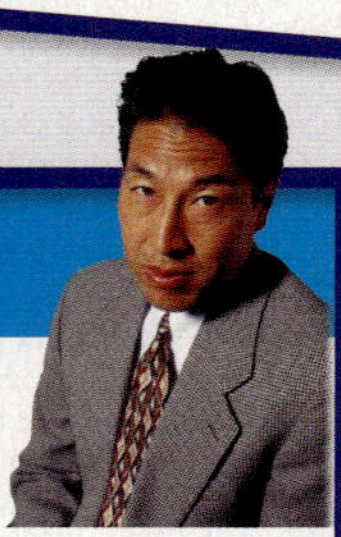

William Johnston, a 42-year-old executive, is newly diagnosed with high blood pressure and high cholesterol. He confides that his health has been the last thing on his mind and that his health habits are less than admirable. "I usually eat on the run, often fast food, or big dinners with lots of alcohol. I can't remember the last time I worked out or did any exercise, unless running from my car to the train counts! I guess it's no wonder I've gained a few pounds over the years!"

Charles Gallagher

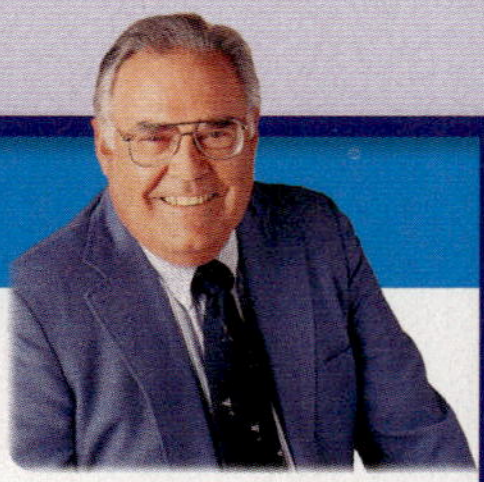

Charles Gallagher is the husband of a 67-year-old woman, Claire, who is in the end stages of advanced dementia. Mrs. Gallagher had a percutaneous endoscopic gastrostomy (PEG) inserted during her last hospitalization 6 weeks ago due to recurrent episodes of aspiration pneumonia from an inability to swallow. Mr. Gallagher states, "I was talking to the chaplain (here, at the long-term care facility) and he questioned the wisdom of this tube. I respect him but we really don't have an option here, do we? I mean, if they take the tube out, she'll starve to death—right?"

Lippincott DocuCare **Additional patient scenarios available in *Lippincott DocuCare*.**

Learning Outcomes

After completing the chapter, you will be able to accomplish the following:

1. Identify six classes of nutrients, explaining the significance of each.
2. Identify risk factors for poor nutritional status.
3. Describe how nutrition influences growth and development throughout the life cycle.
4. Discuss the components of a nutritional assessment.
5. Formulate diagnoses/patient problems that related to nutrition amenable to nursing intervention.
6. Describe nursing interventions to help patients achieve their nutritional goals.
7. Plan, implement, and evaluate nursing care relate to actual and potential health problems and needs associated with alterations in and related to nutrition.
8. Identify nursing interventions to safely deliver enteral nutrition.
9. Identify nursing interventions to safely deliver parenteral nutrition.

Nursing Concepts

- Assessment
- Clinical Decision Making/Clinical Judgment
- Metabolism
- Nutrition
- Safety

Good nutrition is vital for life and health. Poor nutrition can seriously decrease a person's level of wellness, which makes nutrition a vital component of nursing. This chapter provides information about the basic principles of nutrition, focusing on nutrients, energy balance, choices for an adequate diet, and factors affecting nutrition. In addition, components of simple screening and nutritional assessments are outlined. Potential and actual health problems and needs are provided, and patient outcomes for healthy nutrition are discussed. The accompanying Evolving Case Study 37-1 on page 1441 provides an opportunity to develop and apply clinical reasoning and clinical judgment skills. The dietician is the primary nutrition authority, but optimal nutrition care requires collaboration among all health care team professionals (Dudek, 2022). Nurses incorporate nutrition into all aspects of thoughtful, person-centered nursing care and are involved in all aspects of nutritional care. Refer to the accompanying Reflective Practice box on page 1390.

PRINCIPLES OF NUTRITION

The science of **nutrition** is the study of the intake of food and how food nourishes the body. It encompasses the study of nutrients and how they are handled by the body as well as the impact of human behavior and environment on related to food choices and the process of nourishment. As such, nutrition involves chemistry, biology/physiology, psychology, and socioeconomics. Nutrition and health are closely related (U.S. Department of Health and Human Services [DHHS] & U.S. Department of Agriculture [USDA], 2020).

Food is a complex mix of essential and nonessential nutrients (Dudek, 2022). **Nutrients** are specific biochemical substances used by the body for growth, development, activity, reproduction, lactation, health maintenance, and recovery from illness or injury. The metabolic processes involved in these functions are complex. Subsequently, most nutrients work better together than they do alone. Nutrient needs change throughout the life cycle in response to changes in body size, activity, growth, development, and state of health.

Some nutrients are considered *essential* because either they are not synthesized in the body or are made in insufficient amounts. Essential nutrients must be provided in the diet or through supplements. Essential nutrients that supply energy and build tissue (such as carbohydrates, fats, protein) are referred to as *macronutrients. Micronutrients,* such as vitamins and minerals, are required in much smaller amounts to regulate and control body processes.

Nonessential nutrients do not have to be supplied through dietary sources because they either are not required for body functioning or are synthesized in the body in adequate amounts. Some nutrients can be converted to others in the body. For instance, the body converts excess carbohydrates and protein into fat and stores them as triglycerides.

Of the six classes of nutrients, three supply energy (carbohydrates, protein, lipids [fats]) and three are needed to regulate body processes (vitamins, minerals, water).

Current dietary guideline recommendations integrate findings from scientific research, food pattern modeling, and analysis of current intake of the U.S. population (U.S. DHHS & USDA, 2020). Foods are not consumed in isolation, but in various combinations over time, generating an eating pattern (dietary pattern) (U.S. DHHS & USDA, 2020). Dietary patterns are the combination of foods and beverages that make up an individual's dietary intake over time (U.S. DHHS & USDA, 2020). Eating patterns are recognized as having an important role in nutrition; dietary patterns, including nutrient density and diet quality, are linked to health promotion and prevention of disease (Dudek, 2022). Healthy eating patterns are associated with positive healthy outcomes and meet Recommended Dietary Allowances (RDA) and Adequate Intakes for essential nutrients (U.S. DHHS & USDA, 2020). Healthy eating patterns are discussed later in the chapter in the Adequate Diet Selection section on page 1397.

Energy Balance

The body needs energy to function. Energy is derived or obtained from foods consumed. Energy in the diet is measured in the form of kilocalories, commonly abbreviated as calories, or cal. Only carbohydrates, protein, and fat provide energy. Vitamins and minerals, needed for the metabolism of energy, do not provide calories.

QSEN Reflective Practice: Cultivating QSEN Competencies

CHALLENGE TO LEGAL AND ETHICAL SKILLS

Mrs. Constance Gallagher is only 67 years old, but she is in the end stages of advanced dementia. She can no longer swallow and has had several hospitalizations in the past year for aspiration pneumonia. She lives in a long-term care facility (where I am doing a clinical rotation for my gerontologic nursing experience) and has a devoted family—husband, son, and daughter—who all visit regularly. For the last 6 weeks, she has received enteral feedings from a percutaneous endoscopic gastrostomy (PEG) tube that was placed during her last hospitalization. Mrs. Gallagher's husband confided to me that the chaplain at the long-term care facility, whom he respects and likes, questioned the wisdom of the feeding tube. He then asked me, "But we really don't have an option here, do we? I mean, if they take the tube out, she'll starve to death, no?" I had no idea how to respond.

Thinking Outside the Box: Possible Courses of Action

- Simply refer Mr. Gallagher to someone more experienced about these things (since I am clearly over my head).
- Find out more about this myself and then get back to him.
- Request an ethics consult to explore how we can best respond to the husband's questions about what is in his wife's best interests, taking into consideration the role the long-term care facility's chaplain is playing.

Evaluating a Good Outcome: How Do I Define Success?

- The patient's health goals are met, including, if the family/caregiver wishes, a dignified death.
- The Gallagher family feels at peace with their decisions and the results of these decisions.
- An ethically justified decision is made about continuing or withdrawing artificial nutrition and hydration that is respectful of Mrs. Gallagher's wishes (to the extent that these are known) and compatible with her beliefs and interests.
- I develop skill in assisting with tough end-of-life decisions and learn more about how an ethics consult functions.

Personal Learning: Here's to the Future!

When I reported my exchange with Mr. Gallagher to the charge nurse, she said we might want to call an ethics consult because there were actually a few similar situations pending and not everyone on the unit seemed comfortable with the lead role the chaplain was taking in recommending the withdrawal of nutritional support.

The consult was a great experience. All of the patient's family members attended, plus the medical director of the home, the nurses on the patient's unit, the chaplain, the social worker, the long-term care facility's ethicist, and myself. After the medical director described the natural progression of advanced dementia, the ethicist noted that there is a difference between dying of starvation (which only happens if food is withdrawn but fluids continue to hydrate) and dying of dehydration (which will happen if we pull the PEG tube and discontinue all enteral feedings, and which is not believed to be painful). The ethicist then asked the family if they knew how the patient would respond if she could be asked if the benefits of continuing nutritional support outweighed the accompanying burdens of having her wrists restrained so she wouldn't pull out the tube, skin problems, and the like. After some discussion, they were in agreement that she would not want to live this way. Since the Gallaghers were Catholic, the Catholic chaplain was invited to describe what the Roman Catholic Church teaches about this. After a rather lengthy discussion, a decision was made to withdraw enteral feedings. The family seemed at peace with their decision.

Through this experience, I learned how an ethics consult works and can see the advantages of utilizing this resource in the future.

QSEN SELF-REFLECTION ON QUALITY AND SAFETY COMPETENCIES DEVELOPING KNOWLEDGE, SKILLS, AND ATTITUDES FOR CONTINUOUS IMPROVEMENT

How do you think you would respond in a similar situation? Why? What does this tell you about yourself and about the adequacy of your skills for professional practice? Do you agree with the criteria that the nursing student used to evaluate a successful outcome? Are there any other criteria that would be appropriate to use? Did the nursing student meet the criteria? Why or why not? What *knowledge, skills,* and *attitudes* do you need to develop to continuously improve the quality and safety of care for patients like Mrs. Gallagher?

Patient-Centered Care: What resources could you or the nurses offer to provide compassionate and coordinated care based on respect for the patient's preferences, values, and needs? How did the ethics consult facilitate decision making? What ethical and legal principles were maintained? How did the nursing student act as a patient advocate? Was the human dignity of the patient and the patient's family maintained?

Teamwork and Collaboration/Quality Improvement: What communication skills do you need to improve to ensure that you function as a member of the patient-care team? What skills do you need to implement effective strategies for communicating and resolving conflict? What skills do you need to assert your own position/perspective in discussions about patient care? What other services or resources might be available to aid in this type of decision-making process?

Safety/Evidence-Based Practice: What skills do you need to improve to ensure that patients in your care receive the best nursing care possible? What evidence in nursing literature provides guidance for decision making regarding care of this patient?

Informatics: Can you identify the essential information that must be available in Mrs. Gallagher's electronic health record to support safe patient care and coordination of care? Can you identify the appropriate process to protect confidentiality of protected health information in the patient's health records? Can you think of other ways to respond to or approach the situation?

Energy in the body is used to carry on any kind of activity, whether voluntary or involuntary. A person's total daily energy expenditure is the sum of all the calories used to perform physical activity, maintain basal metabolism, and digest, absorb, and metabolize food.

Total energy intake for a meal, a day, or longer can be calculated using food composition tables. The values given for total calories for each food item eaten can simply be added, or the grams of carbohydrate, protein, and fat for each food item eaten can be added and multiplied by the appropriate calorie level (4, 4, and 9 calories, respectively). If a person's daily energy intake is equal to total daily energy expenditure, the person's weight will remain stable. However, if the energy intake is less than the energy expended, the person's weight will decrease. If the energy intake exceeds energy expenditure, weight will increase. Healthy body weight is achieved by balancing calorie intact with calorie expenditure (Dudek, 2022).

Metabolic Requirements

Basal metabolism (**basal metabolic rate [BMR]**) is the energy (number of calories) required to fuel the involuntary activities of the body at rest after a 12-hour fast—the energy needed to sustain the metabolic activities of cells and tissues (Dudek, 2022; Hinkle et al., 2022; Norris, 2020). These activities include actions such as maintaining body temperature and muscle tone, producing and releasing secretions, propelling food through the gastrointestinal (GI) tract, inflating the lungs, and contracting the heart muscle. Sex assigned at birth impacts BMR; men usually have a greater proportion of muscle mass than women of the same age and weight, resulting in a higher BMR (MFMER, 2020d). The less active a person is, the greater the proportion of calories used for BMR (Dudek, 2022).

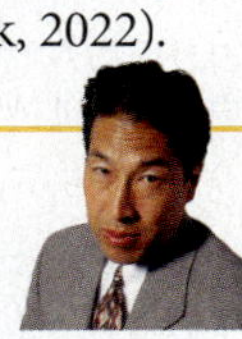

Think back to **William Johnston**, the middle-aged man with hypertension and high cholesterol. Based on the patient's sex assigned at birth, the nurse would anticipate his BMR may be greater than that for a woman. The nurse would need to consider this fact when planning the patient's care.

Other factors that increase BMR include growth, infections, fever, emotional tension, extreme environmental temperatures, and elevated levels of certain hormones, especially epinephrine and thyroid hormones. Aging, prolonged fasting, and sleep all decrease BMR. Fasting or following a very–low-calorie diet may defeat a weight-loss plan because the body interprets this eating pattern as starvation and compensates by slowing down the resting metabolic rate, making it even more difficult to lose weight.

Body Weight Standards

As previously discussed, if a person's energy intake does not equal energy expenditure, weight will fluctuate. Healthy body weight (ideal body weight [IBW]) is an estimate of optimal weight for optimal health. Height and weight tables are commonly used for infants and children. However, the preferred methods to establish weight status include body mass index (BMI) for adults and children and measurement of waist circumference for adults (NHBLI, n.d.a).

BODY MASS INDEX

The **body mass index (BMI)** is a ratio of weight (in kilograms) to height (in meters squared). The BMI provides an estimate of body fat and can be used as an initial assessment of nutritional status. BMI can be calculated with a mathematical formula but is more conveniently determined using a BMI table. One such table from the National Heart, Lung, and Blood Institute (NHLBI, n.d.c) can be accessed at https://www.nhlbi.nih.gov/health/educational/lose_wt/BMI/bmi_tbl.htm. An online calculator is also available from the NHLBI (n.d.e) at https://www.nhlbi.nih.gov/health/educational/lose_wt/BMI/bmicalc.htm. According to the BMI guidelines published by the NHLBI (n.d.b), a person with a BMI below 18.5 is underweight, a BMI of 18.5 to 24.9 is a healthy weight, a BMI of 25 to 29.9 indicates an overweight person, a BMI of 30 to 39.9 indicates **obesity**, and a BMI of 40 or greater indicates extreme obesity.

BMI also provides an estimation of relative risk for diseases that can occur with more body fat, such as heart disease, type 2 diabetes, hypertension, and certain cancers (NHLBI, n.d.d). However, it is important to note that BMI may not be accurate for certain groups of people, such as athletes, people with a muscular build, people with edema or dehydration, and older people and others who have lost muscle mass (Dudek, 2022; NHLBI, n.d.d). In addition, ethnic differences exist in the relationship between BMI and health risks (Tinajero et al., 2021).

Overweight and obesity are defined differently for children and teens than for adults. Children are still growing, and boys and girls mature at different rates. BMIs for children and teens compare their heights and weights against growth charts that take age and sex assigned at birth into account. This is called BMI-for-age percentile. A child or teen's BMI-for-age percentile shows how the individual's BMI compares with children of the same age and biologic sex (NHLBI, n.d.a). Additional information about BMI-for-age and growth charts for children ages 2 through 19 years can be found at the BMI-for-age calculator from the Centers for Disease Control and Prevention (CDC, 2020a). Refer to Box 37-1 for information to interpret the results of a BMI-for-age calculation.

Box 37-1 BMI-for-Age Percentile (Children and Teens)

Percentile Range	Weight Status Category
Less than 5th percentile	Underweight
5th percentile to less than the 85th percentile	Healthy weight
85th percentile to less than the 95th percentile	Overweight
95th percentile or greater	Obese

Source: Centers for Disease Control and Prevention (CDC). (2018, July 3). *Overweight & obesity. Defining childhood obesity. BMI for children and teens.* https://www.cdc.gov/obesity/childhood/defining.html

A significant intentional or unintentional change in the patient's weight can also indicate poor nutritional status and/or health problems. Most clinical screening tools include content addressing recent weight loss, current BMI, recent food intake, and disease severity (Reber et al., 2019).

BODY FAT DISTRIBUTION

Where excess body fat is deposited is thought to be an important and reliable indicator of risk for disease, such as type 2 diabetes, hypertension, stroke, dyslipidemia, and cardiovascular disease (Ashwell & Gibson, 2014; CDC, 2020b). Central or abdominal obesity (centrally located distribution of fat) poses greater risk for cardiovascular disease and diabetes (Johns Hopkins Medicine, 2021). **Waist circumference** is a good indicator of abdominal fat. Waist circumference is measured by placing a measuring tape snugly around the patient's waist, just above the hipbones (CDC, 2020b) (Fig. 37-1). Risk increases with a waist measurement of 40 inches or more for men and 35 inches or more for women (NHLBI, n.d.d). As with BMI, ethnic groups differ in regard to where risk begins in relation to waist circumference (Dudek, 2022). Table 37-1 displays the relationship of the risks of obesity-associated diseases and conditions by BMI and waist circumference. Waist-to-hip ratio (WHR) is another screening tool to identify central obesity. The WHR is calculated by dividing the patient's waist circumference by the hip circumference (Maastricht University Medical Center, 2020). Females should have a waist-to-hip ratio of <0.8 and males <0.95 (Maastricht University Medical Center, 2020).

Caloric Requirements

Just as healthy body weight or IBW can be determined in a variety of ways, so can a person's calorie requirements. The total number of calories a person needs each day

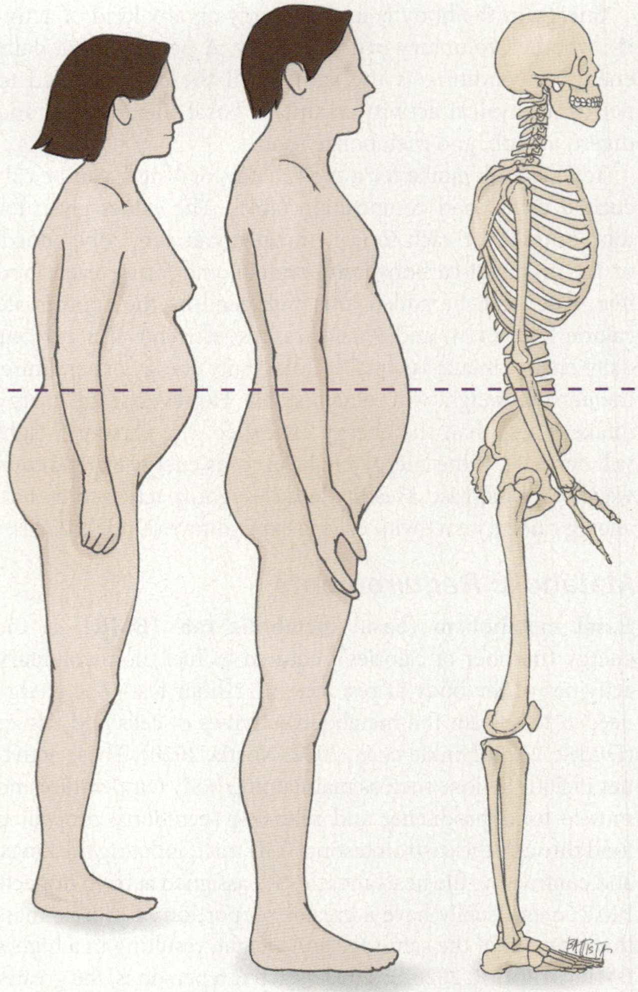

FIGURE 37-1. Positioning of measuring tape at the level of the umbilicus for waist circumference.

Table 37-1 Classification of Overweight and Obesity by Body Mass Index, Waist Circumference, and Associated Disease Risks

	BODY MASS INDEX (BMI) (kg/m^2)	DISEASE RISK[a] RELATIVE TO NORMAL WEIGHT AND WAIST CIRCUMFERENCE	
		Men ≤40 inches (102 cm) Women ≤35 inches (88 cm)	Men >40 inches (102 cm) Women >35 inches (88 cm)
Underweight	<18.5	–	–
Normal	18.5–24.9	–	–
Overweight	25.0–29.9	Increased	High
Obesity (Class I)	30.0–34.9	High	Very high
(Class II)	35.0–39.9	Very high	Very high
Extreme obesity (Class III)	40.0[b]	Extremely high	Extremely high

[a]Disease risk for type 2 diabetes, hypertension, and CVD.

[b]Increased waist circumference also can be a marker for increased risk, even in persons of normal weight.

Source: National Heart, Lung, and Blood Institute (NHLBI). (n.d.b). *Aim for a health weight. Classification of overweight and obesity by BMI, waist circumference, and associated disease risks.* Retrieved September 26, 2020, from https://www.nhlbi.nih.gov/health/educational/lose_wt/BMI/bmi_dis.htm

varies depending on multiple factors, including the person's age, sex, height, weight, and level of physical activity (U.S. DHHS & USDA, 2020). A need to lose, maintain or gain weight also influences the total number of calories that should be consumed. The *Dietary Guidelines for Americans 2020–2025* (U.S. DHHS & USDA, 2020) provides estimated amounts of calories needed to maintain calorie balance based on age, sex assigned at birth, level of physical activity, using average reference heights and weights for each age-sex group. Estimated ranges are provided in Appendix 2 of the 2020–2025 Dietary Guidelines and can be accessed at https://www.dietaryguidelines.gov/.

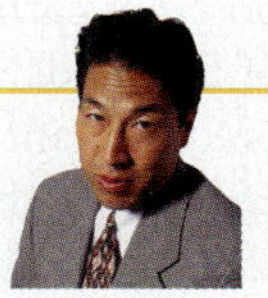

Consider **William Johnston**, the man with poor health habits. The nurse would work with Mr. Johnston and the registered dietician to develop an appropriate weight-loss plan that would contain adequate calories yet still foster a weight loss of 1 to 2 lb/wk. Doing so would promote weight loss while still allowing for adequate nutritional intake.

Energy Nutrients

Carbohydrates, protein, and fats are potential sources of energy for the body.

Carbohydrates

Carbohydrates, commonly known as sugars and starches, are organic compounds composed of carbon, hydrogen, and oxygen. They serve as the structural framework of plants. The only animal source of carbohydrate in the diet is lactose, the sugar present in milk.

Carbohydrates are relatively easy to produce and store, making them the most abundant and least expensive source of calories in the diet worldwide. In countries where grains are the dietary staple, carbohydrates may contribute as much as 90% of total calories. Carbohydrate intake is often correlated to income. As income increases, carbohydrate intake decreases and protein intake, a more expensive form of energy, increases (Kim et al., 2020; Seidelmann et al., 2018). Refer to this text's online resources to view a table that summarizes the sources, functions, and significance of dietary carbohydrates.

CLASSIFICATION AND METABOLISM

The number of molecules within the structure determines the classification of carbohydrates. They are classified as simple (monosaccharide and disaccharide) or complex (polysaccharide) sugars.

Carbohydrates are more easily and quickly digested than protein and fat. Ninety percent of carbohydrate intake is digested. This percentage decreases as fiber intake increases. All carbohydrates are converted to glucose for transport through the blood or for use as energy. Glucose is an efficient fuel that certain tissues, particularly the central nervous system, rely on almost exclusively for energy. Glucose is transported from the GI tract, through the portal vein, to the liver. The liver stores glucose and regulates its entry into the blood. Hormones, especially insulin and glucagon, are responsible for keeping serum glucose levels fairly constant during both feasting and fasting.

Through a series of steps, cells oxidize (burn) glucose to provide energy, carbon dioxide, and water. Depending on a person's state of energy balance, the period between when a carbohydrate is consumed and when it is used for energy may vary from minutes to months or longer. Unlike protein and fat, glucose is burned efficiently and completely and does not leave a toxic product for the kidneys to excrete.

When the supply of glucose exceeds what is needed for energy and for maintaining serum levels, it is stored. If muscle or liver glycogen stores are deficient, glucose is converted to glycogen and stored (glycogenesis). Conversely, glycogen is broken down in time of need to supply a ready source of glucose (glycogenolysis). When glycogen stores are adequate, the body converts excess glucose to fat and stores it as triglycerides in adipose tissue.

FUNCTIONS AND RECOMMENDED DIETARY INTAKE

The primary function of carbohydrates is to supply energy. Except for indigestible fiber, all carbohydrates provide 4 calories per gram, regardless of the source. It is recommended that carbohydrates provide 45% to 65% of total calories for adults, focusing on complex carbohydrates, such as whole grains (U.S. DHHS & USDA, 2020). Sugars added to foods supply calories but few or no nutrients and should be limited. The online Dietary Reference Intake calculator for Healthcare Professionals provides a means to calculate daily nutrient recommendations, including carbohydrates, based on the Dietary Reference Intakes (DRIs) and is available at https://www.nal.usda.gov/fnic/dri-calculator/ (USDA & NAL, n.d.a). Refer to the discussion of DRIs on page 1397.

Protein

Protein is a vital component of every living cell. Within the human body, more than 1,000 different proteins are made by combining various amounts and proportions of the 22 basic building blocks known as amino acids. Proteins are required for the formation of all body structures, including genes, enzymes, muscle, bone matrix, skin, and blood. Refer to this text's online resources to view a table that summarizes the sources, functions, and significance of dietary protein.

CLASSIFICATION AND METABOLISM

Dietary proteins may be labeled complete (high quality) or incomplete (low quality), based on their amino acid composition. Complete proteins contain sufficient amounts and proportions of all the essential amino acids to support growth, whereas incomplete proteins are deficient in one or more essential amino acids. In general, animal proteins (eggs, dairy products, meats) are complete, and plant proteins (grains, legumes, vegetables) are incomplete. There are some plant exceptions; soy and quinoa, for example, are plant proteins that are considered complete proteins (Cedars Sinai, 2019). Because different sources of plant proteins lack different amino acids, a plant protein can be complemented by combining it with a different plant protein or by adding a small amount of an animal protein to supply a complete protein. Examples of complementary vegetable proteins include corn tortilla with refried beans and lentil rice soup. Complementary proteins that use a small amount of animal protein include cereal with milk, rice pudding, and a cheese sandwich. It is not necessary to eat complementary proteins at the same meal; eating a variety of proteins throughout the day will achieve adequate protein intake (Dudek, 2022).

Concept Mastery Alert

Complete protein = animal protein *or* plant protein + small amount of animal protein or two complementary vegetable proteins.

Dietary protein is broken down into amino acid particles by pancreatic enzymes in the small intestine. These are absorbed through the intestinal mucosa to be transported to the liver. In the liver, amino acids are recombined into new proteins or are released into the bloodstream for use in protein synthesis by tissues and cells. Excess amino acids are converted to fatty acids, ketone bodies, or glucose and are stored or used as metabolic fuel.

The body's protein tissues are in a constant state of flux. Tissues are continuously being broken down (catabolism) and replaced (anabolism). Nitrogen balance, a comparison between catabolism and anabolism, can be measured by comparing nitrogen intake (protein intake) and nitrogen excretion (nitrogen lost in urine, urea, feces, hair, nails, skin). When catabolism and anabolism are occurring at the same rate, as in healthy adults, the body is in a state of neutral nitrogen balance (i.e., nitrogen intake equals nitrogen excretion). A positive nitrogen balance occurs when nitrogen intake is greater than excretion, and indicates tissue growth—for example, during childhood, pregnancy, lactation, and recovery from illness. A negative nitrogen balance occurs when more nitrogen is excreted than is ingested, and indicates tissue is breaking down faster than it is being replaced. This undesirable state occurs in situations such as starvation and the catabolism that immediately follows surgery, illness, trauma, and stress. This can result in the wasting of muscle tissue as it is converted to glucose for energy.

FUNCTIONS AND RECOMMENDED DIETARY INTAKE

The major function of protein is to maintain body tissues that break down from normal wear and tear and to support the growth of new tissue. Using protein for energy is more expensive both financially and physiologically than using carbohydrates. The nitrogen remaining after protein is metabolized burdens the kidneys. In addition, energy must be used to excrete the nitrogen. Like carbohydrates, protein consumed in excess of need can be converted to and stored as fat. Protein intake should contribute 10% to 35% of total caloric intake for healthy adults and include a variety of protein foods (U.S. DHHS & USDA, 2020). The online Dietary Reference Intake calculator for Healthcare Professionals provides a means to calculate daily nutrient recommendations, including protein, based on the Dietary Reference Intakes (DRIs) and is available at https://www.nal.usda.gov/fnic/dri-calculator/ (USDA & NAL, n.d.a). Refer to the discussion of DRIs on page 1397.

Fats

Fats in the diet, or lipids, are insoluble in water and, therefore, insoluble in blood. Like carbohydrates, they are composed of carbon, hydrogen, and oxygen. Ninety-five percent of the lipids in the diet are in the form of triglycerides, the predominant form of fat in food and the major storage form of fat in the body. Compound lipids (such as phospholipids, in which a lipid is combined with another substance) and derived lipids (such as cholesterol) constitute the remainder of the lipids ingested. Refer to this text's online resources to view a table that summarizes the sources, functions, and significance of dietary fat.

CLASSIFICATION AND METABOLISM

Food fats contain mixtures of saturated and unsaturated fatty acids. The difference in degree of saturation depends on the amount of hydrogen in fat molecules. Saturated fats contain more hydrogen than unsaturated fats. Most animal fats are considered saturated and have a solid consistency at room temperature. Conversely, most vegetable fats are considered unsaturated, remain liquid at room temperature, and are referred to as oils. Saturated fats tend to raise serum cholesterol levels, whereas unsaturated fats lower serum cholesterol levels. Trans fats (trans-fatty acids) are a form of dietary fat that raise LDL ("bad") cholesterol and lower HDL ("good") cholesterol (MFMER, 2020a). Naturally occurring trans fats are produced by some animals and small amounts of these trans fats made be present in some meat (e.g., beef, lamb) and dairy products (e.g., milk) (American Heart Association, 2017). Most of the trans fat in food is formed when manufacturers partially hydrogenate vegetable (liquid; PHO) oils to solidify the oil and increase stability at room temperature and are found in many manufactured foods (American Heart Association, 2017; MFMER, 2020a). Eating trans fats increases the risk of developing heart disease and stroke and is associated with a higher risk of developing type 2 diabetes (American Heart Association, 2017). Because consumption of trans fat is so unhealthy, the U.S. Food and Drug Administration (FDA) has prohibited food manufacturers from adding major sources of artificial trans fat to foods and beverages, in an attempt to prevent the risks of cardiovascular and other associated diseases (U.S. FDA, 2018; MFMER, 2020a). Trans fats are listed on food nutrition labels so that consumers can make healthy choices in their diet. In the United States, a food with less than 0.5 g of trans fat in a serving can be identified as 0 g of trans fat (MFMER, 2020a).

Cholesterol is a fatlike substance found only in animal products. It is not an essential nutrient; the body makes sufficient amounts (Dudek, 2022). Cholesterol is an important component of cell membranes and is especially abundant in brain and nerve cells. It also is used to synthesize bile acids and is a precursor of the steroid hormones and vitamin D. Although cholesterol serves many important functions in the body, high serum levels are clearly associated with an increased risk for atherosclerosis. To help lower serum cholesterol levels, researchers recommend limiting cholesterol intake, eating less total fat—especially saturated and trans fat—eating more unsaturated fat, and increasing fiber intake, which increases fecal excretion of cholesterol.

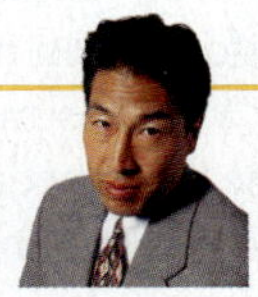

Remember **William Johnston**, the middle-aged executive with hypertension and high cholesterol? Due to Mr. Johnston's "on-the-run" lifestyle, developing an individualized nutritional plan might be somewhat challenging. Based on an assessment of Mr. Johnston's eating habits, likes, and dislikes, the nurse would work with him to develop a plan that promotes weight loss and includes limiting cholesterol and total fat intake and consuming more foods containing unsaturated fats and fiber. Adapting the plan will help to promote adherence to it, thereby increasing the chances for success.

Fat digestion occurs largely in the small intestine. Bile, secreted by the gallbladder, emulsifies fat to increase the surface area so that pancreatic lipase can break down fat more effectively. Through a complex series of events, most fats are absorbed into the lymphatic circulation with the help of a protein carrier and are transported to the liver. Almost all fat consumed is absorbed (about 95%) in the small intestine; a small amount is excreted in the feces (Dudek, 2022).

FUNCTIONS AND RECOMMENDED DIETARY INTAKE

Fats are the most concentrated source of energy in the diet, providing 9 calories for every gram. Fat increases the palatability of the diet (e.g., to most people, filet mignon tastes better than flank steak) and has a high satiety value because it delays gastric emptying time. In the body, fat aids in the **absorption** (the transfer of digested nutrients into the circulation) of the fat-soluble vitamins and provides insulation, structure, and temperature control. The *Dietary Guidelines for Americans 2020–2025* recommends that individuals should limit intake of saturated fats and trans fats, with less than 10% of calories per day from saturated fats and intake of trans fats to as low as possible (U.S. DHHS & USDA, 2020). The online Dietary Reference Intake calculator for Healthcare Professionals provides a means to calculate daily nutrient recommendations, including fats, based on the Dietary Reference Intakes (DRIs) and is available at https://www.nal.usda.gov/fnic/dri-calculator/ (USDA & NAL, n.d.a). Refer to the discussion of DRIs on page 1397.

Regulatory Nutrients

Vitamins, minerals, and water are regulatory nutrients. The body needs them for facilitation of the biochemical reactions within cells to regulate body processes, such as growth and metabolism (Dudek, 2022).

Vitamins

Vitamins are organic compounds needed by the body in small amounts. Most vitamins are active in the form of coenzymes, which, together with enzymes, facilitate thousands of chemical reactions in the body. Although vitamins do not provide energy (calories), they are needed for the metabolism of carbohydrates, protein, and fat. Vitamins are essential in the diet because most are not synthesized in the body or are made in insufficient quantities. The absence or insufficient use of vitamins in the body causes specific deficiency syndromes.

Vitamins are present in foods in only small amounts. Fresh foods are higher in vitamins than processed foods because vitamins may be destroyed by light, heat, air, and during preparation. The exception is when vitamins not naturally occurring in a food are added, such as vitamin D–fortified milk. This process is called fortification.

In the United States, severe vitamin deficiencies are uncommon. Mild or subclinical deficiencies of vitamin A, vitamin C, folate, and vitamin B_6, however, may affect a significant proportion of the population, especially those who (1) are members of certain age groups or patient groups (infants, adolescents, pregnant and lactating women, older people); (2) smoke, abuse alcohol, or use medications on a long-term basis; (3) are chronically ill, either physically or psychologically; or (4) are poor or finicky eaters, such as chronic dieters and food faddists.

Vitamins are classified as either water soluble or fat soluble. Water-soluble vitamins include vitamin C and the B-complex vitamins (ascorbic acid, thiamine, riboflavin, niacin, pyridoxine, biotin pantothenic acid, folate, and cobalamin). They are absorbed through the intestinal wall directly into the bloodstream. Although some tissues are able to hold limited amounts of water-soluble vitamins, they usually are not stored in the body. Deficiency symptoms are apt to develop quickly when intake is inadequate; therefore, a daily intake is recommended. However, because water-soluble vitamins are not stored, amounts consumed in excess of need are excreted in the urine. Toxicities are not likely, although megadoses of certain water-soluble vitamins can be harmful.

Vitamins A, D, E, and K, the fat-soluble vitamins, are absorbed with fat into the lymphatic circulation. Like fat, they must be attached to a protein to be transported through the blood. Secondary deficiencies of the fat-soluble vitamins can occur anytime fat digestion or absorption is altered, such as during malabsorption syndromes and pancreatic and biliary diseases. The body stores excesses of the fat-soluble vitamins mostly in the liver and adipose tissue. Because they are stored, a daily intake is not imperative and deficiency symptoms may take weeks, months, or years to develop. Excessive intake, particularly of vitamins A and D, is toxic.

Although scrutiny and research continue about vitamin supplements and their long-term effects, most nutritionists agree that vitamins will never be a substitute for good nutrition and healthy lifestyle practices (USDA & DHHS, 2020). The *Dietary Guidelines for Americans 2020–2025* (USDA & DHHS, 2020) recommends that nutrient needs be met primarily through consuming foods. However, although the majority of Americans consume sufficient amounts of most nutrients, some vitamins and other nutrients are consumed by many individuals in amounts below the Estimated Average Requirement or Adequate Intake levels (see discussion later in chapter) (USDA & DHHS, 2020). Low intake occurs due to low consumption of the food groups that contain these nutrients (USDA & DHHS, 2020). Supplements may be useful when they fill a specific identified nutrient gap that cannot or is not otherwise being met by the person's intake of food (Dudek, 2022; USDA & DHHS, 2020). Groups that may not be "well nourished" and may benefit from vitamin supplements include dieters consuming less than 1,200 calories/day, vegans, people with alcohol use disorder, older adults, people who are food insecure, and patients with chronic illness (Dudek, 2022, p. 116). Supplementation can also ensure adequate intakes of specific nutrients in patients with physiologic limitations or changes. For example, folate (folic acid) supplementation prior to conception and during pregnancy reduces the risk of neural tube defects (USDA & DHHS, 2020). Refer to this text's online resources to view a table that summarizes water- and fat-soluble vitamins

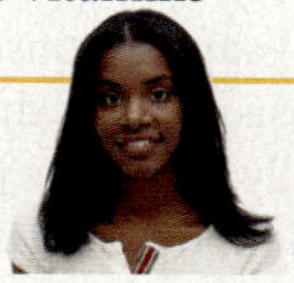

Think back to **Susan Oakland**, the young woman who is pregnant. She will be advised to take a daily multivitamin supplement as part of her prenatal care. Supplements are used in conjunction with an optimal diet to meet the increased nutrient requirements of pregnancy.

Minerals

Minerals are inorganic elements found in all body fluids and tissues in the form of salts (e.g., sodium chloride) or combined with organic compounds (e.g., iron in hemoglobin). Some minerals function to provide structure within the body, whereas others help to regulate body processes. Minerals, which are elements, are not broken down or rearranged in the body but, rather, are contained in the ash that remains after digestion. Excessive soaking and cooking in water can cause loss of minerals from food. However, minerals are commonly not destroyed by food processing.

Major minerals are present in the body in amounts greater than 5 g and include calcium, phosphorus (phosphates), sulfur (sulfate), sodium, chloride, potassium, and magnesium (Dudek, 2022). Trace elements are minerals present in the body in amounts less than 5 g; trace minerals ae not less important than major minerals and include iron, zinc, manganese, chromium, copper, molybdenum, selenium, fluoride, and iodine (Dudek, 2022). Refer to this text's online resources to view a table that summarizes the macrominerals and microminerals that have recommended intake guidelines.

Water

As the major body constituent present in every body cell, water accounts for between 50% and 60% of the adult's total weight. Infants have proportionately more water accounting for body weight. About two thirds of the body's water is contained within the cells (intracellular fluid [ICF]); the remainder is called extracellular fluid (ECF), which includes all other body fluids, such as plasma and interstitial fluid. Total body water and ECF decrease with age; ICF increases with an increase in body mass. Refer to Chapter 41 for more information on water in the body.

Water is more vital to life than food because it provides the fluid medium necessary for all chemical reactions, it participates in many reactions, and it is not stored in the body. Water acts as a solvent that dissolves many solutes, thereby aiding digestion, absorption, circulation, and excretion. Through evaporation from the skin, water helps to regulate body temperature. As a lubricant, water is needed both for mucous secretions and for movement between joints.

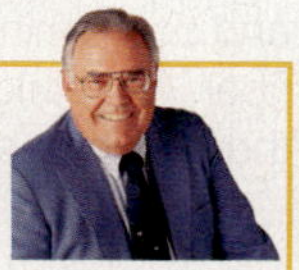

Think back to **Charles Gallagher**, husband of the woman with advanced dementia receiving enteral nutrition. During the group meeting about continuing or withdrawing the enteral nutrition, Mr. Gallagher learns that withdrawal of the feedings would also involve limited water intake. This information is important in helping Mr. Gallagher and his family arrive at an informed decision about whether to continue the enteral feedings.

Sources of water in the diet include not only beverages but also solid foods, which contain between 10% and 98% water. Water is also produced through the metabolism of carbohydrates, protein, and fat. It leaves the body through urine, feces, expired air, and perspiration. Water intake (an average of 2,600 mL/day for adults [Dudek, 2022]) usually equals water output. Water balance may be seriously affected when intake (such as in older adults or people in comatose states) or output (such as in patients with altered renal function, profuse perspiration, diarrhea, vomiting, fistulas, drainage tubes, hemorrhage, severe burns) is altered.

Digestion

The food consumed by a person supplies the essential nutrients needed for cells to perform their necessary functions, but the cells cannot use food in its consumed form. The GI system breaks down the food into particles small enough to pass into the cells and be used by the cells. This breakdown process is called **digestion**. Digestion begins in the mouth where food is taken in, mixes with saliva, is pushed into the pharynx by the tongue, and then continues into the esophagus. Peristalsis moves the food through the esophagus and into the stomach. The stomach churns the ingested food, mixing it with substances to break down the food and convert it to a semiliquid mixture. The food leaves the stomach and enters the small intestine. The small intestine

Box 37-2 Key Recommendations of the Dietary Guidelines for Americans 2020–2025

Consume a healthy eating pattern across the lifespan that accounts for nutrient-dense food and beverage choices to reflect personal preferences, cultural traditions, and budgetary considerations within an appropriate calorie level.

A healthy eating pattern includes:

- A variety of vegetables
- Fruits
- Grains, at least half of which are whole grains
- Fat-free or low-fat dairy
- A variety of protein foods
- Oils

A healthy eating pattern limits:

- Saturated fats, trans fats, added sugars, and sodium
- Calories/day from added sugars to less than 10%
- Calories/day from saturated fats to less than 10%
- Sodium to less than 2,300 mg/day
- Alcohol to moderate consumption

Guidelines for physical activity include:

- Engage in regular physical activity and reduce sedentary activities to promote health, psychological well-being, and a healthy body weight.
- To achieve and maintain a healthy body weight, adults should do the equivalent of 150 to 300 minutes of moderate-intensity aerobic activity each week. If necessary, adults should increase their weekly minutes of aerobic physical activity gradually over time and decrease calorie intake to a point at which they can achieve calorie balance and a healthy weight. Adults should also include muscle-strengthening activities, such as lifting weights or doing push-ups, at least 2 days each week.

Source: Adapted from U.S. Department of Health and Human Services & U.S. Department of Agriculture. (2020). *Dietary guidelines for Americans 2020–2025.* https://www.dietaryguidelines.gov/

secrets enzymes, which, along with secretions from the liver and pancreas, digest the food. The digested nutrients are then transferred into the person's circulation (absorption), to be transported throughout the body. Most absorption of digested food and minerals, and some absorption of water, occurs through the walls of the small intestine. Undigested waste materials continue through the GI tract and are eliminated. Elimination of these waste products is discussed in Chapter 39. Figure 39-1 on page 1519 illustrates the organs of the GI tract.

Adequate Diet Selection

An adequate diet provides a balanced intake of all essential nutrients in appropriate amounts. In the past, defining an adequate diet or healthy eating was less obvious and sometimes difficult. Tools for planning or evaluating a diet for adequacy include dietary recommendations and guidelines issued from health and U.S. governmental facilities, and the Dietary Reference Intakes (DRIs). The task of promoting health through proper nutrition has been made easier by labeling regulations that mandate specific information about food contents and their comparison to recommended daily intakes.

Dietary Recommendations

The *Dietary Guidelines for Americans* (USDA & DHHS, 2020) are science-based strategies compiled by the U.S. Department of Health and Human Services and the U.S. Department of Agriculture. A new edition of the *Guidelines* is published every 5 years to reflect current scientific knowledge and provide sound food-based guidance to promote health (USDA & DHHS, 2020). People are encouraged to choose a healthy eating pattern at an appropriate calorie level to help achieve and maintain a healthy body weight, support nutrient adequacy, and reduce the risk of chronic disease. Key recommendations of the *Dietary Guidelines for Americans* 2020–2025 appear in Box 37-2. The complete guidelines are available at https://www.dietaryguidelines.gov/ (USDA & DHHS, 2020).

Dietary Reference Intakes

The Dietary Reference Intakes (DRIs) provide recommended nutrient intakes that estimate nutrient intakes necessary to ensure that healthy populations meet nutrient needs to maintain health and prevent deficiency diseases (Institute of Medicine, 2006) and are viewed as an average daily intake over at least one week (Dudek, 2022). The DRIs are a set of reference values. The DRIs include:

- **Recommended Dietary Allowance (RDA)** is the average daily dietary intake of a nutrient that is sufficient to meet the requirement of nearly all (97% to 98%) healthy people.
- Adequate Intake (AI) for a nutrient is established when an RDA cannot be determined. Therefore, a nutrient either has an RDA or an AI. The AI is based on observed intakes of the nutrient by a group of healthy people.
- Tolerable Upper Intake Level (UL) is the highest daily intake of a nutrient that is likely to pose no risks of toxicity for almost all individuals. As intake above the UL increases, risk increases.
- Estimated Average Requirement (EAR) is the amount of a nutrient that is estimated to meet the requirement of half of all healthy people in the population.
- Chronic Disease Risk Reduction (CDRR) is the level above which intake reduction is expected to reduce chronic disease risk. At this time, sodium is the only nutrient to be assigned a CDRR (National Academies of Sciences, Engineering, and Medicine, 2019).

Each of these reference values distinguishes between biologic sex and different life stages, providing estimates of nutrient needs for healthy people. Links to information about the DRIs as well as other healthy eating resources can be found at https://www.nutrition.gov/topics/basic-nutrition/healthy-eating (USDA, n.d.a). The online Dietary Reference Intake calculator for Healthcare Professionals provides a means to calculate daily nutrient recommendations based on the Dietary Reference Intakes (DRIs) and is available at https://www.nal.usda.gov/fnic/dri-calculator/ (USDA & NAL, n.d.a).

MyPlate Food Guide

MyPlate food guidance graphic is part of a communication initiative based on the *Dietary Guidelines for Americans* to help consumers make better food choices to follow a healthy heating pattern across the lifespan (USDA & DHHS, 2020; USDA, n.d.b). MyPlate is designed to remind Americans to eat healthfully. MyPlate illustrates the five food groups using a familiar mealtime visual, a place setting (Fig. 37-2). The goals of the recommendations are to balance calories by encouraging consumers to enjoy food, but eat less, and avoid oversized portions. Consumers are also advised to increase the intake a variety of nutrient-dense foods across and within all food groups (USDA & DHHS, 2020). Consumers are encouraged to reduce sodium consumption by comparing sodium in foods such as soup, bread, and frozen meals and choose foods with lower numbers. MyPlate also encourages the consumption of water instead of sugary drinks.

The importance of activity and exercise are also emphasized, including the recommendations for children and adolescents to be physically active for 60 minutes or more a day and adults to engage in activity that requires moderate effort, such as brisk walking for 2 1/2 hours or more a week (USDA, n.d.b). Visitors to the website can personalize nutritional and physical activity plans, track foods consumed and physical activities, and get support to help make healthier choices. The ChooseMyPlate initiative also offers a free mobile app to help patients with daily food goals and track real-time progress (USDA, n.d.b). The MyPlate guidelines are available at https://www.choosemyplate.gov/ (USDA, n.d.b).

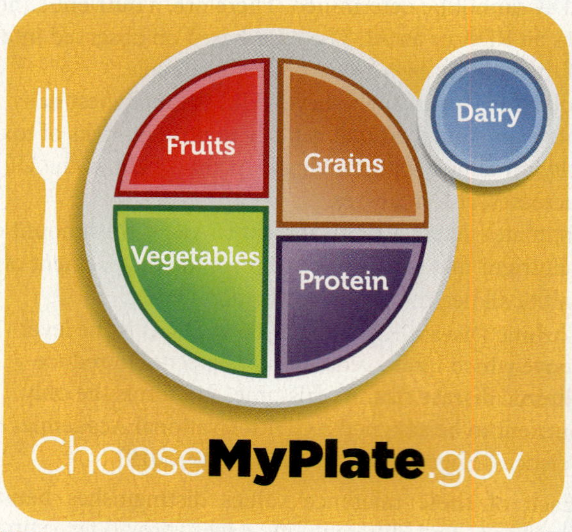

FIGURE 37-2. The MyPlate food guidance graphic. (*Source:* U.S. Department of Agriculture [USDA]. [n.d.]. https://www.choosemyplate.gov/)

Food Labeling

Food labels provide a significant amount of nutritional information for the consumer. Regulations that control food labels have always been controversial. In 1975, the FDA, a federal facility charged with protecting the U.S. food and drug supply, enacted legislation for a standardized label format that was considered a positive step toward educating the consumer about nutrition. Confusion and misinformation resulted as food manufacturers oversimplified or exaggerated health claims for their products. In 1990, Congress passed the Nutritional Labeling and Education Act, which required all foods, including fruits and vegetables, to be clearly labeled. Four broad categories are addressed in this legislation and include nutrition labeling, serving sizes, descriptors, and health claims. In 2006, labels were required to include information related to the amount of trans fat (trans-fatty acids) on nutrition fact labels. Consumers should be easily able to identify the serving size and servings per container; the calories per serving; the amount of total fat, saturated fat and trans fat; the amount of cholesterol and sodium; the total amount of carbohydrates, including dietary fiber and sugars (total sugars and added sugars); and the total amount of protein in the product (U.S. FDA, 2020c). The label also provides information related to vitamin D and potassium because Americans do not always get the recommended amounts (U.S. FDA, 2020c). Diets higher in vitamin D and potassium can reduce the risk of osteoporosis and high blood pressure, respectively (U.S. FDA, 2020c, para. 5). Calcium and iron are also included on the label because Americans do not always get the recommended amounts (U.S. FDA, 2020c). Diets higher in calcium and iron can reduce the risk of osteoporosis and anemia, respectively (U.S. FDA, 2020c, para 5). Figure 37-3 illustrates a sample label with explanation of terms. The food label is a tool to educate the public about nutrition and aid in making informed food decisions to choose a healthy diet (U.S. FDA, 2020b).

FACTORS AFFECTING NUTRITION

A person's food patterns and habits have a great impact on overall food intake. Food habits are a product of many evolving variables, such as physiologic and physical factors that influence nutrient requirements (e.g., stage of development, state of health, medications). Social determinants of health, the conditions (*economic stability, health care access* and quality, social and community context, education access and quality, neighborhood and built environments) in the environments in which people live their lives (U. S. Department of Health and Human Services. Office of Disease Prevention and Health Promotion, n.d.), culture, religion, food ideology (the meaning of food for an individual), and learned aversions also have an impact on food habits.

These variables alone or in combination also can affect food intake and overall nutrition.

Nutrition Facts

4 servings per container
Serving size 1 cup (227g)

Amount per serving	
Calories	**280**
	% Daily Value*
Total Fat 9g	**12%**
Saturated Fat 4.5g	**23%**
Trans Fat 0g	
Cholesterol 35mg	**12%**
Sodium 850mg	**37%**
Total Carbohydrate 34g	**12%**
Dietary Fiber 4g	**14%**
Total Sugars 6g	
Includes 0g Added Sugars	**0%**
Protein 15g	
Vitamin D 0mcg	0%
Calcium 320mg	25%
Iron 1.6mg	8%
Potassium 510mg	10%

* The % Daily Value (DV) tells you how much a nutrient in a serving of food contributes to a daily diet. 2,000 calories a day is used for general nutrition advice.

1. Serving Size

Serving sizes are standardized to make it easier to compare similar foods; they are provided in familiar units, such as cups or pieces, followed by the metric amount (e.g., the number of grams [g]). The serving size reflects the amount that people typically eat or drink. **It is not a recommendation of how much you should eat or drink.** It is important to realize that all the nutrient amounts shown on the label, including the number of calories, refer to the size of the serving. **Pay attention to the serving size, especially how many servings there are in the food package.**

2. Amount of Calories

Calories provide a measure of how much energy you get from a serving of this food. To achieve or maintain a healthy body weight, balance the number of calories you eat and drink with the number of calories your body uses: 2,000 calories a day is used as a general guide for nutrition advice. Your calorie needs may be higher or lower and vary depending on your age, sex, height, weight, and physical activity level. **The number of servings you consume determines the number of calories you actually eat.**

3. Get Enough of these Nutrients

Key nutrients that impact your health. You can use the label to support your personal dietary needs—look for foods that contain more of the nutrients you want to get more of and less of the nutrients you may want to limit. Saturated fat, sodium, and added sugars are nutrients listed on the label that may be associated with adverse health effects. They are identified as nutrients to get less of. Dietary fiber, vitamin D, calcium, iron ad potassium are nutrients on the label that are identified **as nutrients to get more of.** Eating a diet high in dietary fiber can increase the frequency of bowel movements, lower blood glucose and cholesterol levels, and reduce calorie intake. Diets higher in vitamin D, calcium, iron, and potassium can reduce the risk of developing osteoporosis, anemia, and high blood pressure.

4. Percent (%) Daily Value

4.The % Daily Value (%DV) is the percentage of the Daily Value for each nutrient in a serving of the food. The Daily Values are reference amounts (expressed in grams, milligrams, or micrograms) of nutrients to consume or not to exceed each day. The %DV shows how much a nutrient in a serving of a food contributes to a total daily diet. The %DV helps you determine if a serving of food is high or low in a nutrient.

FIGURE 37-3. Sample nutritional label with explanation of terms. (*Source:* U.S. Food and Drug Administration [FDA]. [2020, March 11]. *How to understand and use the nutrition facts label.* https://www.fda.gov/food/new-nutrition-facts-label/how-understand-and-use-nutrition-facts-label)

Physiologic and Physical Factors That Influence Nutrient Requirements

There are various reasons a person's nutrient requirements may differ. Some are permanent, such as chronic illness, whereas others are temporary, such as pregnancy.

Developmental Considerations

Throughout the life cycle, nutrient needs change in relation to growth, development, activity, and age-related changes in metabolism and body composition. Periods of intense growth and development, such as during infancy, adolescence, pregnancy, and lactation, cause an increase in nutrient needs. Nutrient needs stabilize during adulthood, although older people may need more or less of some nutrients. Age influences not only nutrient requirements, but also food intake. The consistency of food consumed, eating patterns, and the significance of food change with physical and psychosocial development.

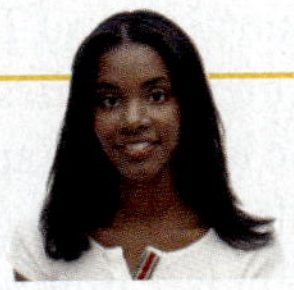

Remember **Susan Oakland**, the student who is pregnant, and William Johnston, the executive with hypertension and high cholesterol, described at the beginning of the chapter. The nurse would need to incorporate knowledge of each patient's developmental level when planning care.

INFANTS

The period from birth to age 1 year is the most rapid period of growth. Birth weight doubles in 4 to 6 months and triples by age 1 year. Length increases 50% in the first year. Muscle control and the development of hand–eye coordination allow the infant to progress to sitting upright and self-feeding. The iron stores present at birth start to become depleted between ages 3 and 4 months. The immune system matures between ages 4 and 6 months.

Nutritional needs per unit of body weight are greater during infancy and childhood than at any other developmental stage (Physicians Committee for Responsible Medicine, n.d.). Breastfeeding is recommended as the major source of nutrition for the first 6 to 12 months of life (NAPNAP, 2019). If the infant is not breastfed, the infant should receive one of the commercially prepared iron-fortified infant formulas. Cow's milk is not recommended for infants younger than age 1 year. Supplemental vitamins may be prescribed. In general, solid foods are not introduced before the infant is developmentally ready, usually at about age 6 months. At this age, the infant gains control of the head, neck, jaw, and tongue; develops hand–eye coordination; and the ability to sit, chew, and drink. New foods should be introduced one at a time for a period of 2 to 3 days so that any allergic reaction, such as rashes, fussiness, vomiting, diarrhea, or constipation, can be easily identified (Dudek, 2022). By age 1 year, infants should be eating a variety of table foods and various textures (Dudek, 2022). Iron-fortified foods are recommended (Dudek, 2022).

TODDLERS AND PRESCHOOLERS

There is continued growth and development during this stage, but the growth rate slows (Kyle & Carman, 2021). Mobility, autonomy, and coordination increase, as do muscle mass and bone density. Language skills improve, and the 3- to 5-year-old child also develops attitudes toward food.

Toddlers and preschoolers can feed themselves, verbalize food likes and dislikes, and occasionally use food to manipulate their parents (Fig. 37-4). Appetite dramatically decreases and becomes erratic. Inappropriate use of food (e.g., to punish, reward, bribe, convey love) may lead to inappropriate food attitudes. Children in this age group often experience

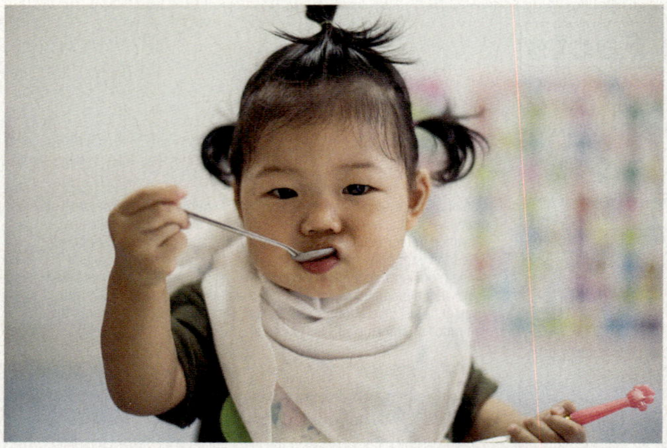

FIGURE 37-4. Toddlers and preschoolers can feed themselves and verbalize food likes and dislikes.

an inadequate intake of fruits and vegetables and/or excessive intake of sweetened fruit drinks.

SCHOOL-AGE CHILDREN

The 6- to 12-year-old child has an uneven, individualized, sometimes erratic slow progressive physical growth pattern (Kyle & Carman, 2021). Permanent teeth erupt as the digestive system matures. Socialization and independence increase. At this stage, the body accumulates reserves in preparation for the upcoming adolescent growth spurt.

Nutritional implications for the school-age child focus on health promotion. Increasing energy requirements need to be balanced with foods of high nutritional value. The appetite improves but still may be irregular. The parents' role as the primary regulator of food intake diminishes, and advertising has more of an impact on the child's food choices.

ADOLESCENTS

Adolescence (ages 11 to 20 years) is a period of rapid physical, emotional, social, and sexual maturation. The growth spurt begins at different ages among individuals. Girls begin menstruation and experience fat deposition, whereas males experience an increase in muscle mass, lean body tissue, and bones. Adolescence is also marked by intense psychosocial growth, family/caregiver conflict, and social and peer pressure. Childhood nutrition problems often worsen during adolescence. Adolescents tend to skip breakfast, contributing to a lower-quality diet and decreased performance in school. Children in this age group tend to consume inadequate amounts of fruits, vegetables, whole grains, and dairy products (USDA & DHHS, 2020).

Nutrient needs, especially for calories, protein, calcium, and iron, increase to support growth. Weight consciousness may become compulsive in teenaged girls, resulting in anorexia nervosa, an eating disorder characterized by extreme weight loss, muscle wasting, arrested sexual development, refusal to eat, and bizarre eating habits. Bulimia, another eating disorder characterized by gorging followed by purging with self-induced vomiting, diuretics, and laxatives, also becomes more common in this age group. Although contrasts exist, there is also some overlap between these diseases. Both conditions are serious health and nutritional problems; individuals with these disorders require professional medical help and counseling. Other unhealthy diet practices include fasting, the use of diet pills, and laxative abuse.

Adolescents often eat their food rapidly, leading to overconsumption before satiety is experienced. Food is often eaten away from home, consisting of products from fast food restaurants, convenience stores, and vending machines—foods high in fat, sugar, and salt. These factors need to be considered when planning dietary interventions for adolescents.

Both the pregnant person and child are at increased nutritional risk during teenage pregnancy due to competition for the nutrients between the adolescent's body and that of the fetus. Nutritional needs may be harder to meet because fewer meals are eaten at home, and peer influence and busy schedules have an impact. Adequate nutrition and appropriate weight gain improve birth outcomes and decrease the incidence of low-birth-weight infants and improve the health of infants born to adolescents (Dudek, 2022; Kyle & Carman, 2021).

ADULTS

With adulthood, growth ceases. This age is also marked by a decline in the BMR with each decade. Adults may become more aware of the preventive role of exercise, or pressures of work and family may lead to a decline in physical activity and exercise.

Nutritional needs level off in adulthood, and fewer calories are required because of the decrease in BMR. Weight gain results if adjustments in caloric intake are not made.

PREGNANT AND LACTATING PERSONS

During pregnancy, the fetus, maternal tissues, and placenta grow dramatically. Weight gain occurs, and GI changes as a result of the pregnancy may result in nausea, vomiting, heartburn, or constipation. The quantity of breast milk produced depends on an adequate supply of nutrients.

Nutrient needs during pregnancy increase to support growth and maintain maternal homeostasis, particularly during the second and third trimesters. During the second trimester, normal-weight pregnant persons need approximately 340 extra calories per day and 450 extra calories per day in the third trimester than when not pregnant (Academy of Nutrition and Dietetics, 2020a). Key nutrient needs include protein, calories, iron, and folic acid. Caloric needs are higher for lactation (approximately 500 cal/day) than nonpregnant calorie needs (Dudek, 2022), and the nutritional quality of breast milk is maintained at the expense of the lactating person's nutrition if dietary intake is inadequate. People who did not gain enough weight during pregnancy may need to increase their calorie intake (Dudek, 2022).

OLDER ADULTS

Because of the decreases in BMR and physical activity and loss of lean body mass, energy expenditure decreases. Loss of teeth and periodontal disease may make chewing more difficult. A decrease in peristalsis can result in constipation. Loss of taste between sweet and salty begins between ages 55 and 59 years, but discrimination between bitter and sour remains intact.

The sensation of thirst also decreases. Degenerative diseases and the use of medications are more common with aging. It is not uncommon for social isolation, poor self-esteem, or loss of independence to affect nutritional intake negatively.

Because of the changes related to aging, the caloric needs of the body decrease. The need for nutrients, however, increases, especially protein, calcium, B_{12}, and vitamin D (Academy of Nutrition and Dietetics, 2020b; Dudek, 2022). Foods that are difficult to chew may need to be eliminated, whereas an increase in fiber and fluid intake can relieve constipation. Older adults are also prone to dehydration, and lack of interest in eating is common. Nutrient intake, digestion, absorption, metabolism, or excretion may be altered because of the physiologic changes common to this age. Dietary restrictions related to chronic illness, limited income, isolation, and age-related physiologic changes place persons in this age group at risk for malnutrition (Bernstein & Munoz, 2020; Touhy & Jett, 2018).

Sex Assigned at Birth

Males differ from females in their nutrient requirements due to differences in body composition and reproductive function. Their larger muscle mass translates into higher caloric and protein requirements (therefore, slightly higher needs for B vitamins that metabolize calories and protein) because muscle is more metabolically active than adipose tissue (females have proportionately more adipose tissue). Females of childbearing age have higher iron requirements related to menstruation. In addition, evidence indicates there are biologic sex—associated differences in metabolism of some nutrients, including fatty acids, proteins, and carbohydrates (Comitato et al., 2015).

State of Health

The alteration in nutrient requirements that results from illness and trauma varies with the intensity and duration of the stress. For instance, fevers increase the need for calories and water. Unlike fevers related to septicemia, however, fevers caused by a mild case of the flu require few dietary adjustments.

Trauma, such as major surgery, burns, and crush injuries, is followed by hormonal changes that profoundly affect the body's use of nutrients. To preserve or replenish body nutrient stores and to promote healing and recovery, nutrient requirements increase dramatically in the adaptive phase after stress. In some cases of severe trauma, such as major burns, the rehabilitative phase of recovery, characterized by the gradual normalization of nutrient needs, may last for years.

Chronic disorders—for example, diabetes, renal disease, hypertension, heart disease, GI disorders, and cancer—can alter nutrient requirements by influencing nutrient intake, digestion, absorption, metabolism, utilization, or excretion.

Mental health problems, such as depression and confusion, can cause a patient to forget to eat or lack the motivation to eat, leading to malnutrition.

Alcohol Use Disorder

Alcohol use disorder is a pattern of alcohol use that includes any alcohol that puts your health or safety at risk or causes other alcohol-related problems and includes binge drinking (a pattern of drinking where a minimum of 4 to 5 drinks are consumed within 2 hours) (MFMER, 2018). Alcohol can alter the body's use of nutrients, and thereby its nutrient requirements, by numerous mechanisms (Gramlich et al., 2021). The toxic effect of alcohol on the intestinal mucosa interferes with normal nutrient absorption; thus, requirements increase as the efficiency of absorption decreases. The need for B vitamins increases because they are used to metabolize alcohol. Alcohol can also influence nutrient metabolism by impairing nutrient storage, increasing nutrient catabolism, and increasing nutrient excretion. Alcohol abuse that results in liver damage has profound effects on the body's nutrient metabolism and requirements.

Medications

Many drugs have the potential to influence nutrient requirements. Nutrient absorption may be altered by drugs that (1) change the pH of the GI tract, (2) increase GI motility, (3) damage the intestinal mucosa, or (4) bind with nutrients, rendering them unavailable to the body. Nutrient metabolism can be altered by drugs that (1) act as nutrient antagonists, (2) alter the enzyme systems that metabolize nutrients, or (3) alter nutrient degradation. Some drugs alter the renal reabsorption of nutrients and, therefore, may increase or decrease nutrient excretion.

Megadoses of Nutrient Supplements

Because some nutrients compete against each other for absorption, an excess of one nutrient can lead to a deficiency (or increase the requirement) of another, especially if one is absorbed preferentially. For instance, a delicate balance exists between zinc and copper. People who take therapeutic levels of zinc run the risk of developing a copper deficiency—which is otherwise rare—unless they also increase their intake of copper.

Dietary supplements can have druglike effects and may interact with food and medications (Karch, 2020). Accurate information regarding the patient's use of dietary supplements is imperative to provide safe and appropriate care. The use of herbs, vitamins, minerals, and other supplements can impact a patient's plan of care and must be considered by all members of the health care team. For example, a patient taking ginkgo biloba (an herbal) and aspirin may have to have surgery postponed due to an increased risk for excessive bleeding, because each of these substances have anticoagulant properties. A list of accurate, reliable sources for the latest information about specific herbs and supplements based on scientific evidence can be found https://www.nutrition.gov/topics/whats-food/vitamins-and-minerals.

Physical, Sociocultural, and Psychosocial Factors That Influence Food Choices

Dietary choices or restrictions also are influenced by social determinants of health (e.g., economics, social supports, literacy, language), culture, religion, and personal feelings and meanings associated with food. The financial income of the patient or the patient's household can directly impact the ability to purchase sufficient food and/or food of high nutritional value. Diverse lifestyles and eating habits directly impact a person's nutritional health and well-being. Religious restrictions and beliefs or cultural practices may affect the patient's acceptance of, response to, and engagement in nutrition therapies. Health care providers need an understanding of a patient's cultural values, beliefs, and practices to provide culturally acceptable care.

Social Determinants of Health

Economic resources and stability affect dietary choices and patterns. Employment and income coupled with the increasing cost of food may result in a decrease in the nutritional quality of the diet. Many variables influence the types of foods purchased. Creative use of the food dollar means using unit pricing to determine cost per serving (e.g., comparing the unit price of 39¢ per serving with a similar product's 45¢ per serving), selecting foods that contain adequate nutrients, and buying seasonal foods that are more economical and can be prepared easily at home. Avoiding convenience foods and meals purchased away from home can save food dollars.

Additional sociocultural factors affecting nutritional intake include:

- Language barriers
- Knowledge of nutrition
  - Literacy
- Lack of caregiver or social support
- Social isolation
- Limited access to food market and ability to obtain food (food deserts)
- Lack of or inadequate cooking and/or food preparation arrangements

Religion

Dietary restrictions associated with religions might affect a patient's nutritional requirements. Many religions eschew certain types of food products. For example, Mormon individuals do not use coffee, tea, or alcohol, and are encouraged to limit meat consumption. Many Hindu people are vegetarian, adhering to the concept of nonviolence as applied to all living being (Andrews et al., 2020; Dudek, 2022). Therefore, alternative food choices or meal patterns may be necessary. Kosher dietary laws require special food preparation techniques and prohibit intake of pork and shellfish (Andrews et al., 2020). Thus, a patient's religious affiliation may affect that individual's nutritional regimen. Question regarding any preferences or restrictions should be included in a nutritional assessment. Vegetarian, kosher, and other special diets are available in hospitals, long-term care facilities, retirement homes, and programs, such as Meals on Wheels.

Meaning of Food

Food means different things to different people, with food playing multiple roles in the lives of most people. In addition to satisfying hunger and providing nutrition, food may signify a celebration, a social gathering, or a reward. Some people use various foods to indicate caring or to give comfort and reassurance during times of stress or unhappiness. Mealtime may evoke memories of family discussions, laughter, and enjoyable times. Some may remember conflicts associated with eating or avoid eating because it reminds them of their loneliness and isolation. Others, because of society's emphasis on being thin, may resort to fad or crash weight-reduction diets to resolve eating conflicts and lose weight rapidly. This initial weight reduction seldom is sustained for an extended period, and a cycle of "yo-yo" dieting frequently results. Drastic weight loss is followed by an eating binge that causes the dieter to regain all the lost weight and, possibly, some additional weight each time the sequence occurs. Nutritional deficiencies may occur and place the person at risk for other diseases. Losing weight and keeping it off require a change in eating habits as part of the overall commitment to health.

Culture

Nutritional diversity is common among cultural or ethnic groups. The variety and selections are unique to each group and represent their personal beliefs and customs. Culture influences what is eaten or considered edible, how it is prepared, and what combinations of food are permitted. Herbal treatments that are popular in some cultures may interfere with or counteract the action of prescribed medication. The variations in food choices within a culture also depend on income levels and availability of foods. General and specific cultural knowledge allows the health care provider to ask the right questions when interacting with patients of varying backgrounds. The U.S. Department of Agriculture and the National Agricultural Library (n.d.b) provides extensive resources for working with various ethnic and cultural groups at https://www.nal.usda.gov/fnic/ethnic-and-cultural-resources-0. Nurses who are aware of the specific needs and beliefs of culturally diverse patient populations are better able to communicate effectively and provide optimal care. Box 37-3 suggests guidelines for effective communication about nutrition with culturally diverse patients.

If a patient of a different culture is to be placed on a specific diet, discussing food choice options is necessary to customize the diet to meet the person's cultural demands. Discussing ways to integrate cultural food preferences into current nutrition guidelines is an important part of nursing care.

Food Intake

At times, a combination of physiologic and physical factors that influence nutrient requirements and, or in combination with, sociocultural and psychosocial factors can affect a person's nutritional intake. Subsequently, these factors can result in a decrease or increase in food intake.

Box 37-3 Communicating Effectively About Nutrition With Culturally Diverse Patients

- Acquire basic information about health beliefs and practices of various cultural groups in your health care setting. This provides a basis for assessing patients' beliefs and practices. Recognize, however, that within all cultures and ethnic groups, there are members who do not hold all the values of the group.
- Ask specifically about the use of folk or home remedies prescribed by a nontraditional healer.
- Determine the patient's language preferences for spoken and written communication.
- Utilize printed or audiovisual information that is in the language spoken by your patients.
- Promote healthy food choices by identifying healthy traditional food practices and encourage their use.
- Encourage cultural sensitivity in health care workers in your particular setting.
- Recognize that diversity exists within cultural groups. For example, the Hispanic/Latino population includes Mexican American, Mexican, Cuban, Puerto Rican, and other groups.
- Emphasize threads or messages in health teaching that are common to all cultures (e.g., concern about family, faith, home).
- Help culturally diverse patients to value and understand the importance of communicating concerns and asking questions about prescribed dietary practices.

Source: Adapted from Andrews, M., Boyle, J. S., & Collins, J. (2020). *Transcultural concepts in nursing care* (8th ed.). Wolters Kluwer; Dudek, S. (2022). *Nutrition essentials for nursing practice* (9th ed.). Wolters Kluwer.

Decreased Food Intake

Food intake may decrease for various reasons. Patients with a BMI of less than 18.5 are considered underweight. **Anorexia**, or the lack of appetite, may be related to systemic and local diseases; numerous psychosocial causes, such as fear, anxiety, depression, or pain; and impaired ability to smell and taste—or it may occur secondary to drug therapy or medical treatments (Dudek, 2022; Jarvis & Eckhardt, 2020). Others who may have limited food intake include those who have difficulty chewing and swallowing, those who experience chronic GI problems or undergo certain surgical procedures, those with certain chronic illnesses (such as cancer), and those with inadequate food budgets.

Concept Mastery Alert

Anorexia is different from anorexia nervosa. *Anorexia* is a general term that involves a lack of appetite that results from numerous causes. *Anorexia nervosa* is an eating disorder that involves varied issues including extreme weight loss, muscle wasting, arrested sexual development, refusal to eat, and bizarre eating habits.

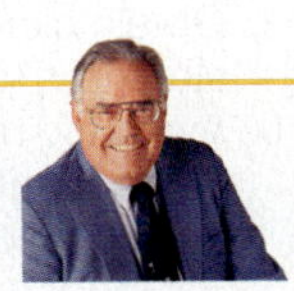

Consider **Charles Gallagher**, whose wife is receiving enteral feedings. The underlying reason for insertion of the PEG tube was her inability to swallow and subsequent development of aspiration pneumonia that required numerous hospitalizations. The nurse would need to communicate this information to Mr. Gallagher to ensure that he understands the rationale for the feeding. This understanding is important for decision making.

Increased Food Intake

Increased food intake may lead to overweight and obesity. Obesity presents a serious health problem physically, socially, and emotionally. Obesity in adults is defined as body weight that is higher than what is considered as healthy weight for a given height or having a BMI of 30 or more (CDC, 2020c; NHLBI, n.d.b). In children and teens, overweight is defined as a BMI at or above the 85th percentile and below the 95th percentile for children and teens of the same age and sex assigned at birth (CDC, 2020c). Obesity in children and teens is defined as a BMI at or above the 95th percentile for children and teens of the same age and sex assigned at birth (CDC, 2018). More than two thirds of adults in the United States are considered to be overweight or have obesity (NIDDK, 2017). In addition, approximately 17% of young people between ages 2 and 19 years are considered to be obese, and about 6% are considered to be extremely obese (NIDDK, 2017).

An imbalance between calories consumed and calories expended, resulting from an excess caloric intake and/or a decrease in energy expenditure, leads to the gradual accumulation of weight (NHLBI, n.d.a). In addition, an increased intake of energy-dense foods that are high in fat and sugars and an increase in physical inactivity due to the increasingly sedentary nature of many forms of work, changing modes of transportation and increasing urbanization are thought to play a role in causing obesity (World Health Organization, 2020). This excess weight increases the risk for numerous health problems, such as metabolic syndrome, cardiovascular diseases, certain cancers, and respiratory problems such as sleep apnea and obesity hypoventilation syndrome (NHLBI, n.d.a); increases the risks associated with surgery (American Society of Anesthesiologists, n.d.); and increases the risk for complications during pregnancy, labor, and delivery (Silbert-Flagg & Pillitteri, 2018). People who are overweight or obese may be the subject of weight bias and stigma and this could lead to feelings of rejection, shame or guilt, depression, isolation, and to perceive oneself as a failure (MFMER, 2020c; NIDDK, n.d.). Obesity is resistant to treatment, and weight loss is temporary at best unless behavior modification and exercise are incorporated into the dietary plan (MFMER, 2020c).

NURSING PROCESS FOR NUTRITION

Assessing

Nutritional status has a significant role in both health. For well patients, good nutritional status can help to maintain health, promote normal growth and development, and protect against disease. During illness, good nutritional status can reduce the risk for complications and speed recovery time. Conversely, poor nutritional status can increase the risk for illness or death.

Like other aspects of nursing care, nutritional assessment is a systematic approach used to identify the patient's actual or potential needs, formulate a plan to meet those needs, initiate the plan or assign others to implement it, and evaluate the effectiveness of the plan. The level of assessment may range from simple screening to a comprehensive, in-depth assessment, depending on individual circumstances. Regardless of the level of assessment, nutritional assessment is appropriate for all patients. Nurses can collect assessment data through history taking (dietary, medical, socioeconomic data), physical assessments (anthropometric and clinical data), and laboratory data. Patients found to be at risk for malnutrition are often referred to a dietitian for comprehensive assessment of their nutritional status (Anderson, 2019a; Dudek, 2022).

Nurses working with patients to promote appropriate behaviors related to nutrition should examine their own behaviors as factors in the success of the plan. Nurses who role model good health behaviors are more effective teachers. Use the display, Promoting Health 37-1: Nutrition, for yourself before using it with others.

Nutritional Data

Collect nutritional data from the patient or family or caregivers and evaluate it according to the *Dietary Guidelines,* DRI, or the MyPlate food guide, depending on the purpose of the assessment and within the context of the patient's health status.

NUTRITIONAL SCREENING

Nutritional screening is an important part of the nursing assessment. Screening looks for cues associated with nutrition problems to determine if a person is malnourished or at risk for malnutrition. The Mini Nutritional Assessment tool (MNA) is one example of a tool frequently used to screen older adults (Fig. 37-5) and is available and regularly updated at www.mna-elderly.com. The MNA is a combination of diverse screening questions, anthropometric measurements, nutritional habits, general condition, and self-evaluation (Reber et al., 2019). The MNA short-form (MNS-SF) is also available and consists of six items, takes less than 5 minutes to complete, and is as effective as the long version (Reber et al., 2019).

After a screening tool identifies a patient at risk it is imperative to complete a nutritional assessment as a follow-up. These patients are usually referred to a dietitian for further nutrition assessment, diagnosis, and intervention (Anderson, 2019a; Dudek, 2022). When this is combined with other methods of assessing nutritional status, the nurse is better prepared to coordinate a focused strategy to combat malnutrition.

Promoting Health 37-1

NUTRITION

Use the assessment checklist to determine how well you are meeting your needs related to nutrition practices. Then develop a prescription for self-care by choosing appropriate behaviors from the list of suggestions.

Assessment Checklist

☐ almost always ☐ sometimes ☐ almost never

☐ ☐ ☐ 1. I know and use the recommended dietary guidelines and servings.

☐ ☐ ☐ 2. My weight is within 10% of the ideal for my height and body frame.

☐ ☐ ☐ 3. I maintain an appropriate balance between exercise and food intake.

☐ ☐ ☐ 4. I limit my fat, sugar, salt, and red meat intake.

☐ ☐ ☐ 5. I limit my caffeine intake.

☐ ☐ ☐ 6. I use alcoholic beverages in moderation.

☐ ☐ ☐ 7. I make an effort to eat high-fiber foods.

Self-Care Behaviors

1. Maintain desirable weight, eating a variety of foods in adequate amounts from each of the food groups.
2. Eat slowly, take smaller portions, and avoid second helpings if trying to control overeating.
3. Eat a variety of foods low in calories and high in nutrients to lose weight.
4. Obtain clearance from a health care provider before starting a weight-loss program.
5. Avoid too many foods high in cholesterol (milk, egg yolk, organ meats, fats, oils); instead choose lean meat, fish, poultry, and beans.
6. Eat foods high in fiber: whole-grain breads and cereals, fruits, vegetables, dry beans.
7. Avoid excess use of salt and sugar.
8. Begin an exercise program and maintain it.
9. Learn healthy eating habits; read labels, become familiar with healthy fast-food and restaurant menus; and drink alcohol moderately (if at all).
10. Substitute healthy rewards for yourself that do not include high-calorie, low-nutrition snacks, and beverages.

Information to promote effective nutrition, dietary supplement use and safety; nutrient recommendations; and database resources are available online.

Mini Nutritional Assessment
MNA®

Nestlé NutritionInstitute

Last name: ____________ First name: ____________

Sex: ______ Age: ______ Weight, kg: ______ Height, cm: ______ Date: ______

Complete the screen by filling in the boxes with the appropriate numbers.
Add the numbers for the screen. If score is 11 or less, continue with the assessment to gain a Malnutrition Indicator Score.

A Has food intake declined over the past 3 months due to loss of appetite, digestive problems, chewing or swallowing difficulties?
0 = severe decrease in food intake
1 = moderate decrease in food intake
2 = no decrease in food intake ☐

B Weight loss during the last 3 months
0 = weight loss greater than 3kg (6.6lbs)
1 = does not know
2 = weight loss between 1 and 3kg (2.2 and 6.6 lbs)
3 = no weight loss ☐

C Mobility
0 = bed or chair bound
1 = able to get out of bed / chair but does not go out
2 = goes out ☐

D Has suffered psychological stress or acute disease in the past 3 months?
0 = yes 2 = no ☐

E Neuropsychological problems
0 = severe dementia or depression
1 = mild dementia
2 = no psychological problems ☐

F Body Mass Index (BMI) = weight in kg / (height in m)^2 ☐
0 = BMI less than 19
1 = BMI 19 to less than 21
2 = BMI 21 to less than 23
3 = BMI 23 or greater ☐

Screening score (subtotal max. 14 points) ☐☐

12-14 points:	Normal nutritional status
8-11 points:	At risk of malnutrition
0-7 points:	Malnourished

For a more in-depth assessment, continue with questions G-R

G Lives independently (not in nursing home or hospital)
1 = yes 0 = no ☐

H Takes more than 3 prescription drugs per day
0 = yes 1 = no ☐

I Pressure sores or skin ulcers
0 = yes 1 = no ☐

J How many full meals does the patient eat daily?
0 = 1 meal
1 = 2 meals
2 = 3 meals ☐

K Selected consumption markers for protein intake
- At least one serving of dairy products (milk, cheese, yoghurt) per day yes ☐ no ☐
- Two or more servings of legumes or eggs per week yes ☐ no ☐
- Meat, fish or poultry every day yes ☐ no ☐

0.0 = if 0 or 1 yes
0.5 = if 2 yes
1.0 = if 3 yes ☐.☐

L Consumes two or more servings of fruit or vegetables per day?
0 = no 1 = yes ☐

M How much fluid (water, juice, coffee, tea, milk...) is consumed per day?
0.0 = less than 3 cups
0.5 = 3 to 5 cups
1.0 = more than 5 cups ☐.☐

N Mode of feeding
0 = unable to eat without assistance
1 = self-fed with some difficulty
2 = self-fed without any problem ☐

O Self view of nutritional status
0 = views self as being malnourished
1 = is uncertain of nutritional state
2 = views self as having no nutritional problem ☐

P In comparison with other people of the same age, how does the patient consider his / her health status?
0.0 = not as good
0.5 = does not know
1.0 = as good
2.0 = better ☐.☐

Q Mid-arm circumference (MAC) in cm
0.0 = MAC less than 21
0.5 = MAC 21 to 22
1.0 = MAC greater than 22 ☐.☐

R Calf circumference (CC) in cm
0 = CC less than 31
1 = CC 31 or greater ☐

Assessment (max. 16 points) ☐☐.☐
Screening score ☐☐.☐
Total Assessment (max. 30 points) ☐☐.☐

Malnutrition Indicator Score

24 to 30 points	☐	Normal nutritional status
17 to 23.5 points	☐	At risk of malnutrition
Less than 17 points	☐	Malnourished

References
1. Vellas B, Villars H, Abellan G, *et al.* Overview of the MNA®-Its History and Challenges. *J Nutr Health Aging.* 2006; **10:**456–465.
2. Rubenstein LZ, Harker JO, Salva A, Guigoz Y, Vellas B. Screening for Undernutrition in Geriatric Practice: Developing the Short-Form Mini Nutritional Assessment (MNA-SF). *J. Geront.* 2001; **56A**: M366-377
3. Guigoz Y. The Mini-Nutritional Assessment (MNA®) Review of the Literature-What does it tell us? *J Nutr Health Aging.* 2006; **10:**466–487.
4. Kaiser Mj, Bauer JM, Ramsch C, et al. Validation of the Mini Nutritional Assessment Short-Form (MNA®-SF): A practical tool for identification of nutritional status. *J Nutr Health Aging* 2009; 13:782–788.

For more information: www.mna-elderly.com

FIGURE 37-5. The Mini Nutritional Assessment tool. (*Source:* Used with permission. ® Société des Produits Nestlé, S.A., Vevey, Switzerland, Trademark Owners © Nestlé, 1994, Revision 2009. N67200 12/99 10M. www.mna-elderly.com)

ASSESSING DIETARY INTAKE

Many different methods can be used to assess actual dietary intake.

24-Hour Recall Method

The easiest way to collect dietary data is to obtain a 24-hour recall of all food and beverages the patient normally consumes during an average day. Ask the patient to recall details related to nutritional intake from the prior 24 hours. This method includes the patient's portion sizes, meal and snack patterns, meal timing, and location where food is eaten. Because this method relies on memory and accurate interpretation of portion sizes, the information may not be reliable.

Food Diaries/Calorie Counts

Food diaries and calorie counts require documentation of actual intake for a specified period of time. In an outpatient setting, ask the patient to record everything the patient has had to eat or drink, including portion size, over a set period of time. In the hospital or other facility settings, documentation is usually completed by the nursing staff. These tools may provide a better overall picture of nutrient intake because all food and beverages consumed in a specified period, usually 3 to 7 days, are recorded.

Food Frequency Record

Food frequency records give a general picture of nutritional consumption. Ask patients questions to elicit an average number of times certain foods or food groups are consumed in a given period of time: per day, per week, or per month. For example, ask, "How many times in the last week have you eaten fresh fruit or fish?" or "How many times in the last week have you had a glass of milk?"

Diet History

A more comprehensive approach to diet assessment is a full diet history. In addition to a 24-hour food recall, calorie counts/food diaries, and food-frequency record, interview questions are geared to provide information on past and present food intake and habits. Sample questions are included in the accompanying Focused Assessment Guide 37-1.

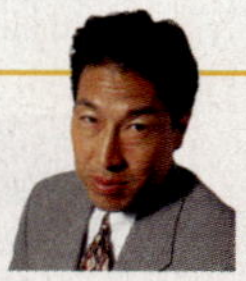

Consider **William Johnston**, the man who has less-than-healthful dietary and health habits. The nurse could use a diet history to obtain specific information about Mr. Johnston's actual intake. Analysis of this information would reveal his actual dietary intake and identify potential and actual nutritional problems.

MEDICAL AND SOCIOECONOMIC DATA

Medical, social determinants of health, as well as cultural and psychological influences, require evaluation for their impact on nutritional requirements and food choices. A nutritional assessment should include the following health, social, and economic information (Dudek, 2022).

Medical data include:

- Current illness as well as health, medical and surgical history
- Past and current drug history

Focused Assessment Guide 37-1

NUTRITION

Factors to Assess	Questions and Approaches
Usual dietary intake	Does your current intake differ from your usual intake? If so, is the reason a loss of appetite, changes in smell or taste, difficulty chewing and swallowing, hospitalization, a modified diet? With whom do you usually eat meals?
Food allergies or intolerances	Do you have any food allergies or intolerances?
Food preparation and storage	Who does the food shopping? Who prepares the meals? How is the food normally prepared? For instance, is food usually fried, baked, or broiled? Do you have adequate food storage space and preparation equipment?
Type of dietary practices	Do you now or have you in the past followed a modified diet prescribed by a health care provider? Do you now or have you in the past used a fad diet, health foods, or self-prescribed supplements?
Eating disorder patterns	Do you view yourself as overweight? Do you weigh yourself frequently during 1 day? How is your appetite? Do you binge on large amounts of food in a short period? Have you ever caused yourself to vomit after eating a meal? Have you used laxatives, diuretics, herbal supplements, or over-the-counter weight-loss pills to lose weight?

- Medications, supplement use, herbal supplement use, complementary, and integrative therapy use
- History of drug dependence or abuse
- Ability to chew and swallow, including condition of mouth, missing teeth, or dentures
- Appetite, food intolerance and allergies, and bowel habits

Social data include:

- Age, sex assigned at birth, family history, lifestyle (e.g., those at extremes in age are most at risk)
- Social determinants of health
  - Educational background
  - Socioeconomic status: occupation, sources of income, food budget
  - Illiteracy
  - Language barriers
  - Caregiver and/or social support
  - Knowledge of nutrition
  - Access to reliable, healthy food options
- Information about exercise, and sleep patterns
- Religious affiliation, cultural and ethnic background
- Use of alcohol and tobacco

ANTHROPOMETRIC DATA

Anthropometric measurements (measurement of the size and proportion of the human body) are used to determine body dimensions. In children, anthropometric measurements are used to assess growth rate and weight gain; in adults, they can give indirect measurements of body protein and fat stores. For the data to be accurate and reliable, use standardized equipment and procedures, and compare the data with the appropriate reference standards for the patient's age and sex assigned at birth.

Obtain height and weight, the most common anthropometric measurements, when the patient is admitted to the health care facility and periodically thereafter and are assessed in community care environments as well. Weigh a patient on the same scale each time and at the same time of day, preferably before breakfast. Height and weight are used to calculate the patient's BMI. Because actual weight may be increased if the patient has edema, consider hydration status. Although self-reported weight may be recorded when actual weight is unobtainable, it is highly inaccurate and must be noted. Record an actual weight as soon as feasibly possible. Self-reported height in the older adult can be inaccurate related to shortening of the spine (MedlinePlus, 2020). Record an actual height as soon as possible.

BODY MASS INDEX AND WAIST CIRCUMFERENCE

Calculate the patient's BMI and measure waist circumference, as discussed earlier in the chapter on page 1391. Compare results with the established guidelines to determine the patient's status and identify potential health risks. Refer to Table 37-1 on page 1392.

CLINICAL DATA

Although signs and symptoms of altered nutrition may be observed during a physical assessment (Table 37-2 on page 1408), they usually do not appear until the condition is advanced. In addition, further investigation is necessary to determine whether abnormal findings are actually caused by a nutritional deficiency, are possibly related to a nutritional deficiency, or are unrelated to nutritional status.

Assess for physical barriers to eating. **Dysphagia** (difficulty swallowing or the inability to swallow) can be the result of poor dental health, cancer, or a neurologic disease, such as stroke, Parkinson disease, or dementia, and may reduce the patient's nutritional intake. Dysphagia also is associated with an increased risk for **aspiration**, the misdirection of oropharyngeal secretions or gastric contents into the larynx and lower respiratory tract (Nazarko, 2020). Dysphagia should be considered if a patient has one or more signs or symptoms of dysphagia or related issues (Holdoway & Smith, 2020; Nazarko, 2020). Refer to Box 37-4 (on page 1409) for signs and symptoms of and risk factors for dysphagia. Assessment tools have been developed to measure patient dysphagia symptoms. These tools may be used to determine the safety of oral feeding, document symptom severity and to monitor the effectiveness of treatment (Oliveirea et al., 2019; Johnson et al., 2018).

Dental problems are associated with impaired chewing and avoidance of foods that may be difficult to chew, such as meat, fruit, and vegetables. Patients who experience weakness and fatigue may find eating to be a chore to avoid. Diminished sensor abilities, such as sight, taste, smell, and hearing, may also impact a patient's nutritional intake.

BIOCHEMICAL DATA

Laboratory tests, which measure blood and urine levels of nutrients or biochemical functions that depend on an adequate supply of nutrients, may be used as part of a nutritional assessment. Most routine biochemical tests measure protein status; measures of body vitamin, mineral, and trace element status are also available. Some evidence suggests, however, that these traditional nutrition indicators do not accurately quantify the degree of malnutrition (Hartwell et al., 2018) and should be avoided as part of assessment of hospitalized patients and patients in critical care settings, in particular, as they do not take the importance of disease severity and inflammation and stress into account (McClave, Taylor, et al., 2016; McClave, DiBaise, et al., 2016).

Hemoglobin, the oxygen-carrying protein of the red blood cells, and hematocrit, the volume of red blood cells packed by centrifugation in a given volume of blood, are measures of plasma protein that also reflect a person's iron status. Protein status can also be determined by measuring serum prealbumin and transferrin levels and by a total lymphocyte count. In the past, serum albumin levels were considered as a marker for malnutrition (Fischbach et al., 2022). However, prealbumin has been suggested as the better reflection of the current nutritional status of within the patient's body (Fischbach et al., 2022). Prealbumin levels provide a timelier picture of a change in dietary status reflecting the current nutritional status within a patient's body (Fischbach et al., 2022). Transferrin acts as an iron-transporting protein, but because it is related to iron levels may not always be an accurate indicator of nutritional status. The total lymphocyte

Table 37-2 Clinical Observations for Nutritional Assessment

BODY AREA	SIGNS OF GOOD NUTRITIONAL STATUS	SIGNS OF POOR NUTRITIONAL STATUS
General appearance	Alert, responsive	Listless, apathetic, and cachectic
General vitality	Has endurance, energetic, sleeps well, vigorous	Easily fatigued, no energy, falls asleep easily, looks tired, apathetic, depressed mood
Weight	Normal for height, age, body build; BMI	Overweight or underweight
Hair	Shiny, lustrous, firm, not easily plucked, healthy scalp	Dull and dry, brittle, loss of color, easily plucked, thin and sparse
Face	Uniform skin color; healthy appearance, not swollen	Dark skin over cheeks and under eyes, flaky skin, facial edema (moon face), pale skin color
Eyes	Bright, clear, moist, no sores at corners of eyelids, membranes moist and healthy pink color, no prominent blood vessels	Pale eye membranes, dry eyes (xerophthalmia); Bitot spots, increased vascularity, cornea soft (keratomalacia), small yellowish lumps around eyes (xanthelasma), dull or scarred cornea
Lips	Good pink color, smooth, moist, not chapped or swollen	Swollen and puffy (cheilosis), angular lesion at corners of mouth or fissures or scars (stomatitis)
Tongue	Deep red, surface papillae present	Smooth appearance, beefy red or magenta colored, swollen, hypertrophy or atrophy
Teeth	Straight, no crowding, no cavities, no pain, bright, no discoloration, well-shaped jaw	Cavities, mottled appearance (fluorosis), malpositioned, missing teeth
Gums	Firm, good pink color, no swelling or bleeding	Spongy, bleed easily, marginal redness, recessed, swollen, and inflamed
Glands	No enlargement of the thyroid, face not swollen	Enlargement of the thyroid (goiter), enlargement of the parotid (swollen cheeks)
Skin	Smooth, good color, slightly moist, no signs of rashes, swelling, or color irregularities	Rough, dry, flaky, swollen, pale, pigmented, lack of fat under the skin, fat deposits around the joints (xanthomas), bruises, petechiae
Nails	Firm, pink	Spoon shaped (koilonychia), brittle, pale, ridged
Skeleton	Good posture, no malformations	Poor posture, beading of the ribs, bowed legs or knock-knees, prominent scapulas, chest deformity at diaphragm
Muscles	Well developed, firm, good tone, some fat under the skin	Flaccid, poor tone, wasted, underdeveloped, difficulty walking
Extremities	No tenderness	Weak and tender, edema of lower extremities
Abdomen	Flat	Swollen
Nervous system	Normal reflexes, psychological stability	Decrease in or loss of ankle and knee reflexes, psychomotor changes, mental confusion, depression, sensory loss, motor weakness, loss of sense of position, loss of vibration, burning and tingling of the hands and feet (paresthesia)
Cardiovascular system	Normal heart rate and rhythm, no murmurs, normal blood pressure for age	Cardiac enlargement, tachycardia, abnormal blood pressure
GI system	No palpable organs or masses (liver edge may be palpable in children)	Enlarged liver or spleen

Source: Adapted from Dudek, S. G. (2022). *Nutrition essentials for nursing practice* (9th ed.). Wolters Kluwer; Jarvis, C., & Echkardt, A. (2020). *Physical examination & health assessment* (8th ed.). Elsevier.

count reflects immune status and is directly affected by impaired nutritional states.

Blood glucose, blood cholesterol, and blood triglycerides are additional laboratory tests relative to nutritional status. Twenty-four-hour urine tests used to measure protein metabolism include urine creatinine excretion and urine urea nitrogen. Urea, a breakdown product of amino acids, can be measured in the urine and blood. It reflects protein intake and the body's ability to detoxify and excrete this metabolic byproduct. Creatinine levels are directly proportional to the body's muscle mass; a reduction in this value reflects severe malnutrition. These biochemical indicators with nutritional implications are summarized in Box 37-5.

Box 37-4 Signs and Symptoms and Risk Factors for Dysphagia

Signs and Symptoms

- Difficulty swallowing foods or fluids; may only be certain foods or liquids
- Coughing or choking when eating or drinking
- Unintentional weight loss
- Frequent throat clearing
- Wet gurgling voice after eating
- Feeling of food or liquids "stuck" in throat
- Leakage of food or saliva from mouth

Risk Factors

- Neurologic condition (e.g., stroke, head injury, brain injury, progressive neurologic disorder [e.g., Parkinson disease, multiple sclerosis])
- Dementia
- Obstructive condition (e.g., head and neck cancer, gastroesophageal reflux disease)
- COPD
- Aging
- Malnutrition
- Childhood syndromes (e.g., Down syndrome, cerebral palsy)

Source: Adapted from Holdoway, A., & Smith, A. (2020). Meeting nutritional need and managing patients with dysphagia. *Journal of Community Nursing, 34*(2), 52–59; Nazarko, L. (2020). Dysphagia: A guide for nurses in general practice. *Practice Nursing, 31*(4), 162–168. https://doi.org/10.12968/pnur.2020.31.4.162.

Diagnosing Actual or Potential Health Problems and Needs

An assessment of a patient's nutrition status may lead to the identification of one or more actual or potential health problems and needs related to nutrition. Following the formulation of the actual or potential health problems and needs, the nurse communicates findings to other nursing and health care professionals through the use of the written and spoken word. The written actual or potential health problem or need becomes a permanent part of the patient's health record. Examples of health problems and needs with related etiology and signs and symptoms can be found in the box Examples of Actual or Potential Health Problems and Needs: Nutrition on page 1410.

Outcome Identification and Planning

Expected outcomes are derived from the actual or potential nutritional problems identified. The goal is to maintain or restore optimal nutritional status using foods the patient likes and tolerates as appropriate for their situation. Goals should also include those to alleviate symptoms or side effects of disease or treatment and to prevent complications or diet-related chronic diseases. General patient outcomes are listed here. Actual patient outcomes should list specific behaviors and criteria individualized for the patient situation. The patient will:

- Attain and maintain ideal body weight, as indicated by BMI and waist circumference.
- Eat a diet adequate but not excessive in all nutrients, based on the *Dietary Guidelines for Americans 2020–2025*, the MyPlate food guideline system, and the DRIs.
- Eat a variety of food in each of three or more meals.
- Follow the appropriate modified diet, when necessary, to restore health, avoid disease recurrences, and prevent or delay potential complications.

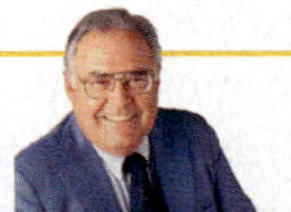

Remember **Charles Gallagher**, the husband of the woman receiving enteral nutrition. Initially, outcomes would focus on maintaining his wife's nutritional status. However, the informed decision made to withdraw the nutritional support would lead the nurse to revise the outcomes. Therefore, the outcomes then would focus on emotional comfort for the Gallagher family and a peaceful, dignified death for Mrs. Gallagher.

Box 37-5 Biochemical Data With Nutritional Implications

Values for Adults

- Hemoglobin (normal = 12–18 g/dL)
  decreased → anemia
- Hematocrit (normal = 46–52%)
  decreased → anemia
- Prealbumin (normal = 19–38 mg/dL)
  decreased → protein depletion, malnutrition
- Transferrin (normal = 250–425 mg/dL)
  decreased → anemia, protein deficiency or loss from burns or malnutrition
- Blood urea nitrogen (normal = 6–20 mg/dL)
  increased → starvation, high-protein intake, severe dehydration
  decreased → malnutrition, low-protein diet, overhydration
- Serum creatinine (normal = 0.6–1.2 mg/dL)
  increased → dehydration
  decreased → reduction in total muscle mass, severe malnutrition

Source: Adapted Fischbach, F. T., Fischbach, M. A., & Stout, K. (2022). *Fischbach's a manual of laboratory and diagnostic tests* (11th ed.). Wolters Kluwer.

Implementing

Providing proper and adequate nourishment to the patient is a collaborative effort implemented in a variety of settings. Diet interventions are prescribed in the inpatient setting based on input from the dietitian, the nurse and other health care providers; nurses often provide dietary education and support for the patient. The nurse may also be responsible for screening patients at home who are at nutritional risk, observing intake and appetite, evaluating the patient's tolerance, and assisting the patient with eating. Other nursing interventions related to meeting patients' nutritional needs may include administering enteral and parenteral feedings, consulting with the dietitian and the health care team when dietary problems

Examples of Actual or Potential Health Problems and Needs

NUTRITION

Actual or Potential Health Problems and Needs	Possible Etiologic Factors	Potential Signs and Symptoms
Impaired Nutritional Status	Insufficient dietary intake, increased metabolic demands	• "Foods just don't taste good anymore." • Reports losing 15 lb within the past 3 weeks. • Several ulcers present on buccal mucosa. • Reports "frequent loose stools" every day for past 2 weeks. • Patient appears fatigued and undernourished; muscle wasting is evident. Laboratory data reveal protein deficiency.
Impaired Swallowing	Neuromuscular impairment, weakness	• "Food seems to get stuck." "Sometimes I can't finish eating because I cough too much." • Swallowing evaluation study reports abnormality in oral and pharyngeal phases. Patient observed to have difficulty chewing; delayed swallow; gags and coughs during meal; gurgly voice quality noted after meal.
Body Weight Problem: Overweight	Excessive food intake in relation to physical activity Sedentary behavior occurring for >2 hours/day BMI 24; waist circumference 39 inches	—

Source: International Council of Nurses (ICN). (2019). *Nursing diagnosis and outcome statements.* https://www.icn.ch/sites/default/files/inline-files/ICNP2019-DC.pdf

arise, addressing the potential for drug–nutrient reactions, obtaining more food or snacks for the patient when appropriate, monitoring food brought by visitors or prepared by family members/caregivers, monitoring food accessibility, and participating in nutrition education efforts.

Patients with increased nutritional requirements, those who are unable to meet their nutritional requirements orally, and those who will be NPO for more than 48 to 72 hours (Jordan & Moore, 2020) may require nutritional support from **enteral nutrition**, administering nutrients directly into the stomach, or **parenteral nutrition (PN)**, providing nutrition via intravenous (IV) therapy, based on individual circumstances.

> **QSEN TEAMWORK AND COLLABORATION**
>
> **Patients, nurses, dieticians, physicians, and other members of the health care team each have key roles in assessing, addressing, and monitoring nutrition and nutrition-related care issues and concerns. Communication and collaboration between the nurse, patient, and other health care professionals result in thoughtful, person-centered nutritional care.**

Teaching Nutritional Information

For the greatest chance of success, tailor nutrition instructions individually to the patient's lifestyle, culture, literacy level, and level of motivation. Although strict guidelines and printed handouts may seem ideal, in practice, simplicity and compromise are often the keys to patient engagement. Educational interventions should reinforce the importance of and rationale for adequate nutrition. Nurses should include basic principles of the prescribed nutritional plan and emphasize positive actions, "things to do" instead of what the patient should not do and/or cannot eat (Tappenden et al., 2013).

In the hospital, shortened stays limit the time available for nutritional screening and intervention. Patients are often acutely ill and may be unable to absorb and retain any nutritional instruction. Educational sessions may be limited and should focus on immediate needs. It may also be difficult to include a family member or caregiver responsible for food preparation in scheduled teaching sessions.

Often, more extensive education is more realistic in community settings. In many situations, the home health care nurse has the opportunity to have a significant impact on nutritional health. Provide instruction in a relaxed setting that allows insight into a patient's cultural orientation and family/caregiver patterns and traditions. This type of environment also encourages modification and adjustments in the nurse's approach to nutritional instruction. Investigate the variety of community services and programs that are available to provide nutritional support to patients at home. The accompanying Focus on the Older Adult includes teaching content and strategies for the specific nutritional challenges facing the older adult. Refer to Chapter 9 for additional information and guidelines related to teaching and counseling.

Focus on the Older Adult

NURSING STRATEGIES TO ADDRESS AGE-RELATED CHANGES AFFECTING NUTRITION

Age-Related Changes	Nursing Strategies
Altered ability to chew related to loss of teeth, ill-fitting dentures, and gingivitis	• Encourage and instruct patient to care for and retain own teeth and dentures. • Encourage proper tooth brushing and use of special toothpaste if gums and teeth are sensitive. • Chop, shred, or puree foods that are difficult to chew. • Select ground meat, fish, or poultry as protein sources more easily chewed.
Loss of senses of smell and taste	• Serve food that is attractive and at proper temperature. • Serve one food at a time rather than mixing foods. • Serve foods with different textures and aromas.
Decreased peristalsis in the esophagus	• Avoid cold liquids. • Avoid emotional upsets and stress-producing situations. • Take anticholinergic drugs as prescribed.
Gastroesophageal reflux	• Avoid overeating. • Avoid juices, chocolate, and fat. • Avoid alcohol and smoking. • Elevate the head of the bed 30 to 40 degrees when sleeping. • Lose weight if necessary. • Avoid bending over. • Take antacids or other medications as prescribed. • Avoid eating right before bedtime.
Decreased gastric secretions	• Chew food thoroughly. • Eat meals on a regular schedule. • Use antacids or other medications as prescribed. • Be alert for symptoms of deficiency of nutrients, particularly iron, calcium, fat, protein, and vitamin B_{12}.
Slowed intestinal peristalsis	• Eat a high-fiber diet. • Remain as active as possible. • Increase fluid intake. • Avoid laxative use. • Eat meals at a regular time. • Drink prune juice or eat prunes every morning.
Lowered glucose tolerance	• Eat more complex carbohydrates. • Avoid sugar-rich foods.
Reduction in appetite and thirst sensation	• Offer fluids at regular intervals and at preferred temperature. • Be alert for symptoms of dehydration and electrolyte imbalance. • Offer small meals at frequent intervals.
Nutritional deficiencies related to alcohol intake	• Encourage diet high in protein and carbohydrates. • Offer small, frequent meals to maintain caloric intake. • Restrict sodium and fluids if edema is present. • Take multivitamin supplements, as prescribed.
Loss of appetite associated with depression and loneliness	• Promote mealtime as a social event. • Set an attractive table in a pleasant setting. • Eat outdoors whenever possible. • Invite guests as often as possible. • Participate in special programs for senior citizens.
Physical disability	• Open cartons and assist with setup of meal. • Arrange for home-delivered meals. • Conserve energy when preparing meals (sit on a stool, etc.). • Provide transportation and assistance to obtain food.
Low income	• Buy specials when available at food store. • Use generic brands. • Use coupons. • Cook larger quantities than necessary and freeze the leftovers for future use. • Substitute eggs, skim milk powder, and beans for meat. • Check for any community resources available to older adult.

(*continued on page 1412*)

Focus on the Older Adult *(continued)*

NURSING STRATEGIES TO ADDRESS AGE-RELATED CHANGES AFFECTING NUTRITION

Age-Related Changes	Nursing Strategies
Malnutrition	• Eat essential foods first. • Select nutrient-dense foods. • Monitor for signs of nutritional deficiencies. • Encourage eating by planning special events.
Increased risk for drug–nutrient interactions	• Avoid unnecessary drugs; monitor for polypharmacy. • Be aware of drug actions and interactions. • Check with pharmacist to determine if medication may or may not be taken with food. • Assess for confusion and inability to manage medication regimen.

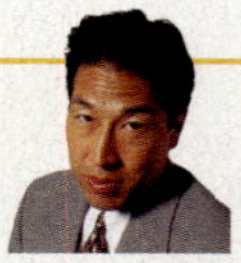

Recall **William Johnston**, the patient with hypertension and high cholesterol. The nurse would need to consider Mr. Johnston's lifestyle when developing a teaching plan for him. As a result of his "on-the-run" lifestyle, the nurse would need to adapt the teaching plan, making sure that it is realistic for his needs. For example, the nurse might teach Mr. Johnston about reading food labels to ensure that his selections, when he is "on the run" are low in fat and cholesterol. In addition, the nurse would also provide Mr. Johnston with appropriate suggestions for choices when dining out. Doing so will help communicate to him that the plan is workable, enhancing the chances of Mr. Johnston complying with the plan, thereby achieving success.

Include information about food safety issues in patient teaching. This includes safe handling of foods, food storage, and preventing food-borne illness. Encourage patients to wash hands and clean food contact surfaces frequently when handling and preparing foods (U.S. DHHS, 2020). Wash fruits and vegetables before eating or preparation but not meat, poultry or eggs (U.S. DHHS, 2020). This helps prevent contamination of food with bacteria and viruses. Teach patients to cook foods to a safe temperature to kill microorganisms. Also, explain that raw, cooked, and ready-to-eat foods should be separated during shopping and preparation and should be stored separately (U.S. DHHS, 2020). This prevents cross-contamination with microorganisms. Chill (refrigerate) perishable food within 2 hours and keep cold foods at 40°F or lower in the refrigerator and 0°F in the freezer to prevent the growth of pathogens. Teach patients to cook food to an internal temperature that is high enough to kill pathogens and keep foods hot (140°F or above) after cooking (U.S. DHHS, 2020). Refer patients and their family/caregivers to a Minimum Cooking Temperature reference to ensure foods are cooked to a safe temperature. The U.S. Department of Health and Human Services (2019) provides one such reference at https://www.foodsafety.gov/food-safety-charts/safe-minimum-cooking-temperature.

Monitoring Nutritional Status

Responsibilities of nurses related to monitoring the patient's nutritional status include (Anderson, 2019a; Dudek, 2022; Tappenden et al., 2013):

- Assessment/observation of food and supplement intake in relation to identified outcomes
- Documentation of appetite and initiating appropriate interventions when the patient does not eat
- Collaborating with the health care team to implement supplements if the patient's intake is low or the patient has increased nutritional requirements
- Collaborating with the health care team to initiate a nutritional consult
- Assess the patient's tolerance of the prescribed diet
- Monitor the patient's weight
- Monitor progression of nothing by mouth (NPO) status and prescribed restrictive diets
- Monitor the patient's understanding of nutritional information and engagement
- Monitor the patient's progress in meeting goals identified in the plan of care for nutrition

Nurses are often involved in the process of diet progression. The decision to advance a patient's diet is based on the return of GI function, the absence of symptoms related to a particular disease process, or the resolution of whatever prompted the dietary restriction. Often, prescribed interventions are written to begin the patient on one diet and advance to another diet as tolerated. This allows the nurse to assess the patient's tolerance of the beginning diet and change, or advance, the diet based on the assessments. Diet tolerance can be assessed by the following: absence of nausea, vomiting, and diarrhea; absence of feelings of fullness; absence of abdominal pain and distention; feelings of hunger; and the ability to consume at least 50% to 75% of the food on the meal tray. For example, a postoperative patient may have an order to begin a clear liquid at breakfast and advance to a house diet as tolerated. The patient would receive a clear liquid diet for breakfast. The nurse would assess the patient's ability to ingest the clear liquids and then make a decision regarding progression of the diet.

Stimulating Appetite

Pain, illness, anxiety, and medications can contribute to anorexia and poor intake when in a health care facility or in the home. To the hospitalized patient, food and eating may take on much greater meaning. Loss of control over food choices, the way food is prepared, when and how food is served, and eating alone may do little to encourage normal eating. Make every effort to ensure that the proper food is not only served, but also eaten. The additional time and attention spent when encouraging a person to eat may have a positive effect on dietary intake. The following measures may help to stimulate appetite in any setting:

- Serve small, frequent meals to avoid overwhelming the person with large amounts of food.
- Solicit food preferences and encourage favorite foods from home or prepared when at home, if possible.
- Provide encouragement and a pleasant eating environment.
- Be sure that any prepared food looks attractive.
- Schedule procedures and medications at times when they are least likely to interfere with appetite.
- Control pain, nausea, or depression with medications.
- Offer alternatives for items that a person cannot or will not eat.
- Encourage or provide good oral hygiene. Ensure that the patient's dentures are well-fitting and in place, if applicable.
- Remove clutter from the eating area.
- Keep eating area free from irritating odors.
- Arrange food tray so that a person can easily reach food.
- Provide a comfortable position.
- Ask about any rituals during mealtimes at home and include them if possible.
- If patients are absent from their rooms during mealtime, order a late food tray or keep food warm until they return.
- Do not disturb mealtime; don't interrupt patients for nonurgent procedures during mealtime.

Technology Alert

Health information technology (HIT) has broadened the ways by which patients can participate and engage in nutrition care, improving dietary intake and outcomes (Roberts et al., 2020). One HIT aims to improve patients' nutrition intakes by engaging patients and enabling patient participation in nutrition care while in the hospital. Patients are provided with patient education related to the importance of meeting energy/protein requirements and training on how to use the HIT, the hospital's electronic foodservice system, access via bedside computer screens. Patients also record their food intake after each meal on the bedside computer and track their intakes relative to their nutritional goals, combined with daily goal-setting sessions with a health care professional (Roberts et al., 2020).

Assisting With Eating

The loss of independence that comes with the inability to self-feed can be a severe blow to a person's self-esteem. The following measures may help a person maintain dignity while being fed:

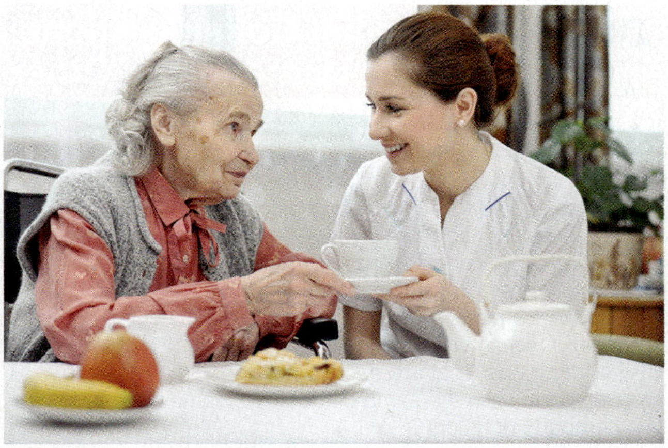

FIGURE 37-6. Creating a relaxed, person-centered atmosphere. (*Source: Photo by Alexander Raths/Shutterstock.*)

- Involve the person as much as possible. Solicit the patient's preferences regarding the order of items eaten and the eating pace.
- Provide appropriate drinks.
- Sit at the patient's eye level and make eye contact to create a more relaxed, person-centered atmosphere (Fig. 37-6).
- Engage the person in pleasant conversation to ease tension.
- Place a napkin, not a bib, over the person's clothes for protection.
- Use straws or special eating utensils whenever possible.
- Ensure that if a person wears dentures, hearing aids, or glasses, they are in place before mealtime.
- Open containers, cut meat, or apply condiments to the prepared food only if the person wishes.

When assisting visually impaired patients:

- Explain placement of foods on plates and food tray. Relating items on plate to the location on a clock face may be helpful.
- Provide special plate guards, utensils, double handles, and compartmentalized plates.
- Place foods and dishes in similar locations at each meal.
- Use straws for beverages, if not contraindicated by the presence of dysphagia.
- Provide supervision as needed.

Box 37-6 (on page 1414) outlines special considerations and interventions for feeding patients with dementia or other alterations in cognition. Box 37-7 (on page 1414) highlights nursing considerations for feeding patients with dysphagia.

Providing Oral Nutrition

A variety of oral diets are available in health care settings and may be prescribed for use at home. Oral diets may be categorized as regular, modified consistency, or therapeutic (Dudek, 2022). Regular, regular vegetarian, and modified consistency diets are outlined here. Information regarding common therapeutic diets is outlined in Table 37-3 on page 1415.

NORMAL OR HOUSE DIETS

Normal, regular, or house diets are designed to achieve or maintain optimal nutritional status by providing adequate

Box 37-6 Special Considerations and Interventions for Feeding Patients With Dementia or Other Alterations in Cognition

- Change the environment in which meals occur.
- Assess the area where meals are served. Create a homelike environment by preparing food close to the place where it will be served to stimulate senses.
- Observe as many former rituals as possible, such as handwashing and saying a blessing.
- Avoid clutter and limit distractions.
- Maintain a pleasant, well-lighted room. Play calming music.
- Keep food as close to its original form as possible; try "finger foods" that are easy to pick up.
- Serve meals in the same place at the same time and in the company of others.
- Provide longer and continuous facilitation at mealtimes.
- Check food temperatures to prevent accidental mouth burns.
- Assist as needed. Be alert for cues from the patient. Turning away may signal that the patient has had enough to eat or that the patient needs to slow down. Leaning forward with an open mouth usually means the patient is ready for more food.
- Stroking the underside of the chin may help promote swallowing.
- Provide one or two food items at a time. Offer small, frequent eating opportunities. A whole tray of food may be overwhelming.
- Ensure that the patient's glasses and hearing aid are working properly.
- Demonstrate what you want the patient to do. State the goal clearly, and then mimic the action with exaggerated motions.
- Provide foods and between-meal snacks that are easy to consume using the hands.
- Use adaptive feeding equipment as needed such as weighted utensils, large-handled cups, and larger or smaller silverware than standard.
- Promote family/caregiver involvement to encourage eating.

Source: Adapted from Alzheimer's Association. Alzheimer's and Dementia Caregiver Center. (n.d.). *Food and eating.* Retrieved September 26, 2020, from https://www.alz.org/help-support/caregiving/daily-care/food-eating; Liu, W., Williams, K., Batchelor-Murphy, M., Perkhounkova, Y., & Hein, M. (2019). Eating performance in relation to intake of solid and liquid food in nursing home residents with dementia: A secondary behavioral analysis of mealtime videos. *International Journal of Nursing Studies, 96,* 18–26. https://doi.org/10.1016/j.ijnurstu.2018.12.010; and Mendes, A. (2018). Optimising nutritional intake in people with dementia on hospital wards. *British Journal of Nursing, 27*(20), 1206. https://doi.org/10.12968/bjon.2018.27.20.1206

amounts of all nutrients. The diet's actual composition and nutritional value varies with the quantity and types of food selected by the patient. No foods are excluded. Portion sizes are not limited. Regular diets are adjusted to meet age-specific needs throughout the life cycle and may also be altered to meet vegetarian, kosher, or other eating preferences for an individual patient (Dudek, 2022).

VEGETARIAN DIETS

Some patients may prefer a vegetarian diet for a variety of reasons, such as religious preference, ethical belief that killing animals for food is unjust, fear of contamination with pesticides, or health concerns about the cholesterol and saturated fats found in meats. There are many different forms of vegetarianism, ranging from avoidance of red meat to complete elimination of all animal products. Meats are usually replaced with legumes, grains, and vegetables, and, if well planned, this type of diet can satisfy all nutritional requirements. Because fewer or no animal products are consumed, vegetarians consume less saturated fat, cholesterol, and animal protein and greater amounts of carbohydrates, fiber, and other important nutrients. Vitamin B_{12}, vitamin A, and iron are nutrients that may require supplementation in some vegetarian diets, but most vegetarian diets are not

Box 37-7 Special Considerations and Interventions for Feeding Patients With Dysphagia

- Provide at least a 30-minute rest period prior to mealtime. A rested person will likely have less difficulty swallowing.
- Sit the patient upright, preferably in a chair. If bedrest is mandatory, elevate the head of the bed to a 90-degree angle. Maintain upright position for 30 minutes after the meal.
- Provide mouth care immediately before meals to enhance the sense of taste.
- Avoid rushed or forced feeding.
- Provide small, frequent meals to help maximize intake.
- Adjust the rate of feeding and size of bites to the patient's tolerance. Allow patient to control the eating process if possible.
- Collaborate to obtain a speech therapy consult for swallowing evaluation.
- Initiate a nutrition consult for appropriate diet modification such as chopping, mincing, or pureeing of foods and liquid consistency (thin, nectar-thick, honeylike, spoon-thick).
- Keep in mind that some patients may find thickened liquids unpalatable and thus drink insufficient fluids.
- Reduce or eliminate distractions at mealtime so that the patient can focus attention on swallowing; discourage chatting during the meal.
- Alternate solids and liquids.
- Assess for signs of aspiration during eating: sudden appearance of severe coughing; choking; cyanosis; voice change, hoarseness, and/or gurgling after swallowing; frequent throat clearing after meals; or regurgitation through the nose or mouth.
- Inspect oral cavity for retained food.
- Avoid or minimize the use of sedatives and hypnotics since these agents may impair the cough reflex and swallowing.

Source: Adapted from Dudek, S. (2022). *Nutrition essentials for nursing practice* (9th ed.). Wolters Kluwer; Holdoway, A., & Smith, A. (2020). Meeting nutritional need and managing patients with dysphagia. *Journal of Community Nursing, 34*(2), 52–59; Metheny, N. (n.d.). *Issue #20. General assessment series. Preventing aspiration in older adults with dysphagia.* From https://hign.org/consultgeri/try-this-series/preventing-aspiration-older-adults-dysphagia; and Nazarko, L. (2020). Dysphagia: A guide for nurses in general practice. *Practice Nursing, 31*(4), 162–168. https://doi.org/10.12968/pnur.2020.31.4.162

Table 37-3 Selected Therapeutic Diets

DIET AND DESCRIPTION	INDICATIONS
Consistent-carbohydrate diet: Total daily carbohydrate content is consistent; emphasizes general nutritional balance. Calories based on attaining and maintaining healthy weight. High-fiber and heart-healthy fats encouraged; sodium and saturated fats are limited.	Type 1 and type 2 diabetes, gestational diabetes, impaired glucose tolerance
Fat-restricted diet: Low-fat diets are intended to lower the patient's total intake of fat.	Chronic cholecystitis (inflammation of the gallbladder) to decrease gallbladder stimulation; cardiovascular disease, to help prevent atherosclerosis
High-fiber diet: Emphasis on increased intake of foods high in fiber.	Prevent or treat constipation; irritable bowel syndrome; diverticulosis
Low-fiber diet: Fiber limited to <10 g/day.	Before surgery; ulcerative colitis; diverticulitis; Crohn disease
Sodium-restricted diet: Sodium limit may be set at 500–3,000 mg/day	Hypertension; heart failure; acute and chronic renal disease, liver disease
Renal diet: Reduce workload on kidneys to delay or prevent further damage; control accumulation of uremic toxins. Protein restriction 0.6–1 g/kg/day; sodium restriction 1,000–3,000 mg/day; potassium and fluid restrictions dependent on patient situation	Nephrotic syndrome; chronic kidney disease; diabetic kidney disease

deficient in any nutrients. Support patients who follow a vegetarian diet by assisting them or their caregiver to select nutritious food items from the large variety of foods available within their dietary framework.

MODIFIED CONSISTENCY DIETS

Liquid diets are used most often as transitional diets when eating resumes after acute illness, surgery, or parenteral nutrition. Because clear-liquid diets are inadequate in calories, protein, and most nutrients, progression to more nutritious alternatives is recommended as soon as possible.

Full-liquid diets contain all the items on a clear-liquid diet. Additional items allowed include milk and milk drinks, puddings, custards, plain frozen desserts, pasteurized eggs, cereal gruels, vegetable juices, and milk and egg substitutes. A full-liquid diet contains liquids that can be poured at room temperature. High-calorie, high-protein supplements are recommended if a full-liquid diet is used for more than 3 days.

Mechanically altered diets are adequate in calories and nutrients and may be used on a long-term basis. Additional information regarding modified-consistency diets (modified-texture diets, texture-modified diets) can be found in Table 37-4.

ORAL NUTRITIONAL SUPPLEMENTS

Oral nutritional supplements (ONSs), foods rich in energy, protein, and macro- and micronutrients are used as part of the plan of care for patients who are unable to meet their nutritional requirements through oral diet alone (Ballesteros-Pomar et al., 2020). Patients whose intake of food is insufficient to meet their requirements, such as patients who are unable or unwilling to eat, or whose nutritional needs are so great that a normal volume of food is insufficient, are often prescribed ONS (Dudek, 2022). ONSs are also indicated as a primary intervention for patients identified at risk of malnutrition (Anderson, 2019a; Holdoway & Anderson, 2019). ONSs are available in a wide range of styles, including clear liquids, milk/dairy-based drinks, specially prepared

Table 37-4 Modified Consistency Diets

DIET AND DESCRIPTION	INDICATIONS
Clear liquid diet: Composed only of clear fluids or foods that become fluid at body temperature. Requires minimal digestion and leaves minimal residue. Includes clear broth, coffee, tea, clear fruit juices (apple, cranberry, grape), gelatin, popsicles, commercially prepared clear liquid supplements.	Preparation for bowel surgery and lower endoscopy; acute gastrointestinal disorders; initial postoperative diet
Puréed diet: Also known as a blenderized liquid diet because the diet is made up of liquids and foods blenderized to liquid form. All foods are allowed.	After oral or facial surgery; chewing and swallowing difficulties
Mechanically altered diet: Regular diet with modifications for texture. Excludes most raw fruits and vegetables and foods with seeds, nuts, and dried fruits. Foods are chopped, ground, mashed, or soft.	Chewing and swallowing difficulties; after surgery to the head, neck, or mouth

foods (puddings, yogurts, shakes, gelatins, nutrition bars), and powders (Dudek, 2022; Holdoway & Anderson, 2019). Patient preferences should be considered when implementing the use of ONSs, and education about the benefits of use should be reinforced to enhance patient understanding and engagement (Dudek, 2022).

NOTHING BY MOUTH

Patients may be prescribed nothing by mouth (**NPO**) for a period of time prior to surgery or before certain diagnostic tests. NPO may also be necessary for patients experiencing severe nausea and vomiting, an inability to chew or swallow, or various acute or chronic GI abnormalities; for those who are comatose; and for women during labor and delivery.

The following measures may provide comfort to patients who are ordered NPO:

- Encourage or provide good oral hygiene.
- Provide the patient with ice chips or sips of water as allowed.
- Urge the patient to avoid watching others eat. Suggest alternate activities at mealtimes.

Well-nourished patients can easily withstand the stress of NPO for a short period, but being NPO for an extended period of time poses a nutritional challenge for many people. Patients who will be NPO for more than 48 to 72 hours may require nutritional support from enteral nutrition (EN) or parenteral nutrition (PN), depending on individual circumstances (Delgado, 2018; Jordan & Moore, 2019). These therapies are discussed in the following sections.

Providing Enteral Nutrition

Oral feeding is the preferred and most effective method of feeding patients. However, at times, a patient may be unable to meet their nutritional needs through oral intake of an adequate diet. In this circumstance, an alternate feeding method may be necessary. Placement of an enteral feeding tube into the stomach (gastric) or small intestine (jejunum) to provide a formula containing adequate nutrients may be appropriate; enteral nutrition is the preferred method of feeding after the oral route for patients who have at least a partially functional GI tract (Dudek, 2022; Hartwell et al., 2018; Pars & Çavuşoğlu, 2019). Enteral nutrition (EN) may be used to supplement an oral diet or provide the only source of nutrition (Dudek, 2022).

Gastric feedings have the advantage of allowing the stomach to be used as a natural reservoir, regulating the amount of foods and liquids released into the small intestine. This alternate feeding method may deliver total or supplemental nutrition over a short-term period or for longer intervals. EN is contraindicated when the GI tract is nonfunctional, in severe short bowel syndrome, intractable vomiting and/or diarrhea, GI ischemia, bowel obstruction, peritonitis, and paralytic ileus (Dudek, 2022). Consider factors related to selection of a feeding tube, including aspiration risk, the anticipated duration of the feeding tube, the function of the GI tract, and the patient's overall condition and prognosis. Also, it is important to consider the ethical implications surrounding initiation of tube feedings, which entail knowledge of the patient's wishes concerning this intervention.

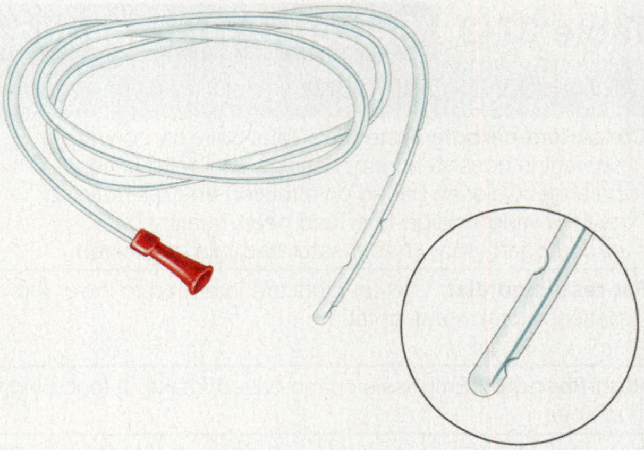

FIGURE 37-7. Levin tube.

The decision to place, maintain, and/or discontinue feeding tubes can be a source of much turmoil in the lives of patients and their families (Hartwell et al., 2018). There are many emotional, physical, psychological, cultural, and quality-of-life aspects to the institution, maintenance, and withdrawal of nutrition (Bischoff et al., 2020). Nurses can be a source of great support and information to aid patients and their families in making nutrition-related health care decisions.

SHORT-TERM NUTRITIONAL SUPPORT

For short-term use (<4 weeks [Bischoff et al., 2020; Dudek, 2022]), a nasogastric or nasointestinal route may be selected. A **nasogastric (NG) tube** is inserted through the nose and into the stomach. However, the patient is at risk for aspirating the tube feeding solution into the lungs, a disadvantage for using this route.

Nasogastric tubes may be firm and large in diameter. One example is a Levin tube. A Levin tube is a flexible rubber or plastic single-lumen tube with holes at the stomach end and a connector at the opposing end (Fig. 37-7). The connector allows for attachment to a feeding apparatus and medication administration. These tubes are fairly inflexible and are associated with patient discomfort (Anderson, 2018a). Smaller, softer, more pliable polyurethane tubes may also be inserted via the nose into the stomach or small intestine. This type of tube is advantageous, providing greater patient comfort and less trauma to the nares (Anderson, 2018a). A Dobbhoff tube is an example of this type of tube (Fig. 37-8). However, the smaller tube diameter makes

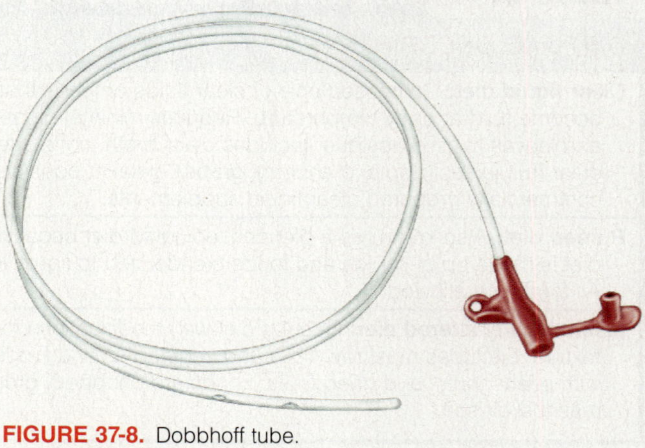

FIGURE 37-8. Dobbhoff tube.

checking tube placement and medication administration more difficult than with the larger-diameter tubes. The methods of inserting and removing a nasogastric tube are described in Skills 39-2 on pages 1560–1565 and 39-3 on pages 1566–1568.

Less commonly, a **nasointestinal (NI) tube** is passed through the nose and into the upper portion of the small intestine (nasoduodenal and nasojejunal). NI may be indicated for a patient with high risk for aspiration or who have shown intolerance to gastric EN (Bischoff et al., 2020; McClave, Taylor, et al., 2016). Some health conditions (e.g., delayed gastroduodenal motility, gastric outlet stenosis) also necessitate the use of a nasointestinal tube (Bischoff et al., 2020; Turner et al., 2020).

CONFIRMATION OF NASOGASTRIC FEEDING TUBE PLACEMENT

Verify correct placement of the nasogastric tube after the initial insertion, before beginning a feeding or instilling medications or liquids, and at regular intervals during continuous feedings. This decreases the risk that the tip of the tube is situated in the stomach or intestine, preventing inadvertent administration of substances into the wrong place. A misplaced feeding tube in the lungs or pulmonary tissue places the patient at risk for aspiration, pneumonia, and even death (Lamont et al., 2011, as cited in Anderson, 2018a). Radiographic examination, measurement of tube length and measurement of tube marking, measurement of aspirate pH, and monitoring of carbon dioxide have been suggested to confirm feeding tube placement (Anderson, 2018a; Irving et al., 2018; Methany et al., 2019). The use of two or more of these techniques in conjunction with each other increases the likelihood of correct tube placement (AACN, 2020; Anderson, 2019b; Anderson, 2018a; Dias et al., 2019; Rahimi et al., 2015). An old technique of auscultation of air injected into a feeding tube has been proved unreliable and is not suggested for use (AACN, 2020; Anderson, 2018a; Boeykens et al., 2014; Boullata et al., 2017; Irving et al., 2018; Metheny et al., 2019). Recommendations for use of visual inspection of gastric aspirate are conflicting; this method should be used cautiously if part of policy and procedure guidelines and with consideration to the potential for inaccuracy (AACN, 2020; Dias et al., 2019; Mak & Tam, 2020; Metheny et al., 2019).

When bedside methods to check placement suggest the tube has been displaced, a radiograph should be requested to determine the tube's location (AACN, 2020).

Technology Alert

The use of ultrasound has been suggested to verify correct positioning of gastric tubes as an alternative for radiologic examination. This visualization technique has shown promise in aiding in confirmation of correct placement of gastric tubes in newborns, pediatric and adult patients, in both inpatient and outpatient settings (Atalay et al., 2016; Dias et al., 2019 ; Mak & Tam, 2020; Tsujimoto et al., 2017). The use of ultrasound to provide accurate imaging of nasogastric tube position and avoid the use of x-ray holds potential to complement other means of verification of placement as well as provide critical information where x-rays are not readily available (Mak & Tam, 2020).

Radiographic Examination

Radiographic examination (x-ray) is the standard procedure to verify initial placement of a feeding tube as it allows the visualization of the entire course and the location of the tip of the tube (AACN, 2020; Boullata et al., 2017; Mueller et al., 2011). However, radiographs expose the patient to radiation, must be interpreted by a radiologist, are costly if done on a routine basis, and may be inaccessible. A radiograph only confirms the position of the tube at the time it was taken. The tube may have moved at any point thereafter. Also, as previously stated, placement must be checked frequently while the tube is in place, and repeated, frequent radiographs are not practical (Boullata et al., 2017). Routine chest and abdominal radiography reports can be reviewed to determine if the radiologist has referred to feeding tube location as part of monitoring tube location (AACN, 2020).

Measurement of Tube Length and Verification of Tube Marking

Another way to verify tube placement is to measure the length of the exposed tube after insertion and document this measurement (AACN, 2020; Dias et al., 2019). Once placement has been confirmed by initial radiograph, mark the exit site of the feeding tube with an indelible marker at the nostril or note the centimeter marking on the tube (AACN, 2020; Irving et al., 2018; Judd, 2020). Observe for a change in the external tube length at regular intervals and before use (AACN, 2020). Any change in the length of the exposed tube may indicate dislodgement (AACN, 2020; Boullata et al., 2017). If a significant change in the external length is observed, use other bedside tests to help determine if the tube has become dislocated (Best, 2013; Boullata et al., 2017). If placement is in doubt, a radiograph should be obtained to verify tube placement (AACN, 2020; Boullata et al., 2017).

Assessment of Aspirate pH

Testing of the pH of gastric secretions aspirated from the tube is recommended to verify gastric tube placement (AACN, 2020; Dias et al., 2019; Irving et al., 2018; Metheny et al., 2019). Fasting gastric pH is usually 5 or less, even in patients receiving gastric-acid inhibitors (AACN, 2020). The pH of feeding tube aspirates is likely to approach fasting levels if nutritional feedings have been off for at least 1 hour (AACN, 2020; Irving et al., 2018). However, when continuous feedings are in use, pH may become less helpful, because the nutritional formula may buffer the pH of GI secretions (Judd, 2020). Refer to Guidelines for Nursing Care 37-1 (on page 1418). Gastric pH ≥ 6 is of no benefit in predicting tube location in the GI tract or in ruling out tracheopulmonary placement (Boullata et al., 2017).

Use of pH test strips calibrated in units of 0.5 and approved for use with human secretions should be used to ensure accuracy (Anderson, 2018; Metheny et al., 2019). There is considerable variation in the evidence guidelines related to the pH values to distinguish between gastric and

Guidelines for Nursing Care 37-1

ASSESSMENT AND pH MEASUREMENT OF GASTRIC CONTENTS

Allow 1-hour interval after patient has received medication or completed an intermittent feeding before testing pH of gastric fluid. Feedings should never be interrupted solely for the purpose of pH testing; however, if a feeding is interrupted as part of preparation for a test or procedure, testing of the pH may be desired.

- Assemble supplies, and provide for privacy. Use of pH test strips calibrated in units of 0.5 and approved for use with human secretions should be used to ensure accuracy.

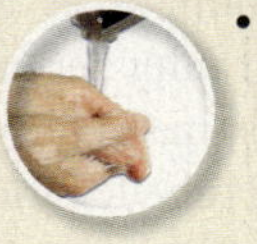

- Explain the procedure to the patient, perform hand hygiene, and put on disposable gloves.
- Attach the syringe to the end of the tube and aspirate a small amount (5 to 10 mL) of gastric secretions.
- If unable to obtain specimen, reposition the patient and flush tube with an air bolus, then apply negative pressure to the plunger. It may be necessary to retry several times.
- Place a drop of gastric secretions onto pH test strip or place small amount in plastic cup and dip pH test strip into it. Within 30 seconds, compare color on test strip with chart supplied by the manufacturer.
- Document results on the patient's flow sheet. The following are indications of placement:

pH

- Stomach: Suggested limits for a safe range are from pH of ≤4.0, ≤5.0, and ≤5.5
- Intestines: pH 7.0 or higher
- Respiratory tract: pH of ≥6.0

This method will not effectively differentiate between intestinal fluid and pleural fluid.

Source: Adapted from American Association of Critical Care Nurses (AACN). (2020, January 29). *AACN Practice Alert. Initial and ongoing verification of feeding tube placement in adults.* https://www.aacn.org/; Anderson, L. (2018). Fine-bore nasogastric tube feeding: Reducing the risks. *British Journal of Nursing, 27*(12), 674–675. https://doi.org/10.12968/bjon.2018.27.12.674; Dias, F. S. B., Almeida, B. P., Alvares, B. R., Jales, R. M., Caldas, J. P. S., & Carmona, E. V. (2019). Use of pH reagent strips to verify gastric tube placement in newborns. *Revista Latino-Americana de Enfermagem, 27*, e3227. https://doi.org/10.1590/1518-8345.3150.3227; Metheny, N. A., Krieger, M. M., Healey, F., & Meert, K. L. (2019). A review of guidelines to distinguish between gastric and pulmonary placement of nasogastric tubes. *Heart & Lung, 48*(3), 226–235. https://doi.org/10.1016/j.hrtlng.2019.01.003

respiratory aspirates (Metheny et al., 2019). The lower the pH, obviously, the stronger the evidence for placement in the stomach and not the respiratory tract (Metheny et al., 2019). Suggested limits for a safe range to identify gastric secretions vary from pHs of ≤4.0, ≤5.0, and ≤5.5 and a pH of ≥6.0 for respiratory secretions (AACN, 2020; Dias et al., 2019; Metheny et al., 2019). Nurses should be certain to follow facility policy, procedure, and practice guidelines. If placement is in doubt, a radiograph should be obtained to verify tube placement (AACN, 2020; Boullata et al., 2017).

Aspiration of fluid through the feeding tubes is sometimes difficult, especially if a smaller diameter tube is used. Because they are less rigid, they may be more likely to collapse when negative pressure is applied during aspiration. More than likely, the difficulty is a result of a blocked tube. In addition, the ports on the tip of the tube may not be positioned in fluid. Several attempts may be necessary to aspirate gastric contents. Inject air boluses into the tube with a large syringe and slowly apply negative pressure to withdraw fluid (AACN, 2020; Metheny et al., 2019). If repeated instillations of air and repositioning prove ineffective and placement is in doubt, a radiograph should be obtained to verify tube placement (AACN, 2020; Boullata et al., 2017).

Carbon Dioxide Monitoring

Monitoring for carbon dioxide to determine nasogastric tube position and/or dislodgement involves the use of a colorimetric end-tidal CO_2 detector to detect the presence of carbon dioxide, which would indicate tube positioning in the patient's airway (Hess et al., 2021). Monitoring for carbon dioxide may be helpful to detect placement of a feeding tube in the tracheobronchial tree (AACN, 2020; Boullata et al., 2017; Hess et al., 2021). However, inaccuracies are possible (Metheny et al., 2019). Carbon dioxide may be detected when the tube is in the mouth and not in the airway and carbon dioxide may not be detected when the tube is in the airway if the ports in the tube are occluded (Gilbert & Burns, 2010, as cited in AACN, 2020). A carbon dioxide sensor cannot determine where a feeding tube's tip ends in the GI tract (esophagus, stomach, or small bowel).

Confirming Nasointestinal Tube Placement

After an initial x-ray for placement, the nurse can validate that the tube is still in the small intestine by checking the pH of the aspirate (pH ≥ 6) and observing the aspirate appearance. During fasting, gastric fluid is typically clear and colorless or grassy green; small-bowel secretions are typically bile-stained, ranging in color from light to golden yellow or brownish green (Metheny et al., 1994, as cited in AACN, 2020). Refer to Guidelines for Nursing Care 37-1.

LONG-TERM NUTRITIONAL SUPPORT

When enteral feeding is required for a longer period (at least 4 to 6 weeks) (Bishcoff et al., 2020), an enterostomal tube may be placed through an opening created into the stomach (**gastrostomy**) or into the jejunum (jejunostomy) (Bischoff et al., 2020; Roveron et al., 2018; Shellnutt, 2019). A gastrostomy may be used for patients who have impaired chewing and swallowing related to neurologic diseases (stroke, multiple sclerosis) or obstruction of the upper respiratory and/or digestive tract, as in head and neck cancers; patients with oncologic health problems associated with malnutrition; and patients with other health issues that lead to malnutrition, such as chronic renal failure, cystic fibrosis, or Crohn disease (Anderson, 2018b; Pars & Çavuşoğlu, 2019). Placement of a tube into the stomach can be accomplished by a surgeon or gastroenterologist via a **percutaneous endoscopic gastrostomy (PEG)**, a surgically (open or laparoscopically) placed **gastrostomy tube**, or gastrostomy placed via interventional radiologic methods (Anderson, 2019b; Roveron et al., 2018). Use of a PEG tube or other type of gastrostomy tube requires an intact, functional GI tract.

The use of a PEG tube is the preferred and most common method of gastrostomy tube insertion for long-term enteral nutrition (Bischoff et al., 2020; Pars & Çavuşoğlu, 2019; Shellnutt, 2019). Unlike a traditional, surgically placed gastrostomy tube, placement of a PEG usually does not require general anesthesia and has lower rate of major complications, such as blocking and dislodgement (Bischoff et al., 2020; Pars & Çavuşoğlu, 2019). Insertion of a PEG tube involves local anesthesia, sedation, passage of an endoscope into the stomach, a small incision or stab wound through the skin of the abdomen, pushing a cannula through the small incision, insertion of a guide wire or suture material through the cannula, and introduction and placement of the PEG tube through one of several methods. PEG tubes are held in place with an internal retention device (bumper or water-filled balloon) which holds it in place in the stomach and an external device (disc) that sits close to the abdominal surface (Anderson, 2019b; Roveron et al., 2018). Figure 37-9 illustrates a PEG tube in place in the stomach.

In long-term feeding situations in which gastric problems exist, the jejunostomy is an alternate method through which nutrition can be delivered. The small bowel may also be used for feeding for patients at high risk for aspiration (McClave, Taylor, et al., 2016). These tubes may be inserted surgically or with endoscopic or laparoscopic guidance. Figure 37-10 illustrates a PEG/J tube in the jejunum. Gastrostomy and jejunostomy tubes are not easily displaced or dislocated (Pars & Çavuşoğlu, 2019).

For patients who are active yet require long-term continuous or intermittent feedings, a low-profile gastrostomy device (LPGD) may be an option (Fig. 37-11 on page 1420). Children are also candidates for LPGDs (Abdelhadi et al., 2020). The external apparatus is minimal and consists of a button or skin disk that is stable, less irritating to the skin, and has no external tubing, making it easier to conceal with clothing (Kyle & Carman, 2021). Additional advantages include that it can be immersed in water, is less noticeable, and is less likely to migrate or become dislodged. The device has a cap, which is opened to access the feeding

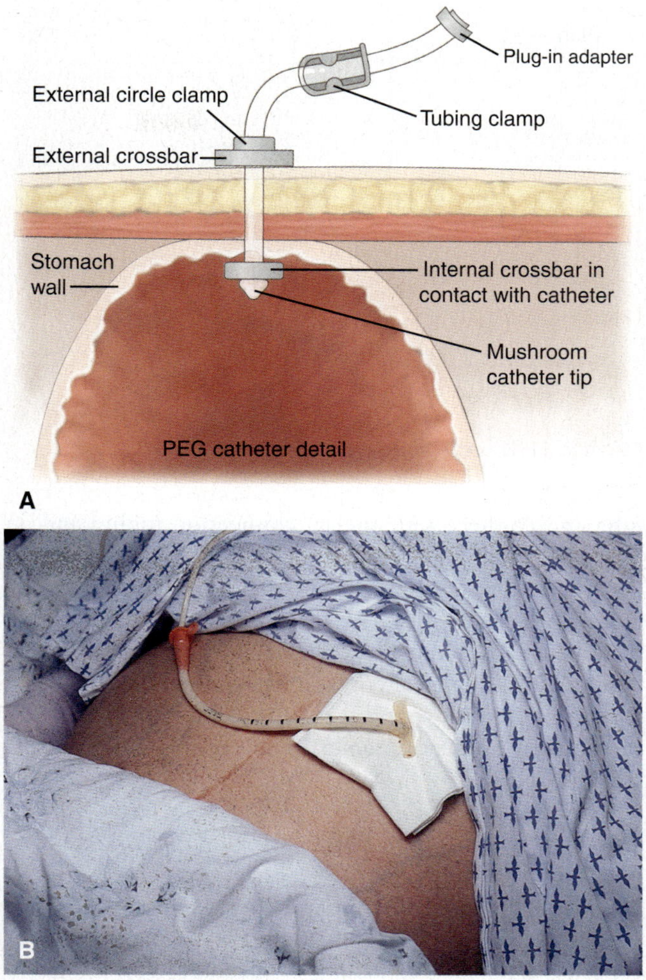

FIGURE 37-9. A. Percutaneous endoscopic gastrostomy tube in place in the stomach. **B.** Percutaneous endoscopic gastrostomy exiting the patient's abdomen.

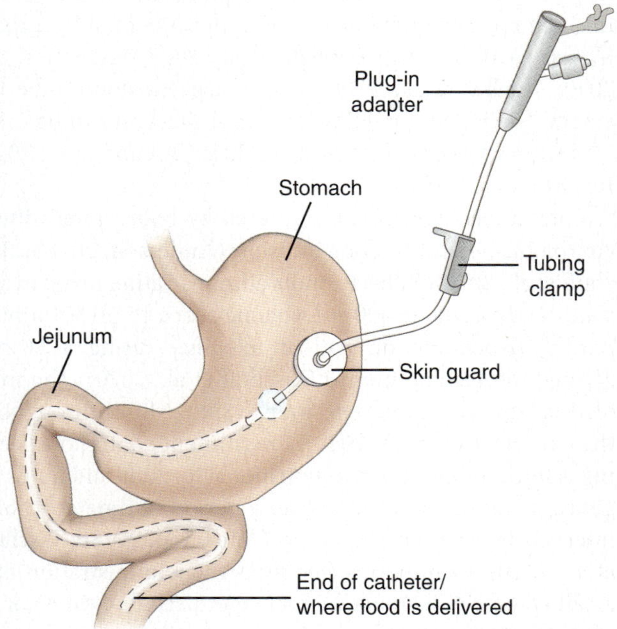

FIGURE 37-10. PEG/J tube inserted in the jejunum.

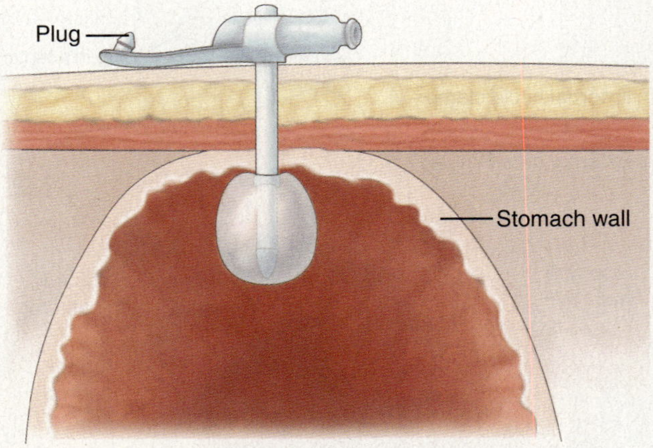

FIGURE 37-11. Low-profile gastrostomy device (LPGD).

tube and connect with special connection tubing and an administration set.

Checking placement of a gastrostomy or jejunostomy tube requires regular comparisons (according to facility policy) of the tube length to the measurement (inches or centimeters) that was documented after placement and status of the external fixation disc (Roveron et al., 2018). An indelible marker can be used to identify the exit point of the tube from the abdominal wall.

ADMINISTRATION OF ENTERAL NUTRITION

Feeding Schedule

Based on the patient's physical, health, and nutritional condition, the nutritionist usually makes recommendations concerning the feeding pattern or schedule, with the intent to deliver a caloric and/or protein goal from enteral nutrition (Anderson, 2018b; Jordan & Moore, 2020). Enteral feeding and medication administration can be initiated using an NGT after insertion once placement is confirmed through radiographic imaging and interpretation by a radiologist (AACN, 2020; Boullata et al., 2017; Bischoff et al., 2020; Mueller et al., 2011). Use of a gastrostomy tube for enteral feeding and medication administration can be initiated within 4 hours after the procedure (Bischoff et al., 2020; Roveron et al., 2018).

Enteral feedings are administered by bolus, intermittent continuous, or continuous infusion (Anderson, 2018b; Bischoff et al., 2020). Bolus formula administration involves administering a 200- to 400-mL volume over a 15- to 60-minute period, depending on patient tolerance, using a 50-mL syringe (no feeding pump) (Bischoff et al., 2020). The total feed volume is divided into four to six feedings throughout the day (Bischoff et al., 2020). Intermittent continuous feeding is the administration of nutritional formula and fluids by giving a volume of formula over a period of time at regular intervals using a feeding pump (Anderson, 2018b; Bischoff et al., 2020). Continuous feeding is the administration of a small volume of formula over a longer period of time, for as much as 12, 18, or 24 hours. Use of a feeding pump delivers nutritional formula and fluid at a set rate over a specified period of time (Anderson, 2018b).

Volume-based feeding protocols in which 24-hour or daily volumes are targeted instead of hourly rates have been shown to increase volume of nutrition delivered (Heyland et al., 2013, as cited in McClave, Taylor, et al., 2016). This type of method empowers nurses to increase feeding rates to make up for volume lost for scheduled and unscheduled interruptions or while enteral nutrition is held and increase attainment of nutritional goals, supporting optimal nutritional intake (Kinikin et al., 2020; McClave, Taylor, et al., 2016). Feedings into the intestine are always continuous and include initiation at a lower rate with a gradual increase in the rate until the target rate identified to meet nutritional goals is met (Bischoff et al., 2020).

For some patients, a combination of methods, such as overnight continuous feeding and bolus feeding during the day best meets their needs and allows for autonomy and lifestyle preferences (Bischoff et al., 2020). For other patients, cyclic feeding may be implemented. This involves administering continuous feeding for a portion of the 24-hour period. The usual routine is to feed the patient for 12 to 16 hours, most often overnight. Cyclic feeding allows the patient to attempt eating regular meals during the day, if this is possible, making ambulation and activity easier. Skill 37-1 on pages 1428–1433 describes the steps used to administer nutrition via a feeding tube.

Enteral Feeding Formulas

Many enteral feeding formulas are available. The nutritional composition of tube feedings depends on the feeding route, the patient's ability to digest and absorb nutrients, and the patient's nutrient and fluid requirements. Other considerations include the availability and cost of the formula, health conditions that require diet modifications, food intolerance, and allergies. Standard formulas contain intact molecules of protein, carbohydrates, and fats, requiring the patient to have normal digestion and absorption. Hydrolyzed formulas contain proteins and other nutrients in simple forms that require little or no digestion. These formulas are used with patients with impaired digestion or absorption. In addition to being nutritionally balanced, formulas may be high in calories; contain fiber; contain additional protein; or be especially formulated for patients with respiratory, renal, or other health problems. Modified enteral formulas are available with lower sugar content and slowly digestible carbohydrates for use by patients with diabetes (Bischoff et al., 2020). Detailed information about their composition and caloric value can be obtained from the product label.

Feedings are initiated at full strength. The previous practice of diluting feedings has not been shown to improve feeding tolerance and prolongs the period of inadequate nutrition support (Bischoff et al., 2020; Dudek, 2022). The rate of infusion begins at the recommended rate, based on guidelines from the dietician or nutrition nurse specialist, and the rate is advanced in increments until the desired rate is achieved (Anderson, 2018b); feeding should be advanced to goal within 48 to 72 hours of initiation (McClave, DiBaise, et al., 2016). Rate advancement is based on patient tolerance. Refer to the discussion Monitoring for Tolerance of Enteral Nutrition on page 1421.

Enteral Feeding Pumps

An enteral feeding pump regulates the amount of feeding solution that is delivered to the patient. A pump should be used when slow rates of enteral formula are required (Boullata et al., 2017; Bischoff et al., 2020). The newer pumps are user friendly, have built-in safeguards that protect the patient from complications, and can be used in both institutions and the home. Safety features include automatic tube flush, cassettes that prevent free flow of formula, safety tips that prevent accidental attachment to an IV setup, and various audible and visible alarms. Most pumps can operate for up to 8 hours on battery. However, manufacturers often recommend using the pump plugged into an electrical outlet for recharging whenever the patient is seated or resting for a period of time. Feeding pumps are also available for mobile use for community-based EN, attaching to a wheelchair or fitting in a specially designed backpack, for example (Bischoff et al., 2020).

NURSING CONSIDERATIONS FOR ENTERAL FEEDING

Nursing actions that contribute to successful enteral tube feedings focus on monitoring patient tolerance of EN, patient safety, monitoring for complications, comfort, and education. Implementation of evidence-based practice guidelines related to these actions provides a means to improve nutritional outcomes.

Monitoring for Tolerance of Enteral Nutrition

Patient tolerance of the volume and type of formula must be monitored daily (Boullata et al., 2017; McClave, Taylor, et al., 2016). Criteria to consider when evaluating patient feeding tolerance include:

- Absence of nausea, vomiting
- Absence of diarrhea and constipation
- Absence of abdominal pain and feelings of fullness
  - Absence of distention
- Presence of bowel sounds within normal limits
  - Achievement of target goal nutrition administration

Evidence related to definition, measurement, monitoring, and management of **gastric residual volume** (feeding remaining in the stomach; GRV) varies. GRV has been used to monitor for tolerance of EN; however, there is little support for this intervention as routine measurement for most patients and is not considered best practice and should not be used as part of routine care to monitor EN (McClave, Taylor, et al., 2016; Ozen et al., 2018; Parker et al., 2019; Pars & Çavuşoğlu, 2019; Rysavy et al., 2020). GRV is not a suitable parameter to determine feeding intolerance (McClave, Taylor, et al., 2016; Pars & Çavuşoğlu, 2019). GRV has been shown to be a poor marker of true gastric volume, gastric emptying, risk of aspiration, pneumonia, and poor outcomes (Hartwell et al., 2018; McClave, DiBaise, et al., 2016). The use of GRVs as a monitor for tolerance increases the risk of tube clogging and decreases attainment of nutritional goals as a result of disruption of delivery of EN (McClave, DiBaise, et al., 2016). Some evidence for practice suggests measurement of GRV may only be necessary during EN initiation and advancement (Roveron et al., 2018; Singer et al., 2019).

If GRV checks are part of facility policy and procedure, automatic cessation of EN should be avoided for GRVs < 500 mL in the absence of other signs of intolerance (Boullata et al., 2017; McClave, Taylor, et al., 2016; Roveron et al., 2018). Evaluate the significance of a single high gastric residual volume in relation to other indicators of GI intolerance, including abdominal distention, abdominal discomfort, nausea, and vomiting (AACN, 2018). Tolerance to gastric feeding can be improved through the use of a prokinetic agent, continuous infusion, and elevation of the head of the bed (McClave, Taylor, et al., 2016).

Promoting Patient Safety

To promote patient safety when administering a tube feeding, be sure to include the following interventions as part of patient care:

- Check tube placement before administering any fluids, medications, or feeding, using multiple techniques: x-ray, external length, external verification marking, pH testing (refer to Guidelines for Nursing Care 37-1, page 1418), and carbon dioxide monitoring. Consistent inability to withdraw fluid from tube may indicate displacement of the tube from the stomach into the esophagus (AACN, 2020).
  - Assess for signs of respiratory distress; coughing, choking, dyspnea may occur when a tube is inadvertently positioned in the airway (AACN, 2020).
- Feeding tubes are prone to blockage, due to protein-rich formula solutions, the viscosity of the feeding formulas, and relatively small diameter of the feeding tube lumens, the use of the tubes for medication administration, and inadequate water flushes (Bischoff et al., 2020; Drummond Hayes & Hayes, 2018). Feeding tubes should be flushed with at least 30 mL of water before starting and after completion of bolus feedings; every 4 to 8 hours during continuous feeding (Bischoff et al., 2020; Boullata et al., 2017; Roveron et al., 2018); and before and after medication administration (Drummond Hayes & Hayes, 2018), based on the patient's fluid needs and restrictions (Boullata et al., 2017).
- Sterile water should be used for tube flushes in immunocompromised or critically ill patients, and for reconstituting powdered enteral formula (Allen, 2015; Boullata et al., 2017).
- Assess the abdomen for abnormalities. Assess for bowel sounds at least once per shift to check for the presence of peristalsis and a functional intestinal tract. Experts, however, have recently concluded that it is common for acutely ill patients to have delayed gastric emptying; therefore, delaying enteral feedings based on hypoactive bowel sounds may place a patient at risk for malnutrition (McClave, Taylor, et al., 2016; McClave, DiBaise, et al.,

2016). Gastric distention, abdominal girth, nausea, vomiting, bloating, or pain are better indicators of how well a patient is tolerating a tube feeding (Bischoff et al., 2020; McClave, Taylor, et al., 2016; Pars & Çavuşoğlu, 2019).

- Make sure the patient is as upright as possible during feeding. Keep the head of the bed elevated at 30 to 45 degrees at all times during administration of enteral feedings and for 1 hour afterward to prevent reflux, aspiration, and pneumonia, unless contraindicated (McClave, Taylor, et al., 2016; Roveron et al., 2018). Patients for whom semi-recumbent position is contraindicated or who cannot tolerate a semi-Fowler position should be placed in a reverse- or anti-Trendelenburg position (Boullata et al., 2017; Roveron et al., 2018). Exceptions to upright supine positioning during feeding are necessary at times. Patients with pulmonary disease who are acutely ill, such as those with acute respiratory distress syndrome (ARDS) or COVID-19-related respiratory failure/ARDS, may be positioned in the prone position on a regular basis to promote improved oxygenation (Guttendorf, 2021; Morata et al., 2021; Siegmeister et al., 2021; Venus et al., 2020). Enteral nutrition during prone positioning is recommended to meet the nutritional needs of the critically ill patient (Behrens et al., 2021; Bruni et al., 2020; Savio et al., 2021). Limited evidence suggests that administration of enteral nutrition while the patient is prone is not associated with substantial increase in complications compared to enteral nutrition administered in a supine position (Boullata et al., 2017; Bruni et al., 2020). Elevation of the head of the bed at 10 to 25 degrees (reverse Trendelenburg) is suggested (Behrens et al., 2021; Boullata et al., 2017; Powers, 2021). Closely monitor abdominal and bowel status at least every 4 hours for feeding tolerance and GI motility status (Boullata et al., 2017; Powers, 2021). Refer to the Research in Nursing display for a discussion of evidence related to enteral feeding in the prone position.
- There is no benefit from stopping feedings during short periods of lowering of the head of the bed (Boullata et al.,

Research in Nursing

BRIDGING THE GAP TO EVIDENCE-BASED PRACTICE

Enteral Feeding in the Prone Position

Integration of evidence-based practice interventions is an important aspect of the provision of effective nursing care. Early enteral nutrition (Behrens et al., 2021; Bruni et al., 2020; Savio et al., 2021) and prone positioning (Guttendorf, 2021; Morata et al., 2021; Venus et al., 2020) may both improve outcomes for patients with pulmonary disease who are acutely ill (Bruni et al., 2020). Is enteral nutrition administration in the prone position safe? Is there increased concern for enteral nutrition intolerance, such as high residual gastric volume, regurgitation, and/or vomiting, during pronation?

Related Research

Bruni, A., Garofalo, E., Grande, L., Auletta, G., Cubello, D., Greco, M., Lombardo, N., Garieri, P., Papaleo, A., Doldo, P., Spagnuolo, R., & Longhini, F. (2020). Nursing issues in enteral nutrition during prone position in critically ill patients: A systematic review of the literature. *Intensive & Critical Care Nursing*, *60*, 102899. https://doi.org/10.1016/j.iccn.2020.102899

The purpose of this systematic review was to assess the occurrence of high residual gastric volume, regurgitation or vomiting in patients receiving enteral nutrition (EN) during pronation. Three databases, MEDLINE, EMBASE, and CINAHL, were searched using keywords and related MeSH terms, from inception until November 19, 2019. All relevant studies enrolling adult patients receiving mechanical ventilation and evaluating early EN during prone positioning were included; case reports or series, literature reviews, systematic reviews, and meta-analyses were excluded. Outcomes investigated included residual gastric volume, EN feeding volume, the need to discontinue EN, rate of episodes of vomiting or regurgitation, rate of ventilator-associated pneumonia (VAP) or secondary infections, ICU and hospital length of stay, and mortality. The search of the databases yielded 111 reports. Fifteen duplicate reports and 89 citations were excluded as a result of the initial screening. One of the remaining 7 reports was excluded as it was a narrative review. Six studies were included in the systematic review. Five of the 6 studies reported no differences with respect to gastric residual volume between supine and prone positioning. Results suggested that administration of EN over 24 hours instead of 18 hours resulted in greater tolerance. The need to hold/stop EN administration and vomiting episodes were higher during prone positioning, with similar rates of high gastric volume between supine and prone positions. The incidence of VAP, length of stay, and mortality were similar between supine and prone positions. One study reported lower mortality in patients receiving EN over 24 hours as compared to an 18-hour administration period. The researchers concluded protocols should be initiated and followed by health care providers to increase the enteral feeding volume, while avoiding EN intolerance. Nurses must be aware of the risk for regurgitation and vomiting during EN in the prone position and closely monitor enteral feeding. The researchers also suggested that, given the limited available evidence, randomized controlled trials are needed to assess if administration of early EN during prone positioning influences major clinical outcomes.

Relevance to Nursing Practice

Adherence to evidence-based guidelines for enteral nutrition contributes to improved nutrition outcomes. Nursing adherence to these guidelines is instrumental in attaining improved patient outcomes. Nurses and facilities should identify best-practice guidelines and incorporate interventions to improve knowledge of and adherence to these guidelines to improve patient outcomes.

2017). If a prolonged procedure will require lowering of the head of the bed, feedings should be stopped during this period; feedings should be promptly restarted when the procedure is ended or as feasible.
- Prevent contamination during enteral feedings by maintaining the integrity of the feeding system and using proper technique. Closed systems, consisting of a sterile, prefilled, ready-to-hang container, reduce the opportunity for bacterial contamination of the feeding formula. An open system exists when formula from a can or bottle is added to a feeding setup. Always check the expiration date of formula. Perform hand hygiene and put on nonsterile gloves before preparing, assembling, and handling any part of the feeding system. Disinfect the opening and rim of any cans to be opened before opening. Label all equipment with the patient's name, date, and time the feeding was hung, and cap or cover any disconnected tubing. Clean a reusable feeding system with soap and hot water every 24 hours; replace a disposable feeding apparatus for open systems every 24 hours. Closed systems can be used up to 48 hours; check the manufacturer's guidelines and facility policy.
- Medications may be administered through a feeding tube, but never give them while a feeding is being infused; feeding must be stopped prior to administration of medications (Boullata et al., 2017).
- Never add medications directly to the formula (Boullata et al., 2017); some drugs become ineffective when mixed with feeding formulas and medications mixed in feeding formulas may cause clogging of the feeding tube.
- Do not mix medications together; administer each medication separately and dilute appropriately prior to administration (Boullata et al., 2017).
- Administer liquid forms of medications whenever possible (Boullata et al., 2017).
- It is very important to flush the tube with water before, between, and after the administration of medications. Purified water (e.g., sterile water, although there is no need for the water to be sterile) should be used for medication administration, as the chemical contaminants in tap water can potentiate drug–drug interactions (Boullata et al., 2017).
- Resume enteral feeding as soon as possible to avoid compromising nutrition status; only hold feeding when time lapse is indicated to avoid potential drug–nutrient interaction in the GI lumen (Boullata et al., 2017).
- Administering medications through an enteral feeding tube is discussed in depth in Chapter 30.

Monitoring for Complications

Patients receiving tube feedings are at risk for several complications. Table 37-5 (on page 1424) summarizes nursing measures to prevent selected complications.

Providing Comfort Measures

Patients with nasogastric tubes often experience discomfort related to irritation to nasal and throat mucosa and drying of the oral mucous membranes. Implement several nursing interventions to ensure the patient's comfort and prevent alterations in the integrity of these tissues.

- Administer oral hygiene frequently (every 2 to 4 hours) to prevent drying of tissues and to relieve thirst. Offer the patient the opportunity to rinse the mouth with warm water and mouthwash solution frequently. Lubricate the lips generously.
- Keep the nares clean, especially around the tube, where secretions tend to accumulate. Using a lubricant after cleaning the nares is recommended.
- Help control local irritation from the tube in the throat. Analgesic throat lozenges or anesthetic sprays may be effective.
- Encourage the patient, if able, to verbalize concerns about tube feeding and presence of the tube. A visit from another person who has learned to cope with this alternate feeding method may prove helpful.
- Secure the nasogastric tube to the patient's nose and cheek, based on facility policy, to prevent tension and tugging on the tube, causing trauma to the nares, and inadvertent displacement or dislodgment (Morton & Fontaine, 2018). Displacement or dislodgement of a tube can lead to aspiration, pneumonia, and sepsis (Powers, 2019). Use of a commercial securement device is recommended (Schroeder & Sitzer, 2019). Refer to Box 37-8 (on page 1424) for methods to secure an NGT.
- Secure the gastrostomy tube to the patient's abdomen in a way that stabilizes the tube and avoids excessive traction (Boullata et al., 2017; Roveron et al., 2018). Excessive friction may result in development of peristomal hypergranulation tissue (Bischoff et al., 2020; Roveron et al., 2018). Excessive traction may contribute to enlargement of the stoma and the development of leakage around the tube (Roveron et al., 2018).

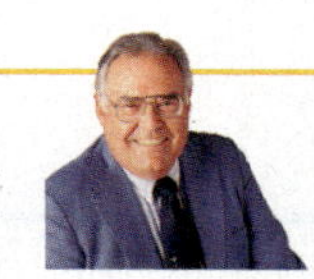

Recall ***Charles Gallagher***, the husband of the woman with advanced dementia receiving enteral nutrition. The nurse could teach Mr. Gallagher how to provide oral hygiene for his wife, including lubricating her lips. Doing so would allow Mr. Gallagher to feel some control over the situation. In addition, he would be helping to meet his wife's comfort needs and his own needs.

Providing Education

Often, patients will continue to receive enteral feedings at home or another community setting. Teaching Tips 37-1 (on page 1425) outlines important points to review with patients and families/caregivers in the home/community setting. Provide individualized instructions in written form as a reference for the patient and family/caregivers. Be sure to include the following in the teaching plan:

- Information about the administration of feedings, amount of fluid to be administered, operation of the pump, formula, instructions regarding rate and frequency and how to check for tube placement, as well as what to do if the tube becomes blocked or dislodged

Table 37-5 Preventing Complications of Enteral Feeding

POTENTIAL COMPLICATION	PREVENTIVE INTERVENTIONS
Aspiration	• Use appropriate measures to check tube placement. • Elevate head of bed at least 30–45 degrees during feeding and for 1 hour afterward. • Give small, frequent feedings. • Avoid over sedation of patient. • Check residual volume per policy.
Clogged tube	• Flush tube before and after feeding, every 4 hours during continuous feeding, and after withdrawing aspirate. • Sterile water should be used for tube flushes in immunocompromised or critically ill patients (Allen, 2015; Boullata et al., 2017). • Attach a 30- or 60-mL piston syringe to the feeding tube and pull back the plunger to help dislodge the clog. Then, fill the syringe with warm water and attempt to flush. If met with resistance, use gentle back and forth motion of the plunger to help loosen the clog. If necessary, clamp the tube to allow the warm water to penetrate the clog for up to 20 minutes and then attempt to flush (Boullata et al., 2017).
Nasal erosion with nasogastric or nasointestinal tubes	• Check nostrils every shift for signs of pressure. • Clean and moisten nares every 4–8 hours. • Secure tube to avoid pulling or pressure
Diarrhea	• Prevent contamination in both open and closed systems. • Change delivery set every 12–24 hours according to facility policy. • Refrigerate opened cans of formula and discard after 24 hours. • Limit hang time to 4 hours when using open system. • Use aseptic technique for patients who are immunosuppressed or acutely ill. • Assess for fecal impaction.
Other GI symptoms (nausea, vomiting, distention)	• Avoid oversedating patient (delays gastric emptying). • Administer GI motility medications, as prescribed.
Unplanned extubation	• Anchor tube appropriately with commercial device, bridle, or tape. • Check on patient frequently. • Measure external length of tubing at regular intervals.
Gastrostomy site infection	• Cleanse stoma and peristomal skin with sterile saline and gauze 24 hours after placement and every day for the first week (Roveron et al., 2018). • Stoma and peristomal skin may be cleansed with skin cleanser/mild soap and warm water 7–10 days after placement (Roveron et al., 2018). • Avoid the use of creams or powders around the stoma (Roveron et al., 2018). • Assess for signs of infection. • Request a consult with a wound care specialist, as needed.

- How to administer medications through the tube
- Care of the tube insertion site and possible complications that need to be communicated to the health care team
- Proper preparation, cleaning, and disposal of equipment

Box 37-8 Methods to Secure a Nasogastric Tube

- Tape
  - Commonly used
  - Associated with the most displacement and dislodgments issues (Powers, 2019)
  - Tape wrapped too tightly around tube may pull tube toward nares and cause erosion or pressure injury
  - Tape in manner to prevent pulling or pressure on nares
- Commercial adhesive devices
- Hydrocolloid dressing and tape to patient's cheek
- Nasal securement devices, such as nasal bridles
  - Associated with significant reduction in dislodgment versus tape (Powers, 2019; Stabler et al., 2018; Taylor et al., 2018)

- Emergency telephone numbers, including the number for the home health care facility and the appropriate members of the health care team
- Arrangements for follow-up from the home health care nurse as soon as possible after discharge

The care of a patient with a gastrostomy tube is outlined in Skill 37-2 on pages 1434–1435.

REMOVAL OF A NASOGASTRIC TUBE

Removing the nasogastric tube as carefully as it is inserted when it is no longer required is important to avoid causing the patient undue discomfort. After the tube is removed, provide for oral hygiene to remove disagreeable tastes and odors. Directions for removing the nasogastric tube are given in Skill 39-3 in Chapter 39.

NASOENTERIC TUBES FOR DECOMPRESSION

In addition to providing enteral feedings, nasogastric tubes can be used for other purposes. They may be inserted to decompress or drain the stomach of fluid, unwanted stomach

Teaching Tips 37-1

HOME ENTERAL FEEDINGS

Health Topic	Teaching Tip	Why Is This Important?
Cleaning around a gastric tube insertion site	Use of soap and water, making sure that area is adequately rinsed and dried. Rotation of the guard after cleaning around it	If soap is left under the gastric tube guard, it can lead to skin irritation. The guard can put pressure on the skin, leading to skin breakdown.
Delivering tube feedings	Head elevation while delivering a gastric feeding and for approximately an hour after the feeding Method of administration such as delivering the feedings via continuous or bolus method, and steps for carrying out the feeding	Keeping the head elevated helps to prevent aspiration of gastric tube feedings. The patient or caregiver should know how to operate the machinery if it is to be delivered via continuous method or how to set up for a bolus feeding.
Leaking of gastric contents	Method of checking for problems (is guard too loose or balloon not filled adequately) if gastric tube is leaking stomach contents around insertion site	If gastric tube is leaking acidic stomach contents, the area around the insertion site can quickly break down.
Placement check	Methods to check placement to ensure that tube has not migrated inward or outward	Gastrostomy tubes can be marked with an indelible marker. The mark should be checked to make sure it is at the level of the abdominal wall. If the mark is not visible, the tube may have migrated inward. If the mark is away from the abdominal wall, the tube may no longer be in the stomach. Patients may also measure the length of the tube from the skin and record the measurement. This measurement should be confirmed to ensure that the tube has not migrated.

contents, such as poison or medication and air, allowing it to rest, or before or after surgery, to promote healing. Tubes used for these purposes and associated nursing care are discussed in detail in Chapter 39.

Providing Parenteral Nutrition

Parenteral nutrition (PN) is the administration of nutritional support via the intravenous route. Use of the enteral route is preferred to the parenteral route for nutrition support whenever feasible (Gorski et al., 2021); patients who cannot meet their nutritional needs by the oral or enteral routes may require intravenous nutritional supplementation. Intravenous supplementation may be prescribed for high-risk patients under specific circumstances, when enteral nutrition is not feasible or sufficient to meet energy or protein goals (McClave, DiBaise, et al., 2016, p. 317). PN may be considered for patients already on EN only after 7 to 10 days, when unable to meet >60% of energy and/or protein requirements by the enteral route alone (McClave, DiBaise, et al., 2016, p. 328).

PN is a highly concentrated, hypertonic nutrient solution. PN provides calories; restores nitrogen balance; and replaces essential fluids, vitamins, electrolytes, minerals, and trace elements. PN can also promote tissue and wound healing and normal metabolic function. It provides the bowel a chance to heal and reduces activity in the gallbladder, pancreas, and small intestine. PN meets the patient's nutritional needs by way of nutrient-filled solutions administered intravenously through a central venous access device, such as a tunneled, multilumen, or nontunneled catheter into the subclavian vein or a peripherally inserted central catheter (PICC).

Peripheral parenteral nutrition (PPN) is a less concentrated nutrient solution that can be administered through a peripheral vein. Peripheral veins cannot tolerate highly concentrated solutions and high fluid volumes, thus the solution used to deliver PPN is not as nutrient dense (Boullata et al., 2014). PPN is associated with a high risk of phlebitis and loss of venous access sites (Boullata et al., 2014; Gorski et al., 2021; McClave, DiBaise, et al, 2016). As a result, the nutritional value of PPN is limited and is most appropriate for patients who need short-term nutritional support (≤7 to 10 days) and to prevent, not correct, nutritional deficits (Dudek, 2022).

PARENTERAL NUTRITION SOLUTIONS AND ADMINISTRATION

PN contains the three primary components necessary to maintain nutrition: amino acids (proteins), carbohydrates (dextrose), and lipids (fats). Additional components of PN include electrolytes, vitamins, and trace elements. The PN formula is tailored to the individual patient's specific needs. Dextrose and lipids caloric value that the body needs to meet energy requirements. Lipids provide essential fatty acids to prevent fatty acid deficiency and support wound healing and red blood cell production. Amino acids provide protein to maintain structure and facilitate tissue repair and wound healing. Vitamins, trace minerals and electrolytes help maintain fluid and electrolyte balance, promote tissue repair/wound healing, maintain biochemical homeostasis, regulate acid–base balance, support metabolism and maintain osmotic pressure (Morton & Fontaine, 2018). Because of the high glucose concentration, usually about 25% (thus, a hypertonic solution), it is important to monitor blood glucose levels based on the patient's clinical status and the PN infusion schedule (cycled vs. continuous) (Ayers et al., 2014). Refer to Skill 37-3 on pages 1437–1440.

PN is administered using an electronic infusion device with anti–free-flow protection and alarms for occlusion, via continuous or cyclic infusion (Gorski et al., 2021). Physical incompatibility between the intravenous nutrition formula and other intravenous solutions, especially medications, is a potential problem that must be addressed. If the patient has a multilumen catheter in place, dedicate one lumen for the administration of the PN. Do not use that lumen or administration set for any other purpose, to prevent incompatibility problems. If the patient's intravenous catheter has only one lumen, attempt to obtain a peripheral intravenous access for the administration of additional solutions. Consider discussing the potential for a midline or peripherally inserted central catheter with the patient's health care team. If an additional access is not available, research the compatibility of the solutions to be administered. Little research exists on the stability and compatibility of PN solutions and most medications. Medications are not added to or coinfused with the PN before or during infusion without consultation with a pharmacist regarding compatibility and stability (Gorski et al, 2021). If compatible medications or other solutions must be given through the same lumen as PN, attach the administration set as close to the catheter hub as possible to limit the amount of contact between the drug (or solution) and the PN solution. A pharmacist can add insulin to PN as part of the plan of care related to glycemic control (Murphy et al., 2020). Never add medication to PN solutions after they are dispensed from the pharmacy (Gorski et al., 2021).

PREVENTING COMPLICATIONS

PN therapy is costly, requires constant monitoring, and has the potential for causing infections as well as metabolic and mechanical complications. It should be used only when enteral intake is inadequate or contraindicated, and should be gradually discontinued as soon as possible (McClave, Taylor, et al., 2016). Prevention of potential complications associated with PN requires vigilance and careful monitoring by the nurse (Guenter et al., 2018). Potential complications include the following (Dudek, 2022; Gorski et al., 2021; Morton & Fontaine, 2018):

- Complications related to the use of central venous access devices, such as pneumothorax, thromboembolism (inflammation of a blood vessel and formation of a thrombus [blood clot]), and air embolism
- Infection and sepsis (central line–associated blood stream infections [CLABSIs])
- Metabolic alterations, such as hyperglycemia or hypoglycemia
- Fluid, electrolyte, and acid–base imbalances
- Hyperlipidemia
- Liver and gallbladder disease
- Refeeding syndrome (life-threatening complication related to overfeeding carbohydrates in nutritionally debilitated patients, characterized by metabolic and physiologic shifts of fluid, electrolytes, and minerals from the extracellular fluid to intracellular fluid) (Dudek, 2022, p. 352).

Guidelines for Nursing Care 37-2 lists nursing guidelines for monitoring administration of PN.

PARENTERAL NUTRITION IN THE HOME SETTING

Many patients require long-term PN and continue such therapy in the home. Individuals with advanced cancer, difficulty swallowing, or chronic bowel problems are candidates for this type of nutritional support. PN is often administered as a cyclic infusion in the home setting. A cyclic infusion is administered during a portion of the day, often overnight, providing periods of freedom from the infusion device and increased mobility. Nurses are involved in educating the patient and caregiver about the techniques and responsibilities associated with PN, providing technical and psychological support, and documenting the assessments that allow PN to be continued in the home. Patient education should specifically include:

- Purpose and expected duration of PN
- Proper storage of PN containers and supplies
- Infection prevention measures, including hand hygiene and maintaining sterile components of the infusion system (Gorski et al., 2021)
  - Safe environment for preparation, including clean workspace
- Signs and symptoms of infection/sepsis and prevention, recognition and management of non–infectious-related complications and/or problems (Pironi et al., 2020).
- Circumstances that require contacting the health care team
- Basic care of the venous access device used to administer
- Use and maintenance of infusion equipment
- Frequency for measuring the patient's weight, intake and output, and monitoring glucose levels

Evaluating

The effectiveness of the plan of care is evaluated as the last step in the nursing process. On an ongoing basis, the nurse accomplishes the following:

- Evaluates the patient's progress toward meeting nutritional outcomes
- Evaluates the patient's tolerance and adherence to the prescribed diet, when appropriate

Guidelines for Nursing Care 37-2

MONITORING ADMINISTRATION OF PARENTERAL NUTRITION

- Use the same catheter lumen for administration of parenteral nutrition each time the tubing is changed.
- Use an electronic infusion device to administer infusion of parenteral nutrition.
- Infusion rate changes are made incrementally to avoid severe hyperglycemia or hypoglycemia. Taper infusion rates gradually (Ayers et al., 2014).
- Discard unused parenteral nutrition solution within 24 hours of starting its administration.
- Check vital signs every 4 hours to monitor for development of infection or sepsis.
- Monitor blood glucose levels as appropriate based on the patient's clinical status (Ayers et al., 2014; Ratliff et al., 2018).
- Use aseptic technique when changing solution, tubing, filter, or dressings according to facility policy.
- Infusion administration sets should include an in-line filter. Change infusion administration sets every 24 hours.
- Avoid blood sampling via the venous access device used for PN when feasible (Gorski et al., 2021).
- Change site dressings according to facility protocol. Transparent semipermeable dressings are changed once per week. Gauze dressings do not allow for inspection of exit site without dressing removal and should be changed every 48 hours. In addition, change dressings immediately if they become wet, soiled, or nonocclusive.
- Check that all connections are securely taped, catheter is clamped before opening the system, and insertion site is covered with sterile dressing.
- Compare the patient's daily weight to fluid intake and output. Total weight gain should not be greater than 3 lb per week. Weight gain greater than 1 lb per day indicates fluid retention.
- Assess serum protein and electrolyte levels for signs of imbalance.

Source: Adapted from Ayers, P., Adams, S., Boullata, J., Gervasio, J., Holcombe, B., Kraft, M. D., Marshall, N., Neal, A., Sacks, G., Seres, D. S., Worthington, P., & American Society for Parenteral and Enteral Nutrition. (2014). A.S.P.E.N. Parenteral nutrition safety consensus recommendations. *Journal of Parenteral and Enteral Nutrition, 38*(3), 296–333. https://doi.org/10.1177/0148607113511992; Infusion Nurses Society (INS). (2016a). *Policies and procedures for infusion therapy* (5th ed.). https://doi.org/10.1097/NHH.0000000000000481.

- Assesses the patient's and family/caregiver's level of understanding of the diet and/or nutrition-related interventions and the need for further instruction or reinforcement
- Communicates findings to other members of the health care team
- Revises the plan of care, as needed, or terminates nursing care

REFLECTIVE PRACTICE LEADING TO PERSONAL LEARNING

Remember that the goal of reflective practice is to look at an experience, understand it, and learn from it. As you begin to develop expertise in implementing measures related to nutrition, reflect on your experiences—successes and failures—in order to improve your practice. How can you do it better next time? What did you learn today that can help you tomorrow? Begin your reflection by paying close attention to the following while performing nutrition interventions and providing nursing care:

- Did your preparation and practice related to performing interventions related to nutrition result in your feeling confident in your ability to provide care? Did your competence and confidence inspire the patient's and family's or caregivers trust?
- How did you prioritize the data you collected? What patterns in the data did you identify? What knowledge from your learning, personal experience and intuition did you use to make decisions and develop your plan of care?
- How confident are you that the nutrition data you communicated and recorded accurately communicates the health status, health problems, issues, risks, and strengths of the patient? How successfully have you communicated this information to other members of the health care team?
- Were you aware of any cultural and/or ethnic beliefs or practices that may have influenced the patient's personal nutrition practices? Were you aware of any stereotypes or prejudices that might have negatively influenced the clinical encounter? If so, how did you address these?
- Did you need to modify the plan of care as a result of ongoing assessments? Did you think of better interventions to produce the expected outcomes?
- As you concluded your care, did the patient and family/caregiver know your name, and know what to expect of you and nursing? Did the patient sense that you are respectful, caring, and competent to provide care?

Perhaps the most important questions to reflect on are: Are your patients and their families/caregivers better for having had *you* share in the critical responsibility of partnering with them to address their nutrition needs? Are your patients now receiving thoughtful, person-centered, prioritized, holistic, evidence-based treatment and care because of your efforts?

Skill 37-1 Administering a Tube Feeding (Open System)

DELEGATION CONSIDERATIONS

The administration of a tube feeding is not usually delegated to assistive personnel (AP) in the acute care setting. The administration of a tube feeding in some settings may be delegated to AP who have received appropriate training, after assessment of tube placement and patency by the registered nurse. Depending on the state's nurse practice act and the organization's policies and procedures, the administration of a tube feeding may be delegated to licensed practical/vocational nurses (LPN/LVNs). The decision to delegate must be based on careful analysis of the patient's needs and circumstances as well as the qualifications of the person to whom the task is being delegated. Refer to the Delegation Guidelines in Appendix A.

EQUIPMENT

- Prescribed tube-feeding formula at room temperature
- Feeding bag or prefilled tube-feeding set
- Stethoscope
- Nonsterile gloves
- Additional PPE, as indicated
- Alcohol preps
- Disposable pad or towel
- Large syringe (20 to 50 mL)
- Enteral feeding pump (if ordered)
- Rubber band
- Clamp (Hoffman or butterfly)
- IV pole
- Water for irrigation and hydration, as needed
- pH test strip (calibrated in units of 0.5 and approved for use with human secretions)
- Tape measure, or other measuring device

IMPLEMENTATION

ACTION	RATIONALE
1. Gather equipment. Check amount, concentration, type, and frequency of tube feeding in the patient's health record. Check the formula expiration date.	This provides for an organized approach to the task. Checking ensures that correct feeding will be administered. Outdated formula may be contaminated.
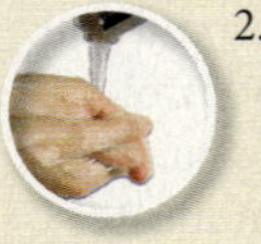 2. Perform hand hygiene and put on PPE, if indicated.	Hand hygiene and PPE prevent the spread of microorganisms. PPE is required based on transmission precautions.
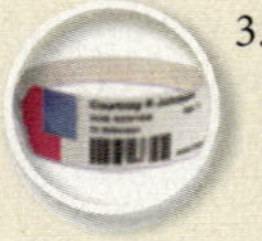 3. Identify the patient.	Identifying the patient ensures the right patient receives the intervention and helps prevent errors.
4. Explain the procedure to the patient. Answer any questions, as needed.	Explanation facilitates patient engagement.
5. Assemble equipment on the overbed table or other surface within reach.	Organization facilitates performance of the task.
6. Close the patient's bedside curtain or door. Raise the bed to a comfortable working position, usually elbow height of the caregiver (VHACEOSH, 2016). Perform respiratory and abdominal assessments as described above.	Closing curtains or the door provides for patient privacy. Having the bed at the proper height prevents back and muscle strain. Assessment is vital to detect changes in the patient's condition before initiating the intervention.
7. **Position the patient as upright as possible with the head of the bed elevated at least 30 to 45 degrees or as near-normal position for eating as possible.** Patient should remain in this position during feeding and for 1 hour afterward. **Patients for whom the semi-recumbent position is contraindicated or who cannot tolerate a semi-Fowler position should be placed in a reverse- or anti-Trendelenburg position** (Boullata et al., 2017; Roveron et al., 2018).	These positions minimize possibility of reflux, aspiration, and pneumonia (McClave, Taylor, et al., 2016; Roveron et al., 2018).
8. Put on gloves. Confirm placement of the nasogastric tube in the patient's stomach using at least two methods.	Gloves prevent contact with blood and body fluids. With the exception of radiographic examination, which is usually done immediately after insertion to verify initial tube placement, the use of two or more of these techniques in conjunction with each other increases the likelihood of correct tube placement (AACN, 2020; Anderson, 2019b; Anderson, 2018a; Dias et al., 2019; Rahimi et al., 2015).

ACTION	RATIONALE
9. If assessments to check placement are inconclusive, the exposed tube length has changed, or there are any other indications that the tube may not be in place, check placement by radiograph (x-ray) of placement of tube, based on facility policy.	Radiographic confirmation is considered the most reliable method for identifying the position of the NG tube (AACN, 2020; Boullata et al., 2017).
10. If gastric residual volume (GRV) checks are part of facility policy and procedure, check GRV: After multiple steps have been taken to ensure that the feeding tube is located in the stomach or small intestine, aspirate all gastric contents with the syringe and measure to check for gastric residual—the amount of feeding remaining in the stomach. Return the residual based on facility policy. Proceed with feeding if the amount of residual does not exceed facility policy or the limit indicated in the health record. Refer to additional information in the Special Considerations below.	GRV has been used to monitor for tolerance of enteral nutrition; however, there is little support for this intervention as routine measurement for most patients, and it is not considered best practice and should not be used as part of routine care to monitor enteral nutrition (McClave, Taylor, et al., 2016; Ozen et al., 2018; Parker et al., 2019; Pars & Çavuşoğlu, 2019; Rysavy et al., 2020). GRV is not a suitable parameter to determine feeding intolerance (McClave, Taylor, et al., 2016; Pars & Çavuşoğlu, 2019). GRV has been shown to be a poor marker of true gastric volume; gastric emptying; and risk of aspiration, pneumonia, and poor outcomes (Hartwell et al., 2018; McClave, DiBaise, et al., 2016). The use of GRVs as a monitor for tolerance increases the risk of tube clogging and decreases attainment of nutritional goals as a result of disruption of delivery of enteral nutrition (McClave, DiBaise, et al., 2016).
11. Flush tube with 30 to 50 mL of water for irrigation. Disconnect syringe from tubing and cap end of tubing while preparing the formula feeding equipment. Remove gloves. Perform hand hygiene.	Flushing the tube prevents occlusion (Bischoff et al., 2020; Boullata et al., 2017; Drummond Hayes & Hayes, 2018). Capping the tube deters the entry of microorganisms and prevents leakage onto the bed linens. Hand hygiene prevents transmission of microorganisms.
12. Put on gloves before preparing, assembling, and handling any part of the feeding system.	Gloves prevent contact with blood and body fluids and deter transmission of contaminants to feeding equipment and/or formula.
13. Administer feeding.	

When Using a Feeding Bag Administration System and Gravity (Bolus; Open System)

ACTION	RATIONALE
a. Label the bag and/or tubing with date and time. Hang the bag on the IV pole and adjust to about 12 inches above the stomach. Clamp tubing.	Labeling date and time of first use allows for disposal of bag and tubing within 24 hours, to deter growth of microorganisms. Proper feeding bag height reduces risk of formula being introduced too quickly.
b. Check the expiration date of the formula. Cleanse top of feeding container with a disinfectant before opening it (Figure 1). Pour formula into the feeding bag and allow solution to run through tubing. Close the clamp.	Cleansing the container top with alcohol minimizes risk for contaminants entering feeding bag. Formula displaces air in the tubing.
c. Attach feeding administration set to the feeding tube (Figure 2), open clamp, and regulate drip according to the prescribed rate or allow feeding to run in over 30 minutes.	Introducing formula at an appropriate rate allows the stomach to accommodate to the feeding and decreases GI distress.

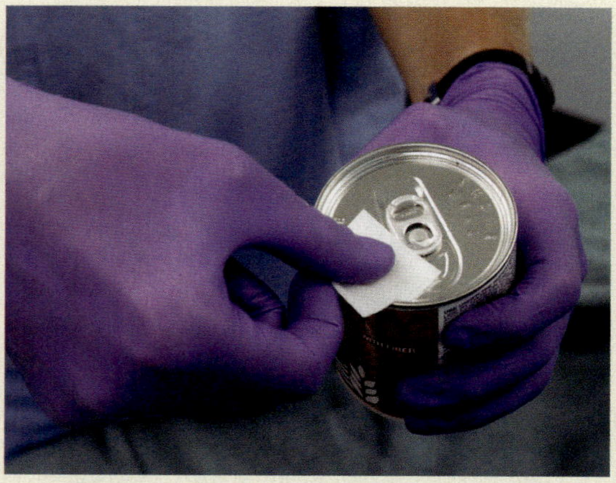

FIGURE 1. Cleaning top of feeding container with alcohol before opening it.

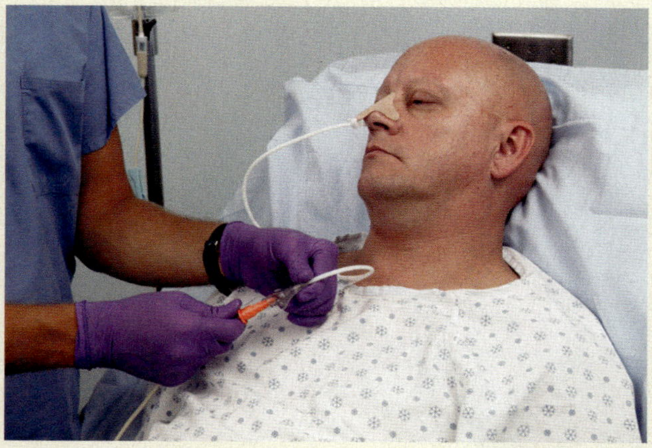

FIGURE 2. Attaching feeding administration set to NG tube.

(continued on page 1430)

Skill 37-1 Administering a Tube Feeding (Open System) *(continued)*

ACTION	RATIONALE
d. **Add 30 to 60 mL (1 to 2 oz) of water for irrigation to feeding bag when feeding is almost completed** (Figure 3) and allow it to run through the tube.	Water rinses the feeding from the tube and helps to keep it patent as well as provides hydration for the patient. Feeding tubes should be flushed with at least 30 mL of water before starting and after completion of bolus feedings and every 4 to 8 hours during continuous feeding (Bischoff et al., 2020; Boullata et al., 2017; Roveron et al., 2018), based on the patient's fluid needs and restrictions (Boullata et al., 2017).
e. Clamp the tubing immediately after water has been instilled. Disconnect the feeding administration set from the feeding tube. Clamp the tube and cover the end with cap (Figure 4).	Clamping the tube prevents air from entering the stomach. Capping the tube deters entry of microorganisms and covering end of tube protects patient and linens from fluid leakage from tube.

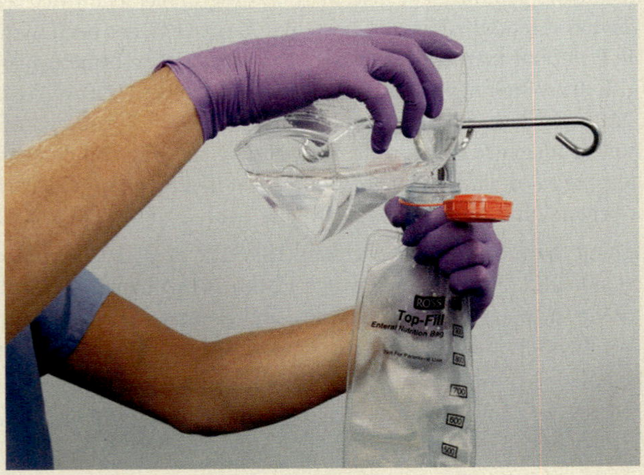

FIGURE 3. Pouring water into feeding bag.

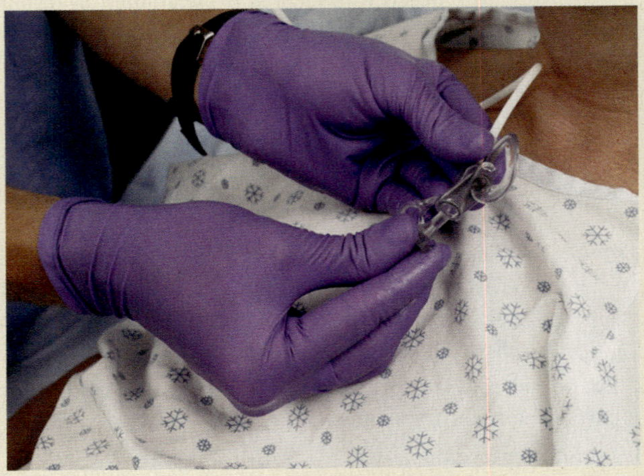

FIGURE 4. Capping NG tube after it is clamped.

When Using a Large Syringe (Bolus; Open System)

ACTION	RATIONALE
a. Remove the plunger from the 30- or 60-mL syringe (Figure 5).	Introducing the formula at a slow, regular rate allows the stomach to accommodate to the feeding and decreases GI distress. The higher the syringe is held, the faster the formula flows.
b. Attach the syringe to the feeding tube and pour a premeasured amount of tube-feeding formula into the syringe (Figure 6). Open the clamp on the feeding tube and allow the formula to enter the tube. Regulate the rate, fast or slow, by the height of the syringe. **Do not push the formula with the syringe plunger.**	

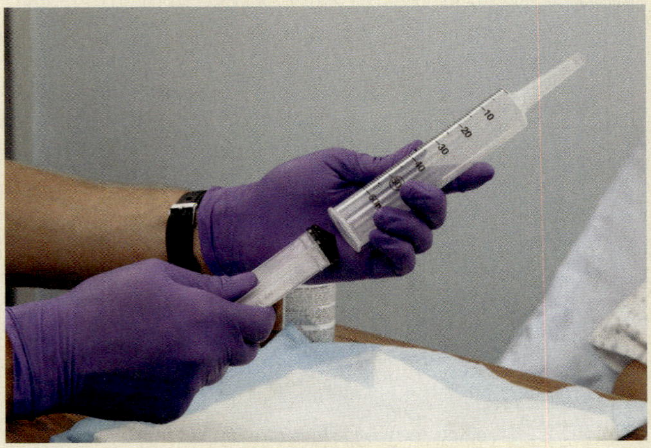

FIGURE 5. Removing plunger from a 60-mL syringe.

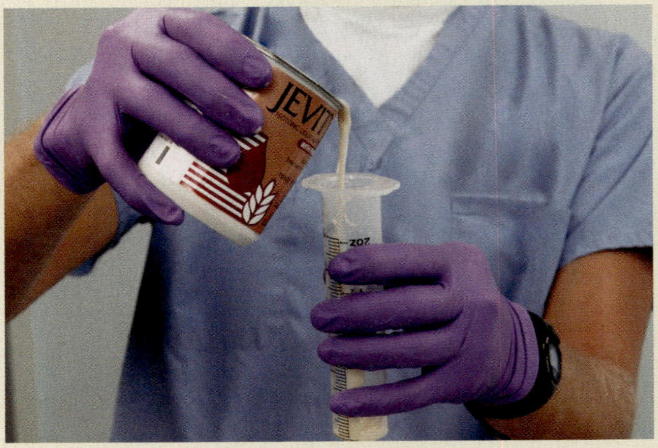

FIGURE 6. Pouring formula into syringe.

ACTION

c. When feeding is almost completed, **add 30 to 60 mL (1 to 2 oz) of water for irrigation to the syringe** (Figure 7) and allow it to run through the tube.

RATIONALE

Water rinses the feeding from the tube and helps to keep it patent as well as provides hydration for the patient. Feeding tubes should be flushed with at least 30 mL of water before starting and after completion of bolus feedings (Bischoff et al., 2020; Boullata et al., 2017; Roveron et al., 2018), based on the patient's fluid needs and restrictions (Boullata et al., 2017).

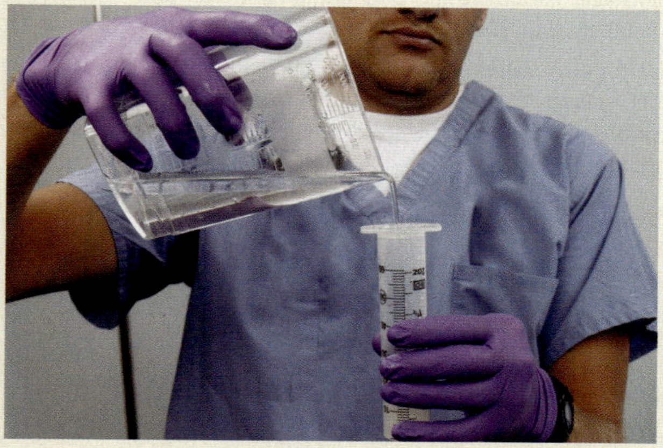

FIGURE 7. Pouring water into almost-empty syringe.

d. When the syringe has emptied, hold it high, clamp the tube, and disconnect it from the tube. Cover the end of the tube with the cap.

By holding syringe high, the formula will not backflow out of tube and onto patient. Clamping the tube prevents air from entering the stomach. Capping end of tube deters entry of microorganisms and prevents fluid leakage from tube.

When Using an Enteral Feeding Pump (Open System)

a. Close the flow-regulator clamp on tubing and fill the feeding bag with prescribed formula, as described in Steps 13a and 13b. Place a label on the bag with patient's name, date, and time the feeding was hung.

Closing the clamp prevents the formula from moving through the tubing until the nurse is ready. Labeling date and time of first use allows for disposal of the bag and tubing within 24 hours, to deter growth of microorganisms.

b. Hang the feeding container on the IV pole. Open the clamp on tubing and allow the solution to flow through the tubing.

This primes the tubing, removing air in the tubing and preventing air from being forced into the stomach or intestines.

c. Connect the administration setup to the feeding pump, following the manufacturer's directions. Set the prescribed rate (Figure 8).

Feeding pumps vary. Some of the newer pumps have built-in safeguards that protect the patient from complications. Safety features include cassettes that prevent free flow of formula, automatic tube flush, safety tips that prevent accidental attachment to an IV setup, and various audible and visible alarms. The rate of infusion begins at the recommended rate, based on guidelines from the dietician or nutrition nurse specialist, and the rate is advanced in increments until the desired rate is achieved (Anderson, 2018b); feeding should be advanced to goal within 48 to 72 hours of initiation (McClave, DiBaise, et al., 2016).

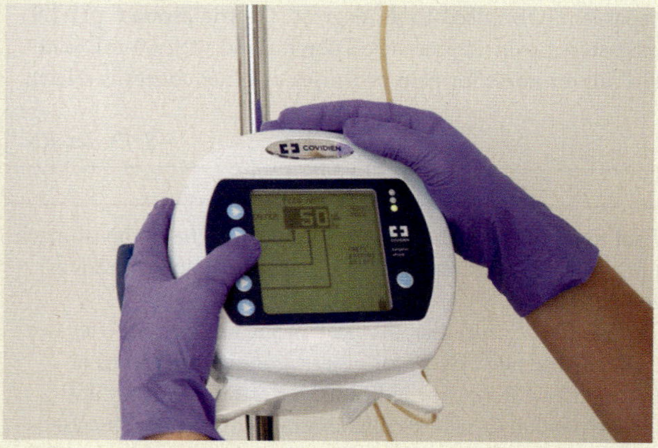

FIGURE 8. Setting infusion rate on pump.

(*continued on page 1432*)

Skill 37-1 Administering a Tube Feeding (Open System) *(continued)*

ACTION	RATIONALE
d. **Flush the tube with at least 30 mL of water at least every 4 to 8 hours during continuous feeding. Verify placement before administering flush.**	Feeding tubes should be flushed with at least 30 mL of water before starting and after completion of bolus feedings; every 4 to 8 hours during continuous feeding (Bischoff et al., 2020; Boullata et al., 2017; Roveron et al., 2018); and before and after medication administration (Drummond Hayes & Hayes, 2018) to prevent blockage, based on the patient's fluid needs and restrictions (Boullata et al., 2017).
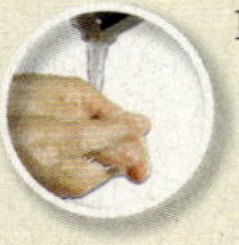 14. Remove equipment and return the patient to a position of comfort. Remove gloves. Perform hand hygiene. Raise the side rail and lower the bed.	This promotes patient comfort and safety. Removing gloves properly reduces the risk for infection transmission and contamination of other items. Hand hygiene prevents transmission of microorganisms.
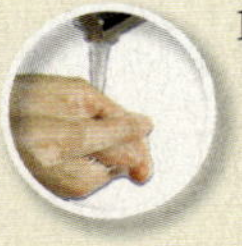 15. Put on gloves. Wash and clean equipment or replace according to facility policy. Remove gloves. Perform hand hygiene.	Gloves prevent contamination and deter spread of microorganisms. Reusable systems are cleansed with soap and water with each use and replaced every 24 hours. Refer to facility policy and manufacturer's guidelines for specifics on equipment care.
16. Monitor patient tolerance of enteral nutrition. Observe the patient's response during and after tube feeding and signs of tolerance at least daily.	Patient tolerance of the volume and type of formula must be monitored daily (Boullata et al., 2017; McClave, Taylor, et al., 2016).
17. **Have the patient remain in an upright position for at least 1 hour after feeding.** Refer to Step 7.	This minimizes possibility of reflux, aspiration, and pneumonia and should be implemented unless contraindicated (McClave, Taylor, et al., 2016; Roveron et al., 2018).
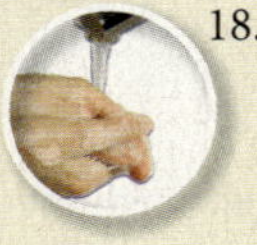 18. Remove additional PPE, if used. Perform hand hygiene.	Proper removal of PPE reduces the risk for infection transmission and contamination of other items. Hand hygiene prevents transmission of microorganisms.

DOCUMENTATION

Guidelines

Document the type of NG tube or gastrostomy/jejunostomy tube that is present. Record the criteria that were used to confirm tube placement before feeding was initiated and during administration, as indicated. Record respiratory and abdominal assessments. If GRVs are part of facility policy and procedure, record the amount of gastric residual volume that was obtained. Document the position of the patient, the type of feeding, and the method and the amount of feeding. Include any relevant patient teaching. Document results of evaluation of tolerance of enteral feeding.

Sample Documentation

Lippincott DocuCare **Practice documenting NG tube insertion in *Lippincott DocuCare.***

10/29/25 1815 Position of NG tube was compared with initial measurement on insertion; no change in measurement. No signs of respiratory distress. Abdomen nondistended and soft; patient denies pain or nausea. HOB raised to 45 degrees. Gastric aspirate pH 3.9. 150 mL of Jevity 1.2 Cal administered over 30 minutes. Tube flushed with 60-mL water with ease. Patient instructed to call for nurse for pain or nausea or other concerns related to feeding.

—S. Essner, RN

UNEXPECTED SITUATIONS AND ASSOCIATED INTERVENTIONS

- *Nasogastric tube is identified not to be in stomach or intestine:* Tube must be in the stomach before feeding. If the tube is in misplaced, the patient is at increased risk for aspiration. Anticipate replacement of feeding tube.
- *Patient reports nausea after tube feeding:* Ensure that the head of the bed remains elevated and that suction equipment is at the bedside. Assess for other signs and symptoms of changes in tolerance to enteral feeding. Check the medication record to see if any antiemetics have been ordered for the patient. Consider collaborating with the health care team to review administration rate, volume, and type of nutritional formula. Monitor for pattern of nausea related to enteral feeding.

- *When attempting to aspirate contents, the nurse notes that tube is clogged:* Feeding tubes are prone to blockage, due to protein-rich formula solutions, the viscosity of the feeding formulas and relatively small diameter of the feeding tube lumens, the use of the tubes for medication administration, and inadequate water flushes (Bischoff et al., 2020; Drummond Hayes & Hayes, 2018). Try to remove the clog: use air bolus or attach a 30- or 60-mL piston syringe to the feeding tube and pull back the plunger to help dislodge the clog. Fill the syringe with warm water and attempt to flush. If met with resistance, use gentle back and forth motion of the plunger to help loosen the clog. If necessary, clamp the tube to allow the warm water to penetrate the clog for up to 20 minutes and then attempt to flush (Boullata et al., 2017). The tube may have to be replaced. To prevent clogs, ensure that adequate flushing is completed after each feeding and before and after medication administration (Bischoff et al., 2020; Drummond Hayes & Hayes, 2018).

DEVELOPING CLINICAL REASONING AND CLINICAL JUDGMENT

SPECIAL CONSIDERATIONS

- There is no benefit from stopping feedings during short periods of lowering of the head of the bed (such as turning the patient) (Boullata et al., 2017). If a prolonged procedure will require lowering of the head of the bed, feedings should be stopped during this period; feedings should be promptly restarted when the procedure is ended or as feasible.
- If GRV checks are part of facility policy and procedure, automatic cessation of enteral nutrition should be avoided for GRVs < 500 mL in the absence of other signs of intolerance (Boullata et al., 2017; McClave, Taylor, et al., 2016; Roveron et al., 2018).
- Volume-based feeding protocols in which 24-hour or daily volumes are targeted instead of hourly rates have been shown to increase volume of nutrition delivered (Heyland et al., 2013, as cited in McClave, Taylor, et al., 2016). This type of method empowers nurses to increase feeding rates to make up for volume lost for scheduled and unscheduled interruptions or while enteral nutrition is held and increase attainment of nutritional goals, supporting optimal nutritional intake (Kinikin et al., 2020; McClave, Taylor, et al., 2016).
- Feedings into the intestine are always continuous and include initiation at a lower rate with a gradual increase in the rate until the target rate identified to meet nutritional goals is met (Bischoff et al., 2020).
- A combination of methods, such as overnight continuous feeding and bolus feeding during the day, may be used for some patients to best meet their needs and allow for autonomy and lifestyle preferences (Bischoff et al., 2020). For other patients, cyclic feeding, administering continuous feeding for a portion of the 24-hour period, may be implemented. The usual routine is to feed the patient for 12 to 16 hours, most often overnight. Cyclic feeding allows the patient to attempt eating regular meals during the day, if this is possible, making ambulation and activity easier.
- Tolerance to gastric feeding can be improved through use of a prokinetic agent, continuous infusion, and elevation of the head of the bed (McClave, DiBaise et al., 2016).
- Sterile water should be used for tube flushes in immunocompromised or critically ill patients (Allen, 2015; Boullata et al., 2017).
- If GRV checks are part of facility policy and procedure, evaluate the significance of a single high gastric residual volume in relation to other indicators of GI intolerance, including abdominal distention, abdominal discomfort, nausea, and vomiting (AACN, 2018).
- Immediately refrigerate formulas reconstituted in advance. Discard unused reconstituted and refrigerated formulas within 24 hours of preparation (Boullata et al., 2017).
- Discard unused reconstituted formulas exposed to room temperature after 4 hours (Boullata et al., 2017).
- Some feeding equipment allows for the addition of water for flushes to a second feeding container, which enters the system through a second set of tubing. The feeding pump will automatically administer the preset volume of flush at the preset frequency.

Skill 37-2 Caring for a Gastrostomy Tube

DELEGATION CONSIDERATIONS

The care of a gastrostomy tube, in the postoperative period, is not delegated to assistive personnel (AP) in the acute care setting. The care of a healed gastrostomy tube site in some settings may be delegated to AP who have received appropriate training, after assessment of the tube by the registered nurse. Depending on the state's nurse practice act and the organization's policies and procedures, the care of a gastrostomy tube may be delegated to licensed practical/vocational nurses (LPN/LVNs). The decision to delegate must be based on careful analysis of the patient's needs and circumstances as well as the qualifications of the person to whom the task is being delegated. Refer to the Delegation Guidelines in Appendix A.

EQUIPMENT

- Nonsterile gloves
- Additional PPE, as indicated
- Washcloth, towel, and skin cleanser or cotton-tipped applicators and sterile saline solution (depending on patient circumstances)
- Gauze (if needed)

IMPLEMENTATION

ACTION	RATIONALE
1. Gather equipment. Verify the prescribed interventions or facility policy and procedure regarding site care.	Assembling equipment provides for an organized approach to the task. Verification ensures the patient receives the correct intervention.
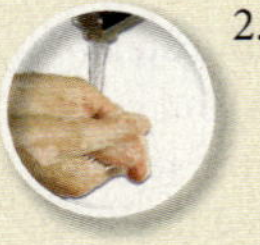 2. Perform hand hygiene and put on PPE, if indicated.	Hand hygiene and PPE prevent the spread of microorganisms. PPE is required based on transmission precautions.
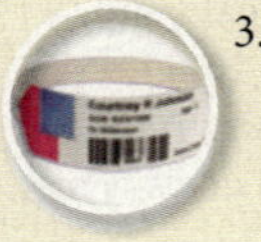 3. Identify the patient.	Identifying the patient ensures the right patient receives the intervention and helps prevent errors.
4. Explain the procedure to the patient. Answer any questions, as needed.	Explanation facilitates patient engagement.
5. Assess for presence of pain at the tube-insertion site. If pain is present, offer the patient analgesic medication per the prescribed interventions and wait for the medication to take effect before beginning insertion-site care.	Feeding tubes can be uncomfortable, especially in the first few days after insertion. Analgesic medication may permit the patient to tolerate the insertion site care more easily. After the first few days, pain at the site should diminish (Roveron et al., 2018).
6. Pull the patient's bedside curtain. Assemble equipment on the bedside table, within reach. Raise the bed to a comfortable working position (VHACEOSH, 2016).	This provides for privacy. Assembling equipment provides for organized approach to the task. An appropriate working height facilitates comfort and proper body mechanics for the nurse.
7. Put on gloves. Assess the gastrostomy site, as described above.	Gloves prevent contact with blood and body fluids. Assessment is vital to detect changes in the patient's condition before initiating the intervention.
8. Measure the length of the exposed tube, comparing it with the initial measurement after insertion. Alternatively, examine the mark on the tube at the skin; the mark should be at skin level at the insertion site.	Tube length should be checked and compared with the initial measurement or marking daily (Roveron et al, 2018). A change in the length of the exposed tube may indicate displacement.

ACTION	RATIONALE
9. Beginning 24 hours after placement of the tube and for the first week, cleanse the stoma and peristomal skin with sterile saline to remove any discharge or material around the tube (Bischoff et al., 2020; Roveron et al., 2018) (Figure 1). Pat the skin around the insertion site dry. If necessary, cover the stoma with sterile gauze to absorb exudate or other fluids (Roveron et al., 2018).	Cleaning the new site with sterile saline solution prevents the introduction of microorganisms into the wound (Roveron et al., 2018). Crust and drainage can harbor bacteria and lead to skin breakdown. Drying the skin thoroughly prevents skin breakdown. Gauze absorbs drainage.
10. After the first week to 10 days, wet a washcloth and apply a small amount of skin cleanser onto the washcloth. Gently cleanse around the insertion, removing any crust or drainage (Bischoff et al., 2020; Roveron et al., 2018) (Figure 2). Rinse the site, removing all cleanser. Pat the skin around the insertion site dry. If necessary, based on facility policy and patient situation, place a gauze dressing above the external fixation device. Alternatively, if the exterior fixation device is 5 mm above the skin, the dressing may be placed under the exterior fixation device, if the dressing is not too thick (Roveron et al., 2018).	Crust and drainage can harbor bacteria and lead to skin breakdown. Removing the cleanser helps to prevent skin irritation. If able, the patient may shower and cleanse the site with soap and water. Drying the skin thoroughly prevents skin breakdown. Placing the dressing above the external fixation device avoids excessive tension (Roveron et al., 2018). Gauze absorbs drainage.

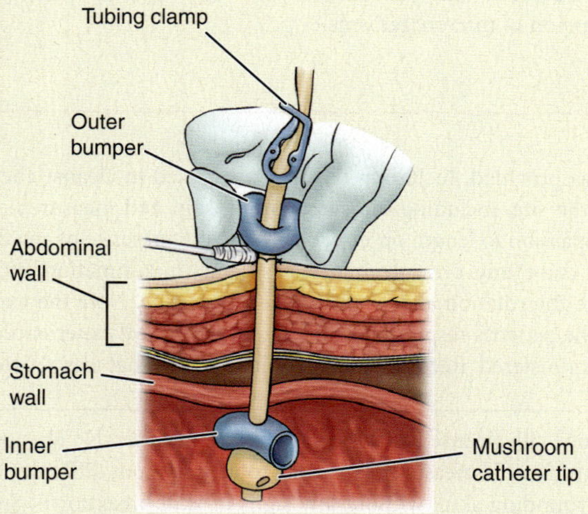

FIGURE 1. Wiping gastric tube site with cotton-tipped applicator and sterile saline.

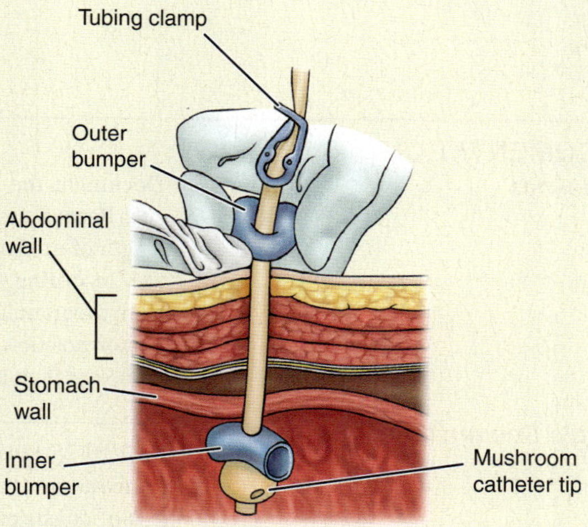

FIGURE 2. Cleaning site with skin cleanser, water, and washcloth.

ACTION	RATIONALE
11. After the first 24 hours, gently rotate the position of the gastrostomy tube 360 degrees. **Rotation of the tube should be done at least once a week and no more than once a day** (Roveron et al., 2018).	Rotation of the tube prevents adherence to the tract and adhesion (Roveron et al., 2018).
12. After the first 7 to 10 days, loosen the exterior fixation device and gently push the tube into the stomach 2 to 3 cm, then gently pull it back until it reaches the area of minimal resistance (the gastric wall). **Push/pull of the tube should be done at least once a week and no more than once a day** (Bischoff et al., 2020; Roveron et al., 2018). Assess that the guard or external bumper is not digging into the surrounding skin. The external fixation device should be 0.5 to 1 cm above the skin (Bischoff et al., 2020; Roveron et al., 2018). **Avoid placing any tension on the tube.**	The gastrocutaneous tract heals in 7 to 10 days (Roveron et al., 2018). This maneuver reduces the risk for buried bumper syndrome (Bischoff et al., 2020; Roveron et al., 2018). Proper placement prevents/avoids excessive tube movement and enlargement of the stoma (Roveron et al., 2018). The external fixation device should be 0.5 to 1 cm above the skin to avoid excessive tension between the interior and exterior fixation devices and to reduce the risk of ischemia, necrosis, infection, and buried bumper syndrome (Bischoff et al., 2020; Roveron et al., 2018). Excessive distance between the external fixation device and the skin could lead to fixation of the gastric wall to the abdominal wall and formation of a gastrocutaneous fistula (Roveron et al., 2018). Excessive traction may contribute to enlargement of the stoma and the development of leakage around the tube (Roveron et al., 2018).

(continued on page 1436)

Skill 37-2 Caring for a Gastrostomy Tube *(continued)*

ACTION	RATIONALE
13. For most patients, the site can be left open to air unless there is drainage. Avoid the use of creams or powders around the stoma (Roveron et al., 2018).	Dressing is not necessary in the absence of drainage (Bischoff et al., 2020; Roveron et al., 2018). Avoiding use of creams or powders around the stoma prevents growth of pathogens (Roveron et al., 2018).
14. If the tube is not in use, check that the cap is securely in place.	The cap should remain closed when the tube is not in use to deter entry of microorganisms and prevent leakage from the tube.
15. Secure the gastrostomy tube to the patient's abdomen in a way that stabilizes the tube and avoids excessive traction (Boullata et al., 2017; Pars & Çavuşoğlu, 2019; Roveron et al., 2018). Assess the integrity of the tape or device used to secure the tube to the stomach.	Excessive friction may result in development of peristomal hypergranulation tissue (Bischoff et al., 2020; Roveron et al., 2018). Excessive traction may contribute to enlargement of the stoma and the development of leakage around the tube (Roveron et al., 2018).
16. Remove gloves. Perform hand hygiene. Lower the bed and assist the patient to a position of comfort, as needed.	Removing gloves reduces the risk for infection transmission and contamination of other items. Hand hygiene prevents transmission of microorganisms. Lowering the bed and assisting the patient ensure patient safety and comfort.
17. Remove additional PPE, if used. Perform hand hygiene.	Proper removal of PPE reduces the risk for infection transmission and contamination of other items. Hand hygiene prevents transmission of microorganisms.

DOCUMENTATION

Guidelines

Document the site care that was provided, including the substance used to cleanse the tube site. Record the assessment of the site, including the surrounding skin and measurement of length of external tube and comparison to length on insertion. Note the presence of any drainage, recording the amount and color, and pressure injury, erythema, inflammation, erosion, or hypergranulation tissue. Note the rotation and/or push/pull of the tube. Note the external fixator position. Comment on the patient's response to the care, if the patient experienced any pain, and if an analgesic was administered. Record any patient instruction that was provided.

Sample Documentation

10/10/25 1145 Gastrostomy tube site cleansed with skin cleanser and water. No change in measurement of tube length from initial measurement. Tube rotated without difficulty. Site is of consistent tone with surrounding skin, without any signs of skin breakdown. Small amount of clear crust noted on tube. Patient tolerated site care without incident. Wife at bedside, actively participating in tube care.

—S. Essner, RN

DEVELOPING CLINICAL REASONING AND CLINICAL JUDGMENT

UNEXPECTED SITUATIONS AND ASSOCIATED INTERVENTIONS

- *Gastrostomy tube is leaking large amount of drainage:* Check tension of tube. If there is a large amount of slack between the internal guard and the external bumper, drainage can leak out of site. Apply gentle pressure to the tube while pressing the external bumper closer to the skin (0.5 to 1 cm from skin [Bischoff et al., 2020; Roveron et al., 2018]). If the tube has an internal balloon holding it in place (similar to a urinary catheter balloon), check to make sure that the balloon is inflated properly.
- *Skin irritation is noted around insertion site:* Investigate the cause of the irritation. Address the cause of the leakage; apply skin barrier or zinc oxide–based skin protectant (Bischoff et al., 2020). If the skin is erythematous and appears to be broken down, gastric fluids may be leaking from the site. Gastric fluids have a low pH and are very acidic. Address the leakage. If the skin has a patchy, red rash, the cause could be candidiasis (yeast). Consult with the health care team regarding the use of an antifungal powder. Ensure that the site is kept dry.

- *Site appears erythematous and patient reports pain at site:* Consult with the health care team; the patient could be developing an infection at the site.
- *Patient reports severe pain that does not respond to routine analgesics when the tube is used for feeding/hydration or when site care is provided during the first 72 hours after placement of the tube:* Discontinue any type of administration through the tube and notify the health care team (Roveron et al., 2018).

SPECIAL CONSIDERATIONS

General Considerations

- Feeding tubes should be flushed with at least 30 mL of water before starting and after completion of bolus feedings, every 4 to 8 hours during continuous feeding, and before and after medication administration (Bischoff et al., 2020; Boullata et al., 2017; Pars & Çavuşoğlu, 2019; Roveron et al., 2018), based on the patient's fluid needs and restrictions (Boullata et al., 2017).
- Avoid occlusive dressings at gastrostomy site; occlusive dressings promote a moist wound environment and can lead to skin maceration (Bischoff et al., 2020).
- Glycerin hydrogel or glycogel dressings may be used as an alternative to gauze dressings (Bischoff et al., 2020). Use of this type of dressing removes the need for daily dressing changes (Bischoff et al., 2020).
- Do not place a dressing between the skin and external fixation device unless drainage is present. Change the dressing immediately when soiled, to prevent skin complications.
- If the length of the exposed tube has changed or marking on tube is not visible, do not use the tube. Consult with the health care team regarding the finding.
- If the patient experiences pain during nutritional infusion, prolonged pain after the procedure, passage of nutritional formula or medications through the stoma, or bleeding from the site, stop the enteral nutrition feeding immediately and consult with the health care team (Roveron et al., 2018, p. 331).

Community-Based Care Considerations

- Advise patients and caregivers to stop the enteral nutrition feeding immediately and contact their health care provider if the patient experiences pain during nutritional infusion, prolonged pain after the procedure, passage of nutritional formula or medications through the stoma, or bleeding from the site (Roveron et al., 2018, p. 331).
- For patients with a well-healed exit site, showering, bathing, and swimming (it is advisable to cover the site with a waterproof dressing when swimming in public pools) is possible after a few weeks (Bischoff et al., 2020).
- All information related to home enteral nutrition should be provided to patients and family members/caregivers verbally and in writing and/or pictures (Bischoff et al., 2020).

Skill 37-3 Obtaining a Capillary Blood Sample for Glucose Testing

DELEGATION CONSIDERATIONS

Obtaining a capillary blood sample for glucose testing may be delegated to assistive personnel (AP) as well as to licensed practical/vocational nurses (LPN/LVNs). The decision to delegate must be based on careful analysis of the patient's needs and circumstances as well as the qualifications of the person to whom the task is being delegated. Refer to the Delegation Guidelines in Appendix A.

EQUIPMENT

- Blood glucose meter
- Sterile lancet
- Cotton balls or gauze squares
- Testing strips for meter
- Nonsterile gloves
- Additional PPE, as indicated
- Skin cleanser and water or alcohol swab

(continued on page 1438)

Skill 37-3 Obtaining a Capillary Blood Sample for Glucose Testing *(continued)*

IMPLEMENTATION

ACTION	RATIONALE
1. Check the patient's health record or plan of care for monitoring schedule. Additional testing may be indicated based on nursing judgment and the patient's condition.	This confirms scheduled times for checking blood glucose. Independent nursing judgment may lead to the decision to test more frequently, based on the patient's condition.
2. Gather equipment. Check the expiration date on blood test strips.	This provides an organized approach to the task. Blood test strips that are past expiration date could cause inaccurate results and should not be used.
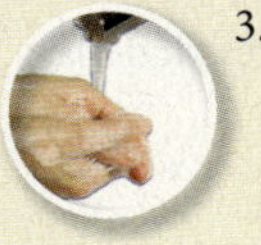 3. Perform hand hygiene and put on PPE, if indicated.	Hand hygiene and PPE prevent the transmission of microorganisms. PPE is required based on transmission precautions.
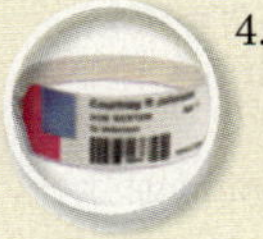 4. Identify the patient. Explain the procedure to the patient and instruct the patient about the need for monitoring blood glucose.	Identifying the patient ensures the right patient receives the intervention and helps prevent errors. Explanation helps to alleviate anxiety and facilitate engagement.
5. Close curtains around the bed and close the door to the room, if possible.	Closing the curtain or door provides for patient privacy.
6. Turn on the monitor.	The monitor must be on for use.
7. Enter the patient's identification number or scan their identification bracelet, if required, according to facility policy.	Use of identification number allows for electronic storage and accurate identification of patient data.
8. Put on gloves.	Gloves protect the nurse from exposure to blood or body fluids.
9. Prepare the lancet using aseptic technique.	Aseptic technique maintains sterility.
10. Remove test strip from the vial. **Recap container immediately.** Test strips also come individually wrapped. **Check that the code number for the strip matches the code number on the monitor screen.**	Immediate recapping protects strips from exposure to humidity, light, and discoloration. Matching code numbers on the strip and glucose monitor ensures that the machine is calibrated correctly.
11. Insert the strip into the meter according to directions for that specific device. Alternatively, strip may be placed in meter after collection of sample on test strip, depending on meter in use.	Correctly inserted strip allows meter to read blood glucose level accurately.
12. **Have the patient wash their hands with skin cleanser and warm water and dry thoroughly. Alternatively, cleanse the skin with an alcohol swab. Allow skin to dry completely.**	Washing with skin cleanser and water or alcohol cleanses the puncture site. Warm water also helps to cause vasodilation. Alcohol can interfere with accuracy of results if not completely dried.
13. Choose a skin site that is intact, warm, and free of calluses and edema (Van Leeuwen & Bladh, 2017).	Areas with lesions are not suitable for capillary sampling. Calluses, edema, and vasoconstriction (cool to palpation) interfere with the ability to obtain a blood sample.
14. Hold the lancet perpendicular to the skin and pierce the skin with the lancet (Figure 1).	Holding the lancet in the proper position facilitates proper skin penetration.

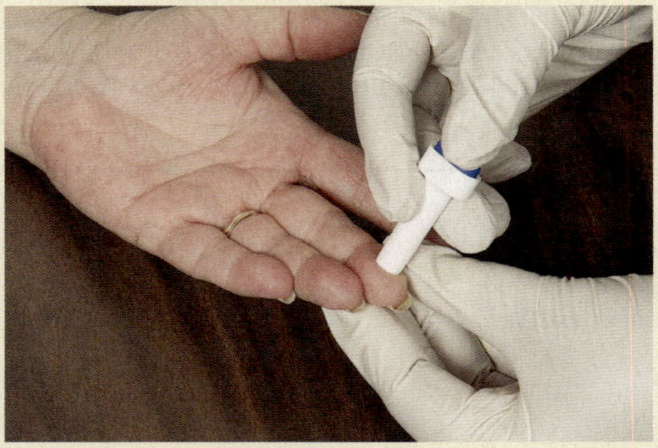

FIGURE 1. Piercing patient's finger with lancet.

ACTION | **RATIONALE**

15. Encourage bleeding by lowering the hand, making use of gravity. Lightly stroke the finger, if necessary, until a sufficient amount of blood has formed to cover the sample area on the strip, based on monitor requirements (check instructions for monitor). If necessary, squeeze from the base of the finger (CDC, 2021d). Take care not to squeeze at the puncture site and not to touch the puncture site or blood.

    Rationale: An appropriate-sized droplet facilitates accurate test results. Squeezing can cause injury to the patient and alter the test.

16. Gently touch a drop of blood to the test strip without smearing it (Figure 2). Depending on the meter in use, insert the strip into the meter after collection of the sample on the test strip.

    Rationale: Smearing blood on the strip may result in inaccurate test results.

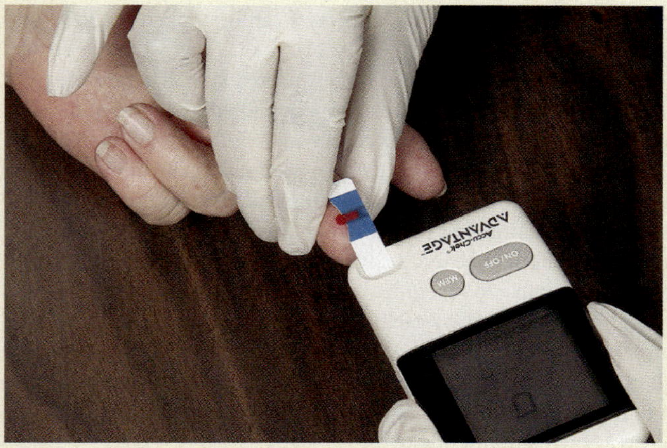

FIGURE 2. Applying blood to test strip.

17. Apply pressure to puncture site with a cotton ball or dry gauze. **Do not use alcohol wipe.**

    Rationale: Pressure causes hemostasis. Alcohol stings and may dry the skin.

18. Read blood glucose results and document the results in the EHR or other designated location, based on facility policy. Inform the patient of the test result.

    Rationale: Timing depends on type of meter.

19. Turn off the meter, remove the test strip, and dispose of supplies appropriately. Place the lancet in a sharps container.

    Rationale: Proper disposal prevents exposure to blood and accidental needlestick.

20. Remove gloves and any other PPE, if used. Perform hand hygiene.

    Rationale: Proper removal of PPE reduces the risk for infection transmission and contamination of other items. Hand hygiene reduces the transmission of microorganisms.

DOCUMENTATION

Guidelines

Document blood glucose level in the patient's health record, according to facility policy. Document pertinent patient assessments, any intervention related to glucose level, and any patient teaching. Communicate abnormal results and/or significant assessments to the health care team.

Sample Documentation

Lippincott DocuCare **Practice documenting blood glucose testing in *Lippincott DocuCare*.**

> 11/1/25 0800 Patient performed own fingerstick blood glucose test with minimal guidance. Verbalized rationale for fasting measurement and able to state symptoms of hypoglycemia. Patient's fingerstick blood glucose level 168. Four units regular Humulin insulin given per sliding scale, in addition to 10 units NPH Humulin insulin scheduled for 0800. Patient encouraged to review written guidelines for subcutaneous insulin administration; will review procedure and plan to have patient administer insulin at dinnertime. Patient verbalized an understanding.
>
> *—B. Clapp, RN*

(continued on page 1440)

Skill 37-3 Obtaining a Capillary Blood Sample for Glucose Testing *(continued)*

DEVELOPING CLINICAL REASONING AND CLINICAL JUDGMENT

UNEXPECTED SITUATIONS AND ASSOCIATED INTERVENTIONS

- *Extremity is pale and cool to the touch:* Begin by warming the extremity. Have adult patients warm their hands by rubbing them together or washing with warm water. Warm, moist compresses may also be used.
- *Blood glucose level results are above- or below-normal parameters:* Assess the patient for signs of hyperglycemia or hypoglycemia, respectively. Check patient's health record for prescribed interventions, such as insulin dosage or glucose-containing carbohydrate administration (ADA, 2021). Notify health care team of results, assessment data, and interventions.

SPECIAL CONSIDERATIONS

General Considerations

- If the selected site feels cool or appears pale, warm compresses can be applied for 3 to 5 minutes to dilate the capillaries.
- Sampling of blood from an alternative site other than fingertips may have limitations. Blood in the fingertips shows changes in glucose levels more quickly than blood in other parts of the body. This means that alternative site test results may differ from fingertip test results when glucose levels are changing rapidly (e.g., after a meal, taking insulin, or during or after exercise) because the results may be inaccurate. Caution patients to use a fingertip sample if it is less than 2 hours after eating, less than 2 hours after injecting rapid-acting insulin, during exercise or within 2 hours of exercise, when sick or under stress, when having symptoms of hypoglycemia, if unable to recognize symptoms of hypoglycemia, or if site results do not agree with the way the patient feels (U.S. FDA, 2019).
- Meters require calibration at least monthly or according to the manufacturer's recommendation, and when a new bottle of test strips is opened. Manufacturer's directions for calibration should be followed. After calibration, the meter is checked for accuracy by testing a control solution containing a known amount of glucose.
- Alternative testing sites, other than fingertips, should not be used to calibrate a continuous glucose monitor or for insulin dosing calculations (U.S. FDA, 2019).
- Inadequate sampling can cause errors in the results. It is very important to be aware of requirements for the specific monitor used.
- Continuous glucose monitoring (CGM) systems use sensors placed just below the skin to check glucose levels in tissue fluid. A transmitter sends information about glucose levels from the sensor to a wireless monitor. These devices provide real-time measurements of glucose levels every few minutes (NIDDK, 2017). These systems provide a way to see glucose trends, and track patterns (NIDDK, 2017).
- Most models of CGMs require confirmation of a CGM reading with a fingerstick blood glucose test before taking insulin or treating hypoglycemia (NIDDK, 2017).

Infant and Child Considerations

- Heel sticks, using the outer aspect of the heel, may be used for infants. Warming the heel for 5 to 10 minutes before the sample is taken dilates the blood vessels in the area and aids in sampling (KarabiyikOğurlu et al., 2020; Vedder, 2021). This technique is not without controversy, as it is painful and can lead to scarring and infection, including infection of bone and cartilage, due to excessive depth of the puncture (Gorski et al., 2021; Vedder, 2021). Venipuncture by a skilled phlebotomist is suggested instead of heel lance methods due to the increased pain from heel lance (Gorski et al., 2021). Automatic lancing devices are preferred over manual devices to control the depth of puncture and to reduce the risk of bone or cartilage infection (Gorski et al., 2021).

Older Adult Considerations

- Blood glucose meters are available with large digital readouts or audio components for patients with visual impairments (Williams, n.d.).

Community-Based Care Considerations

- Patients monitor blood glucose levels routinely at home. Provide education focusing on important elements of diabetes education to assist patients in managing their diabetes, including the signs, symptoms, and management of hypoglycemia and hyperglycemia; correct administration of oral hypoglycemic agents and/or insulin; fingerstick blood glucose monitoring; and the accurate use of fingerstick blood glucose monitoring equipment.
- Many different types of monitors are available. Assist patients to identify desirable features for individual use.

EVOLVING CASE STUDY 37-1

Scenario: Susan Oakland, a 21-year-old student, is pregnant with her first child. She was seen at the prenatal clinical for her first visit at 5 weeks of gestation. On her next visit, 4 weeks later, she reports persistent nausea, vomiting, and fatigue, contributing to a loss of appetite.

QUESTION r/t CUES: Which assessment data are of highest priority for the nurse to collect to provide additional information to address Susan's decreased nutritional intake?

A. Calculate the patient's BMI; measure the patient's waist circumference
B. The patient's plans for childcare
C. Patient's baseline and current weight
D. The patient's decision to breast/chest or bottle feed

Scenario: The patient confides that "Eating food has become pretty unappealing." The patient relays that she is very weight conscious; she appears pale and somewhat withdrawn. The patient and her husband are first-semester graduate students; their source of income is graduate assistantships. She has lost 3 lb since her first visit at 5 weeks of gestation.

QUESTION r/t ANALYZING CUES: What other information (assessment data or evidence) should the nurse obtain related to this issue? Select all that apply.

A. Patient's use of vitamin supplements
B. The patient's living situation
C. The food budget the patient and her husband have established
D. A 24-hour food recall
E. An in-depth psychiatric assessment

Scenario: The patient's 24-hour recall revealed an inadequate intake from the milk food group and marginal intake from grain and meat groups. She skips breakfast because of a "hurried schedule," which is now complicated by nausea. The patient shares that she dislikes red meat and eats it only once or twice a month. She also dislikes milk and substitutes sugar-free soft drinks and water.

QUESTION r/t PRIORITIZING HYPOTHESIS: Based on the assessments of this patient, which priority problem should the nurse identify to guide the plan of care?

A. Anxiety
B. Impaired nutritional intake
C. Risk for impaired skin integrity
D. Fatigue

Scenario: The nurse decides to focus on ways to manage nausea and vomiting and achieve and maintain adequate nutritional intake.

QUESTION r/t GENERATING SOLUTIONS: Which intervention will be most effective to help the patient achieve and maintain improved nutrition?

A. Reinforce the need to consume large amounts of nutrient-dense foods to support the developing fetus
B. Encourage the patient to consume small, frequent meals that include nutrient-dense foods
C. Provide a list of foods that must be eaten during pregnancy, regardless of the patient's preferences
D. Explain that a rigid, fixed schedule of meals is necessary to ensure adequate nutrition

Scenario: Susan's pregnancy continues to progress, but her weight loss persists into week 10 of the pregnancy, and she has lost an additional 4 lb. She has kept a food diary of her intake and has also trended her feelings of nausea and episodes of vomiting. The midwife is concerned and appreciates the need for further intervention.

QUESTION r/t TAKING ACTION: The nurse is preparing teaching materials for the patient. Which materials should the nurse prepare to use for the teaching session with this patient and her husband?

A. Percutaneous endoscopic gastrostomy (PEG) insertion and associated formula administration
B. Megadoses of nutritional supplements including calcium, folic acid, and calcium
C. Prescription for ondansetron, an antinausea agent that blocks the triggers of nausea and vomiting
D. Information on eating disorders such as anorexia nervosa, bulimia, and laxative/diuretic use disorders

Scenario: Susan comes back for her well check-up at 15 weeks and reports that the nausea and vomiting resolved with the use of the medication, but that she has not taken any doses for 2 weeks.

QUESTION r/t EVALUATING OUTCOMES: Although the patient reports feeling better, which of the following objective measures would the nurse use to evaluate the success of the nursing interventions and resolution of the health problem for this particular patient? Select all that apply.

A. The patient is maintaining approximately an extra 340 calories per day in her diet
B. The patient is no longer vomiting after taking her prescribed prenatal supplements
C. The patient reports being able to tolerate a nightly beer with the evening meal
D. The patient divulges the use of nightly suppositories to stimulate a bowel movement
E. The patient's weight is steadily increasing at a rate commensurate with gestational age

DEVELOPING CLINICAL REASONING AND CLINICAL JUDGMENT

1. Work through the Evolving Case Study 37-1 on page 1441 to help develop your clinical reasoning and clinical judgment skills.
2. Prepare a diet for an economically disadvantaged family consisting of a single working mother and her three children, ages 3 to 14 years, taking into consideration the family's culture (specify a minority culture in your locale) and yearly income (below poverty level).
3. Prepare a 1-day menu that meets the recommended daily allowance of essential nutrients for the following patients:
   - An obese teenager
   - A child vegetarian
   - An executive with high blood pressure who dines out frequently with patients
   - A woman running a minimum of 12 miles daily as she trains for a marathon

PRACTICING FOR NCLEX

1. A nurse at a health fair calculates the body mass index (BMI) of a person who weighs 68 kg and is 165 cm (1.65 m) tall. How will the nurse document the BMI?
   a. 25 kg/m^2
   b. 46 kg/m^2
   c. 68 kg/m^2
   d. 165 kg/m^2
2. After administering an enteral feeding, a nurse evaluates the patient's tolerance of the feeding by assessing for the absence of signs and symptoms that indicate intolerance of the feeding. Which findings, if present, suggest potential intolerance of the feeding and require collaboration with the dietician and health care provider? Select all that apply.
   a. Nausea and/or vomiting
   b. Weight gain
   c. Bowel sounds 20/min
   d. 200-mL gastric residual
   e. Absence of diarrhea and constipation
   f. Slight abdominal pain and distention
3. A nurse is feeding an older adult patient with dementia. What intervention will best promote nutritional intake?
   a. Stroke the underside of the patient's chin to promote swallowing.
   b. Serve meals in different places and at different times.
   c. Offer a whole tray of various foods to choose from.
   d. Avoid between-meal snacks to ensure hunger at mealtime.
4. A patient with COPD is experiencing anorexia and weight loss. Which intervention would be most helpful in stimulating appetite in this patient?
   a. Administering pain medication after meals.
   b. Encouraging the patient's family to bring food from home when possible.
   c. Scheduling respiratory therapy nebulizer treatments before each meal.
   d. Reinforcing the importance of eating what is delivered to them.
5. A nurse is feeding a patient who is experiencing dysphagia. Which nursing intervention will best prevent aspiration?
   a. Feed the patient solids first and liquids last.
   b. Place the bed in the semi-Fowler position during feeding.
   c. Provide a 30-minute rest period prior to mealtime.
   d. Provide a straw for the patient's beverages and soups.
6. During interprofessional rounds, the charge nurse and health care provider evaluate patients to determine their need for parenteral nutrition (PN). Which patients will be identified as candidates for this type of nutritional support? Select all that apply.
   a. Patient with irritable bowel syndrome and intractable diarrhea
   b. Patient with celiac disease not absorbing nutrients from the GI tract
   c. Patient who is underweight and needs short-term nutritional support
   d. Patient who is comatose and needs long-term nutritional support
   e. Patient who has anorexia and refuses to take foods via the oral route
   f. Patient with burns who has not been able to eat adequately for 5 days
7. A nurse is feeding a patient who reports feeling nauseated and unable to eat what is being offered. What would be the most appropriate initial action of the nurse in this situation?
   a. Remove the tray from the room.
   b. Administer an antiemetic and encourage the patient to take small amounts.
   c. Explore why the patient does not want to eat the food.
   d. Offer high-calorie snacks such as pudding and ice cream.
8. A nurse is receiving report on a patient with alcoholism who will be transferred to the medical-surgical unit. Due to long-term alcohol exposure, the nurse plans for administration of which nutrient?
   a. B vitamins
   b. Lipids
   c. Fluids
   d. C vitamins
9. A nursing student is caring for a patient who had a gastrostomy tube placement 12 hours ago. Which action by the student is correct?
   a. Using a cotton-tipped applicator dipped into sterile saline solution and gently cleaning around the insertion site
   b. Washing the area surrounding the tube with a wet washcloth and with soap and water.
   c. Adjusting the external disk every 3 hours to avoid crusting around the tube.

d. Taping a gauze dressing over the site after cleansing it.
e. Assessing the gastric residual every 4 hours.
f. Discontinuing feedings when gastric residual volume is 120 mL.

10. A nurse is assessing a patient who has been NPO (nothing by mouth) prior to abdominal surgery. The patient is ordered a clear liquid diet for breakfast, to advance to a house diet as tolerated. Which assessments would indicate to the nurse that the patient's diet should not be advanced?
a. The patient consumed 75% of the liquids on the breakfast tray.
b. The patient tells you they are hungry.
c. The patient's abdomen is soft, nondistended, with bowel sounds.
d. The patient reports fullness and diarrhea after breakfast.

11. A patient hospitalized for a stroke has a prescription for continuous tube feedings through a small-bore nasogastric tube. Following tube placement, which action by the nurse best confirms correct tube placement?
a. Auscultating the bowel sounds
b. Measuring the pH of gastric aspirate
c. Measuring the amount of residual in the stomach
d. Ensuring validation of tube placement by x-ray

12. A nurse specializing in care of older adults speaks to a group of nursing students about that population's challenge with obtaining sufficient nutrition. Which points will the nurse include in the discussion? Select all that apply.
a. An increase in BMR and physical activity require additional calories.
b. Tooth loss and periodontal disease may make chewing more difficult.
c. Decreased peristalsis can result in constipation, requiring additional fiber and fluid.
d. Loss of taste between sweet and salty occurs with a preference for sweets.
e. Older adults express an increase thirst sensation.
f. Caloric needs decrease, and the need for nutrients increases, especially protein.

13. A nurse in the intensive care unit is reviewing diagnostic studies to evaluate a patient's nutritional status. What findings consistent with inadequate nutrition require follow-up by the nurse? Select all that apply.
a. Decreased hemoglobin
b. Low prealbumin level
c. Increased transferrin
d. Anemia
e. Elevated lymphocytes

14. A nurse plans to administer a bolus tube feeding for a patient but is unable to aspirate gastric contents due to a clogged tube. What action will the nurse take next?
a. Use warm water or air, applying gentle pressure to remove the clog.
b. Use the tube's stylet to unclog the tubes.
c. Administer a cola beverage to remove the clog.
d. Replace the tube with a new one.

15. A nurse performs presurgical assessments of patients in an ambulatory care center. Which patient assessment requires collaboration with the surgeon, as the procedure could need to be postponed?
a. 19-year-old patient who is a vegan
b. Older adult patient who takes daily nutritional drinks
c. 43-year-old patient who takes ginkgo biloba and an aspirin daily
d. Infant who is breastfeeding

16. A nurse is caring for a patient with ill-fitting dentures. What modification to their diet will the nurse suggest?
a. Clear liquid
b. Full liquid
c. Mechanically altered
d. Honeylike liquids

ANSWERS WITH RATIONALES

1. **a.** Example: Weight = 68 kg, height = 165 cm (1.65 m), Calculation: $68 \div (1.65)^2 = 24.98$
2. **a, c, e.** Criteria to consider when evaluating patient feeding tolerance include absence of nausea, vomiting, minimal or no gastric residual, absence of diarrhea and constipation, absence of abdominal pain and distention, presence of bowel sounds within normal limits.
3. **a.** To feed a patient with dementia, the nurse should stroke the underside of the patient's chin to promote swallowing, serve meals in the same place and at the same time, provide one food item at a time since a whole tray may be overwhelming, and provide between-meal snacks that are easy to consume using the hands.
4. **b.** Food from home that the patient enjoys may stimulate them to eat. Pain medication should be given before meals, respiratory therapy should be scheduled after meals, and telling the patient what they must eat is no guarantee that they will comply.
5. **c.**The nurse should provide a 30-minute rest period prior to mealtime to promote better swallowing. The nurse alternates solids and liquids when feeding the patient; sits the patient upright or, if on bedrest, elevates the head of the bed at a 90-degree angle; and initiates a nutrition consult for diet modification and food size and/or consistency. Straws are avoided in patients with dysphagia. Assessing breath sounds will help detect aspiration but not prevent it.
6. **a, b, f.** Assessment criteria used to determine the need for PN include an inability to achieve or maintain enteral access, motility disorders, intractable diarrhea, impaired absorption of nutrients from the GI tract, and when oral intake has been or is expected to be inadequate over a 7- to 14-day period. PN promotes tissue healing and is a good choice for a patient with burns who has an inadequate diet with an increased need for calories and nutrients. Oral intake is the best method of feeding; the second-best method is via the enteral route. For short-term use (less than 4 weeks), a nasogastric or

nasointestinal route is usually selected. A gastrostomy (enteral feeding) is the preferred route to deliver enteral nutrition in the patient who is comatose because the gastroesophageal sphincter remains intact, making regurgitation and aspiration less likely than with NG tube feedings. Patients who refuse to take food should not be force fed nutrients against their will.

7. **a.** The first action of the nurse when a patient has nausea is to remove the tray, which may have noxious odor, from the room. The nurse may then offer small amounts of foods and liquids such as crackers or ginger ale. The nurse may also administer a prescribed antiemetic and try small amounts of food when it takes effect.

8. **a.** The need for B vitamins is increased in alcoholism because these nutrients are used to metabolize alcohol, thus depleting their supply. Obesity, dehydration, and vitamin C deficiency may be present, but these are not directly related to the effect of alcohol on the GI tract.

9. **a.** When caring for a new gastrostomy tube, the nurse would use a cotton-tipped applicator dipped in sterile saline to gently cleanse the area, removing any crust or drainage. The nurse would not use a washcloth with soap and water on a new gastrostomy tube but may use this method if the site is healed. Also, once the sutures are removed, the nurse should rotate the external bumper 90 degrees once a day. The nurse should leave the site open to air. If drainage is present, one thickness of precut gauze should be placed under the external bumper and changed as needed to keep the area dry.

10. **d.** Tolerance to a diet can be assessed by the following: absence of nausea, vomiting, and diarrhea; absence of feelings of fullness; absence of abdominal pain and distention; feelings of hunger; and the ability to consume at least 50% to 75% of the food on the meal tray.

11. **d.** Radiographic examination is the most accurate method to validate tube placement in the stomach. In addition, the length of the exposed tube is measured after insertion and documented. Tube length should be checked and compared with this initial measurement, in conjunction with the previous two methods for checking tube placement. Other methods that can be used are aspiration of gastric contents and measurement of the pH of the aspirate. Visual assessment of aspirated gastric contents is also suggested as a tool to check placement. The auscultatory method is considered inaccurate and unreliable. Measurement of residual volume amount does not confirm placement.

12. **b, c, d, f.** Due to age-related changes, caloric needs of the body decrease; however, the need for nutrients, including protein, calcium, vitamin B_{12}, and vitamin D increase. If tooth loss and periodontal disease occur, adequate nutritional intake may become more difficult. An increase in fiber and fluid intake can relieve constipation related to decreased peristalsis. Older adults are also prone to dehydration related to loss of thirst sensation. Loss of taste between sweet and salty occurs with a preference for sweets. Dietary restrictions related to chronic illness, limited income, isolation, and age-related physiologic changes place persons in this age group at risk for malnutrition.

13. **a, b, d, e.** Test results for hemoglobin (normal = 12 to 18 g/dL): decrease indicates anemia. Results for hematocrit (normal = 40% to 50%): decrease indicates anemia; increase indicates dehydration. Serum albumin and prealbumin tests for malnutrition and malabsorption will be decreased, as will transferrin and blood urea nitrogen. Elevated lymphocytes may indicate infection.

14. **a.** To remove a clog in a feeding tube, the nurse should try using warm water or air and gentle pressure to unclog it. The stylet should never be used to unclog a tube, and cola and meat tenderizers have not been shown effective in removing clogs. The nurse should first attempt to remove the clog, and, if unsuccessful, the tube should be replaced.

15. **c.** Patients taking gingko biloba (an herbal), aspirin, and vitamin E (dietary supplement) may have increased risk for excessive bleeding and may requiring surgery to be postponed. Being a vegan should not affect surgery unless the patient has serious nutritional deficiencies. Drinking nutritional drinks and breastfeeding do not adversely affect the outcomes of surgery.

16. **c.** Mechanically altered diets provide adequate in calories and nutrients and contain chopped, ground, or soft foods. Liquid diets are generally used as transitional diets when eating resumes after acute illness, surgery, or parenteral nutrition. Clear-liquid diets are inadequate in calories, protein, and most nutrients; progression to more nutritious alternatives is recommended as soon as possible. Full-liquid diets include clear liquids plus milk and milk drinks, puddings, custards, plain frozen desserts, pasteurized eggs, cereal gruels, vegetable juices, and milk and egg substitutes in addition to clear liquids. A high-calorie, high-protein supplement is recommended if a full-liquid diet is used for more than 3 days.

Bibliography

Abdelhadi, R. A., Dekonenko, C., Dorman, R. M., Oyetunji, T. A., & St. Peter, S. D. (2020). A prospective, randomized cross-over trial of 2 low-profile gastrostomy buttons to determine family preference. *Journal of Pediatric Gastroenterology & Nutrition, 70*(3), 386–388. https://doi.org/10.1097/MPG.0000000000002585

Academy of Nutrition and Dietetics. (2020a, August). *Healthy weight during pregnancy.* https://www.eatright.org/health/pregnancy/prenatal-wellness/healthy-weight-during-pregnancy

Academy of Nutrition and Dietetics. (2020b, July 28). *Healthy lifestyle for healthy older adults.* https://www.eatright.org/food/nutrition/dietary-guidelines-and-myplate/healthy-weights-for-healthy-older-adults

Allen, S. M. (2015). As a flushing agent for enteral nutrition, does sterile water compared to tap water affect the associated risk of infection in critically ill patients? *The Alabama Nurse, 42*(1), 5–6.

Alzheimer's Association. Alzheimer's and Dementia Caregiver Center. (n.d.). *Food and eating.* Retrieved September 26, 2020, from https://www.alz.org/help-support/caregiving/daily-care/food-eating

American Association of Critical Care Nurses (AACN). (2018, May 17). *AACN practice alert. Prevention of aspiration in adults.* https://www.aacn.org/clinical-resources/practice-alerts/prevention-of-aspiration

American Association of Critical Care Nurses (AACN). (2020, January 29). *AACN practice alert. Initial and ongoing verification of feeding tube placement in adults.* https://www.aacn.org/

American Diabetes Association (ADA). (2021). Standards of medical care in diabetes—2021. *Diabetes Care, 44*(Suppl 1), S1–S232. https://care.diabetesjournals.org/content/44/Supplement_1

American Heart Association (AHA). (2017, March 23). *Trans fats.* https://www.heart.org/en/healthy-living/healthy-eating/eat-smart/fats/trans-fat

American Society of Anesthesiologists. (n.d.). *Risks. Obesity.* Retrieved September 26, 2020, from https://www.asahq.org/whensecondscount/preparing-for-surgery/risks/obesity/

Anderson, L. (2018a). Fine-bore nasogastric tube feeding: Reducing the risks. *British Journal of Nursing, 27*(12), 674–675. https://doi.org/10.12968/bjon.2018.27.12.674

Anderson, L. (2018b). Delivering artificial nutrition and hydration safely by feeding pumps. *British Journal of Nursing, 27*(18), 1032–1033. https://doi.org/10.12968/bjon.2018.27.18.1032

Anderson, L. (2019a). Identifying malnutrition in the community. *Journal of Community Nursing, 33*(6), 50–55.

Anderson, L. (2019b). Enteral feeding tubes: An overview of nursing care. *British Journal of Nursing, 28*(12), 748–754. https://doi.org/10.12968/bjon.2019.28.12.748

Andrews, M., Boyle, J. S., & Collins, J. (2020). *Transcultural concepts in nursing care* (8th ed.). Wolters Kluwer.

Ashwell, M., & Gibson, S. (2014). A proposal for a primary screening tool: 'Keep your waist circumference to less than half your height'. *BMC Medicine, 12*, 207. https://doi.org/10.1186/s12916-014-0207-1

Atalay, Y. O., Aydin, R., Ertugrul, O., Gul, S. B., Polat, A. V., & Paksu, M. S. (2016). Does bedside sonography effectively identify nasogastric tube placements in pediatric critical care patients? *Nutrition in Clinical Practice, 31*(6), 805–809. https://doi.org/10.1177/0884533616639401

Atkinson, K. (2019). Neurological conditions and acute dysphagia. *British Journal of Nursing, 28*(8), 490–492. https://doi.org/10.12968/bjon.2019.28.8.490

Ayers, P., Adams, S., Boullata, J., Gervasio, J., Holcombe, B., Kraft, M. D., Marshall, N., Neal, A., Sacks, G., Seres, D. S., Worthington, P., & American Society for Parenteral and Enteral Nutrition. (2014). A.S.P.E.N. Parenteral nutrition safety consensus recommendations. *Journal of Parenteral and Enteral Nutrition, 38*(3), 296–333. https://doi.org/10.1177/0148607113511992

Ballesteros-Pomar, M. D., Cherubini, A., Keller, H., Lam, P., Rolland, Y., & Simmons, S. F. (2020). Texture-modified diet for improving the management of oropharyngeal dysphagia in nursing home residents: An expert review. *The Journal of Nutrition Health & Aging, 24*(6), 576–581. https://doi.org/10.1007/s12603-020-1377-5

Batchelor-Murphy, M., & Amella, E. J. (n.d.). *Eating and feeding issues in older adults with dementia. Part II: Interventions*. Retrieved September 27, 2020, from https://hign.org/consultgeri/try-this-series/eating-and-feeding-issues-older-adults-dementia-part-ii-interventions

Batchelor-Murphy, M. K., Steinberg, F. M., & Young, H. M. (2019). Dietary and feeding modifications for older adults. *American Journal of Nursing, 119*(12), 49–57. https://doi.org/10.1097/01.NAJ.0000615796.40279.9c

Behrens, S., Kozeniecki, M., Knapp, N., & Martrindale, R. G. (2021). Nutrition support during prone positioning: An old technique reawakened by COVID-19. *Nutrition in Clinical Practice, 36*(1), 105–109. https://doi.org/10.1002/ncp.10592

Bernstein, M., & Munoz, N. (2020). *Nutrition for the older adult* (3rd ed.). Jones & Bartlett Learning.

Bischoff, S. C., Austin, P., Boeykens, K., Chourdakis, M., Cuerda, C., Jonkers-Schuitema, C., Lichota, M., Nyulasi, I., Schneider, S. M., Stanga, Z., & Pironi, L. (2020). ESPEN guideline on home enteral nutrition. *Clinical Nutrition, 39*(1), 5–22. https://doi.org/10.1016/j.clnu.2019.04.022

Bishop, A., Witts, S., & Martin, T. (2018). The role of nutrition in successful wound healing. *Journal of Community Nursing, 32*(4), 44–50.

Boeykens, K., Steeman, E., & Dyusburgh, I. (2014). Reliability of pH measurement and the auscultatory method to confirm the position of a nasogastric tube. *International Journal of Nursing Studies, 51*(11), 1427–1433. https://doi.org/10.1016/j.ijnurstu.2014.03.004

Boullata, J. I., Carrera, A. L., Harvey, L., Escuro, A. A., Hudson, L., Mays, A., McGinnis, C., Wessel, J. J., Bajpai, S., Beebe, M. L., Kinn, T. J., Klang, M. G., Lord, L., Martin, K., Pompeii-Wolfe, C., Sullivan, J., Wood, A., Malone, A., & Guenter, P., & ASPEN Safe Practices for Enteral Nutrition Therapy, American Society for Parenteral and Enteral Nutrition. (2017). ASPEN safe practices for enteral nutrition therapy. *Journal of Parenteral and Enteral Nutrition, 41*(1), 15–103. https://doi.org/10.1177/0148607116673053

Boullata, J. I., Gilbert, K., Sacks, G., Labossiere, R. J., Crill, C., Goday, P., Kumpf, V. J., Mattox, T. W., Plogsted, S., Holcombe, B., & American Society for Parenteral and Enteral Nutrition. (2014). A.S.P.E.N. clinical guidelines: Parenteral nutrition ordering, order review, compounding, labeling, and dispensing. *Journal of Parenteral and Enteral Nutrition, 38*(3), 334–377. https://doi.org/10.1177/0148607114521833

Boyd, M. A. (2018). *Psychiatric nursing. Contemporary practice* (6th ed.). Wolters Kluwer.

Bruni, A., Garofalo, E., Grande, L., Auletta, G., Cubello, D., Greco, M., Lombardo, N., Garieri, P., Papaleo, A., Doldo, P., Spagnuolo, R., & Longhini, F. (2020). Nursing issues in enteral nutrition during prone position in critically ill patients: A systematic review of the literature. *Intensive & Critical Care Nursing, 60*, 102899. https://doi.org/10.1016/j.iccn.2020.102899

Cedars Sinai. (2019, January 16). *Are animal proteins better for you than plant proteins?* https://www.cedars-sinai.org/blog/best-protein.html

Centers for Disease Control and Prevention (CDC). (2018, July 3). *Overweight & obesity. Defining childhood obesity. BMI for children and teens.* https://www.cdc.gov/obesity/childhood/defining.html

Centers for Disease Control and Prevention (CDC). (2020a, June 25). *Healthy weight, nutrition, and physical activity. Child & teen BMI calculator.* https://www.cdc.gov/healthyweight/bmi/calculator.html

Centers for Disease Control and Prevention (CDC). (2020b, July 1). *Healthy weight, nutrition, and physical activity. Assessing your weight.* https://www.cdc.gov/healthyweight/assessing/index.html

Centers for Disease Control and Prevention (CDC). (2020c, June 30). *Overweight & obesity. Defining adult obesity.* https://www.cdc.gov/obesity/adult/defining.html

Centers for Disease Control and Prevention (CDC). (2021d, August 10). *Monitoring your blood sugar.* https://www.cdc.gov/diabetes/managing/managing-blood-sugar/bloodglucosemonitoring.html

Chiang, C. K., & Hwu, Y. J. (2018). Feeding experiences of nursing aides for residents with dysphagia. *Geriatric Nursing, 39*(4), 436–442. https://doi.org/10.1016/j.gerinurse.2017.12.016

Comitato, R., Saba, A., Turrini, A., Arganini, C., & Virgili, F. (2015). Sex hormones and macronutrient metabolism. *Critical Reviews in Food Science and Nutrition, 55*(2), 227–241. https://doi.org/10.1080/10408398.2011.651177

Delgado, S. A. (2018). Nutrition is critical. *American Journal of Critical Care, 27*(2), 144. https://doi.org/10.4037/ajcc2018355

Dias, F. S. B., Almeida, B. P., Alvares, B. R., Jales, R. M., Caldas, J. P. S., & Carmona, E. V. (2019). Use of pH reagent strips to verify gastric tube placement in newborns. *Revista Latino-Americana de Enfermagem, 27*, e3227. https://doi.org/10.1590/1518-8345.3150.3227

Dias, F. S. B., Alvares, B. R., Jales, R. M., Franco, A. P. V., Silva, J. E. F. D., Fabene, S. M. S., Caldas, J. P. S., & Carmona, E. V. (2019). The use of ultrasonography for verifying gastric tube placement in newborns. *Advances in Neonatal Care, 19*(3), 219–225. https://doi.org/10.1097/ANC.0000000000000553

Drummond Hayes, K., & Hayes, D. D. (2018). Best practices for unclogging feeding tubes in adults. *Nursing, 48*(6), 66. https://doi.org/10.1097/01.NURSE.0000532744.80506.5e

Dudek, S. (2022). *Nutrition essentials for nursing practice* (9th ed.). Wolters Kluwer.

Dunlap, J. J., & Patterson, S. (2019). Focus on clinical assessment. Assessing dysphagia. *Gastroenterology Nursing, 42*(3), 302–305. https://doi.org/10.1097/SGA.0000000000000472

Eliopoulos, C. (2018). *Gerontological nursing* (9th ed.). Wolters Kluwer Health.

Fetherstonhaugh, D., Haesler, E., & Bauer, M. (2019). Promoting mealtime function in people with dementia: A systematic review of studies undertaken in residential aged care. *International Journal of Nursing Studies, 96*, 99–118. https://doi.org/10.1016/j.ijnurstu.2019.04.005

Fischbach, F. T., Fischbach, M. A., & Stout, K. (2022). *Fischbach's a manual of laboratory and diagnostic tests* (11th ed.). Wolters Kluwer.

Gallotto, M., Rosa, C. M., Takvorian-Bené, M., McClelland, J., Tascione, C., Carey, A., & Raphael, B. P. (2019). Caregiver training for pediatric home parenteral nutrition. A 5-session discharge curriculum. *Journal of Infusion Nursing, 42*(3), 132–136. https://doi.org/10.1097/NAN.0000000000000320

Gorski, L. A., Hadaway, L., Hagle, M. E., Broadhurst, D., Clare, S., Kleidon, T., Meyer, B. M., Nickel, B., Rowley, S., Sharpe, E., & Alexander, M., & Infusion Nurses Society. (2021). Infusion therapy. Standards of practice. (8th ed.). *Journal of Infusion Nursing, 44*(Suppl 1), S1–S224. https://doi.org/10.1097/NAN.0000000000000396

Gramlich, L., Tandon, P., & Rahman, A. (2021, June 8). *Nutritional status in patients with sustained heavy alcohol use*. UpToDate. https://www.uptodate.com/contents/nutritional-status-in-patients-with-sustained-heavy-alcohol-use/print

Guenter, P., Worthington, P., Ayers, P., Boullata, J. I., Gura, K. M., Marshall, N., Holcombe, B., Richardson, D. S., & Parenteral Nutrition Safety Committee, American Society for Parenteral and Enteral Nutrition. (2018). Standardized competencies for parenteral nutrition administration: The ASPEN Model. *Nutrition in Clinical Practice, 33*(2), 295–304. https://doi.org/10.1002/ncp.10055

Guigoz, Y. (2006). The Mini Nutritional Assessment (MNA) review of the literature – What does it tell us? *The Journal of Nutrition Health and Aging, 10*(6), 466–485; discussion 485–487.

Guttendorf, J. (2021). Prone positioning in acute respiratory distress syndrome. *AHC Media Critical Care Alert, 28*(11), 1–6. www.reliasmedia.com/articles/147467-prone-positioning-in-acute-respiratory-distress-syndrome

Harbottle, L. (2019). The effect of nutrition on older people's mental health. *British Journal of Community Nursing, 24*(Sup7), S12–S16. https://doi.org/10.12968/bjcn.2019.24.Sup7.S12

Hartwell, J. L., Cotton, A., & Rozycki, G. (2018). Optimizing nutrition for the surgical patient: An evidenced based update to dispel five common myths in surgical nutrition care. *The American Surgeon, 84*(6), 831–835. https://doi.org/10.1177/000313481808400627

Hess, D. R., MacIntyre, N. R., Galvin, W. F., & Mishoe, S. C. (2021). *Respiratory care. Principles and practice* (4th ed.). Jones & Bartlett Learning.

Hinkle, J. L., Cheever, K. H. & Overbaugh, K. J. (2022). *Brunner & Suddarth's Textbook of medical-surgical nursing* (15th ed.). Wolters Kluwer.

Holdoway, A., & Anderson, L. (2019). What more can community nurses do to manage adult malnutrition. *British Journal of Community Nursing, 24*(Supp7), S6–S10. https://doi.org/10.12968/bjcn.2019.24.Sup7.S6

Holdoway, A., & Smith, A. (2020). Meeting nutritional need and managing patients with dysphagia. *Journal of Community Nursing, 34*(2), 52–59.

Holroyd, S. (2020). Frequency volume charts and fluid balance monitoring: Getting it right. *Journal of Community Nursing, 34*(1), 55–58.

Institute of Medicine. (2006). *Dietary reference intakes: The essential guide to nutrient requirements*. The National Academies Press.

Irving, S. Y., Guenter, P., & Mehta, N. M. (2019). Incorporating the latest pediatric nutrition support guidelines into clinical practice. *Nursing, 49*(2), 38–44. https://doi.org/10.1097/01.NURSE.0000552699.27631.88

Irving, S. Y., Rempel, G., Lyman, B., Sevilla, W. M. A., Northington, L., Guenter, P., & The American Society for Parenteral and Enteral Nutrition. (2018). Pediatric nasogastric tube placement and verification: Best practice recommendations from the NOVEL Project. *Nutrition in Clinical Practice, 33*(6), 921–927. https://doi.org/10.1002/ncp.10189

Jarvis, C., & Echkardt, A. (2020). *Physical examination & health assessment* (8th ed.). Elsevier.

Jennings Dunlap, J., & Patterson, S. (2019). Focus on clinical assessment. Assessing dysphagia. *Gastroenterology Nursing, 42*(3), 302–305. https://doi.org/10.1097/SGA.0000000000000472

Jensen, S. (2019). *Nursing health assessment. A best practice approach* (3rd ed.). Wolters Kluwer.

Johns Hopkins Medicine. (2021). *2021* https://www.hopkinsmedicine.org/health/conditions-and-diseases/metabolic-syndrome

Johnson, K. L., Speirs, L., Mitchell, A., Przybyl, H., Anderson, D., Manos, B., Schaenzer, A. T., & Winchester, K. (2018). Validation of a post-extubation dysphagia screening tool for patients after prolonged endotracheal intubation. *American Journal of Critical Care, 27*(2), 89–96. https://doi.org/10.4037/ajcc2018483

Jordan, E. A., & Moore, S. C. (2020). Enteral nutrition in critically ill adults: Literature review of protocols. *Nursing in Critical Care, 25*(1), 24–30. https://doi.org/10.1111/nicc.12475

Judd, M. (2020). Confirming nasogastric tube placement in adults. *Nursing, 50*(4), 43–46. https://doi.org/10.1097/01.NURSE.0000654032.78679.f1

Kaiser, M. J., Bauer, J. M., Ramsch, C., Uter, W., Guigoz, Y., Cederholm, T., Thomas, D. R., Anthony, P., Charlton, K. E., Maggio, M., Tsai, A. C., Grathwohl, D., Vellas, B., Sieber, C. C., & MNA-International Group. (2009). Validation of the Mini Nutritional Assessment short-form (MNA-SF): A practical tool for identification of nutritional status. *The Journal of Nutrition Health and Aging, 13*(9), 782–788. https://doi.org/10.1007/s12603-009-0214-7

KarabiyikOğurlu, Ö., TuralBüyük, E., & Yildizlar, O. (2020). The effect of warm compression applied before heel lance on pain level, comfort level and procedure time in healthy term newborns: A randomized clinical trial. *Journal of Midwifery & Reproductive Health, 8*(3), 1–8. DOI: 10.22038/jmrh.2020.41747.1475

Karch, A. M. (2020). *Focus on nursing pharmacology* (8th ed.). Wolters Kluwer.

Kim, H., Caulfield, L. E., Rebholz, C. M., Ramsing, R., & Nachman, K. E. (2020). Trends in types of protein in US adolescents and children: Results from the National Health and Nutrition Examination Survey 1999–2010. *PLoS One, 15*(3). e0230686. https://doi.org/10.1371/journal.pone.0230686

Kinikin, J., Phuillipp, R., & Altamirano, C. (2020). Using volume-based tube feeding to increase nutrient delivery in patients on a rehabilitation unit. *Rehabilitation Nursing, 45*(4), 186–194. https://doi.org/10.1097/rnj.0000000000000211

Kisting, M. A., Korcal, L., & Schutte, D. L. (2019). Lose the whoosh: An evidence-based project to improve NG tube placement verification in infants and children in the hospital setting. *Journal of Pediatric Nursing, 46*, 1–5. https://doi.org/10.1016/j.pedn.2019.01.011

Kovacevich, D. S., Corrigan, M., Ross, V. M., McKeever, L., Hall, A. M., & Braunschweig, C. (2019). American Society for Parenteral and Enteral Nutrition guidelines for the selection and care of central venous access devices for adult home parenteral nutrition administration. *Journal of Parenteral and Enteral Nutrition, 43*(1), 15–31. https://doi.org/10.1002/jpen.1455

Kyle, T., & Carman, S. (2021). *Essentials of pediatric nursing* (4th ed.). Wolters Kluwer.

Lin, T., Gifford, W., Lan, Y., Qin, X., Liu, X., Wang, J., Yang, B., You, T., & Chen, K. (2017). Diagnostic accuracy of ultrasonography for detecting nasogastric tube (NGT) placement in adults: A systematic review and meta analysis. *International Journal of Nursing Studies, 71*, 80–88. https://doi.org/10.1016/j.ijnurstu.2017.03.005

Liu, W., Williams, K., Batchelor-Murphy, M., Perkhounkova, Y., & Hein, M. (2019). Eating performance in relation to intake of solid and liquid food in nursing home residents with dementia: A secondary behavioral analysis of mealtime videos. *International Journal of Nursing Studies, 96*, 18–26. https://doi.org/10.1016/j.ijnurstu.2018.12.010

Lyman, B., Peyton, C., & Healey, F. (2018). Reducing nasogastric tube misplacement through evidence-based practice. *American Nurse, 13*(11), 6–11.

Lyman, B., Peyton, C., & Lane, B. (2018). Many hospitals still employ non-evidence based practices, including auscultation, creating a serious patient safety risk in nasogastric tube placement and verification. *Neonatology Today, 13*(7), 3–11.

Maastricht University Medical Center. (2020). *Body composition. Waist-hip ratio (WHR) and waist circumference.* https://nutritionalassessment.mumc.nl/en/waist-hip-ratio-whr-and-waist-circumference

Mak, M. Y., & Tam, G. (2020). Ultrasonography for nasogastric tube placement verification: An additional reference. *British Journal of Community Nursing, 25*(7), 328–334. https://doi.org/10.12968/bjcn.2020.25.7.328

Mayo Foundation for Medical Education and Research (MFMER, July 11). (2018). *Alcohol use disorder.* https://www.mayoclinic.org/diseases-conditions/alcohol-use-disorder/symptoms-causes/syc-20369243

Mayo Foundation for Medical Education and Research (MFMER). (2020a, February 13). *Trans fat is double trouble for your heart health.* https://www.mayoclinic.org/diseases-conditions/high-blood-cholesterol/in-depth/trans-fat/art-20046114

Mayo Foundation for Medical Education and Research (MFMER). (2020b, February 15). *Obesity. Symptoms & causes.* https://www.mayoclinic.org/diseases-conditions/obesity/symptoms-causes/syc-20375742

Mayo Foundation for Medical Education and Research (MFMER). (2020c, February 15). *Obesity. Diagnosis & treatment.* https://www.mayoclinic.org/diseases-conditions/obesity/symptoms-causes/syc-20375742

Mayo Foundation for Medical Education and Research (MFMER). (2020d, November 10). *Metabolism and weight loss: How you burn calories.* https://www.mayoclinic.org/healthy-lifestyle/weight-loss/in-depth/metabolism/art-20046508

McClave, S. A., DiBaise, J. K., Mullin, G. E., & Martindale, R. G. (2016). ACG clinical guideline: Nutrition therapy in the adult hospitalized patient. *The American Journal of Gastroenterology, 111*(3), 315–334; quiz 335. https://doi.org/10.1038/ajg.2016.28

McClave, S. A., Taylor, B. E., Martindale, R. G., Warren, M. M., Johnson, D. R., Braunschweig, C., McCarthy, M. S., Davanos, E., Rice, T. W., Cresci, G. A., Gervasio, J. M., Sacks, G. S., Roberts, P. R., Compher, C., Society of Critical Care Medicine., & American Society for Parenteral and Enteral Nutrition. (2016). Guidelines for the provision and assessment of nutrition support therapy in the adult critically ill patient: Society of Critical Care Medicine (SCCM) and American Society for Parenteral and Enteral Nutrition (A.S.P.E.N.). *Journal of Parenteral and Enteral Nutrition, 40*(2), 159–211. https://doi.org/10.1177/0148607115621863

MedlinePlus. U.S. National Library of Medicine. (2020, August 25). *Aging changes in body shape.* https://medlineplus.gov/ency/article/003998.htm

Mendes, A. (2018). Optimising nutritional intake in people with dementia on hospital wards. *British Journal of Nursing, 27*(20), 1206. https://doi.org/10.12968/bjon.2018.27.20.1206

Metheny, N. (n.d.). *Preventing aspiration in older adults with dysphagia.* Retrieved December 27, 2021, from https://hign.org/consultgeri/try-this-series/preventing-aspiration-older-adults-dysphagia

Metheny, N. A., Krieger, M. M., Healey, F., & Meert, K. L. (2019). A review of guidelines to distinguish between gastric and pulmonary placement of nasogastric tubes. *Heart & Lung, 48*(3), 226–235. https://doi.org/10.1016/j.hrtlng.2019.01.003

Minshall, S., & Pownall, S. (2019). Management of swallowing problems in community settings. *British Journal of Community Nursing, 24*(7), 323–327. https://doi.org/10.12968/bjcn.2019.24.7.323

Morata, L., Sole, M. L., Guido-Sanz, F., Ogilvie, C., & Rich, R. (2021). Manual vs automatic prone positioning and patient outcomes in acute respiratory distress syndrome. *American Journal of Critical Care, 30*(2), 104–112. https://doi.org/10.4037/ajcc2021674

Morris, H. (2018). Adapting mealtimes to residents with dysphagia. *Nursing and Residential Care, 20*(12), 610–614. https://doi.org/10.12968/nrec.2018.20.12.610

Morton, P.G., & Fontaine, D. K. (2018). *Critical care nursing. A holistic approach* (11th ed.). Wolters Kluwer.

Mueller, C., Compher, C., Druyan, M. E., & The American Society for Parenteral and Enteral Nutrition (A.S.P.E.N.) Board of Directors. (2011). A.S.P.E.N. clinical guidelines: Nutrition screening, assessment, and intervention in adults. *Journal of Parenteral and Enteral Nutrition, 35*(1), 16–24. https://doi.org/10.1177/0148607110389335

Murphy, C. V., Saliba, L., MacDermott, J., Soe, K., & Dungan, K. M. (2020). Individualizing glycemic control in the critically ill. *Critical Care Nursing Quarterly, 43*(1), 14–27. https://doi.org/10.1097/CNQ.0000000000000288

National Academies of Sciences, Engineering, and Medicine. (2019). *Consensus study report highlights. Dietary reference intakes for sodium and potassium.* https://www.nap.edu/resource/25353/030519DRISodiumPotassium.pdf

National Association of Pediatric Nurse Practitioners (NAPNAP) (2019). NAPNAP position statement on breastfeeding. *Journal of Pediatric Health Care, 33*(1), A11–A15. https://doi.org/10.1016/j.pedhc.2018.08.011

National Heart, Lung and Blood Institute (NHBLI). (n.d.a). *Overweight and obesity.* Retrieved December 27, 2021, from https://www.nhlbi.nih.gov/health-topics/overweight-and-obesity

National Heart, Lung, and Blood Institute (NHLBI). (n.d.b). *Aim for a health weight. Classification of overweight and obesity by BMI, waist circumference, and associated disease risks.* Retrieved December 27, 2021, from https://www.nhlbi.nih.gov/health/educational/lose_wt/BMI/bmi_dis.htm

National Heart, Lung, and Blood Institute (NHLBI). (n.d.c). *Aim for a health weight. Body mass index Table 1.* Retrieved December 27, 2021, from https://www.nhlbi.nih.gov/health/educational/lose_wt/BMI/bmi_tbl.htm

National Heart, Lung, and Blood Institute (NHLBI). (n.d.d). *Aim for a healthy weight. Assessing your weight and health risk.* Retrieved December 27, 2021, from https://www.nhlbi.nih.gov/health/educational/lose_wt/risk.htm

National Heart, Lung, and Blood Institute (NHLBI). (n.d.e). *Aim for a healthy weight. Calculate your body mass index.* Retrieved December 27, 2021, from https://www.nhlbi.nih.gov/health/educational/lose_wt/BMI/bmicalc.htm

National Institute of Diabetes and Digestive and Kidney Diseases (NIDDK). (n.d.). *Understanding adult overweight & obesity.* Retrieved December 27, 2021, from https://www.niddk.nih.gov/health-information/weight-management/adult-overweight-obesity

National Institute of Diabetes and Digestive and Kidney Diseases (NIDDK). (2017). *Overweight and obesity statistics.* https://www.niddk.nih.gov/health-information/health-statistics/overweight-obesity?dkrd=hispt0880#b

National Institutes of Health, Office of Dietary Supplements. (2020, September 3). *Health information. What you need to know. Dietary supplements.* https://ods.od.nih.gov/factsheets/WYNTK-Consumer/

Nazarko, L. (2018). Fit for life: Improving nutrition in care home residents. *Nursing and Residential Care, 20*(6), 250–255. https://doi.org/10.12968/nrec.2018.20.6.250

Nazarko, L. (2020). Dysphagia: A guide for nurses in general practice. *Practice Nursing, 31*(4), 162–168. https://doi.org/10.12968/pnur.2020.31.4.162

Norris, T. L. (2020). *Porth's essentials of pathophysiology* (5th ed.). Wolters Kluwer.

Oliveira, I. J., Mota, L. A. N., Freitas, S. V., & Ferreira, P. L. (2019). Dysphagia screening tools for acute stroke patients available for nurses: A systematic review. *Nursing Practice Today, 6*(3), 103–115.

Ozen, N., Blot, S., Ozen, V., Donmez, A. A., Gurun, P., Cinar, F. I., & Labeau, S. (2018). Gastric residual volume measurement in the intensive care unit: An international survey reporting nursing practice. *Nursing in Critical Care, 23*(5), 263–269. https://doi.org/10.1111/nicc.12378

Palese, A., Bressan, V., Kasa, T., Meri, M., Hayter, M., & Watson, R. (2018). Interventions maintaining eating independence in nursing home residents: A multicentre qualitative study. *BMC Geriatrics, 18*(1), 292. https://doi.org/10.1186/s12877-018-0985-y

Parker, L. A., Weaver, M., Murgas Torrazza, R. J., Shuster, J., LI, N., Krueger, C., & Neu, J. (2019). Effect of gastric residual evaluation on enteral intake in extremely preterm infants: A Randomized Clinical Trial. *JAMA Pediatrics, 173*(6), 534–543. https://doi.org/10.1001/jamapediatrics.2019.0800

Parker, L. A., Withers, J. H., & Talaga, E. (2018). Comparison of neonatal nursing practices for determining feeding tube insertion length and verifying gastric placement with current best evidence. *Advances in Neonatal Care, 18*(4), 307–317. https://doi.org/10.1097/ANC.0000000000000526

Pars, H., & Çavuşoğlu, H. (2019). A literature review of percutaneous endoscopic gastrostomy. Dealing with complications. *Gastroenterology Nursing, 42*(4), 351–359. https://doi.org/10.1097/SGA.0000000000000320

Physicians Committee for Responsible Medicine (PCRM). (n.d.). *PCRM's nutrition guide for clinicians. Nutritional requirements throughout the life cycle.* Retrieved April 30, 2022, https://nutritionguide.pcrm.org/nutritionguide/view/Nutrition_Guide_for_Clinicians/1342043/all/Nutritional_Requirements_throughout_the_Life_Cycle

Pironi, L., Boeykens, K., Bozzetti, F., Joly, F., Klek, S., Lal, S., Lichota, M., Mühlebach, S., Van Gossum, A., Wanten, G., Wheatley, C., & Bischoff, S. C. (2020). ESPEN guideline on home parenteral nutrition. *Clinical Nutrition, 39*(6), 1645–1666. https://doi.org/10.1016/j.clnu.2020.03.005

Powers, J. (2019). Securing orogastric and nasogastric tubes in intubated patients. *Critical Care Nurse, 39*(4), 61–63. https://doi.org/10.4037/ccn2019542

Powers, J. (2021). *Enteral feeding in the prone position.* American Association of Critical-Care Nurses. [Blog]. https://www.aacn.org/blog/enteral-feeding-in-the-prone-position

Rahimi, M., Farhadi, K., Ashtarian, H., & Changaei, F. (2015). Confirming nasogastric tube position: Methods and restrictions. A narrative review. *Journal of Nursing and Midwifery Sciences, 2*(1), 55–62.

Ratliff, A., Nishnick, A., DeChicco, R., & Lopez, R. (2018). Reducing blood glucose testing is safe in patients receiving parenteral nutrition. *Nutrition in Clinical Practice, 33*(6), 872–878. https://doi.org/10.1002/ncp.10020

Reber, E., Gomes, F., Vasiloglou, M. F., Schuetz, P., & Stanga, Z. (2019). Nutritional risk screening and assessment. *Journal of Clinical Medicine, 8*, 1065. https://doi.org/10.3390/jcm8071065

Roberts, S., Hopper, Z., Chaboyer, W., Gonzalez, R., Banks, M., Desbrow, B., & Marshall, A. P. (2020). Engaging hospitalised patients in their nutrition care using technology: Development of the NUTRI-TEC intervention. *BMC Health Services Research, 20*(1), 148. https://doi.org/10.1186/s12913-020-5017-x

Roveron, G., Antonini, M., Barbierato, M., Calandrino, V., Canese, G., Chiurazzi, L. F., Coniglio, G., Gentini, G., Marchetti, M., Minucci, A., Nembrini, L., Neri, V., Trovato, P., & Ferrara, F. (2018). Clinical practice guidelines for the nursing management of percutaneous endoscopic gastrostomy and jejunostomy (PEG/PEJ) in adult patients: An Executive Summary. *Journal of Wound Ostomy and Continence Nursing, 45*(4), 326–334. https://doi.org/10.1097/WON.0000000000000442

Rubenstein, L. Z., Harker, J. O., Salvà, A., Guigoz, Y., & Vellas, B. (2001). Screening for undernutrition in geriatric practice: Developing the short-form mini-nutritional assessment (MNA-SF). *Journals of Gerontology Series A Biological Sciences and Medical Sciences, 56*(6), M366–M372. https://doi.org/10.1093/gerona/56.6.m366

Rysavy, M. A., Watkins, P. L., Colaizy, T. T., & Das, A. (2020). Is routine evaluation of gastric residuals for premature infants safe or effective? *Journal of Perinatology, 40*(3), 540–543. https://doi.org/10.1038/s41372-019-0582-8

Savio, R. D., Parasuraman, R., Lovesly, D., Shankar, B., Ranganathan, L., Ramakrishnan, N., & Venkataraman, R. (2021). Feasibility, tolerance and effectiveness of enteral feeding in critically ill patients in prone position. *Journal of the Intensive Care Society, 22*(1), 41–46. https://doi.org/10.1177/1751143719900100

Schroeder, J., & Sitzer, V. (2019). Nursing care guidelines for reducing hospital-acquired nasogastric tube-related pressure injuries. *Critical Care Nurse, 39*(6), 54–63. https://doi.org/10.4037/ccn2019872

Seidelmann, S. B., Claggert, B., Cheng, S., Henglin, M., Shah, A., Steffen, L. M., Folsom, A. R., Rimm, E. B., Willett, W. C., & Solomon, S. D. (2018). Dietary carbohydrate intake and mortality: A prospective cohort study and meta-analysis. *The Lancet Public Health, 3*(9), E419–E428. http://dx.doi.org/10.1016/S2468-2667(18)30135-X

Semerdzhieva, E., & Reid, B. (2019). Getting the fundamentals right: Assisting patients with eating and drinking. *Nursing & Residential Care, 21*(10), 562–565. https://doi.org/10.12968/nrec.2019.21.10.562

Shellnutt, C. (2019). The evidence on feeding initiation after percutaneous endoscopic gastrostomy tube placement. *Gastroenterology Nursing, 42*(5), 420–427. https://doi.org/10.1097/SGA.0000000000000393

Siegmeister, D., Pilong, K., Boenisch, A., Brownmiller, E., Foran-Lee, L., Larsen, D. A., Stahre, P., Epstein, H. A. B., & Glasofer, A. (2021). Clinical case report: Prone positioning for non-intubated patients with COVID-19. *MEDSURG Nursing, 30*(3), 201–207, 160.

Silbert-Flagg, J., & Pillitteri, A. (2018). *Maternal and child health nursing* (8th ed.). Wolters Kluwer.

Singer, P., Blaser, A. R., Berger, M. M., Alhazzani, W., Calder, P. C., Casaer, M. P., Hiesmayr, M., Mayer, K., Montejo, J. C., Pichard, C., Preiser, J. C., van Zanten, A. R. H., Oczkowski, S., Szczeklik, W., & Bischoff, S. C. (2019). ESPEN guideline on clinical nutrition in the intensive care unit. *Clinical Nutrition, 38*(1), 48–79. https://doi.org/10.1016/j.clnu.2018.08.037

Stabler, S. N., Brooks, L., Gellatly, R., & Haljan, G. (2018). Implementation of a nasogastric tube securement device in a tertiary care intensive care unit. *The Canadian Journal of Critical Care Nursing, 29*(1), 14–16.

Steinberg, F. M., Batchelor-Murphy, M. K., & Young, H. M. (2019). Eating for healthy aging. *American Journal of Nursing, 119*(11), 43–51. https://doi.org/10.1097/01.NAJ.0000605360.22194.1f

Tappenden, K. A., Quatrara, B., Parkhurst, M. L., Malone, A. M., Fanjiang, G., & Ziegler, T. R. (2013). Critical role of nutrition in improving quality of care: An interdisciplinary call to action to address adult hospital malnutrition. *Journal of the Academy of Nutrition and Dietetics, 113*(9), 1219–1237. https://doi.org/10.1016/j.jand.2013.05.015

Taylor, S. J., Allan, K., Clemente, R., Marsh, A., & Toher, D. (2018). Feeding tube securement in critical illness: Implications for safety. *British Journal of Nursing, 27*(18), 1036–1041. https://doi.org/10.12968/bjon.2018.27.18.1036

Tinajero, M., Jarvis, S., Yu, J., Khan, T., Malik, V., Sievenpiper, J. L., & Hanley, A. (2021). Ethnic differences in the association between body mass index and Type 2 diabetes risk: A meta-analysis of prospective cohort studies. *Current Developments in Nutrition, 5*(Supp 2), 1253. https://doi.org/10.1093/cdn/nzab055_063

Touhy, T. A., & Jett, K. (2018). *Ebersol and Hess' gerontological nursing & healthy aging* (5th ed.). Elsevier.

Trinca, V., Morrison, J., Slaughter, S., & Keller, H. (2020). Making the Most of Mealtimes (M3): Effect of eating occasions and other covariates on energy and protein intake among Canadian older adult residents in long-term care. *Journal of Human Nutrition and Dietetics, 33*(1), 3–11. https://doi.org/10.1111/jhn.12686

Tsujimoto, H., Tsujimoto, Y., Nakata, Y., Akazawa, M., & Kataoka, Y. (2017). Ultrasonography for confirmation of gastric tube placement. *Cochrane Database of Systematic Reviews, 4*(4), CD012083. https://doi.org/10.1002/14651858.CD012083.pub2

Turner, A. D., Hamilton, S. M., Callif, C., Ariagno, K. A., Arena, A. E., Mehta, N. M., & Martinez, E. E. (2020). Bedside postpyloric tube placement and enteral nutrition delivery in the pediatric intensive care unit. *Nutrition in Clinical Practice, 35*(2), 299–305. https://doi.org/10.1002/ncp.10452

U. S. Department of Agriculture (USDA). (n.d.a). *Healthy eating.* Retrieved December 27, 2021, from https://www.nutrition.gov/topics/basic-nutrition/healthy-eating

U.S. Department of Agriculture (USDA). (n.d.b). *ChooseMyPlate.* Retrieved December 27, 2021, from https://www.choosemyplate.gov/

U.S. Department of Agriculture (USDA) and the National Agricultural Library (NAL). (n.d.a). *DRI calculator for healthcare professionals.* Retrieved December 27, 2021, from https://www.nal.usda.gov/fnic/dri-calculator/

U.S. Department of Agriculture (USDA) and the National Agricultural Library (NAL). (n.d.b). *Ethnic and cultural resources.* Retrieved December 27, 2021, from https://www.nal.usda.gov/fnic/ethnic-and-cultural-resources-0

U.S. Department of Health and Human Services (U.S. DHHS). (2019, April 12). *Safe minimum cooking temperatures charts.* https://www.foodsafety.gov/food-safety-charts/safe-minimum-cooking-temperature

U.S. Department of Health and Human Services (U.S. DHHS). (2020, May 19). *Keep food safe.* https://www.foodsafety.gov/keep-food-safe

U.S. Department of Health and Human Services (U.S. DHHS) and U.S. Department of Agriculture (USDA). (2020). *2020–2025 Dietary guidelines for Americans.* https://www.dietaryguidelines.gov/

U. S. Department of Health and Human Services. Office of Disease Prevention and Health Promotion. (n.d.). *Healthy people 2030. Social determinants of health.* Retrieved December 27, 2021, from https://health.gov/healthypeople/objectives-and-data/social-determinants-health

U.S. Food & Drug Administration (FDA). (2018, May 18). *Trans fat.* https://www.fda.gov/food/food-additives-petitions/trans-fat

U. S. Food and Drug Administration (FDA). (2019, April 4). *Blood glucose monitoring devices.* https://www.fda.gov/medical-devices/in-vitro-diagnostics/blood-glucose-monitoring-devices

U.S. Food and Drug Administration (FDA). (2020a, June 29). *The new nutrition facts label.* https://www.fda.gov/food/nutrition-education-resources-materials/new-nutrition-facts-label

U.S. Food and Drug Administration (FDA). (2020b, March 11). *How to understand and use the nutrition facts label.* https://www.fda.gov/food/new-nutrition-facts-label/how-understand-and-use-nutrition-facts-label

U.S. Food and Drug Administration (FDA). (2020c, March 11). *What's new with the nutrition facts label.* https://www.fda.gov/food/new-nutrition-facts-label/whats-new-nutrition-facts-label

Van Leeuwen, A.M., & Bladh, M.L. (2017). *Davis's comprehensive handbook of laboratory & diagnostic tests with nursing implications* (7th ed.). Philadelphia: F.A. Davis Company.

Vedder, T. G. (2021, January 14). *Heel sticks.* Medscape. https://emedicine.medscape.com/article/1413486-overviewn

Vellas, B., Villars, H., ABellan, G., Soto, M. E., Rolland, Y., Guigoz, Y., Morley, J. E., Chumlea, W., Salva, A., Rubenstein, L. Z., & Garry, P. (2006). Overview of the MNA—Its history and challenges. *The Journal of Nutrition, Health and Aging, 10*(6), 456–463; discussion 463-5.

Venus, K., Munshi, L., & Fralick, M. (2020). Prone positioning for patients with hypoxic respiratory failure related to COVID-19. *Canadian Medical Association Journal, 192*(47), E1532-E1537. https://doi.org/10.1503/cmaj.201201

VHA Center for Engineering & Occupational Safety and Health (CEOSH). (2016). *Safe patient handling and mobility guidebook.* http://www.tnpatientsafety.com/pubfiles/Initiatives/workplace-violence/sphm-pdf.pdf

Weber, J. R., & Kelley, J. H. (2018). *Health assessment in nursing* (6th ed.). Wolters Kluwer.

Williams, A. S. (n.d.). Monitoring your diabetes. American Federation for the Blind. https://www.afb.org/blindness-and-low-vision/eye-conditions/diabetes-and-vision-loss-guide-caring-yourself-when-you-2

Wilson, J., Tingle, A., Bak, A., Greene, C., Tsiami, A., & Loveday, H. (2020). Improving fluid consumption of older people in care homes: An exploration of the factors contributing to under-hydration. *Nursing and Residential Care, 22*(3), 139–146. https://doi.org/10.12968/nrec.2020.22.3.139

World Health Organization (WHO). (2020, April 1). *Obesity and overweight.* https://www.who.int/news-room/fact-sheets/detail/obesity-and-overweight

World Health Organization (WHO). (2020). *Nutrition.* https://www.who.int/health-topics/nutrition

38 Urinary Elimination

Elana Jaspers

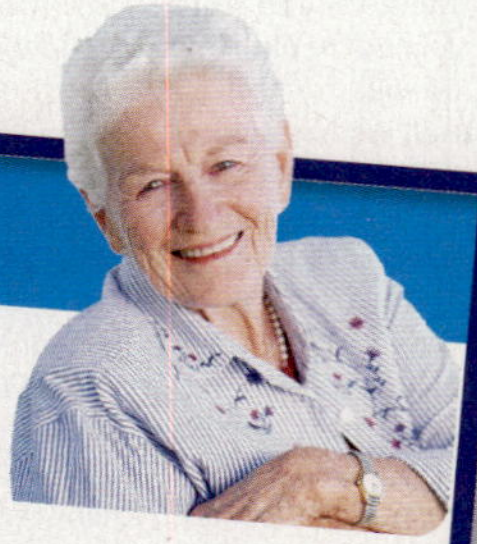

Elana Jaspers, age 83, is experiencing a decreased ability to perform activities of daily living (ADLs) related to arthritis. After being hospitalized for pneumonia, Mrs. Jaspers moved into an extended-care facility. A short time after arrival in their new home, Mrs. Jaspers began having difficulty with urinary incontinence.

Anna Galinski

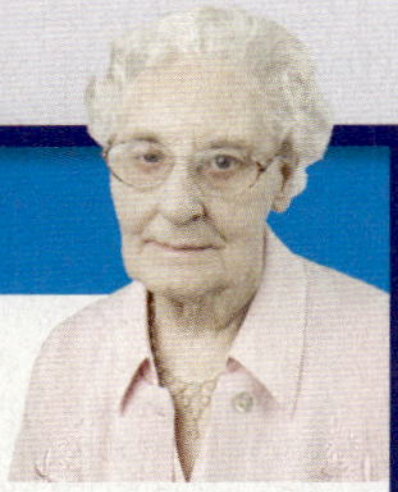

Anna Galinski, age 85, is frail and has numerous medical problems. She lives in a long-term care facility and, like many of the residents, was on a toileting regimen. Not long after a new charge nurse arrived, Anna, and the other residents who used to be on toileting regimens, had indwelling catheters inserted.

Midori Morita

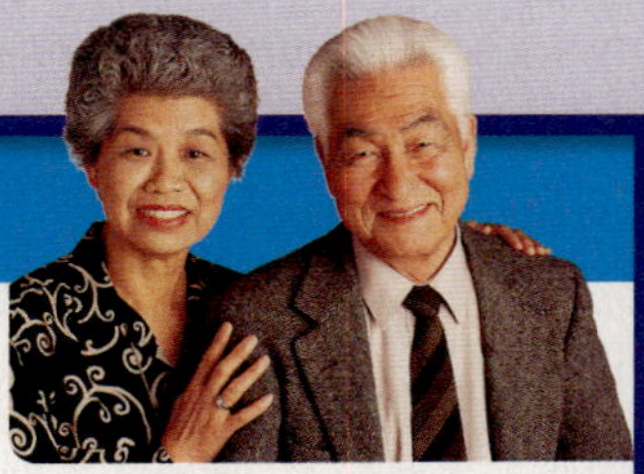

Midori Morita, age 69, is taking care of her 70-year-old husband at home. Mrs. Morita asks, "Should I talk with my husband's doctor about getting a urinary catheter? Ever since he came home from the hospital this last time, he seems unable to use the urinal. He dribbles urine constantly, and I can't keep up with the laundry. He had a catheter in the hospital."

Lippincott DocuCare Additional patient scenarios available in *Lippincott DocuCare.*

Learning Outcomes

After completing the chapter, you will be able to accomplish the following:

1. Describe the anatomy and physiology of the urinary system.
2. Identify variables that influence urination.
3. Assess urinary elimination, using appropriate interview questions and physical assessment skills.
4. Perform the following assessment techniques: measure urine output, collect urine specimens, determine the presence of select abnormal urine constituents, determine urine specific gravity, and assist with diagnostic tests and procedures.
5. Diagnose actual and potential health problems and needs related to urinary elimination that may be addressed through nursing intervention.
6. Demonstrate interventions promote normal urination; facilitate use of the toilet, bedpan, urinal, and commode; perform catheterizations; and assist with urinary diversions.
7. Describe nursing interventions that can be used to manage urinary incontinence effectively.
8. Describe nursing interventions that can prevent the development of urinary tract infections.
9. Plan, implement, and evaluate nursing care related to diagnoses/patient problems involving alterations in and related to nutrition.

Nursing Concepts

- Assessment
- Clinical decision making/clinical judgment
- Elimination
- Safety

Elimination from the urinary tract helps to rid the body of waste products and materials that exceed bodily needs. This chapter describes the anatomy and physiology of the urinary system and factors that affect **urination**, the process of emptying the bladder. A practical guide for assessing urinary elimination is included, along with detailed information on specific assessment measures, such as monitoring fluid intake, collecting urine specimens, testing urine, and assisting with other diagnostic procedures. Potential and actual health problems and needs related to urinary elimination are provided, and patient outcomes related to optimal urinary function are identified. This chapter presents nursing strategies to address these patient outcomes. The concluding care plan illustrates the use of specific nursing interventions to assist patients with urinary elimination problems and needs. Refer also to the accompanying Reflective Practice box (on page 1450).

ANATOMY AND PHYSIOLOGY

Kidneys and Ureters

The kidneys are located on either side of the vertebral column behind the peritoneum, in the upper abdominal cavity. One of the more significant functions of the kidneys is to help maintain the composition and volume of body fluids. About once every 30 minutes, the body's total blood volume passes through the kidneys for waste removal. The kidneys filter and excrete blood constituents that are not needed and retain those that are. Despite varying kinds and amounts of food and fluids ingested, body fluids remain relatively stable if the kidneys are functioning properly. **Urine**, the waste product excreted by the kidneys, contains organic, inorganic, and liquid wastes.

The nephron is the basic structural and functional unit of the kidneys. There are about 1 million nephrons in each kidney. Each nephron consists of a complicated system of arterioles, capillaries, and tubules. Nephrons remove the end products of metabolism, such as urea, creatinine, and uric acid from the blood plasma and form urine. The nephrons maintain and regulate fluid balance through the mechanisms of selective reabsorption and secretion of water, electrolytes, and other substances.

Once formed, urine from the nephrons empties into the pelvis of each kidney. From each kidney, urine is transported by rhythmic peristalsis through the ureters to the urinary bladder. The ureters enter the bladder obliquely. A fold of membrane in the bladder closes the entrance to the ureters so that urine is not forced up the ureters to the kidneys when pressure exists in the bladder. Figure 38-1 (on page 1451) shows the urinary systems for patients with male and female genitalia and the position of the kidneys and ureters in the abdomen.

Bladder

The urinary bladder is a smooth muscle sac that serves as a temporary reservoir for urine. It is composed of three layers of muscle tissue: the inner longitudinal layer, the middle circular layer, and the outer longitudinal layer. These three layers are called the detrusor muscle. At the base of the bladder, the middle circular layer of muscle tissue forms the internal, or involuntary, sphincter, which guards the opening between the urinary bladder and the urethra. The urethra conveys urine from the bladder to the exterior of the body.

The urinary bladder muscle is innervated by the autonomic nervous system. The sympathetic system carries inhibitory impulses to the bladder and motor impulses to the internal sphincter. These impulses cause the detrusor muscle to relax and the internal sphincter to constrict, retaining urine in the bladder. The parasympathetic system carries motor impulses to the bladder and inhibitory impulses to the internal sphincter. These impulses cause the detrusor muscle to contract and the sphincter to relax. The urinary bladder is shown in Figure 38-2 on page 1451.

QSEN Reflective Practice: Cultivating QSEN Competencies

CHALLENGE TO ETHICAL SKILLS

We had a strange experience during our rotation in a community long-term care facility. I was assigned to care for Anna Galinski, an 85-year-old frail adult with numerous medical problems. Like many of the residents, Mrs. Galinski was on a toileting regimen. Interventions to enhance resident safety and reduce health care–associated infections (HAIs) in long-term care facilities are an important focus and include reducing indwelling catheter use and catheter-associated urinary tract infection (CAUTI). In the middle of our 7-week experience, a new charge nurse started working on our unit. All of a sudden, Anna and the other residents who used to be on toileting regimens were given indwelling catheters. Knowing the greatly increased risk of infections with indwelling catheters, we suspected that the decision to rely on indwelling catheters was more a matter of convenience for the staff than what was in the best interests of the residents. How do you advocate for the patients and challenge the actions of a charge nurse?

Thinking Outside the Box: Possible Courses of Action

- Don't rock the boat! In 3 weeks, we'd be out of there. Keep our mouths shut and don't challenge authority.
- Ask for a meeting with the new charge nurse to explain our concerns, bringing our instructor for support. Be willing to go higher if the charge nurse cannot justify their decision and refuses to respond to our concerns.
- Work around the problem and try to get the residents' families to raise the issue.

Evaluating a Good Outcome: How Do I Define Success?

- Decisions are made about indwelling catheters that benefit and do not harm residents.
- I am faithful to my advocacy responsibilities within the current scope of my practice as a third-year student.
- I learn how to make the health care system work for patients/residents.
- I learn how to constructively challenge a health care provider or colleague.

Personal Learning: Here's to the Future!

This turned into a painful experience that made me realize just how difficult it can be to be an effective advocate for patients and residents. I am also newly aware of just how vulnerable long-term care facility residents are. A group of four students and myself asked to meet with the charge nurse. When we told them our concerns, they tried to justify their decision, but we still couldn't see any proof that the decision was made to benefit residents. Regrettably, they didn't respond to our concerns about infections at all. Because they were adamant about keeping the catheters, we told them that we would take the matter higher. Ultimately, we had to go all the way to the medical director, after thoroughly researching our concerns and getting lots of support for the argument we were making. In the process, the charge nurse made horrible accusations about us, threatening to ensure that students from our school would never work in the facility again. Eventually, all was well that ended well. The charge nurse was "relieved of their administrative responsibilities" and our good names were restored. However, the process that we went through was difficult.

QSEN SELF-REFLECTION ON QUALITY AND SAFETY COMPETENCIES DEVELOPING KNOWLEDGE, SKILLS, AND ATTITUDES FOR CONTINUOUS IMPROVEMENT

How do you think you would respond in a similar situation? Why? What does this tell you about yourself and about the adequacy of your skills for professional practice? Do you agree with the criteria that the nursing student used to evaluate a successful outcome? Are there any other criteria that would be appropriate to use? Did the nursing student meet the criteria? Why or why not? What *knowledge, skills,* and *attitudes* do you need to develop to continuously improve the quality and safety of care for patients like Anna Galinski?

Patient-Centered Care: What resources could you or the nurses use as a basis to provide compassionate and appropriate care based on respect for the patient's needs? How did the nursing student act as a patient advocate? Was the human dignity of the patient maintained?

Did the nursing students act appropriately? Legally? Ethically? Why or why not?

Teamwork and Collaboration/Quality Improvement: What communication skills do you need to improve to ensure that you function as a member of the patient-care team? What skills do you need to implement effective strategies for communicating and resolving conflict? What skills do you need to assert your own position/perspective in discussions about patient care? What other services or resources might be available to aid in this type of decision-making process?

Safety/Evidence-Based Practice: What skills do you need to improve to ensure that patients in your care receive the best nursing care possible? What evidence for practice provides guidance for decision making regarding care of this patient? What issues or factors might have played a role in the charge nurse's response? The students' responses? Do you think that the charge nurse would have responded differently if the students had included their instructor in the meeting?

Informatics: Can you identify the essential information that must be available in Mrs. Galinski's electronic health record to support safe patient care and coordination of care? Can you think of other ways to respond to or approach the situation?

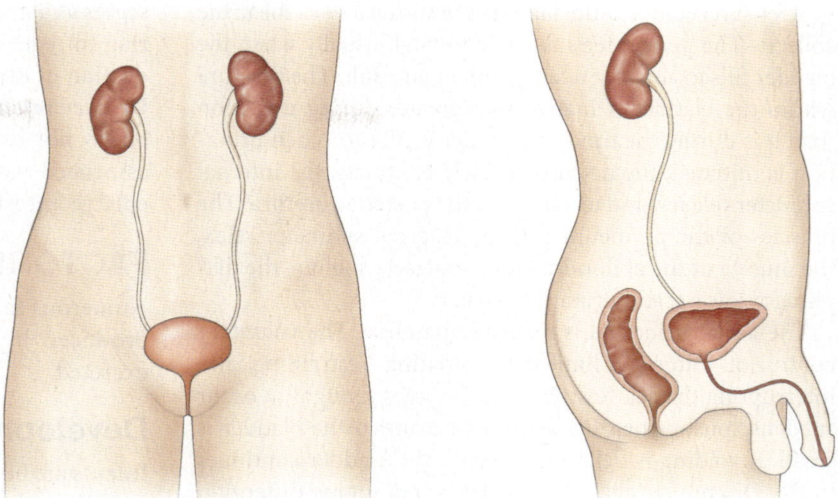

FIGURE 38-1. Frontal view of the female urinary tract **(left)** and lateral view of the male urinary tract **(right)**

The bladder normally contains urine under very little pressure. As the volume of urine increases, the pressure increases only slightly. The bladder wall is able to adapt to this pressure because of the muscle tissue in the bladder. This makes it possible for urine to continue to enter the bladder from the ureters against low pressure. When the pressure becomes sufficient to stimulate nerves in the bladder wall (stretch receptors), the person feels a desire to empty the bladder.

Urethra

The urethra's function is to transport urine from the bladder to the exterior of the body. The anatomy of the urethra differs in patients with male and female genitalia. The male urethra functions in the excretory system and the reproductive system. It is about 8 inches (20 cm) long and consists of three parts: the prostatic, the membranous, and the cavernous portions (Fig. 38-3). The external urethral sphincter consists of striated muscle and is located just beyond the prostatic portion of the urethra. The external sphincter is under voluntary control. The female urethra is about 1.6 inches (4 cm) long (Norris, 2020). The external, or voluntary, sphincter is located in the middle of the urethra (see Fig. 38-2). No portion of the female urethra is external to the body, as in the male.

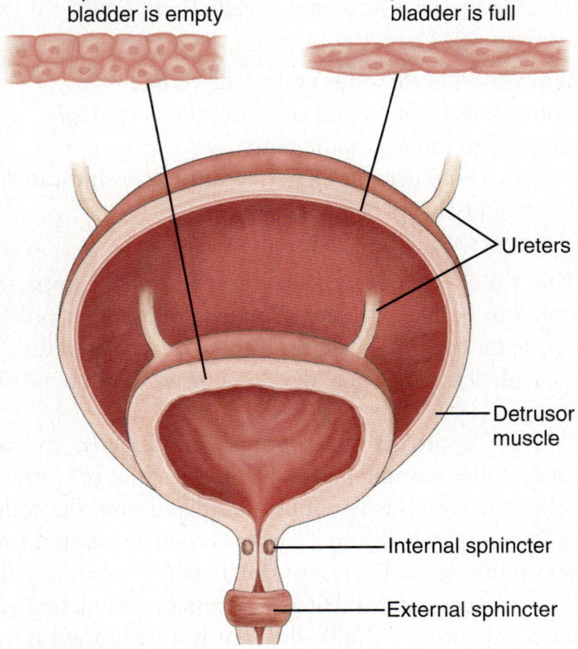

FIGURE 38-2. The urinary bladder.

Act of Urination

The process of emptying the bladder is known as urination, **micturition**, or **voiding** (void). The nerve centers for urination are situated in the brain and the spinal cord. Urinating, or voiding, is largely an involuntary reflex act, but its control can be learned. The voluntary control of urination develops as the higher nerve centers develop after infancy. Until that time, voiding is purely a reflex action. People whose bladders are no longer controlled by the brain because of injury or disease also void by reflex only. This is called **autonomic bladder**.

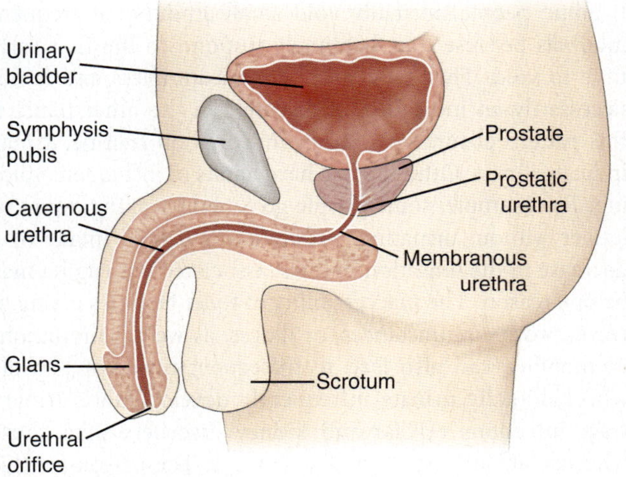

FIGURE 38-3. Parts of the male urethra.

Stretch receptors in the bladder are stimulated as the urine collects. The person feels a desire to void, usually when the bladder fills to about 150 to 250 mL in an adult. The pressure within the bladder is many times greater during urination than it is during the time the bladder is filling. When urination is initiated, the detrusor muscle contracts, the internal sphincter relaxes, and urine enters the posterior urethra. The muscles of the perineum and the external sphincter relax, the muscle of the abdominal wall contracts slightly, the diaphragm lowers, and urination occurs.

The act of urination is normally painless. The voluntary control of voiding is limited to initiating, restraining, and interrupting the act. Restraint of voiding is thought to occur subconsciously when the volume of urine in the bladder is small. If voiding is delayed, however, the bladder continues to fill. Discomfort may then be felt when undue distention occurs, and the urgency to void becomes paramount.

Sometimes, increased abdominal pressure—such as occurs during coughing and sneezing—forces an involuntary escape of urine. This is a particular problem for some people with female genitalia because the urethra is shorter. Any involuntary loss of urine that causes such a problem is referred to as **urinary incontinence**. Urinary incontinence is discussed in detail later in the chapter. Strong psychological factors, such as marked fear, may also result in involuntary urination. Alternatively, in certain conditions, it may be difficult for a person to relax the restraining muscles sufficiently to void, such as when a shy or embarrassed person needs to give a urine specimen.

Frequency of Urination

The frequency of urination depends on the amount of urine being produced. The more urine produced, the more often voiding is necessary. Except when fluid intake is very large, most healthy people do not void during normal sleeping hours. The first voided urine of the day is usually more concentrated than other urine excreted during the day. Because the first urine of the day is not fresh, but rather an accumulation of a number of hours of kidney output, this urine may or may not be used as a specimen for certain tests.

Some people normally void small amounts at frequent intervals because they habitually respond to the first early urge to void. This habit usually is meaningless and is not necessarily an indication of disease. On the other hand, if this pattern occurs as a change in urination routine, it may indicate illness. Other people have habits of infrequent voiding. For example, some people go 8 to 12 waking hours or longer without urinating. A habitual low fluid intake or a decrease in the sensation of thirst associated with aging may be one reason. The inaccessibility of toilet facilities owing to travel, work circumstances, or illness, as well as limitations in mobility, can also lead to infrequent urination. People who habitually urinate infrequently develop more urinary tract infections (UTIs) and kidney disorders than those who urinate at least every 3 to 4 hours. The reason for this is believed to be stagnation of urine in the bladder, which serves as a good medium for bacterial growth. Newly occurring infrequent voiding can also indicate a decreased production of urine caused by a kidney or circulatory disorder. **Urinary retention** occurs when urine is produced normally but is not excreted completely from the bladder. Factors associated with urinary retention include medications, an enlarged prostate, or vaginal prolapse.

FACTORS AFFECTING URINATION

Numerous factors affect the amount and quality of urine produced by the body and the manner in which it is excreted.

Developmental Considerations

Infants are born without voluntary control of urination and with little ability to concentrate urine. An infant's urine is usually very light in' color and without odor. At about age 6 weeks, the infant's nephrons are able to control reabsorption of fluids in the tubules and effectively concentrate urine. As a child grows, the bladder gradually enlarges, with an increase in capacity. Most children develop urinary control between ages 2 and 5 years. Daytime control precedes nighttime control, and girls generally develop control earlier than boys. Older children and adults control urination voluntarily. They seldom wake to void at night because their kidneys are able to concentrate urine and produce less urine at night as a result of decreased renal blood flow.

Toilet Training

Voluntary control of the urethral sphincters occurs between ages 18 and 24 months. However, many other factors are required to achieve conscious control of bladder function. Toilet training usually begins at about age 2 to 3 years.

Assessment of a child's readiness for toilet training includes (American Academy of Pediatrics [AAP], n.d.; Kyle & Carman, 2021):

- Ability to indicate wants and needs verbally
- Motor skills to sit on and rise from the potty chair
- Showing an interest in the potty
- Ability to hold urine for a period of time (as indicated by diapers not always being wet)
- Willingness to follow instructions

The child's desire to gain control is also important. Wanting to be like a parent or older sibling often provides adequate motivation. Lifelong attitudes toward urination, the body, and cleanliness may develop during the time of toilet training.

Cultures approach toilet training differently. In some cultures, toilet training begins before the child is 1 year old; in other cultures, it may not be considered until the child is near 5 years old. It is important to recognize cultural influences on this parenting responsibility while promoting flexibility. Reassure parents that any regression of toileting skills that occurs during a child's illness or hospitalization is to be expected and is usually short-lived.

Occasional daytime incontinence of urine in a child is usually not a cause for concern. Continued incontinence of urine past the age of toilet training is termed **enuresis**. Nocturnal enuresis (nighttime bedwetting) usually subsides by age 6 years (Kyle & Carman, 2021).

Effects of Aging

Physiologic changes that accompany normal aging may affect urination in older adults. These changes include the following:

- The diminished ability of the kidneys to concentrate urine may result in **nocturia** (the need to wake up at night in order to urinate [Weiss, 2020]).
- Decreased bladder muscle tone may reduce the capacity of the bladder to hold urine, resulting in increased frequency of urination.
- Decreased bladder contractility may lead to urine retention and stasis, which increases the likelihood of UTI.
- Neuromuscular problems, degenerative joint problems, alterations in thought processes, and weakness may interfere with voluntary control and the ability to reach a toilet in time.

Medications prescribed for other health problems in the older adult may interfere with bladder function. For example, diuretics cause increased urine production, resulting in the need for increased urination and possibly **urge incontinence** (the involuntary loss of urine that occurs soon after feeling an urgent need to void). Sedatives and tranquilizers may diminish awareness of the need to void.

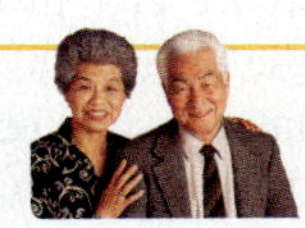

Consider ***Midori Morita's*** 70-year-old husband who has been experiencing urinary problems since their last hospitalization. The nurse would need to keep in mind age-related changes during assessment of Mr. Morita in order to determine if they are experiencing urinary problems related to these changes or if they are due to another cause.

Food and Fluid Intake

When the body is functioning well, the kidneys help the body maintain a careful balance of fluid intake and output, which should be about equal. When the body is dehydrated, the kidneys reabsorb fluid. The urine produced is more concentrated and is decreased in amount. Conversely, with fluid overload, the kidneys excrete a large quantity of dilute urine.

Alcohol produces a diuretic effect by inhibiting the release of antidiuretic hormone, increasing urine production. Foods high in water may increase urine production. Foods and beverages with high sodium content cause sodium and water reabsorption and retention, thereby decreasing urine formation. Certain foods may affect the odor of the urine (asparagus, onions) or its color (beets).

Psychological Variables

Many individual, family, and sociocultural variables influence a person's usual voiding habits. For some people, voiding is a personal and private act—something one does not talk about. Needing assistance with a bedpan or urinal may provoke great embarrassment and anxiety, especially when the bedpan is offered by a nurse of the opposite sex assigned at birth. For others, voiding is a natural act that does not cause embarrassment; these people readily excuse themselves to void whenever the urge presents.

Some people who experience stress void smaller amounts of urine at more frequent intervals. Stress can also interfere with the ability to relax the perineal muscles and the external urethral sphincter. When this happens, the person may feel an urge to void, but emptying the bladder completely becomes difficult or impossible.

Activity and Muscle Tone

Among the many benefits of regular exercise are increased metabolism and optimal urine production and elimination. During prolonged periods of immobility, decreased bladder and sphincter tone can result in poor urinary control and urinary stasis. People with indwelling urinary catheters lose bladder tone because the bladder muscle is not being stretched by the bladder filling with urine. Other causes of decreased muscle tone include childbearing, muscle atrophy due to decreased estrogen levels as seen with menopause, and damage to muscles from trauma.

Pathologic Conditions

Certain renal or urologic problems can affect both the quantity and the quality of urine produced. Diseases associated with renal problems include congenital urinary tract abnormalities, polycystic kidney disease, **urinary tract infection (UTI)**, urinary calculi (kidney stones), hypertension, diabetes, gout, and certain connective tissue disorders. Renal failure is a condition in which the kidneys fail to remove metabolic end products from the blood and are unable to regulate fluid, electrolyte, and pH balance. Acute kidney injury (AKI) is a sudden decline in kidney function (over hours or within a day [Norris, 2020]), and may be caused by conditions such as severe dehydration, anaphylactic shock, sepsis, and ureteral obstruction. AKI is potentially reversible if recognized early, the precipitating factors can be corrected or removed, and it is treated appropriately before permanent kidney damage has occurred (Norris, 2020). Chronic kidney disease (CKD) is the slow loss of kidney function over months or years as a result of irreparable damage to the kidneys. CKD is caused by conditions such as diabetes, hypertension, and glomerulonephritis. Progression of CKD will eventually lead to the final stage of CKD, known as kidney (renal) failure or end-stage renal disease (ESRD). In kidney failure, kidney function drops below 15%, and the kidneys are unable to adequately excrete metabolic waste and regulate fluid and electrolyte balance (NIDDK, 2018a).

Diseases that reduce physical activity or lead to generalized weakness, such as arthritis, Parkinson's disease, and degenerative joint disease, may interfere with toileting. Cognitive deficits and certain psychiatric problems can interfere with a person's ability or desire to control urination voluntarily. Fever and diaphoresis (profuse perspiration) result in body fluid conservation by the kidneys, in which urine production is decreased, and the urine is highly concentrated. Other pathologic conditions, such as heart failure, may lead to fluid retention and decreased urine output. High blood glucose levels, such as with diabetes, may lead to an increase in urine output secondary to an osmotic diuretic effect.

Medications

Medications have numerous effects on urine production and elimination. Of gravest concern are the many prescription and nonprescription drugs known to be **nephrotoxic** (capable of causing kidney damage). Abuse of analgesics, such as aspirin or ibuprofen, can cause nephrotoxicity. Some antibiotics, such as gentamicin, can be nephrotoxic as well.

Diuretics, which commonly are used in the treatment of hypertension and other disorders, prevent the reabsorption of water and certain electrolytes in the tubules. Depending on the dose of the drug, diuretics cause moderate to severe increases in production and excretion of dilute urine. Cholinergic medications stimulate contraction of the detrusor muscle and produce urination. Some analgesics and tranquilizers suppress the central nervous system, interfering with urination by diminishing the effectiveness of the neural reflex.

Certain drugs cause urine to change color, including the following:

- Anticoagulants may cause **hematuria** (blood in the urine), leading to a pink or red color.
- Diuretics can lighten the color of urine to pale yellow.
- Phenazopyridine, a urinary tract analgesic, can cause orange or orange-red urine.
- The antidepressant amitriptyline or B-complex vitamins can turn urine green or blue-green.
- Levodopa (L-dopa), an antiparkinson drug, and injectable iron compounds can lead to brown or black urine.

NURSING PROCESS FOR URINARY ELIMINATION

Assessing

A comprehensive nursing assessment of the functioning of a patient's urinary system includes the following:

- Collection of data about the patient's voiding patterns, habits, and difficulties and a history of current or past urinary problems
- Assessment of the bladder, if indicated, and urethral meatus; assessment of skin integrity and hydration; and examination of the urine
- Correlation of these findings with the results of diagnostic tests and procedures for examining the urine and the urinary tract

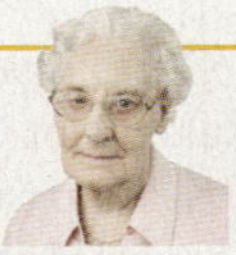

Recall ***Anna Galinski***, the 85-year-old frail individual living in a long-term care facility. Initially, Ms. Galinski was placed on a toileting regimen, but now they and other patients on the unit have indwelling catheters. In determining how to respond to the situation, it would be helpful for the nurse to perform a comprehensive assessment of the patient. Doing so would provide information to substantiate whether or not catheter insertion was indicated or still appropriate.

Nursing History

A nursing history should include questions for the patient (or caregiver) about usual voiding habits and any current or past voiding difficulties. Box 38-1 lists some additional terms that can be used to describe several urinary problems. When interacting with patients, use terminology that the patient and/or the caregiver understands. The accompanying Focused Assessment Guide 38-1 lists elements of a urinary elimination history that should be incorporated into the initial nursing assessment.

When caring for infants, assess the number of wet diapers per day that the infant produces. Newborns should have six to eight wet diapers per day (Kyle & Carman, 2021). With young children, assess whether the child has achieved bladder control during both day and nighttime. Be sure to indicate on the nursing history and care plan the words that the child uses to indicate the need to void.

Decreased bladder tone may be a problem for older adults. Explore any problems, how the person normally handles these problems, and your judgment of the adequacy of the solution while obtaining the nursing history.

Patients with urinary diversions may have established individualized personal care routines. A **urinary diversion** involves the surgical creation of an alternate route for excretion of urine and is discussed later in the chapter. Assess the procedures and equipment used by patients to make sure they follow accepted guidelines and do not predispose themselves to infection or other risk. Record in both the history and the

Box 38-1 Additional Terms Used to Describe Urinary Problems

Anuria: 24-hour urine output is less than 50 mL
Dysuria: Painful or difficult urination
Frequency: Increased incidence of voiding
Glycosuria: Presence of glucose in the urine
Nocturia: Awakening at night to urinate
Oliguria: 24-hour urine output is less than 400 mL
Polyuria: Excessive output of urine (diuresis)
Proteinuria: Protein in the urine
Pyuria: Pus in the urine
Urgency: Strong desire to void
Urinary incontinence: Involuntary loss of urine

Focused Assessment Guide 38-1

URINARY ELIMINATION

Factors to Assess	Questions and Approaches
Usual patterns of urinary elimination	How often do you urinate (pass your water) during the day? Do you awaken at night to empty your bladder? How would you describe your urine?
Recent changes in urinary elimination	Have you noticed any changes in your usual urinary patterns (frequency, amount, force of stream, difficulty, comfort)? Do you ever leak urine (e.g., on your way to the bathroom or when you sneeze or cough)? Do you ever notice that your undergarments are wet or damp?
Aids to elimination	Is there anything you do that helps you to urinate?
Present or past occurrence of voiding difficulties (nature of problem, onset, frequency, causes, severity, symptoms, intervention attempted, results)	Tell me about any problems you are having now when you urinate (urgency, pain or burning, difficulty starting or stopping stream, dribbling, incontinence). If there is a problem, describe what you feel like before you urinate and while you are urinating. Have you had any urinary problems in the past (any history of urinary tract infections, kidney or bladder disease or problems)? Do you use any type of absorbent pad or product to protect your clothes?
Presence of urinary diversion (normal routine, history of problems)	Tell me about your usual routine with your ileal conduit.

care plan any special routine, equipment, or supplies the patient uses for urinary elimination.

When a patient (or caregiver) reports a problem with voiding, explore its duration, severity, and precipitating factors. Also, note the patient's perception of the problem and the adequacy of the patient's self-care behaviors.

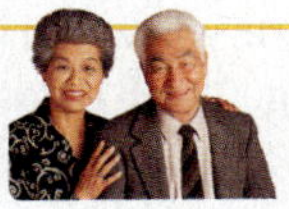

Remember **Midori Morita**, the wife of the 70-year-old individual experiencing problems with "dribbling." The nurse would need to question Mr. and Mrs. Morita about the problem, obtaining specific information such as when it started, how often it occurs, how much the patient is voiding, events of the previous hospitalization, and any factors associated with it such as use of medications, increased fluid intake, or changes in mobility.

Physical Assessment

The physical assessment of urinary functioning includes an examination of the urinary bladder, if indicated, urethral meatus, skin, and urine. The kidneys are normally well protected by considerable fat and connective tissue, making palpation difficult. Palpation of the kidneys is usually performed as part of a more detailed assessment. This technique requires deep palpation and is generally assessed by advanced health care professionals, such as an advanced practice nurse or health care provider.

BLADDER

Assessment of the bladder may be indicated when patients experience difficulty voiding or other alterations in elimination. The bladder is normally positioned below the symphysis pubis and cannot be palpated or percussed when empty. When the bladder is distended, it rises above the symphysis pubis and may reach to just below the umbilicus (Fig. 38-4). Before palpating the bladder, always inquire as to when the patient last voided. Observe the lower abdominal

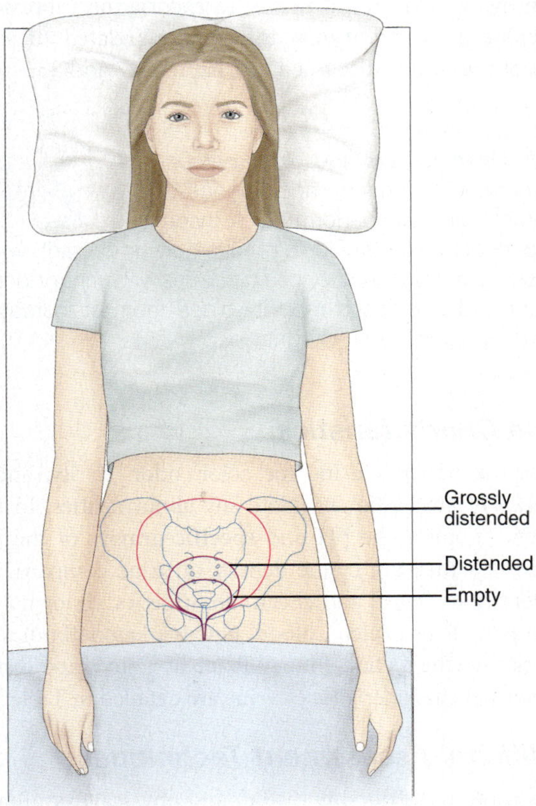

FIGURE 38-4. Position of bladder when empty and distended.

wall, noting any swelling, and palpate this area for tenderness. If distended, note the height of the edge of the bladder above the symphysis pubis.

A bedside scanner is another commonly used method to assess the fullness of the bladder. These portable bladder ultrasound devices create an image of the patient's bladder and calculate urine volume present in the bladder. This method is noninvasive and painless. A bladder scan can be performed at the bedside, poses little risk for infection, and is a safer alternative to catheterization to determine bladder urine volume (Widdall, 2015). Results are most accurate when the patient is in the supine position during the scanning. Skill 38-1 outlines the procedure for assessing bladder volume using an ultrasound bladder scanner.

URETHRAL ORIFICE

Inspect the urethral orifice for any signs of inflammation, discharge, or foul odor. In patients with female genitalia, the urethral meatus is a slit-like opening below the clitoris and above the vaginal orifice. Place patients with female genitalia in the dorsal recumbent position with the inner labia retracted for good visualization of the meatus. In patients with male genitalia, the meatus is at the tip of the penis. If the patient with male genitalia is uncircumcised, retract the foreskin to visualize the meatus.

SKIN INTEGRITY AND HYDRATION

Because problems with urinary functioning may result in disturbances in hydration and excretion of body wastes, assess the skin carefully for color, texture, and turgor. Assess the integrity of the skin in the perineal area. Problems with incontinence may result in severe excoriation (abrasion of the epidermis). Additional information related to assessment of the skin is discussed in Chapters 27 and 33.

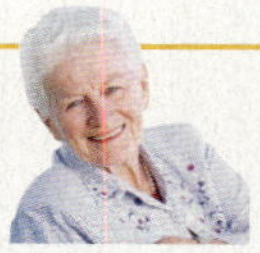

Recall **Elana Jaspers**, the older person who is experiencing urinary incontinence and a decreased ability to perform ADLs. Inspecting the perineal area would be extremely important when assessing Mrs. Jaspers, whose problems with urinary incontinence and decreased mobility place them at increased risk for changes in skin integrity.

Urine Characteristics

Assess the patient's urine for color, odor, clarity, and the presence of any sediment. Note any abnormalities. In select patients, monitor the pH and **specific gravity** of the urine (which is a measure of the density of urine compared with the density of water) and check the urine for abnormal constituents such as protein, blood, glucose, ketone bodies, and bacteria (see the section entitled Point-of-Care Urine Testing). The normal characteristics of urine are detailed in Table 38-1.

Additional Assessment Techniques

In addition to the nursing history and physical examination, the nurse gathers data about urinary elimination through the following assessment measures: measuring urine output, collecting urine specimens, performing point-of-care urine testing, and assisting with diagnostic procedures. These are discussed in the following sections.

MEASURING URINE OUTPUT

Measuring the patient's fluid intake and output is an important nursing responsibility. Accuracy of the total fluid intake and output from all sources aids in identifying potential alterations in fluid balance and is essential for planning the patient's nursing care, as well as medical care. The measurement of fluid intake and output is described further in Chapter 41. Gloves are required when handling urine to prevent exposure to pathogenic microorganisms or blood that may be present in the urine. Goggles also are worn whenever there is a concern of urine splashing. The measurement of fluid intake and output may be delegated to assistive personnel. However, the nurse is responsible for ensuring that staff members understand the required procedures, and the nurse must validate the accuracy of the measurements.

Measuring Urine Output in Patients Who Are Continent

Patients who have self-control over urination are **continent** of urine. Several devices used to collect or measure urine are shown in Figures 38-5A, B. The procedure for measuring the urine output of a patient who is continent is outlined in Box 38-2. To ensure that all voided urine is measured, be sure to tell patients when their urine output is to be measured and recorded. A specimen hat is a valuable device that can be placed under the toilet seat to collect and measure voided urine for patients who use the bathroom (see Fig. 38-5B). Patients who are willing and able can be taught to measure and record their own output. The procedure for measuring the urine output of a patient who is continent is outlined in Box 38-2 on page 1458.

Measuring Urine Output in Patients Who Are Incontinent

Urinary incontinence is the involuntary or uncontrolled loss of urine from the bladder. Patients who experience involuntary or uncontrolled loss of urine are **incontinent**. It is difficult to accurately measure urinary output for incontinent patients. Note the number of times the patient is incontinent and any notable urine characteristics, such as color and odor. Additional nursing interventions are required to collect urine for measurement. Use of scheduled toileting (assisting the patient to the toilet to attempt to void on a regular basis, such as every 2 hours) can assist in obtaining urine for measurement and for required laboratory specimens and in preventing incontinence. External collecting devices are useful in managing urinary incontinence and provide a mechanism to measure urinary output (Vasavada et al., 2019a). An innovative alternative technique has been suggested in the evidence for practice. Measurement of urinary output via weighing of absorbent pads has been used successfully to monitor

Table 38-1 Characteristics of Urine

CHARACTERISTIC	NORMAL FINDINGS	SPECIAL CONSIDERATIONS
Color	A freshly voided specimen is pale yellow, straw-colored, or amber, depending on its concentration.	Urine is darker than normal when it is concentrated. Urine is lighter than normal when it is diluted. Certain drugs, such as cascara, L-dopa, and sulfonamides, alter the color of urine. Some foods can alter the color; for example, beets can cause urine to appear red.
Odor	Normal urine smell is aromatic. As urine stands, it often develops an ammonia odor because of bacterial action.	Some foods cause urine to have a characteristic odor; for example, asparagus causes urine to have a strong, musty odor. Urine high in glucose content has a sweet odor. Urine that is heavily infected has a fetid odor.
Turbidity	Fresh urine should be clear or translucent; as urine stands and cools, it becomes cloudy.	Cloudiness observed in freshly voided urine is abnormal and may be due to the presence of red blood cells, white blood cells, bacteria, vaginal discharge, sperm, or prostatic fluid.
pH	The normal pH is 5–6, with a range of 4.5–8. Urine becomes alkaline on standing when carbon dioxide diffuses into the air. Urine alkalinity or acidity may be promoted through diet to inhibit bacterial growth or urinary stone development or to facilitate the therapeutic activity of certain medications.	A high-protein diet causes urine to become excessively acidic. Certain foods tend to produce alkaline urine, such as citrus fruits, dairy products, and vegetables, especially legumes. Certain foods such as meats tend to produce acidic urine. Certain drugs influence the acidity or alkalinity of urine; for example, ammonium chloride produces acidic urine, and potassium citrate and sodium bicarbonate produce alkaline urine.
Specific gravity	This is a measure of the density of the chemicals and particles in the urine and is a measure of the ability of the kidneys to concentrate urine. The normal range is 1.015–1.025.	Concentrated urine will have a higher-than-normal specific gravity; diluted urine will have a lower-than-normal specific gravity. In the absence of kidney disease, a high specific gravity usually indicates dehydration, and a low specific gravity indicates overhydration.
Constituents	*Organic* constituents of urine include urea, uric acid, creatinine, hippuric acid, indican, urene pigments, and undetermined nitrogen. *Inorganic* constituents are ammonia, sodium, chloride, traces of iron, phosphorus, sulfur, potassium, and calcium.	*Abnormal constituents* of urine include blood, pus, albumin, glucose, ketone bodies, casts, gross bacteria, and bile.

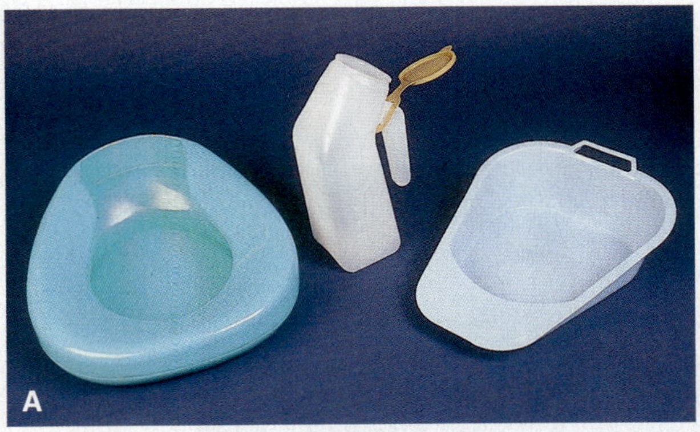

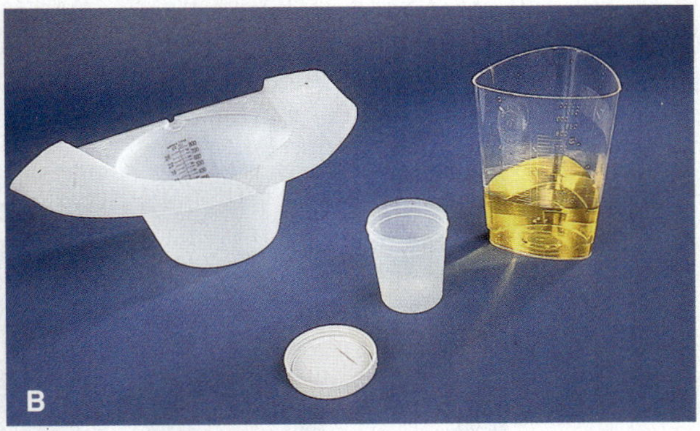

FIGURE 38-5. Devices for collecting and measuring urine. **A.** (**left** to **right**) Bedpan, urinal, and fracture pan. **B.** (**left** to **right**) Specimen hat: container that is placed anteriorly on the toilet, underneath the seat to collect urine; specimen cup: container that holds urine; calibrated measuring device: container to accurately measure urine output.

Box 38-2 Measuring Urine Output in Continent Patients

1. Ask the patient to void into a bedpan, urinal, or specimen hat (container), either in bed or in the bathroom. Urinary devices used to collect or measure urine are shown in Figure 38-5.
2. Put on gloves. Pour the urine from the collection device into the appropriate measuring device provided by the facility (examples are provided in Figure 38-5B). The devices are calibrated in milliliters. Collection devices may be calibrated for measurement, eliminating the need for an additional measuring device.
3. Place the calibrated container on a flat surface, such as a shelf, for an accurate reading. Reading at eye level, note the amount of urine voided and record it in the patient's electronic record. Record the total amount voided during each shift. The total for the 24-hour period is usually calculated by the electronic documentation software.
4. Discard the urine in the toilet unless a specimen is required. If a specimen is required, pour the urine into an appropriate specimen container.

Box 38-3 Measuring Urine Output in Patients With an Indwelling Urinary Catheter

1. Put on gloves.
2. Place a calibrated measuring device (Fig. 38-5) beneath the urine collection bag (Fig. 38-6). To prevent the spread of infection, patients should have their own calibrated measuring device.
3. Place the drainage spout from the collection bag above, but not touching, the calibrated measuring device, and open the clamp.
4. Allow the urine to flow from the collection bag into the measuring device.
5. Reclamp the drainage tube, wipe the spout of the tube with an alcohol pad, and replace the tube into the slot on the drainage bag. Proceed with measurement of urine as described earlier.

urinary output in patients who are incontinent, as well as to reduce use of indwelling urinary catheters (Beuscher, 2014). This initiative is similar to the commonly used practice of weighing diapers to obtain accurate urinary output in nontoilet-trained pediatric settings. The dry pad weight is subtracted from the wet pad weight. The resulting difference in gram weight is then converted to milliliters (1 g = 1 mL) (Beuscher, 2014).

Urinary incontinence and associated nursing care interventions are discussed in more detail later in the chapter.

Measuring Urine Output in Patients With an Indwelling Catheter

Indwelling urethral catheters are connected to a drainage and collection system (see Fig. 38-6), and the urine collected in the drainage bag is measured to calculate urine output. The procedure for measuring the urine output of a patient with an indwelling catheter is outlined in Box 38-3. Catheterized patients who are acutely ill may require hourly or even more frequent measurements of urine. This is facilitated by using a special collection bag that has a built-in calibrated measuring chamber called a urimeter (see Fig. 38-6A). After assessing and recording the amount of urine produced hourly, tilt the measuring chamber on the urimeter so that this urine flows into the general collection bag. This empties the measuring chamber, making it ready to collect the next hour's urine.

COLLECTING URINE SPECIMENS

Various techniques are used for collecting urine specimens. The nurse needs to understand the rationale for the specific test ordered, as well as the correct collection procedure associated with the required test in order to ensure obtaining the appropriate urine sample.

Routine Urinalysis

A sterile urine specimen is not required for a routine urinalysis. Collect urine by having the patient void into a clean bedpan, urinal, or receptacle (e.g., a specimen hat in the toilet bowl). Take care to avoid contamination with feces. If a patient with female genitalia is menstruating when a urine sample is obtained, note this on the laboratory slip because red blood cells may appear in the urine. When patients are voiding into a bedpan or collection device on the toilet, instruct them not to place toilet tissue

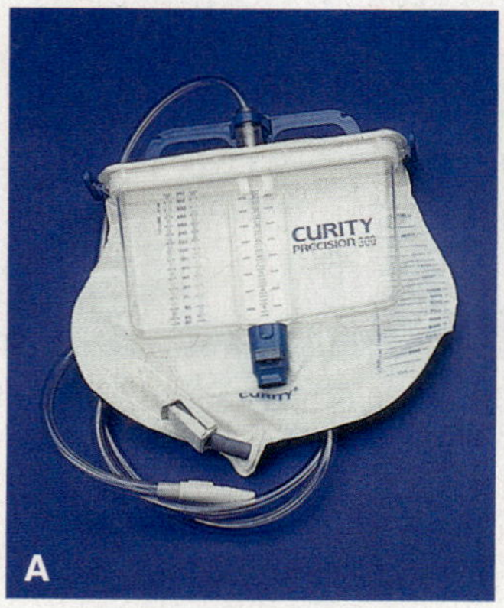

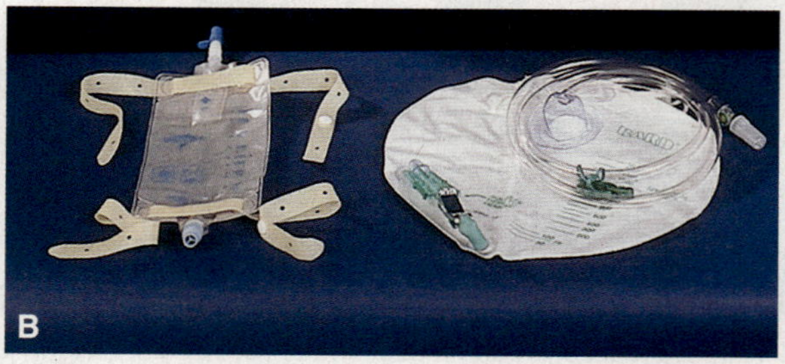

FIGURE 38-6. Urine collection bags. **A.** Large urine collection bag with urimeter. **B.** Small (leg bag) and large urine collection bags.

Guidelines for Nursing Care 38-1

OBTAINING A CLEAN-CATCH OR MIDSTREAM URINE SPECIMEN

Patients With Female Genitalia

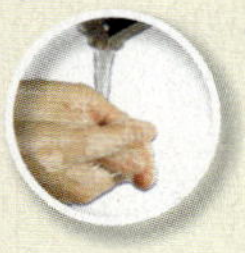

- Perform hand hygiene and put on PPE, if indicated.

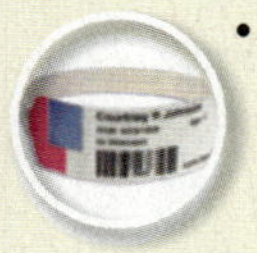

- Identify the patient.
- Explain to the patient what you are going to do and why.
- Put on unsterile gloves.
- Separate the labia. Clean the area at the meatus with soap and water, or according to policy.
- Have the patient void about 30 mL into the toilet or bedpan and discard this urine.
- Position the sterile specimen container near, but not touching, the meatus, and collect at least 3 to 5 mL of urine in the container. If the specimen is being collected while the patient is lying down, ask them to void forcibly to prevent urine from dribbling across the perineum.
- Stop collecting urine before the patient empties their bladder. Allow the patient to continue voiding into a bedpan or the commode and discard this urine.

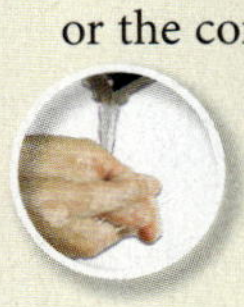

- Remove gloves and other PPE if used. Perform hand hygiene.
- Label the specimen container, package it appropriately, and send it to the laboratory.

Patients With Male Genitalia

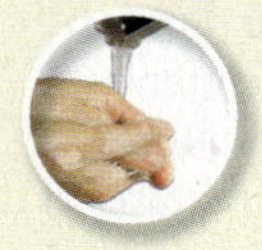

- Perform hand hygiene and put on PPE, if indicated.

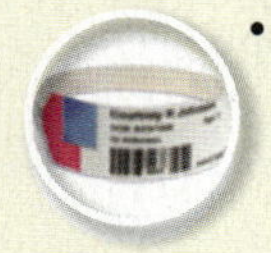

- Identify the patient.
- Explain to the patient what you are going to do and why.
- Put on unsterile gloves
- Retract the foreskin to expose the glans penis in the uncircumcised patient with male genitalia.
- Clean the area of the external meatus with soap and water.
- Have the patient void about 30 mL into the toilet or urinal and discard this urine.
- Have the patient void directly into the sterile container and collect at least 3 to 5 mL of urine in the container.
- Stop collecting urine before the patient empties their bladder. Allow the patient to void the remaining urine into the toilet or urinal and discard it.
- Return the foreskin to its normal position in an uncircumcised patient to prevent swelling and irritation of the glans penis.

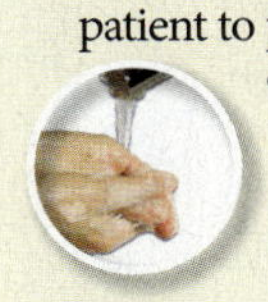

- Remove gloves and other PPE if used. Perform hand hygiene.
- Label the specimen container appropriately and send the specimen to the laboratory.

into the urine. Using aseptic technique, pour the urine into an appropriate container; label it with the patient's name, date, and time of collection; package it appropriately based on facility policy and place it in a sealable biohazard bag; and send it to the laboratory for examination. Do not leave urine standing at room temperature for a long period; transport the specimen to the laboratory. If unable to take the specimen to the laboratory immediately, refrigerate it (Fischbach et al., 2022).

Clean-Catch or Midstream Specimen

A clean-catch specimen of urine is required in some situations. A clean-catch urine specimen is collected during midstream voiding and minimizes bacterial contamination from adjacent anatomic areas (Fischbach et al., 2022). The patient voids a small amount and then collects the urine specimen. Initial voiding of a small amount of urine helps to flush away any organisms near the meatus and minimizes the risk of inaccurate findings if these organisms were to enter the specimen. In addition, it is generally thought that urine voided at midstream is most characteristic of the urine the body is producing. Do not leave urine standing at room temperature for a long period; transport the specimen to the laboratory. If unable to take the specimen to the laboratory immediately, refrigerate it (Fischbach et al., 2022). A patient who can carry out the technique properly may collect their own clean-catch midstream urine specimen and often prefers to do so. The nurse provides the appropriate equipment and instructions for the procedure. Refer to Guidelines for Nursing Care 38-1.

Sterile Specimen

Sterile urine specimens may be obtained by catheterizing the patient's bladder or by taking the specimen from an indwelling catheter already in place. Refer to the Catheterizing the Patient's Bladder discussion and Skill 38-2 on pages 1489–1493 and Skill 38-3 on pages 1493–1499.

When it is necessary to collect a urine specimen from a patient with an indwelling catheter, the specimen should be obtained from the catheter itself using the special port for specimens (see Guidelines for Nursing Care 38-2 on page 1460). Do not collect the specimen from the collecting receptacle; a specimen from the collecting receptacle (drainage bag) may not be fresh urine and could result in an inaccurate analysis. Always observe sterile technique while collecting a urine

Guidelines for Nursing Care 38-2

OBTAINING A URINE SPECIMEN FROM AN INDWELLING URINARY CATHETER

- Gather equipment, including a syringe, an antiseptic swab, a sterile specimen container, nonsterile gloves, and possibly a clamp. The size of the syringe for the specimen depends on the specific laboratory test. A urine culture requires about 3 mL, whereas routine urinalysis requires at least 10 mL of urine.

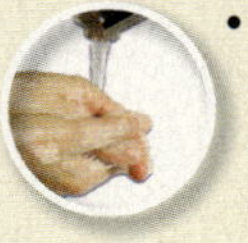

- Perform hand hygiene and put on PPE, if indicated.

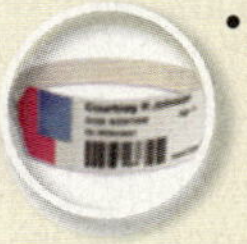

- Identify the patient.
- Explain to the patient what you are going to do and why.
- If urine is not present in the tube, clamp the tube below the access port briefly (not to exceed 30 minutes) to allow urine to accumulate.
- Put on unsterile gloves.
- Clean the access port with an antiseptic swab (Figure A), and carefully attach the syringe to the port.
- Aspirate urine into the syringe (Figure B).
- Remove the syringe. Release the clamp if one was used.
- Transfer the specimen to the appropriate container.

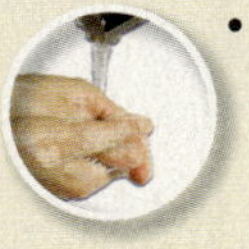

- Remove gloves and other PPE if used. Perform hand hygiene.
- Label the specimen with the patient's name, date, and time of collection
- Package based on facility policy, and place in a sealable biohazard bag. Transport the specimen to the lab according to facility policy.

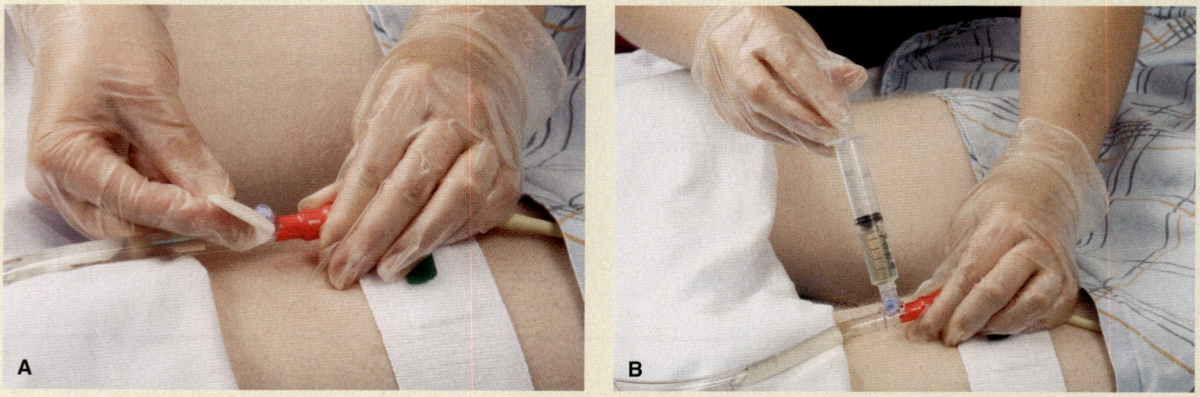

A. Using an antiseptic swab to clean the access port. **B.** Aspirating urine into the syringe. (*Source:* Used with permission from Shutterstock. *Photos by B. Proud.*)

specimen from an indwelling catheter. Guidelines for Nursing Care 38-2 outlines the procedure to collect a urine specimen from an indwelling urinary catheter.

Urine Specimens From a Urinary Diversion

Urine specimens can be obtained from urinary diversions via several methods. Clean urine specimens can be obtained from a urinary diversion appliance into a clean container for a routine urinalysis (Williams, 2012). Specimens for culture should never be obtained directly from an existing urostomy pouch or drainage bag (Mahoney et al., 2013; Wound Ostomy and Continence Nurses Society [WOCN], 2018). If a urine sample is needed for culture and sensitivity, most sources suggest that it should be obtained by sterile catheterization or clean-catch drip collection (Mahoney et al., 2013; Williams, 2012; WOCN, 2018). However, results of at least one study suggest that collection from a clean urostomy pouch is also acceptable (Vaarala, 2018).

In order to collect a specimen using sterile catheterization, remove the stoma appliance and clean the **stoma** (a surgically created opening on the body surface) site with solution, based on facility policy (Mahoney et al., 2013; WOCN, 2018). Using sterile technique, insert the urinary catheter no more than 2 to 3 inches into the stoma site. If there is resistance, rotate the catheter gently until it slides forward. If there is continued resistance, do not force the catheter any further (Mahoney et al., 2013; Williams, 2012; WOCN, 2018). After collection of a sufficient amount of urine, remove the catheter and reapply the stoma appliance.

If a urinary catheter is not available, a specimen may still be obtained (Mahoney et al., 2013; WOCN, 2018)). Remove the stoma appliance and clean the stoma site with solution, based on facility policy (Mahoney et al., 2013; WOCN, 2018). Discard the first few drops of urine by allowing urine to drip onto sterile gauze (Mahoney et al., 2013; WOCN, 2018). Hold a sterile specimen cup under the stoma to collect urine. After collection of a sufficient amount of urine, reapply the stoma appliance.

24-Hour Urine Specimens

For some laboratory studies, 24-hour specimen collection is required. The patient and the entire nursing team must understand the importance of collecting all the urine voided in a 24-hour period. Post a sign on the patient's bathroom door as a helpful reminder not to discard urine. Initiate a collection at a specific time (which is recorded) by asking the patient to empty the bladder. Discard this urine and then collect all urine voided for the next 24 hours. At the end of the 24 hours, ask the patient to void. Add this urine to the previously collected urine, and then send the entire specimen to the laboratory (Fischbach et al., 2022).

Depending on the type of examination, the urine from each voiding may be kept in a separately marked container and the time of each voiding recorded, or all urine voided may be collected in a common receptacle. The laboratory usually specifies whether a preservative is used to retard decomposition and whether the specimen is to be refrigerated or kept on ice. In some situations, the patient may be required to collect the specimen at home. It is very important for the patient and the patient's caregivers to understand the specific collection, storage, timing, and transportation instructions for the prescribed test.

Specimens From Infants and Children

Midstream collection can be accomplished with children older than age 2 years, provided the child is able to follow direction and engage in their care and with the nurse. Try having the child sit facing the back of the toilet, straddling the toilet seat. The nurse or parent can position themselves behind the child, holding the sterile container for urine collection.

The most reliable method to obtain a urine specimen for culture (associated with lower contamination rates) in neonates and young infants is to perform a suprapubic aspiration or transurethral catheterization (American Academy of Pediatrics [AAP], 2016; Cheek et al., 2015). Suprapubic aspiration is not within the scope of practice of registered nurses (May, 2018) and is painful. Pain management during the procedure is important—topical anesthetic cream should be used when time permits as well as age-appropriate distraction techniques (Cheek et al., 2015). Sampling options should be discussed with the health care team and the patient's parents/caregivers.

POINT-OF-CARE URINE TESTING

In some situations, the nurse may perform tests to detect abnormal constituents in urine specimens at the bedside or in the office setting. This is especially true when urine specimens are being tested repeatedly for known abnormalities, when screening tests are being used, or when laboratory facilities are not readily available. For example, a nurse may test urine for the presence of glucose, protein, bilirubin, bacteria, and blood. The results of the test are recorded on the patient's record. Many commercially prepared diagnostic kits are available for such tests and can be used in the home or the health care facility. Although these tests are economical and fast, laboratory analysis is recommended when precise results are needed.

Most commercially prepared diagnostic kits contain all needed equipment and the appropriate reagent (a substance used in a chemical reaction to detect another substance). Reagents are available as tablets, fluids, impregnated paper, and plastic strips with a special coating. When the urine comes in contact with the reagent, a chemical reaction occurs, causing a color change. This color is then compared with an accompanying chart that describes the significance of the color. The precise directions for the amount of the specimen, the time allowed for the chemical reaction, and the interpretation of the color vary with the manufacturer. Therefore, always follow the directions accompanying the diagnostic kit exactly.

The nurse may also determine the specific gravity of urine, which is a measure of the density of urine compared with the density of water (refer to Table 38-1). The higher the number, the more concentrated the urine is, unless there are abnormal components, such as glucose or protein, in the urine. Specific gravity can be determined with manufactured plastic reagent strips, as described previously.

PROVIDING SUPPORT FOR DIAGNOSTIC PROCEDURES

Various diagnostic procedures, which can be performed in a hospital or outpatient facility, are used to study the urinary system. Common diagnostic procedures related to the urinary system include urodynamic studies, cystoscopy, intravenous pyelogram, retrograde pyelogram, computed tomography (CT) scans, renal biopsy, and ultrasound examination. Nurses are responsible for preparing the patient for the procedure and giving appropriate aftercare and providing related patient education. Explaining the procedure helps reduce the patient's anxieties. The preparation and aftercare of the patient for each of these procedures are described in Box 38-4 on page 1462.

Diagnosing Actual or Potential Health Problems and Needs

An assessment of a patient's urinary status may lead to the identification of one or more actual or potential health problems and needs related to urinary elimination. Following the formulation of the actual or potential health problems and needs, the nurse communicates findings to other nursing and health care professionals through the use of the written and spoken word. The written actual or potential health problem or need becomes a permanent part of the patient's health record. Examples of health problems and needs with related etiology and signs and symptoms can be found in the Examples of Actual or Potential Health Problems and Needs: Urinary Elimination on page 1463.

Outcome Identification and Planning

Expected outcomes are derived from the actual or potential urinary elimination problems identified. The goal is to maintain or restore optimum function related to urinary elimination, alleviate symptoms or side effects of disease or treatment, and prevent complications. General patient

Box 38-4 Common Diagnostic Procedures Used to Study the Urinary Tract

Urodynamic Studies

Urodynamic studies are a group of tests that measure how urine flows, is stored, and is eliminated in the lower urinary tract. They are used to identify abnormal voiding patterns in people with incontinence or the inability to void normally.

Preparation

- Usually, no fluid or food restrictions are necessary before the test.
- Bladder should be full before the test.
- Inform the patient that a catheter will be inserted during the test.

Aftercare

- Instruct the patient to drink 8 to 10 8-oz glasses of water in the 24 hours after the test.
- Teach the patient the signs and symptoms of a urinary tract infection and to report any symptoms immediately.

Cystoscopy

Cystoscopy is the direct visual examination of the bladder, ureteral orifices, and urethra with a cystoscope. It is used to view, diagnose, and treat disorders of the lower urinary tract, interior bladder, urethra, male prostatic urethra, and ureteral orifices.

Preparation

- The patient is allowed liquids on the morning of the examination.
- Sedation and analgesics are usually prescribed before the procedure.
- Verify documentation of informed consent (required for the procedure).
- Explain to the patient that the procedure is ordinarily painless.

Aftercare

- Know that tissue swelling, dysuria, and hematuria may occur because of trauma from the procedure.
- Encourage a generous fluid intake and observe and measure urine output for at least 24 hours.
- Observe the patient for urinary retention and for signs of infection; procedure-related infection after a cystoscopy may occur.

Intravenous Pyelogram (Excretory or Intravenous Urography)

Intravenous pyelogram is the radiographic examination of the kidney and ureter after a contrast material is injected intravenously. It is used to diagnose renal disease and urinary tract dysfunction.

Preparation

- Withhold fluids or foods for 12 hours before testing. Obtain patient's allergy history, focusing on prior allergic reaction to contrast substances and sensitivity to iodine, shellfish, or seafood (contrast may contain iodine).
- This test is contraindicated for patients with elevated BUN and creatinine levels and pregnant patients. Some facilities require a recent creatinine level for all patients over 40 years of age prior to performing the procedure (Fischbach et al., 2022).
- Older, debilitated, or young patients may not tolerate this dehydration; compromises may need to be made for those patients.
- Give a laxative the evening before the examination and an enema the morning of the examination so that stool and gas do not interfere with visualization.
- Verify documentation of informed consent (required for the procedure).
- Instruct the patient to void before the examination.

Aftercare

- Offer fluids and food immediately after the examination.
- Provide sufficient fluids to replace those lost during the pretest period and/or encourage a generous fluid intake.
- Observe the patient for and provide patient teaching related to signs of a reaction to the contrast material, such as a rash, nausea, and hives. Contrast may initiate acute renal failure. Monitor intake and output.

Retrograde Pyelogram

Retrograde pyelogram is the radiographic and endoscopic examination of the kidneys and ureters, with placement of ureteral catheter up to the level of the renal pelvis as part of the endoscopic examination. Contrast material is then injected into the renal pelvis through the ureteral catheter, followed by radiographic images.

Preparation

- Do not give fluids or food after midnight before the examination.
- This test is contraindicated for pregnant patients and those with an iodine allergy.
- This test is contraindicated for patients with elevated BUN and creatinine levels and pregnant patients. Some facilities require a recent creatinine level for all patients over 40 years of age prior to performing the procedure (Fischbach et al., 2022).
- Give a laxative the evening before the examination and an enema the morning of the examination so that stool and gas do not interfere with visualization.
- Instruct the patient to void before the examination.
- Verify documentation of informed consent (required for the procedure).

Aftercare

- Offer foods and fluids immediately if no anesthesia has been used. If anesthesia has been used, delay offering foods and fluids for several hours.
- Check the vital signs regularly if anesthesia has been used.
- Observe the patient for signs of a reaction to the contrast material, such as a rash, nausea, and hives.
- Monitor urine output and appearance for at least 24 hours. Hematuria and dysuria can occur.
- Be aware that ureteral catheters may be in place and should be connected to drainage receptacles so that the amount and character of drainage from each catheter can be noted.

Renal Ultrasound

A renal ultrasound is a noninvasive procedure that involves the use of ultrasound to visualize the renal parenchyma and renal blood vessels. It is used to characterize renal masses and infections, visualize large calculi; detect malformed

Box 38-4 Common Diagnostic Procedures Used to Study the Urinary Tract *(continued)*

kidneys; provide guidance during other procedures, such as biopsy; and monitor the status of renal transplants and kidney development in children with congenital processes.

Preparation

- Verify documentation of informed consent (required).
- Food and fluid restriction are usually not necessary but may be required in certain facilities (Fischbach et al., 2022).
- Explain to the patient that the procedure is painless.

Aftercare

- No special care is required after this procedure.

Computed Tomography (CT Scanning)

CT scanning is a noninvasive radiographic procedure whereby a body part can be scanned from different angles with an x-ray beam and a computer that calculates varying tissue densities and records a cross-sectional image.

Preparation

- Verify documentation of informed consent (required).
- The patient is usually NPO for 8 hours before the test if a contrast dye is used.
- Obtain patient's history of any allergic reaction or hypersensitivity to shellfish, iodine, or any contrast dyes (contrast may contain iodine).
- Remove all metal objects from the patient before the test.
- Medications may usually be taken until 2 hours before the test.
- Some patients may receive sedation and/or analgesics to help control feelings of claustrophobia during the procedure.

Aftercare

- Observe for a delayed reaction to the contrast dye (skin rash, urticaria, headache, vomiting). An oral antihistamine may be given for some reactions.
- Instruct the patient to resume usual diet and activity unless otherwise indicated.

outcomes are listed here. Actual patient outcomes should list specific behaviors and criteria individualized for the patient situation. The patient will:

- Produce urine output about equal to fluid intake
- Maintain fluid and electrolyte balance
- Empty the bladder completely at regular intervals
- Report ease of voiding
- Maintain skin integrity
- Demonstrate appropriate self-care behaviors

Implementing

Nursing interventions focus on maintaining and promoting normal urinary patterns, improving or controlling urinary incontinence, preventing potential problems associated with bladder catheterization, and assisting with care of urinary diversions. Nurses can assist the patient and family/caregivers to achieve desirable outcomes for their urination needs.

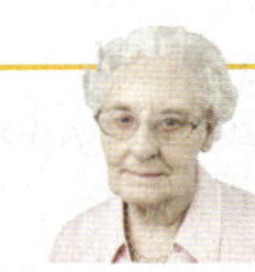

Think back to **Anna Galinski**, the frail person in a long-term care facility. The toileting program focused on maintaining and promoting the patient's normal urinary patterns. However, now that the patient has an indwelling catheter, the nurse needs to focus on preventing problems associated with catheterization. Weighing the risks and benefits of catheterization for this patient would be crucial

Examples of Actual or Potential Health Problems and Needs

URINARY ELIMINATION

Actual or Potential Health Problems and Needs	Possible Etiologic Factors	Potential Signs and Symptoms
Urinary Retention	• Sensory motor impairment • Enlarged prostate • Medications, such as antidepressants, antihistamines, calcium-channel blockers, anticholinergics • Anatomic obstruction	• Postvoid residual of 450 mL via bladder scanner • *"It takes a while for the urine to come and sometimes I have to go every hour!"* • *"I have to get up frequently at night to urinate."*
Stress Incontinence of Urine	• Weak pelvic muscles and structural supports	• Patient reports involuntary leakage of urine with sudden movement, coughing, sneezing, and laughing.
Risk for Urge Incontinence of Urine	• Alcohol and caffeine consumption, fecal impaction, urinary tract infection, ineffective toileting habits	—

Source: International Council of Nurses (ICN). (2019). Nursing diagnosis and outcome statements. https://www.icn.ch/sites/default/files/inline-files/ICNP2019-DC.pdf; Wolters Kluwer. (2022). Problem-based care plans. In *Lippincott Advisor*. Wolters Kluwer. https://advisor.lww.com/lna/home.do

Promoting Health 38-1

URINE ELIMINATION

Use the assessment checklist to determine how well you are meeting your needs related to urinary elimination. Then develop a prescription for self-care by choosing appropriate behaviors from the list of suggestions.

Assessment Checklist

☐ almost always ☐ sometimes ☐ almost never

☐ ☐ ☐ 1. I urinate at regular intervals throughout the day.

☐ ☐ ☐ 2. I have an adequate fluid intake.

☐ ☐ ☐ 3. I limit my sodium intake.

☐ ☐ ☐ 4. My urine volume remains relatively constant.

Self-Care Behaviors

1. Maintain a normal voiding pattern and volume.
2. Respond as soon as possible to the urge to void.
3. Drink six to eight 8-oz glasses of water daily.
4. Avoid foods that contain excess sodium.
5. Monitor use of caffeine, alcohol, or medication schedules that promote voiding and may interfere with sleep.
6. Seek medical assistance for any change in the characteristics of urine or presence of pain on urination.

Information to promote effective urinary elimination—such as information about elimination problems, urinary incontinence, and renal and bladder diseases—is available online.

Promoting Urinary Elimination

Nursing care to promote urinary elimination includes interventions to support voiding habits, fluid intake, strengthening of muscle tone, stimulating urination and resolving urinary retention, and assisting with toileting. Nurses working with patients to promote appropriate behaviors related to urine elimination should examine their own behaviors as factors in the success of the plan. Nurses who role model good health behaviors are more effective teachers. Use the display, Promoting Health 37-1, for yourself before using it with others.

MAINTAINING REGULAR VOIDING HABITS

If the patient's voiding habits are adequate, provide care or teach the patient to maintain these habits to ensure comfort and satisfactory urine output. Attention to the following variables is helpful:

- *Schedule:* Some patients report urinating on demand in no apparent pattern. Others have inflexible patterns that have developed over the years and become anxious if these are interrupted. Some patients need assistance to urinate and may experience urgency. Nursing actions should support the patient's usual urinating pattern as much as possible.
- *Urge to void:* Assist the patient to void when the patient first feels the urge to void. Routinely delaying urination may result in difficulty initiating a stream and/or urinary stasis. Urinary stasis can contribute to the development of UTIs.
- *Privacy:* Many adults and children cannot urinate in the presence of another person. Unless the patient is extremely weak and requires assistance, provide privacy in the health care facility and in the home.
- *Position:* Helping patients assume their usual voiding position may be all that is necessary to resolve an inability to urinate. Some patients with male genitalia cannot use a urinal while lying down or sitting; encourage them to void while standing at the bedside unless this is contraindicated. Similarly, some patients with female genitalia cannot void easily on a bedpan but respond favorably with a bedside commode.
- *Hygiene:* Patients who are confined to bed find it difficult to perform their usual genital hygiene. Careful cleansing of the perineal and genital areas is needed for patient comfort and to prevent infection. This is easily accomplished for patients on bedrest by using warmed, moistened disposable washcloths and skin cleanser or by pouring warm, soapy water over the perineal area while the patient is still on the bedpan, followed by clear water.

Because people customarily wash their hands after toileting and hand hygiene prevents transmission of microorganisms, offer patients confined to bed a moistened towelette or soap and water to wipe their hands after removing the bedpan or urinal. Nursing strategies to address age-related changes affecting urinary elimination are identified in the accompanying Focus on the Older Adult box.

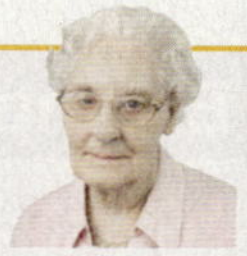

Recall **Anna Galinski**, the frail older person in the long-term care facility. Strategies to promote normal urinary elimination should have been attempted to determine their effectiveness in promoting urinary elimination prior to use of a urinary catheter. In addition, when advocating for the patient, the nurse would strongly urge incorporating strategies to promote normal urinary elimination into the patient's care plan to determine their effectiveness, ultimately substantiating that catheterization was not necessary.

PROMOTING FLUID INTAKE

Many people routinely drink less fluid than is optimal to promote healthy urinary functioning. Adults with no disease-related fluid restrictions should drink an average of six to eight 8-oz glasses of liquid daily (NIDDK, 2017). A common misperception is that drinking this much fluid causes water retention and contributes to weight gain. If a good proportion of the daily fluid intake is water,

Focus on the Older Adult

NURSING STRATEGIES TO ADDRESS AGE-RELATED CHANGES AFFECTING URINARY ELIMINATION

Age-Related Change	Nursing Strategies
Nocturia, frequency, and urgency	• Ensure easy access to the bathroom or commode. • Discourage fluid intake at bedtime. • Discourage alcohol use before bedtime. • Evaluate medication regimen and schedule, particularly diuretics and drugs that produce sedation or confusion. • Use a night light. • Use clothing that is easily removed for voiding. • Keep assistive ambulatory devices (walkers, canes, and the like) readily available. • Evaluate gait and ability to ambulate safely. • Assess for urinary tract infection.
Incontinence	• Maintain a fluid intake (Davis et al., 2020). • Discourage use of alcohol, artificial sweeteners, and caffeine. • Provide easy access to the bathroom. • Assess factors that influence voiding. • Use assistive devices when necessary (raised toilet seat, grab bars, walker). • Use collection devices when necessary (urinal or bedpan). • Ensure safety when ambulating (e.g., skid-proof slippers). • Encourage use of whole, unprocessed, coarse wheat bran to prevent constipation and fecal impaction. • Perform pelvic floor muscle training (PFMT) exercises several times daily. • Encourage participation in a bladder retraining program.
Urinary tract infections	• Maintain a liberal fluid intake (Dudek, 2022; Wu et al., 2020). • Encourage shower instead of tub bath to decrease opportunity for bacteria in bath water to enter urethra. • Encourage appropriate perineal care and frequent changing of incontinence briefs. • Void at frequent intervals; every 2 hours if possible. • Void immediately after sexual intercourse. • Females should avoid use of potentially irritating feminine products, such as deodorant sprays, douches, and powders in the genital area.

the kidneys and urinary structures are well flushed, and waste products, including potentially harmful bacteria, are removed. Monitor fluid intake for excessive amounts of caffeine-containing beverages, high-sodium beverages, and high-sugar beverages.

Provide fresh water, juices, and fluids of preference to patients with alterations in mobility. Remind children and patients who are confused to drink. Fluid restrictions may be ordered for patients with certain health problems. For others, an above-average intake of fluids is prescribed. Incorporate this information in the care plan and provide patient education.

STRENGTHENING MUSCLE TONE

Weakening of the pelvic floor muscles is a common cause of urinary continence problems (Cera & Twiss, 2018; Shin et al., 2016). Pelvic floor muscle training (PFMT) can improve voluntary control of urination and significantly reduce or eliminate problems with **stress incontinence** (involuntary loss of urine related to an increase in intra-abdominal pressure) by strengthening perineal and abdominal muscle tone (Pair & Somerall, 2018; Peate, 2019). PFMT, often referred to as Kegel exercises (Pair & Somerall, 2018), targets the inner muscles that lie under and support the bladder. These muscles can be toned, strengthened, and actually made larger by a regular routine of tightening and relaxing. Often patients have difficulty determining which muscles to exercise. These are the same muscles that the patient contracts to stop urinating in midstream or to control defecation. Instruct patients to contract the pelvic floor muscles for 5 to 10 seconds and to relax them for 10 seconds. Encourage the patient to perform PFMT exercises without involving the muscles in the abdomen, inner thigh, and buttocks. When the patient is familiar with these sensations, these exercises should be performed multiple times a day for at least 3 months, and possibly longer, depending on the response. The exercises can be done anywhere. Assist patients to incorporate them into their daily activities. See the accompanying PICOT in Practice box on page 1466. Urinary incontinence and associated nursing interventions is discussed in more detail later in the chapter.

ASSISTING WITH TOILETING

The amount of assistance provided to a patient in relation to toileting varies, depending on the patient's abilities and health status.

PICOT in Practice

ASKING CLINICAL QUESTIONS: PELVIC FLOOR MUSCLE TRAINING

Scenario: You and your next-door-neighbor Sarah exercise every day after work. Sarah has cancelled several days in a row. They gave birth recently, and you attribute the cancellation to being busy with the infant. Sarah confided with extreme embarrassment that they have been leaking urine when they run or cough over the past few months after childbirth. Sarah has discussed the problem with their OB/GYN, who indicated that Sarah has urinary incontinence. Sarah has seen commercials about drugs available for overactive bladder and hopes that something can help. You remember from class that pelvic floor muscle training (PFMT), or Kegel exercises, were recommended for females after childbirth and wonder if drugs or similar exercises are most appropriate for Sarah.

- **Population:** Adult females with urinary incontinence
- **Intervention:** Drugs used for overactive bladder
- **Comparison:** PFMT
- **Outcome:** Improvement of urinary incontinence
- **Time:** 3 months

PICOT Question: Among postnatal people, are PFMT exercises more effective than drugs used to treat urinary incontinence within 3 months of treatment?

Finding:

Woodley, S. J., Lawrenson, P., Boyle, R., Cody, J.D., Mørkved, S., Kernohan, A., & Hay-Smith, E. J. C. (2020). Pelvic floor muscle training for preventing and treating urinary and faecal incontinence in antenatal and postnatal women. *Cochrane Database of Systematic Reviews, 5*(5), CD007471. https://doi.org/10.1002/14651858.CD007471.pub4

The review included 46 trials involving 10,832 females from 21 countries. The studies included pregnant females and females who had delivered their baby within the last 3 months, and who reported leakage of urine, feces, both urine or feces, or no leakage. They were allocated randomly to receive PFMT, either to try to prevent incontinence or as a treatment for incontinence, or not, and the effects were compared. This review provides evidence that early structured PFMT in early pregnancy for continent females probably prevents the onset of urinary incontinence in late pregnancy and reduces the risk of urinary incontinence slightly postnatally.

Dumoulin, C., Cacciari, L. P., & Hay-Smith, E. J. C. (2018). Pelvic floor muscle training versus no treatment, or inactive control treatments, for urinary incontinence in women. *Cochrane Database of Systematic Reviews, 10*(10), CD005654. https://doi.org/10.1002/14651858.CD005654.pub4

The 31 included trials involved 1,817 females from 14 countries. The studies included females with stress, urgency, or mixed urinary incontinence. They were allocated randomly to either receive or not receive PFMT, and the effects were compared for whether the condition was "cured," or "cured or improved." The review also looked at symptoms, the effect on quality of life, and the frequency and amount of urine lost. Based on the data available, PFMT is better than no treatment, placebo, or inactive control treatments for females with stress urinary incontinence or urinary incontinence (all types). The review reported confidence that PFMT can cure or improve symptoms and may reduce the number of leakage episodes in all types of urinary incontinence.

Level of Evidence I: Systematic review.

Recommendations: You assure Sarah that urinary incontinence is common in females, and the incidence increases with age. You tell Sarah about different types of urinary incontinence with different treatment recommendations and that there is strong evidence that PFMT, also known as Kegel exercises, are effective as a first treatment for females with stress or urinary incontinence (all types). You provide Sarah with information from the U.S. National Library of Medicine, Pelvic Floor Muscle Training Exercises (https://medlineplus.gov/ency/article/003975.htm) and suggest they consistently perform the exercises (10 repetitions three to five times a day) for 3 months.

Toilet

Even when the patient can use the bathroom toilet, the nurse may be responsible for noting any abnormalities of urinary elimination. In some instances, patients may be taught to report abnormalities to the nurse and instructed not to flush the toilet until the nurse checks the urine. In other instances, when the urine volume is to be calculated, the patient may need to urinate in a urinal or a specimen hat placed in the toilet so that the urine can be measured before it is discarded (see Fig. 38-5 on page 1457). Although many patients can easily be taught to measure their urine output, the nurse should assess urine characteristics at least once during a shift in acute care and more frequently if warranted.

Assist weakened patients to the bathroom. If there is any danger of the patient falling, remain in attendance. Never lock the bathroom door. Ensure that a signal bell is within easy reach so that the patient can summon help easily if feeling weak and needing assistance. A handrail near the toilet also is helpful.

Commode

Commodes are chairs—straight-back chairs or wheelchairs with open seats and a shelf or a holder underneath that holds a bucket (Fig. 38-7). Commodes can be used for patients who can get out of bed but cannot use the bathroom toilet. The commode can be placed adjacent to the bed, and the patient can be assisted to it with minimal exertion. If the patient has a roommate, any visitors may be asked to exit the room while the patient uses the commode. Remember to pull the curtain in the room and close the door to provide for patient privacy.

Bedpan and Urinal

In situations in which mobility is compromised or limited, patients with male genitalia usually prefer to use the urinal

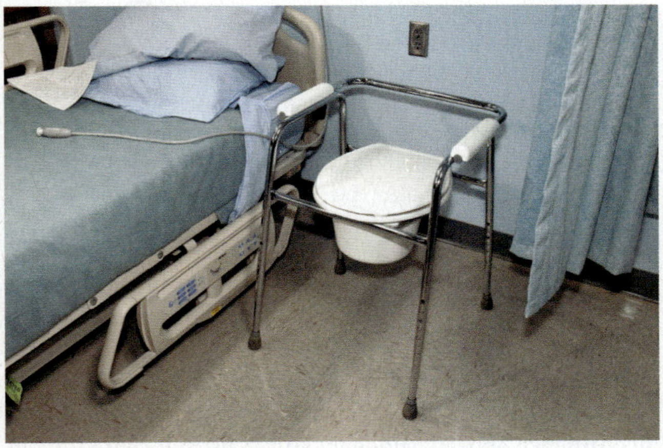

FIGURE 38-7. Bedside commode.

for voiding and the bedpan for defecation; patients with female genitalia usually prefer to use the bedpan for both (see Fig. 38-5 on page 1457). Many patients find it embarrassing and difficult to use the bedpan and/or the urinal. When a patient uses a bedpan or urinal, maintain the patient's privacy.

A fracture bedpan is frequently used by people with fractures of the femur or lower spine. Smaller and flatter than the ordinary bedpan, it is helpful for patients who cannot easily raise themselves onto the regular bedpan. Very thin patients or older adults often find it easier and more comfortable to use the fracture bedpan.

Caring for Patients With Urinary Tract Infections

UTIs are among the most common health care–associated infections and are a common cause of systemic infections in older adults (Clarke et al., 2020; Sepsis Alliance, 2020; Touhy & Jett, 2018). Bladder and urethra infections are the most common type of UTI, but any part of the urinary tract can become infected (Mayo Foundation for Medical Education and Research [MFMER], 2020; National Institute of Diabetes and Digestive and Kidney Diseases [NIDDK], 2017). People with female genitalia are especially vulnerable to UTIs because the urethra is shorter and in closer proximity to the vagina and rectum (NIDDK, 2017). UTIs can affect both the upper urinary tract, involving the kidneys and ureters (pyelonephritis) and lower urinary tract, involving the bladder and urethra (cystitis). *Escherichia coli,* bacteria commonly found in the gastrointestinal tract, are the most common causal organism of infection of the bladder (MFMER, 2020; NIDDK, 2017).

RISK FACTORS

Those at greatest risk for a UTI include the following:

- *Sexually active people with female genitalia:* During intercourse, perineal bacteria can migrate into the urethra and bladder (NIDDK, 2017; National Kidney Foundation [NKF], 2016).
- *People who use diaphragms for contraception:* The spermicide used with a diaphragm decreases the amount of normally protective vaginal flora (NIDDK, 2017).
- *Postmenopausal people:* Urinary stasis, which is common at this age, provides an optimal environment for bacteria to multiply; in addition, decreased estrogen contributes to loss of protective vaginal flora (NIDDK, 2017).
- *People with an indwelling urinary catheter in place:* Bacteria travel through or around the catheter and into the bladder. UTIs are the most common type of health care–associated infection (HAI) reported to the National Healthcare Safety Network, and approximately 75% of these UTIs are associated with a urinary catheter (Centers for Disease Control and Prevention [CDC], 2015). A catheter-associated urinary tract infection (CAUTI) increases health care costs and is associated with increased morbidity and mortality. CAUTIs are considered by the Centers for Medicare and Medicaid Services to represent a reasonably preventable complication of hospitalization. As such, no additional payment is provided to hospitals for CAUTI treatment-related costs (CMS, 2020). Although a break in sterile technique during placement can lead to an infection, most pathogens are introduced via handling of the catheter and drainage device after placement.
- *People with diabetes:* Changes in the body's defense system related to diabetes may increase the risk for UTIs (NKF, 2016).
- *Older adults:* The physiologic changes associated with aging (listed earlier in the chapter) predispose older people to the development of UTIs and other infections (Sepsis Alliance, 2020). In addition, enlargement of the prostate as a person ages can contribute to the development of UTIs (NKF, 2016).

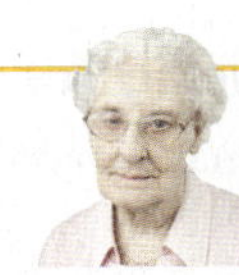

Consider **Anna Galinski**, the frail older adult in the long-term care facility. Their risk for developing a UTI is increased due to their age. This risk now is further increased because of the catheter insertion.

DIAGNOSTIC EVALUATION

In addition to the nursing history and physical examination, laboratory findings can identify the presence of a UTI. A urine sample for urinalysis may be collected and tested for bacteria and white blood cells. A urinalysis suggests the presence of an infection if bacteria and white blood cells are present in the sample (NIDDK, 2017). A urine sample from a clean-catch or sterile specimen may be sent to the laboratory for a culture and sensitivity (C&S) test. A bacterial count of >100,000 colony-forming units (CFU)/mL indicates infection (Fischbach et al., 2022). Lower counts may be considered clinically significant if the patient has signs and symptoms of a UTI (Fischbach et al., 2022). The presence of bacteria in a clean-catch midstream or sterile urine specimen, accompanied by symptoms (e.g., dysuria, urinary frequency or urgency, or cloudy urine with a foul odor), indicates a UTI. Red blood cells and nitrites also may be present in the urine.

TREATMENT AND PATIENT EDUCATION

Various protocols are used to treat UTIs. A short-course antibiotic regimen (one large dose vs. 3 or 7 days of smaller doses) usually eradicates infections of the lower urinary tract; longer antimicrobial therapy is required for upper UTIs (Cleveland Clinic, 2019).

Patient education can help prevent UTIs. Teaching the patient about measures that promote health is an important nursing responsibility. Instruct the patient to:

- Drink six to eight 8-oz glasses of liquid daily (NIDDK, 2017).
- Do not postpone going to the bathroom; urinate when you feel the urge (NKF, 2016). Take enough time to fully empty the bladder when urinating (NIDDK, 2017).
- If you have female genitalia, dry the perineal area after urination or defecation from the front to the back (from the urethra toward the rectum) (MFMER, 2020; NIDDK, 2017).
- Void before and after sex (intercourse) (MFMER, 2020; NIDDK, 2017; NKF, 2016).
- If you have repeat bladder infections and use a diaphragm, unlubricated condoms, or spermicide, talk with your health care professional about switching birth control methods; these methods can increase the chances of developing a bladder infection (NIDDK, 2017).
- Wear underwear with a cotton crotch and avoid clothing that is tight and restrictive on the lower half of the body (MFMER, 2020; NIDDK, 2017).

Nursing interventions to prevent UTIs for a patient with an indwelling catheter are discussed later in the chapter.

Caring for an Incontinent Patient

Urinary incontinence (loss of bladder control with involuntary leakage of urine) is widely underreported and underdiagnosed (Touhy & Jett, 2018; Vasavada et al., 2019b). It is one of the most common chronic health problems. However, it is not an inevitable result of growing old or bearing children (Touhy & Jett, 2018; Yates, 2019). Many people self-manage this life-altering condition for many years before seeking assistance from a health care provider.

Urinary incontinence is more prevalent in females and increases with age (Davis et al., 2020; Vasavada et al., 2019b). It is a special problem for older adults who may experience decreasing control over urination and who may find it more difficult to reach a toilet in time to void because of mobility problems or dexterity problems in undressing. The discomfort, odor, and embarrassment of urine-soaked clothing can greatly diminish a person's self-concept, causing the person to feel like a social outcast.

Age-related changes do affect urinary function, but urinary incontinence can be treated, and individualized interventions can help the patient lead a normal life. Incontinence is a symptom, is treatable, and is often curable (Society of Urologic Nurses and Associates [SUNA], 2019). Specific treatment is based on the specific type on incontinence and its cause (Vasavada et al., 2019b).

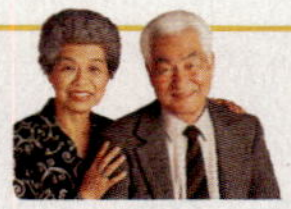

Review the scenario at the beginning of the chapter describing **Midori Morita** and their husband. The nurse should assess the feelings of Midori and her husband related to the problems associated with Mr. Morita's urinary dribbling and incontinence. Mrs. Morita may be feeling overwhelmed and possibly upset or angry. Her husband most likely would be feeling embarrassed and possibly disgusted. Helping them resolve these feelings is essential for effective care.

TYPES OF URINARY INCONTINENCE

There are numerous types of urinary incontinence. **Transient incontinence** appears suddenly and is usually caused by an illness or temporary problem that is short-lived or treatable (Hall, 2018). It is usually caused by treatable factors, such as confusion secondary to acute illness or infection or as a result of medical treatment, such as the use of diuretics or intravenous fluid administration. When the underlying problem is resolved, the patient should regain continence (Hall, 2018). **Stress incontinence** (discussed earlier in the chapter) occurs because of weak pelvic floor muscles and/or a deficient urethral sphincter, causing an involuntary loss of urine related to an increase in intra-abdominal pressure (National Association for Continence [NAFC], n.d.a). This commonly occurs during coughing, sneezing, laughing, lifting, changing position, or exercising (SUNA, 2019). Childbirth, menopause, obesity, or straining from chronic constipation can also result in urine loss (Hooper, 2019; International Continence Society [ICS], 2015). The leakage usually does not occur when the person is supine. Urge incontinence is the involuntary loss of urine that occurs soon after feeling an urgent need to void (urgency). Urge incontinence may be associated with overactive bladder syndrome (ICS, 2015). These patients experience a loss of urine before getting to the toilet and an inability to suppress the need to urinate. **Mixed incontinence** is a combination of stress incontinence and urgency incontinence and is marked by involuntary leakage associated with urgency as well as with exertion, effort, sneezing, and coughing (National Association for Continence [NAFC], n.d.a; SUNA, 2019; Vasavada et al., 2019b). **Overflow incontinence**, or chronic retention of urine, is the involuntary loss of urine associated with overdistention and overflow of the bladder (SUNA, 2019). The signal to empty the bladder may be underactive or absent, the bladder fills, and dribbling occurs. It may be due to a secondary effect of some medications, neurologic conditions, diabetes, and obstruction or injury (SUNA, 2019). **Functional incontinence** is urine loss caused by the inability to reach the toilet because of environmental barriers, physical limitations, loss of memory, or disorientation (National Institute on Aging, 2017; Vasavada et al., 2019b).

Patients with reflex incontinence experience emptying of the bladder without the sensation of the need to void from damage to the nerves that normally signal the brain that the bladder is filling (Harvard Health Publishing, 2014). Spinal cord injuries, multiple sclerosis or damage from surgery or radiation treatment may lead to this type of incontinence (Harvard Health

Publishing, 2014). **Total (continuous) incontinence** is a continuous and unpredictable loss of urine, resulting from surgery, trauma, or physical malformation such as a urogenital fistula (Vasavada et al., 2019c). Urination cannot be controlled.

Urinary incontinence is treatable (SUNA, 2019). Appropriate interventions can significantly reduce the symptoms of urinary incontinence and even prevent its occurrence. Successful treatment of urinary incontinence is tailored to the specific type of incontinence and its cause (National Institute on Aging, 2017; Vasavada et al., 2019b).

ASSESSMENT

Through careful assessment and planned interventions (see upcoming discussion), continence may be restored. A detailed patient history is an important part of the assessment. Refer to the previous discussion regarding nursing assessment on pages 1454–1461. Carefully assess environmental factors for their potential impact on urinary incontinence. Equipment that gives the person better access to toileting facilities, such as a walker, cane, wheelchair, and Velcro closings on clothing, may be necessary. Dietary habits, such as caffeine, artificial sweeteners, or insufficient fluid intake, both of which can irritate the bladder and contribute to incontinence, indicate the need for teaching about nutrition (National Association for Continence, n.d.b).

A voiding record or diary provides information about the frequency, timing, and amount of voiding. By noting any patterns to voiding, either continent or incontinent, the nurse may find correlations with medications, fluid intake, or other causes of incontinence and may be able to prevent any further incontinent episodes. Voiding diaries can also be used to evaluate the effectiveness of interventions.

Physical examination and specific diagnostic tests also aid in identifying urinary incontinence. Palpate the patient's abdomen for a distended bladder, any masses, or tenderness. The **postvoid residual (PVR)** urine (the amount of urine remaining in the bladder immediately after voiding) can be measured by the use of a portable ultrasound device that scans the bladder. Bladder ultrasound poses no risk for infection and is considered a safer alternative to catheterization. A PVR of less than 50 mL indicates adequate bladder emptying. A PVR of greater than 100 mL is an indication the bladder is not emptying correctly (Bauldoff et al., 2020). This measurement can also be obtained by catheterizing the patient. Catheterization, however, involves the increased risk for introduction of microorganisms into the bladder and resulting UTI. Refer to Skill 38-1 (on pages 1489–1493) for the procedure for assessing bladder volume using an ultrasound bladder scanner. Urine specimens are used to screen for UTI, a frequent cause of urinary incontinence (Davis et al., 2020; Hooper, 2019).

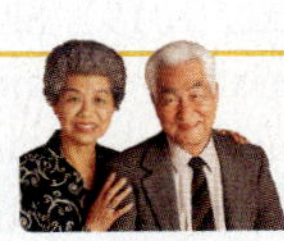

Think back to ***Midori Morita***, the person caring for her husband, who is experiencing urinary problems at home. The nurse would need to carefully assess all aspects of Mr. Morita's current status, including the environment, and develop a patient-specific teaching plan for Mr., and Mrs. Morita.

TREATMENT

Noninvasive, low-risk behavioral interventions are the first line of therapy for urinary incontinence (Newman, 2019a; Pair & Somerall, 2018; Peate, 2019). Community settings are ideally suited for using many of these interventions. Nurses are able to identify patients who are incontinent and use these interventions to help patients manage incontinence. Nurses may also refer a patient to an advanced practice continence nurse or other health care provider expert in the community. All nurses caring for older adults need to be familiar with education about urinary incontinence. Many possible treatment interventions for urinary incontinence fall within the nurse's scope of practice. Many patients incorrectly believe that surgery is the only treatment option for urinary incontinence. Surgical intervention is considered only if behavioral and pharmacologic measures prove ineffective (Davis et al., 2020; Peate, 2019). Indwelling urinary catheters are not recommended because of the associated risk of developing a UTI (Davis et al., 2020; Gould et al., 2019; Payne, 2020). Refer to Box 38-5 on page 1470 for a summary of behavioral and other treatment interventions and to the previous discussion related to strengthening muscle tone on page 1465.

Absorbent products can provide protection for skin and clothing but should not be used in place of definitive interventions to decrease or eliminate urinary incontinence (Vasavada et al., 2019a). These products absorb or contain urine leakage. Many types of disposable and reusable products are available, including perineal pads or liners, protective underwear, pads for furniture and beds, guards and drip collection pouches, and adult briefs (continence pads) (National Institute on Aging, 2017; Vasavada et al., 2019a). When used improperly, such products may cause incontinence-associated dermatitis or skin breakdown and place the patient at risk for a UTI (Nazarko, 2015; Vasavada et al., 2019a). Refer to the following Incontinence-Associated Dermatitis section for more information. Long-term use of these products is not recommended until the following factors have been considered and discussed with a health care provider:

- Functional disability of the patient
- Type and severity of incontinence
- Availability of caregivers
- Failure of previous treatment programs
- Patient preference

Advertisements for adult disposable briefs (undergarments) have increased public awareness about urinary incontinence, but they fail to mention possible treatment strategies. Refer to the accompanying Focused Critical Thinking Guide 38-1 on page 1471. External collecting devices may be useful in managing urinary incontinence (NIDDK, 2018b; Vasavada et al., 2019a). Refer to the External Urine Collection Devices on page 1472.

INCONTINENCE-ASSOCIATED DERMATITIS

Excessive contact of the skin with urine or feces leads to a form of moisture-associated skin damage known as **incontinence-associated dermatitis (IAD)**, inflammation

Box 38-5 Treatment Options for Urinary Incontinence

Behavioral Techniques

- *Pelvic floor muscle training exercises:* Pelvic floor muscle training (PFMT) exercises (Kegel exercises) can be used to strengthen pelvic floor muscles and sphincter muscles. PFMT exercises can be done alone or with biofeedback.
- *Biofeedback:* Measuring devices are used to help the patient become aware of when pelvic floor muscles are contracting.
- *Electrical stimulation:* Electrodes are placed in the vagina or rectum that then stimulate nearby muscles to contract.
- *Scheduled voiding (Timed voiding) Prompted voiding or Bladder training:* May be used with biofeedback. Patient keeps track of when voiding and leaking occur to enable oneself to plan when to void, with increasing length of voiding intervals. Bladder training involves biofeedback and muscle training. Urgency control is addressed using distraction and relaxation techniques. Prompting from a caregiver (reminding the individual to use the toilet and encouraging maintenance of bladder control between voiding) maybe included for individuals who have impaired cognitive function.

Weight Loss

- Obesity is a risk factor for incontinence because of increasing intra-abdominal pressure and pelvic floor weakness. Weight loss should be considered as a lifestyle change to improve incontinence in overweight patients.

Pharmacologic Treatment

- Treatment is dependent on the type of incontinence. Some medications inhibit contractions of the bladder, others may relax muscles, and some tighten muscles at the bladder neck and urethra.
- Collagen may be injected into the tissue around the urethra to add bulk and help close the urethral opening.

Mechanical Treatment

- *Pessaries*: A stiff ring that is inserted into the vagina, where it helps to reposition the urethra. The pessary may be placed by the patient or by a nurse.
- *External barriers*: Adhere to the urethral opening to stop urine leakage. The barrier is a small foam pad placed over the urethral opening. It seals against the body to keep urine from leaking. It is removed and discarded before the patient voids.
- *Urethral insert*: Small device, like a plug, that fits into the urethra. Removed to void, the insert is replaced until the patient needs to void again.
- *Surgical intervention*: Used as a last resort. Type of surgery depends on cause of incontinence.

Source: Davis, N. J., Wyman, J. F., Gubitosa, S., & Pretty, L. (2020). Urinary incontinence in older adults. *American Journal of Nursing, 120*(1), 57–62; Gill, B. C., Firoozi, F., & Rackley, R. R. (2018, June 20). Injectable bulking agents for incontinence. *Medscape.* https://emedicine.medscape.com/article/447068-overview; Hooper, G. L. (2019). Evaluation and current treatments for urinary incontinence. *The Nurse Practitioner, 44*(6), 21–28; Mayo Foundation for Medical Education and Research (MFMER). (2019a, April 13). Urinary incontinence. https://www.mayoclinic.org/diseases-conditions/urinary-incontinence/diagnosis-treatment/drc-20352814#:~:text=Urethral%20insert%2C%20a%20small%2C%20tampon,vagina%20and%20wear%20all%20day; National Institute of Diabetes and Digestive and Kidney Diseases (NIDDK). (2018b, June). *Urologic diseases. Bladder control problems (Urinary incontinence).* https://www.niddk.nih.gov/health-information/urologic-diseases/bladder-control-problems?dkrd=/health-information/urologic-diseases/bladder-control-problems-women; Pair, L. S., & Somerall, W. E. (2018). Urinary incontinence: Pelvic floor muscle and behavioral training for women. *The Nurse Practitioner, 43*(1), 21–25.

of the skin (Lim & Carville, 2019; Mitchell & Hill, 2020; Voegeli, 2018). Excessive moisture can lead to overhydration (maceration) and disruption to the structure of the outer layers of the skin (Voegeli, 2018). Bacteria on the skin act to break down urea in urine to form highly alkaline ammonia, resulting in a shift of the pH of the skin away from normally slightly acidic, thus increasing the disruption to the protective barrier of the skin (Voegeli, 2018). Penetration by bacteria through damaged skin compounds the inflammatory response (Voegeli, 2018). Incontinence and resulting excessive moisture also contribute to pressure injury formation (Gray & Guiliano, 2018; Jacobson & Wright, 2015; Lachenbruch et al., 2016). Symptoms of IAD include erythema with poorly defined edges located in patches on the skin or continuously over large areas, and the skin may feel warmer and firmer than the surrounding unaffected skin (Beeckman et al., 2015; Francis, 2018). In patients with darker skin tones, skin may appear paler, darker, purple, dark red, or yellow when compared with the surrounding area (Beeckman et al., 2015). Lesions may be present, including vesicles, bullae, papules, or pustules. The epidermis may be damaged to varying depths with patients reporting discomfort, pain, burning, itching, or tingling (Beeckman et al., 2015; Francis, 2018; Jacobson & Wright, 2015). In addition to discomfort and pain, patients may experience loss of independence, alterations in activities and sleep, reduced quality of life, and secondary skin infections (bacterial and fungal) (Beeckman et al., 2015; Voegeli, 2018; Yates, 2018b).

Prevention of incontinence is essential to prevent and treat IAD (Yates, 2018b). Skin care and use of containment products for incontinence are also critical pieces of evidence-based nursing care (Beeckman et al., 2015; Jacobson & Wright, 2015; Voegeli, 2018; Yates, 2018a). Appropriate skin care involves a structured skin care regimen that includes regular skin assessment, skin cleansing, moisturizers or emollients to replenish and restore lipids in the skin, and the use of skin barrier protectants to proactively protect the skin from urine-associated irritation, maceration (overhydration), and breakdown (Southgate & Bradbury, 2016; Yates, 2018a).

Cleansing of the skin should be provided daily and after each episode of incontinence. Prompt attention to incontinence events is necessary to prevent IAD (Phipps et al., 2019). Skin cleansers that are specially designed for at-risk or compromised skin and are pH-balanced should be used; many are no-rinse (Beeckman et al., 2015; Southgate & Bradbury, 2016; Voegeli, 2018; Yates, 2018a). Do not use soap and hot water as soap can irritate or dry the skin, or alter the skin's pH (Yates, 2018b). Avoid rubbing, excessive friction, or scrubbing, as this can damage the skin (Jacobson & Wright, 2015; Southgate & Bradbury, 2016; Yates, 2018a).

38-1 Focused Critical Thinking Guide

URINARY INCONTINENCE

You have been assigned to care for an 80-year-old patient, Mrs. Bartowski, who was admitted with a recurrent leg ulcer and is due to be discharged the following day. Their nursing notes indicate that they have had two or three episodes of urinary incontinence every day while in the hospital and their care plan states, "use adult incontinence briefs." You go into the room to answer Mrs. Bartowski's call bell and help them into the bathroom. They are wearing adult disposable briefs (undergarments), and a half-used package is on the chair. After voiding 150 mL of urine, Mrs. Bartowski tearfully begs, "Please don't put that diaper back on me; I'm not a child." According to their chart, Mrs. Bartowski is mentally alert, lives at home with their daughter who has visited Mrs. Bartowski in the hospital frequently and appears able to identify their need to urinate. You are aware that there are effective alternative therapies to resolve or minimize urinary incontinence rather than relying on absorbent products. However, the nurses have obviously made a decision to use disposable undergarments in this situation. You prefer to leave the disposable undergarments off, try some other measures, and possibly discuss this with the patient's daughter, but as a student nurse, you are here for only 2 days. You want to be a patient advocate and do the right thing. What should you do?

1. Identify goal of thinking

Determine whether it is more important to replace the adult briefs against the patient's wishes or leave it off and discuss the possibility of using behavioral strategies with the staff.

2. Assess adequacy of knowledge

Pertinent circumstances: Mrs. Bartowski is alert and oriented and obviously upset that disposable briefs are being used. They have used the call bell when they feel the urge to urinate, but incontinent episodes have also been documented. The nursing staff has decided that disposable briefs are appropriate for this patient. Mrs. Bartowski's daughter, with whom Mrs. Bartowski lives, appears supportive and attentive. Discharge is scheduled for tomorrow.

Prerequisite knowledge: Before you decide what to do in this situation, you need to discuss your options with your instructor. Of primary importance is whether the patient and their daughter are interested in pursuing alternatives. They can also provide invaluable information about their elimination pattern at home. The health care team must be consulted to determine the etiology of the incontinence and validate that their urinary tract is intact and functioning adequately. You will also need to review the various treatment options for incontinence because these will have to be communicated to the patient and their daughter before discharge.

Room for error/time constraints: Absorbent products can provide a sense of security and are widely used for incontinence. There is, however, the possibility that continence can be restored once incontinence is assessed, recognized, and addressed. Early dependence on absorbent products can remove the motivation to seek treatment and promote acceptance of the condition. The treatment options should be discussed with Mrs. Bartowski and their daughter before discharge tomorrow.

3. Address potential problems

Continuing to use absorbent products offers a temporary solution to the problem. They may protect the patient from embarrassment and provide a sense of security, although they do nothing to prevent incontinent episodes. Explore the patient's feelings regarding the use of these products. The use of these products can communicate expectations of an acceptance of incontinence as an inevitable part of aging, which is not true. Absorbent products can also interfere with the patient's ability to use the toilet independently. Using behavioral techniques to control incontinence will require health teaching before discharge and a long-term commitment to follow-up in the home.

4. Consult helpful resources

The patient's motivation to restore continence is your most valuable resource. The primary nurse or case manager, the primary care provider, and your instructor can also help you sort through your priorities in this situation. The latest research recommends use of behavioral techniques first to treat incontinence.

5. Critique judgment/decision

If you decide to reapply disposable briefs against the patient's wishes, you may, in fact, be supporting the myth that incontinence is inevitable and untreatable and are not providing thoughtful person-centered care. Long-term use of absorbent products can place the patient at risk for skin breakdown and a urinary tract infection if used improperly. You decide to leave the disposable briefs off and establish regular intervals for voiding for the 2 days you will be caring for Mrs. Bartowski. In this short time, you hope to demonstrate to the patient, their daughter, and the staff that it is possible for Mrs. Bartowski to maintain a pattern of continence. Because Mrs.Bartowski will most likely be discharged tomorrow, you also discuss the possibility of referral to community-based care or a continence expert who will instruct, support, and follow through with the necessary components of care. When you discuss your situation at postconference, your clinical group supports your decision.

Limit the use of disposable briefs; incontinence products that wick moisture away from the skin may be used as necessary (Jacobson & Wright, 2015). A skin barrier/protectant should be applied to all skin that comes into contact or may potentially come into contact with urine after cleansing to prevent direct contact with urine and to promote resolution of IAD if present (Beeckman et al., 2015; Yates, 2018b). Products are available that are "all-in-one," ensuring all steps of skin care are implemented and include a disposable soft cloth that contains cleanser, moisturizer, and barrier, for example (Francis, 2018). Patients with complicated IAD that does not respond to treatment with 2 weeks should be referred to an advanced practice wound specialist, such as a wound ostomy continence nurse or dermatologist (Francis, 2018).

External collecting devices may be useful in managing urinary incontinence and therefore minimizing and/or preventing IAD (NIDDK, 2018a; Vasavada et al., 2019a). Refer to the following discussion related to External Urine Collection Devices. Additional information and discussion related to incontinence and skin care can be found in Chapters 32 and 33.

External Urine Collection Devices

External urine collection devices adhere to the external genitalia or pubic area and collect urinary output (Gray et al., 2016; Newman, 2020b). There are single-use disposable devices, intended for use for 1 to 2 days, and some that are reusable for multiple times (Newman, 2020a).

EXTERNAL URINARY SHEATH

When voluntary control of urination is difficult or not possible for patients with a penis, an alternative to an indwelling catheter is the condom-type **urinary sheath**, one type of external urine collection device for use on the penis (Newman, 2020a; Panchisin, 2016; Smart, 2014). This soft, pliable sheath made of silicone or latex material is applied externally to the penis and directs urine away from the body (Fig. 38-8). Most devices are self-adhesive. The external urinary catheter is connected to drainage tubing and a collection bag and can be used with a leg bag (refer to Fig. 38-6 [on page 1458] and the Patient Education discussion later in the chapter).

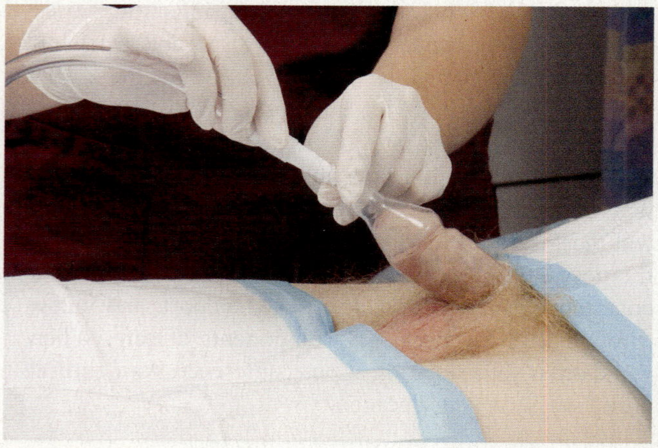

FIGURE 38-8. Urinary sheath applied externally to collect urine.

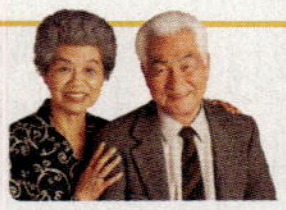

Think back to **Midori Morita**, the person described at the beginning of the chapter who is caring for her husband at home. The nurse might suggest using a urinary sheath for Mr. Morita as a possible intervention to manage his incontinence.

Nursing care of a patient with a urinary sheath includes vigilant skin care to prevent excoriation. Remove the condom daily and wash the penis with soap and water, dry it carefully, and inspect the skin for irritation. In hot and humid weather, more frequent changing may be required. Always follow the manufacturer's instructions for applying the sheath because there are several variations. In all cases, care must be taken to fasten the sheath securely enough to prevent leakage, yet not so tightly as to constrict the blood vessels in the area. When using sheath-type devices, the tip of the tubing should be kept 1 to 2 inches (2.5 to 5 cm) beyond the tip of the penis to prevent irritation to the sensitive glans area. Maintaining free urinary drainage is another nursing priority. Institute measures to prevent the tubing from becoming kinked and urine from backing up in the tubing. Urine can lead to excoriation of the glans; position the tubing that collects the urine from the sheath to draw urine away from the penis.

For some people, the urinary sheath may not be an option because of penis retraction or inadequate length of the penile shaft (Newman, 2020a). For these patients, a non-sheath, glans-adherent device may be appropriate. This external urinary collection device has a hydrocolloid wafer faceplate that attaches to the glans around the meatus to form a seal around the meatus, reducing urine contact with the skin of the penile shaft (Newman, 2020a). An integrated tube attaches to a drainage bag to collect the urine (Newman, 2020a). A male urinary pouch is another option. This is an ostomy-like pouch that holds the penis and has an adhesive skin barrier that secures the device to the pubis (Newman, 2020a). The pouch can then be connected to a drainage bag.

EXTERNAL URINE COLLECTION SYSTEM

When voluntary control of urination is difficult or not possible for patients with female genitalia, an alternative to an indwelling catheter is a female external urine collection device (Beeson & Davis, 2018; Dublynn & Episcopia, 2019; Gentile et al., 2020; Newman, 2020a). Use of this device minimizes the risk for skin injury associated with incontinence and infection associated with an indwelling urinary catheter (Beeson & Davis, 2018; Dublynn & Episcopia, 2019; Gentile et al., 2020). The device consists of a "wick" that conforms to the perineal area between the labia against the urethra (Fig. 38-9B), collection tubing, and a collection canister attached to a pump (Fig. 38-9A). It is connected to low continuous suction providing a sump mechanism to collect and measure urine output. The device also delivers continuous air flow to promote a microclimate environment to the female perineal region (Beeson & Davis, 2018). Patients have reported a sense of cleanliness, increased comfort from remaining dry, and reduced pain and discomfort as a result of less frequent linen changes (Beeson & Davis, 2018). A female urinary pouch is another option. This is an ostomy-like pouch

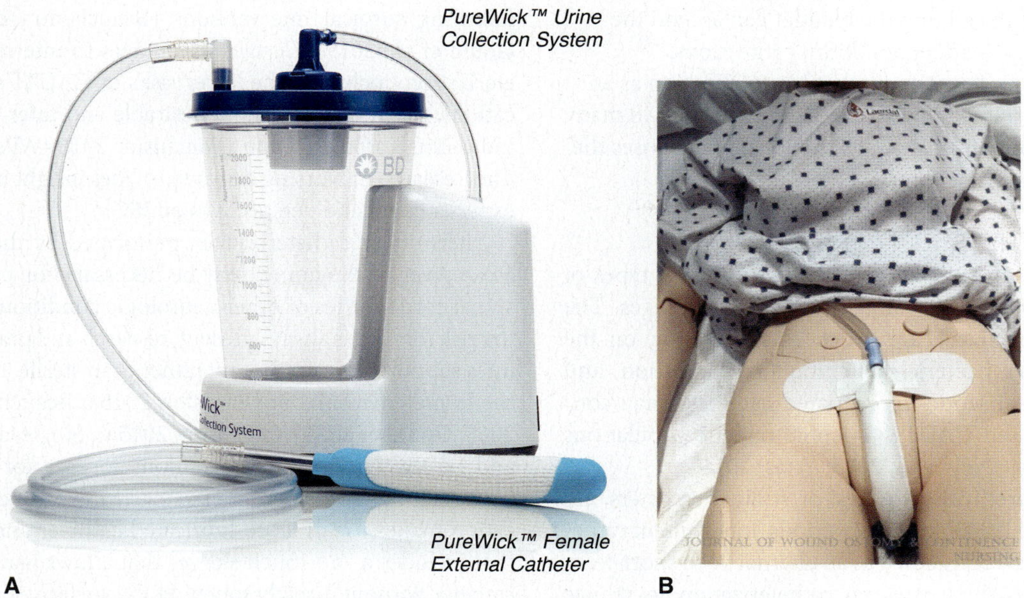

FIGURE 38-9. **A.** External urine collection system (female genitalia). **B.** Device in place, secured to the suprapubic region. **A**, The PureWick™ System includes the PureWick™ Female External Catheter (wick) and the PureWick™ Urine Collection System. © Becton, Dickinson and Company. **B**, Beeson, T., & Davis, C. (2018). Urinary management with an external female collection device. *Journal of Wound, Ostomy and Continence Nursing*, *45*(2), 187–189. Doi: 10.1097/WON.0000000000000417

in which an adhesive skin barrier is cut to fit the vulvar opening and adheres to the labia to secure the pouch in place (Newman, 2020a). The pouch can then be connected to a drainage bag.

Catheterizing the Patient's Bladder

Urinary catheterization is the introduction of a catheter (tube) through the urethra into the bladder for the purpose of withdrawing urine. CAUTIs remain one of the most common causes of health care–associated infections in the United States (Knill et al., 2018). The best way to prevent a CAUTI is to use urinary catheters only when absolutely necessary (American Nurses Association [ANA], n.d.; Panchisin, 2016). The CDC provides parameters to guide the decision to insert an indwelling urinary catheter (Gould et al., 2019). When use of a urinary catheter is deemed necessary, it should be performed using strict aseptic technique, left in place only as long as needed, and removed as soon as possible (ANA, 2014; Gould et al., 2019; Gyesi-Appiah et al., 2020; SUNA, 2015).

APPROPRIATE USE OF URINARY CATHETERIZATION

Appropriate reasons for urinary catheterization include (ANA, 2014; Gould et al., 2019; Meddings et al., 2015):

- Relieving acute urinary retention. Retention is often temporary and is common after surgery involving the lower abdomen, pelvis, bladder, or urethra, especially if ambulation is delayed, fluid intake is minimal, or epidural analgesia is used for pain control. Bladder outlet obstruction, including mechanical obstruction such as swelling at the meatus (which can occur after childbirth), or an enlarged prostate in males may cause retention.
- Some patients who are unable to use any other bladder management method, such as those with neurogenic bladder dysfunction related to a disability (e.g., spinal cord injury) or intractable urinary retention, require long-term use of an indwelling catheter.
- Obtaining a sterile urine specimen when the patient is unable to voluntarily void.
- Accurate measurement of urinary output in critically ill patients.
- Assist in healing open sacral or perineal wounds in incontinent patients.
- Emptying the bladder before, during, or after select surgical procedures and before certain diagnostic examinations.
- Provide improved comfort for end-of-life care.
- Prolonged patient immobilization (potentially unstable thoracic or lumbar spine, multiple traumatic injuries).

Numerous algorithms and decision trees are available to assist nurses in use of best practices and to guide implementation of alternative interventions to an indwelling urinary catheter. Many facilities have adopted plans for standardizing care that outline alternatives to placing a catheter, based on indications for use, allowing nurses to use critical-thinking skills to improve patient safety and outcomes (ANA, 2014; Knill et al., 2018).

RELEVANT CONSIDERATIONS ABOUT THE LOWER URINARY TRACT

When catheterization is planned, consider the following about the lower urinary tract:

- The bladder is normally a sterile cavity.
- The external opening to the urethra can never be sterilized.
- The bladder has defense mechanisms. It empties itself of urine regularly and maintains an acidic environment, which has antibacterial advantages. These help to maintain a sterile bladder under normal circumstances and also help in clearing an infection if it occurs.

- Pathogens introduced into the bladder can ascend the ureters and cause bladder and kidney infections.
- A healthy bladder is not as susceptible to infection as an injured one. A state of lowered resistance, present in many health conditions and stressful situations, predisposes the patient to urinary infection.

TYPES OF CATHETERS

Urinary catheters are available in several different types of materials, with varying advantages and disadvantages. The use of antimicrobial coatings, such as silver alloy, on the catheter to reduce bacterial attachment, colonization, and migration, and antiseptic-impregnated catheters may contribute to decreased CAUTIs in some patient populations (Gould et al., 2019; Newman, 2013; Yates, 2016).

Intermittent urethral catheters, or straight catheters, are used to drain the bladder for short periods. Intermittent catheterization should be considered as an alternative to short-term or long-term indwelling urethral catheterization to reduce CAUTIs (Hooton et al., 2010). Intermittent catheterization is the preferred bladder management method for patients with urinary retention and bladder-emptying dysfunctions and following surgical interventions (Beauchemin et al., 2018; Gould et al., 2019). Certain advantages to intermittent catheterization, including the lower risks of CAUTI and complications, may make it a more desirable and safer option than indwelling catheterization (Panchisin, 2016; Wilson, 2015a). The Research in Nursing display provides insight into patients' experiences of and perspectives on ISC.

Intermittent catheterization, performed by the patient or a caregiver in the home, may be necessary for patients with spinal cord injuries or other neurologic conditions. Although the risk for UTI is always present, research and practice guidelines support the use of clean, rather than sterile, technique in the home environment (Bardsley, 2015a; Beauchemin et al., 2018; Gould et al., 2019; Wilson, 2015a). Single-use catheters and no-touch catheters are options for use for ISC in the home setting (Beauchemin et al., 2018). No-touch catheterization makes use of a pre-lubricated catheter and packaging that includes a "no-touch sleeve" that allows handling of the catheter without directly touching the surface of the catheter (Fig. 38-10) (Gajewski et al., 2017). Due to this construction, no-touch catheterization reduces the risk of external contamination of the catheter, decreasing both the risk for infection

Research in Nursing

BRIDGING THE GAP TO EVIDENCE-BASED PRACTICE

Self-Intermittent Catheterization

Intermittent self-catheterization (ISC) is taught to patients to help reduce complications of incomplete bladder emptying and voiding dysfunction and provides an alternative to the problems associated with indwelling catheterization (Collins, 2019; Lake, 2018). Learning ISC may be challenging, embarrassing, and fear-inducing for a patient and requires lifestyle adjustment and coping mechanisms (Collins, 2019; Logan, 2020). Nurses who have insight into the patient experiences are better equipped to meet patients' needs. What are the experiences of patients using ISC?

Related Research

Goldstine, J., Leece, R., Samas, S., & Zonderland, R. (2019). In their own words. Adults' lived experiences with intermittent catheterization. *Journal of Wound, Ostomy, and Continence Nursing, 46*(6), 513–518. https://doi.org/10.1097/WON.0000000000000591

This qualitative study explored the lived experiences of individuals using ISC to identify themes related to barriers and facilitators to integration of ICS in their daily lives. The sample of 25 adults from five countries had used ISC for at least 1 year and had used at least two different ISC products. Semistructured telephone interviews were conducted to gather information related to participants' reasons for using ISC, details of products in use or used in the past, and problems and/or challenges encountered with ISC products. Participants were also prompted to discuss the frequency and severity of urinary tract infection and ISC-related experiences that had influenced relationships with friends and family, mood and emotions, employment, activities, and other facets of life quality. Interviews were translated and transcribed and then analyzed for themes and subthemes. The researchers derived themes based on information from the transcribed interviews and triangulated selected themes with clinician experts in urology and previously published evidence for practice describing challenges, experiences, and health-related quality of life for ISC users. Analysis revealed nine main themes concerning individuals' lived experiences of ISC: initial fear, urinary tract infection, pain/discomfort, independence, choice, community, life quality, resilience, and acceptance. The researchers concluded that initial resistance to ISC is common, and practical challenges must be overcome. The researchers also concluded that ISC is perceived as a burden by some, but not all, users. The researchers suggested the challenge, and opportunity, for clinicians is to learn more about factors that enhance or hinder successful adaptation to ISC. The researchers suggested clinicians must develop interventions based on these insights as to what has gone right for those who have adapted to enable individuals to integrate ISC into their daily lives.

Relevance to Nursing Practice

The results of this study provide insight into the experiences of patients who use ISC to manage voiding dysfunction. Nurses play an important role in assisting patients with management of ISC. Nurses are in strategic positions to plan interventions to help address the challenges and barriers these patients encounter and to facilitate ISC to assist patients and support their desired quality of life.

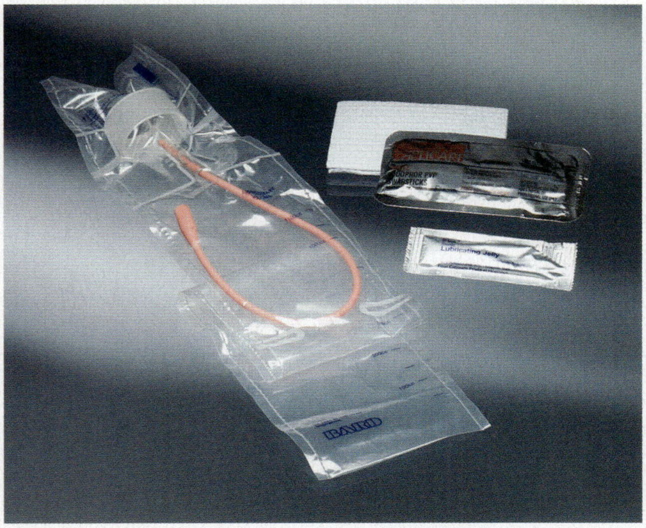

FIGURE 38-10. "No-touch" intermittent urinary catheter. (Courtesy and © Becton, Dickinson and Company)

and the time required to perform the procedure. The past practice of catheter reuse in community settings, instructing patients to wash and reuse the same catheter for multiple catheterizations, is not recommended; no evidence-based guidelines on cleaning or disposing of a reused catheter are available (Beauchemin et al., 2018; Newman, 2019b).

Patients and/or caregivers should be taught to insert and remove intermittent catheters using a clean, nonsterile technique (Collins, 2019; Leach, 2018). The procedure for self-intermittent catheterization is essentially the same as that used by the nurse to catheterize a patient. Initially, a patient with female genitalia may use a mirror to locate the meatus, but eventually they can learn to insert the catheter using just touch. Self-catheterization is recommended at regular intervals to allow the bladder to fill normally before being emptied again and prevent overdistention of the bladder and compromised blood supply to the bladder wall (Beaucheimin et al., 2018). Box 38-6 outlines important information related to ISC.

If a catheter is to remain in place for continuous drainage, an **indwelling urethral catheter** is used. Indwelling catheters are also called retention or Foley catheters. The indwelling urethral catheter is designed so that it does not slip out of the bladder. A balloon is inflated to ensure that the catheter remains in the bladder once it is inserted. Indwelling catheters are used for the gradual decompression of an overdistended bladder, for bladder drainage, and for continuous bladder drainage and irrigation. Several types of indwelling catheters are available, but the principles on which they operate are similar.

The indwelling catheter has more than one lumen (open tube) within the catheter. In a double-lumen catheter, one lumen is connected directly to the balloon, which is inflated with sterile water; the other is the lumen through which the urine drains. The triple-lumen catheter provides an additional lumen for the instillation of irrigating solution. Figure 38-11 on page 1476 illustrates a triple-lumen, double-lumen, and straight (intermittent) catheter. Catheterization using an indwelling urethral catheter is discussed in Skills 38-2 and 38-3 on pages 1493 to 1505.

QSEN EVIDENCE-BASED PRACTICE (EBP)

Urinary catheterization is an intervention that can be associated with many potential adverse effects, including a high risk for catheter-associated infection. Nurses must work to ensure individualized care plans based on patient values, clinical expertise, evidence, and best-practice guidelines related to urinary catheterization.

Box 38-6 Patient Intermittent Self-Catheterization

- Explain the reason for self-catheterization and corresponding health issues related to the need for catheterization.
- Explain the benefits of self-catheterization, including reducing high postvoid residual volumes, reduced risk of urinary tract infection compared to an indwelling urinary catheterization, and improved quality of life.
- Explain potential complications, such as bleeding and the risk of urinary tract infections and what to do if they occur.
- Ensure privacy and dignity.
- Include discussion regarding the frequency of intermittent catheterization and how to incorporate into the patient's usual daily routine.
- Explain the anatomy of the urinary tract, hygiene, and preparation of the catheter.
- Demonstrate how to open, hold, and use the catheter.
- Explain catheterization process, demonstrate process, and observe return demonstration by patient.
- Explore process to obtain supplies and assist with an informed choice of a catheter that suits the patient and their lifestyle.
- Provide information in an appropriate format (such as written materials or video, in appropriate language) to reinforce instruction.
- Allow the patient adequate time to ask questions.
- Provide information about how to recognize a urinary tract infection and other signs/symptoms to report to the health care team.
- Aids are available to help meet the challenges of intermittent self-catheterization for patients with poor eyesight, reduced mobility, and/or reduced manual dexterity.

Source: Adapted from Balhi, S., & Mrabet, M. K. (2020). Teaching patients clean intermittent self-catheterisation: Key points. *British Journal of Community Nursing, 25*(12), 586–593; Bardsley, A. (2015b). Assessing and teaching female intermittent self-catheterization. *British Journal of Community Nursing, 20*(7), 344–346; Collins, L. (2019). Intermittent self-catheterisation: Good patient education and support are key. *British Journal of Nursing, 28*(15), 964–966; Davis, C., & Rantell, A. (2018). Selecting an intermittent self-catheter: Key considerations. *British Journal of Nursing, 27*(15), S11–S16; Hillery, S. (2020). Intermittent self-catheterisation: A person-centred approach. *British Journal of Nursing, 29*(15), 858–860; Leach, D. (2018). Teaching patients a clean intermittent self-catheterisation technique. *British Journal of Nursing, 27*(6), 296–298; Logan, K. (2020). An exploration of men's experiences of learning intermittent self-catheterisation with a silicone catheter. *British Journal of Nursing, 29*(2), 84–90; Mangnall, J. (2015). Managing and teaching intermittent catheterisation. *British Journal of community Nursing, 20*(2), 82–88; and Wilson, M. (2015a). Clean intermittent self-catheterisation: Working with patients. *British Journal of Nursing, 24*(2), 76–85.

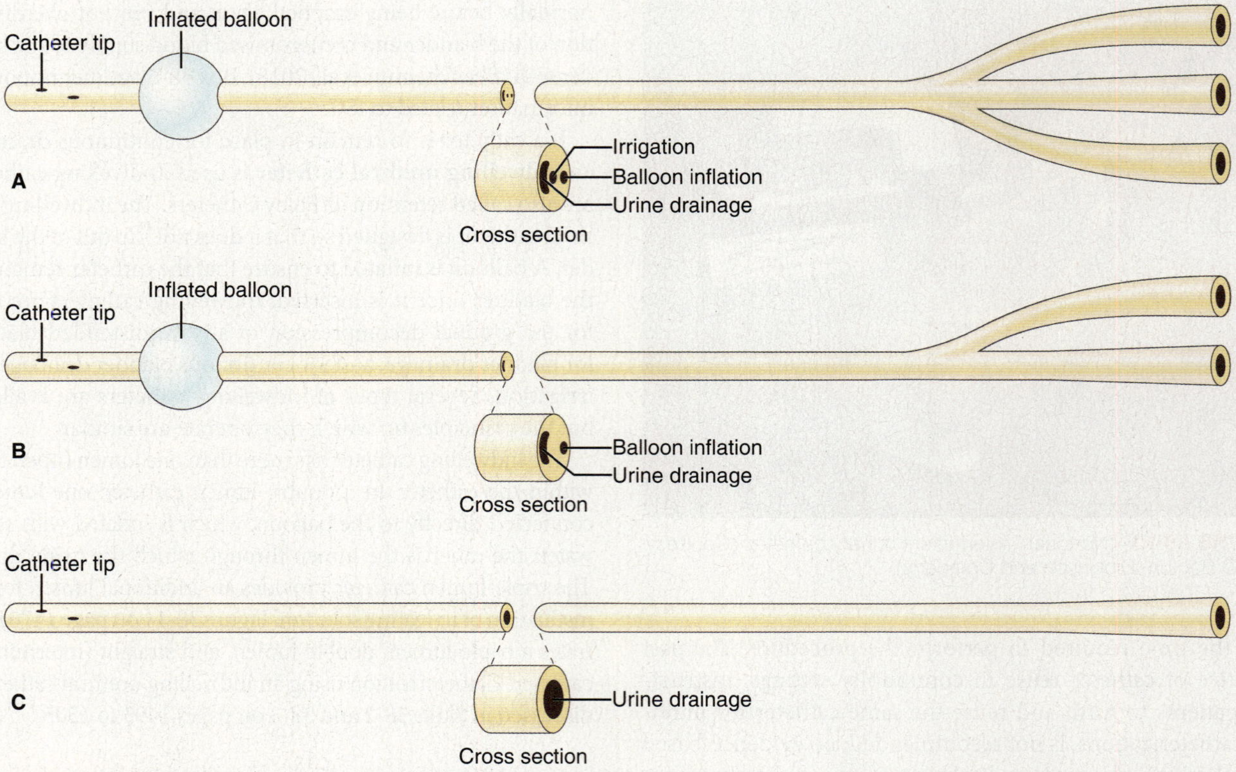

FIGURE 38-11. **A.** Triple-lumen indwelling catheter. **B.** Double-lumen indwelling catheter. **C.** Straight (intermittent) catheter.

A **suprapubic catheter** is an indwelling urinary catheter used for long-term continuous drainage. This type of catheter is inserted surgically through a small incision above the pubic area (Fig. 38-12). Suprapubic bladder drainage diverts urine from the urethra when injury, stricture, prostatic obstruction, or gynecologic or abdominal surgery has compromised the flow of urine through the urethra (Hill & Mitchell, 2018). A suprapubic catheter may be preferred over indwelling urethral catheters for long-term urinary drainage in patients for whom no other alternative is possible (Gibson et al., 2019). Suprapubic catheters are associated with decreased risk of contamination with organisms from fecal material, elimination of damage to the urethra, not interfering with sexual activity, increased comfort for patients with limited mobility, and lower risk of CAUTIs (Buehrle et al., 2020; Gibson et al., 2019; Hooton et al., 2010). The drainage tube may be secured with sutures and should be secured with a catheter fixation device or tape (Holroyd, 2019). Care of the patient with a suprapubic catheter includes skin care around the insertion site; care of the drainage tubing and drainage bag is the same as for an indwelling catheter (see Caring for Patients with an Indwelling Catheter).

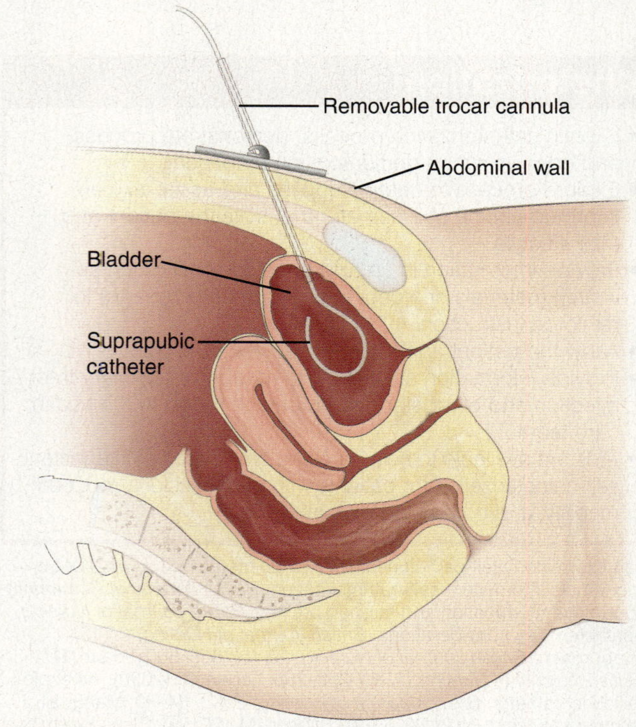

FIGURE 38-12. A suprapubic catheter positioned in the bladder.

CATHETER-ASSOCIATED HARM

UTI, injury, pain and bladder spasm, and sepsis are some of the hazards associated with introducing an instrument such as a catheter into the bladder (Davey, 2015; Fakih et al., 2016; Hill & Mitchell, 2018; Yates, 2017a). The male urethra is especially vulnerable to injury because of its longer length. An object forced through a stricture or an irregular opening from the wrong angle can seriously damage the urethra. Although the female urethra is shorter than the male urethra, it is also susceptible to damage if a catheter is forced through it. The mucous membrane lining the urethra is delicate and damaged easily by the friction resulting from the insertion of a catheter. Bacteria can enter the bladder when the catheter is inserted.

Indwelling catheters are associated with the development of a biofilm, a living layer of bacteria, on the surface of the catheter and drainage system, which may increase the risk of infection; bacteria within biofilms play a role in the development of CAUTI and are a growing concern (Gould et al., 2019; Pelling et al., 2019; Norris, 2020; Sabir et al., 2017). When the catheter is left in place, the organisms may move up the catheter lumen or the space between the catheter and the urethral wall. This asymptomatic condition in which bacteria are present in the urine is known as **bacteriuria**.

EQUIPMENT

The equipment used for catheterization is usually prepackaged in a sterile, disposable tray and is the same for patients with male or female genitalia. Most kits already contain a standard-sized catheter. Catheters are graded on the French (F) scale according to lumen size, with 12 to 16F gauge commonly used (Bardsley, 2015a; Beauchemin et al., 2018; Newman, 2013). The smallest appropriate indwelling urinary catheter that will allow effective drainage should be selected to aid in prevention of CAUTIs in the adult hospitalized patient (ANA, 2014; SUNA, 2021b; Yates, 2017a). A 14F, 5-mL or 10-mL balloon is usually appropriate, unless ordered otherwise (ANA, 2014). Smaller catheters usually are not necessary; a smaller lumen would be so small that it would increase the time necessary for emptying the bladder. Larger catheters distend the urethra and increase the discomfort of the procedure. Large-size catheters (18F or larger) can cause more erosion of the bladder neck and urethral mucosa, cause the formation of strictures, and can cause pain and discomfort (Herter & Wallace Kazer, 2010; Newman, 2013). Sizes 6F to 8F are used for infants and young children; sizes 8F to 12F catheters are commonly used for older children and adolescents (Kyle & Carman, 2021). As mentioned previously, the use of catheters with antimicrobial-coatings has been shown to reduce bacterial colonization and minimize biofilm formation and may be prescribed for use (Gould et al., 2019; Newman, 2013; Yates, 2016).

PATIENT PREPARATION

Before the catheterization, explain the procedure to the patient and the reason for it. Tell the patient that catheter insertion produces a sensation of pressure and some discomfort. Explain that measures will be taken to avoid exposure and embarrassment. The more relaxed the patient is, the easier it will be to insert the catheter.

The most common patient position for catheter insertion is supine with the patient preferably on a solid surface, such as a firm mattress or a treatment table. Catheterizing a patient in a bed with a soft mattress, especially a patient with female genitalia, is not as satisfactory because the patient's pelvic surfaces are not firmly supported, and visualization of the meatus is difficult. Also, the patient may sink into the bed, causing the bladder to be lower than the outlet of the catheter. If the patient is in bed, supporting their buttocks on a firm cushion may be helpful. Patients with female genitalia should lie with their knees bent and legs spread apart (SUNA, 2021a; Yates, 2017b); patients with male genitalia should lie with their legs extended/straight (SUNA, 2021c; Yates, 2017a).

The Sims', or lateral, position is an alternate position for catheter insertion for patients with female genitalia. This position may allow better visualization and be more comfortable for the patient, especially if hip and knee movements are difficult. The smaller area of exposure is also less stressful for the patient. Allow the patient to lie on either side, depending on which position is easiest for the nurse and best for the patient's comfort. Place the patient's buttocks near the edge of the bed with their shoulders at the opposite edge and their knees drawn toward their chest. Lift the upper buttock and labia to expose the urinary meatus (Fig. 38-13).

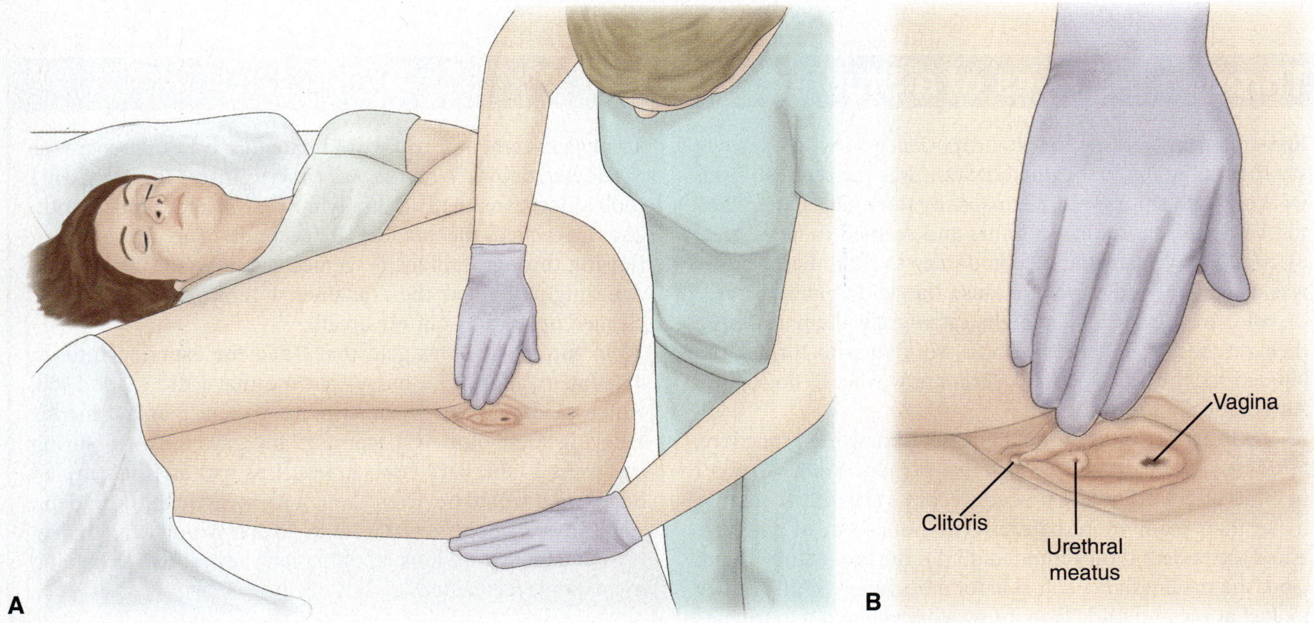

FIGURE 38-13. Demonstration of the side-lying position **(A)** and of how to expose the urinary meatus when catheterizing a patient with female genitalia in the side-lying position **(B)**.

URETHRAL CATHETER INSERTION

Nurses are often responsible for performing urinary catheterization, inserting indwelling catheters and caring for the patient with a catheter. Skill 38-2 (on pages 1493–1499) describes catheterization of the urinary bladder of a patient with female genitalia, and Skill 38-3 (on pages 1500–1505) describes catheterization of the urinary bladder of a patient with male genitalia. Some facilities have adopted a two-person urinary catheter insertion protocol, in which one nurse catheterizes the patient and one observes to ensure that the nurse inserting the catheter follows sterile technique and performs the procedure correctly (Belizario, 2015; Rhone et al., 2017). Implementation of the two-person urinary catheter insertion protocol has been shown to decrease CAUTI (Belizario, 2015; Fletcher-Gutowski & Cecil, 2019; Rhone et al., 2017).

Adhering to surgical asepsis is of utmost importance to help prevent UTIs. An inflated balloon holds the indwelling catheter in position in the bladder. The prefilled syringe included in the catheter kit contains the amount of sterile water needed to inflate the balloon to the desired spherical shape. It is important to use the entire amount provided by the manufacturer to avoid underinflation of the catheter balloon. A balloon that is only partially inflated could cause irritation and erosion to the mucosa in the bladder.

Some institutions' policies/procedures identify use of anesthetic gel should be considered before insertion of the catheter if it is the patient's first catheterization, or if a difficult catheterization is anticipated (SUNA, 2021a; SUNA, 2021d). Check for patient allergy before use of anesthetic gel and allow at least 5 minutes after administration before catheterization to ensure sufficient anesthetic effect (Yates, 2017b).

Properly secure an indwelling catheter to the thigh or abdomen to prevent movement and excessive force on the bladder neck or urethra, which leads to irritation or injury (Holroyd, 2019; SUNA, 2015; Yates, 2016). The indwelling catheter is connected to a drainage and collection system that must be properly positioned and secured to minimize the risk for infection (refer to Fig. 38-6 [on page 1458] for examples of urine collection bags). The following techniques should be used to complete the closed urinary drainage system:

- Maintain a constant downward flow of urine. Check tubing frequently to ensure kinks and dependent loops (low points) are not present in the tubing (ANA, 2014; Gould et al., 2019; Wuthier et al., 2016). Check to see that the patient is not lying on the drainage tubing and compressing it.
- Keep the catheter drainage bag below the level of the bladder at all times (ANA, 2014; Gould et al., 2019).
- Keep the drainage bag off the floor at all times to reduce the risk of infection (ANA, 2014; Gould et al., 2019). The floor is grossly contaminated.
- Check that all connections are secure, and that no leakage is occurring.
- Maintain the closed drainage system (Gould et al, 2017).

See the accompanying Through the Eyes of a Student for a student's account of their experience with urinary catheterization.

CARING FOR PATIENTS WITH AN INDWELLING CATHETER

The following are important nursing measures used to care for patients with an indwelling catheter:

- Wash hands before and after caring for the patient.
- Use mild soap and water or a perineal cleanser to clean the perineal area thoroughly, especially around the meatus, daily and after each bowel movement. Rinse the area well. Do not use powders and lotions after cleaning. Do not use antibiotic or other antimicrobial cleaners or betadine at the urethral meatus (Gould et al., 2019; Herter & Wallace Kazer, 2010).

Through the Eyes of a Student

Remembering my first hospital experiences, I would have to say that doing my first catheterization was the scariest. I was working with a nurse on the maternity floor. Our patient had not voided in more than 8 hours and seemed to be in great discomfort. We palpated their abdomen to see if their bladder was distended, and it was. Because they didn't have an urge to void, we decided to straight catheterize them to lessen their discomfort. The nurse I was working with turned and handed me the kit. They said, "You know what to do, right?" Automatically I replied, "Sure."

My heart began to race. Of course, I knew the procedure, but I never actually did it on a real person. Not only was I nervous about doing the procedure, but I also didn't want to make their labor more painful. The nurse, out of courtesy, asked the patient if they minded if I did the procedure. Thank God, the patient had a soft side for a beginner. Smiling, they looked at me and said, "You know what you're doing, right?" Again, I said, "Sure." I began setting up to start the procedure. To my amazement, I really did remember how to prepare for a catheterization. When it was time to insert the catheter, I took a deep breath. Thankfully, it went in nice and smooth, and I reached the bladder in seconds. The urine began flowing through rapidly. It seemed like it would never stop. Amazingly, it filled the container. I removed the catheter, cleaned up, and let out my breath.

In summary, I was glad that I had the experience to do a catheterization. The nurse told me that I did a good job, which made me feel good. Also, my patient thanked me for relieving some of their discomfort and gave me a reassuring smile. As I look back now, it wasn't as bad as I had myself believing it would be. Even though it's invasive to the patient, sometimes it's necessary. I want to do everything I can to help my patients. Now, I look at all my new adventures as helping my patients feel better.

—Alysia Paxson, Holy Family College, Philadelphia

- Cleanse the catheter by cleaning gently from the meatus outward.
- Make sure that the patient maintains a generous fluid intake, unless contraindicated by other health concerns. This helps prevent infection and irrigates the catheter naturally by increasing urine output.
- Encourage the patient to be up and about, as ordered.
- Note the volume and character of urine, and record observations carefully. Observe the urine through the drainage tubing and in the collection container. Note and record the amount of urine on the patient's intake-and-output record every 8 hours. The collection container is calibrated, but the volume markings are only approximations. Empty the urine into a graduated container that is calibrated accurately for correct determination of output.
- Do not open the drainage system to obtain urine specimens or to measure urine. If the tubing becomes disconnected and the sterile closed drainage system has been compromised, replace the catheter and collecting system (ANA, 2014; SUNA, 2015). When emptying the drainage bag, make sure the drainage spout does not touch a contaminated surface.
- Teach the patient the importance of personal hygiene—especially the importance of careful cleaning after having a bowel movement—and thorough, frequent hand hygiene.
- Promptly communicate any signs or symptoms of infection. These include a burning sensation and irritation at the meatus, cloudy urine, a strong odor to the urine, an elevated temperature, and chills.
- Help the patient take a shower for personal hygiene if possible. Remember to keep the collecting bag lower than the bladder to promote drainage.
- Consider evidence-based practice guidelines and facility policy to ensure that the catheter is removed at the earliest time possible, to limit use to the shortest duration possible (ANA, 2014; Gould et al., 2019; SUNA, 2015).
- Change indwelling catheters only as necessary. The interval between catheter changes varies and should be individualized for the patient, based on clinical symptoms: catheter encrustations, obstruction, leakage, bleeding, and CAUTIs (Gould et al., 2019; Herter & Wallace Kazer, 2010; Palka, 2014; SUNA, 2015).
- Patients who require long-term use of an indwelling catheter may experience self-care practice and catheter challenges. Patients need educational interventions to address fluid intake, bowel management, hygiene, and self-monitoring/management, including potential adverse events (Alex et al., 2020).

PATIENT EDUCATION

Teach patients who have an indwelling catheter how the system functions and how to care for the catheter and drainage system. Teaching points include keeping the tubing free of kinks, maintaining a constant downward flow of urine, maintaining an adequate fluid intake, and promptly reporting any unusual symptoms (Hill & Mitchell, 2018).

Several different urinary drainage systems are available. Nurses need to understand the options in order to provide appropriate patient teaching and support informed patient choice when selecting a drainage option (Yates, 2016). Closed drainage systems include a large, 2-L drainage bag (discussed in previous sections); a smaller drainage bag that can be secured to the leg (leg bag) that is not considered a closed system because of the need to regularly open the leg bag for drainage and connect to an overnight drainage bag (Newman, 2013); or a catheter valve (discussed below). Instruct patients to do the following when handling the drainage system:

- Reinforce the importance of hand hygiene, particularly before and after handling the catheter system, emptying the drainage bag, and personal hygiene.
- Secure the drainage bag below the level of the bladder.
- Empty the leg bag at regular intervals, to allow the bag to become no more than half to two thirds full (Shah, 2019b; Wilson, 2015b). A full drainage bag may cause reflux of urine into the bladder (bags that are not anti-reflux) or may pull away from its attachment on the leg. Use an antiseptic solution to cleanse the bag outlet before and after emptying or changing from a leg bag to a larger overnight drainage bag (Shah, 2019b; SUNA, 2015; Wilson, 2015b).
- Many leg bag systems have a silicone tube attachment that allows for a secure connection between the outlet and to a larger night urine collection bag (Newman, 2013; Yates, 2016).
- Drainage bags should be cleaned between uses according to the manufacturer's recommendations; suggested cleaning solutions vary and include dilute white vinegar or bleach solution (Bradley et al., 2018; Shah, 2019b).
- Leg bags should be changed in accordance with the manufacturer's recommendations; suggested replacement for reusable drainage bags varies from every 5 to 7 days (Wilson, 2015b; Yates, 2016) to every 15 to 30 days (Newman, 2013; Shah, 2019b).
- Leg bags can be used with indwelling urinary catheters, suprapubic catheters, and external urine collection devices.

CATHETER VALVES

Catheter valves are an alternative to use of a large urinary drainage or leg bag (Wilson, 2015b; Yates, 2016). A catheter valve is a small device like an outlet valve on a urine drainage bag that is inserted into the end of an indwelling catheter (Carr, 2019). These valves are used in place of a drainage bag with an indwelling urethral or suprapubic catheter. Urine continues to collect in the bladder instead of a drainage bag. The patient opens the valve to release urine every 3 to 4 hours (Yates, 2017c). Use of a catheter valve promotes bladder health and keeps function as normal as possible, reduces the risk for bladder neck and urethra trauma, and possibly reduces the buildup of biofilm and infection (Carr, 2019). Catheter valves also promote improved patient privacy and dignity, and may be more comfortable for patients (Carr, 2019; Yates, 2016). However, catheter valves may not be appropriate for use by patients with low bladder capacity, detrusor muscle overactivity, reduced sensation of bladder fullness, poor manual dexterity, or with alterations in cognitive function (Carr, 2019; Wilson, 2015b; Yates, 2016). Catheter valves should be changed every 5 to 7 days (Yates, 2017c). The same patient teaching points discussed related to drainage bags and leg bags are relevant to the changing of a catheter valve, as discussed in the previous section (Yates, 2016).

IRRIGATING THE INDWELLING CATHETER

The flushing of a tube, canal, or area with solution is called irrigation. Natural irrigation of the catheter through increased fluid intake by the patient is preferred. The purpose of an external catheter irrigation is to restore or maintain its patency. A bladder irrigation rinses out the bladder and can also instill medication that acts directly on the bladder wall. Routine intermittent irrigation of long-term catheters is not recommended (Gould et al., 2019). Unless obstruction is anticipated, as might occur with bleeding after prostatic or bladder surgery, bladder irrigation is not recommended (Gould et al., 2019; SUNA, 2015). Irrigations might also be used to instill medications that will act directly on the bladder wall. Irrigating a catheter through a closed system is preferred to opening the catheter because opening the catheter could lead to contamination and infection (Gould et al., 2019). Closed-system irrigation via a triple-lumen catheter is suggested to prevent obstruction and maintain a closed system and is recommended to prevent the introduction of pathogens into the bladder (Fig. 38-14) (Gould et al., 2019).

REMOVING THE INDWELLING CATHETER

The removal of an indwelling catheter and the aftercare of the patient should include the following nursing measures:

- Perform hand hygiene before and after the procedure, and wear gloves.
- Check the health record to see how much water was used to inflate the catheter balloon (Yates, 2017d). Empty the catheter drainage bag, taking the time to ensure any urine in the tubing drains into the bag.
- Remove the catheter fixation device. Place a waterproof drape under the catheter where it enters the patient. Deflate the balloon before attempting to remove the catheter by inserting a syringe into the balloon inflation port to remove the same volume of water. Allow the pressure within the balloon to force the syringe plunger back and fill the syringe with water; do not pull on the plunger of the syringe (Yates, 2017d). Do not cut the tubing with scissors.
- Ask the patient to take several deep breaths to relax; ask the patient to exhale, and gently remove the catheter during exhalation (Yates, 2017d). Wrap the catheter in a towel or disposable waterproof drape. Dispose of catheter and drainage system according to facility policy.
- Clean the perineal area after the catheter is removed.
- Ensure that the patient's fluid intake is generous and record the patient's fluid intake as well as time and amount of fluid output for at least 24 hours (or according to facility policy) following catheter removal.
- Instruct the patient to void into a bedpan, urinal, or specimen hat, either in bed or in the bathroom.

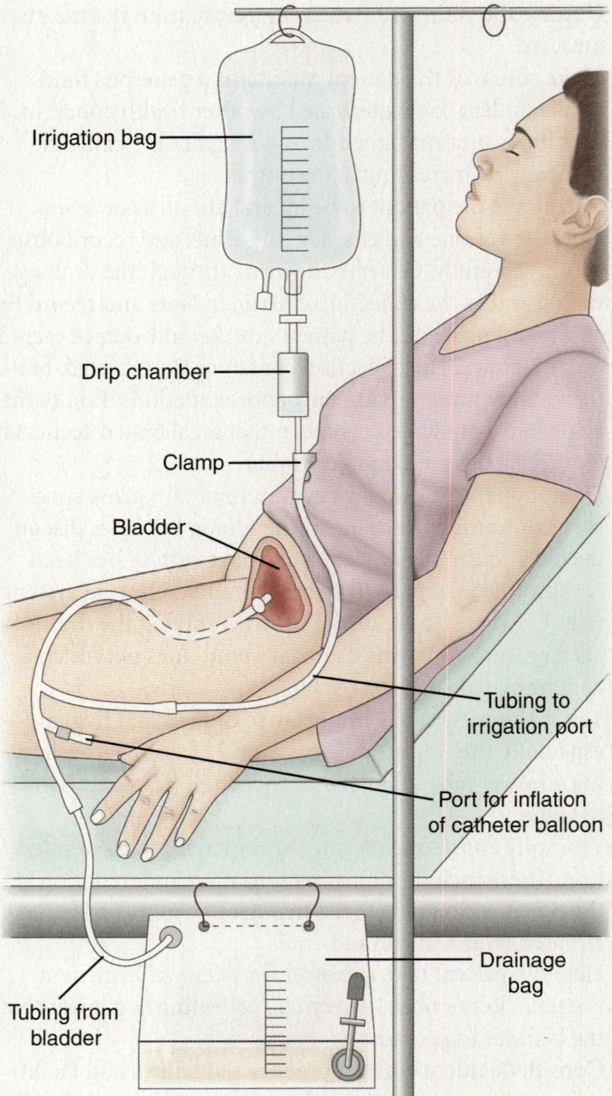

FIGURE 38-14. A continuous bladder irrigation (CBI) setup.

- Inform the patient that it may take a little while for the bladder to reestablish voluntary control and that an accident at this time is not unusual.
- Tell the patient that there may be a slight burning sensation or discomfort when voiding the first time or two after catheter removal as well as urgency and/or frequency.
- If the catheter was in place for more than a few days, decreased bladder muscle tone and swelling of the urethra may cause the patient to experience difficulty voiding or an inability to void. Monitor the patient for urinary retention.
- Check facility policy regarding the length of time the patient is allowed to accomplish successful voiding after catheter removal. If patient does not void within 8 to 10 hours of removal of the indwelling catheter (or timing according to facility policy), notify the health care team.
- Observe the urine carefully for any abnormalities. Document the volume of the first void to validate adequate emptying of the bladder post removal.

- Record and communicate any unusual signs or symptoms, such as discomfort, a burning sensation when voiding, bleeding, or changes in vital signs, especially the patient's temperature. Be alert to any signs or symptoms of infection and communicate them promptly.

Caring for a Patient With a Urologic Stent

Urologic stents are thin, soft hollow tubes inserted into the urinary system to provide drainage of the upper urinary tract, when obstruction of the ureter is present or anticipated (Beysens & Tailly, 2018). Stents are implemented as part of many urologic interventions, such as to facilitate healing after removal of renal calculi and prevent swelling of the ureter, and to facilitate drainage and flow of urine from the kidney to the bladder in the presence of ureteral stricture or obstruction related to cancer or renal calculi (Badawy et al., 2019). The stent may be temporary (e.g., when placed in the ureters) (Fig. 38-15) or permanent (when positioned in the urethra). Temporary stents are usually made of a pliable material such as radiopaque silicone or polyurethane. Permanent stents are stronger and typically are made of a flexible metal mesh. Stents may be placed during surgery or cystoscopy.

Nursing responsibilities for patients with urologic stents include monitoring urine output, including color, consistency, and odor of the urinary output; monitoring for signs of infection or bleeding; and monitoring for decreased urine output, which could indicate obstruction of the stent. The stent could become obstructed because of bleeding or sediment. Obstruction of the stent may result in hydronephrosis (swelling of the kidney) and kidney damage and must be addressed immediately. Never irrigate a stent. If the stent has been brought to the surface of the skin, it is secured to maintain its position (Bauldoff et al., 2020). Instruct the patient with a urologic stent to maintain sufficient fluid intake to maintain adequate urine output. Patients should understand the need to notify the health care team immediately if the urine becomes bright red, severe pain occurs, the drainage pattern changes, or any sign of infection is present. Encourage the patient to wear a medical alert bracelet identifying the presence of a urologic stent at all times.

Caring for a Patient With a Urinary Diversion

Obstructions or tumors in the urinary tract may require some patients to have urinary flow diverted surgically. Urinary diversions may also be used as part of the treatment for patients with a neurogenic bladder, radiation cystitis, or congenital anomalies of the lower urinary tract. An ileal conduit is a type of incontinent cutaneous urinary diversion. An **ileal conduit** (also known as a urostomy) is the most common type of incontinent cutaneous urinary diversion (Berti-Hearn & Elliott, 2019; Goldberg et al., 2018). An ileal conduit involves a surgical resection of the small intestine, with transplantation of the ureters to the isolated segment of small bowel. This separated section of the small intestine is then brought to the abdominal wall, where urine is excreted through a stoma, a surgically created opening on the body surface. Figure 38-16 shows how the ureters are diverted in an ileal conduit. A **cutaneous ureterostomy** is another type of incontinent cutaneous urinary diversion in which the ureters are directed through the abdominal wall and attached to

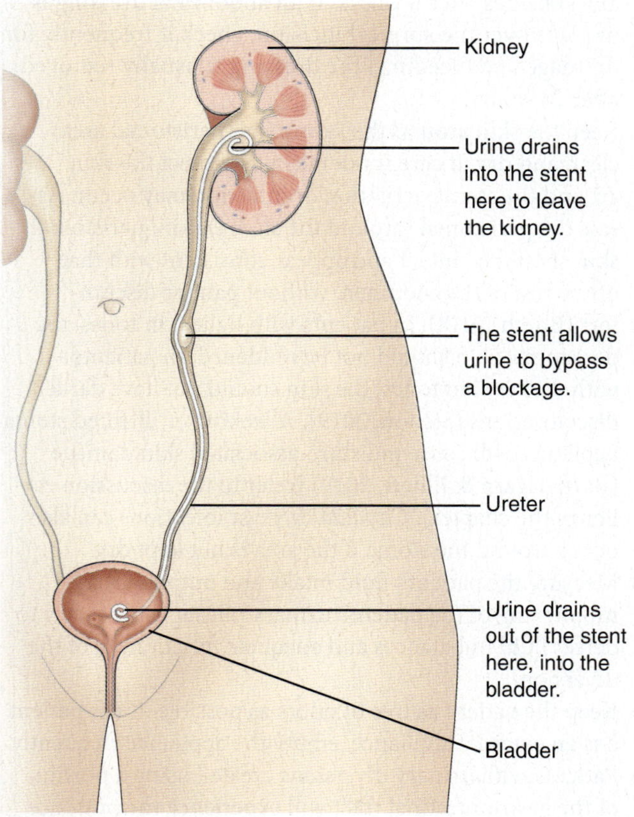

FIGURE 38-15. Ureteral stent.

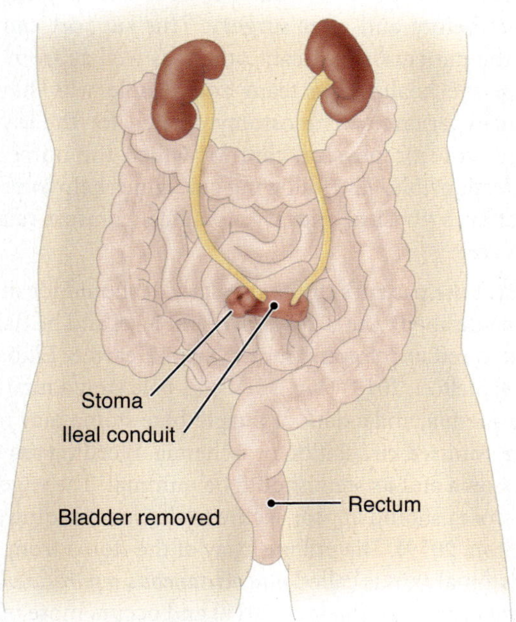

FIGURE 38-16. An ileal conduit. The ureters are brought to the separated segment of the ileum of the small intestine and a stoma is made where the urine is excreted.

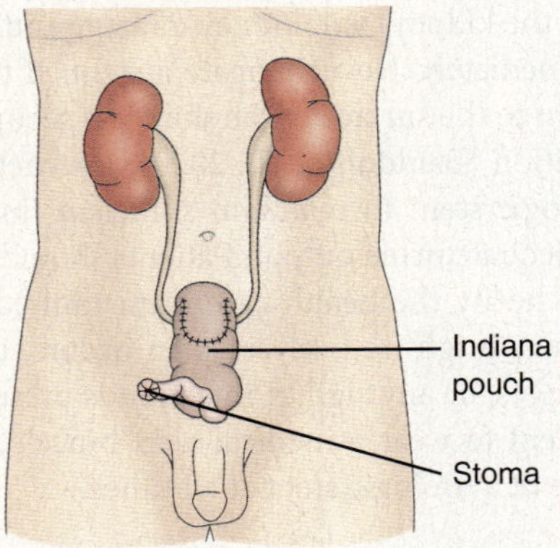

FIGURE 38-17. An Indiana pouch. The ureters are diverted into a segment of ileum and cecum to create an internal reservoir that holds urine and a catheterizable stoma. (*Source:* Reprinted with permission from Hinkle, J. L., Cheever, K. H., and Overbaugh, K. J. [2022]. *Brunner & Suddarth's textbook of medical–surgical nursing* [15th ed.]. Wolters Kluwer.)

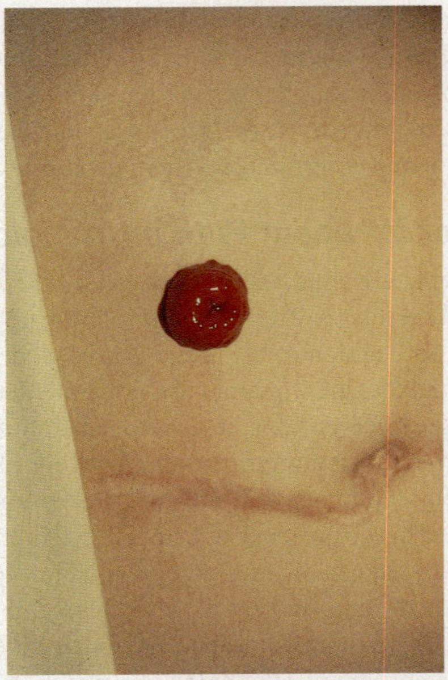

FIGURE 38-18. The appearance of a normal stoma is red and smooth, with a mucous membrane surface.

an opening in the skin. These cutaneous diversions are usually permanent, and the patient wears an external appliance to collect the urine because elimination of the urine from the stoma cannot be controlled voluntarily.

Another option for diversion of urine is a **continent urinary diversion (CUD)** (e.g., the Indiana pouch and the Kock pouch). Figure 38-17 shows how the ureters are diverted into a segment of ileum and cecum in an Indiana pouch. This is a surgical alternative that uses a section of the intestine to create an internal reservoir that holds urine, with the creation of a catheterizable stoma. The external stoma or outlet must be catheterized at regular intervals to drain the urine that has collected in this reservoir.

GENERAL CARE GUIDELINES

Creation of a urinary diversion is a surgical procedure. Therefore, the patient needs physical and psychological support before and after surgery. This support can come from the patient's significant others as well as from members of the health care team and people who have had similar experiences. The ostomy created for the diversion requires specific physical care for which the nurse is initially responsible. The following guidelines help to promote the patient's physical and psychological comfort related to stoma care:

- Inspect the patient's stoma regularly. It should ideally protrude about 1 to 3 cm above skin level and be dark pink to red in color and moist (Berti-Hearn & Elliott, 2019; Stelton, 2019) (Fig. 38-18). A pale stoma may indicate anemia, and a dark or purple-blue stoma may reflect compromised circulation or ischemia. Bleeding around the stoma and its stem should be minimal. The edges of the stoma should appear secure to the surrounding skin (Stelton, 2019). The pulling away of the stoma from the peristomal skin is called *mucocutaneous separation* or *stoma dehiscence* (Stelton, 2019) and occurs more often in patients who are at risk for impaired healing, including patients with diabetes, poor nutritional status or who received high-dose steroid therapy or chemotherapy before surgery (Butler, 2009). Notify the health care team promptly if bleeding persists or is excessive, if color changes occur in the stoma, or if it appears the stoma is separating from the peristomal skin (Stelton, 2019).
- Note the size of the stoma, which usually stabilizes within 6 to 8 weeks (Stelton, 2019). Most stomas protrude 1/2 to 1 inch from the abdominal surface and may initially appear swollen and edematous. The edema usually subsides after 6 weeks. If an abdominal dressing is in place over the surgical incision, check it frequently for drainage and bleeding. The dressing is usually removed after 24 hours.
- Keep the skin around the stoma site (peristomal area) clean and dry. If care is not taken to protect the skin around the stoma, irritation or infection may occur. Assess the peristomal (around the stoma) skin; peristomal skin should be intact and appear consistent with that of the rest of the abdomen, without pain or discomfort (Burch, 2018). In patients with light skin tones, the peristomal skin should not be reddened; in patients with darker skin tones, the skin should not have darker discolorations (Stelton, 2019). A leaking or ill-fitted stoma appliance will cause moisture-associated skin damage (Berti-Hearn & Elliott, 2019) (refer to the discussion earlier in the chapter). *Candida* or yeast infections can also occur around the stoma if the area is not kept dry.
- Measure the patient's fluid intake and output. Careful monitoring of the patient's urinary output is necessary to detect fluid imbalances and adequate functioning of the diversion.
- Keep the patient as free of odors as possible. If the patient has an external appliance, empty the appliance frequently.
- Patients with urinary diversions created using a portion of the gastrointestinal tract will experience the presence of mucus in the urine (Berti-Hearn & Elliott, 2019). The

segment of the gastrointestinal tract continues to produce mucus as part of its normal functioning. This mucus production will decrease over time and is usually not a problem for patients with an ileal conduit (Berti-Hearn & Elliott, 2019). Mucus may be a problem for patients with a continent urinary diversion; mucus retention in the pouch can block the catheter used to empty the pouch. Working with an enterostomal nurse, these patients are taught to irrigate the pouch with normal saline solution using clean technique to clear mucus from the continent urinary diversion (NIDDK, 2020).

- Monitor the return of intestinal function and peristalsis. Initially after surgery, peristalsis is inhibited. Remember, patients with urinary diversions created using a portion of the gastrointestinal tract had a bowel resection as part of the procedure.
- Encourage the patient to participate in care and to look at the stoma. Patients normally experience emotional depression during the early postoperative period. Help the patient to cope by listening, explaining, and being available and supportive. A visit from a representative of the local ostomy support group may be helpful. Patients usually begin to accept their altered body image when they are willing to look at the stoma, make neutral or positive statements concerning the ostomy, and express interest in learning self-care.
- Provide support for the patient's physical, psychological, and social activities. Coping strategies must address body image concerns, permanent body changes, and the underlying health issue(s) that resulted in the surgery (Berti-Hearn & Elliott, 2019; Díaz et al., 2018). Encourage patients and their partners/families/caregivers to discuss concerns and to seek help and support (Berti-Hearn & Elliott, 2019; Chandler, 2020; Hill, 2020).

EXTERNAL APPLIANCES

The external appliance to collect the urine for patients with incontinent urinary diversions is typically a soft pouch that is either reusable or disposable. The upper part of the pouch has a firm faceplate several inches in diameter, with an opening the size of the stoma. Some faceplates are detachable from the pouch, while other appliances are one piece (Fig. 38-19). The plate surface is secured firmly around the stoma opening with a moisture-proof adherent so that no urine leakage occurs. Many patients also wear a supportive accessory, such as an elasticized belt that goes around the waist and connects to each side of the faceplate, for added support (Bird et al, 2019; Goldberg et al., 2018). The lower end of the appliance has a drainage valve, which is used for emptying.

The patient needs to empty the appliance frequently, when it is 1/3 to 1/2 full (Berti-Hearn & Elliott, 2019). This is to prevent the pouch from becoming heavy with the weight of urine, causing tension on the faceplate, and possibly loosening the seal, leading to leakage or a decrease in appliance wear time (Berti-Hearn & Elliott, 2019). For most people, this means emptying the appliance several times a day. The pouch can also be attached to drainage tubing and a large collection bag to avoid having to frequently empty the appliance, such as during the night or when confined to bed. In home situations, urine collection tubing and receptacles designed to be placed under the bed can be used at night.

How frequently the appliance should be changed depends on the type being used and specific patient circumstances, but usually every 3 to 7 days (American Cancer Society, 2019; Berti-Hearn & Elliott, 2019; O'Flynn, 2018; Stelton, 2019). The appliance usually is changed after a time of low fluid intake, such as in the early morning. Urine production is less at this time, making changing the appliance easier. Skill 38-4 (on pages 1505–1509) describes how to change an appliance worn over an incontinent urinary diversion.

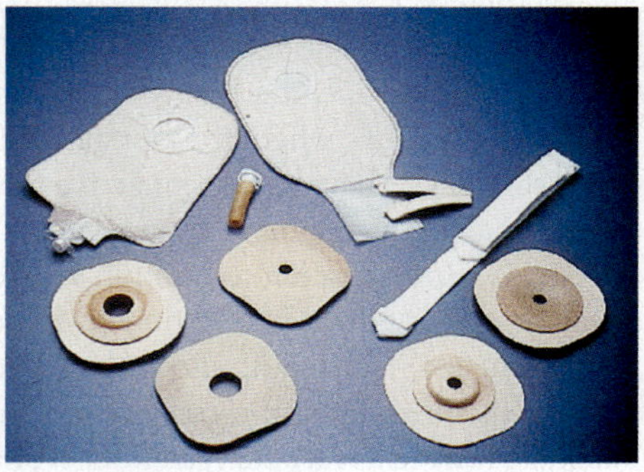

Two-piece pouches

FIGURE 38-19. Two-piece appliances.

PATIENT EDUCATION

Patient teaching is one of the most important aspects of care and should include family members or others identified by the patient when appropriate. Patient education is essential for independence in self-care. Teaching can begin before surgery so that the patient has adequate time to absorb information.

Explain each aspect of care to the patient and what the patient's role will be when beginning self-care. As the patient assumes responsibility for self-care, teach the patient how to make the necessary observations, to be aware of indications of problems, and to recognize when to seek assistance. For these goals to be met, the patient and/or family member/caregivers should be able to:

- Explain the reason for the urinary diversion and the rationale for treatment.
- Identify situations/symptoms that require immediate reporting to the health care provider: the stoma darkens in color or causes unremitting pain; no urine comes from the stoma; or bloating, nausea, vomiting, or loss of appetite occur (Goldberg et al., 2018).
- Demonstrate self-care behaviors that effectively manage the diversion.
- Describe follow-up care and existing support resources.
- Report where supplies may be obtained in the community.
- Verbalize related fears and concerns.
- Demonstrate a positive body image.

The assistance of a wound, ostomy, and continence nurse (WOCN) can help the patient achieve these outcomes (Goldberg et al., 2018; Palmer, 2020). Refer the patient to an outpatient ostomy clinic or a home health care agency to access an ostomy nurse specialist (Goldberg et al., 2018). Refer the patient to a support group or organization like the United Ostomy Associations of America (http://www.ostomy.org/Home.html) for further information, resources, advocacy, and support.

Caring for a Patient Receiving Dialysis

Dialysis is used to treat patients who experience severely decreased or total loss of kidney function. Dialysis is a mechanical way of filtering waste products and excess electrolytes from the blood. There are two categories of dialysis: hemodialysis and peritoneal dialysis.

Hemodialysis involves a machine that does the work healthy kidneys normally perform by filtering harmful wastes, electrolytes, and fluid from the blood that would normally be eliminated in the patient's urine (Fig. 38-20). Patients receive a vascular access in order to receive hemodialysis. This vascular access, an arteriovenous (AV) fistula (a surgically created connection between an artery and a vein; Fig. 38-21A) or AV graft (a surgically created path between an artery and a vein using a flexible, synthetic tube; Fig. 38-21B), allows for access to the bloodstream. A temporary or permanent double-lumen central venous catheter can also be used to provide vascular access for hemodialysis (American Nephrology Nurses Association [ANNA], 2018). These vascular accesses are the point at which blood is removed from the patient's body for dialysis and then returned. The access allows the patient's blood to travel to the hemodialysis machine, which has a semipermeable membrane that filters the blood through diffusion, osmosis, and ultrafiltration (Hinkle et al., 2022). Toxins, wastes, and extra fluid are removed before the blood is returned to the patient (ANNA, 2018).

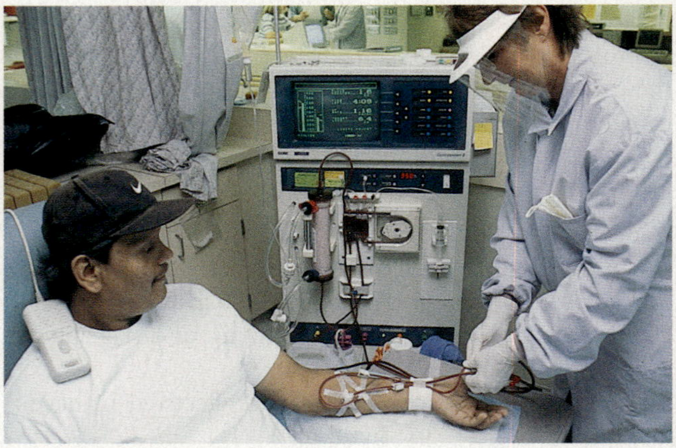

FIGURE 38-20. During hemodialysis, a machine does the work of the kidneys to filter wastes, electrolytes, and fluid from the body. (*Source:* Reprinted with permission from Craven, R., & Hirnle, C. [2017]. *Fundamentals of nursing: Human health and function* [8th ed.]. Wolters Kluwer.)

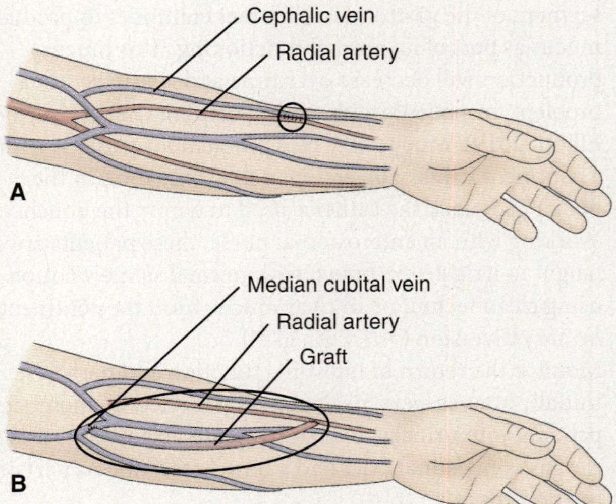

FIGURE 38-21. **A.** Arteriovenous fistula, created by connecting an artery and vein. **B.** Arteriovenous graft created by using a synthetic tube to form a path between an artery and vein. (*Source:* Reprinted with permission from Hinkle, J. L., Cheever, K. H., & Overbaugh, K. J. [2022]. *Brunner & Suddarth's textbook of medical surgical nursing* [15th ed.]. Wolters Kluwer.)

Peritoneal dialysis involves using blood vessels in the abdominal lining (peritoneum) to fill in for the kidneys, with the help of a fluid (dialysate) washed in and out of the peritoneal space. Diffusion and osmosis occur as waste products move from an area of higher concentration (the blood stream) to an area of lesser concentration (the dialysate fluid) through the peritoneum (Hinkle et al., 2022). Patients receive a catheter (a thin, soft, silicone rubber tube) surgically placed through the abdomen into the peritoneal cavity (Fig. 38-22). It is used to carry the dialysis solution in and out of the patient's abdomen (Norris, 2020). Continuous ambulatory peritoneal dialysis (CAPD) is performed manually using small bags of dialysate (dialysis solution), 7 days a week with four to five exchanges of new solution each day (ANNA, 2019). Automated peritoneal dialysis (APD) is performed with the assistance of a machine overnight, while the patient sleeps. The exchange of dialysis solution is cycled by the machine, 7 days a week, for 8 to 10 hours a night (ANNA, 2019).

Patients need a strong sense of support to achieve success and patient teaching is a very important aspect of care for patients who will be receiving peritoneal dialysis (George, 2019a). Education should include family members or others identified by the patient when appropriate. Patients receiving peritoneal dialysis have to take an active role in their therapy, as they may be managing a large part of their care themselves (ANNA, 2019). Patient education is essential for self-management of this chronic condition (George, 2019b; Schaepe & Bergjan, 2015). Teaching should begin as soon as possible prior to the beginning of treatment so that the patient has adequate time to absorb information. Working with a nephrology nurse, these patients are taught to perform peritoneal dialysis, manage exit-site care, take the prescribed

Guidelines for Nursing Care 38-3

CARING FOR A HEMODIALYSIS ACCESS

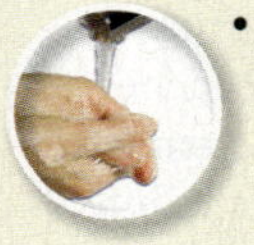

- Perform hand hygiene and put on PPE, if indicated.

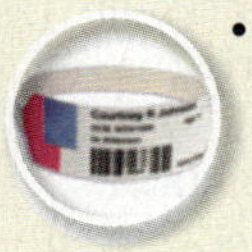

- Identify the patient.
- Close the curtains around the bed and close the door to the room, if possible. Explain to the patient what you are going to do and why.
- Question the patient about the presence of muscle weakness and cramping, changes in temperature, and abnormal sensations.
- Put on gloves, if indicated.
- Inspect the area over the access site for continuity of skin color, muscle strength, and the patient's ability to perform range of motion in the extremity/body part with the hemodialysis access.

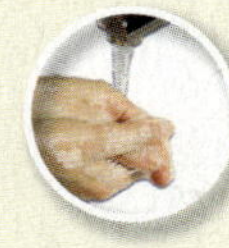

- Palpate over the access site, feeling for a thrill or vibration. Palpate pulses above and below the site. Palpate the continuity of the skin temperature along and around the extremity. Check capillary refill. Remove gloves, if used, and perform hand hygiene.
- Auscultate over the access site with bell of stethoscope, listening for a bruit or vibration.
- Do not measure blood pressure, perform a venipuncture, or start an IV on the access arm.

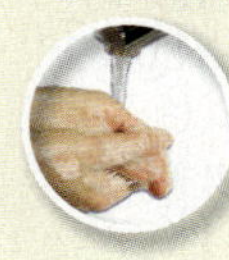

- Remove PPE, if used. Perform hand hygiene.

medication, monitor for complications, and follow dietary and fluid restrictions (George, 2019b). Refer patients to a support group or organization, such as the National Kidney Foundation (https://www.kidney.org/patients) for further information, resources, advocacy, and support (Schaepe & Bergjan, 2015).

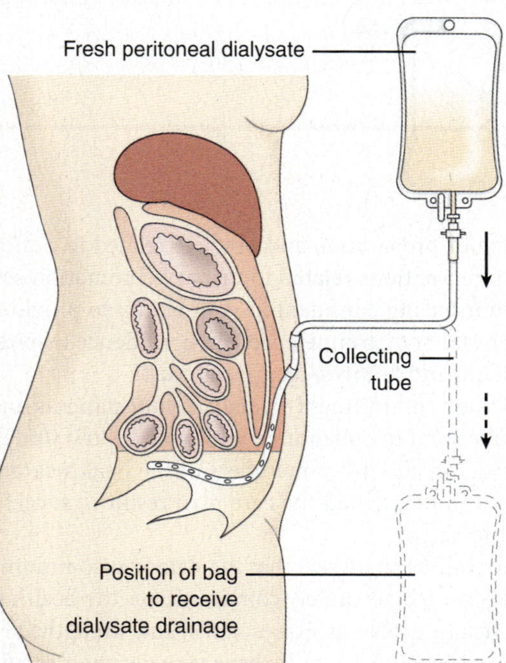

FIGURE 38-22. Peritoneal dialysis. (*Source:* Reprinted with permission from Hinkle, J. L., Cheever, K. H., & Overbaugh, K. J. [2022]. *Brunner & Suddarth's textbook of medical surgical nursing* [15th ed.]. Wolters Kluwer.)

Care of either access site is initially a nursing responsibility and includes assessment of the access site. Guidelines for Nursing Care 38-3 outlines care related to a hemodialysis access. Refer to Guidelines for Nursing Care 38-4 on page 1486 for care related to a peritoneal dialysis catheter.

Evaluating

Evaluation is an ongoing and deliberate part of the nursing process, comparing the patient's health status with previously defined expected outcomes. The nurse reflects on the effectiveness of a care plan to promote healthy urinary functioning by evaluating whether the patient has met the individualized patient goals specified in the plan. Adjustments in the plan of care are made accordingly. See the accompanying Nursing Care Plan 38-1 (on pages 1487–1489) for Mrs. Jaspers. Nursing care is considered effective if the patient expresses satisfaction with the urinary function measures and is able to (as appropriate, based on specific behaviors and criteria individualized for the patient situation):

- Produce a sufficient quantity of urine to maintain fluid, electrolyte, and acid–base balance
- Empty the bladder completely at regular intervals without discomfort
- Provide care for urinary diversion and know when to notify the health care team
- Develop a plan to modify any factors that contribute to current urinary problems or that might impair urinary functioning in the future
- Promote urinary functioning as appropriate for the person

Guidelines for Nursing Care 38-4

CARING FOR A PERITONEAL DIALYSIS CATHETER

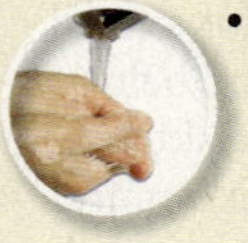

- Perform hand hygiene and put on PPE, if indicated.

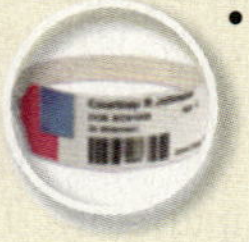

- Identify the patient.
- Close the curtains around the bed and close the door to the room, if possible. Explain to the patient what you are going to do and why.
- Assist the patient to a supine position. Expose the abdomen, draping the patient's chest with the bath blanket, exposing only the catheter site.
- Put on nonsterile gloves. Put on a facemask, and have the patient put a mask.
- Gently remove old dressing, noting odor, amount, and color of drainage; leakage; and condition of the skin around the catheter, then discard.

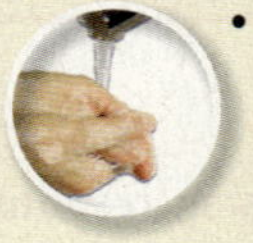

- Remove gloves and discard. Perform hand hygiene. Set up a sterile field. Open packages. Using aseptic technique, place two sterile gauze squares in a basin with antimicrobial agent. Leave two sterile gauze squares opened on the sterile field. Alternatively (based on facility's policy), place sterile antimicrobial swabs on the sterile field. Place the sterile applicator on field. Squeeze a small amount of the topical antibiotic on one of the gauze squares on the sterile field.
- Put on sterile gloves. Pick up the dialysis catheter with your nondominant hand. With the antimicrobial- or sterile normal saline–soaked gauze/swab, cleanse the skin around the exit site using a circular motion, starting at the exit site and then slowly going outward 2 inches (Bridger, 2019). Scabs or crusts should never be removed forcibly to avoid creating open areas susceptible to infection (George, 2019a). Movement of the catheter should be minimal in the immediate postoperative period (Bridger, 2019).
- Continue to hold the catheter with your nondominant hand. After the skin has dried, clean the catheter with an antimicrobial-soaked gauze, beginning at the exit site, going around the catheter, and then moving up to end of the catheter. Gently remove crusted secretions on the tube, if necessary.
- Apply the topical antibiotic to the catheter exit site, if prescribed.
- Place a sterile drain sponge around the exit site. Then place a 4 × 4 gauze over the exit site. Cover with a dressing.

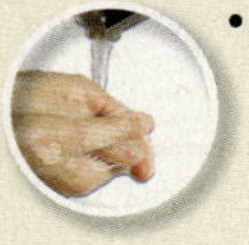

- Remove gloves and then masks. Perform hand hygiene.
- Label the dressing with date, time of change, and your initials.
- Coil the exposed length of tubing and anchor the catheter to the patient's abdomen with tape or a commercial device (Bridger, 2019; George, 2019b).
- Assist the patient to a comfortable position. Cover the patient with bed linens. Place the bed in the lowest position.

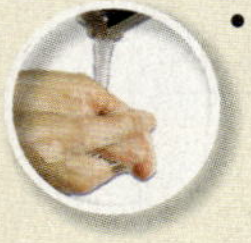

- Remove additional PPE, if used. Perform hand hygiene.

REFLECTIVE PRACTICE LEADING TO PERSONAL LEARNING

Remember that the goal of reflective practice is to look at an experience, understand it, and learn from it. As you begin to develop expertise in implementing measures related to urinary elimination, reflect on your experiences—successes and failures—in order to improve your practice. How can you do it better next time? What did you learn today that can help you tomorrow? Begin your reflection by paying close attention to the following while performing urinary elimination interventions and providing nursing care:

- How did you prioritize the data you collected? What patterns in the data did you identify?
- What knowledge from your learning, personal experience, and intuition did you use to make decisions and develop your plan of care?
- Did your preparation and practice related to performing interventions related to urinary elimination result in your feeling confident in your ability to provide care? Did your competence and confidence inspire the patient's and family's/caregiver's trust?
- Did your commitment to engage your patients and families and to collaborate with your fellow students, instructor, and other members of the health care team as you implemented the care plan result in successful partnerships?
- How confident are you that the data you communicated and recorded accurately communicates the health status, health problems, issues, risks, and strengths of the patient? How successfully have you communicated this information to other members of the health care team?
- Were you aware of any cultural and/or ethnic beliefs or practices that may have influenced the patient's personal

urinary elimination practices? Were you aware of any stereotypes or prejudices that might have negatively influenced the clinical encounter? If so, how did you address these?

- Did you need to modify the care plan as a result of ongoing assessments? Did you think of better interventions to produce the expected outcomes?
- As you concluded your care, did the patient and family/caregivers know your name, and know what to expect of you and nursing? Did the patient sense that you are respectful, caring, and competent to provide care?

Perhaps the most important questions to reflect on are: Are your patients and their families/caregivers better for having had *you* share in the critical responsibility of partnering with them to address their urinary elimination needs? Are your patients now receiving thoughtful, person-centered, prioritized, holistic, evidence-based treatment and care because of your efforts?

Nursing Care Plan for Elana Jaspers 38-1

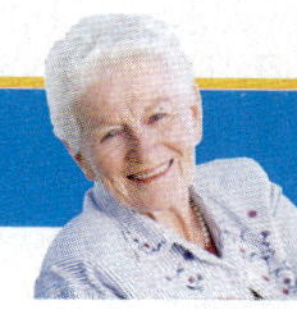

Mrs. Elana Jaspers is an alert, 83-year-old adult whose husband of 59 years died 6 months ago. Although Mrs. Jaspers was adamant about wanting to live independently in their own home, arthritis severely restricted their movement and ability to manage. After a hospitalization for pneumonia, they were transferred to a long-term care facility 1 month ago. The admitting medical diagnoses included hypertension, osteoarthritis, and depression. A comprehensive nursing assessment of Mrs. Jaspers performed 1 month after their admission to a long-term care facility included the following notations:

- Continent of urine on admission
- At present, incontinent of urine one or two times a day; often found wet in the morning; states it is "too much bother to get into the bathroom".
- Sits in chair in room unless encouraged and assisted to walk, although capable of independent ambulation with care; progressive muscle atrophy and joint stiffness
- No identifiable pathology underlying incontinence
- Medications include a diuretic for hypertension and a tricyclic antidepressant
- Reddened skin in the perineal area

ACTUAL OR POTENTIAL HEALTH PROBLEMS AND NEED

Functional urinary incontinence

Etiology: difficult transition to long-term care facility, mobility deficit

Signs and Symptoms: incontinence of urine one or two times a day; feeling toileting is too much bother; mobility deficits secondary to osteoarthritis; diuretic and antidepressant therapy

EXPECTED OUTCOME

By the next monthly assessment, 5/1/25, the patient will:

- Verbalize the importance of getting to bathroom or toilet when they first feel the need to void

NURSING INTERVENTIONS	RATIONALE	EVALUATIVE STATEMENT
Assess the value the patient attaches to voluntary control of urination and urinary continence; counsel appropriately.	Unless the patient is committed to the care plan, goal achievement is impossible.	5/1/25 Outcome partially met. Patient has commented on the importance of regular toileting but still finds this "too much trouble" some days. *Revision:* Reinforce value. *D. Mora, RN*
Teach the importance of complete bladder emptying at regular intervals and the harmful effects of ignoring the urge to void.	Patient understanding of the causes and harmful effects of urinary incontinence may motivate desire for reestablishment of voluntary control.	
Assess patient's normal voiding habits at home and assist the patient to reestablish these. Initial reminders to toilet may be necessary.	Respect for the patient's normal voiding schedule and patterns communicates concern for the person and encourages patient achievement of goals.	

(continued on page 1488)

Nursing Care Plan for Elana Jaspers 38-1 *(continued)*

EXPECTED OUTCOME	By the next monthly assessment, 5/1/25, the patient will: • Demonstrate the ability to walk to the bathroom using a cane to toilet herself	
NURSING INTERVENTIONS	**RATIONALE**	**EVALUATIVE STATEMENT**
Assess the patient's motivation and ability to toilet herself independently. Work consistently with them to increase activity tolerance: encourage short walks throughout the day to increase mobility.	One response to experiencing the multiple losses associated with aging is to surrender all control and become increasingly dependent. Nonpathology-based incontinence is less likely to occur if the daily living of the person keeps them more mobile, flexible, oriented, and motivated. An older adult who seeks to take control and has a positive self-image is more continent.	5/1/25 Outcome met. Patient can safely walk to bathroom using cane and toilet herself when they want to. *D. Mora, RN*
Refer patient to occupational therapy for assistance with diagnosis and treatment if necessary.	The specialized skills of the occupational therapist may facilitate relearning toileting skills.	5/1/25 Outcome not met. Patient repeatedly neglects AM perineal care. *Revision:* Reteach both the importance and procedure of perineal care. Assess each AM. *D. Mora, RN*
EXPECTED OUTCOME	By the next monthly assessment, 5/1/25, the patient will: • Decrease urinary incontinent episodes to less than three or four per week	
NURSING INTERVENTIONS	**RATIONALE**	**EVALUATIVE STATEMENT**
Communicate to patient that the nurses *care* about them reestablishing urinary continence and believe they can do this. Use verbal reinforcement to reward "dry" days.	A common feeling of recently institutionalized older adults is *abandonment* and the sense that no one cares; response: "Why should I?" Communicating that the patient's progress toward goal achievement is valued by the nurses is an excellent encouragement to continue progress.	5/1/25 Outcome met. Patient in last week was completely dry for 4 of 7 days. Recorded four incontinent episodes. *D. Mora, RN*
Chart incontinent episodes and monitor progress; discuss this with patient.	This records progress with incontinent episodes and provides positive reinforcement.	
ACTUAL OR POTENTIAL HEALTH PROBLEMS AND NEED	**Altered skin integrity** **Etiology:** functional urinary incontinence **Signs and Symptoms:** reddened perineal area (skin still intact)	
EXPECTED OUTCOME	By the next monthly assessment, 5/1/25, the patient will: • Demonstrate healing of reddened perineal area	

Nursing Care Plan for Elana Jaspers 38-1 (continued)

NURSING INTERVENTIONS	RATIONALE	EVALUATIVE STATEMENT
Assess skin for breakdown each AM and PM and after each incontinent episode.	Perineal care is often neglected or assigned to the least trained personnel in care settings. Prevention of incontinence-associated dermatitis (IAD) is critical; IAD not detected and treated early may progress to excessive excoriation, skin breakdown, and infection.	5/1/25 Outcome partially met. Perineal area is less inflamed. *Revision:* Continue to monitor perineal hygiene. *D. Mora, RN*
Teach the patient the importance of washing this area carefully with skin cleanser and water each AM and after incontinent episodes. Teach the importance of always cleaning and wiping the perineum from front to back to prevent autoinfection. Until incontinent episodes are eliminated, use of a skin protectant or barrier product after cleansing of the skin is indicated.	The patient who is doing self-care may neglect it entirely or use incorrect technique. Keeping the perineal area clean and dry promotes intact skin around the urinary meatus and the perineal area. Proper hygiene measures also decrease the possibility of bacteria or organisms migrating into the bladder.	
Encourage use of appropriate disposable incontinence products and stress the importance of replacing the briefs or pad as soon as possible after an episode of incontinence. Encourage use of cotton underwear and avoidance of nylon pantyhose, girdles, tight-fitting pants.	Use of appropriate absorbent products designed to wick moisture away from the skin and avoid overhydration of the skin is important to avoid alterations in skin integrity and increased risk of urinary tract infection. Nylon and tight-fitting products tend to hold moisture and may minimize airflow to the perineal area.	

SAMPLE DOCUMENTATION

4/3/25 Nursing

This AM, after an incontinent episode, Mrs. Jaspers began to talk about how hard it is to get adjusted to living here, and commented, "I feel like just giving up." We talked about the importance of being as independent as possible and the dangers of becoming passively dependent. Nursing teaching and counseling included values of independently adhering to usual toileting schedule and importance of perineal hygiene. Two hours later, after lunch, Mrs. Jaspers walked to bathroom and toileted herself. Progress with urinary incontinence will continue to be monitored. Ability definitely present but encouragement needed.

D. Mora, RN

Skill 38-1 Assessing Bladder Volume Using an Ultrasound Bladder Scanner

DELEGATION CONSIDERATIONS

The assessment of bladder volume using an ultrasound bladder scanner is not delegated to assistive personnel (AP). Depending on the state's nurse practice act and the organization's policies and procedures, this procedure may be delegated to licensed practical/vocational nurses (LPN/LVNs). The decision to delegate must be based on careful analysis of the patient's needs and circumstances as well as the qualifications of the person to whom the task is being delegated. Refer to the Delegation Guidelines in Appendix A.

(*continued on page 1490*)

Skill 38-1 Assessing Bladder Volume Using an Ultrasound Bladder Scanner *(continued)*

EQUIPMENT

- Bladder scanner
- Ultrasound gel or bladder scan gel pad
- Alcohol wipe or other sanitizer recommended by the scanner manufacturer and/or facility policy
- Clean gloves
- Paper towel or washcloth

IMPLEMENTATION

ACTION	RATIONALE
1. Review the patient's health record for any limitations in physical activity. Gather equipment.	Physical limitations may require adaptations in performing the skill. Assembling equipment provides for an organized approach to the task.
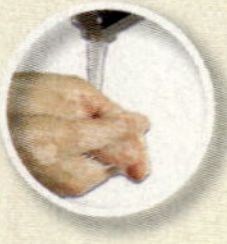 2. Perform hand hygiene and put on PPE, if indicated.	Hand hygiene and PPE prevent the spread of microorganisms. PPE is required based on transmission precautions.
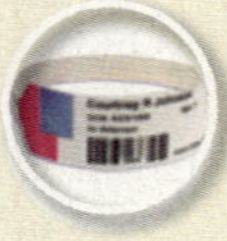 3. Identify the patient.	Identifying the patient ensures the right patient receives the intervention and helps prevent errors.
4. Close the curtains around the bed and close the door to the room, if possible. Discuss the procedure with the patient and assess the patient's ability to assist with the procedure as well as personal hygiene preferences.	This ensures the patient's privacy. Discussion promotes reassurance and provides knowledge about the procedure. Dialogue encourages patient participation and allows for individualized nursing care.
5. Adjust the bed to a comfortable working height (VHACEOSH, 2016). Place the patient in a supine position. Drape the patient. Stand on the patient's right side if you are right-handed or on the patient's left side if you are left-handed.	Having the bed at the proper height prevents back and muscle strain. Proper positioning allows accurate assessment of bladder volume. Keeping the patient covered as much as possible promotes patient comfort and privacy. Positioning allows for ease of use of your dominant hand for the procedure.
6. Put on gloves.	Gloves prevent contact with blood and body fluids.
7. Press the ON button. Wait until the device warms up. Press the SCAN button to turn on the scanning screen.	Many devices require a few minutes to prepare the internal programs.
8. Press the appropriate biologic sex button. The icon for male or female will appear on the screen (Figure 1).	The device must be programmed for the biologic sex of the patient by pushing the correct button on it. If a patient with female genitalia has had a hysterectomy, the male button is pushed (AHRQ, 2020).
9. Clean the scanner head with the appropriate cleaner (Figure 2).	Cleaning the scanner head deters transmission of microorganisms.

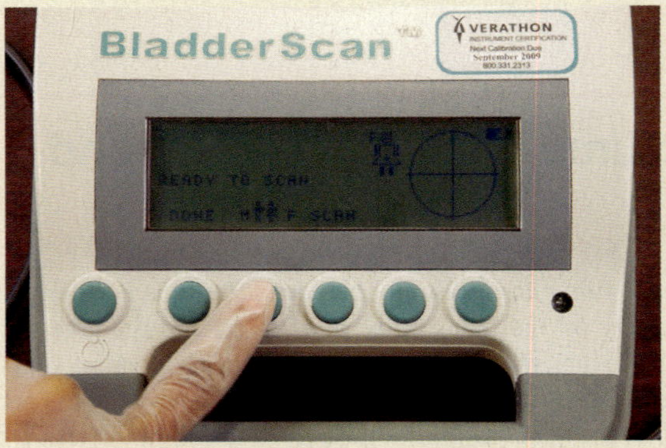

FIGURE 1. Identifying icon for patient's biologic sex. (*Source:* Used with permission from Shutterstock. *Photo by B. Proud.*)

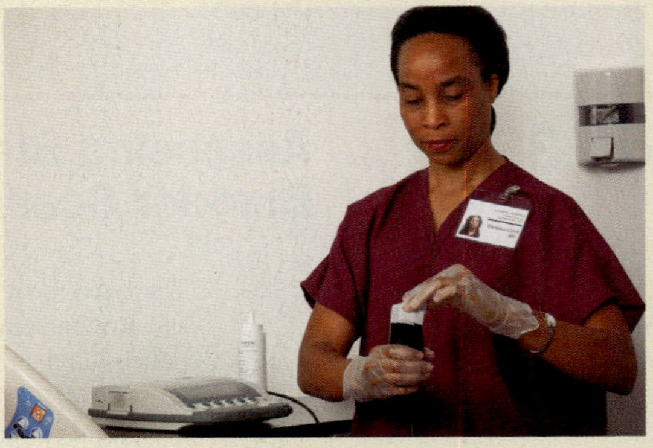

FIGURE 2. Cleaning scanner head. (*Source:* Used with permission from Shutterstock. *Photo by B. Proud.*)

ACTION | **RATIONALE**

10. Gently palpate the patient's **symphysis pubis** (anterior midline junction of pubic bones). Place a generous amount of ultrasound gel (Figure 3A) or gel pad (Figure 3B) midline on the patient's abdomen, about 1 to 1.5 inches above the symphysis pubis. Alternatively, depending on facility policy, apply ultrasound gel to the scanner head (AHRQ, 2020).

    Rationale: Palpation identifies the proper location and allows for correct placement of the scanner head over the patient's bladder.

11. Place the scanner head on the gel or gel pad, **with the directional icon on the scanner head toward the patient's head. Aim the scanner head toward the bladder (point the scanner head slightly downward toward the coccyx)** (Figure 4A). Press and release the scan button (Figure 4B).

    Rationale: Proper placement allows for accurate reading of urine in the bladder (AHRQ, 2020; Widdall, 2015).

12. Observe the image on the scanner screen, which includes the volume measured and an aiming display with crosshairs. **If the crosshairs are not centered on the bladder image, adjust the scanner head and rescan until the bladder image is centered on the crosshairs** (Figure 5).

    Rationale: This action allows for accurate reading of urine in the bladder.

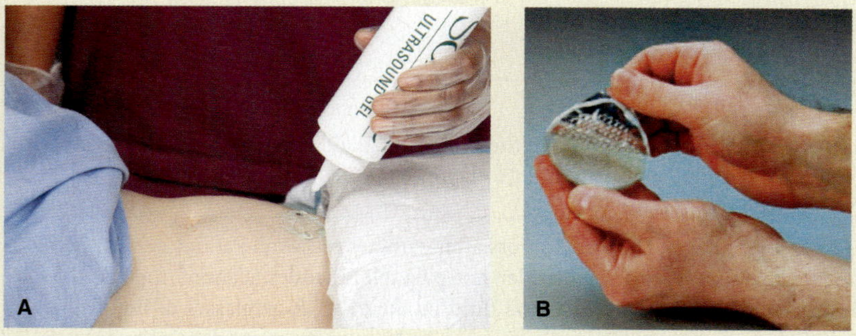

FIGURE 3. **A.** Placing ultrasound gel about 1 to 1.5 inches above symphysis pubis. (*Source:* Used with permission from Shutterstock. *Photo by B. Proud.*) **B.** Gel pad.

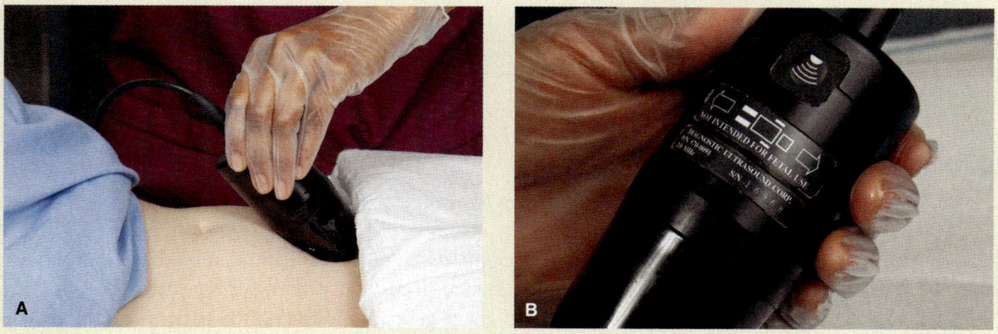

FIGURE 4. **A.** Positioning scanner head with directional icon toward patient's head and aiming the scanner head toward the bladder. **B.** Scan button. (*Source:* Used with permission from Shutterstock. *Photos by B. Proud.*)

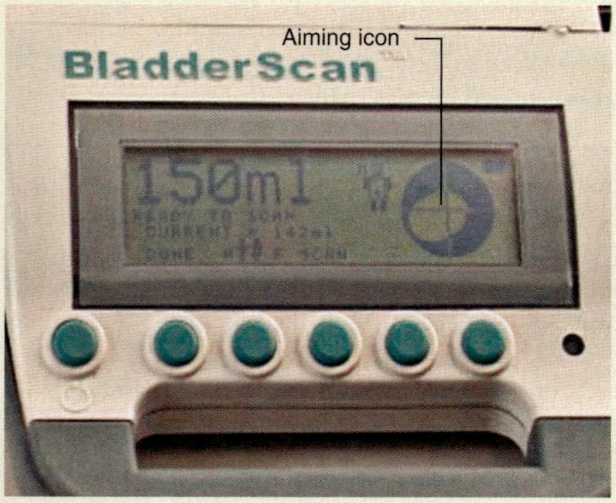

FIGURE 5. Centering image on crossbars.

(*continued on page 1492*)

Skill 38-1 Assessing Bladder Volume Using an Ultrasound Bladder Scanner *(continued)*

ACTION	RATIONALE
13. Once the image is centered, press and hold the DONE button until it beeps. Read the volume measurement on the screen. Print the results, if required, by pressing PRINT.	This action provides for accurate documentation of reading.
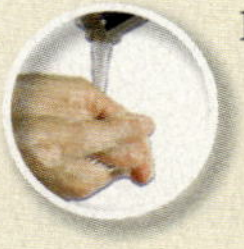 14. Use a washcloth or paper towel to remove the remaining gel from the patient's skin. Alternatively, gently remove the gel pad from the patient's skin. Return the patient to a comfortable position. Remove your gloves and perform hand hygiene. Ensure that the patient is covered.	Removal of the gel promotes patient comfort. Removing contaminated gloves prevents the spread of microorganisms. Hand hygiene prevents the spread of microorganisms.
15. Lower the bed height and adjust the head of the bed to a comfortable position. Reattach the call bell, if necessary.	These actions promote patient safety.
16. Put on gloves. Clean the scanner head according to the manufacturer's instructions and/or facility policy.	Cleaning equipment prevents transmission of microorganisms.
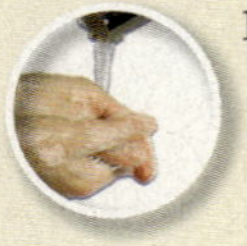 17. Remove gloves and any additional PPE, if used. Perform hand hygiene.	Proper removal of PPE reduces the risk for infection transmission and contamination of other items. Hand hygiene prevents the spread of microorganisms.

DOCUMENTATION

Guidelines

Document the assessment data that led to the use of the bladder scanner, relevant symptoms, the urine volume measured, and the patient's response.

Sample Documentation

7/06/25 1130 Patient has not voided 8 hours after catheter removal. Patient denies feelings of discomfort, pressure, and pain. Bladder not palpable. Bladder scanned for 120 mL of urine. Patient encouraged to increase oral fluid intake to six 8-oz glasses of liquid today. Dr. Liu notified of assessment. Prescribed rescan in 4 hours if patient does not void.

—B. Clapp, RN

DEVELOPING CLINICAL REASONING AND CLINICAL JUDGMENT

UNEXPECTED SITUATIONS AND ASSOCIATED INTERVENTIONS

- *You press the wrong icon when initiating the scanner:* Turn scanner off and back on. Reenter information using the correct icon.
- *You have reason to believe the bladder is full, based on assessment data, but the scanner reveals little to no urine in the bladder:* Ensure proper positioning of the scanner head. Place a generous amount of ultrasound gel or gel pad midline on the patient's abdomen, about 1 to 1.5 inches above the symphysis pubis. Place the scanner head on the gel or gel pad, with the directional icon on the scanner head toward the patient's head. Aim the scanner head toward the bladder (point the scanner head slightly downward toward the coccyx). Ensure that the bladder image is centered on the crossbars.

SPECIAL CONSIDERATIONS

- Ensure use of an adequate amount of ultrasound gel. Do not use lubricant (Widdall, 2015).
- Bladder volume measurements may be inaccurate in the presence of intraabdominal fluid, such as ascites (Schallom et al., 2020).
- If the patient is very thin or obese, use more ultrasound gel (AHRQ, 2020).
- If the patient has a large amount of lower abdominal hair, apply the gel directly to the skin (AHRQ, 2020).
- Ask or assist patients who are overweight or have larger abdominal tissue to hold their abdomen up and away from area to be scanned to reduce risk for interference, resulting in inaccurate measurement (Widdall, 2015).

- The use of bladder scanning can be used to reduce catheterization rates and associated complications (Institute for Healthcare Improvement [IHI], 2011).
- Bladder scanning in combination with intermittent catheterization may be beneficial in the management of postoperative urinary retention to avoid placement of an indwelling catheter (IHI, 2011).

Skill 38-2 Catheterizing the Urinary Bladder of a Patient With Female Genitalia

DELEGATION CONSIDERATIONS

The catheterization of the urinary bladder is not delegated to assistive personnel (AP). Depending on the state's nurse practice act and the organization's policies and procedures, catheterization of the urinary bladder may be delegated to licensed practical/vocational nurses (LPN/LVNs). The decision to delegate must be based on careful analysis of the patient's needs and circumstances as well as the qualifications of the person to whom the task is being delegated. Refer to the Delegation Guidelines in Appendix A.

EQUIPMENT

- Sterile catheter kit that contains:
  - Sterile gloves
  - Sterile drapes (one of which is **fenestrated**)
  - Sterile catheter (use the smallest appropriate-size catheter that will allow effective drainage; a 14F with a 5- to 10-mL balloon is usually appropriate, unless another size is prescribed [ANA, 2014; SUNA 2021b; Yates, 2017a])
- Antiseptic cleansing solution and cotton balls or gauze squares; antiseptic swabs (based on facility policy)
- Lubricant
- Forceps
- Prefilled syringe with sterile water (sufficient to inflate indwelling catheter balloon)
- Sterile specimen container (if specimen is required)
- Anesthetic gel, as prescribed or indicated (see Assessments below)
- Flashlight or lamp
- Waterproof, disposable pad
- Sterile, disposable urine collection bag and drainage tubing (may be connected to catheter in catheter kit)
- Catheter-securing device
- Disposable gloves
- Additional PPE, as indicated
- Washcloth, skin cleanser, and warm water to perform perineal hygiene before and after catheterization

IMPLEMENTATION

ACTION	RATIONALE
1. Review the patient's health record for any limitations in physical activity. Confirm the prescribed intervention for indwelling catheter insertion.	Physical limitations may require adaptations in performing the skill. Verifying the prescribed intervention ensures that the correct intervention is administered to the right patient.
2. Gather equipment. Obtain assistance from another staff member, if necessary or based on facility policy.	Assembling equipment provides for an organized approach to the task. Assistance from another person may be required to perform the intervention safely.
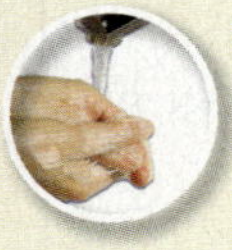 3. Perform hand hygiene and put on PPE, if indicated.	Hand hygiene and PPE prevent the spread of microorganisms. PPE is required based on transmission precautions.
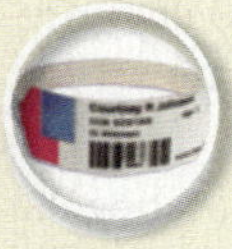 4. Identify the patient.	Identifying the patient ensures the right patient receives the intervention and helps prevent errors.
5. Close the curtains around the bed and close the door to the room, if possible. Discuss the procedure with the patient and assess the patient's ability to assist with the procedure. Ask the patient if they have any allergies, especially to latex or iodine.	This ensures the patient's privacy. Discussion promotes reassurance and provides knowledge about the procedure. Dialogue encourages patient participation and allows for individualized nursing care. Some catheters and gloves in kits are made of latex. Some antiseptic solutions contain iodine.

(continued on page 1494)

Skill 38-2 Catheterizing the Urinary Bladder of a Patient With Female Genitalia *(continued)*

ACTION	RATIONALE
6. Provide good lighting. Artificial light is recommended (use of a flashlight requires an assistant to hold and position it). Place a trash receptacle within easy reach.	Good lighting is necessary to see the meatus clearly. A readily available trash receptacle allows for prompt disposal of used supplies and reduces the risk of contaminating the sterile field.
7. Assemble equipment on the overbed table or other surface within reach.	Arranging items nearby is convenient, saves time, and prevents unnecessary stretching and twisting of muscles on the part of the nurse.
8. Adjust the bed to a comfortable working height (VHACEOSH, 2016). Stand on the patient's right side if you are right-handed or on the patient's left side if you are left-handed.	Having the bed at the proper height prevents back and muscle strain. Positioning allows for ease of use of your dominant hand for catheter insertion.
9. Assist the patient to a dorsal recumbent position with their knees flexed, feet about 2 ft apart, and legs abducted. Drape the patient (Figure 1). Alternatively, the Sims', or lateral, position can be used. Place the patient's buttocks near the edge of the bed with their shoulders at the opposite edge and their knees drawn toward the chest (Figure 2). Allow the patient to lie on either side, depending on which position is easiest for the nurse and best for the patient's comfort. Slide a waterproof pad under the patient.	Proper positioning allows adequate visualization of the urinary meatus. Patients with female genitalia should lie with their knees bent and legs spread apart (SUNA, 2021a; Yates, 2017b). Embarrassment, chilliness, and tension can interfere with catheter insertion; draping the patient will promote comfort and relaxation. The Sims' position may allow better visualization and be more comfortable for the patient, especially if hip and knee movements are difficult. The smaller area of exposure is also less stressful for the patient. The waterproof pad will protect bed linens from moisture.

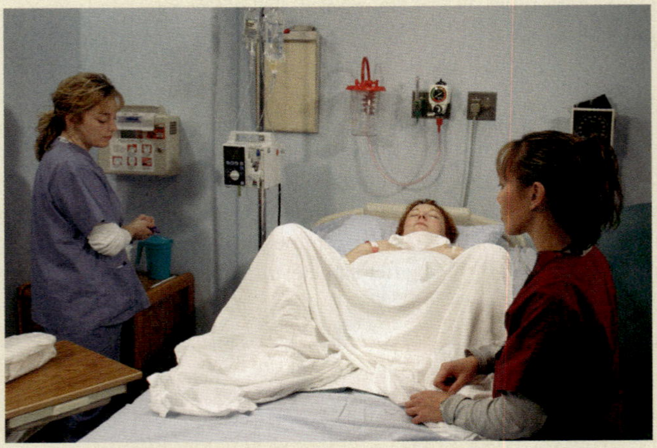

FIGURE 1. Patient in dorsal recumbent position and draped properly.

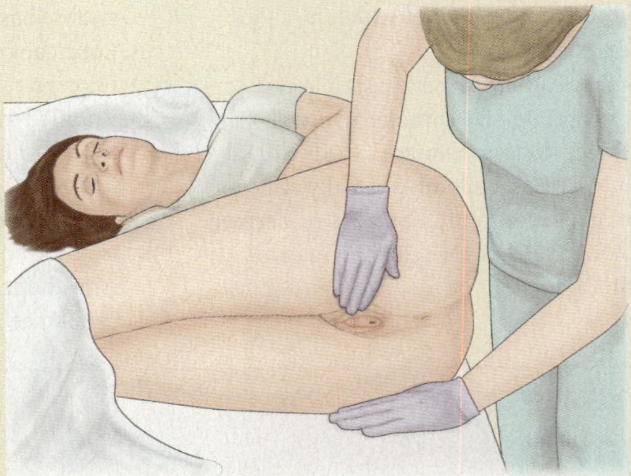

FIGURE 2. Demonstration of side-lying position.

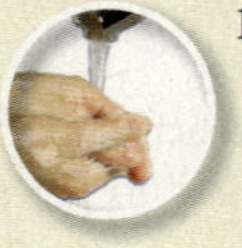

ACTION	RATIONALE
10. Put on clean gloves. Clean the perineal area with a washcloth, skin cleanser, and warm water, using a different corner of the washcloth with each stroke. Wipe from above the orifice downward toward the sacrum (front to back). Rinse and dry. Remove gloves. Perform hand hygiene again.	Gloves reduce the risk of exposure to blood and body fluids. Cleaning reduces microorganisms near the urethral meatus and provides an opportunity to visualize the perineum and landmarks before the procedure. Hand hygiene reduces the spread of microorganisms.
11. Prepare the urine drainage setup if a separate urine collection system is to be used. Secure it to the bed frame, according to the manufacturer's directions.	This facilitates connection of the catheter to the drainage system and provides for easy access.
12. Open the sterile catheterization tray on a clean overbed table using sterile technique.	Placement of equipment near the worksite increases efficiency. Sterile technique protects the patient and prevents transmission of microorganisms.
13. Put on sterile gloves. Grasp the upper corners of the drape and unfold the drape without touching nonsterile areas. Fold back a corner on each side to make a cuff over your gloved hands. Ask the patient to lift their buttocks and slide the sterile drape under them with your gloves protected by the cuff.	The drape provides a sterile field close to the meatus. Covering the gloved hands will help keep the gloves sterile while placing the drape.

ACTION	RATIONALE
14. Based on facility policy, position the fenestrated sterile drape. Place a fenestrated sterile drape over the perineal area, exposing the labia (Figure 3). (*Note:* The fenestrated drape is not shown in the remaining illustrations in order to provide a clear view of the procedure.)	The drape expands the sterile field and protects against contamination. Use of a fenestrated drape may limit visualization and is considered optional by some health care providers and/or facility policies.

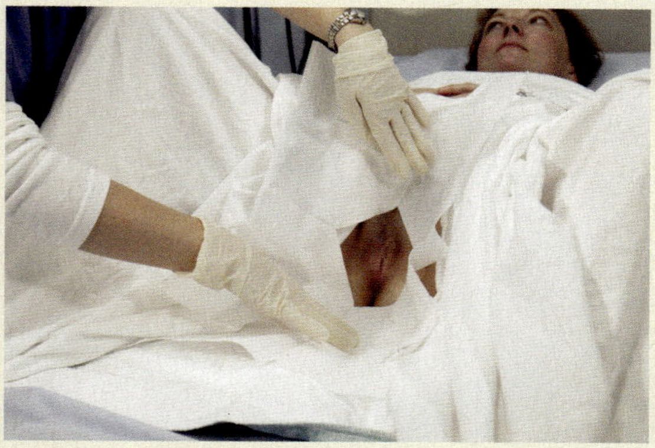

FIGURE 3. Patient with fenestrated drape in place over perineum.

ACTION	RATIONALE
15. Place the sterile tray on the drape between the patient's thighs. If the patient is in the side-lying position, place the sterile tray near the patient's legs close to the sterile drape.	The sterile setup should be arranged so that the nurse's back is not turned to it, nor should it be out of the nurse's range of vision. This provides easy access to supplies.
16. Open all the supplies. Remove the cap from the prefilled sterile saline syringe and attach it to the balloon inflation port on the catheter. Open the package of antiseptic swabs. Alternatively, fluff cotton balls in a tray before pouring antiseptic solution over them. Open the specimen container if a specimen is to be obtained. If using anesthetic gel, remove the cap from the prefilled syringe. Open and squirt lubricant in the tray.	It is necessary to open all supplies and prepare for the procedure while both hands are sterile.
17. Remove the cover from the catheter and lubricate 1 to 2 inches of the catheter tip (SUNA, 2021b).	Lubrication facilitates catheter insertion and reduces tissue trauma (SUNA, 2021a).
18. With the thumb and one finger of your nondominant hand, spread the labia and identify the meatus (Figure 4). **Be prepared to maintain separation of the labia with one hand until the catheter is inserted and urine is flowing well and continuously.** If the patient is in the side-lying position, lift the upper buttock and labia to expose the urinary meatus (Figure 5).	Smoothing the area immediately surrounding the meatus helps to make it visible. Allowing the labia to drop back into position may contaminate the area around the meatus as well as the catheter. The nondominant hand is now contaminated.

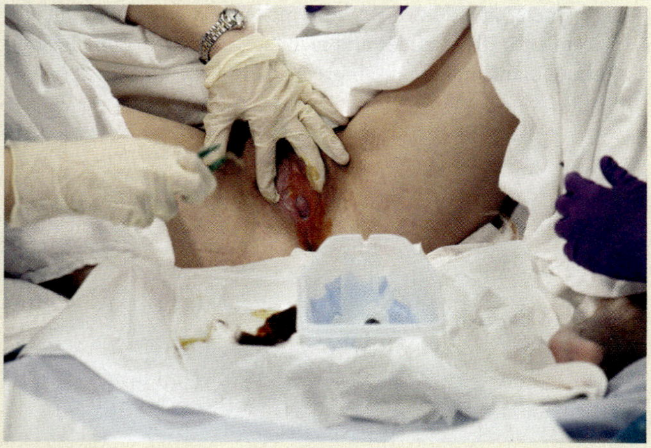

FIGURE 4. Using dominant hand to separate and hold labia open.

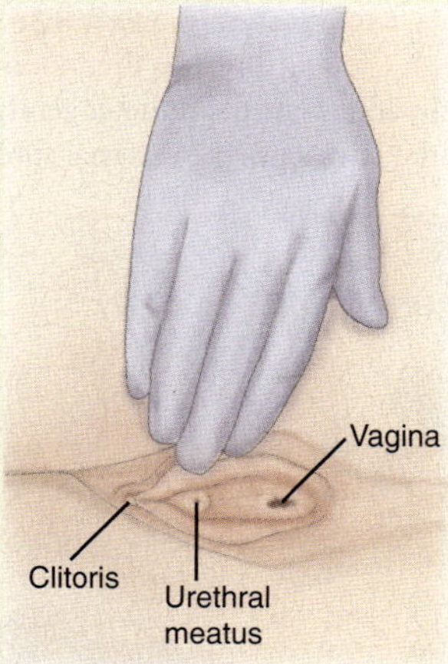

FIGURE 5. Exposing urinary meatus with patient in side-lying position.

(*continued on page 1496*)

Skill 38-2 Catheterizing the Urinary Bladder of a Patient With Female Genitalia *(continued)*

ACTION

19. Use your dominant hand to pick up an antiseptic swab, or use forceps to pick up a cotton ball. **Clean one labial fold, top to bottom (from above the meatus down toward the rectum), then discard the swab/cotton ball** (Figure 6). Using a new swab/cotton ball for each stroke, continue to clean the other labial fold, then use a third to clean directly over the meatus. Discard each swab/cotton ball after one use.

RATIONALE

Moving from an area where there is likely to be less contamination to an area where there is more contamination helps prevent the spread of microorganisms. Cleaning the meatus last helps reduce the possibility of introducing microorganisms into the bladder.

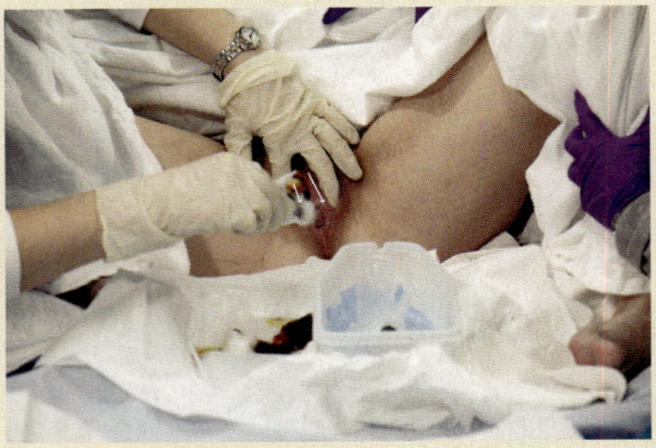

FIGURE 6. Wiping perineum with cotton ball held by forceps. Wipe in one direction—from top to bottom.

20. If using anesthetic gel, with your noncontaminated, dominant hand, pick up the anesthetic syringe. Gently place nozzle of gel near the urethral orifice and apply some gel (SUNA, 2021b). Gently place nozzle at the meatus and slowly squeeze at least 5 mL of gel into the urethra (SUNA 2021b). Allow the gel to dwell for approximately 3 to 5 minutes before starting the catheter insertion (SUNA, 2021b). Additional lubrication with a water-based lubricant may not be needed.

The use of anesthetic gel is usually not necessary for patients with female anatomy but should be considered if it is the patient's first catheterization or if a difficulty catheterization is anticipated (SUNA, 2021a).

21. With your noncontaminated, dominant hand, place the drainage end of the catheter in a receptacle. If the catheter is pre-attached to the sterile tubing and drainage container (closed drainage system), position the catheter and setup within easy reach on the sterile field. Ensure that the clamp on the drainage bag is closed.

This facilitates drainage of urine and minimizes risk of contaminating sterile equipment.

22. **Using your dominant hand, hold the catheter 2 to 3 inches from the tip and insert slowly into the urethra (Figure 7). Advance the catheter until there is a return of urine (approximately 2 to 3 inches [4.8 to 7.2 cm]). Once urine drains, advance the catheter another 2 to 3 inches (4.8 to 7.2 cm). Do not force the catheter through the urethra into the bladder.** Ask the patient to breathe deeply, and rotate the catheter gently if slight resistance is met as the catheter reaches the external sphincter.

The female urethra is about 1.5 to 2.5 inches (3.6 to 6.0 cm) long. Applying force on the catheter is likely to injure mucous membranes. The sphincter relaxes and the catheter can enter the bladder easily when the patient relaxes. Advancing an indwelling catheter an additional 2 to 3 inches (4.8 to 7.2 cm) ensures placement in the bladder and facilitates inflation of the balloon without damaging the urethra.

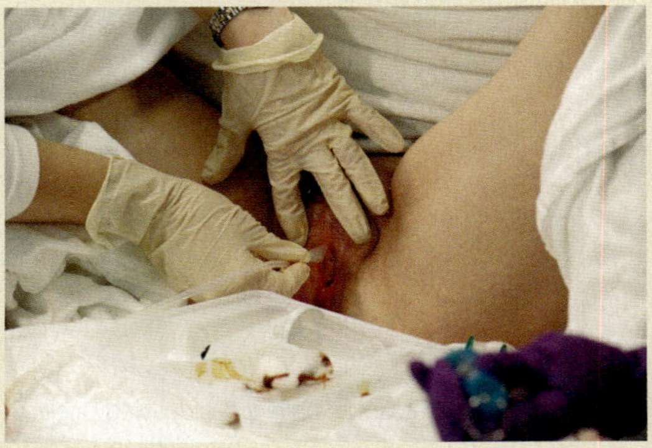

FIGURE 7. Inserting catheter with dominant hand while nondominant hand holds labia apart.

ACTION | **RATIONALE**

23. Hold the catheter securely at the meatus with your nondominant hand. Use your dominant hand to inflate the catheter balloon (Figure 8). Inject the entire volume of sterile water supplied in a prefilled syringe. Remove the syringe from the port.

Bladder or sphincter contraction could push the catheter out. The balloon anchors the catheter in place in the bladder. The manufacturer provides the appropriate amount of sterile water for the size of the catheter in the kit; as a result, use the entire syringe provided in the kit. Removal of the syringe from the injection port prevents the sterile water from pushing back into the syringe and resulting balloon deflation.

24. Pull gently on the catheter after the balloon is inflated to feel resistance.

Improper inflation can cause patient discomfort and malpositioning of the catheter.

25. Attach the catheter to the drainage system if not already preattached (Figure 9).

The closed drainage system minimizes the risk for microorganisms being introduced into the bladder (Gould et al., 2019).

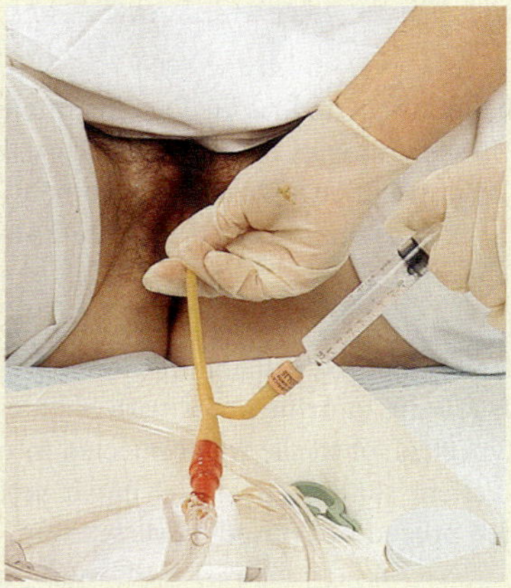

FIGURE 8. Inflating balloon of indwelling catheter.

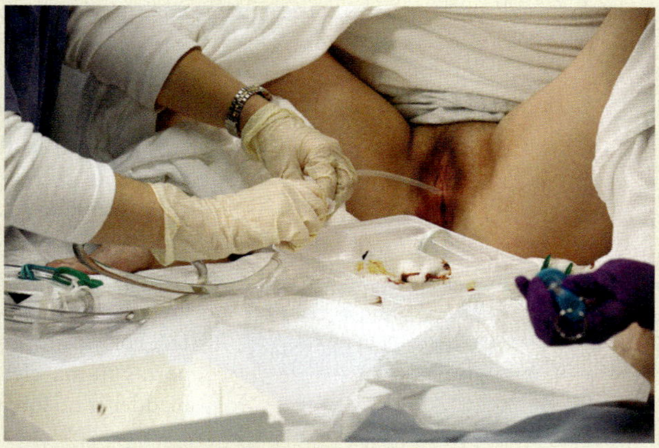

FIGURE 9. Attaching catheter to drainage bag.

26. Remove equipment and dispose of it according to facility policy. Discard the syringe in a sharps container. Wash and dry the perineal area, as needed.

Proper disposal prevents the spread of microorganisms. Placing the syringe in a sharps container prevents reuse. Cleaning promotes comfort and appropriate personal hygiene.

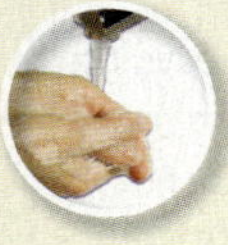

27. Remove gloves. Perform hand hygiene. **Secure the catheter tubing to the patient's inner thigh with a catheter-securing device (Figure 10).** Leave some slack in the catheter for leg movement.

Proper securement prevents tension on the catheter; reduces risk for catheter displacement, expulsion, migration, and trauma; and increases patient comfort (Holroyd, 2019). Hand hygiene prevents the spread of microorganisms. Whether to secure the drainage tubing over or under the leg depends on gravity flow, the patient's mobility, and the patient's comfort.

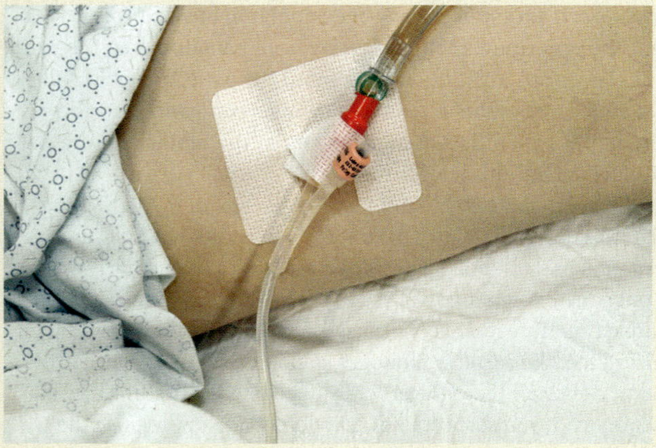

FIGURE 10. Catheter secured to leg.

28. Assist the patient to a comfortable position. Cover the patient with bed linens. Place the bed in the lowest position.

Positioning and covering provides warmth and promotes comfort.

(continued on page 1498)

Skill 38-2 Catheterizing the Urinary Bladder of a Patient With Female Genitalia *(continued)*

ACTION	RATIONALE
29. Secure the drainage bag below the level of the bladder. Check that the drainage tubing is not kinked and that movement of side rails does not interfere with the catheter or drainage bag.	This facilitates drainage of urine and prevents the backflow of urine (ANA, 2014; Gould et al., 2019).
30. Put on gloves. Obtain a urine specimen immediately, if needed, from the drainage bag. Label the specimen. Send the urine specimen to the laboratory promptly or refrigerate it.	The catheter system is sterile. Obtaining a specimen immediately allows access to the sterile system. Keeping the urine at room temperature may cause microorganisms, if present, to grow and distort laboratory findings.
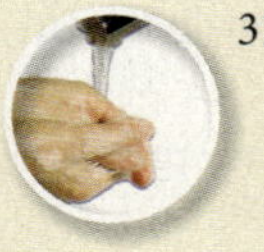 31. Remove gloves and additional PPE, if used. Perform hand hygiene.	Proper removal of PPE reduces the risk for infection transmission and contamination of other items. Hand hygiene prevents the spread of microorganisms.

DOCUMENTATION

Guidelines

Document the type and size of catheter and balloon inserted, as well as the amount of fluid used to inflate the balloon. Document the patient's tolerance of the activity. Record the amount of urine obtained through the catheter and any specimen obtained. Document any other assessments, such as unusual urine characteristics or alterations in the patient's skin. Record urine amount on intake and output record, if appropriate.

Sample Documentation

Lippincott DocuCare DocuCare Practice documenting catheterization of the female urinary bladder in *Lippincott DocuCare*.

7/14/25 0915 Patient's primary care provider notified of palpable bladder (3 cm below umbilicus) and the patient's inability to void; 750 mL of urine noted with bladder scan. A 14F Foley catheter inserted without difficulty; 10 mL of sterile water injected into balloon port; 700-mL clear yellow urine returned. Patient states, "Oh, I feel much better now." Bladder is no longer palpable. Patient tolerated procedure without adverse event.

—B. Clapp, RN

DEVELOPING CLINICAL REASONING AND CLINICAL JUDGMENT

UNEXPECTED SITUATIONS AND ASSOCIATED INTERVENTIONS

- *No urine flow is obtained, and you note that the catheter is in the vaginal orifice:* Leave the catheter in place as a marker. Obtain new sterile gloves and catheter kit. Start the procedure over and attempt to place the new catheter directly above the misplaced catheter. Once the new catheter is correctly in place, remove the catheter in the vaginal orifice. Because of the risk of cross-infection, never remove a catheter from the vagina and insert it into the urethra.
- *Patient moves legs during procedure:* If no supplies have been contaminated, ask the patient to hold still and continue with the procedure. If supplies have been contaminated, stop the procedure and start over. If necessary, get an assistant to remind the patient to hold still.
- *Urine flow is initially well established, and urine is clear, but after several hours flow dwindles:* Check the tubing for kinking. If patient has changed position, the tubing and drainage bag may need to be moved to facilitate drainage of urine.
- *Urine leaks out of the meatus around the catheter:* Do not increase the size of the indwelling catheter. Make sure the smallest-sized catheter with a 10-mL balloon is used. Large catheters cause bladder and urethral irritation and trauma. Large balloon-fill volumes occupy more space inside the bladder and put added weight on the base of the bladder. Irritation of the bladder wall and detrusor muscle can cause leakage. If leakage persists, consider an evaluation for urinary tract infection. Ensure that the correct amount of solution was used to inflate the balloon. Underfilling the balloon can cause the catheter to dislodge into the urethra, causing urethral spasm, pain, and discomfort. If you suspect underfill, do not attempt to push the catheter farther into the bladder. Remove the catheter and replace with a new catheter. Assess the patient for constipation. A bowel full of stool can cause pressure on the catheter lumen and prevent the drainage of urine. Implement interventions to prevent/treat constipation.

SPECIAL CONSIDERATIONS

General Considerations

- Some facilities have adopted a two-person urinary catheter insertion protocol, in which one nurse catheterizes the patient and one observes to ensure that the nurse inserting the catheter follows sterile technique and performs the procedure correctly (Belizario, 2015; Rhone et al., 2017). Implementation of the two-person urinary catheter insertion protocol has been shown to decrease CAUTI (Belizario, 2015; Fletcher-Gutowski & Cecil, 2019; Rhone et al., 2017).
- The use of anesthetic gel is usually not necessary for patients with female anatomy but should be considered if it is the patient's first catheterization or if a difficulty catheterization is anticipated (SUNA, 2021a).
- Check for patient allergy before use of anesthetic gel. Anesthetic gel instilled into the patient's urethra should be administered at 3 to 5 minutes before catheterization to ensure sufficient anesthetic effect (SUNA, 2021b).
- Be familiar with facility policy and/or primary health care provider guidelines for the maximum amount of urine to remove from the bladder at the time of insertion.
- If the patient is unable to lift their buttocks or maintain the required position for the procedure, the assistance of another staff member may be necessary to place the drape under the patient and to help the patient maintain the required position.
- Supplies can be opened and prepared on the overbed table, moving the tray onto the bed just before cleansing the patient.
- If there is not an immediate flow of urine after the catheter has been inserted, several measures may prove helpful:
  - Have the patient take a deep breath, which helps to relax the perineal and abdominal muscles.
  - Rotate the catheter slightly, because a drainage hole may be resting against the bladder wall.
  - Raise the head of the patient's bed to increase pressure in the bladder area.
  - Assess the patient's intake to ensure adequate fluid intake for urine production.
  - Assess the catheter and drainage tubing for kinks and occlusion.
- If the catheter cannot be advanced, have the patient take several deep breaths. Rotate the catheter half a turn and try to advance it. If you are still unable to advance, remove the catheter. Notify the health care team.
- Some catheter kits do not contain the catheter. This allows you to select a catheter and balloon size separately.
- Maintain a constant downward flow of urine. Check tubing frequently to ensure kinks and dependent loops (low points) are not present in the tubing (ANA, 2014; Gould et al., 2019; Wuthier et al., 2016). Check to see that the patient is not lying on the drainage tubing and compressing it.
- Keep the catheter drainage bag below the level of the bladder at all times (ANA, 2014; Gould et al., 2019).
- Keep the drainage bag off the floor at all times to reduce the risk of infection (ANA, 2014; Gould et al., 2019). The floor is grossly contaminated.

Infant and Child Considerations

- Size 6F to 8F is used for infants and young children (Kyle & Carman, 2021). Size 8F to 12F catheters are commonly used for older children (Kyle & Carman, 2021).
- Distraction, such as blowing bubbles, deep breathing, or singing a song, can help the child relax.
- Consider use of lidocaine jelly to anesthetize and lubricate the area before insertion of the catheter, decreasing the child's discomfort and anxiety. Refer to facility policy regarding prescribing requirements and use.

Community-Based Care Considerations

- Intermittent catheterization, performed by the patient or a caregiver in the home, may be necessary for patients with spinal cord injuries or other neurologic conditions. Although the risk for UTI is always present, practice guidelines support the use of clean, rather than sterile, technique in the home environment (Bardsley, 2015a; Beauchemin et al., 2018; Gould et al., 2019; Wilson, 2015a). The procedure for self-intermittent catheterization is essentially the same as that used by the nurse to catheterize a patient, using clean, nonsterile technique (Collins, 2019; Leach, 2018). Box 38-6 outlines important information related to patient intermittent self-catheterization (ISC).
- Single-use catheters and no-touch catheters are options for use for ISC in the home setting (Beauchemin et al., 2018). The past practice of catheter reuse in community settings, instructing patients to wash and reuse the same catheter for multiple catheterizations, is not recommended; no evidence-based guidelines on cleaning or disposing of a reused catheter are available (Beauchemin et al., 2018; Newman, 2019b).

Skill 38-3 Catheterizing the Urinary Bladder of a Patient With Male Genitalia

DELEGATION CONSIDERATIONS

The catheterization of the urinary bladder is not delegated to assistive personnel (AP). Depending on the state's nurse practice act and the organization's policies and procedures, catheterization of the urinary bladder may be delegated to licensed practical/vocational nurses (LPN/LVNs). The decision to delegate must be based on careful analysis of the patient's needs and circumstances as well as the qualifications of the person to whom the task is being delegated. Refer to the Delegation Guidelines in Appendix A.

EQUIPMENT

- Sterile catheter kit that contains:
  - Sterile gloves
  - Sterile drapes (one of which is fenestrated)
  - Sterile catheter (use the smallest appropriate-size catheter, usually a 14F catheter with a 5- to 10-mL balloon [ANA, 2014; SUNA, 2021d; Yates, 2017a])
  - Antiseptic cleansing solution and cotton balls or gauze squares; antiseptic swabs
- Lubricant
- Forceps
- Prefilled syringe with sterile water (sufficient to inflate indwelling catheter balloon)
- Sterile basin (usually base of kit serves as this)
- Sterile specimen container (if specimen is required)
- Anesthetic gel, as prescribed or indicated (See Assessments below)
- Flashlight or lamp
- Waterproof, disposable pad
- Sterile, disposable urine collection bag and drainage tubing (may be connected to catheter in catheter kit)
- Catheter-securing device
- Disposable gloves
- Additional PPE, as indicated
- Washcloth, skin cleanser, and warm water to perform perineal hygiene before and after catheterization

IMPLEMENTATION

ACTION	RATIONALE
1. Review the patient's health record for any limitations in physical activity. Confirm the prescribed intervention for indwelling catheter insertion.	Physical limitations may require adaptations in performing the skill. Verifying the prescribed intervention ensures that the correct intervention is administered to the right patient.
2. Gather equipment. Obtain assistance from another staff member, if necessary.	Assembling equipment provides for an organized approach to the task. Assistance from another person may be required to perform the intervention safely.
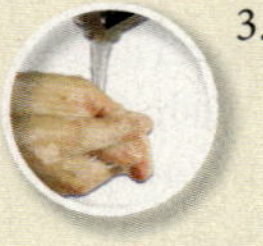 3. Perform hand hygiene and put on PPE, if indicated.	Hand hygiene and PPE prevent the spread of microorganisms. PPE is required based on transmission precautions.
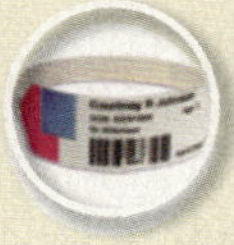 4. Identify the patient.	Identifying the patient ensures the right patient receives the intervention and helps prevent errors.
5. Close the curtains around the bed and close the door to the room, if possible. Discuss the procedure with the patient and assess the patient's ability to assist with the procedure. Ask the patient if they have any allergies, especially to latex or iodine.	This ensures the patient's privacy. Discussion promotes reassurance and provides knowledge about the procedure. Dialogue encourages patient participation and allows for individualized nursing care. Some catheters and gloves in kits are made of latex. Some antiseptic solutions contain iodine.
6. Provide good lighting. Artificial light is recommended (use of a flashlight requires an assistant to hold and position it). Place a trash receptacle within easy reach.	Good lighting is necessary to see the meatus clearly. A readily available trash receptacle allows for prompt disposal of used supplies and reduces the risk of contaminating the sterile field.
7. Assemble equipment on the overbed table or other surface within reach.	Arranging items nearby is convenient, saves time, and prevents unnecessary stretching and twisting of muscles on the part of the nurse.
8. Adjust the bed to a comfortable working height (VHACEOSH, 2016). Stand on the patient's right side if you are right-handed, or the patient's left side if you are left-handed.	Having the bed at the proper height prevents back and muscle strain. Positioning allows for ease of use of your dominant hand for catheter insertion.

ACTION	RATIONALE
9. Position the patient on their back with their thighs slightly apart. Drape the patient so that only the area around the penis is exposed. Slide a waterproof pad under the patient.	Proper positioning allows adequate visualization of the urinary meatus. This prevents unnecessary exposure and promotes warmth. The waterproof pad will protect bed linens from moisture.
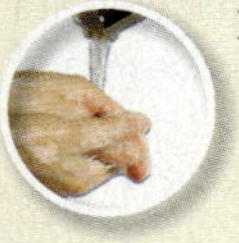 10. Put on gloves. Clean the genital area with a washcloth, skin cleanser, and warm water. Clean the tip of the penis first, moving the washcloth in a circular motion from the meatus outward. Wash the shaft of the penis using downward strokes toward the pubic area. Rinse and dry. Remove gloves. Perform hand hygiene.	Gloves reduce the risk of exposure to blood and body fluids. Cleaning the penis reduces microorganisms near the urethral meatus. Hand hygiene reduces the spread of microorganisms.
11. Prepare the urine drainage setup if a separate urine collection system is to be used. Secure it to the bed frame according to the manufacturer's directions.	This facilitates connection of the catheter to the drainage system and provides for easy access.
12. Open the sterile catheterization tray on a clean overbed table or other flat surface, using sterile technique.	Placement of equipment near the worksite increases efficiency. Sterile technique protects the patient and prevents the spread of microorganisms.
13. Put on sterile gloves. Open the sterile drape and place it on the patient's thighs. Place the fenestrated drape with the opening over the penis (Figure 1).	The drape provides a sterile field close to the meatus.
14. Place the catheter setup on or next to the patient's legs on the sterile drape.	The sterile setup should be arranged so that the nurse's back is not turned to it, nor should it be out of the nurse's range of vision. This provides easy access to supplies.
15. Open all the supplies. Remove the cap from the prefilled sterile saline syringe and attach it to the balloon inflation port on the catheter. Open the package of antiseptic swabs. Alternatively, fluff cotton balls in a tray before pouring antiseptic solution over them. Open the specimen container if a specimen is to be obtained. If using anesthetic gel, remove the cap from the prefilled syringe. Open and squirt lubricant in the tray.	It is necessary to open all supplies and prepare for the procedure while both hands are sterile. The use of anesthetic gel inserted in the urethra prior to catheterization is an option in for patients with male anatomy and should be considered if it is the patient's first catheterization or if a difficulty catheterization is suspected (SUNA, 2021d).
16. Remove the cover from the catheter and lubricate 5 to 7 inches of the catheter tip (SUNA, 2021d).	Lubrication facilitates catheter insertion, reduces urethral trauma, and reduces discomfort during insertion (SUNA, 2021d).
17. Lift the penis with your nondominant hand. Retract the foreskin in an uncircumcised patient. **Be prepared to keep your hand in this position until the catheter is inserted and urine is flowing well and continuously.** Use your dominant hand to pick up an antiseptic swab, or use forceps to pick up a cotton ball. **Using a circular motion, clean the penis, moving from the meatus down the glans of the penis (Figure 2). Repeat this cleansing motion two more times, using a new swab/cotton ball each time. Discard each swab/cotton ball after one use.**	The hand touching the penis becomes contaminated. Cleansing the area around the meatus and under the foreskin in the uncircumcised patient helps prevent infection. Moving from the meatus toward the base of the penis prevents bringing microorganisms to the meatus.

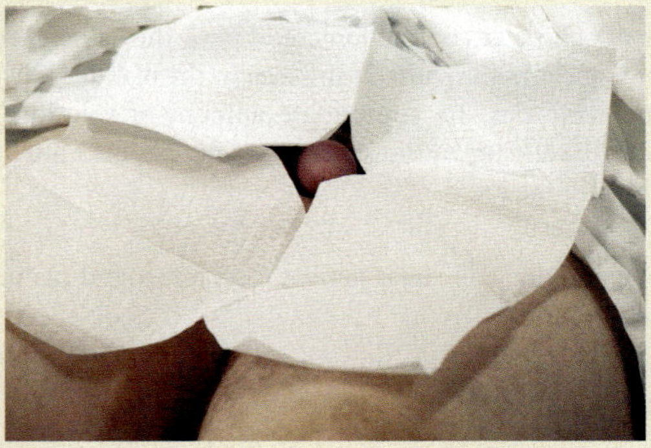

FIGURE 1. Patient lying supine with fenestrated drape +over penis.

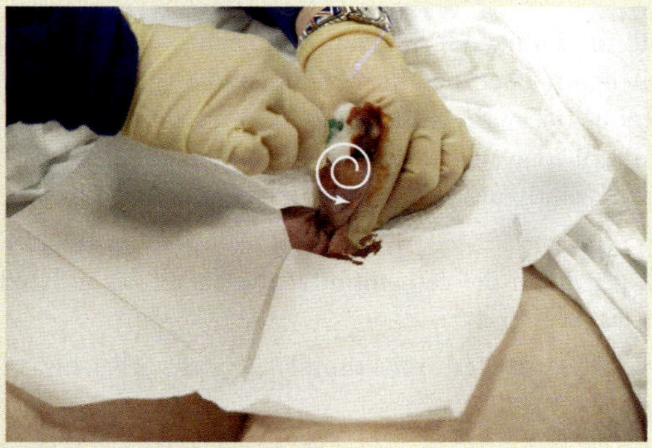

FIGURE 2. Lifting penis with gloved nondominant hand and cleaning meatus with cotton ball held with forceps in gloved dominant hand.

(continued on page 1502)

Skill 38-3 Catheterizing the Urinary Bladder of a Patient With Male Genitalia *(continued)*

ACTION	RATIONALE
18. Hold the penis with slight upward tension and perpendicular to the patient's body at a 90-degree angle to the patient's thighs (SUNA, 2021d). If using anesthetic gel, use your noncontaminated dominant hand to pick up the anesthetic syringe. Gently insert the tip of the syringe with anesthetic into the meatus and inject approximately 5 to 10 mL into the urethra (SUNA, 2021d) (Figure 3). Allow the gel to dwell for approximately 3 to 5 minutes before starting the catheter insertion (SUNA, 2021d).	This position extends the urethra and straightens the curvature of the penis (SUNA, 2021d). The use of anesthetic gel inserted in the urethra prior to catheterization is an option in for patients with male anatomy and should be considered if it is the patient's first catheterization or if a difficulty catheterization is suspected (SUNA, 2021d).
19. With your noncontaminated, dominant hand, place the drainage end of the catheter in a receptacle. If the catheter is preattached to the sterile tubing and drainage container (closed drainage system), position the catheter and setup within easy reach on the sterile field. Ensure that the clamp on the drainage bag is closed.	This facilitates drainage of urine and minimizes risk of contaminating sterile equipment.
20. Use your noncontaminated, dominant hand to pick up the catheter and hold it 3 to 4 inches from the tip. Ask the patient to bear down as if voiding. **Insert the catheter tip into the meatus (Figure 4). Ask the patient to take deep breaths. Advance the catheter about 7 to 10 inches into the urethra; urine should begin to flow through the tubing. Once urine flow is established, insert the catheter two more inches further, to the bifurcation or "Y" juncture of the ports (SUNA, 2021d). Do not use force to introduce the catheter.** If the catheter resists entry, ask the patient to breathe deeply and rotate the catheter slightly.	Bearing down eases the passage of the catheter through the urethra. The male urethra is about 20 cm long. Having the patient take deep breaths or twisting the catheter slightly may ease the catheter past resistance at the sphincters. Insert indwelling catheters in patients with male genitalia to the catheter bifurcation (the "Y" level created by the balloon filling and urinary drainage ports) to assure the balloon is within the bladder and to avoid inadvertent inflation of the balloon in the urethra (ANA, 2014; SUNA, 2021d).

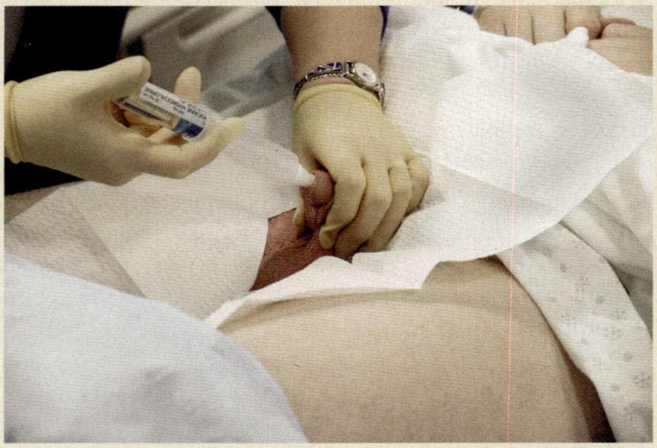

FIGURE 3. Inserting syringe into urethra and instilling lubricant.

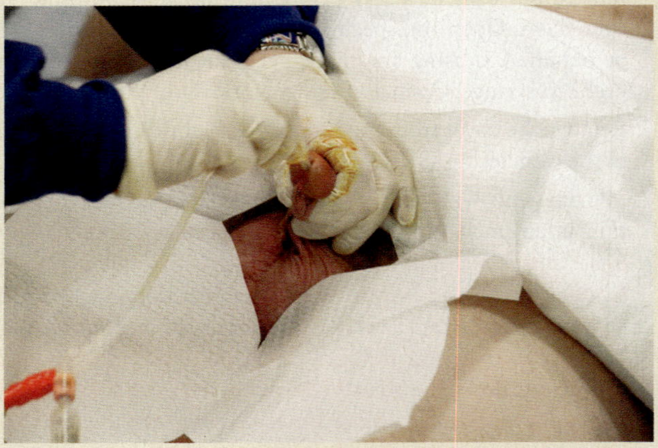

FIGURE 4. Inserting catheter using dominant hand.

ACTION	RATIONALE
21. Hold the catheter securely at the meatus with your nondominant hand. Use your dominant hand to inflate the catheter balloon. Inject the entire volume of sterile water supplied in the prefilled syringe. Once the balloon is inflated, the catheter may be gently pulled back into place. **Replace the foreskin, if present, over the catheter.** Lower the penis.	Bladder or sphincter contraction could push the catheter out. The balloon anchors the catheter in place in the bladder. The manufacturer provides the appropriate amount of solution for the size of the catheter in the kit; as a result, use the entire syringe provided in the kit.
22. Pull gently on the catheter after the balloon is inflated to feel resistance.	Improper inflation can cause patient discomfort and malpositioning of the catheter.
23. Attach the catheter to the drainage system, if necessary.	The closed drainage system minimizes the risk for microorganisms being introduced into the bladder (Gould et al., 2019).

ACTION	RATIONALE
24. Remove equipment and dispose of it according to facility policy. Discard the syringe in a sharps container. Wash and dry the perineal area, as needed.	Proper disposal prevents the spread of microorganisms. Placing the syringe in a sharps container prevents reuse. Cleaning promotes comfort and appropriate personal hygiene.
25. Remove gloves. Perform hand hygiene. **Secure the catheter tubing to the patient's inner thigh or lower abdomen (with the penis directed toward the patient's chest) with a catheter-securing device.** Leave some slack in the catheter for leg movement.	Proper securement prevents tension on the catheter; reduces risk for catheter displacement, expulsion, migration, and trauma; and increases patient comfort (Holroyd, 2019). Hand hygiene prevents the spread of microorganisms. Whether to take the drainage tubing over or under the leg depends on gravity flow, the patient's mobility, and the comfort of the patient.
26. Assist the patient to a comfortable position. Cover the patient with bed linens. Place the bed in the lowest position.	Positioning and covering provides warmth and promotes comfort.
27. Secure the drainage bag below the level of the bladder. Check that the drainage tubing is not kinked and that movement of the side rails does not interfere with the catheter or drainage bag.	This facilitates drainage of urine and prevents the backflow of urine (ANA, 2014; Gould et al., 2019).
28. Put on gloves. Obtain a urine specimen immediately, if needed, from the drainage bag. Label the specimen. Send the urine specimen to the laboratory promptly or refrigerate it.	The catheter system is sterile. Obtaining a specimen immediately allows access to the sterile system. Keeping the urine at room temperature may cause microorganisms, if present, to grow and distort laboratory findings.
29. Remove gloves and additional PPE, if used. Perform hand hygiene.	Proper removal of PPE reduces the risk for infection transmission and contamination of other items. Hand hygiene prevents the spread of microorganisms.

DOCUMENTATION

Guidelines

Document the type and size of catheter and balloon inserted as well as the amount of fluid used to inflate the balloon. Document the patient's tolerance of the activity. Record the amount of urine obtained through the catheter and any specimen obtained. Document any other assessments, such as unusual urine characteristics or alterations in the patient's skin. Record the urine amount on the intake and output record, if appropriate.

Sample Documentation

Lippincott DocuCare **DocuCare Practice documenting catheterization of the male urinary bladder in *Lippincott DocuCare*.**

7/14/25 1830 Patient unable to void for 8 hours and reports, "I feel like I have to go to the bathroom." Bladder scanned for 540-mL urine. Primary care provider notified; 10-mL prescribed 2% lidocaine jelly instilled before catheterization; 14F Foley catheter inserted without difficulty; 10 mL of sterile water injected into 5-mL balloon port; 525-mL clear yellow urine returned. Patient reports decreased bladder pressure. Patient tolerated procedure without adverse event.

—B. Clapp, RN

DEVELOPING CLINICAL REASONING AND CLINICAL JUDGMENT

UNEXPECTED SITUATIONS AND ASSOCIATED INTERVENTIONS

- *You cannot insert the catheter past 3 to 4 inches; rotating the catheter and having the patient breathe deeply are of no help:* If still unable to place the catheter, notify the health care team. Repeated catheter placement attempts can traumatize the urethra. Anticipate the possible insertion of a coudé catheter by a urologist or advanced practice professional.
- *Patient is obese or has a retracted penis:* Have an assistant available to place their fingers on either side of the pubic area and press backward to bring the penis out of the pubic cavity. Hold the patient's penis up and forward. The catheter still needs to be inserted to the bifurcation; the length of the urethra has not changed.

(*continued on page 1504*)

Skill 38-3 Catheterizing the Urinary Bladder of a Patient With Male Genitalia *(continued)*

- *Urine leaks out of meatus around the catheter:* Do not increase the size of the indwelling catheter. Make sure the smallest-sized catheter with a 10-mL balloon is used. Large catheters cause bladder and urethral irritation and trauma. Large balloon-fill volumes occupy more space inside the bladder and put added weight on the base of the bladder. Irritation of the bladder wall and detrusor muscle can cause leakage. If leakage persists, consider an evaluation for urinary tract infection. Ensure that the correct amount of solution was used to inflate the balloon. Underfilling the balloon can cause the catheter to dislodge into the urethra, causing urethral spasm, pain, and discomfort. If you suspect underfill, do not attempt to push the catheter farther into the bladder. Remove the catheter and replace with a new catheter. Assess the patient for constipation. A bowel full of stool can cause pressure on the catheter lumen and prevent the drainage of urine. Implement interventions to prevent/treat constipation.
- *Urine flow is initially well established, and urine is clear, but after several hours, urine flow dwindles:* Check the tubing for kinking. If the patient has changed position, the tubing and drainage bag may need to be moved to facilitate drainage of urine.

SPECIAL CONSIDERATIONS

General Considerations

- Some facilities have adopted a two-person urinary catheter insertion protocol, in which one nurse catheterizes the patient and one observes to ensure that the nurse inserting the catheter follows sterile technique and performs the procedure correctly (Belizario, 2015; Rhone et al., 2017). Implementation of the two-person urinary catheter insertion protocol has been shown to decrease CAUTI (Belizario, 2015; Fletcher-Gutowski & Cecil, 2019; Rhone et al., 2017).
- Assess for the need to use anesthetic gel; the use of anesthetic gel inserted in the urethra prior to catheterization is an option in for patients with male anatomy and should be considered if it is the patient's first catheterization or if a difficulty catheterization is suspected (SUNA, 2021d).
- Check for patient allergy before use of anesthetic gel. Anesthetic gel instilled into the patient's urethra should be administered at least 5 minutes before catheterization to ensure sufficient anesthetic effect (Yates, 2017b).
- Be familiar with facility policy and/or primary health care provider guidelines for the maximum amount of urine to remove from the bladder at the time of insertion.
- Supplies can be opened and prepared on the overbed table, moving the tray onto the bed just before cleansing the patient.
- If there is not an immediate flow of urine after the catheter has been inserted, several measures may prove helpful:
  - Have the patient take a deep breath, which helps to relax the perineal and abdominal muscles.
  - Rotate the catheter slightly because a drainage hole may be resting against the bladder wall.
  - Raise the head of the patient's bed to increase pressure in the bladder area.
  - Assess the patient's intake to ensure adequate fluid intake for urine production.
  - Assess the catheter and drainage tubing for kinks and occlusion.
  - Urethral strictures, false passages, prostatic enlargement, and postsurgical bladder-neck contractures can make urethral catheterization difficult and may require the services of a urologist. If there is any question as to the location of the catheter, do not inflate the balloon. Remove the catheter and notify the health care team (SUNA, 2021c).
- If the catheter cannot be advanced, having the patient take several deep breaths may be helpful. Rotate the catheter half a turn, and try to advance it. If you are still unable to advance it, remove the catheter. Notify the health care team.
- Some catheter kits do not contain the catheter. This allows you to select a catheter and balloon size separately.
- Maintain a constant downward flow of urine. Check tubing frequently to ensure kinks and dependent loops (low points) are not present in the tubing (ANA, 2014; Gould et al., 2019; Wuthier et al., 2016). Check to see that the patient is not lying on the drainage tubing and compressing it.
- Keep the catheter drainage bag below the level of the bladder at all times (ANA, 2014; Gould et al., 2019).
- Keep the drainage bag off the floor at all times to reduce the risk of infection (ANA, 2014; Gould et al., 2019). The floor is grossly contaminated.

Infant and Child Considerations

- Size 6F to 8F is used for infants and young children (Kyle & Carman, 2021). Size 8F to 12F catheters are commonly used for older children (Kyle & Carman, 2021).
- Distraction, such as blowing bubbles, deep breathing, or singing a song, can help the child relax.
- Consider the use of lidocaine jelly to anesthetize and lubricate the area before insertion of the catheter, decreasing the child's discomfort and anxiety. Refer to facility policy regarding prescribing requirements and use.

Older Adult Considerations

- If resistance is met while inserting a catheter, and rotating does not help, it is important to never force the catheter. The resistance may be caused by enlargement of the prostate gland, which is commonly seen in men over age 50 years. A special crook-tipped catheter called a coudé catheter, inserted by the urologist or advanced practice professional, may be required to maneuver past the prostate gland.

Community-Based Care Considerations

- Intermittent catheterization, performed by the patient or a caregiver in the home, may be necessary for patients with spinal cord injuries or other neurologic conditions. Although the risk for UTI is always present, and practice guidelines support the use of clean, rather than sterile, technique in the home environment (Bardsley, 2015a; Beauchemin et al., 2018; Gould et al., 2019; Wilson, 2015a). The procedure for self-intermittent catheterization is essentially the same as that used by the nurse to catheterize a patient, using clean, nonsterile technique (Collins, 2019; Leach, 2018). Box 38-6 (p. 1475) outlines important information related to patient intermittent self-catheterization (ISC).

Skill 38-4 Emptying and Changing a Stoma Appliance on a Urinary Diversion

DELEGATION CONSIDERATIONS

The emptying of a stoma appliance on a urinary diversion may be delegated to assistive personnel (AP) as well as to licensed practical/vocational nurses (LPN/LVNs). The changing of a stoma appliance on a urinary diversion may be delegated to LPN/LVNs. The decision to delegate must be based on careful analysis of the patient's needs and circumstances as well as the qualifications of the person to whom the task is being delegated. Refer to the Delegation Guidelines in Appendix A.

EQUIPMENT

- Premoistened disposable washcloths or
  - Basin with warm water
  - Skin cleanser, towel, washcloth
- Silicone-based adhesive remover
- Gauze squares
- Skin protectant, such as Skin-Prep™
- Ostomy appliance
- Stoma-measuring guide
- Graduated container
- Ostomy belt (optional)
- Disposable gloves
- Additional PPE, as indicated
- Waterproof, disposable pad
- Small plastic trash bag

IMPLEMENTATION

ACTION	RATIONALE
1. Gather equipment.	Assembling equipment provides for an organized approach to the task.
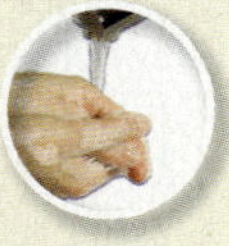 2. Perform hand hygiene and put on PPE, if indicated.	Hand hygiene and PPE prevent the spread of microorganisms. PPE is required based on transmission precautions.
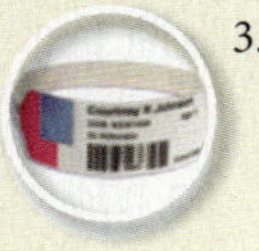 3. Identify the patient.	Identifying the patient ensures the right patient receives the intervention and helps prevent errors.

(*continued on page 1506*)

Skill 38-4 Emptying and Changing a Stoma Appliance on a Urinary Diversion *(continued)*

ACTION / **RATIONALE**

4. Close the curtains around the bed and close the door to the room, if possible. Explain to the patient what you are going to do and why. Encourage the patient to observe or participate, if possible and as appropriate.

This ensures the patient's privacy. Explanation relieves anxiety and facilitates engagement. Having the patient observe or assist encourages self-acceptance and helps the patient develop self-care skills.

5. Assemble equipment on the overbed table or other surface within reach.

Arranging items nearby is convenient, saves time, and prevents unnecessary stretching and twisting of muscles on the part of the nurse.

6. Assist the patient to a comfortable sitting or lying position in bed or a standing or sitting position in the bathroom. If the patient is in bed, adjust the bed to a comfortable working height (VHACEOSH, 2016). Place a waterproof pad under the patient at the stoma site.

Either position should allow the patient to view the procedure in preparation for learning to perform it independently. Lying flat or sitting upright facilitates smooth application of the appliance. Having the bed at the proper height prevents back and muscle strain. A waterproof pad protects linens and the patient from moisture.

Emptying the Appliance

7. Put on gloves. Hold the end of the appliance over a bedpan, toilet, or measuring device. Remove the end cap from the spout. Open the spout and empty the contents into the bedpan, toilet, or measuring device (Figure 1).

Gloves protect the nurse from exposure to blood and body fluids. Emptying the pouch before handling it reduces the likelihood of spilling the excretions.

8. Close the spout. Wipe the spout with toilet tissue. Replace the cap.

Drying the spout removes any urine.

9. Remove equipment. Remove gloves. Perform hand hygiene. Assist the patient to a comfortable position.

Proper removal of PPE prevents the transmission of microorganisms. Positioning ensures patient comfort. Hand hygiene prevents the spread of microorganisms.

10. If the appliance is not to be changed, place the bed in the lowest position. Remove additional PPE, if used. Perform hand hygiene.

Lowering the bed promotes patient safety. Proper removal of PPE reduces the risk for infection transmission and contamination of other items. Hand hygiene prevents the spread of microorganisms.

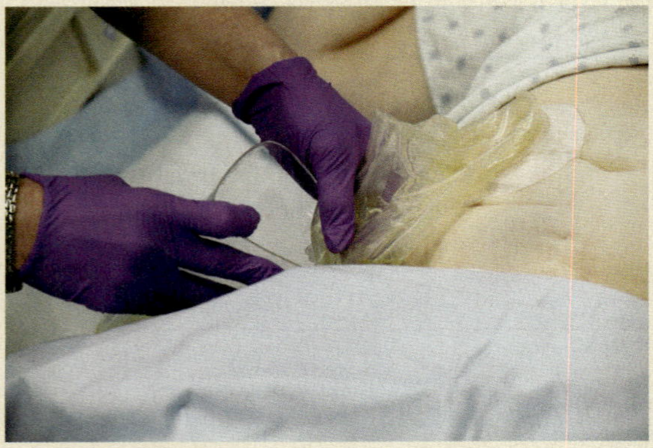

FIGURE 1. Emptying urine into graduated container.

Changing the Appliance

11. Place a disposable waterproof pad on the overbed table or other work area. Open the premoistened disposable washcloths or set up the washbasin with warm water and the rest of the supplies. Place a trash bag within reach.

The pad protects the surface. Organization facilitates performance of the procedure.

12. Put on gloves. Place a waterproof pad under the patient at the stoma site. Empty the appliance, if necessary, as described in Steps 6 to 8.

The waterproof pad protects linens and the patient from moisture. Emptying the contents before removal prevents accidental spillage of fecal material.

ACTION

13. Put on gloves. Use two hands to gently remove the appliance faceplate, starting at the top and keeping the abdominal skin taut (Figure 2). Remove the appliance faceplate from the skin by pushing the skin from the appliance rather than pulling the appliance from the skin (Figure 3). Apply a silicone-based adhesive remover by spraying or wiping with the remover wipe, as indicated.

RATIONALE

Gloves prevent contact with blood and body fluids. The seal between the surface of the faceplate and the skin must be broken before the faceplate can be removed. Harsh handling of the appliance can damage the skin and impair the development of a secure seal in the future. Silicone-based adhesive remover loosens the adhesive bond to make removal easier and less likely to damage the skin and is particularly beneficial for patients with fragile skin and those at increased risk for medical adhesive–related skin injury/stripping (Collier, 2019; LeBlanc et al., 2019; Swift et al., 2020).

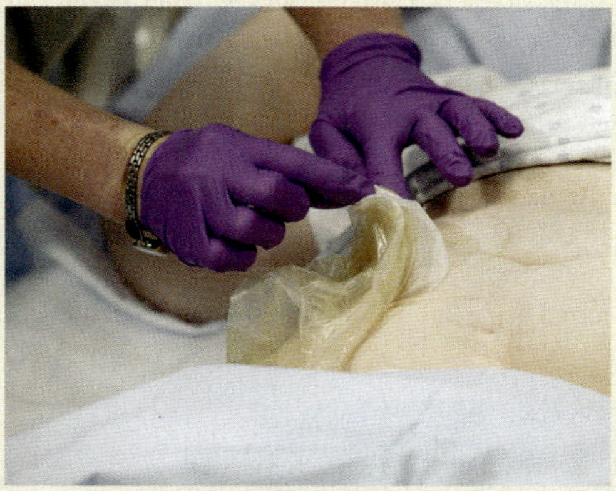

FIGURE 2. Gently removing appliance faceplate from skin.

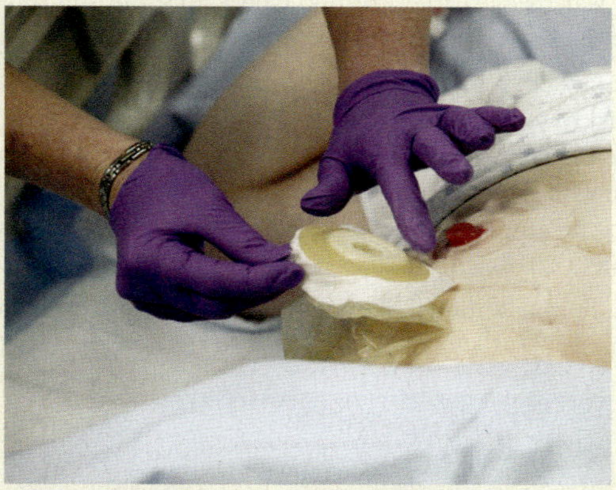

FIGURE 3. Pushing skin from appliance rather than pulling appliance from skin.

14. Place the appliance in the trash bag, if disposable. If reusable, set it aside to wash in lukewarm soap and water and allow it to air dry after the new appliance is in place.

Thorough cleaning and airing of the appliance reduces odor and deterioration of the appliance. For aesthetic and infection control purposes, used appliances should be discarded appropriately.

15. Clean the skin around the stoma with mild skin cleanser and water or a cleansing agent and a washcloth (Figure 4). Remove all old adhesive from the skin; additional adhesive remover may be used. Do not apply lotion to the peristomal area.

Cleaning the skin removes excretions and old adhesive and skin protectant. Excretions or a buildup of other substances can irritate and damage the skin. Lotion will prevent a tight adhesive seal.

16. Gently pat the area dry. **Make sure the skin around the stoma is thoroughly dry.** Assess the stoma and the condition of the surrounding skin.

Careful drying prevents trauma to the skin and stoma. An intact, properly applied urinary collection device protects skin integrity. Any change in color and size of the stoma may indicate circulatory problems.

17. Place one or two gauze squares over the stoma opening (Figure 5).

Continuous drainage must be absorbed to keep the skin dry during appliance change.

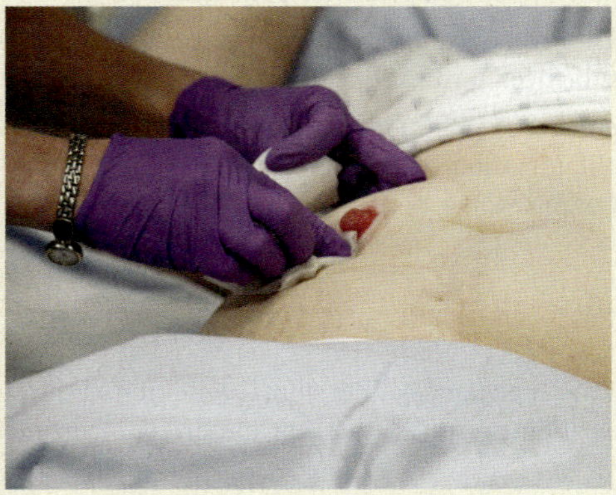

FIGURE 4. Cleaning stoma with cleansing agent and washcloth.

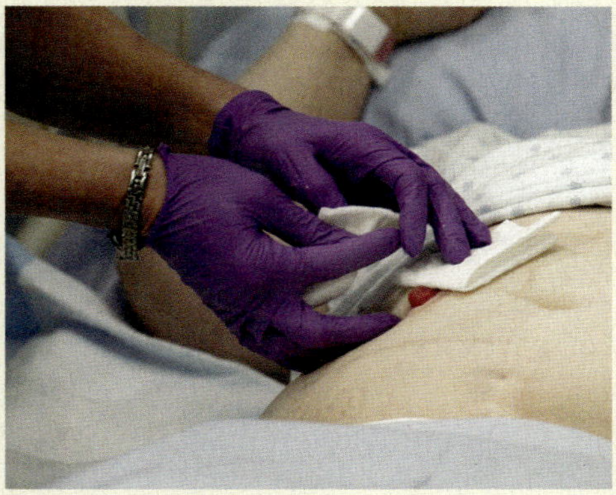

FIGURE 5. Placing one or two gauze squares over stoma opening.

(continued on page 1508)

Skill 38-4 Emptying and Changing a Stoma Appliance on a Urinary Diversion *(continued)*

ACTION	RATIONALE
18. Apply skin protectant/barrier film to a 2-inches (5-cm) radius around the stoma, and allow it to dry completely, which takes about 30 seconds.	The skin needs protection from the potentially excoriating effect of the appliance adhesive (WOCN, 2018). The skin must be perfectly dry before the appliance is placed to get good adherence and to prevent leaks.
19. Lift the gauze squares for a moment and measure the stoma opening, using the measurement guide. Replace the gauze. Trace the same-size opening on the back center of the appliance. Cut the opening 1/8 inch (2 to 3 mm) larger than the stoma size (Hill, 2020) (Figure 6). Use a finger to gently smooth the wafer edges after cutting. Check that the spout is closed, and the end cap is in place.	The appliance should fit snugly around the stoma, with only 1/8 inch of skin visible around the opening. A faceplate opening that is too small can cause trauma to the stoma. If the opening is too large, exposed skin will be irritated by urine. Wafer edges may be uneven after cutting and could cause irritation to and/or pressure on the stoma. A closed spout and secured end cap prevent urine from leaking from the appliance.
20. Remove the paper backing from the appliance faceplate. Quickly remove the gauze squares and discard appropriately; ease the appliance over the stoma. Gently press them onto the skin while smoothing over the surface (Figure 7). Apply gentle, even pressure to the appliance for approximately 30 seconds (Burch, 2019; Hill, 2020).	The appliance is effective only if it is properly positioned and adhered securely. Pressure on the faceplate allows the faceplate to mold to the patient's skin and improves the seal.
21. Secure the optional belt to the appliance and around the patient.	An elasticized belt helps support the appliance for some people.

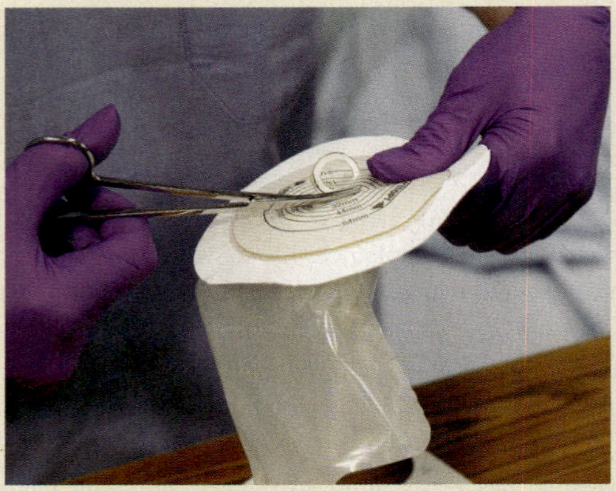

FIGURE 6. Cutting the faceplate opening 1/8 inch larger than stoma size.

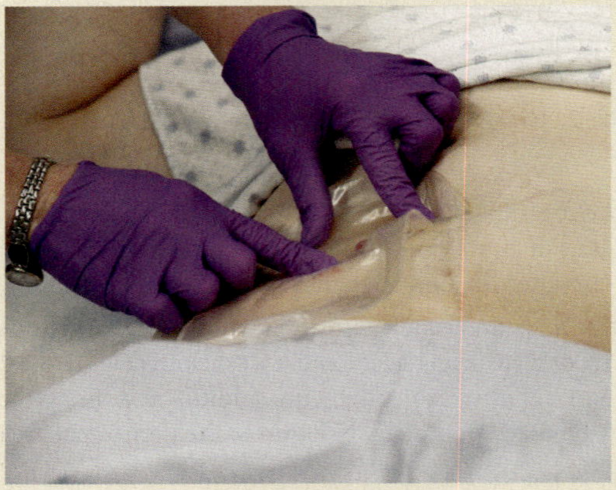

FIGURE 7. Applying faceplate over stoma.

ACTION	RATIONALE
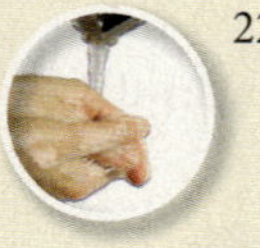 22. Remove gloves. Perform hand hygiene. Assist the patient to a comfortable position. Cover the patient with bed linens. Place the bed in the lowest position.	Removing gloves reduces risk of transmission of microorganisms. Hand hygiene prevents the spread of microorganisms. Positioning and covering provide warmth and promote comfort. The bed in the lowest position promotes patient safety.
23. Put on gloves. Remove or discard any remaining equipment and assess the patient's response to the procedure.	The patient's response may indicate acceptance of the ostomy as well as the need for health teaching.
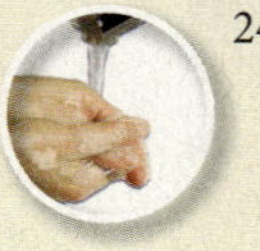 24. Remove gloves and additional PPE, if used. Perform hand hygiene.	Proper removal of PPE reduces the risk for infection transmission and contamination of other items. Hand hygiene prevents the spread of microorganisms.

DOCUMENTATION

Guidelines

Document the procedure, including the appearance of the stoma, condition of the peristomal skin, characteristics of the urine, the patient's response to the procedure, and pertinent patient teaching.

Sample Documentation

7/23/25 1245 Ileal conduit appliance changed. Mr. Jones present. Mrs. Jones asking questions about care for ileal conduit, states, "I don't know if I'll ever be able to care for this thing at home." Tearful at times. Patient encouraged to express feelings. Patient agreed to talk with wound, ostomy, and continence nurse about concerns. Mr. Jones very supportive, also asking appropriate questions. Patient states they would like to watch change one more time before they attempt to do it. Stoma is moist and red, peristomal skin intact, draining yellow urine with small amount of mucus.

—B. Clapp, RN

DEVELOPING CLINICAL REASONING AND CLINICAL JUDGMENT

UNEXPECTED SITUATIONS AND ASSOCIATED INTERVENTIONS

- *You remove appliance and find an area of skin excoriated:* Make sure that the appliance is not cut too large. Skin that is exposed inside of the ostomy appliance will become excoriated. Assess for the presence of a fungal skin infection. Consult with the wound, ostomy, and continence nurse to identify appropriate treatment. Cleanse the skin thoroughly and pat dry. Apply products made for excoriated skin before placing the appliance over the stoma. Frequently check the faceplate to ensure that a seal has formed and that there is no leakage. Document the assessment findings and related interventions in the patient's record.
- *Faceplate is leaking after applying a new appliance:* Remove the appliance, clean the skin, and start over.
- *You are ready to place the faceplate and notice that the opening is cut too large:* Discard the appliance and begin over. A faceplate that is cut too large may lead to excoriation of the skin and leakage.
- *Stoma is dark brown or black:* The stoma should appear pink to red, shiny, and moist. Alterations may indicate compromised circulation. If the stoma is dark brown or black, suspect ischemia and necrosis. Notify the health care team immediately.

SPECIAL CONSIDERATIONS

- Patients with urinary diversions created using a portion of the gastrointestinal (GI) tract will experience the presence of mucus in the urine (Berti-Hearn & Elliott, 2019). The segment of the GI tract continues to produce mucus, as part of its normal functioning. This mucus production does not decrease over time but is usually not a problem for patients with an ileal conduit (Berti-Hearn & Elliott, 2019).
- Key components in postoperative education before the patient is discharged from the hospital include assessment and care of the stoma and peristomal skin, pouch emptying, changing the appliance, drainage collectors, common complications, clothing, fluid guidelines, medications, and obtaining supplies (Goldberg et al., 2018).

DEVELOPING CLINICAL REASONING AND CLINICAL JUDGMENT

1. Review the Nursing Care Plan 38-1 on pages 1487–1489 to help you develop your clinical reasoning and clinical judgment skills.
2. The daughter of an older adult who is about to be discharged to the daughter's home requests that a catheter be inserted in their mother to make home care easier. The patient knows when they need to void but needs assistance to get to the bathroom. How do you respond to the daughter's request?
3. If you encountered the following situations when providing patient care, how would you react and what would you do?
   - A 6-year-old refuses to give a urine sample.
   - Frank blood appears in the urine of a patient who has no history of urinary problems.
   - When you ask for a urine sample, a teenager asks, "This won't reveal drugs, will it?"
   - A young person reports painful urination with burning.
   - An older adult reports frequency and pain when voiding.

PRACTICING FOR NCLEX

1. A new graduate nurse and their preceptor must collect several urine specimens for laboratory testing. Which techniques for urine collection by the graduate nurse are performed incorrectly, requiring the preceptor to intervene? Select all that apply.
   a. Catheterizing a patient to collect a sterile urine sample for routine urinalysis
   b. Collecting a clean-catch urine specimen in the morning and storing it at room temperature until an afternoon pick-up
   c. Collecting a sterile urine specimen from the collection bag of a patient's indwelling catheter
   d. Collecting about 3 mL of urine from a patient's indwelling catheter to send for a urine culture
   e. Planning to collect a sterile specimen from a patient with a urinary diversion by catheterizing the stoma
   f. Discarding the first urine of the day when performing a 24-hour urine specimen collection on a patient
2. A nurse caring for older adults in an extended-care facility performs regular assessments of the patients' urinary functioning. Which patients would the nurse identify as at risk for urinary retention? Select all that apply.
   a. Patient who is diagnosed with an enlarged prostate
   b. Patient who is on bedrest
   c. Patient who is diagnosed with vaginal prolapse
   d. Older adult patient with dementia
   e. Patient who is taking antihistamines to treat allergies
   f. Patient who has difficulty walking to the bathroom
3. A nurse in the gynecology clinic is preparing an educational brochure to teach patients how to prevent UTIs. Which teaching points would the nurse include? Select all that apply.
   a. Wear underwear with a cotton crotch.
   b. Take baths rather than showers.
   c. Drink of six to eight 8-oz glasses of liquid per day.
   d. Urinate before and after intercourse.
   e. After defecation, dry the perineal area from the front to the back.
   f. Observe the urine for color, amount, odor, and frequency.
4. A patient who has pneumonia has had a fever for 3 days. What characteristics would the nurse anticipate related to the patient's urine output?
   a. Decreased amount and highly concentrated
   b. Decreased amount and very pale like water
   c. Increased amount and very concentrated
   d. Increased amount and dilute appearing
5. The health care provider has ordered an indwelling catheter to be inserted to relieve urinary retention in a male patient with prostate enlargement. What consideration will the nurse keep in mind when performing this procedure?
   a. The male urethra is more vulnerable to injury during insertion.
   b. In the hospital, a clean technique is used for catheter insertion.
   c. The catheter is inserted 2 to 3 inches into the meatus.
   d. Since it uses a closed system, the risk for UTI is absent.
6. A nurse is caring for a patient with an enlarged prostate who has had an indwelling catheter for several weeks. A prescription for continuous bladder irrigation (CBI) is written after the patient developed hematuria post cystoscopy. The nurse teaches the patient the purpose of CBI is to prevent what situation?
   a. Catheter infection due to long-term use
   b. Need to flush the catheter of organisms post procedure
   c. Blood clots that could block the catheter
   d. Need for increased fluid intake
7. A nurse is caring for a patient who has a urinary diversion (urostomy) after cystectomy (removal of the bladder) to treat bladder cancer. What interventions are indicated for this patient? Select all that apply.
   a. Measuring the patient's fluid intake and output
   b. Keeping the skin around the stoma moist
   c. Emptying the appliance frequently
   d. Reporting any mucus in the urine to the primary care provider
   e. Encouraging the patient to look away when changing the appliance
   f. Monitoring the return of intestinal function and peristalsis
8. A nurse is changing the stoma appliance on a patient's ileal conduit. Which finding requires the nurse to follow up with the provider?
   a. Stoma is moist.
   b. Skin around the stoma is irritated.
   c. Urine is leaking from the stoma.
   d. Stoma is a purple-black color.
9. A postoperative patient is having difficulty voiding and reports suprapubic pressure. What action can the nurse take to promote voiding?
   a. Pouring cold water over the patient's fingers and perineum
   b. Assessing bladder residual using the bladder scanner
   c. Immediately encouraging the patient to void
   d. Recommending an indwelling catheter
10. A nurse caring for a patient who just began hemodialysis assesses the patient's AV fistula. Nursing documentation includes: "5/10/25 0930 AV fistula in the right forearm negative for thrill and bruit. Patient denies pain and tenderness." Which finding is essential for the nurse report to the health care provider?
   a. Thrill and bruit are absent.
   b. Area is without redness or swelling.
   c. Patient denies pain and tenderness.
   d. Trace edema of the fingers is present.

11. A nurse is caring for an alert, ambulatory, older adult with urinary frequency who has difficulty making it to the bathroom in time. Which nursing intervention is most appropriate to include in the care plan for this patient?
    a. Explaining that incontinence is an expected occurrence with aging
    b. Asking the patient's family/caregivers to purchase incontinence pads for the patient
    c. Teaching the patient how to perform PFMT exercises at regular intervals
    d. Inserting an indwelling catheter to prevent skin breakdown
12. A nurse is caring for a patient who is taking phenazopyridine (a urinary tract analgesic) for a UTI. The patient states, "My urine was bright orange-red today; I think I'm bleeding. Something is terribly wrong." How will the nurse best respond?
    a. "The medication causes a red-orange tinge to the urine; it is expected."
    b. "I will test your urine for blood."
    c. "This may be the result of an injury to your bladder."
    d. "I'll hold the medication and let the provider know you are allergic to the drug."
13. A nurse is caring for a male patient who had a urinary sheath applied following hip surgery. What nursing interventions are appropriate to include when caring for this patient? Select all that apply.
    a. Preventing the tubing from kinking to maintain free urinary drainage
    b. Changing the sheath weekly and provide hygiene
    c. Fastening the sheath tightly to prevent the possibility of leakage
    d. Having the patient maintain bedrest to prevent the sheath from slipping off
    e. Leaving 1 to 2 inches (2.5 to 5 cm) beyond the tip of the penis
    f. Ensuring the device does not restrict blood flow.
14. A nurse receives a prescription to catheterize a patient following surgery. What nursing action reflects correct technique?
    a. Planning to use different equipment for catheterization of male versus female patients
    b. Selecting the smallest appropriate size indwelling urinary catheter
    c. Sterilizing the equipment prior to insertion
    d. Avoiding filling the balloon with sterile water to prevent pressure on tissues
15. A nurse in the emergency room is teaching a patient how to collect a midstream urine specimen. What instructions will the nurse give the patient? Select all that apply.
    a. Wash your hands with soap and water.
    b. Open the container and place the lid face down on the counter.
    c. Separate your labia and wipe with the antiseptic towelettes in the kit.
    d. Without letting go of the labia, void a small amount into the toilet or collection hat.
    e. Lean the collection container against the urinary opening and void into the container.
    f. Void an ounce, then remove the container and finish voiding in the toilet.
16. A nurse on a pediatric surgical unit notes a 10-year-old child has developed nocturnal enuresis. What health concern will the nurse plan for?
    a. Constipation
    b. Bedwetting after the age of toilet training
    c. Patient who is manipulative
    d. Infection
17. A nursing student hears in report that their patient is receiving a nephrotoxic medication. The student plans care to include what action?
    a. Teaching the patient to expect increased voiding
    b. Assessing for kidney damage
    c. Preventing urinary incontinence
    d. Observing for nocturia

ANSWERS WITH RATIONALES

1. **d, e, f.** A urine culture requires about 3 mL of urine, whereas routine urinalysis requires at least 10 mL of urine. The preferred method of collecting a sterile urine specimen from a urinary diversion is to catheterize the stoma. For a 24-hour urine specimen, the nurse should discard the first voiding, then collect all urine voided for the next 24 hours. A sterile urine specimen is not required for a routine urinalysis. Urine chemistry is altered after urine stands at room temperature for a long period of time. A specimen from the collection drainage bag may not be fresh urine and could result in an inaccurate analysis.
2. **a, c, e.** Urinary retention occurs when urine is produced normally but is not excreted completely from the bladder. Factors associated with urinary retention include medications such as antihistamines, an enlarged prostate, or vaginal prolapse. Being on bedrest, having dementia, and having difficulty walking to the bathroom may place patients at risk for urinary incontinence.
3. **a, c, e, f.** It is recommended that a healthy adult drink six to eight 8-oz glasses of fluid daily, dry the perineal area after urination or defecation from the front to the back, and observe the urine for color, amount, odor, and frequency. It is also recommended to wear underwear with a cotton crotch, take showers rather than baths, and drink two glasses of water before and after sexual intercourse and void immediately after intercourse. Observing urine characteristics will not prevent a UTI; however, this observation may help a patient notice an infection.
4. **a.** Fever and diaphoresis cause the kidneys to conserve body fluids. Thus, the urine is concentrated and decreased in amount.
5. **a.** Because of the length of the male urethra and need to insert the catheter 6 to 8 inches, it is more prone to injury. The nurse inserts the catheter for a female patient 2 to 3 inches. This procedure requires surgical asepsis to prevent

introducing bacteria into the urinary tract. The presence of an indwelling catheter places the patient at risk for a UTI.

6. **c.** Post procedure continuous bladder irrigation, in the presence of hematuria, prevents stasis of blood and clot formation potentially obstructing urine output. In the absence of hematuria, clots or debris, natural irrigation of the catheter through increased fluid intake by the patient is preferred. It is preferable to avoid catheter irrigation unless necessary to relieve or prevent obstruction (Gould et al., 2009; SUNA, 2015).

7. **a, c, f.** Urinary diversion involves the surgical creation of an alternate route for excretion of urine. When caring for a patient with a urinary diversion, the nurse should measure the patient's fluid intake and output to monitor fluid balance, change the appliance frequently, monitor the return of intestinal function and peristalsis, keep the skin around the stoma dry, watch for mucus in the urine as a normal finding, and encourage the patient to participate in care and look at the stoma.

8. **d.** The stoma should appear pink to red, shiny, and moist; a dark brown or purple-blue stoma may reflect compromised circulation. The nurse contacts the health care provider immediately. A urostomy is incontinent; urine leakage is expected.

9. **b.** Factors associated with urinary retention include medications, an enlarged prostate, and vaginal prolapse. Assist the patient to void when the patient first feels the urge. Assessing for residual urine will not promote voiding; rather, it will determine the volume of urine in the bladder. Cold water would cause the patient to tighten their muscles.

10. **a.** The nurse palpates and auscultates over the access site, feeling for a thrill or vibration and listening for the bruit or swishing sound. Presence of the thrill and bruit are normal findings, indicating patency of the access. Decreased or absent thrill and/or bruit indicates a that there is an issue with the patency of the access, which could be a result of narrowing or clotting of the access, resulting in poor blood flow. No report of pain, redness, or swelling is a normal finding. A trace of edema is not a priority.

11. **c.** Pelvic floor exercises (Kegel exercises) may help a patient regain control of the micturition. Incontinence is not a normal consequence of aging. Using absorbent products may remove motivation from the patient and caregiver to seek evaluation and treatment of the incontinence; they should be used only after careful evaluation by a health care provider. Due to risk for infection, an indwelling catheter is the last choice of treatment.

12. **a.** Phenazopyridine, a urinary tract analgesic, can cause orange or orange-red urine; the nurse educates the patient to expect this change.

13. **a, e, f.** Maintaining free urinary drainage is a nursing priority. Institute measures to prevent the tubing from becoming kinked and urine from backing up in the tubing. The catheter should be allowed to drain freely through tubing that is not kinked. Nursing care of a patient with a urinary sheath includes skin care to prevent excoriation. Remove the condom daily and wash the penis with soap and water, and dry it carefully. Care must be taken to fasten the sheath securely enough to prevent leakage, yet not so tightly as to constrict the blood vessels in the area. The tip of the tubing should extend 1 to 2 inches (2.5 to 5 cm) beyond the tip of the penis to prevent irritation to the sensitive glans area. Confining a patient to bedrest increases the risk for hazards of immobility.

14. **b.** The smallest appropriate indwelling urinary catheter should be selected to aid in prevention of CAUTIs in the adult hospitalized patient (ANA, 2014; SUNA, 2015). The equipment used for catheterization is usually prepackaged in a sterile, disposable tray and is the same for both male and female patients. Most kits already contain a standard-sized catheter. Catheters are graded on the French (F) scale according to lumen size, with 12 to 16Fr gauge commonly used (Bardsley, 2015a; Beauchemin et al., 2018; Newman, 2013). A 14F, 5-mL or 10-mL balloon is usually appropriate, unless ordered otherwise (ANA, 2014).

15. **a, c, d, e.** The nurse gives these instructions to collect the midstream/clean-catch urine specimen: Wash your hands with soap and water. Open the collection cup, and place the lid face up; do not touch the inside. Separate the labia and cleanse the urinary opening with soap and water or towelettes included in the kit. Void about 1 oz. (30 mL) into the toilet, then move the collection cup close to the urinary opening and void about 1 oz (no less than 2 teaspoons) into the container. Pass the remainder of the urine into the toilet. Without touching the inside of the lid, close the cup and return it to the nurse.

16. **b.** Urinary incontinence of urine past the age of toilet training is termed enuresis. Hospitalization may cause regression of toileting habits.

17. **b.** Nephrotoxic medications are those capable of causing kidney damage. The nurse can assess I&O, quality of the urine, and renal function blood tests to detect this problem. Urinary frequency, incontinence, and getting up at night to void (nocturia) are not effects of nephrotoxic medications.

Bibliography

Agency for Healthcare Research and Quality (AHRQ). (2020, October). *Toolkit for reducing catheter-associated urinary tract infections in hospital units: Implementation guide. Appendix C. Sample Bladder scan policy*. https://www.ahrq.gov/hai/cauti-tools/impl-guide/implementation-guide-appendix-c.html

Alex, J., Salamonson, Y., Ramjan, L. M., Montayre, J., Fitzsimons, J., & Ferguson, C. (2020). The impact of educational interventions for patients living with indwelling urinary catheters: A scoping review. *Contemporary Nurse, 56*(4), 309–330. https://doi.org/10.1080/10376178.2020.1835509

Ambarsari, C. G., Hidayati, E. L., Mushahar, L., & Kadaristiana, A. (2020). Dressing versus non-dressing technique for long-term exit-site care in children on continuous ambulatory peritoneal dialysis: A single-center retrospective cohort study. *Medical Journal of Indonesia, 29*, 290–297. https://doi.org/10.13181/mji.oa.204171

American Academy of Pediatrics (AAP). (n.d.). *Toilet training. Practice guide*. Retrieved December 30, 2020, from https://www.aap.org/en-us/advocacy-and-policy/aap-health-initiatives/practicing-safety/Pages/Toilet-Training.aspx

American Academy of Pediatrics (AAP). (2016). Reaffirmation of AAP Clinical Practice Guideline: The diagnosis and management of the initial urinary tract infection in febrile infants and children 2 to 24 months of age. *Pediatrics, 138*(6), e20163026. https://doi.org/10.1542/peds.2016-3026

American Association of Critical-Care Nurses (AACN). (2016, August 1). *Prevention of CAUTI in adults*. https://www.aacn.org/clinical-resources/practice-alerts/prevention-of-cauti-in-adults

American Cancer Society (ACS). (2019, October 16). *Caring for a urostomy*. https://www.cancer.org/treatment/treatments-and-side-effects/treatment-types/surgery/ostomies/urostomy/management.html

American Nephrology Nurses Association (ANNA). (2018). *Vascular access fact sheet*. https://www.annanurse.org/download/reference/practice/vascularAccessFactSheet.pdf

American Nephrology Nurses Association (ANNA). (2019). *Peritoneal dialysis fact sheet*. https://www.annanurse.org/download/reference/practice/pdFactSheet.pdf

American Nurses Association (ANA). (n.d.). *ANA CAUTI prevention tool*. Retrieved December 16, 2020, from https://www.nursingworld.org/practice-policy/work-environment/health-safety/infection-prevention/ana-cauti-prevention-tool/

American Nurses Association (ANA). (2014). *Streamlined evidence-based RN tool: Catheter associated urinary tract infection (CAUTI) prevention*. https://www.nursingworld.org/~4aede8/globalassets/practiceandpolicy/innovation–evidence/clinical-practice-material/cauti-prevention-tool/anacautipreventiontool-final-19dec2014.pdf

Andrews, M., Boyle, J. S., & Collins, J. (2020). *Transcultural concepts in nursing care* (8th ed.). Wolters Kluwer.

Badawy, A. I., Riad, N. A., & Fareed, M. E. (2019). Effect of nursing staff development regarding ureteral stent management on nurses' knowledge and practice. *American Journal of Nursing Science, 8*(6), 317–323. https://doi.org/10.11648/j.ajns.20190806.15

Balhi, S., & Mrabet, M. K. (2020). Teaching patients clean intermittent self-catheterisation: Key points. *British Journal of Community Nursing, 25*(12), 586–593.

Bardsley, A. (2015a). Safe and effective catheterization for patients in the community. *British Journal of Community Nursing, 20*(4), 166–172. https://doi.org/10.12968/bjcn.2015.20.4.166

Bardsley, A. (2015b). Assessing and teaching female intermittent self-catheterization. *British Journal of Community Nursing, 20*(7), 344–346. https://doi.org/10.12968/bjcn.2015.20.7.344

Bauldoff, G., Gubrud, P., & Carno, M. A. (2020). *LeMone and Burke's Medical-surgical nursing: Clinical reasoning in patient care* (7th ed.). Pearson.

Beauchemin, L., Newman, D. K., Le Danseur, M., Jackson, A., & Ritmiller, M. (2018). Best practices for clean intermittent catheterization. *Nursing, 48*(9), 49–54. https://doi.org/10.1097/01.NURSE.0000544216.23783.bc

Becton, Dickinson and Company (BD). (2020). *BD PureWick™ Urine Collection System. How it works.* https://www.purewickathome.com/howitworks.html#:~:text=The%20PureWick%E2%84%A2%20System%20includes,helping%20to%20keep%20skin%20dry

Beeckman, S., Campbell, J., Campbell, K., Chimentão, D., Coyer, F., Domansky, R., Gray, M., Hevia, H., Junkin, J., Karadag, A., Kottner, J., Long, M. A., McNichol, L., Meaume, S., Nix, D., Sabasse, M., Sanada, H., Yu, P. J., Voegeli, D., & Wang, L. (2015). Proceedings of the Global IAD Expert Panel. Best Practice Principles. Incontinence-associated dermatitis: Moving prevention forward. Addressing evidence gaps for best practice. *Wounds International 2015.* https://www.woundsinternational.com/resources/details/incontinence-associated-dermatitis-moving-prevention-forward

Beeson, T., & Davis, C. (2018). Urinary management with an external female collection device. *Journal of Wound, Ostomy and Continence Nursing, 45*(2), 187–189. https://doi.org/10.1097/WON.0000000000000417

Belizario, S. M. (2015). Preventing urinary tract infections with a two-person catheter insertion procedure. *Nursing, 45*(3), 67–69. https://doi.org/10.1097/01.NURSE.0000460736.74021.69

Berti-Hearn, L., & Elliott, B. (2019). Urostomy care. A guide for home care clinicians. *Home Healthcare Now, 37*(5), 248–255.

Beuscher, T. (2014). Pad weighing for reduction of indwelling urinary use and catheter-associated urinary tract infection. *Journal of Wound Ostomy and Continence Nursing, 41*(6), 604–608. https://doi.org/10.1097/WON.0000000000000068

Beysens, M., & Tailly, T. O. (2018). Ureteral stents in urolithiasis. *Asian Journal of Urology, 5*(4), 274–286. https://doi.org/10.1016/j.ajur.2018.07.002

Bird, A. (2020). Stoma care accessory products: Responsible prescribing and cost-effective use. *Gastrointestinal Nursing, 18*(5), 13–16. https://doi.org/10.12968/gasn.2020.18.5.13

Bird, A., Wilson, K., Bertinara, A., & Amos, L. (2019). Educating patients in stoma care. *Gastrointestinal Nursing, 17*(3), 18–22. https://doi.org/10.12968/gasn.2019.17.3.18

Bradley, S. M., Schweon, S. J., Mody, L., Mahajan, D., & Olmsted, R. N. (2018). Identifying safe practices for use of the urinary leg bag drainage system in the postacute and long-term care setting: An integrative review. *American Journal of Infection Control, 46*(9), 973–979. https://doi.org/10.1016/j.ajic.2018.03.029

Bridger, S. (2019). Peritoneal dialysis access management: More than skin deep. *The Canadian Association of Nephrology Nurses and Technologists Journal, 29*(4), 11–19.

Buehrle, D. J., Clancy, C. J., & Decker, B. K. (2020). Suprapubic catheter placement improves antimicrobial stewardship among Veterans Affairs nursing care facility residents. *American Journal of Infection Control, 48*(10), 1264–1266. https://doi.org/10.1016/j.ajic.2020.01.005

Burch, J. (2018). Stoma-related complications and treatments. *Nursing & Residential Care, 20*(9), 430–433. https://doi.org/10.12968/nrec.2018.20.9.430

Burch, J. (2019). Supporting residents to care for a stoma independently. *Nursing & Residential Care, 21*(5), 276–280. https://doi.org/10.12968/nrec.2019.21.5.276

Butler, D. L. (2009). Early postoperative complications following ostomy surgery. *Journal of Wound, Ostomy and Continence Nursing, 36*(5), 513–519.

Carr, S. (2019). Catheter valves: Retraining the bladder to avoid prolonged catheter use. *Journal of Community Nursing, 33*(3), 46–51.

Centers for Disease Control and Prevention (CDC). (2015, October). *Healthcare-associated infections (HAIs). Catheter-associated urinary tract infections (CAUTI).* https://www.cdc.gov/hai/ca_uti/uti.html

Centers for Disease Control and Prevention (CDC). (2019, November 21). *CDC/STRIVE infection control training. Targeted prevention strategies. Catheter-associated urinary tract infection (CAUTI) – WB4222. CAUTI 103: Alternatives to the indwelling urinary catheter.* https://www.cdc.gov/infectioncontrol/training/strive.html#anchor_CAUTI

Centers for Medicare & Medicaid Services (CMS). (2020, February 11). *Hospital-acquired conditions.* https://www.cms.gov/Medicare/Medicare-Fee-for-Service-Payment/HospitalAcqCond/Hospital-Acquired_Conditions

Cera, J. L., & Twiss, J. J. (2018). Focused integrative review of current continence care and prevention strategies: Expanding the role of the nurse practitioner. *Urologic Nursing, 38*(4), 169–193. https://doi.org/10.7257/1053-816X.2018.38.4.169

Chandler, P. (2020). Lesbian, gay, bisexual and transgender (LGBT) inclusion in nursing services: A reflective case study from stoma care. *European Wound, Ostomy and Continence, 18*(Sup9), S26–S32. https://ecet-stomacare.eu/fileadmin/user_upload/ECET/ECET_org/EWOCS/EWOCS_Issue4_Nov_2020.pdf

Cheek, J. A., Craig, S. S., Seith, R. W., & West, A. (2015). Urine collection in young children. *Emergency Medicine Australasia, 27*(4), 348–350. https://doi.org/10.1111/1742-6723.12442

Chuasuwan, A., Pooripussarakul, S., Thakkinstian, A., Ingsathit, A., & Pattanaprateep, O. (2020). Comparisons of quality of life between patients underwent peritoneal dialysis and hemodialysis: A systematic review and meta-analysis. *Health and Quality of Life Outcomes, 18,* 191. https://doi.org/10.1186/s12955-020-01449-2

Clarke, K., Hall, C. L., Wiley, Z., Chernetsky Tejedor, S., Kim, J. S., Reif, L., Witt, L., & Jacob, J. T. (2020). Catheter-associated urinary tract infections in adults: Diagnosis, treatment, and prevention. *Journal of Hospital Medicine, 15*(9), 552–556. https://doi.org/10.12788/jhm.3292

Cleveland Clinic. (2019, May 22). *Kidney infection (pyelonephritis). Management and treatment.* https://my.clevelandclinic.org/health/diseases/15456-kidney-infection-pyelonephritis/management-and-treatment

Collier, M. (2019). Minimising pain and medical adhesive related skin injuries in vulnerable patients. *British Journal of Nursing, 28*(15), S26–S32. doi: 10.12968/bjon.2019.28.15.S26

Collins, L. (2018). Use of intermittent self-catheterisation for voiding dysfunction. *British Journal of Nursing, 27*(15), 866–868. https://doi.org/10.12968/bjon.2018.27.15.866

Collins, L. (2019). Intermittent self-catheterisation: Good patient education and support are key. *British Journal of Nursing, 28*(15), 964–966. https://doi.org/10.12968/bjon.2019.28.15.964

Colwell, J. C., Bain, K. A., Hansen, A. S., Droste, W., Vendelbo, G., & James-Reid, S. (2019). International consensus results. Development of practice guidelines for assessment of peristomal body and stoma profiles, patient engagement, and patient follow-up. *Journal of Wound, Ostomy and Continence Nursing, 46*(6), 497–504. https://doi.org/10.1097/WON.0000000000000599

Davey, G. (2015). Troubleshooting indwelling catheter problems in the community. *Journal of Community Nursing, 29*(4), 67–74.

Davis, C., & Rantell, A. (2018). Selecting an intermittent self-catheter: Key considerations. *British Journal of Nursing, 27*(15), S11–S16. https://doi.org/10.12968/bjon.2018.27.Sup15.S11

Davis, N. J., Wyman, J. F., Gubitosa, S., & Pretty, L. (2020). Urinary incontinence in older adults: A review of management approaches to a challenging and burdensome problem. *American Journal of Nursing, 120*(1), 57–62. https://doi.org/10.1097/01.naj.0000652124.58511.24

Díaz, C. C., Zambrano, S. M. H., Muñoz, B. M., Crisol, I. S., Marfil, M. N. P., Montoya-Juárez, R., & Montoro, C. H. (2018). Stoma care nurses' perspectives on the relative significance of factors influencing ostomates' quality of life. *Gastrointestinal Nursing, 16*(3), 28–33. https://doi.org/10.12968/gasn.2018.16.3.28

Dublynn, T., & Episcopia, B. (2019). Female external catheter use: A new bundle element to reduce CAUTI. *American Journal of Infection Control, 47*(Supplement), S39–S40. https://doi.org/10.1016/j.ajic.2019.04.093

Dudek, S. (2022). *Nutrition essentials for nursing practice* (9th ed.). Wolters Kluwer.

Eliopoulos, C. (2018). *Gerontological nursing* (9th ed.). Wolters Kluwer Health.

Engberg, S., Clapper, J., McNichol, L., Thompson, D., Welch, V. W., & Gray, M. (2020). Current evidence related to intermittent catheterization. *Journal of Wound, Ostomy and Continence Nursing, 47*(2), 140–165. https://doi.org/10.1097/WON.0000000000000625

Fakih, M. G., Gould, C. V., Trautner, B. W., Meddings, J., Olmsted, R. N., Krein, S. L., & Saint, S. (2016). Beyond infection: Device utilization ratio as a performance measure for urinary catheter harm. *Infection Control and Hospital Epidemiology, 37*(3), 327–333. https://doi.org/10.1017/ice.2015.287

Fischbach, F. T., Fischbach, M. A., & Stout, K. (2022). *Fischbach's a manual of laboratory and diagnostic tests* (11th ed.). Wolters Kluwer.

Fletcher-Gutowski, S., & Cecil, J. (2019). Is 2-person urinary catheter insertion effective in reducing CAUTI? *American Journal of Infection Control, 47*(12), 1508–1509. https://doi.org/10.1016/j.ajic.2019.05.014

Francis, K. (2018). Incontinence-associated dermatitis: Management update. *American Nurse Today, 13*(1), 25–27.

Gajewski, J. B., Schurch, B., Hamid, R., Averbeck, M., Sakakibara, R., Agrò, E. F., Dickinson, T., Payne, C. K., Drake, M. J., & Haylen, B. T. (2017). An International Continence Society (ICS) report on the terminology for adult neurogenic lower urinary tract dysfunction (ANLUTD). *Neurourology and Urodynamics, 37*(3), 1152–1161. https://doi.org/10.1002/nau.23397

Gentile, P., Jacob, J., & Ashraf, S. (2020, November 2). Implementation of a female external urinary catheter reduces indwelling urinary catheter use and catheter-associated urinary tract infections [Poster presentation]. Sixth Decennial International Conference on Healthcare-Associated Infections, Atlanta, GA. In *Infection Control & Hospital Epidemiology, 41*(S1), S482–S483. https://doi.org/10.1017/ice.2020.1158

George, C. (2019a). Caring for patients receiving peritoneal dialysis: Part I. *MedSurg Nursing, 28*(4), 227–233.

George, C. (2019b). Caring for patients receiving peritoneal dialysis: Part II. *MedSurg Nursing, 28*(5), 287–292.

Gibson, K. E., Neill, S., Tuma, E., Meddings, J., & Mody, L. (2019). Indwelling urethral versus suprapubic catheters in nursing home residents: Determining the safest option for long-term use. *Journal of Hospital Infection, 102*(2), 219–225. https://doi.org/10.1016/j.jhin.2018.07.027

Gill, B. C., Firoozi, F., & Rackley, R. R. (2018, June 20). Injectable bulking agents for incontinence. *Medscape.* https://emedicine.medscape.com/article/447068-overview

Goldberg, M., Colwell, J., Burns, S., Carmel, J., Fellows, J., Hendren, S., Livingston, V., Nottingham, C. U., Pittman, J., Rafferty, J., Salvadalena, G., Steinberg, G., Wound Ostomy and Continence Nurses Society, & Guideline Development Task Force. (2018). WOCN Society Clinical Guideline. Management of the adult patient with a fecal or urinary ostomy – An executive summary. *Journal of Wound, Ostomy and Continence Nursing, 45*(1), 50–58. https://doi.org/10.1097/WON.0000000000000396

Goldstine, J., Leece, R., Samas, S., & Zonderland, R. (2019). In their own words. Adults' lived experiences with intermittent catheterization. *Journal of Wound, Ostomy, and Continence Nursing, 46*(6), 513–518. https://doi.org/10.1097/WON.0000000000000591

Gould, C. V., Umscheid, C. A., Agarwal, R. K., Kuntz, G., & Pegues, D. A.; Healthcare Infection Control Practices Advisory Committee (HICPAC). (2019 [update]). *Guideline for prevention of catheter-associated urinary tract infections 2009*. Centers for Disease Control and Prevention. https://www.cdc.gov/infectioncontrol/pdf/guidelines/cauti-guidelines-H.pdf

Gray, M., & Guiliano, K. K. (2018). Incontinence-associated dermatitis, characteristics and relationship to pressure injury: A multisite epidemiologic analysis. *Journal of Wound, Ostomy & Continence Nursing, 45*(10), 63–67. https://doi.org/10.1097/WON.0000000000000390

Gray, M., Skinner, C., & Kaler, W. (2016). External collection devices as an alternative to the indwelling urinary catheter. Evidence-based review and expert clinical panel deliberations. *Journal of Wound Ostomy and Continence Nursing, 43*(3), 301–307. https://doi.org/10.1097/WON.0000000000000220

Gyesi-Appiah, E., Brown, J., & Clifton, A. (2020). Short-term urinary catheters and their risks: An integrated review. *British Journal of Community Nursing, 25*(11), 538–544. https://doi.org/10.12968/bjcn.2020.25.11.538

Hall, S. (2018, September 5). *What causes transient incontinence? Incontinence UK*. https://www.incontinence.co.uk/what-causes-transient-incontinence

Harvard Health Publishing. (2014, December 28). *Types of urinary incontinence*. Harvard Medical School. https://www.health.harvard.edu/bladder-and-bowel/types-of-urinary-incontinence

Herter, R., & Wallace Kazer, M. (2010). Best practices in urinary catheter care. *Home Healthcare Nurse, 28*(6), 342–349. https://doi.org/10.1097/NHH.0b013e3181df5d79

Hill, B. (2020). Stoma care: Procedures, appliances, and nursing considerations. *British Journal of Nursing, 29*(22), S14–S19. https://doi.org/10.12968/bjon.2020.29.22.s14

Hill, B., & Mitchell, A. (2020). Catheter application in the care home. *Nursing and Residential Care, 22*(4), 1–8. https://doi.org/10.12968/nrec.2020.22.4.9

Hill, B., & Mitchell, M. (2018). Urinary catheters. Part 1. *British Journal of Nursing, 27*(21), 1234–1236. https://doi.org/10.12968/bjon.2018.27.21.1234

Hillery, S. (2019). Caring for patients with urinary incontinence-associated dermatitis. *British Journal of Nursing, 28*(9), S26–S28. https://doi.org/10.12968/bjon.2019.28.9.S26

Hillery, S. (2020a). An introduction to urodynamics: Procedure and patient care. *British Journal of Nursing, 29*(12), 710–711. https://doi.org/10.12968/bjon.2020.29.12.710

Hillery, S. (2020b). Intermittent self-catheterisation: A person-centred approach. *British Journal of Nursing, 29*(15), 858–860. https://doi.org/10.12968/bjon.2020.29.15.858

Hinkle, J. L., Cheever, K. H., & Overbaugh, K. J. (2022). *Brunner & Suddarth's Textbook of medical-surgical nursing* (15th ed.). Wolters Kluwer.

Holroyd, S. (2019). The importance of indwelling urinary catheter securement. *British Journal of Nursing, 28*(15), 976–977. https://doi.org/10.12968/bjon.2019.28.15.976

Hooper, G. L. (2019). Evaluation and current treatments for urinary incontinence. *The Nurse Practitioner, 44*(6), 21–28. https://doi.org/10.1097/01.NPR.0000558153.53725.02

Hooton, T. M., Bradley, S. F., Cardenas, D. D., Colgan, R., Geerlings, S. E., Rice, J. C., Saint, S., Schaeffer, A. J., Tambayh, P. A., Tenke, P., Nicolle, L. E., & Infectious Diseases Society of America. (2010). Diagnosis, prevention, and treatment of catheter-associated urinary tract infection in adults: 2009 international clinical practice guidelines from the Infectious Diseases Society of America. *Clinical Infectious Diseases, 50*(5), 625–663. https://doi.org/10.1086/650482

Institute for Healthcare Improvement (IHI). (2011). *How-to guide: Prevent catheter-associated urinary tract infections*. Author. www.ihi.org

International Continence Society (ICS). (2015, August). *International Continence Society (ICS). Fact sheets. A background to urinary and faecal incontinence*. https://www.ics.org/search?q=fact%20sheet

Jacobson, T. M., & Wright, T. (2015). Improving quality by taking aim at incontinence-associated dermatitis in hospitalized adults. *MEDSURG Nursing, 24*(3), 151–157.

Jarvis, C., & Echkardt, A. (2020). *Physical examination & health assessment* (8th ed.). Elsevier.

Jensen, S. (2019). *Nursing health assessment. A best practice approach* (3rd ed.). Wolters Kluwer.

Karch, A. M. (2020). *Focus on nursing pharmacology* (8th ed.). Wolters Kluwer.

Knill, L., Maduro, R., & Payne, J. E. (2018). Targeting zero CAUTIs. *American Nurse Today, 13*(11), 54–57.

Kyle, T., & Carman, S. (2021). *Essentials of pediatric nursing* (4th ed.). Wolters Kluwer.

Lachenbruch, C., Ribble, D., Emmons, K., & VanGilder, C. (2016). Pressure ulcer risk in the incontinent patient: Analysis of incontinence and hospital-acquired pressure ulcers from the International Pressure Ulcer Prevalence Survey. *Journal of Wound Ostomy and Continence Nursing, 43*(3), 1–7. https://doi.org/10.1097/WON.0000000000000225

Lake, H. (2018). Intermittent self-catheterisation: Patient perceptions and experience. *British Journal of Nursing, 27*(18), S4–S6. https://doi.org/10.12968/bjon.2018.27.18.S4

Leach, D. (2018). Teaching patients a clean intermittent self-catheterisation technique. *British Journal of Nursing, 27*(6), 296–298. https://doi.org/10.12968/bjon.2018.27.6.296

LeBlanc, K., Whiteley, I., McNichol, L., Salfadalena, G., & Gray, M. (2019). Peristomal medical adhesive-related skin injury. Results of an international consensus meeting. *Journal of Wound, Ostomy and Continence Nursing, 46*(2), 125–136. DOI: 10.1097/WON.0000000000000513

Lim, Y. S. L., & Carville, K. (2019). Prevention and management of incontinence-associated dermatitis in the pediatric population. An integrative review. *Journal of Wound Ostomy and Continence Nursing, 46*(1), 30–37. https://doi.org/10.1097/WON.0000000000000490

Logan, K. (2020). An exploration of men's experiences of learning intermittent self-catheterisation with a silicone catheter. *British Journal of Nursing, 29*(2), 84–90. https://doi.org/10.12968/bjon.2020.29.2.84

Mahoney, M., Baxter, K., Burgess, J., Bauer, C., Downey, C., Mantel, J., Perkins, J., Rice, M., Salvadalena, G., Schafer, V., & Sheppard, S. (2013). Procedure for obtaining a urine sample from a urostomy, ileal conduit, and colon conduit. A best practice guideline for clinicians. *Journal of Wound Ostomy Continence Nursing, 40*(3), 277–279. https://doi.org/10.1097/won.0b013e31828f1a47

Mangnall, J. (2015). Managing and teaching intermittent catheterisation. *British Journal of Community Nursing, 20*(2), 82–88. https://doi.org/10.12968/bjcn.2015.20.2.82

May, O. W. (2018). Urine collection methods in children: Which is the best? *Nursing Clinics of North America, 53*(2), 137–143. https://doi.org/10.1016/j.cnur.2018.01.001

Mayo Foundation for Medical Education and Research (MFMER). (2019a, April 13). *Urinary incontinence*. https://www.mayoclinic.org/diseases-conditions/urinary-incontinence/diagnosis-treatment/drc-20352814#:~:text=Urethral%20insert%2C%20a%20small%2C%20tampon,vagina%20and%20wear%20all%20day

Mayo Foundation for Medical Education and Research (MFMER). (2019b, April 24). *Tests and procedures. Peritoneal dialysis*. https://www.mayoclinic.org/tests-procedures/peritoneal-dialysis/about/pac-20384725

Mayo Foundation for Medical Education and Research (MFMER). (2019c, July 23). *Tests and procedures. Hemodialysis*. https://www.mayoclinic.org/tests-procedures/hemodialysis/about/pac-20384824

Mayo Foundation for Medical Education and Research (MFMER). (2020, October 14). *Urinary tract infection (UTI)*. https://www.mayoclinic.org/diseases-conditions/urinary-tract-infection/symptoms-causes/syc-20353447#:~:text=The%20most%20common%20UTIs%20occur,sometimes%20other%20bacteria%20are%20responsible

Meddings, J., Saint, S., Fowler, K. E., Gaies, E., Hickner, A., Krein, S. L., & Bernstein, S. J. (2015). The Ann Arbor criteria for appropriate urinary catheter use in hospitalized medical patients: Results obtained by using the RAND/UCLA appropriateness method. *Annals of Internal Medicine, 162*(9), S1–S34. https://doi.org/10.7326/M14-1304

Mitchell, A., & Hill, B. (2020). Moisture-associated skin damage: An overview of its diagnosis and management. *British Journal of Community Nursing, 25*(3), S12–S18. https://doi.org/10.12968/bjcn.2020.25.Sup3.S12

Mitchell, M., & Hill, B. (2018). Urinary catheters: Part 2. Catheterisation in males and females. *British Journal of Nursing, 27*(22), 1306–1310. https://doi.org/10.12968/bjon.2018.27.22.1306

Morton, P. G., & Fontaine, D. K. (2018). *Critical care nursing. A holistic approach* (11th ed.). Wolters Kluwer.

National Association for Continence (NAFC). (n.d.a.). *Urinary incontinence overview*. Retrieved December 26, 2020, from https://www.nafc.org/urinary-incontinence

National Association for Continence (NAFC). (n.d.b.). *Diet and exercise*. Retrieved December 26, 2020, from https://www.nafc.org/diet-and-exercise

National Institute of Diabetes and Digestive and Kidney Diseases (NIDDK). (2014a, February). *Urodynamic testing*. https://www.niddk.nih.gov/health-information/diagnostic-tests/urodynamic-testing

National Institute of Diabetes and Digestive and Kidney Diseases (NIDDK). (2017, March). *Urologic diseases. Bladder infection (Urinary tract infection-UTI) in adults*. https://www.niddk.nih.gov/health-information/urologic-diseases/bladder-infection-uti-in-adults?dkrd=hispt0451

National Institute of Diabetes and Digestive and Kidney Diseases (NIDDK). (2018a, January). *What is kidney failure?* https://www.niddk.nih.gov/health-information/kidney-disease/kidney-failure/what-is-kidney-failure

National Institute of Diabetes and Digestive and Kidney Diseases (NIDDK). (2018b, June). *Urologic diseases. Bladder control problems (Urinary incontinence)*. https://www.niddk.nih.gov/health-information/urologic-diseases/bladder-control-problems?dkrd=/health-information/urologic-diseases/bladder-control-problems-women

National Institute of Diabetes and Digestive and Kidney Diseases (NIDDK). (2020, June). *Urologic diseases. Urinary diversion*. https://www.niddk.nih.gov/health-information/urologic-diseases/urinary-diversion

National Institute on Aging. (2017, May 16). *Urinary incontinence in older adults*. https://www.nia.nih.gov/health/urinary-incontinence-older-adults

National Kidney Foundation (NKF). (2016, August 9). *Urinary tract infections*. https://www.kidney.org/atoz/content/uti

National Kidney Foundation (NKF). (2020, July 2). *Peritoneal dialysis. What you need to know*. https://www.kidney.org/atoz/content/peritoneal

Nazarko, L. (2015). Use of continence pads to manage urinary incontinence in older people. *British Journal of Community Nursing, 20*(8), 378–384. https://doi.org/10.12968/bjcn.2015.20.8.378

Newman, D. K. (2013). Designs – Indwelling urinary catheters. *UroToday*. https://www.urotoday.com/urinary-catheters-home/indwelling-catheters/description/designs.html

Newman, D. K. (2019a). Evidence-based practice guideline. Prompted voiding for individuals with urinary incontinence. *Journal of Gerontological Nursing, 45*(2), 14–26. https://doi.org/10.3928/00989134-20190111-03

Newman, D. K. (2019b, November 28). Urinary catheters. Intermittent catheters. Description. *UroToday*. https://www.urotoday.com/urinary-catheters-home/intermittent-catheters/description/definition-intermittent-catheters.html

Newman, D. K. (2020a). Bladder health. Types and materials – external urine collection devices. *UroToday*. https://www.urotoday.com/library-resources/bladder-health/120651-types-and-materials-external-urine-collection-devices.html

Newman, D. K. (2020b, April 10). Introduction: External urinary catheters. *UroToday*. https://www.urotoday.com/library-resources/bladder-health/120599-introduction-external-urinary-catheters.html

Norris, T. L. (2020). *Porth's essentials of pathophysiology* (5th ed.). Wolters Kluwer.

O'Flynn, S. K. (2018). Care of the stoma: Complications and treatments. *British Journal of Community Nursing, 23*(8), 382–387. https://doi.org/10.12968/bjcn.2018.23.8.382

Pair, L. S., & Somerall, W. E. (2018). Urinary incontinence: Pelvic floor muscle and behavioral training for women. *The Nurse Practitioner, 43*(1), 21–25. https://doi.org/10.1097/01.NPR.0000527571.66854.0d

Palka, M. A. (2014). Evidenced based review of recommendations addressing the frequency of changing long-term indwelling urinary catheters in older adults. *Geriatric Nursing, 35*(5), 357–363. https://doi.org/10.1016/j.gerinurse.2014.04.010

Palmer, S. J. (2020). Overview of stoma care for community nurses. *British Journal of Community Nursing, 25*(7), 340–344. https://doi.org/10.12968/bjcn.2020.25.7.340

Panchisin, T. L. (2016). Improving outcomes with the ANA CAUTI Prevention Tool. *Nursing, 46*(3), 55–59. https://doi.org/10.1097/01.NURSE.0000480603.14769.d6

Payne, D. (2020). Managing incontinence in people with dementia. *British Journal of Community Nursing, 25*(9), 430–436. https://doi.org/10.12968/bjcn.2020.25.9.430

Peate, I. (2019). Urinary incontinence in women: Treatment recommendations. *British Journal of Nursing, 28*(22), 1486–1488. https://doi.org/10.12968/bjon.2019.28.22.1486

Pelling, H., Nzakizwanayo, J., Milo, S., Denham, E. L., MacFarlane, W. M., Bock, L. J., Sutton, J. M., & Jones, B. V. (2019). Bacterial biofilm formation on indwelling urethral catheters. *Letters in Applied Microbiology, 68*(4), 277–293. https://doi.org/10.1111/lam.13144

Phipps, L. A., Gray, M., & Call, E. (2019). Time of onset to changes in skin condition during exposure to synthetic urine. *Journal of Wound Ostomy and Continence Nursing, 46*(4), 315–320. https://doi.org/10.1097/WON.0000000000000549

Razik, A., Das, C. J., Gupta, A., Wanamacher, D., & Verma, S. (2019). Urinary diversions: A primer of the surgical techniques and imaging findings. *Abdominal Radiology, 44*, 3906–3918. https://doi.org/10.1007/s00261-019-02179-w

Rhone, C., Breiter, Y., Benson, L., Petri, H., Thompson, P., & Murphy, C. (2017). The impact of two-person indwelling urinary catheter insertion in the emergency department using technical and socioadaptive interventions. *Journal of Clinical Outcomes Management, 24*(10), 451–456.

Sabir, N., Ikram, A., Zaman, G., Satti, L., Gardezi, A., Ahmed, A., & Ahmed, P. (2017). Bacterial biofilm-based catheter-associated urinary tract infections: Causative pathogens and antibiotic resistance. *American Journal of Infection Control, 45*(10), 1101–1105. https://doi.org/10.1016/j.ajic.2017.05.009

Schaepe, C., & Bergjan, M. (2015). Educational interventions in peritoneal dialysis: A narrative review of the literature. *International Journal of Nursing Studies, 52*(4), 882–898. https://doi.org/10.1016/j.ijnurstu.2014.12.009

Schallom, M., Prentice, d., Sona, C., Vyers, K., Arroyo, C., Wessman, B., & Ablordeppey, E. (2020). Accuracy of measuring bladder volumes with ultrasound and bladder scanning. *American Journal of Critical Care, 29*(6), 458–467. https://doi.org/10.4037/ajcc2020741

Sepsis Alliance. (2020, August 9). *Sepsis. Aging*. https://www.sepsis.org/sepsisand/aging/

Shah, S. M. (2019a, January 31). *Suprapubic catheter care*. MedlinePlus. https://medlineplus.gov/ency/patientinstructions/000145.htm

Shah, S. M. (2019b, January 31). *Urine drainage bags*. MedlinePlus. https://medlineplus.gov/ency/patientinstructions/000142.htm

Shaw, C., & Wagg, A. (2019). Long-term urinary catheterisation in community-dwelling adults. *British Journal of Community Nursing, 24*(6), 258–262. https://doi.org/10.12968/bjcn.2019.24.6.258

Shin, D. C., Shin, S. H., Lee, M. M., Lee, K. J., & Song, C. H. (2016). Pelvic floor muscle training for urinary incontinence in female stroke patients: A randomized, controlled and blinded trial. *Clinical Rehabilitation, 30*(3), 259–267. https://doi.org/10.1177/0269215515578695

Silbert-Flagg, J., & Pillitteri, A. (2018). *Maternal and child health nursing* (8th ed.). Wolters Kluwer.

Slade, S., Hay-Smith, J., Mastwyk, S., Morris, M. W., & Frawley, H. (2018). Barriers and enablers to implementation of pelvic floor muscle training interventions for urinary incontinence. *Australian + New Zealand Continence Journal, 24*(4), 118–125.

Smart, C. (2014). Male urinary incontinence and the urinary sheath. *British Journal of Nursing, 23*(9), S20–S25.

Society of Urologic Nurses and Associates (SUNA). (2015). *Clinical practice guidelines. Care of the patient with an indwelling catheter. [Brochure]*. Author.

Society of Urologic Nurses and Associates (SUNA). (2016). *Clinical practice guidelines. Suprapubic catheter replacement. [Brochure]*. Author.

Society of Urologic Nurses and Associates (SUNA). (2019). *Patient fact sheet. Urinary incontinence*. https://www.suna.org/download/members/incontinenceFactSheet.pdf

Society of Urologic Nurses and Associates (SUNA). (2021a). Clinical practice procedure. Urinary catheterization of the adult female. *Urologic Nursing, 41*(2), 65–69. https://www.suna.org/resource/urinary-catheter-care

Society of Urologic Nurses and Associates (SUNA). (2021b). Clinical practice procedure. Insertion of an indwelling urethral catheter in the adult female. *Urologic Nursing, 41*(2), 76–109. https://www.suna.org/download/catheterInsertionFemaleCCP.pdf

Society of Urologic Nurses and Associates (SUNA). (2021c). Clinical practice procedure. Urinary catheterization of the adult male. *Urologic Nursing, 41*(2), 70–75. https://www.suna.org/download/catheterizationMaleCCP.pdf

Society of Urologic Nurses and Associates (SUNA). (2021d). Clinical practice procedure. Insertion of an indwelling urethral catheter in the adult male. *Urologic Nursing, 41*(2), 86–109.

Southgate, G., & Gradbury, S. (2016). Management of incontinence-associated dermatitis with a skin barrier protectant. *British Journal of Nursing, 25*(9), S20–S29. https://doi.org/10.12968/bjon.2016.25.9.S20

Stelton, S. (2019). Stoma and peristomal skin care: A clinical review. *American Journal of Nursing, 119*(6), 38–45.

Swift, T., Westgate, G., Van Onselen, J., & Lee, S. (2020). Developments in silicone technology for use in stoma care. *British Journal of Nursing, 29*(6), S6–S15. doi: 10.12968/bjon.2020.29.6.S6

Touhy, T. A., & Jett, K. (2018). *Ebersol and Hess' gerontological nursing & healthy aging* (5th ed.). Elsevier.

United Ostomy Associations of America (UOAA). (n.d.). *Support, education, resources advocacy*. Retrieved December 30, 2020, from https://www.ostomy.org/

Vaarala, M. H. (2018). Urinary sample collection methods in ileal conduit urinary diversion patients. *Journal of Wound Ostomy and Continence Nursing, 45*(1), 59–62. https://doi.org/10.1097/WON.0000000000000397

Vasavada, S. P., Carmel, M E., & Rackley, R. R. (2019a, September 23). Urinary incontinence treatment & management. *Medscape*. https://emedicine.medscape.com/article/452289-treatment#d9

Vasavada, S. P., Carmel, M E., & Rackley, R. R. (2019b, September 23). Urinary incontinence. *Medscape*. https://emedicine.medscape.com/article/452289-overview#:~:text=Urinary%20incontinence%20is%20an%20underdiagnosed,in%20females%20than%20in%20males

Vasavada, S. P., Carmel, M. E., & Rackley, R. R. (2019c, September 23). Urology. Urinary incontinence. *Medscape*. https://emedicine.medscape.com/article/452289-overview#a4

VHA Center for Engineering & Occupational Safety and Health (CEOSH). (2016). *Safe patient handling and mobility guidebook*. http://www.tnpatientsafety.com/pubfiles/Initiatives/workplace-violence/sphm-pdf.pdf

Voegeli, D. (2016). Incontinence-associated dermatitis: New insights into an old problem. *British Journal of Nursing, 25*(5), 256–262. https://doi.org/10.12968/bjon.2016.25.5.256

Voegeli, D. (2018). Incontinence-associated dermatitis: Management. *Nursing & Residential Care, 20*(10), 506–512. https://doi.org/10.12968/nrec.2018.20.10.506

Weiss, J. P. (2020, August 25). Nocturia: How to define it, and how to treat it. Urology Times. https://www.urologytimes.com/view/nocturia-how-to-define-it-and-how-to-treat-it

Widdall, D. A. (2015). Considerations for determining a bladder scan protocol. *Journal of the Australasian Rehabilitation Nurses' Association, 18*(3), 22–27.

Williams, J. (2012). Stoma care: Obtaining a urine specimen from a urostomy. *Gastrointestinal Nursing, 10*(5), 11–12.

Wilson, M. (2015a). Clean intermittent self-catheterisation: Working with patients. *British Journal of Nursing, 24*(2), 76–85. https://doi.org/10.12968/bjon.2015.24.2.76

Wilson, M. (2015b). Urine-drainage leg bags: An overview. *British Journal of Nursing, 24*(18), S30–S35. https://doi.org/10.12968/bjon.2015.24.Sup18.S30

Wound Ostomy and Continence Nurses Society (WOCN). (2018). *Catheterization of an ileal or colon conduit stoma: Best practice for clinicians*. https://www.ostomy.org/wp-content/uploads/2018/11/Catheterization-of-Urinary-Stoma-2018.pdf

Wu, M. L., Pu, L., Grealish, L., Johes, C., & Moyle, W. (2020). The effectiveness of nurse-led interventions for preventing urinary tract infections in older adults in residential aged care facilities: A systematic review. *Journal of Clinical Nursing, 29*(9–10), 1432–1444. https://doi.org/10.1111/jocn.15198

Wuthier, P., Sublett, K., & Riehl, L. (2016). Urinary catheter dependent loops as a potential contributing cause of bacteriuria: An observational study. *Urologic Nursing, 36*(1), 7–16. https://doi.org/10.7257/1053-816X.2016.36.1.7

Yates, A. (2016). Indwelling urinary catheterisation: What is best practice? *British Journal of Nursing, 25*(9), S4–S13. https://doi.org/10.12968/bjon.2016.25.9.S4

Yates, A. (2017a). Urinary catheters 1: Male catheterisation. *Nursing Times, 113*(1), 32–34. https://www.nursingtimes.net/clinical-archive/continence/urinary-catheters-1-male-catheterisation-2-05-12-2016/

Yates, A. (2017b). Urinary catheters 2: Inserting a catheter into a female patient. *Nursing Times* [online], *113*(2), 50–20. https://www.nursingtimes.net/clinical-archive/continence/urinary-catheters-2-inserting-a-catheter-into-a-female-patient-16-01-2017/

Yates, A. (2017c). Urinary catheter 5: Teaching patients how to use a catheter valve. *Nursing Times* [online], *113*(5), 25–27. https://www.nursingtimes.net/clinical-archive/continence/urinary-catheters-5-teaching-patients-how-to-use-a-catheter-valve-10-04-2017/

Yates, A. (2017d). Urinary catheters 6: Removing an indwelling urinary catheter. *Nursing Times, 113*(6), 33–35.

Yates, A. (2018a). Incontinence-associated dermatitis in older people: prevention and management. *British Journal of Community Nursing, 23*(5), 218–224. https://doi.org/10.12968/bjcn.2018.23.5.218

Yates, A. (2018b). Incontinence-associated dermatitis: What nurses need to know. *British Journal of Nursing, 27*(19), 1094–1100. https://doi.org/10.12968/bjon.2018.27.19.1094

Yates, A. (2018c). Catheter securing and fixation devices: Their role in preventing complications. *British Journal of Nursing, 27*(6), 290–294. https://doi.org/10.12968/bjon.2018.27.6.290

Yates, A. (2019). Basic continence assessment: What community nurses should know. *Journal of Community Nursing, 33*(3), 52–55.

39 Bowel Elimination

Jeremy Green

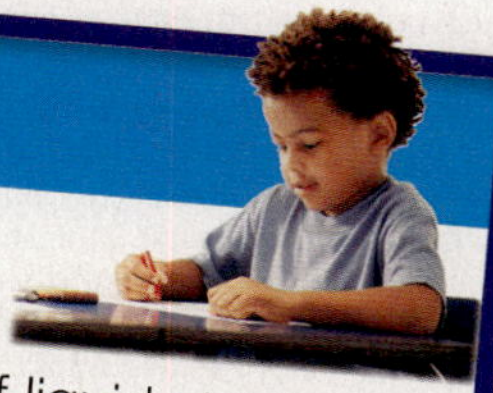

Jeremy, age 4, has been attending day care since his mother returned to work 6 months ago. He presents at the hospital with a history of liquid stools, six to seven times a day, for the last 3 days.

Alberta Franklin

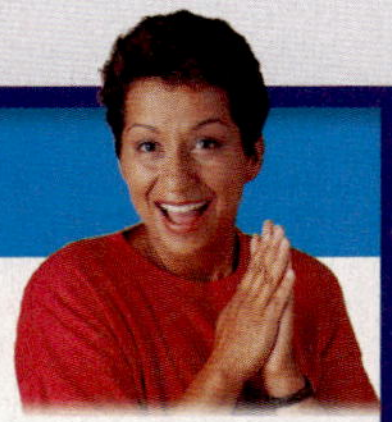

Alberta, age 55, has recently undergone abdominal surgery that resulted in the creation of a sigmoid colostomy. Her stoma is bright red and moist and draining semisoft brown stool. Her ostomy appliance needs to be changed.

Leroy Cobbs

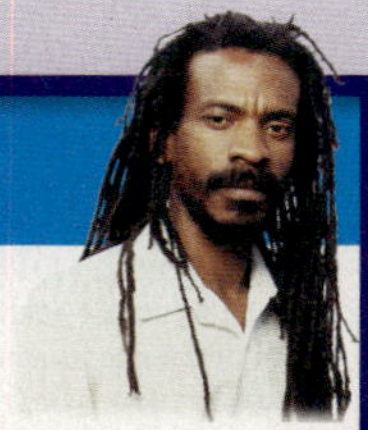

Leroy, newly diagnosed with cancer, is taking acetaminophen with codeine for pain. He comes to the outpatient health center with constipation. “Nobody told me I would get so constipated,” he says. “It's been almost a week, and I'm still not moving my bowels normally. I didn't know anything could hurt so bad. I'll take my chances with the cancer pain in the future rather than take more pain meds and have this happen again.”

Lippincott DocuCare **Additional patient scenarios available in *Lippincott DocuCare*.**

Learning Outcomes

After completing the chapter, you will be able to accomplish the following:

1. Describe the anatomy and physiology of bowel elimination.
2. Identify variables that influence bowel elimination.
3. Assess bowel elimination using appropriate interview questions and physical assessment skills.
4. Assist with stool collection for laboratory analysis and direct and indirect visualization studies of the gastrointestinal tract.
5. Diagnose actual and potential health problems and needs related to bowel elimination that may be addressed through nursing intervention.
6. Describe appropriate nursing interventions to promote regular bowel habits.
7. Describe appropriate nursing interventions when administering laxatives and antidiarrheals.
8. Demonstrate appropriate nursing interventions when administering enemas, rectal suppositories, rectal catheters, and when performing digital removal of stool.
9. Describe appropriate nursing interventions to ease defecation.
10. Plan and provide nursing care for a patient with an ostomy.
11. Plan, implement, and evaluate nursing care related to selected actual and potential health problems and needs associated with alterations in bowel elimination.

Nursing Concepts

- Assessment
- Clinical Decision Making/Clinical Judgment
- Elimination
- Safety

Expectations about bowel elimination, usual patterns of defecation, and the ease with which a person speaks about bowel problems differ widely among people. Although most people have experienced minor acute bouts of diarrhea or constipation, some people experience severe or chronic alterations in bowel elimination that affect their fluid and electrolyte balance, hydration, nutritional status, skin integrity, comfort, and self-concept. Moreover, many illnesses, diagnostic tests, medications, and surgical treatments can affect bowel elimination.

This chapter discusses the anatomy and physiology of bowel elimination and the factors that influence this process. A guide for assessing bowel elimination, including diagnostic studies of the gastrointestinal (GI) tract and their associated nursing responsibilities, is presented. Potential and actual health problems and needs related to bowel elimination are provided, and patient outcomes related to optimal bowel function are identified. In addition, the chapter presents nursing strategies to meet those goals. The accompanying Reflective Practice display illustrates nursing strategies addressing bowel diversions. The concluding care plan illustrates the use of specific nursing interventions to resolve bowel elimination problems and needs.

ANATOMY AND PHYSIOLOGY

The GI tract, also known as the alimentary tract or canal, extends from the mouth to the **anus**, the outlet of the GI tract. The anatomy of the GI tract is shown in Figure 39-1. The stomach and small intestine are discussed briefly. The major organ involved with bowel elimination is the large intestine, which will be discussed in greater detail.

Stomach

The stomach is a hollow, J-shaped, muscular organ located in the left upper portion of the abdomen. The stomach stores food during eating, secretes digestive fluids, churns food to aid in digestion, and pushes the partially digested food, called chyme, into the small intestine. The pyloric sphincter, a muscular ring that regulates the size of the opening at the end of the stomach, controls the movement of chyme from the stomach into the small intestine.

Small Intestine

The small intestine is about 18 to 20 ft (5.5 to 6 m) long and about 1 to 1.5 inches (2.2 to 3.8 cm) wide (Jensen, 2019). The small intestine is made up of three parts: the first is the duodenum, the middle section is the jejunum, and the distal section that connects with the large intestine is the ileum (Fig. 39-2). The small intestine secretes enzymes that digest proteins and carbohydrates. Digestive juices from the liver and pancreas enter the small intestine through a small opening in the duodenum. The small intestine is responsible for digestion of food and absorption of nutrients into the bloodstream.

Large Intestine

The connection between the ileum of the small intestine and the large intestine is the ileocecal, or ileocolic, valve. This valve normally prevents contents from entering the large intestine prematurely and prevents waste products from returning to the small intestine.

The large intestine, the primary organ of bowel elimination, is the lower, or distal, part of the GI tract. The large intestine, also known as the colon, extends from the ileocecal valve to the anus. The large intestine (colon) in adults is about 5 to 6 ft (1.5 to 1.8 m) long, but variations in length are normal (Jensen, 2019; Norris, 2020). Width also varies; at its narrowest point, the colon is about 1 inch (2.5 cm) wide; at its widest point, it is about 3 inches (7.5 cm). The

(text continues on page 1520)

QSEN Reflective Practice: Cultivating QSEN Competencies

CHALLENGE TO TECHNICAL SKILLS

Although nursing students learn the steps of a psychomotor skill in the simulation practice laboratory, it is often quite a different situation when they are asked to perform the skill for the first time on their own. I found this to be true the first time that I had to perform colostomy care independently.

I met Alberta Franklin while working as a nursing extern this summer. Ms. Franklin was a 55-year-old female who had recently undergone abdominal surgery and creation of a sigmoid colostomy. They required a new colostomy bag, and I was asked to change the bag. Although care for a patient with a colostomy does not require the computerized technology found in an ICU, it does require technical skills. I had practiced changing colostomy bags in the nursing skills lab and had observed nurses changing the colostomy bag in the hospital. I had even previously changed a colostomy bag while being supervised by a nurse. Although I was not completely comfortable with the situation, I agreed to change the bag. I quickly reviewed the steps in the protocol book and went into the patient's room. I measured the colostomy and then cut the bag to the appropriate size. Unfortunately, I had measured the colostomy incorrectly, and the bag was too large, so I had to leave the room and get more supplies. After a few more obstacles, I was able to adhere a properly fitting bag to the patient—but not before the patient correctly guessed that this was the first time I had performed this skill! Their ability to guess that I had never performed this skill before illustrates a need to improve my technical competence.

Thinking Outside the Box: Possible Courses of Action

- Refuse to provide the care and ask another nurse to change the colostomy bag.
- Observe a nurse performing the care one more time.
- Check protocol and perform the care, knowing that I could call a nurse if needed.
- "Wing it" and hope that I remember what I had learned in lab.

Evaluating a Good Outcome: How Do I Define Success?

- Patient receives safe care.
- Patient's needs are met.
- Nurse demonstrates technical competency with the skill.

Personal Learning: Here's to the Future!

I think that my actions were appropriate. Although I was unsure about my technical skills regarding colostomy care, I performed the skill adequately. In addition, I reviewed the appropriate steps, and I knew that I could summon the assistance of a nurse in case if I needed to. I also made sure that I knew where the nurse was so that if I did need help, I wouldn't waste any time looking for help. Therefore, I ensured that the patient's safety would not be compromised. Although at that time I would have preferred to have another nurse perform the colostomy change, I am glad that I completed this technical skill independently. Observing another person performing a skill can be beneficial, but there comes a point when you must "spread your wings" and complete the skill on your own. Of course, this philosophy regarding spreading your wings applies only to certain technologies: It would be inappropriate to use this philosophy if it compromised patient safety. However, in instances like this one, where patient safety is not compromised and the appropriate teaching and training have been completed, I think it is appropriate to take action. If you don't, the various skills required to care for patients can become extremely intimidating and overwhelming. As a result, fear increases, which can possibly threaten a patient's safety and lead to injury.

Elizabeth Nalli, Georgetown University

QSEN SELF-REFLECTION ON QUALITY AND SAFETY COMPETENCIES DEVELOPING KNOWLEDGE, SKILLS, AND ATTITUDES FOR CONTINUOUS IMPROVEMENT

How do you think you would respond in a similar situation? Why? What does this tell you about yourself and about the adequacy of your skills for professional practice? Do you agree with the criteria that the nursing student used to evaluate a successful outcome? Are there any other criteria that would be appropriate to use? Did the nursing student meet the criteria? Why or why not? What *knowledge*, *skills*, and *attitudes* do you need to develop to continuously improve the quality and safety of care for patients like Ms. Franklin?

Patient-Centered Care: How could you involve the patient as a partner in coordinating Ms. Fanklin's care to minimize frustration on the part of the patient and student? What interventions should the nursing student implement to provide care based on respect for the patient's preferences, values, and needs? What might you have done to prevent the numerous trips in and out of the patient's room? Did the nursing student's actions adhere to ethical and legal principles? If not, describe what principles were violated.

Teamwork and Collaboration/Quality Improvement: What communication skills do you need to improve to ensure that you function as a member of the patient-care team? What skills do you need to initiate requests for help and to obtain assistance when needed?

Safety/Evidence-Based Practice: What actions or behaviors by the nursing student might have provided clues to the patient that this was the nursing student's first independent attempt at the skill? What skills do you need to improve to ensure that patients in your care receive the best nursing care possible?

Informatics: Can you identify the essential information that must be available in Ms. Franklin's electronic health record to support safe patient care and coordination of care? What information should be documented in the electronic health record regarding the student's assessment and interventions? Can you think of other ways to respond to or approach the situation?

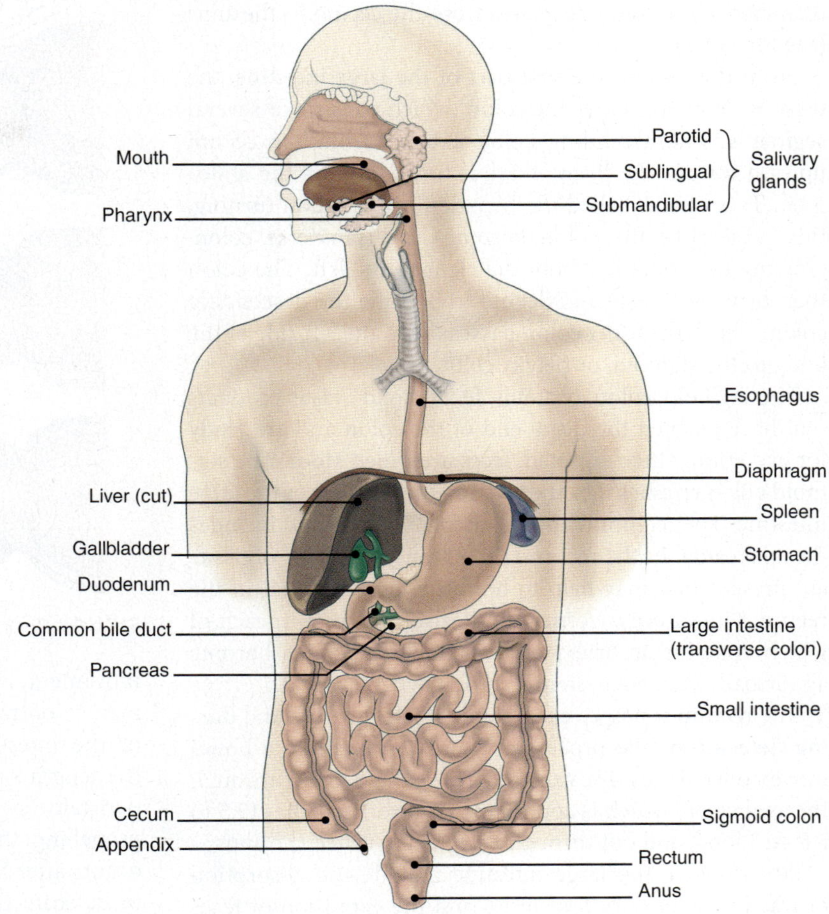

FIGURE 39-1. Organs of the gastrointestinal tract.

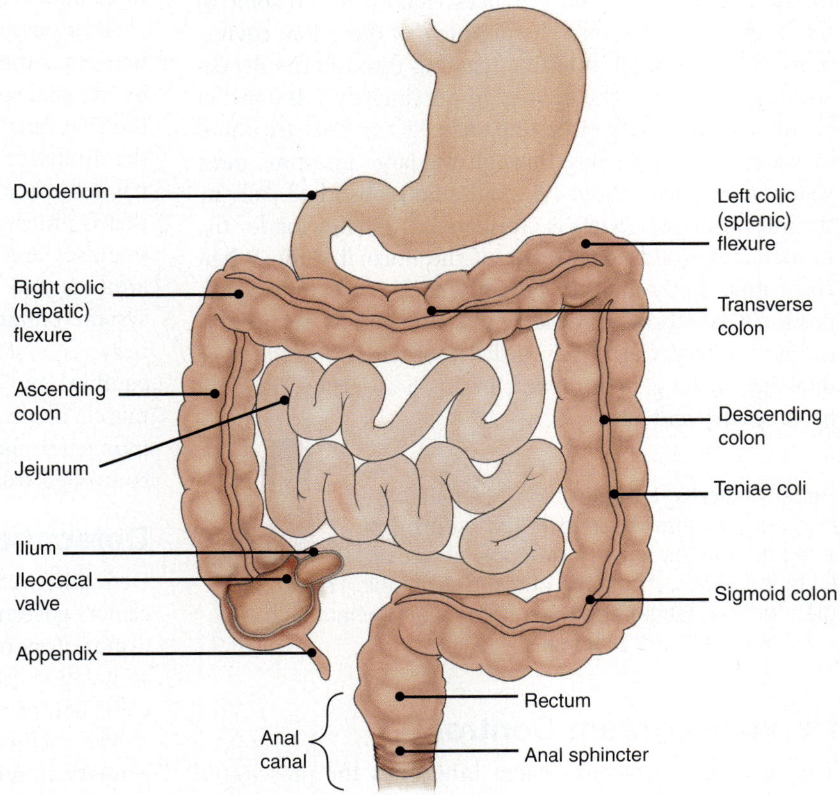

FIGURE 39-2. The small and large intestines.

diameter of the colon decreases from the cecum to the anus (see Fig. 39-2).

From the cecum, the first part of the large intestine, the digestive contents enter the colon, which consists of several segments. The ascending colon extends from the cecum upward toward the liver, where it turns to cross the abdomen. This turn is called the hepatic flexure. Upon turning, this portion of the colon becomes the transverse colon, crossing the abdomen from the right to the left. The colon then turns at the splenic flexure to become the descending colon. The descending colon passes down the left side of the body to the sigmoid, or pelvic, colon.

The sigmoid colon contains **feces**, solid waste products that have reached the distal end of the colon and are ready for excretion. Once excreted, feces are called **stool**. The sigmoid colon empties into the rectum, the last part of the large intestine. The rectum is about 5 inches (12 cm) and includes the anal canal. In the rectum, three transverse folds of tissue are present that may help to hold the fecal material in the rectum temporarily. Vertical folds also are present, each of which contains an artery and a vein. If the veins become abnormally distended, **hemorrhoids** occur.

The rectum is empty except immediately before and during **defecation** (the process of bowel elimination; a bowel movement). Feces are excreted from the rectum through the anal canal, which is approximately 1 to 1.5 inches (2.5 to 3.8 cm) long, and out through an opening called the anus.

Functions of the large intestine include the absorption of water, the formation of feces, and the expulsion of feces from the body. Bacteria that reside in the large intestine act on food residue while it makes its way through the large intestine. Bacterial action produces vitamin K and some of the B-complex vitamins. The products of digestion, chyme, move from the small intestine, passing through the ileocecal valve, and enter the cecum. Approximately 1,500 mL of chyme enters the large intestine daily. Its contents are liquid or watery. While passing through the large intestine, most water is absorbed. About 1.5 L of liquid is absorbed daily by the intestinal tract (Kiela & Ghishan, 2016), allowing for the formed, semisolid consistency of the normal stool. When absorption does not occur properly, such as when the waste products pass through the large intestine rapidly, the stool is soft and watery. Conversely, if the stool remains in the large intestine too long, or if too much water is absorbed, the stool becomes dry and hard.

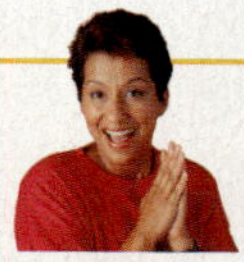

Recall **Alberta Franklin**, the woman who had surgery that resulted in the creation of a sigmoid colostomy. Knowledge of normal GI function would help the nurse in developing a teaching plan for this patient about the ostomy and what to expect in relation to bowel function.

Nervous System Control

The autonomic nervous system innervates the muscles of the colon. The parasympathetic nervous system stimulates movement, while the sympathetic system inhibits movement. Contractions of the circular and longitudinal muscles of the intestine, **peristalsis**, move waste products along the length of the intestine continuously (Fig. 39-3). Mass peristaltic sweeps occur several times a day in most people, propelling the fecal mass forward. Mass peristalsis often occurs after food has been ingested, accounting for the urge to defecate that often occurs after meals. Timing nursing interventions to evacuate bowel contents with this natural urge to defecate is helpful. Normal colonic transit time is 24 to 28 hours (Norris, 2020).

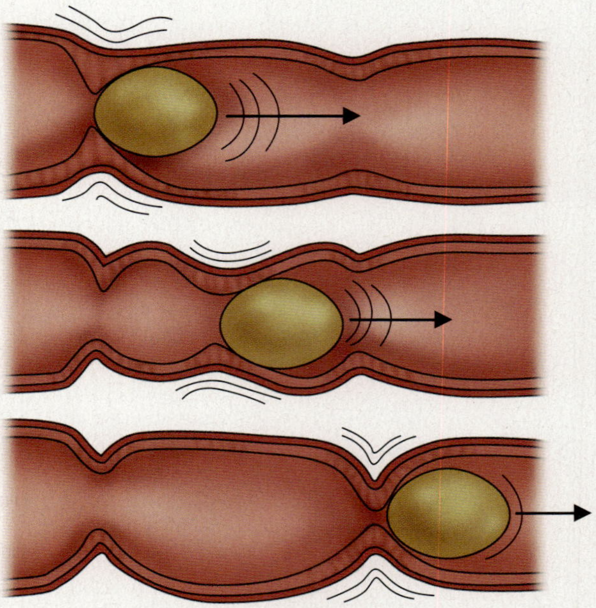

FIGURE 39-3. Peristaltic movements in the intestine.

After passing through the sigmoid colon, the waste products enter the rectum, where they are stopped from exiting by the anal sphincters (Fig. 39-4). The internal sphincter in the anal canal and the external sphincter at the anus control the discharge of feces and **flatus** (intestinal gas). The internal sphincter consists of involuntary smooth muscle tissue that is innervated by the autonomic nervous system. Motor impulses are carried by the sympathetic system (thoracolumbar) and inhibitory impulses by the parasympathetic system (craniosacral). These two divisions of the autonomic nervous system function antagonistically in a dynamic equilibrium. The external sphincter at the anus has striated muscle tissue and is under voluntary control. The levator ani muscle reinforces the action of the external sphincter and is controlled voluntarily.

Defecation

Defecation refers to the emptying of the large intestine. Two centers govern the reflex to defecate, one in the medulla and a subsidiary one in the spinal cord. When parasympathetic stimulation occurs, the internal anal sphincter relaxes and the colon contracts, allowing the fecal mass to enter the rectum.

The rectum becomes distended by the fecal mass, the primary stimulus for the defecation reflex. Rectal distention leads to an increase in the intrarectal pressure, causing the

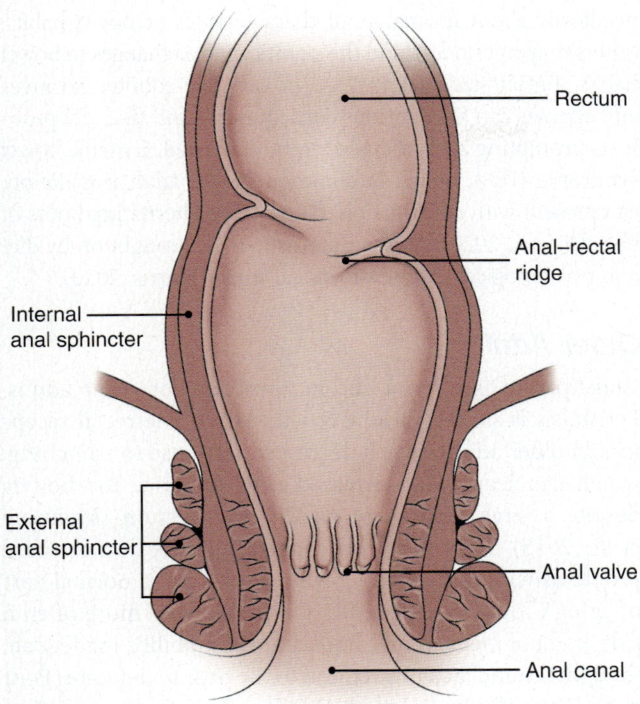

FIGURE 39-4. Interior view of the rectum and anal canal.

muscles to stretch and thereby stimulating the defecation reflex and subsequently the urge to eliminate.

The external anal sphincter, which is under voluntary control, is constricted or relaxed at will. During the act of defecation, several additional muscles aid in the process. Voluntary contraction of the muscles of the abdominal wall by holding one's breath, contracting the diaphragm, and closing the glottis increases intraabdominal pressure up to four or five times the normal pressure, which helps expel feces. Simultaneously, the muscles on the pelvic floor contract and aid in expulsion of the fecal mass. Defecation is eased by flexing the thigh muscles, which increases abdominal pressure, and by the sitting position, which increases downward pressure on the rectum. If the urge to defecate is ignored, defecation often can be delayed voluntarily by contracting the external anal sphincter and pelvic floor muscles.

When a person bears down to defecate, the increased pressures in the abdominal and thoracic cavities result in decreased blood flow to the atria and ventricles, thus temporarily lowering cardiac output. Once bearing down ceases, the pressure is lessened, and a larger-than-normal amount of blood returns to the heart. This act may cause the heart rate to slow (vagal response) and result in syncope in some patients (Hinkle et al., 2022). Therefore, this action of bearing down, termed the **Valsalva maneuver**, may be contraindicated in people with cardiovascular problems and other illnesses.

The act of defecation is usually painless. If the bowels move at regular intervals and the stools are formed and soft, functional problems involving frequency of elimination seldom occur. Many people become concerned if they do not have a daily bowel movement. However, normal elimination patterns can vary widely among people. Although many adults pass one stool each day, other healthy people have more frequent or less frequent bowel movements. Some people have a bowel movement two or three times a week; others, two or three times a day.

FACTORS AFFECTING BOWEL ELIMINATION

Various factors can affect bowel elimination. Interference with the normal functioning of elimination from the intestines can occur in health as well as during illness. Elimination can be affected by a person's developmental stage, daily patterns, the amount and quality of fluid or food intake, the level of activity, lifestyle, emotional states, pathologic processes, medications, and procedures, such as diagnostic tests and surgery.

Developmental Considerations

Age affects what a person eats and the body's ability to digest nutrients and eliminate wastes. The stools of an infant are markedly different from those of an older adult. Because patients are often reluctant to discuss their bowel habits and stool characteristics, nurses need to be familiar with bowel concerns pertinent to each developmental group.

Infant

The stool characteristics depend on whether the infant is being fed breast milk or formula. Breast milk is easier for the infant's intestines to break down and absorb. Breastfed babies have more frequent stools; the stools are yellow to golden and loose, and usually have little odor. The stools of formula-fed infants vary from yellow to brown, are paste-like in consistency, and have a stronger odor because of the decomposition of protein. The stools of both breastfed and formula-fed infants may have curds and mucus. Infants have no voluntary control over bowel elimination.

The number of stools infants pass varies greatly. For example, breastfed infants can pass from 2 to 10 stools daily, whereas bottle-fed infants typically pass 1 or 2 stools daily. At age 1 year, all infants commonly pass 1 or 2 stools a day. Parents may mistakenly interpret the infant's liquid stool as **diarrhea**. Diarrhea is an increase in frequency, and/or a change in consistency of stools (passage of three or more stools a day) (Dunlap & Patterson, 2020; Kyle & Carman, 2021). True diarrhea requires evaluation. Some children have bowel movements only once every 2 to 3 days. Teach parents that as long as the stools are soft, the child is not constipated (Kyle & Carman, 2021). **Constipation** (dry, hard stool; infrequent difficult passage of stool; and/or the incomplete passage of stool) should be reported to the infant's health care provider (Kyle & Carman, 2021). Constipation not related to a health issue is often initially managed with dietary manipulation, such as increased fiber and fluids (Kyle & Carman, 2021).

The consistent use of suppositories and laxatives is discouraged. Infants with persistent constipation require evaluation for structural defects.

Toddler

Between ages 18 and 24 months, the nerve fibers innervating the internal and external anal sphincters become fully developed, at which point voluntary control of defecation becomes possible. Voluntary defecation requires intact muscular, sensory, and nervous structures. Successful bowel training also includes awareness by the toddler of the need to defecate, the ability to communicate this need, the wish to please the significant person involved in bowel training, and praise and reinforcement for the toddler's successful behavior. Daytime bowel control is normally attained by 30 months of age, but the age varies with each child.

Assessment of a child's readiness for toilet training includes (AAP, n.d.; Kyle & Carman, 2021):

- Ability to indicate wants and needs verbally
- Motor skills to sit on and rise from the potty chair
- Showing an interest in the potty
- Willingness to follow instructions

Help parents to understand that physiologic maturity is the first priority for successful bowel training. Discourage the use of punishment or shame for a lack of readiness to become toilet-trained or for elimination accidents. Cultures approach toilet training differently. In some cultures, toilet training begins before the child is 1 year old; in other cultures, it may not be considered until the child is near 5 years old. It is important to recognize cultural influences on this parenting responsibility while promoting flexibility. Reassure parents that any regression of toileting skills that occurs during a child's illness or hospitalization is to be expected and is usually short-lived.

School-Age Child, Adolescent, and Adult

From childhood into adulthood, defecation patterns vary in quantity, frequency, and rhythmicity. Many people worry needlessly about normal stool characteristics or bowel habits; others may not understand the significance of changes in bowel habits. Emphasize that the use of over-the-counter laxatives and enemas can have serious consequences and that any problems prompting such use need to be evaluated. Irritable bowel syndrome (IBS), which is common in the adult population, can present with constipation, diarrhea, or alternating bouts of both (Norris, 2020). The symptoms may be brought on by diet and psychological and physiological stress (Norris, 2020).

Older Adult

Constipation is often a chronic problem for older adults. Peristalsis is slowed (Touhy & Jett, 2018). The rectal receptors in older adults have a decreased response to stretching, which can lead to a decreased urge to move the bowels despite a large amount of stool in the rectum (Mounsey et al., 2015). However, these changes usually do not cause problems with defecation; constipation is not a normal part of aging (Touhy & Jett, 2018). Constipation is more often a side effect of medications, life habits, immobility, inadequate fluid intake and lack of attention to the urge to defecate (Pont et al., 2019; Touhy & Jett, 2018). Diarrhea, **fecal impaction** (prolonged retention or an accumulation of fecal material that forms a hardened mass in the rectum), or **fecal incontinence** (involuntary or inappropriate passing of stool or flatus) can also result from physiologic or lifestyle changes. See the accompanying Focus on the Older Adult box.

Daily Patterns

Most people have individual patterns of bowel elimination involving frequency, timing considerations, position, and place. Changes in any of these patterns may upset a person's routine and lead to constipation. For example, many people defecate

Focus on the Older Adult

NURSING STRATEGIES TO ADDRESS AGE-RELATED CHANGES AFFECTING BOWEL ELIMINATION

Age-Related Changes	Nursing Strategies
Slowing of GI motility with increased stomach-emptying time	• Encourage small, frequent meals. • Discourage heavy activity after eating. • Encourage a high-fiber, low-fat diet. • Encourage adequate fluid intake. • Discourage regular use of laxatives. • Develop a daily routine to move bowels. The optimal time is usually 2 hours after awakening and after breakfast. • Evaluate medication regimen for possible adverse effects.
Decreased muscle tone/incontinence	• Provide easy access to the bathroom. • Use assistive devices when necessary (raised toilet seat, grab bars, walker). • Ensure safety when ambulating (e.g., skid-proof slippers). • Encourage participation in a bowel-retraining program.
Weakening of intestinal walls with greater incidence of diverticulitis	• Encourage a high-fiber diet and adequate fluid intake. • Teach patients not to ignore the urge to have a bowel movement. • Encourage regular exercise.

after breakfast, when the gastrocolic and duodenocolic reflexes cause mass propulsive movements in the large intestine. If this urge to defecate is ignored because the person finds the time or place inconvenient, the feces remain in the rectum until the defecation reflex is initiated again. Meanwhile, water continues to be absorbed from the unexpelled feces, which makes the stool dry, hard, and painful to pass.

In order to defecate, most people assume the squatting or slightly forward-sitting position with the thighs flexed. In either position, increased pressure is placed on the abdomen, as well as downward pressure on the rectum; both facilitate defecation. Obtaining the same results when seated on a bedpan is difficult. Embarrassment may further inhibit defecation. In addition, for most people, defecation is a private affair experienced easily only in the comfort of their own bathroom. Defecation may be difficult in a shared health care facility room with only a curtain for privacy.

Food and Fluid

Both the type and the amount of foods eaten and the amount of fluids ingested affect elimination. A high-fiber diet of 25 to 38 g of fiber (USDA & USDHHS, 2020) and a daily fluid intake of at least 2,000 mL (Academy of Nutrition and Dietetics, 2020, as cited in Dudek, 2022) facilitate bowel elimination. High-fiber foods, such as whole grains and bran, dried peas and beans, and fresh fruits and vegetables, increase the bulk in fecal material. Bulkier feces increase the pressure on the intestinal wall, which serves as a stimulus for peristalsis. As a result, feces move more quickly through the colon, allowing less time for water to be reabsorbed. Subsequently, the stool is soft and easy to pass.

People digest and tolerate foods differently. Food intolerance may alter bowel elimination, possibly resulting in diarrhea, gaseous distention, and cramping. For example, people who lack the enzyme lactase, which helps to break down the simple sugar lactose found in milk and milk products, cannot digest milk; this is called lactose intolerance. These people often experience excessive intestinal gas and diarrhea when they ingest milk, as the small intestine pulls fluid into the bowel through osmosis to assist in moving the dairy product out of the body.

Activity and Muscle Tone

Regular exercise improves GI motility and muscle tone, whereas inactivity decreases both. Adequate tone in the abdominal muscles, the diaphragm, and the perineal muscles is essential for ease of defecation. Patients on prolonged bedrest and those with decreased mobility are prime candidates for constipation (Norris, 2020).

Lifestyle

Many individual, family, and sociocultural variables influence a person's usual elimination habits. The long-term effects of bowel training may result in a person's (1) acceptance of bowel elimination as a normal life process, (2) preoccupation with bowel elimination, or (3) feeling that bowel elimination is a "dirty" process. Rituals associated with bowel elimination, cleanliness considerations, the language used to talk about bowel elimination or reluctance to discuss it, individual responses to involuntary passage of flatus (gas), and so on, vary widely among people. A person's daily schedule, occupation, and leisure activities may contribute to a habit of defecating at regular times or to an irregular pattern. Nurses who role model good health behaviors are more effective teachers. Use the Promoting Health 39-1 display for yourself before using it with others.

Promoting Health 39-1

BOWEL ELIMINATION

Use the assessment checklist to determine how well you are meeting your needs related to bowel elimination. Then develop a prescription for self-care by choosing appropriate behaviors from the list of suggestions.

Assessment Checklist

☐ almost always ☐ sometimes ☐ almost never

☐ ☐ ☐ 1. I have a regular bowel elimination pattern, satisfactory to support comfort and activities of daily living.

☐ ☐ ☐ 2. I eat a diet high in fiber.

☐ ☐ ☐ 3. I exercise regularly.

☐ ☐ ☐ 4. I have an adequate intake of fluids.

Self-Care Behaviors

1. Normal defecation patterns differ in each person. It does not matter how often someone moves their bowels as long as the stool is soft and passes easily. Eat a balanced diet, including high-fiber foods, such as fruits, vegetables, and nuts.
2. Follow a regular exercise program to engage in activity that requires moderate effort, such as brisk walking for a total of 2 ½ hours or more a week.
3. Do not ignore the urge to defecate.
4. Establish a routine, if needed (1 hour after meals is usually best).
5. Avoid prolonged use of over-the-counter medications or enemas to treat constipation.
6. Drink at least 2,000 mL of water per day if approved by your health care provider.
7. Seek medical assistance for any change in the characteristics of or presence of blood in the stool.

Information to promote effective bowel elimination, such as information about elimination problems, fecal incontinence, and GI diseases, is available online.

Psychological Variables

Psychological stress affects the body in many ways. In some people, anxiety seems to have a direct effect on GI motility, and diarrhea accompanies periods of high anxiety. In the fight-or-flight response, when the body mobilizes itself for intense action, blood is shunted away from the stomach and intestines, resulting in a slowing of GI motility. People who chronically worry and those with certain personality types who tend to hold onto problems and negative feelings may experience frequent constipation.

Pathologic Conditions

Numerous pathologic processes may change a person's usual bowel elimination habits. Changes in stool characteristics or frequency may be one of the first clinical manifestations of a disease. For example, when a patient reports stool has become narrower or ribbon-like, a tumor may be obstructing normal stool passage through the colon (Colon Cancer Coalition, n.d.). Similarly, a parent's report that a child's stools are frequent, bulky, greasy, and foul smelling suggests cystic fibrosis. This requires further evaluation and consultation with a health care provider, especially if other clinical manifestations are present.

Medications may also influence the appearance of the stool for a variety of reasons. Any drug with the potential to cause GI bleeding (e.g., anticoagulants, aspirin products) may cause the stool to appear pink to red to black (Karch, 2020). Iron salts result in a black stool from the oxidation of iron (MFMER, 2020a). Bismuth subsalicylate used to treat diarrhea can also cause black stools (MFMER, 2020a). Antidiarrheals may cause a white discoloration or speckling in the stool (MFMER, 2020a). Antibiotics may cause a green-gray color related to impaired digestion.

Diarrhea and constipation may also be a sign of potential disease processes. Diarrhea or constipation may result from pathologic conditions such as diverticulitis (inflammation and/or infection of a diverticulum, a small, bulging pouch in the colon) (Dunlap & Patterson, 2020). Diarrhea may result from bacterial and viral infection, malabsorption syndromes (the inability of the digestive system to absorb one or more of the major vitamins, minerals, or nutrients), neoplastic diseases (tumors), diabetic neuropathy (damage to nerve cells), hyperthyroidism, and chemotherapy (Dunlap & Patterson, 2020; Dunlap, 2021).

Outbreaks of food poisoning can result in severe GI symptoms, including diarrhea. For example, infections caused by certain types of *Escherichia coli,* particularly dangerous for young children (age <10 years) and older adults, can progress quickly to life-threatening hematologic and renal complications (MFMER, 2020b). Severe abdominal cramping followed by watery or bloody diarrhea may signal a microbial infection, which can be confirmed by a stool sample. Supportive treatment, careful monitoring, and attentive nursing care are essential.

Constipation may be the result inadequate fiber in the diet, a change in lifestyle (e.g., lack of exercise), poor fluid intake, and ignoring or delaying the urge to defecate (Bauldoff et al., 2020). Constipation may also occur as a result of metabolic, neurologic, or psychological disorders, such as diseases within the colon or rectum (e.g., tumors), IBS, and injury to, or degeneration of, the spinal cord (Bauldoff et al., 2020). Medications, such as opioid analgesics and calcium-channel blockers, may also cause constipation (Bauldoff et al., 2020; Mitchell, 2019a). Changes in color, contents, odor, and appearance of stool may be related to conditions that traumatize the stomach or intestines, or that interfere with normal digestion. As a result, evaluation of stool may be an important component of the assessment of a patient (Mitchell, 2019a).

Intestinal obstruction occurs when the normal flow of intestinal contents through the intestinal tract is inhibited or blocked (Bauldoff et al., 2020). Mechanical obstructions result from pressure on the intestinal walls. Common causes of mechanical obstruction are tumors of the colon or rectum, diverticulum, adhesions from scar tissue, stenosis, strictures, and hernia and volvulus (twisting of a part of the colon). Nonmechanical (or functional) obstructions result from an inability of the intestinal musculature to move the contents through the bowel. Examples of causes of nonmechanical obstruction include diseases that weaken or paralyze the intestinal walls such as muscular dystrophy, diabetes mellitus, and Parkinson disease. Manipulation of the bowel during surgery may also result in paralytic ileus, a nonmechanical obstruction (Bauldoff et al., 2020). The effects of surgery are further detailed later in the chapter.

Medications

Medications are available that can promote peristalsis (**laxatives**) or inhibit peristalsis (antidiarrheal medications) (Karch, 2020). These are discussed later in the chapter. There are also other types of medications that may affect bowel elimination and stool characteristics. Opioids are a common cause of medication-induced constipation and can result in significant distress for the patient. The enteric neurons control major body functions such as bowel control. Opioid-binding receptors are found in the enteric neurons in the GI tract. The binding of the opioid to these receptor sites interrupts peristalsis, causing slowed movement of stool through the colon, resulting in increased reabsorption of fluid in the large intestine. Antacids containing aluminum, iron sulfate, and anticholinergic medications also decrease GI motility, with the potential to also cause constipation.

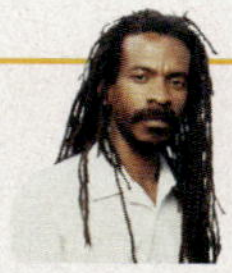

Remember **Leroy Cobbs**, the patient described at the beginning of the chapter who developed severe constipation resulting from the opioid analgesic used to control the cancer pain. Had the possible adverse effects of opioids been addressed in the patient's medication teaching plan when the drug was first prescribed, the risk for constipation could have been reduced. In addition, the teaching plan could have addressed measures to counteract the effects of the medication.

Many medications can cause diarrhea as a side effect. For example, diarrhea is a potential adverse effect of treatment with antibiotics such as amoxicillin clavulanate. In this situation, using antidiarrheal drugs is not recommended because its use would prolong the exposure of the intestinal mucosa to the irritating effect of the antibiotic. Medications with magnesium, such as over-the-counter antacids, can also cause diarrhea. Metformin, a common medication used to treat type 2 diabetes mellitus, can cause diarrhea. The resulting diarrhea can often become bothersome or severe enough with these and other medications that the drugs may need to be discontinued.

Because antibiotics are used so extensively in the health care setting, many patients are at risk for infection with *Clostridioides difficile (C. difficile)* (formerly known as *Clostridium difficile),* a health care–associated infection (HAI) (CDC, 2020a; Ragusa et al., 2018). When a patient is receiving treatment with broad-spectrum antibiotics, there is a disruption in the normal intestinal flora, allowing the microorganism to flourish within the intestine. *C. difficile* causes intestinal mucosal damage and inflammation, resulting in diarrhea and abdominal cramping. *C. difficile* spores are shed in feces and are relatively resistant to disinfectants. These microorganisms can be spread on the hands of health care providers after contact with equipment or surfaces contaminated with the microorganism. It is important to institute contact precautions for infected patients. Consider environmental surfaces and items close to the patient, such as the side rails and overbed table, to be contaminated. The use of gloves and gowns for every patient encounter, even short care intervals, is important to prevent the spread, as well as hand hygiene using soap and water (CDC, 2020b). Gloves are important because hand sanitizer doesn't kill *C. difficile* and handwashing might not be sufficient (CDC, 2020b). Intensified environmental cleaning on a daily basis and upon patient discharge or transfer is required (CDC, 2020b).

Diagnostic Studies

Diagnostic studies may affect a patient's usual bowel elimination pattern. For example, patients may need to fast for diagnostic studies. The ingestion of barium during diagnostic procedures, such as a barium enema, may result in constipation or impaction if it is not completely eliminated after the procedure. In addition, the stress of hospitalization and waiting for the results of studies, combined with changes in food intake, can severely alter a patient's usual elimination patterns. The bowel preparation used for bowel cleansing before certain diagnostic studies of the GI tract can interfere with the normal timing of a patient's bowel movements. Refer to Table 39-2 in the Teaching About Laxatives section for additional information related to the use of laxatives.

Surgery and Anesthesia

Direct manipulation of the bowel during abdominal surgery inhibits peristalsis, causing a condition termed postoperative **paralytic ileus** (Bauldoff et al., 2020). This temporary stoppage of peristalsis normally lasts 3 to 5 days. Many times, the patient is receiving opioids for pain relief, which can exacerbate the situation. If this condition persists, distention and symptoms of acute obstruction may occur, possibly resulting in the need for surgical intervention. Inhaled general anesthetic agents also inhibit peristalsis by blocking the parasympathetic impulses to the intestinal musculature. However, local and regional anesthetics have little effect on peristalsis.

NURSING PROCESS FOR BOWEL ELIMINATION

Assessing

Assessment of the GI tract and bowel elimination includes pertinent patient history, physical assessment, and diagnostic studies.

Nursing History

Patients may be reluctant to initiate a conversation about their bowel status, so include pertinent bowel elimination questions in each comprehensive nursing history. The accompanying Focused Assessment Guide 39-1 provides some appropriate questions for health history assessment related to bowel elimination. If the patient is experiencing any disturbance in bowel elimination, conduct a more detailed assessment, directing attention to the factors described earlier that may influence bowel elimination.

Patients who are critically ill or who have impaired cognition may be incapable of reporting their bowel status accurately. Record the patient's daily bowel status to look for clues to impending problems. While making daily rounds, ask patients who can give reliable answers when they moved their bowels last and chart the response. If the patient cannot provide this information, the nurse or ancillary staff who assists the patient with bowel elimination records any bowel movement.

Physical Assessment

Examination of the abdomen is discussed in Chapter 27. Refer to this chapter for details and additional information related to the assessment of the GI system. An overview of examination techniques that may be helpful when assessing the functioning of the GI tract is described here.

ABDOMEN

The sequence for abdominal assessment proceeds from inspection, auscultation, and percussion to palpation. Inspection and auscultation are performed before palpation because palpation may disturb normal peristalsis and bowel motility. Advanced health care providers usually perform percussion of the abdomen, as this is an advanced assessment skill. Place the patient comfortably in the supine position with the abdomen exposed, the chest and pubic area

Focused Assessment Guide 39-1

BOWEL ELIMINATION

Factors to Assess	Questions and Approaches
Usual patterns of bowel elimination	How often do you move your bowels? Any special time of the day? What does your stool look like? • Frequency • Time of day • Description of usual stool characteristics (amount, consistency, shape, color, odor) • Do you ever have to strain to move your bowels? • Have you ever had to remove hard stool with your finger to help you move your bowels?
Aids to elimination	Do you use anything to help move your bowels? • Natural aids (liquids, food) • Pharmacologic aids (laxatives) • Enemas
Recent changes in bowel elimination	Have you noticed any changes in your stool recently? Have you noticed any change in the color of your stool? Have you noticed any blood in your stool? (May need to ask patient about color blindness.) Have you noted a difference in the appearance of your stool (narrowing, presence of mucus)?
Problems with bowel elimination	Are your bowels causing you any problem now? • Nature of disturbance • Onset and frequency • Causes (*physical:* food and fluid intake, exercise status, history of surgery or illnesses influencing GI tract; psychosocial; medicine related) • Severity • Symptoms • Interventions attempted and results
Presence of a bowel diversion (normal routine, history of problems)	What is your usual routine with your colostomy or ileostomy? Do you have any problems caring for your colostomy or ileostomy? Are there activities you are no longer able to perform because of your colostomy or ileostomy?

draped, and the knees slightly flexed. Encourage the patient to urinate prior to the examination so that the bladder is empty.

Inspection

Observe the contour of the abdomen, noting any masses, scars, or areas of distention. Significant findings may include the presence of asymmetry, swelling, distention (inflation) or protrusion (projection).

Auscultation

Traditionally, bowel sounds are assessed in all four quadrants of the abdomen. Using the diaphragm of a warmed stethoscope, listen for bowel sounds in all abdominal quadrants, using a systematic, clockwise approach. Listen carefully for bowel sounds (gurgles and clicks) and note their frequency and character (usually occur at a rate of 5 to 34 per minute) (Bickley et al., 2021). Current evidence suggests bowel sounds radiate widely over the abdomen and listening in all four quadrants is not necessary; assessment of presence and hypoactivity (decreased; <5/minute)/hyperactivity (increased; >34/minute) is sufficient (Bickley et al., 2021; Jarvis & Eckhardt, 2020). Before deciding that bowel sounds are absent, listen in the epigastric and umbilical area of the abdomen for 2 minutes or longer (Bickley et al., 2021). If the patient has a nasogastric (NG) tube in place, disconnect it from suction during this assessment to allow for accurate interpretation of sounds. Keep in mind that the timing of the patient's most recent meal or a full bladder may also affect the examination.

Significant findings include decreased (hypoactive) bowel sounds; increased (hyperactive) bowel sounds; and absent bowel sounds. Decreased bowel sounds indicate diminished bowel motility, common following abdominal surgery or associated with peritonitis or late bowel obstruction (Bickley et al., 2021; Jarvis & Eckhardt, 2020). Increased bowel sounds indicate increased bowel motility, commonly caused by diarrhea, gastroenteritis, or early/partial bowel obstruction (Jarvis & Eckhardt, 2020).

Palpation

Perform light palpation in each quadrant. Watch the patient's face for nonverbal signs of pain during palpation. Palpate each quadrant in a systematic manner, noting muscular resistance, tenderness, enlargement of the organs, or masses. If the patient reports abdominal pain, palpate the area of pain last. If the patient's abdomen is distended, note the presence of firmness or tautness.

ANUS AND RECTUM

Perform a superficial examination each time you wash a patient's anal area or assist with bowel evacuation. The nurse's skill level determines the extent of further rectal examination. Advanced practice professionals usually conduct physical assessments of the rectum and anus. Refer to a health assessment text for details.

Inspection is used to assess the anal area, which normally has increased pigmentation and some hair growth. Assess for lesions, ulcers, **fissures** (linear break on the margin of the anus), inflammation, and external hemorrhoids (dilated veins appearing as reddened protrusions). Ask the patient to bear down as though having a bowel movement. Assess for the appearance of internal hemorrhoids or fissures. Normally, there is no protrusion of tissue. Inspect the perineal area for areas of skin irritation or breakdown secondary to diarrhea or fecal incontinence.

Stool Characteristics

Nurses are responsible for observing and recording information about the patient's stool. Table 39-1 describes the characteristics of a normal stool, along with special considerations used when observing a stool. Report and record anything unusual, including the passage of little or no gas or unusual amounts of gas.

Note and record, usually in the patient's health record, the frequency, amount, and characteristics of the patient's bowel movements. Describe any additional unusual observations, such as lightheadedness or straining. When assistive personnel or the patient assumes this responsibility, check with the patient and health record at regular intervals to see that the recording is accurate.

Ideally, populations at high risk for bowel elimination problems are identified before problems occur, and such problems are prevented or minimized through vigilant health care. For example, early colorectal cancer usually has no symptoms. Warning signs typically occur with more advanced disease. Refer to Box 39-1, Warning Signs of Colorectal Cancer. For this reason, encourage patients to schedule regular exams with their health care providers. Reinforce the importance of adhering to recommended screening for colorectal cancer, including sigmoidoscopy, colonoscopy, and fecal testing for blood. The American Cancer Society (www.cancer.org) provides guidelines for screening for patients at various risk levels for colorectal cancer.

Box 39-1 Warning Signs of Colorectal Cancer

- Rectal bleeding
- Persistent change in the bowel elimination pattern or consistence of the stool
- Blood in the stool
- Persistent cramping or pain in the lower abdomen or gas
- A feeling that the bowel doesn't empty completely after having a bowel movement
- Weakness or fatigue
- Losing weight without trying

Source: American Cancer Society. (2021). *Do I have colorectal cancer? Signs, symptoms and work-up.* https://www.cancer.org/latest-news/signs-and-symptoms-of-colon-cancer.html; Mayo Foundation for Medical Education and Research (MFMER). (2021). *Colon cancer*. https://www.mayoclinic.org/diseases-conditions/colon-cancer/symptoms-causes/syc-20353669

Unfolding Patient Stories: Marvin Hayes • Part 1

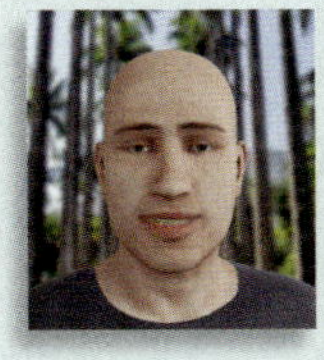

Marvin Hayes, a 43-year-old male, is being seen at the clinic. He has a family history of colorectal cancer. What questions can the nurse ask to identify disturbances in bowel elimination? What are the signs and symptoms of colon and rectal cancer? What patient education would the nurse provide when orders are written to obtain a stool sample and schedule a colonoscopy? (Marvin Hayes' story continues in Chapter 42.)

Care for Marvin and other patients in a realistic virtual environment: ***vSim** for Nursing* (thepoint.lww.com/vSimFunds). Practice documenting these patients' care in DocuCare (thepoint.lww.com/DocuCareEHR).

Diagnostic Studies

The nurse is often responsible for caring for patients with elimination problems who are undergoing diagnostic testing. Specific guidelines for the nurse's role in stool collection and direct and indirect visualization studies follow.

STOOL COLLECTION

The nurse is responsible for obtaining the specimen according to facility procedure, labeling the specimen, and ensuring that the specimen is transported to the laboratory in a timely manner. The institution's policy and procedure manual or laboratory manual identifies specific information about the amount of stool needed, the time frame during which stool is to be collected, and the type of specimen container to use.

Always wear disposable gloves when any contact or handling of a stool specimen is likely. Hand hygiene before and after glove use is essential. Also, take care not to contaminate the outside of the specimen container with stool. Package, label, and transport specimens according to facility policy to ensure that no leakage of the specimen occurs. Patients may need specific instructions about collecting a stool specimen. It is important that health literacy

Table 39-1 Normal Characteristics and Special Considerations for Observation of Stool

CHARACTERISTIC	NORMAL FINDING	SPECIAL CONSIDERATIONS FOR OBSERVATION
Volume	Variable	The volume of the stool depends on the amount the person eats and the nature of the diet. For example, a diet high in roughage produces more feces than a soft, bland diet. Consistently large diarrheal stools suggest a disorder in the small bowel or proximal colon; small, frequent stools with urgency to pass them suggest a disorder of the left colon or rectum.
Color	Infant: Yellow to brown Children and adult: Brown	The brown color of the stool is due to stercobilin, a bile pigment derivative. The rapid rate of peristalsis in the breastfed infant causes the stool to be yellow. Black stool can be as a result of intestinal bleeding. Melena, which is a thick, black, tarry stool, is caused by upper GI bleeding. The black color comes from the changes of hemoglobin during the digestive process. Bleeding low in the intestinal tract or from inflamed hemorrhoids or fissures can result in fresh blood in the stool. The color of the stool can also be influenced by diet. For example, the stool could be dark if the person eats red meat and dark-green vegetables, such as spinach. The stool will be light brown if the diet is high in milk and milk products and low in meat. The absence of bile may cause the stool to appear white or clay-colored. Certain drugs influence the color of the stool. For example, iron salts and bismuth subsalicylate can cause the stool to be black. Antacids cause it to be whitish. The stool darkens with standing.
Odor	Pungent; may be affected by foods ingested	The characteristic odor of the stool is due to indole and skatole, caused by putrefaction and fermentation in the lower intestinal tract. The odor of the stool is influenced by its pH value, which normally is neutral or slightly alkaline. Excessive putrefaction causes a strong odor. The presence of blood in the stool causes a unique odor.
Consistency	Soft, semisolid, and formed	The consistency of the stool is influenced by fluid and food intake and gastric motility. The less time stool spends in the intestine (or the shorter the intestine), the more liquid the stool. Many pathologic conditions influence consistency.
Shape	Formed stool is usually about 1 inch (2.5 cm) in diameter and has the tubular shape of the colon, but may be larger or smaller, depending on the condition of the colon	A GI obstruction may result in a narrow, pencil-shaped stool. Rapid peristalsis thins the stool. Increased time spent in the large intestine may result in a hard, marble-like fecal mass.
Constituents	Waste residues of digestion: bile, intestinal secretions, shed epithelial cells, bacteria, and inorganic material (chiefly calcium and phosphates); seeds, meat fibers, and fat may be present in small amounts	Internal bleeding, infection, inflammation, and other pathologic conditions may result in abnormal constituents. These include blood, pus, excessive fat, parasites, ova, and mucus. Foreign bodies also may be found in the stool.

is assessed, and the terms used regarding the bowel movement are familiar to the patient. For example, many patients may not understand the term "stool." Patients may be embarrassed to ask questions, so it is important the nurse communicates the instructions in a manner which the patient understands (Cinar et al., 2014). Instructions may include the following:

- Void first, because the laboratory study may be inaccurate if the stool contains urine (Fischbach & Fischbach, 2018).

- Defecate into the required container, such as clean or sterile bedpan or the bedside commode (depending on the specimen required), rather than the toilet, because the water in the toilet bowl may affect the analysis results (Fischbach & Fischbach, 2018).
- Do not place toilet tissue in the bedpan or specimen container because contents in the paper may influence laboratory results (Fischbach & Fischbach, 2018).
- Avoid contact with soaps, detergents, and disinfectants as these may affect test results (Fischbach & Fischbach, 2018).
- Notify the nurse when the specimen is available, so that it may be collected and transported to the laboratory as required.

When placing a specimen in a laboratory container, put on gloves and use two clean tongue blades. Usually, 1 inch (2.5 cm) of formed stool or 30 mL of liquid stool is sufficient (Fischbach & Fischbach, 2018). If portions of the stool include visible blood, mucus, or pus, include these with the specimen (Fischbach & Fischbach, 2018). Also, be sure that the specimen is free of any barium or enema solution. Because a fresh specimen produces the most accurate results, send the specimen to the laboratory immediately. If this is not possible, the specimen should be either refrigerated or kept warm; contact the laboratory for instructions based on the type of testing (Fischbach & Fischbach, 2018). Do not refrigerate specimens for ova and parasites (Fischbach & Fischbach, 2018).

Stool Culture

Culture of stool is indicated when there is suspected infection from bacteria, virus, fungi, or parasites. Obtain stool cultures before initiation of antiinfective therapy. If antibiotic or antifungal therapy has already begun, identify the specific medication in the laboratory request (Boruchoff & Weinstein, 2019).

Occult Blood

Certain conditions, such as ulcer disease, inflammatory bowel disorders, and colon cancer, place the patient at high risk for intestinal bleeding. The color of the stool may reflect the source of the bleeding. Black, tarry stools may indicate upper GI bleeding, such as from a peptic ulcer, due to a reaction between hemoglobin and gastric acid. Lower GI bleeding, such as from hemorrhoids or a polyp, may produce bright-red blood in the stool. Certain foods and medications can also cause a black or reddish stool. **Occult blood** in the stool (blood that is hidden in the specimen or cannot be seen on gross examination) can be detected with screening tests.

Fecal occult blood testing (FOBT) may be used to detect occult blood in the stool. It is used for initial/early screening for disorders such as cancer and for GI bleeding in conditions such as ulcer disease, inflammatory bowel disorders, and intestinal polyps (MedlinePlus, 2020). Consecutive stool samples (three to six) should be collected from different stool samples to increase accuracy (Fischbach & Fischbach, 2018). FOBT may be performed within an institution, collected at the bedside, and sent to the laboratory for analysis. The sample may also be collected by the patient at home and delivered or mailed to the health care provider's office or to the laboratory for analysis.

The *guaiac fecal occult blood test* (gFOBT) is a chemical test that detects the enzyme peroxidase in hemoglobin molecules when blood is present in the stool sample. A positive gFOBT result indicates that abnormal bleeding is occurring somewhere in the digestive tract. Certain medications, such as a salicylate intake of more than 325 mg daily, other nonsteroidal antiinflammatory drugs, steroids, iron preparations, and anticoagulants, also may lead to *false-positive* readings (Fischbach & Fischbach, 2018). The evidence for practice is conflicting regarding the impact of ingestion of certain foods and supplements before specimen collection on the accuracy of the test results (Doubeni, 2020, MedlinePlus, 2020). Foods and supplements that are suggested to have a possible effect on test results include red meat, cantaloupe, turnips, radishes, parsnips, horseradish, mushrooms, broccoli, cauliflower, apples, bananas, cantaloupe, and vitamin C–enriched foods and juices as well as vitamin C in excess of 250 mg/day (American Cancer Society, 2020; Colorectal Cancer Alliance, 2019a; Fischbach & Fischbach, 2018; MedlinePlus, 2020). Patients should consult with their health care providers and follow directions provided for the collection test kit provided.

The *fecal immunochemical test* (*FIT*) uses antibodies directed against human hemoglobin to detect blood in the stool. A positive FIT is more specific for bleeding in the lower GI tract (Fischbach & Fischbach, 2018). No drug or dietary restrictions are required for the FIT (American Cancer Society, 2020; Colorectal Cancer Alliance, 2019b).

The following are recommendations for the patient preparing for a fecal occult blood test (Fischbach & Fischbach, 2018):

- Avoid barium enemas for 72 hours before and during stool specimen collection.
- Do not collect samples during or until 3 days after menstrual period.
- Do not collect samples while the patient has bleeding hemorrhoids or hematuria.

In clinical settings, these restrictions are usually not practical. Be sure to note the presence of any of the previously mentioned conditions in the clinical setting.

Figure 39-5 demonstrates the procedure for a gFOBT test. A positive result from either the gFOBT or the FIT requires follow-up testing, such as a sigmoidoscopy or colonoscopy (American Cancer Society, 2020).

Timed Specimens

Consider the first stool passed by the patient as the start of the collection period. Depending on the test, it may require saving the entire stool passed or only a sample. Collect the required volume of every stool passed within the designated period. Follow laboratory instructions for sending stools to the laboratory.

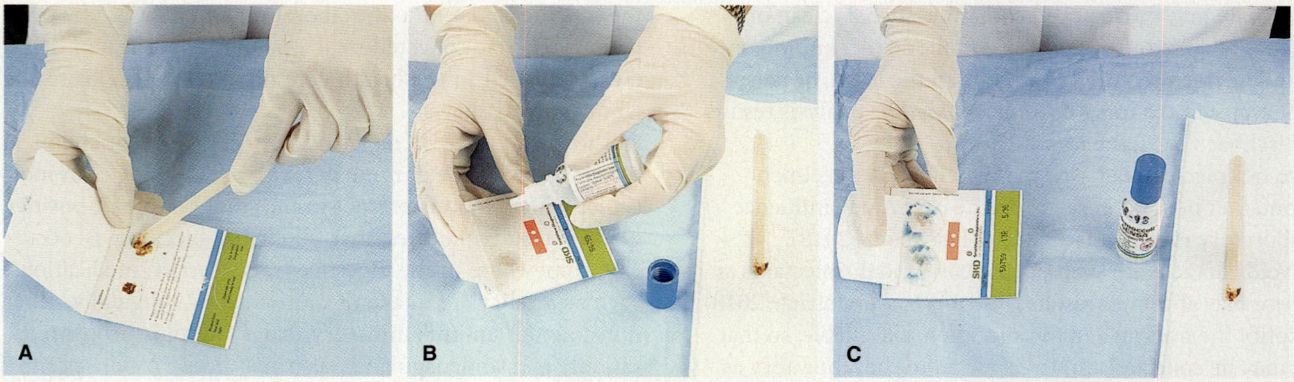

FIGURE 39-5. Testing a stool specimen for occult blood. **A.** Applying a stool specimen to the test paper. **B.** Adding developing solution to the back side of the paper according to directions. **C.** Blue coloration indicating positive results. (*Source:* Used with permission from Shutterstock. *Photos by B. Proud.*)

Specimens for Pinworms

Adult pinworms, parasitic intestinal worms, live in the cecum. Pinworms migrate to the anal area during the night to deposit eggs and retreat into the anal canal during the day. The most common symptom of a pinworm infection is perianal itching. Collect this specimen in the morning, immediately after the patient awakens and before the patient urinates, has a bowel movement, or a bath. Use clear cellophane tape to collect a specimen for pinworms; do not use micropore or adhesive-type tape (Fischbach & Fischbach, 2018). Apply gloves and press the tape against the anal opening, remove it immediately, and then place it on a slide. Pinworm eggs can usually be detected on the tape under a microscope. This test may need to be repeated on 4 to 6 consecutive days before ruling out the presence of pinworms (Fischbach & Fischbach, 2018).

DIRECT VISUALIZATION STUDIES

Endoscopy is the direct visual examination of body organs or cavities. Most commonly, this is done using a fiberoptic endoscope, a long, flexible tube containing glass fibers that transmit light into the organ and return an image that can be viewed. Pincers may be inserted through the tube to obtain a tissue sample for biopsy. An endoscope enables the health care provider to view the integrity of the mucosa, blood vessels, and specific organ parts and is helpful for diagnosing inflammatory, ulcerative, and infectious diseases; benign and malignant neoplasms; and other lesions of the esophageal, gastric, and intestinal mucosa. Endoscopic studies include the following:

- *Esophagogastroduodenoscopy (EGD):* visual examination of the esophagus, the stomach, and the duodenum
- *Colonoscopy:* visual examination of the large intestine from the anus to the ileocecal valve
- *Sigmoidoscopy:* visual examination of the sigmoid colon, the rectum, and the anal canal

Nursing responsibilities before and after these studies are described in Box 39-2.

Virtual enteroscopy (wireless video capsule endoscopy) is a minimally invasive technology that provides diagnostic imaging of the small intestine (American Society for Gastrointestinal Endoscopy, 2020). In this procedure, the patient swallows a capsule, about the size of a vitamin, which contains a small camera that emits a radio signal. The capsule is propelled through the small intestine via peristalsis, taking two pictures per second. Several sensors are attached to the patient's abdomen and pick up the radio signal from the capsule, and the data are recorded on a small recording device worn on a belt. The system captures about 55,000 images in an 8-hour exam. The patient returns to the facility after 8 hours, and the external sensors and data recorder are removed. The information is downloaded from the recorder to a computer and can be transferred to a videotape for easy viewing by the health care provider. The capsule is excreted during the process of normal defecation in 24 to 48 hours and is intended for one-time use only (Cave, 2021).

The patient is normally NPO (fasting) for 10 to 12 hours the evening before capsule ingestion. A bowel prep is usually not needed, but it may be used in some patients (American Society for Gastrointestinal Endoscopy, 2020). During the first 2 hours of the study, the patient is not allowed to eat or drink anything. After the first 2 hours, the patient may consume small amounts of liquids. After 4 hours, the patient may have a small meal (American Society for Gastrointestinal Endoscopy, 2020). The patient should avoid vigorous physical activity such as running or jumping during the study (American Society for Gastrointestinal Endoscopy, 2020). Patients should not be near an MRI device or schedule an MRI examination after ingesting the capsule and until the capsule is excreted (American Society for Gastrointestinal Endoscopy, 2020). Because there is no sedation or discomfort and a relatively normal day can be planned, many patients prefer this method of endoscopy. In addition, no air is needed to expand the small intestine, as it is in traditional endoscopy; therefore, the patient does not feel uncomfortable and bloated. This method, however, does not allow for obtaining biopsies of any suspicious area, so additional endoscopic studies may be required, based on the results.

INDIRECT VISUALIZATION STUDIES

Indirect visualization of the GI tract is commonly performed through radiography. The passage of x-rays through the patient creates a radiograph or film depicting body structures.

Box 39-2 Common Diagnostic Studies for the Gastrointestinal Tract

Esophagogastroduodenoscopy (EGD)

Allows visual examination of the esophagus, stomach, and upper duodenum by means of a long, flexible, fiberoptic-lighted scope.

Preparation

- A signed consent form is required for this procedure.
- Fasting is required 6 to 8 hours before the test (check facility policy).
- Dentures need to be removed before the test.
- Remind patients that they will be awake but sedated and that a local anesthetic will be sprayed into the mouth and throat to depress the gag reflex.

Aftercare

- Withhold food and fluids until the gag reflex returns.
- Check vital signs according to the protocol.
- Observe for signs of perforation: pain, persistent difficulty swallowing, vomiting blood, or black, tarry stools.
- Explain to the patient that it is normal to sense throat soreness and hoarseness for several days; saline gargles and lozenges may be helpful.

Colonoscopy

Allows visual examination of the rectum, colon, and distal small bowel using a long, flexible, fiberoptic-lighted scope.

Preparation

- Ensure that an informed consent is signed.
- Preparation prior to test may involve:
- If possible, a low-residue diet (low fiber) should be followed several days before the procedure. A clear liquid diet is usually ordered for 48 to 72 hours before the procedure (Fischbach & Fischbach, 2018). There are multiple types of bowel preps for this procedure. The provider performing the procedure will decide which is best for the individual patient.
- The prep is usually given as a split dose, with half being given the night before and rest the morning of the procedure. It is recommended the second dose be given at least 5 hours and completed at least 2 hours before the study. There are some who may receive the prep the same day as the procedure, especially if the procedure is scheduled for later in the day.
- The prep may be better tolerated if a straw is used, and the liquid is chilled. Some prep solutions may come with a flavor pack, which may improve the flavor as well.
- Those who cannot tolerate the oral prep or have a contraindication to large volumes of fluid may have an enema prep.
- May be NPO for at least 6 to 8 hours before the study with small sips of water for meds, and nothing for 2 hours before the study.
- Explain to the patient they will be sedated during the test.

Aftercare

- The patient may experience flatulence or gas pains because air was used to distend the intestines for better visibility.
- Usual diet may be resumed once patient recovers from the sedation.
- Check vital signs according to facility protocol.
- Observe for signs of bowel perforation: rectal bleeding, abdominal pain and distention, fever, malaise.

Sigmoidoscopy

Allows visual examination of the distal sigmoid colon, the rectum, and the anal canal through a flexible or rigid sigmoidoscope.

Preparation

- Ensure that an informed consent is signed.
- Preparation may include light meal the night before and two commercially prepared enemas (Fleet). In older adults where these enemas would be contraindicated, an oral preparation could be used. Sedation is not usually required but may be ordered.

Aftercare

- Patient may experience flatulence or gas pains because air was used to distend the intestines for better visibility.
- Observe for signs of bowel perforation.
- If biopsy was performed, patient should be informed that slight rectal bleeding may occur.

Upper Gastrointestinal (UGI) and Small-Bowel Series

Involves fluoroscopic examination of the esophagus, stomach, and small intestine after ingestion of barium sulfate.

Preparation

- Ensure that an informed consent is signed.
- Keep patient NPO after midnight the day of the test.
- Inform patient that a chalky-tasting barium contrast mixture will be given to drink before the test.
- If the patient has diabetes, alert the radiology department, and schedule the exam for early morning. If the patient is taking metformin, special considerations may be necessary. Consult with the health care team to determine if the metformin should be suspended for the day of and several days after the study (Fischbach & Fischbach, 2018).

Aftercare

- A post-test laxative (e.g., milk of magnesia) is usually prescribed to prevent fecal impaction from barium sulfate that has hardened. Notify the health care provider if barium is not passed, usually within 2 days.
- Explain that the barium may lighten the color of stools for the next several days. After the barium is expelled, the stool color will return to normal.

Barium Enema

Involves a series of radiographs that examine the large intestine after rectal instillation of barium sulfate.

Preparation

- An informed consent must be signed.
- Preparation may consist of dietary modifications and a bowel prep.
- Review the patient's history for any history of ulcerative colitis or active GI bleeding that would prohibit the use of the standard bowel preparation.

Aftercare

- Encourage fluids to prevent dehydration.
- Inform the patient that the barium may lighten the color of the stools. A laxative may be prescribed. Notify the health care team if barium is not passed, usually within 2 days.
- Encourage rest because the bowel preparation and the test exhaust many patients.

(*continued on page 1532*)

Box 39-2 Common Diagnostic Studies for the Gastrointestinal Tract *(continued)*

Abdominal Ultrasound

Uses ultrasound waves to visualize organs via a small transducer placed against the skin.

Preparation

- Assure the patient that no radiation is employed and that the test is painless.
- Patient must be NPO for a minimum of 8 hours before the examination.
- Explain that gel will be applied to the skin and that a sensation of warmth or wetness may be felt. The gel does not stain but avoid wearing nonwashable clothing.
- Abdominal ultrasound must be performed before studies involving barium, as retained barium may compromise the study. If this scheduling is not possible, at least 24 hours must elapse between the barium procedure and the ultrasound.

Aftercare

- Ensure that any residual gel is removed from the skin.
- Normal diet and fluids may be resumed, unless contraindicated by the test results.

Magnetic Resonance Imaging (MRI)

Provides physiologic information and detailed anatomic views of tissues using a superconducting magnet and radiofrequency signals.

Preparation

- Evaluate the patient for need for sedation. Patients who are claustrophobic or unable to lie still during study may benefit from sedation.
- Patients with implanted surgical clips or other metallic structures and those with implanted electromechanical devices, such as cardiac pacemakers, drug infusion pumps, and cochlear implants, cannot be exposed to MRI procedures.
- An informed consent is required.
- Pregnant patients are not routinely scanned because an increase in amniotic fluid/fetal temperature may be harmful.

Aftercare

- If intravenous contrast is used during the study, monitor for sensitivity and adverse reactions.
- Monitor contrast injection site for signs of irritation, infection, and bruising.
- If prestudy sedation was given, monitor patient closely until sedation wears off to prevent injury.

Abdominal CT Scan

Thin beams of x-rays are directed at and moved around the abdomen, resulting in computer-manipulated pictures that are not obscured by overlying anatomy.

Preparation

- An oral contrast is consumed before the study
- Intravenous iodine contrast may be administered.
- Assess for patient allergies to iodine, IV contrast, and/or shellfish. Prestudy preparation may be required if allergies are present.
- Assess for renal impairment; check laboratory values for elevated BUN and creatinine levels.
- Patient should not eat solid foods on the day of the study; clear liquids may be consumed up to 2 hours before the study.
- CT scan is contraindicated for pregnant patients.
- An informed consent is required.
- If the patient has diabetes, alert the radiology department, and schedule the exam for early morning. If the patient is taking metformin, special considerations may be necessary. Consult with the health care team to determine if the metformin should be suspended for the day of and several days after the study (Fischbach & Fischbach, 2018).

Aftercare

- If intravenous contrast is used during study, monitor for sensitivity and adverse reactions.
- Monitor contrast injection site for signs of irritation, infection, and bruising.
- If prestudy sedation was given, monitor patient closely until sedation wears off to prevent injury.

Source: Adapted from A-Rahim, Y. I., & Falchuk, M. (2021). UpToDate. *Bowel preparation before colonoscopy in adults.* Wolters Kluwer. https://www.uptodate.com/contents/bowel-preparation-before-colonoscopy-in-adults; Centers for Disease Control and Prevention (CDC). (2021). Colorectal cancer screening continuing education. CRC screening and surveillance: Optimizing quality. Section 3: The role of primary care providers in the delivery of high-quality colonoscopy. https://www.cdc.gov/cancer/colorectal/quality/CRC_Screening_Optimizing_Quality_Primary_Care3.pdf; and Fischbach, F. T., & Fischbach, M. A. (2018). *A manual of laboratory and diagnostic tests* (10th ed.). Wolters Kluwer.

This technique is useful for detecting obstructions, strictures, inflammatory disease, tumors, ulcers, and other lesions, and for diagnosing a hiatal hernia and other structural changes in the GI tract.

Use of a radiopaque contrast medium, such as barium sulfate, accentuates the body structures being visualized. In the upper GI examination and small-bowel series, the patient drinks the barium sulfate like a milkshake. The barium coats the esophagus, stomach, and small intestine to enhance visualization. In the barium enema or lower GI examination, barium sulfate is instilled into the large intestine through a rectal tube inserted through the anus.

Fluoroscopy projects consecutive x-ray images onto a screen for continuous observation of the flow of the barium. During a computerized tomography (CT) scan, thin beams of x-rays are directed at and move around the abdomen, resulting in computer-manipulated pictures that are not obscured by overlying anatomy. Contrast may be given orally or intravenously to enhance the images. Magnetic resonance imaging (MRI) provides physiologic information and detailed anatomic views of tissues using a superconducting magnet and radiofrequency signals. Computers use the signals to construct detailed sectional images of the abdomen. Intravenous contrast can be given to enhance the images. Abdominal ultrasound visualizes all solid upper abdominal organs, including the liver, bile ducts, gallbladder, appendix, pancreas, kidneys, adrenals, spleen, and the abdominal aorta and vena cava. The specific nursing responsibilities related to these studies are included in Box 39-2.

Examples of Actual or Potential Health Problems and Needs

BOWEL ELIMINATION

Actual or Potential Health Problems and Needs	Possible Etiologic Factors	Potential Signs and Symptoms
Diarrhea	Adverse effects of pharmaceutical agents Abuse of laxatives Emotional stress Intestinal infection Colon disease and other diseases Radiation	• At least three loose, liquid stools per day, increased frequency • Urgency • Reports of abdominal pain and/or cramping • Hyperactive bowel sounds
Bowel Incontinence	Dietary habits General decline in muscle tone Laxative abuse Rectal sphincter abnormality Cognitive impairment	• Involuntary passage of stool (stool characteristics vary) • *"I'm sorry, I couldn't get into the bathroom (or onto the bedpan) quickly enough."* • *"It came so fast I couldn't hold it back."* • Constant dribbling of soft stool
Constipation Risk	Insufficient fluid intake Insufficient fiber intake Inactivity Delaying defecation when urge is present Misuse of laxatives	—

Source: International Council of Nurses (ICN). (2019). *Nursing diagnosis and outcome statements.* https://www.icn.ch/sites/default/files/inline-files/ICNP2019-DC.pdf; Wolters Kluwer. (2022). Problem-based care plans. In *Lippincott Advisor.* Wolters Kluwer.

SCHEDULING FOR DIAGNOSTIC STUDIES

Nurses may be involved in scheduling diagnostic studies when a patient is to undergo multiple studies. Use the following guidelines for scheduling studies of the GI tract:

1. Follow a logical sequence when more than one test is required for accurate diagnosis:
   - Fecal occult blood tests: to detect GI bleeding
   - Barium studies: to visualize GI structures and reveal any inflammation, ulcers, tumors, strictures, or other lesions
   - Endoscopic examinations: to visualize an abnormality, locate a source of bleeding, and if necessary, provide biopsy tissue samples
2. A barium enema and routine radiography should precede an upper GI series because retained barium from an upper GI series could take several days to pass through the GI tract and cloud anatomic detail on the barium enema studies.
3. Noninvasive procedures usually take precedence over invasive procedures, such as endoscopic studies, when sufficient diagnostic data can be obtained from them. In some instances, endoscopic studies may be done before barium studies to ensure visualization.
4. It is important to consider any comorbidities, such as diabetes mellitus, that the patient may have in scheduling diagnostic studies that require the patient to have an altered diet or to have nothing by mouth.

Diagnosing Actual or Potential Health Problems and Needs

An assessment of a patient's bowel status may lead to the identification of one or more actual or potential health problems and needs related to bowel elimination. Following the formulation of the actual or potential health problems and needs, the nurse communicates findings to other nursing and health care professionals through the use of written and spoken word. The written actual or potential health problem or need becomes a permanent part of the patient's health record. Examples of health problems and needs with related etiology and signs and symptoms can be found in the Examples of Actual or Potential Health Problems and Needs: Bowel Elimination.

Outcome Identification and Planning

Expected outcomes are derived from the actual or potential bowel elimination problems or needs identified. The goal is to maintain or restore optimum function related to bowel elimination, alleviate symptoms or side effects of disease or treatment, and to prevent complications. General patient outcomes are listed here. Actual patient outcomes should list specific behaviors and criteria individualized for the patient situation. The patient will:

- Have a soft, formed bowel movement without discomfort
- Explain the relationship between bowel elimination and dietary fiber, fluid intake, and exercise
- Relate the importance of seeking medical evaluation if changes in stool color or consistency persist
- Maintain skin integrity

Implementing

Nursing care related to bowel elimination includes interventions to promote regular bowel habits, prevent and treat constipation, prevent and treat diarrhea, decrease flatulence, promote elimination of feces, manage bowel incontinence, and implement bowel-training programs. Nursing care related to caring for a patient with a nasogastric (NG) tube for gastric decompression is also discussed in the following sections.

Promoting Regular Bowel Habits

Promote regular bowel habits in well and ill patients by attention to timing, positioning, privacy, nutrition, and exercise.

TIMING

Encourage toileting at the patient's usual time during the day. Ask the patient to explain what measures are most successful in maintaining regular bowel function. Offer whatever assistance is needed to help the patient to the bathroom, commode, or bedpan at the time that a patient usually experiences the urge to defecate. This is often about an hour after meals, when mass colonic peristalsis occurs. Because many patients feel uncomfortable about requesting time for elimination, educate all patients about the importance of heeding this natural urge, as postponing it could result in constipation and other problems.

POSITIONING

Sitting upright on a toilet or commode promotes defecation. Most patients who are able to use the bedside commode or bathroom toilet have little difficulty assuming this position, although they may need support. An elevated toilet seat may be ordered for patients with orthopedic problems who cannot lower themselves to a toilet seat. Sitting upright promotes a sense of normalcy and the effects of gravity help to promote regular bowel movements. Sitting with the knees higher than the hips (using a small step stool if necessary) instead of resting the feet on the floor may improve defecation by straightening the anorectal junction and easing the evacuation of stool (Mounsey et al., 2015; Queensland Health, 2019).

It is best to avoid bedpan use; encourage use of the toilet or bedside commode, as discussed previously. Patients who need to use a bedpan often benefit from having the head of the bed elevated to as close to a sitting position as possible, at least 30 degrees, unless this is contraindicated. An overhead trapeze may be helpful for patients with weak lower extremities. Offer the patient moistened hand wipes at the bedside to substitute for handwashing after toileting. Always empty, clean, and return the bedpan to the patient's bedside stand or store according to facility policy.

PRIVACY

Many adults and children cannot defecate in the presence of another person. Unless the patient is extremely weak and requires assistance, provide privacy in the health care facility and in the home. Always respect the patient's need to be alone while defecating, unless the patient's condition makes this impossible. Pull the bedside drapes around a patient who is using a bedside commode or bedpan. If any visitors are present, ask them to step outside for a few minutes. When assisting patients to the bathroom, step out of the bathroom as long as it is safe to do so. For well patients who cannot defecate in a public restroom (with multiple toilets) or strange environment, suggest that they use a private restroom with only one toilet.

Hygiene

Patients who are confined to bed or who use a bedside commode find it difficult to perform their usual genital hygiene. Careful cleansing of the perineal and genital areas is needed for patient comfort and to prevent potential alterations in skin integrity. This is easily accomplished for patients by using warmed, moistened disposable washcloths and skin cleanser. Because people customarily wash their hands after toileting and hand hygiene prevents transmission of microorganisms, offer patients a moistened towelette or soap and water to wipe their hands after removing the bedpan or using the bedside commode.

NUTRITION

Patients with bowel elimination problems may need a dietary analysis to determine which foods and fluids are contributing to their problem and which may help in its treatment. General dietary recommendations to promote regular defecation include a fluid intake of 2,000 to 3,000 mL/day (average 2,600 mL) and high-fiber intake (Dudek, 2022; Medline Plus, 2021). It is important to be aware of those patients, particularly older adults with cardiac and renal problems, for whom increased fluid intake may be contraindicated. Increasing fiber intake without sufficient fluid intake can result in severe GI problems, including fecal impaction. Specific recommendations for treating constipation, diarrhea, and excessive flatulence follow.

EXERCISE

Although there is conflicting evidence on the role exercise plays in eliminating constipation, it is known that regular exercise improves GI motility and aids in defecation (Mounsey et al., 2015; Pinto et al., 2020). Encourage those patients who are able to exercise regularly for 2½ hours or more a week (USDHHS, 2018). It is important to get patients out of bed and walking as soon as they are able, instructing them that inactivity can lead to constipation, distention, and impaction. Bedside exercises may be helpful for patients who are immobile. Pelvic floor muscle training exercises (Kegel exercises) strengthen pelvic and rectal muscle tone and may be helpful for weakened patients (Medline Plus, 2021). Refer to Chapter 38 (p. 1465) for details related to use of PFMT exercises.

Providing Comfort Measures

Comfort measures related to defecation include working with the patient to develop a bowel elimination routine that results in the easy passage of a soft, formed stool; being attentive to perineal hygiene and the maintenance of skin integrity; and using warm, moist heat (sitz bath or tub bath) to soothe the perineal area. Additional interventions include the following:

- Encouraging recommended diet (if pertinent) and exercise

- Using medications, such as laxatives and antidiarrheals, only as needed if nonpharmacologic interventions are not effective
- Applying ointments or astringents (witch hazel) to inflamed and irritated tissue around the anal opening

PREVENTING AND TREATING CONSTIPATION

Constipation is dry, hard stool; infrequent difficult passage of stool; and/or the incomplete passage of stool (Bauldoff et al., 2020; Mitchell, 2019a). Decreased gastric motility slows the passage of feces through the large intestine, resulting in increased fluid absorption from the fecal mass and causing dry, hard stool. Straining often accompanies defecation. Some people may be constipated and yet have a daily bowel movement, whereas others who regularly defecate no more than three times a week are not constipated. People at high risk for constipation include patients on bedrest or with decreased mobility (Bauldoff et al., 2020). In addition, those taking medications that cause constipation (e.g., opioids, anticholinergics); patients with reduced fluids, bulk, or fiber in their diet; people who are depressed; and patients with central nervous system disease or local lesions that cause pain while defecating are also at risk (Bauldoff et al., 2020; Mitchell, 2019a; Pont et al., 2019; Touhy & Jett, 2018).

TEACHING ABOUT NUTRITION

Promoting healthy behaviors can assist the patient and family/caregivers to achieve mutually desirable outcomes for preventing constipation. A combination of high-fiber foods (20 to 35 g of fiber), fluid intake of 2,000 to 3,000 mL/day, and exercise has been shown to be effective in controlling constipation in patients with deficiencies in dietary intake of fiber and/or fluid and reduced amounts of exercise (Dudek, 2022; Medline Plus, 2021). It is important to gradually increase the amount of fiber in the diet to avoid bloating and flatulence. It can be trial and error in determining the proper amount of fiber a person needs to maintain regular bowel movements while limiting adverse effects (Dudek, 2022). Caution the patient to avoid increasing fiber intake without drinking enough fluids. Foods that contain high amounts of fiber include bran, fruits, vegetables, and whole grains. Fiber supplements may be necessary if adequate fiber cannot be consumed through food (Dudek, 2022).

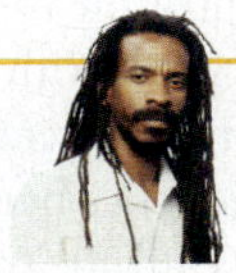

Think back to **Leroy Cobbs**, the patient who developed constipation while using opioid analgesics. The nurse should list in the teaching plan foods that stimulate peristalsis to prevent future episodes of constipation. If the patient knows to include these foods in their diet, they will be less worried about future problems and may be more amenable to using the medication to control their pain.

TEACHING ABOUT LAXATIVES

Laxatives are drugs that induce emptying of the intestinal tract. Bulk-forming laxatives such as psyllium work by absorbing water into the intestine to soften the stool and increasing stool bulk. Osmotic laxatives are not absorbable and work by bringing water into the intestine. Polyethylene glycol is a commonly used, well-tolerated osmotic laxative. Stimulant laxatives, such as bisacodyl and senna, improve defecation by increasing motility through irritation of the intestinal mucosa and increased water in the stool. Other frequently used laxatives are the saline-osmotics, such as magnesium hydroxide or magnesium citrate. Saline-osmotic laxatives act by drawing water into the intestines, stimulating peristalsis, and are effective but should be used in caution in those patients with renal disease. Magnesium hydroxide has antacid properties in small dosages and laxative properties in larger doses. Table 39-2 summarizes the types of laxatives.

Laxatives are sometimes necessary for people with limited activity or poor food intake. They are also used to empty the intestinal tract in preparation for surgery or diagnostic tests. Stool softeners such as docusate sodium may be used in conjunction with some prescribed medications to counteract the medications' constipating properties. Occasional use of laxatives is not harmful for most people, but people should not become dependent on them to induce regular bowel movements. The only laxatives that are appropriate and safe for long-term use are bulking agents, such as psyllium (Bauldoff et al., 2020). Because many laxatives are available as nonprescription drugs, and advertising promotes their use, many people take them frequently on their own initiative, whether they need them or not. Patient education is important in the safe use of over-the-counter medications.

Because of their chemical action, laxatives should not be taken when a patient is experiencing abdominal pain. Increased peristalsis caused by laxative use in the presence of an intestinal pathologic condition such as a bowel obstruction could result in patient harm (Bauldoff et al., 2020). Although many people take laxatives because they believe they are constipated, most are unaware that habitual use of laxatives may be the cause of chronic constipation (Bauldoff et al., 2020).

Nurses play a key role in helping patients who misuse laxatives. Breaking the physical and psychological habit of using laxatives is not easy for a person who has come to depend on them; it often requires much patience, support, and teaching. The person also frequently needs assistance with diet, fluid intake, activity, and regularity of habits (Shen et al., 2018). Overuse of laxatives because of chronic constipation may often be a sign of other disease processes such an eating disorder and requires further investigation (National Eating Disorder Association, 2018).

Preventing and Treating Diarrhea

Diarrhea is an increase in frequency (passage of three or more stools a day) and/or a change in consistency of stools (Dunlap & Patterson, 2020; Kyle & Carman, 2021). It is important to determine the consistency of the stool, as frequent bowel movements alone are not always indicative of diarrhea, but patients with diarrhea usually pass stools more frequently. Diarrhea is often associated with intestinal cramps. Nausea and vomiting may occur, and blood may also be noted. Diarrhea can be a protective response when

Table 39-2 Classification of Laxatives

TYPE	ACTION	ADVANTAGES	CAUTION
Bulk forming Psyllium, methylcellulose	Causes stool to absorb water. Increases stool weight, increases colonic distention, which stimulates peristalsis. Food supplement can take several days to weeks to see changes. Supplements will act within 12–72 hours.	Effects can also be achieved by increasing fiber in the diet to 25–35 g daily.	Can cause bloating and gas. Titrate dose to limit side effects. Not to be used in obstruction. Used cautiously with other swallowing disorders and in those who are immobile. Need to be able to increase water intake as well.
Osmotic Polyethylene glycol (PEG) Lactulose Sorbitol Magnesium citrate Sodium phosphate	Promote secretion of water into the colon. Stimulates bowel movement. Action usually in 12–96 hours.	Products such as polyethylene glycol dissolve completely in any fluid and are well tolerated.	Certain saline osmotic laxatives can lead to fluid and electrolyte imbalances and should not be used in older adults or those with kidney or cardiac disease.
Stimulant Bisacodyl Senna	Increase intestinal motility and colonic secretions Time to action: Oral 6–10 hours Rectal 15–60 minutes	Quick to work	Can cause severe cramping Frequently abused but generally safe Wait 1 hour after ingesting milk and antacids before using
Stool softeners	Agents with surfactant activity that decrease the tension between water and fat and lubricate the stool	Evidence is lacking to demonstrate effectiveness as a laxative. However, still may be seen in combination with use of other products.	Does not stimulate peristalsis, so can make stool soft and mushy but does not assist in evacuation
Lubricants Mineral oil	Lubricates the intestinal tract and slows down absorption of water in the colon, softening the stool and making it easier to pass	Often used in facilitating impaction removal	Serious complications in lungs can occur if aspirated, so avoid oral form in those at risk. Can interfere with absorption of vitamins especially ADEK Avoid use in those taking vitamin D analogs such as calcipotriene

the cause is an irritant in the intestinal tract. Regardless of the cause, however, large amounts of fluids and electrolytes may be lost relatively quickly through diarrhea, especially in infants, young children, and older adults (Bauldoff et al., 2020). If diarrhea is untreated, this loss of fluids and electrolytes places the person at high risk for life-threatening complications, such as vascular collapse and hypovolemic shock, hypokalemia and hypomagnesemia, and metabolic acidosis (Bauldoff et al., 2020). It is particularly important to maintain fluid balance in infants, children, and older adults because of their increased risk for dehydration, fluid overload, and electrolyte imbalances.

NURSING CARE CONSIDERATIONS FOR PATIENTS WITH DIARRHEA

The focus of nursing care is on eliminating the cause of the diarrhea and replacing lost fluids as well as treating the symptoms. Treatment for diarrhea typically depends on whether the problem is acute or chronic. Acute diarrhea may result from a viral or bacterial infection, a reaction to medication, or alterations in diet. It is characterized by its sudden onset and lasts several hours to several days. Rehydration is essential with acute diarrhea. Oral liquids may be used if the patient can tolerate them; otherwise, intravenous fluid replacement may be necessary. Refer to the Teaching about Nutrition discussion below. Stress the importance of hand hygiene with the patient and family/caregivers. Avoid antidiarrheal agents in acute diarrhea until a bacterial causative agent has been ruled out (Bauldoff et al., 2020).

Chronic (persistent) diarrhea typically lasts for more than 2 to 4 weeks (CDC, 2016). A thorough workup is needed in the patient with chronic diarrhea to determine the underlying cause. Chronic diarrhea has many possible causes, such as inflammatory bowel disease (e.g., Crohn disease, ulcerative colitis), irritable bowel syndrome, malabsorption syndromes, bowel tumor, metabolic disease (diabetes, hyperthyroidism), parasitic infection, side effects of drugs, laxative abuse, surgery, alcohol abuse, and radiation and chemotherapeutic agents (Bauldoff et al., 2020; MFMER, 2020c). Chronic diarrhea requires fluid and electrolyte replacement and, if severe and prolonged, may require pharmacologic intervention. Before treatment begins, it is important to make every effort to identify and eliminate the underlying cause (CDC, 2016).

Additional nursing measures for the patient with diarrhea include the following:

- Answer the patient's call bell immediately or ensure that a bedpan or commode is within easy reach. Diarrhea can be embarrassing, and the patient needs to know that the nurse is there to help. This also will decrease the risk of falls if the patient attempts to get out of bed on their own to quickly get to the bathroom to prevent incontinence.
- Whenever possible, address/remove the cause of the diarrhea. For example, discontinuing medications that cause diarrhea usually results in a return to normal defecation within 1 to 3 days.
- Sometimes there can be seepage or leakage of liquid stool in a patient with a fecal impaction. If there is any indication of a fecal impaction, further evaluation is necessary before using antidiarrheal medications.
- Give special care to the region around the anus, where skin irritation is common. Keep the area clean and dry. Use skin creams, moisture barriers, and ointments, as necessary to protect the skin.

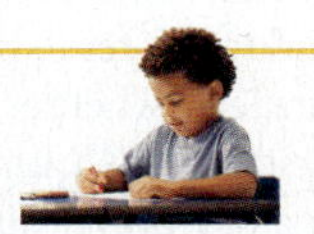

Skin care measures would be important to include in the care plan for ***Jeremy Green***, the young boy experiencing episodes of diarrhea. Doing so reduces Jeremy's risk for perianal excoriation and breakdown, which could further impair his body image and cause additional discomfort and pain.

TEACHING ABOUT NUTRITION

Supportive nutritional interventions depend on the severity of diarrhea and the underlying cause (Dudek, 2022). Encourage liberal fluid intake to replace losses, but clear liquids with high sugar content (high osmolality related to sugar content) should be avoided (Bauldoff et al., 2020; Dudek, 2022). On a short-term basis, a low-fiber, low lactose/sucrose/fructose diet may help decrease bowel stimulation (Dudek, 2022). Teach patients to avoid milk and milk products, raw fruits, gas-producing foods (bran, beans, corn, broccoli, cabbage), coffee, and alcoholic beverages (Bauldoff et al., 2020; Borum & Baumgartner, 2020, as cited in Dunlap and Patterson, 2020, p. 391; Dudek, 2022). Intravenous fluids should be utilized in the presence of severe dehydration and/or intolerance of oral rehydration (Borum & Baumgartner, 2021, as cited in Dunlap and Patterson, 2020, p. 391).

Alterations in fluid and electrolyte balance occur faster and more often in infants and children compared to adults. Therefore, infants and children experiencing diarrhea require more fluid and electrolyte replacement compared to adults. Encourage fluids, especially oral rehydration solutions containing sodium chloride, potassium, and glucose (Pedialyte® and Enfalyte®) and make them accessible for the child. Breast feeding should continue through the diarrhea. Children should resume an age-appropriate diet when tolerated. The diet should be high in complex carbohydrates, meats, fruits, and vegetables. Simple sugars such as fruit juices should be avoided. Special diets such as the BRAT diet (bananas, rice cereal, applesauce, and toast) are no longer recommended because of the lack of nutritional value (O'Ryan, 2020).

The use of probiotics (live microorganisms that are similar to beneficial microorganisms found in the human GI tract) to prevent, limit, and control diarrhea has been suggested as an effective dietary intervention for diarrhea, particularly antibiotic-associated diarrhea and *C. difficile*–associated disease (Cleveland Clinic, 2020a; NIH, 2020). Examples of foods containing probiotics include cheese, yogurt, kefir, tempeh, miso, soymilk, and some commercial dairy drinks. Probiotics can also be ingested through the use of commercially prepared supplements (LaRocque & Harris, 2020). See the accompanying PICOT in Practice box.

TEACHING ABOUT ANTIDIARRHEALS

Antidiarrheal medications should be used sparingly or not at all until the cause of the diarrhea has been identified (Bauldoff et al., 2020). Several types of antidiarrheal medications are available. Antimotility medications such as loperamide and diphenoxylate hydrochloride act directly on the smooth muscle of the GI tract. Bismuth subsalicylate has an antimicrobial action and an antisecretory effect. Refer to the following section on traveler's diarrhea for contraindications to the use of antimotility agents and bismuth subsalicylate. Table 39-3 highlights the major antidiarrheal agents.

TEACHING ABOUT FOOD SAFETY

Ensuring that food is safe for consumption and prepared and stored properly is a priority. Food poisoning, and the diarrhea that frequently accompanies it, can be prevented. The CDC (2020c; CDC, 2020d) recommends these measures related to promoting food safety:

- Take items that require refrigeration home immediately. Refrigerate perishable foods and leftovers within 2 hours (1 hour if it's hotter than 90°F outside). Refrigerator temperatures should be set to 40°F or below. Freezer temperatures should be 0°F or below.
- Wash hands and surfaces often. Wash surfaces and utensils after each use to prevent the spread of microorganisms.
- Use separate cutting boards and plates for produce and for meat, poultry, seafood, and eggs.
- Thoroughly wash all vegetables and fruit before preparing or eating.
- Do not wash meat, poultry, or eggs to prevent spreading microorganisms to the sink, countertops, and other kitchen surfaces.
- Never use raw eggs in any form because of the danger of infection with *Salmonella bacillus*. When cooking eggs, use only fresh ones that have been purchased within 3 to 5 weeks and kept in the refrigerator.
- Do not eat seafood raw or undercooked. Do not eat seafood if it has a strong, unpleasant odor.
- Use a food thermometer to ensure cooking food to the safe internal temperature. Cook whole meats to 145°F,

PICOT in Practice

ASKING CLINICAL QUESTIONS: PROBIOTICS

Scenario: You are a nurse who works in a new gastroenterology clinic. Ulcerative colitis (UC) is an inflammatory condition affecting the colon that cycles from period of exacerbation to remission. The majority of people with UC can be put into remission, leaving a group who do not respond to first- or second-line therapies. You read an article that described the benefits of probiotics in the care of patient with inflammatory bowel disease. You discuss this with the nurse educator who is not familiar with the findings. You both decide to evaluate the literature to see the benefits of probiotics in patients with UC.

- **Population:** Patients with ulcerative colitis
- **Intervention:** Efficacy of probiotics
- **Comparison:** 5-Aminosalicylic acid (5-ASA)
- **Outcome:** Inducing or maintaining of remission
- **Time:** 12 months

PICOT Question: What is the efficacy of probiotics compared to 5-aminosalicylic acid (5-ASA) in inducing or maintaining remission for patient with ulcerative colitis during a 12-month period?

Finding

Two pertinent resources were located:

1. Kaur, L., Gordon, M., Baines, P. A., Iheozor-Ejiofor, Z., Sinopoulou, V., & Akobeng, A. K. (2020). Probiotics for induction of remission in ulcerative colitis. *Cochrane Database of Systematic Reviews*, *3*(3), CD005573. https://doi.org/10.1002/14651858.CD005573.pub3

2. Iheozor-Ejiofor, Z., Kaur, L., Gordon, M., Baines, P. A., Sinopoulou, V., & Akobeng, A. K. (2020). Probiotics for maintenance of remission in ulcerative colitis. *Cochrane Database of Systematic Reviews*, *3*(3), CD007443. https://doi.org/10.1002/14651858.CD007443.pub3

When comparing efficacy of probiotics in the induction of remission 14 studies with 865 randomized participants were included. Twelve of the studies looked at adult participants, and two studies looked at pediatric participants with mild to moderate ulcerative colitis; the average age was between 12.5 and 47.7 years. When comparing efficacy of probiotics in the maintenance of remission, 12 studies with 1,473 randomized participants that met the inclusion criteria were included. Participants were mostly adults. Low-certainty evidence suggests that probiotics may induce clinical remission in active ulcerative colitis (UC) when compared to placebo. There may be little or no difference in clinical remission with probiotics alone compared to 5-ASA. The effectiveness of probiotics for the maintenance of remission in UC remains unclear. Maintenance of remission is low- to very low-certainty evidence from poorly conducted studies, which contribute limited amounts of data from a small number of participants.

Strength of Evidence: Level I: Systematic review

Recommendations: After conducting an assessment of the current literature you note that probiotics may be better at inducing remission than placebo (dummy treatment). It is unclear whether probiotics are better than 5-aminosalicylic acid (5-ASA), an antiinflammatory agent used to treat inflammatory bowel disease; however, there is limited evidence that when both treatments are used as combined therapy, they may be better than 5-ASA alone in inducing remission. It is uncertain as to whether probiotics can maintain remission in people with UC once an exacerbation has subsided. You discussed the findings with the nurse educator and decide to present your findings to the unit during an educational in-service.

ground meats to 160°F, and poultry to 165°F. Microwave food thoroughly; cook to the safe temperature of 165°F or above.

- Keep food hot after cooking; maintain the safe temperature of 140°F or above.
- Give only pasteurized fruit juices to young children (age <5 years) and other people who are at higher risk for food poisoning, such as adults older than age 65, people who are immunocompromised, pregnant women.

PREVENTING AND MANAGING TRAVELER'S DIARRHEA

Traveler's diarrhea (TD) is the most predictable travel-related illness (Connor, 2019). Risk increases when a person travels to a place where the climate or sanitary practices are different from those of their home (MFMER, 2019a). TD is caused by bacterial enteropathogens, viruses, or parasites, acquired from eating contaminated food or drinking contaminated water (MFMER, 2019a). Symptoms usually begin suddenly and may appear during the time of travel or shortly after the person returns home (MFMER, 2019a), and include more than three loose stools in a 24-hour period, fever, nausea, vomiting, and abdominal cramps and/or pain. Diarrhea caused by certain pathogens may also include bloody stools.

Management includes education about prevention and self-treatment strategies. Frequent handwashing with soap and water where available is important. Small containers of alcohol-based hand sanitizer containing ≥60% alcohol should be used when handwashing is not possible (Connor, 2019). Advise patients to peel fruits and vegetables and consume dry foods and foods that are piping hot and cooked thoroughly. Tell travelers to avoid tap water, ice cubes, fruit juice, unpeeled raw fruits and vegetables, unpasteurized dairy products, open buffets, and undercooked or reheated foods. Safe beverages include those that are commercially bottled and factory-sealed (Griffin & Hill, 2019). Boiled beverages and those appropriately chemically treated and disinfected are also safe to drink (Griffin & Hill, 2019).

Bismuth subsalicylate has been shown to reduce the incidence of TD by 50% and is recommended as a prophylaxis for traveler's diarrhea (Connor, 2019). Travelers with aspirin allergy; renal insufficiency and gout; and those taking anticoagulants, probenecid, or methotrexate should not take bismuth subsalicylate (Connor, 2019). It is not recommended for children younger than age 12 years or for pregnant women

Table 39-3 Classification of Antidiarrheal Medications

CATEGORY	NAME	ACTION	ADVANTAGES	CAUTIONS
Opioid-receptor agonists	Diphenoxylate and atropine	Slows gastric motility through local effect on GI wall	Effective	Should not be used if antibiotic-associated diarrhea such as *C. difficile* is suspected The anticholinergic effects can lead to changes in the patient's level of consciousness, increasing the risk for confusion and falls. For this reason, best to avoid in older adults There are also many drug interactions with anticholinergic medications, which can lead to CNS changes Avoid in patients taking opioids as it can increase constipation and urinary retention
	Loperamide	Inhibits peristalsis via direct effect on GI wall muscles; may also have an antisecretory property	Longer duration than diphenoxylate and atropine	Should not be used if antibiotic-related diarrhea such as *C. difficile* is suspected May be used in the older adult Higher-than-recommended doses have been shown to increase serious cardiac events such as prolonged QT, leading to life-threatening arrhythmias May cause drowsiness Should be discontinued if no improvement in 48 hours with acute illness
Antisecretory/antimicrobial	Bismuth subsalicylate	Decreases GI tract secretion Has antimicrobial action against bacterial and viral pathogens	No drowsiness	Requires frequent dosing Contains salicylates. Not to be given to children under 12 years. Check with health care provider in adolescents or when administering to patients using aspirin or other products that contain aspirin. Contraindicated for pregnant women May decrease absorption of some medications Will turn stool black

(Connor, 2019) and should not be taken for longer than 3 weeks (MFMER, 2019a). Use involves four times/day dosing; this inconvenient dosing contributes to decrease practicality of use (Connor, 2019). Prophylactic antibiotics are not recommended for most travelers (Connor, 2019).

Treatment strategies include maintaining hydration with bottled beverages or treated with chlorine, boiled, or otherwise known to be purified and/or oral rehydration solutions; antimotility agents, such as loperamide and diphenoxylate; and antibiotics (Connor, 2019). The use of antibiotics and/or antimicrobials should be based on severity of illness and etiologic agent (Brewer, 2018; Connor, 2019). Antimotility agents should be avoided in those with bloody diarrhea or who have diarrhea and fever.

Adult patients should see a health care professional if the patient (MFMER, 2019a):

- Has diarrhea persisting beyond 2 days
- Becomes dehydrated
- Has bloody or black stools
- Has a fever above 102°F

Children should see a health care professional if the patient has (MFMER, 2019a):

- Persistent vomiting
- Fever of 102°F or more
- Bloody stools or severe diarrhea
- Dry mouth or crying without tears
- Signs of being unusually sleepy, drowsy, or unresponsive
- Decreased volume of urine, including fewer wet diapers in infants

Encourage patients considering travel to underdeveloped countries to discuss their personal risks and the provision of prescription medication with their health care provider before beginning their travels.

Decreasing Flatulence

Formation of gases in the stomach or intestines is a result of normal breakdown of certain undigested foods in the large intestine or from swallowing of air when eating and drinking (Cleveland Clinic, 2020b). Burping or belching is the way most swallowed air leaves the stomach. Some gas moves into the small intestine where it is partially absorbed, and a small amount travels into the large intestine for release through the rectum **flatulence** (Cleveland Clinic, 2020b). Additional gas is produced when undigested carbohydrates move into the large intestine, where harmless and normal bacteria break down the food, producing hydrogen, carbon dioxide and, in about one third of all people, methane (Cleveland Clinic, 2020b). Eventually, these gases exit through the rectum. When the gas is not expelled but accumulates in the intestinal tract, the condition is referred to as intestinal distention. Gas-producing foods include most foods that contain carbohydrates; fats and proteins cause little gas (Cleveland Clinic, 2020b). Foods that often predispose a person to flatulence and distention include beans; vegetables, including broccoli, Brussels sprouts, artichokes, cabbage, onions, asparagus, and cauliflower; fruits, such as pears, apples, and peaches; whole grains, including whole wheat and bran; carbonated drinks and beer; milk and milk products, including cheese and ice cream; and foods containing sorbitol, such as dietetic foods and sugar-free candy and gum (Cleveland Clinic, 2020b; MFMER, 2020d). Foods that produce symptomatic gas in one person may not cause symptoms in another. Continued flatulence associated with unintended weight loss, fever, loss of appetite or feeling full quickly, chest discomfort, or change in bowel habits should be evaluated by the patient's health care provider for the presence of an underlying digestive disorder (MFMER, 2020d).

Teach patients about dietary adjustments through trial and error to avoid foods that cause increased flatulence. Several over-the-counter medications are available to help reduce flatulence. Antacids with simethicone or activated charcoal and supplements with digestive enzymes can help reduce symptoms (Cleveland Clinic, 2020b). Other possible interventions include the use of bismuth subsalicylate for short-term use to reduce odor; probiotics in yogurt and commercial supplements; and exercise to peristalsis and the escape of flatus.

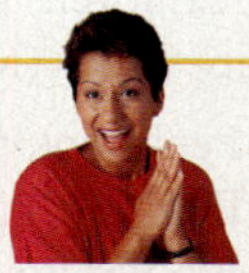

Recall **Alberta Franklin**, the patient described in the Reflective Practice display. The nurse should include information about eliminating gas-producing foods in this patient's teaching plan to avoid excess gas formation and accumulation, which could cause the colostomy bag to overfill and possibly lead to detachment and leakage.

Emptying the Colon of Feces

Several methods are used to help promote elimination of feces: enemas, suppositories, oral intestinal lavage, and digital removal of stool. Discussion of each of these methods follows.

ENEMAS

An **enema** is the introduction of a solution into the large intestine, usually to remove feces. The instilled solution distends the intestine and irritates the intestinal mucosa, thus increasing peristalsis. An enema can also be used to administer certain medications. Enemas are generally classified as cleansing or retention enemas and should only be used occasionally (Mitchell, 2019b). Rectal agents should be avoided in patients at risk of thrombocytopenia, leukopenia, and/or mucositis and manipulation of the rectum and anus, including administration of enemas, should be avoided in immunocompromised patients and/or patients at risk for myelosuppression and mucositis (NCI, 2020). These actions can lead to development of anal fissures or abscesses, which are portals for infection (NCI, 2020). Enemas are also contraindicated for patients with bowel obstruction or paralytic ileus (Mitchell, 2019b) and in situations where administration could cause circulatory overload, mucosal damage, necrosis, perforation, or hemorrhage or following any GI or gynecological surgery in which sutures may be ruptured (Doughery & Lister, 2015, as cited in Mitchell, 2019b, p. 154).

Cleansing (Evacuant) Enemas

Cleansing enemas are given to remove feces from the colon, commonly to:

- Relieve constipation or fecal impaction
- Evacuate the bowel before surgery to prevent involuntary escape of fecal material during surgical procedures
- Promote visualization of the intestinal tract by radiographic or endoscopic examination

The most common types of solutions used for cleansing enemas are tap water, normal saline solution, soap solution, and hypertonic solution. Commonly used enema solutions are described in Table 39-4.

Hypotonic (tap water) and isotonic (normal saline solution) enemas are large-volume enemas that result in rapid colonic emptying. However, using such large volumes of solution (adults, 500 to 1,000 mL; infants, less than 250 mL [Kyle & Carman, 2021]) may be dangerous for patients with weakened intestinal walls, such as those with bowel inflammation or bowel infection.

Hypertonic solution preparations (phosphate and sodium citrate enemas) are available commercially and are administered in smaller volumes (adult, 118 to 197 mL). These solutions draw water into the colon, which stimulates the defecation reflex. They may be contraindicated in patients for whom sodium and/or water retention is a problem (NICE, 2017, as cited in Mitchell, 2019b, p. 154). Phosphate enemas should not be used in older adults (Toughy & Jett, 2018). Hypertonic solution enemas are also contraindicated for patients with renal impairment or reduced renal clearance because such patients have compromised ability to excrete phosphate adequately, with resulting hyperphosphatemia (Dougherty & Lister, 2015, as cited in Mitchell, 2019b, p. 154).

Retention Enemas

Retention enemas are retained in the bowel for a prolonged period for different reasons:

- Oil-retention enemas: soften the stool and lubricate the intestinal mucosa, making defecation easier (Bauldoff et al., 2020). About 150 to 200 mL of solution is administered to adults.

Table 39-4 Commonly Used Enema Solutions

SOLUTION	AMOUNT	ACTION	TIME TO TAKE EFFECT (MINUTES)	ADVERSE EFFECTS
Tap water (hypotonic)	500–1,000 mL	Distends intestine, increases peristalsis, softens stool	15	Can lead to fluid and electrolyte imbalance, water intoxication Should not be used in children
Normal saline (isotonic)	500–1,000 mL	Distends intestine, increases peristalsis, softens stool	15	
Soap	500–1,000 mL (concentrate at 3–5 mL/1,000 mL)	Distends intestine, irritates intestinal, which stimulates peristalsis mucosa, softens stool	10–15	Must only use castile soap, other soaps will cause significant rectal mucosa irritation or damage
Phosphate (hypertonic)	70–130 mL	Draw fluids out of the interstitial space into the colon, leading to distention, which stimulates peristalsis. Commonly used, commercially prepared	5–10	Avoid in patients who are dehydrated or where phosphate retention could be a concern Can be irritating to rectum
Oil (mineral, olive, or cottonseed oil)	150–200 mL	Lubricates stool and intestinal mucosa; often used as a retention enema If able, patient may need to hold solution for 30–60 minutes	30	

- Carminative enemas: help to expel flatus from the rectum and provide relief from gaseous distention. Common solutions include the milk and molasses enema (equal parts) (Wanfui-Verry et al., 2019) and the soap-solution enema (Bauldoff et al., 2020).
- Medicated enemas: provide medications that are absorbed through the rectal mucosa.

Equipment

Commercially prepared enema kits include a flexible bottle containing hypertonic solution with an attached, prelubricated firm tip about 5 to 7.5 cm (2 to 3 inches) long. Its ease of use makes it particularly convenient in the home. In many instances, patients can administer their own enema.

Tap water, saline solution, and soap solution enemas are administered using a container, rubber or plastic tubing with side openings near its distal end, a tubing clamp, lubricant, and the prescribed solution. Regardless of the type of enema to be given, clean technique is used. Always wear or have the caregiver wear disposable gloves to protect from exposure to blood, body fluids, and microorganisms.

Patient Preparation

Some patients already know why enemas are used and how they are administered. Reinforce this information and correct any misconceptions that they may have. For patients who have not previously had an enema, explain the purpose, what they can expect, and how they can participate. In all cases, administration of medications using the rectal route can be embarrassing for the patient; it is essential to provide for patient privacy (Mitchell, 2019b). The procedure offers an excellent opportunity for health teaching because many people are unfamiliar with or uncomfortable talking about the functioning of the intestinal tract. Failure to provide explanations and protect privacy may result in an uncomfortable and disagreeable situation for the patient.

A reclining position is recommended for enema administration—specifically left side-lying with the knees flexed and the upper thigh pulled toward the abdomen if possible (Mitchell, 2019b), but if the patient has a respiratory disorder or is having difficulty breathing, elevate the head of the bed slightly. Avoid Fowler position because the solution will remain in the rectum, and expulsion will occur rapidly, resulting in minimal cleansing. Some patients think the solution should be expelled as soon as possible. Reinforce the need to retain the solution to enhance the evacuant effect (Dougherty & Lister, 2015, as cited in Mitchell, 2019b, p. 156).

Administration Using a Hypotonic or Isotonic (Large-Volume) Solution

The procedure for administering a cleansing enema using a large volume of solution is described in Skill 39-1 (on pp. 1555–1560).

Administration Using a Hypertonic (Small-Volume) Solution

Administering a cleansing enema using a hypertonic solution differs from the procedure described in Skill 39-1 (on pp. 1555–1560) in the following ways:

- The equipment is included in the commercially prepared set. The only additional equipment needed is a bedpan for a bedridden patient; an easily accessible commode in case the patient has an urgent need to expel the enema; and a disposable waterproof pad to protect bed linens (Mitchell 2019b).
- Place the patient in the left side–lying position lying with their knees flexed and the upper thigh pulled toward the abdomen if possible (Mitchell, 2019b). Additional lubrication of the rectal tip is recommended, even though it is prelubricated.
- Slowly insert the nozzle to the depth of 4 to 5 inches (10 to 12.5 cm) (Mitchell, 2019b). Instill the solution into the rectum by applying gentle pressure on the collapsible solution container, squeezing from the bottom to the nozzle (Fig. 39-6). It should take 1 to 2 minutes to administer the enema. Withdraw the nozzle slowly.
- Administer the hypertonic enema solution cautiously to a patient with hemorrhoids. The rigid tip may tear fragile rectal mucosa that is enlarged and inflamed, causing pain, torn rectal tissue, and necrosis. Generous lubrication is recommended before inserting the enema tip.

Administration of an Oil-Retention Enema

The procedure for giving an oil-retention enema differs from that for giving a cleansing enema in the following respects:

- A small nozzle is used. The small size helps to reduce intestinal contractions so that the patient can retain the oil more easily. Oil enemas are available in commercial kits similar to those for hypertonic-solution enemas.
- Administer the oil-retention enema at body temperature to minimize muscle contractions caused by a warmer or cooler solution.
- Instruct the patient to retain the oil for at least 30 minutes for best cleansing results.
- A cleansing enema may be prescribed after an oil-retention enema to facilitate emptying of the bowel.

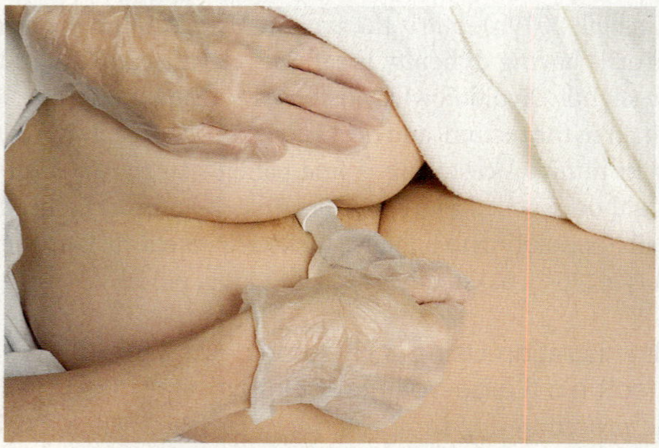

FIGURE 39-6. Technique for compressing a small-volume enema container.

RECTAL SUPPOSITORIES

A **suppository** is a conical or oval solid substance shaped for easy insertion into a body cavity and designed to melt at body temperature. Various rectal suppositories are available. Suppositories can be used to stimulate the bowel in a constipated patient. Suppositories can also be used to deliver drug therapy and can be used to deliver medications such as antipyretics when the patient is unable to take them orally (Mitchell, 2019c). Refer to Chapter 30 for Guidelines for Nursing Care 30-6.

ORAL INTESTINAL LAVAGE

Oral polyethylene glycol solutions (PEG) can be used to cleanse the intestine of feces. This solution is prescribed by the health care provider and can be administered before visual examination of the GI tract, such as with a colonoscopy or sigmoidoscopy, or as a preparation (emptying) of the bowel before intestinal surgery (Karch, 2020). Evacuation of feces may begin within 1 hour after the first glass and is completed within 3 to 6 hours (Karch, 2020). As with an enema, a clear return indicates that the bowel preparation is complete. A clear diet for 24 hours before taking this solution lessens the time needed for completion of the bowel prep, but potassium replacement may be required before surgery because of the limited potassium in a clear diet. The solution has a slightly salty taste and is easier to tolerate if it is cold and consumed quickly. Carefully assess older adults using oral intestinal lavage because they are more prone to electrolyte imbalances (Toughy & Jett, 2018).

DIGITAL REMOVAL OF STOOL

Fecal impaction, most often caused by constipation, prevents the passage of normal stools. Small amounts of fluid may pass around the impacted mass; liquid fecal seepage with no passage of normal feces is a sign of an impaction. Older adults who are hospitalized or under institutional care, patients who are immobile, and patients who have scleroderma, chronic renal failure, spinal cord injury, or other health conditions that damage the nerves that innervate the muscles of the intestines are at high risk for fecal impaction (Falcón et al., 2016; MedlinePlus, 2022a; Setya et al., 2021).

Digital (manual) removal of feces is an invasive procedure that involves the manual removal of feces from the rectum using a gloved finger (Dougherty & Lister, 2015, as cited in Mitchell, 2019d, p. 430). Include dietary interventions, adequate fluids, and adjustment of medication in the patient's care plan before considering digital removal of feces (Mitchell, 2019d). If a patient with a fecal impaction cannot expel the fecal mass voluntarily and oil-retention and cleansing enemas fail to break up the mass, the impaction may need to be removed manually. Digital removal of stool is a prescribed intervention. This procedure is embarrassing and very uncomfortable and may cause great discomfort and pain to the patient as well as irritation of the rectal mucosa and bleeding (Mitchell, 2019d). Digital removal of a fecal mass can stimulate the vagus nerve, resulting in a slowed heart rate (Mitchell, 2019d). If this occurs, stop the procedure immediately, monitor the patient's heart rate and blood pressure, and notify the health care team. Many patients find that a sitz bath or tub bath after this procedure soothes the irritated perineal area. The health care team may order an oil-retention enema to be given before the procedure to soften stool. The procedure for digital (manual) removal of a fecal impaction is outlined in the Guidelines for Nursing Care 39-1.

Guidelines for Nursing Care 39-1

DIGITAL REMOVAL OF FECAL IMPACTION

To manually remove a fecal impaction, the following technique is recommended:

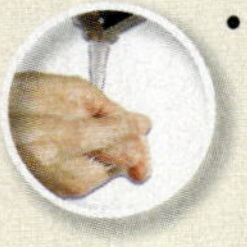

- Perform hand hygiene and put on PPE, if indicated.

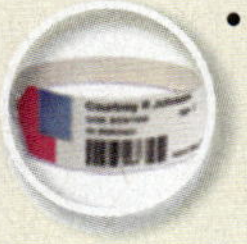

- Identify the patient.
- Close the door to the room and pull the privacy curtain.
- Explain what you are going to do, and why you are going to do it to the patient.
- Have a second person assist with the procedure. The second person can reassure and comfort the patient while the first person works to break up the mass.
- Encourage/assist the patient to empty their bladder.
- Place the patient in a left side-lying position. Drape the patient to preserve privacy yet provide easy access. Place a protective pad under the patient. Remove the patient's clothing from the waist down.
- Place a bedpan on the bed for depositing removed feces. Have toilet paper and personal cleaning supplies on hand for use after the procedure is completed.
- Put on gloves.
- Assess the anal area for evidence of skin soreness, swelling, bleeding, discharge, prolapse, excoriation, and hemorrhoids. If any abnormalities are present, do not continue with the procedure (Mitchell, 2019d). Confer with the health care team.
- Lubricate the index finger generously to reduce irritating the rectum and insert the finger gently into the anal canal (Figure A). The presence of the finger added to the mass tends to cause discomfort for the patient if the work is not done slowly and gently.
- Slowly and gently, work the finger around in circular movements and into the hardened mass to break it up (Figures B and C), then remove pieces of it (Figure D). Instruct the patient to bear down, if possible, while extracting feces to ease in removal. Avoid using a hooked finger to remove feces, as this may cause damage to the rectal mucosa and anal sphincter (Mitchell, 2019d).
- Remove the impaction at intervals if it is severe. This helps to avoid discomfort as well as irritation, which can injure intestinal mucosa.
- Use an oil-retention enema, if necessary. The enema may be given before attempts are made to break up and remove the impaction digitally, or it may be ordered after digital attempts fail. A cleansing enema is often ordered after an oil-retention enema.
- Wash and dry the patient's buttocks and anal area. Assist the patient to a comfortable position.

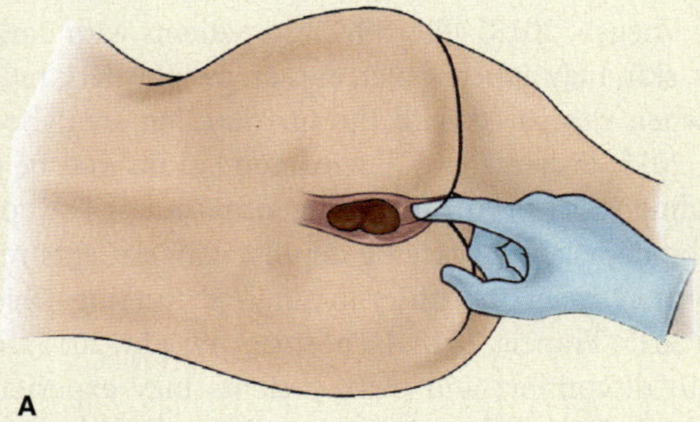

A

A Inserting gloved, lubricated finger into fecal mass.

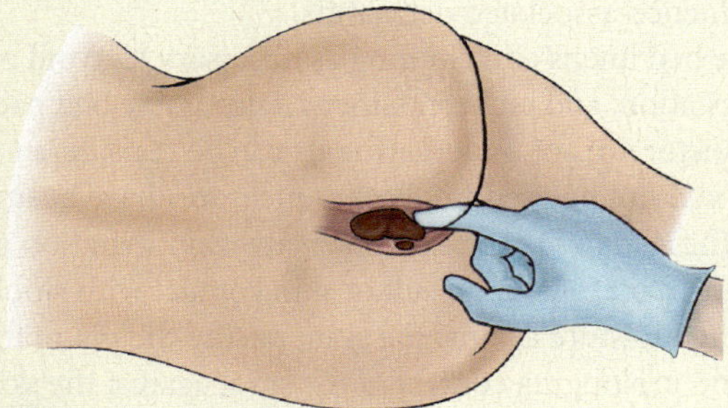

B

B Slowly and gently using finger to break up some of the hardened mass.

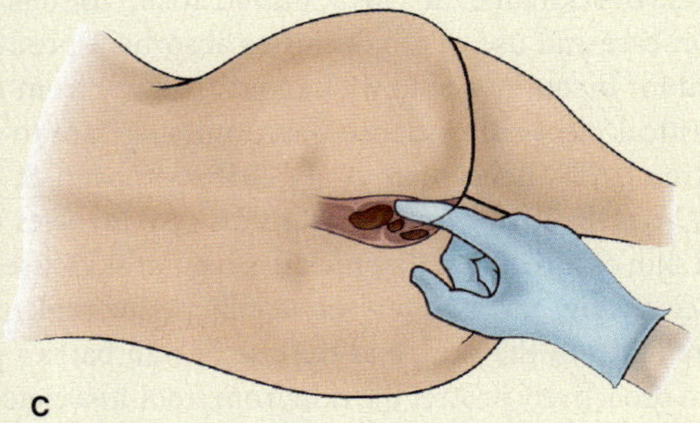

C

C Breaking off a section of the impaction.

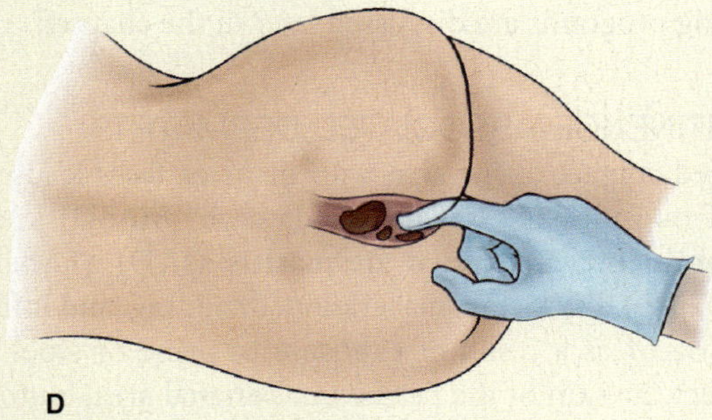

D

D Removing a section of the impaction.

Managing Bowel Incontinence

Bowel incontinence or fecal incontinence is the loss of voluntary control of defecation (Bauldoff et al., 2020), the inability of the anal sphincter to control the discharge of fecal and gaseous material. The cause of incontinence may be related to loss of sphincter tone, such as changes in the function of the rectum and anal sphincter related to aging; neurologic injury or disease; local trauma, such as obstetric tears; inflammation as a result of infection or radiation; and the presence of tumors (Bauldoff et al., 2020; Palmer, 2019; Yates, 2019). The patient may not be able to perceive the urge to move the bowels or completely empty the rectum after a bowel movement, which can also result in incontinence. Alternations in mental health may also cause a patient to be indifferent to the passage of stool. Although bowel incontinence is seldom life threatening, it can be a distressing and undignified experience (Palmer, 2019). Patients with bowel incontinence suffer embarrassment, may become depressed, and may pose a challenge for nurses because of the risk for alterations in skin integrity (Bauldoff et al., 2020; Fisher & Himan, 2020; Voegeli, 2018). (Refer to the discussion regarding incontinence-associated dermatitis in the next section.)

The following nursing interventions are helpful for a patient who experiences bowel incontinence:

- Note when incontinence is most likely to occur and assist the patient to the bathroom or commode at those times. If there is no pattern, offer toileting at regular intervals, such as every few hours (Francis, 2018).
- Keep the skin clean and dry by using proper hygienic measures. Apply a protective skin barrier after cleaning the skin, according to the manufacturer's directions. Impaired skin integrity may develop when such measures are overlooked. Refer to the following discussion regarding incontinence-associated dermatitis.
- Change bed linens and clothing as necessary to avoid odor, skin irritation, and embarrassment. Disposable bed pads and moisture-proof undergarments can be considered but should not be used until other measures have been tried. These materials often worsen any skin irritation or breakdown present as a result of skin contact with stool by retaining moisture against the skin, raising the pH of the skin, and prolonging contact of the stool against the skin, increasing damage from digestive enzymes present in the stool (Gump & Schmelzer, 2016; Voegeli, 2018).
- Bowel-training programs may also be helpful. Bowel-training programs are discussed later in the chapter.

INCONTINENCE-ASSOCIATED DERMATITIS

Prolonged contact of the skin with urine or feces leads to a form of moisture-associated skin damage (MASD) known as **incontinence-associated dermatitis (IAD)** (Fisher & Himan, 2020). Erythema, maceration, denuding, and inflammation occur as a result of exposure to urine or stool and may affect the skin of the perineum, perianal area, buttocks, inner thighs, sacrum, and coccyx (Jacobson & Wright, 2015; Voegeli, 2018). Incontinence and resulting excessive moisture also contribute to pressure injury formation, particularly pressure injury of the sacral area (Gray & Giuliano, 2018; Jacobson & Wright, 2015; Lachenbruch et al., 2016). Symptoms of IAD include erythema with poorly defined edges located in patches on the skin or continuously over large areas and the skin may feel warmer and firmer than the surrounding unaffected skin (Beeckman et al., 2015; Francis, 2018; Voegeli, 2018) (Fig. 39-7). In patients with darker skin tones, skin may appear paler, darker, purple, dark red, or yellow when compared with the surrounding area (Beeckman et al., 2015; Fisher, 2020). Edema and lesions may be present, including vesicles, bullae, papules, or pustules. The epidermis may be damaged to varying depths, with patients reporting discomfort, pain, burning, itching, or tingling (Beeckman et al., 2015; Francis, 2018; Jacobson & Wright, 2015). In addition to discomfort and pain, patients may experience loss of independence, alterations in activities and sleep, reduced quality of life, and secondary skin infections (bacterial and fungal) (Beeckman et al., 2015; Fisher, 2020; Voegeli, 2018).

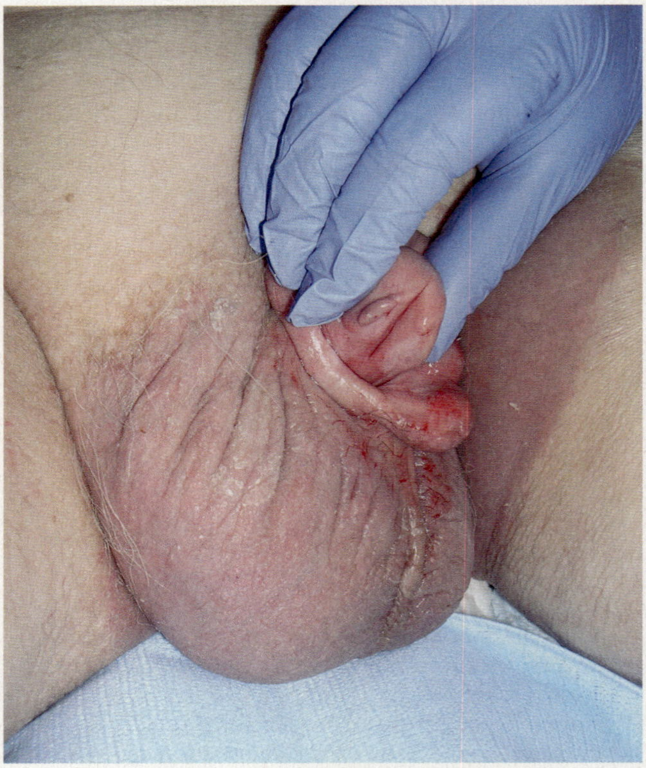

FIGURE 39-7. Incontinence-associated dermatitis (IAD). (*Source:* Wound, Ostomy and Continence Nurses Society®. *Core Curriculum: Continence Management*, 2nd ed.)

Skin care and use of nonocclusive absorbent products designed for incontinence to wick moisture away from the skin are critical pieces of evidence-based nursing care to prevent and treat IAD (Beeckman et al., 2015; Jacobson & Wright, 2015; Voegeli, 2018). Appropriate skin care involves a structured skin care regimen that includes regular skin assessment, skin cleansing, moisturizers or emollients to replenish and restore lipids in the skin, and the use of skin barrier protectants to proactively protect the skin from stool-associated irritation, maceration (overhydration), and breakdown (Southgate & Bradbury, 2016; Voegeli, 2018; Yates, 2018b).

Cleansing of the skin should be provided daily and after each episode of incontinence, using skin cleansers that are specially designed for at risk or compromised skin, are pH balanced and may be no-rinse (Beeckman et al., 2015; Southgate & Bradbury, 2016; Voegeli, 2018; Yates, 2018b). Avoid using soap and water as these can be irritating, drying, and alter the skin's pH, contributing to irritation (Yates, 2018b). Avoid excessive friction on the skin, such as through scrubbing, as this can damage the skin (Jacobson & Wright, 2015; Southgate & Bradbury, 2016). Limit the use of disposable briefs; incontinence products that wick moisture away from the skin may be used as necessary (Jacobson & Wright, 2015). A skin barrier/protectant should be applied to all skin that comes into contact or potentially comes into contact with stool after cleansing to prevent direct contact with stool and to promote resolution of IAD if present (Beeckman et al., 2015; Voegeli, 2018). Products are available that are "all-in-one," ensuring all steps of skin care are implemented and include a disposable soft cloth that contains cleanser, moisturizer, and barrier, for example (Francis, 2018). Patients with complicated IAD that does not respond to treatment with 2 weeks should be referred to an advanced practice wound specialist, such as a wound ostomy continence nurse or dermatologist (Francis, 2018).

Additional information and discussion related to incontinence and skin care can be found in Chapters 32 and 33.

INDWELLING RECTAL TUBE

A fecal management system (or bowel management systems with an indwelling rectal catheter) may be used for patients with uncontrollable diarrhea who are very ill, receiving palliative care at the end of life, or confined to bed (Palmer, 2019). A tube inserted into the rectum directs loose stool into a collection bag (Palmer, 2019). However, relatively little research supports the safety of these systems, and they should be used with caution (Whiteley & Sinclair, 2014). Disadvantages of indwelling rectal tubes include leakage and perirectal skin damage, injury to the rectal mucosa, and injury of the anal sphincter (Continence Product Advisor, 2021). The fecal incontinence device, discussed in the next section, may be a safer alternative.

EXTERNAL ANAL POUCH

Use of an external anal pouch provides the means to protect perianal skin from repeated episodes of fecal incontinence of very loose stool (Powers & Zimmaro Bliss, 2012). This pouch has a flexible wafer with an opening at its center. One side of the wafer adheres to the skin around the anus and the other side is connected to a collection bag (Palmer, 2019). The bag has a port to empty stool without removing the wafer from the skin and the port can be attached to gravity drainage, allowing liquid stool to accumulate in a collection bag (Palmer, 2019) (Fig. 39-8). It is best applied before the perianal area becomes excoriated. If excoriation is already present, application of a skin barrier prior to applying the pouch may be helpful. Disadvantages of these devices include the risk of skin damage from the adhesive on the perianal skin (Continence Product Advisor, 2021).

Nursing responsibilities include careful regular assessment and documentation of the perianal skin condition and attentive management of the drainage system. Change the pouch if it is not intact or leakage has occurred. Provide

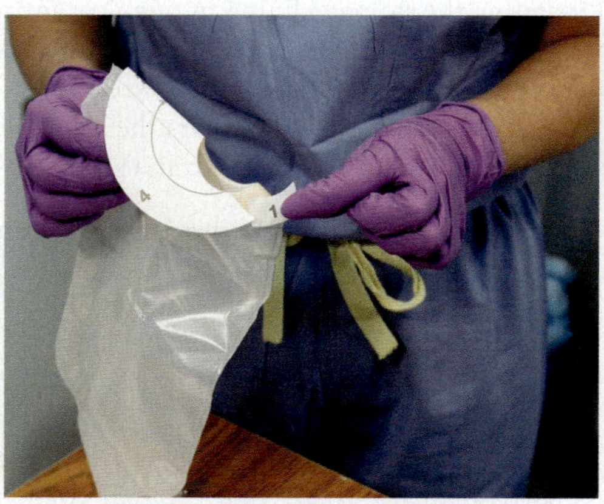

Removing paper backing from adhesive of rectal pouch.

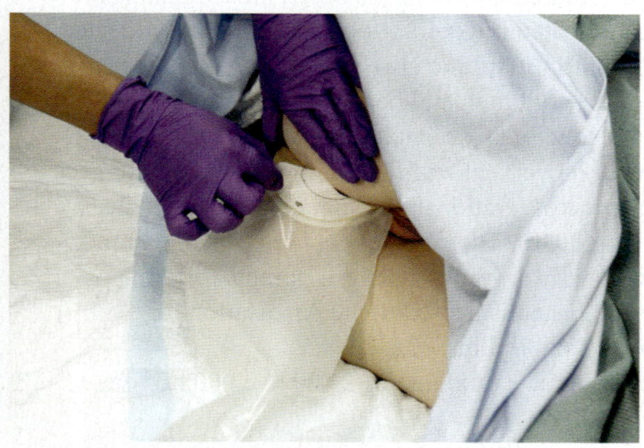

Applying pouch over anal opening.

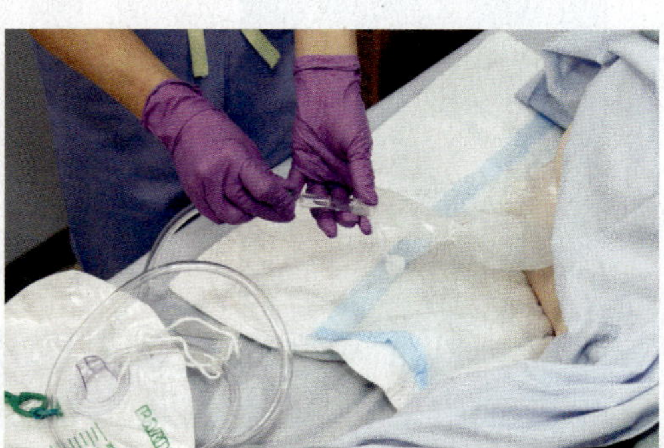

Attaching connector of fecal pouch to tubing of drainage bag.

FIGURE 39-8. Applying a fecal incontinence device.

explanations and support to the patient and family/caregivers so that they understand the use of this system.

Implementing Bowel-Training Programs

Patients with a history of chronic constipation and impaction and those who are incontinent of stool may benefit from a **bowel-training program**. The purpose of this program is to manipulate factors within the person's control (food and fluid intake, exercise, time for defecation) to produce the elimination of a soft, formed stool at regular intervals without a laxative. Kegel exercises (refer to p. 1465 in Chapter 38) and biofeedback may also be used to strengthen pelvic and rectal muscle tone (Phillips, 2020). This effort to regain bowel control may be initiated in the health care setting or the patient's home. When the patient has established a regular pattern of defecation, continue to offer assistance with toileting. A bowel-training program may include the following interventions:

- Plan bowel program with patient and appropriate family members/caregivers.
- Set a regular time for daily bowel movements that is convenient for the patient; consider timing of 20 to 40 minutes after a meal, as eating stimulates bowel activity (Phillips, 2020).
- Monitor bowel movements including frequency, consistency, shape, volume, and color, as appropriate.
- Some patients may benefit from stimulating bowel movements by using a suppository or small enema; drinking warm prune juice or fruit nectar may also be helpful (Phillips, 2020).
- Ensure privacy.
- Use digital stimulation to trigger a bowel movement: Insert a gloved, lubricated finger into the anus and make a circular motion until the sphincter relaxes. Try to contract the muscles of the abdomen and bear down; bending forward on the toilet may be helpful. If the patient does not have a bowel movement within 20 minutes, they should repeat the process (National Association for Continence, n.d.; Phillips, 2020). The patient should perform digital stimulation every day until a pattern of regular bowel movements is established (National Association for Continence, n.d.; Phillips, 2020).
- Encourage adequate fluid intake 2,000 to 3,000 mL/day (Phillips, 2020).
- Teach about foods that promote bowel regularity.

Maintaining a Nasogastric Tube

A **nasogastric (NG) tube** is a pliable single- or double-lumen (inner open space) plastic tube that is hollow, allowing for the removal of gastric secretions and instillation of solutions such as medications or feedings into the stomach. Use of NG tubes for nutritional support is discussed in Chapter 37. Instillation of medications using an NG tube is discussed in Chapter 30.

NG tubes may be inserted to decompress or drain the stomach of fluid or unwanted stomach contents such as poison or medication and air (Burns & Delgado, 2019), and may be used when conditions are present in which peristalsis is absent. Examples include paralytic ileus and intestinal obstruction by tumor or hernia, and adhesive small bowel obstruction (ten Broek et al., 2018). NG tubes may also be used to allow the GI tract to rest before or after abdominal surgery to promote healing (Bauldoff et al., 2020). Historically, an NG tube was often used postoperatively as a routine part of care after major abdominal surgery, to rest the intestinal tract and promote healing. Research now shows the routine use of NG tubes after abdominal surgery may serve no beneficial purpose and may actually delay the patient's progress, increasing the time required for flatus to occur and increasing pulmonary complications (Hodin & Bordeianou, 2020; Kantrancha & George, 2014; Sigmon & An, 2020; Venara et al., 2020). Decompression should be reserved for patients with conditions such as a prolonged postoperative ileus or a small bowel obstruction (Hodin & Bordeianou, 2020).

The NG tube is passed through the nasopharynx into the stomach. Tubes for decompression typically are attached to suction. Suction can be applied intermittently or continuously. When the underlying condition has been resolved and/or the NG tube is no longer indicated, the tube is removed. Skill 39-2 (on pp. 1560–1565) describes the procedure for NG tube insertion. Skill 39-3 (on pp. 1566–1568) outlines for the procedure for removal of an NG tube.

Double-lumen tubes are used for gastric decompression (Sigmon & An, 2020) (Fig. 39-9). One larger lumen empties the stomach via suction, and the other provides for a continuous flow of air (acting as a sump) (Sigmon & An, 2020). The airflow lumen controls suction by preventing the drainage lumen from pulling stomach mucosa into the tube's openings and irritating the stomach lining. A one-way antireflux valve may be used in the airflow lumen to prevent reflux of gastric contents through the airflow lumen (see Fig. 39-9). When pressure from gastric contents enters the airflow tubing, the valve closes to prevent secretions from exiting the tube.

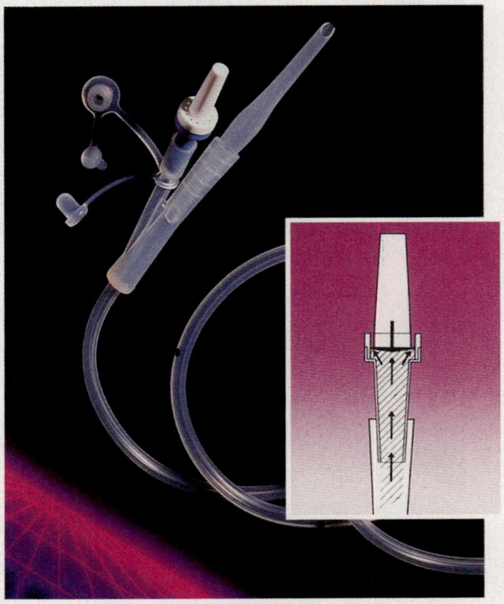

FIGURE 39-9. Double-lumen nasogastric tube. Insert on right shows close up of a one-way antireflux valve.

NG tubes used for decompression require irrigation with 30 to 60 mL of normal saline solution every 4 to 8 hours to maintain patency. Skill 38-4 (on pp. 1568–1572) describes the procedure for irrigating an NG tube connected to suction.

PROMOTING PATIENT SAFETY

Nasogastric tube placement must be verified before administration of any fluids or medications to promote patient safety (Judd, 2020). This decreases the risk that the tip of the tube is situated in the stomach or intestine, preventing inadvertent administration of substances into the wrong place. Radiographic examination, measurement of tube length, measurement of tube marking, measurement of aspirate pH, and monitoring of carbon dioxide have been suggested to confirm feeding tube placement. The use of two or more of these techniques in conjunction increases the likelihood of correct tube placement (AACN, 2020; Anderson, 2019; Anderson, 2018; Dias et al., 2019; Rahimi et al., 2015). Recommendations for use of visual inspection of gastric aspirate are conflicting; this method should be used cautiously if part of policy and procedure guidelines and with consideration to the potential for inaccuracy (AACN, 2020; Dias et al., 2019; Mak & Tam, 2020; Metheny et al., 2019). When bedside methods to check placement suggest the tube has been displaced, a radiograph should be requested to determine the tube's location (AACN, 2020). An old technique of auscultation of air injected into a feeding tube has been proved unreliable and should not be used (AACN, 2020; Anderson, 2018; Boeykens et al., 2014; Boullata et al., 2017; Irving et al., 2018; Metheny et al., 2019).

A detailed discussion of each of these methods to confirm placement is provided in Chapter 37. Radiographic examination (x-ray) to confirm placement is the standard method for checking if the NG tube is in the stomach, but often it is only ordered on initial placement, and many times is not prescribed for NG tubes inserted for decompression. Placement must be checked frequently while the tube is in place, and repeated, frequent radiographs are not practical (Boullata et al., 2017).

Another way to verify tube placement is to mark the tube with an indelible marker at the nostril and measure the length of the exposed tube after insertion. Document this measurement (AACN, 2020; Dias et al., 2019). Check and compare tube length with this initial measurement, in conjunction with the previous two methods for checking tube placement. Observe for a change in the external tube length at regular intervals and before use (AACN, 2020). Any change in the length of the exposed tube may indicate dislodgement (AACN, 2020; Boullata et al., 2017).

Testing of the pH of gastric secretions aspirated from the tube is recommended to verify gastric tube placement (AACN, 2020; Dias et al., 2019; Irving et al., 2018; Metheny et al., 2019). Guidelines for Nursing Care 37-1 outlines the procedure for assessing gastric aspirate pH.

Monitoring for carbon dioxide to determine NG tube position and/or dislodgement has been evaluated (Hess et al., 2021). This involves the use of a colorimetric end-tidal CO_2 detector to detect the presence of carbon dioxide, which would indicate tube positioning in the patient's airway (Hess et al., 2021). However, a carbon dioxide sensor cannot determine where an NG tube's tip ends in the GI tract (esophagus, stomach, or small bowel) (Hodin & Bordeianou, 2020).

Refer to Chapter 37, pages 1417–1421, for a detailed discussion of each of these methods to confirm placement.

PROVIDING COMFORT MEASURES

Patients with NG tubes often experience discomfort related to irritation to nasal and throat mucosa and drying of the oral mucous membranes. Administer oral hygiene frequently, as often as every 2 to 4 hours, to prevent drying of tissues and to relieve thirst. Frequently offer the patient the opportunity to rinse the mouth with warm water and mouthwash solution. Lubricate the lips generously. Keep the nares clean, especially around the tube, where secretions tend to accumulate. Use a lubricant after cleaning the nares. Help control local irritation from the tube in the throat by offering analgesic throat lozenges or anesthetic sprays, as prescribed. Ensure that the tube is secured to patient's nose and cheek, based on facility policy, to prevent tension and tugging on the tube, causing trauma to the nares, and potential inadvertent displacement or dislodgement (Morton & Fontaine, 2018). Displacement or dislodgement of a tube can lead to aspiration, pneumonia, and sepsis (Powers, 2019). Use of a commercial securement device is recommended (Schroeder & Sitzer, 2019). Refer to Box 37-8 in Chapter 37 (p. 1424) for methods to secure an NGT.

Meeting the Needs of Patients With Bowel Diversions

Patients sometimes undergo surgical procedures to create an opening into the abdominal wall for fecal elimination. The word **ostomy** is a term for a surgically formed opening in an organ of the body. In the case of the GI tract, the intestinal mucosa is brought out to the abdominal wall, and a **stoma**, the part of the ostomy that is attached to the skin, is formed by suturing the mucosa to the skin. An **ileostomy** allows liquid fecal content from the ileum of the small intestine to be eliminated through the stoma. A **colostomy** permits formed feces in the colon to exit through the stoma. Colostomies are further classified by the part of the colon from which they originate. Figure 39-10 shows the location of an ileostomy and various colostomies. In many institutions, if the ostomy surgery is not emergent, patients meet with a specially trained registered nurse called a wound, ostomy, and continence nurse (WOCN). Together, they determine the ideal location for the stoma. Stoma site marking is also completed by colorectal surgeons and other clinicians to select an effective stoma site (Salvadalena et al., 2015). Preoperative stoma site marking is associated with reduced occurrence of stoma and perisomal complications and should be considered part of preoperative care (Hsu et al., 2020; Roveron et al., 2016; Salvadalena et al., 2015).

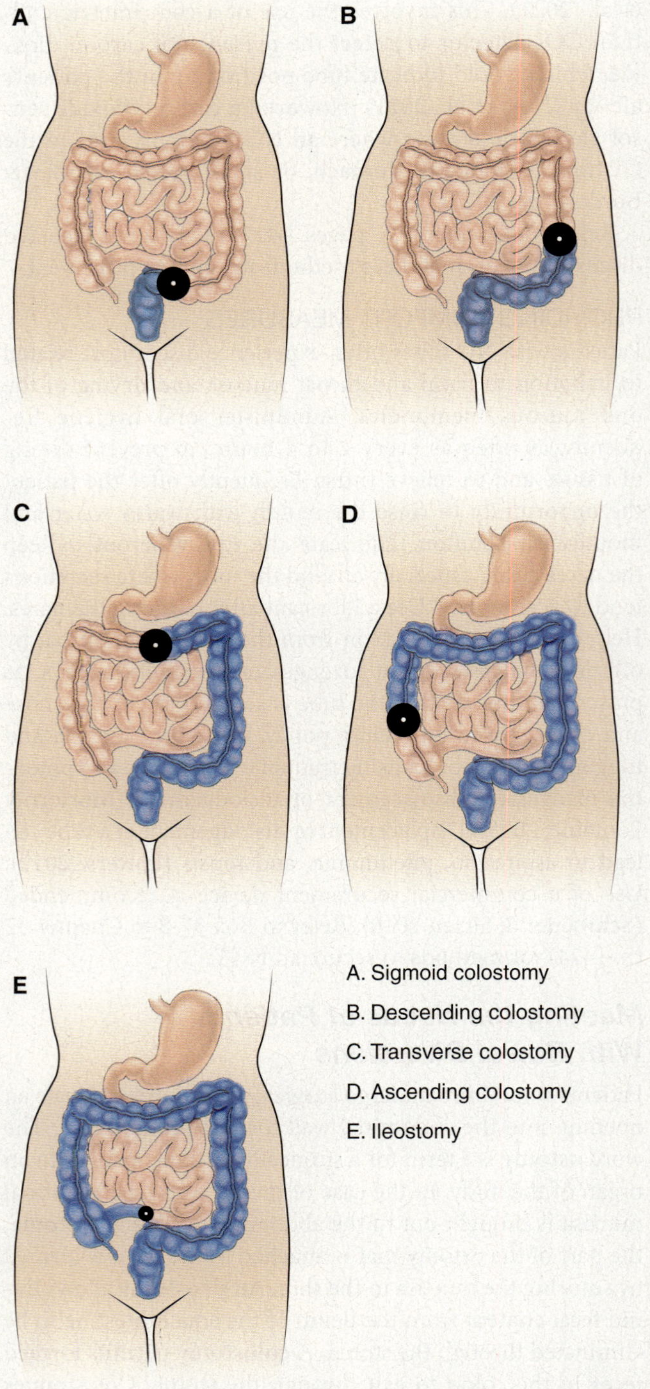

FIGURE 39-10. **A–E.** Location of various colostomies, and location of an ileostomy. The shaded portions represent the sections of the bowel that have been removed or are currently inactive.

An ileostomy or colostomy may be either temporary or permanent. Temporary ostomies are performed to allow the intestine to repair itself after inflammatory disease, some types of intestinal surgery, or injury. The patient returns for a second surgery in several weeks, and the intestine is reconnected. Permanent ostomies are performed for debilitating intestinal diseases or cancer of the colon or rectum. Patients will have these ostomies for the rest of their lives.

A surgical intervention that does not involve an external stoma is the restorative proctocolectomy ileal pouch–anal

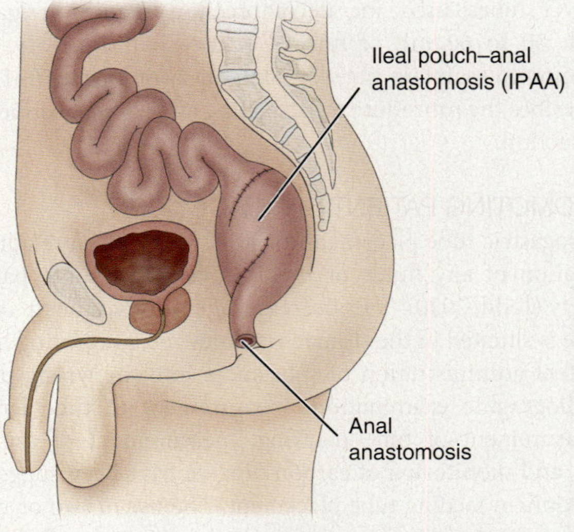

FIGURE 39-11. Ileal pouch–anal anastomosis (IPAA).

anastomosis (IPAA), also called a J pouch or an ileoanal anastomosis. This procedure is an option for use in those patients with inflammatory bowel disease, particularly ulcerative colitis, and patients with hereditary nonpolyposis colorectal cancer and familial adenomatous polyposis (Fichera, 2021). IPAA involves removal of the colon and rectum but leaves the anus sphincter intact. The small intestine is sutured directly to the anus, a colon-like pouch or reservoir is created from the last several inches of the small intestine, and the patient is able to control expulsion of feces through the intact internal and external anal sphincter (Fig. 39-11). The patient often receives a temporary ileostomy, and an adjustment period lasting several months is needed for the newly formed ileoanal reservoir to stretch and adjust to its new function (NIDDK, 2014).

COLOSTOMY AND ILEOSTOMY CARE

The patient with an ostomy needs physical and psychological support both preoperatively and postoperatively (Wasserman & McGee, 2017). Support can come from the patient's family/caregivers, members of the health care team, and from people who have had similar experiences. Evidence shows patients who receive consultation preoperatively and care postoperatively from an enterostomal therapy nurse or a WOCN experience better long-term outcomes (Salvadalena et al., 2015). The following guidelines help to promote the ostomy patient's physical and psychological comfort:

- Keep the patient as free of odors as possible. Empty an ostomy appliance before it is half-full to reduce the risk of separation from the skin and leakage (Blevins, 2019; WOCN, 2018).
- Inspect the patient's stoma regularly. Note the size of the stoma, which usually stabilizes within 6 to 8 weeks (Stelton, 2019). It should ideally protrude about 1 to 3 cm above skin level and be dark pink to red in color and moist (Stelton, 2019) (Fig. 39-12). A pale stoma may indicate anemia (Fig. 39-13A), and a dark or purple-blue stoma may reflect compromised circulation or ischemia and may initially appear swollen and edematous. After 6 weeks, the edema has usually subsided. Bleeding around

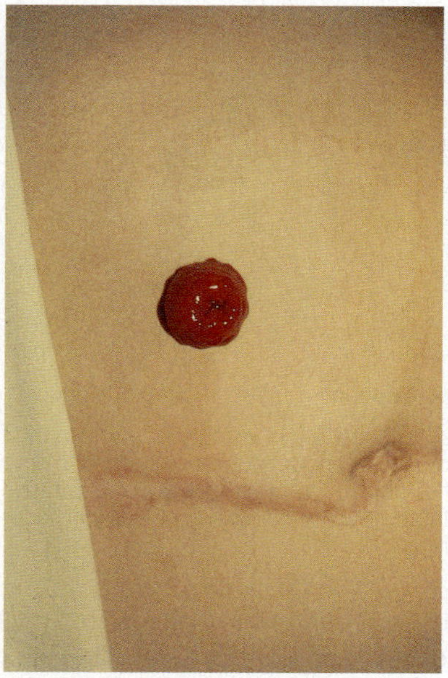

FIGURE 39-12. Stoma should be dark pink to red and moist. (*Source:* Reprinted with permission from Hill, R., Hall, H., & Glew, P. [2022]. *Fundamentals of nursing and midwifery* [4th ed.]. Wolters Kluwer; Fig. 44-33.)

the stoma and its stem should be minimal. The edges of the stoma should appear secure to the surrounding skin (Stelton, 2019). The pulling away of the stoma from the peristomal skin is called mucocutaneous separation or stoma dehiscence (Stelton, 2019) and occurs more often in patients who are at risk for impaired healing, including patients with diabetes, poor nutritional status or who received high-dose steroid therapy or chemotherapy before surgery (Butler, 2009). Notify the health care team promptly if bleeding persists or is excessive, or if color changes occur in the stoma or if it appears the stoma is separating from the peristomal skin (Stelton, 2019).

- Depending on the surgical technique, the final stoma may be flush with the skin. Erosion of skin around the stoma area can also lead to a flush stoma (Fig. 39-13B). If an abdominal dressing is in place at the surgical incision, check it frequently for drainage and bleeding. The dressing is usually removed after 24 hours.
- Keep the skin around the stoma site (peristomal area) clean and dry. If care is not taken to protect the skin around the stoma, irritation or infection may occur. Assess the peristomal (around the stoma) skin; peristomal skin should be intact and appear consistent with that of the rest of the abdomen, without pain or discomfort (Burch, 2018). In patients with light skin tones, the peristomal skin should not be reddened; in patients with darker skin tones, the skin should not have darker discolorations (Stelton, 2019). A leaking or ill-fitted stoma appliance will cause moisture-associated skin damage (Berti-Hearn & Elliott, 2019) (refer to the discussion earlier in the chapter). Candida or yeast infections can also occur around the stoma if the area is not kept dry.
- Measure the patient's fluid intake and output. Check the ostomy appliance for the quality and quantity of discharge. Initially after surgery, peristalsis may be inhibited. As peristalsis returns, stool will be eliminated from the stoma.
- Explain each aspect of care to the patient and explain what the patient's role will be when beginning self-care. Patient teaching is one of the most important aspects of colostomy and ileostomy care and should include family members, caregivers and/or people identified by the patient to include in care, when appropriate. Teaching can begin before surgery so that the patient has adequate time to absorb information.
- Encourage the patient to participate in care and to look at the ostomy. Patients normally experience emotional depression during the early postoperative period. Help the patient cope by listening, explaining, and being available and supportive. A visit from a representative of the local ostomy support group may be helpful. Patients usually begin to accept their altered body image when they are willing to look at the stoma, make neutral or positive statements concerning the ostomy, and express interest in learning self-care.

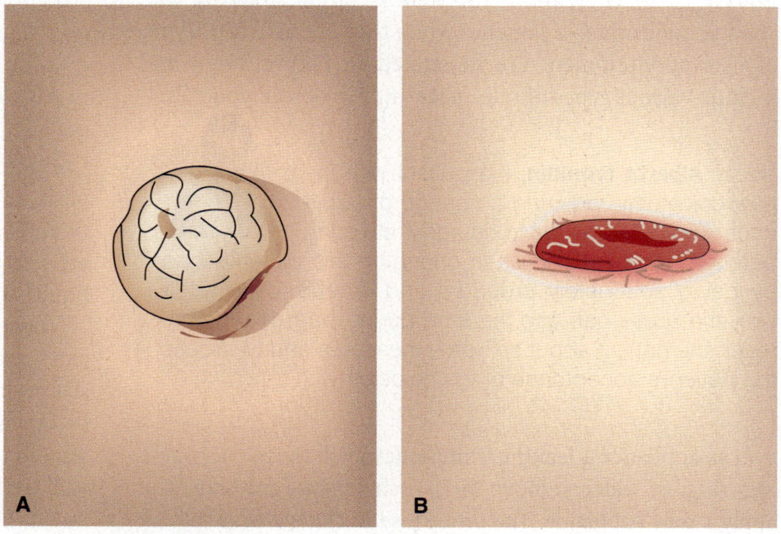

FIGURE 39-13. A. A pale stoma may indicate anemia. **B.** Eroded skin around the area may lead to a flush stoma.

- Provide support for the patient's physical, psychological, and social activities. Coping strategies need to address body image concerns, permanent body changes, and underlying health issue(s) that resulted in the surgery (Berti-Hearn & Elliott, 2019; Díaz et al., 2018).
- Encourage patients and their partner/family/caregiver to discuss concerns and to seek help and support (Berti-Hearn & Elliott, 2019; Chandler, 2020; Hill, 2020).

QSEN INFORMATICS AND PATIENT-CENTERED CARE

Nurses must continually evaluate sources of information to ensure health care decisions based on high-quality resources. Provision of individualized teaching plans that assist patients to select and evaluate appropriate technology and information resources related to bowel elimination support achievement of optimal health care outcomes.

Changing the Ostomy Appliance

The ostomy appliance should protect the skin, collect the fecal discharge, and control odor. Typically, a colostomy does not produce drainage until normal peristalsis returns, usually within 2 to 5 days. An ileostomy drains within 24 to 48 hours because of the liquid contents in the small intestine.

Appliances are either one-piece (barrier backing already attached to the pouch) or two-piece (separate pouch that fastens to the barrier backing). A transparent one-piece appliance is used in the initial postoperative period to allow for visualization of the stoma. For the first few days after surgery, most patients wear an open-ended appliance that allows for drainage of fecal material without removing the appliance. The barrier backing has an adhesive barrier that protects the surrounding skin from the stoma output. Appliances can be either drainable or closed. How frequently a drainable appliance should be changed depends on the type being used and specific patient circumstances, but usually every 3 to 7 days (American Cancer Society, 2019; Berti-Hearn & Elliott, 2019; O'Flynn, 2018; Stelton, 2019). Remove and change nondrainable pouches when they are half-full. Types of ostomy equipment are illustrated in Figure 39-14 and include various types of one-piece and two-piece pouches.

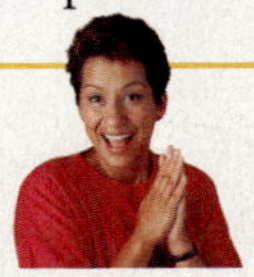

Recall **Alberta Franklin**, the patient with the new colostomy requiring a change of appliance. The nurse needs to demonstrate competence and dexterity when changing this patient's bag by being adequately prepared and organized. In addition, the nurse can use the time during bag changes to teach the patient about self-care measures and to assess the patient's acceptance of the colostomy.

If an appliance is leaking from underneath the barrier backing, ring, or wafer, remove the pouch, cleanse the skin, and apply a new appliance. The procedure to change or empty an ostomy appliance is outlined in Skill 39-5 (on pp. 1572–1577). The act of removing an appliance from the skin can result in mechanical damage to the skin or skin stripping, abrasions, or injury cause by the removal of the outer, loosely bound, epidermal cell layers (peristomal medical adhesive–related skin injury (PMARSI) (Berti-Hearn & Elliott, 2019; Burch, 2019a; LeBlanc et al., 2019). This can be uncomfortable or even very painful for the patient. The cumulative effects of skin stripping over time can result in peristomal skin breakdown. The use of a silicone-based adhesive remover allows for the easy, rapid, and painless removal of a stoma pouch without the associated problems of PMARSI (Berti-Hearn & Elliott, 2019; Chandler, 2015; LeBlanc et al., 2019; Stelton, 2019). A skin barrier film or sealant may be used to protect the skin under the skin wafer or barrier (Goldberg et al., 2018; Landmann & Cashman, 2020; WOCN, 2018).

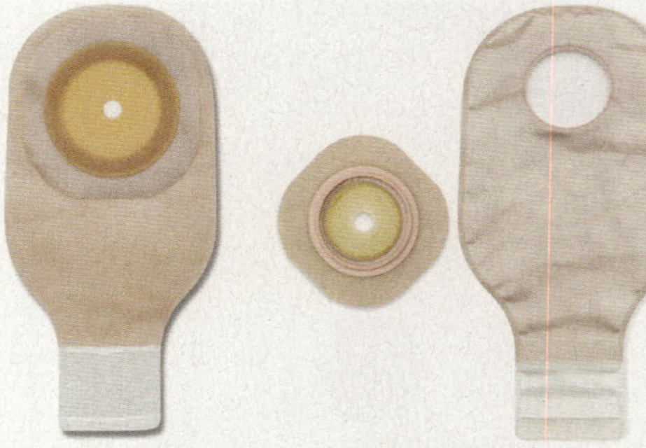

FIGURE 39-14. Examples of ostomy pouches and closures. This equipment comes in various models and sizes. Convex pouches, belts, and other devices to prevent leaks and irritation (not shown) are also available. (*Source:* Courtesy of Hollister Incorporated, Libertyville, Illinois.)

Irrigating a Colostomy

Colostomy irrigation is a way of achieving fecal continence and control (Kent et al., 2015). Irrigations are used to stimulate the colon to empty to promote regular evacuation of stool (up to 24 to 48 hours) from distal colostomies, resulting in reduction or elimination of the need for the patient to use a pouch to collect stool (Cleveland Clinic, 2016; Kent et al., 2015). Colostomy irrigation may be indicated in patients who have a left-sided end colostomy in the descending or sigmoid colon, are mentally alert, have adequate vision, and have adequate manual dexterity needed to perform the procedure (Goldberg et al., 2018; Kent et al., 2015). Contraindications include irritable bowel syndrome (IBS), peristomal hernia, postradiation damage to the bowel, diverticulitis, and Crohn disease (Kent et al., 2015). Ileostomies are not irrigated because the fecal content of the ileum is liquid and cannot be controlled.

Water is inserted into the colostomy, and the water and feces are expelled from the colostomy into the irrigation sleeve and then the toilet. The patient establishes a routine by repeating this process regularly, once a day or once every second day, the colon can be trained to empty with minimal spillage of stool in between irrigations (Cleveland Clinic, 2016). Once the patient has established bowel continence, a small appliance can be worn over the stoma. These "stoma caps" are small-capacity coverings with a pad to soak up discharge and a flatus filter (Kent et al., 2015; Palmer, 2020). If a colostomy irrigation is to be implemented, consult facility policy regarding the accepted procedure and, ideally, consult the WOCN for patient education and support.

Patient Education

The patient can return to an active and full life with an ostomy and may have an improved quality of life as the symptoms of the conditions requiring the ostomy are often eliminated. Make the patient aware of community resources available for assistance, such as home health care nurses, special clinics, wound ostomy and continence nurses, and ostomy support groups. Encourage the patient to seek follow-up health care on a regular basis.

Patient education is essential for independence in self-care. As the patient assumes responsibility for self-care, teach the patient how to make the necessary observations, to be aware of indications of problems, and to recognize when to seek assistance. For these goals to be met, the patient and/or family member/caregiver needs to be able to do the following:

- Explain the reason for bowel diversion and the rationale for treatment.
- Demonstrate self-care behaviors that effectively manage the ostomy.
- Describe follow-up care and existing support resources.
- Report where supplies may be obtained in the community.
- Verbalize related fears and concerns.
- Demonstrate a positive body image.

During the first 6 to 8 weeks after surgery, encourage the patient with an ostomy to consume low-fiber foods, avoiding foods high in fiber to reduce stool output (Palmer, 2020). Urge patients to drink at least 2.5 quarts of fluids, preferably water, daily. Ileostomy output is high in potassium and sodium, so if the patient is experiencing increased output, it is very important that electrolytes are monitored closely.

Patients with ileostomies also need to be aware they may experience a tendency to develop food blockages, especially when high-fiber foods are consumed. This is because scar tissue from the place where the intestine passes through the abdominal muscle tightens the inside diameter of the ileum and can narrow it to much less than its normal diameter. Fiber blockages can cause cessation of gas and/or bowel movements, watery stools with bad odor, abdominal cramping and pain, and distention, along with nausea and vomiting (Burgess-Stocks, 2020; Memorial Sloan Kettering Cancer Center, 2019). Foods that commonly cause blockage to occur include nuts, corn, popcorn, coconuts, mushrooms, stringy vegetables, and foods with skins and casings (Landmann & Cashman, 2020; Memorial Sloan Kettering Cancer Center, 2019).

Additional dietary considerations for patients with an ileostomy or colostomy are outlined in Box 39-3.

Health teaching about medication use is an important intervention for patients with ostomies. The transit time for substances to move through the intestine might change and could affect the absorption of medications (Burgess-Stocks, 2020). Some medications may discolor the stool and cause unusual odors, some may cause constipation, and some may not dissolve or be absorbed completely because the small bowel is where most absorption occurs. Tablets, capsules, or particles of medication found in the appliance pouch when the patient empties it indicate the patient might not be getting the full dose of medication (Burgess-Stocks, 2020). Reinforce with the patient the importance of contacting the health care team if this occurs (Burgess-Stocks, 2020). Long-acting, enteric-coated, or sustained-release medications are designed to be released in the colon. These extended-release medications should be avoided in patients without a colon, and the use of liquid, chewable, or uncoated tablets or injectable forms of

Box 39-3 Dietary Considerations for Patients With an Ileostomy or Colostomy

Foods That May Cause Gas and/or Produce Odor

Apples
Asparagus
Beer
Cucumbers
Dairy products
Dried peas, beans, and lentils
Eggs
Fatty foods
Fish
Garlic
Melons
Nuts
Onions
Pickles
Radish
Vegetables from the cabbage family.
The carbohydrate raffinose in these foods is poorly digested and leads to gas.
This includes foods such as broccoli, Brussels sprouts, cabbage, cauliflower, and turnips.

Foods That May Cause Stomal Blockage

Bean sprouts
Cabbage
Celery
Coconut
Corn
Dried fruit
Mushrooms
Nuts
Peas
Pineapple
Popcorn
Seeds
Skins from fruits and vegetables

Foods That May Help to Thicken Stool

Applesauce
Bananas
Cheese
Creamy peanut butter
Pasta
Potatoes
Rice
Tapioca
Yogurt

Foods That May Decrease Odor

Buttermilk
Kefir
Parsley
Yogurt

Source: Burgess-Stocks, J. (2020). *Eating with an ostomy A comprehensive nutrition guide for those living with an ostomy.* United Ostomy Associations of America. https://www.ostomy.org/wp-content/uploads/2020/07/Eating_with_an_Ostomy_2020-07.pdf

Research in Nursing

BRIDGING THE GAP TO EVIDENCE-BASED PRACTICE

Living with an Ostomy

A stoma operation causes major changes in a patient's life because of the resulting physical damage, disfigurement, loss of bodily function, and change in personal hygiene. Such changes are a cause of major concern for patients and raise important issues for the provision of quality care. Individuals participating in support groups benefit from the social support and information obtained from the group interaction (MFMER, 2020e; MFMER, 2020f). How do support groups impact the life of a person with a stoma?

Related Research

Byfield, D. (2020). The lived experiences of persons with ostomies attending a support group. A qualitative study. *Journal of Wound, Ostomy & Continence Nursing, 47*(5), 489–495. https://doi.org/10.1097/WON.0000000000000696

This study explored how a support groups affect coping and adaptation in those with an ostomy. The purpose of the study was to describe the lived experiences of patients with ostomies participating in a support group. Fifteen adults with different types of ostomies attending an ostomy support group responded to the invitation to participate in the study; data saturation was reached with the final sample of 10 participants. Individual semistructured interviews were conducted by the principal investigator in the classroom where the monthly support group meetings were held. The main open-ended interview question asked participants, "What is your experience of participating in a support group for patients with an ostomy in Georgia?", followed by additional supporting questions. Interviews were recorded, and handwritten field notes were completed that included nonverbal moments, body movements, and facial expressions. Interview recordings were transcribed verbatim. Thematic analysis was performed, and member checking occurred, with individual participants reviewing notes corresponding to their interview. Double coding of the transcripts was done by an independent researcher. Four themes and 10 subthemes emerged regarding the lived experiences of individuals attending an ostomy support group:

Theme 1: support group gives hope and changes lives, with two subthemes of increased knowledge and provided new knowledge and allows open communication.

Theme 2: changes in body image, with two subthemes of some things are different and everyone is the same.

Theme 3: I am not alone, with four subthemes of feeling of belonging, willingness to be helped, being supported, and developing lifelong relationships.

Theme 4: being independent, with two subthemes of confidence in rejoining society and building confidence and decreased shame.

The researchers concluded that participation in an ostomy support group allowed individuals with ostomies to function at more advance levels than they were before participating in the support group. The lived experiences were characterized by hope, willingness to live fully again, participating in different activities, and making new friends. The researchers suggested these findings add to and support the body of knowledge related to the interactions between nurses and individuals with ostomies as well as the care needed to ensure a safe discharge from the acute care facility and may help in the improvement of education provided during hospitalization. Providing this information will equip patients and families with a better understanding of and methods to care for their new ostomies and adjust to their new health status.

Relevance to Nursing Practice

Patients experiencing life-altering surgeries resulting in a stoma require both knowledge and support to adapt and achieve an improved quality of life after surgery. Nurses have a unique opportunity to not only provide the education and support to these patients but to their social support systems as well. This study supports the nurse's role in not only providing hands-on ostomy care but also in helping the patient developing social support systems either through friends, families/caregivers, or outside resources such as a support group or engaging with others who have a colostomy. In addition to assisting patients to learn the physical care needs related to a stoma, nurses must address the psychosocial concerns of patients with ostomies as part of their nursing interventions. Assisting patients to adjust and encouraging social interactions should be part of the care routinely given to stoma patients.

medication may be needed (Burgess-Stocks, 2020). Laxatives and enemas should not be used in patients with an ileostomy or transverse colostomy, as use can cause severe fluid and electrolyte imbalance or severe dehydration (Burgess-Stocks, 2020). Laxatives may sometimes be used by patients with a colostomy who experience constipation, but patients should only do so under the guidance of their health care provider, as effects will vary depending on the type of surgery the patient had (Burgess-Stocks, 2020). The preferred treatment for constipation is an increase in fluid intake and/or dietary fiber as opposed to using laxatives (Palmer, 2020).

Many times, patients are embarrassed when they have to use public restrooms to empty their bag. Teach patients with ostomies about the various methods of odor control. Remind them that if the bag is clean and sealed well, odor usually is not a problem during normal activity. Consuming probiotics, such as yogurt, aids in digestion and can help control odor (Burgess-Stocks, 2020). There are odor eliminators that contain chlorophyll that may be taken orally; reinforce the need for the patient to consult with their healthcare provider prior to use and warn the patient these products may turn the stool green and interfere with absorption of medication (Burgess-Stocks, 2020).

There is some evidence that bismuth subsalicylate can also assist in reducing odors in patients if use is not contraindicated. Use of bismuth can turn the stool black and may also interfere with absorption of medication (Burgess-Stocks, 2020). Patients should consult with their healthcare provider before taking bismuth (Burgess-Stocks, 2020). Commercial odor-control products also are available for purchase. The WOCN can help with the selection of odor-control strategies.

The patient with an ostomy can resume normal activity after healing is completed and their strength returns, including work, swimming, and sexual relations (MFMER, 2020e; Palmer, 2020). However, the patient may need to restrict strenuous activities, such as heavy lifting, during the first 2 to 3 weeks after surgery to avoid increasing the risk of a stoma hernia (MFMER, 2020e; NIDDK, 2014). Physical contact sports such as football or karate and should be avoided (NIDDK, 2014). Patients with an ostomy should talk with their health care provider about timing for resuming their normal activities and possible need for stoma protection devices when participating in sports/activities (Goldberg et al., 2018; MFMER, 2020e; NIDDK, 2014). When traveling, the patient should carry a 1- to 2-day supply of equipment in a carry-on bag in case checked luggage is lost. Nurses play a significant role in providing physical, emotional, and psychological support to help patients, their families, and caregivers others adjust to this major life change. The Research in Nursing display provides insight into the lived experiences of patients with ostomies.

Evaluating

Evaluation is an ongoing and deliberate part of the nursing process, comparing the patient's health status with previously defined expected outcomes. The nurse reflects on the effectiveness of the plan of care to promote healthy bowel functioning by evaluating whether the patient has met the individualized patient goals specified in the plan. Adjustments in the plan of care are made accordingly. Nursing care is considered effective if the patient expresses satisfaction with the bowel elimination measures and is able to (as appropriate, based on specific behaviors and criteria individualized for the patient situation):

- Verbalize the relationships among bowel elimination and nutrition, fluid intake, exercise, and stress management.
- Develop a plan to modify any factors that contribute to current bowel problems or that might adversely affect bowel functioning in the future.
- Promote bowel functioning as appropriate for the person.
- Provide care for bowel diversion and know when to notify the health care team.
- See the accompanying Nursing Care Plan 39-1 for Jeremy Green.

REFLECTIVE PRACTICE LEADING TO PERSONAL LEARNING

Remember that the goal of reflective practice is to look at an experience, understand it, and learn from it. As you begin to develop expertise in implementing measures related to bowel elimination, reflect on your experiences—successes and failures—in order to improve your practice. How can you do it better next time? What did you learn today that can help you tomorrow? Begin your reflection by paying close attention to the following while performing interventions and providing nursing care related to bowel elimination:

- Did your preparation and practice related to performing assessment related to bowel elimination result in your feeling confident in your ability to gather reliable, accurate, and complete data? Did your competence and confidence inspire the patient's and the family/caregiver's trust?
- How did you prioritize the data you collected? What patterns in the data did you identify? What knowledge from your learning, personal experience and intuition did you use to make decisions and develop your plan of care?
- Did your commitment to engage your patients and families/caregivers and to collaborate with your fellow students, instructor, and other members of the health care team as you implemented the care plan result in successful partnerships?
- Were you aware of any cultural and/or ethnic beliefs or practices that may have influenced the patient's personal bowel elimination practices? Were you aware of any stereotypes or prejudices that might have negatively influenced the clinical encounter? If so, how did you address these?
- Was patient/family/caregiver participation in the process at an optimal level? How might you have better engaged the patient and family/caregivers? Did the care plan accurately reflect patient priorities and preferences?
- Did you need to modify the care plan as a result of ongoing assessments? Did you think of better interventions to produce the expected outcomes?

Perhaps the most important questions to reflect on are: Are your patients and their families/caregivers better for having had *you* share in the critical responsibility of partnering with them to address their bowel elimination needs? Are your patients now receiving thoughtful, person-centered, prioritized, holistic, evidence-based treatment and care because of your efforts?

Nursing Care Plan for *Jeremy Green* 39-1

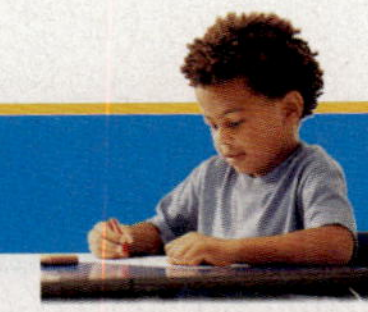

Jeremy Green, age 4 years, was placed in day care when their mother returned to work 6 months ago. Jeremy presents at the hospital with a diagnosis of viral gastroenteritis. A comprehensive nursing assessment included the following notations:

- Admitted with report of diarrhea beginning 3 days ago.
- Seen today by pediatrician, who recommended admission and workup to exclude causes other than viral.
- Mother reports liquid stools (no observable blood, pus, or mucus) six to seven times daily beginning 3 days ago with amounts of "one to two cups."
- Urgency results in soiling of pants.
- Child has sipped boiled skim milk and cola and eaten a small amount of broth and a few pretzels but has no appetite.
- Reports nausea and vomited twice 3 days ago.
- Child is pale and eyes are sunken.
- Skin is warm and dry, with decreased turgor and dry mucous membranes.
- Hyperactive bowel sounds (52/min)
- Height, 45 inches; weight, 36 lb; temperature, 99.8°F (rectally); pulse, 88 beats/min; respiratory rate, 18 breaths/min
- Mother reported several other children in same day care center are out sick with diarrhea.

ACTUAL OR POTENTIAL HEALTH PROBLEMS AND NEED

Diarrhea

Etiology: unknown cause (possibly viral, rule out malabsorption of lactose and other causes)

Signs and Symptoms: passage of liquid stools (1 to 2 cups) for 3 days; urgency with fecal soiling, decreased appetite, transient nausea and vomiting.

EXPECTED OUTCOME

By 5/5/25 the patient will:

- Demonstrate improved fluid and electrolyte balance by maintenance of present weight (36 lb), presence of moist mucous membranes, positive skin turgor, pulse and respiratory rate within normal limits, urine output equal to fluid intake.

EXPECTED OUTCOME

At the time of discharge, the patient will:

- Voluntarily pass a formed stool of usual consistency (experience less or no diarrhea)

NURSING INTERVENTIONS	RATIONALE	EVALUATIVE STATEMENT
Assess and chart frequency and amount of diarrhea, stool characteristics, precipitating factors, and accompanying manifestations (GI symptoms, hyperactive bowel sounds).	This assists in identifying the cause of the diarrhea.	5/8/25 Outcome partially met. No recurrence of liquid stools for 24 hours. Revision: Continue to monitor for return of usual stool *D. Lentsky, RN*

EXPECTED OUTCOME

At the time of discharge, the patient will:

- Exhibit normoactive bowel sounds (occurring every 5 to 15 seconds)

NURSING INTERVENTIONS	RATIONALE	EVALUATIVE STATEMENT
Work collaboratively with the health care provider to identify the cause of the diarrhea. Obtain stool specimens and send to laboratory.	Correct treatment depends on identification of the cause of the diarrhea. Viral diarrhea is usually self-limiting and lasts 24 to 72 hours. Prolonged diarrhea after acute viral illness may be from temporary malabsorption of lactose or other simple sugars.	5/8/25 Bowel sounds are normoactive. *D. Lentsky, RN*

Nursing Care Plan for *Jeremy Green* 39-1 *(continued)*

NURSING INTERVENTIONS	RATIONALE	EVALUATIVE STATEMENT
Instruct Jeremy and their parents (if they want to participate in care) on correct infection control precautions for handling stool.	Proper precautions prevent transmissions of infectious diarrhea to others.	
Increase the frequency and length of rest periods and discourage strenuous activity.	Exercise and activity stimulate peristalsis.	
Assess for the ability to take sips of water and tolerate small servings of food without vomiting or increasing diarrhea.	Antidiarrheal medications are generally not indicated in the care of children with viral gastroenteritis. Therefore, care is symptomatic. The ability to drink sips of water aids in decreasing the risk of dehydration, and if tolerated demonstrates the resolving of the symptoms of the viral gastroenteritis.	

SAMPLE DOCUMENTATION

5/7/25 Nursing

Liquid stools have decreased to two in the past 24 hours. Negative report on stool culture; Dr. Simpson notified of results. Patient denies pain, nausea, and cramping. Patient is playing with toys in bed. Normoactive bowel sounds auscultated in four quadrants.

D. Lentsky, RN

Skill 39-1 Administering a Large-Volume Cleansing Enema

DELEGATION CONSIDERATIONS

The administration of some types of enemas may be delegated to assistive personnel (AP) who have received appropriate training. The administration of a large-volume cleansing enema may be delegated to licensed practical/vocational nurses (LPN/LVNs). The decision to delegate must be based on careful analysis of the patient's needs and circumstances as well as the qualifications of the person to whom the task is being delegated. Refer to the Delegation Guidelines in Appendix A.

EQUIPMENT

- Enema solution as prescribed at or just above body temperature (Dougherty & Lister, 2015, as cited in Mitchell, 2019b, p. 155) in the prescribed amount (amount will vary depending on the type of solution, patient's age, and patient's ability to retain the solution; average cleansing enema for an adult may range from 500 to 1,000 mL)
- Disposable enema set, which includes a solution container and tubing
- Water-soluble lubricant
- IV pole
- Necessary additives, as prescribed
- Waterproof pad
- Bath thermometer (if available)
- Bath blanket
- Bedpan or commode and toilet tissue
- Disposable gloves
- Additional PPE, as indicated
- Paper towel
- Washcloth, skin cleanser, and towel

(continued on page 1556)

Skill 39-1 Administering a Large-Volume Cleansing Enema *(continued)*

IMPLEMENTATION

ACTION	RATIONALE
1. Review the patient's health record for any limitations in physical activity. Verify the prescribed intervention for the enema. Gather equipment.	Physical limitations may require adaptations in performing the skill. Verifying the prescribed intervention ensures that the correct intervention is administered to the right patient. Assembling equipment provides for an organized approach to the task.
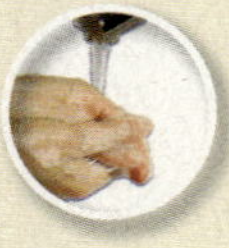 2. Perform hand hygiene and put on PPE, if indicated.	Hand hygiene and PPE prevent the spread of microorganisms. PPE is required based on transmission precautions.
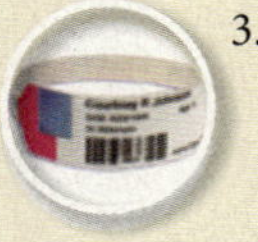 3. Identify the patient.	Identifying the patient ensures the right patient receives the intervention and helps prevent errors.
4. Explain the procedure to the patient and provide the rationale as to why the enema is needed. Discuss the associated discomforts that may be experienced and possible interventions that may allay this discomfort. Answer any questions, as needed.	Explanation facilitates patient engagement and reduces anxiety.
5. Assemble equipment on the overbed table or other surface within reach.	Arranging items nearby is convenient, saves time, and avoids unnecessary stretching and twisting of muscles on the part of the nurse.
6. Close the curtains around the bed and close the door to the room, if possible. Discuss where the patient will defecate. Have a bedpan, commode, or nearby bathroom ready for use.	This ensures the patient's privacy. Explanation relieves anxiety and facilitates patient engagement. The patient is better able to relax and participate if they are familiar with the procedure and know everything is in readiness when the urge to defecate is felt. Defecation usually occurs within 5 to 15 minutes.
7. Warm the enema solution to at or just above body temperature by placing the container with the enema solution in the amount prescribed in a container of warm water, and check the temperature with a thermometer, if available. If a thermometer is not available, warm and test on your inner wrist. If tap water is used, adjust the temperature as it flows from the faucet.	Enema solution should be at or just above body temperature and warmed, if necessary, by placing the container with the enema solution in a container of warm water (Dougherty & Lister, 2015, as cited in Mitchell, 2019b, p. 155). Warming the solution prevents chilling the patient, adding to the discomfort of the procedure. A cold solution could cause cramping; a too-warm solution could cause trauma to intestinal mucosa.
8. Add the enema solution to the enema set solution container. Release the clamp and allow fluid to progress through the tube before reclamping.	This causes any air to be expelled from the tubing. Although allowing air to enter the intestine is not harmful, it may further distend the intestine.
9. Adjust the bed to a comfortable working height (VHACEOSH, 2016). Position the patient on their left side (Sims' position), with the upper thigh pulled toward the abdomen, if possible, or the knee–chest position, as dictated by patient comfort and condition. Fold the top linen back just enough to allow access to the patient's rectal area. Drape the patient with the bath blanket, as necessary, to maintain privacy and warmth. Place a waterproof pad under the patient's hip.	Having the bed at the proper height prevents back and muscle strain. The Sims' or knee–chest position facilitates flow of solution via gravity into the rectum and colon, optimizing solution retention. Folding back the linen in this manner minimizes unnecessary exposure and promotes the patient's comfort and warmth. The waterproof pad will protect the bed.
10. Put on gloves.	Gloves prevent contact with contaminants and body fluids.

ACTION

11. Elevate the solution so that it is no higher than 18 inches (45 cm) above the level of the anus (Figure 1). Plan to give the solution slowly over a period of 5 to 10 minutes. Hang the container on an IV pole or hold it at the proper height.

RATIONALE

Gravity forces the solution to enter the intestine. The amount of pressure determines the rate of flow and pressure exerted on the intestinal wall. Giving the solution too quickly causes rapid distention and pressure, poor defecation, or damage to the mucous membrane.

12. Generously lubricate the end of the rectal tube 2 to 3 inches (5 to 7 cm). A disposable enema set may have a prelubricated rectal tube.

Lubrication facilitates passage of the rectal tube through the anal sphincter and prevents injury to the mucosa.

13. Lift a buttock to expose the anus. Ask the patient to take several deep breaths. Slowly and gently insert the enema tube 4 to 5 inches (10 to 12.5 cm) for an adult. Direct it at an angle pointing toward the umbilicus, not the bladder (Figure 2).

Good visualization of the anus helps prevent injury to tissues. Deep breathing helps relax the anal sphincters. The anal canal is about 1 to 2 inches (2.5 to 5 cm) long. Insertion 4 to 5 inches (10 to 12.5 cm) ensures the tube is inserted past the external and internal anal sphincters (Dougherty & Lister, 2015, as cited in Mitchell, 2019b, p. 155); further insertion may damage the intestinal mucous membrane. The suggested angle follows the normal intestinal contour and thus will help to prevent perforation of the bowel. Slow insertion of the tube minimizes spasms of the intestinal wall and sphincters.

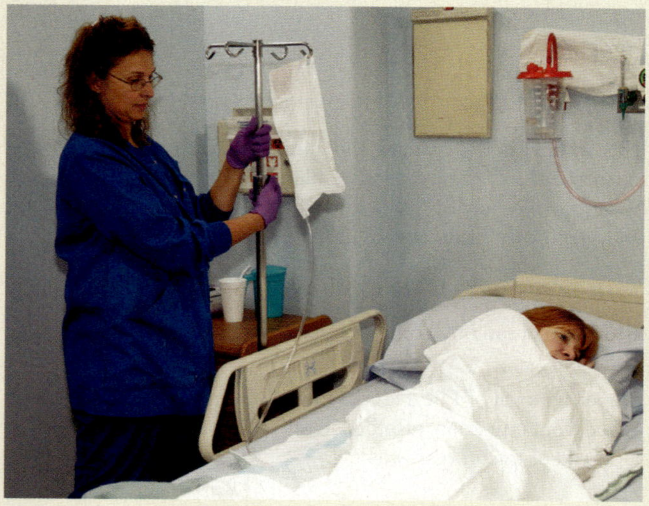

FIGURE 1. Adjusting height of solution container.

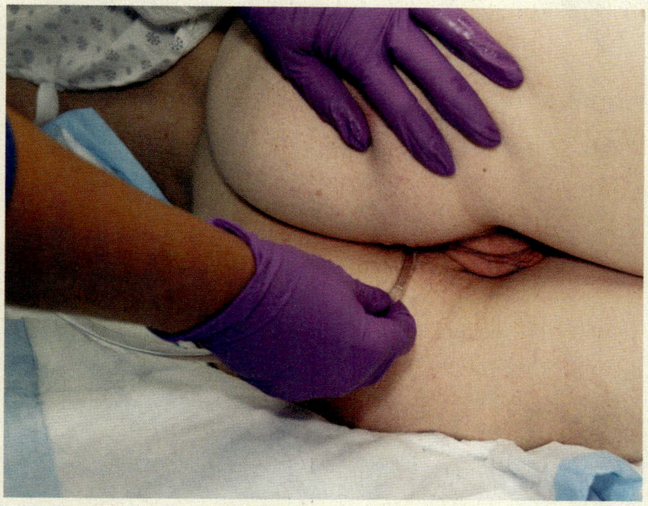

FIGURE 2. Inserting enema tip into anus, directing tip toward umbilicus.

14. If resistance is met while inserting the tube, permit a small amount of solution to enter, withdraw the tube slightly, and then continue to insert it. **Do not force entry of the tube.** Ask the patient to take several deep breaths.

Resistance may be due to spasms of the intestine or failure of the internal sphincter to open. The solution may help to reduce spasms and relax the sphincter, thus making continued insertion of the tube safe. Forcing a tube may injure the intestinal mucosa wall. Taking deep breaths helps relax the anal sphincter.

15. Introduce the solution slowly over a period of 5 to 10 minutes. Hold the tubing all the time that solution is being instilled. Assess for dizziness, lightheadedness, nausea, diaphoresis, and clammy skin during administration. **If the patient experiences any of these symptoms, stop the procedure immediately, monitor the patient's heart rate and blood pressure, and notify the health care team.**

Introducing the solution slowly helps prevent rapid distention of the intestine and a desire to defecate. Assessment allows for detection of a vagal response. The enema may stimulate a vagal response, which increases parasympathetic stimulation, causing a decrease in heart rate.

(continued on page 1558)

Skill 39-1 Administering a Large-Volume Cleansing Enema *(continued)*

ACTION	RATIONALE
16. Clamp the tubing or lower the container if the patient has the urge to defecate or cramping occurs (Figure 3). Instruct the patient to take small, fast breaths or to pant.	These techniques help relax muscles and prevent premature expulsion of the solution.
17. After the solution has been given, clamp the tubing (Figure 4) and remove the tube. Have a paper towel ready to receive the tube as it is withdrawn.	Wrapping the tube in a paper towel prevents dripping of the solution.

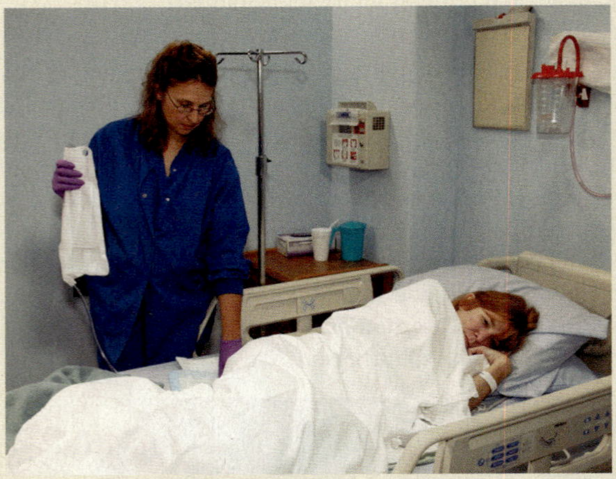

FIGURE 3. Holding bag lower to slow flow of enema solution.

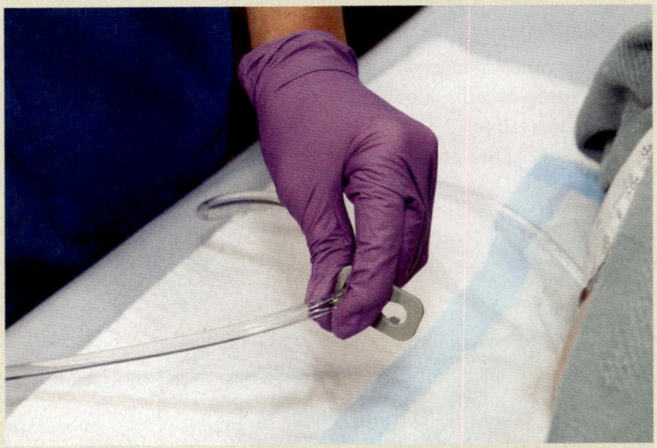

FIGURE 4. Clamping tubing before removing.

ACTION	RATIONALE
18. Return the patient to a comfortable position. Encourage the patient to hold the solution until the urge to defecate is strong, usually in about 10 to 15 minutes. Make sure the linens under the patient are dry. Remove your gloves and ensure that the patient is covered. Perform hand hygiene.	This amount of time usually allows muscle contractions to become sufficient to produce good results. Dry linens promote patient comfort. Removing contaminated gloves and performing hand hygiene prevent the spread of microorganisms.
19. Raise the side rail. Lower the bed height and adjust the head of the bed to a comfortable position.	Positioning promotes comfort and safety.
20. Remove additional PPE, if used. Perform hand hygiene.	Proper removal of PPE reduces the risk for infection transmission and contamination of other items. Hand hygiene prevents the spread of microorganisms.
21. When the patient has a strong urge to defecate, place them in a sitting position on a bedpan or assist them to a commode or a nearby bathroom. Offer toilet tissues, if not in the patient's reach (Figure 5). Stay with the patient or have the call bell readily accessible.	The sitting position is most natural and facilitates defecation. Fall prevention is a high priority due to the urgency of reaching the commode.

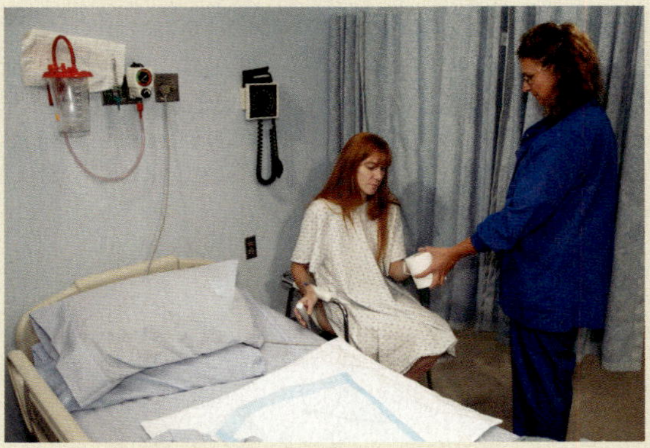

FIGURE 5. Offering toilet tissue to patient on bedside commode.

ACTION	RATIONALE
22. Remind the patient not to flush the commode before you inspect the results of the enema.	The results need to be observed and recorded. Additional enemas may be necessary if the health care provider has prescribed enemas "until clear." Refer to "Special Considerations" below.
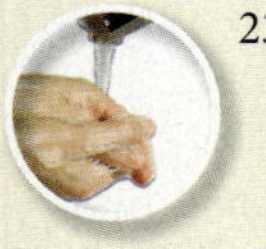 23. Put on gloves and assist the patient, if necessary, with cleaning the anal area. Offer washcloths, skin cleanser, and water for handwashing. Remove gloves. Perform hand hygiene.	Cleaning the anal area and proper hygiene deter the spread of microorganisms. Gloves prevent contact with contaminants and body fluids. Hand hygiene deters the spread of microorganisms.
24. Leave the patient clean and comfortable. Care for equipment properly.	Bacteria that grow in the intestine can be spread to others if equipment is not properly cleaned.
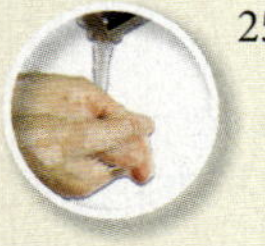 25. Perform hand hygiene.	Hand hygiene deters the spread of microorganisms.

DOCUMENTATION

Guidelines

Document the amount and type of enema solution used; amount, consistency, and color of stool; pain assessment rating; assessment of the perineal area for any irritation, tears, or bleeding; and the patient's reaction to the procedure.

Sample Documentation

> <u>7/22/25</u> 1310 800-mL tap water enema given via rectum. Large amount of soft, brown stool returned. No irritation, tears, or bleeding noted in perineal area. Patient reported "stomach cramping," which was relieved when enema was released. Rates pain as 0 after evacuation of enema.
>
> *—K. Sanders, RN*

DEVELOPING CLINICAL REASONING AND CLINICAL JUDGMENT

UNEXPECTED SITUATIONS AND ASSOCIATED INTERVENTIONS

- *Solution does not flow into rectum:* Reposition the rectal tube. If solution will still not flow, remove the tube, and check for any fecal contents clogging the tube.
- *Patient cannot retain enema solution for adequate amount of time:* The patient may need to be placed on a bedpan in the supine position while receiving the enema. The head of the bed may be elevated 30 degrees for the patient's comfort.
- *Patient cannot tolerate large amount of enema solution:* Amount and length of administration may have to be modified if the patient begins to report pain.
- *Patient reports severe cramping with introduction of enema solution:* Lower the solution container and check the temperature and flow rate. If the solution is too cold or the flow rate too fast, severe cramping may occur.

SPECIAL CONSIDERATIONS

General Considerations

- Rectal agents should be avoided in patients at risk of thrombocytopenia, leukopenia, and/or mucositis, and manipulation of the rectum and anus, including administration of enemas, should be avoided in immunocompromised patients and/or patients at risk for myelosuppression and mucositis (NCI, 2020). These actions can lead to development of anal fissures or abscesses, which are portals for infection (NCI, 2020).
- If the patient experiences fullness or pain, or if fluid escapes around the tube, stop administration. Wait 30 seconds to a minute and then restart the flow at a slower rate. If symptoms persist, stop administration, and contact the health care team.
- If the order states the enema is to be given "until clear," check with the health care team before administering more than three enemas. Severe fluid and electrolyte imbalances may occur if the patient receives more than three cleansing enemas. Results are considered clear whenever there are no more pieces of stool in the enema return. The solution may be colored but still considered a clear return.

(continued on page 1560)

Skill 39-1 Administering a Large-Volume Cleansing Enema *(continued)*

Infant and Child Considerations

- When administering an enema to a child, use isotonic solutions. Plain water is not used because it is hypotonic and can cause rapid fluid shift and fluid overload (Silbert-Flagg & Pillitteri, 2018).
- Appropriate fluid volume for an enema (Silbert-Flagg & Pillitteri, 2018):
- Infant: 250 mL or less
- Toddler or preschooler: 250 to 350 mL
- School-aged child: 300 to 500 mL
- Adolescent: 500 mL
- Position the infant or toddler on their abdomen with knees bent. Position the child or adolescent on their left side with the right leg flexed toward the chest (Cincinnati Children's, 2018).
- Insert the tubing into the rectum 2 to 3 inches (5 to 7.5 cm) for children (ages 2 to 10 years); 1 to 1.5 inches (2.5 to 4 cm) for infants (Cincinnati Children's, 2018).

Older Adult Considerations

- If the older adult cannot retain the enema solution, administer the enema with the patient on the bedpan in the supine position. For comfort, elevate the head of the bed 30 degrees, if necessary, and use pillows appropriately.

Skill 39-2 Inserting a Nasogastric Tube

DELEGATION CONSIDERATIONS

The insertion of an NG tube is not delegated to assistive personnel (AP). Depending on the state's nurse practice act and the organization's policies and procedures, insertion of an NG tube may be delegated to licensed practical/vocational nurses (LPN/LVNs). The decision to delegate must be based on careful analysis of the patient's needs and circumstances as well as the qualifications of the person to whom the task is being delegated. Refer to the Delegation Guidelines in Appendix A.

EQUIPMENT

- NG tube of appropriate size (8F to 18F)
- Stethoscope
- Water-soluble lubricant
- Normal saline solution or sterile water, for irrigation, depending on facility policy
- Tongue blade
- Irrigations set, including a large syringe (20 to 50 mL)
- Flashlight
- Nonallergenic tape (1 inch wide)
- Tissues
- Glass of water with straw
- Topical anesthetic—lidocaine spray or gel (optional)
- Clamp
- Suction apparatus (if prescribed)
- Bath towel or disposable pad
- Emesis basin
- Safety pin and rubber band
- Nonsterile, disposable gloves
- Additional PPE, as indicated
- Tape measure, or other measuring device
- Skin barrier
- pH test strip (calibrated in units of 0.5 and approved for use with human secretions)

IMPLEMENTATION

ACTION	RATIONALE
1. Verify the prescribed intervention for insertion of an NG tube. Gather equipment, including selection of the appropriate NG tube.	This ensures the patient receives the correct treatment. Assembling equipment provides for an organized approach to the task. NG tubes should be radiopaque, contain clearly visible markings for measurement, and may have multiple ports for aspiration.
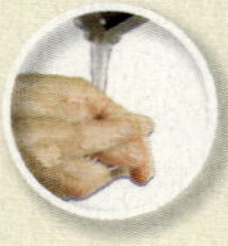 2. Perform hand hygiene and put on PPE, if indicated.	Hand hygiene and PPE prevent the spread of microorganisms. PPE is required based on transmission precautions.
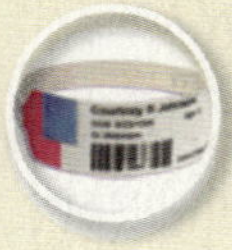 3. Identify the patient.	Identifying the patient ensures the right patient receives the intervention and helps prevent errors.

ACTION	RATIONALE
4. Explain the procedure to the patient, including the rationale for why the tube is needed. Discuss the associated discomforts that may be experienced and possible interventions that may allay this discomfort. Answer any questions, as needed.	Explanation facilitates patient engagement and reduces anxiety.
5. Assemble equipment on the overbed table or other surface within reach.	Arranging items nearby is convenient, saves time, and avoids unnecessary stretching and twisting of muscles on the part of the nurse.
6. Close the patient's bedside curtain or door. Raise the bed to a comfortable working position (VHACEOSH, 2016). Assist the patient to high-Fowler position or elevate the head of the bed 45 degrees if the patient is unable to maintain an upright position. Drape their chest with a bath towel or disposable pad. Have an emesis basin and tissues within reach.	Closing the curtains or the door provides for patient privacy. Having the bed at the proper height prevents back and muscle strain. The upright position is more natural for swallowing and reduces the risk for aspiration if the patient should vomit. Passage of the tube may stimulate gagging and tearing of the eyes.
7. **Refer to facility policy regarding method(s) to determine insertion length.** Measure the distance to insert the tube by placing the tube tip at the patient's nostril and extending it to the tip of the earlobe and then to the point midway between the xiphoid process and umbilicus. Alternatively, measure from the xiphisternum (xiphoid process) to the earlobe, to the nose and add 10 cm (Fan et al., 2019). **Refer to facility policy. Mark the tube with an indelible marker.**	The NEMU (nose-ear-mid-umbilicus) has been suggested as an accurate method of measurement in infants and children (Ellett et al., 2012; Irving et al., 2018). Another method, the xiphisternum-earlobe-nose + 10 cm, has been suggested as the best estimate for the length of NG tube required (Fan et al., 2019). Correct positioning results in tip positioning between 3 and 10 cm under the lower esophageal sphincter (Torsy et al., 2018). Determination of NG tube insertion length is controversial, and recommendations are conflicting; most evidence for practice identifies the need for more research to determine more accurate and reliable ways to determine tube insertion depth (Boeykens, 2018; Fan et al., 2019; Mak & Tam, 2020; Parker et al., 2018; Taylor, 2020; Torsy et al., 2018).
8. Put on gloves. Lubricate the tip of the tube (at least 2 to 4 inches) with water-soluble lubricant. Apply topical anesthetic to the nostril and oropharynx, as appropriate.	Lubrication reduces friction and facilitates passage of the tube into the stomach. Water-soluble lubricant will not cause pneumonia if the tube accidentally enters the lungs. Topical anesthetics act as local anesthetics, reducing discomfort. Consult the health care team for an order for a topical anesthetic, such as lidocaine gel or spray, if needed.
9. After selecting the appropriate nostril, ask the patient to flex their head slightly back against the pillow. Gently insert the tube into the nostril while directing the tube upward and backward along the floor of the nose (Figure 1). The patient may gag when the tube reaches the pharynx. Provide tissues for tearing or watering of the eyes. Offer comfort and reassurance to the patient.	Following the normal contour of the nasal passage while inserting the tube reduces irritation and the likelihood of mucosal injury. The tube stimulates the gag reflex readily. Tears are a natural response as the tube passes into the nasopharynx. Many patients report that gagging and throat discomfort can be more painful than the tube passing through the nostrils.

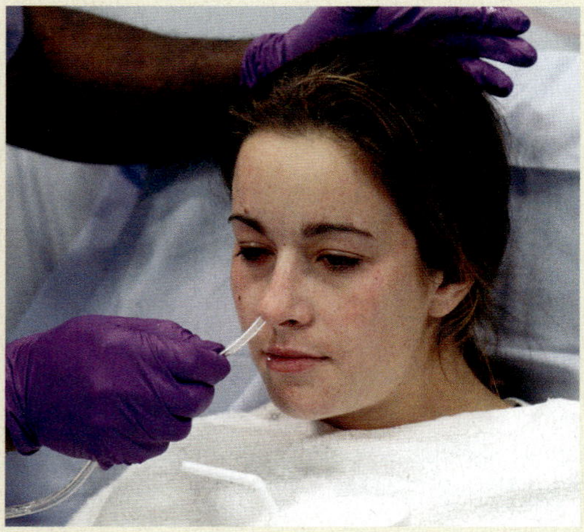

FIGURE 1. Beginning insertion with patient positioned with head slightly flexed back.

(*continued on page 1562*)

Skill 39-2 Inserting a Nasogastric Tube *(continued)*

ACTION	RATIONALE
10. When the pharynx is reached, instruct the patient to touch their chin to their chest. Encourage the patient to sip water through a straw or swallow (Figure 2). Advance the tube in a downward and backward direction when the patient swallows. Stop when the patient breathes. **If gagging and coughing persist, stop advancing the tube and check placement of the tube with a tongue blade and flashlight.** If the tube is curled, straighten the tube and attempt to advance it again. Keep advancing the tube until the pen marking is reached. **Do not use force.** Rotate the tube if it meets resistance.	Bringing the head forward helps close the trachea and open the esophagus. Swallowing helps advance the tube, causes the epiglottis to cover the opening of the trachea, and helps to eliminate gagging and coughing. Excessive coughing and gagging may occur if the tube has curled in the back of the throat. Forcing the tube may injure mucous membranes.
11. **Discontinue the procedure and remove the tube if there are signs of distress, such as gasping, coughing, cyanosis, and inability to speak or hum.**	The tube is in the airway if the patient shows signs of distress and cannot speak or hum. If, after three attempts, NG insertion is unsuccessful, another nurse may try, or the patient should be referred to another health care professional.
12. Secure the tube loosely to the nose or cheek with tape until placement is verified. Confirm placement of the NG tube in the patient's stomach using at least two methods.	Verify correct placement of the NG tube after the initial insertion, before beginning a feeding or instilling medications or liquids, and at regular intervals during continuous feedings (Metheny et al., 2019). A misplaced tube in the lungs or pulmonary tissue places the patient at risk for aspiration, pneumonia, and even death (Lamont et al., 2011, as cited in Anderson, 2018). With the exception of radiographic examination, which is usually done immediately after insertion to verify initial tube placement, the use of two or more techniques in conjunction with each other increases the likelihood of correct tube placement (AACN, 2020; Anderson, 2019; Anderson, 2018; Dias et al., 2019; Rahimi et al., 2015).
13. After confirmation of tube placement, secure the tube. Apply a skin barrier to the tip and end of the nose and allow it to dry. Remove gloves and secure the tube with a commercially prepared securement device (Figure 3) (follow the manufacturer's directions) or tape it to the patient's nose. To secure with tape:	Securing the tube prevents migration of the tube inward and outward. The skin barrier improves adhesion and protects skin. Constant pressure of the tube against the skin and mucous membranes may cause pressure injury (Powers, 2019).

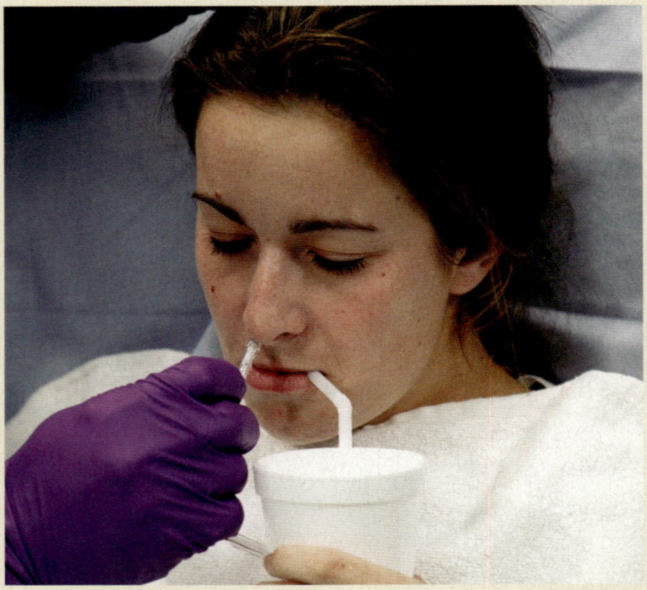

FIGURE 2. Advancing tube after patient drops chin to chest and while swallowing.

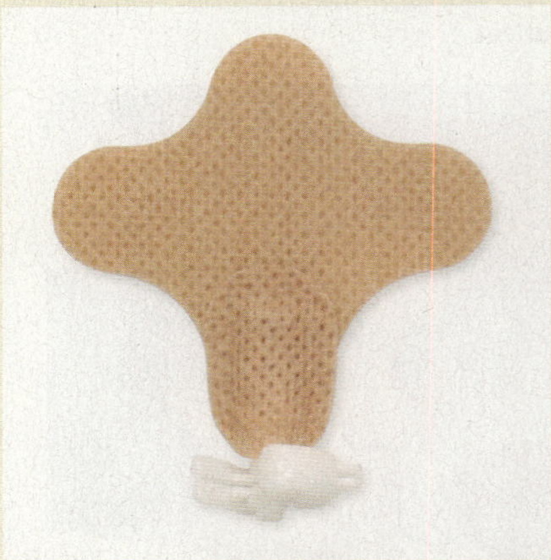

FIGURE 3. Example of a commercially prepared securement device. (*Source:* Courtesy of Hollister, Incorporated, Libertyville, Illinois.)

ACTION

a. Cut a 4-inch piece of tape and split the bottom 2 inches (Figure 4) or use packaged nose tape for NG tubes.

b. Place the unsplit end over the bridge of the patient's nose (Figure 5).

c. Wrap the split ends under and around the NG tube (Figure 6). **Be careful not to pull the tube too tightly against the nose** (Powers, 2019).

RATIONALE

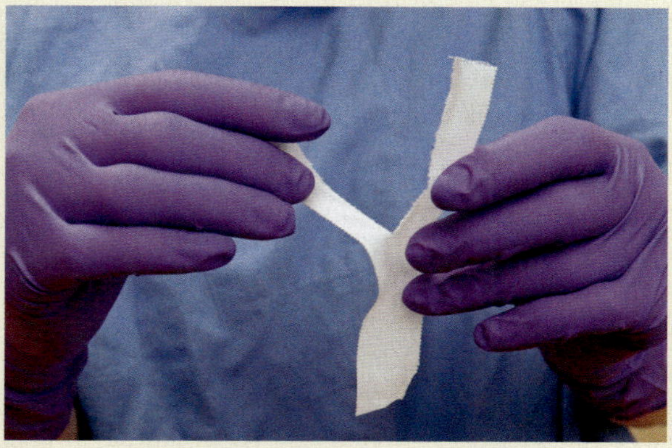

FIGURE 4. Making a 2-inch cut into a 4-inch strip of tape.

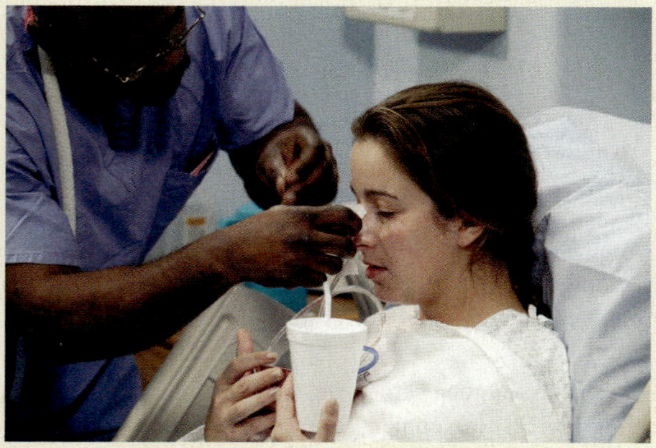

FIGURE 5. Applying tape to patient's nose.

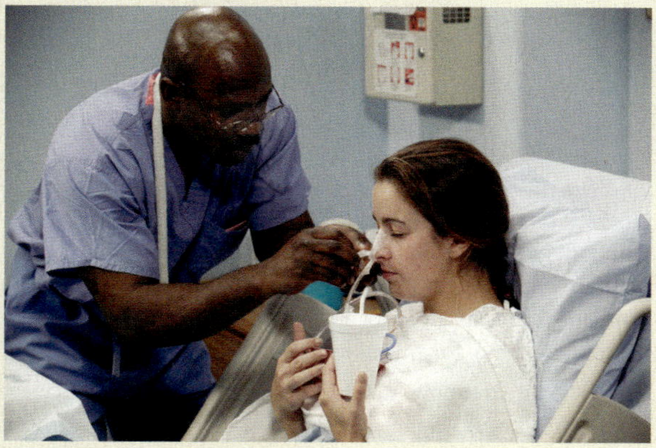

FIGURE 6. Wrapping split ends around NG tube.

14. Put on gloves. Clamp the tube and remove the syringe. Cap or attach the tube to suction (Figure 7), according to the prescribed interventions. Remove gloves. Perform hand hygiene.

Gloves prevent contact with blood and body fluids and transfer of microorganisms. Suction provides for decompression of the stomach and drainage of gastric contents. Removing gloves properly and using hand hygiene reduces the risk for infection transmission and contamination of other items.

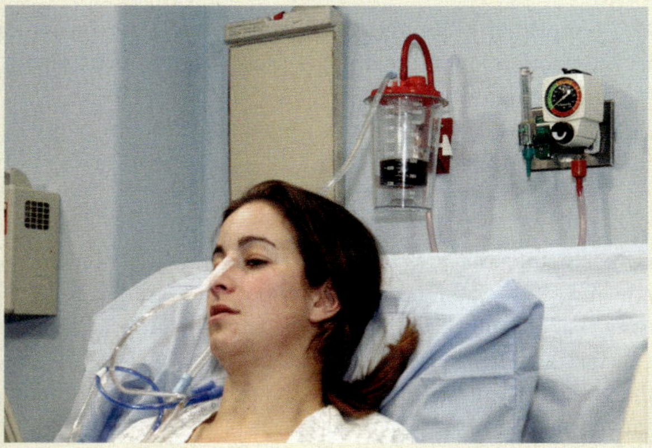

FIGURE 7. NG tube attached to wall suction.

(continued on page 1564)

Skill 39-2 Inserting a Nasogastric Tube *(continued)*

ACTION

15. Measure the length of the exposed tube. Reinforce the marking on the tube at the nostril with indelible ink. Ask the patient to turn their head to the side opposite the nostril in which the tube is inserted. Secure the tube to the patient's gown by using rubber band or tape and a safety pin. For additional support, tape the tube onto the patient's cheek using a piece of tape. **Secure the vent of the double-lumen tube above stomach level.** Attach the vent at shoulder level (Figure 8).

RATIONALE

The tube should be marked with an indelible marker at the nostril. This marking should be assessed each time the tube is used to ensure the tube has not become displaced. Tube length should be checked and compared with this initial measurement, in conjunction with pH measurement and visual assessment of aspirate, at regular intervals. An increase in the length of the exposed tube may indicate dislodgement (AACN, 2020; Boullata et al., 2017). Securing prevents tension and tugging on the tube. Turning the head ensures adequate slack in the tubing to prevent tension when the patient turns the head. Securing the double-lumen tube above stomach level prevents seepage of gastric contents and keeps the lumen clear for venting air.

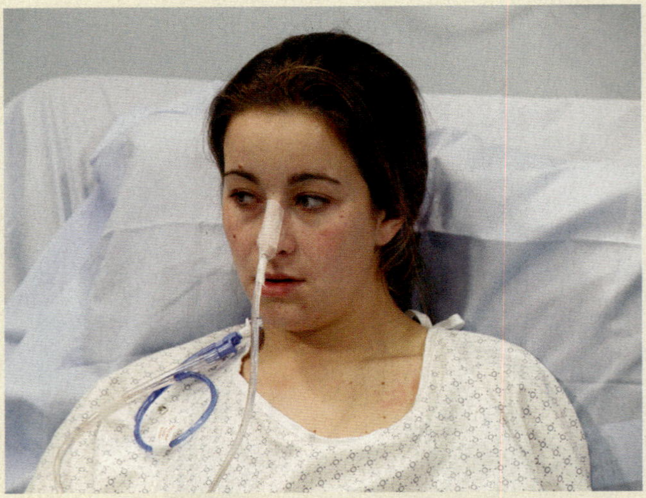

FIGURE 8. Patient with Salem sump tube (NG) secured. Note blue vent at patient's shoulder.

16. Put on gloves. Assist with or provide oral hygiene at 2- to 4-hour intervals. Lubricate the lips generously and clean nares and lubricate, as needed. Offer analgesic throat lozenges or anesthetic spray for throat irritation, if needed.

Gloves prevent contact with blood and body fluids and transfer of microorganisms. Oral hygiene keeps the mouth clean and moist, promotes comfort, and reduces thirst.

17. Remove and reapply the NG tube securement device every 24 hours; assess, clean, and apply a skin barrier to the skin beneath or in contact with the NG tube prior to replacement. Reposition the tube to alleviate pressure. Provide nares hygiene as needed (Schroeder & Sitzer, 2019).

Pressure from the tube can create pressure damage; these actions help prevent development of pressure injury (Baranoski & Ayello, 2020; EPUAP, NPIAP, & PPPIA, 2019a; Schroeder & Sitzer, 2019).

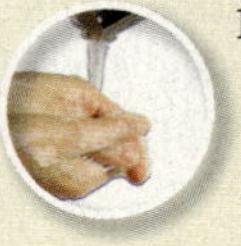

18. Remove equipment and return the patient to a position of comfort. Remove gloves. Perform hand hygiene. Raise the side rail and lower the bed.

Positioning promotes patient comfort and safety. Removing gloves properly and using hand hygiene reduces the risk for infection transmission and contamination of other items.

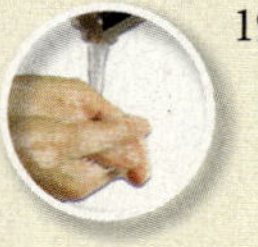

19. Remove additional PPE, if used. Perform hand hygiene.

Proper removal of PPE reduces the risk for infection transmission and contamination of other items. Hand hygiene prevents transmission of microorganisms.

DOCUMENTATION

Guidelines

Document the size and type of the NG tube that was inserted and the postinsertion measurement of the length of the tube from the tip of the nose to the end of the exposed tube. Also, document the results of the x-ray that was taken to confirm the tube position, if applicable. Record the pH of the aspirated gastric contents. Document the naris where the tube was placed and the patient's response to the procedure. Include assessment data related to the abdomen. Record the patient teaching that was discussed.

Sample Documentation

Lippincott DocuCare **Practice documenting NG tube insertion in *Lippincott DocuCare.***

10/4/25 0945 Abdomen slightly distended and taut; hypoactive bowel sounds. Patient reports transient nausea. 14F double-lumen nasogastric tube inserted via right naris, 20 cm of tube from naris to end of tube post insertion; aspirate pH 4; patient tolerated without incident.
—*S. Essner, RN*

DEVELOPING CLINICAL REASONING AND CLINICAL JUDGMENT

UNEXPECTED SITUATIONS AND ASSOCIATED INTERVENTIONS

- *As tube is passing through the pharynx, patient begins to retch and gag:* This is common during placement of an NG tube. Ask the patient if they want to stop the procedure, which will allow the patient to gain composure from the gagging episode. Continue to advance the tube when the patient relates that they are ready. Have the emesis basin nearby in case the patient begins to vomit.
- *You are unable to pass the tube after trying a second time down the one nostril:* If the patient's condition permits, inspect the other nostril and attempt to pass the NG tube down this nostril. If unable to pass down this nostril, consult with the health care team.
- *As the tube is passing through the pharynx, the patient begins to cough and shows signs of respiratory distress:* **Stop advancing the tube.** The tube is most likely entering the trachea. Pull the tube back into the nasal area. Support the patient as they regain normal breathing ability and composure. If the patient feels that they can tolerate another attempt, ask the patient to keep their chin on their chest and swallow as the tube is advanced to help prevent the tube from entering the trachea. Begin to advance the tube, watching for any signs of respiratory distress.
- *No gastric contents can be aspirated:* Reposition the patient and flush the tube with 30 mL of air in a large syringe. Slowly apply negative pressure to withdraw fluid.

SPECIAL CONSIDERATIONS

General Considerations

- A nasal bridle (Figure 9) is another type of commercial device that has been suggested to secure NG tubes (Stabler et al., 2018; Taylor et al., 2018).
- Check tube placement before administering any fluids, medications, or feeding, using multiple techniques: x-ray, external length, external verification marking, pH testing, and carbon dioxide monitoring (if available). Consistent inability to withdraw fluid from tube may indicate displacement of the tube from the stomach into the esophagus (AACN, 2020).
- Signs of respiratory distress may be absent in patients with an impaired level of consciousness when NG tubes are inadvertently positioned in the airway (AACN, 2020).
- Sterile water should be used for tube flushes in immunocompromised or critically ill patients (Allen, 2015; Boullata et al., 2017).
- Gastric pH ≥6 is of no benefit in predicting tube location in the GI tract or in ruling out tracheopulmonary placement (Boullata et al., 2017).

Infant and Child Considerations

- Infants are obligate nose breathers; tubes are usually inserted via the mouth (orogastric tube). Insertion through a nostril is usually more comfortable for older children (Silbert-Falgg & Pillitteri, 2018).

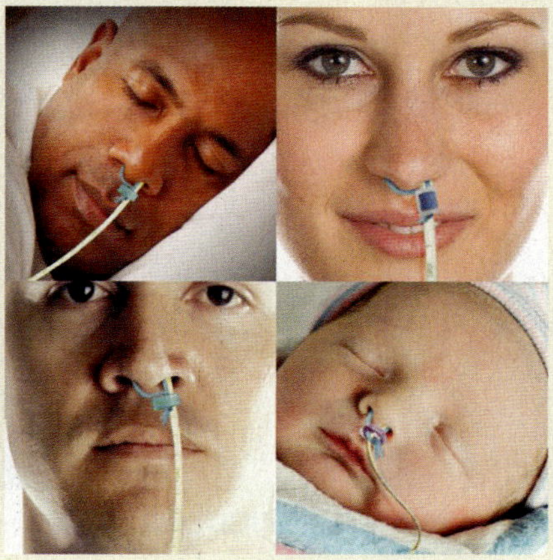

FIGURE 9. Example of a commercially prepared nasal bridle. (*Source:* Images courtesy of Applied Medical Technology, Inc. [AMT]. https://www.appliedmedical.net)

Skill 39-3 Removing a Nasogastric Tube

DELEGATION CONSIDERATIONS

The removal of an NG tube is not delegated to assistive personnel (AP). Depending on the state's nurse practice act and the organization's policies and procedures, removal of an NG tube may be delegated to licensed practical/vocational nurses (LPN/LVNs). The decision to delegate must be based on careful analysis of the patient's needs and circumstances as well as the qualifications of the person to whom the task is being delegated. Refer to the Delegation Guidelines in Appendix A.

EQUIPMENT

- Tissues
- 50-mL syringe
- Nonsterile gloves
- Additional PPE, as indicated
- Stethoscope
- Disposable plastic bag
- Bath towel or disposable pad
- Normal saline solution for irrigation (optional)
- Emesis basin

IMPLEMENTATION

ACTION	RATIONALE
1. Check the health record for the prescribed intervention for removal of the NG tube. Gather equipment.	This ensures the patient receives the correct treatment. Gathering equipment provides for an organized approach to the task.
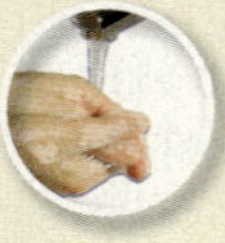 2. Perform hand hygiene and put on PPE, if indicated.	Hand hygiene and PPE prevent the spread of microorganisms. PPE is required based on transmission precautions.
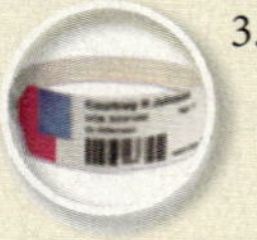 3. Identify the patient.	Identifying the patient ensures the right patient receives the intervention and helps prevent errors.
4. Explain the procedure to the patient and why this intervention is warranted. Describe that it will entail a few moments of discomfort. Perform key abdominal assessments as described above.	Patient engagement is facilitated when explanations are provided. Due to potential changes in a patient's condition, assessment is vital before initiating intervention.
5. Pull the patient's bedside curtain. Raise the bed to a comfortable working position (VHACEOSH, 2016). Assist the patient to a 30- to 45-degree position. Place a towel or disposable pad across the patient's chest (Figure 1). Give tissues and an emesis basin to the patient.	This provides for privacy. An appropriate working height facilitates comfort and proper body mechanics for the nurse. A towel or pad protects the patient from contact with gastric secretions. An emesis basin is helpful if the patient vomits or gags. Tissues are necessary if the patient wants to blow their nose when the tube is removed.
6. Put on gloves. Discontinue suction and separate the tube from suction. Detach the tube from any securement to patient's gown and/or face and carefully remove the securement device or adhesive tape from the patient's nose.	Gloves prevent contact with blood and body fluids. Disconnecting the tube from suction and the patient allows for its unrestricted removal.
7. Check placement (refer to Skill 38-2) and flush the tube with 10 mL of water or normal saline solution (optional) or clear with 30 to 50 mL of air (Figure 2).	Air or saline solution clears the tube of secretions or debris.

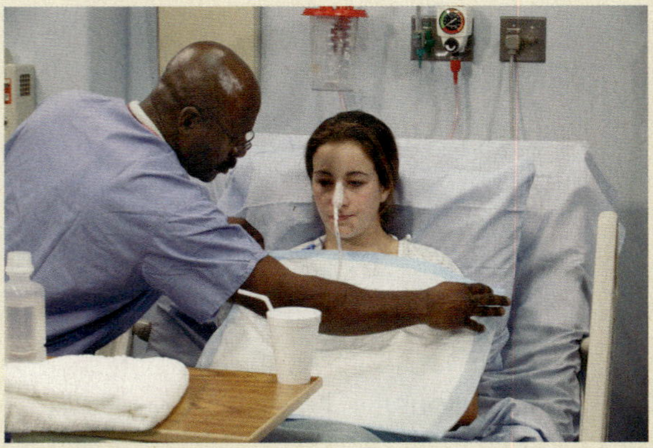

FIGURE 1. Placing towel or disposable pad across patient's chest.

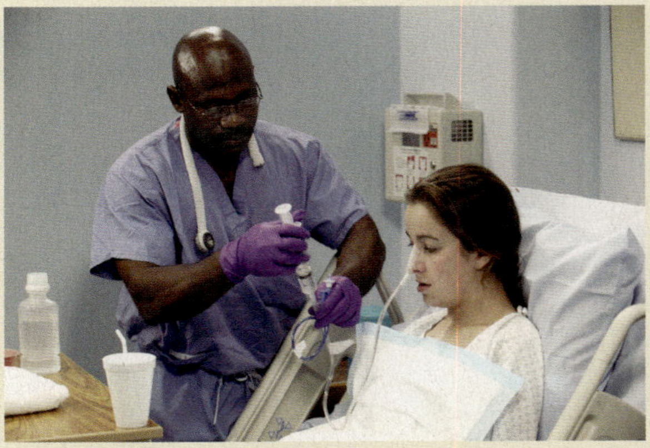

FIGURE 2. Flushing NG tube with 10-mL water.

ACTION

8. Clamp the tube with your fingers by doubling the tube on itself (Figure 3). **Instruct the patient to take a deep breath and hold it. Quickly and carefully remove the tube while the patient holds their breath.** Coil the tube in the disposable pad as you remove it from the patient.

RATIONALE

Clamping prevents drainage of gastric contents into the pharynx and esophagus. The patient holds their breath to prevent accidental aspiration of gastric secretions in the tube. Careful removal minimizes trauma and discomfort for the patient. Containing the tube in a towel while removing it prevents leakage onto the patient.

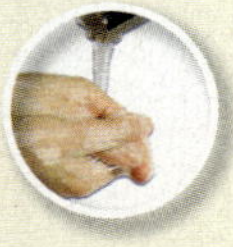

9. Dispose of the tube per facility policy. Remove gloves. Perform hand hygiene.

This prevents contamination with microorganisms.

10. Offer mouth care to the patient and facial tissue to blow their nose. Assist the patient to a position of comfort, as needed.

These interventions promote patient comfort.

11. Remove equipment, raise the side rail, and lower the bed.

Positioning promotes patient comfort and safety.

12. Put on gloves and measure the amount of NG drainage in the collection device. Record the measurement on the output flow record, subtracting irrigant fluids if necessary (Figure 4). Add solidifying agent to the NG drainage and dispose of the drainage according to facility policy.

Irrigation fluids are considered intake. To obtain the true NG drainage, irrigant fluid amounts are subtracted from the total NG drainage. NG drainage is recorded as part of the output of fluids from the patient. Solidifying agents added to liquid NG drainage facilitate safe biohazard disposal.

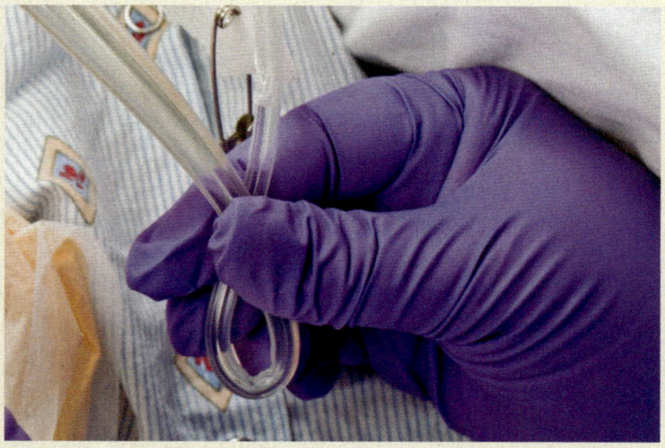

FIGURE 3. Doubling tube on itself.

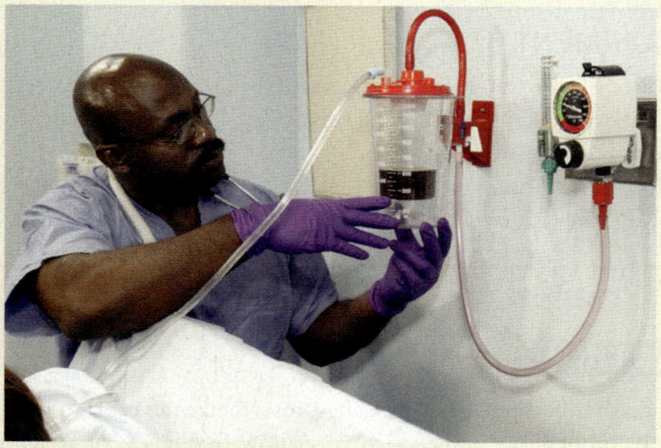

FIGURE 4. Measuring the amount of nasogastric drainage in collection device.

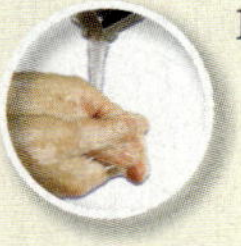

13. Remove gloves and additional PPE, if used. Perform hand hygiene.

Proper removal of PPE reduces the risk for infection transmission and contamination of other items. Hand hygiene prevents transmission of microorganisms.

DOCUMENTATION

Guidelines

Document assessment of the abdomen. If an abdominal girth reading was obtained, record this measurement. Document the removal of the NG tube from the naris where it had been placed. Note if there is any irritation to the skin of the naris. Record the amount of NG drainage in the suction container on the patient's intake-and-output record as well as the color of the drainage. Record any pertinent teaching, such as instructions to the patient to notify the nurse if they experience any nausea, abdominal pain, or bloating.

Sample Documentation

10/29/25 1320 NG tube removed from L naris without incident. 300 mL of dark brown liquid emptied from NG tube. Patient's abdomen is 66 cm; abdomen is soft, nontender with hypoactive bowel sounds in all four quadrants.

—S. Essner, RN

(continued on page 1568)

Skill 39-3 Removing a Nasogastric Tube *(continued)*

DEVELOPING CLINICAL REASONING AND CLINICAL JUDGMENT

UNEXPECTED SITUATIONS AND ASSOCIATED INTERVENTIONS

- Within 2 hours after NG tube removal, the patient's abdomen is showing signs of distention: Notify the health care team. Anticipate an order to reinsert the NG tube.
- Epistaxis occurs with removal of the NG tube: Occlude both nares until bleeding has subsided. Ensure that patient is in upright position. Document the epistaxis in the patient's health record.

Skill 39-4 Irrigating a Nasogastric Tube Connected to Suction

DELEGATION CONSIDERATIONS

The irrigation of an NG tube is not delegated to assistive personnel (AP). Depending on the state's nurse practice act and the organization's policies and procedures, irrigation of an NG tube may be delegated to licensed practical/vocational nurses (LPN/LVNs). The decision to delegate must be based on careful analysis of the patient's needs and circumstances as well as the qualifications of the person to whom the task is being delegated. Refer to the Delegation Guidelines in Appendix A.

EQUIPMENT

- Water, sterile water, or normal saline solution for irrigation (based on facility policy)
- Nonsterile gloves
- Additional PPE, as indicated
- Irrigation set, including a large syringe (20 to 50 mL)
- Clamp
- Disposable waterproof pad or bath towel
- Emesis basin
- Tape measure, or other measuring device
- pH test strip (calibrated in units of 0.5 and approved for use with human secretions)
- Stethoscope (for abdominal assessment)

IMPLEMENTATION

ACTION	RATIONALE
1. Gather equipment. Verify the prescribed intervention or facility policy and procedure regarding frequency of irrigation, solution type, and amount of irrigant. Check expiration dates on the irrigating solution and irrigation set.	Assembling equipment provides for an organized approach to the task. Verification ensures the patient receives the correct intervention. Facility policy dictates safe interval for reuse of equipment.
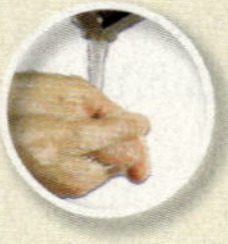 2. Perform hand hygiene and put on PPE, if indicated.	Hand hygiene and PPE prevent the spread of microorganisms. PPE is required based on transmission precautions.
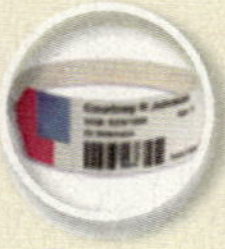 3. Identify the patient.	Identifying the patient ensures the right patient receives the intervention and helps prevent errors.
4. Explain the procedure to the patient and why this intervention is needed. Answer any questions, as needed. Perform key assessments as described above.	Explanation facilitates patient engagement. Due to potential changes in a patient's condition, assessment is vital before initiating an intervention.
5. Assemble equipment on the overbed table or other surface within reach.	Organization facilitates performance of the task.
6. Pull the patient's bedside curtain. Raise the bed to a comfortable working position (VHACEOSH, 2016). Assist the patient to 30- to 45-degree position, unless this is contraindicated. Pour the irrigating solution into container.	This provides for privacy. An appropriate working height facilitates comfort and proper body mechanics for the nurse. This position minimizes risk for aspiration. Preparing the irrigation provides for an organized approach to the task.

ACTION	RATIONALE
7. Put on gloves. Place a waterproof pad on the patient's chest, under the connection of the NG tube and suction tubing. **Check placement of the NG tube.** Refer to Skill 39-2.	Gloves prevent contact with body fluids. The waterproof pad protects the patient's clothing and bed linens from accidental leakage of gastric fluid. Checking placement before the instillation of fluid is necessary to prevent accidental instillation into the respiratory tract if the tube has become dislodged.
8. Draw up 30 mL of irrigation solution (or amount indicated in the order or policy) into the irrigation syringe (Figure 1).	This delivers measured amount of irrigant through the tube. Flushing the tube prevents occlusion (Bischoff et al., 2020; Boullata et al., 2017; Drummond Hayes, 2018).
9. Clamp the NG tube near the connection site using a clamp, or double the tube on itself. Disconnect the tube from the suction apparatus (Figure 2) and lay it on a disposable pad or towel, or hold both tubes upright in your nondominant hand (Figure 3).	Clamping prevents leakage of gastric fluid.
10. Place tip of the syringe in the tube. **If a double-lumen tube is used, make sure that the syringe tip is placed in the drainage port and not in the blue air vent.** Hold the syringe upright and gently insert the irrigant (Figure 4) (or allow solution to flow in by gravity if facility policy or prescribed intervention indicates). **Do not force solution into the tube.**	Gentle insertion of saline solution (or gravity insertion) is less traumatic to gastric mucosa. The blue air vent acts to decrease pressure built up in the stomach when the Salem sump is attached to suction. It is not to be used for irrigation. Flushing the tube prevents occlusion (Bischoff et al., 2020; Boullata et al., 2017; Drummond Hayes, 2018).

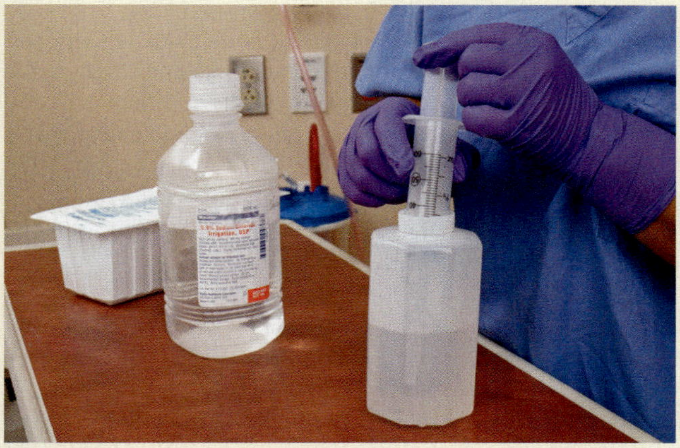

FIGURE 1. Preparing syringe with 30 mL of irrigation solution.

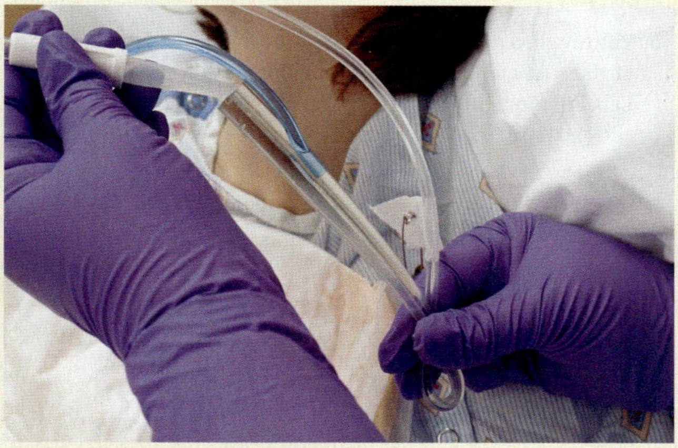

FIGURE 2. Clamping nasogastric tube while disconnecting.

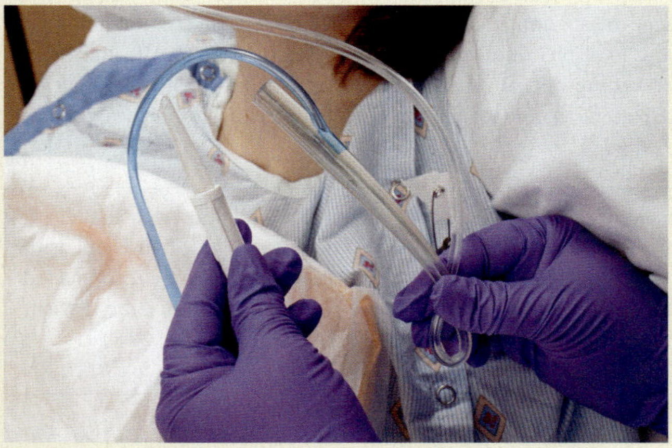

FIGURE 3. Keeping both tubes upright to prevent leakage of gastric fluid.

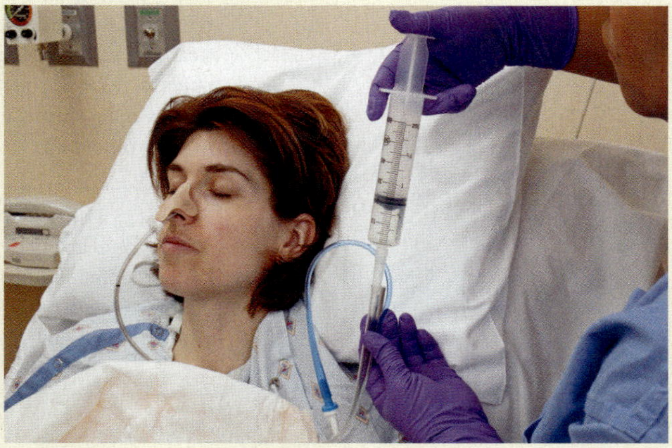

FIGURE 4. Gently instilling irrigation.

(continued on page 1570)

Skill 39-4 Irrigating a Nasogastric Tube Connected to Suction *(continued)*

ACTION	RATIONALE
11. If you are unable to irrigate the tube, reposition the patient and attempt irrigation again. Inject 10 to 20 mL of air and aspirate again. **If repeated attempts to irrigate the tube fail, consult with the health care team or follow facility policy.**	The tube may be positioned against gastric mucosa, making it difficult to irrigate. Injection of air may reposition the end of the tube.
12. After irrigant has been instilled, hold the end of the NG tube over the irrigation tray or emesis basin. Observe for return flow of NG drainage into the container. Alternatively, you may reconnect the NG tube to suction and observe the return drainage as it drains into the suction container.	Return flow may be collected in an irrigating tray or other available container and measured. This amount will need to be subtracted from the irrigant to record the true NG drainage. A second method involves subtracting the total irrigant from the shift from the total NG drainage emptied over the entire shift to find the true NG drainage. Check facility policy for guidelines.
13. If not already done, reconnect the drainage port to suction, if prescribed.	This allows for continued removal of gastric contents, as prescribed.
14. Inject air into the blue air vent after irrigation is complete. Position the blue air vent above the patient's stomach.	Following irrigation, the blue air vent is injected with air to keep it clear. Positioning the blue air vent above the stomach prevents the stomach contents from leaking from the NG tube.
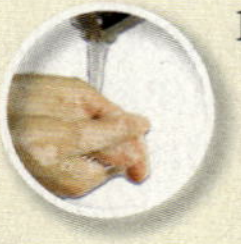 15. Remove gloves. Perform hand hygiene. Lower the bed and raise the side rails, as necessary. Assist the patient to a position of comfort.	Proper removal of gloves and hand hygiene prevent transmission of microorganisms. Lowering the bed and assisting the patient to a comfortable position promote safety and comfort.
16. Put on gloves. Measure returned solution, if collected outside of the suction apparatus. Rinse equipment if it will be reused. Label equipment with the date, patient's name, room number, and purpose (for NG tube/irrigation).	Gloves prevent contact with blood and body fluids. The irrigant placed in the tube is considered intake; solution returned is recorded as output. Record on the intake and output record. Rinsing promotes cleanliness, infection control, and prepares equipment for the next irrigation.
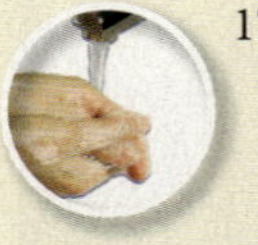 17. Remove gloves and additional PPE, if used. Perform hand hygiene.	Proper removal of PPE reduces the risk for infection transmission and contamination of other items. Hand hygiene prevents transmission of microorganisms.

DOCUMENTATION

Guidelines

Document assessment of the patient's abdomen. Record if the patient's NG tube is clamped or connected to suction, including the type of suction. Document the color and consistency of the NG drainage. Record the solution type and amount used to irrigate the NG tube as well as ease of irrigation or any difficulty related to the procedure. Record the amount of returned irrigant, if collected outside of the suction apparatus. Alternatively, record irrigant amount so it can be subtracted from the total NG drainage amount at the end of the shift. Record the patient's response to the procedure and any pertinent teaching points that were reviewed, such as instructions for the patient to contact the nurse for any feelings of nausea, bloating, or abdominal pain.

Sample Documentation

<u>10/15/25</u> 1100 Abdomen slightly distended but soft; absent bowel sounds, denies nausea. NG tube placement confirmed; aspirate pH 4; exposed NG tube 20 cm, consistent with documented length. NG tube irrigated with 30 mL of normal saline. NG tube reconnected to low intermittent suction. Clear drainage with brown flecks noted from tube. Patient tolerated irrigation without incident.

—S. Essner, RN

DEVELOPING CLINICAL REASONING AND CLINICAL JUDGMENT

UNEXPECTED SITUATIONS AND ASSOCIATED INTERVENTIONS

- *Flush solution is meeting a lot of force when plunger is pushed:* Inject 20 to 30 mL of free air through the NG tube into the stomach in an attempt to reposition the tube and enable flushing of the tube.
- *Tube is connected to suction as prescribed, but nothing is draining from the tube:* First, check the suction canister to ensure that the suction is working appropriately. Disconnect the NG tube from suction and place your gloved thumb over the end of the suction tubing. If there is suction present, the problem lies in the tube itself. Next, attempt to flush the tube to ensure its patency.
- *After flushing the tube, the tube is not reconnected to suction as prescribed:* Reconnect the tube to suction as soon as the error is noticed. Assess the abdomen for distention and ask the patient if they are experiencing any nausea or any abdominal discomfort. Complete any paperwork per institutional policy, such as a variance report.

SPECIAL CONSIDERATIONS

General Considerations

- A one-way, antireflux valve may be used in the airflow lumen to prevent reflux of gastric contents through the airflow lumen (Figure 5). When pressure from gastric contents enters the airflow tubing, the valve closes to prevent secretions from exiting the tube. This valve is removed before flushing the lumen with air and then replaced.
- Check tube placement before administering any fluids, medications, or feeding, using multiple techniques: x-ray, external length, external verification marking, pH testing, and carbon dioxide monitoring (if available). Consistent inability to withdraw fluid from tube may indicate displacement of the tube from the stomach into the esophagus (AACN, 2020).

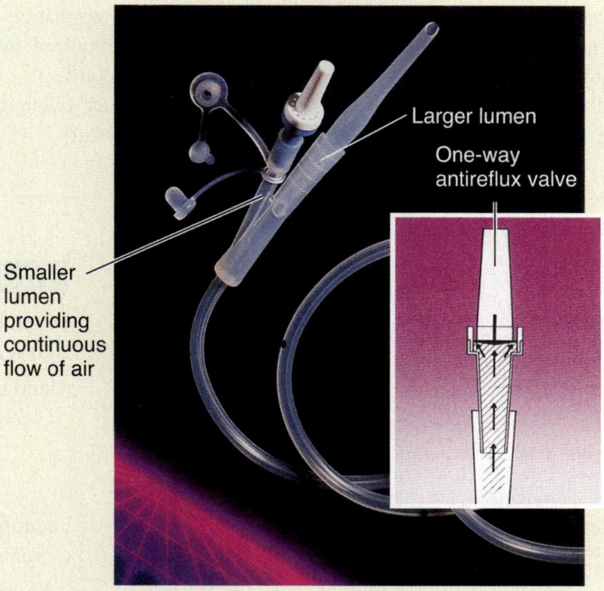

FIGURE 5. Double-lumen nasogastric tube with a one-way antireflux valve in the airflow lumen.

Signs of respiratory distress may be absent in patients with an impaired level of consciousness when NG tubes are inadvertently positioned in the airway (AACN, 2020).

- Sterile water should be used for tube flushes in immunocompromised or critically ill patients (Allen, 2015; Boullata et al., 2017).

(continued on page 1572)

Skill 39-4 Irrigating a Nasogastric Tube Connected to Suction *(continued)*

- Gastric pH ≥6 is of no benefit in predicting tube location in the GI tract or in ruling out tracheopulmonary placement (Boullata et al., 2017).
- Monitoring for carbon dioxide to determine NG tube position and/or dislodgement has been investigated (Hess et al., 2021). This involves the use of a colorimetric end-tidal CO_2 detector to detect the presence of carbon dioxide, which would indicate tube positioning in the patient's airway (Hess et al., 2021). Monitoring for carbon dioxide may be helpful to detect placement of a feeding tube in the tracheobronchial tree (AACN, 2020; Boullata et al., 2017; Hess et al., 2021). However, this technique may be unreliable, as it cannot differentiate placement in the mouth, and carbon dioxide may not be detected when the tube is in the patient's airway if the ports in the tube are occluded (Gilbert & Burns, 2010, as cited in AACN, 2020).

Skill 39-5 Emptying and Changing an Ostomy Appliance

DELEGATION CONSIDERATIONS

Emptying a stoma appliance on an ostomy may be delegated to assistive personnel (AP) as well as to licensed practical/vocational nurses (LPN/LVNs). Changing a stoma appliance on an ostomy may be delegated to an LPN/LVN. The decision to delegate must be based on careful analysis of the patient's needs and circumstances as well as the qualifications of the person to whom the task is being delegated. Refer to the Delegation Guidelines in Appendix A.

EQUIPMENT

- Premoistened disposable washcloths or
  - Basin with warm water
  - Skin cleanser, towel, washcloth
- Toilet tissue or paper towel
- Silicone-based adhesive remover
- Gauze squares
- Skin protectant, such as Skin-Prep™
- One-piece ostomy appliance
- Closure clamp, if required, for appliance
- Stoma measuring guide
- Graduated container, toilet, or bedpan
- Ostomy belt (optional)
- Disposable gloves
- Additional PPE, as indicated
- Small plastic trash bag
- Waterproof disposable pad

IMPLEMENTATION

ACTION	RATIONALE
1. Gather equipment.	Assembling equipment provides for an organized approach to the task.
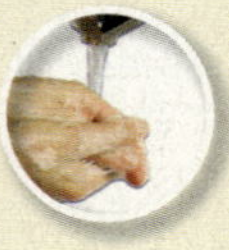 2. Perform hand hygiene and put on PPE, if indicated.	Hand hygiene and PPE prevent the spread of microorganisms. PPE is required based on transmission precautions.
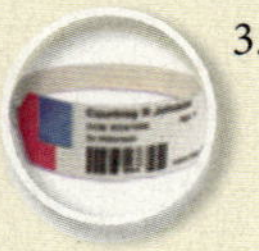 3. Identify the patient.	Identifying the patient ensures the right patient receives the intervention and helps prevent errors.
4. Close the curtains around the bed and close the door to the room, if possible. Explain to the patient what you are going to do and why. Encourage the patient to observe or participate, if possible and as appropriate.	This ensures the patient's privacy. Explanation relieves anxiety and facilitates engagement. Having the patient observe or assist encourages self-acceptance and helps patient develop self-care skills.
5. Assemble equipment on the overbed table or other surface within reach.	Arranging items nearby is convenient, saves time, and avoids unnecessary stretching and twisting of muscles on the part of the nurse.

ACTION	RATIONALE
6. Assist the patient to a comfortable sitting or lying position in bed or a standing or sitting position in the bathroom. If the patient is in bed, adjust the bed to a comfortable working height (VHACEOSH, 2016). Place a waterproof pad under the patient at the stoma site.	Either position should allow the patient to view the procedure in preparation to learn to perform it independently. Lying flat or sitting upright facilitates smooth application of the appliance. Having the bed at the proper height prevents back and muscle strain. A waterproof pad protects linens and the patient from moisture.
Emptying an Appliance	
7. Put on gloves. Remove the clamp (Figure 1) and fold the end of the appliance or pouch upward like a cuff.	Gloves prevent contact with blood, body fluids, and microorganisms. Creating a cuff before emptying prevents additional soiling and odor.
8. Empty the contents into a bedpan, toilet, or measuring device (Figure 2).	Appliances do not need rinsing because rinsing may reduce the appliance's odor barrier.
9. Wipe the lower 2 inches of the appliance or pouch with toilet tissue or a paper towel (Figure 3).	Drying the lower section removes any additional fecal material, thus decreasing odor problems.
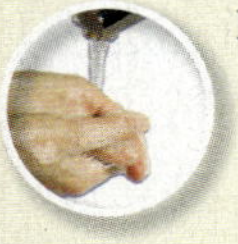 10. Uncuff the edge of the appliance or pouch and apply a clip or clamp, or secure the Velcro closure. Ensure the curve of the clamp follows the curve of the patient's body. Remove gloves. Perform hand hygiene. Assist the patient to a comfortable position.	The edge of the appliance or pouch should remain clean. The clamp secures closure. Hand hygiene deters spread of microorganisms. Positioning ensures patient comfort.
11. If the appliance is not to be changed, place the bed in the lowest position. Remove additional PPE, if used. Perform hand hygiene.	Proper removal of PPE reduces the risk for infection transmission and contamination of other items. Hand hygiene prevents the spread of microorganisms.

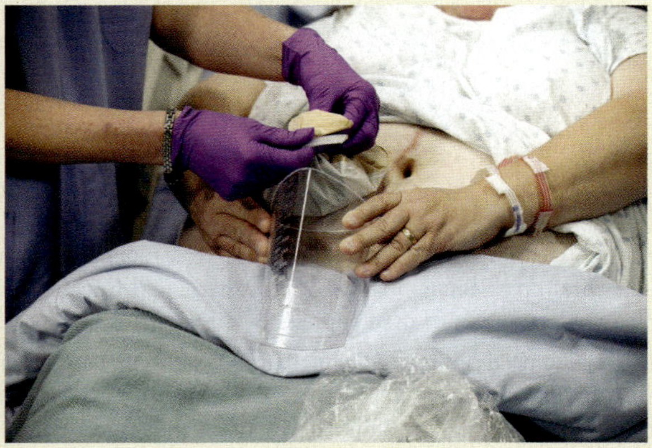

FIGURE 1. Removing clamp, getting ready to empty pouch.

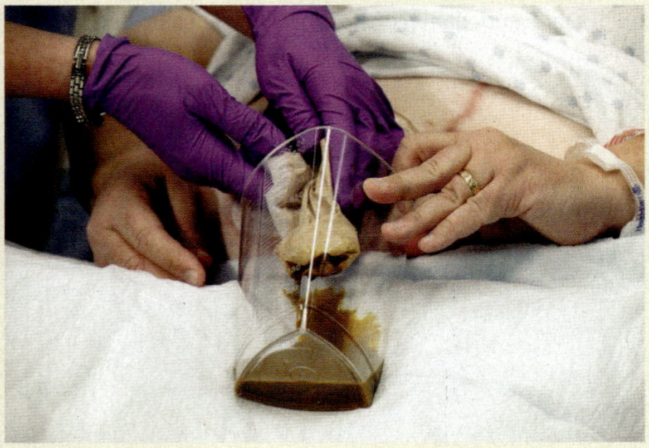

FIGURE 2. Emptying contents of appliance into a measuring device.

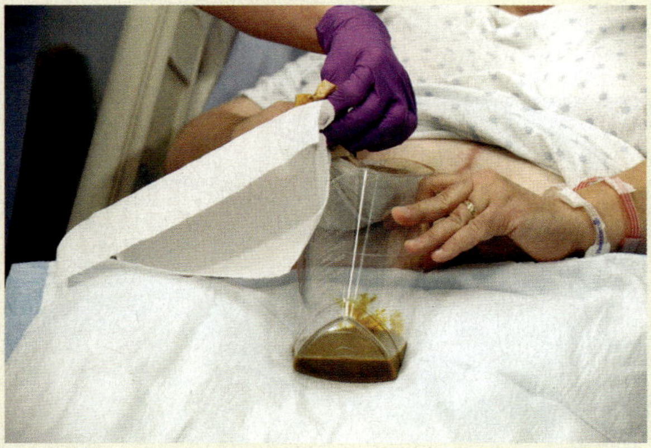

FIGURE 3. Wiping lower 2 inch of pouch with paper towel.

(continued on page 1574)

Skill 39-5 Emptying and Changing an Ostomy Appliance *(continued)*

ACTION	RATIONALE
Changing an Appliance	
12. Place a disposable pad on the work surface. Open the premoistened disposable washcloths or set up the washbasin with warm water and the rest of the supplies. Place a trash bag within reach.	The pad protects the work surface. Organization facilitates performance of the procedure.
13. Put on clean gloves. Place a waterproof pad under the patient at the stoma site. Empty the appliance as described in Steps 7–10.	The pad protects linens and the patient from moisture. Emptying the contents before removal prevents accidental spillage of fecal material.
14. Put on gloves. Use two hands to gently remove the appliance faceplate, starting at the top and keeping the abdominal skin taut. Remove the appliance faceplate from the skin by pushing the skin from the appliance rather than pulling the appliance from the skin (Figure 4). Apply a silicone-based adhesive remover by spraying or wiping with the remover wipe, as indicated.	Gloves prevent contact with blood and body fluids. The seal between the surface of the faceplate and the skin must be broken before the faceplate can be removed. Harsh handling of the appliance can damage the skin and impair the development of a secure seal in the future. A silicone-based adhesive remover loosens the adhesive bond to make removal easier and less likely to damage the skin and is particularly beneficial for patients with fragile skin and those at increased risk for medical adhesive–related skin injury/stripping (Collier, 2019; LeBlanc et al., 2019; Swift et al., 2020).

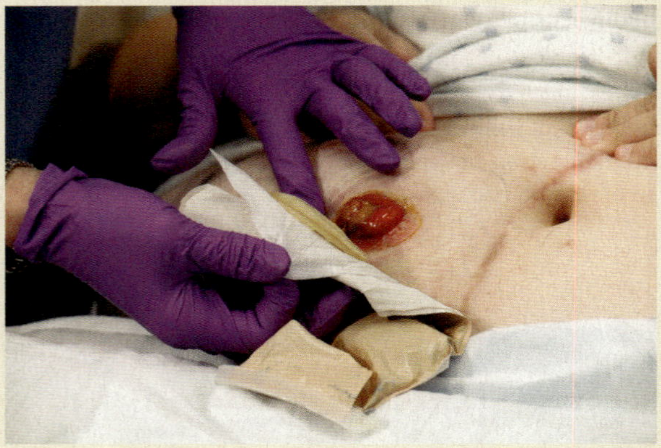

FIGURE 4. Gently removing appliance.

ACTION	RATIONALE
15. Place the appliance in the trash bag, if disposable. If reusable, set it aside to wash in lukewarm soap and water and allow it to air dry after the new appliance is in place.	Thorough cleaning and airing of the appliance reduces odor and deterioration of the appliance. For aesthetic and infection control purposes, discard used appliances appropriately.
16. Use toilet tissue to remove any excess stool from the stoma (Figure 5). Cover the stoma with a gauze pad. Clean the skin around the stoma with skin cleanser and water or a cleansing agent and a washcloth. Remove all old adhesive from the skin; use an adhesive remover, as necessary. Do not apply lotion to the peristomal area.	Toilet tissue, used gently, will not damage the stoma. The gauze absorbs any drainage from the stoma while the skin is being prepared. Cleaning the skin removes excretions, old adhesive, and skin protectant. Excretions or a buildup of other substances can irritate and damage the skin. Lotion will prevent a tight adhesive seal.

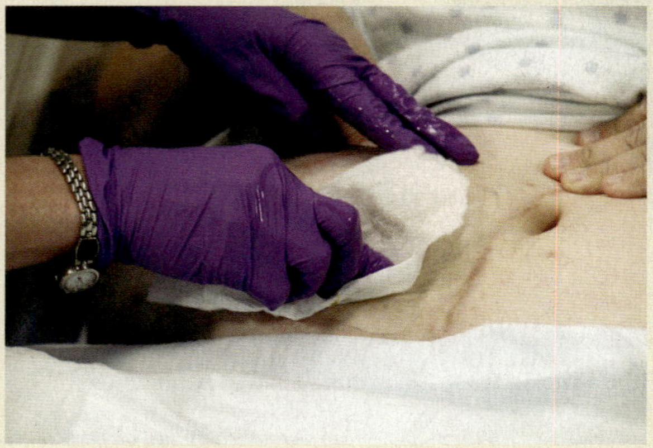

FIGURE 5. Using toilet tissue to remove excess stool from the stoma.

ACTION	RATIONALE
17. Gently pat the area dry. **Make sure the skin around the stoma is thoroughly dry.** Assess the stoma and the condition of the surrounding skin (Figure 6).	Careful drying prevents trauma to the skin and stoma. An intact, properly applied fecal collection device protects skin integrity. Any change in color and size of the stoma may indicate circulatory problems. Refer to Box 39-1.
18. Apply skin protectant/barrier film to a 2-inch (5 cm) radius around the stoma, and allow it to dry completely, which takes about 30 seconds.	The skin needs protection from the excoriating effect of the excretion and potentially from the appliance adhesive (WOCN, 2018). The skin must be perfectly dry before the appliance is placed to get good adherence and to prevent leaks.
19. Lift the gauze squares for a moment and measure the stoma opening, using the measurement guide (Figure 7). Replace the gauze. Trace the same-sized opening on the back center of the appliance (Figure 8). Cut the opening 1/8 inch (2 to 3 mm) larger than the stoma size (Hill, 2020) (Figure 9). Using a finger, gently smooth the wafer edges after cutting.	The appliance should fit snugly around the stoma, with only 1/8 inch of skin visible around the opening. A faceplate opening that is too small can cause trauma to the stoma. If the opening is too large, exposed skin will be irritated by stool. The wafer edges may be uneven after cutting and could cause irritation to, and/or pressure on, the stoma.

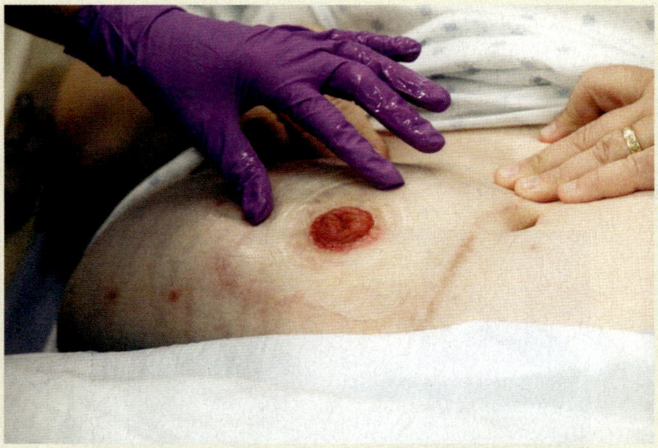

FIGURE 6. Assessing stoma and peristomal skin.

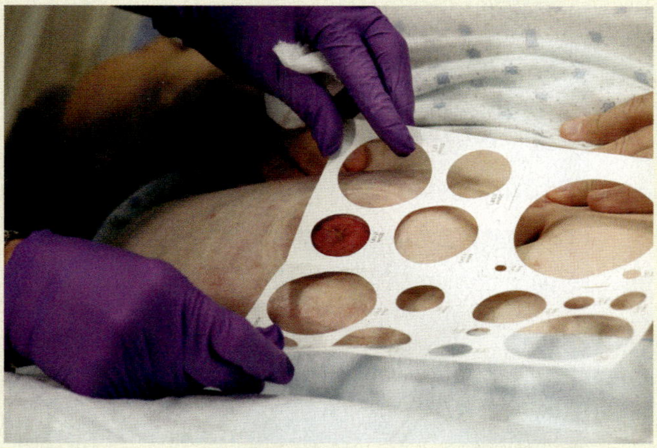

FIGURE 7. Using measurement guide to measure size of stoma.

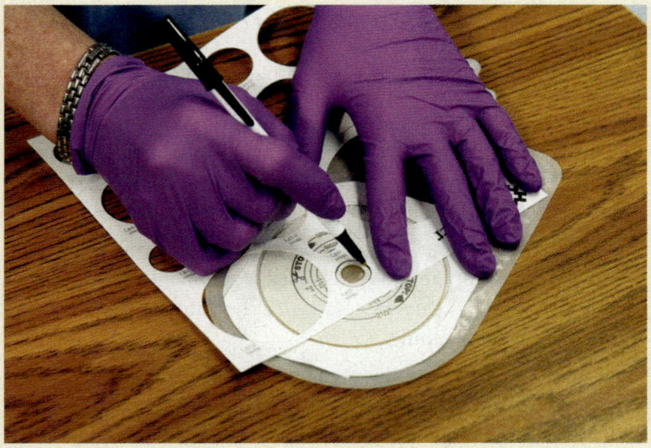

FIGURE 8. Tracing the same-sized circle on back and center of skin barrier.

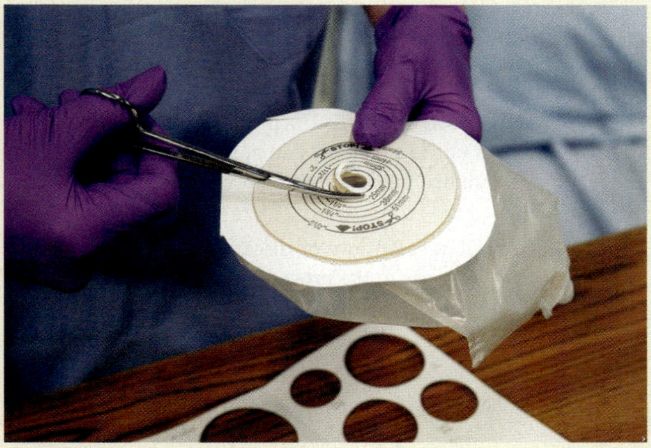

FIGURE 9. Cutting the opening 1/8 inch larger than stoma size.

(continued on page 1576)

Skill 39-5 Emptying and Changing an Ostomy Appliance *(continued)*

ACTION	RATIONALE
20. Remove the paper backing from the appliance faceplate (Figure 10). Quickly remove the gauze squares and ease the appliance over the stoma (Figure 11). Gently press it onto the skin while smoothing over the surface. Apply gentle, even pressure to the appliance for approximately 30 seconds (Burch, 2019a; Hill, 2020).	The appliance is effective only if it is properly positioned and adhered securely. Pressure on the appliance faceplate allows it to mold to the patient's skin and improve adhesion (Burch, 2019a; Hill, 2020).
21. Close the bottom of the appliance or pouch by folding the end upward and using the clamp or clip that comes with the product (Figure 12), or secure the Velcro closure. Ensure the curve of the clamp follows the curve of the patient's body.	A tightly sealed appliance will not leak and cause embarrassment and discomfort for the patient.

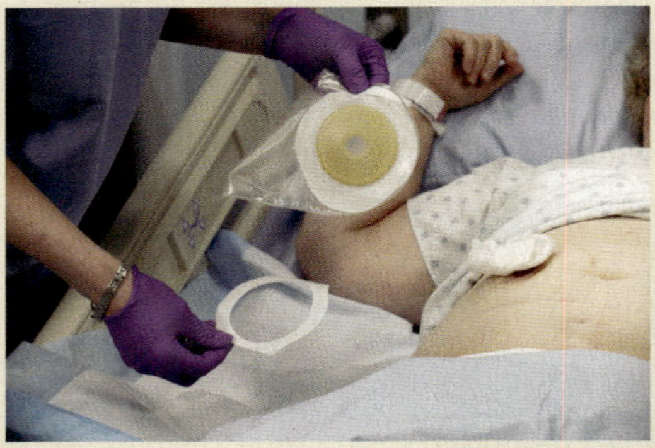

FIGURE 10. Removing paper backing on faceplate.

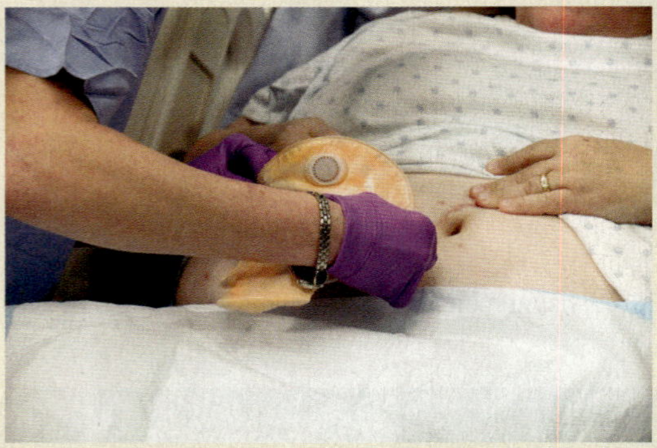

FIGURE 11. Easing appliance over stoma.

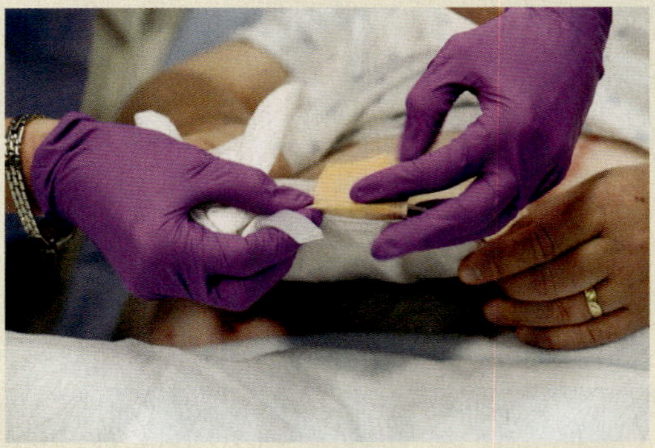

FIGURE 12. Using clip to close bottom of appliance.

ACTION	RATIONALE
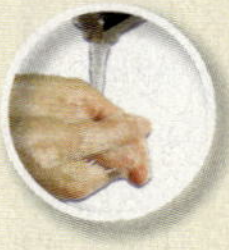 22. Remove gloves. Perform hand hygiene. Assist the patient to a comfortable position. Cover the patient with bed linens. Place the bed in the lowest position.	Removing gloves reduces risk of transmission of microorganisms. Hand hygiene prevents the spread of microorganisms. Covering provides warmth and promotes patient comfort and safety. The bed in the lowest position promotes patient safety.
23. Put on clean gloves. Remove or discard equipment and assess the patient's response to the procedure.	Gloves prevent contact with blood, body fluids, and microorganisms that contaminate the used equipment. The patient's response may indicate acceptance of the ostomy as well as the need for health teaching.
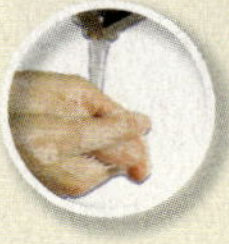 24. Remove gloves and additional PPE, if used. Perform hand hygiene.	Proper removal of PPE reduces the risk for infection transmission and contamination of other items. Hand hygiene prevents the spread of microorganisms.

DOCUMENTATION

Guidelines

Document the appearance of the stoma, the condition of the peristomal skin, characteristics of drainage (amount, color, consistency, unusual odor), the patient's reaction to the procedure, and pertinent patient teaching.

Sample Documentation

DocuCare Practice documenting changing and emptying an ostomy appliance in *Lippincott DocuCare.*

7/22/25 1630 Colostomy appliance changed due to leakage. Stoma is pink, moist, and flat against abdomen. No erythema or excoriation of surrounding skin. Moderate amount of pasty, brown stool noted in bag. Patient asking appropriate questions during appliance application; states, "I'm ready to try changing the next one."

—B. Clapp, RN

DEVELOPING CLINICAL REASONING AND CLINICAL JUDGMENT

UNEXPECTED SITUATIONS AND ASSOCIATED INTERVENTIONS

- *Peristomal skin is excoriated or irritated:* Make sure that the appliance is not cut too large. Skin that is exposed inside of the ostomy appliance will become excoriated. Assess for the presence of a fungal skin infection. If present, consult with the health care team to obtain appropriate treatment. Thoroughly cleanse and dry the skin and apply a product made for excoriated skin before reapplication of the appliance. Allow it to dry completely. Reapply the pouch. Monitor pouch adhesion and change the pouch as soon as there is a break in adhesion. Confer with the health care team for a wound, ostomy, and continence nurse consult to manage these issues. Document the assessment findings and related interventions in the patient's health record.
- *Patient continues to notice odor:* Check the system for any leaks or poor adhesion. Clean the outside of the bag thoroughly when emptying.
- *Bag continues to come loose or fall off:* Thoroughly cleanse the skin and apply a skin barrier. Allow it to dry completely. Reapply the pouch. Monitor pouch adhesion and change the pouch as soon as there is a break in adhesion.
- *Stoma is protruding into bag:* This is called a prolapse. Have the patient rest for 30 minutes. If the stoma is not back to normal size within that time, notify the health care team. If the stoma stays prolapsed, it may twist, resulting in impaired circulation to the stoma.
- *Stoma is dark brown or black:* Stoma should appear pink to red, shiny, and moist. Alterations indicate compromised circulation. If the stoma is dark brown or black, suspect ischemia and necrosis. Notify the health care team immediately.

DEVELOPING CLINICAL REASONING AND CLINICAL JUDGMENT

1. Review the Nursing Care Plan for Jeremy Green on pages 1554–1555.
2. Discuss the appropriate nursing intervention if an assessment revealed the following:
   - Patient has frank blood in stool.
   - Parent reports that child's stool is unusually foul smelling and greasy.
   - Patient's stool is ribbon-like.
   - Patient with cancer and receiving pain medication reports chronic constipation.
   - Teenager reports frequent episodes of diarrhea that leave them weak and dehydrated.
3. A 52-year-old male presents with acute stomach pain and altered bowel elimination: diarrhea. Role-play with another student the interview you would use to assess the patient's bowel elimination status. Identify variables that make you, as either the nurse or patient, uncomfortable talking about elimination. Discuss how you can best address your discomfort.

PRACTICING FOR NCLEX

1. A nurse is performing an abdominal assessment on a patient experiencing frequent bouts of diarrhea. The nurse first observes the contour of the abdomen, noting any masses, scars, or areas of distention. What action will the nurse perform next?
   a. Auscultating the abdomen using an orderly clockwise approach in all abdominal quadrants
   b. Percussing all quadrants of the abdomen in a systematic clockwise manner to identify masses, fluid, or air in the abdomen
   c. Lightly palpating over the abdominal quadrants; first checking for any areas of pain or discomfort
   d. Deeply palpating over the abdominal quadrants, noting muscular resistance, tenderness, organ enlargement, or masses

2. A nurse is administering a large-volume cleansing enema to a patient prior to surgery. When the enema solution is introduced, the patient reports severe cramping. What nursing intervention would the nurse perform next?
   a. Elevating the head of the bed 30 degrees and repositioning the rectal tube
   b. Placing the patient in a supine position and modifying the amount of solution
   c. Lowering the solution container and checking the temperature and flow rate
   d. Removing the rectal tube and notifying the primary care provider
3. A nurse working on a GI unit is caring for a group of patients. In patients with which health problems or issues could the assessment possibly reveal decreased or absent bowel sounds after listening for 2 minutes? Select all that apply.
   a. Peritonitis
   b. Prolonged bedrest
   c. Diarrhea
   d. Gastroenteritis
   e. Early bowel obstruction
   f. Postoperative paralytic ileus
4. A nurse in a long-term care facility is assessing a group of patients. In which patients would the nurse anticipate increased risk for developing diarrhea? Select all that apply.
   a. Patient taking opioids for pain
   b. Patient taking metformin for type 2 diabetes
   c. Patient taking diuretics
   d. Patient who developed dehydration
   e. Patient taking amoxicillin clavulanate for infection
   f. Patient taking magnesium-containing antacids
5. A nurse plans to administer a retention enema to a patient with a fecal impaction. Which nursing action is appropriate for this procedure?
   a. Administering a large volume of solution (500 to 1,000 mL)
   b. Mixing milk and molasses in equal parts for an enema
   c. Instructing the patient to retain the enema for at least 30 minutes
   d. Administering the enema while the patient is sitting on the toilet
6. A nurse prepares to assist a patient with a newly created ileostomy. Which recommended patient teaching points would the nurse stress? Select all that apply.
   a. "When you inspect the stoma, it should be dark purple-blue."
   b. "The size of the stoma will stabilize within 2 weeks."
   c. "Keep the skin around the stoma site clean and moist."
   d. "The stool from an ileostomy is normally liquid."
   e. "Eat dark-green vegetables to control the odor of the stool."
   f. "You may have a tendency to develop food blockages."
7. A nurse is preparing a hospitalized patient for a colonoscopy. Which nursing action is the recommended preparation for this test?
   a. Having the patient consume a low-fiber diet several days before the test
   b. Having the patient take bisacodyl and ingest a gallon oral polyethylene glycol solution (PEG)
   c. Preparing the patient for the use of general anesthesia during the test
   d. Explaining that barium contrast mixture will be given to drink before the test
8. A nurse is performing digital removal of stool on a patient with a fecal impaction. During the procedure, the patient tells the nurse they are feeling dizzy and nauseated and then vomits. What should be the nurse's next action?
   a. Reassuring the patient that this is a normal reaction to the procedure
   b. Stopping the procedure, preparing to administer CPR, and notifying the primary care provider
   c. Stopping the procedure, assessing vital signs, and notifying the health care provider
   d. Pausing the procedure, waiting 5 minutes, and then resuming the procedure
9. A nurse is scheduling tests for a patient who has been experiencing epigastric pain. The health care provider ordered the following tests: (a) barium enema, (b) fecal occult blood test, (c) endoscopic studies, and (d) an upper GI series. What is the correct order for performing the tests?
   a. c, b, d, a
   b. d, c, a, b
   c. a, b, d, c
   d. b, a, d, c
10. A nurse is caring for a patient who had abdominal surgery and has a nasogastric tube attached to low suction. Which nursing actions are appropriate when caring for this patient? Select all that apply.
    a. Irrigating the tube with 30-mL normal saline solution
    b. Confirming tube placement via pH testing of gastric secretions
    c. Positioning the air vent at the level of the patient's umbilicus
    d. Instilling irrigation via the blue air vent
    e. Monitoring the patient's abdomen for distention
    f. Documenting the nasogastric irrigation and drainage with I & O
11. A nurse is planning a bowel program for a patient with frequent constipation after sustaining a spinal cord injury. What is the first step the nurse will take?
    a. Offering a diet that is low in residue
    b. Increasing fluid intake to 3,000 mL daily
    c. Administering daily enemas to stimulate peristalsis
    d. Assessing the patient's bowel patterns

12. A community health nurse is providing an adult education session about colon cancer. Which signs and symptoms of this cancer will the nurse include? Select all that apply.
    a. Blood in the stool
    b. Previous colonoscopy
    c. Passing two large bowel movements daily
    d. Unintentional weight loss
    e. Upper abdominal cramping
    f. Previous opioid use

13. For a patient with which health problem or issue would a nurse expect the health care provider to order colostomy irrigation?
    a. IBS
    b. Left-sided end colostomy in the sigmoid colon
    c. Postradiation damage to the bowel
    d. Crohn disease

14. A nurse is assisting a patient to change an ostomy appliance when they note the stoma is protruding into the bag. What would be the nurse's first action in this situation?
    a. Reassuring the patient that this is a normal with a new ostomy
    b. Notifying the health care provider that the stoma is prolapsed
    c. Having the patient rest for 30 minutes to see if the prolapse resolves
    d. Replacing the appliance with a larger appliance

15. A nurse is caring for an older adult who reports persistent constipation and has a number of laxative prescriptions on the MAR. Which medication would the nurse avoid for this patient?
    a. Saline osmotic laxative
    b. Bulk-forming laxative
    c. Methylcellulose
    d. Stool softener

16. A nurse caring for a patient who reports frequent constipation learns the patient uses phosphate and sodium citrate enemas several times weekly. What education would the nurse provide?
    Electronic Health Record
    PMH: Hypertension, chronic kidney disease
    a. "Avoid consuming fiber or roughage in the diet."
    b. "Sedentary activities will be helpful."
    c. "These enemas should be avoided with kidney failure."
    d. "Restrict your fluids to 1,000 mL daily."

17. A nurse asks a patient for a stool sample to perform the guaiac test. How does the nurse best explain the purpose of this test?
    a. "This test replaces the need for screening colonoscopy."
    b. "We are looking for infectious organisms in your stool."
    c. "The screening assesses for blood in your stool."
    d. "This test assesses for antibodies to colon cancer."

ANSWERS WITH RATIONALES

1. **a.** The sequence for abdominal assessment proceeds from inspection, auscultation, percussion, and then palpation. Inspection and auscultation are performed before palpation because palpation may disturb normal peristalsis and bowel motility.

2. **c.** If the patient reports severe cramping with introduction of an enema solution, the nurse should lower the solution container and check the temperature and flow rate. If the solution is too cold or the flow rate is too fast, severe cramping may occur. The head of the bed may be elevated 30 degrees for the patient's comfort if the patient needs to be placed on a bedpan in the supine position while receiving the enema.

3. **a, b, f.** Decreased or absent bowel sounds—documented only after listening for in the epigastric and umbilical area of the abdomen for 2 minutes or longer (Bickley et al., 2021)—signify the absence of bowel motility, commonly associated with peritonitis, paralytic ileus, and/or prolonged immobility. Hyperactive bowel sounds indicate increased bowel motility, commonly caused by diarrhea, gastroenteritis, or early bowel obstruction.

4. **b, e, f.** Diarrhea is a potential adverse effect of treatment with amoxicillin clavulanate, metformin, or antacids containing magnesium. Opioids, diuretics, and dehydration may lead to constipation.

5. **c.** Instruct the patient to retain the enema solution for at least 30 minutes or as indicated in the manufacturer's instructions. The milk and molasses mixture is a carminative enema that helps to expel flatus. The patient should be instructed to lie on their left side as dictated by patient condition and comfort.

6. **d, e, f.** Ileostomies normally have liquid, foul-smelling stool. The nurse should encourage intake of dark-green vegetables for their chlorophyll content, which helps to deodorize the feces. Explain that patients with ileostomies may tend to develop food blockages, especially when high-fiber foods are consumed. The stoma should be dark pink to red and moist. Stoma size usually stabilizes within 4 to 6 weeks, and the skin around the stoma site (peristomal area) should be kept clean and dry.

7. **a.** If possible, a low-residue diet (low fiber) should be followed several days before the procedure, although some may have a full liquid diet the day before the procedure. There are multiple types of bowel preps for this procedure; the health care provider determines the best regimen for the individual.

   The prep is usually given as a split dose, with half being given the night before and rest the morning of the procedure. It is recommended the second dose be given at least 5 hours before and completed at least 2 hours before the study. Occasionally, some patients may receive the prep the same day as the procedure, especially if it is scheduled for later in the day.

   Conscious sedation, not general anesthesia, will be given for the colonoscopy. A chalky-tasting barium contrast mixture is given to drink before an upper GI and small-bowel series of tests.

8. **c.** When a patient reports dizziness, lightheadedness, nausea, and/or vomiting during digital stool removal, the nurse recognizes the vagus nerve may have been stimulated. The nurse

should stop the procedure, assess heart rate and blood pressure, and notify the health care provider.

9. **d.** A fecal occult blood test is performed first to detect GI bleeding. Lower GI barium studies should be performed next to visualize GI structures and reveal any inflammation, ulcers, tumors, strictures, or other lesions. A barium enema and routine radiography should precede an upper GI series because retained barium from an upper GI series could take several days to pass through the GI tract and obscure anatomic detail on the barium enema studies. Noninvasive procedures usually take precedence over invasive procedures, such as endoscopic studies, when sufficient diagnostic data can be obtained from them.

10. **a, b, d, e, f.** Care of a patient with an NG tube connected to suction includes verifying placement before administration of any fluids or medications to avoid aspiration. Radiographic evidence of the tip of the tube in the stomach, measurement of tube length, measurement of tube marking, measurement of aspirate pH, and carbon dioxide monitoring may be used. The nurse irrigates the tube with 30 mL of saline solution (or as prescribed/ per policy) with an irrigating syringe. The nurse separates the tube from the suction device, clamps the NG tube to prevent gastric secretions from leaking, and places the tip of the syringe in the tube to gently insert the saline solution. The nurse should not place irrigant in the blue air vent of a Salem sump or double-lumen tube; rather, the nurse should instill air through the vent. The air vent decreases any pressure that has built up in the stomach during suction; instilling air promotes drainage. The air vent should be placed above the stomach. Abdominal distention may indicate lack of proper drainage or delayed return of GI function. The nurse documents all irrigation and NG tube output with the I & O. If the nurse allows the irrigant to drain out, that is excluded from intake.

11. **d.** The nurse follows the steps of the nursing process to plan care. First the nurse assesses the patient's bowel movements including frequency, consistency, shape, volume, and color. Based on the assessment findings, the nurse may recommend 3 of fluid daily or administer an enema, as appropriate. The nurse also monitors bowel sounds, teaches about specific foods that promote bowel regularity, ensures privacy, and encourages adequate fluid intake.

12. **a, d.** The nurse discusses signs and symptoms of colon cancer including rectal bleeding or blood in the stool, persistent change in bowel pattern or consistency of stool, persistent cramping or pain in lower abdomen (or gas), a feeling of incomplete bowel emptying, weakness or fatigue, and unintentional weight loss.

13. **b.** Irrigations are used to promote regular evacuation of distal colostomies. Colostomy irrigation may be indicated in patients who have a left-sided end colostomy in the descending or sigmoid colon, are mentally alert, have adequate vision, and have adequate manual dexterity needed to perform the procedure. Contraindications include IBS, peristomal hernia, postradiation damage to the bowel, diverticulitis, and Crohn disease (Kent et al., 2015).

14. **c.** If the stoma protrudes into the bag after changing the ostomy appliance, the nurse should have the patient rest for 30 minutes. If the stoma is not back to normal size within that time, notify the health care provider. If the stoma stays prolapsed, it may twist, resulting in impaired circulation to the stoma.

15. **a.** Certain saline osmotic laxatives can lead to fluid and electrolyte imbalances and should not be used in older adults and those with kidney or cardiac disease.

16. **c.** Hypertonic phosphate and sodium citrate solution enemas are avoided in patients with renal impairment or reduced renal clearance due to their inability to adequately excrete phosphate. This can result in hyperphosphatemia (Dougherty & Lister, 2015, as cited in Mitchell, 2019b, p. 154).

17. **c.** The guaiac fecal occult blood testing (FOBT) is used to detect occult blood in the stool. It is used for initial/early screening for disorders such as cancer and for GI bleeding in conditions such as ulcer disease, inflammatory bowel disorders, and intestinal polyps (MedlinePlus, 2020). A positive FOBT result indicates that abnormal bleeding is occurring somewhere in the digestive tract.

Bibliography

Allen, S. M. (2015). As a flushing agent for enteral nutrition, does sterile water compared to tap water affect the associated risk of infection in critically ill patients? *The Alabama Nurse, 42*(1), 5–6.

American Academy of Pediatrics (AAP). (n.d.). *Toilet training. Practice guide.* https://www.aap.org/en-us/advocacy-and-policy/aap-health-initiatives/practicing-safety/Pages/Toilet-Training.aspx

American Association of Critical Care Nurses (AACN). (2020). *AACN practice alert. Initial and ongoing verification of feeding tube placement in adults.* https://www.aacn.org/

American Cancer Society. (2019, October 16). *Caring for a colostomy.* https://www.cancer.org/treatment/treatments-and-side-effects/treatment-types/surgery/ostomies/colostomy/management.html

American Cancer Society. (2020). *Colorectal cancer screening tests.* https://www.cancer.org/cancer/colon-rectal-cancer/detection-diagnosis-staging/screening-tests-used.html

American Cancer Society. (2021). *Do I have colorectal cancer? Signs, symptoms and work-up.* https://www.cancer.org/latest-news/signs-and-symptoms-of-colon-cancer.html

American Society for Gastrointestinal Endoscopy. (2020). *Understanding capsule endoscopy.* https://www.asge.org/home/for-patients/patient-information/understanding-capsule-endoscopy

Anderson, L. (2018). Fine-bore nasogastric tube feeding: Reducing the risks. *British Journal of Nursing, 27*(12), 674–675.

Anderson, L. (2019). Enteral feeding tubes: An overview of nursing care. *British Journal of Nursing, 28*(12), 748–754. https://doi.org/10.12968/bjon.2019.28.12.748

Andrews, M., Boyle, J. S., & Collins, J. (2020). *Transcultural concepts in nursing care* (8th ed.). Wolters Kluwer.

A-Rahim, Y. I., & Falchuk, M. (2021). UpToDate. *Bowel preparation before colonoscopy in adults.* Wolters Kluwer. https://www.uptodate.com/contents/bowel-preparation-before-colonoscopy-in-adults

Backer, H. D., & Hill, V. (2019). Chapter 2. Preparing international travelers. Water disinfection. In G. W. Brunette and J. B. Nemhauser (Eds.), *CDC Yellow Book 2020. Health information for international travel.* Oxford University Press. https://wwwnc.cdc.gov/travel/yellowbook/2020/preparing-international-travelers/water-disinfection

Baranoski, S., & Ayello, E. A. (2020). *Wound care essentials. Practice principles* (5th ed.). Wolters Kluwer.

Bauldoff, G., Gubrud, P., & Carno, M. A. (2020). *LeMone and Burke's Medical-surgical nursing: Clinical reasoning in patient care* (7th ed.). Pearson.

Beeckman, S., Campbell, J., Campbell, K., Chimentão, D., Coyer, F., Domansky, R., Gray, M., Hevia, H., Junkin, J., Karadag, A., Kottner, J., Long, M. A., McNichol, L., Meaume, S., Nix, D., Sabasse, M., Sanada, H., Yu, P. J., Voegeli, D., & Wang, L. (2015). Proceedings of the Global IAD Expert Panel. Best Practice Principles. Incontinence-associated dermatitis: Moving prevention forward. Addressing evidence gaps for best practice. *Wounds International 2015.* https://www.woundsinternational.com/resources/details/incontinence-associated-dermatitis-moving-prevention-forward

Berti-Hearn, L., & Elliott, B. (2019). Ileostomy care. A guide for home care clinicians. *Home Healthcare Now, 37*(3), 136–144. https://doi.org/10.1097/NHH.0000000000000776

Bickley, L. S., Szilagyi, P. G., & Hoffman, R. M. (2021). *Bates' guide to physical examination and history taking* (13th ed.). Wolters Kluwer.

Bird, A. (2020). Stoma care accessory products: Responsible prescribing and cost-effective use. *Gastrointestinal Nursing, 18*(5), 13–16. https://doi.org/10.12968/gasn.2020.18.5.13

Bird, A., Wilson, K., Bertinara, A., & Amos, L. (2019). Educating patients in stoma care. *Gastrointestinal Nursing, 17*(3), 18–22. https://doi.org/10.12968/gasn.2019.17.3.18

Bischoff, S. C., Austin, P., Boeykens, K., Chourdakis, M., Cuerda, C., Jonkers-Schuitema, C., Lichota, M., Nyulasi, I., Schneider, S. M., Stanga, Z., Pironi, L. (2020). ESPEN guideline on home enteral nutrition. *Clinical Nutrition, 39*(1), 5–22. https://doi.org/10.1016/j.clnu.2019.04.022

Blevins, S. (2019). Colostomy care. *MEDSURG Nursing, 28*(2), 125–126.

Boeykens, K., Steeman, E., & Dyusburgh, I. (2014). Reliability of pH measurement and the auscultatory method to confirm the position of a nasogastric tube. *International Journal of Nursing Studies, 51*(11), 1427–1433. https://doi.org/10.1016/j.ijnurstu.2014.03.004

Boeykens, K. (2018). Verification of blindly inserted nasogastric feeding tubes: A review of different test methods. *Journal of Perioperative & Critical Intensive Care Nursing, 4*(3). DOI: 10.4172/2471-9870.10000145

Boruchoff, S. E., & Weinstein, M. P. (2019). UpToDate. *Microbiology specimen collection and transport.* Wolters Kluwer. https://www.uptodate.com/contents/microbiology-specimen-collection-and-transport?source=search_result&search=stool%20specimen&selectedTitle=1~150

Boullata, J. I., Carrera, A. L., Harvey, L., Escuro, A. A., Hudson, L., Mays, A., Wessel, J. J., Bajpai, S., Beebe, M. L., Kinn, T. J., Klang, M. G., Lord, L., Martin, K., Pompeii-Wolfe, C., Sullivan, J., Wood, A., Malone, A., & Guenter, P., & ASPEN Safe Practices for Enteral Nutrition Therapy, American Society for Parenteral and Enteral Nutrition. (2017). ASPEN safe practices for enteral nutrition therapy. *Journal of Parenteral and Enteral Nutrition, 41*(1), 15–103. https://doi.org/10.1177/0148607116673053

Brewer, C. (2018). Food- and water-borne diseases in travellers. *Practice Nursing, 29*(10), 473–477. https://doi.org/10.12968/pnur.2018.29.10.473

Burch, J. (2018). Stoma-related complications and treatments. *Nursing & Residential Care, 20*(9), 430–433. https://doi.org/10.12968/nrec.2018.20.9.430

Burch, J. (2019a). Supporting residents to care for a stoma independently. *Nursing & Residential Care, 21*(5), 276–280. https://doi.org/10.12968/nrec.2019.21.5.276

Burch, J. (2019b). Peristomal skin care considerations for community nurses. *British Journal of Community Nursing, 24*(9), 414–418. https://doi.org/10.12968/bjcn.2019.24.9.414

Burgess-Stocks, J. (2020). *Eating with an ostomy A comprehensive nutrition guide for those living with an ostomy.* United Ostomy Associations of America. https://www.ostomy.org/wp-content/uploads/2020/07/Eating_with_an_Ostomy_2020-07.pdf

Burns, S. M., & Delgado, S. A. (2019). *AACN essentials of critical care nursing* (4th ed.). McGraw Hill Education.

Butler, D. L. (2009). Early postoperative complications following ostomy surgery. *Journal of Wound, Ostomy and Continence Nursing, 36*(5), 513–519.

Byfield, D. (2020). The lived experiences of persons with ostomies attending a support group. A qualitative study. *Journal of Wound, Ostomy & Continence Nursing, 47*(5), 489–495. https://doi.org/10.1097/WON.0000000000000696

Cave, D. (2021). UpToDate. *Wireless video capsule endoscopy.* Wolters Kluwer. https://www.uptodate.com/contents/wireless-video-capsule-endoscopy?source=search_result&search=small%20bowel%20capsule&selectedTitle=1~150

Centers for Disease Control and Prevention (CDC). (2016). *Hygiene-related diseases. Chronic diarrhea.* https://www.cdc.gov/healthywater/hygiene/disease/chronic_diarrhea.html

Centers for Disease Control and Prevention (CDC). (2020a). *C. diff (Clostridioides difficile).* Your risk of *C. diff.* https://www.cdc.gov/cdiff/risk.html

Centers for Disease Control and Prevention (CDC). (2020b). *C diff (Clostridioides difficile). FAQs for clinicians about C. diff.* https://www.cdc.gov/cdiff/clinicians/faq.html

Centers for Disease Control and Prevention (CDC). (2020c). *Four steps to food safety: Clean, separate, cook, chill.* https://www.cdc.gov/foodsafety/keep-food-safe.html

Centers for Disease Control and Prevention (CDC). (2020d). How to prevent food poisoning. https://www.cdc.gov/foodsafety/prevention.html

Centers for Disease Control and Prevention (CDC). (2021). Colorectal cancer screening continuing education. CRC screening and surveillance: Optimizing quality. Section 3: The role of primary care providers in the delivery of high-quality colonoscopy. https://www.cdc.gov/cancer/colorectal/quality/CRC_Screening_Optimizing_Quality_Primary_Care3.pdf

Chandler, P. (2015). Preventing and treating peristomal skin conditions in stoma patients. *British Journal of Community Nursing, 20*(8), 386–388. https://doi.org/10.12968/bjcn.2015.20.8.386

Chandler, P. (2020). Lesbian, gay, bisexual and transgender (LGBT) inclusion in nursing services: A reflective case study from stoma care. *European Wound, Ostomy and Continence, 18*(Suppl 9), S26–S32. https://doi.org/10.12968/gasn.2020.18.Sup9.S26

Cinar, F. I., Yilmaz, F., Seven, M., Cinar, M., & Gumral, R. (2014). Stool specimen collection: nurses' and patients' perspectives. *International Journal of Caring Sciences, 7*(3), 889–897.

Cincinnati Children's. (2018). *Enema administration.* https://www.cincinnatichildrens.org/health/e/enema

Cleveland Clinic. (2016). *Colostomy irrigation.* https://my.clevelandclinic.org/health/treatments/10747-colostomy-irrigation

Cleveland Clinic. (2020a). *Probiotics.* https://my.clevelandclinic.org/health/articles/14598-probiotics

Cleveland Clinic. (2020b). *Gas.* https://my.clevelandclinic.org/health/diseases/7314-gas

Collier, M. (2019). Minimising pain and medical adhesive related skin injuries in vulnerable patients. *British Journal of Nursing, 28*(15), S26–S32. doi: 10.12968/bjon.2019.28.15.S26

Colon Cancer Coalition. (n.d.). *Colon cancer symptoms.* Retrieved February 27, 2021, from https://coloncancercoalition.org/get-educated/what-you-need-to-know/colon-cancer-symptoms/

Colorectal Cancer Alliance. (2019a). *Guaiac fecal occult blood test.* https://www.ccalliance.org/screening-prevention/screening-methods/guaiac-fecal-occult-blood-test

Colorectal Cancer Alliance. (2019b). *Fecal immunochemical test.* https://www.ccalliance.org/screening-prevention/screening-methods/fecal-immunochemical-test

Colwell, J. C., Bain, K. A., Hansen, A. S., Droste, W., Vendelbo, G., & James-Reid, S. (2019). International consensus results. Development of practice guidelines for assessment of peristomal body and stoma profiles, patient engagement, and patient follow-up. *Journal of Wound, Ostomy and Continence Nursing, 46*(6), 497–504. https://doi.org/10.1097/WON.0000000000000599

Connor, B. A. (2019). Chapter 2. Preparing international travelers. Traveler's diarrhea. In G. W. Brunette and J. B. Nemhauser (Eds.), *CDC yellow book 2020: Health information for international travel.* Oxford University Press. https://wwwnc.cdc.gov/travel/page/yellowbook-home

Continence Product Advisor. (2021). *Faecal devices. Products for faecal incontinence.* https://www.continenceproductadvisor.org/faecaldevices

Dias, F. S. B., Almeida, B. P., Alvares, B. R., Jales, R. M., Caldas, J. P. S., & Carmona, E. V. (2019). Use of pH reagent strips to verify gastric tube placement in newborns. *Revista Latino-Americana de Enfermagem, 27*, 1–8. https://doi.org/10.1590/1518-8345.3150.3227

Díaz, C. C., Zambrano, S. M. H., Muñoz, B. M., Crisol, I. S., Marfil, M. N. P., Montoya-Juárez, R., & Montoro, C. H. (2018). Stoma care nurses' perspectives on the relative significance of factors influencing ostomates' quality of life. *Gastrointestinal Nursing, 16*(3), 28–33. https://doi.org/10.12968/gasn.2018.16.3.28

Doubeni, C. (2020). UpToDate. *Tests for screening for colorectal cancer.* Wolters Kluwer. https://www.uptodate.com/contents/tests-for-screening-for-colorectal-cancer

Drummond Hayes, K. (2018). Best practices for unclogging feeding tubes in adults. *Nursing, 48*(6), 66 DOI-10.1097/01.NURSE.0000532744.80506.5e

Dudek, S. (2022). *Nutrition essentials for nursing practice* (9th ed.). Wolters Kluwer.

Dunlap, J. J. (2021). Assessing chronic diarrhea. *Gastroenterology Nursing, 44*(1), 60–63. https://doi.org/10.1097/SGA.0000000000000579

Dunlap, J. J., & Paterson, S. (2020). Assessing acute diarrhea. *Gastroenterology Nursing, 43*(5), 390–393. https://doi.org/10.1097/SGA.0000000000000560

Ellett, M. L., Cohen, M. D., Perkins, S. M., Croffie, J. M., Lane, K. A., & Austin, J. K. Comparing methods of determining insertion length for placing gastric tubes in children 1 month to 17 years of age. *Journal for Specialists in Pediatric Nursing, 17*(1), 19–32. doi.org/10.1111/j.1744-6155.2011.00302.x

Eliopoulos, C. (2018). *Gerontological nursing* (9th ed.). Wolters Kluwer Health.

European Pressure Ulcer Advisory Panel (EPUAP), National Pressure Injury Advisory Panel (NPIAP), and Pan Pacific Pressure Injury Alliance (PPPIA). Haesler, E. (Ed). (2019). *Prevention and treatment of pressure ulcers/injuries: Clinical Practice guideline. The international guideline.* http://www.internationalguideline.com/

Falcón, B. S., López, M. B., Muñoz, B. M., Sánchez, A. Á., & Rey, E. (2016). Fecal impaction: A systematic review of its medical complications. *BMC Geriatrics, 16*(4). https://doi.org/10.1186/s12877-015-0162-5

Fan, P. E. M., Tan, S. B., Farah, G. I., Cheok, P. G., Cheok, P. G., Chock, W.T., Sutha, W., Xu, D., Chua, W., Kwan, X. L., Li, Ch. L., Teo, W. Q., & Ang, S. Y. (2019). Adequacy of different measurement methods in determining nasogastric tube insertion lengths: An observational study. *International Journal of Nursing Studies, 92*, 73–78. https://doi.org/10.1016/j.ijnurstu.2019.01.003

Fichera, A. (2021). *Restorative proctocolectomy with ileal pouch-anal anastomosis: Laparoscopic approach.* UpToDate. https://www.uptodate.com/contents/restorative-proctocolectomy-with-ileal-pouch-anal-anastomosis-laparoscopic-approach#:~:text=A%20restorative%20proctocolectomy%20with%20ileal,-pelvic%20reservoir%20for%20intestinal%20contents.

Fischbach, F. T., & Fischbach, M. A. (2018). *A manual of laboratory and diagnostic tests* (10th ed.). Wolters Kluwer.

Fisher, P., & Himan, C. (2020). Moisture-associated skin damage: A skin issue more prevalent than pressure ulcers. *Wounds UK, 16*(1), 58–63.

Francis, K. (2018). Incontinence-associated dermatitis: Management update. *American Nurse Today, 13*(1), 25–27.

Goldberg, M., Colwell, J., Burns, S., Carmel, J., Fellows, J., Hendren, S., Livingston, V., Nottingham, C. U., Pittman, J., Rafferty, J., Salvadalena, G., Steinberg, G., & Wound, Ostomy and Continence Nurses Society. Guideline Development Task Force. (2018). WOCN Society Clinical Guideline. Management of the adult patient with a fecal or urinary ostomy – An executive summary. *Journal of Wound, Ostomy and Continence Nursing, 45*(1), 50–58. https://doi.org/doi:10.1097/WON.0000000000000396

Gray, M., & Guiliano, K. K. (2018). Incontinence-associated dermatitis, characteristics and relationship to pressure injury: A multisite epidemiologic analysis. *Journal of Wound, Ostomy & Continence Nursing, 45*(10), 63–67. https://doi.org/10.1097/WON.0000000000000390

Griffin, P. M., & Hill, V. (2019). Chapter 2. Preparing international travelers. Food & water precautions. In G. W. Brunette and J. B. Nemhauser (Eds.), *CDC yellow book 2020: Health information for international travel.* Oxford University Press. https://wwwnc.cdc.gov/travel/page/yellowbook-home

Gump, K., & Schmelzer, M. (2016). Gaining control over fecal incontinence. *Medsurg Nursing, 25*(2), 97–102.

Hess, D. R., MacIntyre, N. R., Galvin, W. F., & Mishoe, S. C. (2021). *Respiratory care. Principles and practice* (4th ed.). Jones & Bartlett Learning.

Hill, B. (2020). Stoma care: Procedures, appliances, and nursing considerations. *British Journal of Nursing, 29*(22), S14–S19. https://doi.org/10.12968/bjon.2020.29.22.s14

Hillery, S. (2019). Caring for patients with urinary incontinence-associated dermatitis. *British Journal of Nursing, 28*(9), S26–S28. https://doi.org/10.12968/bjon.2019.28.9.S26

Hinkle, J. L., Cheever, K. H., & Overbaugh, K. J. (2022). *Brunner & Suddarths's Textbook of medical-surgical nursing* (15th ed.). Wolters Kluwer.

Hodin, R. A., & Bordeianou, L. (2020). *UpToDate. Inpatient placement and management of nasogastric and nasoenteric tubes in adults.* Wolters Kluwer. https://www.uptodate.com/contents/inpatient-placement-and-management-of-nasogastric-and-nasoenteric-tubes-in-adults

Hsu, M. Y., Lin, J. P., Hsu, H. H., Lai, H. L., & Wu, Y. L. (2020). Preoperative stoma site marking decreases stoma and peristomal complications. A meta-analysis. *Journal of Wound, Ostomy and Continence Nursing, 47*(3), 249–256. DOI: 10.1097/WON.0000000000000634

International Continence Society (ICS). (2015). *International Continence Society (ICS). Fact sheets. A background to urinary and faecal incontinence.* https://www.ics.org/search?q=fact%20sheet

International Council of Nurses (ICN). (2019). *Nursing diagnosis and outcome statements.* https://www.icn.ch/sites/default/files/inline-files/ICNP2019-DC.pdf

Irving, S. Y., Rempel, G., Lyman, B., Sevilla, W. M. A., Northington, L., Guenter, P., & The American Society for Parenteral and Enteral Nutrition. (2018). Pediatric nasogastric tube placement and verification: Best practice recommendations from the NOVEL Project. *Nutrition in Clinical Practice, 33*(6), 921–927. https://doi.org/10.1002/ncp.10189

Jacobson, T. M., & Wright, T. (2015). Improving quality by taking aim at incontinence-associated dermatitis in hospitalized adults. *Medsurg Nursing, 24*(3), 151–157.

Jarvis, C., & Echkardt, A. (2020). *Physical examination & health assessment* (8th ed.). Elsevier.

Jensen, S. (2019). *Nursing health assessment. A best practice approach* (3rd ed.). Wolters Kluwer.

Judd, M. (2020). Confirming nasogastric tube placement in adults. *Nursing, 50*(4), 43–46. https://doi.org/10.1097/01.NURSE.0000654032.78679.f1

Kantrancha, E. D., & George, N. M. (2014). Postoperative ileus. *Medsurg Nursing, 23*(6), 387–413.

Karch, A. M. (2020). *Focus on nursing pharmacology* (8th ed.). Wolters Kluwer.

Kent, D. J., Long, M. A., & Bauer, C. (2015). Does colostomy irrigation affect functional outcomes and quality of life in persons with a colostomy? *Journal of Wound, Ostomy & Continence Nursing, 42*(2), 155–161. https://doi.org/10.1097/WON.0000000000000121

Kiela, P. R., & Ghishan, F. K. (2016). Physiology of intestinal absorption and secretion. *Best Practice & Research Clinical Gastroenterology, 30*(2), 145–159. https://doi.org/10.1016/j.bpg.2016.02.007

Kyle, T., & Carman, S. (2021). *Essentials of pediatric nursing* (4th ed.). Wolters Kluwer.

Lachenbruch, C., Ribble, D., Emmons, K., & VanGilder, C. (2016). Pressure ulcer risk in the incontinent patient: Analysis of incontinence and hospital-acquired pressure ulcers from the International Pressure Ulcer Prevalence Survey. *Journal of Wound Ostomy and Continence Nursing, 43*(3), 1–7. https://doi.org/10.1097/WON.0000000000000225

Lacy, B. E., Mearin, F., Chang, L., Chey, W. D., Lembo, A. J., Simren, M., & Spiller, R. (2016). Bowel disorders. *Gastroenterology, 150*(6), 1393–1407. http://dx.doi.org/10.1053/j.gastro.2016.02.031

Landmann, R. G., & Cashman, A. L. (2020). UpToDate. *Ileostomy or colostomy care and complications.* Wolters Kluwer. https://www.uptodate.com/contents/ileostomy-or-colostomy-care-and-complications

LaRocque, R., & Harris, J. B. (2020). UpToDate. *Approach to the adult with acute diarrhea in resource-rich settings.* Wolters Kluwer. https://www.uptodate.com/contents/approach-to-the-adult-with-acute-diarrhea-in-resource-rich-settings?source=machineLearning&search=chronic%20diarrhea%20treatment&selectedTitle=3~150&sectionRank=1&anchor=H13#H224267459

LeBlanc, K., Whiteley, I., McNichol, L., Salfadalena, G., & Gray, M. (2019). Peristomal medical adhesive-related skin injury. Results of an international consensus meeting. *Journal of Wound, Ostomy and Continence Nursing, 46*(2), 125–136. DOI: 10.1097/WON.0000000000000513

Lim, Y. S. L., & Carville, K. (2019). Prevention and management of incontinence-associated dermatitis in the pediatric population. An integrative review. *Journal of Wound Ostomy and Continence Nursing, 46*(1), 30–37. http://dx.doi.org/10.1097/WON.0000000000000490

Mak, M. Y., & Tam, G. (2020). Ultrasonography for nasogastric tube placement verification: An additional reference. *British Journal of Community Nursing, 25*(7), 328–334. http://dx.doi.org/10.12968/bjcn.2020.25.7.328

Mayo Foundation for Medical Education and Research (MFMER). (2019a). *Traveler's diarrhea.* https://www.mayoclinic.org/diseases-conditions/travelers-diarrhea/symptoms-causes/syc-20352182

Mayo Foundation for Medical Education and Research (MFMER). (2019b). *Diseases and conditions. Constipation.* https://www.mayoclinic.org/diseases-conditions/constipation/symptoms-causes/syc-20354253

Mayo Foundation for Medical Education and Research (MFMER). (2020a). *Stool color: When to worry.* https://www.mayoclinic.org/stool-color/expert-answers/faq-20058080

Mayo Foundation for Medical Education and Research (MFMER). (2020b). *E. coli.* https://www.mayoclinic.org/diseases-conditions/e-coli/symptoms-causes/syc-20372058

Mayo Foundation for Medical Education and Research (MFMER). (2020c). *Diarrhea.* https://www.mayoclinic.org/diseases-conditions/diarrhea/symptoms-causes/syc-20352241

Mayo Foundation for Medical Education and Research (MFMER). (2020d). *Belching, gas and bloating: Tips for reducing them.* https://www.mayoclinic.org/diseases-conditions/gas-and-gas-pains/in-depth/gas-and-gas-pains/art-20044739

Mayo Foundation for Medical Education and Research (MFMER). (2020e). Ostomy: Adapting to life after colostomy, ileostomy or urostomy. https://www.mayoclinic.org/diseases-conditions/colon-cancer/in-depth/ostomy/art-20045825

Mayo Foundation for Medical Education and Research (MFMER). (2020f). *Support groups: Make connections, get help.* https://www.mayoclinic.org/healthy-lifestyle/stress-management/in-depth/support-groups/art-20044655

Mayo Foundation for Medical Education and Research (MFMER). (2021). *Laxative (rectal route).* https://www.mayoclinic.org/drugs-supplements/laxative-rectal-route/proper-use/drg-20070715

MedlinePlus. (2020). *Fecal occult blood test (FOBT).* U.S. National Library of Medicine. https://medlineplus.gov/lab-tests/fecal-occult-blood-test-fobt/

MedlinePlus. (2021). *Bowel retraining.* U.S. National Library of Medicine. https://medlineplus.gov/ency/article/003971.htm

MedlinePlus. (2022a). *Fecal impaction.* U.S. National Library of Medicine. https://medlineplus.gov/ency/article/000230.htm#:~:text=A%20fecal%20impaction%20is%20a,constipated%20for%20a%20long%20time.

MedlinePlus. (2022b). *Stool guaiac test.* U.S. National Library of Medicine. https://medlineplus.gov/ency/article/003393.htm

Memorial Sloan Kettering Cancer Center. (2019). *Diet guidelines for people with an ileostomy.* https://www.mskcc.org/cancer-care/patient-education/diet-guidelines-people-ileostomy

Metheny, N. A., Krieger, M. M., Healey, F., & Meert, K. L. (2019). A review of guidelines to distinguish between gastric and pulmonary placement of nasogastric tubes. *Heart & Lung, 48*(3), 226–235. https://doi.org/10.1016/j.hrtlng.2019.01.003

Mitchell, A. (2019a). Carrying out a holistic assessment of a patient with constipation. *British Journal of Nursing, 28*(4), 230–232. https://doi.org/10.12968/bjon.2019.28.4.230

Mitchell, A. (2019b). Administering an enema: Indications, types, equipment and procedure. *British Journal of Nursing, 28*(3), 154–156. https://doi.org/10.12968/bjon.2019.28.3.154

Mitchell, A. (2019c). Administering a suppository: Types, considerations and procedure. *British Journal of Nursing, 28*(5), 288–289. https://doi.org/10.12968/bjon.2019.28.5.288

Mitchell, A. (2019d). Rationale and procedure for performing digital removal of faeces. *British Journal of Nursing, 28*(7), 430–433. https://doi.org/10.12968/bjon.2019.28.7.430

Mitchell, A., & Hill, B. (2020). Moisture-associated skin damage: An overview of its diagnosis and management. *British Journal of Community Nursing, 25*(3), S12–S18. https://doi.org/10.12968/bjcn.2020.25.Sup3.S12

Morton, P. G., & Fontaine, D. K. (2018). *Critical care nursing. A holistic approach* (11th ed.). Wolters Kluwer.

Mounsey, A., Raleigh, M., & Wilson, A. (2015). Management of constipation in older adults. *American Family Physician, 92*(6), 500–504.

National Association for Continence (NAFC). (n.d.). *Bowel retraining.* https://www.nafc.org/bowel-retraining

National Cancer Institute (NCI). (2020). *Gastrointestinal complications (PDQ®)-health professional version. Constipation.* https://www.cancer.gov/about-cancer/treatment/side-effects/constipation/gi-complications-hp-pdq#_8

National Eating Disorder Association (NEDA). (2018). *Laxative abuse.* https://www.nationaleatingdisorders.org/learn/general-information/laxative-abuse

National Institute of Diabetes and Digestive and Kidney Diseases (NIDDK). (2014). *Ostomy surgery of the bowel.* https://www.niddk.nih.gov/health-information/digestive-diseases/ostomy-surgery-bowel#ileonalReservoir

National Institute of Health. (2020). *Probiotics. Fact sheet for health professionals.* Office of Dietary Supplements. https://ods.od.nih.gov/factsheets/Probiotics-HealthProfessional/

National Institute on Aging (NIA). (n.d.). Concerned about constipation? Retrieved February 27, 2021, from https://www.nia.nih.gov/health/concerned-about-constipation

Norris, T. L. (2020). *Porth's essentials of pathophysiology* (5th ed.). Wolters Kluwer.

O'Flynn, S. K. (2018). Care of the stoma: Complications and treatments. *British Journal of Community Nursing, 23*(8), 382–387. https://doi.org/10.12968/bjcn.2018.23.8.382

O'Ryan, M. G. (2020). UpToDate. *Acute viral gastroenteritis in children in resource-rich countries: Management and prevention.* Wolters Kluwer. https://www.uptodate.com/contents/acute-viral-gastroenteritis-in-children-in-resource-rich-countries-management-and-prevention?source=search_result&search=diarrhea%20in%20children&selectedTitle=10~150#H14

Palmer, S. J. (2019). Faecal incontinence in palliative and end-of-life care. *British Journal of Community Nursing, 24*(11), 528–532. https://doi.org/10.12968/bjcn.2019.24.11.528

Palmer, S. J. (2020). Overview of stoma care for community nurses. *British Journal of Community Nursing, 25*(7), 340–344. https://doi.org/10.12968/bjcn.2020.25.7.340

Parker, L. A. Withers, J. H., & Talaga, E. (2018). Comparison of neonatal nursing practices for determining feeding tube insertion length and verifying gastric placement with current best evidence. *Advances in Neonatal Care, 18*(4), 307–317. DOI: 10.1097/ANC.0000000000000526

Phillips, M. M. (2020). *Bowel retraining.* MedlinePlus. U. S. National Library of Medicine. https://medlineplus.gov/ency/article/003971.htm

Pinto, C. F. C. S., Oliveira, P. C. M., Fernandes, O. M. F. S. O., Padilha, J. M. S. C., Machado, P. A. P., Ribeiro, A. L. A., & Ramos, J. L. N. (2020). Nonpharmacological clinical effective interventions in constipation: A systematic review. *Journal of Nursing Scholarship, 52*(3), 261–269. https://doi.org/10.1111/jnu.12555

Pont, L. G., Fisher, M., & Williams, K. (2019). Appropriate use of laxatives in the older person. *Drugs & Aging, 36*(11), 999–1005. https://doi.org/10.1007/s40266-019-00701-9

Powers, J. (2019). Securing orogastric and nasogastric tubes in intubated patients. *Critical Care Nurse, 39*(4), 61–63. https://doi.org/10.4037/ccn2019542

Powers, J., & Bliss, D. Z. (2012). Product options for faecal incontinence management in acute care. *World Council of Enterostomal Therapists Journal, 32*(1), 20–23.

Queensland Health. (2019). *Are you pooing properly?* Queensland Government. The State of Queensland. https://www.health.qld.gov.au/news-events/news/how-to-poo-properly-sit-squat-healthy#:~:text=sitting%20with%20your%20knees%20higher, straighten%20your%20spine

Ragusa, R., Giorgianni, G., Lupo, L., Sciacca, A., Rametta, S., La Verde, M., Mulè, S., & Marranzano, M. (2018). Healthcare-associated Clostridium difficile infection: Role of correct hand hygiene in cross-infection control. *Journal of Preventive Medicine and Hygiene, 59*(2), E145–E152. https://pubmed.ncbi.nlm.nih.gov/30083622/

Rahimi, M., Farhadi, K., Ashtarian, H., & Changaei, F. (2015). Confirming nasogastric tube position: Methods and restrictions. A narrative review. *Journal of Nursing and Midwifery Sciences, 2*(1), 55–62. https://doi.org/10.4103/2345-5756.231420

Rey, E., Bacelo, M., Jiménez-Cebrián, M. J., Alvarez-Sanchez, A., Diaz-Rubio, M., & Rocha, A. L. (2014). A nation-wide study of prevalence and risk factors for fecal impaction in nursing homes. *PLoS One, 9*(8), e105281. https://doi.org/10.1371/journal.pone.0105281

Rogers, B., Ginex, P. K., Anbari, A., Hanson, B. J., LeFebvre, K. B., Lopez, R., Thorpe, D. M., Wolles, B., Moriarty, K. A., Maloney, C., Vrabel, M., & Morgan, R. L. (2020). ONS guidelines for opioid-induced and non-opioid-related cancer constipation. *Oncology Nursing Forum, 47*(6), 671–691. https://doi.org/10.1188/20.ONF.671-691

Roveron, G., De Toma, G., & Barbierato, M. (2016). Italian society of surgery and association of stoma care nurses joint position statement on preoperative stoma siting. *Journal of Wound Ostomy & Continence Nursing, 43*(2), 165–169. https://doi.org/10.1097/WON.0000000000000204

Salvadalena, G., Hendren, S., McKenna, L., Muldoon, R., Netsch, D., Paquette, I., Pittman, J., Ramundo, J., & Steinberg, G. (2015). WOCN Society and ASCRS position statement on preoperative stoma site marking for patients undergoing colostomy or ileostomy surgery. *Journal of Wound, Ostomy & Continence Nursing, 42*(3), 249–252. https://doi.org/10.1097/WON.0000000000000119

Schroeder, J., & Sitzer, V. (2019). Nursing care guidelines for reducing hospital-acquired nasogastric tube-related pressure injuries. *Critical Care Nurse, 39*(6), 54–63. https://doi.org/10.4037/ccn2019872

Setya, A., Mathew, G., & Cagir, B. (2021). *Fecal impaction.* StatPearls [Internet]. https://www.ncbi.nlm.nih.gov/books/NBK448094/

Shen, Q., Zhu, H., Jiang, G., & Liu, X. (2018). Nurse-led self-management educational intervention improves symptoms of patients with functional constipation. *Western Journal of Nursing Research, 40*(6), 874–888. DOI: 10.1177/0193945917701128

Sigmon, D. F., & An, J. (2020). *StatPearls. Nasogastric tube.* National Center for Biotechnology Information. U. S. National Library of Medicine. https://www.ncbi.nlm.nih.gov/books/NBK556063/#:~:text=Nasogastric%20tubes%20are%20typically%20used,unable%20to%20tolerate%20oral%20intake

Silbert-Flagg, J., & Pillitteri, A. (2018). *Maternal and child health nursing* (8th ed.). Wolters Kluwer.

Solomons, J., & Woodward, S. (2013). Digital removal of faeces in the bowel management of patients with spinal cord injury: A review. *British Journal of Neuroscience Nursing, 9*(5), 216–222.

Southgate, G., & Bradbury, S. (2016). Management of incontinence-associated dermatitis with a skin barrier protectant. *British Journal of Nursing, (Urology Supplement), 25*(9), S20–S29. https://doi.org/10.12968/bjon.2016.25.9.S20

Stabler, S. N., Ku, J., Brooks, L., Gellatley, R., & Halijan, G. (2018). Implementation of a nasogastric tube securement device in a tertiary care intensive care unit. *The Canadian Journal of Critical Care Nursing, 29*(1), 14–16.

Stelton, S. (2019). Stoma and peristomal skin care: A clinical review. *American Journal of Nursing, 119*(6), 38–45. https://doi.org/10.1097/01.NAJ.0000559781.86311.64

Swift, T., Westgate, G., Van Onselen, J., & Lee, S. (2020). Developments in silicone technology for use in stoma care. *British Journal of Nursing, 29*(6), S6–S15. doi: 10.12968/bjon.2020.29.6.S6

Taylor, S. J. (2020). Methods of estimating nasogastric tube length: All, including "NEX," are unsafe. *Nutrition in Clinical Practice, 35*(5), 864–870. DOI: 10.1002/ncp.10497

Taylor, S. J., Allan, K., Clemente, R., Marsh, A., & Toher, D. (2018). Feeding tube securement in critical care illness: Implications for safety. *British Journal of Nursing, 27*(18), 1036–1041.

Ten Broek, R. P. G., Krielen, P., Di Saverio, S., Coccolini, F., Biffl, W. L., Ansolani, L., Velmahos, G. C., Sartelli, M., Fraga, G. P., Kelly, M. D., Moore, F. A., Peitzman, A. B., Leppaniemi, A., Moore, E. E., Jeekel, J., Kluger, Y., Sugrue, M., Balogh, Z. J., Bendinelli, C., ... Van Goor, H. (2018). Bologna guidelines for diagnosis and management of adhesive small bowel obstruction (ASBO): 2017 update of the evidence-based guidelines from the World Society of Emergency Surgery ASBO working group. *World Journal of Emergency Surgery, 13*, 24. https://doi.org/10.1186/s13017-018-0185-2

Torsy, T., Saman, R., Boeykens, K., Duysburgh, I., Van Damme, N., & Beeckman, D. (2018). Comparison of two methods for estimating the tip position of a nasogastric feeding tube: A randomized controlled trial. *Nutrition in Clinical Practice, 33*(6), 843–850. DOI: 10.1002/ncp.10112

Toughy, T. A., & Jett, K. (2018). *Ebersol and Hess' gerontological nursing & healthy aging* (5th ed.). Elsevier.

U.S. Department of Agriculture (USDA) and U. S. Department of Health and Human Services (USDHHS). (2020). *Dietary guidelines for Americans, 2020–2025* (9th ed.). DietaryGuidelines.gov

U.S. Department of Health and Human Services (USDHHS). (2018). Office of disease prevention and health promotion. *Physical activity guidelines for Americans* (2nd ed.). https://health.gov/sites/default/files/2019-09/Physical_Activity_Guidelines_2nd_edition.pdf

U.S. Department of Health and Human Services (USDHHS). (2020). *Keep food safe. 4 steps to food safety.* https://www.foodsafety.gov/keep-food-safe/4-steps-to-food-safety

United Ostomy Associations of America (UOAA). (n.d.). *Support, education, resources advocacy.* Retrieved December 30, 2020, https://www.ostomy.org/

Venara, A., Hamel, J. F., Cotte, E., Meillat, H., Sage, P. Y., Slim, K., & GRACE Group. (2020). Intraoperative nasogastric tube during colorectal surgery may not be mandatory: A propensity score analysis of a prospective database. *Surgical Endoscopy, 34*(12), 5583–5592. https://doi.org/10.1007/s00464-019-07359-9

VHA Center for Engineering & Occupational Safety and Health (CEOSH). (2016). *Safe patient handling and mobility guidebook.* http://www.tnpatientsafety.com/pubfiles/Initiatives/workplace-violence/sphm-pdf.pdf

Voegeli, D. (2018). Incontinence-associated dermatitis: Management. *Nursing & Residential Care, 20*(10), 506–512. https://doi.org/10.12968/nrec.2018.20.10.506

Wangui-Verry, J., Farrington, M., Matthews, G., & Tucker, S. J. (2019). Are milk and molasses enemas safe for hospitalized adults? A retrospective electronic health record review. *American Journal of Nursing, 119*(9), 24–28. https://doi.org/10.1097/01.NAJ.0000580148.43193.76

Wasserman, M. A., & McGee, M. F. (2017). Preoperative considerations for the ostomate. *Clinics in Colon and Rectal Surgery, 30*(3), 157–161. https://doi.org/10.1055/s-0037-1598155

Whiteley, I., & Sinclair, G. (2014). Faecal management systems for disabling incontinence or wounds. *British Journal of Nursing, 23*(16), 881–885. https://doi.org/10.12968/bjon.2014.23.16.881

Wolters Kluwer. (2022). Problem-based care plans. In *Lippincott Advisor*. Wolters Kluwer.

Wound, Ostomy and Continence Nurses Society (WOCN). (2018). *Basic ostomy skin care: A guide for patients and health care providers.* https://www.ostomy.org/wp-content/uploads/2018/11/wocn_basic_ostomy_skin_care_2018.pdf

Yates, A. (2018a). Incontinence-associated dermatitis in older people: prevention and management. *British Journal of Community Nursing, 23*(5), 218–224. https://doi.org/10.12968/bjcn.2018.23.5.218

Yates, A. (2018b). Incontinence-associated dermatitis: What nurses need to know. *British Journal of Nursing, 27*(19), 1094–1100. https://doi.org/10.12968/bjon.2018.27.19.1094

Yates, A. (2019). Basic continence assessment: What community nurses should know. *Journal of Community Nursing, 33*(3), 52–55.

40 Oxygenation and Perfusion

Tyrone Jacobs

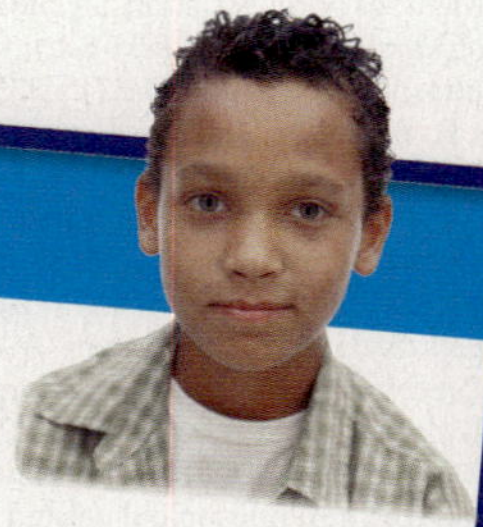

Tyrone Jacobs, age 12, is brought to the emergency department gasping for breath. His parents are frantic. "It just seemed like he had a really bad cold," his mother says. An acute asthma attack is suspected, and measures are instituted immediately to protect the child's airway.

Yan Kim

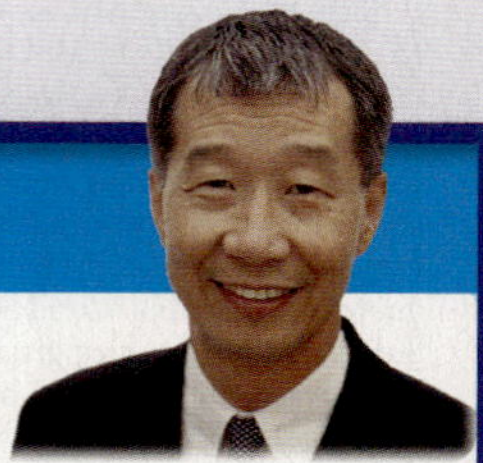

Yan Kim, age 57, developed respiratory failure from complications associated with pulmonary surgery. He is receiving oxygen therapy and mechanical ventilation via an endotracheal tube (airway into the trachea) and undergoing continuous cardiac monitoring.

Joan McIntyre

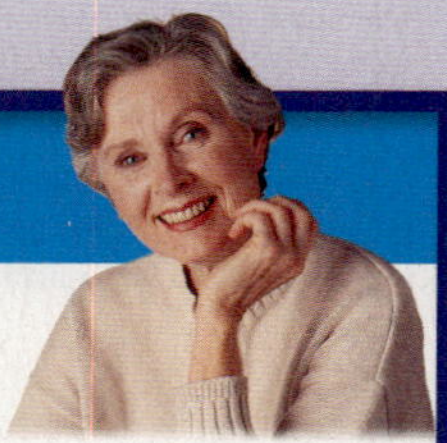

Joan McIntyre, age 72, has been admitted to your medical unit with an acute exacerbation of chronic obstructive pulmonary disease (COPD). This is the fifth time she has been in the hospital this year. She is receiving supplemental oxygen and multiple medications to support her breathing. She is very weak, unable to perform activities of daily living (ADLs) for herself and becomes extremely short of breath with minimal exertion. She has verbalized feelings of despair and has asked the staff, "to let me go if I should stop breathing."

Lippincott DocuCare **Additional patient scenarios available in *Lippincott DocuCare*.**

Learning Outcomes

After completing the chapter, you will be able to accomplish the following:

1. Describe respiratory and cardiovascular anatomy and physiology.
2. Describe the function and role of the respiratory and cardiovascular systems in oxygenation.
3. Describe factors that affect respiratory and cardiovascular function and influence the care of patients with oxygenation problems.
4. Perform a cardiopulmonary assessment using appropriate interview questions and health assessment skills.
5. Diagnose actual and potential health problems and needs related to oxygenation and perfusion that may be addressed through nursing intervention.
6. Describe nursing interventions and strategies to promote adequate oxygenation and perfusion and identify their rationale.
7. Plan, implement, and evaluate nursing care related to selected actual and potential health problems and needs associated with alterations in oxygenation and perfusion.

Nursing Concepts

- Assessment
- Cellular Regulation
- Clinical Decision Making/Clinical Judgment
- Oxygenation/Gas Exchange
- Perfusion
- Safety

Life depends on a constant supply of oxygen. This demand for oxygen is met by the function of the respiratory and cardiovascular systems, also known as the **cardiopulmonary** system. This chapter describes the anatomy and physiology of the respiratory system. Also included is a discussion of the anatomy and physiology of the **cardiovascular** (heart and blood vessels) system as it pertains to its role in **oxygenation**, the process of providing life-sustaining oxygen to the body's cells. Additional information related to the cardiovascular system—including pulse, pulse physiology, blood pressure, and the physiology of blood pressure—is discussed in Chapter 26. In addition, this chapter explores general factors affecting cardiopulmonary functioning and oxygenation. Suggestions for performing a health assessment related to oxygenation are presented, including sample interview questions for both a general and focused history, a description of the nursing examination, and laboratory and radiologic studies related to oxygenation. Additional information related to assessment of these systems is discussed in Chapter 27. Potential and actual health problems and needs related to oxygenation and perfusion are discussed. Expected patient outcomes and specific nursing strategies for implementation are described. The accompanying Evolving Case Study 40-1 on page 1660 provides an opportunity to develop and apply clinical reasoning and clinical judgment skills in caring for a patient with oxygenation and perfusion problems. Refer also to the accompanying Reflective Practice box on pages 1586–1587.

ANATOMY AND PHYSIOLOGY OF OXYGENATION

Oxygenation of body tissues depends on several factors. One is the integrity of the airway system to transport air to and from the lungs. A properly functioning alveolar system in the lungs to oxygenate venous blood and to remove carbon dioxide from the blood is also important. A properly functioning cardiovascular system and blood supply to carry nutrients and wastes to and from body cells is a necessary component of oxygenation.

Knowledge of the basic anatomy and physiology of the respiratory and cardiovascular systems and an understanding of the role of these systems in oxygenation of body tissues provides a foundation for assessing oxygenation and perfusion in patients and for planning and implementing interventions to promote optimal oxygenation and perfusion. This knowledge also helps nurses understand, interpret, and analyze assessment findings and provides the basis for clinical reasoning, clinical judgment, and the rationale for sound nursing interventions.

Respiratory System

Oxygen and carbon dioxide must move through the alveoli as part of the oxygenation process. Thus, an adequately functioning respiratory system is vital for the exchange of gases.

Anatomy of the Respiratory System

The airway, which begins at the nose and ends at the terminal bronchioles, is a pathway for the transport and exchange of oxygen and carbon dioxide. The airway is divided into the upper and the lower airways.

The upper airway is composed of the nose, pharynx, larynx, and epiglottis. Its main function is to warm, filter, and humidify inspired air. The lower airway, known as the tracheobronchial tree, includes the trachea, right and left main stem bronchi, segmental bronchi, and terminal bronchioles (Fig. 40-1 on page 1587). Its major functions are conduction of air, mucociliary clearance, and production of pulmonary surfactant.

The airways are lined with mucus, which traps cells, particles, and infectious debris. This mucus covering also helps to protect the underlying tissues from irritation and infection. **Cilia**, which are microscopic hair-like projections, propel trapped material and accompanying mucus toward the upper airway so they can be removed by coughing. Removal is facilitated when mucus is watery in consistency. An adequate fluid intake is necessary for ciliary action and for the production of watery mucus normally present in the respiratory tract.

QSEN Reflective Practice: Cultivating QSEN Competencies

CHALLENGE TO TECHNICAL SKILLS

Ventilators and telemetry have always intimidated me, so having a patient like Yan Kim was overwhelming. Mr. Kim was a 57-year-old man who had developed respiratory failure from complications secondary to pulmonary surgery. He was receiving oxygen therapy and mechanical ventilation via an endotracheal tube (airway into the trachea) and was also undergoing continuous cardiac monitoring. Providing care for him with all his equipment and so many alarms that could sound seemed insurmountable. The monitor had several different values on it and the continuous ECG monitor always made me feel like the patient was on the verge of dying. We had just recently covered these skills in class, and I felt incompetent for the first 2 weeks of my critical care clinical experience. I could have voiced my concerns with these two machines, and I should have asked the first day what I should and shouldn't be worried about with critical care patients. But I didn't.

Thinking Outside the Box: Possible Course of Action

- Ask my instructor if there was any danger in having a patient who was receiving mechanical ventilation and being monitored by telemetry.
- Ask for someone to explain the ECG waveforms on the monitor and what to be concerned with when looking at them.
- Avoid caring for patients on ventilators and telemetry as part of their care.

Evaluating a Good Outcome: How Do I Define Success?

- Patient is safe and receives care by a competent care provider promoting his health.
- I am confident in my technical skills and able to use technology to deliver the most helpful care.
- I continue to ask questions, challenge my practice, and learn to contribute to improved care, which will lead to enhanced nursing.

Personal Learning: Here's to the Future!

Fortunately, our clinical rotations are planned so that we do not actually assume responsibility for taking care of critical care patients until we learn the necessary skills (telemetry and ventilation). This semester in my critical care clinical experiences, my fears have dissipated. I have learned that having patients that are being monitored continuously via telemetry is quite reassuring: it serves as a constant monitor for me. Although I still assess the patient on my own, having continuous values to check is reassuring. As for the ventilator, I realized I knew a lot more than I thought. My instructor gave me a lesson on the ventilator during my clinical experience and connected the class lectures and bookwork with what I was seeing with my patient. I asked many questions and checked to see if I knew which settings would change with different scenarios. There are several settings and several values constantly being measured with the machine. Once I was able to see what all of these numbers meant and realized that I understood what each was for, I felt much more comfortable with patients on a ventilator. I realized my concerns and made sure that I provided unbiased care so that my concerns did not force me to neglect a patient.

Before, I would have been scared to get too close to the machine for fear of hitting the wrong button, fearing I would harm the patient. Now I am learning how the settings are specific to each patient. I feel comfortable reading the values and setting the controls. Still, I ask questions about the ventilator and telemetry readings because I want to know that I am interpreting them correctly. I feel it is my responsibility to obtain as much understanding and knowledge as I can so that I can provide the best care to these patients. This is very relieving and rewarding: now critical care patients don't seem so critical! My care for these patients is enhanced since I am more confident in my skills, and this enhances the care I deliver. Next time there is something new to me, I will voice my concern early on even if I am not "supposed to know" it yet.

Overall, although I still do not have much experience, I feel technically competent as a senior nursing student. I am confident because I challenge myself and I am self-motivated when it comes to searching for more information when needed.

Carrie Staines, Georgetown University

QSEN SELF-REFLECTION ON QUALITY AND SAFETY COMPETENCIES DEVELOPING KNOWLEDGE, SKILLS, AND ATTITUDES FOR CONTINUOUS IMPROVEMENT

How do you think you would respond in a similar situation? Why? Do you agree with the criteria that the nursing student used to evaluate a successful outcome? Are there any other criteria that would be appropriate to use? Did the nursing student meet the criteria? Why or why not? What *knowledge, skills,* and *attitudes* do you need to develop to continuously improve the quality and safety of care for patients like Mr. Kim?

Patient-Centered Care: What information should be communicated to the patient about the care provided? What interventions should the nursing student implement to provide care based on respect for the patient's preferences, values, and needs?

Teamwork and Collaboration/Quality Improvement: What communication skills do you need to improve to ensure that

QSEN Reflective Practice: Cultivating QSEN Competencies *(continued)*

CHALLENGE TO TECHNICAL SKILLS

you function as a member of the patient-care team? What skills do you need to initiate requests for help and to obtain assistance when needed?

Safety/Evidence-Based Practice: What information did the nursing student receive from the monitors? How did the nursing student use this information? How did the nursing student apply the knowledge obtained through the lessons given by the instructor? What evidence for nursing practice provides guidance for decision making regarding care of this patient? What does this tell you about yourself and about the adequacy of your skills for professional practice? How do you think the nursing student would have responded if the clinical experience were strictly observational?

Informatics: Can you identify the essential information that must be available in Mr. Kim's electronic health record to support safe patient care and coordination of care? Can you think of other ways to respond to or approach the situation?

The lungs, the main organs of respiration, are located within the thoracic cavity on the right and left sides (see Fig. 40-1). The **lungs** extend from the base at the level of the diaphragm to the apex (top), which is above the first rib. The heart lies between the right and left lung.

Each lung is divided into lobes. The right lung has three lobes; the left has two. Each lobe is subdivided into segments or lobules. The main bronchus branches to each lung from the trachea. It immediately subdivides into secondary bronchi, one to each lobe. The bronchi subdivide again and again, becoming smaller and smaller as they branch through the lung. The smallest of these branches are the bronchioles, ending at the terminal bronchioles. The lungs are composed of elastic tissue that can stretch or recoil.

At the end of the terminal bronchioles there are clusters of **alveoli** (singular, alveolus), small air sacs. The alveoli are the site of gas exchange. The wall of each alveolus is made of a single-cell layer of squamous epithelium (see Fig. 40-1). This thin wall allows for exchange of gases with the capillaries covering the alveoli. The average adult has more than 300 million alveoli. **Surfactant**, a detergent-like phospholipid, reduces the surface tension between the moist membranes of the alveoli, preventing their collapse. When surfactant production is reduced, the lung becomes stiff and the alveoli collapse.

The lungs and thoracic cavity are lined with a serous membrane called the pleura. The visceral pleura covers the lungs, and the parietal pleura lines the thoracic cavity. These

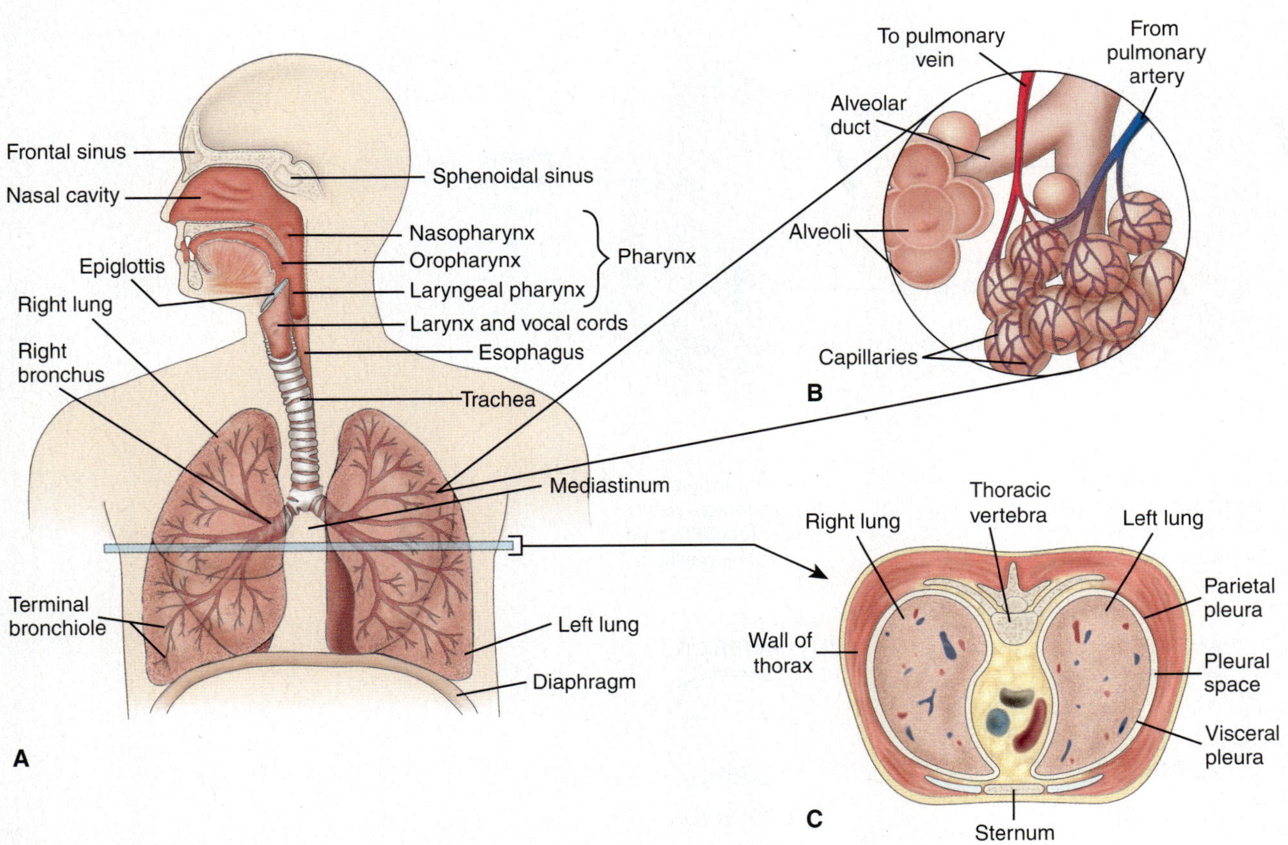

FIGURE 40-1. The organs of the respiratory tract. **A.** Overview. **B.** Alveoli (air sacs) of the lungs and the blood capillaries. **C.** Transverse section through the lungs.

two membranes are continuous with each other and form a closed sac. The pleural space lies between the two layers. Pleural fluid between the membranes acts as a lubricant and as an adhesive agent to hold the lungs in an expanded position. A few milliliters of fluid between the pleural surfaces allow the lungs to move easily along the chest wall as they expand and contract. Without this fluid, filling and emptying of the lungs are difficult.

Pressure within the pleural space (intrapleural pressure) is always subatmospheric (a negative pressure). This constant negative intrapleural pressure, along with the pleural fluid, holds the lungs in an expanded position.

Physiology of the Respiratory System

Living cells require oxygen and the removal of carbon dioxide, a byproduct of oxidation. Gas exchange, the intake of oxygen and the release of carbon dioxide, is made possible by pulmonary ventilation, respiration, and perfusion. **Pulmonary ventilation** refers to the movement of air into and out of the lungs. **Respiration** involves gas exchange between the atmospheric air in the alveoli and blood in the capillaries. **Perfusion** is the process by which oxygenated capillary blood passes through body tissues.

PULMONARY VENTILATION

Pulmonary ventilation (breathing) is the movement of air into and out of the lungs. The process of ventilation has two phases: **inspiration** (inhalation) and **expiration** (exhalation). Inspiration, the active phase, involves movement of muscles and the thorax to bring air into the lungs. Expiration, the passive phase, is the movement of air out of the lungs.

During inspiration, the following events occur: the diaphragm contracts and descends, lengthening the thoracic cavity; the external intercostal muscles contract, lifting the ribs upward and outward; and the sternum is pushed forward, enlarging the chest from front to back. This combination of an increased lung volume and decreased intrapulmonic pressure allows atmospheric air to move from an area of greater pressure (outside air) into an area of lesser pressure (within the lungs). The relaxation, or recoil, of these structures then results in expiration. The diaphragm relaxes and moves up, the ribs move down, and the sternum drops back into position. This causes a decreased volume in the lungs and an increase in intrapulmonic pressure. As a result, air in the lungs moves from an area of greater pressure to one of lesser pressure and is expired (Fig. 40-2).

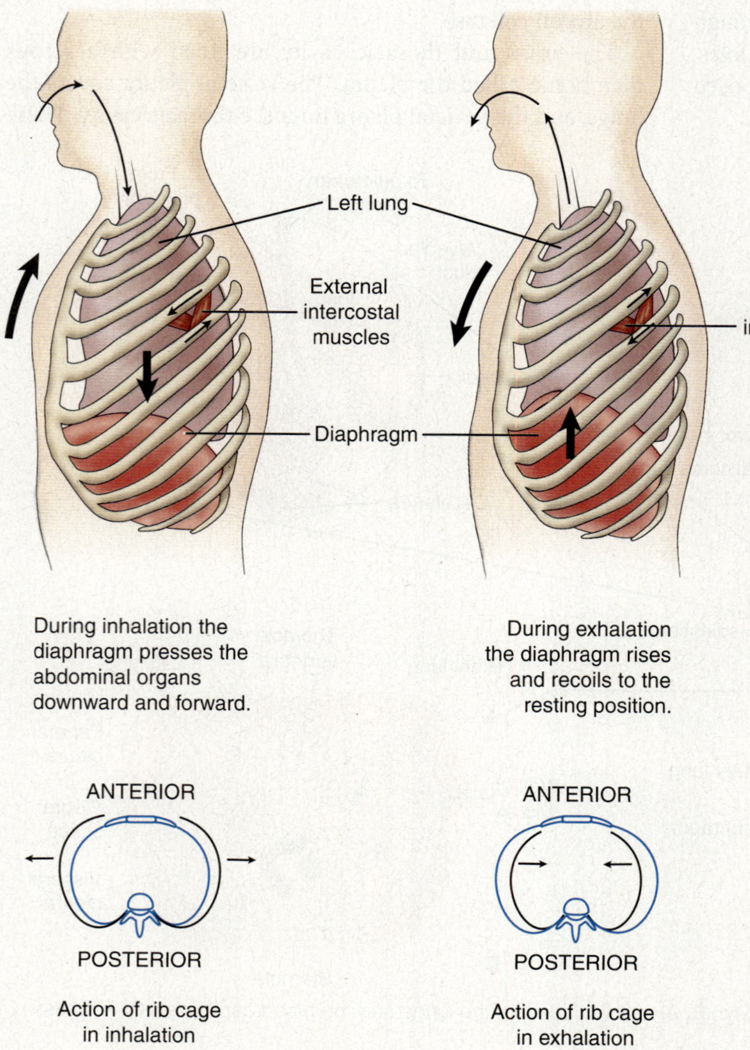

FIGURE 40-2. Pulmonary ventilation.

Other physical factors contribute to airflow in and out of the lungs. These factors include the condition of the musculature, compliance of lung tissue, and airway resistance. The condition of the body's musculature can affect the process of respiration. Weakening of the muscles involved in respiration can contribute to less effective inhalation and exhalation. The accessory muscles of the abdomen, neck, and back are used to maintain respiratory movements at times when breathing is difficult. These muscles are used to facilitate breathing; the movement is called retraction.

Lung compliance refers to the ease with which the lungs can be inflated. The compliance of lung tissue affects lung volume. The ability of the lungs to adequately fill with air during inhalation is achieved by the normal elasticity of lung tissue, aided by the presence of surfactant. The varying changes in lung pressure and resulting lung compliance can be compared to differences in blowing up a new, noncompliant balloon versus one that was inflated previously. A stiff, noncompliant lung (such as a new balloon) requires a greater inspiratory effort to inflate it. Emphysema, a chronic lung condition, and the normal changes associated with aging are examples of conditions that result in decreased elasticity of lung tissue, which, in turn, decreases compliance.

Airway resistance is the result of any impediment or obstruction that air meets as it moves through the airway. Any process that changes the bronchial diameter or width causes airway resistance. Obstruction in any part of the normal passageways impedes respiration. Obstruction can be caused by a foreign substance, such as a piece of food, a coin, or a toy, or by liquids, as in the case of a drowning victim. Obstruction can also result from secretions (e.g., excessive or thickened secretions) or tissues (e.g., tumors or edema of the respiratory tract). A decrease in the size of air passages resulting from constriction or poor neck positioning can also impede respiration. Bronchial constriction in asthma is an example of airway resistance related to a decrease in the size of air passages.

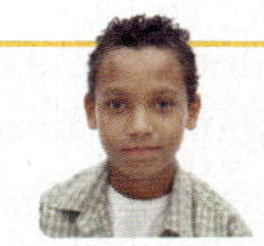

Consider **Tyrone Jacobs**, the 12-year-old boy with suspected asthma. An understanding of the underlying pathophysiologic processes involved with this disorder would provide the basis for the nurse's actions to protect the child's airway.

RESPIRATION

Respiration, gas exchange, occurs at the terminal alveolar capillary system. Gases are exchanged between the air and blood via the dense network of capillaries in the respiratory portion of the lungs and the thin alveolar walls (see Figs. 40-1 on page 1587 and 40-3). Gas exchange occurs via diffusion. **Diffusion** is the movement of gas or particles from areas of higher pressure or concentration to areas of lower pressure or concentration. In respiration, diffusion refers to the movement of oxygen and carbon dioxide between the air (in the alveoli) and the blood (in the capillaries). These gases move passively from an area of higher concentration to an area of lower concentration. The greater pressure of oxygen in the alveoli causes the oxygen to move from the alveoli into the capillaries containing the unoxygenated venous blood. Likewise, the carbon dioxide in the returning venous blood exerts a greater pressure than the carbon dioxide in the alveoli. Therefore, carbon dioxide diffuses across the capillary into the alveoli and ultimately is exhaled.

Diffusion of gases in the lung is influenced by several factors, including changes in the surface area available, thickening of the alveolar–capillary membrane, and partial pressure. Any change in the surface area available for diffusion hinders diffusion. For example, removal of a lung or the presence of a disease that destroys lung tissue can decrease the surface area available, ultimately affecting gas exchange. Incomplete lung expansion or the collapse of alveoli, known as **atelectasis**, prevents pressure changes and the exchange of gas by diffusion in the lungs. Areas of the lung with atelectasis cannot fulfill the function of respiration. Examples of conditions that predispose a patient to atelectasis are obstructions of the airway by foreign bodies, mucus, airway constriction, external compression by tumors or enlarged blood vessels, and

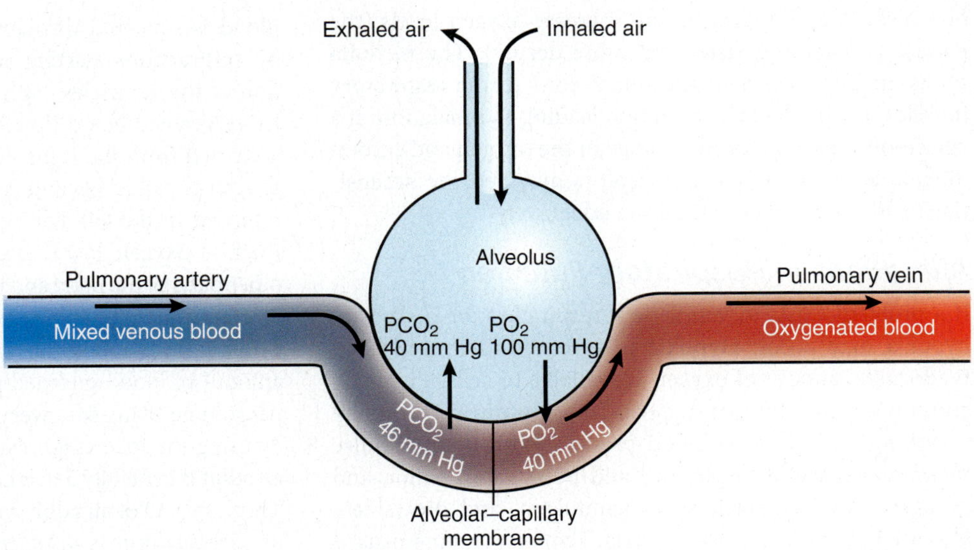

FIGURE 40-3. Gas exchange in the alveolus. The greater pressure of the oxygen in the air inhaled into the alveoli causes the oxygen to move into the capillaries, which contain unoxygenated blood. The carbon dioxide in the returning venous blood moves from the capillaries (area of greater concentration) into the alveoli (area of lesser concentration).

immobility. Any disease or condition that results in thickening of the alveolar–capillary membrane, such as pneumonia or pulmonary edema, makes diffusion more difficult.

The partial pressure, or pressure resulting from any gas in a mixture depending on its concentration, can also affect diffusion. If environmental oxygen is reduced, such as when a person is at higher altitudes or in the presence of toxic fumes, less oxygen is available for diffusion. When oxygen is administered, an increased amount of oxygen is available, resulting in greater diffusion across capillary membranes.

PERFUSION

Oxygenated capillary blood passes through the tissues of the body in the process called perfusion. The amount of blood flowing through the lungs is a factor in the amount of oxygen and other gases that are exchanged. The amount of blood present in any given area of lung tissue depends partially on whether the person is sitting, standing, or lying down. Perfusion is greater in dependent areas. The perfusion of lung tissue also depends on the person's activity level. Greater activity results in an increased need for cellular oxygen by the body's tissues and a subsequent increase in cardiac output (CO) and consequently in increased blood return to the lungs. In addition, perfusion to the body's tissues depends on an adequate blood supply and proper cardiovascular functioning to carry oxygen and carbon dioxide to and from the lungs (discussed later).

Regulation of the Respiratory System

The respiratory center is located in the medulla in the brainstem, immediately above the spinal cord. It is stimulated by an increased concentration of carbon dioxide and hydrogen ions and, to a lesser degree, by the decreased amount of oxygen in the arterial blood. In addition, chemoreceptors in the aortic arch and carotid bodies are sensitive to the same arterial blood gas levels and blood pressure and can activate the medulla. Proprioceptors in the muscles and joints respond to body movements, such as exercise, and cause an increase in ventilation.

Stimulation of the medulla increases the rate and depth of ventilation (both inspiration and expiration) to blow off carbon dioxide and hydrogen and increase oxygen levels (the patient is breathing faster and more deeply). The medulla sends an impulse down the spinal cord to the respiratory muscles to stimulate a contraction leading to inhalation. If a condition causes a chronic change in the oxygen and carbon dioxide levels, these chemoreceptors may become desensitized and not regulate ventilation adequately.

Alterations in Respiratory Function

If a problem exists in ventilation, respiration, or perfusion, hypoxia may occur. **Hypoxia** is a condition in which an inadequate amount of oxygen is available to cells. The most common symptoms of hypoxia are **dyspnea** (difficulty breathing), an elevated blood pressure with a small pulse pressure, increased respiratory and pulse rates, pallor, and cyanosis. Anxiety, restlessness, confusion, and drowsiness also are common signs of hypoxia. Hypoxia is often caused by **hypoventilation** (decreased rate or depth of air movement into the lungs). Hypoxia can also be a chronic condition. The effects of chronic hypoxia can be detected in all body systems and are manifested as altered thought processes, headaches, chest pain, enlarged heart, clubbing of the fingers and toes, anorexia, constipation, decreased urinary output, decreased libido, weakness of extremity muscles, and muscle pain. Additional information related to alterations in respiratory function is discussed in Chapter 26.

Cardiovascular System

Oxygen and carbon dioxide must move through the alveoli and be carried to and from body cells by the blood. Thus, an adequately functioning cardiovascular system is vital for exchange of gases.

Anatomy of the Cardiovascular System

The cardiovascular system is composed of the heart and the blood vessels. The heart is the main organ of **circulation**, the continuous one-way circuit of blood through the blood vessels, with the heart as the pump (Norris, 2020). The heart lies in the thoracic cavity between the lungs, in the center and somewhat to the left of the body's midline (Fig. 40-4). The heart is a cone-shaped, muscular pump, divided into four hollow chambers. The upper chambers, the **atria** (singular, atrium), receive blood from the veins (the superior and inferior vena cava and the left and right pulmonary veins). The lower chambers, the **ventricles**, force blood out of the heart through the arteries (the left and right pulmonary arteries and the aorta). One-way valves that direct blood flow through the heart are located at the entrance (tricuspid and mitral valves) and exit (pulmonary and aortic valves) of each ventricle (Fig. 40-5). The blood vessels form a closed circuit of tubes that carry blood between the heart and the body cells. Arteries and arterioles conduct blood away from the ventricles to the capillaries and the venules and veins and return blood from the capillaries to the atria. Capillaries function in the exchange of substances between the blood and the body cells.

Physiology of the Cardiovascular System

Blood is squeezed through the heart and out into the body by contractions starting in the atria, followed by contraction of the ventricles, with a subsequent resting of the heart. Deoxygenated blood (low in oxygen, high in carbon dioxide) is carried from the right side of the heart to the lungs, where oxygen is picked up and carbon dioxide is released, and then returned to the left side of the heart. This oxygenated blood (high in oxygen, low in carbon dioxide) is pumped out to all other parts of the body and back again (Fig. 40-6 on page 1592). The quantity of blood forced out of the left ventricle with each contraction is called the stroke volume (SV). The CO is the amount of blood pumped per minute and measured in liters per minute (King & Lowery, 2020). This volume is determined by using the following formula: $CO = SV \times \text{heart rate}$. CO in an adult is generally 5 to 6 L/min at rest (King & Lowery, 2020). Thus, the CO of an adult with an SV of 70 mL and a heart rate of 70 beats/min is 4.9 L/min. CO increases during physical

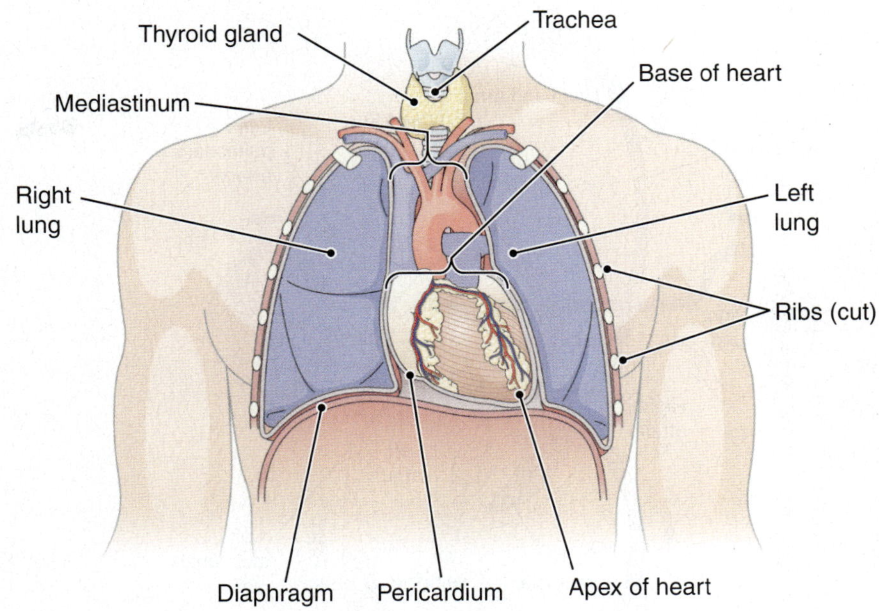

FIGURE 40-4. The heart in position in the thoracic cavity. (*Source:* Reprinted with permission from Cohen, B. J., & Hull, K. L. [2016]. *Memmler's structure and function of the human body* [11th ed.]. Wolters Kluwer.)

activity and decreases during sleep; it also varies depending on the body size and metabolic needs.

Oxygen is carried via plasma and red blood cells (RBCs). It is dissolved in plasma, but because oxygen is insoluble in liquids, little oxygen is carried in this way (2%) (Patel et al., 2021). The majority of oxygen is carried by the RBCs. The hemoglobin in RBCs has a strong affinity for oxygen and most oxygen (98%) is carried in the body by RBCs as part of hemoglobin in the form of oxyhemoglobin (Patel et al., 2021). Hemoglobin also carries carbon dioxide easily in the form of carboxyhemoglobin.

Once the red blood cells reach the tissues, internal respiration must occur. **Internal respiration** is the exchange of oxygen and carbon dioxide between the circulating blood and the tissue cells. Any abnormality in the blood's components affects internal respiration. For example, hemorrhage

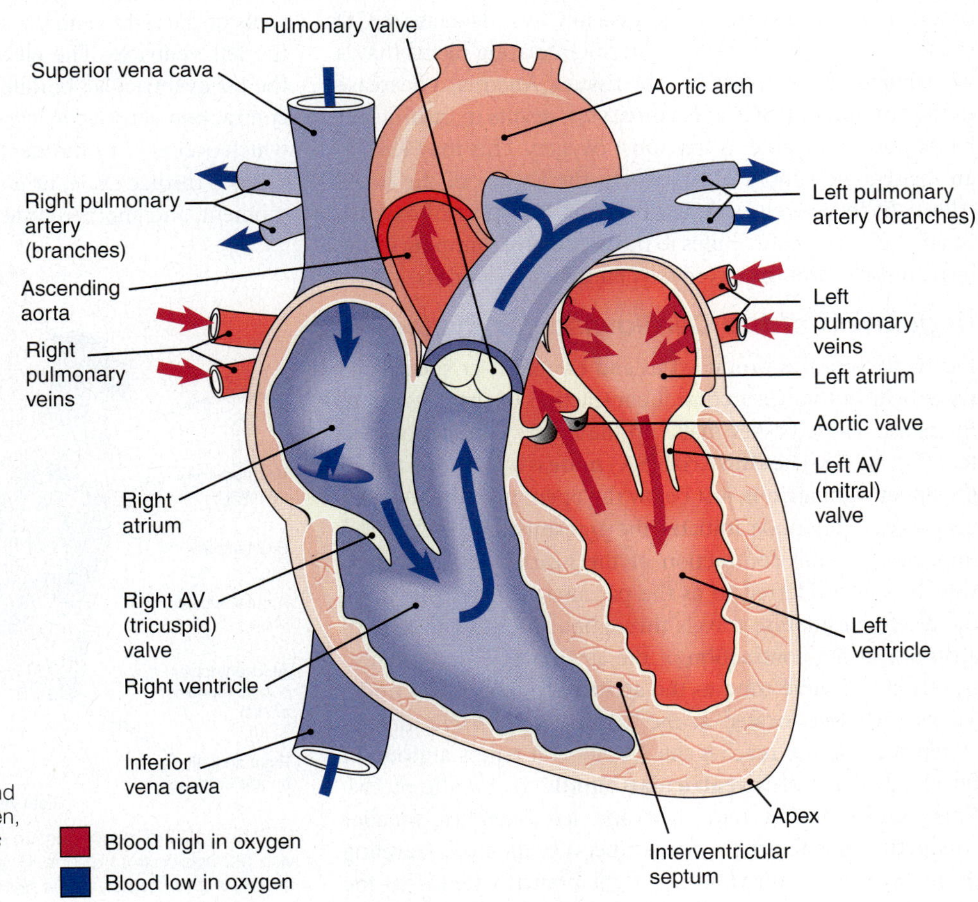

FIGURE 40-5. The heart, valves, and vessels. (*Source:* Adapted from Cohen, B. J., & Hull, K. L. [2016]. *Memmler's structure and function of the human body* [11th ed.]. Wolters Kluwer.)

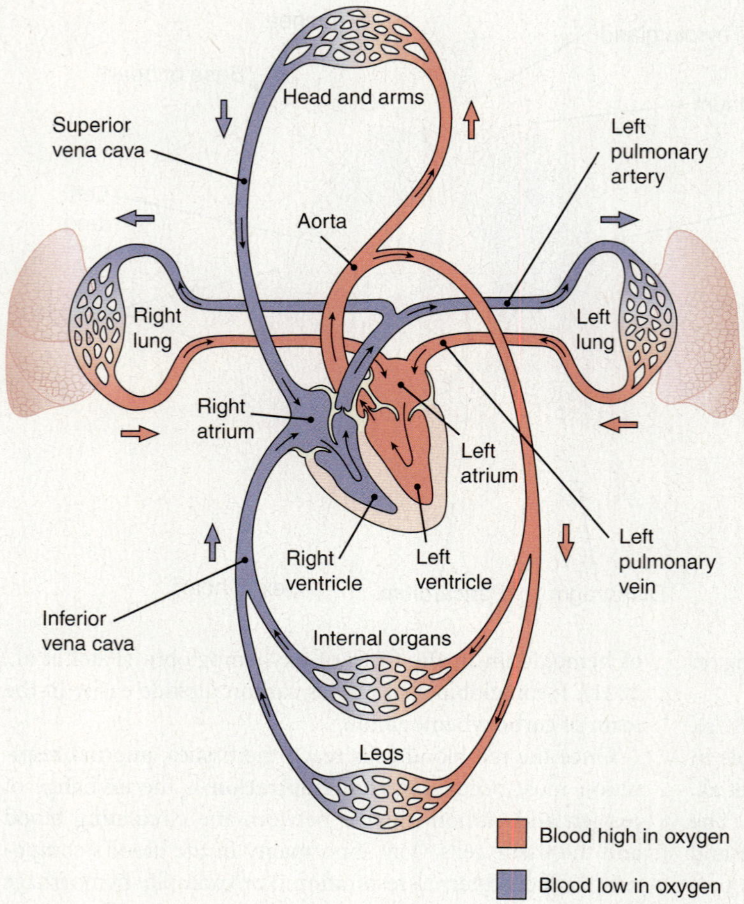

FIGURE 40-6. The right side of the heart pumps deoxygenated blood to the lungs, where oxygen is picked up and carbon dioxide released. The left side of the heart pumps oxygenated blood out to all other parts of the body. (*Source:* Reprinted with permission from Taylor, J. J., & Cohen, B. J. [2013]. *Memmler's structure and function of the human body* [10th ed.]. Wolters Kluwer.)

or loss of blood can cause a decrease in CO. A decrease in CO causes a reduction in the amount of circulating blood that is available to deliver oxygen to the tissues. Anemia, a decrease in the amount of RBCs or erythrocytes, results in insufficient hemoglobin available to transport oxygen. This may lead to an inadequate supply of oxygen to the tissues of the body. Alternatively, exercise can improve the transport of oxygen. Regular exercise contributes to more effective pumping of the heart muscle, and improved oxygen transport to cells.

Regulation of the Cardiovascular System

Electrical impulses produced in and carried over specialized tissue within the heart control contraction of the muscles of the heart. These tissues make up the heart's conduction system (Fig. 40-7). The **sinoatrial (SA) node** is a mass of tissue in the upper right atrium, just below the opening of the superior vena cava. This node initiates the transmission of electrical impulses, causing contraction of the heart at regular intervals. It is also referred to as the pacemaker. After initiation, the electrical impulse travels throughout the muscle of each atrium, causing contraction of the atrium. The impulse also travels at the same time to the **atrioventricular (AV) node,** a mass of tissue located at the bottom of the right atrium. When the impulse reaches the AV node, it enters a group of fibers called the **atrioventricular bundle**, or bundle of His. This bundle divides into right and left branches. Smaller conduction myofibers (Purkinje fibers) branch off, traveling throughout the ventricles. The right branch extends to the walls of the right ventricle and the left branch travels through the left ventricle. The electrical impulse continues through the atrioventricular bundle and the Purkinje fibers, causing contraction of the ventricles. The contraction of the ventricles, which occurs just a moment after the atrial contractions, completes a cardiac cycle, or a single heartbeat. The heart rests a moment, and another cycle begins almost immediately.

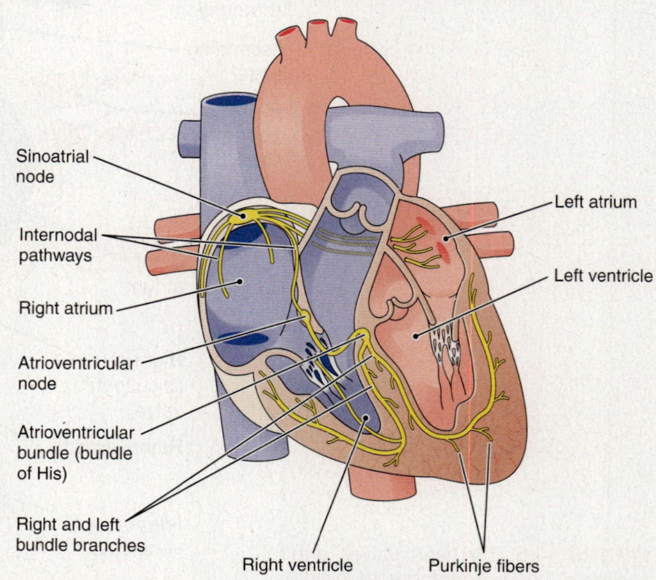

FIGURE 40-7. The conduction system of the heart. (*Source:* Reprinted with permission from Cohen, B. J., & Hull, K. L. [2016]. *Memmler's structure and function of the human body* [11th ed.]. Wolters Kluwer.)

Many things can influence the function of the heart. A person's heart rate can be modified by the nervous system based on the needs of the body. Stimulation of the SA and AV nodes by the sympathetic nerves increases the heart rate and force of contraction in response to increased activity, and as part of the response to real or perceived threats. Parasympathetic stimulation of the SA and AV nodes by the vagus nerve decreases the heart rate. The balance between the parasympathetic and sympathetic effects on the heart is maintained with the help of input from the medulla in the brainstem. Hormones and other chemicals made by the body, as well as drugs, also affect heart action.

Blood Flow to the Cardiovascular System

The muscles of the heart have their own blood vessels that provide oxygen and nourishment and remove waste products. The main blood vessels that provide coronary circulation are the right and left coronary arteries, which branch off the aorta. They encircle the heart and branch out to all regions of the heart. The coronary arteries fill with blood during relaxation of the ventricles. The blood returns to the right atrium after passing through the heart muscle via the cardiac veins.

Alterations in Cardiovascular Function

If a problem exists in the cardiovascular system, alterations in function of the heart may occur, leading to impaired oxygenation. A **dysrhythmia** (also referred to as **arrhythmia**) is a disturbance of the rate and/or rhythm of the heart (Hinkle et al., 2022). Dysrhythmias are caused by an abnormal rate of electrical impulse generation from the SA node, or from impulses originating from a site or sites other than the SA node. They can also be caused by the abnormal conduction of electrical impulses through the heart. Dysrhythmias can occur with heart disease, hypertension, damage to the heart, in the presence of various drugs, with decreased oxygenation of the heart tissues, and with trauma. Dysrhythmias cause disturbances of the heart rate, heart rhythm, or both, and can affect the pumping action of the heart, interfering with circulation, leading to alterations in oxygenation. Symptoms vary, depending on the cause and type of dysrhythmia. Symptoms may include decreased blood pressure, dizziness, palpitations (awareness of throbbing heart beats), weakness, and fainting.

Myocardial **ischemia**, decreased oxygen supply to the heart caused by insufficient blood supply, can lead to impaired oxygenation of tissues in the body. It is most commonly caused by atherosclerosis, the accumulation of fatty substances and fibrous tissue in the lining of arterial blood vessel walls, creating blockages and narrowing the vessels, reducing blood flow. Angina and myocardial infarction can result from myocardial ischemia. Stable **angina** is a temporary imbalance between the amount of oxygen needed by the heart and the amount delivered to the heart muscles, causing chest pain or discomfort. **Myocardial infarction**, one type of acute coronary syndrome characterized by the death of heart tissue due to lack of oxygen, is also known as a heart attack. Myocardial ischemia causes disturbances of the heart rate, heart rhythm, or both, and can affect the pumping action of the heart, interfering with circulation, leading to alterations in oxygenation. Symptoms vary, based on the problem, but include pain, anxiety, nausea, vomiting, indigestion, and shortness of breath.

Heart failure occurs when the heart is unable to pump a sufficient blood supply, resulting in inadequate perfusion and oxygenation of tissues. It can be the result of many heart conditions, including chronic hypertension, coronary artery disease, and disease of the heart valves. Symptoms include shortness of breath, edema (swelling), and fatigue. Additional information related to alterations in cardiovascular function is discussed in Chapter 26.

FACTORS AFFECTING CARDIOPULMONARY FUNCTIONING

A variety of factors affect adequate cardiopulmonary function, leading to impaired oxygenation and perfusion. Important factors are discussed in the following sections.

Level of Health

Acute and chronic illnesses can affect a person's cardiopulmonary function dramatically. For example, people with renal or cardiac disorders often have compromised respiratory functioning because of fluid overload and impaired tissue perfusion. People with chronic illnesses often have muscle wasting and poor muscle tone. These problems affect all the muscles, including those of the cardiopulmonary system. Alterations in muscle function contribute to inadequate pulmonary ventilation and respiration, as well as inadequate functioning of the heart. Anemia can result in impaired cardiopulmonary function. As discussed previously, anemia may lead to an inadequate supply of oxygen to the tissues of the body. Because hemoglobin also carries carbon dioxide to the lungs, anemia results in diminished carbon dioxide exchange. Myocardial infarction causes a lack of blood supply to the heart muscle. Damage to the heart muscle interferes with effective contractions of the heart muscle, leading to decreased perfusion of tissues and decreased gas exchange. Physical changes such as scoliosis (curvature of the spine) influence breathing patterns and may cause air trapping. Research reveals a statistically significant correlation between obesity and obstructive lung disease, including asthma and chronic obstructive pulmonary disease (Ramos-Nino et al., 2021). Moreover, people who are obese are often short of breath during activity, ultimately leading to less participation in exercise. As a result, the alveoli at the base of the lungs are rarely stimulated to expand fully.

Recall **Yan Kim**, the 57-year-old patient who developed respiratory failure from complications associated with pulmonary surgery. The acuity of the situation played a major role in the patient's current condition. The pulmonary surgery most likely reduced his respiratory function. The effects of anesthesia on his lungs and subsequently the development of complications compounded his situation.

Table 40-1 Respiratory Variations in the Life Cycle

	INFANT (BIRTH–1 YEAR)	EARLY CHILDHOOD (1–5 YEARS)	LATE CHILDHOOD (6–12 YEARS)	OLDER ADULT (65+ YEARS)
Respiratory rate	30–60 breaths/min	20–40 breaths/min	15–25 breaths/min	16–24 breaths/min
Respiratory pattern	Abdominal breathing, irregular in rate and depth	Abdominal breathing, irregular	Thoracic breathing, regular	Thoracic, regular
Chest wall	Thin, little muscle, ribs, and sternum easily seen	Same as infant's but with more subcutaneous fat	Further subcutaneous fat deposited, structures less prominent	Thin, structures prominent
Breath sounds	Loud, harsh crackles at end of deep inspiration	Loud, harsh expiration longer than inspiration	Clear inspiration is longer than expiration	Clear
Shape of thorax	Round	Elliptical	Elliptical	Barrel shaped or elliptical

Source: Adapted from Chiocca, E. M. (2019). *Advanced pediatric assessment* (3rd ed.). Springer Publishing Company; Hogan-Quigley, B., Palm, M. L., & Bickley, L. S. (2017). *Bates' nursing guide to physical examination and history taking* (2nd ed.). Wolters Kluwer; and Kyle, T., & Carman, S. (2021). *Essentials of pediatric nursing* (4th ed.). Wolters Kluwer.

Developmental Considerations

There are many age-related developmental considerations affecting cardiopulmonary function. Table 40-1 summarizes respiratory variations in the life cycle. Age-related variations in pulse rate and blood pressure can be found in Chapter 26, Table 26-1 on page 718.

Infants

The normal infant's chest is small, the airways are short, and aspiration is a potential problem. The respiratory rate is more rapid in infants than at any other age (see Table 40-1). As the alveoli increase in number and size, adequate oxygenation is accomplished at lower respiratory rates. Surfactant is formed in utero between 34 and 36 weeks. An infant born before 34 weeks may not have produced sufficient surfactant, leading to collapse of the alveoli and poor alveolar exchange. Synthetic surfactant can be given to the infant to help reopen the alveoli. Infants are at risk for upper respiratory tract infections and asthma as a result of exposure to secondhand smoke. Respiratory activity is primarily abdominal in infants. The pulse rate is more rapid in infancy than in adulthood, limiting the infant's ability to increase CO by increasing the heart rate (Kyle & Carman, 2021).

Toddlers, Preschoolers, School-Age Children, and Adolescents

The preschool child's Eustachian tubes, bronchi, and bronchioles are elongated and less angular. Thus, the average number of routine colds and infections decreases until the child enters day care or school and is exposed more frequently to pathogens. Young children who are not placed in day care usually have not had the opportunity to develop antibodies for the variety of viruses and bacteria they may encounter in a school setting. Encourage good hand hygiene and tissue etiquette. Most children at this age have colds or upper respiratory infections, but some have more serious problems of otitis media, bronchitis, and pneumonia. Children in this age group are also at risk for asthma as a result of exposure to secondhand smoke. By the end of late childhood and during adulthood, the immune system is prepared to protect the person from most infections. A child's blood vessels widen and increase in length over time. The blood pressure increases over time, reaching the adult level in adolescence.

Older Adults

Specific physical changes occur in older adults that are unrelated to any pathology. Refer to the accompanying Focus on the Older Adult box. The tissues and airways of the respiratory tract (including the alveoli) become less elastic. The power of the respiratory and abdominal muscles is reduced; therefore, the diaphragm moves less efficiently. The chest is unable to stretch as much, resulting in a decline in maximum inspiration and expiration. Airways collapse more easily. These alterations increase the risk for disease, especially pneumonia and other chest infections.

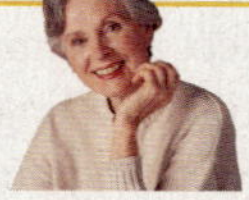

Think back to **Joan McIntyre**, the 72-year-old woman who is having an exacerbation of her chronic COPD. The nurse needs to consider potential age-related changes when planning the patient's care. The nurse also needs to consider that some of these age-related changes may be intensifying some of the patient's symptoms and contributing to their decreased ability to care for themself.

The normal aging heart can maintain adequate CO under ordinary circumstances but may have a limited ability to respond to situations that cause physical or emotional stress, when the demands on the heart are increased (Eliopoulos, 2018; Hinkle et al., 2022). Decreased physical activity, physical deconditioning, decreased elasticity of the blood vessels, and stiffening of the heart valves can lead to a decrease in the overall function of the heart.

Medication Considerations

Many medications affect the function of the cardiopulmonary system. Patients receiving drugs that affect the central

Focus on the Older Adult

NURSING STRATEGIES TO ADDRESS AGE-RELATED CHANGES IN OXYGENATION

Age-Related Changes	Nursing Strategies
Decreased Gas Exchange and Increased Work of Breathing • Decreased elastic recoil of the lungs • Expiration requiring use of accessory muscles • Fewer functional capillaries and more fibrous tissue in alveoli • Decreased skeletal muscle strength in thorax • Reduction in vital capacity and increase in residual volume	• Encourage rest periods, as necessary. • Encourage cessation or moderation of smoking and second-hand smoke exposure. • Teach breathing exercises. • Remind about avoiding air pollutants. • Caution about effect of extreme weather conditions. • Instruct to avoid opioids and sleeping pills. • Discuss home management with patient and family/caregivers. • Teach avoidance of infection and preventive measures (i.e., pneumococcal and flu vaccination). • Use pillows as necessary to sleep.
Decreased Ventilation and Ineffective Cough • Less air exchange; more secretions remain in lungs • Drier mucous membranes • Altered pain sensation • Different norms for body temperature; fever may be atypical • Greater risk for aspiration due to slower gastric motility • Impaired mobility and inactivity, effects of medication	• Encourage increased fluid intake, especially water, as allowed. • Use cool-mist humidifier (teach proper cleaning technique). • Encourage attendance at pulmonary exercise rehabilitation program. • Discourage use of over-the-counter medications. • Teach how to splint thorax and cough effectively. • Instruct in use of supplemental oxygen. • Teach avoidance of milk products if they are troublesome.
Decreased CO and Ability to Respond to Stress • Reduction in the elasticity of the heart's tissues • Heart muscle becomes less efficient—working harder to pump the same amount of blood through the body. • Progressive atherosclerosis (fatty build up or plaques, thickening) in arterial walls and loss of elasticity • Capillary walls thicken slightly, leading to a slower rate of exchange of gases, nutrients, and waste.	• Encourage the inclusion of physical activity in the daily routine; pace activities. • Encourage a healthy low-fat, low-salt diet, including plenty of fruits, vegetables, and whole grains. • Assist with smoking cessation and/or avoid the use of tobacco. • Teach the importance of regular check-ups • Assist with weight control. • Teach the importance of medication compliance. • Teach stress-reduction activities.

nervous system need to be monitored carefully for respiratory complications. For example, opioids are chemical agents that depress the medullary respiratory center. As a result, the rate and depth of respirations decrease. Be alert for the possibility of respiratory depression or arrest when administering any opioid or sedative. Other medications decrease heart rate with associated decreased cardiac output, with the potential to alter the flow of blood to body tissues.

Lifestyle Considerations

Activity levels and habits can dramatically affect a person's cardiopulmonary status. For example, sedentary activity patterns do not encourage the expansion of alveoli and the development of pulmonary exercise patterns (deep breathing). People who exercise (e.g., aerobics, walking, swimming) three to six times per week can better respond to stressors to cardiopulmonary health. Regular physical activity provides many health benefits, including increased heart and lung fitness, improved muscle fitness, and reducing the risk of heart disease. Additional considerations related to the effects of exercise on the cardiopulmonary system are discussed in Chapter 34.

Cultural influences can also play a role in a person's lifestyle, encouraging or discouraging healthy choices. Culture is a strong force in the determinants of health and behavior change. An understanding of a patient's cultural background is necessary to promote health and disease prevention in any population (Andrews et al., 2020). An important part of care would be to assess the impact of any practice and beliefs on a patient's readiness to participate in the proposed plan of care related to the health problem or need.

Cigarette smoking (active or passive) is a major contributor to lung disease and respiratory distress, heart disease, and lung cancer. Cigarette smoking is the most important risk factor for COPD (NHLBI, 2019). Smoking is also one of the key risk factors for heart disease, the leading cause of death in the United States (CDC, 2021a). Use of e-cigarettes, or vaping, is associated with e-cigarette, or vaping, product use–associated lung injury (EVALI) and is an emerging health issue of concern (CDC, 2020d). Several lung diseases, including bronchiolitis obliterans, lipoid pneumonia, and spontaneous pneumothorax, are associated with vaping, and there is concern that the chemicals deposited in the lungs through vaping may lead to the development of cancer (Broderick, 2021). EVALI has been connected with increased emergency room visits, hospitalization, and patient deaths (CDC, 2020d). Evidence related to the impact of e-cigarettes on the lungs continues to evolve.

Nurses working with patients to initiate changes in health habits that affect oxygenation and perfusion must also examine themselves as a factor in the success of the plan. Nurses who role model good health behaviors are more effective teachers. Use the display Promoting Health 40-1: Oxygenation and Perfusion for yourself before using it with others.

Social Determinants of Health

A person's neighborhood and built-environment impact their health and well-being (U.S. DHHS & ODPHP, n.d.). Unsafe air and other toxic environmental pollutants increase the risk for cardiovascular and pulmonary disease, as well as cancer (U.S. DHHS & ODPHP, n.d.). Although it is impossible to pinpoint all the effects of air pollution, researchers have demonstrated a high correlation between air pollution and cancer and lung diseases (Kurt et al., 2016; Turner et al., 2020). Air pollution is the most important environmental cardiovascular risk factor as well (Al-Kindi et al., 2020). For example, a person with adequate respiratory functioning who is exposed to air pollution may experience stinging of the eyes and nasal passages, coughing, choking, headache, and dizziness. Occupational exposure to asbestos, silica, or coal dust, as well as environmental pollution, can lead to chronic pulmonary disease (Johns Hopkins Medicine, 2021). Chronic environmental exposure to radon, radiation, asbestos, and arsenic can lead to lung cancer (MFMER, 2021). In addition, people who have experienced an alteration in respiratory functioning in the past often have difficulty continuing to perform self-care activities in a polluted environment.

Economic resources and stability affect cardiopulmonary health. Employment and income coupled with the increasing cost of food may result in a decrease in the nutritional quality of the diet. People who feel unsafe where they live or have poor street infrastructure may be more likely to stay home, resulting in less physical activity (CDC, 2022). Both these sets of factors may increase the risk for cardiovascular diseases.

Additional sociocultural factors affecting cardiopulmonary health and the risk for cardiopulmonary disease include:

- Language barriers
- Knowledge of nutrition to support cardiopulmonary health; limited access to and/or ability to obtain food
- Literacy
- Social isolation
- Access to physical activity opportunities

Psychological Health Considerations

Many psychological factors and conditions can affect the respiratory system. People responding to stress may sigh excessively or exhibit **hyperventilation** (increased rate and depth of ventilation, above the body's normal metabolic requirements). Hyperventilation can lead to a lowered level of arterial carbon dioxide. Generalized anxiety has been shown to cause enough bronchospasm to produce an episode of bronchial asthma. In addition, patients with respiratory problems often develop some anxiety as a result of the hypoxia caused by the respiratory problem.

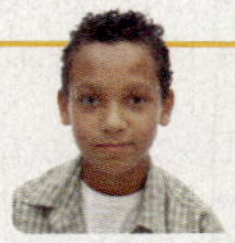

Think back to **Tyrone Jacobs**, the young boy described at the beginning of the chapter. The patient is gasping for breath, which is extremely frightening and anxiety producing. In addition, his parents are frantic; this would increase Tyrone's anxiety level, further limiting his ability to breathe. The nurse needs to incorporate an understanding of this situation and plan interventions that promote oxygenation while reducing anxiety in both Tyrone and his parents.

Promoting Health 40-1

OXYGENATION AND PERFUSION

Use the assessment checklist to determine how well you are meeting your needs related to oxygenation. Then develop a prescription for self-care by choosing appropriate behaviors from the list of suggestions.

Assessment Checklist

☐ almost always ☐ sometimes ☐ almost never

☐ ☐ ☐ 1. I breathe easily, without discomfort and without feeling short of breath.

☐ ☐ ☐ 2. I exercise regularly.

☐ ☐ ☐ 3. I maintain normal weight for my height and body frame.

☐ ☐ ☐ 4. I live in an environment free of pollution.

☐ ☐ ☐ 5. I avoid substances (tobacco, chemicals) that cause respiratory problems.

☐ ☐ ☐ 6. I arrange to receive recommended immunizations.

Self-Care Behaviors

1. Follow a regular exercise program with activities that requires moderate effort, such as brisk walking for 2.5 to 5 hours or more a week (USDHHS, 2018).
2. Maintain healthy body weight.
3. Obtain medical evaluation for chest pain, problems with breathing, and/or chronic cough with sputum or blood.
4. Evaluate personal use of tobacco.
5. Incorporate a plan to reduce smoking, then stop smoking on a specific target date.
6. Avoid exposure to secondhand smoke when possible.
7. Arrange to have a tuberculin test done annually.
8. Receive a yearly influenza vaccine and a pneumococcal vaccine and COVID-19 vaccines, based on current recommendations.
9. Avoid chemical substances that cause respiratory depression.
10. Maintain a pollution-free environment (as much as possible).
11. Support federal and community efforts to keep the air free of pollution.

Information to promote cardiovascular health and oxygenation is available online.

NURSING PROCESS FOR OXYGENATION AND PERFUSION

Assessing

The patient's health history is an essential component for assessing the patient's cardiopulmonary function and ability to maintain adequate oxygenation. This information can be obtained from either the patient or a family member/caregiver. The nursing examination combined with laboratory findings can provide information to identify a patient's strengths; the nature of any problems; their course; related signs and symptoms; and onset, frequency, and effects on activities of daily living (ADLs). The nurse decides, based on these findings, what problems can be treated independently by nursing and which problems should be addressed in collaboration with other health professionals. Additional assessment information is discussed in Chapter 27.

Nursing History

The nursing history, an important clinical tool in the early steps of the nursing process, always includes a cardiopulmonary component. The information gained provides data about why the patient needs nursing care and what kind of care is required to maintain sufficient oxygenation of tissues. Interview questions help identify current or potential health problems or needs, actions performed by the patient for meeting cardiopulmonary needs, and the effects of such actions. They also help identify any contributing factors, the use of any aids to improve oxygenation, and effects of health problems on the patient's lifestyle and relationships with others.

Before starting the interview, make certain that the patient is not in acute distress. If the patient is experiencing any cardiopulmonary distress, initiate appropriate actions immediately to help relieve symptoms. Enlist the aid of family members/caregivers to help answer questions. Interview the patient at a later point, when the patient is able, to expand the initial database. If no emergency interventions are necessary for the patient's clinical condition, obtain a comprehensive history at this time.

Social determinants of health are conditions in the patients environments that may affect the patient's functioning and quality of life (U.S. DHHS & ODPHP, n.d.). Ask about sociocultural factors that may impact a patient's cardiopulmonary status and health, such as:

Access to physical activity opportunities
Safe neighborhoods and environments
Income
Environmental pollutants
Access to a health care provider and health care

This information helps us to understand factors that may influence a patient's health and use of health care and shape more effective interventions (U.S. DHHS & ODPHP, n.d.).

The accompanying Focused Assessment Guide 40-1 on page 1598 provides examples of appropriate questions for health history assessment related to oxygenation and perfusion. If the patient is experiencing any disturbance in cardiopulmonary function, conduct a more detailed assessment, directing attention to the factors described earlier that may influence oxygenation and perfusion.

Physical Assessment

Examinations of the cardiopulmonary systems are discussed in Chapter 27. Refer to this chapter for details and additional information related to the assessment of these systems. Always proceed in a well-organized manner through a sequence of inspection, palpation, percussion, and auscultation. Note the patient's vital sign measurements, particularly the pulse and respiratory rate, as well as the blood pressure. Information related to vital sign assessment is discussed in Chapter 26. Note: Percussion of the thorax is an advanced assessment technique, usually performed by advanced health care providers. Refer to a health assessment text for details.

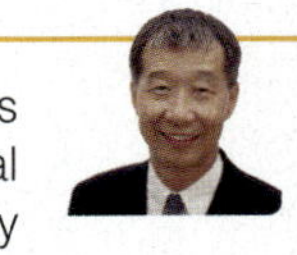

Recall ***Mr. Kim***, the 57-year-old man who is receiving oxygen therapy and mechanical ventilation via an **endotracheal tube** (airway into the trachea). A complete assessment is necessary to identify specific problems related to oxygenation as well as to determine the effectiveness of current treatments.

INSPECTION

Observe the patient's general appearance. Does the patient appear to be in any distress? Is the patient restless or anxious? Note the patient's level of consciousness and orientation to person, place, and time. Alterations in oxygenation to body tissues can be a result of respiratory or cardiac distress and lead to altered mental status. Inspect the patient's skin, mucous membranes, and general circulation, which can be a general indicator of the patient's health status, as well as indicating problems with oxygenation. Pallor (lack of color) of skin and mucous membranes can indicate less than optimal oxygenation. Cyanosis (bluish discoloration) and/or coolness or decreased temperature may indicate decreased blood flow or poor blood oxygenation. Edema may be the result of overhydration, heart failure, kidney failure, trauma or peripheral vascular disease, conditions which may contribute to altered oxygenation.

Note any abnormalities in the structures of the chest. The adult chest contour is slightly convex, with no sternal depression. The anteroposterior diameter should be less than the transverse diameter. Kyphosis (curvature of the spine) contributes to the older adult's appearance of leaning forward and can limit respiratory ventilation. Barrel chest deformity may be a result of aging or COPD. Note the contour of the intercostal spaces, which should be flat or depressed, and the movement of the chest, which should be symmetrical. Observe the respiratory rate, rhythm, and depth. Normally, respirations are quiet and nonlabored, and occur at a rate of 12 to 20 times each minute in healthy adults. Note any flaring of the nostrils, muscular retractions, **tachypnea** (rapid breathing), or **bradypnea** (slow breathing), which are suggestive of a health deviation requiring further evaluation.

Refer to Chapter 27 for a detailed discussion of inspection as part of the assessment of the respiratory and cardiovascular systems.

Focused Assessment Guide 40-1

OXYGENATION AND PERFUSION

Factors to Assess	Questions and Approaches
Usual patterns of respiration	How would you describe your breathing? Do you have allergies? What type(s) of allergies do you have? What relief measures do you use?
Medications	Are you taking any medications for your breathing, your heart, or for your blood pressure? What other medications are you taking?
Health history	Do you have any heart, lung, or breathing conditions? Does anyone in your family/home have any breathing conditions or respiratory infections?
Recent changes	Have you noticed any changes in your breathing (out of breath, cough, wheezing)? Have you noticed any changes in your ability to perform activities of daily living? Do you have any swelling or redness in your arms or legs? Do you have a respiratory infection? If so, what type? What relief measures are you using?
Lifestyle and environment	Do you smoke? If so, how many years have you smoked? How much do you smoke (i.e., how many packs per day or year)? Do you live with a smoker or are there smokers in your workplace? Are you exposed to respiratory irritants in your workplace? Are there other pollutants in your workplace?
Cough	How much and how often do you cough? What is it like (dry, bubbly, hoarse)? Do you cough up mucus? If so, how much and what does it look like? Do you have a history of allergies? Do you ever wheeze? Are you exposed to dust? Fumes?
Sputum	Do you ever cough up and spit out mucus? How much do you spit out and do you associate it with anything (time of day, environment)? What color is it? Is it ever blood tinged? What is its odor?
Pain	Do you have any chest pain? Do you have pain with breathing? Do you have pain in the arms or legs? When did it start? On a scale of 0 to 10 (10 being very painful), how severe is the pain? Where is the pain? Is the pain worse with inspiration? Expiration? Cough? Activity? Does the pain radiate? What measures are you using to relieve the pain?
Dyspnea	Do you have any shortness of breath? Is it constant or remittent or related to any activity? How do different positions affect it? How does it affect your daily activities? Can you sleep lying flat? How many pillows do you use?
Fever	Have you had pneumonia recently? Do you have any contact with people who have tuberculosis? Do you have night sweats? Are others in your household well or ill? Have you traveled anywhere recently?
Fatigue	Have you noticed you feel more tired lately? Are you getting your normal amount of sleep at night? Has your sleep at night been affected by any difficulty breathing? Do you become easily fatigued when you climb stairs?

PALPATION

Palpate the chest. Note skin temperature and color. Skin temperature in this area is typically the same as the rest of the body. Assess chest expansion (thoracic excursion), which should be symmetrical. Note the presence or absence of masses, edema, or tenderness on palpation. Palpate the point of maximal impulse (PMI). Note pulsations in any other area of the chest. Abnormal size or location of the PMI or the presence of vibrations can indicate heart failure, myocardial infarction, disease of the heart valves, or other cardiac diseases. Palpate the patient's extremities. Assess skin temperature and color, pulses, and capillary refill. Note the presence or absence of edema, or tenderness on palpation. The presence of decreased skin temperature, pallor, cyanosis, decreased pulses, and prolonged capillary refill can indicate less than optimal cardiac function and oxygenation. The presence of edema also indicates alterations in cardiovascular function.

Refer to Chapter 27 for a detailed discussion of palpation as part of the assessment of the respiratory and cardiovascular systems.

PERCUSSION

Percussion is used to assess the position of the lungs, density of lung tissue, and identify changes in the tissue. This assessment skill is not used frequently. When used, it is usually included in examinations performed by advanced practice nurses and other advanced practice professionals. Refer to a health assessment text for details.

AUSCULTATION

Auscultation of the lungs assesses air flow through the respiratory passages and lungs. Listen for normal and abnormal lung sounds. Normal breath sounds include **vesicular** (low-pitched, soft sounds heard over peripheral lung fields), **bronchial** (loud, high-pitched sounds heard primarily over the trachea and larynx), and **bronchovesicular** (medium-pitched blowing sounds heard over the major bronchi) sounds. Auscultate as the patient breathes slowly through an open mouth. Breathing through the nose can produce falsely abnormal breath sounds.

In addition to air flow, listen for **adventitious** sounds (extra, abnormal sounds of breathing), such as wheezing or crackles. Abnormal lung sounds can occur as a result of alterations in the respiratory and cardiovascular systems and lead to impaired oxygenation. **Crackles**, frequently heard on inspiration, are soft, high-pitched discontinuous (intermittent) popping sounds. They are produced by air passing through fluid in the airways or alveoli and opening of deflated small airways and alveoli. They occur due to inflammation or congestion and are associated with pneumonia, heart failure, bronchitis, and COPD. **Wheezes** are continuous musical sounds, produced as air passes through airways constricted by swelling, narrowing, secretions, or tumors. They are often heard in patients with asthma, tumors, or a buildup of secretions.

Auscultation of the heart assesses function of the heart, heart valves, and blood flow. Listen for normal and abnormal heart sounds. Listen to the rhythm of the beat and the characteristic "lub–dub." The first sound, the lub, is followed by the second sound, the dub, with a pause before the next lub–dub. These sounds are made by the closure of valves in the heart during the cardiac cycle. The lub correlates with the beginning of systole, the contraction of the ventricles, and is called S_1. The dub correlates with the end of systole and the beginning of diastole, the relaxation of the ventricles, and is called S_2.

In addition to S_1 and S_2, listen for extra and abnormal heart sounds. Abnormal heart sounds occur as a result of alterations in the cardiovascular system that may lead to impaired oxygenation. Refer to Chapter 27 for a detailed discussion of auscultation as part of the assessment of the respiratory and cardiovascular systems.

> *Concept Mastery Alert*
>
> The presence of sputum in the airways can be indicated by coarse crackles that are soft, high-pitched, and discontinuous.

Common Laboratory and Diagnostic Tests

In addition to the nursing history and physical examination, the information provided in Table 40-2 (on page 1600) identifies common laboratory that may be used to assess cardiopulmonary function and can aid in the identification of health problems and needs.

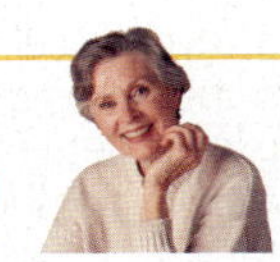

The nurse might anticipate diagnostic procedures such as **arterial blood gas (ABG)** analysis (measurement of blood pH and arterial gases to evaluate acid–base and oxygenation status) for **Joan McIntyre**, the older woman with the acute exacerbation of COPD. This diagnostic test would provide information regarding the adequacy of her oxygenation and ventilation and help titrate (adjust) the administration of supplemental oxygen. It would also be used to evaluate her response to treatment and therapies.

The diagnostic tests described in the next sections are not distinctive for a particular disease but reflect how well the cardiopulmonary systems are functioning.

ELECTROCARDIOGRAPHY

One of the most valuable and frequently used diagnostic tools, electrocardiography, measures the heart's electrical activity. Impulses moving through the heart's conduction system create electric currents that can be monitored on the body's surface. Electrodes attached to the skin can detect these electric currents and transmit them to an instrument that produces a record—the **electrocardiogram (ECG)**—of cardiac activity. The data are graphed as waveforms. ECG can be used to identify myocardial ischemia and infarction, heart damage, rhythm and conduction disturbances, chamber enlargement, electrolyte imbalances, and drug toxicity.

The standard 12-lead ECG uses a series of electrodes placed on the extremities and the chest wall to assess the heart from 12 different viewpoints (leads) by attaching 10 cables with electrodes to the patient's limbs and chest; 4 limb electrodes and 6 chest electrodes. Each lead provides

Table 40-2 Common Laboratory Studies Used to Assess Cardiopulmonary Function

STUDY	PREPARATION	AFTERCARE
Arterial Blood Gas and pH Analysis These examine arterial blood to determine the pressure exerted by oxygen and carbon dioxide in the blood and blood pH. This test measures the adequacy of oxygenation, ventilation, and perfusion. Normal results are: pH, 7.35–7.45; PCO_2, 35–45 mm Hg; PO_2, 80–100 mm Hg; HCO_3, 22–26 mEq/L; and base excess or deficit, −2–+2 mmol/L.	• Explain to the patient that this test requires an arterial puncture and collection of a blood specimen. • The radial, brachial, or femoral arteries are usually the sites of choice. • Perform the Allen test to ensure adequate ulnar blood flow when using the radial artery.	• Record supplemental oxygen or respirator settings on specimen information. • The arterial specimen is immediately placed on ice and taken to the laboratory. • Apply pressure for 5–10 minutes and watch for evidence of bleeding. If the patient is taking anticoagulants, pressure must be applied for a longer interval.
Cardiac Biomarkers Creatine kinase (CK) and isoenzymes are enzymes that are released as a result of injury to tissues, including the heart muscle. Troponin is a protein found in skeletal and cardiac muscle fibers and is also released after injury to the heart. These biomarkers are used to monitor cardiac injury and myocardial infarction. Measuring the levels of these enzymes can help determine the extent and timing of the damage.	• Review the procedure with the patient. Inform the patient that this test can assist in assessing for heart damage. • Inform the patient that a series of samples will be required; based on facility protocol, samples could be taken three to four times, in 3–4-hour intervals. • Inform the patient that specimen collection takes approximately 5–10 minutes. • Address concerns about pain and explain that there may be some discomfort during the venipuncture (puncture of the vein). • There are no food, fluid, or medication restrictions unless prescribed.	• Recognize anxiety related to test results. Provide teaching and information regarding the implications of the test results. • Reinforce information given by the patient's health care team regarding further testing, treatment, or referral to another health care provider. • Depending on the results of this procedure, additional testing may be performed to evaluate or monitor the progression of illness. • Evaluate test results in relation to the patient's symptoms, health care problems, and other tests performed.
Complete Blood Count (CBC)	• Review the procedure with the patient. Inform the patient that this test can assist in evaluating the body's response to illness. • Inform the patient that specimen collection takes approximately 5–10 minutes. • Address concerns about pain and explain that there may be some discomfort during the venipuncture (puncture of the vein). • There are no food, fluid, or medication restrictions unless prescribed.	• Reinforce information given by the patient's health care team regarding further testing, treatment, or referral to another health care provider. • Depending on the results of this procedure, additional testing may be performed to evaluate or monitor progression of illness. • Evaluate test results in relation to the patient's symptoms, health care problems, and other tests performed.
Cytologic Study This involves a microscopic examination of sputum and the cells it contains. It is done primarily to detect cells that may be malignant, determine organisms causing infection, and identify blood or pus in the sputum.	• Collect the specimen, if possible, in the morning before breakfast. The test usually involves 3 successive days of sputum collection. About 1 teaspoon of sputum is needed for a specimen. • The patient should take a deep breath, then expel the air with a deep cough. • Expectorate the specimen into a sterile specimen container with the appropriate preservative, if indicated. • Close the container with a tight-fitting lid.	• Advise the patient to inform the nurse when the specimen has been obtained. • Label and package the specimen and send it to the laboratory as soon as possible.

Source: Adapted from Fischbach, F. T., & Fischbach, M. A. (2018). *A manual of laboratory and diagnostic tests* (10th ed.). Wolters Kluwer; and Hinkle, J. L., Cheever, K. H., & Overbaugh, K. J. (2022). *Brunner & Suddarth's Textbook of medical-surgical nursing* (15th ed.). Wolters Kluwer.

an electrographic snapshot of electrochemical activity of the myocardial cell membrane. The ECG device measures and averages the differences between the electrical potential of the electrode sites for each lead and graphs them over time, creating the standard ECG complex, called PQRST. These electrodes provide views of the heart from the frontal plane as well as the horizontal plane. It is essential that connection or placement of the ECG electrodes/leads is accurate to prevent misdiagnosis.

An ECG is typically accomplished using a multichannel method. All electrodes are attached to the patient at once and the machine prints a simultaneous view of all leads. It is important to reassure the patient that the leads just sense and record and do not transmit any electricity. The patient must be able to lie still and refrain from speaking to prevent body movement from creating artifacts in the ECG. Variations of standard ECG include exercise ECG (stress ECG) and ambulatory ECG (Holter monitoring). Refer to a medical-surgical text for information regarding these tests.

PULMONARY FUNCTION STUDIES

Pulmonary function studies encompass a group of tests used to assess respiratory function to assist in evaluating respiratory disorders. They provide an evaluation of lung dysfunction, diagnose disease, assess disease severity, assist in management of disease, and evaluate respiratory interventions. Most tests are administered by a respiratory therapist, technician, nurses with specialized training, or health care providers. Several tests commonly encountered are described in the next section. More specialized tests and their purposes include:

- Diffusion capacity estimates the patient's ability to absorb alveolar gases and determine if a gas exchange problem exists.
- Maximal respiratory pressures help evaluate neuromuscular causes of respiratory dysfunction.
- Exercise testing helps evaluate dyspnea during exertion.

Refer to Box 40-1: Commonly Measured Values From Pulmonary Function Tests.

Box 40-1 Commonly Measured Values From Pulmonary Function Tests

- Tidal volume (V_T): Total amount of air inhaled and exhaled with one breath during normal breathing
- Vital capacity (VC): Maximum amount of air exhaled after maximum inspiration
- Forced vital capacity (FVC): Maximum amount of air that can be forcefully exhaled after a maximal inspiration
- Forced expiratory volume ($FEV_{[1,2,3]}$): The volume of air exhaled at a specific time interval; for example, in the first, second, and third seconds after a full inspiration (timed vital capacities)
- Total lung capacity (TLC): The volume of air contained within the lungs at maximum inspiration
- Residual volume (RV): The volume of air left in the lungs at maximal expiration
- Peak expiratory flow rate (PEFR): The maximum flow attained during the FVC

Source: Adapted from Fischbach, F. T., & Fischbach, M. A. (2018). *A manual of laboratory and diagnostic tests* (10th ed.). Wolters Kluwer; and Hess, D. R., MacIntyre, N. R., Galvin, W. F., & Mishoe, S. C. (2021). *Respiratory care: Principles and practice* (4th ed.). Jones & Bartlett Learning.

Spirometry

Spirometry measures the volume of air in liters exhaled or inhaled by a patient over time. It evaluates lung function and airway obstruction through respiratory mechanics. Spirometry can be used to measure the degree of airway obstruction and evaluates response to inhaled medications. The patient inhales deeply and exhales forcefully into a **spirometer**, an instrument that measures lung volumes and airflow. Patients also use spirometers to promote deep breathing while recovering from surgery, and to monitor health status in management of chronic asthma. A discussion regarding the use of incentive spirometers can be found later in this chapter.

Peak Expiratory Flow Rate

Peak expiratory flow rate (PEFR) refers to the point of highest flow during forced expiration. PEFR reflects changes in the size of pulmonary airways and is measured using a peak flow meter. It is routinely used for patients with moderate or severe asthma to measure the severity of the disease and degree of disease management. With the patient standing or sitting with the back positioned as straight as possible, the patient takes a deep breath and places the peak flow meter in the mouth, closing the lips tightly around the mouthpiece. The patient forcibly exhales into the peak flow meter, and an indicator on the meter rises to a number. The patient is asked to repeat this three times, and the highest number is recorded. This produces a measurement in liters indicating the maximum flow rate during a forced expiration. Predicted normal values are established in regard to height, age, and biologic sex, but patients with moderate to severe asthma cannot achieve the predicted values (Hess et al., 2021). The individual patient's personal best peak flow provides the benchmark value for their asthma management plan (Hess et al., 2021; MFMER, 2020). The personal best peak flow is identified by measuring the daily peak flow rate over a 2- to 3-week period; the highest peak flow rate over this period is the patient's personal best (MFMER, 2020). Patients with asthma commonly measure PEFR at home to monitor airflow. The results are used to track disease progression and regulate treatment by the patient and health care team.

Pulse Oximetry

Pulse oximetry is a noninvasive technique that measures the peripheral arterial oxyhemoglobin saturation (SpO_2) of arterial blood. The reported result is a ratio, expressed as a percentage, between the actual oxygen content of the hemoglobin and the potential maximum oxygen-carrying capacity of the hemoglobin (Fischbach & Fischbach, 2018). Pulse oximetry is useful for monitoring patients receiving oxygen therapy, titrating oxygen therapy, monitoring those at risk for hypoxia, and monitoring postoperative patients. Pulse oximeter measurements are less accurate at SpO_2 less than 80%, but the clinical importance of this is questionable

(Hess et al., 2021, p. 25). In addition, a patient's SpO_2 may remain relatively normal initially due to an increase in respiratory rate compensating for inadequate oxygen delivery (Dix, 2018; Elliott & Baird, 2019). Pulse oximetry does not replace ABG analysis. Desaturation (decreased level of SpO_2) indicates gas exchange abnormalities. Oxygen desaturation is considered a late sign of respiratory compromise in patients with reduced rate and depth of breathing.

Be aware of the patient's hemoglobin level before evaluating oxygen saturation because the test measures only the percentage of oxygen carried by the available hemoglobin. Thus, even a patient with a low hemoglobin level could appear to have a normal SpO_2 because most of that hemoglobin is saturated. However, the patient may not have enough oxygen to meet body needs (Morton & Fontaine, 2018). Also, take into consideration the presence of preexisting health conditions, such as COPD. Parameters for acceptable oxygen saturation readings may be different for these patients. For patients with chronic lung disease, a level of 88% to 92% may be considered within normal limits or may indicate the need for oxygen therapy (Mirza et al., 2018; Mitchell, 2015). Be aware of any prescribed interventions regarding acceptable ranges and/or check with the patient's health care team.

A range of 90% to 100% is considered the normal SpO_2 (Bauldoff et al., 2020), depending on the patient's health status and health problems and needs; values <90% are considered low (American Thoracic Society, 2021; MFMER, 2018b), indicate that oxygenation to the tissues may be inadequate, and should be investigated for potential hypoxia or technical error (Hinkle et al., 2022). When administering supplemental oxygen, most patients will have a target oxygen saturation of 94% to 98% (O'Driscoll et al., 2017). Refer also to the discussion of provision of supplemental oxygen later in the chapter on page 1613. Figure 40-8 shows a nurse using a pulse oximetry unit. Skill 40-1 on pages 1632–1636 outlines nursing responsibilities when using a pulse oximetry unit.

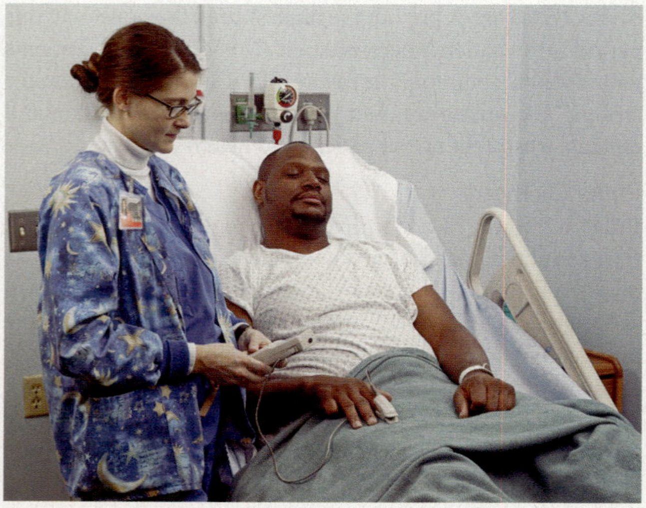

FIGURE 40-8. Using a portable pulse oximetry unit to measure oxygen saturation (SpO_2) of arterial blood.

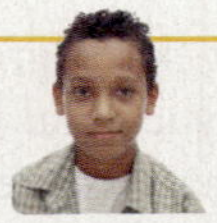

Consider **Tyrone Jacobs**, the young boy with suspected asthma described at the beginning of the chapter. The nurse would use pulse oximetry initially to obtain baseline information about the patient's oxygen saturation level and then as a means to evaluate the effectiveness of therapy.

CAPNOGRAPHY

Capnography is a technique to measure the carbon dioxide level in expired gas (end-tidal CO_2) (Hess et al., 2021) and is a noninvasive method to monitor and evaluate respiratory function and ventilation (Morton & Fontaine, 2018). Exhaled air passes through a sensor that measures the amount of carbon dioxide (CO_2) exhaled with each breath. The reported results also provide information about the respiratory rate and depth, the presence of apnea, and efficiency of gas exchange. The normal range for end-tidal CO_2 is typically 35 to 45 mm Hg (Burns & Delgado, 2019). When carbon dioxide levels are abnormal, either high or low, adverse effects, including death, can occur. Capnography is useful for assessing and monitoring ventilation and aiding in earlier identification of patients who are at risk for respiratory compromise, are experiencing partial or complete airway obstruction or are experiencing hypoventilation (Burns & Delgado, 2019; Seckel, 2018). It may also be used to confirm and monitor placement of endotracheal or tracheostomy tubes, in management of patients receiving mechanical ventilation, and in confirming and monitoring placement of nasogastric tubes as well as identifying patients with low cardiac output (Burns & Delgado, 2019; Hess et al., 2021). Capnography can detect signs of abnormal ventilation, such as respiratory depression and hypoventilation, earlier than pulse oximetry (Bovino et al., 2018; Kummer & Walden, 2019).

A capnometer (device displaying numeric measurement of CO_2) may be incorporated into a bedside monitor, may be a handheld unit (may be incorporated into a pulse oximeter), can be incorporated into a mechanical ventilator, can be a small device attached directly to an artificial airway, and can be incorporated into nasal cannula for nonintubated patients (Fig. 40-9) (Hess et al., 2021). The use of capnography in monitoring placement nasogastric tube placement is discussed in Chapters 37 and 39.

THORACENTESIS

Thoracentesis is the procedure of puncturing the chest wall and inserting a needle into the pleural space to aspirate pleural fluid, air, or both (Morton & Fontaine, 2018). A thoracentesis may be performed to obtain a specimen for diagnostic purposes, to remove fluid or air that has accumulated in the pleural cavity and is causing respiratory difficulty and discomfort, or to instill medications (Hinkle et al., 2022). The physician or other advanced practice professional can perform a thoracentesis at the bedside with the nurse assisting, or it can be performed in a procedure room, in the radiology department, or in an outpatient setting (Bauldoff et al., 2020). The patient is required to sign a permit for this procedure.

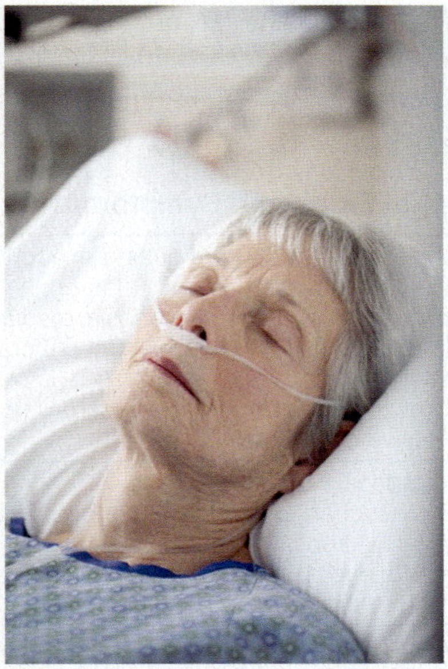

FIGURE 40-9. Nasal cannula designed for oxygen administration with incorporated CO_2 sampling. (*Source:* Nellcor TM Adult/Pediatric Colorimetric CO_2 Detector. 2020 Medtronic. All rights reserved. Used with the permission of Medtronic.)

Because the cavity being entered is sterile, surgical asepsis is required. Standard precautions also are used; transmission-based precautions are implemented as indicated.

Procedure

A thoracentesis is usually carried out with the patient sitting on a chair or the edge of the bed with the legs supported and the arms and shoulders raised (arms folded and resting on a pillow on the bedside table) so the ribs lift and separate, to allow easier needle insertion (Fig. 40-10). If unable to sit up, the patient may lie on the unaffected side with the hand of the affected side raised above the shoulder. A local anesthetic is used to minimize pain and discomfort (Morton & Fontaine, 2018).

The location where the needle is inserted depends on where the fluid is present and where the practitioner can best aspirate it. Once this spot is identified, the skin is cleansed with an antimicrobial agent. After the local anesthetic has taken effect, the needle is inserted between the ribs through the intercostal muscles and fascia and into the pleura. After the procedure, the needle or plastic catheter is removed, and a small sterile dressing is placed over the entry site.

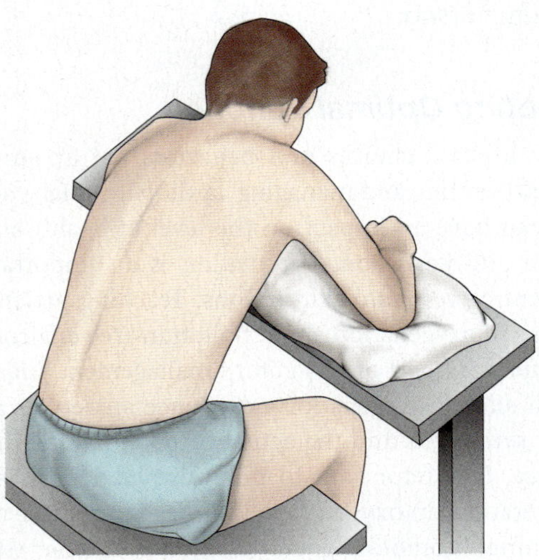

FIGURE 40-10. Position of the patient for thoracentesis.

During thoracentesis, fluid or air can be removed from the pleural cavity with a syringe. Another method for removing fluid is to drain the fluid into a bottle in which a partial vacuum has been created. With this technique, a small plastic catheter may be threaded through the needle, allowing the needle to be withdrawn. This catheter reduces the possibility of puncturing the lung. When this method is used, the tubing connecting the needle and the bottle must be sterile. Commonly, a calibrated bottle is used to collect the drainage, allowing the amount of fluid removed to be determined. The maximum amount of fluid removed at one time is generally 1,200 to 1,500 mL, to reduce the risk of cardiovascular collapse from rapid removal of too much fluid (Bauldoff et al., 2020).

Nursing Responsibilities

The nurse is responsible for collecting baseline data before the procedure and for preparing the patient physically and emotionally for the procedure. Instruct the patient not to cough or breathe deeply during the procedure. Urge the patient to remain as still as possible to diminish the risk for accidental injury to the lung. Administer analgesics before the procedure as ordered.

During the procedure, observe the patient's reactions. Monitor the patient's color, pulse, oxygen saturation, and respiratory rates, communicating immediately to the health care team any deviation from the patient's baseline. Fainting, nausea, and vomiting may occur. If not applied by the practitioner who completed the procedure, dress the wound with a sterile dressing (Morton & Fontaine, 2018), based on prescribed intervention or facility policy. Ensure that specimens, if obtained, are taken to the laboratory immediately.

After the procedure, assess the patient for complications, which could include pneumothorax, pain, hypotension, and pulmonary edema (Morton & Fontaine, 2018). Assess for changes in vital signs, particularly respirations and oxygen saturation; monitor lung sounds; and assess for the presence or worsening of cough or dyspnea. If a large amount of fluid was removed, respirations usually become easier. If the lung was punctured, respiratory distress becomes acute. If blood appears in the sputum or the patient has severe coughing, notify the health care team promptly. Monitor the puncture site. A chest radiograph is usually done after the procedure to verify the absence of complications.

Diagnosing Actual or Potential Health Problems and Needs

An assessment of a patient's oxygenation and perfusion status may lead to the identification of one or more actual or potential health problems and needs related to oxygenation and perfusion. Following the formulation of the actual or potential health problems and needs, the nurse communicates findings to other nursing and health care professionals through the use of written and spoken word. The written actual or

Examples of Actual or Potential Health Problems and Needs

OXYGENATION AND PERFUSION

Actual or Potential Health Problems and Needs	Possible Etiologic Factors	Potential Signs and Symptoms
Ineffective Airway Clearance	Fatigue; retained secretions; a 20-year history of COPD, with recent development of pneumonia	"I never feel as though I am getting enough air." • Thick, yellow secretions • Pale skin with circumoral cyanosis; respiratory rate is 40 breaths/min and shallow. Coarse crackles are auscultated bilaterally. • Cannot sit quietly in chair or on bed. • Ineffective cough
Impaired Gas Exchange	Smokes one pack of cigarettes per day; works with asbestos in auto factory; has had a cold for 7 days	Using pursed-lip breathing • Sitting hunched forward with overbed table supporting arms. • Altered blood gases show respiratory acidosis. • Reports shortness of breath for 1 week.
Impaired Breathing	Anxious about results of cardiac catheterization and possible cardiac surgery	Hyperventilating, tachypneic (40 breaths/min) • "I have a tingling feeling in my fingers." • "I can't catch my breath and I can't lie down in bed."

potential health problem or need becomes a permanent part of the patient's health record. Examples of health problems and needs with related etiology and signs and symptoms can be found in the Examples of Actual or Potential Health Problems and Needs: Oxygenation and Perfusion.

Outcome Identification and Planning

Expected outcomes are derived from the actual or potential oxygenation and perfusion problems identified. The goal is to maintain or restore optimum function related to oxygenation and perfusion, alleviate symptoms or side effects of disease or treatment, and prevent complications. General patient outcomes are listed here. Actual patient outcomes should list specific behaviors and criteria individualized for the patient situation.

When caring for patients with an alteration in oxygenation and perfusion, nursing measures support the following general expected outcomes. The patient will:

- Demonstrate improved gas exchange in the lungs by an absence of cyanosis or chest pain and a pulse oximetry reading more than 95%
- Relate the causative factors, if known, and demonstrate a method of coping with these factors
- Preserve cardiopulmonary function by maintaining an optimal level of activity
- Demonstrate self-care behaviors that provide relief from symptoms and prevent further cardiopulmonary problems

Implementing

Oxygenation and perfusion deficits impair all aspects of daily living. Going to get the mail or cleaning the house may become a monumental task for people with oxygenation and perfusion deficits. Nursing interventions related to oxygenation and perfusion aim to promote optimal functioning of the cardiopulmonary systems, to promote comfort, and to promote and control coughing. Nurses may also need to intervene by suctioning the airway, meeting respiratory needs with medications, providing supplemental oxygen, managing chest tubes, using artificial airways, clearing an obstructed airway, and administering cardiopulmonary resuscitation (CPR).

QSEN TEAMWORK AND COLLABORATION

Patients, nurses, respiratory therapists, physicians, and other advanced practice professionals each have key roles in assessing, addressing, and monitoring oxygenation and perfusion and oxygenation/perfusion-related care issues and concerns. Communication and collaboration between the nurse, patient, and other health care professionals are critical to clarify the roles and responsibilities under conditions of potential overlap in team member functioning.

Promoting Optimal Function

Healthy lifestyle choices and behaviors are an important part of preventing and managing cardiopulmonary diseases, which can have an impact on the level of health and oxygenation and perfusion. Vaccination is an important part of preventing respiratory infections. Teaching patients with problems of oxygenation about pollution-free environments is an important part of respiratory management. Many people with altered oxygenation experience anxiety as a result of their symptoms and the actual or potential loss of independence. It is important to minimize anxiety in patients with alterations in oxygenation in order to promote optimal functioning. Promoting good nutrition is another vital part of promoting optimal cardiopulmonary functioning.

Promoting Health Literacy

IN PATIENTS WITH COPD

Patient Scenario

Nicoli Romanov, age 69, has been experiencing a morning cough for "several years," but states, "It wasn't too bad, so I lived with it." He reports increasing shortness of breath and fatigue over the last few months, with mucus production. He states that he has noticed increased amounts of mucus during the last few weeks, and significantly increased difficulty breathing with activity. Mr. Romanov reports smoking cigarettes for 40 years but has recently been thinking about quitting. After having a medical workup, including pulmonary function studies, Mr. Romanov was diagnosed with COPD. He tells the nurse that he doesn't really think that he can use "all these medications, especially that breathing thing," and doesn't really understand what COPD is. He asks, "Do you think my smoking is making me worse?"

Nursing Considerations: *Tips for Improving Health Literacy*

Provide Mr. Romanov with easy-to-read information about COPD. Encourage him to ask his health care provider as many questions as needed to understand his condition. Explain that it is a breathing problem that comes on over a long time, but there are things he can do to feel better and help keep from getting worse. Reinforce that it is important to take the medications every day and learn the right way to use inhaled medications. Provide information and resources to help him quit smoking. Encourage Mr. Romanov to ask his health care provider the following three questions:

- What is my main problem?
- What do I need to do?
- Why is it important for me to do this?

What additional measures can you take to help increase health literacy in this patient? What other measures would be helpful for Mr. Romanov if he did not speak English, could not read, or had other learning deficits?

Teach patients about their health conditions and provide information and support to improve patient health literacy. Refer to the accompanying Promoting Health Literacy box.

HEALTHY LIFESTYLE

Patients who practice good health-related behaviors can reduce their risk for many cardiopulmonary diseases. Explain that beneficial behaviors should be incorporated into their daily and weekly activities. Encourage patients to eat a healthy diet (see discussion later in the chapter). Encourage patients to maintain a healthy weight. Regular exercise should also be part of a patient's daily activities. Current recommendations suggest adults minimally engage in activity that requires moderate effort, such as brisk walking for 2.5 to 5 hours or more a week (USDHHS, 2018). Teach patients to monitor their cholesterol, triglyceride, high-density lipoprotein (HDL) and low-density lipoprotein levels (LDL) as well as their blood pressure. Encourage patients to limit alcohol intake and stop smoking (see discussion later in the chapter).

VACCINATION

Influenza

Influenza (the flu) is a contagious respiratory illness that causes mild to severe illness, and even death. People at high risk for serious flu complications include young children; pregnant women; people with chronic health conditions like asthma or heart and lung disease; and people ages 65 years and older. The best way to prevent the flu is by getting vaccinated. All people ages 6 months and older should be vaccinated each year (CDC, 2021b).

Pneumococcal Disease

Pneumococcal disease is an infection caused by a type of bacteria called pneumococcus. There are different types of pneumococcal disease, such as pneumococcal pneumonia, meningitis, and otitis media. Pneumococcal disease can be fatal. In some cases, it can result in long-term problems, such as brain damage, hearing loss, and limb loss. Pneumococcal disease is common in young children, but older adults are at greatest risk of serious illness and death (CDC, 2020a). Pneumococcal vaccine is very good at preventing severe disease, hospitalization, and death. Vaccines are recommended for all children younger than 2 years old, all adults ages 65 years and older, adults ages 19 to 64 years who smoke cigarettes, and people ages 2 through 64 years with certain medical conditions (CDC, 2020a). There are two types of pneumococcal vaccines available in the United States, each protecting against different numbers and types of pneumococcal bacteria. Recommendations for use of these vaccines are based on age and health status. Guidelines provided by the Centers for Disease Control can be accessed at http://www.cdc.gov/pneumococcal/vaccination.html

COVID-19

COVID-19 is a disease that became a pandemic in late 2019. COVID-19 is an infection caused by a novel coronavirus (SARS-CoV-2). Most people infected with the COVID-19 virus experience mild to moderate respiratory illness (fever, dry cough, tiredness) and recover without special treatment (CDC, 2021d; WHO, 2021), but some people become severely ill (difficulty breathing or shortness of breath, chest pain or pressure, loss of speech or movement [CDC, 2021d; WHO, 2021]) and/or experience post-COVID conditions. Post-COVID conditions are a wide range of new, returning, or ongoing health problems experienced more than 4 weeks after first being infected with the virus that causes COVID-19 (CDC, 2021d). Various groups of people are at increased risk of getting sick and dying from COVID-19, including many racial and ethnic minority groups and people with disabilities (CDC, 2021e). Patients with underlying alterations in health such as cardiovascular disease, diabetes, chronic respiratory or kidney disease, dementia or other neurologic conditions, immunocompromised state/weakened immune system, overweight or obesity, and cancer as well as those who are older, current or former smokers, or pregnant are more likely to develop serious illness, requiring hospitalization, intensive care, and/or a ventilator to help with breathing, or they may even die (CDC, 2021e). COVID-19 vaccines are effective at protecting patients from getting COVID-19 and significantly decrease the risk of serious illness as a result of infection with the virus (CDC, 2021c). As of this writing (early 2022), scientists and health care providers are still studying and learning about this virus and the impact of the vaccines; however, everyone ages 5 years and older is eligible and encouraged to get a COVID-19 vaccination. Several vaccines are available; the choice of vaccine to be administered and dosing for a particular vaccine depend on the age of the patient and the details of administration identified by the manufacturer of the particular vaccine. Guidelines provided by the Centers for Disease Control can be accessed at https://www.cdc.gov/coronavirus/2019-ncov/vaccines/your-vaccination.html.

TEACHING ABOUT POLLUTION-FREE ENVIRONMENTS

A pollution-free environment is particularly important for people with cardiopulmonary problems. Teach the patient to assess the environment and make adjustments, whenever possible, to factors that impair respiratory functioning ("triggers"). The patient must actively plan to prevent exposure to pollutants and triggers (EPA, 2021). This might involve a job change, use of protective equipment, requesting enforcement of laws by government facilities, or subcontracting jobs. In order to minimize triggers in the home, dusting and vacuuming the office and home must be done at least twice per week. In some situations, the patient may be asked to wear a mask to prevent some symptoms of respiratory distress. Explain to the patient that exposure to industrial or occupational hazards (e.g., paint, varnish, gaseous fumes, asbestos) must also be restricted.

In the United States, fine pollutants—including carbon monoxide, sulfur dioxide, total suspended particulates, ozone, and nitrogen dioxide—that pose a hazard to health are monitored closely. On days when pollutant levels are elevated significantly, morbidity and mortality rates among people with preexisting pulmonary disease are increased greatly. Thus, on days when pollution alerts are announced, people with altered respiratory function should reduce their activities, stay indoors, and use an air conditioner, electronic air cleaner, or air filter (EPA, 2021). If pollen alters the patient's respiratory function, the same principles apply.

Cigarette smoking is a major risk factor in cardiopulmonary diseases. The inhalation of cigarette smoke increases airway resistance, reduces ciliary action, increases mucus production, causes thickening of the alveolar–capillary membrane, and causes bronchial walls to thicken and lose their elasticity. Smoking is the biggest risk factor for COPD (American Lung Association, 2021a), and increases the risk for many types of cancer, including cancers of the oral cavity, throat, larynx, esophagus, lung, urinary bladder, kidneys, colon and rectum, liver, pancreas, and stomach (CDC, 2021f). In addition, cigarette smoking causes reduced circulation by narrowing the blood vessels (arteries). Smoking causes coronary heart disease, the leading cause of death in the United States, and causes a much greater risk for stroke, peripheral vascular disease, and abdominal aortic aneurysm (abnormal dilation of blood vessels) (CDC, 2020b). These effects occur in both smokers and nonsmokers (children and adults) who live with smokers (CDC, 2021b,g). Habitual smokers usually have great difficulty quitting or reducing their smoking and need much encouragement. The American Lung Association (www.lung.org) and the American Heart Association (AHA, www.heart.org) offer free educational materials online to aid and support patients who are trying to stop smoking. Nurses play a key role in presenting accurate information about the effects of smoking. Encourage the decision to never start smoking or to stop smoking. Provide appropriate information, counseling, support, and resources to assist patients to be successful with smoking cessation.

REDUCING ANXIETY

It is important to create an environment that is likely to reduce anxiety. Help institute measures to alleviate discomfort immediately. Use effective listening skills and accurate observation to display a caring attitude. Attempt to understand the patient's life experiences and habits without judging them. Patients with harmful health habits often fear they will be judged, which may impede implementation of the plan of care and reaching collaborative health goals. Patients who believe nurses are genuinely concerned about them and their families are more willing to work toward achieving mutually desirable outcomes. Refer to Chapter 43 for additional discussion related to anxiety and related nursing care.

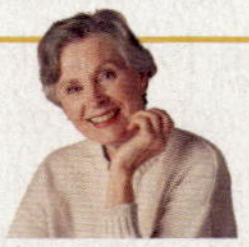

Think back to **Joan McIntyre**, the woman requesting to be "let go" if she should stop breathing. The nurse needs to provide support to the patient, showing genuine concern for her welfare. In addition, the nurse needs to act ethically and legally to ensure the patient's rights.

MAINTAINING GOOD NUTRITION

Beneficial behaviors, such as healthy eating, should be incorporated into a patient's daily activities. Encourage patients to follow healthy eating patterns that include a variety of nutrient-dense foods and beverages across all food groups, including fruits and vegetables, low-fat dairy products, whole grains, a variety of protein foods, and reduced amounts of saturated fats and trans fats, added sugars, and sodium. This diet can help patients reduce their risk for chronic disease such as cardiopulmonary diseases and diabetes, improve health, and reduce the prevalence of overweight and obesity and meet nutrient needs (USDA & USDHHS, 2020).

People who work hard at breathing often do not have much energy for eating. Many of the medications used for treatment can cause anorexia and nausea. However, maintaining an adequate nutritional intake is crucial. Consider the use of small meals at frequent intervals distributed over the course of the day instead of the usual three larger meals. Provide frequent oral hygiene and rest periods before eating to help improve the patient's intake. Encourage patients to eat their meals 1 to 2 hours after breathing treatments and exercises.

Patients who have COPD require a high-protein/high-calorie diet to counter malnutrition. If supplemental oxygen is used, reinforce the importance of wearing the cannula during and after meals. Eating and digestion require energy, which causes the body to use more oxygen.

Promoting Comfort

Interventions to promote patient comfort are an important part of nursing care for patients with alterations in the cardiopulmonary function. Promoting proper positioning, adequate fluid intake, humidification of inspired air, and appropriate breathing techniques are used to maximize the patient's sense of well-being. In addition, encourage the patient to pace physical activities and schedule frequent rest periods to conserve energy.

POSITIONING

Proper positioning is important to ease respirations. A proper position for breathing is a position that allows free movement of the diaphragm and expansion of the chest wall. Alternatively, sitting in a slumped position permits the abdominal contents to push upward on the diaphragm, decreasing lung expansion during inspiration. People with dyspnea and orthopnea are most comfortable in a high-Fowler position because accessory muscles can easily be used to promote respiration.

Research has demonstrated that, in patients with pulmonary disease who are acutely ill, such as those with acute respiratory distress syndrome (ARDS) or COVID-19-related respiratory failure/ARDS, turning to the prone position on a regular basis promotes improved oxygenation (Guttendorf, 2021; Morata et al., 2021; Siegmeister et al., 2021; Venus et al., 2020). In this position, the posterior dependent sections of the lungs are better ventilated and perfused, gravitational pressure on lung structures is decreased, compression of the lungs by abdominal contents is decreased, and chest wall compliance is enhanced (Guttendorf, 2021; Venus et al., 2020). Prone positioning should not be used with patients who have facial fractures, unstable spinal or pelvic fractures, or increased intracranial pressure (Guttendorf, 2021). Patients in the third trimester of pregnancy or patients with open chest or abdominal wounds may be candidates for prone positioning, after evaluation and collaboration with the health care team (Guttendorf, 2021). Coordinated multidisciplinary teams utilizing detailed planning and collaboration are essential to successful implementation of prone positioning (Elpern et al., 2021; Mitchell & Seckel, 2018).

MAINTAINING ADEQUATE FLUID INTAKE

Patients can help keep their secretions thin by drinking at least 1.5 to 2 L of fluids daily (American Lung Association, 2021b; Cleveland Clinic, 2020). Fluid intake should be increased to the maximum that the patient's health state can tolerate. Increased fluids are needed by patients who have an elevated temperature, who are breathing through the mouth, who are coughing, who have thickened respiratory secretions, and who are losing excessive body fluids in other ways. Fluid intake (1 to 2 L/day), along with sodium intake (2,000 to 3,000 mg), is individualized for patients with heart failure (Kuehneman et al., 2018).

PROVIDING HUMIDIFIED AIR

Inspiring dry air removes the normal moisture in the respiratory passages that protect against irritation and infection. Inhalation of dry air also compromises ciliary function and mucous production (Hess et al., 2021). This is especially troublesome for patients who cannot breathe through their nose. When air humidity is low, it may be necessary to humidify the air with room humidifiers or vaporizers to add water vapor (moisture) to the air. A vaporizer heats water and adds steam/warm mist to the air. A humidifier releases a fine cool mist into the air. Either steam or cool mist may be useful in humidifying the air (MFMER, 2019). Cool-mist humidifiers should be used for children to prevent burns from hot water or steam from a vaporizer (MFMER, 2019). It is very important to keep a humidifier clean to prevent mineral buildup and the growth of bacteria and mold (MFMER, 2019). The water tank should be emptied, and all surfaces dried daily to help keep it clean. The use of distilled or purified water instead of tap water can be helpful in preventing mineral buildup (MFMER, 2019). Humidification may also be provided as part of supplemental oxygen therapy, and artificial airway and mechanical ventilation systems. Refer to the discussion of humidification as part of providing supplemental oxygen later in this chapter on page 1613.

Promoting Proper Breathing

Many people, both well and ill, have breathing habits that are not conducive to maximal respiratory functioning. Some people develop a pattern of shallow breathing or walk with a posture that makes the chest wall appear caved in, affecting chest expansion. Ill people may limit their respiratory efforts to compensate for disease symptoms or an illness. Breathing exercises are designed to help patients achieve more efficient and controlled ventilations, decrease the work of breathing, and correct respiratory deficits.

DEEP BREATHING

When hypoventilation occurs, a decreased amount of air enters and leaves the lungs. However, deep-breathing exercises can be used to overcome hypoventilation. Instruct the patient to make each breath deep enough to move the bottom ribs. Unless the patient has a nasal condition that prohibits or prevents normal breathing, have the patient start slowly taking deep ventilations nasally and then expiring slowly through the mouth. Breathing through the nose warms, filters, and humidifies the air. The patient's respiratory status, health problems and clinical status dictate the timing of this exercise; for example, postoperative patients are encouraged to take deep breaths at least every 2 hours to help expel residual anesthetic agents, mobilize secretions, and prevent atelectasis (Hinkle et al., 2022).

USING INCENTIVE SPIROMETRY

Incentive spirometry provides visual reinforcement for deep breathing by the patient (Hess et al., 2021). An incentive spirometer assists the patient to breathe slowly and deeply and to sustain maximal inspiration (Eltorai et al., 2019). Most incentive spirometers direct the patient's inspiratory flow through a tube to lift one or more light balls or disks (Hess et al., 2021). The higher the patient's inspiratory flow, the higher the ball is raised or the greater the number of balls that are raised (Hess et al., 2021). The longer the inspiratory flow is maintained, the larger the volume is and, as a result, the patient is encouraged to take slow, deep breaths (Hess et al., 2021). Visualization of the action of the balls allows the patient to measure one's own progress, providing immediate positive reinforcement. Use of an incentive spirometer encourages the patient to maximize lung inflation and prevent or reduce respiratory complications (Kotta & Ali, 2021). Optimal gas exchange is supported, and secretions can be cleared and expectorated. However, evidence is conflicting in regard to the actual effectiveness of routine use of incentive spirometry, including routine postoperative use; deep breathing without mechanical aids may be as beneficial (Adams, 2018; Eltorai et al., 2018; Hess et al., 2021; Moore et al., 2018). It is important to note that incentive spirometers are not recommended for routine use in postoperative care (Adams, 2018; Eltorai et al., 2018), but may be of more benefit in higher-risk patient populations (Kotta & Ali, 2021).

If the use of incentive spirometry is prescribed for a patient, before use, the patient needs instructions on using the equipment properly. Validate the patient's correct use of this equipment in both health care and community-care environments. See Guidelines for Nursing Care 40-1 for information regarding teaching patients to use this device.

PURSED-LIP BREATHING

Patients who experience dyspnea and feelings of panic can often reduce these symptoms by using pursed-lip breathing. Exhaling through pursed lips creates a smaller opening for air movement, effectively slowing and prolonging expiration. Prolonged expiration is thought to result in decreased airway narrowing during expiration and prevent the collapse of small airways (Lestari et al., 2019). This results in improved air/gas exchange and decreased dyspnea (Hess et al., 2021). Pursed-lip breathing also helps the patient to control the rate and depth of respiration, helping to reduce feelings of dyspnea. It also encourages relaxation, which aids the patient to gain control of dyspnea and reduce feelings of panic. Encourage patients with COPD to try this breathing technique to help manage their daily activities (Hinkle et al., 2022; Mayer et al., 2018; Mendes et al., 2019). Pursed-lip breathing is suggested to increase oxygenation and manage dyspnea in children with ineffective breathing patterns (Lestari et al., 2019).

Instruct the patient to sit upright and inhale through the nose with the mouth closed while counting to two. Then, the patient should pucker or purse their lips, as if they were going to whistle or use a straw, and exhale slowly, gently and

Guidelines for Nursing Care 40-1

TEACHING PATIENTS TO USE AN INCENTIVE SPIROMETER

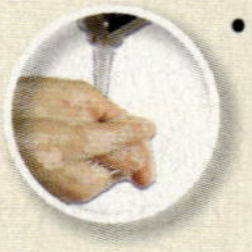

- Perform hand hygiene and put on PPE, if indicated.

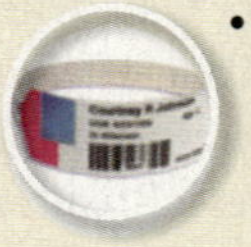

- Identify the patient.
- Establish the volume goal for incentive spirometry.
- Assist the patient to an upright or semi-Fowler position if possible.
- Remove dentures if they fit poorly.
- Assess for pain. Administer pain medication, as prescribed, if needed. **If the patient has recently undergone abdominal or chest surgery, place a pillow or folded blanket over the chest or abdominal incision for splinting.**
- Place the spirometer on a flat surface, like the overbed table, or have the patient hold it in an upright position. Demonstrate how to steady the device with one hand and hold the mouthpiece with the other hand.
- Instruct the patient to exhale normally and then place lips securely around the mouthpiece.
- Instruct the patient not to breathe through their nose. Use a nose clip if necessary. **Instruct the patient to inhale as slowly and as deeply as possible through the mouthpiece without using the nose.** Note the movement of the inhalation indicator on the spirometer.
- When the patient cannot inhale anymore, **the patient should hold their breath for 3 to 5 seconds** (Hess et al., 2021). Check the position of the gauge to determine the progress and level attained.
- Instruct the patient to remove their lips from the mouthpiece and exhale normally. **If the patient becomes lightheaded during the process, tell them to stop and take a few normal breaths before resuming incentive spirometry.**
- Encourage the patient to complete breathing exercises about 5 to 10 times every 1 to 2 hours, if possible. Rest in between breaths as necessary.

evenly against pursed lips while counting to four. The patient should avoid forcing the air out on exhalation; encourage the patient to breathe slowly, easily, and relaxed, breathing out for longer than they breathe in (American Lung Association, 2020a; Cleveland Clinic, 2018a).

DIAPHRAGMATIC BREATHING

Many people with asthma or COPD experience shortness of breath, and people with COPD may sometimes breathe in a shallow, rapid, and exhausting pattern. Use of diaphragmatic breathing can help to slow down the person's breathing and help them "catch their breath" (American Lung Association, 2020b). Diaphragmatic breathing (belly breathing) helps patients to calm down, better control their breathing, and use less energy to breathe (American Lung Association, 2020b).

To do this, the patient should sit upright in a comfortable chair or lie on their back on a flat surface or in bed, with the knees bent and a pillow under the knees to support their legs (American Lung Association, 2020b; Cleveland Clinic, 2018b). The patient should place one hand on their stomach and the other on the middle of their chest. The patient breathes in slowly through the nose, letting their abdomen protrude out against their hand, as far as it will go (filling like a balloon); the hand on their chest should remain as still as possible (Cleveland Clinic, 2018b). The patient should then breathe out through pursed lips while contracting the abdominal muscles, letting the stomach muscles fall inward and keeping the hand on their chest as still as possible (Cleveland Clinic, 2018b). The patient repeats these steps for 5 to 10 minutes three to four times a day, followed by relaxation. Encourage the patient to practice this breathing pattern several times during the day and increase the amount of time spent doing the exercise, so that eventually it becomes automatic (American Lung Association, 2020b; Cleveland Clinic, 2018b).

Promoting and Controlling Coughing

A cough is a cleansing mechanism of the body. It is a means of helping to keep the airway clear of secretions and other debris. A cough that is dry is termed a nonproductive cough. A cough that produces respiratory secretions is termed a productive cough. The respiratory secretion expelled by coughing or clearing the throat is called **sputum**.

When there are excessive fluids or secretions in an organ or body tissue, the patient is said to be congested. Thus, a person with secretions or fluid in the lungs is said to have congested lungs. If the cough is dry, the patient is said to be congested with a nonproductive cough. If the cough produces sputum, the patient is said to be congested with a productive cough. Thick respiratory secretions are sometimes called phlegm. A patient who is coughing and does not have any congestion or secretions produced is said to be noncongested with a nonproductive cough.

A series of events produce a cough. The cough mechanism (Fig. 40-11) consists of an initial irritation; a deep inspiration; a quick, tight closure of the glottis together with a forceful contraction of the expiratory intercostal muscles; and an upward push of the diaphragm. This causes an explosive movement of air from the lower to the upper respiratory tract. To be effective, a cough should have enough muscle contraction to force air to be expelled and to propel a liquid or a solid on its way out of the respiratory tract. Coughing is most effective when the patient is in an upright position. Coughing can be voluntary or involuntary.

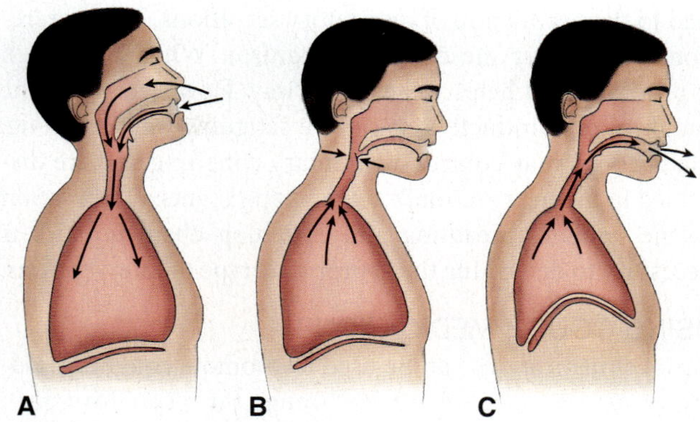

FIGURE 40-11. **A.** A cough begins with a deep inspiration, distending the trachea and hyperinflating the lungs. **B.** After inspiration, the glottis closes while intercostal and abdominal muscles contract forcibly. **C.** When intrathoracic pressure reaches a high level, the glottis opens slightly, and the diaphragm is pushed up, producing an explosive movement of air.

VOLUNTARY COUGHING

When a cough does not occur as a result of reflex stimulation of the cough-sensitive areas, it can be induced voluntarily. Teaching the patient to cough voluntarily is an important aspect of preoperative and postoperative care. Coughing is more effective when combined with deep breathing. Although teaching a patient to cough and deep breathe is relatively easy, experience has shown that it is difficult to motivate patients to follow through and perform coughing on their own. Refer to Guidelines for Nursing Care 31-2: Effective Coughing in Chapter 31 for detailed instructions for teaching this intervention. Frequently remind patients to perform effective coughing throughout the day. Develop a specific schedule for coughing as part of the patient's plan of care. Coughing early in the morning after rising removes secretions that have accumulated during the night. Coughing before meals improves the taste of food and oxygenation. At bedtime, coughing removes any buildup of secretions and improves sleep patterns.

If the patient has a neuromuscular disorder and is unable to cough physically, an assisted cough may be used. For an assisted cough, the caregiver's hands are placed one on top of each other below the diaphragm and above the naval; firm pressure is applied on the abdomen by pushing upward and under the rib cage, in rhythm with exhalation (Frigerio et al., 2015; University of Michigan Health, 2020). This pressure is similar to the Heimlich maneuver, but with less force. This pressure is used to substitute for the weakened or paralyzed abdominal muscles.

INVOLUNTARY COUGHING

Involuntary coughing often accompanies respiratory tract infections and irritations. Many times, respiratory infections lead to the production of respiratory secretions. These secretions can trigger the cough mechanism. When the cough is productive, it helps clear the airway. However, when the cough is nonproductive, it can be fatiguing and irritating. Medications may control involuntary coughing and are discussed in the next section, Cough Suppressants. Observation of the patient's breathing and coughing characteristics is necessary to determine the appropriate type of interventions.

USING COUGH MEDICATIONS

Various medications can be used to promote coughing, aiding in the movement of mucus through the respiratory tract, and in controlling coughing to allow the patient to rest.

Expectorants

Expectorants are drugs that facilitate the removal of respiratory tract secretions by reducing the viscosity of the secretions. Patients with extremely tenacious (thick) secretions may need the secretions liquefied for their cough to be effective. In that way, for example, the nonproductive cough of a person with respiratory congestion can become productive. Use of an expectorant by a person without congestion is inappropriate. Guaifenesin is widely used as an expectorant in cold and cough medications. Adequate fluid intake and air humidification act as effective expectorants as well.

Cough Suppressants

Suppressants are drugs that depress a body function—in this case, the cough reflex. Codeine, which is present in many cough preparations, is generally considered the preferred cough suppressant ingredient. However, codeine can be addictive, and because of possible abuse, most states require a prescription for its use. Drowsiness is a side effect; thus, it may not be safe to use codeine when the person must remain alert, such as when driving a car. A suppressant that is not addictive is dextromethorphan, which can be found in many over-the-counter cold and cough remedies.

An irritating, nonproductive cough in people without congestion may be treated appropriately with suppressants. Suppression of the productive cough is usually not recommended unless the patient is trying to sleep. If a productive cough is suppressed, secretions can be retained, leading to a pulmonary infection.

Lozenges

Cough lozenges can often relieve mild, nonproductive coughs in people without congestion. A lozenge is a small, solid medication intended to be held in the mouth until it dissolves. Lozenges generally control coughs by the local anesthetic effect of benzocaine. The local anesthetic acts on sensory and motor nerves, controlling the primary irritation and inhibiting afferent and efferent impulses.

Teaching about Cough Medications

Cough medications are readily available, and people who purchase them are usually eager for relief. Often, consumers take excessive amounts of more than one type. Teach about the appropriate choice of expectorants and suppressants and about misuse of cough mixtures. For example, cough syrups with a high sugar or alcohol content can disturb the metabolic balance of patients with diabetes or can trigger a relapse for recovering alcoholics. Preparations containing antihistamines have an anticholinergic action, which can cause serious problems for people with glaucoma or cause urinary retention in men with prostate enlargement. Other cough preparations can be detrimental to people with hypertension or thyroid or cardiac diseases. In addition, prolonged use of self-prescribed cough preparations can conceal more serious health problems. If a cough lasts more than 7 days, urge the person to contact their health care provider. In addition, encourage the person to increase fluid intake if the secretions become too thick to expectorate.

Performing Chest Physiotherapy

Conventional chest physiotherapy (CPT) includes percussion, vibration, and postural drainage and is usually performed by respiratory therapists and physical therapists, or nurses with specialized skills, in acute care environments for select patients (Strickland et al., 2013). CPT may help loosen and mobilize secretions, increasing mucus clearance. This is especially helpful for patients with large amounts of secretions or an ineffective cough. Chest physiotherapy has been shown to have short-term effects in increasing mucus transport and expectoration (Warnock & Gates, 2015). Studies suggest active therapies, such as mobilization, deep breathing and incentive spirometry are more effective than chest physiotherapy (passive treatment) (Beningfield & Jones, 2018). Chest physiotherapy has limited evidence for its effectiveness (Hess et al., 2021) and is not recommended for use in numerous patient populations, including patients with head injury, uncontrolled hypertension, and hypotension; for patients at risk for aspiration, children with pneumonia, adults with COPD, and postoperative adults (Andrews et al., 2013; Hess et al., 2021; Lisy, 2014; Strickland et al., 2013).

SUCTIONING THE AIRWAY

Suctioning of the pharynx is indicated to maintain a patent airway and to remove saliva, pulmonary secretions, blood, vomitus, or foreign material from the pharynx. Suctioning of the oropharynx or nasopharynx may be indicated if the patient is able to raise secretions from the airways but unable to clear from the mouth. Refer to Skill 40-2 on pages 1636–1641. The frequency of suctioning varies with the amount of secretions present but should be done often enough to keep ventilation effective and as effortless as possible. If the patient is unable to raise secretions from the airways, tracheal suctioning may be indicated. Tracheal suctioning is discussed later in the chapter on page 1627.

Suctioning irritates the mucosa and removes oxygen from the respiratory tract, possibly causing **hypoxemia** (insufficient oxygen in the blood). Thus, it is important to preoxygenate the patient before suctioning. This is accomplished by applying or increasing supplemental oxygen and having the patient take several deep breaths before inserting the catheter.

When performed correctly, suctioning provides comfort by relieving respiratory distress. When performed incorrectly, it can increase anxiety and pain and cause respiratory arrest. At minimum, it is an uncomfortable procedure, and it can be a very painful and/or distressing experience. Individualized pain management must be performed in response to the patient's needs (Arroyo-Novoa et al., 2008; Chaseling et al., 2014; Düzkaya & Kuğuoğlu, 2015; Wrona et al., 2021). Anticipate the administration of pharmacologic (analgesic medication) and use of nonpharmacologic interventions for the patient before suctioning. Possible complications of suctioning include infection, cardiac arrhythmias, hypoxia, mucosal trauma, and death.

Wear gloves on both hands, goggles or a face shield, and a mask—and a gown, if necessary—for protection from microorganisms. Depending on the patient's health status, N95 or equivalent mask may be indicated, such as for patients with COVID-19 (Pandian et al., 2020). Continuously monitor the patient's color and heart rate and the color, amount, and consistency of secretions. If cyanosis, an excessively slow or rapid heart rate, or suddenly bloody secretions are noted, stop suctioning immediately, administer oxygen, and notify the health care team. Cyanosis and a change in heart rate can indicate hypoxemia. Blood can indicate damage to the mucosa.

Meeting Oxygenation Needs With Medications

Although treating patients with medications is a dependent nursing intervention, monitoring the patient's response and development of side effects to medications is an independent nursing action. Table 40-3 (on page 1612) lists some common medications for improving respiratory functioning, their side effects, and nursing implications. Many of the drugs used to dilate bronchial airways interact with caffeine. Encourage patients to avoid caffeine, which may potentiate the side effects of bronchodilators (Karch, 2020).

ADMINISTERING INHALED MEDICATIONS

Inhaled medications may be administered to open narrowed airways (**bronchodilators**), to liquefy or loosen thick secretions (mucolytic agents), or to reduce inflammation in airways (corticosteroids). These medications typically are administered via nebulizer, metered-dose inhaler (MDI), or dry powder inhaler (DPI). Refer to the discussion of administering medications by inhalation in Chapter 30 and to the Guidelines for Nursing Care 30-8 on pages 961–962 for pictures of these devices and additional use and administration details.

Nebulizers utilize the force of high-glow oxygen or compressed air through a fluid medication to disperse fine particles of liquid medication into the deeper passages of the respiratory tract, where absorption occurs. The treatment continues until all the medication in the nebulizer cup has been inhaled.

An MDI is a handheld inhaler that uses an aerosol spray or mist to deliver a controlled dose of medication with each compression of the canister that is then breathed in by the patient. Common mistakes that patients make when using MDIs include the following:

- Failing to shake the canister
- Holding the inhaler upside down
- Inhaling through the nose rather than the mouth
- Inhaling too rapidly
- Stopping the inhalation when the cold propellant is felt in the throat
- Failing to hold their breath after inhalation
- Inhaling two sprays with one breath

To use an MDI, the patient must activate the device while continuing to inhale. The preferred method of use is with a device called a valved holding chamber or spacer (Center for Disease Control, 2018; Quaranta, 2018). The spacer acts as a reservoir. When the MDI is compressed, the medication is deposited in the reservoir, and the patient then inhales the medication from the spacer device. This makes administration less complicated, the dose more predictable, and enhances the delivery of medication to the lungs. For some patients, young children and older adults for example, a spacer or extender device may be necessary to aid delivery of medication by the inhalation route. An MDI can also be used without a chamber. There are a number of different medication inhaler devices, which increases the risk of administration error (Quaranta, 2018). As a result, using the proper technique for the prescribed inhaler is imperative or therapy will not be effective (Price et al., 2017; Quaranta, 2018).

DPIs are another type of delivery method for inhaled medications. A DPI is a handheld inhaler (diskus) that uses a dry powder form of medication, either in a small capsule or disk inserted into the DPI, or in a compartment inside the DPI. DPIs are breath activated and create aerosols by drawing air through a dose of powdered medication (Hess et al., 2021). A quick deep breath by the patient activates the flow of medication, eliminating the need to coordinate activating the inhaler (spraying the medicine) while inhaling the medicine at the same time. DPIs require less manual dexterity than do MDIs. DPIs are actuated by the patient's inspiration, so there is no need to coordinate the delivery of puffs with inhalation. Many types of DPIs are available with distinctive operating instructions. It is important to understand the particular instructions for the medication being used. One disadvantage of DPIs is that the medication in DPIs will clump if exposed to humidity.

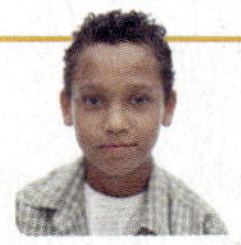

Remember **Tyrone**, the 12-year-old boy with suspected asthma. During this acute attack, the nurse would anticipate administering bronchodilators via a nebulizer. The health care provider may order bronchodilators to be administered at home using a nebulizer or possibly an MDI with a spacer, or DPI.

TEACHING PATIENTS ABOUT INHALED MEDICATIONS

Patients need repeated instruction on how to use inhalers and nebulizers effectively and safely. Overuse may result in

Table 40-3 Selected Medications Used to Improve Respiratory Function

MEDICATIONS	ACTIVITY	ROUTE	SIDE EFFECTS	NURSING IMPLICATIONS
albuterol	Bronchodilator	PO, inhalation	Tremors, anxiety, insomnia, headache, palpitations, hypertension, vomiting	Caution the patient not to increase dosage without consulting their health care provider. Be aware that children ages 2–years more frequently exhibit CNS stimulation.
Theophylline (aminophylline)	Bronchodilator	PO, IV, rectally (not widely used)	Nausea, vomiting, tachycardia, diuresis, irritability, vertigo, convulsions, nervousness	Monitor vital signs closely. Force fluids as clinical status allows. Monitor serum theophylline levels, especially if the patient does not respond to the drug or if severe side effects develop.
Corticosteroids (prednisone, dexamethasone, budesonide, triamcinolone acetonide)	Reduces inflammation	PO, IV, inhalation, intranasal	Fluid retention, hypertension, mood swings, weight gain, gastritis, hyperglycemia, insomnia	Reduce sodium intake. Make the patient and family/caregivers aware of potential for labile emotions. Weigh daily in the morning. Monitor blood pressure and blood sugar.
Diphenhydramine	Antihistamine H_1-receptor antagonist	PO	Drowsiness, anorexia, dry mouth, constipation, blurred vision, urinary retention	Warn the patient to use only on the advice of their health care provider in the presence of bronchial asthma.
Cetirizine	Antihistamine H_1-receptor antagonist	PO	Headache with limited sedative effect, not associated with anticholinergic effects	Monitor effectiveness of the drug. Contraindicated while breastfeeding.
Fexofenadine	Antihistamine H_1-receptor antagonist	PO	Drying of respiratory mucous membranes, dysuria, nausea	Contraindicated during pregnancy and while breastfeeding Use with caution in patients with renal or hepatic impairment
Zafirlukast montelukast	Leukotriene receptor antagonist	PO	Headache, dizziness, nausea, pain, fever, infection, elevated liver enzymes	Remind the patient that this medication is used to prevent asthma attacks, not to treat acute episodes. Inform the patient that the drug is effective only continuously as prescribed Remind the patient to avoid over-the-counter products containing aspirin, which might interfere with effectiveness

CNS, central nervous system; PO, orally; IV, intravenously; MDI, metered-dose inhaler.

serious side effects and eventual ineffectiveness of the medication. Nebulizers require cleaning after use; thus, patients must understand how to do this correctly. Patients must understand that it is important to keep track of dosing with MDIs. Many MDIs have integrated dose counters, but some do not, and it can be difficult to know when the canister is empty. Patients must understand the importance of keeping track of dosing to ensure that they are not using an empty canister. Most DPIs have a dose counter, so patients have accurate information about when to refill the medication. Patients should not exhale into the DPI, as they risk blowing out the medication. Information about how to use MDIs, DPIs, and small-volume nebulizers properly, including patient teaching information, is provided in Chapter 30, Guidelines for Nursing Care 30-8 on pages 961–962. Package inserts with the medication also reinforce correct technique for using inhalers.

To ensure correct administration when a spacer is used, slow, deep inspirations are necessary. To prevent inhaling too quickly, some spacers are equipped with a whistle device that sounds if inhalation is too rapid. A spacer is also recommended for patients using inhaled corticosteroid agents because it reduces the risk of acquiring an oral fungal infection (AIM, n.d.; NHS Inform, 2020).

Providing Supplemental Oxygen

Oxygen, which constitutes 21% of normal air, is a tasteless, odorless, and colorless gas. Oxygen is an essential requirement for cellular respiration and cell function (Rolfe & Paul, 2018a). Oxygen therapy provides a higher concentration of oxygen than ambient air (supplemental oxygen) to increase the pressure difference to aid in the diffusion of gas across the membrane between the alveoli in the lungs and the pulmonary capillaries, with the resulting increased saturation of hemoglobin and delivery of oxygen via the blood to all cells (Hess et al., 2021; Rolfe & Paul, 2018a). Oxygen therapy is indicated when hypoxemia is suspected by history, physical examination or laboratory data and to maintain oxygen saturations within the patient's specified target range (O'Driscoll et al., 2017; Rolfe & Paul, 2018b). Most patients will have a target oxygen saturation of 94% to 98% (O'Driscoll et al., 2017). Patients with chronic obstructive pulmonary disease (COPD) and other risk factors for hypercapnia may have a target oxygen saturation of 88% to 92% (Mirza et al., 2018; Mitchell, 2015; O'Driscoll et al., 2017). Supplemental oxygen is supportive therapy; the cause of the hypoxemia in individual patients should be addressed and corrected (Hess et al., 2021).

Oxygen is considered a medication and must be prescribed by a health care provider. However, in situations where there is a clear clinical indication, such as decreasing oxygen saturations or tachypnea, or an emergency situation, the absence of a prescription should not delay the administration of oxygen to the patient (Higginson et al., 2016; Nippers & Sutton, 2014; O'Driscoll et al., 2017; Rolfe & Paul, 2018b).

Oxygen therapy can be intimidating or frightening for patients. Therefore, provide clear explanations about the procedures and purpose to help reduce anxiety. Encourage patients to discuss concerns. If oxygen is given in an emergency, explanations concurrent with administration are appropriate.

Oxygen supports combustion. To prevent fires and injuries, take the following precautions:

- Check to see that electrical equipment used in the room, such as electric bell cords, razors, radios, and suctioning equipment, is in good working order and emits no sparks.
- Avoid wearing and using synthetic fabrics that build up static electricity.
- Avoid using oils in the area. Oil can ignite spontaneously in the presence of oxygen.
- Avoid contamination of medical devices and medical gas cylinders; contamination with dirt, oil, grease, hand cream, or alcohol hand gel must be avoided. Ensure hands are clean and hand gel has dried completely before handling oxygen equipment (Ford & Robinson, 2021).

Refer to the Teaching Tips 40-1 later in this section for information for patients and families regarding safety measures when oxygen is used in the home.

SOURCES OF OXYGEN

In acute and other clinical care environments, therapeutic oxygen is supplied from a wall outlet or a portable cylinder or tank. A specially designed flow meter is attached to the wall outlet (see Skill 40-3 on pages 1641–1644 for an illustration of a flow meter). A valve regulates the oxygen flow in liters per minute. To release oxygen safely and at the desired rate from a cylinder or tank, a regulator is used. The regulator has two gauges. The one nearest the tank shows the pressure or amount of oxygen in the tank. The other gauge indicates the number of liters per minute of oxygen being released.

Oxygen concentrators are another means to provide supplemental oxygen. This oxygen delivery system concentrates room air to provide the appropriate prescribed concentration of oxygen to the patient. Oxygen concentrators are frequently used in home situations. The concentrator may have a cylinder refill system with a portable oxygen cylinder that can be filled with oxygen for use when the patient leaves the home (McCoy, 2016). Portable oxygen concentrators are available as well, offering the ability to leave home for extended periods of time without the worry of running out of oxygen (Jacobs et al., 2020).

The use of oxygen-conserving devices is another method to deliver oxygen. These systems conserve the oxygen supply, reducing consumption and enabling the use of either smaller and lighter systems or extending the length of time between cylinder refilling (McCoy, 2016; Murphie, 2015). Conservation of oxygen is achieved via various methods, such as integrated reservoirs or by the intermittent flow of oxygen. Further discussion of oxygen-conserving devices is provided in the "Oxygen Therapy in the Home" section on page 1617.

OXYGEN FLOW RATE

The flow rate of oxygen, measured in liters per minute, determines the amount of oxygen delivered to the patient. The rate varies depending on the condition of the patient and the route of administration of the oxygen. The flow rate does not necessarily reflect the oxygen concentration actually inspired by the patient because there is leaking and mixing with atmospheric air. If more precise doses are necessary, they are usually prescribed in terms of percentage of inspired oxygen. To regulate the oxygen percentage concentration accurately, samples of the air mixture the patient is actually inhaling may be analyzed every 4 hours. Several types of commercial oxygen analyzers are available.

HUMIDIFICATION

Supplemental oxygen dries and dehydrates the respiratory mucous membranes, and patients may experience related discomfort, including feelings of dryness and soreness (Hess et al., 2021; Rolfe & Paul, 2018b). Use of humidification is not necessary with very–low-flow oxygen (4 L/min or less), when delivered by nasal cannula (see oxygen delivery systems to follow) to adults, or when anticipated as a therapy for less than 24 hours (O'Driscoll et al., 2017). However, humidifying

Guidelines for Nursing Care 40-2

TRANSPORTING A PATIENT WITH A PORTABLE OXYGEN CYLINDER

Before the Transfer

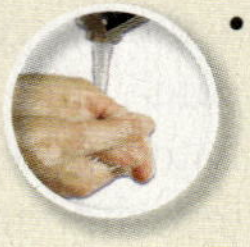

- Perform hand hygiene and put on PPE, if indicated.

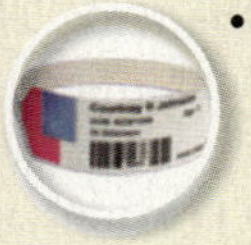

- Identify the patient.

- Check that an additional oxygen source is available where the patient is being transferred.
- Check the amount of oxygen in the cylinder (place the cylinder key or wrench on the valve stem and turn fully counterclockwise until the needle on the gauge indicates the amount of available oxygen; turn the key back a half turn; use the cylinder only if the gauge indicates more than 500 psi).
- If available, use a table that gives the estimated minutes of available oxygen according to the amount of oxygen in the cylinder and the rate of flow ordered for the patient. This can help to determine whether the supply of oxygen is adequate for the transfer (Gardner, 2015).
- Connect the oxygen tubing to the flow meter adapter and adjust the flow-control dial to the prescribed setting.
- Attach the patient's oxygen cannula to transport oxygen.
- Ensure that the cylinder is secured in a holder before transporting the patient (it is a dangerous practice to place the cylinder between the patient's legs or next to the patient during transfer because injury to the patient may result).
- Place the coiled tubing under a pillow or attach it to the linen or the patient's gown.

After the Transfer

- Attach the patient's oxygen cannula to wall oxygen.
- Turn off the oxygen flow from the cylinder by turning the cylinder key clockwise until it is tight.
- Remove any excess oxygen in the pressure gauge by "bleeding" it. Turn the flow-control dial back on until the hissing sound stops and the needle on the gauge has fallen to zero. Turn the flow-control dial off.

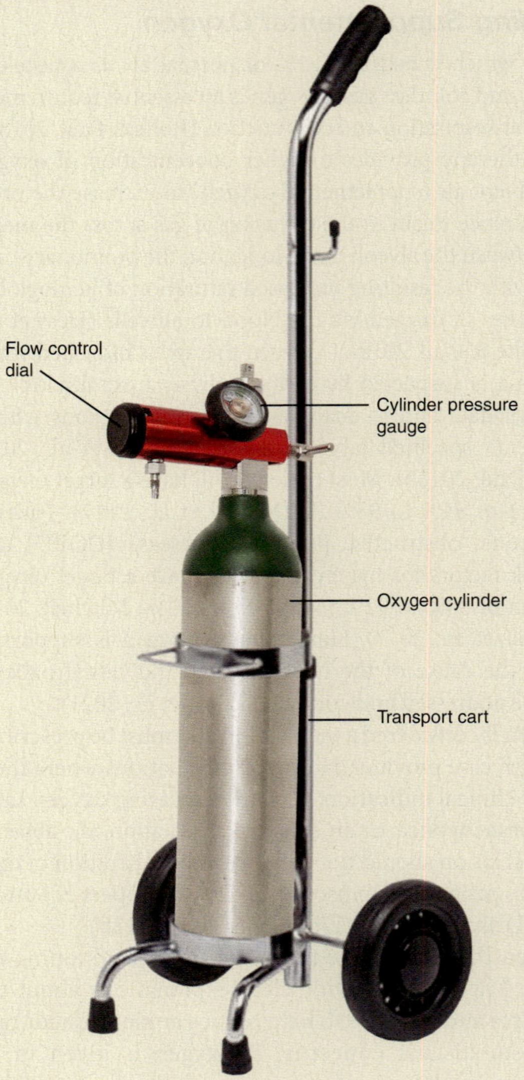

devices is recommended for patients who experience any discomfort associated with dry upper respiratory tract mucosa and when oxygen is delivered at higher flow rates (greater than 35%) (O'Driscoll et al., 2017). Humidification should also be provided with oxygen therapy for patients with a tracheostomy or artificial airway and patients experiencing difficulty expectorating sputum (O'Driscoll et al., 2017). Distilled or sterile water is commonly used in various humidification systems to add molecular water to gas (humidify oxygen) (Ford & Robinson, 2021). When moving patients receiving humidified oxygen, make sure that water from the humidifier does not enter the tubing through which the oxygen is flowing. Additional suggestions for transporting a patient with a portable oxygen tank are given in Guidelines for Nursing Care 40-2.

SUPPLEMENTAL OXYGEN DELIVERY SYSTEMS

Oxygen can be administered by many different delivery systems.

Low-flow/variable performance systems are based on the patient's own inspiratory flow (how deeply and fast the patient is breathing) and the oxygen inhaled is composed of some of the supplemental oxygen mixed with inhalation of some air present in the room, reducing the accuracy of the concentration of oxygen that the patient is actually receiving (Hess et al., 2021; Rolfe & Paul, 2018b). Low-flow devices provide variable performance because the inspired oxygen concentration cannot be accurately known (Hess et al., 2021). Examples of low-flow devices include low-flow nasal cannula/prongs, simple mask, partial rebreather mask, nonrebreather mask, and transtracheal oxygen catheter (discussion of transtracheal

Table 40-4 Oxygen Delivery Systems

METHOD	AMOUNT DELIVERED FiO_2 (FRACTION INSPIRED OXYGEN)	PRIORITY NURSING INTERVENTIONS
Nasal cannula	*Low flow* 1–2 L/min = 24–28% 3–5 L/min = 32–40% 6 L/min = 44%	Check frequently that both prongs are in the patient's nares. For patients with chronic lung disease, limit rate to the minimum needed to raise arterial oxygen saturation to maintain a level of 88–92% (Mitchell, 2015).
Nasal cannula	*High flow* Maximum flow 60 L/min 10 L/min = 65% 15 L/min = 90%	Closely monitor the patient's respiratory status for changes indicating impending respiratory failure. Pharyngeal pressure is affected by mouth-opening or closing, delivered flow, and size of nasal prongs. High-flow nasal cannula oxygen delivery is often better tolerated by children than other noninvasive delivery methods
Simple mask	*Low flow* 5–8 L/min = 40–60% (5 L/min is minimum setting)	Monitor the patient frequently to check placement of the mask. Support the patient if claustrophobia is a concern. Secure a prescribed intervention to replace the mask with a nasal cannula during mealtime.
Nonrebreather mask	*Low flow* 10–15 L/min = 80–95%	Maintain flow rate so that the reservoir bag collapses only slightly during inspiration. Check that the valves and rubber flaps are functioning properly (open during expiration and closed during inhalation). Monitor SaO_2 with pulse oximeter.
Venturi mask	*High flow* 4–6 L/min = 24–40%	Requires careful monitoring to verify FiO_2 at flow rate ordered. Check that air intake valves are not blocked.

Source: Reprinted with permission from Hinkle, J. L., Cheever, K. H., & Overbaugh, K. J. (2022). *Brunner & Suddarths's Textbook of medical-surgical nursing* (15th ed.). Wolters Kluwer; and additional information adapted from Nishimura, M. (2016). High-flow nasal cannula oxygen therapy in adults: Physiological benefits, indication, clinical benefits and adverse effects. *Respiratory Care*, *61*(4), 529–541. https://doi.org/10.4187/respcare.04577

catheters is provided in the Oxygen Therapy in the Home section on page 1617).

High-flow/fixed performance devices produce oxygen flow outputs with a constant mix of air and oxygen as a result of the design of the device (inclusion of a venturi barrel to control the oxygen concentration), rather than the rate and depth of the patient's breathing (Venturi masks) (Rolfe & Paul, 2018b). These devices produce oxygen flow outputs that meet or exceed the patient's full inspiratory flow demand; the flow is such that the patient is not likely to inhale any room air (Hess et al., 2021). Venturi masks are more likely to maintain a fixed concentration of oxygen (fixed-performance) and deliver a more precise amount of oxygen (Hess et al., 2021; Rolfe & Paul, 2018). A high-flow nasal cannula is relatively new supplemental oxygen therapy with an increasing role in patient care (Hess et al., 2021; Messika, 2019; Rolfe & Paul, 2018b; Scott, 2020).

Oxygen enclosures (tents, incubators) have been used historically to deliver supplemental oxygen and provide an oxygen enriched environment (Hess et al., 2021). Current use of oxygen enclosures occurs primarily in infant and pediatric applications, including use of oxygen hoods, incubators, and croup tents; oxygen and aerosol tents, even for children, are, for the most part, not used (Hess et al., 2021, p. 308). An infant oxygen hood is a rigid plastic dome or box with a half-moon cutout that is place over an infant's neck to enclose the entire head (Hess et al., 2021; Medline Plus, 2018). Heated and humidified oxygen is delivered to the hood. While some facilities continue to use infant oxygen hoods, infant nasal cannulas are favored (Hess et al., 2021, p. 308).

Table 40-4 compares several oxygen delivery systems.

Nasal Cannula

A *low-flow nasal cannula*, also called nasal prongs, is a low-flow/variable-performance device and the most commonly used oxygen delivery device for administering low-flow oxygen to infants, children, and adults in the hospital and community settings (Hess et al., 2021). Low-flow nasal cannula can be set to deliver oxygen flows of 1 to 6 L/min in usual circumstances and to deliver an increased flow of 10 to 15 L/min for short-term use (Hess et al., 2021). The cannula is a disposable plastic delivery tubing with two protruding prongs that are inserted into the nostrils; prongs are available in a variety of styles, including curved or straight and tapered or nontapered. The prongs are held in place with an elastic band around the patient's head or by loops of the delivery tubing over the patient's ears, held in place by an adjustable slide placed under the chin (Hess et al., 2021). The delivery tubing is connected to an oxygen source with a flow meter and, many times, a humidifier (refer to the discussion of humidification in the previous section on p. 1613). The cannula does not impede eating or speaking and is used easily in the home. Oxygen may be administered using nasal cannula by a low-flow or high-flow system (refer to the separate discussions of high-flow nasal cannula oxygen therapy). Disadvantages of using a nasal cannula include that it can be dislodged easily, and low-flow rates can cause dryness of the nasal mucosa. There is no evidence that mouth breathing influences the efficiency of oxygen delivery; even when the patient inspires through the mouth oxygen still flows through the nose into the pharynx (O'Driscoll et al., 2017; Hess et al., 2021). Refer as well to Table 40-4 on page 1615. Skill 40-3 (on pp. 1641–1644) describes oxygen administration by nasal cannula.

High-flow nasal cannula (HFNC) is an oxygen therapy that involves the continuous delivery of an air/oxygen mixture through a heater/humidifier to a wide-bore nasal cannula. HFNC delivers oxygen flow greater than 30 L/min up to 60 L/min and up to 100% humidified oxygen (Hernández et al., 2017; Lu et al., 2020; Zemach et al., 2019). The mechanisms of this therapy maintain a small amount of continuous positive pressure during the entire cycle of breath, resulting in a higher level of oxygen delivery, improved breathing and oxygen saturation, reduced dyspnea, and reexpansion of collapsed alveoli (Hernández et al., 2017; Hess et al., 2021; Lu et al., 2020; Zemach et al., 2019). High-flow nasal cannula oxygen therapy reduces patient discomfort and upper airway dryness, improves extubation outcomes and weaning, reduces the risk of intubation, and improves the management of respiratory secretions (Hernández et al., 2017; Liu et al., 2019). It has been used for patients in intensive care units and critical care areas with mild to moderate acute respiratory failure to try to avoid invasive mechanical ventilation and associated risks (Hess et al., 2021; Messika, 2019; Rolfe & Paul, 2018b; Scott, 2020). This therapy is increasingly being investigated for use in other clinical situations as well, such as for the prevention and treatment of respiratory failure, in adult surgical and nonsurgical patients, in patients with COVID-19; and in infants and children with bronchiolitis (Lu et al., 2020; Moreel & Proesmans, 2020; Pruitt, 2020; Scott, 2020; Wang et al., 2020). Close monitoring of the patient's status is critical to avoid the delay of timely airway intervention and intubation in patients who are not doing well on HFNC (Zemach et al., 2019).

Implement medical device–related pressure injury prevention strategies, including appropriate selection, fitting, and securing of the mask; pressure redistribution by frequent repositioning or rotation; and use of a prophylactic cushioning/proactive dressing between the skin and mask (Pittman & Gillespie, 2020). The nasal cannula may cause pressure injuries behind the ears, around the nostril, or in the nasal vestibule; use soft nasal cannulas whenever possible and protect the back of the ears with a hydrocolloid or foam dressing (Camacho-Del Rio, 2018).

Face Masks

Disposable and reusable face masks are available. Fit the mask carefully to the patient's face to avoid leakage of oxygen. It should be comfortably snug but not tight against the face. The most commonly used types of masks are the simple face mask, the partial rebreather mask, the nonrebreather mask, and the Venturi mask. Implement medical device–related pressure injury prevention strategies, including appropriate selection, fitting, and securing of the mask; pressure redistribution by frequent repositioning or rotation; and use of a prophylactic cushioning/proactive dressing between the skin and mask (Pittman & Gillespie, 2020). Masks for oxygen delivery may cause injuries to the cheeks, chin, or bridge of the nose; place silicone border or hydrocolloid dressings over bony prominences or other areas that come in contact with the device and between the device and the skin (Camacho-Del Rio, 2018). Skill 40-4 (on pp. 1644–1648) describes the actions and rationales involved in using face masks.

The *simple face mask* (nonreservoir mask) is a low-flow/variable-performance device and is used when a higher oxygen level is needed than can be attained with a nasal cannula or when a cannula is not appropriate, such as with nasal obstruction (Hess et al., 2021). The simple face mask is connected to oxygen tubing, a humidifier, and a flow meter, just like the nasal cannula, and is used using a flow rate of 5 to 10 L/min (Rolfe & Paul, 2018b). This mask has vents on its sides that allow room air to leak in at many places, thereby diluting the source oxygen. The vents also allow exhaled carbon dioxide to escape. Often a simple mask is used when an increased delivery of oxygen is needed for short periods (e.g., less than 12 hours). The mask should fit closely to the face to deliver this higher concentration of oxygen effectively. Patients may have difficulty keeping the mask in position over the nose and mouth, and because of this pressure and the presence of moisture, skin breakdown is a possibility. Eating or talking with the mask in place can be difficult. Because of the risk of retaining carbon dioxide, never apply the simple face mask with a delivery flow rate of less than 5 L/min (Hess et al., 2021; O'Driscoll et al., 2017). Refer as well to Table 40-4 on page 1615.

The *partial rebreather mask* is a low-flow/variable-performance device and is similar to a simple face mask but is equipped with a reservoir bag for the collection of the first part of the patient's exhaled air. The remaining exhaled air exits through vents. The air in the reservoir is mixed with 100% oxygen and some room air inhaled through the mask ports for the next inhalation. Thus, the patient rebreathes about one third of the expired air from the reservoir bag. This type of mask is used to administer relatively high oxygen concentrations. The oxygen flow rate must be set high when using this type of mask, at 10 to 15 L/min. Monitor the reservoir bag carefully. It should deflate slightly with inspiration; if it deflates completely, the flow rate should be increased until only a slight deflation is noted. An advantage is that the patient can inhale room air through openings in the mask if the oxygen supply is briefly interrupted. The disadvantages are those of any mask: eating and talking are difficult, a tight seal is required, and there is the potential for skin breakdown. Note: partial rebreathing masks are not commonly used in present-day practice (Hess et al., 2021, p. 300).

The *nonrebreather mask,* a low-flow/variable-performance device, delivers the highest concentration of oxygen via a low-flow mask. It is similar to the partial rebreather mask but incorporates valves between the bag and the mask and on at least one of the exhalation side ports on the mask. Supplemental oxygen is directed via tubing into the mask and into the reservoir bag. A one-way valve prevents exhaled gas from entering the reservoir and the entire exhaled volume exits the mask through the mask ports and between the patient's face and mask, preventing the patient from rebreathing exhaled air (Hess et al., 2021).

During exhalation, the reservoir bag refills with oxygen. At the beginning of inspiration, the mask exhalation port valves close, minimizing room air from being drawn in, and the reservoir valve opens, allowing the patient to inhale oxygen from the reservoir in addition to the oxygen flow. The oxygen flow rate must be set high when using this type of mask, not below 10 L/min. Monitor the reservoir bag carefully. It should not deflate with inspiration (Rolfe & Paul, 2018b). A malfunction of the bag or oxygen flow could cause carbon dioxide buildup and suffocation. As a result, manufacturers provide either an antisuffocation valve at the neck of the reservoir bag that opens when the oxygen supply fails or provide only one valve on the mask ports on the side of the mask (Hess et al., 2021). The disadvantages are those of any mask: eating and talking are difficult, a tight seal is required, and there is the potential for skin breakdown. Refer as well to Table 40-4 on page 1615.

The *Venturi mask*, a high-flow/fixed performance device, gets its name from the Venturi effect, which allows the mask to deliver the most precise concentrations of oxygen. This mask has a large tube with an oxygen inlet, a Venturi barrel, to control the oxygen concentration. As oxygen passes through the narrow opening in the barrel, the pressure drops, causing a high velocity stream that draws a constant proportion of room air to be pulled in through the base of the mask (Rolfe & Paul, 2018b). The Venturi barrel on the mask can be changed to deliver a different percentage of oxygen; changing the flow rate of the oxygen alone will not change the percentage of oxygen the patient receives (Rolfe & Paul, 2018b). The barrel is changed according to the prescription for oxygen concentration. Be sure that the ports on the barrel are always open. If these are occluded by linens, clothing, or a patient rolling on the mask, the oxygen delivered might be at an unsafe (too high or too low) concentration. The disadvantages are those of any mask: eating and talking are difficult, a tight seal is required, and there is the potential for skin breakdown. Refer as well to Table 40-4 on page 1615.

MONITORING OF PATIENTS RECEIVING SUPPLEMENTAL OXYGEN THERAPY

The patient's past and current health history are considered when initiating supplemental oxygen therapy (Rolfe & Paul, 2018b). The prescribed intervention should identify the method and rate for supplemental oxygen administration, and the appropriate target saturation range (Rolfe & Paul, 2018b). Initiation and continued administration of oxygen therapy should be based on the patient's target oxygen saturation range and clinical status (Lellouche & L'Her, 2020; O'Driscoll et al., 2017; Rolfe & Paul, 2018b).

Careful observation, monitoring and assessment are necessary when administering oxygen therapy: monitor the flow rate to verify oxygen deliver as prescribed, patient color (signs of cyanosis), respiratory rate (e.g., tachypnea), respiratory depth, increase work of breathing (use of accessory muscles), pulse oximetry measurements, and ABG results closely for changes (Hess et al., 2021; Rolfe & Paul, 2018b). Refer to the discussion of assessment related to oxygenation and perfusion earlier in this chapter as well as assessment information discussed in Chapter 27. Continuous pulse oximetry may also be used to monitor the patient receiving oxygen. Titrate the oxygen flow according to the device and patient requirement. Oxygen therapy should be provide using minimal oxygen to maintain adequate SpO_2 in the patient's target range to avoid complications (Hess et al., 2021; Joint Formulary Committee, 2020, as cited in Ford & Robinson, 2021). Change the oxygen delivery system/device as prescribed or indicated, based on the patient's health status and assessment findings and facility/agency policy.

Assess and monitor the patient's comfort with the delivery device; device comfort can have a direct impact on the patient's acceptance of oxygen therapy (Rolfe & Paul, 2018b). Assess and monitor the oral and nasal mucous membranes, the lips and nose, and face and ears (refer to Chapter 32). Pressure- and moisture-related injuries are possible (Rolfe & Paul, 2018b) (refer to Chapter 33). Monitor fluid status and maintain hydration through adequate fluid intake (refer to Chapters 37 and 41). Provide routine oral hygiene (refer to Chapter 32).

OXYGEN THERAPY IN THE HOME

Liquid oxygen and oxygen concentrators, rather than compressed gas cylinders, are used more commonly in the home setting. Liquid oxygen is kept inside a small container that can be refilled from a larger storage tank kept in the home. An oxygen concentrator removes nitrogen from the room air and concentrates the oxygen left in the air. The oxygen concentrator needs a power source such as an electrical outlet, battery pack, or car charger, but never runs out and does not need to be refilled. Oxygen concentrators are portable, cost-effective, and easy to use (Hanlon, 2014). Refer to the previous discussion related to oxygen concentrators in the "Sources of Oxygen" section of this chapter on page 1613.

Patients with chronic hypoxemia may be treated with transtracheal oxygen delivery (Fig. 40-12). With this type of

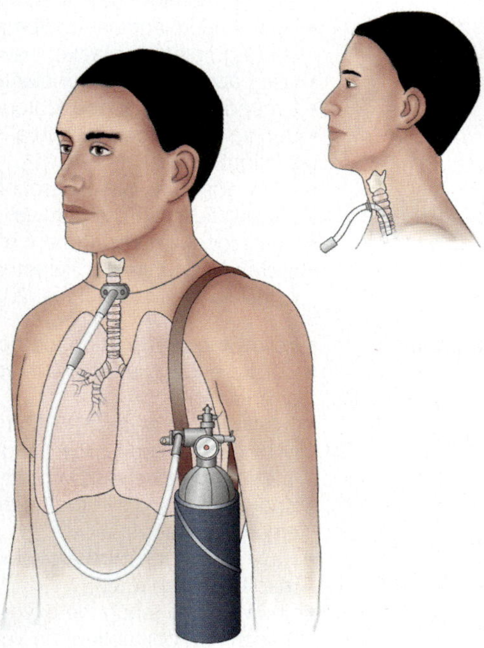

FIGURE 40-12. Transtracheal oxygen.

delivery system, a small catheter is inserted into the trachea under local anesthesia and then the catheter is attached to an oxygen source. A transtracheal catheter does not interfere with talking, eating, or drinking and delivers oxygen throughout the respiratory cycle rather than just at inspiration and is associated with reduced amount of oxygen flow needed at rest and exercise, reduced symptoms of shortness of breath, improved patient mobility, and increased patient adherence with therapy (Hess et al., 2021; University of California San Diego Health, 2021). The patient or family/caregiver must assume responsibility for daily catheter care (Goodman, 2014). Patients usually report improved mobility, comfort, and appearance, and lower cost with this delivery system.

Oxygen-conserving devices (OCDs) are also available for use in community-based settings. Reservoir cannulas are one type of OCD and have a reservoir space that stores oxygen during exhalation. On subsequent inhalation, the patient receives that stored oxygen, essentially adding a bolus volume to the continuous-flow oxygen delivery (Hess et al., 2021). The patient receives the same oxygen therapy at a lower continuous-oxygen flow rate, conserving oxygen use. Intermittent-flow devices operate by turning oxygen delivery on during some portion of inhalation and off for the balance of the breathing cycle (Hess et al., 2021; Jacobs et al., 2020). Patient-exhaled oxygen is conserved, allowing a supply of oxygen to last two to four times as long as if it was delivered continuously (Hess et al., 2021). If an oxygen-conserving device is used, the patient should be tested using the device during exertion, similar to what they would do in daily life, to ensure adequate oxygenation (Jacobes et al., 2020, p. e134). Use of intermittent flow delivery has resulted in much less use of continuous-flow oxygen in community-based settings (Hess et al., 2021).

Patients and families using oxygen at home need education about long-term oxygen use and associated equipment to improve patient adherence and implementation of safety precautions (Henrichs & Makic, 2021). See Teaching Tips 40-1 for information regarding the use of oxygen in the home setting.

Teaching Tips 40-1

USING OXYGEN AT HOME

Health Topic	Teaching Tip	Why Is This Important?
Safety	• Do not smoke in a home where oxygen is in use. Place "No Smoking" signs in conspicuous places in the patient's home. Instruct the patient and family/caregivers about the hazard of smoking when oxygen is in use. • Keep oils, grease, alcohol, and other liquids that can burn away from oxygen. • Keep oxygen at least 6 ft away from any source of fire, such as a stove, fireplace, or candle (MedlinePlus, 2020). • Keep oxygen 6 ft away from toys with electric motors, electric baseboard or space heaters, hairdryers, electric razors, and electric toothbrushes (MedlinePlus, 2020). • Do not use electrical equipment near oxygen administration set (e.g., electric blanket—see also above). • Use caution with gas or electric appliances. • Ground oxygen concentrators. • Secure the oxygen tank in a holder and away from direct sunlight or heat. • Allow adequate airflow around the oxygen concentrator (avoid placing flush against the wall). • Notify local fire department of the use of oxygen in the home. • Have working smoke detectors and a working fire extinguisher in the home (MedlinePlus, 2020).	Oxygen supports combustion; a spark may ignite the oxygen.
Administration	• Follow the prescription for the oxygen flow rate. • Ensure enough available oxygen prior to leaving the house for errands or trips. • Tubing length of up to 98.42 ft (30 m) may be used by patients with flow rates up to 5 L/min for home oxygen delivery to provide freedom of movement within the home. • Know signs and symptoms that indicate the need to call for emergency assistance. • Have the health care provider's and nurse's phone number readily available. • Know how to reach the oxygen equipment vendor and the reasons for contacting the vendor.	• Too much or too little oxygen may be detrimental to the patient. • Tubing length of up to 98.42 ft (30 m) may be used by patients with flow rates up to 5 L/min for home oxygen delivery with no important changes in flow or fraction of inspired oxygen (Aguiar et al., 2015). • This enables the patient and family/caregivers to obtain assistance when necessary.

PICOT in Practice

ASKING CLINICAL QUESTIONS: CONTINUOUS POSITIVE AIRWAY PRESSURE

Scenario: You are a staff nurse in the neonatal intensive care unit working with preterm infants. Those that are born less than 32 weeks' gestation lack surfactant, a detergent-like substance produced by the lung. You notice that early initiation with continuous positive airway pressure (CPAP) decreases mortality in preterm infants. You would like to develop a protocol that highlights signs and symptoms of preterm infants that should have CPAP initiated early or prophylactically.

- **Population:** Preterm infants in the neonatal intensive care unit
- **Intervention:** Early or prophylactically initiation of continuous positive airway pressure
- **Comparison:** Continuous positive airway pressure (or compared to O_2 therapy)
- **Outcome:** Decreased mortality
- **Time:** Duration of hospitalization

PICOT Question: Does initiation of early or prophylactic continuous positive airway pressure (CPAP) compared to continuous CPAP decrease mortality in preterm infants during hospitalization?

Findings:

Level of Evidence: Level I: systematic review

Three pertinent resources were located.

1. Ho, J. J., Subramaniam, P., Davis, P. G. (2020). Continuous positive airway pressure (CPAP) for respiratory distress in preterm infants. *Cochrane Database of Systematic Reviews, 10*(10), CD002271. https://doi.org/10.1002/14651858.CD002271.pub3

In 5 studies involving 322 infants; 2 studies used face mask CPAP, 2 studies used nasal CPAP, and 1 study used endotracheal CPAP and continuing negative pressure for a small number of less ill infants. In preterm infants with respiratory distress, the application of CPAP is associated with reduced respiratory failure, use of mechanical ventilation, and mortality and an increased rate of pneumothorax compared to spontaneous breathing with supplemental oxygen as necessary.

2. Ho, J. J., Subramaniam, P., Sivakaanthan, A., Davis, P. G. (2020). Early versus delayed continuous positive airway pressure (CPAP) for respiratory distress in preterm infants. *Cochrane Database of Systematic Reviews, 10*(10), CD002975. https://doi.org/10.1002/14651858.CD002975.pub2

In 4 studies that recruited a total of 119 infants, all 4 small trials included in this review were performed in the 1970s or the early 1980s and were very uncertain whether early application of CPAP confers clinical benefit in the treatment of respiratory distress, or whether it is associated with any adverse effects. The applicability of these findings to the current practice of neonatal intensive care was uncertain, given that all trials in this Cochrane Review were conducted in the presurfactant era, when antenatal steroid usage was uncommon.

3. Subramaniam, P., Ho, J. J., Davis, P. G. (2016). Prophylactic nasal continuous positive airway pressure for preventing morbidity and mortality in very preterm infants. *Cochrane Database of Systematic Reviews,* (6), CD001243. https://doi.org/10.1002/14651858.CD001243.pub3

Seven trials recruiting 3,123 infants were included in the meta-analysis. Four trials recruiting 765 infants compared CPAP with supportive care and 3 trials (2,364 infants) compared CPAP with mechanical ventilation. In trials comparing CPAP with assisted ventilation with or without surfactant, CPAP resulted in a small but clinically significant reduction in the incidence of bronchopulmonary dysplasia (BPD) at 36 weeks. When compared to mechanical ventilation, prophylactic nasal CPAP in very preterm infants reduces the need for mechanical ventilation and surfactant and also reduces the incidence of BPD and death.

Recommendations: Prophylactic continuous positive airway pressure (CPAP) in very preterm infants reduces the need for mechanical ventilation and surfactant and also reduces the incidence of bronchopulmonary dysplasia (BPD) and death. Furthermore, early application of CPAP does not appear to be associated with any adverse effects. This information is provided to others in the unit through an educational in-service that highlights signs and symptoms of preterm infants that should have CPAP initiated early or prophylactically.

Positive Airway Pressure

Noninvasive positive airway pressure (PAP) therapy uses mild air pressure to keep airways open delivered via a mask. This treatment can help the body to maintain better carbon dioxide and oxygen levels in the blood. PAP therapy may be used to treat many adult disorders, such as sleep apnea, obstructive sleep apnea, obesity hypoventilation syndrome, acute cardiogenic pulmonary edema, heart failure, COPD, and acute hypoxemic respiratory failure (Hess et al., 2021; Martin, 2020; Medline Plus, 2021). It also may be used to treat disorders in infants and children, such as respiratory distress syndrome in preterm infants (Stanford Children's Health, 2021), bronchiolitis in infants (Franklin et al., 2019), and obstructive sleep apnea in children (Al-lede et al., 2018). See the accompanying PICOT in Practice box.

Continuous positive airway pressure (CPAP) provides continuous mild air pressure to keep airways open. *Bilevel positive airway pressure (BiPAP)* changes the air pressure while the patient breathes in and out. *Autotitrating (adjustable) positive airway pressure (APAP)* changes pressure throughout the therapy, based on the patient's breathing patterns (Medline Plus, 2021). All therapies use a mask or other device that fits over the nose or nose and mouth. Straps keep the mask in place. A tube connects the mask to the machine, which blows air into the tube.

Adjusting to the therapy and machine can take time. Patients report feeling strange wearing a mask on the face at night or feeling the flow of air. Some people feel confined by the mask. Nurses can assist patients by reinforcing accurate information about treatment; encourage patients to ease into use of the device. It may help for patients to start by practicing wearing just the mask for short periods of time while awake, for example, while watching TV. Then patients should try wearing the mask and hose with the air pressure on, still during the daytime, while awake. Once patients become accustomed to how the equipment feels, they should shift to using the device every time they sleep—at night and during naps. Inconsistently wearing the device may delay getting used to it.

Provide support and encouragement so that the patient persists with the therapy; it may take several weeks or more to see if the mask and pressure settings will work for the patient. If the device is used in the hospital or other facility or in the community, nursing responsibilities also may include monitoring the settings, ensuring correct use by the patient, and assessment of respiratory status. Careful assessment of the patient's skin on the face, in the areas the mask sits, is an important part of care. Pressure and moisture from the mask can cause alterations in skin integrity (Alqahtani et al., 2018). Implement medical device–related pressure injury prevention strategies, including appropriate selection, fitting and securing of the mask; pressure redistribution by frequent repositioning or rotation; and use of a prophylactic cushioning/proactive dressing between the skin and mask (Pittman & Gillespie, 2020). Masks for oxygen delivery may cause injuries to the cheeks, chin or bridge of the nose; place silicone border or hydrocolloid dressings over bony prominences or other areas that come in contact with the device and between the device and the skin (Camacho-Del Rio, 2018).

MANAGING CHEST TUBES

A chest tube is indicated when negative pressure in the pleural space is disrupted, as from thoracic surgery (postthoracotomy) or unanticipated trauma (Muzzy & Butler, 2015). Patients with fluid (pleural effusion), blood (hemothorax), or air (pneumothorax) in the pleural space require a chest tube to drain these substances, restore the negative intrathoracic pressure, and allow the compressed lung to reexpand (Hinkle et al., 2022). A chest tube may also be indicated for pleurodesis (pleural sclerosing; installation of anesthetic or sclerosing agent to achieve inflammatory adherence of the visceral and parietal pleural to each other) (Burns & Delgado, 2019; Hinkle et al., 2022). A mediastinal chest tube may be placed after cardiac surgery to drain blood from around the heart (Morton & Fontaine, 2018). A tunneled pleural catheter (tunneled under the skin before entering the pleural space) may be used to improve quality of life in patients with recurrent pleural effusions related to some end-stage diseases, such as malignancy (Miller et al., 2018).

A chest tube is a plastic tube with drainage holes in the proximal end that is inserted in the pleural space. Once inserted, the tube is secured with a suture at the insertion site, covered with a dressing, secured with tape a few inches below the insertion site, and attached to a drainage system that may or may not be attached to suction. Other

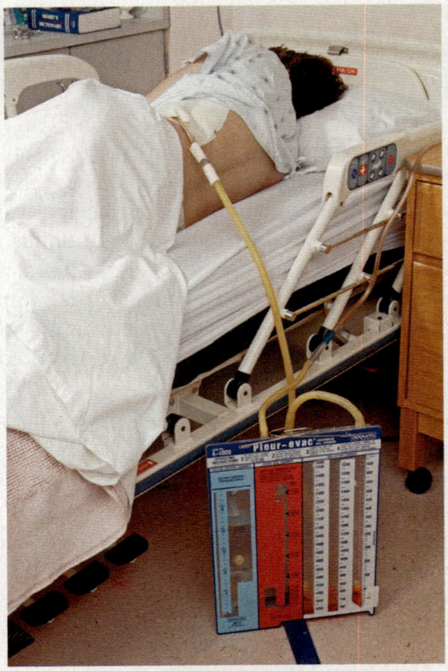

FIGURE 40-13. A chest drainage system. (*Source:* Used with permission from Shutterstock. *Photo by Rick Brady.*)

components of the system may include a closed water-seal drainage system that prevents air from reentering the chest once it has escaped and a suction control chamber that prevents excess suction pressure from being applied to the pleural cavity. The suction chamber may be a water-filled or a dry chamber. A water-filled suction chamber is regulated by the amount of water in the chamber (Fig. 40-13), whereas dry suction has a one-way mechanical valve system that allows air to leave the chest and prevents air from moving back into the chest and is automatically regulated to changes in the patient's pleural pressure. There are also portable drainage systems that utilize gravity for drainage. Table 40-5 compares different types of chest drainage systems.

The type of drainage determines the placement of the chest tube. When air is to be drained, the tube is placed higher in the chest (Morton & Fontaine, 2018). If fluid needs to be drained, the tube is inserted lower in the lung because fluids settle at the base of the lung (Morton & Fontaine, 2018).

Nursing responsibilities include assisting with insertion, monitoring the patient's status and response to the treatment, monitor the patency of the chest drainage system, patient education, and assisting with removal of the chest tube. Once the tube is in place, monitor the patient's response, including respiratory status and vital signs, check the site and site dressing, and maintain the patency and integrity of the drainage system. Guidelines for monitoring and caring for a patient with a chest tube are shown in Guidelines for Nursing Care 40-3 on page 1622.

An advanced practice professional usually performs chest tube removal. The health care provider will determine when the chest tube is ready for removal by evaluating the chest x-ray and assessing the patient and the amount of drainage

Table 40-5 Comparison of Chest Drainage Systems

TYPE	DESCRIPTION	COMMENTS
Traditional water-seal (also referred to as wet-suction) chamber	Has three chambers: a collection chamber, water-seal chamber (middle chamber), and wet-suction control chamber. Generally, used to provide 20 cm H_2O of suction	• Requires that sterile fluid be instilled into the water-seal and suction chambers. • Has positive and negative pressure-release valves. • Intermittent bubbling indicates that the system is functioning properly. • Additional suction can be added by connecting the system to a suction source.
Dry-suction water seal (also referred to as dry suction)	Has three chambers: a collection chamber, water-seal chamber (middle chamber), and dry-suction control chamber. Provides up to 40 cm H_2O of suction	• Requires that sterile fluid be instilled in the water-seal chamber at the 2-cm level. • No need to fill the suction chamber with fluid. • Suction pressure is set with a regulator. • Has positive and negative pressure-release valves. • Has an indicator to signify that the suction pressure is adequate. • Quieter than traditional water-seal systems.
Dry-suction (also referred to as one-way valve system)	Has a one-way mechanical valve that allows air to leave the chest and prevents air from moving back into the chest.	• No need to fill suction chamber with fluid; can be set up quickly in an emergency. • Works even if knocked over, making it ideal for patients who are ambulatory. • Not able to easily observe air leaks, monitor intrapleural pressures, or use suction

Source: Adapted from Hinkle, J. L., Cheever, K. H., & Overbaugh, K. (2022). *Brunner & Suddarth's Textbook of medical–surgical nursing* (15th ed.). Wolters Kluwer; Kane, C. J., York, N. L., & Minton, L. A. (2013). Chest tubes in the critically ill patient. *Dimensions of Critical Care Nursing, 32*(3), 111–117. https://doi.org/1097/DCC.0b013e3182864721; and Sasa, R. I. (2019). Evidence-based update on chest tube management. *American Nurse Today, 14*(4), 10–14.

from the tube. Some facilities are developing programs to train and support nurses and to ensure their continued competency to remove chest tubes. This would improve control of the timing of the procedure and allow for appropriate preprocedure analgesia, reducing the pain and anxiety associated with tube removal (Hood et al., 2014; Muzzy & Butler, 2015). Removal of chest tubes can be a painful and stressful process for patients (Hood et al., 2014; Kane et al., 2013; Muzzy & Butler, 2015; Yarahmadi et al., 2018). Administer analgesics prior to the tube removal, at a sufficient interval to allow for the medication to take effect, based on the medication prescribed. The application of cold to the chest prior to removal may also be implemented to decrease patient discomfort during chest tube removal (Yarahmadi et al., 2018). Nursing responsibilities related to chest tube removal also include providing emotional support for the patient, as well as monitoring the patient's status after removal. Monitor the patient's respiratory status, vital signs, pain, and site dressing.

USING ARTIFICIAL AIRWAYS

Artificial airways are used to preserve a functioning airway in patients who are unable to maintain a patent airway without assistance. Communicating effectively with patients with artificial airways, such as endotracheal tubes or tracheostomies, is essential. Patients with endotracheal tubes, and most tracheostomies, are unable to speak. The communication needs of these patients must be part of the nursing assessment. Identify appropriate alternative communication strategies to ensure that the patient's needs are conveyed. Consider the patient's impaired ability to communicate and keep communication tools (e.g., writing board, letters, vocabulary cards) close at hand, along with the call light or bell. Offer frequent reassurance and explanations and anticipate the patient's needs to promote positive patient outcomes.

Oropharyngeal and Nasopharyngeal Airways

An oropharyngeal or nasopharyngeal airway is a semicircular tube of plastic or rubber inserted into the back of the pharynx through the mouth (oro) or nose (naso) in a patient who is breathing spontaneously (Hinkle et al., 2022). The oropharyngeal airway is used to keep the tongue clear of the airway. It is often used for postoperative patients until they regain consciousness. It is important to ensure use of an airway of the correct size. Incorrect sizing can hinder airway maintenance; using an oropharyngeal airway that is too big will obstruct the airway, and one that is too small will not aid in opening the airway (Higginson et al., 2016). (Refer to Guidelines for Nursing Care 40-4 on page 1623 for details of sizing.) Once the patient regains consciousness, remove the oropharyngeal airway. Do not use tape to hold the airway in place because the patient should be able to expel the airway once they become alert.

A nasopharyngeal airway is inserted through the naris and protrudes into the back of the pharynx. The nasal trumpet allows for frequent nasotracheal suctioning without trauma to the nasal passageway. This airway may be left in place, without much discomfort, in the patient who is alert and conscious. Techniques to use when inserting an oropharyngeal and nasopharyngeal airway are outlined in Guidelines for Nursing Care 40-4 on page 1623.

Guidelines for Nursing Care 40-3

MONITORING A PATIENT WITH A CHEST TUBE

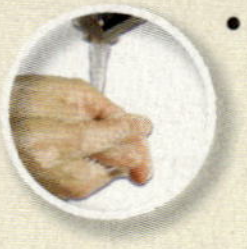

- Perform hand hygiene and put on PPE, if indicated.

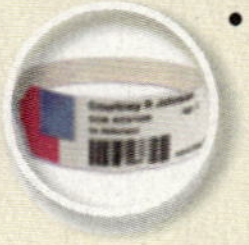

- Identify the patient.
- Assess the patient's vital signs, respiratory status, oxygen saturation, mental status, and breath sounds. Assess for pain. Monitor for any indication of change in the respiratory status.
- Observe the dressing around the chest tube insertion site. Gently palpate around the insertion site, feeling for crepitus, a result of air or gas collecting under the skin (subcutaneous emphysema). Tape all connections securely.
- Check that the drainage tube has no dependent loops or kinks. Make sure the drainage collection device is positioned below the tube insertion site to facilitate drainage.
- Observe the water-seal chamber for fluctuations of the water level with the patient's inspiration and expiration (tidaling). If suction is used, temporarily disconnect the suction to observe for fluctuation. Assess for the presence of bubbling in the water-seal chamber. Add water, if necessary, to maintain the level at the 2-cm mark or the mark recommended by the manufacturer.
- Assess the suction control chamber if suction is in use. If water suction is used, ensure that water is at the appropriate level; add water to ensure that suction is adequate. Gentle bubbling in the suction chamber indicates that suction is being applied to assist drainage.
- Assess the amount and type of fluid drainage. Measure drainage output at the end of each shift by marking the level on the container or placing a small piece of tape at the drainage level to indicate date and time. Document the color and consistency of the drainage. Drainage is never emptied. Drainage that dramatically increases or becomes bright red indicates fresh bleeding. Notify the health care team immediately.
- Keep the drainage collection device secure so that it does not tip over.
- Keep two rubber-tipped clamps and additional dressing material at the bedside for quick access, if needed. If the drainage unit requires changing, engage the clamp integrated on the drainage tubing. (Alternatively, position one clamp 1½ to 2½ inches from the insertion site; position the second clamp 1 inch down from the first one until the unit has been switched.) The chest tube may be clamped before its removal to observe the patient's tolerance when it is discontinued (Sasa, 2019). However, chest tubes are rarely clamped because this increases the risk of causing tension pneumothorax and is a prescribed intervention (Sasa, 2019).
- Keep a bottle of sterile saline or water at the bedside. If the chest tube disconnects from the drainage unit, submerge the end in water, creating a water seal, but allowing air to escape, until a new drainage unit can be attached. This is done instead of clamping to prevent another pneumothorax.
- Never clamp the tube if the patient leaves the unit for a test or moves away from the bed. Disconnect the suction tubing from the drainage system, allowing the unit to continue to collect drainage by gravity.
- **Do not** perform "milking" of the tubing (squeezing and releasing small segments of tubing between the fingers) and "stripping" of the tubing (squeezing the length of the tube without releasing it). This creates excessive negative pressure that can damage delicate lung tissue (Sasa, 2019). Stripping and milking are not necessary to maintain chest tube patency and probably do more harm than good (Makic et al., 2015, p. 44).

Endotracheal Tube

An endotracheal tube is a polyvinyl chloride airway that is inserted through the nose or mouth into the trachea, using a laryngoscope as a guide. It is used to administer oxygen by mechanical ventilator, to suction secretions easily, or to bypass upper airway obstructions (e.g., tongue or tracheal edema). Although uncomfortable and easy to manipulate with the tongue, orotracheal insertion is often the method of choice, especially in an emergency, as it is associated with less trauma and lesser rates of infection and typically accommodates a larger diameter endotracheal tube than the nasal route, making ventilation easier (Hinkle et al., 2022). Placement of the tube through the nasotracheal route, although tolerated better by patients, is more difficult and requires the use of a narrower tube. Most commonly, a cuffed endotracheal tube is used (Fig. 40-14). This type of tube prevents air leakage and bronchial aspiration of foreign material while allowing more precise control of oxygen and mechanical ventilation. However, careful monitoring of cuff pressure is necessary to decrease the risk for tracheal necrosis, tracheal rupture, laryngeal nerve palsy, tracheal stenosis, microaspiration, and/or inadequate ventilation (Turner et al., 2020). The smallest amount of air that results in an airtight seal between the trachea and the tube is desirable and less likely to result in complications; cuff pressures should be checked at least once per shift and maintained between 20 and 30 cm H_2O (AACN, 2018; Hess et al., 2021; Hinkle et al., 2022; Turner et al., 2020). Endotracheal tubes are secured via tape, twill tape, or a commercial device (Hess et al., 2021).

Implement medical device–related pressure injury prevention strategies to reduce the risk for alterations in skin integrity. Interventions may include the use of a prophylactic cushioning/proactive dressing between the skin and securement device, an endotracheal tube repositioning schedule, routine skin and oral assessments, and provision of scheduled skin and oral hygiene interventions (Holdman et al., 2020).

Guidelines for Nursing Care 40-4

INSERTING AN ARTIFICIAL AIRWAY

Inserting an Oropharyngeal Airway

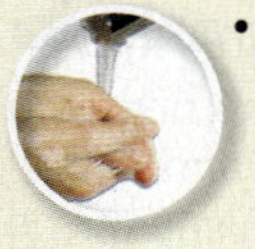

- Perform hand hygiene and put on PPE, if indicated.

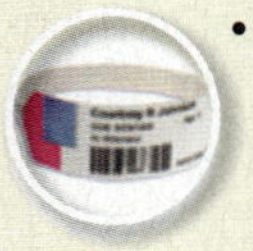

- Identify the patient.
- Use an airway that is the correct size. Measure the oropharyngeal airway by holding the airway on the side of the patient's face. The airway should reach from the opening of the mouth to the back angle of the jaw, and the tip of the airway should reach no farther than the pinna of the ear (Hess et al., 2021).
- Put on gloves; put on a mask and goggles or face shield as indicated.
- Check for loose teeth, dentures, or other foreign material. Remove dentures or material, if present.
- Position the patient in the semi-Fowler position.
- Open the patient's mouth by using your thumb and index finger to gently pry their teeth apart.
- Insert the airway with the curved tip pointing up toward the roof of the mouth.
- Slide the airway across the tongue to the back of the mouth.
- Rotate the airway 180 degrees as it passes the uvula (a flashlight can confirm the position of the airway with the curve fitting over the tongue).
- Ensure accurate placement and adequate ventilation by auscultating breath sounds.
- Position the patient on their side when the airway is in place.
- Remove the airway for a brief period every 4 hours, or according to facility policy. Assess the mouth and provide mouth care and a clean airway before reinserting it.

Inserting a Nasopharyngeal Airway (Nasal Trumpet)

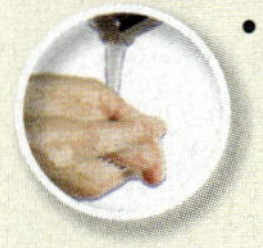

- Perform hand hygiene and put on PPE, if indicated.

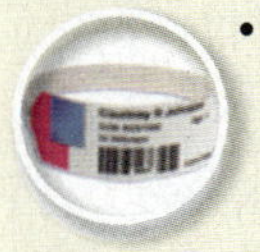

- Identify the patient.
- Put on gloves; put on mask and goggles or face shield as indicated.
- Use an airway that is the correct size. Measure the nasopharyngeal airway for correct size. Measure the nasopharyngeal airway length by holding the airway on the side of the patient's face. The airway should reach from the tip of the nose to the earlobe. The airway with the largest outer diameter that fits the patient's nostril should be used (Morton & Fontaine, 2018).
- **If the patient is awake and alert, position in the semi-Fowler position. If the patient is not conscious or alert, position in a side-lying position.**
- Lubricate the airway with the water-soluble lubricant, covering the airway from the tip to the guard rim.
- Gently insert the airway into the naris, narrow end first, pointing it down, toward the back of the throat, until the rim is touching the naris. If resistance is met, stop and try inserting in the other naris.
- Check placement by closing the patient's mouth and placing your fingers in front of the tube opening to check for air movement. Assess the pharynx to visualize the tip of the airway behind the uvula. Assess the nose for blanching or stretching of the skin.
- Remove the airway, clean it, and place it in the other naris at least every 8 hours, or according to facility policy. Assess for any evidence of alterations in skin integrity.
- The airway may be used for suctioning to prevent trauma to the mucosa.

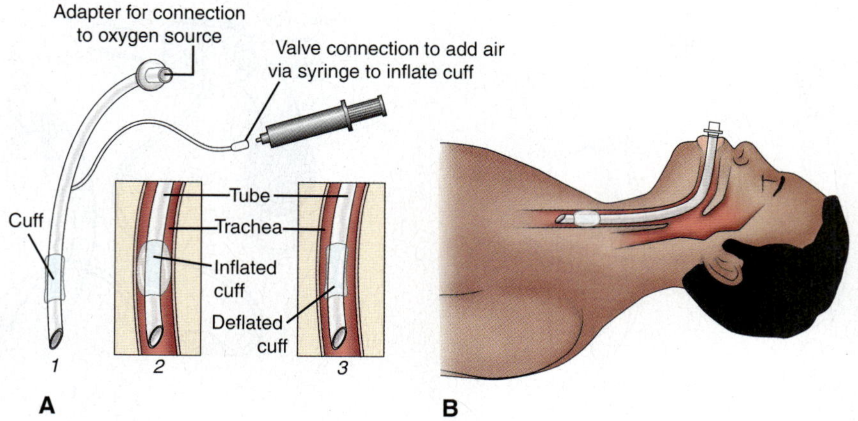

FIGURE 40-14. Endotracheal tube. **A.** (*1*) Parts of a cuffed endotracheal tube; (*2*) tube in place with the cuff inflated; (*3*) tube in place with the cuff deflated. **B.** Endotracheal tube in place.

Technology Alert

Maintaining endotracheal tube cuff pressure within a narrow range is an important part of patient care. Automated cuff pressure regulators and controllers have been developed to provide continuous real-time monitoring and control of optimal cuff pressure. These devices automatically adjust the cuff pressure within preset target, minimum, and maximum pressure values, removing the need for frequent manual monitoring and adjustment of cuff pressure and reducing nursing workload. Cuff pressure regulators have been shown to significantly reduce the drop in cuff pressure observed when pressure is set manually and prevent low and high average pressures (Chenelle et al., 2015; Lorente et al., 2014; Vottier et al., 2016) and reduce the risk of microaspiration (Hess et al., 2021).

Placement of an endotracheal tube results in the inability to speak, which can be frightening and frustrating for the patient and may contribute to ineffective responses to patient concerns and needs. Assess the patient's ability to use alternative methods of communication. Plan for and provide alternative methods of communication. Establishing a rapport with the patient through eye contact and careful attention to nonverbal cues and communication is important.

Patients with endotracheal tubes often require suctioning via the endotracheal tube to remove secretions from the airway. Refer to the discussion related to tracheal suctioning later in the chapter on page 1627. Routine oral suctioning to aspirate secretions that accumulate above the cuff of the tube is also necessary to reduce the risk of pneumonia and provide patient comfort (AACN, 2018; Hess et al., 2021; Morton & Fontaine, 2018). Poor oral hygiene contributes to the colonization of the oropharyngeal secretions by respiratory pathogens. Diligent oral hygiene care can improve oral health and limit the growth of pathogens in the oropharyngeal secretions, decreasing the incidence of aspiration pneumonia, community-acquired pneumonia, nonventilator health care–associated pneumonia (NV-HAP), and ventilator-associated pneumonia (VAP) (AACN, 2017; Chick & Wynne, 2020; Jenson et al., 2018; Quinn et al., 2020). Refer to the previous discussion related to suctioning the airway on page 1610. Oral hygiene measures are discussed in Chapter 32.

Consider **Mr. Kim**, the 57-year-old man receiving oxygen therapy and mechanical ventilation via an endotracheal tube. When developing the patient's plan of care, the nurse needs to assess him closely and frequently for signs and symptoms indicating an increase in secretions. If secretions increase, the nurse needs to suction the patient to maintain a patent airway and minimize his risk for hypoxemia and infection.

TRACHEOSTOMY TUBE

A **tracheostomy** is an artificial opening made into the trachea, usually at the level of the second or third cartilaginous ring. A curved tube, called a **tracheostomy tube**, is inserted through the opening. It is inserted in the operating room or intensive care unit under sterile conditions using local anesthesia and can be temporary or permanent. It may be used to replace an endotracheal tube, to provide a method for mechanical ventilation of the patient, to bypass an upper airway obstruction, in conditions in which endotracheal tube intubation is not possible (e.g., facial trauma, cervical fractures), or to remove tracheobronchial secretions (Hinkle et al., 2022; Morton & Fontaine, 2018).

The tube is made of semi-flexible plastic (polyethylene, polyvinyl chloride, polyurethane or silicone), rigid plastic, rubber, Teflon, or metal and is available in different sizes with varied angles (Hess & Altobelli, 2014; Hess et al., 2021). The most commonly used tubes are made from PVC, silicone or polyurethane (Hess & Altobelli, 2014). As a result of improvements in material design, metal tracheostomy tubes are rarely used today (Hess et al., 2021). The conditions and needs of the patient determine the selection of tube. A tracheostomy tube consists of an outer cannula or main shaft, an inner cannula, and an obturator (Fig. 40-15). An obturator, which guides the direction of the outer cannula, is inserted into the tube during placement and removed once the outer cannula of the tube is in place. Many tubes also have inner cannulas that may or may not be disposable. The outer cannula remains in place in

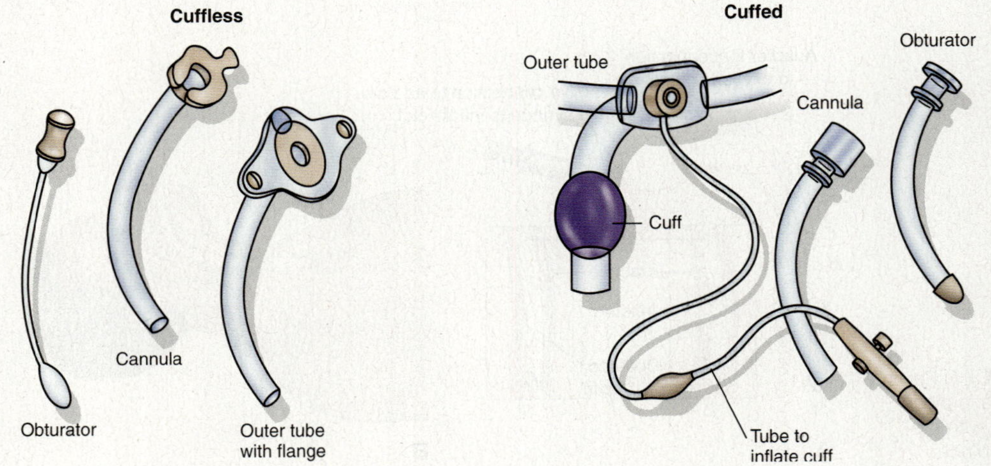

FIGURE 40-15. Two types of tracheostomy sets: cuffless and cuffed.

the trachea, and the inner cannula is removed for cleaning or replaced with a new one (Morton & Fontaine, 2018). Periodic cleaning or replacement of the inner cannula prevents airway obstruction from secretions that have accumulated on the tube's inner surface (Patton, 2019). A tube with an inner cannula is necessary when patients have excessive secretions or have difficulty clearing their secretions. It also may be recommended for a patient who will be discharged with a tracheostomy tube in place.

Tracheostomy tubes may be either cuffed or cuffless (see Fig. 40-15). The inflated cuff seals the opening around the tube to create a seal in the trachea. This prevents air leakage and aspiration and permits mechanical ventilation. Newer tracheal cuffs are low pressure, do not require deflating for short intervals every few hours, and can be maintained at lower than tracheal capillary pressure (Hess et al., 2021). Uncuffed tubes are used in adult patients who do not require invasive respiratory support and have an effective gag and cough reflex; adults who need frequent suctioning but do not need mechanical ventilation; as a method of weaning from the tracheostomy tube; and in pediatric patients under the age of six, to avoid tracheal deformation related to thinner tracheal tissues and softer laryngeal and tracheal cartilage cuff pressure (Hess et al., 2021; Patton, 2019).

A fenestrated tracheostomy tube has one large or several small openings or windows on its outer curve, has an inner cannula, and can be cuffed or cuffless. When the patient is being mechanically ventilated, the inner cannula is in place, blocking the small openings. After the patient is no longer connected to the ventilator, the inner cannula can be removed, the cuff deflated, and the tube plugged, allowing the patient to speak. Because the tube has these openings, it should be considered only for patients with normal upper airway reflexes (Hess et al., 2021).

The tracheostomy is initially held in place with sutures, which are removed after 7 days (O'Toole et al., 2017). After the sutures are removed, the tube is held in place by twill tapes or a commercially available tube holder, which is a wide neck band with elastic to distribute pressure and prevent skin irritation fastened around the patient's neck. Regularly check cuff pressure, although some tubes have a pressure-release valve that prevents pressure from increasing to damaging levels. Careful monitoring of cuff pressure is necessary to decrease the risk for tracheal necrosis, tracheal rupture, laryngeal nerve palsy, tracheal stenosis, microaspiration, and/or inadequate ventilation (Turner et al., 2020). The smallest amount of air that results in an airtight seal between the trachea and the tube is desirable and less likely to result in complications; cuff pressures should be maintained between 20 and 30 cm H_2O (AACN, 2018; Hess et al., 2021; Hinkle et al., 2022; Patton, 2019). Measurement of cuff pressure should occur at least once per shift or following any procedure where movement of the tube may have taken place (e.g., dressing/securement device change, patient repositioning), if there is an audible leak, or following any changes in the volume of the cuff (Hess et al., 2021; Patton, 2019). Continuous cuff monitoring is available and is associated with reduced risk of microaspiration (Hess et al., 2021).

Because the tracheostomy tube bypasses the natural humidifying and heating mechanisms in the nose and mouth, administer heated, humidified oxygen to prevent secretions from becoming dry (Patton, 2019). Keep the tracheostomy tube free from foreign objects and nonsterile materials, such as cotton balls, loose threads from dressings, needles, and other small objects, to reduce the risk of obstruction and infection.

Patients with tracheostomies frequently have an ineffective cough mechanism and copious secretions, which necessitate tracheal suctioning to remove secretions. Refer to the discussion related to tracheal suctioning later in the chapter on page 1627. Routine oral suctioning to aspirate secretions that accumulate above the cuff of the tube and frequent oral hygiene are also necessary to reduce the risk of pneumonia and provide patient comfort (AACN, 2018; Hess et al., 2021; Morton & Fontaine, 2018). Refer to the previous discussion related to suctioning the airway on page 1610. If the patient eats by mouth, it is recommended that the tracheostomy tube be suctioned prior to eating to prevent the need for suctioning during or after meals, which may stimulate excessive coughing and could result in vomiting (Hess et al., 2021, p. 429). Poor oral hygiene contributes to the colonization of the oropharyngeal secretions by respiratory pathogens. Diligent oral hygiene care can improve oral health and limit the growth of pathogens in the oropharyngeal secretions, decreasing the incidence of aspiration pneumonia, community-acquired pneumonia, nonventilator health care–associated pneumonia (NV-HAP), and ventilator-associated pneumonia (VAP) (AACN, 2017; Chick & Wynne, 2020; Jenson et al., 2018; Quinn et al., 2020). Oral hygiene measures are discussed in Chapter 32.

Placement of tracheostomy tube may result in the inability to speak, depending on the type of tube in use. The inability to communicate verbally can be frightening and frustrating for the patient and may contribute to ineffective responses to patient concerns and needs (Tolotti et al., 2018). Assess the patient's ability to use alternative methods of communication. Plan for and provide alternative methods of communication. Establishing a rapport with the patient through eye contact and careful attention to nonverbal cues and communication is important.

Replace a disposable inner cannula or cleaning a nondisposable one at least once per 8 hours; more frequent cleaning may be required based on the patient's status (Patton, 2019). For example, cleaning or replacement may be necessary every 4 hours or more if thick, viscous, or copious secretions are present (Patton, 2019). The inner cannula requires cleaning or replacement to prevent accumulation of secretions that can interfere with respiration and occlude the airway. Because soiled or wet tracheostomy dressings place the patient at risk for the development of skin breakdown and infection, regularly change any dressings and ties. Use gauze dressings that are not filled with cotton to prevent aspiration of foreign bodies (e.g., lint or cotton fibers) into the trachea. The Research in Nursing display (on page 1626) examines the use of a novel tracheostomy dressing applicator to assist in changing tracheostomy dressings and minimizing

Research in Nursing

BRIDGING THE GAP TO EVIDENCE-BASED PRACTICE

Tracheostomy Dressing Changes and Nurse Innovators

Routine tracheostomy care includes cleaning of the stoma site and changing the site dressing, which acts as a cushion and a barrier between the skin and the tube. Changing the site dressing involves placing the new dressing under the tracheostomy tube flanges, which can be difficult due to the presence (immediately postoperatively) of sutures and limited space between the tube flanges and the patient's neck. The process may also be uncomfortable and/or painful for the patient due to manipulation of the surgical site. Nurses must balance the need to avoid injury at the site, the need for interventions to prevent complications, and patient comfort (Morris et al., 2021). Nurses may resort to using forceps, hemostats, their fingers, or another tool in efforts to successfully place site dressings (Morris et al., 2021). Are there better options for tools to assist with dressing placement?

Related Research

Morris, L. L., Kuncis, M., Perleberg, D., Kuczek, A., Kashul, K., Zabel, D., Heinemann, A. W., & Semik, P. (2021). New device makes tracheostomy dressing changes easier and more comfortable. *Rehabilitation Nursing, 46*(2), 95–103. https://doi.org/10.1097/rnj.0000000000000302

The purpose of this quasi-experimental study was to compare the use of a novel tracheostomy dressing applicator (TDA) for tracheostomy dressing changes to the standard procedure for tracheostomy dressing changes regarding nurses' ease of use as well as patient discomfort in an inpatient rehabilitation setting. The TDA was developed and patented by two critical care registered nurses and was designed to assist caregivers in changing tracheostomy dressings quickly and efficiently while minimizing discomfort to the patient. Patients older than age 18 years ($n = 19$) and registered nurses ($n = 117$) at the rehabilitation center participated in the study. The participating nurses were trained on proper use of the device. Nurse participants agreed to change the patients' tracheostomy dressings twice during their usual 12-hour shift: once using the standard method and once using the TDA. The nurses used the same dressing procedure for both dressing changes, but, when completing the dressing with the TDA, used the TDA rather than their fingers alone to apply the dressing. Nurses were randomized into two groups. Group A completed the first dressing change of the shift (completed near the beginning of their shift) without the TDA and the second dressing change (completed near the end of their shift) with the TDA. Group B completed the first dressing change of the shift with the TDA and the second without the TDA. After each dressing change, nurses and patients rated their experience using the TDA compared to the standard method of dressing change via surveys. Nurses rated the ease of dressing change perceived discomfort and also documented their observations of discomfort. Patients who were able to respond were asked to rate discomfort during the dressing changes, and a general description of their neck sized was recorded. Outcome measures were ease of use of the TDA, degree of patient discomfort with the dressing change, and a comparison of ease of use and degree of discomfort on patients with average-sized versus large-sized necks. Nurses rated the TDA easier to use in patients with average-sized necks and more favorably on observed discomfort in patients with average-sized and larger necks. Patients rated less discomfort with the TDA compared with the standard method of dressing change. The researchers concluded the TDA is an effective device to facilitate tracheostomy dressing changes, possibly improving compliance and efficiency and improving outcomes.

Relevance to Nursing Practice

Nursing interventions related to decreasing pain and increasing patient comfort are an important nursing responsibility. Interventions that can improve patient outcomes and improve time management should be considered by nurses. Nurses could easily incorporate this simple intervention as part of nursing care for these patients. This study also reinforces the importance of the role of nurses as innovators, developing, testing, and implementing new and improved products and processes to promote health and deliver optimal care (Spader, 2020).

discomfort to the patient. Clean the skin around a tracheostomy to prevent buildup of dried secretions and skin breakdown. Exercise care when changing the tracheostomy ties to prevent accidental decannulation or expulsion of the tube. Have an assistant hold the tube in place during the change or keep the soiled tie in place until a clean one is securely attached.

Implement medical device–related pressure injury prevention strategies to reduce the risk for alterations in skin integrity. Interventions may include the use of a hydrocolloid dressing under the tracheostomy flange during the postoperative period, removing the tracheostomy plate sutures within 7 days of the procedure, placing a polyurethane foam dressing at the tracheostomy site after suture removal (Dixon et al., 2018; O'Toole et al., 2017), routine skin and oral assessments, and provision of scheduled skin and oral hygiene interventions (Holdman et al., 2020).

Preparation for emergency situations is an important part of nursing care for these patients. The tracheostomy is the patient's only airway, and measures to maintain its patency need to be readily available. Standard bedside equipment for emergency use should include the obturator from the current tube, replacement inner cannula of the same size, suction equipment, oxygen, a manual ventilation bag, a spare tracheostomy tube of the same size, and one a size smaller (Dawson, 2014; Patton, 2019).

Patient condition, nursing assessment and judgment, and facility policy determine specific procedures and schedules, but a newly inserted tracheostomy may require attention every 1 to 2 hours. Skill 40-5 (on pp. 1648–1653) outlines tracheostomy care.

TRACHEAL SUCTIONING

The purpose of suctioning is to maintain a patent airway and remove pulmonary secretions, blood, vomitus, or foreign material from the airway. When performed correctly, suctioning provides comfort by relieving respiratory distress. When performed incorrectly, it can increase anxiety and pain and cause respiratory arrest. Tracheal suctioning may be performed by passing a sterile catheter through a tracheostomy or endotracheal tube. Suctioning to remove secretions is performed using the sterile technique; sterile technique is discussed in Chapter 25.

Tracheal suctioning should be performed only when clinically indicated based on assessment and not routinely (AARC, 2010; Burns & Delgado, 2019; Hess et al., 2021; Morton & Fontaine, 2018). Indications for the need for suctioning include audible and/or visible secretions, reduced oxygen saturation, presence of coarse crackles over the trachea, deterioration of arterial blood gas values, reduced breath sounds, and the patient's inability to generate an effective spontaneous cough, acute respiratory distress, or suspected aspiration of secretions (AARC, 2010; Patton, 2019). The suction catheter should be small enough not to occlude the airway being suctioned but large enough to remove secretions. In adults, use a suction catheter that occludes less than 50% of the lumen of the tracheostomy or endotracheal tube; in infants, the catheter should occlude less than 70% of the lumen (AARC, 2010; Pasrija & Hall, 2020). Several sizes of catheters are available. Wear gloves on both hands, goggles, and a mask—and a gown, if necessary—for protection from microorganisms.

Tracheal suctioning is an uncomfortable procedure at minimum, and it can be a very painful and/or distressing experience. Individualized pain management must be performed in response to the patient's needs (Arroyo-Novoa et al., 2008; Chaseling et al., 2014; Düzkaya & Kuğuoğlu, 2015; Wrona et al., 2021). Anticipate the administration of pharmacologic (analgesic medication) and use of nonpharmacologic interventions for the patient before suctioning (Arroyo-Novoa et al., 2008; Düzkaya & Kuğuoğlu, 2015; Ruan et al., 2017). As mentioned previously, perform suctioning only when clinically necessary because there are many potential risks. Risks include hypoxia, infection, tracheal tissue damage, cardiac dysrhythmias, bronchospasm, and atelectasis (AARC, 2010; Gilder et al., 2020). Sterile technique is used for tracheal suctioning, to reduce the risk of introduction of disease-causing organisms. In the home setting, clean technique is used, as the patient is not exposed to disease-causing organisms that may be found in health care settings, such as hospitals (Johns Hopkins Medicine, n.d.; Sterni et al., 2016; University of Iowa Health Care, 2017). Closely assess the patient before, during, and after the procedure to limit negative effects. In order to prevent hypoxia, hyperoxygenate the patient before and after suctioning for a minimum of 30 seconds (Burns & Delgado, 2019) and limit the application of suction to no more than 10 to 15 seconds (AARC, 2010; Burns & Delgado, 2019; Hess et al., 2021; Pasrija & Hall, 2020). Monitor the patient's pulse frequently to detect potential effects of hypoxia and stimulation of the vagus nerve. Using an appropriate suction pressure (no more than 150 mm Hg for adults) will help prevent atelectasis related to the use of high negative pressure (Hess et al., 2021). Research suggests that insertion of the suction catheter should be limited to a predetermined length (no more than the tip of the artificial airway to no more than 1 cm past the length of the endotracheal tube [adults] and 0.5 cm [pediatric patients] [Boroughs & Dougherty, 2015; Hess et al., 2021; Kendrick, 2020]) to avoid tracheal mucosal damage, including epithelial denudement, loss of cilia, edema, and fibrosis (Boroughs & Dougherty, 2015; Hahn, 2010; Ireton, 2007; Pasrija & Hall, 2020; Pate & Zapata, 2002). The practice of instillation of saline solution directly into the airway during tracheal suctioning is not supported by evidence and is not recommended for inclusion as part of evidence-based practice and suctioning (AARC, 2010; Boroughs & Dougherty, 2015; Burns & Delgado, 2019; Leddy & Wilkinson, 2015; Owen et al., 2016; Wang et al., 2017).

Skill 40-6 (on pp. 1653–1659) describes suctioning a patient with a tracheostomy using the open suctioning system and the procedure is similar for a patient with an endotracheal tube. The open suctioning system requires disconnection of the endotracheal or tracheostomy tube from the ventilator or oxygen therapy source and insertion of a suction catheter each time the patient requires suctioning (Burns & Delgado, 2019). A closed suctioning system (Fig. 40-16) makes use of an in-line suction catheter device that remains attached to the ventilator or oxygen source circuit. The closed suctioning system is another method to provide tracheal suctioning that allows periodic insertion of the suction catheter without disconnection of the endotracheal or tracheostomy tube from the ventilator or oxygen therapy source (Burns & Delgado, 2019). This closed system prevents gas exchange deterioration, atelectasis, and hypoxia; is cost-effective because only one catheter is used daily; and reduces bioaerosol exposure risk for caregivers and contamination of the surrounding environment (Hess et al., 2021; Imbriaco & Monesi, 2021; Yazdannik et al., 2019).

ASSISTING VENTILATION

Mechanical ventilators are used to assist or completely control ventilation. These machines are used with patients who have endotracheal or tracheostomy tubes in place. Mechanical ventilation can be performed in acute care facilities, in extended-care settings, and in the home. Mechanical ventilation improves oxygenation and ventilation and supports the patient's breathing function during emergency or acute care episodes as well as long-term situations.

Many types of ventilators are available. The nurse is responsible for addressing the physical and psychological concerns of the patient and family/caregivers. In addition, key interventions include evaluating the patient's response to ventilation therapy, using safe practices and techniques, and monitoring the patient carefully for complications. (See clinical texts and evidence for practice that discuss the use of mechanical ventilators in greater detail.)

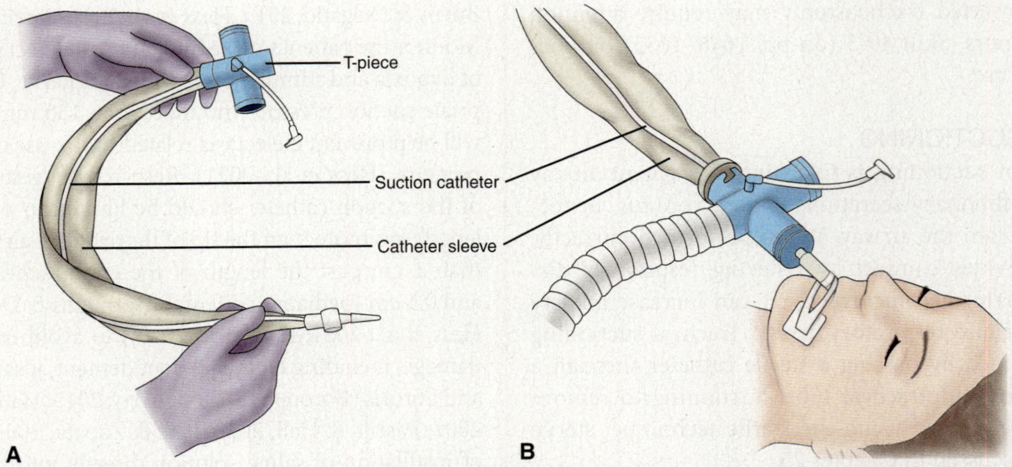

FIGURE 40-16. Closed airway suction system. **A.** Closed tracheal suction system. **B.** Closed system connected by a T-piece to the endotracheal tube and ventilator.

Another mechanical device used to assist ventilation is intermittent positive pressure breathing (IPPB). This is a method of providing a specific amount of air, oxygen, and aerosolized medication under increased pressure to the respiratory tract and is used for short-term hyperinflation therapy. IPPB forces deeper inspiration by positive pressure inhalation and then permits passive exhalation. The amount of pressure varies with each patient. Use of IPPB may be indicated for patients with atelectasis, reduced pulmonary function resulting in an effective cough, neuromuscular disorders, fatigue or muscle weakness with impending respiratory failure, acute severe bronchospasm, and in COPD exacerbations that fail to respond to other therapy (Hess et al., 2021). The use of IPPB is controversial, as evidence supporting its use is weak; in spontaneously breathing patients, it does not appear to have any benefit greater than other lung expansion techniques and its use for lung expansion should be considered after other interventions have been ineffective (Hess et al., 2021).

In emergency situations, the manual resuscitation bag (or bag-mask device) can be used to assist ventilation in patients whose respirations have ceased (Fig. 40-17). With the patient's head tilted back, jaw pulled forward, and airway cleared, the mask is held tightly over the patient's nose and mouth. The bag also fits over tracheostomy and endotracheal tubes. The operator's other hand compresses the bag at a rate of one breath every 6 seconds (about 10 breaths/min, adults) (American Heart Association [AHA], 2020b). The one-way valve in the mask allows exhaled air to escape. Artificial ventilation can be sustained until spontaneous breathing starts, until other mechanical assistance is available, or until death is confirmed. The bag is self-inflating and may be attached to supplemental oxygen (10 to 12 L/min) (Hess et al., 2021) if available.

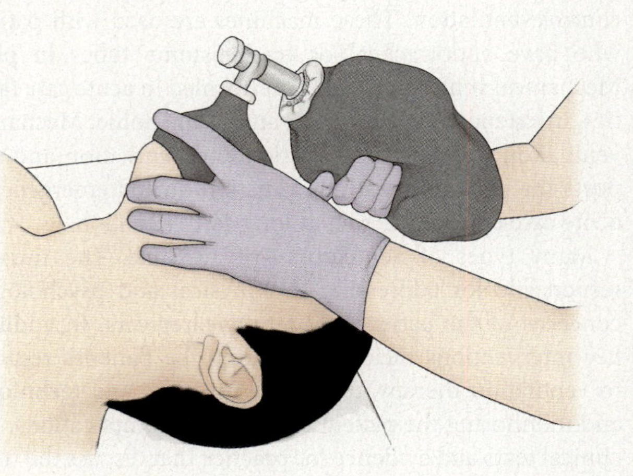

FIGURE 40-17. Manual resuscitation bag.

Clearing an Obstructed Airway

Foreign-body obstruction of the airway often occurs during eating. In adults, meat is the most common food-related cause. In children, any variety of foods or objects can obstruct the upper airway. A patient who is semiconscious or unconscious develops airway obstruction as the tongue falls back, covering the pharynx. In fact, the tongue is the most common cause of airway obstruction.

Foreign bodies can cause a mild or severe airway obstruction. In mild airway obstruction with good air exchange, the patient can cough forcefully. Allow the person to cough and encourage spontaneous breathing. Do not interfere with the patient's efforts to expel the object. With a partial airway obstruction, good air exchange can progress to poor air exchange. Poor air exchange may be indicated by a weak, ineffective cough, high-pitched noises while inhaling, increased breathing difficulties, and cyanosis. When this occurs, it is managed in the same way as complete airway obstruction. If mild airway obstruction continues or progresses, activate the emergency response system.

With a severe airway obstruction, the victim is unable to speak, cry or cough and may demonstrate poor or no air exchange; weak, ineffective cough or no cough; a high-pitched noise while inhaling or no noise at all; increased respiratory difficulty; and/or the universal choking sign (clutching the throat with both hands (AHA, 2020b) (Fig. 40-18). If the victim is an adult or child, ask "Are you choking?" If the victim nods "yes" and cannot talk, severe airway obstruction is present (AHA, 2020b). Immediate action is necessary—take

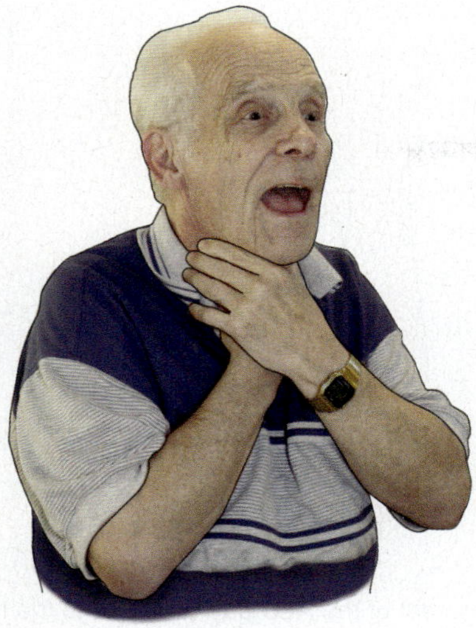

FIGURE 40-18. Universal choking sign.

steps to relieve the obstruction (choking relief). Choking relief in a responsive adult or child includes the use of abdominal thrusts to relieve choking. Do not use abdominal thrusts to relieve choking in an infant. Give each thrust with the intention of relieving the obstruction. It may be necessary to repeat the thrust several times to clear the airway. Follow and refer to the American Heart Association protocols for choking relief, which provide separate guidelines for other patient populations, including infants and pregnant, obese, and unresponsive victims (AHA, 2020b). If severe airway obstruction continues and the victim becomes unresponsive, start CPR. Follow the American Heart Association protocols for cardiopulmonary resuscitation (see next section). These protocols are continually being developed and updated.

Administering Cardiopulmonary Resuscitation

The American Heart Association (AHA, 2020b) identifies interventions to provide emergency cardiovascular care, using the metaphor "Chain of Survival" for the elements of the emergency cardiovascular care systems (AHA, 2022). Elements of this emergency care include cardiopulmonary resuscitation (CPR), which is the combination of chest compressions that circulate blood; mouth-to-mouth breathing, which supplies oxygen to the lungs; and defibrillation, which interrupts or stops an abnormal heart rhythm using controlled electrical shocks. The elements and order of actions in the Chain of Survival differ based on the situation; whether the patient has the cardiac arrest outside the hospital or inside the hospital; and whether the patient is an adult, child, or infant (AHA, 2020b). The brain is very sensitive to hypoxia, and damage to the brain begins to occur within minutes without oxygen; after 5 minutes; permanent anoxic brain injury can occur (Headway, 2021; Lacerte et al., 2020). The faster emergency cardiovascular care (CPR) is initiated, the greater the chance of survival (AHA, 2020b). *The following discussion addresses the main elements in the Chain of Survival and focuses on the interventions for health care providers for the adult patient inside the hospital.* Refer to specific details in the AHA's (2020b) Basic Life Support Provider Manual for further information and details for the other Chains of Survival.

- Verifying scene safety (making sure the environment is safe for rescuers and the victim).
- Check for responsiveness.
- Shout for nearby help.
- Activate the emergency response system.
- Get an automated external defibrillator (AED) or defibrillator and emergency equipment (or send someone to do so).
- Look for no breathing or only gasping and check the carotid pulse (simultaneously) for no more than 10 seconds. If the victim has no breathing or only gasping and no pulse is felt, initiate CPR with the **CAB** sequence. Perform cycles of 30 compressions and two breaths.
- Use the AED as soon as it is available.
- **C** (Chest Compressions): Start compressions within 10 seconds after recognizing cardiac arrest. Push hard (at least 2 inches) and fast (100 to 120/min). Allow complete chest recoil after each compression.
- **A** (Airway): Tilt the head and lift the chin. Check for breathing.
- **B** (Breathing): Deliver two breaths, each over 1 second. Note visible chest rise with each breath. Resume chest compressions in less than 10 seconds.
- Check the rhythm.
  - If it is a shockable rhythm, give one shock. Resume CPR immediately for 2 minutes (until prompted by AED for rhythm check). Continue until ALS (advance life support) provides take over, or the victim starts to move.
  - If it is not a shockable rhythm, resume CPR immediately for 2 minutes (until prompted by AED for rhythm check). Continue until ALS (advance life support) provides take over, or the victim starts to move.

During CPR, standard precautions are followed even though contact with a patient's blood or body fluids does not always occur. Occupational Safety and Health Administration (OSHA) standards require health care facilities to provide an ample supply of ventilation masks along with other protective barriers for staff to use during resuscitation efforts. A barrier device, such as a pocket mask (preferred) (Fig. 40-19) or face shield, should be used by health care providers when giving breaths (AHA, 2020b). Use a bag-mask device if

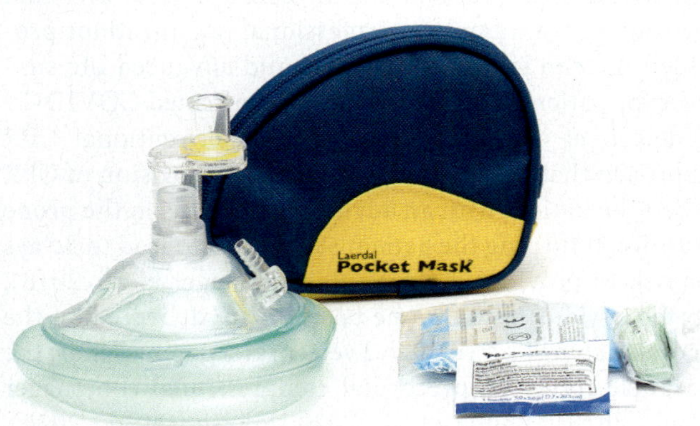

FIGURE 40-19. Pocket mask. (*Source:* Courtesy of Laerdal Medical.)

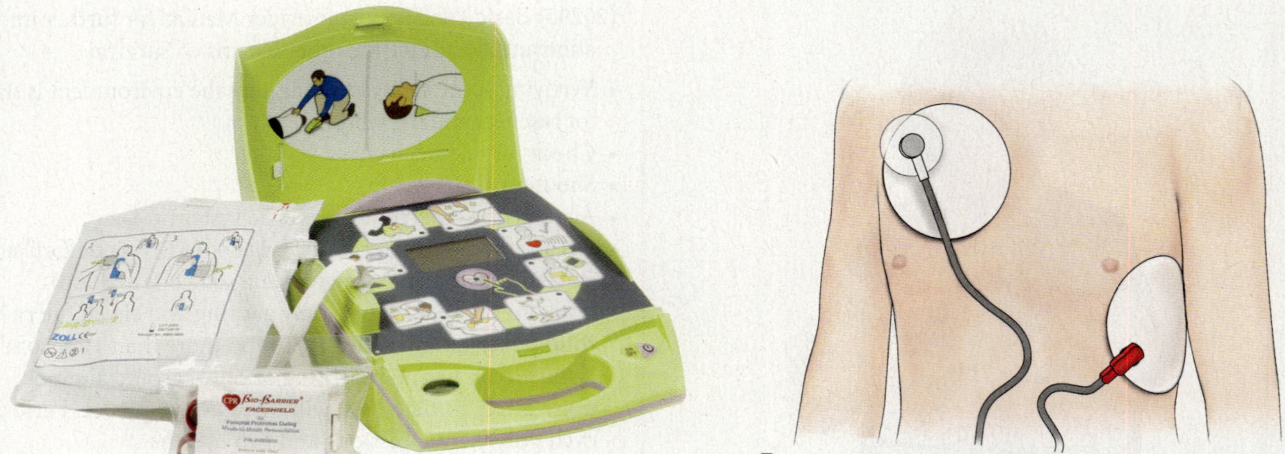

A B

FIGURE 40-20. Automated external defibrillator (AED). **A.** AED device. **B.** Placement of the AED pad attached to the red cable connector to the left of the heart apex. To help remember where to place the pads, think "white right, red ribs." Placement of both electrode pads is the same as it is for manual defibrillation or cardioversion.

available (refer to previous discussion). Bag-mask ventilation during CPR is more effective when two rescuers provide it together, with one rescuer opening the airway and sealing the mask against the face while the other squeezes the bag (AHA, 2020b).

The automated external defibrillator (AED) has proved effective in reducing deaths attributed to cardiac arrest. This easy-to-use, computer-based device is designed to deliver a shock (defibrillation) to the heart muscle quickly to interrupt shockable rhythms that resets the heart's electrical system so a normal (organized) heart rhythm can return (AHA, 2020b). The AED has the ability to analyze the heart's rhythm, direct the operator to deliver a shock when appropriate or deliver one automatically, and then reanalyze the rhythm to determine whether it has returned to normal (Fig. 40-20). Using the AED is an integral part of resuscitation.

Health care providers must use clinical reasoning and judgment and maintain knowledge of current evidence for practice and the patient's health status and circumstances to adapt rescue interventions based on the health status of the patient to balance the immediate needs of the patient with the safety of rescuers. For example, in the setting of the coronavirus disease (COVID-19), the American Heart Association in collaboration with and the support of numerous professional organizations provided interim guidance for basic and advanced life support for patients with suspected or confirmed COVID-19 (Edelson et al., 2020). Another nonconventional CPR approach that has been suggested is the provision of CPR when the patient with an advanced airway is in the prone position if turning the patient supine would lead to delays or risk to providers or patients (Bhatnager et al., 2018). Compressions in the prone position are delivered on the thoracic spine (T7/10), 0 to 2 vertebral segments below the scapulae (reversed precordial compressions) (Bhatnager et al., 2018; Douma et al., 2020; Edelson et al., 2020). Collection of evidence on the provision of CPR in the prone position is ongoing, and further research is needed (Moscarelli et al., 2020).

Most professional organizations recommend and support widespread efforts to teach CPR to laypeople and all health professionals. The nurse is professionally responsible for maintaining proficiency in CPR skills and maintaining CPR certification. CPR must be administered quickly and accurately, without hesitation, when cardiac or pulmonary arrest occurs.

The AHA provides guidelines related to emergency interventions outside of health care facilities. Learning conventional CPR is still recommended, and trained lay rescuers should provide rescue breaths in addition to chest compressions (AHA, 2020b). However, the AHA guidelines recommend that when a teen or adult suddenly collapses, untrained lay bystanders should call 911 (activate the emergency response system) and push hard and fast in the center of the patient's chest (AHA, 2020b). These two steps, called "Hands-Only CPR," can be as effective as conventional CPR (AHA, 2021). Providing Hands-Only CPR to a teen or adult who has collapsed from a sudden cardiac arrest can more than double or triple that person's chance of survival (AHA, 2021).

Evaluating

Evaluation is an ongoing and deliberate part of the nursing process, comparing the patient's health status with previously defined expected outcomes and involves the nurse, patient, family/caregivers, and other health care team members. Refer to the accompanying concept map that illustrates the nursing process and plan of care for Tyrone Jacobs. Everyone involved in the evaluation process reflects on the effectiveness of the plan of care to promote oxygenation and perfusion by evaluating whether the patient has met the individualized patient goals. Adjustments in the plan of care are made accordingly.

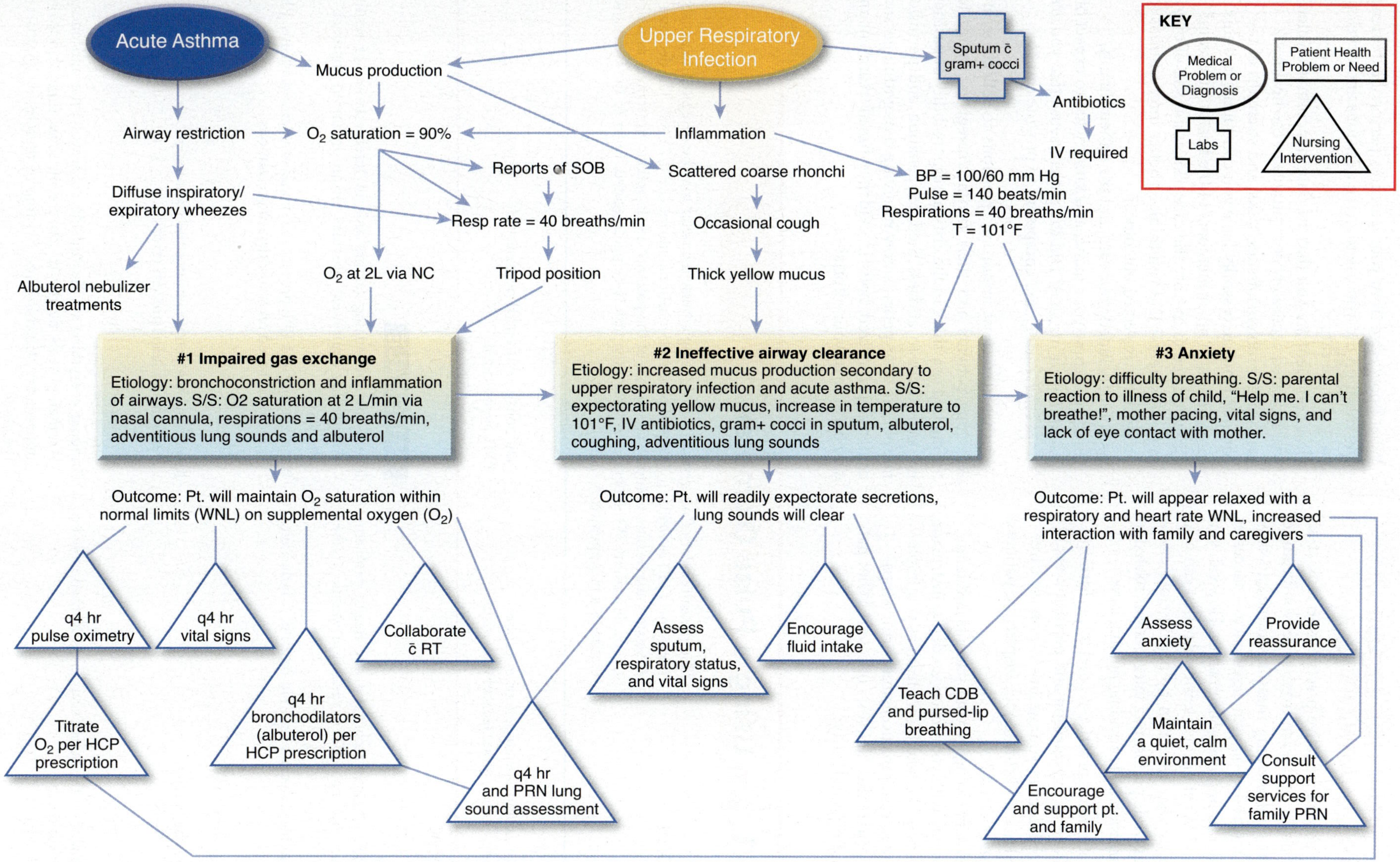

Evaluation

- **Diagnosis #1** Tyrone continues to have oxygen saturation below normal limits, tachypnea, and wheezing. Continue to monitor response to collaborative interventions. Notify physician for an increase in respiratory distress and a decrease in pulse oximetry.
- **Diagnosis #2** Tyrone continues to have audible adventitious sounds. He is readily expectorating secretions. Continue to monitor.
- **Diagnosis #3** Tyrone made eye contact with nurse as she explained the actions of his bronchodilators. Mother stopped pacing and sat beside son to provide comfort and reassurance. Continue interventions.

Concept map that displays the use of the nursing process in designing a care plan for Tyrone Jacobs. c̄ = with; IV = intravenous; pt. = patient; q = each/every (from L., *quaque*).

REFLECTIVE PRACTICE LEADING TO PERSONAL LEARNING

Remember that the goal of reflective practice is to look at an experience, understand it, and learn from it. As you begin to develop expertise in implementing measures related to oxygenation and perfusion, reflect on your experiences—successes and failures—in order to improve your practice. How can you do it better next time? What did you learn today that can help you tomorrow? Begin your reflection by paying close attention to the following while performing interventions related to oxygenation and perfusion and providing nursing care:

- Did your preparation and practice related to performing interventions related to oxygenation and perfusion result in your feeling confident in your ability to provide care? Did your competence and confidence inspire the patient's and family/caregiver's trust?
- Did your commitment to engage your patients and families and to collaborate with your fellow students, instructor, and other members of the health care team as you implemented the care plan result in successful partnerships?
- How did you prioritize the data you collected? What patterns in the data did you identify? What knowledge from your learning, personal experience and intuition did you use to make decisions and develop your plan of care?
- How confident are you that the data you communicated and recorded accurately communicates the health status, health problems, issues, risks, and strengths of the patient? How successfully have you communicated this information to other members of the health care team?
- Did you need to modify the care plan as a result of ongoing assessments? Did you think of better interventions to produce the expected outcomes?
- As you concluded your care, did the patient/family/caregivers know your name, and know what to expect of you and your nursing? Did the patient sense that you are respectful, caring, and competent to provide care?

Perhaps the most important questions to reflect on are: Are your patients and their families/caregivers better for having had *you* share in the critical responsibility of partnering with them to address their oxygenation and perfusion needs? Are your patients now receiving thoughtful, person-centered, prioritized, holistic, evidence-based treatment and care because of your efforts?

Skill 40-1 Using a Pulse Oximeter

DELEGATION CONSIDERATIONS

The measurement of oxygen saturation using a pulse oximeter may be delegated to assistive personnel (AP) as well as to licensed practical/vocational nurses (LPN/LVNs). The decision to delegate must be based on careful analysis of the patient's needs and circumstances as well as the qualifications of the person to whom the task is being delegated. Refer to the Delegation Guidelines in Appendix A.

EQUIPMENT

- Pulse oximeter with an appropriate sensor or probe
- Disposable cleansing cloth or skin cleanser and water
- Nail polish remover (if necessary)
- PPE, as indicated

IMPLEMENTATION

ACTION	RATIONALE
1. Review the patient's health record for any health problems that would affect the patient's oxygenation status. Gather equipment.	Identifying influencing factors aids in interpretation of results. Assembling equipment provides for an organized approach to the task.
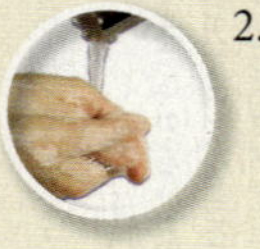 2. Perform hand hygiene and put on PPE, if indicated.	Hand hygiene and PPE prevent the spread of microorganisms. PPE is required based on transmission precautions.
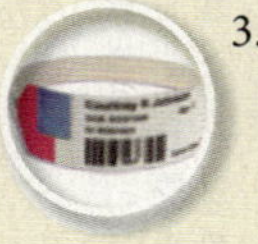 3. Identify the patient.	Identifying the patient ensures the right patient receives the intervention and helps prevent errors.
4. Assemble equipment on the bedside stand or overbed table or other surface within reach.	Bringing everything to the bedside conserves time and energy. Arranging items nearby is convenient, saves time, and avoids unnecessary stretching and twisting of muscles on the part of the nurse.

ACTION	RATIONALE
5. Close the curtains around the bed and close the door to the room, if possible. Explain to the patient what you are going to do and why.	This ensures the patient's privacy. Explanation relieves anxiety and facilitates engagement with care.
6. Select an appropriate site for application of the sensor.	Inadequate circulation can interfere with the oxygen saturation (SpO_2) reading.
a. Use the patient's index, middle, or ring finger (Figure 1).	Fingers are easily accessible.
b. Check the proximal pulse (Figure 2) and capillary refill (Figure 3) closest to the site.	Brisk capillary refill and a strong pulse indicate adequate circulation to the site.
c. If circulation to the site is inadequate, consider using the earlobe or forehead. Use the appropriate oximetry sensor for the chosen site.	These alternative sites are highly vascular. Correct use of appropriate equipment is vital for accurate results.
d. Use a toe only if lower extremity circulation is not compromised.	Peripheral vascular disease is common in lower extremities.

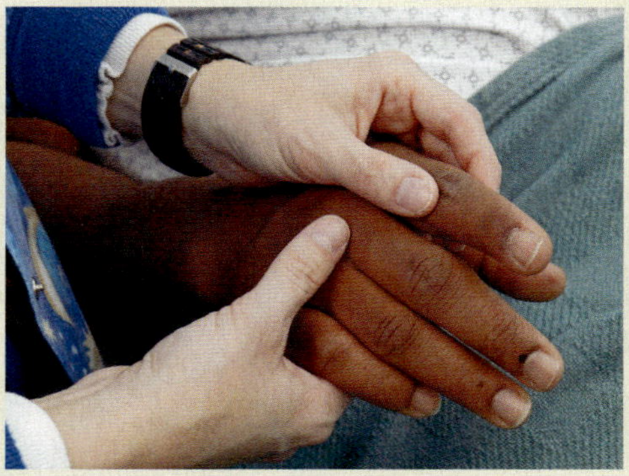

FIGURE 1. Selecting an appropriate finger.

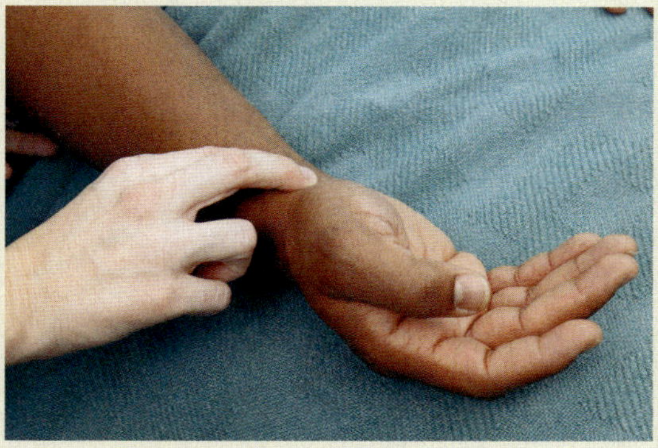

FIGURE 2. Assessing pulse.

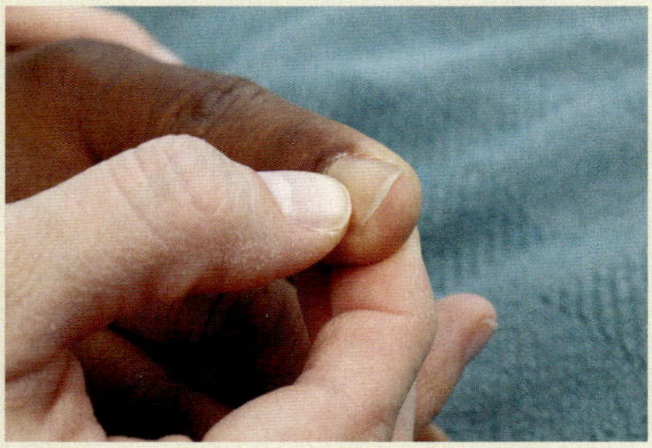

FIGURE 3. Assessing capillary refill.

ACTION	RATIONALE
7. Select the proper equipment:	
a. If one finger is too large for the probe, use a smaller finger.	Inaccurate readings can result if the probe or sensor is not attached correctly.
b. Use probes appropriate for the patient's age and size. Use a pediatric probe for a small adult, if necessary.	Probes come in adult, pediatric, and infant sizes.
c. Check if the patient is allergic to the adhesive. A nonadhesive finger clip or reflectance sensor is available.	A reaction may occur if the patient is allergic to an adhesive substance.
8. Prepare the monitoring site. Cleanse the selected area with a disposable cleansing cloth, as necessary; alternatively, have the patient wash their hands. Allow the area to dry. If necessary, remove any nail polish and artificial nails after checking the pulse oximeter's manufacturer's instructions.	Skin oils, dirt, or grime on the site can interfere with the passage of light waves. Research is conflicting regarding the effect of dark color nail polish and artificial nails. However, it is prudent to remove the nail polish (American Thoracic Society, 2021; USFDA, 2021; World Health Organization [WHO], 2011; Yönt et al., 2014). Refer to facility policy and the pulse oximeter's manufacturer's instructions regarding nail polish and artificial nails for additional information.

(continued on page 1634)

Skill 40-1 Using a Pulse Oximeter *(continued)*

ACTION	RATIONALE
9. Attach the probe securely to the skin (Figure 4). **Make sure that the light-emitting sensor and the light-receiving sensor are aligned opposite each other (not necessary to check if placed on the forehead).**	Secure attachment and proper alignment promote satisfactory operation of the equipment and an accurate recording of the SpO_2.
10. Connect the sensor probe to the pulse oximeter (Figure 5), turn the oximeter on, and check operation of the equipment (audible beep and fluctuation of the bar of light or waveform on the face of the oximeter).	An audible beep represents the arterial pulse, and a fluctuating waveform or light bar indicates the strength of the pulse. A weak signal will produce an inaccurate recording of the SpO_2. The tone of the beep reflects the SpO_2 reading. If SpO_2 drops, the tone becomes lower in pitch.
11. Set alarms on the pulse oximeter. Check the manufacturer's alarm limits for high and low pulse rate settings (Figure 6).	The alarm provides an additional safeguard and signals when high or low limits have been surpassed.

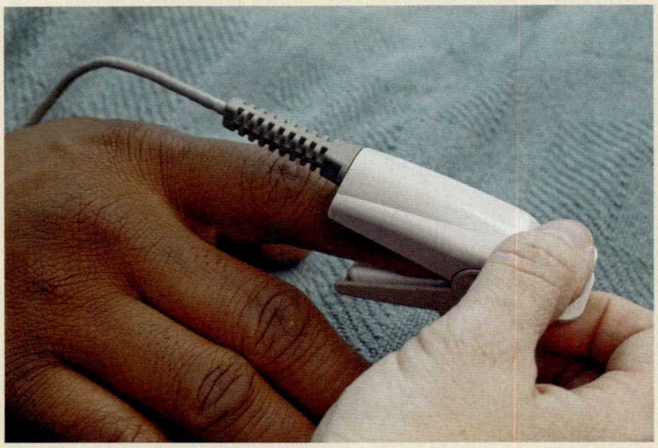

FIGURE 4. Attaching probe to patient's finger.

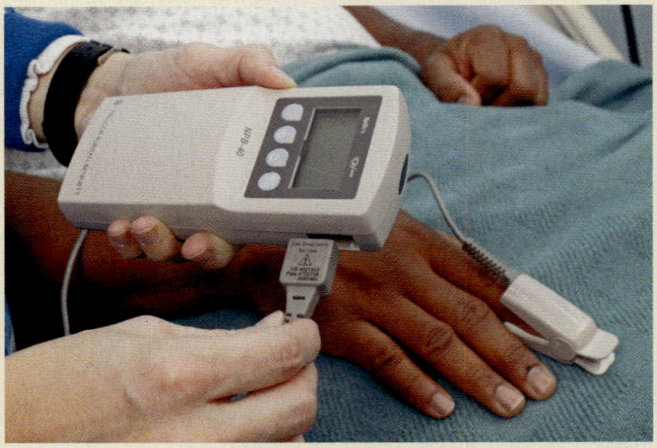

FIGURE 5. Connecting sensor probe to unit.

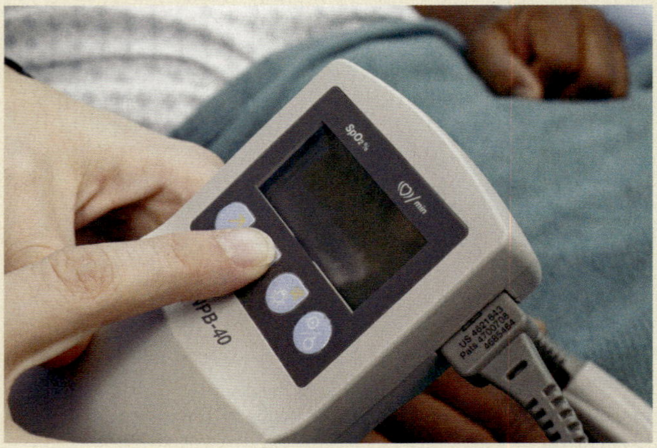

FIGURE 6. Checking alarms.

ACTION	RATIONALE
12. Check oxygen saturation at regular intervals, as prescribed, as per nursing assessment, and as signaled by alarms. Monitor the hemoglobin level.	Monitoring SpO_2 provides ongoing assessment of the patient's condition. A low hemoglobin level may be satisfactorily saturated yet inadequate to meet a patient's oxygen needs.
13. Remove the sensor on a regular basis and check for skin irritation or signs of pressure (every 2 hours for a spring-tension sensor and every 4 hours for an adhesive finger or toe sensor).	Prolonged pressure may lead to tissue necrosis. An adhesive sensor may cause skin irritation.
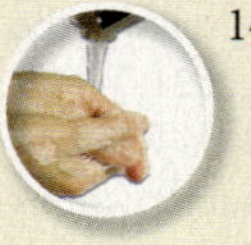 14. Clean nondisposable sensors according to the manufacturer's directions. Remove PPE, if used. Perform hand hygiene.	Cleaning equipment between each patient use reduces the spread of microorganisms. Proper removal of PPE reduces the risk for infection transmission and contamination of other items. Hand hygiene prevents the spread of microorganisms.

DOCUMENTATION

Guidelines

Documentation should include the type of sensor and location used, assessment of the proximal pulse and capillary refill, the pulse oximeter reading, the amount of oxygen, and delivery method if the patient is receiving supplemental oxygen, respiratory status, and any other relevant interventions required as a result of the reading.

Sample Documentation

9/03/25 Pulse oximeter placed on patient's index finger on right hand. Radial pulse presents with brisk capillary refill. Pulse oximeter reading 98% on oxygen at 2 L/min via nasal cannula. Heart rate measured by oximeter correlates with the radial pulse measurement.

—*C. Bausler, RN*

DEVELOPING CLINICAL REASONING AND CLINICAL JUDGMENT

UNEXPECTED SITUATIONS AND ASSOCIATED INTERVENTIONS

- *Absent or weak signal:* Check vital signs and patient condition. If satisfactory, check connections and circulation to site. Hypotension and other conditions that result in low blood flow make an accurate recording difficult (Hess et al., 2021). Equipment such as a restraint or blood pressure cuff may compromise circulation to the site and cause venous blood to pulsate, giving an inaccurate reading. If the extremity is cold, cover it with a warm blanket and/or use another site.
- *Potentially inaccurate reading:* Check prescribed medications and history of circulatory disorders. Try the device on another person to see if the problem is equipment related or patient related. Drugs that cause vasoconstriction interfere with accurate recording of the oxygen saturation.

SPECIAL CONSIDERATIONS

General Considerations

- Review facility procedures for obtaining pulse oximetry readings if the patient's fingers are not suitable. Correct use of appropriate equipment is vital for accurate results. The appropriate ear oximetry sensor should be used to obtain measurements from a patient's ear. A finger sensor should be limited to use on the finger. The oximetry measurement obtained during clinical assessment should include a record of the type of sensor used.
- Accuracy of readings can be influenced by conditions that decrease arterial blood flow, such as peripheral edema, hypotension, and peripheral vascular disease. Bradycardia and irregular cardiac rhythms may also cause inaccurate readings.
- Accuracy of readings may also be affected by skin pigmentation (deeply pigmented skin) (Hess et al., 2021; Sjoding et al., 2020; USFDA, 2021), nail polish, and intravascular dyes (methylene blue and indocyanine green) (Hess et al., 2021; USFDA, 2021).
- Pulse oximetry may be less reliable in patients with chronic bronchitis and emphysema (Amalakanti & Pentakota, 2016).
- Inexpensive, portable over-the-counter pulse oximeters may be less reliable and are not intended for medical purposes, do not undergo FDA review, and should not be used for medical purposes (USFDA, 2021).
- Correlate the pulse reading on the pulse oximeter with the patient's heart rate (American Thoracic Society, 2021). Variation between pulse and heart rate may indicate that not all pulsations are being detected, and another sensor site may be required.
- Excessive motion of the sensor probe site, such as with extremity tremors or shivering, can also interfere with obtaining an accurate reading.
- In patients with low cardiac output, the forehead or ear sensor may be better than the digit sensor for pulse oximetry.

(*continued on page 1636*)

Skill 40-1 Using a Pulse Oximeter *(continued)*

INFANT AND CHILD CONSIDERATIONS

- For infants, the oximeter probe may be placed on the toe or foot (Figure 7).

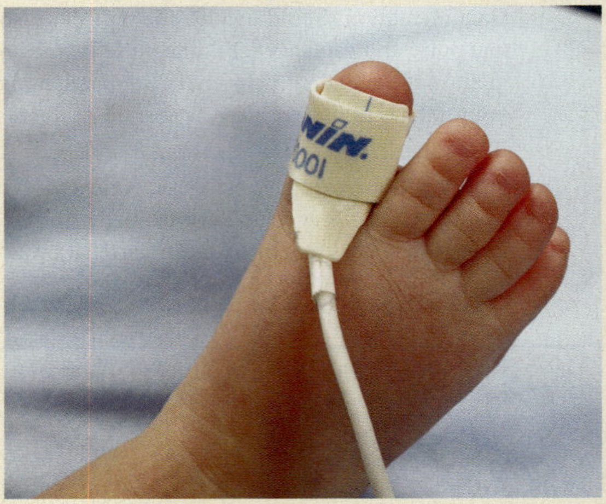

FIGURE 7. Oximetry probe on infant's toe.

OLDER ADULT CONSIDERATIONS

- Careful attention to the patient's skin integrity and condition is necessary to prevent injury. Pressure or tension from the probe, as well as any adhesive used, can damage older, dry, thin skin.

Community-Based Care Considerations

- Portable prescription units are available for use in the home or in an outpatient setting (USFDA, 2021).

Skill 40-2 Suctioning the Oropharyngeal and Nasopharyngeal Airways

DELEGATION CONSIDERATIONS

Suctioning of the oropharyngeal airway may be delegated to assistive personnel (AP) who have received appropriate training. Depending on the state's nurse practice act and the organization's policies and procedures, the suctioning of the oropharyngeal and nasopharyngeal airways may be delegated to licensed practical/vocational nurses (LPN/LVNs). The decision to delegate must be based on careful analysis of the patient's needs and circumstances as well as the qualifications of the person to whom the task is being delegated. Refer to the Delegation Guidelines in Appendix A.

EQUIPMENT

- Portable or wall suction unit with tubing
- A commercially prepared suction kit with an appropriate-size catheter or
  - Sterile suction catheter with Y-port in the appropriate size (adult: 10 to 16 Fr)
  - Sterile disposable container
  - Sterile gloves
- Sterile water or saline
- Towel or waterproof pad
- Goggles and mask or face shield; N95 mask or equivalent, based on patient's health status
- Disposable, clean gloves
- Water-soluble lubricant (nasopharyngeal and nasotracheal suctioning)
- Additional PPE, as indicated

IMPLEMENTATION

ACTION	RATIONALE
1. Gather equipment.	Assembling equipment provides for an organized approach to the task.
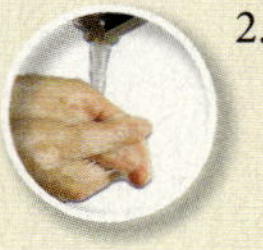 2. Perform hand hygiene and put on PPE, if indicated.	Hand hygiene and PPE prevent the spread of microorganisms. PPE is required based on transmission precautions.

ACTION	RATIONALE
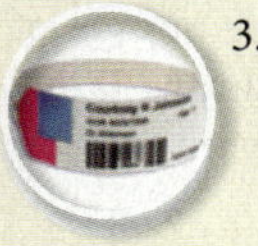 3. Identify the patient.	Identifying the patient ensures the right patient receives the intervention and helps prevent errors.
4. Assemble equipment on the overbed table or other surface within reach.	Bringing everything to the bedside conserves time and energy. Arranging items nearby is convenient, saves time, and avoids unnecessary stretching and twisting of muscles on the part of the nurse.
5. Close the curtains around the bed and close the door to the room, if possible.	This ensures the patient's privacy.
6. Perform assessments to determine the need for suctioning. Verify the prescribed suctioning intervention in the patient's health record, if necessary. Anticipate the administration of pharmacologic (analgesic medication) and use of nonpharmacologic interventions for the patient before suctioning. **Assess for pain or the potential to cause pain. Administer pain medication, as prescribed, before suctioning.**	Suctioning should be performed only when clinically indicated based on assessment and not routinely (AARC, 2010; Burns & Delgado, 2019; Hess et al., 2021; Morton & Fontaine, 2018). Some facilities require that naso- and oropharyngeal suctioning are a prescribed intervention. At a minimum, suctioning is an uncomfortable procedure, and it can be a very painful and/or distressing experience. Individualized pain management must be performed in response to the patient's needs (Arroyo-Novoa et al., 2008; Chaseling et al., 2014; Wrona et al., 2021; Düzkaya & Kuğuoğlu, 2015).
7. Explain to the patient what you are going to do and why, even if the patient does not appear to be alert. Reassure the patient that you will interrupt the procedure if they indicate respiratory difficulty.	Explanation alleviates fears. Even if the patient appears unconscious, explain what is happening. Any procedure that compromises respiration is frightening for the patient.
8. Adjust the bed to a comfortable working height (VHACEOSH, 2016). Lower the side rail closest to you. **If the patient is conscious, place them in a semi-Fowler position. If the patient is unconscious, place them in the lateral position, facing you.** Move the bedside table close to your work area and raise it to waist height.	Having the bed at the proper height prevents back and muscle strain. A sitting position helps the patient to cough and makes breathing easier. Gravity also facilitates catheter insertion. The lateral position prevents the airway from becoming obstructed and promotes drainage of secretions. The bedside table provides a work surface and helps maintain sterility of objects on the work surface.
9. Place a towel or waterproof pad across the patient's chest.	This protects bed linens.
10. **Adjust suction to the appropriate pressure** (Hess et al., 2021) (Figure 1): • No more than 150 mm Hg for adults and adolescents • No more than 125 mm Hg for children • No more than 100 mm Hg for infants **Put on a disposable, clean glove and occlude the end of the connecting tubing to check suction pressure.** Place the connecting tubing in a convenient location.	Higher pressures can cause excessive trauma, hypoxemia, and atelectasis.

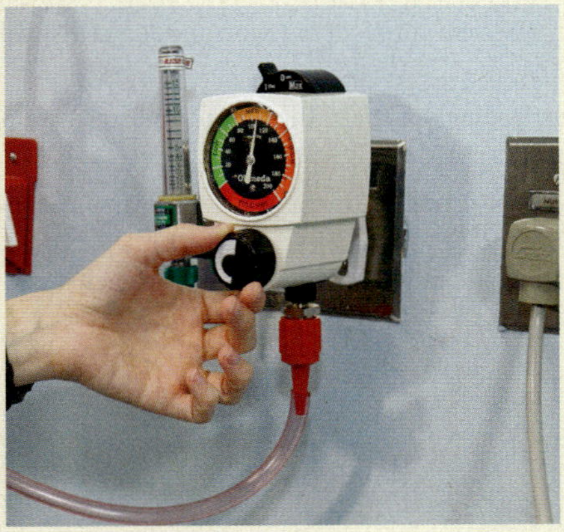

FIGURE 1. Adjusting wall suction.

(continued on page 1638)

Skill 40-2 Suctioning the Oropharyngeal and Nasopharyngeal Airways *(continued)*

ACTION	RATIONALE
11. Open the sterile suction package using aseptic technique. The open wrapper or container becomes a sterile field to hold other supplies. Carefully remove the sterile container, touching only the outside surface. Set it up on the work surface and pour sterile saline into it.	Sterile normal saline or water is used to lubricate the outside of the catheter, minimizing irritation of the mucosa during introduction. It is also used to clear the catheter between suction attempts.
12. Place a small amount of water-soluble lubricant on the sterile field, taking care to avoid touching the sterile field with the lubricant package.	Lubricant facilitates passage of the catheter and reduces trauma to mucous membranes.
13. Increase the patient's supplemental oxygen level, or apply supplemental oxygen per facility policy or prescribed intervention.	Suctioning removes air from the patient's airway and can cause hypoxemia. Hyperoxygenation can help prevent suction-induced hypoxemia (Morton & Fontaine, 2018).
14. Put on a face shield or goggles and mask. Put on sterile gloves. Your dominant hand will manipulate the catheter and must remain sterile. The nondominant hand is considered clean rather than sterile and will control the suction valve (Y-port) on the catheter. In the home setting and other community-based settings, maintenance of sterility is not necessary.	Gloves and other PPE protect the nurse from microorganisms. Handling the sterile catheter using a sterile glove helps prevent introducing organisms into the respiratory tract. In the home setting and other community-based settings, clean (instead of sterile) technique is used because the patient is not exposed to disease-causing organisms that may be found in health care settings, such as hospitals.
15. With your dominant gloved hand, pick up the sterile catheter. Pick up the connecting tubing with the nondominant hand and connect the tubing and suction catheter (Figure 2).	Sterility of the suction catheter is maintained.
16. Moisten the catheter by dipping it into the container of sterile saline (Figure 3). Occlude the Y-tube to check suction.	Lubricating the inside of the catheter with saline helps move secretions in the catheter. Checking suction ensures equipment is working properly.

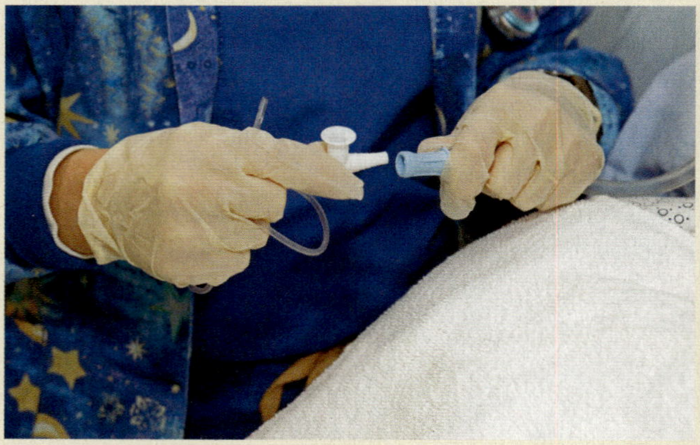

FIGURE 2. Connecting suction catheter to tubing.

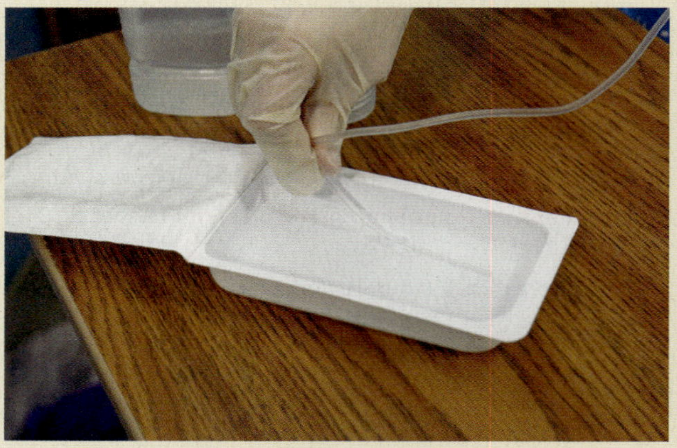

FIGURE 3. Dipping catheter into sterile saline.

ACTION	RATIONALE
17. Encourage the patient to take several deep breaths.	Hyperventilation can help prevent suction-induced hypoxemia (Hess et al., 2021).
18. Apply lubricant to the first 2 to 3 inches of the catheter, using the lubricant that was placed on the sterile field.	Lubricant facilitates passage of the catheter and reduces trauma to mucous membranes.
19. Remove the oxygen delivery device, if appropriate. Do not apply suction as the catheter is inserted. Hold the catheter between your thumb and forefinger.	Suctioning removes air from the patient's airway and can cause hypoxemia. Using suction while inserting the catheter can cause trauma to the mucosa and remove excessive oxygen from the respiratory tract.

ACTION	RATIONALE
20. Insert the catheter: a. **For nasopharyngeal suctioning**, gently insert the catheter through the naris and along the floor of the nostril toward the trachea (Figure 4). Roll the catheter between your fingers to help advance it. Advance the catheter approximately 6 to 8 inches to reach the pharynx (Hinkle et al., 2022). b. **For oropharyngeal suctioning**, insert the catheter through the mouth, along the side of the mouth toward the trachea. Advance the catheter 3 to 4 inches to reach the pharynx.	The correct distance for insertion ensures proper placement of the catheter. The general guideline for determining insertion distance for nasopharyngeal suctioning for an individual patient is to estimate the distance from the patient's earlobe to the nose.
21. **Apply suction by intermittently occluding the Y-port on the catheter with the thumb of your nondominant hand and gently rotating the catheter as it is being withdrawn (Figure 5). Do not suction for more than 15 seconds at a time** (AARC, 2010; Hess et al., 2021).	Turning the catheter as it is withdrawn minimizes trauma to the mucosa. Suctioning for longer than 15 seconds robs the respiratory tract of oxygen, which may result in hypoxemia. Suctioning too quickly may be ineffective at clearing all secretions.
22. Replace the oxygen delivery device using your nondominant hand, if appropriate, and have the patient take several deep breaths.	Suctioning removes air from the patient's airway and can cause hypoxemia. Hyperventilation can help prevent suction-induced hypoxemia.
23. Flush the catheter with saline (Figure 6). Assess the effectiveness of suctioning and repeat, as needed, and according to the patient's tolerance. Wrap the suction catheter around your dominant hand between attempts.	Flushing clears the catheter and lubricates it for next insertion. Reassessment determines the need for additional suctioning. Wrapping prevents inadvertent contamination of the catheter.

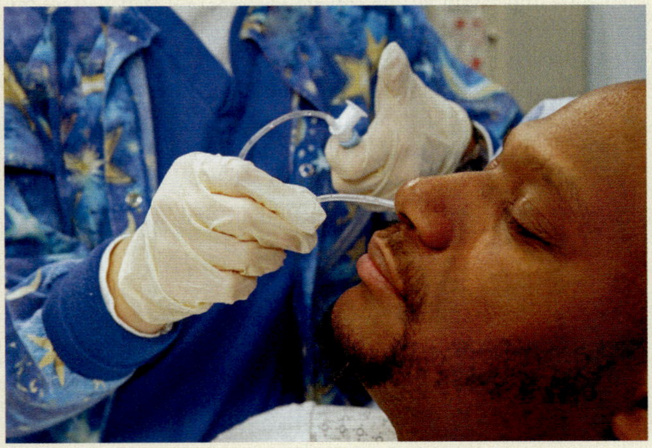

FIGURE 4. Inserting catheter into naris.

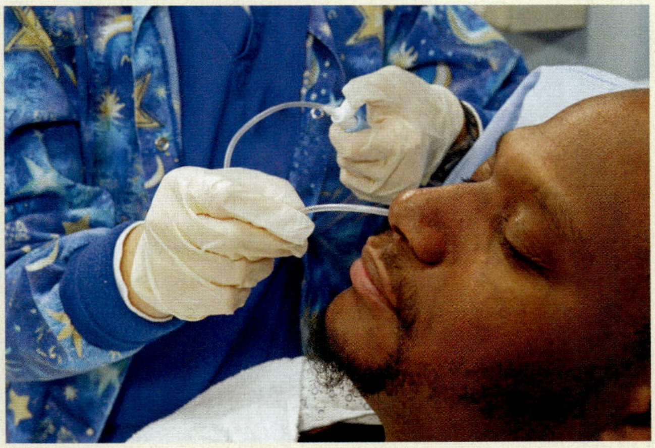

FIGURE 5. Rotating the catheter as it is withdrawn to suction the nasopharynx.

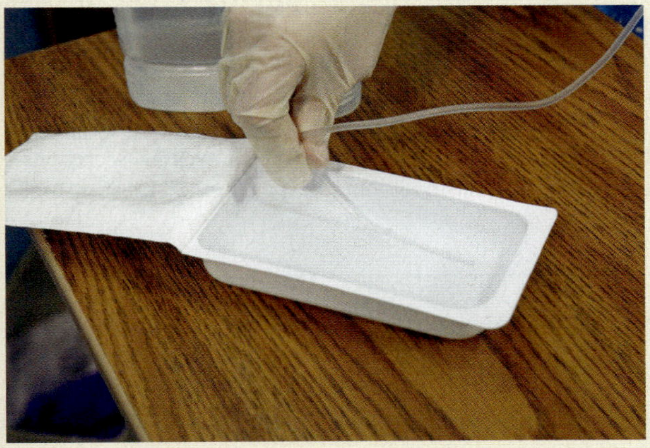

FIGURE 6. Rinsing catheter.

(*continued on page 1640*)

Skill 40-2 Suctioning the Oropharyngeal and Nasopharyngeal Airways *(continued)*

ACTION	RATIONALE
24. **Allow at least a 30-second interval if additional suctioning is needed. Alternate the naris, unless contraindicated, if repeated suctioning is required.** No more than three suction passes should be made per suctioning episode. Do not force the catheter through the naris. Encourage the patient to cough and deep breathe between suctioning. **Suction the oropharynx after suctioning the nasopharynx.**	The interval allows for reventilation and reoxygenation of airways. Excessive suction passes contribute to complications. Alternating the naris reduces trauma. Suctioning the oropharynx after the nasopharynx clears the mouth of secretions. More microorganisms are usually present in the mouth, so it is suctioned last to prevent transmission of contaminants.
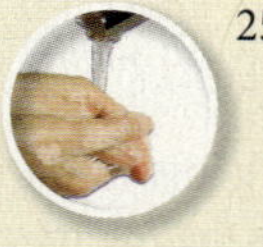 25. When suctioning is complete, remove the glove from your dominant hand over the coiled catheter, pulling it off inside out. Remove the glove from your nondominant hand, and dispose of gloves, catheter, and the container with the solution in the appropriate receptacle. Perform hand hygiene.	This technique of glove removal and hand hygiene reduces transmission of microorganisms.
26. Assist the patient to a comfortable position. Raise the bed rail and place the bed in the lowest position.	Proper positioning with raised side rails and the proper bed height provides for patient comfort and safety.
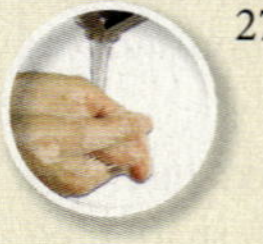 27. Turn off the suction. Remove the supplemental oxygen placed for suctioning, if appropriate. Remove the face shield or goggles and mask. Perform hand hygiene.	Proper removal of PPE and hand hygiene reduce the risk of transmission of microorganisms.
28. Perform oral hygiene after suctioning. Oral hygiene measures are discussed in Chapter 32.	Respiratory secretions that are allowed to accumulate in the mouth are irritating to mucous membranes, pose a risk for aspiration, and are unpleasant for the patient. Diligent oral hygiene care can improve oral health and limit the growth of pathogens in the oropharyngeal secretions, decreasing the incidence of aspiration pneumonia, community-acquired pneumonia, nonventilator health care–associated pneumonia (NV-HAP), and ventilator-associated pneumonia (VAP) (AACN, 2017; Chick & Wynne, 2020; Jenson et al., 2018; Quinn et al., 2020).
29. Reassess the patient's respiratory status, including respiratory rate, effort, oxygen saturation, and lung sounds, and their response to suctioning.	This assesses effectiveness of suctioning and the presence of complications.
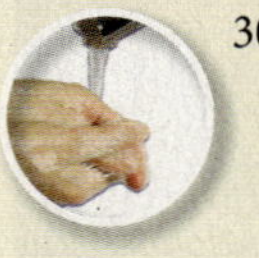 30. Remove additional PPE, if used. Perform hand hygiene.	Proper removal of PPE reduces the risk for infection transmission and contamination of other items. Hand hygiene prevents the spread of microorganisms.

DOCUMENTATION

Guidelines

Document the time of suctioning, assessments before and after the intervention, the reason for suctioning, route used, and the characteristics and amount of secretions.

Sample Documentation

9/17/25 1440 Patient with gurgling on inspiration and weak cough; unable to clear secretions. Lungs with rhonchi (sonorous wheezes) in upper airways. Nasopharyngeal suction completed with 12-Fr catheter. Large amount of thick, yellow secretions obtained. After suctioning, lung sounds clear in all lobes, respirations 18 breaths/min, no gurgling noted.

—C. Bausler, RN

DEVELOPING CLINICAL REASONING AND CLINICAL JUDGMENT

UNEXPECTED SITUATIONS AND ASSOCIATED INTERVENTIONS

- *Patient vomits during suctioning:* If the patient gags or becomes nauseated, remove the catheter; it has probably entered the esophagus inadvertently. If the patient needs to be suctioned again, change the catheter, because it is probably contaminated. Turn the patient to the side and elevate the head of the bed to prevent aspiration.
- *Epistaxis (bleeding) is noted with continued suctioning:* Notify the health care team and anticipate the need for a nasal trumpet. The nasal trumpet will protect the nasal mucosa from further trauma related to suctioning (Morton & Fontaine, 2018).

SPECIAL CONSIDERATIONS

General Considerations

- The use of suction pressure higher than the pressure guidelines presented in the skill have been suggested by some researchers (Maras et al., 2020; Yazdannik et al., 2019).

Infant and Child Considerations

- For infants, use a 5- to 6-Fr catheter.
- For children, use a 6- to 10-Fr catheter.

Skill 40-3 Administering Oxygen by Nasal Cannula

DELEGATION CONSIDERATIONS

The administration of oxygen by nasal cannula is not delegated to assistive personnel (AP). Reapplication of the nasal cannula during nursing care activities, such as during bathing, may be performed by AP. Depending on the state's nurse practice act and the organization's policies and procedures, administration of oxygen by nasal cannula may be delegated to licensed practical/vocational nurses (LPN/LVNs). The decision to delegate must be based on careful analysis of the patient's needs and circumstances as well as the qualifications of the person to whom the task is being delegated. Refer to the Delegation Guidelines in Appendix A.

EQUIPMENT

- Flow meter connected to oxygen supply
- Humidifier with sterile, distilled water (based on circumstances, system, and facility policy)
- Nasal cannula and tubing
- Gauze to pad tubing over ears or commercial padding (optional)
- PPE, as indicated

IMPLEMENTATION

ACTION	RATIONALE
1. Review the prescribed intervention to verify the use of the nasal cannula, flow rate, and administration parameters. Gather equipment.	Verifying the prescribed intervention ensures the patient receives the prescribed amount of oxygen. Assembling equipment provides for an organized approach to the task.
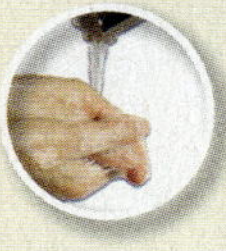 2. Perform hand hygiene and put on PPE, if indicated.	Hand hygiene and PPE prevent the spread of microorganisms. PPE is required based on transmission precautions.
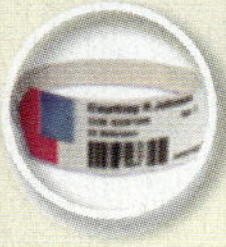 3. Identify the patient.	Identifying the patient ensures the right patient receives the intervention and helps prevent errors.

(continued on page 1642)

Skill 40-3 Administering Oxygen by Nasal Cannula *(continued)*

ACTION | **RATIONALE**

4. Assemble equipment on the overbed table or other surface within reach.

Bringing everything to the bedside conserves time and energy. Arranging items nearby is convenient, saves time, and avoids unnecessary stretching and twisting of muscles on the part of the nurse.

5. Close the curtains around the bed and close the door to the room, if possible.

This ensures the patient's privacy.

6. Explain to the patient what you are going to do and why. Review safety precautions necessary when oxygen is in use.

Explanation relieves anxiety and facilitates engagement with care. Oxygen supports combustion; a small spark could cause a fire.

7. Connect the nasal cannula to the oxygen source (Figure 1), with humidification, if appropriate. Adjust the flow rate as prescribed (Figure 2). Check that oxygen is flowing out of prongs.

Oxygen forced through a water reservoir is humidified before it is delivered to the patient, thus preventing dehydration of the mucous membranes. Low-flow oxygen does not require humidification.

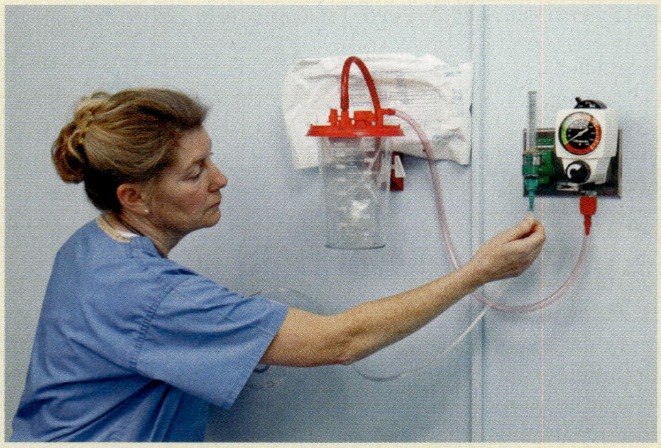

FIGURE 1. Connecting cannula to oxygen source.

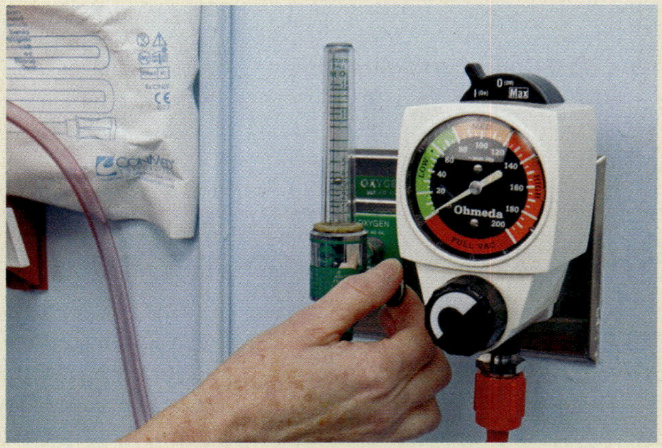

FIGURE 2. Adjusting flow rate.

8. Place the prongs in the patient's nostrils (Figure 3). Place the tubing over and behind each ear with the adjuster comfortably under the chin. Alternatively, the tubing may be placed around the patient's head, with the adjuster at the back or base of the head. Place the gauze (Figure 4) or commercially available pads at the ear beneath the tubing, as necessary.

Correct placement of the prongs and fastener facilitates oxygen administration and patient comfort. Pads reduce irritation and pressure and protect the skin. Pressure injuries may be related to a medical device or other object (EPUAP, NPIAP, & PPPIA, 2019, p. 16; Joint Commission, 2018). Any tube, electrode, sensor, or other rigid or stiff device element under pressure can create pressure damage (Baranoski & Ayello, 2020; EPUAP, NPIAP, & PPPIA, 2019).

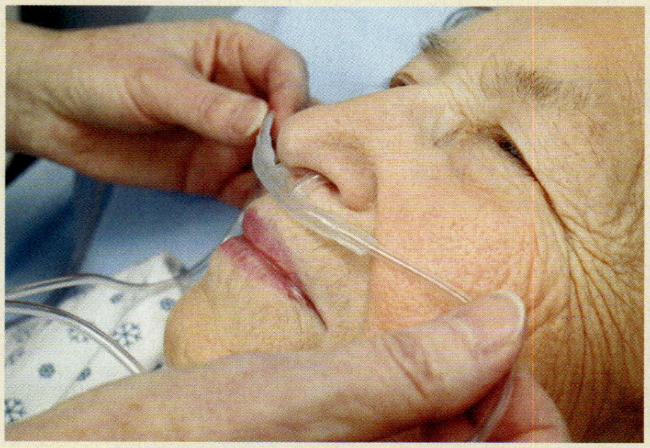

FIGURE 3. Putting the prongs in the patient's nostrils.

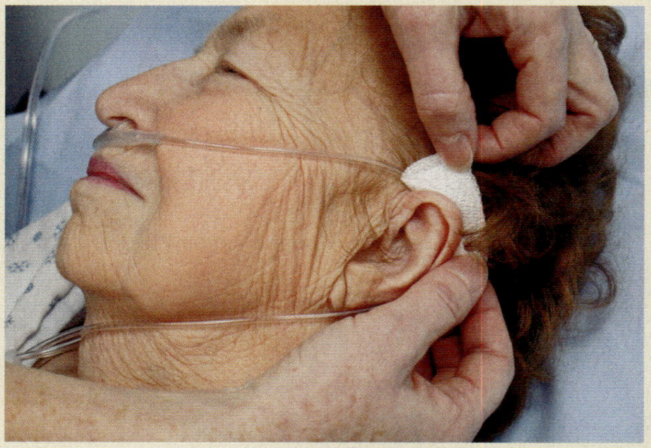

FIGURE 4. Placing gauze pad at ears.

Skill 40-3 Administering Oxygen by Nasal Cannula (continued)

ACTION	RATIONALE
9. Adjust the fit of the cannula, as necessary (Figure 5). The tubing should be snug but not tight against the skin.	Proper adjustment maintains the prongs in the patient's nose. Excessive pressure from the tubing could cause irritation and pressure to the skin. Nasal cannulas may cause pressure injuries behind the ears, around the nostril, or in the nasal vestibule (Camacho-Del Rio, 2018).
10. Reassess the patient's respiratory status, including the respiratory rate, effort, and lung sounds. Note any signs of respiratory distress, such as tachypnea, nasal flaring, use of accessory muscles, or dyspnea.	This assesses the effectiveness of oxygen therapy.
11. Remove PPE, if used. Perform hand hygiene.	Proper removal of PPE reduces the risk for infection transmission and contamination of other items. Hand hygiene prevents the spread of microorganisms.
12. Put on clean gloves. Remove and clean the cannula and assess the nares at least every 8 hours, or according to facility recommendations (Figure 6). Assess the areas of skin contact with the cannula for alterations in skin integrity.	The continued presence of the cannula causes irritation and dryness of the mucous membranes. Nasal cannulas may cause pressure injuries behind the ears, around the nostril, or in the nasal vestibule (Camacho-Del Rio, 2018).

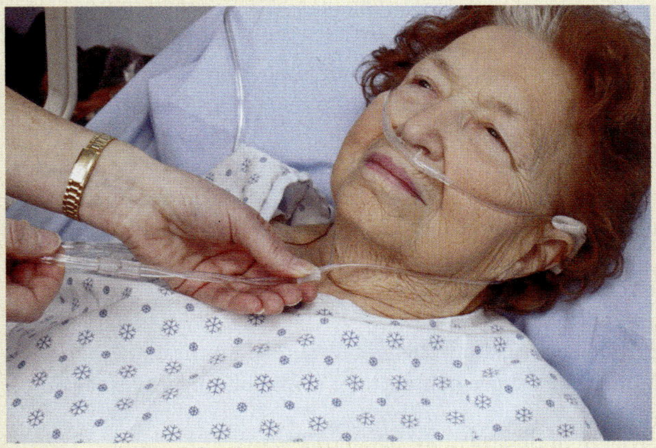

FIGURE 5. Adjusting the fit of the cannula.

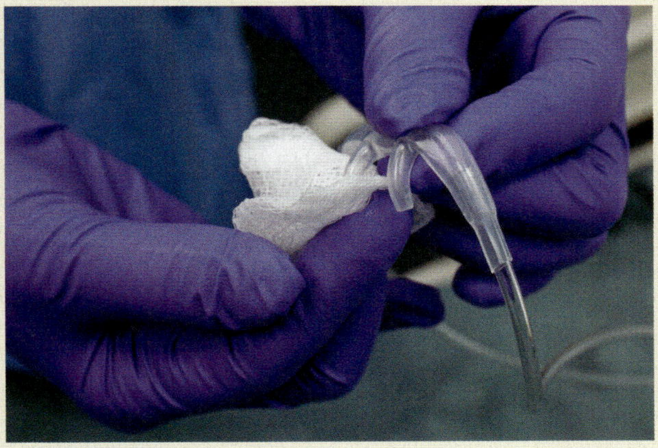

FIGURE 6. Cleaning cannula, when indicated.

DOCUMENTATION

Guidelines

Document your assessment before and after intervention. Document the amount of oxygen applied; the delivery method; and the patient's respiratory rate, oxygen saturation, and lung sounds.

Sample Documentation

DocuCare Practice documenting the administration of oxygen by nasal cannula in *Lippincott DocuCare*.

9/17/25 1300 Oxygen via nasal cannula applied at 2 L/min. Humidification in place. Pulse oximeter before placing oxygen 92%; after oxygen at 2 L/min 98%. Respirations even and unlabored. Chest rises symmetrically. No nasal flaring or retractions noted. Lung sounds clear and equal in all lobes.

—C. Bausler, RN

DEVELOPING CLINICAL REASONING AND CLINICAL JUDGMENT

UNEXPECTED SITUATIONS AND ASSOCIATED INTERVENTIONS

- *Patient was fine on oxygen delivered by nasal cannula but now states they are short of breath, and the pulse oximeter reading is less than 93%:* Check to see that the oxygen tubing is still connected to the flow meter and the flow meter is still on the previous setting. Someone may have stepped on the tubing, pulling it from the flow meter, or the oxygen may have accidentally been turned off. Assess the patient's respiratory status, including respiratory rate, rhythm, effort, and lung sounds. Note any additional signs of respiratory distress. Collaborate with the health care team regarding any changes and assessment findings.

(continued on page 1644)

Skill 40-3 Administering Oxygen by Nasal Cannula *(continued)*

- *Areas over ear or back of head are reddened:* Ensure that areas are adequately padded and that the tubing is not pulled too tight. Consider consultation with the skin care team or wound nurse specialist.

SPECIAL CONSIDERATIONS

General Considerations

- Soft nasal cannulas have been shown to decrease the incidence of pressure injuries (Camacho-Del Rio, 2018).
- When providing oxygen via high-flow nasal cannula, protect the back of the ears with a hydrocolloid or foam dressing (Camacho-Del Rio, 2018).
- There is no evidence that mouth breathing influences the efficiency of oxygen delivery; even when the patient inspires through the mouth, oxygen still flows through the nose into the pharynx (O'Driscoll et al., 2017; Hess et al., 2021).

Community-Based Care Considerations

- Oxygen administration may need to be continued in the home setting. Liquid oxygen in a tank and oxygen concentrators are used frequently in home situations, including portable versions of both sources. Instruct caregivers about safety precautions with oxygen use and make sure they understand the rationale for the specific liter flow of oxygen.
- Oxygen supports combustion. To prevent fires and injuries, patients and families/caregivers should take the following precautions:
  - Do not smoke in a home where oxygen is in use. Place "No Smoking" signs in conspicuous places in the patient's home. Instruct the patient and family/caregivers about the hazard of smoking when oxygen is in use.
  - Keep oils, grease, alcohol, and other liquids that can burn away from the oxygen.
  - Keep the oxygen at least 6 ft away from any source of fire, such as a stove, fireplace, or candle (MedlinePlus, 2020).
  - Keep the oxygen 6 ft away from toys with electric motors, electric baseboard or space heaters, hairdryers, electric razors, and electric toothbrushes (MedlinePlus, 2020).
  - Do not use electrical equipment near oxygen administration set (e.g., electric blanket; see also above).
  - Use caution with gas or electric appliances.
  - Ground oxygen concentrators.
  - Secure the oxygen tank in a holder and away from direct sunlight or heat.
  - Allow adequate airflow around the oxygen concentrator (avoid placing it flush against the wall).
  - Notify the local fire department of the use of oxygen in the home.
  - Have working smoke detectors and a working fire extinguisher in the home (MedlinePlus, 2020).

Skill 40-4 Administering Oxygen by Mask

DELEGATION CONSIDERATIONS

The administration of oxygen by a mask is not delegated to assistive personnel (AP). Reapplication of the mask during nursing care activities, such as during bathing, may be performed by AP. Depending on the state's nurse practice act and the organization's policies and procedures, administration of oxygen by a mask may be delegated to licensed practical/vocational nurses (LPN/LVNs). The decision to delegate must be based on careful analysis of the patient's needs and circumstances as well as the qualifications of the person to whom the task is being delegated. Refer to the Delegation Guidelines in Appendix A.

EQUIPMENT

- Flow meter connected to oxygen supply
- Humidifier with sterile distilled water, if necessary, for the type of mask prescribed (based on circumstances, system, and facility policy)
- Face mask, as prescribed or indicated based on the patient's condition and circumstances
- Gauze to pad elastic band or commercial padding; silicone border or hydrocolloid dressing (optional)
- PPE, as indicated

IMPLEMENTATION

ACTION	RATIONALE
1. Review the prescribed intervention to verify the use of the particular mask, flow rate/concentration, and administration parameters. Gather equipment.	Verifying the prescribed intervention ensures the patient receives prescribed amount of oxygen. Assembling equipment provides for an organized approach to the task.
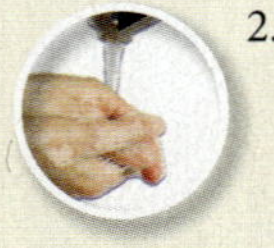 2. Perform hand hygiene and put on PPE, if indicated.	Hand hygiene and PPE prevent the spread of microorganisms. PPE is required based on transmission precautions.
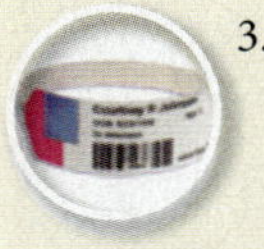 3. Identify the patient.	Identifying the patient ensures the right patient receives the intervention and helps prevent errors.
4. Assemble equipment on the overbed table or other surface within reach.	Bringing everything to the bedside conserves time and energy. Arranging items nearby is convenient, saves time, and avoids unnecessary stretching and twisting of muscles on the part of the nurse.
5. Close the curtains around the bed and close the door to the room, if possible.	This ensures the patient's privacy.
6. Explain to the patient what you are going to do and why. Review safety precautions necessary when oxygen is in use.	Explanation relieves anxiety and facilitates engagement with care. Oxygen supports combustion; a small spark could cause a fire.
7. Attach the face mask to the oxygen source (with humidification, if appropriate, for the specific mask) (Figure 1). Start the flow of oxygen at the specified rate. For a mask with a reservoir, be sure to allow oxygen to fill the bag (Figure 2) before proceeding to the next step.	Oxygen forced through a water reservoir is humidified before it is delivered to the patient, thus preventing dehydration of the mucous membranes. A reservoir bag must be inflated with oxygen because the bag is the oxygen supply source for the patient.

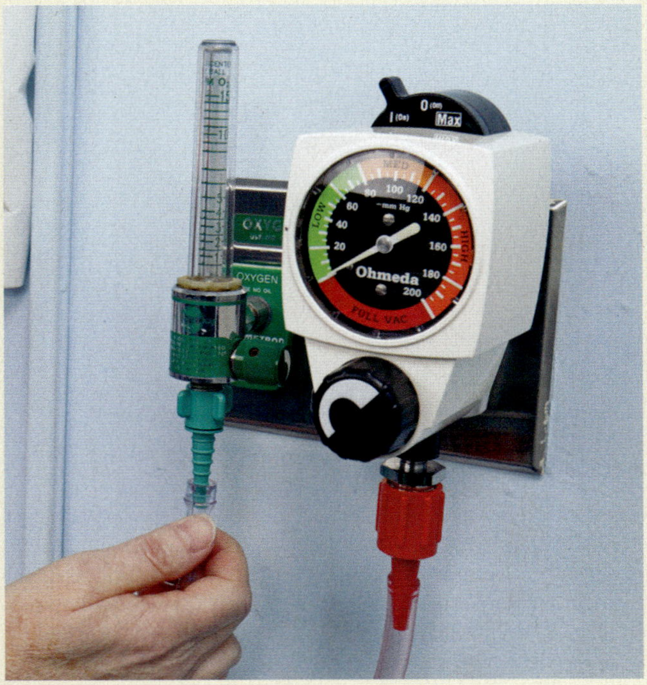

FIGURE 1. Connecting face mask to oxygen source.

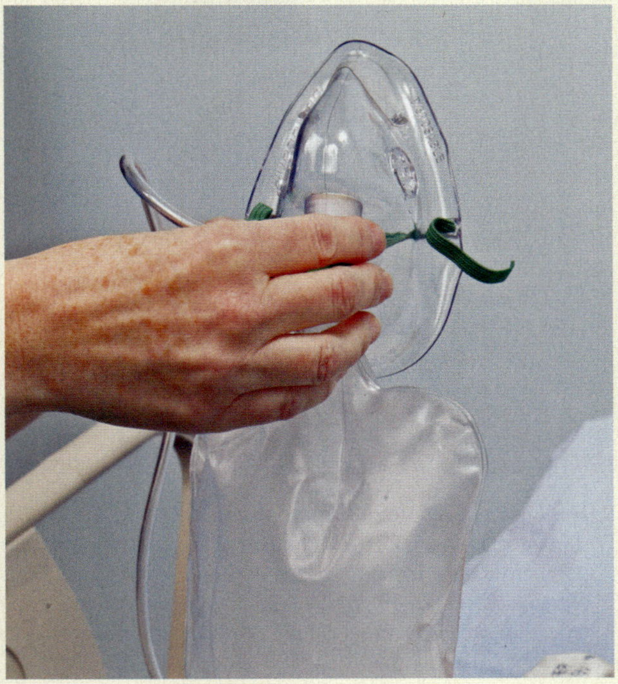

FIGURE 2. Allowing oxygen to fill bag.

(continued on page 1646)

Skill 40-4 Administering Oxygen by Mask *(continued)*

ACTION	RATIONALE
8. Position face mask over the patient's nose and mouth (Figure 3). **Adjust the elastic strap so that the mask fits snugly but comfortably on the face (Figure 4).** Adjust to the prescribed flow rate (Figure 5).	A loose or poorly fitting mask will result in oxygen loss and decreased therapeutic value. Masks may cause a feeling of suffocation, so the patient needs frequent attention and reassurance.

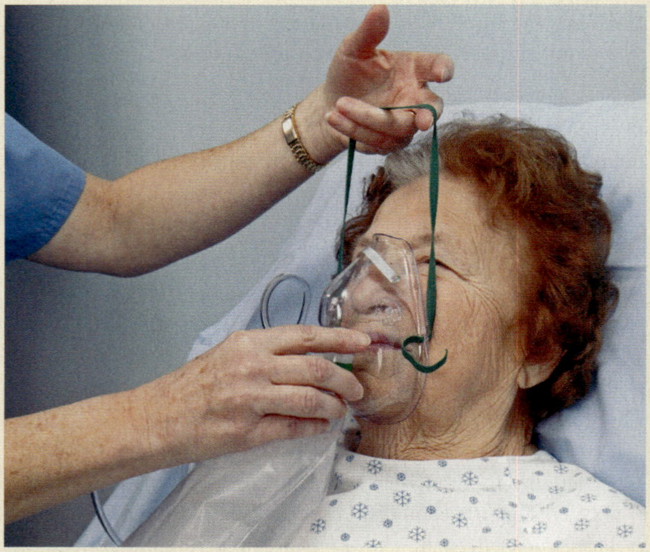

FIGURE 3. Applying face mask over nose and mouth.

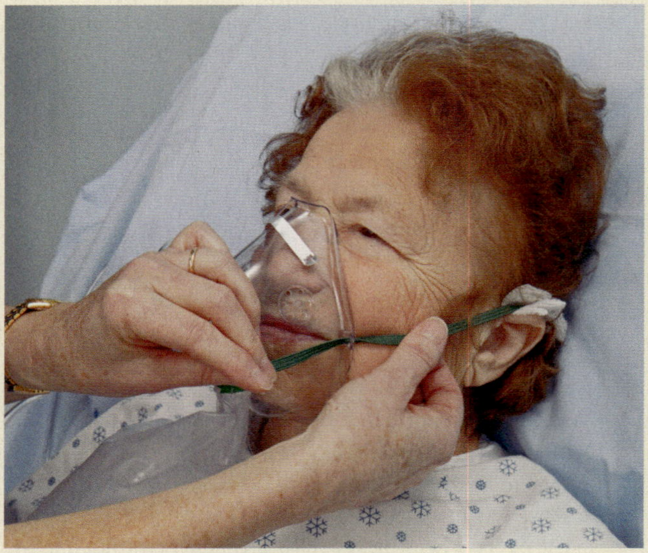

FIGURE 4. Adjusting elastic straps.

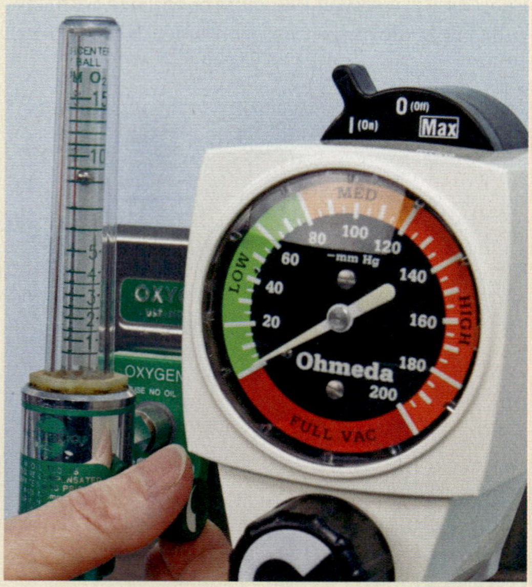

FIGURE 5. Adjusting flow rate.

ACTION	RATIONALE
9. If the patient reports irritation or you note any alteration in skin integrity, use gauze pads under the elastic strap at pressure points to reduce irritation to the ears and scalp. Consider use of a silicone border or hydrocolloid dressings over bony prominences or other areas that come in contact with the device and between the device and the skin (Camacho-Del Rio, 2018).	Pressure injuries may be related to a medical device or other object (EPUAP, NPIAP, & PPPIA, 2019, p. 16; Joint Commission, 2018). Any tube, electrode, sensor, or other rigid or stiff device element under pressure can create pressure damage (Baranoski & Ayello, 2020; EPUAP, NPIAP, & PPPIA, 2019). Pads reduce irritation and pressure and protect the skin.
10. Reassess the patient's respiratory status, including respiratory rate, effort, and lung sounds, and their oxygen saturation. Note any signs of respiratory distress, such as tachypnea, nasal flaring, use of accessory muscles, or dyspnea.	This helps assess the effectiveness of oxygen therapy.

ACTION	RATIONALE
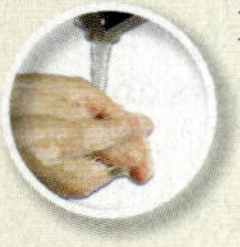 11. Remove PPE, if used. Perform hand hygiene.	Proper removal of PPE reduces the risk for infection transmission and contamination of other items. Hand hygiene prevents the spread of microorganisms.
12. **Remove the mask and dry the skin under the mask every 2 to 3 hours if the oxygen is running continuously. Do not use powder around the mask.** Assess the areas of skin contact with the mask for alterations in skin integrity at least every 8 hours or according to facility recommendations.	The tight-fitting mask and moisture from condensation can irritate the skin on the face. There is a danger of inhaling powder if it is placed on the mask. Masks may cause pressure injuries behind the ears, and to the cheeks, chin, or bridge of the nose (Camacho-Del Rio, 2018).

DOCUMENTATION

Guidelines

Document the type of mask used, the amount of oxygen used, oxygen saturation level, lung sounds, and rate/pattern of respirations. Document your assessment before and after the intervention.

Sample Documentation

DocuCare Practice documenting the administration of oxygen by mask in *Lippincott DocuCare.*

> 9/22/25 Patient reports feeling short of breath. Respirations 30 breaths/min and labored. Lung sounds decreased throughout. Oxygen saturation via pulse oximeter 88%. Findings reported to Dr. Lu. Oxygen via nonrebreather face mask applied at 12 L/min as prescribed. Oxygen saturation increased to 98%. Respirations even and unlabored. Chest rises symmetrically. Respiratory rate 18 breaths/min. Lungs remain with decreased breath sounds throughout. Patient denies dyspnea.
>
> *—C. Bausler, RN*

DEVELOPING CLINICAL REASONING AND CLINICAL JUDGMENT

UNEXPECTED SITUATIONS AND ASSOCIATED INTERVENTIONS

- *Patient was previously fine on oxygen delivered by mask but is now short of breath, and the pulse oximeter reading is less than 93%:* Check to see that the oxygen tubing for the mask is still connected to the flow meter and the flow meter is still on the previous setting. Someone may have stepped on the tubing, pulling it from the flow meter, or the oxygen may have accidentally been turned off. Assess the patient's respiratory status, including respiratory rate, rhythm, effort, and lung sounds. Note any additional signs of respiratory distress. Collaborate with the health care team regarding any changes and assessment findings.
- *Areas over ear, face, or back of head are reddened:* Ensure that areas are adequately padded and that the elastic band for the mask is not pulled too tight. Consider consultation with the skin care team or wound nurse specialist.

SPECIAL CONSIDERATIONS

General Considerations

- Different types of face masks are available for use.
- It is important to ensure the mask fits snugly around the patient's face. If it is loose, it will not effectively deliver the right amount of oxygen.
- The mask may be removed for the patient to eat, drink, and take medications. If appropriate, consult with the health care team regarding the use of oxygen via nasal cannula for use during mealtimes and limit the number of times the mask is removed to maintain adequate oxygenation.

Community-Based Care Considerations

- Oxygen administration may need to be continued in the home setting. Liquid oxygen in a tank and oxygen concentrators are used frequently in home situations, including portable versions of both sources. Instruct caregivers about safety precautions with oxygen use and make sure they understand the rationale for the specific liter flow of oxygen.

(continued on page 1648)

Skill 40-4 Administering Oxygen by Mask *(continued)*

- Oxygen supports combustion. To prevent fires and injuries, patients and families/caregivers should take the following precautions:
  - Do not smoke in a home where oxygen is in use. Place "No Smoking" signs in conspicuous places in the patient's home. Instruct the patient and family/caregivers about the hazard of smoking when oxygen is in use.
  - Keep oils, grease, alcohol, and other liquids that can burn away from the oxygen.
  - Keep the oxygen at least 6 ft away from any source of fire, such as a stove, fireplace, or candle (MedlinePlus, 2020).
  - Keep the oxygen 6 ft away from toys with electric motors, electric baseboard or space heaters, hairdryers, electric razors, and electric toothbrushes (MedlinePlus, 2020).
  - Do not use electrical equipment near oxygen administration set (e.g., electric blanket; see also above).
  - Use caution with gas or electric appliances.
  - Ground oxygen concentrators.
  - Secure the oxygen tank in a holder and away from direct sunlight or heat.
  - Allow adequate airflow around the oxygen concentrator (avoid placing it flush against the wall).
  - Notify the local fire department of the use of oxygen in the home.
  - Have working smoke detectors and a working fire extinguisher in the home (MedlinePlus, 2020).

Skill 40-5 Providing Care of a Tracheostomy Tube and Site

DELEGATION CONSIDERATIONS

Care of a tracheostomy tube is not delegated to assistive personnel (AP). Depending on the state's nurse practice act and the organization's policies and procedures, care of a tracheostomy tube in a stable situation may be delegated to licensed practical/vocational nurses (LPN/LVNs). The decision to delegate must be based on careful analysis of the patient's needs and circumstances as well as the qualifications of the person to whom the task is being delegated. Refer to the Delegation Guidelines in Appendix A.

EQUIPMENT

- Disposable gloves
- Sterile gloves
- Goggles and mask or face shield; N95 mask or equivalent, based on patient's health status
- Additional PPE, as indicated
- Sterile normal saline
- Sterile cup or basin
- Sterile cotton-tipped applicators
- Sterile gauze sponges
- Disposable inner tracheostomy cannula, appropriate size for the patient
- Sterile suction catheter and glove set
- Commercially prepared tracheostomy or drain dressing
- Commercially prepared tracheostomy holder
- Plastic disposal bag
- Assistant (additional nurse or respiratory therapist)

IMPLEMENTATION

ACTION	RATIONALE
1. Gather equipment.	Assembling equipment provides for an organized approach to the task.
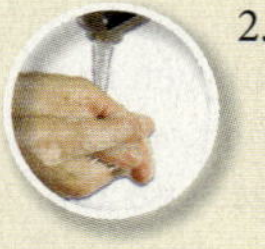 2. Perform hand hygiene and put on PPE, if indicated.	Hand hygiene and PPE prevent the spread of microorganisms. PPE is required based on transmission precautions.
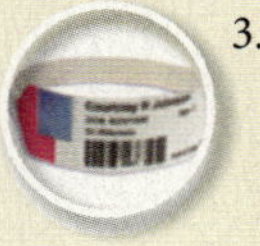 3. Identify the patient.	Identifying the patient ensures the right patient receives the intervention and helps prevent errors.

ACTION	RATIONALE
4. Assemble equipment on the overbed table or other surface within reach.	Arranging items nearby is convenient, saves time, and avoids unnecessary stretching and twisting of muscles on the part of the nurse.
5. Close the curtains around the bed and close the door to the room, if possible.	This ensures the patient's privacy.
6. Determine the need for tracheostomy care. **Assess the patient's pain and administer pain medication, if indicated.**	If the tracheostomy is new or changes in integrity of the site are present, pain medication may be needed before performing tracheostomy care.
7. Explain to the patient what you are going to do and why, even if the patient does not appear to be alert. Reassure the patient that you will interrupt the procedure if they indicate respiratory difficulty.	Explanation alleviates fears. Even if the patient appears unconscious, the nurse should explain what is happening. Any procedure that compromises respiration is frightening for the patient.
8. Adjust the bed to a comfortable working position (VHA-CEOSH, 2016). Lower the side rail closest to you. **If the patient is conscious, place them in a semi-Fowler position. Assist the patient to slightly extend their neck, if not contraindicated. If the patient is unconscious, place them in an appropriate position based on assessment of individual circumstances.** Move the overbed table close to your work area and raise it to waist height. Place a trash receptacle within easy reach of the work area.	Having the bed at the proper height prevents back and muscle strain. A sitting position helps the patient to cough and makes breathing easier. Gravity also facilitates catheter insertion if suctioning is indicated. Having the neck slightly extended can facilitate easier removal of the inner cannula (Patton, 2019). Positioning of the unconscious patient is based on the circumstances of the individual patient, health status, health problems, presence of drains and/or monitoring devices, etc. The overbed table provides a work surface and maintains sterility of the objects on the work surface. A trash receptacle within reach prevents reaching over the sterile field or turning your back to the field to dispose of trash.
9. Put on a face shield or goggles and a mask. Suction the tracheostomy, if necessary. Refer to Skill 40-6. If the tracheostomy has just been suctioned, remove the soiled site dressing and discard it before removal of the gloves used to perform suctioning.	PPE prevents contact with contaminants. Suctioning removes secretions to prevent occluding the outer cannula while the inner cannula is removed.

Cleaning the Tracheostomy: Disposable Inner Cannula

ACTION	RATIONALE
10. Carefully open the package with the new disposable inner cannula, taking care not to contaminate the cannula or the inside of the package (Figure 1). Carefully open the package with the sterile cotton-tipped applicators, taking care not to contaminate them. Open the sterile cup or basin and fill 0.5 inch deep with saline. Open the plastic disposable bag and place it within reach on the work surface.	The inner cannula must remain sterile. Saline and applicators will be used to clean the tracheostomy site. The plastic disposable bag will be used to discard removed inner cannula.
11. Put on disposable gloves.	Gloves protect against exposure to blood and body fluids.

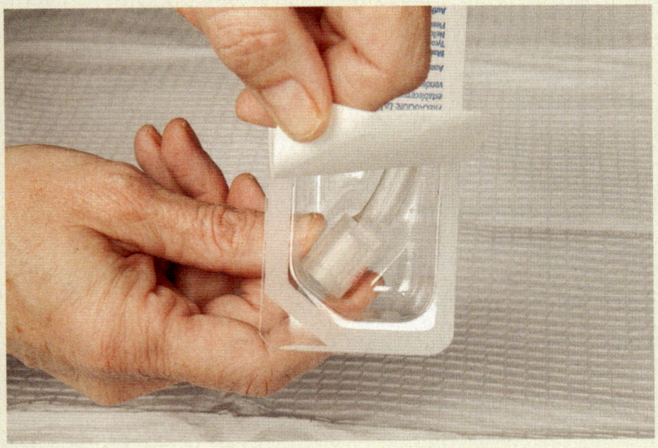

FIGURE 1. Carefully opening package with new disposable inner cannula. (*Source:* Used with permission from Shutterstock. *Photo by B. Proud.*)

(*continued on page 1650*)

Skill 40-5 Providing Care of a Tracheostomy Tube and Site *(continued)*

ACTION	RATIONALE
12. Remove the oxygen source if one is present. Stabilize the outer cannula and faceplate of the tracheostomy with your nondominant hand. Grasp the locking mechanism of the inner cannula with your dominant hand. Press the tabs and release the lock (Figure 2). Gently remove the inner cannula and place it in the disposal bag. If not already removed, remove the site dressing and dispose of it in the trash.	Stabilizing the faceplate prevents trauma to, and pain from, the stoma. Releasing the lock permits removal of the inner cannula.
13. Working quickly, discard your current gloves and put on sterile gloves. Pick up the new inner cannula with your dominant hand; stabilize the faceplate with your nondominant hand and gently insert the new inner cannula into the outer cannula. Press the tabs to allow the lock to grab the outer cannula (Figure 3). Reapply the oxygen source, if one is in use.	Sterile gloves are necessary to prevent contamination of the new inner cannula. Locking to the outer cannula secures the inner cannula in place. Reapplying the oxygen source maintains an oxygen supply to the patient.

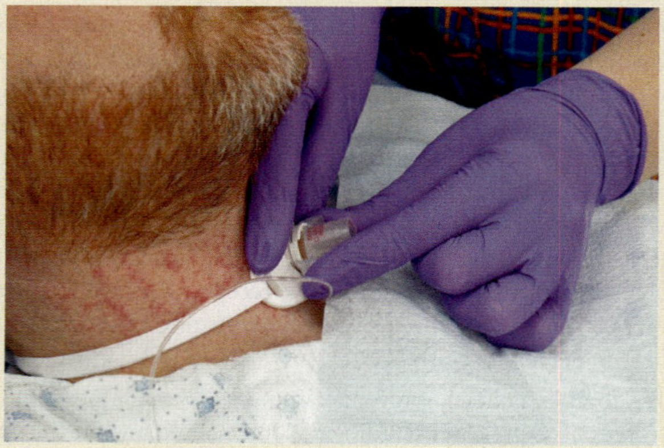

FIGURE 2. Releasing lock on inner cannula.

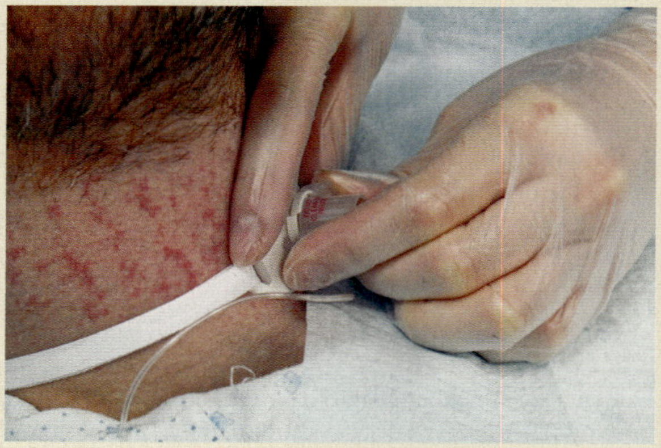

FIGURE 3. Locking new inner cannula in place.

Applying Clean Dressing and Holder

ACTION	RATIONALE
14. Remove the oxygen source, if necessary. Dip the cotton-tipped applicator or gauze sponge in the cup or basin with sterile saline and clean the stoma under the faceplate. Use each applicator or sponge only once, moving from the stoma site outward (Figure 4).	Saline is nonirritating to tissue. Cleansing from the stoma outward and using each applicator only once promotes aseptic technique.

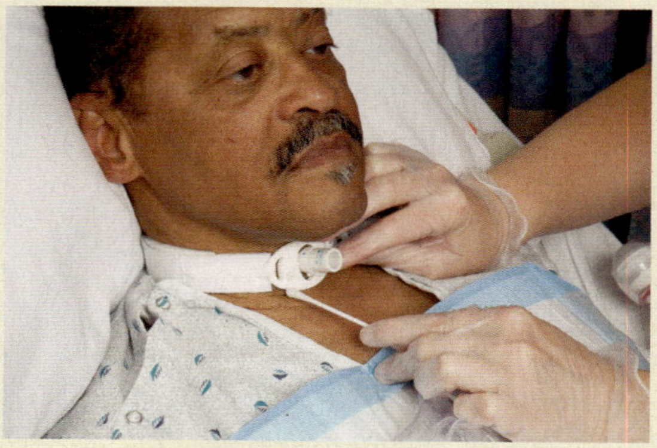

FIGURE 4. Cleaning from stoma site, outward.

ACTION	RATIONALE
15. Pat the skin gently with a dry 4 × 4 gauze sponge.	Gauze removes excess moisture.
16. Slide the commercially prepared tracheostomy dressing or prefolded non–cotton-filled 4 × 4-inch dressing under the faceplate.	Lint or fiber from a cut cotton-filled gauze pad can be aspirated into the trachea, causing respiratory distress, or can embed in the stoma and cause irritation or infection.

ACTION	RATIONALE
17. Alternatively, implement use of a hydrocolloid or polyurethane foam dressing at the tracheostomy site (Dixon et al., 2018; O'Toole et al., 2017). If this type of dressing is already in use, frequency of change is based on the type of dressing in use, assessment of dressing, and facility policy.	Use of a hydrocolloid dressing under the tracheostomy flange during the postoperative period and/or placing a polyurethane foam dressing at the tracheostomy site after suture removal reduces the risk for medical device–related alterations in skin integrity. (Dixon et al., 2018; O'Toole et al., 2017). These types of dressings may remain in place for longer periods of time.
18. Change the tracheostomy tube holder:	
a. **Obtain the assistance of a second person to hold the tracheostomy tube in place while the old collar is removed and the new collar is placed.**	Holding the tracheostomy tube in place ensures that the tracheostomy will not inadvertently be expelled if the patient coughs or moves. Doing so provides attachment for one side of the faceplate.
b. Open the package for the new tracheostomy collar.	This allows access to the new collar.
c. Both nurses should put on clean gloves.	Gloves prevent contact with blood, body fluids, and contaminants.
d. One nurse holds the faceplate while the other pulls up the Velcro tabs. Gently remove the collar.	Holding the tracheostomy tube in place ensures that the tracheostomy will not inadvertently be expelled if the patient coughs or moves. Pulling up the Velcro tabs loosens the collar.
e. The first nurse continues to hold the tracheostomy faceplate.	This prevents accidental extubation.
f. The other nurse places the collar around the patient's neck and inserts first one tab, then the other, into the openings on the faceplate and secures the Velcro tabs on the tracheostomy holder (Figure 5).	Securing the Velcro tabs holds the tracheostomy in place and prevents accidental expulsion of the tracheostomy tube.
g. Check the fit of the tracheostomy collar. You should be able to fit no more than two fingers between the neck and the collar (Cleveland Clinic, 2021; Morton & Fontaine, 2018). Check to make sure that the patient can flex the neck comfortably. Reapply the oxygen source, if necessary (Figure 6).	Allowing one to two fingerbreadths under the collar permits neck flexion that is comfortable and ensures that the collar will not compromise circulation to the area but is sufficiently secure to prevent excessive movement of the tracheostomy tube in the stoma and decannulation. Maintains oxygen supply to the patient.

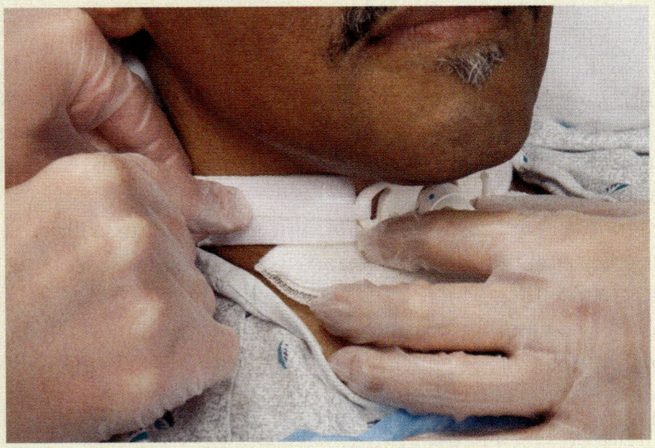

FIGURE 5. Securing tabs on tracheostomy holder.

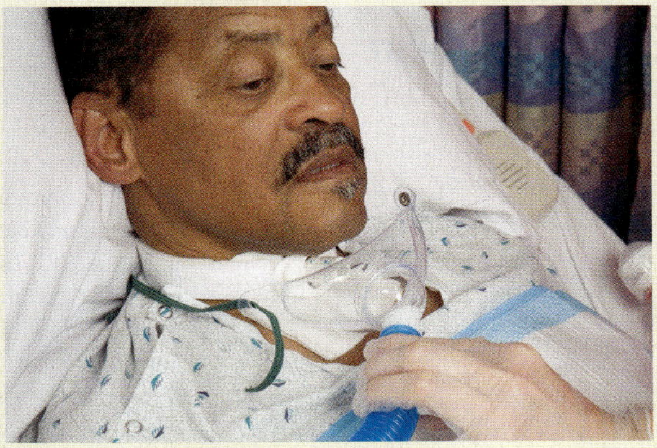

FIGURE 6. Reapplying oxygen source.

ACTION	RATIONALE
19. Remove gloves. Perform hand hygiene. **If the tracheostomy tube is cuffed, check the pressure of the balloon by attaching a handheld pressure gauge to the pilot balloon of the endotracheal tube.**	Removal of gloves and hand hygiene reduce the risk for pathogen transmission and contamination of other items. Careful monitoring of cuff pressure is necessary to decrease the risk for tracheal necrosis, tracheal rupture, laryngeal nerve palsy, tracheal stenosis, microaspiration, and inadequate ventilation (Turner, Feeney, et al., 2020). The smallest amount of air that results in an airtight seal between the trachea and the tube is desirable and less likely to result in complications; maintain pressure between 20 and 30 cm H_2O (AACN, 2018; Hess et al., 2021; Hinkle et al., 2022; Patton, 2019).

(continued on page 1652)

Skill 40-5 Providing Care of a Tracheostomy Tube and Site *(continued)*

ACTION	RATIONALE
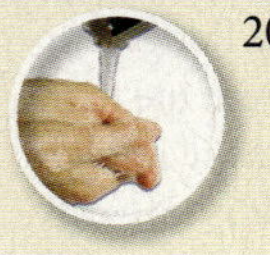 20. Remove the face shield or goggles and mask. Perform hand hygiene. Assist the patient to a comfortable position. Raise the bed rail and place the bed in the lowest position.	Proper removal of PPE reduces the risk for infection transmission and contamination of other items. Hand hygiene prevents the spread of microorganisms. Proper positioning with raised side rails and the proper bed height provides for patient comfort and safety.
21. Reassess the patient's respiratory status, including respiratory rate, effort, oxygen saturation, and lung sounds.	Assessments determine the effectiveness of interventions and the presence of complications.
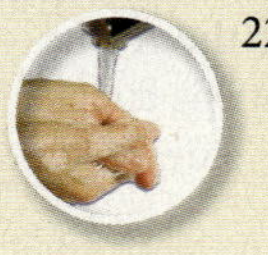 22. Remove additional PPE, if used. Perform hand hygiene.	Proper removal of PPE reduces the risk for infection transmission and contamination of other items. Hand hygiene prevents the spread of microorganisms.

DOCUMENTATION

Guidelines

Document your assessments before and after interventions, including site assessment, skin assessment, the presence of pain, lung sounds, and oxygen saturation levels. Document the procedure, including site care, changing of dressing, and tube securement. Document the presence of any alterations in skin integrity and associated interventions. Document cuff pressure.

Sample Documentation

> 9/26/25 1300 Tracheostomy care completed; lung sounds clear in all lobes; respirations even/unlabored; site without erythema or edema; small amount of thick, yellow secretions noted at site, oxygen saturation 95% on O_2 35% via trach collar, cuff pressure 25 cm H_2O. Site dressing and trach securement collar changed.
>
> —*C. Bausler, RN*

DEVELOPING CLINICAL REASONING AND CLINICAL JUDGMENT

UNEXPECTED SITUATIONS AND ASSOCIATED INTERVENTIONS

- *Patient coughs hard enough to dislodge tracheostomy:* Keep a spare tracheostomy and obturator at the bedside. Insert the obturator into the new tracheostomy and insert the tracheostomy into the stoma. Remove the obturator. Secure the ties and auscultate lung sounds. Palpate for any subcutaneous emphysema.
- *Tracheostomy becomes dislodged and is not easily replaced:* Notify the health care team immediately. This is an emergency situation. Cover the tracheostomy stoma. Assess the patient's respiratory status. Anticipate the possible need for maintaining ventilation using a manual resuscitation device and mask and for possible oro- or nasotracheal intubation.
- *On palpating around the insertion site, you note a moderate amount of subcutaneous emphysema in tissue:* Assess for dislodgment of the tracheostomy tube. If the tube has become displaced, a buildup of air in the subcutaneous portion of the skin is likely. Notify the health care team if the subcutaneous emphysema is a change in the patient's status.

SPECIAL CONSIDERATIONS

General Considerations

- One nurse working alone should always place new tracheostomy ties before removing old ties to prevent accidental extubation of the tracheostomy. If it is necessary to remove the old ties first, obtain the assistance of a second person to hold the tracheostomy tube in place while the old tie is removed and the new tie is replaced.
- Keep emergency equipment easily accessible at the bedside. Keep a bag-valve mask, oxygen, the obturator from the current tracheostomy, a spare tracheostomy of the same size, a spare tracheostomy one size smaller, and suction equipment at the bedside of a patient with a tracheostomy tube at all times (Dawson, 2014; Patton, 2019).

- If the patient is currently using a tracheostomy without a cuff, keep a spare tracheostomy of the same size with a cuff at the bedside for emergency use.
- Monitoring of the cuff pressure using a handheld cuff pressure manometer should take place at the beginning of each shift or following any procedure during which movement of the tube may have taken place (e.g., dressing/tape/collar change, patient repositioning) (Patton, 2019).
- *Pilot balloon is accidentally cut while caring for a tracheostomy tube with a cuff:* Notify the health care team. Obtain a 22-gauge IV catheter and thread it into the pilot balloon tubing, being careful not to puncture the tubing with the needle, below the cut. Remove the needle from the catheter and apply a stopcock or needleless Luer-Lok to the catheter. Alternatively, a blunt needle can be passed into the pilot balloon tubing and a stopcock or Luer-Lok attached to the needle hub (Hess et al., 2021). If air is needed to reinflate the balloon, a syringe can be attached to the stopcock or Luer-Lok so that air may be added. Anticipate the need for a tracheostomy tube change.
- Consider implementation of medical device–related pressure injury prevention strategies to reduce the risk for alterations in skin integrity, including use of a hydrocolloid dressing under the tracheostomy flange during the postoperative period or a polyurethane foam dressing at the tracheostomy site after suture removal instead of a gauze dressing (Dixon et al., 2018; O'Toole et al., 2017).

Community-Based Care Considerations

- Instruct the patient and home caregiver on how to perform tracheostomy care. Observe a return demonstration and provide feedback.
- Clean, rather than sterile, technique can be used in the home setting.
- Sterile saline can be made by mixing 1 teaspoon of table salt in 1 quart of water and boiling for 15 minutes. The solution is cooled and stored in a clean, dry container. Discard the saline at the end of each day to prevent growth of bacteria. In the home, tap water may also be used, but distilled water or homemade saline should be used if the patient has well water (Cleveland Clinic, 2021).
- Instruct the patient who is performing self-care to use a mirror to view the steps in the procedure.

Skill 40-6 Suctioning a Tracheostomy: Open System

DELEGATION CONSIDERATIONS

Suctioning a tracheostomy is not delegated to assistive personnel (AP). Depending on the state's nurse practice act and the organization's policies and procedures, suctioning of a tracheostomy in a stable situation, such as long-term care and other community-based care settings, may be delegated to licensed practical/vocational nurses (LPN/LVNs). The decision to delegate must be based on careful analysis of the patient's needs and circumstances as well as the qualifications of the person to whom the task is being delegated. Refer to the Delegation Guidelines in Appendix A.

EQUIPMENT

- Portable or wall suction unit with tubing
- A commercially prepared suction kit with an appropriate-size catheter (see General Considerations) or
  - Sterile suction catheter with Y-port in the appropriate size
  - Sterile, disposable container
  - Sterile gloves
- Towel or waterproof pad
- Goggles and mask or face shield; N95 mask or equivalent, based on patient's health status
- Additional PPE, as indicated
- Disposable, clean gloves
- Resuscitation bag connected to 100% oxygen

(*continued on page 1654*)

Skill 40-6 Suctioning a Tracheostomy: Open System *(continued)*

IMPLEMENTATION

ACTION	RATIONALE
1. Gather equipment.	Assembling equipment provides for an organized approach to the task.
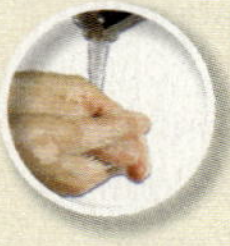 2. Perform hand hygiene and put on PPE, if indicated.	Hand hygiene and PPE prevent the spread of microorganisms. PPE is required based on transmission precautions.
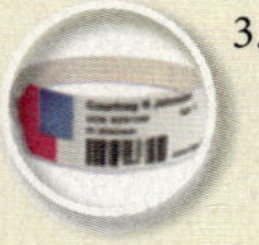 3. Identify the patient.	Identifying the patient ensures the right patient receives the intervention and helps prevent errors.
4. Assemble equipment on the overbed table or other surface within reach.	Arranging items nearby is convenient, saves time, and avoids unnecessary stretching and twisting of muscles on the part of the nurse.
5. Close the curtains around the bed and close the door to the room, if possible.	This ensures the patient's privacy.
6. Determine the need for suctioning. Verify the prescribed suctioning intervention in the patient's health record, if necessary. Anticipate the administration of pharmacologic (analgesic medication) and use of nonpharmacologic interventions for the patient before suctioning. **Assess for pain or the potential to cause pain. Administer pain medication, as prescribed, before suctioning.**	Suctioning should be performed only when clinically indicated based on assessment and not routinely (AARC, 2010; Burns & Delgado, 2019; Hess et al., 2021; Morton & Fontaine, 2018). At a minimum, suctioning is an uncomfortable procedure, and it can be a very painful and/or distressing experience. Individualized pain management must be performed in response to the patient's needs (Arroyo-Novoa et al., 2008; Chaseling et al., 2014; Düzkaya & Kuğuoğlu, 2015; Wrona et al., 2021).
7. Explain to the patient what you are going to do and why, even if the patient does not appear to be alert. Reassure the patient that you will interrupt the procedure if they indicate respiratory difficulty.	Explanation alleviates fears. Even if the patient appears unconscious, the nurse should explain what is happening. Any procedure that compromises respiration is frightening for the patient.
8. Adjust the bed to a comfortable working position (VHACEOSH, 2016). Lower the side rail closest to you. **If the patient is conscious, place them in a semi-Fowler position (Figure 1). If the patient is unconscious, place them in an appropriate position based on assessment of individual circumstances.** Move the overbed table close to your work area and raise it to waist height.	Having the bed at the proper height prevents back and muscle strain. A sitting position helps the patient to cough and makes breathing easier. Gravity also facilitates catheter insertion. Positioning of the unconscious patient is based on the circumstances of the individual patient; health status, health problems, presence of drains and/or monitoring devices, etc. The overbed table provides a work surface and maintains the sterility of the objects on the work surface.

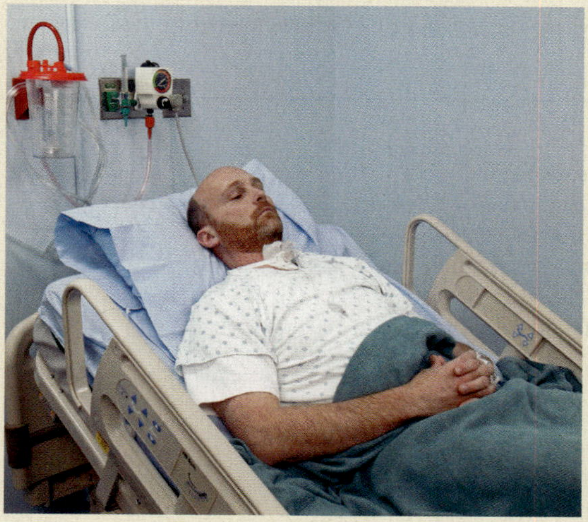

FIGURE 1. Patient in semi-Fowler position.

ACTION	RATIONALE
9. Place a towel or waterproof pad across the patient's chest.	This protects bed linens and the patient.
10. **Adjust suction to the appropriate pressure** (Hess et al., 2021) (Figure 2):	Higher pressures can cause excessive trauma, hypoxemia, and atelectasis.
• No more than 150 mm Hg for adults and adolescents • No more than 125 mm Hg for children • No more than 100 mm Hg for infants	Higher pressures can cause excessive trauma, hypoxemia, and atelectasis.

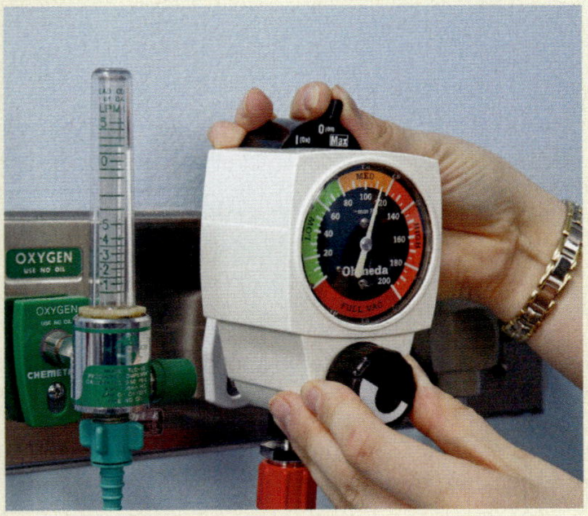

FIGURE 2. Turning suction unit to appropriate pressure.

ACTION	RATIONALE
11. Put on a disposable, clean glove and occlude the end of the connecting tubing to check suction pressure. Place the connecting tubing in a convenient location. If using a resuscitation bag, place it connected to oxygen within convenient reach.	The glove prevents contact with blood and body fluids. Checking pressure ensures that equipment is working properly. Preparation allows for an organized approach to the procedure.
12. Open the sterile suction package using aseptic technique. The open wrapper or container becomes a sterile field to hold other supplies. Carefully remove the sterile container, touching only the outside surface. Set it up on the work surface and pour sterile saline into it.	Sterile normal saline or water is used to lubricate the outside of the catheter, minimizing irritation of the mucosa during introduction. It is also used to clear the catheter between suction attempts.
13. Put on a face shield or goggles and a mask (Figure 3). Put on sterile gloves. Your dominant hand will manipulate the catheter and must remain sterile. The nondominant hand is considered clean rather than sterile and will control the suction valve (Y-port) on the catheter.	Handling the sterile catheter using a sterile glove helps prevent introducing organisms into the respiratory tract; the clean glove protects the nurse from microorganisms.

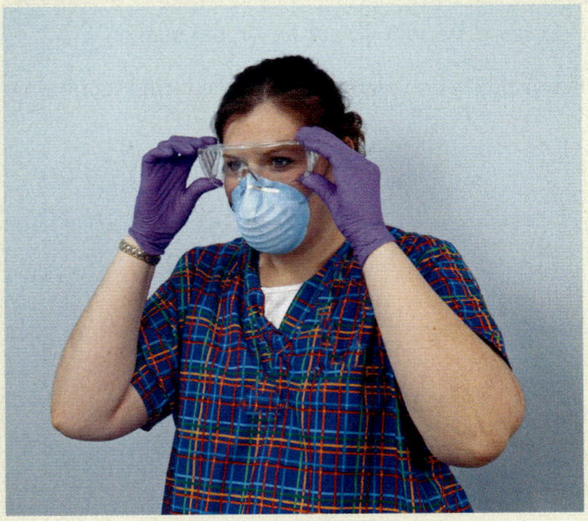

FIGURE 3. Putting on goggles and mask.

(*continued on page 1656*)

Skill 40-6 Suctioning a Tracheostomy: Open System *(continued)*

ACTION	RATIONALE
14. With your dominant gloved hand, pick up the sterile catheter. Pick up the connecting tubing with your nondominant hand and connect the tubing and suction catheter (Figure 4).	This maintains sterility of the suction catheter.

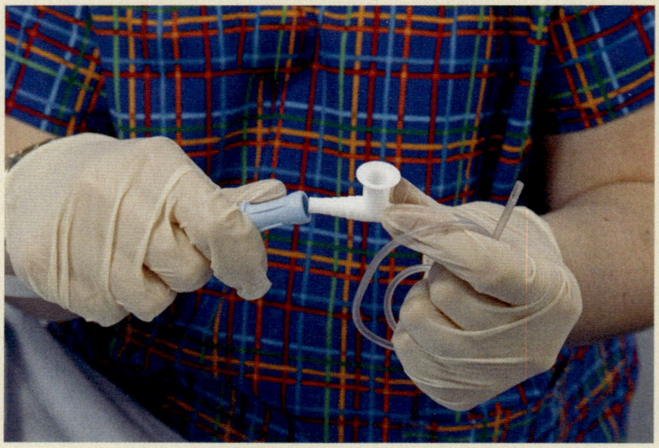

FIGURE 4. Connecting suction catheter to suction tubing.

15. Moisten the catheter by dipping it into the container of sterile saline, unless it is a silicone catheter (Figure 5). Occlude the Y-tube to check suction (Figure 6).	Lubricating the inside of the catheter with saline helps move secretions in the catheter. Silicone catheters do not require lubrication. Checking ensures that equipment is working properly.

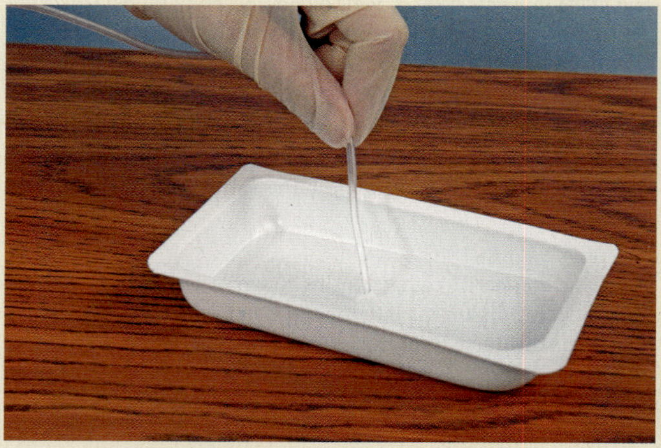

FIGURE 5. Moistening catheter in saline solution.

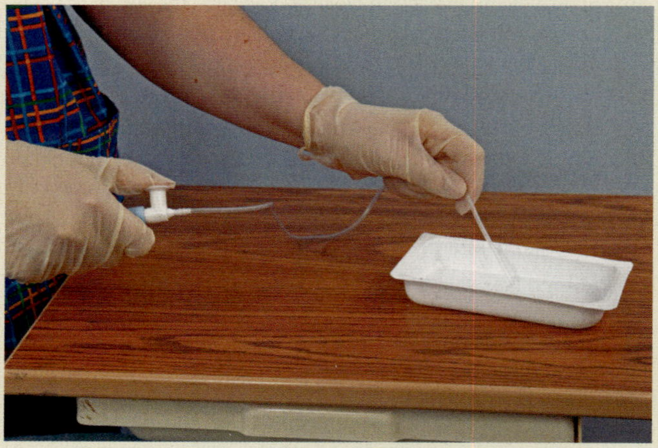

FIGURE 6. Occluding Y-port to check for proper suction.

16. Using your nondominant hand, remove the ventilator tubing or oxygen source (if in use) from the tracheostomy tube and attach the manual resuscitation bag. Hyperoxygenate the patient using your nondominant hand and the manual resuscitation bag for a minimum of 30 seconds (Burns & Delgado, 2019). Alternatively, use the sigh mechanism on a mechanical ventilator.	Hyperoxygenation aids in preventing hypoxemia during suctioning.
17. Using your nondominant hand, remove the manual resuscitation bag from the tracheostomy tube. Alternatively, open the adapter on the mechanical ventilator tubing.	This exposes the tracheostomy tube without contaminating your sterile gloved hand.

ACTION

18. Using your dominant hand, gently and quickly insert the catheter into the tracheostomy tube. **Advance the catheter to the predetermined length. Do not occlude the Y-port when inserting the catheter.**

RATIONALE

Catheter contact and suction cause tracheal mucosal damage, loss of cilia, edema, and fibrosis and increase the risk of infection and bleeding. Insertion of the suction catheter to a predetermined distance, no more than the tip of the artificial airway to no more than 1 cm past the length of the endotracheal tube (adults) and 0.5 cm (pediatric patients) (Boroughs & Dougherty, 2015; Hess et al., 2021; Kendrick, 2020) avoids contact with the trachea and carina, reducing the effects of tracheal mucosal damage (Boroughs & Dougherty, 2015; Hahn, 2010; Ireton, 2007; Pasrija & Hall, 2020; Pate & Zapata, 2002). If resistance is met, the carina or tracheal mucosa has been hit. Withdraw the catheter at least 0.5 inch before applying suction. Occluding the Y-port (i.e., suctioning) when inserting the catheter increases the risk for trauma to the airway mucosa and increases the risk of hypoxemia.

19. Apply suction by intermittently occluding the Y-port on the catheter with the thumb of your nondominant hand, and gently rotate the catheter as it is being withdrawn (Figure 7). **Do not suction for more than 10 to 15 seconds at a time** (AARC, 2010; Burns & Delgado, 2019; Hess et al., 2021; Pasrija & Hall, 2020).

Turning the catheter as it is withdrawn minimizes trauma to the mucosa. Suctioning for longer than 15 seconds robs the respiratory tract of oxygen, which may result in hypoxemia (AARC, 2010; Pasrija & Hall, 2020). Suctioning too quickly may be ineffective at clearing all secretions.

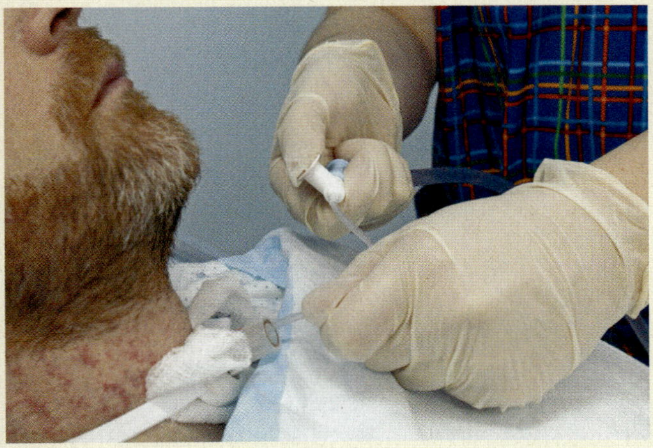

FIGURE 7. Intermittently occluding the Y-port on the catheter to apply suction while withdrawing catheter.

20. Hyperoxygenate the patient using your nondominant hand and a manual resuscitation bag for a minimum of 30 seconds (Burns & Delgado, 2019). Replace the oxygen delivery device, if applicable, using your nondominant hand, and have the patient take several deep breaths. If the patient is mechanically ventilated, close the adapter on the mechanical ventilator tubing and use the sigh mechanism on a mechanical ventilator.

Suctioning removes air from the patient's airway and can cause hypoxemia. Hyperoxygenation can help prevent suction-induced hypoxemia.

21. Flush the catheter with saline. Assess the effectiveness of suctioning and repeat, as needed, according to the patient's tolerance. Wrap the suction catheter around your dominant hand between attempts.

Flushing clears the catheter and lubricates it for the next insertion. Reassessment determines the need for additional suctioning. Wrapping the catheter around your hand prevents inadvertent contamination of the catheter.

22. **Allow at least a 30-second interval if additional suctioning is needed** (Burns & Delgado, 2019). Do not make more than three suction passes per suctioning episode. If the patient is spontaneously breathing, **encourage them to cough and deep breathe between suctioning attempts.** Suction the oropharynx after suctioning the trachea. Do not reinsert the tracheostomy tube after suctioning the mouth.

The interval allows for reventilation and reoxygenation of airways. Excessive suction passes contribute to complications. Suctioning the oropharynx clears the mouth of secretions. Routine oral suctioning to aspirate secretions that accumulate above the cuff of the tube is also necessary to reduce the risk of pneumonia and provide patient comfort (AACN, 2018; Hess et al., 2021; Morton & Fontaine, 2018). More microorganisms are usually present in the mouth, so it is suctioned last to prevent transmission of contaminants.

(continued on page 1658)

Skill 40-6 Suctioning a Tracheostomy: Open System *(continued)*

ACTION	RATIONALE
23. Perform oral hygiene after tracheal suctioning.	Respiratory secretions that are allowed to accumulate in the mouth are irritating to mucous membranes, pose a risk for aspiration, are unpleasant for the patient, and contribute to the colonization of the oropharyngeal secretions by respiratory pathogens. Diligent oral hygiene care can improve oral health and limit the growth of pathogens in the oropharyngeal secretions, decreasing the incidence of aspiration pneumonia, community-acquired pneumonia, nonventilator health care–associated pneumonia (NV-HAP), and ventilator-associated pneumonia (VAP) (AACN, 2017; Chick & Wynne, 2020; Jenson et al., 2018; Quinn et al., 2020).
24. When suctioning is completed, coil the catheter in one hand. Remove the glove from the hand over the coiled catheter (the catheter remains inside the glove), pulling the glove off inside out (Figure 8). Remove the glove from the other hand, pulling inside out, and dispose of gloves, catheter, and container with solution in the appropriate receptacle. Perform hand hygiene. Assist the patient to a comfortable position. Raise the bed rail and place the bed in the lowest position.	This technique of glove removal, disposal of equipment, and hand hygiene reduces transmission of microorganisms. Proper positioning with raised side rails and the proper bed height provides for patient comfort and safety.

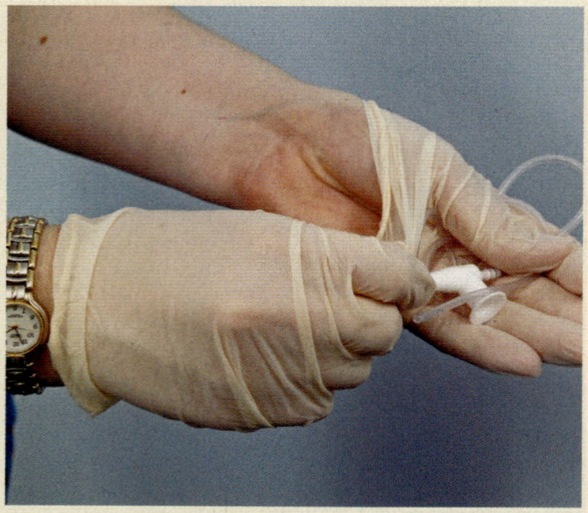

FIGURE 8. Removing gloves while keeping catheter inside.

ACTION	RATIONALE
25. Turn off the suction. Remove the supplemental oxygen placed for suctioning, if appropriate. Remove the face shield or goggles and mask. Perform hand hygiene.	Proper removal of PPE reduces the risk for infection transmission and contamination of other items. Hand hygiene prevents transmission of microorganisms.
26. Reassess the patient's respiratory status, including respiratory rate, effort, oxygen saturation, lung sounds, tracheal sounds, and presence/absence of secretions in artificial airway, and the patient's response to the intervention.	This assesses the effectiveness of suctioning and the presence of complications.
27. Remove additional PPE, if used. Perform hand hygiene.	Proper removal of PPE reduces the risk for infection transmission and contamination of other items. Hand hygiene prevents the spread of microorganisms.

DOCUMENTATION

Guidelines

Document the time of suctioning, assessments before and after interventions, the reason for suctioning, oxygen saturation levels, and the characteristics and amount of secretions.

Sample Documentation

<u>9/1/25</u> 1515 Yellow secretions noted in opening of tracheostomy tube; coarse crackles noted to auscultation over trachea. Lungs auscultated for wheezes in upper and lower lobes bilaterally. Respirations at 24 breaths/min. Weak, ineffective cough noted. Tracheal suction completed with 12-Fr catheter. Large amount of thick, yellow secretions obtained. Specimen for culture collected and sent. After suctioning, no secretions noted in tracheostomy tube, auscultation over trachea clear, faint wheezing persists, oxygen saturation at 97%, respirations 18 breaths/min.

—C. Bausler, RN

DEVELOPING CLINICAL REASONING AND CLINICAL JUDGMENT

UNEXPECTED SITUATIONS AND ASSOCIATED INTERVENTIONS

- *Patient coughs hard enough to dislodge tracheostomy:* Keep a spare tracheostomy and obturator at the bedside. Insert the obturator into the tracheostomy tube and reinsert the tracheostomy into the stoma. Remove the obturator. Secure the ties and auscultate lung sounds. Palpate the tracheostomy site for any **subcutaneous emphysema**, a result of air or gas collecting under the skin (crepitus).
- *Tracheostomy becomes dislodged and is not easily replaced:* Notify the health care team immediately. This is an emergency situation. Cover the tracheostomy stoma. Assess the patient's respiratory status. Anticipate the possible need for maintaining ventilation using a manual resuscitation device and mask and for possible oro- or nasotracheal intubation.
- *Lung sounds do not improve greatly, and oxygen saturation remains low after three suctioning attempts:* Allow the patient time to recover from previous suctionings. If needed, hyperoxygenate again. Suction the patient again and assess whether the oxygen saturation increases, lung sounds improve, and secretion amount decreases.
- *Patient develops signs of intolerance to suctioning; oxygen saturation level decreases and remains low after hyperoxygenation; patient becomes cyanotic; or patient becomes bradycardic:* Stop suctioning. Auscultate lung sounds. Consider hyperventilating the patient with a manual resuscitation device. Remain with the patient. Alert staff to notify the health care team of the change in the patient's status.

SPECIAL CONSIDERATIONS

General Considerations

- Determine the size of the catheter to use by the size of the tracheostomy tube. The suction catheter should be small enough not to occlude the airway being suctioned but large enough to remove secretions; use a suction catheter that occludes less than 50% of the lumen of the endotracheal tube (AARC, 2010; Pasrija & Hall, 2020). Larger catheters can contribute to trauma and hypoxemia.
- If the patient eats by mouth, it is recommended that the tracheostomy tube be suctioned prior to eating to prevent the need for suctioning during or after meals, which may stimulate excessive coughing and could result in vomiting (Hess et al., 2021, p. 429).
- The practice of instillation of saline solution directly into the airway during tracheal suctioning is not supported by evidence and is not recommended for inclusion as part of evidence-based practice and suctioning (AARC, 2010; Boroughs & Dougherty, 2015; Burns & Delgado, 2019; Leddy & Wilkinson, 2015; Owen et al., 2016; Wang et al., 2017).
- Keep emergency equipment easily accessible at the bedside. Keep a bag-valve mask, oxygen, the obturator from the current tracheostomy, a spare tracheostomy of the same size, a spare tracheostomy one size smaller, and suction equipment at the bedside of a patient with a tracheostomy tube at all times (Dawson, 2014; Patton, 2019). If the patient is currently using a tracheostomy without a cuff, keep a spare tracheostomy of the same size with a cuff at the bedside for emergency use.

Infant and Child Considerations

- Insertion of the suction catheter to a predetermined distance, no more than the tip of the artificial airway to no more than 0.5 cm past the length of the endotracheal tube avoids contact with the trachea and carina, reducing the effects of tracheal mucosal damage (Boroughs & Dougherty, 2015; Kendrick, 2020).
- The maximal time for application of negative pressure (suction) for neonates, children, and adolescents should be less than 5 to 10 seconds (Boroughs & Dougherty, 2015; Dawson et al., 2012, as cited in Edwards, 2018, p. 51; Hockenberry et al., 2019).

EVOLVING CASE STUDY 40-1

Scenario: Joan McIntyre, age 72, has been admitted to the medical unit with an acute exacerbation of chronic obstructive pulmonary disease (COPD). This is the fifth time she has been in the hospital this year. She is receiving supplemental oxygen and multiple medications to support her breathing. Her activity level is decreased, and she is reporting fatigue.

QUESTION r/t CUES: Which assessment should the nurse prioritize in caring for this patient?

A. Auscultation of lung/breath sounds and oxygen saturation via pulse oximetry
B. Vital signs: temperature, pulse, respiration, blood pressure
C. General history: subjective and objective
D. Cardiac assessment: heart sounds, peripheral pulses

Scenario: The nurse completes the assessment and notes that the blood pressure, pulse, and respirations are slightly elevated, and the oxygen saturation via pulse oximetry is 86%. Upon auscultation the nurse notes the patient has this loud high-pitched sound that is obvious on expiration, especially end-expiration.

QUESTION r/t ANALYZING CUES: The nurse is completing documentation in the electronic health record (EHR) on this client. How should the nurse document these findings?

A. Expiratory wheezes
B. Coarse rhonchi/coarse crackles
C. Baseline lung/breath sounds
D. Diffuse rales/fine crackles

Scenario: The nurse completes the documentation and asks the patient to describe her breathing. The patient states, "I get like this sometimes, but it's not as bad as it was yesterday…<cough>"

QUESTION r/t PRIORITIZING HYPOTHESIS: Based on the objective and subjective assessment of this patient, which priority problem should the nurse identify to guide the plan of care?

A. Impaired gas exchange
B. Activity intolerance
C. Sensory impairment
D. Ineffective health management

Scenario: The nurse opts to provide teaching on key methods to enhance breathing for this patient.

QUESTION r/t GENERATING SOLUTIONS: Which nonpharmacologic teaching interventions will be most effective for promoting self-care in a patient with COPD?

A. Return demonstration of tripod positioning and use of pursed-lip breathing
B. Review caloric intake and encourage the patient to eat one larger meal per day
C. Encourage the use of home oxygen only when sleeping or resting
D. Teach the patient the signs and symptoms of COPD, with an emphasis on pathophysiology

Scenario: The patient is beginning to have increasing difficulty breathing, and her oxygen saturation via pulse oximetry drops briefly to 84%.

QUESTION r/t TAKING ACTION: The nurse notes the patient is audibly wheezing, has increased use of accessory muscles, and has increasing anxiety. What is the priority nursing intervention?

A. Sit the patient up and increase the oxygen flow rate
B. Call the provider
C. Provide therapeutic touch and soft speech to calm the patient
D. Explain to the patient what is happening in clear terms

Scenario: The patient has returned to baseline respiratory function and has received the annual influenza vaccine (flu shot).

QUESTION r/t EVALUATING OUTCOMES: Which of the following parameters must be in place before discharging a patient with COPD home? Select all that apply.

A. Correct return demonstration of all inhaled and oral medications
B. Ability to complete activities of daily living with frequent rest periods
C. Effective expectoration of secretions using breathing and coughing techniques
D. Articulation of when to call the provider for follow-up and/or intervention
E. Oxygen saturation via pulse oximetry >98% on room air

DEVELOPING CLINICAL REASONING AND CLINICAL JUDGMENT

1. Work through the Evolving Case Study 40-1 Joan McIntyre to help develop your clinical reasoning and clinical judgment skills.
2. Using the Focused Assessment Guide in this chapter, work with a partner to assess the respiratory functioning of the following patients. Discuss ways in which you would modify your assessment to meet the specific needs of individual patients:
   - A 6-year-old who presents in the pediatrician's office with asthma and is experiencing difficulty breathing
   - A 12-year-old who is brought to the emergency department after illicit use of inhalants ("huffing")

- An adult dying of cancer receiving hospice care at home who is receiving increasing doses of narcotics, which depress respiratory functioning
- A hospitalized young adult with a 24-pack/year history of smoking who is noted to have a persistent, hacking cough

3. A postoperative patient who is at high risk for pulmonary complications because of a long history of smoking refuses to use the incentive spirometer or to cooperate with instructions to breathe deeply. How would you respond to this patient? Discuss with other students what nursing response is most likely to secure his engagement in necessary self-care measures.

PRACTICING FOR NCLEX

1. A nurse is assessing a patient with COPD who is experiencing dyspnea. What action will the nurse take first?
   a. Place the patient in Fowler position.
   b. Encourage diaphragmatic breathing.
   c. Ask the patient to cough.
   d. Initiate oral suctioning of secretions.
2. A nurse is maintaining airway patency in an unconscious patient by providing frequent nasopharyngeal suction. When would the nurse anticipate inserting a nasopharyngeal airway (nasal trumpet)?
   a. Vomiting during suctioning occurs.
   b. Secretions appear to contain stomach contents.
   c. The suction catheter touches an unsterile surface.
   d. Epistaxis is noted with continued suctioning.
3. A nurse in the PACU is performing oral suctioning for a patient with an oropharyngeal airway, when the patient begins to vomit. What is the nurse's priority nursing action at this time?
   a. Removing the suction catheter and elevating the head of the bed
   b. Notifying the primary health care provider
   c. Confirming the size of the oral airway is correct
   d. Placing the patient in the supine position
4. A nurse plans to suction a patient's endotracheal tube using the open suction technique. Which intervention is appropriate for this technique?
   a. Using a suction catheter that is the diameter of the endotracheal tube
   b. Maintaining the patient in the supine position
   c. Administering oxygen prior to suctioning
   d. Changing the inline suction device every 24 hours
5. A nurse is caring for a patient admitted for an acute asthma exacerbation. The patient reports extreme dyspnea, stating, "Turn up the oxygen, I'm not getting enough air." Which actions would the nurse take first?
   a. Suction the airway.
   b. Assess the pulse oximetry reading.
   c. Obtain a peak flow meter reading.
   d. Assess for cyanosis of the lips.
6. A patient with COPD is unable to perform personal hygiene without becoming exhausted. What nursing intervention would be appropriate for this patient?
   a. Assisting with all bathing and hygiene
   b. Telling the patient to avoid speaking during hygiene
   c. Teaching the patient to take short shallow breaths during activity
   d. Taking rest periods between activities
7. A nurse working in the pulmonary clinic is providing teaching to patients with altered oxygenation due to conditions such as asthma and COPD. Which measures would the nurse recommend? Select all that apply.
   a. Avoid exercise.
   b. Take steps to manage or reduce anxiety.
   c. Eat meals 1 to 2 hours prior to breathing treatments.
   d. Eat a high-protein/high-calorie diet.
   e. Maintain a high-Fowler position when possible.
   f. Drink 2 to 3 pints of clear fluids daily.
8. A student with a history of asthma visits the school nurse reporting difficulty breathing and wheezing. Which tool would the nurse use to assess the severity of airway resistance?
   a. Peak flow meter
   b. End-tidal CO_2 monitor
   c. Chest tube
   d. Arterial blood gas
9. A nurse is teaching a patient how to use a metered-dose inhaler for asthma. Which comments from the patient assure the nurse that the teaching has been effective? Select all that apply.
   a. "I'll be careful not to shake the canister before using it."
   b. "It's important to hold the canister upside down when using it."
   c. "I have to remember to inhale the medication through my nose."
   d. "I will continue to inhale when the cold propellant is in my throat."
   e. "I won't inhale more than one spray with one breath."
   f. "I will activate the device while continuing to inhale."
10. A nurse is caring for a patient with chronic lung disease who is receiving oxygen through a nasal cannula. What nursing action is performed correctly? Select all that apply.
    a. Making sure the oxygen is flowing into the prongs
    b. Maintaining oxygen saturation between 94% and 98%
    c. Encouraging the patient to breathe through their nose with their mouth closed
    d. Initiating the oxygen flow rate at 6 L/min or more
    e. Protecting the patient's skin from irritation by the oxygen tubing

11. A nurse is securing a patient's endotracheal tube with tape and observes that the tube depth changed during the retaping. Which action would be appropriate related to this incident?
    a. Instructing the assistant to notify the health care team
    b. Assessing the patient's vital signs
    c. Removing the tape, adjusting the depth to the ordered depth, and retaping securely
    d. Taking no action, as the depth will adjust automatically

12. A nurse is providing teaching for a patient who will undergo cardiac surgery and return to the intensive care unit with an endotracheal tube. What education is most important for the nurse to provide?
    a. "The endotracheal tube will drain out excess secretions from the surgical site."
    b. "This tube is used to facilitate breathing; you will not be able to speak while it is in place."
    c. "This is a surgically placed tube in your neck; we will suction it frequently to remove mucus."
    d. "Your oxygenation will be monitored frequently using pulse oximetry."

13. A nurse is caring for a patient who has a pleural chest tube attached to a disposable chest drainage system. Which nursing actions are indicated for this patient? Select all that apply.
    a. Avoiding turning the patient to prevent disconnections in the tubing
    b. Maintaining an occlusive dressing on the site
    c. Assessing the patient for signs of respiratory distress
    d. Keeping the chest drainage device at the level of the patient's thorax
    e. Ensuring there are no dependent loops or kinks in the tubing
    f. Observing for bubbles indicating air leak in the water seal chamber

14. A nurse in the emergency department is caring for a patient who was brought in by fire rescue due to a heroin overdose. The nurse notes the patient is not breathing. What action will the nurse take immediately? Select all that apply.
    a. Tilt the patient's head forward.
    b. Begin ventilation using a manual resuscitation bag (Ambu bag).
    c. Place the mask tightly over the patient's nose and mouth.
    d. Pull the patient's jaw backward.
    e. Compress the bag twice the normal respiratory rate for the patient.
    f. Recommend that a sputum culture for cytology is obtained.

15. Which assessments and interventions should the nurse consider when performing tracheal suctioning? Select all that apply.
    a. Closely assessing the patient before, during, and after the procedure
    b. Hyperoxygenating the patient before and after suctioning
    c. Limiting the application of suction to 20 to 30 seconds
    d. Monitoring the pulse to detect effects of hypoxia and stimulation of the vagus nerve
    e. Using an appropriate suction pressure (80 to 150 mm Hg)
    f. Inserting the suction catheter no further than 1 cm past the length of the tracheal or endotracheal tube

16. A nurse is monitoring a patient with a pleural effusion after a thoracentesis removing 1,400 mL of dark yellow liquid. What is the expected outcome of this procedure?
    a. Tachycardia
    b. Hypotension
    c. Reduced dyspnea
    d. Pulse oximetry of 88%

17. A nursing student attending clinical on a medical-surgical unit receives report from the off-going nurse stating the patient has adventitious breath sounds that clear after expectorating sputum. Which adventitious breath sound will the student expect to auscultate?
    a. Bronchial
    b. Bronchovesicular
    c. Vesicular
    d. Wheezing

18. A nurse in the emergency department is caring for a patient who had eaten shellfish and is now wheezing. The nurse explains to the patient that the health care provider has prescribed a bronchodilator, which will have what action?
    a. Helping the patient cough up thick mucus
    b. Opening narrowed airways and relieving wheezing
    c. Acting as a cough suppressant
    d. Blocking the effects of histamine

19. A nurse is planning to suction a patient's tracheostomy tube the day after its placement. Which action by the nurse is absolutely essential?
    a. Assessing the need to premedicate with an analgesic
    b. Placing the patient in low Fowler position
    c. Inserting the obturator into the outer cannula
    d. Maintaining aseptic technique

ANSWERS WITH RATIONALES

1. **a.** Patients with COPD experience dyspnea related to problems with ventilation and/or hypoxemia. One of the most common symptoms of hypoxia is dyspnea (difficulty breathing). Elevating the head of the bed will improve respiratory expansion and oxygenation. Coughing to facilitate secretion removal, pursed-lip breathing, and/or diaphragmatic breathing may be indicated, after sitting the patient up. Suction is indicated for patients demonstrating the presence of secretions, such as adventitious breath sounds or moist cough with phlegm; there is no indication this patient requires suctioning at this time.

2. **d.** Repeated suctioning may injure or traumatize the nares, resulting in nosebleed (epistaxis). The nurse would recommend insertion of a nasal trumpet, which will facilitate suction while protecting the nasal mucosa from further trauma.

3. **a.** The nurse discontinues suctioning, elevates the head of the bed, and turns the patients to the side to prevent aspiration. Airway protection takes priority; after positioning the patient, the nurse continues to suction the airway and oropharynx. Once airway patency has been established, the nurse will notify the provider of vomiting. There is no indication the oral airway is too large. Placing the patient supine while vomiting is inappropriate, as that could promote aspiration.

4. **c.** To prevent hypoxemia, prior to endotracheal suctioning, the nurse provides 100% oxygen for a minimum of 30 seconds. This is referred to as hyperoxygenation. The nurse limits the application of suction to no more than 10 to 15 seconds (AARC, 2010; Burns & Delgado, 2019; Hess et al., 2021; Pasrija & Hall, 2020). The external diameter of the suction catheter should not exceed half of the internal diameter of the endotracheal tube. An inline suction device is considered a closed, self-contained system used for a "closed technique" for suction; these are changed every 24 hours.

5. **b.** Using the nursing process, the nurse first assesses the oxygen saturation via pulse oximetry before changing the oxygen flow rate. Suctioning is provided to remove respiratory secretions; the nurse would note adventitious breath sounds or phlegm with cough indicating a need for suction. A peak flow meter is used to assess the point of highest flow during forced expiration. It is routinely used for patients with moderate or severe asthma to measure the severity of the disease and degree of disease management. While cyanosis of the lips is a late sign of hypoxemia, the nurse can quickly begin to alleviate or lessen dyspnea by simply repositioning the patient.

6. **d.** To prevent fatigue during activities including hygiene, the nurse should group (personal care) activities into smaller steps and encourage rest periods between activities. The nurse promotes and maintains dignity, independence, and strength by assisting with activities when the patient has difficulty. The nurse should encourage the patient to voice feelings and concerns about self-care deficits and teach the patient to coordinate pursed-lip or diaphragmatic breathing with the activity.

7. **b, d, e.** When caring for patients with COPD, it is important to help create an environment that is likely to reduce anxiety, which increases oxygen demand. A high-protein/high-calorie diet is recommended to meet increased energy needs due to the work of breathing. People with dyspnea and orthopnea are most comfortable in a high-Fowler (upright) position because accessory muscles can easily be used to facilitate respiration and lung expansion. Meals should be eaten 1 to 2 hours after breathing treatments; exercises and drinking 2 to 3 quarts (1.9 to 2.9 L) of clear fluids daily is recommended, rather than 2 to 3 pints.

8. **a.** A peak flow meter is used to assess the point of highest flow during forced expiration. It is routinely used by and for patients with moderate or severe asthma to measure the severity of the disease and degree of disease management. Capnography or end-tidal CO_2 monitoring is used for assessing and monitoring ventilation and placement of artificial airways, predicting patients who are at risk for respiratory compromise, are experiencing partial or complete airway obstruction, or are experiencing hypoventilation (Burns & Delgado, 2019; Seckel, 2018). A chest tube is used to remove air or fluid from the pleural space. The arterial blood gas (ABG) is used to assess oxygenation, ventilation, and acid–base status; it is invasive and not performed in the school setting.

9. **d, e, f.** Common mistakes that patients make when using MDIs include failing to shake the canister, holding the inhaler upside down, inhaling through the nose rather than the mouth, inhaling too rapidly, stopping the inhalation when the cold propellant is felt in the throat, failing to hold their breath after inhalation, inhaling two sprays with one breath, and not activating the device while inhaling.

10. **a, c, e.** The nurse should assure that the oxygen is flowing out of the prongs prior to inserting them into the patient's nostrils. The nurse should encourage the patient to breathe through their nose with the mouth closed. The nurse should adjust the flow rate and maintain the patient's oxygen saturation as prescribed. The nurse should implement pressure injury prevention strategies; pressure from the tubing could result in medical device–related alterations in skin integrity.

11. **c.** The tube depth should be maintained at the same level unless otherwise prescribed. If the depth changes, the nurse should remove the tape or securement device, adjust the tube to the ordered depth, and reapply the tape or securement device.

12. **b.** Patients with an endotracheal tube are unable to speak. Explaining this to the patient preoperatively, along with information that they will be closely monitored, can help decrease anxiety. The endotracheal tube is used during anesthesia or for mechanical ventilation; it is not a surgical drain. A tracheostomy, located in the neck area, is a surgically placed artificial airway. While pulse oximetry will be used to monitor oxygenation, to prevent undue anxiety, it is most important that the patient understands speech will not be possible.

13. **b, c, e, f.** The chest drainage collection device must be positioned below the tube's insertion site. Maintaining an occlusive dressing helps prevent air leak; assess for crepitus around the chest tube site indicating air leak. Avoid dependent loops or kinks in the tubing, which could impede drainage. Assess for bubbling in the water seal, maintaining the water level at the 2-cm mark. When a chest tube becomes separated from the drainage device, the nurse should submerge the tube's end in water, creating a temporary water seal and allowing air to escape until a new drainage unit can be attached.

14. **b, c.** The priority is to establish ventilation using the manual resuscitation bag to provide emergency or rescue breathing. The nurse tilts the head back, pulls the jaw forward, and positions the mask tightly over the patient's nose and mouth. The bag is compressed at a rate that approximates normal respiratory rate (e.g., 12 to 20 breaths/min in adults). Sputum for cytology is done primarily to detect cells that may be malignant, determine organisms causing infection, and identify blood or pus in the sputum. Note that the bag, with the mask removed, also fits easily over tracheostomy and endotracheal tubes.

15. **a, b, d, e, f.** Close assessment of the patient before, during, and after the procedure is necessary to identify complications such as hypoxia, infection, tracheal tissue damage, dysrhythmias, and atelectasis. The nurse should hyperoxygenate the patient before and after suctioning and limit the application of suction

to 10 to 20 seconds. In addition, monitor the patient's pulse frequently to detect potential effects of hypoxia and stimulation of the vagus nerve. Using an appropriate suction pressure (80 to 150 mm Hg) will help prevent atelectasis caused by excessive negative pressure. Research suggests that insertion of the suction catheter should be limited to a predetermined length (no further than 1 cm past the length of the tracheal or endotracheal tube) to avoid tracheal mucosal damage.

16. **c.** Thoracentesis involves inserting a needle into the pleural space to aspirate pleural fluid, air, or both (Morton & Fontaine, 2018). A thoracentesis may be performed to obtain a specimen for diagnostic purposes, to remove fluid or air that has accumulated in the pleural cavity and is causing respiratory difficulty and discomfort, or to instill medications (Hinkle et al., 2022).

17. **d.** Wheezing and crackles represent adventitious or abnormal breath sounds. Bronchial, bronchovesicular, and vesicular breath sounds are normal.

18. **b.** A bronchodilator opens narrowed airways which result in wheezing. An expectorant encourage cough to clear secretions. A cough suppressant reduces, treats, or stops a cough. Medications that block histamine (antihistamine) are often used for allergy but are not specific bronchodilators.

19. **d.** Sterile technique is used for tracheal suctioning, to reduce the risk of introduction of disease-causing organisms. Aseptic technique is imperative to avoid introducing organisms into the lower airway. An obturator, which guides the direction of the outer cannula, is inserted into the tube during placement and removed once the outer cannula of the tube is in place. In the home setting, clean technique is used.

Bibliography

Adams, D. (2018). Is there any incentive? A review on the use of incentive spirometry in postoperative abdominal surgery patients. *Canadian Journal of Respiratory Therapy, 54*(2), 50.

Aguiar, C., Davidson, J., Carvalho, A. K., Iamonti, V. C., Cortopassi, F., Nascimento, O. A., & Jardim, J. R. (2015). Tubing length for long-term oxygen therapy. *Respiratory Care, 60*(2), 179–182. https://doi.org/10.4187/respcare.03454

Al-Kindi, S. G., Brook, R. D., Biswal, S., & Rajagopalan, S. (2020). Environmental determinants of cardiovascular disease: Lessons learned from air pollution. *Nature Reviews Cardiology, 17*(10), 656–672. https://doi.org/10.1038/s41569-020-0371-2

Al-lede, M., Kumaran, R., & Waters, K. (2018). Home continuous positive airway pressure for cardiopulmonary indications in infants and children. *Sleep Medicine, 48*, 86–92. https://doi.org/10.1016/j.sleep.2018.04.004

Alqahtani, J. S., Worsley, P., & Voegeli, D. (2018). Effect of humidified noninvasive ventilation on the development of facial skin breakdown. *Respiratory Care, 63*(9), 1102–1110. https://doi.org/10.4187/respcare.06087

Amalakanti, S., & Pentakota, M. R. (2016). Pulse oximetry overestimates oxygen saturation in COPD. *Respiratory Care, 61*(4), 423–427. DOI: 10.4187/respcare.04435

American Association for Respiratory Care (AARC). (2010). Endotracheal suctioning of mechanically ventilated patients with artificial airways 2010. *Respiratory Care, 55*(6), 758–764. https://www.aarc.org/wp-content/uploads/2014/08/06.10.0758.pdf

American Association of Critical-Care Nurses (AACN). (2017). AACN practice alert. Oral care for acutely and critically ill patients. *CriticalCareNurse, 37*(3), e19–e21. doi:https://doi.org/10.4037/ccn2017179

American Association of Critical-Care Nurses (AACN). (2018). *AACN Practice alert. Prevention of aspiration in adults.* https://www.aacn.org/clinical-resources/practice-alerts/prevention-of-aspiration

American Heart Association (AHA). (2020a, October 20). 2020 American Heart Association guidelines for cardiopulmonary resuscitation and emergency cardiovascular care. Parts 1–7. *Circulation, 142*(16 Suppl 2). https://www.ahajournals.org/toc/circ/142/16_suppl_2

American Heart Association (AHA). (2020b). *2020 CPR & ECC guidelines. BLS provider manual.* AHA product number: 20–1102. https://shopcpr.heart.org/bls-provider-manual

American Heart Association (AHA). (2021). *Hands-only CPR. Fact sheet.* https://cpr.heart.org/-/media/cpr-files/courses-and-kits/hands-only-cpr/2021hocpr-documents/ds17758_cprweek_fact-sheeteng.pdf?la=en

American Heart Association (AHA). (2022). *What is CPR? CPR: Cardiopulmonary resuscitation.* https://cpr.heart.org/en/resources/what-is-cpr

American Lung Association. (2020a, February 27). *Pursed lip breathing.* https://www.lung.org/lung-health-diseases/lung-disease-lookup/copd/patient-resources-and-videos/pursed-lip-breathing-video

American Lung Association. (2020b, February 27). *Belly breathing.* https://www.lung.org/lung-health-diseases/lung-disease-lookup/copd/patient-resources-and-videos/belly-breathing-video

American Lung Association. (2020c, July 21). *Oxygen delivery devices and accessories.* https://www.lung.org/lung-health-diseases/lung-procedures-and-tests/oxygen-therapy/oxygen-delivery-devices

American Lung Association. (2021a, March 5). *COPD causes and risk factors.* https://www.lung.org/lung-health-diseases/lung-disease-lookup/copd/what-causes-copd

American Lung Association. (2021b, June 10). *Nutrition and COPD.* https://www.lung.org/lung-health-diseases/lung-disease-lookup/copd/living-with-copd/nutrition

American Thoracic Society (ATS). (2021). *Patient education/Information series. Pulse oximetry.* https://www.thoracic.org/patients/patient-resources/resources/pulse-oximetry.pdf

Andrews, M., Boyle, J. S., & Collins, J. (2020). *Transcultural concepts in nursing care* (8th ed.). Wolters Kluwer.

Andrews, J., Sathe, N. A., Krishnaswami, S., & McPheeters, M. L. (2013). Nonpharmacologic airway clearance techniques in hospitalized patients: A systematic review. *Respiratory Care, 58*(12), 2160–2186. https://doi.org/10.4187/respcare.02704

Arroyo-Novoa, C., Figueroa-Ramos, M., Puntillo, K., Stanik-Hutt, J., Thompson, C. L., White, C., & Wild, L. R. (2008). Pain related to tracheal suctioning in awake acutely and critically ill adults: A descriptive study. *Intensive & Critical Care Nursing, 24*(1), 20–27. https://doi.org/10.1016/j.iccn.2007.05.002

Asthma Initiative of Michigan (AIM). (n.d.). *Spacers and valved-holding chambers.* https://getasthmahelp.org/spacer-holding.aspx

Baranoski, S., & Ayello, E. A. (2020). *Wound care essentials* (5th ed.). Wolters Kluwer.

Bauldoff, G., Gubrud, P., & Carno, M. A. (2020). *LeMone and Burke's medical-surgical nursing: Clinical reasoning in patient care* (7th ed.). Pearson.

Beningfield, A., & Jones, A. (2018). Peri-operative chest physiotherapy for paediatric cardiac patients: A systematic review and meta-analysis. *Physiotherapy, 104*(3), 251–263. https://doi.org/10.1016/j.physio.2017.08.011

Bhatnager, V., Jinjil, K., Dwivedi, D., Verma, R., & Tandon, U. (2018). Cardiopulmonary resuscitation: Unusual techniques for unusual situations. *Journal of Emergencies, Trauma, and Shock, 11*(1), 31–37. https://doi.org/10.4103/JETS.JETS_58_17

Boroughs, D. S., & Dougherty, J. M. (2015). Pediatric tracheostomy care: What home care nurses need to know. *American Nurse Today, 10*(3), 8–10.

Bovino, L. R., Brainard, C., Beaumier, K., Concetti, V., Lefurge, N., Mittelstadt, E., Wilson, T., & Langhan, M. L. (2018). Use of capnography to optimize procedural sedation in the emergency department pediatric population. *Journal of Emergency Nursing, 44*(2), 110–116. https://doi.org/10.1016/j.jen.2017.10.016

Broderick, S. R. (2021). *Wellness and prevention. What does vaping do to your lungs?* Johns Hopkins Medicine. https://www.hopkinsmedicine.org/health/wellness-and-prevention/what-does-vaping-do-to-your-lungs

Burns, S. M, & Delgado, S. A. (2019). *AACN essentials of critical care nursing* (4th ed.). McGraw Hill Education.

Camacho-Del Rio, G. (2018). Evidence-based practice: Medical device-related pressure injury prevention. *American Nurse Today, 13*(10), 50–52.

Centers for Disease Control and Prevention (CDC). (2018, March 7). *Know how to use your asthma inhaler.* https://www.cdc.gov/asthma/inhaler_video/default.htm

Centers for Disease Control and Prevention (CDC). (2020a, September 1). *Pneumococcal vaccination.* https://www.cdc.gov/pneumococcal/vaccination.html

Centers for Disease Control and Prevention (CDC). (2020b, April 28). *Smoking and tobacco use. Health effects. Heart disease and stroke.* https://www.cdc.gov/tobacco/basic_information/health_effects/heart_disease/index.htm

Centers for Disease Control and Prevention (CDC). (2020c, December 10). *Smoking and tobacco use. Fast facts and fact sheets.* https://www.cdc.gov/tobacco/data_statistics/fact_sheets/index.htm?s_cid=osh-stu-home-spotlight-001

Centers for Disease Control and Prevention (CDC). (2020d, February 25). *Outbreak of lung injury associated with the use of e-cigarette, or vaping,* products. https://www.cdc.gov/tobacco/basic_information/e-cigarettes/severe-lung-disease.html

Centers for Disease Control and Prevention (CDC). (2021a, January 19). *Heart disease.* https://www.cdc.gov/heartdisease/

Centers for Disease Control and Prevention (CDC). (2021b, June 18). *Influenza (flu).* https://www.cdc.gov/flu/index.htm

Centers for Disease Control and Prevention (CDC). (2021c, May 24). *Your COVID-19 vaccination.* https://www.cdc.gov/coronavirus/2019-ncov/vaccines/your-vaccination.html

Centers for Disease Control and Prevention (CDC). (2021d, May 25). *COVID-19. Frequently asked questions.* https://www.cdc.gov/coronavirus/2019-ncov/faq.html#Basics

Centers for Disease Control and Prevention (CDC). (2021e, May 13). *COVID-19. People with certain medical conditions.* https://www.cdc.gov/coronavirus/2019-ncov/need-extra-precautions/people-with-medical-conditions.html

Centers for Disease Control and Prevention (CDC). (2021f, April 2). *Tips from former smokers®. Smoking and cancer.* https://www.cdc.gov/tobacco/campaign/tips/diseases/cancer.html

Centers for Disease Control and Prevention (CDC). (2021g, March 2). Smoking & tobacco use. Secondhand smoke. https://www.cdc.gov/tobacco/basic_information/secondhand_smoke/index.htm

Centers for Disease Control and Prevention (CDC). (2022, April 27). *Physical inactivity*. https://www.cdc.gov/chronicdisease/resources/publications/factsheets/physical-activity.htm

Chaseling, W., Bayliss, S.L., Rose, K., Armstrong, L., Boyle, M., Caldwel, J., Chung, C., Girffiths, K., Johnson, K., Rolls, K., & Davidson, P. (2014). Suctioning an adult ICU patient with an artificial airway. Agency for Clinical Innovation NSW Government. Version 2. NSW, Australia. https://www.aci.health.nsw.gov.au/__data/assets/pdf_file/0010/239554/ACI14_Suction_2-2.pdf

Chaves, G. S. S., Freitas, D. A., Santino, T. A., Angelica, P., Fregonexi, G. A. F., & Mendonça, K. M. P. P. (2019). Chest physiotherapy for pneumonia in children. *Cochrane Database of Systematic Reviews*. https://doi.org/10.1002/14651858.CD010277.pub3

Chenelle, C. T., Oto, J., Sulemanji, D., Fisher, D. F., & Kacmarek, R. M. (2015). Evaluation of an automated endotracheal tube cuff controller during simulated mechanical ventilation. *Respiratory Care, 60*(2), 183–190. https://doi.org/10.4187/respcare.03387

Chick, A., & Wynne, A. (2020). Introducing an oral care assessment tool with advanced cleaning products into a high-risk clinical setting. *British Journal of Nursing, 29*(5), 290–296. DOI: 10.12968/bjon.2020.29.5.290

Cleveland Clinic. (2018a, September 14). *Pursed lip breathing*. https://my.clevelandclinic.org/health/articles/9443-pursed-lip-breathing

Cleveland Clinic. (2018b, September 14). *Diaphragmatic breathing*. https://my.clevelandclinic.org/health/articles/9445-diaphragmatic-breathing

Cleveland Clinic. (2018c, September 14). *Coughing: Controlled coughing*. https://my.clevelandclinic.org/health/articles/8697-coughing-controlled-coughing

Cleveland Clinic. (2020, May 18). *Chronic obstructive pulmonary disease (COPD)*. https://my.clevelandclinic.org/health/diseases/8709-chronic-obstructive-pulmonary-disease-copd

Cleveland Clinic. (2021). *Tracheostomy care*. https://my.clevelandclinic.org/health/treatments/17568-tracheostomy-care

Dawson, D. (2014). Essential principles: Tracheostomy care in the adult patient. *British Association of Critical Care Nurses, 19*(2), 63–72. https://doi.org/10.1111/nicc.12076

Dix, A. (2018). Respiratory rate: The benefits of continuous monitoring. *Nursing Times, 114*(11), 36–37. https://www.nursingtimes.net/clinical-archive/respiratory-clinical-archive/respiratory-rate-6-the-benefits-of-continuous-monitoring-29-10-2018

Dixon, L. M., Mascioli, S., Mixell, J. H., Gillin, T., Upchurch, C. N., & Bradley, K. M. (2018). Reducing tracheostomy-related pressure injuries. *AACN Advanced Critical Care, 29*(4), 426–431. https://dx.doi.org/10.4037/aacnacc2018426

Douma, M. J., MacKenzie, E., Loch, T., Tan, M. C., Anderson, D., Picard, C., Milovanovic, L., O'Dochartaigh, D., & Brindley, P. G. (2020). Prone cardiopulmonary resuscitation? A scoping and expanded grey literature review for the COVID-19 pandemic. *Resuscitation, 155*, 103–111. https://doi.org/10.1016/j.resuscitation.2020.07.010

Dudek, S. (2022). *Nutrition essentials for nursing practice* (9th ed.). Wolters Kluwer.

Düzkaya, D. S., & Kuğuoğlu, S. (2015). Assessment of pain during endotracheal suction in the pediatric intensive care unit. *Pain Management Nursing, 16*(1), 11–19. http://dx.doi.org/10.1016/j.pmn.2014.02.003

Edelson, D. P., Sasson, C., Chan, P. S., Atkins, D. L., Aziz, K., Becker, L. B., Berg, R. A., Bradley, S. M., Brooks, S. C., Cheng, A., Escobedo, M., Flores, G. E., Girotra, S., Hsu, A., Kamath-Rayne, B. D., Lee, H. C., Lehotsky, R. E., Mancini, M. E., Merchant, R. M., … Topjian, A. A. (2020). Interim guidance for basic and advanced life support in adults, children, and neonates with suspected or confirmed COVID-19. *Circulation, 141*(25), e933–e943. https://doi.org/10.1161/CIRCULATIONAHA.120.047463

Eliopoulos, C. (2018). *Gerontological nursing* (9th ed.). Wolters Kluwer.

Elpern, E. H., Nedved, P., Weiss, T., Patel, A. D., & Cerda, F. (2021). Implementing a multidisciplinary prone positioning team. *American Journal of Nursing, 121*(6) 48–53. doi: 10.1097/01.NAJ.0000753652.63203.78

Elliott, M., & Baird, J. (2019). Pulse oximetry and the enduring neglect of respiratory rate assessment: A commentary on patient surveillance. *British Journal of Nursing, 28*(19) 1156–1159. https://doi.org/10.12968/bjon.2019.28.19.1256

Eltorai, A. E. M., Martin, T. J., Patel, S. A., Tran, M., Eltorai, A. S., Daniels, A. H., & Baird, G. L. (2019). Visual obstruction of flow of indicator increases inspiratory volumes in incentive spirometry. *Respiratory Care, 64*(5), 590–594. https://doi.org/10.4187/respcare.06331

Eltorai, A. E. M., Szabo, A. L., Antoci Jr., V., Ventetuolo, C. E., Elias, J. A., Daniels, A. H., & Hess, D. R. (2018). Clinical effectiveness of incentive spirometry for the prevention of postoperative pulmonary complications. *Respiratory Care, 63*(3), 347–352. https://doi.org/10.4187/respcare.05679

European Pressure Ulcer Advisory Panel (EPUAP), National Pressure Injury Advisory Panel (NPIAP), and Pan Pacific Pressure Injury Alliance (PPPIA). Haesler, E. (Ed). (2019). *Prevention and treatment of pressure ulcers/injuries: Clinical Practice guideline. The international guideline*. http://www.internationalguideline.com/

Fischbach, F. T., & Fischbach, M. A. (2018). *A manual of laboratory and diagnostic tests* (10th ed.). Wolters Kluwer.

Ford, C., & Robinson, M. (2021). Oxygen therapy in a hospital setting. *British Journal of Nursing, 30*(2), 96–100. https://doi.org/10.12968/bjon.2021.30.2.96

Franklin, D., Fraser, J. F., & Schibler, A. (2019). Respiratory support for infants with bronchiolitis, a narrative review of the literature. *Paediatric Respiratory Reviews, 30*, 16–24. https://doi.org/10.1016/j.prrv.2018.10.001

Frigerio, P., Longhini, F., Sommariva, M., Stagni, E. G., Curto, F., Redaelli, T., Ciboldi, M., Simonds, A. K., & Navalesi, P. (2015). Bench comparative assessment of mechanically assisted cough devices. *Respiratory Care, 60*(7), 975–982. https://doi.org/10.4187/respcare.03809

Gardner, L. A. (2015). Identify sufficient supplemental oxygen for patient intrahospital transport. *Pennsylvania Patient Safety Advisory, 12*(3), 121–122. http://patientsafety.pa.gov/ADVISORIES/Pages/201509_121.aspx

Gilder, E., McGuinness, S. P., Cavadino, A., Jull, A., & Parke, R. L. (2020). Avoidance of routine endotracheal suction in subjects ventilated for ≤12 hours following elective cardiac surgery. *Respiratory Care, 65*(12), 1838–1846. https://doi.org/10.4187/respcare.07821

Goff, D., & Patterson, J. (2019). Eating and drinking with an inflated tracheostomy cuff: A systematic review of the aspiration risk. *International Journal of Language & Communication Disorders, 54*(1), 30–40. https://doi.org/10.1111/1460-6984.12430

Goodman, J. R. (2014). Treating transtracheal oxygen therapy patients. *RT: The Journal for Respiratory Care Practitioners, 27*(1), 22–25.

Guttendorf, J. (2021). Prone positioning in acute respiratory distress syndrome. *AHC Media. Critical Care Alert, 28*(11), 1–6. www.reliasmedia.com/articles/147467-prone-positioning-in-acute-respiratory-distress-syndrome

Hahn, M. (2010). 10 considerations for endotracheal suctioning. *The Journal for Respiratory Care Practitioners, 23*(7), 32–33.

Halpin, D., Holmes, S., Calvert, J., & McInerney, D. (2014). Improving inhaler technique. *Practice Nursing, 26*(1), 16–20.

Hanlon, P. (2014). Choosing the right portable oxygen concentrator. *RT: The Journal for Respiratory Care Practitioners, 27*(10), 6.

Headway. (2021). *Hypoxic and anoxic brain injury*. https://www.headway.org.uk/about-brain-injury/individuals/types-of-brain-injury/hypoxic-and-anoxic-brain-injury/

Henrichs, K. A., & Makic, M. B. F. (2021). A quality improvement project to increase oxygen therapy adherence in patients newly prescribed oxygen at discharge. *MEDSURG Nursing, 30*(1), 35–40.

Hernández, G., Roca, O., & Colinas, L. (2017). High-flow nasal cannula support therapy: New insights and improving performance. *Critical Care, 21*, 1–11. https://doi.org/10.1186/s13054-017-1640-2

Hess, D. R., & Altobelli, N. P. (2014). Tracheostomy tubes. *Respiratory Care, 59*(6), 956–973. https://doi.org/10.4187/respcare.02920

Hess, D. R., MacIntyre, N. R., Galvin, W. F., & Mishoe, S. C. (2021). *Respiratory care: Principles and practice* (4th ed.). Jones & Bartlett Learning.

Higginson, R., Parry, A., & Williams, M. (2016). Airway management in the hospital environment. *British Journal of Nursing, 25*(2), 94–100. https://doi.org/10.12968/bjon.2016.25.2.94

Hinkle, J. L., Cheever, K. H., & Overbaugh, K. J. (2022). *Brunner & Suddarth's Textbook of medical-surgical nursing* (15th ed.). Wolters Kluwer.

Holdman, J., Rozansky, C., & Baldwyn, T. (2020). Reduction of respiratory device-related pressure injury. *RT*. https://rtmagazine.com/department-management/clinical/reduction-of-respiratory-device-related-pressure-injuries

Hood, B. S., Henderson, W., & Pasero, C. (2014). Chest tube removal: An expanded role for the bedside nurse. *Journal of PeriAnesthesia Nursing, 29*(1), 53–59. http://dx.doi.org/10.1016/j.jopan.2013.11.001

Imbriaco, G., & Monesi, A. (2021). Closed tracheal suctioning systems in the era of COVID-19: Is it time to consider them as a gold standard? *Journal of Infection Prevention, 22*(1), 44–45. https://doi.org/10.1177/1757177420963775

International Council of Nurses (ICN). (2019). *Nursing diagnosis and outcome statements*. https://www.icn.ch/sites/default/files/inline-files/ICNP2019-DC.pdf

Ireton, J. (2007). Tracheostomy suction: A protocol for practice. *Paediatric Nursing, 19*(10), 14–18.

Jacobs, S. S., Krishnan, J. A., Lederer, D. J., Ghazipura, M., Hossain, T., Tan, A. Y. M., Carlin, B., Drummond, M. B., Ekström, M., Garvey, C., Graney, B. A., Jackson, B., Kallstrom, T., Knight, S. L., Lindell, K., Prieto-Centurion, V., Renzoni, E. A., Ryerson, C. J., Schneidman, A., … Holland, A. E. (2020). Home oxygen therapy for adults with chronic lung disease. *American Journal of Respiratory and Critical Care Medicine, 202*(10), e121–e141. https://doi.org/10.1164/rccm.202009-3608ST

Jarvis, C., & Echkardt, A. (2020). *Physical examination & health assessment* (8th ed.). Elsevier.

Jensen, S. (2019). *Nursing health assessment. A best practice approach* (3rd ed.). Wolters Kluwer.

Jenson, H., Maddux, S., & Waldo, M. (2018). Improving oral care in hospitalized non-ventilated patients: Standardizing products and protocol. *MEDSURG Nursing, 27*(1), 38–45.

Johns Hopkins Medicine. (n.d.). Suctioning. https://www.hopkinsmedicine.org/tracheostomy/living/suctioning.html

Johns Hopkins Medicine. (2021). *Occupational lung diseases*. https://www.hopkinsmedicine.org/health/conditions-and-diseases/occupational-lung-diseases

Joint Commission. (2018, July 23). Quick safety 43: Managing medical device-related pressure injuries. https://www.jointcommission.org/resources/news-and-multimedia/newsletters/newsletters/quick-safety/quick-safety-43-managing-medical-devicerelated-pressure-injuries/

Kane, C. J., York, N. L., & Minton, L. A. (2013). Chest tubes in the critically ill patient. *Dimensions of Critical Care Nursing, 32*(3), 111–117. https://doi.org/10.1097/DCC.0b013e3182864721

Karch, A. M. (2020). *Focus on nursing pharmacology* (8th ed.). Wolters Kluwer.

Kendrick, A. (2020). *Clinical guidelines (nursing). Endotracheal tube suction of ventilated neonates*. The Royal Children's Hospital Melbourne. https://www.rch.org.au/rchcpg/hospital_clinical_guideline_index/Endotracheal_tube_suction_of_ventilated_neonates/

King, J., & Lowery, D. R. (2020, September 15). *StatPearls. Physiology, cardiac output*. National Center for Biotechnology Information. U. S. National Library of Medicine. https://www.ncbi.nlm.nih.gov/books/NBK470455/

Kotta, P. A., & Ali, J. M. (2021). Incentive spirometry for prevention of postoperative pulmonary complications after thoracic surgery. *Respiratory Care, 66*(2), 327–333. https://doi.org/10.4187/respcare.07972

Kuehneman, T., Gregory, M., de Waal, D., Davidson, P., Frickel, R., King, C., Gradwell, E., & Handu, D. (2018). Academy of Nutrition and Dietetics evidence-based practice guideline for the management of heart failure in adults. *Journal of the Academy of Nutrition and Dietetics*, *118*(12), 2331–2345. https://doi.org/10.1016/j.jand.2018.03.004

Kummer, D. J., & Walden, B. J. (2019). Capnography monitoring for patients undergoing moderate sedation. *Gastroenterology Nursing*, *42*(1), 49–54. https://doi.org/10.1097/SGA.0000000000000426

Kurt, O. K., Zhang, J., & Pinkerton, K. E. (2016). Pulmonary health effects of air pollution. *Current Opinion in Pulmonary Medicine*, *22*(2), 138–143. https://doi.org/10.1097/MCP.0000000000000248

Kyle, T., & Carman, S. (2021). *Essentials of pediatric nursing* (4th ed.). Wolters Kluwer.

Lacerte, M., Shapshak, A. H., & Mesfin, F. B. (2020, November 19). *Hypoxic brain injury.* StatPearls. https://www.ncbi.nlm.nih.gov/books/NBK537310

Leddy, R., & Wilkinson, J. M. (2015). Endotracheal suctioning practices of nurses and respiratory therapists: How well do they align with clinical practice guidelines? *Canadian Journal of Respiratory Therapy*, *51*(3), 60–64.

Lellouche, F., & L'Her, E. (2020). Usual and advanced monitoring in patients receiving oxygen therapy. *Respiratory Care*, *65*(10), 1591–1600. https://doi.org/10.4187/respcare.07623

Lestari, M. P. L., Wanda, D., & Nurhaeni, N. (2019). The effects of modified pursed lips breathing on oxygenation status in children. *Comprehensive Child & Adolescent Nursing*, *42*(S1), 1–8. https://doi.org/10.1080/24694193.2019.1577920

Lisy, K. (2014). Cochrane corner. Chest physiotherapy for pneumonia in children. *American Journal of Nursing*, *114*(5), 16. Doi: 10.1097/01.NAJ.0000446761.33589.70

Liu, F., Shao, Q., Jiang, R., Zeng, Z., Liu, Y., LI, Y., Liu, Q., Ding, C., Zhao, N., Peng, Z., & Qian, K. (2019). High-flow oxygen therapy to speed weaning from mechanical ventilation: A prospective randomized study. *American Journal of Critical Care*, *28*(5), 370–376. https://doi.org/https://doi.org/10.4037/ajcc2019130

Lorente, L., Lecuona, M., Jiménez, A., Lorenzo, L., Roca, I., Cabrera, J., Llanos, C., Mora, M. L. (2014). Continuous endotracheal tube cuff pressure control system protects against ventilator-associated pneumonia. *Critical Care*, *18*(1), R77. https://doi.org/10.1186/cc13837

Lu, Z., Chang, W., Meng, S., Xue, M., Xie, J., Xu, J., Qiu, H., Yang, Y., & Guo, F. (2020). The effect of high-flow nasal oxygen therapy on postoperative pulmonary complications and hospital length of stay in postoperative patients: A systematic review and meta-analysis. *Journal of Intensive Care Medicine*, *35*(10), 1129–1140. https://doi.org/10.1177/0885066618817718

Makic, M. B., Rauen, C., Jones, K., & Fisk, A. C. (2015). Continuing to challenge practice to be evidence based. *Critical Care Nurse*, *35*(2), 39–50. https://doi.org/http://dx.doi.org/10.4037/ccn2015693

Maraş, G. B., Eşer, I., Şenoğlu, N., Yilmaz, N. Ö., & Derici, Y. K. (2020). Increasing suction pressure during endotracheal suctioning increases the volume of suctioned secretions, but not the procedure-related complications: A comparative study in open system endotracheal suctioning. *Intensive & Critical Care Nursing*, *61*. doi: 10.1016/j.iccn.2020.102928

Martin, T. J. (2020, August 19). *Treatment and prognosis of the obesity hypoventilation syndrome.* UpToDate. https://www.uptodate.com/contents/treatment-and-prognosis-of-the-obesity-hypoventilation-syndrome

Maydick-Youngberg, D., Liao, J., Francis, K., & Kaplan, S. (2020). An evidence-based interprofessional collaborative practice approach to decrease tracheostomy-related pressure injury. *MEDSURG Nursing*, *29*(3), 189–218.

Mayer, A. F., Karloh, M., dos Santos, K., de Araujo, C. L. P., & Gulart, A. A. (2018). Effects of acute use of pursed-lips breathing during exercise in patients with COPD; A systematic review and meta-analysis. *Physiotherapy*, *104*(1), 9–17. https://doi.org/10.1016/j.physio.2017.08.007

Mayo Foundation for Medical Education and Research (MFMER). (2018a, May 17). *CPAP machines: Tips for avoiding 10 common problems.* https://www.mayoclinic.org/diseases-conditions/sleep-apnea/in-depth/cpap/art-20044164

Mayo Foundation for Medical Education and Research (MFMER). (2018b, December 1). *Hypoxemia.* https://www.mayoclinic.org/symptoms/hypoxemia/basics/definition/sym-20050930

Mayo Foundation for Medical Education and Research (MFMER). (2019, March 8). *Warm-mist versus cool-mist humidifier: Which is better for a cold?* https://www.mayoclinic.org/diseases-conditions/common-cold/expert-answers/cool-mist-humidifiers/faq-20058199

Mayo Foundation for Medical Education and Research (MFMER). (2020, April 9). *Peak flow meter.* https://www.mayoclinic.org/tests-procedures/peak-flow-meter/about/pac-20394858

Mayo Foundation for Medical Education and Research (MFMER). (2021, March 23). *Lung cancer.* https://www.mayoclinic.org/diseases-conditions/lung-cancer/symptoms-causes/syc-20374620

McCoy, R. (2016). Home oxygen therapy: Delivery options and clinical issues. *RT: The Journal for Respiratory Care Practitioners*, *29*(6), 18–20.

McLaughlin, M. A. (Ed.). (2020). *Cardiovascular care made incredibly easy!* Wolters Kluwer.

Medline Plus. (2018, November 11). *Oxygen therapy in infants.* https://medlineplus.gov/ency/article/007242.htm

MedlinePlus. (2020, January 12). *Oxygen safety.* https://medlineplus.gov/ency/patientinstructions/000049.htm

MedlinePlus. (2021, June 9). *Positive airway pressure treatment.* https://medlineplus.gov/ency/article/001916.htm

Mendes, L., Moraes, K. S., Hoffman, M., Vieira, D. S. R., Ribeiro-Samora, G. A., Lage, S. M., Britto, R. R., & Parreira, V. F. (2019). Effects of diaphragmatic breathing with and without pursed-lips breathing in subjects with COPD. *Respiratory Care*, *64*(2), 136–144. https://doi.org/10.4187/respcare.06319

Messika, J. (2019). High-flow nasal oxygen therapy outside the intensive care setting: How safe is safe enough? *Respiratory Care*, *64*(11), 1447–1448. https://doi.org/10.4187/respcare.07441

Miller, C., Bridges, E., Laxmanan, B., Cox-North, P., & Thompson, H. (2018). Tunneled pleural catheter: Treatment for recurrent pleural effusion. *AACN Advanced Critical Care*, *29*(4), 432–441. https://dx.doi.org/10.4037/aacnacc2018806

Mirza, S., Clay, R. D., Koslow, M. A., & Scanlon, P. D. (2018). COPD Guidelines: A review of the 2018 GOLD Report. *Mayo Clinic Proceedings*, *93*(10), 1488–1502. https://doi.org/10.1016/j.mayocp.2018.05.026

Mitchell, D. A., & Seckel, M. A. (2018). Acute respiratory distress syndrome and prone positioning. *AACN Advanced Critical Care*, *29*(4), 415–425. https://dx.doi.org/10.4037/aacnacc2018161

Mitchell, J. (2015). Pathophysiology of COPD: Part 2. *Practice Nursing*, *26*(9), 444–449. https://doi.org/10.12968/pnur.2015.26.9.444

Moore, Y., Shotton, E., Brown, R., Gremmel, J., Lindsey, S., & Pankey, J. (2018). Effects of incentive spirometry on perceived dyspnea in patients hospitalized with pneumonia. *MEDSURG Nursing*, *27*(1), 19–37.

Morata, L., Sole, M. L., Guido-Sanz, F., Ogilvie, C., & Rich, R. (2021). Manual vs automatic prone positioning and patient outcomes in acute respiratory distress syndrome. *American Journal of Critical Care*, *30*(2), 104–112. https://doi.org/10.4037/ajcc2021674

Moreel, L., & Proesmans, M. (2020). High flow nasal cannula as respiratory support in treating infant bronchiolitis: A systematic review. *European Journal of Pediatrics*, *179*(5), 711–718. https://doi.org/10.1007/s00431-020-03637-0

Moretta, P., Molino, A., Martucci, M., Fuschillo, S., De Felice, A., Guida, P., Motta, A., Vitacca, M., & Maniscalco, M. (2021). Subject preferences and psychological implications of portable oxygen concentrator versus compressed oxygen cylinder in chronic lung disease. *Respiratory Care*, *66*(1), 33–40. https://doi.org/10.4187/respcare.07829

Morris, L. L., Kuncis, M., Perleberg, D., Kuczek, A., Kashul, K., Zabel, D., Heinemann, A. W., & Semik, P. (2021). New device makes tracheostomy dressing changes easier and more comfortable. *Rehabilitation Nursing*, *46*(2), 95–103. https://doi.org/10.1097/rnj.0000000000000302

Morton, P. G., & Fontaine, D. K. (2018). *Critical care nursing. A holistic approach* (11th ed.). Wolters Kluwer.

Moscarelli, A., Iozzo, P., Ippolito, M., Catalisano, G., Gregoretti, C., Giarratano, A., Baldi, E., & Cortegiani, A. (2020). Cardiopulmonary resuscitation in prone position: A scoping review. *American Journal of Emergency Medicine*, *38*(11), 2416–2424. https://doi.org/10.1016/j.ajem.2020.08.097

Murphie, P. (2015). Home oxygen therapy: An update for community nurses. *Journal of Community Nursing*, *29*(4), 55–59.

Mussa, C. C., Gomaa, D., Rowley, D. D., Schmidt, U., Ginier, E., & Strickland, S. L. (2021). AARC clinical practice guideline: Management of adult patients with tracheostomy in the acute care setting. *Respiratory Care*, *66*(1), 156–169. https://doi.org/10.4187/respcare.08206

Muzzy, A. C., & Butler, A. K. (2015). Managing chest tubes: Air leaks and unplanned tube removal. *American Nurse Today*, *10*(5), 10–13.

National Fire Protection Association. (2016). *NFPA safety tip sheet: Medical oxygen.* https://www.nfpa.org/-/media/Files/Public-Education/Resources/Safety-tip-sheets/OxygenSafety.ashx

National Heart Lung and Blood Institute (NHLBI). (n.d.a). *CPAP. Also known as continuous positive airway pressure.* https://www.nhlbi.nih.gov/health-topics/cpap

National Heart Lung and Blood Institute (NHLBI). (n.d.b). *Obesity hypoventilation syndrome. Also known as Pickwickian syndrome.* https://www.nhlbi.nih.gov/health-topics/obesity-hypoventilation-syndrome

National Heart Lung and Blood Institute (NHLBI). (2019). *COPD. Also known as chronic obstructive pulmonary disease, emphysema.* https://www.nhlbi.nih.gov/health-topics/copd

NHS Inform. (2020, February 26). *Oral thrush in adults.* https://www.nhsinform.scot/illnesses-and-conditions/infections-and-poisoning/oral-thrush-in-adults

Nippers, I., & Sutton, A. (2014). Oxygen therapy: Professional compliance with national guidelines. *British Journal of Nursing*, *23*(7), 382–386. doi: 10.12968/bjon.2014.23.7.382

Nishimura, M. (2016). High-flow nasal cannula oxygen therapy in adults: Physiological benefits, indication, clinical benefits and adverse effects. *Respiratory Care*, *61*(4), 529–541. https://doi.org/10.4187/respcare.04577

Norris, T. L. (2020). *Porth's essentials of pathophysiology* (5th ed.). Wolters Kluwer.

O'Driscoll, B. R., Howard, L. S., Earis, J., & Mak, V., on behalf of the British Thoracic Society Emergency Oxygen Guideline Group. (2017). BTS guideline for oxygen use in adults in healthcare and emergency settings. *Thorax*, *72*(Supp 1), ii1–ii90. https://doi.org/10.1136/thoraxjnl-2016-209729

O'Toole, T. R., Jacobs, N., Hondorp, B., Crawford, L., Boudrereau, L. R., Jeffe, J., Stein, B., & LoSavio, P. (2017). Prevention of tracheostomy-related hospital-acquired pressure ulcers. *Otolaryngology -Head and Neck Surgery*, *156*(4), 642–651. https://doi.org/10.1177/0194599816689584

Owen, E. B., Woods, C. R., O'Flynn, J. A., Boone, M. C., Calhoun, A. W., & Montgomery V. L. (2016). A bedside decision tree for use of saline with endotracheal tube suctioning in children. *Critical Care Nurse*, *36*(1), e1–e10. http://dx.doi.org/10.4037/ccn2016358

Pandian, V., Morris, L. L., Brodsky, M. B., Lynch, J., Walsh, B., Rushton, C., Phillips, J., Rahman, A., DeRose, T., Lambe, L., Lami, L., Wu, S. P. M., Garza, F. P., Maiani, S., Zavalis, A., Okusanya, K. A., Palmieri, P. A., McGrath, B. A., Pelosi, P., … Brenner, M. J. (2020). Critical care guidance for tracheostomy care during the COVID-19 pandemic: A global, multidisciplinary approach. *American Journal of Critical Care*, *29*(6), e116–e127. https://doi.org/10.4037/ajcc2020561

Pasrija, D., & Hall, C. A. (2020, June 2). *Airway suctioning.* StatPearls. https://www.ncbi.nlm.nih.gov/books/NBK557386/

Pate, M., & Zapata, T. (2002). Ask the experts: How deeply should I go when I suction an endotracheal or tracheostomy tube? *Critical Care Nurse, 22*(2), 130–131.

Patel, S., Jose, A., & Mohiuddin, S. S. (2021, March 31). StatPearls. Physiology, oxygen transport and carbon dioxide dissociation curve. National Center for Biotechnology Information. U. S. National Library of Medicine. https://www.ncbi.nlm.nih.gov/books/NBK539815

Patel, V., Peutherer, C., Hodges, E. J., Mariyaselvam, M. Z. A., & Young, P. J. (2019). Unintentional endotracheal tube cuff deflation during routine checks: A simulation study. *Nursing in Critical Care, 24*(2), 83–88. https://doi.org/10.1111/nicc.12397

Patton, J. (2019). Tracheostomy care. *British Journal of Nursing, 28*(16), 1060–1062. https://doi.org/10.12968/bjon.2019.28.16.1060

Pittman, J., & Gillespie, C. (2020). Medical device-related pressure injuries. *Critical Care Nursing Clinics of North America, 32*(4), 533–542. https://doi.org/10.1016/j.cnc.2020.08.004

Price, D. B., Román-Rodríguez, M., McQueen, R. B., Bosnic-Anticevich, S., Carter, V., Gruffydd-Jones, K., Haughney, J., Henrichsen, S., Hutton, C., Infantino, A., Lavorini, F., Law, L. M., Lisspers, K., Papi, A., Ryan, D., Ställberg, B., van der Molen, T., & Chrystyn, H. (2017). Inhaler errors in the CRITIKAL Study: Type, frequency, and association with asthma outcomes. *The Journal of Allergy and Clinical Immunology. In Practice, 5*(4), 1071–1081.e9. https://doi.org/10.1016/j.jaip.2017.01.004

Pruitt, B. (2020). The use of high-flow nasal cannula in patients with COVID-19. *RT: The Journal for Respiratory Care Practitioners, 33*(8), 8–10.

Quaranta, J. (2018). *Asthma management in children and adults* (2nd ed.). S.C. Publishing.

Quinn, B., Giuliano, K. K., & Baker, D. (2020). Non-ventilator health care-associated pneumonia (NV-HAP): Best practices for prevention of NV-HAP. *American Journal of Infection Control, 48*(5), A23–A27. https://doi.org/10.1016/j.ajic.2020.03.006

Ramos-Nino, M. E., MacLean, C. D., & Littenberg, B. (2021). Association between prevalence of obstructive lung disease and obesity: Results from The Vermont Diabetes Information System. *Asthma Research and Practice, 7*(1), 6. https://doi.org/10.1186/s40733-021-00073-1

Rolfe, S., & Paul, F. (2018a). Oxygen therapy in adult patients. Part 1: Understanding the relevant physiology and pathophysiology. *British Journal of Nursing, 27*(14), 798–804. https://doi.org/10.12968/bjon.2018.27.14.798

Rolfe, S., & Paul, F. (2018b). Oxygen therapy in adult patients. Part 2: Promoting safe and effective practice in patients' care and management. *British Journal of Nursing, 27*(17), 988–995. https://doi.org/10.12968/bjon.2018.27.17.988

Ruan, Q., Khasanah, I. H., Kongkeaw, O., & Maneewat, K. (2017). Pain management during endotracheal tube suctioning: An evidence-based approach for nurses. *Nursing & Primary Care, 1*(4), 1–3. https://www.scivisionpub.com/pdfs/pain-management-during-endotracheal-tube-suctioning-an-evidencebased-approach-for-nurses-168.pdf

Sampson, M. (2021). A guide to airway management. *British Journal of Cardiac Nursing, 16*(3), 1–13. https://doi.org/10.12968/bjca.2020.0093

Sasa, R. I. (2019). Evidence-based update on chest tube management. *American Nurse Today, 14*(4), 10–14.

Scott, J. B. (2020, July 1). *Critical care alert. High-flow nasal cannula oxygen therapy in adult acute care.* Relias Media. https://www.reliasmedia.com/articles/146419-high-flow-nasal-cannula-oxygen-therapy-in-adult-acute-care

Seckel, M. A. (2018). Advances in evidence-based pulmonary care. *AACN Advance Critical Care, 29*(4), 394–395. https://dx.doi.org/10.4037/aacnacc2018422

Siegmeister, D., Pilong, K., Boenisch, A., Brownmiller, E., Foran-Lee, L., Larsen, D. A., Stahre, P., Epstein, H. A. B., & Glasofer, A. (2021). Clinical case report: Prone positioning for non-intubated patients with COVID-19. *MEDSURG Nursing, 30*(3), 201–207, 160.

Silbert-Flagg, J., & Pillitteri, A. (2018). *Maternal and child health nursing* (8th ed.). Wolters Kluwer.

Sjoding, M. W., Dickson, R. P., Iwashyna, T. J., Gay, S. E., & Valley, T. S. (2020). Racial bias in pulse oximetry measurement. *New England Journal of Medicine, 383*(25), 2477–2478. DOI: 10.1056/NEJMc2029240

Spader, C. (2020, June 26). *The new normal: Nurses as innovators.* American Nurse. https://www.myamericannurse.com/the-new-normal-nurses-as-innovators/

Stanford Children's Health. (2021). *Respiratory distress syndrome (RDS) in premature babies.* https://www.stanfordchildrens.org/en/topic/default?id=respiratory-distress-syndrome-90-P02371

Sterni, L. M., Collaco, J. M., & Baker, C. D. (2016). An official American Thoracic Society clinical practice guideline: Pediatric chronic home invasive ventilation. *American Journal of Respiratory and Critical Care Medicine, 193*(8), e16–e35. https://doi.org/10.1164/rccm.201602-0276ST

Strickland, S. L., Rubin, B. K., Drescher, G. S., Haas, C. F., O'Malley, C. A., Volsko, T. A., Branson, R. D., Hess, D. R., & American Association for Respiratory Care, Irving, Texas. (2013). AARC clinical practice guideline: Effectiveness of nonpharmacologic airway clearance therapies in hospitalized patients. *Respiratory Care, 58*(12), 2187–2193.https://doi.org/10.4187/respcare.02925

Tasota, F. J., Kress, T. L., Conlin, T. L., & Scarmack, N. M. (2021). Nasal cannula or high-flow oxygen for patients with COPD in acute respiratory distress? *Nursing, 51*(5), 52–57. https://doi.org/10.1097/01.NURSE.0000743096.13461.b6

The Society for Cardiological Science & Technology (SCST). (2017). *Clinical guidelines by consensus: Recording a standard 12-lead electrocardiogram.* An approved methodology by the Society for Cardiological Science & Technology (SCST). https://www.bmj.com/sites/default/files/response_attachments/2016/09/CAC_SCST_Recording_a_12-lead_ECG_final_version_2014_CS2v2.0.pdf

Tolotti, A., Bagnasco, A., Catania, G., Aleo,G., Pagnucci, N., Cadorin, L., Zanini, M., Rocco, G., Stievano, A., Carnevale, F. A., & Sasso, L. (2018). The communication experience of tracheostomy patients with nurses in the intensive care unit: A phenomenological study. *Intensive & Critical Care Nursing, 46*(X), 24–31. https://doi.org/10.1016/j.iccn.2018.01.001

Toughy, T. A., & Jett, K. (2018). *Ebersol and Hess' gerontological nursing & healthy aging* (5th ed.). Elsevier.

Turner, M. A., Feeney, M., & Deeds, J. L. (2020). Improving endotracheal cuff inflation pressures: An evidence-based project in a military medical center. *AANA Journal, 88*(3), 203–208.

Turner, M. C., Andersen, Z. J., Baccarelli, A., Diver, W. R., Gapstur, S. M., Pope III, A., Prada, D., Samet, J., Thurston, G., & Cohen, A. (2020). Outdoor air pollution and cancer: An overview of the current evidence and public health recommendations. *CA: A Cancer Journal for Clinicians, 70*, 460–479. https://doi.org/10.3322/caac.21632

U.S. Department of Agriculture (USDA) and U.S. Department of Health and Human Services (DHHS). (2020, December). *Dietary Guidelines for Americans, 2020–2025* (9th ed.). https://www.dietaryguidelines.gov/sites/default/files/2020-12/Dietary_Guidelines_for_Americans_2020-2025.pdf

U.S. Department of Health and Human Services (USDHHS). Office of Disease Prevention and Health Promotion. (2018). *Physical activity guidelines for Americans* (2nd ed.). https://health.gov/sites/default/files/2019-09/Physical_Activity_Guidelines_2nd_edition.pdf

U. S. Department of Health and Human Services. Office of Disease Prevention and Health Promotion (U.S. DHHS & ODPHP). (n.d.). *Healthy people 2030. Social determinants of health.* Retrieved December 27, 2021, from https://health.gov/healthypeople/objectives-anddata/social-determinants-health

U.S. Environmental Protection Agency (EPA). (2021, April 8). *Particle pollution and your patients' health.* https://www.epa.gov/pmcourse/patient-exposure-and-high-particle-pollution-events

U.S. Food and Drug Administration (USFDA). (2021, February 19). *Pulse oximeter accuracy and limitations: FDA safety communication.* https://www.fda.gov/medical-devices/safety-communications/pulse-oximeter-accuracy-and-limitations-fda-safety-communication

University of California San Diego Health. (2021). *Pulmonary & critical care medicine. Transtracheal oxygen catheter (TTO).* https://health.ucsd.edu/specialties/pulmonary/procedures/pages/transtracheal-oxygen-catheter.aspx

University of Iowa Health Care. (2017, June 5). *Iowa head and neck protocols. Tracheostomy home care booklet.* https://medicine.uiowa.edu/iowaprotocols/tracheostomy-home-care-booklet

University of Michigan Health. (2020, August 4). *Spinal cord injury: Assisted cough.* C. S. Mott Children's Hospital. https://www.mottchildren.org/health-library/ug2709

Venus, K., Munshi, L., & Fralick, M. (2020). Prone positioning for patients with hypoxic respiratory failure related to COVID-19. *Canadian Medical Association Journal, 192*(47), E1532–E1537. https://doi.org/10.1503/cmaj.201201

VHA Center for Engineering & Occupational Safety and Health (CEOSH). (2016). *Safe patient handling and mobility guidebook.* http://www.tnpatientsafety.com/pubfiles/Initiatives/workplace-violence/sphm-pdf.pdf

Vottier, G., Matrot, B., Jones, P., & Dauger, S. (2016). A cross-over study of continuous tracheal cuff pressure monitoring in critically-ill children. *Journal of Intensive Care Medicine, 42*(1), 132–133. https://doi.org/1007/s00134-015-4103-8

Wang, C. H., Tsai, J. C., Chen, S. F., Su, C. L., Chen, L., Lin, C. C., & Tam, K. W. (2017). Normal saline installation before suctioning: A meta-analysis of randomized controlled trials. *Australian Critical Care, 30*(5), 260–265. https://doi.org/10.1016/j.aucc.2016.11.001

Wang, Y., Huang, D., Ni, Y., & Liang, Z. (2020). High-flow nasal cannula vs conventional oxygen therapy for post cardiothoracic surgery. *Respiratory Care, 65*(11), 1730–1737. https://doi.org/10.4187/respcare.07595

Warnock, L., & Gates, A. (2015). Chest physiotherapy compared to no chest physiotherapy for cystic fibrosis. *Cochrane Database of Systematic Reviews. 2015*(12), CD001401. https://doi.org/10.1002/14651858.CD001401.pub3

WoltersKluwer. (2022). Problem-based care plans. In *Lippincott Advisor.* Wolters Kluwer.

Wood, M. S., Powers, J., & Rechter, J. L. (2019). Comparative evaluation of chest tube insertion site dressings: A randomized controlled trial. *American Journal of Critical Care, 28*(6), 415–423. https://doi.org/10.4037/ajcc2019645

World Health Organization (WHO). (2021). *Coronavirus.* https://www.who.int/health-topics/coronavirus#tab=tab_1

Wrona, S. K., Quinlan-Colwell, A., Brown, L., & Enricoso Jannuzzi, R. G. (2021, December 27). Procedural pain management: Clinical practice recommendations American Society for Pain Management Nursing. *Pain Management Nursing, S1524–9042*(21), 00245-9. https://doi.org/10.1016/j.pmn.2021.11.008

Yarahmadi, S., Mohammadi, N., Ardalan, A., Najafizadeh, H., & Gholami, M. (2018). The combined effects of cold therapy and music therapy on pain following chest tube removal among patients with cardiac bypass surgery. *Complementary Therapies in Clinical Practice, 31*, 71–75. https://doi.org/10.1016/j.ctcp.2018.01.006

Yazdannik, A., Saghaei, M., Haghighat, S., & Eghbali-Babadi, M. (2019). Efficacy of closed endotracheal suctioning in critically ill patients: A clinical trial of comparing two levels of suctioning pressure. *Journal of Nursing Practice Today, 6*(2), 60–67.

Yönt, G. H., Korhan, E. A., & Dizer, B. (2014). The effect of nail polish on pulse oximetry readings. *Intensive and Critical Care Nursing, 30*(2), 111–115. DOI: 10.1016/j.iccn.2013.08.003

Zemach, S., Helviz, Y., Shitrit, M., Friedman, R., & Levin, P. D. (2019). The use of high-flow nasal cannula oxygen outside the ICU. *Respiratory Care, 64*(11), 1333–1342. https://doi.org/10.4187/respcare.06611

41 Fluid, Electrolyte, and Acid–Base Balance

Grace Gilligan

Grace, a 28-year-old female, arrives at the emergency department reporting severe episodes of nausea and vomiting over the last 48 hours. She has a medical history of Crohn's disease, a gastrointestinal (GI) problem for which she underwent bowel resection surgery 1 month ago. "I thought the surgery would help my problems," she says. Intravenous (IV) therapy was prescribed to restore her fluid balance.

Jeremiah Stein

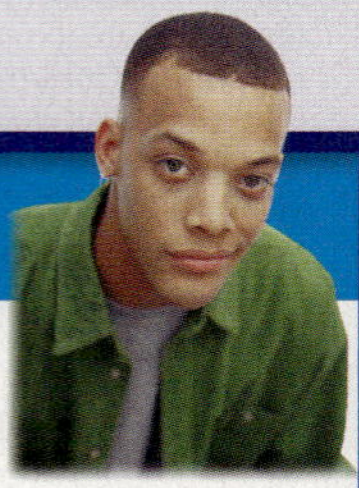

Jeremiah, a 22-year-old student, comes to the campus health center because he has been having two or three loose, watery bowel movements a day for the past week. "I kept thinking I would get better. I didn't have time to come to the clinic because of exams and I have been so busy, but now I don't feel good and I'm weak." Fluid volume deficit and electrolyte imbalances are a concern.

Jack Soo Park

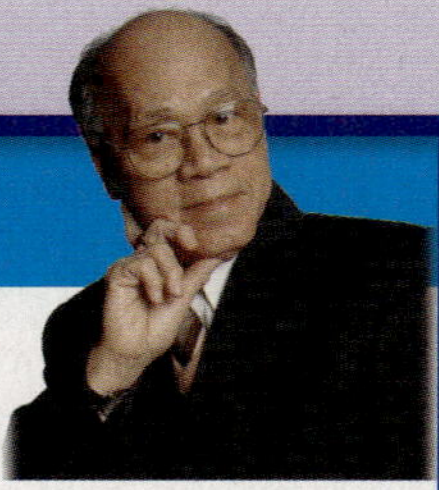

Jack, a 78-year-old male receiving IV therapy with antibiotics, states, "I'm having trouble breathing. It just started a little while ago." Physical examination reveals a bounding pulse, distended neck veins, and crackles and wheezes in the lungs. Excess fluid volume is suspected. Further checking reveals an IV fluid-administration error that has resulted in overhydration.

Lippincott DocuCare **Additional patient scenarios available in *Lippincott DocuCare.***

Learning Outcomes

After completing the chapter, you will be able to accomplish the following:

1. Describe the location and functions of body fluids, including the factors that affect variations in fluid compartments.
2. Describe the functions, regulation, sources, and losses of the main electrolytes of the body.
3. Explain the principles of osmosis, diffusion, active transport, and filtration.
4. Describe how thirst and the organs of homeostasis (kidneys, heart and blood vessels, lungs, adrenal glands, pituitary gland, parathyroid glands) function to maintain fluid homeostasis.
5. Describe the role of buffer systems and respiratory and renal mechanisms in achieving and maintaining acid–base balance.
6. Identify the etiologies and defining characteristics for common fluid, electrolyte, and acid–base imbalances.
7. Perform assessments related to fluid, electrolyte, and acid–base balance.
8. Describe the role of dietary modification, modification of fluid intake, medication administration, IV therapy, blood replacement, and parenteral nutrition (PN) as part of care to address fluid, electrolyte, and acid–base imbalances.
9. Plan, implement, and evaluate nursing care related to selected actual and potential health problems and needs associated with alterations in fluid, electrolyte, and acid–base balance.

Nursing Concepts

- Acid–Base Balance
- Assessment
- Cellular Regulation
- Clinical Decision Making/Clinical Judgment
- Fluids and Electrolytes
- Safety

The balance, or **homeostasis**, of fluid, electrolytes, and acid–base is interrelated and maintained through the functions of almost every organ of the body. In a healthy person, fluid intake and fluid losses are about equal. Abnormalities in fluid, electrolyte, and acid–base balance are also interrelated and may occur together. This chapter provides information about principles of fluid, electrolyte, and acid–base balance and common disturbances. Sample interview questions for performing a fluid-balance assessment are included, with information on related physical assessment techniques and laboratory studies. Potential and actual health problems and needs are provided, and patient outcomes related to fluid and electrolyte balance are described. Appropriate nursing interventions include ongoing assessments, modifying dietary and fluid intake, administering medications, assisting with IV therapy, and blood replacement. The accompanying Concept Map on page 1714 and Evolving Case Study 41-1 on page 1728 provide opportunities to develop and apply clinical reasoning and clinical judgment skills.

Nurses combine knowledge of fluid, electrolyte, and acid–base balance with skilled nursing assessments and interventions to resolve alterations in health status and to improve patient outcomes. Refer to the accompanying Reflective Practice box.

PRINCIPLES OF FLUID, ELECTROLYTES, AND ACID–BASE BALANCE

Fluids and electrolytes are vital to life; adequate balance is imperative to maintain healthy functioning of the body. Fluids and electrolytes are involved in almost every cellular reaction and function. Chemical reactions that occur in the body depend on a regulated acid and base balance.

Body Fluids

The primary body fluid is water, making it the most important nutrient of life. Although life can be sustained for many days without food, humans can survive for only a few days without water. Water in the body functions primarily to:

- Transport nutrients to cells and wastes from cells
- Transport hormones, enzymes, blood platelets, and red and white blood cells
- Facilitate cellular metabolism and proper cellular chemical functioning
- Act as a solvent for electrolytes and nonelectrolytes
- Help maintain normal body temperature
- Facilitate digestion and promote elimination
- Act as a tissue lubricant

The term *total body water* or *fluid* refers to the total amount of water, which is approximately 50% to 60% of body weight in a healthy person (Brinkman et al., 2021).

Body Fluid Compartments

Body fluid is located in two fluid compartments—the intracellular fluid or extracellular fluid, based on its location in the body. **Intracellular fluid (ICF)** is the fluid within cells, constituting about 70% of the total body water or about 40% of the adult's body weight (Brinkman et al., 2021). **Extracellular fluid (ECF)** is all the fluid outside the cells, accounting for about 30% of the total body water or about 20% of the adult's body weight (Brinkman et al., 2021). ECF includes two major areas, the vascular (intravascular) and interstitial compartments. A third, usually minor, compartment is the transcellular fluid compartment. Intravascular fluid, or plasma, is the liquid component of the blood (i.e., fluid found

QSEN Reflective Practice: Cultivating QSEN Competencies

CHALLENGE TO INTERPERSONAL SKILLS

During my clinical rotation in the emergency department, I met Grace Gilligan. She was a 28-year-old woman who came to the emergency department with severe episodes of nausea and vomiting over the last 48 hours. She has a past medical history of Crohn's disease, a GI problem for which she underwent bowel resection surgery 1 month ago. "I thought the surgery would help my problems." The patient was dehydrated and needed IV fluid therapy.

My coassigned nurse attempted to start a peripheral venous access not once, but six times. The patient was already upset by her recurrent abdominal symptoms, but now had to deal with the continuous painful stick of a needle. During the course of attempts to start the IV, the patient stated that a nurse on the IV team always had to be called to insert her IVs. Although my nurse acknowledged the information, she continued trying to start the IV. Finally, on the sixth try, as the patient was in tears, the nurse was successful. It seemed as if the nurse was out to prove her abilities without caring for the patient. By the end, I had difficulty even watching.

Thinking Outside the Box: Possible Courses of Action

- While assisting the nurse to obtain more supplies (outside the patient's room), mention to the nurse that maybe the use of ultrasound to guide placement and/or the IV team should be called (as the patient had requested), since "enough is enough!"
- Tell my clinical instructor that the patient is being abused.
- Ask the doctor if they could address the situation.
- Tell the patient when the nurse was out of the room to refuse any more sticks until the IV team was called.

Evaluating a Good Outcome: How Do I Define Success?

- Patient is benefited by my actions . . . or at least not harmed.
- All actions are supported by rationale.
- The patient's wishes are respected.
- Personal integrity is not compromised.

Personal Learning: Here's to the Future!

Unfortunately, I did not take any actions to protect this patient. This was my first time in the emergency department as well as my first introduction to the nurse. I was intimidated by her. Furthermore, I was scared when she continued to attempt the catheter insertion with the patient in tears. I know that it is my responsibility to advocate for the needs of my patients. In the future, I hope that I will never compromise my integrity, beliefs, and values to prove something to a student. If I fail or am not confident in my skills, I will admit this and stop before my patient is put at risk.

Amy Persinger, Georgetown University

QSEN SELF-REFLECTION ON QUALITY AND SAFETY COMPETENCIES DEVELOPING KNOWLEDGE, SKILLS, AND ATTITUDES FOR CONTINUOUS IMPROVEMENT

How do you think you would respond in a similar situation? What does this tell you about yourself and about the adequacy of your skills for professional practice? Why? Do you agree with the criteria that the nursing student used to evaluate a successful outcome? Are there any other criteria that would be appropriate to use? Did the nursing student meet the criteria? Why or why not? What *knowledge, skills,* and *attitudes* do you need to develop to continuously improve the quality and safety of care for patients like Ms. Gilligan?

Patient-Centered Care: How could you involve Ms. Gilligan as a partner in coordinating her care to minimize frustration on the part of the patient, student, and nurse? What might have prompted the emergency department nurse to act as she did? The nursing student? How could the nursing student have advocated for the patient? What other barriers (other than those listed) might have interfered with the nursing student acting as an advocate?

Teamwork and Collaboration/Quality Improvement: What communication skills do you need to improve to ensure that you function as a member of the patient-care team? What skills do you need to implement effective strategies for communicating and resolving conflict? What skills do you need to assert your own position/perspective in discussions about patient care?

Safety/Evidence-Based Practice: What evidence for practice provides guidance for decision making regarding professional practice and venipuncture?

Informatics: Can you identify the essential information that must be available in Ms. Gilligan's electronic record to support safe patient care and coordination of care? Can you think of other ways to respond to or approach the situation?

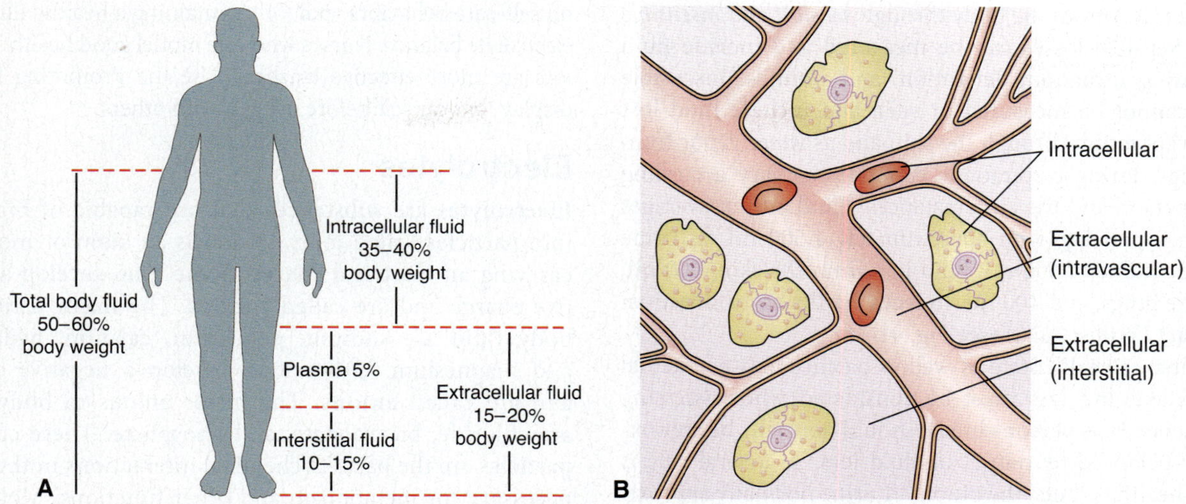

FIGURE 41-1. **A.** Total body fluid represents 50% to 60% of body weight of a normal adult. **B.** Primary fluid compartments.

within the vascular system). Interstitial fluid is the fluid that surrounds tissue cells and includes lymph (Hinkle et al., 2022). Transcellular fluids include cerebrospinal, pericardial, synovial, intraocular, and pleural fluids, as well as sweat and digestive secretions. The capillary walls and cell membranes separate the intracellular and extracellular compartments. Figure 41-1 illustrates the components of total body fluid and the primary fluid compartments.

Variations in Fluid Content

Variations in the fluid content from the normal 50% to 60% of the body's weight can occur, depending on such factors as the person's age, body fat, and biologic sex. Infants have considerably more total body fluid and ECF than adults. Because ECF is more easily lost from the body than ICF, infants are at increased risk for fluid volume deficits (FVDs).

Total body water also differs by biologic sex and the amount of fat cells in the body. Fat cells contain little water, whereas lean tissue is rich in water. Thus, the more obese a person is, the smaller the person's percentage of total body water is when compared with body weight. Because women tend to have proportionally more body fat than men do, they also have less body fluid than men.

Similarly, the decreasing percentage of body fluid in older people is related to an increase in fat cells. In addition, older adults lose muscle mass as a part of aging. The combined increase of fat and loss of muscle results in reduced total body water; after the age 60 years, total body water is about 45% of a person's body weight (Willis, 2020). This decrease in water increases the risk for fluid imbalance in older adults.

Fluid Balance

The human body obtains water from several sources, including ingested liquids, food, and as a byproduct of metabolism. The ingestion of liquids provides the largest amount of water normally taken into the body. Fluid intake is regulated primarily by the thirst mechanism. Located within the hypothalamus, the thirst control center is stimulated by intracellular **dehydration** (the loss of or deprivation of water from the cells [Willis, 2020]) and decreased blood volume. The water contained in food is the second largest source of water for the body. The amount of water ingested depends on the person's dietary intake. For example, melons and citrus fruit are high in water content, whereas cereal and dried fruits have relatively low water content. Water is an end product of the oxidation that occurs during the metabolism of food substances, specifically carbohydrates, fats, and protein. This amount of water obtained varies among the different types of nutrients. In general, fluid intake averages 2,600 mL per day, with approximately 1,500 mL coming from ingested liquids; 800 mL coming from ingested food, and 300 mL from metabolic oxidation (Willis, 2020). Figure 41-2 illustrates daily fluid balance in a healthy person.

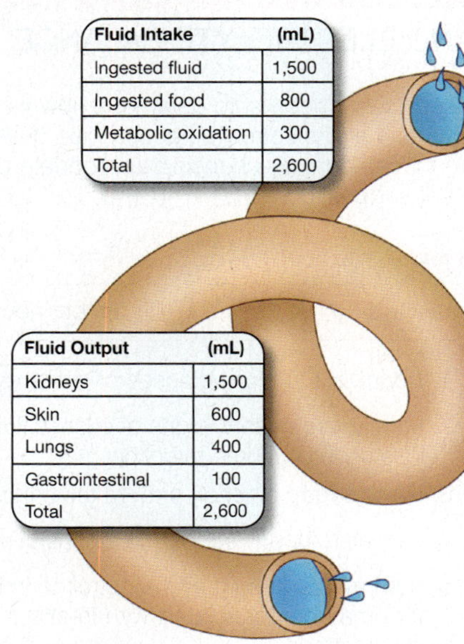

Fluid Intake	(mL)
Ingested fluid	1,500
Ingested food	800
Metabolic oxidation	300
Total	2,600

Fluid Output	(mL)
Kidneys	1,500
Skin	600
Lungs	400
Gastrointestinal	100
Total	2,600

FIGURE 41-2. In health, fluid intake and fluid losses are about equal. The amounts indicated are average adult daily fluid sources and losses.

Fluid is lost from the body through *sensible* and *insensible* losses. Sensible losses can be measured and include fluid lost during urination, defecation, and wounds. Insensible losses cannot be measured or seen and include fluid lost from evaporation through the skin and as water vapor from the lungs during respiration. Water losses vary according to the person and the circumstances. Fluid output averages 2,600 mL per day, with approximately 1,500 mL as urine from the kidneys, 600 mL fluid loss from the skin, 400 mL from the lungs, and 100 mL in feces via the gastrointestinal (GI) tract (Willis, 2020) (see Fig. 41-2).

A person's health state as well as balance between actual fluid intake and loss must be considered when assessing nursing needs. A person's intake should normally be approximately balanced by output or fluid loss. A general rule is that in healthy adults, the output of urine normally approximates the ingestion of liquids, and the water from food and oxidation is balanced by the water loss through the feces, the skin, and the respiratory process. The intake–output balance may not always occur in a single 24-hour period but should normally be achieved within 2 to 3 days.

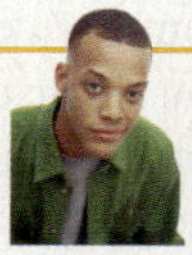

Consider **Jeremiah Stein**, the young student experiencing loose bowel movements for a week. Jeremiah is at increased risk for fluid imbalance related to the increased loss of water via the GI tract. It would be important for the nurse in the health center to teach Jeremiah about the need to increase their fluid intake to compensate for the extra losses.

Any deviations from normal ranges for a balanced water intake and output should alert the nurse to potential imbalances. The accompanying Promoting Health 4-1 display reflects on self-care behaviors vital for maintaining a healthy fluid and electrolyte balance. Nurses who role model good health behaviors are more effective teachers. Use the Promoting Health display for yourself before using it with others.

Electrolytes

Electrolytes are substances that are capable of breaking into particles called ions. An **ion** is an atom or molecule carrying an electrical charge. Some ions develop a positive charge and are called **cations**. The major cations in body fluid are sodium, potassium, calcium, hydrogen, and magnesium. Other ions develop a negative charge and are called **anions**. The major anions in body fluid are chloride, bicarbonate, and phosphate. These charged particles are the basis of chemical interactions in the body necessary for metabolism and other functions. Molecules in the body that remain intact, without a charge, are called nonelectrolytes. In the human body, urea and glucose are examples of nonelectrolytes.

The electrolyte content of the fluids in various compartments of the body differs significantly. Major electrolytes in the ECF include sodium, chloride, calcium, and bicarbonate. Major electrolytes in the ICF include potassium, phosphorus, and magnesium. The functions, sources, means of loss, and regulation of these electrolytes are highlighted in Table 41-1; hydrogen is discussed as part of acid–base balance. Figure 41-3 (on page 1674) illustrates differences in the electrolyte composition of body fluids according to the compartments in which the fluids are found.

Electrolytes are measured in terms of their chemical combining power, or chemical activity. The milliequivalent (mEq) is the unit of measure that describes the chemical activity of electrolytes. One milliequivalent of either a cation

Promoting Health 41-1

FLUID AND ELECTROLYTE BALANCE

Use the assessment checklist to determine how well you are meeting your fluid and electrolyte needs. Then develop a prescription for self-care by choosing appropriate behaviors from the list of suggestions.

Assessment Checklist

☐ almost always ☐ sometimes ☐ almost never

☐ ☐ ☐ 1. I drink six to eight glasses of water every day.

☐ ☐ ☐ 2. I am aware of early signs of excess fluid volume loss or fluid volume retention.

☐ ☐ ☐ 3. I limit sugar, alcohol, and caffeine in my diet.

☐ ☐ ☐ 4. I am alert for any sudden variations in my weight.

☐ ☐ ☐ 5. I am aware of fluid and electrolyte imbalances that may be associated with intake of certain medications

☐ ☐ ☐ 6. I diet sensibly when I need to lose weight.

Self-Care Behaviors

1. Consume about 1½ quarts of water daily.
2. Maintain normal body weight.
3. Avoid consuming excess amounts of products high in salt, sugar, and caffeine.
4. Limit alcohol intake because of its diuretic effect.
5. Obtain medical evaluation for any ongoing indications of fluid imbalance.
6. Monitor side effects of medications, especially diuresis and diarrhea.
7. Identify situations of high risk for fluid and electrolyte imbalance and intervene appropriately.

Information to promote fluid and electrolyte balance is available online.

Table 41-1 Major Electrolytes

ELECTROLYTE	FUNCTIONS	SOURCES AND LOSSES	REGULATION
Sodium (Na^+): chief electrolyte of ECF; normal serum concentration of sodium: 135–145 mEq/L	Regulates extracellular fluid volume; Na^+ loss or gain accompanied by a loss or gain of water Affects serum osmolality Role in muscle contraction and transmission of nerve impulses Regulation of acid–base balance as sodium bicarbonate	Normally enters the body through the gastrointestinal tract from dietary sources, such as salt added to processed foods, sodium preservatives added to processed foods Lost from GI tract, kidneys, and skin	Transported out of the cell by the sodium-potassium pump Regulated by renin–angiotensin–aldosterone system Elimination and reabsorption regulated by the kidneys Sodium concentrations affected by salt and water intake
Potassium (K^+): major cation of ICF; normal serum concentration of potassium: 3.5–5.0 mEq/L	Controls intracellular osmolality Regulator of cellular enzyme activity Role in the transmission of electrical impulses in nerve, heart, skeletal, intestinal, and lung tissue; Regulation of acid–base balance by cellular exchange with H^+	Adequate quantities via a well-balanced diet Leading food sources: fruits and vegetables, dried peas and beans, whole grains, milk, meats Lost via kidneys, stool, sweat, emesis	Regulated by aldosterone Eliminated by the kidneys (no effective method of conserving potassium) Additional regulation via transcellular shift between the ICF and ECF compartments
Calcium (Ca^{2+}): most abundant electrolyte in the body; normal total serum calcium level: 8.6–10.2 mg/dL; normal ionized serum calcium level: 4.5–5.1 mg/dL	Role in blood coagulation and in transmission of nerve impulses Helps regulate muscle contraction and relaxation Major component of bones and teeth	Absorbed from foods in the presence of normal gastric acidity and vitamin D Lost via feces and urine Sources include milk and milk products; dried beans; green, leafy vegetables; small fish with bones; and dried peas and beans	Primarily excreted by GI tract; lesser extent by kidneys Regulated by parathyroid hormone and calcitonin High serum phosphate results in decreased serum calcium; low serum phosphate leads to increased serum calcium
Magnesium (Mg^{2+}): second most abundant ICF cation after potassium; normal serum concentration of magnesium: 1.3–2.3 mEq/L	Metabolism of carbohydrates and proteins Role in neuromuscular function Acts on cardiovascular system, producing vasodilation	Enters the body via GI tract Sources include green, leafy vegetables; nuts; seafood; whole grains; dried peas and beans; cocoa Lost via urine with use of loop diuretics	Eliminated by kidneys Regulated by parathyroid hormone
Chloride (Cl^-): major ECF anion; normal serum level of chloride: 97–107 mEq/L	Major component of interstitial and lymph fluid; gastric and pancreatic juices, sweat, bile, and saliva Acts with sodium to maintain the osmotic pressure Combines with hydrogen ions to produce hydrochloric acid	Enters body via GI tract Almost all chloride in diet comes from salt Found in foods high in sodium, processed foods	Normally paired with sodium; excreted and conserved with sodium by the kidneys Regulated by aldosterone Low potassium level leads to low chloride level
Bicarbonate (HCO_3^-): an anion that is the major chemical base buffer within the body; found in both ECF and ICF; normal serum bicarbonate level: 25–29 mEq/L	Regulates acid–base balance	Losses possible via diarrhea, diuretics, and early renal insufficiency Excess possible via overingestion of acid neutralizers, such as sodium bicarbonate	Bicarbonate levels regulated primarily by the kidneys Bicarbonate readily available as a result of carbon dioxide formation during metabolism
Phosphate (PO_4^-): major ICF anion; a buffer anion in both ICF and ECF; normal serum phosphate level: 2.5–4.5 mg/dL	Role in acid–base balance as a hydrogen buffer Promotes energy storage; carbohydrate, protein, and fat metabolism Bone and teeth formation Role in muscle and red blood cell function	Enters body via GI tract Sources include all animal products (meat, poultry, eggs, milk, bread, ready-to-eat cereal) Absorption is diminished by concurrent ingestion of calcium, magnesium, and aluminum	Eliminated by kidneys Regulation by parathyroid hormone and by activated vitamin D Phosphate and calcium are inversely proportional; an increase in one results in a decrease in the other

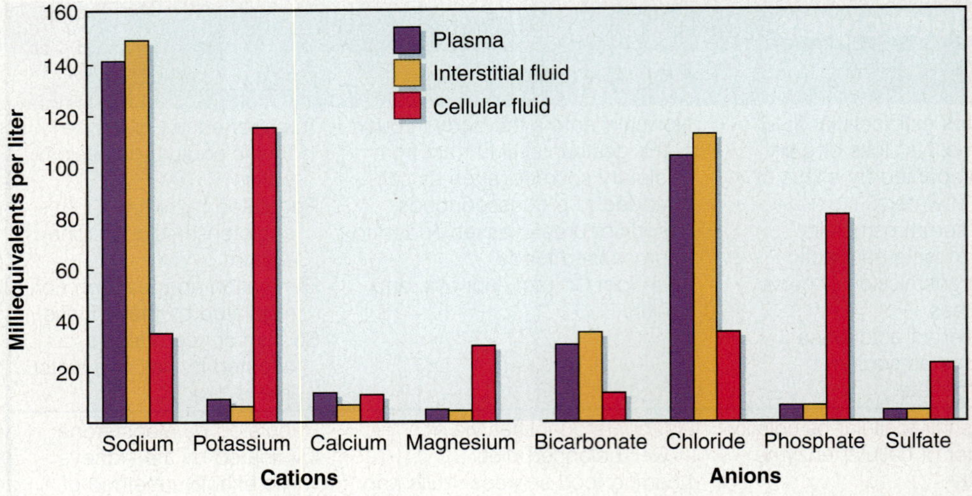

FIGURE 41-3. Electrolyte composition of body fluids according to compartment.

or an anion is chemically equivalent to the activity of 1 mg of hydrogen. Therefore, 1 mEq of any cation is equivalent to 1 mEq of any anion. The total cations in the body are normally equal to the total anions, maintaining homeostasis (balanced state). In healthy people, the milliequivalents per liter for electrolytes in the body vary within a relatively narrow range. When electrolytes are not in balance, the person is at risk for alterations in health.

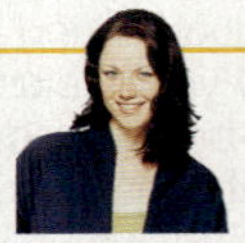

Consider ***Grace Gilligan***, the young female described in one of the beginning chapter scenarios. The nurse would need to be alert for electrolyte imbalances and possible acid–base imbalance due to the loss of gastric secretions from vomiting.

Regulation and Homeostatic Mechanisms of Fluid and Electrolyte Balance

Maintaining homeostasis of fluid volume and electrolytes is essential to healthy body functioning. Fluid and electrolyte homeostasis normally functions automatically and effectively.

Fluid and electrolyte balance is maintained by a number of mechanisms to facilitate fluid and electrolyte movement within the body. **Solvents** are liquids that hold a substance in solution; **solutes** are substances that are dissolved in a solution. Water is the primary solvent in the body. The solutes are electrolytes and nonelectrolytes. The body produces balance by shifting fluids and solutes between the ECF and the ICF. The mechanisms responsible for regulating this shift of fluids and transporting materials to and from intracellular compartments include organs and body systems, osmosis, diffusion, active transport, and capillary filtration, and are described in the following sections.

Organs and Body Systems

Almost every organ and system in the body helps in some way to maintain fluid homeostasis. The specific functions of these organs and body systems related to the regulation of fluid and electrolyte balance are highlighted in Table 41-2.

Osmosis

Cell membranes are semipermeable, allowing some, but not all, solutes to pass through the cell membranes. The cell membrane is permeable to water or fluids. Through the process of **osmosis**, water (the solvent) passes from an area of lesser solute concentration and more water to an area of greater solute concentration and less water until equilibrium is established. As a result, the volume of the more concentrated solution increases, and the volume of the weaker solution decreases. The process of osmosis stops when the concentration of solutes has been equalized on both sides of the cell membrane. The greater the difference in the concentration of the two solutions on each side of a semipermeable membrane, the greater the osmotic pressure of water. Osmosis is the major method of transporting body fluids. Water shifts and balance depend heavily on this route of transport, illustrated in Figure 41-4 on page 1676.

The concentration (number) of particles dissolved in a solution is referred to as the **osmolality** of a solution, which influences the movement of fluid between compartments (Hinkle et al., 2022). A solution that has about the same osmolality as plasma (280 mOsm/L) is considered an isotonic solution (Norris, 2020). An **isotonic** fluid remains in the intravascular compartment without any net flow across the semipermeable membrane. In contrast, a **hypertonic solution** has a greater osmolality than. Because a hypertonic solution has a greater osmolality, water moves out of the cells and is drawn into the intravascular compartment, causing the cells to shrink. A **hypotonic solution** has less osmolality than plasma. Because of a lower osmolality, a hypotonic solution in the intravascular space moves out of the intravascular space and into ICF, causing cells to swell and possibly burst.

Diffusion

Diffusion is the tendency of solutes to move freely throughout a solvent. The solute moves from an area of higher

Table 41-2 Organs and Body Systems Related to the Regulation of Fluid, Electrolyte, and Acid–Base Balance

ORGAN/BODY SYSTEM	FUNCTIONS
Kidneys	• Regulate extracellular fluid (ECF) volume and osmolality by selective retention and excretion of body fluids • Regulate electrolyte levels in the ECF by selective retention of needed substances and excretion of unneeded substances • Regulate pH of ECF by excretion or retention of hydrogen ions • Excrete metabolic wastes (primarily acids) and toxic substances • Normally filter 180 L of blood daily in the adult, while excreting only 1–2 L of urine per day
Heart and blood vessels	• Circulate nutrients and water throughout the body • Circulate blood through the kidneys under sufficient pressure for urine to form (pumping action of the heart) • React to hypovolemia by stimulating fluid retention (stretch receptors in the atria and blood vessels)
Lungs	• Remove approximately 300 mL of water daily through exhalation (insensible water loss) in the normal adult • Eliminate about 13,000 mEq of hydrogen ions (H^+) daily, as opposed to only 40–80 mEq excreted daily by the kidneys • Act promptly to correct metabolic acid–base disturbances; regulate H^+ concentration (pH) by controlling the level of carbon dioxide (CO_2) in the extracellular fluid
Adrenal glands	• Regulate blood volume and sodium and potassium balance by secreting aldosterone, a mineral corticoid secreted by the adrenal cortex, causing sodium retention (and thus water retention) and potassium loss. • Decreased secretion of aldosterone causes sodium and water loss and potassium retention. • Cortisol, another adrenocortical hormone, has only a fraction of the potency of aldosterone. However, secretion of cortisol in large quantities can produce sodium and water retention and potassium deficit.
Pituitary gland	• Stores and releases the antidiuretic hormone (ADH) (manufactured in the hypothalamus), which acts to allow the body to retain water. It acts chiefly to regulate sodium and water intake and excretion. • When osmotic pressure of the ECF is greater than that of the cells (as in hypernatremia—excess sodium—or hyperglycemia), ADH secretion is increased, causing renal retention of water. • When osmotic pressure of the ECF is less than that of the cells (as in hyponatremia), ADH secretion is decreased, causing renal excretion of water. • When blood volume is decreased, an increased secretion of ADH results in water conservation. • When blood volume is increased, a decreased secretion of ADH results in water loss.
Thyroid gland	• Increases blood flow in the body by releasing thyroxine, leading to increased renal circulation and resulting in increased glomerular filtration and urinary output.
Nervous system	• Inhibits and stimulates mechanisms influencing fluid balance; acts chiefly to regulate sodium and water intake and excretion • Regulates oral intake by sensing intracellular dehydration, which triggers thirst (thirst center located in the hypothalamus) • Neurons, called osmoreceptors, are sensitive to changes in the concentration of ECF, sending appropriate impulses to the pituitary gland to release ADH or inhibit its release to maintain ECF volume concentration.
Gastrointestinal tract	Absorbs water and nutrients that enter the body through this route.
Parathyroid glands	• Regulate calcium (Ca^{2+}) and phosphate (HPO_4^{2}–) balance by means of parathyroid hormone (PTH); PTH influences bone reabsorption, calcium absorption from the intestines, and calcium reabsorption from the renal tubules. • Increased secretion of PTH causes elevated serum calcium concentration and lowered serum phosphate concentration. • Decreased secretion of PTH causes lowered serum calcium concentration and elevated serum phosphate concentration.

Source: Adapted from Metheny, N. M. (2012). *Fluid and electrolyte balance. Nursing considerations* (5th ed.). Jones & Bartlett Learning; Norris, T. L. (2020). *Porth's essentials of pathophysiology* (5th ed.). Wolters Kluwer; Willis, L. M. (Ed.). (2020). *Fluids & electrolytes made incredibly easy!* (7th ed.). Wolters Kluwer.

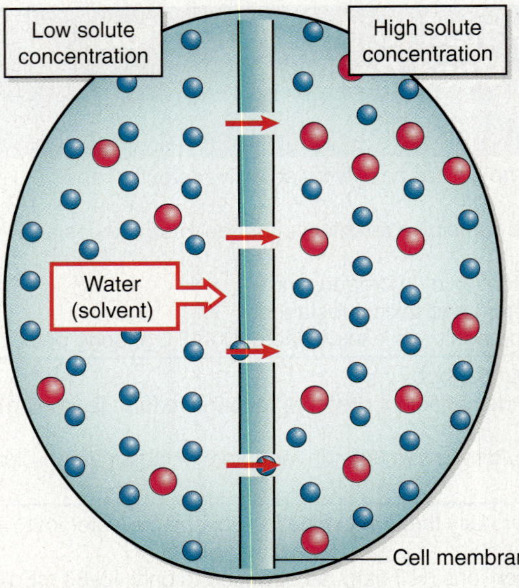

FIGURE 41-4. Osmosis. Body fluids are transported through cell membranes through the process of osmosis. Water, a solvent, moves from an area of lesser solute concentration to one of greater solute concentration, until equilibrium is established.

concentration to an area of lower concentration until equilibrium is established. Figure 41-5 illustrates this mechanism. Gases also move by diffusion. Oxygen and carbon dioxide exchange in the lung's alveoli and capillaries occurs by diffusion.

Active Transport

Active transport is a process that requires energy for the movement of substances through a cell membrane, against the concentration gradient, from an area of lesser solute concentration to an area of higher solute concentration. Adenosine triphosphate (ATP), which is stored in all cells, supplies energy for solute movement in and out of the

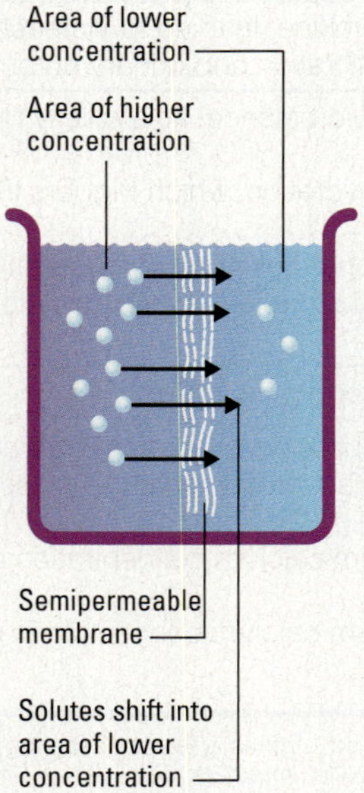

FIGURE 41-5. Diffusion. Solutes move from an area of higher concentration to an area of lower concentration until the concentration is equal in both areas.

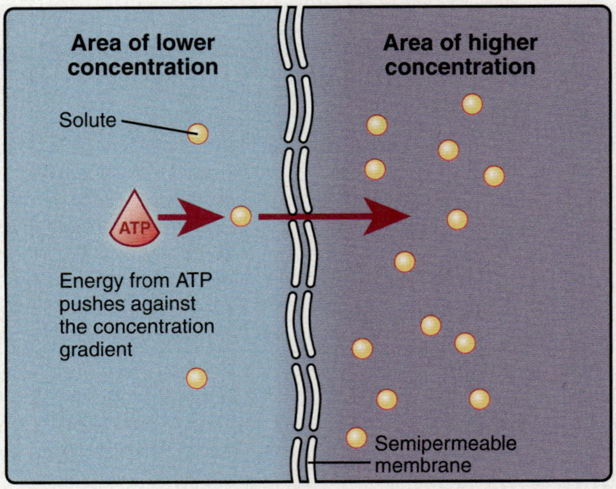

FIGURE 41-6. Active transport. Solutes are moved from an area of lower concentration to an area of higher concentration.

cell. Although this process is not entirely understood, the energy requirements for active transport are affected by characteristics of the cell membrane, specific enzymes, and concentrations of ions. This process explains the so-called pump mechanism, illustrated in Figure 41-6. Substances that require active transport to cross cell membranes include amino acids, glucose (in certain places only, such as in the kidneys and intestines), and ions of sodium, potassium, hydrogen, and calcium (Willis, 2020).

Capillary Filtration

Filtration is the passage of fluid through a permeable membrane. Fluids move from an area of high pressure to one of lower pressure. **Capillary filtration** results from the force of blood "pushing" against the walls of the capillaries. At the arterial end of the capillaries, filtration is dependent primarily on arterial blood pressure; at the venular side of the capillaries, filtration is dependent on venous blood pressure. The "pushing" force is referred to as **hydrostatic pressure**. When the hydrostatic pressure inside the capillary exceeds the surrounding interstitial space, fluids and solutes are forced out of the capillary wall into the interstitial space. In contrast, when the pressure inside the capillary is less than the pressure in the interstitial space, the fluids and solutes will move back into the capillary.

Reabsorption is the process that acts to prevent too much fluid from leaving the capillaries no matter how high the hydrostatic pressure. Plasma proteins, particularly albumin, concentrated in the intravascular space or plasma facilitate this reabsorption process by "pulling" the fluid back into the capillaries. This "pulling" force is known as **colloid osmotic pressure**, or oncotic pressure. Under normal conditions, hydrostatic pressure in the arteriole end of a capillary exceeds plasma colloid pressure. Hydrostatic pressure at the venule end of the capillary is less than plasma colloid pressure. As a result, capillary filtration occurs along the first half of the vessel, and reabsorption occurs along the second half. Filtration pressure is the difference between colloid osmotic pressure and blood hydrostatic pressure.

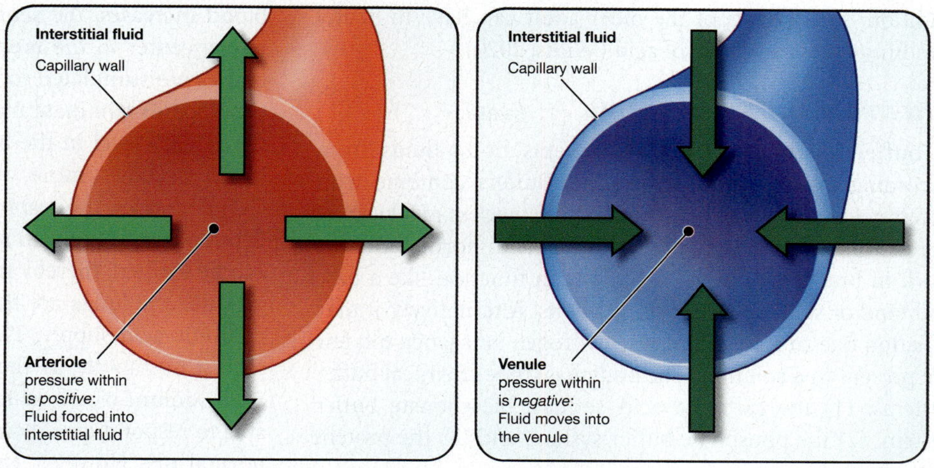

FIGURE 41-7. Capillary filtration.

These pressures are important in understanding how fluid leaves arterioles, enters the interstitial compartment, and eventually returns to the venules. The filtration pressure is positive in the arterioles, helping to force or filter fluids into interstitial spaces; it is negative in the venules and thus helps fluid enter the venules (refer to Fig. 41-7). Filtration is also involved in the proper functioning of the glomeruli of the kidneys.

Acid–Base Balance

Body fluids must maintain an acid–base balance to sustain health, homeostasis, and life. Specific chemical reactions are constantly occurring within the body that influence metabolism and the functions of various bodily systems. These chemical reactions are dependent on a balance of acids and bases. Changes in health such as infection or trauma may alter this delicate acid–base balance. Acidity or alkalinity of a solution is determined by its concentration of hydrogen ions (H^+). An **acid** is a substance containing H^+ that can be liberated or released, such as carbonic acid. An alkali, or **base**, is a substance that can accept or trap H^+ ions, such as the bicarbonate ion.

An acid releases H^+, as follows:

$$\underset{\text{carbonic acid}}{H_2CO_3} \xrightarrow{\text{releases}} \underset{\text{hydrogen ion}}{H^+} \underset{\text{to form}}{+} \underset{\text{bicarbonate base}}{HCO^-_3}$$

A base traps H^+, as follows:

$$\underset{\text{bicarbonate base}}{HCO^-_3} \underset{\text{traps}}{+} \underset{\text{hydrogen ion}}{H^+} \xrightarrow{\text{to form}} \underset{\text{carbonic acid}}{H_2CO_3}$$

A strong acid dissociates (separates) completely in solution and releases all of its H^+ ions, whereas a weak acid releases only a small number. A base that binds or accepts H^+ ions easily is considered a strong base, whereas one that accepts H^+ ions less readily is considered weak.

The unit of measure used to describe acid–base balance is **pH**, which is an expression of H^+ ion concentration and the resulting acidity or alkalinity of a substance. The pH scale ranges from 1 to 14. A neutral solution measures 7; an example of a neutral solution is pure water. Because pH is based on a negative logarithm, as the H^+ ions increase and a solution becomes more acid, the pH becomes less than 7. When the concentration of H^+ ions in a solution is reduced or accepted by another substance and the solution contains more base than acid, it is alkaline, and the pH is greater than 7. Gastric secretions that are strongly acidic have an approximate pH of 1 to 1.3, whereas strongly alkaline pancreatic secretions have an approximate pH of 10.

Normal blood plasma is slightly alkaline and has a normal pH range of 7.35 to 7.45 (Norris, 2020). When the blood plasma pH exceeds the normal pH range in either direction, signs and symptoms of illness develop, and if the condition goes on unabated, death results. **Acidosis** is the condition characterized by an excess of H ions or loss of base ions (bicarbonate) in ECF in which the pH falls below 7.35 (Willis, 2020). **Alkalosis** occurs when there is a loss of H ions or a gain of bases (e.g., bicarbonate) and the pH exceeds 7.45 (Willis, 2020). Refer to the Acid–Base Imbalances discussion on page 1681. Figure 41-8 illustrates normal pH, acidosis, and alkalosis and shows the points at which death typically occurs. The narrow range of normal pH is achieved through three major homeostatic regulators of hydrogen ions: (1) chemical buffer systems, (2) respiratory mechanisms, and (3) renal mechanisms. There are alterations in these systems related to the developmental stage of an individual. Newborns are not able to acidify urine as well as adults (Willis, 2020). As people age, the effectiveness of both the lungs and kidneys can vary. In an older adult, if there is underlying lung disease, the regulation of acid–base balance may be less efficient. In

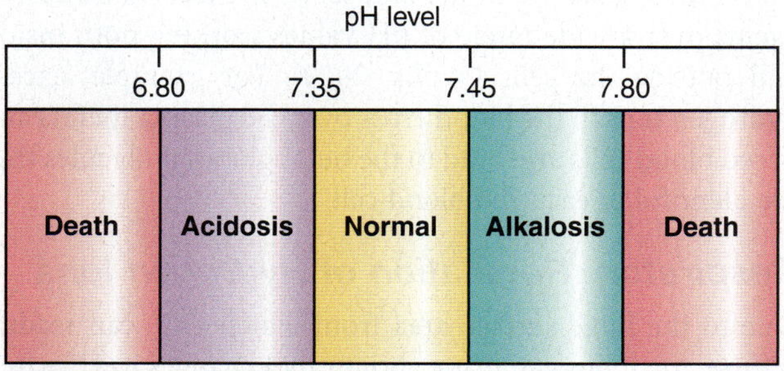

FIGURE 41-8. Acid–base balance. Note that acidosis is used to describe the condition of the pH falling below 7.35, and alkalosis describes a pH above 7.45. When the normal pH is exceeded in either direction, death can occur.

addition, the kidneys of the older adult can have difficulty handling excess amounts of acid (Willis, 2020).

Chemical Buffer Systems

A **buffer** is a substance that prevents body fluids from becoming overly acidic or alkaline. Buffers combine with excess acids or bases to prevent major changes in pH, keeping the pH of body fluids as close as possible to normal. Buffers work in one of two ways. A buffer can function like a base and bind or soak up free hydrogen ions. Alternatively, it may function like an acid and release hydrogen ions when too few are present in a solution. The body has three chemical buffer systems: (1) the carbonic acid–sodium bicarbonate buffer system, (2) the phosphate buffer system, and (3) the protein buffer system.

CARBONIC ACID–SODIUM BICARBONATE BUFFER SYSTEM

The ratio of carbonic acid (H_2CO_3), the most common acid in human body fluid, to the body's most common base, bicarbonate (HCO_3^-), is important for acid–base balance and is the most important buffer system of the body. Normal ECF has a ratio of 20 parts bicarbonate to 1 part carbonic acid (Hinkle et al., 2022). The exact quantities are unimportant for acid–base balance as long as they remain in a 20:1 ratio. Carbonic acid and bicarbonate must be carefully controlled to maintain this ratio; if either is increased or decreased, the 20:1 ratio is no longer in effect and pH will change (Norris, 2020). The lungs help by regulating the production of carbonic acid resulting from the combination of carbon dioxide and water. The kidneys assist the bicarbonate system by regulating the production of bicarbonate.

PHOSPHATE BUFFER SYSTEM

The phosphate buffer system is active in ICFs, especially in the renal tubules. Phosphate buffers react with either acids or bases to form compounds that slightly alter pH to provide effective buffering (Willis, 2020).

PROTEIN BUFFER SYSTEM

The third buffer system is a mixture of plasma proteins and the globin portion of hemoglobin in red blood cells. Because plasma proteins and hemoglobin possess chemical groups that can combine with or liberate hydrogen ions, they tend to minimize changes in pH and serve as excellent buffering agents over a wide range of pH values working both inside and outside the cells (Willis, 2020). For example, excess hydrogen ions in the blood cross over the plasma membrane of red blood cells and bind to the hemoglobin molecules that are plentiful in each red blood cell.

Respiratory Regulation of Hydrogen Ions

Due to the huge surface area from which CO_2 can readily diffuse, the lungs can bring about rapid changes in H^+ when needed. Carbon dioxide, constantly produced by cellular metabolism (carbonic acid [H_2CO_3] yields CO_2 and H_2O), is excreted by exhalation. When the amount of CO_2 in the blood increases, the sensitive chemoreceptors in the respiratory center in the medulla and in the carotid and aortic bodies are stimulated to increase the rate and depth of respirations to eliminate more CO_2. As more CO_2 is exhaled, the H_2CO_3 level in the blood decreases, and the pH of the blood becomes more alkaline. When the blood level of CO_2 decreases, the respiratory center decreases the rate and depth of respirations to retain the CO_2 so that carbonic acid can be formed, thereby maintaining the delicate balance. As a result, the lungs are the primary controller of the body's carbonic acid supply. This total respiratory process occurs almost as rapidly as the buffering action in the carbonic acid–sodium bicarbonate system. The respiratory system is able to respond quickly in a healthy individual to restore the normal pH. However, this response is short term, and the response of the kidneys is needed for long-term adjustment (Willis, 2020).

Renal Regulation of Hydrogen Ions

Essentially, the kidneys excrete or retain hydrogen ions and form or excrete bicarbonate ions in response to the pH of the blood. In the presence of acidosis, the kidneys excrete hydrogen ions and form and conserve bicarbonate ions, thus raising the pH to the normal range. If alkalosis is present, the kidneys retain hydrogen ions and excrete bicarbonate ions in an effort to return to a balanced state. As a result, the concentration of bicarbonate in the plasma is regulated by the kidneys.

Acid–base regulation by the kidneys occurs more slowly than that which occurs by the carbonic acid–sodium bicarbonate system or by respiratory regulation. It may take as long as 3 days for a normal fluid pH to be restored by the kidneys.

DISTURBANCES IN FLUID, ELECTROLYTE, AND ACID–BASE BALANCE

Nurses may encounter actual and potential disturbances in fluid, electrolyte, and acid–base balance while caring for patients in every care setting. Although many of these disturbances are interrelated and may occur together, they are described here separately for learning purposes.

Fluid Imbalances

Fluid imbalances occur when the body's compensatory mechanisms are unable to maintain a homeostatic state. Fluid imbalances involve either the volume or distribution of water or electrolytes. Nursing implications related to fluid volume disturbances—including risk factors, nursing assessments, and interventions—are discussed later in the chapter.

Fluid Volume Deficit

FVD occurs when loss of ECF volume exceeds the intake of fluid (Hinkle et al., 2022). FVD involves a loss of both water and solutes in the same proportion from the ECF space. This state is known as **hypovolemia** or isotonic fluid loss. Both osmotic and hydrostatic pressure changes force the interstitial fluid into the intravascular space in an effort to compensate for the loss of volume in the blood vessels. As the interstitial space is depleted, its fluid becomes hypertonic, and cellular fluid is then drawn into the interstitial space, leaving cells without adequate fluid to function properly. FVDs result from the loss of body fluids, especially if fluid intake is decreased simultaneously.

Young children, older adults, and people who are ill are especially at risk for hypovolemia. FVD can rapidly result in a weight loss of 5% in adults and 10% in infants. A 5% to 10% decrease in weight can indicate mild to moderate fluid loss (Willis, 2020). A 15% weight loss caused by fluid deficiency usually is life threatening.

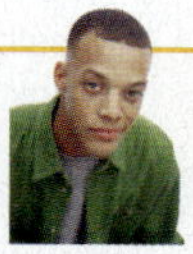

Recall **Jeremiah Stein**, the college student with an increased number of loose, watery stools for a week. Your assessment reveals that they have been limiting their oral intake, further compounding their risk for deficient fluid volume. Weighing Jeremiah would be an important intervention to include as part of the nursing assessment to help determine the extent of fluid loss.

Third-space fluid shift refers to a distributional shift of body fluids into the transcellular compartment, such as the pleural, peritoneal (ascites), or pericardial areas; joint cavities; the bowel; or an excess accumulation of fluid in the interstitial space. The fluid moves out of the intravascular spaces (plasma) to any of these spaces. Once trapped in these spaces, the fluid is not easily exchanged with ECF. With third-space fluid shift, a deficit in ECF volume occurs. The fluid has not been lost but is trapped in another body space for a period of time and is essentially unavailable for use. These fluid shifts may be related to a disruption in the colloid osmotic pressure (decreased albumin), increased fluid volume (excess IV fluid replacement, renal dysfunction), increased capillary hydrostatic pressure (heart failure), hyponatremia, or an increase in the permeability of the capillary membrane (gross tissue trauma). A third-space shift may occur as a result of burns, an acute intestinal obstruction, heart or liver failure, crush injuries, surgical procedures, or acute peritonitis (Willis, 2020). Decreased body weight does not occur as it does with an ECF volume deficit (vomiting or diarrhea), and the fluid loss cannot be measured.

Fluid Volume Excess

Excessive retention of water and sodium in ECF in near-equal proportions results in a condition termed *fluid volume excess (FVE)*. FVE may be a result of fluid overload (excess water and sodium intake) or due to impairment of the mechanisms that maintain homeostasis (Bauldoff et al., 2020). Common causes include malfunction of the kidneys, causing an inability to excrete the excesses, and failure of the heart to function as a pump, resulting in accumulation of fluid in the lungs and dependent parts of the body.

Due to the increased extracellular osmotic pressure from the retained sodium and water, fluid is pulled from the cells to equalize the tonicity. By the time the intracellular and extracellular spaces are isotonic to each other, an excess of both water and sodium is in the ECF, whereas the cells are nearly depleted. The excessive ECF may accumulate in either the intravascular compartments (**hypervolemia**) or interstitial spaces (**edema**). Edema can be observed around the eyes, fingers, ankles, and sacral space, and can also accumulate in or around body organs. Accumulation of fluid may result in a weight gain in excess of 5%. The amount or severity of edema is typically graded (Fig. 41-9 on page 1680). Interstitial-to-plasma shift is the movement of fluid from the space surrounding the cells to the blood. Although the body attempts to maintain normal balance in all fluid spaces, the intravascular fluid is usually protected at the expense of interstitial fluid and ICF.

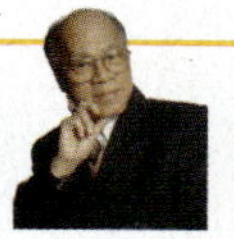

Remember **Jack Soo Park**, the patient who inadvertently received too much IV fluid? In Mr. Park's case, fluid accumulation involved his lungs and heart, exhibited by his bounding pulse, distended neck veins, and abnormal lung sounds.

Electrolyte Imbalances

Electrolyte imbalances commonly involve a deficit or excess of the electrolyte. Abnormalities in electrolyte levels can indicate fluid or acid–base imbalance, or neuromuscular, cardiac, renal endocrine, or skeletal dysfunction. Results from venous blood will provide essential information related to possible electrolyte imbalances. When patients present with deficits or excesses of sodium, potassium, calcium, magnesium, phosphate, or chloride, careful nursing assessment depends on an understanding of the effects of these imbalances.

Hyponatremia and Hypernatremia

Sodium is the most abundant electrolyte in the ECF. Refer to Table 41-1 on page 1673. **Hyponatremia** refers to a sodium deficit in ECF (serum sodium <135 mEq/L) caused by a loss of sodium or a gain of water. Sodium may be lost through vomiting, diarrhea, fistulas, sweating, or as the result of the use of diuretics. The decrease in sodium causes fluid to move by osmosis from the less concentrated ECF compartment to the ICF space. This shift of fluid leads to swelling of the cells, with resulting confusion, hypotension, edema, muscle cramps and weakness, and dry skin. Severe hyponatremia (serum sodium <120 mEq/L) is manifested by signs of increasing intracranial pressure, which may include lethargy, muscle twitching, hyperreflexia, coma, and seizures; death may occur (Bauldoff et al., 2020).

Hypernatremia refers to a surplus of sodium in ECF (serum sodium >145 mEq/L) caused by excess water loss or an overall excess of sodium. Fluid deprivation, lack of fluid consumption (such as in patients who cannot perceive, respond to, or communicate thirst), diarrhea, and

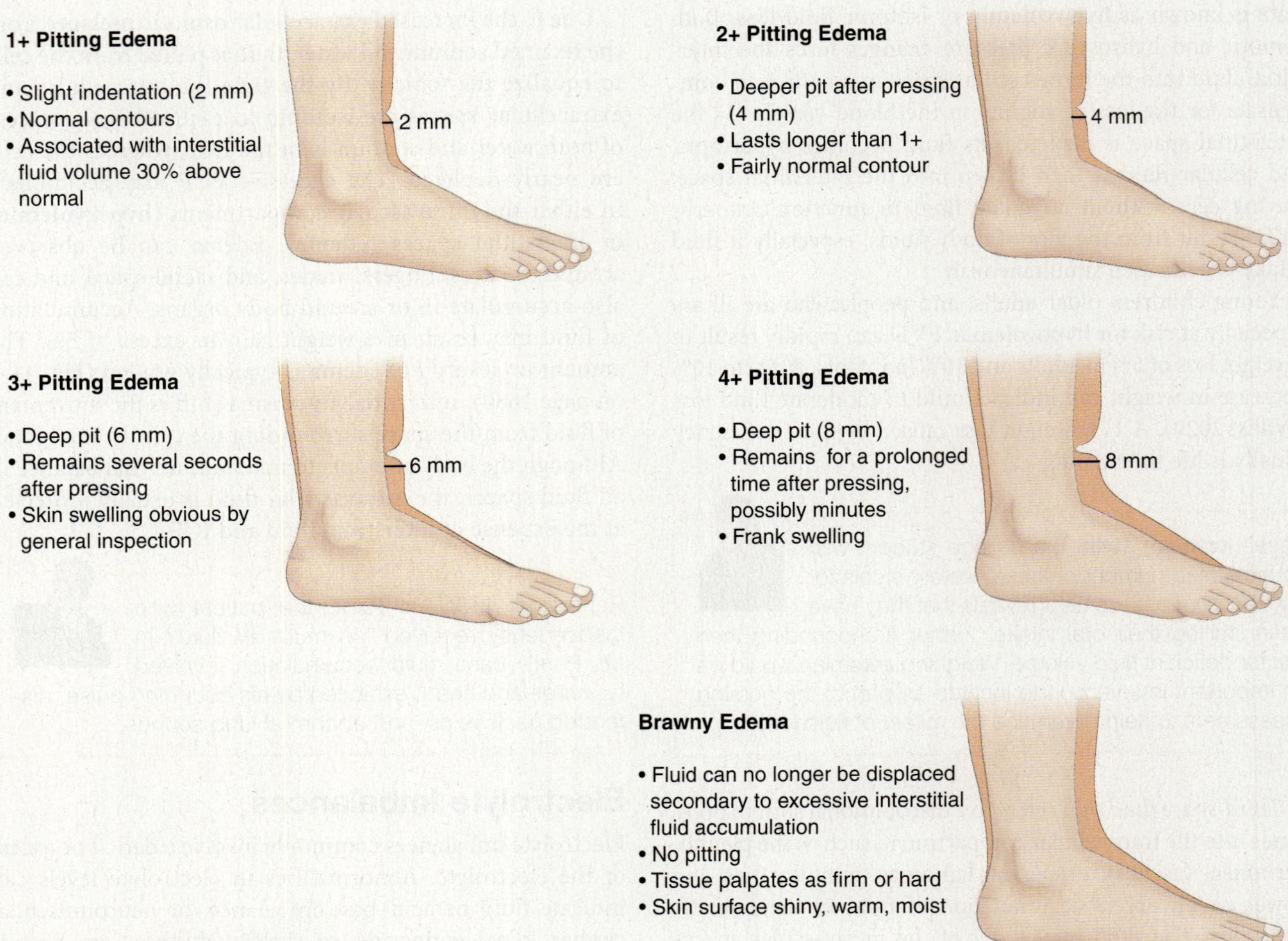

FIGURE 41-9. System for grading edema.

excess insensible water loss (hyperventilation, burns) lead to excess sodium. Rapid or excessive administration of sodium-containing intravenous solutions can also lead to an excess of sodium (Kamel & Halperin, 2017; Norris, 2020). Fluids move from the cells because of the increased extracellular osmotic pressure, causing them to shrink and leaving them without sufficient fluid. The cells of the central nervous system are especially affected, resulting in signs of neurologic impairment, including restlessness, agitation, weakness, disorientation, delusions, hallucinations, and seizures. Permanent brain damage, especially in infants and children, can occur.

Hypokalemia and Hyperkalemia

Potassium is the major intracellular electrolyte. Refer to Table 41-1 on page 1673. **Hypokalemia** refers to a potassium deficit in ECF (serum potassium <3.5 mEq/L) and is a common electrolyte abnormality. Potassium may be lost through vomiting, gastric suction, alkalosis, or diarrhea, or as the result of the use of diuretics. When the extracellular potassium level falls, potassium moves from the cell, creating an intracellular potassium deficiency. Sodium and hydrogen ions are then retained by the cells to maintain isotonic fluids. These electrolyte shifts influence normal cellular functioning, the pH of ECF, and the functions of most body systems, including the cardiovascular system. Skeletal muscles are generally the first to demonstrate a potassium deficiency. Typical signs of hypokalemia include muscle weakness and leg cramps, fatigue, paresthesias, and dysrhythmias (Willis, 2020).

Hyperkalemia refers to an excess of potassium in ECF (serum potassium >5 mEq/L). Excess potassium may result from renal failure, hypoaldosteronism, or the use of certain medications such as potassium chloride, heparin, angiotensin-converting enzyme (ACE) inhibitors, nonsteroidal antiinflammatory drugs (NSAIDs), and potassium-sparing diuretics. Nerve conduction as well as muscle contractility can be affected. Skeletal muscle weakness, paraesthesias, and paralysis may occur. A variety of cardiac irregularities may result, including cardiac arrest if hyperkalemia is not corrected (Norris, 2020).

Hypocalcemia and Hypercalcemia

Calcium is a major component of bones and teeth. Refer to Table 41-1 on page 1673. **Hypocalcemia** refers to a calcium deficit in ECF (serum calcium <8.9 mg/dL, ionized calcium <4.5 mg/dL). Common causes related to a calcium deficit involve inadequate calcium intake, impaired calcium absorption, and excessive calcium loss. Manifestations of hypocalcemia include numbness and tingling of fingers, mouth, or feet; tetany; muscle cramps; and seizures.

Hypercalcemia refers to an excess of calcium in ECF (serum calcium >10.5 mg/dL, ionized calcium >5.6 mg/dL). Two major causes of hypercalcemia are cancer and hyperparathyroidism. Manifestations of hypercalcemia include nausea, vomiting, constipation, bone pain, excessive urination, thirst, confusion, lethargy, and slurred speech. Severe hypercalcemia (serum calcium ≥15 mg/dL) is an emergency situation (Sadiqu et al., 2020).

Hypomagnesemia and Hypermagnesemia

Magnesium is the most abundant intracellular cation after potassium. Refer to Table 41-1 on page 1673. **Hypomagnesemia** refers to a magnesium deficit in the ECF (serum magnesium <1.3 mEq/L). Magnesium loss may occur with nasogastric suction, diarrhea, chronic alcohol use, administration of tube feedings or parenteral nutrition, sepsis, or burns. This abnormality may lead to muscle weakness, tremors, tetany, seizures, cardiac arrhythmias, change in mental status, hyperactive deep tendon reflexes (DTRs), and respiratory paralysis.

Hypermagnesemia refers to a magnesium excess in the ECF (serum magnesium >2.1 mEq/L). It usually occurs with renal failure when the kidneys fail to excrete magnesium or from excessive magnesium intake (use of magnesium-containing antacids or laxatives) (Willis, 2020). Clinical manifestations include nausea, vomiting, weakness, flushing, lethargy, hypoactive DTRs, respiratory depression, coma, and cardiac arrest (Norris, 2020).

Hypophosphatemia and Hyperphosphatemia

Phosphorus is a critical element of all the body's tissues. Refer to Table 41-1 on page 1673. **Hypophosphatemia** refers to a below-normal concentration of phosphorus in the ECF (serum phosphate <2.5 mg/dL or 1.8 mEq/L). Although this may indicate phosphorus deficiency, multiple factors may lower serum phosphate levels while total body phosphorus stores are normal. Hypophosphatemia can result from administration of calories to malnourished patients, alcohol withdrawal, diabetic ketoacidosis, hyperventilation, absorption problems, and diuretic use. Manifestations include muscle weakness, slurred speech, dysphagia, decreased respiratory effort, paresthesias, irritability, confusion, seizures, and coma (Willis, 2020).

Hyperphosphatemia refers to above-normal concentrations of phosphorus in the ECF (serum phosphate >4.5 mg/dL or 2.6 mEq/L). Common causes are impaired kidney excretion and hypoparathyroidism. Hyperphosphatemia can result in hyperreflexia, anorexia, muscle weakness, decreased mental status, and dysrhythmias (Willis, 2020).

Hypochloremia and Hyperchloremia

Chloride is the major anion of the ECF. Refer to Table 41-1 on page 1673. **Hypochloremia** refers to below-normal level of chloride in the ECF (serum chloride <98 mEq/L). A low level of chloride can result from severe vomiting and diarrhea, drainage of gastric fluid (GI tube), metabolic alkalosis, diuretic therapy, and burns. Manifestations include hyperexcitability of muscles, tetany, hyperactive DTRs, weakness, and muscle cramps; severe hypochloremia may result in seizures, coma or respiratory arrest (Willis, 2020).

Hyperchloremia refers to an above-normal level of chloride in the ECF (serum chloride >108 mEq/L). Hyperchloremia can result from metabolic acidosis, hypernatremia, increased chloride retention by the kidneys, and hyperparathyroidism. Signs and symptoms include tachypnea, weakness, lethargy, diminished cognitive ability, decreased cardiac output, dysrhythmias, and coma.

Acid–Base Imbalances

Acid–base imbalances occur when the carbonic acid or bicarbonate levels become disproportionate. When there is a single primary cause, these disturbances are known as respiratory acidosis or alkalosis and metabolic acidosis or alkalosis, which are described in the sections that follow. Some references use the term *nonrespiratory* to refer to metabolic disturbances. Although these disturbances are discussed separately, combined disturbances frequently occur. Complicated clinical situations may occur when respiratory and metabolic imbalances coexist.

Metabolic Acidosis and Alkalosis

Metabolic acidosis and alkalosis occur as the result of metabolic processes. A metabolic or nonrespiratory disturbance alters the bicarbonate level in the ECF. It is reflected in the HCO_3^- level of an arterial blood gas (ABG). Both the lungs and the kidneys attempt to compensate for this disorder by either excreting or retaining $PaCO_2$ (the lungs) and/or HCO_3^- and H^+ ions (the kidneys).

Metabolic acidosis or *nonrespiratory acidosis* is a proportionate deficit of bicarbonate in ECF. The deficit can occur as the result of an increase in acid components or an excessive loss of bicarbonate. It can be produced by a gain of hydrogen ion or loss of bicarbonate. The lungs attempt to increase carbon dioxide excretion by increasing the rate and depth of respirations, which occurs within a short time. However, respiratory compensation is generally not adequate, and the kidneys attempt to compensate by retaining bicarbonate and by excreting more hydrogen. In summary: Metabolic acidosis = low pH (increased hydrogen ion concentration) and a low plasma bicarbonate concentration due to a gain of hydrogen or loss of bicarbonate.

Metabolic alkalosis or *nonrespiratory alkalosis* is associated with an excess of HCO_3, a decrease in H^+ ions, or both, in the ECF. This may be the result of excessive acid losses or increased base ingestion or retention. The body attempts to compensate by retaining carbon dioxide. The respirations become slow and shallow, and periods of no breathing may occur. The kidneys attempt to excrete excess H_2O and Na ions with the excessive bicarbonate and retain H^+ ions. In summary: Metabolic alkalosis = high pH and a high plasma bicarbonate concentration due to a gain of bicarbonate or a loss of hydrogen.

Respiratory Acidosis and Alkalosis

Respiratory acidosis and alkalosis occur as a result of respiratory disturbances. A respiratory disturbance alters the carbonic acid level in the ECF. It is reflected in the $PaCO_2$ level of an ABG. Compensation for a respiratory disturbance occurs when the lungs attempt to either retain or eliminate $PaCO_2$ from the body or when the kidneys attempt to restore balance through the conservation, formation, or excretion of bicarbonate (HCO_3^-).

Respiratory acidosis is a primary excess of carbonic acid in the ECF. It is produced by inadequate excretion of CO_2 with inadequate ventilation, resulting in elevated plasma CO_2 and increased levels of carbonic acid. Any decrease in alveolar ventilation that results in retention of carbon dioxide can cause respiratory acidosis. Initially, the increased amounts of CO_2 stimulate the medulla in the respiratory center to increase the respiratory rate. Due to the increase in respiratory rate, CO_2 is expelled, and the CO_2 level of the blood is reduced. If the respiratory response is not effective, the increasing CO_2 levels will stimulate the kidneys to eliminate H^+ ions (acids) and conserve bicarbonate and sodium ions. The $NaHCO_3$ acts to buffer the free acids and ultimately reduce the CO_2 levels and restore acid–base balance. In summary: Respiratory acidosis = high $PaCO_2$ due to alveolar hypoventilation.

Respiratory alkalosis is a primary deficit of carbonic acid in the ECF. It is the result of alveolar hyperventilation, breathing that is faster and deeper, and the consequent increase in the elimination of CO_2. This loss of CO_2 leads to a decrease in the carbonic acid level in the plasma and an increase in the pH. The chemoreceptors in the medulla sense the increase in pH and the presence of less carbonic acid and stimulate the body to breathe either more slowly or less deeply. If this condition lasts for about 6 hours or longer, the kidneys attempt to alleviate the imbalance by increasing the bicarbonate excretion and by retaining more hydrogen to correct the imbalance. In summary: Respiratory alkalosis = low $PaCO_2$ due to alveolar hyperventilation.

NURSING PROCESS FOR FLUID, ELECTROLYTE, AND ACID–BASE BALANCE

Assessing

Acute and chronic illness, trauma, and certain therapeutic interventions may place a patient at high risk for fluid, electrolyte, and acid–base imbalances. Such imbalances can seriously compromise the patient's health status and may prove life threatening. The nursing assessment can provide information to identify patients at high risk for fluid, electrolyte, and acid–base imbalances and patients with specific imbalances.

Nursing assessment related to fluid, electrolyte, and acid–base balance should include a nursing history, physical assessment, fluid intake and output, daily weights, and laboratory studies. When an imbalance in fluid, specific electrolytes, or acid–base balance is suspected, the nurse needs to incorporate the associated assessments into the patient's care. Physical assessment and clinical assessment parameters, nursing considerations, normal findings in a healthy adult, and possible abnormal or significant findings are outlined in Table 41-3 on pages 1683–1684 and Table 41-4 on page 1685.

Nursing History

A comprehensive nursing history includes questions related to the patient's fluid and electrolyte status and acid–base balance. The accompanying Focused Assessment Guide 41-1 (on page 1686) includes interview questions to help identify the patient's usual pattern of fluid intake and elimination and the patient's self-evaluation of hydration status and awareness of particular problems.

Interview questions are also directed toward identifying patients with health conditions that increase the risk for imbalances. Risk factors include the following:

- Acute and chronic illnesses (e.g., diabetes, congestive heart failure, renal failure)
- Abnormal losses of body fluids (e.g., prolonged or severe vomiting or diarrhea, draining wounds, fistulas)
- Burns
- Trauma
- Surgery
- Therapies that may disrupt fluid and electrolyte balance, for example, medications such as diuretics and steroids, and treatments such as IV therapy and parenteral nutrition (PN)

Physical Assessment

Physical assessment related to fluid, electrolyte, and acid–base balance includes the assessment of multiple body systems. Include assessment of the skin and mucous membranes, vital signs, and a neurologic assessment, as well as identification of relative symptoms or conditions such as excessive thirst, nausea, vomiting, diarrhea, draining wounds, or other fluid losses. Refer to Tables 41-3 (on page 1683–1684) and 41-4 (on page 1685). Assessment of other body systems should be included based on the patient's underlying health conditions.

Fluid Intake and Output

If monitoring of a patient's intake and output is required, alert the patient, family, and all caregivers to the need to measure all fluids entering and leaving the body. Refer to Guidelines for Nursing Care 41-1 (on page 1686) for an explanation of correct measurement of a patient's intake and output.

Daily Weights

The record of a patient's daily weight is an important gauge of fluid balance (Bauldoff et al., 2020). Acute weight loss or gain represents fluid gain or loss (1 liter [L] of water weights 1 kg [2.2 lb]) (Norris, 2020). Weigh the patient at the same time every day. Be alert for other factors that may affect a patient's weight, such as using a different scale and weighing with the patient wearing significantly different clothing.

Table 41-3 Parameters to Be Considered in Physical Assessment for Fluid, Electrolyte, and Acid–Base Balance

ASSESSMENT PARAMETERS	NURSING CONSIDERATIONS	FINDINGS IN HEALTHY ADULT	SIGNIFICANT FINDINGS
Skin turgor (elasticity)	• The patient's skin over the sternum, inner aspect of the thighs, or forehead is pinched. • Some prefer to test skin turgor in children over the abdominal area and on the medial aspect of the thighs. • Skin turgor can vary with age, nutritional state, ethnicity, and complexion.	• Pinched skin immediately falls back to its normal position when released. • Reduced skin turgor is common in older adults because of a primary decrease in skin elasticity.	• In fluid volume deficit, the skin flattens more slowly after the pinch is released; the skin may remain elevated for many seconds. • Severe malnutrition, particularly in infants, can cause depressed skin turgor even in the absence of fluid depletion.
Tongue turgor	• Tongue turgor is not affected appreciably by age and thus is a useful assessment for all age groups. (In an arid climate, this may not be a reliable parameter.)	• Tongue has one longitudinal furrow.	• In fluid volume deficit, there are additional longitudinal furrows, and the tongue is smaller. • Sodium excess causes the tongue to look red and swollen.
Moisture and oral cavity	• A dry mouth may be the result of fluid volume deficit, mouth breathing, or exposure to an arid climate.	• Mucous membranes in oral cavity are moist.	• Dryness of the membrane where the cheek and gum meet indicates fluid volume deficit. • Dry sticky mucous membranes are noted in sodium excess.
Tearing and salivation		• Tearing and salivation decrease normally with age.	• The absence of tearing and salivation in a child is a sign of fluid volume deficit.
Appearance of skin and skin temperature			• Metabolic acidosis can cause warm, flushed skin (due to peripheral vasodilation).
Facial appearance			• A person with a severe fluid volume deficit may have a pinched and drawn facial expression. • A fluid volume deficit of 10% of body weight causes decreased intraocular pressure, causing the eyes to appear sunken and to feel soft to the touch.
Edema (excessive accumulation of interstitial fluid)	• Pitting edema (see Fig. 41-9) • Measurement of an extremity or body part with a millimeter tape, in the same area each day, is a more exact method of measurement. • An excess of interstitial fluid may accumulate predominantly in the lower extremities of ambulatory patients and in the presacral region of bedridden patients.	• No edema	• Clinically, edema is not usually apparent in the adult until the retention of 5–10 lb of excess fluid occurs. • Formation of edema may be localized (as in thrombophlebitis) or generalized (as in heart failure, cirrhosis of the liver, or nephrotic syndrome).
Body temperature	• Fever increases the loss of body fluids. • Body temperature and other vital signs should be assessed as prescribed, indicated in facility policies and procedures, and at the nurse's discretion.	• Baseline temperature	• A temperature elevation between 101°F (38.3°C) and 103°F (39.4°C) increases the 24-hour fluid requirement by at least 500 mL, and a temperature above 103°F increases it by at least 1,000 mL.

(*continued*)

Table 41-3 Parameters to Be Considered in Physical Assessment for Fluid, Electrolyte, and Acid–Base Balance *(continued)*

ASSESSMENT PARAMETERS	NURSING CONSIDERATIONS	FINDINGS IN HEALTHY ADULT	SIGNIFICANT FINDINGS
Pulse		• Baseline pulse rate, rhythm, and quality.	• Tachycardia is usually the earliest sign of the decreased vascular volume associated with fluid volume deficit. • Irregular pulse rates also occur with potassium imbalances and magnesium deficit. • Pulse quality/amplitude is decreased in fluid volume deficit and increased in fluid volume excess.
Respirations		• Baseline respiratory rate, rhythm, and depth	• Deep, rapid respirations may be a compensatory mechanism for metabolic acidosis or a primary disorder causing respiratory alkalosis. • Slow, shallow respirations may be a compensatory mechanism for metabolic alkalosis or a primary disorder causing respiratory acidosis. • Moist crackles may indicate fluid volume excess.
Blood pressure	• Whenever a fluid imbalance is suspected, the patient's blood pressure is measured in the supine, sitting, and standing position to determine the presence of orthostatic changes	• Baseline blood pressure	• A sustained decrease in systolic blood pressure of ≥20 mm Hg or a decrease in diastolic blood pressure of ≥10 mm Hg (postural hypotension) may indicate fluid volume deficit.

Source: Adapted from Hale, A., & Hovey, M. J. (2014). *Fluid, electrolyte, and acid-base imbalances.* F.A. Davis; Hinkle, J. L., Cheever, K. H., & Overbaugh, K. J. (2022). *Brunner & Suddarth's Textbook of medical-surgical nursing* (15th ed.). Wolters Kluwer; and Norris, T. L. (2020). *Porth's essentials of pathophysiology* (5th ed.). Wolters Kluwer.

Laboratory Studies

Laboratory tests are helpful in determining whether fluid, electrolyte, and acid–base balance exist. Descriptions of standard tests follow; tables of normal values are available in Appendix C.

COMPLETE BLOOD COUNT

The complete blood count determines the total number of red blood cells and values for hemoglobin and hematocrit. Significant values include the following:

- Increased hematocrit values: found in severe fluid volume deficit and shock (when hemoconcentration rises considerably)
- Decreased hematocrit values: found with acute, massive blood loss, and with hemolytic reaction after transfusion of incompatible blood or with fluid overload
- Increased levels of hemoglobin: found in hemoconcentration of the blood
- Decreased levels of hemoglobin: found with anemia states, severe hemorrhage, and after a hemolytic reaction

SERUM ELECTROLYTES, BLOOD UREA NITROGEN, AND CREATININE LEVELS

This screening test determines plasma levels of certain electrolytes such as sodium, potassium, chloride, and bicarbonate ions. In addition, the blood urea nitrogen (BUN) and creatinine levels can provide information related to the fluid status and the renal function of the patient. Significant values include the following:

- Below-normal or above-normal levels of sodium, potassium, calcium, magnesium, phosphate, and chloride. Refer to the electrolyte imbalance discussion earlier in the chapter.
- Below-normal or above-normal levels of bicarbonate ions. Refer to the acid–base discussion earlier in the chapter and the ABGs discussion later in this section.
- Increased BUN: found with impaired renal function (such as associated with shock, heart failure, and salt and water depletion), diabetic ketoacidosis, burns
- Increased creatinine: found with impaired renal function, heart failure, shock, fluid volume deficit

Table 41-4 Parameters to Be Considered in Clinical Assessment for Fluid, Electrolyte, and Acid–Base Balance

ASSESSMENT PARAMETERS	NURSING CONSIDERATIONS	FINDINGS IN HEALTHY ADULT	SIGNIFICANT FINDINGS
Comparison of total intake and output of fluids	• Records may be initiated for any patient with a real or potential fluid or electrolyte problem. • Intake should include all fluids taken into the body. • Output should include urine, vomitus, diarrhea, drainage from fistulas, and drainage from suction apparatus. Perspiration and drainage from lesions should be noted	• Fluid intake approximately equals fluid output—when averaged over 2 or 3 days. • Average adult intake and loss per day is 2,600 mL.	• When the total intake is substantially less than the total output, the patient is in danger of fluid volume deficit. • When the total intake is substantially more than the total output, the patient is in danger of fluid volume excess.
Urine volume and concentration	• All fluid losses are measured according to routes. • A device calibrated for small volumes of urine is used when hourly urine volumes need to be measured. • Factors that can alter urinary output must be accounted for, including amount of fluid intake; losses from skin, lungs, and GI tract; renal concentrating ability; blood volume; and influence of aldosterone and ADH	• Normal urinary output for the average adult: 1,500 mL/24 hr.; about 40–80 mL/hr. • The range of specific gravity is from 1.005 to 1.030. Urine osmolality ranges between 500 and 800 mOsm/kg (mmol/kg).	• A low urine volume and high specific gravity indicates fluid volume deficit. • A low urine volume and low specific gravity indicates renal disease. • A high urine volume suggests fluid volume excess. • Hypovolemia causes decreased renal perfusion and oliguria; hypervolemia causes increased urinary volume if the kidneys are functioning normally.
Body weight	• Because of the common inaccuracies in recording intake and output, body weight is believed to be a more accurate indicator of fluid gained and lost. • A patient may have a severe fluid volume deficit even though body weight is essentially unchanged when there is a third-space loss of body fluid.	• A patient's dry weight should remain relatively stable.	• Rapid variations in weight closely reflect changes in body fluid volume. • A rapid gain or loss of 1 kg (2.2 lb) of body weight is about equal to the gain or loss of 1 L of fluid.

Source: Adapted from Hale, A., & Hovey, M. J. (2014). *Fluid, electrolyte, and acid-base imbalances.* F.A. Davis; Hinkle, J. L., Cheever, K. H., & Overbaugh, K. J. (2022). *Brunner & Suddarth's Textbook of medical-surgical nursing* (15th ed.). Wolters Kluwer; and Norris, T. L. (2020). *Porth's essentials of pathophysiology* (5th ed.). Wolters Kluwer.

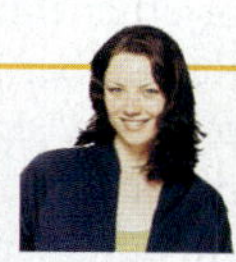

Recall **Grace Gilligan**, the female described in one of the beginning scenarios. Although she needs IV therapy, it would be important for the nurse to determine the patient's electrolyte levels to establish a baseline to aid in determining the best IV solution for the patient and to determine the need for electrolyte replacement.

URINE pH AND SPECIFIC GRAVITY

Both the urine pH and specific gravity may be obtained by dipstick measurement, using a fresh voided specimen or through laboratory analysis. The pH of urine usually ranges between 4.6 and 8.2. Lower-than-normal urinary pH can occur with metabolic acidosis, diabetic ketosis, and diarrhea. Higher-than-normal urinary pH can occur with respiratory alkalosis, potassium depletion, and chronic renal failure. Specific gravity is a measure of the urine's concentration. The range depends on the patient's state of hydration and varies with urine volume and the load of solutes to be excreted. Normal values range from 1.005 to 1.030 (concentrated urine, ≥1.025; dilute urine, ≤1.001 to 1.010). Increased urine specific gravity can occur with dehydration, vomiting, diarrhea, and heart failure. Decreased urine specific gravity can occur with renal damage.

ARTERIAL BLOOD GASES

Arterial blood gases (ABGs) are laboratory tests commonly used to determine the adequacy of oxygenation and ventilation as well as in the assessment and treatment of acid–base imbalance. The ABG findings are obtained through analysis of an arterial blood sample. The pH of the plasma or blood indicates balance or impending acidosis or alkalosis. The blood's oxygen and carbon dioxide gas values are also reported, providing information regarding the effectiveness of the respiratory system. The partial pressures (indicated by "P") of these gases, or their tensions, are determined by the use of a nomogram, which reflects the chemical and physical activities of the two gases. The partial pressure of carbon dioxide is abbreviated $PaCO_2$; for oxygen, it is PaO_2. The "a" indicates an arterial specimen. When the PaO_2 is low, hemoglobin carries less-than-normal amounts of oxygen;

Focused Assessment Guide 41-1

FLUID, ELECTROLYTE, AND ACID–BASE BALANCE

Factors to Assess	Questions and Approaches
Usual patterns of fluid intake	Describe the amount and types of fluids you usually drink in a 24-hour period. Have there been any recent changes?
Usual pattern of fluid elimination	Describe your usual voiding/urination habits. Any recent changes in frequency or amount? Is your body losing fluids in any other major way? • Vomiting • Diarrhea • Excessive perspiration • Fistula
Patient's evaluation of hydration status	Do you think there is an approximate balance between your fluid intake and output? Have you noticed any signs that your body is experiencing too much or too little hydration (difficulty breathing, edema, dry skin and mucous membranes, thirst)?
History of disease process	Is there any history of disease process or injury that might disrupt fluid and electrolyte balance (e.g., diabetes mellitus, cancer, burns)?
Medication/nutrition history	Do you take any medications or treatments that might disrupt fluid and electrolyte balance (e.g., steroids, diuretics, parenteral nutrition, dialysis)? Have you been trying to lose weight by dieting, using diuretics, laxatives, or diet aids? Have you been following a high-protein, low-carbohydrate diet?
Fluid, electrolyte, and acid–base imbalances and contributing factors	Are you aware of any other fluid balance problems you may be experiencing? • Nature • Onset of problem and frequency • Causes • Severity • Symptoms • Intervention attempted and results

Guidelines for Nursing Care 41-1

MEASURING FLUID INTAKE AND OUTPUT

- Instruct the patient and family/caregiver regarding the need for a record of all fluids entering the body and all fluid output. Provide an explanation of the rationale along with instructions for how the patient can help keep measurements accurate. Some patients may need to be reminded each morning that this measurement will continue.
- Use the patient's plan of care to communicate to other nursing personnel the need to measure fluid intake and output.
- A sign posted in the patient's room and a bedside form for recording intake and output are helpful reminders for both the patient and nurses.
- Measure both intake and output whenever possible, rather than estimate.
- Record intake and output totals for each 8-hour shift and total each 24 hours. If the nurse suspects a large difference between intake and output, total the columns earlier so that the health care team can be notified.

Patient's Fluid Intake Includes the Following

- All fluids and foods that are liquid at room temperature (ice cream, gelatin dessert [Jell-O], and the like)
- Use the facility's designation of specific volumes for common food containers (e.g., juice glass, 90 mL; milk carton, 240 mL). Remind the patient that sips of water or other fluids in between meals need to be recorded. Remember that liquid medications or water taken with pills may significantly increase the fluid intake of some patients.
- All parenteral fluids
- Other fluids taken into the body: subcutaneous fluids, gastrointestinal tube feedings and flushes; IV flushes

Patient's Fluid Output Includes the Following

- Urine; vomitus; diarrhea; drainage from fistulas, wounds, and ulcers; and drainage from suctioning devices or other tubes. Calibrated measuring devices should be readily available for accurate measurement. Disposable, calibrated urine collection containers that fit under the toilet seat are available for ambulatory patients. Urine or liquid feces in diapers or bed clothes, vomitus on clothing or bed linens, wound drainage saturating dressings, and so forth, need to be estimated.
- Heavy perspiration, noted on the output record, especially when the patient's clothing or bed linens are soaked.
- Hyperventilation (water vapor loss) also noted on the output record. Record the rate and depth of respirations.

Table 41-5 Acid–Base Parameters for Arterial Blood Gas Studies

	NORMAL	ACID	BASE
pH	7.35–7.45	<7.35	>7.45
$PaCO_2$ (mm Hg)	35–45	>45	<35
HCO_3^- (mEq/L)	22–26	<22	>26

when the PaO_2 is high, the hemoglobin carries more oxygen. The $PaCO_2$ is influenced almost entirely by respiratory activity. When the $PaCO_2$ is low, carbonic acid leaves the body in excessive amounts; when the $PaCO_2$ is high, there are excessive amounts of carbonic acid in the body. Oxygen saturation readings (SaO_2) reveal the percentage of oxygen in the blood that combines with hemoglobin.

The bicarbonate level (HCO_3^-) of the ABG report reflects the bicarbonate level of the body. The kidneys are involved in either reabsorbing bicarbonate or excreting bicarbonate, depending on what is needed to maintain the delicate acid–base balance.

Although compensation is the body's natural attempt to restore balance, correction may also be required. Correction involves using medical and nursing interventions to promote a return to homeostasis (e.g., pharmacologic agents, mechanical ventilation, monitor intake/output, dietary teaching). Table 41-5 outlines acid–base parameters for ABG studies.

Additional ABG values exist but are not included in this simple interpretation of acid–base imbalances. Partial pressure of oxygen (PaO_2) and oxygen saturation (SaO_2) results also directly reflect the adequacy of oxygenation and ventilation. Follow these steps when interpreting ABGs:

1. **Determine whether the pH is alkalotic or acidotic.**
   Remember, the optimal pH is 7.4, but body will tolerate a pH from 7.35 to 7.45. If the pH is lower than 7.35, the patient is acidotic. If the pH is higher than 7.45, the patient is alkalotic. If the pH is within the normal range, determine which side of 7.4 it lies on (lower or higher). This may indicate the patient is acidotic or alkalotic, but the body is compensating to make the pH closer to normal (Woodruff, 2006).
2. **Look at the $PaCO_2$.**
   Remember, carbon dioxide is produced by cellular metabolism and is excreted by the lungs through exhalation. It represents the respiratory component of the blood gas. Normal levels range from 35 to 45 mm Hg. Changes in the $PaCO_2$ reflect lung function. A $PaCO_2$ level below 35 mm Hg can be caused by hyperventilation, resulting in alkalosis. When the patient retains CO_2, as a result of hypoventilation, for example, the $PaCO_2$ level rises above 45 mm Hg, resulting in acidosis.
3. **Look at the HCO_3^-.**
   Remember, bicarbonate is produced by the kidneys. It represents the metabolic component of the blood gas. Normal levels range from 22 to 26 mEq/L. Changes in the HCO_3^- reflect kidney function. A HCO_3^- level below 22 mEq/L indicates acidosis and above 26 mEq/L indicates alkalosis.
4. **Look at the $PaCO_2$ or the HCO_3^- and match either with the pH.**
   If the pH is low and the $PaCO_2$ is high, the patient has respiratory acidosis. If the pH is high and the $PaCO_2$ is low, the patient has respiratory alkalosis. If the pH and HCO_3^- are high but the $PaCO_2$ is normal, the patient has metabolic alkalosis. The patient has metabolic acidosis if the pH and HCO_3^- are low and the $PaCO_2$ is normal (Willis, 2020).
   Respiratory acidosis:
   ↓ pH <7.35 ↑ $PaCO_2$ Normal HCO_3^-
   Respiratory alkalosis:
   ↑ pH >7.45 ↓ $PaCO_2$ Normal HCO_3^-
   In metabolic acid–base imbalances, the pH and HCO_3^- values are both high or both low:
   Metabolic acidosis:
   ↓ pH <7.35 ↓ HCO_3^- Normal $PaCO_2$
   Metabolic alkalosis:
   ↑ pH >7.45 ↑ HCO_3^- Normal $PaCO_2$
5. **Look at the total picture and determine whether compensation has occurred.**
   Determine whether the body is compensating for the pH change. Complete compensation occurs when the body's ability to compensate is so effective that the pH falls within the normal range (Willis, 2020). Partial compensation occurs when the pH remains outside the normal range (Willis, 2020). Compensation involves opposites: for example, in primary metabolic acidosis, compensation involves respiratory alkalosis; in primary respiratory acidosis, compensation involves metabolic alkalosis. Determine which level more closely corresponds with the pH, indicating the primary cause of the problem. The other level reflects the compensation.
   Example:
   pH ↓ 7.29
   $PaCO_2$ ↓ 17 mm Hg
   HC ↓ 19 mEq/L
   The low pH indicates acidosis; the $PaCO_2$ is low, which normally leads to alkalosis, and the bicarbonate level is low, which normally leads to acidosis. In this example, the bicarbonate level more closely corresponds with the pH, making the primary cause of the problem metabolic. The resultant decrease in $PaCO_2$ reflects partial respiratory compensation—metabolic acidosis with partial respiratory compensation (Willis, 2020). When compensation occurs, the $PaCO_2$ and the HCO_3^- will always point in the same direction.
6. **Look at the PaO_2 and SaO_2.**
   The PaO_2 and SaO_2 provide information about the patient's oxygenation status. If the PaO_2 is less than 80, or the SaO_2 is less than 95%, the patient has hypoxemia.

Table 41-6 (on page 1688) identifies risk factors, assessments, and potential nursing interventions related to these acid–base disturbances.

Table 41-6 Acid–Base Disturbances

RISK FACTORS	ASSESSMENTS	NURSING INTERVENTIONS
Respiratory Acidosis		
Acute respiratory disease Pulmonary edema Aspiration of a foreign body Atelectasis Overdose of sedative or anesthetic Cardiac arrest Chronic respiratory disease Emphysema Bronchial asthma Cystic fibrosis Inadequate mechanical ventilation CNS depression Neuromuscular disease	Acute respiratory acidosis Mental cloudiness Dizziness Muscular twitching Unconsciousness ABGs pH <7.35 $PaCO_2$ >45 mm Hg (primary) HCO_3^- normal or only slightly elevated Chronic respiratory acidosis Weakness Dull headache ABGs pH <7.35 or low N $PaCO_2$ >45 mm Hg (primary) HCO_3^- >26 mEq/L (compensatory)	Treatment is directed at improving ventilation Pharmacologic measures Pulmonary hygiene measures Adequate hydration Supplemental oxygen Mechanical ventilation may be necessary to correct disorder but must be used cautiously to decrease $PaCO_2$ slowly.
Respiratory Alkalosis		
Hyperventilation Extreme anxiety (most common cause) Hypoxemia High fever Early sepsis Excessive ventilation by mechanical ventilator CNS lesion involving the respiratory center	Lightheadedness Inability to concentrate Hyperventilation syndrome Tinnitus Palpitations Sweating Dry mouth Tremulousness Convulsions and loss of consciousness ABGs pH >7.45 $PaCO_2$ <35 mm Hg (primary) HCO_3^- <22 mEq/L (compensatory)	If anxiety is the cause, encourage the patient to breathe more slowly (causes accumulation of CO_2) or breathe into a closed system (paper bag). Sedative may also be necessary in extreme anxiety. Treatment of other causes is directed at correcting the underlying problem.
Metabolic Acidosis		
Diarrhea Intestinal fistulas Parenteral nutrition Excessive intake of acids, such as salicylates Diabetic ketoacidosis Renal failure Starvational ketoacidosis	Headache Confusion Drowsiness Increased respiratory rate and depth Nausea and vomiting Peripheral vasodilation ABGs pH <7.35 HCO_3^- <22 mEq/L (primary) $PaCO_2$ <35 mm Hg Hyperkalemia frequently present	Treatment is directed toward correcting the metabolic deficit. If the cause of the problem is excessive intake of chloride, treatment obviously focuses on eliminating the source. When necessary, bicarbonate is administered.
Metabolic Alkalosis		
Vomiting or gastric suction Hypokalemia Potassium-wasting diuretics Alkali ingestion (bicarbonate-containing antacids) Renal loss of H^+ (e.g., from steroid or diuretic use)	Dizziness Tingling of fingers and toes Hypertonic muscles Depressed respirations (compensatory) ABGs pH >7.45 HCO_3^- >26 mEq/L (primary) $PaCO_2$ >45 mm Hg (compensatory) Hypokalemia may be present	Treatment is aimed at reversal of the underlying disorder. Sufficient chloride must be supplied for the kidney to absorb sodium with chloride (allowing the excretion of excess bicarbonate). Treatment also includes administration of NaCl fluids to restore normal fluid volume.

Source: Adapted from Willis, L. M. (Ed.). (2020). *Fluids & electrolytes made incredibly easy!* (7th ed.). Wolters Kluwer.

Examples of Actual or Potential Health Problems and Needs

FLUID, ELECTROLYTE, AND ACID–BASE BALANCE

Actual or Potential Health Problems and Needs	Possible Etiologic Factors	Potential Signs and Symptoms
Fluid overload	Renal failure, decreased cardiac output, excessive IV infusion/fluid intake, excessive sodium intake	• "I've noticed that my wedding ring is tight . . . also my clothes don't fit as well as they used to. I guess I've gained some weight." • Reports dyspnea with exertion, feeling weak and fatigued • Pitting edema in feet, ankles, lower legs, taut, shiny skin • Adventitious breath sounds and increased blood pressure • 10-lb (4.5-kg) weight gain over past month
Fluid imbalance	Inability to obtain or swallow fluids (debilitation, oral pain), extremes of age, vomiting, diarrhea, burns, excessive use of laxative, excessive diaphoresis, fever	• Change in mental status • Increased body temperature and pulse rate, decreased blood pressure • Dry oral mucosa, cracked lips, furrowed tongue, decreased skin turgor • Scanty, dark urine output • Sudden weight loss: 5 lb (2 to 3 kg)
Impaired fluid intake	Inability to access fluids, extremes of age, insufficient knowledge about fluid needs	• "I only drink a little liquid with my meals. I don't want to have to go to the bathroom while I'm out with friends. And I never drink anything after dinner, so I don't have to get up at night!" • Voiding small amounts concentrated urine; urine specific gravity 1.035 • Fluid intake inconsistent and less than 1,500 mL/day • Skin dry, less supple

Source: International Council of Nurses (ICN). (2019). *Nursing diagnosis and outcome statements.* https://www.icn.ch/sites/default/files/inline-files/ICNP2019-DC.pdf; Wolters Kluwer. (2020). Problem-based care plans. In *Lippincott Advisor.* Wolters Kluwer. https://advisor.lww.com/lna/home.do

Diagnosing Actual or Potential Health Problems and Needs

An assessment of a patient's fluid, electrolyte, and acid–base status may lead to the identification of one or more actual or potential health problems and needs related to fluid, electrolyte, and acid–base balance. Following the formulation of the actual or potential health problems and needs, the nurse communicates findings to other nursing and health care professionals through the use of written and spoken word. The written actual or potential health problem or need becomes a permanent part of the patient's health record. Examples of health problems and needs with related etiology and signs and symptoms can be found in the Examples of Actual or Potential Health Problems and Needs: Fluid, Electrolyte, and Acid–Base Balance.

Outcome Identification and Planning

Expected outcomes are derived from the actual or potential fluid, electrolyte, and acid–base balance problems or needs identified. The goal is to maintain or restore optimum function related to fluid, electrolyte, and acid–base balance, alleviate symptoms or side effects of disease or treatment, and prevent complications. General patient outcomes are listed here. Actual patient outcomes should list specific behaviors and criteria individualized for the patient situation.

Nursing care supports the following expected outcomes. The healthy adult patient will:

- Maintain an approximate balance between fluid intake and fluid output (average about 2,500 mL fluid intake and output/day over 3 days)
- Maintain a urine specific gravity within normal range (1.005 to 1.030)
- Practice self-care behaviors to promote fluid, electrolyte, and acid–base balance; maintain adequate intake of fluid and electrolytes; and respond appropriately to the body's signals of impending fluid, electrolyte, or acid–base imbalance.

When an imbalance exists, the patient will:

- Report relief of symptoms (specify) after implementation of treatment regimen (e.g., 1 month after decreasing sodium intake patient reports weight loss of 4 lb [1.8 kg])
- Exhibit signs and symptoms of restored balance or homeostasis after initiation of treatment
- Identify signs and symptoms of recurrence of imbalance with need to notify the health care team.

Implementing

Nursing interventions to prevent or correct fluid, electrolyte, and acid–base imbalances include dietary modification, modification of fluid intake, medication administration, IV therapy, blood and blood products replacement, administration of PN, allaying anxiety as needed, and appropriate patient and family/caregiver teaching.

Preventing Fluid and Electrolyte Imbalances

An adequate fluid intake and a well-balanced, nutritious diet with appropriate adjustments throughout the life cycle are essential to promoting fluid balance. The following are general measures to consider that will help prevent fluid imbalances:

- Be familiar with common life events that can lead to fluid imbalances and observe the patient carefully. Infants are particularly vulnerable to fluid imbalances because body water accounts for a greater percentage of their weight, and fluid fluctuations are more common. Loss of fluid because of an illness can cause serious and life-threatening problems in infants.
- Note the patient's present fluid and food intake and obtain a history of the patient's previous eating and drinking patterns. Learn whether the patient has been using a fad diet, which may lead to imbalances.
- Note whether the patient experiences excessive thirst or little or no thirst. Thirst, a subjective sensation, is an important factor determining water intake and, eventually, output through the kidneys. Although the thirst mechanism is poorly understood, both psychological and physiologic factors appear to be involved. An older adult is more susceptible to fluid-deficient conditions related to a less effective thirst mechanism (Eliopoulos, 2018). Be aware of excessive losses of fluids from the body, and attempt to prevent losses when possible. Vomiting, pronounced perspiration, diarrhea, draining wounds, and excessive urinary output, for example, may cause excessive losses.
- Consider ways in which the patient's medical regimen may lead to fluid and electrolyte imbalances. For example, diuretics that stimulate urine formation may increase the elimination of both fluid and potassium. If food supplements high in potassium are not included in the diet or if potassium supplement drug therapy is not started, hypokalemia often follows.
- Learn whether the patient has been self-administering a treatment that may threaten fluid balance. Common practices that threaten fluid balance include the indiscriminate use of enemas, laxatives, antacids, and over-the-counter drugs or herbal medications to promote urination.
- Consider conditions with destructive effects on the body as threats to fluid balance. Examples include immobilization, trauma, burns, surgical procedures, and exposure to toxic agents.
- Teach patients to observe for signs and symptoms of fluid imbalances and to report them promptly. Examples include rapid weight gains and losses; swollen fingers, feet, and ankles; puffy eyelids; muscle weakness; change in skin sensations; and scanty or profuse urine production.
- Help patients and their families/caregivers understand the significance of maintaining fluid balance and preventing imbalances.
- Be aware that normal physiologic changes associated with aging affect older adults' ability to maintain fluid balance. Fluid volume deficit is a common fluid and electrolyte disorder in this population. The accompanying Focus on the Older Adult box suggests specific nursing strategies to prevent and correct fluid and electrolyte imbalances in older adults.

Focus on the Older Adult

NURSING STRATEGIES TO ADDRESS AGE-RELATED CHANGES AFFECTING FLUID BALANCE

Age-Related Changes	Nursing Strategies
• Decreased sense of thirst • Medical conditions (e.g., heart failure or hypertension, requiring medications such as diuretics)	• Ensure that oral intake is at least 1,500 mL for 24 hours. • Be aware of schedule for diagnostic tests (and associated dietary and fluid restrictions). • Offer fluids at regular intervals. • Replace fluids as necessary, either orally or intravenously. • Investigate individual fluid preferences. • Provide assistance or assistive devices for encouraging fluid intake.
Alterations in Renal Functioning	
• Loss of nephrons • Decreased renal blood flow	• Record accurate intake and output. • Note appearance and specific gravity of urine. • Check laboratory values for abnormal levels.
Alterations in Cardiac Functioning	
• Decreased efficiency as a pump • Volume intolerance	• Monitor breath sounds. • Assess for shortness of breath, wet productive cough, increased respiratory rate and work of breathing, edema. • Monitor chest radiograph.

Promoting Health Literacy

IN PATIENTS WITH FLUID OR ELECTROLYTE IMBALANCES

Patient Scenario

Shamala Johnson, 58, had been experiencing complications from diabetes for the previous 10 years. She tells the nurse, "I really thought that I had things under control until lately. I can't believe one more thing has happened." Ms. Johnson was admitted to the hospital with end-stage renal failure. "I guess I knew this was coming eventually but did not expect it so soon!" She initially received dialysis via a temporary dialysis catheter but had surgery yesterday for placement of an A-V shunt. Her current plan of care includes dietary modifications, including potassium, sodium, protein, and fluid restrictions. The nurse has assisted her with making dietary choices based on the hospital menus and has arranged a consult with the dietitian. The patient asks, "Do you think I will have to keep this up at home? How will I manage to get the right food? And liquids, can I drink anything? I don't understand this at all!"

Nursing Considerations: *Tips for Improving Health Literacy*

Confirm her dietary modifications for after discharge. Provide Ms. Johnson with easy-to-read information about living with renal disease, and managing fluid and electrolytes, as well as protein restrictions. Encourage her to ask her health team members as many questions as needed to understand her condition. Explain that there are things she can do to feel in control and follow the suggested regimen. Provide information and resources for support at home. Encourage Ms. Johnson to ask her primary care provider the following three questions:

- What is my main problem?
- What do I need to do?
- Why is it important for me to do this?

What additional measures can you take to help increase health literacy in this patient? What other measures would be helpful for this patient if she did not speak English, could not read, or had other learning deficits?

Information related to risk factors, related assessments, and specific nursing interventions for fluid volume disturbances and electrolyte disturbances can be found in the Supplemental Resources for this text online.

Developing a Dietary Plan

Teach patients about their health conditions and provide information and support to improve health literacy in patients. Refer to the accompanying Promoting Health Literacy box. Simple dietary changes may help to resolve fluid and electrolyte disturbances. After obtaining a nutritional assessment to identify actual or potential imbalances and food preferences (refer to Chapter 37), initiate teaching based on a nutritional plan that involves both the patient and the person who prepares the patient's meals. Include foods that help to resolve the fluid or electrolyte imbalance and that are acceptable to the patient. For example, for fluid volume deficit, increase foods with high water content (e.g., citrus fruit, melons, celery); for hypokalemia, increase foods with high potassium content (e.g., bananas, citrus fruits, apricots, melons, broccoli, potatoes, raisins, lima beans); and for hypernatremia, avoid foods high in sodium (e.g., processed cheese, lunch meats, canned soups and vegetables, salted snack foods) and eliminate the use of table salt.

When teaching the patient about foods to include or avoid, provide the patient with a written list for reference. Evaluate the patient's understanding of the teaching by having the patient identify foods that can be eaten freely or moderately as well as those to be avoided. Both the patient and person responsible for the patient's food preparation should be able to describe a 24-hour nutrition plan compatible with the recommended modifications.

Modifying Fluid Intake

Depending on the nature of the fluid or electrolyte imbalance, a patient's fluid intake may need to be increased, decreased, or modified in terms of types of fluids ingested. Nursing responsibilities include:

- Identifying the appropriate fluid modification (e.g., with certain illnesses, there may be a prescribed intervention to "Restrict fluids to 1,000 mL daily")
- Determining whether the patient understands the rationale for the fluid modification, is motivated to follow the modification, and is capable of adhering to the plan (e.g., a bedridden patient who needs to increase fluid intake cannot do this independently)
- Developing and implementing a plan of care based on the preceding information

INCREASING FLUIDS

Increasing fluids involves actions to achieve an above-average intake of fluids. A prescribed intervention to encourage or increase fluids indicates the amount of fluid the patient is to have in each 24-hour period. Typically, the plan of care specifies the amount of fluid to be ingested in 24 hours (for hospitalized patients, shift totals are helpful [e.g., 7 to 3, 1,200 mL; 3 to 11, 900 mL; 11 to 7, 300 mL]) and the patient's food preferences. Choose or assist with choosing fluids that best provide the calories and electrolytes needed by the patient.

Several interventions can be implemented to help the patient consume more than average amounts of fluids. Begin by explaining to the patient in understandable terms the rationale for the increased fluids and the specific goal of taking the daily amount of fluid prescribed. This explanation provides the patient with a greater understanding of the reason for the increase in fluid intake. In addition, this information helps motivate the patient to engage in the planned interventions. Together with the patient, develop short-term goals for accomplishing the increased fluid intake. For example, the patient will drink a glass of water every hour, a particular beverage by the time a television program is finished, or a pitcher of water by lunch. In general, patients are more likely to reach set goals when they have been involved in setting these goals.

Ensure that a proportionately larger amount of fluid is offered during the early hours of the patient's waking day, rather than large amounts before bedtime. The patient can usually take fluids relatively easily after having few or no fluids during sleeping hours. However, large amounts of fluid at night interferes with the patient's ability to rest and sleep by being awakened during the night with the need to urinate.

Offering a variety of fluids served at the appropriate temperature is helpful, as is allowing the patient to indicate a preference. The likelihood for success also is increased because the patient is more likely to drink more when some liquids are iced and cold and when coffee or tea is hot. Variety also adds interest and makes increasing fluids more palatable. If patients dislike taking fluids (a common problem with children) or have swallowing difficulties, offering a gelatin dessert, flavored frozen water (popsicles), water ice, or other alternative sources of liquid may meet with more success.

Always have fluids readily available for the patient. Take care to avoid a situation in which patients are unable to secure their own fluids (left with an unfilled water pitcher, an empty glass, a full pitcher out of reach, or a pitcher too heavy to lift). In addition, use attractive, clean, and easy-to-handle cups, glasses, and straws and practices that help to encourage the patient's desire to take fluids.

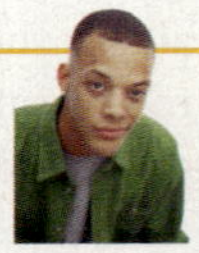

Recall ***Jeremiah Stein***, the student with frequent loose stools. The nurse should discuss the need for increased fluid intake to compensate for fluid lost with the loose stools with Jeremiah. Students are often on tight budgets; it would be important to determine if he has access to or is able to obtain appropriate fluids.

Patient/family/caregiver participation in care promotes autonomy and self-esteem. Therefore, have the patient/family member/caregiver help keep a record of intake when possible. This often serves as a motivating factor to increase fluid intake. Offer support, understanding, and encouragement in providing nursing care because forcing fluid intake for the person experiencing no thirst can be uncomfortable.

Increasing the fluid intake of patients is a common nursing intervention. Use creativity to assist the patient and family/caregiver to reach desired goals. Having a tea party may be a helpful strategy to use when encouraging a child to increase fluids. When determining the patient's increased fluid intake, be sure to include fluids replaced through nasogastric, gastrostomy, or jejunostomy tubes in the fluid balance summary.

RESTRICTING FLUIDS

Restricting the patient's fluid intake is sometimes necessary. A prescribed intervention to decrease or restrict fluids indicates the amount of fluid the patient is to have in each 24-hour period.

Several interventions can be implemented to help patients restrict their intake of fluids. As with the method for increasing fluids, begin by explaining to the patient in understandable terms the rationale for the fluid restriction and the specified daily amount of fluid prescribed. Then work with the patient to develop short-term outcomes for accomplishing the overall task. Discuss with the patient the time intervals at which fluids will be served. Usually, offering fluids at 1- or 2-hour intervals and between meals is best because food often helps to relieve some feelings of thirst. Provide the fluid in small glasses or cups so that the container appears to contain more fluid than it actually does. Using ice chips also is helpful. Ice chips are about twice the volume of water in its liquid state and help to quench thirst. Remember to include the ice chips as part of the patient's fluid intake. If appropriate, encourage the patient/family member/caregiver to participate in their care by helping to keep a record of intake.

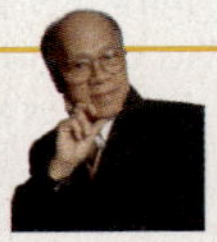

Consider ***Mr. Park***, the patient who received too much IV fluid. As a result of this excess fluid intake and his subsequent development of problems, the nurse would be alert to the possibility that fluid restriction may be appropriate. If this occurs, the nurse needs to ensure that Mr. Park understands the reason for the restriction.

Patients who need to restrict fluid intake often report thirst or dry mouth. Avoid offering patients dry, salty, or sweet foods and fluids because such items tend to increase thirst. Also, attempt to divert the patient's attention from thirst by involving the patient in activities, and keep fluids not intended for the patient out of sight. Provide understanding, support, and encouragement because limiting fluid intake is uncomfortable for a thirsty person.

Provide oral hygiene at regular intervals so that the patient's mouth remains clean and moist. Lubricate the lips and mucous membranes as indicated. If the patient is capable, allow the patient to rinse the mouth with water without swallowing the fluid, to avoid exceeding the intake limit. If appropriate, the patient could try chewing sugar-free gum or sucking on sugar-free hard candy to stimulate the flow of saliva (MFMER, 2017).

Just as with fluid increases, fluid limits should also have shift totals set. This prevents one shift from taking all of the patient's allotted fluid and prepares the patient ahead of time for the fluid limits.

Administering Medications

Patients with fluid, electrolyte, and acid–base imbalances are often prescribed medications as part of the therapeutic regimen. Be knowledgeable about and understand the therapeutic effects of mineral–electrolyte preparations and diuretics and appreciate the potential risk for life-threatening adverse effects. It is also important to consider the impact of other medications, such as steroids and hormone replacements, on fluid and electrolyte balance.

MINERAL–ELECTROLYTE PREPARATIONS

Mineral–electrolyte preparations are frequently prescribed to correct electrolyte imbalances. Nursing responsibilities include:

- Accurate administration of the medications, following the manufacturer's guidelines; for example, diluting potassium supplements to disguise the unpleasant taste and decrease gastric irritation, or monitoring ABGs for increased pH after each 50 to 100 mEq of sodium bicarbonate to avoid overtreatment and metabolic alkalosis.
- Understand the intended therapeutic effect and evaluate the effectiveness of the therapy through patient assessment; for example, when administering magnesium sulfate, assessing for decreased restlessness and irritability, decreased muscle tremors, and control of convulsions.
- Assess for adverse effects; for example, when administering solutions containing sodium chloride, observe for hypernatremia.
- Understand and appreciate the risks associated with administration and the appropriate precautions to avoid adverse outcomes; for example, never administering IV potassium via IV bolus or carefully monitoring the infusion rate for IV potassium chloride solutions. The maximum rate should not exceed 10 mEq/hr (Adams et al., 2020). An administration error can result in sudden hyperkalemia, leading to a fatal cardiac arrhythmia.
- Assess for drug interactions; for example, consider drugs that increase the effects of minerals and electrolytes include acidifying agents, alkalinizing agents, cation exchange resin, iron salts, and potassium salts. Some minerals and electrolytes will enhance the effects of other medications, such as muscle relaxants.
- Teach patients about their prescribed mineral and electrolyte preparations and associated self-care behaviors.

DIURETICS

Diuretics are drugs that increase renal excretion of water, sodium, and other electrolytes. Although helpful in treating patients with FVE, they increase the risk for fluid volume deficit and serious electrolyte deficiencies. Careful monitoring of fluid intake, urine output, and serum electrolytes is essential for patient safety. Direct particular attention toward the patient's serum potassium level. It is important to provide patient education to any patient receiving diuretic therapy, including the rationale for the therapy, precautions, and side effects.

Administering Intravenous Fluid Therapy

The infusion of intravenous (IV) solutions may be prescribed to address fluid and/or electrolyte disturbances. The specific type and volume of solution to be administered is identified by the prescriber. The nurse is responsible for initiating, monitoring, and discontinuing the therapy. The nurse is also responsible for critically evaluating the prescribed intervention prior to administration. Any concerns regarding the type or amount of therapy prescribed should be immediately and clearly communicated to the prescribing practitioner. For example, if a patient's potassium level is noted to be elevated and the patient is prescribed a potassium-containing IV solution such as lactated Ringer's, the nurse should notify the prescribing practitioner of the laboratory result and request a revision of the prescribed intervention.

As with other therapeutic agents, the nurse must understand the rationale for the use of IV therapy for each patient, the type of solution being used, its desired effect, and potential adverse reactions. The contents of selected IV solutions and comments about their use are listed in Table 41-7 on page 1694.

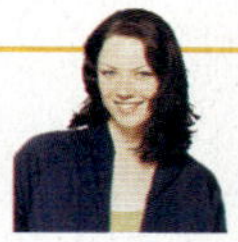

Think back to **Grace Gilligan**, the woman with nausea and vomiting. The nurse could expect that this patient is high risk for fluid and electrolyte imbalances. What would be benefits and risks of administering the various IV solutions in Table 41-7 (on page 1694) to this patient? How would you assess if the IV therapy were having its desired effect (improving the patient's condition)?

EQUIPMENT

Sterile technique must be observed when accessing a vein to avoid possible catheter-related infection. Disposable infusion tubing and needles are used to help eliminate many possible sources of contamination and to reduce the cost of equipment aftercare.

Equipment used to administer IV fluid therapy varies according to the manufacturer. Be familiar with the equipment used in the facility or home setting. Typically, most solutions for infusions are dispensed in 1-L or 500-mL flexible or rigid plastic containers. Because plastic bags collapse under atmospheric pressure as the solution enters the patient's vein, they do not require a vent for air to enter to replace fluid flowing from the container. Small 50-, 100-, and 250-mL solution bags are available to administer intermittent IV medications (such as antibiotics given by IV piggyback).

Some medications bond with the plastic in IV bags. Therefore, glass bottles are required for these medications. Glass bottles do not collapse under atmospheric pressure and thus require a vent to allow air to enter the bottle as the fluid leaves the bottle.

IV administration tubing is used to attach the IV container to the patient's venous access. A basic administration set is illustrated in Figure 41-10 on page 1694. An IV administration set includes a spike or piercing pin to access the IV container, a drip chamber for observing fluid drops, a slide clamp to stop fluid flow, a roller clamp to manually regulate the rate of flow, a filter, several injection ports for administration of medications or additional IV fluids, and a connector at the end of the tubing to connect with the venous access (preferably Luer lock design, with threads that securely screw on) (refer to Fig. 41-10 on page 1694). Electronic infusion devices (infusion pumps) usually require tubing specific for the device; this tubing shares many of the same features as tubing used for gravity infusion. Tubing for an electronic infusion device also includes a mechanism that fits into the electronic device to control the infusion rate. Figure 41-11 (on page 1695) provides an example of an electronic infusion device.

Table 41-7 Selected IV Solutions

SOLUTION	COMMENTS
Isotonic Solutions	
Total osmolality close to that of the ECF; replace the ECF	
0.9% NaCl (normal saline)	Not desirable as routine maintenance solution because it provides only Na^+ and Cl^-, which are provided in excessive amounts. May be used to expand temporarily the extracellular compartment if circulatory insufficiency is a problem; also used to treat hypovolemia, metabolic alkalosis, mild hyponatremia, hypercalcemia. Used with administration of blood transfusions
Lactated Ringer's solution	Contains multiple electrolytes in about the same concentrations as found in plasma (note that this solution is lacking in Mg^{2+}) Used in the treatment of hypovolemia, burns, and fluid lost from GI sources
Hypotonic Solutions	
Hypotonic to plasma; replace ICF	
0.33% NaCl (1/3-strength normal saline)	Provides Na^+, Cl^-, and free water Na^+ and Cl^- allow kidneys to select and retain needed amounts Free water desirable as aid to kidneys in elimination of solutes Used in treating hypernatremia
0.45% NaCl (½-strength normal saline)	A hypotonic solution that provides Na^+, Cl^-, and free water Used as a basic fluid for maintenance needs Often used to treat hypernatremia (because this solution contains a small amount of Na^+, it dilutes the plasma sodium while not allowing it to drop too rapidly)
Hypertonic Solutions	
Hypertonic to plasma	
5% dextrose in lactated Ringer's solution	Supplies fluid and calories to the body Replaces electrolytes; shifts fluid from the intracellular compartment into the intravascular space, expanding vascular volume
5% dextrose in 0.9% NaCl	Used to treat SIADH Can temporarily be used to treat hypovolemia if plasma expander is not available

Source: Adapted from Hale, A., & Hovey, M. J. (2014). *Fluid, electrolyte, and acid-base imbalances.* F.A. Davis Company; Hinkle, J. L., Cheever, K. H., & Overbaugh, K. J. (2022). *Brunner & Suddarth's Textbook of medical-surgical nursing* (15th ed.). Wolters Kluwer; and Willis, L. M. (Ed.). (2020). *Fluids & electrolytes made incredibly easy!* (7th ed.). Wolters Kluwer.

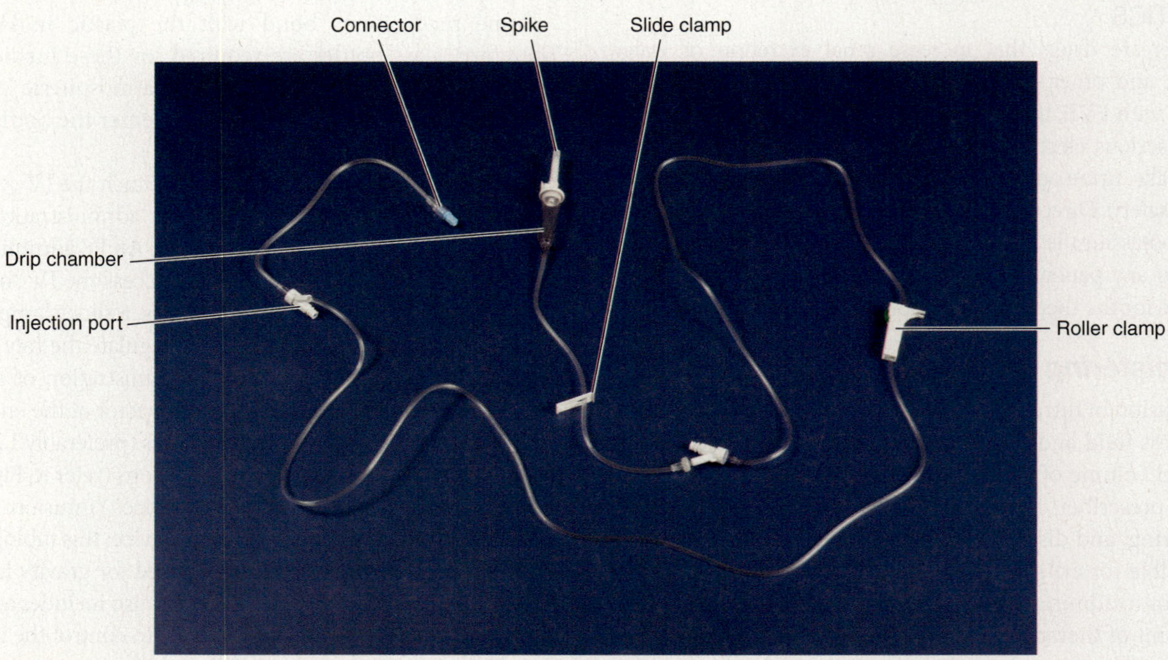

FIGURE 41-10. Basic administration tubing for intravenous therapy. (*Source:* Used with permission from Shutterstock. *Photo by B. Proud.*)

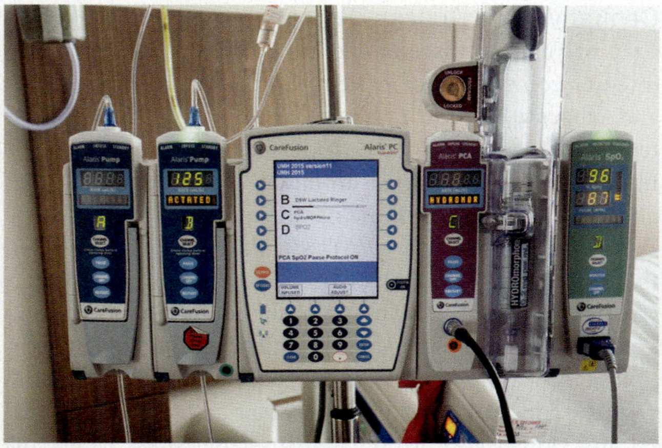

FIGURE 41-11. An electronic infusion device. (*Source:* Used with permission from Shutterstock. *Photo by Rudy Umans.*)

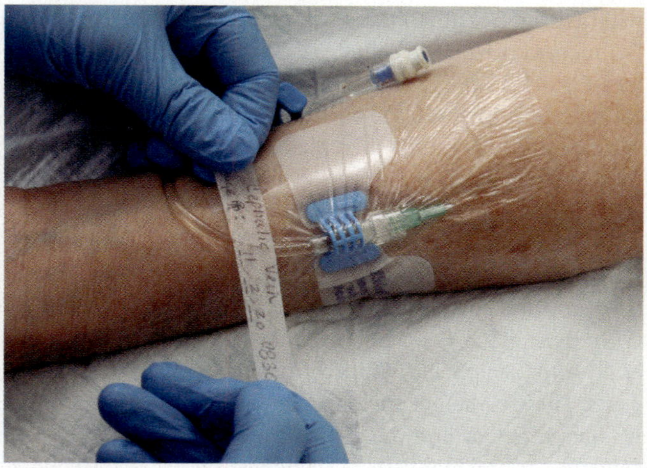

FIGURE 41-12. A peripheral venous access device with short extension tubing and a needleless connector.

A variety of needles and catheters are commonly used for peripheral IV infusions. IV catheters are plastic tubes that have been mounted on a needle or are threaded through a needle for insertion. Once inserted, the needle is withdrawn, and the flexible catheter remains in the vein. The over-the-needle catheter is easy to insert and stable. Single- or double-winged infusion needles (butterflies) are short-beveled, thin-walled needles with plastic flaps and are not flexible, and thus are more likely to infiltrate. They may be used with single-dose administration (Gorski et al., 2021). Refer to the vascular access devices discussion in the next section. Other equipment necessary to start an IV infusion is listed in Skill 41-1 (on pp. 1715–1724).

Many devices are available that minimize the potential for injury and promote safety when connecting, accessing, or disposing of IV equipment, including needleless systems and needle-housing systems in which the needle is recessed and protected. Luer-locking (with threads that securely screw on) needleless connectors are used to connect syringes and/or administration sets to a vascular access device hub or other injection site and should be included as part of vascular access device policies and procedures. The primary purpose of needleless connectors is to protect health care personnel by eliminating needles and reduce associated needlestick injuries when attaching administration sets and/or syringes to the vascular access device (Gorski et al., 2021). A short extension tubing set is often used between the venous access device and the needleless connector to reduce catheter manipulation (Gorski et al., 2021). Closed-system peripheral intravenous catheters integrate the catheter and extension tubing as one piece (Galang et al., 2020), eliminating the need for the addition of separate extension tubing. It is important to follow the manufacturers' recommendations for appropriate sequencing of clamping and final syringe disconnection when flushing and/or using the connector to reduce the amount of blood reflux into the venous access device lumen and subsequent potential occlusion of the venous access device from intraluminal thrombosis (Gorski et al., 2021). Figure 41-12 provides an example of a PIVC with short extension tubing, venous catheter stabilization device, and a needleless connector in place. Additional information regarding needleless connectors is discussed later in the chapter. Additional information regarding closed or closed peripheral intravenous catheters is discussed in the following section.

Refer to Chapter 30 for additional information about protective measures and use of IV equipment related to medication administration.

VASCULAR ACCESS DEVICES

Many different options for vascular access devices (VADs) are available for delivery of solutions and medications into a vein. The length of time the infusion therapy is needed, the type of medication or product that will be delivered intravenously, the patient's vascular condition, and the patient's health status as well as individualized needs determine which option is used (Gorski, et al., 2021). In addition, decisions on insertion site and catheter type should also be guided by what will pose the least risk for IV complications (Gorski et al., 2021; Higginson, 2015; Moureau & Chopra, 2016). Guidelines from the Infusion Nurses Society recommend selection of the least invasive VAD with the smallest outer diameter and fewest number of lumens needed for the prescribed therapy (Gorski et al., 2021). The nursing care that is required will depend on the type of device or IV catheter that is utilized. Vascular access devices include peripheral venous catheters, midline catheters, and central venous access devices (CVADs).

Peripheral Venous Catheters

Peripheral intravenous catheters (PIVCs) are inserted into and reside in veins of the periphery that include all extremities, the external jugular vein and scalp veins in neonates (Gorski et al., 2021). These over-the-needle catheters are the most common type of peripheral vascular catheter used: *short PIVCs* are inserted into superficial veins; *long PIVCs* are inserted in either superficial or deep peripheral veins and are an option when a short PIVC is not long enough to adequately cannulate the available vein, or the vessel is difficult to palpate or visualize with the naked eye (Gorski et al., 2021). When the anticipated duration of infusion therapy will be brief (less than 4 days [Gorski et al., 2021]), a short (<3 inches) peripheral catheter is placed in a peripheral vein (see Fig. 41-12 on page 1695). The tip of a short peripheral catheter terminates in the peripheral vein. This device is not appropriate for certain therapies, such as vesicant chemotherapy, drugs that are classified as irritants, or PN (Gorski et al., 2021).

When the anticipated duration of infusion therapy in hospitalized patients will be 5 to 14 days and peripheral infusion is appropriate, insert a *midline catheter* (Gorski et al., 2021; O'Grady et al., 2017). Midline catheters are inserted peripherally into the upper arm into the basilic, cephalic, or brachial veins. These catheters are longer (>3 inches) than peripheral venous catheters, and the distal tip terminates in the basilic, cephalic, or brachial vein, at or below the axillary level and distal to the shoulder (Gorski et al., 2021). In neonates, midline catheters may also be inserted into a scalp vein with the distal tip located in the jugular vein above the clavicle or in the lower extremity with the distal tip located in the inguinal crease (Gorski et al., 2021). Midlines are not considered to be central lines and should not be used to continuously infuse vesicants, solutions with extremes of pH or osmolarity, or PN (Gorski et al., 2021). Use of midlines should also be avoided for patients with a history of thrombosis, hypercoagulability, decreased venous flow to the extremities, or end-stage renal disease (Gorski et al., 2021).

The smallest-gauge device that will accommodate the prescribed therapy and patient need should be selected (Gorski et al., 2021) (see Chapter 30 for more discussion on gauges). A 20- to 24-gauge catheter is recommended for most infusions to decrease the risk of phlebitis; a 22- to 26-gauge catheter is recommended for neonates, pediatric patients, older adults, and patients with limited venous options to minimize insertion-related trauma (Gorski et al., 2021). In inpatient and nursing facilities, the PIVC insertion site, site dressing and securement device should be assessed every 4 hours at a minimum (Gorski et al., 2021). In community-based settings, assess the PIVC at every visit and teach the patient/family member/caregiver to check the site at least once per day or every 4 hours during waking hours for continuous PIVC infusions (Gorski et al., 2021).

Previously, recommendations suggested routine rotation of insertion sites at various intervals, usually 72 to 96 hours. Current research and guidelines support maintaining peripheral IV access devices until no longer clinically indicated (discontinuation of infusion therapy; not used for 24 hours or more; no longer included in plan of care) or until there is an unresolved complication (presence of site complication [e.g., phlebitis, infiltration, extravasation] or systemic complication [e.g., infection]) (Bolton, 2015; Gorski et al., 2021; Loveday et al., 2014; Tuffaha et al., 2014). Nurses should use clinical assessment and judgment in deciding when to replace or discontinue a peripheral IV catheter. The clinical need for the IV catheter should be assessed on a daily basis in acute inpatient settings and during regular assessment visits in community-based care settings (Gorski et al., 2021).

Central Venous Access Devices

Central venous (vascular) access devices (CVADs) are an integral component of patient care in acute, ambulatory, and subacute care settings, as well as in the home and long-term care facilities. They provide access for a variety of IV fluids, medications, blood products, and PN solutions and allow a means for hemodynamic monitoring and blood sampling. The use of a CVAD should be considered when the anticipated duration of infusion therapy is >15 days (Gorski et al., 2021). The type and duration of infusion therapy, patient preference, the patient's physiologic condition (age, health problems, comorbidities), and the patient's vascular condition (history of vascular access attempts, vessel and skin health at potential insertion sites) determine the type of CVAD used (Gorski et al., 2021). The tip of the CVAD catheter terminates in the central venous circulation, usually in the lower one third of the superior vena cava near its junction with the right atrium (Gorski et al., 2021). The use of ultrasound technology during insertion by a practitioner fully trained in its technique is recommended if available to increase success rates and decrease insertion-related complications (Gorski et al., 2021; O'Grady et al., 2017). **All CVADs require radiographic confirmation of position after insertion and before use** (Gorski et al., 2021). Some CVADs have more than one lumen to allow for multiple concurrent infusions; a CVAD with the minimum number of lumens essential for the management of the patient should be used (O'Grady et al., 2017). The individual patient circumstances and plan of care may result in use of the CVAD for a relatively short period of time or a longer period of time, perhaps years. Insight into the patient experience of living with a CVAD can help nurses provide appropriate support for these patients. Refer to the accompanying Research in Nursing box.

Types of CVADs include the following:

- Peripherally inserted central catheter (PICC)
- Nontunneled percutaneous central venous catheter
- Tunneled percutaneous central venous catheter
- Implanted port

PICCs are a type of CVAD (>20 cm depending on patient size; single or double lumen) that can be introduced into a peripheral vein (the basilic, brachial [preferred], or cephalic veins) above the antecubital fossa (Gorski et al., 2021) (Fig. 41-13). A specially trained registered nurse or other advanced practice professional can insert this type of catheter. A PICC may be inserted in interventional radiology units or, in some institutions, at the bedside. PICCs may have single or multiple lumens. They are used extensively in the home for IV therapy and have become an increasingly common venous access device in acute-care settings, especially for patients requiring long-term IV therapy (6 weeks to 6 months). Indications for use of PICCs include administration of IV antibiotics for an extended period (>1 week), infusion of parenteral nutrition, chemotherapy and other targeted therapy drugs, continuous pain management infusions, vesicants, hyperosmolar solutions, blood

Research in Nursing

BRIDGING THE GAP TO EVIDENCE-BASED PRACTICE

Central Venous Access Devices and Patients' Experiences

Central venous access devices (CVADs) have become an increasingly common in community settings for IV therapy, venous access for blood sampling, especially for patients requiring long-term IV therapy, such as chemotherapy and antibiotics. The use of a CVAD requires patients to make adjustments in daily life situations, such as showering, washing hair and sleeping; possible alterations in body image; and caring for the CVAD. What are patients' experiences of living with a CVAD?

Related Research

Kelly, L., & Snowden, A. (2021). 'Pinholes in my arms': The vicious cycle of vascular access. *British Journal of Nursing, 30*(14), S4–S13. https://doi.org/10.12968/bjon.2021.30.14.S4

The aim of this qualitative study was to explore how patients make sense of living with a CVAD and to explore the experiences of living with an external or implanted vascular access device. Participants were purposefully recruited from a cancer treatment center in Scotland. Patients who had a CVAD in place for longer than 3 weeks were eligible to participate. Eleven patients responded to the recruitment request, and all were enrolled; 5 participants had a PICC, 3 had a tunneled CVAD, and 3 had an implanted CVAD. One-to-one semi-structured interviews were performed and were recorded. The interviews were transcribed verbatim and analyzed. Four superordinate themes, some with subthemes, were identified by the authors, including *The self under attack (subthemes: the violation of vascular access; accepting the ordeals of vascular access), Being rescued/being robbed (subthemes: being thrown a lifeline, device as part of self, better than the rest), Protection of others/protection of self,* and *Bewilderment and dismay at lack of staff competence.* The authors presented a resulting conceptual framework of the "vicious cycle of vascular access." The authors concluded having a CVAD affects the psychological, social, and personal self; impacts on self-esteem and self-image; and that the results suggest that CVADs are accepted by patients and are, in the end, embodied by them.

Relevance to Nursing Practice

Nurses are a key source of support for patients and can provide information, guidance, and support to assist patients in managing life with a CVAD. Nurses should consider patient experiences when developing a plan of care to improve quality of life and support optimal patient outcomes.

components, other specific medications (e.g., vasopressors, anticoagulants), and long-term rehydration. Advantages of using a PICC include that it can remain in place for an extended period of time (6 months to a year or 18 months if no complications arise) and for obtaining blood samples (Memorial Sloan Kettering Cancer Center, 2021). In addition, because the catheter is inserted peripherally, PICCs may be associated with less risk of complications than other CVADs, such as nerve damage, stenosis, and pneumothorax (Moureau & Chopra, 2016).

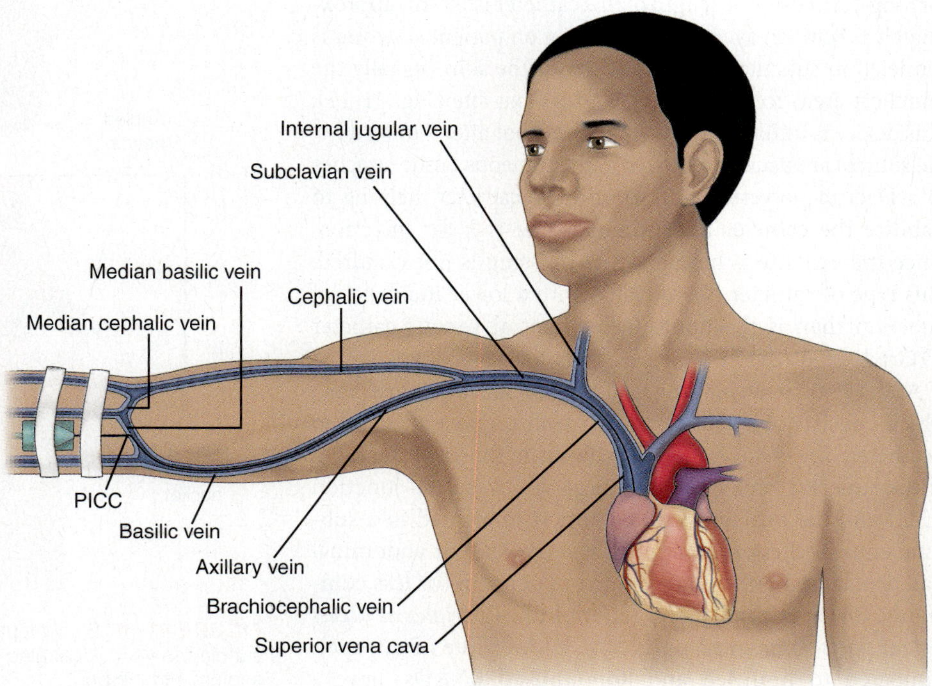

FIGURE 41-13. Placement of a peripherally inserted central catheter (PICC).

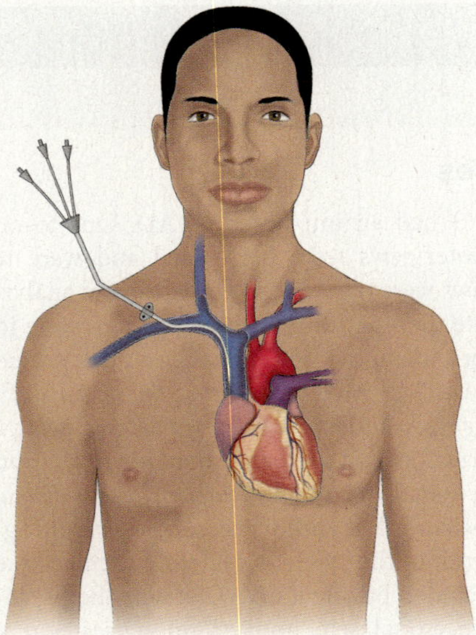

FIGURE 41-14. Placement of a triple-lumen nontunneled percutaneous central venous catheter.

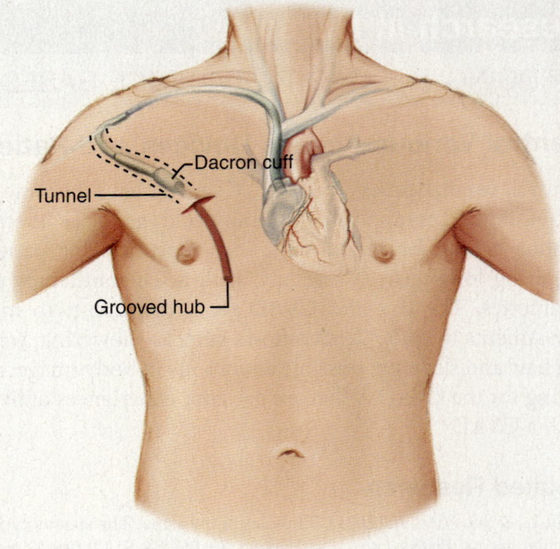

FIGURE 41-15. Placement of a tunneled central venous catheter.

Nontunneled percutaneous central venous catheters (Fig. 41-14) have a shorter dwell time (<14 days). These catheters can have double, triple, or quadruple lumens and are >8 cm, depending on patient size. They are introduced through the skin into the internal jugular, subclavian, or femoral veins. Catheters inserted via the femoral vein should have the distal tip dwell in the thoracic inferior vena cava above the level of the diaphragm (Gorski et al., 2021). They are mainly used short-term critical access with patients who are unstable (Moureau & Chopra, 2016); the CDC recommends avoiding the femoral vein for central venous access in adult patients (O'Grady et al., 2017). Pneumothorax is a potential complication when the catheter is placed in the subclavian vein.

A *tunneled central venous catheter* is implanted into the internal or external jugular or subclavian vein and intended for long-term use. The length of this catheter is >8 cm (approximately 90 cm, on average), depending on patient size, and is tunneled in subcutaneous tissue under the skin (usually the midchest area) for 3 to 6 inches to its exit site (Fig. 41-15). This device is initially sutured into place, but after 7 to 14 days, the sutures are usually removed. Subcutaneous tissue attaches to a Dacron polyester cuff around the catheter, helping to stabilize the catheter and minimize the risk for infection. Once the exit site is healed, a site dressing is not required. This type of catheter is associated with a lower incidence of infection than is the nontunneled central venous catheter (O'Grady et al., 2017).

Another type of long-term CVAD is an *implanted port*, which consists of a subcutaneous injection port attached to a catheter. The distal catheter tip dwells in the lower segment of the superior vena cava at or near the cavoatrial junction (CAJ) and the proximal end or port is implanted in a subcutaneous pocket of the upper chest (typical) or abdominal wall. Implanted ports placed in the upper arm (or less commonly, lower extremity) are referred to as *peripheral access system ports.* Implanted ports have a lower rate of infection compared to tunneled and nontunneled CVADs; have a low risk of complication during treatment, require minimal care and management by the patient, and may be associated with improved body image (Gorski et al., 2021; Kline & Katrancha, 2019; O'Grady et al., 2017). When not in use, no external parts of the system are visible. A special angled noncoring needle is inserted through the skin and rubber septum and into the port reservoir to access the system (Fig. 41-16). Implanted ports require minimal care, but the discomfort related to accessing the port may be a disadvantage for some patients. Surgery is required for catheter removal (O'Grady et al., 2017).

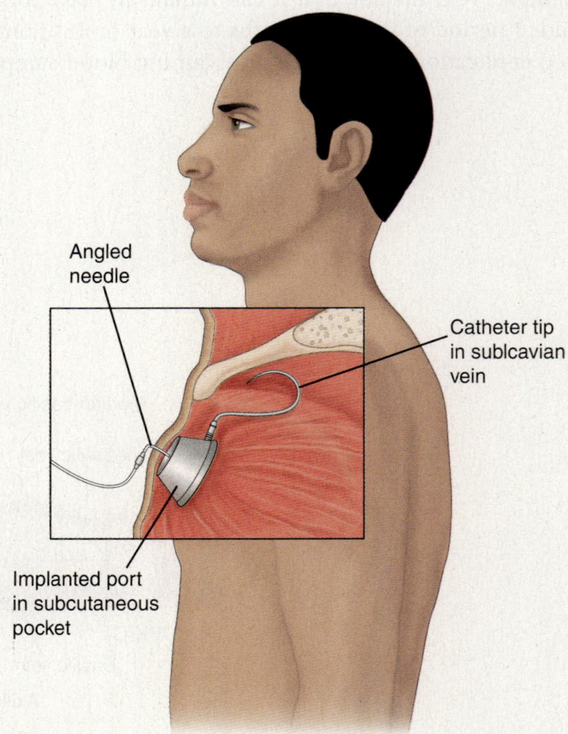

FIGURE 41-16. Placement of an implanted port with the tip in the subclavian vein. An angled needle is inserted through the skin and septum into the port.

In inpatient and nursing facilities, assess the CVAD insertion site, site dressing, and securement device with each infusion and at least daily (Gorski et al., 2021). In community-based settings, assess the CVAD at every visit and teach the patient/family member/caregiver to check the site with each infusion or at least once per day (Gorski et al., 2021). CVADs are not routinely changed in order to reduce the risk of infection (O'Grady et al., 2017). However, any central venous catheter may be removed and/or replaced if suspicion of a catheter-related bloodstream infection or other complication exists. CVAD-related complications include thrombosis, central line–related bloodstream infection (CLABSI), air embolism, phlebitis, and occlusion (Berndt & Steinheiser, 2019; Gorski et al., 2021; McArthur, 2018; Walters & Price, 2019). The continued need for *PICCs* and *nontunneled* CVADs should be assessed on a daily basis and removed when there is a change in the patient's infusion needs or it is no longer needed for the plan of care (Gorski et al., 2021). The continued need for *tunneled* and *implanted* CVADs should be assessed on a regular basis; removal may be indicated when infusion therapy is completed, in the presence of an unresolved complication, or when it is no longer needed for the plan of care; consideration should be given to the possibility for infusion therapy to resume in the future (Gorski et al., 2021).

PERIPHERAL VASCULAR ACCESS CONSIDERATIONS

The nurse initiating a PIVC needs to assess for the safest, most appropriate site for each particular patient. The suitability of particular veins for peripheral IV infusions varies with individual circumstances. The accessibility and condition of the vein and the type of fluid to be infused should be considered when determining the location for intravenous access via a PIVC. Measures to increase insertion success, including consideration of vascular visualization technology and management of insertion pain, should be implemented.

Accessibility of a Vein

Keep in mind the following guidelines related to PIVCs and access sites:

- Discuss the preference for VAD site selection with the patient/family/caregivers (Gorski et al., 2021).
- Determine the most desirable accessible vein. For a short PIVC, use the forearm to prolong dwell time, increase the likelihood of the PIVC lasting the full length of the prescribed therapy, decrease pain during dwell time, promote self-care, and prevent accidental removal and occlusions (Gorski et al., 2021). The dorsal and ventral surfaces of the upper extremities, including the metacarpal, cephalic, basilic, and median veins, are appropriate sites for infusion (Gorski et al., 2021). Avoid the cephalic vein at the radial wrist, inner aspect of the wrist, and sites at/above the antecubital fossa because of the potential risk for nerve damage (Gorski et al., 2021). Figure 41-17A illustrates infusion sites on the arm and hand for adult patients. For a long PIVC, use the veins on the dorsal and ventral surfaces of the upper extremities, including the cephalic, basilic, and median veins; insertion should be in the forearm without crossing into the antecubital fossa (Gorski et al., 2021). Consider use of the basilic, cephalic, or brachial veins when inserting a midline catheter (Gorski et al., 2021).
- In general, either arm may be used for IV therapy. Use of the nondominant arm is preferred for patient comfort and to limit movement in the impacted extremity (Gorski et al., 2021). For example, if the patient is right-handed, the IV is preferably placed on the left extremity to improve the patient's ability to complete activities of daily living. This is particularly important if the duration of infusion is expected to be prolonged.

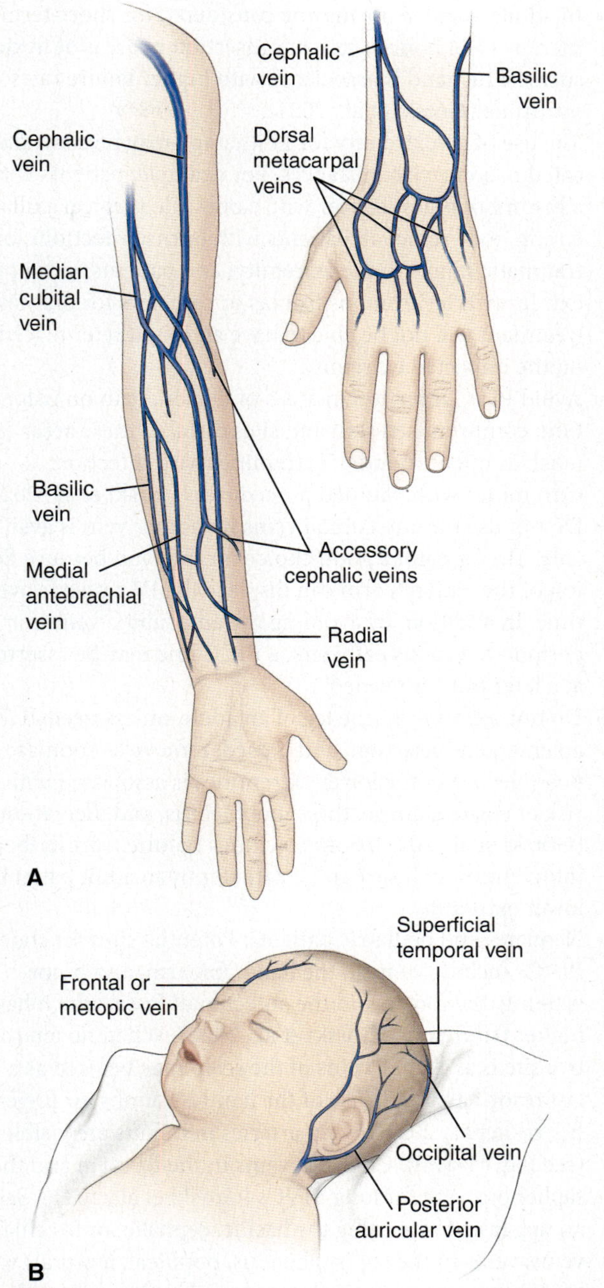

FIGURE 41-17. Peripheral venous access sites. **A.** Infusion sites on the ventral and dorsal aspects of the lower arm and hand. **B.** Infusion sites on the scalp of an infant.

- In adults, hand veins may be considered for short-term therapy (>24 hours); catheter insertion in areas of flexion such as the hand is associated with higher failure rates over time (Gorski et al., 2021).
- The use of an extremity for IV therapy may be contraindicated in some circumstances. For example, patients with a history of breast cancer with same-side surgical axillary lymph node removal; patients with burns, infections, or traumatic injury to the extremity; and patients with upper extremity arteriovenous fistulas or catheters for dialysis treatment will not be able to have an IV catheter placed on the impacted extremity.
- Avoid PIVC insertion in areas of flexion; pain on palpation; compromised skin and sites distal to these areas (such as open wounds); extremities with infection; extremities with planned procedures (Gorski et al., 2021).
- Do not use the antecubital veins if another vein is available. They are not a good choice for infusion because flexion of the patient's arm can displace the IV catheter over time. In addition, by avoiding the antecubital veins for peripheral venous catheters, a PICC line may be inserted at a later time, if needed.
- Do not use veins in the leg of an adult, unless needed for an emergent insertion, and if used, remove as soon as possible; use of the lower extremities is associated with risk of tissue damage, thrombophlebitis, and ulceration (Gorski et al., 2021). Some facilities require a prescribed intervention to insert an IV catheter in an adult patient's lower extremity.
- Neonates and pediatric patients: Potential sites for short PIVCs include veins in the hand, forearm, and if not walking, the foot; avoid the antecubital fossa, which has a higher failure rate (Gorski et al., 2021). When no alternative site is available, veins of the scalp may be used as a last resort; avoid the use of the hands, thumbs, or fingers (Gorski et al., 2021). Scalp arteries in infants are visible (see Fig. 41-17B). Consider veins in the forearm and the saphenous vein for long PIVCs (Gorski et al., 2021). Select an upper arm site using the basilic, cephalic, or brachial veins; veins in the leg (saphenous, popliteal, femoral) with the tip below the inguinal crease; and in the scalp with the tip in the neck, above the thorax for placement of a midline catheter (Gorski et al., 2021).

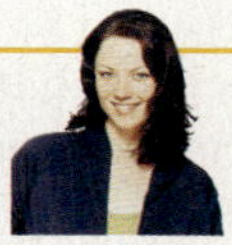

Think back to **Grace Gilligan**, the patient with nausea and vomiting. The nurse would incorporate knowledge of appropriate site selection for adults when determining the location for Grace's venous access.

Condition of the Vein

The ability to assess the condition of the patient's vein and to determine the degree of difficulty for successful insertion of an IV access is an extremely important skill. Experience is necessary to perform these skills. Factors that may interfere with successful evaluation of the condition of the patient's veins and subsequent placement of a peripheral catheter include obesity, diabetes, hypertension, variations in skin between patient populations (e.g., darker skin tones, excessive hair, presence of scars or tattoos), increased patient age, neonates, fluid volume deficit, injection drug use, the presence of multiple chronic health conditions (e.g., diabetes, renal disease), vascular disease, chemotherapy, and/or frequent hospitalizations (Dougherty, 2013; Dychter et al., 2012; Fields et al., 2014; Gorski et al, 2021; Morata & Bowers, 2020; Partovi-Deilami et al., 2016). These factors interfere with use of traditional techniques of direct visualization, anatomic landmarks, and palpation and make placement of PIVC difficult (Gorski et al., 2021; Houston, 2013). In addition, thin-walled and scarred veins, common in older adults, are fragile and prone to infiltration, which can make continued infusion a problem. The size of the vein will also limit the maximum gauge (size) catheter that can be inserted. Insertion of a PIVC in areas of veins that are compromised, such as previous PIVC, bruised, reddened/streaked, infiltrated, sclerosed, and/or engorged should be avoided (Gorski et al., 2021).

Type of Fluid to Be Infused

The type of fluid to be infused should be considered when determining the location for intravenous access via a PIVC. Keep in mind the following about the type of IV fluid to be infused:

- Select a vein and IV catheter size appropriate for the solution. Hypertonic solutions, those containing irritating medications, those administered at a rapid rate, and those with a high viscosity (such as a blood transfusion) should be given in a large vein, ideally using a large-gauge IV catheter to minimize vessel trauma and to facilitate the rate of flow. A larger-gauge catheter should be considered when rapid fluid replacement is required (Gorski et al., 2021). Use a 20- to 24-gauge PIVC based on vein size for blood transfusion; a large-gauge PIVC is recommended when rapid transfusion is required (Gorski et al., 2021). Additional discussion about blood transfusion is provided later in the chapter.
- Advise the patient that some medications administered intravenously in a peripheral vein (e.g., potassium chloride and certain antibiotics) may cause irritation and pain. Use of short PIVCs for continuous infusion of medication with irritant or vesicant properties should be avoided (Gorski et al., 2021). Educate the patient about the need to immediately report any discomfort to allow for timely intervention.

Measures to Increase PIVC Insertion Success

Measures to increase insertion success should be implemented. An individual nurse should not make more than two attempts at vascular access placement when initiating venous access for a patient (Gorski et al., 2021). If unsuccessful after two attempts, a colleague with advanced skills, such as a member of the nurse IV team, should attempt to initiate the venous access (Gorski et al., 2021). Multiple unsuccessful attempts cause pain to the patient and result in delayed treatment, limited future vascular access, increased costs, and increased risk for complications (Gorski et al., 2021). Use of vascular visualization technology may be appropriate after unsuccessful insertion attempts. Refer to the Reflective Practice box on page 1670.

QSEN TEAMWORK AND COLLABORATION

Nurses have a responsibility to function effectively within nursing and interprofessional teams, recognizing the contributions of others to achieve quality patient care. The nurse should collaborate with other members of the health care team and the patient to discuss appropriate options for a patient with difficult vascular access (Gorski et al., 2021; O'Grady et al., 2017).

Assess the patient's health history and current health status to identify factors that may affect the peripheral vasculature and increase difficulty with locating veins by observation. Refer to the previous discussion about vein condition on page 1700. Vascular visualization technology can be used to assist with identification of peripheral veins, with resulting increased insertion success, reduced insertion-related complications, and minimization of the need to escalate to unnecessary, more invasive venous access devices (Gorski et al., 2021). Visible light devices are one technology that can aid in locating superficial veins in neonates, but their usefulness in infants, older children, and adults is limited due to the thickness of subcutaneous tissue and the size of the arm circumference (Çağlar et al., 2019; Gorski et al., 2021; Gümüs & Başbakkal, 2021; Heinrichs et al., 2013; Pitts & Ostroff, 2019). Another vascular visualization technology is near infrared light (nIR). This technology uses infrared light to capture an image of veins and reflect it back to the skin surface or to a screen The use of nIR provides information is recommended to make more informed decisions about vein selection, decreases procedure time for PIVC insertion, and is associated with enhanced first-time insertion success in some patient, such as neonates (Gorski et al., 2021).

Ultrasound is another visualization technology to guide peripheral IV placement. Ultrasound-guided PIVC insertion is a safe, efficient intervention and should be used for placement of short PIVC in difficult-to-access adult patients (Gorski et al., 2021; Houston, 2013), the insertion of long PIVCs (Gorski et al., 2021), and after failed venipuncture attempts (Edwards & Jones, 2018; Egan et al., 2013). Images produced by ultrasound offer a visual advantage for locating the best peripheral veins to access as well as direct measurement of blood vessel diameter and condition (Arbique et al., 2014; Gorski et al., 2021). Use of ultrasound to guide placement also allows visualization of the IV catheter tip inside the vein and verification of placement of the catheter (Arbique et al., 2014). The use of ultrasound-guided PIVC placement has been associated with higher success rates; less time to cannulation; fewer needle sticks; decreased pain; decreased use of more invasive venous access devices, such as PICC and midline catheters; and longer survival time (time from placement to removal) (Desai et al., 2018; Galen et al., 2020; Houston, 2013; Moore, 2013; Vinograd et al., 2018).

Interventions to improve patient experience of PIVC insertion should include pain management strategies. Local anesthetic agents should be used to reduce pain in all adult and pediatric populations (Gorski et al., 2021). Local anesthetic agents to reduce pain associated with PIVC insertion include vapocoolant sprays, topical transdermal agents, jet injection of pressure-accelerated lidocaine (needle-free), application of hot or cold to the site, and intradermal injection of lidocaine or bacteriostatic 0.9% sodium chloride (Gorski et al., 2021; Korkut et al., 2020; Welyczko, 2020). The nurse needs to have knowledge of the anesthetic agent used and correct method of administration, based on the manufacturer's recommendations and facility policy. The use of a local anesthetic requires monitoring for potential allergic reactions, tissue damage, or inadvertent injection of the drug into the vascular system (Gorski et al., 2021). In addition, nonpharmacologic interventions should also be considered to reduce pain associated with PIVC insertion. Nonpharmacologic interventions suggested for use to reduce PIVC insertion-related pain and discomfort include distraction, relaxation, breathing exercises, local application of heat (Korkut et al., 2020), and virtual reality (VR) (Basak et al., 2020; Gorski et al., 2021). The choices of interventions for pediatric patients include swaddling, breastfeeding, pacifiers, rocking, blowing bubbles, reading books, VR, and local vibrating cold devices and should be made with consideration of growth and development level (Gorski et al., 2021).

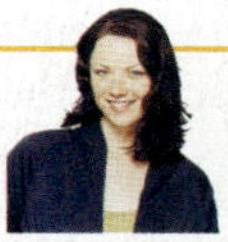

Think back to ***Grace Gilligan***, the patient who experienced several unsuccessful IV catheter insertion attempts, as described in the Reflective Practice box on page 1670. The nurse's ability to palpate the patient's veins before attempting venipuncture might have been helpful in determining the best vein to be used. The information provided by palpation also could have indicated that the patient's veins were scarred, thus suggesting the need for use of ultrasound to guide placement and/or the need for consultation with a more experienced team member, such as an IV nurse specialist (as the patient had requested) to perform the procedure.

INITIATION OF AN INTRAVENOUS INFUSION

Administration of IV solutions requires the same system of checks and rights of administration as for medication administration (refer to Chapter 30). Before the infusion is started, perform a final check of the solution to ensure that it is clear and contains no particles or precipitates. This check is especially important when substances have been added to the solution because some additives create precipitates. Commercially available in-line filters help reduce the risk for contamination by filtering the solution immediately before it enters the patient's vein. Skill 41-1 outlines the procedure for initiating a PIVC and an IV infusion (see p. 1715). Some adults and young children have a fear of needles and/or venipuncture. Provide information about the venipuncture process and infusion therapy procedures in an age-appropriate manner to decrease distress and anxiety (Gorski et al., 2021). Pharmacologic and nonpharmacologic interventions should be implemented to reduce anxiety and pain related to venipuncture. Refer to the discussion of pain management in the previous section (p. 1701).

INFUSION REGULATION AND MONITORING

The nurse is responsible for maintaining the proper IV infusion flow rate while ensuring the comfort and safety of the patient. IV fluid infusions are prescribed interventions, and the prescription identifies the amount of solution to be infused in a specified period of time. The nurse determines the infusion rate based on the amount of solution to be infused over 1 hour to achieve the prescribed infusion volume over the prescribed period of time. If the prescribed intervention is unclear in any way or does not seem appropriate based on the patient's condition and/or status, it is the nurse's responsibility to ask the prescribing practitioner for clarification prior to beginning administration. Maintenance of the flow rate is important because it can directly affect the patient's fluid balance. Too slow a flow may result in a fluid volume deficit because fluid intake is not balancing fluid lost or it may delay the restoration of the balance. Infusing IV fluid too rapidly can overtax the body's capacities to adjust to the increase in the water volume or the electrolytes it contains and may lead to FVE. Allowing an infusion to get behind schedule and then increasing the rate to catch up might seriously jeopardize the patient's compensatory mechanisms and lead to serious complications, such as in a patient with heart failure. Skill 41-2 (on pp. 1725–1727) discusses the monitoring of an IV infusion.

The use of electronic infusion pumps (IV pumps) is suggested best practice (Gorski et al., 2021) and is widely implemented as a standard of care in acute care settings to reduce infusion-related medication errors (ISMP, 2020). These devices can be programmed to infuse a certain amount of fluid over a given time, usually milliliters per hour. When using an electronic device, it is not necessary to calculate the drops per minute, as is necessary with a gravity or free-flowing IV infusion. The pump automatically regulates the flow rate at preset limits. An alarm sounds when air is in the tubing, the flow is obstructed, the solution level of the bottle or bag is getting low, or there is increased pressure in the system, such as occurs when a VAD infiltrates and fluid flows into the tissues. Smart pumps are IV infusion devices that provide computerized dose error-reduction software with IV therapy libraries and corresponding administration rate limits (ISMP, 2020). Smart pumps are used in more than 80% of hospital settings in the United States (ISMP, 2020). The Institute for Safe Medication Practices (ISMP, 2020) suggests "Smart pumps can provide a great deal of data that is useful in driving safe practices" (p. 3). Although the design of these pumps may enhance patient safety, it is important that nurses always remember that they are ultimately responsible for accurate programming of the pump and fluid administration. Check the infusion every hour or more frequently, if indicated, to determine if the solution is being infused at the proper hourly rate.

Administration may be achieved by gravity infusion, which requires the nurse to calculate the infusion rate in drops per minute. If using a gravity or free-flowing IV, calculate the drip rate required to achieve the desired infusion rate. A method for determining flow rate is described in the accompanying Guidelines for Nursing Care 41-2.

Guidelines for Nursing Care 41-2

REGULATING INTRAVENOUS FLOW RATE

Follow facility guidelines to determine if infusion should be administered by electronic infusion device or by gravity.

- Verify the prescribed IV solution.
- Check the patency of IV access.

If the infusion is to be administered by gravity infusion:

- Verify the drop factor (number of drops in 1 mL) of the equipment in use.
- Calculate the flow rate:

EXAMPLE—Administer 1,000 mL D_5W over 10 hours (set delivers 60 drops/1 mL).

a. **Standard formula**

$$\text{gtt (drops)/min} = \frac{\text{volume (mL)} \times \text{drop factor (gtt (drops)/mL)}}{\text{time (in minutes)}}$$

$$\text{gtt (drops)/min} = \frac{1{,}000 \text{ mL} \times 60}{600 \text{ (60 min} \times \text{10 h)}}$$

$$= \frac{60{,}000}{600}$$

$$= 100 \text{ gtt (drops)/min}$$

b. Short formula using milliliters per hour

$$\text{gtt (drops)/min} = \frac{\text{milliliters per hour} \times \text{drop factor (gtt (drops)/mL)}}{\text{time (60 min)}}$$

Find milliliters per hour by dividing 1,000 mL by 10 hours:

$$\frac{1{,}000}{10} = 100 \text{ mL} \times 60$$

$$\text{gtt (drops)/min} = \frac{100 \text{ mL/60}}{60 \text{ min}}$$

$$= \frac{6{,}000}{60}$$

$$= 100 \text{ gtt (drops)/min}$$

This method requires the nurse to know the amount of solution to be delivered, the total infusion time (in minutes), and the drop factor for the infusion tubing in use. The drop factor, or drops per milliliter of solution, is determined by the size of the opening in the infusion apparatus. It varies among different products from different companies. Most health facilities use the products of a single company. The most common drop factors are macrodrop systems (10, 15, 20 drops/mL), a microdrip (60 drops/mL), and a blood administration set (10 drops/mL). Microdrip is used most often when small fluid volumes are administered, such as a rate less than 75 mL/hr. Macrodrop tubing is commonly used for rates greater than 75 mL/hr.

Place a time tape (Fig. 41-18) on the container of solution to provide a quick reference for the nurse to monitor the rate at which the solution is entering the patient. The tape gives an hourly indication of where the fluid level should be at a given time.

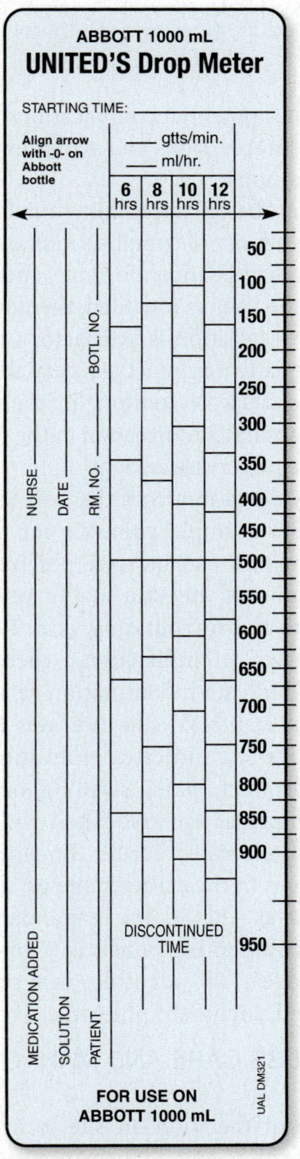

FIGURE 41-18. Sample time tape for an IV solution container.

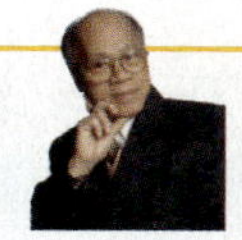

Consider **Jack Soo Park**, the patient who received too much IV fluid. When planning Mr. Park's care, the nurse would need to include frequent assessments of the IV infusion to ensure that it is infusing at the proper flow rate. Ensuring the use of an infusion pump significantly reduces the potential for an infusion error.

A less commonly used volume-control device may be used to reduce the risk for fluid overload or medication overdose. These devices may be used in pediatric settings in which catastrophic fluid overload is possible if adult fluid doses are inadvertently administered. A volume-control device may also be used to deliver intermittent medications that need to be further diluted and given over a specified time. Many facilities have reduced or eliminated the use of volume-control devices as a result of advances in infusion pump technology (Kyle & Carman, 2021). Concerns related to use of these devices include the lack of identification of the drug placed in the device and the potential for chemical inactivation or precipitation that may occur in the device or IV tubing when multiple medications are administered using the same set (Kyle & Carman, 2021).

SOLUTION AND TUBING CHANGES

If more than one container of solution is prescribed for the patient, attach additional containers using the method determined by the facility. The frequency of administration set tubing changes varies. The Infusion Nurses Society (Gorski et al., 2021) provides guidelines related to administration set change and recommends routine changes of administration sets (tubing) based on the type of solution administered via the tubing and frequency of the infusion (continuous vs. intermittent). In addition, infusion administration sets should be changed immediately upon suspected contamination or when the integrity of the administration product or system has been compromised (Gorski et al., 2021, p. S123). Infusion administration sets should also be changed a new VAD is placed (Gorski et al., 2021, p. S124). Table 41-8 (on page 1704) outlines additional recommended infusion administration set changes based on the type of infusion and device, according to INS Standards. It is important to be familiar with the particular policies and procedures of a given facility as well.

COMPLICATIONS OF IV THERAPY

Nurses must maintain current knowledge related to prevention, assessment, recognition, and management of vascular access device-related complications (Gorski et al., 2021; Willis, 2020). Regularly assess venous access sites to detect common complications of IV therapy including infiltration (inadvertent leakage of nonvesicant [agent capable of causing tissue damage] IV solution into surrounding tissue), extravasation (inadvertent leakage of vesicant IV solution into surrounding tissue), phlebitis (inflammation of the wall of a vein), thrombophlebitis (blood clot in a vein, causing inflammation), and infection. Venous access device-related infections are a potentially serious complication related

Table 41-8 Recommended Administration Set Change Schedule

TYPE OF INFUSION/TYPE OF DEVICE	RECOMMENDED FREQUENCY
• Primary and secondary continuous administration sets used to administer fluids other than lipid, blood, or blood products	• Change no more frequently than every 96 hours. • Change at least every 7 days. • Change if VAD is changed • Change if the integrity of the product or system has been compromised • If the first unit of blood requires 4 hours for transfusion, do not reuse toe administration set or filter. Most standard filters have a 4-unit maximum capacity for reuse.
• Intermittent administration sets	• Every 24 hours
• Administration sets with inline or add-on filters used to administer PN	• Change every 24 hours or with each new PN container.
• Administration sets used to administer IV lipid emulsions (ILE)	• Change every 12 hours and/or with each new ILE container.
• Administration sets used to administer blood and blood components	• If the first unit of blood requires 4 hours for transfusion, do not reuse administration set or filter. Most standard filters have a 4-unit maximum capacity for reuse.

Source: Adapted from Gorski, L. A., Hadaway, L., Hagle, M. E., Broadhurst, D., Clare, S., Kleidon, T., Meyer, B. M., Nickel, B., Rowley, S., Sharpe, E., Alexander, M., & Infusion Nurses Society. (2021). Infusion therapy. Standards of practice. (8th ed.). *Journal of Infusion Nursing*, *44*(Suppl 1), S1–S224. https://doi.org/10.1097/NAN.0000000000000396

to IV therapy. The development of venous access device–related infection can range from the minor irritation of a localized site infection to a potentially life-threatening bloodstream infection or septicemia (Berndt & Steinheiser, 2019; Casimero et al., 2020).

Technology Alert

Compliance with evidence-based central venous catheter care bundles to reduce the rate of catheter-associated bloodstream infection can be increased with the use of an electronic dashboard to monitor CABSI bundle-adherence and provide feedback related to compliance (Chemparathy et al., 2021).

Local complications, such as infiltration, phlebitis, and thrombophlebitis, occur more frequently than do systemic complications. However, systemic complications (e.g., fluid overload, embolus, sepsis) are more serious and may be life threatening. Central venous catheters are available that are impregnated with antiseptics and coated with antibiotics (antiinfective CVADs); use of these devices should be considered for patients at high risk for acquiring a catheter-related infection, such as expected dwell time of more than 5 days or those with enhanced risk of infection, including neutropenic, transplant, burn, or critically ill patients (Gorski et al., 2021). Consult facility policy for guidance concerning catheter site care as well as the manufacturer's recommendations and precautions. An additional recommendation to prevent intravascular catheter-related infections is the use of a 2% chlorhexidine wash for daily skin cleansing for patients in the intensive care unit with a CVAD, if other catheter-associated bloodstream infection (CABSI) prevention strategies have not been effective (Gorski et al., 2021; O'Grady et al., 2017).

Table 41-9 outlines potential complications of IV infusions, noting common causes, signs and symptoms, and pertinent nursing considerations.

The patient can be an important source of information regarding the possibility of complications associated with IV therapy. If the patient is uncomfortable, check that the infusion is entering the vein as intended, the flow rate is not too rapid, the patient's position is satisfactory, and the circulatory status of the patient is intact. Anxiety about receiving an infusion can also cause discomfort for the patient. Provide appropriate and accurate information to the patient regarding the infusion to help decrease anxiety.

Assess for any deviation from the normal skin temperature of the site. For example, cool skin can indicate infiltration while warm skin can indicate phlebitis or infection. Also note the tone of the skin at the venous access site in comparison to the surrounding skin. Pale or blanched skin can be a sign of infiltration, whereas red/purple/darker skin can indicate inflammation related to phlebitis or infection. Pus at the IV site indicates infection, while leaking fluid at the site indicates infiltration. Finally, fully investigate discomfort, pain, swelling or edema at the site as these symptoms are associated with all of the five major complications listed earlier. Encourage patients to report any changes in the catheter site or any new discomfort (O'Grady et al., 2017). Use a standardized scale for assessing and documenting phlebitis (Gorski et al., 2021). Box 41-1 (on page 1706) identifies one scale that can be used to assess and document phlebitis.

VENOUS ACCESS CARE AND MANAGEMENT

Site Care

Scrupulous care of the infusion site is necessary to help control contamination and to help prevent the introduction of microorganisms into the bloodstream. Site care and

Table 41-9 Complications Associated With Intravenous Infusions

COMPLICATION/CAUSE	SIGNS AND SYMPTOMS	NURSING CONSIDERATIONS
Infiltration: the escape of fluid into the subcutaneous tissue Dislodged needle Penetrated vessel wall	Swelling, pallor, coldness, or pain around the infusion site; significant decrease in the flow rate	Check the infusion site every hour for signs/symptoms. Discontinue the infusion if symptoms occur. Restart the infusion at a different site. Use site-stabilization device.
Venous access device–related infection: Improper hand decontamination/hand hygiene Frequent disconnection of tubing, access ports, and/or access caps Poor insertion technique, multiple insertion attempts Multilumen catheters Long-term catheter insertion Frequent dressing changes Inadequate/improper decontamination of hub prior to use An IV solution that becomes contaminated when solutions are changed, a medication is added, or the solution is allowed to infuse for too long a period Inappropriate administration set changes	Erythema, edema, induration, drainage at the insertion site Fever, malaise, chills, other vital sign changes	Perform hand hygiene before and after palpating catheter insertion sites; before and after inserting, replacing, accessing, and dressing a venous access device. Assess catheter site routinely. Notify health care team immediately if any signs of infection. Use scrupulous aseptic technique when starting an infusion. Follow best-practice guidelines for site care, changing of administration tubing sets, connectors, caps and other administration equipment. Follow facility protocol for culture of drainage. Consider use of 2% chlorhexidine wash for daily skin cleansing.
Phlebitis: an inflammation of a vein Mechanical trauma from needle or catheter Chemical trauma from solution	Local, acute tenderness; redness, warmth, and slight edema of the vein above the insertion site	Use a phlebitis scale to assess and document phlebitis. Discontinue the infusion immediately. Apply warm compresses to the affected site. Avoid further use of the vein. Restart the infusion in another vein.
Thrombus: a blood clot Tissue trauma from needle or catheter	Symptoms similar to phlebitis IV fluid flow may cease if clot obstructs needle.	Stop the infusion immediately. Apply warm compresses as prescribed or according to facility policy. Restart the IV at another site. *Do not rub or massage the affected area.*
Speed shock: the body's reaction to a substance that is injected into the circulatory system too rapidly Too rapid a rate of fluid infusion into circulation	Pounding headache, fainting, rapid pulse rate, apprehension, chills, back pains, and dyspnea	Use the proper IV tubing. Carefully monitor the rate of fluid flow. Check the rate frequently for accuracy. A time tape is useful for this purpose.
Fluid overload: the condition caused when too large a volume of fluid infuses into the circulatory system Too large a volume of fluid infused into circulation	Engorged neck veins, increased blood pressure, and difficulty in breathing (dyspnea)	If symptoms develop, slow the rate of infusion. Notify the health care team immediately. Monitor vital signs. Carefully monitor the rate of fluid flow. Check the rate frequently for accuracy.
Air embolus: air in the circulatory system Break in the IV system above the heart level, allowing air in the circulatory system as a bolus	Respiratory distress Increased heart rate Cyanosis Decreased blood pressure Change in level of consciousness	Pinch off catheter or secure system to prevent entry of air. Place patient on left side in Trendelenburg position. Call for immediate assistance. Monitor vital signs and pulse oximetry.

dressing changes are performed using aseptic non touch technique (ANTT®) (Gorski et al., 2021); in the nontouch technique, the practitioner touches a site or equipment only as absolutely necessary, even when wearing sterile gloves (ANTT®, 2021). Appropriate skin antisepsis, maintenance of an intact and patent dressing at the insertion site, use of appropriate dressing change regimens, appropriate administration tubing replacements (previously discussed), and appropriate IV needleless connector disinfection are important means of preventing infection. Use of >0.5% chlorhexidine in alcohol

Box 41-1 Phlebitis Scale

Grade and document phlebitis according to the most severe presenting indicator.

Grade	Clinical Criteria
0	No symptoms
1	Erythema at access site with or without pain
2	Pain at access site with erythema and/or edema
3	Pain at access site with erythema and/or edema Streak formation Palpable venous cord
4	Pain at access site with erythema and/or edema Streak formation Palpable venous cord >1 inch in length Purulent drainage

Source: Gorski, L. A., Hadaway, L., Hagle, M. E., Broadhurst, D., Clare, S., Kleidon, T., Meyer, B. M., Nickel, B., Rowley, S., Sharpe, E., Alexander, M., & Infusion Nurses Society. (2021). Infusion therapy. Standards of practice. (8th ed.). *Journal of Infusion Nursing*, *44*(Suppl 1), S139. https://doi.org/10.1097/NAN.0000000000000396

solution is preferred for skin antisepsis (Gorski et al., 2021; Sarani et al., 2018). If there is a contraindication to alcoholic chlorhexidine solution, tincture of iodine, an iodophor (povidone-iodine), or 70% alcohol may instead be used (Gorski et al., 2021; Mimoz et al., 2015; O'Grady et al., 2017). Use chlorhexidine with caution in infants up to age 14 days, premature infants, and low-birth-weight infants due to the risk of skin irritation and chemical burns (Gorski et al., 2021). The use of topical antimicrobial ointment to VAD insertion sites (except hemodialysis catheter sites) as part of routine site care is not recommended because of their potential to promote fungal infections and antimicrobial resistance (Gorski et al., 2021; O'Grady et al., 2017).

Transparent semipermeable membrane (TSM) dressings are commonly used to protect the insertion site. TSM dressings (e.g., Tegaderm™ or OpSite IV™) allow easy inspection of the VAD site and permit evaporation of moisture that accumulates under the dressing. Sterile gauze may also be used to cover the catheter site. A gauze dressing is recommended if the patient is diaphoretic, the site is bleeding or oozing, or there is drainage from the exit site; replace it with a TSM once this is resolved (Gorski, 2020; O'Grady et al., 2017). Chlorhexidine-impregnated dressings are recommended for use as VAD site dressings for certain patient populations, including oncology patients with implanted ports, adult patients with short-term nontunneled CVADs, and patients with an epidural access device (Gorski et al., 2021).

Facility policy generally determines the type of dressing and the intervals for dressing change. Perform site care and replace TSM dressings at least every 7 days (except neonatal patients) or immediately if the dressing becomes damp, loosened, visibly soiled or has a lifted/detached border; blood or drainage is present; or there is compromised skin integrity under the dressing (Gorski et al., 2021). Change sterile gauze dressings at least every 2 days, or if the integrity of the dressing is disrupted (damp, loosened, visibly soiled) (Gorski et al., 2021). Consider the use of sterile adhesive removers and skin barrier film to prevent medical adhesive–related skin injury (MARSI) (Fumarola et al., 2020; Gorski et al., 2021; Zhao et al., 2018). Do not submerge venous catheters and catheter sites in water; showering is permitted with use of impermeable coverings (clear plastic wrap or a device designed for this purpose) to protect the catheter and connections (Gorski et al., 2021; O'Grady et al., 2017). Skill 41-2 (on pp. 1725–1727) reviews how to monitor an IV site.

Entry-Point Disinfection

Venous access device administration set entry points, end caps, and needleless connectors must be vigorously scrubbed and disinfected prior to each access to reduce the risk for introduction of microorganisms and prevent venous access device–related infection (Gorski et al., 2021). Acceptable disinfecting agents include 70% isopropyl alcohol, iodophors, or chlorhexidine in alcohol solution (Berndt & Steinheiser, 2019; Gorski et al., 2021). Friction is needed to physically remove microorganisms from the top, sides, and threads of the access cap. The length of time for the mechanical scrub varies based on the specific device and cleansing agent; recommended time frames include 5 to 15 seconds (Gorski et al., 2021). Allow the antiseptic to dry completely (5 seconds when using alcohol; 20 seconds when using chlorhexidine with alcohol; more than 6 minutes when using povidone iodine) (Gorski et al., 2021).

Passive Disinfection Caps

The use of passive disinfection caps (port protectors) is an effective means to reduce infection associated with central and peripheral VADs (Barton, 2019a; Gorski et al., 2021; Stango et al., 2014). A passive disinfection cap is attached to the venous access end cap, needleless connector, and/or each access site on IV administration set tubing and is left in place between device accesses (Casimero et al., 2020). These caps contain an antiseptic-impregnated sponge that dispenses the antiseptic over the connector's top and threads and protects the hub from contamination by acting as a physical barrier to touch or airborne sources (Barton, 2019a; Casimero et al., 2020). Passive disinfection caps are discarded after removal from the venous access device and should never be reattached (Gorski et al., 2021). Figure 41-19 provides an example of a passive disinfection cap in place on a needleless connector.

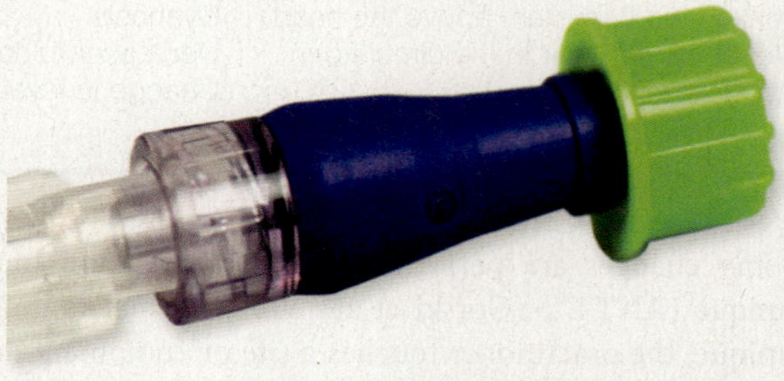

FIGURE 41-19. Disinfection cap in place on a needleless connector. (Courtesy of 3M © 3M 2015. All rights reserved.)

If multiple accesses of the venous access device are required, such as with medication administration (i.e., several flush syringes and administration sets), additional disinfection of the end cap or needleless connector is required before each entry (Gorski et al., 2021). Refer to facility policy for scrub time, technique, and agents.

Needleless Connectors

Needleless connectors should be changed no more frequently than every 96 hours (Gorski et al., 2021). When a needleless connector is used as part of a continuous IV infusion, the connector is changed when the primary administration set is changed. A recommended administration set change schedule is detailed in Table 41-8 on page 1704. Needleless connectors should also be changed if the connector is removed for any reason, it there is residual blood or debris within the connector, prior to drawing a sample for blood culture from the venous access device, upon contamination of the connector, based on the manufacturer's recommendations, and per facility policy and/or procedures (Gorski et al., 2021, p. S106).

It is important to follow the manufacturers' directions for use when flushing, clamping, and disconnecting syringes and IV administration tubing or any other device from needleless connectors. In the absence of the manufacturer's directions, identify the internal mechanism for fluid displacement reported by the manufacturer for the type of needleless connector being used and use the appropriate sequence for flushing, clamping, and disconnecting based on the type of needleless connector to prevent connection/disconnection reflux (Gorski et al, 2021).

Multiple Continuous Infusions

It is important to differentiate and label individual fluid infusions in patients with multiple, continuously infused IV fluids (Gorski et al., 2021). The Infusion Nurses Society recommends tracing all catheters/administration sets/add-on devices between the patient and solution container before connecting or reconnecting any infusion/ device, at each care transition to a new setting or service, and as part of the handoff process (Gorski et al., 2021, p. S123). Some facilities have responded to this challenge by implementing color-coded labeling systems to organize multiple fluids in a visually safe manner and improve accuracy and patient safety (Cho et al., 2013). Commercial devices are also available to organize and label IV tubing and other tubing, cables, wires, and cords that may be present at the bedside in acute care as well as in the patient's home setting. These devices also help keep tubing from dropping to the ground and potential tangles, damage, or contamination (Haynes et al., 2015).

Venous Catheter Securement/Stabilization Devices

Stabilization and securement products are designed to control movement at the catheter hub, decreasing catheter movement internally and externally (Hill & Moureau, 2019, as cited in Barton, 2020, p. S28). Manufactured venous catheter securement/stabilization systems are commercially available. These systems are recommended for use on all venous access sites, particularly central venous access sites, to preserve the integrity of the access device, minimize catheter movement at the hub, and to prevent catheter migration and loss of access (Barton, 2020; Gorski et al., 2021; O'Grady et al., 2017). Many of these devices also function as an integrated dressing product. The use of a stabilization device can also decrease the risk of infiltration, phlebitis, skin damage, occlusion, leaking, catheter-related infection, and unscheduled restart rates/loss of the catheter (Marsh et al., 2015; Smith & Hannum, 2008). There are many devices available, including plastic shields and adhesive anchors. Some securement devices are intended for use with a specific venous access device, such as a subcutaneous anchor for use with PICCs (Rowe et al., 2020).

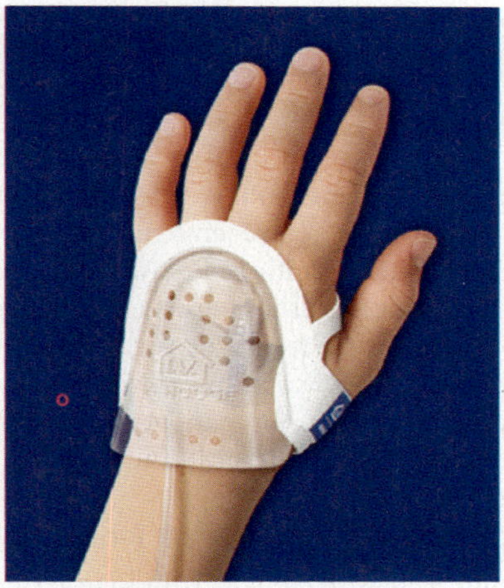

FIGURE 41-20. IV shield in place on the hand.

Hard plastic shields (Fig. 41-20) that are ventilated and secured with tape are often used in pediatric settings. In addition, they are helpful in minimizing venous access complications with geriatric patients (Smith & Hannum, 2008). Adhesive anchors eliminate the need for tape but are costlier and involve the use of strong adhesives that might make it difficult to change the dressing without dislodging the catheter. A skin barrier should be applied to the skin exposed to the adhesive to reduce the risk of medical adhesive–related skin injury (Gorski et al., 2021).

The integrity of the stabilization device should be assessed with each dressing change, and the device itself should be changed according to the manufacturer's directions (Gorski et al., 2021). A dislodged vascular access device should never be readvanced into the vein; a dislodged device should be removed, reinserted at a new site, or exchanged (Gorski et al., 2021).

CAPPING A PRIMARY LINE FOR INTERMITTENT USE

When a continuous IV is no longer necessary, the primary IV line (PIVC or CVAD) can be capped and converted to an intermittent infusion device. A capped line consists of the IV catheter connected to a short length of extension tubing sealed with a cap. Capping of a VAD provides venous access for intermittent infusions or emergency medications. VADs used for intermittent infusions should be flushed with preservative-free 0.9% sodium chloride solution and

PICOT in Practice

ASKING CLINICAL QUESTIONS: CENTRAL VENOUS CATHETERS IN INFANTS AND CHILDREN

Scenario: You are a staff nurse who works on a pediatric medical/surgical unit. You receive report on a patient who was admitted with vomiting 4 days ago. The patient is receiving intermittent flushes to prevent occlusion of a long-term central venous catheter. The patient has a prescription for normal saline (0.9% sodium chloride) flushes. You have seen heparin prescribed for patients with long-term central venous catheters in the past and wonder if there is a difference.

You decide to search the literature for best practice.

- **Population:** Pediatric patients with long-term central venous catheters
- **Intervention:** Normal saline (0.9% sodium chloride) versus heparin flushes
- **Comparison:** Low-molecular-weight heparin injections
- **Outcome:** Occlusions of central venous catheters
- **Time:** Duration of hospitalization.

PICOT Question: Among pediatric patients with long-term central venous catheters, does normal saline (0.9% sodium chloride) when compared to heparin flushes and to low-molecular-weight heparin injections prevent occlusions during the hospitalized stay?

Findings:

1. Bradford, N. K., Edwards, R. M., & Chan, R. J. (2020). Normal saline (0.9% sodium chloride) versus heparin intermittent flushing for the prevention of occlusion in long-term central venous catheters in infants and children. *Cochrane Database of Systematic Reviews, 4*(4), CD010996. https://doi.org/10.1002/14651858.CD010996.pub3
2. Pelland-Marcotte, M.-C., Amiri, N., Avila, M. L., & Brandão, L. R. (2020). Low molecular weight heparin for prevention of central venous catheter-related thrombosis in children. *Cochrane Database of Systematic Reviews, 6*(6), CD005982. https://doi.org/10.1002/14651858.CD005982.pub3.

Four studies with a total of 255 participants were all undertaken in large teaching (tertiary) hospitals and directly compared the use of saline and heparin. The review found that there was not enough evidence to determine the effects of intermittent flushing with normal saline versus heparin to prevent occlusion in long-term central venous catheters in infants and children. It remains unclear whether heparin is necessary to prevent occlusion. Evidence was also insufficient to confirm on the outcomes catheter occlusion, days of catheter patency, episodes of catheter-related bloodstream infection, and other side effects of low-molecular-weight heparin.

Strength of Evidence: Level I systematic review

Recommendations: You write an abstract and submit it to the evidence-based practice committee to discuss your findings. You cite the strength of the evidence in the Cochrane reviews and highlight that there is no difference in intermittent flushing with normal saline versus heparin to prevent occlusion in long-term central. In your proposal, you compare the cost of normal saline versus heparin. The use of heparin incurs costs to health systems with no advantages over normal saline flushes according to the evidence. There is also greater risk with the administration of heparin.

aspirated for a blood return prior to each infusion to assess catheter function (Gorski et al., 2021). Flushing of the device is also required after each infusion to clear the infused medication or other solution from the catheter lumen. Vascular access devices are locked after completion of the flush solution at each use to decrease the risk of occlusion (Gorski et al., 2021). According to the guidelines from the INS, PIVCs are locked with preservative-free 0.9% sodium chloride; CVADs should be locked with either a heparin solution (10 units/mL) or preservative-free 0.9% sodium chloride after each intermittent use, according to the directions for use for the specific CVAD and needleless connector (Gorski et al., 2021). If the device is not in use, periodic flushing according to facility policy is required to keep the catheter patent. Antimicrobial locking solutions are sometimes used in specific situations, such as with patients with long-term CVADs or in high-risk patient populations (Gorski et al., 2021). The accompanying PICOT in Practice box highlights an example of evidence-based decision making regarding flushing of CVADs in infants and children.

DISCONTINUATION OF THE INFUSION

Remove the PIVC when the PIVC is no longer required as part of the plan of care; has not been used for 24 hours or more; or when site assessment and/or clinical signs and symptoms of systemic complications are present (Gorski et al., 2021). Do not remove based solely on length of dwell time (Gorski et al., 2021). After performing hand hygiene, put on gloves, clamp the IV tubing, and remove the tape and sterile dressing. Avoid bending the catheter while it is withdrawn to prevent breakage. Apply pressure immediately to the area just above the insertion site until hemostasis is achieved. Apply pressure using a dry, sterile gauze pad rather than using an alcohol preparation; alcohol tends to burn and does not stop blood flow from the puncture wound. Apply an occlusive dressing to the site. Document the date and time of removal, the name of the person removing the device, and the assessment of the site.

Nurses or specialized IV team nurses may be responsible for removing a midline or PICC line. Other CVADs are usually removed by advanced practice professionals. Specific protocols must be followed to prevent breakage or fracture of the catheter.

HOME INFUSION

Home infusion therapy allows patients to be discharged earlier from acute care and/or avoid hospitalization and return to their home or other community-based care setting

Teaching Tips 41-1

IV THERAPY

Health Topic	Teaching Tip	Why Is This Important?
Aseptic technique	• Proper handwashing technique • Dressing changes and care of site/device • Proper technique for infusing medications	Prevent local and systemic infection
Equipment use	• Proper technique for using all equipment and flushing of CVAD • Safe storage, maintenance, and disposal of solutions, supplies, and equipment • Protection of device/insertion site when showering or bathing	Prevent medication/infusion therapy error and complications such as bleeding, embolus, and/or infection related to improper use of equipment and flushing of CVAD.
Assessment Skills	Assessing for any indications of an infection or other complications and how to report such problems	Understanding of signs of infection and other complications promotes early detection and intervention.
Supplies	Obtaining supplies to continue home infusions	Continued supplies are needed to maintain prescribed home therapy.
Resources	How and why to contact health care team if questions or problems arise Use of educational resources on the Internet that are reputable, usable, and accessible	Understanding of available resources and when it is appropriate to use these resources promotes engagement and maintenance of prescribed therapy. Ensure use of appropriate education sources that incorporate best-practice, support patient safety, and reduce risk of misinformation

Source: Adapted from Gorski, L. A., Hadaway, L., Hagle, M. E., Broadhurst, D., Clare, S., Kleidon, T., Meyer, B. M., Nickel, B., Rowley, S., Sharpe, E., Alexander, M., & Infusion Nurses Society. (2021). Infusion therapy. Standards of practice. (8th ed.). *Journal of Infusion Nursing, 44*(Suppl 1), S1–S224. https://doi.org/10.1097/NAN.0000000000000396

(Gorski, 2020). Portable infusion pumps and the support of community-based care nurses have made this a part of the plan of care for many patients. After a patient has been identified as a candidate for home infusion therapy, begin assessment and education to ensure a successful outcome. Candidates for infusion pump IV therapy in the home should meet certain criteria. They should be medically stable; have support from a motivated, capable, and willing caregiver; have access to a telephone; and have access to electricity and refrigeration (Fields et al., 2020). Patients can receive pain medication, antimicrobials, chemotherapy, parenteral nutrition, or other medications through portable infusion pumps at home.

PICCs and other CVADs are the most common type of catheter used for home health care patients. Home health care nurses play a crucial role in supporting patients and families/caregivers concerning successful management of VADs, IV infusions, and observing for potential complications. The patient and any caregivers should understand the role of the caregiver in giving infusions; monitoring the patient's condition; and managing required medications, equipment, and supplies as well as be able to perform the related skills (Fields et al., 2020). See Teaching Tips 41-1.

Administering Blood and Blood Products

A blood transfusion is the infusion of whole blood or a blood component such as plasma, red blood cells, cryoprecipitate, or platelets into the patient's venous circulation. Red blood cells have the important role of carrying oxygen from the lungs to all body tissues. Oxygen is essential to maintain normal cellular metabolism and cellular integrity. Platelets and the coagulation factors found in cryoprecipitate and plasma are essential for establishing homeostasis following an injury or invasive procedure. These blood components promote normal blood clotting, thus are important in the prevention of excessive blood loss. A blood product transfusion is given when a patient's red blood cells, platelets, or coagulation factors decrease to levels that compromise a patient's health. Blood transfusions are not without risk, however. Potentially life-threatening complications include allergic reaction and anaphylactic reaction, hemolytic reaction, transfusion-related acute lung injury, circulatory volume overload, immunosuppression, and transmission of infectious diseases are a risk associated with blood product transfusion (Carman et al., 2018). It is important that the potential benefits of the transfusion be considered against the potential risks (American Red Cross, 2021; Carman et al., 2018). Blood is a vital but limited resource, and clinical judgment and use of current guidelines and recommendations are crucial in determining whether the associated risks outweigh the patient's need (American Red Cross, 2021; Carman et al, 2018). The person receiving the blood is the recipient. The person giving the blood is the donor.

BLOOD TYPING AND CROSS-MATCHING

Before a blood product can be given to a patient, it must be determined that the blood of the donor is compatible with that of the patient. If incompatible, clumping and hemolysis of the recipient's blood cells result, and death can occur. The laboratory examination to determine a person's blood type is called **blood typing**. The process of determining compatibility between blood specimens is **cross-matching**.

Blood Types

Blood type, an inherited trait, is determined by the type of antigens and antibodies present in the blood. An **antigen** is a substance that causes the formation of antibodies. An **antibody** is a protein substance developed in the body in response to the presence of an antigen that has entered the body. An agglutinin is an antibody that causes a clumping of specific antigens. The four main blood types or groups in the ABO system of blood typing are A, B, AB, and O. Some groups are further broken down into subgroups. People who have type A blood have an A antigen on their red blood cells, those with type B blood have B antigens on their cells, those in the AB group have both A and B antigens, and people with type O blood have neither A nor B antigens on their red blood cells. People in each blood group have the agglutinins to the red blood cell antigens that they lack. Group A people have the agglutinin for B; group AB people have no agglutinins for A and B, whereas group O people have both A and B agglutinins in their blood serum. If a person with type O blood is transfused with blood from a person with either group A or group B blood, there would be destruction of the recipient's red blood cells because the recipient's anti-A or anti-B agglutinins would react with the A or B antigens in the donor's red blood cells. This explains why people with type AB blood are often called universal recipients (because people in this blood group have no agglutinins for either A or B antigens), and group O people are often called universal donors (because they have neither A nor B antigens).

Rh Factor

The Rh factor is an inherited antigen in human blood. There are five antigens in the Rh system, but the one designated D is of first concern. A person whose blood contains a D antigen is called Rh positive; an Rh-negative person lacks this D antigen. An Rh-negative person must receive blood from another Rh-negative person. If Rh-positive blood is administered to an Rh-negative person, the recipient develops anti-Rh agglutinins. Subsequent transfusion with Rh-positive blood may cause serious reactions with clumping and hemolysis of red blood cells.

BLOOD DONORS

Blood donors must be selected with care. Not only must the donor's blood be typed accurately, but it is also important to determine that the donor is free of infectious disease. Transfusion-transmitted infections are infections resulting from the introduction of a pathogen into a person through blood transfusion (CDC, 2020). Transfusion-transmitted infections occur from the transfer of bacteria, viruses, prions, and parasites (CDC, 2020). Donor screening using questionnaires and laboratory tests helps reduce the risk of an infectious organism being transmitted by blood transfusion (CDC). The blood will be tested for Chagas disease, human immunodeficiency virus (HIV), hepatitis B and C virus (HBV and HBC), human T-lymphotropic virus (HTLV), syphilis, West Nile virus, Zika virus, Babesia, cytomegalovirus (CMV), and bacterial contamination (CDC, 2020).

The donor is examined carefully at the time of donation and receives specific information about eligibility and a confidential method to allow or disallow the distribution of the donated blood. Prospective donors must meet minimum requirements for age, height, and weight (American Red Cross, n.d.a). Prospective donors are questioned about their lifestyle and health history, including questions about diseases, health conditions, past surgeries, tattoos, body piercing, travel, sexual habits, and medication/drug use (American Red Cross, n.d.c). People may give blood only if their blood count (hemoglobin or hematocrit), temperature, pulse, and blood pressure are within normal ranges.

Some patients who know in advance that they will need blood can donate their own blood for transfusion, known as **autologous transfusion** or autotransfusion. Autologous transfusion eliminates the danger of transmitting cross-infection from donor to recipient and decreases the risk for complications from mismatched blood. However, this technique requires advance planning; blood can be donated every 4 to 7 days and up to 3 business days before surgery is planned, as long as the patient meets donation guidelines (American Red Cross, n.d.d). Autologous donation is not complication free; administration errors and infection are still possible even with autologous transfusion.

An additional transfusion technique related to autologous transfusion is utilized frequently in surgical settings. It is called intraoperative blood salvage. With this technique, a patient's own blood can be collected from specialized suction canisters, tubes and drains to allow for autologous transfusions.

BLOOD COMPONENTS

Whole blood is rarely used unless blood loss has been massive. This is because whole blood can be easily separated into its components. This allows patients to receive only the blood product they need, decreasing the risk for fluid overload and promoting blood product availability to more patients. Guidelines exist to balance the benefit of treating the patient with the desire to avoid unnecessary transfusion, with associated costs and potential harm (American Red Cross, 2021; Gorski et al., 2021). For example, a patient may need red blood cells but not the blood plasma and its constituents. Red blood cells can therefore be administered in concentrated form, called packed red blood cells (PRBCs). The decision to transfuse is based on laboratory test results and individual patient characteristics, clinical condition, and symptoms.

In situations in which there is a deficit in plasma proteins and/or components of the blood important for normal functioning of coagulation and fibrinolysis (including complement), administration of plasma may be a more appropriate option. Fresh-frozen plasma (FFP) is particularly useful in emergencies that involve massive blood loss because it will restore both coagulation factors and blood volume. It is also an excellent protein containing blood volume expander when a patient develops a sudden critical fluid deficit: for example, in a patient who is severely burned and losing plasma rapidly from burn areas. Separate components of plasma that are also used therapeutically include human albumin (used for hypovolemic shock, albuminemia, liver failure), cryoprecipitate (used to treat bleeding due to hemophilia, disseminated intravascular coagulation, or depletion of coagulation factors such as fibrinogen following massive blood loss), and gamma globulins, the antibody-containing part of plasma (used for immunoglobulin deficiencies).

Platelet infusion is indicated for the treatment or prevention of bleeding associated with deficiencies in the number or quality of a patient's platelets. The demand for platelets has risen noticeably during the past several decades; specialized products and preparation methods have been developed to reduce the risk for complications and improve the patient's response to platelet therapy.

Health care organizations are encouraged to create a patient blood management (PBM) program to optimize the care of patients who might require a blood transfusion (Gorski et al., 2021). These multidisciplinary committees establish, monitor, promote and enforce patient blood management activities (PBM) (American Red Cross, 2021) and assist clinicians to make decisions about appropriate use of transfusion and elimination of unnecessary transfusions (Gorski et al., 2021). Representation by nurses on these types of committees provides the opportunity to advocate for evidence-based changes in practice and wise stewardship of resources (American Red Cross, 2021).

INITIATION AND TRANSFUSION OF BLOOD

Identification of patients at risk for complications and patient monitoring during and after transfusion of blood products is essential because of ongoing risk for transfusion reaction (Carman et al., 2018; DeLisle, 2018). The nurse should always follow facility blood product transfusion policies and protocols. Two adults in the presence of the patient should perform pretransfusion safety checks together prior to blood product administration. In the hospital or outpatient setting, this should be two practitioners trained in the identification of the recipient and blood components, such as registered nurses, advanced practice nurses, or physicians (Gorski et al., 2021). In home settings, it should be the registered nurse and a responsible adult (Gorski et al., 2021). Verify the prescribed transfusion intervention and verify that informed consent was obtained by the prescriber (DeLisle, 2018). Educate the patient about the signs and symptoms of a reaction and the importance of reporting so they will be aware if one develops and take action (DeLisle, 2018; Gorski et al, 2021). Verify the patient's identity by at least two independent identifiers, such as the patient's full name and birthdate. In an in-patient or long-term care setting, the nurse confirms that this information matches the information on the patient's identification band. The patient's blood type and Rh factor should be checked against the blood type and Rh factor of the transfusion product. In addition, the nurse should always confirm the donation identification number (a code to track the blood back to its donor) and the expiration date and date/time of issue of the blood product. Bar codes on blood products provide an additional safety measure to identify, track, and assign data to transfusions. In addition, the facility that prepared the blood must be identified. While such systems offer the potential for improved safety, the nurse must always recognize that there is no replacement for vigilant and consistent safety checks.

The procedure for administering a blood transfusion is similar to the procedure for starting an IV infusion of fluids, with a few differences. Blood or blood components may be transfused via a 20- to 24-gauge PIVC for an adult. When rapid transfusion is required, a larger-sized catheter gauge is recommended (18 to 20 gauge) (Gorski et al., 2021). CVADs may also be used to administer a transfusion (Gorski et al., 2021). Transfusion for infants and children is usually given using a 22- to 24-gauge catheter (umbilical vein in neonates or a peripheral vein large enough to accommodate the catheter) (Gorski et al., 2021).

The Infusion Nurses Society Standards of Practice identifies important components of safe blood transfusion and include (Gorski et al., 2021):

- Baseline assessment prior to obtaining blood for transfusion including measurement of vital signs, lung assessment, identification of conditions that may increase the risk of transfusion-related adverse reactions (e.g., fever, heart failure, renal disease), the presence of an appropriate and patent VAD and current laboratory values.
- Use an in-line filter or an add-on filter that is designated for the specific blood or blood component and for the administration set in use; refer to the manufacturer's guidelines and facility policies.
- Plan to administer the blood or blood component within 4 hours; refer to facility guidelines for infusion times for specific blood components.
- Use an electronic infusion pump labeled for blood transfusion.
- Administer blood or blood component infusions with 0.9% sodium chloride; do not add or infuse any other solutions or medications through the administration set and do not infuse transfusions through other administration sets.
- Start nonemergent transfusions slowly and carefully monitor for complications after getting baseline vital signs; major reactions usually appear before the first 50 mL have been transfused.
- Check the patient's vital signs within 30 minutes prior to transfusion, 15 minutes after initiating the transfusion, after the transfusion is completed, 1 hour after the transfusion has been completed, and as needed based on clinical observation of the patient's condition.

Table 41-10 Transfusion Reactions

REACTION	SIGNS AND SYMPTOMS	NURSING ACTIVITY
Allergic reaction: allergy to transfused blood	Hives, itching Anaphylaxis	• Stop transfusion immediately and keep vein open with normal saline. • Notify health care team immediately. • Administer antihistamine parenterally as necessary.
Febrile reaction: fever develops during infusion	Fever and chills Headache Malaise	• Stop transfusion immediately and keep vein open with normal saline. • Notify health care team. • Treat symptoms.
Hemolytic transfusion reaction: incompatibility of blood product	Immediate onset Facial flushing Fever, chills Headache Low back pain Shock	• Stop infusion immediately and keep vein open with normal saline. • Notify health care team immediately. • Obtain blood samples from site. • Obtain first voided urine. • Treat shock if present. • Send unit, tubing, and filter to lab. • Draw blood sample for serologic testing and send urine specimen to lab.
Circulatory overload: too much blood administered	Dyspnea Dry cough Pulmonary edema	• Slow or stop infusion. • Monitor vital signs. • Notify health care team. • Place in upright position with feet dependent.
Bacterial reaction: bacteria present in blood	Fever Hypertension Dry, flushed skin Abdominal pain	• Stop infusion immediately. • Obtain culture of patient's blood and return blood bag to lab. • Monitor vital signs. • Notify health care team. • Administer antibiotics as prescribed.

- Increase the transfusion rate after 15 minutes when there are no signs of a reaction and to ensure completion of the transfusion within 4 hours.
- Assess the patient for any adverse reactions at least every 30 minutes throughout the transfusion.
- Stop the transfusion immediately if signs and symptoms of a transfusion reaction are present (Table 41-10); notify the prescriber and follow facility policy for additional reporting. Be prepared to administer emergency medications as prescribed.
- Monitor the patient to detect febrile or pulmonary transfusion reactions for at least 4 to 6 hours; educate patients who are not under direct observation after their transfusion about signs and symptoms of delayed transfusion reaction and the importance of reporting.

Consult facility policy regarding the length of time blood or a blood product must be returned after it is obtained from the blood bank/source. Nurses are responsible for monitoring the patient for adverse reactions to the blood transfusion. Short- and long-term complications can occur and ongoing nursing assessment and intervention are a critical part of management of transfusion of blood and blood products (Carman et al., 2018).

Administering Parenteral Nutrition

Parenteral nutrition (PN) is the administration of nutritional support via the IV route. Patients who cannot meet their nutritional needs by the oral or enteral routes may require IV nutritional supplementation. IV supplementation may be prescribed for a variety of patients, such as patients at high risk for malnutrition in specific circumstances or when enteral nutrition is not feasible or sufficient to meet the patient's energy needs or protein goals (McClave et al., 2016). PN is a highly concentrated, hypertonic nutrient solution that can be administered centrally through a central venous access device. A less concentrated nutrient solution is sometimes prescribed for a patient and is administered through a short-term IV access in a peripheral vein (peripheral parenteral nutrition [PPN]). The basic difference between the two types is the concentration of the solutions infused. Assess for potential complications of PN such as catheter-related infection and electrolyte imbalances. Parenteral nutrition is discussed in Chapter 37 in further detail, including the procedure for PN administration and related nursing responsibilities.

Evaluating

Ongoing evaluation of the plan of care is integral. Collaborate with the health care team and the patient and family/caregivers to evaluate and readjust the plan of care and interventions. Refer to the accompanying concept map for an illustration of the nursing process for Grace Gillian. Evaluate the effectiveness of the plan of care to promote healthy fluid, electrolyte, and acid–base balance based on the following parameters:

- Is the patient making progress toward meeting identified outcomes related to fluid, electrolyte, and acid–base balance?
- Are the patient's drinking and eating patterns supplying the needed fluid and electrolytes?
- Is the patient having any difficulties with oral fluids, tube feedings, IV therapy, or PN?
- Is the patient's urine output about equal to the fluid intake? Do the patient's weight and record of fluid intake and output indicate fluid balance?
- Are abnormal sources of fluid loss (e.g., vomiting, diarrhea, draining wounds, fistula) responding to prescribed interventions? Are the signs of fluid volume deficit improving?
- Are the signs and symptoms that initially manifested the fluid, electrolyte, or acid–base imbalances absent or improved? Has therapy led to any troublesome new signs or symptoms?
- Is the patient now able to practice self-care behaviors to maintain fluid, electrolyte, and acid–base balance? Can the patient describe appropriate responses to potential future problems?

This evaluation should be ongoing as the plan of care is implemented. As the patient achieves the expected outcomes, these should be noted and reinforced. Before nursing care is terminated, the patient and family/caregivers should be able to independently promote fluid, electrolyte, and acid–base balance.

REFLECTIVE PRACTICE LEADING TO PERSONAL LEARNING

Remember that the goal of reflective practice is to look at an experience, understand it, and learn from it. As you begin to develop expertise in implementing measures related to fluid, electrolyte and acid–base balance, reflect on your experiences—successes and failures—in order to improve your practice. How can you do it better next time? What did you learn today that can help you tomorrow? Begin your reflection by paying close attention to the following while performing interventions and providing nursing care related to fluid, electrolyte and acid–base balance:

- Did your preparation and practice related to performing interventions related to fluid, electrolyte, and acid–base balance result in your feeling confident in your ability to provide care? Did your competence and confidence inspire the patient's and family/caregiver's trust?
- How did you prioritize the data you collected? What patterns in the data did you identify? What knowledge from your learning, personal experience and intuition did you use to make decisions and develop your plan of care?
- How confident are you that the data you communicated and recorded related to fluid, electrolyte, and acid–base balance accurately communicate the health status, health problems, issues, risks, and strengths of the patient? How successfully have you communicated this information to other members of the health care team?
- Were you aware of any cultural and/or ethnic beliefs or practices that may have influenced the patient's personal practices impacting fluid, electrolyte, and acid–base balance? Were you aware of any stereotypes or prejudices that might have negatively influences the clinical encounter? If so, how did you address these?
- Was the patient/family/caregiver participation in the process at an optimal level? How might you have better engaged the patient and family/caregivers?
- Did the patient/family/caregivers know your name, and know what to expect of you and nursing? Did the patient sense that you are respectful, caring, and competent to provide care?

Perhaps the most important questions to reflect on are: Are your patients and their families/caregivers better for having had *you* share in the critical responsibility of partnering with them to address their fluid, electrolyte, and acid–base balance needs? Are your patients now receiving thoughtful, person-centered, prioritized, holistic, evidence-based treatment and care because of your efforts?

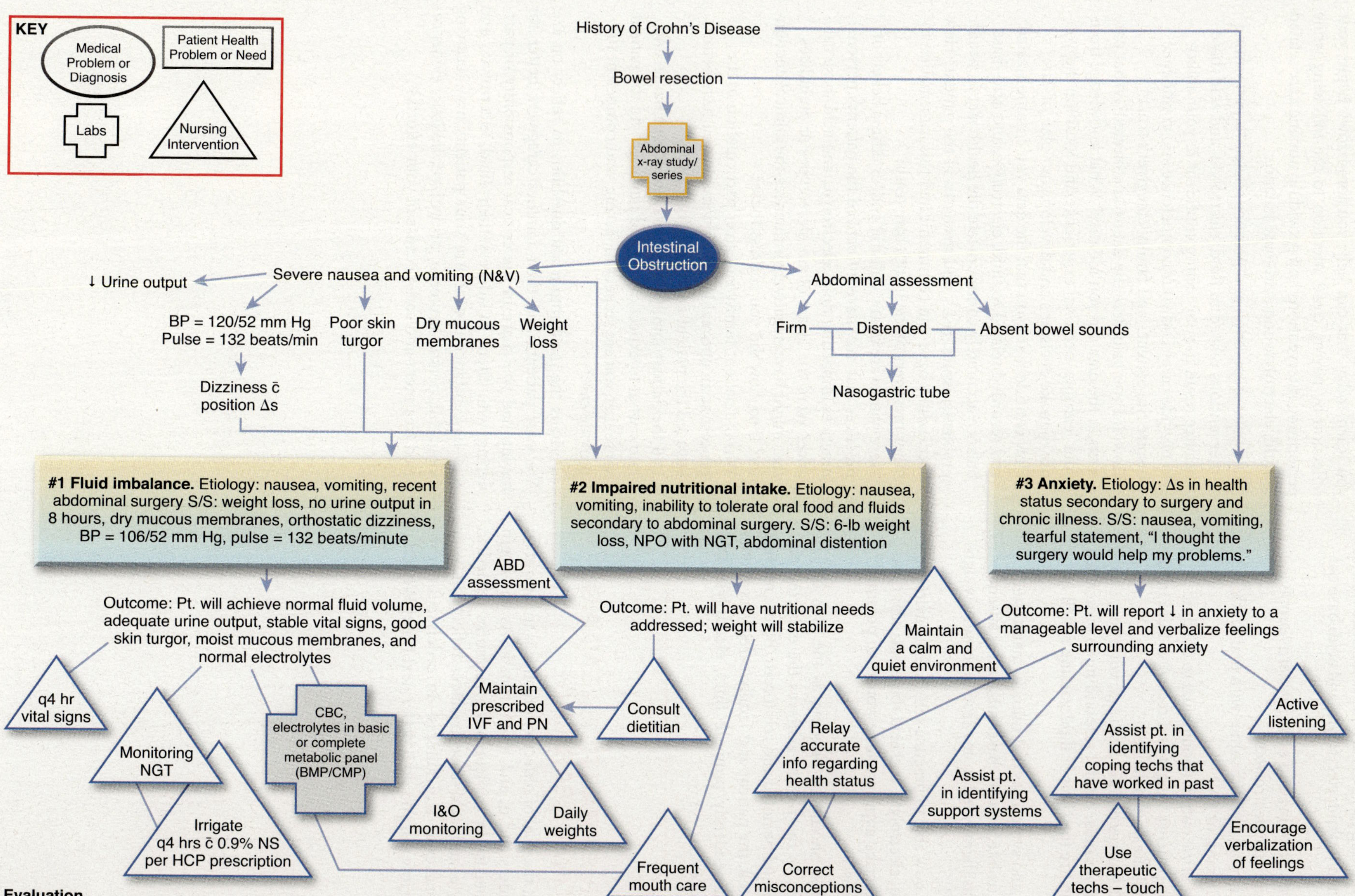

Evaluation

- **Diagnosis #1** Intravenous therapy is maintained. Grace voided 250 mL of urine after 4 hours of IV therapy. Vital signs stabilized. Her abdomen remains distended without bowel sounds. A surgical consult was prescribed to evaluate the need for abdominal surgery.
- **Diagnosis #2** Grace's abdomen remains distended with absent bowel sounds. She remains NPO and is being evaluated for surgery. Collaborate with dietitian and physician to determine need for TPN.
- **Diagnosis #3** Grace verbalizes and understanding of rationales for interventions. She is participating in the plan of care and asking questions regarding plan of care.

Skill 41-1 Initiating a Peripheral Intravenous Catheter Access and Intravenous Infusion

DELEGATION GUIDELINES

The initiation of a PIVC and IV infusion is not delegated to assistive personnel (AP). Depending on the state's nurse practice act and the organization's policies and procedures, initiation of a PIVC and IV infusion may be delegated to licensed practical/vocational nurses (LPN/LVNs). The decision to delegate must be based on careful analysis of the patient's needs and circumstances as well as the qualifications of the person to whom the task is being delegated. Refer to the Delegation Guidelines in Appendix A.

EQUIPMENT

- IV solution, as prescribed
- Electronic MAR (eMAR) or medication administration record (MAR)
- Towel or disposable pad
- Nonallergenic tape
- IV administration set
- Label for infusion set (for next change date)
- Transparent semipermeable membrane (TSM) dressing
- Electronic infusion device (if appropriate)
- Tourniquet
- Time tape and/or label (for IV container)
- Cleansing swabs (>0.5% chlorhexidine in alcohol solution is preferred; tincture of iodine, an iodophor [povidone-iodine], or 70% alcohol may also be used) (Gorski et al., 2021; Mimoz et al., 2015; O'Grady et al., 2017)
- IV securement/stabilization device, as appropriate
- Clean gloves
- Additional PPE, as indicated
- IV pole
- Local anesthetic (based on facility policy and/or if prescribed)
- PIVC
- Short extension tubing, if not permanently attached to the PIVC
- Needleless connector or end cap for extension tubing
- Antimicrobial wipes
- Passive disinfection caps (based on facility policy)
- Skin barrier protectant wipe (e.g., Skin-Prep®)
- Single-use clippers or scissors for hair removal (as indicated)
- Single-use, commercially prepared, prefilled syringe with sterile normal saline for injection, minimum volume equal to twice the internal volume of the catheter system (Gorski et al., 2021), according to facility policy.

IMPLEMENTATION

ACTION	RATIONALE
1. Verify the prescribed IV solution on the eMAR/MAR. Consider the appropriateness of the prescribed therapy in relation to the patient. Clarify any inconsistencies. Check the patient's health record for allergies. Know techniques for IV insertion, precautions, and the purpose of the IV solution administration, if prescribed. Check the solution for color and the container for leaking and expiration date, if prescribed. Gather the necessary supplies.	This ensures that the correct IV solution and rate of infusion and/or medication will be administered. The nurse is responsible for critically evaluating all prescribed interventions prior to administration. Any concerns regarding the type or amount of therapy prescribed should be immediately and clearly communicated to the prescribing health care provider. This knowledge and skill are essential for safe and accurate IV and medication administration. Preparation promotes efficient time management and an organized approach to the task.
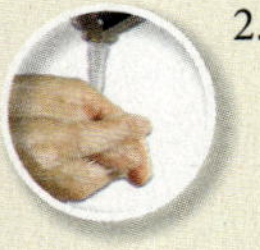 2. Perform hand hygiene and put on PPE, if indicated.	Hand hygiene and PPE prevent the spread of microorganisms. PPE is required based on transmission precautions.
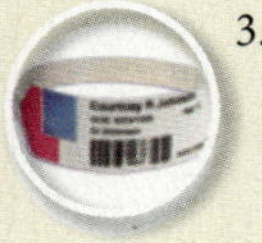 3. Identify the patient.	Identifying the patient ensures the right patient receives the intervention and helps prevent errors.
4. Assemble equipment on the bedside stand or overbed table or other surface within reach.	Bringing everything to the bedside conserves time and energy. Arranging items nearby is convenient, saves time, and avoids unnecessary stretching and twisting of muscles on the part of the nurse.

(continued on page 1716)

Skill 41-1 Initiating a Peripheral Intravenous Catheter Access and Intravenous Infusion *(continued)*

ACTION	RATIONALE
5. Close the curtains around the bed and close the door to the room, if possible. Explain to the patient what you are going to do and why. Ask the patient about allergies to medications, tape, or skin antiseptics, as appropriate. If considering using a local anesthetic, inquire about allergies for these substances as well. Consider use of nonpharmacologic interventions to reduce pain associated with PIVC insertion.	This ensures the patient's privacy. Explanation relieves anxiety and facilitates engagement. Possible allergies may exist related to medications, tape, or local anesthetic. Injectable anesthetic can result in allergic reactions and tissue damage. Nonpharmacologic interventions suggested for use to reduce PIVC insertion–related pain and discomfort include distraction, relaxation, breathing exercises, and virtual reality (VR) (Basak et al., 2020; Gorski et al., 2021). The choices of interventions for pediatric patients include swaddling, breastfeeding, pacifiers, rocking, blowing bubbles, reading books, use of VR, and local vibrating cold devices and should be made with consideration of growth and development level (Gorski et al., 2021).
6. If using a local anesthetic, explain the rationale and procedure to the patient. Apply the anesthetic to a few potential insertion sites. Allow sufficient time for the anesthetic to take effect.	Explanations provide reassurance and facilitate engagement. Local anesthetic agents should be used to reduce pain in all adult and pediatric populations (Gorski et al., 2021). Local anesthetic agents to reduce pain associated with PIVC insertion include vapocoolant sprays, topical transdermal agents, jet injection of pressure-accelerated lidocaine (needle-free), application of hot or cold to the site, and intradermal injection of lidocaine or bacteriostatic 0.9% sodium chloride (Gorski et al., 2021; Korkut et al., 2020; Welyczko, 2020). Some anesthetics take up to an hour to become effective.
Prepare the IV Solution and Administration Set	
7. Compare the IV container label with the eMAR/MAR. Remove the IV bag from the outer wrapper, if indicated. Check expiration dates. Scan the bar code on container, if necessary. Compare the patient identification band with the eMAR/MAR. Alternatively, label the solution container with the patient's name, solution type, additives, date, and time. Complete a time strip for the infusion and apply to the IV container.	Checking the label with eMAR/MAR ensures the correct IV solution will be administered. Identifying the patient ensures the right patient receives the medications and helps prevent errors. The time strip allows for quick visual reference by the nurse to monitor infusion accuracy.
8. Maintain aseptic technique when opening sterile packages and the IV solution. Remove the administration set from the package (Figure 1). Apply the label to the tubing reflecting the day/date for the next set change, per facility guidelines.	Asepsis is essential for preventing the spread of microorganisms. Labeling the tubing ensures adherence to facility policy regarding administration set changes and reduces the risk of the spread of microorganisms. Refer to Table 41-8 for recommended administration set change guidelines.

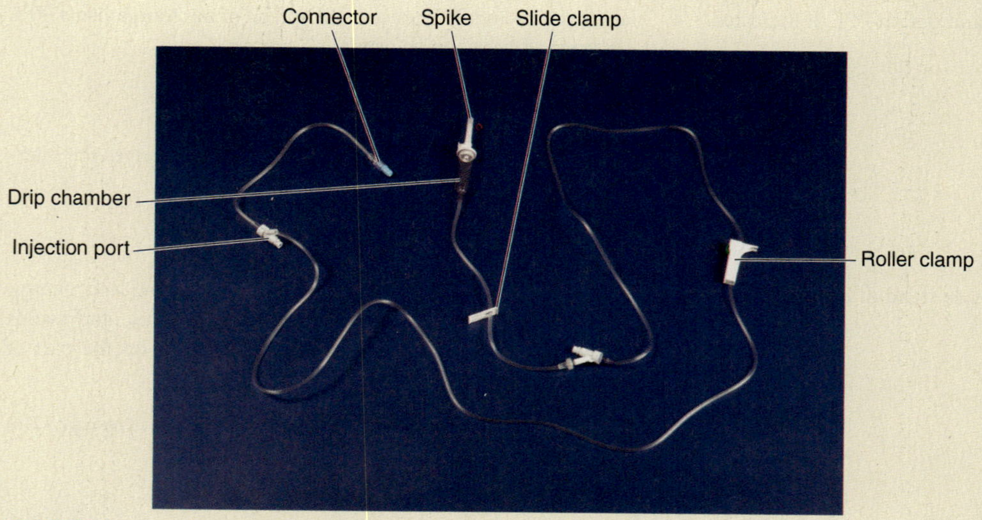

FIGURE 1. Basic administration set for gravity/free-flow infusion.

ACTION

9. Close the roller clamp or slide the clamp on the IV administration set (Figure 2). Invert the IV solution container and remove the cap on the entry site, taking care not to touch the exposed entry site. Remove the cap from the spike on the administration set. Using a twisting and pushing motion, insert the administration set spike into the entry site of the IV container (Figure 3). Alternatively, follow the manufacturer's directions for insertion.

RATIONALE

Clamping the IV tubing prevents air and fluid from entering the IV tubing.

Inverting the container allows easy access to the entry site. Touching the opened entry site on the IV container and/or the spike on the administration set results in contamination, resulting in the need to discard the container/administration set. Inserting the spike punctures the seal in the IV container and allows access to the contents.

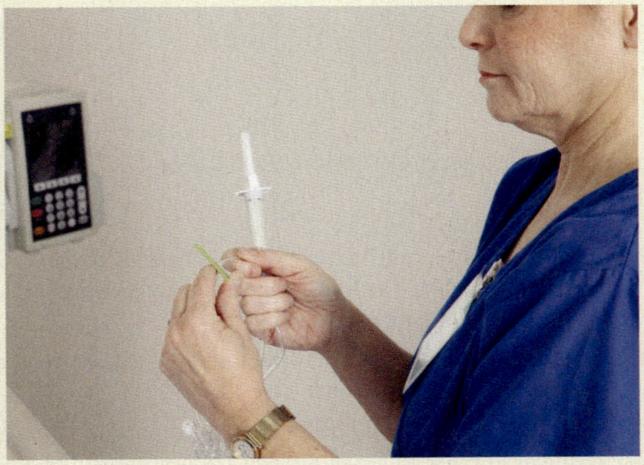

FIGURE 2. Closing clamp on administration set.

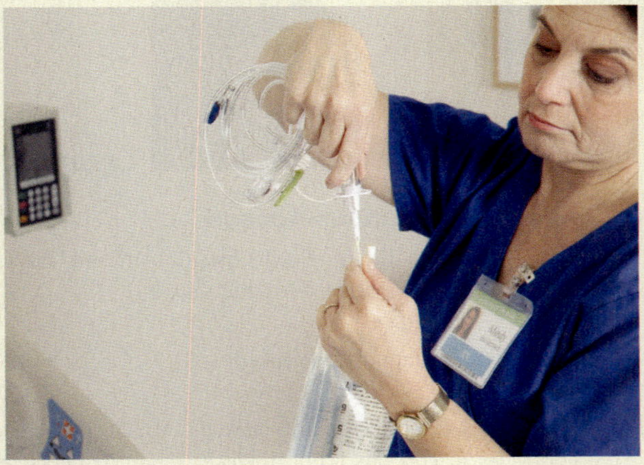

FIGURE 3. Inserting administration set spike into entry site of IV fluid container.

10. Hang the IV container on the IV pole. Squeeze the drip chamber and fill it at least halfway (Figure 4).

Suction causes fluid to move into the drip chamber. Fluid prevents air from moving down the tubing.

11. Open the IV tubing clamp and allow fluid to move through the tubing. Follow the additional manufacturer's instructions for the specific electronic infusion pump, as indicated. **Allow fluid to flow until all air bubbles have disappeared, and the entire length of the tubing is primed (filled) with IV solution (Figure 5).** Close the clamp. Alternatively, some brands of tubing may require removal of the cap at the end of the IV tubing to allow the fluid to flow. Maintain its sterility. After the fluid has filled the tubing, recap the end of the tubing.

This technique prepares for IV fluid administration and removes air from the tubing. Air should be purged from all administration sets to prevent air embolism (Gorski et al., 2021). Touching the open end of the tubing results in contamination, resulting in the need to discard the administration set.

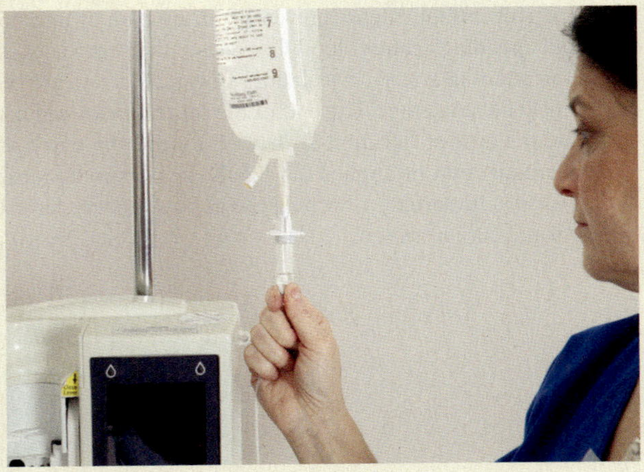

FIGURE 4. Squeezing drip chamber to fill at least halfway.

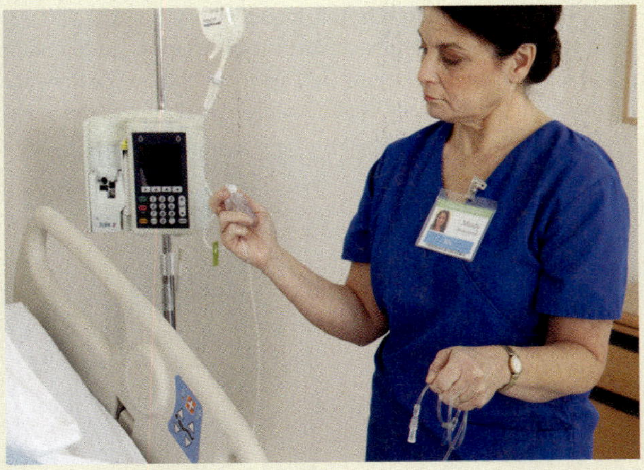

FIGURE 5. Priming administration set.

(continued on page 1718)

Skill 41-1 Initiating a Peripheral Intravenous Catheter Access and Intravenous Infusion *(continued)*

ACTION	RATIONALE
12. If an electronic device is to be used, follow the manufacturer's instructions for inserting the tubing into the device (Figure 6).	This ensures proper use of equipment.

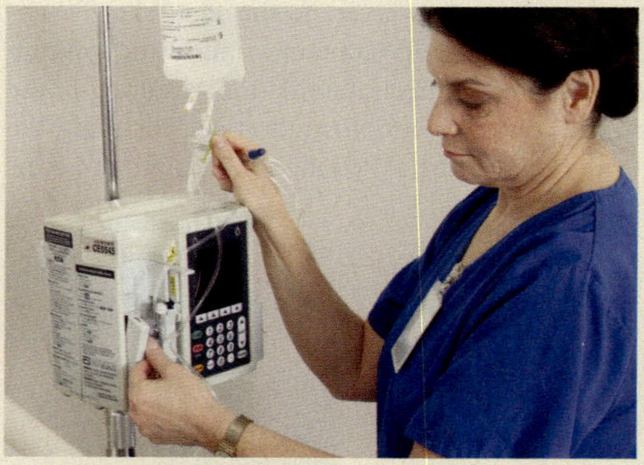

FIGURE 6. Inserting administration set into electronic infusion device.

Initiate Peripheral Venous Access

ACTION	RATIONALE
13. Place the patient in the low-Fowler position in bed. Place a protective towel or pad under the patient's arm.	The supine position permits either arm to be used and allows for good body alignment. The towel protects the underlying surface from blood contamination.
14. Provide emotional support, as needed.	The patient may experience anxiety because they may, in general, fear needlestick or IV infusion.
15. Open the short extension tubing package. Attach the needleless connector or end cap, if not in place. Clean the needleless connector or end cap with an alcohol wipe. Insert a syringe with normal saline into the extension tubing. Fill the extension tubing with normal saline and place the extension tubing and syringe back on the package, within easy reach.	A needleless connector should be attached to the extension tubing to eliminate the use of needles when connecting to the VAD (Gorski et al., 2021). Priming the extension tubing removes air from the tubing and prevents administration of air when connected to venous access. Having the tubing within easy reach facilitates accomplishment of procedure.
16. Select and palpate for an appropriate vein. Refer to the guidelines in the previous Assessment section. If the intended insertion site is visibly soiled, clean the area with soap and water (Gorski et al., 2021).	The use of an appropriate vein decreases discomfort for the patient and reduces the risk for damage to body tissues.
17. Remove excess hair at the insertion site, if needed, to facilitate application of the site dressing. Use single-patient-use scissors or disposable-head surgical clippers to remove hair at the insertion site and dressing area.	Hair can inhibit adhesion of the site dressing. Shaving causes microabrasions and may increase the risk for infection (Gorski et al., 2021).
18. Put on gloves.	Gloves prevent contact with blood and body fluids.
19. Apply a single-patient-use tourniquet (Gorski et al., 2021) 3 to 4 inches above the venipuncture site to obstruct venous blood flow and distend the vein (Figure 7). Direct the ends of the tourniquet away from the entry site. Make sure the radial pulse is still present.	A single-patient-use tourniquet prevents transmission of microorganisms. Impeding venous blood flow causes the vein to distend while maintaining arterial circulation. Distended veins are easy to see, palpate, and enter. The end of the tourniquet could contaminate the area of injection if directed toward the entry site. The tourniquet may be applied too tightly, so assessment for the radial pulse is important. Checking radial pulse ensures arterial supply is not compromised.

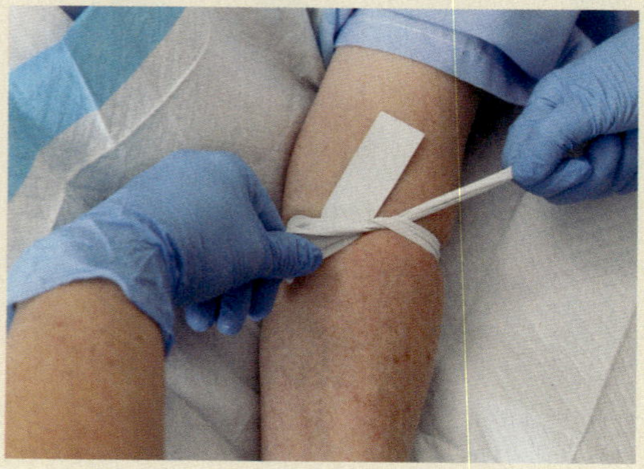

FIGURE 7. Applying tourniquet.

ACTION	RATIONALE
20. Instruct the patient to hold their arm lower than their heart.	Lowering the arm below the heart level helps distend the veins by filling them.
21. Ask the patient to open and close their fist. Observe and palpate for a suitable vein. If a vein cannot be felt, consider the use of vascular visualization technology or ultrasound to assist with identification of peripheral veins (Gorski et al., 2021).	Contracting the muscles of the forearm forces blood into the veins, thereby distending them further. Vascular visualization technology can be used to assist with identification of peripheral veins, with resulting increased insertion success; reduced insertion-related complications; and minimization of the need to escalate to unnecessary, more invasive VADs (Gorski et al., 2021). Ultrasound-guided PIVC insertion is a safe, efficient intervention and should be used for placement of a short PIVC in difficult-to-access adult patients (Gorski et al., 2021; Houston, 2013), the insertion of long PIVCs (Gorski et al., 2021), and after failed venipuncture attempts (Edwards & Jones, 2018; Egan et al., 2013).
22. Use a single-use sterile applicator containing sterile antiseptic solution to **cleanse the site with >5% chlorhexidine in alcohol solution or the solution identified by facility policy. Follow the manufacturer's directions for use to determine the product application process and dry times** (Gorski et al., 2021). **Allow the antiseptic to dry naturally; do not wipe, fan, or blow on the skin** (Gorski et al., 2021).	Cleansing is necessary because organisms on the skin can be introduced into the tissues or the bloodstream with the needle. Use of >0.5% chlorhexidine in alcohol solution is preferred for skin antisepsis (Gorski et al., 2021; Sarani et al., 2018). If there is a contraindication to alcoholic chlorhexidine solution, tincture of iodine, an iodophor (povidone-iodine), or 70% alcohol may instead be used (Gorski et al., 2021; Mimoz et al., 2015; O'Grady et al., 2017).
23. **Do not touch/palpate the insertion site after skin antisepsis. Use sterile gloves if repalpation of the vein is necessary after skin antisepsis.**	Touching the site after skin antisepsis recontaminates the insertion site. Use of sterile gloves for palpation prevents contamination of the insertion site.
24. Using your nondominant hand placed about 1 or 2 inches below the entry site, hold the patient's skin taut against the vein. **Avoid touching the prepared site.** Ask the patient to remain still while performing the venipuncture.	Pressure on the vein and surrounding tissues stabilizes the vein and helps prevent movement of the vein as the needle or catheter is being inserted. The planned IV insertion site is not palpated after skin cleansing unless sterile gloves are worn to prevent contamination (Gorski et al., 2021). Patient movement may prevent proper technique for IV insertion.
25. Align the IV catheter on top of the vein; enter the skin gently, holding the catheter by the hub in your dominant hand, bevel side up, at a 10- to 15-degree angle (Figure 8). Insert the catheter from directly over the vein or from the side of the vein. While following the course of the vein, advance the needle or catheter into the vein. A sensation of "give" can be felt when the needle enters the vein.	This allows the needle or catheter to enter the vein with minimal trauma and deters passage of the needle through the vein.

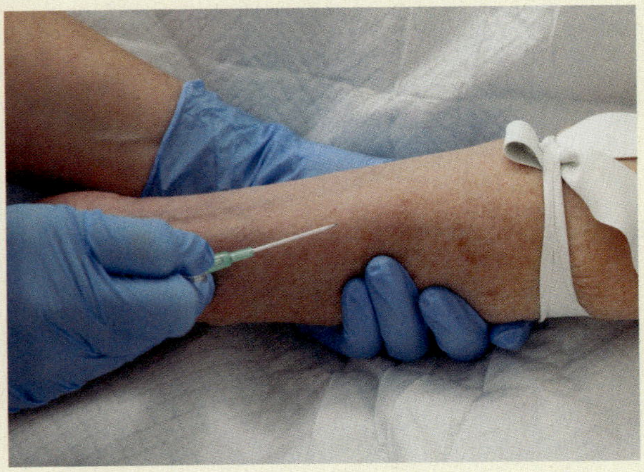

FIGURE 8. Stretching skin taut and inserting needle.

(continued on page 1720)

Skill 41-1 Initiating a Peripheral Intravenous Catheter Access and Intravenous Infusion *(continued)*

ACTION	RATIONALE
26. Continue to hold the skin taut. When blood returns through the catheter and/or the flashback chamber of the catheter, use the push-off tab to separate the catheter from the needle stylet and advance the catheter into the vein until the hub is at the venipuncture site. The exact technique depends on the type of device used.	The tourniquet causes increased venous pressure, resulting in automatic backflow. Placing the access device well into the vein helps to prevent dislodgment.
27. Release the tourniquet. Activate the safety mechanism on the needle stylet. Compress the skin well above the catheter tip to stop the flow of blood. Quickly remove the protective cap from the extension tubing, attach it to the catheter hub, and tighten the Luer lock. Stabilize the catheter or needle with your nondominant hand.	Bleeding is minimized and the patency of the vein is maintained if the connection is made smoothly between the catheter and extension tubing.
28. Continue to stabilize the catheter or needle and pull back on the syringe to assess for blood return, then flush gently with the saline, observing the site for infiltration and leaking. Remove the syringe from the end cap.	Presence of a blood return upon aspiration and lack of resistance when flushing indicate patency of the VAD (Gorski et al., 2021). Infiltration and/or leaking and the patient reports of pain and/or discomfort indicate that the insertion into the vein is not successful and should be discontinued. The syringe is no longer needed once flushing is complete.
29. Open the skin protectant wipe. Apply the skin protectant to the site, making sure to apply—at a minimum—the area to be covered with the dressing. Place a sterile transparent dressing and/or catheter securing/stabilization device over the venipuncture site. Loop the tubing near the entry site, and anchor it with tape (nonallergenic) close to the site.	The skin protectant aids in adhesion of the dressing and decreases the risk for skin trauma when the dressing is removed. A transparent dressing allows easy visualization and protects the site. Stabilization/securing devices preserve the integrity of the access device, minimize catheter movement at the hub, and prevent catheter dislodgement and loss of access (Gorski et al., 2021). Some stabilization devices also act as a site dressing. The weight of the tubing is sufficient to pull it out of the vein if it is not well anchored. Nonallergenic tape is less likely to tear fragile skin.
30. Label the IV dressing with the date, time, site, and type and size of the catheter placed (Figure 9).	Other personnel working with the infusion will know the site, type of device being used, and when it was inserted.

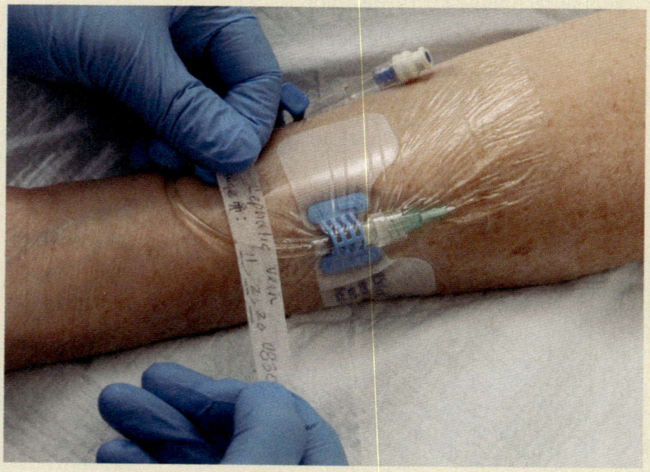

FIGURE 9. Venous access site with labeled dressing.

ACTION	RATIONALE
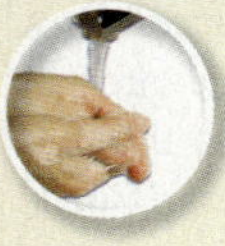 31. Using an antimicrobial swab, vigorously disinfect the connection surface and sides of the needleless connector or end cap on the extension tubing and allow it to dry. Remove the end cap from the administration set. Insert the end of the administration set into the needleless connector or end cap (Figure 10). Loop the administration set tubing near the entry site, and anchor it with tape (nonallergenic) close to the site. Remove your gloves. Perform hand hygiene.	Venous access device (VAD) administration set entry points, end caps, and needleless connectors must be disinfected prior to each access to reduce the risk for introduction of microorganisms and prevent VAD-related infection (Frimpong et al., 2015; Gorski et al., 2021; Harper, 2014; Loveday et al., 2014). Friction is needed to physically remove microorganisms from the top, sides, and threads of the needleless connector or end cap. Allow the antiseptic to dry completely following the manufacturer's directions for use (Gorski et al., 2021). Inserting the administration set allows initiation of the fluid infusion. The weight of the tubing is sufficient to pull it out of the vein if it is not well anchored. Nonallergenic tape is less likely to tear fragile skin. Removing gloves properly reduces the risk for infection transmission and contamination of other items. Hand hygiene prevents transmission of microorganisms.

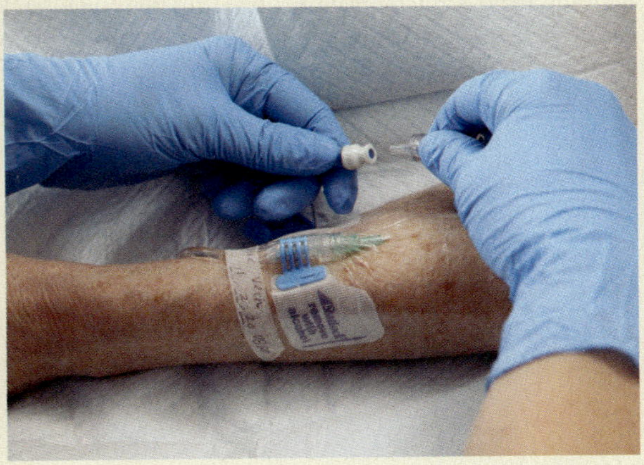

FIGURE 10. Inserting administration set into the end cap of venous access device.

ACTION	RATIONALE
32. Open the clamp on the administration set. Set the flow rate and begin the fluid infusion (Figure 11). Alternatively, start the flow of solution by releasing the clamp on the tubing and counting the drops. Adjust until the correct drop rate is achieved. Assess the flow of the solution and function of the infusion device. Inspect the insertion site for signs of infiltration (Figure 12).	Verifying the rate and device settings ensures the patient receives the correct volume of solution. If the catheter slips out of the vein, the solution will accumulate (infiltrate) into the surrounding tissue.

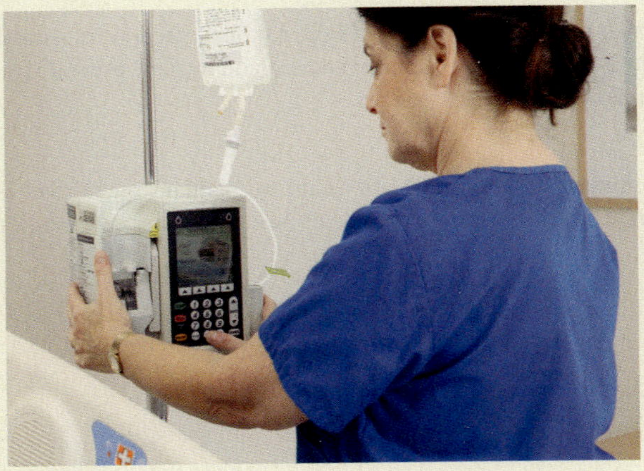

FIGURE 11. Initiating IV fluid infusion.

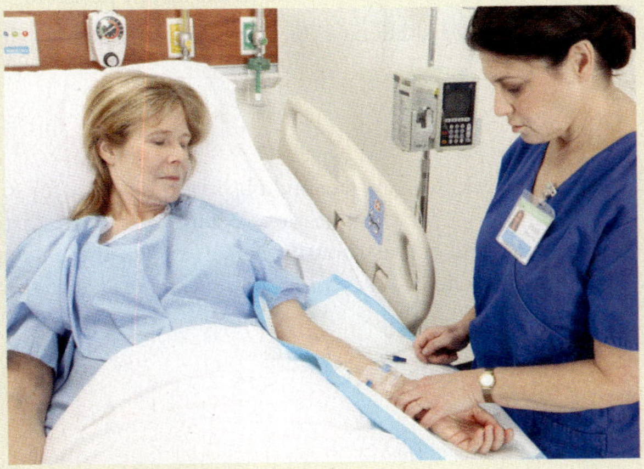

FIGURE 12. Inspecting insertion site.

(continued on page 1722)

Skill 41-1 Initiating a Peripheral Intravenous Catheter Access and Intravenous Infusion *(continued)*

ACTION

33. Apply an IV securement/stabilization device if not already in place as part of the dressing, as indicated, based on facility policy. Explain to the patient the purpose of the device and the importance of safeguarding the site when using the extremity.

RATIONALE

These systems are recommended for use on all venous access sites, particularly central venous access sites, to preserve the integrity of the access device, minimize catheter movement at the hub, and prevent catheter dislodgement and loss of access (Gorski et al., 2021). Some devices also act as a site dressing and may already have been applied.

34. Apply a passive disinfection cap to each access site on the administration set; use an antimicrobial swab to vigorously disinfect the connection surface and sides of each access site and allow it to dry. Attach a passive disinfection cap to each site (Figure 13).

Passive disinfection caps contain an antiseptic-impregnated sponge that dispenses the antiseptic over the connector's top and threads and protects the hub from contamination by touch or airborne sources (Gorski et al., 2021; Stango et al., 2014). VAD administration set entry points, end caps, and needleless connectors must be vigorously scrubbed and disinfected prior to each access to reduce the risk for introduction of microorganisms and prevent VAD-related infection (Frimpong et al., 2015; Gorski et al., 2021; Harper, 2014; Loveday et al., 2014). Friction is needed to physically remove microorganisms from the top, sides, and threads of the needleless connector or end cap. Allow the antiseptic to dry completely to ensure complete effectiveness.

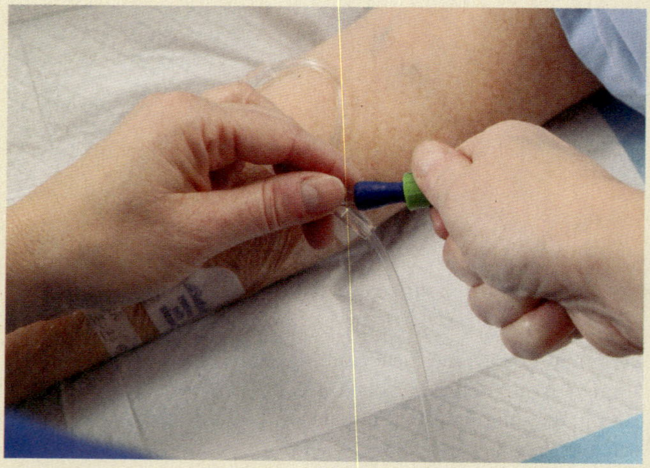

FIGURE 13. Attaching a passive disinfection cap to each access site.

35. Remove the equipment and return the patient to a position of comfort. Lower the bed, if it is not in the lowest position.

Positioning promotes patient comfort and safety.

36. Remove additional PPE, if used. Perform hand hygiene.

Proper removal of PPE reduces the risk for infection transmission and contamination of other items. Hand hygiene prevents transmission of microorganisms.

37. Return to check the flow rate and observe the IV site for infiltration and/or other complications 30 minutes after starting the infusion and at least hourly thereafter. Ask the patient if they are experiencing any pain or discomfort related to the IV infusion.

Continued monitoring is important to maintain the correct flow rate. Early detection of problems ensures prompt intervention.

DOCUMENTATION

Guidelines

Document the date and time of insertion, number of attempts, and location (anatomical descriptors, laterality, landmarks) where the IV access was placed as well as the type, length and gauge/size of the PIVC inserted, type of anesthetic (if used), type of IV solution, rate of the IV infusion (often done in the eMAR/MAR), and the use of a securing or stabilization device. Document the use of visualization technology (if used). Document the condition of the site. Record the patient's reaction to the procedure and pertinent patient teaching, such as alerting the nurse if the patient experiences any pain from the IV or notices any swelling at the site. Document the IV fluid solution on the intake and output record.

Sample Documentation

Lippincott DocuCare **Practice documenting peripheral venous access infusion in *Lippincott DocuCare*.**

11/02/25 0830 20-gauge IV started in dorsal surface of the L forearm via the cephalic vein; positive blood return, lack of resistance when flushed. Transparent dressing and peripheral stabilization device applied. Site without redness, drainage, or edema; patient denies discomfort. $D_5$1/2 NS with 20 mEq KCl begun at 110 mL/hr. Patient instructed to call with any pain, discomfort, or swelling and verbalizes an understanding of instructions.

—S. Barnes, RN

DEVELOPING CLINICAL REASONING AND CLINICAL JUDGMENT

UNEXPECTED SITUATIONS AND ASSOCIATED INTERVENTIONS

- *An artery is inadvertently accessed or the patient reports paresthesias, numbness, or tingling upon insertion:* Immediately remove the catheter, apply pressure to the insertion site, and notify the health care team (Gorski et al., 2021).
- *Fluid does not easily flow into the vein:* Reposition the extremity because certain positions that the patient may assume may prevent the IV from infusing properly. If the IV is a free-flowing IV, raise the height of the IV pole. This may promote an increase in IV flow. Attempt to flush the PIVC with saline. Check the IV connector to ensure that the clamp is fully open. If fluid still does not flow easily, or if resistance is met while flushing, the IV may be against a valve and may need to be restarted in a different location.
- *Fluid does not flow easily into the vein, and the skin around the insertion site is edematous and cool to the touch:* The IV has infiltrated. Put on gloves and remove the catheter. Use a skin marker to outline the area with visible signs of infiltration to allow for assessment of changes (Gorski et al., 2021). Secure the gauze with tape over the insertion site without applying pressure. Assess the area distal to the VAD for capillary refill, sensation, and motor function Gorski et al., 2021). Restart the IV in a new location. Estimate the volume of fluid that escaped into the tissue based on the rate of infusion and length of time since the last assessment. Notify the health care team and use an appropriate method for clinical management of the infiltrate site, based on the infused solution and facility guidelines (Gorski et al., 2021). Record the site assessment and interventions as well as the site for new venous access.
- *A small hematoma is forming at the site while you are inserting the catheter:* The vein is "blowing," which means a small hole has been made in the vein, and blood is leaking out into the tissues. Remove and discard the catheter and choose an alternative insertion site.
- *Fluids are leaking around the insertion site:* Check connections. Change the dressing on the site. If the site continues to leak, remove the IV and restart it in a new location.
- *IV infusion set becomes disconnected from IV:* Discard the administration set to prevent infection. Assess patency and attempt to flush the PIVC. If the PIVC is still patent, the site may still be used as long as the catheter hub has not been contaminated.
- *IV catheter is partially pulled out of the insertion site (migrates externally):* Do not readvance the catheter. Whether the access is salvageable depends on how much of the catheter remains in the vein. Assess for proper placement in the vein before further use and consider the infusion therapy and circumstances to determine viability and secure at the current location (Gorski et al., 2021). Removal and reinsertion at a new site might be the most appropriate intervention if the PIVC is no longer in an appropriate position for the prescribed infusion (Gorski et al., 2021). If the PIVC is not removed, monitor it closely for signs of infiltration and infection.

(continued on page 1724)

Skill 41-1 Initiating a Peripheral Intravenous Catheter Access and Intravenous Infusion *(continued)*

SPECIAL CONSIDERATIONS

General Considerations

- The smallest-gauge PIVC that will accommodate the prescribed therapy and patient need should be selected (Gorski et al., 2021). A 20- to 24-gauge catheter is recommended for most infusions to decrease the risk of phlebitis (Gorski et al., 2021).
- A 22- to 26-gauge catheter is recommended for patients with limited venous options to minimize insertion-related trauma (Gorski et al., 2021).
- An individual nurse should not make more than two attempts at vascular access placement when initiating venous access for a patient (Gorski et al., 2021). If unsuccessful after two attempts, a colleague with advanced skills, such as a member of the nurse IV team, should attempt to initiate the venous access (Gorski et al., 2021). Multiple unsuccessful attempts cause pain to the patient and result in delayed treatment, limited future vascular access, increased costs, and increased risk for complications (Gorski et al., 2021).
- Factors that may interfere with successful evaluation of the condition of the patient's veins and subsequent placement of a peripheral catheter include obesity, diabetes, hypertension, variations in skin between patient populations (e.g., darker skin tones, excessive hair, presence of scars or tattoos), increased patient age, neonates, fluid volume deficit, injection drug use, the presence of multiple chronic health conditions (e.g., diabetes, renal disease), vascular disease, chemotherapy, and/or frequent hospitalizations (Dougherty, 2013; Dychter et al., 2012; Fields et al., 2014; Gorski et al, 2021; Morata & Bowers, 2020; Partovi-Deilami et al., 2016). These factors interfere with use of traditional techniques of direct visualization, anatomic landmarks, and palpation and make placement of the PIVC difficult (Gorski et al., 2021; Houston, 2013).
- Ultrasound-guided PIVC insertion is a safe, efficient intervention and should be used for placement of a short PIVC in difficult-to-access adult patients (Gorski et al., 2021; Houston, 2013), the insertion of long PIVCs (Gorski et al., 2021), and after failed venipuncture attempts (Edwards & Jones, 2018; Egan et al., 2013).
- Closed-system peripheral intravenous catheters are available. These systems integrate the catheter and extension tubing as one piece (Galang et al., 2020), eliminating the need for the addition of separate extension tubing, reducing potential contamination.
- Drying time with 70% isopropyl alcohol is 5 seconds; alcohol-based chlorhexidine requires 20 seconds. Povidone iodine requires longer than 6 minutes to be thoroughly dry, making it less favorable to clinical practice (Gorski et al., 2021).
- Transparent semipermeable membrane (TSM) dressings are commonly used to protect the insertion site. A gauze dressing is recommended if the patient is diaphoretic, the site is bleeding or oozing, or there is drainage from the exit site; replace it with a TSM once this is resolved (Gorski et al., 2021; O'Grady et al., 2017).
- Avoid blood pressure measurement or placement of a tourniquet over the site/upper extremity with a peripheral VAD during periods of infusion (Gorski et al., 2021).
- When the patient is showering or bathing, protect the peripheral VAD with clear plastic wrap or a device designed for this purpose. Cover the connections and protect the hub connections from water contamination (Gorski et al., 2021).

Infant and Child Considerations

- Potential sites for short PIVCs for neonates and pediatric patients include veins in the hand; forearm; and, if not walking, the foot. Avoid the antecubital fossa, which has a higher failure rate (Gorski et al., 2021). Consider veins in the forearm and the saphenous vein for long PIVCs (Gorski et al., 2021). Select an upper arm site using the basilic, cephalic, or brachial veins; veins in the leg (saphenous, popliteal, femoral) with the tip below the inguinal crease; and in the scalp with the tip in the neck, above the thorax for placement of a midline catheter (Gorski et al., 2021).
- When no alternative site is available, veins of the scalp may be used as a last resort; avoid the use of the hands, thumbs, or fingers (Gorski et al., 2021).
- A 22- to 26-gauge catheter is recommended for neonates and pediatric patients to minimize insertion-related trauma (Gorski et al., 2021).
- Use chlorhexidine with caution in infants up to age 14 days, premature infants, and low-birth-weight infants due to the risk of skin irritation and chemical burns (Gorski et al., 2021).

Older Adult Considerations

- A 22- to 26-gauge catheter is recommended for older adults to minimize insertion-related trauma (Gorski et al., 2021).
- Insert the PIVC using a 5- to 15-degree angle for older adults (Gorski et al., 2021).

Skill 41-2 Monitoring an Intravenous Site and Infusion

DELEGATION CONSIDERATIONS

The monitoring of an IV site and infusion is not delegated to assistive personnel (AP). Depending on the state's nurse practice act and the organization's policies and procedures, these procedures may be delegated to licensed practical/vocational nurses (LPN/LVNs). The decision to delegate must be based on careful analysis of the patient's needs and circumstances as well as the qualifications of the person to whom the task is being delegated. Refer to the Delegation Guidelines in Appendix A.

EQUIPMENT

- PPE, as indicated
- Standardized scale for assessing and documenting phlebitis

IMPLEMENTATION

ACTION	RATIONALE
1. Verify the IV prescribed solution on the eMAR/MAR with the health record. Consider the appropriateness of the prescribed therapy in relation to the patient. Clarify any inconsistencies. Check the patient's health record for allergies. Check solution for color and the container for leaking and expiration date. Know the purpose of the IV administration.	This ensures that the correct IV solution and rate of infusion and/or medication will be administered. The nurse is responsible for critically evaluating all prescribed interventions. Any concerns regarding the type or amount of therapy prescribed should be immediately and clearly communicated to the prescribing health care provider. This knowledge and skill are essential for safe and accurate IV and medication administration.
2. **Monitor the IV infusion every hour or per facility policy. More frequent checks may be necessary if medication is being infused.**	This promotes safe administration of IV fluids and medication.
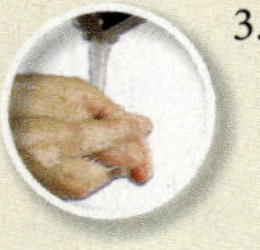 3. Perform hand hygiene and put on PPE, if indicated.	Hand hygiene and PPE prevent the spread of microorganisms. PPE is required based on transmission precautions.
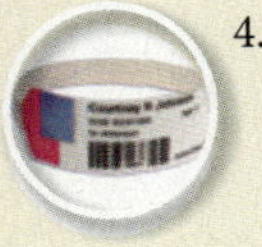 4. Identify the patient.	Identifying the patient ensures the right patient receives the intervention and helps prevent errors.
5. Close the curtains around the bed and close the door to the room, if possible. Explain to the patient what you are going to do and why.	This ensures the patient's privacy. Explanation relieves anxiety and facilitates engagement.
6. If an electronic infusion device is being used, check settings, alarm, and indicator lights. Check the set infusion rate (Figure 1). Note the position of fluid in the IV container in relation to the time tape. Teach the patient about the alarm features on the electronic infusion device.	Observation ensures that the infusion control device and the alarm are functioning. Lack of knowledge about "alarms" may create anxiety for the patient.

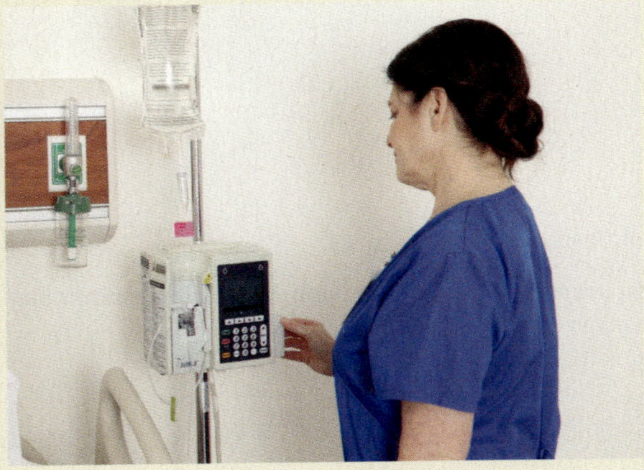

FIGURE 1. Checking infusion device settings.

(continued on page 1726)

Skill 41-2 Monitoring an Intravenous Site and Infusion *(continued)*

ACTION	RATIONALE
7. If the IV is infusing via gravity/free flow, check the drip chamber and time the drops (Figure 2). Refer to Guidelines for Nursing Care 41-2 to review calculation of IV flow rates for gravity/free-flow infusion.	This ensures that the flow rate is correct. Use a watch with a second hand for counting the drops in regulating a gravity/free-flow drip IV infusion.
8. Check the tubing for anything that might interfere with the flow (Figure 3). Be sure the clamps are in the open position.	Any kink or pressure on the tubing may interfere with the flow.

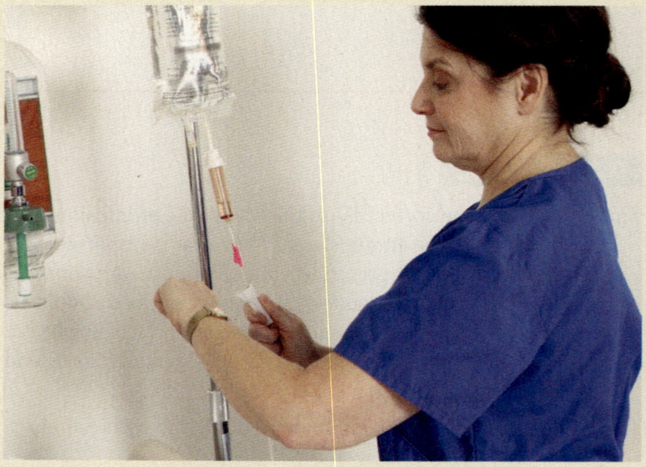

FIGURE 2. Checking drip chamber and timing drops.

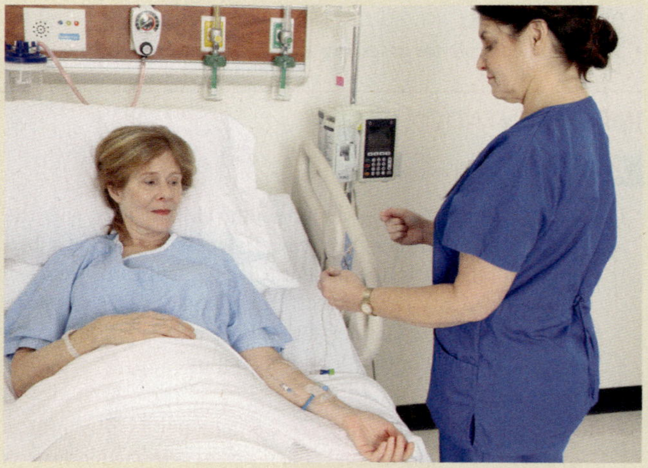

FIGURE 3. Checking tubing for anything that might interfere with flow rate.

ACTION	RATIONALE
9. Observe the dressing for leakage of the IV solution.	Leakage may occur at the connection of the tubing with the hub of the catheter and allow for loss of the IV solution.
10. Inspect the site for swelling, leakage at the site, coolness, or pallor, which may indicate infiltration (Figure 4). Ask if the patient is experiencing any pain or discomfort. If any of these symptoms are present, the IV will need to be removed and restarted at another site. Check facility policy for treating infiltration. Refer to Table 41-9.	The catheter may become dislodged from the vein, and IV solution may flow into the subcutaneous tissue.

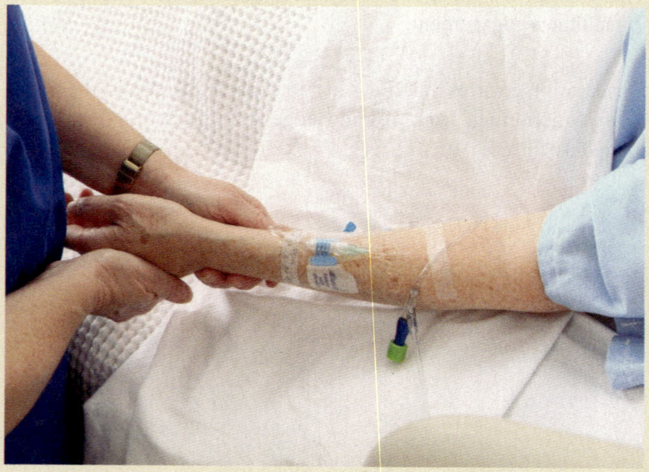

FIGURE 4. Inspecting IV site.

ACTION	RATIONALE
11. Inspect the site for redness, swelling, and heat. Palpate for induration. Ask if the patient is experiencing pain. These findings may indicate phlebitis, making it necessary to discontinue and restart the IV at another site. Grade phlebitis. Refer to Table 41-9 and Box 41-1. Check facility policy for treatment of phlebitis.	Chemical irritation, mechanical trauma, and microorganisms may cause injury to the vein and can lead to phlebitis.

ACTION	RATIONALE
12. Check for local manifestations (redness, pus, warmth, induration, and pain) that may indicate an infection is present at the site. Also check for systemic manifestations (chills, fever, tachycardia, hypotension) that may accompany local infection at the site. If signs of infection are present, discontinue the IV and notify the health care team. Be careful not to disconnect the IV tubing when putting on the patient's hospital gown or assisting the patient with movement to avoid contamination.	Poor aseptic technique may allow bacteria to enter the catheter insertion site or the tubing connection and may occur with manipulation of equipment.
13. Be alert for additional complications of IV therapy, such as fluid overload or bleeding. Refer to Table 41-9.	Infusing too much IV solution results in an increase of circulating fluid volume.
a. Fluid overload can result in signs of cardiac and/or respiratory failure. Monitor intake and output and vital signs. Assess for edema and auscultate lung sounds. Ask if the patient is experiencing any shortness of breath.	Older adults are most at risk for this complication due to possible decrease in cardiac and/or renal functions.
b. Check for bleeding at the site.	Bleeding may be caused by anticoagulant medication. Bleeding at the site is most likely to occur when the IV is discontinued.
14. If appropriate, instruct the patient to call for assistance if any discomfort is noted at the site, the solution container is nearly empty, the flow has changed in any way, or if the electronic pump alarm sounds.	This facilitates patient engagement and safe administration of IV solution.
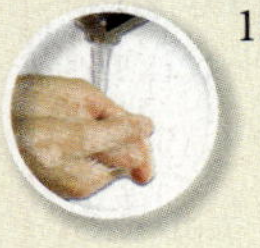 15. Remove PPE, if used. Perform hand hygiene.	Proper removal of PPE reduces the risk for infection transmission and contamination of other items. Hand hygiene prevents transmission of microorganisms.

DOCUMENTATION

Guidelines

Document the type of IV solution as well as the infusion rate. Note the insertion site location and site assessment. Document the patient's reaction to the IV therapy as well as the absence of subjective reports that they are not experiencing any pain or other discomfort, such as coolness or heat associated with the infusion. In addition, record that the patient is not demonstrating any other IV complications, such as signs or symptoms of fluid overload. Document pertinent patient teaching. Document the IV fluid solution on the intake and output record.

Sample Documentation

> 11/6/25 1020 IV site right forearm/cephalic vein intact without swelling, redness, or drainage; dressing and stabilization device intact. D_5 0.9% NS with 20 mEq KCl continues to infuse at 110 mL/hr. Patient and partner instructed to call nurse with any swelling, discomfort or pain and verbalize an understanding of instructions.
>
> —*S. Barnes, RN*

DEVELOPING CLINICAL REASONING AND CLINICAL JUDGMENT

UNEXPECTED SITUATIONS AND ASSOCIATED INTERVENTIONS

- *Patient's lung sounds were previously clear, but now some crackles in the bases are auscultated, and the patient reports some shortness of breath:* Notify the health care team immediately. The patient may be exhibiting signs of fluid overload. Be prepared to tell the health care provider what the past intake and output totals were as well as the patient's vital signs and pulse oximetry assessment findings.
- *IV is not flowing as easily as it previously had been:* Check all clamps on the tubing, and check the tubing for any kinking. Check that the patient is not lying on the tubing. If the IV is over a joint, reposition the extremity and see if this helps the flow. Attempt to flush the PIVC with normal saline. If the IV is painful, you meet resistance when attempting to flush, or fluid still does not flow easily, discontinue the IV and restart it in another place.

EVOLVING CASE STUDY 41-1

Scenario: Jack Soo Park, a 78-year-old adult with a history of renal failure, is being treated for urosepsis. When Mr. Park was admitted 24 hours ago, he was disoriented, febrile, and had not been eating or drinking for several days as a result of "not feeling well" and is receiving intravenous fluid replacement and intravenous antibiotics. You have just finished receiving report and answer the patient's call bell. Mr. Park tells you, "I'm having trouble breathing."

QUESTION r/t CUES: Based on the patient's current situation, what assessment information is most important for the nurse to collect first?

A. Observe for edema in the lower extremities.
B. Review the complete metabolic panel results from earlier in the day.
C. Review the patient's baseline and current weight.
D. Assess the patient's lung sounds and oxygen saturation.

Scenario: While you are conducting your assessment, Mr. Park shares that he didn't sleep "at all" last night. Your assessment reveals the patient is very thin with a bounding pulse of 118, BP 142/90, crackles and wheezes in their lungs, and an oxygen saturation of 92%. You note that Mr. Park has a peripheral intravenous access device in his right forearm.

QUESTION r/t ANALYZING CUES: What other information (assessment data or evidence) should the nurse obtain to aid in determining the plan of care? Select all that apply.

A. Intake and output measurements
B. IV infusion site assessment
C. IV infusion solution and rate
D. The patient's usual sleep routine
E. 24-hour recall of dietary intake

Scenario: Mr. Park's intravenous infusion was prescribed to infuse at 125 mL/hr for the first 8 hours after admission and then be decreased to 40 mL/hr. A fluid-administration error resulted in the rate not being adjusted and your assessment reveals that the intravenous infusion has a current rate of 125 mL/hr.

QUESTION r/t PRIORITIZING HYPOTHESIS: Based on the assessment data for this patient, which ***priority*** patient problem should the nurse identify to guide the plan of care?

A. Impaired sleep
B. Fluid imbalance
C. Impaired nutritional intake
D. Fatigue

Scenario: After collaborating with the interprofessional team, you convert the intravenous to a capped peripheral venous access device and prepare to administer the prescribed 20-mg furosemide IV bolus.

QUESTION r/t GENERATING SOLUTIONS: Which action should be taken to evaluate or verify the integrity of the peripheral IV access site?

A. Remove the securement device to assess the site.
B. Document a negative aspiration for a blood return
C. Rotate the site every 72 hours.
D. Assess the skin temperature and tone at the site.

Scenario: Mr. Park's breathing has improved; he denies shortness of breath, dyspnea and pain, and his vital signs and oxygen saturation values are within expected limits. During one of your conversations, Mr. Park shares that "I don't always take my medications the way I'm supposed to. And, to tell the truth, I try not to drink a lot of liquids. I don't like to have to rush to the bathroom all the time!" After speaking with Mr. Park, you identify that problems with fluid balance occur at home as well. You and the patient agree there is a need for review and reinforcement of self-management strategies related to fluid balance.

QUESTION r/t TAKING ACTION: A second patient problem of deficient knowledge is identified. The nurse is preparing teaching materials for the patient. Which interventions should the nurse focus on with this patient? Select all that apply.

A. Monitoring of fluid intake and output.
B. Measuring weight at the same time each day.
C. Taking prescribed diuretics early in the day.
D. Keeping track of changes in breathing, weight, and urinary output to report at his 6-week check-up.
E. Restricting fluid intake to as little volume as possible.

Scenario: Mr. Park has been afebrile, and his vital signs and laboratory values have remained within expected parameters. His antibiotics have been changed to oral medications. Mr. Park is scheduled to be discharged home.

QUESTION r/t EVALUATING OUTCOMES: Based on the identified health problem, how will the nurse and Mr. Park *best* know that the plan of care has been effective?

A. The patient reports getting sufficient sleep at night.
B. The patient reports he is not experiencing dyspnea and his weight has remained stable.
C. The patient shares that he plans to take his diuretic every other day to avoid problems.
D. The patient's weight steadily increases over the next several weeks.

DEVELOPING CLINICAL REASONING AND CLINICAL JUDGMENT

1. Work through the Concept Map for on page 1714 and the Evolving Case Study 41-1 for Jack Soo Park on page 1728 to help develop your clinical reasoning and clinical judgment skills.
2. Assess a healthy person and a patient whose fluid and electrolyte or acid–base balance is altered using Tables 40-3 and 40-4, which describe parameters to be considered in physical and clinical assessments for fluid, electrolyte, and acid–base balance. Compare and contrast your findings.
3. Review the record of a patient who has been receiving IV fluids over a period of 3 or more days. Note the daily intake and output records, pertinent laboratory values, and clinical behaviors, and make a judgment about the patient's fluid, electrolyte, and acid–base balance. What factors complicate a hospitalized patient's usual ability to remain in balance?

PRACTICING FOR NCLEX

1. A nurse on the respiratory unit is interpreting ABGs for several patients. The patient with which problem will the nurse suspect may have developed respiratory alkalosis?
   a. Hypoxia
   b. Atelectasis
   c. Chronic respiratory illness
   d. Sedative overdose
2. A nurse is caring for a group of patients. The patient with which problem would the nurse identify is at high risk for fluid volume excess?
   a. Renal failure
   b. Vomiting
   c. Hypernatremia
   d. NPO for surgery
3. A nurse is caring for a patient who has developed hypernatremia. For which intravenous solution would the nurse anticipate a prescription?
   a. 5% dextrose in 0.9% NaCl
   b. 0.9% NaCl (normal saline)
   c. 0.45% NaCl (½-strength normal saline)
   d. 5% dextrose in lactated Ringer's solution
4. A nurse is assessing infants in the NICU for fluid balance status. Which nursing action would the nurse depend on as the most reliable indicator of a patient's fluid balance status?
   a. Recording intake and output
   b. Testing skin turgor
   c. Reviewing the complete blood count
   d. Measuring weight daily
5. A nurse is caring for a patient in the intensive care unit. How will the nurse interpret the patient's arterial blood gas values: pH, 7.30; $PaCO_2$, 36 mm Hg; HCO_3^-, 14 mEq/L?
   a. Respiratory acidosis
   b. Respiratory alkalosis
   c. Metabolic acidosis
   d. Metabolic alkalosis
6. A patient with dehydration has been encouraged to increase fluid intake. Which measure would be most effective for the nurse to implement?
   a. Explaining the mechanisms of fluid transport in cellular compartments
   b. Keeping the patient's preferred fluids readily available for the patient
   c. Emphasizing the long-term benefit of increasing fluids
   d. Planning to offer most daily fluids in the evening
7. A nurse is flushing a patient's peripheral venous access device. The nurse finds that the access site is leaking fluid during flushing. What action will the nurse take next?
   a. Removing the IV from the site and start at another location
   b. Immediately notifying the primary care provider
   c. Outlining the affected area in ink and monitoring for changes
   d. Aspirating the catheter and attempting to flush again
8. A nurse is monitoring a patient who is receiving an IV infusion of normal saline at 250 mL /hr. The patient is apprehensive and presents with a pounding headache, rapid pulse, chills, and dyspnea. What would be the nurse's priority intervention related to these symptoms?
   a. Discontinuing the infusion immediately, monitoring vital signs, and reporting findings to the primary care provider immediately
   b. Slowing the rate of infusion, notifying the primary care provider immediately, and monitoring vital signs
   c. Pinching off the catheter or securing the system to prevent entry of air, placing the patient in the Trendelenburg position, and calling for assistance
   d. Discontinuing the infusion immediately, applying warm compresses to the site, and restarting the IV at another site
9. A nurse carefully assesses the acid–base balance of a patient whose bicarbonate (HCO_3^-) level is decreased on the ABG results. This typically occurs in patients with damage to which organ?
   a. Kidneys
   b. Lungs
   c. Adrenal glands
   d. Brain
10. A nurse is monitoring a patient who is diagnosed with hypokalemia. Which nursing intervention would be appropriate for this patient?
    a. Encouraging foods and fluids with higher sodium content
    b. Administering oral potassium supplements as prescribed
    c. Cautioning the patient about eating foods high in potassium content
    d. Discussing calcium-losing aspects of nicotine and alcohol use

11. A nurse has begun administering an intravenous antibiotic via the patient's peripheral venous access. Immediately, the nurse observes that the fluid does not flow easily into the vein and the skin around the insertion site is edematous and cool to the touch. What would be the nurse's next action related to these findings?
    a. Repositioning the extremity and raise the height of the IV pole
    b. Applying pressure to the dressing on the IV
    c. Pulling the catheter out slightly and reinserting it
    d. Putting on gloves; removing the catheter
12. When caring for a patient receiving hemodialysis through an arteriovenous fistula, which action is essential for the nurse to take?
    a. Avoiding IM injections
    b. Not assessing the radial pulse on the same side as the access
    c. Performing BP and venipuncture on the opposite extremity
    d. Using the distended portion of the fistula for IV medications
13. A nurse is administering a blood transfusion for a patient following surgery. During the transfusion, the patient displays signs of dyspnea, dry cough, and pulmonary edema. What would be the nurse's priority actions related to these symptoms?
    a. Slowing or stopping the infusion; monitoring vital signs, notifying the health care provider, and placing the patient in an upright position with their feet dependent
    b. Stopping the transfusion immediately and keeping the vein open with normal saline, notifying the health care provider immediately, and administering antihistamine parenterally as needed
    c. Stopping the transfusion immediately and keeping the vein open with normal saline, notifying the health care provider, and treating symptoms with acetaminophen
    d. Stopping the infusion immediately, obtaining a culture of the patient's blood, monitoring vital signs, notifying the health care provider, and administering antibiotics immediately
14. A nurse is performing physical assessments for patients with fluid imbalance. Which findings indicate a fluid volume excess? Select all that apply.
    a. Pinched and drawn facial expression
    b. Deep, rapid respirations
    c. Moist crackles heard upon auscultation
    d. Tachycardia
    e. Distended neck veins
    f. Sluggish skin turgor
15. A nurse is caring for a patient experiencing a fluid volume deficit. What should be included in the recorded intake and output for the patient? Select all that apply.
    a. Urine
    b. Carbonated beverage
    c. Formed stool
    d. Vomitus
    e. Chicken noodle soup
    f. Pressure wound irrigant
16. A nurse is caring for an older adult with a fluid volume deficit related to decreased thirst sensation. For which signs and symptoms of this health problem will the nurse assess?
    a. Dependent edema
    b. Crackles in the lungs
    c. Neck vein distention
    d. Weight loss
17. A nurse on the IV team is making rounds to assess patients receiving IV therapy. Under which circumstance will the nurse recommend an intravenous catheter be discontinued?
    a. The area surrounding the catheter is bruised.
    b. The patient's extremity is cool to touch.
    c. The site is red, warm, and swollen.
    d. Part of the catheter (1 mm) is visible under the dressing.

ANSWERS WITH RATIONALES

1. **a.** Patients experiencing hypoxia will breathe rapidly, "blowing off" CO_2. This drives the pH up reflecting alkalosis related to the respiratory system.
2. **a.** Patients with renal (kidney) failure are unable to excrete fluids; they typically have oliguria and fluid volume excess. The other patient scenarios typically occur in patients with fluid volume deficit.
3. **c.** A solution of 0.45% NaCl (½-strength normal saline) or 0.33% NaCl (⅓-strength normal saline) are hypotonic fluids used to treat hypernatremia. As there are less particles in the ½-strength saline than in the bloodstream, infusing this fluid will cause the sodium level to decrease. Normal saline (0.9% NaCl) is used to treat hypovolemia, metabolic alkalosis, hyponatremia, and hypochloremia. Lactated Ringer's solution is used in the treatment of hypovolemia, burns, and fluid lost from gastrointestinal sources. Dextrose (5%) in lactated Ringer's solution replaces electrolytes and shifts fluid from the intracellular compartment into the intravascular space, expanding vascular volume.
4. **d.** Daily weight is the most reliable indicator of fluid balance. Intake and output are not always as accurate and may involve a subjective component. Testing skin turgor may not be totally accurate due to loose skin; measurement of skin turgor is subjective. The complete blood count itself does not necessarily reflect fluid balance; however, a high hematocrit can provide further support for fluid excess or deficit.
5. **c.** The first step is to analyze the pH; low pH indicates acidosis. This, coupled with a low bicarbonate (regulated by the kidney), indicates metabolic acidosis. The pCO_2 is normal, indicating the acid–base disturbance is nonrespiratory in origin. The pH and bicarbonate would be elevated with metabolic alkalosis. Decreased $PaCO_2$ in conjunction with a low pH indicates respiratory acidosis; increased $PaCO_2$ in conjunction with an elevated pH indicates respiratory alkalosis.

6. **b.** Having fluids the patient prefers readily available and within reach helps promote intake. Explanation of the fluid transport mechanisms is inappropriately complex and does not address dehydration. Meeting short-term outcomes rather than long-term outcomes is the priority at this time provides further reinforcement, and additional fluids should be taken earlier in the day.
7. **a.** If the peripheral venous access site leaks fluid when flushed, the nurse should remove it from the site; evaluate the need for continued access; and, if clinically necessary, restart the IV in another location. This action is a nursing intervention; the primary care provider does not need to be notified first. The nurse should use a skin marker to outline the area with visible signs of infiltration to allow for assessment of changes or aspirate and attempt to flush again if the IV does not flush easily.
8. **a.** The nurse is observing the signs and symptoms of speed shock: the body's reaction to a substance that is injected into the circulatory system too rapidly. The nursing interventions for this condition are discontinue the infusion immediately, report symptoms of speed shock to primary care provider immediately, and monitor vital signs once signs develop. The other choices are interventions for fluid overload; air embolus; and phlebitis, respectively.
9. **b.** The kidney primarily controls the bicarbonate level and, if damaged, can affect acid–base balance. The adrenal glands secrete catecholamines and steroid hormones. The brain may regulate respiration and therefore CO_2, not the bicarbonate level.
10. **b.** Nursing interventions for a patient with hypokalemia include encouraging foods high in potassium and administering (oral) potassium supplements as prescribed. Encouraging foods with high sodium content is appropriate for a patient with hyponatremia. Cautioning the patient about foods high in potassium is appropriate for a patient with hyperkalemia and discussing the calcium-losing aspects of nicotine and alcohol use is appropriate for a patient with hypocalcemia.
11. **d.** The IV fluid is infiltrating the tissue, suggested by lack of flow, swelling, and the area feeling cool to the touch. The nurse should put on gloves and remove the catheter. The nurse should also use a skin marker to outline the area with visible signs of infiltration to allow for assessment of changes and secure gauze with tape over the insertion site without applying pressure. The nurse should assess the area distal to the venous access device for capillary refill, sensation and motor function and restart the IV in a new location. Finally, the nurse should estimate the volume of fluid that escaped into the tissue based on the rate of infusion and length of time since last assessment, notify the primary health care provider and use an appropriate method for clinical management of the infiltrate site, based on infused solution and facility guidelines, and record site assessment and interventions, as well as site for new venous access. Raising the height of the IV pole will increase the pressure causing fluid to flows; however, that will promote further infiltration of fluid.
12. **c.** When caring for a patient with an arteriovenous fistula for dialysis, it is essential the nurse does not compress the area. Therefore, no BP or venipuncture is performed in that extremity. The patient may receive IM injections in an area of the body without the access. Taking a radial pulse in the arm with the access will not harm the fistula. The nurse does not use the fistula for any reason other than dialysis; damage to the fistula delays lifesaving dialysis.
13. **a.** The patient is displaying signs and symptoms of circulatory overload: too much fluid volume as a result of the infusion of blood. In the other choices, the nurse is providing interventions for an allergic reaction; responding to a febrile reaction; and providing interventions for a bacterial reaction, respectively.
14. **c, d, e.** Moist crackles, neck vein distention, and tachypnea typically indicate fluid volume excess. A person with a severe fluid volume deficit may have a pinched and drawn facial expression. Deep, rapid respirations may be a compensatory mechanism for metabolic acidosis or a primary disorder causing respiratory alkalosis. Tachycardia is usually the earliest sign of the decreased vascular volume associated with fluid volume deficit. Sluggish skin turgor is present with fluid volume deficit.
15. **a, b, d, e.** The nurse includes urine, emesis, liquid stool, drainage from wounds, and drains in the output. Intake includes IV fluids, foods, and liquid at room temperature. The liquid portion of the chicken noodle soup can be measured; however, the nurse excludes the solids. Irrigation to a pressure wound is not absorbed; rather, it drains out after cleansing the wound.
16. **d.** Assessing weight is the most sensitive indicator of fluid balance. As fluid is lost, the patient's weight will decrease. The other options are indicative of fluid excess.
17. **c.** The IV nurse will assess the IV fluids, rate, and site. A site that is red, warm, and swollen may have developed phlebitis, and the IV catheter should be removed. A bruised area surrounding the insertion site is likely associated with the initial insertion and can be monitored. A patient with a cool extremity may be chilly or hypothermic; the nurse assesses the IV site. Having 1 mm of the catheter visible from the insertion site that is covered with an occlusive, transparent dressing does not require immediate action.

Bibliography

AABB. (n.d.) *Clinical Resources. Clinical Guidelines and Guidance.* Retrieved August 4, 2021, from https://www.aabb.org/news-resources/resources/clinical-resources

Adams, M. P., Holland, N., & Urban, C. Q. (2020). *Pharmacology for nurses. A pathophysiologic approach* (6th ed.). Pearson.

American Red Cross. (2021, January). *A Compendium of transfusion practice guidelines* (4th ed.). https://www.redcrossblood.org/content/dam/redcrossblood/hospital-page-documents/334401_compendium_v04jan2021_bookmarkedworking_rwv01.pdf

American Red Cross. (n.d.a). *Requirements by donation type.* Retrieved August 4, 2021, from https://www.redcrossblood.org/donate-blood/how-to-donate/eligibility-requirements.html

American Red Cross. (n.d.b). *Why give blood.* Retrieved August 4, 2021, from https://www.redcrossblood.org/donate-blood/how-to-donate/common-concerns/first-time-donors.html

American Red Cross. (n.d.c). *Blood donation process. Frequently asked questions.* Retrieved August 4, 2021, from https://www.redcrossblood.org/faq.html

American Red Cross. (n.d.d). *Autologous and directed donations.* Retrieved August 4, 2021, from https://www.redcrossblood.org/donate-blood/how-to-donate/types-of-blood-donations/autologous-and-directed-donations.html

Andrews, M., Boyle, J. S., & Collins, J. (2020). *Transcultural concepts in nursing care* (8th ed.). Wolters Kluwer.

Arbique, D., Boredelon, M., Dragoo, R., & Huckaby, S. (2014). Ultrasound-guided access for peripheral intravenous therapy. *Med-Surg Matters, 23*(3), 1–15.

Aseptic Non Touch Technique (ANTT®). (2021). ANTT® procedures and environments. Retrieved May 11, 2022, https://www.antt.org/antt-procedures-settings.html#anchor2

Barton, A. (2018). Clinical use of closed-system safety peripheral intravenous cannulas. *British Journal of Nursing, 27*(8), S22–S27. https://doi.org/10.12968/bjon.2018.27.8.S22

Barton, A. (2019a). The case for using a disinfecting cap for needle free connectors. *British Journal of Nursing, 28*(14), S22–S27. https://doi.org/10.12968/bjon.2019.28.14.S22

Barton, A. (2019b). Intravenous infusion drug administration: Flushing guidance. *British Journal of Nursing, 28*(8), S16–S17. https://doi.org/10.12968/bjon.2019.28.8.S16

Barton, A. (2020). Universal adhesive vascular access securement with Grip-Lok devices. *British Journal of Nursing, 29*(8), S28–S33. https://doi.org/10.12968/bjon.2020.29.8.S28

Basak, T., Duman, S., & Demirtas, A. (2020). Distraction-based relief of pain associated with peripheral intravenous catheterisation in adults: A randomised controlled trial. *Journal of Clinical Nursing, 29*(5–6), 770–777. https://doi.org/10.1111/jocn.15131

Bauldoff, G., Gubrud, P., & Carno, M. A. (2020). *LeMone and Burke's Medical-surgical nursing: Clinical reasoning in patient care* (7th ed.). Pearson.

Berndt, D., & Steinheiser, M. (2019). Central vascular access device complications. *American Nurse, 14*(10), 6–13.

Bolton, D. (2015). Clinically indicated replacement of peripheral cannulas. *British Journal of Nursing, 24*(19), S4–S12. https://doi.org/10.12968/bjon.2015.24.Sup19.S4

Brinkman, J. E., Dorius, B., & Sharma, S. (2021, May 9). *Physiology, body fluids.* StatPearls. https://www.ncbi.nlm.nih.gov/books/NBK482447/

Çağlar, S., Büyükyilmaz, F., Bakoğlu, İ., İnal, S., & Salihoğlu, Ö. (2019). Efficacy of vein visualization devices for peripheral intravenous catheter placement in preterm infants: A randomized clinical trial. *Journal of Perinatology & Neonatal Nursing, 33*(1), 61–67. https://doi.org/10.1097/JPN.0000000000000385

Carman, M., Uhlenbrock, J. S., & McClintock, S. M. (2018). A review of current practice in transfusion therapy. *American Journal of Nursing, 118*(5), 36–44. https://doi.org/10.1097/01.NAJ.0000532808.81713.fc

Carson, J. L., & Kleinman, S. (2021, June 23). *Indications and hemoglobin thresholds for red blood cell transfusion in the adult.* UpToDate. Wolters Kluwer. https://www.uptodate.com/contents/indications-and-hemoglobin-thresholds-for-red-blood-cell-transfusion-in-the-adult#H430736130

Casimero, C., Ruddock, T., Hegarty, C., Barber, R., Devine, A., & Davis, J. (2020). Minimising blood stream infection: Developing new materials for intravascular catheters. *Medicines, 7*(9), 49. https://doi.org/10.3390/medicines7090049

Centers for Disease Control and Prevention (CDC). (2020, March 18). *Blood safety basics.* https://www.cdc.gov/bloodsafety/basics.html

Chemparathy, A., Seneviratne, M. G., Ward, A., Mirchandani, S., Li, R., Mathew, R., Wood, M., Shin, A. Y., Donnelly, L. F., Scheinker, D., & Lee, G. M. (2021). Development and implementation of a real-time bundle-adherence dashboard for central line-associated bloodstream infections. *Pediatric Quality and Safety, 6*(4), e431. https://doi.org/10.1097/pq9.0000000000000431

Cho, J., Chung, H. S., & Hong, S. H. (2013). Improving the safety of continuously infused fluids in the emergency department. *International Journal of Nursing Practice, 19*(1), 95–100. https://doi.org/10.1111/ijn.12022

Corley, A., Ullman, A. J., Mihala, G., Ray-Barruel, G., Alexandrou, E., & Rickard, C. M. (2019). Peripheral intravenous catheter dressing and securement practice is associated with site complications and suboptimal dressing integrity: A secondary analysis of 40,637 catheters. *International Journal of Nursing Studies, 100*, 103409. https://doi.org/10.1016/j.ijnurstu.2019.103409

DeLisle, J. (2018). Is this a blood transfusion reaction? Don't hesitate; check it out. *Journal of Infusion Nursing, 41*(1), 43–51. https://doi.org/10.1097/NAN.0000000000000261

Desai, K., Vinograd, A. M., Abbadessa, M. K. F., & Chen, A. E. (2018). Longevity and complication rates of ultrasound guided versus traditional peripheral intravenous catheters in a pediatric emergency department. *Journal of the Association for Vascular Access, 23*(3), 149–154. https://doi.org/10.1016/j.java.2018.06.002

Dougherty, L. (2013). Intravenous therapy in older patients. *Nursing Standard, 28*(6), 50–58. https://doi.org/10.7748/ns2013.10.28.6.50.e7333

Dudek, S. (2022). *Nutrition essentials for nursing practice* (9th ed.). Wolters Kluwer.

Duncan, M., Warden, P., Bernatchez, S. F., & Morse, D. (2018). A bundled approach to decrease the rate of primary bloodstream infections related to peripheral intravenous catheters. *Journal of the Association for Vascular Access, 23*(1), 15–22. https://doi.org/10.1016/j.java.2017.07.004

Dychter, S., Gold, D., Carson, D., & Haller, M. (2012). Intravenous therapy: A review of complications and economic considerations of peripheral access. *Journal of Infusion Nursing, 35*(2), 84–91. https://doi.org/10.1097/NAN.0b013e31824237ce

Edwards, C., & Jones, J. (2018). Development and implementation of an ultrasound-guided peripheral intravenous catheter program for emergency nurses. *Journal of Emergency Nursing, 44*(1), 33–36. http://dx.doi.org/10.1016/j.jen.2017.07.009

Egan, G., Healy, D., O'Neill, H., Clarke-Maloney, M., Grace, P. A., & Walsh, S. R. (2013). Ultrasound guidance for difficult peripheral venous access: A systematic review and meta-analysis. *Emergency Medicine Journal, 30*(7), 521–526. https://doi.org/10.1136/emermed-2012-201652

Eliopoulos, C. (2018). *Gerontological nursing* (9th ed.). Wolters Kluwer.

Fields, J. M., Piela, N. E., Au, A. K., & Ku, B. S. (2014). Risk factors associated with difficult venous access in adult ED patients. *American Journal of Emergency Medicine, 32*(10), 1179–1182. https://doi.org/10.1016/j.ajem.2014.07.008

Fields, B. E., Whitney, R. L., & Bell, J. F. (2020). Managing home infusion therapy. *American Journal of Nursing, 120*(12), 53–59. https://doi.org/10.1097/01.naj.0000724252.22812.a2

Fischbach, F. T., & Fischbach, M. A. (2018). *A manual of laboratory and diagnostic tests* (10th ed.). Wolters Kluwer.

Flynn, J. M., Larsen, E. N., Keogh, S., Ullman, A. J., & Rickard, C. M. (2019). Methods for microbial needleless connector decontamination: A systematic review and meta-analysis. *American Journal of Infection Control, 47*(8), 956–962. https://doi.org/10.1016/j.ajic.2019.01.002

Fowler, S. B., Penoyer, D. A., & Bourgault, A. M. (2018). Insertion and removal of PIVCs: Exploring best practices. *Nursing, 48*(7), 65–67. https://doi.org/10.1097/01.NURSE.0000534108.88895.e2

Frimpong, A., Caguioa, J., & Octavo, G. (2015). Promoting safe IV management in practice using H.A.N.D.S. *British Journal of Nursing (IV Therapy Supplement), 24*(2), S18–S23. DOI: 10.12968/bjon.2015.24.Sup2.S18

Fumarola, S., Allaway, R., Callaghan, R., Collier, M., Downie, F., Geraghty, J., Kiernan, S., Spratt, F., Bianchi, J., Bethell, E., Downe, A., Griffin, J., Hughes, M., King, B., LeBlanc, K., Savine, L., Stubbs, N., & Voegeli, D. (2020). Overlooked and underestimated: Medical adhesive-related skin injuries. Best practice consensus document on prevention. *Journal of Wound Care, 29*(Sup3c), S1–S24. https://doi.org/10.12968/jowc.2020.29.Sup3c.S1

Galang, H., Hubbard-Wright, C., Hahn, D. S., Yost, G., Yoder, L., Maduro, R. S., Morgan, M. K., & Zimbro, K. S. (2020). A randomized trial comparing outcomes of 3 types of peripheral intravenous catheters. *Journal of Nursing Care Quality, 35*(1), 6–12. https://doi.org/10.1097/NCQ.0000000000000421

Galen, B., Baron, S., Young, S., Hall, A., Berger-Spivack, L., & Southern, W. (2020). Reducing peripherally inserted central catheters and midline catheters by training nurses in ultrasound-guided peripheral intravenous catheter placement. *BMJ Quality & Safety, 29*(3), 245–249. https://doi.org/10.1136/bmjqs-2019-009923

Gorski, L. A. (2020). Infusion therapy: A model for safe practice in the home setting. *American Nurse Today, 15*(6), 12.

Gorski, L. A., Hadaway, L., Hagle, M. E., Broadhurst, D., Clare, S., Kleidon, T., Meyer, B. M., Nickel, B., Rowley, S., Sharpe, E., Alexander, M., & Infusion Nurses Society. (2021). Infusion therapy. Standards of practice. (8th ed.). *Journal of Infusion Nursing, 44*(Suppl 1), S1–S224. https://doi.org/10.1097/NAN.0000000000000396

Gümüs, M., & Başbakkal, Z. (2021). Efficacy of Veinlit PEDI in pediatric peripheral intravenous access: A randomized controlled trial. *Pediatric Emergency Care, 37*(3), 145–149. https://doi.org/10.1097/PEC.0000000000001515

Hale, A., & Hovey, M. J. (2014). *Fluid, electrolyte, and acid-base imbalances.* F.A. Davis Company.

Harper, D. (2014). I.V. Rounds. Infusion therapy: Much more than a simple task. *Nursing, 44*(7), 66–67. DOI: 10.1097/01.NURSE.0000446643.87747.1f

Harrold, K. (2018, December). Guide to the safe use of needle free connectors. *British Journal of Nursing,* 28(Sup14b). [Online]. https://www.magonlinelibrary.com/doi/abs/10.12968/bjon.2019.28.Sup14b.1

Haynes, J., Bowers, K., Young, R., Sanders, T., & Schultz, K. E. (2015). Managing spaghetti syndrome in critical care with a novel device: A nursing perspective. *Critical Care Nurse, 35*(6), 38–45. https://doi.org/10.4037/ccn2015321

Heinrichs, J., Fritze, Z., Klassen, T., & Curtis, S. (2013). A systematic review and meta-analysis of new interventions for peripheral intravenous cannulation of children. *Pediatric Emergency Care, 29*(7), 858–866. https://doi.org/10.1097/PEC.0b013e3182999bcd

Higgins, N., Iu, P., Carr, P., Ware, R., & Van Zundert, A. (2021). Techniques to select site of insertion for a peripheral intravenous catheter with vessel locating devices using light, sounds or tactile actions (or pulsations). *Journal of Clinical Nursing, 30*(7–8), 1091–1098. https://doi.org/10.1111/jocn.15654

Higginson, R. (2015). Intravenous therapy: Guidance and implications for practice. *British Journal of Healthcare Management, 21*(6), 264–268. https://doi.org/10.12968/bjhc.2015.21.6.264

Hill, B., & Derbyshire, J. (2021). Blood transfusions: Ensuring patient safety. *British Journal of Nursing, 30*(9), 520–524. https://doi.org/10.12968/bjon.2021.30.9.520

Hill, S., & Moore, S. (2018). Arterial blood gas sampling: Using a safety and pre-heparinised syringe. *British Journal of Nursing, 27*(14), S20–S26. https://doi.org/10.12968/bjon.2018.27.14.S20

Hinkle, J. L., Cheever, K. H., & Overbaugh, K. J. (2022). *Brunner & Suddarth's textbook of medical-surgical nursing* (15th ed.). Wolters Kluwer.

Holroyd, S. (2020). Frequency volume charts and fluid balance monitoring: Getting it right. *Journal of Community Nursing, 34*(1), 55–58.

Houston, P. A. (2013). Obtaining vascular access in the obese patient population. *Journal of Infusion Nursing, 36*(1), 52–56. https://doi.org/10.1097/NAN.0b013e31827989d8

Institute for Safe Medication Practices (ISMP). (2020, February 10). *Guidelines for optimizing safe implementation and use of smart infusion pumps.* https://www.ismp.org/guidelines/safe-implementation-and-use-smart-pumps

Jarvis, C., & Echkardt, A. (2020). *Physical examination & health assessment* (8th ed.). Elsevier.

Jensen, S. (2019). *Nursing health assessment. A best practice approach* (3rd ed.). Wolters Kluwer.

The Joint Commission. (2021). *National patient safety goals.* https://www.jointcommission.org/standards/national-patient-safety-goals/

Kamel, K. & Halperin, M. L. (2017). *Fluid, electrolyte, and acid-base physiology. A problem-based approach* (5th ed.). Elsevier.

Karch, A. M. (2020). *Focus on nursing pharmacology* (8th ed.). Wolters Kluwer.

Kelly, L., & Snowden, A. (2021). 'Pinholes in my arms': The vicious cycle of vascular access. *British Journal of Nursing, 30*(14), S4–S13. https://doi.org/10.12968/bjon.2021.30.14.S4

Kline, M., & Katrancha, E. D. (2019). Central venous access devices: An overview for nursing students. *Nursing, 49*(7), 63–64. https://doi.org/10.1097/01.NURSE.0000559922.99814.f8

Korkut, S., Karadağ, S. & Doğan, Z. (2020). The effectiveness of local hot and cold applications on peripheral intravenous catheterization: A randomized controlled trial. *Journal of PeriAnesthesia Nursing, 35*(6), 597–602. https://doi.org/10.1016/j.jopan.2020.04.011

Kyle, T., & Carman, S. (2021). *Essentials of pediatric nursing* (4th ed.). Wolters Kluwer.

Loveday, H. P., Wilson, J. A., & Pratt, R. J. (2014). Epic3: National evidence-based guidelines for preventing healthcare-associated infections in NHS hospitals in England. *Journal of Hospital Infection, 86*(S1), S1–S70. https://doi.org/10.1016/S0195-6701(13)60012-2

Marsh, N., Larsen, E., Genzel, J., Mihala, G., Ullman, A. J., Kleidon, T., Cadigan, S., & Rickard, C. M. (2018). A novel integrated dressing to secure peripheral intravenous catheters in an adult acute hospital: A pilot randomised controlled trial. *Trials, 19*(1), 596. https://doi.org/10.1186/s13063-018-2985-9

Marsh, N., Webster, J., Mihala, G., & Rickard, C. M. (2015). Devices and dressings to secure peripheral venous catheters to prevent complications. *Cochrane Database of Systematic Reviews,* (6), CD011070. https://doi.org/10.1002/14651858.CD011070.pub2

Mayo Foundation for Medical Education and Research (MFMER). (2017, February 28). Dry mouth treatment: Tips for controlling dry mouth. https://www.mayoclinic.org/diseases-conditions/dry-mouth/expert-answers/dry-mouth/faq-20058424

McArthur, B. (2018). Peripherally inserted central catheters (PICCs): A review of complications and innovative solutions. *Vascular Access, 12*(1), 32–37.

McClave, S. A., DiBaise, J. K., Mullin, G., & Martindale, R. G. (2016). ACG clinical guideline: Nutrition therapy in the adult hospitalized patient. *The American Journal of Gastroenterology, 111*(3), 315–334. doi: 10.1038/ajg.2016.28

Memorial Sloan Kettering Cancer Center. (2021, March 29). *About your peripherally inserted central catheter (PICC).* https://www.mskcc.org/cancer-care/patient-education/about-your-peripherally-inserted-central-catheter-picc

Metheny, N. M. (2012). *Fluid and electrolyte balance: Nursing considerations* (5th ed.). Jones & Bartlett Learning.

Mimoz, O., Lucet, J. C., & Kerforne, T. (2015). Skin antisepsis with chlorhexidine-alcohol versus povidone iodine-alcohol, with and without skin scrubbing, for prevention of intravascular-catheter-related infection (CLEAN): An open-label, multicenter, randomized, controlled, two-by-two factorial trial. *Lancet, 386*(10008), 2069–2077. https://doi.org/10.1016/S0140-6736(15)00244-5

Moore, C. (2013). An emergency department nurse-driven ultrasound-guided peripheral intravenous line program. *Journal of the Association for Vascular Access, 18*(1), 45–51.

Morata, L., & Bowers, M. (2020). Ultrasound-guided peripheral intravenous catheter insertion: The nurse's manual. *CriticalCareNurse, 40*(5), 38–46. https://doi.org/10.4037/ccn2020240

Morrell, E. (2020). Reducing risks and improving vascular access outcomes. *Journal of Infusion Nursing, 43*(4), 222–228. https://doi.org/10.1097/NAN.0000000000000377

Morton, P. G., & Fontaine, D. K. (2018). *Critical care nursing. A holistic approach* (11th ed.). Wolters Kluwer.

Moureau, N. (2013). Safe patient care when using vascular access devices. *British Journal of Nursing, 22*(2), S14–S21.

Moureau, N., & Chopra, V. (2016). Indications for peripheral, midline and central catheters: Summary of the MAGIC recommendations. *British Journal of Nursing, IV Therapy Supplement, 25*(8), S15–S24. https://doi.org/10.12968/bjon.2016.25.8.S15

Nailon, R. E., Rupp, M. E., & Lyden, E. (2019). A day in the life of a CVAD. *Journal of Infusion Nursing, 42*(3), 125–131. https://doi.org/10.1097/NAN.0000000000000321

Norris, T. L. (2020). *Porth's essentials of pathophysiology* (5th ed.). Wolters Kluwer.

O'Grady, N. P., Alexander, M., Burns, L. A., & The Healthcare Infection Control Practices Advisory Committee (HICPAC). (2017). *Guidelines for the prevention of intravascular catheter-related infections.* https://www.cdc.gov/infectioncontrol/guidelines/bsi/index.html

Oncology Nursing Society (ONS). Infusion of antineoplastic therapies in the home. *Oncology Nursing Forum, 47*(6), 629–630. https://doi.org/10.1188/20.ONF.629-630

Otani, T., Morikawa, Y., Hayakawa, I., Atsumi, Y., Tomari, K., Tomobe, Y., Uda, K., Funakoshi, Y., Sakaguchi, C., Nishimoto, S., & Hataya, H. (2018). Ultrasound-guided peripheral intravenous access placement for children in the emergency department. *European Journal of Pediatrics, 177*(10), 1443–1449. https://doi.org/10.1007/s00431-018-3201-3

Partovi-Deilami, K., Nielsen, J. K., Møller, A. M., Nesheim, S. S., & Jørgensen, V. L. (2016). Effect of ultrasound-guided placement of difficult-to-place peripheral venous catheters: A prospective study of a training program for nurse anesthetists. *AANA Journal, 84*(2), 86–92.

Paterson, R. S., Chopra, V., Brown, E., Kleidon, T. M., Cooke, M., Richard, C. M., Berstein, S. J., & Ullman, A. J. (2020). Selection and insertion of vascular access devices in pediatrics: A systematic review. *Pediatrics, 145*(e3), e20193474H.

Pitts, S., & Ostroff, M. (2019). The use of visualization technology for the insertion of peripheral intravenous catheters. *The Journal of the Association for Vascular Access, 24*(3), 10–14. https://doi.org/10.2309/j.java.2019.003.007

Pompey, J., & Abraham-Settles, B. (2019). Clarifying the confusion of arterial blood gas analysis: Is it compensation or combination? *American Journal of Nursing, 119*(3), 52–56. https://doi.org/10.1097/01.NAJ.0000554035.74335.59

Rickard, C. M., Flynn, J., Larsen, E., Mihala, G., Playford, E. G., Shaw, J., Keogh, S., Ullmann, A., Zhang, L., Gavin, N., Kleidon, T., Chopra, V., McCarthy, A. L., Rocha, P. K., & Marsh, N. (2021). Needleless connector decontamination for prevention of central venous access device infection: A pilot randomized controlled trial. *American Journal of Infection Control, 49*(2), 269–273. https://doi.org/10.1016/j.ajic.2020.07.026

Rowe, M. S., Arnold, K., & Spencer, T. R. (2020). Catheter securement impact on PICC-related CLABSI: A university hospital perspective. *American Journal of Infection Control, 48*(12), 1497–1500. https://doi.org/10.1016/j.ajic.2020.06.178

Sadiqu, N. M., Naganathan, S., & Badireddy, M. (2020, September 10). *Hypercalcemia.* StatPearls. https://www.ncbi.nlm.nih.gov/books/NBK430714

Sarani, H., Moulaei, N., Tabas, E. E., Safarzai, E., & Jahani, S. (2018). Comparison of the effects of alcohol, chlorhexidine and alcohol-chlorhexidine on local catheter-related infections rate: A double-blind clinical trial study. *Medical-Surgical Nursing Journal, 7*(2), e85962. https://doi.org/10.5812/msnj.85962

Sengul, T., Guven, B., Ocakci, A. F., & Kaya, N. (2020). Connectors as a risk factor for blood-associated infections (3-way stopcock and needleless connector): A randomized-experimental study. *American Journal of Infection Control, 48*(3), 275–280. https://doi.org/10.1016/j.ajic.2019.08.020

Sharp, R., Childs, J., Bulmer, A. C. & Esterman, A. (2018). The effect of oral hydration and localised heat on peripheral vein diameter and depth: A randomised controlled trial. *Applied Nursing Research, 42*, 83–88. https://doi.org/10.1016/j.apnr.2018.06.013

Sharp, R., Turner, L., Altschwager, J., Corsini, N., & Esterman, A. (2021). Adverse events associated with home blood transfusion: A retrospective cohort study. *Journal of Clinical Nursing, 30*(11–12), 1751–1759. https://doi.org/10.1111/jocn.15734

Shaw, S. J. (2017). Use of closed cannulae in peripheral intravenous cannulation. *Nursing Standard, 31*(36), 54–62. https://doi.org/10.7748/ns.2017.e10713

Silbert-Flagg, J., & Pillitteri, A. (2018). *Maternal and child health nursing* (8th ed.). Wolters Kluwer.

Slater, K., Cooke, M., Fullerton, F., Whitby, M., Hay, J., Lingard, S., Douglas, J., & Rickard, C. M. (2020). Peripheral intravenous catheter needleless connector decontamination study- Randomized controlled trial. *American Journal of Infection Control, 48*(9), 1013–1018. https://doi.org/10.1016/j.ajic.2019.11.030

Slater, K., Cooke, M., Scanlan, E., & Rickard, C. M. (2019). Hand hygiene and needleless connector decontamination for peripheral intravenous catheter care – time and motion observational study. *American Journal of Infection Control, 47*(8), 1017–1019. https://doi.org/10.1016/j.ajic.2019.01.022

Slater, K., Fullerton, F., Cooke, M., Snell, S., & Rickard, C. M. (2018). Needleless connector drying tome—how long does it take? *American Journal of Infection Control, 46*(9), 1080–1081. https://doi.org/10.1016/j.ajic.2018.05.007

Smith, B., & Hannum, F. (2008). Optimizing IV therapy in the elderly. *Advance for Nurses, 10*(18), 27–28.

Spencer, T. R. (2018). Securing vascular access devices. *American Nurse Today, 13*(9), 29–31.

Stango, C., Runyan, D., Stern, J., Macri, I., & Vacca, M. (2014). A successful approach to reducing bloodstream infections based on a disinfection device for intravenous needleless connector hubs. *Journal of Infusion Nursing, 37*(6), 462–465. https://doi.org/10.1097/NAN.0000000000000075

Thorpe, M., Berry, W., & Soper, J. (2021). Duration of peripheral intravenous catheter patency in children. *Paediatrics & Child Health, 26*(1), 32–34. https://doi.org/10.1093/pch/pxaa038

Toughy, T. A., & Jett, K. (2018). *Ebersol and Hess' gerontological nursing & healthy aging* (5th ed.). Elsevier.

Tuffaha, H. S., Rickard, C. M., Weber, J., Marsh, N., Gordon, L., Wallis, M., & Scuffham, P. A. (2014). Cost-effectiveness analysis of clinically indicated versus routine replacement of peripheral intravenous catheters. *Applied Health Economics and Health Policy, 12*(1), 51–58.

VHA Center for Engineering & Occupational Safety and Health (CEOSH). (2016, January). *Safe patient handling and mobility guidebook.* http://www.tnpatientsafety.com/pubfiles/Initiatives/workplace-violence/sphm-pdf.pdf

Vinograd, A. M., Zorc, J. J., Dean, A. J., Abbadessa, M. K. F., & Chen, A. E. (2018). First-attempt success, longevity, and complication rates of ultrasound-guided peripheral intravenous catheters in children. *Pediatric Emergency Care, 34*(6), 376–380. https://doi.org/10.1097/PEC.0000000000001063

Walters, B., & Price, C. (2019). Quality improvement initiative reduces the occurrence of complications in peripherally inserted central catheters. *Journal of Infusion Nursing, 42*(1), 29–36. https://doi.org/10.1097/NAN.0000000000000310

Welyczko, N. (2020). Peripheral intravenous cannulation: Reducing pain and local complications. *British Journal of Nursing, 29*(8), S12–S19. https://doi.org/10.12968/bjon.2020.29.8.S12

Wiencek, C. A., Kleinpell, R., Moss, M., & Sessler, C. N. (2019). Choosing wisely in critical care: A national survey of critical care nurses. *American Journal of Critical Care, 28*(6), 434–440. https://doi.org/https://doi.org/10.4037/ajcc2019241

Willams, A. (2018). Catheter occlusion in home infusion. *Journal of Infusion Nursing, 41*(1), 52–57. https://doi.org/10.1097/NAN.0000000000000259

Willis, L. M. (Ed.). (2020). *Fluids & electrolytes made incredibly easy!* (7th ed.). Wolters Kluwer.

WoltersKluwer. (2022). Problem-based care plans. In *Lippincott Advisor*. Wolters Kluwer.

Woodruff, D. W. (2006). Take these 6 easy steps to ABG analysis. *Nursing Made Incredibly Easy, 4*(1), 4–7.

York, N., Angell-Barrick, N., & Carter, J. (2020). Avoiding contamination of CVADs when bathing and showering. *Journal of Kidney Care, 5*(2), 71–78. https://doi.org/10.12968/jokc.2020.5.2.71

Zhao, H., He, Y., Wei, Q., & Ying, Y. (2018). Medical adhesive-related skin injury prevalence at the peripherally inserted central catheter insertion site. *Journal of Wound, Ostomy, and Continence Nursing, 45*(1), 22–25. https://doi.org/10.1097/WON.0000000000000394

UNIT VII

Promoting Healthy Psychosocial Responses

Every person is a composite of interrelated physiologic, psychosocial, and spiritual dimensions; alterations in one dimension affect the others. Unit VII discusses psychosocial considerations in holistic, person-centered care, focusing on sense of self; stress and adaptation; loss, grief, and dying; sensory stimulation; sexuality; and spirituality.

Each person's sense of self is critical to that person's attitudes toward health and may affect self-care abilities positively or negatively. Additionally, developmental or experiential stressors can motivate or thwart psychosocial growth and self-actualization. Nursing interventions to promote healthy psychosocial responses—including maintaining, strengthening, or changing self-concept—are basic to all aspects of patient care. Because a person's sense of self shapes their ability to respond to health care interventions, nurses include assessment and intervention to promote a positive sense of self.

Loss, grief, and dying are universal human experiences that most nurses encounter in some form on a daily basis. Effective nurses are competent and willing to assist people struggling with loss, grief, and dying.

Intact, functioning senses are necessary for life, normal growth and development, communication, and pleasurable experiences. Alterations in any of the senses require caring, knowledgeable, and individualized nursing interventions to meet needs, enhance individual independence, and prevent further overload or deprivation.

Sexuality and spirituality are also important components of human functioning. These dimensions are an integral part of each person's identity and are critical elements in holistic patient care. Nurses recognize the importance of these areas for optimal health and use their knowledge and skills to assist patients to enhanced wellness in these areas.

To facilitate wellness in each of these psychosocial spheres, nurses must develop self-awareness, including knowledge of their own personal attitudes, values, perceptions, and practices, as well as understand how others differ in these characteristics. Nurses' own personal biases, including the ability to accept others who have cultural, spiritual, racial, ethnic, or sexual identity characteristics that differ from their own, affect their ability to plan and provide optimal care. Nursing interventions and therapeutic interpersonal skills are used to elicit concerns, identify needs, implement teaching, make referrals, and demonstrate empathic caring and acceptance.

"The unique function of the nurse is to assist the individual . . . in the performance of those activities contributing to health or its recovery (or to peaceful death) that he would perform unaided if he had the necessary strength, will or knowledge . . . in such a way as to help him gain independence as rapidly as possible."

Virginia Henderson (1897-1996), *the "first lady of nursing," whose career spanned almost 70 years as both author and researcher; her works on nursing principles are research based and have been translated into 25 languages*

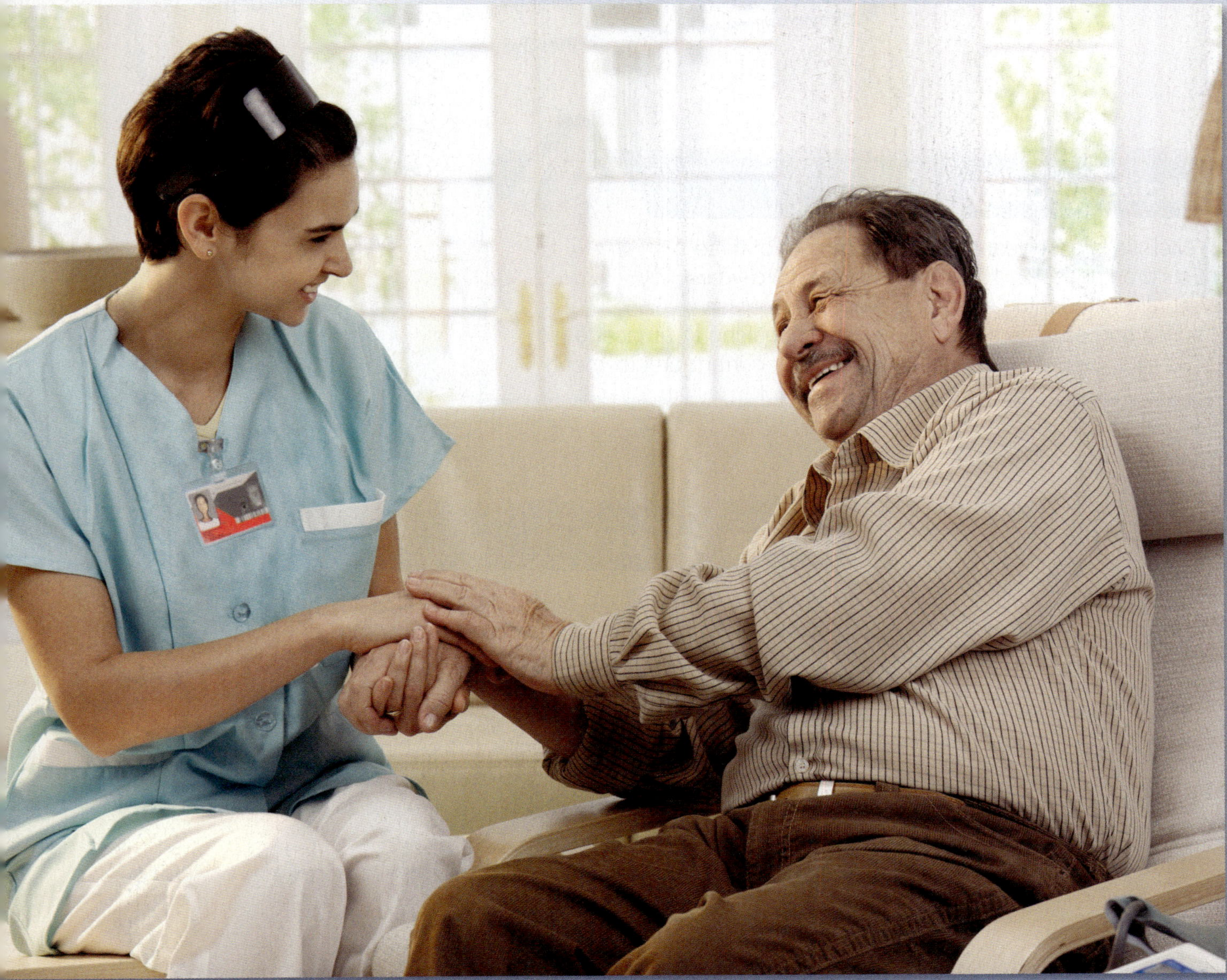

42 Self-Concept

Anthony Santorini

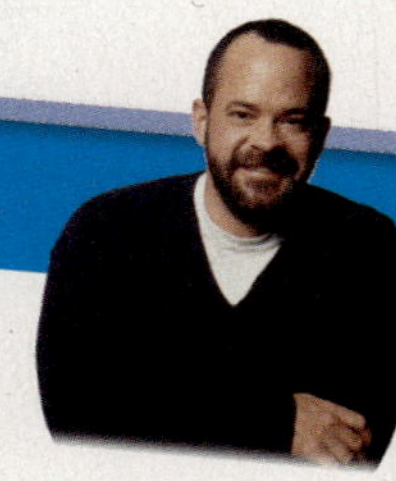

Anthony is a 44-year-old male with a history of diabetes. He recently underwent a below-the-knee amputation because of complications resulting from poor glucose control. One morning, he states, "I feel like damaged goods. I'm not a whole man anymore."

Melissa Motsky

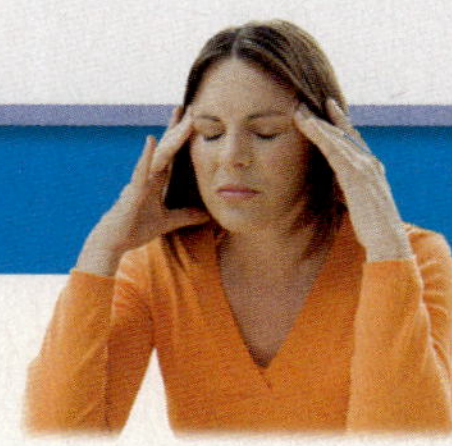

Melissa is a 31-year-old married mother of three children ages 12, 10, and 8. She is a third-year nursing student in academic jeopardy. Melissa cries and calls herself a failure when speaking to an academic advisor, seeing no way to get out of her current predicament.

Delores Sparks

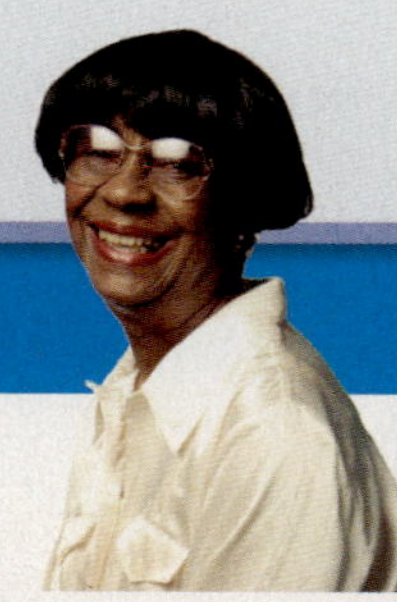

Delores is a 72-year-old widow diagnosed with advanced lung cancer 14 months ago. She had been living alone in a small apartment until 9 months ago, when she moved in with her daughter after a lengthy hospital stay because she was no longer capable of living alone. Delores has a probable prognosis of 3 months to live at most. A recent home visit reveals that the patient is increasingly depressed and feels like a burden to her daughter. She states, "I'm just an old dish rag, not good for anything anymore."

Learning Outcomes

After completing the chapter, you will be able to accomplish the following:

1. Describe three dimensions of self-concept: self-knowledge, self-expectations, and self-evaluation (self-esteem).
2. Identify major steps in the development of self-concept.
3. Differentiate positive and negative self-concept and high and low self-esteem.
4. Identify six variables that influence self-concept.
5. Use appropriate interview questions and observations to assess a patient's self-concept.
6. Describe how the experience of aging, illness, trauma, disability, loss, diagnostic testing, and treatment can threaten a patient's self-concept.
7. Develop nursing diagnoses/health problems to identify disturbances in self-concept (body image, self-esteem, role performance, personal identity).
8. Describe nursing strategies that are effective in resolving self-concept problems.
9. Plan, implement, and evaluate nursing care related to select diagnoses/health problems for disturbances in self-concept.

Nursing Concepts

- Self-concept
- Self-esteem

Self-concept, or self-image, is crucial to a person's health and well-being throughout life. A person's **self-concept**, which is the mental image or picture of self, has the power to either encourage or thwart personal growth. People with deficient self-concept may lack the motivation to learn self-care behaviors in response to illness, injury, or trauma. Nursing efforts aimed at teaching new health behaviors may fail until the patient values themselves enough to want to invest energy in self-care. Some patients may be aware that their negative self-concept affects their health behaviors, and may desperately want to make modifications, but have no idea how to do so. In addition, the experience of aging, illness, disability, trauma, loss, diagnostic testing, and treatment can severely threaten a patient's self-concept. Nurses who are sensitive to patients' expressions of self-concept can use each nurse–patient interaction to enhance a patient's sense of self and to assist the patient in resolving self-concept disturbances (see the Reflective Practice box on page 1738 for an example).

Several variables contribute to self-concept. As discussed in Chapter 4, as people move through the hierarchy of human needs to higher levels, needs for self-esteem and self-actualization arise. The need for **self-esteem** is the need that people have to feel good about themselves and to believe that others hold them in high regard. The need for **self-actualization** is the need for people to reach their full potential through development of their unique capabilities. Disturbances in self-concept may occur for a number of reasons. **Identity diffusion** is the failure to integrate various childhood identifications into a harmonious adult psychosocial identity, which can lead to disruptions in relationships and problems of intimacy. **Depersonalization** is a person's subjective experience of the partial or total disruption of the ego and the disintegration and disorganization of self-concept (Stuart, 2013). Figure 42-1 illustrates the continuum of self-concept responses.

OVERVIEW OF SELF-CONCEPT

Dimensions of Self-Concept

All of the feelings, beliefs, and values associated with "I" or "me" compose self-concept. Specific components of self-concept include personal identity, body image, self-esteem, and role performance. Crucial to each component are the dimensions of self-concept, which include self-knowledge, self-expectations, and self-evaluation.

People with a positive self-concept usually have greater and more diversified self-knowledge, more realistic perceptions and expectations, and a higher evaluation of themselves or higher self-esteem, whereas those with negative self-concept tend to exhibit poorer self-knowledge, less realistic perceptions and expectations, and lower self-esteem.

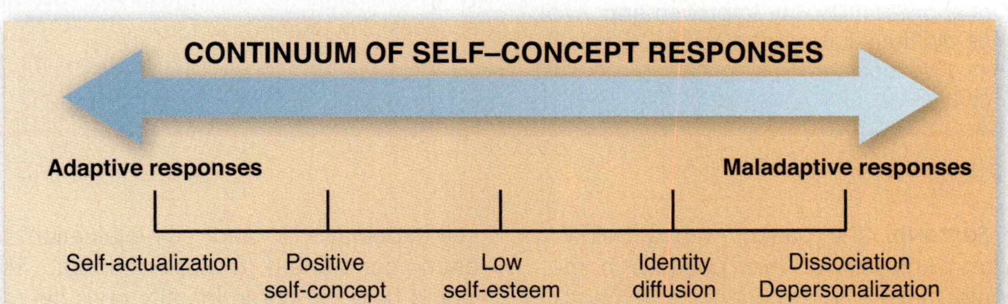

FIGURE 42-1. Continuum of self-concept responses. (*Source:* Reprinted with permission from Stuart, G. W. [2013]. *Principles and practice of psychiatric nursing* [10th ed., p. 264]. Elsevier/Mosby.)

QSEN Reflective Practice: Cultivating QSEN Competencies

CHALLENGE TO INTERPERSONAL SKILLS

Mrs. Delores Sparks is a 72-year-old, widowed, African American female. Before her diagnosis of advanced lung cancer 14 months ago, she lived alone in a small apartment. Nine months ago, following a lengthy hospital stay, she moved in with her daughter when it was determined that she was no longer capable of living alone and probably had, at most, 3 months to live. I was visiting her during my home health care nursing experience and growing more and more concerned with her depression. Mrs. Sparks verbalized that she felt like a burden to her daughter, who has three children herself and was currently taking care of a granddaughter as well. Mrs. Sparks was being treated for her depression, but I was concerned about the effects all this was having on her self-concept. She told me she was like "an old dish rag" that wasn't good for anything anymore.

Thinking Outside the Box: Possible Courses of Action

- Try to cheer her up at each visit.
- Ignore her deteriorating self-concept, since focusing on it may only make her feel worse; it is certainly true that she has enough bad stuff going on in her life to make her feel bad.
- Explore sources of positive affirmations of her worth; try to use my professional relationship with her to communicate "You are a person of worth and I care about you!"

Evaluating a Good Outcome: How Do I Define Success?

- Mrs. Sparks' self-concept improves.
- I learn how to communicate a sense of worth to vulnerable patients.
- I learn how to address problems with self-concept.

Personal Learning: Here's to the Future!

Unfortunately, this situation got worse before it got better. Mrs. Sparks did not always take her meds for depression, and her daughter voiced increasing frustration with her mother's mood. "Mom talks all the time now about how even God doesn't want her. She says that she may have to take her own life since God doesn't seem to be doing it!" The daughter also said that Mrs. Sparks apologized to her constantly for being such a bother. Things didn't start to change until I learned that Mrs. Sparks used to be a very important member of her church community. She stopped attending services when she got too weak to go out. This was clearly a major loss for her. When I successfully got her minister to visit, he literally turned her life around, providing her with lots of positive reinforcement for how she could use her illness to do God's work. She seems much more peaceful now. I've also encouraged her to tell me stories about the church work she did in the past and these reminiscences seem to be helpful.

QSEN SELF-REFLECTION ON QUALITY AND SAFETY COMPETENCIES DEVELOPING KNOWLEDGE, SKILLS, AND ATTITUDES FOR CONTINUOUS IMPROVEMENT

Do you agree with the criteria that the nursing student used to evaluate a successful outcome? Why or why not? What *knowledge, skills,* and *attitudes* do you need to develop to continuously improve the quality and safety of care for patients like Mrs. Sparks?

Patient-Centered Care: How would you develop a respectful and successful partnership with Mrs. Sparks and her daughter? How might your interpersonal skills influence her self-concept?

Teamwork and Collaboration/Quality Improvement: What special competence did the minister bring to Mrs. Sparks? What other members of your caregiving team can you consult? What does quality care for this family "look like"?

Safety/Evidence-Based Practice: Describe the patient's self-concept in the dimensions of self-knowledge, self-expectations, and self-evaluation. What does the evidence point to as "best practice" for Mrs. Sparks? What safety needs does she have, and how can you meet them?

Informatics: Can you identify the essential information that must be available in Mrs. Spark's electronic record to support safe patient care and coordination of care? Can you think of other ways to respond to or approach the situation? What else might the nursing student have done to ensure a successful outcome?

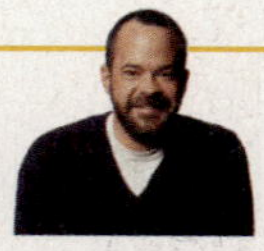

Consider Anthony Santorini, the patient with a below-the-knee amputation. Analysis of this patient's comments would indicate that he is experiencing a negative self-concept. The nurse would need to assess Mr. Santorini more closely to determine their self-knowledge, self-expectations, and self-evaluation for each component of self-concept. This would help the nurse identify possible factors contributing to their status and gain a fuller picture of Mr. Santorini's current condition.

Self-Knowledge: "Who am I?"

Global self is the term used to describe the composite of all the basic facts, qualities, traits, images, and feelings people hold about themselves. These factors strongly influence a person's ability to manage life events and ensure emotional stability. A person's self-knowledge includes:

- basic facts (sex assigned at birth, age, ethnicity, occupation, cultural background, sexual orientation);
- the person's position within social groups; and
- qualities or traits that describe typical behaviors, feelings, moods, and other characteristics (e.g., generous, hotheaded, ambitious, intelligent).

Although some labels cannot be changed (e.g., age and ethnicity), most are subjective and sensitive to change. Some conditions associated with alterations in self-concept or global self-worth include developmental changes, life crisis, illness, disability, and loss.

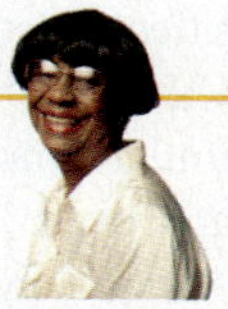

Think back to **Delores Sparks**, the older woman with advanced lung cancer who feels like a burden. When assessing her global self-worth, the nurse would need to identify any developmental changes Mrs. Sparks is experiencing that may be contributing to her current status, such as changes related to her increasing age. In addition, information about role changes, including the inability to care for herself and the need to be dependent owing to her illness, in conjunction with the knowledge of her terminal condition and anticipatory grieving related to her death, would be essential for determining her feelings of global self-worth.

Self-Expectations: "Who or What Do I Want to Be?"

Expectations for the self flow from various sources. The **ideal self** constitutes the self one wants to be. These self-expectations develop unconsciously early in childhood and are based on images of role models such as parents, other caregiving figures, and public figures. These personal expectations may be healthy or unhealthy. Contrast the significance of a child's identifying a television "bad boy" or a drug dealer as their hero rather than parents, civic leaders, or other professional people. A **false self** may develop in people who have an emotional need to respond to the needs and ambitions significant people, such as parents, have for them.

Self-Evaluation: "How Well Do I Like Myself?"

Self-esteem is the evaluative and affective component of the self-concept, sometimes termed *self-respect, self-approval,* or *self-worth.* According to Maslow (1954, p. 90), all people "have a need or desire for a stable, firmly based, usually high evaluation of themselves, for self-respect or self-esteem, and for the esteem of others." Accordingly, he identified two subsets of esteem needs: (1) self-esteem needs, such as strength, achievement, mastery and competence, confidence in the face of the world, independence, and freedom; and (2) respect needs or the need for esteem from others, such as status, dominance, recognition, attention, importance, and appreciation. For Maslow, self-esteem comes from two major sources: how competent children think they are in various aspects of life and how much social support they receive from other people. A person's self-esteem, like the various self-images that make up a person's self-concept, varies considerably in relation to specific relationships or situations.

Coopersmith (1967) identified the four bases of self-esteem as (1) *significance*, or the way people feel they are loved and approved of by the people important to them; (2) *competence*, or the way tasks that are considered important are performed; (3) *virtue*, or the attainment of moral–ethical standards; and (4) *power*, the extent to which people influence their own and others' lives. According to Coopersmith, people with high, medium, and low self-esteem differ in their expectations of the future, in their affective reactions, and in their basic styles of adapting to environmental demands. People with high self-esteem, for example, are accustomed to being well received and successful. They are able to approach people, tasks, and new situations freely, with confidence in their ability to interact and to get along with people and to respond successfully to life's challenges. With healthy self-esteem, you are:

- Assertive in expressing your needs and opinions
- Confident in your ability to make decisions
- Able to form secure and honest relationships—and less likely to stay in unhealthy ones
- Realistic in your expectations and less likely to be overcritical of yourself and others
- More resilient and better able to weather stress and setbacks (Mayo Clinic, 2020a)

Three major self-evaluation feelings or affects found in people are (1) *pride*, based on a positive self-evaluation, (2) *guilt*, based on behaviors incongruent with ideal self, and (3) *shame*, associated with low global self-worth. These affects are learned in early childhood within relationships with significant others and maintained through practice.

Sullivan (1953) proposed the self-representations of "good-me" and "bad-me" based on reflected appraisals of the self, learned in the context of a child's early relationship with significant others, especially parents. The child's feelings of self-esteem and self-worth develop out of that child's perceptions of the parenting figure's feelings, or affects, expressed in caring for the child. Sullivan posited that children perceived their parents' relative anxiety through a process he termed "empathy." Children exposed to higher levels of parental anxiety are at risk for developing lower self-esteem and a greater self-representation of "bad-me." As the child developed further, that child would begin to behave in ways that confirmed the earlier self-appraisals.

Sullivan and their most important interpreter within nursing, Hildegard Peplau (1952, 1997), emphasized the fluidity of self-appraisals throughout the life span. They taught that positive interaction at any point in a person's life with new significant others (such as nurses) who are less anxious and more accepting and nurturing than prior figures can have a positive, growth-promoting effect on that person's self-esteem and self-concept.

Bowlby (1969) developed attachment theory, which describes modes by which a young child develops and maintains feelings about the self as well as values and beliefs about the world. Attachment is a process by which the child maintains felt security via an interpersonal bond with close caregivers, most notably parents. Through a learning process based on children's perception of their caregivers' thoughts and reactions toward them, children form a sense of self as secure or insecure, calm or anxious, likable or not. Through this process, a child also develops beliefs and feelings about others as well as individual perceptions of situations and events. The growing child's self-esteem is affected by how healthy the child's attachment experience is with the early caregiver. If the attachment is secure, the child's thoughts and feelings about events are likely to closely match reality; if the attachment is insecure, the child's thoughts and feelings about events may be distorted and out of touch with reality. Such patterns tend to remain relatively fixed into adulthood.

Formation of Self-Concept

Although self-concept is largely considered to be a social creation that develops as a result of interactions with others (Fig. 42-2), contemporary nursing researchers and others recognize that certain inborn tendencies, such as temperament, when interacting with social and interpersonal experiences, are crucial in the formation of self-concept. Psychoanalysts have also emphasized the importance of inborn traits, such as innate aggression, because they affect a child's interpersonal experiences and shape self-concept (Freud, 1961). According to the theoretical formulations previously stated, the formation of self-concept includes the following:

1. An infant learns that the physical self is different from the environment. If basic needs are met, warmth and affection are experienced, and the caregivers' anxiety is minimized, then the child begins life with positive feelings about self.
2. The child next internalizes (incorporates into self) other people's attitudes toward self, including attitudes directed toward the child's innate tendencies, such as temperament and aggression. This internalization forms the foundation of self-concept. Parents or other direct caregivers play the most influential role; peers play the second most influential role. Later, the child continues to behave in ways that confirm this early self-concept. How loved you felt as a child is a great predictor of how you manage all sorts of difficult situations later in life (Zimmeran, 2020).
3. The child or adult internalizes the standards of society.

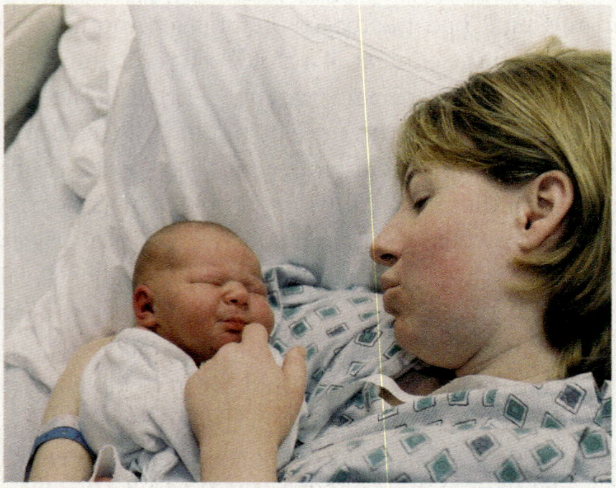

FIGURE 42-2. Interaction between caregiver and infant, such as feeding, holding, cuddling, and cooing, are important to the child's development.

Stages in the development of the self include self-awareness (infancy), self-recognition (18 months), self-definition (3 years), and self-concept (6 to 7 years). Psychological conditions that foster healthy development of the self in children include:

- Emotional warmth and acceptance
- Effective structure and discipline
- Clearly defined standards and limits, so that children understand what goals, procedures, and conduct are approved
- Adequately defined roles for both older and younger members of the family
- Established methods of handling children that produce the desired behavior, discourage misbehavior, and deal with infractions when they occur
- Encouragement of competence and self-confidence (Fig. 42-3)

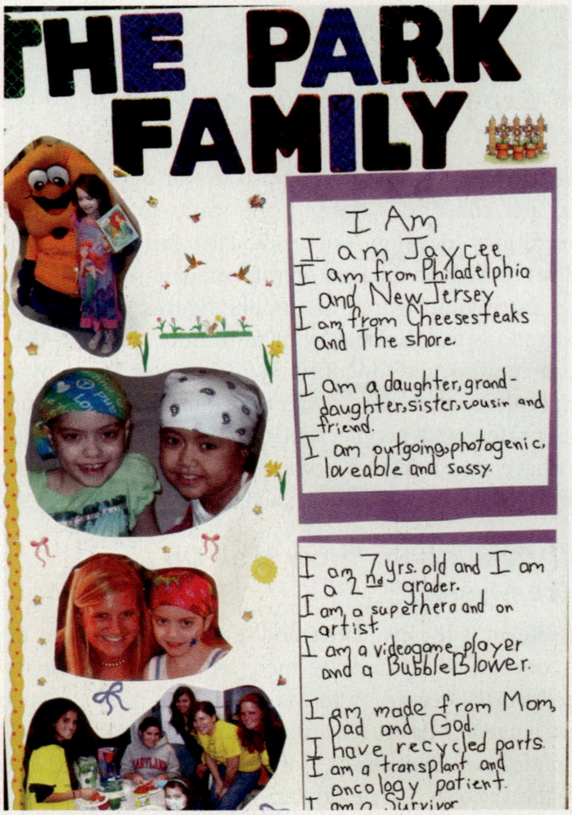

FIGURE 42-3. Jaycee's artwork illustrates a healthy self-concept. (Used with permission.)

- Helping children meet challenges
- Appropriate role models
- Stimulating and responsive environment

Formation of self-concept is further described in developmental theories, especially in Erikson's stages of development, Piaget's cognitive developmental stages, and Havighurst's developmental tasks (see Chapters 22 and 23).

Preventing Adverse Child Experiences

According to the Centers for Disease Control and Prevention (CDC) adverse childhood experiences, or ACEs, are potentially traumatic events that occur in childhood (ages 0–17 years). For example:

- Experiencing violence, abuse, or neglect
- Witnessing violence in the home or community
- Having a family member attempt or die by suicide

Also included are aspects of the child's environment that can undermine their sense of safety, stability, and bonding such as growing up in a household with:

- Substance misuse
- Mental health problems
- Instability due to parental separation or household members being in jail or prison.

It is critically important for every nurse to understand that ACEs are linked to chronic health problems, mental illness, and substance misuse in adulthood. ACEs can also negatively impact education and job opportunities. See Box 42-1 for strategies to prevent ACEs, and check the CDC website to learn more about the consequences of ACEs (https://www.cdc.gov/violenceprevention/aces/fastfact.html?CDC_AA_refVal=https%3A%2F%2Fwww.cdc.gov%2Fviolenceprevention%2Facestudy%2Ffastfact.html).

Box 42-1 Preventing Adverse Childhood Experiences

ACEs are preventable. Creating and sustaining safe, stable, nurturing relationships and environments for all children and families can prevent ACEs and help all children reach their full potential. The CDC has produced a resource, Preventing Adverse Childhood Experiences (ACEs): Leveraging the Best Available Evidence (https://www.cdc.gov/violenceprevention/pdf/preventingACES.pdf), to help states and communities take advantage of the best available evidence to prevent ACEs. It features six strategies from the CDC Technical Packages to Prevent Violence (https://www.cdc.gov/violenceprevention/communicationresources/pub/technical-packages.html).

Strategy	Approach
Strengthen economic supports to families	• Strengthening household financial security • Family-friendly work policies
Promote social norms that protect against violence and adversity	• Public education campaigns • Legislative approaches to reduce corporal punishment • Bystander approaches • Men and boys as allies in prevention
Ensure a strong start for children	• Early childhood home visitation • High-quality childcare • Preschool enrichment with family engagement
Teach skills	• Social–emotional learning • Safe dating and healthy relationship skill programs • Parenting skills and family relationship approaches
Connect youth to caring adults and activities	• Mentoring programs • After-school programs
Intervene to lessen immediate and long-term harms	• Enhanced primary care • Victim-centered services • Treatment to lessen the harms of ACEs

Raising awareness of ACEs can help:

- Change how people think about the causes of ACEs and who could help prevent them.
- Shift the focus from individual responsibility to community solutions.
- Reduce stigma around seeking help with parenting challenges or for substance misuse, depression, or suicidal thoughts.
- Promote safe, stable, nurturing relationships and environments where children live, learn, and play.

Let's help all children reach their full potential and create neighborhoods, communities, and a world in which every child can thrive.

Source: Centers for Disease Control and Prevention. (2019). *Preventing adverse childhood experiences.* https://www.cdc.gov/violenceprevention/aces/fastfact.html?CDC_AA_refVal=https%3A%2F%2Fwww.cdc.gov%2Fviolenceprevention%2Facestudy%2Ffastfact.html

Factors Affecting Self-Concept

Almost any life experience can influence a person's self-concept. Key factors include developmental considerations, culture, internal and external resources, history of success and failure, stressors, and illness or trauma.

Developmental Considerations

As a person matures, the criteria that mark the experiences necessary for a positive self-concept change. Although the infant needs a supportive environment in which all human needs are met, the growing child needs the freedom to explore and develop the ability to meet increasing personal needs. Table 42-1 highlights developmental changes affecting self-concept, related implications for nursing, and potential causes of self-concept disturbances. Box 42-2 on page 1744 invites you to test your clinical reasoning and judgment. See also Chapters 22–24.

Culture

As a child internalizes the values of parents and peers, culture begins to influence a sense of self. If the culture is relatively stable, little tension may be experienced between what culture expects of the child and what the child expects of self. When parents, peers, and the adult world confront the child with different cultural expectations, however, the sense of self may become confused. For example, an adolescent might realize their parents live by the work ethic and believe it is necessary to rise early every day and put in a full day's work. That adolescent's peer group, however, has few demands placed on it and encourages the adolescent to hang out with the group. The adolescent's vocational aptitudes, meanwhile, are leading them to consider a music career in a rock group, which will keep the adolescent out late many nights doing something the parents do not classify as work.

Children of immigrants whose values and practices of their culture of origin vary from the culture of adoption face cultural dissonance. Parents may expect children to behave according to their own cultural norms, whereas peers and society, as well as the adolescent's wish to "belong," may create the desire to abandon old cultural beliefs, attitudes, and practices. Conflict between parents and children, as well as cultural confusion, may occur.

Refer to the accompanying Research in Nursing box for a study concerning how acculturation into the nursing profession affected the self-esteem in nursing students.

Internal and External Resources

The personal strengths a person recognizes, develops, and uses are powerful but subjective determinants of self-concept. For example, one person may use humor as both an effective coping mechanism and a successful interpersonal tool. Another person may use humor to avoid facing conflict but may feel badly about being known as a "joker" or "clown." The degree to which a person integrates healthy, useful internal resources or personal strengths is associated with how well a person has been able to establish a positive self-concept in the context of nurturing experiences.

Self-concept is also associated with the ability to identify and use external resources, such as a network of support people, adequate finances, and organizational supports. People who feel more positive about themselves tend to feel connected to others and to society; they can identify and use more external resources. People who feel disconnected and alone tend to perceive and use fewer environmental resources.

Research in Nursing

BRIDGING THE GAP TO EVIDENCE-BASED PRACTICE

Nursing Students' Understanding of the Concept of Self-Esteem

Positive self-esteem helps students academically and facilitates development of the role of the professional nurse. That said, little study has been done on nursing students' self-esteem.

Related Research

Zamanzadeh, V., Valizadeh, L., Gargari, R. B., Ghahramanian, A., Tabriz, F. J., & Crowley, M. (2016). Nursing students' understanding of the concept of self-esteem: A qualitative study. *Journal of Caring Science*, 5(1), 33–41.

This study aimed to discover the extent and characteristics of the concept of self-esteem from the perspective of Iranian nursing students through a qualitative approach. Purposive sampling was used to recruit participants and data were collected through in-depth semistructured interviews and analyzed simultaneously. The results revealed that from the nursing students' perspective, self-esteem referred to the value they gave to being a nursing student. From the findings, three main themes emerged and related to "enthusiasm about being a nursing student," "socialization into the profession," and "sense of worth related to perceived professionalism level."

Relevance to Nursing Practice

This study revealed that the nursing students' self-esteem is influenced greatly by their professionalization and socialization. Faculty should give more attention to the factors that facilitate the development of higher levels of self-esteem among nursing students during curriculum development. The study authors noted that the concept of self-esteem is affected by different cultural influences and contexts. This study was conducted in northwest Iran, and it would be helpful to replicate it in other countries.

Table 42-1 Developmental Changes Affecting Self-Concept

DEVELOPMENTAL PERIOD	CHANGES AFFECTING SELF-CONCEPT	IMPLICATIONS FOR NURSING	POTENTIAL CAUSES OF DISTURBANCES IN SELF-CONCEPT
Infancy	• No self-concept at birth • Beginning differentiation of self and nonself	• Teach parents the critical importance of providing consistent and affectionate parenting. • Assess whether the parents have reasonable expectations of the infant: sleeping, eating, other awake behaviors.	• Unmet basic human needs • Lack of adequate body and sensory stimulation • Parents' lack of acceptance of the infant's appearance or behavior • Poor match between parent's and child's temperament or needs
Childhood	• An intact body is important to the young child, who fears bodily mutilation. • During middle childhood, a sense of being trusted and loved, of being competent and trustworthy develops. • Differences between self and others are strong.	• If invasive procedures are indicated, explain simply to the child what is being done and offer the child support. • Assess the parents' ability to provide the type of developmental environment in which the child's self-concepts can evolve positively.	• Dysfunctional family • Too much or too little structure • Sensory perceptual impairments
Adolescence	• Development of secondary sex characteristics; rapid body changes • Sense of self is consolidated. • Emphasis on sexual identity • Parental influences on self-concept are often rejected; peers become more important; movement is toward development of own identity.	• Assess adolescent's self-knowledge and understanding of body changes. • Counsel adolescents regarding mature and healthy use of independence they crave. • Provide anticipatory guidelines regarding hazards to life, health, human functioning.	• Inability to accept body • Inability to resolve competing pulls to be both a child and an adult • Unhealthy peer pressure • Identity confusion
Adulthood	• Society places emphasis on intactness of body, fitness, energy, sexuality, style, productivity, sophistication, beauty. • Important to meet role expectations well.	• Assess how realistic the adult's expectations are and the incentive they provide for growth and development. • Assist patient to deal constructively with negative influences in self-image. • Preretirement counseling.	• Inability to fulfill conflicting role expectations • Failure to accept role responsibility (e.g., parenting responsibilities) • Unreasonable expectations • Irreversible body change related to trauma, illness • Unsatisfying job • Failure to develop new goals to give meaning and purpose to life • Multiple stressors
Later Adult Years	• Declining physical and possibly mental abilities • Multiple losses • Increasing dependency • Impending death • Diminished choices/options	• Assess how the older adult is adjusting to effects of aging. • Counsel regarding meaningful use of time. • Explore resources. • Assess depression, substance abuse. • Recognize and value older adults' life experience.	• Loss of significant work (retirement); feelings of uselessness • Death of spouse, significant others • Diminished physical attractiveness, strength, overall health • Multiple stressors • Fear of dependency • Change may be more difficult

Box 42-2 Test Your Clinical Reasoning and Judgment

Reflective Practice: Worries grow about the treatment of children who say they are transgender

In 2008, Andrea Davidson's 12-year-old daughter, Meghan, announced that they were "definitely a boy." Ms. Davidson says Meghan was never a tomboy, but the family doctor congratulated Meghan and asked what pronouns they have chosen, before writing a referral to the British Columbia Children's Hospital. "We thought we were going to see a psychologist, but it was a nurse and a social worker" says Ms. Davidson. "Within 10 minutes they had offered our child Lupron"—a puberty blocking drug. "They brought up the drug directly with our child, in front of us, without discussing it with us privately first." There was no mention of other mental health issues, which are known to increase the likelihood of gender dysphoria, the feeling that you are in the wrong body. "There was no therapy on offer, and we were just brushed aside when we raised it."

Meghan belongs to a wave of children across the Western world who have identified as transgender in recent years. America had 1 gender clinic in 2007; now it has more than 50. An increasing number of children are also de-transitioning, choosing to revert to their previous gender. Unfortunately, if children have already begun a medical transition, including hormone treatment, it can leave them infertile and unable to have a full sex life. [(December 12, 2020). Boys and girls. *The Economist*, 60–62.]

If you were caring for Meghan, what would your assessment priorities be, and which interventions/treatment plans should be offered?

History of Success and Failure

People with a history of repeated failure (in school, friendships, work, or marriage) may perceive themselves as failures and actually perpetuate this image by unconsciously encouraging others to treat them this way. They may come to fear success, and actually find it easier to fail even though they do not like themselves that way. Thus, failure influences a person's self-concept negatively (e.g., Sullivan's "bad-me" self-representation), and that negative self-concept causes the person to continue to fail. On the other hand, a series of successful experiences—especially when occurring in the context of an accepting, nurturing, caring relationship—may condition a person to strive for the next success, forging a positive self-concept that fosters an expectation of success and encourages the person to "make it happen."

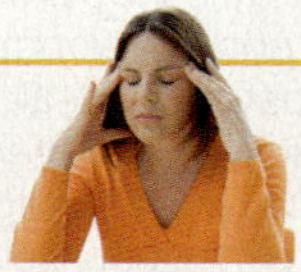

Think back to **Melissa Motsky**, the struggling nursing student. Consider how multiple less-than-satisfactory life experiences may culminate in Ms. Motsky's sense of personal failure in areas such as academics, relationships, role performance in their family, and work experience.

Crises or Life Stressors

Life stressors or crises (e.g., cyber bullying, marriage, divorce, acute or chronic illness, an exam, a new job or job loss, a gray hair, a fire) may call forth a personal response and mobilize a person's talents, resulting in good feelings about oneself, or it might result in emotional paralysis with diminished self-concept. People vary greatly in their perception of what constitutes a crisis or stressor, as well as the degree to which such experiences disrupt or diminish self-concept. However, major stressors place anyone at relative risk for maladaptive responses, such as withdrawal, isolation, depression, extreme anxiety, substance abuse, or exacerbation of physical illness. How the person perceives the stressor (threat, challenge, defeat) and the person's ability to mobilize personal strengths and other resources are determined largely by that person's self-concept, which, in turn, is influenced by the response the person chooses.

Aguilera (1998) described three factors that determine a person's response to crisis: (1) the person's perception of the event or situation, (2) the person's situational supports (external resources), and (3) the coping mechanisms the person possesses (internal resources). All of these factors are related to self-concept. The degree of strength a person has in each area is related to the person's pre-crisis self-concept. Similarly, each of these factors can alter self-concept either positively or negatively during or after the crisis. Intervention to strengthen any of these three areas can help people better cope with crisis and emerge with enhanced self-concept.

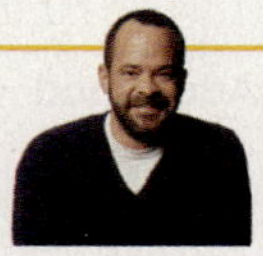

Recall **Anthony Santorini**, the patient who had an amputation. To promote an enhanced self-concept, the nurse would need to assess their perception of the situation and their coping mechanisms to gain further insight into Mr. Santorini's self-concept. In addition, the nurse would need to investigate the support systems available to Mr. Santorini, such as family, friends, and community resources, which might be helpful in fostering a more positive self-concept.

Aging, Illness, Disability or Trauma

Many people take a healthy body for granted. Society encourages a kind of denial of the eventuality of aging, chronic illness, and the necessity to integrate crisis and change throughout each person's lifetime. Society emphasizes and rewards youth, health, and narrow norms for physical attractiveness while devaluing seniors, those with chronic illness, and those whose appearance does not correspond to celebrity standards. Thus, a sudden illness, trauma, or bodily disfigurement, or even the suggestion of disease, as well as signs of the aging process may pose serious threats to the self. People vary greatly in their response to aging, illness, disability, and trauma (Fig. 42-4). This is due to the threats to self-concept and internal beliefs about the self that these conditions may pose. See the accompanying Vulnerable Population Alert and reflect on your ability

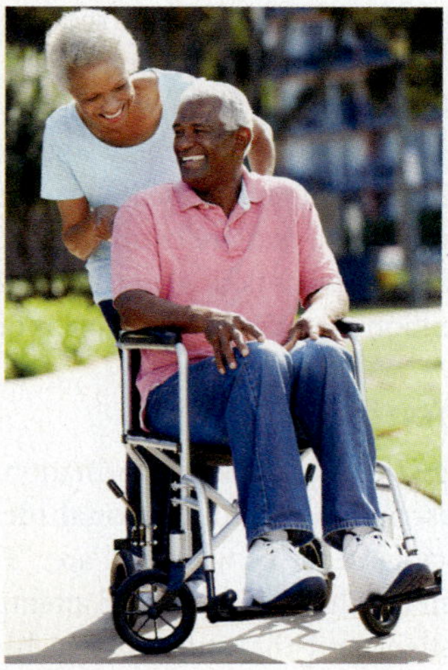

FIGURE 42-4. An illness or alteration in function may present challenges that affect a patient's self-concept. Changes may be positive or negative. How family and professional caregivers respond is critical.

to competently and compassionately care for persons with disabilities.

Unfolding Patient Stories: Marvin Hayes • Part 2

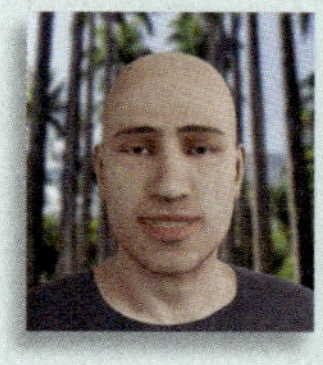

Think back to **Marvin Hayes** from Chapter 39, who is 43 and married. He underwent surgery for rectal cancer requiring a permanent colostomy. What effect can a colostomy have on his self-concept? How would the nurse assess for a disturbance in self-image caused by the colostomy? If a body image disturbance, low self-esteem, or ineffective role performance is identified, what nursing interventions can help Marvin modify a negative self-concept and adapt to his colostomy?

Care for Marvin and other patients in a realistic virtual environment: ***vSim** for Nursing* (thepoint.lww.com/vSimFunds). Practice documenting these patients' care in DocuCare (thepoint.lww.com/DocuCareEHR).

Vulnerable Population Alert: Persons With Disabilities

Approximately 61 million adults in the United States live with a disability. A disability is any condition of the body or mind (impairment) that makes it more difficult for the person with the condition to do certain activities (activity limitation) and interact with the world around them (participation restrictions). According to the World Health Organization, disability has three dimensions:

- **Impairment** in a person's body structure or function, or mental functioning; examples of impairments include loss of a limb, loss of vision or memory loss.
- **Activity limitation**, such as difficulty seeing, hearing, walking, or problem solving.
- **Participation restrictions** in normal daily activities, such as working, engaging in social and recreational activities, and obtaining health care and preventive services.

Disability is especially common in these groups:

- 2 in 5 adults ages 65 years and older have a disability
- 1 in 4 women have a disability
- 2 in 5 Non-Hispanic American Indian/Alaska Native individuals have a disability

Adults living with disabilities are more likely to have obesity (38.2%), smoke (28.2%), have heart disease (11.5%), and have diabetes (16.3%).

Health care access barriers for working-age adults include:

- 1 in 3 adults (18 to 44 years) with disabilities do not have a usual health care provider
- 1 in 3 adults with disabilities have an unmet health care need because of cost in the past year
- 1 in 4 adults with disabilities did not have a routine checkup in the past year. (*Source*: Centers for Disease Control and Prevention. *Disability impacts all of us.* https://www.cdc.gov/ncbddd/disabilityandhealth/infographic-disability-impacts-all.html)

Have you ever cared for an individual with disabilities? How competent and confident are in meeting their needs? What does thoughtful person-centered care "look like" for individuals with mobility, cognition, independent living, hearing, vision, and/or self-care disabilities? Are there particular challenges to their self-esteem? You may want to check out these resources:

- Core Competencies on Disability for Healthcare Education: https://nisonger.osu.edu/education-training/ohio-disability-health-program/corecompetenciesondisability/ (Ohio State)
- The US Centers for Disease Control and Prevention: http://www.cdc.gov/ncbddd/disabilityandhealth/women.html/
- Women's Health.gov: http://www.womenshealth.gov/search/node?keys=disabilities

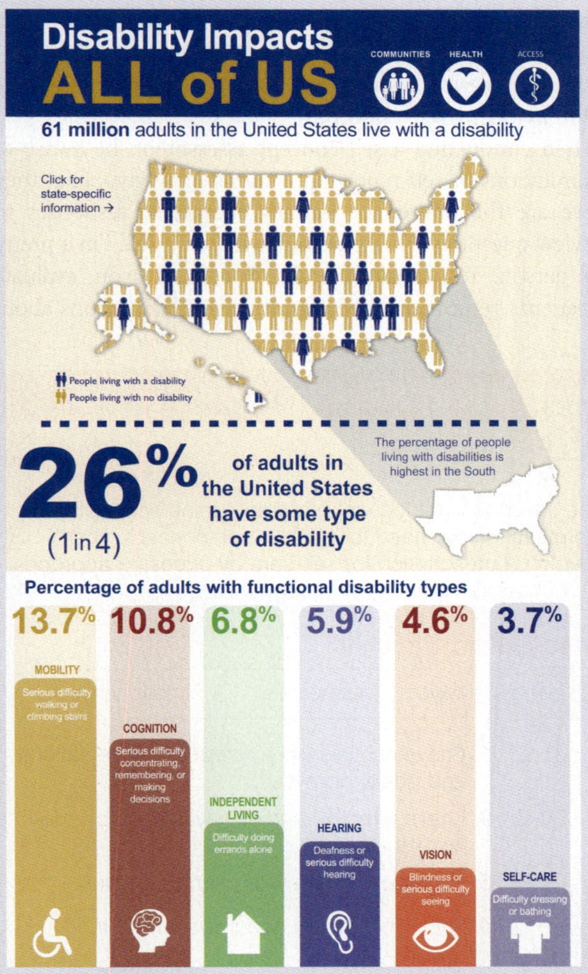

NURSING PROCESS FOR PATIENTS WITH ALTERATIONS IN SELF-CONCEPT

Nurses who role-model good health behaviors are more effective teachers. Use the display, Promoting Health 42-1, for yourself before using it with others. Before you can successfully identify and resolve self-concept disturbances in patients, you must be comfortable with yourself and possess an adequate self-concept.

Assessing

The nurse assessing a patient's self-concept focuses on personal identity, personal strengths, body image, self-esteem, and role performance. A general assessment of self-concept should be included in every comprehensive nursing assessment. It is as important to identify and label a patient's positive self-concept as it is to note actual or potential problems.

Patients experiencing illness or trauma resulting in body disfigurement, altered functioning, or life crises that arrest development and thwart the achievement of life goals are at high risk for problems related to self-concept and should be assessed more carefully. If potential problems surface during the interview, a more thorough assessment should be carried out.

The accompanying Focused Assessment Guide highlights elements common to any self-concept assessment and high-risk factors, as well as questions and approaches that can be used in assessing self-concept.

When conducting a self-concept assessment, be aware of the limitations of self-reporting. Patients may give what they believe are the desired or socially acceptable responses to interview questions. "Why, of course I like myself. I'm a pretty good person. Yes, I have friends." For this reason, evaluate the patient's responses in relation to your observations about the patient and what you know about the patient from other sources. When the nursing assessment reveals a clustering of these behaviors, discuss this finding with the patient. This is especially true when there is a discrepancy between the patient's words and behavior. "You've told me that you feel in control of your situation right now and are committed to the treatment plan, but I notice you're not taking your medications regularly, and you did mention that you are drinking more heavily...."

Personal Identity

When assessing self-concept, the information needed first is the patient's description of self. **Personal identity** describes a person's conscious sense of who they are. "How would you describe yourself to others?" Pay special attention to the labels used by the patient and the order in which they appear. A simple exercise consists of asking patients to "make a list of 10 labels that you believe identify yourself (e.g., gay man, student, Italian American person, opera fan, premedicine major). Put the most important label first, and then list the others in order of decreasing importance. What if the order were reversed? To what extent do you think your way of organizing information about yourself affects your behavior?"

It is important to discover whether people are comfortable with their perceived identity. Developmental changes, trauma, and cultural and gender dysphoria may all place a patient at risk for personal identity disturbances.

Personal Strengths

Many patients focus naturally on their deficiencies; asking pointed questions about personal strengths can help a patient identify positive factors:

"What are some of your personal strengths ... qualities you are proud of ... things you do well?"

"What has helped you cope in the past when things were tough?"

Promoting Health 42-1

SELF-CONCEPT

Use the assessment checklist to determine how well you are meeting your need for positive self-concept. Then develop a prescription for self-care by choosing appropriate behaviors from the list of suggestions.

Assessment Checklist

☐ almost always ☐ sometimes ☐ almost never

☐ ☐ ☐ 1. I have established appropriate expectations and goals for myself.

☐ ☐ ☐ 2. I have effective and satisfying relationships with others.

☐ ☐ ☐ 3. I cope effectively with change and loss.

☐ ☐ ☐ 4. I accept and feel good about myself.

Self-Care Behaviors

1. Accept normal variations in physical appearance and capabilities.
2. Use problem-solving and decision-making strategies to define expectations and set goals.
3. Set priorities and accept that no one person can be all things to all people.
4. Learn from past mistakes and then forget them; carrying around "excess baggage" is unhealthy.
5. Emphasize strengths and abilities in self.
6. Take an active part in group activities in school, work, church, or the community.
7. Volunteer time, talents, or services.
8. Avoid excessive alcohol and drugs.
9. Live life one day at a time.
10. Get help for self-concept disturbances that interfere with healthy social and professional activities.

Focused Assessment Guide 42-1

SELF-CONCEPT

Factors to Assess	High-Risk Factors	Questions and Approaches
Personal identity	• Developmental changes • Trauma • Gender dysphoria • Cultural dissonance	*How would you describe yourself to others?* • Personal characteristics and traits • Strengths • Fears
Body image	• Loss of body part or function • Disfigurement • Developmental changes	*Describe your body to me.* *What do you like most/least about your body?* *Is there anything about your body that you would like to change?*
Self-esteem	• Unhealthy interpersonal relationships • Failure to achieve developmental milestones • Failure to achieve life goals • Failure to live up to personal moral code • Sense of powerlessness	*Tell me something about your sense of satisfaction with yourself.* *Tell me about your relationships with others.* *Who would you like to be?* *Who or what has influenced your self-expectations?* *Are these expectations realistic?* Significance: *What is your response when you feel unloved or unappreciated by those who are important to you?* Competence: *How do you feel about your ability to do the things in life that are important to you?* Virtue: *To what degree are you satisfied with the way you are able to live up to your moral standards?* Power: *To what extent do you feel able to control what happens to you in life? How does this make you feel?*
Role performance	• Loss of valued role • Ambiguous role expectations • Conflicting role expectations • Inability to meet role expectations	*Many of us "wear many hats." What roles (spouse, parent, student, athlete, nursing aide, dancer) are most important to you?* *How do you feel about your ability to do all the things your roles demand of you?* *Are these roles satisfying for you?*

Body Image

Body image is the person's subjective view of their physical appearance. Body image disturbances can be expected with any alteration in bodily appearance, structure, or function.

When a disturbed body image is suspected, carefully interview and observe the patient to identify the nature of the threat to the person's body image (functional significance of the part involved, importance of physical appearance, visibility of the part involved), the meaning the patient attaches to the threat, the adequacy of the patient's coping abilities, response of family members and significant others, and help available to the patient and patient's family.

Assess the patient's response to the deformity or limitation, including changes in independence–dependence patterns and in socialization and communication.

RESPONSE TO MALFORMATION OR LIMITATION

- *Adaptive responses:* Patient exhibits signs of grief and mourning (shock, disbelief, denial, anger, guilt, acceptance).
- *Maladaptive responses:* Patient continues to deny and to avoid dealing with the deformity or limitation, engages in self-destructive behavior, talks about feelings of worthlessness or insecurity, equates deformity or limitation with whole person, shows a change in ability to estimate relationship of body to environment.

INDEPENDENCE–DEPENDENCE PATTERNS

- *Adaptive responses:* Patient assumes responsibility for care (makes decisions), develops new self-care behaviors, uses available resources, interacts in a mutually supportive way with family.
- *Maladaptive responses:* Patient assigns responsibility for their care to others, becomes increasingly dependent, or stubbornly refuses necessary help.

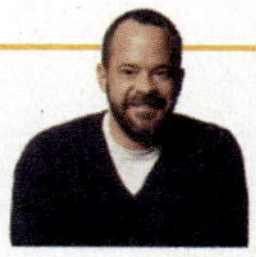

Recall **Anthony Santorini**, the 44-year-old man who had an amputation. The patient voiced concerns that he was not "whole" anymore. The nurse would need to assess the underlying factors associated with this feeling. Is the feeling related to the actual loss of a body part, fear of further disfiguration from continued complications, inability to function independently, or fear of how others will react to the loss? Additional inquiry is needed to determine the value Mr. Santorini places on physical appearance and the meaning he attaches to their extremities, such as ability to walk, work, or just get around the house or their environment. The nurse could then work with the patient and assist with adapting to the loss of their leg. Incorporating information about the use of a prosthesis may be helpful as they begin to adapt to their body change.

Self-Esteem

When patients share their self-perceptions, use the opportunity to ask questions about whether patients like themselves, and whether they are pleased with their expectations and the progress they are making to realize these expectations. For example, you might state:

"Tell me what you like about yourself."

"What would you change about yourself if you could?"

You can obtain a quick indication of a patient's self-esteem by using a graphic description of self-esteem as the discrepancy between the "real self" (who we think we really are) and the "ideal self" (who we think we would like to be). Have the patient plot two points on a line—real self and ideal self (Fig. 42-5). The greater the discrepancy, the lower the self-esteem; the smaller the discrepancy, the higher the self-esteem.

A person's ideal self may differ dramatically from the current sense of self and may positively or negatively influence behavior and personal development. If indicated, question the patient about self-expectations:

"You've told me something about who you are and how you view yourself now. Tell me who you would like to be in the future."

"What life goals are important to you?"

"Where do you see yourself 5 years from now? In 10 years?"

"Are these expectations realistic?"

"Are your expectations stemming from who you would like to be or from who you think you should be?"

"Who or what has influenced your self-expectations?"

Such questions help assess whether the patient possesses life goals that are positively motivating personal development.

Identify any unrealistic expectations and explore their source with the patient. For example:

"You seem to feel that it is necessary to be all things to all people—no matter what this costs you. How might this belief have developed? Is it helpful to you?"

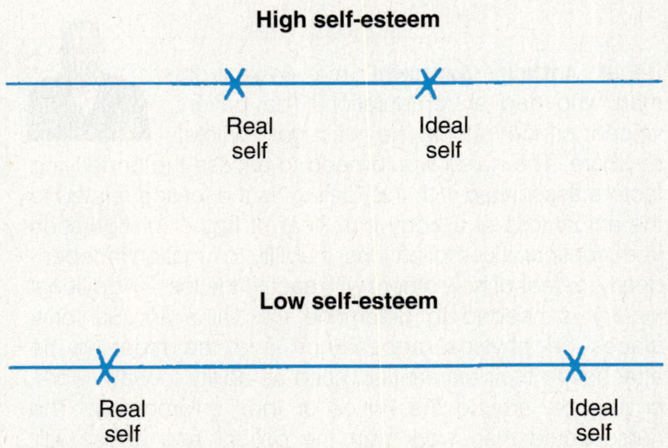

FIGURE 42-5. Patients who perceive their real self as relatively close to the ideal self have high self-esteem. Patients who perceive their real self as far from the ideal self have low self-esteem.

"What I'm hearing is that your performance must always be perfect, that although you allow others to make mistakes, you cannot allow yourself this luxury. Tell me more about this."

"You state you have no goals for the future. When you wake up each morning, what gets you out of bed? What keeps you moving?"

If a more detailed assessment is needed, the concepts of socialization and communication, significance, competence, virtue, and power should be explored next.

SOCIALIZATION AND COMMUNICATION

Responses to socialization and communication may be adaptive or maladaptive:

- *Adaptive responses:* Maintains usual social patterns, communicates needs and accepts offers of help, serves as support for others.
- *Maladaptive responses:* Isolates self, exhibits superficial self-confidence, is unable to express needs (becomes hostile, ashamed, frustrated, depressed).

To assess the quantity and quality of the patient's interpersonal relationships, which helps identify the person's level of social support and relatedness, you might ask:

"Who do you feel is important to you?"

"Is there anyone you feel you can depend on for help if you need it?"

"How do you feel about your relationships?"

"Tell me about changes you've noticed in your ways of meeting and interacting with others."

"Many people have 'people' problems. Are your relationships causing you any problems right now?"

SIGNIFICANCE

To assess the patient's feelings of significance, you might ask:

"Are there people in your life with whom you share a close relationship?"

"To what extent do you feel loved and approved of by the key people in your life?"

"Does it bother you when you feel unloved or when others fail to appreciate you?"

"In what ways do you let family members and friends know that you like them or are proud of their accomplishments?"

COMPETENCE

To assess the patient's feelings of competence, you might ask:

"What are the things you need to do to feel important?"

"Is anything interfering with your ability to execute these tasks? How does this make you feel?"

"How important to you is it to feel that others value your work?"

VIRTUE

To assess the patient's sense of virtue, you might ask:

"Tell me something about the moral–ethical principles that govern your life."

"How must you live to describe yourself as a 'good' person?"

"Describe any difficulties you experience in living up to your moral principles that you would like to discuss."

"In what ways can the nurses help you to live better according to your moral standards?"

POWER

To assess the patient's sense of power, you might ask:

"How important is it to you to 'be in control' of your life (health)?"

"To what extent did you feel 'in control' of your life (health) before this illness (trauma, crisis)?"

"To what extent do you feel 'in control' of your life (health) currently?"

"What is it that makes you feel not in control?"

"How might you change this? How can nurses help you to develop and gain more control?"

Role Performance

We all play many roles. Life roles such as our occupation or profession can constitute a major portion of our identity. Our ability to successfully live up to societal as well as our own expectations regarding role-specific behaviors, or our **role performance**, is easily compromised by illness and injury. Often, illness or developmental processes such as aging make it necessary to alter or relinquish previous roles. In general, people experience such alterations as major losses. Thus, all people whose roles are altered or compromised are at risk for disturbances in self-concept. Role performance may also be affected by role ambiguity (failure to completely and accurately understand what a role demands), role stress (disparity between what one believes the role demands and what one is able to offer), and role overload (limited time because of other commitments makes it impossible to meet realistic role expectations). With any patient who has experienced compromised role performance, use the following questions:

"What major roles describe you—son, daughter, spouse, parent, employer or employee, student, club member, and so on?"

"How important is it to you to be good in each of these roles?"

"Tell me how successful you think you are in each of these roles."

"What roles or expectations would you change if you could?"

"What new skills or behaviors might be necessary to help you resume or modify current roles?"

"What is it like for you to lose a role that's been important to you?"

"How can I help you identify other role options or direction?"

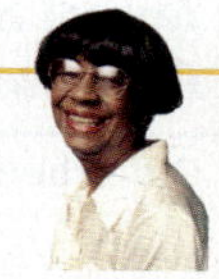

Think back to **Delores Sparks**, the woman with advanced lung cancer now living with her daughter. The change in living situation and dependence on her daughter for everyday activities has definitely affected the patient's role performance. Once living alone and fairly self-sufficient, Mrs. Sparks now relies on her daughter. The role performance questions would be extremely important to ask Mrs. Sparks to determine the actual impact her illness and change in living situation has had on her self-concept.

Diagnosing Actual or Potential Health Problems and Needs

An assessment of a patient's self-concept may lead to the identification of one or more actual or potential health problems and needs related to self-concept. Following the formulation of the actual or potential health problems and needs, the nurse communicates findings to other nursing and health care professionals through the use of the written and spoken word. The written actual or potential health problem or need becomes a permanent part of the patient's health record.

The International Classification for Nursing Practice (ICNP) identifies several actual or potential health problems that may be identified by nurses:

- Negative Self-Image
- Disturbed Body Image
- Disturbed (or Risk for Disturbed) Personal Identity
- Chronic (or Risk for Chronic) Low Self-Esteem or Situational (or Risk for Situational) Low Self-Esteem
- Impaired Role Performance

Common etiologic factors and potential signs and symptoms for some of these health problems are found in the accompanying box, Examples of Actual or Potential Health Problems and Needs: Self-Concept on page 1750.

The ICNP lists as a positive diagnosis and health outcome Positive Self Image (body image, personal identity, and self-esteem.

Important Distinctions

When assessment data point to an alteration in self-image, the first task is to determine whether the altered self-concept is the problem, the cause of the problem (etiology), or merely a sign that a problem exists. It is important to make an accurate determination because this directs the outcomes developed for the patient and related nursing interventions.

Examples of Actual or Potential Health Problems and Needs

DISTURBANCES IN SELF-CONCEPT

Actual or Potential Health Problems and Needs	Possible Etiologic Factors	Potential Signs and Symptoms
Disturbed Body Image	• Illness • Trauma • Disability • Aging	• "I don't recognize my body anymore and it certainly doesn't work like it should!" • "I can't even imagine my husband wanting to have sex with me. I feel so different after losing a breast." • Avoids looking at their body • Avoids touching their body
Risk for Situational Low Self-Esteem	• Sudden alteration in body image or functioning • Alteration in social role • Behavior inconsistent with values • Decrease in control over environment • Inadequate recognition from significant others • Unrealistic self-expectations	—
Positive Self-Image	—	• Acceptance of limitations • Acceptance of strengths • Actions congruent with verbal expressions • Expresses confidence in abilities • Expresses desire to enhance role performance or self-concept • Expresses satisfaction with sense of worth

Source: International Council of Nurses. (2019). *Nursing diagnosis and outcome statements.* International Classification for Nursing Practice (ICNP) Catalogue. https://www.icn.ch/sites/default/files/inline-files/icnp2017-dc.pdf

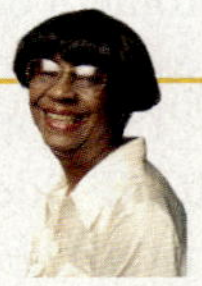

Consider **Delores Sparks** and the following problem statements:

Situational Low Self-Esteem related to perceived failure in role of mother and grandmother; signs and symptoms: feelings of being a bother and not good for anything anymore. Assessment data point to a disturbance in self-esteem as the priority problem. Nursing energies will be directed to helping the patient evaluate herself positively despite the stress of the illness and loss of independence.

Impaired Health Maintenance related to decreased self-esteem; signs and symptoms: feelings of depression. Here, low self-esteem is contributing to the patient's problem of failing to maintain her health as much as possible by following through with actions, and by voicing thoughts of ending her own life. Nursing energies will be best directed to improving the patient's use of health resources, including helping her to value herself enough to choose healthy behaviors.

Difficulty Coping related to difficulty accepting changes in health status and role resulting from terminal illness; Signs and symptoms: low self-esteem statements ("I feel like an old dish rag, not good for anything anymore") and thoughts about ending her life ("since God isn't doing it"). Here, low self-esteem statements are the cues that led to the identification of the problem statement. One of the criteria used to evaluate nursing intervention to increase the patient's coping skills will be a reduction in or elimination of low self-esteem statements.

Outcome Identification and Planning

With all patients, nursing interventions need to be supportive of the following patient outcomes:

The patient will:

- Describe self realistically, identifying both strengths and deficiencies
- Verbalize realistic expectations for self, based on who the patient would like to be
- Verbalize that self is liked, or at least "OK"
- Communicate feelings and needs in a way that is comfortable and effective in meeting needs
- Nurture relationships in which needs for love and worth are mutually met (significance)
- Assume role-related responsibilities with confidence (competence)
- Express satisfaction with ability to live according to their moral–ethical standards (virtue)
- Demonstrate confidence in ability to accomplish what is desired (power)

The following are sample outcomes for patients with specific disturbances in self-concept:

The patient will:

- Describe the relation between self-concept and behavior
- Identify faulty thinking that reinforces a negative self-concept (distortions and denials, faulty categorizing, inappropriate standards)

- Integrate positive self-knowledge into self-concept
- Report feeling better about himself or herself

Implementing

Nursing interventions to assist patients to develop and maintain a positive self-concept can vary tremendously from one patient to another.

Nurse Self-Care Alert

Remember: You must be comfortable with your own self-concept before you can address problems in patients.

Specific nursing strategies addressed in this section include helping patients identify and use personal strengths, helping at-risk patients maintain a sense of self, enhancing or modifying the self-concept, developing a positive body image, and working with parents and educators to develop self-esteem in children, adolescents, and older adults.

Helping Patients Identify and Use Personal Strengths

When confronted with a major stressor, many people forget that they have histories of successful coping and numerous personal strengths. Patients at high risk for giving up are those with low self-esteem or multiple stressors they perceive as overwhelming.

Although attributing strength to a patient sounds like something nurses would do naturally, nurses frequently fall into the trap of "doing" for patients (i.e., solving their problems rather than helping them to identify and tap their personal power and strengths). Moreover, patients continually instruct nurses about how they should be perceived, and some patients successfully communicate a manipulative helplessness that encourages the nurse to take charge. An appropriate nursing response in this case is, "I wonder why you want me to speak with your health care provider about treatment alternatives. I'm sure you would feel much better hearing this information firsthand. If you'd like, I will stay here while you talk with the health care provider."

Patients experiencing powerlessness may need help to recognize their strengths (Fig. 42-6). Examples of personal strengths that might better equip a person to respond to life's challenges include:

- Healthy, functioning body
- Ability to adjust to or function with chronic bodily malfunction
- Cognitive abilities
- Positive self-concept
- Interpersonal skills
- Sense of meaning and purpose in life
- Belief system
- Social support network
- Meaningful work

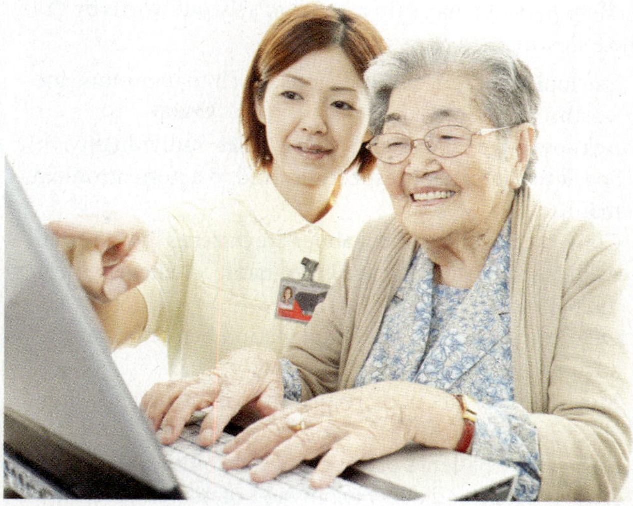

FIGURE 42-6. The nurse helps the patient recognize their self-worth and strengths.

- Hobbies and other interests
- Education
- Life experience and a past history of effective coping
- Good sense of humor
- Spirituality
- Healthy nutritional state
- Ability to make decisions

If you search for "Self-Esteem Worksheets" online, you will find many resources to help your patients build their self-esteem.

Specific strategies that can be used to help patients identify and use personal strengths include the following:

- Encourage patients to identify their strengths.
- Replace self-negation with positive thinking.
- Notice and reinforce patient strengths.
- Encourage patients to will for themselves the strengths they desire and to try them on.
- Help patients cope with necessary dependency resulting from aging or illness.

Helping At-Risk Patients Maintain a Sense of Self

People who are acutely ill are often separated not only from their strengths, but also from any real sense of self. This occurs largely because, as patients in health care facilities, they are removed from their personal roles, environments, and belongings, and stripped of their individuality by staff caring for them. One patient, a college president who was recovering from serious complications after surgery for ovarian cancer, shared the following:

> When I first got sick, it didn't matter how people treated me because I knew who I was. As I've grown sicker and weaker, I become whatever people make me. If a nurse walks in here and moves me like meat, I become a slab of meat. My sense of self seems more and more dependent on how people respond to me.

Help patients maintain a sense of self and worth by doing the following:

- Use looks, speech, and judicious touch to communicate worth.
- Acknowledge the patient's status, roles, individuality.
- Speak to the patient respectfully and in a nonpatronizing manner.
- Converse with the patient about the patient's life experience.
- Address the patient by preferred name whenever entering the patient's room.
- Offer the patient a simple explanation before initiating any procedure.
- Move the patient's body respectfully if the patient is unable to do this.
- Respect the patient's privacy and sensibilities.
- Acknowledge and allow expression of negative feelings.
- Help the patient to recognize strengths and explore alternatives.

QSEN PATIENT-CENTERED CARE

You can help patients by respecting them and encouraging them to express their values, preferences, and expressed needs. This enables you to communicate patient values, preferences, and expressed needs to other members of the health care team.

Always keep in mind that patients are *people*, first and foremost. See Through the Eyes of a Nurse. A person's illness does not define who that person is. Too often, health care professionals tend to focus primarily on a patient's illness, and the whole person is forgotten or ignored, with potential negative consequences for that patient's sense of self, such as lack of motivation to learn or execute important health care behaviors. The way nurses care for patients can directly affect self-concept; self-concept, in turn, directly affects health. Thoughtful person-centered nursing care does not require additional nursing time or energy. It does require from the nurse continual reaffirmation that nursing is a thoughtful, person-centered profession, and that nothing is more important at any moment of a nurse's workday than the person being served. Be sure to check out Box 47-2, Steps for being a healing presence, in the chapter on Spirituality.

Teaching Self-Compassion

Self-compassion is a powerful tool that nurses can use for themselves and for patients. When we see others who are suffering and feel their plight, when we are moved by the suffering of others and want to respond in a helpful way, we are being compassionate.

Nurse Self-Care Alert

Self-compassion scholar Dr. Kristin Neff writes that **self-compassion** involves acting the same way toward yourself when you are having a difficult time, fail, or notice something you don't like about yourself. "Instead of just ignoring your pain with a 'stiff upper lip' mentality, you stop and tell yourself, 'this is really difficult right now; how can I comfort and care for myself in this moment?'" Instead of mercilessly judging and criticizing yourself for various inadequacies or shortcoming, self-compassion means you are kind and understanding when confronted with personal failings—after all, who ever said you were supposed to be perfect?"

Through the Eyes of a Nurse

Picture Those You Love

Over the course of my nursing career, I've seen many different approaches used to instill a focus on improving patient satisfaction, some far better than others. I just experienced what was, for me, the best one yet. Our speaker asked all attendees to take out their cell phones and find a picture of a loved one. She then asked participants to partner with someone else and, in turn, tell each other about their loved ones.

Knowing the session topic was on patient experience, many of us had a sense of foreboding about what might happen next. The speaker smiled and reminded us that every person we contact in health care is pictured in someone's cell phone or wallet. She simply suggested that we keep in mind the feeling we have for those *we* love when we encounter others.

In our health care world, we often erect walls around our hearts to enable enough professional distance to keep us focused and objective despite difficult or tragic circumstances. Those walls are a survival strategy. They reduce our vulnerability to emotional pain from constantly being immersed in situations that those outside of health care can hardly fathom. Much like scar tissue, however, the walls can become too thick.

Each of whom has had the unfortunate experience of being on the other side of the bed rails, whether as a patient or as a family member, wants to feel a caring connection. Our patients do, too. We can't lose sight of that. Distance and vulnerability are on two different ends of the caring spectrum. We each need to find a balance that doesn't exclude patients. When in doubt, consider whose picture is on your cell phone.

—Linda Laskowski-Jones, Christiana Care Health System

Source: Used with permission. Laskowski-Jones, L. (2018). Picture those you love. *Nursing, 48*(2), 6.

You may want to try out the official self-compassion website (http://self-compassion.org) for helpful self-compassion practices (guided meditations and exercises).

Modifying a Negative Self-Concept

The time is ripe for change when a patient realizes that a negative self-concept is hindering personal development related to health and wellness care. One option is using a cognitive-behavioral approach to assist the patient in modifying self-concept. The general principle is to help the patient alter their perspective of a situation from a more negative view to a more positive view, a process known as "reframing." Once a person can view their situation more positively, a wider variety of behavioral options, coping mechanisms, or internal or external supports can be identified and activated. While any person's self-concept is usually firmly entrenched and naturally resists change, you should remain optimistic that change is possible, if even in small increments. Helpful nursing interventions include the following:

- Help the patient identify and describe in detail how the patient thinks and feels about situations related to self-concept. Identify the patient's faulty thinking patterns.
- Explore with the patient alternative ways of viewing the same situation—that is, reframe the patient's thinking about the situation.
- Teach the patient to "red flag" faulty thinking behavior as soon as the patient is aware of it. The goal is to replace the negative thinking and self-talk with thinking and self-talk that will develop a more positive self-image.
- Help the patient explore the positive dimensions of the self that the patient wishes to develop, and incorporate this new knowledge into the self-concept.

Developing a Positive Body Image

Interventions for body image disturbances vary according to the nature of the disturbance. Interventions may include a combination of the following:

- Express interest in and acceptance of the patient through verbal and nonverbal expression. Allow the patient to share their feelings openly. Sitting quietly by the patient for a few minutes, with a few words such as, "How are things?" or "Tell me what's going on with you" communicates to the patient your willingness and readiness to share the patient's experience.
- Explore with the patient their feelings about altered body image and the patient's perceptions about the meaning and consequences of such alteration.
- Support the patient through the various stages of loss, grief, and mourning (shock, disbelief, denial, anger, guilt, acceptance), remembering that there is no one right way to proceed through these stages. Rather, patients may move fluidly in and out of various stages, sometimes returning to earlier stages. Some patients may need to learn that it is okay to cry, to be angry, or to feel depressed.
- Use play therapy with children so that they can describe their feelings and work through their grief using the nonthreatening medium of dolls or animals.
- Use self-reflection to gain awareness of your attitudes and feelings toward the patient. Be careful not to let facial expressions, words, or body positioning communicate to the patient disgust, fear, or rejection.
- While communicating support to the patient who is slow to develop and use appropriate self-care behaviors, firmly insist that the patient participate in their care to the extent that the patient is able. Whenever possible, provide the patient with honest answers to questions or put the patient in touch with the appropriate person to give the answers.
- Strengthen the patient's decision-making ability by honestly exploring alternatives; help the patient to imagine living with the consequences of different courses of action.
- Reinforce the patient's personal strengths and help the patient and family to identify all possible resources.
- Assess the response of the patient's significant others and intervene if they negatively influence the patient.

Developing Self-Esteem in Children and Adolescents

Nurses who work in practice settings where they have access to groups of parents, adult caregivers, or teachers can offer specific guidelines for creating developmental environments that build high self-esteem. Box 42-3 (on page 1754) offers five strategies for building self-esteem in children. Because some parents and educators may not have experienced these aids to personal growth themselves, it is beneficial to role-model these behaviors when interacting with children.

Important learning tasks for children include understanding and accepting themselves, their feelings, and others; independence; goals and purposeful behavior; mastery, competence, and resourcefulness; emotional maturity; and choices and consequences.

Enhancing Self-Esteem in Older Adults

The many losses associated with aging (e.g., diminished strength and physical health, interpersonal losses, retirement, shrinking income) make older adults especially vulnerable to disturbances in self-concept, particularly chronic low self-esteem. Society's generally negative view of aging compounds the problem. When interacting with older adults, employ the following interventions to enhance and maintain self-esteem in this population:

- Identify your own attitudes and feelings about aging and older adults.
- Address seniors respectfully, communicating that you take their concerns seriously.
- Respect and affirm seniors' intellect, individuality, personal strengths, culture, and spirituality.
- Adjust your communication style to accommodate any sensory or cognitive deficits.
- Encourage sharing of life experiences.
- Assist the person to identify strengths and coping mechanisms to deal with problems.

Box 42-3 Building Self-Esteem in Children

Strategy 1: Looking at the Positive and the Negative

Instruct parents to write an honest description of their child for a stranger. Next, have the parents underline the child's positive and negative qualities.

To reinforce the positive qualities, encourage the parents to (1) notice examples of ability in many different circumstances and point this out to the child; (2) find occasions to frequently and honestly praise the child; and (3) give the child frequent opportunities to show their abilities.

To address the negative qualities constructively, have the parents ask themselves: (1) What need is being expressed by this behavior? (2) Can I see a positive quality being expressed by this behavior? (3) How can I help my child express this quality and meet their needs in a more positive way?

Advise the parents to reexamine the list of negative qualities and ignore those that are merely a matter of taste, preference, or personal style—and not really negative in a harmful manner.

Strategy 2: Listening

The following guidelines can help parents use listening to communicate to a child, "You are important. What you say matters to me. You matter to me."

1. Make sure that you are ready to listen.
2. Give your child your full attention.
3. Minimize distractions.
4. Be an active listener.
5. Invite your child to talk.

Listen for the point of a child's story: "What is she trying to tell me? Why is this important to him?" Don't feel that you have to fix things. Listen for and respond to the feelings.

Strategy 3: Using the Language of Self-Esteem

The following concepts may help parents understand how to use language that builds self-esteem:

Feedback that enhances self-esteem has three components: (1) a description of the behavior (describe the behavior without judging it); (2) your reaction to the behavior (language that shares something about yourself); and (3) acknowledgment of the child's feelings. For example: "Thanks for playing with your brother tonight [*description*]. I was wondering how I was going to pay attention to our guests if he got fussy and was really grateful when I noticed that you kept him occupied and happy [*reaction*]. I know that there were other things you might have enjoyed doing more [*acknowledgment*]."

To give correction using the language of self-esteem, (1) describe the problematic behavior, (2) state a reason for the behavior change, (3) acknowledge the child's feelings, and (4) offer a clear statement of what is expected.

- *Attacking communications:* "Don't let me ever hear you talk that way to your mother again."
- *Language of self-esteem:* "I overheard you telling your mom that she should 'Get a life and get off your case.' (*description*). When you talk like that it just makes people angry or sad, which isn't very helpful (*reason for behavior change*). You probably feel like you are being picked on, and we may have some expectations that are different from those of your friends' parents. I hope you know that this is because we love you and want the best for you [*acknowledgment*]. In the future, try to talk to others with the same respect you'd like others to show you [*statement of expectation*]."

Avoid using the following destructive language styles, which tear down self-esteem: overgeneralizations ("You *never* come home on time!"), the silent treatment, and vague or violent threats.

Strategy 4: Helping Children Meet Expectations

To help children meet expectations, advise parents as follows: (1) Be sure that your expectations are reasonable and appropriate for your child's age. (2) Plan ahead. (3) Be clear about your expectations. (4) Focus on the positive. (5) Provide choices when possible. (6) Provide rewards.

Strategy 5: Promoting a Feeling of Success

To help children have the courage to try new types of experiences, which results from successfully meeting challenges, advise parents to (1) let a child know what to expect; (2) let your child practice the necessary skills; (3) be patient; and (4) make it safe to fail.

Source: Republished with permission of New Harbinger Publications; from McKay, M., & Fanning, P. (2016). *Self-esteem: A proven program of cognitive techniques for assessing, improving, and maintaining your self esteem* (4th ed.). New Harbinger Publications; permission conveyed through Copyright Clearance Center, Inc.

- Provide a safe environment for older adults to communicate such concerns as interpersonal or physical loss, feelings about illness and death, sexuality, or financial issues.
- Advocate for seniors needing help in attaining services necessary to meet their health care needs.
- Explore the personal meaning of dependency for the person, and help seniors adapt both physically and emotionally to any necessary dependency.

The Focus on the Older Adult box describes nursing interventions to promote self-esteem in older adults.

Evaluating

Nurses who are sensitive to the relationship between self-concept and general well-being consistently evaluate the effect the nursing care plan has on the patient's self-concept. When the care plan includes specific interventions to assist patients with disturbances in body image, self-esteem, role performance, and personal identity, listen carefully to the patient's self-report and observe patient behaviors to see if the disturbances are being resolved. Basically, the patient should be able to meet the following outcomes:

- Is comfortable with body image and able to use it effectively to meet human needs
- Is able to describe self positively
- Is able to meet realistic role expectations without undue anxiety and fatigue
- Is capable of interacting appropriately with environment while recognizing self to be a separate and distinct entity

See the accompanying Nursing Care Plan 42-1 on pages 1756–1758, for Ms. Motsky.

Focus on the Older Adult

PROMOTING SELF-ESTEEM IN OLDER ADULTS

Area of Concern	Nursing Strategies
Personal identity	• When an older adult's sense of self is threatened, assist the person to find meaning in the experience, to regain mastery to the extent that this is possible, and to evaluate realistically the adequacy of the person's coping strategy. • Teach older adults to identify and develop a game plan for confronting anxiety-producing situations. • Help to identify and secure intervention for treatable depressions. • Treat causes of self-identity disturbances such as pain, abusive living arrangements, and substance abuse.
Body image	• Notice and affirm positive physiologic characteristics of older adults. • Teach preventive self-care measures that reduce discomforting signs of aging (e.g., exercise, which maintains muscle mass and joint flexibility; proper nutrition; basic hygiene and skin care measures). • Explore new activities (including hobbies) that are within the changing physical capabilities of the older adult.
Self-Esteem	• Assist older adults to identify and use personal strengths. • Communicate that you value older adults simply for who they are (unconditional affirmation); know and use the name they prefer; ask them questions about their life, interests, or values. • Reinforce loving relationships, "It's obvious your son and grandchildren love you." "You must be a VIP—look at these flowers!" • When appropriate, use the expertise of older adults and ask their advice; let them know you value their life experiences. • Engage older adults in activities in which they can be successful. • Allow older adults to make tough decisions and confront challenging situations when appropriate; teach protective family members the value of older adults confronting situations that invite continued growth. • Empower older adults to meet their own needs; provide necessary knowledge, teach new behaviors, instill the belief that they "can manage."
Role performance	• Explore with older adults the many roles they have fulfilled throughout their lifetime; invite reminiscences. • Facilitate grieving over valued roles that can no longer be performed. • Remedy, whenever possible, factors that prevent older adults from engaging in valued roles. • Explore new roles.

REFLECTIVE PRACTICE LEADING TO PERSONAL LEARNING

Remember that the object of reflective practice is to look at an experience, understand it, and learn from it. As you begin to develop your expertise in identifying and responding to self-concept needs, reflect on your experiences—both successes and failures—in order to improve your practice. We all need to feel good about ourselves, but a healthy self-concept may take real work.

- Have you encountered patients or their family/caregivers whose self-concept and self-esteem needs are unmet? If you identified such needs, did you feel confident and comfortable responding to these needs?
- Have your care plans ever identified and addressed self-concept needs? Did your presence communicate respect and affirmation to each person you encountered today?
- Are you aware of any subtle messages you may be sending others that diminishes or violates their sense of worth? This may be a good time for some personal reflection about your own self-concept and self-esteem. Clinical practice challenges all of us, and some people are good at "pushing our buttons" and making us feel inadequate. How do you respond when this happens?

Perhaps the most important questions to reflect on are: Are your patients and their families/caregivers better for having had *you* share in the critical responsibility of partnering with them to nurture self-concept? Are your patients now receiving thoughtful, person-centered, prioritized, holistic, evidence-based treatment and care because of your efforts?"

Nursing Care Plan for *Melissa Motsky* 42-1

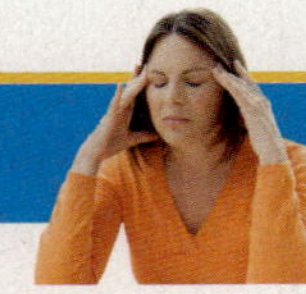

PATIENT CARE STUDY

Melissa Motsky is a 31-year-old married woman, mother of three children (ages 12, 10, and 8 years), and junior-level nursing student. She works every other weekend as a nurse's aide. She has just received a letter from the nursing division head informing her that she is in academic jeopardy and will fail out of the program unless her grades improve. She presents this to her adviser.

After talking with Ms. Motsky, who calls herself "a failure" and who cries as she describes her situation at home, her faculty adviser suspects a serious self-esteem problem, and helps her to list factors contributing to her current sense of failure and low self-esteem. The following list is generated:

SIGNIFICANCE

– Receives little understanding, affection, approval from husband. "I stay with him because of the kids. I started back to school because I had to get out of the house and want to make something of myself. He doesn't understand this."

+ "The children are very supportive but get impatient when I have to study and can't spend time with them."

– Feels a failure in all the roles that are important to her—wife, mother, and, now, student. "I jeopardized everything to go back to school—if I fail, it's all over for me. There just isn't enough time or energy to do anything well."

+ "They do love me at work, though, which makes me feel like nursing is what I should be doing."

VIRTUE

– "I've always believed that hard work pays off, and that if you were faithful to your duty you'd be rewarded by the good life—I'm beginning to doubt that. Maybe I'm a fool for trying so hard."

+ "I do still try to live according to my beliefs and feel okay about this. I treat others as I'd like to be treated."

POWER

– "I always believed I could do anything I put my heart and soul into. But I can't seem to change my marriage, and if I fail out of school, that will be the end of all my dreams."

Key indicators of low self-esteem that also surfaced in the interview include overeating (10-lb weight gain during the past year), difficulty sleeping, fatigue, new sensitivity to criticism, and expressions of feeling unloved, alone, and no longer able to manage. Personal strengths include history of "can do" mentality, high motivation to succeed, and past history of success as mother and nurse's aide.

ICNP NURSING DIAGNOSIS

Situational Low Self-Esteem related to decreased sense of significance, competence, virtue, and power; signs and symptoms: expressions of being a failure, powerlessness, fatigue, tears, weight gain, low academic performance (test grades 68, 74)

EXPECTED OUTCOME

By this time next month, 11/2/25, the patient will demonstrate increased self-esteem by:
- Expressing positive statements about herself

NURSING INTERVENTIONS	RATIONALE	EVALUATIVE STATEMENT
Assist the patient to rediscover her "own" personal strengths: identify personal qualities and strengths that have pleased her in the past and explore why this has changed; recommend that she make at least one positive statement about herself each morning and evening.	Patients can lose touch with their strengths, especially when multiple stressors seem to create impossible demands.	11/3/25 Outcome partially met. Patient's statements are of the "This is good, *but*…" variety. "I think I'm doing better in school but I don't know if it will continue." *Recommendation:* Continue to identify and reinforce personal strengths. *C. Taylor, RN*
Consistently interact with the patient as if she had the power to weather the crisis successfully (i.e., "will" strength to her). Role-model positive self-concept behaviors.	Once the patient senses that an authority believes in her power and expects her to use it, she may internalize this knowledge and act on it.	

EXPECTED OUTCOME

By this time next month, 11/2/25, the patient will demonstrate increased self-esteem by:
- Reporting ability to receive negative feedback without falling apart

Nursing Care Plan for *Melissa Motsky* 42-1 *(continued)*

NURSING INTERVENTIONS	RATIONALE	EVALUATIVE STATEMENT
Explore with the patient to what degree she allows the opinions of others to influence her self-concept.	Significance—sense of being loved and approved of by significant others—is a critical component of self-esteem.	11/3/25 Outcome partially met. Patient reports being able to handle everything except put-downs from her husband. *Recommendation:* Explore origin of power she has given to her husband to influence her sense of self and what she wants to do about this. *C. Taylor, RN*
Teach how self-concept filters life experiences; thus, if I feel that I am a failure, I may interpret the words and behaviors of others as confirming this, even though that was not their intention.	Principle of self-consistency: once I am down, I may reinforce this by distorting what I feel, hear, and experience.	
Explore with the patient ways she can enhance her self-concept independently of others (e.g., take time each day for herself). Encourage the patient to draw on personal strengths.	This facilitates internal locus of control versus external. Spending time on self communicates that self is valuable.	
Teach the patient how to analyze feedback constructively and respond appropriately; *cancel negative thinking.* For example, the patient receives care plan back with many corrections and the notation, "sloppy work." *Maladaptive response:* "She hates me. See, this proves I'll never be a good nurse. I wasted my time even doing this." *Adaptive response:* "I spent as much time as I had on this …now let me see what I did wrong. Maybe I should make an appointment with my instructor so she can show me how to improve."	It is important to break the cycle of negative thinking, which reinforces negative self-concept.	

EXPECTED OUTCOME By this time next month, 11/2/25, the patient will demonstrate increased self-esteem by:

- Getting a passing grade on her next quarterly examination

NURSING INTERVENTIONS	RATIONALE	EVALUATIVE STATEMENT
Explore study skills with the patient; recommend a study group.	Poor study skills may also be contributing to her low academic performance. A study group will meet both her social and academic needs.	11/3/25 Outcome met. Grade: 82 *C. Taylor, RN*
Discuss the importance of how she *perceives* present situation. If present failures are equated with *defeat,* she may be unable to mobilize her resources to succeed; if present failures represent *challenge,* it may call forth her best efforts and result in success.	The meaning given to present stressor can dramatically affect the patient's response to it and condition her for success or failure.	
Discuss the importance of breaking the cycle of failure leading to another failure.	If this short-term goal is met, it will set the stage for future successes and contribute to the patient's positive self-concept.	

EXPECTED OUTCOME By this time next month, 11/2/25, the patient will demonstrate increased self-esteem by:

- Verbalizing that the way she is living her life is okay

(continued on page 1758)

Nursing Care Plan for *Melissa Motsky* 42-1 *(continued)*

NURSING INTERVENTIONS	RATIONALE	EVALUATIVE STATEMENT
Assist the patient to examine her moral–ethical standards; explore sources of these standards and whether the patient feels comfortable with them.	Moral–ethical standards may be uncritically internalized and place the patient in conflict.	11/3/25 Outcome met. Patient stated: "I guess I'm living the best way I know how right now. If things are meant to be different, someone is going to have to show me how." *Recommendations:* Reinforce self-acceptance. *C. Taylor, RN*
Identify unrealistic standards; the patient may need "permission" to be human.	Unrealistic standards (perfectionism, conventionality) may constantly undermine the patient's self-esteem.	
Refer for counseling, if appropriate.	Support groups on campus (counseling centers, ministries) may be able to meet the patient's needs.	

EXPECTED OUTCOME

By this time next month, 11/2/25, the patient will demonstrate increased self-esteem by:

- Reporting two recent instances when personal power was effective in accomplishing desired goals

NURSING INTERVENTIONS	RATIONALE	EVALUATIVE STATEMENT
Identify and affirm the patient's use of personal power to accomplish goals.	A negative self-concept may deny or distort personal successes; outside intervention may be necessary to bring these to consciousness.	11/3/25 Outcome met . . . with difficulty. Needed considerable prompting to identify successful use of her personal power. Was ready to attribute passing grade to luck rather than her own efforts. *Recommendations:* Have patient make daily record of her use of personal power and results. *C. Taylor, RN*

SAMPLE DOCUMENTATION

10/2/25 Nursing

Melissa Motsky presented today after receiving academic jeopardy letter. She is strongly motivated to complete nursing program successfully and seems to have the ability to do this. Current multiple life stressors—lack of support from husband, need to mother three children (12, 10, 8), part-time nurse's aide job (necessary for financial reasons), and current academic jeopardy (test grades 68, 74)—are all contributing to her low self-esteem and overwhelming sense of being a failure. We together developed a care plan that it is hoped will help her to do better academically, as well as begin to feel better about herself. See attached. She will return 11/2/25 at 1000 for follow-up.

C. Taylor, RN

SOAP Format

10/2/25, 1230, Nursing

Academic jeopardy—Melissa Motsky

S: "I jeopardized everything to go back to school—if I fail, it's all over for me." Reports lack of support from husband, grief that she does not have enough time for children, failure of personal work ethic ("hard work pays off"), and sense of powerlessness.

O: Nursing II quarterly exam grades: 68, 74; weight gain of 10 lb during past year; facial and body expressions of fatigue, profuse tears

A: Low Self-Esteem related to decreased sense of significance, competence, virtue, and power

P: See attached care plan.

C. Taylor, RN

DEVELOPING CLINICAL REASONING AND CLINICAL JUDGMENT

1. Work through the Nursing Care Plan 42-1 for Melissa Motsky on pages 1756–1758 to help develop your clinical reasoning and clinical judgment skills.
2. The personal strengths a person recognizes, develops, and uses are powerful but subjective determinants of self-concept. Identify the strengths that have been major determinants of your self-concept (e.g., power, intelligence, physical attractiveness, goodness, humor, "can do" attitude), and explore how these help you to succeed in nursing. Discuss with another student ways that nurses can assist patients to recognize, develop, and use personal strengths to cope better with the stress of injury and illness.
3. Role-play with another student your responses to the following patients, then reverse roles. Reflect on the effects different types of nursing presence and response have on a patient's self-concept. Discuss the nursing responses that would be most helpful to patients at risk for self-concept disturbances.
   - A man who was recently passed over for a promotion states, "I can't believe I've got to deal with this ulcer. It's just one more thing holding me back from succeeding in this business."
   - An anorexic teenager tells you that she can't possibly eat the dinner you brought her, and states, "I can't do my usual workout in here, and look how fat I'm getting."
   - A middle-aged patient confides, "I need to talk with someone about how it feels to be a woman trapped in a man's body."
   - A woman, after mastectomy, refuses to look at the incision site, and notes, "If I can't bring myself to look at this, how can I ever expect my husband to want me again?"
   - Your patient confides that they lost their job during the pandemic, live in fear of being evicted because they can no longer pay the rent, knows their children are losing out because they have difficulty helping them with online classes, and hates that they can no longer afford the food and medicine they need. "What good am I?"
   - A resident in a long-term care facility says, "Don't trouble yourself about me. I'm sure you have lots of people to take care of who are more deserving of your time and attention."
4. What is your experience in relation to the self-concept and self-esteem of professional nurses? How does society affirm or challenge nursing's self-concept?
5. You are the school nurse for a large middle school, and are approached by the parents of a 7th-grade transgender student whose sex assigned at birth was male, but who identifies as a female and wants permission to use the female bathroom. How do you respond? What informs your response?
6. A young mother asks your opinions about parenting and the best way to develop their child's self-esteem. You know that "helicopter parenting"—a tendency to hover over children and swoop in to rescue them at the first sign of trouble—is producing higher rates of general anxiety in children. Children with overly controlling parents have higher levels of depression and report feeling less satisfied with family life. How do you respond to this mother, and what informs your response?

PRACTICING FOR NCLEX

1. A nurse is performing a psychological assessment of an adolescent patient who has Down syndrome with mild intellectual disability. The patient tells the nurse, "I'm a good helper. I can carry things because I'm strong, but I'm not real smart, so I help with things I know how to do." What findings for self-concept and self-esteem would the nurse document for this patient?
   a. Negative self-concept and low self-esteem
   b. Negative self-concept and high self-esteem
   c. Positive self-concept and fairly high self-esteem
   d. Positive self-concept and low self-esteem
2. A nurse asks a 25-year-old patient to describe themself with a list of 20 words. After 15 minutes, the patient listed, "25 years old, male, named Joe," then declared he could not think of anything else. What should the nurse document regarding this patient?
   a. This patient presents with lack of self-esteem.
   b. The patient does not possess self-knowledge.
   c. This person has unrealistic expectations of themselves.
   d. There is an inability to evaluate himself realistically.
3. A nurse asks a patient who has few descriptors of themselves to list facts, traits, or qualities that they would like to apply to themselves. The patient quickly lists 25 traits of a successful person, stating, "My father is like this; I wish I were like him." How does the nurse best interpret the discrepancy between the patient's description of themselves as they are and how they would like to be seen?
   a. The patient suffers from a negative self-concept.
   b. This person demonstrates modesty (lack of conceit).
   c. This individual has a disturbed body image.
   d. The patient likely has a low self-esteem.
4. A nurse is counseling a couple who have decided that the wife will provide financial support for the family while the husband attends pharmacy school. The husband plans to work 16 hours weekly, while attending school and states, "I was always an A student, but I might have to settle for Bs now because I don't want to neglect my family." How would the nurse document the husband's self-expectations?
   a. Realistic and positively motivating their development
   b. Unrealistic and negatively motivating their development
   c. Unrealistic but positively motivating their development
   d. Realistic but negatively motivating their development

5. A school nurse is teaching parents how to foster a healthy development of self in their children. Which statement made by one of the parents requires further teaching?
   a. "I love my child so much I 'hug him to death' every day."
   b. "I think children need challenges, don't you?"
   c. "My partner and I grew up in restrictive families; we want our children to be free to do whatever they want."
   d. "We have different ideas about discipline, but we've continued our discussions so we can be consistent."
6. A mother of an outspoken school-aged child tells the nurse: "I feel incompetent as a parent and have difficulty disciplining my child." What should be the nurse's first action when counseling this patient?
   a. Recommending that she discipline her child more strictly and consistently
   b. Making a "to-do" list for the child's father to allow her more time to focus on improving her parenting skills
   c. Assisting the mother to identify both what she thinks is successful and what she can do to improve
   d. Exploring how the child can improve their behavior and make the mother's role as a parent easier
7. A nurse is conducting a parent workshop on how to build self-esteem in children. Which teaching points would the nurse include to help parents achieve this goal? Select all that apply.
   a. Reinforce their child's positive qualities.
   b. Overlook occasional negative behavior.
   c. Ignore neutral behavior that is a matter of personal preference.
   d. Listen and "fix things" for their children.
   e. Describe the child's behavior and judge it.
   f. Let their children practice skills and make it safe to fail.
8. A nurse practicing in a health clinic assesses patient's self-concept during the patient intake. Which of these patients would the nurse identify has risk for problems related to self-concept?
   a. Older adult scheduled for a hysterectomy next week
   b. Young adult pastor whose vocal cords were paralyzed after a surgical procedure
   c. Young accountant who survives a heart attack and near-death experience
   d. Model who just learned that they have breast cancer
   e. Adolescent recovering from a spinal cord injury who will be wheelchair "mobile"
9. A patient who has been in the United States only 3 months has recently suffered the loss of partner and job. They state that nothing feels familiar—"I don't know who I am supposed to be here"—and says "I miss home terribly." For what alteration in self-concept is this patient most at risk?
   a. Disturbed (or Risk for Disturbed) Personal Identity
   b. Disturbed Body Image
   c. Chronic (or Risk for Chronic) Low Self-Esteem or Situational (or Risk for Situational) Low Self-Esteem
   d. Impaired Role Performance
10. A sophomore in high school has missed a great deal of school due to treatment of leukemia. They stated they feel that they are falling behind in everything, and miss "hanging out at the mall" with friends most of all. What statement by the nurse is most appropriate?
   a. "It sounds like you don't know who you are anymore..."
   b. "Have the changes in your body since your diagnosis affected you?"
   c. "How are you viewing yourself these days?"
   d. "This must be difficult as adolescents' friends are very important to them."
11. A college student visits the health clinic for a refill of a prescription for acne medication. In response to the nurse's question about how her semester is going the student bursts into tears and cries, "No one will ever ask me out on a date. I just want to be thin and pretty like the other girls." What response by the nurse could promote the student's examination of their self-esteem?
   a. "You seem to have a negative body image and poor self-esteem."
   b. "What are some things you'd like to change about your body."
   c. "Most college students want to fit in; tell me what you enjoy doing."
   d. "You are quite pretty and have a lovely figure."
12. A young adult businessperson attends counseling, attempting to deal with a history of sexual abuse by their father. "I should feel satisfied with what I've achieved, but nothing I accomplish makes me feel good about myself. . . . I hate my father for making me feel like I'm no good. This is an awful way to live." What statement by the nurse would be most helpful?
   a. "You've managed to overcome a lot since your childhood."
   b. "Can you identify some positive attributes about yourself."
   c. "Perhaps it's time to accept you're an adult and the abuse is in the past."
   d. "What might make you feel more content? Go after it!"
13. A patient is admitted through the emergency department with severe facial burns and cuts to the face after a car accident in in which their fiancé was the driver. Three weeks later, their fiancé has not yet contacted them. The patient states that they are too tired to have visitors anyway and frequently lies with their eyes closed and head turned away. Based on this information, what action would the nurse take first?
   a. Identify a disturbance in self-concept.
   b. Question the patient about disturbances of body image.

c. Ask the patient how the accident has affected her.
d. Explain that the wounds are healing well, but she can consult a plastic surgeon after discharge if needed.

14. A nurse is providing care for a patient with cancer who is approaching the end of life. Which nursing interventions will the nurse use to help the patient to maintain a positive sense of self? Select all that apply.
   a. Making a point to address the patient by name upon entering the room
   b. Avoiding fatiguing the patient by performing all procedures in silence
   c. Performing care in a manner that respects the patient's privacy and preferences
   d. Offering the patient a simple explanation before moving them in any way
   e. Ignoring the patient's negative feelings since they are part of the grieving process
   f. Avoiding conversing with the patient about their life, family, and occupation

15. An older adult patient has a health problem of Disturbed Body Image documented on their care plan. The nurse discovers that patient feels they look old and feeble when ambulating with an assistive device often walking without it. The patient has fallen several times. What is an appropriate goal for this patient?
   a. The patient will state the need to use the assistive device both inside and outside the house.
   b. The patient will demonstrate proper use of the assistive device as observed by the nurse and physical therapist.
   c. The patient will discuss their feelings about the device and compare that with the need for safety.
   d. The patient will be given a wheelchair for mobility, as it is safer.

16. A school nurse is meeting with the parent of a child who stated the child's other parent has been given a lengthy prison sentence. Which action by the nurse would be most helpful to mitigate an adverse child experience?
   a. Assessing the student's grades and ability to complete class work
   b. Suggesting a mentoring program for children of incarcerated parents
   c. Asking the parent to tell you what happened
   d. Suggesting the parent help the child identify their strengths

ANSWERS WITH RATIONALES

1. **c.** The data point to the patient's positive self-concept ("I'm a good helper") and fairly high self-esteem (realizes their strengths and limitations). Stating, "But I'm not really smart" is likely accurate compared to non-disable peers and is not an indication of a negative self-concept.

2. **b.** The patient's inability to list more than three items about themselves indicates deficient self-knowledge and lack of familiarity with their own qualities and traits. There is insufficient data to determine whether they lack self-esteem, have unrealistic self-expectations, or are unable to evaluate themselves.

3. **d.** The nurse can obtain a quick indication of a patient's self-esteem by using a graphic description of self-esteem as the discrepancy between the "real self" (what we think we really are) and the "ideal self" (what we think we would like to be). The greater the discrepancy, the lower the self-esteem; the smaller the discrepancy, the higher the self-esteem.

4. **a.** The patient's self-expectations are realistic, given their multiple commitments, and seem to be positively motivating their self-development.

5. **c.** Each option with the exception of c correctly addresses some aspect of fostering healthy development in children. Because children need effective structure and development, giving them total freedom to do as they please may actually hinder their development.

6. **c.** The nurse assesses the issue first, helping the mother identify what they believe is working and what is preventing them from being an effective parent. Next the nurse can explore solutions aimed at improving their parenting skills. Without assessment, there is no indication the child needs more strict discipline or assistance of the father. The child is not responsible for making the mother's parental role easier.

7. **a, c, f.** The nurse should include the following teaching points for parents: (1) reinforce their child's positive qualities; (2) address negative qualities constructively; (3) ignore neutral behavior that is a matter of taste, preference, or personal style. Parents should allow children to be challenged or fail, rather than "fix things" for their children; avoid judgmental observations and let their child know what to expect, practice the necessary skills, be patient, and make it safe to fail.

8. **b, c, d, e.** Based on the data, those who are at risk for negative self-concept include the pastor who will face challenges without his voice, the survivor of the near-death experience, and the model, whose work and livelihood depends on their physical appearance. The older adult would be least likely to experience body image or role performance disturbance because they are beyond childbearing years, and the surgery should not impair their functional ability. The young clergyperson's inability to preach, the 32-year-old's massive myocardial infarction, and the model's breast resection have much greater potential to result in self-concept problems.

9. **a.** An unfamiliar culture, coupled with traumatic life events such as loss of husband and job, result in this patient's total loss of their sense of self, supported by the statement: "I don't know who I am supposed to be here."

10. **d.** Important roles for this adolescent include student and a friend; the illness is preventing them from doing either of these well, which reflects a disturbance in role performance. Stating that it sounds like you don't know who you are anymore is a question related to personal identity disturbance; asking about changes in the body would relate to disturbed body image; asking how are you viewing yourself these days relates to self-esteem disturbance.

11. **b.** This patient is likely expressing concern with body image and self-esteem. The nurse seeks further information to support this, rather than suggesting the student has a negative

body image or glossing over the student's concern and offering their opinion about the student's appearance or suggesting that their body needs changing. The nurse identifies the etiology of the student's concern, needing to fit in and be desired.

12. **d.** This patient's self-concept disturbance is mainly one of devaluing themselves and thinking that they are no good. The nurse assists the patient in reframing their negative thoughts into positive thoughts.

13. **c.** The nurse first assesses the patient's response to the accident before documenting a health problem and etiology. The nurse takes cues from the patient regarding their traumatic injuries, their fiancé's failure to contact them, and their withdrawal, which point to potential problems with both body image and self-esteem. The burn/trauma team would likely recommend plastic surgery, if indicated.

14. **a, c, d.** Interventions to assist the patient to maintain a positive sense of self include addressing the patient by name when entering the room; performing care in a manner that respects the patient's privacy; offering simple explanations before moving the patient; acknowledging the patient's status, role, and individuality; and conversing with the patient about the patient's life experiences.

15. **b.** The patient is demonstrating a maladaptive response. Patients who deny and avoid dealing with limitations or deformity, engage in self-destructive behavior, or fail to estimate relationship of body to environment are experiencing a disturbed self-concept. The patient will need to grieve the loss of mobility as they age as well as realize that safety is a priority to prevent injury. The other interventions focus on the negative without helping the patient reframe the situation or allowing the patient to discuss their feelings.

16. **b.** Factors that can mitigate adverse child experiences include strengthening economic support to families; promoting social norms that protect against violence and adversity; and ensuring a strong start for children including support groups, mentoring, and teaching needed skills.

Bibliography

Aguilera, D. C. (1998). *Crisis intervention: Theory and methodology* (8th ed.). Elsevier/Mosby.

Baldwin, D., & Parsh, B. (2020). Assessing self-image in patients with type 1 diabetes. *Nursing 2020, 50*(3), 13–14.

Bowlby, J. (1969). *Attachment and loss: Vol I: Attachment* (2nd ed.). Basic Books.

Brene Brown on Empathy. https://www.youtube.com/watch?v=1Evwgu369Jw

Centers for Disease Control and Prevention. (April 2, 2020). *Preventing adverse childhood experiences*. https://www.cdc.gov/violenceprevention/aces/fastfact.html?CDC_AA_refVal=https%3A%2F%2Fwww.cdc.gov%2Fviolenceprevention%2Facestudy%2Ffastfact.html

Cleveland Clinic's Empathy Videos. (2013). *Empathy: The human connection to patient care*. Published on February 27, 2013. https://www.youtube.com/watch?v=dYhpxn81xus

Coopersmith, S. (1967). *The antecedents of self-esteem*. Freeman.

Freud, S. (1961). The ego and the id. In J. Strachey (Ed.). *The standard edition of the complete psychological works of Sigmund Freud* (Vol. *XIX*, pp. 3–63). The Hogarth Press.

International Council of Nurses. (2017). *Nursing diagnosis and outcome statements*. International Classification for Nursing Practice (ICNP) Catalogue. https://www.icn.ch/sites/default/files/inline-files/icnp2017-dc.pdf

LeMone, P. (1991). Analysis of a human phenomenon: Self concept. *Nursing Diagnosis, 2*(3), 126–130.

Maslow, A. (1954.) *Motivation and personality*. Harper & Row.

Mayo Clinic. (2020a). *Range of self-esteem*. http://www.mayoclinic.org/healthy-lifestyle/adult-health/in-depth/self-esteem/art-20047976?pg=2

Mayo Clinic. (2020b). *Self-esteem: Take steps to feel better about yourself*. https://www.mayoclinic.org/healthy-lifestyle/adult-health/in-depth/self-esteem/art-20045374?pg=1

McKay, M., & Fanning, P. (2016). *Self-esteem* (4th ed.). New Harbinger Publications.

Metzler, M., Merrick, M. T., Klevens, J., Ports, K. A., & Ford, D. C. (2017). Adverse childhood experiences and life opportunities: Shifting the narrative. *Children and Youth Services Review, 72*, 141–149.

Neff, K. D. & Germer, C. (2017). *Self compassion and psychological wellbeing*. In J. Doty (Ed.), Oxford Handbook of Compassion Science.

Neff, K. D., & Germer, C. (2019). *The mindful self-compassion workbook*.

Peplau, H. E. (1952). *Interpersonal relations in nursing*. G. P. Putnam & Sons.

Peplau, H. E. (1997). Peplau's theory of interpersonal relations. *Nursing Science Quarterly, 10*(4), 162–167.

Stuart, G. W. (2013). *Principles and practice of psychiatric nursing* (10th ed.). Elsevier/Mosby.

Sullivan, H. S. (1953). *The interpersonal theory of psychiatry*. W. W. Norton & Co.

Zimmerman, E. (June 21, 2020). *Build your resilience toolbox*. The New York Times.

43 Stress and Adaptation

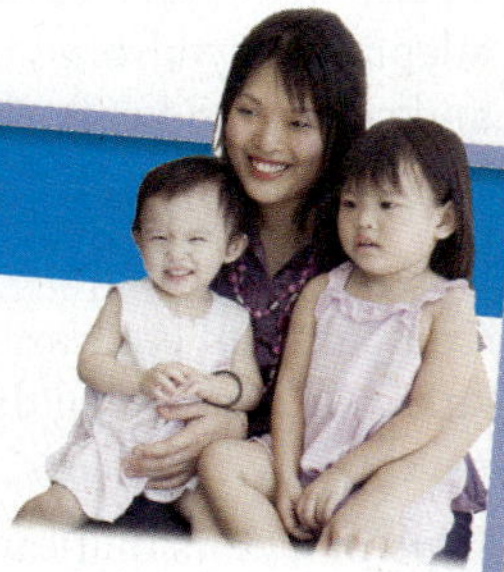

Mei Fu

Mei Fu is a 24-year-old graduate student. She is married, has two small children, and is taking courses toward a degree in physical therapy. Her husband is also a graduate student. Although she lived in China until 3 years ago, she speaks English well. After several months of headaches and diarrhea, Mei Fu made an appointment at the student health clinic.

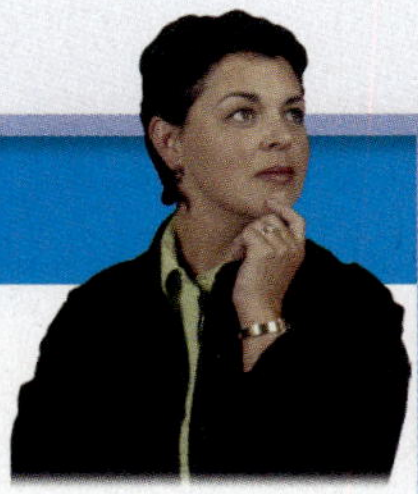

Joan Rogerrio

Joan, a 48-year-old woman with a history of inflammatory bowel disease, comes to the outpatient clinic with reports of increasing episodes of diarrhea. She says, “I think my bowel disease is flaring up again.” Further assessment reveals she started a new job a month ago after being out of the workforce for the past 15 years. “Since the children are in school most of the day, my spouse and I decided it was time for me to go back to work to help out financially,” she says.

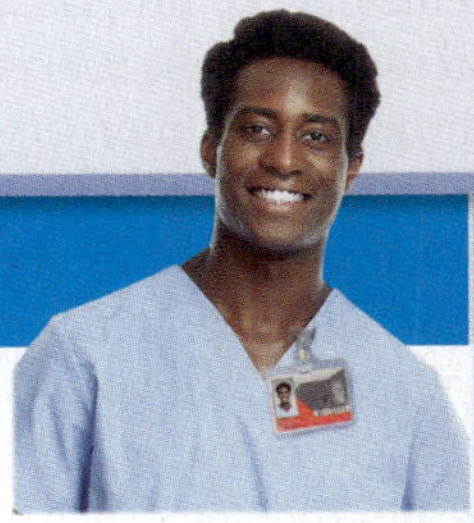

Christopher Weiss

Christopher, a nursing student, comes to the student health center saying that he feels sick. He states, “I'm supposed to start my critical care rotation tomorrow, and I'm terrified not only of the tubes and machines, but also of my instructor. I had her for my health assessment class, and it was really a disaster. I feel sick, and I am just shaking all over.”

Learning Outcomes

After completing the chapter, you will be able to accomplish the following:

1. Summarize the mechanisms involved in maintaining physiologic and psychological homeostasis.
2. Explain the interdependent nature of stressors, stress, and adaptation.
3. Differentiate the physical and emotional responses to stress, including local adaptation syndrome, general adaptation syndrome, mind–body interaction, anxiety, and coping and defense mechanisms.
4. Discuss the effects of short- and long-term stress on basic human needs, health and illness, and the family.
5. Compare and contrast developmental and situational stress, incorporating the concepts of physiologic and psychosocial stressors.
6. Explain factors that cause stress in the nursing profession.
7. Integrate knowledge of healthy lifestyle, support systems, stress management techniques, and crisis intervention into hospital- and community-based care.

Nursing Concepts

- Anxiety
- Mood and Affect
- Stress and Coping

Stress—a word taken from the term *distress*—is a part of life: Everyone feels stress at one time or another. Books and magazines are full of articles about stress that discuss everything from the stressful effects of performing your job to the positive (or negative) stress of holidays. Television and online advertisements for over-the-counter remedies promise fast relief from stress headaches and upset stomachs. Stress is blamed for obesity, drug and alcohol use, divorce, and interpersonal violence. Feeling *stressed out* is common and taking *stress breaks* to do physical exercise is recommended in many work settings. Nursing emphasizes self-care, well-being, mental health, and building resilience (American Nurses Association, n.d.). With stress such a part of everyday life, it is easy to see that an additional health problem, such as an illness or injury, can increase the physical and psychological effects of stress. However, keep in mind that not all stress is negative. *Eustress* (Selye, 1976) is the term used for short-term stress that promotes positive emotional, intellectual, and physiologic adaptation and development.

The experience of stress and the responses to it are unique to each person. The process of responding to stress is constant and dynamic, and is essential to a person's physical, emotional, and social well-being. Stress is a major factor in health and illness. Nurses need to understand the concepts and levels of stress when providing nursing care to patients in all settings. Nurses themselves are subject to stress from the demands of their career and need to know healthy ways of responding (see the Reflective Practice display for an example).

BASIC CONCEPTS OF STRESS AND ADAPTATION

The basic concepts of stress and adaptation include stress, stressors, adaptation, and homeostasis.

Stress

Stress is a condition in which the human system responds to changes in its normal balanced state. Stress results from a change in a person's internal or external environment that is perceived as a challenge, a threat, or a danger. The major sources of stress in our society arise from interpersonal relationships and performance demands rather than from actual physical threats (Murdaugh et al., 2019). Stress is a part of the everyday human experience and our responses to stress shape who we are as people. Stress affects the whole person in all the human dimensions (physical, emotional, intellectual, social, spiritual) positively and negatively.

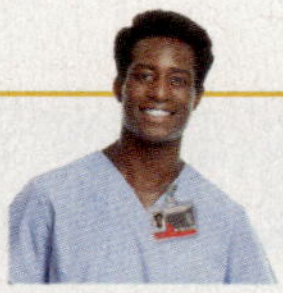

Think back to **Christopher Weiss,** the nursing student who reports feeling ill. He admitted feeling overwhelmed and extremely anxious about his upcoming critical care clinical rotation. His stressors included lack of confidence in manipulating the equipment and machines of the unit, and the demands that might be placed on him by the instructor. As a result, he exhibited physiologic responses to these stressors. These stressors could also affect his ability to function intellectually and socially.

The perception of stress and the responses to it are highly individualized. Responses vary not only from person to person, but also within a person depending on the specific circumstances, established coping mechanisms, available resources, and timing of the stress in that person's life. In addition, each person's perception of and responses to stress are influenced by that person's culture, family, history, and life experiences.

Stressors

A **stressor** is anything that is perceived as challenging, threatening, or demanding that triggers a stress reaction. Stressors may be internal (e.g., an illness, a hormonal change, or fear) or external (e.g., loud noise or cold temperature). As with stress, the perception and effects of the stressor are highly individualized. Stressors themselves are neither positive nor negative, but they can have positive or negative effects that may be short- or long-term.

QSEN Reflective Practice: Cultivating QSEN Competencies

CHALLENGE TO ETHICAL AND LEGAL SKILLS

I went to the student health center this afternoon because I was feeling sick. Tomorrow, I am supposed to begin my critical care rotation. My instructor is the same one that I had for health assessment, and that rotation was really a disaster. She has a reputation for being the hardest instructor in the school, and I struggled with the content that semester. I learned quite a bit but can't shake the nerves. I do not work in a hospital like many of my peers, and I'm pretty terrified of the tubes and machines that I'm going to be faced with in the critical care unit. I'm still working on developing dexterity, and my hands shake when I get nervous—not a good combination. I actually tried to switch rotations and get on a less acute unit but had no luck. Now, I have to decide what to do tomorrow. I already feel a migraine starting.

Thinking Outside the Box: Possible Courses of Action

- Call in sick. Obviously, this can't be a long-term strategy.
- Grin and bear it. Just try to do my job and not stand out from my peers.
- Try to find a mentor in critical care to whom I can explain my fears and have the preceptor help me develop the skills I definitely need.
- Be honest with my instructor about my fears and the stress I am experiencing and ask for help.

Evaluating a Good Outcome: How Do I Define Success?

- I develop the technical and coping skills I need to effectively provide care in a high-tech environment.
- No patient is harmed because of my lack of skill and confidence.
- I learn to manage my stress and use it to my advantage.
- I pass this rotation with flying colors.

Personal Learning: Here's to the Future!

After some hard reflection (and the wise counsel of my mother), I decided I was giving my fear of this rotation (and instructor) way too much power over me. I realized that nursing would continue to put me in new and frightening situations, and I had better learn to deal with it now. Escape just couldn't be my modus operandi. I made it to clinical on time but was feeling jittery and queasy. Immediately after preconference, I literally grabbed my instructor and told her I had to talk to her before I began giving care. While she'll never be called warm and fuzzy, she surprised me by being understanding. Then she spent some extra time orienting me to the unit and helping me develop comfort with a lot of equipment I'd be using that day. I learned an important lesson in confronting fear and not letting it get the best of me. Hopefully, I can remember this the next time *flight* seems more attractive than *fight*!

Christopher Weiss, Georgetown University

QSEN SELF-REFLECTION ON QUALITY AND SAFETY COMPETENCIES DEVELOPING KNOWLEDGE, SKILLS, AND ATTITUDES FOR CONTINUOUS IMPROVEMENT

How do you think you would respond in a similar situation? Why? What does this tell you about yourself and about the adequacy of your skills for professional practice? Can you think of other ways to respond? What *knowledge, skills,* and *attitudes* do you need to develop to continuously improve quality and safety in situations like the one experienced by this student nurse?

Patient-Centered Care: Can you identify a beneficial aspect of the stress experienced by this student nurse? Did his handling of this stressful situation facilitate his ability to deliver effective care and treatment to his patients in a new environment? Did this student nurse's interaction with his instructor reinforce his commitment to treating patients with dignity and respect?

Teamwork and Collaboration/Quality Improvement: How important are effective communication skills when collaborating with team members? Did the acknowledgment of the student's personal stress and his decision to share these concerns with his instructor facilitate his understanding of the value of working in a nonpunitive environment? Explain the autonomic nervous system responses the nursing student was experiencing. How did the nursing student use task-oriented reactions and attack behavior? Propose some strategies that would be appropriate for him to use in the future to cope with stress and facilitate his role as an effective team member.

Safety/Evidence-Based Practice: Is there anything more the nursing student could have done to confront his fears, contribute to a safe patient care environment, and promote a positive outcome? Do you agree with his criteria to evaluate a successful outcome? Did the nursing student meet the criteria? What evidence in nursing literature provides guidance for managing stress in the work environment and finding effective methods to deal with it and care for yourself?

Informatics: Can you think of other ways to respond or to approach this situation? Do you think self-confidence gained from dealing effectively with stressful situations improves your ability to care for patients effectively and accurately document this care?

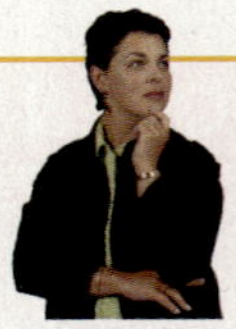

Consider **Joan Rogerrio,** the middle-aged woman who is returning to the workforce and experiencing a recurrence of her inflammatory bowel disease. The decision to return to work was fostered by the family's financial need, which could also be a stressor for her. The stress of returning to work after a 15-year absence exerted a negative effect, resulting in frequent episodes of diarrhea.

Stressors can be physiologic or psychosocial. A physiologic stressor may cause psychosocial stress, and vice versa.

Physiologic Stressors

Physiologic stressors have both a specific effect and a general effect. The specific effect is an alteration of normal body structure and function. The general effect is the stress response. Primary physiologic stressors include chemical agents (drugs, poisons), physical agents (heat, cold, trauma), infectious agents (viruses, bacteria), nutritional imbalances, hypoxia, and genetic or immune disorders.

Psychosocial Stressors

There are an almost infinite variety of psychosocial stressors. They become such a part of our daily lives that we often minimize or overlook them. The environment, interpersonal relationships, or a life event can lead to the stress response if a person does not have the resources to adequately respond to the perceived or actual stressor. To illustrate the many types of psychosocial stressors, consider those listed in Box 43-1. Psychosocial stressors include both real and perceived threats. The person's responses are continuous and include individualized coping mechanisms for responding to anxiety, guilt, fear, frustration, and loss. Coping mechanisms serve to maintain psychological homeostasis.

Adaptation

When a person is in a threatening or otherwise stressful situation, immediate responses occur. Those responses, which are often involuntary, are called coping responses. The change that takes place as a result of the response to a stressor is referred to as **adaptation**. Adaptation is, to some degree, an ongoing process as a person strives to maintain balance in the internal and external environments (Fig. 43-1). Adaptation also occurs in families and groups. Adaptation is necessary for maintaining normal growth and development, tolerating changing situations, and responding to physical and emotional stressors.

Homeostasis

Our bodies are always interacting with a constantly changing environment, including the external environment that surrounds our bodies and the internal environment that includes the mechanisms that regulate body functions and the fluids that surround body cells. To maintain health, the

Box 43-1 Examples of Psychosocial Stressors

- Accidents, which cause stress for the victim, the person who caused the accident, and the families of both
- Stressful or traumatic experiences of family members and friends
- Horrors of history, such as Nazi concentration camps, the dropping of the atomic bomb on Hiroshima, the September 11, 2001 or Orlando Pulse nightclub (2016) terrorist attacks, any of the school shootings of 2018 (e.g., Parkland, FL), or the murder of George Floyd in May 2020 that fueled the Black Lives Matter movement
- Fear of aggression or mutilation, such as muggings, rape, shootings, and terrorism
- Events of history that are brought into our homes through television and the Internet, such as wars, earthquakes, violence in schools, and civil unrest
- Rapid changes in our world and the way we live, including changes in economic and political structures, rapid advances in technology, and shifting values and priorities
- The inherent stressors, social isolation, political divides, change in work-life separation, and public health crisis brought about by the COVID-19 pandemic that began in 2020

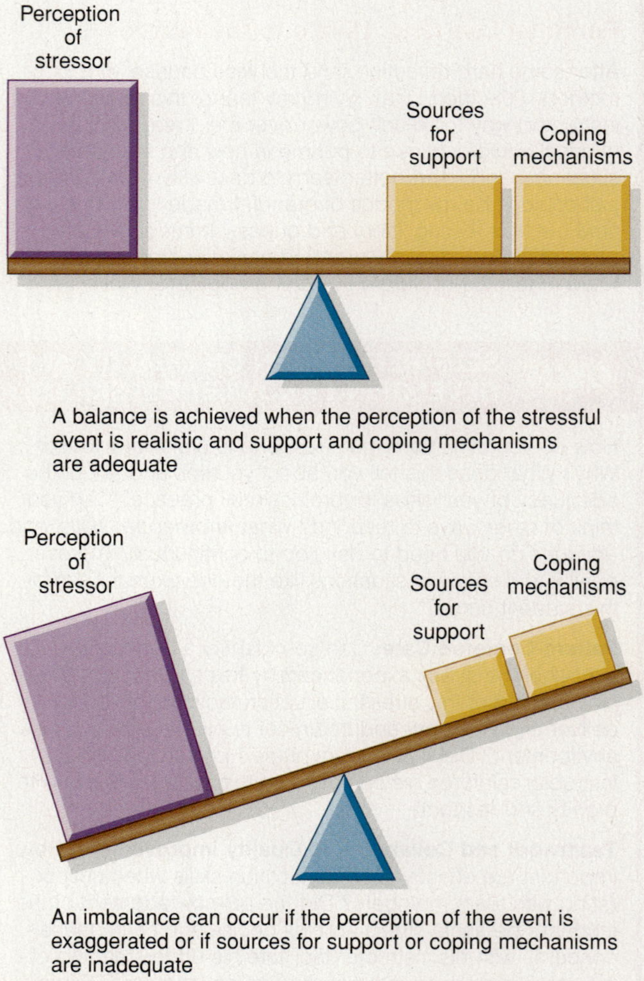

FIGURE 43-1. A realistic perception of a stressful event, sources for emotional support, and appropriate coping mechanisms are components of a system of balances during stress.

body's internal environment must remain in a balanced state. Various physiologic mechanisms within the body respond to internal changes to maintain **homeostasis**, a relative constancy in the internal environment.

Throughout history, people have believed that health is the result of a balanced state. Some of the most important people in medical history, including Hippocrates (modern medicine) and Claude Bernard (homeostasis physiology), believed in and wrote about this balanced state. Originally, the focus was on life processes that occur within the body such as heart rate, blood pressure, and water balance. The concept of homeostasis has been expanded to include both physiologic and psychological balance.

MAINTENANCE OF PHYSIOLOGIC AND PSYCHOLOGICAL HOMEOSTASIS

The effects of physiologic and psychological stress are interrelated, as are the mechanisms that are consciously or unconsciously used to maintain homeostasis in response to stress. For example, the mechanisms described later, including the general adaptation syndrome (GAS) and mind–body interaction, are physiologic responses to either physical or emotional stressors.

Physiologic Homeostasis

The autonomic nervous system and the endocrine system primarily control homeostatic mechanisms. The respiratory, cardiovascular, gastrointestinal, and renal systems are involved to a lesser degree. These mechanisms are self-regulating, organized, and coordinated; they occur without conscious thought, and defend against change to the body's internal environment. On a simple level, these self-regulating mechanisms are like a thermostat regulating a furnace. When the temperature in a house falls below the preset temperature on the thermostat, the thermostat turns on the furnace, which heats the house to the desired temperature and then shuts off. This is a classic example of a negative feedback system, which is the primary means by which homeostasis is maintained (Norris, 2020).

The regulatory mechanisms of the body are reacting constantly to internal changes to maintain homeostasis and health. The homeostatic mechanisms of the body systems are summarized in Table 43-1 on page 1768. These mechanisms explain the consequences of both short- and long-term stress, which can threaten physiologic homeostasis and result in illness. In the 1980s, some investigators began using the term **allostasis** to describe this process of achieving stability or homeostasis through physiologic or behavioral change. The cumulative negative effects of these physical responses to prolonged environmental and psychosocial stressors are referred to as an *allostatic load*. This represents the consequences of ongoing stress on the body with its resultant risks for a variety of diseases (McEwen & Stellar, 1993; Norris, 2020). Box 43-2 provides examples of illnesses known to be associated with stress.

Box 43-2 Examples of Physical Illnesses Associated With Stress

Autoimmune Disorders

Graves disease (hyperthyroidism)
Myasthenia gravis
Psoriasis
Rheumatoid arthritis
Systemic lupus erythematosus (SLE)
Ulcerative colitis

Cardiovascular and Hematologic Disorders

Coronary artery disease
Hypertension
Sickle cell disease

Gastrointestinal Disorders

Constipation
Diarrhea
Esophageal reflux

Respiratory Disorders

Asthma

Local Adaptation Syndrome

The **local adaptation syndrome (LAS)** is a localized response of the body to stress. It involves only a specific body part (such as a tissue or organ) instead of the whole body. The stress precipitating the LAS may be traumatic or pathologic. LAS is a primarily homeostatic, short-term adaptive response. Although the body has many localized stress responses, the two most common responses that influence nursing care are the reflex pain response and the inflammatory response.

REFLEX PAIN RESPONSE

The **reflex pain response** is a response of the central nervous system to pain. It is rapid and automatic, serving as a protective mechanism to prevent injury. The reflex depends on an intact, functioning neurologic reflex arc and involves both sensory and motor neurons. For example, if you step into a bathtub of dangerously hot water, sensors in your skin detect the heat and immediately send a message to the spinal cord. A message is then sent to a motor nerve, which activates the muscles in your leg to pull back your foot. All of this happens before you consciously realize that the water is too hot to be safe. The pain response is discussed in Chapter 36.

INFLAMMATORY RESPONSE

The **inflammatory response** is a local response to injury or infection. It serves to localize and prevent the spread of infection and promote wound healing. When you cut your finger, for example, you often develop the symptoms of the inflammatory response: pain, swelling, heat, redness, and changes in function. The inflammatory response is discussed in Chapter 33.

Table 43-1 Homeostatic Regulators of the Body

SYSTEM	ACTION	EFFECT
Autonomic Nervous System		
Parasympathetic—Functions under normal conditions and at rest (cranial and sacral nerves)		
	Regulates heart rate	Slows rate
	Stimulates secretion of digestive juices and digestive tract smooth muscle	Improves digestion, increases peristalsis
	Stimulates insulin secretion	Increases uptake of glucose by cells
Sympathetic—Functions under stress conditions to bring about the fight-or-flight response		
	Stimulates heart rate and force	Increases rate, strengthens contractions, increases cardiac output
	Dilates skeletal muscle blood vessels	Increases muscle strength
	Dilates blood vessels to the brain	Increases mental alertness
	Stimulates release of glycogen stores	Increases blood glucose levels
Endocrine System		
Pituitary	Secretes hormones:	
	• Adrenocorticotropic hormone (ACTH)	Stimulates the adrenal cortex
	• Thyroid-stimulating hormone (TSH)	Stimulates the thyroid
Adrenals	Medulla produces epinephrine and norepinephrine	Prepares the person for emergencies; supports the sympathetic system
	Cortex secretes mineralocorticoids, glucocorticoids, and androgens	Mineralocorticoid aldosterone regulates fluid and electrolytes Glucocorticoids (cortisol) raise glucose levels (for energy) and increase resistance to physical stress Androgens control the development and maintenance of male characteristics and are the primary precursor of natural estrogens
Thyroid	Secretes thyroid hormone and calcitonin	Regulates metabolic rate and growth
Other		
Cardiovascular	Serves as transport system and pump	Provides oxygen and nutrients and removes carbon dioxide and wastes from cells
Renal	Filters, excretes, and reabsorbs metabolic products and water	Maintains fluid, electrolyte, and acid–base balance
Respiratory	Regulates inhalation of oxygen and exhalation of carbon dioxide	Necessary for metabolism; helps maintain acid–base balance
Gastrointestinal	Digests and metabolizes food and fluids Eliminates waste products	Energy sources; maintains fluids and electrolytes

General Adaptation Syndrome

The **general adaptation syndrome (GAS)** is a biochemical model of stress developed by Selye (1976). The GAS describes the body's general response to stress, a concept that impacts all facets of nursing care. The three stages in the GAS are alarm reaction, stage of resistance, and stage of exhaustion (Fig. 43-2). Although the alarm stage is short term (minutes to hours), the length of the resistance and exhaustion stages varies greatly, depending on such variables as the severity and duration of the stressor, the person's previous health and coping mechanisms, and the immediacy and effectiveness of health care interventions.

The GAS is a physiologic response to stress, but it is important to remember that the response results from either physical or emotional stressors, and the stages occur with either physical or psychological damage to the person. Obvious examples are seen in patients with severe injury or an illness, but GAS is also a factor in mental illness, social isolation, and loss of (or lack of) human relationships.

ALARM REACTION

Alarm is initiated when a person perceives a specific stressor and various defense mechanisms are activated. The perception of threat may be conscious or unconscious. The hypothalamic–pituitary–adrenal (HPA) axis controls the neuroendocrine response, and hormone and catecholamine levels rise to prepare the body to react. The sympathetic nervous system initiates the **fight-or-flight response**, preparing the body to either fight off the stressor or to run away from it (usually not literally in the modern world). This phase of the alarm reaction, called the shock phase, is characterized by an increase in energy levels, oxygen intake, cardiac output, blood pressure, and mental alertness. (If you recall the

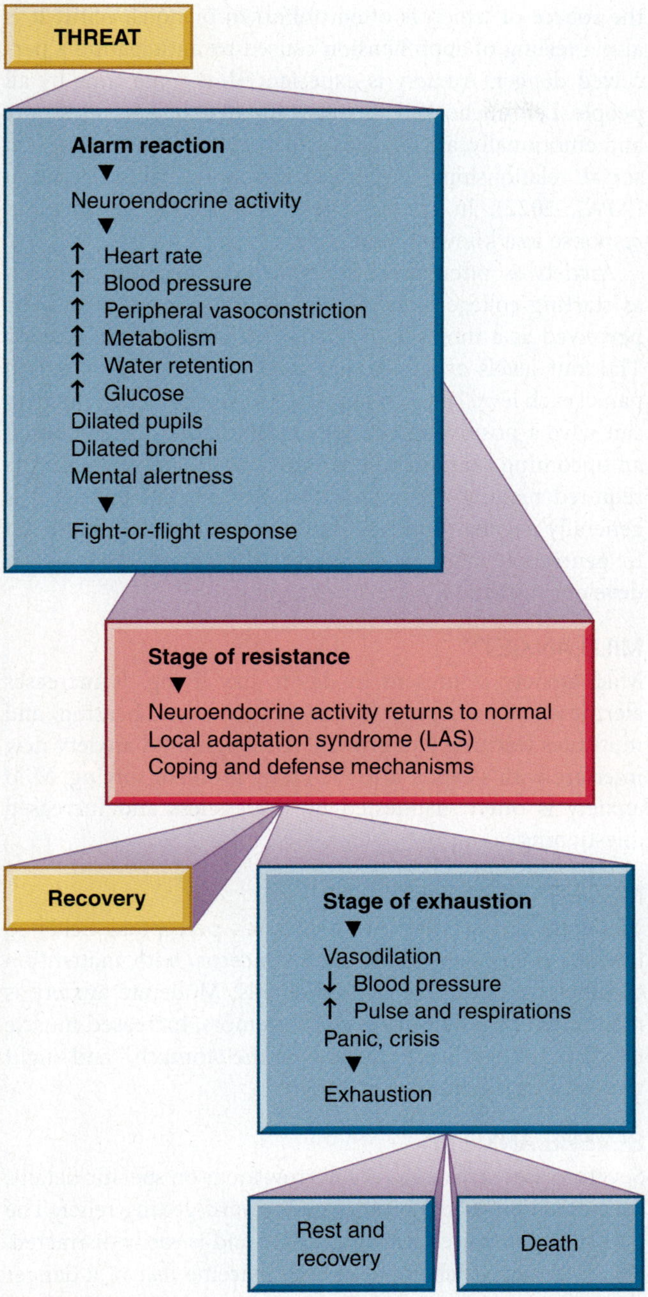

FIGURE 43-2. The general adaptation syndrome (general response to stress).

last time you almost had a car crash, you can easily identify these body reactions!) During the second phase of the alarm reaction, countershock, there is a reversal of body changes.

STAGE OF RESISTANCE

Having perceived the threat and mobilized its resources, the body now attempts to adapt to the stressor. Vital signs, hormone levels, and energy production return to normal. If the stress can be managed or confined to a small area (LAS), the body regains homeostasis. If the stressor is prolonged or strong enough to overwhelm the body's ability to defend itself (e.g., severe injury and bleeding or a major illness such as cancer or a heart attack), the adaptive mechanisms become exhausted.

STAGE OF EXHAUSTION

Exhaustion results when the adaptive mechanisms can no longer provide defense. This depletion of resources results in damage to the body in the form of *wear and tear* or systemic damage (Norris, 2020). Without defense against the stressor, the body may either rest and mobilize its defenses to return to normal or reach total exhaustion and die.

Psychological Homeostasis

To maintain mental well-being, humans also must maintain psychological homeostasis. As discussed in Chapter 4, every person needs to feel loved and a sense of belonging, to feel safe and secure, and to have self-esteem. When these needs are not met or a threat to need fulfillment occurs, homeostatic measures in the form of coping or defense mechanisms help return the person to emotional balance.

Individuals frequently encounter physical, psychological, and social changes in their internal and external environments. A person's perception of these changes may be conscious or unconscious. If the person has the necessary resources, adaptation takes place and balance is maintained. If the resources cannot reestablish balance, a state of stress results. The person's responses and the degree of stress depend in part on the nature, intensity, timing, number, and duration of stressors. Adaptation to stress also depends on a person's age, developmental level, past experiences, support systems, and coping mechanisms (see Box 43-3 for sources of stress with aging). Adaptive responses include the mind–body interaction, anxiety, and coping or defense mechanisms.

Mind–Body Interaction

Consider the following examples of mind–body interaction:

- Tomorrow, you are scheduled to take a final examination, and you must earn a passing score to pass the course and

Box 43-3 Sources of Stress With Aging

Stress, with resultant anxiety, is a known risk for individuals in the older population. As the number of older adults increases in the population, anxiety is now, and increasingly will be, a significant problem. Not all older adults will experience stress to the point of anxiety, but anxiety should be kept in mind as a possible problem when providing nursing care for older adults in the following situations:

- Invasive or health-related tests or examinations
- Surgical procedures
- Diagnosis of chronic illnesses, including diabetes, cancer, and cardiovascular diseases
- Declining physical and/or mental capabilities
- Retirement
- Loss of spouse or significant other
- Increased social isolation
- Chronic pain
- Alcohol abuse
- Loss of independence in living arrangements, driving, or activities of daily living

remain in the nursing program. After being awake most of the night, you cannot swallow any food at breakfast, you have a rapid heartbeat, you are filled with feelings of apprehension, and you have diarrhea.

- Since his wife was killed in a car crash, Tom Green has been the sole support of his 4-year-old son, who is developmentally disabled and hyperactive. Tom has been coming to the neighborhood health clinic with increasing frequency over the past 5 months, reporting weight loss, headaches, and stomach pain.

These examples illustrate the relationship between psychological stressors and the physiologic stress response (the GAS). In the first example, as you begin the test and discover that you know most of the answers, your stress decreases and your symptoms disappear rapidly. Tom's stress, however, is always present and is long term, increasing his risk for developing an illness.

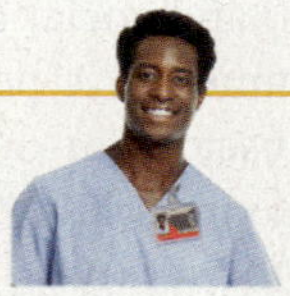

Remember **Christopher Weiss,** the nursing student who said he felt he was getting sick from fears about his upcoming clinical rotation in the critical care unit and anticipation of having a strict instructor. As a result of his anticipated fears and lack of confidence, he physiologically responded to the stressors by feeling sick.

What causes this link between psychological stressors and the physiologic stress response? Although the exact cause is not well understood, it is thought that humans react to threats of danger as if they were physiologic threats. A person perceives the threat on an emotional level, and the body prepares itself either to resist the danger or to run away from it (the fight-or-flight response); see Figure 43-3.

Each person reacts in their own way to prolonged stress. Some may develop chronic diarrhea, while others may develop nausea or heart palpitations. Such illnesses are real and are called **psychosomatic disorders** because the physiologic alterations are thought to be at least partially caused by psychological influences.

Another component of mind–body interaction is the effect of life changes on a person. Researchers have found that the number of changes a person has in life (both positive and negative) can be correlated with illness. A life change is defined as an event in a person's life that requires energy for adaptation. When energy is expended to adapt to the event, the person's resistance to illness is lowered. For example, although a holiday celebration with family and friends is considered a positive event in a person's life, factors including the time necessary to prepare for the party, worrying about how everyone will get along, and trying to decide how much money to spend can generate stress.

Anxiety

The most common human response to stress is anxiety. **Anxiety** is a vague, uneasy feeling of discomfort or dread, the source of which is often unknown or nonspecific. It is also a feeling of apprehension caused by anticipating a perceived danger. Anxiety is experienced at some time by all people. Left unchecked, anxiety can affect person physically and emotionally, alter their self-perceptions, and impact on social relationships (American Psychological Association [APA], 2022). In contrast, **fear** is a feeling of dread in response to a known threat.

Anxiety is often present before new experiences, such as starting college or beginning a new job, which may be perceived as a threat to a person's identity and self-esteem. The four levels of anxiety are mild, moderate, severe, and panic; each level has different effects. At a mild level, anxiety can have a positive effect; for example, mild anxiety about an upcoming examination can motivate a student to do the required reading and review. Anxiety beyond that level is generally negative and has unpleasant effects. In an attempt to neutralize, deny, or counteract the anxiety, the person develops individual patterns of coping.

MILD ANXIETY

Mild anxiety is present in day-to-day living. It increases alertness and perceptual fields (e.g., vision and hearing) and motivates learning and growth. Although mild anxiety may interfere with sleep, it also facilitates problem solving. Mild anxiety is often manifested by restlessness and increased questioning.

MODERATE ANXIETY

Moderate anxiety narrows a person's perceptual fields so that the focus is on immediate concerns, with inattention to other communications and details. Moderate anxiety is manifested by a quavering voice, tremors, increased muscle tension, a report of "butterflies in the stomach," and slight increases in respirations and pulse.

SEVERE ANXIETY

Severe anxiety creates a very narrow focus on specific details, causing all behavior to be geared toward getting relief. The person has impaired learning ability and is easily distracted. Severe anxiety is characterized by extreme fear of a danger that is not real, emotional distress that interferes with everyday life, and avoidance of situations that cause anxiety. It is manifested by difficulty communicating verbally, increased motor activity, a fearful facial expression, headache, nausea, dizziness, tachycardia, and hyperventilation. At this point, anxiety is no longer functioning as a signal for danger or motivation for a needed change, but instead results in maladaptive behaviors and emotional instability that signal the presence of an anxiety disorder.

PANIC

Panic causes the person to lose control and experience dread and terror. The resulting disorganized state is characterized by increased physical activity, distorted perception of events, and loss of rational thought. Panic is manifested by difficulty communicating verbally, agitation, trembling, poor motor control, sensory changes, sweating, tachycardia,

Here are ways in which some key body systems react.

1 NERVOUS SYSTEM
When stressed — physically or psychologically — the body suddenly shifts its energy resources to fighting off the perceived threat. In what is known as the "fight or flight" response, the sympathetic nervous system signals the adrenal glands to release adrenaline and cortisol. These hormones make the heart beat faster, raise blood pressure, change the digestive process and boost glucose levels in the bloodstream. Once the crisis passes, body systems usually return to normal.

2 MUSCULOSKELETAL SYSTEM
Under stress, muscles tense up. The contraction of muscles for extended periods can trigger tension headaches, migraines and various musculoskeletal conditions.

3 RESPIRATORY SYSTEM
Stress can make you breathe harder and cause rapid breathing — or hyperventilation — which can bring on panic attacks in some people.

4 CARDIOVASCULAR SYSTEM
Acute stress — stress that is momentary, such as being stuck in traffic — causes an increase in heart rate and stronger contractions of the heart muscle. Blood vessels that direct blood to the large muscles and to the heart dilate, increasing the amount of blood pumped to these parts of the body. Repeated episodes of acute stress can cause inflammation in the coronary arteries, thought to lead to heart attack.

5 ENDOCRINE SYSTEM
Adrenal glands
When the body is stressed, the brain sends signals from the hypothalamus, causing the adrenal cortex to produce cortisol and the adrenal medulla to produce epinephrine — sometimes called the "stress hormones."

Liver
When cortisol and epinephrine are released, the liver produces more glucose, a blood sugar that would give you the energy for "fight or flight" in an emergency.

6 GASTROINTESTINAL SYSTEM
Esophagus
Stress may prompt you to eat much more or much less than you usually do. If you eat more or different foods or increase your use of tobacco or alcohol, you may experience heartburn, or acid reflux.

Stomach
Your stomach can react with "butterflies" or even nausea or pain. You may vomit if the stress is severe enough.

Bowels
Stress can affect digestion and which nutrients your intestines absorb. It can also affect how quickly food moves through your body. You may find that you have either diarrhea or constipation.

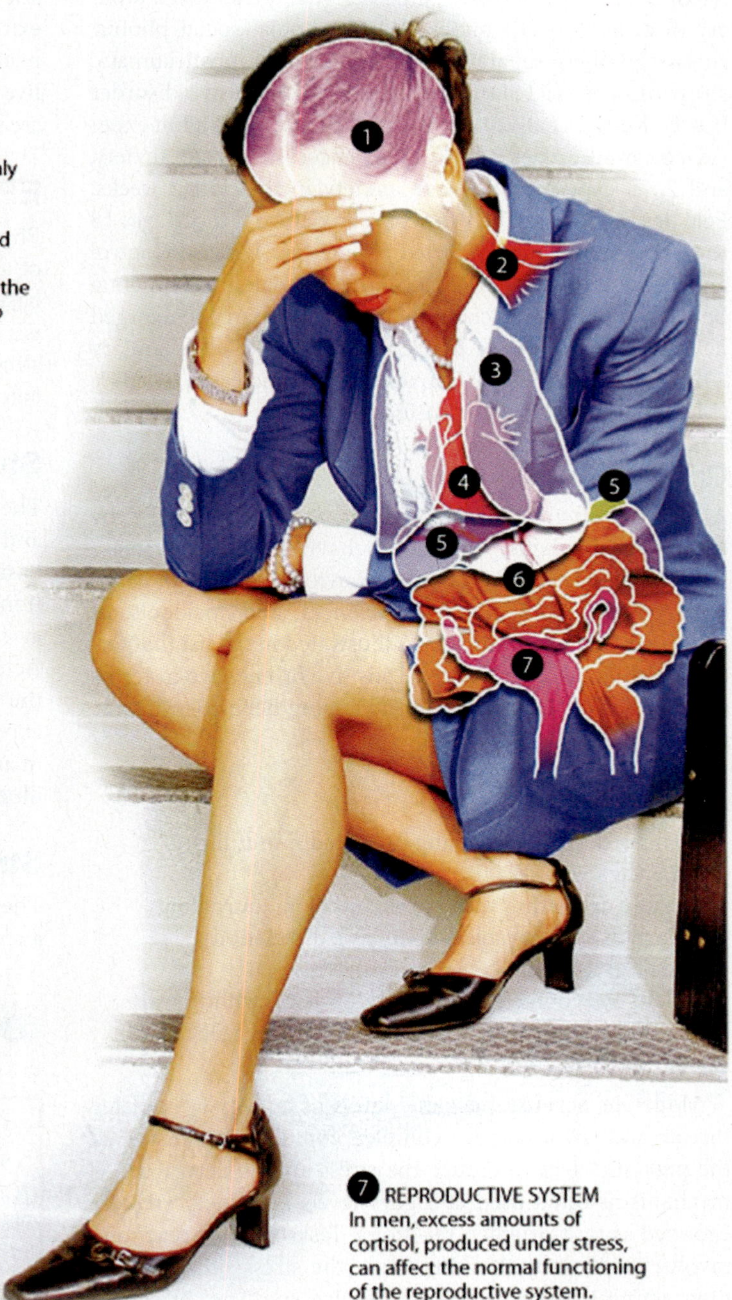

7 REPRODUCTIVE SYSTEM
In men, excess amounts of cortisol, produced under stress, can affect the normal functioning of the reproductive system. Chronic stress can impair testosterone and sperm production and cause impotence.

In women stress can cause absent or irregular menstrual cycles or more-painful periods. It can also reduce sexual desire.

FIGURE 43-3. The effects of stress. (Courtesy of the American Institute of Stress. https://www.stress.org/the-effects-of-stress)

hyperventilation, dyspnea, palpitations, a choking sensation, and sensations of chest pain or pressure. The person is unable to learn, concentrates only on the present situation, and often experiences feelings of impending doom. This level of anxiety can lead to exhaustion and death.

ANXIETY DISORDERS

Anxiety disorders are a group of conditions in which excessive anxiety is the key feature. This type of anxiety is persistent and affects responses from a cognitive, behavioral, emotional, and physiologic perspective (Videbeck, 2019).

Anxiety disorders include panic disorder, generalized anxiety disorder (GAD), phobias (agoraphobia, social phobia, specific phobia), separation anxiety disorder, posttraumatic stress disorder (PTSD), and obsessive-compulsive disorder (OCD; Kessler et al., 2012). During 2019, 9.5% of adult experienced mild anxiety, 3.4% experienced moderate anxiety, and 2.7% experienced severe anxiety in the past 2 weeks. Females were more likely to report anxiety and those ages 18 to 29 years were most affected (Center for Disease Control and Prevention [CDC], 2020b). The prevalence of mental health disorders, especially depression and anxiety, surged nationwide in response to the pandemic. Between January 2020 and September 2020, anxiety screens increased by 634% (Mental Health America, 2020).

Coping Mechanisms

Anxiety is often managed without conscious thought by **coping mechanisms**, which are behaviors used to decrease stress and anxiety. Many coping behaviors are learned, based on a person's family, past experiences, and sociocultural influences and expectations. As illustrated in the list that follows, coping behaviors may be positive or negative in terms of how they affect health. Typical coping behaviors include the following:

- Crying, laughing, sleeping, cursing
- Physical activity, exercise
- Taking a deep breath, using practiced mindfulness/centering exercises
- Verbally debriefing with another person, journaling
- Engage in an enjoyable activity as a distraction
- Smoking, drinking
- Lack of eye contact, ignoring the stressor, withdrawal
- Limiting relationships to those with similar values and interests

Moderate, severe, and panic levels of anxiety are greater threats and involve more complex coping mechanisms as the person strives to reduce the stress and anxiety. Coping mechanisms often used at higher levels of anxiety are categorized as task-oriented reactions. Task-oriented reactions involve consciously thinking about the stress situation and then acting to solve problems, resolve conflicts, or satisfy needs. These reactions include attack behavior, withdrawal behavior, and compromise behavior.

Attack behavior occurs when a person attempts to overcome obstacles to satisfy a need; it may be constructive, with assertive problem solving, or destructive, with feelings and actions of aggression and hostility. Withdrawal behavior involves physical withdrawal from the threat, or emotional reactions such as admitting defeat, becoming apathetic, or feeling guilty and isolated. Compromise behavior is usually constructive, often involving the substitution of goals or negotiation to partially fulfill needs.

Defense Mechanisms

Other unconscious reactions to stressors, called **defense mechanisms**, often occur. These mechanisms protect a person's self-esteem and are useful in mild to moderate anxiety. When extreme, however, they distort reality and create problems with relationships. At that point, the mechanisms become maladaptive instead of adaptive. Some common defense mechanisms are summarized in Table 43-2.

EFFECTS OF STRESS

Physiologic and psychological stress affects all dimensions of a person. Stress strongly influences how a person attains basic human needs, it is a factor in health and illness, and it is a component in family reactions to illness. Both long-term stress and crisis situations may seriously affect physical and emotional health.

Stress and Basic Human Needs

The drive to meet basic human needs (described in Chapter 4) and address stress are universal human experiences. Meeting basic needs and adapting to stress requires energy and intentional action. As a person strives to meet basic human needs at each level, stress can be either a stimulus or a barrier. Actions to achieve balance are individualized and depend on the person's sociocultural background, priorities, and past experiences. In all people, the failure to meet needs results in an imbalance in homeostatic mechanisms and, eventually, illness (Box 43-4).

Stress in Health and Illness

The health–illness continuum (described in Chapter 3) is affected by stress. Health and homeostatic balance are at one

Box 43-4 Effects of Stress on Basic Human Needs

Physiologic Needs

Change in appetite, activity, or sleep
Change in elimination patterns
Increased pulse, respirations, blood pressure

Safety and Security

Feels threatened or nervous
Uses ineffective coping mechanisms
Is inattentive

Love and Belonging

Is withdrawn and isolated
Blames others for own faults
Demonstrates aggressive behaviors
Becomes overly dependent on others

Self-Esteem

Becomes a workaholic
Exhibits attention-seeking behaviors

Self-Actualization

Refuses to accept reality
Centers on own problems
Demonstrates lack of control

Table 43-2 Commonly Occurring Defense Mechanisms

DEFENSE MECHANISM	CAUSES	EXAMPLE
Compensation	A person attempts to overcome a perceived weakness by emphasizing a more desirable trait or overachieving in a more comfortable area.	A student who has difficulty with academics may excel in sports.
Denial	A person refuses to acknowledge the presence of a condition that is disturbing.	Despite finding a lump in her breast, a woman does not seek medical treatment.
Displacement	A person transfers (displaces) an emotional reaction from one object or person to another object or person.	An employee who is angry with a coworker kicks a chair.
Dissociation	A person subconsciously protects themself from the memories of a horrific or painful event by allowing the mind to forget the incident.	An adult cannot recall childhood memories surrounding the traumatic death of a sibling.
Introjection	A person incorporates qualities or values of another person into their own ego structure. This mechanism is important in the formation of conscience during childhood.	An older sibling tells his preschool sister not to talk to strangers, expressing his parents' values to his younger sister.
Projection	A person attributes thoughts or impulses to someone else.	A person who denies any sexual feelings for a coworker accuses them of sexual harassment.
Rationalization	A person tries to give a logical or socially acceptable explanation for questionable behavior ("behavior justification").	A patient who forgot to keep a health care appointment says, "If patients didn't have to wait 3 months to get an appointment, they wouldn't forget them."
Reaction formation	A person develops conscious attitudes and behavior patterns that are opposite to what they would really like to do.	A married woman is attracted to her husband's best friend but is constantly rude to him.
Regression	A person returns to an earlier method of behaving.	Children may regress to soiling diapers or demanding a bottle when they are ill.
Repression	A person voluntarily excludes an anxiety-producing event from conscious awareness.	A father may not remember shaking his crying baby.
Sublimation	A person substitutes a socially acceptable goal for one whose normal channel of expression is blocked.	A person who is aggressive toward others may become a star football player.
Undoing	A person uses an act or communication to negate a previous act or communication.	A husband who was physically abusive to his wife may bring her an expensive present the next day.

extreme of the continuum; exhaustion and death are at the other extreme.

Stress in a healthy person may promote health and prevent illness. For example, the fear of developing lung cancer may motivate a person to stop smoking, or anxiety about baby care may prompt prospective parents to attend prenatal classes and read childcare books. Stressors in health also facilitate normal growth and development, provide the stimulus for learning constructive adaptive behaviors, stimulate problem-solving abilities, encourage social relationships, and help develop spiritual strength and resilience.

The effects of stress on a sick or injured person are, in contrast, usually negative. Stress can make illness worse, and illness can cause stress. The presence of an illness or a disability demands new coping skills at a time when homeostasis is challenged. People who enter health care settings as patients are also subjected to situational stressors.

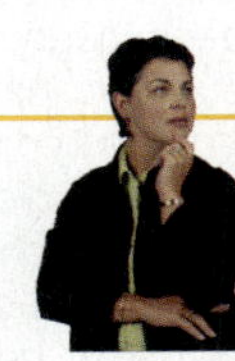

Remember **Joan Rogerrio,** the woman experiencing an exacerbation of her bowel disease. The negative effects of stress exacerbated her illness. As a result, Joan needs to develop new coping skills to deal with the demands of working to minimize the negative effects of this stressor on her illness.

Adaptation to acute and chronic illness or to traumatic injury involves two sets of adaptive tasks:

1. General tasks (as in the case of any situational stress) involve maintaining self-esteem and personal relationships while preparing for an uncertain future.
2. Illness-related tasks include such stressors as losing independence and control, managing pain and disability, and carrying out the prescribed medical regimen.

Every situation is different, and each person perceives and reacts to stressors in an individual manner. There is no one *best* way to cope with a given situation. Nursing considerations include the person's major concern, specific illness, sociocultural background, and available resources. For example, an older patient may be anxious about the cost of treatment for a hip fracture, whereas another patient with the same injury may be seriously worried about the care of their cats while she is in the hospital. As another example, Kristin and Jane have both entered the hospital for treatment of breast cancer. Kristin is worried about possible disfigurement and death, but she believes that with the help of surgery and chemotherapy, she can overcome the cancer. Jane, on the other hand, comes from a community that has strong fundamental religious beliefs. She believes that the cancer is a punishment from God and refuses treatment, even though she fears death.

Long-Term Stress

Long-term stress poses a serious threat to physical and emotional health. As the duration, intensity, or number of stressors increases, a person's ability to adapt is lessened. The failure of adaptive mechanisms is also influenced by a person's state of health and past experiences with stress. In 2020, with the pandemic continuing well past initial predictions, 77% of adults reported the *future of the nation* as a significant source of stress, and almost 65% specified the *current amount of uncertainty* as the primary source of stress. Health care (66%), mass shootings (62%), and climate change (55%) represent the top three, specific, societal stressors identified. The prolonged state of stress experienced by the world constitutes a mental health crisis that could result in long-lasting health and societal issues (APA, 2020).

Long-term stress affects physical status, increasing the risk for disease or injury. Recovery and return to normal function are also compromised. High levels of ongoing stress are associated with multiple health disorders (see Box 43-2 on page 1767). Alcoholism and drug abuse, depression, suicide, accidents, and eating disorders have also been associated with chronic stress (Norris, 2020). It is believed that these diseases are the result of various factors, including the effects of the fight-or-flight response, eating patterns, lifestyle, and coping mechanisms. Stress alone does not cause autoimmune diseases such as rheumatoid arthritis, but it is believed to contribute to the progression of these diseases. Researchers have confirmed that chronic stress affects the ability of immune cells to respond to the hormones that normally regulate inflammation, thus allowing the development and progression of some diseases.

Stress has negative effects on the entire body—the cardiovascular, respiratory, musculoskeletal, endocrine, gastrointestinal, nervous, and reproductive systems (see Fig. 43-3 on page 1771). Under normal circumstances, cortisol, an antiinflammatory hormone released by the adrenal glands, regulates the inflammatory response, but prolonged stress may decrease the effectiveness of cortisol, or the immune cells may be resistant to its effects (American Institute of Stress, 2020; American Psychological Association, 2018; Norris, 2020). A person who reacts to stress by overeating, smoking, using alcohol or illicit drugs, or becoming hyperactive puts additional strain on the body. See the Promoting Health Literacy box for tips useful for patients experiencing long-term stress.

Promoting Health Literacy

IN PATIENTS EXPERIENCING LONG-TERM STRESS

Patient Scenario

Eva Weber is a 34-year-old single mother of twin boys. Both boys, now age 6, have had developmental delays and have been diagnosed with attention-deficit disorder. Eva has a job at a dry cleaner but worries constantly that she will not be able to keep her job since she has been late frequently because her car is old and breaks down often. Her former husband only pays child support about half the time, often because he has lost his construction job due to chronic alcoholism. When he drinks, he calls her constantly and sometimes comes to her house, beating on the door until she calls the police. She has problems sleeping and has lost 25 lb; she is 5 ft 9 inches tall and now only weighs 120 lb. She admits she drinks and smokes too much, but says, "It's the only thing that makes me feel better for a while." Although the nurse practitioner at the local clinic has talked to her about stopping smoking and gaining weight, Eva has not been able to do so.

Nursing Considerations: *Tips for Improving Health Literacy*

Ask Eva to keep a stress diary, noting when and how often something triggers her stress, how it makes her feel, and listing the things in her life that make her happy. Teach her how to take one day at a time, encouraging her to believe that she has control over some aspects of her life, but acknowledging that other aspects are uncontrollable. Work with Eva to do a computer search, using reputable sites, to assess her ability to access resources for her children and herself. Suggest that she ask her primary health care provider for some help in stopping smoking in the form of medications. She needs to identify appropriate support systems and create a plan to stop smoking. Explain and provide written guidelines for relaxation exercises that Eva identifies as potentially useful. Discuss methods of reducing stress other than through alcohol and nicotine, including taking time to relax, talking with a friend, and intentionally identifying positive aspects of a situation. Suggest other activities that are known to reduce stress, such as regular exercise, eating a nutritious diet, learning to say "no," avoiding people who are stressful, being more assertive, and doing something enjoyable each day. Encourage Eva to make an appointment at the clinic and to be prepared to ask her provider the following three questions:

- What is my main problem?
- What do I need to do?
- Why is it important for me to do this?

What additional measures can you take to help maintain health literacy in this patient? What other measures would be helpful for Eva if she did not speak English, could not read, or had other learning deficits?

Unfolding Patient Stories: Vernon Russell • Part 2

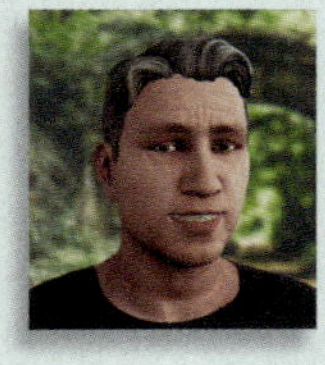

Recall **Vernon Russell** from Chapter 12, a 55-year-old with a 5-year history of hypertension, coronary artery disease, and diabetes who has mild left hemiplegia from a right-sided stroke. He is divorced and living with his son, and both work at an oil refinery. What are potential sources of stress for Vernon and his son? Describe interventions the nurse can use to assist them with coping skills and stress reduction. What risks may be present for ineffective adaptation to, and coping with, his current condition?

Care for Vernon and other patients in a realistic virtual environment: ***vSim** for Nursing* (thepoint.lww.com/vSimFunds). Practice documenting these patients' care in DocuCare (thepoint.lww.com/DocuCareEHR).

Family Stress

The stress that affects an ill person also affects the person's family members or significant others. When the family is viewed as a system, the behavior of the individual is influenced by family, and any alterations in the individual's behavior affect the family. Stressors for the family include changes in family structure and roles, anger and feelings of helplessness and guilt, loss of control over normal routines, and concern for financial stability.

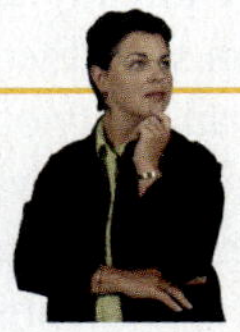

Consider ***Joan Rogerrio,*** the woman with an exacerbation of her bowel disease. Her family is already experiencing changes related to her return to work. These changes could be possible stressors for the family. These family stressors are increased by Joan's illness, which may ultimately affect her role performance. Thus, the nurse would need to assess the family situation for the effect of these stressors on the family.

The family, both as individuals and as a unit, uses many of the same coping and defense mechanisms described previously. Family members may be overly protective, deny the seriousness of the illness, or blame health care providers for the patient's condition or behaviors. On the other hand, the family can provide the social support necessary to help the patient manage and adapt to stress. Emotional support from family members fosters open expression of feelings, and helps meet love and belonging needs. The inclusion of family members in problem solving, teaching and learning activities, and physical care helps both the patient and the family maintain their self-esteem and feelings of worth.

Caring for a family member at home for long periods can also cause prolonged stress. This stress response, called **caregiver burden**, or caregiver stress, includes chronic fatigue, sleep problems, and an increased incidence of stress-related illnesses, such as high blood pressure and heart disease. Prolonged stress can seriously threaten mental health. As coping or defense mechanisms become ineffective, a person may try less effective coping patterns or maladaptive defense mechanisms. As anxiety increases despite these measures, the person may experience difficulties on the job, with personal relationships, and with self-esteem. Although caregiving is hard work, stressful, and provokes a wide range of both positive and negative emotions, when support systems are sufficient, advocating for another person builds what is often a reciprocal, bonded relationship (Turner & Finch-Guthrie, 2020).

People who were neglected or abused as children are more vulnerable to stress as adults. An ongoing study of adverse childhood experiences (ACEs) by the CDC (2020a) and Kaiser Permanente documents and tracks the development of chronic diseases, mental health disorders, health risk behaviors, and other health and social behaviors associated with negative childhood experiences. When the abuse occurs early in a child's life and is ongoing, changes in the brain's structure and function can occur, resulting in an altered immune response to inflammation and wound healing. The family is an integral part in the assessment, planning, nursing interventions, and evaluation of actions to prevent ACEs and promote adaptation to stress.

Crisis

A **crisis** is a disturbance caused by a precipitating event, such as a perceived loss, a threat of loss, or a challenge, that is interpreted as a threat to self. In a crisis, the person's usual methods of coping are ineffective. This failure produces high levels of anxiety, disorganized behavior, and an inability to function adequately. The crisis and associated anxiety initially activate the person's usual methods of coping. If these are not effective, the person experiences more anxiety because the coping mechanisms are not working. As the crisis continues, the person tries new methods of coping or redefines the threat. This may lead to resolution of the crisis or, if not effective, may result in severe or panic levels of anxiety. The crisis is more likely to be successfully resolved if the person views the event realistically, effective coping mechanisms are present, and situational support systems are available.

Crises may be maturational, situational, or adventitious. Maturational crises occur during developmental events that require role change, such as when a teenager transitions into adulthood. Situational crises occur when a life event disrupts a person's psychological equilibrium, such as loss of a job or death of a loved family member. Adventitious crises include accidental and unexpected events resulting in multiple losses, and major environmental changes—such as fires, earthquakes, and floods—that involve not only individuals but also entire communities. Preparation for an adventitious crisis, such as active shooter drills in elementary schools, can cause stress, even with proper framing, education, and support. The stress experienced during the pandemic led to periods of fatigue and inactivity, restlessness, an inability to concentrate, loneliness, and general feelings of unhappiness in all age groups. Generation Z (ages 13 to 23 years in 2020) reported the greatest impact, with 34% of Generation Z adults reporting worse mental health than the previous year (APA, 2020). This prolonged period of crisis presented unique challenges and opportunities. This global crisis led to a collective moral fatigue and general unrest that is likely to have long-term impact on the psychological, social, and physical well-being of individuals and communities for years to come.

FACTORS AFFECTING STRESS AND ADAPTATION

Stress and adaptation are affected by the sources of stress (i.e., the types of stressors experienced) and personal factors.

Sources of Stress

Although there are an almost infinite number of sources of stress, they can be categorized into two broad areas: developmental stress and situational stress. Both require adaptive responses.

Developmental Stress

Developmental stress occurs as a person progresses through the normal stages of growth and development from birth to old age (described in Chapters 22, 23, and 24). Within each stage, certain tasks must be resolved to reduce the stress. Examples of stages of growth and development associated with developmental stress include the following:

- The infant learning to trust others
- The toddler learning to control elimination
- The school-aged child socializing with peers
- The adolescent striving for independence
- The middle-aged adult accepting physical signs of aging
- The older adult reflecting on past life experiences with satisfaction

Situational Stress

Situational stress is different from developmental stress. It does not occur in predictable patterns as a person progresses through life. Situational stress can occur at any time, although the person's ability to adapt may be strongly influenced by their developmental level. Examples of situational stress, which may be either positive or negative, include the following:

- Illness or traumatic injury
- Marriage or divorce
- Loss (of belongings, relationships, family member)
- New job
- Role change

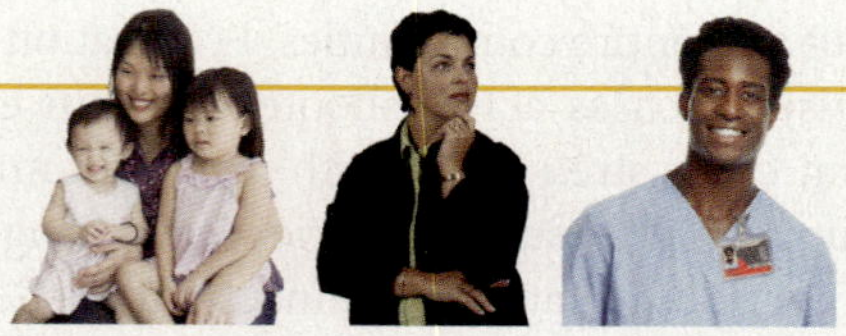

Recall the three people described at the beginning of the chapter. All three are experiencing situational stress, but each is responding differently. **Mei Fu** is having headaches and diarrhea, **Joan** is experiencing an exacerbation of her bowel disease, and **Christopher** is feeling sick and shaky.

Consider pregnancy as an example of a situational stress. A young married couple may be overjoyed at the prospect of becoming parents, whereas an unmarried adolescent may be panic-stricken when told the pregnancy test is positive. The situations and the developmental levels of the young couple and the adolescent will have a major effect on the adaptations they will make. A person's physical and psychosocial capacities to cope with the situation depend not only on stage of maturation, but also on the support systems available.

Personal Factors

Adaptation to stress, whether positive or negative, is influenced by a number of personal factors. A person's physiologic reserve, genetics, epigenetic changes, and psychosocial factors influence a person's ability to maintain homeostasis and adapt to stressors. The ability to adapt is lower in the very young, the very old, and those with altered physical health who do not have the necessary physiologic reserves to cope with physical changes such as dehydration or fluid excess. Adequate nutrition and sleep are necessary for enzyme function, immune responses, wound healing, and energy production and restoration. Malnutrition, dietary deficits or excess, and sleep deprivation all impair a person's ability to adapt to stress. People with mental health issues may lack adaptability and flexibility because their resources, both internal and external, are already dedicated to maintaining balance; a new stressor can send them into crisis. Genetics influences the number and availability of adaptive responses and the ability to choose the most effective response. For example, although the sickle cell gene is prevalent in some communities in Africa, the gene provides some resistance to malaria, which may be adaptive for those communities (Norris, 2020). Social factors and life events also affect a person's adaptation to stress. People who have strong support systems and relationships are better able to adapt to stress and remain healthy.

STRESS AND ADAPTATION IN NURSING

Nursing involves activities and interpersonal relationships that are often stressful (Fig. 43-4). Activities and situations identified as highly stressful include the following:

- Assuming responsibilities for which you are not prepared
- Working with unqualified or an insufficient number of personnel
- Working in an environment in which supervisors and administrators are not supportive
- Experiencing conflict with a peer or other member of the interprofessional team
- Caring for a patient who is suffering while also supporting the patient's family
- Caring for a patient during a cardiac arrest or for a patient who is dying
- Providing care to a patient who is disengaged, nonadherent, or lacks the resources to participate in their care
- Knowing the correct, right, or ethical course of action in a situation, but being unable to take that action (moral distress)

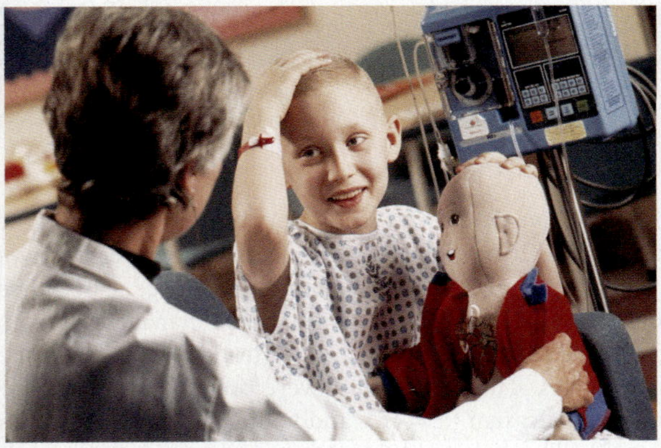

FIGURE 43-4. Some nursing specialties can be more stressful than others. To prevent burnout and alleviate personal stress, a nurse may need to work in another area of nursing temporarily or permanently.

This kind of stress is even greater for two specific groups of nurses: new graduates, who must adjust to an environment and role different from that experienced as students, and nurses who work in settings such as intensive care and emergency care.

Patients in hospitals are more acutely ill today than in the past. This situation, combined with a shortage of nurses, the increasing number of people older than age 65 years, technologic advances, and health care policies that impact on health care access and resources, has resulted in more stressful conditions for nurses in the workplaces. Nurses often need to work longer hours or more overtime.

In addition, nurses may have concerns about incivility, bullying, or workplace violence (American Nurses Association [ANA], 2015). Incivility encompasses rude or discourteous actions that negatively affect others. Incivility can escalate to bullying, which can be defined as repeated, ongoing actions that intend to harm another person, such as humiliation, offensive speech or actions, or other methods of causing distress. Workplace violence, which consists of actions that cause psychological or physical damage, can be perpetrated by: (1) someone who has no relationship with the victim (crime-based); (2) a customer, client, or patient; (3) a co-worker, who may or may not be a peer; or (4) someone involved in a personal relationship with the victim (ANA, 2015). Nurses may worry not only about the future of their positions, but also about the safety of their patients, and may harbor concerns about their own personal safety. The anxiety is complicated by the expectations of nurses to provide compassionate, person-centered care in sometimes challenging situations. Creating a culture of respect within the profession and our workplaces promotes positive interpersonal and interprofessional relationships, and improves the physical and psychological well-being of nurses (ANA, 2015).

Student nurses also experience stress related to the difficulty of adapting to the requirements and responsibilities of caring for others. Other factors causing stress in student nurses include the following:

- Fear of failing the classroom or clinical laboratory components of each course
- Fear of failing the licensure examination after graduation
- The physical, emotional, cognitive, and psychological demands of the nursing program
- Fear of injuring patients
- The need to balance work, home, and school
- The need to meet financial and family responsibilities

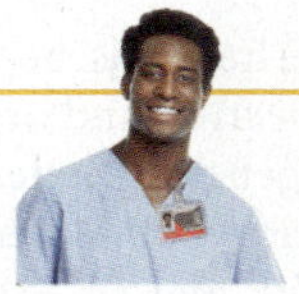

Recall **Christopher Weiss,** the nursing student described in the Reflective Practice display. He was feeling overwhelmed with the responsibilities of caring for patients in a high-tech environment. This feeling was compounded by his concerns about the assigned instructor. Subsequently, Christopher began to feel ill.

Most nurses and student nurses enjoy their education and work, coping with physical and emotional demands effectively. Some, however, become overwhelmed and develop symptoms of stress, or a complex set of behaviors and emotions called **burnout**. Burnout can be compared with the exhaustion stage of anxiety and is characterized by a wide range of behaviors. Some nurses try to become "supernurses," expecting perfection in themselves and others. Some withdraw and do only minimal work, while still others resort to drugs or alcohol. Nurses must acknowledge their stress and secure the necessary personal and professional resources to adapt and cope or they may end up leaving the profession. Refer to the Research in Nursing box (on page 1778) for a discussion of resilience practices.

What can graduate and student nurses do to help reduce stress and prevent burnout? The first step in preventing a stress level high enough to cause burnout is to identify and accept the stress. The same stress-reduction techniques that are used for patients have positive benefits for nurses. Nurses must accept that they have the same needs and are as individual as their patients. Largely in response to the pandemic, the American Nurses Foundation of the ANA, in partnership with the Emergency Nurses Association (ENA, https://www.ena.org/), the American Association of Critical-Care Nurses (AACN, https://www.aacn.org/), the American Psychiatric Nurses Association (APNA, https://www.apna.org/i4a/pages/index.cfm?pageid=1), and the Association of periOperative Registered Nurses (AORN) launched the *Well-Being Initiative*. The site links to free tools and apps designed to support the mental health and well-being of nurses. Specific topics include cultivating gratitude, narrative expressive writing, sleep assistance, access to therapy, suicide prevention, and other topics designed to support nurses and foster resilience (ANA Enterprise, 2021). By recognizing the early signs of stress and taking steps to reduce it, nurses can continue to be effective, productive, and satisfied in the profession (see Focused Critical Thinking Guide 43-1 on page 1782).

Nurse Self-Care Alert

Check out Moodfit at https://www.getmoodfit.com/. The app provides tools to help build your mental health fitness.

Research in Nursing

BRIDGING THE GAP TO EVIDENCE-BASED PRACTICE

Resilience in Nursing

There has been an emphasis on building individual, collective, and organizational resilience in nursing. Resilience generally refers to the ability to withstand or adapt to adversity, stress, or trauma. It requires a responsive flexibility and includes neurobiologic, psychological, and social ecologic components (Rushton, 2018). Although wellness initiatives, an emphasis on self-care, and the integration of concrete mindful and reflective practices support nurses in developing their individual resilience, individual resilience is not enough to mitigate the complexities in health care systems that often lead to moral distress (Rushton, 2018; Wocial, 2020). A systems approach holds health care organizations, professional organizations, governing and regulatory bodies, and the public accountable for the health and well-being of health care professionals. This approach supports the development of viable processes to mitigate moral distress, decrease microaggressions, and eliminate burnout. Nurse leaders are crucial for the successful implementation of initiatives focused on changes at the systems level that foster nurse resilience and, ultimately, lead to improved patient outcomes.

Related Research

Wei, H., Roberts, P., Strickler, J., & Corbett, R. W. (2019). Nurse leaders' strategies to foster nurse resilience. *Journal of Nursing Management, 27*(4), 681–687. https://doi.org/10.1111/jonm.12736

This qualitative descriptive study from November 2017–June 2018 involved 20 nurse leaders and explored their perspectives on effective strategies to foster nurse resilience. The nurse leaders were charge nurses ($n = 8$), nurse managers ($n = 8$), and nurse executives ($n = 4$) from a tertiary hospital in the United States. The participants were predominantly female ($n = 18$), Caucasian ($n = 16$), and younger than age 56 years ($n = 17$). Through qualitative interviews and the associated phenomenologic-based analytical framework, seven resilience-cultivating strategies were identified: (1) facilitating social connections and acts of kindness, (2) promoting positivity through role modeling and practicing gratitude, (3) capitalizing on nurses' strengths and creativity, (4) nurturing nurses' growth personally and professionally, (5) encouraging nurses' self-care and establishing a supportive work environment, (6) fostering mindfulness practice, and (7) conveying altruism through the creation of caring connections and meaningful recognition.

Relevance to Nursing Practice

Nurse leaders make a difference in building resilience in their teams. The specific initiatives described in the interviews were generally simple, focused on the nurses, and were collaborative in nature. A systems approach to building resilience in the workplace can begin with nurse leaders.

NURSING PROCESS FOR THE PATIENT WITH STRESS AND ANXIETY

Self-awareness of stress and anxiety is essential when caring for patients. Nurses who role-model good health behaviors are more effective teachers. Use the tool found in Promoting Health 43-1 for yourself before using it with others.

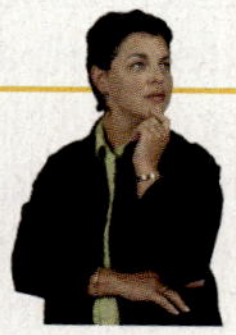

Remember **Joan Rogerrio,** the woman returning to work after an absence of 15 years. The nurse could use the tool in Promoting Health 43-1 (on page 1780) as part of the patient's assessment. Then the nurse could use those items identified as *sometimes* and *almost never* as a basis for teaching Joan measures to adapt and cope with her stressors.

Assessing

Stress and anxiety are problems that nurses encounter in patients of all ages and in all settings. Stress is assessed through a health assessment, which includes a nursing history and physical assessment. Risk factors for, or indicators of, stress may be identified through standardized tests or open-ended questions to elicit information. The patient's willingness to share information is affected by the level of stress experienced as well as the coping or defense mechanisms in use.

Nursing History

The nursing history assists the nurse in identifying stressors and how the person perceives and copes with stress. Manifestations of anxiety, as well as questions and leading statements to identify stress and anxiety, are listed in the Focused Assessment Guide 43-1 on page 1780.

Physical Assessment

There are no specific guidelines for the physical assessment of stress. Physical indicators of stress, in addition to those listed in the Focused Assessment Guide, may include cardiac dysrhythmias, chest pain, headache, hyperventilation, diarrhea, tense muscles, and skin lesions, such as eczema. These manifestations are the result of the mind–body interaction described earlier.

Diagnosing

Assessment data may reveal stress to be the actual or potential problem, or stress may be the etiology of another problem.

Promoting Health 43-1

STRESS AND ADAPTATION

Nurses who design care plans for patients to reduce stress must also consider themselves a factor in the success of that care plan. The nurse who wishes to encourage healthy adaptation to stress must demonstrate behaviors that support a healthy lifestyle. Use the assessment checklist to determine how well *you* are adapting to stress. Then develop a prescription for self-care by choosing the appropriate behaviors from the list of suggestions.

Assessment Checklist

☐ almost always ☐ sometimes ☐ almost never

☐ ☐ ☐ 1. I have realistic perceptions of new situations, self, and others.

☐ ☐ ☐ 2. I understand my own personal physical and emotional responses to stress.

☐ ☐ ☐ 3. I anticipate and prepare for change.

☐ ☐ ☐ 4. I have the ability to satisfactorily solve problems and make decisions.

Self-Care Behaviors

1. Accept the changes that come with different parts and stages of life as positive indicators of growth.
2. Maintain an open mind about change—change what you can and accept what you cannot change.
3. Avoid self-defeating behaviors to cope with stress such as smoking, alcohol, and drugs.
4. Avoid confrontational and unprofessional interactions with other staff members—engage in civil discourse.
5. Develop a greater awareness of potential risks in the workplace that can result in violence.
6. Practice methods of stress management that work best for you: relaxation techniques, exercise, hobbies.
7. Set realistic goals.
8. Develop problem-solving strategies for use in stressful situations.
9. Accept help from others.
10. Take life one day at a time—embrace the concepts of mindfulness and centering.

See the accompanying display, Examples of Actual or Potential Health Problems and Needs: The Patient Experiencing Stress on page 1780.

Stress as the Problem

The following problems may be identified when stress is the problem (International Council of Nurses [ICN], 2019):

- Stress overload related to single parenthood, inadequate economic resources, and chronic illness
- Moral distress related to cultural conflicts, end-of-life decisions, conflicting information about ethical decision making, or treatment decisions

Stress as the Etiology

Stress and anxiety may affect many other areas of human functioning. In the following problems, stress and anxiety are involved in the etiologies of other problems (ICN, 2019):

- "Caregiver stress related to the long-term stress of caring for a parent with dementia, as evidenced by the statement," "I am just at my wits ends trying to keep mom safe!"
- "Impaired spiritual status related to the stress of a new terminal diagnosis, as evidenced by the statement," "God has forsaken me"
- Hopelessness related to presence of disabling physical injuries, as evidenced by statement, "I give up . . . it's just not worth it," apathy, visible lack of engagement

Outcome Identification and Planning

The nurse plans and implements care to decrease anxiety and facilitate adaptation in the patient with stress. The expected outcomes of the plan must be mutually determined with the patient or family members. Examples of expected outcomes are as follows:

The patient will:

- Decrease the level of anxiety by verbalizing feelings and using support systems.
- Develop effective methods of coping through problem-solving skills and anxiety-reducing techniques.
- Describe a reduction in anxiety and an increase in comfort.
- Identify three concrete stress-reduction techniques that are of interest.
- Identify resources to manage moral distress (see Chapter 6) and spiritual distress.

Implementing

Nurses may use a variety of interventions to help patients decrease stress and to facilitate coping. Methods should be selected carefully based on the person's physical and emotional characteristics, family and social structure, and previously used successful coping mechanisms. Guidelines for Nursing Care 43-1 on page 1781 list nursing interventions to reduce stress and anxiety for patients as they enter a health care setting.

If the patient's anxiety seems too great or if the nurse is uncomfortable with the interventions, a referral should be made to a professional counselor. The patient may also be helped by meeting with a spiritual advisor (rabbi, minister, priest, etc.) or people who have experienced the same type of surgery or health problem. (see Focused Critical Thinking Guide 43-1 on page 1782).

Focused Assessment Guide 43-1

ANXIETY PRECIPITATED BY STRESS

Factors to Assess	Questions and Approaches
Subjective data Heart palpitations Difficulty breathing Problems with appetite or sleep Feelings of sadness, apprehension, anger, mistrust, helplessness, hopelessness Changes in sexual desire	• "Have you noticed that you sometimes feel your heart beating or have difficulty breathing?" • "Tell me about your appetite and sleep." • "Of the following, which best describes how you are feeling: sad, apprehensive, angry, mistrustful, helpless, hopeless?" • "Tell me about any changes you have noticed in your sexual desire." • "How does your body feel when you are upset?"
Objective data Dry mouth Increased perspiration Tremors Tachycardia Increased blood pressure Dilated pupils Crying Restlessness Rapid speech Pacing around the room Lack of facial expression	• Note body posture and movements. • Inspect skin and mucous membranes. • Take and record vital signs. • Note general affect.
Ability to verbalize anxiety	• "You have been very quiet today. Has something happened since our last visit?" • "It must be very frightening to be told that you have cancer." • "I notice you seem upset. Would you like to talk about it?" • "What has caused you to feel stressed in the past?" • "What do you do to feel better when you feel anxious?"

Examples of Actual or Potential Health Problems and Needs

THE PATIENT EXPERIENCING STRESS

Actual or Potential Health Problem or Need	Possible Etiologic Factors	Potential Signs and Symptoms

Anxiety	• Conflicts about values and goals in life
	  • Threat to self-concept, threat of death, threat of change in health status, threat to environment or role
	  • Situational/maturational crisis
	• Unmet needs
		• Verbalizations of anxiety
		• Impaired decision making
		• Nervous behaviors: pacing, twitching, picking, frequent movements, or shaking
		• Impatience or anger
		• Physiologic changes such as tachycardia or tachypnea

		—
Coping Impairment	• Previous coping mechanisms ineffective or insufficient • Inability to identify coping strategies • Inability to identify or employ internal or external resources • Lack of experience with stress • Decreased adaptability	• Signs of anxiety or depression • Verbalization of coping issues • Negative physical, psychological, emotional, or behavioral changes

Source: International Council of Nurses (ICN). (2019). *Nursing diagnosis and outcome statements.* https://www.icn.ch/sites/default/files/inline-files/ICNP2019-DC.pdf; Wolters Kluwer. (2022). Problem-based care plans. In *Lippincott Advisor.* Wolters Kluwer. https://advisor.lww.com/lna/home.do

Guidelines for Nursing Care 43-1

REDUCING ANXIETY ON ADMISSION TO A HEALTH CARE FACILITY

1. Assess physical status, sensory status, and cognitive status.
2. Assess cultural/ethnic background, including beliefs about health care, dietary restrictions, and language spoken.
3. Assess past experiences with the health care system, including medical-surgical treatment for illness or injury.
4. Assess concerns and stressors.
5. Assess number and type of support systems available.
6. Provide information about the environment:
   a. Ensure that all health care providers introduce themselves by name and title.
   b. Explain policies and routines.
   c. If the hospital is the setting, provide verbal and written guidelines for use of equipment, telephone, and television. Also provide information about meals and visiting hours.
7. Provide and discuss the patient's rights specific to care in the facility.
8. Mutually determine expected outcomes of the plan of care.
9. Provide information about all diagnostic procedures, surgical procedures, activity, and diet.

Teaching Healthy Activities of Daily Living

A person's usual lifestyle greatly influences that person's perceptions of and reactions to stressors. Exercise, rest, and good nutrition are important components of stress reduction, so it follows that a person who is overweight, sedentary, and chronically sleep-deprived is at increased risk for developing an illness as a result of stress.

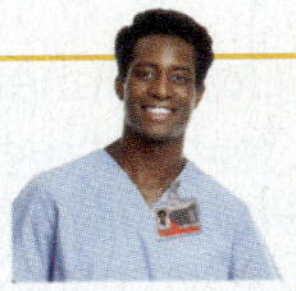

Think about **Christopher Weiss's** lifestyle as a student nurse. His school-related workload places Christopher at risk for stress. In addition, other factors, such as demands from family members or a need to work part-time, decrease his ability to maintain a healthy lifestyle that includes regular exercise, rest, and good nutrition.

EXERCISE

Regular exercise helps maintain physical and emotional health. The benefits of exercise include an improved musculoskeletal system, more effective cardiovascular function, weight control, and relaxation. Exercise improves a person's general sense of well-being, relieves tension, and enables coping with day-to-day stressors. General health guidelines recommend that an exercise program consists of 30 to 45 minutes of moderate activity above usual activity on most days of the week. People who are overweight, chronically ill, or older than age 35 years should have a physical examination before beginning such a program. The type of exercise depends on what the person enjoys—for example, walking, jogging, bicycling, swimming, or sports such as golf or tennis.

REST AND SLEEP

Rest and sleep help the body maintain homeostasis and restore energy levels. Adequate rest can provide insulation against stress, but stress may interfere with a person's ability to sleep. Each person has individual sleep needs, but 7 to 9 hours of sleep a day is the usual recommendation. Relaxation techniques can be used during both health and illness to facilitate rest and sleep. Hospitalized patients may require additional nursing interventions to relieve pain and promote comfort to get needed rest.

NUTRITION

Overeating food that is not nutrient-dense, severely limiting intake, and craving a specific food are common (often negative) coping strategies that need to be considered when addressing stress and coping mechanisms. Nutrition plays an active role in maintaining the body's homeostatic mechanisms and in increasing resistance to stress. (Nutrition is discussed in detail in Chapter 37.) Obesity and malnutrition are major stressors and greatly increase the risk for illness. New 2020–2025 Dietary Guidelines for Americans includes a call to action, "Make Every Bite Count with the Dietary Guidelines" (U.S. Department of Agriculture & U.S. Department of Health and Human Services, 2020). This initiative focuses on choosing nutrient-dense foods and portion control to stay within the stage-of-life-specific calorie recommendations. This means limiting sugars, saturated fat, and alcohol intake to about 15% of calories. In the United States, there is public health concern over the dietary intake of calcium, potassium, fiber, vitamin D, and iron, so standard portions and smaller portions of nutrient-dense foods are specifically addressed in the recommendations. To allow for cultural, budgetary, and lifestyle choices, the guidelines are adaptable and not prescriptive, but they do encourage assessing and developing a pattern of healthy eating and not focusing on a specific food or meal (U.S. Department of Agriculture & U.S. Department of Health and Human Services, 2020). Check out the specific guidelines and teaching materials for you and the populations you serve at https://www.dietaryguidelines.gov/resources/2020-2025-dietary-guidelines-online-materials

Encouraging Use of Support Systems

Families and support groups provide emotional support that can help a person identify and verbalize feelings associated with stress. In addition, families and support groups provide an accepting environment, allowing the person to explore problem-solving methods and try out new coping skills. Support groups, aside from providing information and services, may help a person maintain a positive self-concept and establish an avenue for new relationships and social roles. There are support groups for almost every situation; examples are listed in Box 43-5 on page 1783.

43-1 Focused Critical Thinking Guide

STRESS AND ANXIETY

You are a senior nursing student in a community health course. You have been assigned to visit and provide ongoing assessments for Charles Obedide, a 28-year-old man who was involved in a serious motorcycle crash a year ago and is paralyzed from the waist down. Charles initially participated fully in his rehabilitation, and has been living independently in an apartment that is wheelchair accessible. However, a month ago, Charles was ill for 2 weeks, lost his job, and broke up with his girlfriend. When you made your last home visit, Charles was restless, had an increased pulse, and did little talking. At today's visit, Charles is wearing dirty clothes and has a strong body odor. There are several empty beer cans on the table in the kitchen. Charles begins to cry, saying, "I am so upset—I can't sleep or eat—I need help." What would you do?

1. Identify goal of thinking

Identify the level of anxiety experienced by Charles and begin interventions to help Charles decrease his level of anxiety.

2. Assess adequacy of knowledge

Pertinent circumstances: Charles has had numerous losses in the past year, including loss of body function and changes in body image. He has recently lost his job, a major source of economic support and self-concept. He separated from his girlfriend, a major source of support. Previously, Charles was clean and well groomed. There was no previous evidence of drinking. His parents live nearby and are supportive and loving. These stressors are manifesting as anxiety in Charles.

Prerequisite knowledge: Before you decide what to do in this situation, you need to assess the level of stress and associated anxiety experienced by Charles. You need to know the typical behaviors of each level and be able to recognize that Charles has severe anxiety. You must recognize that Charles needs interventions to regain equilibrium.

Room for error: Charles requires and has asked for help. You are unsure of your abilities to help him deal effectively with his anxiety. You realize that his frustration with the situation could make him angry. You also know that depression and the potential for self-violence are risks unless something is done to reduce his anxiety.

Time constraints: Although you are not certain about how serious his problem is, you understand that Charles needs help in reducing his anxiety soon. There is time for you to ask for guidance from your instructor.

3. Address potential problems

There are several potential barriers to critical thinking in this situation. You realize Charles needs help in reducing his level of stress, which in turn causes you anxiety. You are also somewhat frightened about his appearance and behavior. You do not believe your own abilities are developed well enough to help Charles adequately, but at the same time, you do know he needs help. You are comfortable sitting with Charles, making eye contact, and being present with him. Although he is not very talkative, making sure he is not alone and receives compassionate care in this moment is important.

4. Consult helpful resources

Your best source of information is Charles himself. You ask him what you can do to help him. He replies, "Just get someone here to help me." You ask his permission to call his mother and he agrees. His mother says she will be there in 5 minutes. You call your instructor, and she tells you to call the home health care facility for further instructions.

5. Critique judgment/decision

When his mother arrives, she says she had no idea he was so distressed. She talks to the home health care facility staff, who report that they have called Charles's health care provider and will continue to follow up on needed care and referrals for professional counseling. You believe you made the right decisions: you identified that Charles needed help, you provided compassionate support in the moment, you contacted his mother to provide support, you contacted your instructor, and you contacted the home health care facility. You also remained calm during the situation, despite your own anxiety.

Encouraging Use of Stress Management Techniques

Stress creates emotional distress that often produces physical signs and symptoms. One person may have tension headaches, another may become irritable, and yet another may clench both fists. Some people take legal or illegal drugs, smoke, drink to excess, or eat compulsively. These behaviors can be modified, and adaptive mechanisms can be strengthened through specific techniques aimed at managing stress. Only a few techniques are included here, but the literature describes many stress reduction methods, including exercise, prayer, art therapy, music therapy, massage, and therapeutic touch. Chapter 29 provides more information. Students should learn different methods they can use for themselves and in varied clinical situations.

RELAXATION

Relaxation techniques are useful in many situations, such as childbirth, pain, anxiety, sleeplessness, illness, and anger. Relaxation promotes a body reaction opposite to that of the fight-or-flight response: respiratory, pulse, and metabolic rates, as well as blood pressure and energy use, can all be decreased using relaxation methods.

Box 43-5 Examples of Support Groups

- Alcoholics anonymous
- Assertiveness training groups
- Child abuse support groups
- Ostomy clubs
- Overeaters anonymous
- Parents without partners
- Reach to recovery (cancer)
- Stroke clubs
- Sudden infant death support groups
- Weight Watchers

Look also for online support groups sponsored by professional organizations or individuals with similar issues. See Healthfinder.gov, a website of the Office of Disease Prevention and Health Promotion, U.S. Department of Health and Human Services, to locate a support group.

Relaxation can be taught to individuals or groups. It is especially helpful because it allows people to control their feelings and behaviors. Relaxation techniques include progressive relaxation (tensing, then relaxing), autogenic training (focused mental exercises), guided imagery, biofeedback-assisted relaxation, self-hypnosis (uses suggestions), and breathing exercises (diaphragmatic breathing; National Center for Complementary and Integrative Health [NCCIH], 2021). Relaxation is discussed as a comfort measure in Chapter 36. See Guidelines for Nursing Care 43-2 for a description of deep breathing and progressive muscle relaxation.

MINDFULNESS

Mindfulness practice has been widely implemented in health care in the past few years. Mindfulness requires intentional presence and focus on the moment. Curiosity, openness, and acceptance without judgment support the centering. Meditation and breathing exercises may be used to support the mindfulness practice. Forest bathing or *shinrin-yoku*, the Japanese-based practice of opening the five senses to connect with the natural world in the present moment, provides another method of engaging in mindfulness. Psychological and physical benefits include stress and anxiety reduction; improvement in cardiovascular and immune health; and increases in energy, concentration, and creativity (Li, 2018). Mindfulness practices may positively impact nurses by decreasing their stress, anxiety, depression, and burnout while increasing their well-being and capacity for empathy (Chmielewski et al., 2021).

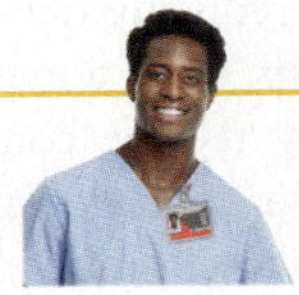

Christopher Weiss, the student nurse, could learn to perform relaxation exercises or practice meditation. Both techniques would be helpful in reducing his stress.

ANTICIPATORY GUIDANCE

Anticipatory guidance focuses on psychologically preparing a person for an unfamiliar or painful event. Nurses use this technique when they teach patients about procedures and the surgical experience. When patients know what to expect, their anxiety is reduced and their coping mechanisms are more effective. For example, before performing a painful procedure (such as ambulating for the first time after surgery), teaching would include information about the pain involved, including onset, severity, cause, and methods of relief. With this knowledge, the patient feels less threatened and tolerates the procedure more easily.

A related process is anticipatory socialization, in which people prepare themselves for roles to which they aspire but do not yet occupy. Parenting classes taken before the birth of a child or an internship/externship provide good examples of this activity.

GUIDED IMAGERY

In guided imagery, a person creates a mental image, concentrates on the image, and becomes less responsive to other stimuli (including pain). The nurse sits by the patient and reads a description of a scene or an experience that the patient has described as happy, pleasant, or peaceful. The patient is then "guided" through the image. For example, using a soothing, soft voice, the nurse might start as follows: "You are floating in your swimming pool. The water is cool and comfortable. Birds are singing in the trees. The roses are perfuming the air." As the patient becomes more and more focused on the scene, the nurse needs only to verbally "paint the picture" at intervals.

Guidelines for Nursing Care 43-2

RELAXATION ACTIVITIES

Deep Breathing

1. Sit comfortably and place your hands on your stomach. Inhale slowly and deeply, letting your abdomen expand as much as possible. Hold your breath for a few seconds.
2. Exhale slowly through your mouth, blowing through puckered lips. When your abdomen feels empty, begin again with a deep inhalation.

Progressive Muscle Relaxation

1. Tighten your hand into a fist and notice how it feels. Hold the tension for a few seconds.
2. Loosen your grip, relax the muscles in your hand, and let the tension slip away.
3. Continue to tighten–hold–relax each muscle group, moving head to toe: face, shoulders, arms, chest, back, abdomen, legs, and feet.

Providing Crisis Intervention

A crisis is a situation that cannot be resolved by usual coping mechanisms. As a result, the person cannot function normally and requires interventions to regain equilibrium. **Crisis intervention** is a short-term management technique focused on reducing damage to an individual or group affected by a crisis, often a mental or medical health emergency. The crisis may require community resources, such as a local mobile crisis team, to diffuse. The need for crisis intervention may arise with individuals or groups of any age and may be triggered by internal psychological processes or external factors, such as natural or manmade disasters (Wang & Gupta, 2021). Although there are several models of crisis intervention and the contextual elements of the crisis need to be considered, the SAFER-R model is often used as a beginning framework for individual crisis intervention (Everly & Mitchell, 2017):

1. *Stabilization.* Introduce yourself and establish your role and that of the other people involved. Meet basic needs, consider safety of all parties, and mitigate any acute stressors if possible.
2. *Acknowledgment.* Acknowledge the precipitating event and the reactions of the individual.
3. *Facilitation of understanding.* Paraphrase and reflect back to the individual what they are experiencing. Normalize their reaction to a stressful event and work to minimize feelings of personal weakness.
4. *Encourage effective coping.* Tap into their existing coping tools and resources and identify external sources of support to facilitate coping.
5. *Recovery.* Assess and establish the person's ability to function safety.
6. *Referral.* Make referrals as needed.

The major factor in helping patients adapt to high levels of stress is to identify and plan individually for situations causing the stress. Maintaining immediate safety is a priority. Facilitate the patient's recognition of their own stress level and specific responses to stress. Encourage adoption of a philosophy of accepting what cannot be changed and changing what cannot be accepted. Emphasize the importance of accepting help from others and giving support to others when needed as well as being actively involved in problem solving and decision making. Nurses must use therapeutic communication skills in all interactions but must be especially cognizant of their words and actions in a crisis situation.

QSEN SAFETY

Promoting safety is an overriding priority in crisis management. Consider whether the individual (or group) is in danger of self-harm or harm from others. Also consider environmental safety and whether the person (or group) in crisis is a danger to others. Once any immediate safety concerns are addressed, engage in crisis-management techniques that are appropriate for the situation.

Crisis Standards of Care

Crisis standards of care may be considered during times of mass crisis when resources (equipment, space, or trained personnel) are insufficient to meet the demands. It involves careful consideration of the circumstances and available resources, and equitable allocation of available resources. In a crisis, the health care system may not be able to maintain usual approaches to care. We may be forced to implement contingency care that requires reworking strategies, including staffing decisions, space designation, and resource conservation to maintain the delivery of functionally equivalent care. If the system is taxed further, crisis standards of care may be implemented, which requires a systems approach (The Commonwealth of Massachusetts, Executive Office of Health and Human Services Department of Public Health, 2020). It is important to remember that these processes stress the individuals involved, but the stress experienced by the entire system can be mitigated by planning and regularly reevaluating processes and decisions.

Evaluating

The evaluation of the plan of care is based on the mutually established expected outcomes. Be sure to observe both verbal and nonverbal cues when evaluating the usefulness of the plan. In general, the plan is considered successful if the patient and those important to them have been able to do the following:

- Verbalize causes and effects of stress and anxiety
- Identify and use sources of support
- Use problem solving to find solutions to stressors
- Practice healthy lifestyle habits and anxiety-reducing techniques
- Verbalize a decrease in anxiety and an increase in comfort

REFLECTIVE PRACTICE LEADING TO PERSONAL LEARNING

Remember that the object of reflective practice is to look at an experience, understand it, and learn from it. As you begin to develop your expertise in identifying and responding to stress and adaptation needs, reflect on your experiences—successes and failures—in order to improve your practice. How can you do it better next time? What did you learn today that can help you tomorrow? Begin your reflection by paying close attention to the following:

- How aware are you of developmental and situational stressors and stress? Are you able to articulate key manifestations of stress?
- What value do you attach to involving the patient in stress management techniques? How do you individualize the care for patients?
- How do you plan to hone your skills in managing the complexities of stress that can involve psychological and physiologic aspects?

Keeping up with the latest evidence-based practice guidelines can be challenging. New technology and techniques in stress management continue to be developed to combat perceived stressors. Developing a working knowledge of the core principles of stress and stress management provides a foundation for your nursing practice.

Perhaps the most important questions to reflect on are: Are your patients and families/caregivers better for having had *you* share in the critical responsibility of partnering with them to ensure appropriate skin and wound care? Are your patients now receiving thoughtful, person-centered, prioritized, holistic, evidence-based treatment and care because of your efforts?

Nursing Care Plan for *Mei Fu* 43-1

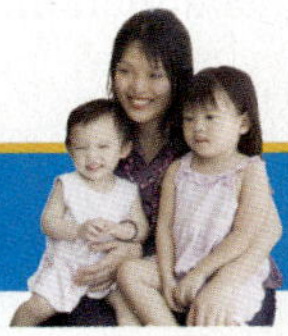

Remember Mei Fu, the 24-year-old graduate student with a husband and two small children. At her clinic appointment, the nurse conducted a health history and physical assessment of Mei Fu and noted the following data:

- Patient is a thin woman who appears her stated age. She is currently in school and expects herself to make the highest grades. She also cares for her two children and her husband. Although her husband encourages her to go to school, he believes it is the wife's responsibility to provide all child and house care. She has had no previous serious illnesses or surgery.
- Patient reports having frequent headaches, rating the pain as a 3 on a scale of 0 (no pain) to 10 (worst possible pain). She also reports having four to six bowel movements each day, sometimes with abdominal cramping. The diarrhea does not seem to be related to any type of foods eaten. Both the headaches and the diarrhea have been present for the past 2 months. During the interview, the patient appeared restless and talked rapidly. Questions often had to be repeated.
- Physical assessment reveals slight tachycardia, a fine hand tremor, and visible perspiration. Large muscle groups are tense and fists clenched. No tenderness is noted on abdominal palpation. Pupils are equal in size and react to light and accommodation. Nasal mucosa is normal.

ACTUAL OR POTENTIAL HEALTH PROBLEMS OR NEED

Anxiety

Etiology: stress of achievement in school and care of family

Signs and Symptoms: rapid speech, tachycardia, tremor, tense muscles, headache, and diarrhea

Goal: Patient reports experiencing a decrease in anxiety.

EXPECTED OUTCOME

By her return appointment in 2 weeks, 10/20/25, Mei Fu will:

- Identify sources of and responses to stress

NURSING INTERVENTIONS	RATIONALE	EVALUATIVE STATEMENT
Ask Mei Fu to keep a diary of hours spent in school-related activities and family care, number and times of headaches, and circumstances that occurred before diarrhea.	Identifying sources of stress and the physical responses to stress is the first step in planning coping strategies to reduce stress.	10/20/25 Outcome met. Mei Fu kept a diary as requested. She identified that she does not have any time for herself. Her headaches are worse during the week. She often has diarrhea when papers are due or when her husband and children are demanding of her time. *S. Aird, RN, FNP*

EXPECTED OUTCOME

By her return appointment, 10/20/25, Mei Fu will:

- Identify sources of personal strength and support

(continued on page 1786)

Nursing Care Plan for *Mei Fu* 43-1 *(continued)*

NURSING INTERVENTIONS	RATIONALE	EVALUATIVE STATEMENT
Ask Mei Fu to make a list of the people who are important to her and provide her comfort and discuss how these people can help her cope with her situation.	Identifying support people provides the patient with the means to manage stress and enhances self-concept.	10/20/25 Outcome met. Mei Fu stated that her family is her greatest source of support, but they are in China and she misses them very much. She does have a very good friend who is also a good listener. She identified her strengths as being a person who cares for others and a good student. She said she is also a good artist but has not had time for art for months. *S. Aird, RN, FNP*
Ask Mei Fu to create a list of her strengths as a woman, a mother, a wife, and a student.	Recognizing strengths provides an opportunity to build confidence and mobilize internal coping mechanisms	

EXPECTED OUTCOME

By her return appointment, 10/20/25, Mei Fu will:

- Describe lifestyle changes that include eating a well-balanced diet with three meals a day, walking for 20 to 30 minutes four times a week, and sleeping restfully 7 hours a night

NURSING INTERVENTIONS	RATIONALE	EVALUATIVE STATEMENT
Provide Mei Fu the Dietary Guidelines for Americans and review the importance of healthy eating patterns that include eating three meals a day and include any specific cultural preferences.	Adequate nutrition helps maintain the homeostatic mechanisms of the body and increases resistance to stress.	10/20/25 Outcome met. Mei Fu was given a copy of the Dietary Guidelines for Americans and food preparations were discussed. Although the Fu family has a healthy diet, Mei Fu often was too busy to eat more than a few bites. She said that she is making a big effort to eat three times a day. She is walking to school and enjoys the time by herself. She arranged this time by asking her husband to take the children to school. She is sleeping better, and averages 7 hours most nights. *S. Aird, RN, FNP*
Teach Mei Fu about the physiologic and psychological effects of regular exercise in reducing stress.	Exercise improves well-being, relieves tension, and facilitates coping with daily stressors.	
Discuss with Mei Fu the importance of sleep in reducing stress.	Adequate rest and sleep restore energy and facilitate coping with stressors.	

EXPECTED OUTCOME

By her return appointment, 10/20/25, Mei Fu will:

- Practice relaxation for 20 minutes each day

Nursing Care Plan for *Mei Fu* 43-1 *(continued)*

NURSING INTERVENTIONS	RATIONALE	EVALUATIVE STATEMENT
Teach and have Mei Fu practice progressive muscle relaxation.	Relaxation promotes a response opposite to the stress response; it decreases heart rate, respiratory rate, blood pressure, and metabolic processes.	10/20/25 Outcome met. Mei Fu said that at first she had difficulty in finding time to be alone, but she feels so much better after she relaxes that she insists on the time. She found an online site she "really likes" and says it helps her "very much." *S. Aird, RN, FNP*
Teach Mei Fu how to access and use free online resources for relaxation techniques.	Free resources that are easily accessible are more likely to be used by this busy college student.	
Create a calendar with Mei Fu outlining time for intentional, mindful relaxation exercises.	Time constraints are the primary concern for this patient. Writing things into a calendar promotes accountability and provides a means to communicate with her family when she needs to block time for relaxation.	

EXPECTED OUTCOME

By her return appointment, 10/20/25, Mei Fu will:
- Report a decrease in signs and symptoms of stress, headaches, and diarrhea

NURSING INTERVENTIONS	RATIONALE	EVALUATIVE STATEMENT
Assess frequency and severity of headaches and bowel movements.	Decreasing stress in daily life often is effective in decreasing physical responses. Self-care of stress is critical in effective management.	10/20/25 Outcome met. Mei Fu reports she has noticed fewer headaches in the past week, and the diarrhea is almost gone. Mei Fu verbalized the importance of continuing to practice a healthy lifestyle and relaxation. She said she has spent time with her friend and has gotten out her sketch pad. She stated that she believes she can manage her life much better now. *S. Aird, RN, FNP*
Create a log to track use of coping mechanisms and their effect on managing stress.	Tracking the short- and long-term effectiveness of stress management techniques provides the patient the opportunity to reflect on time spent and efficacy of individual measures taken.	

SAMPLE DOCUMENTATION

10/06/25, 1000, nursing

Initial visit to student health center by Mei Fu to discuss physical problems of headache and diarrhea. History and physical assessment findings indicated large number of personal stressors, manifested by physical signs and symptoms. Assessment data supported problem identification: Anxiety related to stress of achievement in school and care of family. Discussion centered on identifying sources of stress, physical responses to stress, sources of support, and personal strength. Teaching strategies included diet, exercise, sleep, and progressive muscle relaxation. Patient to keep a log/diary of stressors and coping mechanisms. Patient's progress will be monitored at next visit on 10/20/25.

DEVELOPING CLINICAL REASONING AND CLINICAL JUDGMENT

1. Review the Nursing Care Plan 43-1 on pages 1785–1787 to help you hone your clinical reasoning and clinical judgment skills.
2. Identify the nursing activities and relationships that cause you the most stress. What are your personal warning signs that a situation is becoming stressful? What do you do to decrease your level of stress? Who is most important in helping you do this?
3. List nursing interventions you would use to reduce stress in the following situations:
   - A newly married young woman who found a lump in her breast and is undergoing a breast biopsy.
   - The parents of a 2-year-old who are sitting in the surgical waiting room as their child undergoes brain surgery.
   - The daughter (and caregiver) of a woman with severe Alzheimer disease.

PRACTICING FOR NCLEX

1. A nurse is assessing a patient who reports their migraines have become "unbearable." The patient states, "I got laid off from my job last week, and I have two kids in college. I don't know how I'm going to pay for it all." Which effects of physiologic effects of stress would the nurse expect to find in this patient? Select all that apply.
   a. Increased or decreased appetite
   b. Changes in elimination patterns
   c. Decreased pulse and respirations
   d. Use of ineffective coping mechanisms
   e. Withdrawal
   f. Attention-seeking behaviors
2. A nurse who performs preoperative assessments and teaching prepares patients for postoperative discomfort using anticipatory guidance. What interventions would this nurse use to decrease postoperative stress?
   a. Teaching rhythmic breathing to perform prior to the procedure
   b. Telling the patient to mentally place themselves in a pleasant place and breathe in and out slowly
   c. Explaining about expected incisional discomfort or nausea and describing relief methods
   d. Suggesting the patient create and focus on a mental image during the procedure to be less responsive to the pain
3. A nurse in a medical practice has assessed a patient reporting abdominal pain, diarrhea, and anxiety. When the health care provider finds no identifiable cause for the symptoms, which actions would the nurse recommend? Select all that apply.
   a. Keeping a diary identifying sources of stress
   b. Sleeping 4 hours per night
   c. Considering previous strengths and coping
   d. Asking whom the patient relies on for support
   e. Asking if the patient's partner is abusive
   f. Assessing for prior psychiatric conditions
4. A nurse is assessing the developmental levels of patients in a pediatric office. Which person would a nurse document as experiencing developmental stress?
   a. Infant who learns to turn over
   b. School-aged child learning to add and subtract
   c. Adolescent who is a "loner"
   d. Young adult who has a variety of friends
5. A nurse in a long-term care facility is caring for patient with a spinal cord injury affecting their sensory and motor reflexes below the waist. Based on the patient's condition, what would be a priority intervention for this patient?
   a. Taking care with hot beverages to prevent burns
   b. Providing adequate pain relief measures to reduce stress
   c. Monitoring for depression related to social isolation
   d. Offering meals high in carbohydrates to promote healing
6. A nurse in the emergency department receives a patient rescued from a building fire. The firefighter giving the handoff report tells the nurse the building collapsed immediately after they removed the patient from the building. The nurse notes the patient is experiencing the alarm phase of the fight-or-flight response. What assessment findings support the nurse's observation? Select all that apply.
   a. Rapid breathing
   b. Hypotension
   c. Restlessness
   d. Withdrawn demeanor
   e. Tachycardia
7. Nurses working in a trauma intensive care unit state they experience a high level of stress. Which stressor are they likely to encounter?
   a. Nurse manager support for equitable assignments
   b. Health care benefits
   c. Debriefings after the death of a patient
   d. Incivility by team members or bullying
8. A college student visits the school's health center reporting extreme fatigue and slight restlessness. The student states, "Exams are right around the corner, and all I feel like doing is sleeping." There are no abnormal physical assessment findings. How does the nurse best help the student frame their desire to sleep?
   a. Asking the student if they are worried about failing exams
   b. Telling them they must strive to sleep 7 to 9 hours nightly
   c. Evaluating their use of recreational drugs
   d. Explaining that some people use sleep as a coping mechanism

9. A nurse is interviewing a patient who just received a diagnosis of pancreatic cancer. The patient tells the nurse, "I'm a vegetarian. I'm not the type to get cancer; this must be a mistake." Which defense mechanism is this patient demonstrating?
   a. Projection
   b. Denial
   c. Displacement
   d. Repression
10. A visiting nurse is assessing a family that includes a young couple and their infant who has cerebral palsy. The nurse notes that the mother is unkempt, the house is untidy, and the mother states she is "so busy with the baby that I don't have time to do anything else." What priority intervention would the nurse set for this family?
    a. Arranging to have the infant removed from the home
    b. Informing other members of the family of the situation
    c. Increasing the number of visits by the visiting nurse
    d. Recommending respite care for the parent(s)
11. A nurse is teaching a patient who is experiencing stress how to perform a relaxation technique. Which statement by the patient indicates the need for additional teaching?
    a. "I must breathe in and out in rhythm."
    b. "I should expect my pulse to be faster."
    c. "I can expect my muscles to feel less tense."
    d. "I will be more relaxed and less aware."
12. A nurse in the obstetrics clinic is teaching pregnant patients techniques to manage pain during labor. Which stress reduction activities would be most effective? Select all that apply.
    a. Progressive muscle relaxation
    b. Meditation
    c. Anticipatory socialization
    d. Biofeedback
    e. Rhythmic breathing
    f. Guided imagery
13. A nurse at the university health clinic has assessed a student reporting an inability to concentrate and a pounding heart. The student states, "my boyfriend just dumped me out of the blue. They were supposed to be my date at my sister's wedding this weekend. How can I go now?" Which response would the nurse make?
    a. "Can you tell me what part of this is most problematic right now?"
    b. "What alternatives can you think of at this late date?"
    c. "You might start by evaluating your relationship."
    d. "It may be best to not think about this person until after the wedding."
14. A nurse is performing an assessment of a patient who is 8 months' pregnant. The patient states, "I worry about being able to handle becoming a mother." The nurse plans interventions for which problem?
    a. Poor coping skills
    b. Denial about the impending birth
    c. Uncertainty and anxiety due to change in role
    d. Low self-esteem and fear of parenting
15. A parent bringing their toddler for a visit to the pediatric clinic tells the nurse that after work their partner yelled at the child for dropping a fork. Later the patient learned the partner's supervisor had been angry about the contents of a report that was submitted. The nurse explains it is likely their partner was using which coping mechanism?
    a. Denial
    b. Sublimation
    c. Displacement
    d. Dissociation
16. A nursing student tells the clinical professor that they hate when they feel anxious before performing new procedures. They state they do not sleep well the night before, feel restless, and have increased alertness. How does the professor best respond to this concern?
    a. Suggesting the student seems worried about failing clinical and should seek professional help
    b. Stating that we cannot diagnose students, but these symptoms of mild anxiety can aid in learning and growth
    c. Suggesting the student is in denial about the need to increase their clinical grade and should meet with the course faculty
    d. Asking if they have considered speaking to someone about their panic disorder and recommend a provider
17. A nurse in a medical practice has assessed a patient reporting abdominal pain, diarrhea, and anxiety. With no identifiable cause for the pain, which actions to reduce stress would the nurse recommend? Select all that apply.
    a. Keeping a diary identifying sources of stress
    b. Sleeping 4 hours per night
    c. Considering previous strengths and coping mechanisms
    d. Asking whom the patient relies on for support
    e. Asking if their partner is abusive
    f. Assessing for prior psychiatric conditions
18. When caring for an older adult in a geriatric practice who seems anxious and inattentive, the nurse plans to discuss stressors particular to the older adult. For which stressors will the nurse assess? Select all that apply.
    a. Concern over memory loss
    b. Acting as the designated driver for friends
    c. Death of spouse last month
    d. Inappropriate use of alcohol
    e. Successful cataract surgery
    f. Recent mobility issues

ANSWERS WITH RATIONALES

1. **a, b.** Physiologic effects of stress include changes in appetite and elimination patterns as well as increased pulse and respirations. Using ineffective coping mechanisms, becoming withdrawn and isolated, and exhibiting attention-seeking behaviors are psychological effects of stress.
2. **c.** Anticipatory guidance focuses on psychologically preparing a person for an unfamiliar or painful event. When the patient knows what to expect through advanced explanation about discomfort, nausea, or pain and available relief measures, the patient's anxiety can be reduced. Rhythmic breathing is a relaxation technique, focusing on a pleasant place and breathing slowly in and out is a meditation technique, and focusing on a mental image to reduce responses to stimuli is a guided imagery technique. While these might be addressed, the other options do not reflect anticipatory guidance or focus on postoperative discomfort.
3. **a, c, d.** The sympathetic nervous system reacts to stress with the fight-or-flight response. This response causes increased the heart rate, muscle strength, cardiac output, blood glucose levels, and mental alertness. Increased peristalsis is brought on by the parasympathetic nervous system under normal conditions and at rest.
4. **c.** The adolescent who is a loner is not meeting a major task (being a part of a peer group) for that level of growth and development.
5. **a.** A patient with a damaged neurologic reflex arc has a diminished pain reflex response. This diminished sensation and motor response places the patient at risk for burns. All patients should be provided adequate pain relief, but this is not a priority. Monitoring for depression would be an intervention for this patient but is not related to the damaged neurologic reflex arc. A patient who is immobile should eat a well-balanced diet.
6. **a, c, e.** The sympathetic nervous system initiates the fight-or-flight response, preparing the body to fight a stressor or run from it. This phase of the alarm reaction, called the shock phase, is characterized by an increase in energy levels, oxygen intake, cardiac output, blood pressure, and mental alertness. During the second phase, called the countershock phase, there is a reversal of body changes. Hypotension and withdrawn demeanor represent the countershock phase.
7. **d.** Incivility encompasses rude or discourteous actions that negatively affect others. Incivility can escalate to bullying, which is defined as repeated, ongoing actions that intend to harm another person. This includes humiliation, offensive speech or actions, or other methods of causing distress. The other options exist in a positive work environment.
8. **a.** Fatigue and mild anxiety are often handled without conscious thought through the use of coping mechanisms, such as sleeping. These coping mechanisms are protective behaviors used to decrease stress and anxiety.
9. **b.** Denial, a coping mechanism, occurs when a person refuses to acknowledge the presence of a condition that is disturbing. Projection involves attributing thoughts or impulses to someone else. Displacement occurs when a person transfers an emotional reaction from one object or person to another object or person. Repression is used by a person to voluntarily exclude an anxiety-producing event from conscious awareness. This patient is not blocking out the fact that the diagnosis was made, but refusing to believe it.
10. **d.** A person providing care at home for a family member for long periods of time often experiences caregiver burden, manifested by chronic fatigue, sleep disorders, and an increased incidence of stress-related illnesses, such as hypertension and heart disease. The nurse could recommend a consultation with a social worker or suggest community resources including possible respite care for the parent(s).
11. **b.** No matter what the technique, relaxation involves rhythmic breathing, a slower (not a faster) pulse, reduced muscle tension, and an altered state of consciousness.
12. **a, b, e, f.** Relaxation techniques are useful in many situations, including childbirth, and consist of rhythmic breathing and progressive muscle relaxation. Meditation and guided imagery could also be used to distract a patient from the pain of childbirth. Anticipatory socialization helps to prepare people for roles they don't have yet, but aspire to, such as parenthood. Biofeedback is a method of gaining mental control of the autonomic nervous system and thus regulating body responses, such as blood pressure, heart rate, and headaches.
13. **a.** Although identifying the problem may be difficult, a solution to a crisis situation is impossible until the problem is identified.
14. **c.** The nurse prepares a care plan focusing on anxiety, which can develop in a situational/maturational crises or changes in role status. There is insufficient data to determine whether the patient is demonstrating poor coping, referring to an inability to appraise stressors or use available resources. The patient is not displaying denial, as she is consciously discussing the anxiety rather than attempting to disavow the knowledge or meaning of the impending birth. There is no indication the patient has feelings of worthlessness (poor self-esteem) but rather expresses concern about the role change as she becomes a mother.
15. **c.** The nurse can explain that the patient's partner used the coping mechanism displacement, by transferring (displacing) their anger to a "safe" target. Another example is an angry person kicking a chair or slamming a door. The nurse can encourage the patient to discuss this with their partner.
16. **b.** The professor can normalize the student's experience by explaining that mild anxiety is present in day-to-day living. It can increase alertness and perceptual fields (e.g., vision and hearing) and motivate learning and growth. Although mild anxiety may interfere with sleep, it also facilitates problem solving. Mild anxiety is often manifested by restlessness and increased questioning. The other options call attention to problems that may not exist.
17. **a, c, d.** Keeping a diary of sources of stress can help identify the problem, which is the first step in stress management. The nurse can help the patient identify supports and their strengths. The nurse should recommend sleeping 7 to 9 hours nightly. The nurse would not infer there is a problem of abuse or a psychiatric condition as a cause of their symptoms. Abuse is assessed for routinely, often at the start of the interview, but not in the context of this situation.
18. **a, c, d, f.** Stressors of the older adult include declining physical and/or mental capabilities; invasive or health-related tests, examinations, or surgeries (even those with a positive outcome can produce stress, especially related to declining vision); alcohol abuse; diagnosis of chronic illnesses; loss of spouse or significant other; retirement; increased social isolation; loss of independence in living arrangements, driving, or activities of daily living; and chronic pain. The ability to still drive is not considered a stressor.

Bibliography

American Institute of Stress. (2022). *Stress effects.* Retrieved May 14, 2022, from https://www.stress.org/stress-effects

American Nurses Association (ANA). (2015, July 22). *Position Statement: Incivility, bullying, and workplace violence.* http://www.nursingworld.org/MainMenuCategories/WorkplaceSafety/Healthy-Nurse/bullyingworkplaceviolence/Incivility-Bullying-and-Workplace-Violence.html

American Nurses Association (ANA). (n.d.). *Well-being initiative.* Retrieved May 14, 2022, from https://www.nursingworld.org/practice-policy/work-environment/health-safety/disaster-preparedness/coronavirus/what-you-need-to-know/the-well-being-initiative/

American Nurses Association Enterprise. (2021, September 12). Well-being initiative. https://www.nursingworld.org/practice-policy/work-environment/health-safety/disaster-preparedness/coronavirus/what-you-need-to-know/the-well-being-initiative/

American Psychological Association. (2018, November 1). *Stress effects on the body.* http://www.apa.org/helpcenter/stress-body.aspx

American Psychological Association. (2020, October 20). *Stress in America™ 2020: A national mental health crisis.* https://www.apa.org/news/press/releases/stress/2020/sia-mental-health-crisis.pdf

American Psychological Association (APA). (2022). *Anxiety.* Retrieved May 14, 2022, from https://www.apa.org/topics/anxiety

Centers for Disease Control and Prevention (CDC). (2020a, April 3). *Adverse childhood experiences (ACEs).* https://www.cdc.gov/violenceprevention/acestudy/index.html

Centers for Disease Control and Prevention (CDC). (2020b, September). *Symptoms of generalized anxiety disorder among adults: United States, 2019.* https://www.cdc.gov/nchs/products/databriefs/db378.htm

Chmielewski, J., Łoś, K., & Łuczyński, W. (2021). Mindfulness in healthcare professionals and medical education. *International Journal of Occupational Medicine and Environmental Health, 34*(1), 1–14. https://doi.org/10.13075/ijomeh.1896.01542

The Commonwealth of Massachusetts, Executive Office of Health and Human Services Department of Public Health. (2020, April 7). Crisis standards of care: Planning guidance for the COVID-19 pandemic. https://archives.lib.state.ma.us/bitstream/handle/2452/825300/on1149151040.pdf

Everly, G., & Mitchell, J. (2017). The SAFER-R model: *Psychological Crisis Intervention.* International critical incident stress foundation, incorporated.

Kessler, R. C., Petukhova, M., Sampson, N. A., Zaslavsky, A. M., & Wittchen, H. U. (2012). Twelve-month and lifetime prevalence and lifetime morbid risk of anxiety and mood disorders in the United States. *International Journal of Methods in Psychiatric Research, 21*(3), 169–184. https://doi.org/10.1002/mpr.1359

Li, Q. (2018). Forest bathing: How trees can help you find health and happiness. *Penguin Life.*

McEwen, B. S., & Stellar, E. (1993). Stress and the individual. Mechanisms leading to disease. *Archives of Internal Medicine, 153*(18), 2093–2101.

Mental Health in America. (2020, October 20). *2021 The state of mental health in America.* https://mhanational.org/issues/state-mental-health-america

Murdaugh, C. L., Parsons, M. A., & Pender, N. J., (2019). *Health promotion in nursing practice* (8th ed.). Pearson Education, Inc.

National Center for Complementary and Integrative Health (NCCIH). (2021, June). *Relaxation techniques: What you need to know.* https://www.nccih.nih.gov/health/relaxation-techniques-what-you-need-to-know

Norris, T. L. (2020). *Porth's essentials of pathophysiology* (5th ed.). Wolters Kluwer.

Rushton, C. (2018). *Moral resilience: Transforming moral suffering in healthcare.* Oxford University Press.

Selye, H. (1976). *The stress of life* (rev. ed.). McGraw-Hill.

Turner, C., & Finch-Guthrie, P. (2020). Experiences of caregivers caring for a family member who is using hemodialysis. *Nephrology Nursing Journal, 47*(1), 23–34. https://doi.org/10.37526/1526-744X.2020.47.1.23

U.S. Department of Agriculture, & U.S. Department of Health and Human Services. (2020, December). *Dietary guidelines for Americans.* 2020–2025 (9th ed.). https://www.dietaryguidelines.gov/resources/2020-2025-dietary-guidelines-online-materials

Videbeck, S. L. (2019). *Psychiatric-mental health nursing* (8th ed.). Wolters Kluwer.

Wang, D., & Gupta, V. (2021, May 3). Crisis Intervention. *In StatPearls.* StatPearls Publishing.

Wei, H., Roberts, P., Strickler, J., & Corbett, R. W. (2019). Nurse leaders' strategies to foster nurse resilience. *Journal of Nursing Management, 27*(4), 681–687. https://doi.org/10.1111/jonm.12736

Wocial, L. D. (2020). Resilience as an incomplete strategy for coping with moral distress in critical care nurses. *Critical Care Nurse, 40*(6), 62–66. https://doi.org/10.4037/ccn2020873

44 Loss, Grief, and Dying

Yvonne Malic

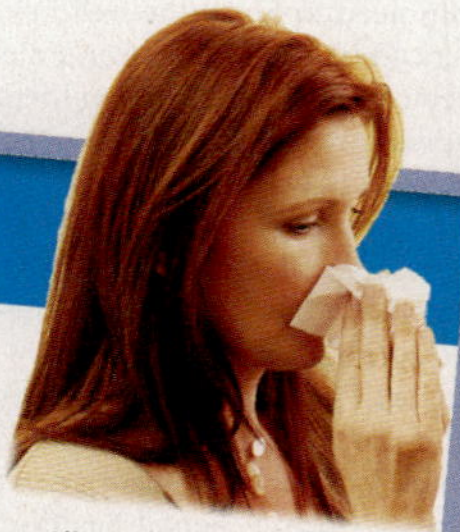

Yvonne, a 20-year-old single woman, has just given birth to a baby, 11 weeks premature. The newborn weighs 2 lb 2 oz (1,021 g) and is immediately admitted to the neonatal intensive care unit because of severe respiratory distress. Up until this point, Yvonne had a normal pregnancy and was expecting a healthy baby girl. "I was so happy to be pregnant and I wanted to be a mother so much. But my baby is so tiny! And now the doctors are telling me that she has less than a 50% chance of surviving the next 24 hours."

Anna Maria Esposita

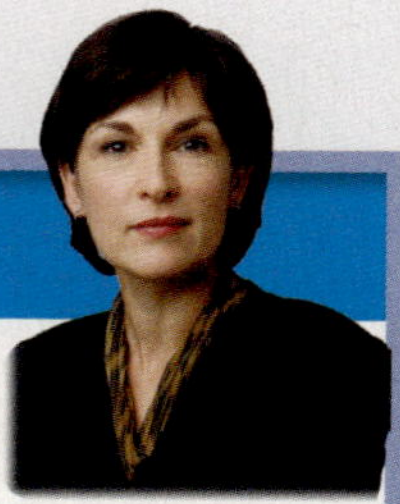

The Espositas have been married for 19 years and have two children, Jorge, who is 16, and Marita, who is 13. It has been 2 years since Mrs. Esposita was diagnosed with ovarian cancer, and this period has been difficult for the entire family. At present, she is extremely cachexic (thin) and in the end stage of her illness. She initially tried aggressive treatment, and several chemotherapy regimens failed. During her last hospitalization 2 months ago, a decision was made not to continue treatment, and Mrs. Esposita told her family she wanted to die at home.

Manuel Perez

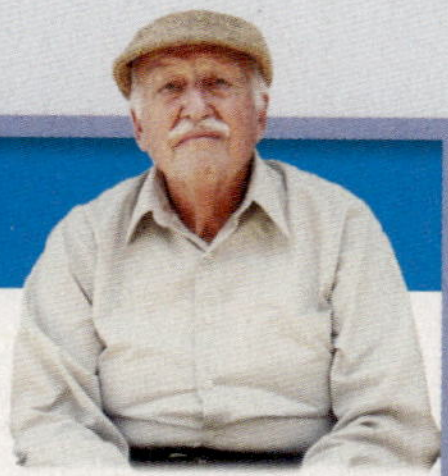

Manuel, 68 years old, moved to a retirement community with his 69-year-old wife 2 months ago. "We were looking forward to traveling and playing lots of golf. But she had this stroke, and now she has massive irreversible brain damage." Mr. Perez is sitting at his wife's bedside, holding her hand, and crying. "The doctors are asking me if I want to continue treatments that are keeping her alive. They mentioned donating her organs. I don't know what to do. We never talked about what we would want."

Learning Outcomes

After completing the chapter, you will be able to accomplish the following:

1. Explain the concepts of loss and grieving, including types of loss and grief reactions.
2. Describe the signs of impending death.
3. Compare and contrast the five emotional stages of dying defined by Kübler-Ross.
4. Identify ethical and legal issues in end-of-life care, including advance directives, physician orders, assisted suicide/medically assisted dying, and euthanasia.
5. Articulate and defend a personal response to a patient's plea, "Please help me die."
6. Explain six factors that affect loss, grief, and dying.
7. Describe physiologic, psychological, and spiritual care of a seriously ill and/or dying patient and family.
8. Use the nursing process to plan and implement care for seriously ill and/or dying patients and their families.
9. Outline nursing interventions when providing postmortem care.
10. Discuss the role of the nurse in caring for the family/caregivers of a dying patient.

Nursing Concepts

- Grief and loss
- End of life
- Dying and death

The potential for loss, grief, and death exists at any stage of life. This is especially true for people experiencing altered health and for members of their families. A wide variety of losses may occur, including loss of a body part or function, loss of the ability to care for oneself or to perform valued family or work roles, and death, which may be the most difficult loss of all. Death may be as difficult for health care professionals as it is for surviving family members. The goals of nursing include promoting a respectful and peaceful death through compassionate palliative care and facilitating the patient's and family's coping with disability and death. The nurse is often the person providing support and care when loss or death occurs. To provide effective care, the nurse must have accepted their own feelings about death and understood the stages of grieving and dying. Care of the seriously ill and dying became increasingly challenging during the COVID-19 pandemic when many critically ill patients were deprived of the comfort of family because of revised visitation policies. Nurses not only provided the physical care that seriously ill patients needed but used smartphones and tablets to facilitate communication between patients and their families. All too often it was only the nurse holding the hand of a hospitalized dying patient. For an example, see the Reflective Practice box on pages 1794–1795.

CONCEPTS OF LOSS AND GRIEF

The types of loss, as well as the varied responses to a loss, are important concepts when planning and implementing nursing interventions to facilitate effective coping and adaptation.

Loss

Loss occurs when a valued person, object, or situation is changed or becomes inaccessible such that its value is diminished or removed. There are several types of loss, all of which everyone may experience at some time. **Actual loss** can be recognized by others as well as by the person sustaining the loss—for example, loss of a limb, a child, a valued object such as money, and a job. **Perceived loss**, such as loss of youth, financial independence, or a valued environment, is experienced by the person but is intangible to others. Directly related to actual and perceived loss are physical and psychological loss. A person who loses an arm in an automobile crash suffers from both the physical loss of the arm and the psychological loss that may be caused by an altered self-image and the inability to return to their occupation or other activities. These losses are simultaneously physical, psychological, and actual. A person who is scarred but does not lose a limb may suffer a perceived and psychological loss of self-image.

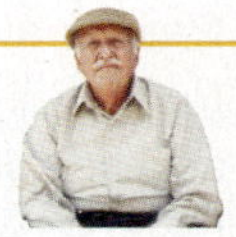

Remember **Mr. Perez**, whose wife has brain damage from a recent stroke. The nurse could use knowledge of the types of loss to help Mr. Perez deal with all the recent changes in his life, including the loss of his wife as an active partner.

Other types of loss are maturational loss, situational loss, and anticipatory loss. Maturational loss is experienced as a result of natural developmental processes. As examples, a first child may experience a loss of status when a sibling is born, and the parent of a single child may experience a sense of loss when the child begins school. Situational loss is experienced as a result of an unpredictable event, including traumatic injury, disease, death, or national disaster. **Anticipatory loss** occurs when a person displays loss and grief behaviors for a loss that has yet to take place (Fig. 44-1 on page 1795). Anticipatory loss is often seen in the families of patients with serious and life-threatening illnesses and may lessen the effect of the actual loss of the family member.

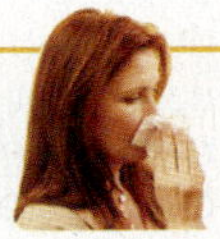

Think back to **Yvonne Malic**, the 20-year-old single mother of the premature neonate described at the beginning of the chapter. The nurse could use knowledge of anticipatory loss to assist Yvonne in coping with the seriousness of her neonate's condition.

QSEN Reflective Practice: Cultivating QSEN Competencies

CHALLENGE TO ETHICAL AND LEGAL SKILLS

Anna Maria Giordano was a 49-year-old attorney who had recently suffered a major cerebral hemorrhage. I came in contact with Ms. Giordano on one of my off-site clinical rotations when I accompanied a social worker for a day at a large medical center. According to most of the nurses and physicians, and the documentation in her chart, her prognosis looked very poor. Due to the fact that she was a lawyer, her advance directives were very clear, appearing to say exactly what she wanted. In essence, her advance directives stated that if she was in a comatose condition and that it appeared as if there was no hope for recovery, she did not want life-sustaining treatment. Although testing did not reveal brain death, almost all the health care providers agreed that her condition had little to no hope for improvement. However, one neurosurgeon felt that her condition was improving, with hopes for her recovery; therefore, he had no intention of stopping the life-sustaining treatment. Her family members from Boston had come earlier in the week to discuss treatment options and were given two points of view by two different health care providers. Upon hearing the determination of a poor prognosis, seeing no improvement in the patient's condition over the past few weeks, and being familiar with her expressed preferences in the advance directive, I felt certain that she would not want life-sustaining treatment continued.

Thinking Outside the Box: Possible Courses of Action

- Ignore the entire situation: It didn't entirely concern me, since I was only observing as a nursing student for 1 day.
- Talk to the social worker about what I thought was stated in the advance directives, and ask why it wasn't being followed.
- Challenge the doctor as to why he was telling the family that the patient was improving when her assessments for the past 3 weeks had shown no improvement.

Evaluating a Good Outcome: How Do I Define Success?

- The patient is properly diagnosed and her wishes from her advance directives are followed as clearly as they are stated.
- Since the patient is unable to speak, her power of attorney is able to convey what the patient would want.
- The family and the patient's power of attorney are fully informed about the patient's condition so that they can make an educated decision based on what the patient would want.
- My personal and professional integrity are affirmed.

Personal Learning: Here's to the Future!

I chose to talk to the social worker about the patient's advance directives. The social worker was very aware of the situation; she explained that, in the past, this neurosurgeon had given other patients' families more optimistic views of their situations and had refused to stop life-sustaining treatment. The social worker explained that she was in the process of bringing this issue to an ethics committee to discuss the situation and hoped that something would be resolved. She also explained that advance directives are often difficult to follow precisely. If the patient is unable to communicate, then the person designated with power of attorney takes over and tries their best to do what the patient would want. In such situations, decision making can become very subjective. Therefore, following the advance directives is not as simple as one would think it would be.

Although my actions were not extraordinary in this situation, I felt that I learned quite a bit about advance directives, especially trying to honor the patient's and family's wishes. I had learned about advance directives in the past in my previous classes. However, this was the first time I had ever had to deal with one in actual practice. I was able to see how difficult it can be to make such an important decision. I was impressed by the way the social worker was handling the case; I only hope that I would act in a similar fashion if I were ever faced with a situation like this in the future.

Kathryn Southerton, Georgetown University

QSEN SELF-REFLECTION ON QUALITY AND SAFETY COMPETENCIES DEVELOPING KNOWLEDGE, SKILLS, AND ATTITUDES FOR CONTINUOUS IMPROVEMENT

How do you think you would respond in a similar situation? Why? Are there any factors that might affect your response? If so, explain what these factors are and their possible effect. Do you agree with the criteria that the nursing student used to evaluate a successful outcome? Why or why not? What *knowledge, skills,* and *attitudes* do you need to develop to continuously improve the quality and safety of care for patients like Ms. Giordano? Was professional integrity affirmed? Explain.

Patient-Centered Care: How can you deliver thoughtful, person-centered care for patients with whom you cannot communicate? How can you best communicate empathy and respect for this patient and her family?

Teamwork and Collaboration/Quality Improvement: What do you think might be influencing the neurosurgeon's refusal to end the life-sustaining treatment? How would you respond to this neurosurgeon? What does this tell you about

QSEN Reflective Practice: Cultivating QSEN Competencies *(continued)*

CHALLENGE TO ETHICAL AND LEGAL SKILLS

yourself and about the adequacy of your skills for professional practice? The neurosurgeon is in what stage of grief, in your opinion? The nursing student? The social worker? What communication and interpersonal skills do you need to improve to ensure that you function as an effective member of the patient care team and are able to obtain assistance when needed? What does quality care for Ms. Giordano "look like"?

Safety/Evidence-Based Practice: What does the evidence point to as "best practice" for Ms. Giordano? What safety needs does Ms. Giordano have and how can you meet them? Have you ever been involved in a situation involving an advance directive? If so, were the patient's wishes followed? If not, why not?

Informatics: Can you identify the essential information that must be available in Ms. Giordano's electronic record to support safe patient care and coordination of care? Can you think of other ways to respond to or approach the situation? What else might the nursing student have done to ensure a successful outcome?

Grief

Grief is an internal emotional reaction to loss. It occurs with loss caused by separation or by death. For example, many people who divorce experience grief. Loss of a body part, job, house, or pet may also cause grief. Normal expressions of grief may be physical (crying, headaches, difficulty sleeping, fatigue), emotional (feelings of sadness and yearning), social (feeling detached from others and isolating yourself from social contact), and spiritual (questioning the reason for your loss, the purpose of pain and suffering, the purpose of life and the meaning of death). **Mourning** is the actions and expressions of that grief, including the symbols and ceremonies (e.g., a funeral or final celebration of life) that make up the outward expressions of grief. **Bereavement** is a state of grieving due to loss of a loved one.

Grief Reactions

Grief reactions and reactions to dying are similar. The stages of these reactions overlap and vary among people (see Factors That Affect Grief and Dying, later in this chapter). One person may skip a reaction stage, whereas another may repeat an earlier stage. Each person is different, and patients and family members may be at different reaction stages. Several theories explain the stages of grief reactions and reactions to dying; two discussed here are by Engel and Kübler-Ross. More important than the actual stages of any given grief reaction is the idea that grief is a process that varies from person to person.

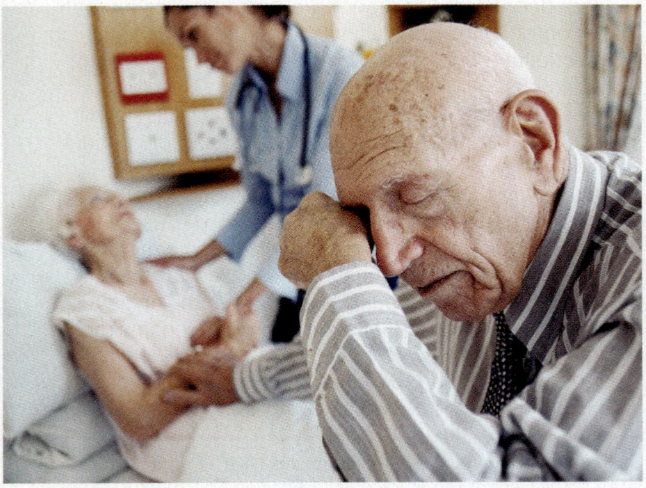

FIGURE 44-1. A terminally ill patient's husband begins the grieving process.

Engel (1964) was among the first to define stages of grief. Engel's six stages are (1) shock and disbelief, (2) developing awareness, (3) restitution, (4) resolving the loss, (5) idealization, and (6) outcome. Shock and disbelief are usually defined as refusal to accept the fact of loss, followed by a stunned or numb response: "No, not me." Developing awareness is characterized by physical and emotional responses such as anger, feeling empty, and crying: "Why me?" Restitution involves the rituals surrounding loss; with death, it includes religious, cultural, or social expressions of mourning, such as funeral services. Resolving the loss involves dealing with the void left by the loss. Idealization is the exaggeration of the good qualities of the person or object, followed by acceptance of the loss and a lessened need to focus on it. Outcome, the final resolution of the grief process, includes dealing with loss as a common life occurrence.

Kübler-Ross (1969), a pioneer in the study of grief and death reactions, defined five stages of reaction similar to Engel's. These stages—(1) denial and isolation, (2) anger, (3) bargaining, (4) depression, and (5) acceptance—are discussed later in the chapter.

Dysfunctional Grief

Dysfunctional grief is abnormal or distorted; it may be either unresolved or inhibited. In unresolved grief, a person may have trouble expressing feelings of loss or may deny them; unresolved grief also describes a state of bereavement that extends over a lengthy period. With inhibited grief, a person suppresses feelings of grief and may instead manifest somatic (body) symptoms, such as abdominal pain or heart palpitations.

DYING AND DEATH

Death may occur suddenly as a result of an accident, injury, or illness or it may occur after a prolonged experience of a debilitating disease such as cancer, acquired immunodeficiency syndrome (AIDS), or Alzheimer's disease.

Definitions of Death

The accurate definition of death has proven difficult over time, as technologic advances, such as cardiopulmonary resuscitation, have been able to restore lost functions and "bring a person back to life." The Uniform Determination of Death Act (1981) provides a legal definition of **death** as either (1) irreversible cessation of circulatory and respiratory functions, or (2) irreversible cessation of all functions of the entire brain, including the brainstem. A determination of death must be made in accordance with accepted medical standards.

A Harvard University Medical School committee later added that the irreversible loss of brain function, accompanied by the more traditional signs, should be the definitive definition of death. These "Harvard criteria" are generally accepted with the understanding that errors in certification of death could occur in conditions that may not permanently suspend life processes, such as hypothermia (extreme cold), drug or metabolic intoxication, or circulatory shock. In addition, special attention must be paid when establishing death in a child younger than age 5 years.

Most protocols for establishing death require two separate clinical examinations. The medical criteria used to certify a death are as follows:

- Breathing cessation
- No response to deep painful stimuli
- Lack of reflexes (such as the gag or corneal reflex) and spontaneous movement
- Flat encephalogram (brain waves)

You may hear clinicians refer to heart–lung death (cessation of the apical pulse, respirations, and blood pressure) and cerebral or higher brain death (when the cerebral cortex is irreversibly destroyed). These clinical signs may be further confirmed by an electroencephalogram or cerebral blood flow study. See Milliken and Uveges (2020) for a discussion of brain death, its history, updates, and implications for nurses.

Signs of Impending Death

The clinical signs of impending or approaching death include:

- Difficulty talking or swallowing
- Nausea, flatus, and abdominal distention
- Urinary or bowel incontinence or constipation
- Loss of movement, sensation, and reflexes
- Decreasing body temperature with cold or clammy skin
- Weak, slow, or irregular pulse
- Decreasing blood pressure
- Noisy, irregular, or Cheyne–Stokes respirations
- Restlessness or agitation
- Cooling, mottling, and cyanosis of the extremities and dependent areas

As death nears, the patient may have a decreased level of consciousness or agitated delirium. Although decreased consciousness and agitation are both normal at the end of life, they are very distressing to the patient's family. It is important for nurses to prepare family members when death is imminent and to determine if they are more comfortable being alone with a dying loved one or supported by a nurse or other member of the professional caregiving team.

A "Good Death"

A good death is one that allows a person to die on their own terms, relatively free of pain, and with dignity. It is free from avoidable distress and suffering for patients, families, and caregivers; in general accord with patients' families' wishes; and reasonably consistent with clinical, cultural, and ethical standards (Institute of Medicine [IOM], 1997). The characteristics of a good death vary for each patient; several important factors include control of symptoms, preparation for death, opportunity for the person to have a sense of completion of their life, and a good relationship with health care professionals. The indicators for care that promotes a good death are listed in Box 44-1; although they were developed by the American Geriatrics Society (AGS) Ethics Committee (2007), they apply to people of all ages. Nurses play a critical role in focusing the health care team's attention on meeting the needs of dying people and their families. Broden et al. (2020) define what a "good death" looks like in the pediatric intensive care unit (ICU).

In 2015, the IOM (now the National Academy of Sciences, Engineering, and Medicine) issued a report, *Dying in America: Improving quality and honoring individual*

Box 44-1 Providing Care to Facilitate a Good Death

Although death occurs at any age, the probability of death increases as a person grows older. These selected statements from the American Geriatrics Society Ethics Committee provide guidance for all health care providers in providing excellent care for dying patients of any age.

- The care of the dying patient should be guided by the values and preferences of the individual patient. Independence and dignity are central issues for many dying patients, particularly in older adults. Maintaining control and not being a burden can also be relevant concerns.
- Palliative care of dying patients is an interdisciplinary undertaking that attends to the needs of both patient and family.
- Care for dying patients should focus on the relief of symptoms, not limited to pain, and should use both pharmacologic and nonpharmacologic means.
- Physicians and other health care professionals, at all levels of training, should receive in-depth, insightful, and culturally sensitive instruction in the optimal care of dying patients.
- Adequate funding for research on the optimal care of dying patients is essential to improving end-of-life care.

Source: From American Geriatrics Society (AGS) Ethics Committee. (2007). *The Care of Dying Patients: A Position Statement from the American Geriatrics Society. 43*(5) Author; with permission from John Wiley and Sons.

preferences near the end of life. The IOM recommended that comprehensive care should:

- Be seamless, high quality, integrated, patient centered, family oriented, and consistently accessible around the clock.
- Consider the evolving physical, emotional, social, and spiritual needs of individuals approaching the end of life as well as those of their family and caregivers.
- Be competently delivered by professionals with appropriate expertise and training.
- Include coordinated, efficient, and interoperable information transfer across all providers and all settings.
- Be consistent with individuals' values, goals, and informed preferences.

Responses to Dying and Death

People have varying attitudes about death. Increasing numbers are choosing to die at home surrounded by loved ones. Others die alone or in ICUs surrounded by health care professionals and technologic equipment. Although each person reacts to the knowledge of impending death or to loss in their own way, there are similarities in the psychosocial responses to the situation. Kübler-Ross (1969) studied the emotional responses to death and dying in depth, and nursing and other helping professions have used her findings extensively.

The stages of dying, much like the stages of grief, may overlap, and the duration of any stage may range from as little as a few hours to as long as months. The process varies from person to person. Some people may be in one stage for such a short time that it seems as if they skipped that stage. Sometimes a person returns to a previous stage. According to Kübler-Ross, the five stages of dying, with common reactions, are:

1. *Denial:* The patient denies the reality of death and may repress what is discussed. The patient may think, "They made a mistake in the diagnosis. Maybe they mixed up my records with someone else's."
2. *Anger:* The patient expresses rage and hostility and adopts a "why me?" attitude: "Why me? I quit smoking and I watched what I ate. Why did this happen to me?"
3. *Bargaining:* The patient tries to barter for more time: "If I can just make it to my son's graduation, I'll be satisfied. Just let me live until then." Many patients put their personal affairs in order, make wills, and fulfill last wishes, such as trips, visiting relatives, and so forth. It is important to meet these wishes, if possible, because bargaining helps patients move into later stages of dying.
4. *Depression:* The patient goes through a period of grief before death. The grief is often characterized by crying and not speaking much: "I waited all these years to see my daughter get married. And now I may not be here to see her walk down the aisle. I can't bear the thought of not being there for the wedding—and of not seeing my grandchildren."
5. *Acceptance:* When the stage of acceptance is reached, the patient feels tranquil. The patient has accepted the reality of death and is prepared to die. The patient may think, "I've tied up all the loose ends: made the will, made arrangements for my daughter to live with her grandparents. Now I can go in peace knowing everyone will be fine."

Terminal Illness

In the case of a **terminal illness**, an illness in which death is expected within a limited period of time, the health care provider is usually responsible for deciding what, when, and how the patient should be told. The nurse, along with members of the clergy and other health care professionals, may be involved with these decisions and in discussing the condition with the patient. Most patients want to know their diagnosis and prognosis as soon as possible so that they can begin appropriate planning and take care of business and personal affairs. It is critical for terminally ill patients and their families to have some sense of how the disease is most likely to progress and what this will mean for the patient. All who are involved with the patient's care should know exactly what the patient and the family have been told; members of the patient's health care team need to communicate among themselves. *Cultural influences may dictate how much information is desired and which family members are to be informed.* For example, in some cultures it is still the norm that the patient's family—not the patient—is told the diagnosis and prognosis. Since this is now changing, nurses must check local practice standards and policies as well as the preferences of individual patients and families. You can never go wrong if you ask patients how much information they would like about their medical condition. "We will be learning things about your health as a result of the diagnostic testing we are doing. Do you want to receive this information or would you prefer that we give this to a family member or someone else of your choosing?"

Effect on the Patient

Many patients realize without being told that they have a terminal illness, picking up this knowledge from nonverbal communication by their families and by health care professionals. Patients must be allowed to go through the stages of the grieving process and be supported in their decision making. Competent patients have the right to consent to or refuse any and all indicated medical treatment—even life-sustaining treatment—and should be made aware of this right. In the past, patients and family members complained about receiving care they did not want and of not being allowed to die. In today's climate of cost-conscious decision making, some patients and family members are complaining that they are being denied costly life-sustaining treatment because of inadequate personal funds or insurance or because they are deemed a poor "investment" of scarce resources. Remember that a patient's wishes should, if possible, be followed. Box 44-2 (on page 1798) lists the rights of people who are dying.

Box 44-2 The Dying Person's Bill of Rights

I have the right to be treated as a living human being until I die.
I have the right to maintain a sense of hopefulness, however changing its focus may be.
I have the right to be cared for by those who can maintain a sense of hopefulness, however changing this might be.
I have the right to express my feelings and emotions about my approaching death in my own way.
I have the right to participate in decisions concerning my care.
I have the right to expect continuing medical and nursing attention even though "cure" goals must be changed to "comfort" goals.
I have the right not to die alone.
I have the right to be free from pain.
I have the right to have my questions answered honestly.
I have the right not to be deceived.
I have the right to have help from and for my family in accepting my death.
I have the right to die in peace and dignity.
I have a right to retain my individuality and not be judged for my decisions, which may be contrary to beliefs of others.
I have the right to discuss and enlarge my religious and/or spiritual experiences, whatever these may mean to others.
I have the right to expect that the sanctity of the human body will be respected after death.
I have the right to be cared for by caring, sensitive, knowledgeable people who will attempt to understand my needs and will be able to gain some satisfaction in helping me face my death.

Source: The Bill of Rights was created at a workshop on 'The Terminally Ill Patient and the Helping Persons,' in Lansing, Michigan, sponsored by the Southwestern Michigan Inservice Education Council and conducted by Amelia J. Barbus, associate professor of nursing, Wayne State University, Detroit.

Effect on the Family

Whenever possible, with the patient's permission, encourage the family and significant others of terminally ill patients to participate in planning the patient's care. Orsatti and Colbert (2020) offer helpful advice when siblings are conflicted about a parent's end-of-life care. Health care personnel should be available to discuss the patient's condition with family members and should offer support and care as the family begins the grieving process (Fig. 44-2). The family may want to make arrangements with the patient for funeral or memorial services, depending on which stage of grief both the patient and the family members are in.

Palliative Care and Hospice

Palliative care involves taking care of the whole person—body, mind, and spirit; heart and soul. It views dying as something natural and personal. The goal of palliative care is to give patients with life-threatening illnesses the best quality of life they can have by the aggressive management of symptoms. In January 2016, The American Nurses Association (ANA) and the Hospice and Palliative Nurses Association (HPNA) partnered to develop *Call for Action: Nurses Lead and Transform Palliative Care*. They concluded that seriously ill and injured patients, families, and communities should receive quality palliative care in all care settings. This was to be achieved by the delivery of primary palliative care nursing by every nurse regardless of setting. Since nurses are frequently the source of palliative care consults, you will want to be familiar with palliative care screening tools to identify patients for whom palliative care will be helpful (Martz et al., 2020; Venis & Dodek, 2020).

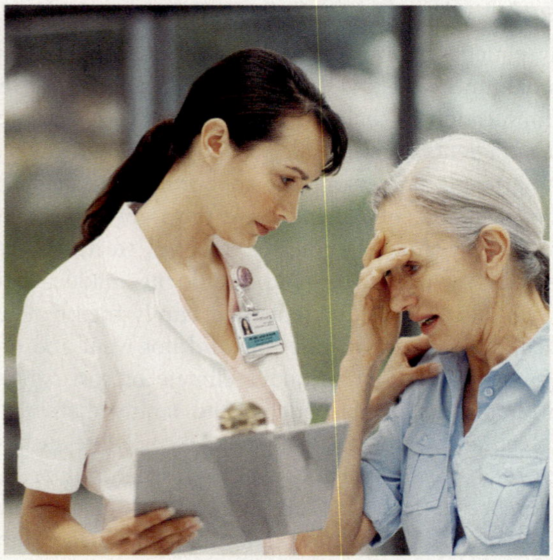

FIGURE 44-2. A nurse offers support to a patient's grieving spouse.

As you begin your clinical practice, you will want to be intentional about developing the knowledge, skills, and attitudes necessary to provide excellent palliative care. Roy (2020) answers frequently asked questions about palliative care. Be sure to check out the Clinical Practice Guidelines for Quality Palliative Care, published by the National Consensus Project for Quality Palliative Care, available online at http://keyweb24.com/nchpc/wp-content/uploads/2017/04/NCP_Clinical_Practice_Guidelines_3rd_Edition.pdf. Also of interest, in 2017, the ANA issued a call for public comment on a position statement, The Ethical Responsibility to Manage Pain and Suffering. See Chapter 36 for further information.

Hospice care is care provided for people with limited life expectancy, often in the home. When considering whether a patient is a candidate for hospice care, ask yourself, "Would I be surprised if this person died within the next 6 months?" Indicators for hospice referral (Puffenbarger, 2014) include:

- Poor performance status
- Declining cognitive status
- Advanced age
- Poor nutritional intake
- Pressure injuries
- Comorbidities
- Previous hospital admissions for acute decompensation

While hospice care focuses on the needs of the dying, palliative care is appropriate across the spectrum of disease and illness. Both palliative care and hospice care are discussed in Chapter 11. Also see the National Hospice and Palliative Care Organization's (2019) "Palliative care or hospice? The right service at the right time for seriously ill individuals" available at https://www.nhpco.org/wp-content/uploads/2019/04/PalliativeCare_VS_Hospice.pdf.

Established in 1986, the HPNA (www.hpna.org) is the nation's largest and oldest professional organization dedicated to promoting excellence in palliative nursing care. Among its aims are assisting members of the nursing team with ensuring quality nursing care delivery, managing complex symptoms along with grief and bereavement, and having difficult conversations.

Ethical and Legal Dimensions

Multiple treatment options and sophisticated life support technologies may make it difficult to draw the line between promoting life and needlessly prolonging the dying process. This complicates health care decision making for patients and health care professionals alike. Patients have a legally and morally protected right to consent to or refuse medical therapies. Legal foundations for the patient's freedom to choose include the common law right of self-determination and the constitutionally supported right of privacy (discussed in Chapters 6 and 7). Discussions about legalizing physician-assisted suicide and physician-administered lethal injections (euthanasia) pose new ethical challenges. As patients and families struggle with end-of-life treatment decisions, they are increasingly looking to nurses for information, advice, and support. It is important for you to clarify your own beliefs about suicide and euthanasia before attempting to counsel patients and the public. Take time to work through your answers to the questions in Box 44-4 on page 1804. Articles addressing the moral distress nurses experience when helping patients and their families make these decisions include the following: Altaker et al. (2018), Esfahani et al. (2020), Wolf et al. (2019).

Advance Care Planning

Decisions about health care are becoming increasingly complex. Patients, family members, and health care professionals are voicing frustration as they grapple with complex decisions about prolonging life. Some of the most difficult cases involve patients who are no longer able (competent) to indicate their treatment preferences. **Advance care planning (ACP)** is a process of planning for future care in the event a person becomes unable to make their own decisions. Because such events can occur in healthy people as well as in older adults or patients with serious illnesses, ACP is recommended for all adults, whatever their age or health status (Izumi, 2017, p. 57).

Two kinds of written **advance directives**—a *living will* and a *durable power of attorney for health care*—can minimize difficulties by allowing people to state in advance what their choices would be for health care should certain circumstances develop. Living wills provide specific instructions about the kinds of health care that should be provided or foregone in particular situations. A durable power of attorney for health care appoints an agent the person trusts to make decisions in the event of subsequent incapacity. A combination directive is illustrated in Figure 44-3 (on pages 1800–1801). The organization Aging with Dignity offers a popular living will titled *Five Wishes* (available at https://www.agingwithdignity.org) that allows people to specify the following:

- The person I want to make care decisions for me when I can't
- The kind of medical treatment I want or don't want
- How comfortable I want to be
- How I want people to treat me
- What I want my loved ones to know

Many methods have been suggested to ensure that adult patients have an opportunity to learn about and use advance directives to indicate their wishes about life-prolonging treatment and to appoint surrogate decision makers should they lose decision-making capacity. Nurses play an important role in facilitating this dialogue. In the United States, the Patient Self-Determination Act of 1990 requires all hospitals to inform patients about advance directives.

Legal Alert

Because the status of advance directives varies from state to state, nurses must be familiar with federal and state laws concerning these directives.

Nurses can also be instrumental in developing institutional policies that ensure that patients on admission are encouraged to talk with family, significant others, and health care professionals about their treatment preferences. Important resources for ACP include the National Hospice and Palliative Care Organization's CaringInfo program (www.caringinfo.org); the American Bar Association's Tool Kit for Health Care Advance Planning (https://www.americanbar.org/groups/law_aging/resources/health_care_decision_making/consumer_s_toolkit_for_health_care_advance_planning.html); and The Conversation Project (http://theconversationproject.org).

A Physician Order for Life-Sustaining Treatment form, or **POLST form**, is a medical order indicating a patient's wishes regarding treatments commonly used in a medical crisis. Because it is a medical order, a POLST form must be completed and signed by a health care professional and cannot be filled out by a patient. These forms are always completed in close consultation with the patient to ensure that the patient's values and goals of care are accurately represented. These brightly colored forms (see the POLST website, www.polst.org) always remain with the patient, regardless of whether the patient is in the hospital, at home,

(text continued on page 1802)

D.C., Maryland and Virginia

ADVANCE DIRECTIVE

My Durable Power of Attorney for Health Care, Living Will and Other Wishes

I, ______________________, write this document as a directive regarding my medical care.

Put the initials of your name by the choices you want.

PART 1. MY DURABLE POWER OF ATTORNEY FOR HEALTH CARE.

_______ I appoint this person to make decisions about my medical care if there ever comes a time when I cannot make those decisions myself:

NAME ______________________ PHONE HOME __________ WORK __________

ADDRESS ____

____

If the person above cannot or will not make decisions for me, I appoint this person:

NAME ______________________ PHONE HOME __________ WORK __________

ADDRESS ____

____

_______ I have not appointed anyone to make health care decisions for me in this or any other document.

I want the person I have appointed, my doctors, my family, and others to be guided by the decisions I have made below:

PART 2. MY LIVING WILL.

These are my wishes for my future medical care if there ever comes a time when I can't make these decisions for myself.

A. **These are my wishes if I have a *terminal condition:***

Life-Sustaining Treatments

_______ I do not want life-sustaining treatments (including CPR) started. If life-sustaining treatments are started, I want them stopped.

_______ I want life-sustaining treatments that my doctors think are best for me.

_______ Other wishes: ______________________________

Artificial Nutrition and Hydration

_______ I do not want artificial nutrition and hydration started if it would be the main treatment keeping me alive. If artificial nutrition and hydration is started, I want it stopped.

_______ I want artificial nutrition and hydration even if it is the main treatment keeping me alive.

_______ Other wishes: ______________________________

Comfort Care

_______ I want to be kept as comfortable and free of pain as possible, even if such care prolongs my dying or shortens my life.

_______ Other wishes: ______________________________

B. **These are my wishes if I am ever in a *persistent vegetative state:***

Life-Sustaining Treatments

_______ I do not want life-sustaining treatments (including CPR) started. If life-sustaining treatments are started, I want them stopped.

_______ I want life-sustaining treatments that my doctors think are best for me.

_______ Other wishes: ______________________________

FIGURE 44-3. Example of an advance directive. (*Source:* Used with permission of District of Columbia Hospital Association, Washington, DC.)

Artificial Nutrition and Hydration

_______ I do not want artificial nutrition and hydration started if it would be the main treatment keeping me alive.
If artificial nutrition and hydration is started, I want it stopped.

_______ I want artificial nutrition and hydration even if it is the main treatment keeping me alive.

_______ Other wishes: ____________________

Comfort Care

_______ I want to be kept as comfortable as possible, even if such care prolongs my dying or shortens my life

_______ Other wishes: ____________________

C. **Other Direction**

You have the right to be involved in all decisions about your medical care, even those parts not dealing with terminal conditions or persistent vegetative states. If you have wishes not covered in other parts of this document, please indicate them here.

____

____

PART 3. OTHER WISHES.

A. **Organ Donation**

_______ I do not wish to donate any of my organs or tissues.

_______ I want to donate all of my organs and tissues.

_______ I only want to donate these organs and tissues: ____________________

_______ Other wishes: ____________________

Autopsy

_______ I do not want an autopsy.

_______ I agree to an autopsy if my doctors wish it.

_______ Other wishes: ____________________

If you wish to say more about any of the above choices, or if you have any other statements to make about your medical care, you may do so on a separate sheet of paper. If you do so, put here the number of pages you are adding: ____________________

PART 4. SIGNATURES.

You and two witnesses must sign this document for it to be legal.

A. **Your Signature**

By my signature below I show that I understand the purpose and the effect of this document.

SIGNATURE ____________________ DATE ________

ADDRESS ____________________

B. **Your Witnesses' Signatures**

I believe the person who has signed this advance directive to be of sound mind, that he/she signed or acknowledged this advance directive in my presence, and that he/she appears not to be acting under pressure, duress, fraud or undue influence. I am not related to the person making this advance directive by blood, marriage or adoption, nor, to the best of my knowledge, am I named in his/her will. I am not the person appointed in this advance directive. I am not a health care provider or an employee of health care provider who is now, or has been in the past, responsible for the care of the person making this advance directive.

Witness #1

SIGNATURE ____________________ DATE ________

ADDRESS ____________________

Witness #2

SIGNATURE ____________________ DATE ________

ADDRESS ____________________

FIGURE 44-3. *(continued)*

Box 44-3 Advance Directive Versus POLST Form: Primary Differences

Advance Directive

- For anyone 18 and older
- Provides instructions for **future** treatment
- Appoints a Health Care Representative
- Does not guide Emergency Medical Personnel
- Guides inpatient treatment decisions when made available

Physician Order for Life-Sustaining Treatment (POLST) Form

- For persons with serious illness—at any age
- Provides medical orders for **current** treatment
- Guides actions by Emergency Medical Personnel when made available
- Guides inpatient treatment decisions when made available

Source: Data from National POLST Paradigm. (n.d.). *POLST and advance directives.* http://www.polst.org/advance-care-planning/polst-and-advance-directives

or in a long-term care facility. See Box 44-3 for a description of the differences between an advance directive and POLST form. POLST forms are not available in every state. In some states, such as Maryland, they are called Medical Orders for Life-Sustaining Treatment forms, or **MOLST forms**.

Allow Natural Death, Do-Not-Resuscitate, or No-Code Order

To prevent the improper use of cardiopulmonary resuscitation, which is designed to prevent unexpected death, some health care providers write **Do-Not-Resuscitate (DNR) order**, or No Code, on the medical record of a patient if the patient or surrogate has expressed a wish that there be no attempts to resuscitate the patient. A DNR order means that no attempts are to be made to resuscitate a patient whose breathing or heart stops. Some facilities use the term **Allow Natural Death (AND) order** instead of DNR because it is easier for families to authorize doing something positive rather than preventing something (i.e., a resuscitative effort) that is usually perceived to be helpful. You may also see a Do-Not-Intubate (DNI) order. Many health care providers are reluctant to write these orders, however, especially when the issue is a source of conflict between the patient and family or between individual family members. See the accompanying Research in Nursing box.

In some cases, a health care provider who believes the patient will not benefit from resuscitative measures may indicate verbally to the nurse that only a Slow Code (or "Show Code") should be called—that is, in the case of cardiopulmonary or respiratory arrest, calling a code and resuscitating the patient are to be delayed until these measures will be ineffectual. Many health care institutions have policies forbidding this, and a nurse could be charged with negligence in the event of a Slow Code and resulting patient death. Be sure to check your facility's policies.

The standard of care still obligates health care professionals to attempt resuscitation if a patient's breathing or heart stops (cardiopulmonary arrest) and there is no AND or DNR order to the contrary. For this reason, nurses must clarify a patient's code status if the probable benefits of resuscitation are negligible or if the nurse has reason to believe a patient would not want to be resuscitated. Many states now allow patients living at home to craft POLST/MOLST orders that allow emergency medical technicians called to the home in the event of cardiopulmonary arrest to respect the patient's wishes not to be resuscitated.

Comfort Measures Only and Other Special Orders

When a discussion is taking place about resuscitation, it is also appropriate to question the use of other life-sustaining interventions, such as dialysis, ventilatory support, artificial nutrition and hydration, blood transfusions, antibiotics and other medications, and surgery. Whereas some patients may want aggressive life-sustaining treatment and such treatment may be medically beneficial, other patients may be at a point in their illness at which they choose to terminate all life-sustaining measures and allow the disease to progress naturally

Research in Nursing

BRIDGING THE GAP TO EVIDENCE-BASED PRACTICE

Interpreting Do-Not-Resuscitate Orders

Misinterpretations of do-not-resuscitate (DNR) orders (including the belief that it means "do not treat") are common but there is a paucity of research concerning nurses' perspectives on DNR orders.

Related Research

Kelly, P. A., Baker, K. A., Hodges, K. M., Vuong, E. Y., Lee, J. C., & Lockwood, S. W. (2021). Nurses' perspectives on caring for patients with Do-Not-Resuscitate orders. *American Journal of Nursing, 121*(1), 26–36.

This mixed-methods study was designed to explore nurses' perspectives on the meaning and interpretation of DNR orders in relation to caring for hospitalized adults with such orders. Most of the 35 nurses who responded to the case study survey chose to prioritize palliative care, despite no indication that any plan of care was in place. Analysis of interview data revealed this overarching theme: varying interpretations of DNR orders among nurses were common, resulting in unintended consequences. Participants also reported perceived variances among health care team members, patients, and family members. Such misinterpretation resulted in shifts in care, varying responses to deteriorating status, tension, and differences in role expectations for health care team members.

to death. There is no moral obligation to initiate or continue the use of life-sustaining treatment that is minimally effective or is a burden. However, laws may place constraints on those who decide to withhold or withdraw life-sustaining treatment for incompetent patients and, in some states, for patients who are pregnant. Nurses should know pertinent federal and state laws and the policies in their institution or facility concerning the withholding or withdrawing of life-sustaining treatment. Nurses should also be familiar with the forms used to indicate patient preferences about end-of-life care.

Patients or their surrogates may request a **Comfort Measures Only order**, which indicates that the goal of treatment is a comfortable, dignified death and that further life-sustaining measures are no longer indicated. A Do-Not-Hospitalize order is often used for patients in long-term care and other residential settings who have elected not to be hospitalized for further aggressive treatment.

Terminal Weaning

Terminal weaning is the gradual withdrawal of mechanical ventilation from a patient with a terminal illness or an irreversible condition with a poor prognosis. In some cases, competent patients wish their ventilatory support to be ended; more often, the surrogate decision makers for an incompetent patient determine that continued ventilatory support is futile. Although it may be expected that a patient will not survive the weaning, death is never a certain outcome, and it is not unusual for a patient to begin spontaneous respirations once ventilatory support is withdrawn and live for several hours to several days. Competent patients and family members should be prepared for all possibilities. A nurse's role in terminal weaning is to participate in the decision-making process by offering helpful information about the benefits and burdens of continued ventilation and a description of what to expect if terminal weaning is initiated. Supporting the patient's family, monitoring symptoms, and administering medications as available to manage symptoms are critical nursing responsibilities. The goal should be the minimum dose of medication necessary to manage the symptoms. The goal is not sedation. Unfortunately, many facilities and institutions do not have policies covering this issue. Nurses involved in terminal weaning should consult the literature and be familiar with the latest research.

Voluntary Stopping of Eating and Drinking (VSED)

As seriously ill, competent patients make end-of-life treatment decisions, they may also choose to refuse food and fluid with the intention of hastening death. It is important to distinguish the voluntary act of a patient who is still capable of eating and drinking, making the decision to refuse food and fluids from the natural anorexia and loss of thirst that frequently accompany the end stages of dying. While some consider refusal of food and fluid to be a form of suicide, others view this as a decision to forego life-sustaining treatment. When nurses care for patients who want to refuse food and fluids, they must ensure that this is an informed and voluntary choice and remember that honoring this preference requires the support of the family, physician, and health care team who focus on palliative measures as the dying process unfolds (Quill & Byock, 2000, p. 410).

Active and Passive Euthanasia

Euthanasia literally means "good dying." **Active euthanasia** is taking specific steps to cause a patient's death, while *passive euthanasia* is defined as withdrawing medical treatment with the intention of causing the patient's death. In other words, active euthanasia is *doing something* to end a patient's life, whereas passive euthanasia is *not doing something* to preserve a patient's life. In assisted suicide (which could be considered a form of active euthanasia), the clinician provides the patient with the means to cause their own death (e.g., a prescription for a lethal dose of barbiturates). In active euthanasia, the clinician acts directly to cause the death of the patient (e.g., administers a lethal dose of medication).

Until recently, most societies maintained that the distinction between "killing" and "allowing to die" was morally relevant. This meant that passive euthanasia, the withholding or withdrawing of medically ineffective or disproportionately burdensome therapies, was morally and legally justified even when this hastened or directly caused a patient's death. On the other hand, making a lethal combination of drugs available to a patient wishing to die (assisted suicide) or administering a lethal injection or carbon monoxide, even when performed with compassionate intent at the request of a patient (active euthanasia), was deemed both immoral and illegal. Some are questioning this distinction today, and efforts are underway to legalize assisted suicide and active euthanasia in numerous countries. Another area of significant debate is whether the inclusion criteria for assisted suicide and active euthanasia should be broadened to include intractable psychological suffering.

Nurses are often the first to hear a patient's plea, "Please help me die." It is critical for nurses to reflect carefully on what they believe about assisted suicide and active euthanasia and how this influences the responses they make to patients. As of 2020, six states (Oregon, Washington, Colorado, Vermont, Hawaii, and California) and the District of Columbia have passed laws legalizing assisted suicide in certain limited circumstances. Laws and rulings in Montana and New Mexico are less clear but have allowed assisted suicide. If practicing in one of these states, be sure you understand your state's requirements. Talk with your classmates about your responses to the following questions and the reflection questions in Box 44-4 (on page 1804).

- Should the principle of respect for autonomy be expansive enough to embrace respect for, and acquiescence to, a competent patient's request for assistance in dying?
- Does the right to privacy entail a person's right, in effect, to decide the time and manner of their own death and to gain assistance in implementing that decision?
- Is there such a thing as *rational* suicide?
- If assisted suicide and active euthanasia were to become accepted practices, would this simply represent a logical, defensible extension of the well-established moral basis for refusal of treatment and withholding or withdrawing treatment?

Box 44-4 Ethical Challenges: Thinking Critically About Aid in Dying: Personal, Professional, and Facility Responsibilities

For many years, professional caregivers knew exactly how to respond when a patient expressed suicidal ideation. We "knew" that healthy minds didn't choose to end life and our responsibility was to prevent suicide, so we placed these people on suicide precautions. Today, many accept the concept of rational suicide as an autonomous choice; this opens the question of what our roles should be if someone chooses to end life sooner rather than later. This question is vitally important for professional caregivers, given the hospice philosophy to do nothing to hasten or postpone dying, and the ANA Code of Ethics for Nursing's (2015) statement: "The nurse should provide interventions to relieve pain and other symptoms in the dying patient consistent with palliative care practice standards and may not act with the sole intent to end life."

Questions for Reflection and Discussion

1. If a patient expresses the wish to commit suicide, what are my personal, professional, and facility obligations?
   - Should I compassionately counsel the person about choosing to live and initiate suicide precautions?
   - Must I share this information with the team—even if the patient requests that it be kept confidential?
   - Should I ask the patient to talk more about why they are feeling this way, using nondirective counseling to help the person clarify what they want to do?
   - May I counsel the person about safe, effective, legal ways to achieve this goal (i.e., should I become the patient's advocate)?
   - Should I develop and implement a care plan that honors the person's wishes?
2. Many people consider suicide to be a private decision. Is suicide ever private? What is the impact of a patient's successful suicide on family and staff?
3. How confident am I that I can distinguish a rational suicide from a mental health crisis?
4. How confident am I that I'm meeting the physical, psychological, social, and spiritual needs of patients? If unmet patient needs are prompting the request to die sooner rather than later, what are my responsibilities?
5. How can professional caregivers better respond to attempted suicide and successful suicide? What strategies will best meet the needs of families and staff?
6. Recent reports indicate that the U.S. suicide rate has been rising. What is my obligation as a nurse to prevent suicide?
7. How would I respond if my personal beliefs about suicide differ from those of a patient, or from a facility's philosophy and policies?
8. How would I feel about a patient's voluntarily stopping consumption of food and drink to cause their death? Is this suicide? Am I obligated to mention this as an option to patients wanting to die? If I recommend this, or even tacitly allow it, am I participating in a suicide?
9. Is there an ethical difference between attempting suicide with a gun, an overdose of liquid morphine, or cessation of eating and drinking?
10. Should facilities be more careful about limiting a patient's access (or a family member's access) to liquid morphine or other medications if the facility suspects the medications are being stockpiled to cause the patient's death? What would I do if I suspect a family member is stealing a patient's medication?
11. What about palliative sedation to unconsciousness? If someone wants to "go to sleep and never wake up," is that an option? Are policies that require that the patient be imminently dying appropriate? What about policies that exclude emotional angst or existential suffering as criteria? Since people choosing this option will die if we do not feed them, is this a "back door" to euthanasia?

- Are assisted suicide and active euthanasia acts of mercy, morally grounded in the principles of benefiting and not harming patients and expressive of the virtues of compassion and beneficence?
- Is it possible to conceive of situations in which a nurse or a health care provider has a duty to help a patient die (specifically via active euthanasia or assisted suicide)?
- Is refusal to accede to a patient's request for assisted suicide or active euthanasia a form of abandonment, or are there limits to the duty to respect autonomy, right to privacy, and self-determination?
- Are calls for assisted suicide and active euthanasia emblematic of failure to provide adequate palliative care and to address the suffering of the dying?
- If medicine and nursing possess an "internal" morality, are assisted suicide and active euthanasia consistent with that morality?
- Should assisted suicide and euthanasia be limited to those with a terminal illness with 6 months or less to live, or should it also be an option for those with intractable psychological suffering?

The ANA Code of Ethics states that the nurse "should provide interventions to relieve pain and other symptoms in the dying patient consistent with palliative care practice standards and may not act with the sole intent to end life" (2015, p. 3). Yet nurses may be confronted by patients who seek assistance in ending their lives. Unless you think through this issue carefully, you will be unprepared to respond to the request, "Nurse, please help me die." The ANA's position statement on The Nurse's Role When a Patient Requests Medical Aid in Dying can be reviewed at: http://www.nursingworld.org/~49e869/globalassets/practiceandpolicy/nursing-excellence/ana-position-statements/social-causes-and-health-care/the-nurses-role-when-a-patient-requests-medical-aid-in-dying-web-format.pdf.

Palliative Sedation

Palliative sedation is the lowering of patient consciousness using medication for the express purpose of limiting patient awareness of suffering that is intractable and intolerable (Kirk et al., 2010). When patients who are imminently dying have pain and suffering that is unresponsive to other palliative interventions, palliative sedation to unconsciousness may be considered. Some are concerned that palliative sedation to unconsciousness offers a "back door" to euthanasia, since death is hastened for an unconscious patient who is not being artificially fed. Be sure to check your facility policies. Most restrict palliative sedation to unconsciousness to the imminently dying and exclude patients asking for such sedation for existential suffering or angst.

Death Certificate

U.S. law requires that a death certificate be prepared for each person who dies and specifies what information must be included. Death certificates are sent to local health departments, which compile many statistics from the information. The mortician assumes responsibility for handling and filing the death certificate with proper authorities. A clinician's signature is required on the certificate (check your state law to see if nurses can sign death certificates), as well as that of the pathologist, the coroner, and others in special cases. The nurse is responsible to ensure that the death certificate is signed.

Organ Donation

Patients who express a wish to donate functional organs, such as heart, corneas, liver, lungs, and kidneys, can fill out an organ donor consent card. In addition, depending on state law, a person may sign the back of their driver's license indicating approval of organ donation. The family of a deceased patient may also decide to donate the patient's functional organs. The nurse should be able to review options and provide consent forms to interested patients and their families.

Until recently, most organs were retrieved from totally brain-dead patients. New protocols for retrieving organs from non–heart-beating cadavers are raising multiple practice concerns. Comprehensive attention to optimal patient and family care at the time of withdrawal of life-sustaining therapy must remain the nurse's priority.

The scarcity of organs has resulted in legislation mandating hospitals and other health care facilities to notify transplantation programs of potential donors. Consult the United Network for Organ Sharing (UNOS; https://unos.org/), the private, nonprofit organization that manages the nation's organ transplant system under contract with the federal government, to learn more about donation and transplantation.

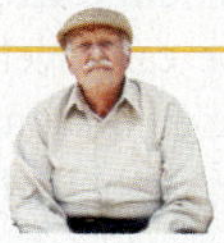

Think back to **Mr. Perez**, who was asking about advance directives and organ donation after his wife was found to have massive, irreversible brain damage. The nurse could incorporate knowledge of organ donation to provide appropriate information for Mr. Perez so that he could make the most informed decision possible.

Autopsy

An autopsy is an examination of the organs and tissues of a human body after death. Consent for autopsy is legally required. The closest surviving family member or members usually have the authority to give or refuse consent. Some religious groups prohibit autopsies except for legal purposes.

It is usually the health care provider's responsibility to obtain permission for an autopsy. Sometimes the patient may grant this permission before death. The nurse can assist by explaining the reasons for an autopsy. Many relatives find comfort when they are told that the knowledge gained from an autopsy may contribute to advances in medical science as well as establish the exact cause of death.

If death is caused by accident, suicide, homicide, or illegal therapeutic practice, the coroner must be notified according to law. The coroner may decide that an autopsy is advisable and can order that one be performed, even if the patient's family has refused consent. In some cases, a death that occurs within 24 hours of admission to the hospital must be reported to the coroner.

FACTORS THAT AFFECT GRIEF AND DYING

Many factors, including age, family relationships, socioeconomic position, and cultural and religious influences, affect a person's reaction to death and expression of grief. Like the stages of grief reaction, these factors vary from person to person.

Developmental Considerations

Children do not understand death on the same level as adults do, but their sense of loss is just as great. Both terminally ill children and their siblings are likely to talk about and ask questions about death in an attempt to understand it. Terminally ill children require parental love and support as well as social interaction with other children. Death of a parent or another significant person can retard a child's development or may cause the child to regress developmentally. Children need to go through the same grief reactions as adults to accept such a loss and maintain emotional well-being.

The loss of a parent by a middle-aged adult helps to prepare the adult for the loss of a spouse or significant other and to accept their own eventual death. Older adults may lose a spouse or friends and relatives their own age. As this happens, they reminisce about life, put their lives and the purpose of living in perspective, and prepare themselves for their own inevitable death.

Family

Family roles have an important effect on a person's reactions to and expressions of grief. For example, the eldest sibling may feel a need to "be strong" and therefore may not grieve openly; a person who loses a spouse may display the same type of behavior to "protect the children."

The death of a child is a devastating experience for the family. The family needs time to accept the reality of the situation, opportunities to talk and to be listened to, and the experience of being able to express themselves behaviorally in a nonjudgmental environment. For example, the family of a terminally ill child may express feelings of guilt by wondering if they were responsible for the impending death.

A sibling may suppress a guilt feeling for having wished the ill child (or a parent) dead. See Ganz (2019) for a discussion of how to improve family ICU experiences at the end of life.

Socioeconomic Factors

A bereaved family may suffer more acutely if there is no health or life insurance or pension after the death of the family provider. Such families face not only the loss of a loved one, but also an economic loss that may further disrupt family life. Older adults especially may be placed in a difficult position because the death of a spouse may result in the decrease or even elimination of a source of retirement income for the surviving spouse. This reduction in income may lead to loss of home, community, and support systems.

Cultural, Gender, and Religious Influences

Culture influences a person's expression of grief. In many families in the Western culture, grief is a private matter shared only with the family. As such, many people internalize their feelings of grief and may not express their feelings of loss to others. On the other hand, cultural background may necessitate that the patient's and family's public display be emotional and distressed, with loud weeping and moaning.

Although sex assigned at birth roles have become less differentiated in the past few decades, male and female reactions to death may differ. Although men are often expected to be stoic and not cry in public, women may be judged as "cold" if they do not grieve publicly. A widow who has a job may not be as emotionally distraught as a woman who needed her husband for financial and other support. Likewise, a widower who has not taken care of the children or the house may view the future more bleakly than a man who has cooked meals and changed diapers. Some ethnic traditions may be ingrained in certain people. For example, the woman may be expected to be weak and need support, whereas the man may be expected to be emotionally supportive. This varies from culture to culture and from person to person.

Faith and religious practices play an important role in the expression of grief and may provide comfort and solace to the person experiencing loss. However, some people may blame God for their suffering and the death of their loved one and turn away from God. Many people who have put spiritual matters in the background of their lives have found death to be an impetus for a return to earlier practices of religion. The thought of death also invites many to contemplate life's big questions: Is there life after death? Is there a supreme being? And if there is a supreme being, where do I stand in relationship to that being? What is the ultimate source of meaning in my life? See Chapter 47 for a discussion of spiritual care.

Cause of Death

The grief response often depends on the cause of death. Many deaths are sudden and involve shock as well as normal grieving in the survivors. Death from disease may generate several types of responses, including the belief that death is a punishment (e.g., when AIDS was first diagnosed in homosexuals and drug users); terror and panic (e.g., when people are reminded of the devastation caused by plagues of earlier centuries); and guilt (e.g., when family and friends believe that they could have prevented the death).

Accidental death is often associated with feelings of bad luck. The guilt response can be enormous, especially when children die as the result of an accident. Death while defending a country usually is viewed by most of society as honorable and necessary. Violent deaths occur daily, especially in larger cities. Suicide accounts for a great number of violent deaths; in fact, among teenagers, it has become a major concern. It is also believed that many accidental deaths are actually suicides.

SUICIDE PREVENTION: MENTAL HEALTH FIRST AID

A 2016 New York Times article (Tavernise, 2016) reported that the U.S. suicide rate surged to a 30-year high, with increases in every age group except older adults. The rise was particularly steep for women. It was also substantial among middle-aged Americans, sending a signal of deep anguish from a group whose suicide rates had been stable or falling since the 1950s. Causative factors linked to the increase in suicides include economic recession, increased drug addiction, "gray divorce," increased social isolation, and the rise of the Internet and social media. During the pandemic, significant increases in feeling isolated and lonely increased the number of deaths by suicide in all ages.

What are our obligations to prevent suicide? It can be difficult for nurses to discern when someone is freely and knowingly choosing to end their life and when a genuine mental health crisis is operative. Mental Health First Aid USA teaches the risk factors and warning signs for mental health crises and discusses additional concerns and strategies for helping someone in both crisis and noncrisis situations. It focuses on a five-step action plan that you can remember with the acronym ALGEE:

- **A**ssess for risk of suicide or harm
- **L**isten nonjudgmentally
- **G**ive reassurance and information
- **E**ncourage appropriate professional help
- **E**ncourage self-help and other support strategies

Visit the Mental Health First Aid USA website (https://www.mentalhealthfirstaid.org) to access valuable resources for frontline caregivers. The *American Nurse Journal* has a three-part series that aims to highlight the work of the ANA Building Strength Through Resilience Committee. To promote the mental health of nurses, the committee has developed web content that focuses on mental health promotion and prevention, suicide prevention, and grief. A full list of the committee's work can be found at https://www.nursingworld.org/practice-policy/nurse-suicide-prevention/ (Melnyk et al., 2021). Also see the Challenging Topic on Nurse Suicide in Chapter 9.

NURSE AS ROLE MODEL

Holistic care of the terminally ill patient and family almost always involves some personal emotional investment. It is

Promoting Health 44-1

GRIEVING

If a past or current loss is influencing your everyday functioning, use the assessment checklist to see how well you are responding to the losses in your life. Then develop a prescription for self-care by choosing appropriate behaviors from the list of suggestions.

Assessment Checklist

☐ almost always ☐ sometimes ☐ almost never

☐ ☐ ☐ 1. I can name the personal losses that are currently influencing my state of well-being.

☐ ☐ ☐ 2. I have a plan that is in place for coping with these losses and helping me to cope.

☐ ☐ ☐ 3. I understand the importance of grieving, and I actually set time aside for this self-care measure.

☐ ☐ ☐ 4. I am comfortable with my feelings and am able to give them expression.

☐ ☐ ☐ 5. There is someone who knows and accepts me well enough to allow me to share openly and honestly.

☐ ☐ ☐ 6. I value being a supportive presence for people with life-threatening illnesses.

☐ ☐ ☐ 7. I respond genuinely to the concerns and feelings of dying patients and their families; I am not afraid to cry with patients and to allow my feelings to show.

Self-Care Behaviors

1. Make a list of the losses that are interfering with your present state of well-being. These may include the loss of health, valued role, image or reputation, relationship, material object, job, or person.
2. Determine whether or not you are addressing these losses in a conscious fashion, and identify coping strategies that may be of help.
3. Try implementing a "tried and true" or new coping strategy.
4. Talk about one of these losses with a friend, religious leader, counselor, or therapist. Assess your comfort level in sharing your feelings openly. Ask the person you are sharing with how that person thinks you are responding.
5. Be honest about any maladaptive coping strategies you may be using, such as addictions, apathy ("Who cares?"), withdrawal and passivity, depression, and acting out. Get any help you need to replace these maladaptive coping measures.
6. Reflect on what your level of comfort in being with people who are dying reveals about your own acceptance of the fact that we will all die.

unrealistic and unfair to expect nurses to handle circumstances surrounding death without feelings. The best policy seems to be taking the time to explore your own feelings and to express them (see Promoting Health 44-1).

Nurse Self-Care Alert

A nurse who neglects to deal with personal feelings about life, dying, and death is in a questionable position for analyzing and considering the needs of patients facing death. A nurse's own feelings play a major role in determining the care given to a patient with a terminal illness. Some questions nurses should use to help clarify their thinking and feelings about dying and death include:

- If I could control the events that result in my own death, where would I want to be? What cause of death would I choose? Whom would I want to have present during my terminal illness?
- What fears do I have about death?
- How would I answer these same questions for a patient for whom I have been caring?
- How could I improve the quality of care for a terminally ill patient for whom I am caring?
- If I were a member of the patient's family, what things would I want a nurse to do for me?

Nurses who care for a patient for an extended period may undergo a grief reaction when the patient dies (Fig. 44-4). Grief after the death of a patient is natural; nurses should allow themselves to go through the grieving process rather than shut off the grief. Work pressures can make it difficult to create the time and space to respond to a patient's

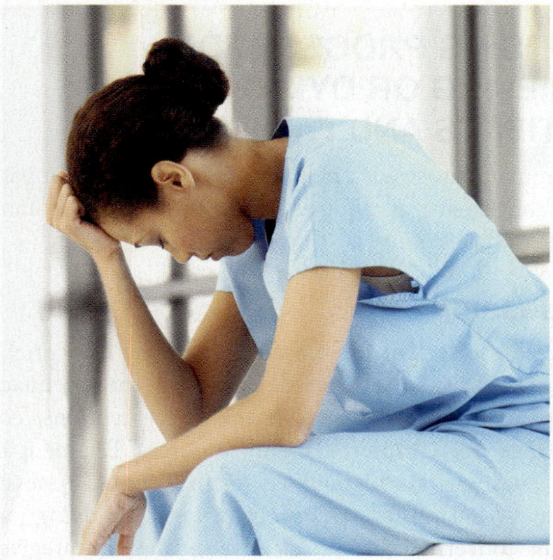

FIGURE 44-4. A nurse grieves the loss of a patient.

Through the Eyes of a Nurse

Honoring Our Fallen Colleagues and Ourselves: Taking Time to Grieve

Sadly, at the time of writing, an estimated 7,000 or more health care workers from around the world have died from COVID-19…Of the 1,361 U.S. health care providers who died, more people of color and nurses (85) have died compared with other races and health care disciplines. The majority of media reports speak about the *number* of deaths. We hear about aggregate losses in the news but often lose sight of the individuals who lost their lives. What we have lost are people, real people who were valuable and meaningful to our critical care community. We lost a considerable amount of critical care knowledge, experience, and talent that cannot be easily replaced. We have lost trusted colleagues who had our back, who mentored us, and who shared laughs and cried with us. Not only were the deceased your colleagues, in many cases, they were your friends and, in some cases, they were family or loved ones.

You may have already honored fallen colleagues in your own way on an individual basis or with your team. Honoring those who have died through a short observance known as The Pause is a practice you may want to be familiar with. The Pause was developed by critical care nurse Jonathan Bartels for critical care nurses and their teams… It was also a way for health care providers to take a breath and reflect on their contribution rather than rushing away to another complex and busy emergency immediately following resuscitation efforts.

According to the Institute for Healthcare Improvement, grief is a near-universal aspect of disasters. Grief during the pandemic may be due to a variety of sources, such as loss of general safety; loss of autonomy; separation from family; financial loss; lack of patient visitation; social distancing; social isolation; and death of patients, colleagues, and loved ones…We each cope with death and dying in our own personal way, yet it is necessary to openly acknowledge our grief to begin dealing with pain and loss. Talking about your experiences, including end-of-life care, with friends, families, and/or colleagues has been found to help validate feelings, share grief, and provide healing support. Strategies to enhance positive coping mechanisms include self-care such as exercise, sleep, healthy diet, leisure activities, and spiritual or religious support. Although self-care during the midst of a pandemic may seem counterintuitive, it helps health care workers to cope with death and continue to provide compassionate, empathetic, and effective care.

…The year 2020 has been a year like no other. I hope you will join me as I pause to take a big breath, reflect, and honor our fallen colleagues. I will also be thinking about all of you and how much you have given of yourselves during the past year. I honor each of you…Please take good care and know you are deeply appreciated.

Annette M. Bourgault, PhD, RN, CNL, FAAN
Editor, CriticalCareNurse

death, but nursing leadership is increasingly affirming the need to do this. *CriticalCareNurse* editor Annette M. Bourgault wrote a poignant editorial about the importance of nurses taking the time to grieve all the colleagues we lost to COVID-19. See the accompanying Through the Eyes of a Nurse.

Nurses should also address their personal health needs.

NURSING PROCESS FOR GRIEVING OR DYING PATIENTS AND FAMILIES

The nursing process is a helpful tool when caring for patients who are grieving or dying as well as caring for their families and significant others.

Assessing

Focused assessment for those experiencing loss, grief, and dying is directed toward determining the adequacy of the patient's and family's knowledge, perceptions, coping strategies (see Chapter 43), and resources. Pertinent interview questions are highlighted in the Focused Assessment Guide 44-1. Holistic assessment of both the dying patient and of concerned family, friends, and family/caregivers is essential to diagnosing problems.

Diagnosing Actual or Potential Health Problems and Needs

An assessment of a grieving, seriously ill, or dying patient may lead to the identification of one or more actual or potential health problems and needs. Following the formulation of the actual or potential health problems and needs, the nurse communicates findings to other nursing and health care professionals through the use of the written and spoken word. The written actual or potential health problem or need becomes a permanent part of the patient's health record.

The International Classification for Nursing Practice (ICNP) identifies several actual or potential health problems that may be identified by nurses:

- Conflicting Attitude toward Treatment
- Despair
- Difficulty Coping
- Dysfunctional Grief
- Fear about Being a Burden to Others
- Fear about Death
- Hopelessness
- Impaired Ability of Caregiver to Perform Caretaking
- Impaired Health Maintenance
- Risk for Suicide

Common etiologic factors and potential signs and symptoms for some of these health problems are found in

Focused Assessment Guide 44-1

EXPERIENCE OF LOSS, GRIEF, DYING, AND DEATH

Assessment Priorities

- Patient and family's understanding of medical condition, prognosis, and dying process
- Patient and family's attitude toward death and dying and knowledge of the dying process
- Patient's preferences for end-of-life treatment and care, such as desire to be at home or in a hospital, and decisions concerning treatment, resuscitation, advanced life support, organ donation, and so forth
- Documented evidence of advance care planning
- Existence of an advance directive **(It is critical that the authorized decision maker be known to all members of the health care team.)**
- Religious beliefs
- Cultural influences
- Stage of grief and death reaction
- Adequacy of coping behaviors
- Adequacy of resources
- Physiologic needs of the patient, for example, personal hygiene, pain control, nutritional and fluid needs
- Psychological needs of the patient and family, for example, fear of the unknown, pain, separation
- Spiritual needs of the patient and family: need for meaning and purpose, for love and relatedness, for forgiveness, for hope

Factors to Assess	Questions and Approaches
Adequacy of knowledge base	What have you been told about your condition? What do you know about this condition? Please describe what you have been told about your treatment options. Is there anything you don't understand about what your doctor is recommending? What else would you like to know about your present condition and treatment options? Do you know how to contact your doctor and to get the information you need or desire? *OBJECTIVE: to identify whether the patient's and family's knowledge will allow them to make informed decisions that will serve their best interests.*
Realism of expectations and perceptions	Have you had any previous experiences with this condition or with the death of someone you love? What are your expectations in this case? How do you see the next few weeks (days) playing out? What are your fears, hopes, concerns, worries? What good do you think might be happening in the midst of all this? *OBJECTIVE: to discover whether the patient and family have unrealistic expectations or misperceptions about the diagnosis, prognosis, and care options that will interfere with their decision making and coping.*
Adequacy of coping strategies	Dealing with our own dying is a once-in-a-lifetime experience, and sometimes we begin the process feeling totally unprepared. Tell me something about how you think you are coping with all this. How well do you think those around you are coping? How can I help you develop or tap the resources that will help you to cope better? *OBJECTIVE: to identify whether the patient and family are using effective coping strategies. If you detect problems, try to identify coping strategies they have used effectively in the past. Also, identify and address destructive habits that have not served them well in the past such as addictions, destructive relationships, passivity, and acting out. Creatively problem solve about new strategies they might try.*
Adequacy of resources	What is helping you to get through this? Do you think the resources available to you are adequate? If the sky was the limit, what help would you wish for? What is interfering with your getting the help you need? What community resources might be of help to you? Are you using these? *OBJECTIVE: to assess the adequacy of the human, financial, spiritual, and psychological resources available to the patient. Questions should be directed to determining what, if anything, is interfering with the patient using whatever resources are available to facilitate coping.*
Signs and symptoms	A holistic assessment of the patient and the patient's family and caregivers should be performed. *OBJECTIVE: to detect problems with coping that result in fatigue, decreased energy, decreased self-care (deficient grooming, unplanned weight loss), and other maladaptive responses.*

Examples of Actual or Potential Health Problems and Needs

LOSS AND IMPENDING DEATH

Actual or Potential Health Problems and Needs	Possible Etiologic Factors	Potential Signs and Symptoms
Fear about Being a Burden **Conflicting Attitude toward Treatment**	• Patient's increasing dependence on family, especially spouse, to meet activities of daily living (hygiene, nutrition, medication administration, mobility, etc.) • History of being fiercely independent • Patient has rejected a lung transplant • Transplant team wants to list them for a second lung transplant • Family wants the patient to live.	• Talks frequently about not wanting to be a burden • Decreased requests for assistance • Expressions of sadness, "I'm not good for anything anymore…" • "I don't want to give up, I've never been a quitter, but I don't think I can go through all of this again." • "It's true that there is still so much I want to do, but maybe not in this life."
Risk for Impaired Ability of Caregiver to Perform Caregiving	• Patient's increasing dependency • Discharged home with significant needs • Increase in care needs • Caregiver's unstable health condition	—
Readiness for Enhanced Coping	—	• Verbalizes that he knows his days are few and begins to express how he wants to spend his time.

Source: International Council of Nurses (ICN). (2019). *Nursing diagnosis and outcome statements.* https://www.icn.ch/sites/default/files/inline-files/ICNP2019-DC.pdf

the accompanying box, Examples of Actual or Potential Health Problems and Needs: Loss and Impending Death. Box 44-5 provides an overview of the nursing process related to the seriously ill or dying person's impaired health maintenance.

Outcome Identification and Planning

Nursing care should be directed toward the achievement of the following goals or outcomes for grieving and dying patients and their families.

The patient or family will:

- demonstrate freedom to express feelings, needs, fears, and concerns.
- identify and use effective coping strategies.
- accept the need for help as appropriate and use available resources.
- make health care decisions reflecting personal values and goals; ultimately feel peaceful about their role in decision making.
- declare and record preferences regarding treatment options.
- report sufficient relief of pain to interact meaningfully with family and to attend to everyday concerns.
- experience a dignified and comfortable death.
- resolve grief after a suitable period of mourning and resume meaningful roles and daily activities (family or significant others).

The patient and the family should take an active role in planning for care. Such planning takes the patient's preferences into consideration, facilitates the acceptance of death by the patient and the family, and provides interventions to meet holistic needs.

Implementing

In addition to promoting a comfortable, dignified death, the nurse's aims in caring for dying patients and their families include facilitating coping of the dying person and family and promoting health and preventing illness of the family. The display box titled Focus on the Older Adult (on page 1812) provides indicators for a comfortable, dignified, and peaceful death. See Jensen et al. (2020) for a discussion of practice recommendations for end-of-life care.

Developing Trusting Nurse–Patient and Nurse–Family Relationships

Communication is a lifelong need up to the moment of death and should be maintained at all times with the patient and family. To develop meaningful communication, the nurse must develop a trusting relationship with the patient. The nurse needs listening skills and the ability to recognize both verbal and nonverbal cues given by the patient and family. These skills are discussed in Chapter 8.

Be willing to discuss the patient's fears and doubts openly and to serve as a nonjudgmental listener. However, talking with dying patients is often difficult. The following observations and suggestions by P. Rancour (personal communication, 2008) are helpful:

- Often, when patients initiate conversations about dying, you may feel unprepared for their questions. They can take you by surprise and can often lead you to believe that the patient expects a crystal ball response. Remember that the purpose of all such discussions is to keep the lines of communication open with the patient. The idea is to keep the subject of dying open to discussion and to communicate

Box 44-5 Nursing Process Related to the Seriously Ill or Dying Person's Impaired Health Maintenance

Patients and the surrogate decision makers for incompetent patients frequently feel overwhelmed when they need to make life-and-death decisions about end-of-life care.

Assessment Priorities

The objective of assessment is to identify patients and families who are at high risk for impaired health outcomes because of their difficulty making end-of-life decisions and to provide the support they need to make appropriate end-of-life care decisions that advance the patient's interests before problems develop. Potential problems when this need is overlooked include postponement of decision making, which interferes with the patient receiving optimal care; vacillation in decision making, which disturbs continuity of care for the patient; and escalation of conflict concerning decision making, which may result in a standoff between participating parties—the patient, individual family members, and health care professionals.

- Detect difficulties with making decisions: fear; insufficient or erroneous information; inadequate support; conflict between religious convictions, personal moral beliefs, and choice one wants to make; and reluctance to assume responsibility for making life-and-death decision.
- Identify what is causing the decision making to be hard for the patient or family and what type of information or support could reverse this.
- Identify potential conflicts between what the patient wants and what the patient's family or caregivers believe should be done.
- Observe the patient or the patient's surrogate decision makers for physical signs of distress that reflect feeling overwhelmed by the decision that needs to be made: signs of fatigue and general exhaustion, signs of agitation and distress, and signs of growing anger and alienation.
- Read the chart carefully to identify decisions that are pending and note the lack of movement toward a decision or toward resolution of existing conflict.

Expected Outcomes

The ethically and legally valid decision maker will achieve the following:

- Describe care options (including the option of nontreatment), listing the advantages and disadvantages of each.
- Seek clarification of options, if necessary, and whatever support is needed.
- Express fears, concerns, and hopes.
- Make an informed and voluntary choice.
- Make end-of-life decisions that reflect the patient's values and goals, advancing the patient's interests.
- Make end-of-life decisions that are consistent with the aims of medicine and nursing.

Interventions

Nursing measures revolve around identifying and supporting the morally and legally valid decision maker. The following should be considered:

- Competent patients—those who can (1) understand the information needed to make the decision, (2) reason in accord with a relatively consistent set of values, and (3) communicate a preference—have the right to consent to and to refuse any and all indicated medical treatment.
- Surrogates of previously competent patients are to be guided by what is known about the patient's values and preferences. These surrogates may be designated in an advance directive, or there may be state or province law designating a hierarchy of surrogates, such as spouse, parent, adult child, sibling; the morally valid surrogate is the one who best knows the patient and the patient's preferences.
- Surrogates deciding for a never-competent patient (child or profoundly retarded adult) must be guided by a determination of what is in the patient's best interests by referring to more objective and socially shared values.

The nurse clarifies the goal of treatment (cure, stabilization of functioning, preparation for a comfortable and dignified death) and makes sure that treatment decisions are consistent with this goal. Nursing intervention may be helpful in making sure that everyone is clear about the goal of care and changes in the goal of care as the patient's condition changes.

Because some health care providers are reluctant to accept preparation for a comfortable, dignified death as an appropriate goal of medicine, some patients have received unwanted care that needlessly prolonged their dying. Conversely, decisions are being made today for financial and other reasons that deprive patients of wanted end-of-life care. The nurse serves as an advocate for the patient and the family unless what the patient or family wants violates the profession of nursing and nursing's code of ethics or the nurse's own conscience. If your beliefs and convictions do not allow you to advocate for a patient or family when what the patient wants is legal and clinically appropriate, you should immediately seek the advice of your supervisor.

Interventions include the following:

- Providing whatever information and support the patient or family needs to make an informed and voluntary decision
- Referring the patient or family to sources that can clarify problematic aspects of the decision, such as religious authority, ethicist, legal counsel
- Identifying and addressing coercive influences on decision making, being sensitive to cultural norms; for example, whereas a controlling husband may be violating his wife's freedom to make autonomous choices in one culture, in another, it is customary for the husband (or male elder in the family) to make choices for a woman

Documentation of end-of-life care preferences of competent, or previously competent, patients is important. This includes a written record of communication, a living will, durable power of attorney for health care, and a medical advance directive. These preferences must be communicated to those who are ordering care.

- Mediating sources of conflict
- Referring patient or family to an ethics consult team or ethics committee if conflict cannot be resolved

Focus on the Older Adult

MEASURING QUALITY OF CARE AT THE END OF LIFE

The American Geriatrics Society developed the following statement of principles about quality care at the end of life, but these indicators work well for persons of all ages:

1. *Physical and emotional symptoms.* Pain, shortness of breath, fatigue, depression, fear, anxiety, nausea, skin breakdown, and other physical and emotional problems often destroy the quality of life at its end. Symptom management is regularly deficient. Care systems should focus on these needs and ensure that people can count on a comfortable and meaningful end of their lives.
2. *Support of function and autonomy.* Even with an inevitable and progressive decline with fatal illness, much can be done to maintain personal dignity and self-respect. Achieving better functional outcomes and greater autonomy should be valued.
3. *Advance care planning.* Often, the experience of patient and family can be improved just by planning ahead for likely problems, so that decisions can reflect the patient's preferences and circumstances rather than responding to crises.
4. *Aggressive care near death—site of death, CPR, and hospitalization.* Although aggressive care is often justified, most patients would prefer to have avoided it when short-term outcome is death. High rates of medical interventions near death should prompt further examination of provider judgment and care system design.
5. *Patient and family satisfaction.* The dying patient's peace of mind and the family's perception of the patient's care and comfort are extremely important. In the long run, we can hope that the time at the end of life will be especially precious, not merely tolerable. We must measure both patient and family satisfaction with these elements: the decision-making process, the care given, the outcomes achieved, and the extent to which opportunities were provided to complete life in a meaningful way.
6. *Global quality of life.* Often a patient's assessment of overall well-being illuminates successes and shortcomings in care, which are not apparent in more specific measures. Quality of life can be good despite declining physical health, and care systems that achieve this should be valued.
7. *Family burden.* How health care is provided affects whether families have serious financial and emotional effects from the costs of care and the challenges of direct caregiving. Current and future pressures on funding health care are likely to displace more responsibility for services and payment onto families.
8. *Survival time.* With pressures on health care resources likely to increase, there is a new reason to worry that death will be accepted too readily. Purchasers and patients need to know survival times vary across plans and provider systems. In conjunction with information about symptoms, satisfaction, and the other domains listed here, such measures will allow insights into the priorities and trade-offs within each care system.
9. *Provider continuity and skill.* Only with enduring relationships with professional caregivers can patient and family develop trust, communicate effectively, and develop reliable plans. The providers must also have the relevant skills, including rehabilitation, symptom control, and psychological support. Care systems must demonstrate competent performance on continuity and provider skill.
10. *Bereavement.* Often health care stops with the patient's death, but the suffering of the family goes on. Survivors may benefit with relatively modest interventions.

Source: From American Geriatrics Society (AGS) Ethics Committee. (1995). *The Care of Dying Patients: A Position Statement from the American Geriatrics Society. 43*(5). Author; with permission from John Wiley and Sons.

to the patient that it does not make you afraid to talk about it. An open-ended statement, such as, "Tell me what concerns you the most," provides a means of encouraging communication.

- Some patients may be too fearful to ask health care providers questions about dying. They often approach staff whom they perceive as less intimidating or more approachable. The question often comes in the middle of the night, when there are no distractions, when anxiety or pain may keep the patient awake, and when the patient may feel most alone with psychospiritual distress. In any case, it is often on the nurse's watch when questions about dying may arise.
- Because of the surprising nature of such questions, you may feel tempted to escape ("I've got to go take that patient's vital signs right now…") or pass the buck ("That sounds like a question for your doctor."). Be vigilant to prevent such reactions, keeping in mind that avoidance would only help reduce your own anxiety and would do nothing to assist with the patient's anxiety. It is well within the scope of your professional practice as a competent nurse to provide counseling and death education, especially when the patient asks you for it or indicates an unmet need for such information and support. *When in doubt, ask a question in response*, such as "What do you feel about that?" or "What have you been told already?" This will accomplish several things. It will help you regain your composure and will give you more information about what is on the patient's mind so that your intervention can be as specific and responsive to that patient as possible.
- Do not provide false reassurance. Remember that avoiding discussions about death robs the patient of precious time to accomplish goals that produce hope (Box 44-6). People who are dying hope for many things even when they cannot hope for a cure, such as hope for freedom from pain, to be surrounded by loved ones, and for the rest of their allotted time to be spent in meaningful pursuits.

A caring nurse feels at ease in crying with the grieving person and sharing experiences with fears, loneliness, and death.

Box 44-6 Enabling Hope in the Terminally Ill

These guidelines are the product of an interdisciplinary team of those providing care for the terminally ill. They are presented to encourage anyone providing care for the terminally ill to consider the crucial place of hope in their caring and also their own potential to enable such hope.

What Is Hope?

Hope is the ingredient in life that enables a person both to consider a future and to actively bring that future into being. Hope originates in imagination but must become a valued and realistic possibility for that person in order to energize action. Hope has the capacity to embrace the reality of a person's suffering without escaping from it (false hope) or being suffocated by it (despair, helplessness, hopelessness).

Hope is unique to each person. During terminal illness, the future being considered will become more focused, yet hope is essential for a person to transcend despair and complete crucial life tasks.

Enabling Hope

Acknowledging Individual Uniqueness

To enable hope, the care provider must acknowledge *the uniqueness of the person* and take seriously the dreams of the terminally ill person within the changing nature of the illness. Steps that can be taken to translate hope into accomplishment must be considered. For this to happen, care providers need to do the following:

- Consider all language used, and appreciate how easily hopes can be disabled by such terms as "hopeless situation" or "nothing more can be done."
- Encounter the person's feelings at their own level; be willing to stay at that person's level and allow them to lead.
- Be willing to take the necessary time to establish rapport with the person in order that their hopes can be shared in a supportive atmosphere. Where appropriate, use physical contact to build trust.
- Realize the changing nature of both the disease and the accompanying hopes. At one point, a hope for a cure may be the necessary activating force for a person to undergo treatment; at another, the person's acceptance of impending death may give them the energy to complete crucial life tasks or endure the many losses of terminal illness.

Granting Control

A factor crucial to the nourishing of hope within a person is that of *control.* A person must be willing to take the necessary action to achieve what is hoped for. Terminal illness places many restrictions upon a person and often robs that person of a feeling of being able to control the situation, thus leading to increasing helplessness and hopelessness. To counter this, efforts must be made not only to support a person in hoping, but also to grant the person control in bringing realistic hopes into being.

To help support a person's sense of control in order to enable active hoping, care providers need to do the following:

- Provide honest and accessible information regarding the progress of the illness.
- Allow a person to express and work through many hopes in order to develop those hopes appropriate to them in the present context.
- Allow for freedom of choice regarding treatment options to the degree possible within the setting.
- Maximize the present possibilities for achieving hopes while allowing for the changing realities of terminal illness.

Being Aware of Your Own Feelings

Hope is strengthened by those who care for and support a terminally ill person. Within the context of illness and suffering, hope may be fragile, and must be nurtured in relationships with professional caregivers, family, and friends. To enable hope, care providers must be aware of their own hope for that person.

As a care provider, you need to do the following:

- Recognize your own assumptions regarding the particular person and how those assumptions may inhibit the enabling of hope for that person.
- Be aware of how your own hope for that person may differ from the hope being expressed by that person.
- Resist judging expressed hope and be willing to explore such hope further.
- Accept the person's present suffering. Avoid giving "false hope" that minimizes the reality of the situation ("It can't be that bad," or "Don't worry, everything will be fine"); at the same time, avoid encouraging despair by focusing only upon the illness ("God can't possibly heal you now. That cancer's all through you!").

Supporting Spirituality

A component of hope is *spirituality.* Supported by faith in God, hope is the capacity of the person to transcend present suffering, to lift their perspective to future possibilities, and so to enable the person to accomplish important life tasks. This capacity to transcend is facilitated by belief in the presence of God within the changing context of terminal illness.

To enable this spiritual aspect of hope, care providers need to do the following:

- Accept the person's own spiritual journey and present level of faith (or lack of faith).
- Be open to expressed hopes that link with religious belief (e.g., "God will cure me" or "I pray that God will take me home soon").
- Allow for spiritual struggle and its resultant emotions (e.g., anger when "the cancer is back and God has failed to cure me!"). Recognize that the level of spiritual struggle during terminal illness may increase to enable the accomplishment of crucial hope for life tasks such as reconciliation and forgiveness.
- Be prepared to accept the reality of death as an aspect of hope. Accept a person who has shifted hope to how they wish to die, to life after death, to a meeting with deceased loved ones, and so on.
- Enable a person to have access to whatever means and rites of religion that will encourage their hope.

Source: Courtesy of Ted Creen, D. *Min., Palliative Care Pastoral Consultant,* 865 2nd Ave. West, Owen Sound, Ontario, Canada.

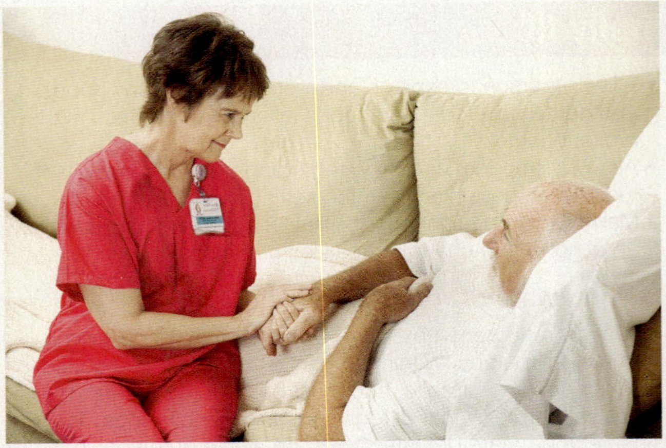

FIGURE 44-5. A nurse displays empathy and compassion. (*Source:* Used with permission from Shutterstock. *Photo by Lisa F. Young.*)

This allows the griever the freedom to express their deepest concerns. Nonverbal communication is equally important. A smile, holding a hand, and eye-to-eye contact are all meaningful (Fig. 44-5). The warmth behind the gesture and the honest concern of the nurse are what count.

Hearing is believed to be the last sense to leave the body; many patients retain their hearing almost to the moment of death. Demonstrate kindness and thoughtfulness by speaking to a comatose patient and encouraging family members to do likewise. Explain to the patient the nursing care being given and the people and sounds in the environment.

Explaining the Patient's Condition and Treatment

All involved health care personnel should know exactly what the patient and family have been told. Conflicting information puts the nurse and other team members at cross-purposes and causes the family to distrust the patient's caregivers. Because patients and families often direct questions about the patient's prognosis to the nurse, the nurse should take the initiative in ensuring that terminology, prognosis, and the description of the progress are consistently presented and explained.

Explain the patient's condition and treatment to both the patient and the family. Patience is required during explanations. The patient and family members may be so overwhelmed by the diagnosis that they do not hear all the information that is shared with them. Question them to learn how much they have retained, then repeat the information they missed. Explain care options, as well as the expected outcomes of each option, fully.

Sadly, many health care professionals do not embrace "good dying" as a legitimate aim of medical and nursing care. As a result, the dying of many patients is painfully prolonged because no one initiates a patient or family conference to clarify the treatment goals when cure is no longer an option (see Promoting Health Literacy in Caregivers of Terminally Ill Patients). The nurse plays a key role in helping the patient and family prepare for a comfortable and dignified death. Here, the primary focus

Promoting Health Literacy

IN CAREGIVERS OF TERMINALLY ILL PATIENTS

Patient Scenario

Marlene Bough is the 47-year-old wife of a 49-year-old man who is nearing the end of his life as a result of widely metastasized thyroid cancer. Mr. Bough was initially diagnosed almost 5 years ago, but treatment is no longer able to control the growth of malignant tumors throughout his body. He has almost constant pain, is unable to walk, and has severe pulmonary and cardiovascular impairments. The doctors have told the couple that no more can be done to prolong Mr. Bough's life and that he has, at the most, less than 6 months to live. Mrs. Bough has taken a family leave from her job as a third-grade teacher so she can care for Mr. Bough at home, even though she is very concerned about being able to care for him and afraid she will cause him further pain.

Nursing Considerations: *Tips for Improving Health Literacy*

Schedule a home care planning meeting for Marlene and others who have indicated a desire to be helpful (daughter, sister-in-law, brother, colleagues at her school) and discuss how each person can help. Include times for family and friends to stay with Mr. Bough so that Marlene can have some time away from the care responsibilities. Demonstrate and have Marlene practice moving Mr. Bough in bed, providing hygiene, and administering pain medications. Discuss the responsibilities of the hospice provider and the goals of palliative care. Provide a written list of phone numbers for health care providers, including those that would be available at any time. Encourage Marlene to ask her husband, "What concerns you most?" and then to talk openly about what kind of treatment he wants for his final days. Include the following questions:

- "Where do you want to die?"
- "What kind of medical treatment do you want and do not want?"
- "What do you consider a good death?"
- "What kind of funeral service do you want?"
- "Where do you want to be buried?"

Ensure that advanced planning documents are completed. Encourage Marlene to take some time for herself, to recognize the stress of her husband's care, to welcome the help of others, and to use support people and groups after her husband's death. At that time, ask her to be prepared to ask the following three questions to herself and her health care provider:

- What is my main problem?
- What do I need to do?
- Why is it important for me to do this?

What additional measures can you take to help maintain health literacy in this woman? What other measures would be helpful for Marlene if she did not speak English, could not read, or had other learning disabilities?

Research in Nursing

BRIDGING THE GAP TO EVIDENCE-BASED PRACTICE

Helping Patients and Families Make Decisions About End-of-Life Treatment and Care

Needing to provide ineffective and sometimes actually harmful interventions to seriously ill and dying patients in intensive care units (ICUs) troubles many nurses. Too often, no one calls for a family conference to clarify the patient's and family's understandings of the medical condition, reasonable expectations, and goals of care.

Related Research

Edward, K. L., Galletti, A., & Huynh, M. (2020). Enhancing communication with family members in the intensive care unit: A mixed methods study. *Critical Care Nurse, 40*(6), 23–32.

ICU nurses have particularly challenging and intense interactions with patients and their families, acting as confidantes, educators, advocates, cultural liaisons, and translators. According to Edward, Galletti, & Huynh (2020), family members rate their satisfaction with the ICU admission according to the quality of communication they received, more than the level of care given to their loved one.

Brooks, L. A., Manias, E., & Nicholson, P. (2017). Communication and decision-making about end-of-life care in the intensive care unit. *American Journal of Critical Care, 26*(4), 336–341.

This study used an interpretive, qualitative inquiry method with focus groups to explore the experiences and perspectives of nurses and physicians when initiating end-of-life care in the ICU. Five focus groups were conducted with 17 nurses and 11 physicians participating. The key aspects discussed included communication and shared decision making. Researchers concluded that multidisciplinary implementation and acceptance of end-of-life care plans in the ICU need improvement. Clear organizational processes that support the introduction of nurse and physician end-of-life care leaders are essential to optimizing outcomes for patients, family members, and clinicians.

Watson, A. C., & October, T. W. (2016). Clinical nurse participation at family conferences in the pediatric intensive care unit. *American Journal of Critical Care, 25*(6), 489–497.

Realizing that clinical nurses attend family conferences in the ICU, but that their role during these meetings is not yet fully understood, researchers surveyed nurses and reviewed 40 audio-recorded family conferences conducted in the 44-bed pediatric ICU of an urban pediatric hospital. Most nurses surveyed thought it important to attend family conferences but identified workload as a barrier to attendance. Audio recordings revealed that bedside nurses attended 20 (50%) of 40 family conferences and spoke in 5 (25%) of the 20. Nurses verbally contributed 4% to 6% to the overall speech at the family conference.

Relevance to Nursing Practice

Clearly, nurses could be playing a larger role in helping patients and families make critical decisions about treatment and end-of-life care. Family conferences need to happen earlier, and strategies to improve the physical and verbal participation of clinical nurses are needed, especially in the context of previous research demonstrating the need for more attention in family conferences to social–emotional support and patient advocacy.

is palliative, such that the patient and family accept that death is inevitable and now focus on how to spend the remaining days. For some, this means a referral to hospice or a palliative care program. Nurses play an important role in ensuring that timely prognostic information is given to patients and families so that they can decide how to spend their last days together. Some patients want to "die fighting" and will insist on intensive, life-sustaining treatment until every system fails. Others will choose not to have further treatment and will want to spend their last days in a comfortable setting (see the Research in Nursing box). See the Care Coordination Checklist (Box 44-7 on page 1816) for helpful hints on thoughtful, person-centered care at the end of life and the accompanying Thoughtful, Person-Centered Practice: Challenging Topics: Medically Assisted Dying on pages 1816–1817.

Teaching Self-Care and Promoting Self-Esteem

Encourage the patient to retain independence and make decisions as long as possible. Allow the patient to manage personal hygiene practices and self-feeding for as long as possible. After the patient is confined to bed, the creative nurse and family caregivers should attempt to find self-care activities the patient can perform. When physical abilities fail, determining when to take medication, for example, may be all the control the patient can retain.

Having familiar objects in view can help make the patient feel more comfortable and secure. Whether the patient is at home or in a health care facility, it is desirable to have the environment reflect personal preferences. This gives the patient some degree of control when health and other activities of daily living have slipped out of the patient's reach. It also supports self-esteem.

In the transition from independence to interdependence and ultimately to dependence, the patient may experience depression and express frustration and grief about "being a burden." It is crucial for professional and nonprofessional caregivers to respond to the dying patient as a person of worth whose life has meaning and value. Chapter 8 discusses practical ways in which nurses can use looks, touch, words, and actions to communicate respect and caring.

Teaching Family Members to Assist in Care

Preparing family members to help provide care yields benefits to both the patient and family members. Having

(text continues on page 1818)

Box 44-7 End-of-Life Care Coordination Checklist

Consider These Suggestions as You Coordinate End-of-Life Care

☐ **Know the patient and the person**

- Include the patient and family in developing specific patient-centered goals.
- Communicate and collaborate as a health care team member.
- Provide thoughtful, person-centered care.
- Reflect as a nurse and with patient/family about plans.
- Use available resources to support the patient and family during transitions.
- Listen to the patient and family.

☐ **Assessment questions to ask the patient**

- "What activities are you having difficulty doing now that you were able to do 3 months ago?"
- "Describe your pain and how it's different now than 3 months ago."
- "How does your pain (shortness of breath, fatigue, other symptoms) affect your activities of daily living?"
- "What work/hobbies does your illness prevent you from doing?"
- "What coping strategies do you use when stressed?"
- "What are your concerns (or fears) for the future?"

☐ **Exploring the patient's goals**

- "If you were given a 3-month life expectancy, what would you want to accomplish?"
- "What plans have you made to do when you return home?"
- "What resources do you have to accomplish your goals?"
- "What resources will you need to accomplish your goals?"
- "Who have you included to be with you as a part of your goals?"

☐ **Developing patient-centered goals**

- "It sounds like you want (fill in with restatement of patient's goals)."
- "What resources are available to help you meet your goal?"
- "What, if any, changes will your family need to consider to help you meet your goal?"
- "How will you accomplish your goal?"
- "What modifications might be needed (such as home, job, family obligations, cultural influences, spiritual considerations) to meet your goal?"

☐ **Involving the family**

- "What help will you need when (call the patient by name) is discharged?"
- "How do you cope with stress (anxiety, change)?"
- "What's your understanding regarding the plan of care?"
- "What concerns (or fears) do you have?"

Source: Used with permission. Wittenberg-Lyles, E., Goldsmith, J., Ferrell, B., & Ragan, S. L. (2013). *Communication in palliative nursing.* By Permission of Oxford University Press, USA; Ferguson, R. (2018). Care coordination at the end of life: The nurse's role. *Nursing, 48*(2), 11–13; Wolters Kluwer Health, Inc.

Thoughtful, Person-Centered Practice: Challenging Topics

Medically Assisted Dying

Many controversial issues make it challenging to know how to respond as a professional nurse in select scenarios. Often, the nurse's personal and/or professional values may conflict with options desired by patients, families, employers, and communities. Not infrequently, nurses must make clinical judgments balancing, promoting, and safeguarding personal integrity and respecting the values and preferences of patient. The *Essentials* competencies for nurses includes 9.5b, Demonstrate the core values of professional nursing identity, 9.5c, Demonstrate sensitivity to the values of others, and 9.5d, Demonstrate ethical comportment and moral courage in decision making and actions (American Association of Colleges of Nursing [AACN], 2021).

Read the scenario below and see if you can articulate what you believe, why you believe this, and how these beliefs are likely to inform the decisions you make and your behavior, especially when you are confronted with competing obligations. Based on Tanner's Clinical Judgment Model (2006), consider reflection-in-action and reflection-on-action (Nielson et al., 2007).

Reflection-in-Action

As you read, consider what the student is thinking at the moment—what happened? How did the patient, family, and/or health care provider respond? What did the nurse do next?

Scenario

Mr. Sam Wallner was diagnosed with extensive stage small cell lung cancer and was told that the cancer had spread too far for surgery or radiation therapy to be useful as the initial treatment. Since until this time he had been in fairly good health, chemotherapy, possibly with an immunotherapy drug was suggested in hopes of shrinking the cancer, treating symptoms, and helping to live longer. The nursing student was shocked when Mr. Wallner asked their opinion about the likelihood that the chemotherapy and immunotherapy would have any benefit. "I've heard horror stories about all sorts of cancer treatments, and I don't want to start something that will just make me feel more miserable. Maybe it's time to pack it in?" Since this happened on the first day of their rotation in the oncology unit, they could not answer the question about the likely benefits of the proposed treatment, but promised to get an answer for Mr. Wallner. The nurse left the room wondering if Mr. Wallner had been serious about "packing it in," and what exactly was meant by this.

Effective Noticing (Cues)

1. What did you notice about the situation initially? What information/observations are significant? What information deviates from what is expected/normal/usual?

Thoughtful, Person-Centered Practice: Challenging Topics (*continued*)

Effective Interpreting

2. How would you prioritize this data? What other assessment data, evidence, and/or information would you need to consider the situation? How would you obtain this additional information?
3. What do you think about this situation? Consider personal and previous nursing experiences that you have had and formal knowledge (physiology, psychology, communication skills) that may be of assistance in providing care in this situation.

Scenario

The student was able to find the oncology nurse practitioner, and she shared Mr. Wallner's questions. The nurse practitioner promised to accompany the student back to his room to answer his questions about the probable benefits of treatment, but he asked the student what she thought Mr. Wallner meant about "packing it in." The student replied, "He seems pretty scared, and I thought he was asking me if dying sooner rather than later was a good option." She shared with the nurse practitioner, "I don't believe I'd feel comfortable talking with him about that option—I'm not sure what I believe. I was raised as a Christian, and suicide was never an approved option." Medically assisted dying legislation was recently passed in this state, and the student knew that its legalization was a heated topic. She had never been asked by a patient to help them die before and she wasn't sure how she should respond. "You'll talk to the patient about this, too, right? I need to do more research before I understand my professional responsibilities."

Now, consider the nurses' decisions and reflect on your learning. See if you can articulate what you believe, why you believe this, and how these beliefs are likely to inform the decisions you make and your behavior, especially when you are confronted with competing obligations.

Effective Responding

4. How would you describe the obligations the student has in this scenario to her patient, to herself, and to her team?
5. If you cannot fulfill each of these obligations, how will you prioritize them? What basis/rationale do you use for prioritization? Remember that the ANA *Code of Ethics for Nurses* reminds us that "the nurse's primary commitment is to the patient," while, at the same time, states that "the nurse owes the same duties to self as to others, including the responsibility to promote health and safety, preserve wholeness of character and integrity, maintain competence, and continue personal and professional growth."

Effective Reflecting

When the student talks with her faculty, her preceptor, other nurses on the unit, and other students, she is not surprised to learn that there are many opinions about what a competent and compassionate response to the patient's questions should look like. These range from being a cheerleader for aggressive treatment to being an advocate for his right to use the new legislation to obtain the means to end his life when he is ready. Several nurses have already read the legislation and are ready to coach patients on how to meet the criteria, and to "accompany them" on this stage of their life journey. Because the legislation is so new, the hospital has yet to draft a policy on how to respond to a request for medically assisted dying, should this be what the patient wants. The student also realizes that there are many palliative care options to explore before the patient chooses medically assisted dying. Given her unfamiliarity with this topic, the student is happy to defer to the experience of the nurse practitioner and promises to continue to educate herself. She is eager to observe the nurse practitioner's conversation with Mr. Wallner. She realizes in a more poignant way, the importance of what she says to patients and the power her words may have in life-and-death decisions.

6. Do you agree with the choice the student made? Would you have made the same choice, why or why not? What would inform your decision?
7. Do you agree with the criteria the nurse used to evaluate her decision? How do you evaluate your clinical and moral judgments?
8. What resources can you access to better inform your decision?
9. Whether or not you decide to try and respond to Mr. Wallner, how might you use reflective practice to evaluate your decision so you can respond more confidently in the future? What criteria will you use to evaluate a good response?
10. What personal attributes and competencies are most likely to lead to a good response?

Reflection-on-Action

Then look back at the student's decisions and reflect on your learning—how did your knowledge and/or skills expand based on this scenario? What attitude, value, or belief shifts did you experience (if any) after reading this scenario? What would you do differently if you were in this situation? What more do you need to know to be able to manage this or a similar situation in the future?

Nielson, A., Stragnell, S., & Jester, P. (2007). Guide for reflection using the clinical judgment model. *Journal of Nursing Education*, *46*(11), 513–516.

Olsen, D. P., Chan, R., & Lehto, R. (2017). Ethical nursing care when the terminally ill patient seeks death. *American Journal of Nursing*, *117*(7), 50–55

Tanner, C. A. (2006). Thinking like a nurse: A research-based model of clinical judgment in nursing. *Journal of Nursing Education*, *45*(6), 204–211.

loved ones near comforts the patient. Family members, too, are comforted by knowing that they helped comfort the patient. Teach family members how to provide care to the patient. Family members may not want to provide physical care themselves but may want to know what to expect and how they can psychologically aid the patient. Provide assistance in this area by explaining the patient's condition, what treatment the patient is undergoing, and what result the family can expect from the treatment. Knowing the facts may help family members to cope better with impending loss.

Meeting the Needs of the Dying Patient

There are many ways you can intervene to meet the needs of the dying patient. Many hospice professionals use the nonpharmacologic side to guide family education. Please refer to online Student Resources for this text for a helpful four-page nonpharmacologic/pharmacologic symptom management guide (used with permission, Hospice of the Valley, Phoenix, AZ).

ADDRESSING PHYSIOLOGIC NEEDS

Physiologic care of the patient involves meeting physical needs such as personal hygiene, pain control, nutritional and fluid needs, movement, elimination, and respiratory care. Personal hygiene includes cleanliness of the skin, hair, mouth, nose, and eyes. Frequent baths and linen changes may be necessary. The mouth and nose should be kept free of mucus, and secretions should be wiped from the eyes.

The health care provider determines the medication and dosage needed for pain control, but the patient's wishes should be considered (see Chapter 36 for further discussion of pain control). Some patients prefer and are able to control their own medication. A patient requiring nutritional support should be encouraged to take sips of water or ice chips if still able to swallow. The dying patient may elect to forego artificial nutrition and hydration because the burdens of feeding and hydrating artificially may outweigh the benefits. Problems with elimination include the development of incontinence, constipation, and urinary retention. Absorbent pads or a nearby bedpan or urinal may be used for patients experiencing incontinence; laxatives or enemas may be used for relieving constipation; and catheterization may be required for urinary retention. Bed linens should be changed often. Periodic movement should also be assisted; regular changes of position help prevent pressure injuries. Repositioning the conscious patient in semi-Fowler's position can facilitate respirations; positioning the unconscious patient in a semiprone position allows drainage of saliva and mucus. Oxygen therapy may be necessary for some patients.

ADDRESSING PSYCHOLOGICAL NEEDS

When people speak of their fears of death, responses typically include fear of the unknown, pain, separation, leaving loved ones, loss of dignity, loss of control, and unfinished business. Kübler-Ross believes that there is still another, more overwhelming and more significant fear that often is repressed and unconscious: that of the catastrophic, destructive force that has befallen a person and that the person cannot change. Kübler-Ross points out that terminally ill people communicate this fear of a destructive force but do so largely through symbolic language. A person may use nonverbal language, such as a facial expression, a particular kind of handclasp, or, in the case of children, drawings and manner of play with toys. Verbal communication may also be used symbolically.

A fear of isolation, of having to face death alone, is a primary concern of the dying patient. Support the patient by indicating your presence, giving full attention, and showing that you care. Encourage the presence of family members in the room and sharing of reminiscences. There is now a national volunteer program designed to provide companionship and support for dying persons so that no patient dies alone (http://www.eskenazihealth.edu/programs/noda). Check to see if your hospital has a "No one dies alone" program.

ADDRESSING NEEDS FOR INTIMACY

Terminally ill patients and their sexual partners may feel uncomfortable discussing their needs for intimacy. Partners may wish to be physically intimate with the dying person but are afraid of "hurting" them and may also be afraid that an open expression of sexuality is somehow "inappropriate" when someone is dying. Encourage discussion and suggest ways to be physically intimate that will meet the needs of both partners. A loving foot massage or a tender, cradling body embrace may be exactly what a dying person needs in their last moments.

ADDRESSING SPIRITUAL NEEDS

Although not all patients follow specific spiritual or religious beliefs, most require some form of spiritual care. Many terminally ill patients find great comfort in the support they receive from their religious faith. Help obtain the services of clergy or pastoral care workers as the situation indicates. Most patients need to feel that their lives have meaning; many feel a need for hope in the face of death. Spiritual needs are discussed more fully in Chapter 47.

Meeting the Needs of the Family

The nurse can provide care for the family facing loss by listening to their concerns. Family members need to verbalize their worries and fears; nurses and other health care personnel can provide support by being nonjudgmental listeners. Likewise, nursing care of the grieving family involves communication and listening. Use the communication skills discussed in Chapter 8 and earlier in this section to be a nonjudgmental listener. Feedback to the family can be provided by summarizing or paraphrasing, without questioning the validity of the family's emotions. Be sure that all family members, including children, are able to participate in the grieving process. Family members may need to be reminded to get rest and to eat. Too many visitors may tire the patient; when explanations are offered, most relatives readily understand this.

The reality of death can be made less painful by preparing the family ahead of time. When the process has been explained to the family, they are better prepared to understand the needs of the dying person and how to support the person.

Explain the steps of the grieving process to all family members ahead of time so that they will recognize the specific stages as they experience them and understand that the process is normal. They can then recognize that other members of the family are going through the same stages, perhaps at different times. This preparation promotes better understanding and communication within the family.

Death creates a change in family roles. As one person (the dying person) leaves a role, adjustments must be made within the family to compensate. Each member plays a part in that compensation, and the nurse can help with these adjustments.

Providing Postmortem Care

When a patient dies, the nurse's responsibilities include caring for the patient's body, caring for the family, and discharging specific legal responsibilities. The last involves ensuring that a death certificate is issued and signed, labeling the body, and reviewing organ donation arrangements, if any.

CARING FOR THE BODY

After the patient has been pronounced dead, the nurse is responsible for preparing the body. The body is placed in normal anatomic position to avoid pooling of blood, soiled dressings are replaced, and tubes are removed. In most cases, it is unnecessary to wash the body; the mortician normally attends to this. Some religions strictly forbid washing of the body, whereas in others a special person must perform it. In cultures in which the family's washing of the deceased's body is considered the last service a family can give a loved one, the family should be given the necessary supplies and left alone in the room with the body. If an autopsy is to be performed, any tubes that were in place should not be removed. In such cases, the nurse should follow the facility's policy.

The nurse is legally responsible for placing identification tags on either the shroud or garment the body is clothed in and on the ankle to ensure that the body can be identified even if it is separated from its shroud. The nurse also places an identification tag on the patient's dentures or other prostheses to ensure that the mortician receives these. The importance of proper and complete identification cannot be overemphasized. The patient's body may be placed in the hospital's morgue refrigerator if mortuary arrangements were not made before the patient's death. If the patient died of a communicable disease, the body may require special handling to prevent the spread of disease. Requirements for such handling are usually specified by local laws and depend on the disease-causing organism, mode of transmission, and other characteristics.

CARING FOR THE FAMILY

After a patient has died, the nurse provides support and care to the patient's family (see Through the Eyes of a Student). In most cases, this involves listening to the family's expressions of grief, loss, and helplessness. Because comforting words are often difficult to find, offer solace and support by being an attentive listener. Family members may need to see the patient's body to accept the death fully; in such cases, arrange for family members to view the body before it is discharged to the mortician.

Sudden death creates unique problems for the family. In the case of sudden injury or illness, the physical needs of the patient are paramount to the health care team. This means that family members are not provided as much emotional support or information as they would be if the patient's illness were prolonged, nor are they permitted to exercise as many options regarding the patient's care. The family that loses a member unexpectedly has not had an opportunity to begin the grieving process or to share in grieving with the

Through the Eyes of a Student

We had had several day-shift clinical rotations, but this was our first evening clinical experience. We were unsure as to what the evening would be like. We knew the evening would provide us with a new outlook on nursing, but we were not prepared for what unfolded.

I had been taking care of a patient when another nursing student asked if I would check in on her patient while she had her dinner break. Each of the students knew this patient because we all had the pleasure of caring for him. I was told he was lying in bed watching television and that he had changed his code status to "DNR" (do not resuscitate) just that day. When I went to check on him, I found him lying in bed but not watching television. His eyes were closed as if he were sleeping peacefully. His mouth was open, and his respirations were slow. I spoke his name several times without a response. At the same time, I was also checking for a radial pulse. When I couldn't find his pulse, I swiftly walked to find the instructor. Together we went back to him and assessed his condition. There were no radial or carotid pulses. His chest was now not rising, and the instructor listened to his heart with a stethoscope. There wasn't a heartbeat. I stood there feeling helpless and low spirited. This was a man to whom we had all grown close. His family came to see him and to say a few final words. Tears were shed not only by his family but also by those of us who had cared for him.

Our first evening clinical was an extremely emotional night. We were all quiet as we walked down the hallway to go home. The student who was caring for him that night was stopped by his daughter and two young granddaughters. One granddaughter was wearing his hat and the other was carrying his belt. This man's daughter was brokenhearted by his death yet needed to know that he wasn't alone when he died. The student told her that I had been the one with him. The daughter seemed relieved to know that he was not by himself when he died.

As I look back on that evening, I'm sad that this man is no longer with us. I did not know him for very long, but he touched me in a way that helped me understand the true meaning of nursing: not only to care for the sick, disabled, or enfeebled, but also to be human and offer support for grieving families.

—Joyce A. Shearman, Delaware County Community College, Media, Pennsylvania

deceased person. Allow family members to express grief and provide emotional support. Often the family is in the emergency department waiting room when death is confirmed. They are stunned, bewildered, and numb. Do not rush them from the waiting room, but rather provide them with a private place to begin their grieving. Acknowledge their shock and listen to their grief. The family needs guidance in making plans and help in making decisions.

It is appropriate for the nurse who was caregiver or who took care of the patient for a prolonged period to attend the funeral. It also is appropriate for the nurse to make a follow-up call to the patient's family after the funeral or memorial service to offer both concern and care for the family's well-being. Follow-up visits are important to give support to the family. If the nurse assesses that the family is not coping well, appropriate referrals should be made. If the patient was cared for by a hospice, the family is offered grief support for up to a year following the death.

CARING FOR OTHER PATIENTS

Because nurses in institutional settings often provide care to more than one patient at a time, after the death of one patient, the nurse must continue to provide care to the other patients. Other patients are often aware of a death and may need to be consoled; this is particularly true of a patient who has shared a room with the deceased patient. Other patients may have grief reactions and should be supported through the grief process. Death of a patient may cause depression in other patients and may make them more aware of their own future deaths.

CARING FOR ONESELF

Witnessing the deaths of patients we have cared for can take a toll on health care professionals who can become numb or burned out. Nurses are now being encouraged to "pause" after a patient dies to silently reflect and honor the life. It is also a good time to be grateful for the care that you provided the patient. "Pause" guidelines are now being implemented in many settings that stop professional caregivers in a reflective moment of silence to honor the newly dead (Mason & Warnke, 2017).

Evaluating

The nursing care plan for dying patients is effective if patients meet the outcome of a comfortable, dignified death and family members resolve their grief after a suitable time of mourning and resume meaningful life roles and activities. See the Evolving Case Study 44-1 for Mrs. Esposita and Her Family.

REFLECTIVE PRACTICE LEADING TO PERSONAL LEARNING

Remember that the object of reflective practice is to look at an experience, understand it, and learn from it. As you begin to develop your expertise in identifying and responding to needs related to loss, grief, and dying, reflect on your experiences—successes and failures—in order to improve your practice. I don't think any nurse forgets the first time they cared for a patient who died. It can be scary and make us feel uncomfortable.

- What are your experiences with the seriously ill and dying and their families?
- Have you encountered patients or their family caregivers whose holistic needs are unmet?
- If you identified such a need, did you feel confident and comfortable responding to these needs?
- Have your care plans ever identified and addressed needs specifically related to loss, grief, and dying?
- Are you familiar with the palliative care resources available in your practice settings?
- Have you tried to learn more about these members of the interprofessional team and how you can develop collaborative relationships that will best serve your patients?
- Have you ever consulted with a palliative care or hospice professional?

Remember, we create the memories families will live with for the rest of their lives.

EVOLVING CASE STUDY 44-1

Scenario: The Espositas have been married for 19 years and have two children, Jorge, who is 16, and Marita, who is 13. It has been 2 years since Mrs. Esposita was diagnosed with ovarian cancer, and this period has been difficult for the entire family. At present, she is extremely cachexic (thin) and in the end stage of her illness. She initially tried aggressive treatment, and several chemotherapy regimens failed. During her last hospitalization 2 months ago, a decision was made not to continue cancer treatments and to transition to purely palliative goals, and Mrs. Esposita told her family she wanted to die at home.

QUESTION r/t CUES: Which assessment data is of highest priority for the nurse to collect to provide additional information to address the family's ability to care for Mrs. Esposita at home?

A. The family's knowledge about ovarian cancer and appropriate therapies.
B. The condition of Mrs. Esposita's skin.
C. Mrs. Esposita's mental health and well-being.
D. The adequacy of the husband's and children's coping strategies.
E. The availability of community resources.

EVOLVING CASE STUDY 44-1 (*continued*)

Scenario: Until now, Mrs. Esposita wanted nothing to do with the local hospice because of a reported "bad experience" a neighbor had. Her insurance will not provide for all the home nursing care she needs, and her husband and children have been trying to meet her needs for nursing as well as run the house and meet their own needs. A demanding woman, Mrs. Esposita never seems satisfied with anything anyone does, and the family is looking utterly frustrated, angry, and fatigued. Her son Jorge is coping by "opting out"; he frequently spends the night with friends and doesn't even call home to report on his whereabouts. Daughter Marita's grades have fallen, and she has dropped out of cheerleading and other school activities so that she can take care of her mother.

QUESTION r/t ANALYZING CUES: What other information (assessment data or evidence) should the nurse obtain related to this issue? Select all that apply.

A. Did Mrs. Esposita have a case manager or social worker who explored and recommended community resources?
B. Medication record.
C. Degree to which Mrs. Esposita understands the effect she is having on the well-being of her family.
D. Family's willingness to sacrifice their interests to care for their mother.

Scenario: Mr. Esposita, who has been silent until now, recently confided that he doesn't know how much longer he can go on this way, and seemed horrified to hear himself say, "I just wish she would die already and get this all over with!" He is very concerned about the changes in his children and feels powerless to change what is happening.

QUESTION r/t PRIORITIZING HYPOTHESIS: Based on the assessments of this patient, which priority problem should the nurse identify to guide the plan of care?

A. Conflicting Caregiver Attitude
B. Impaired Family Coping
C. Death Anxiety
D. Despair
E. Helplessness

Scenario: The nurse decides to focus on each member of the family's coping strategies and to explore the possibility of there being untapped community resources to supplement their reserves.

QUESTION r/t GENERATING SOLUTIONS: Which intervention will be most effective to help each member of the family develop healthier coping strategies? Select all that apply.

A. Reassure Mr. Esposita and the children that their mother's death is imminent and that they will be able to return to their usual lives in good time.
B. Compliment Marita for the sacrifices she is making and suggest at some level her mother must understand and be grateful.
C. Help Mr. Esposita develop clearer guidelines for Jorge and effective punishments.
D. Communicate clearly that many families facing similar struggles find it difficult to be patient with themselves and with one another. Normalize their responses.
E. Encourage each family member to identify helpful and nonhelpful coping behaviors and to devise positive coping strategies.

Scenario: Marita tells the nurse that her mother seems much sleepier now. "When I come home from school, I can hardly wake her. It also seems like her liquid morphine is disappearing quickly. You don't think dad might be overdosing her, do you?"

QUESTION r/t TAKING ACTION: The nurse confirms what Marita is telling her and realizes that a response is indicated. What is the priority nursing intervention?

A. Assess if the changes in Mrs. Esposita are the result of her worsening condition as death nears and if she has been receiving more morphine in response to worsening pain.
B. Call 911 and ask for an ambulance.
C. Call the police and report your suspicions.
D. Confront Mr. Esposita with Marita's concerns and ask for an explanation of what is happening.
E. Allow the family dynamics to play out.

QUESTION r/t EVALUATING OUTCOMES: The nurse visits the family upon learning that Mrs. Esposita died and makes a follow-up bereavement call 6 months after her death. Which of the following parameters indicates a successful implementation of the plan of care? Select all that apply.

A. Mr. Esposita thanks you for your assistance during a hard time for everyone.
B. Marita's grades have started to improve, and she is eager to go back to cheerleading next year.
C. Mr. Esposita thanks you for being patient with all of them. "I can't believe I wanted this all to be over, but I guess I'm glad she's in a better place now. Have to admit I miss her a lot."
D. Jorge is still that absent family member who says he is too angry to spend time at home and pretend that everything is OK.
E. Mr. Esposita shyly asks you if you'd like to come over for dinner some Sunday evening.

DEVELOPING CLINICAL REASONING AND CLINICAL JUDGMENT

1. Work through the Thoughtful, Person-Centered Practice: Challenging Topics: Medically Assisted Dying 44-1 and Evolving Case Study 44-1, Mrs. Esposita and Her Family, to help develop your clinical reasoning and clinical judgment skills.
2. Recall personal losses (death of a family member or friend; loss of a significant relationship, job, or opportunity) and recollect what you were experiencing at the time. Try to remember what your expectations were for those to whom you looked for support and how your ability to cope was influenced by whether those expectations were met. Remembering that no two people respond to loss in exactly the same way, develop a list of nursing measures to help patients who are dealing with loss. Compare your list with other students' lists and incorporate their ideas.
3. Compare and contrast the care a patient dying of cancer would receive in a critical care unit with the care they would receive at home with hospice care. Identify the advantages and disadvantages of each. Talk with family members and friends about their preferences. Use your analysis to help describe these options to prospective patients.
4. Role-play a situation with a peer in which you counsel a woman with cancer who is told that cure is no longer an option and that she has less than 6 months to live. What will you say to elicit the patient's preferences for treatment and care? Reflect on how your experiences, beliefs, and values might affect what you say to patients and how you say it.
5. You have to call the family of a patient who died alone in a nursing home. What do you say? Would you matter-of-factly report, "I am sorry to tell you that your mother died this evening," or would you use terms like "passed" or "is no longer suffering"?
6. How would you respond if the woman described in Item 4 above asks you to "Please help me die"? What knowledge, skills, and attitudes do you need to respond well to this question?
7. You meet a couple who has never "gotten over" the death of their 22-year-old daughter. The 2022 edition of the *Diagnostic and Statistical Manual of Mental Disorders*, Fifth Edition, includes a controversial new diagnosis: prolonged grief disorder. Many have argued to see intense grief as a target for medical treatment. Its inclusion in the DSM-5 means that clinicians can now bill insurance companies for treating people for the condition. Opponents warn that the designation risks pathologizing a fundamental aspect of the human experience. Some people actually emerging slowly but naturally from their losses may be told by their doctors that they have mental illnesses. What are the potential benefits and harms of adding intense grief to the manual of mental disorders? What resources can you tap to answer this question? Do you believe it would be helpful for this couple to have prolonged grief disorder medical diagnosis? (Barry, E. March 18, 2022. How long should it take to grieve? Psychiatry has come up with an answer. *The New York Times*. https://www.nytimes.com/2022/03/18/health/prolonged-grief-disorder.html.)

PRACTICING FOR NCLEX

1. A nurse midwife is assisting a patient whose birth plan states she is firmly committed to natural childbirth. When informed the infant is in distress and a cesarean delivery is necessary, the pregnant patient sobs inconsolably, calling herself a failure. The nurse offers emotional support based on what likely types of losses? Select all that apply.
   a. Actual
   b. Perceived
   c. Psychological
   d. Anticipatory
   e. Physical
   f. Maturational
2. A hospice nurse who cared for a dying patient and their family documents that the family is experiencing a period of mourning. Which behaviors would the nurse expect to see at this stage? Select all that apply.
   a. The family arranges for a funeral for their loved one.
   b. The family arranges for a memorial scholarship for their loved one.
   c. The coroner pronounces the patient's death.
   d. The family arranges for hospice for their loved one.
   e. The patient is diagnosed with terminal cancer.
   f. The patient's daughter writes a poem expressing her sorrow.
3. An older adult who recently moved into a long-term care facility tells the nurse their only son died 20 years ago, and they haven't enjoyed life since. When giving report to the next shift, the nurse tells the oncoming nurse the resident seems to be suffering from which type of grief?
   a. Somatic
   b. Anticipatory
   c. Unresolved
   d. Inhibited
4. A home health care nurse has been caring for a patient with advanced AIDS who is working through the stages of death and dying. The nurse documents the patient has entered the acceptance phase of death when the patient makes which statement?
   a. "I've made peace with everyone, and I'm actually ready to move on."
   b. "God cannot possibly be good if He allows people to get this horrible disease."
   c. "I just want to get better. A friend of mine had success with a plant-based diet."
   d. "The test results must be mixed up with someone else's; I feel better now."
5. A patient tells the nurse it is unfair that they should have to die now when they have finally made peace

with their family. Which response by the nurse would be most appropriate?
a. "I'm sorry you're feeling this way when death is inevitable."
b. "It does seem unfair. Tell me more about how you are feeling."
c. "You'll come to acceptance soon; no one knows how much time they have."
d. "Tell me about your pain. Did it keep you awake last night?"

6. A nurse is caring for a terminally ill patient who says, "I just can't sleep. I keep worrying about what my family will do when I am gone." What response by the nurse is most appropriate?
a. "You need your sleep for your visitors tomorrow."
b. "What seems to be concerning you the most?"
c. "Your family told me they will be fine."
d. "I suggest you discuss this with your family."

7. A patient tells a nurse that their daughter has been appointed to make decisions for them should they become incapacitated. What follow-up question would the nurse ask?
a. "Did the health care provider complete a Physician Order for Life-Sustaining Treatment (POLST) form?"
b. "Do we have a copy of your durable power of attorney for health care?"
c. "Have you prepared a living will?"
d. "Should I phone your provider for you to sign an Allow Natural Death (AND) form?"

8. A group of nursing students in a leadership course are studying the ANA position regarding assisted suicide. The professor asks the students for the best response to a note written by a ventilator-dependent patient "help me end my suffering, I don't want to live anymore." Which nursing response is consistent with the ANA's position?
a. "I will do everything possible to keep you comfortable but will not administer medication to cause your death."
b. "Being removed from the ventilator is a form of active euthanasia, which is not supported by the nurses' code of ethics."
c. After exhausting every intervention to keep a dying patient comfortable, the nurse says, "Let's talk about when and how you want to die."
d. "I'm personally opposed to assisted suicide, but I'll find you a colleague who can help you."

9. A patient with end-stage breast cancer has been in the medical intensive care unit for 3 weeks. Her husband tells the nurse that his wife was very clear about not wanting aggressive treatment that would merely prolong her dying. Which type of order could the nurse suggest the husband discuss with his wife's health care provider?
a. Comfort Measures Only
b. Do Not Hospitalize
c. Living Will
d. Slow Code Only

10. A nurse in the intensive care unit is preparing a patient's family for terminal weaning from mechanical ventilation. What nursing actions would facilitate this process? Select all that apply.
a. Offering the family information about the advantages and disadvantages of continued ventilatory support
b. Explaining to the family what will happen at each phase of the weaning and offer support
c. Validating orders for sedation and analgesia to promote comfort and dignity
d. Explaining that death occurs quickly after the patient is removed from the ventilator
e. Teaching the family that the decision for terminal weaning must be made by the primary care provider
f. Arranging mandatory counseling for the patient and family to assist them in making this end-of-life decision

11. The parents of an infant in the neonatal intensive care unit (ICU) for several months also have a 22-month-old child at home. The nurse notes the parents seem chronically fatigued, express guilt about neglecting their child at home, have been short tempered, and express anxiety about their continued ability to manage their family. The nurse plans to address which of these health problems in the plan of care?
a. Dysfunctional Grief
b. Fear about Being a Burden to Others
c. Impaired Ability of Caregiver to Perform Caretaking
d. Impaired Health Maintenance

12. A nurse is caring for terminally ill patients in a long-term care setting. Which nursing action is appropriate during end-of-life care?
a. Avoiding disturbing a comatose patient by speaking to them while providing care
b. Holding the hand of a dying patient and crying with the patient and family
c. Requesting a social work consult for family members with multiple complaints about the care
d. Performing hygiene for the patient because it is easier than having the patient help

13. After validating an autopsy is not planned, a new graduate nurse provides postmortem care. Which action requires the preceptor to correct the graduate?
a. Leaving the patient in a sitting position at the family's request
b. Placing identification tags on both the shroud and the ankle
c. Removing soiled dressings and tubes, while washing the body
d. Ensuring a death certificate is issued and signed

14. The family of a patient who has just died asks for privacy and supplies to wash their loved one's body. How does the nurse best respond?
    a. Inform the family that there is no need for them to wash the body since the funeral home typically does this.
    b. Explain that hospital policy forbids their being alone with the deceased patient.
    c. Provide the requested the supplies and maintain a watchful eye to ensure they maintain the patient's dignity.
    d. Provide the requested supplies, assess if this request is linked to religious or cultural customs, and offer assistance.
15. An older adult who has had multiple strokes is refusing artificial nutrition and hydration against medical advice and in opposition to their daughter. The patient's nurse advocates for the patient, stating which party is the most appropriate decision maker?

    Electronic Health Record (EHR), Consultations Tab
    Psychiatric Consult: Patient is competent, understands the consequences of her actions, no depression noted. Patient persists in refusing treatment. Suggest ethics consultation.
    a. Patient
    b. Patient's daughter
    c. Health care provider
    d. Ethics consult team
16. A nurse receives information in a shift report that a patient who has rapidly progressing terminal illness is in the denial phase of death and dying. The nurse expects a patient in this stage to make which statement?
    a. "I can't wait to get out of the hospital and plan next year's beach vacation."
    b. "I've chosen my favorite music and readings for my memorial service."
    c. "The people in this hospital are so incompetent, what a bunch of idiots!"
    d. "I cry every time I wonder how my children will get along when I'm gone."
17. A nurse notes a hospice patient is increasingly agitated, with noisy, irregular breathing and periods of apnea. The skin of their feet appears mottled. The nurse takes which action?
    a. Activates the rapid response team to treat shock
    b. Contacts the respiratory therapist for a nebulizer treatment
    c. Prepares the patient's family for imminent death
    d. Inserts an oropharyngeal airway for suctioning

ANSWERS WITH RATIONALES

1. **a, b, c.** The losses experienced by the pregnant patient are actual, perceived, and psychological. Actual loss can be recognized by others as well as by the person sustaining the loss; perceived loss is experienced by the person but is intangible to others; and psychological loss is a loss that is felt emotionally as opposed to physically. Anticipatory loss occurs when one grieves prior to the actual loss; physical loss is tangible and perceived by others; and maturational loss is experienced as a result of natural developmental processes.
2. **a, b, f.** Mourning refers to the actions and expressions of grief, including the symbols and ceremonies (e.g., a funeral or final celebration of life) that make up the outward expressions of grief. It is a period of grief and acceptance, as the person learns to deal with their loss. A diagnosis of cancer and the coroner's pronouncing the patient's death are not behaviors of the family during a period of mourning. Arranging for hospice care precedes a patient's death.
3. **c.** Dysfunctional grief is abnormal or distorted; it may be either unresolved or inhibited. In unresolved grief, a person may have trouble expressing feelings of loss or may deny them; it may also describe a state of bereavement that extends over a lengthy period. With inhibited grief, a person suppresses feelings of grief and may instead manifest somatic (body) symptoms, such as abdominal pain or heart palpitations. Anticipatory loss or grief occurs when a person displays loss and grief behaviors for a loss that has yet to take place.
4. **a.** According to Kübler-Ross, when the patient reaches the stage of acceptance, they feel tranquil. This patient has accepted the reality of death and is prepared for the transition to death.
5. **b.** This response by the nurse validates the patient's feelings, saying they have been heard, and invites them to share more of their feelings, concerns, and fears. The other responses either deny the patient's feelings or change the subject.
6. **b.** Using an open-ended question, such as, "What seems to be concerning you the most?" encourages communication. False reassurances or side-stepping the statement are not helpful. The nurse then would assess the patient's restlessness and consider possible comfort measures.
7. **b.** A durable power of attorney for health care appoints an agent the person trusts to make decisions in the event of subsequent incapacity. Living wills provide specific instructions about the kinds of health care that should be provided or foregone in particular situations. A POLST form is a medical order indicating a patient's wishes regarding treatments commonly used in a medical crisis. The living will is a document whose purpose is to allow people to record specific instructions about the type of health care they would like to receive in particular end-of-life situations. AND on the medical record of a patient indicates the patient or surrogate has expressed a wish that there be no attempts to resuscitate the patient.
8. **a.** The ANA Code of Ethics states that the nurse "should provide interventions to relieve pain and other symptoms in the dying patient consistent with palliative care practice standards and may not act with the sole intent to end life" (2015, p. 3). Removing mechanical ventilation or other life support at the patient's request or request of the surrogate when treatment is futile is not performed with the sole intent to end life but to promote dignity and comfort. Nurses should be prepared to respond to the request: "Nurse, please help me die…."
9. **a.** The nurse could suggest that the husband speak to the health care provider about a Comfort Measures Only order in which the goal of treatment is a comfortable, dignified death, and further life-sustaining measures have been declined. A Do-Not-Hospitalize order is often used for patients in long-term care and other residential settings who refuse hospitalization

for further aggressive treatment. A living will is a document in which the patient provides specific instructions about the kinds of health care that should be provided or foregone in particular situations in which they are unlikely to recover. A Slow Code refers to a delay in calling a code and beginning resuscitation efforts until these measures will be ineffective. This is not consistent with current best practice and may be forbidden in certain facilities. A nurse could be charged with negligence in the event of a Slow Code and resulting patient death.

10. **a, b, c.** A nurse's role in terminal weaning is to assist patients and families in the decision-making process by offering helpful information about the benefits and burdens of continued ventilation. The nurse teaches what to expect if terminal weaning is initiated, including the use of sedation and analgesia for patient comfort. Supporting the patient and family and managing sedation and analgesia are critical nursing responsibilities. In some cases, competent patients decide that they want to discontinue their ventilatory support; more often, the surrogate decision makers determine that continued ventilatory support is futile. The nurse would not predict the time until death. Once removed from the ventilator, a patient may not resume spontaneous breathing or may breathe on their own, living for hours, days, or rarely, longer. Counseling may be arranged if requested but is not mandatory for decision making.

11. **c.** Impaired ability of a caregiver to perform caretaking applies to these parents. Even with a positive outcome, the infant in the ICU is likely to be discharged with many needs, which may still impact them and their other child. Grief is an expression of loss, but the focus here is on the parents' exhaustion and coping. The health problem of being a burden refers to a patient's fear, rather than the caregiver. There is no specific information about the health maintenance needs of the child, rather, in this situation, the parents are the focus of care.

12. **b.** The nurse should not be afraid to show compassion and empathy for the dying person, including crying with the patient or family. The sense of hearing is believed to be the last sense to leave the body before death; therefore, the nurse should explain care to comatose or unresponsive patients. The nurse should address caregiver role endurance by actively listening to family members. Encouraging the dying patient to remain active and participate in care for as long as possible is appropriate, rather than taking over self-care measures.

13. **a.** Because the body should be placed in normal anatomic position to avoid pooling of blood, leaving the body in a sitting position is contraindicated. The other actions are appropriate nursing responsibilities related to postmortem care.

14. **d.** The family may want to wash the body for personal, religious, or cultural reasons and should be allowed to do so. This action may reflect caring, the last service to a loved one, or promote acceptance of death.

15. **a.** Because this patient is competent, they have the right to refuse treatment felt to be disproportionately burdensome, even if this hastens their death. Neither her daughter nor her doctor has authority to assume decision-making responsibilities unless appointed as surrogates. The ethics consult team is not a decision-making body; they can make recommendations but have no prescription authority.

16. **a.** In the denial phase, the patient denies the reality of death and may repress what is discussed. The patient may think, "They made a mistake in the diagnosis" or "they mixed up my records with someone else's." Planning a vacation for the following year indicates the patient is not ready to take in the information. When the stage of acceptance is reached, the patient feels tranquil and has accepted the reality of and is prepared for death. The patient may think, "I've tied up all the loose ends." In the anger phase, the patient expresses rage and hostility and may adopt a "why me?" attitude. During the depression phase, the patient goes through a period of grief before death. The grief is often characterized by crying and not speaking much.

17. **c.** Signs of imminent death include difficulty talking or swallowing; urinary or bowel incontinence or constipation; loss of movement, sensation, and reflexes; decreasing body temperature with cold or clammy skin; weak, slow, or irregular pulse and decreasing blood pressure; noisy, irregular, or Cheyne–Stokes respirations; restlessness or agitation and/or; cooling, mottling, and cyanosis of the extremities and dependent areas. The purpose of hospice care is to provide comfort as death approaches rather than invasive interventions. As death approaches, the irregular noisy breathing is expected; nebulizer treatments are not the priority.

Bibliography

Adams, K. M., & Warshaw, H. (2017). Respecting end-of-life care wishes. *Healthcare Executive*, 68–70. https://theconversationproject.org/wp-content/uploads/2017/09/RepectingEndofLifeCareWishes_HCExec_Sept2017.pdf

Aging with Dignity. (n.d.). *Five wishes*. Retrieved January 31, 2021, from www.agingwithdignity.org/five-wishes.php

Altaker, K. W., Howie-Esquivel, J., & Cataldo, J. K. (2018). Relationships among palliative care, ethical climate, empowerment, and moral distress in intensive care unit nurses. *American Journal of Critical Care, 27*(4), 295–302.

American Association of Colleges of Nursing (AACN). (2021). *The essentials: Core competencies for professional nursing education*. https://www.aacnnursing.org/Portals/42/AcademicNursing/pdf/Essentials-2021.pdf

American Bar Association. (n.d.). *Tool kit for health care advance planning*. Retrieved January 31, 2021, from https://www.americanbar.org/groups/law_aging/resources/health_care_decision_making/consumer_s_toolkit_for_health_care_advance_planning.html

American Geriatrics Society (AGS) Ethics Committee. (2007). *Position statement: The care of dying patients*. Author.

American Nurses Association. (2015). *Code of ethics for nurses*. Author.

American Nurses Association (ANA). (2016a). *Call for action: Nurses lead and transform palliative care*. http://nursingworld.org/MainMenuCategories/ThePracticeofProfessionalNursing/Palliative-Care-Call-for-Action

American Nurses Association (ANA). (2016b). *Nurses' roles and responsibilities in providing care and support at the end of life*. https://www.nursingworld.org/practice-policy/nursing-excellence/official-position-statements

American Nurses Association (ANA). (2017). *Nutrition and hydration at the end of life*. https://www.nursingworld.org/practice-policy/nursing-excellence/official-position-statements

American Nurses Association (ANA). (2018). *The ethical responsibility to manage pain and the suffering it causes*. https://www.nursingworld.org/practice-policy/nursing-excellence/official-position-statements

American Nurses Association (ANA). (2019). *The nurse's role when a patient requests medical aid in dying*. https://www.nursingworld.org/practice-policy/nursing-excellence/official-position-statements

American Nurses Association (ANA). (2020). *Nursing care and do-not-resuscitate (DNR) decisions*. https://www.nursingworld.org/practice-policy/nursing-excellence/official-position-statements

Anderson, W. G., Puntillo, K., Cimino, J., Noort, J., Pearson, D., Boyle, D., Grywalski, M., Meyer, J., O'Neil-Page, E., Cain, J., Herman, H., Barbour, S., Turner, K., Moore, E., Liao, S., Ferrell, B., Mitchell, W., Edmonds, K., Fairman, N., … Pantilat, S. Z. (2017). Palliative care professional development for critical care nurses: A multicenter program. *American Journal of Critical Care, 26*(5), 361–371.

Bauchner, H., & Fontanarosa, P. B. (2016). Death, dying and end of life. *JAMA, 315*(3), 270–271.

Bourgault, A. M. (2020). Honoring our fallen colleagues and ourselves: Taking time to grieve. *Critical Care Nurse, 40*(6), 10–12.

Bowdoin, C. T. (2017). Easing the final journey. *Nursing, 47*(9), 42–44.

Broden, E. G., Deatrick, J., Ulrich, C., & Curley, M. A. Q. (2020). Defining a "good death" in the pediatric intensive care unit. *American Journal of Critical Care, 29*(2), 111–121.

Brooks, L. A., Manias, E., & Nicholson, P. (2017). Communication and decision-making about end-of-life care in the intensive care unit. *American Journal of Critical Care, 26*(4), 336–341.

Bui, N., Halifax, E., David, D., Hunt, L., Uy, E, Ritchie, C., & Stephens, C. (2020). Original Research: Understanding nursing home staff attitudes toward death and dying: A Survey. *American Journal of Nursing,* 120(8), 24–31.

Chichester, M., & Harding, K. M. (2021). Early pregnancy loss: Invisible but real. *Nursing, 51*(12), 28–32.

Czekanski, K. (2017). The experience of transitioning to a caregiving role for a family member with Alzheimer's disease or related dementia. *American Journal of Nursing, 117*(9), 24–32.

Delgado, S. A. (2017). Increasing nurses' palliative care communication skills. *American Journal of Critical Care, 26*(5), 372.

Edward, K. L., Galletti, A., & Huynh, M. (2020). Enhancing communication with family members in the intensive care unit: A mixed-methods study. *Critical Care Nurse, 40*(6), 23–32.

Engel, G. L. (1964). Grief and grieving. *American Journal of Nursing, 64*(9), 93–98.

Esfahani, S., Yi, C., Madani, C. A., Davidson, J. E., Edmonds, K. P., & Wynn, S. (2020). Exploiting technology to popularize goals-of-care conversations and advance care planning. *Critical Care Nurse, 40*(4), 32–41.

Fahlberg, B. (2016). My patient needs palliative care: Now what? *Nursing, 46*(11), 14–16.

Fahlberg, B. (2017). Why attitudes matter in palliative care. *Nursing, 47*(11), 11–12.

Ferguson, R. (2018). Care coordination at the end of life: The nurse's role. *Nursing, 48*(2), 11–13.

Ferrell, B., & Coyle, N. (2008). *The nature of suffering and the goals of nursing.* Oxford University Press.

Ganz, F. D. (2019). Improving family intensive care unit experiences at the end of life: Barriers and facilitators. *Critical Care Nurse, 39*(3), 52–58.

Goldsborough, J. L., & Matzo, M. (2017). Palliative care in the acute care setting. *American Journal of Nursing, 117*(9), 64–67.

Halsted, C., & Hart, V. T. (2021). Mental health in nursing: A student's perspective. *Nursing, 51*(1), 52–55.

Hammond, L., & Pullen, R. L. Jr. (2020). Managing loneliness and chronic illness in older adults. *Nursing, 50*(12), 22–28.

Hartjes, T. M., Baron-Lee, J., Hester, J. M., & Kittelson, S. M. (2017). Improving care at the end of life: Creating hospice in place. *Critical Care Nurse, 37*(5), 93–96.

Hold, J. L. (2017). A good death. *Nursing Ethics, 24*(1), 9–19.

Institute of Medicine (IOM). (1997). *Approaching death: Improving care at the end of life.* National Academies Press.

Institute of Medicine (IOM). (2015). *Dying in America: Improving quality and honoring individual preferences near the end of life.* National Academies Press.

International Council of Nurses (ICN). (2019). *Nursing diagnosis and outcome statements. International Classification for Nursing Practice (ICNP) Catalogue.* https://www.icn.ch/sites/default/files/inline-files/ICNP2019-DC.pdf

Izumi, S. (2017). Advance care planning: The nurse's role. *American Journal of Nursing, 117*(6), 56–61.

Jensen, H. I., Halvorsen, K., Jerpseth, H., Fridh, I., & Lind, R. (2020). Practice recommendations for end-of-life care in the intensive care unit. *Critical Care Nurse, 40*(3), 14–22.

Jones, C., Puntillo, K., Donesky, D., & McAdam, J. L. (2018). Family members' experiences with bereavement in the intensive care unit. *American Journal of Critical Care, 27*(4), 312–321.

Kelly, P. A., Baker, K. A., Hodges, K. M., Vuong, E. Y., Lee, J. C., & Lockwood, S. W. (2021). Nurses' perspectives on caring for patients with Do-Not-Resuscitate orders. *American Journal of Nursing, 121*(1), 26–36.

Kirk, T. W., Mahon, M. M., & Palliative Sedation Task Force of the National Hospice and Palliative Care Organization Ethics Committee. (2010). National Hospice and Palliative Care Organization (NHPCO) position statement and commentary on the use of palliative sedation in imminently dying terminally ill patients. *Journal of Pain and Symptom Management, 39*(5), 914–923.

Krochmal, R. L., Blenko, J. W., Afshar, M., Netzer, G., Roy, S. C., Wiegand, D. L., & Shanholtz, C. B. (2017). Family presence at first cardiopulmonary resuscitation and subsequent limitations on care in the medical intensive care unit. *American Journal of Critical Care, 26*(3), 221–228.

Kübler-Ross, E. (1969). *On death and dying.* Macmillan.

Kübler-Ross, E. (1978). *To live until we say goodbye.* Prentice Hall.

Kübler-Ross, E. (2014). *On death and dying: What the dying have to teach doctors, nurses, clergy and their own families. Anniversary Edition to the title.* Simon & Schuster.

Lehto, R. H., Olsen, D. P., & Chan, R. R. (2016). When a patient discusses assisted dying: Nursing practice implications. *Journal of Hospice & Palliative Nursing, 18*(3), 184–191.

Lowey, S. E. (2008). Communication between the nurse and family caregiver in end-of-life care: A review of the literature. *Journal of Hospice & Palliative Nursing, 10*(1), 35–45.

MacFarquhar, L. (2016, July 4). A tender hand in the presence of death. *The New Yorker*, 62–73. https://www.newyorker.com/magazine/2016/07/11/the-work-of-a-hospice-nurse

Martz, K., Alderden, J., Bassett, R., & Swick, D. (2020). Outcomes associated with a nurse-driven palliative care screening tool in the intensive care unit. *Critical Care Nurse, 40*(3), 23–29.

Mason, T. M., & Warnke, J. (2017). Finding meaning after a patient's death. *American Nurse Today, 12*(9), 66–68.

Melnyk, B. M., Hsieh, A. P., Davidson, J., Carpenter, H., Choflet, A., Heath, J., Hess, M. E., Lee, P., Link, T., Marcus, J., Pabico, C., Poindexter, K., & Stand, L. (2021). Promoting nurse mental health. *American Nurse Journal, 16*(1), 20–22, 59.

Mending mortality. (2017, April 29–May 5). *The Economist.* 45–48. https://www.economist.com/international/2017/04/29/a-better-way-to-care-for-the-dying

Milliken, A., & Uveges, M. (2020). CE: Brain death: History, updates, and implications for nurses. *American Journal of Nursing, 120*(3), 32–38.

National Consensus Project for Quality Palliative Care. (2013). *Clinical practice guidelines for quality palliative care* (3rd ed.). https://www.nationalcoalitionhpc.org/ncp-guidelines-2013

National Hospice and Palliative Care Organization. (n.d.). *Advance care planning.* Retrieved January 31, 2021, from http://www.caringinfo.org/i4a/pages/index.cfm?pageid=3277

National Hospice and Palliative Care Organization. (2019). *Palliative care or hospice? The right service at the right time for seriously ill individuals.* https://www.nhpco.org/wp-content/uploads/2019/04/PalliativeCare_VS_Hospice.pdf

Nelson, R. (2017). Discussing death over coffee and cake: The emergence of the death café. *American Journal of Nursing, 117*(2), 18–19.

Nelson, A., & Lewis, A. (2017). Determining brain death: Basic approach and controversial issues. *American Journal of Critical Care, 26*(6), 496–500.

Olmstead, J. A., & Dahnke, M. D. (2016). The need for an effective process to resolve conflicts over medical futility: A case study and analysis. *Critical Care Nurse, 36*(6), 13–23.

Olsen, D. P., Chan, R., & Lehto, R. (2017). Ethical nursing care when the terminally ill patient seeks death. *American Journal of Nursing, 117*(7), 50–55.

Orentlicher, D., Pope, T. M., & Rich, B. A. (2016). Clinical criteria for physician aid in dying. *Journal of Palliative Medicine, 19*(3), 259–262. https://www.ncbi.nlm.nih.gov/pmc/articles/PMC4779271

Orsatti, G. W., & Colbert, A. M. (2020). Sibling conflict over a parent's end-of-life care: A legal perspective. *Nursing, 50*(11), 17–20.

Perrin, K. O., & Kazanowski, M. (2015). Overcoming barriers to palliative care consultation. *Critical Care Nurse, 35*(5), 44–52.

President's Commission for the Study of Ethical Problems in Medicine and Biomedical and Behavioral Research. (1981). *Defining death: A report on the medical, legal and ethical issues in the determination of death.* [Publication No. 81–600150]. Government Printing Office.

Price, D. M., & Knotts, S. E. (2017). Communication, comfort, and closure for the patient with cystic fibrosis at the end of life: The role of the bedside nurse. *Journal of Hospice & Palliative Nursing, 19*(4), 298–302.

Puffenbarger, E. (2014). When to refer patients for hospice care. *American Nurse Today, 9*(9), 42–44.

Quill, T. E., & Byock, I. R. (2000). Responding to intractable terminal suffering: The role of terminal sedation and voluntary refusal of food and fluids. *Annals of Internal Medicine, 132*(5), 408–414.

Roy, K. M. (2020). Frequently asked questions about palliative care. *American Nurse Journal, 15*(7), 6–10.

Serious Illness Conversation Guide. (2016). https://www1.nyc.gov/assets/doh/downloads/pdf/chi/chi-36-1.pdf

Skelley, B. H. (2016). When families ask about an autopsy. *American Journal of Nursing, 116*(8), 11.

Tavernise, S. (2016, April 22). U.S. suicide rate surges to a 30-year high. *The New York Times.* https://www.nytimes.com/2016/04/22/health/us-suicide-rate-surges-to-a-30-year-high.html

The Conversation Project. (2017). http://theconversationproject.org/

Thomas, R., Wilson, D. M., Justice, C., Birch, S., & Sheps, S. (2008). A literature review of preferences for end-of-life care in developed countries by individuals with different cultural affiliations and ethnicity. *Journal of Hospice & Palliative Nursing, 10*(3), 142–161. https://journals.lww.com/jhpn/Abstract/2008/05000/A_Literature_Review_of_Preferences_for_End_of_Life.12.aspx

Ufema, J. (2006). *Insights on death & dying.* Wolters Kluwer Health/Lippincott Williams & Wilkins.

Venis, J., & Dodek, P. (2020). Feasibility and acceptability of a palliative approach screening tool in the intensive care unit. *American Journal of Critical Care, 29*(3), 214–220. VITALtalk. https://www.vitaltalk.org/clinicians/

Watson, A. C., & October, T. W. (2016). Clinical nurse participation at family conferences in the pediatric intensive care unit. *American Journal of Critical Care, 25*(6), 489–497.

Wiegand, D. L., MacMillan, J., dos Santos, M. R., & Bousso, R. S. (2015). Palliative and end-of-life ethical dilemmas in the intensive care unit. *AACN Advanced Critical Care, 26*(2), 142–150.

Wittenberg-Lyles, E., Goldsmith, J., Ferrell, B., & Ragan, S. L. (2013). *Communication in palliative nursing.* Oxford University Press.

Wolf, A. T., White, K. R., Epstein, E. G., & Enfield, K. B. (2019). Palliative care and moral distress: An institutional survey of critical care nurses. *Critical Care Nurse, 39*(5), 38–49.

45 Sensory Functioning

Ori Soltes

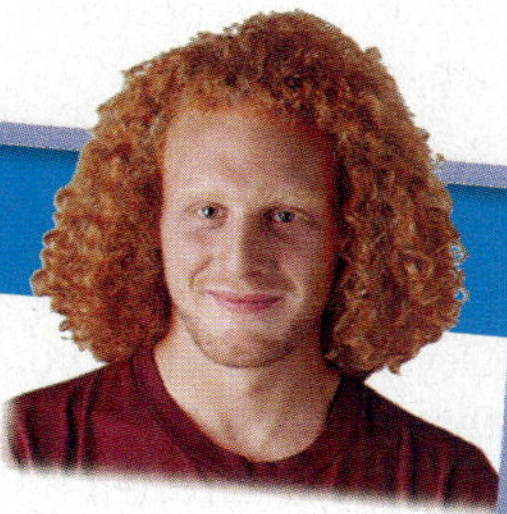

Ori, a 28-year-old man, is in the intensive care unit (ICU) after a motor vehicle crash that resulted in multiple internal injuries as well as fractures. He is being monitored continuously and receiving mechanical ventilation. On the fifth day after the crash, he begins to exhibit transient episodes of acute confusion.

Muriel Hao

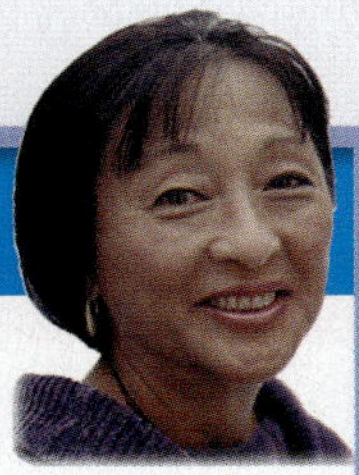

Muriel is a 56-year-old woman who had surgery 2 days ago. She denies any complaints of pain or discomfort. She is receiving intravenous (IV) therapy via an infusion pump. She states, "Please stop that beeping. It's driving me nuts and I can't rest."

Dolores Pirolla

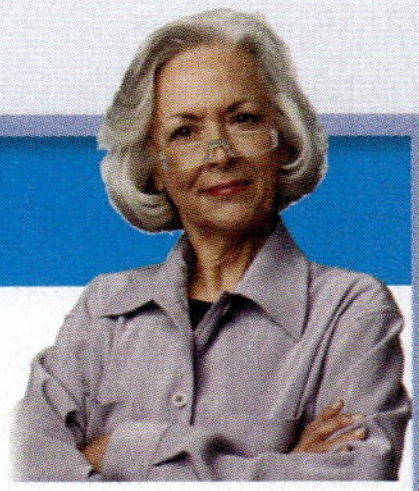

Dolores, a 74-year-old woman, comes to the older adult clinic with her 77-year-old husband who was diagnosed with macular degeneration and progressive vision loss. She states, "Now I've noticed he's also having difficulty hearing me. I'm worried because he doesn't want to leave the house and we hardly see any of our friends anymore. We used to go out to the movies or dinner at least once a week. Lately, if we get out once a month, that's a lot!"

Learning Outcomes

After completing the chapter, you will be able to accomplish the following:

1. Describe the four conditions that must be met in each sensory experience.
2. Explain the role of the reticular activating system in sensory experience.
3. Identify etiologies and perceptual, cognitive, and emotional responses to sensory deprivation and sensory overload.
4. Perform a comprehensive assessment of sensory functioning using appropriate interview questions and physical assessment skills.
5. Develop actual and potential health problem statements that correctly identify sensory/perceptual alterations that may be treated by nurses.
6. Describe specific nursing interventions to prevent sensory alterations, stimulate the senses, promote health literacy, and assist patients with sensory difficulties.
7. Develop, implement, and evaluate a plan of nursing care to help patients safely meet individualized sensory/perceptual outcomes.

Nursing Concepts

- Sensory perception

A person's senses are vital to survival, growth and development, and the experience of bodily pleasure and pain. Nurses encounter many patients who have impaired sensory functioning that places them at risk for injury, disturbed growth and development, and decreased well-being. Moreover, the stress of illness or trauma and the need for diagnosis and treatment may quickly result in sensory deprivation or overload, with serious disturbances in visual, perceptual, cognitive, or emotional functioning (see the Reflective Practice box for an example). Nurses are in the position to use knowledge of sensory functioning to support positive outcomes for patients (see Box 45-1). For example, awareness of the intensities and sources of sound, ways to control noise, and the assessment of patients' perceptions of and responses to sound can provide nurses with a basis for therapeutic manipulation of the environment.

SENSORY EXPERIENCE

Reception and Perception

The sensory experience consists of two components: reception and perception.

Sensory reception is the process of receiving data about the external or internal environment through the senses. The senses by which people maintain contact with the external environment are vision, hearing, smell, taste, and touch. The terms used to describe the senses are **visual** (pertaining to sight), **auditory** (pertaining to hearing), **olfactory** (pertaining to smell), **gustatory** (pertaining to taste), and **tactile** (pertaining to touch). In addition, **stereognosis** is the sense that perceives the solidity of objects and their size, shape, and texture. See Figure 45-1 on page 1830.

People orient themselves internally by the kinesthetic and visceral senses. **Kinesthesia** refers to awareness of positioning of body parts and body movement; **visceral** pertains to inner organs. The kinesthetic and visceral senses arise internally from muscles and hollow organs, respectively, and are the body's basic orienting systems. **Proprioception** is the term used to describe the sense, usually at a subconscious level, of the movements and position of the body and especially its limbs, independent of vision. This sense is gained primarily from input from sensory nerve terminals in muscles and tendons and the fibrous capsules of joints combined with input from the vestibular apparatus.

Sensory perception is the conscious process of selecting, organizing, and interpreting data from the senses into meaningful information. Perception is influenced by the intensity, size, change, or representation of stimuli, as well as by past experiences, knowledge, and attitudes.

Box 45-1 Healthy People 2030 Goal

Overview

Many people in the United States will have a sensory or communication disorder in their lifetime. This includes problems with vision, hearing, balance, smell, taste, voice, speech, or language. Healthy People 2030 focuses on preventing, diagnosing, and treating these disorders in people of all ages.

Sensory or communication disorders can have a major impact on social, emotional, and physical well-being. Some groups have a higher risk of these disorders, including people with low incomes, people who work in certain industries, and older adults. People who are diagnosed or treated later often have worse outcomes.

Preventive care such as hearing screenings for newborns and comprehensive eye exams in adults are critical for finding and treating these disorders early. Strategies to increase use of eye and hearing protection can help prevent new cases.

See the Healthy People 2030 website for specific objectives: https://health.gov/healthypeople/objectives-and-data/browse-objectives/sensory-or-communication-disorders

Source: Reprinted from HealthyPeople.gov. (n.d.). *Healthy People 2030: Hearing and other sensory or communication disorders.* Retrieved January 15, 2022, from https://health.gov/healthypeople/objectives-and-data/browse-objectives/sensory-or-communication-disorders

QSEN Reflective Practice: Cultivating QSEN Competencies

CHALLENGE TO TECHNICAL SKILLS

All throughout nursing school, we are taught theory, and from that theory we are to use clinical reasoning and clinical judgment to determine how to care for a particular patient, focusing on the patient, not the machines surrounding them. "You'll learn that later," they say.

I was assigned to care for Muriel Hao, a 56-year-old woman who had surgery 2 days ago. As I walk into her room, I check to see if she is comfortable and whether she needs anything at that particular point in time. She asks me one favor. "Please stop that beeping. It's driving me nuts and I can't rest." So, I look at the machine, dumbfounded, and worried that the patient is going to think I am incompetent because I cannot even work a simple machine. No theory from a classroom is going to teach me how to make the machine stop beeping. To make things worse, every facility has different machines. As nursing students, we go from one facility to another, trying to get accustomed to the equipment and technologies of each one. I assume that things will get easier once I have steady employment in a facility. If that particular facility changes its technologies, I would hope that there would be an in-service on the new technology. But what do I do now, as a nursing student?

Thinking Outside the Box: Possible Courses of Action

- Press the buttons on the machine, and hope that the beeping goes away.
- Seek out someone who does know how to work the machine and have that person fix it so I don't do more damage.
- Find someone who knows how to work the machine, have that person fix it, and then have the person explain to me how to fix it so I can do it next time.

Evaluating a Good Outcome: How Do I Define Success?

- Personal integrity is maintained (if I can't fix it, I feel stupid, and that's an insult to my integrity).
- Professional integrity remains intact (if I can't fix it, I will feel incompetent as a nurse—if I can't even fix a machine, how am I supposed to help a person?).
- The patient expresses relief that the beeping has stopped, and she is now able to rest.

Personal Learning: Here's to the Future!

Although this does not seem like a huge or very troublesome problem, every nursing student can probably attest to feeling this way at least once. The first few times it happened to me, I just asked someone to fix it for me, thinking it was a one-time problem. Then I realized that this is something that I was facing over and over again. So, I asked someone to show me how to fix the problem if it should occur again. I understood what to do and knew how to do it. Then we switched hospitals and I was confused once again. In today's environment of ever-changing technology, I realized that it is not just the students who feel this way. Nurses, too, have these same feelings. We all learn new things every day, whether it's from a patient, another nurse, a doctor, or a technical specialist. We just need to know that it's okay to ask questions. Moreover, not knowing how to work with a piece of equipment does not mean that you are incompetent with people. Learning in the health care field is an ongoing process.

Michele Jordan, Georgetown University

QSEN SELF-REFLECTION ON QUALITY AND SAFETY COMPETENCIES DEVELOPING KNOWLEDGE, SKILLS, AND ATTITUDES FOR CONTINUOUS IMPROVEMENT

Do you agree with the criteria that the nursing student used to evaluate a successful outcome? Why or why not? What *knowledge, skills,* and *attitudes* do you need to develop to continuously improve the quality and safety of care for patients like Ms. Hao? Was professional integrity affirmed? Explain.

Patient-Centered Care: How can you deliver thoughtful, person-centered care for patients while feeling overwhelmed by their equipment?

Teamwork and Collaboration/Quality Improvement: Who on your team is most likely to help you? What communication and interpersonal skills do you need to improve to ensure that you function as a competent and confident member of the patient care team? What does quality care for Ms. Hao "look like"?

Safety/Evidence-Based Practice: What does the evidence point to as "best practice" for Ms. Hao? If you stop the machine from beeping in response to her requests, will you be silencing critical alarms? What safety needs does she have and how can you meet them?

Informatics: Can you identify the essential information that must be available in Ms. Hao's electronic record to support safe patient care and coordination of care? Can you think of other ways to respond to or approach the situation? What else might the nursing student have done to ensure a successful outcome?

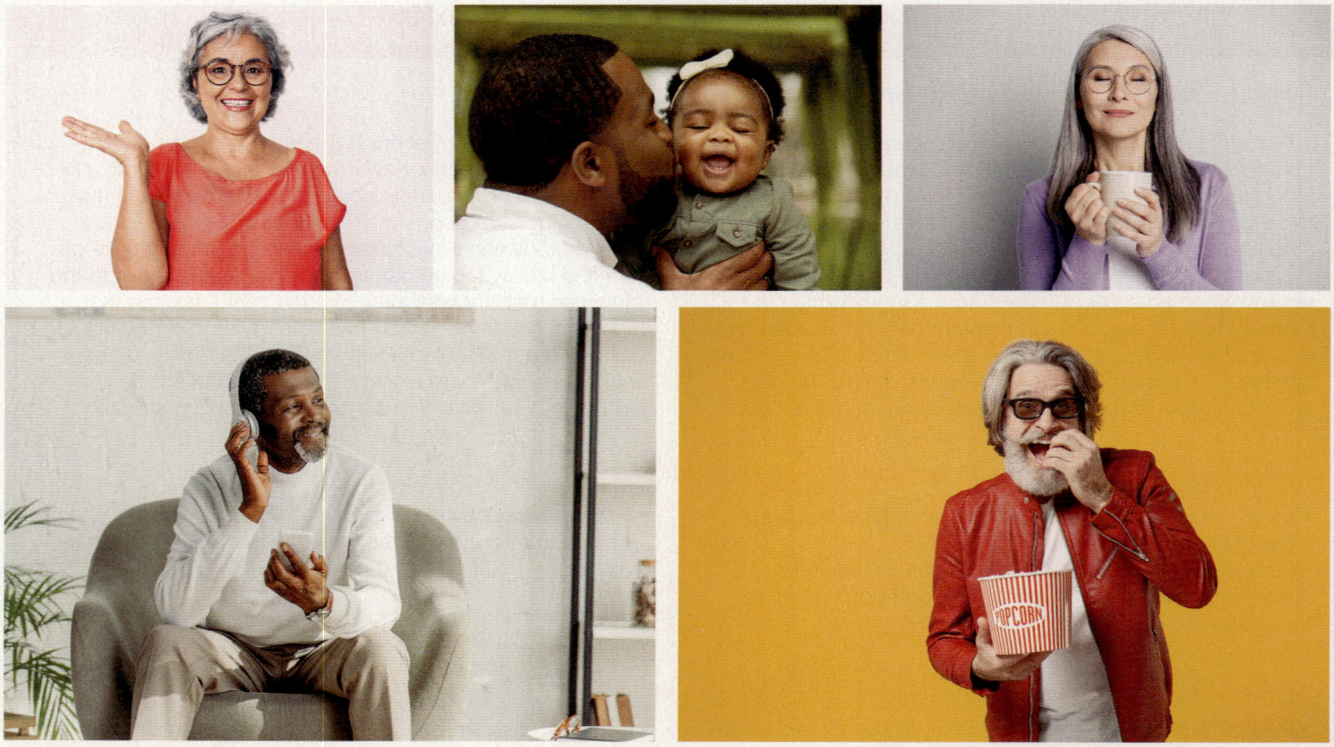

FIGURE 45-1. People delight in their abilities to see, touch, smell, hear, and taste. (*Source*: Used with permission from *Shutterstock. Photos by Krakenimages.com, pixelheadphoto digitalskillet, Roman Samborskyi, LightField Studios, and ViDI Studio.*)

For a person to receive the necessary data to experience the world, four conditions must be met:

1. A **stimulus**—an agent, act, or other influence capable of initiating a response by the nervous system—must be present.
2. A receptor or sense organ must receive the stimulus and convert it to a nerve impulse.
3. The nerve impulse must be conducted along a nervous pathway from the receptor or sense organ to the brain.
4. A particular area in the brain must receive and translate the impulse into a sensation.

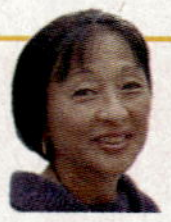

Think back to ***Muriel Hao***, the 56-year-old woman unable to rest because of the machine's beeping. The nurse would incorporate knowledge of sensory reception and perception to determine that the patient is experiencing a continuous and large amount of auditory stimuli from the beeping of the machine. In addition, the nurse would need to keep in mind other sources of stimuli, such as possible visual stimuli from the lighted numbers on the machine, tactile stimuli from being touched to determine the possible problem associated with the machine, and internal stimuli associated with pain and discomfort from surgery.

Arousal Mechanism

To receive stimuli and respond appropriately, the brain must be alert or aroused. The **reticular activating system (RAS)**, a poorly defined network that extends from the hypothalamus to the medulla, mediates **arousal**. The optimal arousal state of the RAS is a general drive state called **sensoristasis**. Nerve impulses from all the sensory tracts reach the RAS, which then selectively allows certain impulses to reach the cerebral cortex and be perceived. The mesencephalic portion of the RAS appears to be the center of the system. Stimulation of this area produces the most pronounced and long-lasting effects on the cerebral cortex (Fig. 45-2). With its many ascending and descending connections to other

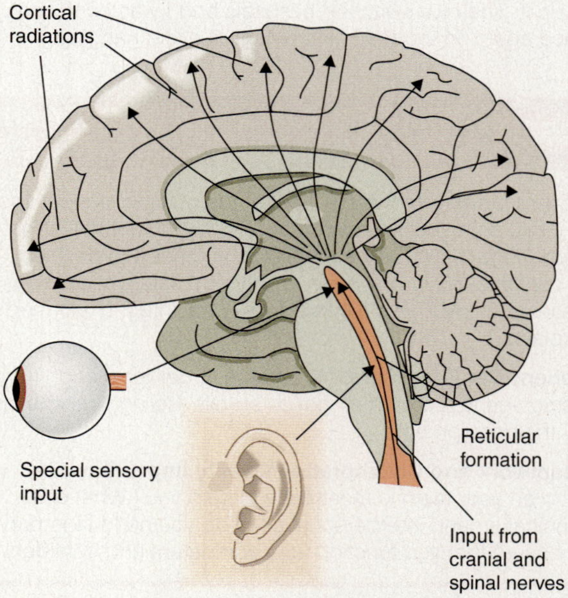

FIGURE 45-2. Nerve impulses from all the sensory tracts reach the reticular activating system (RAS), which then selectively allows certain impulses to reach the cerebral cortex and to be perceived.

Box 45-2 States of Arousal/Awareness

Conscious States

Delirium: Disorientation, restlessness, confusion, hallucinations, agitation, alternating with other conscious states

Dementia: Difficulties with spatial orientation, memory, language; changes in personality

Confusion: Reduced awareness, easily distracted, easily startled by sensory stimuli, alternates between drowsiness and excitability; resembles minor form of delirium state

Normal consciousness: Aware of self and external environment, well oriented, responsive

Somnolence: Extreme drowsiness, but will respond normally to stimuli

Minimally conscious states: Part consciousness; sleep–wake cycles present; some motor function, including automatic movements; inconsistently follows commands

Locked-in syndrome: Full consciousness; sleep–wake cycles present; quadriplegic, auditory and visual function preserved; emotion preserved

Unconscious States

Asleep: Can be aroused by normal stimuli (light touch, sound, and the like)

Stupor: Can be aroused by extreme and/or repeated stimuli

Coma: Cannot be aroused and does not respond to stimuli (coma states can be further subdivided according to the effect on reflex responses to stimuli; see Glasgow Coma Scale, Chapter 27)

Vegetative state: Cannot be aroused. Sleep–wake cycles, postures or withdraws to noxious stimuli, occasional nonpurposeful movement, random smiling or grimacing.

See the Glasgow coma scale and full outline of unresponsiveness (four) coma scale in Chapter 27.

areas of the brain, the RAS serves to monitor and to regulate incoming sensory stimuli, thus maintaining, enhancing, or inhibiting cortical arousal. States of arousal or awareness are described in Box 45-2.

The body quickly adapts to constant stimuli. For example, the repeated stimulus of a continuing noise, such as city traffic, or a noxious odor eventually goes unnoticed. This phenomenon is termed **adaptation**. Therefore, a stimulus must be variable or irregular to evoke a response. Impulses that are not acted on when received may be used at a later date in response to the same or similar stimuli. The memory process involves the storage of that material. For example, thought and memory are used when a new sensory experience occurs, and the person uses a response based on previous knowledge and experience. For example, if a toddler remembers a painful visit to a pediatrician, that memory can trigger avoidance behaviors with future visits.

DISTURBED SENSORY PERCEPTION

When patients are admitted to a health facility, they are confronted with stimuli that are different in quality and quantity from those to which they are accustomed. For example, a patient confined to bed rest may receive many fewer stimuli, whereas someone undergoing multiple diagnostic tests may receive a greater-than-normal level of sensory input. These and other typical experiences are likely to result in **disturbed sensory perceptions** experienced by the patient. Being sensitive to how visual stimuli, noises, and touch are stimulating to the patient, combined with paying attention to the patient's need for privacy and for social interaction, can significantly reduce disturbances in sensory perception.

Severe sensory alterations can occur, especially in certain areas of a facility, such as the critical care or intensive care units; this type of sensory alteration is sometimes termed *intensive care unit (ICU) psychosis*. Factors contributing to severe sensory alteration include sensory overload, sensory deprivation, sleep deprivation, and cultural care deprivation.

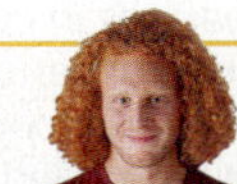

Consider **Ori Soltes**, the young man in the ICU. The nurse would need to assess Mr. Soltes closely for underlying reasons for his confusion. Although the possible causes are numerous and most likely multiple in nature, the nurse would need to address the possibility of sensory deprivation and overload contributing to the patient's confusion.

Box 45-3 (on pages 1832–1833) provides an overview of sensory deprivation and sensory overload with related nursing interventions.

Sensory Deprivation

Sensory deprivation occurs when a person experiences decreased sensory input or input that is monotonous, unpatterned, or meaningless. With decreased sensory input, the RAS is no longer able to project a normal level of activation to the brain. As a result, the person may hallucinate simply to maintain an optimal level of arousal. During the COVID-19 pandemic, many people who sheltered in place experienced sensory deprivation, especially those in nursing homes who were confined to their rooms. Patients at high risk for sensory deprivation include:

- Patients in an environment with decreased or monotonous stimuli (such as institutionalized patients, or those confined to a small living area at home, on bed rest, or in isolation)
- Patients with impaired ability to receive environmental stimuli (e.g., patients with impaired vision or hearing; with bandages or casts that interfere with vision, hearing, or tactile stimulation; or with affective disorders who "close out" the environment)
- Patients who are unable to process environmental stimuli (e.g., patients with spinal cord injuries or brain damage, those who are confused or disoriented, and those who are taking prescribed or recreational drugs affecting the central nervous system)

Box 45-3 Overview of Sensory Deprivation and Sensory Overload

Sensory Deprivation

Sensory deprivation is insufficient quantity or quality of stimuli; may result from decreased sensory input or monotonous, unpatterned, and unmeaningful input.

Signs and Symptoms	Contributing Factors	Patients at Risk
Physical behaviors: drowsiness, excessive yawning *Escape behaviors:* eating, exercising, sleeping, running away to escape the deprived environment *Changes in perception:* unusual body sensations; preoccupation with somatic complaints (dry mouth, palpitations, difficulty breathing, nausea); change in body image; illusions and hallucinations *Changes in cognitive behavior:* decreased attention span, inability to concentrate, decreased problem solving and task performance *Changes in affective behavior:* crying, increased irritability and annoyance over small matters, confusion, panic, depression	*Decreased environmental stimuli:* institutionalized environment; separation from significant others and usual sources of stimuli; treatments that decrease access to stimuli, such as bed rest or isolation *Impaired ability to receive environmental stimuli:* impaired vision, hearing, taste, smell, touch resulting from treatments such as bandages or body casts that interfere with reception of stimuli, or as a result of depression and other affective disorders *Inability to process environmental stimuli:* spinal cord injuries, brain damage, confusion, dementia, medications that depress the central nervous system	Institutionalized patients, especially those in long-term care settings Patients with communicable diseases (e.g., COVID-19, AIDS) Patients confined to bed Patients with sensory alterations (e.g., impaired vision or hearing, or patients with eye patches or body casts) Patients who are depressed Patients from a different culture Patients with a disturbance of the nervous system

Nursing Interventions

Maintain sufficient level of arousal by increasing sensory stimuli from all sensory modalities:

- Instruct the patient in self-stimulation methods: counting, singing, reading, reciting poetry.
- Structure meaningful tangible stimuli into the patient's external environment; include a variety of people, ideas, sensations; a pet may provide excellent stimulation.

Visual Stimulation
- Colorful sheets, pajamas, robes
- Colorful uniform tops for the nurse
- Face-to-face human contact
- Clocks, calendars, wristwatches
- Pictures, flowers, greeting cards

Auditory Stimulation
- Calling the person by name
- Conversation that communicates caring as well as orients the patient
- Reading to the patient
- Television, radio, iPod

Gustatory and Olfactory Stimulation
- Attention to oral hygiene and properly fitting dentures
- Food of different textures, colors, temperatures, served attractively
- Smelling food before eating it and recalling pleasurable aromas from the past
- Seasoning foods or having favorite foods brought from home

Tactile Stimulation
- Back rubs and foot soaks
- Turning and repositioning
- Passive range-of-motion exercises
- Hair brushing, combing, washing
- Hugs
- Touching arms or shoulders

Cognitive Input
- Orient the patient to the environment.
- Encourage patient participation in self-care.
- Discuss current events or the patient's occupation, hobbies, or interests.
- Reinforce reality without arguing with a patient who is hallucinating. "No, I don't see a man standing there, but the linen hamper may be confusing you."

Emotional Input
- Encourage the patient to share fears, concerns, and perceptions.
- Reassure the patient that illusions and misperceptions do occur with sensory deprivation.
- Incorporate culturally assistive, supportive, facilitative acts into nursing care.
- *Caution:* Because it can be difficult to distinguish the behavioral manifestations of sensory deprivation from sensory overload, introduce more stimulation cautiously. If the added stimulation only increases the patient's maladaptive behaviors, consider reducing sensory input because the patient may be experiencing sensory overload.

Box 45-3 Overview of Sensory Deprivation and Sensory Overload *(continued)*

Sensory Overload

Sensory overload is excessive stimuli over which a person feels little control; the brain is unable to meaningfully respond to or ignore stimuli.

Signs and Symptoms	Contributing Factors	Patients at Risk
Similar to those observed in sensory deprivation Older patients and patients who have suffered a stroke are more likely to experience confusion or agitation. Young patients are more likely to seek the comfort of their parents' embrace to block out sensory overload.	*Increased internal stimuli:* pain, pressure and discomfort of intrusive tubes (e.g., intravenous [IV] lines, catheters; endotracheal tubes; nasogastric tubes), worry about state of health or need to make treatment decisions *Increased external stimuli:* unfamiliar health care environment, such as lights, noises, sounds, odors, movement, and constant presence of strangers, many of whom touch the body; intrusive procedures such as diagnostic tests and treatments; scratchy linens *Inability to perceptually disregard or selectively ignore some stimuli:* nervous system disturbances, substances such as caffeine that stimulate the central nervous system arousal mechanism	Acutely or chronically ill patients Patients in pain Patients with intrusive monitoring or treatment equipment Hospitalized patients, especially those in critical care settings Patients with disturbances of the nervous system

Nursing Interventions

- Provide a consistent, predictable pattern of stimulation to help the patient develop a sense of control over the environment.
- Offer simple explanations before procedures, tests, and examinations.
- Establish a schedule with the patient for routine care such as eating, bathing, turning, positioning, coughing, and exercising.
- Speak calmly with the patient and move slowly; communicate confidence.
- Explore with the patient what stimuli are most distressing and develop a plan to reduce or eliminate them (e.g., incoming phone calls, visitors); earplugs or pain medication may be indicated. Noise-reducing headphones may be helpful.
- Be careful not to cause sensory deprivation.
- Identify and, wherever possible, eliminate culturally inappropriate stimuli.

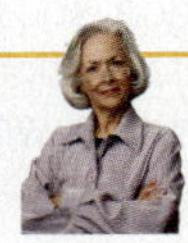

Remember **Dolores Pirolla**, the wife of the older man with vision deficits who was developing hearing deficits. The nurse would incorporate knowledge of risk factors for sensory deprivation when developing the patient's care plan. In this case, Mr. Pirolla's sensory deficits involving vision and now hearing are affecting his ability to receive environmental stimuli. Thus, the nurse would develop a care plan with measures to ensure that the patient and his wife receive adequate stimulation from the environment.

Sensory deprivation can lead to perceptual, cognitive, and emotional disturbances. *Perceptual responses* result from inaccurate perception of sights, sounds, tastes, smells, and body position, coordination, and equilibrium. These responses can range from mild distortions such as daydreams, to gross distortions such as hallucinations. *Cognitive responses* involve the patient's inability to control the direction of thought content. Typically, attention span and ability to concentrate are decreased. The patient may demonstrate difficulty with memory, problem solving, and task performance. *Emotional responses* typically are manifested by apathy, anxiety, fear, anger, belligerence, panic, or depression. Rapid mood changes may also occur (see Box 45-2 on page 1831 for additional information).

Sensory Overload

Sensory overload occurs when a person experiences so much sensory stimuli that the brain is unable to either respond meaningfully or ignore the stimuli. The person feels out of control and may exhibit all of the manifestations observed in sensory deprivation. The amount and quality of stimuli necessary to produce overload may differ greatly from one person to another and is influenced by factors such as age, culture, personality, and lifestyle.

In some patients, especially those coming from a quiet environment with unvarying stimuli, the experience of being hospitalized quickly results in sensory overload (Fig. 45-3 on page 1834). In such patients, the brain is assaulted by the constant presence of strangers who not only demand to

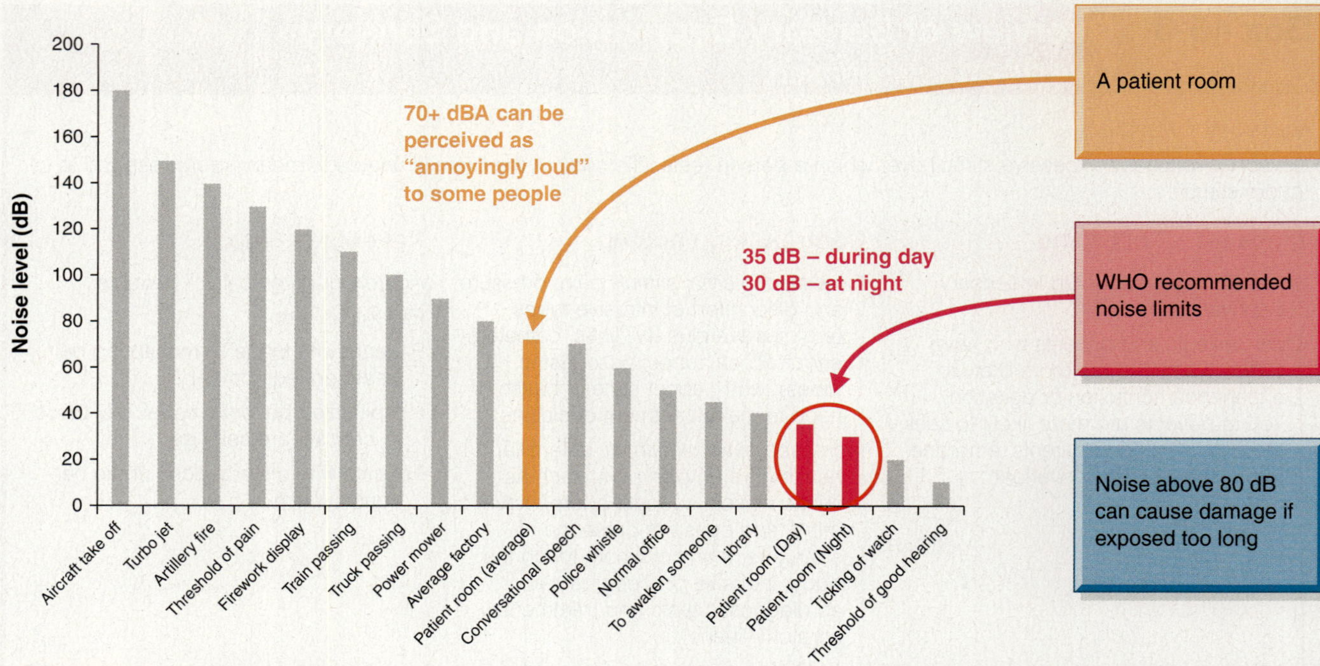

FIGURE 45-3. A noisy hospital room can contribute to patient sensory overload among other problems. (*Source:* Adapted from https://blog.schneider-electric.com/healthcare/2015/05/28/the-hidden-dangers-of-hospital-noise)

be spoken to, but also touch and poke at the body; by the strange sights, odors, sounds, and feels of the unfamiliar environment; by the constant presence of pain or discomfort from dressings, IV lines, drainage tubes, or endotracheal tubes; and by the ever-present worries about the meaning and course of the illness. Nursing care focuses on reducing distressing stimuli and helping the patient to gain control over the environment (see Box 45-3 on pages 1832–1833).

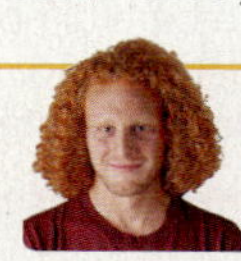

Now consider **Ori Soltes**, the young man in the ICU. When assessing Mr. Soltes and his confusion, the nurse needs to be alert for factors that would contribute to sensory overload, such as bright lights, noises from the various monitoring devices, and frequent examinations. In addition, the nurse needs to assess for possible factors contributing to sensory deprivation. For example, the patient is receiving mechanical ventilation. As a result, health care team members may limit verbal communication with the patient, thus reducing some auditory stimuli that he would receive. In addition, the patient is in bed with multiple injuries, also restricting his ability to interact with the environment.

Sensory Deficits

Impaired or absent functioning in one or more senses is termed **sensory deficit**. Examples of sensory deficits include impaired sight and hearing, altered taste, numbness and paralysis that result in altered tactile perception, and impaired kinesthetic sense. These deficits may be reversible or permanent, may occur gradually or all at once, and may be present at birth or evolve later.

Awareness of a patient's sensory deficits is necessary to determine whether the patient is able to compensate for the deficit. Illness and hospitalization may threaten a patient's usual adaptive patterns and require new self-care abilities. Patients with evolving deficits will require assistance with coping and learning to compensate skillfully.

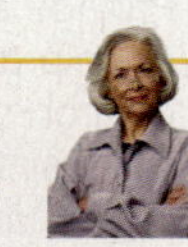

Think again of **Dolores Pirolla**, the wife of the man with vision and hearing deficits. The nurse needs to assess both the patient and his wife to determine how each is coping. From the description at the beginning of the chapter, Mr. Pirolla appears to be experiencing problems coping with vision changes. As a result, both Mr. and Mrs. Pirolla are beginning to experience social isolation. The nurse would incorporate this information when developing a plan of care for the patient and his wife.

Sensory Processing Disorder

A **sensory processing disorder** is difficulty in the way the brain takes in, organizes, and uses sensory information, causing a person to have problems interacting effectively in the everyday environment (Kranowitz, 2005, p. 68). Children with sensory processing disorders may experience a range of sensory processing issues:

- The child's central nervous system may not receive or detect sensory information.
- The brain may not integrate, modulate, organize, and discriminate sensory messages efficiently.
- The disorganized brain may send out inaccurate messages to direct the child's actions. As a result, the child may not behave in a purposeful way (e.g., they may have trouble listening, paying attention, interacting with others, processing new information, and learning).

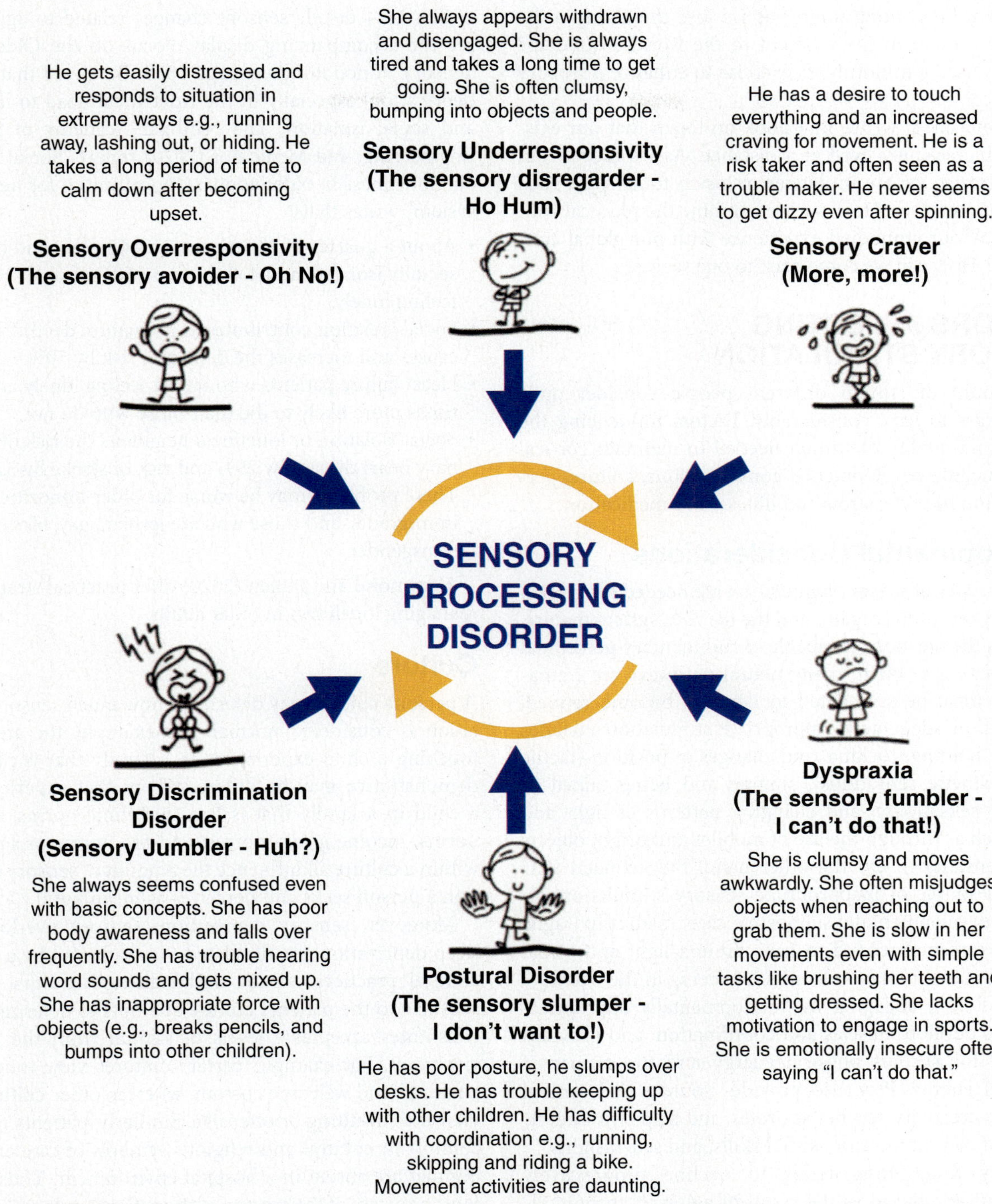

FIGURE 45-4. This poster was designed to guide parents and educators to recognize the characteristics and signs of sensory processing disorder. (*Source:* Reprinted with permission from Emmaly Rowley, Calm the Chaos.)

It is important for parents, educators, and nurses to identify a child's specific type of processing disorder in order to secure appropriate treatment. See Figure 45-4 for a description of characteristics and signs of common disorders (Kranowitz, 2005).

Sensory Poverty

Diane Ackerman (1990), poet, essayist, and naturalist, believes that we are now living in an age of **sensory poverty**. High-tech devices deliver a bewildering array of assaults on our senses every day. Yet we are learning about our world without experiencing it up close, right here, right now, in "all its messy, majestic, riotous detail." You have probably often heard the advice to stop and take time to smell the roses. But when was the last time you cradled a rose bloom, inhaled its perfume, and marveled at its color? When did you last lie on freshly mown and fragrant grass and look up at the night sky mesmerized by the moon and stars? When did you last marvel at the complex aromas and flavors coming from a new culinary experience? Do you agree with Ackerman that our lives are becoming poorer as we lose the ability to be sensually present in the moment to the world around us? Have you used a mindfulness exercise to enhance a sensory experience?

Kearney (2021) writes in a book on touch that our existence is increasingly lived at a distance. As we move from flesh to image, we are in danger of losing touch with each other and ourselves. How can we combine the physical with the virtual, our embodied experience with our global connectivity? How can we come back to our senses?

FACTORS AFFECTING SENSORY STIMULATION

The amount of stimuli different people consider optimal appears to vary considerably. Factors influencing the amount and quality of stimuli needed to maintain cortical arousal include developmental considerations, culture, personality and lifestyle, stress and illness, and medication.

Developmental Considerations

Different types of sensory stimulation are needed for growth as sensory receptors, organs, and the nervous system mature. Although the newborn is capable of rudimentary perceptual discrimination at birth, many neural pathways are immature and must be stimulated to develop, become refined, and function adequately. Appropriate stimulation includes soothing, holding, rocking, and changes of position (tactile and kinesthetic sensations), singing and being talked to (auditory sensations), and changing patterns of light and shade, such as through the use of mobiles and bright objects (visual sensations). On the other hand, the neonatal ICU may be a source of inappropriate sensory stimulation. To facilitate developmentally supportive care, medically fragile infants are recommended to have limited light and visual and vestibular stimulation to simulate being in the womb.

For children, engaging in developmentally appropriate play helps develop muscles and coordination, and provides an outlet for surplus physical energy and the release of emotional energy. Play also provides sources of learning, stimulates creativity, teaches sex roles, and helps with development of communication, social skills, and self-insights.

Sensory functioning tends to decline progressively throughout adulthood as the result of aging or chronic illness. Adults may experience the need to compensate for the loss of one type of stimulation by increasing other sources of sensory stimuli. Touch becomes increasingly important as we age. Paturel (2017) offers the following advice to stimulate touch:

- If you like to dance, then dance. If you like to walk, walk. The more your body has experience of moving in space, the more those receptors will stay active and useful.
- Wear body-hugging clothing to stimulate touch receptors.
- Be generous with physical affection. Hug your spouse, kiss your grandkids, and ask them to reciprocate. Pet the dog. Schedule a massage. Touch boosts well-being and helps you feel in tune with the people around you.

Box 45-4 details sensory changes related to aging. Also see the accompanying display, Focus on the Older Adult: Sensory Functioning on page 1838. Be aware that sensory deprivation, especially in the elderly, can lead to loneliness and social isolation. The National Academy of Sciences, Engineering, and Medicine's (2020) report "Social isolation and loneliness in older adults: Opportunities for health care system" writes that:

- About a quarter of Americans ages 65 years and older are socially isolated, and 43% of those 60 and older report feeling lonely.
- Social isolation contributes to premature death from all causes and increases the dementia risk by 50%.
- Heart failure patients who report feeling lonely are four times more likely to die than those who do not.
- Social isolation or loneliness heightens the risk of coronary heart disease by 29% and risk of stroke by 32%. These problems may be worse for older minorities, immigrants, and those who are lesbian, gay, bisexual, or transgender.

Hammond and Pullen (2020) offer practical strategies for managing loneliness in older adults.

Culture

A person's culture may determine how much sensory stimulation is considered normal. For example, the amount of touching a child experiences in a family that is physically demonstrative may be different from that experienced by a child in a family that is less so. Ethnic norms, religious norms, income group norms, and the norms of subgroups within a culture all influence the amount of sensory stimulation a person seeks and perceives as meaningful.

Moreover, sensory deprivation, sensory overload, and sleep deprivation are all related to or affected by a person's cultural practices, values, and beliefs. The nurse who is sensitive to the patient's culture attempts to determine what constitutes acceptable levels of stimuli from the patient's viewpoint. For example, certain cultures view touching as a natural and welcome custom, whereas other cultures may view it as insulting or offensive. Similarly, patients may find comfort in cultural and religious symbols of care and healing that are absent in a hospital environment. Thus, nurses must be aware of the aspects of the patient's culture to deliver culturally competent care.

Personality and Lifestyle

Apart from a person's culture, different personality types demand different levels of stimulation. One person may thrive on a steady stream of fast-paced changes and excitement, whereas another may feel best when daily routines are rigidly structured, and life sends no challenges necessitating changes. Lifestyle choices can dramatically influence the quantity and quality of stimuli a person receives. The nurse who elects to work in the emergency department of a large city hospital is exposed to stimuli vastly different from those of the nurse making home visits in a rural setting.

Box 45-4 Sensory Changes Related to Aging

As a normal part of aging, most older adults will experience some changes in their sensory capacity that can have a severe impact on communication skills. The following are common changes seen with advancing age and the disease states and injuries that occur more frequently in aging.

Vision Changes Common in Older Adults

Presbyopia: A loss of elasticity in the lens of eye leading to a decrease in the eye's ability to change the shape of the lens to focus on near objects such as fine print and decreased ability to adapt to light.

Diseases That Alter Vision Seen More Frequently as People Age

- *Cataracts:* Clouding of the crystalline lens presents as painless, progressive loss of vision; can be unilateral or bilateral.
- *Macular degeneration:* The most common cause of legal blindness in the older adult. The development of drusen deposits in the retinal pigmented epithelium is the leading cause of central vision loss in older adults. More common in fair-haired, blue-eyed people. Other risk factors include smoking and excessive sunlight exposure. There are wet and dry forms of macular degeneration.
- *Glaucoma:* A potentially serious form of eye disease. The majority of cases of glaucoma are open-angle glaucoma (95%). Increased intraocular pressure causing atrophy and cupping of the optic nerve head causing visual field deficits that can progress to blindness. Vision changes include loss of peripheral vision, intolerance to glare, decreased perception of contrast, and decreased ability to adapt to the dark.
- *Diabetic retinopathy:* End-organ damage from diabetes causing retinopathy and spotty vision. Risk can be reduced by tight blood sugar control. Starts as nonproliferative and progresses to proliferative that should be treated with laser photocoagulation.
- *Hypertensive retinopathy:* End-organ damage from poorly controlled hypertension causing background and eventual proliferative retinopathy. Usually treated with laser photocoagulation and tight blood pressure control.
- *Temporal arteritis:* Autoimmune disorder that causes inflammation of the temporal artery. It presents as malaise, scalp tenderness, unilateral temporal headache, jaw claudication, and sudden vision loss (usually unilateral). This vision loss is a medical emergency but is potentially reversible if identified immediately. The patient should see an ophthalmologist, or go to the emergency room immediately if symptoms develop.
- *Detached retina:* Can occur in patients with cataracts or recent cataract surgery, trauma, or be spontaneous. Presents as a curtain coming down across vision. Should see an ophthalmologist or proceed to the emergency room immediately.

Hearing Changes Common in Older Adults

- *Presbycusis:* Loss of high-frequency, sensorineural hearing loss. Has a gradual onset, is progressive, and is bilateral. Due to gradual loss of hair cells and fibrous changes in the small blood vessels that supply the cochlea. Difficulty hearing high-pitched sounds such as *s, z, sh,* and *ch.* Background noise further aggravates hearing deficit.
- *Conductive hearing loss:* Involves the outer and/or middle ear. Causes of conductive hearing impairment include cerumen impactions or foreign bodies, ruptured eardrum, otitis media, and otosclerosis.
- *Sensorineural hearing loss:* Involves damage to the inner ear, the cochlea, or the fibers of the eighth cranial nerve. Causes of sensorineural hearing loss include hereditary causes, viral or bacterial infections, trauma, tumors, noise exposure, cardiovascular conditions, ototoxic drugs, and Ménière disease.

Diseases That Alter Hearing Seen More Frequently as People Age

- *Central auditory processing disorder:* An uncommon disorder that includes an inability to process incoming signals and is often found in stroke patients and older adults with Alzheimer dementia. The person's hearing is intact but their ability to process the sound is impaired.
- *Tinnitus:* Ringing in the ears may fluctuate, can be due to damage to the hair receptors of the cochlear nerve and age-related changes in the organs of hearing and balance. Patients with tinnitus should be referred to ENT.
- *Ménière disease:* Characterized by fluctuating hearing loss, dizziness, and tinnitus. Possible causes of Ménière disease include hypothyroidism, diabetes, and neurosyphilis.

Changes in Smell and Taste Common to Older Adults

- Common changes in smell include a decline in the sensitivity to airborne chemical stimuli with aging.
- Common changes in taste include a decreased ability to detect foods that are sweet. Most changes in taste are thought to occur due to decreased sense of smell, medications, diseases, and tobacco use.

Diseases That Alter Smell and Taste Seen More Frequently as People Age

Burning mouth syndrome: This is a sensation that the tongue is tingling or burning. There may be several contributing factors: Vitamin B deficiencies, local trauma, gastrointestinal disorders causing reflux, allergies, salivary dysfunction, and diabetes.

Changes in Peripheral Sensation Common to Older Adults

- Peripheral nerve function that controls the sense of touch declines slightly with age.
- Two-point discrimination and vibratory sense both decrease with age.
- The ability to perceive painful stimuli is preserved in aging. However, there may be a slowed reaction time for pulling away from painful stimuli with aging.

Diseases That Alter Peripheral Sensation Seen More Frequently as People Age

- *Peripheral neuropathy:* Nerve pain in the distal extremities related to nerve damage from circulatory problems or vitamin deficiencies. Common vitamin deficiencies which impact peripheral nerves include B_6, B_{12}, and folate.
- *Diabetic neuropathy:* End-organ damage to the peripheral nerves from microvascular changes which occur with diabetes. Often leads to loss of sensation in the feet of diabetics leading to undetected trauma to the extremities

(*continued*)

Box 45-4 Sensory Changes Related to Aging *(continued)*

which can lead to refractory infections due to poor vascular supply to the extremity. It is extremely important to teach diabetics and patients with peripheral neuropathy to provide special care to their feet.

- *Phantom limb pain:* The experience of pain that can range from dull ache to crushing pain where an amputated limb once was. The sensory cortex of the brain has influence in this mechanism. This pain is often chronic and requires special interventions to control and manage the pain including electronic prosthetics, analgesics, and psychosocial support.
- *Acute sensory loss:* May be due to a stroke, acute nerve entrapment in the spine, or compartment syndrome due to trauma to a limb. Will present with acute onset of numbness, tingling, or lack of sensation and function in the affected extremity.

Source: Reprinted with permission from Boltz, M., Capezuti, E., Fulmer, T., & Zwicker, D. (2016). *Evidence-based geriatric nursing protocols for best practice* (5th ed.). Springer Publishing Company.

Stress and Illness

Increased sensory stimulation may be sought during periods of low stress simply to maintain cortical arousal. During high-stress periods, multiple stressors may already be overloading the sensory system, and the person desires decreased sensory stimulation. Illness, a time of stress, can affect the reception of sensory stimuli and their transmission and perception. Therefore, the stress of physical illness, pain, hospitalization, testing, surgery, or treatment may provide more stimulation than a person can process and respond to without assistance.

One of the surprising symptoms of COVID-19 that was recognized early was the loss of smell. See the accompanying "Through the Eyes (Nose) of the Patient." While some also reported a loss of taste, Jarvis (2021) explains why this was complicated thanks to a process called oral referral, which causes us to perceive what is happening in the nose as if it were happening in the mouth.

Smell is integral to our experience of taste. People often struggle to separate the two, certain that they have lost their sense of taste when the taste buds—which detect only sweet, salty, bitter, sour, and umami

Focus on the Older Adult

SENSORY FUNCTIONING

Age-Related Changes	Nursing Strategies
Decrease in vision	• Ensure that the patient is using corrective lenses such as contacts, glasses, and/or magnifiers. • Administer medications that enhance vision, such as medications that lower intraocular pressure in older adult patients with glaucoma. • Provide adequate lighting and clear pathways of clutter to prevent injury. • Provide enlarged print. • Encourage the patient to visit the ophthalmologist annually.
Decrease in hearing	• Ensure that the patient is using appropriate and functioning hearing assistive devices. • When communicating with the patient, use a lower tone. • Speak so that the patient can see your mouth movements. • Explore the use of an approved clear mask or plastic shield so that the patient can see your mouth movements.
Decreased sense of touch	• Protect the patient's skin from temperature extremes. • Assess the extremities for breaks in the skin, blisters, drainage, or open wounds. • Use moisturizers to keep the patient's skin supple. • Ensure that the patient is ambulating with assistive devices. • Use massage, shampoos, foot rubs, etc. as desired by the patient.
Sensory deprivation	• Discourage the use of sedatives. • Assess the effect of medications on the patient's central nervous system. • Provide interaction with children and pets. • Encourage the patient to participate in exercise classes and provide activity therapy. • Ensure that institutionalized older adults share meals with four people per table. • Ensure that homebound older adults have frequent visits from family and community resources such as Meals on Wheels or church volunteers.
Sensory overload	• Orient the patient to person, place, and time. • Decrease environmental noise. • Encourage the patient to participate in nursing care.

Through the Eyes (Nose) of the Patient

As the COVID-19 pandemic progressed, many began to talk about a loss of smell and the symptoms—known as parasomnia, incorrect smells; phantosomia, phantom smells—went from nearly unknown to incredibly common.

"I doused a worryingly bland breakfast with hot sauce to no effect."

"Meat smells like it is rotting, and mint toothpaste is so off-putting I had to switch to a bubble gum flavor."

"Nothing is savory anymore, coffee is just bitter, a cake is just sweet, a burger is just salty."

"I [a sommelier] failed to notice that the cat's litter box was full."

"All of a sudden, life is newly dangerous: food poisoning, gas leaks, not noticing that dinner is burning."

"I feel like I'm living my life in black and white, trapped behind a sheet of glass."

"My sense of normalcy and well-being disappeared with my olfaction. I feel alien from myself, detached from normality. Lonely in my body. It's so hard to explain."

"I feel discombobulated—like I don't exist."

As the sense of smell seemed to be returning, many reported something new.

"My sense of smell was coming back broken. Food smells like gasoline or cigarettes, scented body wash was like burning rubber."

"My boyfriend no longer smells or tastes right, and I've begun to avoid kissing him, but I haven't told him why."

"Poo smells better than coffee."

"But what is life without taste, without smell? If I never regain these abilities, will the question 'What do you want for dinner?' mean anything? Will a nice restaurant still have value? How will it feel when someone cooks for me, watches me take the first bite, and waits for my reaction? What is the point of perfume, or piney mountain air?"

Source: These comments are extracted from Chiu, A. (2020, November 5). COVID-19, in addition to stealing sense of smell, may also warp it, *The Washington Post*, p 12; Diamond, K. (2020, September 6). The Strange Grief of Losing My Sense of Taste. *The New York Times*, A23; Jarvis, B. (2021, January 31). The forgotten sense. *The New York Times Magazine*, pp. 20–25, 46–47, 49.

flavors—remain fully functional. There was also the question of the sensations we experience through neither olfaction nor taste, but via the nerves of the trigeminal system, the coolness of mint, the spice of peppers, the bubble of carbonation. Were these also affected? (The three, together, are known as our chemosensory senses, those we use to detect the presence of chemicals in our environment [p. 24]).

Lindsay (2021) describes the following smell and taste disorders:

- Anosomia: inability to smell
- Dysomia: altered smell perception
- Hyposomia: decreased ability to smell
- Ageusia: complete loss of taste
- Dysageusia: distorted taste perception
- Hypogeusia: reduced ability to taste

Nomosomia and nomogeusia refer to the normal ability to smell and taste, respectively.

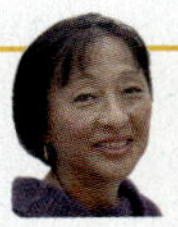

Think back to **Muriel Hao**, the woman who had surgery 2 days ago. Most likely, Ms. Hao is experiencing sensory overload from all of the events of the past several days. The constant beeping of the equipment is adding to this overload.

Medication

Medications that alert or depress the central nervous system may interfere with the perception of sensory stimuli. Narcotics and sedatives decrease awareness of sensory stimuli. Antipsychotics can influence how sensory stimuli are perceived and processed. Certain medications may also contribute to the impairment of sensory functioning by decreasing reception (e.g., captopril, an antihypertensive agent, can cause taste alteration). Examples of medications that are ototoxic and can impair auditory function if taken over a long period of time include furosemide, some cancer chemotherapies, and aspirin. Be sure to review patients' medication records when assessing for sensory alterations.

NURSING PROCESS FOR SENSORY FUNCTIONING

Assessing

When assessing a patient for disturbed sensory perceptions, interview the patient and assess for sensory deficits and manifestations of sensory deprivation or overload. Be sure to include an assessment of the patient's environment to determine whether it is providing adequate sensory stimulation for healthy development.

Identifying At-Risk Patients

Patients may be at risk for sensory disturbances for different reasons. Often there are physiologic reasons that place patients at risk. Aging, for example, is often accompanied by diminished senses. Diseases can also diminish senses. Diabetes-related neuropathies can result in a loss of sensation in limbs, rendering the diabetic unable to feel hot objects such as bath water, which can result in burns. Certain drugs affect taste. Social and environmental factors likewise place people at risk. Humans need appropriate human and environmental stimulation. When either or both are deficient or excessive, problems may result. Lifestyle factors may also place people at risk, such as engaging in work or leisure activities that are potentially harmful to the eyes or ears—for example, exposure to chemicals, flying objects, and loud noises.

With all of us spending more time during the pandemic staring at a computer screen, phone, or other digital device, especially children doing distance learning, more people than ever before are experiencing computer vision syndrome (CVS), or digital eye strain. Symptoms of CVS include eye fatigue and discomfort, dry eyes, headaches, blurred vision, neck and shoulder pain, eye twitching, and red eyes. All About Vision suggests these 10 easy steps you can take to reduce your risk of eye strain and other common symptoms of CVS. See Box 45-5.

Assessment of the Sensory Experience

When assessing a patient's sensory experience, structure the history using the components of the sensory experience—stimulation, reception, and transmission–perception–reaction (see Focused Assessment Guide 45-1 on pages 1842–1843). Because patients may adapt to sensory impairments, it may be helpful to include someone the patient knows well (e.g., a partner or parent) in the assessment to see if that person has noticed behavioral characteristics in the patient that suggest a sensory disturbance (e.g., "I've noticed he turns the television volume much louder than ever before."). Also, recognize that people may develop acuity in certain senses to compensate for losses in others. For example, many people who are blind have acute hearing. Begin by asking patients to evaluate their sensory functioning: "How would you rate your vision (hearing, and the like): Excellent, good, fair, poor, or bad?"

The mental status exam is included in assessments of sensory functioning. Chapter 27 provides a detailed description of how to assess levels of awareness (also see Box 45-2 on page 1831), levels of consciousness, memory, abstract reasoning, and language. The Mini-Mental State Examination (MMSE), available at https://www.dementia.org/diagnosing-dementia-mini-mental-status-exam, is one of the most widely used clinical instruments for quickly detecting cognitive impairment and assessing its severity, as well as for monitoring cognitive changes over time.

STIMULATION

Assess for any recent changes in sensory stimulation, for example, reduction of stimulation from one or more sensory modalities ("Since my husband died, no one touches me anymore. It sounds crazy, but I'm hungry to be touched!") or new or unusual stimulation ("Ever since my granddaughter moved in with me, my house is always noisy. I can't stand the constant noise and her smoking."). Assess whether the type of stimulation present is developmentally appropriate. Patients at high risk for problems related to stimulation include children in nonstimulating environments, older people, terminally ill patients, patients on bed rest, patients in isolation, and patients requiring intensive nursing in a critical care setting.

RECEPTION

Assess for anything that may interfere with sensory reception and identify any corrective devices the patient uses for sensory impairments, such as eyeglasses, contact lenses, or hearing aids. If corrective devices are necessary, assess whether the patient is actually using them, has the proper equipment, and understands related care. For example, ask the patient, "When were your eyes last examined?" or "Are there batteries for your hearing aid?" The reception section of the Focused Assessment Guide 45-1 (on page 1842–1843) highlights assessment strategies for each sense. Patients at high risk for reception problems include people with visual, auditory, or other sensory impairments.

Box 45-5 Computer Eye Strain: 10 Steps for Relief

Get a comprehensive eye exam

Having a routine comprehensive eye exam every year is the most important thing you can do to prevent or treat computer vision problems. During your exam, be sure to tell your eye doctor how often you use a computer and digital devices at work and at home.

Measure how far your eyes are from your screen when you sit at your computer, and bring this measurement to your exam so your eye doctor can test your eyes at that specific working distance.

Use proper lighting

Eye strain often is caused by excessively bright light either from outdoor sunlight coming in through a window or from harsh interior lighting. When you use a computer, your ambient lighting should be about half as bright as that typically found in most offices.

Eliminate exterior light by closing drapes, shades, or blinds. Reduce interior lighting by using fewer light bulbs or fluorescent tubes, or use lower-intensity bulbs and tubes.

Also, if possible, position your computer screen so windows are to the side, instead of in front or behind it.

Many computer users find their eyes feel better if they can avoid working under overhead fluorescent lights. If possible, turn off the overhead fluorescent lights in your office and use floor lamps that provide indirect "soft white" LED lighting instead.

Box 45-5 Computer Eye Strain: 10 Steps for Relief *(continued)*

Minimize glare	Glare from light reflecting off walls and finished surfaces, as well as reflections on your computer screen also can cause computer eye strain. Consider installing an antiglare screen on your display and, if possible, paint bright white walls a darker color with a matte finish. If you wear glasses, purchase lenses with antireflective (AR) coating. AR coating reduces glare by minimizing the amount of light reflecting off the front and back surfaces of your eyeglass lenses.
Upgrade your display	If you have not already done so, replace your old tube-style monitor (called a cathode ray tube or CRT) with a flat-panel LED (light-emitting diode) screen with an antireflective surface. When choosing a new flat panel display, select a screen with the highest resolution possible. Resolution is related to the "dot pitch" of the display. In general, displays with a lower dot pitch have sharper images. Choose a display with a dot pitch of .28 mm or smaller. Also, choose a relatively large display. For a desktop computer, select a display that has a diagonal screen size of at least 19 inches.
Blink more often	Blinking is very important when working at a computer; blinking moistens your eyes to prevent dryness and irritation. When staring at a screen, people blink less frequently—only about one third as often as they normally do—and many blinks performed during computer work are only partial lid closures, according to studies. Tears coating the eye evaporate more rapidly during long nonblinking phases and this can cause dry eyes. Also, the air in many office environments is dry, which can increase how quickly your tears evaporate, placing you at greater risk for dry eye problems. If you experience dry eye symptoms, ask your eye doctor about artificial tears for use during the day. To reduce your risk of dry eyes during computer use, try this exercise: Every 20 minutes, blink 10 times by closing your eyes as if falling asleep (very slowly). This will help rewet your eyes.
Exercise your eyes	Another cause of computer eye strain is focusing fatigue. To reduce your risk of tiring your eyes by constantly focusing on your screen, look away from your computer at least every 20 minutes and gaze at a distant object (at least 20 feet away) for at least 20 seconds. Some eye doctors call this the "20-20-20 rule." Looking far away relaxes the focusing muscle inside the eye to reduce fatigue. Another exercise is to look far away at an object for 10 to 15 seconds, then gaze at something up close for 10 to 15 seconds. Then look back at the distant object. Do this 10 times. This exercise reduces the risk of your eyes' focusing ability to "lock up" (a condition called accommodative spasm) after prolonged computer work. Both of these exercises will reduce your risk of computer eye strain. Also, remember to blink frequently during the exercises to reduce your risk of computer-related dry eye.
Take frequent breaks	To reduce your risk for computer vision syndrome and neck, back, and shoulder pain, take frequent screen breaks during your workday (at least one 10-minute break every hour). During these breaks, stand up, move about and stretch your arms, legs, back, neck, and shoulders to reduce tension and muscle fatigue.
Modify your workstation	If you need to look back and forth between a printed page and your computer screen, place the written pages on a copy stand adjacent to your screen. Poor posture also contributes to computer vision syndrome. Adjust your workstation and chair to the correct height so your feet rest comfortably on the floor. Position your computer screen so it's 20 to 24 inches from your eyes. The center of your screen should be about 10 to 15 degrees below your eyes for comfortable positioning of your head and neck.
Consider computer glasses	For the greatest comfort at your computer, you might benefit from having your eye doctor modify your eyeglasses prescription to create customized computer glasses. This is especially true if you normally wear contact lenses, which may become dry and uncomfortable during extended screen time. Computer glasses also are a good choice if you wear bifocals or progressive lenses, because these lenses generally are not optimal for the distance to your computer screen. Also, you may want to consider photochromic lenses or lightly tinted lenses for computer eyewear to reduce your exposure to potentially harmful blue light emitted by digital devices. Ask your eye doctor for details and advice.

Source: Adapted from Heiting, G., & Wan, L. K. (2022, April). *Computer eye strain: 10 steps for relief.* https://www.allaboutvision.com/cvs/irritated.htm

Focused Assessment Guide 45-1

SENSORY STIMULATION

Factors to Assess	Questions and Approaches
Stimulation	"Does your current environment overly, insufficiently, or appropriately stimulate you?" "Are you bored? Why?" "Are you able to read? Watch television? Knit? Why not?" "Are there other people in your home during the day? Do you spend much time together? How do you spend the time?" "Who visits you while you are in the hospital?" Note reduction in the patterns or meaningfulness of stimulation in each sensory modality, changes in stimulation other than decreases (e.g., new or unusual stimulation), or developmental appropriateness of stimulation.
Reception	"Does anything interfere with the functioning of your senses?" (You may need to list these.) "Describe any corrective devices you use for sensory impairments."
Visual disturbances	"Please read my name tag (or this page of print)." Note if the patient can correctly identify objects directly in front of the eyes as well as those requiring peripheral vision. Note eye rubbing, squinting, movements indicating faulty vision (bumping into furniture, over-reaching or underreaching for objects), changes in the appearance of the eye (cataracts, swelling), and complaints of eye pain, spots, halos, or other visual disturbances.
Auditory disturbances	"Repeat the words that I will speak softly close to each ear." Note if the patient is able to hear equally well from both ears, distinguish voices, locate the direction of a sound; if the patient needs to face the person speaking and relies on lip reading; if the patient's responses to questions include blank looks, many nods, smiling, or inappropriate responses indicating faulty hearing. Note complaints of ringing or buzzing in the ears.
Gustatory (taste) disturbances	"Close your eyes, stick out your tongue, and tell me if what I place on your tongue is sweet, sour, bitter, salty or umami." "Have you been experiencing any strange tastes (bitter, metallic) or aftertastes lately?" Note if the patient is able to differentiate sweet, sour, bitter, salty or umami tastes or reports unusual, persistent taste sensations. Note deficient oral hygiene, ill-fitting dentures, braces, or anything else that might contribute to gustatory disturbances.
Olfactory (smell) disturbances	"Close your eyes and tell me what you smell." "Have you smelled odors lately that others cannot smell, or have you been especially sensitive to odors?" Note if the patient can correctly identify common odors (coffee, vanilla) or has noticed increased sensitivity to odors.
Tactile (touch) disturbances	"Close your eyes and tell me when you feel something (brush skin with cotton ball), if what you feel is dull or sharp (use both ends of a safety pin), hot or cold (use items from the food tray). Now, keep your eyes closed and tell me what I am placing in your hand (coin, cotton ball, paper clip)." Note if the patient can correctly sense touch and distinguish sharp and dull, hot and cold, and different shapes. Note if the patient reports decreased sensation in any part of the body; numbness, pins, and needles; tingling or abnormal sensitivity to pain or touch.
Kinesthetic and visceral disturbances	Note if the patient withdraws from being touched. "Have you noticed any changes in the way you perceive your body?" "Do you feel any unusual pressure or pain inside your body?" Note if the patient seems unsure of their body parts or body position and if the patient experiences new internal sensations (fullness, pressure, pain).
Transmission–perception–reaction	"Are you aware of any problems with your nervous system?" "Have you found it difficult to communicate verbally?" Note consciousness, orientation, appropriateness of responses, ability to perform usual self-care activities, ability to follow simple commands, decision-making abilities, pathology affecting the central nervous system, or prescribed or recreational drug use that affects the central nervous system.

Focused Assessment Guide 45-1 *(continued)*

SENSORY STIMULATION

Factors to Assess	Questions and Approaches
Behavioral manifestations of sensory deprivation or overload	
Perceptual responses	Mild to gross sensory distortions (illusions, hallucinations)
Cognitive responses	Thought disorganization, slowness of thought, decreased attention/concentration, difficulty with problem solving and task performance
Emotional responses	Rapid mood changes, anxiety, panic

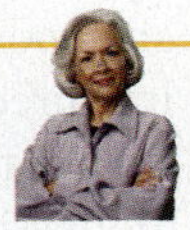

Consider **Dolores Pirolla**, and her husband who has visual and hearing deficits. The nurse needs to assess the amount and type of stimulation Mr. Pirolla is receiving. In addition, the nurse needs to investigate what measures the couple uses to adapt to the progressive visual changes. Doing so would provide a sound basis on which to build the care plan. See Box 45-6 for sample documentation of Mr. Pirolla's assessment of sensory functioning.

TRANSMISSION–PERCEPTION–REACTION

Be alert for patients at high risk for transmission–perception–reaction problems, such as the patient who is confused or who has a nervous system impairment. Use everyday interactions as multiple opportunities to assess patients' abilities to transmit, perceive, and react to stimuli.

SIGNS AND SYMPTOMS OF SENSORY DEPRIVATION AND OVERLOAD

Complete the assessment of the patient's sensory functioning by assessing for specific indicators of sensory deprivation or overload (see Box 45-2). Observe for boredom, inactivity, slowness of thought, daydreaming, increased sleeping, thought disorganization, anxiety, panic, illusions, and hallucinations. Know the patient's usual state so that you can identify changes stemming from sensory deprivation or overload.

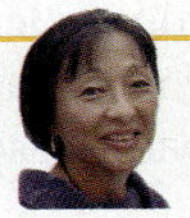

Think back to **Muriel Hao**, the woman who had surgery 2 days ago. The patient's complaints of being unable to rest because of the machine's beeping should alert the nurse to the possibility of sensory overload. To confirm the suspicion, the nurse needs to review the patient's medical record to gather more data about the patient's usual state and behavior.

Physical Assessment

Physical examination skills related to the senses are discussed in Chapter 27. Ear and eye tests, whether performed by a physician or nurse, should be considered when planning care. Problems with the neurologic system require further assessment of the sensory experience (Fig. 45-5 on page 1844).

Assessment of the Ability to Perform Self-Care

Alterations in sensory functioning may limit a person's ability to perform everyday activities safely. Exercise empathy by trying to imagine how you would get through a day if you lacked sight, hearing, or other senses. Ideally, this exercise will help you fashion a care plan responsive to the needs of patients. Patients with new sensory alterations and their family caregivers need to be instructed about practical ways to modify their home environment for safety. In addition, recognize that patients who are out of their home

Box 45-6 Sample Documentation of a Targeted Assessment

Mr. Anthony Pirolla came to the clinic with his wife who reported a new concern about his hearing.

Chief complaint: Difficulty hearing.

Signs and symptoms: According to his wife, Mr. Pirolla frequently fails to answer her questions or answers inappropriately. She also reports that he plays the radio and television louder than before. He complains that people seem to be "mumbling" more than usual—especially in church. Patient denies ringing or buzzing in ears.

Onset/duration: Mr. Pirolla states that he has had difficulty hearing since Christmas (2 months ago)—when the whole family came to visit. Mrs. Pirolla believes he had difficulty starting in the summer.

Predisposing factors: In his youth, Mr. Pirolla worked construction and was frequently around loud equipment. He is 77.

Effect on patient: Patient no longer enjoys going out or being with friends and has become more reclusive.

Self-remedies: None.

Intervention: Referred Mr. Pirolla to the clinic's audiologist.

02/24/24
C. Taylor, RN

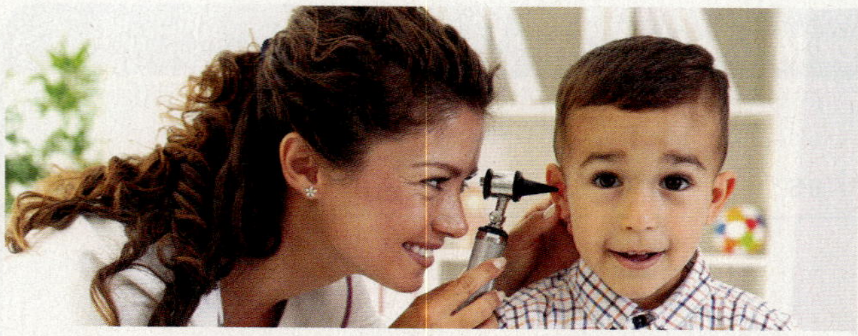

FIGURE 45-5. Preventive care such as hearing screenings and comprehensive eye exams are critical for finding sensory disorders early.

environment need to be oriented to their new surroundings. Patients need to know how to call the nurse, how to use the lights and television, and how to navigate safely to the bathroom. Before leaving a patient's room, do a quick check to ensure that the environment is safe—especially for patients with sensory impairments.

Diagnosing Actual or Potential Health Problems and Needs

An assessment of sensory functioning may lead to the identification of one or more actual or potential health problems and needs. Following the formulation of the actual or potential health problems and needs, the nurse communicates findings to other nursing and health care professionals through the use of the written and spoken word. The written actual or potential health problem or need becomes a permanent part of the patient's health record.

The International Classification for Nursing Practice (ICNP) identifies several actual or potential health problems related to sensory functioning that may be identified by nurses, among them Impaired Cognition, Confusion, Impaired Memory, Risk for Delirium, Disorientation, and Altered Perception. Different types of Sensory Deficits are among the most common. A sensory deficit is a state in which a person or group experiences or is at risk for a change in the amount, pattern, or interpretation of incoming stimuli. These alterations may be further specified as visual, auditory, gustatory, olfactory, tactile, or kinesthetic. Sensory deprivation, sensory overload, and uncompensated sensory loss may also be used to further specify the disturbed sensory perception and in some cases may be the etiology.

Common etiologies for disturbed sensory perception include the following:

- Altered environmental stimuli: excessive or insufficient
- Altered sensory reception, transmission, or integration
- Chemical alterations: endogenous (e.g., electrolytes) or exogenous (e.g., drugs)
- Psychological stress

Common etiologic factors and potential signs and symptoms for some of these health problems are found in the accompanying box, Examples of Actual or Potential Health Problems and Needs: Sensory Deficits.

Because disturbed sensory perceptions affect many other areas of human functioning, they serve as etiologies for multiple problem statements. Examples may include the following:

- Activity intolerance related to impaired balance and coordination (kinesthetic alteration)
- Anxiety related to paranoia stemming from hearing impairment, sensory deprivation (specify setting), sensory overload
- Communication barrier related to difficulty receiving, transmitting, and perceiving sensory stimuli
- Ineffective coping related to sensory overload (multiple stressors)
- Deficient diversional activity related to impaired vision or hearing
- Delayed growth and development related to nonstimulating home environment
- Impaired physical mobility related to impaired balance and coordination (kinesthetic alteration)
- Impaired parenting associated with failure to provide stimuli for growth related to lack of knowledge, decreased motivation to provide for child's growth and development
- Impaired health maintenance (specify) related to visual impairment, auditory impairment, tactile impairment
- Ineffective role performance related to sensory/perceptual alteration (blindness, deafness, and so forth)
- Sexual dysfunction related to decreased sensation
- Impaired skin integrity related to absent tactile sensation (injury)
- Disturbed sleep pattern related to sensory deprivation or overload
- Impaired social Interaction related to inability to receive and process interactional stimuli
- Social isolation related to visual or auditory impairment
- Disorientation (specify illusions, hallucinations, decreased attention or concentration, and the like) related to sensory deprivation or overload

Outcome Identification and Planning

In all settings in which nurses care for patients, optimal sensory stimulation is a priority. Nursing care focuses on the following patient outcomes:

The patient will:

- live in a developmentally stimulating and safe environment.
- exhibit a level of arousal that enables the brain to receive and meaningfully organize patterns of stimulation.
- demonstrate intact functioning of the senses: vision, hearing, taste, smell, touch, and kinesthetic and visceral awareness.
- schedule appropriate health screening exams for sensory functioning.
- maintain orientation of time, place, and person.
- respond appropriately (verbally and nonverbally) to sensory stimuli while executing self-care activities.

Patients with impaired sensory functioning require individualized outcomes similar to the following:

The patient will:

- report feeling safe and in control of the environment.
- describe different types of meaningful stimuli present in the environment.

Examples of Actual or Potential Health Problems and Needs

SENSORY FUNCTIONING

Actual or Potential Health Problem	Possible Etiologic Factors	Signs and Symptoms
Impaired vision	Eye patches after surgery	"I never realized before how sight-dependent I am. I don't know what time of day it is now unless I have the radio on or smell food coming in." "It's frightening not to know who is in my room and what they are doing." Patient observed sitting in room with blank facial expression; frequently comments on how bored they are and how slowly time is passing; hesitant to move about room without assistance despite having been oriented repeatedly.
Impaired hearing	Effects of aging	"You're right. I don't always hear what people are saying anymore so I try not to get involved in conversations. If people insist on talking, I just nod and hope I'm giving the right response." Able to hear moderately spoken word close to right ear; cannot hear same from left ear; often startled when someone approaches from left side. Sits close to television and radio; loud volume, no history of hearing testing.
Impaired taste	Chemotherapy	"I always seem to have a bitter taste in my mouth now and can't stomach certain foods at all that I used to enjoy, like beef, tomatoes, coffee…. I also can't take sweets, and I used to be a real sweets junkie." "Sometimes the very smell of certain foods or even the thought of eating nauseates me." Patient has been receiving vincristine (cancer chemotherapeutic agent) for past 3 months; some nausea and vomiting; history of poor oral hygiene.
Impaired tactile perception	Psychological stress	"I don't know why I feel this way, but I'm hypersensitive to touch. If anyone even brushes against me, I feel burning pain. Even the weight of my clothes against my skin bothers me. I'm trying to move my body as little as possible and keep it protected—but that's obviously impossible when even a breeze assaults me." Patient observed holding the body stiffly looking like they do not know what to do with their arms and legs; dressed only in a loose-fitting outfit; reports sitting at home all day afraid to go out.
Impaired kinesthetic functioning	Clinitron bed therapy	"I've been in this bed for 2 weeks now and I've lost all sense of my body… it's a curious weightless feeling that I have … sort of like floating in Jell-O. I'm no longer sure where my body begins and ends, and when I try to lift an arm or leg, I feel like I'm in slow motion. I hope I'll be able to walk when I get out of here."
Sensory deprivation	Isolation	"One of the worst things that has happened to me since I found out I had COVID-19 is that everyone is afraid of me—and no one touches me. I'm so lonely. I've always needed a lot of people around." "Here in the hospital, I think I'm going crazy. I can't leave this room. Everyone who comes in looks the same, dressed in those yellow gowns. Lately, I've seen some bizarre things that I know can't be real. I look at the clock and it turns into a swirling sun with a sad face that keeps coming closer and closer to me and I'm terrified I'll burn up if it gets too close. That's crazy, isn't it? I'm really losing it now." Disturbed sleep for past 2 weeks; during the day, yawns excessively and catnaps; limited attention span; states they are unable to concentrate on anything.
Sensory overload	Trauma of rape and aftercare	"When is everyone going to stop touching me? First, he wouldn't stop. Now, everyone here is poking at me, looking at me, asking me hundreds of questions…. Why did I have to report this and come to the hospital? Oh, please leave me alone. Get out of here, everyone."

Source: International Council of Nurses. (2019). *Nursing diagnosis and outcome statements.* International Classification for Nursing Practice (ICNP) Catalogue. https://www.icn.ch/sites/default/files/inline-files/ICNP2019-DC.pdf

- demonstrate (describe) appropriate self-care behaviors for visual impairment, hearing impairment, or other sensory impairment.
- verbalize acceptance of the sensory deficit.

Implementing

The nurse can assist patients to improve sensory functioning by teaching them and their significant others some methods for stimulating the senses; teaching patients with intact and impaired senses, appropriate self-care behaviors; and interacting therapeutically with patients experiencing sensory impairments. Safety is always a special concern for patients with sensory alterations. Ensure that the patient's environment is as free of danger as possible, and assist the patient to develop new self-care behaviors to compensate for sensory impairments. Safety considerations are discussed in Chapter 28 in more detail. The nursing interventions described here relate to preventing sensory alteration, stimulating the senses, meeting the needs of vision- and hearing-impaired people, communicating with a confused person, and communicating with an unconscious person. Communication guidelines for patients with sensory deficits are also highlighted in Chapter 8.

Preventing Disturbed Sensory Perception and Stimulating the Senses

Prevention is the most effective means to manage sensory alteration. The key to prevention is to create a functional and meaningful environment with the patient's help, while keeping limitations in mind. The creation of such an environment requires careful observation, analysis, and creative planning.

Although numerous nursing measures can be considered when planning care, their appropriateness depends on the circumstances. Promote the patient's well-being by offering care that provides rest and comfort (see Chapters 35 and 36). Attempt to control patient discomfort whenever possible.

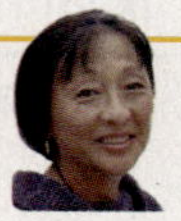

Recall **Muriel Hao**, the woman who had surgery 2 days ago. The patient verbalizes an inability to rest because of the "beeping of the machine." The initial priority is to stop the machine from beeping. The nurse needs to investigate the underlying problem related to the machine's beeping, such as a low battery or an occlusion. The nurse can then focus on comfort measures.

Be aware of a patient's need for sensory aids and prostheses, such as eyeglasses, contact lenses, hearing aids, dentures, canes, and artificial limbs, ensuring that they are available as needed. See the accompanying Research in Nursing box to see how one group of nurses organized to meet the needs of visually impaired people (VIPs) in the hospital. Social activities help stimulate the senses and mind (Fig. 45-6). Enlist the aid of family members to participate in or encourage these activities. Also encourage physical activity and exercise, which help maintain normal sensory perceptions and decrease the likelihood of sensory alteration. (Exercises are discussed in Chapter 34.)

TEACHING ABOUT SENSORY EXPERIENCES

Teaching is a significant nursing responsibility that helps prepare patients for sensory experiences. An informed patient

Research in Nursing

BRIDGING THE GAP TO EVIDENCE-BASED PRACTICE

Caring for Visually Impaired Patients in the Hospital

People with low vision may understandably experience anxiety, fear, and depression when seeking health care.

Related Research

Carlson, C., Howe, T., Pedersen, C., & Yoder, L. H. (2020). Caring for visually impaired patients in the hospital: A multidisciplinary quality improvement project. *American Journal of Nursing, 120*(5), 48–55.

A group of nurses did a literature search on the needs of visually impaired people (VIPs) but could not find a comprehensive program that health care facilities could use to meet the needs of this vulnerable population. The aims of this study were to determine the needs of hospitalized VIPs, develop educational and other resources that would help clinicians and other ancillary hospital staff in their interactions with VIPs, and assemble a toolbox of useful materials for VIPs themselves. The team conducted an education program, developed bracelets and room identifiers to alert staff to VIPs needs, introduced a braille version of the hospital menu, and provided VIP toolboxes at each nurses' station. Patient and staff member responses were overwhelmingly positive.

Relevance to Nursing Practice

Provide stimulation for as many senses as possible. Sights, sounds, smells, body positions, and textures help provide a variety of sensations. For example, music therapy has been found to benefit select physiologic variables such as pulse rate, respiratory rate, and mood state in patients receiving mechanical ventilation. Listening to music can ameliorate the stress response and promote nonpharmacologically induced relaxation for the study subjects. All nurses, especially critical care nurses, can confidently implement this nonpharmacologic, independent intervention to promote relaxation without concern about the untoward side effects sometimes caused by pharmacologic sedation (see the next Research in Nursing box). Consider cultural factors when stimulating the patient's senses and when offering nursing care, especially when caring for patients from cultures different from your own (see Chapter 29 for a discussion of common complementary and alternative therapies).

Research in Nursing

BRIDGING THE GAP TO EVIDENCE-BASED PRACTICE

Music, Sleep, and Well-Being

Adequate sleep is a critical component of illness recovery, and the majority of hospitalized patients, especially those in critical care, experience difficulty sleeping. These sleep disturbances may endure beyond hospitalization. Researchers are now seeking nonpharmacologic interventions to address these and other disturbances.

Related Research

Golilno, A. J., Leone, R., Gollenberg, A., Christopher, C., Stanger, D., Davis, T. M., Meadows, A., Zhang, Z., & Friesen, M. A. (2019). Impact of an active music therapy intervention on intensive care patients. *American Journal of Critical Care, 28*(1), 48–55.

This study examined the effect of an active music therapy intervention on physiologic parameters and self-reported pain and anxiety levels of patients in the intensive care unit. The study was conducted using a pretest–posttest, within-subject, single-group design. The study population consisted of a convenience sample of 52 patients. Study participants received a 30-minute music therapy session consisting of either a relaxation intervention or a "song choice" intervention. The music therapist recorded the patients' vital signs before and after the intervention, and patients completed self-assessments of their pain and anxiety levels before and after the intervention. After the intervention, significant decreases were found in respiratory rate, breaths per minute, heart rate, and self-reported pain and anxiety levels. No significant change in oxygen saturation level was observed. Outcomes differed between the two intervention groups: patients receiving the relaxation intervention often fell asleep.

Hetland, B., Lindquist, R., Weinert, C. R., Peden-McAlpine, C., Savik, K., & Chlan, L. (2017). Predictive associations of music, anxiety, and sedative exposure on mechanical ventilation weaning trials. *American Journal of Critical Care, 26*(3), 210–220.

In this study of 307 patients, listening to music, anxiety levels, and sedative exposure did not influence time to initial weaning trial or duration of trials. Clinical factors of illness severity, days of weaning trials, and tracheostomy placement influenced weaning patterns in this sample.

Bush, H. I., LaGasse, A. B., Collier, E. H., Gettis, M. A., & Walson, K. (2021). Effect of live versus recorded music on children receiving mechanical ventilation and sedation. *American Journal of Critical Care, 30*(5), 343–349.

Relevance to Nursing Practice

Listening to music is an inexpensive intervention without negative effects. Prospective studies of music intervention and other psychophysiologic factors are needed to determine best practices to address sleep disturbances and facilitate physiologic outcomes and well-being.

is better able to handle fears, frustration, and confusion. Therefore, explain procedures before performing them or having the patient experience them. Explanations also help prevent patients feeling that their personal space and body are being invaded.

Allow patients experiencing perceptual and thought distortions the opportunity to acknowledge that fact. Discussing such experiences and reassuring the patient that these experiences are normal and usually temporary generally eases anxiety.

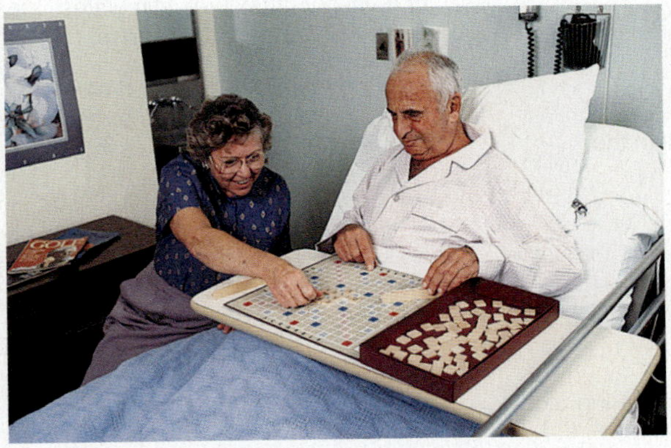

FIGURE 45-6. The nurse helps the patient find methods for stimulating the senses. Family members may participate in sensory activities.

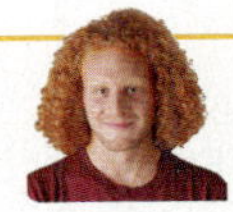

Remember **Ori Soltes**, the young man in the ICU who becomes confused. The nurse needs to acknowledge the patient's confusion, reorienting him frequently. In addition, the patient's ability to communicate is limited because of the ventilator. Therefore, the nurse should provide the patient with alternative means to communicate, such as paper and pencil or a blackboard to write on, to make his needs known. The nurse also needs to reinforce explanations about all the equipment and technologies to which the patient is being exposed, to help alleviate some of his anxiety.

Patients and family members can be guided in sensory self-stimulation, and parents can be aided in stimulation of newborns, infants, and children. The Teaching Tips 45-1 (on page 1848) display gives helpful suggestions for teaching patients about protecting and stimulating sensory function and includes suggestions that the nurse can use in a variety of situations. Table 45-1 (on page 1849) provides additional information on stimulating the senses for patients and nurses.

PROMOTING HEALTH LITERACY

Risk factors for inadequate health literacy include advanced age, low educational level, poverty, inability to read, learning

(text continues on page 1850)

Teaching Tips 45-1

SENSORY FUNCTIONING

Health Topic	Teaching Tip	Why Is This Important?
Hearing	• Avoid loud noise that is concentrated at the ear canal, such as with earphones. • Decrease background or loud noises. • Use earplugs when using loud machinery, including lawn mowers, grass trimmers, or industrial equipment. • Have regular hearing assessments. Children should be assessed in school yearly. • Do not insert objects such as cotton-tipped applicators into the ear. • Do not clean inside the ear. • Have ear pain evaluated by a physician or nurse practitioner. • Be aware of the signs and symptoms of hearing loss.	Hearing loss occurring as a person ages is called presbycusis. Presbycusis involves the deterioration of nerves and structures within the inner ear. Many occupations result in hearing loss due to increased noise. Thus, the use of ear-protective devices can decrease the development of hearing loss. Instructing the patient on signs and symptoms of hearing loss and interventions to be implemented can help to slow the development of hearing loss.
Vision	• Protect the eye from damage due to ultraviolet rays with sunglasses and tinted windows. • Provide adequate light for working or reading. • Stimulate vision with colors and shapes. • Use large print to assist in readability. • Have an annual eye examination. • Do not rub the eyes. • Use cleaning products or aerosol products safely in a well-ventilated area. • Use eye shields when in contact with harmful or toxic products, such as blood or body fluids or cleaning products. • Do not use nonprescription eye drops.	The education of the patient to maintain adequate eye function enhances the patient's quality of life. The avoidance of strain on the eye stimulates vision, thus enhancing sensory perception.
Taste (gustatory)	• Practice oral care three times per day to prevent infection and decay. • Visit the dentist biannually for dental cleaning and examination. • Notify the dentist about pain or sensitivity to hot or cold. • Provide nutritional foods that are high in fiber, and low in fat and sugar. • Enhance taste with the use of spices.	Prevention of mouth disease enhances the taste and enjoyment of foods.
Smell	• Use aromatherapy to reduce stress. • Protect the nose from noxious fumes. • Eliminate disturbing odors with adequate ventilation. • Visit the physician or nurse practitioner when experiencing nasal congestion or diminished sense of smell. • Do not wear heavy colognes or perfumes. • Enhance the sense of smell by remembering pleasant odors.	The sense of smell is important in assisting the person to relax, particularly during times of stress. It is important to evaluate any difficulty with the sense of smell and nasal congestion, since the nose lies in close proximity to the ear and the brain. Thus, the prevention of infection is a primary aspect of care.
Touch	• Protect the skin from extremes in temperature. • Provide various textures in the environment. • Provide touch such as during the bath or massage therapy. • Instruct on all aspects of invasive procedures.	Protecting the skin from temperature changes decreases damage to the skin and underlying tissues. The use of a variety of textures stimulates nerve fibers and tactile sense.
Sensory Overload	• Reduce the number and type of stimuli. • Provide periods of rest. • Provide explanation of sounds and activities within the environment. • Use relaxation techniques to enhance rest.	Sensory overload can be prevented by using these measures. As a result, the patient is able to organize stimuli to decrease anxiety and stress.
Sensory Deprivation	• Provide reading material, audiovisual stimulation, and interactive activities. • Provide stimulation through visitors, phone conversations, and e-mail. • Use therapeutic touch. • Encourage the use of assistive devices such as hearing aids and glasses. • Provide a radio and television. • Orient to time, place, and person.	Increasing sensory perception enhances the patient's responses, helping to create a meaningful environment.

Table 45-1 Stimulating the Senses

SENSE	TEACHING PATIENTS	NURSING INTERVENTIONS
Vision	Surround yourself with different colors and with an environment that changes (walk through a mall, sit by a window where you see people come and go). Develop a sensitivity to changes in nature (weather patterns, dawn-to-night cycle, changing seasons, changes in a plant or animal). Use visual devices to keep oriented (watches, calendars, newspaper, television). Use crossword puzzles and games to stimulate mental activities. Create favorite scenes in your mind, paying attention to tiny details.	Wear visually stimulating and comforting colors. Keep meaningful visual stimuli such as photos, greeting cards, toys, or flowers near the patient. Position patients with impaired mobility where they can see out a window or watch local traffic on the unit.
Hearing	Decrease or eliminate distressing auditory stimuli (change bedroom, talk with family members about noise of stereos and other such equipment, use earplugs, use headphones to listen to soft music). Develop a sensitivity to different sounds (music, chirping birds, night sounds, different voices). Use the telephone to maintain contact with family and friends. Use television, radio, CDs to keep current and to stimulate mental activities. Recall favorite sounds of the past with the situations in which they were heard.	Speak in a warm and pleasant tone and communicate caring to the patient. Use your voice to orient the patient to the environment and current situation (e.g., procedure, treatment). Avoid speaking about the patient to others within the patient's hearing. Remember that patients overhearing snatches of conversation outside their room often presume it is about *them!* Decrease extraneous noise (intercom, movement of carts, loud conversations of staff); use carpets and sound-absorbing material whenever possible.
Taste	Experiment with foods of different tastes (seasonings), colors, temperature, and textures; realize that as taste buds age, things will no longer taste the same. Practice thorough oral hygiene and have regular dental examinations. Recall foods that tasted especially good in the past and the events surrounding these tastes (e.g., grandparent baking cookies or homemade bread).	Consult with the dietitian about preparing meals with varied taste sensations; serve meals attractively. Perform routine oral hygiene for patients who are unable to do this for themselves.
Smell	Consciously savor smells that are pleasant; decrease or eliminate noxious odors. Recall pleasant aromas or smells from the past and the events surrounding them (e.g., smell of the ocean when nearing the vacation house, smell of fresh pine in the house at Christmas, the body scent of a loved person or animal).	Keep the patient's room well ventilated, using opportunities when the patient is out of the room to air it out. Remove dressings, drainage, and any equipment with odors from the patient's room as quickly as possible. Encourage patients to focus on pleasant or familiar smells, such as coffee, newspaper, or flowers. Avoid wearing heavy perfumes.
Touch	Consciously surround yourself with different textures and let yourself feel and enjoy them (scratchy afghan; a puppy's moist, wet tongue; soft petal of a flower; smooth silk scarf; mug of hot chocolate). Allow these textures to evoke memories of past tactile experiences (grandchild's hug may bring back memories of hugs from own children, scrap of fabric may recall a prom dress or wedding gown or baby blanket). Recognize the need to be touched and tell someone, "I need a hug today!" Receive tactile stimulation from a pet.	Include different textures in the patient's environment (silky pillow sham from home, soft sheepskin, wooly blanket). Respect the patient's need and desire to be touched or not touched (touch the patient's forearm or shoulder, hug the patient). Use physical care (bath time, foot soaks, hair care, back massages, turning and positioning, passive range of motion) to provide tactile stimulation. Limit intrusive procedures and times when the patient needs to be uncomfortably manipulated.

Promoting Health Literacy

IN PATIENTS WITH HEARING DEFICITS

Patient Scenario

Mr. Rosato is 84 years old, and until recently had no difficulty hearing. He lives in a long-term care facility because of complications from several serious diseases: diabetes, congestive heart failure, high blood pressure, and degenerative joint disease. His daughter, who visits frequently, informs you, the nurse manager, that Mr. Rosato seems to be having increasing difficulty with hearing, although he denies this. She shares that he sometimes answers questions inappropriately or asks people to speak louder, and she noticed that his television volume is always loud. She made an appointment for him with an audiologist but shares that she does not know the first thing about hearing disorders.

Nursing Considerations: *Tips for Improving Health Literacy*

Compliment the daughter's keen observation, report that sensory disorders are common among older adults, and tell her how important the visit with the audiologist is. Give her an information sheet about hearing disorders and tips on finding out more information about the disorder online from a credible source. Encourage her to be prepared to ask the audiologist three questions:

- What is her father's main problem?
- What do they need to do?
- Why is it important for them to do this?

What additional measures can you take to help increase health literacy in this patient and his family? What other measures would be helpful if Mr. Rosato or his daughter does not speak English, cannot read, or has other learning deficits?

disabilities, and lack of English proficiency. Patients may also be at risk for inadequate health literacy because of hearing or visual impairments or confusion and inability to process or remember what is heard. See the Promoting Health Literacy box for ideas on how to help a patient with a hearing deficit. You can also download The Joint Commission white paper, "What Did the Doctor Say?": Improving Health Literacy to Protect Patient Safety, at https://www.jointcommission.org/assets/1/18/improving_health_literacy.pdf

MEETING THE NEEDS OF PATIENTS WITH REDUCED VISION

Always check with the health care provider to learn whether a patient's visual problem is temporary, permanent, partial, or complete, and the degree to which the problem is likely to affect the patient's everyday functioning. This information is vital to developing a realistic teaching plan or care plan.

The first priority is to teach patients self-care behaviors for maintaining vision and preventing blindness, such as the following:

- Know that regular exercise maintains blood flow to the eyes.
- Plentiful sleep keeps eyes lubricated and helps remove irritants.
- Do not rub the eyes.
- Avoid eyestrain (e.g., reading in poor light or viewing television or smart devices when tired).
- Avoid damage from ultraviolet rays.
- Protect eyes from foreign bodies.
- Keep eyeglasses clean, protected, and adjusted.
- Do not use nonprescription eye drops, and seek attention for symptoms.
- Do not clean eyes or contact lenses with soiled articles.
- Use caution with aerosol sprays.
- Use caution with ammonia, lye, and other chemical agents.
- Visit your health care provider frequently if you are prone to eye problems.
- Know the danger signals that indicate serious eye problems, including persistent eye redness; pain or discomfort, especially after injury; visual disturbances; crossing eyes; a growth on or near the eyes; discharge or increased tearing; and pupil irregularities.

When communicating with patients with reduced vision, follow these guidelines:

- Acknowledge your presence in the patient's room. Identify yourself by name.
- Speak in a normal tone of voice. Remember that the blind person is unable to pick up most nonverbal cues during communication.
- Explain the reason for touching the person before doing so.
- Keep the call light or bell within easy reach of the person and place the bed in the lowest position.
- Orient the person to sounds in the environment.
- Orient the person to the arrangement of the room and its furnishings. Clear pathways for the person, and do not rearrange furnishings; clarify this policy with housekeeping personnel.
- Assist with ambulation by walking slightly ahead of the person, allowing the person to grasp your arm.
- Stay in the person's field of vision if they have partial or reduced peripheral vision.
- Provide diversions using other senses.
- Indicate to the person when the conversation has ended and when you are leaving the room.

MEETING THE NEEDS OF PATIENTS WITH REDUCED HEARING

Temporary hearing losses are most often conductive in nature, that is, due to a problem with the external or middle ear (wax buildup, foreign-body obstruction, infection). However, sensorineural hearing losses caused by inner ear or central nervous system problems may not be totally correctable. Health teaching to prevent hearing problems includes the following recommendations for patients:

- Watch your weight, blood sugar level, and blood pressure to keep the tiny arteries that fuel hair cells in your ears healthy.
- Avoid excessive noise.
- Do not insert sharp objects into ears.
- Do not clean the ears excessively.
- Avoid practices that can cause infection; treat infection early.
- Use devices or aids to amplify the sound of your TV.
- Know the symptoms of hearing loss: asking others frequently to repeat what they said, an inability to hear at a distance, need to see the person who is talking, leaning forward or turning an ear toward the speaker, answering inappropriately, talking too loudly, inability to carry on a phone conversation, strained facial expression.

When communicating with patients who have hearing deficits or impairments, follow these guidelines:

- Orient the person to your presence before initiating conversation, such as by moving so you can be seen or by gently touching the person.
- Decrease background noises (television, radio), if possible, before you speak.
- Make sure that the patient's hearing aids (if applicable) are working optimally.
- Position yourself so that the light is on your face and the person can see your lips and expressions.
- Talk directly to the person while facing them, or angle your chair so that your voice reaches the ear that hears best. If the person can lip-read, use simple sentences and speak in a quiet, natural manner and pace. Be aware of nonverbal communication.
- Do not chew gum, cover your mouth, or turn away when talking with the person.
- Demonstrate or pantomime ideas you wish to express, as appropriate.
- Use sign language or finger spelling, as appropriate.
- Write any statement that you cannot convey to the person in another manner.

Aids for people with reduced hearing include telecommunication devices (TDDs), infrared systems, computers, voice amplifiers, amplified telephones, low-frequency doorbells and telephone ringers, closed-caption TV decoders, flashing alarm clocks, and flashing smoke detectors. The Centers for Disease Control and Prevention has numerous resources to prevent hearing loss (search for "hearing loss" at www.cdc.gov).

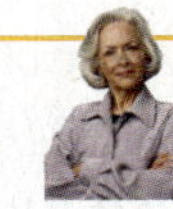

Dolores Pirolla, the wife of the patient who has a visual deficit and is now demonstrating signs of a hearing deficit. The nurse would incorporate knowledge of the guidelines (for communicating with people with reduced vision and hearing) when developing a teaching plan to assist Mrs. Pirolla in dealing with her husband's condition. In addition, the nurse could enlist the aid of social services to help Mrs. Pirolla obtain supportive services for her husband's visual impairment and obtain assistive devices for her husband to minimize the effects of the hearing deficit.

COMMUNICATING WITH A PATIENT WHO IS CONFUSED

Some patients who lack the mental ability to process environmental stimuli may be aware of this inability and find it frustrating. Such patients need support to make adjustments to this limitation. Other patients in a similar situation may be oblivious to their deficiency. In both instances, always protect the safety of the patient while providing optimal sensory stimulation.

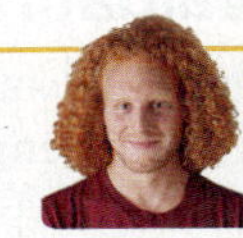

Ori Soltes, the patient in the ICU who becomes confused, most likely is experiencing a high level of frustration. Because of his accident, he suddenly is thrust into an environment filled with unfamiliar sights, sounds, and activities, leading to feelings of being overwhelmed physically and emotionally. His level of frustration may be further increased by his inability to speak while receiving mechanical ventilation.

Nursing interventions for the patient who is confused include the following:

- Use frequent face-to-face contact to maintain the patient's social dimension. Use touch when appropriate (e.g., walk arm in arm, hug, give a back rub).
- Speak calmly, simply, and directly to the patient and allow sufficient time for the patient to think before responding.
- Orient and reorient the patient to the environment, and fill the patient's personal space with as many personal objects as possible.
- Use conversation, watches, clocks, calendar, newspaper, television, radio, and other such devices to help orient the patient to time, place, and person.
- Clearly communicate that the patient is expected to perform all the self-care activities they can.
- Emphasize the patient's strengths rather than deficiencies, and verbally reinforce strengths.
- Offer the patient simple explanations for care, new activities, and so on.
- Vary environmental stimuli gradually while keeping the environment structured enough that the patient feels comfortable and at home.
- Use objects from the patient's past (e.g., a favorite baseball, a picture of a train, a photograph) to spark reminiscences and discussions.
- Reinforce reality if the patient is delusional.

A list of selected cognitive stimulation activities may be found in Chapter 8.

COMMUNICATING WITH A PATIENT WHO IS UNCONSCIOUS

The following are recommended guidelines for communicating with a patient who is unconscious:

- Be careful of what you say in the person's presence. Hearing is believed to be the last sense lost; therefore, the person is often likely to hear what is being said, even if there does not appear to be a response.
- Assume the person can hear you. Talk with the person in a normal tone of voice about things you would ordinarily discuss.
- Speak to the person before touching. Remember that touch can be an effective means of communicating with the unconscious person.
- Keep environmental noises at as low a level as possible. This helps the person focus on the communication.

Evaluating

While implementing a nursing care plan designed to decrease excessive sensory stimuli or increase meaningful stimuli, evaluate the plan's effectiveness by observing for a decrease in the behavioral manifestations of sensory deprivation or overload. You may conclude that the care plan is working if a patient who had begun to withdraw and spend most of the day lying in bed with a blank facial expression appears more alert and begins to initiate conversations and to take an interest in personal care. Also evaluate the patient's ability to interact appropriately with the environment while practicing necessary self-care behaviors, as well as the patient's need for nursing care versus the person's ability to manage the care plan independently.

Ideally, the patient and family learn to manipulate the environment to promote optimal sensory stimulation for growth and development. Patients with specific sensory impairments are evaluated for their knowledge of the impairment, acceptance and management of the treatment regimen, and their ability to perform necessary self-care activities. See the accompanying concept map for Ori Soltes and Evolving Case Study 45-1 for the Pirollas on pages 1854–1855.

REFLECTIVE PRACTICE LEADING TO PERSONAL LEARNING

Remember that the objective of reflective practice is to look at an experience, understand it, and learn from it. As you begin to develop your expertise in identifying and responding to sensory alterations, reflect on your experiences—successes and failures—in order to improve your practice. Are you routinely aware of your patients' environments and the degree to which these stimulate the senses? Have you ever identified sensory deprivation or overload and developed evidence-based strategies to address these problems. Have you encountered patients or their family caregivers whose sensory needs are unmet? Have you created partnerships with family caregivers to identify ways to stimulate senses of at-risk patients? Equally important, do you take mini-breaks and focus on your own experience, savoring the taste and texture of a summer tomato, marveling at the tenacity of a newborn grasping your finger, or quieting to listen to the next crack of thunder during a summer storm?

Perhaps the most important questions to reflect on are: Are your patients and their families/caregivers better for having had *you* share in the critical responsibility of partnering with them to stimulate their senses or improve their alterations in sensory perception? Are your patients now receiving thoughtful, person-centered, prioritized, holistic, evidence-based treatment and care because of your efforts?

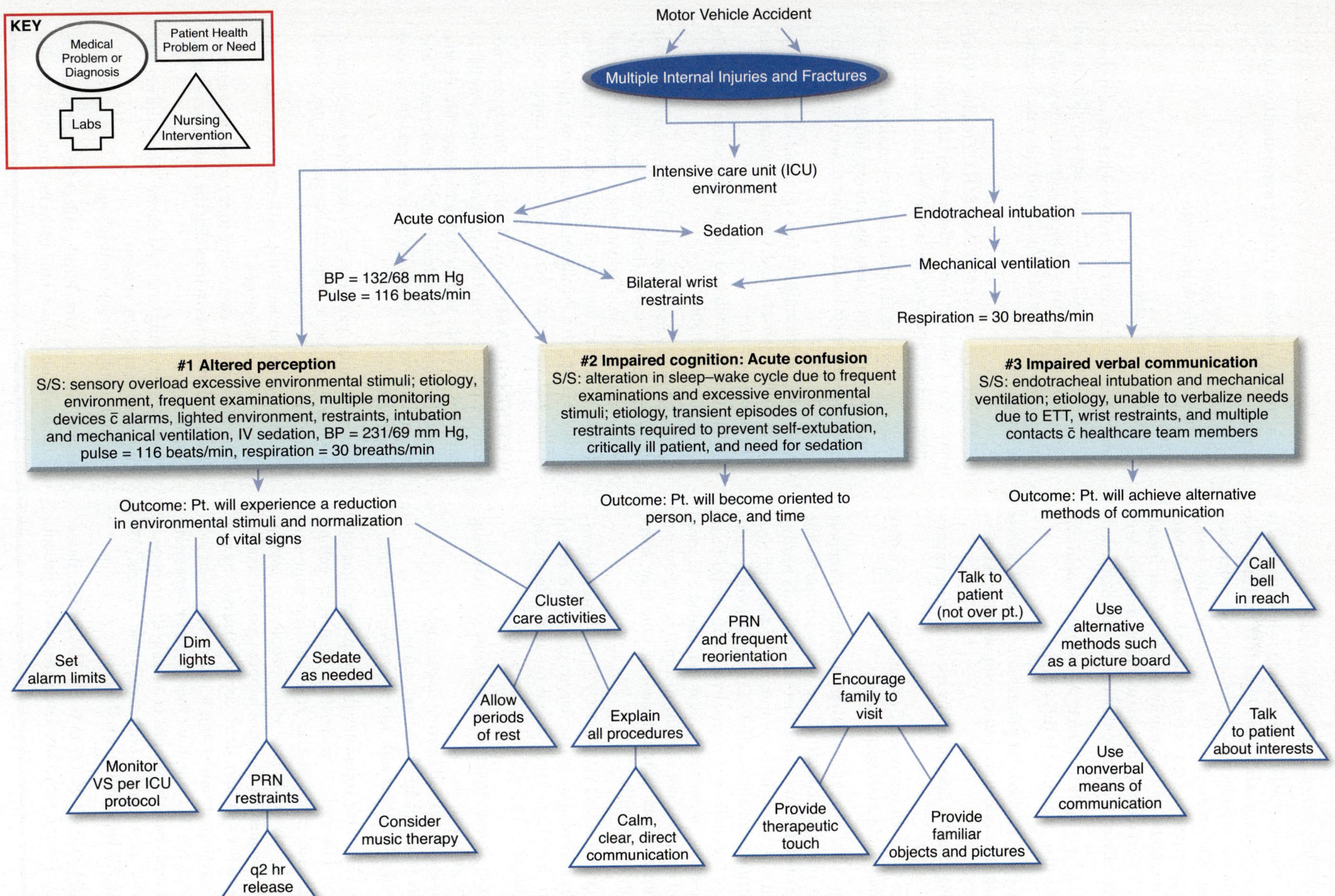

Evaluation

- **Diagnosis #1** Ori's environment has been managed to reduce stimuli. Sedation has only been required every 4 hours. Vital signs have returned to normal.
- **Diagnosis #2** Ori continues to exhibit transient periods of confusion but with decreasing frequency. Continue interventions.
- **Diagnosis #3** Ori has been unable to use picture board due to his weakened condition. Continue interventions.

Concept map that displays the use of the nursing process in designing a care plan for Ori Soltes. BP, blood pressure; c̄, with; ETT, endotracheal tube; HCP, health care provider; IV, intravenous; PRN, when necessary (from L. pro re nata); Pt., patient; q2, each/every (from L. *quaque*); S/S, signs and symptoms; VS, vital signs.

EVOLVING CASE STUDY 45-1

Scenario: Dolores Pirolla, a 74-year-old woman, comes to the older adult clinic with her 77-year-old husband, who was diagnosed with macular degeneration and progressive vision loss. She states, "Now I've noticed he's also having difficulty hearing me. I'm worried because he doesn't want to leave the house and we hardly see any of our friends anymore. We used to go out to the movies or dinner at least once a week. Lately, if we get out once a month, that's a lot!"

QUESTION r/t CUES: Which assessment should the nurse prioritize in caring for this couple?

A. Vision exam to check for progression in visual defects
B. Vital signs: temperature, pulse, respiration, blood pressure
C. Hearing exam to determine degree of hearing impairment
D. Degree to which sensory deficits are impacting ability to socialize and meet social needs

Scenario: After a brief discussion to establish rapport and flesh out their concerns, the nurse completes the physical assessment and notes that the husband's hearing on the left side is verifiably compromised, although he is not admitting to any difficulties hearing. Dolores is quite vocal about the challenges of now living with her husband who frequently cannot see or hear her, and she is most concerned about his not wanting to admit to any deficits and resulting serious diminishment of time they spent with family and friends.

QUESTION r/t ANALYZING CUES: The nurse is completing documentation in the electronic health record (EHR) on this client. How should the nurse document these findings?

A. Increasing social isolation as a result of increasing sensory impairment
B. Progressive visual and hearing impairment
C. Inability to accept aging and its decline
D. Impaired self-esteem with self-protective behaviors

Scenario: The nurse completes the documentation and says to the husband, "I understand that it is getting harder and harder for you to read and see your surroundings clearly and hear what people are saying, Mr. Pirolla. Frequently when this happens, people tend to isolate themselves so they don't get embarrassed by not hearing a question or answering it incorrectly, or by not seeing something. Do you think this might be happening to you? I know that Mrs. Pirolla is missing the frequency of times you used to meet with family and friends." He slowly nods his head that this is the case.

QUESTION r/t PRIORITIZING HYPOTHESIS: Based on the objective and subjective assessment of this patient, which priority problem should the nurse identify to guide the plan of care?

A. Sensory Deficit: Vision
B. Ineffective Health Maintenance
C. Social Isolation
D. Decreased Self Esteem

Scenario: The nurse opts to explore what visual or hearing aids might be tried to reduce the sensory deficits and to also explore what type of social interactions would be most comfortable for Mr. Pirolla and his wife, together and separately.

QUESTION r/t GENERATING SOLUTIONS: Which interventions will be most effective for addressing the sensory deficits and their impact on social interactions?

A. Making sure that his vision and eye exams are recent and accurately document his sensory deficits
B. Investigating their insurance plan to see what devices they can afford
C. Assessing which auditory and visual aids best improve Mr. Pirolla's sensory and social functioning and that he is willing to try
D. Identifying the family and friends with whom Mr. Pirolla is most comfortable

Scenario: When you next see the Pirollas, you notice that Mr. Pirolla seems more withdrawn—he responds only when pressed and only in one-word answers; he is not holding eye contact but instead looks down at his folded hands in his lap. Mrs. Pirolla remains animated, talks over her husband, and voices her frustration and impatience.

QUESTION r/t TAKING ACTION: Mr. Pirolla does not readily respond to questioning, leaving Mrs. Pirolla to speak for him. While you are trying to engage Mr. Pirolla, Mrs. Pirolla launches a tirade about his "stubbornness" and "insensitivity" to her needs. What is the priority nursing intervention?

A. Counsel both partners that accepting age-related changes can be a huge challenge and not solved quickly.
B. Remind both partners that, as Bette Davis said, "Old age is no place for sissies."
C. Use motivational counseling to try to identify each of their commitments to resolving the challenge of social isolation.
D. Repeat everything you told them before during the previous counseling session.
E. Recommend marriage counseling.

Scenario: Mr. and Mrs. Pirolla reflect on their situation and have articulated potential paths forward. Mrs. Pirolla

EVOLVING CASE STUDY 45-1 *(continued)*

is no longer visibly upset and is focused on attending to her husband. Mr. Pirolla is still formulating his thoughts and indicates he will discuss them with his wife at home.

QUESTION r/t EVALUATING OUTCOMES: Which of the following parameters must be in place to ensure a successful resolution of the reason for the Pirolla's initial visit? Select all that apply.

A. Mr. Pirolla is looking into adaptive devices (hearing aid, new glasses) to make socializing more possible for him.

B. Mrs. Pirolla reports that she no longer has to yell to get her husband's attention and that the TV can be kept at a moderate volume.

C. Mr. Pirolla regains 20/20 vision.

D. Mrs. Pirolla reports that her husband seems to be enjoying family visits more and no longer withdraws to his study.

E. Mrs. Pirolla reports that they both seem content with their "new normal" social life.

F. Mrs. Pirolla reports that they have pretty much resumed their active social life.

DEVELOPING CLINICAL REASONING AND CLINICAL JUDGMENT

1. Work through the Evolving Case Study 45-1, The Pirollas, to help develop your clinical reasoning and clinical judgment skills.
2. Describe the practical measures you would take to stimulate the senses of the following sensory-impaired patients. Think carefully about the special sensory needs that accompany different conditions.
   - A deaf child
   - A confused older adult
   - An adult man who has just lost his sight
   - A premature infant whose skin is extremely fragile
3. Visit a critical care unit with other students and list all the factors that contribute to sensory overload or deprivation. Try to identify how the critical care culture evolved in ways that are actually harmful to patients. Discuss which of these factors are unavoidable and which could be modified to better meet patient needs. Identify individualized nursing strategies to minimize sensory overload and deprivation.
4. Dolores Pirolla expresses concern about her husband's safety at home—especially when she is not present—because of his increasingly limited vision. What resources can you recommend to her to "safety proof" their house?
5. How do you respond to the following questions?
   a. My daughter seems bright enough, but her grades are barely passing. Could it be her eyesight?
   b. My mother who lives alone has been complaining of hearing music when there is no source for the music. I'm afraid she may be getting Alzheimer disease.
   c. I'm worried I might have COVID-19 because, all of a sudden, I've lost my sense of smell… what do you think?
   d. I am really worried about my children spending all their time in front of a screen now that the schools are closed. If it's not their schoolwork, it's their phones. This can't be good for their eyes, can it?

PRACTICING FOR NCLEX

1. A nurse in a long-term care facility notes that a patient with limited activity related to severe rheumatoid arthritis is at risk for sensory deprivation. Based on this information, which interventions will the nurse include in the care plan? Select all that apply.
   a. Using a lower tone when communicating with the patient
   b. Providing interaction with children and pets
   c. Decreasing environmental noise
   d. Ensuring that the patient shares meals with other patients
   e. Discouraging the use of sedatives
   f. Providing adequate lighting and clear pathways of clutter
2. A nurse in the neonatal intensive care unit (ICU) is planning care to reduce inappropriate sensory stimulation to their patients. Which interventions could the nurse include in the care plan? Select all that apply.
   a. Providing bright mobiles and objects for the neonate to look at
   b. Rocking the neonate frequently, especially when crying
   c. Maintaining reduced ambient light, similar to conditions in the womb
   d. Reducing vestibular stimulation, such as rocking
   e. Playing music or singing to the neonate to stimulate hearing
3. A nurse is assessing a patient for gustatory disturbances. Which question asked by the nurse would be appropriate for this assessment?
   a. "Have you been experiencing any loss of taste or strange tastes lately?"
   b. "Have you smelled odors lately that others cannot smell?"
   c. "Can you tell me what object I am placing in your hand right now?"
   d. "Have you found it difficult to communicate verbally?"

4. A nurse observes that a patient with a history of cataracts is sitting closer to the television than usual. When assessing the patient, which additional findings will the nurse anticipate?
   a. Clouding of the lens in one or both eyes
   b. Eye pain when performing close work
   c. Abrupt loss of vision
   d. Loss of central vision
5. A nurse supervises APs in a long-term care facility where many residents have presbycusis. What directions will the nurse give the APs to best promote communication with these patients?
   a. Provide patients with large-print written menus.
   b. Speak clearly and distinctly, using a lower tone of voice.
   c. Decrease tactile stimulation.
   d. Remind all patients to "call, not fall."
6. A patient is in the late stages of AIDS, which has affected their brain function and memory. The patient reports loneliness because his friends "are afraid to visit." Based on this data, what nursing intervention would best help meet the patient's need for sensory stimulation?
   a. Providing stimulation through music, television, or movies
   b. Assessing the patient's hearing and vision to ensure optimal function
   c. Ensuring the patient is able to transmit their message to others
   d. Arranging for a volunteer to sit with the patient each day
7. A home care nurse is visiting a group of patients. Which patient does the nurse identify as having the highest risk for sensory deprivation?
   a. Older adult confined to bed at home after a stroke
   b. Adolescent in an oncology unit working on homework
   c. Pregnant patient in active labor
   d. Toddler awaiting same-day surgery in a playroom
8. A nurse is caring for a patient with a traumatic spinal cord injury that resulted in paraplegia (paralysis) and sensory loss from the waist down. When obtaining data about this patient, what component of sensory function does the nurse plan to assess?
   a. Transmission of tactile stimuli
   b. Adequate stimulation in the environment
   c. Reception of visual and auditory stimuli
   d. General orientation and ability to follow commands
9. A school nurse is performing vision screenings on middle-school children. The nurse notes a student squinting and that their visual acuity using a Snellen's eye chart is 20/160. When questioned, the student states their grades have dropped, and they are having difficulty completing work on time. What is the best recommendation for the nurse to make to the student's guardian(s)?
   a. Purchase or prepare a calendar to organize assignments.
   b. Ensure the student understands what is expected of them in each class.
   c. Seek medical attention if the student has eye pain while at home.
   d. Obtain an appointment with an eye professional for further evaluation.
10. A nurse is caring for a patient with a severe hearing deficit who reads lips and uses sign language. Which nursing intervention would best prevent sensory alterations for this patient?
    a. Turning the radio or television volume up very loud and closing the door to his room
    b. Preventing embarrassment and emotional discomfort as much as possible
    c. Providing daily opportunities for them to participate in a social hour with six to eight people
    d. Encouraging daily participation in exercise and physical activity
11. In a group home where most residents have varying degrees of visual or hearing impairments and some are periodically confused, what nursing action is essential?
    a. Maintaining safety and preventing sensory deterioration
    b. Insisting that residents participate in as many self-care activities as possible
    c. Emphasizing and reinforcing individual patient strengths
    d. Encouraging reminiscence and life review in groups
12. A visiting nurse conducts a visit for an 11-month-old infant. The nurse finds the infant lying on the floor, rocking back and forth with a flat expression, and few vocalizations. Which nursing action would be appropriate at this time?

    Electronic Health Record 1/2/2025, 1000, Nurses note, age 8 months: infant not vocalizing or babbling; parents admit they do not know how to provide stimulation to the infant. The infant is cared for during working hours by the grandmother who has reduced vision. Parenting classes recommended to help promote sensory stimulation. S. Smith, RN 4/2/2025, 1300, Nurses note, age 11 months (follow-up visit): parents stated they attended parenting classes and that they provide sensory stimulation after work, as taught in the parenting classes. The infant is still cared for by the grandmother during working hours. S. Smith, RN

    a. Assessing the type of stimulation the infant has been receiving
    b. Removing the infant from the grandmother's care as the child has not progressed.

c. Explaining that their negligence has resulted in the child's speech delays
d. Taking no action, as this is expected behavior for an 11-month-old infant

13. A nurse is providing information on smoking cessation at a hospital health fair. The nurse teaches that smoking cessation may help prevent what problem?
a. Reduced vision due to macular degeneration
b. Glare from cataracts
c. Presbyopia and the need for corrective lenses
d. Reduced auditory senses

14. A nurse is caring for an older adult who has a severe visual deficit related to glaucoma. Which nursing action is most appropriate when providing care for this patient?
a. Assisting the patient to ambulate by walking slightly behind them and grasping the arm
b. Concentrating on the patient's sense of sight and limit diversions that involve other senses
c. Staying outside of the patient's field of vision when performing personal hygiene for them
d. Cueing the patient when the conversation has ended and when leaving the room

15. A school nurse is teaching a group of high school students about preventing hearing loss. What preventative actions does the nurse recommend? Select all that apply.
a. Use earphones when listening to music, podcasts, or other programs.
b. Do not insert objects such as cotton-tipped applicators into the ear.
c. Avoid playing contact sports.
d. Use ear protection when performing tasks with loud sounds.
e. It is best to begin screening for hearing loss at age 18 years.

16. A home care nurse is visiting an older adult with longstanding diabetes who reports pain and numbness in their feet. What education is most appropriate for this patient?
a. Take acetaminophen or over-the-counter analgesic when pain occurs.
b. Increase intake of foods containing vitamins B_6, B_{12}, and folate.
c. Explain that phantom limb pain can become chronic, but psychosocial support can help.
d. Validate the patient's understanding of foot care for patients with diabetes.

17. When caring for an older adult who repeatedly states their food does not taste as good as it used to, a nurse explains that which factors can contribute to loss of taste as patients age? Select all that apply.
a. Decreased sense of smell
b. Presbycusis
c. Medications
d. Diseases
e. Tobacco use
f. Presbyopia

18. During shift report, a nurse is told that their patient admitted with an electrolyte imbalance is experiencing delirium. For which finding consistent with delirium will the nurse assess?
a. Statements that they plan to harm themselves or take their own life
b. Chronic memory loss and personality changes
c. Acute confusion, disorientation, restlessness, or agitation
d. Ability to be aroused by extreme and/or repeated stimuli

ANSWERS WITH RATIONALES

1. **b, d, e.** For a patient who has sensory deprivation, the nurse provides interaction with children and pets, ensures that the patient shares meals with other patients, and discourages the use of sedatives. Using a lower tone (pitch) of voice is appropriate for a patient with a hearing deficit. Decreasing environmental noise helps relieve sensory overload. Providing adequate lighting and removing clutter is an intervention for a vision deficit; additionally, this promotes safety.

2. **c, d.** The neonatal ICU may be a source of excess sensory stimulation. It is recommended that medically fragile infants receive limited light (visuals stimuli) to simulate being in the womb as well as reduced vestibular stimulation. The nurse avoids activities that promote stimulation in this population including soothing, holding, rocking, and changes of position (tactile and kinesthetic sensations), singing and speaking to the neonate (auditory sensations), and changing patterns of light and shade, such as through the use of mobiles and bright objects (visual sensations).

3. **a.** When the nurse asks: "Have you been experiencing any strange tastes lately?" the nurse is assessing for gustatory disturbances. The question: "Have you smelled odors lately that others cannot smell?" assesses for olfactory disturbances. When the nurse asks: "Can you tell me what I am placing in your hand right now?" the nurse is assessing for tactile disturbances. The question "Have you found it difficult to communicate verbally?" assesses for transmission–perception–reaction.

4. **a.** Cataracts, clouding of the crystalline lens, cause altered sensory reception by interfering with the patient's ability to receive visual stimuli. The other options are not characteristic of cataracts.

5. **b.** Presbycusis is an expected decrease or loss of hearing as a result of the aging process. Speaking distinctly in lower frequencies is indicated. Obtaining large-print written material is appropriate for visual alterations. Decreasing tactile stimulation is appropriate for a patient with a sensory overload, and initiating a safety program to prevent falls is appropriate for a patient experiencing kinesthetic/visceral alterations.

6. **d.** This patient is receiving decreased environmental stimuli (e.g., from lack of visitors) and may experience problems with reception because of brain involvement. The other options

do not alleviate the sensory deprivation of loneliness and isolation.

7. **a.** The patient confined to bed rest at home has a high risk for greatly reduced environmental stimuli. The other patients are in environments in which environmental stimuli are present.

8. **a.** Trauma to the spinal cord can cause both motor and sensory loss, interfering with transmission of tactile stimuli. Although the other options may be assessed, they do not relate to the spinal cord injury.

9. **d.** Visual acuity of 20/160 indicates myopia; this student sees at 20 feet what a person with normal vision can see at 160 feet. The impaired vision is interfering with their academic performance, and further assessment by an eye care professional is indicated. Corrective lenses or a prescription change may be needed. Eye pain is not a symptom of myopia. Although the other options may represent appropriate interventions, they do not flow from the data presented.

10. **c.** Providing opportunities for the patient to socialize builds on their strength of being able to lip-read and helps prevent sensory deprivation from hearing loss. Although all the options may be appropriate, they do not address improving sensory deprivation from hearing loss.

11. **a.** Safety is a basic physiologic need that must be met before higher-level needs—such as love and belonging, self-esteem, and self-actualization—can be met.

12. **a.** Using the first step of the nursing process, assessment, the nurse determines if the types of stimulation given by the infant's parents validate that they understand the education provided at the parenting classes. The grandmother's reduced vision would not impact the child's speech. While the infant's development is not progressing, accusing the parents of negligence is premature; further evaluation by a health care provider may be indicated. It is not the nurse's role to remove a child from a family's care.

13. **a.** Macular degeneration is the leading cause of blindness in older adults. Glare from cataracts is an expected symptom, not caused by smoking. There is no indication that smoking is related to the other options.

14. **d.** When caring for a patient who has a visual deficit, the nurse should indicate when the conversation is over and when they are leaving the room. When assisting with ambulation, the nurse should walk slightly ahead of (rather than behind) the patient and allow them to grasp the nurse's arm. The nurse should provide, rather than limit, diversions using other senses, and remain in the person's field of vision if partial or reduced peripheral vision is present.

15. **b, d.** To prevent hearing loss, the nurse teaches students to avoid concentrating sound in the ear canal, such as when using earphones. In addition, they should not insert objects such as cotton-tipped applicators into the ear canal. For occupations or activities with load sounds, ear protection should be worn. Contact sports are not typically associated with hearing loss. Screening for hearing loss should be performed annually in school-age children.

16. **d.** Patients with diabetes can develop peripheral neuropathy resulting in loss of sensation and reduced blood flow. The loss of sensation can promote injury the patient does not readily notice. Therefore, those with diabetes must perform special foot care and visual inspection. The nurse does not prescribe analgesics (medications). Vitamins are indicated when the underlying cause of numbness is identified as a vitamin deficiency. While a decrease in gustatory senses is expected in the older adult, it is unrelated to numbness and pain in the feet.

17. **a, c, d, e.** As the patient ages, gustatory senses, along with sense of smell, some medications, and smoking can blunt the taste (gustatory sense). Presbycusis refers to the reduced ability to hear, and presbyopia refers to the inability of the lens to accommodate to near (or far) objects.

18. **c.** Delirium is a state of acute confusion manifested by disorientation, restlessness, hallucinations, and agitation. Dementia is a chronic progressive illness characterized by difficulties with spatial orientation, memory, language, and changes in personality. Option a describes a patient who has thoughts of suicide, and option d describes a patient who is displaying stupor. A stuporous state indicates the patient can be aroused briefly by extreme and/or repeated stimuli.

Bibliography

Ackerman, D. (1990). *A natural history of the senses*. Vintage Books.

Allard, M. E., & Katseres, J. (2016). Using essential oils to enhance nursing practice and for self-care. *American Journal of Nursing, 116*(2), 42–49.

Boltz, M., Capezuti, E., Fulmer, T., & Zwicker, D. (2016). *Evidence-based geriatric nursing protocols for best practice* (5th ed.). Springer Publishing Company.

Bush, H. I., LaGasse, A. B., Collier, E. H., Gettis, M. A., & Walson, K. (2021). Effect of live versus recorded music on children receiving mechanical ventilation and sedation. *American Journal of Critical Care, 30*(5), 343–349.

Carlson, C., Howe, T., Pedersen, C., & Yoder, L. H. (2020). Caring for visually impaired patients in the hospital: A multidisciplinary quality improvement project. *American Journal of Nursing, 120*(5), 48–55.

Chiu, A. (2020, November 5). COVID-19, in addition to stealing sense of smell, may also warp it. *The Washington Post*, p. 12.

Diamond, K. (2020, September 8). The Strange Grief of Losing My Sense of Taste. *The New York Times*, A23.

Ding, Q., Redeker, N. S., Pisani, M. A., Yaggi, H. K., & Knauert, M. P. (2017). Factors influencing patients' sleep in the intensive care unit: Perceptions of patients and clinical staff. *American Journal of Critical Care, 26*(4), 278–286.

Goeren, D., John, S., Meskill, K., Iacono, L., Wahl, S., & Scanlon, K. (2018). Quiet time: A noise reduction initiative in a neurosurgical intensive care unit. *Critical Care Nurse, 38*(4), 38–44.

Golino, A. J., Leone, R., Gollenberg, A., Christopher, C., Stanger, D., Davis, T. M., Meadows, A., Zhang, Z., & Friesen, M. A. (2019). Impact of an active music therapy intervention on intensive care patients. *American Journal of Critical Care, 28*(1), 48–55.

Gorisek, R., Mayer, C., Hicks, W. B., & Barnes, J. (2021). An evidence-based initiative to reduce alarm fatigue in a burn intensive care unit. *Critical Care Nurse, 41*(4), 29–37.

Hammond, L., & Pullen, R. L. Jr. (2020). Managing loneliness and chronic illness in older adults. *Nursing, 50*(12), 22–28.

HealthyPeople.gov. (n.d.). *Healthy People 2030: Sensory and communication disorders*. https://health.gov/healthypeople/objectives-and-data/browse-objectives/sensory-or-communication-disorders

Heiting, G., & Wan, L. K. (2022, April). *Computer eye strain: 10 steps for relief*. https://www.allaboutvision.com/cvs/irritated.htm

Hetland, B., Lindquist, R., Weinert, C. R., Peden-McAlpine, C., Savik, K., & Chlan, L. (2017). Predictive associations of music, anxiety, and sedative exposure on mechanical ventilation weaning trials. *American Journal of Critical Care, 26*(3), 210–220.

Jarvis, B. (2021, January 31). The forgotten sense. *The New York Times Magazine*, pp. 20–25, 46–47, 49.

The Joint Commission. (2007). *"What did the doctor say?": Improving health literacy to protect patient safety*. https://www.jointcommission.org/assets/1/18/improving_health_literacy.pdf

Kearney, R. (2021). *Touch: Recovering our most vital sense*. Columbia University Press.

Koomar, J., Kranowitz, C., Szklut, S., Balzer-Martin L., Haber E., & Sava D. I. (2001). *Answers to questions teachers ask about sensory integration: Forms, checklists, and practical tools for teachers and parents*. Sensory World.

Kranowitz, C. S. (2005). *The out-of-sync child. Recognizing and coping with sensory processing disorder*. Penguin Group.

Lane, K. R., & Conn, V. S. (2013). To hear or not to hear. *Research in Gerontological Nursing, 6*(2), 79–80.

Lindsay, L. (2021). COVID-19-related smell and taste disorders: A guide for nurses. *Nursing, 51*(4), 50–53.
Miller, C. R., Patmon, F. L., & Knapp, H. (2021). Music to reduce stress in hospitalized patients. *Nursing, 51*(8), 62–66.
National Academy of Sciences, Engineering, and Medicine. (2020). *Social isolation and loneliness in older adults: Opportunities for health care system.* https://www.nap.edu/catalog/25663/social-isolation-and-loneliness-in-older-adults-opportunities-for-the
Navarro-Ruiz, N. E. (2020). Prevention of platinum-induced hearing loss in children with cancer. *American Journal of Nursing, 120*(6), 21.
Parker, A. M., Aldabain, L., Akhlaghi, N., Glover, M., Yost, S., Velaetis, M., Lavezza, A., Mantheiy, E., Albert, K., & Needham, D. M. (2021). Cognitive stimulation in an intensive care unit: A qualitative evaluation of barriers to and facilitators of implementation. *Critical Care Nurse, 41*(2), 51–60.
Paturel, A. (July–August 2017). *Saving our 5 senses as we age.* AARP Bulletin. https://www.aarp.org/health/conditions-treatments/info-2017/hearing-loss-senses-decline-age.html
Purvis, K. B., McKenzie, L. B., Cross, D. R., & Razuri, E. B. (2013). A spontaneous emergence of attachment behavior in at-risk children and a correlation with sensory deficits. *Journal of Child and Adolescent Psychiatric Nursing, 26*(3), 165–172.
Quach, J., & Lee, J. A. (2017). Do music therapies reduce depressive symptoms and improve QOL in older adults with chronic disease? *Nursing, 47*(6), 58–63.
Shaw, R. (2016). Using music to promote sleep for hospitalized adults. *American Journal of Critical Care, 25*(2), 181–184.
Spiegelberg, J., Song, H., Pun, B., Webb, P., & Boehm, L. M. (2020). Early identification of delirium in intensive care unit patients: Improving the quality of care. *Critical Care Nurse, 40*(2), 33–44.

46 Sexuality

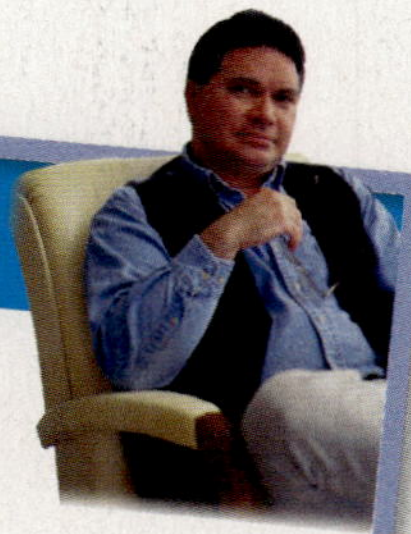

Jefferson Smith

Jefferson, a middle-aged man with a history of diabetes and hypertension, is receiving numerous medications as treatment. During a routine visit to his primary care provider, Mr. Smith confides that he has been having problems "in the bedroom." He reports difficulty attaining and maintaining an erection.

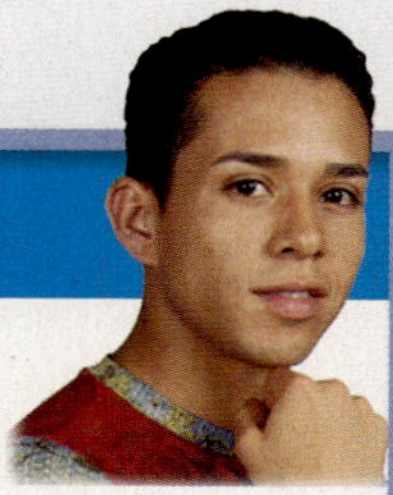

Paul Rojas

Paul, a young adult man who has told the health care team he is gay, was diagnosed with AIDS. He comes to the clinic today for infusion therapy, which usually takes several hours. Mr. Rojas comments to the nurse, "You don't feel comfortable with me, do you?"

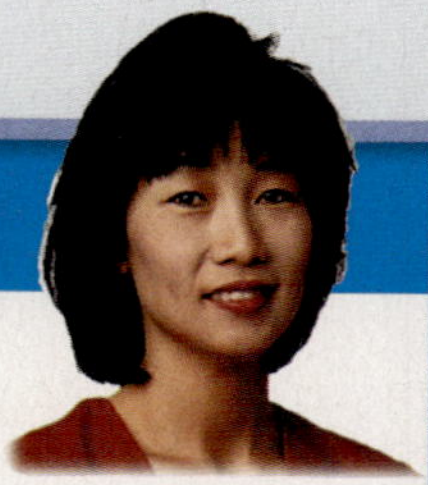

Amy Liu

Amy is a middle-aged woman who had a hysterectomy about a year ago for excessive uterine bleeding due to multiple uterine fibroids. She comes to the clinic for a checkup and begins to cry during the assessment. She says, "I don't feel like a woman anymore. My husband and I used to have a wonderful sexual relationship, but now I rarely want to have sexual intercourse, and when I do, it hurts. My husband is being so patient, but I don't know how much longer he'll put up with me! What's wrong with me?"

Learning Outcomes

After completing the chapter, you will be able to accomplish the following:

1. Describe reproductive anatomy and physiology.
2. Describe the sexual response cycle, differentiating individual responses.
3. Describe the concepts of sexuality, gender, gender identity, sexual orientation, and sexual health.
4. Perform a sexual assessment, using suggested interview questions and appropriate physical assessment skills.
5. Describe types of sexual dysfunction and the assessment priorities for each.
6. Identify actual and potential health problems with sexuality that may be addressed by independent nursing actions.
7. Plan, implement, and evaluate nursing care related to selected identification of problems involving facets of sexuality.
8. Assess how your personal beliefs and values about human sexuality affect your ability to deliver competent, compassionate, and respectful care to patients with challenges, differences, or problems with sexuality.
9. Describe effective responses to sexual harassment by patients or colleagues.

Nursing Concepts

- Diversity
- Identity
- Reproduction
- Sexuality

A critical component of human identity and well-being, **sexuality** encompasses biological sex or sex assigned at birth, sexual activity (including pleasure, intimacy, and reproduction), gender identities and roles, and sexual orientation (World Health Organization [WHO], 2006, 2021). It involves how a person both exhibits and experiences sexuality physically, emotionally, and mentally. Edelman and Kudzma (2022) define sexuality as the "behavioral expression of sexual identity" (p. 161). Sexuality includes learned behaviors that affect how people respond to their own sexuality and how they behave in relationships with others. Cultural, biological, sociopolitical, legal, economic, religious, spiritual, and historical factors influence sexuality (WHO, 2006, 20121). Sexuality can be an integral part of a person's identity and is present in a person's demeanor through actions, communications, and physical appearance (see the Reflective Practice box on page 1862 for an example).

SEXUAL HEALTH

Sexual health represents the integration of the somatic, emotional, intellectual, and social aspects of sexual being, in ways that are positively enriching and that enhance personality, communication, and love. Because our sexuality is so basic to our sense of self, nurses need to value sexuality as a critical element of general health and well-being. The WHO (2021) identifies the following critical elements of positive, holistic sexual health:

- Sexual health is about well-being, not merely the absence of disease.
- Sexual health involves respect, safety, and freedom from discrimination and violence.
- Sexual health depends on the fulfillment of certain human rights.
- Sexual health is relevant throughout the individual's lifespan, not only to those in the reproductive years, but also to both the young and the elderly.
- Sexual health is expressed through diverse sexualities and forms of sexual expression.
- Sexual health is critically influenced by gender norms, roles, expectations, and power dynamics.
- Sexual health needs to be understood within specific social, economic, and political contexts.

Nurses must be skilled in identifying and addressing problems related to sexual self-concept, body image, sexual identity, sexual activity, and sexual discrimination or violence.

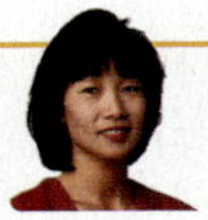

Think back to **Amy Liu,** the woman who reported changes in sexual desire and pain with intercourse. As a result of these changes, she reported, "not feeling like a woman anymore." The nurse would interpret her statements as reflecting a change in her self-concept and body image secondary to her sexual health issues.

Sexual identity encompasses a person's self-identity, biological sex, gender identity, gender role behavior or expression, and sexual orientation. Biological sex or the sex assigned/documented at birth, is the term used to denote chromosomal sexual development: male (XY) or female (XX), external and internal genitalia, secondary sex characteristics, and hormonal states.

There are instances of difference in sex/sexual development (DSD) that may result in contradictions among chromosomal sex, gonadal sex, internal organs, and external genital appearance (previously referred to as intersex; Dwyer & Greenspan, 2021). Sex assignment with these infants presents a very difficult decision for parents and the entire interprofessional team. Should the parents make the decision based on advice from the provider, or should the decision be postponed until the child is old enough to participate? Challenges exist with the timing of assigning sex (along with the gender implications), physical changes that occur at puberty, and the potential for gender identity disorder (GID). Each patient with DSD is unique and often benefits from ongoing psychosexual care and support (Babu & Shah, 2021).

QSEN Reflective Practice: Cultivating QSEN Competencies

CHALLENGE TO INTERPERSONAL SKILLS

During my clinical experience in the HIV/infectious disease clinic, I met Paul Rojas, a single young adult man who is gay and was diagnosed with AIDS. One day, he came to the clinic for infusion therapy, which usually takes several hours.

I was a 20-year-old, single woman who identifies as heterosexual. I had no personal experience with gay or lesbian friends, or with people who identify as bisexual or use other terms to describe their sexual orientation. I was confused and uncertain about how to respond to Paul. How should I approach him? What would we talk about during these several hours at the clinic? I was sure my instructor thought this would be a "great learning experience," but what was I supposed to learn? Usually quite self-confident, I was confused, uncomfortable, and uncertain as to how to act.

Thinking Outside the Box: Possible Courses of Action

- Hide my discomfort and simply provide the technical nursing care Paul needs; spend as little time as possible in his room.
- Refuse this assignment because I am unsure I can provide the care Paul needs.
- Talk with my instructor or another experienced nurse who I respect about my questions and concerns.
- Share with Paul that this is my first experience working with a gay patient and ask him what I should know; spend extra time getting to know him and his experiences with other health care professionals.

Evaluating a Good Outcome: How Do I Define Success?

- Provide the nursing care he needs in a manner that is respectful.
- Learn from this experience how to be respectful of all patients and to interact in a way that affirms their human dignity.
- Gain knowledge about sexual orientation through this experience.

Personal Learning: Here's to the Future!

I met Paul and did exactly what I didn't want to do: I completed the technical nursing care such as vital signs and intravenous care, and then got out of the room as quickly as possible. It wasn't until almost the end of his treatment that he asked me, "You don't feel comfortable with me, do you?" When I answered truthfully that I was very uncertain how to best interact with him due to my lack of exposure and experience, Paul took the lead and began to share stories about his life. When I look back now and realize I almost allowed my fear to prevent me from providing person-centered care to Paul, I could kick myself. Not all patients are willing or need to talk about their sexuality, but Paul recognized that I was an inexperienced student nurse and took the time to explain that his sexuality was integral to who he was as a person. For Paul, it was important I learn to consider sexuality when providing patient care. He opened the door to new perspectives. I hope I always remember to treat patients how they want to be treated and appreciate when they teach me about themselves and their experiences.

QSEN SELF-REFLECTION ON QUALITY AND SAFETY COMPETENCIES DEVELOPING KNOWLEDGE, SKILLS, AND ATTITUDES FOR CONTINUOUS IMPROVEMENT

Do you agree with the criteria that the student nurse used to evaluate a successful outcome? Why or why not? What *knowledge, skills,* and *attitudes* do you need to develop to continuously improve the quality and safety of care for patients?

Patient-Centered Care: How would you develop a respectful and successful partnership with Paul, given your initial fears? How can you best communicate empathy and respect and use this opportunity to learn about Paul and his experiences? How will this experience affect your ability to consider sexuality when interacting with patients? Explain how the nursing student's truthful response to the patient's question affected the therapeutic relationship.

Teamwork and Collaboration/Quality Improvement: What communication and interpersonal skills do you need to improve to ensure that you function as a member of the patient care team? Who might the student have turned to for help when first acknowledging her discomfort? What does quality care for Paul look like?

Safety/Evidence-Based Practice: What does the evidence point to as best practice for Paul? What safety needs does he have and how can you meet them?

Informatics: Can you identify the essential information that must be available in Paul's electronic record to support safe patient care and coordination of care? Are smart devices available for you to use to learn more about Paul and his experiences? Can you think of other ways to respond to or approach the situation? What else might the nursing student have done to ensure a successful outcome?

Gender is not the same as biological sex or sexual orientation; they are distinct concepts. **Gender identity** is the inner sense a person has of being male, female, or nonbinary, which may be the same as or different from that person's biological sex or sex assigned at birth. **Gender expression** is how a person presents themselves to the world, is often expressed on a continuum, and may or may not correspond to gender identity. **Gender diverse** is a term that represents a wide range of gender identities that may vary from expected developmental norms; it includes nonbinary, genderqueer, and gender fluid identities (American Psychological Association [APA], 2020; Dwyer & Greenspan, 2021). People who experience clinically significant distress or impairment because their biological sex or sex assigned at birth is contrary to their gender identity are diagnosed with **gender dysphoria**, a concept designated in the *Diagnostic and Statistical Manual of Mental Disorders* (*DSM-5*). It is important to note that not all transgender or gender diverse individuals experience gender dysphoria (American Psychiatric Association, 2021). **Cisgender** refers to a gender identity or role performance that matches society's expectations based on biological sex. For example, a woman who identifies as cisgender would have a vagina and clitoris (biologically female) and would identify as female (gender).

Transgender, frequently shortened to *trans*, is a term that describes a wide range of experiences or identities where gender identification and expression differ from societal expectations that are based on a person's biological sex. For example, a person born biologically male (penis and scrotum) may identify as female (gender). More specifically, transgender is an inclusive term used to describe those who feel that the sex that was assigned to them at birth incompletely describes or fails to describe them at all. This term includes:

- People who have a gender expression that differs from their biological sex or sex assigned at birth (according to societal norms)
- People who have DSD where their reproductive or sexual anatomy does not fit the typical definition of male or female
- People who identify outside the female/male binary
- People who identify as having no gender or multiple genders

For many transgender people, the solution is to change their bodies, through surgery, hormone therapy, or both, to match their inner feelings; this process is referred to as *transitioning*. The surgery is frequently referred to as *gender affirmation surgery* or *gender confirmation surgery*. The terminology used for the surgery is significant because it reinforces the belief that the surgery is realigning a person with their actual gender.

Teens who are transgender face the reality of puberty, where their body will go through biological changes that betray who they feel they are or who they want to be. Puberty blockers, medications that pause puberty, may be taken to block secondary sex characteristics for a few years. They are generally safe, and their effects are reversible. Exogenous hormones (testosterone or estrogen) may also be administered. When the teen reaches the age of consent and has solidified their gender identification, surgery may be a viable, even medically necessary option (WPATH, 2016). Typically, genital surgery requires two mental health evaluations to confirm gender dysphoria, capacity for informed consent, 12 continuous months of hormone use, control of significant medical or mental health concerns, and living in the gender to which a person is transitioning (WPATH, 2012).

Gender binary (male or female identification) is not the only option. *Gender fluid* describes a person whose gender identification and behaviors shift from time to time, whether within or outside of societal, gender-based expectations. There is an emerging understanding that external genitalia do not always dictate gender identification or gender expression. Some people identify as nonbinary and may prefer the gender-neutral pronouns *they* and *their* rather than *him/her* or *his/her*. For inclusivity and to promote bias-free language in published works, the American Psychological Association (2020) now integrates gender-neutral language into their format and style guidelines (which is reflected in this textbook). Each person's experience is individual, and the vocabulary and terms continue to evolve. There is a growing understanding that asking people their pronouns is appropriate, but a nuanced approach is helpful to maintain rapport in the healthcare environment (Das, 2021). For a current glossary, check out the University of California—Davis Lesbian, Gay, Bisexual, Transgender, Queer, Intersex, Asexual (LGBTQIA) Resource Center at https://lgbtqia.ucdavis.edu/educated/glossary.html.

People experience sexual satisfaction in many ways; what is considered normal differs from one person to another and among cultures. **Sexual orientation** refers to romantic, emotional, affectionate, or sexual attraction to other people (Regents of the University of California, Davis campus, 2020). In general, gender identity is one's psychological self-identification, whereas sexual orientation is who one is attracted to physically, emotionally, and/or romantically. The origins of sexual orientation are unknown, but many studies claim a genetic basis. Some sexual preferences are culturally determined or may be dictated by opportunity.

Although there is possible fluidity and ongoing debate regarding the human sexuality spectrum, commonly identified sexual orientations are as follows:

- **Heterosexual** or *straight* refers to a person who is attracted to a person of the opposite gender.
- **Gay** (males or females) or **lesbian** (females) refers to a person attracted to members of the same gender. (Note that the term *homosexual* is outdated and no longer considered appropriate [GLAAD, n.d.].)
- **Bisexual** refers to a person who is attracted to both males and females. A bisexual relationship or encounter does not necessarily mean a person is gay.
- *Asexual* refers to a person who lacks romantic or sexual attraction to others.
- *Questioning* refers to a person who is unsure of their sexual orientation.

GLAAD's Accelerating Acceptance 2021 survey of more than 2,517 adults provides insight into some trends. Non-LGBTQ Americans recognize that gender is not limited to female and male; the vast majority polled (81%) identified that transgender and nonbinary identities will become an even more familiar part of life, similar to gay and lesbian orientations. Reports of discrimination against LGBTQ persons have increased since 2020, with 6 in 10 LGBTQ people (59%) reporting discrimination based on their sexual orientation and/or gender identity (GLAAD, 2021). Education of children in the history of LGBTQ individuals remains a point of discomfort with non-LGBTQ people. Cultural and sociopolitical trends will continue to impact on the acceptance of the LGBTQ community (GLAAD, 2021).

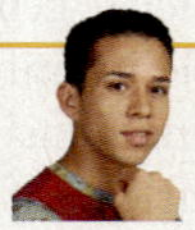

Consider **Paul Rojas,** the patient with AIDS, who is gay. The nurse would need to also consider his gender identity and gender role behaviors to gain a fuller understanding of his sexual identity and to provide appropriate care.

SEXUAL EXPRESSION

The methods by which people gain satisfaction through sexual stimulation are varied. Touches, smells, sights, sounds, feelings, thoughts, and fantasies can all contribute to sexual fulfillment in any form of expression chosen by people. Feelings of love for another person are closely associated with desire (Fig. 46-1).

Forms of sexual stimulation include kissing, hugging, stroking, squeezing, breast stimulation, manual stimulation of the genitals, oral–genital stimulation, and anal stimulation. Sexual stimulation may be physical or psychological. Erotic stimulation through the use of films, magazines, and photographs is common. Fetishism, more often practiced by males, is sexual arousal with the aid of an inanimate object not generally associated with sexual activity. Items such as shoes, leather, rubber, and women's undergarments might be used.

On a continuum, sexual behavior ranges from adaptive to maladaptive. Adaptive responses meet the following criteria:

- Between two consenting adults
- Mutually satisfying to both
- Not psychologically or physically harmful to either
- Lacking in force or coercion
- Conducted in private

Maladaptive sexual responses are behaviors that do not meet one or more of the criteria for adaptive responses (Boyd & Luebbert, 2022; Stuart, 2013).

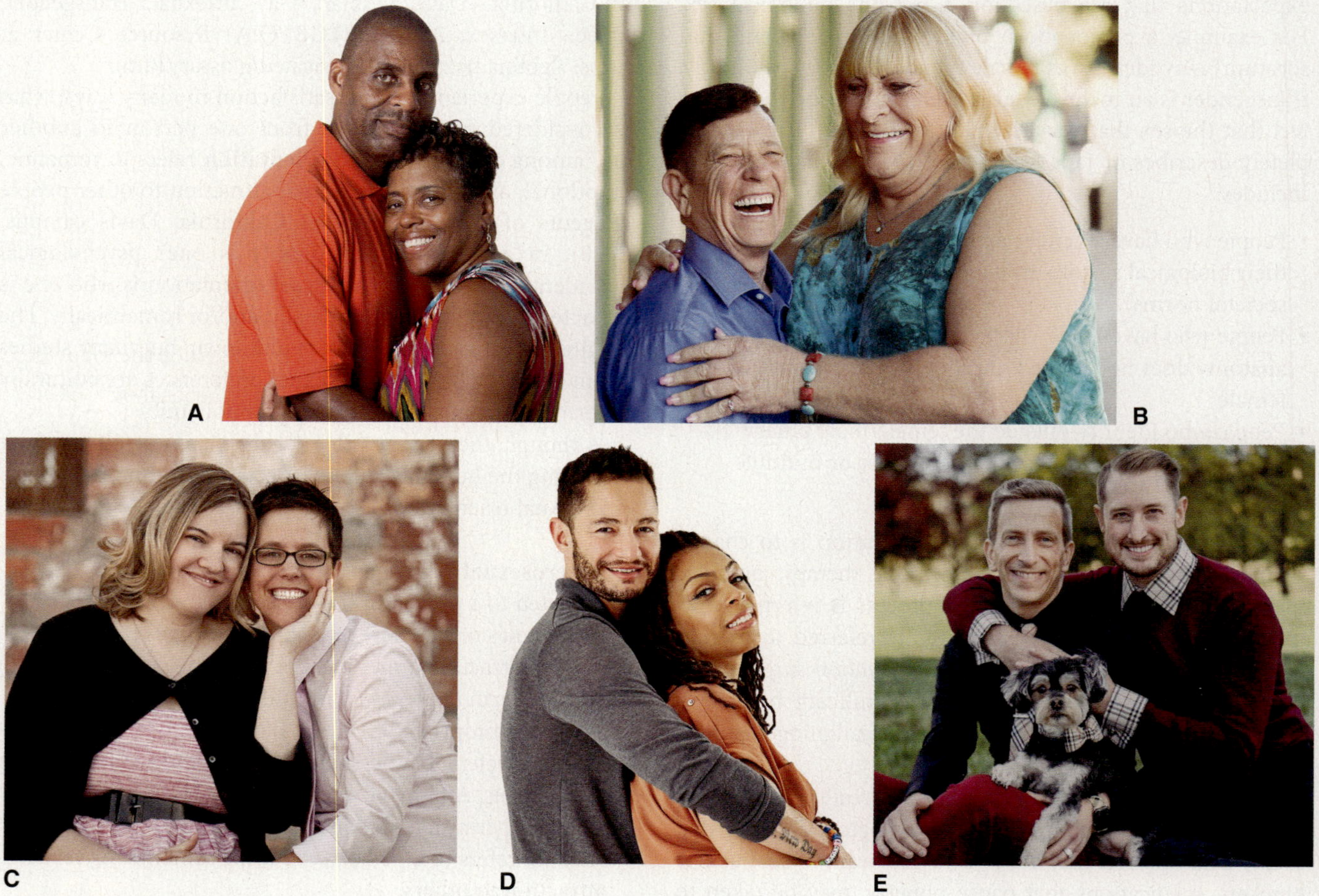

FIGURE 46-1. Gender identity, biological sex or sex assigned at birth, and sexual preference may vary, but here are just a few examples of self-identified couples. (*Source:* Used with permission from Shutterstock. *Photos by Hogan Imaging* [**A**], *CREATISTA* [**B**, **C**], and *Monsterstock* [**D**]. **E** courtesy of Paul Harwerth.)

Masturbation

Masturbation is a technique of sexual expression in which a person practices self-stimulation. It is a way for people to learn what they prefer during stimulation and what feels good. Males masturbate by holding and stroking the shaft of the penis. Females find manual stimulation of the clitoris enjoyable, although variations of technique are numerous. Many myths and misinformation surround masturbation. The reality is that people masturbate regardless of sex, gender, age, or marital status. People might not masturbate if they feel guilty about it or believe self-stimulation is wrong. Masturbation is not dirty and will not lead to blindness or insanity.

Sexual Intercourse

The act of **intercourse** (coitus or copulation) is the insertion of the penis into the partner's vagina, anus, or mouth. It usually begins by stimulation of the senses in some way, followed by a period of activity known as foreplay. *Petting* is part of foreplay; it can involve simple stroking of the breasts, arms, back, and neck without genital involvement or may lead to mutual masturbation and orgasm.

Vaginal Intercourse

The act of placing the penis in the vagina, penile–vaginal intercourse, can be accomplished in various positions. The most common position in Western cultures is the *missionary position*, in which the female lies horizontally underneath the male. You may find it interesting that the Polynesians named this position because it was the preferred position for intercourse used by religious missionaries. Couples may find other positions to be more stimulating and comfortable. Clitoral stimulation is difficult to achieve in the missionary position. Lying side by side, female on top, and rear entry are some examples of coital positions that enable clitoral stimulation. Sexually inhibited people may believe they need permission to engage in alternative sexual positions.

When the penis is pushed into the vagina, the male begins rhythmic thrusting movements of the hips to move the penis back and forth along the vaginal walls. The female may match their partner's hip movements with movements of their own body. These movements continue until orgasm is attained by one person or both. Similar vaginal stimulation for the female can be performed with fingers or a synthetic sex toy.

Simultaneous orgasms, or both people attaining orgasm at the same moment, are difficult to achieve. A preoccupation with attaining simultaneous orgasms might disrupt the ultimate intimacy and satisfaction possible during coitus.

The period after coitus is just as significant as the events leading up to it. Caressing, hugging, and kissing deepen the couple's intimacy and should be nurtured, not rushed.

Anal Intercourse

Anal intercourse, the act of inserting the penis into the anus and rectum of a partner, is another form of intercourse. Commonly practiced by gay men, it is also used by lesbians and heterosexual couples. Once the penis (or any object) is placed in the rectum, it should not be introduced into the vagina without thorough cleansing because many microorganisms present in the rectum can cause vaginal infections. Care should be used to avoid injury to the delicate rectal mucosa, and lubrication is essential for comfort.

Condoms are now recommended for both vaginal and anal intercourse to prevent sexually transmitted infections (STIs).

Oral–Genital Stimulation

Stimulation of the genitals by the mouth and tongue might be used during foreplay or as a way to reach orgasm. Cunnilingus is stimulation of the female genitals by licking and sucking the clitoris and surrounding structures. Fellatio is stimulation of the male genitals by licking and sucking the penis and surrounding structures. One partner or both may use these techniques simultaneously (commonly known as *69* or *sixty-nine*). Some people may use oral–genital stimulation as a replacement for vaginal intercourse to avoid pregnancy.

Abstinence

Abstinence is not having sex. It is the most effective form of birth control, preventing pregnancy 100% of the time when practiced consistently. Abstinence also prevents the transmission of STIs 100% of the time when practiced appropriately and consistently (Centers for Disease Control and Prevention [CDC], 2021a). Some STIs spread through oral–genital sex, anal sex, or even intimate skin-to-skin contact without actual penetration (genital warts and herpes can be spread this way). Therefore, only avoiding all types of intimate genital contact can prevent these STIs. Avoiding all types of intimate genital contact—including anal and oral sex—is complete abstinence. There are no side effects or health risks related to abstinence.

Alternative Forms of Sexual Expression

Alternative forms of sexual expression include the following:

- *Voyeurism*: the achievement of sexual arousal by looking at the body of someone other than one's sexual partner. Although voyeurism itself is not inherently wrong, some voyeurs develop complex means to spy on others that involve violations of privacy that are illegal.
- *Sadism*: the practice of gaining sexual pleasure while inflicting abuse on another person.
- *Masochism*: gaining sexual pleasure from the humiliation of being abused.
- *Sadomasochism*: practicing sadism and masochism together. It might involve being tied up, biting, hitting, spanking, whipping, pinching, and other activities.
- *Pedophilia*: the practice of adults gaining sexual fulfillment by performing sexual acts with children. Unlike the other items on this list that (depending on the circumstances) may be considered adaptive sexual responses, pedophilia involves children who, by nature of their age and maturity, cannot consent to sexual activity. Pedophilia is wrong, illegal, and maladaptive in all cases.

FACTORS AFFECTING SEXUALITY

Many factors influence a person's sexuality and contribute to personal feelings regarding sexuality. The brain, rather than the genitals, plays the most significant role in how people perceive themselves as sexual beings.

Developmental Considerations

The process of human development affects the psychosocial, emotional, and biological aspects of life, which in turn affect a person's sexuality. Biological sex is the only distinguishing trait present at conception. From birth onward, biological sex and gender influence behavior throughout life. Table 46-1 summarizes sexuality throughout the lifespan and the nursing implications for each stage. Individuals with intellectual and developmental disabilities (IDDs) may require additional, individualized support and counseling regarding contraception, preconception planning, pregnancy, and sex education to ensure respect and protection of their autonomy (American Nurses Association [ANA] Ethics Advisory Board, 2020). Although those with IDD report similar rates of sexual activity as those without IDD, they often receive limited education on sex, reproductive health, and methods to prevent pregnancy and STIs. Females with IDD are at greater risk for sexual abuse and benefit from critical education (CDC, 2020b). Always involve the patient in their care and consider any privacy, confidentiality, and informed consent implications.

Culture

The manner in which a society perceives sexuality influences the person. Every culture has its own norms regarding sexual identity and behavior. To some degree, culture dictates the choice of sexual partner, duration of sexual intercourse, methods of sexual stimulation, and sexual positions. In some cultures, women may be expected to merely tolerate sex; in others, the woman's participation is encouraged. To gain an appreciation for all the ways that culture can influence sexual expression and health, ask people from different cultures the following questions:

- What type of dress is appropriate for children, men, and women? How is nudity viewed?
- What role behaviors and social responsibilities are expected of men and women?
- Is masturbation acceptable?
- At what age is genital sexual intimacy appropriate? With whom is it appropriate?
- What sexual practices are accepted?
- What are the rules for marriage? Is premarital sex, extramarital sex, or polygamy accepted?

The fact that a practice is common in a culture does not mean that it is healthy or ethical. **Female genital mutilation (FGM)**, for example, includes procedures that intentionally injure or alter the female genital organs for nonmedical reasons. It is a procedure that has no health benefits for girls and women and can cause severe bleeding and problems urinating. Later in life, it can cause cysts, infections, and infertility, as well as complications in childbirth and increased risk of newborn deaths. About 200 million girls and women worldwide, primarily in Africa, the Middle East, and Asia, are currently living with the consequences of FGM. The WHO (2020) writes that:

> "FGM is recognized internationally as a violation of the human rights of girls and women. It reflects deep-rooted inequality between the sexes, and constitutes an extreme form of discrimination against women. It is nearly always carried out on minors and is a violation of the rights of children. The practice also violates a person's rights to health, security, and physical integrity, the right to be free from torture and cruel, inhuman or degrading treatment, and the right to life when the procedure results in death" (para. 3).

There are four major types of FGM:

- *Clitoridectomy:* partial or total removal of the clitoris and, in very rare cases, only the prepuce (the fold of skin surrounding the clitoris)
- *Excision:* partial or total removal of the clitoris and the labia minora, with or without excision of the labia majora
- *Infibulation:* narrowing of the vaginal opening through the creation of a covering seal. The seal is formed by cutting and repositioning the inner, or outer, labia, with or without removal of the clitoris.
- *Other:* all other harmful procedures to the female genitalia for nonmedical purposes—for example, pricking, piercing, incising, scraping, and cauterizing the genital area

Religion

Some people view organized religion as having a generally negative effect on the expression of sexuality. For example, in many religions, the concept of virginity came to be synonymous with purity, and sex became synonymous with sin. In addition, many forms of sexual expression other than male–female coitus are considered unnatural by some religions. As a result of the rigid regulations and negative connotation of sex dictated by some religious groups, a number of sexual dysfunctions can be related to a person's resulting guilt and anxiety. Most major religions are reexamining their teachings on sexuality in response to challenges posed by their members. Organized religions, such as Catholicism, have public figures who are moving toward gender inclusivity by accepting and having frank conversations with and about the LGBT communities (Martin, 2017). Many people have recognized the importance of accurate sex education within the realm of the church and organized religions. There is also a new interest in the spirituality of marriage: churches and organized religions are examining their role in supporting the intimate sexual relationship of married couples.

Ethics

Healthy sexuality depends on freedom from guilt and anxiety. What one person believes is wrong may be perfectly natural and correct to another. Some people may feel that certain

Table 46-1 Developmental Aspects of Sexuality Through the Lifespan

STAGE	CHARACTERISTICS	NURSING IMPLICATIONS AND TEACHING GUIDELINES
Infancy: Birth to 18 months	• Needs affection and tactile stimulation • Males have penile erections, and females have orgasmic potential • Gradually can differentiate self from others • Obtains pleasure from touching genitals • Often dressed according to social norms based on biological sex or sex assigned at birth	• Avoid early weaning to prevent oral deprivation. • Encourage parents/caregivers to provide ample physical touch, deprivation of which may cause physical and mental underdevelopment. • Self-manipulation of genitals is normal behavior; avoid denoting this as bad or wrong.
Toddler: Ages 1–3 years	• Establishes control over bowels and bladder • All toddlers enjoy fondling genitals • Able to identify own sex and gender • Develops vocabulary related to anatomy	• Allow toddlers to designate readiness for toilet training. Strict measures may lead to compulsive behaviors later. • Punishment of genital fondling may lead to guilt and shame regarding sexual behavior later in life. • Use proper terms for body parts.
Preschooler: Ages 4–6 years	• Becomes increasingly aware of self • Enjoys exploring body parts of self and playmates • Engages in masturbation • Gender identity is formed	• Parents/caregivers may cause anxiety in the child by intolerance of inconsistency of sex-role behavior. • Negative overreaction by parents to child's masturbating behavior can lead to a belief that the genitals and sex are bad and dirty.
School-age: Ages 6–10 years	• Tendency toward attachment to the parent of the opposite sex (when this fits the family model) • Tendency toward having same-sex friends • Curiosity about sex and sharing of fears • Increasing self-awareness	• Same-sex preference for relationships is not related to heterosexual, lesbian, or gay tendencies. • Give child the information (intercourse, abstinence, STI prevention, pregnancy) in a clear, factual form. May look to peers for information that may be incorrect.
Preadolescence: Ages 10–13 years	• Puberty begins for most adolescents with development of secondary sex characteristics • Menarche takes place • May test behavioral limits	• Information is necessary regarding body changes to alleviate fears. This information should be given to the young person before pubertal changes begin. • Parents/caregivers need to find a satisfactory middle ground for rule setting. Rules that are either too rigid or too lenient can interfere with the development of self-confidence and an internal value system. • Treat body image changes with a positive attitude to prevent poor self-image.
Adolescence: Ages 13–19 years	• Primary and secondary sex characteristics develop • Sexual fantasies are common • Masturbation is common • May begin to partake in sexual activity ranging from light to heavy petting to full genital intercourse • May experiment with same-sex relationships (even if they don't identify as gay) • At risk for pregnancy and sexually transmitted infections • Gender expression and identification is often solidified during adolescence	• Parents/caregivers share their beliefs and moral value systems with their children. • Teenagers may share their feelings with parents/caregivers. Not taking them seriously may lead to lack of trust and a communication gap. • Teens need information regarding contraceptive measures and the potential for contracting sexually transmitted infections. • Review receiving and giving consent prior to engaging in sexual activity.
Young adulthood: Ages 20–35 years	• Premarital sex is common • Knowledge regarding sexual response and activity increases pleasure of relationship • May experiment with various sexual expressions • Develops own value system and respects values of other people • Many couples share financial responsibilities as well as household tasks	• Encourage communication between partners regarding sexual needs and differences. • Reinforce the use of abstinence and contraceptive measures to prevent unwanted pregnancies. • Counsel against promiscuous behavior to guard against sexually transmitted infections and loss of trust of partner. • Daily communication is necessary to vent stresses and work out difficulties.

(*continued*)

Table 46-1 Developmental Aspects of Sexuality Through the Lifespan *(continued)*

STAGE	CHARACTERISTICS	NURSING IMPLICATIONS AND TEACHING GUIDELINES
Adulthood: Ages 35–55 years	• Bodily changes as a result of menopause • Couples focus on quality rather than quantity of sexual experiences • Divorce is common • Grown children begin their own lives and sexual experiences • Sexual satisfaction may actually increase because of loss of fear of pregnancy	• People need positive reinforcement of what is good about themselves and their relationships. • Teach parents/caregivers that empty nest syndrome (feelings of loss caused by children leaving) is common. Accentuate positive aspects of this situation. • Encourage couple to use this period as one of renewal for themselves.
Late adulthood: Ages 55 years and older	• Orgasms may become shorter and less intense in both males and females • Vaginal secretions decrease, and period of resolution in males lengthens • May feel need to conform to stereotypes regarding the aging process, and cease sexual activity • Fear of loss of sexual abilities	• Sexual activity need not be hindered by age. • Teach couples that adaptation to bodily changes is possible with use of comfortable positions for intercourse and increased time for stimulation. • Teach alternatives to coitus, such as caressing, hugging, and stroking, when coitus is impossible because of illness or disability. • Couples who have been consistently sexually active throughout their lives may continue their intimate relationship for as long as they desire.

forms of sexual expression are bizarre, and the people who participate in them are perverted. If the sexual expression is performed by consenting adults, is not harmful to them, and is practiced in privacy, it should not be considered a deviant behavior. People should personally decide which aspects of sexual expression are comfortable for them. There are times that education and support from a health care professional to engage in a different form of expression may effectively alleviate guilt and enhance sexual satisfaction.

Lifestyle

Modern lifestyles greatly affect sexuality and its expression. All adults are exposed to stress, and many are under considerable strain to perform and function in the workplace as well as at home. Stressors may be external, such as job and financial demands, or internal, such as a person's competitive nature. Varied responsibilities may place a time constraint on communication between a couple, as well as on the energy level and motivation for sexual satisfaction. Although some couples view sexual activity as a release from the stressors of everyday life, most place nurturing relationships and sexual expression far from the top of the list of things-to-do. It is crucial to a relationship's survival that a couple set aside priority time for their relationship—if not for lovemaking, then for intimate, quiet contact. Lifestyle variables can also influence the sexual expression of adolescents and young adults. Young people who receive accurate, direct information regarding sex and develop associated skills to protect themselves are less likely to engage in sexual behavior that involves multiple partners and increases the risk of STIs, unwanted pregnancy, HIV, and other unintended health outcomes (CDC, 2021a).

Menstruation

Menstruation, often referred to as a *period* or menses, is the normal vaginal bleeding that takes place for 2 to 7 days during the monthly menstrual cycle if pregnancy has not occurred. During the menstrual cycle, the body prepares for the presence of a fertilized ovum; if fertilization does not occur, the body sheds the lining of the uterus during menstruation. Cycles are about 28 days long but may vary from 21 to 40 days. The first menstrual period, called **menarche**, is experienced at about age 12 years, but the age of menarche is particular to the person and may occur anywhere between 8 and 17 years. **Menopause**, the cessation of menstrual activity, occurs between the ages 48 and 55 years. There may be irregular menses over time before menstruation ends (Norris, 2019).

The Menstrual Cycle

The menstrual cycle is controlled by a series of reactions that rely on a complex interaction between the hypothalamic–pituitary axis, the ovaries, and the uterus (Norris, 2019). Two cycles occur simultaneously: one in the ovaries and one in the endometrium of the uterus (Fig. 46-2).

In the ovaries, in a typical 28-day cycle, the phase from day 4 to 14 is called the follicular phase. During this phase, a number of follicles mature, but only one produces a mature ovum. At the same time, in the uterus, the endometrium is becoming thick and velvety in preparation for receiving a fertilized egg. This phase in the uterus is called the proliferation phase. Ovulation generally occurs on day 14 when the mature ovum ruptures from the follicle and the surface of the ovary and is swept into the fallopian tube. If sperm are present, the ovum is fertilized at this time. Some individuals can detect ovulation by the presence of a sharp, cramping

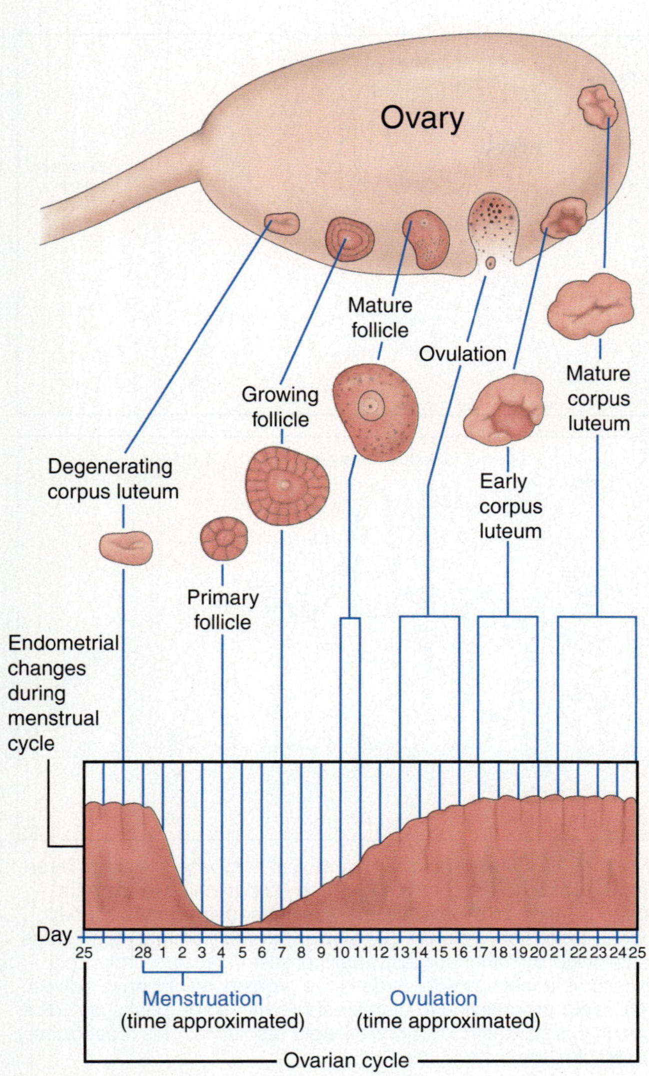

FIGURE 46-2. Schematic representation of one ovarian cycle and the corresponding changes in the endometrium.

pain over the ovulating ovary; this pain is called *mittelschmerz*, or middle pain, because it occurs in the middle of the cycle (Norris, 2019).

From day 15 to day 28, the phase in the ovaries is called the luteal phase. The leftover empty follicle fills up with a yellow pigment and is then called the corpus luteum, or yellow body. The purpose of the corpus luteum is to produce hormones that encourage a fertilized egg to grow. If fertilization does not occur, the corpus luteum begins to disintegrate. During the luteal phase in the ovaries, the uterus also undergoes changes; this phase is called the secretory phase. The endometrial lining thickens. However, in the absence of a fertilized egg, the corpus luteum dies and the endometrial lining disintegrates (Norris, 2019).

At day 28, menses, or the menstrual flow, begins as a result of the uterus shedding the useless portion of its endometrium. Menses lasts for 2 to 7 days (Norris, 2019), with flow averaging 5 days. The menstrual discharge is a bloody fluid that also contains endometrial debris, mucus, and enzymes. Normal blood loss averages 30 to 80 mL. Usually, the flow is the heaviest and is bright red on the first day or two of menses, gradually tapering off to light-brown staining. Many individuals experience some degree of discomfort either premenstrually or during menses.

Menstrual discharge is odorless until exposed to the air, when a person may notice a light, fleshy, pungent odor. Deodorized pads and tampons do little to minimize odor and can cause chemical irritation to the vulva and vagina. Good hygiene and regular bathing are much more effective during menses to prevent odor. Pads and tampons should be changed frequently to prevent odor and irritation from wetness. Individuals using tampons should read and follow the manufacturer's suggestions to reduce the risk for toxic shock syndrome (TSS).

Menstrual cycle irregularities can have many different causes, including the following (Mayo Clinic Staff, 2021; Norris, 2019):

- *Pregnancy or breastfeeding.* A delayed or missed period can be an early sign of pregnancy. Breastfeeding typically delays the return of menstruation after pregnancy.
- *Eating disorders, extreme weight loss, or excessive exercising.* Eating disorders (such as anorexia nervosa), extreme weight loss, malnutrition, and increased physical activity can disrupt menstruation.
- *Polycystic ovary syndrome (PCOS).* This common hormonal disorder can cause small cysts (fluid-filled sacs) to develop on the ovaries and irregular menstruation.
- *Premature ovarian failure.* Premature ovarian failure refers to the loss of normal ovarian function before age 40 years. Individuals who have premature ovarian failure, also known as primary ovarian insufficiency, may have irregular or infrequent periods for years.
- *Pelvic inflammatory disease (PID).* This infection of the upper reproductive organs (uterus, fallopian tubes, or ovaries) can cause pain, discharge, and irregular menstrual bleeding.
- *Uterine fibroids.* Uterine fibroids are noncancerous growths of the uterus. They can cause heavy, prolonged menstrual periods and bleeding between periods.

There is no scientific rationale supporting abstinence from sexual activity during menses. Many females enjoy sex during menses owing to the increase in vascularity in the pelvic region, which heightens enjoyment. Males may also enjoy the warm wetness the menstrual flow provides to the vagina. If flow is heavy, a diaphragm can be used to hold it back during sexual activity, or a towel can be used to protect bedding. Some females who experience abdominal cramping during menses, called *dysmenorrhea,* find that sexual activity and orgasm relieve their discomfort.

In May 2007, the U.S. Food and Drug Administration (FDA) approved the first oral contraceptive designed to be taken 365 days a year by those who want to avoid menstruating altogether. Females who use the drug do not have regular menstrual periods, although they may have breakthrough bleeding (spotting or light bleeding). While there are obvious advantages to not having menstrual periods, females should be counseled that there are no long-term safety data on these drugs. Risks are thought to be similar to those of conventional oral contraceptives: an increased incidence of blood clots, heart attacks, and stroke, especially in those who smoke. Positive benefits may include lowering the risk for ovarian cancer and endometrial cancer (National Cancer Institute, National Institutes of Health, 2018; FDA, 2021).

Premenstrual Syndrome and Premenstrual Dysphoric Disorder

Premenstrual syndrome (PMS) is characterized by the appearance of one or more of the following symptoms several days before the onset of menstruation: (1) emotional symptoms such as depression, irritability, anxiety, changes in sleep habits, changes in sexual desire, poor concentration, crying, anger, and social withdrawal; and (2) physical symptoms such as appetite changes, breast tenderness, bloating and weight gain, aches and pains, swelling, acne, gastrointestinal issues, and fatigue (The American College of Obstetricians and Gynecologists [ACOG], 2021). An estimated 85% of menstruating females experience at least one PMS symptom with their monthly cycle; up to 12% of menstruating females present with premenstrual disorders (Hofmeister & Bodden, 2016; Office on Women's Health, U.S. Department of Health & Human Services [USDHHS], 2018). PMS is diagnosed by a health care provider by establishing a pattern of symptoms that are associated with menstruation. In order to establish a pattern, providers frequently ask the patient to keep a log of their symptoms and menstrual cycle.

Premenstrual dysphoric disorder (PMDD) differs from PMS primarily in that it is a DSM-5-classified diagnosis by the American Psychiatric Association, and its symptoms are primarily psychiatric in nature. Some studies have shown that PMDD is related to serotonin levels, and the symptoms reported are more disabling than symptoms reported with PMS.

Management of PMS and PMDD are primarily symptom-management focused, with individuals diagnosed with PMDD benefitting from antidepressants that address serotonin levels (ACOG, 2021; Hofmeister & Bodden, 2016; Office on Women's Health, USDHHS, 2018). Nurses have a great role to play in researching PMS and PMDD and ensuring that females and the public correctly understand their effects.

Sexual Response Cycle

The physiologic responses to sexual activity of females and males can be more similar than different (Fig. 46-3). The body's response is essentially the same regardless of the source of stimulation; that is, fantasy, masturbation, and sexual intercourse can all bring about the same body reactions. The sexual response cycle is not limited to the genital organs but is a total body response that causes many physiologic changes throughout the body. The classic sexual response cycle outlined by Masters and Johnson (1966) is linear in nature and has four phases: excitement, plateau, orgasm, and resolution; there is a smooth progression from one phase to the next. Although only physiologic responses are discussed here, the emotional and mental involvement of sexual response contributes a great deal to the pleasure and satisfaction of sexual activity.

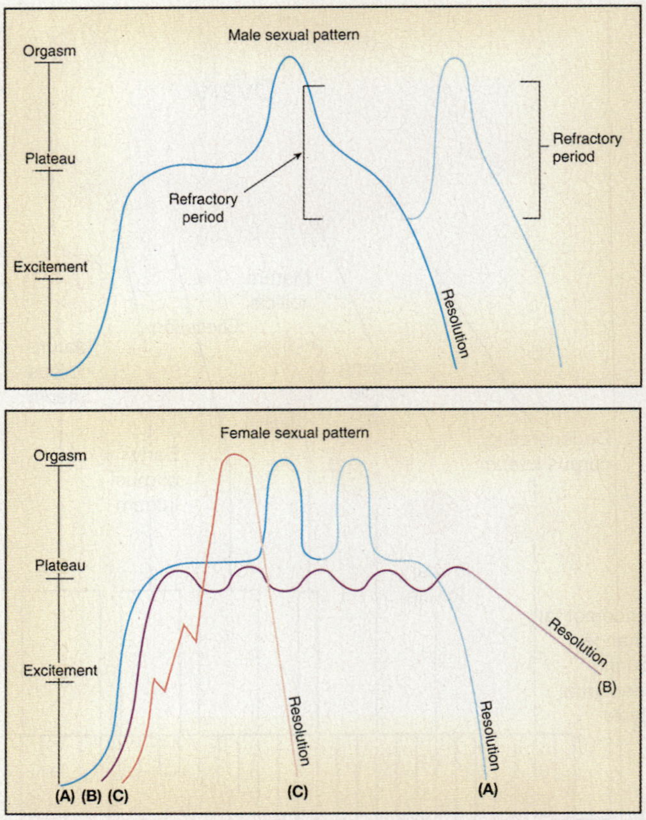

FIGURE 46-3. Male and female sexual response patterns. Three female patterns are shown: **(A)** Steady progression to plateau stage is followed by intense orgasm; subsequent orgasms may occur; resolution is slower. **(B)** Slower progression to plateau stage is followed by minor surges toward orgasm, causing prolonged pleasurable feelings without definitive orgasm; resolution is slowest. **(C)** Rapid progression to plateau stage with some peaks and dips; one intense orgasm follows with rapid resolution. This most closely resembles the male pattern.

The human body contains many **erogenous zones**, areas that when stimulated cause sexual arousal and desire. The genitals are an obvious source of sexual pleasure for all people, but other areas of the body are also considered erogenous zones. The skin is the largest erogenous zone. Other areas include the ears, lips, thighs, and breasts. Some people can reach orgasm simply by stimulation of nongenital erogenous zones.

The most important body organ for sexual arousal and stimulation is the brain. Engagement of the brain in arousal allows people the freedom to enjoy a sexual experience but may also prevent satisfaction because of inhibitions, doubts, and guilt.

Excitement

The excitement phase is initiated by erotic stimulation and arousal. Some of the physiologic changes common in all people include an increase in heart rate and blood pressure, and the appearance of a pink to red flush to the skin. This sex flush, which is more evident in females than in males, spreads over the face, neck, back, and upper torso. Congestion of the genitals with increased blood flow begins in the excitement phase and causes even more arousal. The length of the excitement phase varies greatly among people and even from one experience to another.

During the excitement phase, the female breasts swell, and the nipples become erect and hard to the touch. Lubrication of the vagina seeps to the outside of the body along the vulvar creases and makes stimulation of the genitals more pleasurable by decreasing friction. The upper two thirds of the vagina enlarge and expand. The clitoris enlarges and emerges slightly from the clitoral hood. The labia also enlarge and separate and turn a deep rosy red with arousal.

The first obvious sign of arousal in the male is an erection of the penis caused by increased pelvic congestion of blood. The scrotum noticeably elevates, thickens, and enlarges. The skin of the penis and scrotum turns a deep reddish purple in response to congestion and arousal. Male nipples may also harden and become erect.

Plateau

The intensity of the plateau phase is greater than that of excitement, but not enough to begin orgasm. Desire and arousal continue to build and intensify. This phase varies from a few minutes to 15 to 20 minutes. In the female, the clitoris retracts and disappears under the clitoral hood. It is thought that the clitoris performs in this mysterious way as the body's protection against overstimulation. In the male, secretions from Cowper's glands may appear at the glans of the penis during the plateau phase.

Orgasm

The term **orgasm** defines the climax and sexual explosion of the tension that has been building over the preceding phases. Orgasm lasts only seconds but is an extremely intense reaction. Characteristics of the orgasm phase are the involuntary spasmodic contractions of the genital organs. The number of contractions felt by the person depends on the intensity of the orgasm.

The orgasm phase in the female begins with a heightened feeling of physical pleasure, followed by overwhelming release and involuntary contractions of the genitals. Loss of muscular control may cause spastic contractions and twitching of the arms and legs. The number of contractions can be as few as 4 or as many as 20. Areas of the body that contract spasmodically are the uterus, anal sphincter, rectum, and urethral sphincter. It is believed that females achieve orgasm in a variety of ways. Although some females can achieve orgasm by penile thrusting in the vagina alone, most individuals need clitoral stimulation to reach orgasm.

During orgasm in the male, involuntary spasmodic contractions occur in the penis, epididymis, vas deferens, and rectum. The male orgasm is most often accompanied by ejaculation of semen from the urinary meatus of the penis. Ejaculation and orgasm usually, but not necessarily, occur at the same time.

Resolution

The resolution phase is characterized by a return to the normal body functioning present before the excitement phase. Feelings of relaxation, fatigue, and fulfillment are common. Some people have a need to be held, fondled, and caressed. Physical demonstrations of affection may initiate the sexual response cycle once again. The female body is physiologically capable of immediate response to sexual stimulation. Because of this, many females can achieve multiple orgasms. Males experience a period during which the body does not respond to continued sexual stimulation, called the refractory period. The length of the refractory period varies from a few minutes to longer, even days.

Female Sexual Response: A Nonlinear Model

Basson's (2000) Nonlinear Model of female sexual response is important because it acknowledges differences in the sexual responses of women, especially those who have been in a long-term relationship. Basson specifically focuses on distinguishing *different* from *dysfunction*. According to her model, women who do not have traditional sexual desire (thoughts and fantasies), but who are able respond to sexual stimulation, do not necessarily have a sexual dysfunction. Sexual desire differs among women—for some it may revolve around the desire for intimacy or manifest as responsive desire (i.e., desire that is responsive to cues, behaviors, and other stimuli). This means a woman may engage in sex based on their choice to respond to other needs (such as emotional closeness), not necessarily the biological need to experience sexual arousal or release. Vaginal lubrication and other genital changes that are frequently considered signs of arousal may not be considered important by the woman, but this does not mean they have a sexual dysfunction. Orgasm is not essential for sexual satisfaction for many women. Basson's Nonlinear Model emphasizes the effect of emotional intimacy, sexual stimuli, mental excitement, and relationship satisfaction on the female sexual response.

Childbearing Considerations

All sorts of questions surround childbearing, and the ability (or lack of ability) to procreate can put great pressure on a sexual relationship: Are we ready to be parents? What does it mean to be a responsible parent—especially in this age when an increasing number of prenatal interventions are available to maximize fetal outcomes? Should we choose life partners only if genetic testing reveals a good match for reproduction? If we choose to be sexually active and not have children, what are the best means to prevent unwanted pregnancies? If we become pregnant and choose not to continue the pregnancy, what are our options? If we desperately want a child and discover one or both to be infertile, what are our options? What are our options if we are a same-sex couple? Who donates sperm or eggs and who carries the baby to term? The age of biotechnology promises *designer babies* and raises difficult questions for individuals and society. People frequently look to nurses for help in sorting through how to respond to these challenges. Experienced nurses are good at detecting when a fear of pregnancy or inability to conceive is interfering with a couple's normal sexual expression, or when a changing developmental stage (e.g., menopause) is interfering with normal sexual expression.

Sexually Transmitted Infections

Sexually transmitted infections (STIs), or sexually transmitted diseases (STDs) are infections that are spread primarily through sexual contact. Although *STIs* and *STDs* are often used interchangeably, in health care, STI is more commonly used because not every STI results in disease or has active symptoms.

STIs are among the most common infectious diseases in the United States today. Each of these infections is a potential threat to a person's immediate and long-term health and well-being, and can lead to severe reproductive health complications, such as infertility. Prevention and counseling involve obtaining a sexual history focused on the 5Ps: partners, practices, protection from transmitted infections, past history of STIs, and pregnancy intention (CDC, 2021c). Check out this guide from the CDC that walks through the 5Ps and taking a sexual history: https://www.cdc.gov/std/treatment/SexualHistory.pdf

According to the National Institute of Allergy and Infectious Diseases (NIAID, 2015–2022), understanding the basic facts about STIs—the ways in which they are spread, their common symptoms, and how they can be treated—is the first step toward prevention. News releases, fact sheets, research studies, and other NIAID-related materials are available on the NIAID website at www.niaid.nih.gov. NIAID recommends understanding at least five key points about all STIs in the United States today:

1. STIs affect people of all backgrounds and economic levels. They are most prevalent among teenagers and young adults.
2. The incidence of STIs is rising, in part because in the last few decades, young people have become sexually active earlier yet are marrying later. In addition, divorce is more common. The net result is that sexually active people today are more likely to have multiple sex partners during their lives and are potentially at risk for developing STIs.
3. STIs frequently cause no symptoms, particularly in women. When symptoms develop, they may be confused with those of other diseases not transmitted through sexual contact. Even when an STI causes no symptoms, a person who is infected may be able to pass the disease on to a sex partner. That is why many doctors recommend periodic testing or screening for people who have more than one sex partner.
4. Health problems caused by STIs tend to be more severe and more frequent for females than for males, in part because the frequency of asymptomatic infection means that many females do not seek care until serious problems have developed.
   - Some STIs can spread into the uterus and fallopian tubes to cause pelvic inflammatory disease (PID), which is a major cause of both infertility and ectopic (tubal) pregnancy. The latter can be fatal.
   - STIs in anyone with a cervix may also be associated with cervical cancer. One STI, human papillomavirus (HPV) infection, causes genital warts and cervical/other genital cancers.
   - STIs can be passed from a female to their baby before, during, or immediately after birth; some of these infections of the newborn can be cured easily, but others may cause a baby to be permanently disabled or even die.
5. When diagnosed and treated early, many STIs can be treated effectively. Some infections have become resistant to the drugs used to treat them and now require newer types of antibiotics. Experts believe that having STIs other than HIV increases a person's risk for becoming infected with the HIV virus (NIAID, 2015–2022).

Prevention counseling for STIs and HIV is essential and should be provided in a nonjudgmental, empathetic manner that accounts for the person's culture, primary language, sex, gender identity, sexual orientation, age, and intellectual development level. It should be offered to all sexually active adolescents and to all adults who have an active STI, have had an STI in the past year, or who report multiple sex partners (CDC, 2021c). There is a renewed emphasis on partner services, which includes clinical evaluation, counseling, diagnostic testing, and treatment for individuals in a sexual network. Expedited partner therapy, focused specifically on chlamydia and gonorrhea, permits a patient to obtain prescribed medication for their partner(s) who are unlikely to seek clinical evaluation. Partner services require collaboration between patients, providers, and public health partners (CDC, 2021c). Primary prevention strategies aim to reduce the spread and potentially devastating effects of untreated STIs. Recent guidelines outline specific strategies for prevention and treatment of STIs in specific populations including adolescents, children, men who have sex with men (MSM), women who have sex with women (WSW), women who have sex with women and men (WSWM), transgender or gender diverse persons, and those who are pregnant or incarcerated (CDC, 2021c). Table 46-2 lists common types of STIs and their signs and symptoms.

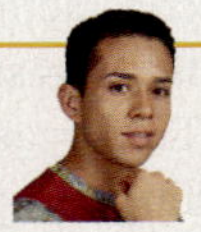

Consider ***Paul Rojas,*** a young adult man who has told the health care team he is gay, was diagnosed with AIDS. The nurse would need to assess the patient's sexual practices and instruct him about methods to prevent the transmission of HIV/AIDS. In addition, the nurse would need to assess for potential STIs that could increase his ability to transmit HIV to a HIV-negative sexual partner.

Sexual Dysfunction

Sexual dysfunction is a problem that prevents a person or couple from engaging in or enjoying sexual intercourse and orgasm. Dysfunctions might occur as a result of physiologic malfunctions, conflicts with cultural norms, interpersonal problems, or any combination of these. Anxieties and fears concerning the sexual act are almost always present. Patients with severe sexual dysfunctions require intensive professional therapy from a qualified sex therapist.

Male Primary Sexual Dysfunctions

ERECTILE DYSFUNCTION

Erectile dysfunction (ED), also called **impotence**, is the inability of a male to attain or maintain an erection to such

Table 46-2 Sexually Transmitted Infections

DISEASE/ INFECTION	CHARACTERISTICS
Human immunodeficiency virus (HIV)[a]	• HIV-1/HIV-2 Ag/Ab combination assay—begin antiretroviral therapy (ART) as soon as possible for all people • Higher risk in those who engage in needle-sharing and sexually active gay, bisexual, and other men who have sex with men (MSM)—recommend at least annual testing • Recommend testing for all pregnant persons in the United States at the first prenatal visit; test when another STI is diagnosed • Consider pre-exposure prophylaxis (PrEP) and post-exposure prophylaxis (PEP) with any STI diagnosis; begin ART and behavioral/psychosocial services as soon as possible with HIV infection • Asymptomatic or fatigue, diarrhea, weight loss, enlarged lymph nodes, fever, anorexia, and night sweats
Bacterial vaginosis (BV)	• Imbalance of bacteria (alters flora in the vagina) • Symptoms in females: foul-smelling, thin, grayish white vaginal discharge • Males typically asymptomatic • Treat with metronidazole (abstain from alcohol when taking)
Chlamydia[a]	• *Chlamydia trachomatis*—intracellular bacteria • Primarily affects young people ages 15–24 years • Many people are asymptomatic • Symptoms in females: vaginal discharge, burning on urination, urinary frequency, dysuria, and urethral soreness • Symptoms in males: penile discharge, burning sensation with urination, pain and swelling in testicles
Cytomegalovirus (CMV)	• A virus in the same family as herpes and Epstein–Barr • A first-time infection may cause mononucleosis, a mild illness with fever and swollen glands, liver, and spleen • May be asymptomatic • Not exclusively sexually transmitted; can be associated with certain pelvic inflammatory disease (PID) cases
Genital herpes	• Herpes simplex virus type 2 (HSV-2) typically causes genital herpes • Can be caused by HSV-1 through oral sex; HSV-1 typically leads to cold sores • Chronic, lifelong viral infection—systemic antiviral medications • Lesions develop around the genitals, rectum, or mouth • Appear as single or multiple painful vesicles, which rupture and form ulcer-like lesions; these form scabs as they heal • First infections last about 10–14 days, whereas subsequent infections are shorter in duration • Recurrences are usually preceded by prodromal symptoms of tingling and fullness
Gonorrhea[a]	• Gram-negative bacteria *Neisseria gonorrhoeae* • Primarily affects young people ages 15–24 years • Many people are asymptomatic • Symptoms in females: most have no symptoms; dysuria, abnormal menses, vaginal discharge, pelvic inflammatory disease • Symptoms in males: purulent penile discharge, dysuria, frequency of urination • Symptoms of pharyngitis if oral sex was practiced • May be accompanied by chlamydial infection • Newborns exposed at birth are at risk for blindness and pneumonia • Untreated gonorrhea can result in infertility, skin rash with lesions, and acute arthritis
Human papillomavirus (HPV)	• A DNA virus; vaccine recommended for everyone • Most people who have had sex acquire HPV, but are asymptomatic; HPV resolves spontaneously • Genital warts: pale, soft, papillary lesions found around the internal and external genitalia and perianal and rectal areas of the body; vary in size • Females with HPV are at risk for cervical (and other) cancer

Syphilis[a]	• *Treponema pallidum*, a spirochete detected through serologic blood test
	• Syphilis rates rising among gay and bisexual males and pregnant people
	• Stages of disease if left untreated:
	  • *Primary:* Single painless genital lesion 10 days to 3 months after exposure
	  • *Secondary:* Generalized skin rash, enlarged lymph nodes, fever that may appear 2–4 weeks after appearance of primary lesion; may last for several years
	  • *Latent:* Usually no clinical symptoms present for as long as 20 years
	  • *Tertiary:* If left untreated, syphilis can lead to severe medical problems that affect the heart, brain, nervous system, and blood vessels

Trichomoniasis ("Trich")	• *Trichomonas vaginalis*, a protozoan with flagella • May be identified on Pap smear • Males typically asymptomatic • Symptoms in females: foul-smelling vaginal discharge, thin, foamy, and green in color, causes itching of vulva and vagina, burning on urination and dyspareunia; strawberry-appearing cervix may be seen on colposcopy.

[a]Reportable diseases in every state.

Source: Data from Centers for Disease Control and Prevention (CDC). (2021c, July 23). *Sexually transmitted infections treatment guidelines, 2021. Morbidity and Mortality Weekly Report, 70*(4). https://www.cdc.gov/std/treatment-guidelines/STI-Guidelines-2021.pdf; National Institute of Allergy and Infectious Diseases (NIAID). (2015-2022). *Sexually transmitted diseases.* https://www.niaid.nih.gov/diseases-conditions/sexually-transmitted-diseases

an extent that they cannot have satisfactory intercourse. Common causes of impotence (which may be physiologic or psychological) include various illnesses, treatments for these illnesses, and personal anxieties. New medications have revolutionized treatment for erectile dysfunction.

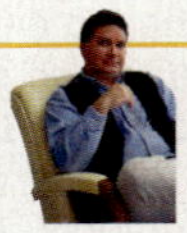

Recall **Jefferson Smith,** the patient with diabetes and hypertension who is having problems with erections. The nurse would review the pathophysiologic effects of diabetes and hypertension on sexual response. The nurse would also evaluate his current status, including a review of all medications that he is taking, to determine possible contributory factors.

PREMATURE EJACULATION

Premature ejaculation is a condition in which a male consistently reaches ejaculation or orgasm before, or soon after entering the vagina or other orifice. The result is that the partner usually does not have time to reach sexual satisfaction. Causes of this problem are rarely physical. See the Nursing Care Plan 46-1 for Pete Manheim on pages 1896–1899 for a discussion of a related phenomenon, nocturnal ejaculation.

DELAYED EJACULATION

Delayed ejaculation, also called ejaculatory incompetence, refers to a male's inability to ejaculate in an expected time frame. The causes of this problem are similar to those of impotence. When it occurs after experiencing normal ejaculations, the cause is most likely due to interpersonal problems.

Female Primary Sexual Dysfunctions

INHIBITED SEXUAL DESIRE

Inhibited sexual desire consists of an inhibition in sexual arousal so that congestion and vaginal lubrication are absent or minimal. Causative factors may be anxiety, negative emotions, fear, interpersonal problems, or physical factors. Orgasmic dysfunction is defined as the inability of a female to reach orgasm. The causes are similar to those of inhibited sexual desire.

DYSPAREUNIA

Dyspareunia is painful intercourse. Although it is most often described by females, some males may also suffer from this disorder. The cause is usually physical, although psychological problems such as fear and anxiety can cause pain.

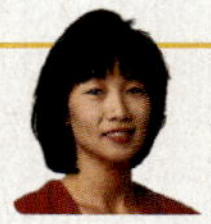

Consider **Amy Liu,** the woman who had a hysterectomy and is experiencing pain on intercourse. The nurse would review the patient's history to determine if the problem is physiologic, secondary to changes in the reproductive tract from surgery, or psychological, secondary to the changes in self-concept and her report of not feeling "like a woman anymore."

VAGINISMUS

Vaginismus is a rare condition in which the vaginal opening closes tightly and prevents penile penetration. Vaginismus is due to involuntary spastic contractions of the muscles at and around the vaginal opening and the levator ani muscles. The cause of vaginismus may be physical, psychological, or both.

VULVODYNIA

Vulvodynia, a chronic vulvar discomfort or pain characterized by burning, stinging, irritation, or rawness of the female genitalia that interferes with sexual activity, is particularly problematic because little is known about its cause or treatment.

Effects of Illness, Injury, and Medications

A healthy body, mind, and emotions are necessary for sexual wellness. A primary sexual dysfunction can affect a person's sexual expression. Similarly, any trauma or stress that interferes with a person's ability to perform daily functions will also affect the expression of sexuality. Illness is no exception.

Diabetes Mellitus

Diabetes mellitus (DM) is a hormonal disease in which an inadequate amount of insulin is secreted by the pancreas. Although almost all hormonal disorders affect sexuality in some way, diabetes is the most prevalent and well known. ED, or impotence, is a great concern among those with type 2 diabetes. Treatment to date depends largely on the degree of erectile ability lost. Some individuals may be candidates for a penile prosthesis, which was developed in 1973. The prosthesis is surgically implanted below the base of the penis, and inflation of the device produces an erection when sexual activity is desired. Pharmacologic management (e.g., sildenafil, vardenafil, or tadalafil) may also be indicated.

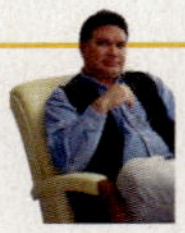

Think back to **Jefferson Smith,** the patient with diabetes and hypertension. The nurse would explore with Mr. Smith his feelings about the effect of his disorder on his sexual function and sexuality. Additional consultation with other members of the health care team would be necessary to determine the most appropriate plan for treatment of Mr. Smith's impotence.

Females with type 2 diabetes may also experience loss of capacity for orgasm (orgasmic dysfunction). Difficulty experiencing arousal and loss of vaginal lubrication have also been reported. Females with diabetes are more prone to urinary tract or vaginal infections, which can cause discomfort during coitus.

Cardiovascular Disease

Cardiovascular disease is prevalent in North America, and the sexual response cycle can greatly increase the demands on the heart and other structures. A person with a cardiovascular disease may experience much anxiety over the effect the illness will have on sexuality and sexual functioning.

HYPERTENSION

The most significant difficulty a person diagnosed with hypertension faces regarding sexuality is that the medication used to control the disease frequently causes a change in sexual functioning. These sexual dysfunctions may be relieved by modifying the dose of the medication or switching to a different medication.

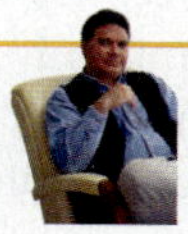

Consider **Jefferson Smith,** the patient with a history of diabetes and hypertension. The nurse would obtain a complete medication history from the patient to determine if his pharmacologic therapy is the underlying cause of his impotence or if the medication is contributing to a preexisting problem associated with his diabetes. This investigation would provide information about whether an adjustment in medication dosage might minimize or alleviate Mr. Smith's impotence.

MYOCARDIAL INFARCTION

The primary goal after a myocardial infarction (MI), or heart attack, is to allow the heart ample time to heal. Activities of daily living, including sexual activity, should be resumed gradually, and stressors such as overexertion, alcohol consumption, and emotional upheavals should be avoided. After an uncomplicated MI, sexual activity may begin at about the third week of recovery, beginning with masturbation to partial erection in the male. In general, this activity is gradually increased until 3 months after the MI, when sexual intercourse may be resumed. A comfortable position that places the least stress on the affected partner should be used.

Diseases of the Joints and Mobility

Joint diseases and disorders affect people of all ages. Pain, fatigue, stiffness, and loss of range of motion can accompany any of the dozens of known diseases of the joints. The disease itself does not affect sexual functioning, although the manifestation of it can cause discomfort and anxiety.

Surgery and Body Image

Surgery is performed to remove diseased tissue and repair body organs, usually requiring an incision with resulting scars. The most devastating kinds of surgery are those used to remove cancerous tissue and surrounding structures. Patients are almost always distressed about a diagnosis of cancer and possible death. After surgery, patients need to adjust to major alterations in their bodies. Changes in body image also affect a person's self-perception as a sexual being.

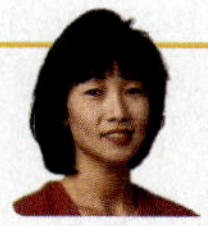

Remember **Amy Liu,** the woman who had had a hysterectomy. The uterus, because it is a female reproductive organ, is often associated with childbearing and may trigger a specific grieving response. The nurse would interpret the significance of the uterus to the patient's self-concept and how the surgery to remove it has affected her overall feelings of femininity and womanhood. Using this information, the nurse would then correct any misconceptions that Mrs. Liu may have about this reproductive organ and develop an appropriate teaching plan.

Mastectomy is a surgical procedure to remove a breast and surrounding tissue. After such a surgery, the return to sexual functioning depends on many factors, such as support of a sexual or life partner(s), the value placed on the breast by either partner, and fear of discomfort during sexual activity. Allowing the patient time to grieve the loss of the uterus or breast(s) is appropriate and may help with long-term coping.

An ostomy is a surgical opening placed on the outside of the body to allow for the passage of secretions and elimination into a closed drainage bag. Grieving over the loss of the natural means to eliminate waste, such as urine or feces, accompanies learning to live with an obvious artificial device. Many people are anxious as to how this apparatus will affect their sex lives and how accepting their partners will be of it. Odor and leakage concerns need to be addressed to increase comfort with the device.

Spinal Cord Injuries

Thousands of people are victims of spinal cord injuries each year as a result of various types of accidents. This type of injury almost always results in some degree of permanent disability. People with SCI face multiple adaptations in their lifestyles, including those related to mobility, bowel and bladder control, sexual functioning, and role expectations. The extent of sexual response that remains after a spinal cord injury depends primarily on the level and extent of the injury. Ejaculation and orgasm are most likely to remain with low spinal injuries. Females are more likely to experience orgasm than males, but they more frequently report a lack of physical sensations during the excitement phase than do males. Many people find that other erogenous zones become more easily stimulated after the injury.

Chronic Pain

Many chronic illnesses are accompanied by constant pain, and a person with persistent pain may not desire any sexual contact. However, the desire for human warmth and contact does not cease because of pain. Altered or modified positions for coitus are sometimes necessary; discussing these positions with patients can be an important part of implementing the nursing process, reviewed later in this chapter.

Mental Illness

Various psychological and physical disorders can cause mental illness. The mind plays a powerful role in sexuality; any disruption of its functioning will no doubt cause some disturbance in sexual functioning. Even mild depression can affect desire and sexual functioning. At times, patients with mental illness act out in a sexual manner, such as touching themselves or removing their clothing at inappropriate times and places. Sometimes, it is difficult for the partner of a patient who has developed a mental illness to continue the sexual relationship. People afflicted with Alzheimer disease can lose the memory of any contact with a partner or spouse.

Medications

Some medications have side effects that may affect sexual functioning. These include nitrates, anticonvulsants, antidepressants, antihistamines, antihypertensives, antipsychotics, antispasmodics, barbiturates, and narcotics. Recreational drugs including cocaine, alcohol, and marijuana are used by some to heighten the sexual experience. These drugs can have serious and even deadly side effects. While some use alcohol to release inhibitions and to increase sexual arousal and desire, heavy drinking can decrease libido and negatively affect sexual functioning.

SEXUAL HARASSMENT

Harassment is any annoying or distressing comment or conduct that is known, or should be known to be unwelcome. **Sexual harassment** is unwelcome behavior that is based on a person's sex or gender. This type of harassment usually occurs in the context of an asymmetrical relationship in which one person has more formal power than the other (e.g., a faculty member over a student) or more informal power (e.g., one peer over another). Sexual harassment can be directed toward people of any age, any gender, and any sexual orientation. There are two forms of sexual harassment: quid pro quo and environmental harassment (also called a *hostile environment*). Quid pro quo means something given or withheld in exchange for something else. *Quid pro quo harassment* occurs when a person's employment or well-being is dependent on agreeing to unsolicited and unwelcome sexual demands. This type of harassment is typically initiated by a person in a position of authority who offers either direct or indirect reward or punishment based on the granting of sexual favors. Quid pro quo harassment is a clear abuse of power and is legally, morally, and ethically wrong.

Hostile work environment occurs when sex- or gender-based behaviors create a hostile, intimidating environment that hurts a person's work performance, classroom performance, or general sense of well-being. In the workplace, for example, the negative behaviors in hostile environment harassment are not directly linked to job-related consequences; instead, the employee's willingness to suffer the experience of the demeaning environment becomes a condition of employment. This type of harassment is not necessarily caused by a person with formal power. A hostile environment is sometimes difficult to identify, as it is not always easy to determine when offensive speech or behavior actually turns to true harassment. In order to be considered a hostile work environment, the behaviors must be unwanted, frequent (not a one-time event), and pervasive. Coworkers and peers can create a hostile environment for a member of the group through the following:

- Unwelcome sexually oriented and gender-based behaviors
- Sexual bantering
- Sexual jokes
- Offensive pictures and language
- Sexual innuendoes
- Sexual behavior
- Unwanted attention such as asking for dates constantly, physically blocking movement, or creating unwanted interactions

Effects of Harassment

Harassment can cause feelings of helplessness, worthlessness, and guilt in the victim. This can often lead to less career satisfaction and feelings of loss of control. Anger is commonly experienced by those who have been harassed, which may lead to requests for transfer, resignation, or withdrawal from the environment where the harassment occurs. In many cases, job performance is affected due to reduced levels of concentration. Loss of job motivation and skill confidence, along with reduced job satisfaction and organizational commitment, are common.

Responding to Harassment in the Nursing Environment

Inappropriate sexual behavior by a patient may cause the nurse to respond with a range of actions from passive avoidance to aggressive retaliation. An assertive response that supports the nurse in maintaining self-respect, while encouraging the patient to accept responsibility for their behavior, is recommended.

1. *Be self-aware*: Do not deny feelings about being harassed.
2. *Confront:* Provide feedback to the patient in a nonthreatening way and clearly state what behavior is or is not acceptable.
3. *Set limits*: Define clear and reasonable consequences that will be enforced if the behavior continues.
4. *Enforce the stated limits*: Maintain boundaries.
5. *Report*: Document the incident and submit to supervisor.

Colleagues may also be a source of harassment. The objective of employers should be to create a positive work environment that is characterized by mutually respectful behavior. Many have taken steps to eliminate hostile work environments by educating employees, developing policies against workplace harassment, and outlining guidelines for responding to sexual harassment.

1. If harassed by a coworker, confront the behavior immediately. An assertive statement is sometimes sufficient to stop the behavior.
2. If the harassment continues, document the date and time, and describe the behavior.
3. Consult a supervisor not involved in the harassment.
4. If the harassment still does not stop, file a grievance with administration.
5. Seek legal advice if all previous efforts to stop the behavior have been unsuccessful. Sexual harassment is illegal and you have the right to ask for legal representation.

NURSE AS ROLE MODEL

Nurses' attitudes, biases, and prejudices regarding sexuality are readily transmitted to patients through their actions, manner of speech, and avoidance of certain circumstances or types of discussion (see Focused Critical Thinking Guide 46-1). A nurse's knowledge about sexual issues can inhibit or promote discussions of sexual health. The nurse who does not have a sound knowledge base of reproductive anatomy and physiology, sexual response, sexual expression,

46-1 Focused Critical Thinking Guide

SEXUALITY AND NONJUDGMENTAL NURSING CARE

A 33-year-old man with AIDS who is living alone at home asks you, the visiting nurse, about the nurse who was substituting for you during your vacation. "I don't like to complain, but he was overly friendly—if you get what I mean.... I wasn't comfortable with the way he was touching me, and I'd rather not have help with my bath than have him back here." You have to decide how to respond.

1. Identify goal of thinking

Clarify what the patient is saying and make a judgment about the behavior behind his concern so that you can respond appropriately.

2. Assess adequacy of knowledge

Pertinent circumstances: You have been visiting the patient for the last 2 months following his discharge from a local hospital because of AIDS-related complications. Apart from his clinical picture, you know very little about the patient, who has always seemed private and reserved during your visits. You feel sorry that the patient is as sick as he is at this point in his life, and your instinct is to trust him. You really don't know the colleague who was substituting for you because he was newly hired.

Prerequisite knowledge: Before you can make a judgment about the patient's concern, you need to know more about what actually happened between your colleague and him. You do not know your colleague well because he is a new hire and has been working in the facility for only 3 months. You have heard reports that he is gay. You know that the patient is single, but do not know his sexual orientation. You need to talk with your colleague to get his description of his encounter with the patient. You also need to know more about what touch means to both the patient and your colleague because culture and individual preference can profoundly influence the meaning different people give to touch.

Room for error: Life and death do not hinge on how you respond to this patient. However, the well-being of the patient and your colleague's reputation are at stake, so the matter is grave.

Time constraints: You must make some immediate response to the patient. Because you do not have sufficient information to evaluate what happened, you should not feel pressured to make a definitive response. The patient's well-being will not be jeopardized if you postpone a complete response until you have investigated the complaint.

3. Address potential problems

The most serious obstacles to critical thinking in this situation would be forgoing a systematic reasoning process and immediately moving to make false assumptions about sexuality, sexual expression, and gay male nurses. Your tendency to "go to bat" for patients and to believe whatever a patient tells you (no matter what) may result in your unfairly and prematurely judging a colleague.

4. Consult helpful resources

Your colleague is the first resource you should consult because you need to hear his side of the event before you can think critically about what happened. When you do meet with him, he thanks you for bringing up the subject because he was similarly disturbed by his encounter with this patient. "I guess I'm a touchy-feely kind of guy and generally find that patients respond well to human touch. In the past, patients have told me how much it means to them to have someone massage their back, stroke a forearm, or greet them with a hug. Touch is certainly an integral part of my therapeutic style. I did sense rather quickly, though, that Jim didn't like to be touched and so I modified my approach. My sense, from a few comments he made, is that he's probably homophobic" (afraid of gay or lesbian people).

After listening to your colleague, you decide you need to learn more about touch, touch as a therapeutic intervention, and homophobia. You can consult the literature or local experts.

5. Critique judgment/decision

Wanting to explore the situation more fully, you responded to the patient initially by saying, "I am sorry that you felt uncomfortable by my colleague's care. I want to talk with him about his sense of what happened and will then discuss this with you when I return on Wednesday." After talking with your colleague, you are reasonably assured that he was not intending, inappropriately, to communicate anything of a sexual nature to the patient. On your return visit to the patient, you inform him about your research and judgment and say, "Touch can mean different things to different people. My sense is that Dave simply wanted to communicate that he cares. If he is going about this in the wrong way, he wants to know what he should be doing differently. He recognized that you weren't responding to touch, so he did alter his style, but your rapport was likely already negatively affected. We certainly don't want this to be a problem for you or any other patient. Would you like to talk more about this or to file a report?"

You initially thought you had four options: (1) agree at the outset that your colleague has behaved in a sexually inappropriate and unprofessional manner; (2) defend your colleague on principle alone; (3) investigate the incident and conclude that your colleague was in the wrong; or (4) investigate the incident and conclude that your colleague was in the right. You chose the fourth option and are relieved when the patient seems to accept your explanation. You are a bit bothered by the fact the nurse immediately labeled the patient homophobic, without providing any rationale, and you make a mental note to follow up on that comment. Two months later, when you receive a similar complaint from another male patient, you are troubled. You realize now that there was a fifth option, and that this is the one you should have taken. Irrespective of the fact you were convinced by your colleague's sincerity and good intent, you should have informed Dave, the nurse, that you needed to communicate this patient's concern to your supervisor so that if future incidents were reported, there would be a record of repeat complaints.

and other issues surrounding sexuality will be unable to assess, teach, or counsel patients with sexual concerns.

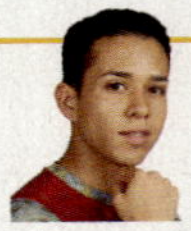

Recall **Paul Rojas,** the patient described in the Reflective Practice box on page 1862. The nurse caring for Mr. Rojas needs to be comfortable with their own sexuality to provide nonjudgmental care. In addition, the nurse needs knowledge about sexual orientation to develop an appropriate, unbiased plan of care that meets Mr. Rojas' needs.

Nursing goals to enhance interactions with patients and to promote individual sexual health are as follows:

The nurse will be able to:

- Feel comfortable as a sexual being.
- Develop self-awareness regarding sexual topics.
- Develop communication skills that promote discussion of sexual concerns with patients.
- Identify patients with problems related to sexuality and intervene competently and comfortably to meet these needs.
- Practice responsible sexual expression and respect the sexual expression of others.

NURSING PROCESS FOR THE PATIENT WITH A SEXUAL HEALTH NEED

Nurses who role model good health behaviors are more effective teachers. Use the display, Promoting Health 46-1, for yourself before using it with others.

Assessing

Sexual History

The comprehensive health history should include information regarding a patient's reproductive and sexual health, depending on the circumstances in which the patient is receiving care. As a rule, three general categories of patients should have a sexual history recorded by the nurse:

- Any inpatient or outpatient receiving care for pregnancy, STI, infertility, or contraception
- Any patient experiencing sexual dysfunction
- Any patient whose illness will affect sexual functioning and behavior in any way

Information is best obtained from the patient by beginning with nonthreatening questions and progressing to more sensitive concerns (see Focused Assessment Guide 46-1). Patients usually have no difficulty answering questions regarding their bodies and general reproductive issues, such as, "When did your menstrual periods first begin?" Explain to patients that this information may help you develop the plan of care and identify any sexual problems or concerns. The assessment provides an excellent opportunity to teach by helping the patient confront fears.

Four general levels of sexual history are:

Level 1: Sexual history as part of a comprehensive health history—obtained by a nurse

Level 2: Sexual history—obtained by a nurse with education and training in sexuality

Level 3: Sexual problem history—obtained by a sex therapist

Level 4: Psychiatric/psychosocial history—obtained by a psychiatric nurse clinician

Each level acquires more specific information from the patient regarding sexual health, and thus requires the interviewer to have more sophisticated preparation and skills. The clinical nurse usually performs a sexual history on level 1.

The nurse sets the tone or atmosphere for the interview. The nurse's attitudes will greatly affect the patient's response to the sexual history; patients will be more cooperative if they sense the nurse's security and ease during the interview. Privacy is essential for the sexual history; doors should be closed, and no interruptions allowed. Sit close to the patient

Promoting Health 46-1

SEXUALITY

Use the assessment checklist to determine how well you are meeting your sexuality needs. Then develop a prescription for self-care by choosing appropriate behaviors from the list of suggestions.

Assessment Checklist

☐ almost always ☐ sometimes ☐ almost never

☐ ☐ ☐ 1. I feel positive about my sexual identity.

☐ ☐ ☐ 2. I have satisfying relationships with others.

☐ ☐ ☐ 3. I accept sexual needs as a normal part of life.

☐ ☐ ☐ 4. I am comfortable with physical actions that indicate love and belonging (such as touching and hugging).

Self-Care Behaviors

1. Avoid stereotyping gender roles.
2. Learn the biological aspects of sexual functioning and consider the implications for those who are transgender.
3. Ask questions about sexual needs and sexual activity when necessary.
4. Enjoy close relationships with others who love you.
5. Give a hug to someone you love.
6. Accept touch from others as a sign of caring and affection.
7. Use contraceptives, condoms, and other barrier devices, and choose sexual partner(s) carefully.
8. Recognize how age, illness, or disability influences sexual needs and expression.

Focused Assessment Guide 46-1

SEXUALITY

Factors to Assess	Questions and Approaches
Reproductive history	Ask females their date of menarche, date of last menstrual period, duration and length of flow in days, number of pregnancies, living children, miscarriages, abortions, method of birth control. Ask males the number of children they have produced and method of birth control used. Ask all persons of childbearing age if they have any concerns about their fertility and determine whether there is any interest in the new reproductive technologies and genetic testing options. Consider the unique needs of persons who are transgender and integrate a holistic assessment.
History of sexually transmitted infections	"Do you or a sexual partner have a history of sexually transmitted infections?" "Many people today have questions about sexually transmitted infections that they are reluctant to express. Do you have any questions? Have you noticed any signs that might indicate a problem?"
History of sexual dysfunction	"Have you ever experienced a problem such as erectile dysfunction, failure to achieve orgasm, or pain during intercourse?"
Sexual self-care behaviors	"Do you know what your breasts (testicles) feel and look like normally?" "When was your last gynecologic (urologic) examination (Pap smear, mammogram)?" "Is there a family history of breast disease, ovarian cancer, testicular cancer, colon cancer?" "With all the attention on safer sex today and responsible parenting, many people have questions about their sexual self-care behaviors. Do you have any such concerns?" (It is important to ascertain whether patients possess the knowledge, attitudes, and skills necessary to promote their own sexual health and that of others.)
Sexual self-concept	
Sexual identity	"How do you feel about yourself as a man or woman? Is anything changing the way you feel about yourself?" Use appropriate terms and be open to conversations regarding gender when, for example, the individual does not consider gender in relation to their sexual identity or when gender and sex assigned at birth are not the same.
Sexual body image	"Many people have concerns about their sexual body image. Are you comfortable with your physical, sexual presentation?" "Have you experienced any physical changes (e.g., baldness, weight loss or gain, impotence, menopause, mastectomy, hysterectomy, sterilization) that are troubling to you?"
Sexual self-esteem	"We all have certain expectations of ourselves. Are you comfortable with the way you are currently expressing yourself sexually and meeting your sexual needs?"
Sexual role performance	"Has anything interfered with your ability to be a spouse, sexual partner, or other valued sex-related role?"
Sexual functioning	"It's not unusual for people with health concerns (name specific medical problem, if appropriate) to have questions related to sexuality and sexual functioning. Do you have any questions or concerns that I can help you with?" "Has anything (substitute the name of a specific disease, surgery, or medication, if appropriate) changed your ability to function sexually?" Asking patients if they have questions about resuming their usual sexual activity is an appropriate part of discharge planning for many patients.

and speak in a quiet, relaxed, objective tone of voice. Use eye contact and open body posture. Explain to the patient that only providers directly involved with the care of the patient will have access to this information.

Obtain reproductive health information first, followed by the sexual health history. The best approach is to begin with general open-ended questions and progress to more specific ones. Try to use the terminology used by the patient because the patient may be reluctant to admit not understanding certain terms for fear of appearing ignorant or foolish. For example, the patient may use the term "come" or "cum" to mean climax or orgasm. Although gender identity is different from biological sex or sexual identify, it may need to be discussed if working with a patient whose gender is different from their sex assigned at birth. For example, gender discussion will help determine preferred pronouns and ensure the appropriate biological questions are asked. Keep in mind that using "they" as a pronoun is becoming more common; checklists and other facility intake forms are evolving to reflect an expanding list of options. Use appropriate terms and allow the patient to provide whatever information the patient is comfortable sharing.

It is useful to begin questions with phrases such as "many people like" or "many people feel." This gives patients security in knowing they are not alone in how they feel and will encourage them to talk about their problems or concerns. For example, "Many people feel that it's helpful to discuss their concerns about sex with their partner. What do you think about this?"

One helpful structure for obtaining information about sexual problems follows:

- *Description of the problem:* "How would you describe the problem?"
- *Onset and cause of the problem:* "What do you think caused the problem, or what was happening when you first noticed it?"
- *Past attempts at resolution:* "What have you tried in the past to correct the problem?"
- *Goals of the patient:* "What do you wish to accomplish?"

A narrative format is generally used for recording a sexual history because it allows the interviewer to document the data in many of the patient's own words. If a patient is seeking help for a sexual problem, a more specific format is used to record information obtained by a skilled therapist.

Unfolding Patient Stories: Jared Griffin • Part 2

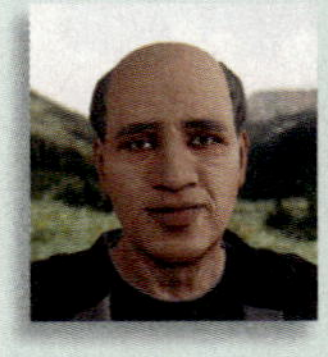

Recall **Jared Griffin** from Chapter 7, a 63-year-old male who has undergone a right total knee arthroplasty. He is in a private room on contact precautions because he is a carrier of methicillin-resistant *Staphylococcus aureus* (MRSA). He is concerned about resuming sexual activity and transmitting the infection to his wife when he is discharged home. What communication characteristics portray professionalism and competency when the nurse is assessing sexual health? How can the nurse promote discussion of his sexual concerns? What patient education would the nurse provide for Jared?

Care for Jared and other patients in a realistic virtual environment: ***vSim** for Nursing* (thepoint.lww.com/vSimFunds). Practice documenting these patients' care in DocuCare (thepoint.lww.com/DocuCareEHR).

THE BETTER MODEL

The BETTER model was created to help oncology nurses conduct sexual assessments with their patients more effectively. The acronym BETTER (Mick et al., 2004) stands for the following:

Bring up the topic of sexuality so that patients know they can discuss sexuality openly.

Explain that you are concerned with all aspects of patients' lives affected by disease.

Tell patients sexual dysfunction can happen and that you will find appropriate resources to address their concerns.

Timing is important to address sexuality with each visit to let patients know they can ask for information at any time.

Educate patients about the side effects of their treatments and that side effects may be temporary.

Record your assessment and interventions in patients' medical records.

A few of the major dysfunctions and assessment priorities are briefly discussed in Table 46-3. Also see the Focus on the Older Adult display on page 1882.

Physical Assessment

Physical examination of the reproductive or genitourinary system is necessary for patients under the following circumstances:

- As part of a routine physical examination
- Annual gynecologic health care examination, including a Pap smear
- Suspected STI
- Suspected pregnancy
- Workup for infertility
- Unusual lump, discharge, or appearance of the genital organs noticed by the patient
- Request for birth control
- Change in urinary function

The examiner may routinely perform a complete physical examination along with assessment of the reproductive system if the patient has not had contact with the health care system within 1 year, or if the assessment findings from a complete examination would be useful in diagnosing something reported by the patient. See Chapter 27 for a detailed description of how to examine the female and male genitalia.

Initially, ask whether the patient has had this type of examination in the past (if this information is not evident in the patient's records). Depending on the patient's knowledge base, explain the progressive steps of the examination and what the patient may feel during the examination. This will give the patient some feeling of control and security during the examination. The nurse's responsibilities during an examination of the reproductive system are as follows:

- Provide information about the examination.
- Teach the patient.
- Provide support to the patient during the examination.
- Perform the examination or assist the examiner, if appropriate, with any procedures or laboratory studies.

Keeping the patient comfortable and respecting the patient's privacy and modesty should be primary nursing considerations. Some female patients may be uncomfortable with a male examiner, or vice versa, for religious, cultural, or other reasons. The examiner can adapt to such concerns, for example, by ensuring that a female nurse is in the room when a female patient is undergoing a pelvic examination by a male provider. Some patients who are transgender prefer to be seen by a provider who is known to be *LGBTQIA+ welcoming* or who provides transgender care specifically, particularly when seeking a gynecologist or endocrinologist.

Diagnosing

The International Council of Nurses (ICN, 2019) groups sexual problems into several categories:

- *Problematic Sexual Behavior:* This problem arises when a person experiences or is at risk for a change in sexual

Table 46-3 Sexual Dysfunction and Nursing Assessment

SEXUAL DYSFUNCTION	ASSESSMENT PRIORITIES
Male	
Erectile dysfunction (impotence)	• Assess for history of diabetes, spinal cord trauma, cardiovascular disease, surgical procedure, or alcoholism. • Assess for use of certain medications such as antihypertensives, antidepressants, or illicit drugs. • Determine degree of mental depression that may be present. • Obtain specific information regarding the degree of impotence, length of time of disorder, or continuing life factors.
Premature ejaculation	• Assess what patient defines as the dysfunction and ability to control ejaculation. • Assess any causative relationship factors such as anxiety, guilt, lack of time, or new partner.
Delayed ejaculation	• Assess for history of neurologic disorders, Parkinson disease, or use of certain medications. • Use the same assessment priorities as for premature ejaculation.
Female	
Inhibited sexual desire	• Assess for use of oral contraceptives or other hormonal therapy, use of alcohol or certain medications. • Assess for history of sexual abuse, rape or incest, depression, or other sexual dysfunctions. • Assess any other contributing or relationship factors.
Orgasmic dysfunction	• Assess knowledge regarding sexual response cycle and anatomy. • Assess the communication pattern between the patient and partner(s). • Assess the usual sexual pattern and behavior between the patient and partner(s). • Assess any other contributing factors.
Dyspareunia	• Assess for history of diabetes, hormonal imbalance, vaginal infection, endometriosis, urethritis, cervicitis, or rectal lesions. • Assess for use of antihistamines, alcohol, tranquilizers, or illicit drugs. • Assess the patient's ability for vaginal lubrication during the sexual act. • Assess the patient's use of coital positions. • Assess the use of cosmetic or chemical irritants to the genitals, such as deodorant tampons, contraceptive creams or jellies, or condoms. • Perform physical assessment of internal and external genitalia. • Assess any other contributing factors.
Vaginismus	• Assess knowledge regarding anatomy and sexual response. • Assess the pattern of sexual activity: how often, level of arousal, orgasm. • Assess the presence of other sexual dysfunctions. • Assess for history of sexual abuse, trauma, or rape. • Assess the patient's feelings regarding partner(s). • Assess any other causative factors, such as fear of pregnancy, anxiety, or guilt. • Perform physical assessment of internal and external genitalia.

health, which results in concern regarding their own sexuality. Sexual health is the integration of somatic, emotional, intellectual, and social aspects of sexual being in ways that are enriching and that enhance personality, communication, and love. This problem may result from problematic behavior or may be based on a knowledge deficit.

- *Impaired Sexual Functioning*: This problem presents when a person experiences or is at risk for change in sexual function (desire, excitation, or orgasm) that does not meet the sexual needs of the individual.
- *Victim of Sexual Assault* and subsequent *Effective Recovery from Sexual Assault*: Problem identification of this nature is very patient-specific and may involve the interprofessional team, law enforcement, and specific counseling. Progression to effective recovery is rarely linear, and is based on existing and developed coping mechanisms and resources.

Before a sexual-based issue is identified as a problem, carefully review the assessment data to determine whether the situation can be corrected by independent nursing interventions. Although many problems of sexuality experienced by a patient in a health care situation are amenable to nursing action, some require the expertise of other specialties.

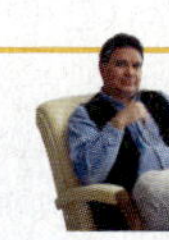

A patient with impotence and diabetes who would benefit from a penile implant—such as **Jefferson Smith,** described at the beginning of the chapter—needs medical consultation. A patient with a serious sexual dysfunction or one who practices destructive sexual expression needs intensive therapy by a clinical psychologist, sex therapist, or counselor. Appropriate referrals by the nurse should follow the identification of such problems.

Sexual patterns can be further specified by loss of desire (to abstinence), increased desire (to promiscuity), or change in sexual expression. Common etiologies for a change in sexual behaviors include stress (lifestyle, job, family, finances, marital

Focus on the Older Adult

NURSING STRATEGIES TO ADDRESS AGE-RELATED CHANGES IN SEXUALITY AND SEXUAL FUNCTION

Factors that contribute to sexual dysfunction in the older adult are essentially the same as those that affect performance at any age: disease or mutilating surgery of the genitourinary tract, diverse systemic diseases, and emotional disturbances coupled with societal attitudes.

Age-Related Changes	Nursing Strategies
Use of multiple medications may impact on sexual desire and performance.	• Educate older adult patients, intimate partners, and family about the sexual side effects of specific medications. Sometimes a change in medication dosage or modification in the treatment regimen can reduce sexual dysfunction.
Dependence on alcohol or marijuana to cope with discomforts of aging may result in weakened erection, reduced desire, or delayed ejaculation.	• Before the patient can decide to stop using alcohol or drugs, the patient must realize the need to change the behavior. The nurse can assist in attitude and value clarification about substance use, sexuality, and sexual behavior. Refer the older adult patient to a counselor who can assist with sexual performance problems as well as emotional and dependence problems.
Age-related metabolic disorders such as anemia, diabetes, malnutrition, and fatigue or depression may affect the quality of life and cause impotence.	• Symptoms may be initially discussed with the nurse. The patient may be hesitant to discuss sexual problems openly. Listen carefully. Acknowledge that sexual problems in the older adult are not unusual. Even if the nurse does not know all the answers, active listening on the nurse's part may encourage the patient to visit a health care provider or a counselor. Encourage older adult patients to have a thorough physical evaluation by a health care provider.
Obesity may damage cardiac and vascular integrity and reduce self-esteem, resulting in decreased sexual performance and interest.	• Encourage the patient to seek the advice of a health care provider and to explore weight reduction and health promotion programs.
Many older adult people are concerned that sexual activity might increase the risk for illness or even death due to stress on the heart or blood pressure.	• Teach the patient that sexual intercourse and similar forms of sexual expression are not considered dangerous for anyone able to walk around a room and may actually offer physiologic benefits. Although there is no risk of pregnancy for females after menopause, both partners need to engage in wellness strategies to prevent STIs.
Radical surgery or dysfunction of the genitourinary tract affects sexual capacity and libido. Extensive surgery due to malignancy may make intercourse difficult or impossible.	• Patients need support and guidance in adjusting to these changes. Provide specific suggestions for how to accommodate to the surgical changes while still maintaining a sexually satisfying relationship. Acknowledge the need for sexual expression in some form or another and provide an open, nonjudgmental response when patients articulate a need for warmth, close contact, and companionship. Touch is particularly important. An atmosphere of trust between the nurse and the older adult patient is essential.
Loss of a spouse or committed partner	• Explore alternative forms of sexual expression with patients who lose their primary sexual partner. Encourage them to attend a support group and become active socially. Acknowledge that human sexuality crosses a wide spectrum and that the pattern for each person is an outcome of their development, experiences, and sense of personal identity. The basic pattern is not altered by age or loss of a spouse or committed partner. It continues to influence one's capacity for involvement in all life activities.

Source: Adapted from Edelman, C. L., & Kudzma, E. C. (2022). *Health promotion throughout the life span* (10th ed.). Elsevier; Murray, R. B., Zentner, J. P., & Yakimo, R. (2009). *Health promotion strategies through the life span* (8th ed.). Prentice Hall, Inc./Pearson Education.

conflict), isolation from partner, effects of pregnancy, feelings of depression, loss of privacy, loss of communication with partner, relationship change (new partner), effects of disease process (sexual position, frequency, mode of expression), change in body image, change in self-concept, or loss of partner.

Sexual function issues may include erectile failure (impotence), premature ejaculation, delayed ejaculation, inhibited sexual desire, orgasmic dysfunction, vaginismus, or dyspareunia. Common etiologies for sexual dysfunction include effects of medication, effects of alcohol consumption, effects of disease process, history of abuse, feelings of depression, guilt, anxiety, fear of rejection, miscommunication with partner, fear of pain, effects of birth control method, lack of knowledge, or effects of surgical procedure.

Changes in sexuality can affect other areas of human functioning. Sexual functioning and expression may be a primary problem for a patient. Examples of these patient problems and needs with related etiology and signs and symptoms can

Examples of Actual or Potential Health Problems and Needs

PATIENT EXPERIENCING SEXUAL ALTERATIONS OR DYSFUNCTION

Actual or Potential Health Problems and Needs	Possible Etiologic Factors	Potential Signs and Symptoms
Problematic Sexual Behavior	• Sexual behavior that does not match developmental or expressed comfort level • Lack of exposure, lack of knowledge, or lack of experience	• Verbalizations of feeling pressured to engage in sexual activities with a partner that cause unwanted pain or discomfort • Engagement in vaginal, anal, or oral sex without a condom to prevent the spread of STIs
Impaired Sexual Functioning	• Underlying medical issue(s) • Medications known to cause sexual dysfunction • History of trauma or abuse • Change in libido—may be physical and/or psychological	• Change in sexual performance that is unacceptable to the person • Inability to engage in wanted, meaningful sexual encounters • Loss of/decrease in sexual desire and drive

Source: International Council of Nurses (ICN). (2019). *Nursing diagnosis and outcome statements.* https://www.icn.ch/sites/default/files/inline-files/ICNP2019-DC.pdf

be found in the box titled Examples of Actual or Potential Health Problems and Needs: Patient Experiencing Sexual Alterations or Dysfunction. In the following examples, problems of sexuality are the etiology of another problem (ICN, 2019):

- Anxiety related to fear of pregnancy, loss of sexual functioning or desire, or effects of disease process on sexual functioning
- Difficulty Coping related to effects of body image on sexual expression or change in sexual partner
- Disturbed Body Image (specify: surgical excision of genital body part, loss of or gain in body weight) related to fear of rejection
- Disturbed Personal Identity related to alteration in social role, cultural incongruence, discrimination, or stages of growth
- Fear related to pain during sexual intercourse or history of sexual abuse
- Grief related to loss of sexual functioning or effects of surgical excision of genital body part
- Impaired Human Development related to sexual exploitation or abuse, sexual guilt, effects of hormonal imbalance, or lack of information about sexuality
- Lack of Knowledge (specify: contraceptive methods, spread of STIs, sexual response, genital anatomy, modes of sexual expression, self-examination, effects of disease or medications) related to misinformation, sexual myths, lack of interest in learning, or cognitive limitation
- Pain related to sexual position, penile penetration, effects of genital surgery, or lack of vaginal lubrication
- Social Isolation related to effects of marital separation or divorce

Outcome Identification and Planning

Nurses should value sexuality as an important component of who the patient is and how the patient identifies as a unique human. Specific patient outcomes to promote sexual health are identified below.

The patient will:

- Define individual sexuality
- Establish open patterns of communication with significant others
- Develop self-awareness and body awareness
- Describe responsible sexual health self-care practices, identifying appropriate resources
- Practice responsible sexual expression (e.g., by 5/1/25, the patient will use condoms during all sexual encounters)

Specific patient outcomes depend on the nature of the patient's problem or concern. Expected outcomes should be patient-oriented—that is, something the patient desires to do or has the ability to accomplish. For example, it is not enough to advise a method of birth control; rather, the nurse needs to know which method the patient is motivated and able to use.

Implementing

Establishing a Trusting Nurse–Patient Relationship

It is impossible to address a patient's sexuality if trust has not been developed between you and the patient (see Through the Eyes of a Student on page 1884). To develop trust, project an objective, nonthreatening, and nonjudgmental attitude, and emphasize that the information the patient gives will be kept confidential. You need to be aware of your own behavior and verbal and nonverbal cues. You also need to anticipate the patient's concerns to help the patient trust you with information of an intimate nature. Be sure to establish respect for the patient and empathy before discussing sexual issues. Consider all of the patient's circumstances and life experiences using a therapeutic approach. Only when you are accepted as a trusted, caring person will the patient reveal details of their private life, including sexual concerns.

Through the Eyes of a Student

I knew it was going to happen sooner or later, but I admit that I was glad this happened my first clinical rotation with Miss Ethel. Male nurses are not unheard of in this day and age, but some people just aren't yet ready for us—especially Miss Ethel, an 88-year-old woman with a deep religious conviction. I concluded this because she called on Jesus for help when I told her that I was her student nurse for the day, and that I would be giving her a bath.

"You're my nurse?" she said. "Help me, Jesus…. No, no, you just go on and help somebody else, honey. I've already had my bath," she insisted.

I told her she was mistaken and that I understood her anxiety. I proceeded to exaggerate the truth by saying that I had done this before, when really I had given baths before, but not to an older woman. She thought *she* was having anxiety!

Next, I asked my instructor, Mrs. Anderson, for help. She quickly assessed the situation and tried to reassure Miss Ethel (and me) by vouching for my professional character and abilities, but Miss Ethel still was unconvinced. Then I tried using logic with Miss Ethel.

"This is a hospital where male doctors examine you all the time. Why is this any different?" I asked. "Because you are not a doctor," was her logical reply.

I felt inadequate. I could not give this woman the care she needed because of my gender. Luckily, in the next bed, Michele was about to give her patient a bath. Michele offered to give Miss Ethel a bath if I would help her with her patient.

Consequently, Miss Ethel got her bath, and I learned that a nurse has to be flexible as well as willing to ask for and accept help when the patient's quality of care is at stake. Changing assignments is not always possible, but we were able to make it work and honor the patient's request. This is something I hope to remember throughout my nursing career. The good news is that because I maintained a positive attitude and respected her wishes, Miss Ethel and I worked together the rest of the day. I was able to provide detailed teaching and form a rapport with her. Although she was not comfortable with being exposed in front of me, I was able to provide effective nursing care in other ways.

—Daniel E. Zirolli
Delaware County Community College, Media, Pennsylvania

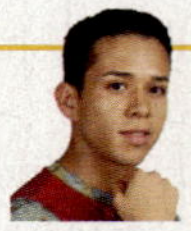

Review the Reflective Practice display for this chapter. Note how the nursing student initially avoided interpersonal contact with **Paul Rojas**, performing the technical aspects of care, but ignoring Paul (the patient) as a person. Communication and trust did not occur until Paul asked the nursing student about her level of discomfort and the nursing student responded truthfully.

Teaching About Sexuality and Sexual Health

Most nursing interventions pertaining to a patient's sexuality involve teaching to promote sexual health. Major goals of patient teaching involve effecting change in knowledge, attitude, or behavior. In some situations, patients need help defining or redefining their sexuality and its importance to their lives. Offering information, dispelling fears, and providing positive reinforcement are some ways to help patients increase their knowledge about their bodies and sexual functioning. Patients may need assistance in modifying behaviors or learning new skills to increase the quality of sexual health and functioning. See the Promoting Health Literacy box.

Part of teaching also includes correcting sexual myths and promoting body awareness. Many people believe things

Promoting Health Literacy

IN PATIENTS RECEIVING THE HPV VACCINE

Patient Scenario

Mrs. Smith, mother of 15-year-old Diane Smith, was told by her daughter's high school that all girls must get the HPV vaccine. Mrs. Smith knows that Diane has been dating a boy from school for almost a year but insists that her daughter "is not sexually active and should not have to get the vaccine." She is primarily concerned that this new vaccine is not safe.

Nursing Considerations: *Tips for Improving Health Literacy*

Tell Mrs. Smith that one in four young females between ages 14 and 19 years is infected with at least one of the most common STIs, which include HPV. According to the Centers for Disease Control and Prevention (CDC), adolescents between ages 11 and 26 years should receive the HPV vaccine.[a] Give both Mrs. Smith and her daughter an information sheet about HPV and the HPV vaccine. Encourage the mother and daughter to be prepared to ask the clinician these questions:

- What problem is the HPV vaccine trying to prevent?
- What do I need to know in order to make an informed decision about getting the vaccine?
- Why does the school think it is important for all girls to get the vaccine?

What additional measures can you take to help increase health literacy in this mother and daughter? What other measures would be helpful if they did not speak English, could not read, or had other learning deficits? What other measures could you take if the daughter confided in you that she is sexually active? What additional measure would be necessary if the primary reason for refusing the HPV vaccine was religious?

[a]Centers for Disease Control and Prevention (CDC). (2020a, March 17). *HPV vaccine recommendations.* https://www.cdc.gov/vaccines/vpd/hpv/hcp/recommendations.html

Table 46-4 Sexual Myths and Facts to Refute Them

SEXUAL DYSFUNCTION	ASSESSMENT PRIORITIES
Each person is born with a certain amount of sexual drive, which if overdrawn in youth, leaves little reserve for later years.	Actually, the correlation between sexual activity and length of time it persists throughout life is just the opposite. The more consistently sexually active a person is, the longer the activity continues into the later years of life.
A person's need for sexual expression becomes less important in the latter half of life.	Physiologically, sexual desire and ability do not decrease markedly after middle age. The expression of sexuality as an integral part of development follows the overall pattern of health and physical performance.
Sexual abstinence is necessary in training for sports.	Physiologically, the achievement of orgasm is rarely more demanding than most activities encountered in daily life. The desire for sleep that often follows is most commonly due to factors other than physical exhaustion from sexual activities. There is no scientific evidence that sex weakens a person.
Excessive sexual activity can lead to mental illness.	The biological significance of human sexuality has no greater effect on total development than any other necessary biological function. There is no scientific basis for believing that a person will develop a mental or physical illness with excessive or no sexual activity.
Wet dreams are indicators of sexual disorders.	Erotic dreams that culminate in orgasms are normal and common physiologic phenomena in at least 85% of males. They can occur at any age after puberty. Some females also report in clinical studies that their sexual dreams culminate in orgasm. In females, this phenomenon is believed to increase with advancing age.
Because of the anatomical nature of the sex organs, females are passive and males are aggressive.	Physiologic studies disprove this myth by showing females to be far from passive. Sexual satisfaction requires each partner to be both passive and aggressive while participating mutually and cooperatively.
It is unnatural for a woman to have as strong a desire for sex as a man. Women should not enjoy sex as much as men.	These myths have been reinforced by a society that has traditionally taught women that they are to suppress sexual desires to gain love, security, and social respect, based on the assumption that it is the basic nature of women to be submissive, dependent, and subordinate. Physiologic studies indicate that, in some respects, a woman's sex drive is not only as strong, but may be even stronger than that of a man.
Women who have multiple orgasms or who readily come to climax are nymphomaniacs or promiscuous.	Physiologic studies suggest that we do not know women's sexual potential; these studies indicate that there is a wide range of intensity and duration of orgasmic experience, and the potential for multiple or frequent orgasms within a brief period is not at all uncommon. Therefore, women normally may have greater orgasmic capacity than men with regard to duration and frequency of orgasm.
There is a difference between vaginal orgasm and clitoral orgasm.	Physiologic misunderstanding has produced the myth of separate clitoral and vaginal orgasms rather than their interrelations. Female orgasm is normally initiated by clitoral stimulation, but because orgasm is a total body response, there are marked variations in intensity and timing. There is no reason to believe that the female response to the sex act is due to a vaginal rather than a clitoral orgasm.
A mature sexual relationship requires both partners to achieve simultaneous orgasm.	Although simultaneous orgasm may be desirable, it is unrealistic. Often, it is possible only under the most ideal circumstances and is not a determinant of sexual achievement or of satisfaction (except to someone who accepts this as dogma).
The larger penis has greater possibilities for producing orgasm in a partner.	Physiologically, there is practically no relation between the size of a man's penis and their ability to satisfy a partner sexually. Furthermore, there is little correlation between penile or body size and sexual potency.
The face-to-face coital position is the proper, moral, and healthy one.	Knowledge of human sexual practices dispels this myth with the recognition that there is no normal or single most acceptable sexual position. Whatever position offers the most pleasure and is acceptable to both partners is correct for them. Any variation is normal, healthy, and proper if it satisfies both partners.
The ability to achieve orgasm is an indicator of a person's sexual responsiveness.	Achievement of a satisfactory sexual response is the result of numerous physical, psychological, and cultural influences. Too often, the physical fact of orgasm (or lack of orgasm) is taken to be symbolic of sexual responsiveness and seen out of context of the entire relationship.

about sex that they have heard from family or friends that are not true or are not based on scientific data. During the assessment, or while providing care, take the opportunity to refute sexual myths and teach factual information (Table 46-4).

Patients may need assistance in becoming familiar with what they believe and feel about their sexual selves. Be helpful to patients who have difficulty accepting or developing their sexuality by promoting their self-confidence and a positive self-concept. When patients feel comfortable about themselves and their sensual feelings, they can begin to focus on how they feel about their sexual functioning and specific sexual expressions.

Getting to know your physical body is important to healthy sexual development. All people, sexually active or not, need to be aware of the appearance of their genitalia. Some people, because of their background, feel ashamed and repulsed by their bodies; others feel that touching the body is dirty and may feel guilt and anxiety in stimulating themselves. Patients need assistance in improving body awareness if any of these issues are present. Patients can become accustomed to looking at their bodies by looking at nonthreatening anatomy first and then proceeding to the genitals. This can be done in the shower or with the use of a mirror. Knowing what looks normal can be of great importance so that patients can report the development of an unusual appearance later.

After patients have developed some degree of comfort in looking at their bodies, they can progress to experiencing touch. Again, patients should progress from nonthreatening parts of the body until the genitals can be touched without stress.

A good exercise for anyone with a vagina in developing body awareness is the use of Kegel exercises. These exercises promote good vaginal tone by localizing and strengthening the pubococcygeal muscle. A person can locate this muscle by stopping a stream of urine midway through urination. Contracting this muscle can be repeated at any time of the day in any circumstance because its performance is undetectable. Some women who practice Kegel exercises have found that their sexual satisfaction is improved.

Promoting Responsible Sexual Expression

Patients need to know how to gain satisfactory sexual experiences while behaving responsibly in their activities. Responsible sexuality encompasses sexual expression, prevention of unwanted pregnancy, prevention of STIs, and sex education.

FORM OF SEXUAL EXPRESSION

The form of sexual expression used by patients should not inflict unwanted harm on themselves or others. When sexual expression encroaches on the rights of others, it is neither healthy nor desirable. Sexual acts that violate another's rights are usually considered to be acts of aggression or hostility rather than stemming from sexual need or desire. Rape, in particular, is motivated by a need to dominate and humiliate the victim—it is an act of violence.

PREVENTION OF UNWANTED PREGNANCY

Contraception is a process or technique for preventing pregnancy by means of a medication, device, or method that blocks or alters one or more of the processes of reproduction in such a way that sexual intercourse can occur without impregnation. The prevention of unwanted pregnancy must be a conscious decision. Anyone who is unprepared for pregnancy should refrain from intercourse or obtain a contraceptive method from a health care provider or from the pharmacy; it is too late to think about contraception during sexual intercourse. To practice responsible sex, the contraceptive method must be used consistently and according to instructions.

PREVENTION OF STIs

As described earlier, STIs are widespread. The only sure way to avoid an STI is to avoid all types of intimate genital contact. When this is impractical, there are other practices that can decrease a patient's risk for STIs (Box 46-1). In the United States, Black/African American people account for 42% of new HIV diagnoses in 2018. Black women account

Box 46-1 What Can You Do to Prevent STIs?

The best way to prevent STIs is to avoid sexual contact with others. If you decide to be sexually active, there are things that you can do to reduce your risk of developing an STI.

- Have a mutually monogamous sexual relationship with an uninfected partner.
- Correctly and consistently use a male condom.
- Use clean needles if injecting intravenous drugs.
- Prevent and control other STIs to decrease susceptibility to HIV infection and to reduce your infectiousness if you are HIV infected.
- Delay having sexual relations as long as possible. The younger people are when having sex for the first time, the more susceptible they become to developing an STI. The risk of acquiring an STI also increases with the number of partners over a lifetime.

Anyone who is sexually active should:

- Have regular checkups for STIs even in the absence of symptoms, and especially if having sex with a new partner. These tests can be done during a routine visit to the provider's office.
- Learn the common symptoms of STIs. Seek medical help immediately if any suspicious symptoms develop, even if they are mild.
- Use a male condom if practicing anal intercourse.
- Avoid douching because it removes some of the normal protective bacteria in the vagina and increases the risk of getting some STIs.

Anyone diagnosed as having an STI should:

- Be treated to reduce the risk of transmitting an STI to a sex partner or from birthing person to baby.
- Discuss with a doctor the possible risk of transmission in breast milk and whether commercial formula should be substituted.
- Notify all recent sex partners and urge them to get a checkup.
- Follow the provider's orders and complete the full course of medication prescribed. A follow-up test to ensure that the infection has been cured is often an important step in treatment.
- Avoid all sexual activity while being treated for an STI.

Sometimes people are too embarrassed or frightened to ask for help or information. Most STIs are readily treated. The earlier a person seeks treatment and warns sex partners about the disease, the less likely the disease will do irreparable physical damage, be spread to others, or, in the case of a female, be passed on to a newborn baby.

for most new cases of HIV and AIDS among women, and are second only to Black, White, and Hispanic/Latino MSM (CDC, 2021d). Most Black/African American women acquire the disease from heterosexual contact, often from a partner who has undisclosed risk factors for HIV infection. A combination of testing, education, socioeconomic support, and behavioral interventions can help reduce the rate of HIV infection and its complications among women of color.

SEX EDUCATION

Sex education is critical to healthy sexual development and safe sexual behaviors. Information received from peers and friends is almost always inadequate and may be erroneous. Parents/caregivers should be taught to answer children's questions immediately and accurately. Evidence-based, age-appropriate teen pregnancy programs are funded by Congress through Teen Pregnancy Prevention (TPP) Program grants (Office of the Assistant Secretary for Health, U.S. Department of Health & Human Services, n.d.). Abstinence-only programs that do not include more comprehensive approaches have limited (if any) impact on reducing sexual activity. Abstinence-only programs do not influence the number of sexual partners, use of contraceptives, incidence of STIs, or even pregnancy rates. Comprehensive sex education programs improve knowledge, change attitudes and behaviors, and affect outcomes; abstinence-only programs have not been shown to have this positive effect (Chin et al., 2012; Denford et al., 2017; Russell et al., 2020).

Considering Contraception

Unintended pregnancy remains a significant women's health issue in the United States as well as a critical social issue. Healthy People 2020 (2021a) and Healthy People 2030 (n.d.a) aim to improve pregnancy planning and spacing, and to prevent unintended pregnancy, especially in adolescents. Many unintended pregnancies result from the use of less effective methods of contraception, such as condoms, spermicide, or barrier methods. The past several years have seen the development of new, easier to use, and more effective methods of contraception. Nurses and nurse practitioners have a responsibility to provide information to individuals regarding their many contraceptive options (Fig. 46-4 on page 1888).

Patients choose contraception for many reasons and may contact health care providers specifically to obtain information about birth control. Some people use contraception for the orderly spacing of pregnancies in a family; others may want to prevent pregnancy from occurring until a family is desired. Some people choose a permanent method to prevent pregnancy from ever occurring. Factors that affect a person's choice of a contraceptive method include age, marital status, desire for future pregnancy, religious beliefs, level of education, cost, and ease of use. Other considerations include knowledge about available methods, perceptions of various methods, and in many cases, previous experience with contraception.

All contraceptive methods have advantages and disadvantages. Understanding and explaining the available methods thoroughly is a must so that patients can choose the one that will best meet their situation and needs (Box 46-2).

When choosing a contraceptive method, the patient should consider the following:

- How well will it fit into my lifestyle?
- How convenient will it be?
- How effective will it be?
- How safe will it be?
- How affordable will it be?
- How reversible will it be?
- Will it protect against STIs?

Box 46-2 Knowledge Deficit: Contraceptive Methods

Assessment Priorities

- Determine the patient's past use of contraceptive methods.
- Assess the effectiveness and satisfaction with past methods.
- Assess the patient's current knowledge of contraceptive methods.
- Assess the frequency of the patient's sexual activity.
- Identify any methods that are unacceptable to the patient.
- Assess the motivation of the patient to use certain methods.
- Assess the patient's level of comfort with manipulation of genital body parts.
- Obtain a complete patient history and perform a physical examination, if indicated.

Expected Outcomes

The patient will achieve the following:

- Choose a contraceptive method that the patient is motivated to use.
- List the adverse effects or danger signs associated with the contraceptive method.
- List the steps needed to use the contraceptive method effectively.
- Use the contraceptive with every act of sexual intercourse.
- Choose a backup method.
- Report back to the health care setting for follow-up as directed.

Nursing Interventions

- Describe in terms at the patient's level of understanding, each contraceptive method for which the patient needs information (give objective information in a matter-of-fact manner to avoid bias by nurse).
- Describe the effectiveness of each method and side effects or possible complications.
- Instruct the patient in the use of a chosen method, giving step-by-step instructions.
- Advise the patient of the importance of having a backup method on hand.
- Instruct the patient in the use of the backup method.
- Have the patient obtain a physical examination if required for the chosen contraceptive method (e.g., the pill).
- Instruct the patient to report back in a specified period for follow-up if indicated (follow-up visits to a health care facility are important, particularly if a patient elects to use oral contraceptives).

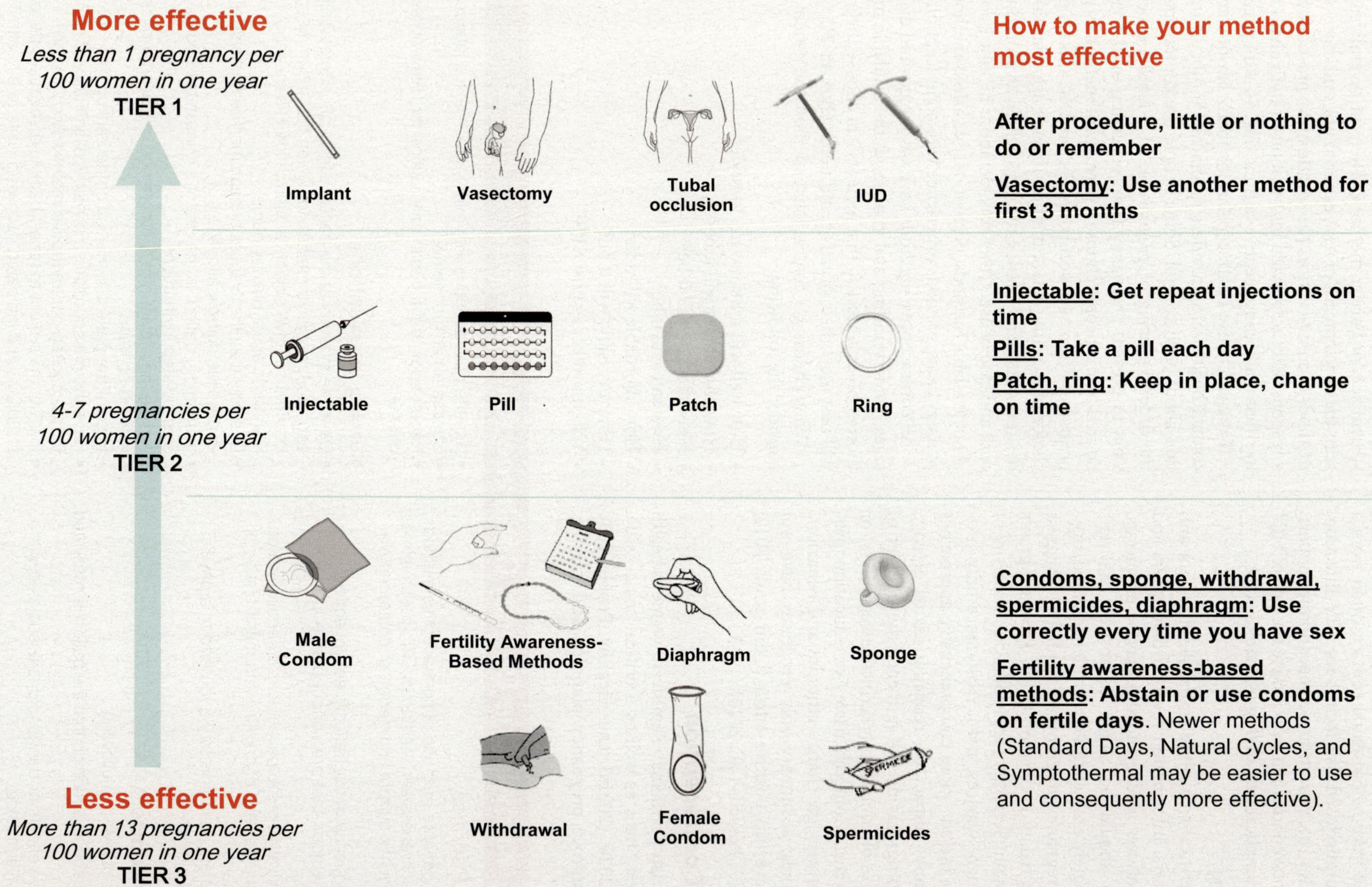

FIGURE 46-4. Contraceptive effectiveness. (*Source:* Trussell, J., Aiken, A. R. A., Micks, E., & Guthrie, K. A. [2018]. Efficacy, safety, and personal considerations. In: Hatcher, R. A., et al. [Eds.], *Contraceptive technology* [21st ed.]. Ayer Company Publishers, Inc. https://www.cdc.gov/reproductivehealth/contraception/index.htm#Contraceptive-Effectiveness)

BEHAVIORAL METHODS

Abstinence is a behavioral method of contraception. There are two types of abstinence: continuous and periodic. Choosing abstinence does not mean that a person is sexless. Most people are abstinent at some point in their lives. Abstinence can be a positive way of dealing with sexuality when it represents a well-thought-out decision regarding the person's mind, body, spirit, and sexual health.

Continuous abstinence involves not having any sex with a partner at all. It is 100% effective in preventing pregnancy and STIs. However, people may find it difficult to abstain for long periods of time. Ending abstinence without first being prepared to protect against an unplanned pregnancy or infection may cause additional problems.

Periodic abstinence and fertility awareness methods (FAMs) are two methods of contraception that involve charting a female's fertility pattern. Periodic abstinence is a method used by some sexually active people to prevent pregnancy. They become familiar with their fertility patterns and abstain from vaginal intercourse on the days they think they could become pregnant. Those who monitor their fertility to prevent pregnancy either abstain from vaginal intercourse for at least one third of each menstrual cycle or use barrier methods during the fertile or unsafe period.

Three basic charting methods can be used to predict ovulation to plan or prevent pregnancy (Planned Parenthood Federation of America Inc., 2021):

- *Temperature method:* The female takes her temperature every morning before getting out of bed. The temperature will rise between 0.4°F and 0.8°F on the day of ovulation and will remain at that level until the next period.
- *Cervical mucus method:* The female observes the changes in the cervical mucus throughout the first part of the menstrual cycle, until after ovulation. Cervical mucus is normally cloudy, but a few days before ovulation it becomes clear and slippery and can be stretched between the fingers. This indicates the most fertile phase of the cycle. The couple must abstain from vaginal intercourse or use a barrier method during this period to avoid pregnancy.
- *Calendar method:* The menstrual cycle is charted on a calendar. The couple must refrain from intercourse or use a barrier method during days when pregnancy is more likely.

The best approach to monitoring fertility is a combination of all three methods, called the symptothermal method. FAMs are 76% to 88% effective (Planned Parenthood Federation of America Inc., 2021). Using the methods carefully and consistently, and avoiding unprotected vaginal intercourse during the fertile phase can give better results.

Coitus interruptus, the withdrawal of the penis from the vagina before ejaculation, is one of the oldest and most widely used contraceptive methods. Pregnancy cannot occur if sperm are kept out of the vagina. Although the withdrawal or *pull-out* method is 78% effective if timed correctly, it does not protect against STIs (Planned Parenthood Federation of America Inc., 2021). Preejaculate can contain enough sperm to cause a pregnancy, and preejaculate or semen may spill onto the vulva.

BARRIER METHODS

Barrier methods include the condom, diaphragm, cervical cap, and vaginal sponge used in combination with a spermicidal agent (Planned Parenthood Federation of America Inc., 2021). Cost and the commitment to adhere to a specific regimen affect the choice and efficacy of each option.

Diaphragm

Diaphragm approaches have been used in various forms since ancient times. The current diaphragm is a dome-shaped device made of latex rubber that mechanically prevents semen from coming into contact with the cervix. It is also used to hold a spermicidal jelly in place against the cervix. The diaphragm is placed in the vagina before sexual activity. It fits between the pelvic notch at the front of the vagina to behind the cervix at the back. It is not felt by either partner when correctly situated in the vagina.

A diaphragm must be individually sized during a pelvic examination. Placement and removal of a diaphragm requires a familiarity with the genitals and a level of comfort touching and manipulating the vulva and vagina. The diaphragm must be worn during each episode of sexual activity and consistently used with a spermicidal agent. If used perfectly, a diaphragm is 94% effective; in most real-life situations, a diaphragm is 88% effective (Planned Parenthood Federation of America Inc., 2021).

Condom

The traditional condom is applied to a penis, but it is not unusual for a partner not wearing the condom to have one available. The condom is rolled over the erect penis and collects the semen after ejaculation occurs. If the condom does not have a nipple receptacle end, a small space should be left at the end of the condom to collect sperm (this prevents breakage). Condoms are available over the counter and have become more widely used because of the incidence of HIV/AIDS and other STIs.

A female condom, often called an internal condom, is also available. The female condom is a ringed pouch that unrolls in the vagina. Advantages include the fact that the male does not need to first have an erection for the pouch to be used, and it offers significant protection from STIs.

If used perfectly, condoms are 98% effective at preventing pregnancy; in most real-life situations, condoms are 85% effective at preventing pregnancy (Planned Parenthood Federation of America Inc., 2021). The latex condom protects against STIs, including HIV. The latex condom offers better protection against STIs than any other birth control method because it blocks the exchange of body fluids that may be infected.

Cervical Cap

The cervical cap is a thimble-shaped rubber device that is placed over the cervix and may be left there for up to 3 days at a time. Its mechanism of action is similar to that of the diaphragm. Not all females can wear a cervical cap because of individual anatomic differences. There is some evidence to suggest that the cervical cap can cause cervical inflammation and increase the risk for pelvic infection.

Spermicides

Spermicides are used with barrier methods but can also be used alone. Spermicides come in creams, jellies, foams, and suppositories. Although readily available, spermicides are not as effective alone as when combined with another method, such as a diaphragm or a condom.

Vaginal Sponge

The vaginal sponge is a barrier method that contains a spermicide. The sponge acts not only as a barrier between the semen and the cervix but also as a reservoir to hold semen. The vaginal sponge carries some risk of toxic shock syndrome (TSS) and is contraindicated for use in females who have a past history of TSS. Anyone who uses the vaginal sponge must follow package directions carefully and remove the sponge within 24 hours. The vaginal sponge is about as effective as the diaphragm.

HORMONAL METHODS

Hormonal methods are based on the feedback mechanism of hormones of the menstrual cycle. Synthetic estrogens and progestin chemical compounds are used in the form of a pill, shot, or implant to prevent ovulation.

Oral Contraceptives

The birth control pill (*the pill*) is the most common contraceptive method and the most popular method for females in their 20s. Most of the harmful side effects and dangers associated with taking the pill are related to the estrogen component. However, most pills currently available contain a small dose of estrogen. The pill also has many beneficial noncontraceptive effects. It has been shown to protect against the development of breast, ovarian, and endometrial cancer. Taken consistently and as prescribed (at the same time every day), the pill is almost 100% effective in guarding against pregnancy. However, based on insurance and access, the ongoing expense may be cost-prohibitive. A health history and physical examination by a health care provider are necessary to obtain a prescription for oral contraceptives. Some females should not take the pill if they have certain physiologic disorders or diseases. Smoking increases the risks associated with oral contraceptives. Remind those who are taking the pill to take measures to protect themselves from STIs.

Nexplanon

In the Nexaplanon system, a single etonogestrel-containing rod is implanted in the upper arm through the use of a disposable insertion kit. Removal, which should occur at the 3-year mark, requires a small incision and takes about 3 minutes. The single-rod system contains 68 mg of etonogestrel in an ethylene vinyl acetate (EVA) copolymer core surrounded by an EVA membrane. This method of contraceptive is 99% effective (Organon Connect, 2022). The most common reason for discontinuation is weight gain.

Depo-Provera

Depo-Provera is the brand name of a progestin-only hormonal birth control system. It uses depot medroxyprogesterone acetate (DMPA), a hormone similar to progesterone (one of the hormones made by the ovaries that regulates the menstrual cycle). An injection of DMPA in the buttock or arm can prevent pregnancy for 12 to 13 weeks and is 99% effective when taken in the prescribed timeframe and 94% effective for those who are late getting their injections. Protection is immediate if the injection is given within the first 7 days of the start of a period. Irregular bleeding is the most common side effect for females using DMPA (Planned Parenthood Federation of America Inc., 2021).

Transdermal Contraceptive Patch

The transdermal contraceptive patch supplies continuous daily circulating levels of ethinyl estradiol (20 mcg) and norelgestromin (150 mcg). The patch is applied weekly on the same day of each week for 3 weeks, followed by a patch-free week. It may be applied to any of four sites: lower abdomen, upper outer arm, buttock, or back. Because it is applied weekly and does not require daily consideration (like the pill), some people prefer the patch, but they have to consider daily time spent in the water (swimming, soaking) and their use of lotions and powders. When used perfectly, the patch is 99% effective at preventing pregnancy, but only 91% effective with mistakes (Planned Parenthood Federation of America Inc., 2021). This contraceptive method has the same contraindications as oral contraceptives. The most common side effects include breast symptoms, headache, application site reactions, nausea, upper respiratory tract infection, and dysmenorrhea.

Vaginal Ring

The vaginal ring is a soft, flexible, transparent ring made of EVA copolymer. It releases approximately 120 mcg of etonogestrel and 15 mcg of ethinyl estradiol daily. After self-insertion into the vagina, the ring generally stays in place for one menstrual cycle, and then may be either disposed of or reused, depending on the specific ring. It does not need to be fitted, nor does it require particular placement within the vagina. The ring works by inhibiting ovulation in much the same way as oral contraceptives. Used appropriately, the vaginal ring is 99% effective in protecting against pregnancy; real-world application shows it to be 91% in preventing pregnancy (Planned Parenthood Federation of America Inc., 2021). Benefits of the vaginal ring include ease of use, self-insertion, high degree of effectiveness, and low incidence of negative or adverse effects. The most common side effects include headache, vaginal discharge, vaginitis, vaginal discomfort, foreign body sensation, coital problems, and ring expulsion.

INTRAUTERINE DEVICES

The intrauterine device (IUD) is an object that is placed by a physician or nurse practitioner within the uterus to prevent implantation of a fertilized ovum. IUDs are small, T-shaped, flexible plastic devices inserted into the vagina through the cervix (using a speculum) that provide reversible birth control. IUDs are classified as copper IUDs or hormonal IUDs (progestin). IUDs seem to affect the way the sperm or egg moves, making it impossible for the sperm to reach the egg. IUDs that contain copper are more effective for two reasons: the copper affects the behavior of enzymes in the lining of the uterus to prevent implantation and causes the production of increased amounts of prostaglandin. Copper IUDs can be used as emergency contraception within five days of sex without a condom. Both types of IUDs have a filament string that serves two purposes: it allows for easier removal by a clinician, and it assists in verifying placement. IUDs are the best, yet sometime cost-prohibitive, birth control option. They are 99% effective primarily because there is nothing to remember to insert, take, or change for 3 to 12 years (Planned Parenthood Federation of America Inc., 2021).

EMERGENCY CONTRACEPTION METHODS

Emergency contraception, often called the *morning after pill*, is designed to reduce the risk of pregnancy after intercourse (without a condom or other birth control method) that could result in a pregnancy. Emergency contraception is provided in two ways (Planned Parenthood Federation of America Inc., 2021):

1. Emergency contraceptive pills delay ovulation and reduce the risk of pregnancy when taken up to 120 hours after intercourse (ideally within 72 hours). Most are up to 89% effective when taken within 72 hours and can be purchased, by an adult, without a prescription.
2. Insertion of a copper IUD within up to 5 days after intercourse.

STERILIZATION

Sterilization should be regarded as permanent and irreversible in males and females. Although sterilization can sometimes be surgically reversed, the results are not always satisfactory. Sexual desire and ability are unaffected by sterilization.

Sterilization in females is accomplished by surgically severing the fallopian tubes. This procedure, known as tubal ligation, prevents the ovum from traveling down the tube. Tubal ligation is usually performed on an outpatient basis, sometimes under local anesthesia. Postoperative care and recovery time are required after a tubal ligation. Sterilization is safe and, because it lasts for life, is simple and convenient.

Sterilization in males is accomplished by surgically severing the vas deferens, which prevents sperm from entering the semen. The vasectomy is usually performed in a health care provider's office under local anesthesia. Vasectomy is the most effective birth control for males—nearly 100% effective. An alternative form of contraception is necessary until two semen analyses show zero sperm. It usually takes about 4 to 6 weeks for all stored sperm to be eliminated from the ductal system.

FUTURE TRENDS

Private industry remains a driving force behind contraceptive research and development. More than 100 experimental contraceptive methods are being studied around the world. The U.S. government contributes to contraceptive research primarily by funding research conducted at the National Institutes of Health.

About 43% of the pregnancies in the United States are unintended. To decrease the negative effect of unintended pregnancy on the birthing person and the infant, current initiatives center on increasing the use of and access to birth control, providing family planning services, and linking adolescents to targeted health care that may help prevent pregnancy and STIs (Healthy People 2030, n.d.a). Future trends in contraception are likely to be shaped in part by increased awareness of STIs and continuation of the AIDS pandemic.

Female Contraceptives

Most of the contraceptive products that will soon be available are refinements of products already available. New barrier methods will include enhanced cervical caps and vaginal sponges with microbicides to protect against STIs. New contraceptive pills, patches, and rings will use varied combination of hormones. Injectable progestin products may one day protect against pregnancy for up to 90 days. Oral and injectable vaccines may one day immunize females against pregnancy. These vaccines might produce antibodies to attack egg or sperm, or the immune system might create antibodies to a crucial type of protein molecule found on the head of sperm. Contraceptive implants designed to remain effective for 2 or 3 years, as well as biodegradable implants with efficacy of up to 18 months, are in development. Computerized fertility monitors that predict ovulation will offer couples who use FAMs of contraception a much more sophisticated and accurate charting method. Methods for permanent sterilization will expand to include chemical scarring techniques and insertion of fallopian tube chemical plugs and cryosurgery. Temporary sterilization may be achieved by the use of silicone plugs.

Unisex Reversible Contraceptives

The concept of unisex reversible contraception is being explored. This method involves a group of drugs called gonadotropin-releasing hormone (GnRH) agonists and can be used to prevent the release of follicle-stimulating hormone (FSH) and luteinizing hormone (LH) from the pituitary gland. The release of FSH and LH triggers ovulation and spermatogenesis. Blocking the release of these hormones will temporarily suppress fertility for females and males.

Male Contraceptives

Methods of contraception for males continue to be explored. The challenge of developing a reversible method of contraception for males is complicated because they are always producing sperm. Because of this continuous fertility, the opportunities for reversible intervention that are permitted by females' fertility cycles are not available for males. Various contraceptive injections, implants, and vaccines for males are being researched.

Effective contraceptive methods that do not permanently impair fertility have proven elusive, but research continues. Most research has focused on a hormonal approach to decrease spermatogenesis. The major problem is that interference with steroidogenesis may also interfere with the other actions of testosterone such as sexual function, bone and muscle growth, kidney function, and protein anabolism.

Research in Nursing

BRIDGING THE GAP TO EVIDENCE-BASED PRACTICE

Transphobia

Transgender women experience high rates of gender-based violence (GBV), such as transphobic hate crimes, which can negatively impact their health outcomes. Exploring self-reported experiences with these crimes provides insight into the lived experience of these women.

Related Research

Gyamerah, A. O., Baguso, G., Santiago-Rodriguez, E., Sa'id, A., Arayasirikul, S., Lin, J., Turner, C. M., Taylor, K. D., McFarland, W., Wilson, E. C., & Wesson, P. (2021). Experiences and factors associated with transphobic hate crimes among transgender women in the San Francisco Bay Area: Comparisons across race. *BMC Public Health*, *21*(1), 1053. https://doi.org/10.1186/s12889-021-11107-x

An interprofessional team engaged in a secondary analysis of data collected in a longitudinal cohort study of HIV (n = 629). This analysis focused on self-reported experiences of transphobic hate crimes in the San Francisco Bay area. Demographic and sociocultural factors including race and ethnicity along with gender identity factors were examined in relation to transphobic experiences and whether or not the crime was reported to the police. Not surprisingly, 45.8% of these transgender women reported they had experienced a hate crime, but only 51.1% of those cases were reported to the police. This analysis supports the assertion that these crimes are underreported, especially when the women felt their gender identity was questioned, which makes tracking transphobic hate crimes difficult. Structural factors and social determinants of health including poverty, unemployment, sex work, incarceration, immigration status, housing discrimination, and unhomed status are all associated with trans women's risk for experiencing a hate crime. The intersectionality of race, ethnicity, gender, and transphobia increase the risk of violence for Black and Latina trans women. Although the overall hate crime rate did not show significant differences based on race or ethnicity, Black and Latina transgender women were more likely to experience battery with a weapon than their White counterparts.

Relevance for Nursing Practice

Trans women who have their gender identity questioned in the context of a hate crime are less likely to report the crime. Nurses have an obligation to provide a safe space for women to express themselves and advocate for their individualized needs. Policies that address structural issues related to racial disparities, intersectionality, and other social determinants of health would benefit the trans population directly.

Facilitating Coping With Special Sexual Needs

The nurse can help patients cope with sexual concerns generated by diseases and their treatments. See the accompanying Research in Nursing box. Offer anticipatory guidance and information to patients, stressing the importance of open communication with the patient's partner. Include the partner in teaching when appropriate.

When indicated, start a discussion about possible sexual positions that can reduce pain during coitus. Show the patient drawings of possible sexual positions. Inform the patient that intercourse may be more comfortable if pain medication is taken before beginning sexual activity.

When teaching patients about medications, mention any sexual side effects that may occur to prevent anxiety and depression. Patients should alert the health care provider if these side effects occur because the drug dosage may be able to be modified or the drug changed. If patients are unaware of this, they may discontinue the medication on their own rather than sacrifice sexual functioning, especially if this is an important aspect of life for them.

Health Care Needs of Lesbian, Gay, Bisexual, and Transgender People

The health and well-being of lesbian, gay, bisexual, and transgender (LGBT) people has been made a priority by major federal health care facilities. The term LGBT has been expanded to LGBTQIA+ (lesbian, gay, bisexual, transgender, questioning/queer, intersex, ally/asexual), but the terms associated with the acronym vary slightly depending on the source. The plus sign is often used to include those whose personal identity is not represented by any of the other terms. The Institute of Medicine's consensus report (IOM, 2011; since renamed the National Academy of Sciences, Engineering, and Medicine), Healthy People 2020 (2021b), Healthy People 2030 (n.d.b), and USDHHS (2016) all highlight the need for better science-based knowledge on how best to address the existence of health disparities of the LGBTQIA+ community and the lack of compassionate services. Stigma and a range of other social and cultural factors affect the health of LGBTQIA+ people, as well as the ability of the health care system and providers to care for them. LGBTQIA+ people come from diverse cultural backgrounds, have varied ethnic or racial identity, and differ in terms of education, age, income, and place of residence. LGTBQIA+ may be defined by their sexual orientation, but this definition is complex and variable. Sexual behavior, cultural factors, disclosure of sexual orientation and/or gender identity, prejudice and discrimination, and concealed sexual identity each present unique health challenges to this population (Box 46-3).

Other issues that affect health care delivery to the LGBTQIA+ population include the following:

- *Public health infrastructure:* Efforts to research and address the health care needs of LGBTQIA+ people are hindered

Box 46-3 Health Disparities in the Gay, Lesbian, Bisexual, and Transgender (LGBT) Population

Healthy People 2020 (2021b) identified significant LGBT health disparities and sought much-needed collaboration from health care professionals and policy makers to address them. Among its findings are the following:

- LGBT youth are two to three times more likely to attempt suicide.
- LGBT youth are more likely to be homeless.
- Lesbians are less likely to get preventive services for cancer.
- Gay men are at higher risk of HIV and other sexually transmitted infections, especially among communities of color.
- Lesbians and bisexual females are more likely to be overweight or obese.
- Transgender people have a high prevalence of HIV and sexually transmitted infections, victimization, mental health issues, and suicide: They are less likely to have health insurance than heterosexual, lesbian, gay, or bisexual people.

Based on the progress on the 2020 initiatives, *Healthy People 2030* (n.d.c) focuses on LGBT adolescents and related school- and family-based interventions to address the specific challenges faced by these adolescents.

- Older LGBT people, referred to as *elders* by the LGBT community and *trans elders* in the transgender community, face additional barriers to health due to isolation and a lack of social services and culturally competent providers.[a]
- LGBT populations have the highest rates of tobacco, alcohol, and other drug use. These health issues are partly thought to be the effects of chronic stress resulting from stigmatization.[b]

[a]Harley, D. A., & Teaster, P. B. (2016). *Handbook of LGBT elders: An interdisciplinary approach to principles, practices, and policies.* Springer International Publishing.

[b]Institute of Medicine, Committee on Lesbian, Gay, Bisexual, and Transgender Health Issues and Research Gaps and Opportunities. (2011). *The health of lesbian, gay, bisexual, and transgender people: Building a foundation for better understanding.* National Academies Press.

by an inadequate infrastructure to support and fund population-specific initiatives.

- *Access to quality health services:* Financial, structural, personal, and cultural barriers limit access to screening and prevention services and cause delays in care for acute conditions in the LGBTQIA+ population.
- *Health communication:* Negative provider attitudes, lack of provider education regarding unique aspects of lesbian and gay health, and exclusion of same-sex partners in care planning seriously hamper therapeutic communication between members of the LGBTQIA+ community and those who provide care.
- *Educational and community-based programs:* Some government facilities, professional organizations, and health care organizations address health issues of the LGBTQIA+ community, but this population still relies heavily on self-created community-based programs to address their special health care requirements.

Clearly, significant research is needed regarding the unique experience and health care needs of the LGBTQIA+ population, along with increased education for health care providers. Issues of prejudice and inequitable service distribution in the health care system need to be addressed to improve the health of this population.

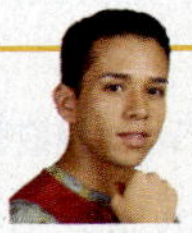

Think back to **Paul Rojas,** a young adult man who is gay and was diagnosed with AIDS. The nurse needs to be acutely aware of the health care delivery system in the community to ensure that Mr. Rojas has access to the most appropriate and needed services. Depending on his specific needs, consultation with social services may be helpful for initiating referrals for appropriate services as Mr. Rojas's condition changes.

Advocating for Patients' Sexuality Needs

A hospital experience or institutionalization puts a strain on a person's individuality and sexual self. Illness may diminish feelings of sexual desire, and the desire for sexual interaction can signal a patient's improving health. The nurse should provide anticipatory guidance because many patients may hesitate to request help for fear of being ridiculed. Often, a patient merely desires privacy to hold and caress their partner. The intimacy of this act often fulfills the patient's feelings of longing to be needed and loved.

There are many ways to advocate for a patient's sexual needs (Box 46-4 on page 1894). Some may seem obvious and commonplace, whereas others may first require coming to terms with your own sexuality.

Counseling the Patient Regarding Sexuality

Not all patients with sexual concerns need intensive therapy. Some patients benefit greatly from simply having someone listen to their concerns. Voicing their concerns allows patients to put the information into perspective and focus on what the problem is and how to solve it. When counseling patients, do not offer your own advice, because what is right for one person may be wrong for another. Also, offering false reassurances, such as, "It'll be all right," is unproductive. Rather, adopt an objective, nonjudgmental, empathic, and receptive attitude to facilitate open communication with the patient.

Abortion Counseling

Abortion remains an issue that deeply divides people. Many believe it is a woman's right to choose whether to continue a pregnancy or to take safe and legal action on a decision to terminate. Others believe that from fertilization onward, the embryo and fetus is a human being deserving of the full

Box 46-4 Advocating for Patients' Sexual Needs

- All patients should be accepted as sexual beings with the right to be treated with dignity and with sensitivity to their feelings.
- All patients have the right to some degree of privacy.
  - Anticipate the patient's desire for privacy by the simple act of drawing a curtain or closing a door.
  - Give patients the option of wearing their own sleepwear to promote sexual identity.
- Anticipate potentially shaming situations for the patient. Give information regarding the procedure and why it needs to be done, and acknowledge that the patient's embarrassment is normal and understandable.
- Health care providers should not simply take for granted that patients do not mind intrusive or embarrassing procedures performed on their bodies and private parts.
- Patients have a right to question the heath care provider regarding sexual needs or future sexual functioning.
  - Anticipate these questions for the patient.
  - Ask patients if they have any concerns regarding sexuality that can be answered by the nurse.
  - Interface with the health care provider to obtain information required by the patient.
- The atmosphere in health care settings needs to allow for sexual expression between patients and their partners.
- Confidentiality is a right of every patient.
  - Do not promise confidentiality if that promise cannot be kept.
  - Do not allow anyone not directly involved with the patient's care access to a patient's personal records.
  - Allow no information regarding patients to escape into idle conversation.
- Patients should be referred to formally by whatever name or title the identified by the patient. Use appropriate pronouns.
- Patients should be allowed to keep some personal possessions, if it is practical to do so.

respect and protection we afford humans after birth; these people view abortion as always wrong. Some would allow abortion only if it is indicated for a birthing person's health or in cases of rape. You should examine what you believe, why you believe this, and how your beliefs are likely to influence your ability to counsel individuals and couples of childbearing age.

Counseling in Cases of Abusive Relationships and Rape

Nurses encounter children, adolescents, women, and sometimes men who have experienced sexual abuse or rape. Sexual violence (rape, forced sodomy, sexual child abuse, incest, fondling, sexual harassment, or any unwanted sexual contact) is *not* about love or sex; it is about power, violence, and control. The Rape, Abuse & Incest National Network (RAINN, 2022) reports that:

- One out of every six American women has been a victim of an attempted or completed rape in her lifetime (14.8% completed rape; 2.8% attempted rape).
- About 3% of American men—or 1 in 33—have experienced an attempted or completed rape in their lifetime.
- Every 68 seconds, an American is sexually assaulted.
- Approximately 15% of victims of sexual assault and rape are ages 12 to 17 years; 54% are ages 18 to 34 years.
- The majority of sexual assaults occur at or near the victim's home; 48% of victims were sleeping or at home doing something else when the crime occurred.
- Approximately 21% of transgender college students have been sexually assaulted (compared to 18% of nontransgender females and 4% of nontransgender males).

Date rape occurs when there is forced or coerced sex within a dating relationship. With acquaintance rape, the act is committed by someone known to the victim. Nearly two thirds of all victims between ages 18 and 29 years report that they had a prior relationship with their attacker. More than 13% of college women report they have been forced to have sex while in a dating situation (Center for Family Justice, 2021).

Victims of sexual assault are 3 times more likely to suffer from depression, 6 times more likely to suffer from post-traumatic stress disorder, 13 times more likely to abuse alcohol, 26 times more likely to abuse drugs, and 4 times more likely to contemplate suicide. Clearly, nurses need to be alert to evidence of sexual abuse while taking the history and conducting physical examinations. Abuse crosses all socioeconomic and ethnic groups. Become familiar with your legal and clinical responsibilities when a victim is identified. The first priority is getting the victim into a safe environment and mobilizing support for the victim and family. Multiple parties may need therapy. Be familiar with local resources and make appropriate referrals. The National Sexual Assault Online Hotline is a free, confidential, secure service that provides live help over the RAINN website (https://www.rainn.org/get-help).

Human trafficking is a form of abuse and a human rights violation. Although data collection on human trafficking is difficult to collect, the public is aware of this issue through public service announcements at airports, online, and on television. There is even a TikTok video on a hand signal to alert others: put your hand up with the palm facing out, tuck the thumb, and then trap the thumb with the other four fingers (making a fist with the thumb inside). See the Vulnerable Populations Alert on Human Trafficking for more information.

Evaluating

The nurse works with the patient to evaluate the effectiveness of sexual counseling or intervention. Several factors can be considered when evaluating the sexual health of an individual (Boyd & Luebbert, 2022; Stuart, 2013):

- *Wellness.* Has the patient's sense of well-being improved during the treatment? Have issues regarding access and disparities been addressed?

Vulnerable Population Alert: Human Trafficking Victims

Identifying Victims of Human Trafficking Fact Sheet: https://www.acf.hhs.gov/sites/default/files/orr/fact_sheet_identifying_victims_of_human_trafficking.pdf.

Who Is a Human Trafficking Victim? Human trafficking is a form of modern-day slavery in which victims are subjected to force, fraud, or coercion for the purpose of commercial sex, debt bondage, or involuntary labor. Victims of human trafficking can be young children, teenagers, and adult males and females. They can be U.S. citizens, Lawful Permanent Residents (LPRs), or foreign nationals, and they can be found in urban, suburban, and rural areas. Minors (younger than age 18 years) who are induced to perform commercial sex acts are victims of trafficking, regardless of whether their traffickers used force, fraud, or coercion.

Human trafficking may occur in the following situations:

- Prostitution and escort services;
- Pornography, stripping, or exotic dancing;
- Massage parlors;
- Sexual services publicized on the Internet or in newspapers;
- Agricultural or ranch work;
- Factory work or sweatshops;
- Businesses like hotels, nail salons or home-cleaning services;
- Domestic labor (cleaning, childcare, eldercare, etc. within a home);
- Restaurants, bars, or cantinas; or
- Begging, street peddling, or door-to-door sales.

Victims of human trafficking may exhibit any of the following:

- Evidence of being controlled either physically or psychologically;
- Inability to leave home or place of work;
- Inability to speak for oneself or share one's own information;
- Information is provided by someone accompanying the individual;
- Loss of control of one's own identification documents (ID or passport);
- Have few or no personal possessions;
- Owe a large debt that the individual is unable to pay off; or
- Loss of sense of time or space, not knowing where they are or what city or state they are in.

If you think you have come into contact with a victim of human trafficking, call the National Human Trafficking Resource Center at 1.888.3737.888. The NHTRC can help you identify and coordinate with local organizations that protect and serve trafficking victims. For more information on human trafficking visit: www.acf.hhs.gov/trafficking

- *Functional ability.* If the person was dysfunctional, has functional ability improved or been restored? Have medical and behavioral strategies been implemented?
- *Satisfaction with treatment.* Does the patient believe the treatment was helpful? Were the patient's goals and expectations met? Does the patient feel seen, heard, and supported without bias or discrimination? Has the health care team partnered with the individual to develop a plan?

To evaluate the plan of care, the nurse needs to use information from the patient for most outcomes. The nurse cannot evaluate patients by observing their expression of sexuality, but the nurse can evaluate how patients are progressing toward sexuality-oriented goals by their appearance, self-confidence, and manner. For example, a patient who has expressed feelings of anxiety in the past over a sexual concern should be observably more confident and exhibit less anxiety if the patient outcomes are being met. Ask the patient about progress toward outcomes. Some outcomes need to be incrementally addressed because not all problems are easily resolved with one-time intervention and direction.

When evaluating a patient's progress, it may help to ask these questions: "In what ways have you been able to achieve your goal (orgasm, increased desire, comfortable intercourse, erection)?" "What methods seemed most effective? Which were not?" "What do you think should be the next step?" Determine from this interaction with the patient whether something more needs to be accomplished. It is not enough to assume that because a set of outcomes has been met, the patient is satisfied with the results.

REFLECTIVE PRACTICE LEADING TO PERSONAL LEARNING

Remember that the object of reflective practice is to look at an experience, understand it, and learn from it. As you begin to develop your expertise in evaluating the care plan, reflect on your experiences—successes and failures—in order to improve your practice. How can you do it better next time? What did you learn today that can help you tomorrow? Begin your reflection by paying close attention to the following:

- How aware are you of the components of sexuality: biological sex or sex assigned at birth, sexual activity (including pleasure, intimacy, and reproduction), gender identities and roles, and sexual orientation?
- What value do you attach to sexuality? How will you begin to approach discussing these personal concepts with your patients? How do you individualize the care for patients?
- How do you plan to hone your skills in managing the complexities of sexuality that can involve psychological and physiologic aspects?

Keeping up with the latest evidence-based practice guidelines, evolving terms, public opinion, and legal protections can be challenging. Developing a working knowledge of the core principles of sexuality and identity provides a foundation for your nursing practice.

Perhaps the most important questions to reflect on are : Are your patients and families/caregivers better for having had *you* share in the critical responsibility of partnering with them to explore and embrace their sexuality? Are your patients now receiving thoughtful, person-centered, prioritized, holistic, evidence-based treatment and care because of your efforts?

Nursing Care Plan for *Pete Manheim* 46-1

Pete Manheim is a 13-year-old adolescent boy attending the area health clinic. His mother consented to the nurse conversing with Pete and agreed to leave the room to provide her son privacy. Pete tells you his pronouns are *he* and *his* and that he identifies as straight. He is nervous as he explains to the nurse his need for health care. He has noticed "sticky white stuff" around his penis and bedclothes on arising some mornings and fears he may be ill. Pete has also expressed concern about his lack of knowledge regarding sexuality. He has heard a lot of stories from his friends but does not feel he can talk to his parents because the subject has never been broached at home. Also, although Pete is "a virgin", he is beginning to feel pressured by his friends, who boast of many sexual experiences.

After spending time in conversation with Pete, the nurse gathered the following data:

- Pete is experiencing nocturnal emissions and has little scientific knowledge about their source.
- Pete is anxious because of the stories regarding sex he has heard from his friends.
- There is no communication or dialogue at home with parents about issues of sexuality.
- Pete is having feelings of insecurity and anxiety about his present virginal status, which he feels he should change.
- Peer pressure from friends is also a concern.

The nurse will work with Pete to develop a care plan to correct misinformation and relieve his anxiety. Planning will be directed toward correcting myths and supplying Pete with accurate information. Because Pete has a negligible knowledge base on sexuality, the care plan will allow for ongoing sessions to augment the initial information. The nurse should outline this plan with Pete to be certain it is acceptable to him.

ACTUAL OR POTENTIAL HEALTH PROBLEMS AND NEEDS

Knowledge Deficit: Adolescent Sexuality Concerns

Etiology: misinformation and absent family-based sex education

Signs and symptoms: the patient's self-report.

EXPECTED OUTCOME

By the end of the teaching session, the patient will:

- Describe the nature of nocturnal emissions

NURSING INTERVENTIONS	RATIONALE	EVALUATIVE STATEMENT
Assess patient's present knowledge base on nocturnal emission and the source of his information.	It is necessary to discover what the patient does know and to build on that knowledge.	8/1/25 Outcome met. Patient able to describe the source of nocturnal emissions. *N. Hill, RN*
Use terms that the patient has used and language at the level of the patient's understanding.	This facilitates comprehension.	
Teach the patient about nocturnal emissions: • Nocturnal emissions, or "wet dreams," are normal in males of all ages, and they are particularly common in the teenage years. They are not the result of disease. • They occur during sleep as the result of erotic dreams. The "white sticky stuff" is the result of ejaculation of semen from the penis. • This is an involuntary action over which the male has no control.	Knowledge decreases anxiety.	

EXPECTED OUTCOME

By the end of the teaching session, the patient will:

- Differentiate sexual myths from sound knowledge

Nursing Care Plan for Pete Manheim 46-1 *(continued)*

NURSING INTERVENTIONS	RATIONALE	EVALUATIVE STATEMENT
Assess what the patient has heard from peers regarding sexual information:	The nurse can then specifically address the myths to which the patient has been exposed. This enables the patient to develop a positive sexual body image based on fact.	8/1/25 Outcome met. Patient was able to differentiate between truth in sexual issues and what is myth. *N. Hill, RN*
Myth 1: "A large penis is better for sex than a small one." *Truth:* No relation exists between the size of a penis and the male's ability to perform sexually. When a penis becomes erect, it reaches sufficient size to engage in sexual intercourse. *Myth 2:* "Jerking off causes blindness. It is a dirty habit."		
Truth: Masturbation, or self-stimulation, is a natural and healthy outlet for sexual urges. People of all ages masturbate. Masturbation can also teach the person what feels good and what does not. Every person has the right to masturbate if desired. *Myth 3:* "It looks bad for a guy to be a virgin—everybody's doing it" (having sex).	The patient is given permission to engage in a sexual activity of a masturbatory nature.	
Truth: No one, whether male or female, should feel pressured into sexual activity at any age. Engaging in sexual activity carries with it a great deal of responsibility and concerns of pregnancy and spread of sexually transmitted infections (STIs). No one needs to know of another person's status if the person chooses not to discuss it.	The patient is given permission to abstain from sexual activity and not to feel pressured by friends. Almost 39% of teens have had sex by age 16 years.	

EXPECTED OUTCOME By the end of the teaching session, the patient will:

- List the positive aspects of abstinence in a sexual relationship

NURSING INTERVENTIONS	RATIONALE	EVALUATIVE STATEMENT
Assess the patient, including previous discussion of sexual myths and knowledge. Instruct the patient on the positive aspects of abstinence, including the following: • Engagement in any sexual activity should be a personal decision and not the result of pressure from friends.	Giving the patient all the information necessary allows him to make an informed decision.	8/1/25 Outcome partially met. Patient able to list verbally all positive aspects of abstinence but is still undecided. *Revision:* Reinforce to patient that this is a personal decision that he can make for himself with a good knowledge base. Also, he does not have to make a firm decision for or against abstinence immediately. He should take time to think about this information. *N. Hill, RN*

(continued on page 1898)

Nursing Care Plan for Pete Manheim 46-1 *(continued)*

NURSING INTERVENTIONS	RATIONALE	EVALUATIVE STATEMENT
• Abstinence will guarantee protection from pregnancy and from most STIs.	Many young people think they are immune to the consequences of their actions. Therefore, it is important to stress that pregnancy and STIs are very probable results of sexual intercourse.	
• People can show affection for each other without sexual involvement.	It is difficult to understand and undertake all the implications of a sexual relationship during the teenage years. The patient learns that a successful sexual relationship requires intimacy, love, and sharing; it should not be merely an outlet for sexual feelings.	
• Every person has the right to say no.	The patient has permission to refuse an activity in which he is not sure he wishes to engage.	

EXPECTED OUTCOME By the end of the teaching session, the patient will:
- Describe the correct use of rubber condoms

NURSING INTERVENTIONS	RATIONALE	EVALUATIVE STATEMENT
Assess what the patient knows about condoms and their use.	Since the patient is undecided about whether to initiate a sexual relationship in the future, it is prudent to give him information to protect against pregnancy and STIs.	8/1/25 Outcome met. Patient successfully listed the steps in using a condom. *N. Hill, RN*
Inform the patient that condoms are available over the counter in drugstores. Prices vary according to type and style.	Patient should know where to purchase condoms and the variety available.	
Teach the patient the steps in using rubber condoms:	Patient should know how to use condoms safely.	
• Roll condom onto the penis as soon as it becomes erect.	Protects against sperm from secretions from Cowper's glands	
• If condom does not have a nipple receptacle end, leave a small space at end of condom to collect semen.	Provides a pocket to collect semen and prevents breakage	
• Immediately after ejaculation, remove penis and condom from vagina by holding onto base of condom.	Prevents spillage of semen into the vagina	
• Discard condom.	Condoms are not meant to be reused. A new condom is used for each act of intercourse.	
Advise the patient to use a condom with every act of intercourse. Spermicides used with the condom increase effectiveness.	To be as effective as possible, the condom should be used with every act of intercourse. The rubber condom used with spermicide is effective against pregnancy and the spread of STIs. The use of a spermicide foam in the vagina increases effectiveness.	

Nursing Care Plan for Pete Manheim 46-1 (continued)

EXPECTED OUTCOME	By the end of the teaching session, the patient will: • Express a decrease in anxiety	
NURSING INTERVENTIONS	**RATIONALE**	**EVALUATIVE STATEMENT**
Assess the patient's anxiety level by verbal and nonverbal behavior.	The patient was anxious when he came into the clinic. It is important to evaluate his level of anxiety before he leaves. If he is still anxious, reassessment should occur because the care plan may have been unsuccessful.	8/1/25 Outcome met. Patient expressed relief that he is normal. Would like to bring a friend to next session. Future teaching sessions to include these topics identified by patient: • STIs, particularly AIDS • Pregnancy—occurrence and prevention • Sexual expression • Further discussion of sexual myths *N. Hill, RN*
SAMPLE DOCUMENTATION	8/1/25, 1100, nursing Nursing consultation with 13-year-old patient regarding anxiety about cause and source of nocturnal emissions. Patient also expressed concern about sexual myths he has heard from friends. Stated that much peer pressure exists to become sexually active. Patient admits to possessing little knowledge regarding sexual issues. Feels he cannot discuss sexuality with parents (who consented to this conversation) because it is not a topic that has been brought up in the past at home. Will conduct initial teaching session with patient to provide information and decrease anxiety about priority concerns. Patient is willing to return to clinic for at least three more teaching sessions to expand knowledge base of sexuality. *N. Hill, RN*	

DEVELOPING CLINICAL REASONING AND CLINICAL JUDGMENT

1. Review the Nursing Care Plan 46-1 on pages 1896–1899 to help you hone your clinical reasoning and clinical judgment skills.
2. Role-play with another student and perform the interview you would use to obtain a sexual history from the following people. Think about how you modified the interview in each situation and why. Identify what made you feel uncomfortable as either the nurse or the patient. Discuss how you can best address this discomfort.
   - A mother voices concern that her 9-year-old son is frequently playing with his penis.
   - An adult man appears distressed when they note that they have suddenly become impotent with their partner of many years.
   - A high school girl says that her mother tells her something is wrong with her because she is attracted only to women.
   - A new resident in a long-term care facility complains that he misses his privacy and has nowhere to make love.
3. Describe how you would respond to a newly diagnosed woman with HIV who has had multiple partners and tells you that it is none of your business how she acquired the virus or what she plans to do now that she has it. Think carefully about what is at stake in terms of your response.
4. You know a woman is uncomfortable about undergoing a pelvic examination, and you ask the male provider to wait for you before he begins the examination. He tells you he can't wait and doesn't need your assistance. You know the patient wants another woman in the room. How would you respond, and what is at stake? Does it matter if the reason for the patient's request to have you present is simply preference, is linked to a history of abuse, or is related to her cultural or religious beliefs?

PRACTICING FOR NCLEX

1. A nurse is teaching parents about expected developmental aspects of sexuality in children. Which statements from parents indicate further teaching is needed? Select all that apply.
   a. "When my 2-year-old son touches his genitals, I push his hand away and tell him 'No.'"
   b. "I should wean my infant by 4 months and encourage him to use a sippy cup."
   c. "I should explain sexuality to my 9-year-old in a factual manner when they ask questions about their body."
   d. "I should explain about body changes to my 11-year-old prior to them happening to alleviate their fears."
   e. "I should teach my 10-year-old about contraception and ways to avoid sexually transmitted diseases."
   f. "I should allow my teenager to establish their own beliefs and moral value system rather than sharing my own beliefs."
2. A nurse is counseling an older couple regarding sexuality. Which statement from the couple should the nurse address?
   a. "We're at the age when we should consider stopping sexual activity."
   b. "We need more time for sexual stimulation than we used to."
   c. "If we are unable to have sex, we can still have an intimate relationship."
   d. "If we change our position, we can still have sex and be more comfortable."
3. A nurse in a urology practice performs sexual health assessments of male older adults. Which patients would the nurse identify as having an increased risk for erectile dysfunction? Select all that apply.
   a. Patient with a history of diabetes
   b. Patient with a new partner
   c. Patient with Parkinson disease
   d. Patient with alcoholism
   e. Patient taking antihypertensive medication
   f. Patient who is a tobacco smoker
4. A school nurse is providing sex education classes for adolescents. Which statement would the nurse include when describing normal sexual functioning?
   a. "People are born with a certain amount of sexual drive, which can be depleted in later years."
   b. "If you want to be a great athlete, sexual abstinence is necessary during training."
   c. "A nocturnal emission (wet dream), is an indicator of a sexual disorder."
   d. "It is natural for women to have as strong a desire for sex and enjoy it as much as men."
5. During a checkup in a pediatric office, the mother of a school-aged boy tells the nurse that she is worried because she has occasionally found him masturbating. She asks the nurse how she should handle this "problem." How would the nurse best respond to this mother's concern?
   a. "Children should be taught not to masturbate because most people believe self-stimulation is wrong."
   b. "Masturbation is a means of learning what a person prefers sexually; overreacting can lead the child to believe sex is bad or dirty."
   c. "There are serious health risks associated with frequent masturbation, and the practice should be discouraged in children."
   d. "Children who masturbate demonstrate sexual dysfunction and should be seen by a child psychologist."
6. A patient who developed a pulmonary embolism (blood clot in the lung) after using oral contraceptives asks the nurse what she should do if she can no longer use "the pill." The nurse suggests which mechanical barrier for birth control?
   a. Diaphragm
   b. Transdermal contraceptive patch
   c. Depo-Provera
   d. Evra patch
7. A 17-year-old college student calls the emergency department (ED) and tells the nurse they were raped by a professor. They want to come to the ED, but only if the nurse promises their parents will not be contacted. What should be the nurse's first priority?
   a. Getting the patient into a safe environment and mobilizing support for them
   b. Encouraging the student to disclose the name of the professor
   c. Ensuring the student is assessed for pregnancy, STIs, and other complications
   d. Convincing the student to tell their parents to receive their support
8. A nurse is teaching patients about contraception methods. Which statement by a patient indicates a need for further teaching?
   a. "Depo-Provera is not effective against sexually transmitted infections, but contraceptive protection is immediate if I get the injection on the first day of my period."
   b. "The hormonal contraceptive, NuvaRing, protects against pregnancy by suppressing ovulation, thickening cervical mucus, and preventing implantation of the fertilized eggs."
   c. "Abstinence is an effective method of contraception and may be used as a periodic or continuous strategy to prevent pregnancy and STIs."
   d. "Withdrawal is an effective method of birth control that reduces risk for STIs."
9. A nurse in a gynecology practice is assessing a patient reporting vaginal discharge that "smells bad and is green and foamy." She also reports burning upon

urination and dyspareunia. The nurse suggests the patient and partner will need treatment for which STI?
a. Human papillomavirus (HPV)
b. Syphilis
c. Trichomoniasis
d. Herpes simplex virus

10. A school nurse is providing information for parents of teenagers regarding the human papillomavirus (HPV) and the recommended HPV vaccination. What teaching point would the nurse include?
a. "HPV causes genital warts and cervical and other cancers."
b. "HPV causes a single painless genital lesion and can lead to sterility."
c. "Fifty percent of females between ages 14 and 19 years are infected with HPV."
d. "The HPV vaccination is only recommended for the female population."

11. Students enrolled in a sexuality course are discussing people who achieve sexual arousal by looking at the body of someone other than a sexual partner. How would the students correctly name this behavior?
a. Masochism
b. Pedophilia
c. Voyeurism
d. Sadism

12. An 18-year-old presents at a women's health care clinic seeking oral contraceptives before having heterosexual intercourse for the first time. She tells the nurse she doesn't know what to expect. What accurate statements by the nurse would be helpful? Select all that apply.
a. "During the excitement phase, your breasts swell and the nipples invert."
b. "Lubrication of the vagina seeps outside of the body making stimulation more pleasurable by decreasing friction."
c. "Your clitoris enlarges and emerges slightly from the clitoral hood."
d. "The first obvious sign of arousal in your partner is an erection of the penis caused by increased blood flow."
e. "The man's scrotum noticeably elevates, thickens, and enlarges."
f. "The skin of the penis and scrotum become pale in color."

13. A nurse working in a gynecology practice screens patients for menstrual irregularities. Which patients would a nurse identify are at risk for menstrual cycle irregularities? Select all that apply.
a. Breastfeeding mother
b. Adolescent with anorexia
c. Individual abstaining from sexual intercourse
d. Patient diagnosed with pelvic inflammatory disease
e. Patient obsessed with exercising
f. Patient with a spinal cord injury

14. A nurse in a gynecology clinic is obtaining a health history on a patient reporting pain during sexual activity. Which assessment question would be most appropriate for a patient who is experiencing dyspareunia?
a. "Do you currently have a new partner?"
b. "Have you been diagnosed with a neurologic disorder?"
c. "Do you take antihypertensive medication?"
d. "Do you regularly use antihistamines?"

15. A nurse is providing health care for patients in a clinic located in a predominately LGBTQIA+ community. Which health disparities should the nurse keep in mind when planning care for this population? Select all that apply.
a. LGBTQIA+ youth are more likely to attempt suicide.
b. LGBTQIA+ youth are more likely to be homeless.
c. Lesbians are less likely to get preventive services for cancer.
d. Lesbians and bisexual females are more likely to be underweight.
e. Transgender people have a high prevalence of HIV and sexually transmitted infections.
f. LGBTQIA+ populations have low rates of tobacco, alcohol, and other drug use.

16. Nurses in the emergency department (ED) have received education on identification of victims of human trafficking. Which patients would the ED nurse identify may be at risk? Select all that apply.
a. Those who work in hotels, nail salons, or home-cleaning services
b. Those who perform agricultural or ranch work
c. Those who show evidence of being controlled physically or psychologically
d. Those accompanied by someone who encourages them to share their own information
e. Those who produce identification documents (ID or passport)
f. Those who show the loss of the sense of time or space or not do know what city or state they are in

17. A parent brings their preteen daughter to the pediatric office for an annual checkup. The parent asks when they should tell the child about menses. What information will the nurse provide?
a. "You can discuss this when you are ready."
b. "It isn't necessary to discuss menstruation until age 13."
c. "Most preteens have heard about menses from their friends. There is no rush."
d. "Menses begins between ages 10 and 13 years, so now is a good time."

ANSWERS WITH RATIONALES

1. **a, b, c, e, f.** Self-manipulation of genitals is a normal behavior; parents should avoid telling a child this as "bad." Parents should avoid early weaning of infants to prevent oral

deprivation. Parents should explain contraception and STIs to their adolescent children; it would be premature to do so for a 10-year-old. Parents should share their beliefs and moral system with their children. Parents should also give their children the desired information about sexuality in a clear, factual form and give them information about body changes before they experience them, to alleviate fears.

2. **a.** Sexual activity need not be hindered by age, and couples who have been consistently sexually active throughout their lives may continue their intimate relationship for as long as they desire. Nurses should teach couples that adaptation to bodily changes is possible with use of comfortable positions for intercourse and increased time for stimulation as well as teach alternatives to coitus, such as caressing, hugging, and stroking, when coitus is impossible because of illness or disability.

3. **a, d, e.** Risk factors for erectile dysfunction include history of diabetes, spinal cord trauma, cardiovascular disease, surgical procedure, alcoholism, and use of antihypertensives, antidepressants, or illicit drugs. Having a new partner may be a risk factor for premature ejaculation, and a history of Parkinson disease may predispose the patient to delayed ejaculation. Smoking is not a risk factor for impotence.

4. **d.** Physiologic studies indicate that, in some respects, the female's sex drive is not only as strong but may be even stronger than that of the male. The more consistently sexually active a person is, the longer the activity continues into the later years of life. Physiologically, the achievement of orgasm is rarely more demanding than most activities encountered in daily life; there is no scientific evidence that sex "weakens" a person. Erotic dreams that culminate in orgasms are normal common physiologic phenomena in at least 85% of men.

5. **b.** Masturbation is a technique of sexual expression in which a person practices self-stimulation. It is a way for people to learn what they prefer during stimulation and what feels good. People masturbate regardless of sex, age, or marital status. Negative reaction or overreaction by parents to a child's masturbating can lead to a belief that the genitals and sex are bad or dirty, causing guilt or a feeling they are wrong. People may not masturbate due to guilt about it or believe self-stimulation is wrong. It is important to let patients know masturbation is not "dirty" and will not lead to blindness or insanity.

6. **a.** The diaphragm is the only barrier method of contraception listed; all the other methods are hormonal.

7. **a.** While the remaining options may be indicated, the priority is to ensure the safety of the woman and to get her the support she needs at this moment.

8. **d.** Withdrawal offers no protection against sexually transmitted infections. An injection of depot medroxyprogesterone acetate (DMPA) can prevent pregnancy for 12 weeks, is 99.7% effective, and provides contraception immediately if administered on the first day of the female's period. The NuvaRing works by inhibiting ovulation in much the same way as oral contraceptives. Used appropriately, the vaginal ring is 99.3% effective in protecting against pregnancy. Abstinence is the most effective form of birth control, preventing pregnancy and STIs 100% of the time when practiced consistently and appropriately.

9. **c.** Trichomoniasis causes a foul-smelling vaginal discharge that is thin, foamy, and green in color; it also causes itching of the vulva and vagina, burning on urination, and dyspareunia. HPV causes a profuse watery vaginal discharge, dyspareunia, intense pruritus, and vulvar irritation. Syphilis causes a single painless genital lesion 10 days to 3 months after exposure and generalized skin rash, enlarged lymph nodes, and fever that may appear 2 to 4 weeks after appearance of primary lesion and may last for several years. Herpes presents as single or multiple painful vesicles that rupture and form ulcer-like lesions, which form scabs as they heal.

10. **a.** HPV causes genital warts and cervical and other cancers. It manifests as pale, soft, papillary lesions found around the internal and external genitalia, perianal and rectal areas of the body. One in four young females between ages 14 and 19 years is infected with at least one of the most common STIs, which include the human papillomavirus (HPV). The HPV vaccination is recommended for males and females.

11. **c.** Voyeurism is the achievement of sexual arousal by looking at the body of someone other than a person's own sexual partner. Masochism refers to gaining sexual pleasure from the humiliation of being abused. Pedophilia is a term used to describe the practice of adults gaining sexual fulfillment by performing sexual acts with children. Sadism refers to the practice of gaining sexual pleasure while inflicting abuse on another person.

12. **b, c, d, e.** It is appropriate to provide education about sexuality and sexual responses. The nurse could teach that during the excitement phase, the female breasts swell and the nipples become erect and hard to the touch. Lubrication of the vagina seeps along the vulvar creases decreasing friction and making stimulation of the genitals more pleasurable. The upper two thirds of the vagina enlarge and expand. The clitoris enlarges and emerges slightly from the clitoral hood. The labia also enlarge and separate and turn a deep rosy-red with arousal. The first obvious sign of arousal in the male is an erection of the penis caused by increased pelvic congestion of blood. The scrotum noticeably elevates, thickens, and enlarges. The skin of the penis and scrotum turns a deep reddish purple in response to congestion and arousal. Male nipples may also harden and become erect. The nurse should also discuss contraception, preventing STIs, and the patient's right to say no if she chooses.

13. **a, b, d, e.** Causes of menstrual cycle irregularities include pregnancy or breastfeeding, eating disorders, extreme weight loss, excessive exercising, and pelvic inflammatory disease, as well as many other causes. Abstaining from sex and spinal cord injuries are not causes of menstrual irregularities.

14. **d.** Factors contributing to dyspareunia include diabetes; hormonal imbalances; vaginal, cervical, or rectal disorders; antihistamine, alcohol, tranquilizer, or illicit drug use; and cosmetic or chemical irritants to genitals.

15. **a, b, c, e.** LGBTQIA+ youth are two to three times more likely to attempt suicide and be homeless. Lesbians are less likely to get preventive services for cancer. Transgender people have a high prevalence of HIV and sexually transmitted infections. LGBTQIA+ youth are two to three times more likely to attempt suicide. Lesbians and bisexual females are more likely to be overweight or obese. LGBTQIA+ populations have

the highest rates of tobacco, alcohol, and other drug use in the country. These health issues are partly thought to be the effects of chronic stress resulting from stigmatization.

16. **a, b, c, e, f.** Victims of human trafficking can be any age. The nurse observes for those engaging in sex work, agricultural, or ranch work; working in hotels, massage parlors, nail salons, or home-cleaning services; performing domestic labor (cleaning, childcare, eldercare, etc.); working in restaurants, bars, or cantinas; and begging, street peddling, or door-to-door sales. Victims of human trafficking may exhibit evidence of being controlled either physically or psychologically, an inability to leave home or their place of work, or an inability to speak for themselves or share their own information. Information is provided by someone accompanying the individual, and they do not have control of their own identification documents (ID or passport). They have few or no personal possessions, may owe a large debt that they are unable to pay off, and may demonstrate loss of sense of time or whereabouts.

17. **d.** Puberty begins for most girls with development of secondary sex characteristics, and menarche begins at about age 12 years but may occur anywhere between ages 8 and 17 years. Information regarding body changes is needed to alleviate fears and should be given to the child before puberty begins. The focus should be on the daughter's needs, not the parent's need.

Bibliography

The American College of Obstetricians and Gynecologists (ACOG). (2021, May). *Premenstrual syndrome (PMS)*. https://www.acog.org/womens-health/faqs/premenstrual-syndrome?utm_source=redirect&utm_medium=web&utm_campaign=otn

American Nurses Association (ANA) Ethics Advisory Board. (2020, October 20). ANA position statement: Nurse's role in providing ethically and developmentally appropriate care to people with intellectual and developmental disabilities. *The Online Journal of Issues in Nursing, 26*(1). https://doi.org/10.3912/OJIN.Vol26No01PoSCol01

American Psychological Association (APA). (2020). *Publication manual of the American Psychological Association: The official guide to APA style* (7th ed.). American Psychological Association.

American Psychiatric Association (APA). (2021). *What is gender dysphoria?* Retrieved May 18, 2022, from https://psychiatry.org/patients-families/gender-dysphoria/what-is-gender-dysphoria

Babu, R., & Shah, U. (2021). Gender identity disorder (GID) in adolescents and adults with differences of sex development (DSD): A systematic review and meta-analysis. *Journal of Pediatric Urology, 17*(1), 39–47. https://doi.org/10.1016/j.jpurol.2020.11.017

Basson, R. (2000). The female sexual response: A different model. *Journal of Sex & Marital Therapy, 26*(1), 51–65. https://doi.org/10.1080/009262300278641

Boyd, M. A., & Luebbert, R. (2022). *Psychiatric nursing: Contemporary practice* (7th ed.). Wolters Kluwer.

Centers for Disease Control and Prevention (CDC). (2020a, March 17). *HPV vaccine recommendations*. https://www.cdc.gov/vaccines/vpd/hpv/hcp/recommendations.html

Centers for Disease Control and Prevention (CDC). (2020b, September 14). *Tips for communicating with female patients with intellectual disabilities*. https://www.cdc.gov/ncbddd/disabilityandhealth/materials/communicating-with-female-patients.html

Centers for Disease Control and Prevention (CDC). (2021a, June 14). *Sexual risk behaviors can lead to HIV, STDs, & teen pregnancy*. https://www.cdc.gov/healthyyouth/sexualbehaviors/index.htm

Centers for Disease Control and Prevention (CDC). (2021b, June 17). *Sexually transmitted diseases (STDs)*. https://www.cdc.gov/std/default.htm

Centers for Disease Control and Prevention (CDC). (2021c, July 23). *Sexually transmitted infections treatment guidelines, 2021. Morbidity and Mortality Weekly Report, 70*(4). https://www.cdc.gov/std/treatment-guidelines/STI-Guidelines-2021.pdf

Centers for Disease Control and Prevention (CDC). (2021d, September 23). *HIV and African American people*. https://www.cdc.gov/hiv/group/racialethnic/africanamericans/index.html

Center for Family Justice. (2021). *Statistics*. https://www.centerforfamilyjustice.org/community.-education/statistics

Chin, H. B., Sipe, T. A., Elder, R., Mercer, S. L., Chattopadhyay, S. K., Jacob, V., Wethington, H. R., Kirby, D., Elliston, D. B., Griffith, M., Chuke, S. O., Briss, S. C., Ericksen, I., Galbraith, J. S., Herbst, J. H., Johnson, R. L., Kraft, J. M., Noar, S. M., Romero, L. M., … Community Preventive Services Task Force. (2012). The effectiveness of group-based comprehensive risk-reduction and abstinence education interventions to prevent or reduce the risk of adolescent pregnancy, human immunodeficiency virus, and sexually transmitted infections: two systematic reviews for the Guide to Community Preventive Services. *American Journal of Preventive Medicine, 42*(3), 272–294. https://doi.org/10.1016/j.amepre.2011.11.006

Das, L. T. (2021, February 19). The inclusivity trap. *The Washington Post*.

Denford, S., Abraham, C., Campbell, R., & Busse, H. (2017). A comprehensive review of reviews of school-based interventions to improve sexual-health. *Health Psychology Review, 11*(1), 33–52. https://doi.org/10.1080/17437199.2016.1240625

Dwyer, A. A., & Greenspan, D. L. (2021). Endocrine Nurses Society position statement on transgender and gender diverse care. *Journal of the Endocrine Society, 5*(8), bvab105. https://doi.org/10.1210/jendso/bvab105

Edelman, C. L., & Kudzma, E. C. (2022). *Health promotion throughout the life span* (10th ed.). Elsevier.

GLAAD. (n.d.). *GLAAD media reference guide—Terms to avoid*. https://www.glaad.org/reference/offensive

GLAAD. (2021). *Accelerating acceptance 2021*. https://www.glaad.org/publications/accelerating-acceptance-2021

Gyamerah, A. O., Baguso, G., Santiago-Rodriguez, E., Sa'id, A., Arayasirikul, S., Lin, J., Turner, C. M., Taylor, K. D., McFarland, W., Wilson, E. C., & Wesson, P. (2021). Experiences and factors associated with transphobic hate crimes among transgender women in the San Francisco Bay Area: Comparisons across race. *BMC Public Health, 21*(1), 1053. https://doi.org/10.1186/s12889-021-11107-x

Harley, D. A., & Teaster, P. B. (2016). *Handbook of LGBT elders: An interdisciplinary approach to principles, practices, and policies*. Springer International Publishing.

Healthy People 2020. (2021a, October 27). *Family planning*. U.S. Department of Health and Human Services, Office of Disease Prevention and Health Promotion. https://www.healthypeople.gov/2020/topics-objectives/topic/family-planning

Healthy People 2020. (2021b, October 27). *Lesbian, gay, bisexual, and transgender health*. U.S. Department of Health and Human Services, Office of Disease Prevention and Health Promotion. http://www.healthypeople.gov/2020/topics-objectives/topic/lesbian-gay-bisexual-and-transgender-health

Healthy People 2030. (n.d.a). *Family planning*. U.S. Department of Health and Human Services, Office of Disease Prevention and Health Promotion. Retrieved November 21, 2021, from https://health.gov/healthypeople/objectives-and-data/browse-objectives/family-planning

Healthy People 2030. (n.d.b). *Lesbian, gay, bisexual, and transgender health workgroup*. U.S. Department of Health and Human Services, Office of Disease Prevention and Health Promotion. Retrieved November 21, 2021, from https://health.gov/healthypeople/about/workgroups/lesbian-gay-bisexual-and-transgender-health-workgroup

Healthy People 2030. (n.d.c). *LGBT*. U.S. Department of Health and Human Services, Office of Disease Prevention and Health Promotion. Retrieved February 22, 2022, from https://health.gov/healthypeople/objectives-and-data/browse-objectives/lgbt

Hofmeister, S., & Bodden, S. (2016). Premenstrual syndrome and premenstrual dysphoric disorder. *American Family Physician, 94*(3), 236–240.

Institute of Medicine, Committee on Lesbian, Gay, Bisexual, and Transgender Health Issues and Research Gaps and Opportunities. (2011). *The health of lesbian, gay, bisexual, and transgender people: Building a foundation for better understanding*. National Academies Press.

Martin, J. (2017). *Building a bridge: How the Catholic church and the LGBT community can enter into a relationship of respect, compassion, and sensitivity*. HarperCollins Publishers.

Masters, W. H., & Johnson, V. E. (1966). *Human sexual response*. Little, Brown.

Mayo Clinic Staff. (2021, April 29). *Menstrual cycle: What's normal, what's not*. http://www.mayoclinic.org/healthy-living/womens-health/in-depth/menstrual-cycle/art-20047186?pg=1

Mick, J., Hughes, M., & Cohen, M. Z. (2004). Using the BETTER model to assess sexuality. *Clinical Journal of Oncology Nursing, 8*(1), 84–86. https://doi.org/10.1188/04.CJON.84-86

National Cancer Institute, National Institutes of Health. (2018, February 22). *Oral contraceptives and cancer risk*. https://www.cancer.gov/about-cancer/causes-prevention/risk/hormones/oral-contraceptives-fact-sheet

National Institute of Allergy and Infectious Diseases (NIAID). (2015-2022). *Sexually transmitted diseases*. https://www.niaid.nih.gov/diseases-conditions/sexually-transmitted-diseases

Norris, T. L. (2019). *Porth's pathophysiology: Concepts of altered health states* (10th ed.). Wolters Kluwer.

Office of the Assistant Secretary for Health (OASH), U.S. Department of Health & Human Services (USDHHS). (n.d). *Teen pregnancy prevention (TPP) program*. Retrieved November 20, 2021, from https://opa.hhs.gov/grant-programs/teen-pregnancy-prevention-program-tpp

Office on Women's Health, U.S. Department of Health & Human Services (USDHHS). (2018, March 16). *Premenstrual syndrome (PMS)*. https://www.womenshealth.gov/menstrual-cycle/premenstrual-syndrome

Organon Connect. (2022). *Professional resources*. Retrieved on May 18, 2022, from https://www.organonconnect.com/nexplanon/professional-resources/

Planned Parenthood Federation of America Inc. (2021). *Birth control*. Retrieved November 20, 2021, from https://www.plannedparenthood.org/learn/birth-control

Rape, Abuse & Incest National Network (RAINN). (2022). *Statistics*. Retrieved May 18, 2022, from https://www.rainn.org/statistics

Regents of the University of California, Davis campus. (2020, January 14). *Lesbian, gay, bisexual, transgender, queer, intersex, asexual resource center: LGBTQIA resource center glossary*. https://lgbtqia.ucdavis.edu/educated/glossary.html

Russell, S., Mallory, A., Bishop, M., & Dorri, A. (2020). Innovation and integration of sexuality in family life education. *Family Relations, 69*(3), 595–613. https://doi.org/10.1111/fare.12462

Stuart, G. W. (2013). *Principles and practice of psychiatric nursing* (10th ed.). Elsevier/Mosby.

U.S. Department of Health & Human Services (USDHHS). (2016). *Advancing LGBT health and well-being: 2016 report of the HHS LGBT policy coordinating committee*. Retrieved May 18, 2022, from https://www.hhs.gov/sites/default/files/2016-report-with-cover.pdf

U.S. Food & Drug Administration (FDA). (2021, June 18). *Birth control*. https://www.fda.gov/consumers/free-publications-women/birth-control

World Health Organization (WHO). (2006). *Defining sexual health: Report of a technical consultation on sexual health 28–31 January 2002*. http://www.who.int/reproductivehealth/publications/sexual_health/defining_sexual_health.pdf

World Health Organization (WHO). (2020, February 3). *Female genital mutilation*. https://www.who.int/news-room/fact-sheets/detail/female-genital-mutilation

World Health Organization (WHO). (2022). *Defining sexual health*. Retrieved May 18, 2022, from https://www.who.int/teams/sexual-and-reproductive-health-and-research/key-areas-of-work/sexual-health/defining-sexual-health

World Professional Association for Transgender Health (WPATH). (2012). *Standards of care for the health of transsexual, transgender, and gender nonconforming people* (7th ed.). The World Professional Association for Transgender Health. Retrieved on May 18, 2022, from https://s3.amazonaws.com/amo_hub_content/Association140/files/Standards%20of%20Care%20V7%20-%202011%20WPATH%20(2)(1).pdf

World Professional Association for Transgender Health (WPATH). (2016, December 21). *Position statement on medical necessity of treatment, sex reassignment, and insurance coverage in the U.S.A.* https://www.wpath.org/newsroom/medical-necessity-statement

47 Spirituality

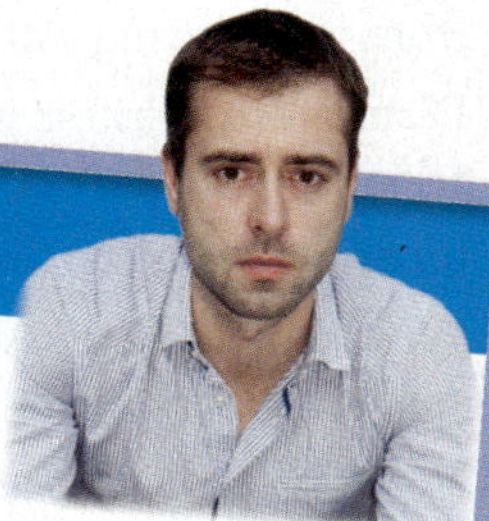

Kevin Gargan

Kevin, a 38-year-old divorced man on a step-down unit after treatment for a myocardial infarction, asks the night nurse, "Did you ever give much thought to whether or not there is a God?" Kevin listed his religion as Protestant but says it's been a long time since he went to church or prayed.

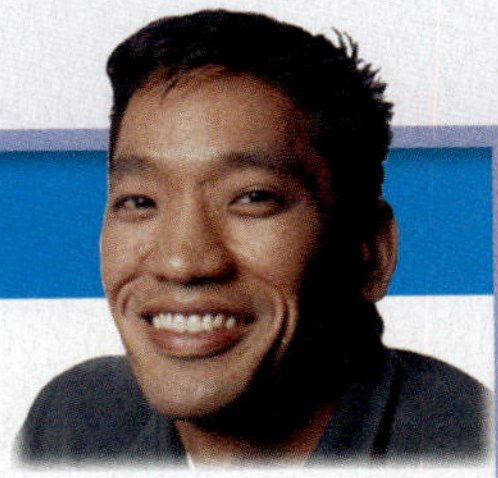

Choi Min Lai

Choi, a member of the Hmong culture from Laos, is refusing to allow health care providers to perform a series of surgical repairs to correct severe deformities of his 8-year-old son's feet. "In our culture, the deformity is a sign of spiritual favor and good luck. Because of Kou's condition, a warrior ancestor whose feet were wounded in battle will no longer be spiritually trapped. You see, Kou is special."

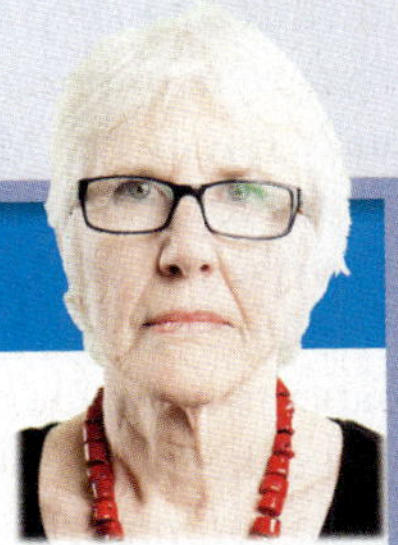

Margot Zeuner

Margot, a 75-year-old woman, is taking care of her 80-year-old husband with advanced Alzheimer's disease, who was just discharged from the hospital and requires constant supervision. When visited at home, she says, "I really miss going to church and seeing everyone. They're so supportive. That was the one thing that helped to keep me going."

Learning Outcomes

After completing the chapter, you will be able to accomplish the following:

1. Identify the three spiritual needs believed to be common to all people.
2. Describe the influences of spirituality on everyday living, health, and illness.
3. Differentiate life-affirming influences of religious beliefs from life-denying influences.
4. Distinguish spiritual beliefs and practices of major religions practiced in the United States.
5. Identify five factors that influence spirituality.
6. Perform a nursing assessment of spiritual health, using appropriate interview questions and observation skills.
7. Develop problem identifications that correctly identify spiritual problems.
8. Describe nursing strategies to promote spiritual health, and state their rationale.
9. Plan, implement, and evaluate nursing care related to select problem identifications involving spiritual problems.

Nursing Concepts

- Spirituality

Paying attention to the spiritual dimension of health and well-being is integral to holistic person-centered care. Patients facing the losses and limits related to injury, disease, or aging begin to evaluate what is important in life, and often ask the "big questions": Is there a God or transcendent being? Does life have meaning and purpose? Am I dying? Is there anyone I can trust to be with me during this hard time? Nurses skilled in spiritual care are able to identify and elicit the inner resources of patients and family caregivers to promote health and healing with sensitivity to such questions. Many nurses who describe themselves as professional healers use the terms "vocation" or "calling" to describe the work of nursing. They claim to be "standing on holy ground" when they create that hospitable place where patients can expose their vulnerabilities and face their biggest concerns. We learn, with great humility, that sometimes the most important things we do are accomplished simply by being present to those we serve (see Through the Eyes of a Caregiver on pages 1908–1909). A Baptist woman with a life-threatening cancer who had shared the importance of her spirituality with me recently wrote to me:

> When you made a cross on my forehead with your thumb, it felt unfamiliar—but perfect. Like a blessing with no conditions—no strings. How liberating. Affirming. Loving. And to think you did it with just your thumb. And your heart. Thank you.

SPIRITUAL DIMENSION

The human "spirit" dimension was first recognized in ancient cultures. One person often played the roles of both priest and health care provider, ministering to the spirit and the body. Over the years, however, medicine and religion evolved separately. Not until the holistic health movement took root was the person once again viewed as an integrated whole of body, mind, and spirit. Health care practitioners began again to probe the relationships among physical, psychological, social, and spiritual health. Two models are currently used to illustrate these relationships (Fig. 47-1 on page 1908). In the integrated approach, the physio-psycho-socio-spiritual model has four equal dimensions, each of which influences the other. In the unifying approach, the spiritual dimension grounds the physiologic, psychological, and sociologic dimensions. While it is interesting to interview professional healers about which model is more consistent with their experience, both demand from the nurse greater competence in identifying and meeting spiritual needs than most practicing nurses today display. National guidelines now mandate spiritual care—see the Joint Commission requirements and the National Consensus Project for Palliative Care (2018). In 2016, the Health Care Chaplaincy Network developed the most comprehensive evidence-based indicators that demonstrate the quality of spiritual care in health care in a move aimed at advancing spiritual support and meeting the needs of patients, their families, and health care institutions.

According to Shelly and Fish (1988), three **spiritual needs** underlie all religious traditions and are common to all people regardless of whether or not they belong to a particular religious tradition:

1. Need for meaning and purpose
2. Need for love and relatedness
3. Need for forgiveness

Although nurses may differ in their beliefs about how involved they should become in meeting patients' spiritual needs, it is impossible to nurse patients well while ignoring the spiritual dimensions of health. Nurses can assist patients to meet spiritual needs by offering a compassionate presence; assisting in the struggle to find meaning and purpose in the face of suffering, illness, and death; fostering relationships (with a higher being or other people) that nurture the spirit; and facilitating the patient's expression of religious or spiritual beliefs and practices (e.g., see the Reflective Practice box).

CONCEPTS RELATED TO SPIRITUALITY AND SPIRITUAL HEALTH

Spirituality, faith, religion, and the influence of these elements on everyday living and health and illness are important concepts to understand when caring for patients. Although some use the words *spirituality, faith,* and *religion* interchangeably, there are distinctions. These and other concepts are explored in the following sections.

QSEN Reflective Practice: Cultivating QSEN Competencies

CHALLENGE TO INTELLECTUAL SKILLS

During my pediatric rotation, I encountered a Hmong family from Laos whose 8-year-old son, Kou, had severe deformations in his feet. It seemed as if the entire health care team was united to persuade, cajole, and if necessary, force Choi Min Lai, Kou's father, and his mother to authorize a series of surgical repairs. But the parents were adamant in their refusal. In their culture, the deformity was a sign of spiritual favor and good luck. They believed that a warrior ancestor whose own feet were wounded in battle would be released from a form of spiritual entrapment because of their son's condition. This made Kou special in their community. I admired their fierce championing of their beliefs, but my heart ached for Kou because of the difficulties he would face in the U.S. society if his feet were not repaired. I didn't know anything about the Hmong culture or their beliefs. As a result, I didn't know which side I should support. I also didn't know much about the legal rights of the parents to refuse a procedure that, although not lifesaving, would clearly benefit their son.

Thinking Outside the Box: Possible Courses of Action

- Remain detached from the conflict and just observe.
- Try to learn more about the family's cultural and religious beliefs to see if this information could be helpful.
- Contact the hospital attorney to find out about the legal rights of the parents to refuse a procedure that, while not lifesaving, would clearly benefit their son.
- Use my relationship with the family to try to persuade them to comply.
- Use my knowledge of Kou and his family to try to persuade the health care team to respect their wishes.

Evaluating a Good Outcome: How Do I Define Success?

- The health care team chooses a course of action that is beneficial to Kou and simultaneously respects the family's religious and cultural beliefs.
- We respect the legal rights of this family.
- My knowledge of the Hmong religion and culture is increased.
- I am faithful to my advocacy obligations.

Personal Learning: Here's to the Future!

Unfortunately, this issue was not resolved during my rotation. In fact, the conflict continued to grow. When I completed my rotation, the hospital was appealing to the court to force the parents to accept surgery. I came to believe that the rights of the parents should be respected. Their cultural community was so strong, and they clearly did not see Kou's condition as a correctable "health problem" but rather a blessing to be enjoyed. While a few other nurses felt the way I did, the health care providers and the social worker felt strongly that the parents were wrong. I learned much about the Hmong culture, realizing that my practice will continue to surprise me as I encounter patients and families with beliefs and practices very different from mine. As a result of this experience, I hope I will keep an open mind and always be ready to learn.

QSEN SELF-REFLECTION ON QUALITY AND SAFETY COMPETENCIES DEVELOPING KNOWLEDGE, SKILLS, AND ATTITUDES FOR CONTINUOUS IMPROVEMENT

Do you agree with the criteria that the nursing student used to evaluate a successful outcome? Why or why not? What *knowledge, skills,* and *attitudes* do you need to develop to continuously improve the quality and safety of care for patients like Kou and his family?

Patient-Centered Care: How would you develop a respectful and successful partnership with Kou and his family, given that their culture is so different? How can you best communicate empathy and respect given the conflict created by their wishes?

Teamwork and Collaboration/Quality Improvement: What communication and interpersonal skills do you need to improve to ensure that you function as a member of the patient-care team when members of the team are so divided? The social worker? Other members of the health care team? What other team members can be called upon to provide needed assistance in clarifying this family's legal rights? What does quality care for Kou and his family "look like"?

Safety/Evidence-Based Practice: What does the evidence point to as "best practice" for Kou? What safety needs does he have and how can you meet them?

Informatics: Can you identify the essential information that must be available in Kou's electronic record to support safe patient care and coordination of care? Are there smart devices or online resources you can use to learn more about the Hmong culture? Can you think of other ways to respond to or approach the situation? What else might the nursing student have done to ensure a successful outcome?

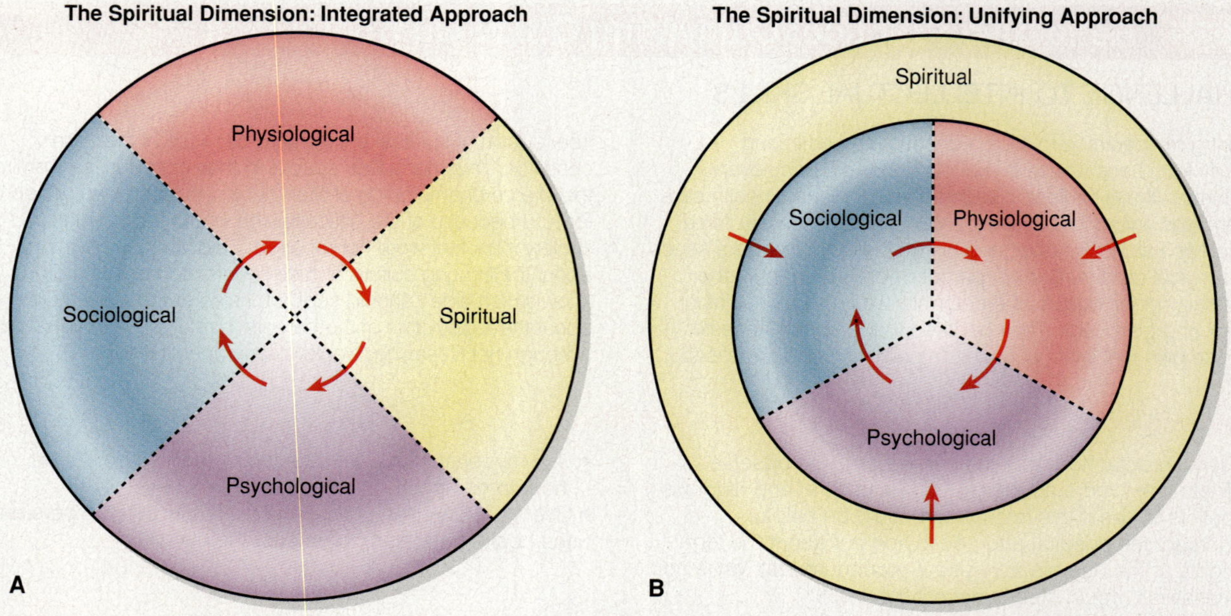

FIGURE 47-1. Spiritual dimensions. No consensus exists about the role of the spiritual dimension in health. **A.** The integrated approach views each of the four dimensions as equal and influencing one another. **B.** The unifying model grounds the physiologic, psychological, and social dimensions in the spiritual dimension. (*Source:* Redrawn by permission from Springer Nature from Farran, C. J., Fitchett, G., Quiring-Emblen, J. D., & Burk, J. R. [1989]. Development of a model for spiritual assessment and intervention. *Journal of Religion and Health*, *28*[3], 185–194.)

Through the Eyes of a Caregiver

My name is Janine Landry and I love nursing! I especially have a passion for emergency department (ED) nursing, and I'm pleased to be employed in a faith-based community hospital. I don't feel like I have a job, but rather I look at it as an amazing opportunity to meet people from diverse cultures and beliefs. My work has enabled me to learn and grow both professionally and personally. My dream has always been to become a nurse, to have the opportunity to follow my heart and the purpose of my life—that is, to "*make a difference.*" I strive to create an environment of hope and healing and to have an impact on the people from the vulnerable population we serve. I would like to recount a true story that encompasses all that I believe in, and live, as a registered nurse.

I'll never forget the day I walked into the Grey Nuns Hospital and noticed the mission statement posted on the wall. It began with "Healing the Body, Enriching the Mind, Nurturing the Soul," and went on to express the hospital's values and beliefs, all of which I truly support. This mission statement helps to guide my decisions and actions I make every day, and in all areas in which I work. As a clinical nurse educator, I have made it my habit to instruct our newly hired staff to locate the mission statement; read, understand, and respect it; and most importantly, to live it!

In the ED, we often have repeat visitors and one particular gentleman comes to mind. Fred (not his real name) was a "high-maintenance" kind of guy who always appeared cranky. He had silky white hair, bright blue eyes, wore a constant frown on his face, and often demanded a lot of attention. Fred had a chronic condition, which resulted in him visiting us on a regular basis. At that time, I was working on the floor, and I was often assigned to be his nurse. Fred was somewhat gruff when he spoke to people, and he never called me by my given name, Janine. Although I would remind him, he still chose to call me a myriad of other names.

One day while Fred was in the department awaiting admission to the medical unit, I served him his breakfast tray. He snarled and refused to eat it. I looked at him and said "Fred, you're not eating." He grumbled under his breath and said, "No, I don't want to eat this." "Fred, may I remind you that you're at the Grey Nuns Hospital, and did you know that every meal prepared here is made with love… and this breakfast was made especially for you?" "Really… it was made with love?" "Absolutely!" Not surprisingly, Fred ate all his breakfast, and later on, he ate his entire lunch. When his wife and friends came to visit him, he would tell them how amazed he was to find out that all his meals were made with love. Every time his wife and daughter would come and visit him, I would look at them and wink; this always made them smile and giggle.

A few months later, Fred was a patient once again. Guess which nurse was assigned to him? You're right… it was me again. While I was busy changing a wound dressing on his leg, a message came over the hospital intercom system. Fred asked, "What's that noise I hear every morning in this hospital?" "Fred, what may be noise to your ears, is known as a prayer or a reflection to others." He asked, "What do you call it?" "I personally call it Hope!" "Hope?" "Yes, let me explain. Do you like Neapolitan ice cream?" "Yeah!" "What's your favorite flavor?" "I like all the flavors, but I especially enjoy chocolate and my wife and daughter like the vanilla and strawberry flavors. Why do you ask?" "Imagine this; we'll compare Hope to an entire brick of Neapolitan ice cream that

Through the Eyes of a Caregiver *(continued)*

has three individual flavors, right?" Fred nodded and agreed. "For some people, in order to have hope, they need to taste that vanilla flavor, which represents *faith,* and depending on what their beliefs are or what they're faced with at that particular moment, having faith may require *courage;* that would be the strawberry flavor. Most importantly, to have hope, you need *love*—a sense of love for yourself, to be able to receive love and to love others unconditionally, and for some people it also means loving God. So, just think how lucky you are Fred, knowing your favorite flavor is chocolate… that's awesome because everyone knows that chocolate and love are both really good for your heart! You can enjoy each flavor individually…and that's o.k.…or you can swirl the ice cream and mix it all together to make one flavor; a delicious flavor called HOPE!"

Fred really didn't know how to respond. He looked up at me with his big bright blue eyes and a puzzled look on his face. He then asked me "Are you a tree hugger?" I said no! "Would you ever hug a tree?" I thought about it, and I said, "You know, for the right reason and at the right time, yes, I guess I would hug a tree, because a tree symbolizes creation, growth, and change." Fred looked up at me and said, "If I was a tree, what type of a tree would I be?" I quickly replied "Oh…without a doubt…you would be an ol' crabapple tree!" Fred started to laugh, it was the first time I had ever heard him laugh, and this laughter came from his toes.

A few weeks later, as I was walking in the main lobby of the hospital, I heard a familiar gruff voice calling out to me. I turned around, and sure enough it was Fred and his wife. He asked me to close my eyes and to put out my hand. When I opened up my eyes, Fred had placed the shiniest, most perfect red apple in my hand. I was speechless but realized that we really had no need for words: our eyes spoke volumes. I'll never forget that moment.

A few months later, when Fred returned to the ED, I learned that his wife had recently passed away. Fred was depressed and acutely ill; his chronic condition had worsened, and the cardiologist informed me that Fred was dying and that he was made aware of this. I quickly notified his daughter and then went to his bedside to support him, but he shouted, "get out, get away from me, and leave me alone!" I respected his wishes by leaving the room; but I intentionally left the curtain slightly open so that I could continue to monitor him from the nursing desk. While I was charting, I sensed that he was watching me, so I looked up and just like the time before, our eyes silently spoke to each other.

Fred was deteriorating quickly, and his daughter hadn't arrived yet. My shift was over but I couldn't imagine leaving him alone, so I went into his room to say goodnight. Although we both knew it wasn't really "goodnight," I asked him if I could come and sit next to him, and he simply raised his finger and nodded his head. I sat next to him, and for the longest time neither one of us said anything. I held his hand and looked into his blue eyes and said, "what do you need?" His response was "this ol' tree needs a hug!" So, I held him tightly in my arms for the longest time, and when his daughter arrived, I gently laid him back and said "good bye." Next, when I stood up, the most amazing thing happened: Fred looked up at me, and despite his labored breathing, he whispered, "Thank you…thank you, Janine." This was truly a precious moment for me because it was the first and only time Fred called me by my given name.

Shortly thereafter, he died. I will never forget this experience because when I walked away, I was thinking about the time we had spent together, and although there were many challenging times with this gentleman, I realized that I had grown to respect him. He died with dignity, because I knew who he was, I took the time to get to know what was truly at the "core" of this man. In essence, I got to know what was in his heart…and he was truly a gift to me!

—Janine Landry

Spirituality

Spirituality is anything that pertains to a person's relationship with a nonmaterial life force or higher power. While one person describes spirituality in terms of coming to know, love, and serve God, another speaks of transcending the limits of body and experiencing a universal energy.

Aspects of spirituality include the following:

- Spirituality is experienced as a unifying force, life principle, essence of being.
- Spirituality is expressed and experienced in and through connectedness with nature, the earth, the environment, and the cosmos.
- People express and experience spirituality in and through connectedness with other people.
- Spirituality shapes self-becoming and is reflected in a person's being, knowing, and doing.
- Spirituality permeates life, providing purpose, meaning, strength, and guidance, and shaping the journey.

While analyzing concepts of spirituality through a review of related literature, nurse scholar Bernice Golberg (1998) identified the following phenomena: meaning, **presencing** (standing in the presence of another consciously believing in—and affirming—their capacity for wholeness), empathy/compassion, giving hope, love, religion/transcendence, and touch and healing. All appeared to be products of relationships, some physical (presencing, touch, and healing), and others emotional (meaning, empathy/compassion, hope, love, and religion/transcendence). Golberg combined these and gave spirituality the label "connection" (1998, p. 836). In 2021, the American Nurses Association highlighted the importance of compassionate presence by including it in their definition of nursing. "Nursing integrates the art and science of caring and focuses on the protection, promotion, and optimization of health and human functioning; prevention of illness and injury; facilitations of healing; and alleviation of suffering through compassionate presence" (p. 1).

In the words of theologian Karl Rahner, spirituality is…simply the ultimate depth of everything spiritual creatures do when they realize themselves—when they laugh or cry, accept responsibility, love, live and die, stand up for truth, break out of preoccupation with themselves to help the neighbor, hope against hope, cheerfully refuse to be embittered by the stupidity of daily life, keep silent, not so that evil festers in their hearts, but so that it dies there—when, in a word, they live as they would like to live in opposition to selfishness and to the despair that always assails us (1971, p. 229).

Faith

Faith generally refers to a confident belief in something for which there is no proof or material evidence. It can involve a person, idea, or thing, and is usually followed by action related to the ideals or values of that belief. For example, if I have faith in my doctor, parish nurse, or healer, I am more likely to adhere to a prescribed regimen or plan of care and to experience benefits. Similarly, patients who believe in a loving and all-powerful being who knows them and cares for them are often better able to cope with the suffering related to injury and illness. The declaration made by the World Conference of the Religions for Peace in Kyoto, Japan, in 1970 is an excellent example of a confident belief in something for which there is no proof or material evidence. At this conference, Baha'i, Buddhist, Confucianism, Christian, Hindu, Jain, Judaism, Muslim, Shintoist, Sikh, and others discovered that the beliefs that unite them were more important than those that divided them. They discovered that they shared:

- A conviction of the fundamental unity of the human family, of the quality and dignity of all human beings
- A sense of the sacredness of the individual person and the person's conscience
- A sense of the value of the human community
- A belief that love, compassion, unselfishness, and the force of inner truthfulness and of the spirit have ultimately greater power than hate, enmity, and self-interest
- A sense of obligation to stand on the side of the poor and the oppressed and against the rich and the oppressors
- A profound hope that good will finally prevail

Faith is a term also used to describe a cultural or institutional religion, such as Judaism, Islam, or Confucianism. An **atheist** is a person who denies the existence of a higher power; an **agnostic** is one who holds that nothing can be known about the existence of a higher power. Atheists and agnostics deserve respect for what they choose to believe, just as do those who accept a particular religious creed.

Religion

Religion can be defined as an organized system of beliefs about a higher power that often includes set forms of worship, spiritual practices, and codes of conduct. Although it is impossible for nurses to be knowledgeable about all religions, we are better able to meet patients' spiritual needs when we understand their religious beliefs and practices. These can directly influence patients' responses to illness and suffering, self-care practices such as diet and hygiene, birth and death rituals, biologic sex roles, spiritual practices, and moral codes. The beliefs and health practices of major religious traditions in the United States are briefly described in Table 47-1. Please remember that these are generalizations and that not all members of religious traditions hold the same beliefs or practices. Also understand that this is not a comprehensive list, especially as the U.S. population becomes increasingly diverse.

The U.S. Religious Landscape Survey of 35,000 Americans by the Pew Research Center's Forum on Religion & Public Life (2015) found that most Americans were religious and most had a nondogmatic approach to faith. At the time of the survey, the largest percentage of Americans—70.6%—were Christian, and 5.9% belonged to non-Christian faiths (Jewish, Muslim, Buddhist, Hindu, and other world religions). Religious "nones" (those unaffiliated with a religion) represented 22.8% of Americans, and of these 3.1% were atheist and 4% were agnostic.

This study found a modest drop between 2007 and 2014 in the percentages of those who say they believe in God, pray daily, and regularly go to church or other religious services. This recent decrease in religious beliefs and behaviors is largely attributable to the "nones"—the growing underrepresented group of Americans, particularly in the Millennial generation, who say they do not belong to an organized religion. In addition:

- Most Americans who are affiliated with a religion do not believe their religion is the only way to salvation. Most also believe that there is more than one true way to interpret the teachings of their religion.
- More than half of Americans rank the importance of religion very highly in their lives, attend religious services regularly, and pray daily.
- A plurality of adults who are affiliated with a religion want their religion to preserve its traditional beliefs and practices rather than either adjust to new circumstances or adopt modern beliefs and practices.
- Significant minorities across nearly all religious traditions see a conflict between being a devout person and living in a modern society.
- The relationship between religion and politics is particularly strong with respect to political ideology and views on social issues such as abortion LGBTQIA, with the more religiously committed adherents across several religious traditions expressing more conservative political views.
- Americans are very similar in some basic religious beliefs. For instance, Americans are nearly unanimous in saying they believe in God (91%); large majorities believe in life after death (74%) and believe that Scripture is the word of God (63%).
- More than three quarters of American adults (78%) believe there are absolute standards of right and wrong,

Table 47-1 Beliefs and Health Care Practices of Major Religious Traditions in the United States

RELIGION	BELIEFS	SELECT HEALTH CARE PRACTICES
Adventist	Believe in the person's choice and God's sovereignty. The body is believed to be the temple of the Holy Spirit.	• The taking of all narcotics and stimulants is prohibited because the body is the temple of the Holy Spirit and should be protected. Many groups prohibit meat. • Many regard Saturday as the Sabbath. • Approach to health care is holistic.
American Muslim Mission	Accept the *Koran* as their sacred scripture (see Islam); most stress the importance of cooperation among Black individuals in business and education to build self-esteem.	• Members are encouraged to obtain health care provided by members of the Black community. • Major tenets involve prayer rituals, dietary restrictions (prohibitions against pork and alcohol), hygiene (extreme cleanliness), lifestyle modifications, and marital faithfulness.
Baha'i International Community	Believe in a basic harmony between religion and science	• Seek out competent medical care and pray for health. • Obligatory prayers, holy days, and the 19-day fast. • Permanent sterilization is prohibited, and abortion is discouraged.
Buddhism	Buddha—or "the Great Physician"—taught the Four Noble Truths to indicate the range of "suffering," its "origin," its "cessation," and the "way" that leads to its cessation. The real cause of human suffering is ignorant craving. The Noble Eightfold Path—which consists of right views, aspirations, speech, conduct, mode of livelihood, effort, mindfulness, and concentration—leads to the cessation of suffering.	• Buddhists do not outwardly proclaim healing through faith. However, spiritual peace and liberation from anxiety attained through the awakening to Buddha's wisdom may be an important factor in expediting healing and the recovery process. • Accepts modern science. The doctrine of avoidance of extremes is applied to the use of drugs, blood, vaccines. • Buddhism does not condone taking lives of any form. • Check with the patient about any special diet restrictions and the observance of holy days.
Christian Scientist	They deny the existence of health crises; sickness and sin are errors of the human mind and can be overcome by altering thoughts, not by using drugs or medicines.	• They will use orthopedic services to set a bone but decline drugs and, in general, other medical or surgical procedures. • They do not allow hypnotism or any form of psychotherapy, which alters the "Divine Mind." • A Christian Science Practitioner may be called to administer spiritual support. • Alcohol and tobacco are not used.
Church of Jesus Christ of Latter Day Saints (Mormons)	Devout adherents believe in divine healing through the "laying on of hands," though many do not prohibit medical therapy. The Church maintains an extensive and well-funded welfare system, including financial support for the sick.	• Mormons who have served a full-time mission are more likely than those who have not served a mission to see believing Joseph Smith saw God, helping the poor and avoiding coffee and tea are essential for being a good Mormon. • Church leaders encourage Mormons to keep at least three months of food supplies on hand.
Confucianism	Inherent in Confucianism is the appreciation of life and the desire to keep the body from untimely or unnecessary death.	• Appreciate life and desire to keep the body from untimely or unnecessary death. • Historically emphasized public health solutions to impending health problems.
Daoism (Taoism)	Health is a manifestation of the harmony of the universe, obtained through the proper balancing of internal and external forces. Implicit throughout the Daoist tradition is the tendency to understand salvation in the biomedical sense of health and qualitative improvement and prolongation of human life. The universal principle of the Tao is the mysterious biologic and spiritual life rhythm or order of nature.	• There is a "medicinal" concern for maintaining and prolonging human health and life (sheng). Knowing and living a natural life—following the Tao—is the secret of both health and sagehood. • Long tradition of seeking pragmatic medical techniques, along with its religious techniques of meditation and ritual for establishing a harmony of body and spirit, humanity, and nature (holistic approach).
Hinduism	Doctrine of Transmigration. Moral factors, linked with the all-embracing doctrine of "karma," are believed to be significant in promoting health or causing disease.	• Hindu medicine shows a surprising openness to new ideas, at least in respect to practical treatment. • Many Hindu dietary restrictions conform to individual sect doctrine. • The nurse administering medications should avoid touching the patient's lips. • Certain prescribed rites are followed after death; disposal of the body is by cremation.

(*continued*)

Table 47-1 Beliefs and Health Care Practices of Major Religious Traditions in the United States *(continued)*

RELIGION	BELIEFS	SELECT HEALTH CARE PRACTICES
Islam	Allah, one God, who is only one, all seeing, all hearing, all speaking, all knowing, all willing, all powerful. Must be able to practice the Five Pillars of Islam. May have a fatalistic view of health.	• Obligatory prayers, holy days, fasting (Ramadan), and almsgiving. • Koranic law and customs that influence birth, diet (eating pork and drinking alcohol are forbidden), care of women, death and prayer rituals. • Some Muslim women are not allowed to make independent decisions; husbands may need to be present when consent is sought.
Jehovah's Witnesses	They oppose the "false teachings" of other sects; opposition often extends to modern science, including medicine.	• Blood transfusions violate God's laws and therefore are not allowed. • The courts have not supported the right of Jehovah's Witness parents to refuse lifesaving treatment for their children. • Use of alcohol and tobacco are discouraged.
Judaism	Formation closely bound with a divine revelation and with commitment to obedience to God's will. The Hebrew Bible is the authority, guide, and inspiration of the many forms of religion of the Jewish people (currently Reform, Conservative, Orthodox).	• For observant Jewish: special needs in the areas of diet, birth rituals, male and female contact, and death. • Treatment and procedures should not be scheduled on the Sabbath.
Native American Religions	Difficult to generalize; notion of cosmic harmony, emphasis on directly experiencing powers and visions and a common view of the cycle of life and death. Death is not the end but the beginning of new life (reincarnation or transcendent hereafter).	• Rituals mark important life changes: birth, puberty, initiation rites, death. • Medicine men and women have specialized spirits from whom they receive the mission to cure. • Common therapeutic measures: sucking, blowing, and drawing out with a feather fan.
Protestantism	Worship of the one God revealed to the world through Jesus Christ. Love of neighbor is a central tenet. Other beliefs include sin, redemption, salvation, and a final accounting with God. Care of the sick is encouraged. God the author and giver of life is also the healer. Most accept modern medical science.	• Religious practices vary according to denomination; may include prayer, faith healing, "laying on of hands," and anointing. • Sacraments: baptism, communion, confirmation.
Roman Catholicism	Worship of the one God revealed to the world through Jesus Christ. Love of neighbor is a central tenet. Other beliefs include sin, redemption, salvation, and a final accounting with God. Care of the sick is encouraged. God the author and giver of life is also the healer. Human life is a gift of God. Many take an antiabortion stance; most accept modern medical science.	• Importance of private devotions and Mass attendance on Sunday. • Seven sacraments (importance of baptism, Eucharist, penance, and the anointing of the sick). • Dietary habits. • Sexual ethical norms. • Only natural means of birth control; abortion, euthanasia, and sterilization are forbidden.
Sikhism	Draws on features from Islam and Hinduism to establish a reformist movement with the aim of creating a new world order based on equality and social justice for all. The holy book is a code of conduct for daily life and an instruction for reaching true understanding and unity with God, the ultimate goal.	• Respect the special dress code including "Kesh," uncut hair for both men and women, and "Kara," a steel bangle worn on the right wrist. Removing a turban without permission, except in an emergency, is considered an insult. • Sexual activity is allowed only within marriage. Large families are encouraged, more for cultural than religious reasons. • Sikh individuals prefer a nurse or doctor of the same sex.
Unitarian Universal Association of Churches and Fellowships	Encourage creativity, reason, and living an ethical life. No member is required to adhere to a given creed or set of religious beliefs. The inherent worth and dignity of every person is affirmed.	• Free to accept what they take to be best for their health.

Disclaimer: Please note not all individuals within any tradition subscribe to the same beliefs.

with a majority (52%) saying they rely primarily on practical experience and common sense for guidance regarding right and wrong. Far fewer say they rely mainly on their religious beliefs (29%), and fewer still say they rely on philosophy and reason (9%) or scientific information (5%).

- The United States has largely avoided the secularizing trends that have reshaped the religious scene in recent decades in European and other economically developed nations—but not entirely. The Landscape Survey documents, for example, that the number of Americans who are not affiliated with a religion has grown significantly in recent decades, with the number of people who today say they are unaffiliated with a religious tradition (16% of U.S. adults) more than double the number who say they were not affiliated with a religion as children (7%).

This chapter is being written during the COVID-19 pandemic, during which in-person religious services were suspended for many different religious groups, and in-person wedding and funeral or memorial services were suspended. Many are wondering if the changes during the pandemic will affect the practice of religion once people can return safely to their places of worship.

Nurses who are unfamiliar with a patient's religion can gain valuable knowledge by discussions with the patient and the patient's family and spiritual advisor.

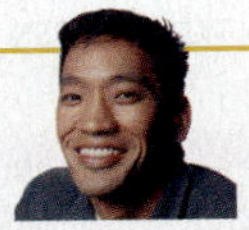

Recall **Choi Min Lai**, the father of the 8-year-old boy with foot deformities who is refusing surgical repair based on his cultural and religious beliefs. Researching information about the patient's beliefs would be essential in planning this family's care and advocating for the patient and his family.

Never presume to know what a patient's religious beliefs or practices are just because you have learned the patient's faith tradition. Many religious groups and people work out their own set of beliefs and practices, which may or may not be compatible with the tradition at large. Also, you should not interpret the fact that a patient does not belong to an organized religion to mean that the patient has no spiritual needs; a person may be deeply spiritual yet not profess to belong to an organized religion.

Hope

Closely related to spirituality, faith, and religion, **hope** is the ingredient in life responsible for a positive outlook, even in life's bleakest moments. It enables a person both to consider a future and to work to actively bring that future into being. Hope originates in imagination but must become a valued and realistic possibility in order to energize action. Hope allows a person to embrace the reality of suffering without escaping from it (false hope) or being suffocated by it (despair, helplessness, hopelessness). Hope is unique to each person. Box 44-6 on page 1813 contains a set of suggestions, developed by an interdisciplinary team, for enabling hope in the terminally ill that can apply to any situation in which people feel hopeless (Creen, 2002).

Love

Earlier, we noted that people express and experience spirituality in and through connectedness with other people. There is a basic human need to love and be loved, and we cannot be spiritually whole, spiritually healthy, unless this need is met. Mother Teresa wrote:

> "The greatest disease in the West today is not TB or leprosy; it is being unwanted, unloved, and uncared for. We can cure physical diseases with medicine, but the only cure for loneliness, despair and hopelessness is love. There are many in the world who are dying for a piece of bread but there are many more dying for a little love. The poverty in the West is a different kind of poverty—it is not only a poverty of loneliness but also of spirituality."

Suffering

Eric Cassell (1991), a physician who has written eloquently on human **suffering** describes suffering as a specific state of distress that occurs when the intactness or integrity of the person is threatened or disrupted. It lasts until the threat is gone or integrity is restored. Suffering involves some symptom or process that threatens the patient because of fear, the meaning of the symptom, and concerns about the future. The meanings and the fear are personal and individual, so that even if two patients have the same symptoms, their suffering would be different. While it has taken health care professionals decades to get serious about managing physical pain, too many of us remain unskilled in identifying and responding to human suffering. Have you practiced your own key phrases to elicit the human fears and sufferings of your patients? "I can only try to imagine how difficult this time must be for you and your family. How can we better help you?" See accompanying Box 47-1 (on page 1914) in which two nurse researchers outline the tenets of human suffering. Remember, an analgesic will not "fix" human suffering. Your presence, however, has the power to comfort and heal. See Box 47-2 Steps for Being a Healing Presence on page 1914. A friend once wrote:

> *"...Here is the hardest thing I know: I am alone. The kind of alone that even having such good and plentiful friends can't fix. Ultimately alone. When they said, "You have cancer," they did not mean, "You and your friends have cancer" or just "You and your family have cancer." They meant "You, Laurie, have cancer." Well. Darn. I don't have much practice doing things alone. I don't have any desire either. I'm a team player....Where's my "You have cancer" team? I looked around. The room was empty. They meant just me....They say there is a pill for making the sad more tolerable. I'll take that pill, but I'll keep wishing for the one that makes being alone less lonely."*

Box 47-1 Tenets of Suffering

by Betty Ferrell and Nessa Coyle

- Suffering is a loss of control that creates insecurity. Suffering people often feel helpless and trapped, unable to escape their circumstances.
- In most instances, suffering is associated with loss. The loss may be of a relationship, of some aspect of the self, or of some aspect of the physical body. The loss may be evident only in the mind of the sufferer, but it nonetheless leaves a person diminished and with a sense of brokenness.
- Suffering is an intensely personal experience.
- Suffering is accompanied by a range of intense emotions, including sadness, anguish, fear, abandonment, despair, and myriad other emotions.
- Suffering can be linked deeply to recognition of one's own mortality. When threatened by serious illness, people may fear the end of life. Conversely, for others, living with serious illness may result in a yearning for death.
- Suffering often involves asking the question "why?" Illness or loss may be seen as untimely and undeserved. Suffering people frequently seek to find meaning and answers for that which is unknowable.
- Suffering often is associated with separation from the world. Individuals may express intense loneliness and yearn for connection with others while also feeling intense distress about dependency on others.
- Suffering often is accompanied by spiritual distress. Regardless of religious affiliation, individuals experiencing illness may feel a sense of hopelessness. When life is threatened, people may conduct self-evaluation of what has been lived and what remains undone. Becoming weak and vulnerable and facing mortality may cause a person to reevaluate their relationship with a higher being.
- Suffering is not synonymous with pain but is closely associated with it. Physical pain is closely related to psychological, social, and spiritual distress. Pain that persists without meaning becomes suffering.
- Suffering occurs when an individual feels voiceless. This may occur when a person is unable to give words to their experience or when their "screams" are unheard.

Source: Ferrell, B. R., & Coyle, N. (2008). The Nature of Suffering and the Goals of Nursing. *Oncology Nursing Forum, 35*(2), 241–247.

Spiritual Health and Healing

Defined most simply, **spiritual health**, or spiritual well-being, is the condition that exists when the person's universal spiritual needs for meaning and purpose, love and belonging, and forgiveness are met. O'Brien's conceptual model of spiritual well-being in illness (Fig. 47-2) identifies three empirical referents of spiritual well-being: personal faith, spiritual contentment, and religious practice. **Spiritual healing** is the movement toward integration, from brokenness to wholeness.

Box 47-2 Steps for Being a Healing Presence

Inasmuch as it's more art than science, you'll have your own ways of bringing healing presence into your life and the lives of others. Following is a rough order for how you might proceed.

1. Open Yourself

Begin not with the other person but with you. Become present to yourself in a way that is honest, insightful, and accepting. Open to your uniqueness, humanness, prejudices, brokenness, and wholeness. Do this by owning your life story, continually fathoming who you are in a holistic manner, and developing or using a support system to which you hold yourself accountable.

2. Intend to Be a Healing Presence

Be aware that the healing presence doesn't just occur out of the blue, you intentionally decide to be such a presence with another. Intend to promote healing in its many forms, while being understanding of yourself as you emerge in the day-to-day intricacies of this practice.

3. Prepare a Space for Healing Presence to Take Place

Clear a space to interact with the other or others, assuring as much privacy as possible and creating an atmosphere of calm. Prepare a space also within by placing yourself out of the way and clearing away your personal expectations for what the other should be or do.

4. Honor the One in Your Care

Approach those you accompany as people with dignity and worth. Show your regard for them by honoring their individuality, equality, humanness, separateness, and sacredness. Respect their natural and unique healing capacity.

5. Offer What You Have to Give

Freely and simply make available what you have to offer, realizing it is up to the other or others to accept or not. Offer presence, loving acceptance, empathy, dependability, an unselfish focus on them, your firm belief in them, your willingness to follow their lead, and, as much as anything, hope.

6. Receive the Gifts That Come

Accept with a grateful heart what is yours to receive. This may include living your life more fully as a result of this practice. Other gifts may include uncovering your genuine self, enjoying wonderful relationships, finding personal satisfaction, realizing you have made a difference, receiving your own healing, and exploring some of life's most valuable lessons.

7. Live a Life of Wholeness and Balance

There is more to life than being a healing presence. So, live your days fully, caring for your own needs, setting appropriate boundaries, encouraging your own growth, and nurturing a loving attitude toward life, including the sacred dimension. Affirm and live out the truth of the transforming potential of healing presence. Be grateful for the possibilities.

Source: Reprinted with permission from Miller, J. E., & Cutshall, S. C. (2001). *The art of being a healing presence: A guide for those in caring relationships.* Willowgreen Publishing.

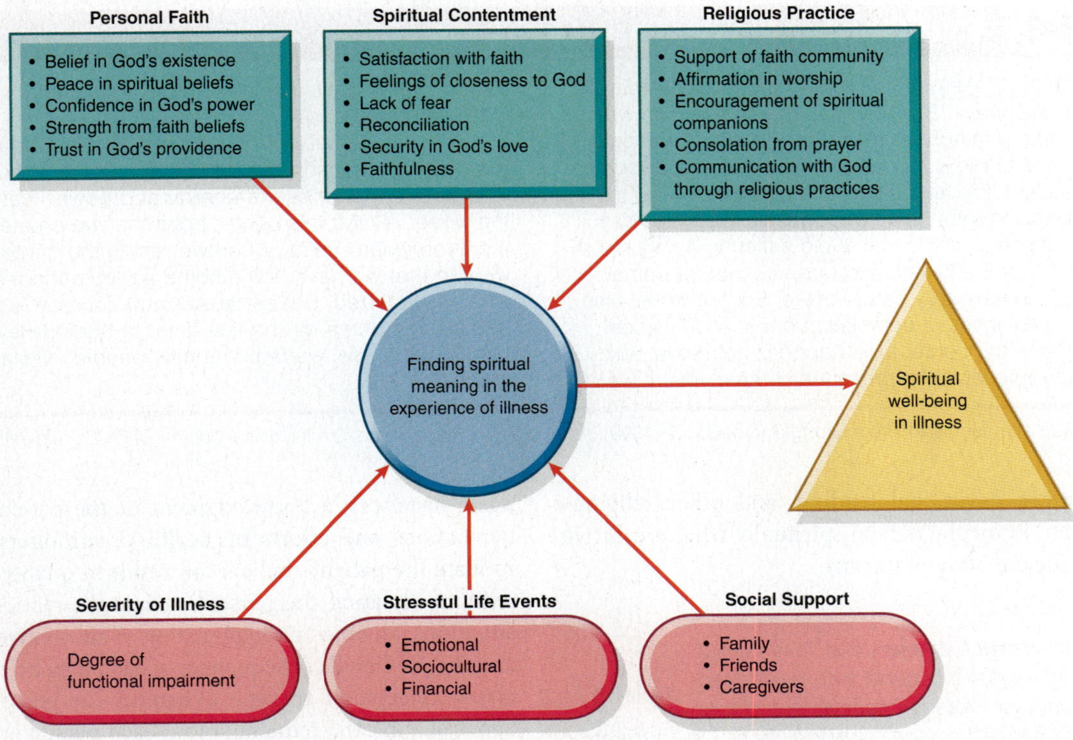

FIGURE 47-2. A conceptual model of spiritual well-being in illness. (*Source:* Redrawn from O'Brien, M. E. [2013]. *Spirituality in nursing: Standing on holy ground* [p. 81]. Jones and Bartlett.)

Spirituality and Everyday Living

Spiritual beliefs and practices are associated with all aspects of a person's life, including health and illness. The major wisdom traditions address the invisible Spirit—a creative, mysterious guiding power—by creating principles and practices that:

- Cultivate love for ourselves, our neighbors, of a higher being, and of nature
- Cultivate wisdom that helps us find meaning in life; be in relationships with others; be true to ourselves; live in uncertainty and mystery; deal with suffering, sickness, and death; and honor life's transitions (birth, marriage, death)
- Cultivate awareness of the sacred dimension of life through practices such as worship, prayer, meditation, and singing (Fig. 47-3)

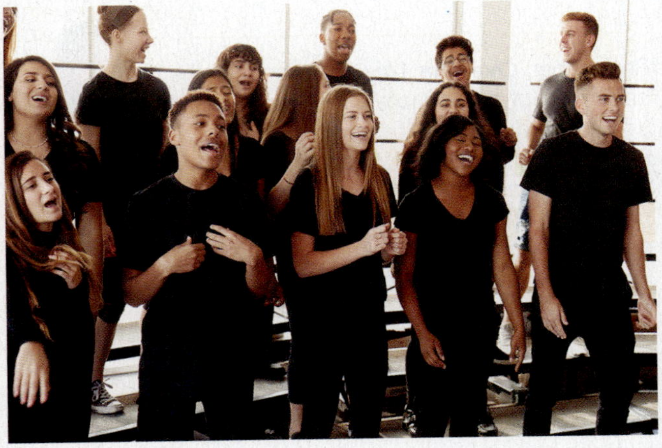

FIGURE 47-3. Members of a Gospel choir put their whole selves into a song. (Courtesy of Shutterstock.)

- Respect our connectedness as fellow human beings while acknowledging our differences
- Help us be generous in service to others

Religious influences may be life affirming or life denying. Life-affirming influences enhance life, give meaning and purpose to existence, strengthen a person's feelings of self-worth, encourage self-actualization, and are health giving and life sustaining. Life-denying influences restrict or enclose life patterns, limit experiences and associations, place burdens of guilt on people, encourage feelings of unworthiness, and are generally health denying and life inhibiting.

Spirituality, Health, and Illness

Spiritual beliefs are of special importance to nurses because of the many ways they can influence a patient's level of health, sense of well-being, and self-care behaviors.

Guide to Daily Living Habits

Certain practices generally associated with health care may have religious significance for a patient. For example, many religions have dietary requirements and restrictions. Acceptable birth-control practices are determined by some religious faiths, as are some types of medical treatments (refer back to Table 47-1).

Source of Support

Many people seek support from their religious faith during times of stress. This support is often vital to the acceptance of an illness, especially if the illness brings with it a prolonged period of convalescence or may lead to a questionable

Box 47-3 The Center Point That Grounds Us...

I could scarcely make out the large sitting Buddha near the entrance of the house. But what caught my attention was the metal circle with spokes resembling a wheel, hanging over the Figure of the Buddha....I asked our host about the wheel. I was told it represented our eternal journey in this life and continuing into the next. Buddha's teachings say that life is suffering. We cannot avoid suffering as we move around the rim of the wheel, which represents perpetual change and the transitory nature of life. But the wheel also symbolizes wholeness or completion because the wheel revolves around the center axis that does not move. That center point represents the presence of the divine. If we remain aware of this center point, we are strengthened for whatever lies ahead.

...It is this center point that grounds us in the midst of the many changes in our lives. It is at the center point where we experience the energy and power that turns the wheel. It is at this center point that we connect with the Everywhere Spirit. When we rest in the center point, we find that we have come home again to the place from which we started. But because of the journey, it is as if we had arrived home for the first time. In our journey around the circles of life, we become new people over and over again.

Source: Reprinted with permission from Gregg-Schroeder, S. (1999). A transforming experience: Circles of life. *Journal of Fellowship in Prayer*, 23–25.

outcome. Prayer, devotional reading, and other religious practices often do for the person spiritually what protective exercises do for the body physically.

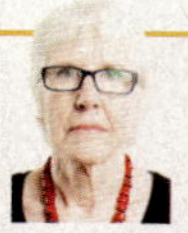

Think back to **Margot Zeuner**, the 75-year-old woman caring for her husband with advanced Alzheimer's disease. Assessment revealed that Mrs. Zeuner derived much support from her church group. The nurse, acknowledging the importance of this aspect, could work with Mrs. Zeuner to arrange for assistance at home so that she can attend church activities and continue to receive the support she needs. A referral to the church might also result in church members seeking out the Zeuners and offering assistance.

Box 47-3 describes how one religion, Buddhism, sees the divine grounding for all human experience, including suffering.

Source of Strength and Healing

The value of religious faith cannot be enumerated or evaluated easily. However, the effects attributable to faith are constantly in evidence to health care workers. People have been known to endure extreme physical distress because of strong faith. Patients' families have taken on almost unbelievable rehabilitative tasks because they had faith in the eventual positive results of their effort. In the Through the Eyes of a Patient box, a woman facing life-threatening events describes what she means by healing. She paints a robust vision of living fully, not in spite of illness, but rather because of it.

Source of Conflict

Sometimes religious beliefs conflict with prevalent health care practices (see Table 47-1 on pages 1911–1912). For example, the doctrine of the Jehovah's Witnesses prohibits blood transfusions. Some Navajos use a lengthy religious ceremony to cure certain diseases, such as tuberculosis. For some people, illness is viewed as punishment for sin and is therefore inevitable.

Such beliefs may require the health care worker to modify a treatment plan to accommodate the person's religion. In some instances, acknowledgment of the patient's religious convictions and efforts by health practitioners to accommodate the patient's beliefs can result in quality health care without violating the person's religious practices. In other situations, an objective explanation of alternative treatments and the predicted consequences of each may help the patient choose acceptable therapy. Whatever the person's decision about health care, remember that each person is unique and has a right to pursue their own convictions, even though they may differ from those of the health care provider.

Health care professionals can reduce conflict by attempting to understand how a particular religious culture influences people's thinking about basic questions of biology and ethics. Some of the major questions that religious beliefs, attitudes, and values can affect include:

- What is the meaning of suffering?
- How should we regard the physical body and its functions?
- What are the meaning and role of biologic sex differences, sexuality, and reproduction?
- How are we to understand and respond to birth, aging, and death?
- What constitutes the self, and how is selfhood assessed?
- How are sin and moral culpability understood? What makes something sinful, and how is sin relieved or absolved?
- What are the tradition's specific bioethical teachings?

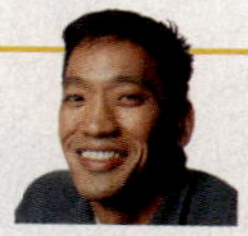

Remember **Choi Min Lai**, described at the beginning of this chapter. The nurse could use these questions to assess the family's beliefs in greater depth, providing significant data for the health care team to incorporate when discussing the possibility of surgery to repair Kou's deformities. Doing so could be helpful in minimizing the conflict between the family and health care team.

FACTORS AFFECTING SPIRITUALITY

Among the many factors that can influence a person's spirituality, the most important are developmental considerations, family, ethnic background, formal religion, and life events.

Through the Eyes of a Patient

Seven years ago, I was faced with three life-threatening events in a period of 3 years. Those life-threatening experiences taught me that it is possible to "heal" and to live fully even when we are in the abyss of suffering. I believe everyone would benefit if we redefined "healing." Here are elements I now include in my definition.

Healing is:

- Becoming whole, a life-long journey of becoming fully human, involving the totality of our being: body, mind, emotion, spirit, social, and political context, as well as our relationships with others and with the Divine. Healing does not necessarily mean being happy or getting what we think we want out of life; it means growth, often with pain.
- Becoming our authentic self, releasing old unreal self-images, discovering who we really are, not what we think we should be, knowing why we are here and what we really value, restoring our ability to heed our aspirations.
- Reconnecting lost aspects of ourselves, paying attention to buried feelings and places inside us that are distressed or sick, enabling us to express our self in fullness, both the light and shadow sides.
- Being open to change and new possibilities, responding to problems by changing the picture, being willing to let in more life, to open up to what may have been previously closed or destroyed for us and that which holds promise of giving us new life and fulfillment.
- Facing our fears and refusing to be injured or wounded, changing our belief systems, breaking unnecessary taboos, letting go of what is familiar, and stepping into the unknown.
- Accepting that problems, pain, and suffering are part of life and inseparable from us—not a peripheral relationship, not something isolated and avoidable—enabling us to enter into problems and use suffering, pain, and life-threatening events to enrich our lives.
- Being empowered by the Divine; discovering meaning in our defects, disorders, problems, and disease; experiencing new degrees of creativity and life forces that we might never have imagined before our difficulty; finding that our pains and fears are transformed into relief and confidence.
- Recognizing the value and preciousness of life, knowing that every moment is unique and significant, which usually leads to greater appreciation of the wonder of our minds, bodies, and spirits and of the Divine.
- Having faith and hope—important preconditions for mental and physical health; having a belief in the Divine, the meaning of human life, and the universe; helping us to claim our capacity to create and make something new.
- Finding inner peace, contentment, and tranquility amid the realities of daily life, including its problems, changes, and chaos; experiencing a sense of fullness that makes the burdens of pain or illness lighter.
- Being forgiving of ourselves and others and being forgiven; giving ourselves and others the freedom to let go of rivalry, strife, anger, hatred, fear, and limitations.
- Feeling connected to one another, a sense of interdependence; knowing we are not isolated or autonomous, giving up the illusions of boundaries in life; taking responsibility, acting justly, and accepting that we share our humanity.
- Being loving and loved; loving one's self and wanting to love and serve others, as well as being capable of receiving love; having an ability to trust, a feeling of aliveness, and a sense of greater participation in life.

Source: Reprinted with permission. Carol, J. (2002). What is healing? *Sacred Journey, 53*(4), 33–35.

Developmental Considerations

Because spirituality involves the nonmaterial realm of being, a child must have developed some capacity for abstraction in order to understand the spiritual self. However, this is not to say that spirituality is meaningless for children. For example, David Heller (1985) interviewed 40 children between 4 and 12 years old who were affiliated with one of four major religions (Judaism, Roman Catholicism, Protestantism, or Hinduism) and discovered that the children had definite perceptions of God. Central themes in all the children's descriptions included the following:

- Notion of a God who works through human intimacy and the interconnectedness of lives
- Belief that God is involved in self-change and growth and transformations that make the world fresh, alive, and meaningful
- Attributing to God tremendous and expansive power and then showing considerable anxiety in the face of this power
- Image of light

As the child matures, life experiences usually influence and mature the child's spiritual beliefs. With advancing years, the tendency to think about life after death prompts some people to reexamine and reaffirm their spiritual beliefs. Chapter 22 describes the stages of faith development.

Family

A child's parents play a key role in the development of the child's spirituality. What parents explicitly teach a child about spirituality and religion is generally less important than what the child learns about spirituality, life, and self from the parents' behavior.

Ethnic Background

Religious traditions differ among ethnic groups. There are clear distinctions between Eastern and Western spiritual traditions as well as among those of individual ethnic groups, such as Native Americans. A person's culture and formal religion significantly affect whether the person's approach to religion is doing something, being someone, or continually striving for harmony.

Formal Religion

Each of the major religious groups discussed earlier in this chapter shares several characteristics:

- Basis of authority or source of power
- Scripture or sacred word
- An ethical code that defines right and wrong
- A psychology and identity, so that its adherents fit into a group, and the world is defined by the religion
- Aspirations or expectations
- Ideas about what follows death

Life Events

Both positive and negative life experiences can influence spirituality, and they in turn are influenced by the meaning a person's spiritual beliefs attribute to them. For example, if two women who believe in a loving God both lose a child in a car accident, one may bitterly deny God's existence, whereas the other may spend more time in prayer, asking God to help her. Similarly, a chain of successful life experiences (marriage, promotion) may cause one person to assume success and experience no need for God, whereas for another it occasions deep gratitude and rejoicing.

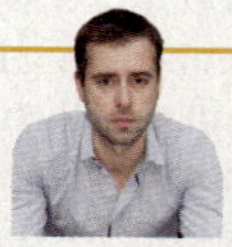

Recall **Kevin Gargan**, who recently experienced a heart attack. The experience of his own mortality and the thought that he might have died now have him questioning whether there is a God and where he stands in relationship to God.

RELIGION AND LAW, ETHICS, AND MEDICINE

Christian Scientists, Jehovah's Witnesses, and members of certain faith-healing groups are among those challenging the intricate web of rights and responsibilities that links people, society, church, and state. These religious bodies are asking for protection, under the umbrella of religious freedom, of the believer's right to exercise individual decisions in accordance with scriptural interpretations, even though those decisions may result in a person's own death or that of a family member, including a child. Most troubling are those cases in which treatable problems, such as bacterial meningitis, diabetes, or bowel obstruction, resulted in the death of minors whose parents choose religious means of healing over traditional medicine. (See Focused Critical Thinking Guide 47-1.) The American Academy of Pediatrics urges that all child abuse, neglect, and medical neglect statutes be applied without potential or actual exemption for religious beliefs.

Perhaps even more troubling for nurses are situations in which family members insist on painful care that is deemed medically futile (i.e., the likelihood of medical benefit is virtually nonexistent) because they believe that God is going to work a miracle. In these cases, simple nursing measures, such as turning or bathing patients, can become occasions of pain and torment to both the patient and nurse. Nurses are forced to administer care that they take to be cruel and abusive to patients capable of experiencing pleasure and pain. This nursing care can needlessly prolong a patient's painful dying. Unfortunately, there are no clear guidelines for drawing a line between promoting life and prolonging the dying process. Although nurses always have the moral right to withdraw from administering care that violates their personal moral code, this does not resolve the problem for the patient. More dialogue is needed on the interaction between religion and law, ethics, and medicine. Ideally, the religious freedom of patients and their families is respected, as is the moral autonomy of caregivers and the integrity of the healing professions. Nurses in these situations should seek the assistance of the ethics committee or ethics consultation service.

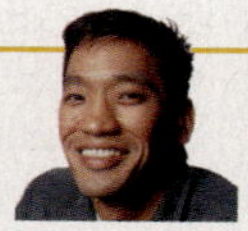

Consider the situation of **Choi Min Lai**, the father described at the beginning of this chapter. The nurse is required to respect the family's religious freedom and advocate for them while at the same time acting as a professional member of the health care team.

PARISH NURSING

Parish nurse programs are a relatively new movement in faith communities in many denominations. They seek to reclaim the church's role in the ministry of healing and focus again on the impact that spirituality, caring relationships, and a responsibly balanced life can have on health and wellness. Parish nurses (also called faith community nurses) and health ministry teams work to reintegrate the healing tradition into the life of faith communities by:

- Interpreting the relationship between faith and health
- Promoting personal responsibility for health and wellness
- Serving as health counselors and educators
- Staying aware of available resources and making appropriate referrals
- Acting as advocates for people who have health needs but only limited resources
- Recruiting and training volunteers
- Visiting church members
- Initiating caring relationships with older adults, the chronically ill, and the "worried well"

Parish nurses are not visiting nurses or home health care nurses who provide direct bedside care. The key roles of the parish nurse are health educator, personal health counselor, referral agent, trainer of volunteers, developer of support groups, integrator of faith and health, and health advocate. Nurses who wish to be parish nurses must be registered and compliant with both the state practice act and Faith Community Nursing: Scope and Standards of Practice (American Nurses Association, 2012). Check out the website of the Westberg Institute for Faith Community Nursing at http://www.parishnurses.org for more information on parish nursing.

47-1 Focused Critical Thinking Guide

SPIRITUALITY

A 16-year-old student approaches you, the school nurse, and confides that she is worried about her brother, who is sick and getting sicker. "My parents are Christian Scientists and have had Christian Science Practitioners in to pray for him, but he seems to be getting worse. I'm afraid he'll die if we don't get him to the hospital." Your first impulse is to visit the student's home to try to see her brother and parents. You immediately remember an article in the paper about the Supreme Court's decision to let stand a Minnesota Court of Appeals ruling upholding an award of $1.5 million to the father of a boy who died in 1989 after his mother, stepfather, and two Christian Scientist Practitioners tried to use prayer to heal his diabetes. Despite their efforts, the boy slipped into a coma and died. What is troubling you is the following comment by Stephen Carter: "By refusing to intervene in *McKown v. Lundman*, the Supreme Court has reinforced a societal message that has grown depressingly common: It is perfectly OK to believe in the power of prayer, so long as one does not believe in it so sincerely that one actually expects it to work—a peculiar fate indeed for our 'most inalienable' right" (Carter, S. L. [1996, January 31]. The power of prayer, denied. *The New York Times*, A17). You do believe in the power of prayer and are not sure how you should respond to the student's plea for help for her brother.

1. Identify goal of thinking

Clarify (1) what I believe about prayer's power to heal, and (2) what I believe about a parent's right to substitute prayer for modern medicine when a child is seriously ill. Decide how I should respond. What are my professional obligations?

2. Assess adequacy of knowledge

Pertinent circumstances: This is the first time I have encountered a family of Christian Scientists. As a school nurse, I am not responsible for my student's brother if he is not in my school and place of employment. That said, I have been asked to help and have the resources to do so.

Prerequisite knowledge: I have no knowledge of what Christian Scientists believe. Moreover, I do not know how the law in our state responds to situations like these. I do not know if any nursing or medical groups have guidelines for situations like these. I immediately get on the Internet to address these deficiencies and also contact my professional nursing organization to see what the law is and if any professional organizations have addressed this issue. I also have to find out how sick the student's brother is and the probable consequences of his not seeking traditional medical care.

Room for error: The student's brother's very life may depend on whether and how I choose to respond.

Time constraints: Until I learn the exact nature of the boy's medical problems, I cannot know how urgent the need to intervene is.

3. Address potential problems

In a situation like this, the most obvious impediments to critical thinking would be (1) the unexamined belief that religion trumps all other considerations ("by golly, this country is founded on respect for religious freedom") and (2) the belief that modern medicine is owed to everyone with a life-threatening illness, no matter what other considerations are present.

4. Consult helpful resources

I decide to visit the boy's home with the student and call first to seek the parents' permission. After talking with the parents and seeing the boy, I believe that the boy is in a life-threatening situation because the parents were told that their son has diabetes. I am struck by the love and devotion of both parents, and I learn via internet research that they are doing exactly what their religion prescribes. I later consult with a local Christian Scientist group that confirms this. I learn from my professional nursing organization that there is no consensus about how society should respond in situations like these. Many believe that what these parents are doing is neglect and that if the boy dies, they should be held criminally accountable for manslaughter. Others respect their right to practice their religion. Uncertain of how I should respond, I decide to call Child Protective Services and tell them that I am willing to help if they think my relationship with the daughter would be helpful. I explain to my student what I am doing and tell her to keep me informed and to come back for help if she is not getting the assistance she needs.

5. Critique judgment/decision

Child Protective Services did intervene immediately, and the boy was hospitalized and treated against the parents' wishes. While I was happy that the boy's condition was stabilized, I did feel uncomfortable about the disrespect shown to these obviously intelligent, devout, and loving parents. I decided to learn more about how different states are responding to these challenges and to see if nursing can get involved in some way.

NURSING PROCESS FOR SPIRITUAL HEALTH

Nurses who role model good health behaviors are more effective teachers. Many nurses approach professional practice as more than a "job" and use the language of "sacred calling" or "vocation" to describe their career choice. Refer to the display, Promoting Health 47-1; use the assessment checklist for yourself before using it with others.

Assessing

Nursing History

Because a person's spirituality and religious beliefs can influence every aspect of being, an assessment of the patient's spirituality—including beliefs and practices, the effect of these beliefs on everyday living, spiritual distress, and spiritual needs—should be included in each comprehensive nursing history. However, nurses often need guidance in assessing spirituality in their patients, and in providing spiritual care; the accompanying Research in Nursing box highlights two studies related to spiritual care. Many guides are available for eliciting a spiritual history, such as those from O'Brien (1982), Shelly and Fish (1988), and Puchalski and Romer (2000). One simple guide is Anandarajah and Hight's (2001) HOPE acronym:

- **H—**Sources of **H**ope, meaning, comfort, strength, peace, love, and connection
- **O—O**rganized religion
- **P—P**ersonal spirituality and practice
- **E—E**ffects on medical care and end-of-life issue

Sample questions are listed in the Focused Assessment Guide 47-1.

If the patient reveals a spiritual problem, use interview questions to determine the specific nature of the problem, its probable causes, its related signs and symptoms, when it began and how often it occurs, how it affects everyday living, its severity and whether it can be treated independently by nursing or needs to be referred, and how well the patient is coping.

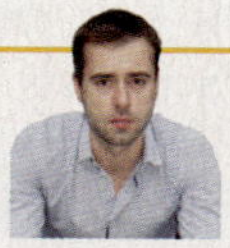

Think back to **Kevin Gargan**, the man who experienced the heart attack. The nurse could use the questions in the Focused Assessment Guide to determine Mr. Gargan's beliefs and thereby develop a care plan that addresses his current needs. In addition, this assessment would provide valuable information about how the patient is coping with the current situation.

Nursing Observation

Because many patients find it difficult to talk about their spiritual beliefs and problems, also observe the patient's behavior for signs of spiritual distress. A family member or close friend may share significant observations:

- "He's been awfully moody since his heart attack. I can't believe how hopeless he seems now."
- "I've never seen my father so depressed. He's never in his life been away from the synagogue at Passover. I don't know how to help him."

Significant behavioral observations include sudden changes in spiritual practices (rejection, neglect, fanatical devotion), mood changes (frequent crying, depression, apathy, anger), sudden interest in spiritual matters (reading religious books or watching religious programs on television, visits to clergy), and disturbed sleep. If you observe these

Promoting Health 47-1

SPIRITUALITY

Use the assessment checklist to determine how well you are meeting your spirituality needs. Then develop a prescription for self-care by choosing appropriate behaviors from the list of suggestions.

Assessment Checklist

☐ almost always ☐ sometimes ☐ almost never

☐ ☐ ☐ 1. I am comfortable with my spiritual beliefs and values.

☐ ☐ ☐ 2. My beliefs meet my needs for love and belonging, forgiveness, and meaning and purpose.

☐ ☐ ☐ 3. I respect the belief systems of others.

☐ ☐ ☐ 4. I derive sufficient strength from my religious beliefs to meet each day's challenges, especially when confronting pain, suffering, and death.

Self-Care Behaviors

1. Explore personal values and beliefs of self and others.
2. Set aside regular periods to nurture spiritual self.
3. Explore practices that are spiritually supportive.
4. Demonstrate in interaction with others peace, inner strength, warmth, joy, caring, creativity.
5. Respect the belief systems of others.
6. Practice loving relationships with self and others.
7. Seek spiritual assistance to help cope with stress, crisis, or loss.

Research in Nursing

BRIDGING THE GAP TO EVIDENCE-BASED PRACTICE

Critical Care Nurses' Perceived Need for Guidance in Addressing Spirituality in Critically Ill Patients

The term *spirituality* is defined in different ways by different people. No common or universally accepted definition for the term exists.

Related Research

Canfield, C., Taylor, D., Nagy, K., Strauser, C., VanKerkhove, K., Wills, S., Sawicki, P., & Sorrell, J. (2016). Critical care nurses' perceived need for guidance in addressing spirituality in critically ill patients. *American Journal of Critical Care, 25*(3), 206–211. https://doi.org/10.4037/ajcc2016276

The researchers interviewed 30 nurses who worked in a critical care unit at a large Midwestern teaching hospital. Their objectives were to examine individual critical care nurses' definitions of spirituality, their comfort in providing spiritual care to patients, and their perceived need for education in providing care. They found that nurses generally feel comfortable providing spiritual care to critically ill patients but need further education about multicultural considerations. Nurses identified opportunities to address spiritual needs throughout a patient's stay but noted that these needs are usually not addressed until the end of life.

Ernecoff, N. C., Curlin, F. A., Buddadhumaruk, P., & White, D. B. (2015). Health care professionals' responses to religious or spiritual statements by surrogate decision makers during goals-of-care discussions. *JAMA Internal Medicine, 175*(10), 1662–1669.

Researchers recorded conversations between health care professionals and patient surrogates to determine how frequently religion and spirituality were discussed, by whom, and with what responses. Of 249 analyzed conversations, discussions of religion or spirituality occurred in 40 (16.1%), and the surrogates raised the subject in 26 of those (65%). In only eight conferences did health care professionals ask questions in response to the raised religious issues to gain deeper understanding. More often they switched the conversation back to medical issues. The study authors concluded, "It may be that clinicians do not know how to navigate these conversations or that they were taught to avoid discussion of such topics in favor of prioritizing discussions of medical facts."

Relevance for Nursing Practice

Clearly, more guidance must be offered to nurses and other health care professionals about how to recognize and respond to spiritual needs. Evidence-based interventions coupled with clear standards of care that hold nurses accountable for meeting spiritual needs and promoting spiritual health are needed. This research is still in its infancy.

Focused Assessment Guide 47-1

SPIRITUALITY

Factors to Assess	Questions and Approaches
Spiritual beliefs	"Are there particular spiritual or religious beliefs that are important to you? Have these beliefs changed recently? Is your illness challenging these beliefs? Do your religious beliefs in any way dictate a course of action that puts you in conflict with what your health care providers are recommending?"
Spiritual practices	"Describe your usual spiritual practices and anything interfering with your ability to perform them. Can I help in any way to secure the aids necessary for these practices (prayer shawl, Bible, crystals, amulets, beads, icons)?"
Relation between spiritual beliefs and everyday living	"Describe ways your spiritual beliefs affect everyday living (daily schedule, diet, hygiene, sense of self and the world, relationships). Do you find this influence to be healthy (life affirming) or destructive (life denying)?"
Spiritual deficit or distress	"Are your spiritual beliefs currently causing you any distress?"
Spiritual needs	"In what ways can I and the other nurses help you to meet your spiritual needs?" "Would you like me to contact your spiritual advisor or the hospital's pastoral care minister?"
Need for meaning and purpose	"In what ways do your religious beliefs help or hinder you to understand your current situation and face it with peace and courage?"
Need for love and relatedness	"In what ways do your religious beliefs help or hinder you to meet your need to love and be loved?"
Need for forgiveness	"In what ways do your religious beliefs help or hinder you to feel at peace?"
Significant behavioral observations	Be alert to sudden changes in spiritual practices, mood changes, sudden interest in spiritual matters, and sleep disturbances—any of which may point to unresolved spiritual needs.

behaviors, you should follow up with appropriate interview questions.

"Often, problems with spiritual distress do not surface until well after a patient's diagnosis of serious illness." This would be applicable in a home as well as hospital setting. Effective questions include the following:

- "You've been lying there so quietly. What are you thinking about?"
- "After all you've been through, you must have done a good bit of soul searching. Experiences like these are enough to shake anyone's faith—how is yours holding up?"

Diagnosing Actual or Potential Health Problems and Needs

An assessment of a patient's spirituality and spiritual health may lead to the identification of one or more actual or potential health problems and needs related to spirituality. Following the formulation of the actual or potential health problems and needs, the nurse communicates findings to other nursing and health care professionals through the use of the written and spoken word. The written actual or potential health problem or need becomes a permanent part of the patient's health record.

The International Classification for Nursing Practice (ICNP) identifies several actual or potential health problems that may be identified by nurses:

- Impaired Spiritual Status
- Spiritual Distress
- Suffering
- Risk for Conflicting Religious Belief

Spiritual distress may be further specified as spiritual pain, alienation, anxiety, guilt, anger, loss, or despair (O'Brien, 1982). Common etiologies for spiritual distress include inability to reconcile a current life situation (e.g., illness, death of loved person, divorce) with spiritual beliefs ("God is all-powerful, all-loving, all-wise, and He cares about me") or separation from the religious community or supports. Common etiologic factors and potential signs and symptoms for some of these health problems are found in the accompanying box, Examples of Actual or Potential Health Problems and Needs: Spiritual Distress.

Outcome Identification and Planning

Enhancing Spiritual Health

Show you value spiritual health by being sensitive to the role that spiritual beliefs play in influencing both a person's thoughts about self and the world and their interactions with the world. Your interactions with any patient who values spirituality support the following patient outcomes.

The patient will:

- Identify spiritual beliefs that meet needs for meaning and purpose, love and relatedness, and forgiveness
- Derive from these beliefs strength, hope, and comfort when facing the challenge of illness, injury, or other life crisis
- Develop spiritual practices that nurture communion with inner self, with God or a higher power, and with the world
- Express satisfaction with the compatibility of spiritual beliefs and everyday living

Addressing Spiritual Distress

Goals and expected outcomes for patients in spiritual distress need to be individualized and may include a patient achieving some of the following:

- Exploring the origin of spiritual beliefs and practices
- Identifying factors in life that challenge spiritual beliefs
- Exploring alternatives given these challenges: denying, modifying, or reaffirming beliefs; developing new beliefs
- Identifying spiritual supports (e.g., spiritual reading, faith, community)
- Reporting or demonstrating a decrease in spiritual distress after successful intervention

Implementing Spiritual Care

A variety of interventions are available to help patients meet their spiritual needs. Like other nursing skills, these interventions need to be practiced before they can be used confidently, competently, and at the right moment. These interventions can be used in the home, hospital, or care center to help patients meet their spiritual needs. When implementing spiritual care, nurses work closely with other spiritual caregivers, including chaplains and pastoral care workers. Often the most important intervention is a well-timed referral to a professional spiritual caregiver.

Ethical and Professional Boundaries

Before exploring spiritual care strategies, remind yourself of the importance of discussing spiritual concerns in a respectful manner and as directed by patients. While the PEW landmark religion survey shows the importance of religion to many Americans, it is also true that religion means very different things to different people. A nurse's offer to pray for a patient may be received gratefully by one person and dismissed angrily by another who associates prayer with a "last resort" intervention when everything else has failed. The fact that some health care professionals confuse spiritual care with proselytizing (trying to convert others to their own religion) is another source of concern. Puchalski (2006) offers the following hints about professional boundaries:

- Keep the spiritual history patient centered.
- Recognize pastoral care professionals as experts in this field and consult them appropriately.
- Proselytizing is never acceptable in professional settings. Addressing spiritual issues should not be coercive.
- More in-depth spiritual counseling should be under the direction of chaplains and other spiritual leaders.
- Praying with patients should not be initiated by the nurse unless there is no pastoral care available and the patient requests it, or in situations in which the nurse and patient have a long-standing relationship or share a similar belief system. The nurse can stand in silence as the patient prays in her or his tradition. The nurse can always make a referral to pastoral care for chaplain-led prayer.

Examples of Actual or Potential Health Problems and Needs

SPIRITUAL DISTRESS

Actual or Potential Health Problems and Needs	Possible Etiologic Factors	Potential Signs and Symptoms
Spiritual Pain	Inability to accept death of son	A 46-year-old woman, agnostic, only son died 6 months ago (lung cancer) "I've often wondered throughout my life if there is a God—thought maybe if I had tried harder, I'd have recognized him. Now, I don't care if God exists or not because if he allows this, I don't want to know him." "My son was my whole life; there's nothing left for me to live for." Lost 10 lb in 6 months since son died; leaves home only when necessary to purchase food, go to bank, and engage in other routine activities.
Spiritual Alienation	Separated from "faith community"	A 72-year-old Orthodox Jewish man, recently admitted to Protestant long-term care facility following 3-week hospitalization for stroke "I guess Yahweh has written me off; first the stroke that killed half my body and then I'm abandoned here where I can't even observe the Sabbath." "I want to go home."
Spiritual Anxiety	Challenged belief and value system	A 37-year-old previously healthy executive recovering from massive myocardial infarction "My parents were strict Methodists, but when I left home for college, I stopped going to church…never gave it much thought…there was always something else to do. I started going again but it never meant much." "I haven't exactly done anything awful, but I've also not been a saint and I find myself wondering if there is a God, what does he think of me." "Funny, I guess I thought I'd live forever. I sure never thought about dying and what happens after that." Often observed lying quietly in bed awake; asked to see minister.
Spiritual Guilt	Failure to live according to religious rules	A 23-year-old, single, Baptist woman being treated for premenstrual syndrome "I was raised in a strict Baptist home but had to leave…I needed more room to be me. I like life here at the university but there's a restlessness in me I can't describe. I've dated several men, one or two I really liked, but I always do something to mess up the relationship. It would kill my mother if she knew I lived with Gary for 3 months." "What it really comes down to is my own sense of betraying myself, my family, and my religion. Who am I anyway?"
Spiritual Anger	Inability to accept illness	A 38-year-old gay man recently diagnosed with AIDS "My parents are fundamentalists…all I ever heard at home was how much Jesus loves me…all the while my mom was beating the daylights out of me.…Does He love me? Does He love me so much that He had my parents throw me out when I finally told them I was gay? Does He love me so much that I got AIDS and now no one comes near me?" Facial features are tight; body held rigidly; speech is sharp, appears angry with God, the world, himself.
Spiritual Loss	Terminal illness; anticipatory grieving; inability to find comfort in religion	A 40-year-old mother of three sons who was diagnosed with ovarian cancer 18 months ago; currently in advanced stage of disease "I've tried hard to do it all right…I read my Bible, prayed every day, went to church each Sunday, loved my husband and kids…why is this all happening to me? Why must I lose it all? Where is God now that I need him? Some mornings I wish I could shoot myself and end it all—instead another day drags on. Who can help me?" Cries frequently, no longer interested in everyday activities of family, no interest in praying, told family not to have pastor call anymore. "No one can help now."

(*continued*)

Examples of Actual or Potential Health Problems and Needs *(continued)*

SPIRITUAL DISTRESS

Actual or Potential Health Problems and Needs	Possible Etiologic Factors	Potential Signs and Symptoms
Spiritual Despair	Feeling that no one (not even God) cares	A 92-year-old frail widow who lives alone in a two-room apartment; crippled with arthritis; has two married sons she has not seen for years. Says to community nurse who visits every week, "No one should have to live like this. If it weren't for the neighbor who comes on Saturday with a few groceries and you, I'd be dead. I guess that would be for the best. It's been a long time since I felt like my living or dying would matter to anyone. Because I'm 92 now, I guess even God doesn't want me. Couldn't you do something to put me out of my misery?"

Source (for Actual or Potential Health Problems or Needs): O'Brien, M. E. (1982). The need for spiritual integrity. In H. Yura, & M. B. Walsh (Eds.). *Human needs and the nursing process* (pp. 81–115). Appleton-Century-Crofts.

Offering Supportive or Healing Presence

A nurse's gift of supportive presence must underlie all other types of intervention to meet the patient's spiritual needs. The aim of this intervention is to create a hospitable and sacred space ("holy ground") in which patients can share their vulnerabilities without fear. Supportive presence communicates value and respect (Fig. 47-4). Chapter 8 presents basic communication skills helpful in establishing this type of presence. Box 47-3 (on page 1916) outlines helpful steps for nurses who are intent on developing the art of healing presence. Never was presencing more important than during the COVID-19 pandemic. Patients with COVID-19 who were admitted to the hospital were often allowed no visitors and nurses helped facilitate communication with families using smartphones or social media. Too often, the only person present to a dying patient was a nurse, a nurse newly valuing their ability to be present in a respectful, affirming way.

The patient who senses that the nurse is sincerely concerned and committed to helping meet human needs is better able to participate in the care plan. Patients who experience respect and affirmation from other humans find it easier to hold spiritual beliefs that meet their needs for meaning and purpose, love and relatedness, and forgiveness.

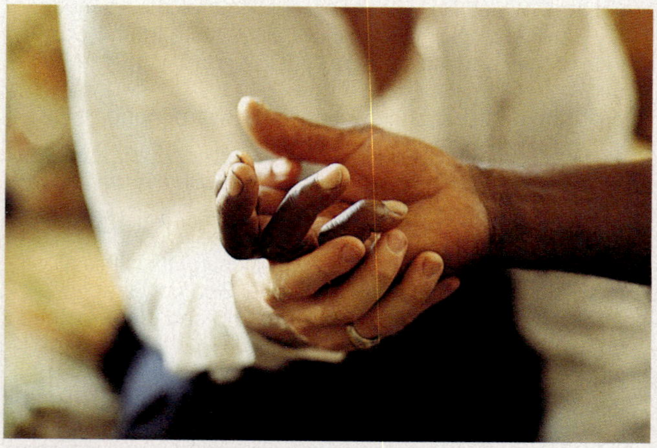

FIGURE 47-4. The nurse offers supportive presence by holding the patient's hand to show sincere concern, or simply by being present to communicate value and respect.

Facilitating the Practice of Religion

Ways that the nurse can help the patient continue normal spiritual practices in the unfamiliar environment of the hospital or care center are as follows:

- Familiarize the patient with the pastoral and religious services and materials available within the institution.
- Respect the patient's need for privacy or quiet during periods of prayer.
- Assist the patient to obtain devotional objects and protect them from loss or damage.
- Arrange for the patient wishing to receive the sacraments to do so.
- Attempt to meet the patient's religious dietary restrictions.
- Arrange for the patient's minister, priest, healer, or rabbi to visit if the patient so wishes.

If the patient has a conflict between spiritual beliefs and the proposed medical therapy, assist the patient in discussing this with the health care provider. For ill patients in the home who cannot attend services or meetings to which they are accustomed, help them find ways to meet their spiritual needs.

Nurturing Spirituality

Some patients who experience a need to get in touch with their spiritual self and to nurture their spiritual development look to the nurse for direction. Someone who lives life enmeshed in the action and noises of society may feel strange and uncomfortable when illness forces introspection. Be helpful by recommending methods a person might use to develop a relationship with their own inner world (such as prayer, reflection, dream analysis, nature walks, enjoying art) and ways to manifest spiritual energy in the outer world (such as loving relationships, compassion, forgiveness, joy, service).

Spiritual nurturing for the patient's family caregivers is also important. Recent research findings support the importance and value of caregivers' spirituality, yet this resource is often overlooked. Consider using interventions that enhance a caregiver's ability to take part in church activities to satisfy spiritual needs and to work with church groups to secure helpful services. Using clergy, prayer, forgiveness, and spiritual reading materials as resources for caregivers may also be helpful.

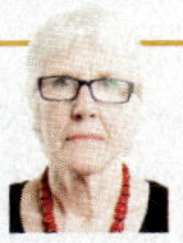

Knowledge of the supportive services provided by the church group of **Mrs. Zeuner**, the 75-year-old woman taking care of her husband with advanced Alzheimer's disease, would be important to include in the care plan for Mrs. Zeuner and her husband. Supportive services, such as respite care, parish nursing, and meals, in addition to the emotional support provided by the group, could be extremely helpful for Mrs. Zeuner in her role as caregiver.

Nurse Self-Care Alert

Finally, remember that, as nurses, we cannot give what we do not have. Unless our own spiritual needs are met, we will never be able to be truly present to another. Thus, the art of being a healing presence requires a lifestyle that supports our being a healing presence. Reflect on this proverb: *A happy heart is like good medicine. But a broken spirit drains your strength (dries your bones).—Proverbs 17:22*

The nurse can help patients to nurture their own spirituality by promoting meaning and purpose, love and relatedness, and forgiveness.

PROMOTING MEANING AND PURPOSE

In the book *Man's Search for Meaning,* psychiatrist Victor Frankl, who survived the horrors of the Nazi concentration camps, writes, "Once an individual's search for meaning is successful, it not only renders him happy, but also gives him the capability to cope with suffering" (1985, p. 163). To help patients searching for meaning, explore with them what has given their life meaning and purpose up to the present, sources of meaning for other people, and possible meanings for patients' current experience of illness, pain, suffering, or impending death. If a patient desires, arrange for referral to a spiritual advisor. Explore with patients some spiritual practices that may give them strength and hope (e.g., prayer or reading scripture or other spiritual books). You might also want to recommend that patients read spiritual biographies or Harold Kushner's book When Bad Things Happen to Good People (1983), Kathleen Brehony's book *After the Darkest Hour: How Suffering Begins the Journey to Wisdom* (2000), Oliver Sack's Gratitude (2015), or Dr. Paul Kalanithi's *When Breath Becomes Air.* Referring patients to appropriate support groups (e.g., self-help groups for people with stroke, cancer) also is helpful.

PROMOTING LOVE AND RELATEDNESS

First and foremost, always treat the patient with respect, empathy, and genuine caring. Encourage the patient to talk about relationships with others and to identify the origin of any negative beliefs about people. Box 47-4 may be a good starting point for reflection on loving kindness.

Box 47-4 Loving Kindness Meditation

May you be at peace.
May your heart remain open.
May you awaken to the light of your own true nature.
May you know the power of your higher self.
May peace of mind be your only goal and forgiveness your only task.
May you be healed of all pain and hurt.
May you be a source of healing for others.
May you know the inner beauty of the person you truly are.
May you be at peace.

Source: unknown.

Encourage conversation about how a patient experiences God or a higher being if that is part of the patient's spiritual beliefs. If appropriate, introduce or reinforce the belief that God is a loving and personal God who is concerned about the patient. Whenever possible, encourage and facilitate visits from the patient's family, friends, and spiritual advisor.

PROMOTING FORGIVENESS

Offer a supportive presence to the patient that demonstrates your acceptance of the patient. Explore with the patient the importance of learning to accept self and others, including both strengths and limitations. Explore negative feelings that make it difficult for the patient to seek forgiveness and to believe that he or she is forgiven.

Explore the patient's self-expectations and assist the patient to determine how realistic these are. Allow the patient to verbalize shame, guilt, and anger, and counsel about the importance of expressing negative emotions in healthy ways. Refer the patient to a spiritual advisor, if appropriate. Offer the patient examples of how not forgiving others can end up hurting only the person who cannot forgive.

The Spiritual Needs of Younger Generations

Younger generations, such as Millennials, Millennials are less religiously affiliated than ever before. See the 2012 Pew Research Center report, "Nones on the Rise," which reports that nearly 1 in 3 millennials do not belong to a faith community, and, of those, only 10% are looking for one. This is especially troubling when we consider that rates of isolation, loneliness, and depression continue to rise and that suicide is the third leading cause of death among youth (Centers for Disease Control and Prevention, 2020). All of this, of course, was exacerbated during the COVID-19 pandemic. The Thurston-ter Kuile study, "How We Gather," notes that millennials are flocking to a host of new organizations that deepen community in "ways that are powerful, surprising, and perhaps even religious." The six themes central to their study of 10 organizations meeting the needs of millennials are

- Community
- Personal transformation
- Social transformation
- Purpose finding
- Creativity
- Accountability

Thurson-ter Kuile ask a formative question:

> What does it mean to touch the world in 2015? This is a moment when Brene Brown's TED Talks on vulnerability and Taylor Swift's random acts of kindness go viral. It's a moment when virtual connectivity is more immediate than the "real" world, so that an American millennial feels more comfortable setting up a Kiva loan to a farmer in Kenya than bringing chicken soup to a neighbor. Is it possible to harness these new tools of global engagement to deepen our everyday experience of community as well?

If you belong to a traditional religion, have you reflected on the ways our changing generations and culture meet universal spiritual needs? You may also want to check out the Sacred Design Lab (Box 47-5). Learning that a patient does not claim membership in a traditional religion does not mean that they have no spiritual needs.

Box 47-5 Sacred Design Lab

Sacred Design Lab is a soul-centered research and development lab devoted to understanding and designing for 21st-century spiritual well-being. We translate ancient wisdom and practices to help our partners develop products, programs, and experiences that ground people's social and spiritual lives.

We envision a world in which every person is connected to their inherent goodness, known and loved in communities of care, and bountifully giving their gifts toward beauty, justice, and wholeness.

And yet, interlocking systems of oppression pull us apart. Unmet needs for meaning and connection play out in the way we live, love, work, and lead. The problem is soul-deep. So too must be our response.

Our Approach

Belonging Knowing and being known, loving and being loved.	We belong to each other. The experience of belonging changes the way we show up, stimulating loyalty, compassion, and joy, and diminishing anxiety, loneliness, and fear. But belonging is not a passive state. It's something we nurture, express, renew, savor, and pass down. So much in our culture works against us meeting our need for deep connection: to ourselves, other people, place, story, and time. The more we reclaim the power of knowing, loving, and caring for one another, the more our hearts open and our society heals.
Becoming Growing into the people we are called to be.	We each carry gifts the world needs. Yet too many of us face barriers to tending our inner gifts, sharing them in community, and bountifully receiving the gifts of others. To design for becoming is to disrupt productivity culture. It means listening for where we are each needed, addressing what stands in the way of our shared growth, and cultivating each other's courage to say "yes" to the soul's call. Soul-centered design fuels collective becoming.
Beyond Experiencing ourselves as part of something more.	When our soul is fed, we remember that we are bound up in something larger than ourselves. Stretching across generations, ineffable and yet as solid as the ground, this is the larger story of which we are a part. What would it take to create a rhythm of life in which we have space in our days to feel fully big and fully small? When we design for the soul, we create pathways to move closer to the beyond, to the endlessly renewable resource at the heart of all things.
Ancient Wisdom, Emergent World Applying ancient practices to emergent challenges.	How do we meet the needs of the soul and move toward flourishing? Luckily, humans have been responding to this question all over the world for thousands of years. Their wisdom is our collective inheritance. Now our work is to apply it, while honoring the origins and custodians of these traditions. We tap into ancient best practices to design for belonging, becoming, and beyond, and we work with partners to remix the wisdom of our ancestors to create soul-centered solutions.
Collective Liberation Never forgetting that justice is what love looks like in public.	We long for a world in which every person is cared for and free from oppression. Without love as our means, and commitment beyond our self-interest, we can't build the resolve to dismantle systems of domination. Collective liberation is more than something we think; it's something we do. So we commit ourselves to constant learning, reflection, action, and practice. Refusing to use shame as a strategy, we invite our partners to lead with justice-seeking love, that all might flourish.
Means and Ends Cohere How we are together shapes what we do together.	We envision a world of justice, beauty, healing, and wholeness. Though interlocking systems of oppressions impact us differently, they keep all of us from fully living in that world. To design products, programs, and experiences that meet the soul's needs, our means must themselves be soul-centered. We center relationships even as we focus on outcomes, reject grind culture, and embrace our justice commitments. We show up with joy, integrity, and care.
Witness the Meantime Holding space for all that emerges.	This work is not easy. Our culture devalues presence, patience, kindness, and care. Few opportunities exist for lament, atonement, and reconciliation, despite long histories of suffering. Deepening meaning and connection takes courage, perseverance, and trust. We accompany the leaders we work with through the inevitable challenges of soul-centered work, drawing on practices of witness and reflection to encourage and embolden them.

Source: Used with permission from Sacred Design Lab: https://sacred.design/how-we-work

Praying With Patients

Patients accustomed to regular periods of prayer but who feel too ill to pray as they would like or who enjoy praying with others may ask the nurse to pray with them or hope that the nurse will suggest this. Because there are many forms of prayer—quiet reflection, silent communion with God or a higher power, reading or recitation of formal prayers, silent or loud calling on God or a higher power or conversation with God or a higher power, lamentations, or reading a holy book or other religious materials—the nurse can take the lead from the patient by asking, "How would you like us to pray?" Consider the patient's religious background along with the type of prayers that have been meaningful in the past. Ask whether the patient has a particular prayer request.

A nurse unaccustomed to praying aloud or in public may find it helpful to have a Bible passage or formal prayer readily available. The prayer may also be a simple expression aloud of the patient's needs and hopes. A sample follows:

> Lord God, our Creator and Healer, I entrust Mrs. Smith and her family to your loving care. Bring peace to her mind and health and strength to her body. Be with her [as her treatment begins today, as she goes for surgery, and so on]. We remember all your blessings to us in the past and thank you. We are confident of your help now as we claim your promises.

Prayer should not block communication with the patient. Praying before a patient feels ready to pray may communicate to the patient a lack of interest in the patient's feelings. Because prayer often evokes deep feelings, the nurse should be prepared to spend time with the patient after sharing prayer to respond to these feelings.

Praying for Patients

With research suggesting links between prayer and physical, mental, and spiritual health, some have argued that health care professionals should pray for, as well as with, their patients. At the present time, no one is claiming that health care professionals are negligent if they fail to pray for patients. Prayer may, however, be an effective intervention strategy. At the very least, nurses ought to be mediators of the spiritual resources patients and their families need.

Counseling Patients Spiritually

The patient who feels that the nurse is sensitive to spiritual needs and comfortable with their own spirituality may choose to share spiritual concerns with the nurse rather than with a religious counselor. A nurse who feels competent to counsel the patient may assist the patient to accomplish the following:

- Articulate spiritual beliefs.
- Explore the origin of the patient's spiritual beliefs and practices.
- Identify life factors that challenge the patient's spiritual beliefs (cause spiritual distress).
- Explore alternatives given these challenges (e.g., modify lifestyle; deny, modify, or reaffirm beliefs; develop new beliefs).
- Develop spiritual beliefs that meet needs for meaning and purpose, care and relatedness, forgiveness.

To be an effective spiritual counselor, the nurse must be open to different spiritual beliefs and forms of spiritual expression and should be supportive of the patient's efforts to nurture spiritual growth.

Contacting a Spiritual Counselor

Not every nurse feels comfortable in the role of spiritual counselor. If you do not, suggest that the patient talk to a pastoral caregiver or spiritual counselor. When a patient expresses a desire to speak to a spiritual counselor, help make the appropriate referral or offer to contact the patient's own spiritual advisor. Other options are to contact the health care facility's pastoral ministry department or use a referral list of clergy in the local community. If no representative of the patient's own religion can visit in the hospital at a particular time, suggest a visit from a member of the clergy from another faith. The patient, depending on the situation and the immediacy of the need, may welcome such a suggestion.

In a health care setting, you can assist the spiritual counselor by making the counselor feel welcome, directing the counselor to the patient, and ensuring that the patient is ready to receive the counselor. Preparations of the patient's room for the visit may vary, but the following are generally recommended practices:

- The room should be orderly and free of unnecessary equipment and items.
- There should be a seat for the religious counselor at the bedside or near the patient so that both can be comfortable. Ideally, the room will allow a private conversation.
- The bedside table should be free of items and covered with a clean, white cover if a sacrament is to be administered.
- The bed curtains should be drawn for privacy if the patient can't be moved to a more private setting.

Some patients and spiritual advisors may value the nurse's participation in prayers, rituals, or the administration of sacraments. By having good working relations with chaplains and pastoral caregivers, you can quickly direct them to patients most likely to benefit from their visits.

Resolving Conflicts Between Spiritual Beliefs and Treatments

Both the patient and members of the patient's family may experience conflict between a particular spiritual belief or religious law and a proposed medical treatment or health option. The patient may want assistance when conferring with the spiritual advisor about a particular procedure. The nurse's role is to help the patient obtain the information needed to make an informed decision and to support the patient's decision making. Because what the nurse says and the way it is said may powerfully influence the patient's decision, it is important to maintain objectivity. Conflicts that resist resolution may be referred to an ethics committee or consult team (see Chapter 6).

Nursing, Religion, and Conscientious Objection

In recent years, some pharmacists attracted media attention by refusing to fill prescriptions for contraceptives. These pharmacists supported their refusals by claiming that fulfilling such a prescription would violate their religious beliefs and convictions. In this situation, the woman's right to access medications is pitted against the pharmacist's right to practice with personal integrity. Nurses can also find themselves in situations in which their professional or institutional responsibilities involve participation in activities, such as abortion, assisted suicide, and counseling about birth control, that may violate their personal integrity. Nurses therefore must ensure that they can fulfill the responsibilities of their job or that they are free to exercise the right of conscientious objection. As legislation addressing these conflicts is in a state of flux, you should be familiar with federal and state guidelines. For example, in September of 2011, the University of Medicine and Dentistry of New Jersey announced that all nurses employed in its hospital would have to help with abortion patients before and after the procedure, "reversing a long-standing policy exempting employees who refuse based on religious or moral objections." After a group of objecting nurses filed a federal lawsuit, the hospital backed down, agreeing that nurses with conscientious objections do not have to assist with pre- or postoperative care for abortions except when the mother's life is threatened and no other nonobjecting staff are available to assist (Galston & Rogers, 2012, p. 1).

Evaluating

The nurse working with a patient and family to achieve specified goals or outcomes to meet spiritual needs evaluates the care plan in each patient interaction. Necessary to the evaluation are sensitivity to what the patient is saying and not saying, and observation of the patient when alone as well as when interacting with the family and nurses.

In general, the nurse evaluates the patient's ability to accomplish the following:

- Identify some spiritual belief that gives meaning and purpose to everyday life
- Move toward a healthy acceptance of the current situation: illness, pain, suffering, impending death
- Develop mutually caring relationships
- Reconcile any interpersonal differences causing the patient anguish
- Verbalize satisfaction with their relationship with God or a higher being (if important to the patient)
- Express peaceful acceptance of limitations and failings
- Express the ability to forgive others and to live in the present
- Demonstrate an "interior state of peace and joy; freedom from abnormal anxiety, guilt, or a feeling of sinfulness; and a sense of security and direction in the pursuit of one's life goals and activities" (O'Brien, 1982, p. 98)

The nurse helps the patient to determine whether their spiritual beliefs are generally life affirming or life denying, and whether there is harmony between these beliefs and the patient's everyday life experiences. See Nursing Care Plan 47-1 for Mr. Gargan on pages 1929–1930.

REFLECTIVE PRACTICE LEADING TO PERSONAL LEARNING

Remember that the object of reflective practice is to look at an experience, understand it, and learn from it. As you begin to develop your expertise in identifying and responding to spiritual needs, reflect on your experiences—successes and failures—in order to improve your practice. Universal spiritual needs, shared by all humans, are to find meaning and purpose, love and relatedness, and forgiveness.

- Have you encountered patients or their family caregivers whose spiritual needs are unmet?
- If you identified such needs, did you feel confidant and comfortable responding to these needs?
- Have your care plans ever identified and addressed spiritual needs?
- Are you familiar with the spiritual health resources, including professional spiritual caregivers, available in your practice settings?
- Have you tried to learn more about these members of the interprofessional team and how you can develop collaborative relationships that will best serve your patients?
- Have you ever consulted with a professional spiritual caregiver?

Perhaps the most important questions to reflect on are: Are your patients and their families/caregivers better for having had *you* share in the critical responsibility of partnering with them to respond to their spiritual needs? Are your patients now receiving thoughtful, person-centered, prioritized, holistic, evidence-based treatment and care because of your efforts?

Nursing Care Plan for *Mr. Gargan* 47-1

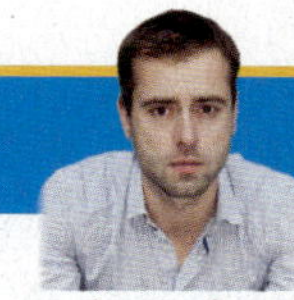

Mr. Gargan is a 38-year-old divorced man on a step-down unit after treatment for a myocardial infarction. He owns a small car dealership. His religion is listed as Protestant. Frequently unable to sleep at night, Mr. Gargan often talks with the night nurse, and once asked, "Did you ever give much thought to whether or not there is a God?" Sensing much concern behind this question, the nurse asks specific questions to determine whether the patient has spiritual needs that are not being met.

12/26/25, 0200

Patient again unable to sleep and initiated discussion about God. States that he was raised in a Lutheran home where everyone went to church on Sunday and tried to live according to God's commandments. Upon leaving home, he stopped going to church (was never a value for his wife) and simply has not given much thought to religion—too busy running his business. Until now, has not experienced any need for God. "But when I think how close I was to dying and that I've no idea what to expect after death—I'm actually scared. Do others feel this way?" Wants to explore religious beliefs—feels lack in his life. Said he would like to talk with hospital minister—will arrange for tomorrow.

E. Nolan, RN

ACTUAL OR POTENTIAL HEALTH PROBLEM Spiritual Distress: Anxiety related to concerns about relationship with God as manifested by self-report

EXPECTED OUTCOME Before discharge, the patient will:

- Identify his religious beliefs

NURSING INTERVENTIONS	RATIONALE	EVALUATIVE STATEMENT
Assist the patient to (1) identify the spiritual beliefs he had as a child and the origin of these beliefs, (2) evaluate these beliefs in terms of his life experiences, and (3) reaffirm, modify, or reject these beliefs or develop new spiritual beliefs.	Life experiences may challenge religious beliefs that were uncritically held as a child.	12/30/25 Outcome partially met. Patient states he has a much clearer concept of God and no longer fears that God will reject him for ignoring him for so long … but believes he also has a lot to learn. *E. Nolan, RN*
Assist the patient to assess whether his newly articulated spiritual beliefs are life affirming or life denying and the degree to which they meet his needs for meaning and purpose, love and relatedness, and forgiveness.	Because spiritual beliefs can exert positive (life-affirming) and negative (life-denying) influences on a person's life, people should have some criteria to use when evaluating their beliefs.	
Refer the patient to the hospital minister for assistance with the problem.	Patient may value speaking with a minister.	

EXPECTED OUTCOME Before discharge, the patient will:

- Reconcile his life up until the present with God

NURSING INTERVENTIONS	RATIONALE	EVALUATIVE STATEMENT
Reassure the patient that many people get involved in day-to-day living to the extent that they forget about God, and that in some religions, people believe that God uses illness and other stressors to invite people to rethink their spiritual beliefs. In these traditions, God is often pictured with open arms waiting to welcome a child home.	Images of a stern and unyielding God ready to strike down transgressors may contribute to a patient's spiritual distress. The need for forgiveness is a universal spiritual need.	12/30/25 Outcome met. "This minister has really helped. I wish I had talked to him a long time ago. I've carried so much guilt about my divorce and some other things—thought God would never forgive me. I feel so much more at peace now." *E. Nolan, RN*

(continued on page 1930)

Nursing Care Plan for *Mr. Gargan* 47-1 *(continued)*

NURSING INTERVENTIONS	RATIONALE	EVALUATIVE STATEMENT
Refer the patient to a spiritual advisor for help in experiencing forgiveness if he mentions guilt feelings.	Guilt often inhibits people from seeking and experiencing the forgiveness they desire.	
Communicate to the patient the importance of people accepting themselves—with all their strengths and weaknesses.	Many people have unrealistic self-expectations.	

EXPECTED OUTCOME

Before discharge, the patient will:

- Verbalize that his spiritual beliefs have become a source of strength and peace rather than anxiety

NURSING INTERVENTIONS	RATIONALE	EVALUATIVE STATEMENT
Encourage the patient to compare the role of spiritual beliefs in his life before, during, and after hospitalization.	This highlights the positive and negative roles spiritual beliefs can play. It may motivate the patient to continue searching if he values his present experience.	12/30/25 Outcome met. "It's good to be able to feel more peaceful about whatever the future brings. I'm anxious to get out of here because there's a lot I want to do with God's help." *E. Nolan, RN*

EXPECTED OUTCOME

Before discharge, the patient will:

- Increase night sleep to at least 6 undisturbed hours

NURSING INTERVENTIONS	RATIONALE	EVALUATIVE STATEMENT
Nurse on the night shift checks on the patient at the beginning of the shift to make sure he is comfortable and ready for sleep.	Nursing supervision of the patient at bedtime rules out other factors that may interfere with sleep.	12/30/25 Outcome met. Patient slept last night from midnight to 0600. Will continue to monitor. *E. Nolan, RN*
Use power of suggestion to enhance sleep: *"I'm sure when I check back you'll be sound asleep."*	Suggestion has been shown to enhance the therapeutic effect of other interventions.	
If sleep remains disturbed, try relaxation exercises or guided imagery (see Chapter 35).	As spiritual anxiety decreases, sleep should improve. If sleep does not improve, other contributing factors and interventions will need to be explored.	

SAMPLE DOCUMENTATION

12/27/25, 1500, nursing

B. Hanks, Protestant minister, here to see patient at 1300. Afterward, patient said he felt "a whole lot better." Reported minister had assured him that many people in the hospital with a serious illness go through exactly what he is experiencing now—this thought seemed to decrease much of his anxiety. Minister had reinforced nurse's suggestion that he explore his religious beliefs and he has already jotted down some thoughts. "I knew you fixed bodies in hospitals but didn't know you fix souls, too." Patient looking forward to minister's visit tomorrow.

E. Nolan, RN

DEVELOPING CLINICAL REASONING AND CLINICAL JUDGMENT

1. Assess your spiritual well-being. To what extent are you able to meet your needs for love and belonging, meaning and purpose, and forgiveness? If confronted with a life-threatening or chronic illness, would you be able to draw on religion or spirituality as a source of strength? Do you believe you need any special skills to develop to better meet the spiritual needs of your patients? Compare your responses to those of your classmates and explore reasons for differences.
2. Poll your classmates and see if they agree strongly, agree, disagree, or disagree strongly with the following statements. Discuss reasons for the differences in your answers and how this is likely to affect your professional practice.
   - Prayer has the power to heal physical, mental, and spiritual illness.
   - Nurses who do not pray for their patients are deficient professional caregivers.
   - Nurses who do not offer to pray with their patients are deficient professional caregivers.
3. How would you respond to a patient who tells you that he isn't very religious but is now wondering if there is a God, and if so, wonders where he stands in relation to God now that his life is in jeopardy? Think about how your personal experience of religion or spirituality colors your response, and determine whether your personal experience of religion or spirituality has prepared you well to respond to these queries.
4. You are a male nurse. The husband of your female patient requests that you get a female nurse to provide her care because their Muslim religion demands this. You are short-staffed and not sure you can accommodate this request. Do you make honoring his request a priority? Why or why not?
5. When a nurse is caring for a scared, possibly mechanically ventilated, and dying patient with COVID-19 who is isolated from friends, family, personal clergy, and even hospital chaplains, should they ever initiate an offer of prayer? If so, under what circumstances might a nurse ethically do so? And practically, how could a nurse do this in a therapeutic manner? (Taylor, E. J., 2020).
6. Your patient with advanced stage cancer is in danger of bleeding out and may require a life-saving blood transfusion. She is a practicing Jehovah's Witness. Do you inform the team that she cannot receive blood transfusions, even if these would be life-saving?
7. Your 26-year-old patient on an inpatient mental health unit is 13 weeks' pregnant and undecided about continuing the pregnancy. You are working in a Catholic hospital and know that abortion is not an option on site. Do you explore more with the patient how committed she is to continuing the pregnancy, ready to offer abortion options if she chooses to terminate?

PRACTICING FOR NCLEX

1. A hospice nurse is caring for a patient who is dying of pancreatic cancer. The patient tells the nurse, "I feel no connection to God" and "I'm worried that I've found no real meaning in life." What is the nurse's best response to this patient?
   a. Give the patient a hug and tell them that their life still has meaning.
   b. Arrange for a spiritual advisor to visit the patient.
   c. Ask if the patient would like to talk about their feelings.
   d. Call in a close friend or relative to talk to the patient.

2. A nurse who was raised as a strict Roman Catholic but is no longer practicing stated they could not assist patients with spiritual distress because they recognize only a "field of power" in each person. The nurse says to her colleague, "My parents and I hardly talk because I've deserted my faith. Sometimes I feel really isolated from them and God—if there is a God." These statements reveal which unmet spiritual need?
   a. Meaning and purpose
   b. Forgiveness
   c. Love and relatedness
   d. Strength for everyday living

3. A nurse in a long-term care facility is performing spirituality assessments of residents on their unit. What is the best question the nurse could use to assess for spiritual needs?
   a. "Can you describe your usual spiritual practices and how you maintain them daily?"
   b. "Are your spiritual beliefs causing you any concern?"
   c. "How can I and the other nurses help you maintain your spiritual practices?"
   d. "How do your religious beliefs help you to feel at peace?"

4. A patient who stated their religion as Jewish at the intake interview was served a kosher meal ordered from a restaurant on a paper plate because the hospital had no provision for kosher food or dishes. The patient became angry and accused the nurse of insulting him, emphatically stating, "I want to eat what everyone else does—and give me decent dishes." After analyzing the data, the nurse returns to the patient and makes which of these statements?
   a. "I'm terribly sorry, I should have ordered kosher food and dishes as well."
   b. "Did someone on the staff behave condescendingly or critically?"
   c. "It seems difficult to please you today."
   d. "We did not ask about your dietary preferences; tell me what you usually eat."

5. A surgeon tells a patient who is a Jehovah's Witness that they need emergency surgery to repair an aortic aneurysm, which will require blood transfusions. The patient states, "If I receive blood, I will not go to paradise. It is against my religion." What nursing response to the patient is appropriate?
   a. "I understand you will not receive blood products, even if it means you will die."
   b. "Please listen to the surgeon; I've seen many aneurysms successfully repaired"
   c. "Have you discussed your decision to refuse surgery with your family?"
   d. "What can I say to help you through this difficult decision?"

6. The Roman Catholic family of an infant born with hydrocephalus requests a baptism for their infant. The nurse advocates for the family's wishes to be honored for which reason?
   a. Baptism frequently helps postpone or prevent death or suffering.
   b. It is legally required that the nurse provide for this care when requested.
   c. It is a nursing function to assure the salvation of the infant.
   d. Not facilitating the baptism may increase the family's sorrow and suffering.

7. A nurse is caring for patients in a long-term care facility. Which nursing actions are appropriate based on the religious beliefs of these patients? Select all that apply.
   a. Asking a Buddhist if they have any diet restrictions related to the observance of holy days
   b. Asking a Christian Scientist who is in traction if they would like to try nonpharmacologic pain measures
   c. Administering medications to a Muslim patient and avoiding touching the patient's lips
   d. Asking a Roman Catholic patient if they would like to attend Mass in the common room on Sunday
   e. Avoiding scheduling treatment and procedures on Saturday for a Hindu patient
   f. Consulting with the medicine man of a Native American patient and incorporating their suggestions into the care plan

8. A nurse who is caring for patients on a pediatric unit is assessing children's spiritual needs. Which is the most important source of learning for a child's own spirituality?
   a. Child's church or religious organization
   b. What their parents say about God and religion
   c. Their parents' behavior in relationship to the family, others, and to God
   d. Family's spiritual advisor

9. A nursing student is caring for a patient admitted with chest pain related to aortic valve stenosis. The student notes the patient, who had been calm and cooperative the day before, has become contemplative and withdrawn, stating, "I've never thought much about dying, but my chances of making it through tomorrow's surgery are 50-50." How does the student best respond when the clinical professor asks the student why this behavior likely surfaced later in the patient's admission?
   a. Patients usually want to maintain privacy about their spiritual needs.
   b. People are better able to focus on spiritual needs after their spiritual advisor visits.
   c. Family members and close friends often initiate spiritual concerns.
   d. Illness increases spiritual concerns, which may initially be difficult to verbalize.

10. A nurse who is comfortable with spirituality is caring for a patient who needs spiritual counseling. What action will the nurse take first?
    a. Calling the patient's own spiritual advisor
    b. Asking if the patient has a spiritual advisor they wish to consult
    c. Counseling the patient and, if unsuccessful, making a referral to a spiritual advisor
    d. Explaining the best health options for the patient to the spiritual advisor

11. A patient states they feel very isolated from their family and church, and even from God, "in this huge medical center so far from home." When preparing expected outcomes for this patient, which most appropriately measures relief of the patient's spiritual distress?
    a. The patient will express satisfaction with the compatibility of their spiritual beliefs and everyday living.
    b. The patient will identify spiritual beliefs that meet their need for meaning and purpose.
    c. The patient will express peaceful acceptance of limitations and failings.
    d. The patient will identify spiritual supports available to them in this medical center.

12. A patient who lost their home, spouse, and children in a fire is depressed and states that they have no reason to live. The patient states, "My family was my life." The nurse documents a health problem of Spiritual Distress based on the patient's inability to find meaning and purpose in their current situation. What is the priority nursing action for this patient?
    a. Asking the patient which spiritual advisor they would like you to call
    b. Recommending that the patient engage in spiritual or religious readings
    c. Determining what has given the patient meaning and purpose in the past
    d. Reminding the patient that God is a loving and personal God

13. After terminating a pregnancy, a patient tells the nurse, "I shouldn't have had that abortion because I'm Catholic, but what else could I do? I'm afraid I'll never get close to my mother or back in the Church again." They then talk with their priest about this feeling of guilt.

Which evaluation statement shows a solution to the problem?

a. Patient stated, "I wish I had talked with the priest sooner. I now know God has forgiven me, and my mother is beginning to understand."
b. Patient has slept from 10 pm to 6 am for 3 consecutive nights without medication.
c. Patient has developed mutually caring relationships with others.
d. Patient has identified several spiritual beliefs that give purpose to their life.

14. A parish nurse is speaking to a congregant whose adolescent child was arrested for shoplifting. The congregant is very angry, stating they cannot face the child, let alone discuss the situation: "I just will not tolerate a thief." What nursing action will best assist the congregant at this time?
    a. Assuring the congregant that many parents feel the same way
    b. Reassuring the congregant that many teenagers act rebelliously and that it will pass
    c. Assisting the congregant to identify how withholding forgiveness hurts them
    d. Asking the congregant if they have spent sufficient time with their child
15. A hospice nurse who provides pastoral care is teaching nursing students about the three spiritual needs believed to be common to all people. Which of these will the nurse include in the discussion? Select all that apply.
    a. Food, clothing, and shelter
    b. Meaning and purpose
    c. Family
    d. Love and relatedness
    e. Forgiveness
    f. Rules to live by

ANSWERS WITH RATIONALES

1. **c.** When caring for a patient who is in spiritual distress, the nurse should listen to the patient first, then ask whether the patient would like to visit with a spiritual advisor. Arranging for a spiritual advisor first may not be respectful of the patient's wishes. A hug and false reassurances do not address the problem of spiritual distress. Talking to friends or relatives may be helpful, but only if the patient agrees.
2. **c.** The data point to an unmet spiritual need to experience love and belonging, given the nurse's estrangement from their family and God after leaving the church. The other options may represent other needs this nurse has, but the nurse's statements do not support them.
3. **c.** Questioning how the staff can meet patients' spiritual practices assesses spiritual needs. Asking the patient to describe spiritual practices is an assessment of spiritual practices. Asking about concerns assesses spiritual distress, and asking about feeling at peace assesses the need for forgiveness.
4. **d.** On the basis of the patient's stated religion, the nurse assumed they would want a kosher diet. This is a form of stereotyping. When evaluating the outcome of the situation, the nurse returns to the first step of the nursing process and assesses the patient's dietary practices and preferences.
5. **c.** Patients who practice the Jehovah's Witness faith believe blood transfusions violate God's laws and do not allow them. The nurse supports the patient's beliefs. It is disrespectful of the nurse to attempt to coerce a decision or impose their beliefs on the patient.
6. **d.** Failure to ensure that an infant baptism is performed when parents desire it may greatly increase the family's sorrow and suffering. Whether baptism postpones or prevents death and suffering is a religious belief that is insufficient to bind all nurses. There is no legal requirement regarding baptism, and although some nurses may believe part of their role is to ensure the salvation of the infant, this function could be rejected by many.
7. **a, b, d, f.** The nurse should ask a Buddhist if they have any diet restrictions related to the observance of holy days. Since Christian Scientists avoid the use of pain medications, the nurse should offer nonpharmacologic pain relief measures. A nurse administering medications to a Hindu patient avoids touching the patient's lips. A nurse should ask a Roman Catholic if they would like to attend Mass on Sunday. The nurse is careful not to schedule treatment and procedures on Saturday for a Jewish patient who observes the Sabbath. The nurse would appropriately consult with the medicine man of a Native American patient and incorporate their suggestions into the care plan.
8. **c.** Children learn most about their own spirituality from how their parents behave in relationship to one another, their children, others, and God (or a higher being). What parents say about God and religion, the family's spiritual advisor, and the child's church or religious organization are less important sources of learning.
9. **d.** Illness may increase spiritual concerns, which many patients find difficult to initially express. The other options presume patients are purposefully secretive or must speak with a spiritual advisor, friends, or family to promote discussion of spiritual concerns. Spirituality is anything that pertains to a person's relationship with a nonmaterial life force or higher power; there is no universal definition, as the experience is individual and personal.
10. **b.** Even when a nurse feels comfortable discussing spiritual concerns, they should always determine whether the patient has a spiritual advisor they would like to consult. Calling the patient's spiritual advisor may be premature if it is a matter the nurse can handle. The other two options deny the patient's right to speak privately with their spiritual advisor from the outset, if that is their preference.
11. **d.** Each of the four options represents appropriate spiritual goals, but identifying spiritual supports available to this patient in this medical center at this point in time, is the most appropriate and realistic.
12. **c.** The nurse prioritizes determining what, in addition to their family, has given the patient's life meaning and purpose in the past. This helps the patient focus on their strengths. This assessment data can be used to further plan individualized spiritual care.
13. **a.** The patient's statements indicate feelings of guilt, which has caused spiritual distress. Only option a clearly evaluates whether the patient's feelings of guilt have resolved after speaking to the priest.

14. c. Helping the congregant identify how their unforgiving feelings may be harmful to themselves is the only intervention that directly addresses forgiveness, a universal spiritual need. Assuring the congregant that many parents would feel the same way or that many teenagers shoplift out of rebelliousness may make them feel better initially, but this does not address the benefits of forgiveness. Suggesting the congregant may not have spent enough time with their child may be untrue and could promote guilty feelings, when they may be unwarranted.

15. b, d, e. Meaning and purpose, love and relatedness, and forgiveness are the three spiritual needs believed to be common to all people. Option a is a human need as described by Maslow, as is family (love and belonging). Many people live by a set of rules, but this is not a common spiritual need.

Bibliography

Albom, M. (1997). *Tuesdays with Morrie.* Broadway Books.

American Nurses Association (ANA). (2012). *Faith community nursing: Scope and standards of practice* (2nd ed.). Author.

American Nurses Association (ANA). (2021). *Nursing: Scope and standards of practice* (4th ed.). Author.

Anandarajah, G., & Hight, E. (2001). Spirituality and medical practice: Using the HOPE questions as a practical tool for spiritual assessment. *American Family Physician, 63*(1), 81–89.

Ausar, K., Lekhak, N., & Candela, L. (2021). Nurse spiritual self-care: A scoping review. *Nursing Outlook, 69*(4), 660–671.

Bone, N., Swinton, M., Hoad, N., Toledo, F., & Cook, D. (2018). Critical care nurses' experiences with spiritual care: The SPIRIT study. *American Journal of Critical Care, 27*(3), 212–219.

Borneman, T., Ferrell, B., & Puchalski, C. M. (2010). Evaluation of the FICA tool for spiritual assessment. *Journal of Pain and Symptom Management, 40*(2), 163–173.

Brehony, K. A. (2000). *After the darkest hour: How suffering begins the journey to wisdom.* Henry Holt and Company.

Canfield, C., Taylor, D., Nagy, K., Strauser, C., VanKerkhove, K., Wills, S., Sawicki, P., & Sorrell, J. (2016). Critical care nurses' perceived need for guidance in addressing spirituality in critically ill patients. *American Journal of Critical Care, 25*(3), 206–211.

Carol, J. (2002). What is healing? *Sacred Journey, 53*(4), 12–17.

Carson, V. B., & Koenig, H. G. (2004). *Spiritual caregiving: Healthcare as a ministry.* Templeton Foundation Press.

Carson, V. B., & Koenig, H. G. (2008). *Spiritual dimensions of nursing practice* (revised edition). Templeton Foundation Press.

Cassell, E. J. (1991). *The nature of suffering and the goals of medicine (2nd ed).* Oxford University Press.

Centers for Disease Control and Prevention. (2020). *Suicide prevention.* https://www.cdc.gov/violenceprevention/suicide/index.html

Cobb, M., Puchalski, C. M., & Rumbold, B. (2012). *Spirituality in healthcare.* Oxford University Press.

Creen, T. (2002). Enabling hope in the terminally ill. In R. C. Anderson (Ed.). *Palliative care patient and family counseling manual* (2nd ed., pp. 16–17). Aspen Publishers.

Diego-cordero, R., Lopez-Gomez, L., Lucchetti, G., & Badanta, B. (2022). Spiritual care in critically ill patients during COVID-19 pandemic. *Nursing Outlook, 70*, 64–77.

Dossey, B. (Ed.). (1989). Spirituality and healing. *Holistic Nursing Practice, 3*(3), entire issue.

Drews, M. F. (2017). The evolution of hope in patients with terminal illness. *Nursing, 47*(1), 13–14.

Ernecoff, N. C., Curlin, F. A., Buddadhumaruk, P., & White, D. B. (2015). Health care professionals' responses to religious or spiritual statements by surrogate decision makers during goals-of-care discussions. *JAMA Internal Medicine, 175*(10), 1662–1669.

Ferrell, B. R., & Coyle, N. (2008). The nature of suffering and the goals of nursing. *Oncology Nursing Forum, 35*(2), 241–247.

Ferrell, B. R., & Munevar, C. (2012). Domain of spiritual care. *Progress in Palliative Care, 20*(2), 66–71.

Fowler, J. W. (1981). *Stages of faith: The psychology of human development and the quest for meaning.* Harper & Row.

Frankl, V. E. (1984). *Man's search for meaning.* Beacon Press.

Frush, B. W., & Curlin, F. A. (2022). Is it ethically appropriate for physicians to offer to pray with patients in ICU? Yes. Point and Counterpoint. *Chest, 161*(4), 882–887.

Galanti, G. A. (2018). *Cultural and religious sensitivity: A pocket guide for health care professionals* (3rd ed.). Joint Commission Resources.

Galston, W. A., & Rogers, M. (2012). *Health care providers' consciences and patients' needs: The quest for balance.* Governance Studies at Brookings. https://www.brookings.edu/wp-content/uploads/2016/06/0223_health_care_galston_rogers.pdf

Golberg, B. (1998). Connection: An exploration of spirituality in nursing care. *Journal of Advanced Nursing, 27*(4), 836–842.

Gregg-Schroeder, S. (1999). A transforming experience: Circles of life. *Journal of Fellowship in Prayer*, 23–25.

Hauerwas, S. (1990). *Naming the silences: God, medicine, and the problem of suffering.* Eerdmans.

Hawthorne, D. M., & Gordon, S. C. (2020). The invisibility of spiritual nursing care in clinical practice. *Journal of Holistic Nursing, 38*(1), 147–155. https://doi.org/10.1177/0898010119889704

HealthCare Chaplaincy Network. (2016). *What is quality spiritual care in health care and how do you measure it*? https://www.spiritualcareassociation.org/docs/research/evidence_base/quality_indicators_document_1_7_2021.pdf

Heller, D. (1985). The children's God. *Psychology Today, 19*(12), 22–27.

Hickman, J. S. (2006). *Faith community nursing.* Wolters Kluwer Health/Lippincott Williams & Wilkins.

The Joint Commission. (2020). *Spiritual beliefs and preferences-Evaluating a patient's spiritual needs.* https://www.jointcommission.org/standards/standard-faqs/home-care/provision-of-care-treatment-and-services-pc/000001669/

Kalanithi, P. (2016). *When breath becomes air.* Random House.

Koenig, H. G. (2013). *Spirituality in patient care: Why, how, when and what* (3rd ed.). Templeton Press.

Kushner, H. S. (1983). *When bad things happen to good people.* Avon.

Lazenby, M., McCorkle, R., & Sulmasy, D. P. (2014). *Decisions at the end of life: A spiritual sourcebook.* Oxford University Press.

Lepianka, J. (2020). Contemplation, connection, collaboration: Keys to compassionate spiritual care. *American Nurse Journal, 15*(4), 59–62.

Lichter, D. (2018, May–June). Chaplaincy: Identity, focus and trends. *Health Progress*, 65–69.

Macrae, J. (1995). Nightingale's spiritual philosophy and its significance for modern nursing. *Image: The Journal of Nursing Scholarship, 27*(1), 8–10.

Magelssen, M. (2012). When should conscientious objection be accepted? *Journal of Medical Ethics, 38*(1), 18–21.

McDonnell-Naughton, M., Gaffney, L., & Fagan, A. (2020). Spirituality and caring for the older person: A discussion paper. *Journal of Religion and Health, 59*(6): 2775–2793. https://doi.org/10.1007/s10943-020-01027-2

Miller, J. E., & Cutshall, S. C. (2001). *The art of being a healing presence: A guide for those in caring relationships.* Willowgreen Publishing.

Miller, L. J. (2012). *The Oxford handbook of psychology and spirituality.* Oxford University Press.

Mother Teresa. (1995). *A simple path.* Ballantine Books.

NANDA International (2017). *NANDA international nursing diagnoses—definitions and classification (2018–2020) Thieme.*

National Consensus Project for Quality Palliative Care. (2018). *Clinical practice guidelines for quality palliative care* (4th ed.). http://www.nationalcoalitionhpc.org/guidelines-2018

O'Brien, M. E. (1982). The need for spiritual integrity. In H. Yura & M. B. Walsh (Eds.). *Human needs and the nursing process* (pp. 81–115). Appleton-Century-Crofts.

O'Brien, M. E. (1999). *Spirituality in nursing: Standing on holy ground.* Jones and Bartlett.

O'Brien, M. E. (2001). *The nurse's calling: A Christian spirituality of caring for the sick.* Paulist Press.

O'Brien, M. E. (2003). *Parish nursing: Healthcare ministry within the church.* Jones and Bartlett.

O'Brien, M. E. (2008). *A sacred covenant: The spiritual ministry of nursing.* Jones and Bartlett.

Pew Forum on Religion and Public Life. (2012). *"Nones" on the rise: One-in-five adults have no religious affiliation.* https://www.pewresearch.org/wp-content/uploads/sites/7/2012/10/NonesOnTheRise-full.pdf

Pew Research Center. (2015). *America's changing religious landscape.* http://www.pewforum.org/2015/05/12/americas-changing-religious-landscape

Puchalski, C. M. (2006). *A time for listening and caring: Spirituality and the care of the chronically ill and dying.* Oxford University Press.

Puchalski, C. M., & Ferrell, B. (2010). *Making health-care whole: Integrating spirituality into patient care.* Templeton Press.

Puchalski, C., Ferrell, B., Virani, R., Otis-Green, S., Baird, P., Bull, J., Chochinov, H., Handzo, G., Nelson-Becker, H., Prince-Paul, M., Pugliese, K., & Sulmasy, D. (2009). Improving the quality of spiritual care as a dimension of palliative care: The report of the consensus conference. *Journal of Palliative Medicine, 12*(10), 885–904.

Puchalski, C., & Romer, A. L. (2000). Taking a spiritual history allows clinicians to understand patients more fully. *Journal of Palliative Medicine, 3*(1), 129–137.

Rahner, K. (1971). How to receive a sacrament and mean it. *Theology Digest, 19*(3), 227–234.

Sacks, O. (2015). *Gratitude.* Alfred A. Knopf.

Sacred Design Lab. https://sacred.design/

Shelly, J. A., & Fish, S. (1988). *Spiritual care: The nurse's role* (3rd ed.). InterVarsity Press.

Simmons, A. M., Rivers, F. M., Gordon, S., & Yoder, L. H. (2018). The role of spirituality among military en route care nurses: Source of strength or moral injury. *Critical Care Nurse, 38*(2), 61–67.

Taylor, C. (2012). Rethinking hopelessness and the role of spiritual care when cure is no longer an option. *Journal of Pain and Symptom Management, 44*(4), 626–630.

Taylor, E. J. (2020). During the COVID-19 pandemic, should nurses offer to pray with patients? *Nursing, 50*(7), 42–46.

Tennyson, C. D., Oliver, J. P., & Jooste, K. R. (2021). A descriptive study of chaplains' code blue responses. *American Journal of Critical Care, 30*(6), 419–425.

Thurston, A., & Ter Kuile, C. *How we gather.* https://sacred.design/wp-content/uploads/2019/10/How_We_Gather_Digital_4.11.17.pdf

Walker, S., & Taylor, C. (2012). Compassion and health-care: Luxury or necessity? In M. Cobb, B. Rumbold, & C. Puchalski (Eds.). *Spirituality in Health Care* (pp. 135–143). Oxford University Press.

INDEX

Note: Page numbers followed by b, f, or t indicate text in box, figure, or table, respectively.

H

I

N

P

Q

U

List of Nursing Skills